WITHDRAWN

AVERY'S DISEASES OF THE NEWBORN

AVERY'S DISEASES OF THE NEWBORN

Ninth Edition

Christine A. Gleason, MD
W. Alan Hodson Endowed Chair in Pediatrics
Professor of Pediatrics
Head, Division of Neonatology
Department of Pediatrics
University of Washington
Seattle Children's Hospital
Seattle, Washington

Sherin U. Devaskar, MD
Mattel Endowed Executive Chair and Distinguished Professor
Department of Pediatrics
David Geffen School of Medicine
Assistant Vice Chancellor for Children's Health
University of California, Los Angeles Health System
Physician in Chief
Mattel Children's Hospital
Los Angeles, California

ELSEVIER
SAUNDERS

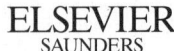
ELSEVIER
SAUNDERS

1600 John F. Kennedy Blvd.
Ste 1800
Philadelphia, PA 19103-2899

Library of Congress Cataloging-in-Publication Data

Avery's diseases of the newborn. -- 9th ed. / [edited by] Christine A. Gleason, Sherin U. Devaskar.
   p. ; cm.
  Diseases of the newborn
  Includes bibliographical references and index.
  ISBN 978-1-4377-0134-0 (pbk. : alk. paper) 1. Newborn infants--Diseases. I. Gleason, Christine A. II. Devaskar, Sherin U. III. Avery, Mary Ellen, 1927- IV. Title: Diseases of the newborn.
  [DNLM: 1. Infant, Newborn, Diseases. WS 421]
  RJ254.S3 2012
  618.92'01--dc23   2011020667

Acquisitions Editor: Judith Fletcher
Developmental Editor: Dee Simpson
Publishing Services Manager: Anne Altepeter
Associate Project Manager: Jessica L. Becher
Design Direction: Steve Stave

Printed in the United States of America

Last digit is the print number: 9 8 7 6 5 4 3 2 1

CONTRIBUTORS

Steven H. Abman, MD
Professor
Department of Pediatrics
University of Colorado School of Medicine
Director
Pediatric Heart Lung Center
Co-Director
Pulmonary Hypertension Program
The Children's Hospital
Aurora, Colorado

Amina Ahmed, MD
Pediatric Infectious Disease
Department of Pediatrics
Carolinas Medical Center
Levine Children's Hospital
Charlotte, North Carolina
Adjunct Clinical Associate Professor
Department of Pediatrics
University of North Carolina
Chapel Hill, North Carolina

Marilee C. Allen, MD
Professor of Pediatrics
Johns Hopkins University School of Medicine
Co-Director
Neonatal Intensive Care Unit Developmental
   Clinic
Kennedy Krieger Institute
Baltimore, Maryland

David Askenazi, MD, MSPH
Assistant Professor
Division of Nephrology and Transplantation
Department of Pediatrics
University of Alabama at Birmingham
Birmingham, Alabama

Stephen A. Back, MD, PhD
Associate Professor of Pediatrics and
   Neurology
Oregon Health and Science University
Clyde and Elda Munson Professor of
   Pediatric Research
Director
Neuroscience Section
Papé Family Pediatric Research Institute
Portland, Oregon

H. Scott Baldwin, MD
Professor of Pediatrics and Cell and
   Developmental Biology
Vanderbilt University Medical Center
Chief
Division of Pediatric Cardiology
Co-Director
Pediatric Heart Institute
Monroe Carell Jr. Children's Hospital
   at Vanderbilt
Nashville, Tennessee

Roberta A. Ballard, MD
Professor
Department of Pediatrics and Neonatology
University of California, San Francisco School
   of Medicine
San Francisco, California

Eduardo Bancalari, MD
Professor of Pediatrics
Director
Division of Neonatology
University of Miami Miller School
   of Medicine
Chief
Newborn Service
Jackson Memorial Hospital
Miami, Florida

Carlton M. Bates, MD
Associate Professor
Department of Pediatrics
University of Pittsburgh School of Medicine
Chief and Program Director
Pediatric Nephrology
Children's Hospital of Pittsburgh
Rangos Research Building
Pittsburgh, Pennsylvania

Donald L. Batisky, MD
Associate Professor of Pediatrics
Division of Pediatric Nephrology
Emory University School of Medicine
Director
Pediatric Hypertension Program
Children's Healthcare of Atlanta
Atlanta, Georgia

Stephen Baumgart, MD
Professor of Pediatrics
Department of Neonatology
George Washington University School
   of Medicine and Health Sciences
Children's National Medical Center
Washington, DC

Thomas J. Benedetti, MD, MHA
Professor
Department of Obstetrics and Gynecology
University of Washington School of Medicine
Seattle, Washington

Gerard T. Berry, MD
Professor
Department of Pediatrics Harvard Medical
   School
Director
Metabolism Program
Division of Genetics
Children's Hospital Boston
Boston, Massachusetts

Diana W. Bianchi, MD
Natalie V. Zucker Professor of Pediatrics,
   Obstetrics and Gynecology
Tufts University School of Medicine
Vice Chair for Research
Department of Pediatrics
Floating Hospital for Children
Boston, Massachusetts

Gil Binenbaum, MD, MSCE
Assistant Professor
Department of Ophthalmology
University of Pennsylvania School of
   Medicine
Attending Surgeon
Department of Ophthalmology
The Children's Hospital of Philadelphia
Philadelphia, Pennsylvania

Sureka Bollepalli, MD
Assistant Professor
Department of Pediatrics
University of South Florida Diabetes Center
Tampa, Florida

Sonia L. Bonifacio, MD
Assistant Adjunct Professor
Department of Pediatrics and Neonatology
University of California, San Francisco School
   of Medicine
Co-Director
Neurological Intensive Care Nursery
University of California, San Francisco
   Medical Center
Benioff Children's Hospital
San Francisco, California

Mitchell S. Cairo, MD
Professor of Pediatrics and Medicine
   and Pathology
Chief
Division of Blood and Marrow
   Transplantation
Department of Pediatrics
New York-Presbyterian Morgan Stanley
   Children's Hospital
Columbia University Medical Center
New York, New York

Katherine H. Campbell, MD, MPH
Fellow
Department of Obstetrics, Gynecology,
   and Reproductive Sciences
Yale School of Medicine
New Haven, Connecticut

Michael Caplan, MD
Chairman
Department of Pediatrics
NorthShore University HealthSystem
Evanston, Illinois
Professor
Department of Pediatrics
University of Chicago Pritzker School
  of Medicine
Chicago, Illinois

Stephen Cederbaum, MD
Professor Emeritus
Departments of Psychiatry and Pediatrics
  and Human Genetics
University of California, Los Angeles
Attending Physician
Department of Pediatrics
Ronald Reagan UCLA Medical Center
Los Angeles, California
Consulting Physician
Department of Pediatrics
Santa Monica UCLA Medical Center
Santa Monica, California

Sudhish Chandra, MD, FAAP
Medical Director
Department of Neonatology
Neonatal Intensive Care Unit
St. Anthony Medical Center
Crown Point, Indiana

Ming Chen, MD, PhD
Assistant Professor
Department of Pediatrics
University of Michigan
Ann Arbor, Michigan

Nelson Claure, MSc, PhD
Research Associate Professor of Pediatrics
Director
Neonatal Pulmonary Research Laboratory
Department of Pediatrics
Division of Neonatology
University of Miami Miller School
  of Medicine
Miami, Florida

Ronald I. Clyman, MD
Professor
Department of Pediatrics
Senior Staff
Cardiovascular Research Institute
University of California, San Francisco
San Francisco, California

Bernard A. Cohen, MD
Professor of Pediatrics and Dermatology
Johns Hopkins University School of Medicine
Director
Pediatric Dermatology
Johns Hopkins Children's Center
Baltimore, Maryland

F. Sessions Cole, MD
Park J. White, MD, Professor of Pediatrics
Assistant Vice Chancellor for Children's
  Health
Director
Division of Newborn Medicine
Washington University School of Medicine
Chief Medical Officer
St. Louis Children's Hospital
St. Louis, Missouri

Lawrence Copelovitch, MD
Assistant Professor
University of Pennsylvania School of
  Medicine
Attending in Nephrology
Department of Pediatrics
The Children's Hospital of Philadelphia
Philadelphia, Pennsylvania

Michael Cunningham, MD, PhD
Professor and Chief
Division of Craniofacial Medicine
Department of Pediatrics
University of Washington
Medical Director
Craniofacial Center
Seattle Children's Hospital
Seattle, Washington

**Alejandra G. de Alba Campomanes,
MD, MPH**
Assistant Professor of Ophthalmology
Division of Pediatric Ophthalmology and
  Strabismus
University of California, San Francisco
Director
Department of Pediatric Ophthalmology
  and Strabismus
San Francisco General Hospital
San Francisco, California

Ellen Dees, MD
Assistant Professor of Pediatrics
Division of Pediatric Cardiology
Monroe Carell Jr. Children's Hospital
  at Vanderbilt
Nashville, Tennessee

Scott C. Denne, MD
Professor of Pediatrics
Indiana University School of Medicine
Riley Hospital for Children
Indianapolis, Indiana

Sherin U. Devaskar, MD
Mattel Endowed Executive Chair and
  Distinguished Professor
Department of Pediatrics
David Geffen School of Medicine
Assistant Vice Chancellor for Children's
  Health
University of California, Los Angeles Health
  System
Physician in Chief
Mattel Children's Hospital
Los Angeles, California

Robert M. DiBlasi, RRT-NPS, FAARC
Respiratory Research Coordinator
Center for Developmental Therapeutics
Seattle Children's Research Institute
Seattle, Washington

Reed A. Dimmitt, MD, MSPH
Associate Professor of Pediatrics and Surgery
Director
Division of Neonatology and Pediatric
  Gastroenterology and Nutrition
University of Alabama at Birmingham
Birmingham, Alabama

Eric C. Eichenwald, MD
Associate Professor
Vice Chair and Division Director
Neonatology
Department of Pediatrics
University of Texas Health Science Center
Texas Children's Hospital
Houston, Texas

Eli M. Eisenstein, MD
Senior Pediatrician
Department of Pediatrics
Hadassah-Hebrew University Medical Center
Mount Scopus, Jerusalem, Israel

Jacquelyn R. Evans, MD
Medical Director
Newborn/Infant Intensive Care Unit
The Children's Hospital of Philadelphia
Associate Division Chief
Department of Neonatology
University of Pennsylvania School of
  Medicine
Philadelphia, Pennsylvania

Kelly Evans, MD
Fellow
Division of Craniofacial Medicine
Department of Pediatrics
University of Washington
Craniofacial Center
Seattle Children's Hospital
Seattle, Washington

Diana L. Farmer, MD, FAAP, FACS, FRCS
Professor of Surgery, Pediatrics, and
  Obstetrics, Gynecology, and
  Reproductive Sciences
Chief
Division of Pediatric Surgery
Vice Chair
Department of Surgery
University of California, San Francisco School
  of Medicine
Surgeon-in-Chief
University of California, San Francisco
  Medical Center
Benioff Children's Hospital
San Francisco, California

Patricia Ferrieri, MD
Professor
Chairman's Fund Endowed Chair in Lab
   Medicine and Pathology
Division of Infectious Diseases
Department of Pediatrics
University of Minnesota Medical School
Minneapolis, Minnesota

Donna M. Ferriero, MS, MD
Professor and Interim Chair of Pediatrics
Professor of Neurology
Co-Director
Newborn Brain Research Institute
University of California, San Francisco School
   of Medicine
Physician-in-Chief
University of California, San Francisco
   Medical Center
Benioff Children's Hospital
San Francisco, California

Neil N. Finer, MD
Division of Neonatal-Perinatal Medicine
Department of Pediatrics
University of California, San Diego
San Diego, California

Maria Victoria Fraga, MD
Fellow
Division of Neonatology and Pediatrics
The Children's Hospital of Philadelphia
Philadelphia, Pennsylvania

Lydia Furman, MD
Associate Professor of Pediatrics
Case Western Reserve University School
   of Medicine
Rainbow Babies and Children's Hospital
Cleveland, Ohio

Susan Furth, MD, PhD
Associate Professor
Department of Pediatrics
Johns Hopkins University School of Medicine
Associate Professor
Department of Epidemiology
Johns Hopkins Bloomberg School of Public
   Health
Baltimore, Maryland

Estelle B. Gauda, MD
Professor
Department of Pediatrics
Division of Neonatology
Johns Hopkins University School of Medicine
Baltimore, Maryland

Bertil Glader, MD, PhD
Professor of Pediatrics (Hematology/
   Oncology) and Pathology
Stanford University School of Medicine
Stanford, California

Christine A. Gleason, MD
W. Alan Hodson Endowed Chair in Pediatrics
Professor of Pediatrics
Head, Division of Neonatology
Department of Pediatrics
University of Washington
Seattle Children's Hospital
Seattle, Washington

Michael J. Goldberg, MD
Clinical Professor
Department of Orthopedics and Sports
   Medicine
University of Washington
Director
Skeletal Health Program
Department of Orthopedics
Seattle Children's Hospital
Seattle, Washington

Fernando Gonzalez, MD
Assistant Professor
Department of Pediatrics
Division of Neonatology
University of California, San Francisco
   Medical Center
Benioff Children's Hospital
San Francisco, California

Sameer Gopalani, MD
Clinical Assistant Professor
Department of Obstetrics and Gynecology
University of Washington School of Medicine
Division of Perinatal Medicine
Swedish Medical Center
Seattle, Washington

P. Ellen Grant, MD
Associate Professor
Department of Radiology
Harvard Medical School
Founding Director
Center for Fetal-Neonatal Neuroimaging
   and Developmental Science Center
Chair
Department of Neonatology
Children's Hospital Boston
Boston, Massachusetts

Carol L. Greene, MD
Professor
Departments of Pediatrics and Obstetrics,
   Gynecology, and Reproductive Sciences
Division of Genetics
University of Maryland School of Medicine
Baltimore, Maryland

Salvador Guevara-Gallardo, MD
Surgeon
University of California, San Francisco
   Medical Center
Benioff Children's Hospital
San Francisco, California

Jean-Pierre Guignard, MD
Honorary Professor of Pediatrics
Lausanne University Medical School
Lausanne, Switzerland

Susan Guttentag, MD
Associate Professor
Department of Pediatrics
University of Pennsylvania School
   of Medicine
The Children's Hospital of Philadelphia
Philadelphia, Pennsylvania

Chad R. Haldeman-Englert, MD
Assistant Professor
Department of Pediatrics
Section on Medical Genetics
Wake Forest University School of Medicine
Winston-Salem, North Carolina

Thomas Hansen, MD
Professor
Department of Pediatrics
University of Washington School of Medicine
Chief Executive Officer
Seattle Children's Hospital
Seattle, Washington

Anne V. Hing, MD
Associate Professor
Division of Craniofacial Medicine
Department of Pediatrics
University of Washington
Craniofacial Center
Seattle Children's Hospital
Seattle, Washington

A. Roger Hohimer, PhD
Associate Professor
Department of Obstetrics
Division of Perinatology
Oregon Health and Science University
Portland, Oregon

Margaret K. Hostetter, MD
Professor and Chair
Department of Pediatrics
Yale School of Medicine
New Haven, Connecticut

Andrew D. Hull, MD, FRCOG, FACOG
Professor of Clinical Reproductive Medicine
University of California, San Diego
Director
Maternal Fetal Medicine Fellowship
University of California, San Diego Medical
   Center
La Jolla, California

J. Craig Jackson, MD, MHA
Professor
Department of Pediatrics
Division of Neonatology
University of Washington
Neonatal Intensive Care Unit Medical
   Director
Seattle Children's Hospital
Seattle, Washington

Lucky Jain, MD, MBA
Executive Vice Chairman
Department of Pediatrics
Emory University
Medical Director
Emory Children's Center
Atlanta, Georgia

Vandana Jain, MD
Associate Professor
Division of Pediatric Endocrinology
Department of Pediatrics
All India Institute of Medical Sciences
New Delhi, India

Halima Saadia Janjua, MD
Pediatric Nephrology Fellow
Department of Pediatrics
Ohio State University
Nationwide Children's Hospital
Columbus, Ohio

Sandra E. Juul, MD, PhD
Professor
Department of Pediatrics
University of Washington
Seattle, Washington

Satyan Kalkunte, MPharm, PhD
Research Associate
Superfund Basic Research Program
Department of Pediatrics
Women and Infants' Hospital of Rhode Island
Warren Alpert Medical School of Brown
    University
Providence, Rhode Island

Bernard S. Kaplan, MB, BCh
Professor of Pediatrics
University of Pennsylvania School
    of Medicine
Attending in Nephrology
Department of Pediatrics
The Children's Hospital of Philadelphia
Philadelphia, Pennsylvania

Roberta L. Keller, MD
Assistant Professor of Clinical Pediatrics
University of California, San Francisco
Director
Neonatal Extracorporeal Membrane
    Oxygenation Program
University of California, San Francisco
    Medical Center
Benioff Children's Hospital
San Francisco, California

Thomas F. Kelly, MD
Clinical Professor and Chief
Division of Perinatal Medicine
Department of Reproductive Medicine
University of California, San Diego School
    of Medicine
La Jolla, California
Director
Maternity Services
University of California, San Diego Medical
    Center
San Diego, California

Steven E. Kern, PhD
Associate Professor of Pharmaceutics,
    Anesthesiology, and Bioengineering
University of Utah
Salt Lake City, Utah

Nanda Kerkar, MD
Department of Pediatrics
Division of Pediatric Hepatology
Recanati-Miller Transplantation Institute
The Mount Sinai Medical Center
New York, New York

John P. Kinsella, MD
Professor of Pediatrics
Section of Neonatology
University of Colorado School of Medicine
Medical Director
Newborn/Young Child Transport Service
Co-Director
Newborn Extracorporeal Membrane
    Oxygenation Service
The Children's Hospital
Aurora, Colorado

Roxanne Kirsch, MD, FRCPC, FAAP
Cardiac Intensivist
Departments of Anesthesia and Critical Care
The Children's Hospital of Philadelphia
Philadelphia, Pennsylvania

Monica E. Kleinman, MD
Associate Professor of Anesthesia
Department of Pediatrics Harvard Medical
    School
Clinical Director
Medical-Surgical Intensive Care Unit
Department of Anesthesia
Division of Critical Care Medicine
Department of Anesthesia, Perioperative,
    and Pain Medicine
Medical Director
Critical Care Transport Program
Children's Hospital Boston
Boston, Massachusetts

Thomas S. Klitzner, MD, PhD
Jack H. Skirball Professor and Chief
Pediatric Cardiology
David Geffen School of Medicine
University of California, Los Angeles
Los Angeles, California

Sarah M. Lambert, MD
Assistant Professor of Surgery in Urology
University of Pennsylvania School of
    Medicine
The Children's Hospital of Philadelphia
Philadelphia, Pennsylvania

John D. Lantos, MD
Professor of Pediatrics
University of Missouri at Kansas City
Director
Children's Mercy Bioethics Center
Children's Mercy Hospital
Kansas City, Missouri
Visiting Professor of Pediatrics
University of Chicago
Chicago, Illinois

Tina A. Leone, MD
Assistant Professor of Pediatrics
University of California, San Diego
San Diego, California

Mary Leppert, MB, BCh
Assistant Professor of Pediatrics
Johns Hopkins University School of Medicine
Attending Physician
Neurodevelopmental Medicine
Kennedy Krieger Institute
Baltimore, Maryland

Harvey L. Levy, MD
Professor
Department of Pediatrics
Harvard Medical School
Senior Physician in Medicine and Genetics
Department of Medicine
Children's Hospital Boston
Boston, Massachusetts

Mark Lewin, MD
Professor and Chief
Pediatric Cardiology
University of Washington School of Medicine
Co-Director
Heart Center
Seattle Children's Hospital
Seattle, Washington

Karen Lin-Su, MD
Clinical Associate Professor of Pediatrics
Pediatric Endocrinology
Weill Cornell Medical College
New York, New York

Mignon L. Loh, MD
Professor of Clinical Pediatrics
Department of Pediatrics
University of California, San Francisco
Pediatric Hematological Oncologist
University of California, San Francisco
    Medical Center
Benioff Children's Hospital
San Francisco, California

Scott A. Lorch, MD, MSCE
Assistant Professor
Department of Pediatrics
University of Pennsylvania School
    of Medicine
Attending Neonatologist
Division of Neonatology and Center
    for Outcomes Research
The Children's Hospital of Philadelphia
Philadelphia, Pennsylvania

Ralph A. Lugo, PharmD
Professor and Chair
Department of Pharmacy Practice
Bill Gatton College of Pharmacy
East Tennessee State University
Johnson City, Tennessee

Volker Mai, PhD
University of Florida Microbiology and Cell
    Sciences
Emerging Pathogens Institute
Gainesville, Florida

Bradley S. Marino, MD, MPP, MSCE
Associate Professor of Pediatrics
University of Cincinnati College of Medicine
Director
Heart Institute Research Core
Attending Physician
Cardiac Intensive Care Unit
Divisions of Cardiology and Critical Care
    Medicine
Cincinnati Children's Hospital Medical
    Center
Cincinnati, Ohio

Barry Markovitz, MD, MPH
Professor of Clinical Anesthesiology and
    Pediatrics
University of Southern California Keck
    School of Medicine
Director
Critical Care Medicine
Children's Hospital Los Angeles
Los Angeles, California

Kerri Marquard, MD
Clinical Fellow
Reproductive Endocrinology and Infertility
Department of Obstetrics and Gynecology
Division of Reproductive Endocrinology and
    Infertility
Washington University School of Medicine
St. Louis, Missouri

Camilia R. Martin, MD, MS
Assistant Professor of Pediatrics
Harvard Medical School
Associate Director
Neonatal Intensive Care Unit
Director
Cross-Disciplinary Research Partnerships
Division of Translational Research
Beth Israel Deaconess Medical Center
Boston, Massachusetts

Richard J. Martin, MD
Drusinsky-Fanaroff Chair in Neonatology
Professor
Rainbow Babies and Children's Hospital
Professor of Pediatrics
Case Western Reserve University
Cleveland, Ohio

Katherine K. Matthay, MD
Mildred V. Strouss Professor of Translational
    Research
Chief of Pediatric Hematology-Oncology
University of California, San Francisco
    Medical Center
Benioff Children's Hospital
San Francisco, California

Dana C. Matthews, MD
Associate Professor
University of Washington School of Medicine
Director
Clinical Hematology
Pediatric Hematology and Oncology
Seattle Children's Hospital
Seattle, Washington

Dennis E. Mayock, MD
Professor
Division of Neonatology
Department of Pediatrics
University of Washington School of Medicine
Seattle, Washington

William L. Meadow, MD, PhD
Professor
Department of Pediatrics
University of Chicago
Chicago, Illinois

Ram K. Menon, MD
Professor of Pediatrics and Molecular
    and Integrative Physiology
Director
Division of Endocrinology
Department of Pediatrics
University of Michigan Medical School
Ann Arbor, Michigan

Eugenio Mercuri, MD, PhD
Professor of Pediatric Neurology
Department of Pediatrics
Catholic University
Rome, Italy

Sowmya S. Mohan, MD
Neonatal-Perinatal Medicine Fellow
Department of Pediatrics
Division of Neonatology
Emory University
Atlanta, Georgia

Kelle Moley, MD
James P. Crane Professor of Obstetrics and
    Gynecology
Division of Reproductive Endocrinology and
    Infertility
Vice Chair
Basic Science Research
Washington University School of Medicine
St. Louis, Missouri

Thomas J. Mollen, MD
Associate Medical Director
Infant Breathing Disorder Center
The Children's Hospital of Philadelphia
Philadelphia, Pennsylvania

Jeremy P. Moore, MD
Assistant Professor of Pediatrics
Division of Pediatric Cardiology
Mattel Children's Hospital
David Geffen School of Medicine
University of California, Los Angeles
Los Angeles, California

Thomas R. Moore, MD
Professor and Chairman
Department of Reproductive Medicine
University of California, San Diego
San Diego, California

David A. Munson, MD
Assistant Professor of Clinical Pediatrics
University of Pennsylvania School of Medicine
Associate Medical Director
Newborn and Infant Intensive Care Unit
The Children's Hospital of Philadelphia
Philadelphia, Pennsylvania

Jeffrey C. Murray, MD
Professor
Departments of Pediatrics, Biology, Nursing,
    and Epidemiology
University of Iowa
Iowa City, Iowa

Josef Neu, MD
Professor of Pediatrics
Division of Neonatology
University of Florida College of Medicine
Gainesville, Florida

Maria I. New, MD
Professor of Pediatrics
Director
Adrenal Steroid Disorders Program
Mount Sinai School of Medicine
New York, New York

Annie Nguyen-Vermillion, MD, FAAP
Department of Neonatology
Northwest Permanente, PC
Providence St. Vincent Medical Center
Neonatal Intensive Care Unit
Portland, Oregon

Victoria Niklas, MD
Associate Professor of Pediatrics
Division of Neonatal Medicine
University of Southern California Keck
    School of Medicine
Children's Hospital Los Angeles
Los Angeles, California

Saroj Nimkarn, MD
Assistant Professor of Pediatrics
Associate Director
Pediatric Endocrinology
Weill Cornell Medical College
New York, New York

James F. Padbury, MD
Oh-Zopfi Professor of Pediatrics and
    Perinatal Biology
Vice Chair for Research
Department of Pediatrics
Warren Alpert Medical School of Brown
    University
Women and Infants' Hospital of Rhode Island
Providence, Rhode Island

Marika Pane, MD, PhD
Institute of Neurology
Catholic University
Rome, Italy

Nigel Paneth, MD, MPH
University Distinguished Professor
Departments of Epidemiology and Pediatrics
    and Human Development
College of Human Medicine
Michigan State University
East Lansing, Michigan

Thomas A. Parker, MD
Associate Professor of Pediatrics
Director
Training Program in Neonatal-Perinatal
    Medicine
University of Colorado School of Medicine
Aurora, Colorado

Janna C. Patterson, MD, MPH
Assistant Instructor
Department of Pediatrics
Division of Neonatology
University of Washington
Seattle, Washington

Christian M. Pettker, MD
Assistant Professor
Department of Obstetrics, Gynecology,
and Reproductive Sciences
Yale School of Medicine
New Haven, Connecticut

Lauren L. Plawner, MD
Acting Assistant Professor of Neurology
University of Washington
Pediatric Neurologist
Seattle Children's Hospital
Seattle, Washington

Dan Poenaru, BSc, MD, MHPE
Adjunct Professor
Department of Surgery
Queen's University
Kingston, Ontario, Canada
Medical Director
BethanyKids at Kijabe Hospital
Kijabe, Kenya

Brenda B. Poindexter, MD, MS
Associate Professor of Pediatrics
Section of Neonatal-Perinatal Medicine
Indiana University School of Medicine
Indianapolis, Indiana

Michael A. Posencheg, MD
Assistant Professor of Clinical Pediatrics
University of Pennsylvania School of
Medicine
Associate Medical Director
Intensive Care Nursery
Medical Director
Newborn Nursery
Division of Neonatology and Newborn
Services
Hospital of the University of Pennsylvania
Attending Neonatologist
The Children's Hospital of Philadelphia
Philadelphia, Pennsylvania

Sanjay P. Prabhu, MBBS, DCH, MRCPCH, FRCR
Instructor
Department of Radiology
Harvard Medical School
Director
Advanced Image Analysis Lab
Department of Radiology
Children's Hospital Boston
Boston, Massachusetts

Katherine B. Püttgen, MD
Assistant Professor
Departments of Dermatology and Pediatrics
Johns Hopkins University School of Medicine
Baltimore, Maryland

Graham E. Quinn, MD, MSCE
Professor of Ophthalmology
Division of Pediatric Ophthalmology
The Children's Hospital of Philadelphia
University of Pennsylvania School of
Medicine
Philadelphia, Pennsylvania

Tonse N.K. Raju, MD, DCH
Medical Officer
Eunice Kennedy Shriver National Institute of
Child Health and Human Development
National Institutes of Health
Bethesda, Maryland

Gladys A. Ramos, MD
Associate Physician
Department of Reproductive Medicine
Division of Perinatology
University of California, San Diego
San Diego, California

Benjamin E. Reinking, MD
Clinical Assistant Professor
Department of Pediatrics
University of Iowa
Iowa City, Iowa

C. Peter Richardson, PhD
Associate Research Professor
Department of Pediatrics
University of Washington
Associate Research Professor
Department of Pulmonary and Newborn Care
Seattle Children's Hospital
Principal Investigator
Center for Developmental Therapy
Seattle Children's Research Institute
Seattle, Washington

David L. Rimoin, MD, PhD
Professor of Pediatrics, Medicine, and
Medical Genetics
David Geffen School of Medicine
University of California, Los Angeles
Director
Medical Genetics Institute
Steven Spielberg Chair
Cedars-Sinai Medical Center
Los Angeles, California

Elizabeth Robbins, MD
Clinical Professor
Department of Pediatrics
University of California, San Francisco
San Francisco, California

Richard L. Robertson, MD
Associate Professor of Radiology
Harvard Medical School
Radiologist-in-Chief
Children's Hospital Boston
Boston, Massachusetts

Mark D. Rollins, MD, PhD
Associate Professor
Department of Anesthesia and Perioperative
Care
University of California, San Francisco
San Francisco, California

Susan R. Rose, MEd, MD
Professor of Pediatrics and Endocrinology
University of Cincinnati
Pediatric Endocrinologist Cincinnati
Children's Hospital Medical Center
Cincinnati, Ohio

Mark A. Rosen, MD
Professor
Departments of Anesthesia and Periopera-
tive Care and Obstetrics, Gynecology, and
Reproductive Sciences
University of California, San Francisco
Director
Obstetric Anesthesia
University of California, San Francisco
San Francisco, California

Lewis P. Rubin, MPhil, MD
Pamela and Leslie Muma Endowed Chair
in Neonatology
Professor of Pediatrics, Obstetrics and
Gynecology, Pathology and Cell Biology,
and Community and Family Health
University of South Florida
Medical Director
Newborn Service Line
Tampa General Hospital
Tampa, Florida

Inderneel Sahai, MD, FACMG
Assistant Professor
Department of Pediatrics
University of Massachusetts
Chief Medical Officer
New England Newborn Screening Program
Division of Genetics and Metabolism
Massachusetts General Hospital
Department of Pediatrics
Harvard Medical School
Boston, Massachusetts

Sulagna C. Saitta, MD, PhD
Assistant Professor of Pediatrics
Division of Genetics
The Children's Hospital of Philadelphia
University of Pennsylvania School of
Medicine
Philadelphia, Pennsylvania

Pablo J. Sánchez, MD
Professor of Pediatrics
University of Texas Southwestern Medical
Center
Children's Medical Center Dallas
Dallas, Texas

Gary M. Satou, MD
Associate Clinical Professor
David Geffen School of Medicine
University of California, Los Angeles
Director
Pediatric Echocardiography
Co-Director
Fetal Cardiology Program
Mattel Children's Hospital
Los Angeles, California

Richard J. Schanler, MD
Professor
Department of Pediatrics
Hofstra North Shore-LIJ School of Medicine
Hempstead, New York
Associate Chairman
Department of Pediatrics
Chief
Neonatal-Perinatal Medicine
Steven and Alexandra Cohen Children's
    Medical Center of New York
New Hyde Park, New York

Mark S. Scher, MD
Professor of Pediatrics and Neurology
Case Western Reserve University School
    of Medicine
Chief of Pediatric Neurology
Rainbow Babies and Children's Hospital
University Hospitals of Cleveland
Cleveland, Ohio

Mark R. Schleiss, MD
Professor of Pediatrics
Director
Division of Pediatric Infectious Diseases and
    Immunology
Associate Chair for Research
Department of Pediatrics
University of Minnesota Medical School
American Legion Endowed Chair in Pediatric
    Infectious Diseases
Co-Director
Center for Infectious Diseases and
    Microbiology Translational Research
Minneapolis, Minnesota

Thomas D. Scholz, MD
Children's Miracle Network Professor
    of Pediatrics
Director
Division of Pediatric Cardiology
University of Iowa Carver College
    of Medicine
Iowa City, Iowa

Andrew L. Schwaderer, MD
Assistant Professor
Department of Pediatrics
Ohio State University
Columbus, Ohio

Istvan Seri, MD, PhD, HonD
Professor and Chief
Division of Neonatal Medicine
Department of Pediatrics
University of Southern California Keck
    School of Medicine
Director
Center for Fetal and Neonatal Medicine
Children's Hospital Los Angeles
Los Angeles, California

Surendra Sharma, MD, PhD
Professor
Department of Pediatrics
Warren Alpert Medical School of Brown
    University
Women and Infants' Hospital of Rhode Island
Providence, Rhode Island

Evan B. Shereck, MD
Assistant Professor of Pediatrics
Division of Pediatric Hematology and
    Oncology
Oregon Health and Science University
Doernbecher Children's Hospital
Portland, Oregon

Eric Sibley, MD, PhD
Associate Professor of Pediatrics
Stanford University School of Medicine
Stanford, California

Caroline Signore, MD, MPH
Medical Officer
Pregnancy and Perinatology Branch
Eunice Kennedy Shriver National Institute of
    Child Health and Human Development
Bethesda, Maryland

Rebecca Simmons, MD
Associate Professor of Pediatrics
Children's Hospital Philadelphia
University of Pennsylvania School of
    Medicine
Philadelphia, Pennsylvania

Jeffrey B. Smith, MD, PhD
Professor
Department of Pediatrics
David Geffen School of Medicine
University of California, Los Angeles
Medical Director
Newborn Nursery
Mattel Children's Hospital
Los Angeles, California

Lorie B. Smith, MD, MHS
Staff Pediatric Nephrologist
Walter Reed National Military Medical
    Center
Bethesda, Maryland

Clara Song, MD, FAAP
Assistant Professor of Pediatrics
Division of Neonatal-Perinatal Medicine
The University of Oklahoma Health Sciences
    Center
Children's Hospital at Oklahoma University
    Medical Center
Oklahoma City, Oklahoma

Robin H. Steinhorn, MD
Professor and Division Head
Department of Pediatrics
Children's Memorial Hospital
Northwestern University Feinberg School
    of Medicine
Chicago, Illinois

Frederick J. Suchy, MD
Professor of Pediatrics
Associate Dean for Child Health Research
University of Colorado School of Medicine
Chief Research Officer and Director
The Children's Hospital Research Institute
The Children's Hospital
Aurora, Colorado

Endre Sulyok, MD, PhD, DSc
Professor of Pediatrics
Faculty
Health Sciences University of Pecs
Institute of Public Health and Health
    Promotion
Pecs, Vorosmarty, Hungary

Peter Tarczy-Hornoch, MD, FACMI
Head and Professor
Division of Biomedical and Health
    Informatics
Department of Medical Education and
    Biomedical Informatics
Professor
Division of Neonatology
Department of Pediatrics
Adjunct Professor
Computer Science and Engineering
University of Washington
Seattle, Washington

George A. Taylor, MD
John A. Kirkpatrick Professor of Radiology
Department of Pediatrics
Harvard Medical School
Radiologist-in-Chief Emeritus
Children's Hospital Boston
Boston, Massachusetts

James A. Taylor, MD
Professor
Department of Pediatrics
University of Washington
Seattle, Washington

Janet A. Thomas, MD
Associate Professor
Department of Pediatrics
Section of Clinical Genetics and Metabolism
University of Colorado School of Medicine
The Children's Hospital
Aurora, Colorado

George E. Tiller, MD, PhD
Regional Chief
Department of Genetics
Southern California Permanente Medical
    Group
Los Angeles, California

Mark M. Tran, MD
Resident Physician
Department of Dermatology
Johns Hopkins Hospital
Baltimore, Maryland

Michael Stone Trautman, MD
Clinical Professor of Pediatrics
Section of Neonatal-Perinatal Medicine
Indiana University School of Medicine
Riley Hospital for Children
Indianapolis, Indiana

Jeffrey S. Upperman, MD
Associate Professor of Surgery
Department of Pediatric Surgery
Program Director
Pediatric Surgery Fellowship
Children's Hospital Los Angeles
Los Angeles, California

Carmella van de Ven, MA
Department of Pediatrics
Columbia University
Senior Research Staff Associate
Pediatric Blood and Marrow Transplantation
New York-Presbyterian Morgan Stanley
  Children's Hospital
Columbia University Medical Center
New York, New York

Margaret M. Vernon, MD
Assistant Professor
Department of Pediatrics
Division of Cardiology
University of Washington School of Medicine
Children's Heart Center
Seattle Children's Hospital
Seattle, Washington

W. Allan Walker, MD
Conrad Taff Professor of Pediatrics and
  Nutrition
Harvard Medical School
Mucosal Immunology Laboratory
Boston, Massachusetts

Linda D. Wallen, MD
Clinical Professor of Pediatrics
Associate Division Head
Neonatal Clinical Operations
University of Washington
Associate Medical Director
Neonatal Intensive Care Unit
Seattle Children's Hospital
Seattle, Washington

Sarah A. Waller, MD
Maternal Fetal Medicine Fellow
Department of Obstetrics and Gynecology
University of Washington
Seattle, Washington

Bradley A. Warady, MD
Professor of Pediatrics
University of Missouri at Kansas City
  School of Medicine
Senior Associate Chairman
Department of Pediatrics
Chief
Section of Pediatric Nephrology
Director
Dialysis and Transplantation
Pediatric Nephrology
Children's Mercy Hospitals and Clinics
Kansas City, Missouri

Robert M. Ward, MD
Professor
Department of Pediatrics
Attending Neonatologist
Adjunct Professor
Pharmacology and Toxicology
Director
Pediatric Pharmacology Program
University of Utah
Salt Lake City, Utah

Jon F. Watchko, MD
Professor of Pediatrics, Obstetrics,
  Gynecology, and Reproductive Sciences
Division of Newborn Medicine
Department of Pediatrics
University of Pittsburgh School of Medicine
Senior Scientist
Magee-Women's Research Institute
Pittsburgh, Pennsylvania

Gil Wernovsky, MD
Professor of Pediatrics
Department of Pediatric Cardiology
University of Pennsylvania School of
  Medicine
Medical Director
Neurocardiac Care Program
Associate Chief
Department of Pediatric Cardiology
Director
Program Development and Staff Cardiac
  Intensivist
The Cardiac Center
The Children's Hospital of Philadelphia
Philadelphia, Pennsylvania

Klane K. White, MD, MSc
Assistant Professor
Department of Orthopedics and Sports
  Medicine
University of Washington
Seattle, Washington
Pediatric Orthopedic Surgeon
Department of Orthopedics and Sports
  Medicine
Seattle Children's Hospital
Seattle, Washington

Calvin B. Williams, MD, PhD
Professor of Pediatrics
Chief
Section of Pediatric Rheumatology
Medical College of Wisconsin
D.B. and Marjorie Reinhart Chair in
  Rheumatology
Children's Hospital of Wisconsin
Milwaukee, Wisconsin

David Woodrum, MD
Professor of Pediatrics
Division of Neonatology
University of Washington School of Medicine
Seattle, Washington

George A. Woodward, MD, MBA
Professor
Department of Pediatrics
University of Washington School of Medicine
Chief
Emergency Medicine
Medical Director
Transport Services
Seattle Children's Hospital
Seattle, Washington

Dakara Rucker Wright, MD
Pediatric Dermatologist
Johns Hopkins University School of Medicine
Johns Hopkins Children's Center
Baltimore, Maryland

Jeffrey A. Wright, MD
Associate Professor
Department of Pediatrics
University of Washington
Seattle, Washington

Linda L. Wright, MD
Deputy Director
Center for Research for Mothers
  and Children
Director
Global Network for Women's and Children's
  Health Research
Eunice Kennedy Shriver National Institute of
  Child Health and Human Development
National Institutes of Health
Bethesda, Maryland

Christopher M. Young, MD
Fellow
Neonatal-Perinatal Medicine
Department of Pediatrics
Division of Neonatology
University of Florida
Gainesville, Florida

Guy Young, MD
Associate Professor of Pediatrics
University of Southern California Keck
  School of Medicine
Director
Hemostasis and Thrombosis Center
Center for Cancer and Blood Disorders
Children's Hospital Los Angeles
Los Angeles, California

Elaine H. Zackai, MD
Division of Genetics
Department of Pediatrics
The Children's Hospital of Philadelphia
Philadelphia, Pennsylvania

Stephen A. Zderic, MD
Professor of Surgery in Urology
University of Pennsylvania School of
  Medicine
John W. Duckett Endowed Chair
The Children's Hospital of Philadelphia
Philadelphia, Pennsylvania

PREFACE

"The neonatal period ... represents the last frontier of medicine, territory which has just begun to be cleared of its forests and underbrush in preparation for its eagerly anticipated crops of saved lives."

Introduction from the first edition of
Schaffer's Diseases of the Newborn

The first edition of *Diseases of the Newborn* was published in 1960 by Dr. Alexander J. Schaffer, a well-known Baltimore pediatrician who coined the term *neonatology* to describe this emerging pediatric subspecialty that concentrated on "the art and science of diagnosis and treatment of disorders of the newborn infant." Schaffer's first edition was used mainly for diagnosis, but also included reference to neonatal care practices (i.e., the use of antibiotics, temperature regulation, and attention to feeding techniques)—practices that had led to a remarkable decrease in the infant mortality rate in the United States, from 47 deaths per 1000 live births in 1940 to 26 per 1000 in 1960. But a pivotal year for the new field of neonatology came 3 years later in 1963, with the birth of President John F. Kennedy's son, Patrick Bouvier Kennedy, at 36 weeks' gestation (i.e., late preterm). His death at 3 days of age, from complications of hyaline membrane disease, accelerated the development of infant ventilators that, coupled with micro-blood gas analysis and expertise in the use of umbilical artery catheterization, led to the development of intensive care for newborns in the 1960s on both sides of the Atlantic. Advances in neonatal surgery and cardiology, along with further technological innovations, stimulated the development of neonatal intensive care units and regionalization of care for sick newborn infants over the next several decades. These developments were accompanied by an explosion of neonatal research activity that led to improved understanding of the pathophysiology and genetic basis of diseases of the newborn, which in turn has led to spectacular advances in neonatal diagnosis and therapeutics—particularly for preterm infants. These efforts led to continued improvements in the infant mortality rate in the United States, from 26 deaths per 1000 livebirths in 1960 to 6.5 per 1000 in 2004. Current research efforts are focused on decreasing the striking global disparities in infant mortality rates, decreasing neonatal morbidities, advancing neonatal therapeutics, and preventing prematurity and newborn diseases. We neonatologists would like to be put out of business one day!

Dr. Mary Ellen Avery joined Dr. Schaffer for the third edition of *Diseases of the Newborn* in 1971. For the fourth edition in 1977, Drs. Avery and Schaffer recognized that their book now needed multiple contributors with subspecialty expertise and they became co-editors, rather than sole co-authors, of the book. In the preface to that fourth edition, Dr. Schaffer wrote, "We have also

seen the application of some fundamental advances in molecular biology to the management of our fetal and newborn patients"—referring to the new knowledge of hemoglobinopathies. Dr. Schaffer died in 1981, at the age of 79, and Dr. H. William Taeusch joined Dr. Avery as co-editor for the fifth edition in 1984. Dr. Roberta Ballard joined Drs. Taeusch and Avery for the sixth edition in 1991, with the addition of Dr. Christine Gleason for the eighth edition in 2004. Drs. Avery, Taeusch, and Ballard retired from editing the book in 2009, and became "editors emeriti." Dr. Gleason was joined by Dr. Sherin Devaskar as co-editor for this, the ninth edition.

What's new and different about this edition? The book has been completely (and often painfully) revised and updated by some of the best clinicians and investigators in their field. Some chapters required more extensive revision than others, particularly those that deal with areas in which we have benefitted from new knowledge and/or its application to new diagnostic and therapeutic practices. This is particularly true in areas such as the genetic basis of disease, neonatal pain management, information technology, and the fetal origins of adult disease—an area that is now embedded within many of the chapters of this book. Some of the book's sections were reorganized to reflect our field's continued evolution. For example, Chapter 52, Persistent Pulmonary Hypertension, previously in Part X, Respiratory System, has found a new home in Part XI, Cardiovascular System. Finally, we've added new chapters that reflect the continued growth and development of our subspecialty. These include Chapter 4, Global Neonatal Health; Chapter 29, Stabilization and Transport of the High-Risk Infant; Chapter 33, Care of the Late Preterm Infant; Chapter 74, Disorders of the Liver; and Chapter 95, Craniofacial Malformations.

With the incredible breadth and depth of information immediately available to neonatal caregivers and educators on multiple internet sites, what's the value of a textbook? We, the co-editors of this ninth edition, believe that textbooks such as *Diseases of the Newborn* and all forms of integrative scholarship, will always be needed—by clinicians striving to provide state-of-the-art neonatal care, by educators striving to train the next generation of caregivers, and by investigators striving to advance neonatal scholarship. A textbook's content is only as good as its contributors and this textbook, like the previous editions, has awesome contributors. They were chosen for their expertise and ability to integrate their knowledge into a comprehensive, readable, and useful chapter. They did this despite the demands of their day jobs in the hopes that their syntheses could, as Ethel Dunham wrote in the foreword to the first edition, "spread more widely what is already known ... and make it possible to apply these facts." Textbooks of the future will undoubtedly take advantage of online, interactive publishing technologies, making their content readily accessible and more real-time, with continued revision and updating. However, in 2011—a full 50 years after the publication of the first edition of this book—we continue to find copies of this and other textbooks important to our subspecialty lying dog-eared, coffee-stained, annotated, and broken-spined in all of the places where neonatal caregivers congregate. These places, these congregations of neonatal caregivers, are now present in every country around the world. The tentacles of neonatal practice and education are spreading—ever deeper, ever wider—to improve the outcome of pregnancy worldwide. Textbooks connect us to the past, bring us up to date with the present, and prepare and excite us for the future. We will always need them, in one form or another, at our sites of practice. To that end, we have challenged ourselves to meet, and hopefully exceed, that need—for our field, for our colleagues, and for the babies.

We wish to thank key staff at Elsevier—Deidre Simpson, senior developmental editor, and Judith Fletcher, publishing director, both of whom demonstrated patience, guidance, and persistence, and Jessica Becher, associate project manager, for our book. We also wish to thank our academic institutions and our administrative assistants, Mildred Hill at the University of Washington and Kristie Smiley at the University of California, Los Angeles. They kept us grounded, on track, and basically saved our lives! We are indebted to our contributors, who actually *wrote* the book and did so willingly, enthusiastically, and (for the most part) in a timely fashion—despite the myriad of other responsibilities in their lives. And we are deeply grateful for the support of our families throughout the long, and often challenging, editorial process. Finally, we thank the editors emeriti of this book, Drs. Mary Ellen Avery, Bill Taeusch, and Roberta Ballard, for their enormous contributions to the field of neonatology and to the lives of babies throughout the world, and their wise influence on us, the editors of the ninth edition of this text.

Christine A. Gleason
Sherin U. Devaskar

CONTENTS

PART VII

CARE OF THE HEALTHY NEWBORN

PART VIII

CARE OF THE HIGH-RISK INFANT

PART IX

IMMUNOLOGY AND INFECTIONS

PART X

RESPIRATORY SYSTEM

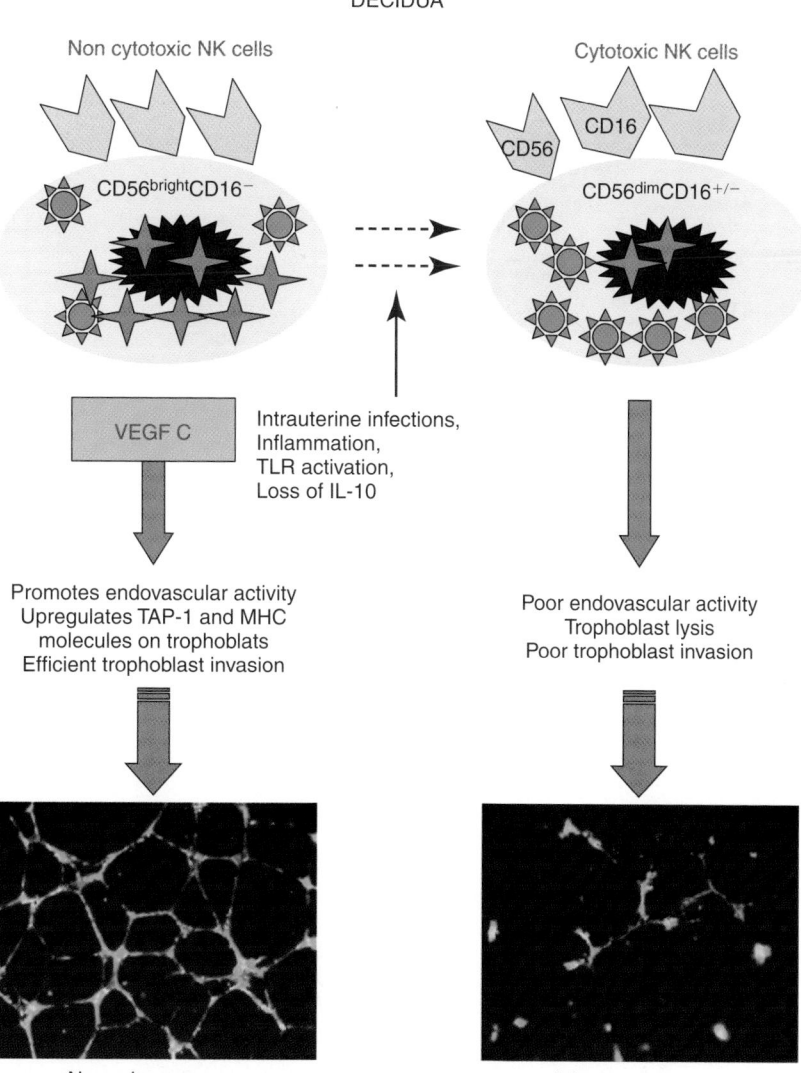

COLOR PLATE 1 *(See Chapter 5, p. 46.)* Angiogenic features of natural killer (NK) cells render them immune tolerant at the maternal-fetal interface. Vascular endothelial growth factor (VEGF) C-producing noncytotoxic uterine NK cell clones similar to decidual NK cells support endovascular activity in a coculture of endothelial cells (*red*) and first-trimester trophoblast HTR8 cells (*green*) on matrigel. By contrast, cytotoxic uterine NK cell clones similar to peripheral blood NK cells disrupted the endovascular activity because of endothelial and trophoblast cell lysis. This distinct functional feature determines whether optimal trophoblast invasion takes place and can result in normal or adverse pregnancy outcomes.

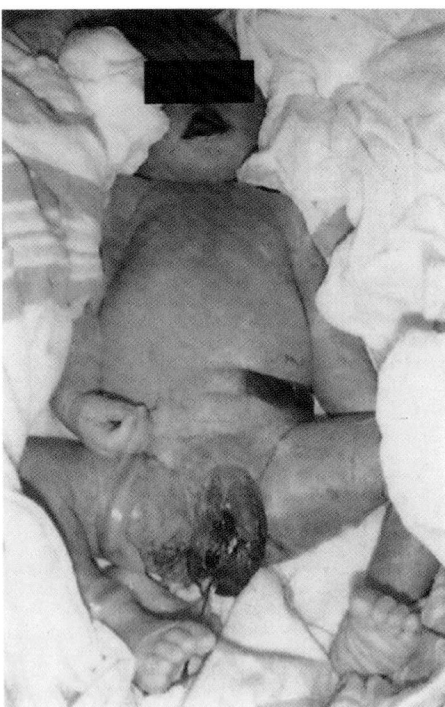

COLOR PLATE 2 *(See Chapter 15, p. 158.)* A 28-year-old woman was admitted to the labor and delivery department with an intrauterine demise. Examination of the fetus shows the cord wrapped tightly around the torso, leg, and ankle, suggesting cord accident as a cause of death. No other pathologic abnormalities were found on autopsy. *(Courtesy Thomas R. Easterling.)*

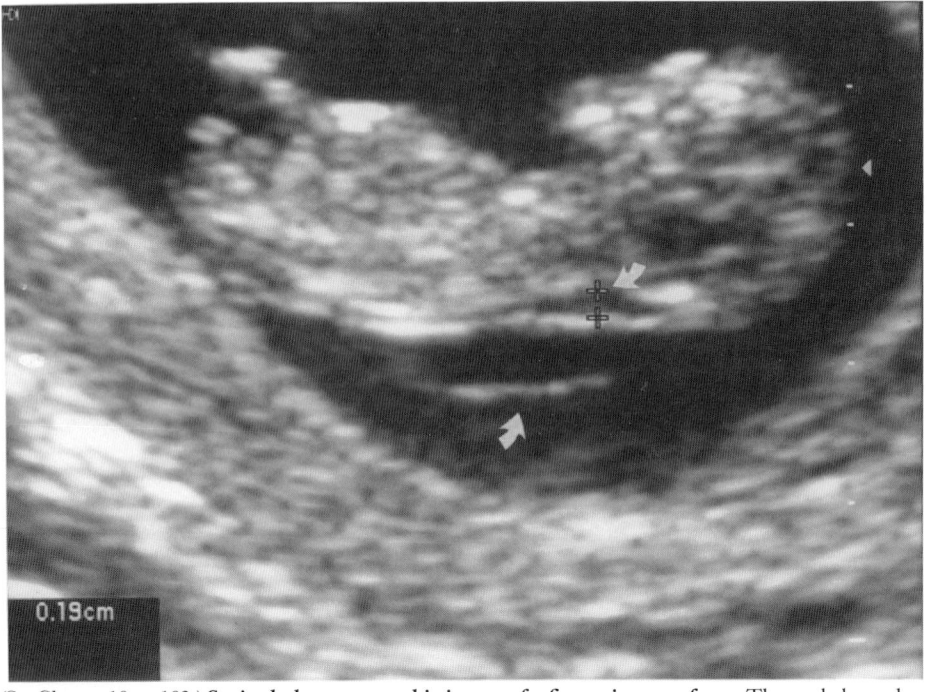

COLOR PLATE 3 *(See Chapter 18, p. 182.)* **Sagittal ultrasonographic image of a first-trimester fetus.** The nuchal translucency measurement is the distance between the two crosses. A measurement larger than normal standards for gestational age indicates that the fetus is at high risk for Down syndrome, congenital heart disease, or both. *(Courtesy Dr. Fergal Malone.)*

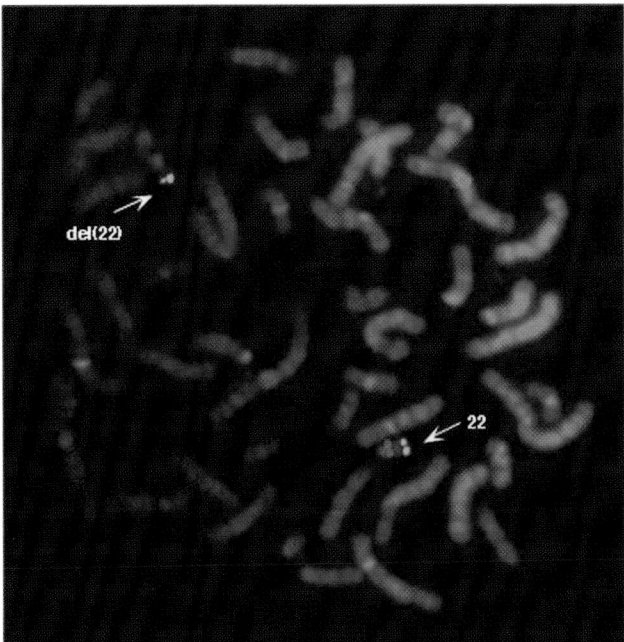

COLOR PLATE 4 *(See Chapter 20, p. 205.)* Fluorescence in situ hybridization study of a 22q deletion. *(Courtesy Beverly S. Emanuel.)*

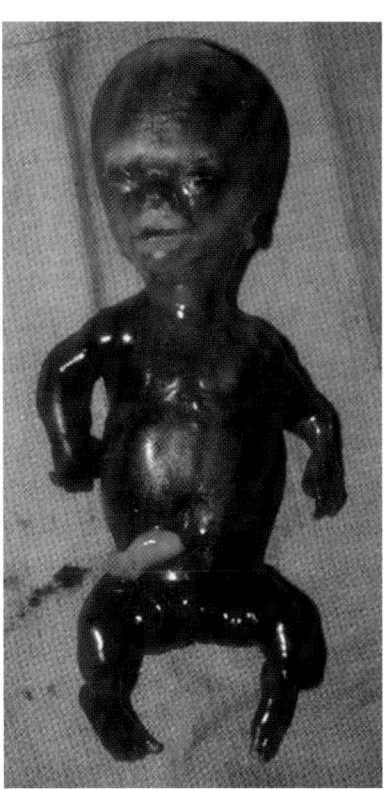

COLOR PLATE 5 *(See Chapter 24, p. 262.)* **Osteogenesis imperfecta type II.** A 20-week fetus with limbs that are angulated and deformed from multiple fractures.

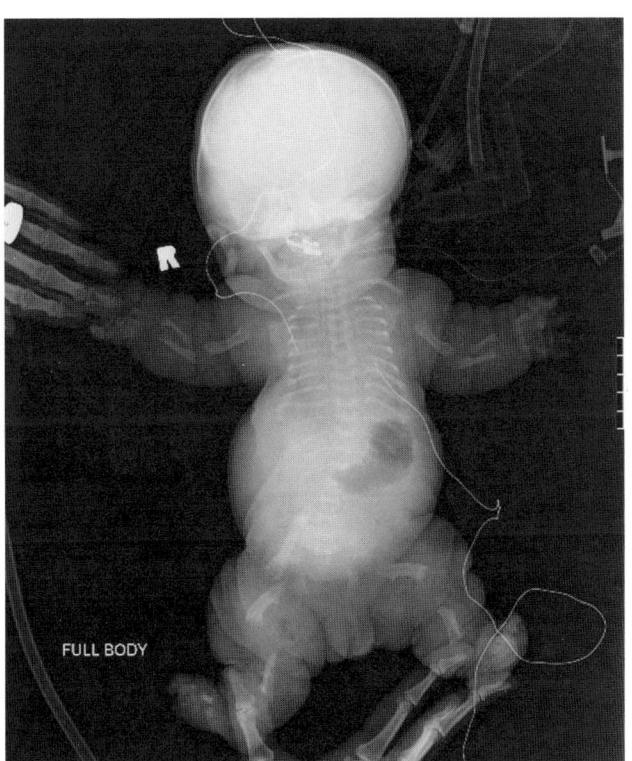

COLOR PLATE 6 *(See Chapter 24, p. 267.)* **Thanatophoric dysplasia.** Radiograph of an infant with thanatophoric dysplasia demonstrates a large calvarium, short ribs with anterior splaying, flat vertebral bodies (platyspondyly), and short bowed femurs with medial metaphyseal spike.

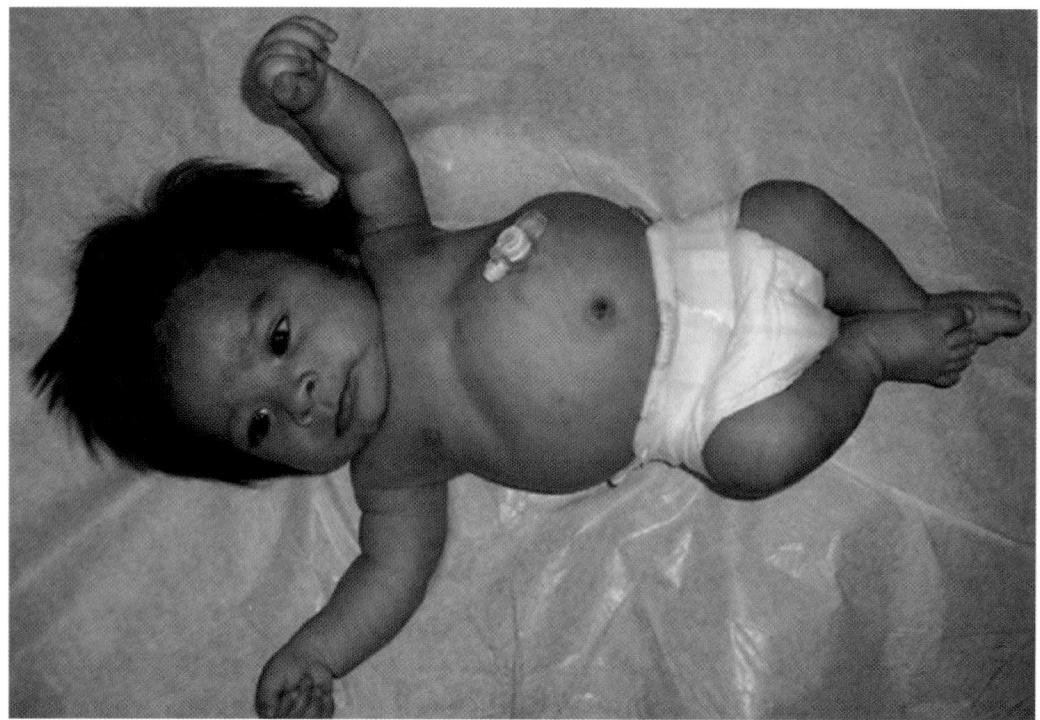

COLOR PLATE 7 *(See Chapter 24, p. 268.)* **Spondyloepiphyseal dysplasia congenita.** A 2-month-old infant demonstrating short neck, trunk, and limbs. Note the flat facial profile and normal size of hands and feet.

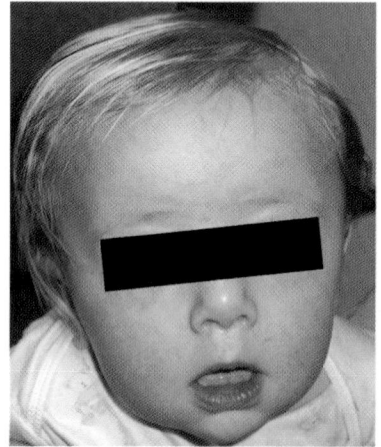

COLOR PLATE 8 *(See Chapter 24, p. 276.)* **Menkes syndrome.** Note blonde hair, fair complexion, and epicanthal folds in this 11-month-old Hispanic boy.

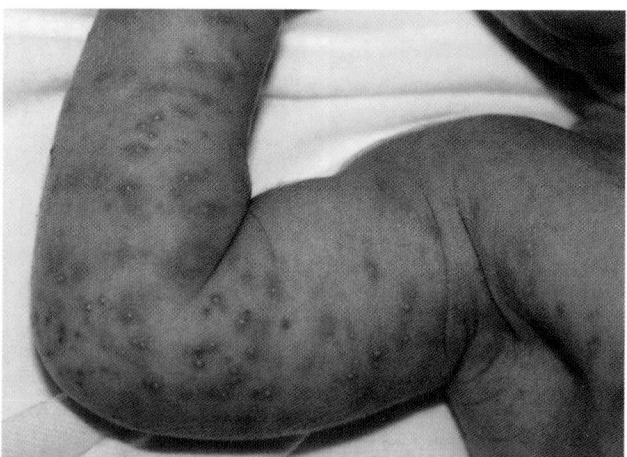

COLOR PLATE 9 *(See Chapter 25, p. 284.)* **Erythema toxicum neonatorum with erythematous macules, wheals, and pustules.** Pustules predominate in this example. At times, patchy or confluent areas of erythema occur without pustules. *(Reprinted from Eichenfield LF, et al, editors:* Neonatal dermatology, *Philadelphia, 2008, Saunders, p 88.)*

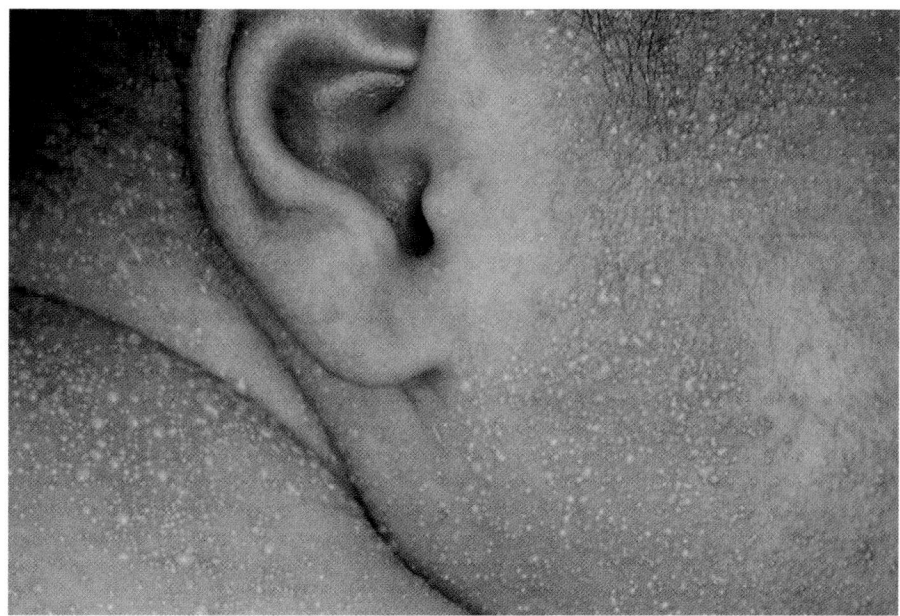

COLOR PLATE 10 *(See Chapter 25, p. 285.)* **Miliaria crystallina.** The tiny, clear vesicles resemble water droplets, with no signs of inflammation. *(Reprinted from Rudolph AJ:* Atlas of the newborn, *vol 4, Hamilton, Ontario, Canada, 1997, BC Decker, p 13.)*

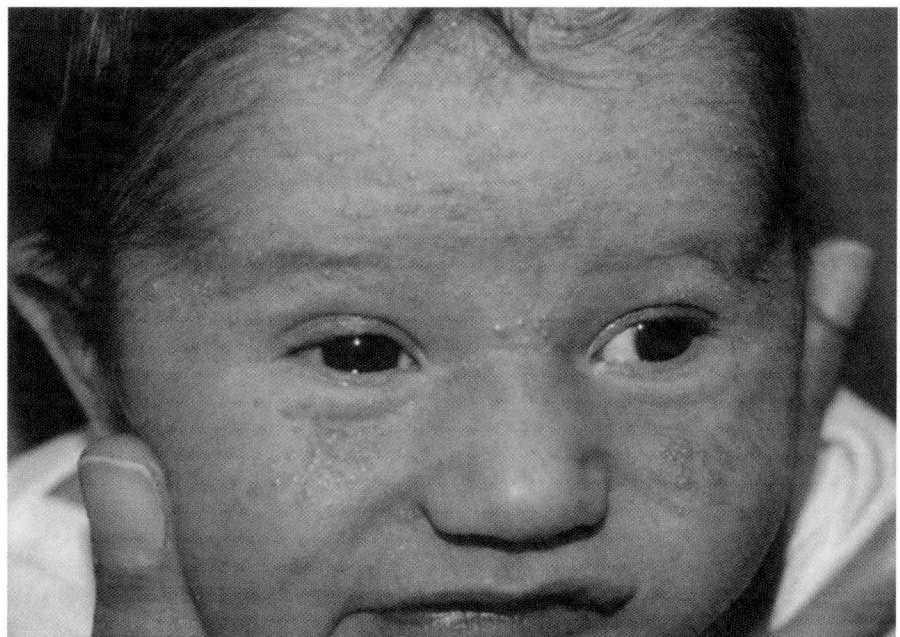

COLOR PLATE 11 *(See Chapter 25, p. 285.)* **Neonatal cephalic pustulosis (neonatal acne).** Small red papules and pustules are seen on the cheeks and forehead, with some extension into the scalp. Comedones are absent. *(Reprinted from Eichenfield LF, et al, editors:* Neonatal dermatology, *Philadelphia, 2008, WB Saunders, p 90.)*

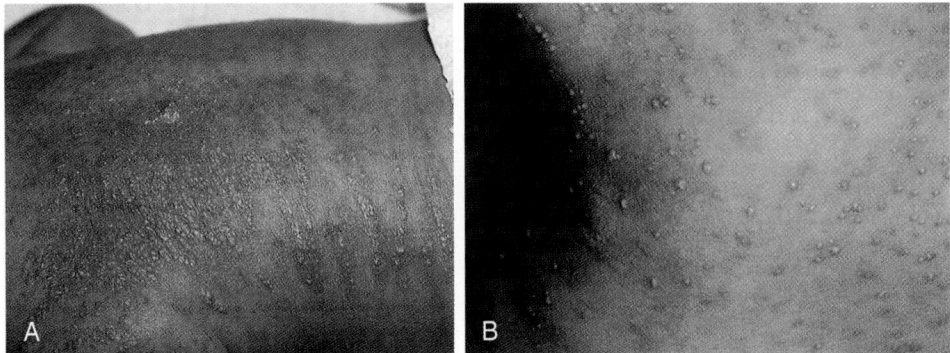

COLOR PLATE 12 *(See Chapter 25, p. 286.)* **Congenital candidiasis.** The rash may be a diffuse, erythematous pustular eruption **(A)** or have diffusely distributed but distinct pustules **(B)**. In premature infants, a diffuse scaldlike erythematous dermatitis may be seen (not shown). *(Reprinted from Eichenfield LF, et al, editors:* Neonatal dermatology, *Philadelphia, 2008, Saunders, p 214.)*

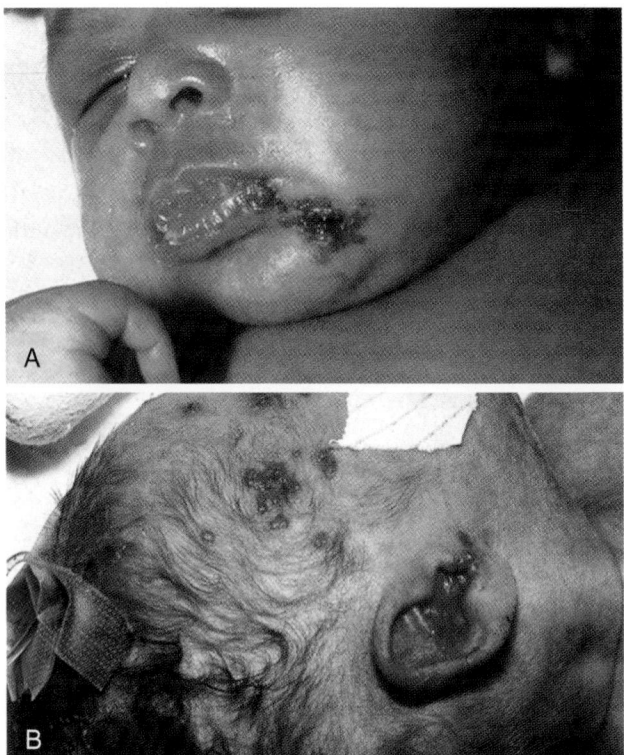

COLOR PLATE 13 *(See Chapter 25, p. 286.)* **Herpes simplex. A,** The first signs of herpes infection in this neonate were eroded vesicles at the corner of the mouth. **B,** Herpetic vesicles on the face, scalp, and ear of an infant with respiratory distress and hepatitis. *(Reprinted from Cohen B:* Pediatric dermatology, *ed 3, Philadelphia, 2005, Mosby, p 36.)*

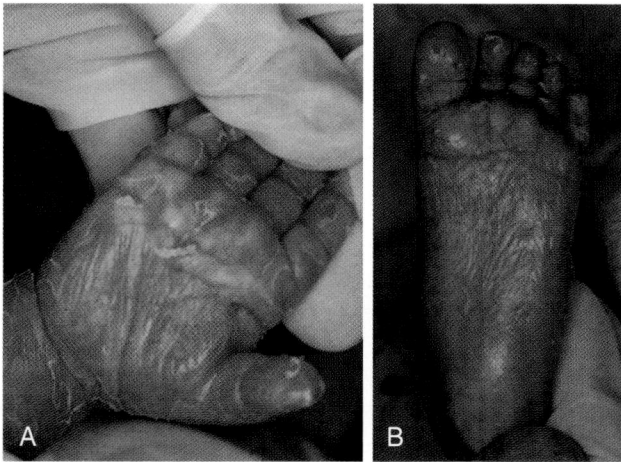

COLOR PLATE 14 *(See Chapter 25, p. 286.)* Desquamation on the palms **(A)** and soles **(B)** of an infant with congenital syphilis. *(Reprinted from Rudolph AJ: Atlas of the newborn, vol 4, Hamilton, Ontario, Canada, 1997, BC Decker, p 108.)*

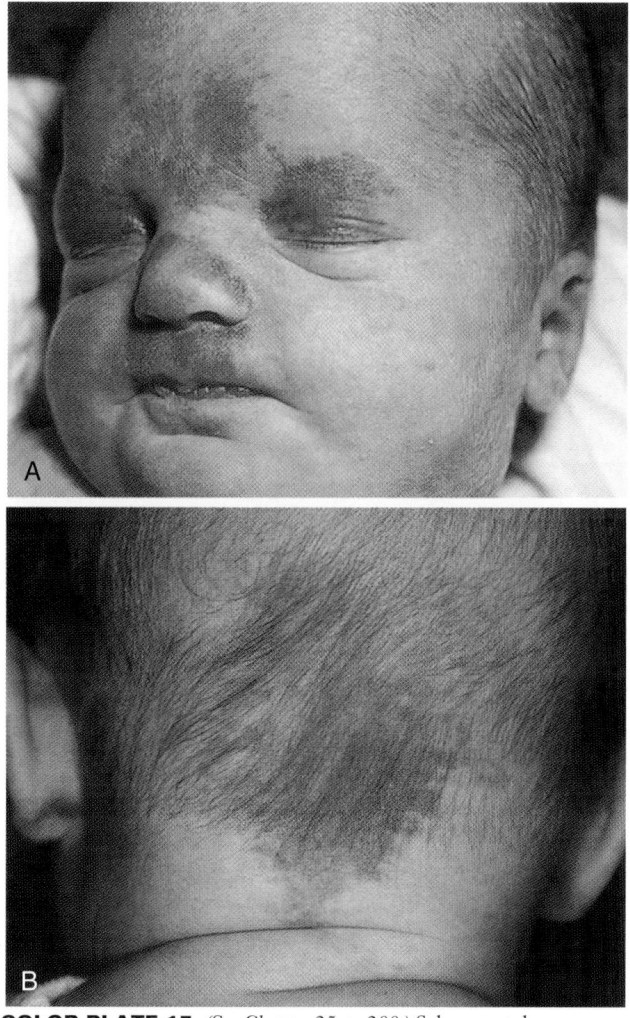

COLOR PLATE 15 *(See Chapter 25, p. 288.)* Salmon patches are commonly seen on the glabella, eyelids, nose, or upper lip, either singly or in all these locations **(A)**, and on the nape of the neck **(B)**. *(Reprinted from Eichenfield LF, et al, editors:* Neonatal dermatology, *Philadelphia, 2008, Saunders, p. 95.)*

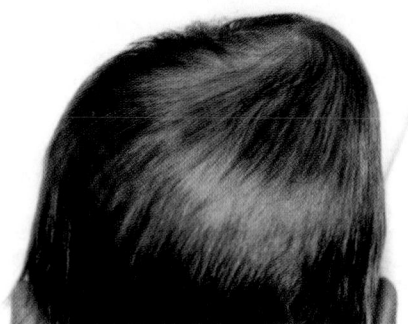

COLOR PLATE 16 *(See Chapter 25, p. 289.)* Posterior view of a large cephalohematoma under the periosteum of the right parietal bone. *(Reprinted from Fletcher MA:* Physical diagnosis in neonatology, *Philadelphia, 1998, Lippincott-Raven, p 185.)*

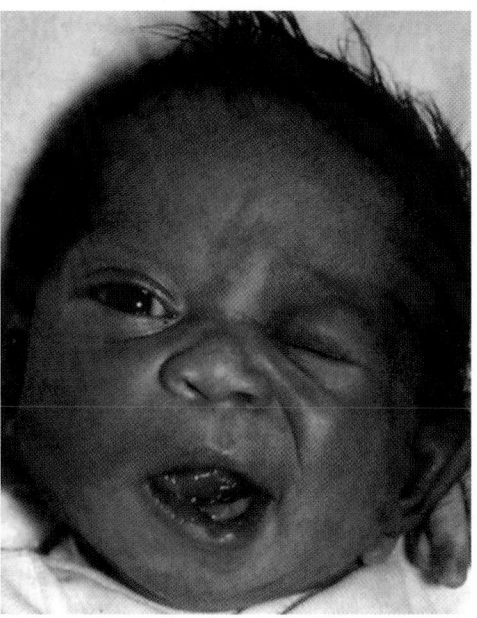

COLOR PLATE 17 *(See Chapter 25, p. 299.)* **Unilateral facial weakness.** There are obvious asymmetries of the grimace and eye closing during crying; the weakness is shown on the right side here. *(Reprinted from Fletcher MA:* Physical diagnosis in neonatology, *Philadelphia, 1998, Lippincott-Raven, p 457.)*

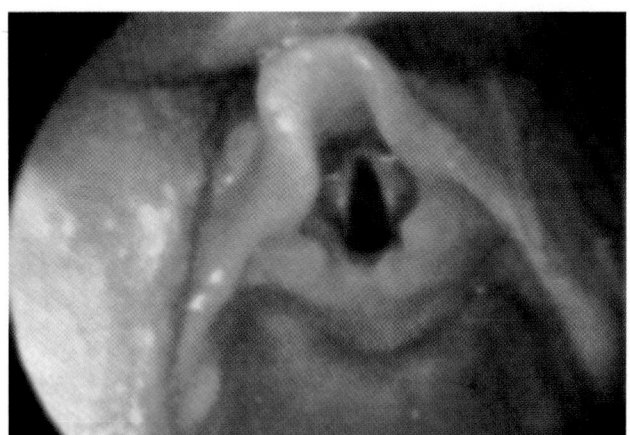

COLOR PLATE 18 *(See Chapter 28, p. 336.)* View of the glottis and vocal cords as the laryngoscope is gently lifted. *(From American Heart Association, American Academy of Pediatrics: Kattwinkel J, editor:* Neonatal resuscitation textbook, *ed 5, Elk Grove Village, Ill, 2006, American Academy of Pediatrics.)*

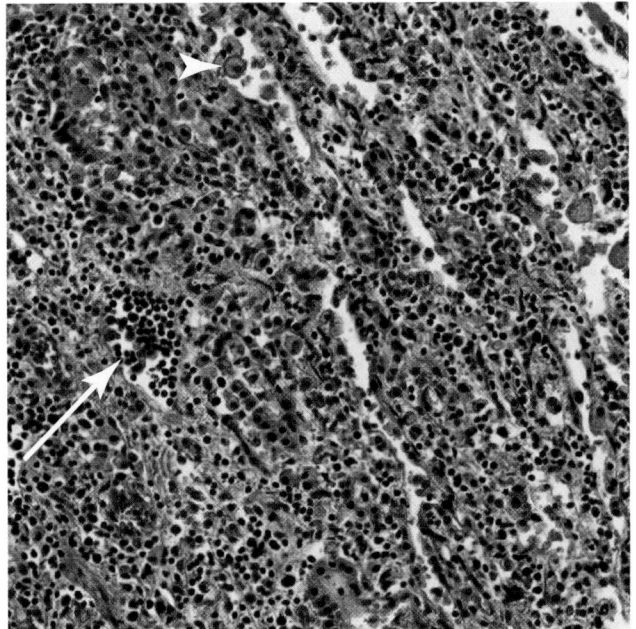

COLOR PLATE 19 *(See Chapter 37, p. 503.)* Postmortem histology from infant who expired from disseminated adenovirus infection at 2 weeks of age. H & E stain of lung demonstrating inflammatory infiltrates (*arrow*) and intranuclear inclusions (*arrowhead*). This infant had a viral sepsis syndrome characterized by hepatic failure, DIC, and pneumonitis from adenovirus infection, presumed to have been acquired intrapartum.

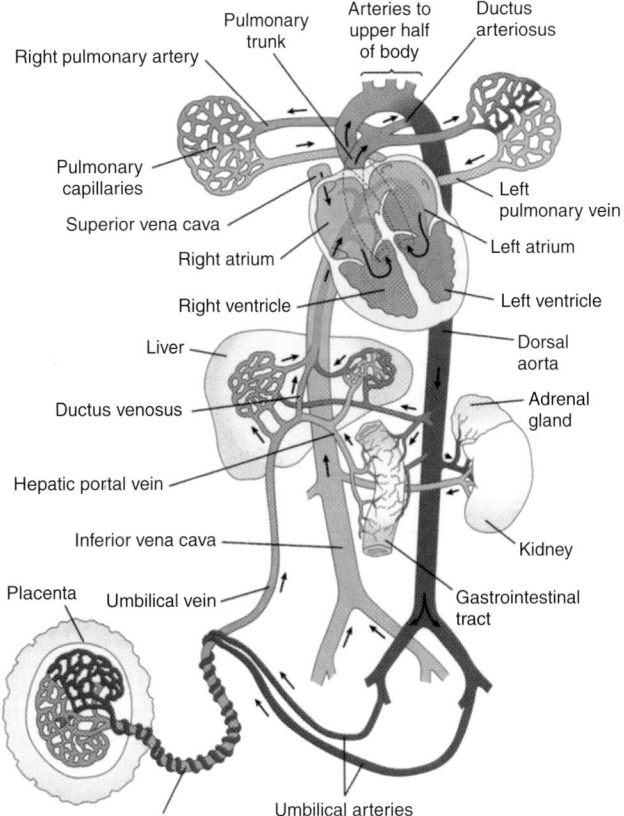

COLOR PLATE 20 *(See Chapter 50, p. 712.)* **The fetal circulation at term.** The path of oxygenated blood returning from the placenta is shown in orange. It mixes with deoxygenated blood returning from the fetal systemic veins shown in light blue. There is intracardiac mixing of blood as shown. The upper body receives higher oxygen content than the lower body, as deoxygenated blood enters the descending aorta via right-to-left flow at the ductus arteriosus. *(From Carlson BM: Human embryology and developmental biology, ed 4, Philadelphia, 2009, Mosby, p 466.)*

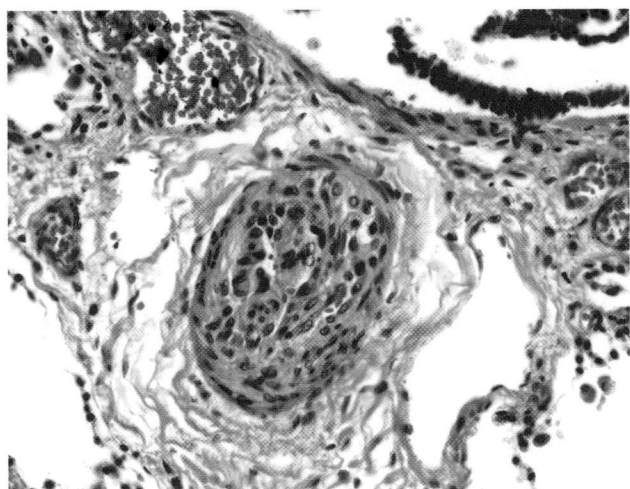

COLOR PLATE 21 *(See Chapter 52, p. 734.)* Histology of a pulmonary vessel from an infant with fatal PPHN illustrating the dramatic remodeling that can be associated with severe PPHN.

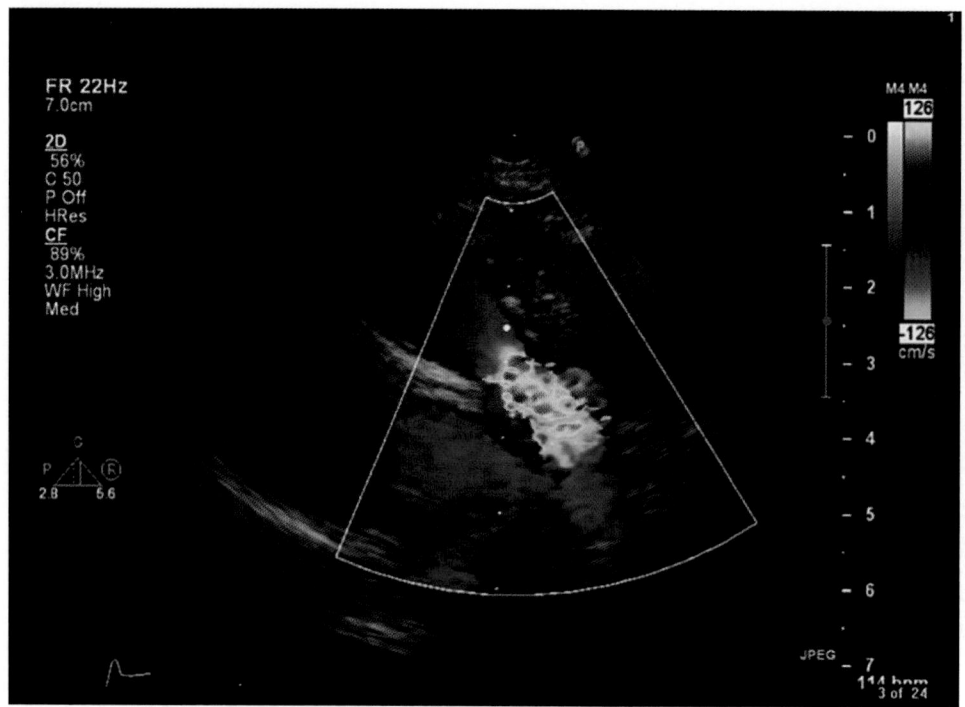

COLOR PLATE 22 *(See Chapter 55, p. 771.)* **Pulmonic stenosis.** Using color Doppler imaging, turbulence in the main pulmonary artery is seen above the pulmonic valve.

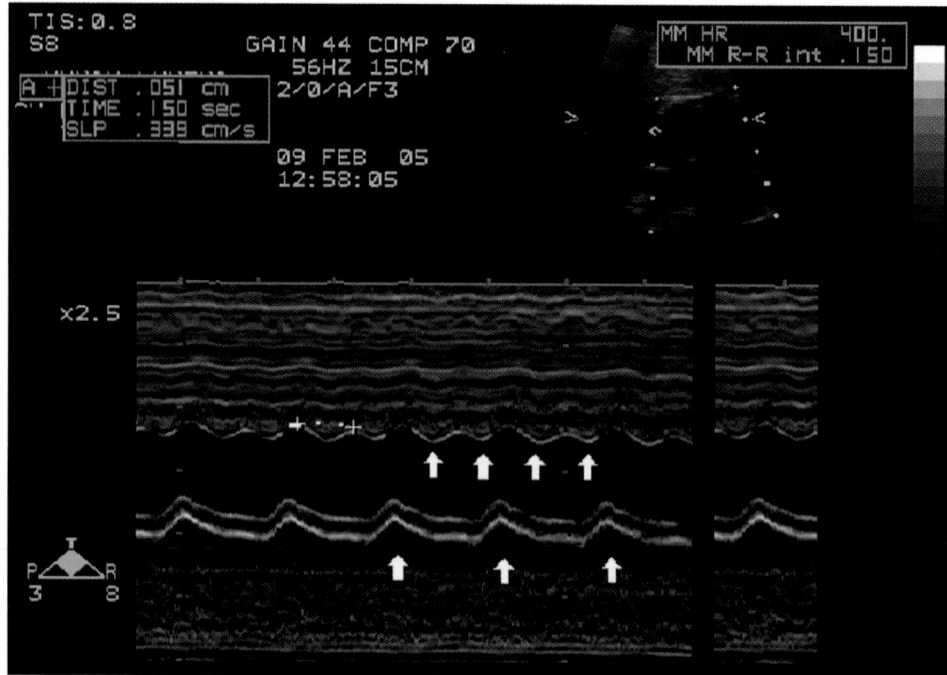

COLOR PLATE 23 *(See Chapter 56, p. 797.)* **Fetal m-mode echocardiogram recording of a late second-trimester fetus with atrial flutter.** The ultrasound cursor is positioned through the right atrium, tricuspid valve, and the right ventricle *(upper right corner)*. The top row of four arrows delineates the mechanical right atrial contraction rate, which is faster than the tricuspid valve/right ventricle contraction rate *(bottom three arrows)*.

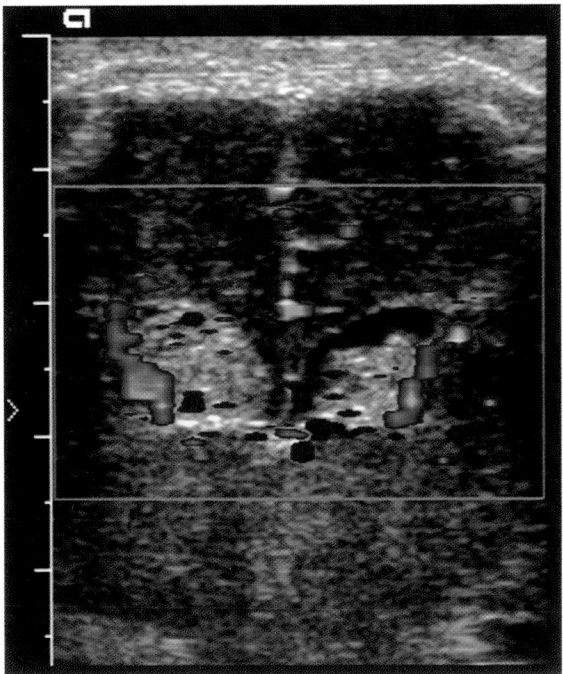

COLOR PLATE 24 *(See Chapter 59, p. 828.)* **Coronal color Doppler image of bilateral grade I germinal matrix hemorrhages.** The hemorrhages are echogenic. Although flow is confirmed within the terminal veins (*blue*), the veins are laterally displaced by the subependymal hemorrhages.

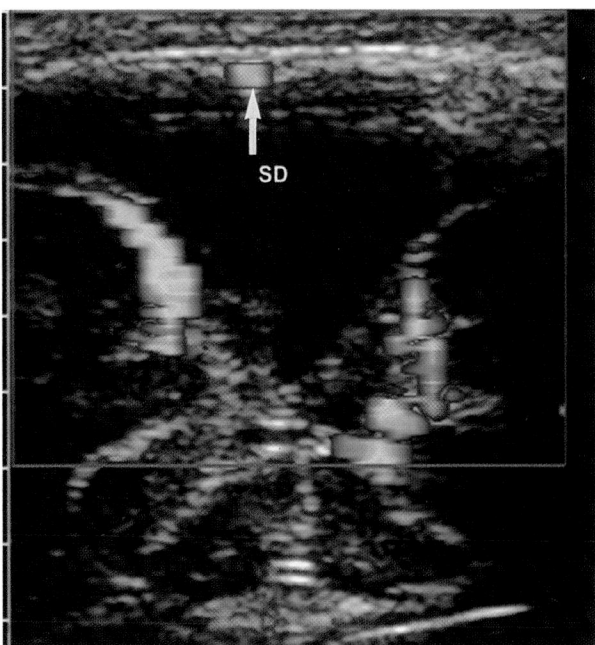

COLOR PLATE 25 *(See Chapter 59, p. 830.)* Coronal color Doppler ultrasound study shows that the vessels (color) are displaced toward the brain parenchyma by the subdural fluid (SD). Note flow in the superior sagittal sinus (*arrow*).

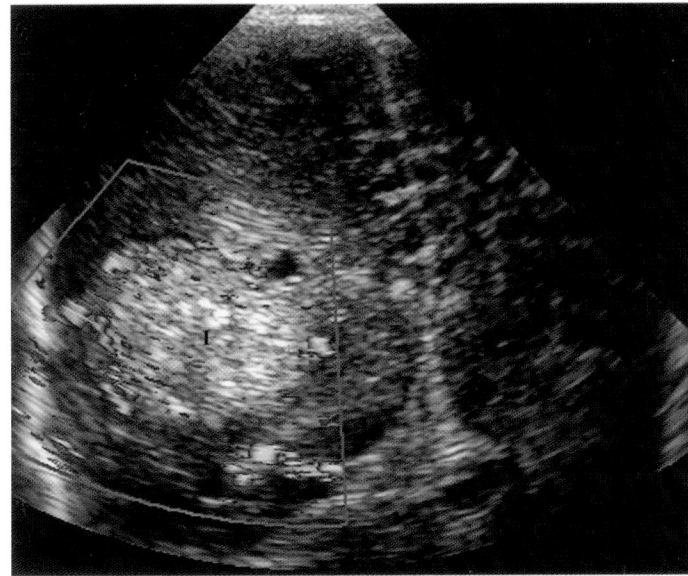

COLOR PLATE 26 *(See Chapter 59, p. 832.)* **The patient was a neonate with a focal right occipital infarction with surrounding "luxury perfusion."** A coronal ultrasound image obtained through the anterior fontanel shows a hyperechoic right occipital infarction (I) surrounded by increased flow on color Doppler examination.

GASTRULATION

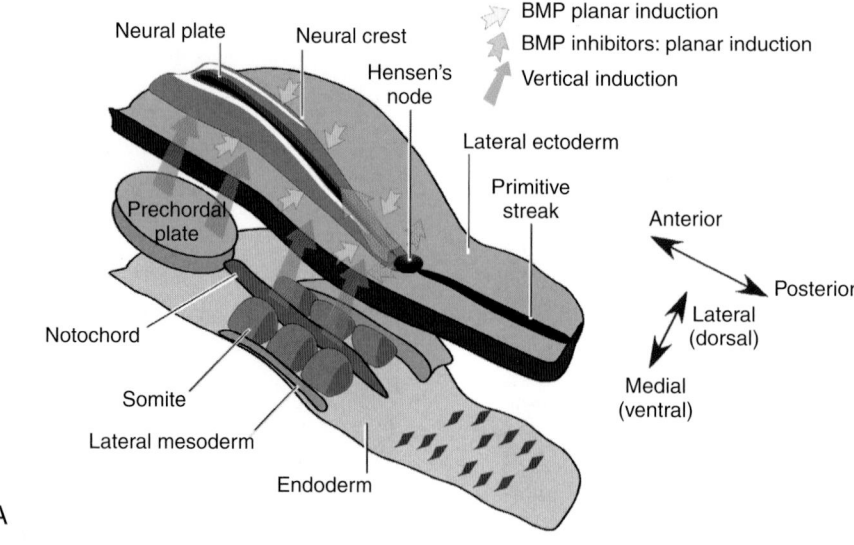

Neural plate   Neural crest
                        Hensen's
                        node
                        Lateral ectoderm
                        Primitive
                        streak

Prechordal
plate

Notochord

Somite

Lateral mesoderm

Endoderm

A

BMP planar induction
BMP inhibitors: planar induction
Vertical induction

Anterior

Posterior

Lateral
(dorsal)

Medial
(ventral)

NEURULATION

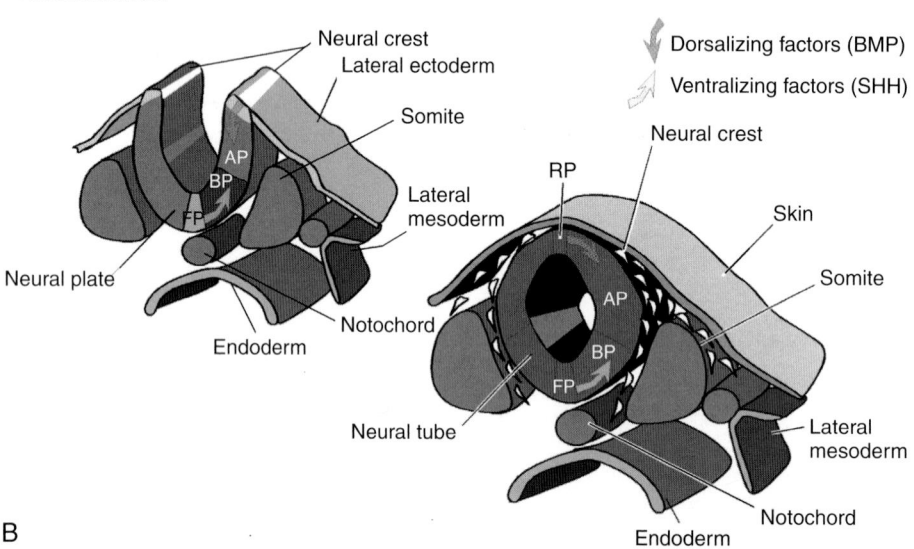

Neural crest
Lateral ectoderm
Somite

AP
BP
FP

Lateral
mesoderm

Neural plate

Notochord

Endoderm

Dorsalizing factors (BMP)
Ventralizing factors (SHH)

Neural crest

RP

Skin

AP

Somite

BP

FP

Neural tube

Lateral
mesoderm

Notochord

Endoderm

B

COLOR PLATE 27 *(See Chapter 60, p. 846.)* **Formation of the neural tube. A,** During gastrulation, at the neural plate stage, dorsoventral polarity and early anteroposterior regionalization is defined by a process of vertical induction by fibroblast growth factor-8 (FGF-8) and other factors *(long gray arrows)* derived from mesendoderm (notochord and prechordal plate). Planar induction occurs via BMPs and BMP inhibitors that are derived from lateral ectoderm *(short light gray arrows)* and Hensen's node *(short dark gray arrows),* respectively. **B,** The process of neurulation proceeds with the approximation of the neural folds toward the dorsal midline. Before closure of the neural tube, neural crest cells delaminate and migrate from the neural folds. Dorsalizing factors (BMPs; *dark gray arrow)* derived from the dorsal midline roofplate (RP) and ventralizing factors (SHH; *light gray arrow)* from the floor plate (FP) establish dorsal-ventral gradients of these key signaling molecules that induce formation of the alar plate (AP) and the basal plate (BP) from the lateral wall of the neural tube. *(From: Vieira C, Pombero A, Garcia-Lopez R, et al: Molecular mechanisms controlling brain development: an overview of neuroepithelial secondary organizers, Int J Dev Biol 54:7-20, 2010; courtesy Dr. Salvador Martinez, Institute of Neuroscience, Universidad Miguel Hernandez, San Juan de Alicante, Spain.)*

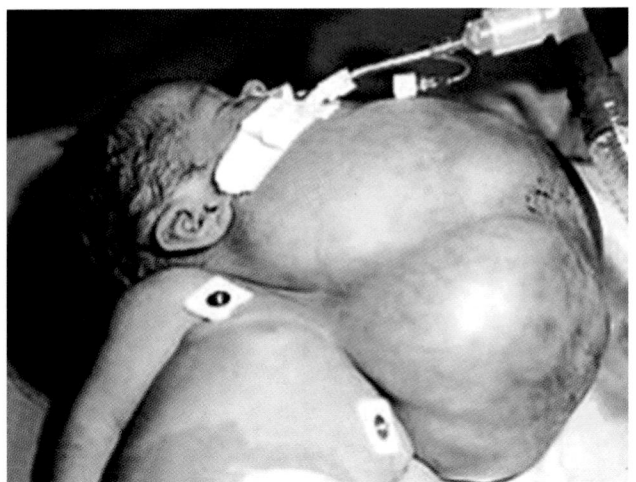

COLOR PLATE 28 *(See Chapter 69, p. 980.)* **Cystic hygroma of the face and neck.** Prenatal diagnosis of this large lesion led to the delivery of this infant using EXIT. *(From American Medical Association:* Archives of pediatrics and adolescent medicine, *155:1271–1272, 2001. All rights reserved.)*

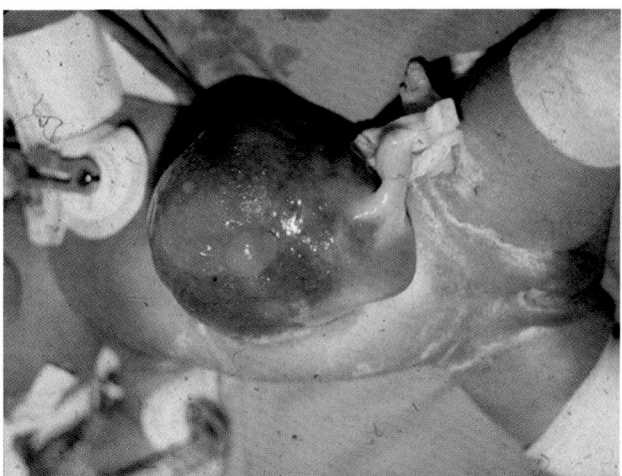

COLOR PLATE 29 *(See Chapter 71, p. 1008.)* **Female newborn with omphalocele.** The fascial defect is large, situated at the base of the umbilical cord, covered by a glistening membrane, and contains both liver and bowel.

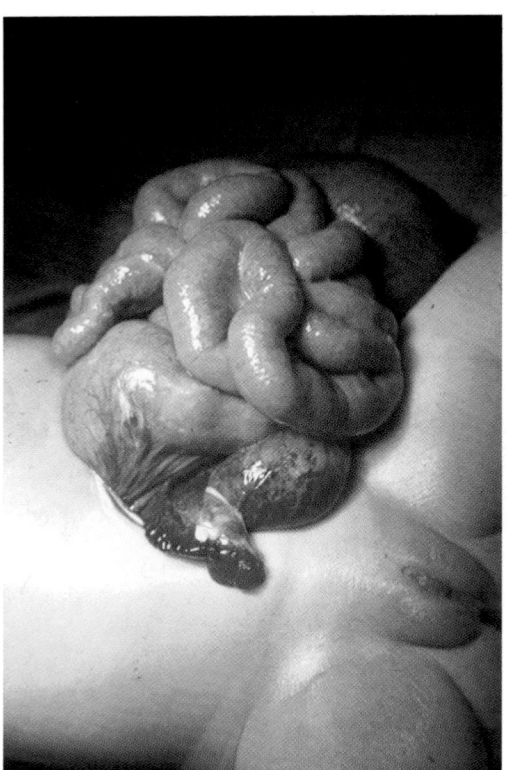

COLOR PLATE 30 *(See Chapter 71, p. 1010.)* **Female newborn with gastroschisis.** The fascial defect is relatively small, situated to the right of the umbilical cord, and contains exposed bowel (as well as an ovary in this instance).

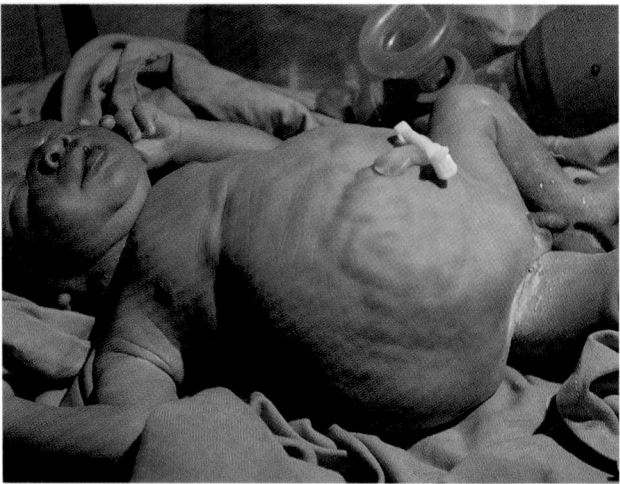

COLOR PLATE 31 *(See Chapter 71, p. 1011.)* **Newborn with prune belly syndrome.** The laxity of the abdominal wall musculature is obvious.

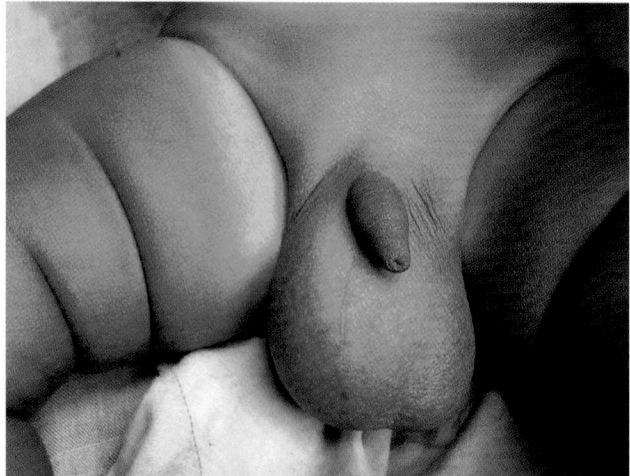

COLOR PLATE 32 *(See Chapter 71, p. 1012.)* **Bilateral infantile hydroceles.** The scrotum is distended by fluid, while the inguinal canals are normal.

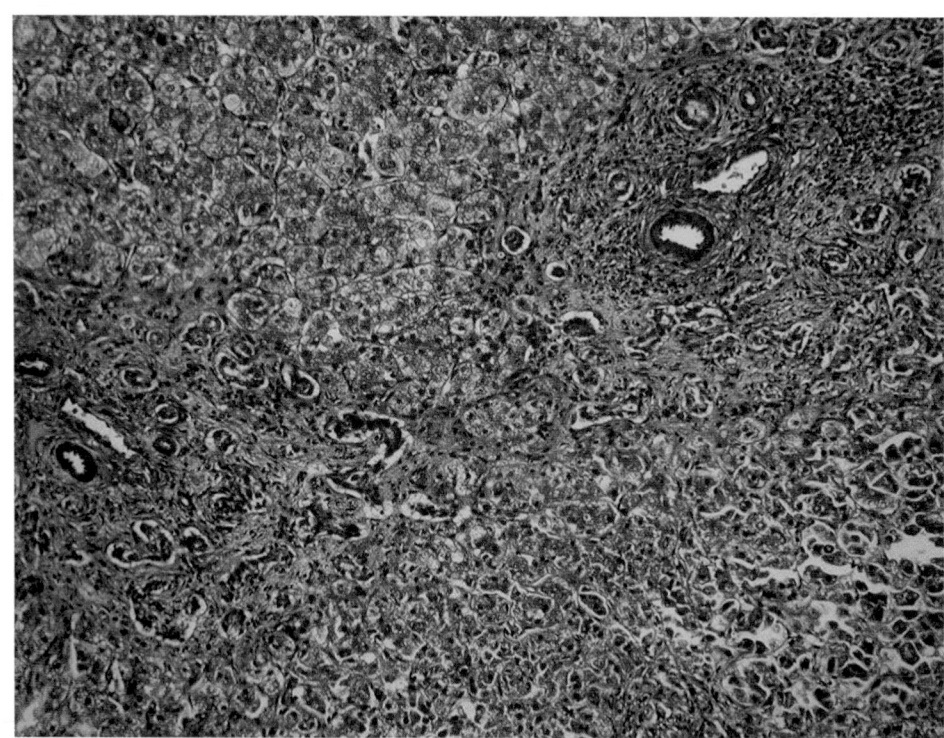

COLOR PLATE 33 *(See Chapter 74, p. 1035.)* **Liver biopsy from an infant with biliary atresia.** Trichrome stain demonstrates portal tract fibrosis.

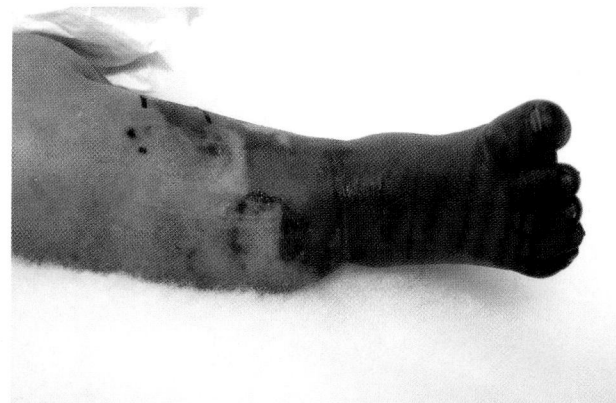

COLOR PLATE 34 *(See Chapter 76, p. 1078.)* Arterial thrombosis with skin necrosis.

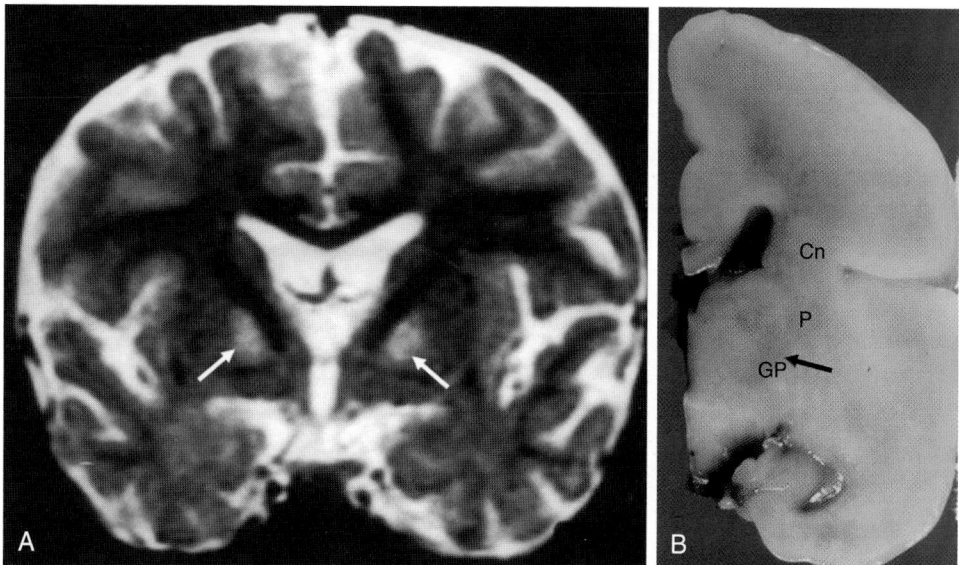

COLOR PLATE 35 *(See Chapter 79, p. 1135.)* **A,** Coronal T1-weighted magnetic resonance image at the level of the basal ganglia in one infant is shown on the left, demonstrating bilateral, symmetric high-intensity globus pallidus *(GP)* signals *(arrows).* **B,** Deep orange-yellow staining of the globus pallidus (GP) of the coronal section at postmortem in another neonate. Note unstained putamen *(P)* and caudate nucleus *(Cn).* These findings illustrate the selective vulnerability and regional nature of kernicterus and concordancy of neuroimaging and neuropathology in this disorder. *(A, Reprinted with permission from Coskun A, Yikilmaz A, Kumandas S, et al: Hyperintense globus pallidus on T1-weighted MR imaging in acute kernicterus: is it common or rare?* Eur Radiol 15:1263-1267, 2005; **B,** reprinted with permission from Monographs in Clinical Pediatrics 11:78, 2000. Available at www.tandf.co.uk.)

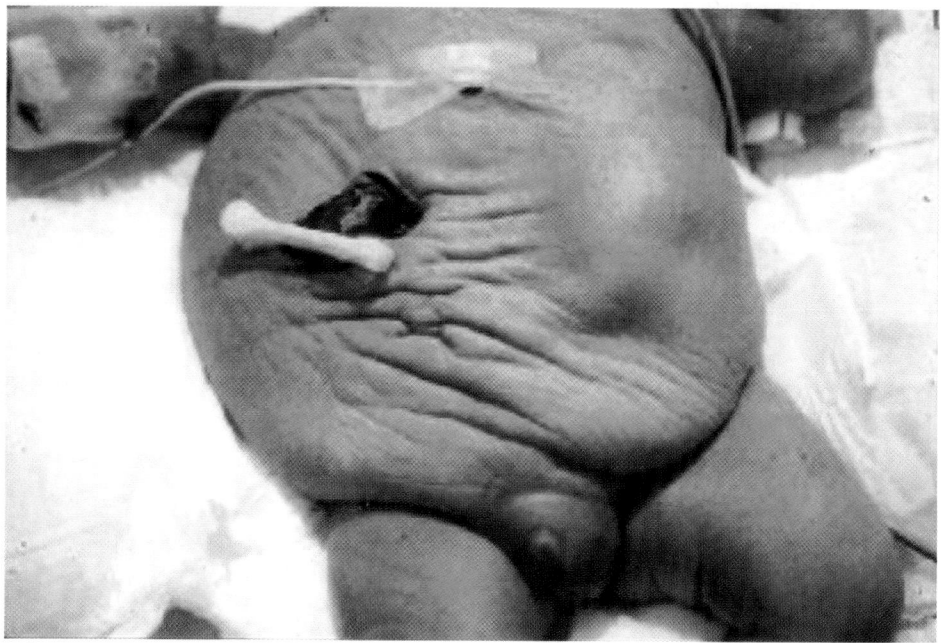

COLOR PLATE 36 *(See Chapter 84, p. 1197.)* The classic wrinkled abdominal wall seen in the prune-belly syndrome is accompanied by bilateral undescended testes.

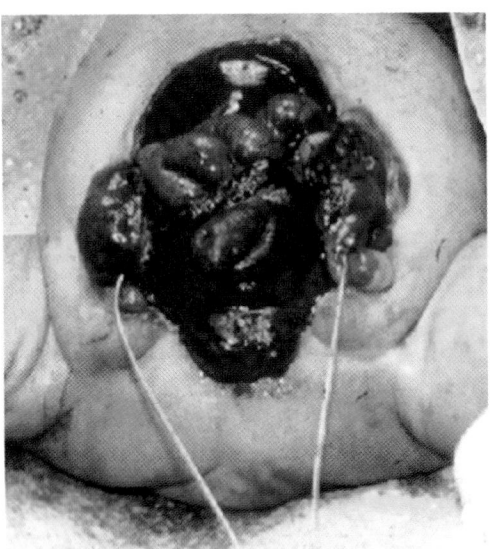

COLOR PLATE 37 *(See Chapter 84, p. 1198.)* **Dramatic appearance of cloacal exstrophy.** In cloacal exstrophy, the bladder halves are separated by the presence of a large cecal plate and a protruding ileal stump. In this intraoperative photograph, the omphalocele has been removed to expose the small bowel and liver.

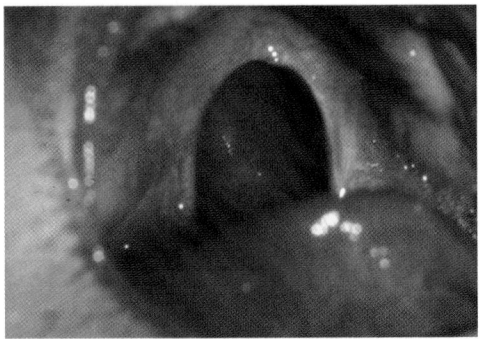

COLOR PLATE 38 *(See Chapter 95, p. 1332.)* U-shaped cleft palate.

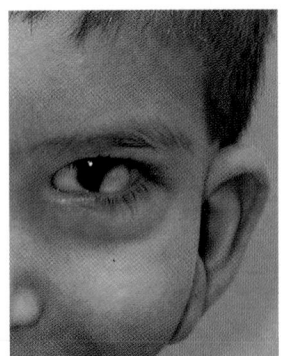

COLOR PLATE 39 *(See Chapter 95, p. 1344.)* A child with an epibulbar lipodermoid and craniofacial microsomia.

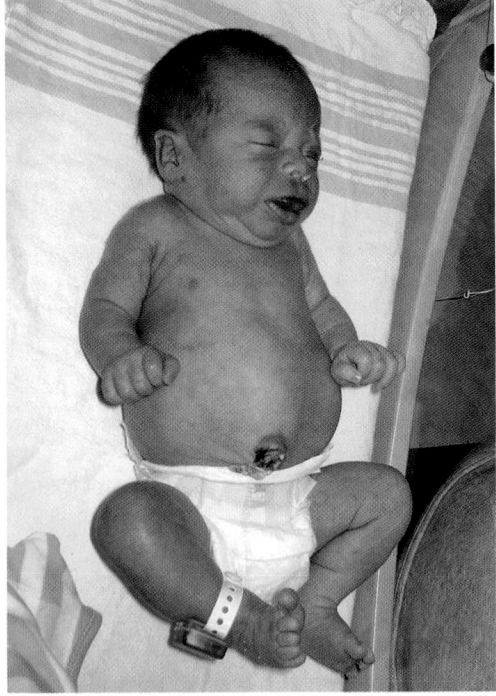

COLOR PLATE 40 *(See Chapter 95, p. 1348.)* A premature newborn with Beckwith-Wiedemann syndrome, macroglossia, and rectus diastasis.

PART I

OVERVIEW

CHAPTER 1

NEONATAL AND PERINATAL EPIDEMIOLOGY

Nigel Paneth

EPIDEMIOLOGIC APPROACHES TO THE PERINATAL AND NEONATAL PERIODS

The period surrounding the time of birth (the perinatal period) is a critical episode in human development, rivaling only the period surrounding conception in its significance. During this period, the infant makes the critical transition from its dependence on maternal and placental support—oxidative, nutritional, and endocrinologic—and establishes independent life. The difficulty of this transition is indicated by mortality risks that are higher than any occuring until old age (Kung et al, 2008) and by risks for damage to organ systems, most notably the brain, that can be lifelong. Providers of care in the perinatal period recognize that the developing human organism cannot always demonstrate the immediate effects of even profound insults. Years must pass before the effects on higher cortical functions of insults and injuries occurring during the perinatal period can be detected reliably. Epidemiologic approaches to the perinatal period must therefore be bidirectional—looking backward to examine the causes of adverse health conditions that arise or complicate the perinatal period, and looking forward to see how these conditions shape disorders of health found later in life.

Traditionally the perinatal period was described as from 28 weeks' gestation until 1 week of life, but the World Health Organization has more recently antedated the onset of the perinatal period to 22 weeks' gestation (World Health Organization, 2004). For this discussion we will view the term *perinatal* more expansively, as including the second half of gestation—by which time most organogenesis has occurred, but growth and maturation of many systems have yet to occur—and the first month of life. The neonatal period, usually considered as the first month of life, is thus included in the term *perinatal*, reflecting the view that addressing the problems of the neonate requires an understanding of intrauterine phenomena.

HEALTH DISORDERS OF PREGNANCY AND THE PERINATAL PERIOD

KEY POPULATION MORTALITY RATES

Maternal and child health in the population have traditionally been assessed by monitoring two key rates—maternal mortality and infant mortality. Maternal mortality is defined by the World Health Organization as the death of a woman from pregnancy-related causes during pregnancy or within 42 days of pregnancy, expressed as a ratio to 100,000 live births in the population being studied (World Health Organization, 2004). Because pregnancy can contribute to deaths beyond 42 days, some have argued for examining all deaths within 1 year of a pregnancy (Hoyert, 2007). When the cause of death is attributed to pregnancy-related causes, it is described as *direct*. When pregnancy has aggravated an underlying health disorder, the death is termed an *indirect maternal death*. Deaths unrelated to pregnancy that occur within 42 days of pregnancy are termed *incidental maternal deaths* or sometimes *pregnancy-related deaths* (Khlat and Guillaume, 2006). These distinctions are not always easy to make. Homicide and suicide, for example, are sometimes found to be more common in pregnancy, and thus might not be entirely incidental (Samandari et al, 2010; Shadigian and Bauer, 2005).

Since 2003, the U.S. Standard Certificate of Death has included a special requirement for identifying whether the decedent, if female, was pregnant or had been pregnant in the previous 42 days, or from 43 days to 1 year before the death, thus enhancing the monitoring of all forms of maternal death (Centers for Disease Control and Prevention, 2003). This addition has added to the number of recorded maternal deaths.

In most geographic entities, *infant mortality* (IM) is defined as all deaths occurring from birth to 365 days of age in a calendar year divided by all live births in the same year. This approach is imprecise, because some deaths in the examined year occurred to the previous year's birth cohort, and some births in the examined year may die as infants in the following year. In recent years, birth-death linkage has permitted vital registration areas in the United States to provide IM rates that avoid this imprecision. The standard IM rate reported by the National Center for Health Statistics links deaths for the index year to all births, including those taking place the previous year. This form of IM is termed *period infant mortality*. An alternative procedure is to take births for the index year and link them to infant deaths, including those taking place the following year; this is referred to as *birth cohort infant mortality*, and it is not used for regular annual comparisons because it cannot be completed in as timely a fashion as period IM (Mathews and MacDorman, 2008).

Infant deaths are often divided into deaths in the first 28 days of life (neonatal death) and deaths later in the first year (postneonatal death). Neonatal deaths, which are largely related to preterm birth and birth defects, tend to reflect the circumstances of pregnancy. Postneonatal deaths, when frequent, commonly result from infection, often in the setting of poor nutrition. Thus in underdeveloped countries, postneonatal deaths predominate; in industrialized countries the reverse is true. In the United States, neonatal deaths have been more frequent than postneonatal deaths since 1921. In recent years, the ratio of neonatal to postneonatal deaths in the United States has consistently been approximately 2:1.

Perinatal mortality is a term used for a rate that combines stillbirths and neonatal deaths in some fashion (World Health Organization, 2004). Stillbirth reporting before 28 weeks' gestation is probably incomplete, even in the United States, where such stillbirths are required to be reported in every state. Nonetheless, stillbirths continue to be reported at a levels not much lower those of neonatal deaths, and our understanding of the causes of stillbirth remains very limited.

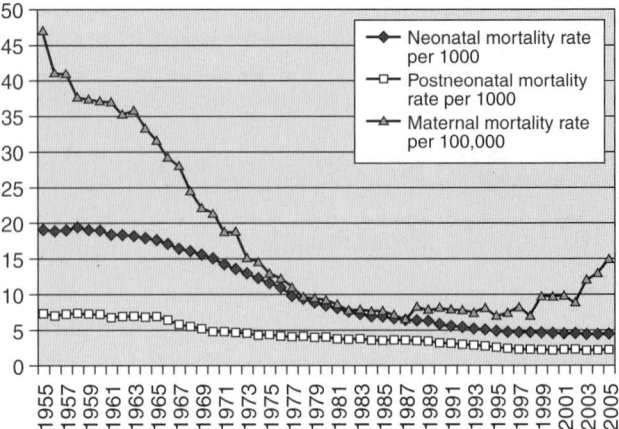

FIGURE 1-1 Neonatal, postneonatal, and maternal mortality, 1955 to 2005.

TIME TRENDS IN MORTALITY RATES IN THE UNITED STATES

Maternal mortality and IM declined steadily through the twentieth century. By 2000, neonatal mortality was 10% of its value in 1915, and postneonatal mortality less than 7%. Maternal mortality in this interval declined 74-fold; the rate in 2000 was less than 2% of the rate recorded in 1915. The contribution to these changes of a variety of complex social factors including improvements in income, housing, birth spacing, and nutrition have been documented widely, as has the role of ecologic-level public health interventions that have produced cleaner food and water (Division of Reproductive Health, 1999). Public health action at the individual level, including targeted maternal and infant nutrition programs and immunization programs, have made a lesser but still notable contribution. Medical care was, until recently, less critically involved, except for the decline in maternal mortality, which was highly sensitive to the developments in blood banking and antibiotics that began in the 1930s. To this day, hemorrhage and infection account for a large fraction of the world's maternal deaths (Khan et al, 2006).

A notable feature of the past 50 years is the sharp decline in all three mortality rates, beginning in the 1960s after a period of stagnation in the 1950s (Figure 1-1). The decline began with maternal mortality, followed by postneonatal and then by neonatal mortality. The contribution of medical care of the neonate was most clearly seen in national statistics in the 1970s, a decade that witnessed a larger decline in neonatal mortality than in any previous decade of the century (Division of Reproductive Health, 1999). All of the change in neonatal mortality between 1950 and 1975 was in mortality for a given birthweight; no improvement was seen in the birthweight distribution (Lee et al, 1980). The effect of newborn intensive care on mortality in extremely small babies has been striking. In 1960, 142 white singletons weighing less than 1000 g in the United States survived to age 1, less than 1% of births of that weight. In 2005, the survival rate for infants weighing 501 to 999 g was 70%, and the number of survivors at age 1 was almost 18,000 (Mathews and MacDorman, 2008).

In retrospect, three factors seem to have played critical roles in the rapid development of newborn intensive care programs. These programs that largely accounted for the rapid decline in birthweight-specific neonatal mortality that characterized national trends in the last third of the twentieth century. The first factor was the willingness of medicine to provide more than nursing care to marginal populations such as premature infants. It has often been noted that the death of the mildly premature son of President John F. Kennedy in 1963 provided a stimulus to the development of newborn intensive care, but it should be noted that the decline in IM that began in the 1970s was paralleled by a similar decline in mortality for the extremely old (Rosenwaike et al, 1980). A second factor was the availability of government funds, provided by the Medicaid program adopted in 1965, to pay for the care of premature newborns, among whom the poor are overrepresented. Whereas these two factors were necessary, they would have been insufficient to improve neonatal mortality had not new medical technologies, especially those supporting ventilation of the immature newborn lung, been developed at approximately the same time (Gregory et al, 1971).

Advances in newborn care have ameliorated the effects of premature birth and birth defects on mortality. Unfortunately, the underlying disorders that drive perinatal mortality and the long-term developmental disorders that are sometimes their sequelae have shown little tendency to abate. With the important exception of neural tube defects, whose prevalence has declined with folate fortification of flour in the United States and programs to encourage intake of folate in women of child-bearing age (Mathews et al, 2002), the major causes of death—preterm birth and birth defects—have not declined, nor has the major neurodevelopmental disorder that can be of perinatal origin, cerebral palsy (Paneth et al, 2006). Progress has come from improved medical care of the high-risk pregnancy and the sick infant, rather than through understanding and preventing the disorders themselves.

The period since 1990 has witnessed much less impressive mortality improvement. While infant, neonatal, and postneonatal mortality have declined since 1990, in the 1995-2005 decade these rates were at a near standstill

TABLE 1-1 U.S. Perinatal Mortality, Morbidity, Interventions, Health Conditions, and Behaviors, 1990 to 2005

	1990	1995	2000	2005	Net Change 1990-2005 (%)
Death Rates and Ratios					
Maternal mortality ratio (per 100,000 live births)	8.2	7.1	9.8	15.1	+84%
Infant mortality rate (per 1000 live births)	9.2	7.6	6.9	6.9	−25%
Neonatal mortality rate (per 1000 live births)	5.8	4.9	4.6	4.5	−22%
Postneonatal mortality rate (per 1000 live births)	3.4	2.6	2.3	2.3	−32%
Fetal mortality ratio (per 1000 live births)*	7.5	6.9	6.6	6.2	−17%
Morbidity Rates					
Preterm birth (<37 weeks' gestation) per 100 live births	10.6%	11.0%	11.6%	12.7%	+20%
Very preterm birth (<32 weeks' gestation) per 100 live births	1.9%	1.9%	1.9%	2.0%	+5%
Extremely preterm birth (<28 weeks' gestation) per 1000 live births	7.1	7.0	7.2	7.6	+7%
Low birthweight (<2500 g) per 100 live births	7.0%	7.3%	7.6%	8.2%	+12%
Very low birthweight (<1500 g) per 100 live births	1.3%.	1.4%	1.4%	1.5%	+15%
Extremely low birthweight (<1000 g) per 1000 live births	6.3	6.6	7.1	7.3	+16%
Cesarean Section					
Per 100 live births	22.6%	20.8%	22.9%	30.3%	+34%
Health Behaviors (per 100 live births)					
Cigarette smoking[†]	17.7%	13.7%	12.2%	10.7%	−40%
Alcohol intake[‡]	3.2%	1.5%	0.9%	0.7%	−78%
Late or no prenatal care	6.1%	4.2%	3.9%	3.5%	−42%
Inadequate weight gain (<16 lb) at 40 weeks' gestation[§]	7.9%	9.3%	11.6%	11.4%	+44%
Unmarried	28.0%	32.1%	33.2%	36.9%	+32%
Multiple Births					
Per 1000 live births	23.3	26.1	31.1	33.8	+45%
Fertility Rate					
Per 1000 women aged 15-44 years	70.9	64.6	65.3	66.7	−5.9%

*Fetal deaths with stated or presumed period of 20 weeks' gestation or more.
[†]1990-2000 smoking data based on 45 states and Washington, D.C.; 2005 data based on 36 states, New York City, and Washington, D.C., which used pre-2003 smoking definitions.
[‡]1990-2000 alcohol data based on 46 states and Washington, D.C.; 2005 data based on 36 states, New York City, and Washington, D.C., which used pre-2003 drinking definitions.
[§]1990 weight gain data based on 48 states and Washington, D.C. Remaining data based on 49 states and Washington, D.C.

(Table 1-1). Infant mortality actually rose in 2002, the first 1 year since 1958. Data from the Vermont Oxford Neonatal Network encompassing hundreds of neonatal units show stability in weight-specific mortality rates for all categories of infants weighing less than 1500 g, beginning in approximately 1995 (Horbar et al, 2002). It appears that the pace of advancement in newborn medicine and the expansion of newborn intensive care to previously underserved populations, factors that have exerted a constant downward pressure on infant mortality since the 1960s, have lessened greatly in the past decade.

Maternal mortality has actually climbed substantially, but this is almost certainly the effect of improved reporting (Hoyert, 2007). Two key changes were the implementation of the *International Classification of Diseases, Tenth Revision*, in 1999, which was less restrictive in including indirect maternal deaths, and the introduction of the separate pregnancy question on the U.S. Standard Certificate of Death in 2003.

The risk of preterm birth has been increasing in recent years. This increase is mostly noted in moderately preterm babies, and is likely to reflect increased willingness on the part of obstetricians to deliver fetuses earlier in gestation who are not doing well in utero, in addition to the increased prevalence of twins and triplets, who are generally born preterm, resulting from in vitro fertilization. The small rise in extremely small and preterm babies is likely to reflect trends toward increased reporting of marginally viable immature babies as live births rather than stillbirths (MacDorman et al, 2005).

The cesarean section rate continues its long-term increase, from 5% in 1970 to 23% in 1990 to 32% in 2005. The reasons for this unprecedented trend are multifactorial and include pressures from patients, physicians, and the medical malpractice system. The steady reduction in smoking during pregnancy is likely to be real, whereas trends in the self-reporting of alcohol use in pregnancy may be influenced by societal norms and expectations. Fewer women seem to have late or no prenatal care in recent years, but more women have been found to have inadequate pregnancy weight gain at term. A slight increase in the fertility rate follows a long-term (since approximately

1960) decline in fertility in the United States. One third of mothers in the United States are now unmarried when they give birth.

International Comparisons

The United States lags in IM compared with other developed nations; the United States ranked thirtieth in the world in IM in 2005 (MacDorman and Mathews, 2009). This surprising finding, in light of more favorable socioeconomic and medical care circumstances in the United States than in many nations with lower IM, cannot be attributed to inferior neonatal care. Mortality rates for low-birthweight infants are generally lower in the United States than in European and Asian nations, although mortality at term may be higher. The key difference, however, is that the United States suffers from a striking excess of premature births. Whereas the U.S. African American population is especially vulnerable to premature birth, and especially severe prematurity, premature birth rates are also considerably higher in white Americans than in most European populations. It is likely that the recording of marginally viable small infants as live births rather than stillbirths is more pronounced in the United States than in Europe (Kramer et al, 2002). Although this practice makes a contribution to our higher prematurity and IM rates, it cannot fully explain them.

Premature birth, fetal growth retardation, and IM are tightly linked, in every setting in which they have been studied, to most measures of social class and especially to maternal education; however, uncovering precisely why lower social class drives these important biologic differences has been elusive. Factors such as smoking have at times been implicated, but can only explain a small fraction of the social class effect. It is unlikely that this situation will change until a better understanding of the complex social, environmental, and biologic roots of preterm birth is achieved.

Health Disparities in the Perinatal Period

In 2005, 55.1% of all U.S. births were to non-Hispanic white mothers, 23.8% were to Hispanic mothers, 14.1% were to African American mothers, and 7% were to mothers of other ethnic groups. Health disparities are especially prominent in the perinatal period, with African American IM stubbornly remaining about double that of white IM in the United States, even as rates decline in both populations (Table 1-2). Preterm birth is the central contributor to this racial disparity in IM, and the more severe the degree of prematurity, the higher the excess risk for African American infants. The risk of birth before 37 weeks' gestation was 76% higher in African American mothers than among non-Hispanic whites in 2005, but the risk of birth before 32 weeks' gestation was 310% higher. Reduction in IM disparities in the United States thus requires a better understanding of the causes and mechanisms of preterm birth. Birth defect mortality shows a less pronounced gradient by ethnic group, and it does not contribute in a major way to overall IM disparities (Yang et al, 2006).

The *Hispanic paradox* is a term often used to describe the observation that IM is the same or lower in U.S. citizens classified as Hispanic than in non-Hispanic whites, despite the generally lower income and education levels of U.S. Hispanics (Hessol and Fuentes-Afflick, 2005). The IM experience of Hispanic mothers in the United States reflects the principle that premature birth and low birthweight are key determinants of IM, because these parameters are also favorable in Hispanics. Smoking is much less common among Hispanics in the United States, but this factor alone does not fully explain the paradox.

MAJOR CAUSES OF DEATH

Analyzing the cause of death, a staple of epidemiologic investigation, has limitations when applied to the perinatal period. Birth defect mortality is probably reasonably accurate, but causes of deaths among premature infants are divided among categories such as respiratory distress syndrome, immaturity, and a variety of complications of prematurity. Choosing which particular epiphenomenon of preterm birth to label as the primary cause of death is arbitrary to some extent. Some maternal complications, such as preeclampsia, are also occasionally listed as causes of newborn death. However categorized, prematurity accounts for at least one third of infant deaths (Callaghan et al, 2006).

Before prenatal ultrasound examination could be used to estimate gestational age with reasonable accuracy, a high fraction of neonatal deaths were attributed to low birthweight, but most of these deaths occurred in premature infants, because premature birth is much more important as a cause of death than is fetal growth restriction. Extreme prematurity makes a contribution to IM well beyond its frequency in the population; 1.9% of births, that occurred before 32 weeks' gestation, accounted for 54% of all infant deaths in 2005.

Following premature birth, another important group of causes of death is congenital anomalies (Mathews and MacDorman, 2008). With the exception of folate supplementation to prevent neural tube defects, there is no clearly effective primary prevention program for any birth defect. Pregnancy screening and termination of severe defects, however, is an option for many mothers, and there is evidence that this practice contributes to a reduced prevalence of chromosomal anomalies at birth (Khoshnood et al, 2004).

The major postneonatal cause of death since the 1970s in the United States is sudden infant death syndrome. This cause of death has declined substantially in the United States in parallel with successful public health efforts to discourage sleeping in the prone position during infancy (Ponsonby et al, 2002).

MAJOR MORBIDITIES RELATED TO THE PERINATAL PERIOD

The principal complications of preterm birth involve five organs: the lung, heart, gut, eye, and brain. Management of respiratory distress syndrome and its short- and long-term complications is the centerpiece of neonatal

TABLE 1-2 Ethnic Disparities in Key Perinatal Outcomes and Exposures in 2005

	Non-Hispanic White	African American		Hispanic	
	Prevalence rate	Prevalence rate	RR*	Prevalence rate	RR*
Deaths Rates and Ratios					
Maternal mortality ratio (per 100,000 live births)	11.7	39.2	3.4	9.6	0.8
Infant mortality rate (per 1000 live births)	5.7	13.7	2.4	5.8	1.0
Neonatal mortality rate (per 1000 live births)	3.8	9.1	2.4	3.9	1.0
Postneonatal mortality rate (per 1000 live births)	1.9	4.6	2.4	1.8	1.0
Fetal mortality ratio (per 1000 live births)[†]	4.8	11.1	2.3	5.4	1.1
Morbidity (percent of live births)					
Preterm birth	11.6%	18.3%	1.6	11.6%	1.0
Very preterm birth	1.6%	4.1%	2.6	1.8%	
Extremely preterm birth	5.6	18.9	3.4	6.2	1.2
Low birthweight	7.3%	14.0%	1.4	6.9%	0.9
Very low birthweight	1.2%	3.3%	2.8	1.2%	1.0
Extremely low birthweight	5.5	1.8%	3.3	5.9	1.1
Pregnancy-associated hypertension	4.5%	4.6%	1.0	2.8%	0.6
Diabetes in pregnancy	3.6%	3.5%	1.0	3.8%	1.1
Interventions (percent of live births)					
Cesarean section	30.4%	33.6%	1.1	29.0%	1.0
Induction of labor	26.6%	19.7%	0.7	15.5%	0.6
Health Behaviors					
Smoking[‡]	13.9%	8.5%	0.7	2.9%	0.2
Alcohol intake					
Late or no prenatal care[§]	2.2%	5.6%	2.5	5.1%	2.3
Inadequate weight gain (<16 lb) at 40 weeks' gestation[¶]	9.4%	16.3%	1.7	14.2%	1.5
Unmarried	25.3%	69.9%	2.8	48.0%	1.9
Fertility rate (women 15-44 years old)	58.3	67.2	1.2	99.4	1.7
Multiple births	38.2	37.5	1.0	22.8	0.6

*Relative risk compared with non-Hispanic white (rounded to nearest decimal point).
[†]Fetal deaths with stated or presumed period of 20 weeks' gestation or more.
[‡]Based on 36 states, New York City, and Washington, D.C., which used pre-2003 smoking definitions
[§]Based on 37 states, Washington, D.C. and New York City
[¶]Based on 49 states, New York City, and Washington, D.C.

medicine. Surgical or medical management of symptomatic patent ductus arteriosus is the major cardiac challenge in premature infants, and there is limited understanding of the striking variations, by time and place, of necrotizing enterocolitis—a disorder that in its most extreme forms can cause death or substantial loss of bowel function. Retinopathy of prematurity is closely related to arterial oxygen levels. The epidemic level of this disorder encountered in the 1950s, when oxygen was freely administered without monitoring, was a major setback for neonatal medicine (Silverman, 1980). However, even with more careful management of oxygen, retinopathy of prematurity continues to occur.

The largest unsolved problem in neonatal medicine remains the high frequency of brain damage in survivors of premature birth. The extraordinary decline in mortality rates has not been paralleled by similar declines in rates of neurodevelopmental disabilities in survivors. The key epidemiologic feature of cerebral palsy rates in population registries toward the end of the twentieth century was a modest overall increase in the prevalence of that disorder, which was attributable entirely to the increasing number of survivors of very low birthweight. There are suggestions that this rise may now be leveling (Paneth et al, 2006).

FACTORS AFFECTING PERINATAL HEALTH

HEALTH STATES IN PREGNANCY

The major causes of neonatal morbidity, prematurity and birth defects, generally occur in pregnancies free of antecedent complications. Having a previous birth with an anomaly or a previous preterm birth raises the risk for recurrence of the condition. For preterm birth, no other known risk factor carries as much risk for the mother as having previously delivered preterm.

More than a quarter of preterm birth is iatrogenic, the result of induced labor in pregnancies in which the fetus is severely compromised (Morken et al, 2008). Generally the reason is preeclampsia with attendant impairments in uterine blood flow and poor fetal growth, but poor uterine blood flow and impaired fetal growth can also occur independently of diagnosed preeclampsia; the other major complication of pregnancy is diabetes, most often gestational but sometimes preexisting. Insulin resistance in the mother promotes the movement of nutrients towards the fetus, and typically the infant of the diabetic mother is large for gestational age. Severe diabetes, however, can be accompanied by fetal growth retardation.

HEALTH BEHAVIORS

The most carefully studied and well-established health behavior affecting newborns is maternal cigarette smoking, which has a consistent effect in impairing fetal growth (Cnattingius, 2004). Infants with growth retardation from maternal cigarette smoking paradoxically survive slightly better than do infants of the same weight whose mothers did not smoke, but the net effect of smoking, which also shortens gestation slightly, is to increase perinatal mortality. Although the subject is much debated, it has not been conclusively shown that prenatal maternal smoking has independent long-term effects on children's cognitive capacity (Breslau et al, 2005).

Alcohol is less clearly a growth retardant, but mothers who drink heavily during pregnancy are at risk of having infants with the cluster of defects known as *fetal alcohol syndrome*. Cocaine use in pregnancy is almost surely a severe growth retardant, and it may affect neonatal behavior, but the long-term effects of this exposure on infant cognition and behavior are not as grave as initially feared (Bandstra et al, 2010).

PERINATAL MEDICAL CARE

In light of the potent effects of medical care on the neonate, it has been important to develop systems of care that ensure, or at least facilitate, provision of care to neonates in need. This concept was first promoted by the March of Dimes Foundation, which in its committee report of 1976 recommended that all hospitals caring for babies be classified as level 1 (care for healthy and mildly sick newborns), level 2 (care for most sick infants born in the hospital, but not accepting transfers), or level 3 (regional centers caring for complex surgical disease and receiving transfers) (The Committee on Perinatal Health, 1976). This concept of a regional approach to neonatal care, with different hospitals playing distinct roles in providing care, was endorsed by organizations such as American College of Obstetricians and Gynecologists and the American Academy of Pediatrics and by many state health departments. Whereas it is important to transfer sick babies to level 3 centers when needed, it is preferable to transfer mothers at risk of delivering prematurely or of having a sick neonate, because transport of the fetus in utero is superior to any form of postnatal transport. Birth at a level 3 center has been shown consistently to produce lower mortality rates than birth in other levels of care (Paneth, 1992). The overall system of care, which includes selecting mothers and babies for transfer to other hospitals, is highly dependent on cooperative physicians and health systems. Concern has been raised that economic considerations may threaten ideal systems of regionalization of newborn intensive care (Bode et al, 2001).

EPIDEMIOLOGIC STUDY DESIGNS IN THE PERINATAL PERIOD

Epidemiologic studies have contributed substantially to better understanding the patterns of risk and prognosis in the perinatal period, to tracking patterns of mortality and morbidity, to assessing regional medical care, and to assisting physicians and other providers in evaluating the efficacy of treatments. A variety of study designs have been used in this research.

VITAL DATA ANALYSES

Routinely collected vital data serve as the nation's key resource for monitoring progress in caring for mothers and children. All data presented in this chapter's figures and tables are derived from the annual counts of births and deaths collected by the 52 vital registration areas of the United States (50 states, Washington, D.C., and New York City) and then assembled into national data sets by the National Center for Health Statistics. Unlike data collected in hospitals, in clinics, or from nationally representative surveys, birth and death certificates are required by law to be completed for each birth and death. Birth and death registration has been virtually 100% complete for the entire United States since the 1950s. The universality of this process renders the findings from vital data analyses stable and generalizable. Figure 1-2 illustrates the most recent nationally recommended standard for birth certificate data collection, which has been adopted by most states. Birth certificates contain valuable information for neonatologists. Especially of note are variables such as to whether the mother or infant was transferred for care (not shown), breastfeeding plans, alcohol and cigarette smoking histories, and patterns of maternal weight gain and prenatal care.

The limitations of vital data are well known. Causes of death are subject to certifier variability and, perhaps more importantly, to professional trends in diagnostic categorization. The accuracy of recording of conditions and measures on birth certificates is often uncertain and variable from state to state and hospital to hospital; however, the frequencies of births and deaths in subgroups defined objectively, such as birthweight, are likely to be valid.

COHORT STUDIES IN PREGNANCY AND BIRTH

Studies that follow populations of infants over time, beginning at birth or even before birth and continuing to hospital discharge, early childhood, and adult life, are the leading sources of information about perinatal risk factors for disease and adverse outcomes. As with all observational studies, cohort studies produce associations of exposures and

28. MOTHER TRANSFERRED FOR MATERNAL MEDICAL OR FETAL INDICATIONS FOR DELIVERY? ☒ Yes ☒ No
IF YES, ENTER NAME OF FACILITY MOTHER TRANSFERRED FROM:
_____

29a. DATE OF FIRST PRENATAL CARE VISIT	29b. DATE OF LAST PRENATAL CARE VISIT	30. TOTAL NUMBER OF PRENATAL VISITS FOR THIS PREGNANCY
____/____/____ ☒ No Prenatal Care MM DD YYYY	____/____/____ MM DD YYYY	_____ (If none, enter A0".)

31. MOTHER'S HEIGHT _____ (feet/inches)	32. MOTHER'S PREPREGNANCY WEIGHT _____ (pounds)	33. MOTHER'S WEIGHT AT DELIVERY _____ (pounds)	34. DID MOTHER GET WIC FOOD FOR HERSELF DURING THIS PREGNANCY? ☒ Yes ☒ No

35. NUMBER OF PREVIOUS LIVE BIRTHS (Do not include this child)

36. NUMBER OF OTHER PREGNANCY OUTCOMES (spontaneous or induced losses or ectopic pregnancies)

37. CIGARETTE SMOKING BEFORE AND DURING PREGNANCY
For each time period, enter either the number of cigarettes or the number of packs of cigarettes smoked. IF NONE, ENTER A0".

38. PRINCIPAL SOURCE OF PAYMENT FOR THIS DELIVERY

35a. Now Living	35b. Now Dead	36a. Other Outcomes
Number _____	Number _____	Number _____
☒ None	☒ None	☒ None

Average number of cigarettes or packs of cigarettes smoked per day.

	# of cigarettes	# of packs
Three Months Before Pregnancy	_____ OR	_____
First Three Months of Pregnancy	_____ OR	_____
Second Three Months of Pregnancy	_____ OR	_____
Third Trimester of Pregnancy	_____ OR	_____

☒ Private Insurance
☒ Medicaid
☒ Self-pay
☒ Other
  (Specify) _____

35c. DATE OF LAST LIVE BIRTH ____/____ MM YYYY	36b. DATE OF LAST OTHER PREGNANCY OUTCOME ____/____ MM YYYY	39. DATE LAST NORMAL MENSES BEGAN ____/____/____ MM DD YYYY	40. MOTHER'S MEDICAL RECORD NUMBER

41. RISK FACTORS IN THIS PREGNANCY (Check all that apply)
Diabetes
  ☒ Prepregnancy (Diagnosis prior to this pregnancy)
  ☒ Gestational (Diagnosis in this pregnancy)

Hypertension
  ☒ Prepregnancy (Chronic)
  ☒ Gestational (PIH, preeclampsia)
  ☒ Eclampsia

☒ Previous preterm birth

☒ Other previous poor pregnancy outcome (Includes perinatal death, small-for-gestational age/intrauterine growth restricted birth)

☒ Pregnancy resulted from infertility treatment-If yes, check all that apply:
  ☒ Fertility-enhancing drugs, Artificial insemination or intrauterine insemination
  ☒ Assisted reproductive technology (e.g., in vitro fertilization (IVF), gamete intrafallopian transfer (GIFT))

☒ Mother had a previous cesarean delivery
  If yes, how many _____

☒ None of the above

42. INFECTIONS PRESENT AND/OR TREATED DURING THIS PREGNANCY (Check all that apply)

☒ Gonorrhea
☒ Syphilis
☒ Chlamydia
☒ Hepatitis B
☒ Hepatitis C
☒ None of the above

43. OBSTETRIC PROCEDURES (Check all that apply)

☒ Cervical cerclage
☒ Tocolysis

External cephalic version:
☒ Successful
☒ Failed

☒ None of the above

44. ONSET OF LABOR (Check all that apply)

☒ Premature Rupture of the Membranes (prolonged, ☒12 hrs.)

☒ Precipitous Labor (<3 hrs.)

☒ Prolonged Labor (☒ 20 hrs.)

☒ None of the above

45. CHARACTERISTICS OF LABOR AND DELIVERY (Check all that apply)

☒ Induction of labor
☒ Augmentation of labor
☒ Non-vertex presentation
☒ Steroids (glucocorticoids) for fetal lung maturation received by the mother prior to delivery
☒ Antibiotics received by the mother during labor
☒ Clinical chorioamnionitis diagnosed during labor or maternal temperature > _38°C (100.4°F)
☒ Moderate/heavy meconium staining of the amniotic fluid
☒ Fetal intolerance of labor such that one or more of the following actions was taken: in-utero resuscitative measures, further fetal assessment, or operative delivery
☒ Epidural or spinal anesthesia during labor
☒ None of the above

46. METHOD OF DELIVERY

A. Was delivery with forceps attempted but unsuccessful?
  ☒ Yes ☒ No

B. Was delivery with vacuum extraction attempted but unsuccessful?
  ☒ Yes ☒ No

C. Fetal presentation at birth
  ☒ Cephalic
  ☒ Breech
  ☒ Other

D. Final route and method of delivery (Check one)
  ☒ Vaginal/Spontaneous
  ☒ Vaginal/Forceps
  ☒ Vaginal/Vacuum
  ☒ Cesarean
    If cesarean, was a trial of labor attempted?
    ☒ Yes
    ☒ No

47. MATERNAL MORBIDITY (Check all that apply) (Complications associated with labor and delivery)
☒ Maternal transfusion
☒ Third or fourth degree perineal laceration
☒ Ruptured uterus
☒ Unplanned hysterectomy
☒ Admission to intensive care unit
☒ Unplanned operating room procedure following delivery
☒ None of the above

NEWBORN INFORMATION

48. NEWBORN MEDICAL RECORD NUMBER

49. BIRTHWEIGHT (grams preferred, specify unit)
_____
9 grams   9 lb/oz

50. OBSTETRIC ESTIMATE OF GESTATION:
_____ (completed weeks)

51. APGAR SCORE:
Score at 5 minutes:_____
If 5 minute score is less than 6,
Score at 10 minutes: _____

52. PLURALITY - Single, Twin, Triplet, etc.
(Specify)_____

53. IF NOT SINGLE BIRTH - Born First, Second, Third, etc. (Specify) _____

54. ABNORMAL CONDITIONS OF THE NEWBORN (Check all that apply)

☒ Assisted ventilation required immediately following delivery

☒ Assisted ventilation required for more than six hours

☒ NICU admission

☒ Newborn given surfactant replacement therapy

☒ Antibiotics received by the newborn for suspected neonatal sepsis

☒ Seizure or serious neurologic dysfunction

☒ Significant birth injury (skeletal fracture(s), peripheral nerve injury, and/or soft tissue/solid organ hemorrhage which requires intervention)

☒ None of the above

55. CONGENITAL ANOMALIES OF THE NEWBORN (Check all that apply)
☒ Anencephaly
☒ Meningomyelocele/Spina bifida
☒ Cyanotic congenital heart disease
☒ Congenital diaphragmatic hernia
☒ Omphalocele
☒ Gastroschisis
☒ Limb reduction defect (excluding congenital amputation and dwarfing syndromes)
☒ Cleft Lip with or without Cleft Palate
☒ Cleft Palate alone
☒ Down Syndrome
  ☒ Karyotype confirmed
  ☒ Karyotype pending
☒ Suspected chromosomal disorder
  ☒ Karyotype confirmed
  ☒ Karyotype pending
☒ Hypospadias
☒ None of the anomalies listed above

56. WAS INFANT TRANSFERRED WITHIN 24 HOURS OF DELIVERY? 9 Yes 9 No IF YES, NAME OF FACILITY INFANT TRANSFERRED TO:_____	57. IS INFANT LIVING AT TIME OF REPORT? ☒ Yes ☒ No ☒ Infant transferred, status unknown	58. IS THE INFANT BEING BREASTFED AT DISCHARGE? ☒ Yes ☒ No

FIGURE 1-2 U.S. national standard birth certificate, 2003 revision.

outcomes whose strength and consistency must be carefully judged in the light of other biologic evidence, and with attention to confounding and bias. Collaborations across centers in assembling such data are highly valuable. One notable collaboration is the Vermont-Oxford Network, which provides continuous information on the frequency of conditions observed and diagnoses made in hundreds of U.S. and overseas hospitals, with a particular emphasis on using these data for improving care (Horbar et al, 2010). The neonatal network supported by the National Institute of Child Health and Human Development (NICHD) has been a rich source of randomized trials and has produced observations about prognosis based on large samples of low-birthweight babies (Fanaroff, 2004). These collaborations focus mainly on the period until hospital discharge.

Multicenter cohort studies focusing on diagnosis and follow-up of brain injury in premature infants—such as the Developmental Epidemiology Network (Kuban et al, 1999), Neonatal Brain Hemorrhage (Pinto-Martin et al, 1992), and Extremely Low Gestational Age Newborns (O'Shea et al, 2009) studies—have contributed to our understanding of the prognostic value of brain injury imaged by ultrasound in the neonatal period, because they include follow-up to the age of 2 years or later. Of particular value have been regional or population-wide studies of low-birthweight infants with follow-up to at least school age, among which are included the Neonatal Brain Hemorrhage study from the United States and important studies from Germany (Wolke and Meyer, 1999), the Netherlands (Veen et al, 1991), the United Kingdom (Wood et al, 2000), and Canada (Saigal et al, 1990).

Newborn intensive care has been in place long enough that the first reports of adult outcomes in small infants are now emerging (Saigal and Doyle, 2008). These reports paint a picture that is perhaps less dire than anticipated.

From 1959 to 1966, the National Collaborative Perinatal Project assembled data on approximately 50,000 pregnancies in 12 major medical centers and followed them to age 7 (Niswander and Gordon, 1972). This highly productive exercise, one of whose major contributions was to show that birth asphyxia is a rare cause of cerebral palsy, has now been followed by the development of even larger birth cohort studies starting in pregnancy. For reasons that are not entirely clear, a sample size of 100,000 has been adopted in studies in Norway (Magnus et al, 2006), Denmark (Olsen et al, 2001), and the United States (Lyerly et al, 2009). A major difference from the National Collaborative Perinatal Project is that each of the studies aims to obtain some degree of national representativeness. The U.S. National Children's Study, currently underway, plans to enroll women in early pregnancy and possibly before conception and to follow the offspring to age 21 in 105 locations in the United States, selected by a stratified random sampling of all 3141 U.S. counties.

RANDOMIZED CONTROLLED TRIALS

Few areas of medicine have adopted the randomized trial as wholeheartedly as has newborn medicine. The number of trials mounted has been large and have created a strong influence on practice. A notable influence on this field has been the National Perinatal Epidemiology Unit at Oxford University, established in 1978, which prioritized randomized trials among their several investigations of perinatal care practices and other circumstances affecting maternal and newborn outcomes. The NICHD neonatal research network was established in 1986, principally to support trials. Hundreds of trials have been mounted by these two organizations, but many other centers have contributed to the trial literature.

Trials in pregnancy or in labor have also been supported by the National Perinatal Epidemiology Unit and by NICHD, who support a network of obstetric centers to conduct trials in pregnancy and labor, the NICHD maternal-fetal research network. These trials have often had important implications for newborns and mothers, most notably for showing that the risk of preterm birth can be reduced by administering 17-OH hydroxyprogesterone caproate in midgestation to high-risk women (Meis et al, 2003).

Most newborn trials have focused on outcomes evident in the newborn period, such as mortality, chronic lung disease, brain damage visualized on ultrasound exam, and duration of mechanical ventilation or hospital stay. Recently however, trials extending into infancy or early childhood that incorporate measures of cognition or neurologic function have been a welcome addition to the trial arena. In the past few years, such trials have shown that moderate hypothermia can reduce mortality and brain damage in asphyxiated term infants (Shankaran et al, 2005), and that both caffeine for apnea treatment (Schmidt et al, 2007) and magnesium sulfate administered during labor can reduce the risk of cerebral palsy (Rouse et al, 2008).

Trials in which both mortality and later outcome are combined raise complex methodologic issues. Imbalance in the frequency of the two outcomes being combined can result in a random variation in the more common outcome, overwhelming a significant finding in the other. Precisely how best to conduct such dual- or multiple-outcome trials is the subject of discussion and debate in the neonatal and epidemiology communities.

As the number of trials increases, not all of them sufficiently powered, the methodology for summarizing them and drawing effective conclusions has become increasingly important to neonatologists. The terms *systematic review* and *metaanalysis* have firmly entered the research lexicon, especially the randomized trial literature. The Cochrane Collaboration is an international organization that uses volunteers to systematically review trial results in all fields of medicine. The collaboration, established in 1993, began in the field of perinatal medical trials. Systematic reviews of neonatal trials reviewed by the Cochrane Collaboration are hosted on the website of the NICHD (http://www.nichd.nih.gov/cochrane).

SUMMARY

The patterns of disease, mortality, and later outcome in the perinatal period are complex. Some factors are reasonably stable (e.g., long-term trends in preterm birth and birthweight), whereas others can undergo rapid change (e.g., the rates of cesarean section and twinning). The success of newborn intensive care is well established. No other organized medical care program, targeted at a broad patient population, has had such remarkable success in lowering mortality rates in such a short period of time. Much of that success is due to the evidence-based nature of neonatal practice.

Nonetheless, this success has opened the door to new problems as survivors of intensive care face the challenges of the information age. Resource allocations similar to those that permitted the development of newborn intensive care are now needed to address the educational and rehabilitative needs of survivors. A hopeful sign is the success of some recently studied interventions in reducing the burden of brain damage.

On the nontechnologic front, targeted epidemiologic efforts to address perinatal disorders have yielded progress. Careful study of the circumstances surrounding infant sleep patterns led to active discouragement of sleeping in the prone position, which has reduced mortality from sudden infant death syndrome by half (The Committee on Perinatal Health, 1976). Observational research, followed by two important randomized trials in Europe, led to interventions that increased folate intake in women of child-bearing age and a substantial reduction in the birth prevalence of neural tube defects (Czeizel and Dudás, 1992; Medical Research Council, 1991).

The population-level study of health events occurring in pregnancy and infancy, their antecedents, and their long-term consequences have been an important component to the success of newborn care. Careful self-evaluation through monitoring of vital data and collaborative clinical data, rigorous assessment of new treatments through randomized trials, and alertness to opportunities to implement prevention activities after discovering important risk factors should continue to guide the care of the newborn.

ACKNOWLEDGMENTS

The author thanks Ariel Brovont and Kimberly Harris for assisting in the preparation of the figures and tables.

SUGGESTED READINGS

Division of Reproductive Health: National Center for Chronic Disease Prevention and Health Promotion: achievements in public health, 1900-1999: healthier mothers and babies, *MMWR* 48:849-858, 1999.

Fanaroff A: The NICHD neonatal research network: changes in practice and outcomes during the first 15 years, *Semin in Perinatol* 27:281-287, 2004.

Horbar JD, Soll RF, Edwards WH: The Vermont Oxford Network: a community of practice, *Clin Perinatol* 37:29-47, 2010.

Hoyert DL: National Center for Health Statistics: maternal mortality and related concepts, *Vital Health Stat* 33:1-13, 2007.

Khan KS, Wojdyla D, Say L, et al: WHO analysis of causes of maternal death: a systematic review, *Lancet* 367:1066-1074, 2006.

MacDorman MF, Mathews TJ: Centers for Disease Control and Prevention National Center for Health Statistics: behind international rankings of infant mortality: how the United States compares with Europe, *NCHS Data Brief* 23:1-8, 2009.

Niswander KR, Gordon M, editors: *The Collaborative Perinatal Study of the National Institute of Neurological Diseases and Stroke: the women and their pregnancies*, Philadelphia, 1972, WB Saunders.

Saigal S, Szatmari P, Rosenbaum P, et al: Intellectual and functional status at school entry of children who weighed 1000 grams or less at birth: a regional perspective of births in the 1980s, *J Pediatr* 116:409-416, 1990.

Silverman WA: *Retrolental fibroplasias: a modern parable*, New York, 1980, Grune & Stratton.

World Health Organization: *International statistical classification of diseases and related health problems, Tenth Revision*, vol 2, ed 2, Geneva, 2004.

Complete references and supplemental color images used in this text can be found online at www.expertconsult.com

Evaluation of Therapeutic Recommendations, Database Management, and Information Retrieval

Peter Tarczy-Hornoch

BACKGROUND

At a fundamental level, the practice of neonatology can be considered an information management problem. The care provider is combining patient-specific information (history, findings of physical examination, and results of physiologic monitoring, laboratory tests, and radiologic evaluation) with generalized information (medical knowledge, practice guidelines, clinical trials, and personal experience) to make medical decisions (diagnostic, therapeutic, and management). The Internet has made possible a revolution in the sharing and disseminating of knowledge in all fields, including medicine, with continued growth and maturation of online clinical information resources and tools. Although medicine remains a quintessentially human endeavor, computers are playing a growing role in information management, particularly in neonatology. Patient-specific and generalized information (medical knowledge) are becoming increasingly available in electronic form. In the United States, a growing number of hospitals are adopting electronic medical record systems to manage patient-specific information, with the approaches ranging from electronic flow sheets in the intensive care unit to entirely paperless hospitals. The American Recovery and Reinvestment Act of 2009 (ARRA; i.e., the federal economic stimulus plan) has a provision for the investment of $19 billion in health information technology to motivate physicians to adopt electronic health records (in the Health Information Technology for Economic and Clinical Health [HITECH] act, a part of AARA) and $1.1 billion to research the effectiveness of certain health care treatments. These ARRA provisions are predicated on the belief that quality, safety, and efficiency of clinical care can be improved through electronic medical records and through evidence-based practice.

Parallel with and related to the adoption of information technology is the growth of societal pressures to improve the quality of medical care while controlling costs. These changes are beginning to affect the way in which medicine and neonatology are practiced. In turn, it is becoming important for neonatologists to understand basic principles related to biomedical and health informatics, databases and electronic medical record systems, evaluation of therapeutic recommendations, and online information retrieval.

This expansion of information technology in clinical practice and the concurrent growth of medical knowledge have great promise in addition to potential pitfalls. One pitfall that must not be underestimated, and which is as great a danger today as when Blois (1984) first cautioned

against it, is the unquestioning adoption of information technology: "And, since the thing that computers do is frequently done by them more rapidly than it is by brains, there has been an irresistible urge to apply computers to medicine, but considerably less of an urge to attempt to understand where and how they can best be used." A present and real challenge is information overload. Bero and Rennie (1995) observed, "Although well over 1 million clinical trials have been conducted, hundreds of thousands remain unpublished or are hard to find and may be in various languages. In the unlikely event that the physician finds all the relevant trials of a treatment, these are rarely accompanied by any comprehensive systematic review attempting to assess and make sense of the evidence." The potential of just-in-time information at the point of care is thus particularly appealing, especially considering that the growth in published literature continues at an accelerating rate, with a flood of new knowledge coming from the latest research in genomics, proteomics, metabolomics, and systems biology. A vision to address this was articulated by one of the editors of the *British Medical Journal:* "New information tools are needed: they are likely to be electronic, portable, fast, easy to use, connected to both a large valid database of medical knowledge and the patient record" (Smith, 1996). Although these goals are close to being achieved, there is still progress to be made before this vision is a reality. This chapter aims to provide an overview of the current progress in this direction.

BIOMEDICAL AND HEALTH INFORMATICS

In the 1970s, clinicians with expertise in computers became intrigued by the potential of these tools to improve the practice of medicine, and thus the field of medical informatics was born. The importance of this field addressing the issues of information management in health care is growing rapidly, as seen in the activities of the American Medical Informatics Association (AMIA; www.amia.org). *Medical informatics* can be concisely defined as "the rapidly developing scientific field that deals with storage, retrieval, and optimal use of biomedical information, data, and knowledge for problem solving and decision making" (Shortliffe and Blois, 2006). A more extensive definition can be found at the AMIA Web site under About AMIA, including professional and training opportunities. The University of Washington

Web site (www.bhi.washington.edu) contains a review of the discipline (found under History, About Us, Vision). The field includes both applied and basic research, with the focus in this chapter being on the applied aspects. Examples of basic research are artificial intelligence in medicine, genome data analysis, and data mining (sorting through data to identify patterns and establish relationships). As our knowledge of the genetic mechanisms of disease expands and more data about patients and outcomes are available electronically, the role of informatics in medicine will expand, particularly in the field of neonatology.

The applied focus of the field in the 1960s and 1970s was data oriented, focusing on signal processing and statistical data analysis. In neonatology, the earliest applications of computers were for physiologic data monitoring in the neonatal intensive care unit (NICU). As the field matured in the 1980s, applied work focused on systems to manage patient information and medical knowledge on a limited basis. Examples are laboratory systems, radiology systems, centralized transcription systems, and, probably the best-known medical knowledge management system, the database of published medical articles maintained by the National Library of Medicine known first as MEDLARS, then as MEDLINE and currently as PubMed (www.ncbi.nlm.nih.gov/pubmed). For example, neonatologists began to develop tools to aid in the management of patients in the NICU, such as computer-assisted algorithms to help manage ventilators, although the algorithms have not been successfully deployed on a large scale in the clinical setting.

As computers and networking became mainstream in the workplace and home in the 1990s, informatics researchers began to develop integrated and networked systems (Fuller, 1992, 1997). With the explosion of information from the Human Genome Project, the intersection between bioinformatics and medical informatics began to blur, leading to the adoption of the term *biomedical informatics*. The 1990s saw the development of a number of important systems. In terms of patient-specific information retrieval, these systems included integrated electronic medical record systems that in their full implementation can encompass—in a single piece of easy-to-use software—interfaces to physiologic monitors; electronic flow sheets; access to laboratory and radiology data; tools for electronic documentation (charting), electronic order entry, and integrated billing; and modules to help reduce medical errors. The Internet has permitted ready access and sharing of this information within health care organizations and limited secured remote access to this information from home. In terms of patient population information retrieval, a number of tools were developed to help clinicians and researchers examine aggregate data in these electronic medical records to document outcomes and help to improve quality of care. The Internet, particularly the World Wide Web, has transformed access to medical knowledge (Fuller et al, 1999). Health sciences libraries are becoming digital and paper repositories. Journals are available online. Knowledge is now available at the point of care in ways that were not previously possible (Tarczy-Hornoch et al, 1997). In 2004, in recognition of the unfulfilled potential of health care information technology, the Office of the National Coordinator for Health Information Technology (ONC) was established (www.healthit.hhs.gov) to achieve the following vision:

Health information technology (HIT) allows comprehensive management of medical information and its secure exchange between health care consumers and providers. Broad use of HIT has the potential to improve health care quality, prevent medical errors, increase the efficiency of care provision and reduce unnecessary health care costs, increase administrative efficiencies, decrease paperwork, expand access to affordable care, and improve population health.

In the upcoming decade, the focus will be shifting from demonstrating the potential of electronic medical record and information systems toward implementing them more broadly to realize their benefit (e.g., the ARRA legislation). Evidence-based medicine is considered by many as a part of informatics as an approach to the evaluation of therapeutic recommendations and their implementation (see later discussion), and it is part of the ARRA and some approaches to health care reform being proposed in 2009.

Neonatologists have been involved in informatics for a long time. Duncan (2010) maintains an excellent continually updated bibliographic database on the literature about computer applications in neonatology. In 1988, as one of the earlier groups to develop national databases of clinical care, neonatologists established and expanded the Vermont Oxford Network (www.vtoxford.org) to improve the quality and safety of medical care for newborn infants and their families. As part of the activities, the Vermont established and maintained Oxford Network a nationwide database about the care and outcome of high-risk newborn infants. In 1992, Sinclair et al (1992) published one of the earlier evidence-based textbooks, *Effective Care of the Newborn Infant*.

DATABASES

In broad terms, a database is an organized, structured collection of data designed for a particular purpose. Thus, a stack of 3 × 5 cards with patient information is a database, as is the typical paper prenatal record. Most frequently, the term *database* is used to refer to a structured electronic collection of information, such as a database of clinical trial data for a group of patients in a study. Databases come in a variety of fundamental types, such as single-table, relational, and object-oriented.

A simple database can be built using a single table by means of a spreadsheet program such as Microsoft Excel, or a database program such as Microsoft Access (Microsoft, Redmond, Washington). The advantage of such a database is that it is easy to build and maintain. For an outcomes database in a neonatology unit, each row can represent a patient and each column represents information about the patients (e.g., name, medical record number, gestational age, birth date, length of stay, patent ductus arteriosus [yes/no], necrotizing enterocolitis [NEC; yes/no]). The major limitation of such a database is that a column must be added to store the information each time the researcher wants to track another outcome (e.g., maple syrup urine disease [MSUD]). This limitation can result in tables with dozens to hundreds of columns, which then become difficult to maintain. The challenges can be illustrated with a few examples. The first example of a challenge is that which results from adding a new column (e.g., MSUD); one must either review all records (rows) already in the spreadsheet for the presence or absence of MSUD or flag all existing records (rows) in the spreadsheet as *unknown* for MSUD status. The second example of a challenge results from the logistics of managing an extremely wide spreadsheet—imagine not adding the tenth column but the 1000th column.

The majority of databases and electronic medical records in neonatology are built using relational database software. To build a simple outcomes relational database that permits easy adding of new outcome measures, one could use a three-table database design (Figure 2-1). The first table contains all the information for each patient (e.g., name, medical record number, gestation in weeks, birth date, admit date, discharge date). The second table is a dictionary that assigns a code number to each diagnosis or outcome being tracked (e.g., patent ductus arteriosus = 1; NEC = 2; MSUD = 10234). The third table is the diagnosis-tracking table; it links a patient number to a particular code and assigns a value to that code. Adding a new diagnosis to track would require adding an entry to the diagnosis dictionary table. To add a diagnosis to a patient, one would add an entry to the tracking table. For example, Girl Smith (medical record number 00-00-01) has a diagnosis of NEC. To add the diagnosis, add to the diagnosis table an entry that has a value of 00-00-01 in the medical record column, a value of 2 (the code for NEC) in the code column, and a value of 2 in the value column (the code for surgical). Although relational

databases are harder to build, they provide greater flexibility for expansion and maintenance and thus are the preferred implementation for clinical databases. They address the challenges in a simple spreadsheet by tracking dates that new diagnostic codes were added and by user interfaces that allow one to easily view only diagnoses present for a given patient rather than all potential diagnoses for a patient.

The distinction between an NICU quality assessment–quality improvement (i.e., outcomes) database and an electronic medical record is largely a matter of degree. Some characteristics typical of a neonatal outcomes database are data collection and data entry after the fact, limited amount of data collected (a small subset of the information needed for daily care), lack of narrative text, lack of interfaces to laboratory and other information systems, and the episodic (e.g., quarterly) use of the system for report generation. Some characteristics typical of an electronic medical record are real-time (daily or more frequent) data entry, a large amount of data collected (approximating all the information needed for daily care in a fully electronic care environment), narrative text (e.g., progress notes, radiology reports, pathology reports), interfaces to laboratory and other information systems, and, most important, the use of the system for daily patient care, including features such as results review, messaging or alerting for critical results, decision support systems (drug dosage calculators, drug-drug interaction alerts, among others), and computerized electronic order entry.

In the past, the majority of neonatal databases and first-generation NICU electronic medical record systems were

Tables in the database:

DEMOGRAPHIC DATA
  Name
  Hospital_Number
  Gestational_Age
  Birthdate
  Admit_Date
  Discharge_Date

DIAGNOSES
  Hospital_Number
  Diagnosis_Code
  Value

DIAGNOSIS DICTIONARY
  Diagnosis_Code
  Description

Example Entries in the Tables:

DEMOGRAPHIC DATA

Name	Hospital_Number	Gestational_Age	Birthdate	Admit_Date	Discharge_Date
John Smith	00-00-01	27	1/1/2003	1/1/2003	3/21/2003
Jane Doe	00-00-02	24	1/2/2003	1/3/2003	4/15/2003

DIAGNOSES

Hospital_Number	Diagnosis_Code	Value
00-00-01	1	1
00-00-01	2	1
00-00-02	1	2
00-00-02	10234	

DIAGNOSIS DICTIONARY

Diagnosis_Code	Description
1	PDA (1=small, 2=large)
2	NEC (1=medical, 2=surgical)
….	
10234	Maple Syrup Urine Disease

FIGURE 2-1 Example of a relational database.

developed locally by and for neonatologists. The literature describing these efforts is available online (Duncan, 2010). Unfortunately the majority of these systems were never published or publicly documented, and thus a number of important and useful innovations are lost or must be repeatedly rediscovered. Anybody thinking about building their own neonatology database would be well advised to review the existing literature and existing commercial products before embarking on this path. That said, there is room for improvement of the existing products, and neonatologists continue to develop their own databases today. With the national push toward interoperable electronic medical records through U.S. Department of Health and Human Services Office of the National Coordinator for Health Information Technology (ONC; since 2004) and ARRA HITECH (since 2009), it is likely that the market will consolidate into a smaller number of neonatology practice tailored systems that are certified and that interoperate with the National Health Information Network (2010). The largest neonatal outcomes database is the centralized database maintained by the Vermont Oxford Network with the mission of improving the quality and safety of medical care for infants and their families. One of the key activities of the network is their outcomes database, which involves more than 800 participating intensive care nurseries both in the United States and internationally collecting data on approximately 55,000 low-birthweight infants each year. Other activities of the network are clinical trials, follow-up of extremely low–birthweight infants, and NICU quality and safety studies. The focus of the database initially was very low–birthweight infants (401 to 1500 g), but this focus has expanded to include data on infants weighing more than 1500 g. Presently the network collects data on more than two thirds of the very low–birthweight infants born in the United States. Participants in the network submit data and in return receive outcome data for their own institution and comparative data from other nurseries nationwide, including custom reports, comparison groups, and quality management reports. Members also have the ability to participate in collaborative research projects and collaborative multi-center quality-improvement collaborations. All data except their own are anonymous for all participants. The network does have access to both the individual and aggregate data. The network database is maintained centrally, and data quality monitoring and data entry are centralized. Initially the process involved paper submission of data by participating nurseries. Currently a number of the commercial and custom NICU databases and electronic medical record systems can export their data in the format required by the Vermont Oxford Network as well as the option to submit data directly using the custom eNICQ software developed by Vermont Oxford. Submissions of data are thus a combination of paper forms and reports generated by commercial and custom software packages.

The database focuses on tracking outcomes. With the passage of the Health Insurance Portability and Accountability Act of 1996 (HIPAA) and federal regulations governing the confidentiality of electronic patient data, some of the anonymous demographic data that were collected by the network in the past have decreased. This change has grown from concerns that, in combination with identity of the referring center, these data could be used to uniquely identify patients, which is a violation of the HIPAA.

ELECTRONIC HEALTH RECORD

An electronic health record (EHR; also known as an *electronic medical record*) is much more complex than an outcomes database, because the system is intended to be used continually on a daily basis to replace electronically some, if not all, of the record keeping, laboratory result review, and order writing that occur in a neonatal intensive care nursery (or more generically in any inpatient or outpatient clinical setting). The complexity of this task becomes evident if one imagines that, for a paperless medical record environment, every paper form in a nursery would need to be replaced with an electronic equivalent, which is also true for every paper-based workflow and process. Organizations are moving in this direction because of a combination of forces, such as the desire to reduce error and to control the spiraling costs of health care. These reasons are addressed at great length in two reports from the Institute of Medicine (Institute of Medicine Committee on Improving the Patient Record, 1997; Kohn et al, 2000). These benefits are typically achieved when information is available electronically (e.g., results of laboratory tests, radiology procedures, transcription) and input into the system (e.g., problem lists, allergies), and when both sets of information are combined and checked against electronic orders. Only with electronic orders has it been shown that errors can be reduced and care provider behavior clearly changed. Combining just electronic laboratory results (e.g., creatinine level) and electronic order entry (e.g., a drug order), for example, enables one to verify that drug dosages have been correctly adjusted for renal failure. This approach would work well in adults, but in neonates, whose renal function is more difficult to assess and for whom drug dosage norms depend on gestational age and post-delivery age, additional information must be entered into the system (e.g., urine output, gestational age), requiring a more sophisticated EHR. Despite more than one decade of work deploying EHRs, the proportion of acute care hospitals that are members of the American Hospital Association and have a comprehensive EHR is remarkably low (1.5%), and computerized order entry has been implemented in only 17% of hospitals (Jha et al, 2009).

Results review systems include basic demographic data, such as name, age, and address from the hospital registration system. These systems require a moderate amount of work to tie them to the various laboratory, radiology, and other systems and to train users. The benefits are hard to quantify, but users typically prefer them to the paper alternative because of the more rapid access to information. The challenge in moving beyond the results review level to the integrated system level is that the documentation level and order entry level are essentially prerequisites for the integrated system level, but they have marginal benefit, particularly given the human and financial costs. Integrated systems require significant work to implement, including the presence of computers at each bedside, as well as significant work to train users. The benefits accrue mainly to the organization, in the form of reduced costs of filing, printing, and maintaining paper records and, if providers are forced to enter notes instead of dictate them, significant savings in transcription costs.

The challenge is that the end users often find that it takes much longer to do their daily work with electronic documentation. Without moving to electronic order entry, if not an integrated system, the users do not realize major day-to-day benefits. The ARRA HITECH provisions noted earlier essentially are designed to create incentives for provider adoption of EHRs to overcome this activation barrier.

The benefits start to accrue more clearly at the next level—electronic order entry. The complexity of implementing and deploying an electronic order entry system cannot be overstated. Interfaces need to be built with all the systems that are part of results review in addition to other systems. Furthermore, a huge database of possible orders must be created to allow users to pick the right orders. This database and the menu of choices are needed because computers are poor at recognizing and interpreting a narrative text typed by a human. Finally and most important, there is a huge training challenge, because writing orders electronically is more complex and time consuming than writing them by hand. The change management issues become apparent when one considers that typically these systems take the unit assistant out of the loop; therefore much of the oversight that can occur at the unit assistant level does not, or the burden of oversight is borne by the person entering the orders.

After overcoming the barriers to electronic order entry, organizations can start to benefit from integrated systems. For this reason, the trend today is not a stepwise move from results review to documentation of integrated systems. Instead, organizations are moving from results review directly to integrated systems. Interestingly, the technical complexities and the training and usage complexities of integrated systems are not much higher than those for order entry. Integrated systems add tools to make life easier for care providers using all the data in the system. As an analogy, an integrated EHR system is like an office software suite that encompasses a word processor, a spreadsheet, a slide presentation tool, a graphic drawing tool, and a database, all of which can communicate with one another, making it easy to put a picture from the drawing tool or a graph from a spreadsheet into a slide show. Integrated systems include (1) checking orders for errors, (2) alerts and reminders triggered by orders or by problems on the problem list or other data in the system, (3) care plans tied to patient-specific information, (4) charting modules customized to the problem list, (5) charting and progress notes that automatically import information (e.g., from laboratory tests, flow sheets) and that help generate orders for the day as the documentation occurs, (6) modules to facilitate hyperalimentation ordering, and (7) modules to assist in management. For example it is possible to imagine a system in which reminders for screening studies (e.g., for retinopathy of prematurity, intraventricular hemorrhage, and brainstem auditory evoked response) were triggered by gestational age, a problem list, and previous results of screening studies. Similarly, admitting a neonate at a particular gestational age with a particular set of problems could trigger pathways, orders, and reminders specific to that clinical scenario. An important caveat is that all such systems are only as good as the data and rules put into them. The issues raised in the section on evaluation of therapeutic recommendations are important to consider in the context of electronic order entry and integrated systems.

The EHR market is still relatively young and continually evolving; this is true of products designed specifically for the NICU and more generic products designed to be used throughout a hospital or health care system. The ONC was established in part to address this young marketplace by creating standards and certification bodies. In particular, the ONC created the Certification Commission for Healthcare Information Technology (CCHIT) and the Health Information Technology Standards Panel to begin to bring more standardization to the marketplace. The CCHCIT examines criteria for certifying systems, including functionality, security, and interoperability. Order entry and documentation systems are beginning to be more widely adopted, however truly integrated systems are much less broadly implemented. The major reason for this situation is that the needs of different health care systems vary significantly, and the existing products are not flexible enough to meet all these needs in one system. Furthermore, there is a trend among health care organizations, EHR developers, and vendors to move away from niche systems tailored to particular subsets of care providers, such as neonatology, and toward a focus on systems that are generically useful. There are two important drivers behind this trend.

The first and most important reason for adopting a single integrated system is that the benefits of an EHR system begin to accrue only when an entire organization uses the same one. Consider the following scenario: a woman receives prenatal care in the clinic of an institution and is then admitted to the emergency department in preterm labor. Her infant is delivered in the labor and delivery department, hospitalized in the neonatal intensive care nursery, and discharged to an affiliated pediatric follow-up clinic. In the current era of paper medical records, paper is used to convey information from one site to the other. In an integrated EHR system, all the information for both mother and infant is in one place for all providers to see. Interoperability is important as well if the care described crosses organizational boundaries, such as an outpatient-focused health maintenance organization contracting inpatient obstetric care to one hospital system and neonatal or pediatric care to a children's hospital in a different health care system. If a single unified institution were to adopt niche software tailored to the needs of each site, a provider caring for the infant might need to access an emergency department system, an obstetric system, an NICU system, and an outpatient pediatric system to gather all the pertinent information. Each system would require the user to learn a separate piece of software. Learning a site-specific piece of software is a considerably greater burden on care providers than learning to use a site-specific paper form. If care crosses organizations and electronic systems are not interoperable, then care transitions most often remain on paper.

The second factor driving adoption of integrated systems is economies of scale. The ideal EHR system contains electronic interfaces that automatically import the system data from laboratory, pharmacy, radiology, transcription, integrated electronic orders, error checking, and electronic documentation by care providers. Given that development of these interfaces, training, and maintenance cost more than the purchase of the system itself, it is far more cost effective to install one system with one set of interfaces and one set of training and maintenance issues than to replicate the process multiple times.

The neonatal intensive care environment poses some unique challenges for EHRs. As a result, it is important to ensure that when health care systems are making decisions about the purchase of an EHR, neonatologists and other neonatal health care providers are involved in the process. An excellent source of information about NICU medical record systems and databases is an article by Stavis (1999). Neonatologists in the position of helping to select an EHR system must acquire the necessary background through reading some basic introductory texts on medical informatics, focusing on EHRs. It is then critical that they survey other organizations similar to their own to discover which systems have worked and which ones have not. For example, the needs of a level III academic nursery that performs extracorporeal membrane oxygenation are different from those of a community level II hospital that does not perform mechanical ventilation. Systems that work well in teaching hospitals with layers of trainees may not work well in private practice settings and vice versa. Most important, when using a medical informatics framework, the neonatologists must develop a list of prioritized criteria specific to their institution and compare available products in the marketplace with this list, while also considering the recommendations of the CCHIT as described earlier.

All end user needs must also be considered. If residents, nurse practitioners, nutritionists, pharmacists, and respiratory therapists are expected to use the system, their input must be solicited. Ensuring broad-based input is especially relevant if the goal is an EHR system into which a lot of data will be entered by health care providers (e.g., electronic charting, note writing, medication administration records, order entry). The reason to ensure acceptance by all users of systems that require data entry is that a significant percentage of systems requiring data entry has ultimately been unsuccessful because of lack of user acceptance. Unfortunately there is little literature on this issue, because institutions rarely publicize and publish their failures in this arena, although the situation is beginning to change. A review of some of these challenges and a theoretical framework for looking at them is provided by Pratt et al (2004).

The final step in evaluating a potential system is to develop a series of scenarios and to have potential users test the scenarios. Evaluating usage scenarios typically involves visits to sites that have installed the EHR system under consideration. An example of a scenario might be for a nurse, a respiratory therapist, a resident, and an attending physician to try to electronically replicate, on a given system under consideration, the bedside charting, progress note charting, and order writing for a critically ill patient who undergoes extracorporeal membrane oxygenation and then decannulation. The reason for developing and testing such scenarios is that this approach is the best way to ensure that aspects of charting, note writing, and documentation unique to the NICU are supported by the system.

EVALUATING THERAPEUTIC RECOMMENDATIONS

Once all the data about a patient, whether in electronic or paper form, are in hand, the clinician is faced with the challenge of medical decision making and applying all that he or she knows to the problem. It is vital that the clinician understand what is known and what is still uncertain in terms of the validity of therapeutic recommendations. The evaluation of new recommendations arising from a variety of sources, including journal articles, metaanalyses, and systematic reviews, is a critical skill that all neonatologists must master. Broadly speaking, this approach has been termed *evidence-based medicine*. A full discussion of this approach to evaluation of new approaches in clinical medicine is beyond the scope of this chapter. Two outstanding sources of information are the works by Guyatt and Rennie (2002) and Straus et al (2005). An excellent overview of the progress in evidence-based medicine over the last 15 years is provided by Montori and Guyatt (2008). An important caveat is that evidence-based medicine is not a panacea. It is not helpful when the primary literature does not address a particular clinical situation, such as one that is rare or complex. This approach also does not necessarily address broader concerns, such as clinical importance or cost effectiveness, although it sometimes does. There are potential challenges when combining evidence-based medicine with the emerging humanistic approach to health care, which can heavily weight patient preferences potentially over the evidence base.

In the early days of medicine, the standard practice was observation of individual patients and subjective description of aggregate experiences from similar patients. As the science of medicine evolved, formal scientific methods were applied to help to assess possible therapeutic and management interventions. Important tools in this effort are epidemiology, statistics, and clinical trial design. Currently medicine in general and neonatology in particular are faced with an interesting paradox. For some areas, there is a wealth of information in the form of randomized controlled clinical trials, whereas there is scant information to guide clinical practice for others. A wealth of well-designed clinical trials on the use of surfactant has been published, for example, but there are essentially no trials addressing the management of chylothorax. One might assume that the practice of medicine reflects the available evidence, but this is not the case. McDonald (1996) summarized the problem as follows: "Although we assume that medical decisions are driven by established scientific fact, even a cursory review of practice patterns shows that they are not." A study of 2500 treatments in the British Medical Journals Clinical Evidence Database (http://clinical-evidence.bmj.com), shows that, as of the summer of 2009, 49% of treatments are of unknown effectiveness, 12% are clearly beneficial, 23% are likely to be beneficial, 8% are a tradeoff between beneficial and harmful, 5% are unlikely to be beneficial, and 3% are likely to be ineffective or harmful. As a result, neonatologists have a responsibility to identify what knowledge is available in the literature and elsewhere and to critically evaluate this information before applying it to practice. Furthermore, because this information is constantly evolving, practitioners must continually revisit the underlying literature as it expands (e.g., the recommendations regarding the use of steroids for chronic lung disease).

The evidence-based practice of medicine is an approach that addresses these issues. It is helpful to consider the process as involving two steps—the critical review of the primary literature and the synthesis of the information offered in the primary literature. Critical review of the primary literature is an area in which most neonatologists have significant experience, with journal clubs and other similar forums. The approach involves systematically reviewing each section of an article (i.e., background, methods, results, discussion) and asking critical questions for each section (e.g., for the methods section: Is the statistical methodology valid? Were power calculations made? Was a hypothesis clearly stated? Do the methods address the hypothesis? Do the methods address alternative hypotheses? Do the methods address confounding variables?). The formal evaluation of each section must then be synthesized into conclusions. A helpful question to ask is, "Does this paper change my clinical practice, and if so, then how?" Additional resources for systematic review of the primary literature are listed in the Suggested Readings. It is important to note that guidelines for systematic review of a single article differ according to whether it describes a preventive or therapeutic trial (e.g., use of nitric oxide for chronic lung disease), evaluation of a diagnostic study (e.g., use of C-reactive protein level for prediction of infection), or prognosis (e.g., prediction of outcome from a Score for Neonatal Acute Physiology score).

The second, and arguably more important, step is to determine not the effect of one article on one's practice, but the overall effect of the body of relevant literature on one's practice. For example, if the preponderance of the literature favors one therapeutic recommendation, then a single article opposing the recommendation must be weighed against the other articles that favor it. This task is complex, and the most complete and formal statistical approach to combining the results of multiple studies (i.e., metaanalysis) requires significant investment of time and effort. Part of the evidence-based practice of medicine approach therefore involves the collaborative development of evidence-based systematic reviews and metaanalyses by communities of care providers. Within the field of neonatology, Sinclair et al (1992) laid the seminal groundwork for this approach; their textbook *Effective Care of the Newborn* remains an important milestone, but it illustrates the problem of information currency. Because the book was published in 1992, none of the clinical trials in neonatology in the last decade and a half are included. The Internet has permitted creation and continual maintenance of up-to-date information by a distributed group of collaborators, lending itself well to the maintenance of a database of evidence-based medicine reviews of the literature. This international effort is the Cochrane Collaboration, and the *Cochrane Neonatal Review* is devoted to neonatology (Cochrane Neonatal Collaborative Review Group). A limitation of the Cochrane approach is illustrated by the relatively restricted scope of topics covered at the National Institute of Child Health and Human Development Web site (www.nichd.nih.gov/cochrane/cochrane.htm). The existence of a review requires adequate literature on a topic and a dedicated and committed clinician to create and update the review.

It is important to distinguish between these formal approaches to reviewing the literature (i.e., systematic literature reviews and metaanalyses) that have specific methodologies and more ad hoc reviews of the literature. Evidence-based medicine aggregate resources such as the Cochrane Collaboration take a more systematic approach, but review articles published in the literature vary in their approach. Metaanalyses are easy to distinguish, but systematic reviews versus ad hoc reviews are harder to distinguish. Systematic reviews focus on quality primary literature (e.g., controlled studies rather than case series or case reports) and must include (1) a methods section for the review article that explicitly specifies how articles were identified for possible inclusion and (2) what criteria were used to assess the validity of each study and to include or exclude primary literature articles in the systematic review. Systematic reviews also tend to present the literature in aggregate tabular form, even when metaanalyses of statistics of all the articles cannot be done. One commonly used source of overview information in neonatology—the *Clinics in Perinatology* series—is a mix of opinion (written in the style of a book chapter), ad hoc literature review, systematic literature review, and metaanalysis. Guidelines (e.g., screening recommendations for group B streptococcal infection), although based on primary literature review, are typically neither metaanalyses nor systematic reviews of the literature. Whereas formal methods are used to derive conclusions with metaanalyses and systematic reviews, guidelines are developed frequently instead by consensus among committee members; this is true of both national and local practice guidelines. General textbooks of neonatology are typically based on ad hoc literature review that includes both primary literature and systematic literature review. When reading overviews of the aggregate state of current knowledge on a given topic in neonatology, it is important to keep these distinctions in mind.

Anyone interested in developing evidence-based reviews on a particular topic should review some of the textbooks on evidence-based practice listed at the end of this chapter. Initially, it is a good idea to collaborate with someone who has experience in systematic review and metaanalysis. The process consists of the following steps: (1) identifying the relevant clinical question (e.g., management of bronchopulmonary dysplasia); (2) narrowing the question to a focus that enables one to determine whether a given article in the primary literature answers it (e.g., does prophylactic high-frequency ventilation have positive or negative effects on acute and chronic morbidity—pulmonary and otherwise?); (3) extensively searching the primary literature (frequently in collaboration with a librarian with expertise searching the biomedical literature) and retrieving the articles; (4) critically, formally, and systematically reviewing each article for inclusion, validity, utility, and applicability; and (5) formally summarizing the results of the preceding process, including conclusions valid throughout the body of included primary literature.

ONLINE INFORMATION RETRIEVAL

Because of the rapid growth of biomedical information and because it changes over time, investigators in informatics and publishers believe that print media will soon no longer be used for sharing and distributing biomedical information (Smith, 1996; Weatherdall, 1995). Economic realities will dictate, however, that quality information will generally come at a price. The medical digital library at the University of Washington (www.healthlinks.washington.edu, under Care Provider) serves to illustrate the current state of the art. The information available is a combination of locally developed material (e.g., University of Washington faculty writing practice guidelines), material developed by institutions elsewhere (faculty elsewhere writing such guidelines), material developed by organizations (e.g., the neonatal Cochrane Collaboration), and electronic forms of journals, textbooks, and evidence-based medicine databases. The last (journals, textbooks, databases) generally are not free, and the University of Washington pays a subscription fee (termed a *site license*) to provide access to these resources for their faculty, staff, and students. Libraries will likely remain the primary source of information, but will shift their attention from paper to electronic records. Health sciences libraries can provide invaluable training in the efficient use of online medical resources, and most offer training sessions and consultation.

A number of online resources are valuable for neonatologists. For accessing the primary literature, the most valuable resource is the National Library of Medicine's database of the published medical literature accessible (PubMed; www.ncbi.nlm.nih.gov/entrez) along with many other databases accessible from the Health Information Web site (www.nlm.nih.gov/hinfo.html). The PubMed system is continually being enhanced; therefore it is useful to review the help documentation online and regularly check the New/Noteworthy section to see what has changed. One of the most powerful yet underused tools is the Find Related Link that appears next to each article listed on PubMed. This link locates articles that are related to the one selected (Liue and Altman, 1998). The PubMed system applies a powerful statistical algorithm with complex weightings to the article selected to each word in the title, to each author, to each major and minor keyword (Medical Subject Heading terms), and to each word in the abstract and then finds statistically similar articles in the database. In general, this system outperforms novice to advanced health care providers performing a complex search, and it begins to approach the accuracy of an experienced medical librarian. Another powerful search tool within PubMed is the Clinical Query (www.ncbi.nlm.nih.gov/corehtml/query/static/clinical.shtml). This tool facilitates searches for papers by clinical study category (e.g., etiology, diagnosis, therapy, prognosis), focuses on systematic reviews, and performs medical genetics searches—the last of which is useful in the context of neonatology. All the major pediatric journals are available online either through a package at local hospital libraries or by subscription, instead of or in addition to a print subscription. The value of having an electronic subscription to a journal is that it provides access to current and past issues. The best free online source of information on evidence-based practice is the *Cochrane Neonatal Review*. Subscriptions to the full Cochrane database can be purchased online as well.

Given the growing role of genetics in health care, and in particular the importance of genetic diseases in infants, there are two notable genetics databases that are available free of charge online (in addition to the Medical Genetics Searches mentioned previously). The first is Online Mendelian Inheritance in Man (www.ncbi.nlm.nih.gov/omim). This database, which is a catalog of human genes and genetic disorders, is an online version of the textbook by the same name. It is a diachronic collection of information on genetic disorders, meaning that each disease entry chronologically cites and summarizes key papers in the field. The second is the GeneTests database (www.genetests.org), which is a directory of genetic testing (what testing is available on a clinical and research basis, where, and how one sends a specimen) and a user's manual (how to apply genetic testing). The user's manual section consists of entries for a growing number of diseases or clinical phenotypes of particular importance. Entries are written by experts, peer reviewed both internally and externally, subjected to a formal process similar to a systematic review, and updated regularly online. As of the winter of 2011, the GeneTests database includes GeneReviews (user's manual entries) for 527 diseases, and the directory includes 1189 genetics clinical, 595 laboratories, and information on testing for 2270 diseases (2005 clinically and 265 on a research basis). An excellent site that maintains links to the majority of locally developed, neonatology-specific content around the country is the site maintained by Duncan (2010). In addition to a database of links to clinical resources around the country, the site also has a job listing and a database of the literature on computer applications in medicine.

The clinician must realize that, unlike journals, textbooks, and guidelines, the material on the World Wide Web (whether accessed from Duncan's site or based on a search) is not necessarily subject to any editorial or other oversight as to what is published; therefore, as stated by Silberg et al (1997), "caveat lector" (reader beware). A number of articles and Web sites address criteria for assessing the validity and reliability of material on a Web site. (Health on the Net Foundation, www.hon.ch Mitretek Systems). With caution in mind, a search on the entire World Wide Web using a sophisticated search engine (e.g., Google, Google Scholar) can yield valuable information, though search results typically include a lower proportion of quality resources compared with curated resources. Google also has a sophisticated statistical algorithm that allows a user to find similar Web pages after identifying a particular one of interest.

SUGGESTED READINGS

Cochrane Neonatal Collaborative Review Group: Cochrane neonatal review. Available from www.nichd.nih.gov/cochrane.

Jha AK, DeRoches CM, Campbell EG, et al: Use of electronic health records in U.S. hospitals, *NEJM* 360:1628-1638, 2009.

Montori VM, Guyatt GH: Progress in evidence-based medicine, *JAMA* 300:1814-1816, 2008.

Norris T, Fuller SL, Goldberg HI, et al: *Informatics in primary care: strategies in information management for the healthcare provider*, New York, 2002, Springer-Verlag.

Pratt W, Reddy MC, McDonald DW, et al: Incorporating ideas from computer supported cooperative work, *J Biomed Inform* 37:128-137, 2004.

Shortliffe EH, Cimino JJ, editors: *Biomedical informatics: computer applications in health care and biomedicine*, ed 3, New York, 2006, Springer Science+Business Media.

Straus SE, Richardson WS, Glasziou P, et al: *Evidence-based medicine: how to practice and teach EBM*, ed 3, London, 2005, Churchill Livingstone.

Complete references used in this text can be found online at www.expertconsult.com

CHAPTER 3

ETHICS, DATA, AND POLICY IN NEWBORN INTENSIVE CARE

William L. Meadow and John D. Lantos

PHILOSOPHY

Ethics in the neonatal intensive care unit (NICU), as in all clinical contexts, starts with the traditional triangular framework of autonomy (do what the patient, or in this case the parent, thinks is right), paternalism (do what the doctor thinks is right), and beneficence and nonmaleficence (do the right thing). These concepts, independent of context or data, are timeless.

The problem with timeless concepts, of course, comes in knowing what to do in real time. What exactly is the right thing? What facts should be brought to bear in the decision? What weight should each fact be given? And whose opinion should count in the end? Nonetheless, some applications of traditional ethical concepts in the NICU are already universally adopted (e.g., avoid futility, do not torture, and intervene when the data provide compelling evidence to do so).

Unfortunately, much of NICU care falls between not resuscitating 21-week births, obligatory support of 28-week births, and not performing cardiopulmonary resuscitation on infants with lethal anomalies. The traditional ethical solution to medical dilemmas is to ground concerns in context, take data into account, and be sympathetic to patient preferences when the balance of benefits and burdens is not clear. The precise problem in the NICU is that the burdens are real, immediate, long term, and significant—months of painful procedures such as intubation, ventilation, intravenous catheterization, and any permanent sequelae that might ensue—whereas the benefits of NICU interventions are distant, statistical, and unpredictable. Moreover, NICU success is often viewed as "all or none"—that is, in most of the NICU follow-up literature a Bayley mental developmental index MDI or psychomotor developmental index PDI greater than 70 is classified as *normal*, whereas an MDI or PDI less than 70 is classified as an *adverse outcome*.

Faced with a difficult case, it is rare that simply applying principles will help to devise a solution. Difficult cases are usually ones in which the principles themselves are in conflict, or their application to the case is ambiguous.

DATA

What kind of information would parents, physicians, or judges want to know about the NICU? The essential truth at the intersection of NICU epidemiology and ethics is that survival depends sharply on gestational age (GA), within relatively precise boundaries. In the United States, as in virtually all the industrialized world, infants born after 27 weeks' gestation have, from any ethical perspective, no increased mortality over infants born at term. Consequently, for these infants, the ethical principle of best interests requires their resuscitation, in the same way that sick children born at term deserve resuscitation.

Conversely, for infants born before 22 weeks' gestation, survival is essentially zero. Consequently, these infants and their parents deserve our compassion, but not our interventions, on the ethical grounds of strict futility.

In between, spanning roughly one gestational month, from 23 to 26 weeks, we will require not just data, but interpretation. First, there is the intriguing finding that GA-specific mortality for infants resuscitated in this gestational range has more or less reached a plateau. Within 10 to 20 years ago, the "border of viability" was steadily decreasing, thus improving outcomes for infants in the gray zone. Not so much, recently, and there is little reason to think that things will change for infants born in this gestational range in the foreseeable future.

Nonetheless, epidemiologic progress has been made. Tyson et al (2008), using the vast data base of the National Institute of Child Health and Human Development network, attempted to go "beyond gestational age" and quantify additional risk factors for both mortality and neurologic morbidity in infants born on the cusp of viability. The analysis revealed that singleton status, appropriate in utero growth, antenatal steroids, and female gender all improve the likelihood of survival and intact neurologic outcome, independent of GA. Tyson's algorithm, using information available at the time of birth, significantly improved predictive value and sensitivity of prognostication over GA alone.

However, two problems remain. First, for many infants the predictive value of the Tyson algorithm is still not very good—that is, many of the lower-risk patients will still die, and many of the higher-risk patients will survive. Second, the Tyson algorithm, like GA, ignores a potentially important feature of NICU care—time. The algorithm stops accumulating data at the time of birth, and it does not account for prognostic features that might become available as the infant's course unfolds in the NICU. In theory, making decisions over the course of time offers two advantages over prognostication in the delivery room. First, parents often appreciate the opportunity to get to know their baby as an individual, as opposed to evaluating anonymous population-based prognostications at the time of birth. Second, there is valuable information to learn while the baby is in the NICU.

Two time-sensitive prognostic features have been evaluated in the context of infants born at the border of viability—serial illness severity algorithms (Score for Neonatal Acute Physiology [SNAP] scores) and serial that intuitions that the patient would "die before NICU discharge" (Meadow et al, 2008). Unfortunately, although SNAP scores on the first day of life have good prognostic power for death or survival, their power diminishes over time. Intriguingly, serial intuitions that an individual baby will die before discharge—offered by medical caretakers for

18

patients who require mechanical ventilation and for whom there is an ethical alternative to continued ventilation, namely extubation and palliative care—are remarkably accurate in predicting a combined outcome of either death or survival with neurologic impairment (MDI or PDI <70). Children with abnormal results from a cranial ultrasound examination and corroborated predictions of death have a less than 5% chance of surviving with both MDI and PDI greater than 70 at 2 years, independent of their gestational age. The predictive power of these data, acquired over time during an individual infant's NICU course, though not perfect, is greater than any algorithm available at the time of birth.

What do prospective parents or medical caretakers consider when they are asked to decide whether or not to resuscitate their micro-premie? A fascinating insight has been offered by Janvier et al, (2008), who have done extensive surveys comparing responses to requests for resuscitation of sick micro-premies with resuscitation of comparably sick patients at other ages (from term infants to 80-year-olds). Consistently, it appears that micro-premies are devalued—that is, for comparable likelihood of survival and comparable likelihood of neurologic morbidity in survivors, more people would let a micro-premie die first, or at least offer to resuscitate them last. There is no theory to account for these findings.

Indeed, for male infants born at 23 weeks' gestation, the likelihood of intact survival (i.e., neither death in the NICU nor permanent neurologic morbidity) is less than 10%. Given that the likelihood of burdensome therapy is 100%, how can resuscitation be justified? Intriguingly, combining the outcomes of death in the NICU with abnormal neurologic function in later life may not reflect the emotional reality of many NICU parents. For these parents, death in the NICU is not necessarily the worst outcome, because acknowledging that the baby was too small might be better consolation than not ever giving the baby a chance at life.

If trying and failing is seen as a positive process, then the long-term burden of NICU care for parents should perhaps be calculated not as a function of all live births (the current practice), but as a function of infants who survive to discharge. Numerous studies analyzing various populations in several countries have converged on the same surprising observation: the incidence of neurologic morbidity in NICU survivors is not very different when comparing infants at 23, 24, 25, and 26 to 27 weeks' gestation. The essential epidemiologic difference for infants born in this gestational range appears to be whether the baby will survive at all. Once the baby leaves the NICU, the risk of severe morbidity is largely the same; this is true in single-center and multicenter studies, in the United Kingdom, Canada, Europe, and the United States (Johnson et al, 2009; Tyson et al, 2008). Paradoxically, if avoiding survival with permanent crippling neurologic injury is the driving force behind resuscitation decisions, it appears that we should not be worrying about 23- and 24-weekers–rather we should not be resuscitating 26- or 27-weekers, since many more of them will survive, and survive with disability. But that seems very odd.

Finally, there is epidemiologic difficulty in assigning value to morbidity in surviving infants in the NICU. Verrips et al (2008) have attempted to assess the effects of permanent

residual disability for NICU survivors and their immediate families; they have demonstrated consistently that children with disabilities and their parents place a much higher value on their lives, and the quality of those lives, than do either physicians or NICU nurses. The vast majority of infants who survive the NICU, even those with significant permanent neurologic compromise, have "lives worth living," as judged by the people most affected by those lives.

GA-specific mortality seems to preclude resuscitation for infants born before 22 weeks' gestation and require resuscitation for infants born after 27 weeks' gestation. In between, the outcomes are murky, prognostic indices are imperfect, and sociologic analyses of human behaviors (of parents and physicians) appear inadequate to develop any uniform approach that is satisfactory.

POLICY

Neonatologists in the United States are sued for medical negligence approximately once every 10 years, and the average U.S. neonatologist will be sued more than once during his or her career (Meadow et al, 1997). Other than case-specific failures or oversights, are there any overarching themes that have arisen from medical malpractice cases in neonatology?

In the United States most malpractice allegations are state based, as opposed to federal cases. Consequently, the decisions of lower state courts, or even state supreme courts, are not binding in any other state, but they can be informative. The first important legal case in neonatology in the United States was *Miller v HCA* (2003). In 1990, Mrs. Miller came to the Hospital Corporation of America (HCA) in Texas in labor at 23 weeks' gestation. The fetus was estimated to weigh 500 to 600 g. No baby born that size had ever survived at that hospital. Mrs. Miller, her husband, and the attending physicians agreed that the baby was previable and that no intervention was indicated. The baby was born, but a different physician performed resuscitation, and the infant survived with brain damage. As a result, the Millers sued the hospital for a breach of informed consent, and they were awarded $50 million by a trial jury. The case wound its way to the Texas Supreme Court, which dismissed the verdict and articulated an "emergency exception" for physicians—that is, if a Texas physician finds himself or herself in the emergency position of needing to resuscitate a patient to prevent immediate death, the physician can try to perform resuscitation without being obligated to obtain consent from anyone. Whether it would be acceptable for a physician not to perform resuscitation in an emergency was left unarticulated by the Texas court.

In Wisconsin, the case of *Montalvo v Borkovec* (2002) took the legal obligations of neonatologists and parents to a different place. The case derived from the resuscitation of a male infant born between 23 4/7 and 24 2/7 weeks' gestation, weighing 679 g. The parents claimed a violation of informed consent, arguing that the decision to use "extraordinary measures" should have been relegated to the parents. The Wisconsin Appellate Court disagreed, holding that "in the absence of a persistent vegetative state, the right of a parent to withhold life-sustaining treatment from a child does not exist." Because virtually no infant is born in a persistent vegetative state, this decision would apparently eliminate the ethical possibility in Wisconsin of a "gray zone" of parental discretion. No other jurisdiction in the United States has adopted this position. The Wisconsin Appellate Court, like the Texas Supreme Court, was silent on whether physicians have discretion not to resuscitate. However, in Texas and Wisconsin, physicians are apparently not liable if they choose to do so.

A number of other state courts have addressed issues of treatment or nontreatment. In general, the courts are permissive of physicians who resuscitate infants. If courts are asked to sanction decisions to allow infants to die, most will do so only if there is consensus among physicians and parents, and occasionally ethics committees. Courts are not eager to punish physicians who treat infants over parental objections or to empower physicians to stop treatment when parents want it to continue.

BABY DOE REGULATIONS

Of course, state-by-state civil malpractice cases are not the only administrative means for redrawing the interface between neonatal medicine and the law. The federal government has contributed as well. The Baby Doe Regulations were one of the first attempts to codify and impose a federal vision of appropriate ethical behavior in the NICU.

In 1982, a baby with Down syndrome and esophageal atresia was born in Bloomington, Indiana. At that time, the standard of care for babies with Down syndrome was shifting. A decade or two earlier, most babies with Down syndrome who survived infancy were institutionalized. If babies needed surgery for an anomaly like Baby Doe's atresia, the parents were given the option. Approximately half chose surgery and half chose palliative care (Shaw, 1973). Similarly, half of pediatricians thought that palliative care, rather than surgery, was the better option (Todres et al, 1977). By the early 1980s, this practice had started to change. More parents opted for active intervention to save their babies (Shepperdson, 1983), and more physicians believed that withholding treatment was medical neglect (Todres et al, 1988). Baby Doe was born into this shifting cultural milieu.

Baby Doe's parents refused to consent to surgery and chose palliative care instead. The pediatrician alerted the state child protection agency, which investigated the case. At a court hearing, the parents claimed that they were following the advice of their obstetrician and not their pediatrician. The court found that parents only had to follow the advice of a licensed physician and that, since they were doing so, they were not neglectful. The court did not take protective custody. The doctor and hospital appealed. The Indiana Supreme Court refused to hear the appeal, and the baby died after 8 days (Lantos, 1987).

These facts became publicly known and led to a national controversy that eventually reached the Oval Office. President Reagan demanded federal action. It was difficult to decide which action should be taken, because the federal government has no jurisdiction over child abuse and neglect; it is the domain of the states. The federal government oversees civil rights enforcement, however, and the Reagan administration devised a legal strategy that defined not treating babies with Down syndrome or other congenital anomalies as discrimination against people with disabilities, rather than medical neglect. This strategy gave the federal government a justification for oversight. The new regulations were implemented, and bright red signs containing federal hotline telephone numbers were posted in NICUs across the country. These signs proclaimed that withholding treatment on the basis of disability was a federal civil rights violation (Annas, 1984) and that federal investigative squads could review medical records to determine whether discrimination had taken place. These regulations were challenged and eventually struck down by the U.S. Supreme Court (Annas, 1984).

A diluted version of the original Baby Doe guidelines was eventually incorporated into the federal Child Abuse and Treatment Act (Annas, 1986; Kopelman, 1988). That law, however, is primarily a funding mechanism to channel federal funds to state child protection agencies; it is not a regulation that can be enforced for physicians or hospitals. The Baby Doe regulations do not exist today and have not existed since 1984; however, they still hold symbolic power. The mention of Baby Doe strikes fear in the hearts of pediatricians who lived through the events, in part because pediatricians had made pediatricians into villains in the societal battle over child protection.

There is a certain irony in the controversy over Baby Doe regulations. The original goal—to decrease the range of cases in which withholding treatment of newborns is permissible—did not need federal input. Progress was already being made. Many diseases that used to be considered incompatible with life or that were seen as leading to an unacceptable quality of life were being treated routinely. Metabolic therapies for genetic diseases (phenylketonuria [PKU], hypothyroidism, Gaucher disease) and surgical therapies for organ dysgenesis (congenital heart corrections, congenital diaphragmatic hernia (CDH) repair, extra corporeal membrane oxygenation (ECMO), dialysis) have been forcefully advanced by medical subspecialists in their corresponding fields (e.g., genetics, cardiac surgery, general surgery). With few exceptions (hypoplastic left ventricle being one of the best recognized), these advances have been relatively uncontroversial. Once sufficient data are gathered to demonstrate moderate efficacy, the innovations are widely and rapidly adopted.

There is still controversy when treatments enable survival but have a high likelihood, or certainty, that survival will be accompanied by severe neurologic impairment. As a result, two questions must be asked. First, how severe will the neurologic impairment be? Second, what is the likelihood that the child will have the most severe possible impairment? The prognostic spectrum of Down syndrome is broad, but few infants with trisomy 21 are severely impaired. In contrast, almost all infants with trisomy 13 or 18 either die in infancy or are left with profound neurologic impairment. The outcomes for these chromosomal anomalies can be used to define the spectrum within which clinical decisions are made. For babies whose outcomes are likely to be similar to those seen in trisomy 21, it is no longer permissible to withhold life-sustaining treatment. For babies whose outcomes are likely to be similar to babies with trisomy 13, it is permissible to withhold or withdraw life-sustaining treatment and offer palliative care instead. The calculus becomes more complex in conditions associated with a wider range of outcomes, such as extreme prematurity or high myelomenigocele with hydrocephalus.

The shift in moral standards regarding babies with Down syndrome was not related to technology, but rather sociology. The capacity to repair Arnold–Chiari malformation and duodenal atresia existed long before it was applied to children with myelomeningocele and Down syndrome. What has changed the mood of the country is a growing recognition that disability is as much a social construct as a medical construct, although it is always both and not one or the other.

BORN ALIVE INFANT PROTECTION ACT

In 2002, the U.S. Congress passed a law called the *Born Alive Infant Protection Act* (BAIPA). BAIPA, like the discredited Baby Doe regulations, was an attempt to insert federal values into medical deliberations. There are some interesting similarities and distinctions between Baby Doe and BAIPA. The Baby Doe regulations addressed disability, whereas BAIPA applies to abortion. BAIPA declares that "for the purposes of Federal law, the words 'person', 'human being', 'child', and 'individual' shall include every infant who is born alive at any stage of development." As Sayeed (2005) noted, "The agency arguably substitutes a nonprofessional's presumed sagacious assessment of survivability for reasonable medical judgment." It is unclear what the implications of this law have been. On the one hand, all infants born alive before BAIPA were also treated as human beings; however, that did not necessarily mean that they received all available life support and resuscitation. After all, patients can have do-not-resuscitate orders or receive palliative care rather than intensive care. Still, the purpose of BAIPA seemed to be less about the treatment of babies and more about restrictions on abortion. Although some authors have expressed concern that the influence of BAIPA may transform neonatal care of infants born at, or even below, the threshold of viability, it appears to have had little measurable effect to date. Partridge et al (2009) surveyed neonatologists in California and found that they were concerned about the implications of BAIPA. They write, "If this legislation were enforced, respondents predicted more aggressive resuscitation potentially increasing risks of disability or delayed death." There have been no cases to date in which BAIPA has been invoked or in which physicians and hospitals have been found to be in violation of its requirements.

FUTURE DIRECTIONS

There is no new technology in development that appears likely to affect outcomes significantly. Consequently, for infants who receive resuscitation in the delivery room, birthweight-specific mortality and morbidity are unlikely to change much in the near future. Nonetheless, three developments may change the way we think about newborns, and consequently shift the terrain of neonatal bioethics.

HIGH RISK MATERNAL-FETAL MEDICINE CENTERS

Many children's hospitals are now developing high-risk, maternal-fetal medicine centers. The goal of these centers is to identify fetuses at risk—particularly those with congenital anomalies—and to care for those fetuses and their mothers in centers where there is expertise in fetal diagnosis, therapy, and neonatal care. The hope is that such centers will allow more timely, and therefore more effective, intervention for babies with congenital heart disease, congenital diaphragmatic hernia, or other anomalies.

The medical effectiveness of fetal centers will depend on two distinct developments. First, on a population basis, these centers will only be as effective as fetal screening and diagnosis. The existence of these centers will almost certainly create an expectation and a demand for better fetal screening. Such screening is likely to include both better imaging and better screening tests that can be performed on maternal blood; both will lead to earlier diagnosis of fetal anomalies. These diagnoses will create more complex dilemmas for perinatologists and parents who will need to decide, in any particular case, whether to terminate the pregnancy, offer fetal therapy, or offer either palliative care or interventions after birth. Ironically, better fetal diagnosis may increase the likelihood of pregnancy termination, even when postnatal treatment is possible, such as in hypoplastic left heart syndrome.

Second, the effectiveness of fetal centers will depend on the effectiveness of fetal interventions. Perhaps surprisingly, other than in utero transfusion for Rhesus disease or vascular ablation for twin-twin transfusion syndromes—neither of which are particularly new and neither of which is performed by pediatric surgeons or pediatricians—there is little evidence that any fetal intervention has had any effect on any neonatal outcome. This lack of demonstrated effectiveness has, thus far, not suppressed the proliferation of fetal intervention centers. There may be other factors, including institutional prestige, finances, and recruitment of "desirable" patients.

EXPANDED NEWBORN SCREENING

In recent years, the number of diseases and conditions that can be diagnosed through newborn screening has expanded dramatically. Such screening is under the purview of states, rather than the federal government, and there is wide variation in the number of tests that are performed. In 1995 the average number of tests per state was five (range: zero to eight disorders). Between 1995 and 2005 most states added tests, so that the average number of screening tests done by 2005 was 24 (Tarini et al, 2006). The expansion of newborn screening raises three problems. First, even the most accurate test has false positives. For rare conditions, the percentage of positive tests that are false positives is increased. Thus, the more rare conditions that are added to a newborn screening panel, the more false positives there will be. False positives are associated with considerable parental anxiety and can lead to potentially dangerous and unnecessary diagnostic procedures or treatments. Second, expanded newborn screening costs money. Interestingly, the tests themselves are astoundingly inexpensive, which is why policy makers are tempted to add more to the panels. However, the follow-up counseling and testing after positive tests are expensive, and without such follow-up the screening programs will not work. The Centers for Disease Control and Prevention has recently expressed concern about these costs (Centers for Disease Control and Prevention, 2008). Finally, there is the potential for discrimination against patients for whom documented heterozygous carrier status conveys no recognized medical infirmity, but social or psychological stigma may be real. There is little funding available to assist or counsel these patients.

FINANCIAL CONSTRAINTS

The American Academy of Pediatrics guidelines on neonatal resuscitation suggest that resuscitation should be obligatory at 25 weeks' gestation or greater, optional at 24 weeks' gestation, and unusual at 23 weeks' gestation. These recommendations are thought to reflect the best understanding of both the ethical discussion and the epidemiologic facts surrounding NICU outcomes. The recommendations purport to reflect the traditional paradigm that data drive policy. However, particularly in the context of NICU survival for infants at 23 to 25 weeks' gestation, there is good evidence that causation can work in the reverse direction—that is, policy drives data. In the Netherlands, Canada, and some parts of Oregon, survival at 25 weeks' gestation is comparable and comparably good; more than 50% of infants born at 25 weeks' gestation will survive to discharge. However, in the Netherlands, virtually no infant survives birth at 24 weeks' gestation, whereas in Canada and Oregon the survival rate is 40%. In addition, in Oregon and some parts of Canada, survival at 23 weeks' gestation is close to zero, whereas in other parts of Canada and the United States the survival rate is 20% or greater. Why? Certainly not because the Dutch, Canadians, or Oregonians have forgotten how to resuscitate small infants. Rather, they have chosen not to. Why not? Perhaps it is non-maleficence–the fear that survival with permanent neurologic morbidity may be cruel to the child, the family, or society at large. However, the incidence of neurologic morbidity in survivors is not different when comparing infants at 23, 24, 25, and 26 to 27 weeks' gestation. If the fear of a permanent crippling neurologic injury is the driving force, we should not be resuscitating 26 or 27 weekers, since many more of them will survive, and survive with disability. But that seems odd.

The approach in the Netherlands is consistent; there is a limited budget and a communitarian ethic. There is a certain rationale behind spending money on all pregnant women, instead of 1% of micro-premies. The United States appears ambivalent–we value individuals over community, are fascinated with high-technology, and claim to prize our children. On the other hand, we will not spend money to prevent unwanted teen pregnancy or to provide visiting nurses for new mothers.

Finally the concept of generational conflict must be considered. We appear quite comfortable calling delivery-room resuscitation of 24 weekers "optional," based on gestational age alone. It is difficult to imagine the AMA recommending that resuscitation for 85-year-olds who come to the emergency department is "optional," based on age alone. NICU care is often criticized as "too expensive." We ask, "Compared to what?"

Fewer than 5% of infants will be in the NICU for more than a short stay. The vast majority of these patients will survive. Only 24,000 infants of 4 million births die each year in the United States, and half of these will die within fewer than 7 days. In contrast, nearly 3 million adults will die in the United States each year and one third of these will have been admitted to an medical intensive care unit (MICU) in the 6 months before dying. MICU costs outpace NICU costs by at least 100 to 1.

SUMMARY

Ethical philosophy is a place to start, not a place to finish. Data are relatively easy to acquire and agree on. Policy is intriguingly insensitive to data, but that may reflect social and political realities that exist beyond the NICU—perceptions of disability, abortion politics, individual versus communitarian emphasis, fascination with technology, discrimination, publicity, financial constraints—so that an ethical course of action in one country, one city, or one family might seem perverse elsewhere.

SUGGESTED READINGS

Annas GJ: The Baby Doe regulations: governmental intervention in neonatal rescue medicine, *Am J Public Health* 74:618-620, 1984.

Born-Alive Infants Protection Act of 2001: Report together with additional and dissenting views of the House Committee on the Judiciary, 107th Congress, 1st Session, August 2, 2001. 1-38, 3. (Purpose and Summary).

Centers for Disease Control and Prevention: Impact of expanded newborn screening: United States, 2006, *MMWR Morb Mortal Wkly Rep* 57:1012-1015, 2008.

Janvier A, Leblanc I, Barrington KJ: The best-interest standard is not applied for neonatal resuscitation decisions, *Pediatrics* 121:963-969, 2008.

Johnson S, Fawke J, Hennessy E, et al: Neurodevelopmental disability through 11 years of age in children born before 26 weeks of gestation, *Pediatrics* 124:E249-E257.

Lantos J: Baby Doe five years later: implications for child health, *N Engl J Med* 317:444-447, 1987.

Meadow W, Lagatta J, Andrews B, et al: Just in time: ethical implications of serial predictions of death and morbidity for ventilated premature infants, *Pediatrics* 121:732-740, 2008.

Miller v HCA, Inc, 118 S.W. 3d 758, 771 (Texas 2003).

Montalvo v Borkovec, 647 N.W. 2d 413 (Wis. App. 2002).

Shepperdson B: Abortion and euthanasia of Down's syndrome children: the parents' view, *J Med Ethics* 9:152-157, 1983.

Todres ID, Guillemin J, Grodin MA, et al: Life-saving therapy for newborns: a questionnaire survey in the state of Massachusetts, *Pediatrics* 81:643-649, 1988.

Tyson JE, Parikh NA, Langer J, et al: National Institute of Child Health and Human Development Neonatal Research Network. Intensive care for extreme prematurity: moving beyond gestational age, *N Engl J Med* 358:1672-1681, 2008.

Complete references used in this text can be found online at www.expertconsult.com

GLOBAL NEONATAL HEALTH

Linda L. Wright

CHILD MORTALITY

In 2000, the 192 United Nations member states and many international partners adopted the Millennium Development Goals (MDGs) in response to morbidity and mortality rates in the developing world that were alarmingly high. These eight international development goals were to eradicate extreme hunger and poverty; achieve universal primary education; promote gender equality and empower women; reduce child mortality; improve maternal health; combat HIV/AIDS, malaria, and other diseases; ensure environmental sustainability; and develop a global partnership for development. The agreement included 18 specific targets and 48 technical indicators to measure progress toward the MDGs between 1990 and 2015 (United Nations General Assembly, 2001).

Although significant progress has been made toward achieving many of the MDGs, progress has been uneven, with huge disparities across the goals and among countries. This disparity is especially true for MDG 5 (i.e., improving indicators of maternal health, including maternal mortality during pregnancy or the 42 days following the end of pregnancy, per 100,000 deliveries) and MDG 4 (i.e., reducing child mortality, expressed as deaths before 5 years per 1000 live births). Regions and countries that have the highest maternal mortality rates also have the highest child mortality rates (Table 4-1).

Twenty percent of all deaths in the world are child deaths (Save the Children, 2007; United Nations Children's Fund, 2007), and greater than 99% of deaths occurring in children aged 5 years or younger are in the developing world. Of the 136 million babies born in 2007, an estimated 9.7 million died before the age of 5 years (approximately 26,000 per day) (Save the Children, 2007; United Nations Children's Fund, 2007). This staggering number equals approximately half of all U.S. children younger than 5 years (Save the Children, 2007; U.S. Census Bureau's American Community Survey, 2007). The latest estimates suggest that 8.8 million children died in 2008 (United Nations Children's Fund, 2008b). The rate of decline in mortality in children younger than 5 years is grossly insufficient to meet the MDG 4 goal by 2015, particularly in Sub-Saharan Africa and South Asia (United Nations Children's Fund, 2009). At the current rate, the target of fewer than 5 million annual child deaths will not be met until 2045. To meet the goal of fewer than 5 million child deaths in 2015, deaths in children younger than 5 years must be cut in half between 2008 and 2015 (Table 4-2) (United Nations Children's Fund, 2007, 2009a).

The regions with the highest numbers of child deaths are Sub-Saharan Africa (which has high fertility rates and the highest child mortality rates [144 deaths per 1000 live births], and 4.8 million children [1 in 7] dies before the age of 5 years) and South Asia (3.1 million deaths [1 in 13] before the age of 5 years) (United Nations Children's

Fund, 2007). Sub-Saharan Africa accounts for 51% of all deaths among children younger than 5 years, followed by Asia with 42% (You et al, 2009).

In 2008, 75% of deaths in children younger than 5 years occurred in only 18 countries, and 40% occurred in only three countries: India, Nigeria, and the Democratic Republic of the Congo. Of the 34 countries with mortality rates exceeding 100 per 1000 live births in 2008, all were in Sub-Saharan Africa, except for Afghanistan (You et al, 2009). Equally troubling, only 10 of the 67 countries with high mortality rates (at least 40 per 1000 live births) were on track to meet MDG 4 before the 2009 economic crisis (You et al, 2009). However, a number of relatively poor countries with low gross national incomes have made considerable progress in improving survival, including Malawi, Tanzania, Madagascar, Nepal, Bangladesh (Save the Children, 2007), Eretria, the Lao People's Democratic Republic, Mongolia, and Bolivia (Figure 4-1) (You et al, 2009).

More than 70% of deaths in children younger than 5 years are caused by newborn problems, pneumonia, and diarrhea. Pneumonia kills more children than any other illness—more than HIV, malaria, and measles combined (Figure 4-2). Pneumonia results in death for more than 2 million children younger than 5 years each year, or approximately 20% of child deaths worldwide. More than 95% of all new pneumonia cases, representing an estimated 150 million episodes of pneumonia annually, occur in children younger than 5 years in developing countries. Sub-Saharan Africa and South Asia together have more than half the total number of pneumonia cases. Effective prevention strategies include immunization against measles, whooping cough, *Haemophilus influenzae* type b, and *Streptococcus pneumoniae*; exclusive breastfeeding and improved nutrition or low birthweight; zinc supplementation; reducing indoor air pollution; and prevention and management of HIV infection (Qazi et al, 2008); however, the protection afforded by immunizations will not prevent neonatal pneumonia. Universal use of simple standardized management guidelines for identifying and treating pneumonia in communities and primary health care centers, with the World Health Organization (WHO) Integrated Management of Childhood Illness (Niessen et al, 2009), may reduce the child pneumonia fatality rate (Niessen et al, 2009). Sazawal and Black (1992) suggested that community-based acute respiratory infection case management might reduce mortality by more than 20% in children younger than 4 years. Failing prevention, prompt diagnosis and treatment are necessary to improve pneumonia mortality and morbidity; however, prompt diagnosis and effective treatment of pneumonia and hypoxemia are often not available. Radiology, laboratory tests, and pulse oximetry, which can predict response to antibiotic therapy in cases of severe pneumonia (Fu et al, 2006), are not available in most first-level (i.e., rural)

TABLE 4-1 Countries With the Highest Numbers of Child Deaths Also Have High Rates of Maternal Death

Country	Ranking for Number of Child Deaths	Number of Child Deaths	Ranking for Number of Maternal Deaths	Number of Maternal Deaths
India	1	1,919,000	1	136,000
Nigeria	2	1,043,000	2	37,000
DR Congo	3	589,000	4	24,000
Ethiopia	4	509,000	4	24,000
Pakistan	5	473,000	3	26,000
China	6	467,000	9	11,000
Afghanistan	7	370,000	7	20,000
Bangladesh	8	274,000	8	16,000
Uganda	9	200,000	12	10,000
Angola	10	199,000	9	11,000
	6,043,000 child deaths Approximately 60 percent of global total		315,000 maternal deaths Approximately 60 percent of global total	

Sources: Child deaths UNICEF. State of the World's Children 2007, Table 1; Maternal deaths: World Health Organization, United Nations Children's Fund and United Nations Population Fund, Maternal Mortality in 2000: Estimates Developed by WHO, UNICEF and UNFPA.
From *Save the Children*: State of the world's mothers, 2007: saving the lives of children under 5.

TABLE 4-2 Global Progress in Reducing Child Mortality is Insufficient to Reach Millennium Development Goal 4*
Average annual rate of reduction (AARR) in the under 5 mortality rate (U5MR) observed for 1990–2006 and required during 2007–2015 in order to reach MDG 4

	U5MR No. of Deaths per 1,000 Live Births		AARR Observed %	Required %	Progress Toward the MDG Target
	1990	2006	1990–2006	2007–2015	
Sub-Saharan Africa	187	160	1.0	10.5	Insufficient progress
Eastern and Southern Africa	165	131	1.4	9.6	Insufficient progress
West and Central Africa	208	186	0.7	11.0	No progress
Middle East and North Africa	79	46	3.4	6.2	Insufficient progress
South Asia	123	83	2.5	7.8	Insufficient progress
East Asia and Pacific	55	29	4.0	5.1	On track
Latin America and Caribbean	55	27	4.4	4.3	On track
CEE/CIS	53	27	4.2	4.7	On track
Industrialized countries/territories	10	6	3.2	6.6	On track
Developing countries/territorries	103	79	1.7	9.3	Insufficient progress
World	**93**	**72**	**1.6**	**9.4**	Insufficient progress

United Nations Children's Fund: The state of the world's children 2008: child survival, 2007, New York.
*Progress towards MDG 4, with countries classified according to the following thresholds:
On track: U5MR is less than 40, or U5MR is 40 or more and the average annual rate of reduction (AARR) in under 5 mortality rate observed from 1990 to 2006 is 4.0% or more.
Insufficient progress: U5MR is 40 or more and AARR observed for the 1990-2006 period is between 1.0% and 3.9%.
No progress: U5MR is 40 or more and AARR observed for 1990-2006 is less than 1.0%.
Source: UNICEF estimates based on the work of the interagency Child Mortality Estimation Group.

hospitals, despite high mortality rates in children who have hypoxemia or HIV. Randomized controlled trials of parenteral antibiotic treatment in hospitals compared with home-based treatment have demonstrated the safety and efficacy of treating pneumonia with oral antibiotics outside of a hospital setting in older children. New evidence regarding home treatment of severe pneumonia is changing concepts about the need for hospitalization. The first randomized trial to compare outcomes of hospital treatment of severe pneumonia, without underlying complications, with home-based oral antibiotics in Pakistan demonstrated that home-based antibiotics are safe and effective. Of 2037 children with severe pneumonia aged 3 to 59 months, randomized to either parenteral ampicillin for 48 hours followed by 3 days of oral ampicillin or home-based oral amoxicillin for 5 days, there were equal numbers of failures in the hospitalized group (8.6%) and in the ambulatory group (7.5%) by day 6. Just 0.2% children died within 14 days of enrollment and none of the deaths were considered to be associated with treatment

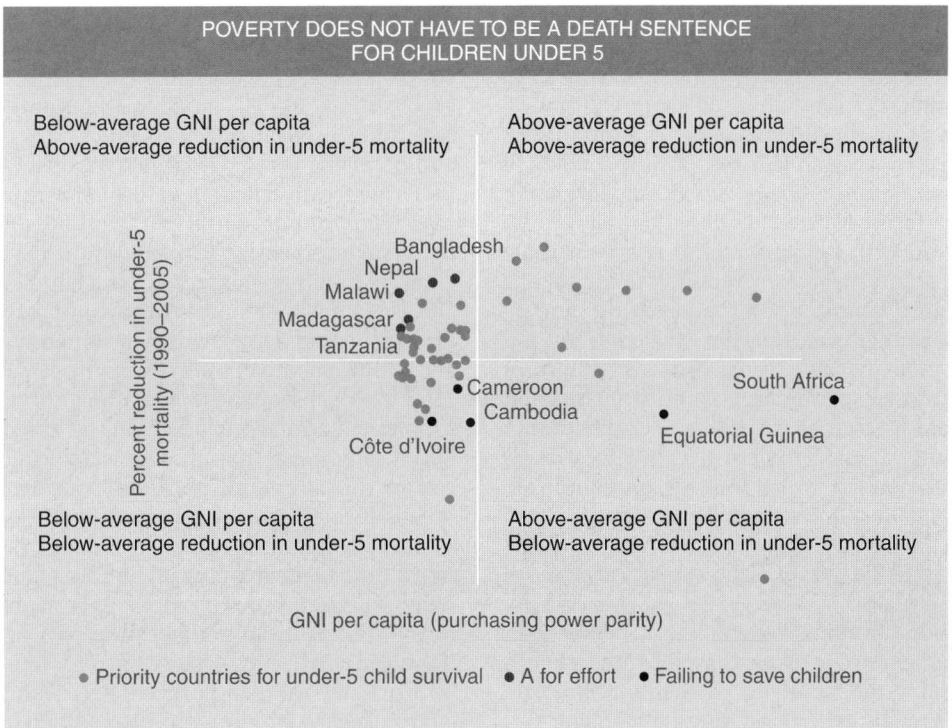

FIGURE 4-1 Poverty does not have to be a death sentence for children under 5. (*From* Save the Children: *State of the world's mothers 2007: saving the lives of children under 5, 2007.*)

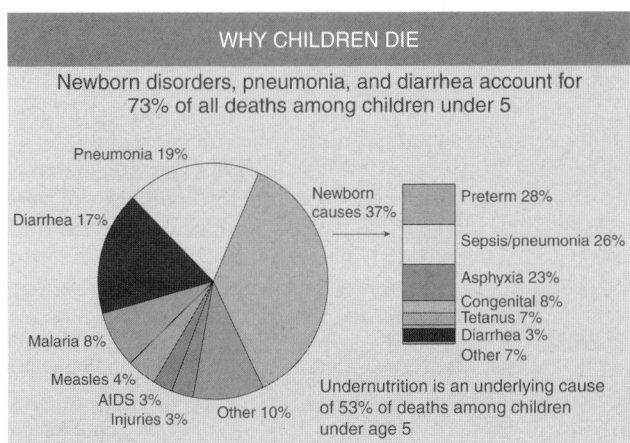

FIGURE 4-2 Why children die. (*From* Save the Children: *State of the world's mothers 2007: saving the lives of children under 5, 2007.*)

allocation (Hazir et al, 2008). A small percentage (approximately 2% to 3%) of severely ill children will still require early community detection and transport to a hospital for evaluation of hypoxia, infection, pneumonia, malaria, and parenteral antibiotics with or without oxygen (Mwaniki et al, 2009). The WHO has spearheaded efforts to reduce the global burden of child pneumonia with the Integrated Management of Childhood Illness, a Global Action Plan for Control and Prevention of Pneumonia (GAPP) (Qazi et al, 2008), publication of new comprehensive global, regional, and national disease burden statistics for pneumococcal and hepatitis b disease, the Global Coalition against Childhood Pneumonia, and the first World Pneumonia Day on November 2, 2009 (United Nations Children's Fund, 2009b).

Diarrheal diseases are the second most common cause of child deaths globally. Worldwide, diarrhea accounts for 18% of deaths among children younger than 5 years, or an estimated 1.7 million child deaths every year, and it accounts for 10% to 80% of growth retardation in the first few years of life (Baqui and Ahmed, 2006). Exclusive breastfeeding provided significant protection from diarrheal diseases before the WHO-recommended introduction of complementary feeds at 6 months. Children in poverty are especially prone to diarrheal diseases after the introduction of complementary feeding, because diarrhea is spread by poor hygiene and sanitation facilities; contaminated water, formula, food, or utensils; low rates of vitamin A supplementation; low zinc intake; and limited access to rotavirus immunization. Most diarrhea-related deaths in children are due to dehydration. The WHO recommendations for oral rehydration therapy (ORT) for childhood diarrheal diseases have changed. Research has demonstrated that homemade fluids that contain lower concentrations of sodium and glucose, sucrose, or other carbohydrates (e.g., cereal-based solution) can be as effective as ORT. Current recommendations include increased fluid intake and continued feeding, as well as the use of zinc and low-osmolarity ORT to prevent and treat diarrheal episodes (Fischer-Walker et al, 2009; World Health Organization and United Nations Children's Fund, 2004). Lower-osmolarity ORT reduces stool output, vomiting, and unscheduled intravenous therapy (Baqui and Ahmed, 2006). In Sub-Saharan Africa there has been little progress in diarrhea prevention and treatment in the last decade—the percentage of children younger than 5 years who received the recommended treatment increased from 32% in 2000 to only 38% in 2008 (United Nations Children's Fund, 2009). Progress on case management of childhood pneumonia, diarrhea, and malaria will depend on strengthening the integrated community-based prevention and treatment of these pervasive childhood diseases within the health system (United Nations Children's Fund, 2009).

Undernutrition is another major factor in mortality of children younger than 5 years; it is responsible for 7% of the total disease burden in any age group, making it the highest of any risk factor for overall global burden of disease (Black et al, 2008b). Undernutrition is a contributing factor in more than half of infectious disease deaths in children (Save the Children, 2007) and is the underlying cause of more than one third of all deaths among children younger than 5 years (United Nations Children's Fund, 2008a). The effects of undernutrition reach beyond the individual child. Maternal or child undernutrition is a complex intergenerational problem that includes intrauterine growth restriction, severe wasting, and stunting. Virtually no progress has been made toward overcoming undernutrition in the last 25 years (United Nations Children's Fund, 2008a). Wasting (weight-for-height Z score less than −2) is associated with acute weight loss. Of the estimated 55 million children younger than 5 years with wasting (10% of all children), more than half are in south central Asia or Sub-Saharan Africa; 19 million children have severe acute malnutrition or wasting (weight-for-height Z score less than −3) and are in need of urgent therapeutic feeding (United Nations Children's Fund, 2008a). Stunting (height-for-age Z score less than −2), which is more common, indicates chronic restriction of a child's potential growth. An estimated 178 million children younger than 5 years have stunting—almost one third of children in low- to middle-resource settings. Ninety percent of them (160 million) live in just 36 countries and represent almost half of the children in those countries. India's 61 million children with stunting represent more than half of all Indian children younger than 5 years and 34% of all children with stunting worldwide (Bhutta et al, 2008a). This urgent problem must be solved, because the period between birth and 24 months old is critical. If children do not grow appropriately before 2 years old, they are more likely to be short as adults, have lower educational achievement and economic productivity, and give birth to smaller infants who repeat the cycle in the next generation. Although the problem of undernutrition has been overshadowed by concerns over obesity, there is no evidence that rapid weight or linear growth in the first 2 years of life increases the risk of chronic disease in adults (fetal origin of adult disease), even in children with poor fetal growth (Victora et al, 2008).

A recent review of interventions that affect maternal and child undernutrition suggested that counseling about breastfeeding and supplementation with vitamin A and increased zinc intake have the greatest potential to reduce the burden of child morbidity and mortality (Bhutta et al, 2008a). The promotion of breastfeeding has had an effect on the improved survival of infants and young children, but its effect on stunting has been negligible. Among populations with inadequate food, food supplements are beneficial with or without educational interventions (increased height-for-age Z scores by 0.41; 95% confidence interval [CI], 0.05-0.76) and can reduce stunting and the related burden of disease. In populations with sufficient food,

complementary feeding education increased height-for-age Z scores by 0.25 (95% CI, 0.01-0.49) compared with controls. Facility management of severe acute malnutrition, according to WHO guidelines, reduced the case fatality rate by 55% (relative risk [RR], 0.45; 95% CI, 0.32-0.62), and observational data suggest that ready-to-use prepared foods in treatment of severe malnutrition may be effective in community settings as well. Recommended micronutrient interventions for children include strategies for vitamin A supplementation, zinc supplements to prevent and treat diarrhea and lower respiratory tract infections, iron supplements in areas where malaria is not endemic, and universal promotion of iodized salt (Bhutta et al, 2008a). A subsequent metaanalysis of neonatal vitamin A supplementation concluded, on the basis of six trials in the developing world, that there was no evidence for a reduced risk of mortality and morbidity during infancy and thus no justification for neonatal vitamin A supplementation as a public health measure to reduce infant mortality and morbidity in developing countries (Gogia and Sachdev, 2009). The efficacy of zinc supplementation in reducing overall mortality in neonates has been questioned as well (Sazawal et al, 2007). Existing interventions designed to improve nutrition and prevent related disease may reduce stunting at 36 months old by as much as 36% and mortality between birth and 36 months old by approximately 25%. However, elimination of stunting will require long-term investment in improved nutrition and interventions to improve early childhood education, maternal education, and women's economic status (Black et al, 2008a). Growth (length, height, and weight) should be monitored routinely and regularly in view of its importance as a marker for undernutrition and stunting (Victora et al, 2009).

The nutrition of the children of India and Sub-Saharan Africa are of greatest concern. India is a concern because it represents 34% of the world's children with stunting, who often start life with intrauterine growth retardation and as adults are members of families with intergenerational stunting that live on less than $2 per day. In Africa, neonates are born with normal birthweight, but develop stunting and wasting because of poverty and civil unrest. Although exclusive breastfeeding protects the neonate, providing adequate amounts of nourishing food in early infancy is critical to the future of children from these two continents. Among the areas needing further research are assessments of the effectiveness and cost-effectiveness of a national health system's nutritional interventions on stunting rates and weight gain; long-term effects of maternal nutritional interventions on maternal and child health and cognitive outcome; research on the reversibility of stunting and cognitive impairment in children aged 36 to 60 months; studies of community-based prevention and treatment strategies for severe acute malnutrition; and studies of the effectiveness of various zinc delivery strategies.

EPIDEMIOLOGY OF NEONATAL MORTALITY (BEFORE 28 DAYS)

Developed countries have experienced significant declines in child mortality in the last 30 years, but only 1% of the world's neonatal deaths occur in 39 high-income countries whose average neonatal mortality rates are 4 to 6 per 1000

TABLE 4-3 Regional or Country Variations in Neonatal Mortality Rates and Numbers of Neonatal Deaths, Showing the Proportion of Deaths in Children Younger than Age 5 Years

	NMR per 1000 Livebirths (range across countries)	Number (%) of Neonatal Deaths (1000s)	Percentage of Deaths in Children Aged Younger than 5 Years in the Neonatal Period	Percentage Change in NMR between 1996 and 2005 Estimates[*]
Income groups				
High-income countries[†]	4 (1–11)	42 (1%)	63%	−29%
Low-income and middle-income countries	33 (2–70)	3956 (99%)	38%	−8%
WHO regions				
Africa	44 (9–70)	1128 (28%)	24%	5%
Americas	12 (4–34)	195 (5%)	48%	−40%
Eastern Mediterranean	40 (4–63)	603 (15%)	40%	−9%
Europe	11 (2–38)	116 (3%)	49%	−18%
Southeast Asia	38 (11–43)	1443 (36%)	50%	−21%
Western Pacific	19 (1–40)	512 (13%)	56%	−39%
Overall	30 (1–70)	3998 (100%)	38%	−16%

From Lawn JE, Cousens S, Zupan J: 4 Million neonatal deaths: when? where? why? *Lancet* 365:891-900, 2005.
[*]The data inputs cover at least a 5-year period before each set of estimates. Period of change may be assumed to be up to 15 years.
[†]Thirty-nine countries with NMR data of 54 countries with gross national income per person of US$9386.10.

live births. In contrast, little progress has been made in reducing maternal and neonatal deaths in the developing world, where the disparity is large and growing (Lawn et al, 2005) and the average neonatal mortality rate (deaths in the first 28 days of life per 1000 live births) in 2000 was 33, with a range of 2 to 70. Together Africa and Southeast Asia account for approximately two thirds of neonatal deaths (Table 4-3) (Lawn et al, 2005).

More than half of all maternal and newborn deaths occur at birth or in the first few days after birth, when health coverage is the lowest. Cultural norms, financial constraints, and small fetuses that are considered nonviable also limit the reporting of neonatal deaths. As a consequence, the births of an estimated 51 million children per year go unrecorded in any formal registration system (United Nations Children's Fund, 2007). These children are often born in slums or rural poverty to very young or older mothers who lack access to education and basic health and reproductive services, and who also live in countries that have experienced recent political unrest (United Nations Children's Fund, 2007). As a result, fewer than 3% of neonatal deaths occur in countries that have high-coverage vital registration data or recent, reliable data on causes of neonatal death; therefore global analysis is based on estimates (Lawn et al, 2005) derived from statistical modeling. Until the middle to late 1990s, estimates of neonatal deaths were drawn from historical data. More rigorous estimates using demographic and health surveys of newborn deaths at a national level were available in 1995 and 2000 (Lawn et al, 2005; United Nations Children's Fund, 2008a), which produced more reliable neonatal mortality rates. The lack of reliable data from most high-risk countries, and the complex methods for developing estimates and for estimating uncertainty, makes even these improved neonatal mortality data inherently uncertain (United Nations Children's Fund, 2008a). As a result, data from different sources are difficult to compare and interpret; this will be especially true when comparing data from before and after 2008, when the Inter-agency Group for Child Mortality Estimation (IGME) incorporated a substantial amount of new data and developed a new method to adjust mortality related to HIV/AIDS (You et al, 2009).

The latest available data suggest that 3.7 million deaths (40% of deaths in children younger than 5 years) occur in the first month and that there are almost as many stillbirths per year worldwide (3.3 million) (Stanton et al, 2006; United Nations Children's Fund, 2008a; World Health Organization, 2006). The first hours and days of a baby's life are the most critical (Figure 4-3). Every year 2 million babies die on the day they are born (Save the Children, 2007), representing almost 50% of all neonatal deaths, and an astounding 75% of neonatal deaths occur within the first 7 days of life (Murray et al, 2007; Save the Children, 2007).

As a result, a neonate is approximately 500-fold more likely to die in the first day of life than at 1 month of age (United Nations Children's Fund, 2007). Without a major reduction in early (7 days) deaths in high-mortality countries, it will be impossible to meet the MDG 4 (Figure 4-4) (World Health Organization, 2006).

MATERNAL RISK FACTORS FOR NEONATAL DEATH

Because 40% to 90% of women in low-resource settings deliver their baby in the home without a skilled birth attendant or access to facility care for themselves or their newborn, intrapartum complications put the fetus or neonate at increased risk for death, especially maternal bleeding after the eighth month, hypertensive disorders, obstructed labor, prolonged second-stage of labor or malpresentation, maternal fever or rupture of membranes for longer than 24 hours, multiparity, malaria or syphilis, meconium staining, and maternal HIV (Lawn et al, 2005).

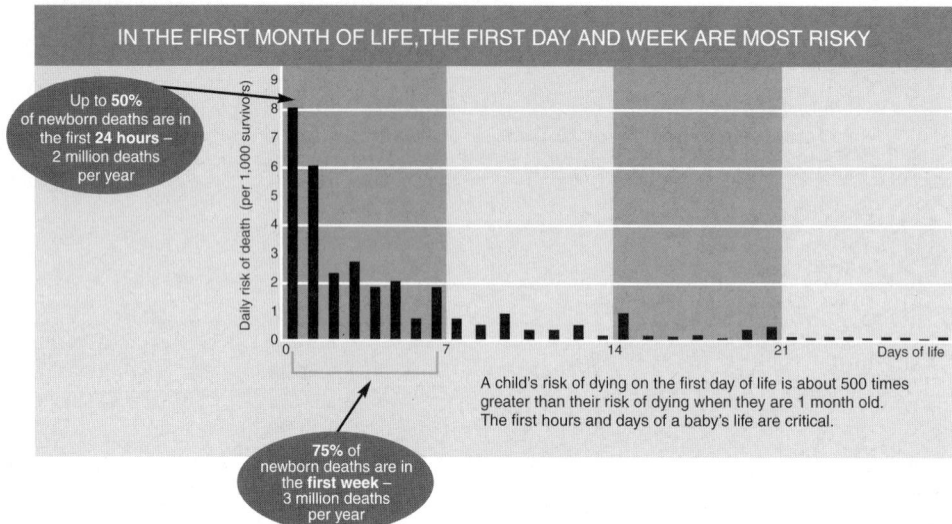

FIGURE 4-3 In the first month of life, the first day and week pose the highest risk. *(Modified from ORC Macro: Measure Demographic Health Survey STAT compiler, 2006. Available at www.measuredhs.com. Accessed April 6, 2006. Based on the analysis by J. Lawn of 38 DHS datasets [2000 to 2004] with 9022 neonatal deaths.)*

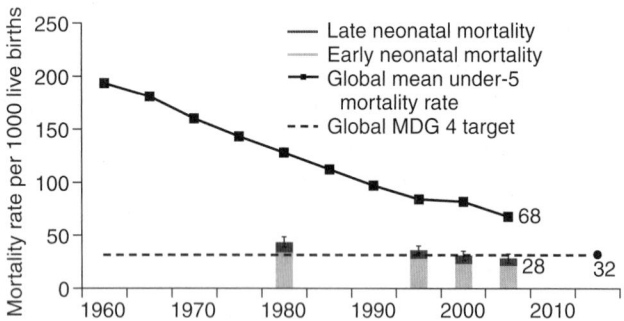

FIGURE 4-4 Progress toward Millennium Development Goal 4 for child survival showing the increasing proportion of deaths in children younger than 5 years. *(Modified from Lawn JE, Kerber K, Enweronu-Laryea C, et al: Newborn survival in low resource settings: are we delivering? BJOG 116[Suppl 1]:49-59, 2009.)*

STILLBIRTHS

Current estimates attribute at least 3.2 million deaths worldwide to stillbirth—defined as having no signs of life at delivery in a fetus at 28 weeks' gestation or greater—ranging from 5 per 1000 in wealthy countries to 32 per 1000 in South Asia and sub-Saharan Africa (Lawn et al, 2009c; Stanton et al, 2006); however, stillbirths are largely unrecorded and uncounted. Although differentiating a macerated stillbirth from a recent stillbirth seems simple, differentiating a stillbirth from an early neonatal death is challenging, especially in community settings with weak health systems and limited access to facility care. The task requires training in monitoring fetal heart rate and early signs of life, prompt and appropriate resuscitation, and emergency caesarian section, as required (McClure et al, 2007). Lack of training of birth attendants in resuscitation and careful assessment for signs of life, variability in what is considered the lower limit of viability, gender bias, and the influence of financial or other burdens with an assignment can result in the misclassification of early deaths as stillbirths. Cultural norms that discourage the weighing of dead infants and dictate prompt burial may serve to perpetuate misclassification. *Stillbirth* is commonly defined as fetal death within the last 12 weeks of pregnancy (i.e., at least 28 weeks' gestation or weighing 1000 g); however, some community and national standards define *stillbirth* as fetal death after 22 weeks' gestation or weighing 500 g. Because most of these deaths occur in settings where women have limited access to skilled birth attendants, it is likely that the current estimates of stillbirth numbers are too low and that a cause of death may not be established in the majority of stillbirths that occur in the developing world. Better data on the number and causes of stillbirth are urgently needed to prioritize action to reduce avoidable stillbirths in high-mortality settings, where rates are at least 10-fold higher than in wealthy countries (Stanton et al, 2006). Stillbirths are included in the mortality tables of the 2009 *Global Burden of Disease* for the first time (Lawn et al, 2009c).

DIRECT CAUSES OF NEONATAL DEATH

The proportion of neonatal deaths among children younger than 5 years varies, but the absolute number of neonatal deaths is determined by the size of the population and the neonatal mortality rate (NMR). Africa and Southeast Asia represent approximately two thirds of neonatal deaths, with the largest number of newborn deaths in South Asia and the highest rates of neonatal mortality in Sub-Saharan Africa, similar to child deaths. India contributes 25% of the world's neonatal deaths (United Nations Children's Fund, 2007).

Three causes of neonatal death are responsible for approximately 75% of neonatal deaths: prematurity (28%), sepsis and pneumonia (26%), and asphyxia (23%) (Save the Children, 2007). Prematurity (birth before 37 weeks' gestation) and asphyxia (failure to initiate and sustain spontaneous respiration) can result in long-term neurologic injury and cognitive impairment among survivors in countries and families that are least able to provide appropriate care. For every newborn that dies, another 20 suffer birth injury, preterm birth complications, or other neonatal conditions (United Nations Children's Fund, 2007). Determining cause-specific perinatal and neonatal mortality would allow the development of focused interventions and evaluation of their effects on perinatal and neonatal survival. However, establishing a primary cause of stillbirth and neonatal death in the 50% (2 million) of neonates that die in the first day—often in homes without access to health care systems, skilled birth attendants, or diagnostic techniques—is extremely challenging. To overcome these problems, verbal autopsy techniques have been developed to assign a cause of death in such cases, usually based on an interview with the infant's mother or caretaker within 6 months of the child's death. The cause of death is assigned by a panel of physicians or compared to a reference standard from prospective hospital-assigned causes of death. The diagnostic accuracy of verbal autopsy techniques to establish neonatal cause of death is limited because of the lack of standardization of case definitions, cause of death classifications, methods of assigning cause of death, and the limited generalizability of hospital reference standards to infants who die in the community (Edmond et al, 2008; World Health Organization, Development of Verbal Autopsy Standards). In the absence of critical vital registry data (Setel et al, 2007), global estimates of the causes of neonatal deaths are possible only through statistical modeling.

The cause-specific distribution of neonatal deaths correlates with the NMR. In high-mortality settings (>45 per 1000 live births), the risk of neonatal death because of severe sepsis and pneumonia is approximately 11-fold higher, and the risk of dying because of birth asphyxia is approximately eightfold higher than the risk in low-mortality countries (<15 per 1000 live births). The proportion of deaths as a result of prematurity drops in countries with a high NMR because of the deaths due to infection; however, the risk of death attributable to the complications of prematurity is still threefold higher than in low-mortality countries (Lawn et al, 2005). In addition to significant differences in cause-of-death distribution between countries, there is often substantial variation within countries (Lawn et al, 2005), especially between urban and rural areas.

CONSEQUENCES OF PRETERM DELIVERY AND LOW BIRTHWEIGHT

Prematurity and low birthweight are often not distinguished because of the lack of gestational age dating and failure to weigh all babies at birth. As many as 18 million babies worldwide may be born annually at a low birthweight (<2500 g). Although low birthweight affects approximately 15% of births, preterm delivery and low birthweight may account for up to 60% to 80% of neonatal deaths (Awasthi et al, 2006). South Asia contributes 50% of the world's babies with low birthweight, because 29% of babies have a low birthweight. In contrast, only 14% of Sub-Saharan African babies have a low birthweight (United Nations Children's Fund, 2007).

In developed countries, preterm birth is the leading cause of morbidity and mortality, and the percentage of deaths attributed to preterm delivery is more than twofold the percentage of deaths due to asphyxia, sepsis and pneumonia, and congenital anomalies (death from diarrhea does not occur) (Lawn et al, 2005). The current rate of 12.5% in the United States represents an increase of more than 30% since 1981 and is almost double the 5% to 9% frequency in other developed countries. The highest rates of preterm birth in the United States occur among racial and ethnic minorities and in older women who conceive by artificial reproductive technology (Preterm birth: crisis and opportunity, 2006). Whether the number of preterm deliveries is rising in the developing world is unknown.

Despite 30 years of research, little is known about the etiology and prevention of preterm delivery, but improved management in neonatal intensive care units has increased the survival of extremely immature fetuses in the developed world. Complex technology is not required to prevent deaths attributable to prematurity and birth asphyxia in the developing world. Low-cost interventions, including resuscitation training (Deorari et al, 2001), nutritional and thermal support through kangaroo-mother care (Charpak et al, 2005), and exclusive breastfeeding may reduce deaths attributable to asphyxia and preterm delivery after 34 weeks' gestation. The WHO has developed an Essential Newborn Care package, which includes clean delivery practices, neonatal delivery care (including prompt stimulation and bag-mask resuscitation as required), thermoregulation with skin-to-skin care, early initiation of exclusive breastfeeding, care of the moderately small baby at home, and recognition of common illnesses (World Health Organization and Department of Reproductive Health and Research, 1996). The addition of neonates to the WHO–United Nations Children's Fund *Integrated Management of Childhood Illnesses* package, which has been adopted by India, represents a significant resource to improved neonatal survival. The package provides skill-based training with elements similar to the Essential Newborn Care package, but it adds immunization and several postpartum home visits by health workers to help mothers recognize and manage minor conditions and refer severe cases in a timely manner (World Health Organization, 2003a). The Global Alliance to Prevent Prematurity and Stillbirth (GAPPS) has recently been launched to address stillbirth and prematurity with a comprehensive review of published and unpublished data on preterm birth and stillbirth research and interventions. In collaboration with diverse global partners in science, public health, and policy, GAPPS plans to advance research on the etiology of preterm delivery and stillbirth, accelerate delivery of low-cost effective interventions, and raise awareness of the effects of prematurity and stillbirth (www.gapps.org).

NEONATAL SEPSIS AND PNEUMONIA

Neonatal infections are responsible for more than 1 million of the 3.7 million annual deaths in the developing world. More than 95% of all deaths from birth to 2 months of age occur in developing countries. Risk factors include chorioamnionitis, low birthweight, unhygienic delivery, skin care, cord care, and environments. Ideally, simple preventive strategies such as clean delivery kits, hand washing, and cord care would be effective, but such data are not available, and the effectiveness of using chlorhexidine to prevent community-acquired neonatal sepsis and mortality is still unsettled (Cutland et al, 2009; Mullany et al, 2006). The quality and quantity of data on neonatal deaths caused by infections in the developing world are extremely limited. The estimated total is at least 1.6 million annual deaths (26% for sepsis and pneumonia, excluding tetanus and diarrhea) (Lawn et al, 2005). The majority of births and deaths are thought to occur at home without coming to medical attention (Lawn et al, 2004), because of cultural norms that prescribe seclusion for mothers and neonates; lack of trained caretakers and facilities; high out-of-pocket costs for transport, hospitalization, and medications; and loss of wages for the mother, the father, and often another family member. As a result, the current WHO recommendation of 10 to 14 days of inpatient treatment with broad-spectrum parenteral antibiotics is unavailable or unacceptable to most families (Zaidi et al, 2005).

Among those babies born in hospitals, the risk of nosocomial infection is threefold to 20-fold higher (6.5 to 38 per 1000) than in industrialized countries because of poor intrapartum and postnatal infection-control practices (Zaidi et al, 2005). Many hospitals are overcrowded and understaffed and lack even basic infection control procedures, despite the guidelines of WHO–United Nations Children's Fund *Integrated Management of Pregnancy and Childbirth* and the *Newborn Problems Handbook: A Guide for Doctors, Nurses, and Midwives* (World Health Organization, 2003a, 2003b; Zaidi et al, 2005). The major pathogens among babies born in a hospital (11,471 isolates) are *Klebsiella pneumonae*, other gram-negative rods (*Escherichia coli, Pseudomonas* spp., *Acinetobacter* spp.), and *Staphylococcus aureus* (8% to 22%) (Zaidi et al, 2009). Newborns in a hospital often receive empiric therapy with broad spectrum parenteral antibiotics (imipenem and amikacin), because of the lack of culture facilities and concerns about resistance.

Data from community settings during the first week of life are almost nonexistent. A 2009 *Pediatric Infectious Disease* supplement (Qazi and Stoll, 2009) reviewed evidence on community-acquired neonatal sepsis in the developing world from 32 studies published since 1990. The tremendous heterogeneity in studies, suggesting that infections may be responsible for 8% to 80% of all neonatal deaths and up to 42% of deaths in the first week, make the data difficult to interpret. Among neonates from 0 to 60 days old, rates of clinically diagnosed neonatal sepsis were as high as 170 per 1000 live births versus 5.5 blood-culture confirmed sepsis cases per 1000 live births (Thaver and Zaidi, 2009). Gram-negative rods (*Klebsiella* spp. [25%], *E. coli* [15%]) and *S. aureus* were the major community-acquired pathogens. Group B streptococcus was relatively uncommon (7%) in the first week, but group B streptococcus, *S. aureus*, and nontyphoid *Salmonella* spp. infection rates increased to 12% to 14% after the first week. Only 170 isolates, predominantly gram negative, were reported among home-delivered babies. The authors concluded that hospital-based and community studies suggest that most infections in the first week are attributable to gram-negative pathogens that may be environmentally acquired during unhygienic deliveries, rather than maternally acquired. As with hospital-born infants, empiric therapy with broad spectrum antibiotics was the norm, based on clinical

diagnosis or on algorithms, because advanced technology was neither available nor affordable. Because the signs and symptoms of neonatal sepsis and pneumonia are nonspecific and medical systems are weak, delays in recognition, referral, and treatment were common and were reflected in both the high mortality rate (22%) (Bang et al, 2005) and frequent prescription of broad-spectrum antibiotics.

A recent population-based nested observational study of community and hospital-born neonates randomized to a package of neonatal and maternal interventions in Mirzapur, Bangladesh, represents the difficulty of obtaining reliable infection data in the developing world. Of the 239 neonates who died without being enrolled, 59% and 87% died within the first 2 and 7 days, respectively, and were thought to be the result of birth asphyxia, prematurity, or both. Among the 7310 neonates who were assessed at least once by community health workers, the incidence of early neonatal sepsis was only 3 in 1000 live births. The 29 positive blood cultures represent an incidence of bacteremia of only 2.9 cases per 1000 live births; 38% of these cultures were obtained in the first three postnatal days. Fifty percent of the organisms were gram negative and 50% were gram positive; 10 in 15 gram-positive organisms were *S. aureus*, and one was group B streptococcus. The case fatality rate was 13% (2/15) in the gram-positive and 27% in the gram-negative infections. Seventy percent of the isolates were sensitive to the combination of ampicillin plus gentamicin or ceftriaxone. The authors noted that the incidence rate was roughly comparable to reported early-onset neonatal sepsis in the United States; however, the reported rates are likely to be low because infants who died early were not enrolled, parents were not compliant with referrals, and the intervention package may have prevented some infections.

For the many reasons noted, the current recommendations for hospitalization and parenteral therapy are simply not feasible in the developing world. Therefore several multicenter trials have been launched in Asia (2009) and (2010) Africa to test the safety and efficacy of simplified antibiotic regimens to treat possible serious bacterial infections in 0- to 59-day-old infants in the community or first-level facilities (S. Qazi, personal communication, 2010). Studies evaluating the effect of prenatal and postnatal home visits by community health workers to improve newborn care practices, and identification and referral of positive serious bacterial infection were completed in 2010 in Ghana and Uganda. Studies are ongoing in Tanzania (R. Bahl, personal communication, 2011). Such research is a priority to guide community management of infections and prevent unacceptably high neonatal mortality rates in developing countries.

Effective and simple interventions for the prevention and treatment of neonatal infections exist, but poor coverage of health services, a shortage of health care providers, access to referral services, and lack of knowledge on how to implement existing cost-effective interventions at scale in low-resource settings prevent them from reaching community neonates in the developing world. A methodology developed by the WHO Department of Child and Adolescent Health and Development (CAH) provides a systematic method, the Child Health and Nutrition Research Initiative (CHNRI) methodology, for setting priorities in health research investments at any level (institutional to global) (Rudan et al, 2007, 2008). Applying the CHNRI methodology to the prevention and treatment of neonatal infection identified the need for health policy and systems research to understand the barriers to implementation, effectiveness, and optimized use of available interventions (Bahl et al, 2009). The need for point-of-care diagnostics for neonatal pneumonia, hypoxia, bacterial sepsis, and antibiotic resistance is urgent because standard laboratory and radiologic technology are not available. To clarify the contribution of vertical transmission to neonatal mortality, sepsis data during the first 3 days of life are also a high priority.

Malaria and HIV infection are threats to neonatal health in Sub-Saharan Africa. The burden of malaria in pregnancy is exacerbated by HIV, which increases susceptibility in pregnancy, in addition to reducing the efficacy of antimalaria interventions and complicating their use because of potential drug interactions. Important progress has been made in preventing malaria with intermittent preventive treatment in pregnancy and insecticide-treated nets, but coverage of these treatments with funds is still unacceptably low (Menendez et al, 2007). HIV has devastated Sub-Saharan Africa, but progress is being made. The latest guidelines are available on the WHO Web site (www.who.int/hiv). Other useful, sites for current recommendations for treating pregnant women, reducing mother-to-child transmission, and infant feeding include http://AIDSinfo.nih.gov (for U.S. guidelines and access to information on trials and drugs), http://unaidstoday.org, www.accessdata.fda-gov, and www.cdc.gov/hiv/dhap.htm.

ASPHYXIA

The major causes of stillbirth and early neonatal death (during the first 7 days after birth) are birth asphyxia (defined by the WHO as the failure to initiate and maintain spontaneous respiration), low birthweight, and preterm delivery. Concerns about identifying stillbirth prevention strategies, the appropriate timing for such interventions, misclassification of early neonatal deaths as stillbirths, and the limitations of verbal autopsy have led to proposals to use terms that describe the timing of an insult (*intrapartum deaths* and *intrapartum-related neonatal deaths*) and specific adverse outcome (*neonatal encephalopathy*) rather than the term *asphyxia* (Lawn et al, 2009b, 2009c). Classification of the timing of death as previable versus antepartum (macerated) or intrapartum (fresh stillbirth) may be possible, even among the 60 million annual home births; however, the consequences of intrapartum fetal organ damage caused by poor oxygenation are often difficult to distinguish from those associated with infection and trauma; therefore differentiating the specific outcomes associated with each condition might not be important. Intrapartum fetal organ damage caused by poor oxygenation may be the final common pathway for many stillbirths and early neonatal deaths (Goldenberg and McClure, 2009).

Several studies suggest that improved neonatal resuscitation skills reduce misclassification of stillbirths and improve neonatal survival (Cowles, 2007; Daga et al, 1992), including a before-and-after study that provided college-educated Zambian midwives equipment and training in essential newborn care and resuscitation. The training resulted in a reduction of stillbirths from 23 to 16 per 1000 births without an increase in neonatal deaths (Chomba et al, 2008), suggesting that resuscitation training of providers can decrease misclassification of stillbirths and improve neonatal survival.

Of the approximately 136 million babies born every year, approximately 10% (14 million) require only stimulation at birth to establish regular respiration. As many as 3% to 6% (4 million) require stimulation and basic resuscitation with room air and a self-inflating resuscitation bag and mask, and less than 1% (1.4 million) require advanced resuscitation and postresuscitation care (Wall et al, 2009). Because less than 1% of neonates require advanced resuscitation, and few of those would survive without mechanical ventilation, advanced neonatal resuscitation is not a priority unless neonatal intensive care is available. The 1997 *WHO Basic Newborn Resuscitation: A Practical Guide*, which will be revised and published in 2011, provides guidelines for resuscitation training that are appropriate for first-referral level facilities in low-resource settings. A new educational resuscitation training program, *Helping Babies Breathe*, by the American Academy of Pediatrics and others (Niermeyer, 2009), is designed to support resuscitation training in low-resources settings. It emphasizes the "golden moment," provides clear graphics for decision making in basic resuscitation and hands-on exercises. It is being rolled out globally by USAID and partners. New low-cost resuscitation bags and infant resuscitation models will facilitate hands-on resuscitation training initiatives.

A recent review of resuscitation in low-resource settings describes the available evidence for which newborns should be resuscitated, when resuscitation should not be initiated, and when it should be stopped; management of meconium-stained infants; equipment needed for ventilation during resuscitation; evidence to support resuscitation with room air; evidence of the effects of resuscitation training in facilities and communities; postresuscitation management; and considerations for improving neonatal resuscitation in low- and middle-income countries (Wall et al, 2009). Improvement will require providing essential newborn care to newborns in all settings and frequent retraining to maintain resuscitation knowledge and skills. The authors estimate that systematic implementation of personnel using standard neonatal and competency-based training could avert an estimated 192,000 intrapartum-related neonatal deaths per year and an additional 5% to 10% of deaths as a result of complications of preterm birth (Lawn et al, 2009; Wall et al, 2009).

Among critical issues neonatal resuscitation are:
- How to deliver neonatal resuscitation in settings with the highest burden, but the weakest health systems
- How to implement and sustain national vital registries
- How to document the actual number of births
- How to document the number of intrapartum stillbirths
- Whether improved survival is associated with increased numbers of disabled survivors
- How to improve monitoring of the proportion of infants requiring resuscitation and their outcome
- How to deliver cost-effective neonatal care, resuscitation training methods, and maintenance of resuscitation skills by different levels of providers in facilities and communities
- How to determine whether infants should be suctioned, including those with meconium staining

- Early infant stimulation methods to ameliorate the effects of perinatal hypoxia

Equally important are methods to improve the quality of care for mothers and neonates, including maternal and perinatal death reviews, criterion-based audits, and emergency drills (van den Broek and Graham, 2009). Dissemination of the new *Helping Babies Breathe* curriculum represents an important opportunity for implementation research to improve newborn survival in the developing world.

PROVIDING A CONTINUUM OF CARE

Early efforts to improve neonatal mortality focused on high coverage levels of a few simple and cost-effective interventions in low-resource settings. Because simple interventions did not decrease neonatal mortality, the emphasis has subsequently shifted to comprehensive packages of community interventions and to a continuum of levels of care from home to hospital.

Interventions that improve access to qugality health care systems and can provide training, skilled birth attendants, transportation, timely emergency obstetric and neonatal care, and early postnatal care are likely to simultaneously reduce stillbirths and early neonatal deaths, as well as maternal morbidity and mortality; however, they have only been achieved in the context of research. The proposed components include:

- Empowerment of women
- Increased training of all levels of birth attendants in essential newborn care and resuscitation
- Emphasis on increased institutional deliveries

- Mobilization of communities to identify and transfer high-risk pregnancies and neonates
- Improved strategies for community treatment of postpartum hemorrhage, eclampsia, and sepsis
- Increased postpartum home visits
- The *Safe Childbirth Checklist* (World Health Organization, Safe Childbirth Checklist)

The joint statement from the WHO and United Nations Children's Fund recommending several early postpartum visits to deliver effective elements of care to newborns and their mothers is based on studies in Bangladesh and Pakistan, where such visits have been associated with reductions in newborn deaths and improved care practices. However, postpartum visits in a large-scale community-based integrated nutrition and health program in Uttar Pradesh, India, improved care practices but did not reduce the primary outcome (i.e., neonatal mortality) at the population level (Baqui et al, 2008a).

A 2007 review of the effects of packaged interventions on neonatal health (Haws et al, 2007) found no true effectiveness trials among 19 randomized controlled trials. No trial targeted women before pregnancy, and antenatal interventions were largely micronutrient supplementation. Intrapartum interventions were limited principally to clean delivery, and few increased the demand for care or improved the delivery of interventions to large populations. Subsequent trials using existing human and material resources and documenting external input are limited, but there is an increased emphasis on rural community-based interventions that could be improved. The early Bang Gadchiroli trial in Mahrashtra, India—which achieved a greater than 60% reduction in

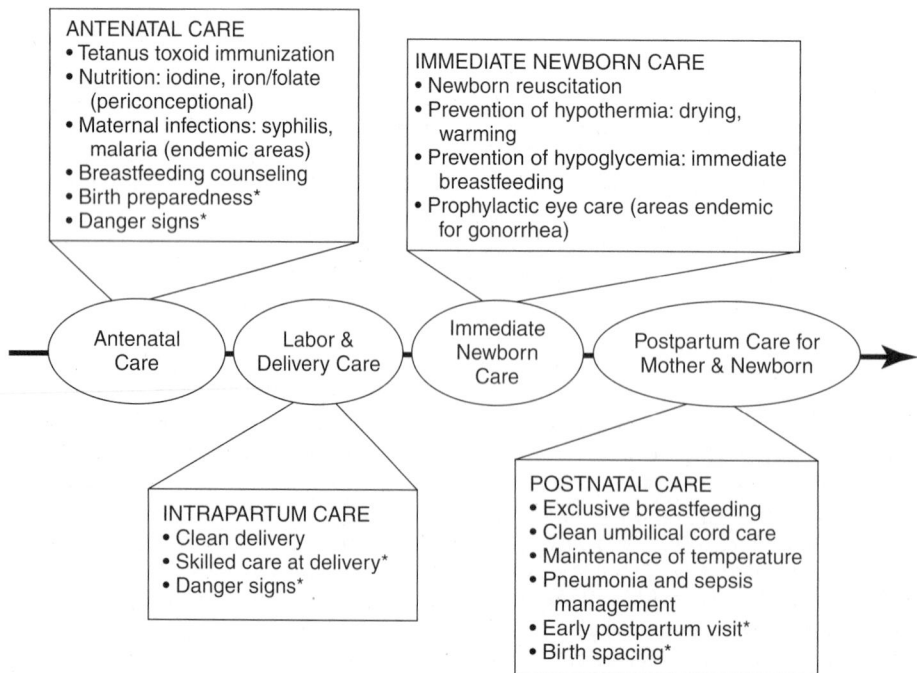

CONTINUUM OF CARE

FIGURE 4-5 Summary of priority antepartum, intrapartum, and postnatal interventions. (*Modified from Bhutta ZA, Darmstadt GL, Hasan BS, et al: Community-based interventions for improving perinatal and neonatal health outcomes in developing countries: a review of the evidence,* Pediatrics 115[Suppl 2]:519-617, 2005.)

neonatal mortality by intensive training of community health workers to resuscitate asphyxiated infants, manage infants with low birthweight, and treat suspected bacterial infections with oral and injectable antibiotics (Bang et al, 1999, 2005)—has not been replicated in other communities. However, community mobilization training (women's support groups with little additional input of health system strengthening) in rural Nepal between 2001 and 2003 reduced the neonatal mortality rate in intervention clusters by 30% (adjusted odds ratio, 0.70; 95% CI, 0.53–0.94) to 26.2 per 1000 (76 deaths per 2899 live births) compared with 36.9 per 1000 (119 deaths per 3226 live births) in controls (Manandhar et al, 2004). More recently, a community-based mobilization and education trial of care of newborn babies in rural India was associated with improved household care behaviors (early initiation of breastfeeding, delayed bathing, and skin-to-skin care) and a reduction of neonatal mortality (Kumar et al, 2008). This 30-month, community-based unmasked cluster randomized trial was conducted through government and nongovernmental organization infrastructures. The trial provided home care visits (two prenatal and four postnatal care home care and referral or treatment of sick neonates by a female community health worker [CHW]) or community-based promotion of care-seeking and birth or newborn care preparedness through group sessions with female and community mobilizers, in addition to a comparison arm. Neonatal mortality was reduced in the home-care arm by 34% (adjusted RR, 0.66; 95% CI, 0.47–0.93) over the last 6 months of the intervention versus the comparison arm. The community-care arm documented improved care practices, but no reduction in neonatal mortality. These favorable results were achieved despite a much lower community health worker (CHW) density and 30% of the CHW postnatal care visits, compared with the Gadcharoli trial (Bang et al, 2005). Improvement of the home care service delivery strategy for essential newborn care is underway in Bangladesh (Baqui et al, 2008b). Although it appears that community-based preventive strategies for newborn care can improve newborn survival and care practices, it is not clear that government health care workers and CHWs can duplicate these research results (Bhutta and Soofi, 2008). Because each setting is unique, such efforts are likely to be improved after local formative research with the communities, CHW, and birth attendants (Bahl et al, 2008).

Key research gaps in community management include:
- How best to create the political will to prioritize community maternal and neonatal health
- How to provide a continuum of care from home to hospital (effectiveness trials carefully tailored to local health needs and conducted at scale)
- How to mobilize communities to identify, stabilize, and transfer at-risk pregnancies and neonates
- What strategies should be used to ensure quality of care
- How to manage birth asphyxia, preterm delivery, and serious neonatal bacterial infections in the community

Finally, it is important to test whether the community strategies that were effective in rural Southern Asia will be equally effective in Africa and in urban slums (Bhutta and Soofi, 2008; Bhutta et al, 2008b; Kumar et al, 2008).

RESOURCES

Some of the key challenges to global health initiatives are information, communication, and assessment. Although the data are not always available or consistent, a number of important resources are available. The United Nations Children's Fund reports progress in maternal and child survival in the *The State of the World's Children*, based on the work of the Inter-agency Group for Child Mortality Estimation (United Nations Children's Fund, 2007). The *State of the World's Children* provides summary tables of basic, health, education, demographics, economics, and progress indicators with national rankings. The detailed text discusses when, where, and why mothers and neonates die, and it documents interventions to improve outcomes. The 2009 *State of the World's Children* emphasizes maternal health.

The WHO Department of Child and Adolescent Health and Development is the Secretariat for the Child Epidemiology Reference Group (CHERG) that quantifies the burden of child illnesses, supports and disseminates research to understand the determinants of childhood illnesses, and develops and evaluates interventions of new delivery strategies and large-scale interventions (Bryce et al, 2005; World Health Organization, 2009).

A number of other important partnerships publish current data, including *The Countdown to 2015* (United Nations Children's Fund, 2005, 2008a), which assembles and summarizes the latest published data on 68 priority countries that represent 97% of child and maternal mortality worldwide. A unique feature is data on coverage rates for interventions that are feasible for universal implementation in poor countries and have been empirically proven to reduce mortality in mothers, children, and neonates. The 2008 edition included approaches such as delivery care and reproductive health services, which can serve as platforms for delivering multiple, proven interventions to reduce maternal and neonatal mortality (United Nations Children's Fund, 2008a); it is intended to assist policy makers, development agencies, and donors in making performance-based policy and decisions. An explicit goal is to hold governments, development partners, and the international health community accountable for the lack of progress (United Nations Children's Fund, 2008a).

In 2003 a group of technical experts published The Child Survival Series in *The Lancet* (United Nations Children's Fund, 2007), which went on to become a unique series of special editions on perinatal health in the developing world. The series has played a critical role in drawing attention and resources to improved neonatal survival, which is important to the future of the developing world.

The comprehensive Disease Control Priorities Project (DCPP)—a joint effort of the National Institutes of Health Fogarty International Center, the WHO, and the World Bank—was launched in 2001 to identify policy changes and intervention strategies for the health problems of countries in need. The aim of the DCPP was to generate knowledge to assist decision makers in developing countries to realize the potential of cost-effective interventions to rapidly improve the health and welfare of their populations and to detail prevalent investments that are not cost

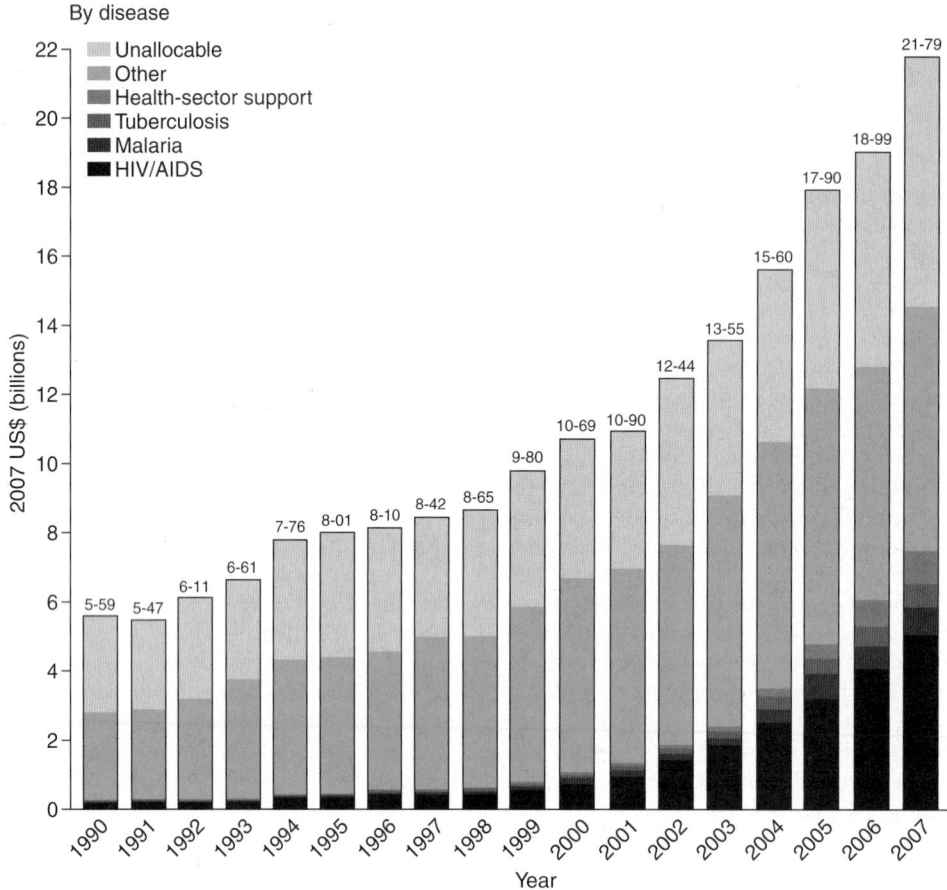

FIGURE 4-6 Development assistance for health from 1990 to 2007, by disease. (*Modified from Ravishankar N, Gubbins P, Cooley RJ, et al: Financing of global health: tracking development assistance for health from 1990 to 2007,* Lancet *373:2113-2124, 2009.*)

effective. The DCPP published an expanded and updated second edition that addresses disease conditions, their burdens and risk factors, strategy and intervention effectiveness and health systems, and financing (Laxminarayan et al, 2006).

FUNDING

There is no comprehensive system for tracking total amounts of developmental assistance for health or how they are spent. However, recent analyses have documented a fourfold increase in developmental assistance, from $5.6 billion in 1990 to $21.8 billion in 2007. The WHO estimated that the 10-year incremental global costs for universal health coverage of maternal and child health services ranged from $39.3 billion for a moderate improvement scenario to $551.7 billion for a rapid improvement scenario. These projections did not include the cost of health system reforms, such as recruiting, training, and retaining a sufficient number of personnel (Johns et al, 2007).

Global assistance rose sharply after 2002 because of increases in public funding, especially from the United States, and from increased philanthropic donations and in-kind contributions from corporations. (The Bill and Melinda Gates Foundation is the largest single source of private developmental health assistance.) Donor funding from the United States for HIV/AIDS has increased from $300 million in 1996 to $8.9 billion in 2006 (Oomman,

et al, 2007). The proportion of developmental assistance from United Nations agencies and development banks decreased between 1990 and 2007 as targeted funding increased for the Global Alliance for Vaccines and Immunization; Medicines for Malaria, the Global Fund to Fight AIDS, Tuberculosis and Malaria; and the United States President's Emergency Plans for AIDS Relief (PEPFAR). The influx of funds has been accompanied by major changes in the institutional landscape of global health, with global health initiatives such as the Global Fund and the GAVI assuming a central role in mobilizing and channeling global health funds. Nongovernmental organizations have become a major conduit for an increasing share of developmental assistance (Ravishankar et al, 2009).

The pattern is similar for research and development for drugs: Global Funds and GAVI HIV/AIDS, tuberculosis, and malaria initiatives accounted for approximately 80% of the $2.5 billion that was spent on research and drug development in 2007 for neglected diseases in developing countries (Moran et al, 2009). Drugs and vaccines—rather than diagnostics, platform technologies, or country-specific products—are also funded preferentially (Moran et al, 2009). Research and development in neglected diseases—such as pneumonia and diarrheal illness, two major causes of mortality in developing countries–are severely underfunded at less than 6% of the budgeted funding. Increasing attention has been focused on the large amount of funding being earmarked for HIV, malaria, and tuberculosis and

TABLE 4-4 The Research Pipeline of Description and Determinants, Discovery, Development, and Delivery

	Description and Determinants	Discovery	Development	Delivery
Research aim	Descriptive epidemiology and understanding determinants, advancing definitions	New science for the discovery of mechanisms and causes of neonatal disease that provides foundation for developing new interventions	Developing new or adapting existing interventions to reduce the cost, increase effect, improve deliverability	Delivering existing interventions in new ways or in new settings. Includes monitoring and evaluation as feedback to additional discovery and development science
Types of research (research instrument)	Epidemiology	New drugs and vaccines. Biochemical and genetic basis for disease	Refining or adapting existing technology or drugs	Effectiveness trials or implementation research for scale-up in health systems
Typical timeline before impact is seen	Variable	5 to 15 years	5 to 10 years	2 to 5 years
Investment level	Variable	Very high	Moderate	Low to moderate depending on size of trial and rigor of evaluation
Probability of major impact	Variable, if new epidemiology leads directly to program or intervention	Very high	Moderate	Very high if high impact intervention and currently low coverage
Risk of failure	Low	High	Moderate	Low to moderate
Specific examples for global newborn health	Cohort studies to better delineate preterm birth and term small for gestational age and define short-and long-term outcomes	Discovering a marker for preterm birth amenable to intervention	Adapting technology for head or body cooling to be effective, lower cost, feasible and safe in low-income settings	Impact and cost to provide early postnatal care package using different cadres of workers in a range of varying health system contexts especially in Africa

From Lawn JE, Rudan I, Rubens C: Four million newborn deaths: is the global research agenda evidence-based? *Early Hum Dev* 84:809-814, 2008.

the missed opportunities to save more lives—especially young lives—at a lower cost by focusing on simpler interventions (Gostin, 2008).

CAREER OPPORTUNITIES

American universities are experiencing an unprecedented surge in interest in global health. Students and faculty have become actively engaged in operational research, project analysis, workforce training, and policy debates. A number of American universities have made long-term commitments to specific countries in the developing world, including formal opportunities for faculty and residents to work in targeted countries in low-resource settings. Opportunities range from in-depth experiences to volunteer research and service projects. The newly launched Consortium of University for Global Health 2009 survey of 37 universities found that the number of students enrolled in global health programs in universities across the United States and Canada doubled in just 3 years and that universities have established 302 training and education programs in 97 countries. Although there is currently no official "bulletin board" for international global opportunities at the faculty level, a number of Web sites offer a range of opportunities for individuals seeking additional training, career opportunities, and interaction with other global health professionals, including the American Medical Students Association (www.amsa.org); the Global Health Council career network (careers.globalhealth.org); the United States Agency for International Development (USAID) (www.usaid.gov); and the National Institutes of Health Fogarty International Center (www.nih.fogarty.org). A number of Web sites also

provide research updates, including the WHO, USAID, Save the Children Newborn Research e*Updates*, and *Medical News Today*. The Federation of Pediatric Organizations is working in the areas of international certification, cataloging international rotations, creating a checklist of requirements for international rotations, and creating global partnerships.

THE WAY FORWARD: DATA, COLLABORATION, EVALUATION, AND INVOLVEMENT

There is a consensus in the global research community regarding the importance of providing a continuum of care from home to hospital for mothers and neonates and evaluating the effectiveness of packages of interventions that have proved effective in smaller trials (Madon et al, 2007). Much attention has been focused on the lack of quality data; social and cultural limitations; the need for large community randomized trials and their high cost; the lack of coordination of efforts to maximize current data by prioritizing and strengthening existing programs with proven, low-cost, high-impact interventions; and the need to systematically establish research priorities (Lawn et al, 2008, 2009a).

The need for a change in the design, implementation, and evaluation of programs has received less attention, to meet the needs of national governments and donors for rigorous assessment of child survival and health in general. Victora, Black, and Bryce (2009) emphasize the need for nationwide improvement and nationwide assessments of multiple programs, in collaboration with the government and other concurrent programs. They suggest three initial steps for an ecologic evaluation platform: (1) develop and regularly update a district database from multiple sources, (2) conduct an initial survey to be repeated every 3 years to measure coverage for proven interventions and health status, and (3) establish a continuous monitoring system to document provision, use, and quality of interventions at the district level, with mechanisms for prompt and transparent reporting. Although this ambitious plan would support the analysis of combinations of interventions and delivery strategies with the ability to adjust for confounders, there is no precedent for undertaking such a massive effort. Short of their comprehensive strategy, there is increasing recognition of the need for national vital registries and recurrent surveys to provide the basis for changes in health policy. There is also clear evidence of the need for a new emphasis on implementation science and the urgency of strengthening the independent capacity for health research in the developing world (Whitworth et al, 2008), which will enable collaborators to solve their own national problems. Finally, everyone has the power to advocate for political change to support maternal and child health. Shiffman (2009) emphasizes the need to build a strong policy community to generate political attention for global maternal and neonatal health; to develop issue frames that resonate with politicians to move them to act; to cultivate strategic alliances within women's groups, key ministers, and congressional aides; to link the health of women and neonates in the developing world with other problems; and to remember that medical professionals carry great moral authority because of their expertise and pursuit of a humanitarian cause, if they choose to exert their political power in a strategic way.

SUGGESTED READINGS

Baqui A, Williams EK, Rosecrans AM, et al: Impact of an integrated nutrition and health programme on neonatal mortality in rural northern India, *Bull World Health Organ* 86:796-804, 2008.
Bhutta ZA, Ali S, Cousens S, et al: Alma-Ata. Rebirth and revision 6 interventions to address maternal, newborn, and child survival: what difference can integrated primary health care strategies make?, *Lancet* 372:972-989, 2008.
Himawan B: *State of the world's mothers 2007: saving the lives of children under 5*, 2007, New York, Save the Children.
Jamison DT, Breman JG, Measham AR, et al: *Disease control priorities in developing countries: a copublication of The World Bank and Oxford University Press*, ed 2, New York, 2006, Oxford University Press.
Madon T, Hofman KJ, Kupfer L, et al: Public health: implementation science, *Science* 318:1728-1729, 2007.
Martines J, Paul VK, Bhutta ZA, et al: Neonatal survival: a call for action , *Lancet* 365:1189-1197, 2005.
Morris SS, Cogill B, Uauy R: Effective international action against undernutrition: why has it proven so difficult and what can be done to accelerate progress? *Lancet* 371:608-621, 2008.
Save the Children: Serious bacterial infections among neonates and young infants in developing countries: evaluation of etiology and therapeutic management strategies in community settings, *Pediatr Infect Dis J* 28:S1-S48, 2009.
United Nations Children's Fund: *Countdown 2015: tracking progress in maternal, newborn & child survival, the 2008 report*, vol 2, New York, 2008a.
United Nations Children's Fund: *The state of the world's children 2008: child survival*, New York, 2007.
United Nations Children's Fund: *The state of the world's children 2009: maternal and newborn health*, New York, 2008b.

Complete references used in this text can be found online at www.expertconsult.com

PART II

FETAL DEVELOPMENT

CHAPTER
5

IMMUNOLOGIC BASIS OF PLACENTAL FUNCTION AND DISEASES: THE PLACENTA, FETAL MEMBRANES, AND UMBILICAL CORD

Satyan Kalkunte, James F. Padbury, and Surendra Sharma

Complex yet intricate interactions between maternal and fetal systems promote fetal growth and normal pregnancy outcomes. Throughout embryonic development, organogenesis and functional maturation are taking place. This period of development coincides with a high rate of cellular proliferation and organ development, which creates critical periods of vulnerability. Adverse factors, disruption, or impairment during these critical periods of fetal development can alter developmental programming, which can lead to permanent metabolic or structural changes (Baker, 1998). For example, triggers such as undernutrition can elicit placental and fetal adaptive responses that can lead to local ischemia and metabolic, hormonal, and immune reprogramming, resulting in small for gestational age (SGA) fetuses. Maternal health, dietary status, and exposure to environmental factors, uteroplacental blood flow, placental transfer, and fetal genetic and epigenetic responses likely all contribute to in utero fetal programming (Figure 5-1). Adult diseases such as coronary heart disorders, hypertension, atherosclerosis, type 2 diabetes, insulin resistance, respiratory distress, altered cell-mediated immunity, cancer, and psychiatric disorders are now thought to be a consequence of in utero life (Sallour and Walker, 2003). It is a matter of considerable interest that, in addition to maternal predisposing factors, cytokines, hormones, growth factors, and the intrauterine immune milieu also contribute to in utero programming. Adaptations of the maternal immune system exist to modulate detrimental effects on the fetus and additional mechanisms and factors actively cross the placenta and induce regulatory T cells in the fetus to suppress fetal antimaternal immunity. These effects persist at least through adolescence (Burlingham, 2009; Mold et al, 2008). Excessive restraint of maternal immune responses could lead to a lethal infection in the newborn. On the other hand, too little modulation of maternal immune response to the fetal allograft could lead to autoimmune-mediated fetal-placental rejection. Moreover, placental growth resembles that of a tumor, evading immune surveillance and initiating its own angiogenesis. Therefore a healthy mother with healthy placentation is critical to healthy fetal outcomes.

MAMMALIAN PLACENTATION

The immune tolerance of the semiallograft fetus and de novo vascularization are two highly intriguing processes that involve direct interaction of maternal immune cells,

invading trophoblast cells, and arterial endothelial cells. Pregnancy is considered an immunologic paradox, in which paternal antigen-expressing placental cells interact directly with and coexist with the maternal immune system (Medawar, 1953). This anatomic distinction of the immunologic interface that arises from hemochorial placentation that occurs in humans and rodents is distinct from epitheliochorial placentation as seen in marsupials, horses, and swine or the endotheliochorial placentation seen in dogs and cats. Understanding the anatomic and physiologic events that occur during placentation is the key to appreciate the uniqueness of human placentation in the phylogenetic evolution. Typically, in hemochorial placentation, maternal uterine blood vessels and decidualized endometrium are colonized by trophoblast cells, derived from trophectoderm of the implanting blastocyst. These cells come in direct contact with maternal blood and uterine tissue. A similar phenomenon is evident in murine pregnancy, except the trophoblast invasion is deeper in humans (Moffett and Loke, 2006). In epitheliochorial placentation, trophoblast cells of the placenta are in direct contact with the surface epithelial cells of the uterus, but there is no trophoblast-cell invasion beyond this layer. In endotheliochorial placentation, the trophoblast cells breach the uterine epithelium and are in direct contact with endothelial cells of maternal uterine blood vessels.

EMBRYOLOGIC DEVELOPMENT OF THE PLACENTA

Shortly after fertilization takes place in the ampullary portion of the fallopian tube, the fertilized ovum or zygote begins dividing into a ball of cells called a *morula*. As the morula enters the uterus (by the fourth day after fertilization), it forms a central cystic area and is called a *blastocyst* (Figure 5-2). The blastocyst implants within the endometrium by day seven (Moore, 1988).

The blastocyst has two components: an inner cell mass, which becomes the developing embryo, and the outer cell layer, which becomes the placenta and fetal membranes. The cells of the developing blastocyst, which eventually become the placenta, are differentiated early in gestation (within 7 days after fertilization). The outer cell layer, the trophoblast, invades the endometrium to the level of the decidua basalis. Maternal blood vessels are also invaded. Once entered and controlled by the trophoblast, these

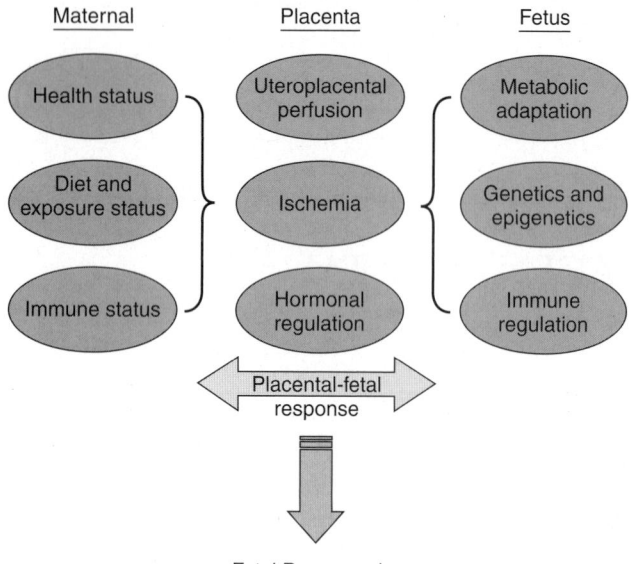

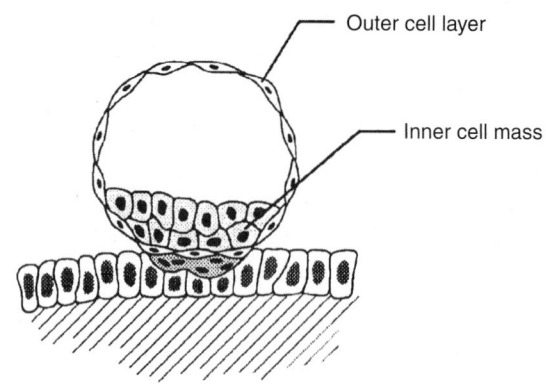

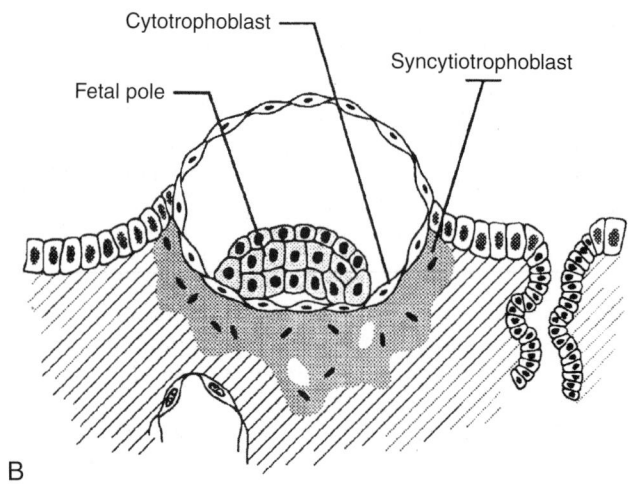

FIGURE 5-1 Fetal programming. Maternal health and the placenta influence fetal adaptations. Dietary status, exposure to environmental factors, uteroplacental blood flow, placental transfer, and genetic and epigenetic changes contribute to the in utero fetal programming.

FIGURE 5-2 A, The human blastocyst contains two portions: an inner cell mass, which develops into the embryo, and an outer cell layer, which develops into the placenta and membranes. **B,** The outer acellular layer is the syncytiotrophoblast, and the inner cellular layer is the cytotrophoblast. (*From Moore TR, Reiter RC, Rebar RW, et al, editors:* Gynecology and obstetrics: a longitudinal approach, *New York, 1993, Churchill Livingstone.*)

maternal blood vessels form lacunae, which provide nutrition and substrates for the developing products of conception. The trophoblast differentiates into two cell types, the inner cytotrophoblast and the outer syncytiotrophoblast (Figure 5-3); the former has distinct cell walls and is thought to represent the more immature form of trophoblast. The syncytiotrophoblast, which is essentially acellular, is the site of most placental hormone and metabolic activity. Once the trophoblast has invaded the endometrium, it begins to form outpouchings called *villi*, which extend into the blood-filled maternal lacunae or further invade the endometrium to attach more solidly with the decidua, forming anchoring villi.

PLACENTAL ANATOMY AND CIRCULATION

At term, the normal placenta covers approximately one third of the interior portion of the uterus and weighs approximately 500 g. The appearance is of a flat circular disc approximately 2 to 3 cm thick and 15 to 20 cm across (Benirschke and Kaufmann, 2000). Placental and fetal weights throughout gestation are presented in Table 5-1. During the first trimester and into the second, the placenta weighs more than the fetus; after that period, the fetus outweighs the placenta. With the formation of the tertiary villi (19 days after fertilization), a direct vascular connection is made between the developing embryo and the placenta (Moore, 1988). Umbilical circulation between the placenta and the embryo is evident by 5½ weeks' gestation. Figure 5-4 demonstrates aspects of the maternal and fetal circulation in the mature placenta. The umbilical arteries from the fetus reach the placenta and then divide repetitively to cover the fetal surface of the placenta. Terminal arteries then penetrate the individual cotyledons, forming capillary beds for substrate exchange within the tertiary villi. These capillaries then reform into tributaries of the umbilical venous system, which carries oxygenated blood back to the fetus.

EXAMINATION OF THE PLACENTA

A renaissance in placental pathology has led to a new relevance of the placenta to neonatology and early infant life, including issues of preterm birth, growth restriction, and cerebral, renal, and myocardial diseases. The placenta can give some clues to the timing and extent of important adverse prenatal or neonatal events as well as to the relative effects of sepsis and asphyxia on the causation of neonatal diseases. Placental disorders can be noted immediately in the delivery room, and others can be diagnosed through detailed gross and microscopic examinations over the ensuing 48 hours. Every placenta should be examined at the time of birth regardless of whether the newborn has any immediate problems. Most placentas invert with traction at the time of delivery, and the fetal membranes cover the maternal surface. It is important to reinvert the membranes and examine all surfaces of the placenta and membranes, looking for abnormalities. Table 5-2 lists pregnancy complications or conditions that are diagnosable at birth through examination of the placenta.

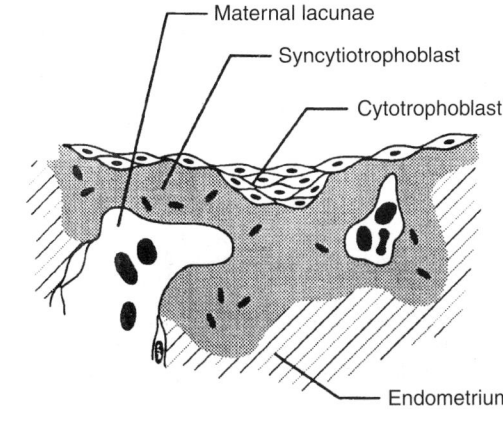

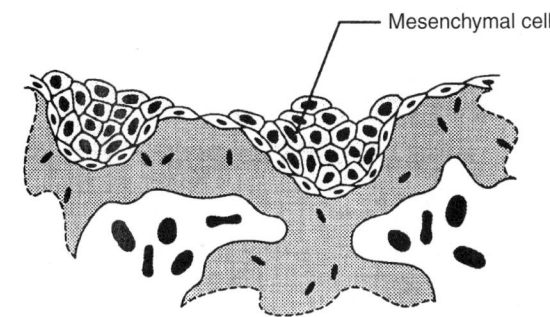

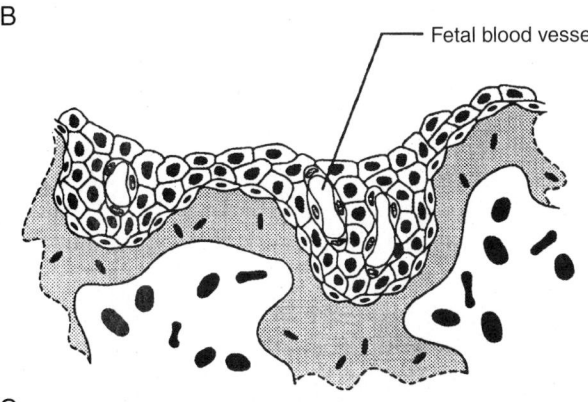

FIGURE 5-3 A, The cytotrophoblast indents the syncytiotrophoblast to form primary villi. **B,** Mesenchymal cells invade the cytotrophoblast 2 days after formation of the primary villi to form secondary villi. **C,** Blood vessels arise de novo and eventually connect with blood vessels from the embryo, forming tertiary villi. (*From Moore TR, Reiter RC, Rebar RW, et al, editors:* Gynecology and obstetrics: a longitudinal approach, *New York, 1993, Churchill Livingstone.*)

The initial placental examination should include checking the edges for completeness. The membranes and fetal surface should be shiny and translucent. An odor may suggest infection, and cultures of the placenta may be beneficial (Benirschke and Kaufmann, 2000). Greenish discoloration may represent meconium staining or old blood; placentas with such discoloration should be sent to the pathologist for complete histologic examination. The finding of deep meconium staining of the membranes and umbilical cord suggests that the meconium was passed at least 2 hours before delivery; this fact may be helpful in

TABLE 5-1   Fetal and Placental Weight Throughout Gestation

Gestational Age (wk)	Placental Weight (mg)	Fetal Weight (g)
14	45	—
16	65	59
18	90	155
20	115	250
22	150	405
24	185	560
26	217	780
28	250	1000
30	282	1270
32	315	1550
34	352	1925
36	390	2300
38	430	2850
40	470	3400

Adapted from Benirschke K, Kaufmann P: *Pathology of the human placenta*, ed 4, New York, 2000, Springer-Verlag.

cases of meconium aspiration syndrome, for which legal questions may arise as to whether the aspiration occurred before or during labor. If the membranes are deeply stained, the passage of meconium by the fetus may have predated onset of labor; therefore aspiration could have occurred before labor. The umbilical cord should also be examined for the number of vessels and their insertion into the placenta. Vessels on the fetal surface of the placenta should be examined for evidence of clotting or thrombosis.

FUNCTIONS OF THE PLACENTA

To ensure normal fetal growth and development, the placenta behaves as an efficient organ of gas and nutrient exchange and as a robust endocrine and metabolic organ. Besides mediating the transplacental exchange of gases and nutrients, the placenta also synthesizes glycogen with a significant turnover of lactate. Hormones secreted by the placenta have an important role for the fetus and the mother. Placental trophoblasts are a rich source of cholesterol and peptide hormones, including human chorionic gonadotrophin (HCG), human placental lactogen, cytokines, growth hormones, insulin-like growth factors, corticotrophin-releasing hormones, and angiogenic factors such as vascular endothelial growth factor (VEGF) and placental growth factor (PlGF). HCG, which is detected as early as day 8 after conception, is secreted by syncytiotrophoblasts into the maternal circulation, reaches maximal levels by week 8 of pregnancy and diminishes later during gestation. HCG is essential to promote estrogen and progesterone synthesis during different stages of pregnancy. Human placental lactogen mobilizes the breakdown of maternal fatty acid stores and ensures an increased supply of glucose to the fetus. VEGF and PlGF are secreted by trophoblasts and specialized natural killer (NK) cells in the decidua, and they promote angiogenesis and vascular activity, particularly during early stages of pregnancy when spiral

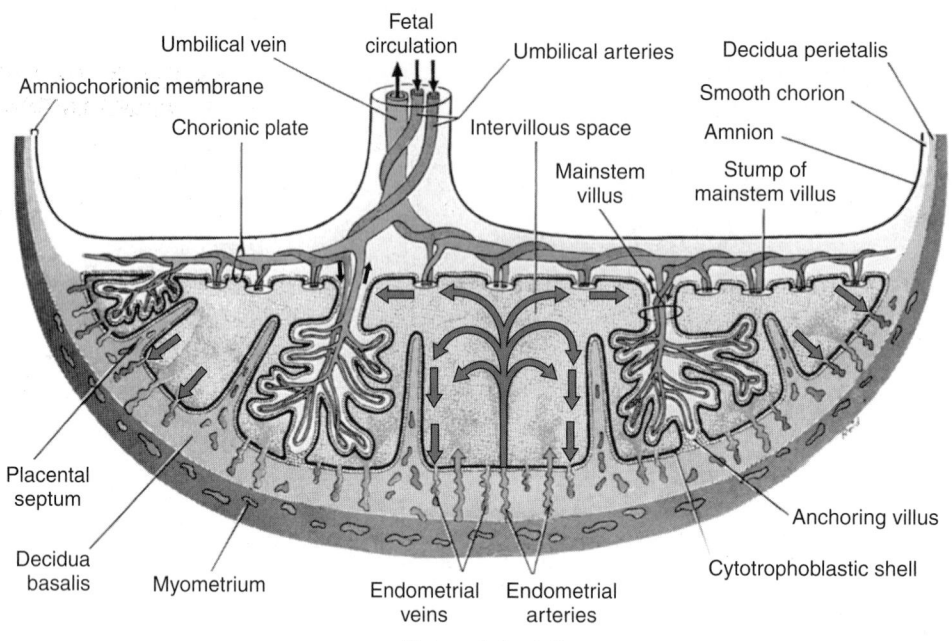

FIGURE 5-4 Schematic drawing of a section of a mature placenta showing the relation of the villous chorion (fetal part of the placenta) to the decidua basalis (maternal part of the placenta), the fetal placental circulation, and the maternal placental circulation. Maternal blood flows into the intervillous spaces in funnel-shaped spurts, and exchanges occur with the fetal blood as the maternal blood flows around the villi. Note that the umbilical arteries carry deoxygenated fetal blood to the placenta, and the umbilical vein carries oxygenated blood to the fetus. In addition, the cotyledons are separated from each other by decidual septa of the maternal portion of the placenta. Each cotyledon consists of two or more mainstem villi and their main branches. In this drawing, only one mainstem villus is shown in each cotyledon, but the stumps of those that have been removed are shown. (*From Moore KL:* The developing human: clinically oriented embryology, *ed 5, Philadelphia, 1993, WB Saunders.*)

TABLE 5-2   Pregnancy Conditions Diagnosable at Birth by Gross Placental Examination and Associated Neonatal Outcomes

Pregnancy Conditions	Fetal/Neonatal Outcomes
Monochorionic twinning	TTT syndrome donor/recipient status, pump twin in TRAP, survivor status after fetal demise, selective termination, severe growth discordance without TTT
Dichorionic twinning	Less likelihood of survivor brain disease in the event of demise of one fetus
Purulent acute chorioamnionitis	Risk of fetal sepsis, fetal inflammatory response syndrome, cerebral palsy
Chorangioma	Hydrops, cardiac failure, consumptive coagulopathy
Abnormal cord coiling	IUGR, fetal intolerance of labor
Maternal floor infarction	IUGR, cerebral disease
Abruption	Asphyxial brain disease
Velamentous cord	IUGR, vasa previa
Cord knot	Asphyxia
Chronic abruption oligohydramnios syndrome	IUGR
Single umbilical artery	Malformation, IUGR
Umbilical vein thrombosis	Asphyxia
Amnion nodosum	Severe oligohydramnios leading to pulmonary hypoplasia
Meconium staining	Possible asphyxia, aspiration lung disease
Amniotic bands	Fetal limb reduction abnormalities
Chorionic plate vascular thrombosis	Asphyxia, possible thrombophilia
Breus mole	Asphyxia, IUGR

IUGR, Intrauterine growth retardation; *TRAP,* twin-reversed arterial perfusion; *TTT,* twin-to-twin transfusion.

artery transformation and trophoblast invasion occurs. In addition, the placenta is a rich source of estrogen, progesterone, and glucocorticoids. Whereas progesterone maintains a quiescent, noncontractile uterus, it also has a role in protecting the conceptus from immunologic rejection by the mother. Glucocorticoids promote organ development

and maturation. Placental transport is another important function, efficiently transferring nutrients and solutes that are essential for normal fetal growth. The syncytiotrophoblast covering the maternal villous surface is a specialized epithelium that participates in the transport of gases, nutrients, and waste products and the synthesis of hormones

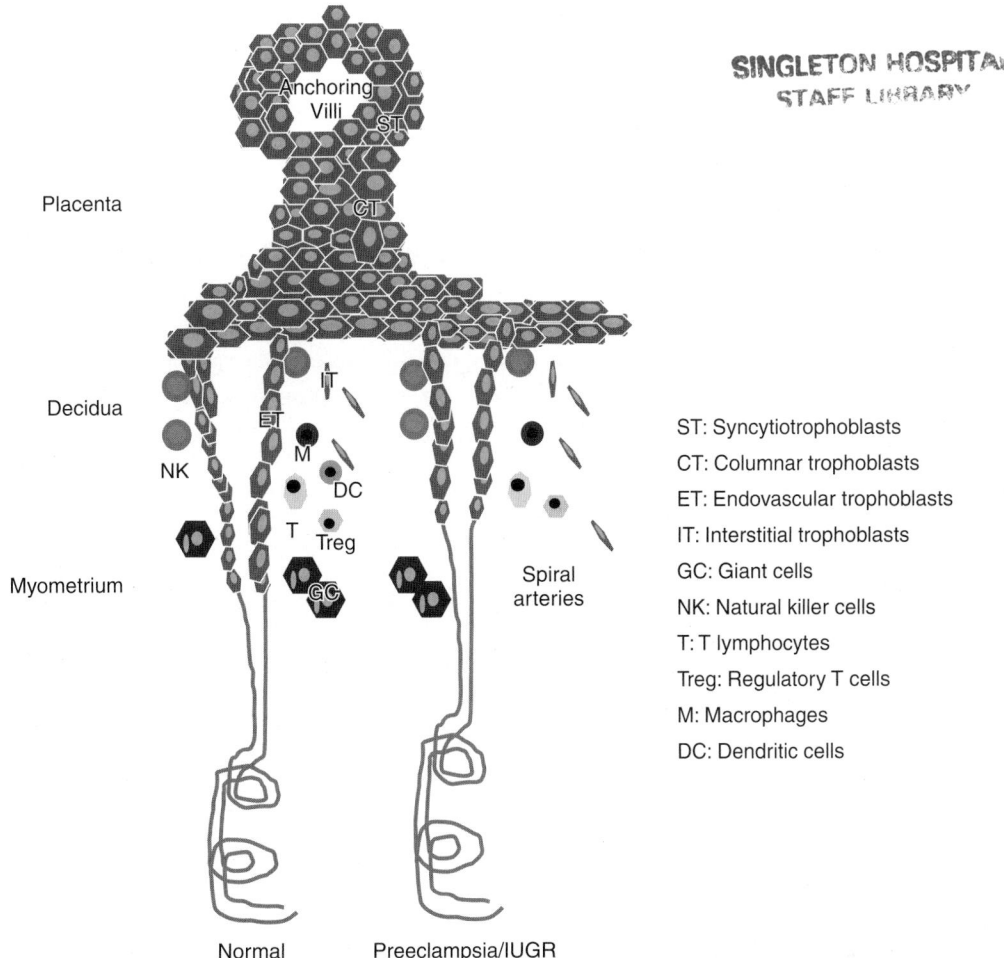

ST: Syncytiotrophoblasts

CT: Columnar trophoblasts

ET: Endovascular trophoblasts

IT: Interstitial trophoblasts

GC: Giant cells

NK: Natural killer cells

T: T lymphocytes

Treg: Regulatory T cells

M: Macrophages

DC: Dendritic cells

FIGURE 5-5 **Trophoblast differentiation and spiral artery remodeling.** Progenitor trophoblast cells from villi differentiate into syncytiotrophoblasts and the extravillous cytotrophoblasts (EVTs). EVTs migrate out in columns as columnar trophoblasts and anchor the placenta to the decidua. Further differentiation takes place into invasive or proliferative EVTs. The invasive EVTs invade the decidua known as *interstitial trophoblasts*, and some of them fuse to form the multinucleated gaint cells. Endovascular transformation ensues as endovascular trophoblasts migrate into and colonize the spiral arteries, almost reaching the myometrium. This results in wide-bore, low-resistant capacitance blood vessels as observed in normal pregnancy. In contrast, shallow trophoblast invasion and incomplete transformation of spiral arteries is a common feature of preeclampsia and intrauterine growth restriction.

that regulate placental, fetal, and maternal systems. The syncytiotrophoblast layer of the placenta is an important site of exchange between the maternal blood stream and the fetus. In addition to simple diffusion, syncytiotrophoblasts facilitate exchange by transcellular trafficking that utilizes transport proteins such as the water channels (aquaporins). Facilitated diffusion for molecules such as glucose and amino acids are performed by glucose transporters (GLUT) and amino acid transporters. In addition, adenosine triphosphate (ATP)-mediated active transport, such as the Na^+, K^+-ATPase or the Ca^{2+}-ATPase, besides endocytosis and exocytosis, participates in transplacental exchange (Hahn et al, 2001; Malassiné and Cronier, 2002; Randhawa and Cohen, 2005; Siiteri, 2005).

In healthy women who are not pregnant, uterine blood vessels receive approximately 1% of the cardiac output to maintain the uterus. During pregnancy, these same vessels must support the rapidly growing and demanding placenta and fetus. This evolutionary challenge is addressed by remodeling of the spiral arteries, converting them into large, thin-walled, dilated vessels with reduced vascular resistance.

TROPHOBLAST DIFFERENTIATION AND REMODELING OF SPIRAL ARTERIES

The placental-decidual interaction through invading trophoblasts determines whether an optimal transformation of the uterine spiral arteries is achieved. Trophoblast-orchestrated artery remodeling is an essential feature of normal human pregnancy. As shown in Figure 5-5, progenitor trophoblast cells from villi differentiate along two pathways: terminally differentiated syncytiotrophoblasts and the extravillous cytotrophoblasts (EVTs) that migrate out in columns and anchor the placenta to the decidua.

From these anchoring layers of EVTs further differentiation takes place into invasive or proliferative EVTs. The invasive EVTs invade the decidua and shallow parts of the myometrium and are known as interstitial EVTs. Thereafter endovascular transformation ensues as invasive EVTs migrate into and colonize the spiral arteries, almost reaching the myometrium. These trophoblasts are known as *endovascular EVTs*. Insufficient uteroplacental interaction characterized by shallow trophoblast invasion and incomplete transformation of spiral arteries is a common feature of preeclampsia and intrauterine growth restriction (IUGR) (Brosens et al, 1977; Meekins et al, 1994). The precise period when trophoblast invasion of decidua and spiral arteries ceases is not clear. Nevertheless it is widely believed to be completed late in the second trimester.

Although our understanding of the molecular events underlying spiral artery remodeling in pregnancy remains poor, efficient trophoblast invasion is an essential feature. There are two waves of trophoblast invasion that follow implantation. The first wave is during the first trimester, when the invasion is limited to the decidual part of the spiral artery. The second wave is during the late second trimester involving deeper trophoblast invasion, reaching the inner third of myometrial segment. The initial invasion of EVTs into the endometrium initiates the decidualization process, which is characterized by replacement of extracellular matrix, loss of normal musculoelastic structure, and deposition of fibrinoid material. Displacement of the endothelial lining of spiral arteries by the invading trophoblasts further results in uncoiling and widening of the spiral artery, ensuring the free flow of blood and nutrients to meet the escalating demands of the growing fetus (Kham et al, 1999; Pijnenborg et al, 1983). A lack of spiral artery remodeling with shallow trophoblast invasion has been associated with preeclampsia. During the process of invasion in a normal pregnancy, cytotrophoblasts undergo phenotypic switching, with a loss of E-cadherin expression, and they acquire vascular endothelial-cadherin, platelet-endothelial adhesion molecule-1, vascular endothelial adhesion molecule-1, and α4 and αvβ3 integrins (Bulla et al, 2005; Zhau et al, 1997). Along with a repertoire of facilitators for invasion, trophoblasts express a nonclassic major histocompatibility complex (MHC) human leukocyte antigen (HLA) G, which has gained widespread interest because of providing noncytotoxic signals to uterine NK cells. It still needs to be evaluated whether intrinsic HLA-G inactivation by polymorphic changes influences the dysregulated trophoblast invasion seen in preeclampsia (Hiby et al, 1991; Le Bouteiller et al, 2007).

Although the exact gestational age at which trophoblast invasion ceases is not known, recent studies have shown that late pregnancy trophoblasts loose the ability to transform the uterine arteries. Using a novel dual-cell in vitro culture system that mimics the vascular remodeling events triggered by normal pregnancy serum, we have shown that first- and third-trimester trophoblasts respond differentially to interactive signals from endothelial cells when cultured on the extracellular matrix, matrigel. Term trophoblasts not only fail to respond to signals from endothelial cells, but they inhibit endothelial cell neovascular formation. In contrast, trophoblast cells representing first-trimester trophoblasts with invasive properties undergo spontaneous migration and promote endothelial cells to form a capillary network (Figure 5-6).

This disparity in behavior was confirmed in vivo using a matrigel plug assay. Poor expression of VEGF-C and VEGF receptors coupled with high E-cadherin expression by term trophoblasts contributed to their restricted migratory and interactive properties. Furthermore, these studies showed that the kinase activity of VEGF receptor 2 is essential for proactive crosstalk by invading first-trimester trophoblast cells (Kalkunte et al, 2008b). This unique maternal and fetal cell interactive model under the pregnancy milieu offers a potential approach to study cell-cell interactions and to decipher inflammatory components in the serum samples from adverse pregnancy outcomes (Kalkunte et al, 2010). One of the inimitable contributors to trophoblast cell invasion is the specialized NK cell of the pregnant uterus.

IMMUNE PROFILE AND IMMUNO VASCULAR BALANCE DURING PLACENTATION

During pregnancy, trophoblast cells directly encounter maternal immune cells at least at two sites. One site is the syncytiotrophoblasts covering the placental villi that are bathed in maternal blood, and the other is by the invading trophoblasts in the decidua. Although the syncytiotrophoblasts do not express MHC antigens, the invading trophoblasts express nonclassic HLA-G and HLA-C and would elicit immune responses in the decidua. The decidua is replete with innate immune cells including T cells, regulatory T cells, macrophages, dendritic cells and NK cells (Table 5-3). Interestingly, NK cells peak and constitute the largest leukocyte population in the early pregnant uterus, accounting for 60% to 70% of total lymphocytes. These cells diminish in proportion as pregnancy proceeds.

PHENOTYPIC AND FUNCTIONAL FEATURES OF UTERINE NATURAL KILLER CELLS

Peripheral blood NK (pNK) cells constitute 8% to 10% of the CD45+ population in circulation. All NK cells are characterized by a lack of CD3 and expression of CD56 antigen. Based on the intensity of CD56 antigen, NK cells are further divided into CD56^{bright} and CD56^{dim} populations. The presence or absence of FcγRIII or CD16 further differentiates subpopulations of uterine NK (uNK) cells. Thus the majority of peripheral NK cells are of the CD56^{dim}CD16+ phenotype (approximately 90%), and the remaining cells are CD56^{bright}CD16$^-$ (approximately 10%). The majority of uterine NK cells (approximately 90%) are CD56^{bright}CD16$^-$. In the uterine decidua, uNK cell numbers cyclically increase and decrease in tandem with the menstrual cycle—low in the proliferative phase (10% to 15%), which amplifies during the early, middle and late secretory phases (25% to 30%)—falling to a basal level with menstruation (Figure 5-7) (Kalkunte et al, 2008a; Kitaya et al, 2007).

With successful implantation, the uNK cell population further increases in the decidualized endometrium, reaches a peak in first-trimester pregnancy, and dwindles thereafter by the end of the second trimester. The origin of uNK cells that peak during the secretory phase of the menstrual cycle and early pregnancy is currently not well established, and the evidence indicates multiple different possibilities. These possibilities include recruitment of CD56^{bright}CD16$^-$ pNK cells, recruitment and tissue specific terminal differentiation of CD56^{dim}CD16+ pNK cells, development of NK cells from Lin$^-$CD34+CD45+ progenitor cells, or proliferation of resident CD56^{bright}CD16$^-$ NK cells. Comparative surface expression of antigens, natural cytotoxicity receptors, inhibitory receptors, and

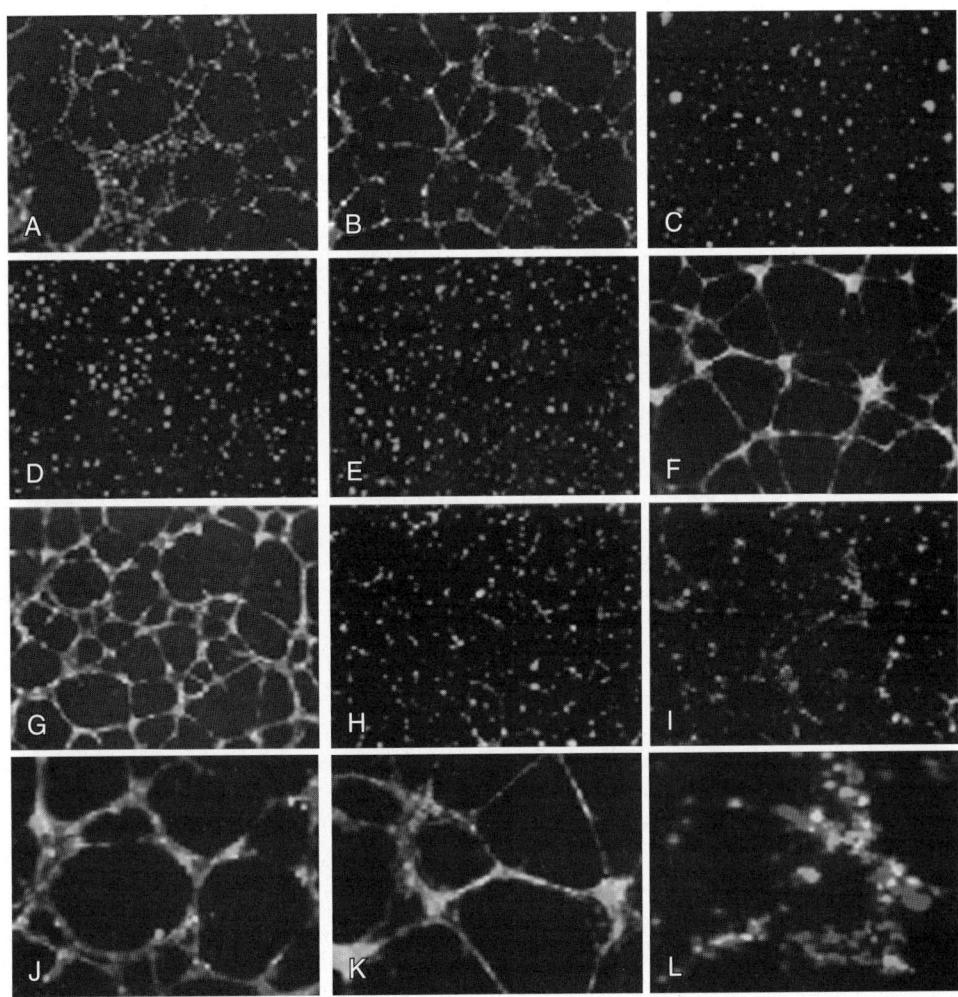

FIGURE 5-6 *(Supplemental color version of this figure is available online at www.expertconsult.com.)* **Differential endovascular activity of first- and third-trimester trophoblasts in response to normal pregnancy serum.** A representative micrograph of trophoblasts-endothelial cell interactions on matrigel is shown. Endothelial cells and trophoblasts are labeled with red and green cell tracker respectively, were independently cultured (**A** to **E**) or cocultured (**F** to **I**) on matrigel. Capillary-like tube structures were observed with human uterine endothelial cells (HUtECs) (**A**) and umbilical vein endothelial cells (HUVECs) (**B**), but not with first-trimester trophoblast HTR8 cells (**C**), third trimester trophoblast TCL1 cells (**D**), and primary term trophoblasts (**E**). However, in cocultures, HTR8 cells fingerprint the HUtECs (**F**) and HUVECs (**G**), while TCL1 cells (**H**) and primary term trophoblasts (**I**) inhibit the tube formation by endothelial cells (magnification ×4). Panels **J** to **L** show the cocultures of HTR8 with HUVECs (**J**), HUtECs (**K**), and term trophoblasts with HUVECs (**L**) at higher magnification (×10). *(Reproduced with permission from Kalkunte S, Lai Z, Tewari N, et al: In vitro and in vivo evidence for lack of endovascular remodeling by third trimester trophoblasts, Placenta 29:871-878, 2008.)*

TABLE 5-3   Comparison of Peripheral Blood and Decidual Immune Cell Profiles

Immune Cells	Peripheral blood (%)	Decidua (%)
T cells	65-70	9-12
γδT cells	2-5	7-10
Macrophages	7-10	15-20
B cells	7-10	ND
NKT cells	2-5	0.5-1.0
Tregs	2-4	6-10
NK cells	7-12	65-70 (CD56^{bright}CD16$^-$)

ND, Not detected.

chemokines and cytokines on human pNK and uNK cells are provided in Table 5-4. Furthermore, CD56^{bright} uNK cells are different from the CD56^{bright} minor population of pNK cells because of the expression of CD9, CD103, and killer immunoglobulin-like receptors (KIRs). Despite

being replete with cytotoxic accessories of perforin, granzymes A and B and the natural cytotoxicity receptors NKp30, NKp44, NKp46, NKG2D, and 2B4 as well as LFA-1, uNK cells are tolerant cytokine-producing cells at the maternal-fetal interface (Kalkunte et al, 2008a). The temporal occurrence around the spiral arteries and timed amplification of these specialized uNK cells observed during the first trimester implicate its role in spiral artery remodeling.

NK cell–deficient mice display abnormalities in decidual artery remodeling and trophoblast invasion, possibly because of a lack of uNK cell–derived interferon γ (Ashkar et al, 2000). Other studies have shown that unlike pNK cells, uNK cells are a major source of VEGF-C, Angiopoietins 1 and 2 and transforming grwoth factor (TGF-β1) within the placental bed that decrease with gestational age (Lash et al, 2006). These observations implicate uNK cells in promoting angiogenesis. Studies have provided further evidence that uNK cells, but not pNK cells, regulate trophoblast invasion both in vitro and in vivo through the production of interleukin-8 and interferon-inducible

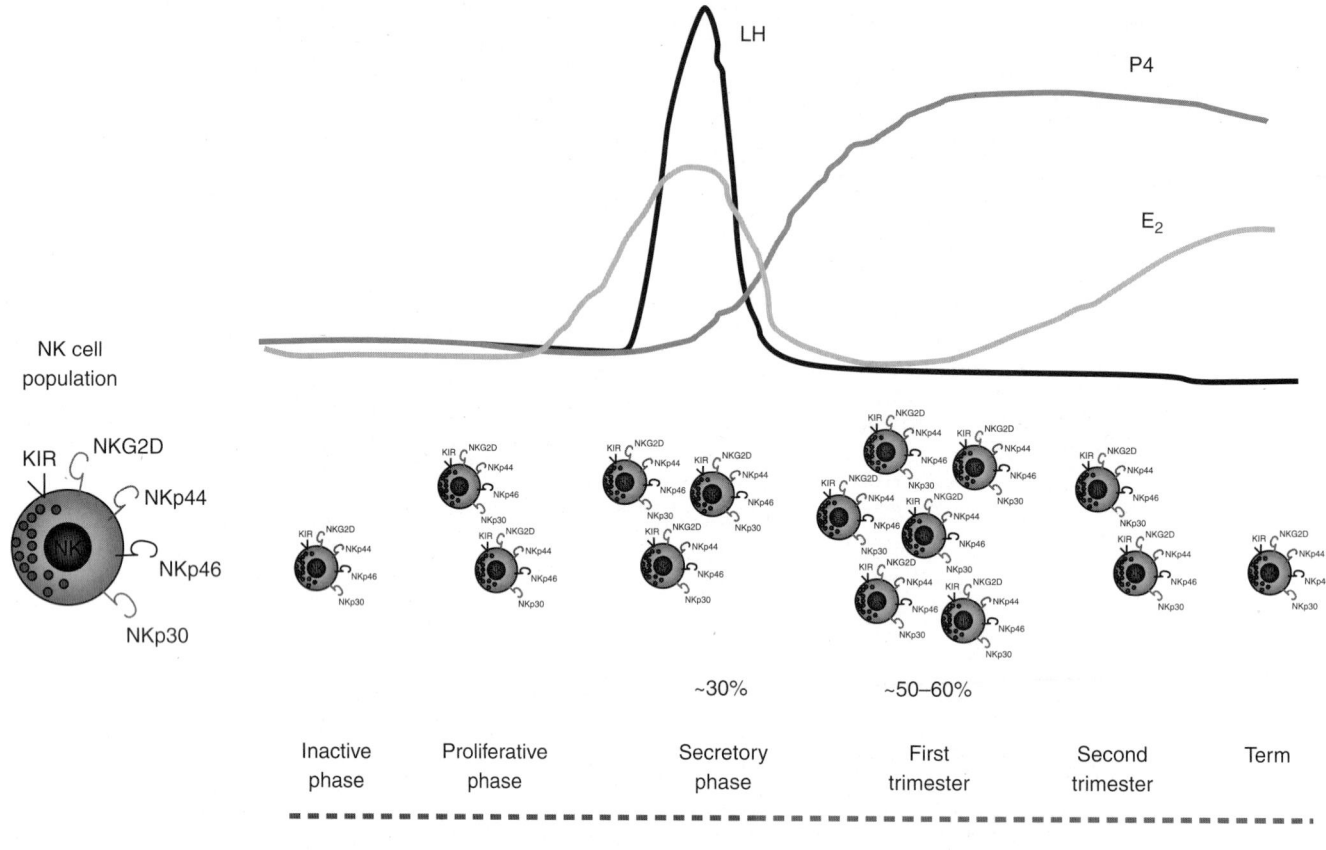

FIGURE 5-7 **Biologic pattern of natural killer (NK) cells in the human endometrium and the decidua.** The uterine NK cell population characterized by natural cytotoxicity receptors (Nkp30, Nkp44, Nkp46, NKG2D), killer immunoglobulin-like receptors, and cytolytic machinery (perforin and granzyme) cyclically increases and decreases in tandem with the hormonal changes during menstrual cycle. With successful implantation, uterine NK cells further increase in the decidua and dwindle thereafter by the end of second trimester. *E₂*, Estradiol; *LH*, luteinizing hormone; *P4*, progesterone.

protein-10, in addition to other angiogenic factors (Hanna et al, 2006). Recent studies suggest that VEGF-C, a pro-angiogenic factor produced by uNK cells, is responsible for the noncytotoxic activity (Kalkunte et al, 2009). As noted previously, VEGF-C–producing uNK cells support endovascular activity in a coculture model of capillary tube formation on matrigel (Figure 5-8). Peripheral blood NK cells fail to produce VEGF-C and remain cytotoxic. This function can be reversed by recombinant human VEGF-C. Cytoprotection by VEGF-C is related to induction of the transporter associated with antigen processing 1 and MHC assembly in target cells. Overall, these findings suggest that expression of angiogenic factors by uNK cells keeps these cells noncytotoxic, which is critical to their pregnancy compatible immunovascular role during placentation and fetal development (Kalkunte et al, 2009).

Although uNK cells seem to play a role that is compatible with pregnancy, retention of their cytolytic abilities suggests their role as sentinels at the maternal-fetal interface in situations that threaten fetal persistence. This facet of uNK cell function was elegantly demonstrated in animal models when pregnant mice were challenged with toll-like receptor (TLR) ligands that mimic bacterial and viral infections. These observations raise an important question whether uNK cells can harm the fetal placental unit and, if so, under what conditions?

The antiinflammatory cytokine interleukin (IL)-10 plays a critical role in pregnancy because of its regulatory relationship with other intrauterine modulators and its wide range of immunosuppressive activities (Moore et al, 2001). IL-10 expression by the human placenta depends on gestational age, with significant expression through the second trimester followed by attenuation at term (Hanna et al, 2000). IL-10 expression is also found to be poor in decidual and placental tissues from unexplained spontaneous abortion cases (Plevyak et al, 2002) and from deliveries associated with preterm labor (Hanna et al, 2006) and pre-eclampsia (S. Kalkunte et al, unpublished observations). However, the precise mechanisms by which IL-10 protects the fetus remains poorly understood. IL-10$^{-/-}$ mice suffer no pregnancy defects when mated under pathogen-free conditions (White et al, 2004), but they exhibit exquisite susceptibility to infection or inflammatory stimuli compared with wild type animals. It is then plausible that in addition to IL-10 deficiency, a "second hit" such as an inflammatory insult resulting from genital tract infections, environmental factors, or hormonal dysregulation during gestation can lead to adverse pregnancy outcomes (Tewari et al, 2009; Thaxton et al, 2009). Our recent studies provide direct evidence that uNK cells can become adversely activated and mediate fetal demise and preterm birth in response to low doses of TLR ligands

Antigen	Peripheral blood	Decidua
CD56	Dim (>90%)	Bright
CD16	+	–
CD45	+	+
CD7	+	+
CD69	–	+
L-Selectin	–	–/+
NK Receptors		
KIR	+	+
NKp30	+	+
NKp44	–*	+
NKp46	+	+
NKG2D	+	+
CD94/NKG2A	–/+	+
Chemokine Receptors		
CXCR1	+	+
CXCR2	+	–
CXCR3	–	+
CXCR4	+	+
CX3CR1	+	–
CCR7	–	+

Data from Kalkunte S, Chichester CO, Sentman CL, et al: Evolution of non-cytotoxic uterine natural killer cells, *Am J Reprod Immunol* 59:425-432, 2008.
+, Present; –, absent; –/+, variable expression; *KIR*, killer immunoglobulin receptor; *CXCR*, CX-chemokine receptor; *CX3CR1*, CX3-C–chemokine receptor 1; *CCR7*, CC-chemokine receptor 7.
*Expression seen on activation with interleukin 2.

resulting in placental pathology (Murphy et al, 2005; Murphy et al, 2009). Moreover, spontaneous abortion is associated with an increase in $CD56^{dim}CD16^+$ cells and a decrease in $CD56^{bright}CD16^-$ NK cells in the preimplantation endometrium during the luteal phase (Michimata et al, 2002; Quenby et al, 1999). Therefore a fine balance between maternal activating and inhibitory KIRs and their ligand HLA-C on fetal cells seems to be maintained in normal pregnancy. Insufficient inhibition of uNK cells can activate the cytolytic machinery, resulting in spontaneous abortion, intrauterine growth restriction, or preterm labor, depending on the timing of the insult (Varla-Leftherioti et al, 2003). In the setting of IVF, the implantation failure has been associated with high uNK cell numbers, but direct evidence for their role in abnormal implantation is not clear (Quenby et al, 1999). Nevertheless current understanding strongly implies that uNK cells retain the ability to become foes to pregnancy under the axis of genetic stress and inflammatory trigger.

REGULATORY T CELLS AND PREGNANCY

The existence of regulatory mechanisms that suppress the maternal immune system was proposed in the early 1950 (Medawar, 1953). For several years, maternal tolerance toward fetal alloantigens was explored in the context of Th1/Th2 balance, with Th2 cells and cytokines proposed to predominate over Th1 cellular immune response under normal pregnancy. Recently the role of specialized T lymphocytes, termed *regulatory T cells* (Tregs), in tolerogenic mechanisms has emerged. Tregs are potent suppressors of T cell–mediated inflammatory immune responses and prevent autoimmunity and allograft rejection. Tregs act by controlling the autoreactive T cells that have escaped negative selection from the thymus, and they restrain the intensity of responses by T cells reactive with alloantigens and other exogenous antigens. This unique functional capability to suppress responses to tissue-specific self-antigens that escape recognition by T cells during maturation is due to tissue specific expression and alloantigens, particularly in the epithelial surfaces where tolerance to nondangerous foreign antigen is essential to normal function. This capability enables Tregs to play a unique role at the maternal-fetal interface. Tregs are typically characterized by a $CD4^+CD25^+$ surface phenotype and expression of the hallmark suppressive transcription factor Foxhead Box P3 ($Foxp3^+$). Their cell numbers increase in blood, decidual tissue, and lymph nodes draining the uterus during pregnancy. These cells are implicated in successful immune tolerance of the conceptus, mainly by producing IL-10 and TGF-β. Recent evidence suggests that fetal Tregs also play a vital role in suppressing fetal antimaternal immunity against maternal cells that cross the placenta (Mold et al, 2008).

In the absence of Tregs the allogeneic fetus is rejected, suggesting their critical role in normal pregnancy. Unexplained infertility, spontaneous abortion, and preeclampsia are associated with proportional deficience, functional Treg deficiency, or both. In the context of pregnancy, the local milieu, particularly during the first trimester, that includes hCG, TGF-β, IL-10, granulocyte-macrophage colony-stimulating factor, and indoleamine 2,3-dioxygenase expression has now been shown to induce $CD4^+CD25^+$ Tregs with Foxp3 expression with immunosuppressive features. This induction is thought to occur through the immature dendritic cells. In addition to immune suppressive and anti-inflammatory properties, TGF-β is recognized as inducing differentiation of naïve CD4 T cells into suppressor T-cell phenotype, expressing Foxp3, and promoting the proliferation of mature Tregs. In addition to the suppressive effects of cytokines produced by these cells, contact-mediated immune suppression by Tregs results from ligation of inhibitory cytotoxic T-lymphocyte antigen (CTLA-4) and its ability to induce tolerogenic dendritic cells and influence T-cell production of IL-10 (Aluvihare et al, 2004; Schumacher et al, 2009; Shevach et al, 2009). Therefore the pregnant uterus may be a natural depot for Tregs.

EPIGENETIC REGULATION IN THE PLACENTA

The regulation of gene expression is a crucial process that defines phenotypic diversity. Switching off or turning on genes as well as tissue-specific variation in gene expression contributes to this diversity. Besides the genetic make-up (i.e, sequence) of the individual, the regulation of gene expression is also influenced by epigenetic factors. Epigenetic changes include the noncoding changes in DNA and chromatin, or both, that mediate the interactions between genes and their environment. Epigenetic regulation generates a wider

DECIDUA

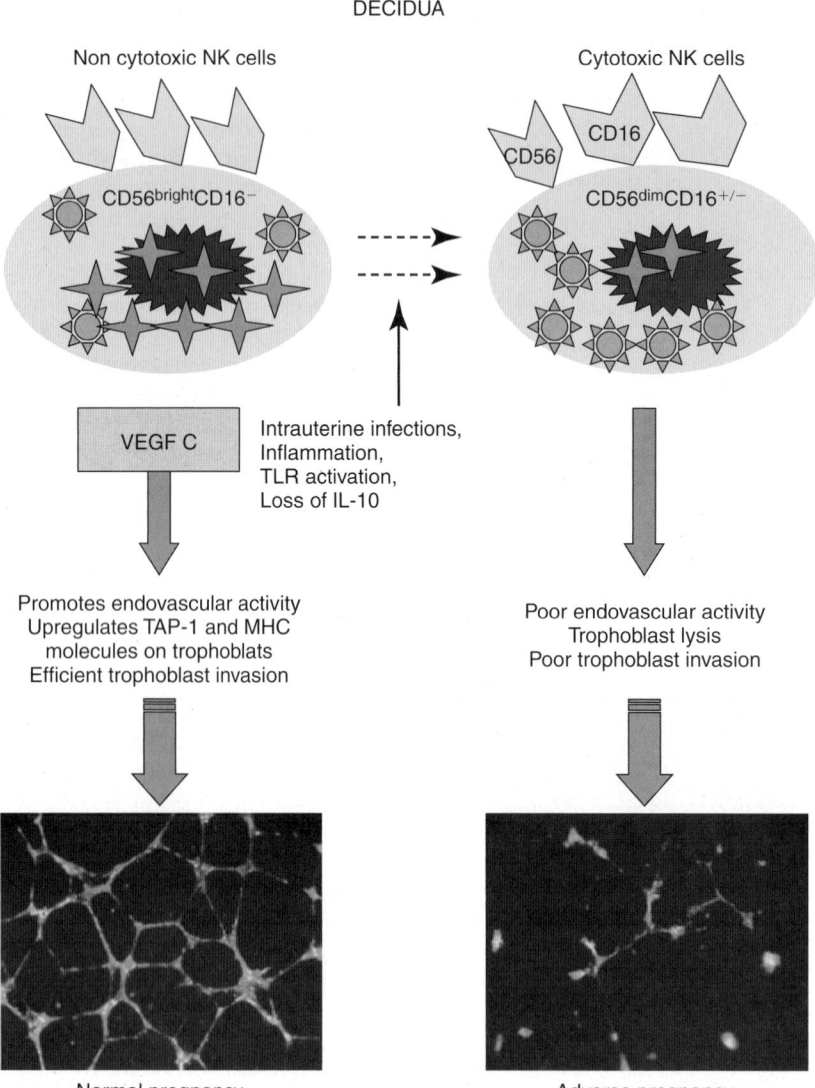

FIGURE 5-8 *(See also Color Plate 1.)* Angiogenic features of natural killer (NK) cells render them immune tolerant at the maternal-fetal interface. Vascular endothelial growth factor (VEGF) C–producing noncytotoxic uterine NK cell clones similar to decidual NK cells support endovascular activity in a coculture of endothelial cells and first-trimester trophoblast HTR8 cells on matrigel. By contrast, cytotoxic uterine NK cell clones similar to peripheral blood NK cells disrupted the endovascular activity because of endothelial and trophoblast cell lysis. This distinct functional feature determines whether optimal trophoblast invasion takes place and can result in normal or adverse pregnancy outcomes.

diversity of cell types during mammalian development and sustains the stability and integrity of the expression profiles of different cell types and tissues. This regulation is choreographed by changes in cytosine-phosphate-guanine (CpG) islands of the DNA promoter region by methylation, histone modification, genomic imprinting, and expression of noncoding RNAs such as micro RNA (miRNA).

Gene-environment interactions resulting in epigenetic changes in the placenta during the critical window of development can influence fetal programming in utero, with predisposing health consequences later in life. Using a micro-array-based approach to compare chorionic villous samples from the first trimester of pregnancy with gestational age–matched maternal blood cell samples, recent studies show tissue-specific differential CpG methylation patterns that identify numerous potential biomarkers for the diagnosis of fetal aneuploidy on chromosomes 13, 18 and 21 (Chu et al, 2009). Human placentation displays many similarities

with tumorigenesis, including rapid mitotic cell division, migration, angiogenesis and invasion, and escape from immune surveillance. Indeed, there are striking similarities in the DNA methylation pattern of tumor-associated genes between invasive trophoblast cell lines and first-trimester placenta and tumors (Christensen et al, 2009). This finding suggests that a distinct pattern of tumor-associated methylation can result in a series of epigenetic silencing events necessary for normal human placental invasion and function (Novakovic et al, 2008). Other studies using the placenta as a source suggest that the specific loss of imprinting because of altered methylation and subsequent gene expression can result in small for gestational age (SGA) newborns. Moreover, unbalanced expression of imprinted genes in IUGR placenta when compared with non-IUGR placenta was observed suggesting a differential expression pattern of imprinted genes as a possible biomarker for IUGR (Guo et al, 2008; McMinn et al, 2006).

The unique cytokine and hormonal milieu in utero may influence the trophoblast function and differentiation as well as immune cell regulation through histone posttranslational modification. In this regard, interferon γ produced by uNK cells and essential for spiral artery remodeling fails to induce MHC class II expression in trophoblast cells because of hypermethylation of regulatory class II MHC transactivator (CIITA) regions (Morris et al, 2002). This inability to upregulate classical MHC class II molecules by trophoblasts is essential for maintaining immune tolerance at the maternal-fetal interface. Moreover, the transcription factor regulating trophoblastic fusion protein syncytin, which is essential for the syncytialization of trophoblasts, is regulated by histone acetyl transferase and histone deacetylase activity (Chuang et al, 2006). miRNAs are small regulatory RNA molecules that can alter gene and protein expression without altering the underlying genetic code. Expression of miRNA is tissue specific, and several are expressed in the placenta. In placental pathology associated with preeclampsia, there is differential expression of miRNA (such as miR-210 and miR-182) compared with normal pregnancy placenta. This finding suggests that signature differences in placental miRNA and their detection in maternal serum may potentially be used as a biomarker for preeclampsia. Because implantation and early placentation is under the regulation of low oxygen tension, it is possible that miRNA are differentially expressed under different oxygen levels, as suggested by recent observations (Maccani and Marsit, 2009; Pineles et al, 2007).

PLACENTAL DISEASES

The placenta provides a wealth of retrospective information about the fetus and prospective information regarding the infant. Healthy development of the placenta requires efficient metabolic, immune, hormonal, and vascular adaptation by the maternal system as well as the fetus. Abnormal placentation and placental infections can lead to maternal or fetal anomalies as seen in preeclampsia, preterm birth, and SGA, which can have lifelong bearing on the development and health of infants. Maternal factors such as ascending infections, obesity, hypertension, genetic predisposition such as gene polymorphism of the pregnancy-compatible cytokine milieu, and environmental exposure could also contribute to the placental pathology. The following sections contain an abbreviated discussion of the pathogenesis of some of these placenta-associated disorders.

PREECLAMPSIA

Hypertensive disorders of pregnancy are enigmatic. They pose a major public health problem and affect 5% to 10% of human pregnancies. Preeclampsia is clinically associated with maternal symptoms of hypertension, proteinuria, and glomeruloendotheliosis. This disorder is strictly a placental condition because of its clearance after delivery. It causes morbidity and mortality in the mother, fetus, and newborn. *Pregnancy-associated hypertension* is defined as blood pressure greater than 140/90 mm Hg on at least two occasions and at 4 to 6 weeks apart after 20 weeks'

gestation. *Proteinuria* is defined by excretion of 300 mg or more of protein every 24 hours or 300 mg/L or more in two random urine samples taken at least 4 to 6 hours apart (ACOG Committee on Practice Bulletins, 2002). The fetal problems most commonly associated with preeclampsia include fetal growth restriction, reduced amniotic fluid, and abnormal oxygenation (Sibai et al, 2005). However, the onset of clinical signs and symptoms can result in either near-term preeclampsia without affecting the fetus or its severe manifestation that is associated with low birthweight and preterm delivery (Vatten and Skjaerven, 2004). The heterogeneous manifestation of this disease is further confounded by preexisting maternal vascular disease, multifetal gestation, metabolic syndrome, obesity, or previous incidence of the disease. In addition, the pathophysiology of the disorder could differ from the onset before 24 weeks' gestation and its diagnosis at later stages of pregnancy:

Abnormal remodeling of spiral arteries and shallow trophoblast invasion are two hallmark features of preeclampsia. Preeclampsia is considered a two-stage disease where a poorly perfused placenta (stage I) causes the release of factors leading to maternal symptoms (stage II). However, it is also now being recognized that the maternal factors may contribute to programming of stage I of preeclampsia, suggesting that the intrinsic maternal factors stemming from genetic, behavioral, and physiologic conditions may contribute to placental pathology. Stage I initiated pathology may be particularly apparent in the oxidative stress-induced release of causative factors from the poorly perfused placenta and their effects on the maternal syndrome (Roberts and Hubel, 1999).

Despite a poor mechanistic understanding of placental pathology leading to preeclampsia, several critical features are common to this disease. Multiple studies have shown that reduced vascular activity could be a major factor contributing to preeclampsia. In normal pregnancy, the circulating PlGF levels steadily increase in the first and second trimesters, peak at 29 to 32 weeks, and decline thereafter. However, free VEGF remains low and unchanged during this window. Reduced placental expression of VEGF and PlGF is consistently observed in preeclampsia. Furthermore, preeclampsia is frequently accompanied by enhanced circulation and placental expression of the anti-angiogenic soluble VEGF receptor 1 (sFlt-1), which is a decoy receptor titrating out VEGFs and PlGF (Levine et al, 2004; Romero et al, 2008; Thadhani et al, 2004). A lack of available VEGF and increased sFlt-1 expression has been associated with trophoblast injury. The soluble form of endoglin (CD105), a coreceptor involved in TGF-β signaling is reported to enhance the antiangiogenic effects of sFlt-1. Soluble endoglin has been found to be elevated in the serum of preeclamptic women and is accompanied by an increased ratio of sFlt-1:PlGF and correlates with the severity of the disease. Soluble endoglin is thought to inhibit TGF-β1 signaling in endothelial cells and blocks activation of endothelial nitric oxide synthase and vasodilatation (Venkatesha et al, 2006). Several recent studies have suggested an increase in apoptosis within villous trophoblast from preeclampsia and IUGR deliveries (Allaire et al, 2000; Heazell and Crocker, 2008; Levy et al, 2002). Unlike normal pregnancy, villous placental explants from preeclamptic placenta have an increased sensitivity and susceptibility to apoptosis on exposure to proinflammatory cytokines, suggesting altered programming of apoptotic cascade pathway (Crocker et al, 2004; Levy et al, 2002). It is possible that incomplete spiral artery transformation resulting in reduced placental perfusion (stage I) in preeclampsia leads to focal regions of hypoxia with increase in apoptosis, oxidative stress, shedding of villous microparticles, and release of antiangiogenic factors such as sFlt-1.64 (Hung et al, 2002; Nevo et al, 2006; Redman and Sargent, 2000).

Another pathway that may contribute to the etiology of preeclampsia is unscheduled and excessive activation of the complement cascade; this is highly likely as a result of the maternal immune system responding to paternal antigens and inflammation. However, in normal pregnancy the placenta expresses complement regulatory proteins such as DAF, CD55, and CD59 and may control activation of complement factors (Tedesco et al, 1993). Despite the positioning of complement inhibitory proteins for protective roles, increasing evidence supports the involvement of complement activation in the pathogenesis of preeclampsia (Lynch et al, 2008). Interestingly, recent in vitro studies suggest that hypoxia enhances placental deposition of the membrane attack complex and apoptosis in cultured trophoblasts (Rampersad et al, 2008). The upstream factors that trigger complement activation are not yet known.

Recent studies also suggest increased serum levels of agonistic autoantibodies against angiotensin type 1 receptor (AT-1-AA) in preeclampsia as compared with healthy women (Zhou et al, 2008). Importantly, studies from our laboratory have shown that the full spectrum of preeclampsia-like symptoms can be reproduced in mice by injecting human preeclampsia serum containing subthreshold levels of AT-1-AA immunoglobulin G, suggesting that pregnancy serum contains some unknown causative factors. Therefore serum can be used as a blueprint to identify functional biomarkers for preeclampsia (Kalkunte et al, 2009).

PRETERM BIRTH

Preterm birth is the leading cause of infant morbidity and mortality in the world. Babies born before 37 weeks' gestation are considered premature. In the United States, approximately 12.8% of births are preterm, and the rate of premature birth has increased by 36% since early 1980s (Martin et al, 2009). Babies from preterm birth face an increased risk of lasting disabilities such as mental retardation, learning and behavioral problems, autism, cerebral palsy, bronchopulmonary dysplasia, vision and hearing loss, and risk for diabetes, hypertension, and heart disease in adulthood. The majority of preterm deliveries are due to preterm labor. Other factors leading to premature birth are preterm premature rupture of membranes (PPROM), intervention for maternal or fetal problems, preeclampsia, fetal growth restriction, cervical incompetence, and antepartum bleeding. Additional risk factors for preterm birth include stress, occupational fatigue, uterine distention by polyhydramnios or multifetal gestation, systemic infection such as periodontal disease, intrauterine placental pathology such as abruption, vaginal bleeding, smoking,

substance abuse, maternal age (<18 or >40 years), obesity, diabetes, thrombophilia, ethnicity, anemia, and fetal factors such as congenital anomalies and growth restriction.

Activation of the hypothalamic-pituitary-adrenal (HPA) as a result of major maternal physical or psychological stress is thought to increase the release of corticotrophin-releasing hormone. In addition to the hypothalamus as a source of corticotrophin-releasing hormone, placental trophoblasts, amnion, and decidual cells also express this hormone during pregnancy. Corticotrophin hormone regulates the release of adrenocorticotropic hormone from pituitary and cortisol from adrenal glands, and it can also influence the activity of matrix metalloproteinases (MMPs). Premature activation of the HPA axis can eventually stimulate the prostaglandins, ultimately resulting in parturition via activation of proteases. In addition, activation of the HPA axis promotes the release of estrone, estradiol, and estriol that can activate the myometrium by increasing oxytocin receptors, prostaglandin activity, and enzymes such as myosin light chain kinase and calmodulin, which are responsible for muscle contraction. Concomitantly, progesterone withdrawal is expected with the raising concentration of myometrial estrogen receptors, further enhancing estrogen-induced myometrial activation and preterm birth (Dole et al, 2003; Grammatopoulos and Hillhouse, 1999; McLean et al, 1995).

There is increasing evidence that approximately 50% of preterm births are associated with infection of the decidua, amnion, or chorion and amniotic fluid caused by either systemic or ascending genital tract infection. Both clinical and subclinical chorioamnionitis are implicated in preterm birth. Maternal or fetal inflammatory responses to chorioamniotic infection can trigger preterm birth. Activated neutrophils and macrophages and the release of cytokines IL-1β, IL-6, IL-8, tumor necrosis factor alpha (TNF-α) and granulocyte colony-stimulating factor can lead to an enhanced cascade of signaling activity, causing release of prostaglandins and expression of various MMPs of fetal membranes and the cervix. Furthermore, elevated levels of TNF-α and apoptosis are associated with PPROM. Non–infection-related inflammation caused by placental insufficiency and apoptosis can also cause preterm birth. In addition to augmented inflammatory responses to infections, pathogenic microbes (e.g. *Staphylococcus, Streptococcus, Bacteroides,* and *Pseudomonas* spp.) are thought to directly degrade fetal membranes by releasing proteases, collagenases, and elastases, produce phospholipase A2, and release endotoxin that stimulate uterine contractions and cause preterm birth (Goldenberg et al, 2000, 2008; Romero et al, 2006; Slattery and Morrison, 2002).

The innate immune system and trophoblasts during pregnancy recognize bacterial and viral infections using TLRs. Placental transcripts for TLRs 1 to 10 have been detected in human placental tissue, and placental choriocarcinoma cell lines reportedly express TLR-2, TLR-4, and TLR-9 (Abrahams and Mor, 2005). Studies have demonstrated functionality for TLR-2, TLR-3, and TLR-4 in first- and third-trimester placental tissue (Patni et al, 2007). Decidual expression in humans has demonstrated functional receptors in term decidua of TLR-1, TLR-2, TLR-4, and TLR-6 (Canavan and Simhan, 2007). Our recent studies using mice have shown that extremely small doses of the TLR-4 ligand lipopolysaccharide can cause preterm birth or fetal demise in pregnant IL-10–deficient mice by activating and promoting infiltration of uterine NK cells into the placenta and inducing apoptosis by secretion of TNF-α (Murphy et al, 2005, 2009). Similarly, activation of TLR-3 or TLR-9 has been shown to induce spontaneous abortion or preterm birth in IL-10–deficient pregnant mice that is attributed to immune infiltration and proinflammatory cascade in the placenta (Thaxton et al, 2009).

Decidual hemorrhage leading to vaginal bleeding increases the risk for preterm birth and PPROM. Increased occult decidual hemorrhage, hemosiderin deposition, and retrochorionic hematoma formation is seen between 22 and 32 weeks' gestation as a result of PPROM and preterm birth after preterm labor. The development of PPROM in the setting of abruption could be caused by high decidual concentration of tissue factors, which eventually generate thrombin. Thrombin activation as measured by serum thrombin-antithrombin III complex levels are elevated on preterm birth. Thrombin binds to decidual protease-activated receptors (PAR1 and PAR2), induces the production of IL-8 in decidua, attracts neutrophils, and promotes degradation of the fetal membrane MMPs that can result in PPROM (Lockwood et al, 2005; Salafia et al, 1995).

Polyhydramnios is also a high risk factor for preterm birth. It was shown recently that exposure of IL-10–deficient pregnant mice to polychlorinated biphenyls, an environmental toxicant, can lead to preterm birth with IUGR. The IUGR was due to increased amniotic fluid volume (polyhydramnios) and placental insufficiency caused by poor spiral artery remodeling associated with reduced expression of water channel aquaporin-1 in the placenta (Tewari et al, 2009). Increasing evidence also suggests impaired vascular activity because of an increase in antiangiogenic factors such as sFlt-1 and decreased VEGF in PPROM and preterm birth (Kim et al, 2003).

INTRAUTERINE GROWTH RESTRICTION

IUGR is used to designate a fetus that has not reached its growth potential; it can be caused by fetal, placental, or maternal factors. Disparities between fetal nutritional or respiratory demands and placental supply can result in impaired fetal growth. Chromosomal abnormalities (aneuploidy, partial deletions, gene mutation particularly on the gene for insulin-like growth factors), congenital abnormalities, multiple gestation, and infections can also result in IUGR. Preterm birth, preeclampsia, and abruption because of placental ischemia can result in IUGR. Reduced placental weight with identifiable placental histologic abnormalities (e.g, impaired development or obstruction in uteroplacental vasculature, chronic abruption, chronic infections, maternal floor infarction, thrombosis in uteroplacental vasculature or fetoplacental vasculature) are common findings in IUGR. In addition, a single umbilical artery, velamentous umbilical cord insertion, bilobate placenta, circumvallate placenta, and placental hemangioma are some of the other structural anomalies seen in the placenta. Maternal factors such as nutritional deficiency; severe anemia; pulmonary disease leading to maternal hypoxemia; smoking; exposure to

toxins such as warfarin, anticonvulsants, folic acid antagonists, and caffeine; and pregnancies conceived through assisted reproductive techniques have a higher prevalence of IUGR. IUGR results in the birth of an infant who is SGA. Mortality and morbidity are increased in SGA infants compared with those who are appropriate for gestational age. SGA infants at birth have many clinical problems that include impaired thermoregulation; difficulty in cardiopulmonary transition with perinatal asphyxia, pulmonary hypertension, hypoglycemia, polycythemia and hyperviscosity; impaired cellular immune function; and increased risk for perinatal mortality. SGA infants in their childhood and adolescence are at higher risk for impaired physical growth and neurodevelopment. Adolescents born SGA at term were reported to have learning difficulties with attention deficits. Cognitive performance is generally lower in SGA infants at the ages of 1 to 6 years compared with those whoe are appropriate for gestational age. Adults who were SGA infants could be at higher risk for ischemic heart diseases and essential hypertension (Figueras et al, 2007; Kaijser et al, 2008; Lapillonne et al, 1997; Norman and Bonamy, 2005; O'Keefe et al, 2003; Spence et al, 2007).

FETAL MEMBRANES AND THEIR PATHOLOGY

The fetal tissue–derived membrane structure surrounds the fetus and forms the amniotic cavity. This membrane, which lacks both vascular and nerve cells, is composed of an inner layer adjacent to the amniotic fluid and is called the *amnion*. The outer layer that is attached to the decidua is called the *chorion*. Amnion is composed of inner epithelial cells, and the mesenchymal cell layer is composed of fibroblast and an outer spongy layer. Intact, healthy fetal membranes are required for normal pregnancy outcome. Chorion is composed of an outer reticular cell layer composed of fibroblasts and macrophages and an inner cytotrophoblast layer. The elasticity and strength of these membranes are maintained by extracellular matrix proteins such as collagens, fibronectin, laminins, and the activity of MMP-2 and MMP-9 and their inhibitors until the initiation of parturition when the membranes are susceptible to rupture. During parturition, when contractions begin or membranes rupture, MMP activity in the amnion and chorion increases with a concurrent fall in tissue inhibitors of metalloproteinases. This change is followed by apoptosis in the amnion epithelial and chorion trophoblast layers of fetal membrane. Interestingly, some evidence suggests that fetal membranes have antimicrobial activity and are known to express TLR-2 and TLR-4, which are pattern recognition receptors and help in initiating a protective host response to infection.

The histopathology of amnion and chorion includes infections, amniotic fluid contaminants, and fetal diseases. In addition to the membranes, whose infection can lead to chorioamnionitis, another vulnerable portal for infection to occur is the placental intervillous space and fetal villi that provide hematogenous access. Hematogenous sources of infection are typically associated with inflammation of villi (villitis) and intervillous space (intervillositis). Viral pathogens (cytomegalovirus, HIV, herpes simplex virus) commonly produce hematogenous infection of the placenta in addition to bacteria, spirochetes, fungi, and protozoa (Gersell, 1993; Goldenberg et al, 2000; Lahra and Jeffery, 2004).

UMBILICAL CORD

The connecting cord from the developing embryo or fetus to the placenta is the umbilical cord, or funiculus umbilicalis. During prenatal development in humans, the normal umbilical cord contains two umbilical arteries and one umbilical vein buried within Wharton's jelly. The umbilical vein supplies the fetus with oxygenated blood from the placenta while the arteries return the deoxygenated, nutrient-depleted blood to the placenta. In the fetus, the umbilical vein branches into the ductus venosus and another branch that joins the hepatic portal vein. Shortly after parturition, physiologic processes cause the Wharton's jelly to swell with the collapse of blood vessels, resulting in a natural halting of the flow of blood. Within the infant, the umbilical vein and ductus venosus close and degenerate into remnants known as the *round ligament of the liver* and the *ligamentum venosum*, while the umbilical arteries degenerate into what is known as *medial umbilical ligaments*.

Abnormalities associated with the umbilical cord can affect both the mother and the child. Pathology of umbilical cord is generally grouped as congenital remnants, infections, meconium, and masses. Abnormalities that have clinical significance are nuchal cord, single umbilical artery, umbilical cord prolapse, umbilical cord knot, umbilical cord entanglement, vasa previa, and velamentous cord insertion. Common intrauterine infections can result in the umbilical cord being invaded by fetal cells and bacteria infiltrated from the decidua to amniotic fluid, or they can elicit fetal inflammatory response. Umbilical cord inflammation, known as *funisitis* or *vasculitis*, poses a higher risk for development of neurologic compromise in the fetus. Funisitis is predictive of a lower median Bayley psychomotor developmental index in infants. Meconium pigment at high concentrations can damage the umbilical cord by triggering apoptosis of smooth muscle cells. Vascular necrosis caused by meconium is associated with

oligohydramnios, low Apgar scores, and significant neurodevelopmental delay. Interruption of normal blood flow in the cord can cause prolonged hypoxia in utero. Clamping of the umbilical cord within minutes of birth is hospital-based obstetric practice. A Cochrane review studying the effects of the timing of umbilical cord clamping in hospitals showed that infants whose cord clamping occurred later than 60 seconds after birth had a significantly higher risk of neonatal jaundice requiring phototherapy. However, randomized, controlled studies have shown that delayed cord clamping in preterm infants reduces the incidence of intraventricular hemorrhage and late-onset sepsis. Furthermore, premature clamping can increase the risk of ischemia and hypovolemic shock, which can lead to fetal complications (McDonald and Middletone, 2008; Mercer et al, 2006).

SUGGESTED READINGS

Aluvihare VR, Kallikourdis M, Betz AG: Regulatory T cells mediate maternal tolerance to the fetus, *Nat Immunol* 5:266-271, 2004.

Ashkar AA, Di Santo JP, Croy BA: Interferon γ contributes to initiation of uterine vascular modification, decidual integrity, and uterine natural killer cell maturation during normal murine pregnancy, *J Exp Med* 192:259-269, 2000.

Baker DJP: In utero programming of chronic disease, *Clin Sci* 95:115-128, 1998.

Christensen BC, Houseman EA, Marsit CJ, et al: Aging and environmental exposures alter tissue-specific DNA methylation dependent upon CpG island context, *PLoS Genet* 5:e1000602, 2009.

Goldenberg RL, Culhane JF, Iams JD, et al: Epidemiology and causes of preterm birth, *Lancet* 371:75-84, 2008.

Hanna J, Goldman-Wohl D, Hamani Y, et al: Decidual NK cells regulate key developmental processes at the human fetal-maternal interface, *Nat Med* 12:1065-1074, 2006.

Kalkunte S, Mselle TF, Norris WE, et al: VEGF C facilitates immune tolerance and endovascular activity of human uterine NK cells at the maternal-fetal interface, *J Immunol* 182:4085-4092, 2009.

Moffett A, Loke C: Immunology of placentation in eutherian mammals, *Nat Rev Immunol* 6:584-594, 2006.

Murphy SP, Hanna NN, Fast LD, et al: Evidence for participation of uterine natural killer cells in the mechanisms responsible for spontaneous preterm labor and delivery, *Am J Obstet Gynecol* 200:308, 2009.

Paria BC, Reese J, Das SK, et al: Deciphering the cross-talk of implantation: advances and challenges, *Science* 296:2185-2188, 2002.

Roberts JM, Hubel CA: Is oxidative stress the link in the two–stage model of preeclampsia? *Lancet* 354:788-789, 1999.

Slattery MM, Morrison JJ: Preterm delivery, *Lancet* 360:1489-1497, 2002.

Thadhani R, Sachs BP, Epstein FH, et al: Circulating angiogenic factors and the risk of preeclampsia, *N Engl J Med* 350:672-683, 2004.

Complete references and supplemental color images used in this text can be found online at www.expertconsult.com

ABNORMALITIES OF FETAL GROWTH

Rebecca Simmons

Fetal growth and size at birth are critical in determining mortality and morbidity, both immediately after birth and in later life. Normal fetal growth is determined by a number of factors, including genetic potential, the ability of the mother to provide sufficient nutrients, the ability of the placenta to transfer nutrients, and intrauterine hormones and growth factors. The pattern of normal fetal growth involves rapid increases in fetal weight, length, and head circumference during the last half of gestation. During the last trimester, the human fetus accumulates significant amounts of lipid. The birthweight for gestational measurements among populations has been shown to increase over time; therefore, standards for normal fetal growth require periodic reevaluation for clinical relevance. These increases in birthweight for gestational age over time are attributed to improvements in living conditions and maternal nutrition and changes in obstetric management. Variations in fetal growth have been identified in diverse populations and are associated with geographic locations (sea level versus high altitude), populations (white, African American, Latino), maternal constitutional factors, parity, maternal nutrition, fetal gender, and multiple gestations. In this chapter, we discuss these factors in greater detail and critically review the long-term effects of abnormal fetal growth.

DEFINITIONS

Most approaches for defining fetal growth use gestational age-based norms. The duration of pregnancy has become an integral component of prenatal growth assessment, and all currently prevailing definitions of fetal growth are specific for gestational age. Assessing the gestational age accurately, however, can be challenging. Any error in dating will lead to misclassification of the infant, which can have significant clinical implications. In many instances, the method of gestational age determination has contributed to variations in the gestational age–specific reference growth curves. For example, some nomograms are based on approximating the gestational age to the nearest week, whereas others use the completed weeks. The birthweight charts are also affected by other variables that may limit their reliability. Many of these variables, such as fetal gender, race, parity, birth order, parental size, and altitude, contribute to the normal biologic variations in human fetal growth. There is continuing controversy regarding whether the reference growth charts should be customized by multiple variables or developed from the whole population. The customized approach predicts the optimal growth in an individual pregnancy and therefore specifically defines suboptimal growth for that pregnancy. However, it has been argued that such an approach can lead to a profusion of standards and might not contribute to improving the outcome of infants who

are small for gestational age (SGA). In recognition of the utility of a national standard, a population-based reference chart for fetal growth has been developed from all the singleton births (more than 3 million) in the United States in 1991 (Alexander, 1996). More recently, a similar national population-based fetal growth chart, which is also sex specific, has been developed in Canada (Kramer et al, 2001). There is insufficient evidence about whether one approach is superior to the other in improving the perinatal outcome.

There is no universal agreement on the classification of an SGA infant. Various definitions appear in the medical literature, making comparisons between studies difficult. In addition, investigators have shown that the prevalence of fetal growth restriction varies according to the fetal growth curve used (Alexander et al, 1996). The most common definition of SGA refers to a weight less than the 10th percentile for gestational age or birthweight less than 2 standard deviations (SDs) from the mean. Some investigators also use measurements less than the 3rd percentile to define SGA. However, these definitions do not make a distinction among infants who are constitutionally small, growth restricted and small, and not small but growth restricted relative to their potential. As an example, as many as 70% of fetuses with a weight less than the 10th percentile for gestational age at birth are small simply because of constitutional factors such as female sex or maternal ethnicity, parity, or body mass index; they are not at high risk of perinatal mortality or morbidity. In contrast, true fetal growth restriction is associated with numerous perinatal morbidities. This has clinical relevance to perinatologists and neonatologists, because many of the tiniest premature neonates in the neonatal intensive care units are probably growth restricted. McIntire et al (1999) reported a threshold of increased adverse outcomes in infants born with measurements less than the 3rd percentile and suggested that this level of restriction represents a clinically relevant measurement. Other researchers have found higher rates of neonatal complications when the 15th percentile of birthweight is used as a cutoff level (Seeds and Peng, 1998).

There is an important distinction in identifying the fetus with intrauterine growth restriction (IUGR), and the fetus that is constitutionally small (i.e., SGA). IUGR is a condition in which a fetus is unable to achieve its genetically determined potential size and represents a deviation and a reduction in the expected fetal growth pattern. IUGR complicates approximately 5% to 8% of all pregnancies and 38% to 80% of all neonates with low birthweight (LBW). This discrepancy underscores the fact that no uniform definition of IUGR exists. Even when a normal intrauterine growth pattern is established for a population, somewhat arbitrary criteria are used to define growth restriction.

PATTERNS OF ALTERED GROWTH

Neonates with intrauterine growth retardation can be classified as demonstrating either symmetrical or asymmetrical growth. Infants with symmetric IUGR have reduced weight, length, and head circumference at birth. Weight (and then length) of infants with asymmetric growth retardation is affected, with a relatively normal or "head-sparing" growth pattern. Factors intrinsic to the fetus in general cause symmetrical growth restriction, whereas asymmetric IUGR is often associated with maternal medical conditions such as preeclampsia, chronic hypertension, and uterine anomalies. Asymmetric patterns generally develop during the third trimester, a period of rapid fetal growth. However, now that fetal surveillance is more common, asymmetric growth restriction is often diagnosed in the second trimester. Furthermore, many extremely premature neonates (<750 g) probably have IUGR.

Factors that are well recognized to limit the growth of both the fetal brain and body include chromosomal anomalies (e.g., trisomies), congenital infections (toxoplasmosis, rubella, cytomegalovirus, herpes simplex, malaria, HIV, and parvovirus), dwarf syndromes, and some inborn errors of metabolism. Cardiac and renal structural anomalies are common fetal conditions associated with SGA. These conditions retard fetal growth primarily by impaired cell proliferation. Recognized causes of IUGR are listed in Table 6-1.

Etiologies of Fetal Growth Restriction

The epidemiology of fetal growth restriction varies internationally (Keirse, 2000). In developed countries, the most frequently identified cause of growth restriction is smoking, whereas in developing countries, maternal nutritional factors (prepregnancy weight, maternal stature) and infections (malaria) are the leading identified causes (Krampl, 2000; Robinson et al, 2000). In addition, in developing countries there is a direct correlation between the incidence of LBW (<2500 g) and IUGR. In developing countries, the high incidence of infants with LBW is almost exclusively caused by the incidence of IUGR. Data from developed countries show the opposite, with rates of LBW being explained almost exclusively by prematurity rates. In the United States, the cause of IUGR is identified in approximately 40% of cases, with the remaining cases labeled as *idiopathic*.

Numerous factors have been identified as influencing size at birth. In a simplified manner, these factors can be grouped as fetal, placental, or maternal in origin. These factors will be discussed in detail in the following sections.

Fetal Causes of Growth Restriction

Fetal factors affecting growth include gender, familial genetic inheritance, chromosomal abnormalities, and dysmorphic syndromes. In one large, population-based study, the frequency of IUGR among infants with congenital malformations was 22%. The majority of the infants affected had chromosomal abnormalities. Other studies have similarly found that fetal growth restriction is more common among infants with malformations. Fetal gender also influences size, with male infants showing greater intrauterine growth than female infants (Glinianaia et al, 2000; Skjaerven et al, 2000; Thomas et al, 2000).

Placental Causes of Growth Restriction

In mammals, the major determinant of intrauterine growth is the placental supply of nutrients to the fetus (Fowden et al, 2006). In many species, fetal weight near term is positively correlated to placental weight, as a proxy measure of the surface area for maternal-fetal transport of nutrients. Fetal weight near term is positively correlated to placental weight, and the nutrient transfer capacity of the placenta depends on its size, morphology, blood flow, and transporter abundance (Fowden et al, 2006). In addition, placental synthesis and metabolism of key nutrients and hormones influences the rate of fetal growth (Fowden and Forhead, 2004). Changes in any of these placental factors can, therefore, affect intrauterine growth; however, the fetus is not just a passive recipient of nutrients from the placenta. The fetal genome exerts a significant acquisitive drive for maternal nutrients through adaptations in the placenta, particularly when the potential for fetal and placental growth is compromised.

Placental maturation at the end of pregnancy is associated with an increase in substrate transfer, a slowing (but not cessation) of placental growth, and a plateau in fetal growth near term (Fox, 1997). Abnormalities of placental growth, senescence, and infarction have been shown to affect fetal growth. The placentas from pregnancies complicated by poor fetal growth have a higher incidence of vascular damage and abnormalities (Pardi et al, 1997). Fetal size and placental growth are directly related, and placentas from pregnancies yielding growth-restricted infants demonstrate a higher incidence of smallness and abnormality than do those from

TABLE 6-1 Causes of Intrauterine Growth Restriction

Genetic	Inheritance, chromosomal abnormalities, fetal gender
Maternal constitutional effects	Low maternal pre-pregnancy weight, low pregnancy weight gain, ethnicity, socioeconomic status, history of intrauterine growth restriction
Nutrition	Low pre-pregnancy weight (body mass index), low pregnancy weight gain, malnutrition (macronutrients, micronutrients), maternal anemia
Infections	TORCH infections (toxoplasmosis, rubella, cytomegalovirus, syphilis)
Decreased O_2-carrying capacity	High altitude, maternal congenital heart disease, hemoglobinopathies, chronic anemia, maternal asthma
Uterine and placental anatomy	Abnormal uterine anatomy, uterine fibroid, vascular abnormalities (single umbilical artery, velamentous umbilical cord insertion, twin-twin transfusion), placenta previa, placental abruption
Uterine and placental function	Maternal vasculitis (system lupus erythematosus), decreased uteroplacental perfusion, maternal illness (preeclampsia, chronic hypertension, diabetes, renal disease)
Toxins	Tobacco, ethanol, lead, arsenic

pregnancies with appropriately grown infants. The difference in size is seen even in a comparison of placentas associated with growth-restricted infants and those associated with appropriate for gestational age (AGA) infants of the same birthweight (Heinonen et al, 2001). Placental growth in the second trimester correlates with placental weight and function and, thus, with weight at birth (Godfrey et al, 1996). Clinical conditions associated with reduced placental size (and subsequent reduced fetal weight) include maternal vascular disease, uterine anomalies (uterine fibroids, abnormal uterine anatomy), placental infarctions, unusual cord insertions, and abnormalities of placentation.

Multiple gestations are associated with greater risk for fetal growth restriction. The higher risk stems from crowding and from abnormalities with placentation, vascular communications, and umbilical cord insertions. Divergence in fetal growth appears from approximately 30 to 32 weeks in twin gestation compared with singleton pregnancies (Alexander et al, 1996; Glinianaia et al, 2000; Skjaerven et al, 2000). Others have identified differences in fetal growth between twins and singletons as occurring earlier in gestation, at approximately 21 weeks' gestation (Devoe and Ware, 1995). Larger effects on fetal growth are seen with increasing number of fetal multiples. Abnormalities in placentation are also more common with multiple gestations (Benirschke, 1995). Monochorionic twins can share placental vascular communication (twin-twin transfusion), leading to fetal growth restriction during gestation. Fetal competition for placental transfer of nutrients raises the incidence of growth restriction and discordance in growth between fetuses. The rate of birthweights less than the 5th percentile is higher in monochorionic twins. Placental growth is restricted in utero because of limitation in space, leading to a higher incidence of placenta previa in multiple-gestation pregnancies. In addition, abnormalities in cord insertions (marginal and velamentous cord insertions) and occurrence of a single umbilical artery are more frequently found in multiple gestations. The higher incidence of growth restriction in multiple-gestation pregnancies is strongly associated with monochorionic gestations, the presence of vascular anastomoses, and discordant fetal growth (Hollier et al, 1999; Sonntag et al, 1996; Victoria et al, 2001). Placentas of smaller fetuses with discordant growth are significantly smaller than those of their larger twin counterparts (Victoria et al, 2001).

Investigators have shown an effect of altitude on fetal growth, with infants born at high altitudes having lower birthweights (Galan et al, 2001). Differences in fetal growth are detected from approximately 25 weeks' gestation with pregnancies at 4000 m. In these high-altitude pregnancies, the abdominal circumference is most affected (Krampl et al, 2000). At tremendously high altitudes, the incidence of LGA infant births is markedly reduced. In the United States (and at less severe altitudes), infants born at higher altitudes are lighter at birth, but those differences are not pronounced. Interestingly, investigators have shown that adaptation to high altitude during pregnancy is also possible. Tibetan infants have higher birthweights than infants of more recent immigrants of ethnic Chinese living at the same high-altitude (2700 to 4700 m) region of Tibet (Moore et al, 2001). Tibetan infants also have less IUGR than do infants born to more recent immigrants to the area.

Maternal Causes of Growth Restriction

Maternal health conditions associated with chronic decreases in uteroplacental blood flow (maternal vascular diseases, preeclampsia, hypertension, maternal smoking) are associated with poor fetal growth and nutrition. Preeclampsia has been shown to be associated with fetal growth restriction (Ødegård et al, 2000; Spinillo et al, 1994; Xiong et al, 1999). Investigators have shown that the extent of growth restriction correlates with the severity and the onset during pregnancy of the preeclampsia. Ødegård et al (2000) showed that fetuses exposed to preeclampsia from early in pregnancy had the most serious growth restriction, and more than half of these infants were born SGA. Chronic maternal diseases (cardiac, renal) may decrease the normal uteroplacental blood flow to the fetus and thus may also be associated with poor fetal growth (Spinillo et al, 1994).

Maternal constitutional factors have a significant effect on fetal growth. Maternal weight (pre-pregnancy), maternal stature, and maternal weight gain during pregnancy are directly associated with maternal nutrition and correlate with fetal growth (Clausson et al, 1998; Doctor et al, 2001; Goldenberg et al, 1997; Mongelli and Gardosi, 2000). Numerous studies show that these findings are often confounded by highly associated cultural and socioeconomic factors. The woman with a previous SGA infant has a higher risk of a subsequent small infant (Robinson et al, 2000). Investigators have shown a higher incidence of SGA infants to be associated with lower levels of maternal education (Clausson et al, 1998). Parity of the mother also affects fetal size; nulliparous women having a higher incidence of SGA infants (Cnattingius et al, 1998). A large population-based study in Sweden found that women who were older than 30 years, were nulliparous, or had hypertensive disease were at increased risk of preterm and term growth-restricted infants.

Studies have shown differential fetal growth for women of diverse ethnicities, with Latina and white women having higher rates of LGA infants, and African American women having a higher incidence of SGA infants (Alexander et al, 1999; Collins and David, 2009; Fuentes-Afflick et al, 1998). These gender and ethnic differences in birthweight become pronounced after 30 weeks' gestation (Thomas et al, 2000). Investigators in California have shown that U.S.-born black women have higher rates of prematurity and LBW infants than do foreign-born black women. Other researchers have found that even among women with low risk of LBW infants (married, age 20 to 34 years, 13 or more years of education, adequate prenatal care, and absence of maternal health risk factors and tobacco or alcohol use), the risk of delivering an SGA infant is still higher for African American women than for white women (Alexander et al, 1999; Collins and David, 2009). It is unclear whether these differences in fetal growth are caused by inherent differences or by differential exposure to environmental factors.

Maternal nutrition and supply of nutrients to the fetus affect fetal growth significantly, primarily in developing countries (Doctor et al, 2001; Godfrey et al, 1996; Neggers et al, 1997; Robinson et al, 2000; Zeitlin et al, 2001). Although numerous factors interact with and affect fetal development, maternal malnutrition is assumed to be a major cause of IUGR in developing countries. Furthermore, pre-pregnancy weight may be a potential marker for intergenerational effects on infant weight in developing countries. A woman's birthweight has been shown to correlate with her infant's weight as well as the placental weight during pregnancy. In the United States, Strauss and Dietz (1999) report that low maternal weight gain in the second and third trimesters is associated with a twofold risk of IUGR, whereas poor maternal weight gain in the first trimester has no such effect on fetal growth (Strauss and Dietz, 1999). These investigators also showed that older women (older than 35 years) and smokers were at increased risk of IUGR associated with lower weight gains in late pregnancy.

Teen pregnancy represents a special condition in which fetal weight is highly influenced by maternal nutrition. Teen mothers (younger than 15 years) have been shown to have a higher risk for delivering a growth-restricted infant (Ghidini, 1996). Teen pregnancies are complicated by the additional nutritional needs of a pregnant mother, who is still actively growing, as well as by socioeconomic status of pregnant teens in developed countries (Scholl and Hediger, 1995). Maternal nutrition and maternal weight gain are adversely affected by inadequate or poorly balanced intake in conditions such as alcoholism, drug abuse, and poverty.

The effects of micronutrients on pregnancy outcomes and fetal growth have been less well studied. Maternal intake of certain micronutrients has also been found to affect fetal growth. Zinc deficiency has been associated with fetal growth restriction and other abnormalities, such as infertility and spontaneous abortion (Jameson, 1993; Shah and Sachdev, 2001). In addition, dietary intake of vitamin C during early pregnancy has been shown to be associated with an increase in birthweight (Mathews et al, 1999). Others have shown strong associations between maternal intake of folate and iron and infant and placental weights (Godfrey et al, 1996). In developing countries, the effects of nutritional deficiencies during pregnancy are more prevalent and easier to detect. Rao et al (2001) have estimated that one third of infants in India are born weighing less than 2500 g, mainly because of maternal malnutrition. These investigators have shown significant associations between infant birthweight and maternal intake of milk, leafy greens, fruits, and folate during pregnancy.

Although toxins such as cigarette smoke and alcohol have a direct effect on placental function, they may also affect fetal growth through an associated compromise in maternal nutrition. Other environmental toxins (lead, arsenic, mercury) are associated with IUGR and are believed to affect fetal growth by entering the food chain and depleting body stores of iron, vitamin C, and possibly other nutrients (Iyengar and Nair, 2000; Srivastava et al, 2001).

Numerous studies have shown associations between birthweight and maternal intake of macronutrients and micronutrients, but the effects of nutritional supplements used during pregnancy on fetal growth are equivocal (de Onis et al, 1998; Jackson and Robinson, 2001; Rush, 2001; Say et al, 2003). This finding is underscored by the results of a recent, large, double-blind, randomized controlled trial including 1426 pregnancies in rural Burkina

Faso (Roberfroid et al, 2008). Pregnant women were randomly assigned to receive either iron and folic acid or the UNICEF-WHO-UNU[*] international multiple micronutrient preparation (UNIMMAP) daily until 3 months after delivery, with the UNIMMAP thereafter in both groups. Birthweight was increased by 52 g, and length was increased by 3.6 mm. Unexpectedly, the risk of perinatal death was marginally significantly increased in the UNIMMAP group (odds ratio, 1.78; 95% confidence interval, 0.95 to 3.32; $p = 0.07$).

Maternal socioeconomic status and ethnicity have also been identified as risk factors for IUGR and poor health outcomes in infants. Numerous investigators have shown a significant effect of socioeconomic status on birth outcomes, including fetal growth restriction, in both developing and developed countries (Wilcox et al, 1995). In the United States, low levels of maternal and paternal education, certain maternal and paternal occupations, and low family income are associated with lower birthweights in children of African American and white women (Parker et al, 1994). In a large population-based study in Sweden, investigators have shown a higher incidence of fetal growth restriction in association with low maternal education (Clausson et al, 1998). Researchers have also shown that rates of compromised birth outcome are higher among African American women than among Mexican American and non-Hispanic white women (Collins and Butler, 1997; Frisbie et al, 1997; Thomas et al, 2000). Some of these studies also show that the risk of IUGR is higher in women without medical insurance. In the United States, the incidence of IUGR is significantly higher among African American women than among white women; this higher incidence is seen even among African American women with higher socioeconomic status (Alexander et al, 1999).

In a study in Arizona, the incidence of IUGR was found to be lower in Mexican American women than in white women (Balcazar, 1994). Other researchers have shown that Mexican-born immigrants in California have better perinatal outcomes (including birthweight) than African Americans and U.S.-born women of Mexican descent (Fuentes-Afflick et al, 1998). The reasons for this apparent paradox are unclear, but one postulate is the tendency of recent immigrants to maintain the favorable nutritional and behavioral characteristics of their country of origin (Guendelman and English, 1995). These studies support the speculation that the differences in fetal growth between groups do not reflect inherent differences in fetal growth, but rather stem from inequalities in nutrition, health care, and other environmental factors (Keirse, 2000; Kramer et al, 2000).

Smoking

Cigarette smoking is consistently found to adversely affect intrauterine growth in all studies in which this factor is considered. In developed countries, cigarette smoking is the single most important cause of poor fetal growth (Kramer et al, 2000). The incidence of IUGR in smokers

---

[*]United Nations Children's Fund, World Health Organization, United Nations University.

is estimated to be threefold to 4.5-fold higher than in nonsmokers (Nordentoft et al, 1996). Cigarette smoking has a significant effect on abdominal circumference and fetal weight, but not on head circumference (Bernstein et al, 2000). Lieberman et al (1994) reported that cigarette smoking also appears to have a dose-dependent effect on the incidence of IUGR, with this effect being seen especially with heavy smoking and smoking during the third trimester. These investigators have shown that if women stop smoking during the third trimester, their infants' birthweights are indistinguishable from those of infants born to the normal population. Other researchers have shown that even a reduction in smoking is associated with improved fetal growth (Li et al, 1993; Walsh et al, 2001). Numerous potential causes of the effects of smoking on fetal growth have been suggested, including direct effects of nicotine on placental vasoconstriction, decreased uterine blood flow, higher levels of fetal carboxyhemoglobin, fetal hypoxia, adverse maternal nutritional intake, and altered maternal and placental metabolism (Andres and Day, 2000; Pastrakuljic et al, 1999).

SHORT-TERM OUTCOMES

IUGR alters many physiologic and metabolic functions in the fetus and neonate that result in a number of morbidities. A large cohort study of 37,377 pregnancies found a fivefold to sixfold greater risk of perinatal death for both preterm and term fetuses that had IUGR (Cnattingius et al, 1998; Lackman et al, 2001; Mongelli and Gardosi, 2000). Predictive factors for perinatal mortality in preterm fetuses with IUGR reveals that of all antenatal factors examined, only oligohydramnios and abnormal umbilical artery Dopplers with absent or reversed diastolic flow were predictive of perinatal mortality (Scifres et al, 2009). Although the growth-restricted fetus may show symmetric or asymmetric growth at birth, it is unclear whether the proportionality of the fetus with IUGR truly affects outcomes or is related to the timing or the severity of the insult. Lin et al (1991) found that symmetric IUGR resulted in higher levels of prematurity and higher rates of neonatal morbidity. In contrast, Villar et al (1990) have shown that infants with asymmetric IUGR have higher morbidity rates at birth. They found that infants with low ponderal index measurements (which they defined as Weight $\div$ Length^3) had a higher risk of low Apgar scores, long hospitalization, hypoglycemia, and asphyxia at birth than infants with symmetric IUGR. There is evidence to suggest that infants with asymmetric IUGR show better gains in weight and length in the postnatal period than symmetrically restricted infants (May et al, 2001). Other investigators propose that IUGR represents a continuum, with symmetric IUGR occurring as the severity of growth retardation increases. Data also suggest that the more severe the growth restriction, the worse the neonatal outcomes, including risk of stillbirth, fetal distress, neonatal hypoglycemia, hypocalcemia, polycythemia, low Apgar scores, and mortality (Kramer et al, 1990; Spinillo et al, 1995).

Fetal growth restriction is associated with intrauterine demise. Almost 40% of term stillbirths and 63% of preterm stillbirths are SGA (Mongelli and Gardosi, 2000). Both short-term and long-term effects of abnormalities in SGA fetuses have been described. Perinatal mortality for intrauterine SGA infants is higher overall than that for appropriately grown term and preterm infants (Clausson et al, 1998). The risk of perinatal death is estimated to be fivefold to sixfold greater for both preterm and term fetuses with IUGR (Lackman et al, 2001). Overall, intrauterine death, perinatal asphyxia, and congenital anomalies are the main contributing factors to the higher mortality rate in SGA infants. The effects of acute fetal hypoxia may be superimposed on chronic fetal hypoxia, and placental insufficiency may be an important etiologic factor in these outcomes. Investigators have described higher incidences of low Apgar scores, umbilical artery acidosis, need for intubation at delivery, seizures on the first day of life, and sepsis in SGA infants (McIntire et al, 1999). The incidence of adverse perinatal effects correlates with the severity of the growth restriction, the highest rates of respiratory distress syndrome, metabolic abnormalities, and sepsis being found in the most severely growth-restricted infants (Spinillo et al, 1995). As previously described, Villar et al (1990) reported that infants with asymmetric IUGR and low ponderal index measurements had a higher risk of low Apgar scores, hypoglycemia, asphyxia, and long hospitalization.

Preterm infants with growth abnormalities have a much higher risk of adverse outcomes. Preterm SGA infants have a higher incidence of a number of complications, including sepsis, severe intraventricular hemorrhage, respiratory distress syndrome, necrotizing enterocolitis, and death, than do normally grown preterm infants (Gortner et al, 1999; McIntire et al, 1999; Simchen et al, 2000). In addition, SGA infants have a higher incidence of chronic lung disease at corrected gestational ages of 28 days and 36 weeks.

Neonatal hypoglycemia and hypothermia occur more frequently in growth-restricted infants (Doctor et al, 2001). These metabolic abnormalities presumably occur from decreased glycogen stores, inadequate lipid stores, and impaired gluconeogenesis in the growth-restricted neonate. Growth-restricted neonates have inadequate fuel stores and are at increased risk for hypoglycemia during fasting, and these risks are increased in preterm SGA infants. Infants with IUGR also have a higher incidence of hypocalcemia, with the incidence correlating strongly with the severity of growth restriction (Spinillo et al, 1995).

Developmental Outcomes: Early Childhood

Neurologic outcomes, including intellectual and neurologic function, are affected by growth restriction. Overall, neurologic morbidity is higher for SGA infants than for AGA infants. Without identified perinatal events, SGA infants have a higher incidence of long-term neurologic or developmental handicaps. Investigators have found the incidence of cerebral palsy to be greater in IUGR infants than in a population with normal fetal growth (Blair and Stanley, 1990; Spinillo et al, 1995; Uvebrant and Hagberg, 1992). SGA infants born at term appear to have double or triple the risk for cerebral palsy, between 1 to 2 per 1000 live births and 2 to 6 per 1000 live births (Goldenberg et al, 1998). The rate of cerebral palsy is also higher in preterm growth-restricted infants than in preterm infants with appropriate fetal growth (Gray et al, 2001). At 7 years of age, children whose birth was associated with hypoxia-related factors had a higher risk for adverse neurologic outcomes. Infants with symmetric IUGR, or perhaps more severe restriction, were at higher risk than infants with asymmetric IUGR. Other researchers have shown higher rates of learning deficits, lower intelligence quotient scores, and increased behavioral problems in children with a history of fetal growth restriction, even at 9 to 11 years of age (Low et al, 1992).

LONG-TERM CONSEQUENCES: THE DEVELOPMENTAL ORIGINS OF ADULT DISEASE

Programming

The period from conception to birth is a time of rapid growth, cellular replication and differentiation, and functional maturation of organ systems. These processes are highly sensitive to alterations in the intrauterine milieu. The term *programming* describes the mechanisms whereby a stimulus or insult at a critical period of development has lasting or lifelong effects. The "thrifty phenotype" hypothesis proposes that the fetus adapts to an adverse intrauterine milieu by optimizing the use of a reduced nutrient supply to ensure survival; but because this adaptation favors the development of certain organs over that of others, it leads to persistent alterations in the growth and function of developing tissues (Hales and Barker, 1992). In addition, although the adaptations may aid in survival of the fetus, they become a liability in situations of nutritional abundance.

Epidemiology

It has been recognized for nearly 70 years that the early environment in which a child grows and develops can have long-term effects on subsequent health and survival (Kermack, 1934). The landmark cohort study of 300,000 men by Ravelli et al (1976) showed that men who were exposed in utero to the effects of the Dutch famine of 1944 and 1945 during the first half of gestation had significantly higher obesity rates at the age of 19 years. Subsequent studies demonstrated relationships among LBW, the later development of cardiovascular disease (Barker et al, 1989), and impaired glucose tolerance (Fall et al, 1995) in men in England. Men who were smallest at birth (2500 g) were nearly sevenfold more likely to have impaired glucose tolerance or type 2 diabetes than those who were largest at birth. Barker et al (1993) also found a similar relationship between lower birthweight and higher systolic blood pressure and triglyceride levels.

Valdez et al (1994) observed a similar association between birthweight and subsequent glucose intolerance, hypertension, and hyperlipidemia in a study of young adult Mexican American and non-Hispanic white men and women participants in the San Antonio Heart Study. Normotensive individuals without diabetes whose birthweights were in the lowest tertile had significantly higher rates of insulin resistance, obesity, and hypertension than subjects whose birthweights were normal. In the Pima Indians, a population with extraordinarily high rates of type 2

diabetes, McCance et al (1994) found that the development of diabetes in the offspring was related to both extremes of birthweight. In their study, the prevalence of diabetes in subjects 20 to 39 years old was 30% for those weighing less than 2500 g at birth, 17% for those weighing 2500 to 4499 g, and 32% for those weighing 4500 g or more. The risk of developing type 2 diabetes was nearly fourfold higher for those whose birthweight was less than 2500 g. Other studies of populations in the United States (Curhan et al, 1996), Sweden (Lithell et al, 1996; McKeigue et al, 1998), France (Jaquet et al, 2000; Leger et al, 1997), Norway (Egeland et al, 2000), and Finland (Forsen et al, 2000) have all demonstrated a significant correlation between LBW and the later development of adult diseases.

Studies controlling for the confounding factors of socioeconomic status and lifestyle have further strengthened the association between LBW and a higher risk of coronary heart disease, stroke, and type 2 diabetes. In 1976, the Nurses' Health Study was initiated, and a large cohort of American women born from 1921 to 1946 established. The association between LBW and increased risks of coronary heart disease, stroke, and type 2 diabetes remained strong even after adjustment for lifestyle factors such as smoking, physical activity, occupation, income, dietary habits, and childhood socioeconomic status (Rich-Edwards et al, 1999).

Role of Catch-up Growth

Many studies have suggested that the associations between birth size with later disease can be modified by body mass index (BMI) in childhood. The highest risk for the development of type 2 diabetes is among adults who were born small and become overweight during childhood (Eriksson et al, 2000). Insulin resistance is most prominent in Indian children who were SGA at birth, but had a high fat mass at 8 years of age (Bavdekar et al, 1999). Similar findings were reported in 10-year-old children in the United Kingdom (Whincup et al, 1997). In a Finnish cohort, adult hypertension was associated with both lower birthweight and accelerated growth in the first 7 years of life. In contrast, in two preliminary studies from the United Kingdom, catch-up growth in the first 6 months of life was not clearly related to blood pressure in young adulthood, although birthweight was (McCarthy et al, 2001).

Interpreting the findings of these studies is complicated by the vague definitions of *catch-up growth*. The term, which can encompass either the first 6 to 12 months only or as much as the first 2 years after birth, usually refers to realignment of genetic growth potential after IUGR. This definition allows for fetal growth retardation at any birthweight; large fetuses can be growth retarded in relation to their genetic potential. However, postnatal factors can obviously affect infant growth in the first few months of life. For example, breastfeeding appears to protect against obesity later in childhood, but breastfed infants usually exhibit higher body mass during the first year of life than formula-fed infants. Although it is likely that accelerated growth confers an additional risk to the growth-retarded fetus, these conflicting results demonstrate the need for additional, carefully designed studies to determine how childhood growth rates affect the later development of cardiovascular disease and type 2 diabetes.

Size at Birth, Insulin Secretion, and Insulin Action

The mechanisms underlying the association between size at birth and impaired glucose tolerance or type 2 diabetes are unclear. A number of studies in children and adults have shown that nondiabetic or prediabetic (abnormal glucose tolerance) subjects with LBW are insulin resistant and thus are predisposed to development of type 2 diabetes (Bavdekar et al, 1999; Clausen et al, 1997; Flanagan et al, 2000; Hoffman et al, 1997; Leger et al, 1997; Li et al, 2001; Lithell et al, 1996; McKeigue et al, 1998; Phillips et al, 1994; Yajnik et al, 1995). IUGR is known to alter the fetal development of adipose tissue, which is closely linked to the development of insulin resistance (Lapillonne et al, 1997; Widdowson et al, 1979). In a well-designed case-control study of 25-year-old adults, Jaquet et al (2000) demonstrated that individuals who were born SGA at 37 weeks' gestation or later had a significantly higher percentage of body fat (15%). Insulin sensitivity, after adjustment for BMI or total fat mass, was markedly impaired in these SGA subjects. There were no significant differences between the SGA and control groups regarding parental history of type 2 diabetes, cardiovascular disease, hypertension, or dyslipidemia. Of importance when generalizing the findings to other populations, the causes of IUGR in these subjects were gestational hypertension (50%), smoking (30%), maternal short stature (7%), congenital anomalies (7%), and unknown (6%).

The adverse effect of IUGR on glucose homeostasis was originally thought to be mediated through programming of the fetal endocrine pancreas. Growth-retarded fetuses and newborns have been shown to have a reduced population of pancreatic β cells (Van Assche et al, 1977). LBW has been associated with reduced insulin response after glucose ingestion in young men without diabetes; however, a number of other studies have found no effect of LBW on insulin secretion in humans (Clausen et al, 1997; Flanagan et al, 2000; Lithell et al, 1996). However, none of these earlier studies adjusted for the corresponding insulin sensitivity, which has a profound effect on insulin secretion. Jensen et al (2002) measured insulin secretion and insulin sensitivity in a well-matched population of 19-year-old, glucose-tolerant white men whose birthweights were either less than the 10th percentile (i.e., SGA) or between the 50th and 75th percentiles (controls). To eliminate the major confounding factors, such as "diabetes genes," the researchers ensured that none of the participants had a family history of diabetes, hypertension, or ischemic heart disease. They found no differences between the groups in regard to current weight, BMI, body composition, and lipid profile. When data were controlled for insulin sensitivity, insulin secretion was found to be lower by 30%. However, insulin sensitivity was normal in the SGA subjects. These investigators hypothesized that defects in insulin secretion precede defects in insulin action, and that SGA individuals demonstrate insulin resistance once they accumulate body fat.

Epidemiologic Challenges

The data described in the preceding section suggest that LBW is associated with glucose intolerance, type 2 diabetes, and cardiovascular disease. However, the question remains whether these associations reflect fetal nutrition or other factors that contribute to birthweight and the observed glucose intolerance. Because of the retrospective nature of the cohort identification, many confounding variables were not always recorded, such as lifestyle, socioeconomic status, education, maternal age, parental build, birth order, obstetric complications, smoking, and maternal health. Maternal nutritional status, either directly in the form of diet histories, or indirectly in the form of BMI, height, and pregnancy weight gain, were usually not recorded. Instead, birth anthropometric measures were used as proxies for presumed undernutrition in pregnancy.

Size at Birth Cannot Be Used as a Proxy for Fetal Growth

Birthweight is determined by the sum of multiple known and unknown factors, including gestational age, maternal age, birth order, genetics, maternal pre-pregnancy BMI, and pregnancy weight gain, plus multiple environmental factors, such as smoking, drug use, infection, and maternal hypertension. Some of these determinants may be related to susceptibility to adult disease, and others may not. Conversely, some prenatal determinants of adult outcomes may not be related to fetal growth. A good example of how size at birth may potentially be a proxy for an underlying causal pathway is the hypothesis that essential hypertension in the adult is caused by a congenital nephron deficit (Brenner and Chertow, 1993). This study shows that kidney volume is smaller in adults who were thinner at birth, after adjustment for current body size. In contrast, maternal cigarette smoking is a good example of a prenatal exposure that restricts fetal growth, but to date no association has been found between cigarette smoking and adverse long-term outcome in offspring.

Genetics versus Environment

Several epidemiologic and metabolic studies of twins and first-degree relatives of patients with type 2 diabetes have demonstrated an important genetic component of diabetes (Vaag et al, 1995). The association between LBW and risk of type 2 diabetes in some studies could theoretically be explained by a genetically determined reduced fetal growth rate. In other words, the genotype responsible for type 2 diabetes may itself restrict fetal growth. This possibility forms the basis for the fetal insulin hypothesis, which suggests that genetically determined insulin resistance could result in insulin-mediated low growth rate in utero as well as insulin resistance in childhood and adulthood (Hattersley et al, 1999). Insulin is one of the major growth factors in fetal life, and monogenic disorders that affect the fetus's insulin secretion or insulin resistance also affect fetal growth (Elsas et al, 1985; Froguel et al, 1993; Hattersley et al, 1998; Stoffers et al, 1997). Mutations in the gene encoding glucokinase have been identified that result in LBW and maturity-onset diabetes of the young. Such mutations are rare, and no analogous common allelic variation has been discovered, but it is likely that some variations exist that, once identified, will help to explain a proportion of the cases of diabetes in LBW subjects.

There is obviously a close relationship between genes and the environment. Maternal gene expression can alter the fetal environment, and the maternal intrauterine environment also affects fetal gene expression. An adverse intrauterine milieu is likely to have profound long-term effects on the developing organism that might not be reflected in birthweight.

Cellular Mechanisms

Fetal malnutrition has two main causes: poor maternal nutrition and placental insufficiency. In the extensive literature about the fetal origins hypothesis, these two concepts have not been discerned clearly. Such a distinction is necessary, because maternal nutrition has probably been adequate in the majority of populations in which the hypothesis has been tested. Only extreme maternal undernutrition, such as occurred in the Dutch famine, reduces the birthweight to an extent that could be expected to raise the risk of adult disease (Lumey et al, 1995). To a lesser extent but equally important is the LBW in populations with low resources, resulting in maternal undernutrition. Overall, in most populations it is reasonable that placental insufficiency has been a main cause of LBW. The oxygen and nutrients that support fetal growth and development rely on the entire nutrient supply line, beginning with maternal consumption and body size, but extending to uterine perfusion, placental function, and fetal metabolism. Interruptions of the supply line at any point could result in programming of the fetus for the future risk of adult diseases.

The intrauterine environment influences development of the fetus by modifying gene expression in both pluripotential cells and terminally differentiated, poorly replicating cells. The long-range effects on the offspring (into adulthood) are determined by which cells are undergoing differentiation, proliferation, or functional maturation at the time of the disturbance in maternal fuel economy. The fetus also adapts to an inadequate supply of substrates (e.g., glucose, amino acids, fatty acids, and oxygen) through metabolic changes, redistribution of blood flow, and changes in the production of fetal and placental hormones that control fetal growth.

The fetus's immediate metabolic response to placental insufficiency is catabolism, consuming its own substrates to provide energy. A more prolonged reduction in availability of substrates leads to slowed growth, which enhances the fetus's ability to survive by reducing the use of substrates and lowering the metabolic rate. Slowed growth in late gestation leads to disproportionate organ size, because the organs and tissues that are growing rapidly at the time are affected the most. For example, placental insufficiency in late gestation can lead to reduced growth of the kidney, which is developing rapidly at that time. Reduced replication of kidney cells can permanently reduce cell numbers, because there seems to be no capacity for renal cell division to catch up after birth.

Substrate availability has profound effects on fetal hormones and on the hormonal and metabolic interactions among the fetus, placenta, and mother. These effects are most apparent in the fetus of the mother with diabetes. Higher maternal concentrations of glucose and amino acids stimulate the fetal pancreas to secrete exaggerated amounts of insulin and stimulate the fetal liver to produce higher levels of insulin-like growth factors. Fetal hyperinsulinism stimulates the growth of adipose tissue and other insulin-responsive tissues in the fetus, often leading to macrosomia. However, many offspring of mothers with diabetes with fetal hyperinsulinism are not overgrown by usual standards, and many with later obesity and glucose intolerance were not macrosomic at birth (Pettitt et al, 1987; Silverman et al, 1995). These observations suggest that birthweight is not a good indication of intrauterine nutrition.

MACROSOMIA

Excessive fetal growth (macrosomia, being large for gestational age) is found in 9% to 13% of all deliveries and can lead to significant complications in the perinatal period (Gregory et al, 1998; Wollschlaeger et al, 1999). Maternal factors associated with macrosomia during pregnancy include increasing parity, higher maternal age, and maternal height. In addition, the previous delivery of an infant with macrosomia, prolonged pregnancy, maternal glucose intolerance, high pre-pregnancy weight or obesity, and large pregnancy weight gain have all been found to raise the risk of delivering an infant with macrosomia (Mocanu et al, 2000).

Maternal complications of macrosomia include morbidities related to labor and delivery. Prolonged labor, arrest of labor, and higher rates of cesarean section and instrumentation during labor have been reported. In addition, the risks of maternal lacerations and trauma, delayed placental detachment, and postpartum hemorrhage are higher for the woman delivering an infant with macrosomia (Lipscomb et al, 1995; Perlow et al, 1996). Complications of labor are more pronounced in primiparous women than in multiparous women (Mocanu et al, 2000). The neonatal complications of macrosomia include traumatic events such as shoulder dystocia, brachial nerve palsy, birth trauma, and associated perinatal asphyxia. Other complications for the neonate are elevated insulin levels and metabolic derangements, such as hypoglycemia and hypocalcemia (Wollschlaeger et al, 1999). In a large population-based study in the United States, macrosomia (defined as birthweight greater than 4000 g) was detected in 13% of births. Of these, shoulder dystocia was noted in 11% (Gregory et al, 1998).

Macrosomia is often not detected during pregnancy and labor. The clinical estimation of fetal size is difficult and has significant false-positive and false-negative rates. Ultrasonography estimates of fetal weight are not always accurate, and there are a wide range of sensitivity estimates for the ultrasound detection of macrosomia. In addition, there is controversy regarding how to define macrosomia and which ultrasound measurement is most sensitive in predicting macrosomia. Smith et al (1997) demonstrated a linear relation between abdominal circumference and birthweight. They showed that the equations commonly used for estimated fetal weight have a median error rate of 7%, with greater errors seen with larger infants. Using receiver operating characteristics curves to measure the diagnostic accuracy of ultrasound,

O'Reilly-Green and Divon (1997) reported sensitivity and specificity rates of 85% and 72%, respectively, for estimation of birthweight exceeding 4000 g. In their study, the positive predictive value (i.e., a positive test result represents a truly macrosomic infant) was approximately 49%. Chauhan et al (2000) found lower sensitivity for the use of ultrasound measurement of abdominal and head circumference and femur length (72% sensitivity), similar to the sensitivity of using clinical measurements alone (73%). Other investigators have shown that clinical estimation of fetal weight (43% sensitivity) has higher sensitivity and specificity than ultrasound evaluation in predicting macrosomia (Gonen et al, 1996). In a retrospective study, Jazayeri et al (1999) showed that ultrasound measurement of abdominal circumference of greater than 35 cm predicts macrosomia in 93% of cases and is superior to measurements of biparietal diameter or the femur. Other researchers have reported that an abdominal circumference of more than 37 cm is a better predictor (Al-Inany et al, 2001; Gilby et al, 2000).

Numerous investigators have also questioned whether antenatal diagnosis improves birth outcomes in macrosomic infants. Investigators indicate the low rates of specificity of antenatal tests resulting in high rates of false-positive results (Bryant et al, 1998, O'Reilly-Green and Divon, 1997). Antenatal identification of macrosomia or possible macrosomia can lead to a higher rate of cesarean section performed for infants with normal birthweights (Gonen et al, 2000; Mocanu et al, 2000; Parry et al, 2000). Macrosomia is a risk factor for shoulder dystocia, but the majority of cases of shoulder dystocia and birth trauma occur in infants with macrosomia (Gonen et al, 1996). A retrospective study of infants weighing more than 4200 g at birth showed a cesarean section rate of 52% in infants predicted antenatally to have macrosomia, compared with 30% in infants without such an antenatal prediction. The antenatal prediction of fetal macrosomia is also associated with a higher incidence of failed induction of labor and no reduction in the rate of shoulder dystocia (Zamorski and Biggs, 2001). Using retrospective data from a 12-year period, Bryant et al (1998) estimated that a policy of routine cesarean section for all infants with estimated fetal weight greater than 4500 g would require between 155 and 588 cesarean sections to prevent a single case of permanent brachial nerve palsy.

SUMMARY

This chapter has described many identified biologic and genetic factors associated with fetal growth and with abnormalities of fetal growth. Physicians are limited in the ability to identify a causative agent in every case. Modification of fetal growth is possible and occurs from diverse influences such as socioeconomic status, maternal nutrition, and maternal constitutional factors. Abnormal fetal growth influences acute perinatal outcomes and health during infancy, childhood, and adulthood. In schools of public health, students are taught to search "up river" for solutions to health problems. Solutions for ill health in adulthood may reside in the identification of methods to improve the health of the fetus.

SUGGESTED READINGS

Alexander GR, Himes JH, Kaufman R, et al: A United States national reference for fetal growth, *Obstet Gynecol* 87:163-168, 1996.
Dahri S, Snoeck A, Reusens-Billen B, et al: Islet function in off-spring of mothers on low-protein diet during gestation, *Diabetes* 40:115-120, 1991.
Wilson MR, Hughes SJ: The effect of maternal protein deficiency during pregnancy and lactation on glucose tolerance and pancreatic islet function in adult rat offspring, *J Endocrinology* 154:177-185, 1997.
Zeitlin J, Ancel P, Saurel-Cibizolles M, Papiernik E: The relationship between IUGR and preterm delivery: an empirical approach using data from a European case-control study, *Brit J Obstet Gynecol* 107:750-758, 2000.

Complete references used in this text can be found online at www.expertconsult.com

MULTIPLE GESTATIONS AND ASSISTED REPRODUCTIVE TECHNOLOGY

Kerri Marquard and Kelle Moley

EPIDEMIOLOGY OF MULTIPLES

Since the birth of the first in vitro fertilization (IVF) baby in 1978, the numbers of IVF clinics, ovarian stimulation cycles, and live births from assisted reproductive technology (ART) have all steadily increased. Between 1998 and 2003, total births in the United States increased by 4%, while ART births grew by 67% (Dickey, 2007). The growing use of ART, in addition to delayed childbearing until age-related fertility issues become apparent, has contributed greatly to multiple birth rates. In 2006 ART infants accounted for 1% of all U.S. births, but represented 17% of twins and 38% of triplets or greater (Centers for Disease Control and Prevention et al, 2008; Sunderam et al, 2009). Three percent of all U.S. births are multiples, yet in 2003 ART multiple live birth rates from fresh nondonor, donor oocyte, and frozen embryo transfer cycles were 34%, 40%, and 25%, respectively (Centers for Disease Control and Prevention et al, 2008).

The assisted conception and spontaneous rates associated with twins, triplets, and higher-order multiples (HOMs; i.e., four or more fetuses) are as follows. In 2003, 62.7%, 16.3%, and 21% of twins were conceived naturally, from ART, and from non-ART ovulation induction, respectively. For triplets in the same year, 17.7% were natural conceptions, 45.4% were from ART, and 36.9% were from non-ART ovulation induction. HOM rates from spontaneous conception, ART, and non-ART ovulation induction were 8%, 30%, and 62.4%, respectively (Dickey, 2007). Given the maternal, perinatal, and neonatal complications associated with multiples, the goal of infertility treatment is one healthy child. Multifetal pregnancies drastically affect individuals, families, and the public health system. Of particular importance in both maternal and fetal outcomes are fetal number and placentation.

DIAGNOSING ZYGOSITY AND CHORIONICITY

Determining zygosity and chorionicity is important medically, genetically, and psychosocially for the individual and family. More immediately, the chorion-amnion arrangement is crucial to antepartum management in cases of one fetal demise or selective reduction, and because of potential associated problems such as twin-twin transfusion syndrome (TTTS), growth discordance, intrauterine growth restriction (IUGR), congenital anomalies, and cord accidents. Diagnosing zygosity is possible using ultrasound markers including the number of placental sites, thickness of dividing membrane, the lambda sign, and fetal gender in addition to postpartum placental examination, physical similarity questionnaires, blood type, and DNA analysis (Hall, 2003; Ohm Kyvik and Derom, 2006; Scardo

et al, 1995) At 10 to 14 weeks' gestation, ultrasound criteria correctly diagnosed chorionicity in 99.3% of cases as confirmed by postpartum placental examination and gender (Carroll et al, 2002). Assessment of zygosity and chorionicity in 237 same-sex twins with physical likeness questionnaires, DNA analysis, and placental inspection accurately diagnosed 96% of twin pairs (Forget-Dubois et al, 2003).

ZYGOSITY AND CHORIONICITY

Zygosity and placentation affect fetal morbidity and mortality in multifetal pregnancies. Dizygotic twins (DZTs), which comprise 67% of spontaneous twins, arise from the fertilization of two separate eggs by different sperm (Gibbs et al, 2008), and with few exceptions they lead to a dichorionic diamniotic arrangement in which the placenta can be separate or fused. A rare case of dizygotic monochorionic (MC) diamniotic (DA) twins has been reported (Souter et al, 2003). The overall DZT rate varies from 4 to 50 per 1000 worldwide: 1.3% in Japan, 7.1% to 11% in the United States, 8.1% in India, 8.8% in England and Wales, and 49% in Nigeria (Table 7-1) (MacGillivray, 1986). Risk factors for DZT include advancing maternal age, increased parity, female relatives with DZT, taller height, and larger body mass index (Hoekstra et al, 2008; MacGillivray, 1986).

The true incidence of monozygotic twins (MZTs) is difficult to ascertain because of its rarity, inaccuracies in diagnosis, and lack of confirmatory studies at birth, but spontaneous MZT rates are estimated to occur in 0.3% to 0.5% of all pregnancies and in 30% of all twins (Bulmer, 1970; MacGillivray, 1986). Unlike DZT, it is unclear whether MZT is related to genetics or environment (Bortolus et al, 1999; Hoekstra et al, 2008), although familial components may play a role (Hamamy et al, 2004). Chorionicity in monozygotic gestations is determined by the

TABLE 7-1 Twinning Rates per 1000 Births by Zygosity

Country	Monozygotic	Dizygotic	Total
Nigeria	5.0	49	54
United States			
African American	4.7	11.1	15.8
Caucasian	4.2	7.1	11.3
England and Wales	3.5	8.8	12.3
India	3.3	8.1	11.4
Japan	3.0	1.3	4.3

From MacGillivray I: Epidemiology of twin pregnancy, *Semin Perinatol,* 10:4-8, 1986; and Cunningham FG, Hauth JC, Wenstrom KD, et al, editors: *Williams obstetrics,* ed 22, New York, 2005, McGraw-Hill.

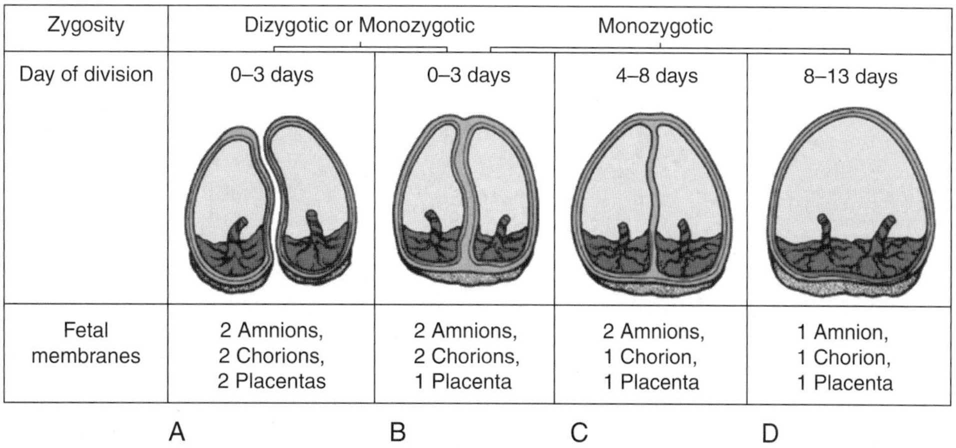

Zygosity	Dizygotic or Monozygotic		Monozygotic	
Day of division	0–3 days	0–3 days	4–8 days	8–13 days
Fetal membranes	2 Amnions, 2 Chorions, 2 Placentas	2 Amnions, 2 Chorions, 1 Placenta	2 Amnions, 1 Chorion, 1 Placenta	1 Amnion, 1 Chorion, 1 Placenta
	A	B	C	D

FIGURE 7-1 Placentation and membranes based on timing of embryonic division. A, Two amnions, two chorions, and separate placentas from the division of either a dizygotic or monozygotic embryo within 3 days of fertilization. **B,** Two amnions, two chorions, and one fused placenta from the division of either a dizygotic or monozygotic embryo within 3 days of fertilization. **C,** Two amnions, one chorion, and one placenta from monozygotic embryonic cleavage, days 4 to 8 after fertilization. **D,** One amnion, one chorion, and one placenta from a monozygotic embryo splitting, days 8 to 13 after fertilization. *(Modified from Gibbs R, Karlan B, Haney A, et al:* Danforth's obstetrics & gynecology, *ed 10, Philadelphia, 2008, Lippincott, Williams & Wilkins.)*

timing of the embryonic division (Figures 7-1 and 7-2) (Benirschke and Kim, 1973; Hall, 2003). In 18% to 36% of MZTs, the zygote divides within 72 hours of fertilization resulting in dichorionic (DC) DA gestation (the placenta can be separate or fused); 60% to 75% split between days 4 and 8, leading to an MC-DA unit, and 1% to 2% separate between days 8 and 13, leading to an MC monoamniotic (MA) pregnancy. Embryonic division after day 13 results in conjoined twins with an MC/MA placenta (Cunningham et al, 2005; Gibbs et al, 2008; Hall, 2003).

Although the majority of ART MZTs are MC/DA, any of the three MZ placental arrangements can transpire after ART, implying that the timing and mechanism of embryonic splitting are variable (Aston et al, 2008; Knopman et al, 2009). Monozygotic DCDA twins can occur after inner cell mass (ICM) splitting and atypical hatching in a blastocyst embryo (Meintjes et al, 2001; Van Langendonckt et al, 2000). In addition, MA twinning may be increased after IVF (Alikani et al, 2003) and zona pellucida (ZP) manipulation (Slotnick and Ortega, 1996). Contributing factors to MZT in ART include ICM damage and other ZP abnormalities (Hall, 2003).

INCREASE IN MONOZYGOTIC TWINS WITH ASSISTED REPRODUCTIVE TECHNOLOGY

The first reported association between ART and MZT (Yovich et al, 1984) preceded numerous accounts of similar findings. The majority (>90%) of ART twins are dizygotic (Gibbs et al, 2008) secondary to transferring multiple embryos; however, the rate of MZTs per pregnancy after fertility treatment is higher (0.9% to 4.9%) (Alikani et al, 2003; Blickstein et al, 2003; Elizur et al, 2004; Knopman et al, 2009; Papaniklaou et al, 2009; Schachter et al, 2001; Sharara and Abdo, 2010; Sills et al, 2000; Vitthala et al, 2009; Wenstrom et al, 1993) versus the general population (0.3% to 0.5%) (Bulmer, 1970; MacGillivray, 1986). Several theories to explain the mechanism responsible for elevated MZTs with ART have been proposed.

AGE

Maternal age affects fertility and reproductive outcomes. Spontaneous dizygotic twinning increases with advancing maternal age (Bortolus et al, 1999; Bulmer, 1970; MacGillivray, 1986), but the connection between age and MZTs is controversial. Some studies reported trends toward elevated MZT rates in older women (Abusheikha et al, 2000; Alikani et al, 2003; Bulmer, 1970), whereas others found no association with increasing maternal age and MZT (Bortolus et al, 1999; Skiadas et al, 2008), and one study found that the MZT risk doubles in women younger than 35 years (Knopman et al, 2009). Overall, the correlation between age and MZT in ART remains unclear.

ZONA PELLUCIDA MANIPULATION

The ZP, an acellular protein surrounding the ovum, provides a species-specific sperm barrier and decreases polyploidy by inhibiting penetration by multiple sperm (Speroff and Fritz, 2005). Components of both ART and non-ART procedures are capable of modifying this barrier. Stimulation protocol, elevated follicle-stimulating hormone or estradiol levels, and prolonged culture conditions can change ZP thickness (Loret et al, 1997). In addition, ZP manipulations performed during IVF all potentially affect MZT risk.

Manipulation of the ZP in IVF occurs via both intracytoplasmic sperm injection (ICSI) and AH (assisted hatching). The injection of one sperm into a mature oocyte (i.e., ICSI) is most commonly performed for male factor infertility. AH is achieved with an artificial breach in the ZP by laser, chemical, or mechanical methods and is indicated in patients with a poor prognosis (Practice Committee of Society for Assisted Reproductive Technology and Practice Committee of American Society for Reproductive Medicine, 2008c). Some studies indicate no association with ICSI or AH and MZT (Behr et al, 2000; Elizur et al, 2004; Knopman et al, 2009; Meldrum et al, 1998; Milki et al, 2003; Sills et al, 2000), whereas others imply that

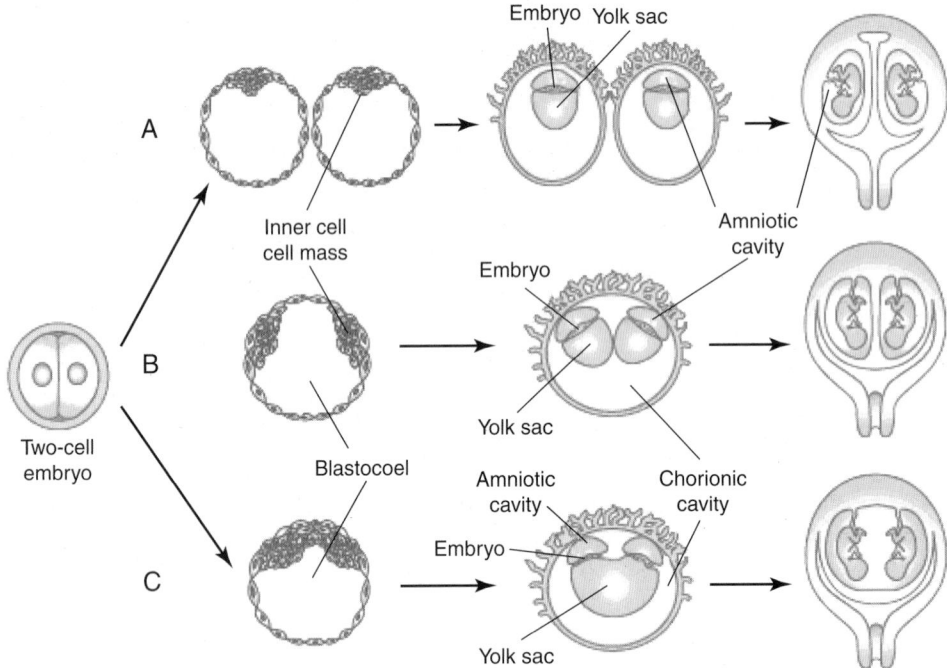

FIGURE 7-2 Types of monozygotic placentation. A, Dichorionic diamniotic pregnancy. **B,** Monochorionic diamniotic pregnancy. **C,** Monochorionic monoamniotic pregnancy. *(Adapted from Hall JG: Twinning,* Lancet *362:735-743, 2003; and Benirschke K, Kim CK: Multiple pregnancy,* N Engl J Med *288:1276-1284, 1973.)*

ZP manipulation increases the risk of MZT (Alikani et al, 1994; Saito et al, 2000; Schieve et al, 2000; Skiadas et al, 2008; Vitthala et al, 2009), particularly if multiple embryos undergo hatching before transfer (Alikani et al, 2003; Schieve et al, 2000). The results of a Cochrane review on the risk of multiples with AH and ICSI reported increased multiples with both ICSI and AH, and elevated MZT with AH versus no manipulation (0.8%) (Das et al, 2009). Alterations in ZP thickness or abnormal ICM splitting or embryo hatching in both animal (Cohen, 1991; Malter and Cohen, 1989) and human embryos may explain this increase in MZT after ZP manipulation (Alikani et al, 1994; Cohen, 1991; Malter and Cohen, 1989; Sheen et al, 2001).

BLASTOCYST TRANSFER

After oocyte retrieval and insemination, embryos undergo intrauterine transfer at either the cleavage stage (day 2 to 3 after retrieval) or the blastocyst stage (day 5 to 6 after retrieval). Blastocyst-stage embryo transfer produces higher pregnancy rates (29.4% vs 36%) (Blake et al, 2007) and may lower overall multiple rates (Frattarelli et al, 2003), but evidence supports the increased incidence of MZTs (Behr et al, 2000; Chang et al, 2009; Jain et al, 2004; Knopman et al, 2009; Peramo et al, 1999; Practice Committee of American Society for Reproductive Medicine and Practice Committee of Society for Assisted Reproductive Technology, 2008a; Sheiner et al, 2001; Skiadas et al, 2008; Wright et al, 2004) compared with cleavage-stage embryos. One institution initially noted increased MZT after blastocyst transfer (5.6% vs 2%; Milki et al, 2003), but a follow-up study 3 years later demonstrated similar MZT rates between blastocyst and day 3 embryos (2.3% vs 1.8%), indicating that changes in

culture media and an experienced embryology team may affect the rate of MZTs (Moayeri et al, 2007).

Culture media or prolonged culture may influence MZTs with blastocyst transfer in both human and animal models. Elevated glucose levels in extended culture and subsequent glucose-induced apoptotic remodeling of the ICM (Cassuto et al, 2003; Menezo and Sakkas, 2002), and ICM splitting in extended culture in murine and human embryos are both explanations for the phenomenon of MZTs in blastocysts (Chida, 1990; Hsu and Gonda, 1980; Payne et al, 2007). Whether MZT rates are elevated with blastocyst transfer (Behr et al, 2000; Chang et al, 2009; Jain et al, 2004; Knopman et al, 2009; Peramo et al, 1999; Practice Committee of American Society for Reproductive Medicine and Practice Committee of Society for Assisted Reproductive Technology, 2008a; Sheiner et al, 2001; Skiadas et al, 2008; Wright et al, 2004), or similar to cleavage-stage transfer (Frattarelli et al, 2003; Papanikolaou et al, 2006, 2010; Sharara and Abdo, 2010), the explicit role of culture media remains to be determined. Another environmental factor that may affect MZTs is temperature variation in frozen-thawed embryo cycles. Although minute evidence links frozen embryo transfers and temperature fluctuations to MZTs (Belaisch-Allart et al, 1995; Faraj et al, 2008; Toledo, 2005), most studies show no difference between fresh and frozen-thawed embryos and multiple rates (Blickstein et al, 2003) or MZT rates (Alikani et al, 2003; Knopman et al, 2009; Sills et al, 2000a, 2000b).

OVARIAN STIMULATION

Human studies of ovarian stimulation with clomiphene citrate and gonadotropins reveal a higher rate (1.2%) of MZTs compared with the expected rates in the general population (Derom et al, 1987). MZT incidences of 1.5% after ovulation induction with gonadotropins, 0.72% after IVF, and 0.87% with IVF ICSI-AH suggests that gonadotropins elevate MZTs regardless of ZP manipulation (Schachter et al, 2001). Ovulation induction medications may cause uneven hardening of the ZP and atypical blastocyst hatching thereby increasing the chance of MZTs (Derom et al, 1987).

FETAL COMPLICATIONS ASSOCIATED WITH MULTIPLES

Singleton pregnancies after assisted conception have increased complications, including preterm delivery (<37 weeks' gestation), low birthweight (LBW) (Helmerhorst et al, 2004; Schieve et al, 2007), prolonged hospital stay (Schieve et al, 2007), cesarean deliveries, neonatal intensive care unit (NICU) admission, and mortality compared with spontaneous singletons (Helmerhorst et al, 2004). Some risk persists in an IVF singleton pregnancy, even after spontaneous reduction from two to three initial heartbeats to one heartbeat (Luke et al, 2009). Although singleton IVF births are associated with morbidity and mortality, assisted-conception multiple gestations comprise the majority of adverse maternal, perinatal, and neonatal outcomes.

Multiple pregnancies account for a small percentage of overall live births, but are responsible for a disproportionate amount of morbidity and mortality, largely because of intrauterine growth restriction and prematurity (Garite et al, 2004), including 13% of all preterm deliveries, 21% of all LBW infants, and 25% of all very LBW infants (Robinson et al, 2001). Compared with a singleton pregnancy, fetal and maternal complications are elevated in twins, and pregnancies with three fetuses or more have even greater morbidity and mortality rates (Table 7-2) (ACOG Practice Bulletin #56, 2004; Albrecht and Tomich, 1996; Elliott and Radin, 1992; Ettner et al, 1997; Grether et al, 1993; Kiely et al, 1992; Luke, 1994; Luke and Keith, 1992; Luke et al, 1996; Martin et al, 2003; Mauldin and Newman, 1998; McCormick et al, 1992; Newman et al, 1989; Seoud et al, 1992). Higher fetal number correlates with increased risk of growth restriction, earlier delivery, LBW, neonatal intensive care unit admission, length of stay, risk of major handicap and cerebral palsy, and death in first year of life (ACOG Practice Bulletin #56, 2004; Gardner et al, 1995; Garite et al, 2004).

The average gestational ages for twin, triplet, and quadruplet deliveries are 35.3, 32.2, and 29.9 weeks, respectively (ACOG Practice Bulletin #56, 2004), corresponding to NICU admission rates fivefold higher in twins and 17-fold higher in triplets and HOMs (Ross et al, 1999). Twins have an increased risk of intrauterine fetal demise (fourfold), intraventricular hemorrhage, sepsis, necrotizing enterocolitis, respiratory distress syndrome and neonatal death (sixfold) versus singletons, and surviving infants of preterm multifetal pregnancies have higher rates of developmental handicap (Gardner et al, 1995). A review of 100 triplet gestations (88 with assisted conception) revealed that 78% experienced preterm labor (PTL), 14% delivered before 28 weeks, 5% had congenital anomalies, and 9.7% died in the perinatal period (Devine et al, 2001).

TABLE 7-2 Morbidity and Mortality by Fetal Number

Characteristic	Twins	Triplets	Quadruplets
Average birthweight	2347 g	1687 g	1309 g
Average gestational age at delivery	35.3 wk	32.2 wk	29.9 wk
Percentage with growth restriction	14-25	50-60	50-60
Percentage requiring admission to neonatal intensive care unit	25	75	100
Average length of stay in neonatal intensive care unit	18 days	30 days	58 days
Percentage with major handicap	-	20	50
Risk of cerebral palsy	4 times more than singletons	17 times more than singletons	-
Risk of death by age 1 year	7 times higher than singletons	20 times higher than singletons	-

From ACOG Practice Bulletin #56: Multiple gestation: complicated twin, triplet, and high-order multifetal pregnancy, *Obstet Gynecol* 104:869-883, 2004.

Similar to ART singleton versus spontaneous singleton outcomes, ART multiples may have higher morbidity compared with spontaneous multiples. Assisted-conception twins are at increased risk for LBW (Luke et al, 2009), preterm delivery (Luke et al, 2009; Nassar et al, 2003), cesarean delivery (Helmerhorst et al, 2004; Nassar et al, 2003), NICU admission (Helmerhorst et al, 2004; Nassar et al, 2003; Pinborg et al, 2004), longer length of stay, respiratory distress syndrome (Nassar et al, 2003), and birthweight discordance (Pinborg et al, 2004) versus spontaneously conceived twins. Oftentimes with IVF, because of multiple embryos transferred or MZ splitting, there are multiple heartbeats on an initial ultrasound examination that ultimately spontaneously reduce; however, these pregnancies are still at risk for an adverse outcome. In twin IVF cycles with two initial heartbeats on early ultrasound versus three heartbeats that spontaneously reduced to two heartbeats, pregnancies with three heartbeats on an early examination had increased rates of preterm delivery (35%) and LBW (47%) (Luke et al, 2009).

In contrast, other studies suggest comparable outcomes in assisted conception and spontaneous multiples. Rates of pregnancy-induced hypertension, gestational diabetes mellitus (GDM), preterm premature rupture of membranes (PPROM), placenta previa, placental abruption (Nassar et al, 2003), congenital malformations (Nassar et al, 2003; Pinborg et al, 2004), and mortality (Pinborg et al, 2004) were similar in IVF twins versus spontaneous twins. Similarly, morbidity and mortality in ART triplets versus spontaneous triplets were comparable regarding the rates of PPROM, PTL, pregnancy-induced hypertension, GDM, gestational age at delivery, birthweight, and NICU admissions (Fitzsimmons et al, 1998).

Besides fetal number, another important factor in pregnancy outcome is placental arrangement. MC multiples

TABLE 7-3   Incidence of Twin Pregnancy Zygosity and Chorionicity With Corresponding Complications

Type of Twinning	Incidence (%)	Complication (%)		
		IUGR	Delivery <37 Weeks' Gestation	Perinatal Mortality
Dizygotic	67-70	25	40	10-12
Monozygotic	30-33	40	50	15-18
Diamniotic-dichorionic	18-36	30	40	18-20
Diamniotic-monochorionic	60-75	50	60	30-40
Monoamniotic-monochorionic	1-2	40	60-70	30-70

From Cunningham FG, Hauth JC, Wenstrom KD, et al, editors: *Williams obstetrics*, ed 22, New York, 2005, McGraw-Hill; originally from Manning FA: Fetal biophysical profile scoring. In *Fetal medicine: principles and practices*, Norwalk, Conn, 1995, Appleton & Lange.
IUGR, Intrauterine growth restriction.

experience higher rates of morbidity and mortality, largely because of placental factors (Table 7-3) (Cunningham et al, 2005; Gaziano et al, 2000; Hack et al, 2008; Manning, 1995). When Dube et al (2002) studied different chorionicity–zygosity groups (monozygotic monochorionic [MZMC], dizygotic dichorionic [DZDC], and monozygotic dichorionic [MZDC]) they found smaller birthweight, and IUGR, congenital anomalies, and perinatal death in the MZMC versus DZDC twins, whereas MZDC and DZDC risks were similar, implying that poor outcomes are related more to chorionicity than zygosity. Negative outcomes such as cerebral palsy, mental retardation, and death, measured at 1 year of life in MC twins, are elevated (10%) compared with DC twins (3.7%), the majority of which are caused by complications from TTTS (Minakami et al, 1999).

Both placental asymmetry and abnormal vascular anastomosis affect fetal morbidity and mortality. IUGR and growth discordance afflict both DC and MC pregnancies, but MC twins are more likely to have cord abnormalities, unequal placental distribution, and TTTS (Cleary-Goldman and D'Alton, 2008). TTTS, ranging in severity from oligohydramnios to hydrops and fetal death (Cleary-Goldman and D'Alton, 2008; Gaziano et al, 2000) occurs in 15% to 32% of MC pregnancies (Hack et al, 2008; Minakami et al, 1999). Mortality rates vary from 22% to 100% (Bajoria et al, 1995; Cleary-Goldman and D'Alton, 2008; Hack et al, 2008), and surviving infants are at risk for long-standing adverse neurologic outcomes (Cleary-Goldman and D'Alton, 2008).

MC-MA twins occur in 1 in 10,000 pregnancies, but they suffer the highest risk of perinatal morbidity and mortality (Cordero et al, 2006). Similar to other MC twins, MC-MA twins are susceptible to TTTS, growth discordance, IUGR, preterm delivery, and congenital anomalies, but they also face the unique complication of cord entanglement. These factors historically account for perinatal mortality rates of 30% to 70%; however, lower morbidity and mortality rates (8% to 23%) reported in recent articles (Allen et al, 2001; Cordero et al, 2006; Heyborne et al, 2005; Rodis et al, 1997; Roque et al, 2003) may be

attributed to increased prenatal diagnosis and fetal surveillance (Allen et al, 2001; Heyborne et al, 2005; Rodis et al, 1997).

MATERNAL COMPLICATIONS

Approximately 80% of multiples experience antepartum complications versus 25% of singletons (Norwitz et al, 2005), and hospitalization for hypertensive disorders, PTL, PPROM, placental abruption, and postpartum hemorrhage are elevated sixfold (ACOG Practice Bulletin #56, 2004). Mothers with two or more fetuses are at increased risk for myocardial infarction, left ventricular heart failure, pulmonary edema, GDM, operative vaginal or cesarean delivery, hysterectomy, blood transfusion, longer hospital stay, and the three major causes of maternal mortality: post partum hemorrhage, venous thromboembolism, and hypertensive disorders (Walker et al, 2004).

Stratified by fetal number, plurality correlates with maternal morbidity where quadruplets and other HOMs experience significantly increased maternal morbidity versus twins and triplets (Wen et al, 2004). Hypertensive disorders occur in 12% to 20% of twins, triplets, and quadruplets compared with 6.5% of singletons, HELLP syndrome increases with higher numbers of fetuses (Day et al, 2005), and twins with preeclampsia experience more complications than singletons with preeclampsia (Sibai et al, 2000). Results of a triplet cohort showed that 96% had maternal complications, 96% required antenatal hospitalization, one in four were diagnosed with preeclampsia, and 44% encountered postpartum complications (Devine et al, 2001).

PSYCHOSOCIAL FACTORS

As fetal number in an assisted conception pregnancy increases, parents report decreased quality of life, increased social stigma, increased difficulty meeting material family needs (Ellison et al, 2005; Roca de Bes et al, 2009), increased depression (Ellison et al, 2005; Olivennes et al, 2005; Sheard et al, 2007), decreased marital satisfaction (Roca de Bes et al, 2009), increased fatigue (Sheard et al, 2007) and stress (Golombok et al, 2007; Olivennes et al, 2005; Sheard et al, 2007). Part of this challenge lies in the fact that there are 168 hours in 1 week, but adequately caring for 6-month-old triplets and household activities requires 197.5 hours per week (Bryan, 2003). Multiple fetuses themselves face an increased risk of long-term disabilities that contribute to increased parental fatigue and depression, and overall siblings of multiples are more at risk for behavioral issues (Bryan, 2003).

Psychosocial consequences between naturally conceived multiples versus IVF multiples might differ. On the one hand, parents of IVF multiples can experience significantly more stress, increased child difficulty (Cook et al, 1998; Glazebrook et al, 2004), and increased dysfunctional parent-child interactions (Glazebrook et al, 2004) compared with spontaneous multiples. On the other hand, both ART and non-ART twin conceptions are more stressful for parents, creating higher levels of anxiety and depression compared with singletons (Vilska et al, 2009). Regardless of conception mode, multiples potentially have negative psychosocial effects on parents and families.

COST

Multiple gestations economically influence both the family and society. Preterm delivery, LBW, and postdischarge hospitalization are increased in multiple fetuses, all of which have a role in short- and long-term cost (Cuevas et al, 2005). Annually, neonatal health care consumes $10.2 billion in the Unites States, 57% of which comes from preterm infants (<37 weeks' gestation) who comprise less than 10% of live births (St. John et al, 2000). According to gestational age, the mean initial hospital charge for infants born between 26 and 28 weeks' gestation is approximately $240,000 compared with approximately $4800 for a term infant. By birthweight, infants weighing less than 1250 g cost approximately $250,000 compared with infants weighing more than 2500 g, who cost $5800 (Cuevas et al, 2005).

ART multiples and their associated comorbidities have a significant role in health care expenditures. In the United Kingdom, IVF-induced multiples account for 27% of pregnancies yearly, but represent 54% of expenditures (Ledger et al, 2006); this is due largely to IVF triplets and twins, which are remarkably more costly than IVF singletons from both neonatal and maternal standpoints. Estimated maternal cost ratios for IVF singleton:twin and singleton:triplet are approximately 1:1.94 and 1:3.96, respectively, and neonatal cost ratios for IVF singleton:twin and singleton:triplet are 1:16 and 1:109, respectively (Ledger et al, 2006). The cost for IVF triplets from diagnosis through 1 year of life is tenfold (Ledger et al, 2006), and IVF twin cost up to 6 weeks postpartum is fivefold versus IVF singletons (Lukassen et al, 2004). ART singletons are more costly than spontaneous singletons, possibly because of increased rates of LBW (Chambers et al, 2007) or the underlying infertility contributing to these outcomes (Koivurova et al, 2004). An Australian study comparing IVF singletons, twins, and HOMs to control counterparts revealed no significant cost differences between ART twins and non-ART twins or between ART HOMs and non-ART HOMs, but combined neonatal-maternal cost was 57% higher for ART births than for non-ART births (Chambers et al, 2007).

Because of the extreme economic cost of multiples, one proposed mechanism to reduce multifetal pregnancies is single embryo transfer (SET). Elective SET in first-cycle IVF patients costs less than double embryo transfer (DET) (Fiddelers et al, 2006; Gerris et al, 2004), and although SET produced lower live birth rates than DET in an unselected population (20.8% versus 39.6%) (Fiddelers et al, 2006), when stratified to less than 38 years age, SET and DET generate similar live birth rates (Gerris et al, 2004).

DECREASING THE RISK OF MULTIPLES

ART procedures and the rate of multiple pregnancies are rising concordantly. Although ART triplets and the incidence of HOMs has declined since 1996, ART twin rates

are unchanged.[2] Primary forms of preventing multiples include canceling ovulation induction cycles or converting to IVF, and in IVF cycles limiting the number of embryos transferred. Worldwide differences exist in medical practice and laws regarding restrictions on the number of embryos transferred.

The American Society for Reproductive Medicine (ASRM) and the Society for Assisted Reproductive Technology established transfer guidelines to assist in determining the appropriate embryo number in an attempt to decrease multiples. Recommended limits are based on age, prognosis, and embryo stage and further differentiate between a favorable patient (first IVF cycle, good quality embryos, number of embryos for potential cryopreservation, successful past IVF cycles) and less favorable conditions. To date there are no embryo transfer guidelines for frozen embryo cycles. Transfer recommendations by the ASRM are not legally binding, and they are subject to interpretation or adjustment based on clinical experience and unique patient instances (Practice Committee of Society for Assisted Reproductive Technology and Practice Committee of American Society for Reproductive Medicine, 2008b). Reduction of the number of embryos transferred and the incidence of triplets or greater in women aged 37 years or less from 1996 to 2003 may be attributed to a change in the 1998-1999 ASRM guidelines (Stern et al, 2007).

The most important factor involved in creating multiple fetuses is the number of embryos transferred. Given the emotional, physical, and financial burden of ART and the concern that only one embryo might lower pregnancy rates, multiples fetuses were previously accepted as a known risk in an effort to ensure a pregnancy. More recently, however, practitioners across the globe are stressing the impact of multiples and are encouraging SET (Gerris, 2005).

A Swedish study in women aged less than 36 years undergoing their first or second IVF cycle with two or more good-quality embryos were randomized to DET or SET followed by frozen-thawed embryo transfer if unsuccessful. Live birth rates were lower in the SET-alone versus the DET group, but SET followed by frozen-thawed embryo transfer resulted in a 38.8% live birth rate and a 0.8% multiple rate, compared with a 42.9% live birth rate and a 33.1% multiple rate in the DET group, showing that with SET pregnancy rates were acceptable and multiple pregnancy rates were significantly lower (Thurin et al, 2004). Women aged 36 to 39 years may also be candidates for SET, because similar live birth rates between SET and DET and significantly higher cumulative multiple rates occur in the DET (16.6%) versus SET (1.7%) groups (Veleva et al, 2006). Superb cryopreservation technique with frozen embryo transfer after SET in the appropriate patient lowers multiple fetus rates (Gerris, 2005) and leads to comparable cumulative LBR compared with DET (Veleva et al, 2009).

Consideration of multiples from non-ART ovulation induction by controlled ovarian hyperstimulation also merits discussion. Twenty-two percent of twins, 40% of triplets, and 71% of HOMs in 2004 were a result of non-ART ovulation induction (Dickey, 2009). During gonadotropin stimulation, follicular growth is supervised via ultrasound examination, and estradiol levels are monitored in an attempt to minimize overstimulation. Ovulation induction risk factors for multiples have revealed that HOMs are positively correlated with gonadotropin dose and stimulation length, estradiol levels greater than 1000 pg/mL, and seven or more follicles measuring 10 mm or greater, whereas negative predictors were age less than 32 years, lower body mass index, and a higher number of prior treatment cycles (Dickey, 2009). Techniques to reduce the chance of multiple fetuses include minimizing gonadotropin dose, canceling the cycle by discontinuing medications for excess follicles or high estradiol levels, or converting to IVF (Dickey, 2009; Nakhuda and Sauer, 2005); however, the specific criteria warranting cycle cancelation are not uniform between centers (Practice Committee of the American Society for Reproductive Medicine, 2006).

MULTIFETAL PREGNANCY REDUCTION

As the rates of ART procedures, multiple fetuses, and prematurity-related sequelae have increased, so has the use of selective reduction. Primary prevention of multiple fetuses by limiting the number of embryos transferred or canceling an overstimulated ovulation induction cycle is optimal; however, in reality multifetal pregnancies continue to occur. Multifetal pregnancy reduction (MFPR) provides another option to enhance overall survival and decrease the risk of fetal or neonatal morbidity and mortality by decreasing pregnancy loss rates and prematurity (Evans and Britt, 2005). First developed in the 1980s, selective termination of one or more fetuses is performed to reduce the final fetal number. The majority of patients reduce to twins, followed by singletons; few reduce to triplets (Stone et al, 2008). A discussion of the ethical, medical, and psychosocial factors involved in MFPR are important counseling points for any patient undergoing ovulation induction (Committee on Ethics, 2007).

Improvements in MFPR techniques have enhanced success rates such that quadruplet or triplets reduced to twins have equal outcomes compared with natural twins (Evans and Britt, 2005; Evans et al, 2001). Success rates correlate with both beginning and ending fetal number (Evans et al, 2001). The average loss rate in one series of 1000 MFPR cases was 4.7% (Stone et al, 2008). Loss rates are higher after reducing to a singleton versus reducing to twins, but twins overall have higher morbidity than do singletons (Evans and Britt, 2005, 2008; Evans et al, 2001; Stone et al, 2008). Reduction of twins to singletons may be considered given a lower loss rate after reduction versus continuing with twins (Evans et al, 2004). Benefits after MFPR are apparent in preterm delivery rates, because half of twins and almost 90% of singletons are delivered full term, and 95% were delivered after 24 weeks' gestation in one series (Stone et al, 2008). Although beneficial in certain cases, MFPR is not without medical and psychological risk. It might not be an option for some women; therefore primary prevention should be the focus for reducing the risk of multiple fetuses.

SUMMARY

Over the last 30 years, advances in ART have helped countless infertile couples achieve a pregnancy. The percentage of ART live births will likely continue on an upward trend because of increased accessibility of ART and delayed childbearing. These factors in addition to ART techniques will continue to contribute to multiple gestation rates. Multiple gestations are associated with increased maternal, fetal, and neonatal complications that generate a medical, psychological, and economic burden to families and society. Efforts to decrease multifetal pregnancies and prematurity-related sequelae include prevention-based practice policies and further knowledge regarding the mechanisms involved with MZT and ART.

SUGGESTED READINGS

ACOG Practice Bulletin #56: Multiple gestation: complicated twin, triplet, and high-order multifetal pregnancy, *Obstet Gynecol* 104:869-883, 2004.

Aston KI, Peterson CM, Carrell DT: Monozygotic twinning associated with assisted reproductive technologies: a review, *Reproduction* 136:377-386, 2008.

Chambers GM, Chapman MG, Grayson N, et al: Babies born after ART treatment cost more than non-ART babies: a cost analysis of inpatient birth-admission costs of singleton and multiple gestation pregnancies, *Hum Reprod* 22:3108-3115, 2007.

Dickey RP: The relative contribution of assisted reproductive technologies and ovulation induction to multiple births in the United States 5 years after the Society for Assisted Reproductive Technology/American Society for Reproductive Medicine recommendation to limit the number of embryos transferred, *Fertil Steril* 88:1554-1561, 2007.

Ellison MA, Hotamisligil S, Lee H, et al: Psychosocial risks associated with multiple births resulting from assisted reproduction, *Fertil Steril* 83:1422-1428, 2005.

Evans MI, Britt DW: Fetal reduction, *Semin Perinatol* 29:321-329, 2005.

Hack KE, Derks JB, Elias SG, et al: Increased perinatal mortality and morbidity in monochorionic versus dichorionic twin pregnancies: clinical implications of a large Dutch cohort study, *BJOG* 115:58-67, 2008.

Hall JG: Twinning, *Lancet* 362:735-743, 2003.

Knopman J, Krey LC, Lee J, et al: Monozygotic twinning: an eight-year experience at a large IVF center, *Fertil Steril* 94:502-510, 2010.

Practice Committee of the American Society for Reproductive Medicine: Multiple pregnancy associated with infertility therapy, *Fertil Steril* 86(Suppl 1): S106-S110, 2006.

Norwitz ER, Edusa V, Park JS: Maternal physiology and complications of multiple pregnancy, *Semin Perinatol* 29:338-348, 2005.

Thurin A, Hausken J, Hillensjo T, et al: Elective single-embryo transfer versus double-embryo transfer in vitro fertilization, *N Engl J Med* 351:2392-2402, 2004.

Complete references and supplemental color images used in this text can be found online at www.expertconsult.com

NONIMMUNE HYDROPS

Scott A. Lorch and Thomas J. Mollen

An infant with hydrops has an abnormal accumulation of excess fluid. The condition varies from mild, generalized edema to massive edema, with effusions in multiple body cavities and with peripheral edema so severe that the extremities are fixed in extension. Fetuses with severe hydrops may die in utero; if delivered alive, they may die in the neonatal period from the severity of their underlying disease or from severe cardiorespiratory failure.

The first description of hydrops in a newborn, in a twin gestation, may have appeared in 1609 (Liley, 2009). Ballantyne (1892) suggested that the finding of hydrops was an outcome for many different causes, in contrast to the belief at that time that hydrops was a single entity. Potter (1943) first distinguished between hydrops secondary to erythroblastosis fetalis and nonimmune hydrops, by describing a group of infants with generalized body edema who did not have hepatosplenomegaly or abnormal erythropoiesis. Potter's description of more than 100 cases of hydrops included two sets of twins in which one had hydrops and the other did not, thus presenting the first description of twin-twin transfusion syndrome. With the nearly universal use of anti-D globulin and refinement of the schedule and doses for its administration, the occurrence of immune-mediated hydrops has steadily declined, such that later studies found that immune-mediated causes accounted for only 6% to 10% of all cases of hydrops (Heinonen et al, 2000; Machin, 1989). The reported incidence of nonimmune hydrops in the general population has been highly variable, ranging from 6 per 1000 pregnancies in a high-risk referral clinic in the United Kingdom between 1993 and 1999 (Sohan et al, 2001) to 1 in 4000 pregnancies (Norton, 1994); other published rates are 6 per 1000 pregnancies (Santolaya et al, 1992), 1.3 per 1000 pregnancies (Wafelman et al, 1999), and 1 per 1700 pregnancies (Heinonen et al, 2000). However, all the published studies come from single institutions, with the at-risk populations ranging from that of a high-risk pregnancy clinic to infants in a neonatal intensive care unit. No study has monitored all pregnant women in one geographic area to calculate the true population incidence of nonimmune hydrops, especially monitoring infants who died in utero. Geography also affects the incidence; several causes of nonimmune hydrops, such as α-thalassemia, are more common in certain areas of the world. Finally, the incidence of nonimmune hydrops may be rising because of the more routine use of ultrasound investigation in the late first trimester of pregnancy (Iskaros et al, 1997).

ETIOLOGY

Nonimmune hydrops has been associated with a wide range of conditions (Table 8-1). In many of these conditions, edema formation results from one of the following possible processes:

- Elevated central venous pressure, in which the cardiac output is less than the rate of venous return

- Anemia, resulting in high-output cardiac failure
- Decreased lymphatic flow
- Capillary leak

The actual pathophysiology of hydrops for many of the conditions in Table 8-1, however, is still not understood.

The most common causes of nonimmune hydrops are chromosomal, cardiovascular, hematologic, thoracic, infectious, and related to twinning (Abrams et al, 2007; Bellini et al, 2009; Wilkins, 1999). As with reported incidence rates, the relative contribution of these causes varies by study. The studies that focus on early fetal presentation of hydrops (postconceptional age of less than 24 weeks' gestation) have found that chromosomal abnormalities, such as Turner syndrome and trisomies 13, 18, and 21, are the causes of 32% to 78% of all cases of hydrops (Boyd et al, 1992; Heinonen et al, 2000; Iskaros et al, 1997; McCoy et al, 1995; Sohan et al, 2001). For infants whose hydrops becomes evident after 24 weeks' gestation, cardiovascular and thoracic causes are most prevalent, with rates ranging between 30% and 50% (Machin, 1989; McCoy et al, 1995; Shan et al, 2001). Studies from Asia have noted a higher percentage of cases from hematologic causes, probably because of the higher rates of α-thalassemia in the population (Lin et al, 1991; Nakayama et al, 1999).

The percentage of infants with "idiopathic" hydrops, or hydrops of unknown etiology, varies from 5.2% to 50%, depending on the ability of the clinicians to complete their diagnostic evaluation and the inclusion of fetal deaths in the analysis (Bellini et al, 2009; Heinonen et al, 2000; Iskaros et al, 1997; Machin, 1989; McCoy et al, 1995; Nakayama et al, 1999; Santolaya et al, 1992; Sohan et al, 2001; Wafelman et al, 1999; Wy et al, 1999). Yaegashi et al (1998) used enzyme-linked immunosorbent assay and polymerase chain reaction techniques to improve the detection of parvovirus infection. In both their own institution, and in eight other series of patients, these investigators found evidence of parvovirus infection in 15% to 19% of all infants previously diagnosed with idiopathic hydrops. It is likely that, as there is increased understanding of and testing for many of the conditions listed in Table 8-1, the number of infants diagnosed with idiopathic, nonimmune hydrops will continue to decline.

PATHOPHYSIOLOGY

NORMAL FLUID HOMEOSTASIS

Abnormal body fluid homeostasis is the underlying cause of edema, whether local or generalized. To understand the pathogenesis of hydrops, the clinician must consider the forces underlying normal fluid homeostasis. The regulation of net fluid movement across a capillary membrane depends on the Starling forces, which were first described by E.H. Starling in 1896 (Starling, 1896). Flow between intravascular and interstitial fluid compartments is

TABLE 8-1 Conditions Associated With Hydrops Fetalis

Condition Type	Specific Conditions	Condition Type	Specific Conditions
Hemolytic anemias	Alloimmune, Rh, Kell, α-Chain hemoglobinopathies (homozygous α-thalassemia) Red blood cell enzyme deficiencies (glucose phosphate isomerase deficiency, glucose-6-phosphate dehydrogenase)	Nervous system lesions	Absence of corpus callosum Encephalocele Cerebral arteriovenous malformation Intracranial hemorrhage (massive) Holoprosencephaly Fetal akinesia sequence
Other anemias	Fetomaternal hemorrhage Twin-twin transfusion Diamond-Blackfan	Pulmonary conditions	Cystic adenomatoid malformation of the lung Mediastinal teratoma Diaphragmatic hernia Lung sequestration syndrome Lymphangiectasia
Cardiac conditions	Premature closure of foramen ovale Ebstein anomaly Hypoplastic left or right heart Subaortic stenosis with fibroelastosis Cardiomyopathy, myocardial fibroelastosis Atrioventricular canal Myocarditis Right atrial hemangioma Intracardiac hamartoma or fibroma Tuberous sclerosis with cardiac rhabdomyoma	Renal conditions	Urinary ascites Congenital nephrosis Renal vein thrombosis Invasive processes and storage disorders Tuberous sclerosis Gaucher disease Mucopolysaccharidosis Mucolipidosis
Cardiac arrhythmias	Supraventricular tachycardia Atrial flutter Congenital heart block	Chromosome abnormalities	Trisomy 13, trisomy 18, trisomy 21 Turner syndrome XX/XY
Vascular malformations	Hemangioma of the liver Any large arteriovenous malformation Klippel-Trenaunay syndrome Idiopathic infantile arterial calcification	Bone diseases	Osteogenesis imperfecta Achondroplasia Asphyxiating thoracic dystrophy
Vascular accidents	Thrombosis of umbilical vein or inferior vena cava Recipient in twin-twin transfusion	Gastrointestinal conditions	Bowel obstruction with perforation and meconium peritonitis Small bowel volvulus Other intestinal obstructions Prune-belly syndrome
Infections	Cytomegalovirus, congenital hepatitis, human parvovirus, enterovirus, other viruses Toxoplasmosis, Chagas disease Coxsackie virus Syphilis Leptospirosis	Tumors	Neuroblastoma Choriocarcinoma Sacrococcygeal teratoma Hemangioma or other hepatic tumors Congenital leukemia Cardiac tumors Renal tumors
Lymphatic abnormalities	Lymphangiectasia Cystic hygroma Noonan syndrome Multiple pterygium syndrome Congenital chylothorax	Maternal or placental conditions	Maternal diabetes Maternal therapy with indomethacin Multiple gestation with parasitic fetus Chorioangioma of placenta, chorionic vessels, or umbilical vessels Toxemia Systemic lupus erythematosus
		Miscellaneous	Neu-Laxova syndrome Myotonic dystrophy
		Idiopathic	

determined by the balance among (1) capillary hydrostatic pressure, (2) serum colloid oncotic pressure, (3) interstitial hydrostatic pressure or tissue turgor pressure, and (4) interstitial osmotic pressure, which depends on lymphatic flow. The Starling equation defines the relationship among these forces and their net effect on net fluid movement, or filtration, across a semipermeable membrane (such as the capillary membrane) as:

$$\text{Filtration} = K[(P_c - P_t) - R(O_p - O_t)]$$

where K = capillary filtration coefficient, representing the extent of permeability of a membrane to water and thus describing capillary integrity; P_c = capillary hydrostatic pressure; P_t = interstitial hydrostatic pressure or tissue turgor pressure; R = reflection coefficient for a solute, representing the extent of permeability of the capillary wall to that solute; O_p = plasma oncotic pressure as determined by plasma proteins and other solutes; and O_t = interstitial osmotic pressure (Figure 8-1).

Although an abnormality of any of the components of this equation may, in theory, result in the accumulation of edema fluid, the fetal-placental unit presents a unique physiologic condition that effectively eliminates two of the factors, assuming unimpeded fetal-placental flow and an appropriately functioning maternal-placental interface. Because approximately 40% of fetal cardiac output is allocated to the placenta, there is rapid transport of water

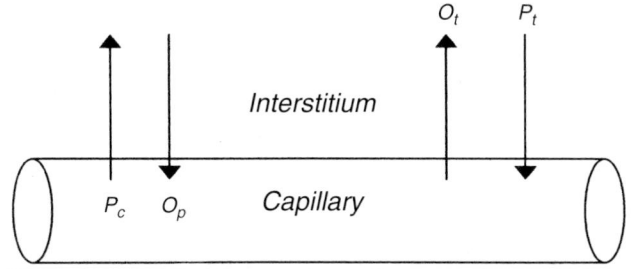

FIGURE 8-1 **Starling forces and net effect on fluid homeostasis.**
Arrows represent net effect of movement of fluid across the capillary membrane for each factor under normal conditions. P_c, Capillary hydrostatic pressure; P_t, interstitial hydrostatic pressure or tissue turgor pressure; O_p, plasma oncotic pressure as determined by plasma proteins and other solutes; O_t, interstitial osmotic pressure.

between the fetus and mother. Any condition resulting in elevated fetal capillary hydrostatic pressure or low plasma colloid oncotic pressure would likely cause the net flow of water from fetal villi in the placenta to the maternal blood stream, where it can be effectively eliminated. This elimination of fluid would counteract the accumulation of interstitial fluid by the fetus. Although the placenta of a fetus with hydrops is also edematous, these changes are believed to occur with, and not before, fetal fluid accumulation.

DERANGEMENTS IN FLUID HOMEOSTASIS

Diamond et al (1932) suggested three possible mechanisms that might be relevant in infants with hydrops: anemia, low colloid osmotic pressure with hypoproteinemia, and congestive heart failure with hypervolemia. Others have reviewed these potential mechanisms (Phibbs et al, 1974), which remain among the central hypotheses addressed by investigators in this area. The causes of hydrops appear to be multifactorial, with mechanisms that produce elevated central venous pressure (CVP), capillary leakage, and impaired lymphatic drainage all contributing to its development.

Infants with alloimmune hydrops (and several of the nonimmune hydrops conditions as well) have significant anemia. It has been proposed that anemia leads to congestive heart failure with increased hydrostatic pressure in the capillaries, causing vascular damage that results in edema. However, the hematocrit values of infants with and without hydrops overlap significantly, suggesting that anemia alone is not the complete explanation. A rapidly lowered hemoglobin concentration results in greater cardiac output to maintain adequate oxygen delivery. This output results in higher oxygen demands by the myocardium, which may be difficult to meet because of the anemia. The hypoxic myocardium can become less contractile and less compliant, with ventricular stiffness causing increased afterload to the atria. High-output congestive heart failure may then exist, resulting in elevated CVP. Raised CVP leads to increased capillary filtration pressures and impairment of lymphatic return (Weiner, 1993). In addition, reduced compliance of a right ventricle may result in flow reversal in the inferior vena cava, which may in turn cause end-organ damage to the liver, with consequent hypoalbuminemia and portal hypertension enhancing formation of both edema and ascites. Hydrops has been produced in fetal lambs

(Blair et al, 1994) in which the hemoglobin content was lowered in 12 fetuses through exchange transfusion using cell-free plasma; six became hydropic. Anemia developed more rapidly with a higher CVP in fetuses with hydrops than in the fetuses without hydrops. In the most severely anemic fetuses, it is probable that decreased oxygen transport causes tissue hypoxia, which in turn increases capillary permeability to both water and protein. These changes in capillary permeability also likely contribute to the development of hydrops.

Infants who have erythroblastosis and hydrops seem to demonstrate a correlation between serum albumin concentration and the severity of hydrops (Phibbs et al, 1974). Initial therapy after birth, however, tends to rapidly raise the serum albumin value toward normal, and with diuresis the albumin concentrations normalize. This finding suggests that hypoalbuminemia may be the result of dilution rather than the cause of hydrops.

To elucidate the role of isolated hypoproteinemia in the genesis of hydrops, Moise et al (1991) have induced hypoproteinemia in sets of twin fetal lambs. One twin from each set underwent serum protein reduction through repeated removal of plasma and replacement with normal saline; the other twin served as the control. Over 3 days, plasma protein concentrations were reduced by an average of 41%, with a 44% reduction in colloid osmotic pressure, in experimental subjects. No fetuses became edematous, and total body water content values were similar in experimental and control animals. Thus hypoproteinemia alone was insufficient to cause hydrops fetalis over the course of the study. Transcapillary filtration probably increased with hypoproteinemia, but was compensated by lymphatic return. Human fetuses with hypoproteinemia as a result of nephrotic syndrome or analbuminemia rarely experience hydrops, further supporting the hypothesis that hypoproteinemia alone is not sufficient to cause hydrops. Hypoproteinemia may, however, lower the threshold for edema formation in the presence of impaired lymphatic return or increased intravascular hydrostatic pressures.

The most commonly diagnosed causes of nonimmune hydrops that appears in fetuses older than 24 weeks' gestation are cardiac disorders. Any state in which cardiac output is lower than the rate of venous return results in an elevated CVP. Increased CVP raises capillary filtration pressures and, if high enough, restricts lymphatic return. Both of these mechanisms may then contribute to interstitial accumulation of fluid. Structural cardiac causes of elevated CVP include right-sided obstructive lesions and valvular regurgitation. The most common and easily reversible cause of nonimmune hydrops is supraventricular tachycardia (SVT). In general, cardiac output rises with heart rate. At the increasingly high rates seen in SVT, however, cardiac output plateaus and then diminishes. The heart rates observed with SVT are often associated with decreased cardiac output. Impaired cardiac output results in elevated CVP, which can give rise to edema through mechanisms discussed previously (Gest et al, 1990). Myocardial hypoxia (most often caused by severe anemia) and myocarditis (usually infectious) reduce both the contractility and compliance of the myocardium and can also cause an increase in CVP.

A fourth factor that contributes to hydrops is decreased lymph flow. If the rate of fluid filtration from plasma to tissues exceeds the rate of lymph return to the central venous system, then edema and effusions may form. A structural impediment or increased CVP that opposes lymphatic return to the heart can impair lymph flow. To determine the effects of alterations in CVP on lymphatic return, Gest et al (1992) applied an opposing hydrostatic pressure to the thoracic duct in fetal lambs; they inserted catheters into the thoracic ducts of 10 fetuses. Varying the height of the catheter altered the thoracic duct outflow pressure. Thoracic duct flow was nearly constant over the physiologic range of CVP, but sharply decreased at elevated pressures; therefore lymphatic flow may be reduced or essentially blocked in pathologic states associated with elevated CVP.

PRENATAL DIAGNOSIS

The initial presentation of fetal hydrops varies by report. Watson and Campbell (1986) found that two thirds of prenatally diagnosed cases were discovered on routine ultrasonographic examinations, and one third was referred for evaluation because of suspected polyhydramnios. Graves and Baskett (1984) reported that hydrops was more commonly discovered after referral for polyhydramnios, fetus large for dates, fetal tachycardia, or pregnancy-induced hypertension. Despite the underlying cause of hydrops or the clinical presentation, the prenatal diagnosis is made via the ultrasonographic finding of excess fluid in the form of ascites, pleural or pericardial effusions, skin edema, placental edema, or polyhydramnios. Several definitions for ultrasonographic diagnosis based on quantity and distribution of excess fluid have been proposed. One widely accepted set of criteria consists of the presence of excess fluid in any two of the previously listed compartments. Because this definition is based on the presence of excess fluid alone, the degree of severity is generally subjective.

Swain et al (1999) outlined a multidisciplinary approach to the evaluation and management of the mother and fetus with hydrops. Table 8-2 provides recommendations for the investigation of fetal hydrops. Patient history should focus on ethnic background, familial history of consanguinity, genetic or congenital anomalies, and complications of pregnancy, including recent maternal illness and environmental exposures. Maternal disorders such as diabetes, systemic lupus erythematosus, myotonic dystrophy, and any type of liver disease should also be noted. Initial laboratory investigation includes blood typing and a Coombs' test to rule out immune-mediated hydrops. Other blood tests are a screening for hemoglobinopathies, a Kleihauer-Betke test to eliminate fetal-maternal hemorrhage, and testing for the TORCH diseases (i.e., toxoplasmosis, other infections, rubella, cytomegalovirus infection, and herpes simplex), including syphilis and parvovirus B19.

Further evaluation is directed at identifying possible causes (Forouzan, 1997). Rapid evaluation is necessary to determine whether fetal intervention is possible and to estimate the prognosis for the fetus. Many conditions, such as arrhythmias, twin-twin transfusion, large vascular masses, and congenital diaphragmatic hernias and other chest-occupying lesions, are discovered during the initial ultrasonographic evaluation (Coleman et al, 2002). Middle cerebral artery peak systolic velocity measurement can

TABLE 8-2 Antenatal Investigation of Fetal Hydrops

Area	Testing
Maternal	History, including: Age, parity, gestation Medical and family histories Recent illnesses or exposures Medications Complete blood count and indices Blood typing and indirect Coombs antibody screening Hemoglobin electrophoresis Kleihauer-Betke stain of peripheral blood Syphilis, TORCH, and parvovirus B19 titers Anti-Ro and anti-La, systemic lupus erythematosus preparation Oral glucose tolerance test Glucose-6-phosphate dehydrogenase, pyruvate kinase deficiency screening
Fetal	Serial ultrasound evaluations Middle cerebral artery peak systolic velocity Limb length, fetal movement Echocardiography
Amniocentesis	Karyotype Alpha-fetoprotein Viral cultures; polymerase chain reaction analysis for toxoplasmosis, parvovirus 19 Establishment of culture for appropriate metabolic or DNA testing Lecithin-to-sphingomyelin ratio to assess lung maturity
Fetal blood sampling	Genetic testing Complete blood count Hemoglobin analysis Immunoglobulin M test; specific cultures Albumin and total protein measurements Measurement of umbilical venous pressure Metabolic testing

Adapted from Swain S, Cameron AD, McNay MB, et al: Prenatal diagnosis and management of nonimmune hydrops fetalis, *Aust N Z J Obstet Gynaecol* 39:285-290, 1999. *TORCH,* Toxoplasmosis, other infections, rubella, cytomegalovirus, and herpes simplex.

aid in detecting the presence of fetal anemia (Hernandez-Andrale et al, 2004). If the initial ultrasonic examination is not helpful in identifying a cause, it may be helpful to repeat it at a later date to reassess fetal anatomy, monitor progression of the hydrops, and evaluate well-being of the fetus.

Fetal echocardiography should also be performed to evaluate for cardiac malformations and arrhythmia. Amniotic fluid can be obtained for fetal DNA analysis, cultures, and lecithin-to-sphingomyelin ratio to assess lung maturity. Fetal blood sampling allows for other tests, such as a complete blood cell count, routine chemical analyses, DNA analysis, bacterial and viral cultures, metabolic studies, and serum immunoglobulin measurements.

PRENATAL MANAGEMENT

The goals of antenatal evaluation of fetal hydrops depend on the underlying cause. In diagnoses in which therapy is futile, the goal is to avoid unnecessary invasive testing and cesarean section. The prognosis should be discussed frankly with the parents, who should be given the option of terminating the pregnancy. If the underlying cause is amenable to fetal therapy, the risks and benefits of such therapy, as well as the warning that diagnostic error is possible, should be discussed with the family.

SVT is one of the most common known causes of nonimmune hydrops, and it is the most amenable to treatment (Huhta, 2004; Newburger and Keane, 1979). Usually the mother is given antiarrhythmic agents, and the fetus is monitored closely for resolution of the SVT. Digoxin is most commonly administered, although other antiarrhythmics have been used, such as sotolol or flecainide, because transplacental transfer of digoxin may be impaired in the setting of hydrops. In extreme circumstances, such as fetal tachyarrhythmia refractory to maternal treatment, direct fetal administration of antiarrhythmic agents via percutaneous umbilical blood sampling or intramuscular injection, although untested and highly risky, has met with some success.

If anemia is the cause of hydrops, transfusions of packed red blood cells may be administered to the fetus. Often a single transfusion reverses the edema, although serial transfusions may be necessary. Parvovirus B19 (Anand et al, 1987) and fetal-maternal hemorrhage are examples of diagnoses that are amenable to this therapy. Other diagnoses involving anemias that are refractory to transfusions, such as α-thalassemia, may require neonatal stem cell transplantation. Transfusions should be given, with the use of ultrasonographic guidance, into the intraperitoneal space or umbilical vein. Blood instilled into the abdominal cavity is taken up by lymphatics, but elevated CVPs present in hydropic fetuses may impair this uptake. If uptake of intraperitoneal blood is incomplete, treatment for the hydrops is less successful; degeneration of the remaining hemoglobin may create a substantial bilirubin load, necessitating phototherapy or exchange transfusion after the infant is delivered.

Surgery continues to evolve as a promising therapy for select cases of fetal hydrops (Azizkhan and Crombleholme, 2008; Kitano et al, 1999). Fetal lung lesions such as congenital cystic adenomatoid malformation (CCAM) and pulmonary sequestration can, in the most extreme cases, result in mediastinal shift, pulmonary hypoplasia, cardiovascular compromise, and hydrops. A recent review of 36 fetuses with CCAM found higher rates of hydrops in infants whose mass-to-thorax ratio was greater than 0.56, in whom the lesion had a cystic predominance, or in whom the hemidiaphram was everted (Vu et al, 2007). Adzick et al (1998) reported on the outcome of 175 cases of fetal lung masses, including 134 cases of CCAM and 41 of extralobar pulmonary sequestration. The 76 fetuses with CCAM lesions without associated hydrops were all managed expectantly (maternal transport to a high-risk center, planned delivery near term, and resection in the newborn period). CCAMs frequently involute and may disappear before delivery; therefore there were no deaths in the nonhydropic group of fetuses in this study. Twenty-five fetuses with hydrops were managed expectantly, and all 25 died before or after preterm labor at 25 to 26 weeks' gestation. These results highlight the fact that fetuses with lung lesions leading to hydrops have high mortality rates. Thirteen fetuses with CCAM and associated hydrops underwent open fetal resection or lobectomy. Eight survived and were reported as healthy at 1 to 7 years of follow-up. Maternal morbidities related to fetal intervention ranged from uterine wound infection with dehiscence to

mild postoperative interstitial pulmonary edema, which was treated with diuretics.

High morbidity and mortality rates in severe twin-twin transfusion with associated hydrops led to multiple international trials of laser photocoagulation of interfetal vascular connections. Although the trials met with varying results, metanalysis involving the three major trials demonstrates improvement in perinatal and neonatal outcomes. However, the current level of evidence is limited in the reported effect on neurodevelopmental outcomes in survivors. A 2008 Cochrane review recommends considering treatment with laser coagulation at all stages of twin-twin transfusion (Roberts et al, 2008).

Fetal intervention has met with some success in other diagnoses with associated hydrops. Thoracoamniotic shunts for large unicystic lesions and pleuroamniotic shunts for hydrothorax have reportedly enhanced survival in extreme cases. Similarly, in cases of massive urinary ascites, urinary diversion via peritoneal shunts has been reported, but with a poor long-term prognosis (Crombleholme et al, 1990).

However, as with other invasive interventions, there are potential risks with fetal surgery. A review of the reproductive outcomes of future pregnancies after a pregnancy complicated by maternal-fetal surgery found a complication rate of 35%: 12% affected by uterine dehiscence, 6% with uterine rupture, 3% requiring hysterectomy; and 9% with hemorrhage requiring transfusion (Wilson et al, 2004). These longer-term complications suggest that the potential benefit of fetal surgical intervention must be balanced by the potential complications of the procedure experienced by the mother.

In cases in which the cause can be corrected by appropriate care at the time of delivery, such as elimination of a chorioangioma, and in cases in which no cause can be ascertained, close observation for fetal demise is the focus of prenatal management. Many cases of nonimmune hydrops manifest in the third trimester as preterm labor. It is difficult to decide whether to attempt tocolysis and delay delivery so as to allow the potentially beneficial administration of steroids before birth or to deliver the fetus immediately. If tocolysis is possible, expectant management should include usual biophysical testing, although fetal decompensation may be difficult to measure. Abnormal fetal heart tracings, oligohydramnios, decreased fetal movement, and poor fetal tone are all ominous signs. There is no indication to prolong pregnancy beyond attainment of a mature lung profile unless available evidence indicates improvement or resolution of the hydrops.

NEONATAL EVALUATION

Table 8-3 summarizes the diagnostic evaluations recommended for newborn infants with nonimmune hydrops of unknown cause.

INTENSIVE CARE OF THE INFANT WITH HYDROPS FETALIS

After successful resuscitation, including intubation, administration of surfactant, and placement of umbilical catheters, the clinical management can address both the cause and the complications of hydrops. Morbidity and

TABLE 8-3 Diagnostic Evaluation of Newborns With Nonimmune Hydrops

System	Type of Evaluation
Cardiovascular	Echocardiogram, electrocardiogram
Pulmonary	Chest radiograph, pleural fluid examination
Hematologic	Complete blood cell count, differential platelet count, blood type and Coombs' test, blood smear for morphologic analysis
Gastrointestinal	Abdominal radiograph, abdominal ultrasonography, liver function tests, peritoneal fluid examination, total protein and albumin levels
Renal	Urinalysis, blood urea nitrogen and creatinine measurements
Genetic	Chromosomal analysis, skeletal radiographs, genetic consultation
Congenital infections	Viral cultures or serologic testing, including TORCH agents and parvovirus
Pathologic	Complete autopsy, placental examination

Adapted from Carlton DP, McGillivray BC, Schreiber MD: Nonimmune hydrops fetalis: a multidisciplinary approach, *Clin Perinatol* 16:839-851, 1989.
TORCH, Toxoplasmosis, other infections, rubella, cytomegalovirus, and herpes simplex.

mortality may result from the hydropic state, the underlying conditions giving rise to hydrops, or both. A fetus with hydrops that is delivered prematurely is subject to the additional complications of prematurity. If there is massive ascites or pleural effusions, initial resuscitation may require thoracentesis or peritoneal tap. Because of pulmonary edema, infants with hydrops are susceptible to pulmonary hemorrhage and require high levels of positive end-expiratory pressure.

RESPIRATORY MANAGEMENT

Virtually all infants with hydrops require mechanical ventilation because of pleural and peritoneal effusions, pulmonary hypoplasia, surfactant deficiency, pulmonary edema, poor chest wall compliance caused by edema, or persistent pulmonary hypertension of the newborn. The presence of persistent pleural effusions may necessitate the placement of chest tubes. Ascites may also compress the diaphragm and impair lung expansion. Breath sounds, chest movement, blood gas levels, and radiographs must all be monitored frequently, so that ventilator support can be reduced in response to improvements in lung compliance and water clearance. Pneumothoraces and pulmonary interstitial emphysema remain potential complications as long as ventilator support is continued. Infants who need a prolonged course of ventilation, particularly those born prematurely, may develop bronchopulmonary dysplasia. Chronic lung disease results in a longer and more complicated hospital course and contributes to the late mortality of hydrops.

FLUID AND ELECTROLYTE MANAGEMENT

A primary goal of fluid management is resolution of the hydrops itself. Maintenance fluids should be restricted, with volume boluses given only in response to clear signs of inadequate intravascular volume. The hydropic

newborn has an excess of free extracellular water and sodium. Fluids given during resuscitation further increase the amount of water and sodium that must be removed during the immediate neonatal period. Initial maintenance fluids should contain minimal sodium. Serum and urine sodium levels, urine volume, and daily weights should be monitored carefully to guide administration of fluids and electrolytes. Urinary sodium levels may help differentiate between hyponatremia caused by hemodilution and urinary losses.

CARDIOVASCULAR MANAGEMENT

Shock may be a prominent feature of patients with hydrops. Hydropic infants may have hypovolemia as a result of capillary leakage, poor vascular tone, and impaired myocardial contractility from hypoxia or infection, impaired venous return caused by shifting or compression of mediastinal structures, or pericardial effusion. Adequate intravascular volume must be maintained, and correctable causes of impaired venous return should be addressed. Peripheral perfusion, heart rate, blood pressure, and acid-base status should be monitored carefully.

CLINICAL COURSE AND OUTCOME

Despite improvements in diagnosis and management, mortality from nonimmune hydrops remains high. Reported survival rates for all fetuses diagnosed antenatally with hydrops range from 12% to 24% (Heinonen et al, 2000; McCoy et al, 1995; Negishi et al, 1997). Higher survival rates have been reported in infants born alive, but the highest rates are still only 40% to 50% (Wy et al, 1999). Improved ultrasonography techniques and earlier testing may actually lead to lower survival rates as hydrops is diagnosed in more first-trimester infants. These infants are more likely to have chromosomal abnormalities that are incompatible with survival, but were previously not included in populations of hydropic fetuses. The best predictor of survival is the cause of the hydrops and the gestational age of the child at delivery. Highest survival rates are seen in infants with parvovirus infection, chylothorax, or SVT. The lowest survival rates are for hydrops from chromosomal cause, although the figures may be biased because a significant number of the pregnancies in such cases are terminated (Heinonen et al, 2000; Sohan et al, 2001). A recent review of 598 patients with nonimmune hydrops found other risk factors for increased mortality including younger gestational age, lower 5-minute Apgar score, and the need for increased respiratory support (Abrams et al, 2007). A smaller study from Taiwan also found that lower albumin levels were associated with a higher mortality rate (Huang et al, 2007).

Interventions to improve outcomes in hydrops are limited by the rarity of the disease. Carlton et al (1989) reported on a group of 36 infants with nonimmune hydrops and noted that 90% of the infants who died within 24 hours had pleural effusions, compared with only 50% of those who survived. More than one third of the infants in this study required thoracentesis in the delivery room to aid in lung expansion. All the infants who lived more than 24 hours were treated with mechanical ventilation and received supplemental oxygen; they needed ventilation for an average of 11 days (range, 2 to 48 days). Most hydropic infants lose a minimum of 15% of their birthweight, and some lose as much as 30%. Ordinarily, diuresis begins on the second or third day after birth and continues for a period of 2 to 4 days. Once the edema has resolved, the infants have normal levels of circulating protein and eventually recover from their apparent capillary leak syndrome. No specific management strategies during the neonatal period, such as the use of high-frequency oscillatory ventilation, have been shown to improve outcome, although the published studies are powered to detect small survival differences (Wy et al, 1999).

For infants who survive the immediate neonatal period, long-term outcomes appear to be excellent. Nonimmune hydrops by itself does not seem to lead to residual developmental delay. A small study from Japan found that 13 of 19 surviving infants with nonimmune hydrops had normal development at 1 to 8 years (Nakayama et al, 1999). The six infants with mild or severe delays in this study had other morbidities, such as extreme prematurity, structural cardiac lesions, or chromosomal anomalies. Thus long-term morbidities from nonimmune hydrops appear to result from the underlying cause of the hydrops, gestational age at delivery, and complications arising immediately after delivery.

SUGGESTED READINGS

Abrams ME, Meredith KS, Kinnard P, et al: Hydrops fetalis: a retrospective review of cases reported to a large national database and identification of risk factors associated with death, *Pediatrics* 120:84-89, 2007.

Anand A, Gray ES, Brown T, et al: Human parvovirus infection in pregnancy and hydrops fetalis, *N Engl J Med* 316:183-186, 1987.

Azizkhan RG, Crombleholme TM: Congenital cystic lung disease: contemporary antenatal and postnatal management, *Pediatr Surg Int* 24:643-657, 2008.

Huhta JC: Guidelines for the evaluation of heart failure in the fetus with or without hydrops, *Pediatr Cardiol* 25:274-286, 2004.

Bellini C, Hennekam RCM, Fulcheri E, et al: Etiology of nonimmune hydrops fetalis: a systematic review, *Am J Med Genet* 149A:844-851, 2009.

Machin GA: Hydrops revisited: literature review of 1414 cases published in the 1980s, *Am J Med Genet* 34:366-390, 1989.

Swain S, Cameron AD, McNay MB, et al: Prenatal diagnosis and management of nonimmune hydrops fetalis, *Aust N Z J Obstet Gynaecol* 39:285-290, 1999.

Complete references used in this text can be found online at www.expertconsult.com

PART III

MATERNAL HEALTH AFFECTING NEONATAL OUTCOME

ENDOCRINE DISORDERS IN PREGNANCY

Gladys A. Ramos and Thomas R. Moore

DIABETES IN PREGNANCY

Currently, 17 million people in the United States have a form of diagnosed diabetes. Alarmingly, the data for 2003 to 2006 indicate that approximately 10.2% (11.5 million) of women older than 20 years have diabetes. Data indicate that new cases of type 2 diabetes mellitus are occurring at an increasing rate among American Indian, African American, Hispanic, and Latino children and adolescents (http://diabetes.niddk.nih.gov/dm). Continued immigration among populations with high rates of type 2 diabetes mellitus and the effects of changes in diet (increases in number of calories and fat content) and lifestyle (sedentary) portend marked rises in the percentage of patients with preexisting diabetes who will become pregnant in the future. There is also an epidemic of childhood obesity currently under way in the United States, with approximately 23 million (30%) children and youth who are overweight. This trend will have a profound effect on obstetrics and pediatric practice in the future. Expanded efforts to reach the populations at risk are necessary if a significant increase in maternal and neonatal morbidity is to be avoided (Persson and Hanson, 1998).

Depending on the population surveyed, abnormalities of glucose regulation occur in 3% to 8% of pregnant women. Although more than 80% of this glucose intolerance arises only during pregnancy (gestational diabetes) and involves relatively modest episodes of hyperglycemia, the attendant fetal and newborn morbidity is disproportionate. Compared with weight-matched controls, infants of diabetic mothers (IDMs) have double the risk of serious birth injury, triple the likelihood of cesarean section, and quadruple the incidence of admission to a newborn intensive care unit. Studies indicate that the magnitude of risk of these maloccurrences is proportional to the level of maternal hyperglycemia. Therefore, to some extent, the excessive fetal and neonatal morbidity of diabetes in pregnancy is preventable or at least reducible through meticulous prenatal and intrapartum care.

MATERNAL-FETAL METABOLISM IN NORMAL PREGNANCY AND DIABETIC PREGNANCY

Normal Maternal Glucose Regulation

With each meal, a complex combination of maternal hormonal actions, including the secretion of pancreatic insulin, glucagon, somatomedins, and adrenal catecholamines, ensures an ample but not excessive supply of glucose to the mother and fetus during pregnancy. The key effects of pregnancy on maternal metabolic regulation are as follows:

- Because the fetus continues to draw glucose from the maternal bloodstream across the placenta, even during periods of fasting, the tendency toward maternal hypoglycemia between meals becomes increasingly marked as pregnancy progresses and fetal glucose demand grows.
- Placental steroid and peptide hormone production (estrogens, progesterone, and chorionic somatomammotropin) rises linearly throughout the second and third trimesters, resulting in a progressively increasing tissue resistance to maternal insulin action.
- Progressive maternal insulin resistance requires a significant augmentation in pancreatic insulin production (more than twofold nonpregnant levels) during feeding to maintain euglycemia. Twenty-four–hour mean insulin levels are 30% higher in the third trimester than in the nonpregnant state.
- If pancreatic insulin output is not adequately augmented, maternal hyperglycemia and then fetal hyperglycemia result. The severity of hyperglycemia and its timing depend on the relative inadequacy of insulin production.

Fetal Effects of Maternal Hyperglycemia
Congenital Anomalies

A major threat to IDMs is the possibility of a life-threatening structural anomaly. In the normoglycemic pregnancy, the risk of a major birth defect is 1% to 2%. Among women with pregestational diabetes, the risk of a fetal structural anomaly is fourfold to eightfold higher. In a recent cohort study of 2359 pregnancies in women with pregestational diabetes, the rate of anomalies was more than doubled. Major congenital anomalies occurred in 4.6% overall with 4.8% for type 1 diabetes mellitus and 4.3% for type 2 diabetes mellitus. This is a significant increase over the expected rate of birth defects in the general population (approximately 1.5%). Neural tube defects in IDM were increased 4.2-fold (Figure 9-1), and congenital heart disease by 3.4-fold. Prenatal diagnosis of these anomalies was accomplished in 65% of neonates (Macintosh et al, 2006). The typical defects and their frequency of occurrence,

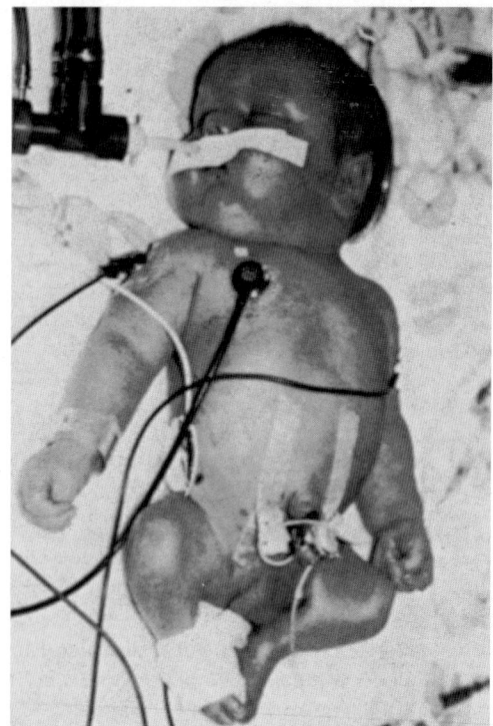

FIGURE 9-1 Newborn with caudal regression syndrome, macrosomia, and respiratory distress. The mother had type 1 diabetes and a glycosylated hemoglobin concentration of 13.5% when first seen for prenatal care at 12 weeks' gestation. *(From Creasy RK, Resnik R, editors: Maternal-fetal medicine: principles and practice, ed 2, Philadelphia, 1989, WB Saunders.)*

TABLE 9-1   Congenital Malformations in Infants of Mothers With Insulin-Dependent Diabetes

Anomaly	Appropriate Risk Ratio	Risk (%)
All cardiac defects	18×	8.5
All central nervous system anomalies	16×	5.3
Anencephaly	13×	–
Spina bifida	20×	–
All congenital anomalies	8×	18.4

Becerra JE, Khoury MJ, Cordero JF, et al: Diabetes mellitus during pregnancy and the risks for specific birth defects: a population based case-control study, *Pediatrics* 85:1, 1990.

noted in a prospective study of infants with major malformations, are listed in Table 9-1. The majority of lesions involve the central nervous and cardiovascular systems, although other series have reported an excess of genitourinary and limb defects (Cousins, 1991).

There is no increase in birth defects among offspring of diabetic fathers, nondiabetic women, or women in whom gestational diabetes develops after the first trimester. These findings suggest that glycemic control during embryogenesis is a critical factor in the genesis of diabetes-associated birth defects. In a study by Miller et al (1981), the frequency of congenital anomalies was proportional to the maternal glycohemoglobin (HbA_{1c}) value in the first trimester (rate of anomalies 3.4% with HbA_{1c} <8.5%, and 22.4% with HbA_{1c} >8.5%). Lucas et al (1989) reported a similar

experience with 105 diabetic patients, finding an overall malformation rate of 13.3%. A recent study conducted in the United Kingdom from 1991 to 2000 in patients with type 1 diabetes mellitus found similar results (Temple et al, 2002). Adverse outcome was significantly higher in the poor control group ($HbA_{1c} \geq 7.5$) than in the fair control group ($HbA_{1c} <7.5$), with a ninefold increase in the congenital malformation rate (relative risk, 9.2; 1.1 to 79.9) (Temple et al, 2002). For a woman with an HbA_{1c} value of less than 7.1%, the risk of delivering a malformed infant was equivalent or slightly less than that for the normoglycemic population. However, the anomaly rate rose progressively with increasing HbA_{1c}, 14% with an HbA_{1c} value of 7.2% to 9.1%, 23% with an HbA_{1c} value of 9.2% to 11.1%, and 25% with an HbA_{1c} value of greater than 11.2%.

Pathogenesis

The specific mechanisms by which hyperglycemia disturbs embryonic development are incompletely elucidated, but reduced levels of arachidonic acid and *myo*-inositol and accumulation of sorbitol and trace metals in the embryo have been demonstrated in animal models (Pinter et al, 1986). Fetal hyperglycemia may promote excessive formation of oxygen radicals in the mitochondria of susceptible tissues, leading to the formation of hydroperoxides, which inhibit prostacyclin. The resulting overabundance of thromboxanes and other prostaglandins may then disrupt vascularization of developing tissues. In support of this theory, the addition of prostaglandin inhibitors to mouse embryos in culture medium prevents glucose-induced embryopathy. Furthermore, the addition of dietary antioxidants in the form of high doses of vitamins C and E decreased fetal dysmorphogenesis to nondiabetic levels in rat pregnancy and rat embryo culture (Cederberg and Eriksson, 2005; El-Bassiouni et al, 2005).

Prevention

Because the critical period for teratogenesis is the first 3 to 6 weeks after conception, normal glycemic control must be instituted before pregnancy to prevent these birth defects. Several clinical trials of meticulous preconception glycemic control in women with diabetes have resulted in malformation rates equivalent to those in the general population (Fuhrmann et al, 1983). A recent metaanalysis of these trials demonstrated that the pooled risk of malformations was lower in women with preconception care compared with those without preconception counseling (Ray et al, 2001). The threshold level of glycemic control, as evidenced by the HbA_{1c} value, necessary to normalize a patient's risk of congenital anomalies appears to be a near-normal value. Thus any elevation of the HbA_{1c} above normal increases the risk of teratogenesis proportionately.

Macrosomia

Fetal overgrowth is a major problem in pregnancies complicated by diabetes, leading to unnecessary cesarean sections and potentially avoidable birth injuries. A 1992 study of birthweights in the previous 20 years indicated that 21% of infants with birthweights of 4540 g or greater were born to mothers who were glucose intolerant, a rate clearly disproportionate to the only 2% to 5% of gravidas with some form of diabetes (Shelley-Jones et al, 1992). Thus the problem of abnormal fetal growth in diabetic pregnancy remains an important clinical challenge.

Macrosomia is defined variously as birthweight above the 90th percentile for gestational age or birthweight greater than 4000 g; it occurs in 15% to 45% of diabetic pregnancies. Excessive fetal size contributes to a greater frequency of intrapartum injury (shoulder dystocia, brachial plexus palsy, and asphyxia). Macrosomia is also a major factor in the higher rate of cesarean delivery among diabetic women. Because the risk of macrosomia is fairly constant for all classes of diabetes, it is likely that first-trimester metabolic control has less of an effect on fetal growth than does glycemic regulation in the second and third trimesters.

Growth Dynamics

IDMs with macrosomia follow a unique pattern of in utero growth compared with fetuses in euglycemic pregnancies. During the first and second trimesters, differences in size between fetuses born to diabetic and nondiabetic mothers are usually undetectable with ultrasound measurements. After 24 weeks, however, the growth velocity of the IDM fetus' abdominal circumference typically begins to rise above normal (Ogata et al, 1980). Reece et al (1990) demonstrated that the IDM fetus has normal head growth, despite marked degrees of hyperglycemia. Landon et al (1989) have reported that although head growth and femur growth of IDM fetuses were similar to those of normal fetuses, abdominal circumference growth significantly exceeded that of controls beginning at 32 weeks' gestation (abdominal circumference growth in IDM fetuses is 1.36 cm/week, versus 0.901 cm/week in normal subjects).

Morphometric studies of the IDM newborn indicate that the greater growth of the abdominal circumference is caused by deposits of fat in the abdominal and interscapular areas. This central depositing of fat is a key characteristic of diabetic macrosomia and underlies the pathology associated with vaginal delivery in these pregnancies. Acker et al (1986) showed that although the incidence of shoulder dystocia is 3% among infants weighing more than 4000 g, the incidence in infants from diabetic pregnancies who weigh more than 4000 g is 16%. Finally, despite our emphasis on birthweight, this alone may not be a sensitive measure of fetal growth. Catalano et al (2003) conducted body composition studies on infants born to mothers with diabetes and found that even when appropriate for gestational age, these infants have increased fat mass and percent body fat compared with a normoglycemic control group.

Childhood Effects

Higher growth velocity, begun in fetal life during a pregnancy complicated by diabetes, may extend into childhood and adult life. Silverman et al (1995) reported follow-up of IDMs through age 8 years in which half the infants weighed more than the 90th percentile for gestational age at birth. By age 8 years, approximately half of the IDMs weighed more than the heaviest 10% of the nondiabetic children. The asymmetry index was 30% higher in diabetic offspring than in the controls by age 8 years. These investigators also showed that offspring with diabetes have permanent derangement of glucose-insulin kinetics, resulting in a higher incidence of impaired glucose tolerance. In addition, Dabelea et al (2000) also reported that the mean adolescent body mass index was 2.6 kg/m^2 greater in sibling offspring of diabetic pregnancies compared with the index siblings born when the mother previously had normal glucose tolerance.

Pathophysiology

The pathophysiology of excessive fetal growth is complex and reflects the delivery of an abnormal nutrient mixture to the fetoplacental unit, regulated by an abnormal confluence of growth factors. Pedersen (1952) hypothesized that maternal hyperglycemia stimulates fetal hyperinsulinemia, which in turn mediates acceleration of fuel utilization and growth. The features of the abnormal growth in diabetic pregnancy include excessive adipose deposition, visceral organ hypertrophy, and acceleration of body mass accretion (Ogata et al, 1980).

Data from the Diabetes in Early Pregnancy project suggest that maternal metabolic control is a critical factor leading to fetal macrosomia (Jovanovic-Peterson et al, 1991). In this study, in which meticulous glycemic care was maintained in early pregnancy and beyond, fetal weight did not correlate significantly with fasting glucose levels. During the second and third trimesters, however, postprandial blood glucose levels were strongly predictive of both birthweight and the overall percentage of macrosomic infants. With postprandial glucose values averaging 120 mg/dL, approximately 20% of infants had macrosomia; a 30% rise in postprandial levels to 160 mg/dL resulted in a predicted percentage of macrosomia of 35%. In contrast, Persson et al (1996) showed that fasting glucose concentrations account for 12% of the variance in birthweight and correlated best with estimates of neonatal fat. Similarly, Uvena-Celebrezze et al (2002) found that the strongest correlation was between fasting glucose and neonatal adiposity rather than postprandial measures.

The Pedersen hypothesis (Pedersen, 1977) presumes that abnormal fuel milieu in the maternal bloodstream is reflected contemporaneously in the fetal compartment: *Maternal hyperglycemia = Fetal hyperglycemia*. Studies by Hollingsworth and Cousins (1981) have confirmed much of Pedersen's hypothesis and note the following features of normal pregnancy:

- Maternal fasting blood glucose levels decline from approximately 85 mg/dL to 75 mg/dL. Mean blood glucose also declines.
- At night, maternal glucose levels drop markedly as the fetus continues to draw glucose stores from the maternal circulation.
- Postprandial peaks in maternal blood glucose rarely exceed 120 mg/dL at 2 hours or 130 mg/dL at 1 hour.

In addition, in diabetic pregnancies:

- If maternal glucose levels surge excessively after a meal, the consequent fetal hyperglycemia is accompanied by fetal pancreatic beta-cell hyperplasia and hyperinsulinemia.
- Fetal hyperinsulinemia, lasting only episodically for 1 to 2 hours, has detrimental consequences for fetal growth and well-being, in that it (1) promotes storage of excess nutrients, resulting in macrosomia, and (2) drives catabolism of the oversupply of fuel, using energy and depleting fetal oxygen stores.

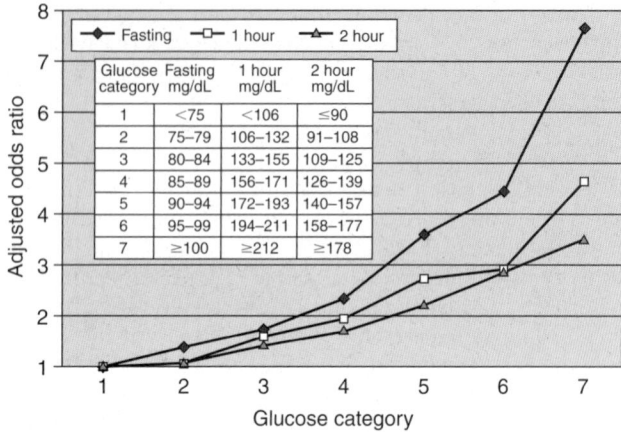

FIGURE 9-2 Adjusted odds ratios for cord C-peptide levels at >90th percentile at different glucose categories based on a 2-hour oral glucose challenge test. (*Adapted from HAPO Study Cooperative Research Group, Metzger BE, Lowe LB, et al: Hyperglycemia and adverse pregnancy outcomes,* N Engl J Med *358:1991-2002, 2008.*)

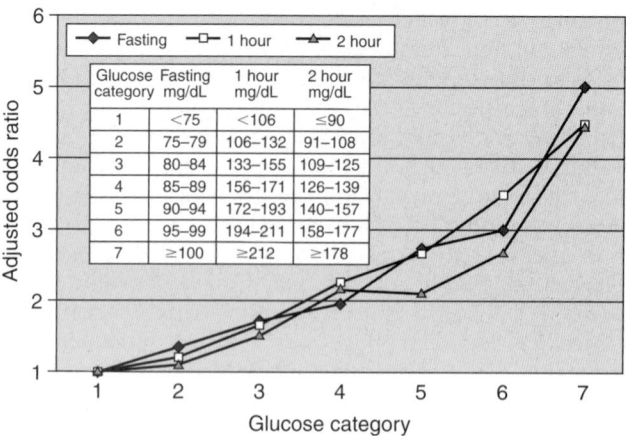

FIGURE 9-3 Adjusted odds ratios for macrosomia at >90th percentile at different glucose categories based on a 2-hour oral glucose challenge test. (*Adapted from HAPO Study Cooperative Research Group, Metzger BE, Lowe LB, et al: Hyperglycemia and adverse pregnancy outcomes,* N Engl J Med *358:1991-2002, 2008.*)

- Episodic fetal hypoxia stimulated by episodic maternal hyperglycemia leads to an outpouring of adrenal catecholamines, which in turn causes hypertension, cardiac remodeling, and cardiac hypertrophy.

The Hyperglycemia and Adverse Pregnancy Outcomes (HAPO) study provided additional evidence in support of the Pedersen hypothesis. In this well-designed, multicenter prospective trial, women underwent a 75-g oral glucose challenge test between 28 and 32 weeks' gestation. Providers were blinded to test results if the fasting value was 105 mg/dL or less and the 2-hour plasma glucose level was 200 mg/dL or less. The women did not receive any therapeutic intervention. The study found a continuous association between maternal glucose values, cord C-peptide levels (Figure 9-2) and birthweight above the 90th percentile (Figure 9-3) (HAPO Study Cooperative Research Group et al, 2008). A followup analysis of the same cohort evaluating neonatal anthropometric measurements, found a link between maternal hyperglycemia, cord C-peptide levels and neonatal adiposity (HAPO Study Cooperative Research Group et al, 2009). This study suggested that maternal hyperglycemia results in neonatal adiposity that is mediated by fetal insulin production (C-peptide level >90th percentile) (HAPO Study Cooperative Research Group et al, 2009).

Prevention of Macrosomia

Because macrosomic fetuses are at an increased risk for immediate complications related to birth injury and for potential long-term consequences such as late childhood obesity and insulin resistance, measures for prevention of macrosomia have been recommended. As described previously, fetal hyperinsulinemia, which acts as a fetal growth factor, occurs in response to fetal hyperglycemia, which in turn reflects the maternal hyperglycemic condition. Therefore, measures that promote consistent maternal euglycemia may prevent macrosomia. Several prospective trials have shown that strict maternal glycemic control using insulin and dietary therapy and fastidious blood glucose monitoring can reduce the incidence of macrosomia

(Coustan and Lewis, 1978; Langer et al, 1994; Thompson et al, 1990). Langer et al (1994) compared the outcomes of diabetic pregnancies managed conventionally (four blood glucose measurements per day) or intensely (seven blood glucose measurements per day). Fasting blood glucose values were maintained between 60 and 90 mg/dL and 2-hour postprandial values at less than 120 mg/dL. Outcomes were compared to nondiabetic control pregnancies. The rate of infants born weighing more than 4000 g was 14% in the conventionally managed group, 7% in the intensely managed group, and 8% in nondiabetic controls. Similarly, the rate of shoulder dystocia was 1.4% in the conventionally managed group, 0.4% in the intensely managed group, and 0.5% in the control group. Thus, like the reduction of congenital anomalies in mothers with diabetes by means of first-trimester euglycemia, strict glycemic control in the second and third trimesters may reduce the fetal macrosomia rate to near baseline.

Fetal Hypoxic Stress

As noted previously, episodic maternal hyperglycemia promotes a fetal catabolic state in which oxygen depletion occurs. Several fetal metabolic adaptive responses to this episodic hypoxia occur. For example, the drop in fetal oxygen tension causes stimulation of erythropoietin, red cell hyperplasia, and elevation in fetal hematocrit. Polycythemia can lead to poor circulation and postnatal hyperbilirubinemia. Profound episodic hyperglycemia in the third trimester causing severe fetal hypoxic stress has been theorized as the cause of sudden intrauterine fetal demise in poorly controlled diabetes.

CLASSIFYING AND DIAGNOSING DIABETES IN PREGNANCY

The classification system for diabetes in pregnancy recommended by White has been replaced by a scheme based on the pathophysiology of hyperglycemia and developed by the National Diabetes Data Group (NDDG) in 1979 (Hare and White, 1980). The two types are summarized in Table 9-2. This nomenclature is useful because it categorizes patients according to the underlying pathogenesis of their diabetes—insulin-deficient (type 1) and insulin-resistant (type 2 and gestational). One must remember that the diagnosis of gestational diabetes applies to any woman who is found to have hyperglycemia during pregnancy. A certain percentage of such women actually have type 2 diabetes, but the diagnosis cannot be confirmed until postpartum testing.

Pregestational Diabetes

Patients with type 1 diabetes mellitus typically exhibit hyperglycemia, ketosis, and dehydration in childhood or adolescence. Often the diagnosis is made during a hospital admission for diabetic ketoacidosis and coma. Rarely is the diagnosis of type 1 diabetes mellitus made during pregnancy. Conversely, it is not unusual for women with a tentative diagnosis of gestational diabetes to be found to have overt, type 2 diabetes mellitus after delivery. The American Diabetic Association has outlined three criteria for diagnosing type 2 diabetes mellitus in nonpregnant subjects. They include the finding of a casual plasma glucose of 200 mg/dL or greater, a fasting plasma glucose of 126 mg/dL or greater, or a 2-hour glucose value of 200 mg/dL or greater on a 75-g, 2-hour glucose tolerance test (GTT). Diagnostic criteria are listed in Box 9-1.

Gestational Diabetes

Gestational diabetes mellitus (GDM) is defined as glucose intolerance that begins or is first recognized during pregnancy (American Diabetes Association, 2002). Almost

uniformly, GDM arises from significant maternal insulin resistance, a state similar to type 2 diabetes mellitus. In many cases, GDM is simply preclinical type 2 diabetes mellitus unmasked by the hormonal stress imposed by the pregnancy. Although GDM complicates no more than 5% to 6% of pregnancies in the United States, the prevalence of GDM in specific populations varies from 1% to 14% (American Diabetes Association, 2002). Clinical recognition of GDM is important because therapy—including medical nutrition therapy, insulin when necessary, and antepartum fetal surveillance—can reduce the well-described perinatal morbidity and mortality associated with GDM.

Traditionally, universal screening for GDM has been recommended (Metzger, 1991). However, the Fourth International Workshop-Conference on Gestational Diabetes and the American College of Obstetricians and Gynecologists have now indicated that either a risk-factor approach or universal screening can be considered (American College of Obstetricians and Gynecologists, 2001; Metzger and Coustan, 1998). This recommendation is based on the findings of Sermer et al (1994), who reported the results of screening Canadian women at 26 weeks' gestation with the 100-g, 3-hour GTT. They identified several risk factors as significantly increasing the likelihood of GDM, among which were maternal age of 35 years or more, body mass index higher than 22 kg/m², and Asian or other ethnicity than white. Women with one or no risk factors had a 0.9% risk of GDM, whereas the risk for those with two to five factors was 4% to 7%. By limiting screening for GDM to patients with more than one risk factor, these investigators were able to reduce testing by 34% while retaining a sensitivity rate of approximately 80%, with a false-positive result rate of 13%. Therefore in patients meeting all criteria listed in Table 9-3 and Box 9-2, it may be cost effective to avoid screening. Currently a multicenter trial is underway by National Institute of Child Health and Human Development Maternal Fetal Medicine Unit Network in which women with GDM will be randomized to standard therapy versus no therapy (Landon et al, 2009). This randomized study will address whether identification and treatment of GDM decrease perinatal morbidity.

Notwithstanding these findings, multiple studies from more heterogeneous U.S. populations have demonstrated

TABLE 9-2 Classification of Diabetes Mellitus

Type	Old Nomenclature	Clinical Features
Type 1	Juvenile-onset diabetes	Insulin-deficient, ketosis-prone; virtually all patients with type 1 diabetes mellitus are insulin dependent
Type 2	Adult-onset diabetes	Insulin-resistant, not ketosis-prone; few patients with type 2 diabetes mellitus are truly insulin dependent
Gestational	—	Occurs during and resolves after pregnancy; insulin-resistant; not ketosis-prone

BOX 9-1 Criteria for the Diagnosis of Type 2 Diabetes Mellitus

- Symptoms of diabetes (polyuria, polydipsia, and unexplained weight loss) and a casual plasma glucose level >200 mg/dL (11.1 mmol/L). *Casual* is defined as any time of day without regard to time of last meal, or
- Fasting glucose level >126 mg/dL (7.0 mmol/L). *Fasting* is defined as no caloric intake for at least 8 hours, or
- Two-hour plasma glucose >200 mg/dL (11.1 mmol/L) during a 75-g oral glucose challenge test.

Adapted from the American Diabetes Assoication: Clinical practice recommendations: Standards of medical care for diabetes, 2007, *Diabetes Care* 30:s4-s41, 2007.

TABLE 9-3 Oral Glucose Tolerance Test for Gestational Diabetes

	Venous Plasma Glucose Level*			
	100-g Glucose Load		75-g Glucose Load	
	mg/dL	mmol/L	mg/dL	mmol/L
Fasting value	95	5.3	95	5.3
1-hr value	180	10.0	180	10.0
2-hr value	155	8.6	155	8.6
3-hr value	140	7.8	—	—

*Test prerequisites: 1-hr, 50-g glucose challenge result >135 mg/dL; overnight fast of 8 to 14 hours; carbohydrate loading for 3 days, including >150 g carbohydrate; seated and not smoking during the test; two or more values must be met or exceeded; either a 2-hr (75-g glucose) or 3-hr (100-g glucose) test can be performed.

BOX 9-2   Criteria for Low Risk of Gestational Diabetes*

- Age <25 years
- Normal prepregnancy body weight
- No first-degree relatives with diabetes
- Not a member of an ethnic group at high risk for GDM
- No history of GDM in prior pregnancy
- No history of adverse pregnancy outcome

Data from Metzger BE, Coustan DR: Summary and Recommendations of the Fourth International Workshop-Conference on Gestational Diabetes Mellitus. The Organizing Committee, *Diabetes Care* 21(Suppl 2):B161-B167, 1998.
GDM, Gestational diabetes mellitus.
*Screening for GDM may be omitted only if all criteria are met.

BOX 9-3   Indications for the First-Trimester 50-g Glucose Challenge

- Maternal age >25 years
- Previous infant >4 kg
- Previous unexplained fetal demise
- Previous pregnancy with gestational diabetes
- Strong immediate family history of type 2 or gestational diabetes mellitus
- Maternal obesity (>90 kg)
- Fasting glucose level >140 mg/dL (7.8 mmol/L) or random glucose reading >200 mg/dL (11.1 mmol/L)

the inadequacy of risk factor based screening of patients for GDM. Lavin et al (1981) noted that if only those with risk factors were screened, the percentage of GDM cases detected was similar to the detection rate in those without risk factors (1.4%). A later study (Weeks et al, 1995), which assessed the effect of screening only patients with risk factors, reported that selective screening would have failed to detect 43% of cases of GDM. Moreover, 28% of the women with undiagnosed GDM would have required insulin and had a several-fold higher risk of cesarean section because of macrosomia.

Universal screening should be performed in women in ethnic groups at a higher risk for glucose intolerance during pregnancy, namely those of Hispanic, African, Native American, South or East Asian, Pacific Islands, or Indigenous Australian ancestry. For simplicity of administration, universal screening, with the possible exception of the lowest risk category, is probably best. The universal screening method for GDM has been shown to result in earlier diagnosis and improved pregnancy outcomes, including lower rates of macrosomia and a decrease in neonatal admissions to neonatal intensive care units (Griffin et al, 2000).

The timing of screening for GDM is important. Because maternal insulin resistance rises progressively during pregnancy, screening too early can miss some patients who will become glucose intolerant later. Screening too late in the third trimester can limit the time during which metabolic interventions can take place. Thus, risk factors for GDM should be assessed at the initial prenatal visit. Factors that should lead to a first-trimester glucose challenge test are listed in Box 9-3. In the remaining patients, screening should be performed with the use of 50 g of glucose at 26 to 28 weeks' gestation.

Various threshold levels for the 50-g glucose challenge are in use, including 140 mg/dL, 135 mg/dL, and 130 mg/dL. The sensitivity of the GDM testing regimen depends on the threshold value used. The most commonly used threshold, 140 mg/dL, detects only 80% of patients with GDM and results in requiring a 3-hour oral GTT in approximately 10% to 15% of patients. Using a challenge threshold of 135 mg/dL improves sensitivity to more than 90% but increases the number of 3-hour oral GTTs by 42% (Ray et al, 1996). Thus, the clinician encountering a newborn with multiple stigmata of an IDM, yet whose mother had a negative diabetes screening test result, should realize that this result during pregnancy does not rule out GDM. This is also why every patient who delivered an

infant with macrosomia in a prior pregnancy should be screened early in all subsequent pregnancies.

Definitive diagnosis of gestational diabetes is made with a GTT. Either 100 g of glucose and 3 hours of testing, or 75 g of glucose and 2 hours of testing can be used. The diagnostic criteria are shown in Box 9-1. Two or more values must be met or exceeded for the diagnosis of GDM to be made. A GTT should be performed after overnight fasting and with modest carbohydrate loading before the test.

PERINATAL COMPLICATIONS OF DIABETES DURING PREGNANCY

Fetal Morbidity and Mortality

Perinatal Mortality

Perinatal mortality in diabetic pregnancy has decreased 30-fold since the discovery of insulin in 1922 and the advent of intensive obstetric and infant care in the 1970s (Figure 9-4). Improved techniques for maintaining maternal euglycemia have led to later timing of delivery and have reduced the incidence of iatrogenic respiratory distress syndrome (RDS).

Nevertheless, the currently reported perinatal mortality rates among women with diabetes remain approximately twice those observed in nondiabetic women (Table 9-4). Congenital malformations, RDS, and extreme prematurity account for most perinatal deaths in contemporary diabetic pregnancy. Figure 9-5 shows the different rates of RDS in diabetic and euglycemic pregnancies. In the past decade, fewer intrauterine deaths have been reported, probably reflecting more careful fetal monitoring. Nevertheless, intrapartum asphyxia and fetal demise remain persistent problems.

Birth Injury

Birth injury, including shoulder dystocia (Keller et al, 1991) and brachial plexus trauma, is more common among IDMs, and macrosomic fetuses are at the highest risk (Mimouni et al, 1992). Shoulder dystocia, defined as difficulty in delivering the fetal body after expulsion of the fetal head, is an obstetric emergency that places the fetus and mother at great risk. Shoulder dystocia occurs in 0.3% to 0.5% of vaginal deliveries among normal pregnant women; the incidence is twofold to fourfold higher in women with diabetes, probably because the hyperglycemia in a diabetic pregnancy causes the fetal shoulder and abdominal widths

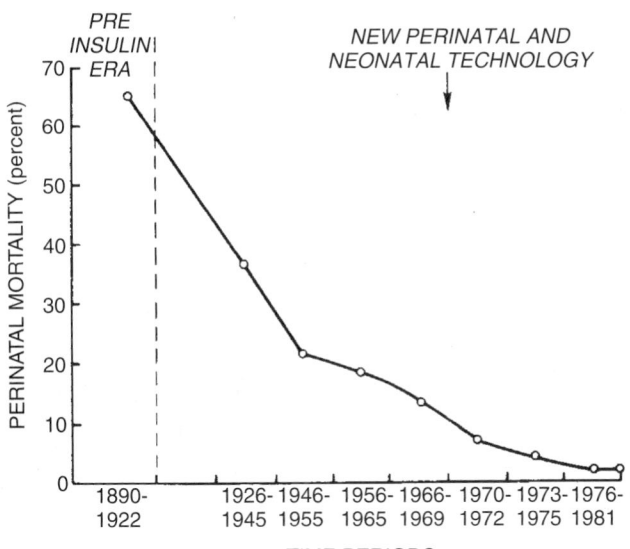

FIGURE 9-4 Perinatal mortality rate (percentage) among infants of diabetic mothers from 1890 to 1981. *(From Creasy RK, Resnik R, editors: Maternal-fetal medicine: principles and practice, ed 2, Philadelphia, 1989, WB Saunders. Data from Craigin EB, Ryder GH: Obstetrics: a practical textbook for students and practitioners, Philadelphia, 1916, Lea and Febiger; DeLee JB: The principles and practice of obstetrics, ed 3, Philadelphia, 1920, WB Saunders; Jorge CS, Artal R, Paul RH, et al: Antepartum fetal surveillance in diabetic pregnant patients, Am J Obstet Gynecol 141:641-645, 1981; Pedersen J: The pregnant diabetic and her newborn, ed 2, Baltimore, 1977, Williams and Wilkins; and Williams JW: Obstetrics: a textbook for the use of students and practitioners, New York, 1925, D Appleton.)*

TABLE 9-4 Perinatal Mortality Rates (No. of Deaths per 100 Births) in Diabetic and Normal Pregnancies

Mortality	Mothers With Gestational Diabetes	Mothers With Preexisting Diabetes	Healthy Mothers*
Fetal	4.7	10.4	5.7
Neonatal	3.3	12.2	4.7
Perinatal	8.0	11.6	10.4

*California data for 1986, corrected for birthweight, sex, and race.

to become massive (Nesbitt et al, 1998). This relationship was investigated by Athukorala et al, (2007), who found a strong association with fasting hyperglycemia such that with each 1-mmol increase in the fasting value in the oral glucose-tolerance test there was an increasing relative risk (RR) of 2.09 (95% confidence interval [CI], 1.03 to 4.25) for shoulder dystocia. Although half of shoulder dystocias occur in infants of normal birthweight (2500 to 4000 g), the incidence of shoulder dystocia is 10-fold higher (5% to 7%) among infants weighing 4000 g or more and rises to 31% for infants whose mothers have diabetes (Gilbert et al, 1999; see also Chapter 15 for a discussion of complicated deliveries and Chapter 64 for a discussion of the neurologic consequences of birth injury.)

Neonatal Morbidity and Mortality

For a complete discussion of neonatal morbidity and mortality, see Chapter 94.

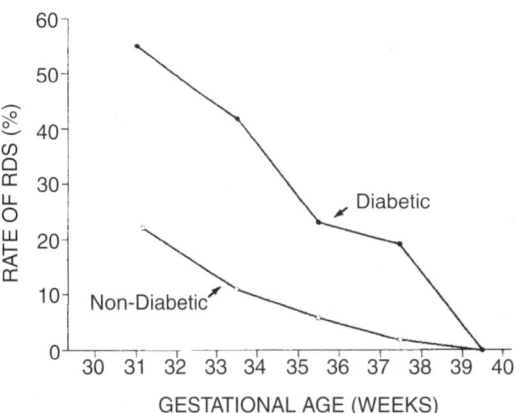

FIGURE 9-5 Rate of respiratory distress syndrome (RDS) versus gestational age. Improved management of maternal glycemic control permits delaying delivery until after 38 weeks' gestation, when the risk of RDS approaches that in nondiabetic pregnancy. *(From Moore TR: A comparison of amniotic fluid fetal pulmonary phospholipids in normal and diabetic pregnancy, Am J Obstet Gynecol 186:641-650, 2002.)*

Polycythemia and Hyperviscosity

Polycythemia (defined as central venous hemoglobin concentration >20 g/dL or hematocrit >65%) is not uncommon in IDMs and is apparently related to glycemic control. Widness et al (1990) demonstrated that hyperglycemia is a powerful stimulus to fetal erythropoietin production, probably mediated by decreased fetal oxygen tension. Neonatal polycythemia may promote vascular sludging, ischemia, and infarction of vital tissues, including the kidneys and central nervous system.

Neonatal Hypoglycemia

Approximately 15% to 25% of neonates delivered from women with diabetes during gestation will develop hypoglycemia during the immediate newborn period (Alam et al, 2006). This complication is usually much milder and less common in the infant of a woman whose insulin-dependent diabetes is well controlled throughout the entire pregnancy and who exhibits euglycemia during labor and delivery. Unrecognized postnatal hypoglycemia can lead to neonatal seizures, coma, and brain damage; therefore, it is imperative that the nurseries receiving IDMs have a protocol for frequent monitoring of the infant's blood glucose level until metabolic stability is ensured.

Hyperbilirubinemia

The risk of hyperbilirubinemia is higher in IDMs than in normal infants. There are multiple causes of hyperbilirubinemia in IDMs, but prematurity and polycythemia are the primary contributing factors. Increased destruction of red blood cells contributes to the risks of jaundice and kernicterus. This complication is usually managed using phototherapy, but exchange transfusions may be necessary for marked bilirubin elevations.

Hypertrophic and Congestive Cardiomyopathy

In some infants with macrosomia of mothers with poorly controlled diabetes, a thickened myocardium and significant septal hypertrophy have been described (Gutgesell et al, 1976). Although the prevalence of myocardial hypertrophy in IDMs may exceed 30% at birth, almost all cases have resolved by 1 year of age (Mace et al, 1979).

Hypertrophic cardiac dysfunction in a newborn IDM often leads to respiratory distress, which may be mistaken for hyaline membrane disease. IDMs with cardiomegaly may have either congestive or hypertrophic cardiomyopathy. Echocardiograms show a hypercontractile, thickened myocardium, often with septal hypertrophy disproportionate to the ventricular free walls. The ventricular chambers are often smaller than normal, and there may be anterior systolic motion of the mitral valve, producing left ventricular outflow tract obstruction.

The pathogenesis of hypertrophic cardiomyopathy in IDMs is unclear, although it is recognized to be associated with poor maternal metabolic control. There is evidence that the fetal myocardium is particularly sensitive to insulin during gestation, and Susa et al (1979) reported a doubling of cardiac mass in hyperinsulinemic fetal rhesus monkeys. The myocardium is known to be richly endowed with insulin receptors. Recently maternal insulin-like growth factor-1 (IGF-1), which is elevated in suboptimally controlled diabetic pregnancies, has been shown to be significantly elevated among neonates with asymmetrical septal hypertrophy. Because IGF-1 does not cross the placenta, it can exert its action through binding to the IGF-1 receptor on the placenta (Hayati et al, 2007). Halse et al (2005) noted that B-type natriuretic peptide, a marker for congestive cardiac failure, is elevated in neonates whose mothers had poor glycemic control during the third trimester.

IDMs can also have congestive cardiomyopathy without hypertrophy. Echocardiography shows the myocardium to be overstretched and poorly contractile (Jaeggi et al, 2001). This condition is often rapidly reversible with correction of neonatal hypoglycemia, hypocalcemia, and polycythemia; it responds to digoxin, diuretics, or both. In contrast, treatment of hypertrophic cardiomyopathy with an inotropic or diuretic agent tends to further decrease the size of the ventricular chambers and leads to obstruction of blood flow. Prenatal echocardiogram can identify septal hypertrophy and other structural abnormalities, but routine fetal echocardiogram in diabetics has not been proved to be cost-effective or to improve outcomes (Bernard et al, 2009).

Respiratory Distress Syndrome

Since the 1970s, improved maternal management and better protocols for timing of delivery have resulted in a dramatic decline in the incidence of RDS from 31% to 3%. Nevertheless, respiratory dysfunction in the newborn IDM continues to be a common complication of diabetic pregnancy; it may be because of surfactant deficiency or another form of pulmonary distress. Surfactant production occurs late in diabetic pregnancies. Studies of fetal lung ion transport in the diabetic rat by Pinter et al (1991) demonstrated decreased fluid clearance and a lack of thinning of the lung's connective tissue in diabetic rats compared with controls. In humans, Kjos et al (1990) noted respiratory distress in 18 of 526 infants delivered after diabetic gestations (3.4%). Surfactant-deficient airway disease accounted for fewer than one third of cases, with transient tachypnea, hypertrophic cardiomyopathy, and pneumonia responsible for the majority.

As a result, the near-term infant of a mother with poorly controlled diabetes is more likely to have neonatal RDS than the infant of a mother without diabetes at the same gestational age. This circumstance further compounds the diabetic infant's metabolic and cardiovascular difficulties after birth. The fetus without diabetes achieves pulmonary maturity at a mean gestational age of 34 to 35 weeks. By 37 weeks' gestation, more than 99% of normal newborn infants have mature lung profiles as assessed by phospholipid assays. In a diabetic pregnancy, however, it is unwise to assume that the risk of respiratory distress has passed until after 38.5 weeks' gestation (Moore, 2002). Any delivery contemplated before 38.5 weeks' gestation for other than the most urgent fetal and maternal indications should be preceded by documentation of pulmonary maturity through amniocentesis.

OBSTETRIC COMPLICATIONS

Pregnancy complicated by diabetes is subject to a number of obstetric disorders, including ketoacidosis, preeclampsia, polyhydramnios, and abnormal labor, at higher rates than in nondiabetic pregnancy.

Preeclampsia

Preeclampsia is an unpredictable multisystem disorder in which maternal neurologic, renal, and cardiovascular status can decline precipitously, which can threaten fetal health through placental ischemia and abruptio placentae. Preeclampsia is more common among women with diabetes, occurring two to three times more frequently in women with pregestational diabetes than in nondiabetic women (Moore et al, 1985; Sibai et al, 2000). However, the risk of developing preeclampsia is proportional to the duration of diabetes before pregnancy and the existence of nephropathy and hypertension; preeclampsia develops in more than one third of women who have had diabetes for more than 20 years. Patients with type 2 diabetes mellitus without complications have a risk profile similar to that of patients without diabetes, but the risk of hypertensive complications is 50% higher in women with evidence of renal or retinal vasculopathy than in those with no hypertension. The rate of fetal death is higher in women with diabetes and preeclampsia. In the patient with diabetes and chronic hypertension, preeclampsia may be difficult to distinguish from near-term blood pressure elevations. The onset is typically insidious and not confidently recognized until it is severe. Renal function assessment (creatinine, blood urea nitrogen, uric acid, and 24-hour urine collection) should be performed each trimester in women with evidence of pregestational diabetes and vascular disease.

When a patient with diabetes experiences preeclampsia, she should be evaluated for delivery. If signs of severe disease are present (e.g., blood pressure >160 mm Hg systolic and 110 mm Hg diastolic, neurologic symptoms, or significant renal dysfunction), delivery should be performed promptly. In mild cases, the patient may be observed if the fetal lungs are immature. Preeclampsia after 38 weeks' gestation, however, is appropriate grounds for initiating delivery.

Polyhydramnios

Polyhydramnios is defined as excess amniotic fluid. The precise clinical definition varies, encompassing the recording of more than 2000 mL of amniotic fluid at delivery and various measures of amniotic fluid pocket depths as observed on ultrasonography. In practice, polyhydramnios is usually diagnosed when any single vertical pocket of amniotic fluid is deeper than 8 cm (equivalent to the 97th percentile) or when the sum of four pockets, one from each quadrant of the uterus (amniotic fluid index), exceeds approximately 24 cm (95th percentile; Moore and Cayle, 1990). The principal cause of hydramnios in diabetic pregnancies is usually poor glycemic control, although fetal gastrointestinal anomalies (e.g., esophageal atresia) need to be excluded. A rapid increase in fundal height should prompt a thorough ultrasound examination by a skilled examiner. The main clinical problems associated with hydramnios are fetal malposition and preterm labor.

Management of the patient with hydramnios is predominantly symptomatic, focused on improving glycemic control and preventing premature labor. Enhanced patient awareness of contractions and the signs and subtle sensations of preterm labor is essential.

MANAGEMENT

Preconception Management

Preconception counseling and a detailed medical risk assessment are recommended for all women with overt diabetes as well as for those with a history of gestational diabetes in a previous pregnancy. The significant effects on the maternal and neonatal complications of diabetic pregnancy cannot be realized until meticulous preconception metabolic control is achieved in all women contemplating pregnancy.

The important elements to be considered in preconception counseling of patients with diabetes are the patient's level of glycemic control; current status of the patient's retinal and renal health; and any medications being taken, especially antihypertensive or thyroid medications. A realistic assessment of the patient's risk of complications during pregnancy, including worsening of renal or ophthalmologic function, should be provided.

Preconception management should lead to a comprehensive program of glucose control. The major goals of the prepregnancy metabolic program are as follows:

- Establishing a regimen of frequent, regular monitoring of capillary blood glucose levels
- Adopting an insulin dosing regimen that results in a smooth interprandial glucose profile (fasting blood glucose value 90 to 99 mg/dL, 1-hour postprandial glucose level of less than 140 mg/dL or 2-hour postprandial glucose level less than 120 mg/dL, no reactions between meals or at night)
- Bringing HbA_{1c} level into the normal range
- Developing family, financial, and personal resources to assist the patient if pregnancy complications require that she lose work time or assume total bed rest

This preconception care has been shown to decrease congenital anomalies and to result in fewer hospitalizations, fewer infants requiring intravenous glucose after delivery, and a substantial reduction in total costs (Herman et al, 1999).

Prenatal Metabolic Management

The goals of glycemic monitoring, dietary regulation, and insulin therapy in diabetic pregnancy are to prevent the postnatal sequelae of diabetes in the newborn—macrosomia, shoulder dystocia, and postnatal metabolic instability. These measures must be instituted early and aggressively if they are to be effective.

Principles of Dietary Therapy

Because women with diabetes have inadequate insulin action after feeding, the goal of dietary therapy is to avoid single, large meals and foods with a large proportion of simple carbohydrates. Three major meals and three snacks are prescribed. The use of nonglycemic foods that release calories into the gut slowly also improves metabolic control.

Nutritional therapy should be supervised by a trained professional who performs formal dietary assessment and counseling at several points during the pregnancy. The dietary prescription should provide adequate quantity and distribution of calories and nutrients to meet the needs of the pregnancy and support achieving the plasma glucose targets that have been established. For obese women (body mass index >30 kg/m^2), a 30% to 33% restriction in caloric intake (to 25 kcal per kilogram of actual weight per day or less) has been shown to reduce hyperglycemia and plasma triglycerides with no increase in ketonuria. Moderate restriction of dietary carbohydrate intake to 35% to 40% of calories has been shown to reduce maternal glucose levels and improve maternal and fetal outcomes (Major et al, 1998). In a nonrandomized study, subjects with low carbohydrate intake (<42% of calories) had lower requirements for insulin for glucose control and significantly lower rates of macrosomia and cesarean deliveries for cephalopelvic disproportion and macrosomia. Recently, a randomized trial was performed in which 958 women with gestational diabetes were randomized to usual prenatal care or treatment (Landon, 2009). Women randomized to treatment underwent nutritional counseling, diet therapy, and insulin if indicated. Among those who underwent treatment there was lower mean birthweight, neonatal fat mass, rates of large for gestational age and macrosomic (>4000 g) infants. There was also a trend toward lower cord C-peptide levels in the treatment group. Maternal outcomes were significant for lower rates of cesarean delivery, preeclampsia, and shoulder dystocia (Landon et al, 2009).

Principles of Glucose Monitoring

The availability of chemical test strips for capillary blood glucose measurements has revolutionized the management of diabetes, and their use should now be considered the standard of care for pregnancy monitoring. The discipline of measuring and recording blood glucose levels before and after meals may have the effect of improving glycemic control (Goldberg et al, 1986).

Controversy exists as to whether the target glucose levels to be maintained during diabetic pregnancy should be designed to limit macrosomia or to closely mimic nondiabetic pregnancy profiles. The Fifth International Workshop Conference on Gestational Diabetes (Metzger et al, 2007) recommended the following: fasting plasma glucose less than 90 to 99 mg/dL (5.0 to 5.5 mmol/L) and 1-hour postprandial plasma glucose less than 140 mg/dL (7.8 mmol/L), or 2-hour postprandial plasma glucose less than 120 to 127 mg/dL (6.7 to 7.1 mmol/L).

The glycemic control profiles from Cousins et al (1980) were derived from highly controlled studies in which volunteer subjects were fed test meals with specific caloric content on a rigid schedule. Parretti et al (2001) profiled normal pregnant women twice monthly, preprandially, and postprandially during the third trimester. Testing was conducted with capillary glucose meters, and the women followed an ad libitum diet. The data demonstrate that fasting and premeal plasma glucose levels are usually less than 80 mg/dL and often less than 70 mg/dL. Peak postprandial plasma glucose values rarely exceed 110 mg/dL. Yogev et al (2004) used a sensor that monitored interstitial fluid glucose levels to obtain continuous glucose information from pregnant women without diabetes and found similar results to those of Parretti et al (2001). The range of normal glucose levels in nondiabetic pregnancy is summarized in Table 9-5.

Postprandial values must be assessed because they have the strongest correlation with fetal growth (Jovanovic-Peterson et al, 1991). The Diabetes in Early Pregnancy Study found that postprandial glucose levels were strongly predictive of both birthweight and the overall percentage of macrosomic infants. With postprandial glucose values averaging 120 mg/dL, approximately 20% of infants were macrosomic; a 30% rise in postprandial levels to 160 mg/dL resulted in a predicted percentage of macrosomia of 35%.

Similar results were reported by de Veciana et al (1995). Compared with the group who performed preprandial glucose monitoring, the group performing postprandial glucose monitoring demonstrated a greater mean change in the HbA_{1c} value (3.0% vs. 0.6%; p <0.001), lower birthweights (3469 g vs. 3848 g; p = 0.01), and lower rates of both neonatal hypoglycemia (3% vs. 21%, p = 0.05) and macrosomia (12% vs. 42%; p = 0.01).

A typical schedule involves performing blood glucose checks upon rising in the morning, 1 or 2 hours after breakfast, before and after lunch, before and after dinner, and before bedtime. The goal of physiologic glycemic control in pregnancy, however, is not met by simply avoiding hypoglycemia. The data summarized here regarding fetal macrosomia and postnatal morbidity emphasize the key role of excessive postprandial excursions in blood glucose values. Therefore, close attention must be paid to preprandial and postprandial glycemic profiles.

Principles of Insulin Therapy

No available insulin delivery method approaches the precise secretion of the hormone from the human pancreas. The therapeutic goal of exogenous insulin therapy during pregnancy is to achieve diurnal glucose excursions similar to those of nondiabetic pregnant women. Normal pregnant women maintain postprandial blood glucose excursions within a relatively narrow range (70 to 120 mg/dL). As pregnancy progresses, the fasting and between-meal blood glucose levels drop progressively lower as a result of the continual uptake of glucose from the maternal circulation by the growing fetus. Any insulin regimen for pregnant women must be designed to avoid excessive unopposed insulin action during the fasting state.

Insulin type and dosage frequency should be individualized. Use of regular insulin before each major meal helps to limit postprandial hyperglycemia. To provide basal insulin levels between feedings, a longer-acting preparation is necessary, such as isoprotane insulin (NPH) or insulin zinc (Lente). Typical subcutaneous insulin dosing regimens are two thirds of total insulin in the morning, of which two thirds as intermediate-acting and one third as regular insulin. The remaining third of the total insulin dose is given in the evening, with 50% as short-acting insulin before dinner and 50% as intermediate-acting given at bedtime.

The use of an insulin pump for type 1 diabetes mellitus during pregnancy has become more widespread (Gabbe et al, 2000). An advantage of this approach is the more physiologic insulin release pattern that can be achieved with the pump.

Ultrasonography has also been used to direct insulin management (Rossi et al, 2000). Kjos et al (2001) showed that serial normal fetal abdominal circumference measurements can be used to avoid insulin therapy without increasing neonatal morbidity.

Oral Hypoglycemic Therapy

Historically, insulin has been the mainstay of therapy for gestational diabetes because of early reports that oral hypoglycemic drugs are a potential cause of fetal anomalies and neonatal hypoglycemia. Sulfonylurea compounds are contraindicated during pregnancy because of a high level of transplacental penetration and clinical reports of prolonged and severe neonatal hypoglycemia (Zucker and Simon, 1968). An increased rate of congenital malformations, particularly ear anomalies, has been reported from a small case-control study (Piacquadio et al, 1991).

TABLE 9-5 Ambulatory Glucose Values in Pregnant Women With Normal Glucose Tolerance

Study	No. of Subjects	Fasting (mg/dL)	Postprandial Level at 60 min (mg/dL)	Postprandial Peak (mg/dL)
Parretti et al, 2001	51	69 (57-81)	108 (96-120)	—
Yogev et al, 2004	57	75 (51-99)	105 (79-131)	110 (68-142)*

Adapted from Metzger BE, Buchanan TA, Coustan DR, et al: Summary and recommendations of the Fifth International Workshop-Conference on Gestational Diabetes Mellitus, *Diabetes Care* 30:S251-S260, 2007.
*The time of the peak postprandial glucose concentration was 70 minutes (range, 44 to 96 minutes).

However, when Towner et al (1995) evaluated the frequency of birth defects in patients who took oral hypoglycemic agents during the periconception period, they noted that first-trimester HbA$_{1c}$ level and duration of diabetes were strongly associated with fetal congenital anomalies, but that use of oral hypoglycemic medications was not.

Glyburide, a second-generation sulfonylurea, has been shown to cross the placenta minimally in laboratory studies (Elliott et al, 1994) and in a large clinical trial. The prospective, randomized trial conducted by Langer et al (2000) compared glyburide and insulin in 404 women with gestational diabetes and showed equivalently excellent maternal glycemic control and perinatal outcomes.

Beyond this single, encouraging study, experience with glyburide during pregnancy is limited (Coetzee and Jackson, 1985; Lim et al, 1997). Chmait et al (2004), reporting experience with 69 patients with gestational diabetes who were given glyburide, found a failure rate of 19% (>10% glucose values above target). Glyburide failure rate was higher in women receiving a diagnosis earlier in pregnancy (20 vs. 27 weeks' gestation; p <0.003) and whose average fasting glucose in the week before starting glyburide was higher (126 vs. 101 mg/dL).

Following the publication of the randomized control trial, several retrospective series have been published comprising 504 glyburide-treated patients, summarized recently by Moore (2007). Jacobson et al (2005) performed a retrospective cohort comparison of glyburide and insulin treatment of gestational diabetes. The insulin group (n = 268) consisted of those diagnosed in 1999 through 2000 and the glyburide group (n = 236) was diagnosed in 2001 through 2002. Glyburide dosing was begun with 2.5 mg in the morning and increased by 2.5 to 5.0 mg weekly. If the dose exceeded 10 mg daily, twice daily dosing was considered. If glycemic goals were not met on a maximum daily dose of 20 mg, treatment was changed to insulin. There were no statistically significant differences in gestational age at delivery, mode of delivery, birthweight, large for gestational age (LGA), or percent macrosomia. The rate of preeclampsia doubled in the glyburide group (12% vs 6%; p = 0.02). Women in the glyburide group also had significantly lower posttreatment fasting and postprandial blood glucose levels. The glyburide group was also superior in achieving target glycemic levels (86% vs. 63%; p <0.001). The failure rate (transfer to insulin) was 12%. The study size, however, was insufficient to detect less than a doubling of the rate of macrosomia/LGA and a 44% increase in neonatal hypoglycemia.

Conway et al (2004) reported a retrospective cohort of 75 glyburide-treated patients with GDM. Good glycemic control was achieved by 84% of the subjects with glyburide, and treatment for 16% was switched to insulin. The rate of fetal macrosomia was similar between women successfully treated with glyburide and those who received insulin (11.1% vs. 8.3%; p = 1.0), and mean birthweight was also similar. Of note, a nonsignificantly higher proportion of infants in the glyburide group required intravenous glucose infusions because of hypoglycemia (25.0% vs. 12.7%; p = 0.37). Currently there is a growing acceptance of glyburide use as a primary therapy for GDM (Coustan, 2007).

OTHER AGENTS

Metformin is frequently used in patients with polycystic ovary syndrome and type 2 diabetes mellitus to improve insulin resistance and fertility (Legro et al, 2007). Metformin therapy has been demonstrated to improve the success of ovulation induction (Vandermolen et al, 2001) and may reduce first-trimester pregnancy loss in women with polycystic ovary syndrome (Jakubowicz et al, 2002). However, the effects of continuing metformin treatment during pregnancy are currently being studied. Older studies evaluating the efficacy and safety of the treatment of pregestational and gestational diabetics with metformin raised concerns regarding a higher perinatal mortality, a higher rate of preeclampsia, and failure of therapy (Coetzee and Jackson 1979; Hellmuth et al, 2000). However, the metformin-treated women were older, more obese, and treated later in pregnancy.

A more recent cohort study of metformin in pregnancy by Hughes and Rowan (2006) included 93 women with metformin treatment (only 32 continued until delivery) and 121 controls. There was no difference in perinatal outcomes between the groups. Glueck et al (2002) compared women without diabetes but with polycystic ovary syndrome who conceived while taking metformin and continued the agent through delivery (n = 28) to matched women without metformin therapy (n = 39). Gestational diabetes developed in 31% of women who did not take metformin versus 3% of those who did (odds ratio, 0.115; 95% CI, 0.014 to 0.938).

Recently a large randomized controlled trial was performed comparing metformin to insulin for the treatment of gestational diabetes (Rowan et al, 2008). This study was powered to detect a 33% increase in composite outcome (neonatal hypoglycemia, respiratory distress, need for phototherapy, birth trauma, 5-minute American Pediatric Gross Assessment Record score of less than 7, or prematurity) in neonates born to mothers treated with metformin. Seven hundred fifty-one women with gestational diabetes between 20 and 30 weeks' gestation were randomized to metformin or insulin. Of these, 363 women were assigned to metformin and 370 were assigned to insulin. Forty-six percent of women receiving metformin required the addition of insulin to obtain adequate glycemic control. There were no differences in the rate of the primary composite outcome. There was a lower rate of severe neonatal hypoglycemia in the metformin-treated group and no differences in neonatal anthropometric measurements. There was, however, a higher rate of prematurity in the metformin-treated group (12.1%) versus the insulin group (7.6%). A follow-up study is currently under way to assess the offspring of these women at 2 years of age.

Prenatal Obstetric Management

The overall strategy for managing a diabetic pregnancy in the third trimester involves two goals: (1) preventing stillbirth and asphyxia and (2) monitoring growth of the fetus to select the proper time and route of delivery to minimize maternal and infant morbidity. The first goal is accomplished by testing fetal well-being at frequent intervals, and the second through ultrasonographic monitoring of fetal size.

Periodic Biophysical Testing of the Fetus

A variety of biophysical tests of the fetus are available to the clinician, including fetal heart rate testing, fetal movement assessment, ultrasound biophysical scoring, and fetal umbilical Doppler studies. Most of these tests, if applied properly, can be used with confidence to provide assurance of fetal well-being while awaiting fetal maturity; they are summarized in Table 9-6.

Testing should be initiated early enough to avoid significant risk of stillbirth, but not so early that the risk of a false-positive result is high. In patients with poor glycemic control or significant hypertension, testing should begin as early as 28 weeks' gestation. In lower-risk patients, most centers begin formal fetal testing by 34 to 36 weeks' gestation. Counting of fetal movements is performed in all pregnancies from 28 weeks' gestation onward.

Assessing Fetal Growth

Monitoring of fetal growth continues to be a challenging and highly inexact process. Although the current tools, consisting of serial plotting of fetal growth parameters, are superior to earlier clinical estimations, accuracy is still ±15%. Single and multiple longitudinal assessments of fetal size have been attempted.

Calculation of Estimated Fetal Weight

Several polynomial formulas using combinations of head, abdominal, and limb measurements have been proposed to predict the weight of the macrosomic fetus from ultrasonography parameters (Ferrero et al, 1994; Tongsong et al,

1994). Unfortunately, in such formulas, small errors in individual measurements of the head, abdomen, and femur are typically multiplied together. In the obese fetus, the inaccuracies are further magnified. Bernstein and Catalano (1992) observed that a significant correlation exists between the degree of error in the ultrasonographically estimated fetal weight and the percentage of body fat on the fetus ($r = 0.28$; $p <0.05$). Perhaps this problem explains why no single formula has proved to be adequate in identifying the macrosomic fetus (Tamura et al, 1985).

Shamley and Landon (1994) reviewed the relative accuracy of the various available formulas. Approximately 75% of the fetal weight predictions were within 10% of actual birthweight, with sensitivity for detecting macrosomia varying greatly (11% to 76%). In another study, McLaren et al (1995) found that 65% of weight estimates based on a simple abdominal circumference and femur length formula were within 10% of actual weight. A similar accuracy was achieved with more complex models (53% to 66% of estimates within the range).

The formula developed by Shepard et al (1982), which uses biparietal diameter and abdominal circumference, is readily available in textbooks and is used most commonly in current ultrasonographic equipment software. The formula has accuracy levels similar to the statistics quoted previously.

Serial Estimated Fetal Weight Assessments

Because prediction of fetal weight from a single set of measurements is inaccurate, serial estimates showing the trend of ultrasonographic parameters (typically made every 1.5 to 3 weeks) might theoretically offer a better estimate of actual weight percentile. A comparison of the efficacy of serial estimated fetal weight calculations to a single measurement, however, did not show better predictive accuracy. Larsen et al (1995) reported that predictions based on the average of repeated weight estimates, on linear extrapolation from two estimates, or on extrapolation by a second-order equation fitted to four estimates were no better than the prediction from the last estimate before delivery. Similar findings (that a single estimate is as accurate as multiple assessments) were reported by Hedriana and Moore (1994).

Choosing the Timing and Route of Delivery

Timing of delivery should be selected to minimize maternal and neonatal morbidity and mortality. Delaying delivery to as near as possible to the due date helps to maximize cervical ripeness and improve the chances of spontaneous labor and vaginal delivery. Yet the risks of fetal macrosomia, birth injury, and fetal death rise as the due date approaches (Rasmussen et al, 1992). Although earlier delivery at 37 weeks' gestation might reduce the risk of shoulder dystocia, the higher rates of failed labor inductions and poor neonatal pulmonary status at this time must be considered. Therefore an optimal time for delivery of most diabetic pregnancies is between 39.0 and 40 weeks' gestation.

Delivery of a diabetic patient before 39 weeks' gestation without documentation of fetal lung maturity should be performed only for compelling maternal or fetal reasons. Fetal lung maturity should be verified in such cases from the presence of more than 3% phosphatidyl glycerol or the equivalent in amniotic fluid as ascertained from an amniocentesis

TABLE 9-6   Tests of Fetal Well-Being

Test	Frequency	Reassuring Result	Comment
Counting of fetal movements	Every night from 28 weeks' gestation	Ten movements in <60 min	Performed in all patients
Nonstress test	Twice weekly	Two heart rate accelerations in 20 min	Begin at: 28-34 wk in patients with insulin-dependent diabetes, 36 wk in patients with diet-controlled gestational diabetes
Contraction stress test	Weekly	No heart rate decelerations in response to ≤3 contractions in 10 min	Same as for nonstress test
Ultrasound biophysical profile	Weekly	Score of 8 in 30 min	The following findings are given 2 points each: 3 movements 1 flexion 30 sec breathing 2 cm amniotic fluid

specimen. After 39 weeks' gestation, the obstetrician can await spontaneous labor if the fetus is not macrosomic and results of biophysical testing are reassuring. In patients with gestational diabetes and superb glycemic control, continued fetal testing and expectant management can be considered until 41 weeks' gestation (Lurie et al, 1992).

Given the previous data, the decision to attempt vaginal delivery or perform a cesarean section is inevitably based on limited data. The patient's obstetric history from previous pregnancies, the best estimation of fetal weight, the fetal adipose profile (abdomen larger than head), and results of clinical pelvimetry should all be considered. A policy of elective cesarean section for suspected fetal macrosomia (ultrasonographically estimated fetal weight of greater than 4500 g) would require 443 cesarean deliveries to avoid one permanent brachial plexus injury (Rouse et al, 1996). Most large series of diabetic pregnancies report a cesarean section rate of 30% to 50%. The best means by which this rate can be lowered is early and strict glycemic control in pregnancy. Conducting a long labor induction in the patient with a large fetus and marginal pelvis may increase rather than decrease morbidity and costs.

Intrapartum Glycemic Management

Maintenance of intrapartum metabolic homeostasis is essential to avoid fetal hypoxemia and promote a smooth postnatal transition. Strict maternal euglycemia during labor does not guarantee newborn euglycemia in infants with macrosomia and long-established islet cell hypertrophy. Nevertheless, the use of a combined insulin and glucose infusion during labor to maintain maternal blood glucose in a narrow range (80 to 110 mg/dL) during labor is a common and reasonable practice. Typical infusion rates are 5% dextrose in lactated Ringer's solution at 100 mL/hr and regular insulin at 0.5 to 1.0 U/hr. Capillary blood glucose levels are monitored hourly in such patients.

For patients with diet-controlled gestational diabetes in labor, avoiding dextrose in all intravenous fluids normally maintains excellent blood glucose control. After 1 to 2 hours, no further assessments of capillary blood glucose are typically necessary.

Neonatal Management
Neonatal Transitional Management

One of the metabolic problems common to IDMs is hypoglycemia, which is related to the level of maternal glycemic control over the 6 to 12 weeks before birth. Neonatal hypoglycemia is most likely to occur between 1 and 5 hours after birth, as the rich supply of maternal glucose stops with ligation of the umbilical cord and the infant's levels of circulating insulin remain elevated. These infants therefore require close monitoring of blood glucose concentration during the first hours after birth. IDMs also appear to have disorders of catecholamine and glucagon metabolism as well as diminished capability to mount normal compensatory responses to hypoglycemia.

In the past, IDMs were treated with glucagon; however, this treatment frequently results in high blood glucose levels that trigger insulin secretion and repeated cycles of hypoglycemia and hyperglycemia. Current

recommendations, therefore, consist of early oral feeding, when possible, with infusion of intravenous glucose.

Ordinarily, blood glucose levels can be controlled satisfactorily with an intravenous infusion of 10% glucose. If greater amounts of glucose are required, bolus administration of 2 mL/kg of 10% glucose is recommended. Close monitoring to correct hypoglycemia while avoiding hyperglycemia and consequent stimulation of insulin secretion is important.

Breastfeeding

Most authorities prefer to maintain strict monitoring of newborn IDM glucose levels for at least 4 to 6 hours, which frequently necessitates admission to a newborn special care unit. IDMs who are delivered atraumatically and are well oxygenated, however, can be kept with their mothers while undergoing close glycemic monitoring for the first 1 to 2 hours of life. This approach permits early breastfeeding, which may reduce the need for intravenous glucose therapy.

Summary

Intensive management of women with glucose intolerance during pregnancy has resulted in markedly improved pregnancy outcomes. Despite these advances, care of the IDM continues to require vigilance and meticulous monitoring with a full understanding of the quality of the glycemic milieu in which the infant developed.

DISORDERS OF THE THYROID
INCIDENCE

Thyroid disorders, in general, are more common in women than in men and represent a common endocrine abnormality during pregnancy. Both hyperthyroidism and hypothyroidism in the mother put the infant at risk and require careful management by the perinatal-neonatal team. Table 9-7 presents an overview of the approach to infants who are thought to be at risk for abnormal thyroid function because of maternal thyroid abnormalities. The most frequently described problem is the syndrome of postpartum thyroiditis, which has been reported to complicate as many as 5% of all pregnancies. The diagnosis of thyroid disease in pregnancy is complicated by the natural changes that occur in immunologic status of the mother and fetus and that variously affect the assessment of any of the autoimmune thyroid disorders.

MATERNAL-FETAL THYROID FUNCTION IN PREGNANCY

Maternal Thyroid Function

Several pregnancy-related physiologic conditions affect maternal thyroid function, and the appropriate interpretation of thyroid function test results during pregnancy must take these normal physiologic factors into account. One important modification that occurs during pregnancy is the estrogen-dependent increase in thyroid-binding globulin. This results in an increase in total thyroxine and total triiodothyronine levels throughout pregnancy. The

TABLE 9-7   Approaches for Infants Judged to be at Risk for Abnormal Thyroid Function

Possible Thyroid Abnormality	Cord Blood Analyses	Assessment at Birth	Assessment at 2-7 Days of Life
Congenital hyperthyroidism because mother has any of the following: Graves' disease with hyperthyroidism and may have been treated with PTU, methimazole, ^{131}I, iodides, or surgery; history of Graves' disease; history of Hashimoto's disease	T_4, TSH, TSAb	Physical examination for intrauterine growth restriction, goiter, exophthalmos, tachycardia, bradycardia, size of anterior fontanel, synostosis, congenital anomalies; determination of gestational age by dates, ultrasonography during pregnancy, or Dubovitz examination; neurologic examination; determination of bone age (knee); for selected cases: electrocardiogram, auditory and visual evoked potentials, motor conduction, velocity tests, skull radiographs	T_4, TSH, TSAb (if available) determinations: If results normal, give no treatment; observe and repeat T_4, T_3, TSH determinations at 7-10 days[*]; if results indicate hypothyroidism, repeat T_4, TSH; if results are abnormal, begin treatment at 7-10 days[†]; if results indicate hyperthyroidism, begin treatment with PTU (8 mg/kg) and propranolol
Congenital or early childhood hypothyroidism because mother has any of the following: Graves disease with excessive PTU therapy; Hashimoto's disease; acute (subacute) thyroiditis; familial genetic defect in thyroxine synthesis; treatment with iodides or lithium for nonthyroidal illness; exposure to ^{131}I while pregnant	T_4, TSH, ThyAb	Same as for hyperthyroidism	T_4, TSH, ThyAb determinations: If results indicate hypothyroidism, perform ultrasound scan to define presence, size, location of thyroid tissue; if hypothyroidism confirmed, begin treatment with levothyroxine sodium (Synthroid), 0.05 mg/day

Adapted from Creasy RK, Resnik R, editors: *Maternal-fetal medicine: principles and practice,* ed 2, Philadelphia, 1989, WB Saunders.
I, Radioactive iodine; *PTU,* propylthiouracil; *T₄,* thyroxine; *TSAb,* thyroid-stimulating antibody; *T₃,* triiodothyronine; *ThyAb,* thyroid antibody; *TSH,* thyroid-stimulating hormone.
[*]Graves disease does not develop at 7 to 10 days in children whose mothers receive PTU.

levels of unbound (free) thyroxine (FT_4) and free triiodothyronine (FT_3), as well as levels of thyroid-stimulating hormone (TSH), in general remain unchanged. However, human chorionic gonadotropin, a second factor in pregnancy that may modify thyroid function, has a stimulatory effect on the thyroid and may transiently effect the FT_4, FT_3, and TSH levels in the first trimester and early in the second trimester. This stimulatory affect of human chorionic gonadotropin rarely causes aberrations of the thyroid function parameters into the thyrotoxic range (American College of Obstetricians and Gynecologists, 2001).

Fetal Thyroid Function

The fetal thyroid actively concentrates iodide after 10 weeks' gestation, releases thyroxine (T_4) after 12 weeks' gestation, and becomes responsive to pituitary TSH at 20 weeks' gestation. Although maternal TSH does not cross the placenta, maternal thyroid hormones and thyrotropin-releasing hormone are transferred to the fetus throughout gestation. Early studies found that cord blood thyroid function testing of neonates with congenital thyroid agenesis revealed hormone levels that were 30% of normal (Vulsma et al, 1989), suggesting a maternal source. Recent studies show that by 4 weeks after conception, small amounts of T_4 and triiodothyronine (T_3) from the maternal origin are found in the fetal compartment, with T_4 levels increasing throughout gestation. Free T_4 levels reach concentrations of biologic significance in the adult by midgestation. Studies using rat models have demonstrated that this thyroid hormone is important for corticogenesis early in the pregnancy (Morreale de Escobar et al, 2004). Transplacental transfer of thyroid-stimulating immunoglobulin (TSI) may occur, causing fetal

thyrotoxicosis. Other substances that may be transferred from the maternal compartment to the fetal compartment and affect fetal thyroid function are iodine, a radioactive isotope of iodine, propylthiouracil (PTU), and methimazole. The fetal effects of these agents are reviewed later.

Hyperthyroidism

Hyperthyroidism occurs in approximately 0.2% of pregnancies and results in a significant increase in the prevalence of both low-birthweight delivery and a trend toward higher neonatal mortality. The most common cause of thyrotoxicosis (85% of cases) in women of child-bearing age is Graves' disease; other causes are acute (or subacute) thyroiditis (transient), Hashimoto's disease, hydatidiform mole, choriocarcinoma, toxic nodular goiter, and toxic adenoma. Graves' disease has a peak incidence during the reproductive years, but patients with the disorder may actually have remissions during pregnancy, followed by postpartum exacerbations. The unique feature of these pregnancies is that the fetus may also be affected, regardless of the mother's concurrent medical condition. Thyroid function is difficult to evaluate in the fetus, and the status of the fetus may not correlate with that of the mother.

Diagnosis

The differential diagnosis of thyrotoxicosis becomes more difficult during pregnancy because normal pregnant women may have a variety of hyperdynamic signs and symptoms—intolerance to heat, nervousness, irritability, emotional lability, increased perspiration, tachycardia, and anxiety. Laboratory data are also difficult to evaluate because total serum thyroxin values are normally elevated during pregnancy as a result of estrogen-induced increases in thyroxine-binding globulin. Therefore if thyroxine-binding globulin is increased, then T_3 resin uptake may be in the euthyroid to slightly increased range in a patient who has true hyperthyroidism. Hollingsworth (1989) has reviewed the assessment of thyroid function tests in nonpregnant and pregnant women, along with the differential diagnosis of hyperthyroidism during pregnancy.

Pathogenesis of Graves' Disease

The pathogenesis of Graves' disease is not completely understood, but it probably represents an overlapping spectrum of disorders that are characterized by the production of polyclonal antibodies. It has been appreciated since the 1960s (Sunshine et al, 1965) that abnormal TSIs, which appear to be immunoglobulin G, are present in pregnant women with Graves' disease and cross the placenta easily to cause neonatal hyperthyroidism in some infants (McKenzie and Zakarija, 1978). The clinical spectrum of Graves' disease in utero is broad and may result in stillbirth or preterm delivery. Some affected infants have widespread evidence of autoimmune disease, including thrombocytopenic purpura and generalized hypertrophy of the lymphatic tissues. Thyroid storm can occur shortly after birth, or the infant may have disease that is transient in nature, lasting from 1 to 5 months. Infants born to mothers who have been treated with thioamides may appear normal at birth, but demonstrate signs of thyrotoxicosis at 7 to 10 days of age, when the effect of thioamide suppression of thyroxine synthesis is no longer present. The measurement of thyroid-stimulating antibodies is useful in predicting whether the fetus will be affected.

Management of the Mother

Because radioactive iodine therapy is contraindicated during pregnancy, treatment of the pregnant woman with thyrotoxicosis involves a choice between antithyroid drugs and surgery. The therapeutic goal is to achieve a euthyroid, or perhaps slightly hyperthyroid, state in the mother while preventing hypothyroidism and hyperthyroidism in the fetus. Either PTU or methimazole can be used to treat thyrotoxicosis during pregnancy. Because methimazole therapy can be associated with aplasia cutis in the offspring of treated women, and because PTU crosses the placenta more slowly than methimazole, PTU has become the drug of choice for use during pregnancy. Ordinarily, thyrotoxicosis can be controlled with doses of 300 mg per day. Once the disorder is under control, however, it is important to keep the dose as low as possible, preferably less than 100 mg daily, because this drug crosses the placenta and blocks fetal thyroid function, possibly producing hypothyroidism in the fetus.

In women with cardiovascular effects, the use of beta-blockers may be appropriate to achieve rapid control of thyrotoxicosis. Because administration of propranolol to pregnant women has been associated with intrauterine growth restriction and impaired responses of the fetus to anoxic stress as well as postnatal bradycardia and hypoglycemia, the doses must be closely controlled. Iodides have also been used, particularly in combination with beta-blocking agents, to control thyrotoxicosis. Long-term iodide therapy presents a risk to the fetus. Because of the inhibition of the incorporation of iodide into thyroglobulin, a large, obstructive goiter can develop in the fetus. Surgery during pregnancy is best reserved for cases in which the mother is hypersensitive to antithyroid drugs, compliance with medication is poor, or drugs are ineffective in controlling the disease.

Effects on the Newborn

Approximately 1% of infants born to mothers with some level of thyrotoxicosis have thyrotoxicosis (Figure 9-6). Assessment of fetal risk in utero includes measurement of TSIs, with the expectation that if the titers are high, there is a higher risk of thyrotoxicosis. Additional assessment of the fetus should pay particular attention to elevated resting

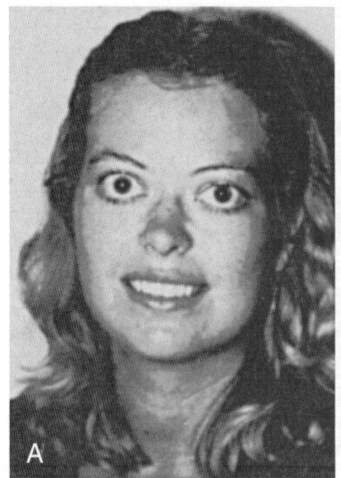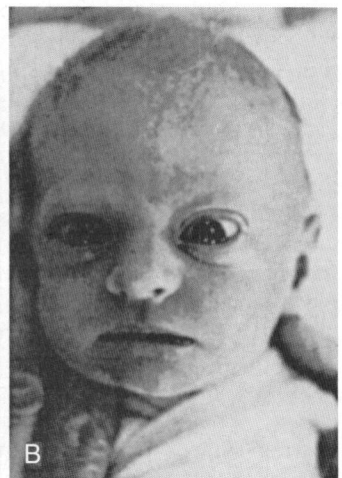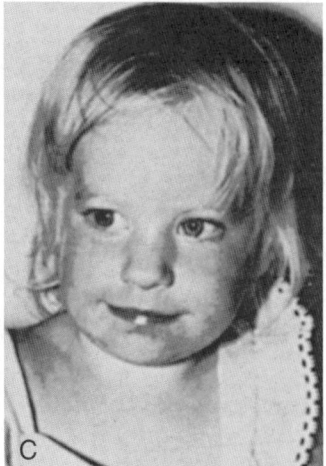

FIGURE 9-6 A, Hypothyroid 21-year-old mother who experienced Graves' disease at age 7 years and was treated by subtotal thyroidectomy. She was given maintenance therapy with daily levothyroxine sodium (Synthroid; 0.15 mg) throughout pregnancy. **B,** Her infant girl was born at term with severe Graves' disease, goiter, and exophthalmos that persisted for 6 months. **C,** The child was healthy at 20 months old. *(From Creasy RK, Resnik R, editors:* Maternal-fetal medicine: principles and practice, *ed 2, Philadelphia, 1989, WB Saunders.)*

heart rate and poor fetal growth. Daneman and Howard (1980) reported on the outcome of nine infants with neonatal thyrotoxicosis and noted normal growth, but a high incidence of craniosynostosis and intellectual impairment. It may be necessary to treat the asymptomatic mother with thioamides and propranolol (and thyroid replacement) during pregnancy to treat the infant and prevent serious neonatal morbidity and long-term problems.

Mothers with thyrotoxicosis who are taking normal doses of thioamide can safely breastfeed their infants, although thioamide appears in breast milk in low amounts. Currently there does not appear to be any long-term adverse outcome for infants whose mothers have received PTU during pregnancy.

HYPOTHYROIDISM

Hypothyroidism complicates about 1 to 3 per 1000 pregnancies. The leading cause of hypothyroidism in pregnancy is Hashimoto's thyroiditis, which is a chronic autoimmune thyroiditis characterized by painless inflammation and enlargement of the thyroid gland (Casey and Leveno, 2006). Other causes of primary hypothyroidism include iodine deficiency, thyroidectomy, or ablative radioiodine therapy for hyperthyroidism. Secondary causes of hypothyrodism include Sheehan's syndrome caused by obstetric hemorrhage leading to pituitary ischemia, necrosis and abnormalities in all pituitary hormones, lymphocytic hypophysitis, and hypophysectomy (Casey and Leveno, 2006). Women with over hypothyroidism are at increased risk of pregnancy complications, such as a higher rate of miscarriage, preeclampsia, placental abruption, growth restriction, and stillbirth (Casey and Leveno, 2006).

Diagnosis

The finding of a goiter may be associated with cases of Hashimoto's thyroiditis or iodine deficiency. The signs and symptoms of hypothyroidism are usually insidious and easily confused with those of normal pregnancy including fatigue, cold intolerance, cramping, constipation, weight gain, hair loss, insomnia, and mental slowness. The serum TSH level is an accurate and widely clinically available test to diagnose hypothyroidism. If the serum TSH is elevated, a free T_4 level should be obtained. In the classic definition of hypothyroidism, the serum TSH is elevated and the free T_4 is low. Other forms of hypothyroidism have also been described, including subclinical hypothyroidism, which is defined as an elevated TSH with a normal free T_4, or hypothyroxinemia defined as a normal TSH but a low free T_4; these have no clinical significance to the mother, but may be associated with neonatal effects discussed later in the neonatal neurologic development section.

Management of the Mother

Levothyroxine is the treatment of choice. Adults with hypothyroidism require approximately 1.7 µg/kg of body weight and should be initiated on full replacement (www.thyroidguidelines.org). The goal of therapy is normalization of the TSH level; therefore the TSH is checked at 4- to 6-week increments, and the dose of levothyroxine is adjusted by 25- to 50-µg increments.

Neonatal Neurologic Development

In humans, early epidemiologic data from iodine-deficient areas of Switzerland suggested a link between mental retardation in the children of women with abnormal thyroid function (Gyamfi et al, 2009). Studies performed by Haddow et al (1999) found that in women with overt, untreated hypothyroidism, the intelligence quotient (IQ) points of children aged 7 to 9 years (using the Wechsler Intelligence Scale IQ test) were 7 points lower in cases than in controls ($p = 0.005$). The percentage of children with IQ scores less than 85 was higher in the cases than in controls (19% versus 5%; $p = 0.007$; Haddow et al, 1999).

It has been demonstrated that early transplacental passage of thyroid hormone is important for normal neurodevelopment of the fetus. T_3 is made from the conversion of maternal T_4. If maternal T_4 levels are low, fetal T_3 in the brain will be low even if the maternal and fetal serum T_3 are normal (Morreale de Escobar et al, 2004). Studies involving rats—which, like humans, are dependent on maternal thyroid hormone early in development—have demonstrated that thyroid hormone receptor is present in the brain before neural tube closure, suggesting a biologic role (Morreale de Escobar et al, 2004). Furthermore in humans, thyroid hormone concentrations in the cerebral cortex at 20 weeks' gestation are comparable to those found in adults (Morreale de Escobar et al, 2004). Lavado-Autric et al (2003) have demonstrated that in iodine-deficient rat pups, there is aberrant neuronal migration, blurring of the cytoarchitecture, and abnormal morphology in the somatosensory cortex and hippocampus. Early in human development there is expression of nuclear thyroid receptors, which are already occupied by T_3, suggesting that normal maternal T_4 levels are necessary for normal cortical development (Morreale de Escobar et al, 2004).

Given the increased risk of adverse perinatal and neurodevelopmental outcomes, all women with overt hypothyroidism should be treated in pregnancy. However, controversy still exists as to whether subclinical hypothyroidism (defined as an elevated TSH level, but normal free T_4) or hypothyroxinemia (defined as a normal TSH level, but a low free T_4) warrant treatment in pregnancy. In 1969, Man and Jones were the first to evaluate offspring of mothers with hypothyroxinemia and found that they had lower IQ scores than normal controls or of those born to mothers with adequately treated hypothyroidism (Gyamfi et al, 2009). Studies performed by Pop et al (1999) in the iodine-deficient areas of the Netherlands have shown that free T_4 levels below the 10th percentile at 12 weeks' gestation were associated with lower scores on the Dutch version of the Bayley Scale of Infant Development at 10 months old. The study included women with a low free T_4 (hypothyroxinemia) and excluded women with elevated TSH. A follow-up study on these same infants, tested in both motor and mental scores at 1 and 2 years of age, found significantly lower scores in infants born to mothers with low free T_4 levels (Pop et al, 2003). Casey et al (2005) performed a study on

Parkland Hospital patients with subclinical hypothyroidism defined as a TSH at 97.5th percentile or higher and a normal free T_4 level. Approximately 2.3% of women screened (404 women) were identified as having subclinical hypothyroidism; compared with normal controls, they had a higher incidence of placental abruption (RR, 3.0; 95% CI, 1.1 to 8.2) and preterm birth before 34 weeks' gestation (RR, 1.8; 95% CI, 1.1 to 2.9) (Casey et al, 2005). The authors concluded that the reduction in IQ in children born to women with subclinical hypothyroidism may be caused by prematurity. Based on the available animal and clinical data, the American Association of Clinical Endocrinologists, the American Thyroid Association, and the Endocrine Society recommend universal screening for all pregnant women. However, the American College of Obstetricians and Gynecologist (2001) recommend that screening should be performed only in women who have risk factors, such as pregestational diabetes, or who are symptomatic. Universal screening is not recommended by the American College of Obstetricians and Gynecologist, given that decision and cost effectiveness studies on the effects of such a strategy are currently lacking. Furthermore, data are lacking regarding therapy dosing, efficacy, or whether medication should be stopped after pregnancy in otherwise asymptomatic women with subclinical hypothyroidism and hypothyroxinemia. A multicenter randomized trial is currently underway to examine whether screening and treatment of hypothyroxinemia or subclinical hypothyroidism have a long-term effect on neurodevelopment of offspring (http://clinicaltrials.gov; study identifier number NCT00388297).

SUGGESTED READINGS

Alam M, Raza SJ, Sherali AR, et al: Neonatal complications in infants born to diabetic mothers, *J Coll Physicians Surg Pak* 16:212-215, 2006.

American College of Obstetricians and Gynecologists: ACOG Practice Bulletin. Clinical management guidelines for obstetrician-gynecologists: gestational diabetes, *Obstet Gynecol* 98:525-538, 2001.

American Diabetes Association: Expert Committee on the Diagnosis and Classification of Diabetes Mellitus: Report of the Expert Committee on the Diagnosis and Classification of Diabetes Mellitus, *Diabetes Care* 25(Suppl 1):S5-S20, 2002.

Casey BM, Dashe JS, Wells CE, et al: Subclinical hypothyroidism and pregnancy outcomes, *Obstet Gynecol* 105:239-245, 2005.

Casey BM, Leveno KJ: Thyroid disease in pregnancy, *Obstet Gynecol* 108:1283-1292, 2006.

Coustan DR: Pharmacological Management of Gestational Diabetes: an overview, *Diabetes Care* 30:S206-S208, 2007.

Study Cooperative Research Group HAPO, Metzger BE, Lowe LP, et al: Hyperglycemia and adverse pregnancy outcomes, *N Engl J Med* 358:1991-2002, 2008.

HAPO Study Cooperative Research Group: Hyperglycemia and adverse pregnancy outcomes: associations with neonatal anthropometrics, *Diabetes* 58:453-459, 2009.

Landon MB, Thom E, Spong CY, et al: A multicenter, randomized trial of treatment for mild gestational diabetes, *N Engl J Med* 361:1339-1348, 2009.

Langer O, Conway D, Berkus M, et al: A comparison of glyburide and insulin in women with gestational diabetes mellitus, *N Engl J Med* 343:1134-1138, 2000.

Morreale de Escobar, Obregon MJ, Escobar del Rey F: Role of thyroid hormone during early brain development, *Eur J Endocrinol* 151(Suppl 3):U25-U37, 2004.

Pop VJ, Browthers EP, Vader HL, et al: Maternal hypothyroxinaemia during early pregnancy and subsequent child development: a 3-year follow-up study, *Clin Endocrinol (Oxf)* 59:282-288, 2003.

Ray JG, O'Brien TE, Chan WS: Preconception care and the risk of congenital anomalies in the offspring of women with diabetes mellitus:a meta-analysis, *QJM* 94:435-444, 2001.

Rowan JA, Hague WM, Gao W, et al: Metformin versus insulin for the treatment of gestational diabetes, *N Engl J Med* 358:2003-2015, 2008.

Temple R, Aldridge V, Greenwood R, et al: Association between outcome of pregnancy and glycaemic control in early pregnancy in type 1 diabetes: population based study, *BMJ* 325:1275-1276, 2002.

Complete references and supplemental color images used in this text can be found online at www.expertconsult.com

MATERNAL MEDICAL DISORDERS OF FETAL SIGNIFICANCE: SEIZURE DISORDERS, ISOIMMUNIZATION, CANCER, AND MENTAL HEALTH DISORDERS

Thomas F. Kelly and Thomas R. Moore

A significant spectrum of maternal medical disorders may complicate pregnancy. Some of these disorders, although readily manageable in nonpregnant patients, can be lethal to pregnant women. As a result, two questions arise for the specialist caring for a pregnant woman with a medical complication. First, is the condition affected by the patient's normal adaptations to pregnancy? Second, how does the medical problem affect the woman and her fetus? Although many medical conditions during pregnancy can be managed much like they would be in a nonpregnant woman, there are usually nuances in care during gestation to which the obstetrician must be attuned and that will potentially affect the fetus and neonate.

During pregnancy, any potential medical therapy should be considered carefully to minimize fetal risk. For example, thalidomide and diethylstilbestrol were prescribed in the past for morning sickness and recurrent miscarriages, respectively, on the basis of the reasonable hypotheses that maternal sedation would decrease nausea and increased estrogens would support the placenta and reduce the likelihood of first-trimester loss. Unfortunately, the use of both of these agents led to significant and tragic congenital anomalies in the offspring. In view of the profusion of new drugs available today, the importance of assessing the expected risk-to-benefit ratio for each medication prescribed to a pregnant woman is increasingly important. An example is phenytoin treatment for maternal seizures. If there is a less teratogenic alternative that is effective, it should be prescribed; however, for most women taking phenytoin, other agents are unable to control their seizures, and the risks to the fetus must be accepted.

The altered pharmacokinetics of many drugs during pregnancy must be considered, because the dosing of familiar medications may have to be adjusted if toxicity is to be avoided. Classic examples are thyroid hormone replacement (a higher level of thyroid-binding globulin in pregnancy increases total thyroxin, but leaves the serum free thyroxin value unchanged) and aminoglycoside antibiotic therapy (increased glomerular filtration in pregnancy results in lower serum drug levels).

This chapter discusses four maternal conditions that can influence fetal growth, development, and outcome: seizure disorders, red blood cell isoimmunization, cancer, and mental disorders. The basics of management, the potential effects of pregnancy on the condition, and the effects of the condition on the mother and fetus are considered.

MATERNAL SEIZURE DISORDERS

Epilepsy is the most common major neurologic disorder in pregnancy. Approximately 18 million women are affected worldwide, and 40% of those are of childbearing age. The estimated prevalence in pregnancy is 0.2% to 0.7% (Chen et al, 2009). The pattern of maternal seizures ranges from complex partial to generalized tonic clonic (grand mal) and generalized absence (petit mal) seizures. Physiologically, seizures arise from paroxysmal episodes of abnormal brain electrical discharges; when associated with motor activity, they are termed *convulsive*.

The effect of pregnancy on the frequency and severity of the seizure disorder has been difficult to ascertain because of limited prospective data. The International Registry of Antiepileptic Drugs and Pregnancy (EURAP) recently reported on more than 1800 patients whose seizure frequency and treatment were recorded. Fifty-eight percent of patients had no seizures during their pregnancy. When using first-trimester seizure activity as a reference, 64% had no change in frequency in the second and third trimester, 6% improved, and 12% deteriorated (EURAP Study Group, 2006). The only exception was that tonic-clonic seizures occurred more frequently in women using oxcarbazepine monotherapy; this has been confirmed by an Australian registry in which seizures occurred in 50% of pregnant women with epilepsy who were receiving therapy. However, in a subset that had no seizures for 12 months before pregnancy, there was a 50% to 70% reduced frequency during gestation (Vajda et al, 2008). In patients in whom higher numbers of seizures occur during gestation, decreased plasma concentrations of antiepileptic medications have been hypothesized as causative. The fall in plasma drug levels during pregnancy may be due in part to increased protein binding, reduced absorption, and increased drug clearance. The adequacy of prepregnancy seizure control can influence a patient's course during gestation. Patients whose seizures were poorly controlled tended to have more frequent seizures during pregnancy, whereas patient who had no seizures for 2 years before pregnancy had only a 10% chance of experiencing seizures during gestation. These latter patients may be candidates for stopping therapy or considering monotherapy if they have previously required multiple antiepileptic drugs (Schmidt et al, 1983; Walker et al, 2009).

PERINATAL RISK

For reasons that are not clear, women with seizures have more obstetric complications during pregnancy and a higher rate of poor perinatal outcomes. Rates of preeclampsia, preterm delivery, small-for-gestational-age infants, congenital malformations, cerebral palsy, and perinatal mortality have all been reported as higher in women with an antecedent seizure disorder (Lin et al, 2009; Nelson and Ellenberg, 1982). Pregnancy outcome is also greatly influenced by the mother's socioeconomic status and age as well as by the prenatal care received.

Earlier publications suggested an increased risk of congenital malformations in children of mothers with epilepsy even without prenatal use of antiepileptic drugs (Bjerkedal, 1982). More recent data appear to refute this, and the malformation risk apparently correlates with the number of medications used. A study comparing patients with epilepsy to matched controls revealed that women receiving no medication had no increased rate of congenital malformations; however, monotherapy was associated with and increased risk of embryopathy (odds ratio of 2.8). Furthermore the frequency was even higher with use of two or more drugs (odds ratio of 4.2) (Homes et al, 2001). Recent updates from five international registries have reported malformation rates ranging from 3.7% to 8.0% (with monotherapy) and 6% to 9.8% (with polytherapy) (Meador et al, 2008). Specific malformations include a fivefold rise in the rate of orofacial clefts (Friis et al, 1986), an increase in the rate of congenital heart disease, particularly with trimethadione (Friis and Hauge, 1985), and a 3.8% incidence of neural tube defects in fetuses exposed to valproic acid (Samrén et al, 1997). Facial abnormalities (e.g., midface hypoplasia) are not specific to any particular antiepileptic drug; they have been seen with phenytoin, carbamazepine, and trimethadione. Some antiepileptic medications can adversely affect postnatal cognitive development. Although conclusive data are lacking, there may be an increased adverse effect, particularly with valproate (Meador et al, 2008; Tomson and Battino, 2009).

FETAL HYDANTOIN SYNDROME

The classic features of the fetal hydantoin syndrome are facial clefting, a broad nasal ridge, hypertelorism, epicanthal folds, distal phalangeal hypoplasia, and growth and mental deficiencies; however, these effects also result from the use of other antiseizure medications (Table 10-1). The postulated cause of this syndrome is the teratogenic action of a common epoxide intermediate of these medications. The hydantoin syndrome was found to develop in fetuses with inadequate epoxide hydrolase activity (Buehler et al, 1990). This enzymatic deficiency appears to be recessively inherited. It appears that preconception folic acid supplementation can reduce the risk of major congenital malformations in women taking antiepileptic medication (Harden et al, 2009).

MANAGEMENT

Management of the pregnant patient with epilepsy is based on keeping her free of seizures. Theoretically, this goal reduces maternal physical risk and lowers the incidence of fetal complications. Preconception counseling is preferable and should entail (1) adjusting medication doses into the therapeutic range, (2) attempting to limit the patient to one drug if possible, and (3) choosing an agent with the least risk of teratogenesis. Frank discussion of the various risks of each agent should be conducted, particularly the risks associated with valproic acid and trimethadione. Usually if the patient's disease is adequately controlled with one agent, it rarely needs to be changed, because the risks of increasing seizure activity are believed to outweigh the potential for reducing congenital malformations.

Patients taking antiepileptic medications should also take folic acid supplements (800 to 1000 μg) before conception, because inhibition of folate absorption has been proposed as a teratogenic mechanism, particularly with phenytoin. During gestation, the anticonvulsant levels should be checked monthly, and the dose should be adjusted accordingly, particularly with the use of lamotrigine, carbamazepine, and phenytoin (Harden et al, 2009). Although the evidence is less clear with other agents such as phenobarbital, valproate, primidone, and ethosuximide, serial level assessment should not be discouraged. Medications should not be changed unless they prove ineffective at the optimal serum level. If a patient reports greater seizure activity, the serum drug level should be checked immediately. A common reason for increased seizures is that the patient is not taking her medication, usually because she fears its teratogenicity.

Mothers taking phenytoin, phenobarbital, or primidone may have a higher incidence of neonatal coagulopathy as a result of vitamin K–dependent clotting factor deficiency. Although maternal vitamin K supplementation in the third trimester may be reasonable, there is insufficient evidence to determine whether it will reduce neonatal hemorrhagic complications (Harden et al, 2009).

RED BLOOD CELL ISOIMMUNIZATION

Hydrops fetalis, a condition associated with abnormal fluid collections in various body cavities of the fetus, was first described in 1892. The causes are many but can be divided into two categories: immune causes and nonimmune causes. In immune-mediated hydrops, circulating immunoglobulins lead to the destruction of fetal red blood cells and hemolytic anemia. Landsteiner and Weiner first elucidated the Rhesus factor (Rh) in 1940. Levine et al, showed pathogenesis of erythroblastosis to be due to maternal isoimmunization in 1941. Rh immune globulin was developed in the middle 1960s. Prophylaxis protocols using Rh immune globulin significantly reduced the incidence of D isoimmunization, increasing the relative frequency of alloimmunization against atypical red blood cell antigens such as E, Duffy, and Kell (Figure 10-1). The pathophysiology of immune-mediated fetal hemolytic disease is similar, regardless of the blood group antigen involved; therefore this discussion focuses on the Rh system.

GENETICS

The Rh blood group actually represents a number of antigens, designated D, Cc, and Ee. The genes for these antigens, located on the short arm of chromosome 1, are inherited in a set of three from each parent. The presence of D determines whether the individual is Rh positive, and the absence of D (there is no recessive allele, so "d" does not exist) yields the Rh-negative type. Rarely, a patient exhibits a Du variant and should be considered D positive. The combinations of these various antigens occur with different frequencies. For example, prevalence of Cde (41%) is higher than that of CDE (0.08%) (Lewis et al, 1971). Although the Rh phenotype is the result of D status, the various genotype combinations help to predict the zygosity of an individual. Approximately 45% of Rh-positive individuals are homozygous and therefore will always produce an Rh-positive offspring; 55% are heterozygous and may have an Rh-negative child if paired with an Rh-negative partner.

TABLE 10-1   Clinical Features of the Fetal Hydantoin Syndrome

Craniofacial abnormalities	Broad nasal ridge
	Wide fontanel
	Low-set hairline
	Broad alveolar ridge
	Metopic ridging
	Short neck
	Ocular hypertelorism
	Microcephaly
	Cleft lip with or without palate
	Abnormal or low-set ears
	Epicanthal folds
	Ptosis of eyelids
	Coloboma
	Coarse scalp hair
Limb abnormalities	Smallness or absence of nails
	Hypoplasia of distal phalanges
	Altered palmar crease
	Digital thumb
	Dislocated hip

Data from Briggs GC, Freeman RK, Yaffe SJ: *Drugs in pregnancy and lactation*, ed 7, Baltimore, 2005, Lippincott Williams & Wilkins.

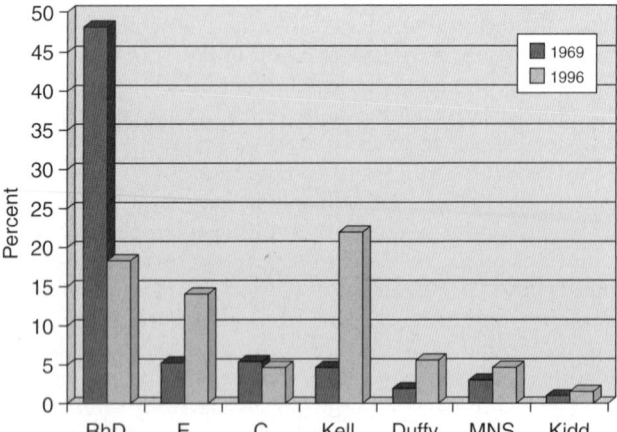

FIGURE 10-1 Differences in incidence of maternal red cell antibodies over time. (*Adapted from Queenan JG, Smith BD, Haber JM, et al: Irregular antibodies in the obstetric patient, Obstet Gynecol 34:767-770, 1969; and Geifman-Holtzman O, Wojtowycz M, Kosmas E, et al: Female alloimmunization with antibodies known to cause hemolytic disease, Obstet Gynecol 89:272-275, 1997.*)

There are no sex differences in the frequency of Rh negativity; however, racial variations are striking. Rh negativity is common in the Basque population (30% to 35%), but rare in Chinese, Japanese, and North American Indian populations (1% to 2%). The average incidence in white populations is approximately 15%. North American blacks have a higher incidence (8%) than African blacks (4%).

PATHOGENESIS

Before modern blood banking, Rh-negative patients became immunized from the transfusion of Rh-positive blood. In the case of atypical red blood cell antigens (e.g., Duffy, Kidd), blood transfusion is still a significant cause of isoimmunization. Currently, fetal transplacental hemorrhage is the primary cause of Rh isoimmunization. Rh immune globulin prophylaxis protocols have reduced but not eliminated this problem. Transplacental hemorrhage of fetal cells into the maternal circulation is surprisingly common, with 75% of women showing evidence of this event at some time during gestation (Bowman et al, 1986). Using sensitive Kleihauer-Betke testing, 0.01 mL or more fetal cells are found in 3%, 12% and 46% of women in the first, second and third trimesters, respectively. The amount of fetal blood is usually small, but approximately 1% of women have 5 mL. In 0.25% of women, 30 mL or more of fetal cells are noted after delivery. Obstetric events increase the chance of transplacental hemorrhage (Box 10-1). As little as 0.3 mL of Rh-positive blood produces immunization, and the risk is dose dependent. ABO blood group incompatibility between fetus and mother affords some protection, reducing the risk from 16% to 2%.

The primary maternal immune response is slow and can take as long as 6 months to develop. The first appearance of immunoglobulin (Ig) M class anti-D antibodies is weak; they do not cross the placenta, but are soon followed by smaller IgG antibodies that are capable of traversing the placental barrier. Therefore the initial event causing sensitization rarely results in fetal hemolysis. A second transplacental hemorrhage leads to the more rapid and abundant amnestic IgG response that, in the presence of fetal D-positive cells, can cause significant hemolysis and fetal anemia.

The severity of hemolytic disease is related to the maternal antibody titer, the affinity for the red blood

---

BOX 10-1   Obstetric Events Associated With Increased Risk of Fetal-Maternal Hemorrhage

- Unexplained vaginal bleeding
- Abruptio placentae
- External breech version
- Amniocentesis
- Chorionic villus sampling, placental biopsy
- Umbilical cord sampling
- Manual removal of the placenta
- Abdominal trauma
- Ectopic pregnancy

cell membrane, and the ability of the fetus to compensate for the red blood cell destruction. Table 10-2 summarizes the severity levels of fetal and neonatal disease and their incidence. Most cases are mild and result in normal outcomes; the cord blood is strongly Coombs positive, but the infants do not exhibit significant anemia or hyperbilirubinemia. Moderate disease results from the red blood cell destruction and the greater production of indirect bilirubin. Although the mother is able to clear this product for the fetus in utero, the neonate is deficient in the liver glucuronyl transferase enzyme, leading to the buildup of this water-insoluble molecule. Albumin carries the indirect bilirubin, but if the binding capacity is exceeded, diffusion of the bilirubin into the fatty tissues occurs. Neural tissue is high in lipid content. Ultimate destruction of neurons can occur, resulting in kernicterus. Treatment depends on the recognition of the hyperbilirubinemia and usually entails phototherapy and possible exchange transfusion in the nursery (see Chapter 79).

Severe disease occurs when the fetus is unable to produce sufficient red blood cells to compensate for the increased destruction of these cells. Extramedullary hematopoiesis, which is prominent in the liver, ultimately leads to enlargement, hepatocellular damage, and portal hypertension. This process is believed to be the etiology of placental edema and ascites. Albumin production diminishes because of hepatocellular damage and results in anasarca, giving rise to hydrops fetalis. The theory that hydrops is due to fetal heart failure no longer holds, as a result of observations that these infants are neither hypervolemic nor in failure. The relationship between fetal anemia and hydrops is variable, but most hydropic fetuses have hemoglobin levels less than 4 g/dL or have a hemoglobin concentration deficit greater than 7 g/dL (Nicolaides et al, 1988).

MANAGEMENT

Management of the sensitized patient, for both Rh and atypical red blood cell antigens, requires an understanding of the mechanism of disease and the skill and experience to

predict its severity. Although management schemes follow some basic guidelines, successful management requires access to a blood bank with expertise in antibody typing and individuals skilled in prenatal diagnostic procedures (e.g., cordocentesis). Referral to experienced high-risk centers for the management of this problem is common in the United States.

MONITORING

At their first prenatal visit, all pregnant patients should undergo a blood type and antibody screen (indirect Coombs' test), which identifies the Rh-negative woman and screens for the presence of anti-D antibody and other immunoglobulins that are associated with atypical red blood cell antigens and capable of causing fetal hemolytic disease (Table 10-3). Any positive result on antibody screening should be evaluated aggressively to identify the antibody and quantify its amount by titer. A consultation with a blood bank pathologist may be necessary for atypical antibodies.

The amount of the anti-D antibody present according to indirect antibody titer is important. For a titer that is less than 16 and remains at that level throughout the pregnancy, most centers consider the fetus to be at negligible risk of hydrops or stillbirth. Each blood bank sets different standards for this critical titer, which depend on the assay used. At a titer of 16, the risk is 10%; at 128, it is 75%. For a woman with a previously affected fetus, no titer is predictive; therefore management based on its result may underestimate the severity of fetal disease.

Once the patient has been identified as isoimmunized, obtaining her obstetric history is important. All of her prior pregnancies and their outcomes must be documented to attempt to elucidate the timing and cause of the sensitization and to assess the risk in the current pregnancy. In general, the condition is worse with each pregnancy. In a first sensitized pregnancy, the risk of hydrops is approximately 10%. More than 90% of patients who have delivered one hydropic baby will deliver another one subsequently.

Paternal blood typing and Rh genotyping should be performed to calculate the fetal risk of Rh positivity. Given

TABLE 10-2   Classification of the Severity of Hemolytic Disease

Severity	Description	Incidence (%)
Mild	Indirect bilirubin result, 16-20 mg/dL No anemia No treatment needed	45-50
Moderate	Fetal hydrops does not develop Moderate anemia Severe jaundice with risk of kernicterus unless treated after birth	25-30
Severe	Fetal hydrops develops in utero Before 34 weeks' gestation After 34 weeks' gestation	20-25 10-12 10-12

Data from Bowman JM: Maternal blood group immunization. In Creasy R, Resnik R, editors: *Maternal-fetal medicine: principles and practice*, Philadelphia, 1984, WB Saunders.

TABLE 10-3   Examples of Atypical Red Blood Cell Antigens Associated With Fetal Hemolytic Disease

Blood Group System	Antigen	Severity of Hemolytic Disease
Kell	K	Mild to severe
Duffy	Fya	Mild to severe
Kidd	JKa	Mild to severe
	JKb	Mild to severe
MNSs	M	Mild to severe
	N	Mild
	S	Mild to severe
	s	Mild to severe
	U	Mild to severe
P	PP	Mild to severe
Public antigens	Yta	Moderate to severe

the high percentage of heterozygosity in Rh-positive individuals, assays utilizing free DNA in the maternal circulation are used to determine a potentially D+ fetus. Accuracy with this technique can approach 97% (Geifman-Holtzman et al, 2006). For atypical blood group immunization, a history of prior obstetric outcomes plus transfusions (a significant cause of such antibodies) and determination of the father's antigen status are of similar importance. For example, a woman with an anti-Kell antibody titer of 128 would be at moderate risk of hydrops, unless the father of the baby were found to be Kell negative. No invasive procedures for isoimmunization should be performed until the father's antibody status is established, unless the fetus's paternity is in question or the partner is unavailable.

Ultrasonographic screening to identify the prehydropic fetus is notoriously unreliable, in that significantly anemic fetuses may not be grossly hydropic. However, clues that have been proposed to suggest impending hydrops are polyhydramnios, skin thickening, early ascites (particularly around the fetal bladder), and placental thickening. Ultrasonographic measurements of the liver and spleen have been suggested as aids in predicting anemia in nonhydropic fetuses, but lack sensitivity and specificity (Bahado-Singh et al, 1998; Vintzileos et al, 1986).

Antibody titers should be followed monthly to predict which fetus is at risk (in the absence of a history of a prior infant with hydrops). If the indirect antibody titer value is less than 16, the development of hydrops is unlikely. Most centers consider the critical value to be 16, because above this level, one cannot ensure the absence of hydrops. When a patient's antibody titer value is equal to or greater than 16, more invasive testing is needed. Such testing is usually accomplished with amniocentesis and, less commonly, through direct fetal blood sampling.

Amniocentesis is the standard screening technique for fetal anemia, because amniotic fluid contains hemolytic products excreted from the fetal kidneys and lungs, including bilirubin. The unconjugated form of bilirubin is secreted across the respiratory tree and therefore into the amniotic fluid. The supernatant is analyzed with a spectrophotometer, and the bilirubin peak corresponding to the level of absorbance (or optical density [OD]) of these hemoglobin products (450 nm) is quantified. The magnitude of the peak is calculated after subtracting the mean baseline value surrounding the peak. The difference from baseline to peak is the ΔOD_{450} value.

The amount of the increase in the ΔOD_{450} value correlates reasonably well with severity of hemolysis. In 1961, Liley developed a graph that has been used to predict the severity of fetal hemolytic disease using the ΔOD_{450} value. The graph is divided into three zones. Zone I represents the lowest risk and indicates an unaffected fetus, whereas zone III strongly suggests a severely affected fetus, in which fetal hydrops and death can ensue if disease is not treated within the next 7 to 10 days. The Liley curve is authoritative in the third trimester, but its reliability before 26 weeks' gestation has been questioned (Queenan et al, 1993). At less than 20 weeks' gestation, the ΔOD_{450} value must be greater than 0.15 or less than 0.09 to be predictive

of severe or mild disease, respectively, with a "gray zone" between the two values that is nonpredictive (Ananth and Queenan, 1989). Thus, the clinician must integrate clinical history and ultrasonography clues for possible impending hydrops or consider fetal blood sampling in a fetus at risk between 18 and 25 weeks' gestation.

Amniocytes can be obtained during the amniocentesis procedure. Through polymerase chain reaction analysis, fetal D antigen typing can be obtained as early as 14 weeks' gestation (Dildy et al, 1996). This process allows the identification of the fetus that is not at risk for hemolytic disease caused by maternal antibody isoimmunization. Isoimmunization with atypical red blood cell antigens other than D can be detected similarly, reducing the amount of unnecessary invasive procedures on an otherwise unaffected fetus.

A recent advance in ultrasound technology has dramatically altered the assessment of the potentially affected fetus. Doppler blood flow measurements in the umbilical vein (Iskarios et al, 1998) and in the middle cerebral artery have shown to be altered in anemia, with the latter revealing an elevated peak systolic velocity. Using a developed reference range with a cutoff of 1.5 multiples of the median, Mari (2000), was able to predict which nonhydropic fetuses had moderate or severe anemia (Figure 10-2). A prospective multicenter trial compared the use of middle cerebral artery Doppler against the "gold standard" amniotic fluid ΔOD_{450}. One hundred sixty-five fetuses were studied, and almost half were found to have severe fetal anemia at cordocentesis. Middle cerebral artery Doppler was noted to have a sensitivity of 88%, a specificity of 85%, and an accuracy of 85%. Doppler outperformed ΔOD_{450} analysis using the Liley curve, with a 9% improvement in the accuracy. Furthermore, it has been suggested that 50% of invasive procedures could have been averted with the use of Doppler (Oepkes et al, 2006). Direct ultrasound-guided fetal umbilical blood sampling provides valuable

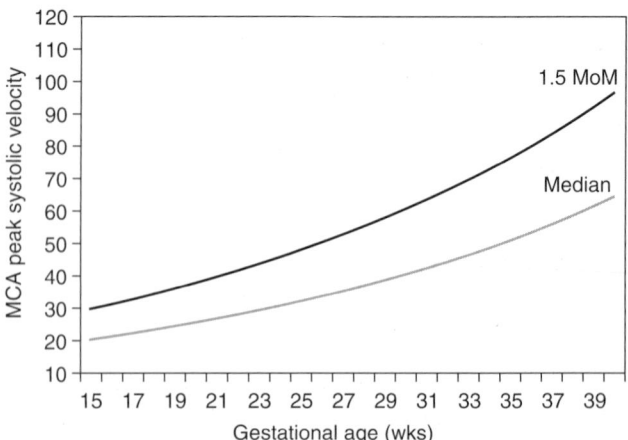

FIGURE 10-2 Peak velocity of systolic blood flow in the middle cerebral artery (MCA) with advancing gestation. The *bottom curve* indicates the median peak systolic velocity in the middle cerebral artery, and the *top line* indicates 1.5 multiples of the median (MoM; the threshold for significant fetal anemia). (*Adapted from Mari G, Hanif F: Fetal Doppler: umbilical artery, middle cerebral artery, and venous system,* Semin Perinatol *32:254, 2008.*)

data for the fetus at risk, particularly after 18 weeks' gestation. Cordocentesis is used most often when the risk determined from history, indirect antibody titer values, Liley curve comparisons, or ultrasonographic clues are significant. Cordocentesis also provides vascular access if fetal transfusion becomes necessary. Although most obstetricians are skilled in amniocentesis, cordocentesis is usually performed in tertiary centers by perinatologists. The latter procedure carries a higher risk of fetal loss and morbidity, and it is associated with a more significant chance of worsening maternal sensitization (Bowman and Pollock, 1994).

THERAPY

Fetal transfusion therapy is the mainstay of treatment for the severely affected but premature fetus. In most centers, for pregnancies beyond 33 weeks' gestation with suspected fetal anemia, administration of steroids and delivery are preferable to an invasive procedure with significant morbidity and mortality. Intraperitoneal transfusions, the primary therapy in the past, are still a useful treatment. O-negative, tightly packed, irradiated blood is infused percutaneously into the fetal peritoneal cavity via an amniocentesis needle with real-time ultrasound guidance. Approximately 10 mL is transfused for each week of gestation beyond 20 weeks. Red blood cell absorption occurs promptly through the subdiaphragmatic lymphatics, although it may be erratic in the hydropic fetus. Overall survival rates with fetuses requiring transfusion approaches 89% (Van Kamp et al, 2005). However, hydrops was associated with a decreased survival rate of 78% (Van Kamp et al, 2001), with severely hydropic fetuses having a survival rate of 55%. Problems associated with intraperitoneal transfusions include injury to vascular or intraabdominal organs and the inability to obtain fetal blood type and blood count. This procedure should be avoided if possible in the hydropic fetus, because the resulting higher abdominal pressure can precipitate venous compression and lead to circulatory collapse.

Direct intravascular transfusions are currently the first line of treatment. The advantages of this procedure include assessing the severity of fetal anemia and documenting the fetal blood type. Ultimate success does not appear to be affected by the presence of hydrops (Ney et al, 1991). The overall success rate is approximately 85%. Limitations are usually related to the procedure. The most accessible site usually requires an anterior placenta, in which the cord root can be visualized; posterior placentation makes the technique more difficult. In addition, risks include bleeding from the cord puncture site, fetal exsanguination, cord hematoma, rupture of membranes, and chorioamnionitis.

Additional transfusions are required every 2 to 3 weeks to compensate for the falling hematocrit associated with fetal growth, the finite life of the transfused red blood cells, and ongoing hemolysis of the existing fetal erythrocytes. Ultimately the entire fetal blood supply is replaced with Rh-negative blood by successive transfusions. A major neonatal side effect is bone marrow depression, which may require postnatal transfusions for 1 to 3 months (De Boer et al, 2008).

As the pregnancy proceeds through the third trimester, frequent fetal testing is performed either with nonstress tests and amniotic fluid index or with biophysical profiles. Delivery is planned for 3 to 6 weeks before term, usually after demonstration of a mature fetal lung profile. Preterm delivery may be indicated in a severely affected fetus, regardless of lung profile, if the risk of transfusion is deemed to exceed the morbidity of a delivery of a near-term yet premature baby.

CANCER

PRINCIPLES

Cancer complicating pregnancy is rare, with an estimated frequency of 1 case per 1000 live births. The trend of delaying childbearing to later maternal age may have influenced this rate. The sites or types of cancer in pregnancy, in descending order of frequency, are cervical, breast, ovarian, lymphoma, melanoma, brain, and leukemia (Table 10-4) (Haas et al, 1984; Jacob and Stringer, 1990). Finding a malignancy during gestation poses a unique set of issues that must be addressed with care. Will the pregnancy accelerate the malignant process? Are the accepted therapies appropriate for the mother, and are they safe for the unborn fetus? Will delay of therapy adversely affect the mother? Should the pregnancy be terminated, or should the child be delivered prematurely to maximize treatment of the mother with no resultant risk to the child?

Few conditions in pregnancy require as meticulous a multidisciplinary approach as cancer. Oncologists who are unaccustomed to interacting with a pregnant woman commonly wish to have the child delivered before giving definitive cancer therapy, for fear of the teratogenic risks to the fetus. Therefore input regarding the situation must be acquired not only from an oncologist but also from the obstetrician, perinatologist, pediatrician, neonatologist, and dysmorphologist. The patient and her family must be involved in decision making, being given information not only about the risks of the disease and its potential therapies, but also about the limitations of current knowledge about cancer in pregnancy and the uncertainties of outcomes.

TABLE 10-4 Cancers that Can Complicate Pregnancy

Site/Type	Incidence (per number of gestations)
Cervix	1:2000 to 1:10,000
Breast	1:3000 to 1:10,000
Melanoma	1:1000 to 1:10,000
Ovary	1:10,000 to 1:100,000
Colorectal	1:13,000
Leukemia	1:75,000 to 1:100,000
Lymphoma	1:1000 to 1:6000

Data from Pentheroudakis G, Pavlidis N, Castiglione M: Cancer, fertility and pregnancy: ESMO clinical recommendations for diagnosis, treatment and followup, *Ann Oncol* 20(Suppl 4):S178-S181, 2009.

SURGERY

Patients can undergo indicated surgery during pregnancy safely. The risk of fetal loss does not seem to rise with uncomplicated anesthesia and surgery. However, if there are any complications from either the anesthesia or the operation, the risk of fetal and maternal mortality increases. For example, fetal loss is rarely related temporally to maternal appendectomy, but is common when the mother's appendix has ruptured. The most comprehensive series of pregnant patients undergoing surgery was collected in Sweden (Mazze and Kallen, 1989). Although these researchers found a slight increase in the rates of low birthweight and neonatal death by 7 days of life, the rates of stillbirth and congenital malformation were similar to the outcomes expected without surgery. Anesthetic agents are not believed to be teratogenic.

A few management guidelines help to optimize outcome for the pregnant patient undergoing surgery. If general anesthesia is used, the maternal airway must be protected to avoid aspiration. Gastrointestinal motility is reduced during pregnancy, and the stomach may contain significant residual contents after many hours without eating. A left lateral decubitus position on the operating table is preferred to maximize uteroplacental blood flow. If the fetus is viable, monitoring of the fetal heart rate should be performed to assist the anesthesia team in optimizing fetal status. Preoperative counseling with the patient is important to allow the surgical team to make appropriate choices in regard to any interventions for fetal distress.

CHEMOTHERAPY

Administering agents that impair cell division in pregnancy is a concern for both the mother and the care team. Often the patient is more concerned about this issue than about the underlying cancer. Cytotoxic chemotherapy should be avoided in the first trimester because of the high incidence of spontaneous abortion and the potential teratogenic effects on the fetus (Table 10-5). For a few agents with confirmed teratogenic effects (e.g., methotrexate, amethopterin, chlorambucil), chemotherapy must be avoided during organogenesis. The use of folic acid antagonists in first-trimester cancer treatment raises the specific problem of possible induction of neural tube defects, because these lesions are known to be folate sensitive.

The literature regarding most other chemotherapeutic agents is limited, consisting of a few collected series; therefore these agents should be used cautiously, with their potential harm to the fetus balanced against their benefit to the maternal condition. Little is also known regarding the long-term outcomes of fetuses exposed to chemotherapeutic agents in utero. The National Cancer Institute in Bethesda, Maryland, maintains a registry in the hopes of determining the delayed effects. A small series of fetuses exposed to chemotherapeutic agents for acute leukemia revealed normal mental development with follow-up between 4 and 22 years (Aviles and Niz, 1988).

The risk of teratogenicity does not appear to be higher with combination chemotherapy than with single-agent therapy (Doll et al, 1989). Studies performed thus far involve small numbers of patients, with power insufficient

to show a statistic difference, but there seems not to be a trend. Low birthweight is found in approximately 40% of babies whose mothers received cytotoxic drugs during pregnancy (Nicholson, 1968). Theoretical consequences, such as bone marrow suppression, immune suppression, and anemia, could occur in the fetus. As a result, the timing of chemotherapy should account for the anticipated date of delivery. Data regarding safety for breastfeeding the neonate of a mother receiving cancer chemotherapy are limited. For this reason, the majority of agents are contraindicated in nursing mothers.

TABLE 10-5 Common Chemotherapy Agents and Uses

Class or Drug	Risk Category	Common Uses
Alkylating Agents		
Busulfan	Dm	Leukemias
Chlorambucil	Dm	Lymphomas, leukemias
Cyclophosphamide	Dm	Breast, ovary, lymphomas, leukemias
Melphalan	Dm	Ovary, leukemia, myeloma
Procarbazine	Dm	Lymphomas
Antimetabolites		
5-Fluorouracil	D*	Breast, gastrointestinal
6-Mercaptopurine	Dm	Leukemias
Methotrexate	Xm	Trophoblastic disease, lymphomas, leukemias, breast
6-Thioguanine	Dm	Leukemias
Antibiotics		
Bleomycin	Dm	Cervix, lymphomas
Daunorubicin	Dm	Leukemias
Doxorubicin	Dm	Leukemias, lymphomas, breast
Other Agents		
All-*trans*-retinoic acid	X	Leukemias
L-Asparaginase	Cm	Leukemias
Cisplatin	Dm	Ovary, cervix, sarcoma
Hydroxyurea	D	Leukemias
Prednisone	C*	Lymphomas, leukemias, breast
Tamoxifen	Dm	Breast, uterus
Paclitaxel	Dm	Breast, ovarian
Vinblastine	Dm	Breast, lymphomas, choriocarcinoma
Vincristine	Dm	Leukemias, lymphomas

Data from Neoplastic diseases. In Cunningham FG, MacDonald PC, Gant NF, et al, editors: *Williams obstetrics*, ed 20, Stamford, Conn., 1997, Appleton and Lange; and Briggs GC, Freeman RK, Yaffe SJ: *Drugs in pregnancy and lactation*, ed 7, Philadelphia, 2005, Lippincott Williams & Wilkins.
*Risk factor D if used in the first trimester.

RADIATION THERAPY

The deleterious effects of irradiation on the fetus have been both theorized and actual. Fortunately, the amount of concern about the former far exceeds the incidence of the latter. Irradiation promotes genetic damage and thus the potential for congenital malformations. The risk depends on both dose and time (Table 10-6). A dose of less than 5 rad is believed to be of little consequence (Brent et al, 1989). If radiation exposure occurs before implantation, the adverse outcomes are usually a small increase in miscarriage.

The major concern is high-dose radiation (>10 rad) received during the period of organogenesis (embryonic weeks 1 to 10). The central nervous system is the most radiation-sensitive organ, and the complications most often observed are microcephaly and mental retardation. Cataracts and retinal degeneration are also seen. After organogenesis is complete, there is still a risk of central nervous system abnormalities. However, the sequelae most often seen are skin changes and anemia. Because of the highly variable yet potentially grave consequences of irradiation greater than 10 rad, patients should be counseled accordingly, and termination of pregnancy should be offered as an alternative if exposure has occurred in the previable period (Orr and Shingleton, 1983).

There are several other considerations for a pregnant woman undergoing radiation therapy. First, the dose used in estimating risk should be the amount that the fetus actually receives. For example, axillary or neck irradiation for lymphoma involves a lower direct fetal exposure than direct pelvic irradiation for cervical cancer. The latter treatment, if given in the second trimester, will likely cause fetal demise. Second, the magnitude of radiation scatter to the pelvis must be considered. External shielding does not prevent internal reflection of the ion beam. Third, the advancing size of the uterus actually increases the amount of radiation exposure of the fetus, because of the closer proximity of the nonpelvic irradiation. Therefore an 8-week-old fetus may actually receive a smaller radiation dose from supraclavicular irradiation than a 30-week-old fetus. Fourth, will the fetus concentrate the radiation, and therefore increase its dose? This is exemplified by the use of radioactive iodine (^{131}I) for maternal thyroid conditions.

The actual rad dose is markedly higher in the fetus, because the fetal thyroid concentrates the iodine.

Diagnostic tests such as radiography may also be associated with radiation exposure for the fetus (Table 10-7). The doses involved are usually much smaller than those used for cancer therapy. Nonetheless, the practitioner should limit the amount of radiographic testing if at all possible. Inadvertent imaging of a patient who is not known to be pregnant continues to occur despite sensitive pregnancy tests, thus creating significant concerns. Indicated radiographs should never be withheld because of pregnancy, but lead shielding of the patient's abdomen and careful selection of the type of study should be performed to minimize the pelvic dose. Usually the amount of fetal exposure is much less than 5 rad, with no significantly greater risk of malformations. There does appear to be a slightly higher incidence of childhood cancer if the fetus is exposed to doses on the order of 10 mGy (Doll and Wakeford, 1997).

CERVICAL CANCER

Cervical cancer is the most common malignancy found in pregnancy. The incidence is approximately 1 in 2500 gestations. A Papanicolaou test smear should be performed for all patients at their first prenatal visit. However, approximately 30% of cervical cancers can be associated with negative cytologic smear results. Although the evaluation for

TABLE 10-6 Radiation Dose Thresholds for Deleterious Fetal Effects

Weeks Since LMP	Fetal Dose (mGy)	Potential Fetal Effects
2-4 (preimplantation)	>50-100	Spontaneous abortion, but generally not malformation
2-8 (organogenesis)	>200	Malformations
8-15	100-1000	Severe mental retardation
>15	>1000	Mental retardation

Adapted from Doyle S, Messiou C, Rutherford JM, et al: Cancer presenting during pregnancy: radiological perspectives, *Clin Radiol* 64:857-871, 2009.
LMP, Last menstrual period.

TABLE 10-7 Estimated Radiation Dose to the Fetus With Common Diagnostic Imaging Procedures

Test	Fetal Dose (rad)
Radiograph	
Upper extremity	<0.001
Lower extremity	<0.001
Upper gastrointestinal series (barium)	0.048-0.360
Cholecystography	0.005-0.060
Lumbar spine	0.346-0.620
Pelvis	0.040-0.238
Hip and femur series	0.051-0.370
Chest (two views)	<0.010
Retropyelography	0.800
Abdomen (kidneys, ureter, bladder	0.200-0.245
Urography (intravenous pyelography)	0.358-1.398
Barium enema	0.700-3.986
Computed Tomography Scan	
Head	<0.050
Chest	0.100-0.450
Abdomen (10 slices)	0.240-2.600
Abdomen and pelvis	0.640
Pelvis	0.730
Lumbar spine	3.500
Other	
Ventilation perfusion scan	0.06-1.00

From Bentur Y: Ionizing and nonionizing radiation in pregnancy. In: Koren G: *Medication safety in pregnancy and breastfeeding*, Philadelphia, 2007, McGraw Hill.

an abnormal Papanicolaou test result should not be altered because of pregnancy, many physicians are reluctant for fear of cervical hemorrhage. Cervical biopsy remains the mainstay of diagnosis. The greater vascularity of the cervix during pregnancy predisposes bleeding. An experienced colposcopist may be able to defer actual biopsy in cases of possible visual findings of a noninvasive process. However, if cancerous invasion is suspected or if the physician is uncertain of the visual findings, biopsy is necessary. If microinvasive disease is confirmed by biopsy, cone biopsy is required to rule out frankly invasive disease. This procedure is undertaken with caution during pregnancy, because of the associated high rate of bleeding complications and miscarriage. Cervical conization may raise the risk of incompetence or preterm labor. The assistance of a gynecologic oncologist is preferred, given these unique sets of potential consequences. A shallow cone biopsy will reduce the risk of subsequent cervical weakness.

The therapy for invasive cervical cancer is based on the stage of disease and the gestational age of the fetus. Therapy can involve external beam radiation, internal radiotherapy (brachytherapy), or surgery (Table 10-8). In most cases, delay of definitive therapy by 4 to 14 weeks may be acceptable. Pregnancy does not seem to accelerate the growth of the tumor. However, patient counseling is important. In the extremely previable gestation, the likelihood of achieving a safe gestational age for the fetus without worsening the stage or spread of the cancer in the mother must be balanced against parental desires based on ethical or religious beliefs. Conversely, it might be reasonable to delay definitive therapy until a time when delivery would not likely result in a long-term disability because of extreme prematurity.

BREAST CANCER

Breast cancer is the most common malignancy of women, with approximately 1 in 8 women affected in their lifetimes (Goldman and O'Hair, 2009). The incidence of breast cancer in pregnancy is estimated to be 10 to 30 per 100,000 pregnancies (Isaacs, 1995). Pregnancy does not seem to influence the actual course of the disease; however, there appears to be a higher risk of delay in diagnosis and a trend toward more advanced stages at diagnosis in pregnant women than in nonpregnant controls.

The diagnostic procedures for breast cancer should not be altered during pregnancy. Any suspicious mass should undergo biopsy. Mammography, although discouraged for routine screening in pregnancy, can be used safely if indicated. The amount of radiation is negligible—approximately 0.01 cGy (Liberman et al, 1994). Mammography imaging may be hampered by physiologic changes because of pregnancy, and ultrasound examination may be a useful alternative. Metastatic evaluation may be hampered somewhat because of a reluctance to use bone and liver scans during pregnancy. Magnetic resonance imaging can be used safely in the second and third trimesters.

Surgical therapy for breast cancer should not be delayed because of pregnancy. The risks of mastectomy and axillary node dissection appear to be low (Isaacs, 1995). Radiation therapy is usually not recommended during pregnancy because of the risk of beam scatter to the pregnant uterus. If the pregnancy is to continue and the patient has evidence of tumor invasion in the lymph nodes, adjuvant chemotherapy is often given. The timing of delivery should account for the following factors:

- When would the fetus have a reasonable chance for survival with a low risk of severe permanent morbidity?
- Can the number of cycles of chemotherapy be minimized with an earlier delivery? In addition, avoiding delivery just before or just after administration of chemotherapy is important to reduce the risk of immunosuppression and infection.
- How long can radiotherapy be delayed without increasing the risk of metastatic spread of the tumor?

Approximately 10% of women treated for breast cancer become pregnant, the majority within 5 years of diagnosis. Data from small series suggest that pregnancy does not influence the rate of recurrences or of distal metastasis (Dow et al, 1994). However, women should be encouraged to delay childbearing for at least 2 to 3 years, which is the time of the highest rate of recurrence. Breastfeeding may be possible in women who have undergone conservative breast cancer surgery.

TABLE 10-8 Treatment Options for Cervical Cancer in Pregnancy

Gestational Age (weeks)	Stage I to IIa	Stage IIb to IIIb
<20	4500 cGy Wide pelvic irradiation If no spontaneous abortion: modified radical hysterectomy If spontaneous abortion: brachytherapy or radical hysterectomy with lymphadenectomy	5000 cGy Wide pelvic irradiation If no spontaneous abortion: type II radical hysterectomy If spontaneous abortion: brachytherapy or cesarean section at fetal viability Subsequent wide pelvic radiation (±5000 cGy) and brachytherapy (±5000 cGy)
>20	Cesarean section at fetal viability Subsequent wide pelvic radiation (5000 cGy) and brachytherapy (5000 cGy) or cesarean radical hysterectomy with lymphadenectomy	Cesarean section at fetal viability Subsequent wide pelvic radiation (±5000 cGy) and brachytherapy (±5000 cGy)

Data from Berman ML, Di Saia PJ, Brewster WR: Pelvic malignancies, gestational trophoblastic neoplasia and nonpelvic malignancies. In Creasy RK, Resnik R, editors: *Maternal-fetal medicine*, ed 4, Philadelphia, 1999, WB Saunders.

OVARIAN CANCER

Most ovarian cancer occurs in women older than 35 years. Delayed childbearing has been more widely accepted, exemplified by British birth rates doubling in women older than 30 years and tripling in women older than 40 years since 1975 (Palmer et al, 2009), in addition to a twofold increased birth rate among U.S. women older than 40 years since 1981 (Martin et al, 2009). It would not be surprising for the rate of ovarian and other cancers during pregnancy to increase. However, the current estimate of actual ovarian malignancies in pregnancy is low and estimated to range from 1 in 10,000 to 1 in 50,000 deliveries (Jacob and Stringer, 1990; Palmer et al, 2009). Whereas most ovarian cancers are epithelial in origin, borderline epithelial and germ cell tumors (dysgerminomas and malignant teratomas) are more common in pregnancy.

The widespread use of ultrasonography, particularly in the first two trimesters, has been helpful in identifying adnexal masses. Fortunately, most are benign functional cysts. Actual malignancy is rare and is estimated at 5% of the ovarian masses found. The risk is higher in non-pregnant females, approaching 15% to 20%. Surgery for a suspected ovarian mass occurs in approximately 1 per 1000 pregnancies. Most procedures are performed not for suspected malignancy, but because of concern about torsion and rupture. The incidence of adnexal torsion ranges from 1% to 50%, and there appears to be a trend with increasing rates in masses greater than 6 cm (Yen et al, 2009). The maximal times of risk of these events are at the end of the first trimester, when the uterus elevates beyond the true pelvis, and at the time of delivery. The characterization of an ovarian process can be aided by ultrasonography or magnetic resonance imaging, but these modalities are not definitive. Ultrasound scoring systems that use size and character poorly predict malignancy, but have a better negative predictive value (Lerner et al, 1994). Although an ovarian cyst, particularly if it is simple in nature, is likely not malignant, the patient must be cautioned that histologic diagnosis is more definitive. Indications for surgical exploration include a complex mass, a persistent simple cyst 8 cm or larger, or one that is symptomatic (Leiserowitz, 2006). The optimal time for laparotomy is in the second trimester. At that time, there is minimal interference from the gravid uterus and less of a risk of fetal loss, and the theoretical concerns of teratogenic exposure to anesthetic agents are avoided. Some patients opt for more conservative management; they should be counseled that they have a 40% chance of needing urgent intervention with either surgery or percutaneous drainage (Platek, 1995).

If a malignancy is confirmed at the time of laparotomy, treatment and staging are no different than for a nonpregnant woman. Frozen-section diagnosis, peritoneal washings, omentectomy, and subdiaphragmatic biopsy are performed. Depending on the cell type and the stage, treatment can range from removal of the affected adnexa to complete hysterectomy and bilateral oophorectomy. Chemotherapy may be given during pregnancy if necessary. Fortunately, most epithelial ovarian cancers found in pregnant women are usually of a lower stage, with 59% of reported cases being stage I (Palmer et al, 2009).

SURVIVORS OF CHILDHOOD CANCER

Given the improvements of therapy for childhood cancer, a large number of these individuals have survived into adulthood. Some are unable to conceive because of high-dose radiation or cytotoxic chemotherapy. The risk of decreased fertility for patients exposed to pelvic radiation therapy may as high as 32% (Geogeseu et al, 2008). Those who remain fertile may have concerns regarding whether their treatment increases the risk of adverse pregnancy outcomes. Although data are limited, female cancer survivors treated with radiation therapy appear to have increased risks of premature delivery, low birthweight, and miscarriage. There is no evidence that female partners of male cancer survivors treated with radiation have these excess risks (Reulen et al, 2009).

MENTAL DISORDERS

Pregnancy can be a stressful process. At times, it may induce a psychotic event. Women experiencing a mental disorder during pregnancy who have no history of a mood disorder usually exhibit a milder constellation of symptoms. Serious disorders such as mania and schizophrenia that are antecedent to pregnancy may not be so benign. In women with all types of mental illness, and in previously nonaffected women, the postpartum state is a time of greater maternal risk. Ten percent to 15% of new mothers experience a depressive disorder (Weissman and Olfson, 1995). Furthermore, there appears to be an increased perinatal risk with mental disorders and pregnancy (Table 10-9). Women with preexisting mental illness have a higher recurrence risk in the puerperium. Patients with suspected mental illness should be assessed for substance abuse and thyroid dysfunction. A multidisciplinary approach is advantageous. If the patient's mental competency is an issue, the caregiver should obtain legal assistance to be able to make medical decisions for the patient.

DEPRESSION

Depression ranks as the fourth leading cause of disability worldwide, and recognized prevalence appears to be increasing (Dossett, 2008). A study by Dietz et al (2007) suggests that the prevalence of depression during pregnancy or postpartum, as defined by onset within 3 to 6 months after delivery, to be approximately 10%.

The predisposing risk factors for depression include early childhood loss, physical or sexual abuse, socioeconomic deprivation, genetic predisposition, and lifestyle stress caused by multiple roles (McGrath et al, 1990). These factors can exaggerate or prolong symptoms and, if not addressed, can lengthen the duration of depression. The obstetrician must be aware that life events such as miscarriage, infertility, and complicated pregnancy in patients with risk factors are likely to precipitate depression; therefore there is a low threshold for diagnosis and treatment of mood alterations in such patients.

TABLE 10-9 Impact of Psychiatric Illness on Pregnancy Outcome

Illness	Teratogenic Effects	Impact on Outcome Obstetric	Impact on Outcome Neonatal	Treatment Options
Anxiety disorders	N/A	Increased incidence of forceps deliveries, prolonged labor, precipitate labor, fetal distress, preterm delivery, and spontaneous abortion	Decreased developmental scores and inadaptability; slowed mental development at 2 years of age	Benzodiazepines Antidepressants Psychotherapy
Major depression	N/A	Increased incidence of low birthweight, decreased fetal growth, and postnatal complication	Increased newborn cortisol and catecholamine levels, infant crying, rates of admission to neonatal intensive care units	Antidepressants Psychotherapy ECT
Bipolar disorder	N/A	Increased incidence of low birthweight, decreased fetal growth, and postnatal complication	Increased newborn cortisol and catecholamine levels, infant crying, rates of admission to neonatal intensive care units	Lithium Anticonvulsants Antipsychotics ECT
Schizophrenia	Congenital malformations, especially cardiovascular	Increased incidence of preterm delivery, low birthweight, small for gestational age, placental abnormalities and placental hemorrhage	Increased rates of postnatal death	Antipsychotics

From ACOG Practice Bulletin: Clinical management guidelines for obstetrician-gynecologists number 92, April 2008 (replaces practice bulletin number 87, November 2007): use of psychiatric medications during pregnancy and lactation, *Obstet Gynecol* 111:1001-1020, 2008.
ECT, Electroconvulsive therapy.

Alternatively, perinatal loss experienced by a woman without predisposing risk factors will probably lead to a grief reaction or adjustment disorder, which may be misdiagnosed as depression.

Chronic medical conditions that are associated with a high prevalence of depression and may occur in women of childbearing age include renal failure, cancer, AIDS, and chronic fatigue or pain. Antihypertensives, hormones, anticonvulsants, steroids, chemotherapeutics, and antibiotics can cause depression. Alcoholism and substance abuse may manifest as depression. Underlying personality disorders complicate the diagnosis of depression by confusing the clinical situation, in addition to contributing to the secondary effect of many physicians' avoidance of patients suffering from such disorders.

Therapeutic interventions for depression include psychotherapy and medication. Electroconvulsive therapy has been shown to be an effective and relatively safe treatment in refractory cases (Rabheru, 2001). However, there remains controversy and some degree of concern because of published series and case reports suggesting a risk of fetal cardiac arrhythmias, vaginal bleeding, and premature uterine contractions (Bhatia et al, 1999); therefore it should be reserved for refractory cases and performed in a setting with immediate access to obstetric care (Pinette et al, 2007; Richards, 2007). Treatment of depression is effective in approximately 70% of cases. Supportive treatment alone is rarely effective in major depressive episodes. Most antidepressant medications currently prescribed during pregnancy are selective serotonin reuptake inhibitors (SSRIs). SSRIs have an advantage over the tricyclic antidepressants by not causing orthostatic hypotension. Unfortunately, and although limited series suggest that the SSRIs are relatively safe, little is known about long-term consequences for children exposed to SSRIs in utero (Altshuler et al, 1996; Chambers et al, 1996; Karasu et al, 2000). Fluoxetine is the best-studied SSRI in terms of safety. Alternatively, paroxetine has been associated with an increased risk of congenital heart defects (Kallen et al, 2007). Although data remain inconsistent, they suggest avoiding paroxetine as a first-line agent. However, if a certain agent is controlling the patient's symptoms, it would seem reasonable not to change medications for the sake of these concerns.

A recent issue has been raised regarding the use of SSRIs and persistent pulmonary hypertension of the newborn; however, the incidence remains low at approximately 10 in 1000 fetuses exposed after 20 weeks' gestation (Chambers et al, 2006). Currently, there is no consensus regarding the use of SSRIs during breastfeeding. Fluoxetine has an active metabolite with a long half-life and is found in higher concentrations in infants (Eberhard-Gran et al, 2006). Short-term neonatal effects have been reported, including increased crying, decreased sleep, and irritability, particularly with fluoxetine and citalopram. Reasonable guidelines regarding the use of SSRIs and other psychotropic medications are listed in Table 10-10. The long-term side effects are currently listed as "unknown" (Briggs et al, 2005; Dodd et al, 2000). The theoretical concerns are that such drugs may affect the developing central nervous system of the newborn and that abnormalities may not be readily apparent in the short term. Therefore SSRIs should be prescribed for a nursing mother only if the benefit clearly exceeds the risk, and after the patient has been counseled regarding the potential yet currently ill-defined risks. Given current medical knowledge, bottle feeding should be offered as an acceptable alternative if antidepressants must be used.

TABLE 10-10   Summary of Current Knowledge of Drug Excretion into Breast Milk, Drug Concentrations in Infant Serum, Adverse Effects in the Child, and Breastfeeding Recommendations for Different Psychotropic Drugs

Class or Drug	Drug Transfer into Breast Milk	Infant Plasma Concentrations	Adverse Effects in the Child	Breastfeeding Recommendations
SSRIs	Low transfer	Low plasma concentrations	Case reports of adverse effects in infants exposed to fluoxetine and citalopram	Compatible with breastfeeding; however, fluoxetine and citalopram may not be drugs of first choice
TCAs	Low transfer	Low plasma concentrations (except doxepin)	No suspected immediate adverse effects observed (except doxepin)	Compatible with breastfeeding; however, doxepin should be avoided
Other antidepressants	Limited data	Limited data	Limited data	None able to be made
Benzodiazepines	Low transfer	High plasma concentrations with longer acting drugs with active metabolites	Case reports of CNS depression reported for diazepam	Sporadic use of short-acting benzodiazepines unlikely to cause adverse effects
Lithium	Low transfer	Dose received by the infant is high	Limited data; some reports of toxicity in the infant	Limited data; however, breastfeeding should be avoided
Carbamazepine, sodium valproate	Low transfer	Low plasma concentrations	Some case reports of various adverse effects in the infant	Generally more compatible with breastfeeding than lithium
Lamotrigine	High transfer	High plasma concentrations	Limited data	None able to be made
Novel antipsychotics	Moderate transfer	Variable plasma concentrations	Limited data	None able to be made

Modified from Eberhard-Gran M, Esklid A, Opjordsmoen S: Use of psychotropic medications in treating mood disorders during lactation: practical recommendations, *CNS Drugs* 20:187-198, 2006.
CNS, Central nervous system; *SSRI,* selective serotonin reuptake inhibitor; *TCA,* tricyclic antidepressants.

POSTPARTUM PSYCHOSIS

A severe disorder, postpartum psychosis is fortunately rare, occurring in 1 to 4 per 1000 births (Weissman and Olfson, 1995). This condition is more worrisome than postpartum depression, because of the patient's inability to discern reality from the periods of delirium. Patients at risk for postpartum psychosis may have underlying depression, mania, or schizophrenia. Other risks are younger age and family history. The recurrence rate is approximately 25%. The peak onset of symptoms is between 10 and 14 days after delivery. Recognition of this disorder is extremely important to the protection of the patient and her family.

SCHIZOPHRENIA

The prevalence of schizophrenia is approximately 1% in the general population (Myers et al, 1984); it is associated with delusions, hallucinations, and incoherence. Morbidity due to this mental illness is higher than that due to any other. There appears to be a genetic component to the etiology; schizophrenia develops in approximately 10% of offspring of an affected person. Concordance of schizophrenia in identical twins reaches 65%. There is some speculation and controversy as to whether low birthweight (Smith et al, 2001) and obstetric complications (Kendell et al, 2000) are associated with a higher rate of schizophrenia.

Because the peak age of incidence is approximately 20 years and women are affected more often than men, it is unrealistic to assume that obstetricians will never encounter patients with schizophrenia. There appear to be higher rates of cesarean section and surgical vaginal delivery in affected patients (Bennedsen et al, 2001b). Children of women with schizophrenia may have a higher rate of sudden infant death syndrome and congenital malformations (Bennedsen et al, 2001a). However, it is difficult to ascertain whether these risks are independent of other factors such as smoking, poor socioeconomic status, and use of certain medications.

Treatment is achieved primarily through the use of psychotropic medication. The potential for teratogenesis appears low with the older-generation medications in the phenothiazine class, but most data for this issue were derived from the use of lower doses given to patients with hyperemesis gravidarum. Antipsychotic medication does cross the placenta. Current recommendations include avoiding use in the first trimester if possible, the use of lower doses or higher-potency alternatives, and cessation of medication 5 to 10 days before delivery (Herz et al, 2000). The use of most antipsychotics in breastfeeding is associated with an unknown risk (Briggs et al, 2005).

Lithium, used primarily in mania, is associated with a higher rate of Ebstein anomaly. Although the incidence of this consequence is low, either discontinuing the medication in the first trimester or continuing its use with careful counseling is a viable alternative. Fetal echocardiography should be performed in women who have used lithium in early pregnancy.

SUGGESTED READINGS

ACOG Committee on Practice Bulletin–Obstetrics: ACOG Practice Bulletin: Clinical management guidelines for obstetrician-gynecologists, number 92, April 2008. Use of psychiatric medications during pregnancy and lactation, *Obstet Gynecol* 111:1001-1020, 2008.

Bent RL: Saving lives and changing family histories: appropriate counseling of pregnant women and men and women of reproductive age, concerning the risk of diagnostic radiation exposures during and before pregnancy, *Am J Obstet Gynecol* 200:4-24, 2009.

Cohn D, Ramaswamy B, Blum K, et al: Malignancy in pregnancy. In Creasy RK, Resnik R, Iams JD, editors: *Maternal-fetal medicine*, ed 6, Philadelphia, 2009, WB Saunders, pp 885-904.

Moise KJ: Management of rhesus alloimmunization in pregnancy, *Obstet Gynecol* 112:164-176, 2008.

Walker S, Permezal M, Berkovic S: The management of epilepsy in pregnancy, *BJOG* 116:758-767, 2009.

Complete references and supplemental color images used in this text can be found online at www.expertconsult.com

HYPERTENSIVE COMPLICATIONS OF PREGNANCY

Andrew D. Hull and Thomas R. Moore

Hypertension is the most common medical problem in pregnancy, affecting 10% to 15% of all pregnant women. As the third most common cause of maternal mortality after thromboembolic disease and hemorrhage, hypertension accounts for almost 16% of maternal deaths in the United States (Berg et al, 2003). Complications arising from hypertensive disorders have profound effects on the fetus and neonate and thus are a major source of perinatal mortality and morbidity. Preeclampsia is also the primary cause of iatrogenic prematurity.

CLASSIFICATION OF HYPERTENSIVE DISORDERS OF PREGNANCY

Any discussion of hypertension and pregnancy must begin with a set of definitions. Although many classifications are in use worldwide, perhaps one of the more useful comes from the Report of the National High Blood Pressure Education Program Working Group on High Blood Pressure in Pregnancy (2000) (Table 11-1). Although this classification scheme appears to be somewhat pedantic, it is of paramount importance because pregnancy outcome varies according to the type of hypertension involved. For practical purposes, hypertension in pregnancy can be divided into the following categories: chronic hypertension, gestational hypertension, and preeclampsia.

Hypertension is defined as a systolic blood pressure of 140 mm Hg or higher or a diastolic pressure of 90 mm Hg or higher, measured on two separate occasions. Korotkoff phase V (disappearance of sound) is used rather than Korotkoff phase IV (muffling of sound) to define *diastolic pressure*, because Korotkoff IV is poorly reproducible in pregnancy. The term *severe hypertension* identifies a population at significantly increased risk for stroke and cardiac decompensation, and it is defined as a systolic blood pressure of 160 mm Hg or a diastolic pressure of 110 mm Hg or higher.

CHRONIC HYPERTENSION

Up to 5% of pregnant women have chronic hypertension, which is diagnosed when hypertension is present before pregnancy or recorded before 20 weeks' gestation. However, when hypertension is first noted in a patient after 20 weeks' gestation, it may be difficult to distinguish chronic hypertension from pregnancy-induced hypertension or preeclampsia. In such cases, the precise diagnosis might not be made until after delivery. Hypertension that is first diagnosed during the second half of pregnancy and persists more than 12 weeks postpartum is diagnosed as chronic hypertension.

Chronic hypertension has an adverse effect on pregnancy outcome. Women with the disorder are at higher risk for

preterm delivery and placental abruption, and their fetuses are at risk for intrauterine growth restriction (IUGR) and demise (Ferrer et al, 2000). Superimposed preeclampsia complicates up to 50% of pregnancies in women with pre-existing severe chronic hypertension (Sibai and Anderson, 1986), and it occurs before 34 weeks' gestation in 50% of cases (Chappell et al, 2008). The adverse effects on fetal and maternal perinatal outcomes are directly related to the severity of the preexisting hypertension. When chronic hypertension is secondary to maternal renal disease, the risks of poor outcome are further increased, with as much as a tenfold rise in fetal loss rate (Jungers et al, 1997). Women with untreated severe chronic hypertension are at increased risk for cardiovascular complications during pregnancy, including stroke (Brown and Whitworth, 1999).

The majority of cases of chronic hypertension seen in pregnancy are idiopathic (essential hypertension), but causes of secondary hypertension should always be sought because pregnancy outcome is worse in women with secondary hypertension. Renal disease (e.g., chronic renal failure, glomerulonephritis, renal artery stenosis), cardiovascular causes (coarctation of the aorta, Takayasu arteritis), and, rarely, Cushing disease, Conn syndrome, and pheochromocytoma should be excluded through physical examination, history, and more detailed testing if needed.

All patients with chronic hypertension should be evaluated periodically with serum urea, creatinine, and electrolyte measurements, urinalysis, and 24-hour urine collection for protein and creatinine clearance determinations. Typically this assessment should be performed in each trimester and more frequently if the patient's condition deteriorates.

ANTIHYPERTENSIVE TREATMENT OF CHRONIC HYPERTENSION IN PREGNANCY

Except in cases of severe hypertension, randomized trials have shown that antihypertensive treatment of chronic hypertension in pregnancy does not improve fetal outcome (Sibai and Anderson, 1986). Rates of preterm delivery, abruption, IUGR, and perinatal death are similar in treated and untreated women. Therefore treatment is usually reserved for patients whose hypertension places them at a significant risk of stroke (systolic blood pressure of 180 mm Hg or higher or diastolic pressure of 110 mm Hg or higher). Patients with less severe hypertension who were taking medications before conception might be able to discontinue therapy with close surveillance. The risk of superimposed preeclampsia is not changed by antihypertensive therapy, so its development should be tracked carefully.

TABLE 11-1   Classification of Hypertensive Disorders of Pregnancy*

Category	Definition
Chronic hypertension	Hypertension present before pregnancy or diagnosed before 20 weeks' gestation, or diagnosed for the first time during pregnancy that persists postpartum
Gestational hypertension	Transient if blood pressure returns to normal by 12 weeks after delivery, and preeclampsia was not diagnosed before delivery Chronic if blood pressure does not resolve by 12 weeks after delivery
Preeclampsia-eclampsia	Usually occurs after 20 weeks' gestation Hypertension accompanied by proteinuria in a woman normotensive before 20 weeks' gestation Strongly suspected if nonproteinuric hypertension is accompanied by systemic symptoms such as headache, visual disturbance, abdominal pain, or laboratory abnormalities such as low platelet count and elevated liver enzyme values (HELLP syndrome)
Preeclampsia superimposed on chronic hypertension	Preeclampsia occurring in a chronically hypertensive woman

Adapted from the Report of the National High Blood Pressure Education Program Working Group on High Blood Pressure in Pregnancy, Am J Obstet Gynecol 183:S1-S22, 2000.
HELLP, Hemolysis, elevated liver enzymes, and low platelets.
*Hypertension is defined as a systolic blood pressure ≥140 mm Hg systolic or diastolic blood pressure ≥90 mm Hg.

TABLE 11-2   Drugs Commonly Used to Treat Chronic Hypertension in Pregnancy and Their Modes of Action

Drug	Mode of Action
Methyldopa	Centrally acting antihypertensive
Labetalol	Mixed alpha- and beta-adrenergic blocker
Nifedipine	Calcium channel blocker
Hydralazine	Peripheral vasodilator
Prazosin	Alpha-blocker

The choice of antihypertensive agent for use in pregnancy is governed by a desire to adjust blood pressure without having ill effects on the fetus. Because excessive lowering of maternal blood pressure below 140 mm Hg systolic or 90 mm Hg diastolic (140/90 mm Hg) can compromise uterine perfusion, with consequent slowing of fetal growth, fetal hypoxia, or both, the therapeutic goal is to maintain maternal pressures at 140 to 155 systolic and 90 to 105 diastolic. The drugs most commonly used in pregnancy are listed in Table 11-2.

Methyldopa, a centrally acting antihypertensive agent, formerly was the most widely used drug in this setting. Many obstetricians remain faithful to the use of this agent because of extensive clinical and research experience demonstrating its safety for both mother and fetus during pregnancy (Report of the National High Blood Pressure Education Program Working Group on High Blood Pressure in Pregnancy, 2000). This agent does not impair uteroplacental perfusion and has a wide therapeutic margin before side effects are seen. However, methyldopa has the disadvantage of a rather slow onset of action with prolonged time to therapeutic effect (days), and compliance with methyldopa therapy may be impeded by side effects such as sedation in some patients.

Labetalol is a mixed alpha$_1$-adrenergic and beta$_1$- and beta$_2$-adrenergic blocking agent, and it is the most frequently used alternative to methyldopa. Some pure beta-blockers have been associated with a significant increase in the risk of IUGR (e.g., atenolol), and the mixed adrenergic blockade produced by labetalol is thought to mitigate this unwanted effect (Pickles et al, 1989). Labetalol is also used intravenously to manage severe hypertension accompanying preeclampsia.

Calcium channel blockers (e.g., nifedipine) are used mainly as second-line drugs, usually in long-acting, extended-release forms. Calcium channel blockers appear to be as effective as methyldopa and labetalol with minimal fetal side effects (Levin et al, 1994).

Hydralazine, a potent peripheral vasodilator, is frequently used intravenously to treat acute hypertensive emergencies in pregnancy (blood pressure of >160/110 mm Hg). Its role as an oral agent in the management of chronic hypertension is limited to a second- or third-line choice. Long-term use of hydralazine may be associated with a lupuslike syndrome in some patients.

Prazosin, an alpha-adrenergic blocker, has been used as a second- or third-line drug in pregnant women whose hypertension is difficult to control or is severe with an early onset. This agent appears to be similar in efficacy to nifedipine in such a setting (Hall et al, 2000).

Although diuretics are used extensively in adults with hypertension, there appears to be little role for them in the treatment of chronic hypertension in pregnancy. Diuretics have been alleged to reduce or prevent the normal plasma volume expansion seen in pregnancy (Sibai et al, 1984), an effect that theoretically might impede fetal growth, although the evidence for this is mixed. Most authorities restrict the use of diuretics in pregnant patients to those with cardiac dysfunction or pulmonary edema.

Angiotensin-converting enzyme inhibitors and angiotensin receptor blockers should not be used during pregnancy. In the second and third trimesters, these agents are associated with malformation of the fetal calvarium, fetal renal failure, oligohydramnios, pulmonary hypoplasia, and fetal and neonatal death (Buttar, 1997). Angiotensin-converting enzyme inhibitors appear to be safe when taken in the first trimester (Steffensen et al, 1998), but a patient who conceives while taking an angiotensin receptor blocker or angiotensin-converting enzyme inhibitor should be switched to a safer alternative as soon as possible. Similar precautions apply to the use of angiotensin receptor blockers in pregnancy.

ANTENATAL FETAL SURVEILLANCE IN CHRONIC HYPERTENSION

As the third trimester progresses, patients with chronic hypertension are at an increasing risk of slowing of fetal growth and superimposed preeclampsia. Antenatal surveillance in women with chronic hypertension should include careful screening for signs and symptoms of superimposed preeclampsia, which constitutes the greatest perinatal risk. Fetal growth should be followed with serial ultrasonography evaluations (every 3 to 6 weeks). All patients should perform fetal movement counts from 28 weeks' gestation onward, and cases with suspected fetal growth impairment should be followed with twice-weekly non-stress tests with amniotic fluid index or weekly ultrasound biophysical profile. Although the optimum interval for these tests is controversial (every 3 to 7 days), and their role is unproven in the absence of fetal IUGR or other evidence of fetal compromise, most centers begin regular fetal biophysical testing at 32 to 34 weeks' gestation and continue until delivery.

If fetal growth tapers below expectations (typically sonographic estimated fetal weight [EFW] falls below the tenth percentile or abdominal circumference much smaller percentile than head), more intensive fetal surveillance is indicated. In cases with IUGR, serial sonography should be performed at 10- to 21-day intervals with attention paid to amniotic fluid volume, careful profiling of each biometric parameter, and cerebral and umbilical Doppler waveforms. Typical indications for delivery in the setting of IUGR and hypertension include no growth of the head and abdomen over a 10-day interval, severe oligohydramnios, biophysical score of less than 6, or reversal of end-diastolic velocity on the umbilical Doppler waveform. However, individualization of management in these cases is important.

Women with renal impairment and chronic hypertension have a markedly higher risk of poor perinatal outcome than normotensive women and women with hypertension without renal impairment. In addition, moderate or severe renal disease (serum creatinine level ≥1.4 mg/dL) may accelerate the loss of renal function during pregnancy (Cunningham, 1990; Hou, 1999). The incidence of impaired fetal growth is directly related to the degree of renal impairment, and women undergoing dialysis are at particular risk for fetal growth failure, preterm delivery, and fetal death, even with optimal management. Those who start dialysis during pregnancy are at the greatest risk, with only a 50% chance of a surviving infant (Hou, 1999).

GESTATIONAL HYPERTENSION

The diagnosis of gestational hypertension can be made with confidence only after delivery; it is defined as hypertension occurring in the second half of pregnancy in the absence of any other signs or symptoms of preeclampsia. Because a woman with apparent gestational hypertension at 36 weeks' gestation can rapidly evolve into preeclampsia at 39 weeks' gestation, the diagnosis of gestational hypertension should always evoke caution and vigilance. Only if the patient's blood pressure returns to normal postpartum without development of signs of preeclampsia during the pregnancy should the final diagnosis of gestational hypertension be applied. During pregnancy, gestational hypertension is indistinguishable from preeclampsia in evolution. Therefore all patients with gestational hypertension should be regarded as being at risk for progression to preeclampsia.

The earlier gestational hypertension is evident, the greater the risk of preeclampsia. When the diagnosis is made before 30 weeks' gestation, more than one third will develop preeclampsia, whereas the risk is less than 10% when the diagnosis is made after 38 weeks' gestation. Decisions to treat patients with gestational hypertension with antihypertensive agents must be carefully considered, given the risk of concurrent preeclampsia and the lack of evidence supporting improved fetal outcome. Gestational hypertension tends to recur in subsequent pregnancies and predisposes women to hypertension in the future (Marin et al, 2000).

PREECLAMPSIA-ECLAMPSIA

Preeclampsia is one of the most enigmatic diseases affecting humans. Apparently unique to humans, preeclampsia has proved difficult to simulate in animal experiments. Despite years of intensive research, the underlying causes of the disease are only recently becoming clearer. It is evident that the clinical manifestations of preeclampsia arise from vascular endothelial dysfunction that ultimately may involve the central nervous, renal, hepatic, and cardiovascular systems. In its full-blown form, preeclampsia can produce a profound coagulopathy and liver, respiratory, or cardiac failure.

The classic symptom triad of hypertension, proteinuria, and edema defines preeclampsia. Most classifications of preeclampsia no longer include edema, because this common finding affects approximately 80% of pregnant women near term. Preeclampsia is divided into mild and severe forms (Box 11-1). This distinction is important, because in the presence of severe disease at any gestational age, the only appropriate treatment option is delivery, whereas expectant management may be acceptable in a woman who has mild disease and is remote from term.

Although the precise etiology of preeclampsia remains uncertain, numerous factors are associated with elevated the risk (Table 11-3). Up to 10% of primigravid patients have mild preeclampsia, and approximately 1% have severe disease.

PREECLAMPSIA

Etiology

The most widely accepted theory for the pathophysiology of preeclampsia is based on a model of impaired placental implantation that results in placental hypoperfusion and hypoxia. The placenta then releases substances into the maternal circulation that adversely affect endothelial function, leading to the clinical syndrome of widespread vascular dysfunction, which is recognized as the syndrome of preeclampsia (Myers and Baker, 2002). Individual responses to the process of progressive vascular dysfunction vary in severity and timing in a manner that seems to have genetic, familial, and immunologic components. For example, preeclampsia occurring in a first-degree relative confers a fourfold increase in risk of the disease in siblings and children (Chesley and Cooper, 1986). Women born to mothers with preeclampsia have a higher risk. There is some evidence that the presence of certain genotypes, such as factor V Leiden and thrombophilia (de Vries et al, 1997), or metabolic defects such as hyperhomocystinemia secondary to methylenetetrahydrofolate reductase deficiency (Kupferminc et al, 1999), predispose women to

BOX 11-1   Features of Mild and Severe Preeclampsia

MILD

- Systolic blood pressure ≥140 mm Hg or diastolic pressure of 90 mm Hg
- Proteinuria ≥300 mg/24 hr

SEVERE*

- Systolic blood pressure ≥160 mm Hg or diastolic pressure of 100 mm Hg
- Proteinuria ≥5 g/24 hr
- Elevated serum creatinine value
- Eclampsia
- Pulmonary edema
- Oliguria <500 mL/hr
- HELLP syndrome
- Intrauterine growth restriction
- Symptoms suggestive of end-organ involvement: headache, visual disturbance, epigastric or right upper quadrant pain

Modified from ACOG practice bulletin: Diagnosis and management of preeclampsia and eclampsia. Number 33, January 2002. American College of Obstetricians and Gynecologists, Int J Gynaecol Obstet 77:67-75, 2002.
HELLP, Hemolysis, elevated liver enzymes, and low platelets.
*Any single feature in the severe definition satisfies criteria for the diagnosis of severe preeclampsia.

TABLE 11-3   Risk Factors for Development of Preeclampsia

Factor	Relative Risk
Primigravida	3
Age >40 years	3
African American race	1.5
Family history	5
Chronic hypertension	10
Chronic renal disease	20
Antiphospholipid syndrome	10
Insulin-dependent diabetes mellitus	2
Multiple gestation	4

preeclampsia, although a true candidate gene is yet to be established and probably never will be. Population studies have suggested that women exposed to the antigenic effects of sperm before conception have a lower rate of preeclampsia than do women who conceive with lesser degrees of exposure, although the evidence is inconclusive (Koelman et al, 2000).

The endothelial dysfunction that characterizes preeclampsia (Roberts, 1999) manifests as greater vascular reactivity to circulating vasoconstrictors such as angiotensin, reduced production of endogenous vasodilators such as prostacyclin and nitric oxide (Ashworth et al, 1997), increased vascular permeability, and an increased tendency toward platelet consumption and coagulopathy. The end result is hypertension, proteinuria secondary to glomerular injury, edema, and a tendency toward extravascular fluid overload with intravascular hemoconcentration.

Predictors

Perhaps one of the most important contributions that prenatal care makes to maternal and fetal outcomes is the detection of preeclampsia and the prevention of eclampsia (Backe and Nakling, 1993; Karbhari et al, 1972). A wide variety of biochemical and physical tests has been proposed as screening tools for the early detection of preeclampsia (Dekker and Sibai, 1991). Most physical tests have been discredited, and even the most widely used biochemical tests have poor predictive values. Uric acid levels are elevated in many cases of preeclampsia, but the sensitivity of the measurement is low (Lim et al, 1998). Early detection of proteinuria is possible with the use of more sensitive tests, such as gel electrophoresis (Winkler et al, 1988), rather than conventional urinalysis, but such tests do not lend themselves to routine use. Clinicians should be aware of the limitations of routine urine testing for detection of proteinuria, with standard dipstick testing being notoriously inaccurate (Bell et al, 1999).

Doppler ultrasonographic assessment of the vascular dynamics in the uterine arteries during the second trimester has been proposed as a valuable screening tool in populations in which obstetric ultrasonography is routine (Kurdi, 1998). Up to 40% of women who develop preeclampsia have abnormal waveforms, and this finding was reported to be associated with a sixfold rise in the risk of preeclampsia (Papageorghiou et al, 2002). Other researchers have obtained less impressive results (Goffinet et al, 2001).

Recently the role of angiogenic factors in the pathophysiology of preeclampsia has been explored. Vascular endothelial growth factor (VEGF) and placental growth factor bind to Flt-1 and sFlt-1 receptors and have a critical role in angiogenesis and placental development. The interactions among FLt-1, VEGF, and placental growth factor promote angiogenesis and placental vasculogenesis, whereas those among sFLT-1, VEGF, and placental growth factor lead to the inactivation of those proteins and disordered angiogenesis and endothelial dysfunction. sFlt-1 levels have been found to be elevated in women with preeclampsia, and such elevated levels of sFlt-1 precede the features of clinical preeclampsia. Recent reviews of the state of the art in this area (Wang et al, 2009; Widmer et al, 2007) concluded that sFlt-1 and placental growth factor levels were significantly different after 25 weeks' gestation between women destined to develop preeclampsia and those with a normal pregnancy course. Measurements of these factors earlier in pregnancy do not appear to have the same predictive value. There is no doubt that angiogenic factors are intimately involved in the pathophysiology of preeclampsia, but alterations in their levels do not seem to be the cause of the disease. Several large studies are ongoing to further explore the role of these factors and their potential use in the prediction of disease. On balance, no effective screening test to predict preeclampsia currently exists, and clinicians are faced with the necessity of diagnosing the disease early and managing it as adroitly as possible.

Prevention

If an accurate predictor of preeclampsia could be identified, the next logical step would be the application of a preventive or ameliorative treatment. Unfortunately attempts to identify an effective treatment have proved equally difficult. Given the recognized association between vascular endothelial dysfunction and preeclampsia (in particular, vasoconstriction and excessive clotting in the maternal placental arteries), prostaglandin inhibitors have been viewed as a likely candidate for prophylaxis or treatment. Numerous trials (Duley et al, 2001) have been conducted with low-dose aspirin, based on the idea that the ability of aspirin to irreversibly inhibit production of the vasoconstrictive prostaglandin thromboxane would promote greater activity of prostacyclin, a vasodilatory prostaglandin. This ability of aspirin would help to maintain patency in the maternal placental vascular bed and limit or prevent the evolution of preeclampsia. Unfortunately, although a modest reduction in the frequency of preeclampsia (approximately 15%) was documented, no improvement in key measures of perinatal outcome was demonstrable in a metaanalysis of the results of available studies (Duley et al, 2001).

Calcium supplementation was briefly in vogue as a preventive treatment in the 1990s, on the basis of the known vasodilatory effect of calcium and impressive results in earlier, small studies (Atallah et al, 2000); however, its worth was not supported in a metaanalysis (Atallah et al, 2000). Similarly, it has been suggested that antioxidants may have a role in preeclampsia prevention, but the only available trial to date showed mixed results, with improvements in biochemical indices in women receiving vitamins C and E, although perinatal outcomes were not different in treated and untreated groups (Chappell et al, 1999). Of concern was the finding that women in whom preeclampsia developed despite vitamin therapy had markedly worsened preeclampsia than controls in whom the disease developed. Therefore, at present, an ideal preventive measure for preeclampsia does not exist.

Antepartum Management

Given the current inability to predict or prevent preeclampsia, clinicians are left to address established disease and to try to prevent maternal and fetal morbidity. The division of established preeclampsia into mild and more severe forms is of great worth in determining management and minimizing morbidity (see Box 11-1). Mild disease is generally managed conservatively (bed rest and frequent fetal and maternal biophysical assessments) until term is reached or there is evidence of maternal or fetal compromise. The appearance of severe preeclampsia mandates delivery in all but highly selected cases regardless of gestational age.

Patients with a diagnosis of mild preeclampsia should be evaluated for signs of maternal or fetal compromise, which would make their disease severe. Evaluation should include a 24-hour urine collection to evaluate for proteinuria; full blood count and platelet measurements; determination of serum uric acid, blood urea nitrogen, and creatinine levels; and evaluation of liver transaminases. Fetal size should be estimated with ultrasonography; the presence of IUGR (less than the tenth percentile) is a sign of severe preeclampsia. Patients with mild disease at 37 weeks' gestation or more should be delivered, because prolonging pregnancy has no material benefit and increases the risks of maternal and fetal morbidity. Patients at earlier gestational stages should be closely monitored with sequential clinical

TABLE 11-4 Drugs for Acute Treatment of Hypertension in Severe Preeclampsia

Drug	Dosage
Hydralazine	1-2 mg test dose 5-10 mg IV followed by 5-10 mg every 20 min as required, to a total of 30 mg
Labetalol	10-20 mg IV followed by 20-80 mg every 10 min to a total of 300 mg
Nifedipine	10 mg PO every 10-30 min up to three doses

IV, Intravenous; *PO*, by mouth.

and laboratory evaluations. Such monitoring often begins in the hospital and may be continued in an outpatient or home setting with appropriate supervision. If the clinical picture deteriorates or term is reached, the baby should be delivered. There is no evidence that antihypertensive therapy influences progression of preeclampsia, and its use may actually be dangerous by masking worsening hypertension. Fetal well-being should be evaluated until delivery by means of kick counts and regular non-stress tests or modified biophysical profiles.

Patients with severe disease should be delivered. The only exception to this approach is the diagnosis of severe preeclampsia, in a patient remote from term (<28 weeks' gestation), on the basis of proteinuria and transiently (unsustained) severe hypertension alone. Such patients may be managed conservatively under close supervision while antenatal corticosteroids are administered without adversely affecting maternal or fetal outcome (Sibai et al, 1990). There is no reason for conservative management in any other circumstance. The patient with severe preeclampsia at less than 24 weeks' gestation should be offered termination of the pregnancy; all others should be delivered by the most expedient means. Cesarean section should be reserved for obstetric indications.

Severe hypertension requires treatment with fast-acting antihypertensive agents if stroke and placental abruption are to be avoided. Intravenous hydralazine is well established as a first-line drug for this purpose, although there is a growing experience with other agents, including intravenous labetalol and oral nifedipine (Duley and Henderson-Smart, 2000a) (Table 11-4). The aim of treatment is to lower blood pressure into the mild preeclampsia range (140/90 mm Hg) to reduce the risk of stroke and other maternal cardiovascular complications. There is evidence to support the use of parenteral magnesium sulfate to prevent eclampsia in all cases of severe disease (Duley et al, 2003).

Severe preeclampsia can manifest as classic disease with severe proteinuric hypertension, or it can cause atypical findings such as pulmonary edema or severe central nervous system symptoms, including blindness. More commonly, patients show evidence of microangiopathy leading to the hemolysis, elevated liver enzymes, and low platelets (HELLP) syndrome. The full-blown clinical syndrome of HELLP carries a significant maternal risk. Earlier reports suggested that the disease carries a grave prognosis (Weinstein, 1982). This suggestion remains true for florid clinical cases, but most patients now have "laboratory" HELLP and never experience major clinical features of the syndrome because delivery is initiated before their condition deteriorates to that point.

Preeclampsia and Fetal Risk

Because the only recourse in severe preeclampsia is delivery, the disease has a corresponding effect on prematurity and its attendant complications. IUGR is not uncommon in severe preeclampsia, and there may be evidence of progressive deterioration in fetal well-being with worsening disease. Infants delivered at less than 34 weeks' gestation will benefit from antenatal steroid therapy—even as little as 8 hours of therapy before delivery may have benefit. Many patients are able to deliver vaginally, but fetal compromise may preclude aggressive induction and mandate delivery by cesarean section. The incidence of respiratory distress syndrome is lower in infants of mothers with preeclampsia who are delivered preterm than in those of age-matched controls without antenatal steroid exposure (Yoon et al, 1980). Nonetheless, the morbidity of such infants is greater because of hypoxemic insults received in utero. Infants born to mothers with preeclampsia may also have thrombocytopenia or neutropenia, which further complicates their newborn course (Fraser and Tudehope, 1996).

Intrapartum Management

All women in labor with a diagnosis of preeclampsia should receive magnesium sulfate as seizure prophylaxis (Box 11-2). Although the absolute risk of seizure is low (1 in 2000 to 3000), the occurrence of seizures is unpredictable, and the efficacy of magnesium sulfate and margin of safety has been validated in multiple randomized trials (Duley et al, 2003). The mechanism of action of $MgSO_4$ in the prevention of seizures is still unresolved, with various theories being advanced, including peripheral neuromuscular blockade, membrane stabilization, N-methyl D-aspartate (NMDA) receptor blocking activity, cerebral vasodilation, and calcium channel blocking action (Belfort et al, 2006).

Blood pressure should be maintained in the mild preeclampsia range using intravenous antihypertensive agents (labetalol, hydralazine). Epidural anesthesia is indicated for pain control and to aid in blood pressure management. Vaginal delivery should be possible in most cases. Delivery by cesarean section should be reserved for obstetric indications. Careful attention to fluid balance should be maintained. After delivery, the preeclamptic process should begin to resolve rapidly.

ECLAMPSIA

Eclampsia is the occurrence of generalized tonic-clonic seizures in association with preeclampsia. It affects approximately 1 in 2500 deliveries in the United States and may be much more common in developing countries, affecting as many as 1% of parturients. Up to 10% of maternal deaths are due to eclampsia (Duley, 1992).

> **BOX 11-2   Magnesium Sulfate Therapy for Prevention of Eclampsia**
>
> - Bolus 4-6 g IV over 20 min
> - Continuous infusion 1-2 g/hr
> - Follow up levels every 6-8 hours to target 4-6 mEq/L
> - Continue infusion 24 hours after delivery or 24 hours after seizure if seizure occurs despite magnesium therapy

Most cases of eclampsia occur within 24 hours of delivery. Almost 50% of seizures occur before the patient's admission to the labor and delivery department, approximately 30% are intrapartum, and the remainder are postpartum. There is a considerable drop in the risk of eclampsia by 48 hours postpartum, with seizures occurring in less than 3% of women beyond that time. Most patients have antecedent features that are suggestive of preeclampsia, although in some cases eclampsia may occur without warning. If eclampsia is left untreated, repetitive seizures become more frequent and of longer duration, and ultimately status eclampticus develops. Maternal and fetal mortality may be as high as 50% in severe cases, especially if the seizures occur while the patient is far from medical care.

Randomized controlled trials have demonstrated the clear superiority of magnesium sulfate for the treatment of eclampsia over all other anticonvulsants (Duley and Gulmezoglu, 2002; Duley and Henderson-Smart, 2002b, 2002c). Intravenous magnesium sulfate is given as a 4-g bolus over 5 minutes followed by a maintenance infusion of 1 to 2 g/hr for 24 hours after delivery. Subsequent seizures can be treated with further bolus injections. In refractory cases, second-line treatment with other anticonvulsants may be required, or the patient may have to be paralyzed and their lungs ventilated.

Delivery after an eclamptic seizure should take place in a controlled, careful manner. There is little to be added by performing an emergency cesarean section (Coppage and Polzin, 2002). The patient's condition should be stabilized first. Vaginal delivery is possible in most cases, although cesarean delivery may be indicated if the status of the cervix is unfavorable or if fetal compromise is ongoing despite control of seizures and maternal stabilization. Infants born to mothers after eclampsia require careful observation after birth.

SUGGESTED READINGS

ACOG Practice Bulletin: Chronic hypertension in pregnancy, ACOG Committee on Practice Bulletins, *Obstet Gynecol* 98(Suppl l):177-185, 2001.

Chappell LC, Enye S, Seed P, et al: Adverse perinatal outcomes and risk factors for preeclampsia in women with chronic hypertension: a prospective study, *Hypertension* 51:1002-1009, 2008.

Myers JE, Baker PN: Hypertensive diseases and eclampsia, *Curr Opin Obstet Gynecol* 14:119-125, 2002.

Wang A, Rana S, Karumanchi SA: Preeclampsia: the role of angiogenic factors in its pathogenesis, *Physiology* 24:147-158, 2009.

Complete references used in this text can be found online at www.expertconsult.com

PERINATAL SUBSTANCE ABUSE

Linda D. Wallen and Christine A. Gleason

Substance abuse during pregnancy has been recognized as a problem for more than a century. Psychotropic substances, both legal (alcohol, cigarettes, and prescription drugs such as opioids and benzodiazepines) and illegal (opioids, amphetamines, cocaine, and marijuana), can cause obstetric, fetal, and neonatal complications. These complications include poor intrauterine growth, prematurity, abruptio placenta, fetal distress, spontaneous abortion, stillbirth, fetal (and maternal) cerebral infarctions and other vascular accidents, malformations, and neonatal neurobehavioral dysfunction. Although substance abuse occurs in all socioeconomic classes, illegal drug abuse is more frequently associated with unhealthy lifestyles, poor access to prenatal care, untreated health problems, poverty, stress, and psychological disorders. Because of these socioeconomic confounders as well as the confounders of polysubstance exposure and the influence of various postnatal environmental factors, it is often difficult to determine the effects of maternal use of one specific drug on the fetus and newborn. This chapter addresses the epidemiology of perinatal substance use and abuse; the effects of specific drugs on the fetus and newborn; maternal issues and their effects on the newborn; identification of pregnancies and babies at risk; neonatal management; and long-term effects and follow-up. The discussion will focus on abused substances that are known or suggested to be associated with significant perinatal and neonatal morbidity: alcohol, tobacco, nicotine, opioids, cocaine, marijuana, and methamphetamine.

EPIDEMIOLOGY OF PERINATAL SUBSTANCE EXPOSURE

PREVALENCE

Prevalence rates for perinatal substance exposure have been determined by using a number of different definitions, survey methods, and drug use detection procedures (Lester et al, 2004). One of the most comprehensive geographically based prevalence studies on substance use and abuse by pregnant women was undertaken in California in the early 1990s by the Perinatal Substance Exposure Study Group (Vega et al, 1993). In that study, urine was collected at the time of delivery from more than 30,000 pregnant women. The prevalence rates for illicit drug use were 3.5% (overall), 8.8% (tobacco), and 7.2% (alcohol). The authors concluded that if these results could be extrapolated to the United States at large, an estimated 450,000 infants per year (11% of 4 million live births) would be exposed to alcohol, illicit drugs, or both in the days before delivery.

Rates of perinatal substance exposure have not changed substantially over the past 20 years, although there is wide geographic variation. The U.S. Department of Health and Human Services Pregnancy Risk Assessment Monitoring System is designed to monitor maternal behaviors and experiences among women who deliver live-born infants. Data collected during 2000 to 2003 from 19 states revealed that during the last 3 months of pregnancy, tobacco use ranged from 4.9% to 27.5%, and alcohol use ranged from 2% to 8.7%. Data from a 2005-2006 National Survey on Drug Use and Health revealed that of pregnant women aged 15 to 44, 4% reported using illicit drugs, 16.5% reported using tobacco, and 12% reported using alcohol sometime within the past month (Substance Abuse and Mental Health Services Administration, 2007). These rates are significantly lower than the rates reported by women aged 15 to 44 years who were not pregnant (10% reported using illicit drugs, 29.5% reported using tobacco, and 53% reported using alcohol within the past month), confirming that the prevalence of substance use among pregnant women remains less than among nonpregnant women.

The Maternal Lifestyle Study was developed in the early 1990s by the National Institute of Child Health and Human Development (NICHD) and National Institute on Drug Abuse (NIDA) to follow pregnant women known to be using opioids or cocaine and to follow their offspring. The study followed 11,800 pregnant women who received prenatal care during 1993 to 1995 at four teaching hospital sites. Women were followed from initial presentation throughout their offspring's childhood, with a planned evaluation at 8 to 11 years. Meconium analyses were used to confirm maternal substance use; there was 66% agreement between meconium analyses and positive maternal reports. The prevalence of cocaine and opioid exposure was 10.7%; 98% of cocaine users also used other drugs; and only 2% of women used cocaine alone (Shankaran et al, 2007).

EPIDEMIOLOGY OF SPECIFIC SUBSTANCES

Nicotine—in the form of cigarettes, smokeless tobacco, and nicotine replacement patches—remains the substance used most often during pregnancy. Although cigarette smoking in the United States has decreased significantly over the last 20 years, 26% of reproductive-aged women still smoke, and 15% to 20% of women smoke during their pregnancies (Andres and Dar, 2000). Women who smoke during pregnancy are more likely to use opioids, alcohol, cocaine, amphetamines, and marijuana during pregnancy than women who do not smoke (Vega et al, 1993). Cigarette smoking has been associated with numerous perinatal complications, often in a dose-dependent fashion. Smoking has been shown to raise the risk of spontaneous abortion, stillbirth, fetal growth retardation, prematurity, perinatal mortality, and sudden infant death syndrome (Andres and Day, 2000; Kallen, 2001; Lambers and Clark, 1996; Tuthill et al, 1999). Cigarette smoking represents the most influential and most common factor adversely affecting perinatal outcomes. In a 2008, Rogers "estimated that if all the women in the United States stopped smoking, there would be an 11% reduction in stillbirths and 5% reduction in neonatal deaths."

Before 1970, the detrimental effects of alcohol abuse during pregnancy were believed to be related only to drunkenness, such as an increased risk for accidents. There was a widely held belief that the placenta formed a protective barrier between alcohol and the fetus. This belief repudiated by studies in the United States (Jones and Smith, 1973) and France (Lemoine et al, 1967) describing fetal alcohol syndrome. These studies led to the 1989 U.S. federal law requiring that warning labels be placed on all alcoholic beverage containers regarding alcohol-related birth defects. Despite this extensive public health campaign designed to inform and warn women about the dangers of alcohol consumption during pregnancy, approximately 10% of pregnant women still report using alcohol (Centers for Disease Control and Prevention, 2009). A smaller percentage of these women are alcoholics, but their infants are at significantly higher risk for fetal alcohol syndrome or alcohol-related neurobehavioral disorders compared with the infants of nonalcoholic pregnant women who use alcohol.

Opium derivatives have been used as analgesics for centuries and remain the most effective analgesics available. Opioids of clinical interest are morphine, heroin, methadone, meperidine, oxycodone, and codeine. Perinatal problems associated with opium were first reported in the late 1800s. Since the 1950s, heroin use, particularly among women, has been endemic in most major American cities. Compared with cocaine, marijuana, alcohol, and tobacco abuse, opioid addiction during pregnancy is rare (Shankaran et al, 2007). The prevalence of opioid use among pregnant women is reported to range from 1% to 2% (Vega et al, 1993; Yawn et al, 1994) to as much as 21% in a highly selected group of women (Behnke and Eyler, 1993; Nair et al, 1994; Ostrea et al, 1992b). One multicenter study found that the prevalence of opioid use varied by center and ranged from 1.6% to 4.5% at the different sites (Lester et al, 2001). In addition, these centers reported higher rates of opioid use by mothers of low-birthweight and very low-birthweight infants. Rates for heroin use are higher in metropolitan areas and cities and are more concentrated in northeastern and west coast cities. Opioid abuse is more common in groups of lower socioeconomic status, and women using opioids during pregnancy are more likely to use other drugs (Bauer, 1999; Brown et al, 1998; van Baar and de Graaff, 1994). Investigators have also reported that 93% of women identified as using opioids and cocaine during pregnancy had also used a combination of alcohol, nicotine, or marijuana (Bauer, 1999). Of the opioid drugs known to be abused during pregnancy, heroin and methadone have been studied the most extensively. Heroin can be ingested through smoking or by the intranasal or intravenous route. Reports from European countries suggest a trend away from intravenous injection of opioids (Hartnoll, 1994). The use of noninjectable heroin may reduce the risk of transmission of human immunodeficiency virus (HIV); however, its wider use ensures the emergence of new groups of heroin users for whom the risk of intravenous use is a major deterrent.

The euphoria-producing effect of cocaine was exploited extensively in the United States in the late nineteenth and early twentieth centuries, when the agent was an active ingredient in a number of widely used over-the-counter elixirs and tonics. Cocaine use markedly decreased after the Harrison Narcotic Act of 1914 and the supervening Comprehensive Drug Abuse Prevention and Control Act of 1970, which classified cocaine as a schedule II drug (i.e., one of "high abuse potential with restricted medical use," similar to opioids, barbiturates, and amphetamines). Cocaine's reputation as a glamour drug, the widely held misconception that cocaine is not addictive, and the development and marketing of crack, a cheap version of cocaine, were major factors in the resurgence of drug use. Growing concern regarding the effects of maternal cocaine use on pregnancy outcomes was one of the reasons that the U.S. Congress passed the 1986 Narcotics Penalties and Enforcement Act, which imposed severe penalties on any person convicted of either possessing or distributing effects; however, this law did not appreciably alter the fact that cocaine and other stimulants had become the drugs of choice for women in the United States. In the 1990s, studies based on urine toxicology screening reported a prevalence of cocaine use among pregnant women of 5% in New York City, 1.1% in a geographic sample in California, and less than 0.5% in private hospitals in Denver, Colorado (Burke and Roth, 1993). Prevalence increases to 18% when both self-reporting and urine testing are used, and the highest prevalence rates are reported from studies using meconium testing.

Amphetamines have surpassed cocaine as the primary illicit drugs used by pregnant women in many areas of California and other states. Methamphetamine (or "crystal") has been the primary form abused, because it can be produced locally and fairly cheaply. Greater restrictions on the importing of cocaine have also contributed to resurgence in amphetamine use. Amphetamines have always been popular among adolescents, especially females, and accordingly women of child-bearing age are at high risk for perinatal abuse. A California study of drug-exposed infants in the social welfare system documented a higher prevalence of amphetamine use among white pregnant women than in women of other ethnicities (Sagatun-Edwards et al, 1995). The Infant Development, Environment, and Lifestyle (IDEAL) study chose four major U.S. cities with known methamphetamine abusing populations and reported methamphetamine use in 5.2% of pregnant women. As in previous reports, these women frequently used other substances: 25% used tobacco, 22.8% used alcohol, 6% used marijuana, and 1.3% used barbiturates (Arria et al, 2006).

According to the 2003 National Survey on Drug Use and Health, marijuana is the most widely used illegal drug used in the United States, with approximately 14.6 million people reporting that they use the drug. In a 1986 study, the most frequent age of marijuana use for women included the childbearing ages, with 50% of 18- to 35-year-old women reporting that they used marijuana at least once and 8% reporting that they used marijuana a minimum of 10 of the past 30 days (Clayton et al,

1986). The 2002-2006 National Household Survey on Drug Abuse included information on drug use in the last 30 days from over 94,000 women aged 18 to 44 years, of whom 5017 were pregnant. Marijuana use was reported in 7.3% of nonpregnant women and 2.8% of pregnant women with moderate to heavy use (more than five times per month) in 1.8% of pregnant women compared with 3.7% in nonpregnant women. Marijuana use declined over the course of pregnancy, from 4.5% in the first trimester to 1.5% in the third trimester (Muhuri and Gfroerer, 2009).

HEALTH POLICY

In the 1980s, with rising cocaine use and the emergence of crack cocaine, national attention turned to drug use during pregnancy, with a general public outcry being the result. Children born to crack addicts were widely believed to be irrevocably damaged and public opinion was that mothers should be punished. As the foster care system became overwhelmed and as evidence to the contrary has emerged, public opinion regarding prenatal drug use has shifted more toward maternal treatment and prevention rather than punishment. As Lester et al (2004) stated, the initial overreaction of the public "in which drug-exposed children were characterized as irrevocably and irreversibly damaged" has shifted "to a perhaps equally premature excessive 'sigh of relief' that drugs such as cocaine do not have lasting effects, especially if children are raised in appropriate environments." This statement has led to a change in the public discourse regarding health policy interventions for substance use and abuse during pregnancy.

The focus of current policy is to provide appropriate medical care for substance-using pregnant women, including medical management of their chemical dependency and programs to decrease substance use during pregnancy. However, there remains the important step of recognizing that "the idea that illegal drugs are more harmful to the unborn fetus than legal drugs is incorrect" (Thompson et al, 2009). Future research and intervention need to include programs to educate women of childbearing age of the significant effects of both legal and illegal substance use on the early-gestation fetus, starting even before pregnancy may be recognized.

PERINATAL EFFECTS OF SPECIFIC DRUGS (Table 12-1)
ETHANOL (ALCOHOL)
Pharmacology and Biologic Actions

Alcohol is a mood-altering substance that enhances the effects of the inhibitory neurotransmitter gamma-aminobutyric acid and lessens the effect of the excitatory neurotransmitter glutamate, thus acting as a central nervous system (CNS) depressant or sedative. Alcoholic beverages come in many forms, and for centuries they have been consumed for diverse reasons: celebrations, relaxation, religious ceremonies, and medicinal purposes (alcohol is an excellent sedative and tocolytic agent). The alcohol contained in alcoholic beverages is ethanol. Ethanol is absorbed in the digestive tract and into the body fat and bloodstream. Ethanol is metabolized to acetaldehyde by alcohol dehydrogenase (ADH), primarily in the liver. ADH is then metabolized to acetate by aldehyde dehydrogenase (ALDH) and eventually eliminated as water and CO_2. Although acetaldehyde is short-lived, it can cause significant tissue damage, which is particularly evident in the liver, where most alcohol metabolism takes place. Pregnant women have slower rates of alcohol clearance, likely related to hormonal alterations in the activity of the alcohol-metabolizing enzymes; this leads to slower clearance of alcohol compared with nonpregnant women consuming the same amount of alcohol (Shankaran et al, 2007).

Complications of Pregnancy

Heavy drinking carries a higher risk of cardiovascular and hepatic complications in women compared with men, and the alcohol-associated mortality rate is also considerably higher (Smith and Weisner, 2000). These factors alone can clearly complicate a woman's pregnancy. In addition, nutritional deficiencies and poor diet can affect general health and dentition, which can negatively affect a pregnancy. Alcoholism is a chronic disease that is often progressive and can be fatal. Pregnant alcoholics often have related medical disorders such as cirrhosis, pancreatitis, and alcohol-related neurologic problems. These disorders can affect the health and well-being of their fetus.

TABLE 12-1 Enhanced Risk for Various Events or Processes after Substance Use during Pregnancy*

Event or Process	Ethanol	Cigarettes	Marijuana	Opiates	Cocaine	Amphetamines
Malformations	+	–	–	–	–	–
Abortion/stillbirth	+	+	?	+	+	+
Intrauterine growth restriction	+	+	–	+	+	+
Prematurity	–	+	?	+	+	+
Withdrawal	?	+	+/–	+	–	–
Central nervous system sequelae	+	?	+	?	+	?
Sudden infant death syndrome	+	+	?	+	?	?
Foster care	+	–	–	+	+	+

+, Causes event or process; –, does not cause event or process; ?, not known whether agent causes event or process.
*Although risk is increased, the risk ratio ranges for many from 1 to 2 for these associations.

Alcohol affects prostaglandin levels, increasing levels of its precursors in human placental tissue and thus affecting fetal development and parturition. In fact, researchers have used this knowledge to test the effect of aspirin, which inhibits alcohol-induced increases in prostaglandin levels, on reducing alcohol-induced fetal malformations in a mouse model (Randall, 2001). Specific obstetric complications of heavy drinking may relate to alterations in prostaglandin levels, including an increased risk for spontaneous abortion, abruptio placenta, and alcohol-related birth defects such as fetal alcohol syndrome.

Fetal Alcohol Syndrome

Fetal alcohol syndrome (FAS) was first described by Lemoine (1967), a Belgian pediatrician who observed a common pattern of birth anomalies in children born to alcoholic mothers in France. This description was followed by a landmark article by Jones and Smith (1973) reporting similar features in several children born to alcoholic mothers in the United States.

It is unclear how much alcohol exposure is necessary to cause fetal teratogenicity, and even high consumption levels do not always result in the birth of a child with FAS (Abel and Hannigan, 1995). However, a woman with a previous affected child is at increased risk for having a child with FAS if she consumes alcohol during a subsequent pregnancy. The adverse effects of alcohol on the fetus are related to gestational age at exposure, the amount of alcohol consumed, and the pattern of consumption (e.g., binge drinking), maternal peak blood alcohol concentrations, maternal alcohol metabolism, and the individual susceptibility of the fetus. Studies show that maternal peak blood alcohol levels are affected by maternal nutrition, age, body size, and genetic disposition (Eckardt et al, 1998; Maier and West, 2001). In addition, various risk factors increase susceptibility to FAS, including advanced maternal age and confounding factors such as nonwhite race, poverty, and socioeconomic status (Abel, 1995; Bagheri et al, 1998; May and Gossage, 2001). In the United States, the incidence of FAS is tenfold higher for African Americans living in poverty than for white middle-class women (Abel, 1995). Despite the differences in incidence of FAS worldwide, reports consistently indicate poverty or socioeconomic status as major determinants of FAS (Abel, 1995; May et al, 2000).

Features of FAS include characteristic facial dysmorphology (short palpebral fissures, midface hypoplasia, broad flat nasal bridge, flat philtrum, and thin upper lip; Figure 12-1), prenatal and postnatal growth deficiency, and variable CNS abnormalities. Skeletal anomalies, abnormal hand creases, and ophthalmologic, renal, and cardiac anomalies have been described in children with FAS, but less frequently than the facial dysmorphology and CNS abnormalities that include structural brain defects (e.g., dysgenesis of the corpus callosum and cerebellar hypoplasia), cognitive abnormalities, delayed brain development, and signs of neurologic impairment, including lifelong behavioral and psychosocial dysfunction. In 1996, the Institute of Medicine further defined the criteria for the diagnosis of FAS and proposed a new term—alcohol-related neurodevelopmental disorder (ARND).

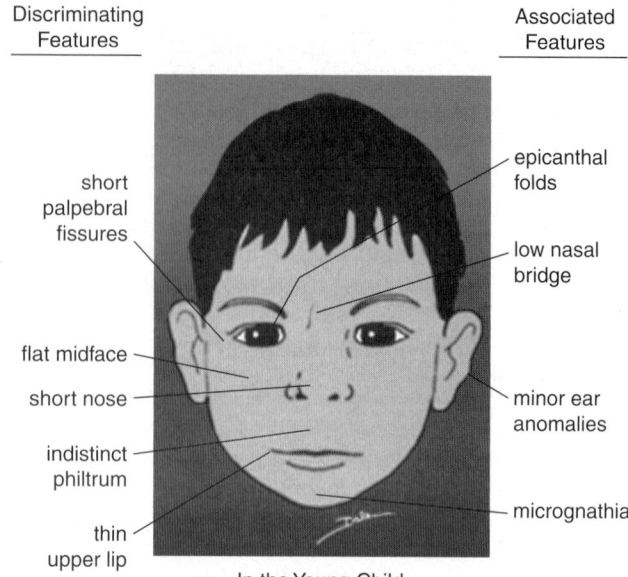

FIGURE 12-1 Facies in fetal alcohol syndrome. (*From Streissguth AP, Little RE: Alcohol, pregnancy, and the fetal alcohol syndrome, ed 2, unit 5 of* Alcohol use and its medical consequences: a comprehensive slide teaching program for biomedical education. *Developed by Project Cash of the Dartmouth Medical School. Reproduced with permission from Milner-Fenwick, Inc., Timonium, Michigan, 1994.*)

This term includes structural CNS and cognitive abnormalities in children with confirmed fetal exposure to alcohol. Unlike FAS, a diagnosis of ARND does not require the presence of facial or other physical abnormalities. In 2000, the American Academy of Pediatrics Committee on Substance Abuse published these new definitions with an explanatory drawing (Figure 12-2).

The incidence of FAS in the United States has been estimated to vary from 1.95 to 5 cases per 1000 live births (Abel, 1995; American Academy of Pediatrics Committee on Substance Abuse and Committee on Children with Disabilities, 2000; Bertrand et al, 2005; Sampson et al, 1997). FAS is recognized more frequently in the United States than in other countries and is most common (4.3%) among women who report heavy drinking (Abel, 1995). Accurate incidence and prevalence rates of FAS are difficult to obtain because of wide variations in methodologies used for estimation of rates, and because the clinical diagnosis is often missed in the neonatal period. In fact, most cases (up to 89%) are not diagnosed until after a child is age 6 (Centers for Disease Control and Prevention [CDC], 1997).

FAS is diagnosed from the history and physical findings. No laboratory tests are available for clinical use to quantify the extent of alcohol exposure during fetal life. There are also no clinical methods for validating maternal self-reporting of alcohol use, quantifying the level of fetal exposure, or predicting future disability after fetal exposure (Jones and Chambers, 1999). Koren et al (2002) have proposed meconium fatty acid ethyl ester levels as a potential biologic marker for fetal alcohol exposure. Whether this finding is shown to correlate with childhood outcomes remains to be studied. Investigators have shown that pediatricians fail to recognize FAS in the newborn and do not always inquire about alcohol exposure during pregnancy

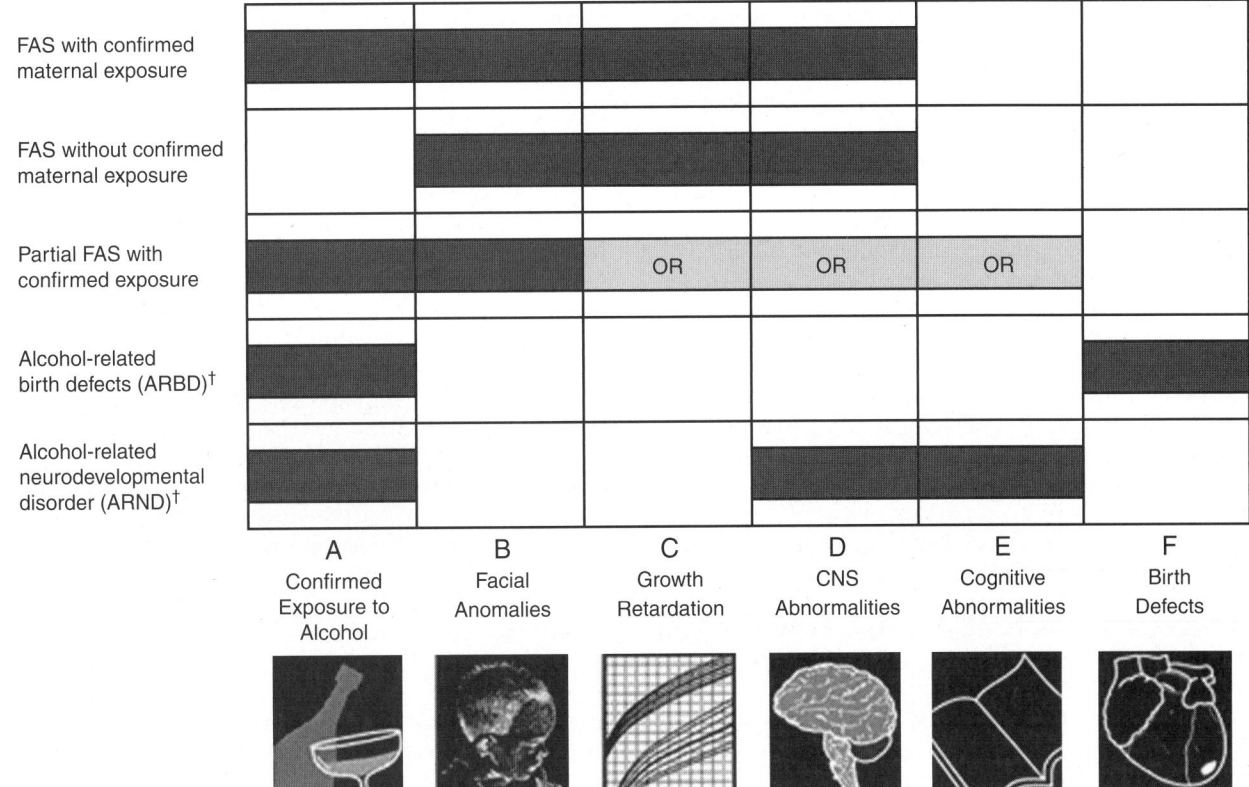

	A Confirmed Exposure to Alcohol	B Facial Anomalies	C Growth Retardation	D CNS Abnormalities	E Cognitive Abnormalities	F Birth Defects

*Adapted from *Fetal Alcohol Syndrome; Diagnosis, Epidemiology, Prevention, and Treatment.* 1996;4–5. Letter designations in the figure indicate the following:

A. Confirmed maternal alcohol exposure indicates a pattern of excessive intake characterized by substantial, regular intake or heavy episodic drinking. Evidence of this pattern may include frequent episodes of intoxication, development of tolerance or withdrawal, social problems related to drinking, legal problems related to drinking, engaging in physically hazardous beavior while drinking, or alcohol-related medical problems such as hepatic disease.

B. Evidence of a characteristic pattern of facial anomalies that includes features such as short palpebral fissures and abnormalities in the premaxillary zone (e.g., flat upper lip, flattened philtrum, and flat midface).

C. Evidence of growth retardation, including at least one of the following:
 • low birthweight for gestational age
 • decelerating weight over time not caused by nutrition
 • disproportional low weight to height

D. Evidence of CNS neurodevelopmental abnormalities, including at least one of the following:
 • decreased cranial size at birth
 • structural brain abnormalities (e.g., microcephaly, partial or complete agenesis of the corpus callosum, cerebellar hypoplasia)
 • neurological hard or soft signs (as age appropriate), such as impaired fine motor skills, neurosensory hearing loss, poor tandem gait, poor eye-hand coordination

E. Evidence of a complex pattern of behavior or cognitive abnormalities that are inconsistent with developmental level and cannot be explained by familial background or environment alone, such as learning difficulties; deficits in school performance; poor impulse control; problems in social perception; deficits in higher level receptive and expressive language; poor capacity for abstraction or metacognition; specific deficits in mathematical skills; or problems in memory, attention, or judgment

F. Birth defects associated with alcohol exposure include:

Cardiac	Atrial septal defects Ventricular septal defects	Aberrant great vessels Tetralogy of Fallot
Skeletal	Hypoplastic nails Shortened fifth digits Radioulnar synostosis Flexion contractures Camptodactyly	Clinodactyly Pectus excavatum and carinatum Klippel-Feil syndrome Hemivertebrae Scoliosis
Renal	Aplastic, dysplastic, hypoplastic kidneys Horseshoe kidneys	Ureteral duplications Hydronephrosis
Ocular	Strabismus Retinal vascular anomalies	Refractive problems Secondary to small globes
Auditory	Conductive hearing loss	Neurosensory hearing loss
Other	Virtually every malformation has been described in some patient with FAS. The etiologic specificity of most of these anomalies to alcohol teratogenesis remains uncertain.	

†Alcohol-related effects indicate clinical conditions in which there is a history of maternal alcohol exposure, and where clinical or animal research has linked maternal alcohol ingestion to an observed outcome. There are two categories, alcohol-related neurodevelopmental disorder and alcohol-related birth defects, which may co-occur. If both diagnoses are present, then both diagnoses should be rendered.

FIGURE 12-2 **Diagnostic classification of fetal alcohol syndrome and alcohol-related effects.** *(From the American Academy of Pediatrics Committee on Substance Abuse and Committee on Children with Disabilities: Fetal alcohol syndrome and alcohol-related neurodevelopmental disorders,* Pediatrics *106:359. Reproduced with permission from the American Academy of Pediatrics, 2000.)*

(Stoler and Holmes, 1999). One promising screening tool is the use of averaged cranial ultrasound images to examine the size and shape of the corpus callosum, which is typically dysgenic in FAS (Bookstein et al, 2005). Guidelines to aid in the earlier recognition and referral of infants and children with FAS and fetal alcohol spectrum disorder have been published recently (Bertrand et al, 2005; Hoyme et al, 2005). FAS is not a problem just for neonatologists. Adolescents who were exposed prenatally to alcohol have a different approach to alcohol than their nonexposed peers, with an increased risk for earlier use and subsequent alcohol abuse (Baer et al, 2003). One study in rodents suggests that fetal ethanol exposure increases ethanol intake later in life by making it smell and taste better (Youngentob and Glendinning, 2009). Children with FAS continue to have serious disabilities into adulthood (Streissguth et al, 1991; Streissguth, 1993). Although the facial features and growth restriction are no longer as distinctive as during childhood, mental retardation continues to have a significant effect. Adults with FAS have behavior, socialization, and communication dysfunction, and on average they function at the second- or third-grade level. A significant number of FAS patients do not achieve fully independent living. Earlier recognition and intervention for children with FAS and its variants may help to minimize eventual adulthood disabilities and help to prepare adolescents and young adults with the disorder for independent living (Bertrand et al, 2005).

Fetal Growth

Intrauterine growth restriction (IUGR) is one of the most consistent findings of prenatal exposure to alcohol (Hannigan and Armant, 2000). Growth deficit begins in utero and continues throughout childhood (American Academy of Pediatrics Committee on Substance Abuse and Committee on Children with Disabilities, 2000). The facial features and the growth restriction become less noticeable during adolescence and puberty (Streissguth et al, 1991; Streissguth, 1993).

CIGARETTE SMOKING AND NICOTINE

Pharmacology and Biologic Actions

Cigarette smoke contains a complex mixture of approximately 4000 compounds, including nicotine and carbon monoxide, which can adversely affect the fetus (Lester et al, 2004). In rodents, nicotine releases chemicals in the reward center of the brain, which likely triggers the euphoria that smokers experience. Nicotine activates nicotinic acetylcholine receptors, and these receptors remain depressed for a longer time after their activation stops, which likely accounts for compulsive smoking (Cohen, 2007). Nicotine crosses the placenta and concentrates in fetal blood and amniotic fluid, where its levels significantly exceed maternal blood concentrations (Haustein, 1999). The serum concentration of cotinine, the primary metabolite of nicotine, is used to quantitate the level of smoking and fetal exposure. Cotinine has a half-life of 15 to 20 hours, and because its serum levels are tenfold higher than those of nicotine, this substance may represent a better

marker for intrauterine exposure (Lambers and Clark, 1996).

Complications of Pregnancy

Although the exact mechanism of the adverse effects of smoking on pregnancy is unknown, cigarettes contain numerous potentially toxic compounds that affect fetal health in a number of ways. Nicotine and its metabolites can act as vasoconstrictors, and a study in pregnant rhesus monkeys demonstrated a nicotine-associated decrease in uterine blood flow (Suzuki et al, 1980), which might provide a partial explanation for the association between maternal cigarette smoking and low birthweight. Theories regarding mechanisms for the adverse effects of smoking on fetal health include direct vasoconstrictive effects of nicotine on uteroplacental blood flow, the induction of fetal hypoxia from carbon monoxide production, direct toxic effects and indirect effects of altered maternal nutritional intake, and altered maternal and placental metabolism (Andres and Day, 2000; Pastrakuljic et al, 1999). When pregnant women smoke cigarettes, the resulting increased levels of carbon monoxide cross the placenta and form carboxyhemoglobin in the fetus, with resulting hypoxemia (Lambers and Clark, 1996). Supporting this theory, serum erythropoietin levels are higher in tobacco smoke–exposed infants at delivery, a finding that is presumed to reflect fetal hypoxia (Beratis et al, 1999; Jazayeri et al, 1998). In addition to the fetal hypoxia theory, there have recently been studies demonstrating that nicotine may act as a developmental neurotoxin targeting nicotinic acetylcholine receptors (Lester et al, 2004; Levin and Slotkin, 1998) and may disturb protein metabolism during gestation, leading to decreased serum amino acids in umbilical cord blood (Jauniaux et al, 2001).

Maternal smoking has also been show to affect the length of gestation in a dose-dependent manner, with a higher risk of preterm delivery (Jaakkola et al, 2001; Savitz et al, 2001) and a twofold increase in the incidence of placental abruption (Ananth et al, 1996). Perinatal mortality is increased in pregnant smokers, likely reflecting the increases in rates of prematurity, placental abruption, and placenta previa in women who smoke. Mothers who smoke during pregnancy commonly continue to smoke during their infants' childhood. Asthma and recurrent otitis media are more common in infants who are exposed to passive smoking (Ey et al, 1995; Martinez et al, 1995).

Fetal Growth

The effect of smoking on fetal growth is significant and dose dependent (Kyrklund-Blomberg et al, 1998; Nordentoft et al, 1996). Studies have shown lower birthweights associated with levels of nicotine exposure, with a 1-g reduction in birthweight observed for every microgram per milliliter increase in maternal serum cotinine level (Eskenazi et al, 1995; Perkins et al, 1997). Investigators have shown a dose-dependent relationship between the amount of smoking and the extent of fetal growth restriction and birthweight reduction (Horta et al, 1997; Jaakkola et al, 2001; Savitz et al, 2001; Sprauve et al, 1999).

Both reducing and ceasing cigarette smoking during pregnancy have been shown to be beneficial and to lead to improved fetal growth. Lieberman et al (1994) have shown that if pregnant women stop smoking during the third trimester, their infants' weights are indistinguishable from those of a nonsmoking population. Other investigators report that even a modest reduction in smoking is associated with improved fetal growth (Li et al, 1993; Walsh et al, 2001).

MARIJUANA

Pharmacology and Biologic Actions

Marijuana, the dried material from the hemp plant *Cannabis sativa*, is most often smoked but can be ingested with food. Its most active ingredient is delta-9-tetrahydrocannabinol (THC), which binds to cannabinoid receptors in the brain and modifies the release of several neurotransmitters. Its primary biologic effects include euphoria; relaxation; increased heart rate, blood pressure, and appetite; and impaired coordination, decision-making, short-term memory, concentration, and learning. Although controversial, there is increasing evidence that regular marijuana use can cause respiratory difficulties, cognitive impairments, withdrawal, and dependence (Khalsa et al, 2002). THC crosses the placenta and collects in the amniotic fluid.

Complications of Pregnancy

Marijuana use during pregnancy is inconsistently reported to have effects on birth outcomes. The inconsistency likely stems from the fact that marijuana is often used in combination with other substances, thus potentiating the risks for prematurity and low birthweight. Day et al (1991) reported a higher incidence of meconium-stained amniotic fluid and other pregnancy and delivery complications after maternal marijuana use, but subsequent studies have not replicated this finding. The IDEAL study did not find any relation between marijuana use and altered fetal growth parameters (Smith et al, 2006). Frequent use of marijuana was associated with a small decrement in birthweight in a study that did not control for other illicit drug use (Schempf, 2007).

OPIOIDS (INCLUDING PRESCRIPTION PAIN KILLERS)

Pharmacology and Biologic Actions

Opioids are either drugs derived from the opium poppy or synthesized compounds that have similar biologic actions. The prototype opioid is morphine, and all opioids relate to it. For example, heroin (diacetylmorphine) exerts its effects by being metabolized to morphine, as does codeine, which is methylated morphine. Other opioids, such as methadone and oxycodone, are structurally unlike morphine but share its pharmacologic properties, because they stimulate similar opioid receptors. Specific opioid receptors (μ, δ, κ) have been identified in the nervous system and bowel that are activated by endogenous opioids, such as the naturally

occurring endorphins and enkephalins (Vaccarino and Kastin, 2000). As modulators of the sympathoadrenal system, endogenous opioids are important during periods of diverse forms of stress. Activation of these receptors by the endogenous opioids has physiologic effects, including analgesia, drowsiness, respiratory depression, decreased gastrointestinal motility, nausea, vomiting, and alterations in the endocrine and autonomic nervous systems. Activation of these same endogenous opioid receptors by exogenous opioid drugs has similar clinical effects, producing euphoria, sleepiness, and decreased sensitivity to pain, as well as adverse effects such as constipation and nephrotic syndrome (ACOG, 2005).

The use of opioid drugs can result in the development of tolerance, physiologic dependence, and addiction. Tolerance leads to a shortened duration of the action of opioids and a decrease in the intensity of the drug action, followed by the need for a higher dose to obtain the same clinical effect. Tolerance is believed to result from continued occupancy of the opioid receptor. Continuous administration of opioids, therefore, leads to the more rapid onset of tolerance (Anand and Arnold, 1994; Suresh and Anand, 2001). With physiologic dependence, there is a need for further drug administration to prevent withdrawal symptoms (agitation, dysphoria, temperature instability). Addiction is a more severe form of dependence that involves a complex pattern of drug-seeking behavior (Christensen, 2008).

Complications of Pregnancy

Obstetric complications associated with maternal use of opioids include a higher incidence of spontaneous abortion, premature delivery, preterm labor, abruptio placentae, chorioamnionitis, impaired fetal growth, and fetal distress. In women who use opioids during pregnancy, the incidence of preterm labor and premature delivery ranges from 25% to 41% (Chiriboga, 1993; Lam et al, 1992; Little et al, 1990). Maternal opioid use is also associated with higher rates of meconium-stained amniotic fluid, lower American Pediatric Gross Assessment Record (Apgar) scores, longer duration of membrane rupture (Gillogley et al, 1990), and increased incidence of syphilis and HIV infection at birth (Bauer, 1999). The rates of maternal complications of pregnancy are further increased when drug use is added to infection with HIV. Women infected with HIV who also use opioids, particularly methadone, have higher rates of miscarriage, preterm deliveries, and small-for-gestational-age infants, and more vaginal and urinary tract infections than women with HIV who do not use drugs (Mauri et al, 1995).

The etiology of these opioid-associated pregnancy complications is multifactorial. Maternal lifestyle, malnutrition, infections, and polydrug effects are likely to result in poor perinatal outcomes, including poor intrauterine growth and prematurity. Because the drug supply is often episodic, the pregnant addict is subject to episodes of withdrawal and overdose, thereby subjecting the fetus to intermittent episodes of hypoxia in utero, hindering growth and raising the risk of spontaneous abortion, stillbirth, fetal distress, and prematurity. Infants born to mothers who are addicted to opioids are more likely to be of low birthweight, to be premature, and to suffer from infection and perinatal asphyxia (Christensen, 2008).

Fetal Growth

Initial reports from studies addressing the effects of maternal opioid use on the fetus suggested that infants exposed to opioids in utero have a higher incidence of IUGR (Lam et al, 1992) and smaller head circumference (Bauer, 1999; Boer et al, 1994). Hulse et al (1997) reported an association with heroin abuse and increased prematurity, low birthweight, and reduced fetal growth. However, more recent work controlling for confounding factors has not demonstrated a significant relationship between opioid use and prematurity, low birthweight, or IUGR (Minozzi et al, 2008; Sharpe and Kuschel, 2004).

COCAINE

Pharmacology and Biologic Actions

Cocaine is a highly psychoactive stimulant with a long history of abuse. A naturally occurring anesthetic of the tropane family of alkaloids, cocaine is obtained from the *Erythroxylon coca* plant, which is indigenous to the mountain slopes of Central and South America. The coca leaf has been chewed or made into a stimulant tea by the natives of these areas to decrease fatigue and hunger. The pharmacologic actions of cocaine include inhibition of postsynaptic reuptake of norepinephrine, dopamine, and serotonin neurotransmitters by sympathetic nerve terminals, thus allowing higher concentrations of these neurotransmitters. In adults, cocaine binds strongly to neuronal dopamine reuptake transporters, thereby increasing postsynaptic dopamine at the mesolimbic and mesocortical levels and producing the addictive cycle of euphoria and dysphoria (Malanga and Kosofsky, 1999). Tryptophan uptake is similarly inhibited, altering serotonin pathways with resultant effects on sleep.

Cocaine use leads to a sense of well-being, increased energy, increased sexual achievement, and an intense euphoria or "high." The sympathomimetic action can have potentially devastating physiologic effects on the cardiovascular system. In adults, cocaine has been associated with cerebral hemorrhage, cardiac arrest, cardiac arrhythmias, myocardial infarction, intestinal ischemia, and seizures. Chronic use is associated with anorexia, nutritional problems, and paranoid psychosis and can ultimately result in neurotransmitter depletion and a "crash," characterized by lethargy, depression, anxiety, severe insomnia, hyperphagia, and cocaine craving.

Two forms of cocaine are commonly used—cocaine hydrochloride and cocaine base, which are either extracted by organic solvents or precipitated as "crack" through the use of ammonia and baking soda). Cocaine hydrochloride is a water-soluble white powder that is used orally, intranasally ("snorting"), or intravenously ("running"). Intravenous users are more likely to have a history of heroin abuse and often use the drug in combination with heroin (known as *speedballing*). Cocaine hydrochloride decomposes on heating and is, therefore, cocaine converted to

the free base for inhalation. "Freebasing" involves extracting cocaine from aqueous solution into an organic solvent such as ether. Crack, the most widely available form of freebase, is almost pure cocaine; when smoked, it readily enters the bloodstream to produce levels similar to those occurring with intravenous use. Crack cocaine is popular in urban minority communities, where it may be smoked in combination with PCP (known as *spacebasing*). Crack smoking appears to be particularly reinforcing and is associated with compulsive use, binges, and acceleration of the addictive process.

Cocaine and some of its metabolites readily cross the placenta and achieve pharmacologic levels in the fetus (Schenker et al, 1993). Amniotic fluid may serve as a reservoir for cocaine, and its metabolites and prolong exposure to vasoactive compounds. The extent to which cocaine or its metabolites are responsible for aberrant fetal growth, neurodevelopmental sequelae in exposed infants, and the range of congenital malformations reported in the literature may be less than suggested by uncontrolled case reports early in the cocaine-epidemic era. The confounding effects of increased use of multiple drugs, tobacco, alcohol, nutritional deficits, and decreased use of prenatal care among cocaine users make interpretation of the causal relationships between gestational cocaine exposure and intrauterine growth and subsequent neurobehavioral development difficult (Chiriboga, 1993). These identified confounders might serve to explain the reported effects attributed to cocaine in clinical series (Dempsey et al, 1996), although significant effects on the fetus and newborn have been reported in more recent studies that controlled for many confounders (Bada et al, 2002; Shankaran et al, 2007).

Complications of Pregnancy

Adverse perinatal outcomes associated with cocaine use are believed to be largely because of the vasoconstrictive effects of cocaine on uterine blood supply (Woods et al, 1987). An increase in maternal mean arterial blood pressure, a decrease in uterine blood flow, and a transient rise in fetal systemic blood pressure after an intravenous cocaine infusion have been described in fetal sheep along with significant fetal hypoxemia associated with changes in uterine blood flow (Moore et al, 1986; Woods et al, 1987). Maternal hypertension and intermittent fetal hypoxia contribute to the higher risks for abruptio placentae and IUGR seen in cocaine-exposed infants.

To date, no well-defined cocaine-associated syndrome has been identified, and the teratogenic potential of cocaine remains controversial. Earlier reports had suggested that cocaine-exposed infants had a higher rate of limb reduction anomalies, heart defects, ocular anomalies, intestinal atresia or infarction, and other vascular disruption sequences. However, the preponderance of more recent data from multiple studies has failed to demonstrate higher rates of other congenital anomalies among cocaine-exposed infants (Behnke et al, 2001). Any association between fetal cocaine exposure and malformations is likely to be confounded by higher rates of maternal tobacco, marijuana, or alcohol use among the cocaine-exposed groups.

Women who use cocaine during pregnancy are at higher risk for stillbirths, spontaneous abortions, abruptio placentae, IUGR, anemia and malnutrition, and maternal death from intracerebral hemorrhage. Cocaine directly stimulates uterine contractions because of its alpha-adrenergic, prostaglandin, or dopaminergic effects, with resulting greater risk for fetal distress and premature deliveries. Abruptio placentae appears to be related to cocaine only when the drug is used shortly before delivery (Ostrea et al, 1992b). Pregnant women who use cocaine are also at high risk for premature labor, low-birthweight infants, premature rupture of the membranes, and perinatal infections. Cocaine use significantly increases the odds ratio for prematurity, low birthweight, premature rupture of membranes, and IUGR (Bada et al, 2002, 2005; Shankaran et al, 2007) as well as perinatal infections.

Overall, because of the higher risks of premature delivery, the frequency of respiratory distress syndrome is greater in cocaine-exposed infants. Cocaine-exposed infants less frequently require surfactant administration and intubation for respiratory distress syndrome; however, the risks of bronchopulmonary dysplasia are similar in infants who have and those who have not been exposed to cocaine during gestation (Hand et al, 2001).

Fetal Growth

Infants exposed to cocaine in utero have lower birthweight, smaller birth length, and smaller head circumference (Bada et al, 2002, 2005; Behnke et al, 2001). Cocaine is hypothesized to reduce fetal growth via vasoconstriction of uteroplacental vessels with consequent decreased fetal substrate and oxygen delivery (Schempf, 2007). Several studies have shown a dose-response effect of cocaine exposure on fetal growth. In the Maternal Lifestyle Study, cocaine-exposed infants were 1 week younger in gestational age, and after controlling for confounders, cocaine exposure was associated with decrements in birthweight (151 g), length (0.71 cm), and head circumference (0.43 cm) at 40 weeks' gestation (Shankaran et al, 2007). After adjusting for the effects of birthweight, gestational age, sex, maternal height, maternal weight gain, and other drug use, newborns with a high exposure to cocaine, as measured by radioimmunoassay of cocaine metabolites in maternal hair, had a disproportionately smaller head circumference even for their birthweight, resulting in "head wasting" (Bateman and Chiriboga, 2000).

AMPHETAMINES

Pharmacology and Biologic Actions

Amphetamine (methylphenethylamine) was synthesized in 1887 and introduced in the United States in 1931. The N-methylated form, methamphetamine (or "crystal"), is increasingly abused because it readily dissolves in water for injection and it sublimates (converts directly from a solid to gas) when smoked (known as *ice*). The amphetamine isomers have similar clinical effects and can be distinguished only in the laboratory. Amphetamines were initially marketed for the treatment of obesity and narcolepsy and continue to be used for the treatment of attention deficit disorders in children. Amphetamines are classified as schedule II drugs, like cocaine and narcotics. Amphetamines are taken orally, inhaled, or injected. The clinical effects and toxicity of these agents are often indistinguishable from those of cocaine. The primary difference is in the duration of action. The psychotropic effects of cocaine are of a short duration—5 to 45 minutes. The effects of amphetamines may last from 2 to 12 hours. Methamphetamine exposure has direct and indirect effects on the fetus, with increases in maternal blood pressure and restrictions in delivering nutrients and oxygen to the fetus (Smith et al, 2003). The clinical effects of amphetamines resemble those of cocaine. Like cocaine, amphetamines are sympathomimetics, and they potentiate the actions of norepinephrine, dopamine, and serotonin. In contrast to cocaine, amphetamines appear to exert their CNS effects primarily by enhancing the release of neurotransmitters from presynaptic neurons. Amphetamines can block reuptake of released neurotransmitters; they can also exert a weaker direct stimulatory action on postsynaptic catecholamine receptors.

Complications of Pregnancy

The medical and obstetric complications of amphetamine use are similar to those described for cocaine use. Amphetamine toxicity has been described as more intense and prolonged than cocaine toxicity. Visual, auditory, and tactile hallucinations are common, and microvascular damage has been seen in the brains of chronic users. Amphetamine withdrawal is characterized by prolonged periods of hypersomnia, depression, and intense, often violent paranoid psychosis. Obstetric complications include a higher incidence of stillbirth. Methamphetamine use is also associated with an increased incidence of premature delivery and placental abruption. Methamphetamine users who stop using earlier in gestation have rebound weight gain, suggesting that the anorexic effects are limited to continuous use (Smith et al, 2003). Like the pregnancies of cocaine users, the pregnancies of amphetamine users are characterized by poor prenatal care, sexually transmitted diseases, and cardiovascular problems including abruptio placentae and postpartum hemorrhage. The risk of cerebrovascular accidents is lower in pregnant amphetamine users than in pregnant cocaine users, but the mechanism for this difference is not understood.

Perinatal problems associated with maternal amphetamine use include prematurity and IUGR (Smith et al, 2006). Fetal growth restriction, leading to smaller head circumference and lower birthweight, can result from the vasoconstrictive effects of norepinephrine or other vasoactive amines or from diminished maternal nutrient delivery as a consequence of the anorectic effect of amphetamine. Systemic effects from altered norepinephrine metabolism explain the transient bradycardia and tachycardia reported in exposed infants. Studies have failed to show consistent patterns of malformations in amphetamine-exposed infants, although several studies report cleft lip and cleft palate in association with amphetamine and methamphetamine exposure during early gestation (Plessinger, 1998).

Fetal Growth

The IDEAL study followed 84 methamphetamine-exposed and 1534 unexposed infants (confirmed by screening for meconium). Both groups included alcohol, tobacco, and marijuana use, but excluded opioids, PCP, and LSD (Arria et al, 2006; Smith et al, 2003, 2006). Cocaine and methamphetamine use occurred together in 13% of the methamphetamine users, and tobacco, alcohol, and marijuana use were also more frequent in the methamphetamine users. Methamphetamine-exposed infants were 3.5-fold more likely to be small for gestational age (less than the tenth percentile; 18% incidence). Methamphetamine contributed significantly to low birthweight, even after correcting for confounders such as low socioeconomic status, gestational age, and tobacco exposure.

IDENTIFYING PREGNANCIES AND BABIES AT RISK

PREGNANCIES

Identification of perinatal substance abuse to intervene and protect the health and well-being of both mother and child has been a goal of practitioners for decades, ever since the scope of the problem became known—particularly for alcohol. Urine toxicology testing was initially believed to be the best approach, and the universal approach was used in many busy labor and delivery units, particularly in urban centers. In 1994, an American College of Obstetricians and Gynecologists (ACOG) Technical Bulletin concluded that urine toxicology testing had limited ability to detect substance abuse and therefore recommended against universal toxicology screening and for alternative screening methods. In 2003, the U.S. Congress passed the Keeping Children and Family Safe Act. This law requires each state (as a condition of receiving federal funds under the Child Abuse Prevention and Treatment Act) to develop policies and procedures designed "to address the needs of infants born and identified as being affected by illegal substance abuse or withdrawal symptoms resulting from prenatal drug exposure." This law included a requirement that health care providers notify child protective services regarding prenatal substance exposure, but differed from the providers' legal responsibility to report suspected child abuse or neglect because the former "shall not be construed to be child abuse" and "shall not require prosecution of the mother" (Washington State Department of Health, 2009). Each state was expected to develop their own guidelines for identification of at-risk pregnancies. A 2004 ACOG Committee Opinion stated that best practices included universal screening questions followed by brief interventions or referrals. A number of screening tools have been developed including tolerance, annoyed, cut down, eye-opener (T-ACE), tolerance, worried, eye-opener, amnesia, K/cut down (TWEAK), and parents, partner, past, pregnancy (4 *P*'s Plus) (Chang, 2001; Chasnoff et al, 2005; Sokol et al, 1989). Identification of at-risk pregnancies concentrated on the maxim "if you don't ask, they won't tell." In 2008, ACOG issued a committee opinion entitled *At-Risk Drinking and Illicit Drug Use: Ethical Issues in Obstetric and Gynecologic Practice*, which reaffirmed the 2004 ACOG

TABLE 12-2 Risk Indicators for Gestational Substance Exposure

Maternal	No prenatal care Precipitous labor Placental abruption Repeated spontaneous abortions Hypertensive episodes Severe mood swings Previous unexplained fetal demise Myocardial infarction or stroke
Newborn	Jittery with normal blood glucose level Marked irritability Unexplained seizures or apneic spells Unexplained IUGR NEC in an otherwise healthy term infant Neurobehavioral abnormalities Signs of neonatal abstinence syndrome

IUGR, Intrauterine growth restriction; *NEC*, necrotizing enterocolitis.

statement. The opinion stated that "as a result of intensive research in addiction over the past decade, evidence-based recommendations have been consolidated into a protocol for universal screening questions, brief intervention and referral to treatment." This approach—in particular, the use of standard screening questionnaires—was strongly recommended for obstetricians. Therefore a history of drug and alcohol use should be routinely included in the initial contact with every pregnant patient. To be effective, the history taking must be nonjudgmental and must occur in the context of other lifestyle questions. When a positive history of use is obtained, intervention should begin immediately. The person taking the history should be prepared to offer preliminary counseling on risk reduction and concrete referrals for treatment programs, although access to drug programs is often restricted, inadequate, or delayed.

Although the screening questionnaire approach works well for women who seek prenatal care, it is not useful for the significantly higher percentage of substance-using pregnant women who do not seek or actively avoid prenatal care. For these women, it is more helpful to identify maternal risk indicators for perinatal substance abuse at the time of delivery. Use of one of the screening questionnaires in addition to drug testing increases the likelihood of identifying at-risk pregnancies and neonates, allowing for earlier referral for treatment or specialized interventions. Several of these maternal risk indicators for perinatal substance abuse were identified in the 2004 ACOG statement (Table 12-2) (American College of Obstetricians and Gynecologists, 2004).

BABIES

It is important for practitioners to know the difference between a substance-exposed newborn and a substance-affected newborn. The Washington State Department of Health defines them as follows:
- Substance exposed:
  - Tests positive for substances at birth or
  - Mother tests positive for substances at time of delivery or
  - Is identified by medical practitioner as having been prenatally exposed to substances

- Substance affected:
  - Has withdrawal symptoms resulting from prenatal substance exposure or
  - Demonstrates physical and behavioral signs that can be attributed to prenatal exposure to substances and is identified by a medical practitioner as affected

For the identification of either of these groups of infants, assessment of both maternal and newborn risk indicators (see Table 12-2) is essential. If risk indicators suggest perinatal substance abuse, then consideration should be given to newborn drug testing. For urine testing, there is a poor correlation between maternal and newborn tests. The earliest newborn urine will contain the highest concentration of substances, but the first urination may be missed and urine output in the first day is often scant. However, some drug metabolites such as cocaine are present for 4 to 5 days, and marijuana metabolites may persist for weeks. The disadvantages of newborn urine drug testing are that it primarily reflects substance exposure during the preceding 1 to 3 days, and alcohol is nearly impossible to detect. Meconium drug testing (at term) reflects substance exposure during the second half of gestation, has a high sensitivity for opioids and cocaine, and can assess for more drugs than urine testing. The cost is similar to newborn urine testing, but it generally takes longer to obtain results. Other newborn drug tests include hair—which is costly and has a high sensitivity for cocaine, amphetamines, and opioids but not for marijuana—and umbilical cord segments, which is an evolving technology that is not widely available (Kuschel, 2007).

PREGNANCY MANAGEMENT

Ideally, perinatal substance use or abuse should be identified by universal screening procedures during prenatal visits; this gives the practitioner an opportunity to intervene, with the goal being prevention of significant obstetric and neonatal complications related to substance abuse. Screening procedures and counseling should include the following topics:

Antepartum
- Initial screening for hepatitis, HIV, and tuberculosis (if not part of routine prenatal care) and ongoing screening for sexually transmitted infections
- Referring to methadone treatment program, if appropriate
- Discussing possible drug effects on the fetus and newborn
- Discussing contraception and prevention of sexually transmitted disease
- Discussing breastfeeding issues related to alcohol and drug use

Intrapartum
- Effects of recent drug use on labor and fetal well-being
- Pain management (women in methadone or alternative opioid treatment programs will be less responsive to opioid pain medications)
- Intrapartum prophylaxis for HIV, herpes simplex virus infections
- Need for social services involvement

Postpartum
- Breastfeeding issues (related to both drug use and infection)
- Contraception and pregnancy prevention including tubal ligation

- Support for continuation in, or initiation of, a drug treatment program
- Child Protective Services notification

MATERNAL METHADONE MAINTENANCE

The potential benefits of maternal methadone maintenance are numerous (Kandall and Doberczak, 1999; Ward et al, 1999) and include the prevention of opioid withdrawal symptoms in the mother, better medical and prenatal care, improved health and growth of the fetus, and maintenance of opioid levels in the mother to decrease both the use of illicit drugs and the potential for perinatal infections. Methadone maintenance programs associated with comprehensive medical and psychosocial services for the pregnant woman are of additional benefit. Methadone maintenance has been shown to be associated with higher birthweight in some but not all studies (Brown et al, 1998; Kandall and Doberczak, 1999). Detoxification of a pregnant heroin user is infrequently attempted, because maternal drug withdrawal is believed to be associated with subsequent fetal withdrawal, fetal asphyxia, and spontaneous abortions (Barr and Jones, 1994). Dashe et al (1998) reported on a small study of opioid-using pregnant women undergoing safe maternal detoxification. Close to 60% of the women completed detoxification, but almost 30% resumed opioid use. McCarthy et al (1999) showed that women who reduced their methadone dose during pregnancy had infants with higher birthweights than a control group who continued on the same or increased methadone dose throughout pregnancy. In the United States, most pregnant, narcotic-addicted women are treated with daily methadone rather than a program of detoxification. Some authorities, however, have urged the reappraisal and reevaluation of the benefits of methadone maintenance in pregnancy (Brown et al, 1998; Hulse and O'Neil, 2001), and there are recent studies comparing methadone with buprenorphine in pregnancy (Jones et al, 2008; Minozzi et al, 2008).

In the Netherlands, women enrolled in a methadone program had higher rates of prenatal care, which were associated with higher birthweights and reduced prematurity in the offspring (Soepatmi, 1994). When women in a methadone maintenance program were enrolled in an enhanced prenatal care program, their infants' birthweights were significantly larger than those in the control group of women receiving regular methadone maintenance during pregnancy (Chang et al, 1992). Others have shown that higher methadone doses are associated with improved head circumference and increased gestational age at delivery (Hagopian et al, 1996). Using a metaanalysis design, Hulse et al (1997) found that low infant birthweight was associated with heroin use and that birthweights were improved with methadone treatment during pregnancy. These favorable outcomes are believed to be to the result of a stable intrauterine environment uncomplicated by periods of intoxication and withdrawal, as well as less stress and better nutrition in the mother.

Several investigators have found that neonatal withdrawal symptoms, birthweight, length of pregnancy, and the number of days infants require treatment for abstinence do not correlate with maternal methadone dosage (Brown et al, 1998; Finnegan, 1991; Madden et al, 1977; Rosen and Pippenger, 1976). In contrast, others have reported a correlation between the severity of neonatal withdrawal and maternal methadone dose (Dryden et al, 2009; Harper et al, 1977; Maas et al, 1990; Malpas et al, 1995). Studying maternal and neonatal serum levels of methadone does not help clarify this dilemma. Investigators have found no correlation between neonatal serum levels of methadone and the maternal methadone dose at delivery, the maternal serum levels, or the severity of withdrawal symptoms in the neonates (Harper et al, 1977; Mack et al, 1991). Other researchers have reported that neonatal signs of withdrawal correlate with the rate of decline of the neonatal plasma level during the first few days of life (Doberczak et al, 1993).

There are no definitive guidelines for methadone doses during pregnancy, and there is continuing controversy over the most appropriate dose of methadone maintenance during pregnancy. The divergent findings noted previously have been used to argue either for weaning a pregnant woman to a low methadone maintenance dose or for attempting complete maternal detoxification during pregnancy. Some authorities believe in maintaining high methadone doses to keep the mother from "chipping" with additional street drugs, which would put her at risk for greater complications of pregnancy and for a higher risk of infections transmitted by intravenous use of drugs (HIV, hepatitis) or sexually transmitted disease. High-dose methadone maintenance ranges between 60 and 150 mg/day. Despite reports of the safe detoxification of pregnant women, there are still concerns that the fetus is placed at risk during maternal detoxification. The medical management of pregnant women who are addicted to opioids remains controversial (Christensen, 2008).

There is a growing body of literature promoting breastfeeding for infants of mothers in methadone maintenance programs as both beneficial and safe. Studies have shown that breastfed infants tend to have less need for pharmacotherapy for neonatal abstinence syndrome, despite low and unpredictable levels of methadone in breast milk and in infant serum. Maternal serum levels, breast milk levels, and infant serum levels do not correlate with maternal methadone dose (Jansson et al, 2008).

Buprenorphine (Suboxone, Subutex)

Buprenorphine is an alternative opioid substitute that was first introduced in France in 1996. It is increasingly being used with or instead of methadone for the treatment of opioid addiction, because it has fewer autonomic side effects than methadone as well as improved compliance and treatment efficacy. Recent trials have compared methadone with buprenorphine treatment during pregnancy and found no difference in the neonatal outcome or incidence of withdrawal symptoms (Jones et al, 2008; Minozzi et al, 2008).

Human Immunodeficiency Virus and Other Viral Infections

Nationwide, intravenous drug abusers are the second largest risk group for HIV infection. Drug abusers also may be the primary source of infection for non–drug-using heterosexuals and children (Chamberland and Dondero, 1987). Seventy-five percent of cases of acquired immunodeficiency syndrome (AIDS) in children are perinatally acquired. The seropositivity rate varies across the country; the rate among female intravenous drug users in New York City and northern New Jersey is estimated at 50% to 70%, compared with 5% to 20% in California. Heroin and cocaine addicts often resort to prostitution to support their habits, and amphetamine and methamphetamine users often inject drugs several times daily. Alcohol decreases sexual inhibition, impairs judgment, and increases the incidence of unsafe sexual activity. Every infant born to a substance abuser should be evaluated for HIV infection, and universal precautions should be observed. The American Academy of Pediatrics Committee on Infectious Diseases (2009) recommends rapid HIV testing of any mother whose HIV status is not known, with appropriate consent as required by local law.

Intravenous drug use places the woman at risk for multiple infectious complications, including cellulitis, thrombophlebitis, hepatitis, endocarditis, syphilis, gonorrhea, and AIDS. In a prospective study undertaken in Canada, a 5-year incidence of HIV seroconversion was 13.4%; the rate of conversion associated with injection of heroin or cocaine was 40% higher in women than in men (Spittal et al, 2002). Opioid abusers are also less likely to receive prenatal care or to obtain late prenatal care (Bauer, 1999). Heroin-addicted mothers are often poorly nourished, and iron-deficiency anemia is more common in pregnant opioid users than in nonusers. Bauer (1999) found that maternal hepatitis infections were fivefold higher in opioid-using women than in a control group of nonusers.

Hepatitis C virus (HCV) is another chronic infectious condition that is spread by parenteral exposure to infected blood and can be perinatally acquired by the newborn. The most common risk factors for acquiring infection are injection drug use, having multiple sexual partners, or having received blood products before 1992. The 2009 American Academy of Pediatrics Red Book (American Academy of Pediatrics Committee on Infectious Diseases, 2009) states that "seroprevalence [of hepatitis C] among pregnant women in the United States has been estimated at 1% to 2%," and the risk of perinatal transmission averages 5% to 6% from women who are HCV-RNA positive at the time of delivery. Maternal coinfection with HIV has been associated with increased risk of perinatal transmission of HCV. Antibodies to HCV and HCV RNA have been detected in colostrum, but the risk of HCV transmission is similar in breastfed and bottle-fed infants, so breastfeeding is currently allowed.

NEONATAL MANAGEMENT AFTER GESTATIONAL SUBSTANCE ABUSE

GENERAL

Although at higher risk for medical complications, the majority of infants of drug-using women do not require intensive neonatal care; however, symptomatic infants often need more nursing care. Physical examination on admission should document a gestational age assessment, birthweight, head circumference, and length. Infants should be examined carefully for evidence of malformations, dysmorphic facial features, or both. Studies such as electroencephalography and brain imaging may add diagnostic or prognostic information when physical or neurologic abnormalities are not clearly consistent with drug exposure, but these procedures are not indicated for most drug-exposed infants. If indicated by neonatal or maternal risk indicators, toxicology testing should be performed on neonatal urine, meconium, or both as soon as possible after birth. Infants whose mothers were not screened for HIV should undergo screening for perinatal HIV exposure and other infections such as hepatitis and syphilis, as clinically indicated. In some states, rapid testing of the newborn for HIV is "required by law if the mother refuses to be tested," so that appropriate treatment of the infant can be started before 12 hours of age. Rapid screening detects only HIV-1, the most common serotype of HIV in the United States, but it can miss HIV-2, so measurement of HIV antibodies should also be performed (American Academy of Pediatrics Committee on Infectious Diseases, 2009).

Cocaine-exposed infants weighing more than 1500 g have longer hospital stays and increased need for therapies, procedures, intravenous fluid, and formula feeding. These infants also undergo more investigations for sepsis, more neonatal intensive care unit (NICU) admissions, and more social and family problems delaying discharge (Bada et al, 2002). In the Maternal Lifestyle Study, cocaine-exposed infants had a higher frequency of infection (odds ratio [OR], 3.1; 99% confidence interval [CI], 1.8 to 5.4) and neurologic signs and symptoms (adjusted OR, 1.7; 99% CI, 1.0 to 2.1). Neurologic signs were highest in the infants exposed to opioids and cocaine, but remained significantly increased in infants exposed to cocaine alone. Smoking also increased the risk for neurologic signs and symptoms (Shankaran et al, 2007). The association between cocaine exposure and fetal hypoxic ischemic episodes creates special concerns. Maternal cocaine use exposes infants to a higher than expected risk of problems with postasphyxial syndrome, and organ dysfunction from hypoxic-ischemic injury should be investigated and treated. Feedings in premature infants with cocaine exposure should be started cautiously, because premature infants exposed to cocaine may be at increased risk for necrotizing enterocolitis. In addition, after controlling for gender, gestational age, birthweight, maternal parity, ethnicity, and polydrug use, heavy cocaine use during pregnancy was associated with a slightly higher risk of subependymal hemorrhage (Shankaran et al, 2007).

Using the NICU Network Neurobehavioral Scale (NNNS), subtle differences in behavior were detected in drug-exposed infants (Lester et al, 2002; Smith et al, 2008). Cocaine-exposed infants showed lower arousal, and with heavy cocaine use they showed lower regulation and higher excitability than did unexposed infants (Lester et al, 2002). There were no stress or abstinence signs associated with cocaine exposure. Marijuana use was associated with more stress and abstinence signs and higher excitability scores (Lester et al, 2002). Low birthweight was also significantly correlated with poorer regulation and higher excitability. Methamphetamine exposure was also associated with increased stress signs, especially in first-trimester use. Heavy methamphetamine use was related to lethargy, lower arousal, and increased physiologic stress (Smith et al, 2008). Neonatal neurologic abnormalities similar to a mild withdrawal syndrome, consisting of hypertonicity, irritability, and jitteriness, have been reported after in utero marijuana exposure, but without documented evidence of long-term sequelae (Cornelius et al, 1995). Finally, gestational nicotine exposure definitely altered the newborn neurobehavioral scores and has also been reported to elevate neonatal abstinence scores (Godding et al, 2004; Law et al, 2003).

In the Maternal Lifestyle Study, only 100 women were identified as isolated users of opioids, and a similar number used cocaine and opioids. Transient but dramatic neurobehavioral signs are present in the first week of life as symptoms of opioid withdrawal (increased irritability, jitteriness, poor feeding, sweating, sneezing; Shankaran et al, 2007). See the discussion under Neonatal Abstinence Syndrome.

BREASTFEEDING AND DRUG EXPOSURE

Breastfeeding has the benefit of improved bonding, but the risks of HIV and continued drug exposure may outweigh this benefit. Women who wish to breastfeed despite these potential risks should undergo drug monitoring and sequential HIV antibody testing. Close observation of mother-infant interactions should be documented in the infant's chart. Parenting and childcare skills should be stressed as part of the discharge education for the mother. All physician interactions with the family should be documented in detail.

Most illicit drugs of abuse that are of low molecular weight and lipophilic, are readily excreted in breast milk, but have varying degrees of bioavailability (Howard and Lawrence, 1998). Cocaine has been detected in breast milk and Chasnoff et al described a two-week-old breastfed infant who had clinical signs of cocaine intoxication. Both the baby's urine and the mother's milk contained cocaine (Chasnoff et al, 1987). A widely-referenced report of cocaine seizures in a breastfed infant actually resulted from topical coacine applied to sore nipples, not from cocaine-laced breast milk (Chaney et al, 1988). Because of the potential risk of toxicity, breastfeeding is generally discouraged in women who are known abusers of these drugs and who are not willing to engage in substance abuse treatment and monitoring. Breastfeeding may be supported for women who are engaged in substance abuse treatment and who have received good prenatal care with a confirmed period of sobriety prior to delivery. Breastfeeding by women using methadone is recommended. Concentrations of methadone in human milk are low, and there are other significant advantages for the mother and infant (Jansson et al, 2008).

Alcohol use while breastfeeding is not listed as a contraindication by the American Academy of Pediatrics, but excessive maternal alcohol intake during breastfeeding can be deleterious for the infant and should be avoided. Smoking in the postnatal period and during breastfeeding also has deleterious effects on the newborn. Smoking is associated with measurable levels of nicotine and cotinine in maternal breast milk.

NEONATAL ABSTINENCE SYNDROME

Clinical Findings

Classic neonatal withdrawal or abstinence syndrome consists of a wide variety of CNS signs of irritability, gastrointestinal and feeding problems (diarrhea, hyperphagia or poor feeding), autonomic signs of dysfunction (fever, sweating, sneezing), and respiratory symptoms (Tables 12-3 and 12-4). These symptoms are most often related to gestational opioid exposure, but are relatively nonspecific, with the differential diagnosis including infection, meningitis, hypocalcemia, hyponatremia, intracranial hemorrhage, seizures, and stroke. The signs of neonatal serotonin syndrome (or selective serotonin reuptake inhibitor withdrawal) may also mimic the signs of neonatal opioid abstinence syndrome (Boucher et al, 2008; Moses-Kolko et al, 2005). The timing of withdrawal signs from specific drug exposures can often be anticipated; for example, heroin withdrawal usually occurs within 24 hours of birth, whereas methadone withdrawal symptoms typically begin later, at approximately 48 to 72 hours after birth. The incidence of neonatal abstinence syndrome (NAS) in infants of women using heroin or methadone is high, with wide ranges reported between 16% and 90% (Agarwal et al, 1999; Boer et al, 1994; Maas et al, 1990; van Baar et al, 1994), and between 30% and 91% of infants with signs of NAS receive pharmacologic treatment for NAS with inpatient stays averaging 3 weeks (Dryden et al, 2009; Kuschel, 2007). Premature infants generally have milder signs of withdrawal and often show alternating periods of hyperactivity and lethargy, with tremors seen less commonly. The mortality rate for these infants is less than 1% (Boer et al, 1994). Death is rarely associated with withdrawal alone, but usually occurs as a consequence of prematurity, infection, and severe perinatal asphyxia.

A number of evaluation tools are used to assess the severity of opioid withdrawal after birth. The neonatal abstinence score is a scale based on nursing observations of the severity of signs of withdrawal (Finnegan et al, 1975) and is the most widely used scale. The Lipsitz score was developed at the same time and is simpler to use, with a score greater than 4 indicating withdrawal. Green and Suffet (1981) introduced the Neonatal Narcotic Withdrawal Index as a rapid physician-based evaluation for neonatal signs of withdrawal. The use of these scoring systems allows more objective quantification of the severity of the infant's withdrawal and the response to treatment. These scoring systems have shown good interobserver reliability and can improve clinicians' ability to treat the withdrawing infant appropriately (Anand and Arnold, 1994; Franck and Vilardi, 1995).

The goal of medical management of opioid withdrawal is to avoid serious symptoms of NAS, such as seizures, and to maintain the infant's comfort while enabling the infant to feed, sleep, and gain weight in an appropriate manner. There are a number of reported threshold scores for initiating pharmacologic treatment (Finnegan NAS scores between 7 and 12) (Kuschel, 2007), but none of these choices have been examined in a scientific manner. The decision to begin treatment or to wean treatment should be influenced by the absolute score and other factors, such as the infant's age, comorbidities, other conditions leading to abnormal behavior, and a daily evaluation of the abnormal clinical elements observed in the scoring system (Kuschel, 2007). Standard medical practice is to combine both developmental and behavioral methods with pharmacologic interventions as necessary to control symptoms and signs of narcotic abstinence.

TABLE 12-3   Clinical Signs of Neonatal Withdrawal Syndrome (Narcotic Abstinence Syndrome)

Central nervous system dysfunction	Excoriation (from frantic movement) Hyperactive reflexes Increased muscle tone Irritability, excessive crying, high-pitched cry Jitteriness, tremulousness Myoclonic jerks Seizures Sleep disturbance
Autonomic dysfunction	Excessive sweating Frequent yawning Hyperthermia
Respiratory symptoms	Nasal stuffiness, sneezing Tachypnea
Gastrointestinal and feeding disturbances	Inadequate oral intake Diarrhea (loose, watery, frequent stools) Excessive sucking Hyperphagia Regurgitation

These signs were abstracted from Finnegan L, Connaughton J, Kron R: Neonatal abstinence syndrome: assessment and management, *Addict Dis* 2:141-158, 1975.

TABLE 12-4   Neonatal Neurobehavioral Symptoms after Fetal Drug Exposure

Drug	Onset (days)	Peak (days)	Duration	Relative Severity	Likely NICU Admission	Symptoms
Alcohol	0-1	1-2	1-2 days	Mild	No	?
Amphetamine	0-3	—	2-8 wk	Mild	No	Neuro
Cocaine	0-3	1-4	? mo	Mild	No	Neuro
Heroin	0-3	3-7	2-4 wk	Mild to severe	Yes	Neuro, Resp, GI
Methadone	3-7	10-21	2-6 wk	Mild to severe	Yes	Neuro, Resp, GI
SSRI	0-3	1-3	2-10 days	Mild to moderate	No	Neuro, Resp, GI
Tobacco	0-1	1-2	2-3 days	Mild	No	Neuro

GI, Gastrointestinal symptoms including poor weight gain; *Neuro,* neurobehavioral symptoms; *NICU,* neonatal intensive care unit; *Resp,* respiratory symptoms; *SSRI,* selective serotonin reuptake inhibitor.

Treatment

Treatment for opioid withdrawal should always begin with supportive, nonpharmacologic measures such as soothing including swaddling, rocking, decreased environmental stimulation, avoiding unnecessary handling and irritation, and progressing to pharmacologic management only when medically necessary. Between 30% and 91% of infants exhibiting signs of NAS will receive pharmacologic treatment (Kuschel, 2007). The mainstay of treatment for opioid withdrawal is the use of opioids, either alone or in combination with other medications (American Academy of Pediatrics Committee on Drugs, 1998; Osborn et al, 2002, 2005). Medication is titrated for each infant according to the severity of the signs of withdrawal and abstinence scoring.

A recent survey in the United States showed that opioids are the most common medication used for narcotic withdrawal, and phenobarbital is frequently used or added for polydrug exposure (Sarkar and Donn, 2006). A metaanalysis of seven studies found that opioid treatment reduced the time to regain birthweight and the duration of supportive care compared with supportive care alone; however, the length of hospital stay was increased (Osborn et al, 2005). Phenobarbital was also shown to be superior to diazepam for treating NAS, but small, randomized, controlled trials comparing morphine to phenobarbital for treatment of NAS suggested that opioids are superior at decreasing treatment duration and lowering NAS scores (Ebner et al, 2007; Jackson et al, 2004; Osborn et al, 2002).

Morphine is the opioid most often used in treating NAS. The only study comparing an oral preparation of morphine to dilute tincture of opium (DTO), a concentrated morphine solution that also contains alcohol, recommends oral morphine to avoid problems with dilution of highly concentrated DTO and the unwanted effects of the alcoholic extracts with various alkaloids (Langenfeld et al, 2005). A standard starting dose of morphine is 0.04 to 0.05 mg/kg given orally every 3 to 4 hours. This dose can be increased in increments of 0.05 to 0.1 mg until the symptoms are controlled. The usual dose for infants experiencing withdrawal at birth ranges from 0.08 to 0.2 mg every 3 to 4 hours (American Academy of Pediatrics Committee on Drugs, 1998; Anand and Arnold, 1994; Burgos and Burke, 2009; Levy and Sino, 1993). Higher doses may be needed to control significant physiologic signs of withdrawal such as diarrhea, pyrexia, hypertension, and significant hypertonicity.

Although preparations of oral morphine are most commonly used in recent studies, methadone has also been reported as an option for treatment of NAS (Burgos and Burke, 2009; Kuschel, 2007). There is one retrospective report of methadone use for neonatal abstinence syndrome (Lainwala et al, 2005) and more extensive experience with methadone in the treatment of opioid withdrawal in older infants and children (Tobias, 2000; Tobias et al, 1990). Methadone has a long duration of action and can be administered by either the oral or the parenteral routes. The initial recommended methadone dose is 0.05 to 0.1 mg/kg followed by 0.025 to 0.05 mg/kg every 4 to 12 hours until abstinence scores are controlled. The total daily dose given to control symptoms is then divided into two doses and given every 12 hours. Tobias et al (1990) showed that methadone could be given every 12 to 24 hours because of its longer half-life. There were no advantages to methadone over morphine in neonatal abstinence (Lainwala et al, 2005). In addition, sublingual buprenorphine has been reported as a treatment for NAS (Kraft et al, 2008).

Phenobarbital has been used for signs of acute opioid withdrawal. Phenobarbital does not, however, reduce significant physiologic signs of withdrawal, such as diarrhea and seizures. At higher doses, phenobarbital has also been shown to impair infant sucking and cause excessive sedation. The doses of phenobarbital used are 5 to 20 mg/kg in the first 24 hours, followed by 2 to 4 mg/kg every 12 hours; the therapeutic blood level of phenobarbital for control of opioid withdrawal signs is not known. Combining oral morphine solution (i.e., DTO) and phenobarbital treatment was found to shorten duration of hospitalization and lessen the severity of withdrawal symptoms, compared with morphine treatment alone (Coyle et al, 2002, 2005). Compared with those treated with morphine alone, infants treated with morphine and phenobarbital were more interactive, had smoother movements, were easier to handle, and were less stressed. Dual treatment resulted in improved neurobehavioral organization during the first 3 weeks of life, which may indicate a more rapid recovery from opioid withdrawal (Coyle et al, 2005). In these studies, however, the infants were discharged home on phenobarbital therapy, from which they were slowly weaned throughout infancy. Some of these infants received phenobarbital for prolonged times.

Clonidine, an α_2-adrenergic receptor antagonist, is used treating opioid withdrawal symptoms in older children and adults. A recent randomized, controlled trial showed that adding clonidine to opioid treatment (i.e., DTO) significantly reduced the median length of therapy with opioids and the number of infants requiring high dose opioids, and it eliminated infants who met their definition of treatment failure (Agthe et al, 2009). During hospitalization, there were no significant adverse events (i.e., hypertension, hypotension, bradycardia, desaturations) related to clonidine use. A German group has also retrospectively reported their experience using clonidine and chloral hydrate for NAS compared to a larger group treated with morphine and phenobarbital; they also reported decreased duration of treatment, decreased length of stay, and reduction of symptoms in the clonidine group (Esmaeili et al, 2010). Before clonidine is used widely, a larger trial is indicated to investigate appropriate dosing regimens and to determine long-term safety.

Once medications have been titrated to a level that controls the severity of opioid withdrawal and lowers the NAS scores, then tapering of the dosage should be started. A common method is to decrease the opioid dose by 10% to 20% of the highest dose, with continued surveillance of NAS scores to assure the infant tolerates the decrease. It is not unusual to note increased signs of opioid withdrawal during the medication tapering. The goal of weaning is to allow the infant to acclimate to a new and lower dose of medication while ensuring that he or she is comfortable and consolable and is able to sleep, eat, and gain weight appropriately. Objective measurements using established withdrawal scoring systems should be used to determine the rate and efficacy of medication tapering. Most often opioid medications are weaned every 24 to 48 hours as long as NAS scores remain low and the infant's clinical condition is unchanged (Burgos and Burke, 2009; Coyle et al, 2002; Jackson et al, 2004). Whether narcotics can safely be weaned more rapidly in infants has not been studied. One small study reported good results using oral morphine on an as-needed basis for elevated individual withdrawal scores, rather than providing regular doses of morphine every 3 to 4 hours (Ebner et al, 2007). No specific protocols for weaning phenobarbital or clonidine have been reported.

The average length of hospital stay for infants with NAS who are treated with medications varies from 8 to 78 days, with a stay of 21 to 30 days being common (Coyle et al, 2002; Ebner et al, 2007; Jackson et al, 2004; Kuschel, 2007). Investigation of outpatient management of detoxification may result in a shorter hospital stay, but with a more prolonged duration of neonatal treatment (Kuschel, 2007).

LONG-TERM EFFECTS OF PERINATAL SUBSTANCE ABUSE

SUDDEN INFANT DEATH SYNDROME IN DRUG-EXPOSED INFANTS

The incidence of sudden infant death syndrome (SIDS) is greater in drug-exposed infants, although the increase appears less significant for cocaine-exposed infants (Chasnoff et al, 1989b; Kandall et al, 1993) than for methadone-exposed or heroin-exposed infants (Bauchner and Zuckerman, 1990). A metaanalysis of 10 studies demonstrated a 4.1 OR for SIDS among cocaine-exposed infants (Fares et al, 1997) compared with infants not exposed to perinatal drugs. However, after data were controlled for concurrent use of other drugs, the increased risk for SIDS could not be attributed to intrauterine cocaine alone, but was believed to be caused by exposure to other illicit drugs and smoking.

There is a significant relationship between exposure to tobacco smoke and SIDS. A higher risk for SIDS is reported in infants exposed to maternal smoking with either antenatal or postnatal exposure (Blair et al, 1996; Mitchell et al, 1993; Schoendorf and Kiely, 1992). Additional evidence supporting a causal role includes a dose-response relationship (Rogers, 2008). With recent substantial decreases in SIDS risk (after "back to sleep"), maternal smoking is calculated to account for an increasing proportion of SIDS risk. Mitchell and Millerad (2006) suggest that one third of all SIDS deaths might be prevented by eliminating in utero exposure to maternal smoking. Despite the increased risks of SIDS among drug- and tobacco-exposed infants, home apnea monitoring is not indicated in the absence of other risk factors.

POSTNATAL GROWTH AND MEDICAL PROBLEMS

There are no documented long-term effects of substance exposure on postnatal growth. In the Maternal Lifestyle Study, cocaine-exposed infants were lighter than non–cocaine-exposed infants at birth, but there were no differences in weight between ages 1 and 6 years. For height, cocaine-exposed infants were shorter at birth through 2 years, but the difference disappeared by age 3, and cocaine-exposed infants had a smaller head circumference from birth to 1 year old, but this difference subsequently disappeared (Shankaran et al, 2007). A previous systematic review concluded that there is no consistent effect of cocaine exposure on physical growth in children younger than 6 years (Frank et al, 2001). Opioid-exposed infants also show no difficulties with postnatal growth through 3 years (Hunt et al, 2008). Infants with IUGR at birth remained significantly lighter (by 2.1 kg) and shorter (by 1.8 cm) at 6 years, and they continued to have a smaller head circumference (by 0.9 cm). There was no interaction between cocaine exposure and IUGR status (Shankaran et al, 2007).

There were also no differences in medical diagnoses, blood pressure, hospitalizations, or overall health status associated with opioid exposure (Shankaran et al, 2007). The effect of cocaine on subsequent blood pressure is unclear. IUGR status at birth was significantly associated with hypertension after correcting for in utero drug exposures, maternal race, and child's body mass index.

NEUROBEHAVIORAL ABNORMALITIES

Detailed studies have identified both neurologic soft signs and a higher risk of cognitive, behavioral, and psychiatric problems linked to gestational substance exposure. However, significant confounding factors make it difficult to attribute specific deficits directly to substance exposures. No major neurologic deficits in motor development are found after in utero exposure to cocaine (Shankaran et al, 2007) or opioids (Hunt et al, 2008). Infants exposed to cocaine were reported to have lower motor skills at 1-month testing, but they displayed significant improvements over time. Both higher and lower levels of tobacco use were related to poor motor performance (Shankaran et al, 2007).

Subtle neurobehavioral abnormalities have been reported in older studies and more recently using the NNNS to evaluate infants in the month after birth. Cocaine-exposed infants manifest a range of neurobehavioral abnormalities that were initially described as drug withdrawal, but are more likely caused by acute intoxication (Dempsey et al, 1996). Signs are present at birth and wane as cocaine and the metabolite, benzoylecgonine, are cleared from plasma. The infants are hypertonic, irritable, and tremulous (Chiriboga, 1993), and they may have abnormal crying, sleep, and feeding patterns. Tachycardia, tachypnea, and apnea have been noted in two blinded, controlled studies, with significant elevations in cardiac output, stroke volume, mean arterial blood pressure, and cerebral artery flow velocity resolving by day 2, which is consistent with an intoxicant effect of cocaine (van de Bor et al, 1990a, 1990b) Cocaine-exposed infants may have abnormal electroencephalograms or clinical seizures, perhaps the result of toxicity from the metabolite, benzoylecgonine (Konkol et al, 1994); however, neonatal seizures attributable directly to maternal use of cocaine are rare (Legido et al, 1992).

A number of studies suggest that exposure to exogenous opioids during fetal development may produce lifelong alterations in the developing brain. Infants who have been exposed to opioids in utero have a higher risk for fetal growth retardation and smaller head circumference than those who have not (Bauer, 1999). In addition, significant developmental and learning deficits have been described in both methadone-exposed and heroin-exposed children (Soepatmi, 1994; van Baar and de Graaff, 1994; van Baar et al, 1994), and Bunikowski et al (1998) have reported a higher incidence of abnormalities in intellectual performance, developmental retardation, and neurologic abnormalities in a group of opioid-exposed infants compared with a control group of infants. However, the treated infants in the study had an unusually high incidence of seizures during withdrawal treatment with phenobarbital alone, as well as a higher incidence of prematurity than the control infants. These important considerations temper the findings of that study.

Early neurobehavioral changes have been associated with maternal methamphetamine use; heavy use was associated with lower arousal, increased lethargy, and increased CNS stress (Smith et al, 2008). However, a detailed analysis in a subgroup of the same population found that these same abnormalities on the NNNS were associated with maternal depression and that prenatal methamphetamine exposure was not associated with additional neurodevelopmental differences (Paz et al, 2009).

Persisting behavioral, neurologic, and rearing problems are reported in children exposed to both cocaine and opioids (Chasnoff et al, 1989; Hunt et al, 2008). No significant differences in mean developmental scores were noted in a group of children exposed to cocaine plus polydrugs compared to a group without drug exposure (Chasnoff et al, 1992). Other investigators reported no differences between infants who have and those who have not been exposed to cocaine in mean cognitive, psychomotor, or language quotients at age 36 months (Kilbride et al, 2000). A recent report following a cohort of opioid exposed infants documented lower Bayley mental development index (MDI) scores at 18 months old, lower Stanford Binet Intelligence Scale scores at 3 years, and decreased scores on the Vineland Social Maturity Scale and Reynell Language Scale at 3 years (Hunt et al, 2008). However, a similar evaluation at 3 years showed no mental, motor, or behavioral deficits after controlling for birthweight and environmental risk factors (Messinger et al, 2004).

The neurodevelopmental problems among children exposed to cocaine may occur either from a direct teratogenic drug effect during gestation or from the effects of the social environment in which the developing infant is reared. Singer et al (2002) reported that cocaine-exposed infants are twice as likely to have significant cognitive but not motor delays at 2 years, and they demonstrated a downward trend in mean developmental scores by 2 years, which is consistent with a deleterious effect of the environment, parental stimulation, socioeconomic status, or possibly other, indirect effects of drugs on the developing CNS. Other studies have not consistently demonstrated this association (Frank et al, 2001). In contrast, the Maternal Lifestyle Study, after controlling for covariates, found no differences in Bayley scores between cocaine-exposed,

opioid-exposed, and control infants for the first 3 years of life (Shankaran et al, 2007), although subtle effects on cognitive subscales were reported at 3 years (Messinger et al, 2004).

Other investigators have shown normal development for opioid-exposed infants during the first 2 years of life after data have been controlled for socioeconomic status and birthweight (Bauer, 1999). Using regression analysis, researchers have shown that the amount of prenatal care obtained by the mother and the postnatal home environment were more predictive of the infant's future intellectual performance. Conversely, the amount of maternal opioid use during pregnancy was not found to be predictive. Ornoy et al (2001) have shown that children exposed to heroin but adopted at an early age performed better on intelligence testing than did opioid-exposed infants who were raised in the homes of their biologic parents. The same investigators found a higher rate of attention deficit disorders in children exposed to opioids regardless of home environment, with the highest incidence in children who were raised in the homes of their biologic parents. Numerous studies point also to the importance of the home environment in optimizing child development. Variable outcomes of these studies may depend on the amount and type of drug use, or on other covariates such as nutritional status, poverty, psychosocial problems, and parental educational level.

With the lack of major neurologic deficits, recent studies have focused on neurologic soft signs, nonfocal signs with no localized findings that are more often associated with cognitive deficits, and increased prevalence of attention deficit hyperactivity disorder and behavior problems. Neurologic soft signs including speech, balance, coordination, and tone were markedly stable over a 1-year period in 6- to 9-year-olds. Soft signs are a marker for increased risk of cognitive and psychiatric problems. In the Maternal Lifestyle Study, 23.5% of children exposed to cocaine had more than two soft neurologic signs, similar to rates in the comparison group. Soft signs were more common in infants born weighing less than 1500 g. Both cocaine and alcohol use significantly increased the incidence of soft signs in exposed infants weighing less than 1500 g, and this effect persisted after controlling for other substances used, birthweight, sex, and race (Shankaran et al, 2007).

Childhood behavior problems were more common in infants with heavy cocaine exposure than in those with no or some cocaine exposure. Prenatal tobacco and alcohol exposure were also significantly associated with behavioral problems until 7 years, with a significant dose-response relationship (Shankaran et al, 2007). Evaluation at 7 years demonstrated behavior problems in cocaine- and substance-exposed infants that suggested direct effects resulting in neurobehavioral dysregulation, which was tracked through serial assessments beginning at an early age. This work on a model of early abnormalities predictive of later behavioral problems may allow for early identification and possible prevention of later behavioral problems (Lester et al, 2009).

Follow-up studies have been reported at 9 to 15 years. Cognitive outcomes at 10 years were not abnormal in opioid-exposed children (Shankaran et al, 2007). Cocaine-exposed children were more likely to be referred for special education services in school than unexposed children, with an estimated additional cost to the United States of $25,248,384 per year (Shankaran et al, 2007). Prenatal marijuana exposure is reported to be associated with deficiencies in executive function in 9 to 12 year olds (Fried and Smith, 2001; Fried et al, 1998), and recent reports have found that prenatal marijuana exposure has a significant effect on school-age intellectual performance (Goldschmidt et al, 2004, 2008; Richardson et al, 2002).

In methamphetamine-exposed infants, neurodevelopmental abnormalities have been described to persist as late as 14 years (Cernerud et al, 1996). Intellectual capacity does not appear to be diminished among exposed infants. These children are described as exhibiting disturbed behavior, including hyperactivity, aggressiveness, and sleep disturbances. Eriksson et al (2000) reported that neurobehavioral abnormalities appear to be associated with the extent and duration of fetal exposure and with the severity of head growth restriction. In this study, children with the most severe problems were those born to mothers who abused amphetamines throughout pregnancy and were reared in homes with an addicted parent. Alterations in growth have been reported after prenatal exposure, with striking gender differences (Cernerud et al, 1996). Drug-exposed boys in Sweden were taller and heavier, and girls were smaller and lighter, than national standards. This finding suggests that fetal amphetamine exposure affects the onset of puberty and amphetamines may interfere with neurodevelopment of the adenohypophysis. Children of amphetamine abusers appear to be at high risk for social problems, including abandonment, abuse, and neglect. In two Swedish studies, only 22% of 10-year-old children who had been exposed to amphetamine in utero remained in the care of their biologic mothers, whereas 70% were in foster care (Cernerud et al, 1996; Eriksson and Zetterstrom, 1994).

Considering all the data, it is still difficult to create a coherent picture and provide a prognosis for a newborn after gestational substance exposure. A recent report of volumetric magnetic resonance imaging in thirty five 12-year-old children exposed to cocaine in utero found smaller total parenchymal volumes, lower cortical gray matter volumes, and smaller head circumferences with prenatal substance exposure. The decreases were statistically significant only for prenatal cigarette exposure and for infants exposed to all substances studied (cocaine, tobacco, marijuana and alcohol) (Rivkin et al, 2008). As in other studies, exposure to multiple substances clearly has detrimental effects on the developing brain.

SUMMARY

The magnitude of observed perinatal outcomes after illicit maternal substance use pales in comparison to the established health and developmental risks associated with tobacco and alcohol exposure (Schempf, 2007). The greatest impact of illicit substance use may be the increased postnatal risks of neglect, maltreatment, and disruptions in the home environment. Health policy must be directed at reducing all these complex factors associated with perinatal substance abuse.

SUGGESTED READINGS

American Academy of Pediatrics Committee on Substance Abuse and Committee on Children with Disabilities: Fetal alcohol syndrome and alcohol-related neurodevelopmental disorders, *Pediatrics* 106:358-361, 2000.

Burgos AE, Burke BL: Neonatal abstinence syndrome, *NeoReviews* 10:e222, 2009.

Chasnoff IJ, McGourty RF, Bailey GW, et al: The 4P's Plus screen for substance use in pregnancy: clinical application and outcomes, *J Perinat* 25:368-374, 2005.

Jones HE, Martin PR, Heil SH, et al: Treatment of opioid-dependent pregnant women: clinical and research issues, *J Subst Abuse Treat* 35:245-259, 2008.

Messinger DS, Bauer CR, Das A, et al: The Maternal Lifestyle Study: cognitive, motor, and behavioral outcomes of cocaine-exposed and opiate-exposed infants through three years of age, *Pediatrics* 113:1677-1685, 2004.

Mitchell EA, Millerad J: Smoking and the sudden infant death syndrome, *Rev Environ Health* 21:81-103, 2006.

Moses-Kolko EL, Bogen D, Perel J, et al: Neonatal signs after late in utero exposure to serotonin reuptake inhibitors, literature review and clinical applications, *JAMA* 293:2372-2383, 2005.

Rogers JM: Tobacco and pregnancy: overview of exposure and effects, *Birth Defects Res C Embryol Today* 84:1-15, 2008.

Schempf AH: Illicit drug use and neonatal outcomes: a critical review, *Obstet Gynecol Surv* 62:749-757, 2007.

Shankaran S, Lester BM, Das A, et al: Impact of maternal substance use during pregnancy on childhood outcome, *Semin Fetal Neonatal Med* 12:143-150, 2007.

Smith LM, LaGasse LL, Derauf C, et al: The infant development, environment, and lifestyle study: effects of prenatal methamphetamine exposure, polydrug exposure, and poverty on intrauterine growth, *Pediatr* 118:1149-1156, 2006.

Thompson BL, Levitt P, Stanwood GD: Prenatal exposure to drugs: effects on brain development and implications for policy and education, *Nat Rev Neurosci* 10:303-312, 2009.

Complete references and supplemental color images used in this text can be found online at www.expertconsult.com

PART IV

LABOR AND DELIVERY

ANTEPARTUM FETAL ASSESSMENT

Christian M. Pettker and Katherine H. Campbell

A primary objective of obstetric care is the assessment and prevention of adverse fetal and neonatal outcomes. Maternal care is an integral step toward this goal. Optimization of the maternal state, through careful monitoring and treatment of chronic conditions such as diabetes or hypertension or acute states like preeclampsia or preterm labor, is one important facet of care to achieve desirable perinatal outcomes. Monitoring and management of the fetus, although a more obvious step toward this goal, are somewhat less straightforward. Fetal assessment demands a view into the intrauterine environment, which is somewhat inaccessible. Our ability to gain access to this space to gauge the needs and health of the fetus has improved dramatically with the developments in technology, as well as the increased understanding of fetal physiology over the past 50 years. As a result, perinatal morbidity and mortality have decreased substantially (Figure 13-1).

In general, antepartum fetal assessment encompasses the screening and diagnosis of fetal disorders and fetuses that are at risk. Selecting appropriate patients at risk for adverse perinatal events can enhance the prediction of these events, although some tests may be appropriate even for a low-risk population. The assessment may allow for certain therapeutic options—often, timely delivery—to prevent fetal harm. The overall goal of these efforts is to reduce perinatal mortality, although the reduction of morbidities such as cerebral palsy or preventable birth injury is intertwined with this objective. In antenatal assessment in the third trimester, the prediction and detection of fetal acidemia and hypoxemia form a central principle underlying these efforts.

It is important to make the distinction between antepartum and intrapartum fetal assessment. The latter is specifically related to monitoring the fetus during labor. The nature of labor affords certain advantages (e.g., dilation allows blood samples from the fetus) and restrictions (the lack of fluid after rupture of membranes creates difficulties for ultrasound examination) that do not occur in the antenatal period. As a result, this chapter focuses only on events and assessment preceding labor.

GENERAL PRINCIPLES

PRINCIPLES OF TESTING

Many of the tests used for antepartum fetal assessment are screening tests that will lead to further testing allowing for diagnosis and decision-making; therefore it is important

to note the principles guiding such tests. The outcome, principally perinatal morbidity and mortality, is a significant burden to both the individual and the overall health care system. The primary tools for assessment, ultrasound examination, and fetal heart rate monitoring, are generally easy, safe, and acceptable to patients. Screening has the potential to allow important and timely interventions, such as antenatal steroid administration or delivery. The predominant difficulty with fetal testing comes in the unproven utility of testing to improve outcomes. Furthermore, some tests, such as the nonstress test (NST), have high false-positive rates; therefore, when used as a diagnostic test (e.g., to decide on delivery), they can lead to the overuse of interventions. The specificity and sensitivity of the tests vary and the critical step to enhancing test performance is patient selection. The utility of fetal surveillance involves the judicious application of the tests in patients with specific risk profiles.

FETAL PHYSIOLOGY AND BEHAVIOR

The first trimester (≤14 weeks' gestation) is mainly a time of system development and organogenesis. The hyperplastic enlargement during the first 11 weeks produces standard rates of growth, with deviation being rare. At the completion of the first trimester, the major organ systems have developed, allowing the opportunity during the second trimester to assess for anomalies in development. The second and third trimesters involve maturation of these systems. Because antenatal fetal assessment is primarily concerned with the prediction or detection of fetal hypoxemia and acidemia, the integration of the neurologic and cardiovascular systems, particularly as reflections of fetal acid-base status, is the cornerstone of this assessment. We are thus able to monitor the manifestations of hypoxemia and acidemia as shown by neurologic and cardiovascular changes.

TECHNOLOGY

The technology underpinning fetal assessment is ultrasound. Fetal heart rate monitoring during the antepartum period depends on a Doppler cardiogram; movements of the fetal heart, in particular the sounds of the valves, are detected by this monitor. The time between the beats is translated into a heart rate, which is then graphically represented on a chart over time. This process produces the

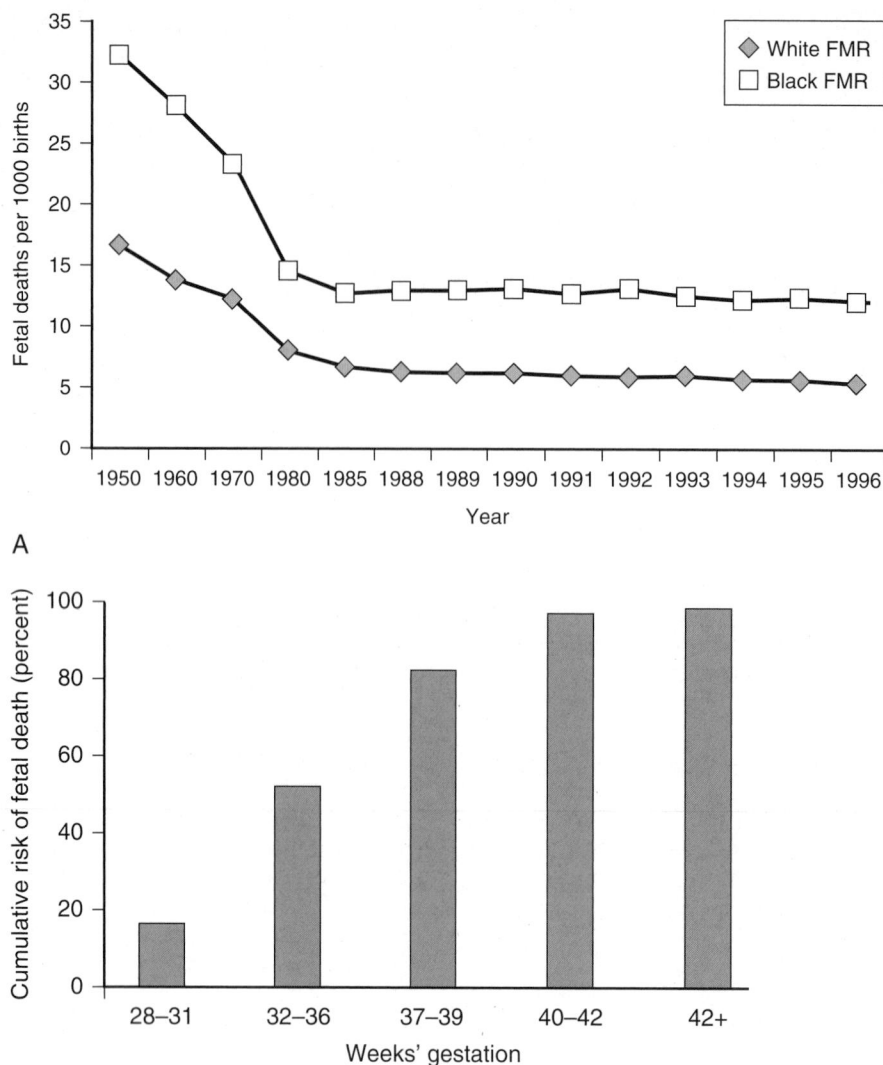

FIGURE 13-1 Fetal mortality rate (FMR) in the United States, 1959 to 1996. *(Adapted from McIlwaine GM, Dunn FH, Howat RC, et al: A routine system for monitoring perinatal deaths in Scotland,* Br J Obstet Gynaecol *92:9-13, 1985.)*

fetal heart rate monitoring strip that becomes the NST or contraction stress test (CST).

Contemporary ultrasound technology involves a wide array of features, including B-mode (basic imaging), M-mode (mapping the movement of structures over time), pulsed Doppler (demonstrating flow velocity in a particular area, such as a vessel), color Doppler (showing intensity and direction of flow through shades of red and blue), and power Doppler (a more sensitive form of colorized Doppler).

INDICATIONS AND TIMING

Most fetal testing protocols involve a stepwise approach, and the first step is the selection of the appropriate patient. Suggested assessments for low-risk pregnancies include one ultrasound examination for dating and one for the basic anatomic survey. Prenatal risk assessments for chromosomal disorders, such as first-trimester risk assessment with maternal serum analysis and fetal nuchal translucency assessment or the second-trimester maternal quadruple serum screen, are additional options. Whereas up to 30%

of perinatal morbidity may occur in low-risk patients, routine fetal testing beyond that described previously in a low-risk pregnancy is an ineffective use of resources.

High-risk pregnancies are those at greater peril for perinatal morbidity and mortality. These pregnancies often have more justification for targeted or detailed anatomic ultrasound examinations and for regular assessment of fetal growth or heart rate assessment. Common conditions requiring increased fetal surveillance are shown in Box 13-1.

Pregnancy dating should be confirmed at the earliest possible moment, and fetal anatomic screening is best accomplished in the second trimester, specifically at 18 to 20 weeks' gestation, when visualization of the anatomic features is adequate. However, standards for the timing of antepartum fetal assessment to survey for fetal compromise do not exist. Certainly assessment with NST or biophysical profiles would have little utility before viability (approximately 24 weeks' gestation). Guidelines for initiating fetal testing for specific indications are largely based on the risk of fetal loss at a particular gestational age.

BOX 13-1 Typical Indications for Antepartum Fetal Assessment: High-Risk Pregnancies

FETAL
- Abnormal fetal testing, fetal distress
- Anatomic anomaly
- Decreased fetal movement
- Heart block
- Intraamniotic infection
- Intrauterine growth restriction
- Multiple gestation
- Oligohydramnios

MATERNAL-FETAL
- Abruptio placenta
- Anemia, fetal (e.g., parvovirus, Rh alloimmunization, NAIT)
- Abnormal serum screening (low PAPP-A, high MSAFP)
- Placenta previa, vasa previa
- Postterm or postdates premature rupture of fetal membranes
- Threatened preterm delivery

MATERNAL
- Advanced maternal age
- Cardiac disease (severe)
- Cholestasis of pregnancy
- Diabetes, gestational
- Diabetes, pregestational
- Hemoglobinopathies
- HIV (receiving medication)
- Hypertension, chronic
- Hypertension, gestational
- History of IUFD
- Obesity
- Preeclampsia
- Pulmonary disease (severe)
- Renal disease
- Seizure disorder
- Substance abuse
- Systemic lupus erythematosis
- Thyroid disease
- Thrombophilia or thromboembolic disease

IUFD, Intrauterine fetal demise; *MSAFP,* maternal serum alpha-fetoprotein; *NAIT,* neonatal alloimmune thrombocytopenia; *PAPP-A,* pregnancy associated plasma protein

FETAL ASSESSMENT IN LOW RISK PREGNANCIES

ULTRASOUND: PREGNANCY DATING

The *estimated date of delivery* is defined at the beginning of pregnancy based on the best available information, including menstrual history, ultrasound data, and assisted reproduction technology. The median duration of a singleton pregnancy is 280 days (40 weeks) from the first day of the last menstrual period or 266 days (38 weeks) from the time of ovulation. *Term* is defined as 37 to 42 weeks' (259 to 294 days) gestation. Given that the preterm and postterm periods are associated with increased risks to the fetus and newborn, pregnancy dating provides an approximate expectation for the completion of the pregnancy and serves as a basis for the efficient and appropriate use of fetal surveillance, testing, and treatment. Accurate pregnancy dating by ultrasound has been associated with

reduced diagnoses of growth restriction (Waldenstrom et al, 1992), reduced use of tocolysis for preterm labor (LeFevre et al, 1993), and a reduced need to intervene in postterm pregnancies (Neilson, 2000).

In a spontaneous pregnancy in a woman with regular cycles and normal menstrual periods, the last menstrual period is often an accurate way of dating a pregnancy. Menstrual dating is less accurate in women who are taking oral contraceptives, were recently pregnant, or have irregular periods or intermenstrual bleeding. In these cases, and others in whom there is uncertainty, ultrasound dating in the first trimester is accurate and effective. A fetal pole may be seen beginning at 5 weeks' gestation, and the fetal heartbeat should be visualized at 6 to 8 weeks' gestation. In the first trimester, measurement of the crown-rump length is accurate to within 3 to 5 days; therefore this measurement should take priority in dating a pregnancy when the timing of the last menstrual period suggests a gestational age outside this range of variation (Drumm et al, 1976; Robinson and Fleming, 1975). A first-trimester ultrasound examination is indicated to confirm an intrauterine pregnancy (i.e., exclude ectopic pregnancy), confirm fetal viability, document fetal number, estimate gestational age, and evaluate the maternal pelvis and ovaries.

In the second trimester, ultrasound dating is less accurate, but can nonetheless be helpful. Measurement of the biparietal diameter (BPD) of the fetal head, the most accurate parameter, can be accurate to within 7 to 10 days (Campbell et al, 1985; Waldenstrom et al, 1990). The BPD is also a parameter of choice because it is less affected by chromosomal anomalies, in particular Down syndrome (Cuckle and Wald, 1987). Usually in the second or third trimesters, several biometric measurements—such as cerebellar distance, femur and humerus length, and abdominal circumference—are recorded and a computerized algorithm can generate an estimated gestational age.

ULTRASOUND: SECOND AND THIRD TRIMESTERS

Perinatal ultrasound examination in the second and third trimesters can be classified broadly into three types: the basic or standard examination, the specialized (detailed) examination, and the limited examination. The standard examination (level I) includes the determination of fetal number, fetal viability, fetal position, gestational age, placental location, amniotic fluid volume, the presence or absence of a maternal pelvic mass, and the presence of gross fetal malformations (American College of Obstetricians and Gynecologists, 2009). Most pregnancies can be evaluated adequately by this basic examination. If the patient's history, physical examination, or basic ultrasound examination suggest the presence of a fetal malformation, a specialized examination (level II) should be performed by a sonographer who is skilled in fetal evaluation. During a detailed ultrasound, which is best performed at 18 to 20 weeks' gestation, fetal structures are examined in detail to identify and characterize any fetal malformation. In addition to identifying structural abnormalities, a specialized ultrasound examination can identify sonographic markers of fetal aneuploidy. In some situations, a limited examination may be appropriate to answer a specific clinical question (such as fetal viability, amniotic fluid volume, fetal presentation, placental location, or cervical length) or to provide sonographic guidance for an invasive procedure (such as amniocentesis).

Current debate centers on who should undergo sonographic examination and what type of evaluation these patients should have. Advocates of routine sonography cite several advantages of universal ultrasound evaluation, including more accurate dating of pregnancy and earlier and more accurate diagnosis of multiple gestation, structural malformations, and fetal aneuploidy (discussed later in ultrasound section). Opponents of routine sonographic examination argue that it is an expensive screening test ($100 to $250 for a standard examination) and that the cost is not justified by published research, which suggests that routine ultrasound examinations do not significantly change perinatal outcome (Crane et al, 1994; Ewigman et al, 1993; LeFevre et al, 1993)

Second-trimester ultrasound examination is indicated in patients with uncertain dating, uterine size larger or smaller than expected for the estimated gestational age, a medical disorder that can affect fetal growth and development (e.g., diabetes, hypertension, collagen vascular disorder), a family history of an inherited genetic abnormality, or a suspected fetal malformation or growth disturbance (American College of Obstetricians and Gynecologists, 2009). In the United States, most patients undergo a standard examination at 18 to 20 weeks' gestation to screen for structural defects. An understanding of normal fetal physiology is critical to the diagnosis of fetal structural anomalies. For example, extraabdominal herniation of the midgut into the umbilical cord occurs normally in the fetus at 8 to 12 weeks' gestation and can be misdiagnosed as an abdominal wall defect. Placental location should be documented with the bladder empty, because overdistention of the maternal bladder or a lower uterine contraction can give a false impression of placenta previa. If placenta previa is identified at 18 to 22 weeks' gestation, serial ultrasound examinations should be performed to follow placental location. Only 5% of placenta previa identified in the second trimester will persist to term (Zelop et al, 1994). The umbilical cord should also be imaged, and the number of vessels, placental insertion, and insertion into the fetus should be noted.

The indications for third-trimester ultrasound examination are similar to that for second-trimester ultrasound. Fetal anatomy survey examinations and estimates of fetal weight become less accurate as gestational age increases, especially in obese women or in pregnancies complicated by oligohydramnios. However, fetal biometry and an anatomic survey should still be performed, because certain fetal anomalies, such as achondroplasia, will become evident for the first time later in gestation.

FETAL MOVEMENT COUNTING

Fetal movement (quickening) is typically perceived by the mother at 16 to 22 weeks' gestation. Fetal hypoxemia is typically associated with a reduction in fetal activity; the fetus is essentially conserving energy and oxygen for vital activities. A typical procedure for fetal movement counting

consists of having the patient record the interval taken to feel 10 fetal movements, usually after a meal when the fetus is more active. If 10 movements are not detected in 1 hour, further testing is often recommended. The data supporting fetal movement counting are mixed. A large international cluster randomized trial involving more than 68,000 patients demonstrated no benefit (Grant et al, 1989), and a Cochrane analysis found insufficient evidence to support this technique to prevent stillbirth (Mangesi and Hofmeyr, 2007). Fetal movement counting represents a low-technology screening test that can be applied easily to all pregnancies. Although its effectiveness in improving perinatal outcomes is debatable, it can be used as a cost-effective first line strategy

FETAL ASSESSMENT IN HIGH-RISK PREGNANCIES

CARDIOTOCOGRAPHY

Cardiotocography is the visual representation of fetal heart rate and uterine contractions. Fetal heart rate has been recognized as an important indicator of fetal status since the nineteenth century, with Lejumeau Kergaradec of Switzerland being credited with the first accounts of direct fetal auscultation and the uterine soufflé in 1821. Fetal heart rate monitoring is based on the principle that the fetal neurologic system, through its afferent and efferent networks, serves as a key mediator to demonstrate fetal well-being. Oxygenation, acidemia, and other vital functions are monitored by peripheral chemoreceptors and baroreceptors, which provide input on fetal status through afferent neurologic networks to the central nervous system (CNS). This information is processed by the CNS, and signals are conducted through efferent networks to produce peripheral changes, particularly to the heart via direct parasympathetic vagal neurons, direct sympathetic signals, or indirect sympathetic stimulation of catecholamine release. In this way, fetal cardiac activity can be seen as a surrogate for fetal oxygenation and acid-base status.

For many years, assessment of the fetal heart rate was limited to the fetoscope, a direct stethoscope attributed to Adolphe Pinard in 1876. In 1957, Orvan Hess and Ed Hon at Yale University introduced electronic fetal heart rate monitoring as a window into the status of the fetus (Hon and Hess, 1957). This technology relied on direct monitoring through a scalp electrode; only years later would Doppler technology allow cardiac signals to be detected noninvasively. Fetal heart rate monitoring became a tool for fetal assessment as it was recognized that certain fetal heart rate patterns were associated with fetal compromise and poor fetal outcomes.

The basic elements of a fetal heart rate strip are baseline, variability, accelerations, and decelerations. A baseline of 110 to 160 beats per minute is normal. Variability is determined by the irregular fluctuations in amplitude and frequency in the baseline, and variability of fewer than 6 beats per minute is often abnormal. Accelerations are classified as visually apparent abrupt increases that peak at 15 beats per minute or more above the baseline that last 15 seconds or longer. Fetal movements often coincide with fetal heart rate (FHR) accelerations. Finally decelerations,

TABLE 13-1 Interpretation of Antepartum Cardiotocography

Term	Characteristic	Description
Baseline	Definition	Mean fetal heart rate, rounded to increments of 5 beats/min (e.g. 140, 145); need baseline duration of ≥2 min during a 10-min segment, between periodic or episodic changes, to determine baseline
	Bradycardia	<110 beats per minute for >10 min
	Tachycardia	>160 beats per minute for >10 min
Variability	Definition	Fluctuations of the baseline heart rate; measured from peak to trough
	Absent	Undetectable
	Minimal	Undetectable to ≤5 beats/min
	Moderate	6-25 beats/min
	Marked	>25 beats/min
Acceleration	Definition	Abrupt increase ≥15 beats/min lasting ≥15 s
	Prolonged	≥2 min and <10 min (≥10 min is a baseline change)
Deceleration	Definition	Decreases in the fetal heart rate
	Variable	Abrupt decrease onset to nadir <30 s; decrease ≥15 beats/min lasting ≥5 s to <2 min
	Early	Gradual decrease onset to nadir ≥30 s with contraction
	Late	Gradual decrease onset to nadir ≥30 s; nadir of deceleration occurring after peak of contraction
	Prolonged	Decrease ≥15 beats/min lasting ≥2 min, but <10 min (≥10 min is a baseline change)
	Recurrent	Occur with ≥50% of uterine contractions in any 20-min window
	Intermittent	Occur with <50% of uterine contractions in any 20-min window
Contractions	Considerations	Frequency, duration, intensity, and relaxation
	Normal	≤5 contractions per 10 minutes averaged over a 30-min window
	Tachysystole	>5 contractions per 10 minutes averaged over a 30-min window; should always be qualified as to the presence or absence of associated FHR decelerations

often classified as early, variable, or late, are decreases in the fetal heart rate that have specific pathologic and physiologic associations. Although primarily focused on intrapartum monitoring, the 2008 National Institute of Child Health and Human Development workshop report on fetal monitoring provides an excellent summary of the nomenclature and interpretation involved (Table 13-1) (Macones et al, 2008).

NONSTRESS TEST

A normal result of an NST is defined as a 20-minute fetal heart rate tracing that contains two heart rate accelerations lasting 15 seconds or longer that peak 15 beats or more above the baseline. Often this is called a *reactive NST* (Figure 13-2). Modifications are made in reference to gestational age. NSTs for fetuses at less than 32 weeks' gestation are often considered reactive if the acceleration is 10 beats per minute or more above the baseline and lasts for at least 10 seconds. Furthermore, to account for the periodicity of 20- to 30-minute sleep cycles in the fetus, an NST that is not reactive over the first 20 minutes may be continued an additional 20 to 40 minutes. A nonreactive NST or an NST with specific abnormalities (e.g., high or low baseline, decelerations) should be followed by a biophysical profile (BPP). It is important to note that some abnormal states, such as a fetal CNS abnormality or maternal drug ingestion, may contribute to a nonreactive NST. In these cases, ultrasound examination may provide appropriate information to determine the diagnosis or required management.

Falsely reassuring NSTs occur at a rate of 3 to 5 per 1000 tests, although this does not account for a baseline rate of unpreventable fetal deaths (Freeman et al, 1982b). The difficulty with the NST really lies in its lack of specificity for fetal death or compromise; the false-positive rate may be as high as 50% (Freeman et al, 1982b).

The rather modest false-negative rate is likely because of the NST being a measurement of short-term hypoxemia. Indeed, longer-term fetal status can be measured through amniotic fluid assessment, because the amniotic fluid is correlated with fetal urinary output, which is a surrogate for renal perfusion. When combined with an assessment of amniotic fluid level, the false-negative rate of the NST is reduced to 0.8 per 1000, although a 60% false-positive rate remains (Miller et al, 1996). Indeed, when combined with the NST and amniotic fluid assessment—sometimes known as the *modified biophysical profile*—reduces the risk of fetal death to negligible levels in high-risk populations (Clark et al, 1989). For these reasons, the NST combined with amniotic fluid assessment is a modality of choice for monitoring the high-risk pregnancy.

CONTRACTION STRESS TEST

The CST assesses the fetal heart rate response in the presence of contractions. This test improves on the specificity and sensitivity of the NST by assessing the fetal response to stress. In fact, the CST preceded the NST, although the NST became more favorable because of fewer contraindications, ease of administration, and reduced time and supervision necessary. Compared with the NST, there is a much lower incidence of falsely reassuring tests (0.4 per 1000), representing an eightfold reduction in the risk of fetal loss in one study (Freeman et al, 1982a).

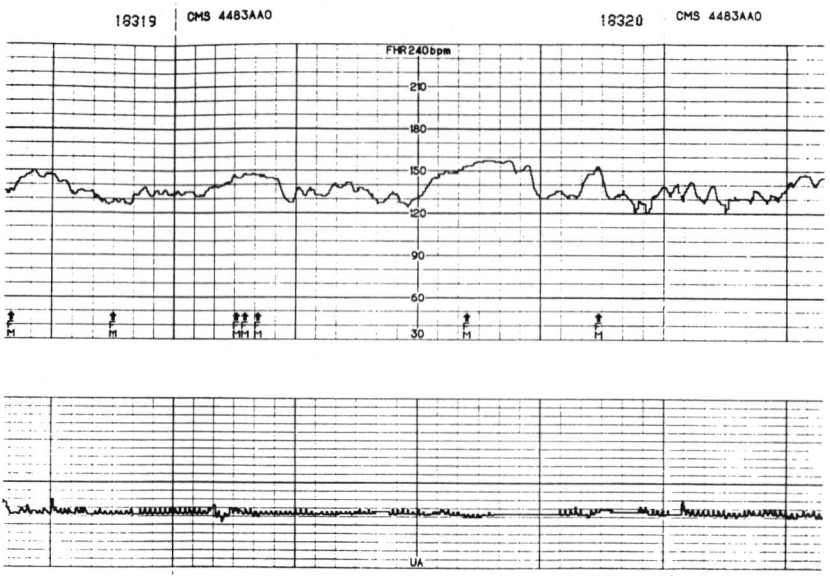

FIGURE 13-2 A reassuring nonstress test. Note two fetal heart rate accelerations exceeding 15 beats/min and lasting at least 15 seconds during the monitoring period.

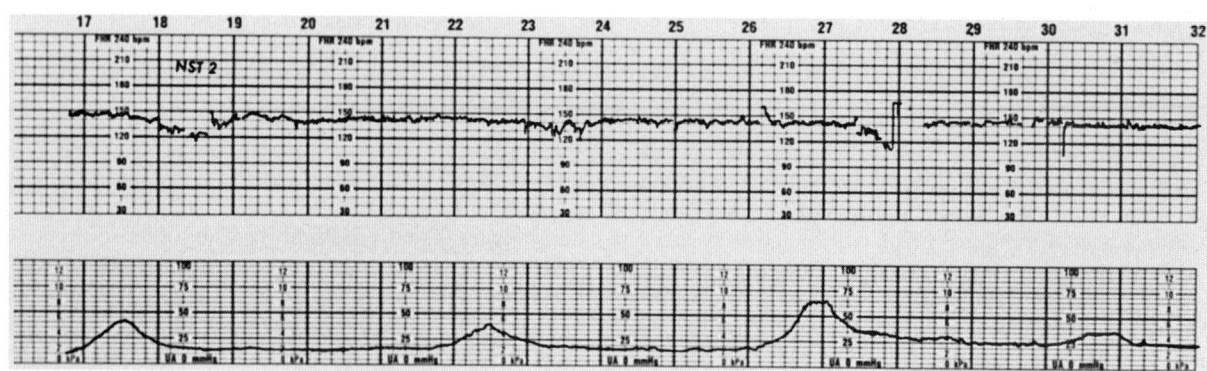

FIGURE 13-3 A contraction stress test. The fetal heart rate is plotted above the uterine contraction signal. Note the late deceleration after a contraction; this is a positive, or abnormal, test result.

Contractions are stimulated by the administration of intravenous oxytocin or through maternal nipple stimulation. Of course, the CST is contraindicated in patients in whom contractions should not be provoked, such as threatened preterm delivery or preterm premature rupture of membranes, prior classical cesarean delivery, or placenta previa. A minimum of three contractions over a 10-minute period of continuous fetal heart rate assessment are necessary for a satisfactory test interpretation. An unsatisfactory test should be followed by continued testing with a modification of the mode of contraction stimulation. A negative (i.e., normal) test result demonstrates no late decelerations, whereas a positive test result shows late decelerations after 50% or more of contractions (Figure 13-3). A positive test result requires immediate further testing or evaluation, if not delivery. An equivocal test demonstrates late decelerations with less than 50% of contractions and requires further testing or monitoring. A test that encompasses a hyperstimulatory contraction pattern (e.g., five contractions within 10 minutes or contractions lasting longer than 90 seconds) is also considered equivocal and requires further testing.

ULTRASOUND

Although routine sonography for low-risk pregnant women is controversial, few would disagree that the benefits far outweigh the costs for high-risk patients. Given the higher risk for fetal complications such as anatomic anomalies or growth disturbances, a specialized examination is performed between 18 and 20 weeks' gestation in most high-risk pregnancies.

Additional ultrasound modalities are also available, including fetal echocardiography, three-dimensional (3D) sonography, and Doppler. Cardiac anomalies are the most common major congenital defects encountered in the antepartum period. A four-chamber view of the heart at the time of fetal anatomy survey at 18 to 20 weeks' gestation will detect only 30% of congenital cardiac anomalies, although the detection rate can be increased to approximately 60% to 70% if the outflow tracts are adequately visualized (Kirk et al, 1994), but this still leaves 30% to 40% of all congenital cardiac anomalies undiagnosed. For this reason, fetal echocardiography should be performed by a skilled and experienced sonologist at 20 to 22 weeks' gestation in all pregnancies at high-risk of a fetal cardiac anomaly; this includes pregnancies complicated by pregestational diabetes mellitus, a personal or family history of congenital cardiac disease regardless of the nature of the lesion or whether it has been repaired), maternal drug exposure (e.g., lithium and paroxetine) (Bérard et al, 2007), and pregnancies conceived by in vitro fertilization, but not if the pregnancy was conceived using clomiphene citrate or ovarian stimulation or intrauterine insemination alone (Olson et al, 2005).

Compared with standard two-dimensional (2D) ultrasound, 3D ultrasound (or four-dimensional if fetal movements are included) allows for visualization of fetal structures in all three dimensions concurrently for the improved characterization of complex fetal structural anomalies and for storage of scanned images with 3D reconstruction at a later date or remote location (telemedicine). Unlike 2D ultrasound, 3D images are greatly influenced by fetal movements and are subject to more interference from structures such as fetal limbs, umbilical cord, and placental tissue. Because of movement interference, visualization of the fetal heart with 3D ultrasound is suboptimal.

In addition to rapid acquisition of images that can be later reconstructed and manipulated, 3D ultrasound has other potential advantages:
- Surface rendering mode can provide clearer images of many soft tissue structures. Such images can improve the diagnosis of certain fetal malformations, especially craniofacial anomalies (cleft lip and palate, micrognathia, ear anomaly, facial dysmorphism, club foot, finger and toe anomalies), intracranial lesions, spinal anomalies, ventral wall defects, and fetal tumors.
- 3D ultrasound may be useful in early pregnancy by providing more accurate measurements of the gestational sac, yolk sac, and crown-rump length. It may also allow for a more accurate midsagittal view of the fetus for measuring nuchal translucency.
- 3D ultrasound can also be used to measure tissue volume. Preliminary data suggest that the assessment of cervical volume may predict the risk of cervical insufficiency (Rovas et al, 2005), and measurement of placental volume in the first trimester may predict fetuses at risk of intrauterine growth restriction (IUGR) (Schuchter et al, 2001).

Despite these advantages and the fact that 3D ultrasound has been available since the early 1990s, it has yet to live up to its promises. Although 3D ultrasound is unlikely to replace standard 2D imaging in the near future, it is a valuable complementary modality in obstetric imaging. As the technology improves, it is likely that perinatal ultrasound will evolve to resemble computed tomography and magnetic resonance imaging.

GROWTH ASSESSMENT

Normal fetal growth is a critical component of a healthy pregnancy and the subsequent long-term health of the child. A systematic method of examination of the gravid abdomen was first described by Leopold and Sporlin (1894). Although abdominal examination has several limitations, particularly in the setting of maternal obesity, multiple pregnancy, uterine fibroids, or polyhydramnios,

it is safe, free, and well tolerated and may add valuable information to assist in antepartum management. Palpation is divided into four separate Leopold maneuvers. Each maneuver is designed to identify specific fetal landmarks or to reveal a specific relationship between the fetus and mother. For example, the first maneuver involves measuring fundal height. The uterus can be palpated above the pelvic brim at approximately 12 weeks' gestation. Thereafter, fundal height should increase by approximately 1 cm per week, reaching the level of the umbilicus at 20 to 22 weeks' gestation. Between 20 and 32 weeks' gestation, the fundal height (in centimeters, from the superior edge of the pubic symphysis) is approximately equal to the gestational age (in weeks) in healthy women of average weight with an appropriately grown fetus. However, there is a wide range of normal fundal height measurements. One study has shown a 6-cm difference between the 10th and 90th percentiles at each week of gestation after 20 weeks (Belizan et al, 1978). Moreover, fundal height is maximal at approximately 36 weeks' gestation, at which time the fetus drops into the pelvis in preparation for labor and the fundal height decreases. For these reasons, reliance on fundal height measurements alone will fail to identify more than 50% of fetuses with IUGR (Gardosi and Francis, 1999). Serial fundal height measurements by an experienced obstetric care provider are more accurate than a single measurement, and they will lead to an improved diagnosis of fetal growth restriction with reported sensitivities as high as 86% (Belizan et al, 1978).

If the clinical examination is not consistent with the stated gestational age, an ultrasound examination is indicated to confirm gestational age and to establish a more objective measure of fetal growth. Ultrasound examination may also identify an alternative explanation for the discrepancy, such as multiple pregnancy, polyhydramnios, oligohydramnios, fetal demise, or uterine fibroids.

For many years, obstetric sonography has used fetal biometry to define fetal size by weight estimation, although this approach has a number of key limitations. For example, regression equations used to create weight estimation formulas are derived primarily from cross-sectional data that rely on infants delivering within an arbitrary period of time after the ultrasound examination, and they assume that body proportions (i.e., fat, muscle, bone) are the same for all fetuses. Moreover, growth curves for healthy infants from 24 to 37 weeks' gestation rely on data collected from pregnancies delivered preterm, which should not be regarded as normal pregnancies and are likely to be complicated by some element of uteroplacental insufficiency regardless of whether the delivery was spontaneous or iatrogenic. Despite these limitations, if the gestational age is well validated, the prevailing data suggest that prenatal ultrasound can be used to verify an alteration in fetal growth in 80% of cases and exclude abnormal growth in 90% of cases (Sabbagha, 1987).

Sonographic estimates of fetal weight are commonly derived from mathematical formulas that use a combination of fetal measurements, especially the BPD, abdominal circumference (AC), and femur length (Hadlock et al, 1984). Whereas the BPD may be the most accurate indicator of gestational age in the second or third trimesters, fetuses gain weight in their abdomen, making the AC the single most important measurement for fetal size. The AC is thus given more weight in these formulas. Unfortunately the AC is also the most difficult measurement to acquire, and a small difference in the AC measurement will result in a large difference in the estimated fetal weight (EFW). The accuracy of the EFW depends on a number of variables, including gestational age (in absolute terms, EFW is more accurate in preterm or IUGR fetuses than in term or macrosomic fetuses), operator experience, maternal body habitus, and amniotic fluid volume (measurements are more difficult to acquire if the amniotic fluid volume is low). Although objective, sonographic EFW estimations are not particularly accurate and have an error of 15% 20%, even in experienced hands (Anderson et al, 2007). Indeed, a sonographic EFW at term is no more accurate than a clinical estimate of fetal weight by an experienced obstetric care provider or the mother's estimate of fetal weight if she has delivered before (Chauhan et al, 1992). Sonographic estimates of fetal weight must therefore be evaluated within the context of the clinical situation and balanced against the clinical estimate of fetal weight. Serial sonographic evaluations of fetal weight are more useful than a single measurement in diagnosing abnormal fetal growth. The ideal interval to evaluate fetal growth is every 3 to 4 weeks, with a minimum 10- to 14-day interval necessary to see significant differences. Because of the inherent error in fetal biometric measurements, more frequent ultrasound determinations of EFW may be misleading. Similarly, the use of population-specific growth curves, if available, will improve the ability of the obstetric care provider to identify abnormal fetal growth. For example, growth curves derived from a population that lives at high altitude, where the fetus is exposed to lower oxygen tension, will be different from those derived from a population at sea level. Abnormal fetal growth can be classified as insufficient (i.e., IUGR) or excessive (fetal macrosomia).

The definition of IUGR has been a long-standing challenge for modern obstetrics. Distinguishing the healthy, constitutionally small-for-gestational-age fetus, defined as an EFW below the 10th percentile for a given week of gestation, from the nutritionally deprived, truly growth-restricted fetus has been particularly difficult. Fetuses with an EFW less than the 10th percentile are not necessarily pathologically growth restricted. Conversely, an EFW greater than the 10th percentile does not mean that an individual fetus has achieved its growth potential, and such fetuses may still be at risk of perinatal mortality and morbidity. As such, IUGR is best defined as either an EFW of less than the 5th percentile for gestational age in a well-dated pregnancy or an EFW of less than the 10th percentile for gestational age in a well-dated pregnancy with evidence of fetal compromise, such as oligohydramnios or abnormal umbilical artery Doppler velocimetry.

Fetal growth restriction has traditionally been classified into asymmetric or symmetric IUGR. Asymmetric IUGR is characterized by normal head growth, but suboptimal body growth, and is seen most commonly in the third trimester. It is thought to result from a late pathologic event, such as chronic placental abruption leading to uteroplacental insufficiency, in an otherwise uncomplicated pregnancy and healthy fetus. In cases of symmetric IUGR, both the fetal head size and body weight are reduced, indicating a global insult that likely occurred early in gestation. Symmetric IUGR may reflect an inherent fetal abnormality (e.g., fetal chromosomal anomaly, inherited metabolic disorder, early congenital infection) or long-standing severe placental insufficiency caused by an underlying maternal disease (e.g., hypertension, pregestational diabetes mellitus, collagen vascular disorder). In practice, the distinction between asymmetric and symmetric IUGR is not particularly useful.

Early and accurate diagnosis of IUGR coupled with appropriate intervention will lead to an improvement in perinatal outcome. If IUGR is suggested clinically and by ultrasound examination, thorough evaluations of the mother and fetus are indicated. Referral to a maternal-fetal medicine specialist should be considered. Every effort should be made to identify the cause of IUGR and to modify or eliminate contributing factors. Up to 20% of cases of severe IUGR are associated with fetal chromosome abnormalities or congenital malformations, 25% to 30% are related to maternal conditions characterized by vascular disease, and a smaller proportion are the result of abnormal placentation. However, in a substantial number of cases (50% or more in some studies), the cause of the IUGR will remain uncertain even after a thorough investigation (Resnik, 2002). Fetal macrosomia is defined as an EFW (not birthweight) of 4500 g or greater, measured either clinically or by ultrasound, and is independent of gestational age, diabetic status, or actual birthweight (American College of Obstetricians and Gynecologists, 2000). Fetal macrosomia refers to a single cutoff EFW; this should be distinguished from the large-for-gestational age fetus, which is one in whom the EFW is greater than the 90th percentile for gestational age. By definition, 10% of all fetuses are large for gestational age at any given gestational age. Fetal macrosomia is associated with an increased risk of cesarean delivery, operative vaginal delivery, and birth injury to both the mother (including vaginal, perineal, and rectal trauma) and the fetus (orthopedic and neurologic injury) (American College of Obstetricians and Gynecologists, 2000, 2001; Kjos and Buchanan, 1999; Magee et al, 1993; O'Sullivan et al, 1973; Widness et al, 1985). Shoulder dystocia with resultant brachial plexus injury (Erb's palsy) are a serious consequence of fetal macrosomia and are further increased in the setting of diabetes, because of the increased diameters in the upper thorax and neck of fetuses of mothers with diabetes.

Fetal macrosomia can be determined clinically, by abdominal palpation using the Leopold's maneuvers, or by ultrasound examination; these two techniques appear to be equally accurate (Watson et al, 1988). However, EFW measurements are less accurate in large (macrosomic) fetuses than in normally grown fetuses, and factors such as low amniotic fluid volume, advancing gestational age, maternal obesity, and the position of the fetus can compound these inaccuracies. Clinical examination has been shown to underestimate the birthweight by 0.5 kg or more in almost 80% of fetuses with macrosomia (Niswander et al, 1970). For these reasons, the prediction of fetal macrosomia is not particularly accurate, with a false-positive rate of 35% and a false-negative rate of 10% (Niswander et al, 1970; Watson et al, 1988). A number of alternative sonographic measurements have therefore been proposed in an attempt to better identify the macrosomic fetus, including fetal AC alone, umbilical cord circumference, cheek-to-cheek diameter, and upper arm circumference; however, these measurements remain investigational and should not be used clinically.

Despite the inaccuracy in the prediction of fetal macrosomia, an EFW should be documented either by clinical estimation or ultrasound examination in all women at high risk at approximately 38 weeks' gestation. Suspected fetal macrosomia is not an indication for induction of labor, because induction does not improve maternal or fetal outcomes (American College of Obstetricians and Gynecologists, 2000). However, if the EFW is excessive, an elective cesarean delivery should be considered to prevent fetal and maternal birth trauma. Although controversy remains as to the precise EFW at which an elective cesarean delivery should be recommended, a suspected birthweight in excess of 4500 g in women with diabetes or 5000 g in women without diabetes is a reasonable threshold (American College of Obstetricians and Gynecologists, 2000, 2001, 2002).

AMNIOTIC FLUID ASSESSMENT

Amniotic fluid plays a key role in the health and development of a growing fetus. Once considered an afterthought during the ultrasound examination of the fetus, evaluation of the amniotic fluid is now considered an integral part of ultrasound evaluation for fetal well-being. Amniotic fluid serves a number of important functions for the developing embryo and fetus. It provides cushioning against physical trauma; creates an environment free of restriction and or distortion, allowing for normal growth and development of the fetus; provides a thermally stable environment; allows the respiratory, gastrointestinal, and musculoskeletal tracts to develop normally; and helps to prevent infection (Hill et al, 1984).

The chorioamnion acts as a porous membrane early in pregnancy, allowing the passage of water and solutes across the membrane; there is little contribution from the small embryo. As the pregnancy progresses into the late first trimester, the diffusion of fluid across the fetal skin occurs, increasing the volume of amniotic fluid. In the second half of the pregnancy, the main sources of amniotic fluid come from fetal kidneys and lungs. The primary sources for removal of fluid are from fetal swallowing and absorption into fetal blood perfusing the surface of the placenta. As more fluid is produced than is resorbed by the fetal-placental unit, the volume of amniotic fluid increases throughout the first 32 weeks of pregnancy (Figure 13-4). The volume peaks at approximately 32 to 33 weeks' gestation, and at this gestational age equal amounts of fluid are produced and resorbed. After term, the amniotic fluid declines at a rate of 8% per week (Brace and Wolf, 1989).

Because amniotic fluid plays a critical role in the normal development of a fetus, the assessment of amniotic volume is an essential component of the ultrasound evaluation for fetal well-being. Subjective estimates of the amniotic fluid volume have been validated, but two ultrasound measurements—amniotic fluid index (AFI) and maximum vertical pocket—have been developed to quickly and accurately assess the quantity of amniotic fluid surrounding the fetus.

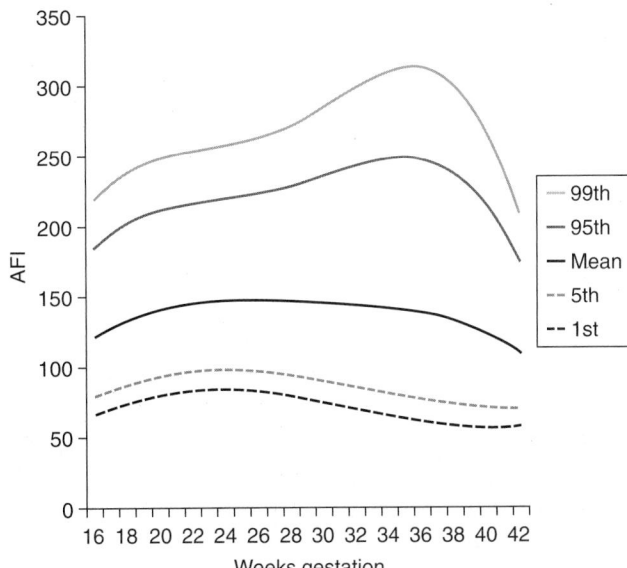

FIGURE 13-4 Amniotic fluid index (AFI; in mm) plotted against gestational age. The lines represent percentiles.

The AFI is a semiquantitative method for assessing the amniotic fluid volume with ultrasound. The gravid uterus is divided into four quadrants using the umbilicus, linea nigra, and external landmarks (Rutherford et al, 1987). The deepest amniotic fluid pocket is measured in each quadrant with the ultrasound transducer perpendicular to the floor. The four measurements are added together and the sum is regarded as the AFI. Pockets filled with umbilical cord or fetal extremities should not be used for generating the AFI (Hill, 1997). Researchers and clinicians have used a variety of measurements to define abnormalities in amniotic fluid volume. However, the normal range of the AFI most commonly used in clinical practice is 5 to 20 cm of fluid. Pregnancies with AFIs less than 5 cm can be described as having oligohydramnios, and pregnancies with measurements greater than 20 cm can be described as having polyhydramnios.

The maximal vertical pocket is another semiquantitative method for assessing the fluid volume. The technique involves scanning the gravid uterus for the single deepest pocket of amniotic fluid that is free of umbilical cord and fetal parts and with the transducer perpendicular to the floor, measuring the pocket of fluid (Manning et al, 1981b). Currently this method is used mostly in multiple gestation pregnancies in which the AFI is not technically feasible. Oligohydramnios can be defined as a single measurement less than 2 cm. Polyhydramnios can be defined as a single measurement greater than 10 cm.

BIOPHYSICAL PROFILE

An NST alone might not be sufficient to confirm fetal well-being; in such cases, a biophysical profile (BPP) may be performed. The BPP refers to a sonographic scoring system performed over a 30- to 40-minute period designed to assess fetal well-being. The BPP was initially described for testing postterm fetuses, but has since been validated for use in both term and preterm fetuses (Manning et al,

1981a, 1985, 1987; Vintzileos et al, 1983, 1987a, 1987b). Notably, BPP is not validated for use in active labor. The five variables described in the original BPP were: gross fetal body movements, fetal tone (i.e., flexion and extension of limbs), amniotic fluid volume, fetal breathing movements, and NST (summarized in Table 13-2) (Manning, 1989). More recently, however, BPP is interpreted without the NST.

The individual variables of the BPP become apparent in healthy fetuses in a predictable sequence: fetal tone appears at 7.5 to 8.5 weeks, fetal movement at 9 weeks, fetal breathing at 20 to 22 weeks, and FHR reactivity at 24 to 28 weeks' gestation. Similarly, in the setting of antepartum hypoxia, these characteristics typically disappear in the reverse order in which they appeared (i.e., FHR reactivity is lost first followed by fetal breathing, fetal movements, and finally fetal tone) (Vintzileos et al, 1987a). The amniotic fluid volume, which is composed almost entirely of fetal urine in the second and third trimesters, is not influenced by acute fetal hypoxia or acute fetal central nervous system dysfunction. Rather, oligohydramnios (decreased amniotic fluid volume) in the latter half of pregnancy and in the absence of ruptured membranes is a reflection of

chronic uteroplacental insufficiency, increased renal artery resistance leading to diminished urine output, or both (Oz et al, 2002); it predisposes to umbilical cord compression, thus leading to intermittent fetal hypoxemia, meconium passage, or meconium aspiration. Adverse pregnancy outcome (including nonreassuring FHR tracing, low Apgar score, and neonatal intensive care unit admission) is more common when oligohydramnios is present (Bochner et al, 1987; Morris et al, 2003; Oz et al, 2002; Tongsong and Srisomboon, 1993). Serial (weekly) screening of high-risk pregnancies for oligohydramnios is important, because amniotic fluid can become drastically reduced within 24 to 48 hours (Clement et al, 1987).

Although each of the five features of the BPP are scored equally (2 points if the variable is present or normal, and 0 points if absent or abnormal, for a total of 10 points), they are not equally predictive of adverse pregnancy outcome. For example, amniotic fluid volume is the variable that correlates most strongly with adverse pregnancy events. The recommended management based on the BPP is summarized in Table 13-3 (Manning, 1989). A score of 8 to 10 out of 10 is regarded as reassuring; a score of 4 to 6 is suspicious and requires reevaluation, and a score of 0 to 2 suggests nonreassuring fetal testing—previously referred to as *fetal distress* (Manning et al, 1981a, 1981b). Evidence of nonreassuring fetal testing or oligohydramnios in the setting of otherwise reassuring fetal testing should prompt evaluation for immediate delivery (Vintzileos et al, 1987a, 1987b).

DOPPLER

Doppler velocimetry shows the direction and characteristics of blood flow, and it can be used to examine the maternal, uteroplacental, or fetal circulations. Because of placental capacitance, the umbilical artery is one of the few arteries that normally has forward diastolic flow, and it is one of the most frequently targeted vessels during

TABLE 13-2 Fetal Biophysical Profile

Element	Criterion (2 points for each element satisfied)
Breathing	≥1 episode of breathing movements lasting 30 seconds
Movement	≥3 discrete body or limb movements
Tone	≥1 episode of active extension and flexion of limbs or trunk
Amniotic fluid	≥1 pocket of amniotic fluid measuring ≥2 cm in two perpendicular planes
Nonstress test	≥2 fetal heart rate accelerations lasting ≥15 seconds over 20 minutes

TABLE 13-3 Interpretation and Management of Biophysical Profile

Score	Comment	Perinatal Morbidity or Mortality Within 1 week (no intervention)	Management
10/10	Normal	<1/1000	No intervention
8/8	Normal	—	No intervention
8/10 (abnormal NST)	Normal	—	No intervention
8/10 (abnormal amniotic fluid)	Suspect chronic fetal compromise, renal anomaly, or rupture of membranes	89/1000	Rule out renal abnormality or rupture of membranes; consider delivery or prolonged observation if dictated by gestational age
6/8 (other)	Equivocal, possible asphyxia	Variable	If fetus is mature, deliver; if immature, repeat test within 4-6 hours
6/8 (abnormal amniotic fluid)	Suspect asphyxia	89/1000	Repeat 4-6 hours; consider delivery
4/8	Suspect asphyxia	91/1000	If ≥36 weeks' gestation or documented pulmonary maturity, deliver immediately; if not, repeat within 4-6 hours
2/8	High suspicion of asphyxia	125/1000	Immediate delivery
0/8	High suspicion of asphyxia	600/1000	Immediate delivery

Adapted from Manning FA, Morrison I, Harman CR, et al: Fetal assessment based on fetal biophysical profile scoring: experience in 19,221 referred high-risk pregnancies, *Am J Obstet Gynecol* 157:880, 1987.
NST, Nonstress test.

pregnancy. Umbilical artery Doppler velocimetry measurements reflect resistance to blood flow from the fetus to the placenta. Factors that affect placental resistance include gestational age, placental location, pregnancy complications (placental abruption, preeclampsia), and underlying maternal disease (chronic hypertension).

Doppler velocimetry of umbilical artery blood flow provides an indirect measure of placental function and fetal status (Giles et al, 1985). Decreased diastolic flow with a resultant increase in systolic-to-diastolic ratio suggests increased placental vascular resistance and fetal compromise. Severely abnormal umbilical artery Doppler velocimetry (defined as absent or reversed diastolic flow) is an especially ominous observation and is associated with poor perinatal outcome, particularly in the setting of IUGR (Ducey et al, 1987; McCallum et al, 1978; Rochelson et al, 1987; Trudinger et al, 1991; Wenstrom et al, 1991; Zelop et al, 1996). The overall mortality rate for fetuses with absent or reversed flow may be near 30% (Karsdorp et al, 1994). It should be noted that abnormal Doppler studies are often seen in cases of anatomic anomalies or chromosomal abnormalities, which should be noted when managing a case.

The role of ductus venosus and middle cerebral artery (MCA) Doppler in the management of IUGR pregnancies is not well defined. As such, urgent delivery should be considered in IUGR pregnancies when the results of umbilical artery Doppler studies are severely abnormal regardless of gestational age. However, it is unclear how to interpret these findings in the setting of a normally grown fetus. For these reasons, umbilical artery Doppler velocimetry should not be performed routinely on low-risk women. Appropriate indications include IUGR, cord malformations, unexplained oligohydramnios, suspected or established preeclampsia, and possibly fetal cardiac anomalies. Umbilical artery Doppler velocimetry has not been shown to be useful in the evaluation of a variety of high-risk pregnancies, including diabetic and postterm pregnancies, primarily because of its high false-positive rate (Baschat, 2004; Farmakides et al, 1988; Landon et al, 1989; Stokes et al, 1991).

As such, in the absence of IUGR, obstetric management decisions are not usually made on the basis of Doppler velocimetry studies alone. Nonetheless, new applications for Doppler technology are currently under investigation. A recent application that has proved extremely useful is the noninvasive evaluation of fetal anemia resulting from isoimmunization. When a fetus develops severe anemia, cardiac output increases and there is a decline in blood viscosity, resulting in an increase in MCA blood flow, which can be demonstrated by measuring the peak velocity using MCA Doppler velocimetry (Mari et al, 1995). This demonstration can help the perinatologist to better counsel such patients about the need for cordocentesis and fetal blood transfusion. Doppler studies of other vessels—including the uterine artery, fetal aorta, ductus venosus, and fetal carotid arteries—have contributed considerably to our knowledge of maternal-fetal physiology, but as yet have resulted in few clinical applications.

SUMMARY

There are a variety of testing modalities available to the obstetrician for assessing fetal well-being in the antepartum period, each with specific applications, advantages, and disadvantages. As such, it is difficult to apply generalized protocols to the assessment of the fetus. A stepwise approach entails applying the appropriate tests for low-risk patients and identifying those patients, from the results of those tests or from historical factors, for whom further testing is needed. Although many tests, including NST, fetal weight assessment, and uterine artery Doppler, may be somewhat nonspecific and may have misleading false-positive rates, combining those tests with others increases the specificity. Test results that raise concerns require further investigation or active management.

SUGGESTED READINGS

American College of Obstetricians and Gynecologists (ACOG): *Fetal macrosomia*, Washington, DC, 2000, ACOG Practice Bulletin No. 22, ACOG.

American College of Obstetricians and Gynecologists (ACOG): *Gestational diabetes*, Washington, DC, 2001, ACOG Practice Bulletin No. 30, ACOG.

American College of Obstetricians and Gynecologists (ACOG): *Shoulder dystocia*, Washington, DC, 2002, ACOG Practice Bulletin No. 40, ACOG.

American College of Obstetricians and Gynecologists (ACOG): *Ultrasonography in pregnancy*, Washington, DC, 2009, ACOG Practice Bulletin No. 101, ACOG.

Anderson NG, Jolley IJ, Wells JE: Sonographic estimation of fetal weight: comparison of bias, precision and consistency using 12 different formulae, *Ultrasound Obstet Gynecol* 30:173-179, 2007.

Baschat AA: Doppler application in the delivery timing of the preterm growth-restricted fetus: another step in the right direction, *Ultrasound Obstet Gynecol* 23:111-118, 2004.

Brace RA, Wolf EJ: Normal amniotic fluid volume changes throughout pregnancy, *Am J Obstet Gynecol* 161:382-388, 1989.

Freeman RK, Anderson G, Dorchester W: A prospective multi-institutional study of antepartum fetal heart rate monitoring: I. risk of perinatal mortality and morbidity according to antepartum fetal heart rate test results, *Am J Obstet Gynecol* 143:771-777, 1982.

Freeman RK, Anderson G, Dorchester W: A prospective multi-institutional study of antepartum fetal heart rate monitoring: II. contraction stress test versus nonstress test for primary surveillance, *Am J Obstet Gynecol* 143:778-781, 1982.

Macones GA, Hankins GD, Spong CY, et al: The 2008 National Institute of Child Health and Human Development workshop report on electronic fetal monitoring: update on definitions, interpretation, and research guidelines, *Obstet Gynecol* 112:661-666, 2008.

Manning FA, Morrison I, Harman CR, et al: Fetal assessment based on fetal biophysical profile scoring: experience in 19,221 referred high-risk pregnancies, *Am J Obstet Gynecol* 157:880-884, 1987.

Manning FA, Morrison I, Lange IR, et al: Fetal assessment based on fetal biophysical profile scoring: experience in 12,620 referred high-risk pregnancies: I. Perinatal mortality by frequency and etiology, *Am J Obstet Gynecol* 151:343-350, 1985.

Complete references and supplemental color images used in this text can be found online at www.expertconsult.com

PREMATURITY: CAUSES AND PREVENTION

Tonse N.K. Raju and Caroline Signore

BURDEN OF PRETERM BIRTH

Despite major advances in perinatal medicine, preterm births (PTBs) in the United States have been increasing over the past two decades, reaching a high of 12.8% of live births in 2006 (Martin et al, 2009). This rate amounts to one PTB occurring at each minute of every day, throughout the year. From the perspective of a societal health care burden, these data are sobering, because infants born even 1 or 2 weeks before full term suffer higher rates of morbidity and mortality throughout life. Thus even a minimal increase in the PTB rate has a major effect on the societal burden of disease. Conversely, even a modest reduction in the PTB rate can have a major positive effect on the societal health care burden. In this chapter we focus on the etiology, prediction, and prevention of PTB.

DEFINITIONS

The World Health Organization defines *preterm birth* as a birth occurring either before 37 completed weeks of gestation or on or before the 259th day, counting from the first day of the last menstrual period. Only completed weeks of gestation are reported; therefore an infant born 6 days after completing 35 weeks of gestation is noted as 35 weeks, not rounded up to 36 weeks. However, one can precisely denote the exact gestational age by using a superscript for the number of days after the completion of the gestational week. Thus, the infant in the example can be noted as being born at $35^{6/7}$ weeks' gestation.

PTBs can be categorized into three major gestational age strata: those occurring at <32 weeks' (on or before 224 days) gestation, usually referred to as *very preterm births*; those occurring between $32^{0/7}$ and $33^{6/7}$ weeks' (between 225 and 238 days) gestation (a group with no specific name, but can be termed *moderate preterm births*); and those occurring between $34^{0/7}$ and $36^{6/7}$ weeks' (239 to 259 days) gestation, referred to as *late preterm births* (Figure 14-1). It is worth noting that the phrase *near term* is no longer used to refer to the third group, because the phrase falsely conveys a message that such "borderline" preterm infants are almost as mature as term infants (Raju et al, 2006).

EPIDEMIOLOGY

In the United States, the PTB rate increased from 10.6% in 1990 to 12.8% in 2006—a 21% increase (Goldenberg et al, 2008; Martin et al, 2009). This increase was part of a general trend in the distribution of gestational age at delivery, which showed a dramatic, leftward shift by 1 week, such that the peak modal week (the gestational week at which most deliveries occurred) shifted from 40 weeks in 1992 to 39 weeks in 2002 (Davidoff et al, 2006). Whereas this shift has decreased births at 41 weeks' gestation or later, it has also led to an increase in the number of all PTBs.

Preliminary data in the United States for 2007 showed that among the total number of live births, 2.04% were very preterm, 1.59% were moderate preterm, and 9.03% were late preterm (Hamilton et al, 2009). Thus, of all the PTBs the late PTB stratum was the largest at 71%, the very PTB stratum was intermediate at 16.1%, and the moderate PTB stratum was the smallest at 12.6%.

The U.S. 2007 preliminary data also suggest a slight decline in the total PTB rate to 12.7%, from 12.8% in 2006. The 2007 decline was predominantly among late PTB, from 9.1% in 2006 to 9.0% in 2007 (Hamilton et al, 2009). However, trends over longer periods need to be examined to confirm these preliminary findings and to judge whether the PTB rates in the United States have leveled or begun to decline.

ETIOLOGY AND RISK FACTORS

Individual PTBs can be categorized into two major groups: (1) spontaneous PTB (accounting for up to 60% of all PTBs), which occur after the spontaneous onset of preterm labor, and in some cases, after spontaneous preterm rupture of the fetal membranes before the onset of labor; and (2) indicated PTB (accounting for about 40% of PTBs), which arise from interventions by the health care team to reduce poor outcomes in the presence of specific medical, surgical, or obstetric conditions and indications in the mother or fetus.

SPONTANEOUS PRETERM BIRTHS

In most spontaneous PTBs, the precise cause for the onset of labor remains unknown; however, a variety of risk factors have been identified (Behrman and Butler, 2007) (Table 14-1).

BEHAVIORAL AND PSYCHOLOGICAL CONTRIBUTORS

Behavioral and psychological contributors, especially when occurring in constellation, tend to increase the risk for PTB. Some of these factors include excessive consumption of alcohol, smoking, use of cocaine, unfavorable diet, prolonged and stressful physical labor during pregnancy, shorter interval between pregnancies, and a variety of psychosocial stressors (Goldenberg et al, 2008).

Sociodemographic and Community Contributors

Increased risk for PTB has been associated with extremes of maternal age (<17 or >35 years), unmarried status, poverty, adverse neighborhood conditions, and lower educational attainment. The causal pathways for the

CATEGORIZATION OF GESTATIONAL
AGE AT BIRTH

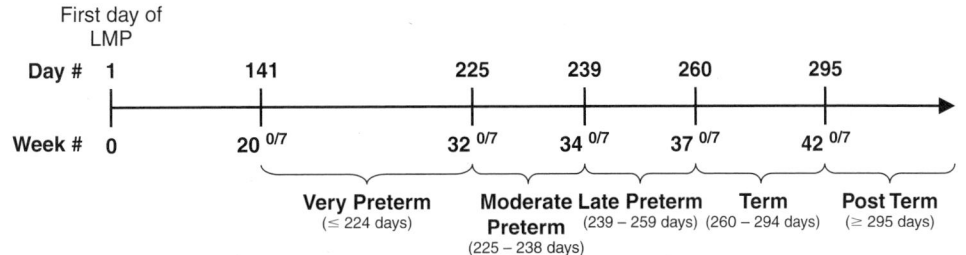

FIGURE 14-1 Categorization of gestational age at birth.

TABLE 14-1   Risk Factors for Preterm Birth*

Category	Specific Variable	Effect Size and Comments
Behavioral and psychological contributors	Tobacco and alcohol	Inconsistent effect; these variables may be confounders with lower socioeconomic status
	Other drugs	Cocaine users experience a twofold increase in PTB; other drugs (e.g., marijuana) have inconsistent effects
	Nutrition	Low prepregnancy weight and lower weight gain increase PTB risk; these factors may be confounders with other medical conditions
	Physical activity, employment	Inconsistent effect of employment per se; but long work hours and stress have been associated with increased risk of PTBs
	Douching	Frequent and prolonged vaginal douching during pregnancy can alter vaginal flora and enhance the risk for PTB
	Stress (chronic, acute, life events)	Emotional stress, living conditions, major stressful life events, discrimination, and racism, and other forms of stress experiences may act through diverse mechanistic pathways, affect many body functions, such as the HPA, immune defense mechanisms, and autonomic nervous system, leading to PTB
Sociodemographic contributors	Maternal age	U-shaped relationship with maternal age and PTB rate, with increased risk in women <17 and >35 years; in black women, risk seems to increase by age 30
	Marital status	Although unmarried mothers have higher rates of PTB, the protective effects of marital status on the PTB rate may vary across different ethnic groups
	Race and ethnicity	Non-Hispanic black women have high rates of PTB; the causes are likely to multifactorial
	Socioeconomic conditions	Disparities in PTB rates by SES (high rates with low SES) are well documented, although the etiologic pathways for such effects are unclear
	Community and neighborhood	Adverse neighborhood conditions influence health outcomes, including PTB rates, through direct and indirect pathways
Medical and pregnancy conditions	Maternal medical illnesses and conditions	Indicated PTBs may occur with chronic hypertension, hypertensive disorders of pregnancy, systemic lupus, hyperthyroidism, pregestational diabetes mellitus, cardiac disease, asthma, renal disorders, and gestational diabetes mellitus
	Underweight and low weight gain	Low prepregnancy weight and lower-than-average increase in weight during pregnancy have been documented with higher rates of PTB
	Fetal conditions	In vitro fertilization, assisted reproductive technology, multifetal pregnancy, congenital anomalies, umbilical cord accidents
	Pregnancy conditions	Placenta previa, first-trimester vaginal bleeding, abruption of the placenta, uterine malformations
	Infections	Maternal-fetal infections, bacterial vaginosis
	Other	Interpregnancy interval of less than 6 months is estimated to increase PTB rate by 30% to 60%; family history of PTB is associated with higher rates of PTB; it is unclear if the effect is caused by genetic factors, environmental factors, or a combination of both
Environmental toxins	Lead, air pollution	Exposures linked to higher PTB rates include lead, tobacco smoke, air pollution (sulfur dioxide, particulates, carbon monoxide), and arsenic in drinking water; however, interactions between such exposures and confounding factors such as SES, race, and ethnicity need to be studied
Gene-environment interactions		Genetic susceptibility and gene environmental interactions is a rapidly evolving field; according to some experts, epigenetic mechanisms are the final common pathway to explain diverse sociodemographic, racial, and ethnic factors and their effects on PTB rates

HPA, Hypthalamopituitary axis; *PTB*, preterm birth; *SES*, socioeconomic status.
*For a comprehensive discussion of various factors noted in this table, please see Behrman RE, Butler AS: *Preterm birth, causes, consequences, and prevention*, Washington, DC, 2007, The National Academies Press.

association between adverse sociodemographic and community contributors are complex and poorly understood. It should be noted, however, that these factors are interrelated and often coexist with other medical or obstetric conditions.

Racial Disparity

African American women are consistently found to have higher PTB rates than women of other racial and ethnic groups (16% to 18% versus 5% to 9%; Goldenberg et al, 2008). Black women are also more likely to experience preterm premature rupture of membranes (PPROM) and very PTB. The reason for this persistent racial disparity is unknown.

Previous Preterm Birth

The prior history of a PTB is consistently identified as one of the strongest predictors of preterm delivery, elevating the risk to more than twofold the background rate (Mercer et al, 1999). Risk is further elevated if there is a history of multiple PTBs, consecutive previous PTBs, and births at earlier gestational ages (Spong, 2007).

Short Cervix

Among asymptomatic women, cervical length less than 25 mm at 24 weeks' gestation, as measured by transvaginal ultrasound, in singleton pregnancy is associated with a sixfold increase in the risk of delivery before 35 weeks' gestation (Iams et al, 1996). Among women in suspected preterm labor, a cervical length of less than 15 mm may discriminate between women who are likely to deliver preterm and those whose pregnancies will continue (Tsoi et al, 2003).

Genetic Factors

The risk of PTB is increased in women with a positive family history of PTB. Single nucleotide polymorphisms in a number of maternal and fetal candidate genes involved in inflammatory pathways have been associated with PPROM and PTB (Varner and Esplin, 2005). Studies using genomic and proteomic approaches to further investigate molecular risk factors for PTB are in progress.

Infections

Overt or subclinical intrauterine infection, which might lead to rupture of the membranes before onset of labor, has been hypothesized to etiologically contribute to onset of labor, especially among very PTBs. The most common route of intrauterine infection is ascension of vaginal bacteria. Bacterial vaginosis (BV) is a common vaginal infection characterized by a shift in vaginal flora toward anaerobic species, accompanied by an abnormally high pH. Risk of PTB is increased up to twofold in women with BV (Hillier et al, 1995; Meis et al, 1995). Periodontal disease has also been linked to PTB (Jeffcoat et al, 2001); however, the biologic pathway is not well understood.

Multifetal Gestation

Twin and higher-order pregnancies account for 3% of all births. Multiple pregnancies are at increased risk of preterm delivery, with approximately 40% of twins delivered spontaneously before 37 weeks' gestation. Uterine overdistention is believed to be the major etiologic factor in these births. An additional 20% of twins will develop maternal or fetal complications leading to indicated PTB. The mean gestational age at delivery is 35 weeks' gestation for twins, 32 weeks' gestation for triplets, and 29 weeks' gestation for quadruplets (Elliott, 2005; Martin et al, 2003).

Infertility Treatment

The use of assisted reproductive technology (ART), in which gametes are manipulated outside the body, is steadily increasing. In 2006, 41,000 American women delivered after successful infertility treatment with ART, accounting for approximately 1% of all live births (Sunderam et al, 2009). The use of ART is strongly associated with multifetal pregnancies, dramatically increasing the risk for PTBs. However, even singleton pregnancies following ART have a twofold higher risk for PTB (Jackson et al, 2004), suggesting a complex relationship between a history of infertility, ART, and reproductive outcomes. Medical treatment of infertility (i.e., ovulation induction) is also associated with multiple gestation and PTB. In 2003, 21% of twin, 37% of triplet, and 62% of quadruplet and higher-order multiple births were attributable to non-ART ovulation induction (Dickey, 2007).

Maternal Body Habitus: Underweight and Obesity

Low prepregnancy body mass index (<18.9 kg/m^2) is associated with a 1.5- to 2.5-fold increase in the risk of PTB and has previously been a target of PTB prevention efforts (Goldenberg et al, 1998; Siega-Riz et al, 1996). Currently there is an epidemic of overweight and obesity in all U.S. populations. Maternal obesity is not associated with an increased risk of spontaneous PTB (Hendler et al, 2005). However, maternal obesity is a risk factor for a variety of pregnancy complications, including congenital anomalies, preeclampsia, and macrosomia, which may result in the need for indicated PTB (Aly et al, 2010).

Fetal Fibronectin

Fetal fibronectin (FFN) is a glycoprotein involved in the adherence of the fetal membranes to the uterine wall. The presence of FFN in the cervicovaginal secretions has been considered a risk factor for PTB and has been evaluated for its predictor value of preterm delivery in large cohort studies. A positive test result for FFN at 22 to 24 weeks' gestation in asymptomatic women is significantly associated with PTB (Goldenberg et al, 1998); however, because of its low positive predictive value, it is not a reliable universal screening tool in low-risk women. The most useful aspect of FFN assessment is its high negative predictive value: among women with signs and symptoms of preterm labor and a negative FFN, 99% will not deliver over the next 7 days (Lu et al, 2001).

INDICATED PRETERM BIRTHS

Medical and Pregnancy Conditions

Well-recognized medical and pregnancy-related conditions are noted in Table 14-1. Many of these conditions are also encountered to a greater extent among women in lower socioeconomic strata and among those living under adverse conditions.

Maternal and fetal conditions that can lead to indicated preterm deliveries include diabetes; hypertension; preeclampsia or eclampsia; maternal cardiovascular and pulmonary disorders; multifetal gestations; uterine structural disorders; polyhydramnios or oligohydramnios; placenta previa, abruption, and other uterine hemorrhagic events; chorioamnionitis and fetal infection; fetal distress; and congenital anomalies.

Causes for Increasing Preterm Birth

The precise reasons for increasing rates of PTB are unclear. The contribution of many factors is noted in Table 14-2 (Behrman and Butler, 2007; Raju, 2006; Raju et al, 2006).

Etiologic Pathways

Preterm labor and delivery arise from abnormal activation of parturition. No single mechanism describes all cases of PTB; rather, preterm parturition can be viewed as an obstetric syndrome with multiple etiologies, a long preclinical phase, frequent fetal involvement, and genetic factors that modify risk. Contributing pathologic processes may include intrauterine inflammation or infection, uterine

TABLE 14-2 Possible Causes for Increasing Preterm Birth*

Variable	Comments
Increasing maternal age at first pregnancy	Number of pregnant women 35-39 years nearly doubled between 1993 and 2003
Increasing infertility treatment and multifetal gestations	Number of women seeking infertility treatment increased twofold between 1996 and 2002
Change in practice parameters or guidelines	Improved surveillance and increased medical interventions to prevent still births
Increasing cesarean section rates and decreasing VBAC	—
Increasing maternal overweight and obesity	Errors in estimating gestational age of macrosomic fetus
Inaccuracy in estimating gestational age	Lack of early ultrasound examination
Iatrogenic or nonmedical reasons	Maternal request for early delivery or other logistical considerations of the patient, family or health care team

VBAC, Vaginal birth after cesarean.
*For a review, please see Goldenberg et al (2008), Raju (2006), and Reddy et al (2007, 2009).

ischemia, uterine over distension, abnormal allograft reaction, allergy, cervical insufficiency, and hormonal dysregulation (Romero et al, 2006).

Allostatic Load

Recent studies of the pathophysiology of and biologic responses to stress have uncovered a series of causal pathways for adverse outcomes caused by stresses at multiple levels and from different sources. The biologic responses to stressors have been collectively called *allostatic load*, a summary measure of major perturbations in the autonomic, endocrine, and immune systems. Allostatic load has been linked to accelerated aging, worsened immunologic tolerance, ineffective defense systems, and increased cardiovascular morbidity. Abnormal allostatic load during the entire life span of a woman can potentially modulate her biologic systems and worsen perinatal outcomes (Groer and Burns, 2009; Herring and Gawlik, 2007; Latendresse, 2009; Lu and Halfon, 2003; McEwen, 2006; Shannon et al, 2007). Studies are under way to understand the complex relationship between the effects of sociodemographic and biologic stressors on organ systems and their influence on perinatal outcomes.

PREVENTION OF PRETERM BIRTH

Despite intense research efforts, few widely effective strategies for preventing PTB have been identified. Because of the multifactorial nature of preterm labor and birth, it is unlikely that any single intervention could serve to prevent all cases of prematurity. In the United States, efforts have focused on addressing specific risk factors to prevent PTB (i.e., secondary prevention), such as treatment of infection, and interventions to mitigate the morbidity and mortality of PTB (i.e., tertiary prevention), such as administration of tocolytic drugs to women in preterm labor (Iams et al, 2008). A better understanding of the complex mechanisms leading to preterm labor and birth is needed to advance development of interventions to prevent PTB. In this section, a number of strategies—both encouraging and disappointing in terms of effectiveness—are described.

Progesterone

Progesterone is thought to have antiinflammatory effects and to be a smooth muscle relaxant that inhibits uterine contractions. Administration of progesterone has shown the most promise as an effective intervention for preventing PTB in women with certain risk factors for PTB. In a recent metaanalysis of 11 trials, progesterone significantly decreased PTB of singleton gestations less than 34 weeks in women with a prior spontaneous preterm birth (SPTB) by 85%, with a number needed to treat of seven (Dodd et al, 2005). However, progesterone does not prevent PTB in women carrying twins (Rouse et al, 2007) or triplets (Caritis et al, 2009). Petrini et al, (2005) estimated that if all eligible women with a history of prior SPTB were treated with progesterone, then 10,000 PTBs per year could be prevented. Progesterone treatment does not appear to pose a developmental risk to the fetus or infant. In a follow-up study of children exposed to 7-alpha hydroxy-progesterone caproate versus placebo in utero, there were no differences in growth or neurodevelopmental measures between groups at age 4 years (Northen et al, 2007).

Cerclage

Cervical cerclage is a purse-string suture of the cervix intended to mechanically prevent cervical dilation. A number of investigators have evaluated the use of cerclage to prevent PTB in women with shortened cervical length, and they have not demonstrated a significant effect (Berghella et al, 2004; To et al, 2004). A more recent trial indicated a significant beneficial effect (adjusted odds ratio, 0.23; 95% confidence interval, 0.08 to 0.66) of cerclage in women with a history of previous SPTB and cervical length less than 15 mm (Berghella et al, 2008; Owen et al, 2009).

Limited Embryo Transfer

Preterm delivery of multifetal pregnancies arising from ART can be prevented in many cases by limiting the number of embryos transferred to the uterus. The proportion of in vitro fertilization cycles in which three or more fresh embryos were transferred declined significantly in the United States between 1996 and 2002 (92% to 54%; p <0.001); however, the proportion of single-embryo transfer cycles remained small (2.5% in 2002) (Reynolds and Schieve, 2006). Recent practice guidelines from the American Society for Reproductive Medicine call for wider consideration of single-embryo transfer in many clinical situations (American Society for Reproductive Medicine, 2008).

Multifetal Pregnancy Reduction

Reduction of multifetal pregnancy, or the selective termination of one or more fetuses in a high-order pregnancy, has been proposed as a means to reduce the risk of prematurity and other pregnancy complications. Although effective at preventing some very PTBs, the procedure carries an approximately 1% risk of loss of the entire pregnancy (Stone et al, 2002) and can create profound ethical dilemmas (American College of Obstetricians and Gynecologists, 2007).

Treatment of Vaginal Infections

Despite consistent associations between lower genital tract infection and PTB, multiple randomized trials have failed to demonstrate a benefit of screening and antibiotic treatment for vaginitis or genital tract colonization on the PTB rates (Carey et al, 2000; Iams et al, 2008; Klebanoff et al, 2001; McDonald et al, 2007).

Treatment of Periodontal Disease

PTB has been associated with maternal periodontal disease in a number of studies, and early clinical trials suggested that treatment of periodontitis reduces the risk of PTB (Jeffcoat et al, 2003; Lopez et al, 2002). On the other hand, a recent multicenter clinical trial in the United States found that, whereas periodontal disease improved in pregnant women randomized to treatment, there were no differences in rates of PTB, low birthweight, or fetal growth restriction in the treatment group compared with controls (Michalowicz et al, 2006).

Tocolytics: Acute and Maintenance

Preterm labor (PTL), is defined as the onset before 37 weeks' gestation of regular uterine contractions that result in cervical change. Although numerous pharmacologic and nonpharmacologic treatments have been aimed at arresting PTL and preventing PTB, none have been shown to prolong pregnancy for more than 2 to 7 days (Iams et al, 2008). Nevertheless, tocolytic drugs are often used to allow for the administration of steroids and maternal transfer to a facility capable of caring for a preterm neonate. Drugs commonly used to treat PTL are summarized in Table 14-3. Maintenance tocolysis after an acute episode of PTL has not been shown to prevent PTB (Dodd et al, 2006; Gaunekar and Crowther, 2004; Nanda et al, 2002).

MANAGEMENT OF PRETERM PREMATURE RUPTURE OF MEMBRANES

Preterm premature rupture of membranes (PPROM) is defined as the prelabor rupture of membranes before 37 weeks' gestation. The period between initial leakage of

TABLE 14-3 Drugs Commonly Used to Treat Preterm Labor*

Agent	Class, Mechanism	Maternal Side Effects	Fetal and Neonatal Effects
Magnesium sulfate	Decreases intracellular calcium, inhibits contractile response	Flushing, lethargy, nausea, muscle weakness	Lethargy, decreased tone, respiratory depression
Terbutaline	β-Mimetic	Tachycardia, hyperglycemia, myocardial ischemia, pulmonary edema	Tachycardia, hyperinsulinemia, hyperglycemia
Nifedipine	Calcium channel blocker	Hypotension, flushing	None reported
Indomethacin	NSAID, prostaglandin synthase inhibitor	Gastrointestinal upset	Decreased renal function, oligohydramnios, closure of the ductus arteriosus
Atosiban (not available in the United States)	Oxytocin inhibitor	Hypersensitivity, injection site reaction	Increased risk of fetal or infant death if administered before 28 wk

NSAID, Nonsteroidal antiinflammatory drug.
*For a review, see American College of Obstetricians and Gynecologists (2007), Dodd et al (2006), Gaunekar and Crowther (2004), Nanda et al (2002), Simhan and Caritis (2007), and Stone et al (2002).

fluid and the onset of labor and delivery is known as the *latency period*. Without treatment, the latency period after PPROM is usually less than 1 week, with an inverse relationship between the gestational age at rupture and length of the latency period. In a large multicenter trial, a 7-day course of broad-spectrum antibiotics was shown to prolong the latency period for up to 3 weeks in women who had experienced PPROM at 24 to 32 weeks' gestation. In addition, antepartum antibiotic treatment decreased the incidence of chorioamnionitis and major morbidity (respiratory distress syndrome, early sepsis, severe intra ventricular hemorrhage, or severe necrotizing enterocolitis) in the infants (Mercer et al, 1997).

SUMMARY

PTBs are occurring at epidemic proportions in the United States. With more than 4.3 million live births each year, a prematurity rate of 12.5% results in more than 537,000 PTBs annually. As described in other chapters, preterm infants are at greater risk for mortality, and short- and long-term morbidities compared with term infants. A recent study from Norway on the adult-age outcomes of preterm infants reported that even mild prematurity was associated with significantly elevated risk for long-term adverse medical, behavioral, psychological, and vocational outcomes (Moster et al, 2008). In addition to the families' burden of illness, death, and disability, society bears a large burden of health care costs related to PTBs. The collective economic burden from prematurity was more than $26 billion in 2005 (Behrman and Butler, 2007). Given the complex nature of the risk factors and causal pathways for PTBs, and the difficulties in diagnosing, preventing, and treating them, there have been renewed calls in support of multidisciplinary research to address the problems of PTBs. The Institute of Medicine of the National Academies of Science issued a major publication providing specific recommendations and guidelines for research, surveillance, and education on this topic (Behrman and Butler, 2007). The U.S. Senate approved the PREEMIE

Act on August 1, 2006. This bill called for efforts to reduce preterm labor and delivery and the risk of pregnancy-related deaths and complications, and to reduce infant mortality caused by prematurity. The U.S. House of Representatives passed the bill unanimously on December 9, 2006, and the president signed it into law on December 22, 2006 (March of Dimes Foundation, 2006). The March of Dimes Foundation initiated the *Prematurity Campaign*, designed to educate and inform health care professionals, industry, government agencies, and the general public about prematurity-related issues. These and other efforts have begun recently and will take time to yield positive results. Their collective effect on reducing the burden of PTBs needs to be monitored on a long-term basis.

SUGGESTED READINGS

Behrman RE, Butler AS: *Preterm birth, causes, consequences, and prevention*, Washington, DC, 2007, The National Academies Press.
Dodd JM, Crowther CA, Cincotta R, et al: Progesterone supplementation for preventing preterm birth: a systematic review and meta-analysis, *Acta Obstet Gynecol Scand* 84:526-533, 2005.
Goldenberg RL, Culhane JF, Iams JD, et al: Epidemiology and causes of preterm birth, *Lancet* 371:75-84, 2008.
Goldenberg RL, Iams JD, Mercer BM, et al: The preterm prediction study: the value of new vs standard risk factors in predicting early and all spontaneous preterm births. NICHD MFMU Network, *Am J Public Health* 88:233-238, 1998.
Iams JD, Romero R, Culhane JF, et al: Primary, secondary, and tertiary interventions to reduce the morbidity and mortality of preterm birth, *Lancet* 371:164-175, 2008.
Owen J, Hankins G, Iams JD, et al: Multicenter randomized trial of cerclage for preterm birth prevention in high-risk women with shortened midtrimester cervical length, *Am J Obstet Gynecol* 201:375, 2009.
Raju TN, Higgins RD, Stark AR, et al: Optimizing care and outcome for late-preterm (near-term) infants: a summary of the workshop sponsored by the National Institute of Child Health and Human Development, *Pediatrics* 118:1207-1214, 2006.
Romero R, Espinoza J, Kusanovic JP, et al: The preterm parturition syndrome, *BJOG* 113(Suppl 3):17-42, 2006.
Simhan HN, Caritis SN: Prevention of preterm delivery, *N Engl J Med* 357:477-487, 2007.
Spong CY: Prediction and prevention of recurrent spontaneous preterm birth, *Obstet Gynecol* 110:405-415, 2007.
Varner MW, Esplin MS: Current understanding of genetic factors in preterm birth, *BJOG* 112(Suppl 1):28-31, 2005

Complete references used in this text can be found online at www.expertconsult.com

COMPLICATED DELIVERIES: OVERVIEW

Sarah A. Waller, Sameer Gopalani, and Thomas J. Benedetti

Historically, child birth was often regarded as a perilous undertaking. However, over the past century in the United States, perinatal and maternal mortality have dramatically fallen with advances in modern obstetric care, such as widespread use of antibiotics, easy access to expedient cesarean delivery, and better understanding of the proper use of instruments such as forceps and vacuum extraction (Ali and Norwitz, 2009). Indeed, adverse outcomes are generally uncommon in modern obstetrics, and unlike in the past, most labor and delivery concludes with a healthy mother and neonate. Nevertheless, complicated deliveries still exist, and knowledge of their conduct and sequelae is still required for the administration of proper maternal and infant care.

In this chapter we will first address the complicated vaginal delivery, with particular attention to neonatal outcomes. We will then discuss cesarean delivery and vaginal birth after a prior cesarean delivery (VBAC) and what neonatal implications these may have. Before discussing complicated labor and its neonatal effects, it is important to have a brief understanding of the conduct of normal labor and delivery. A comprehensive discussion of labor and delivery is beyond the scope of this chapter, and the interested reader is directed *Williams Obstetrics*, ed 23, chapter on normal labor.

The first stage of labor begins with the onset of regular uterine contractions with concomitant cervical dilation and effacement, and it ends with complete cervical dilation. The first stage is further subdivided into a latent phase, the length of which is variable and can last for several hours, and an active phase, which usually begins when the cervix is dilated 3 to 4 cm and is marked by further rapid, progressive cervical dilation and effacement. Often the diagnosis of the transition from latent to active phase labor is retrospective, because the time of onset of active labor is variable by patient. The second stage begins with complete cervical dilation and terminates with the expulsion of the fetus from the birth canal. The third stage of labor concludes with the delivery of the placenta.

Disorders of the conduct of labor are of either protraction, in which cervical dilation or fetal descent occurs but is at a rate much less than expected, or arrest. Both disorders are addressed by operative delivery if they are unresponsive to active medical management; this can be performed abdominally through cesarean section or vaginally by obstetric forceps or vacuum extraction if the cervix is fully dilated and specific criteria are fulfilled (see later discussion on operative vaginal delivery). All these modalities can have neonatal and maternal effects, and the choice of instrument or mode of delivery must always be selected taking these potential morbidities into account.

CESAREAN SECTION

Neonatal mortality within 7 days of birth was 17.8 per 1000 live births in 1950; it is currently 3.8 per 1000 (Ali and Norwitz, 2009). Certainly much of the improvement in neonatal survival stems from advances in neonatal intensive care and resuscitative techniques. Along with improved technology available to the pediatricians, however, is the fact that the last 50 years have also seen a dramatic increase in the universal access to safe cesarean section, which affords quick and timely fetal delivery. However, a cause-and-effect relationship between cesarean delivery and improved neonatal outcome has never been demonstrated, and recent evidence suggests that some current obstetric cesarean delivery practices may actually cause harm (Bates, 2009). Currently almost one mother in three is giving birth by cesarean section, a record level for the United States. Recommendations from the U.S. Department of Health and Human Services Healthy People 2010 recommend a cesarean section rate of less than 15% for a first pregnancy and 63% for previous cesarean sections. In addition, there are wide variations in cesarean delivery rates among hospitals in a given state or region, suggesting that factors other than pregnancy risk factors may be responsible for the current cesarean delivery rate. This rise in cesarean delivery has been associated with a parallel drop in the vaginal operative delivery rate to less than 10%. These two trends have increased the cost of childbirth in the United States and are now threatening many state budgets, because almost 50% of obstetric care cost is paid with public funds (i.e., Medicaid). In response as the result of a budget crisis, the state of Washington reduced hospital payment for uncomplicated cesarean delivery (DRG 371: Cesarean section) by reimbursing only the equivalent of a complicated vaginal birth (DRG 372: Normal delivery with problems), a projected savings of $2 million per year. Many states are actively working to safely reduce the rate of cesarean delivery. Projects are under way to reduce elective delivery before 39 weeks' gestation, safely promote VBAC and limit the occurrence of higher-order multiple gestations.

Cesarean section is usually performed through either a Pfannenstiel or vertical skin incision. The uterine incision is often made transversely in the lower uterine segment, because it minimizes intraoperative blood loss and future risk of rupture during subsequent labor, compared with a vertical or classical incision. The risk of rupture in future labor is thought to be 0.5% to 1.0% for a low transverse incision, compared to 4% to 9% for a classical incision (Feingold et al, 1988).

Cesarean delivery is also performed for disorders of protraction or arrest in the first stage of labor when conservative measures fail to augment delivery, such as oxytocin or amniotomy, or in the second stage when assisted or operative vaginal delivery is deemed unfeasible or unsafe.

Accepted obstetric indications for operative delivery are as follows:

1. Fetal malpresentation (e.g., shoulder or breech)
2. Placenta previa
3. Prior classical uterine incision

4. Fetal status not reassuring, remote from vaginal delivery
5. Higher-order multiple gestation (triplet or greater)
6. Fetal contraindications to labor (alloimmune thrombocytopenia, neural tube defect)
7. Maternal contraindication to labor (e.g., history of rectal or perineal fistulas from inflammatory bowel disease, large lower-uterine segment, cervical leiomyoma preventing vaginal delivery)
8. Maternal choice after counseling regarding risks versus benefits

COMPLICATED VAGINAL DELIVERY: OBSTETRIC FORCEPS AND VACUUM EXTRACTION

DESCRIPTION OF THE OBSTETRIC FORCEPS

Obstetric forceps have been used to facilitate vaginal deliveries since 1500 BC. Most commonly, the invention is credited to Peter Chamberlen and his brother of England. Designed originally as a means of extracting fetuses from women who were at high risk of dying during childbirth, forceps now are an alternative to cesarean delivery in women with a protracted second stage of labor. Originally, many of these instruments were furnished with hooks and other accessories of destruction, and they were intended to save the mother but not the fetus. Over the last 500 years, the modern instruments in current use have been through hundreds of modifications, safer techniques have been established, and the overriding goal now includes delivering an intact, living baby and a healthy mother (Meniru, 1996; O'Grady et al, 2002).

Current obstetric forceps were first devised for practical use in the sixteenth and seventeenth centuries and were perfected over the past 300 years into the models in current use. Although there are many variations on the standard blueprint depending on the indication for its use, all obstetric forceps have a similar design.

Forceps are made of stainless steel and consist of two blades (each approximately 37.5 cm long, crossing each other), a lock at the site of crossing, and a handle, whereby the instrument is grasped by the obstetrician. The long blades are parallel, divergent, or convergent, depending on the type of instrument; the lower 8 cm comprises the shank, which is the part between the blade proper and the handle, giving a length for the forceps that is sufficient to be locked easily outside the vagina. The four most common types of lock are the sliding lock, which can articulate anywhere along the shanks of the blade (Kielland and Barton's forceps); the English, which is fixed, a double slot lock; the French, which is a screw lock; and the German, which is a combination of the English and French. The part of the forceps that grasps the fetal head is the blade; this is further divided into the heel, which is the part closest to the lock, and the toe, which is the most distal part of the blade. The blade can be either fenestrated—meaning the body of the blade is hollow—or solid to prevent fetal head compression. A further modification is pseudofenestration, in which a solid blade has a ridged edge, combining the advantages of easier applicability and less fetal trauma that a solid blade affords with the ease of traction of a

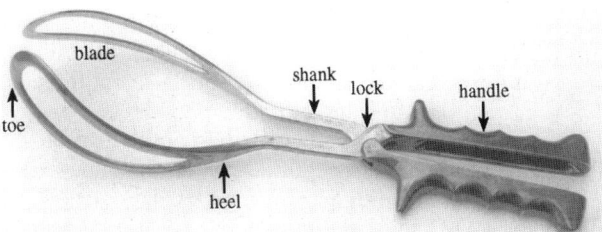

FIGURE 15-1 Simpson forceps: a standard obstetric forceps with features common to all such instruments.

TABLE 15-1 Types of Obstetric Forceps in Most Common Use

Type	Anatomic Modification	General Use
Classic		
Tucker-McClane	Solid blade	Nonmolded vertex
Simpson	Parallel shanks	Molded vertex or significant caput
Elliot	Convergent shanks	Nonmolded vertex
Laufe	Pseudofenestrated blade; divergent shanks	For preterm infants or EFW <2500 g
Rotational		
Kielland	English lock; absent pelvic curve	For rotation of fetal vertex ≥45 degrees
Breech		
Piper	Long handles with no pelvic curvature	For after-coming head in breech vaginal delivery

EFW, Estimated fetal weight

fenestrated blade. Obstetric forceps also possess a rounded cephalic curve, which accommodates the fetal vertex, and a pelvic curve that mirrors the maternal pelvic curve (Figure 15-1).

There are more than 60 different types of obstetric forceps described in the literature, but most of are not used currently. The forceps used most commonly today are described in Table 15-1, along with their indications for use and the variations in anatomy, which distinguish one from the other.

INDICATIONS FOR USE OF OBSTETRIC FORCEPS

To an individual without obstetric training, the use of forceps can be a dangerous and difficult undertaking, fraught with potential trauma for both the mother and fetus. It is true that the use of this instrument, if not performed carefully or appropriately, can have serious consequences. Nevertheless, with properly trained hands, and a proper appreciation of its use, forceps can be lifesaving for both mother and fetus.

The criteria for the safe application of obstetric forceps are as follows:

1. The cervix must be fully dilated.
2. The position of the fetal vertex must be known. Forceps should not be applied when the fetal presentation is in doubt.

3. The fetal vertex must be engaged within the maternal pelvis. Often in difficult or challenging labors, significant caput can lead to the false impression that fetal station is lower than it actually is. For this reason, the obstetrician must be confident that the actual biparietal diameter has passed the pelvic inlet and that the leading part of the fetal skull is beyond the level of the ischial spines. In addition, when the presentation is occiput posterior, the leading point of the fetal skull may appear to be lower in the pelvis although the biparietal diameter has not yet passed through the pelvic inlet; this can also lead to an erroneous conclusion about fetal station.

4. When the forceps are properly applied, the sagittal suture must be exactly midway between the blades, and the lambdoidal sutures should be equidistant (usually one fingerbreadth) from the edge of the blade.

If these conditions are not met, application of the forceps should be reconsidered. Furthermore, in 1988 the American College of Obstetricians and Gynecologists (ACOG) revised its classification of the type of forceps delivery, according to the station of the fetal vertex before forceps application (Ali and Norwitz, 2009), which is as follows:

1. Outlet forceps—the fetal vertex is visible at the labia without manually separating them, and the fetal skull has reached the pelvic floor
2. Low forceps—the leading point of the fetal skull is greater than 2 cm beyond the ischial spines
3. Mid forceps—the fetal head is engaged and is beyond the level of the ischial spines; the forceps should be applied only if cesarean delivery is not quickly or imminently possible, and the fetus is in distress; or there should be a high likelihood that the forceps operation will be successful
4. High forceps—the vertex is not engaged (i.e., not at the level of the ischial spines or beyond); under these circumstances, the forceps must never be applied.

The forceps are further divided into whether they are rotational (sagittal suture is ≥45 degrees from the midline) or nonrotational (sagittal suture <45 degrees from the midline).

The indications for use of the obstetric forceps are:

1. Maternal exhaustion or inability to push (endotracheal intubation with sedation or paralysis; neuromuscular disease)
2. Fetal heart tracing not reassuring or fetal distress
3. Maternal contraindications to pushing (cardiopulmonary disease, cerebrovascular aneurysm)
4. After-coming head in a vaginal breech delivery
5. Facilitate difficult extraction of the fetal vertex during cesarean delivery

FORCEPS AND POTENTIAL NEONATAL MORBIDITY

As stated previously, forceps were used for hundreds of years without regard to fetal survival and were primarily needed to facilitate or terminate difficult labors for maternal benefit. Today, with the widespread availability of cesarean delivery, considerations turn to providing the best neonatal outcome possible; therefore the difficult forceps deliveries of the past have been abandoned. Nevertheless, forceps still play a crucial role in modern obstetrics, and if judiciously used can provide a safer alternative to cesarean delivery for both mother and baby.

The difficulty in interpreting the obstetric literature, in regard to neonatal morbidity incurred by forceps, is that the classification for type of forceps was revised by the ACOG in 1988; therefore prior studies do not use the same clinical criteria used currently to select appropriate candidates for forceps use. Furthermore, residency training in operative vaginal delivery has dramatically decreased over the past 30 years, potentially increasing fetal risk (Benedetto et al, 2007). Consequently, for proper interpretation of adverse outcomes, one must look to studies performed after the ACOG revised the classifications.

The incidence of operative vaginal delivery in the United States is approximately 5% (1 in 20 deliveries), ranging from 1% to 23% with a 99% success rate (Menacker and Martin, 2008). The prevalence of forceps use varies widely by region (highest in the South), and recent estimates show that it accounts for approximately 25% (1:4 ratio with vacuum extractions) of all operative vaginal deliveries (Benedetto et al, 2006). National statistics show that of the 1,268,502 deliveries in 12 states (31% of U.S. deliveries) in 2005, 1% were forceps assisted and 3.7% were vacuum assisted, for a estimated total national operative vaginal delivery rate of 4.7% (Menacker and Martin, 2008). Unfortunately, the prevalence of low, outlet, and mid-forceps (the application of forceps when the head is engaged but the leading point of the skull is more than +2 cm station) deliveries nationally is not known, nor is the rate of rotational and nonrotational forceps use. Neonatal outcome by type of forceps application is also not generally known and is hindered by the fact that even with the universal ACOG classification scheme, the determination of fetal station and type of forceps can be subjective and dependent on the experience and examining skill of the obstetrician. Moreover the indication for forceps use varies widely by clinical situation, and the neonatal morbidity that can result from a "difficult pull" in a patient with a transverse arrest with marked fetal asynclitism may be different from the quick delivery of a 2600-g fetus whose mother is unable to push, even if both deliveries are by low-forceps.

Nevertheless, what large studies show that long-term and short-term neonatal morbidity from outlet or low-forceps delivery is uncommon? In 2009, Prapas et al (2009) noted that the rate of vacuum- versus forceps-assisted deliveries had increased and that different maternal and neonatal outcomes have been proposed. The aim of their study was to compare the short-term maternal and neonatal outcomes between vacuum and forceps delivery. They conducted a medical record review of live born singleton, vacuum- and forceps-assisted deliveries. Of 7098 deliveries, 374 were instrument assisted, 324 were conducted by vacuum (86.7%), and 50 were assisted by forceps (13.3%). The incidence of third-degree lacerations and periurethral hematomas was similar between vacuum and forceps (3.4% vs. 2% and 0.3% vs. 0%, respectively), whereas perineal hematomas were more common in forceps compared with vacuum application (2% vs. 0.3%, respectively), albeit not significantly. The rate of neonates with Apgar scores ≤6 at 1 min was significantly higher after forceps compared with vacuum delivery (18% vs. 5.2%, respectively; $p = 0.0003$). The rate of neonatal trauma and respiratory distress syndrome did not differ significantly between the two groups. The conclusion was that both modes of instrumental vaginal delivery are safe in regard to maternal morbidity and neonatal trauma (Prapas et al, 2009).

Alternatively, Benedetto et al, (2007) found that in healthy women with antenatally normal singleton pregnancies at term, instrument-assisted deliveries are associated with the highest rate of short-term maternal and neonatal complications. Of the 332 women who underwent an operative vaginal delivery, 201 met study criteria and were analyzed, with 54% forceps-assisted deliveries. Maternal complications were mostly associated with forceps-assisted and vacuum-assisted instrumental deliveries (odds ratio [OR], 6.9; 95% confidence interval [CI], 2.9 to 16.4; and OR, 3.0; 95% CI, 1.1 to 8.8, respectively, versus spontaneous deliveries). Neonatal complications were also mostly correlated with forceps-assisted and vacuum-assisted instrumental deliveries (OR, 3.5; 95% CI, 1.9 to 6.7; and OR, 3.8; 95% CI, 2.0 to 7.4, respectively, versus spontaneous deliveries) (Table 15-2) (Bendetto et al, 2007).

There are few randomized prospective trials specifically addressing the issue of neonatal morbidity arising from forceps operations, yet those that exist suggest no significantly increased risk from operative vaginal delivery when compared with spontaneous birth. Yancey et al (1991) randomized 364 full-term women at +2 station to elective outlet forceps delivery or unassisted birth. Women with suspected fetal macrosomia or chorioamnionitis were excluded. Neonates were examined at birth and 72 hours of age, and cranial ultrasound examinations were performed by neonatologists 24 to 72 hours after birth. The spontaneous and forceps-assisted births had no statistically significant differences in the incidence of scalp abrasions, facial bruising, cephalhematoma, subconjunctival hemorrhage, or abnormal cranial sonograms (Herbst and Källén, 2008).

Several retrospective, population-based studies have further examined the issue of potential adverse neonatal sequelae arising from forceps procedures. Robertson et al

(1991) reclassified forceps operations in accordance with the 1988 revised ACOG guidelines and examined neonatal outcomes by type of forceps operation, matched to cesarean section with a second stage of at least 30 minutes, from a similar station. They found that mid-forceps operations compared with a cesarean section from a comparable station resulted in greater neonatal resuscitation requirements, lower umbilical artery pH, and *birth trauma*, defined as nerve injuries or fractures. There was no increased risk of trauma from low forceps procedures compared with cesarean delivery, although the prevalence of arterial cord pH less than 7.10 was increased (Keith et al, 1988). It must be noted, however, that this study was not randomized and that an abdominal delivery group is not necessarily an appropriate control for operative vaginal delivery. Nevertheless, this large population-based study (from a database of 20,831) emphasizes the relative safety of outlet and low-forceps procedures, casting some doubt as to the safety of mid-forceps operations.

The role of mid-forceps delivery in modern obstetrics, specifically in regard to rotation of 45 degrees or greater, has incited much controversy. The difficulty lies in the fact that no randomized trials exist comparing mid-forceps operations and other modes of delivery, and it is unlikely that any will be done in the near future given that training in this type of delivery has declined among obstetric residents in the United States (Kozak and Weeks, 2002; Learman, 1998).

Hankins et al reported a case-control study of 113 rotational forceps of 90 degrees or greater matched to 167 controls with rotation 45 degrees or less. They found no significant differences in major injuries, defined as skull fracture, brachial plexus, facial or sixth nerve palsy, and subdural hemorrhage. There were also no differences in the prevalence of cephalhematoma, clavicular fracture, or superficial laceration. All deliveries were performed with Kielland forceps by resident staff members, with attending supervision as required. The prevalence of nerve injury in these forceps-assisted operations ranged from 2% to 3%; there were no skull fractures (Lipitz et al, 1989).

The available literature supports the fact that neonatal morbidity from outlet or low forceps is exceedingly low, and comparable to spontaneous vaginal delivery. This finding comes from prospective data and large, population-based investigations. The evidence concerning neonatal safety from more advanced forceps operations (mid-forceps and rotations) shows that there is some degree of increased morbidity from these procedures, although whether this arises from the operative vaginal delivery itself or from difficult labor is not currently possible to discern (Meniru, 1996; O'Grady et al, 2002). In well-trained hands, the benefit of appropriately selected candidates for mid-forceps or rotational forceps may be justifiable, although the number of physicians in the United States who are facile and comfortable with attempting these procedures is steadily declining.

VACUUM DELIVERY: INDICATIONS, USES, AND COMPARISON WITH FORCEPS PROCEDURES

Operative vaginal delivery for the indications listed previously can also be performed by the vacuum extractor. Vacuum extraction was first described in 1705 by Dr. James

TABLE 15-2 Risk of Intracranial Injury According to Type of Delivery

Mode of Delivery	Incidence of Intracranial Injury
Vacuum	1 in 860
Forceps	1 in 664
Combined vacuum and forceps	1 in 256
Cesarean, in labor	1 in 907
Cesarean, not in labor	1 in 2750
Spontaneous vaginal delivery	1 in 1900

Adapted from Towner D, Castro MA, Eby-Wilkens E, Gilbert WM: Effect of mode of delivery in nulliparous women on intracranial injury, *N Engl J Med* 341:1709-1714, 1999.

Yonge, an English surgeon, several decades before the invention of the obstetric forceps. However, it did not gain widespread use until the 1950s, when it was popularized in a series of studies by the Swedish obstetrician Dr. Tage Malmström. By the 1970s, the vacuum extractor had almost completely replaced forceps for assisted vaginal deliveries in most northern European countries, but its popularity in many English-speaking countries, including the United States and the United Kingdom, was limited. By 1992, however, the number of vacuum-assisted deliveries surpassed the number of forceps-assisted deliveries in the United States, and by the year 2000 approximately 66% of operative vaginal deliveries were by vacuum (Ali and Norwitz, 2009; Hillier and Johanson, 1994).

The situations that indicate the use of the vacuum and the requirements that must be fulfilled for its correct use are identical to those for the obstetric forceps. The device consists of a metal or plastic cup (flexible or semirigid) that is applied to the fetal vertex. Care is taken in its application to ensure that an adequate seal has been created, and that no maternal soft tissue is trapped between the suction device and the fetus. Traction is then applied to the fetal head in the line of the birth canal in an effort to assist delivery. It is also cautioned that rocking movements or torque to the cup are not used. The premature infant is a relative contraindication to vacuum application. It is generally advised that no more than three detachments occur before attempts at vacuum extraction are abandoned (Ali and Norwitz, 2009).

In a laboratory experiment, Duchon et al (1988) compared the maximum force at suggested vacuum pressures (550-600 mm Hg) prior to detachments for different types of vacuum devices. They found that the average force of traction exerted before detachments ranged from 18 to 20 kg (Benedetto et al, 2007). This result is interesting to bear in mind when one considers the older data of Wylie who estimated the average tractive force required for delivery of infants weighing 15.95 kg for a primigravida and 11.33 kg for a multipara (Feingold et al, 1988) (Figure 15-2).

The original vacuum device developed in the 1950s by the Swedish obstetrician Dr. Tage Malmström was a disc-shaped stainless steel cup attached to a metal chain for traction. Because of technical problems and lack of experience with this instrument, vacuum devices did not gain popularity in the United States until the introduction of the disposable cups in the 1980s. There are two main types of disposable cups, which can be made of plastic, polyethylene, or silicone. The soft cup is a pliable, funnel- or bell-shaped cup, which is the most common type used in the United States. The rigid cup is a firm mushroom-shaped cup (M cup) similar to the original metal disc-shaped cup and is available in three sizes.

A metaanalysis of 1375 women in nine trials comparing soft and rigid vacuum extractor cups demonstrated that soft cups were more likely to fail to achieve a vaginal delivery, because of more frequent detachments (OR, 1.65; 95% CI, 1.19 to 2.29), but were associated with fewer scalp injuries (OR, 0.45; 95% CI, 0.15 to 0.60) and no increased risk of maternal perineal injury (Benedetto et al, 2007; Hillier and Johanson, 1994). For example, the risk of scalp laceration with the rigid Kiwi OmniCup (Clinical Innovations, Murray, Utah) was reported to be 14.1% compared with 4.5% using a standard vacuum device ($p = 0.006$). These and other authors concluded that handheld soft bell cups should be considered for more straightforward occiput-anterior deliveries, and that rigid M cups should be reserved for more complicated deliveries, such as those involving larger infants, significant caput succedaneum (scalp edema), occiput-posterior presentation, or asynclitism.

The vacuum extractor is widely used in the United States, but is not free of preventing neonatal injury. Other than superficial scalp lacerations or abrasions, which usually heal without incident, as well as local soft tissue swelling or bruising, the use of the vacuum has been associated with cephalhematoma and subgaleal hemorrhages.

Cephalhematoma occurs when the force created by the vacuum results in the rupture of diploic or emissary vessels between the periosteum and outer table of the skull; this fills the potential space that exists between the two with blood. Although cephalhematomas are often cosmetically alarming, they are limited to traveling along one cranial bone, because the firm periosteal attachments limit further extravasation of blood across suture lines. Thus large amounts of blood cannot usually collect in this space, and serious neonatal compromise from this bleeding is rare. In a randomized trial of continuous and intermittent vacuum application, Bofill examined factors associated with increasing the risk of cephalhematoma; they found that only asynclitism and traction time were independently related to this complication (Hartley and Hitti, 2005). There was a clear relationship between increasing time of vacuum application (up to 6 minutes) and cephalhematoma. Interestingly, Hartley and Hitti did not find a significant independent association of neonatal injury with continuous versus intermittent vacuum, or with decreasing gestational age or increasing birthweight. Furthermore, the number of detachments was not correlated with cephalhematoma. These results were further corroborated by Teng who conducted a prospective observational study of 134 vacuum extractions and found that only increasing total duration of vacuum application was associated with neonatal injury (Feingold et al, 1988). Metaanalysis of randomized trials comparing vacuum to forceps extractions showed that vacuums are more likely to fail to deliver the baby and lead to increased rates of cephalhematoma and retinal hemorrhage (Figure 15-3) (Vacca, 2007).

Subgaleal hemorrhage poses much more of a potential risk for the neonate; it occurs when emissary veins above

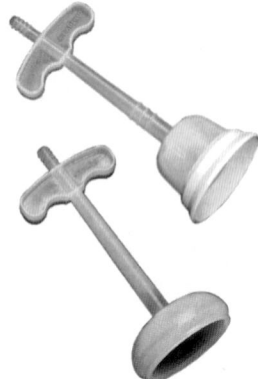

FIGURE 15-2 A soft, bell-shaped vacuum extractor (*top*) and a rigid, mushroom-shaped vacuum extractor (*bottom*). (*Courtesy Cooper Surgical.*)

the skull and periosteum rupture, with blood dissecting through the loose tissue underlying the cranial aponeurosis, unimpeded by suture lines. A tremendous amount of blood, potentially the entire neonatal blood volume (approximately 250 mL) can fill this space, and thus can significantly compromise the neonate's condition (Hillier and Johanson, 1994). Much of the literature about this rare complication of vacuum extraction was published in the 1970s and early 1980s, with few recent studies to detail associated risk factors. Plauche, in his classic paper on vacuum related neonatal injury, identified only 18 cases of subgaleal hematomas among 14,276 cases of vacuum-assisted births, in contrast to a mean incidence of cephalhematoma of 6% (Keith et al, 1988). These morbidity

estimates are derived from data that are approximately 30 to 40 years old; nevertheless, Teng noted an incidence of cephalhematoma of 8%, and 0.7% for subgaleal hemorrhage in their more recent investigation, which agrees well with Plauche's estimates (Herbst and Källén, 2008).

A recent study from Australian investigators evaluated 37 cases of subgaleal hemorrhage at a single tertiary care center accrued over a period of 23 years, with an estimated prevalence of 1.54/10,000 total births. The finding was that this complication occurred most often in primigravidae, and that a large proportion of these infants (89.1% compared with 9.8% of the general control population) had an attempted vacuum extraction (Figure 15-4) (Hillier and Johanson, 1994; Kozak and Weeks, 2002).

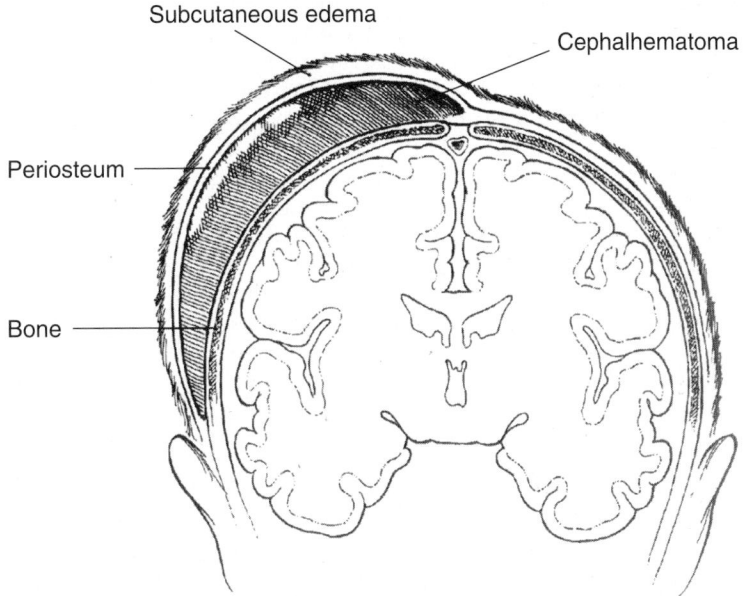

FIGURE 15-3 A cephalhematoma is a hemorrhage that occurs under the periosteum of the skull and is thus confined to a defined space with limited capacity for expansion. (*Adapted from Gilstrap LC, Cunningham FG, Hankins GDV, et al: Operative obstetrics, ed 2, Stamford, Conn, 2002, Appleton and Lange.*)

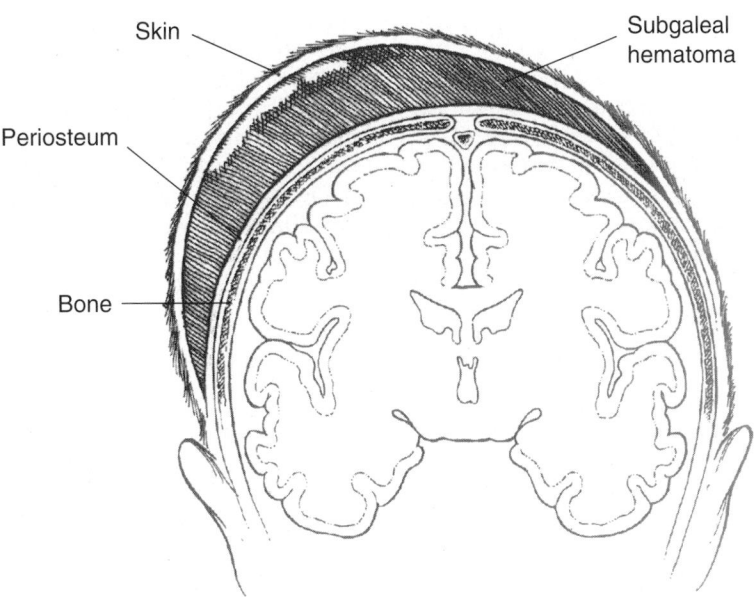

FIGURE 15-4 A subgaleal hematoma spreads along subcutaneous soft tissue planes and has no immediate barrier to expansion, creating the potential for significant neonatal hemodynamic compromise. (*Adapted from Gilstrap LC, Cunningham FG, Hankins GDV, et al: Operative obstetrics, ed 2, Stamford, Conn, 2002, Appleton and Lange.*)

It must be kept in mind that the overall neonatal morbidity of the vacuum extractor is low, as ascertained from the large population-based study by Towner showed that the risk of intracranial injury is only 1 in 664 (Learman, 1998). Yet as outlined previously, there are definite neonatal risks associated with the use of vacuum extraction. The U.S. Food and Drug Administration has suggested that infants delivered with the vacuum have close monitoring for subgaleal or subaponeurotic hematoma, and that a high index of suspicion be maintained for this rare complication.

It must be emphasized that the overall risk of adverse events attributable to the vacuum is extremely low, because the U.S. Food and Drug Administration estimated five serious complications per year of recent use during a time period when 228,354 vacuum deliveries were performed. However, it is likely that sequelae related to vacuum extraction often go underreported (Menacker and Martin, 2008).

The choice of which instrument to use, forceps or vacuum, is usually determined by the obstetric care provider depending on the skill level and experience with either method. There have been several randomized trials exploring this issue (Menacker and Martin, 2008, Meniru, 1996; O'Grady et al, 2002; Prapas et al, 2009). The Cochrane Library has pooled the results from 10 randomized trials comparing neonatal morbidity and successful vaginal delivery between these two devices (Roberts et al, 2002). This analysis found that the vacuum was more likely than forceps to fail (OR, 1.69; 95% CI, 1.31 to 2.19), and was associated with a greater likelihood of Apgar scores less than 7 at 5 minutes (OR, 1.67; 95% CI, 0.99 to 2.81), cephalhematoma (OR, 2.38; 95% CI, 1.68 to 3.37), and retinal hemorrhage (OR, 1.99; 95% CI, 1.35 to 2.98). However the overall serious complication rate was low, and there was no difference in long-term morbidity between groups (Johnson and Menon, 2003).

The greatest danger in the use of either vacuum or forceps comes in the combination of both instruments together. Towner showed that the use of one instrument after the other had failed and carried a neonatal intracranial injury risk of 1 per 256, significantly greater than that of either modality alone (Learman, 1998). This finding was further supported by the work of Gardella et al, (2001), who matched 11,223 women (a third of whom had combined instruments, vacuum alone, or forceps alone, respectively) to an equivalent number of spontaneous vaginal deliveries. These investigators found no statistically significant difference in intracranial hemorrhage when a single instrument was compared to spontaneous vaginal delivery; however, the combined use of both instruments markedly increased the risk of intracranial hemorrhage, seizures, and low 5-minute Apgar scores (Ron-El et al, 1981). The overall risk of nerve and scalp injury was greater when single-instrument delivery was compared with spontaneous delivery, but the overall incidence of each complication is rare.

The vacuum extractor is an acceptable instrument if used judiciously and in the proper circumstances, carrying an overall minimal risk of serious neonatal complications. Its safety is comparable to the obstetric forceps, although it has a higher incidence of cephalhematoma, but a lower potential for facial nerve injury. The chance of failure is greater with the vacuum, which could then potentially tempt the health care provider to subsequently use the forceps. The use of both forceps and vacuum after one instrument has failed carries a higher risk of adverse outcomes, and it should be undertaken only with an understanding of the higher likelihood of neonatal morbidity.

SHOULDER DYSTOCIA

Shoulder dystocia is arguably the most dreaded complication in obstetrics. The problem posed by this entity is that although it is highly anticipated, it is unpredictable and can appear despite the most cautious measures taken to prevent it. *Shoulder dystocia* is defined as the delivery of the fetal head with an impaction of the fetal shoulder girdle or trunk against the pubic symphysis, making subsequent delivery either difficult or impossible without performing auxiliary delivery maneuvers. In some cases the posterior shoulder may be lodged behind the sacral promontory—a bilateral shoulder dystocia.

Once shoulder dystocia occurs, a series of maneuvers—which have never been tested in a prospective fashion, because of the sporadic and unpredictable nature of this complication—are used to resolve it. The first step is usually the McRoberts maneuver, which consists of hyperflexing the maternal thighs onto the abdomen. This maneuver flattens the pubic symphysis and sacral promontory and facilitates delivery of both the anterior and posterior shoulders. If unsuccessful, this maneuver is usually followed by suprapubic pressure to remove the anterior shoulder from its impacted state behind the pubic symphysis. If these two maneuvers fail, either rotational maneuvers or extraction of the posterior fetal arm are usually tried. The Woods-Screw maneuver, or the Rubin's rotational maneuver, is used in an attempt to rotate the infant's shoulders in an effort to relieve the impaction of the shoulder against the pubic bone. Alternatively, delivery of the posterior arm can be accomplished by inserting the operator's hand into the vagina and grasping the posterior fetal wrist and guiding it across the fetal chest and through the vaginal introitus. It is often necessary to perform an episiotomy to have sufficient room in the vagina to accomplish this maneuver. An alternative maneuver to fetal manipulation is the all-fours position, or Gaskin maneuver. With this maneuver, the mother is moved from the lithotomy position to a hands and knees position. Next the posterior fetal shoulder, which is now at the 12 o'clock position, is delivered with gentle downward traction. If the dystocia continues unresolved, the Zavanelli maneuver or cephalic replacement can be performed. After the fetal head is rotated from occiput transverse to occiput anterior, it is flexed and pushed back in the birth canal, and the child was delivered by emergent cesarean section. McRoberts maneuver, suprapubic pressure, or both will relieve greater than 50% of instances. Cephalic replacement should be necessary in rare cases. Recent data have focused on enhanced practitioner training for shoulder dystocia by means of simulation. It is estimated that almost 50% of currently practicing obstetric birth attendants have never successfully performed maneuvers other than the McRoberts maneuver and suprapubic pressure. Draycott et al (2008) have published data showing that the annual compulsory training of all attending obstetric physicians in Southmead Hospital in the United Kingdom reduced the incidence of fetal injury and brachial plexus injury within 3 years of introduction. These data await confirmation in the United States or other countries.

The prevalence of shoulder dystocia varies depending on the population studied and the presence of various risk factors known to predispose women to this obstetric emergency. Estimates range from 0.2% to 1% in a low-risk population to 20% in higher-risk groups (Ali and Norwitz, 2009; Benedetto et al, 2007; Feingold et al, 1988; Hartley and Hittii, 2005; Herbst and Källén, 2008). Maternal obesity, fetal macrosomia, history of prior shoulder dystocia, and maternal diabetes mellitus are the most common associated variables, but are not of sufficient prognostic power to be clinically useful in predicting should dystocia (Ali and Norwitz, 2009; Benedetto et al, 2007; Herbst and Källén, 2008).

Because shoulder dystocia has the potential to cause significant neonatal morbidity and mortality, efforts have been made to predict its occurrence; unfortunately, no clinical guidelines have been clinically tested or proved. Ultrasound examination is commonly used in patients with suspected fetal macrosomia or diabetes to detect large birthweight in infants who might be more likely to suffer shoulder dystocia. Third-trimester sonographic examination has an accuracy of 10% to 15% in the prediction of fetal weight, and is thus not highly reliable (Feingold et al, 1988; Hillier and Johanson, 1994; Keith et al, 1988). In addition, if ultrasound examination were completely reliable, the fetal weight cut-off that would prompt an elective cesarean section has not been determined.

Lipscomb evaluated the deliveries of 227 mother-infant pairs at their institution with birthweights greater than 4500 g and found a shoulder dystocia rate of 18.5%; therefore the majority of those delivering vaginally did so without any adverse event occurring (Hartley and Hitti, 2005). In those with a shoulder dystocia, 51.7% infants had a neurologic injury, but at 2 months, all the infants had a normal neurologic examination. Therefore the occurrence of brachial plexus injury at birth does not necessarily guarantee permanent neurologic morbidity.

This conclusion has been reinforced by several other studies. Gherman et al (2006) reviewed 285 cases of shoulder dystocia and found that 77 (24.9%) suffered fatal injury, most commonly of the brachial plexus (16.8%) or clavicular (9.5%) or humeral (4.2%) fractures. Almost half of the shoulder dystocias resolved with use of the McRoberts maneuver alone; the rest required Woods' maneuver, posterior arm extraction, or the Zavanelli maneuver. The requirement of additional fetal manipulative procedures increased the risk of humeral fracture only and not clavicular or brachial plexus injury. The incidence of permanent musculoskeletal injury was only 1.4% (Kozak and Weeks, 2002).

A prospective investigation evaluated the natural history of recovery following a birth-related brachial plexus injury of infants referred to a tertiary care, multidisciplinary neurological center. Enrollment required identification of injury in the newborn period, initial evaluation at the center between 1 and 2 months of age, and lack of antigravity movement in the shoulder or elbow persisting until 2 weeks of age. In this group of children subject to ascertainment bias (as those injuries resolving before 2 weeks of age would not have been included in the results), complete

neurologic recovery was documented in 66%, and only 14% had persistent, severe weakness (Learman, 1998). In the best systematic review of brachial plexus injury to date, the risk of permanent brachial plexus impairment, if recognizable at birth, was 15% to 20% (Pondaag et al, 2004). Rouse et al (1996) elaborated further on these concepts in their decision analysis, which showed that if one chose to perform an elective cesarean section for all women without diabetes and with sonographically predicted macrosomia (estimated fetal weight >4000 g), 2345 cesarean sections would need to be performed to prevent one permanent brachial plexus injury. If the 4500-g cutoff were selected, 50% more cesarean deliveries would be needed to prevent one permanent brachial plexus injury. In the mother with diabetes, if one chose a cut-off of 4500 g or greater, 443 cesareans would need to be done to prevent one permanent injury (Keith et al, 1988)—a tradeoff that most practitioners now believe is acceptable. The conclusions from this decision analysis have been borne out by several other investigators who have established that the risk of nerve injury certainly increases with rising birthweight, but the large number of macrosomic infants who have a normal, spontaneous vaginal delivery without sequelae does not justify a policy of elective cesarean for macrosomia alone in a nondiabetic population (Lipitz et al, Loucopoulos and Jewewicz, 1982; Menacker and Martin, 2008; Meniru, 1996; O'Grady et al, 2002; Pondaag et al, 2004; Roberts et al, 2002).

Therefore at present there is no universally accepted method to prevent shoulder dystocia. Studies have shown that operative vaginal delivery, especially vacuum delivery, of a fetus suspected to have macrosomia either clinically or sonographically could increase the risk of shoulder dystocia (Ron-El et al, 1981). It seems wise to avoid difficult forceps or vacuum delivery if a patient is thought to have an infant weighing more than 4000 g, especially if she has diabetes or a past history of shoulder dystocia. In addition, the ACOG states that "for pregnant women with diabetes who are suspected of carrying macrosomic fetuses, a planned cesarean delivery may be a reasonable course of action, depending on the incidence of shoulder dystocia, the accuracy of predicting macrosomia, and the cesarean delivery rate within a specific population" (Ali and Norwitz, 2009; Benedetto et al, 2007).

The documentation of the events surrounding shoulder dystocia are important, as is the discussion of current status and future status of an infant delivered with a birth injury after shoulder dystocia. Both obstetric and pediatric providers should debrief the shoulder dystocia event immediately after the delivery. In the case of fetal injury, it is optimal for both obstetric and pediatric providers to discuss the delivery events and subsequent newborn treatment plans with the mother before discharge.

VAGINAL BREECH DELIVERY

Three percent to 4% of all infants at term will be in the breech presentation at the time of delivery. There are three main types of breech presentations. The footling breech has one (single footling) or both (double footling) lower extremities presenting. The frank breech has both thighs flexed, but legs extended. The complete breech has both thighs and legs flexed. The vaginal delivery of a singleton footling breech carries attendant risks of cord prolapse and head entrapment, and the consensus among obstetricians is that this presentation should be delivered operatively (unless the fetus is a second twin, see later discussion on Twin Delivery). The frank breech with buttocks presenting has a lower risk of these adverse events occurring, and thus could potentially deliver vaginally. The complete breech presentation will convert to frank or footling during labor, and the appropriate management scheme for delivery depends on which leading fetal part will descend.

The mechanics of vaginal breech delivery are as follows. The frame of reference for the presenting part is the sacrum (i.e., sacrum anterior, posterior, or transverse). In the absence of urgent fetal indications, the singleton breech is allowed to deliver passively with maternal expulsive efforts until the infant has been delivered past the umbilicus. At this point the legs are gently reduced, and the trunk and body are gently rotated to bring the sacrum anteriorly. With the appearance of the scapula below the maternal symphysis, the arms are then delivered by gently sweeping them across the chest. Every effort is then made to keep the neck from extending during the delivery of the aftercoming head; this is accomplished during delivery of the body by an assistant exerting suprapubic pressure on the fetal head to keep it flexed. Once the body has delivered, the delivery of the head is accomplished by either the Mariceau-Smellie-Veit maneuver, in which one hand extends along the posterior neck and occiput and applies pressure to prevent hyperextension, while the other hand gently applies downward traction against the maxilla to flex the head forward as the head is delivered, or with Piper forceps directly applied to the fetal vertex.

The feasibility of vaginal breech delivery and its safety have been the subject of much debate throughout the past half century. With the advent of safe, expedient cesarean delivery in the United States, many obstetricians have favored the operative approach as the method of choice for management of the breech presentation at term. The literature to support this point of view has produced conflicting conclusions, and its interpretation is consequently difficult. There has been an extensive body of literature over the past half century examining this issue. Unfortunately, there are only two randomized trials that have explored the question of which delivery route is best for the term singleton frank breech fetus (Ali and Norwitz, 2009; Benedetto et al, 2007), but there are several large retrospective series describing neonatal outcomes with the vaginal approach, most of which suggest that vaginal delivery in carefully selected patients carries a low risk of long-term neonatal morbidity and mortality. Diro et al (1999) evaluated 1021 term singleton breech deliveries occurring at their institution over a 4-year period. Infants with a clinically adequate pelvis and frank breech presentation less than 3750 g were allowed a trial of labor. They found an overall cesarean rate of 85.6%; however, for women allowed to deliver vaginally, the success rate, defined as vaginal delivery, was 50% (19 of 38 patients) for nulliparous women and 75.8% (116 of 153 patients) for multiparous women. The length of neonatal intensive care unit (NICU) stay was higher for the group delivered vaginally (17.4% vs. 12.1%; $p = 0.036$), but major morbidities between operative and vaginal delivery were not

significantly different (Feingold et al, 1988). Long-term outcome was not evaluated. Of note, the women in this cohort had pelvic dimensions evaluated clinically, and not by x-ray or computed tomography pelvimetry, as has been performed in other studies.

Norwegian investigators examined their similar policy of vaginal breech delivery and evaluated maternal and neonatal outcomes in a large cohort of women (Fang and Zelop, 2006). Patients were allowed a trial of vaginal delivery if they had adequate x-ray pelvimetry, and they were excluded if they had an estimated fetal weight greater than 4500 g or a footling presentation. Each vaginal breech was matched to a term vaginal vertex birth; each cesarean delivery was matched to the appropriate vertex control; 1212 breech deliveries were evaluated, 639 (52.7%) of which were vaginal, 172 (11.4%) were intrapartum cesarean section, and 138 (11.4%) were planned cesarean section. Once major or lethal anomalies and fetal disorders not related to delivery were excluded, there were no perinatal deaths attributable to mode of delivery. When births planned vaginally were compared with operative deliveries, there was an increased risk of 1-minute Apgar score less than 7 and traumatic morbidity in the vaginal group, but no significant differences in NICU admissions, 5-minute Apgar scores, or normal neonatal course. The conclusion reached was that short-term morbidity was worse in the group delivered vaginally, but long-term outcome was similar between groups. It must be remembered, however, that this study was not randomized, and the infants selected for vaginal delivery versus cesarean section were intrinsically different. In addition, all deliveries occurred in a tertiary care institution.

The truly interesting point raised by these investigators is that, aside from the issue of cesarean versus trial of labor, singleton breech infants regardless of mode of delivery have an increased risk of morbidity compared with their vertex counterparts. Breech infants had higher incidences of NICU admissions, eventful courses, hip dislocation, and traumatic morbidity (soft tissue trauma, fracture, facial nerve paralysis, and brachial plexus palsy). Thus both the obstetrician and pediatrician must be aware that the infant in breech presentation requires careful attention upon birth for the presence of these potential factors.

Christian evaluated their policy of offering a trial of vaginal breech delivery to women with an estimated fetal weight between 2000 and 4000 g and having computed tomographic pelvimetry documenting adequate pelvic dimensions (Herbst and Källén, 2008). Of 122 women evaluated, 85 were judged appropriate by these standards for vaginal delivery, of which 81.2% had a successful vaginal delivery. The only indices of neonatal outcome evaluated were the Apgar score, which was not different between groups, and neonatal cord pH, which was lower in a statistically but not clinically significant manner in the vaginal delivery group.

The largest difficulty in interpreting the large number of retrospective studies examining the issue of vaginal breech delivery in the obstetric literature is that even the best designed reports have relatively small numbers of patients, and the possibility of a type II or beta error is high. In addition, the groups being compared (planned cesarean section and vaginal delivery) are different because the patients are not randomized (Herbst and Källén, 2008; Hillier and Johanson, 1994). Often the women chosen to have a cesarean section tend to have factors that would place their neonates at higher risk than those allowed a trial of labor. A metaanalysis evaluating seven cohort studies and two randomized trials compared 1825 trial of labor patients to 1231 elective cesarean patients and found a statistically significant, but clinically questionable, increased risk with vaginal breech delivery of 1.10% (Keith et al, 1988).

There is a paucity of randomized trials to specifically address the role of the vaginal breech delivery in modern obstetrics. Collea et al randomized 208 women with a singleton frank breech presentation at term to vaginal delivery or cesarean section; they found a low overall risk of permanent birth injury or neonatal morbidity in the vaginal delivery group, although the incidence of neonatal morbidity was higher in the vaginal delivery group (Ali and Norwitz, 2009). Of note, a majority of conditions listed as morbidities (hyperbilirubinemia, meconium aspiration, mild brachial plexus injury) had resolved by hospital discharge. In addition, decreased neonatal morbidity with cesarean section was offset by a striking increase in higher maternal risk in the operative group. It must be remembered that this study was published in 1979, and standards of maternal and neonatal care have changed dramatically since then. Until 2001, no additional randomized investigations were available to settle the long raging debate of the optimal mode of delivery for term singleton breech.

This controversy has recently been clarified by a large, multicenter, multinational trial that randomized 2088 women at 121 centers in 26 countries to planned vaginal birth or planned elective cesarean section (Benedetto et al, 2007). Criteria for enrollment were frank or complete term singleton breech with no evidence of fetal macrosomia. The investigation was halted when preliminary results showed that there was significantly increased neonatal mortality and severe morbidity in the vaginal breech arm compared with the cesarean arm (5.0% vs. 1.6%). This conclusion was not altered by the experience of the delivering obstetrician or maternal demographic factors such as parity and race. Maternal morbidity between both groups was comparable. The difference in outcome was even more striking in countries, such as the United States, with a low national perinatal mortality rate (5.7% vs. 0.4%).

Criticisms of this study are that patients enrolled did not have computed tomography pelvimetry performed, which in some institutions is standard practice before considering a vaginal breech delivery. Furthermore, subjects did not have continuous fetal monitoring, but rather intermittent fetal auscultation every 15 minutes. In addition, the capability of various centers to perform emergent cesarean sections differs markedly, and this could have potentially affected the neonatal morbidity and mortality rate. Nevertheless, it is unlikely that another large study will ever be performed to examine this issue again, and the ultimate results are difficult to dispute given the excellent study design and adequate sample size. Indeed the ACOG recently issued a statement that "planned vaginal delivery of a term singleton breech may no longer be appropriate … patients with a persistent breech presentation at term in a singleton gestation should undergo a planned cesarean delivery" (Kozak and Weeks, 2002). As will be discussed later in Multifetal Delivery, this statement

does not apply to the vaginal delivery of a nonvertex second twin.

The delivery of the vaginal breech is also an emotional issue; physicians trained in the art of the vaginal breech delivery maintain that for an appropriately selected candidate, vaginal breech delivery has acceptable neonatal risk and has the advantage of sparing the mother significant operative morbidity. Proponents of cesarean delivery further state that the level of resident training in the art of the singleton vaginal breech delivery has markedly diminished, with most graduating senior residents having performed few such births. Nonetheless, many practitioners will be required to assist in vaginal birth of a breech infant in unplanned situations. The acquisition of skills necessary to competently perform this procedure may need to be learned and practiced with simulation-based training, because the opportunities for training in most residency programs are few.

MULTIFETAL DELIVERY

With the advent of in vitro fertilization and the sophisticated assisted reproductive technologies (ARTs), the incidence of multifetal pregnancies has dramatically increased, particularly higher-order multiples. The incidence of twin gestations in patients undergoing in vitro fertilization is currently more than 30%, and it is 1% to 3% in higher-order multiples. As a result, the frequency of twin gestation in the United States has increased 65% since 1980; twins now account for 3% of births. Of these, 80% are dizygotic and 20% are monozygotic. This 3% of births accounts for 17% of preterm births and approximately 25% of infants of low birthweight and very low birthweight. The perinatal mortality rate of twins is sevenfold that of singletons, of which a small fraction is due to problems during labor and at delivery. The mode of delivery for twins is well delineated by several studies, and the issues surrounding the choice of vaginal birth versus cesarean is outlined in the following sections (Smith et al, 2005).

TWIN DELIVERY

Vertex-Vertex

It is almost universally accepted that the appropriate method of delivery is vaginal if both twins are vertex. The first infant is delivered like a singleton infant. The second infant is delivered in a similar fashion, but care must be taken not to rupture membranes before the head is well engaged, because this may increase the risk of cord accident. Of note, the delivery of the second twin does not necessarily occur immediately after the first.

Vertex-Nonvertex

The first twin is usually delivered vaginally. The options for delivery of the second twin are as follows: cesarean section, breech extraction, or attempts at external cephalic version and vertex delivery of the second twin if successful. The subject of the optimal delivery choice for the second twin has been the subject of much controversy. Many obstetricians claim that cesarean section is the safest approach to the nonvertex twin, whereas others claim that vaginal delivery affords equivalent neonatal outcome, sparing the mother from an unnecessary surgical procedure (Usta et al, 2005). Fortunately there is a large body of evidence in the literature addressing these issues.

If the vaginal approach is chosen, once the first twin is delivered the obstetrician inserts a hand into the uterine cavity and, under sonographic guidance if necessary, finds the feet of the second twin. Once the feet are firmly grasped, they are brought down into the vagina, and the membranes are then ruptured. Traction is applied to the fetus along the pelvic curve; once the body has been delivered through the introitus, delivery of the arms, shoulders, and aftercoming head proceed in a fashion similar to that of a singleton breech.

In 2003, Hogle et al performed a metaanalysis to determine whether a policy of planned cesarean or planned vaginal birth is preferable for twins. They found only four studies with a total of 1932 infants met their inclusion criteria. There were no significant differences in maternal morbidity, perinatal or neonatal mortality, or neonatal morbidity between the two groups. They did find significantly fewer low 5-minute Apgar scores in the planned cesarean group, principally because of a reduction among breech first twins. They concluded that, if twin A is vertex, "there is no evidence to support planned cesarean section for twins." In contrast, Smith et al (2005) published a retrospective cohort study of 8073 twin births after 36 weeks of gestation in Scotland between 1985 and 2001. There was a death of either twin in two of 1472 (0.14%) deliveries by planned cesarean and in 34 of 6601 (0.52%) deliveries by other means ($p = 0.05$; OR for planned cesarean, 0.26; 95% CI, 0.03 to 1.03). They concluded that planned cesarean may reduce the risk of perinatal deaths of twins at term by 75% despite the lack of statistical significance in outcomes between the two groups. The data also suffer from the fact that 30 of the 36 deaths were in second twins, and there were no data regarding fetal presentation (Smith et al, 2004).

There are several large cohort studies examining the issue of feasibility and safety of total breech extraction of the nonvertex second twin. These studies have almost unanimously reached the similar conclusion that the neonatal outcome for nonvertex second twins delivered vaginally is similar to the vertex first twin, but is not statistically different from those second twins delivered by cesarean section, regardless of birthweight or gestational age (Ali and Norwitz, 2009; Benedetto et al, 2007; Feingold et al, 1988; Hartley et al, 2005; Herbst and Källén, 2008; Hillier and Johanson, 1994; Keith et al, 1988). Hartley et al (2005) conducted a retrospective analysis of birth certificates and fetal and infant death certificates for 5138 twin pairs selected from those born in Washington State from 1989 to 2001. They concluded that if prompt vaginal delivery of twin B does not occur, the benefits of vaginal delivery for twin A might not outweigh the risks of distress and low Apgar scores in twin B and vaginal plus cesarean delivery for the mother (Hartley and Hitti, 2005).

Although there are several retrospective studies evaluating the outcome of vaginally born nonvertex second twins, there is only one randomized trial (Hillier and Johanson, 1994). Rabinovici et al (1987) allocated 60 women with vertex-nonvertex twins to either operative or vaginal delivery.

Maternal morbidity and hospital stay were increased in the surgical group, but there were no differences in neonatal outcome. In addition, Acker et al (1982) retrospectively reviewed 150 nonvertex second twins of all birthweights, 74 delivered by cesarean and 76 by breech extraction, and they found no mortality in either group and a 3.9% incidence of low Apgar scores in the breech extraction group, which was no different from that in the cesarean group. Chervenak et al (1986) reviewed 76 breech extractions for second twins, found no morbidity or mortality in the 60% weighing more than 1500 g, and concluded "for birthweights >1500 gm, routine cesarean for vertex/nonvertex twins may not be necessary."

The available body of evidence supports attempts at vaginal delivery of the nonvertex second twin. Of course the responsible obstetrician must choose a management plan most compatible with his or her experience and training. For those not versed in the techniques of successful vaginal breech extraction, cesarean delivery might be a more prudent plan. As in the case of the singleton vaginal breech, simulation training may play a role in the acquisition and maintenance of skills for safe vaginal breech birth.

In addition to abdominal delivery and total breech extraction, there is the option of external cephalic version (i.e., attempting to turn a nonvertex fetus to vertex by abdominal manipulation). Studies have shown that this option is associated with a higher failure rate at successful vaginal delivery and other complications (such as cord accidents and malpresentations not amenable to vaginal delivery) when compared with primary breech extraction or cesarean section (Hillier and Johanson, 1994; Learman, 1998).

Nonvertex-Nonvertex

Because of to the theoretical risk of interlocking twins, as well as the recent data showing the greater morbidity for the singleton vaginal breech (see the preceding discussion), cesarean section is the recommended choice for delivery of the nonvertex-nonvertex presentation.

Monochorionic, Monoamniotic Twins

Monochorionic, monoamniotic twins share a single intraamniotic space, and thus have a higher risk of cord and extremity entanglement during the course of delivery. It is commonly accepted that the optimal mode of delivery is a planned cesarean section before labor ensues.

HIGHER-ORDER MULTIPLE GESTATIONS

Most perinatologists would suggest cesarean delivery for triplets and higher-order multiples (Lipitz et al, 1989). Although this practice is common, the data mandating operative delivery are far from conclusive.

A Dutch study compared the outcomes of triplets delivered vaginally and abdominally at two institutions (Learman, 1998). One hospital favored cesarean section, whereas at another trial of labor was offered to all appropriate candidates. The success of vaginal delivery was relatively high (34 of 39 women [87%]). There was a higher incidence of neonatal mortality and postdelivery depression (as estimated by Apgar score) in the hospital favoring operative delivery compared with the vaginal delivery group. The biases inherent in this study are obvious, although the reported findings have been corroborated by several other reports from single institutions that offer trial of vaginal delivery to triplet gestations (Menacker and Martin, 2008; Meniru, 1996; O'Grady et al, 2002). Vintzileos et al (2005) attempted to estimate the risks of stillbirth and neonatal and infant deaths in triplets, according to mode of delivery; they used the "matched multiple birth" data file that was composed of triple births that were delivered in the United States during 1995 through 1998 and found that 95% of all triplets were delivered by cesarean delivery. Vaginal delivery (all vaginal) was associated with an increased risk for stillbirth (relative risk, 5.70; 95% CI, 3.83 to 8.49) and neonatal (relative risk, 2.83; 95% CI, 1.91 to 4.19) and infant (relative risk, 2.29; 95% CI, 1.61 to 3.25) deaths. They concluded that cesarean delivery of all three triplet fetuses is associated with the lowest neonatal and infant mortality rate and that vaginal delivery among triplet gestations should be avoided (Vintzileos et al, 2005). Most of the data on triplet births consists of small cohort studies and not randomized trials, and the possibility of type II or beta errors exists in the interpretation of many of these studies (Feingold et al, 1988; Keith et al, 1988). Thus delivery of triplet gestations vaginally while not an unreasonable approach has nearly disappeared from the practice of modern obstetrics in favor of routine cesarean delivery. Currently quadruplets and other higher-order multiples are usually delivered by cesarean section (Ron-El et al, 1981).

VAGINAL BIRTH AFTER CESAREAN: NEONATAL ISSUES

Cesarean section accounts nationally for one quarter of all deliveries (Ali and Norwitz, 2009). Surgery carries the maternal risks of increased blood loss, prolonged hospital stay, and longer recovery period compared with vaginal delivery. During the 1980s to 1990s, efforts were made to encourage women to attempt vaginal birth after a prior cesarean delivery, because success rates vary from 60% to 80% for vaginal delivery, dependent on the indications for the prior cesarean delivery (Benedetto et al, 2007). Whereas VBAC rates remain relatively high in the United Kingdom at 33% (range, 6% to 64%), the rates are decreasing rapidly in the United States from a high rate of 28.3% in 1996 to less than 10 per 1000 deliveries in 2006 (Caughey, 2009; Fang and Zelop, 2006). This decrease occurred primarily because VBAC can result in uterine dehiscence, in which the prior scar asymptomatically separates or, more seriously, uterine rupture occurs. This decrease has significantly affected the United States cesarean section rate of 31.1% (Caughey, 2009; Fang and Zelop, 2006). A full discussion of VBAC, studies supporting its safety, and controversies surrounding its feasibility is beyond the scope of this chapter, and the interested reader is urged to consult *Williams Obstetrics*, ed 23, for further details. This discussion instead focuses on neonatal risks from VBAC, particularly from its most dreaded complication, uterine rupture.

Studies have uniformly shown a risk of uterine rupture with VBAC on the order of 0.5% to 1% (Benedetto et al, 2007; Caughey, 2009; Feingold et al, 1988). A recent large, retrospective study evaluated 20,095 women with a history of prior cesarean delivery and found that rupture risk was 0.16% if the woman elected a repeated, elective operative delivery; 0.52% if VBAC occurred as a result of spontaneous labor; 0.77% if labor was induced without prostaglandins; and 2.5% if labor was induced with prostaglandins (Feingold et al, 1988). Thus VBAC carries the lowest risk if labor is spontaneous and not augmented.

There are few large, well-designed studies specifically evaluating neonatal rather than maternal outcomes in VBAC. Most recently, Kamath et al (2009) performed a retrospective cohort study of 672 women with one prior cesarean section undergoing trial of labor. They found that infants born by cesarean delivery had higher rates of admission to the NICU (9.3% compared with 4.9%) and higher rates of oxygen supplementation for delivery room resuscitation (41.5% compared with 23.2).

Yap retrospectively evaluated 38,027 deliveries occurring at a single tertiary care institution and found 21 cases of uterine rupture; 17 occurred after a history of a prior cesarean delivery (Herbst and Källén, 2008). The two neonatal deaths that occurred were a result of prematurity (23-week-old fetus) and multiple congenital anomalies; all live born infants were discharged from the hospital without neurologic sequelae. Thus the ultimate neonatal outcome despite uterine rupture was favorable. However, all deliveries occurred in a tertiary care institution with readily available obstetric anesthesiologists, neonatologists, and obstetricians. Most deliveries after diagnosis of rupture occurred within 26 minutes.

A third group of investigators retrospectively identified 99 cases of uterine rupture occurring over a period including 159,456 births (Hillier and Johanson, 1994). Thirteen of these ruptures occurred before the onset of labor. There were six neonatal deaths, but four of these occurred in women with uterine rupture at admission, and thus were never given a trial of labor. There were five cases of perinatal asphyxia, but once again it is not detailed whether these occurred in women allowed a trial of labor or in those who had ruptured on presentation to the hospital. Moreover, many of these women had an undocumented prior scar, which in some institutions would warrant an elective repeated cesarean section. The aforementioned recent study evaluating 20,095 women with a prior cesarean delivery and their subsequent risk of rupture found a neonatal mortality of 5.5% (Feingold et al, 1988). However, because this was a population based study, it was not specified whether these deliveries occurred in tertiary care institutions with the capability of performing emergent operative rescue procedures in the event of uterine rupture.

Finally Fang et al (2006) reviewed all of the literature to date in regard to adverse neonatal outcomes and found that the combined rates of intrapartum stillbirth and neonatal death were not statistically different between trial of labor and those who elected for repeated cesarean section. Thus the true neonatal risk of VBAC, especially in the event of uterine rupture, cannot be precisely estimated at the current time. There are no studies adequately evaluating long-term outcomes of surviving infants after uterine rupture (Fang and Zelop, 2006).

It appears that the risk of uterine rupture after a prior cesarean delivery is low, but this risk increases when labor is augmented with oxytocin or prostaglandins. It is appropriate to offer women VBAC, but they must be counseled carefully about the potential risk of uterine rupture. Careful documentation of the informed consent and labor management must be completed. Moreover, VBAC should ideally occur in a tertiary care institution or in facilities capable of rapidly performing an emergent cesarean section, because this improves the likelihood of minimizing adverse neonatal sequelae.

CORD ACCIDENTS

The term *cord accident* usually refers to adverse events affecting the fetus that occur as a result of a problem with the umbilical cord. This heterogeneous term encompasses umbilical cord prolapse, in which the cord delivers through the cervix and compression by a fetal part results in a significantly increased risk of asphyxia; it also includes such entities as cord entanglements or "true knots," which can lead to fetal compromise.

The incidence of such events is not clearly known, because the diagnosis is often one of exclusion. One large population-based study compared 709 cases of cord prolapse occurring among 313,000 deliveries to matched controls and found that low birthweight, male sex, multiple gestations, breech presentation, and congenital anomalies all increased the risk of umbilical cord prolapse (Ali and Norwitz, 2009). Not surprisingly, cord prolapse was associated with a high mortality rate (10%) that was reduced if cesarean rather than vaginal delivery was performed.

The standard of care in cases of cord prolapse is to proceed immediately with cesarean section as quickly as possible while an assistant elevates the presenting fetal part with a vaginal hand to prevent compression of the umbilical cord. It is also of paramount importance to have appropriate pediatric support available at the time of delivery, because the newborn is likely to be depressed and require resuscitation.

Cord accident, or in utero compromise, secondary to entanglement of the umbilical cord as a clinical entity is difficult to understand. Often in cases of in utero fetal demise (IUFD), a diagnosis or cause of fetal death is never found. It is tempting to attribute the demise to an event that compromises umbilical blood flow to the developing pregnancy. The literature on this subject is scarce. Hershkovitz et al (2001) identified 841 cases of true knots from a population of 69,139 deliveries (for a prevalence of 1.2%) and in a case-controlled study found that grand multiparity (>10 deliveries), chronic hypertension, history of genetic amniocentesis, male gender, and umbilical cord prolapse were all independently associated with true knots of the umbilical cord. The presence of a true knot was associated with both in utero fetal demise and greater

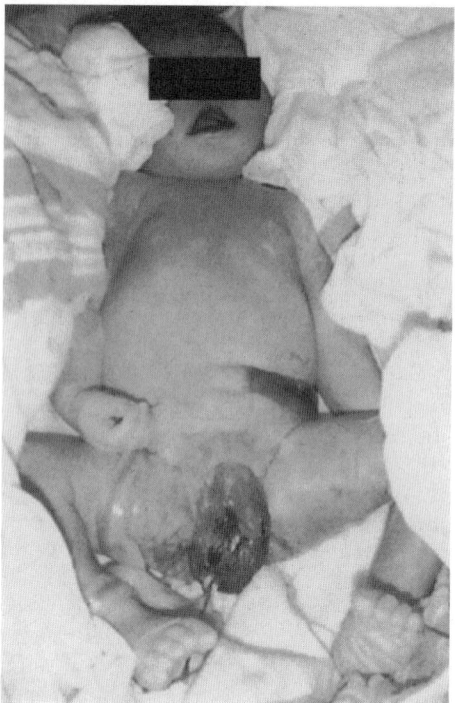

FIGURE 15-5 *(See also Color Plate 2.)* A 28-year-old woman was admitted to the labor and delivery department with an intrauterine demise. Examination of the fetus shows the cord wrapped tightly around the torso, leg, and ankle, suggesting cord accident as a cause of death. No other pathologic abnormalities were found on autopsy. (*Courtesy Thomas R. Easterling.*)

likelihood of cesarean delivery (Figure 15-5) (Benedetto et al, 1994).

SUGGESTED READINGS

American College of Obstetricians and Gynecologists: *ACOG Committee Opinion No. 340: Mode of term singleton breech delivery,* 108:235-237, 2006.
American College of Obstetricians and Gynecologists: Fetal macrosomia. ACOG Practice Bulletin No. 22, *Obstet Gynecol* 96 , 2000.
American College of Obstetricians and Gynecologists: Operative vaginal delivery. ACOG Practice Bulletin No. 17, *Obstet Gynecol* 95 , 2000.
American College of Obstetricians and Gynecologists: Shoulder dystocia. ACOG Practice Bulletin No. 40, *Obstet Gynecol* 100:1045-1050, 2002.
American College of Obstetricians and Gynecologists: Vaginal birth after cesarean section. ACOG Practice Bulletin No. 54, *Obstet Gynecol* 104:203-212, 2004.
Draycott TJ, Crofts JF, Ash JP, et al: Improving neonatal outcome through practical shoulder dystocia training, *Obstet Gynecol* 112:14-20, 2008.
Fang YM, Zelop CM: Vaginal birth after cesarean: assessing maternal and perinatal risks: contemporary management, *Clin Obstet Gynecol* 49:147-153, 2006.
Hartley RS, Hitti J: Birth order and delivery interval: analysis of twin pair perinatal outcomes, *J Matern Fetal Neonatal Med* 17:375-380, 2005.
Johanson RB, Menon BK: Vacuum extraction versus forceps for assisted vaginal delivery, *Cochrane Database Syst Review* (2):CD000224, 2000.
Kamath BD, Todd JK, Glazner JE, et al: Neonatal outcomes after elective cesarean delivery, *Obstet Gynecol* 113:1231-1238, 2009.
Prapas N, Kalogiannidis I, Masoura S, et al: Operative vaginal delivery in singleton term pregnancies: short-term maternal and neonatal outcomes, *Hippokratia* 13:41-45, 2009.
Thorngren-Jerneck K, Herbst A: Low 5-minute Apgar score: a population-based register study of 1 million term births, *Obstet Gynecol* 98:65-70, 2001.

Complete references and supplemental color images used in this text can be found online at www.expertconsult.com

OBSTETRIC ANALGESIA AND ANESTHESIA

Mark D. Rollins and Mark A. Rosen

This chapter introduces some of the scientific background and clinical techniques used in providing obstetric analgesia and anesthesia. These practices provide substantial benefit to the patient in labor and are essential for operative delivery. Although the effects of obstetric analgesia and anesthesia on the fetus and neonate are typically benign, there is potential for significant neonatal effects.

HISTORY OF OBSTETRIC ANESTHESIA

Modern obstetric anesthesia began in Edinburgh, Scotland, on January 19, 1847, when the professor of obstetrics James Young Simpson used diethyl ether to facilitate child delivery by anesthetizing a woman with a contracted pelvis. Morton's historic demonstration of the anesthetic properties of ether at the Massachusetts General Hospital in Boston had occurred only 3 months earlier. Fanny Longfellow, wife of Henry Wadsworth Longfellow, was the first American to receive anesthesia for childbirth, publicly proclaiming in 1847, "This is certainly the greatest blessing of this age" (Longfellow and Wagenknecht, 1956).

Although anesthesia for surgery was rapidly and widely accepted, most of Simpson's contemporaries in the United States, France, and England were critical of using anesthesia in obstetrics, presenting both medical and religious arguments in outspoken opposition. However, the public outcry in support of labor analgesia was vehement. In 1853, the negative reaction from Thomas Wolsley, editor of *The Lancet*, after John Snow administered ether for Queen Victoria's eighth child was so strong that court physicians denied anesthesia had been used. The great debate was largely settled 4 years later when Victoria delivered her ninth and last child, and the use of a royal anesthetic was acknowledged. Although many physicians had remained opposed, public opinion had changed and women were requesting labor analgesia from their doctors.

During the second half of the twentieth century, anesthesiologists made significant advances in techniques and improved safety for delivering labor analgesia. Hingson and Edwards (1943) developed the continuous caudal catheter that preceded development of the epidural catheter. Apgar (1953) initially proposed a simple neonatal scoring system as a guide for evaluating the effects of obstetric anesthesia and later as a guide for neonatal resuscitation. Other early pioneers in the emerging specialty of obstetric anesthesia were Gertie Marx (Marx and Orkin, 1958), John Bonica (1967), and Sol Shnider et al (1963). These pioneers helped to characterize the normal changes in maternal physiology related to pregnancy, confirm the safety and efficacy of obstetric analgesia, determine the effects of these techniques on uterine blood flow and placental transfer of anesthetic agents, and evaluate the effects of these techniques and agents on newborn well-being.

ANATOMY OF LABOR PAIN

Contraction of the uterus, dilatation of the cervix, and distention of the perineum cause pain during labor and delivery. Somatic and visceral afferent sensory fibers from the uterus and cervix travel with sympathetic nerve fibers to the spinal cord (Figure 16-1). These fibers pass through the paracervical tissue and course with the hypogastric nerves and the sympathetic chain to enter the spinal cord at T10 to L1. During the first stage of labor (cervical dilation), the majority of painful stimuli are the result of afferent nerve impulses from the lower uterine segment and cervix, as well as contributions from the uterine body causing visceral pain (poorly localized, diffuse, and usually described as "a dull but intense aching"). These nerve cell bodies are located in the dorsal root ganglia of levels T10 to L1. During the second stage of labor (pushing and expulsion), afferents innervating the vagina and perineum cause somatic pain (well localized and described as "sharp"). These somatic impulses travel primarily via the pudendal nerve to dorsal root ganglia of levels S2 to S4. Pain during this stage is caused by distention and tissue ischemia of the vagina, perineum, and pelvic floor muscles, associated with descent of the fetus into the pelvis and delivery. Neuraxial analgesic techniques that block levels T10 to L1 during the first stage of labor must be extended to include S2 to S4 for efficacy during the second stage of labor.

Labor pain can have significant physiologic effects on the mother, fetus, and the course of labor. Pain stimulates the sympathetic nervous system, elevates plasma catecholamine levels, creates reflex maternal tachycardia and hypertension, and reduces uterine blood flow. In addition, changes in uterine activity can occur with the rapid decrease in plasma epinephrine concentrations associated with onset of neuraxial analgesia. Oscillations in epinephrine can result in a range of uterine effects from a transient period of uterine hyperstimulation (Clarke et al, 1994) to a transient period of uterine quiescence, or conversion of dysfunctional uterine activity patterns associated with poorly progressive cervical dilation to more regular patterns associated with normal cervical dilation (Leighton et al, 1999).

CHANGES IN MATERNAL PHYSIOLOGY AND THE IMPLICATIONS

During pregnancy, labor, and delivery, women undergo fundamental changes in anatomy and physiology. These alterations are caused by changing hormonal activity, biochemical shifts associated with increasing metabolic demands of a growing fetus, placenta, and uterus, and mechanical displacement by an enlarging uterus (Cheek and Gutsche, 2002; Parer et al, 2002).

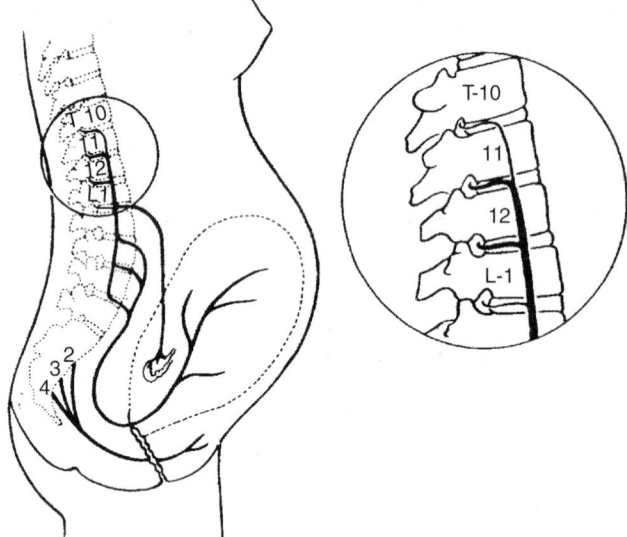

FIGURE 16-1 Parturition pain pathways. Nerves that accompany sympathetic fibers and enter the neuraxis at the *T10, T11, T12,* and *L1* spinal levels carry afferent pain impulses from the cervix and uterus. Pain pathways from the perineum travel to *S2, S3,* and *S4* via the pudendal nerve. *(From Bonica JJ:* Principles and practice of obstetric analgesia and anesthesia, *Philadelphia, 1967, F.A. Davis Co.)*

MATERNAL CIRCULATORY SYSTEM

Hypotension can occur when a pregnant woman is in the supine position because of compression of the vena cava by the gravid uterus. Significant aortoiliac artery compression occurs in 15% to 20% of parturients and vena caval compression is universal, often as early as 13 to 16 weeks' gestation. Vena caval compression contributes to lower extremity venous stasis and can cause ankle edema and varices despite increased collateral circulation. Venous compression by the gravid uterus diverts some blood returning from the lower extremities through the internal vertebral venous plexus, the azygos, and the epidural veins. This increases the likelihood of entering an epidural vein with spinal or epidural anesthetic techniques. Anesthetic interventions that diminish sympathetic tone can further exacerbate the effects of vena caval compression induced by supine positioning, potentially causing profound hypotension. Therefore supine positioning is avoided during anesthetic administration in the second and third trimesters. Significant lateral tilt is used in all operative deliveries and frequently during labor analgesia to help preserve uterine blood flow and fetal circulation.

Cardiac output increases during pregnancy, reaching an output 50% greater than the prepregnant state by the third trimester. During labor, maternal cardiac output increases during the first and second stages, reaching an additional 40% above prelabor values in the second stage (Robson et al, 1987). Each uterine contraction results in the autotransfusion of 300 to 500 mL of blood back into the maternal central circulation. The greatest increase in cardiac output occurs immediately after delivery, when values can increase as much as 75% above predelivery levels. This abrupt increase in cardiac output is secondary to the loss of aortocaval compression, autotransfusion from the contracted uterus, and decreased venous pressure in the lower extremities (Kjeldsen, 1979).

Physiologic (dilutional) anemia of pregnancy occurs as a result of a greater increase in plasma volume (45%) than in red blood cell volume (20%) at term. Average blood loss at delivery—Approximately 500 mL for vaginal delivery and 1000 mL for cesarean section—is well tolerated because of this expanded blood volume and autotransfusion (normally in excess of 500 mL) from the contracted uterus after delivery (Cheek and Gutsche, 2002).

MATERNAL AIRWAY AND RESPIRATORY SYSTEMS

During pregnancy, the maternal airway has significantly increased mucosal edema and tissue friability throughout the pharynx, larynx, and trachea. These changes make laryngoscopy and intubation more challenging. In addition, the presence of comorbidities such as preeclampsia, upper respiratory tract infections, and the active pushing and increased venous pressure during the second stage further exacerbate airway tissue edema (Munnur et al, 2005).

At term, minute ventilation is increased approximately 50%, oxygen consumption is increased by more than 20%, and functional residual capacity is decreased by 20%. The combination of these changes (increased oxygen consumption and decreased oxygen reserve) results in a state promoting rapid desaturation during periods of apnea. The changes in both airway and respiratory physiology during pregnancy make ventilation and intubation more difficult and increase the potential for complications.

MATERNAL GASTROINTESTINAL SYSTEM

The gravid uterus displaces the stomach cephalad and anterior and the pylorus cephalad and posterior. These changes reposition the intraabdominal portion of the esophagus into the thorax and result in decreased competence of the esophageal sphincter. Higher progesterone and estrogen levels further reduce esophageal sphincter tone. Gastric pressure is increased by the gravid uterus and by the lithotomy position used during vaginal delivery. Maternal gastric reflux symptoms increase with the gestational age of the pregnancy and ultimately affect the majority of parturients (Marrero et al, 1992).

Beyond midgestation, women are at increased risk for pulmonary aspiration of acidic gastric contents; this is caused by decreased tone and competence of the lower esophageal sphincter as well as delayed gastric emptying with onset of labor or administration of opioids. This risk has important implications for induction of general anesthesia and airway management by the anesthesiologist, and it is discussed in detail under General Anesthesia.

UTERINE AND FETAL CIRCULATION

Uterine weight and blood flow increase throughout gestation from approximately 100 mL/min before pregnancy to approximately 700 mL/min (10% of cardiac output) at term gestation, with 50% to 80% of the uterine blood flow perfusing the intervillous space (placenta) and 20% to 50% supporting the myometrium. Uterine vasculature has limited autoregulation and remains (essentially) maximally dilated under normal conditions during pregnancy.

Maternal uterine blood flow decreases as a result of either decreased uterine arterial perfusion pressure or increased arterial resistance. Decreased perfusion pressure can result from systemic hypotension secondary to hypovolemia, aortocaval compression, or significant decreases in vascular resistance from the initiation of neuraxial anesthesia or induction of general anesthesia. Uterine perfusion pressure can also decrease from increased uterine venous pressure associated with vena caval compression (e.g., supine position), uterine contractions (particularly uterine hypertonus by oxytocin hyperstimulation), or significant increase in intra-abdominal pressure (pushing during second stage or seizure activity). Stress-induced endogenous catecholamines and exogenous vasopressors can increase uterine artery resistance and decrease uterine blood flow. Despite these potential effects, phenylephrine (alpha-adrenergic) is useful for treating maternal hypotension secondary to neuraxial anesthesia, and it has been demonstrated to result in less fetal acidosis and base deficit compared to treatment with ephedrine (primarily beta-adrenergic) in many clinical trials (Lee et al, 2002a; Ngan Kee et al, 2009; Smiley, 2009).

ANALGESIC OPTIONS FOR LABOR AND VAGINAL DELIVERY

The pain of labor is highly variable and described by many women as severe. Factors influencing the patient's perception of labor pain include duration of labor, maternal pelvic anatomy in relation to fetal size, use of oxytocin, parity, participation in childbirth preparation classes, fear and anxiety about childbirth, attitudes about and experience of pain, and coping mechanisms. Labor analgesia prevents autonomic reflex effects that can be deleterious for certain high-risk patients and their fetuses (e.g., patients with severe preeclampsia, valvular heart disease, myasthenia gravis). The American College of Obstetricians and the American Society of Anesthesiologists issued a joint statement indicating that a maternal request for pain relief is sufficient justification for administration of analgesics during labor (American College of Obstetricians and Gynecologists, 2002). Although older observational studies associate increased cesarean delivery rates with early administration of epidural analgesia, more recent randomized studies found no difference in the rate of cesarean delivery or instrument-assisted vaginal delivery between women in whom analgesia was initiated early in labor versus later (Eltzschig et al, 2003; Wong et al, 2005). Consequently the American Society of Anesthesiology stated in its 2007 Practice Guidelines, "Neuraxial analgesia should not be withheld on the basis of achieving an arbitrary cervical dilation, and should be offered on an individualized basis. Patients may be reassured that the use of neuraxial analgesia does not increase the incidence of cesarean delivery" (American Society of Anesthesiologists Task Force on Obstetric Anesthesia, 2007).

The choice of analgesic method resides primarily with the patient. The medical condition of the parturient, stage of labor, urgency of delivery, condition of the fetus, and availability of qualified personnel are also factors. Many different techniques are available to alleviate labor and delivery pain. *Analgesia* refers to pain relief without loss of consciousness; *regional analgesia* denotes partial sensory

---

BOX 16-1   Techniques for Labor Analgesia

Nonpharmacologic analgesia
Systemic medications
 Opioid analgesics
 Sedatives and anxiolytics
 Dissociative analgesics
Inhalation analgesia
Regional analgesia
 Epidural
 Spinal
 Combined spinal-epidural
 Paracervical block
 Pudendal block

---

blockade in a specific area of the body, with or without partial motor blockade. *Regional anesthesia* is the loss of sensation, motor function, and reflex activity in a limited area of the body. *General anesthesia* results in the loss of consciousness and the goals for providing general anesthesia typically include hypnosis, amnesia, analgesia, and skeletal muscle relaxation.

Techniques for labor analgesia must be safe for mother and fetus and individualized to satisfy the analgesic requirement and desires of the parturient; they also must accommodate the changing nature of labor pain and the evolving, varied course of labor and delivery (e.g., spontaneous vaginal delivery, instrumentally assisted vaginal delivery, and cesarean delivery). The current approaches to pain relief are outlined in Box 16-1.

NONPHARMACOLOGIC ANALGESIA

There is a variety of nonpharmacologic techniques for labor analgesia. These techniques include hypnosis, the breathing techniques described by Lamaze, acupuncture, acupressure, the LeBoyer technique (LeBoyer, 1975), transcutaneous nerve stimulation, massage, hydrotherapy, vertical positioning, presence of a support person, intradermal water injections, and biofeedback. A metaanalysis reviewing the effectiveness of a support individual (e.g., doula, family member) noted that parturients with a support individual used fewer pharmacologic analgesia methods, had a decreased length of labor, and had a lower incidence of operative deliveries (Hodnett et al, 2007). In a 2006 retrospective national survey of women's childbearing experiences, although neuraxial methods of pain relief were rated as the most helpful and effective, nonpharmacologic methods of tub immersion and massage were rated more or equally helpful in relieving pain compared with the use of opioids (Declercq et al, 2006). Although many nonpharmacologic techniques seem to reduce labor pain perception, most studies lack the rigorous scientific methodology for the useful comparison of these techniques to pharmacologic methods.

SYSTEMIC MEDICATIONS

Systemic medications for labor and delivery are widely used, but are administered with limitations on both dose and timing because they readily cross the placenta and are associated with a risk of neonatal respiratory depression in a dose-dependent fashion. Although the use of systemic opioid analgesics is common (e.g., fentanyl, meperidine, morphine, nalbuphine, butorphanol), the use of sedatives and anxiolytics (e.g., barbiturates, phenothiazine derivatives and benzodiazepines), and dissociative agents (e.g., ketamine, scopolamine) is rare.

Opioid Analgesics

Opioids are the most frequently used systemic analgesic, but for many patients opioids do not provide adequate analgesia during labor and delivery (Bricker and Lavender, 2002; Olofsson et al, 1996). Opioids are inexpensive, easy to administer, and do not require a trained anesthesia provider. However, they have a high rate of maternal side effects (sedation, respiratory depression, dysphoria, nausea, pruritus), can decrease fetal heart rate variability and fetal movements, and carry a potential risk of neonatal respiratory depression and changes in neurobehavior. Systemic administration of opioids at doses that are safe for mother and newborn provides some analgesia, but it is not a substitute for the analgesia provided by regional techniques. Systemic opioids are recommended for administration in the smallest doses possible with minimization of repeated dosing to reduce the accumulation of drug and metabolites in the fetus. Systemic opioids are most useful for patients with minimal pain, precipitous labor, or contraindications to neuraxial blockade, such as a coagulopathy.

The opioid analgesics act by binding to opiate receptors located throughout the central nervous system. Although this is the main site of action, opioid receptors have also been identified in other peripheral tissues. Four main types of receptor have been identified: mu (μ), kappa (κ), delta (δ), and sigma (σ). The analgesic effects, side effects, and pharmacodynamic characteristics depend on the receptor affinity of each individual opioid. These receptors are also responsible for the associated respiratory depression, sedation, and dysphoria and may affect thermoregulation. Binding of opiate agonist agents (e.g., meperidine, morphine, and fentanyl) and subsequent receptor activation alters neural transmission of pain by inhibiting the presynaptic and postsynaptic release of neurotransmitters. The opioid antagonists (e.g., naloxone, naltrexone) are competitive antagonists and bind with high affinity to the μ receptor more so than the κ or δ opioid receptors. These drugs do not produce analgesia and are capable of displacing other agonist drugs from the receptor and reversing their effects. A third class of agents interacts with the receptors and results in both agonist and antagonist activity depending on the receptor type. These drugs, with high receptor affinity, are capable of analgesic effect (e.g., pentazocine, nalbuphine, and butorphanol).

Opioids differ in pharmacokinetics, pharmacodynamics, method of elimination, and the presence of active metabolites, but all readily cross the placental barrier through passive diffusion. In order for systemic opioids to effectively alleviate labor pain, larger doses would be necessary. This dosing would risk excessive maternal sedation, maternal respiratory depression, loss of protective airway reflexes, newborn respiratory depression, and impairment of both early breastfeeding and neurobehavior. Consequently,

large doses of opioids are avoided, and the doses used routinely for labor analgesia typically do not have significant adverse effects on either the mother or neonate.

Meperidine remains the most widely used opioid worldwide. Maternal half-life of meperidine is 2 to 3 hours, with the half-life in the fetus and newborn being significantly greater and more variable at values between 13 and 23 hours (Kuhnert et al, 1979). In addition, meperidine is metabolized to an active metabolite (normeperidine) that can significantly accumulate after repeated doses. With increased dosing and shortened time interval between dose and delivery, there is greater neonatal risk of decreased Apgar scores, lowered oxygen saturation, prolonged time to sustained respiration, abnormal neurobehavior, and more difficulty initiating successful breastfeeding (Nissen et al, 1997).

Morphine was used more frequently in the past, but currently is rarely used. Like meperidine it has an active metabolite (morphine-6-glucuronide) and a prolonged duration of analgesia (3 to 4 hours). The half-life is longer in neonates compared with adults, and it produces significant maternal sedation.

Fentanyl is a synthetic opioid with a short duration of action (approximately 30 minutes), no active metabolites, and a ratio of fetal to maternal plasma concentrations of approximately 1:3. In small intravenous (IV) doses of 50 to 100 μg/hr there were no significant differences in Apgar scores, respiratory depression, or neurobehavior scoring compared with newborns of mothers who did not receive fentanyl (Rayburn et al, 1989a). In addition, a comparison of equianalgesic doses of IV fentanyl compared with IV meperidine (Rayburn et al, 1989b) demonstrated a decreased frequency of maternal nausea, vomiting, and prolonged sedation in the fentanyl group. In addition, neonates whose mothers received meperidine required naloxone more often compared with the fentanyl-exposed infants. There was no difference in the neuroadaptive testing scores of the two groups of infants.

Opioids can be given by intramuscular (IM) or IV administration. IM injection of opioids is technically easy but leads to uneven analgesia, the possibility of late respiratory depression, and profound neonatal effects if not properly timed (Shnider and Moya, 1960). IM administration is associated with a high incidence of neonatal depression 2 to 4 hours after injection in some of the less lipid soluble opioids. IV administration is the most widely used technique to give opioids to a woman in labor, with effects that are more predictable and doses more easily timed. However, achievement of a steady blood level of opiate sufficient to provide analgesia is difficult, with the parturient frequently suffering underdosage (rarely overdosage). In an effort to improve pain relief and maternal satisfaction, continuous IV infusion of short-acting opiates (e.g., alfentanil, remifentanil) or self-administration of IV opiates is increasingly used for systemic opioid delivery during labor.

Patient-controlled analgesia (PCA) has the implied advantage of allowing the patient to titrate her dose to the minimum required for analgesia with the lowest blood levels of opiates, resulting in considerably less placental transfer and fewer side effects with increased patient satisfaction (McIntosh and Rayburn, 1991). Remifentanil, an ultra-short–acting opioid rapidly metabolized by nonspecific serum esterases, is significantly metabolized by the fetus with umbilical artery–to–vein ratios of approximately 0.3 (Kan et al, 1998). It can be used effectively for labor PCA, but it appears difficult to achieve satisfactory analgesia without significant potential of maternal respiratory depression (Olufolabi et al, 2000; Thurlow and Waterhouse, 2000; Volikas, 2001). In a prospective randomized controlled trial comparing the effectiveness of epidural analgesia to a remifentanil PCA with optimized settings, epidural analgesia was significantly more effective than PCA in regard to labor pain, but no differences were noted in neonatal outcome measures (Volmanen et al, 2008).

Although there are individual differences among opioids, all readily cross the placental barrier and exert neonatal effects in typical clinical doses, including decreased fetal heart rate variability and dose-related neonatal respiratory depression. All opioids can have maternal side effects, including nausea, vomiting, pruritus, and decreased gastrointestinal motility and stomach emptying.

Sedatives and Anxiolytics

Sedatives and anxiolytics are administered infrequently to pregnant patients because they increase risks of sedation and respiratory depression in both mother and newborn, especially when used with opioids. Sedatives and anxiolytics were used more frequently in the past to diminish the adverse motivational-affective component of labor pain. Examples of such drugs are barbiturates and benzodiazepines.

Diazepam and midazolam are benzodiazepines used as anxiolytic agents in obstetrics. They rapidly cross the placenta, yielding approximately equal maternal and fetal blood levels within minutes of IV administration (Cree et al, 1973). In addition, the neonate has a limited ability to excrete diazepam, so the drug and its active metabolite may persist in significant amounts in the neonate for up to 1 week (Scher et al, 1972). Diazepam can result in neonatal hypotonia, lethargy, and hypothermia when used in large maternal doses (30 mg) (Cohen et al, 1993). However, when it is used in small doses (2.5 to 10 mg IV), minimal sedation and hypotonia have been observed (McAllister, 1980). Midazolam has a shorter duration of activity, but rapidly crosses the placenta and is associated with neonatal hypotonia in larger doses. The use of benzodiazepines remains somewhat controversial, but these agents can reduce maternal anxiety and are useful for treating convulsions associated with local anesthetic toxicity or eclampsia. However, all benzodiazepines are amnestics, and therefore may not be appropriate in many childbirth situations, depending on the desires of the parturient.

Dissociative Analgesia

The IM or IV administration of low-dose ketamine (0.25 mg/kg) produces a state called *dissociative analgesia*, which is characterized by analgesia and unreliable amnesia without loss of consciousness or protective airway reflexes (Galloon, 1976). This state is accompanied by a dreaming phenomenon, which may be unpleasant but can be minimized by coadministration of benzodiazepines to improve amnesia. In divided doses totaling less than 1 mg/kg, ketamine provides adequate analgesia for vaginal delivery and episiotomy repair. Although these low doses are not associated with neonatal depression, higher doses are associated with decreased Apgar scores (Akamatsu et al, 1974). With larger doses, maternal airway protection cannot be guaranteed, increasing the risk of gastric content aspiration. Ketamine is best reserved for use as a supplement (in low doses) to other techniques or for situations in which (1) more reliable and safer agents or techniques are contraindicated or ineffective or (2) when rapid control is required because the mother's pain is compromising the fetus (e.g., mother is moving uncontrollably, unable to effectively push, and jeopardizing delivery while the fetal head is presenting during a prolonged fetal heart rate deceleration).

INHALATION ANALGESIA

The use of nitrous oxide is widespread in Canada, Australia, the United Kingdom and other parts of the world, but its use in the United States as a labor analgesic is uncommon. It is usually administered as a 50% mixture with oxygen. At a 50% concentration (without coadministration of opioids), nitrous oxide is insufficient to cause unconsciousness or loss of protective airway reflexes. Appropriate equipment and trained personnel are essential to ensure safety (i.e., limiting the nitrous oxide concentration, avoiding administration of a hypoxic mixture, avoiding coadministration of other agents). Nitrous oxide is a weak analgesic but can provide satisfactory pain relief for some parturients. It can be used during the first, second, or third stage of labor either alone or as a supplement for a regional block or local infiltration (Rosen, 1971). The use of 50% nitrous oxide in a supervised fashion is safe and rapid acting, causes minimal maternal cardiovascular or respiratory depression, and does not affect uterine contractility. The effects of nitrous oxide are rapidly reversed with discontinuation, and it does not cause neonatal depression regardless of duration of administration (Rosen, 2002a). Although the use of inhaled halogenated agents such as sevoflurane in low-inspired concentrations was found to be safe and effective at reducing labor pain in a small study (Yeo et al, 2007), barriers to routine use include the need for specialized vaporizers, scavenging systems, and the lack of larger studies.

NEURAXIAL (REGIONAL) ANALGESIA

Neuraxial analgesia, including epidural, spinal, and combined spinal-epidural (CSE) techniques, has become the most widely used method for labor analgesia in the United States (Bucklin et al, 2005). Neuraxial techniques typically involve epidural and spinal administration of local anesthetic agents, and often the co-administration of epidural and spinal opioid analgesics. Other adjuvant agents, such as clonidine and neostigmine, can decrease the dose of local anesthetics or opioids required for effective analgesia; however, they are not routinely used and do not appear to offer a significant advantage when compared to local anesthetics with or without opioids (Eisenach, 2009; Parker et al, 2007; Roelants, 2006).

Neuraxial Local Anesthetics

Local anesthetic agents consist of amine moieties linked by an intermediate chain containing an ester or amide. Local anesthetics reversibly block nerve impulse conduction via voltage-gated sodium channels. Their chemical structures are secondary or tertiary amines, which are weak bases, marketed as the hydrochloride salts to achieve aqueous solubility.

The ester-linked local anesthetics (e.g., chloroprocaine, procaine, tetracaine) are rapidly metabolized by plasma cholinesterase, decreasing the risk of maternal toxicity and placental drug transfer (O'Brien et al, 1979). Amide-linked local anesthetics (e.g., lidocaine, bupivacaine, ropivacaine) are degraded by P-450 enzymes in the liver. Local anesthetics differ in their onset, peak plasma concentration, potency and duration based on their lipid solubility, protein binding, site of injection, and concentration. Vascular absorption of local anesthetics limits the safe dose that can be administered. Elevated plasma concentrations produce neurologic toxicity (seizures) or cardiovascular toxicity (myocardial depression, ventricular arrhythmia). Bupivacaine and ropivacaine are the most commonly used local anesthetics for labor analgesia. Ropivacaine is a pure amide-linked S-isomer, unlike bupivacaine, which is a racemic mixture. Because the R-isomer of bupivacaine can bind strongly to cardiac sodium channels, ropivacaine can decrease the possibility of severe cardiac toxicity associated with accidental intravascular injection of large doses of bupivacaine. However, ropivacaine is less soluble than bupivacaine and may be slightly less potent. Regardless of differences, bupivacaine and ropivacaine are extremely safe when appropriately used for epidural or intrathecal administration. An accidental, large intravascular dose of any local anesthetic can result in significant maternal morbidity or mortality.

As with all drugs, placental transfer is determined by molecular size, lipid solubility, protein binding, and maternal drug concentration. Local anesthetics are weak bases with high lipid solubility and a low ionized fraction. However, the lower pH of the fetus has the potential to increase the fraction of ionized molecules, decrease lipid solubility, and result in ion trapping. Therefore in an acidotic fetus, higher concentrations of local anesthetic can accumulate (ion trapping). Increased concentrations of local anesthetics result in decreased neonatal neuromuscular tone similar to that seen with magnesium. If a direct intravascular or intrafetal injection of local anesthetics occurs, significant toxicity and depression can develop, signified by bradycardia, ventricular arrhythmia, and severe cardiac depression with acidosis.

Neuraxial Opioids

Although intraspinal (intrathecal) opiates were demonstrated in 1979 to be capable of producing profound analgesia in humans (Behar et al, 1979; Wang et al, 1979), the epidural injection of opioids as sole agents has proved to be of limited use for effective labor analgesia. In one study, high doses of epidural morphine (7.5 mg) provided satisfactory but not excellent analgesia for 6 hours in the first stage of labor, whereas 2 to 5 mg produced barely satisfactory analgesia in fewer than half the patients (Hughes et al, 1984). Besides the inadequate analgesia and the long onset

time (approximately 1 hour), the side effect of pruritus was significant. In contrast, when lipid-soluble opioids (e.g., sufentanil, fentanyl) are administered in the epidural space as sole agents, analgesia is rapid and equivalent to that of systemic administration (Camann et al, 1992), but remains inferior to that of dilute concentrations of local anesthetics, and less effective for somatic pain associated with the second stage of labor. When lipid-soluble opioids are administered as an adjunctive agent with local anesthetics in the epidural space, they decrease the total local anesthetic dose required and lower the minimum local anesthetic concentration needed to achieve adequate labor analgesia (Buyse et al, 2007; Celleno and Capogna, 1988; Lyons et al, 1997). The most common maternal side effect of conventional doses of epidural fentanyl or sufentanil is pruritus. After maternal epidural administration, the lipid-soluble, poorly ionized opioid analgesics rapidly enter the fetal circulation. An epidural bolus injection of an opioid results in peak neonatal depression at 30 to 60 minutes (similar to an IV bolus dose). Although typical doses used for labor analgesia adversely affect the neonate, the potential for respiratory depression is a function of the amount and timing of drug administered.

Subarachnoid (i.e., spinal, intrathecal) injections of fentanyl, sufentanil, meperidine, and morphine as sole agents are more promising for effective maternal labor analgesia. Analgesic effects of spinal opioids are more potent than epidural or systemic administration, but are of limited duration (2 hours) and are less effective than dilute epidural solutions of local anesthetics for analgesia in the second stage (Honet et al, 1992; Leighton et al, 1989). Spinal opioid administration is often performed as part of a CSE technique (discussed in the following section), with fentanyl or sufentanil being the most commonly used agents. The intrathecal opioid is often combined with a small dose of local anesthetic (e.g., 2.5 mg bupivacaine), decreasing the dose of opioid needed and incidence of pruritus (Wong et al, 2000). Reports of fetal heart rate changes after intrathecal administration of fentanyl or sufentanil (Cohen et al, 1993) may be caused by rapid onset of analgesia and rapid decrease in circulating catecholamines, with epinephrine decreasing faster than norepinephrine, resulting in an unopposed oxytocic effect on the uterus. This effect would increase uterine tone and decrease uterine blood flow. This mechanism is speculative, but it is suggested by observed cases and case reports (Friedlander et al, 1997). Some prospective randomized studies have found no difference in incidence of fetal bradycardia between epidural administration of local anesthetics and intrathecal opioids administered with the CSE technique (Fogel et al, 1999; Nageotte et al, 1997). A systematic review of studies comparing intrathecal opioids to other methods of labor analgesia noted an increase in fetal bradycardia (odds ratio [OR], 1.8; 95% CI, 1.0 to 3.1) and increased maternal pruritus (RR, 29.6; 95% CI, 13.6 to 64.6), but the risk of cesarean section because of FHR abnormalities was similar (Mardirosoff et al, 2002).

NEURAXIAL TECHNIQUES FOR LABOR ANALGESIA

Neuraxial techniques represent the most effective form of labor analgesia, and they achieve the highest rates of maternal satisfaction (Declercq et al, 2006). The patient remains awake and alert without sedative side effects, maternal catecholamine concentrations are reduced (Shnider et al, 1983), hyperventilation is avoided (Levinson et al, 1974), cooperation and capacity to participate actively during labor are facilitated, and predictable analgesia can be achieved, superior to the analgesia provided by all other techniques. Before initiating any neuraxial blockade, anesthesiologists assess the patient's gestational and health history, perform a focused physical examination, discuss the risks, benefits, and alternatives, and obtain consent. In otherwise healthy parturients, routine laboratory tests are not required (American Society of Anesthesiologists Task Force on Obstetric Anesthesia, 2007). Resuscitation equipment and drugs must be immediately available to manage serious complications secondary to initiation of epidural or spinal blocks (discussed under Contraindications and Complications of Neuraxial Techniques). During initiation of the neuraxial blockade, mother and fetus are closely monitored.

EPIDURAL ANALGESIA

Epidural labor analgesia is a catheter-based technique to provide continuous analgesia during labor. The technique involves insertion of a specialized needle and catheter (Figure 16-2) between vertebral spinous processes in the back, into the epidural space. Most commonly, the needle is inserted at a lumbar space between L1 and L4. The needle traverses the skin and subcutaneous tissues, supraspinous ligament, interspinous ligament, and the ligamentum flavum, and it is advanced into the epidural space (Figure 16-3). The tip of the needle does not penetrate the dura, which forms the boundary between the intrathecal or subarachnoid space and the epidural space. To locate the epidural space, a tactile technique called *loss of resistance* is used. The tactile resistance noted with pressure on the plunger of an air- or saline-filled syringe dramatically decreases as the tip of the needle is advanced through the ligamentum flavum (dense resistance) into the epidural space (no resistance), which has an average depth of approximately 5 cm from the skin. Once the needle is properly positioned, a catheter is inserted through the needle.

The catheter remains in the epidural space and the needle is removed. The catheter is secured with adhesives and used for intermittent or continuous injections. Once the catheter is placed, analgesia is achieved by administration of local anesthetics, opioids, or both (see Neuraxial Local Anesthetics and Neuraxial Opioids, earlier) and maintained throughout the course of labor and delivery. The catheter can also be used for operative anesthesia (cesarean delivery) and postoperative analgesia, when necessary.

After an incremental local anesthetic bolus to initiate reliable analgesia, local anesthetics are typically infused continuously with similar or lower blood drug levels compared with repetitive, intermittent boluses of local anesthetics (Hicks et al, 1988; Rosenblatt et al, 1983). Most importantly, the possibility of disastrous complications is reduced with continuous infusions, such as total spinal anesthesia or massive intravascular injections with cardiovascular collapse secondary to large bolus doses of local anesthetics (D'Athis et al, 1988). If the catheter enters the subarachnoid space instead, the level of sensory and motor blockade increases slowly without the sudden onset of complete subarachnoid blockade that can occur with large bolus techniques (Li et al, 1985). Patient-controlled epidural anesthesia is a delivery technique allowing the patient to self-administer small boluses of epidural analgesics with or without a background infusion. Studies comparing patient-controlled epidural anesthesia with continuous infusion technique have found decreased local anesthetic requirements, less anesthesia provider intervention, equivalent or improved patient satisfaction, equivalent or decreased motor blockade, and no significant differences in effects on the fetus or neonate (Halpern, 2005; van der Vyver et al, 2002).

The choices for local anesthetics for epidural infusion include dilute solutions of bupivacaine, ropivacaine, lidocaine, or chloroprocaine (Lee et al, 2002b). The concentration and volume of the loading dose, which is administered before initiating the continuous infusion, and the volume and concentration of the infusion are highly variable. With higher concentrations of local anesthetics, the density of the motor blockade increases. With larger volumes, a greater dermatomal spread of analgesia is achieved. Most practitioners routinely use low concentrations of local

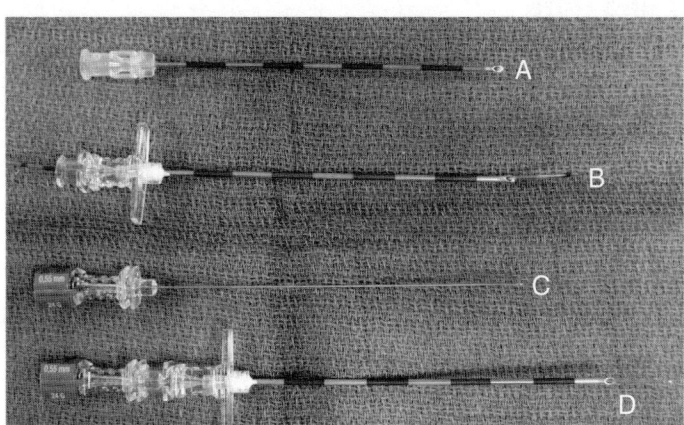
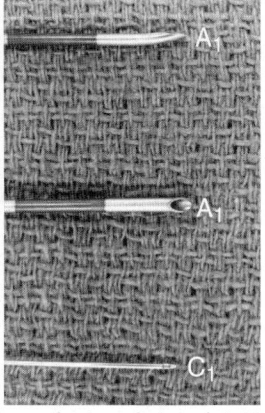

FIGURE 16-2 **Photograph of typical needles and catheters used for neuraxial analgesia and anesthetic techniques. A,** Epidural needle (18-gauge Tuohy) with magnification of tip shown at right (A_1). **B,** Epidural needle (Tuohy) with catheter inserted through needle. **C,** Spinal needle (24-gauge Whitacre) with magnification of tip shown at right (C_1). **D,** Spinal needle inserted through epidural needle for use in combined spinal-epidural technique.

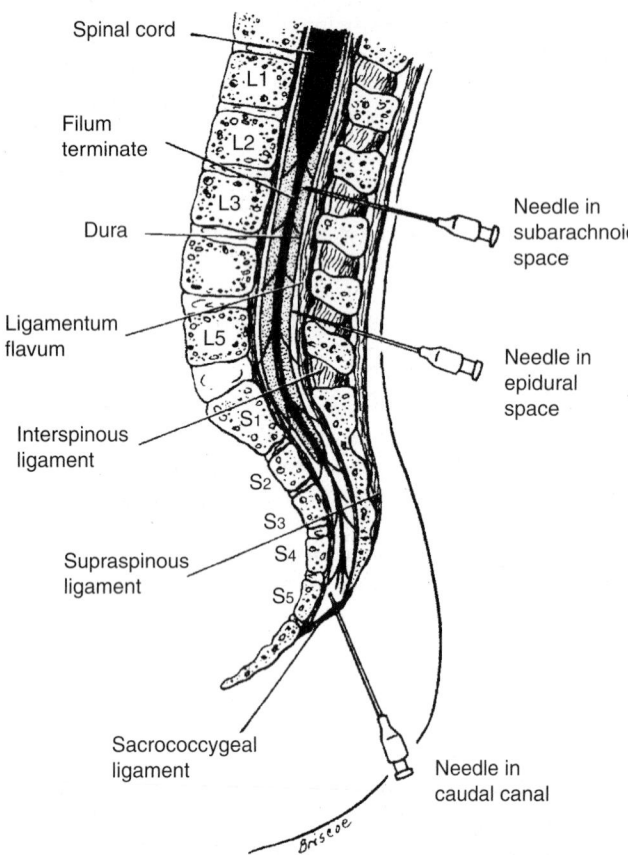

FIGURE 16-3 Schematic diagram of lumbosacral anatomy showing needle placement for subarachnoid, lumbar epidural, and caudal blocks. *(From Rosen MA, Hughes SC, Levinson G: Regional anesthesia for labor and delivery. In Hughes SC, Levinson G, Rosen MA, editors:* Shnider and Levinson's anesthesia for obstetrics, *ed 4, Baltimore, 2002, Lippincott Williams and Wilkins, p 125.)*

anesthetics and many coadminister an opioid with both the initial bolus and the infusion (e.g., 2 μg/mL fentanyl) for its synergistic effect. Dilute solutions of local anesthetics (0.0625% to 0.125% bupivacaine or ropivacaine) minimize the motor blockade and preserve the perception of pelvic pressure with descent of the fetus.

Effects on the Progress of Labor and Rate of Operative Delivery

The use of epidural analgesia has been associated with prolonged labor and increased rates of assisted delivery and cesarean section. Retrospective studies are difficult to interpret, because higher pain scores are predictive of increased labor duration (Wuitchik et al, 1989), and higher analgesic requirements are predictive of increased rates of cesarean section (Alexander et al, 2001). A Cochrane review of the effects of epidural analgesia, including CSE, compared with nonepidural analgesia or no analgesia during labor (Anim-Somuah et al, 2005) concluded that, although there was an increased risk of instrumental vaginal birth (RR, 1.38; 95% CI, 1.24 to 1.53; 17 trials including 6162 women), there was no evidence of a significant difference in the risk of caesarean delivery (RR, 1.07; 95% CI, 0.93 to 1.23; 20 trials including 6534 women). A recent meta-analysis summarized the results of studies addressing the

timing of neuraxial analgesia in labor on operative deliveries in nulliparous women (Marucci et al, 2007). Cesarean delivery rates (OR, 1.00; 95% CI, 0.82 to 1.23) and instrumental vaginal delivery rates (OR, 1.00; 95% CI, 0.83 to 1.21) were similar in the early neuraxial analgesia and later control groups. Neonates of patients with early neuraxial analgesia had a higher umbilical artery pH and received less naloxone than did patients when using other methods. The timing and use of neuraxial labor analgesia have differing effects on the length of labor. Compared with opioids for labor analgesia, the use of epidural analgesia minimally lengthens the first stage in some women and shortens it in others, but overall appears to lengthen the second stage by approximately 15 minutes (Anim-Somuah et al, 2005; Ohel et al, 2006; Sharma et al, 2004; Wong et al, 2005).

SPINAL ANALGESIA

Spinal analgesia is typically administered near the time of anticipated delivery. A small dose of a local anesthetic, opioid, or both is injected into the subarachnoid space. This dose of local anesthetic is far lower than that used for spinal anesthesia for cesarean section, and it has minimal effects on motor nerve function. Compared with epidural analgesia, it has the benefits of a more rapid onset, a lower failure rate, and being technically easier and quicker to perform. It has the significant disadvantage of a finite effective duration (approximately 90 minutes), but can be extremely useful for certain circumstances such as forceps-assisted delivery for a woman without epidural analgesia.

COMBINED SPINAL-EPIDURAL ANALGESIA

One variation of the lumbar epidural technique is a CSE analgesic. After placement of the epidural needle, but before insertion of the epidural catheter, a longer spinal needle is passed through the indwelling epidural needle (see Figure 16-2), puncturing the dura, and a small dose of local anesthetic or opioid is administered. If opioid alone is administered and the epidural catheter is placed but no local anesthetic is given, some analgesia can be achieved without motor blockade or sympathectomy. This method can allow the patient to walk safely (i.e., a "walking epidural"), but the analgesia is limited in efficacy and duration (approximately 2 hours in the first stage) and is rarely effective for the second stage of labor.

If small doses of local anesthetics are administered through the spinal needle, segmental analgesia results more rapidly than with epidural administration of local anesthetics. Specifically, the onset of analgesia in the sacral root distribution is much more rapid with CSE compared with epidural alone. The epidural placement of the catheter allows continuation of the segmental analgesia initiated by the spinal technique. In a metaanalysis of 19 trials (2658 women) comparing CSE to epidural labor analgesia (Simmons et al, 2007), CSE had a faster onset of effective analgesia (especially in spread to sacral roots), was associated with more pruritus, and was associated with a clinically insignificant lower umbilical arterial pH. No differences were seen for maternal satisfaction, walking in labor, type of delivery, maternal hypotension, postdural puncture headache rate, or need for blood patch.

CONTRAINDICATIONS AND COMPLICATIONS OF NEURAXIAL TECHNIQUES

Certain conditions contraindicate neuraxial procedures; these include patient refusal, infection at the needle insertion site, significant coagulopathy, hypovolemic shock, increased intracranial pressure from mass lesion, and inadequate provider expertise. Other conditions such as systemic infection, neurologic disease, and mild coagulopathies should be evaluated on a case-by-case basis. Human immunodeficiency virus infection is not a contraindication to regional technique in the pregnant patient (Hughes et al, 1995).

Infrequent but occasionally life-threatening complications can result from administration of regional anesthesia. The most serious complications are from accidental IV or intrathecal injections of local anesthetics. A prospective study of 145,550 epidurals in the United Kingdom noted unintended intravascular injection rates of 1 in 5000 and high spinal rates of 1 in 16,000 (Jenkins, 2005). An unintended bolus of IV local anesthetic causes dose-dependent consequences ranging from minor side effects (e.g., tinnitus, perioral tingling, mild blood pressure, heart rate changes) to major complications (e.g., seizures, loss of consciousness, severe arrhythmias, cardiovascular collapse). The severity depends on the dose, type of local anesthetic, and preexisting condition of the parturient. Measures that minimize the likelihood of accidental intravascular injection include careful aspiration of the catheter before injection, test dosing, and incremental administration of therapeutic doses. If a local anesthetic overdose occurs, consider using a 20% IV lipid emulsion to bind the drug and decrease toxicity. Successful resuscitation and support of the mother will reestablish uterine blood flow; this will provide adequate fetal oxygenation and allow time for excretion of local anesthetic from the fetus. The neonate has an extremely limited ability to metabolize local anesthetics and may have prolonged convulsions if emergent delivery is required (Morishima and Adamsons, 1967; Ralston and Shnider, 1978).

A "high spinal" (or total spinal) can result from an unrecognized epidural catheter placed subdural, migration of the catheter during its use, or an overdose of local anesthetic in the epidural space (i.e., high epidural). Both high spinals and high epidurals can result in severe maternal hypotension, bradycardia, loss of consciousness, and blockade of the motor nerves to the respiratory muscles (Yentis and Dob, 2001).

Treatment of complications resulting from both intravascular injection and high spinal is directed at restoring maternal and fetal oxygenation, ventilation, and circulation. Intubation, vasopressors, fluids, and advanced cardiac life support algorithms are often required. In any situation of maternal cardiac arrest with unsuccessful resuscitation, the fetus should be delivered by cesarean section if the mother is not resuscitated within 4 minutes of the arrest. This guideline for emergent operative delivery increases the chances of survival for both the mother and neonate (American Heart Association, 2005; Katz et al, 1986).

In addition, a variety of less severe complications and side effects can occur with neuraxial blockade. The retrospective rates of inadequate epidural analgesia or inadequate CSE analgesia requiring catheter replacement were 7% and 3%, respectively, at a U.S. academic center (Pan et al, 2004). The rate of accidental dural puncture during epidural catheter placement is 1.5%, and approximately half of these will result in a severe headache (Choi et al, 2003), which are typically managed with analgesics or a blood patch if necessary. Hypotension (decrease in systolic blood pressure greater than 20%) secondary to sympathetic blockade is the most common complication of neuraxial blockade for labor analgesia, with rates between 10% and 24% (Brizgys et al, 1987; Simmons et al, 2007). Prophylactic measures include left uterine displacement and hydration. Although standards for timing, amount, and hydration fluid remain controversial, dehydration should be avoided (Hofmeyr et al, 2004; Kinsella et al, 2000; Ko et al, 2007). Treatment of hypotension consists of further uterine displacement, IV fluids, and vasopressor administration. Small boluses of either phenylephrine or ephedrine can be used to treat hypotension. Although ephedrine (primarily β-adrenergic) was historically used, phenylephrine (primarily α-adrenergic) is associated with less fetal acidosis (Lee et al, 2002a; Ngan Kee et al, 2009; Smiley, 2009). If treated promptly, maternal hypotension does not lead to fetal depression or neonatal morbidity.

A rise in core maternal body temperature is associated with labor epidural analgesia and may be influenced by several factors; these include duration, ambient temperature, administration of systemic opioids, and the presence of shivering. During the first 5 hours of epidural analgesia, there is no significant rise in body temperature (Mercier and Benhamou, 1997). In a retrospective study, temperature increases approximately 0.10° C per hour, and may reach 38° C in as many as 15% of parturients with a labor epidural compared with 1% without an epidural (Lieberman et al, 1997). Although Lieberman et al suggest a significant increase in the rate of newborn evaluation for sepsis (i.e., sepsis work-up [SWU]) with epidural analgesia, 67.3% of the noted SWUs were ordered in infants born to mothers without fever. Kaul et al (2001) found no association between epidural analgesia and SWU. However, patients who received epidural analgesia and their neonates had an increased body temperature at delivery, and approximately 6% of these women had temperatures equal to or exceeding 38° C. Although maternal temperature had no predictive value for the SWU, Kaul et al (2001) found other risk factors associated with the SWU, including low birthweight, gestational age, meconium, or respiratory distress requiring intubation at birth, hypothermia at birth, group-B β-hemolytic *streptococcus* colonization, and maternal preeclampsia or hypertension. Although the etiology of the maternal temperature rise remains uncertain, it need not affect the neonatal SWU. Epidural analgesia during labor does not increase the incidence of neonatal sepsis. Although it is suggested that the fever is associated with noninfectious inflammatory activation or altered thermoregulation, the fever is not associated with a change in white blood cell count or with an infectious process, and treatment is not necessary.

Other potential side effects from neuraxial blockade include pruritus, nausea, shivering, urinary retention, motor weakness, low back pain, and a prolonged block. More serious complications of meningitis, epidural hematoma, and nerve or spinal cord injury are extremely rare.

A retrospective Swedish study of severe neurologic complications from neuraxial blockade included 200,000 obstetric epidurals and 50,000 obstetric spinals. Rates of serious neurologic events (i.e., neuraxial hematoma or abscess, nerve or cord damage) were 1:29,000 for obstetric epidural and 1:25,000 for obstetric spinal anesthetic procedures (Moen et al, 2004).

PARACERVICAL BLOCK

A paracervical block is used to provide pain relief during the first stage of labor in up to 3% of patients (Bucklin et al, 2005). The technique consists of submucosal administration of local anesthetics immediately lateral and posterior to the uterocervical junction, which blocks transmission of pain impulses at the paracervical ganglion. Analgesia is not as profound as with epidural or spinal regional block, and the duration of analgesia is short (45 to 60 minutes), but the complications and side effects of epidural analgesia, such as hypotension, hypoventilation, and motor blockade, are avoided. Complications from systemic absorption or transfer of local anesthetic can occur. There is also the possibility of direct fetal trauma or injection. Paracervical block is associated with a 15% rate of fetal bradycardia based on a metaanalysis of studies (Rosen, 2002b). The mechanism of this phenomenon is unclear, and close fetal monitoring is warranted. The bradycardia may occur secondary to decreased uterine blood flow from the vasoconstrictor properties of local anesthetics, greater uterine activity, or transfer of the local anesthetic across the placenta to the fetus, causing direct toxic effects on the fetal heart. The bradycardia is usually limited to less than 15 minutes, and treatment is supportive, consisting of lateral positioning and administration of oxygen.

PUDENDAL BLOCK

The obstetrician performs a pudendal block with a transvaginal technique, guiding a sheathed needle to the vaginal mucosa and sacrospinous ligament just medial and posterior to the ischial spine. The technique primarily blocks sensation of the lower vagina and perineum, and it is typically placed just before vaginal delivery. Although the technique provides analgesia for vaginal delivery or uncomplicated instrumental delivery, the rate of failure is high. In many centers, this technique is used when epidural or spinal techniques are unavailable. Complications in addition to failure include systemic local anesthetic toxicity, ischiorectal or vaginal hematoma, and, rarely, fetal injection of local anesthetic.

ANESTHESIA FOR CESAREAN DELIVERY

In the United States, the vast majority of cesarean deliveries are performed with neuraxial anesthesia. It offers the advantages of less anesthetic exposure to the neonate, has the benefit of an awake mother at the delivery, allows for placement of neuraxial opioids to decrease postoperative pain, and avoids the risks of maternal aspiration and difficult airway associated with general anesthesia. However, the use of general anesthesia is sometimes required if regional anesthesia is contraindicated (e.g., coagulopathy, hemorrhage) or if a rapid onset is needed for emergent deliveries (e.g., fetal bradycardia, uterine rupture). Benefits of general anesthesia compared with regional anesthesia include a secure airway, controlled ventilation, rapid and dependable onset, and potential for less hemodynamic instability.

EPIDURAL ANESTHESIA

Epidural anesthesia is an excellent choice for surgical anesthesia when an indwelling, functioning epidural catheter had been placed for labor analgesia. Epidural anesthesia provides the ability to titrate the desired level of anesthesia and extend the block time, if needed for a prolonged procedure. Epidural anesthesia is also ideal for patients in a nonemergent delivery who would not tolerate the abrupt onset of a sympathectomy from spinal anesthesia, such as some patients with cardiac disease. The volume and concentration of local anesthetic agents used for surgical anesthesia are larger than those used for labor analgesia. However, the technique of catheter placement, test dosing, and potential complications are similar. A typical dose regimen of epidural anesthesia for cesarean delivery could include 2% lidocaine (20 mL). Typically the anesthesiologist attempts to provide a dense block from the T4 level to the sacrum. This technique might not completely alleviate the visceral pain and pressure sensation associated with peritoneal manipulation, and adjuvant drugs are occasionally necessary. IV ondansetron and metoclopramide are frequently given to decrease nausea and vomiting associated with the operative delivery and hemodynamic effects from the dense neuraxial blockade (Lussos et al, 1992; Pan and Moore, 2001). Epidural morphine (3 to 5 mg) is typically given near the end of the procedure to decrease postoperative pain for up to 24 hours (Cohen et al, 1991).

SPINAL ANESTHESIA

For the patient without an epidural catheter, spinal anesthesia is the most common regional anesthetic technique used for cesarean delivery. The block is technically easier than epidural blockade, more rapid in onset, and more reliable in providing surgical anesthesia from the midthoracic level to the sacrum (Riley et al, 1995). The risk of profound hypotension is higher with spinal anesthesia than with epidural anesthesia, because the onset of the sympathectomy is more rapid. However, this risk can be nearly eliminated by avoidance of aortocaval compression, prehydration, and appropriate use of vasopressors. Colloid is significantly more effective than crystalloid (Ko et al, 2007). Historically, ephedrine was recommended as the vasopressor of choice, but more recent data confirm that a phenylephrine infusion at the time of spinal placement is effective at preventing hypotension and is associated with less fetal acidosis compared to ephedrine (Ngan Kee et al, 2004, 2009). Data also suggest that spinal anesthesia can be used safely for patients with preeclampsia (Hood and Curry, 1999; Wallace et al, 1995). A typical spinal anesthetic could consist of bupivacaine (12.5 mg) with morphine (200 μg) added to decrease postoperative pain. A large variety of other combinations of local anesthetics and opioids are used. A hyperbaric solution of local anesthetic is often used to facilitate anatomic and gravitational control of the block distribution. The medication will flow with the spinal curvature to a position near T4, and a head-down position can enhance the rostral spread of the block if needed. The duration of a single shot spinal anesthetic is variable, but normally provides adequate surgical anesthesia for greater than 90 minutes. In selected circumstances, the use of a CSE technique offers the advantage of a spinal anesthetic, with rapid onset of a dense block and the ability to administer additional local anesthetic through the epidural catheter if the procedure lasts for an extended time. A continuous spinal anesthetic technique with deliberate subdural catheter placement is a rarely used alternative, but is sometimes chosen in cases of accidental dural puncture during attempts to place an epidural catheter. This technique allows the advantage of a titratable, reliable, dense anesthetic, but carries the risks of high spinal if the intrathecal catheter is mistaken for an epidural catheter, or if the provider is unfamiliar with the technique. The rates of rare complications of meningitis or neurologic impairment from local anesthetic toxicity with the use of a spinal catheter may be somewhat higher than the other neuraxial techniques, but they remain unknown. Some data suggest that leaving the spinal catheter in place for 24 hours decreases the risk of postdural puncture headache (Ayad et al, 2003; Cohen et al, 1994).

LOCAL ANESTHESIA

Although cesarean delivery can be performed with local infiltration, it is accompanied with considerable discomfort to the woman and risks the possibility of local anesthetic overdose. Most obstetricians are not trained to perform the technique. However, local infiltration is useful in rare circumstances, such as acute fetal distress without an available anesthesia provider.

GENERAL ANESTHESIA

General anesthesia is used in obstetric practice for cesarean section typically when regional anesthesia is contraindicated or for emergencies, because of its rapid and predictable action. The major risks for maternal morbidity are pulmonary aspiration and failed intubation. Appropriate airway examination, preparation for unanticipated events, and familiarity with techniques and the algorithm for difficult intubation (American Society of Anesthesiologists Task Force on Management of the Difficult Airway, 2003) are critical for providing a safe general anesthetic.

After denitrogenation of the lungs (i.e., preoxygenation), general anesthesia is induced by rapid-sequence administration of an IV induction agent, followed by a rapidly acting muscle relaxant. The trachea is intubated with a cuffed endotracheal tube, and a surgical incision is made after confirmation of tracheal intubation and adequate ventilation. Anesthesia is maintained by administering a combination of inhaled nitrous oxide and a potent inhaled halogenated agent (e.g., isoflurane), as well as sedative-hypnotics, opioid analgesics, and additional muscle relaxants if needed. During typical general anesthesia for cesarean delivery, opioids and benzodiazepines are administered after the baby is delivered, to avoid placental transfer of these agents to the neonate. Before delivery of the baby, the primary anesthetic for the incision and delivery is the induction agent, because there is little time for uptake and distribution of the inhaled agents into the mother or fetus (Dwyer et al, 1995). If intubation attempts fail, the operative delivery may proceed if the anesthesiologist communicates that it is possible to reliably ventilate the mother's lungs with either facemask or laryngeal mask airway (American Society of Anesthesiologists Task Force on Management of the Difficult Airway, 2003).

Induction Agents

Anesthesiologists use a variety of agents to rapidly induce unconsciousness. Among the most common are thiopental, propofol, etomidate, and ketamine. Each agent represents a different biochemical class, and each has specific advantages and cardiovascular effects.

Sodium thiopental is a highly lipid-soluble, protein-bound barbiturate that can cause decreased cardiac output and hypotension and rapidly crosses the placenta. Historically, it was the most common induction agent for cesarean section under general anesthesia. In a study of healthy volunteers undergoing uncomplicated cesarean section, the mean umbilical artery (UA)–to–umbilical vein (UV) ratio of thiopental concentrations was 0.87 (Morgan et al, 1981). IV administration of an appropriate dose (4 to 6 mg/kg) renders the patient unconscious within a circulation time (30 seconds), peaks in the UV blood in 1 minute and in the UA blood in 2 to 3 minutes, and has no significant clinical effect on neonatal well-being. However, doses of 8 mg/kg can result in neonatal depression (Finster et al, 1972), and higher doses may require cardiorespiratory supportive techniques until the neonate can excrete the drug. This elimination may take up to 2 days (Fox et al, 1979). The lack of neonatal effects is unclear, but may be caused by first-pass metabolism by the neonatal liver, rapid redistribution into maternal vascular-rich tissue beds, additional dilution by the fetal circulation, and higher fetal brain water content.

Propofol is a diisopropylphenol that is available as a 1% aqueous solution in an oil-in-water emulsion containing soybean oil, glycerol, and egg lecithin. Like thiopental, propofol is rapid in onset and can cause significant hypotension with a similar UA:UV ratio of 0.7 (Dailland et al, 1989). Unlike thiopental, propofol is preservative free and must be drawn up only hours before use. Other differences are that propofol decreases the incidence of nausea and vomiting, and it is currently not a controlled substance. Propofol has not been demonstrated to be superior to thiopental in maternal or neonatal outcome. Propofol administration has no significant effect on neonatal behavior scores with induction doses of 2.5 mg/kg, but larger doses (9 mg/kg) are associated with newborn depression (Gregory et al, 1990).

Etomidate contains a carboxylated imidazole ring that provides water solubility in acidic solutions and lipid solubility at physiologic pH. Like thiopental, etomidate has a rapid onset of action because of its high lipid solubility, it rapidly crosses the placenta, and redistribution results in a relatively short duration of action. Unlike thiopental and propofol, etomidate has minimal effects on the cardiovascular system, but it is painful on injection, can cause involuntary muscle tremors, has higher rates of nausea and vomiting, and can increase the risk of seizures in patients with decreased thresholds. At typical induction doses (0.3 mg/kg), etomidate administration can cause decreased neonatal cortisol production (<6 hours), but the clinical significance remains uncertain (Crozier et al, 1993).

Ketamine, a structural analogue to phencyclidine, is more lipid soluble and less protein bound than thiopental. It is an analgesic, hypnotic, and amnestic with minimal respiratory depressive effects. Ketamine is biotransformed in the liver to active metabolites, such as norketamine. In contrast to thiopental, sympathomimetic characteristics of ketamine increase arterial pressure, heart rate, and cardiac output through central stimulation of the sympathetic nervous system, making it an ideal choice for a patient in hemodynamic compromise. Doses that are higher than those appropriate for induction of general anesthesia (1 mg/kg) can increase uterine tone, reducing uterine arterial perfusion. No neonatal depression is noted with typical induction doses (Little et al, 1972). In low doses (0.25 mg/kg), ketamine has profound analgesic effects, unlike barbiturates, but has been associated with undesirable psychomimetic side effects (e.g., illusions, bad dreams), which can be lessened by coadministration of benzodiazepines.

Nitrous Oxide

Inhaled nitrous oxide is often used as part of maintenance for general anesthesia, because of its minimal effects on maternal hemodynamics and uterine tone. As a sole agent, it is insufficient to provide an appropriate level of anesthesia for an operative procedure. It rapidly crosses the placenta with increasing UV-to–maternal artery ratios of 0.37 in the first 2 to 9 minutes increasing to 0.61 at 9 to 14 minutes (Karasawa et al, 2003). The effects of nitrous oxide on the neonate are not significant. Additional information about nitrous oxide is found in the previous section under Inhalation Analgesia.

Inhaled Halogenated Anesthetics

Isoflurane, sevoflurane, desflurane, and halothane are all halogenated hydrocarbons that differ in chemical composition, physical properties, biotransformation, potencies, and rates of uptake and elimination. In clinical use, specialized vaporizers deliver these volatile liquid agents, so that the inhaled concentrations can be carefully titrated by anesthesiologists because of the relatively profound cardiovascular effects and potential for uterine muscle relaxation. These agents are important components of general anesthesia for cesarean section, but readily cross the placenta. Without the use of these agents, the incidence of maternal recall of intraoperative events is unacceptably high (Schultetus et al, 1986; Tunstall, 1979).

Placental transfer of inhalation agents is rapid because these are nonionized, highly lipid-soluble substances of low molecular weight. The concentrations of these agents in the fetus depend directly on the concentration and duration of anesthetic in the mother. Clinicians often confuse the use of general anesthesia and the terms *fetal distress*

and *depressed neonate*. A depressed fetus will likely become a depressed neonate, and general anesthesia may be used because it is the most rapidly acting anesthetic to allow cesarean delivery. For a healthy fetus, the use of general anesthesia is not contraindicated. A Cochrane review of 16 studies comparing neuraxial blockade versus general anesthesia in otherwise uncomplicated cesarean deliveries found that "no significant difference was seen in terms of neonatal Apgar scores of six or less and of four or less at one and five minutes and need for neonatal resuscitation" (Afolabi et al, 2006). The authors concluded that there was no evidence to show that neuraxial anesthesia was superior to general anesthesia for neonatal outcome. Recent experimental animal studies have demonstrated neuronal apoptosis in the developing brain when a variety of agents are administered to induce and maintain general anesthesia (Istaphanous and Loepke, 2009; Loepke and Soriano, 2008). Implications for the fetus and neonate from brief anesthetic exposures are currently unknown because of a lack of human studies and difficulties extrapolating animal study methodology to humans.

The induction–delivery interval is not as important in neonatal outcome as the uterine incision–delivery interval, during which uterine blood flow may be compromised and fetal asphyxia may occur. A long induction–delivery time may result in a neonate who is lightly anesthetized but not asphyxiated. If excessive concentrations of anesthetic are given for inordinately long times, neonatal anesthesia, evidenced by flaccidity, cardiorespiratory depression, and decreased tone, can be anticipated (Moya, 1966). It cannot be overemphasized that if the neonatal depression is caused by transfer of anesthetic drugs, the infant is merely lightly anesthetized and should respond easily to basic treatment measures. Treatment should include and focus on effective ventilation; cardiopulmonary resuscitation is rarely necessary. Ventilation will allow elimination of the inhalation anesthetic by the infant's lungs. Rapid improvement of the infant should be expected. Otherwise, a search for other causes of depression is imperative. For these reasons, it is critical that clinicians experienced with neonatal ventilation are present at operative deliveries under general anesthesia in which the time from skin incision to delivery may be longer (i.e., known percreta, large fibroids), or maternal condition necessitates an atypical induction and maintenance of anesthesia (e.g., a patient with critical aortic stenosis undergoing an opioid-based induction). A discussion of the operative and anesthetic plan by the neonatologist, obstetrician, and anesthesiologist is crucial for optimizing the outcome of neonates in these situations.

Neuromuscular Blocking Agents

Succinylcholine remains the skeletal muscle relaxant of choice for obstetric anesthesia, because of its rapid onset and short duration of action. In doses of 1.5 mg/kg, appropriate intubating conditions are present within 45 seconds. Because it is highly ionized and poorly lipid soluble, only small amounts cross the placenta. Side effects include increased maternal potassium levels, myalgias, and succinylcholine is a known trigger agent for malignant hyperthermia in susceptible individuals. This depolarizing neuromuscular blocking agent is normally hydrolyzed in maternal plasma by pseudocholinesterase and usually does not interfere with fetal neuromuscular activity. If the hydrolytic enzyme is present either in low concentrations (Shnider, 1965) or in a genetically determined atypical form (Baraka, 1975), prolonged maternal or neonatal respiratory depression secondary to muscular paralysis can occur.

Rocuronium is a rapid-acting, nondepolarizing neuromuscular blocker that is an acceptable alternative to succinylcholine. It provides adequate intubating conditions in approximately 90 seconds at doses of 0.6 mg/kg and in less than 60 seconds at doses of 1.2 mg/kg (Abouleish et al, 1994; Magorian et al, 1993). Unlike succinylcholine, it has a much longer duration of action, decreasing maternal safety in the event the anesthesiologist is unable to intubate or ventilate the patient. It has the benefit of not being a triggering agent of malignant hyperthermia or elevating serum potassium levels.

During the operation, nondepolarizing neuromuscular blocking agents can be titrated to improve operating conditions. Under normal circumstances, the poorly lipid-soluble, highly ionized, nondepolarizing neuromuscular blockers (i.e., rocuronium, vecuronium, *cis*-atracurium, pancuronium) do not cross the placenta in amounts significant enough to cause neonatal muscle weakness (Kivalo and Saaroski, 1972). This placental impermeability is only relative, however, and neonatal neuromuscular blockade can occur when large doses are given (Older and Harris, 1968).

The diagnosis of neonatal depression secondary to neuromuscular blockade can be made on the basis of the maternal history (e.g., prolonged administration of neuromuscular blockers, history of atypical pseudocholinesterase), the response of the mother to neuromuscular blocking drugs, and the physical examination of the newborn. The paralyzed neonate has normal cardiovascular function and good color, but lacks spontaneous ventilatory movements, has muscle flaccidity, and shows no reflex responses. The anesthesiologist can place a nerve stimulator on the neonate and demonstrate the classic signs of neuromuscular blockade (Ali and Savarese, 1976). Treatment consists of ventilatory support until the neonate excretes the drug, up to 48 hours. Reversal of nondepolarizing relaxants with cholinesterase inhibitors

may be attempted (e.g., neostigmine, 0.06 mg/kg), but adequate ventilatory support is the mainstay of treatment. Concomitant administration of an anticholinergic (e.g., atropine, glycopyrrolate) is normally necessary to prevent severe bradycardia from muscarinic side effects of the increased acetylcholine.

SUMMARY

This chapter serves as a general overview of the changes in maternal physiology during pregnancy and briefly discusses options and techniques for both labor analgesia and anesthesia for operative delivery. Its purpose is to allow the pediatrician and neonatologist a better understanding of the decisions and concerns of the anesthesiologist and the implications of his or her interventions. To provide the best care for mother and child, excellent communication is required between the obstetrician, pediatrician, anesthesiologist, and nurse. Only by facilitating these lines of communication and obtaining input from each discipline can patient care and safety become optimized.

SUGGESTED READINGS

Afolabi BB, Lesi FE, Merah NA: Regional versus general anaesthesia for caesarean section, *Cochrane Database Syst Rev* (4):CD004350, 2006.
American Society of Anesthesiologists Task Force on Obstetric Anesthesia: Practice guidelines for obstetric anesthesia: an updated report by the American Society of Anesthesiologists Task Force on Obstetric Anesthesia, *Anesthesiology* 106:843-863, 2007.
Anim-Somuah M, Smyth R, Howell C: Epidural versus non-epidural or no analgesia in labour, *Cochrane Database Syst Rev* (4):CD000331, 2005.
Chestnut DH: *Obstetric anesthesia: principles and practice*, ed 4, Philadelphia, 2009, Mosby.
Eltzschig HK, Lieberman ES, Camann WR: Regional anesthesia and analgesia for labor and delivery, *N Engl J Med* 348:319-332, 2003.
Hughes SC, Levinson G, Rosen MA, et al: *Shnider and Levinson's anesthesia for obstetrics*, ed 4, Philadelphia, 2002, Lippincott Williams & Wilkins.
Marucci M, Cinnella G, Perchiazzi G, et al: Patient-requested neuraxial analgesia for labor: impact on rates of cesarean and instrumental vaginal delivery, *Anesthesiology* 106:1035-1045, 2007.
Simmons SW, Cyna AM, Dennis AT, et al: Combined spinal-epidural versus epidural analgesia in labour, *Cochrane Database Syst Rev* (3):CD003401, 2007.
Ngan Kee WD, Khaw KS, Tan PE, et al: Placental transfer and fetal metabolic effects of phenylephrine and ephedrine during spinal anesthesia for cesarean delivery, *Anesthesiology* 111:506-512, 2009.
Wong CA, Scavone BM, Peaceman AM, et al: The risk of cesarean delivery with neuraxial analgesia given early versus late in labor, *N Engl J Med* 352:655-665, 2005.

Complete references used in this text can be found online at www.expertconsult.com

PART V

GENETICS

IMPACT OF THE HUMAN GENOME PROJECT ON NEONATAL CARE

Jeffrey C. Murray

HISTORY OF THE HUMAN GENOME PROJECT

Within 50 years of the discovery of the structure of DNA by Watson and Crick, the Human Genome Project achieved a major milestone with its description of an almost complete sequence of the approximately 3 billion nucleotides (A,C,G,T) contained within the human haploid genome. This effort was the result of an early vision by a group of scientists that with advances in technology and sequence analysis this task could be achieved (Watson and Cook-Deegan, 1991). The central goal was to provide a reference sequence of the human genome that could serve as a framework on which to better understand disease pathogenesis. Eventually, it was hoped, this would lead to improved treatments and prevention.

There have been numerous spin-offs from the technology and analytic platforms developed. A wide range of other organisms have now had their genomes sequenced from pathogenic viruses to complex plants and animals. These sequences provide insights into disease pathogenesis that are infectious or immunologic and open new doors to therapies. Comparing DNA sequences across species to look for evolutionary conservation has also provided tremendous insights into the protein structure of genes and the regulatory elements that control the cell type, timing, and amount for the synthesis of any individual protein. The nature of how a gene is defined has been substantially altered by these insights, so that the gene is now recognized as a far more complex structure with elements dispersed sometimes 1 million nucleotides or more from the protein coding components classically thought of as "the gene" (Gerstein et al, 2007).

Understanding the genetic relationships between individuals of different ancestral origins has led to the current effort to describe genetic variation across the human species as an essential aspect of understanding predisposition to or resistance from disease. Because the identification that carriers of sickle cell trait had increased resistance to malaria, or the identification of genetic factors conferring persistence of lactose tolerance into adult life as a mechanism associated with the advantages of dairy farming (Bersaglieri et al, 2004), it has been evident that individual genetic variation is an important contributor to health and disease. The hemoglobin system has provided an evolving paradigm for our understanding of the molecular nature of genetic disease beginning in the 1940s (Neel, 1949; Pauling et al, 1949) and onward to serving as a model for gene therapy in the modern era. The conception of the genome project led to wide ranging concerns about ethical, legal, and social aspects and resulted in the development of the Ethical, Legal and Social Issues (ELSI) Project to investigate these areas and to anticipate future concerns and problems. Finally, as part of the social and legal component, the work has led to legislation in the United States and abroad that is designed to protect individuals from discrimination based on their genetic background.

The Human Genome Project has been an international effort from its beginnings and had critical predecessors in the human gene mapping (HGM) meetings that had an initial focus on identifying the chromosomal location of normal and disease causing genetic variants. The community established by the HGM meetings provided an infrastructure that enabled the more comprehensive sequence-based maps developed in the wake of the HGM meetings. One early outcome of these meetings and the recognized need to convert research findings to clinical utility was creation of *Mendelian Inheritance in Man* by Victor McKusicks, which has now evolved into *Online Mendelian Inheritance in Man* (www.ncbi.nlm.nih.gov/omim/)—a comprehensive catalogue of single-gene disorders that is an essential reference tool for learning about the genetic aspects of both rare and common disease.

The international effort continues with many individual countries now focusing on genome efforts that are specifically relevant to their own high-risk medical conditions (e.g., malaria, HIV, hemoglobinopathies). These early collaborative international efforts also created the framework for one of the greatest successes of the Human Genome Project—that is, information generated relevant to the human DNA sequence and its variation should be held in public trust and there should be open access to DNA sequence and its annotation. This spirit of open access has, in turn, led to a stronger community ethic for the sharing of scientific and medical data that may be a legacy that will exceed the value of the sequence itself.

There have been many technical and analytic advances that have enabled the sequence, and more recently its variation, to be understood and applied. Currently these advances extend to the characterization of hundreds of thousands of genetic variants on large populations of individuals. In the last few years this characterization has led to dramatic advances in the understanding of how common genetic variation can contribute to human genetic disease. This chapter will provide some detail on the various aspects of the Human Genome Project that are of current relevance.

The interval of more than 50 years between the elucidation of DNA as the information-containing macromolecule and its structural description by Watson and Crick has also spanned the embedding of medical genetics as an important specialty in health care. This same time interval has seen the identification, treatment, and in some cases prevention of a wide range of disorders that have a strong genetic component (including Rh incompatibility and phenylketonuria) and a variety of other neonatal biochemical disorders and the hemoglobinopathies. Discussed in Chapters 3 and 27 are the details of the current state of our knowledge of these important advances in prenatal and neonatal screening. It now seems apparent that the past focus on adding one disease at a time to the armamentarium of those that can be studied and treated using genetic tools will soon give way to a comprehensive analysis available at the level of the individual genome. Much of the current effort in human genome work is devoted toward individualized medicine, in which physicians will have the ability to treat not just a disease but a specific person with a disease and to account for their genetic and environmental variation in response to therapy or risks associated with prevention. Motulsky (1957) recognized this pharmacogenetic (or pharmacogenomic when applied globally) approach in the early days of human genetic study as being essential to understanding the significant variation in response to therapeutic agents or toxins. Pharmacogenetics is already being applied clinically to identify patients at risk for toxic reactions to some chemotherapeutic agents as well as anti-infectious compounds. Individualization of diet and nutritional approaches is also on the immediate horizon, and it seems likely that over the next few years there will be in place high-throughput genotyping platforms that will provide comprehensive information to the pediatrician and neonatologist for providing direct alterations and care beginning in early infancy. These individualized genome-wide profiles are already available to early adopters and are creating new models for how physicians will anticipate health care needs and outcomes for their patients.

The history of the Human Genome Project, both its scientific and social basis, has been published widely in review articles and books. Its central conceit arose in the middle 1980s, when it became apparent that technology was advancing so that an undertaking could at least be considered (Watson and Cook-Deegan, 1991). By the early 1990s there were formal projects devoted to its implementation in academic settings (e.g., the U.S. Department of Energy, the National Institutes of Health [NIH] and the Medical Research Council in the United Kingdom) as well as several commercially based entities that had an interest in gene identification as a mechanism to developing therapeutic products. Besides the primary emphasis on DNA sequencing, preliminary steps that entailed the development of physical and genetic maps also proved critical to assembling the DNA sequence of humans into its linear order on each of the individual chromosomes. These steps were also necessary for the conversion of DNA sequence data into useful tools for gene identification and mutation

discovery. The combination of academic and commercial interests led to a competition that in the end provided the stimulus to develop large-scale, high-throughput methodologies and the analysis tools that in 2001 enabled the project to reach one of its primary goals ahead of some of even the most aggressive predictions for when a complete human sequence might be in place (Lander et al, 2001; Venter et al, 2001). These successes and their resulting technologies and algorithmic advances were based on trials in less complex organisms (e.g., *Escherichia coli*, yeast, fruit fly) and were then quickly applied to model and experimental organisms and to identify the sequences of plants and animals of commercial and nutritional importance. At the time of this writing, there are 998 microorganisms (www.ncbi.nlm.nih.gov/genomes/lproks.cgi), as well as many higher organisms, whose sequences have been completed.

SCIENCE AND THE HUMAN GENOME

In the years since the description of the primary human sequence, a deeper understanding of the nature of the DNA sequence and its regulation has developed. Phenomena that are still relatively new in 2011 (e.g., copy number variants, micro-RNA, epigenetic regulation) are important aspects of how the human genome functions and interacts. There is doubtless much more to learn about our DNA sequence, but this chapter will review some current understandings. There are enormous numbers of highly conserved DNA sequences outside of traditional DNA-encoded protein sequences for which function is completely unknown. The next decades will be, in part, devoted to developing and understanding how these conserved sequences play a role in human health and disease. A few current features will be discussed, with many more evolving almost daily in the primary literature. The effects of these approaches have been reviewed recently for neonatology, and this chapter will expand on those themes (Cotten et al, 2006).

SINGLE NUCLEOTIDE POLYMORPHISMS

Single nucleotide polymorphisms (SNPs) are the workhorses of human genetic variation and indeed are only a more specific term and characterization of restriction fragment length polymorphisms (RFLPs), which were the original DNA variants studied in the human genome. The advent of the polymerase chain reaction eliminated the need for RFLP studies. SNPs are specific nucleotide sites in the human genome, where it is possible to have one of two different nucleotides, or polymorphisms, at that position on one of the DNA strands. For example, there might be either a T or a G at a specific site. These variant sites are common with up to 1% of the human DNA sequence being potentially variable between any two individuals, resulting in tens of millions of SNPs across the genome. Most variation is found across all human populations, although some variants appear to be highly population specific. These variants are usually normal, in the sense that they do not appear to be disease causing, although they may lie adjacent to DNA changes that do contribute to disease predisposition. Chip-based DNA sequence detection allows the assay of up to 1 million SNPs simultaneously on one individual at a cost of a few hundred dollars.

COPY NUMBER VARIANTS

A relatively recent discovery in human genetic variation has been the importance of copy number variants as contributors to human inherited disorders. Although both small and large deletion and duplication events of the human DNA sequence have been known since the 1970s, based on cytogenetic banding, only recently has the role that these play in disease been recognized widely. Early copy number variants ranged in length from one to five nucleotides and proved to be useful in characterizing common genetic variation used in family linkage studies. In parallel with these were variants of which the central element might be 15 to 50 nucleotides in length—so-called mini satellites, which were also used in family-based linkage studies. The new class of variation is thousands to occasionally hundreds of thousands (or millions) of base pairs in length. These variations may contain one or multiple genes that can exist in two, three, or more copies arrayed in tandem at particular chromosomal positions. When these tandem arrays of largely identical sequences align themselves during meiosis, there is occasionally a misalignment that can result in the deletion or duplication of one or more of the copies. This event in turn can create a range of the number of copies present from zero to many (Zhang et al, 2009). When functional genes are contained within the copied element or functional regulatory elements, the amount of gene product made may be increased or decreased from a reference level. Early examples in which copy number variants contributed to disease include the Di George syndrome 22q- deletion and deletions associated with spinal muscular atrophy and Charcot-Marie-Tooth disease. New microdeletion syndromes are now being characterized with great precision using array-based DNA analysis that is rapidly replacing the traditional karyotype as the first line of chromosomal analysis. The recognizable syndromes that are found recurrently, and with an identifiable phenotype such as 22q-, are complemented by rare deletion or duplication events that result in congenital anomalies, developmental delay, or both, and where their etiologic nature can be inferred from the normal structure of the parental chromosomes. Finally, in areas such as autism, it is clear that these microdeletion duplication events are a major explanation for the sometimes sporadic, as well as familiar nature, of these disorders. Their contribution to human genetic disease is now suggested to be in the vicinity of 10% of all variant-contributed disease, and thus they form an important class for investigation. Despite their clear importance, there remains to be resolved many technical and clinical issues related to their identification and meaning (Aki-Khan et al, 2009).

MITOCHONDRIAL DNA

Mitochondria are the energy-producing organelles present in thousands of copies within each cell. Each mitochondrion has its own genome, distinct from the nuclear genome and thought to arise from incorporation of bacterial DNA by a eukaryotic cell. Although the mitochondrial genome is approximately 16,500 bp in length (compared with the 3 billion bp of the nuclear genome), there is a wide range of disorders associated with variation in mitochondrial sequence. In addition, because mitochondria reside in the cytoplasm and are not found in sperm, they have a unique pattern of maternal-only inheritance, in which mothers pass their mitochondria to all of their offspring with their daughters in turn passing that on to subsequent generations and with no passing of mitochondrial DNA from males to their children.

GENE IDENTIFICATION

One of the primary benefits of the reference human DNA sequence is our ability to move quickly from finding the location of a gene on a chromosome to identifying the specifics of that gene and the disease-causing mutations. Gene discovery can provide immediate clinical benefit in the form of more accurate diagnoses and risk predictions and longer-term benefits when gene discovery leads to an understanding of gene function and physiology that can be converted into treatment and prevention. Gene mapping approaches to human gene identification have been in use since the late 1970s, and the first successes were the identification of single-gene disorders, sometimes termed *monogenic* or *Mendelian* because their inheritance patterns follow the traditional modes of autosomal dominant, autosomal recessive, and sex linked. Currently there are three primary methodologies under use for gene identification (Altshuler et al, 2008). The first involves linkage studies using large families with genetic disorders or many small families with the same disorder than can be studied and their data pooled. These linkage-based approaches can provide a relatively well-defined chromosomal location for single-gene conditions and has led to successful gene finding for cystic fibrosis, neurofibromatosis, and hundreds of additional, mostly rare, conditions. This approach can also be applied to common but genetically complex traits for which there are no simple inheritance pattens. This technique may require many hundreds of small families, and the resultant gene localization is imprecise. A second method for gene localization can make use of small chromosome rearrangements, such as balanced translocations or small deletions or duplications, that result in a phenotype for a known disorder. In these cases, the location of the chromosomal rearrangement immediately suggests that a gene at or near that rearrangement is etiologic and can be used to again directly search for evidence of a specific gene and mutation in that region. A third approach now in great favor is described next in some detail, and it is exerting a major influence on disease gene finding.

HAPMAP AND GENOME-WIDE ASSOCIATION

As noted previously, it is particularly challenging to find genes associated with complex traits that have multiple genetic and environmental contributors. This heterogeneity creates substantial difficulties in both finding and confirming that any particular gene plays a role in the disorder of interest. A new approach, enabled by advances in technology (i.e., DNA chips) and statistical analysis is proving to be remarkably successful. This approach takes the form of the genome-wide association (GWA) study in which a panel of genetic variants are densely arrayed on DNA chips and characterized in large case and control populations (Manolio and Collins, 2009). GWA can also be applied successfully to case-parent approaches, as will be described in more detail.

The prerequisite to this comprehensive search for variation was the development of the human HapMap (http://hapmap.ncbi.nlm.nih.gov/). The HapMap project developed a comprehensive understanding of the relationship of SNPs across multiple human ancestral groups including Europe, Africa, and Asia (International HapMap Consortium, 2007). HapMap is an essential component of a GWA study because it provides a comprehensive reference listing of the relationships of SNPs and copy number variants to enable their careful characterization in case and control populations. By looking for evidence of DNA sequence variation or allelic variation in which one allele is found significantly overrepresented in a case compared with a control population, there is a strong suggestion that the etiologic gene and variant lies in the vicinity of the surrogate or marker gene allele. In the last 2 years this approach has greatly extended the gene discovery process. Because these common complex traits have a far greater population impact, they are the ones that hold the greatest promise for providing information about the common contributors to pediatric disease. As of this writing approximately 100 associations have been identified (Manolio et al, 2009), but to date the emphasis has largely been on adult complex disorders (e.g., type 2 diabetes, cardiovascular disease, mental health disorders such as schizophrenia), with only a handful applied to pediatric traits. Autism (Wang et al, 2009), asthma (Himes et al, 2009), and cleft lip or palate (Birnbaum et al, 2009) have had new loci identified with the hope that this will provide insights into their pathogenesis. One challenge of the GWA study is that at present, whereas it can identify one or more loci associated with the disease, implementation of a GWA requires expensive technology and large (usually numbering in the thousands), well-phenotyped case and control populations. Thousands of cases and controls must be available to have sufficient power to detect the small effects seen. A second caveat is that the loci found usually have low relative risks or odds ratios, so that the clinical effect of any one identified locus is very small (Hardy and Singleton, 2009). However, collections of loci can have a combined substantial impact, and even a low odds ratio may identify a new biologic pathway that could provide great insights into etiology and treatment (Hirschhorn, 2009). As analytic approaches improve and as costs drop, it seems likely that the GWA study will become a common approach to a wide range of neonatal disorders in which either genetic risks or pharmacogenetic variation important in drug choice and dosing will be unraveled.

Besides detecting disease-associated genetic risk factors, these studies also contribute to knowledge of the genetics of normal trait variation, such as height and skin color. Substantial advances in this area have also occurred with more than 50 genes found to have a role in factors such as height determination (Hirschhorn and Lettre, 2009). However, although identical twin studies tell us that height is almost entirely genetically determined across a broad range of environmental variation, the genetic findings to date explain only a small amount of the contributors to height. There is still much to learn in regard to normal

trait variation and the ability to make predictions about a child's future physical traits or cognitive behavioral range. New approaches beyond GWA are still critically needed to find this large amount of unexplained genetic contributors (Manolio et al, 2009).

The final, and in some ways ultimate, strategy for identifying gene variation associated with disease will be to perform comprehensive genome-wide sequencing. In the last few years, completely new technologies have been applied to DNA sequencing, and the costs of DNA sequencing of a specific individual have dropped by four or five factors of 10 from the original cost of assembling the reference human genome. The reference genome was an amalgamation of many individuals and cost approximately $3 billion, or $1 per nucleotide of sequence. The goal is to eventually reduce this cost by $1000 per individual genome sequenced, which would place it well within the realm of current medical investigations, such as imaging, and well below the cost of many therapeutic approaches. At the time of this writing, several individuals have had their individual genome sequence reported (Wheeler et al, 2008). There is a newly initiated project under way to sequence the genome from approximately 1000 individuals around the world to provide a catalog of DNA sequence variation that can be used as a reference point for comparisons in the future for normal and disease trait variation studies.

The high-throughput sequencing projects have an initial focus on the sequencing of all exons or conserved elements in the genome that are known to be at higher risk for containing disease-causing mutations. Nonetheless, mutations can also reside in the intergenic regions and outside of regions of conservation. Eventually whole-genome sequencing will be required for a comprehensive view of contributors to human inherited disorders. This high-throughput sequencing approach, when performed in sufficient numbers of individuals, can identify disorders in which there are common variants contributing to the disease process as well as individually rare variants that also compose a portion of the disease risk panel. Cystic fibrosis provides an example of this model in that of the single mutation (the ΔF508) consisting of a three-nucleotide deletion, which explains approximately 70% of the allelic variants that result in cystic fibrosis. The remaining 30%, however, are divided across an additional 20 to 50 that are relatively common, and then more than 1000 others that may be rare or family specific. Therefore to identify all the mutations associated with cystic fibrosis risk, one would need to perform comprehensive DNA sequencing.

COMPARATIVE GENOMIC HYBRIDIZATION

Comparative genomic hybridization (CGH), or array-based hybridization, is another technical advance that is now providing, in many cases, a replacement for traditional karyotype-based chromosomal analysis. CGH has already had a substantial influence on prenatal and newborn testing for genetic disease and is discussed in more detail in Chapter 20. Although these array approaches cannot yet detect every form of chromosomal abnormality (e.g., balanced translocations are not detected), they are highly successful in detecting major structural whole chromosomal aneuploidy such as Turner syndrome (45X) or trisomy 21, and they are also effective in identifying small deletions and duplications with a high degree of resolution. These approaches are increasingly becoming a first-line screen for chromosomal structural abnormalities, with the potential for replacing standard karyotypes almost entirely. The arrays also benefit from being able to use DNA directly, so that live cells are not required as they have been for traditional karyotypes. Thus material obtained from even a deceased infant or fetus can be used in the analysis. Because the amount of DNA required is also small, minimal DNA quantity further facilitates its technical application. There are a variety of competing approaches available for such CGH. The current generation of array-based tools use fragments of DNA that are far smaller than prior versions; therefore the resolution is in the range of thousands of nucleotides. This resolution provides detection of very small deletions or duplication events of potential etiologic importance and begins to approach the level of direct sequence comparison. At some point, direct genome sequencing may replace these tiled-array approaches for detection of deletions and duplications.

In parallel with this improvement in resolution has been the recognition that there is no comprehensive catalog of the normal range of variation for rare deletion and duplication events. When new deletions or duplications are identified for which there is not a strong prior track record for their clinical importance (as would be the case for 22q- for example), then the interpretation as to whether they are causal for disease can be challenging. This challenge can sometimes be aided by examining parental samples in which the presence of a de novo deletion or duplication event may be more strongly indicative of contributing to a disease etiology than when the event is also identified in one or more other family members. However, caution needs to be exercised when such deletion-duplications are found in other family members, because there can be a range of penetrance for such abnormalities as well as other co-contributors that might be necessary for the full disease phenotype to be expressed (van Bon et al, 2009). Therefore caution must be exercised in family counseling, and it is essential to have the most accurate and up-to-date information on the nature and role of such variants when using them in a clinical setting. Fortunately these catalogs of normal variation are becoming available (Shaikh et al, 2009). With these caveats, it is still clear that there is an enormous amount to learn about how these structural variants can contribute to disease of the neonate.

PHARMACOGENOMICS

Pharmacogenomics, although originally described in the 1950s as a result of genetic variation associated with commonly recognized enzymes such as G6PD (Motulsky, 1957), is now a highly active area for the clinical application of genome studies. The U.S. Food and Drug Administration has already identified more than a dozen genes for which characterization of allelic variation of those genes may be an important component of therapeutic decision making, including several that have a pediatric application. Perhaps one of the best understood is the role of thiopurine methyltransferase and its genetic variation associated with

major adverse events associated with chemotherapeutic agents such as 6-mercaptopurine (Weinshiboum, 2006). It is now standard care to study pediatric patients preparing to begin chemotherapy for their risks associated with these allelic variants that affect thiopurine methyltransferase drug metabolism. These current pharmacogenetic variants are the beginnings of a much larger group of variants that will tie individual response to therapeutics and will eventually result in direct individualized medicine on an individual basis. In neonatology, many potentially toxic medications are used routinely; these include indomethacin or ibuprofen for treatment of patent ductus arteriosus, antibacterial and antifungal agents that have potential serious adverse consequences such as gentamicin, medications to treat pulmonary or systemic hypertension, antiarrhythmic agents, and others for which individual patient response may be based in part on enzyme allelic variation in those individuals.

By identifying individual risk beforehand, one can either adjust medication doses or choose alternative medications to minimize complications and maximize therapy. In some cases it may be that larger doses of medication will be required based on pharmacogenetic variation as well. It is in the area of this pharmacogenetic variation that perhaps the greatest advances will come in the application of the genome project to neonatal care in the next decade.

With the availability of large clinical trials, such as those overseen by the Neonatal Network and others, improved understanding of the role of genetic variation in drug response will almost certainly be obtained. Because the cost of studies of genetic variation are modest, and the consequences of using the wrong drug or the wrong dose potentially devastating, it will be critical for neonatologists and pediatricians to understand the evidence for which variants can contribute in a proven way to improved therapeutic approaches. Just as measuring drug levels has become a routine part of care in many settings, so will testing beforehand for genetics risk identification and dosage plans also become a part of neonatal care.

INDIVIDUALIZED GENETIC INFORMATION

One of the most dramatic recent advances has been the application of the SNP-based association technologies to commercial entities that are now providing direct consumer testing to interested parties. Currently there are multiple commercial organizations that, for a fee of between $100 and $1000, will extract DNA from a saliva sample and perform high throughout SNP analysis. The results are then provided to the individual with the whole array of GWA risks that have been published in peer-review journals. Although currently controversial (Ng et al, 2009), it seems likely that the use of these technologies will expand in the private or "recreational" setting, directly in the clinical care setting, and eventually into newborn screening. A challenge for clinicians is presented when families have obtained this information but have little context for its meaning, and anecdotal examples of its application to neonates in terms of risk are already arising. This example is yet another example of why clinicians need to remain current with the rapidly advancing genomic capabilities.

MICROBIOMES AND THE METAGENOME

As described previously, there have been approximately 1000 bacterial and viral genomes sequenced, as well as more complicated pathogenic eukaryotic species. These microbial and viral sequences can be used to establish the genetic framework of the many organisms that are found in or on an individual. Because the newborn infant is largely thought to be sterile at birth, but rapidly acquires its microbial flora through environmental exposures, an understanding of the relationships of these many microbial species and how they participate in maintaining health or contributing to disease will be critical to an understanding of neonatal health and disease. Humans have tens of thousands of microbial and viral species contained in or on their bodies in locations such as the gut, mouth, and skin (Turnbaugh et al, 2007). A few obvious disease states, such as necrotizing enterocolitis (Neu et al, 2008) or presumed sepsis, are already under active study for the role in which microbial communities might have a role in predisposition or disease prevention.

It would seem likely that probiotic therapy at sometime in the future might be targeted to provide a milieu that would optimize the microbial flora or the neonatal gut to prevent or limit disease and to assist in nutrition. Our understanding of the transmittal of microbiomes to the infant from maternal and environmental sources is still limited (Palmer et al, 2007), but the capacity of the Human Genome Project and its DNA sequencing capabilities allows identification of the organisms involved with a high degree of precision. It is already apparent that there are many organisms present in and on newborns that have been previously unknown to science, because the identification of species has been limited by the ability to characterize them initially through culture or antigen characterization. For organisms for which appropriate culture media have not been identified, their existence was not known until the development of the ability to perform direct genome sequencing of material collected from the stool, urine, or elsewhere (DiGiulio et al, 2008).

By bypassing the culture step and sequencing biologic samples with DNA sequenced directly, it is possible to establish the identification of new organisms that may be contributing directly to disease in ways that were not previously identifiable. This concept of the microbiome also suggests that in the future—whereas the core DNA sequence will need to be sequenced only once because it is relatively unchanging, except in the case of rare somatic events—the metagenome sequence is constantly evolving based on alterations in factors such as nutrition and antibiotic exposure. In the pediatric population, it may be that DNA sequences sampled from the metagenome will be performed repeatedly as a way of assaying responses to therapy or risks to disease.

EPIGENETICS

Epigenetic regulation or the modification of DNA sequences through environmental exposures, such as altered nutrition or drug exposure, is also an evolving part of the Human Genome Project's contributions to our understanding of how genes function and work

(Devaskar and Raychaudhuri, 2007). Many of these epigenetic changes are thought to arise in utero. As a result, a new field of inquiry into the developmental origins of adult disease (Joss-Moore and Lane, 2009; Simmons, 2009) is now expanding to help better understand the consequences of how DNA can be modified and gene function altered, whereas the linear DNA sequence remains the same. Alterations of DNA can include methylation of individual nucleotides or acetylation or other modifications that take place in the histones that help to establish the chromosomal and chromatin-based structure of DNA sequences.

The developmental origins of disease hypothesis posits that in utero changes can be induced by altered exposure states such as malnutrition, and these exposure states can imprint on the DNA a modified form that is then transmitted cell to cell and established in the infant, with continuing effects on gene regulation into childhood and adulthood. For example, if this imprinting results in a more effective storage capacity for calories, then in adult life when calories are more readily accessible, adults may be predisposed to obesity and its consequences. Similarly, such changes might also regulate cell division and transfer and play a role in childhood leukemias. Because these effects may occur in utero and in the premature infant, it seems likely that in the future a better understanding of our nutritional and drug exposure to infants will be important, which could have direct consequences on the predisposition of neonates to later disease. Although there are some technologies in place to develop an understanding of epigenetic modifications and changes, their application in a clinical setting is still relatively modest.

GENE THERAPY

Although not a direct consequence of the Human Genome Project, the idea of gene therapy has developed in parallel with our understanding of the human genome. Early efforts to use direct gene replacement are continuing, and although many challenges still remain it seems likely that these forms of therapy will continue to expand and eventually be commonly applied in the pediatric setting. Enzyme replacement therapy for several biochemical disorders is now widely available and, for those disorders for which earlier treatment results in better outcomes, recognition of such disorders early in life becomes critical. In other settings direct gene replacement has begun to suggest it may be both safe and efficacious (Maguire et al, 2009), opening an important door to future therapies. In parallel with projects that examine gene replacement, there is also the development of a better understanding of how related phenomena such as micro RNAs or small interfering RNAs also function. These small interfering RNAs, for example, may prove to be highly effective therapeutic agents, and a wide range of pediatric disorders are now under study to determine whether these can be used in a therapeutic or preventive sense. The genome sequence is likely to contribute to an understanding of undiscovered elements that may have an important role in gene regulation that could be effective in therapeutic settings as well, and these advances are eagerly anticipated.

Finally, advances in stem cell research and its therapeutic potential have now been enabled by new legislation that is affording the NIH an opportunity to make stem cell lines available to investigators for studies using NIH funding (Collins, 2009). More readily available stem cells will likely increase the pace of research into the use of these potentially powerful therapeutic agents.

ETHICAL ASPECTS OF HUMAN GENETICS

The ethical, legal, and social aspects of the Human Genome Project have been of at least equal importance to the technology developments that have provided the advances in basic science and translational science described elsewhere in this chapter. It was Watson's insight early on in the process of establishing the Human Genome Project to allot 3% to 5% of the NIH Genome Institute budget directly for ELSI Project activities. The goal was to anticipate the controversies that might develop and to address them proactively whenever possible. In addition, the ELSI Project has also been involved in a wide range of concerns about genetic discrimination. ELSI Project investigators and their colleagues worked hard to develop model legislation that could eliminate genetic discrimination in the job and for health insurance purposes.

The successful passage of the Genetic Information Nondiscrimination Act (Tan, 2009) in the summer of 2008 was a major milestone at the federal level in providing protection for all citizens from workplace and health insurance discrimination. While many states had already addressed these issues, this federal assurance provides a greater level of national protection that is likely to facilitate the ease with which individuals enroll in both clinical genetics studies and research-oriented studies. The second critical aspect of the ELSI Project is addressing the need to have common forms and formats for enrolling research subjects in what are now the highly complex and large genetic investigations required to perform GWA studies described elsewhere in this chapter. It was recognized early that obtaining informed consent for participation in a genetics study was a constantly moving target, because technologies often outstripped the ability of social scientists to be prepared for the scale and possibilities of what might come next. These issues have been dramatically highlighted in recent years during which the scale of genetic characterization is being performed on the SNP ChIP assays, and the recognition that even aggregate data might be able to result in individual identification (Homer et al, 2008) has dramatically altered the clinical and research landscape for genetics.

GWA studies in particular have been scrutinized in great depth, and the NIH has detailed guidelines in place for how consent documents should be worded and the information that must be provided to research subjects. Similar oversight is provided for external users of the GWA data, which, to the benefit of the research community, have been deposited in readily accessible databases after appropriate scientific and ethical review. Another area of influence of the genome project has been on forensic DNA analysis. Although such a discussion is beyond the scope of this chapter, the ability to identify family relationships or ancestral origins has now made DNA analysis a widely used legal investigative and as a commercial tool. It has had spectacular successes in freeing convicts whose DNA evidence has exonerated them from being a participant in major crimes. DNA analysis is also applied widely to assess paternity and to help suggest the ancestral origin of an individual when it might be unknown, as with adoptees or descendants of slaves.

SUMMARY

The advances in the genome project have now begun to be evident at the bedside. Individualized or personalized medicine already has applications in pharmacogenetic variation, and risk profiles can also be generated for common diseases. These risk profiles may one day assist in anticipatory guidance for common disorders such as asthma, diabetes, or preterm birth. The microbiome will also represent an opportunity to better identify disease etiology and to improve therapeutic specificity. As long as protections against discrimination continue to be aggressively implemented, detailed genetic information will greatly improve patient care.

SUGGESTED READINGS

Altshuler D, Daly MJ, Lander ES: Genetic mapping in human disease, *Science* 322:881-888, 2008.

Christensen K, Murray JC: What genome-wide association studies can do for medicine, *N Engl J Med* 356:1094-1097, 2007.

Devaskar SU, Raychaudhuri S: Epigenetics: a science of heritable biological c adaptation, *Pediatr Res* 61:1R-4R, 2007.

Hardy J, Singleton A: Genome-wide association studies and human disease, *N Engl J Med* 360:1759-1768, 2009.

Hirschhorn JN: Genome-wide association studies: illuminating biologic pathways, *N Engl J Med* 360:1699-1701, 2009.

Joss-Moore LA, Lane RH: The developmental origins of adult disease, *Curr Opin Pediatr* 21:230-234, 2009.

Manolio TA, Collins FS, Cox NJ, et al: Finding the missing heritability of complex diseases, *Nature* 461:747-753, 2009.

Complete references used in this text can be found online at www.expertconsult.com

PRENATAL GENETIC DIAGNOSIS

Diana W. Bianchi

As a result of the expanding number of prenatal diagnostic tests that are performed on pregnant women, clinicians know a lot about their patients long before they even touch them. To date, prenatal genetic diagnosis has focused broadly on detection of fetal structural abnormalities. Whereas in the past the major indication for prenatal diagnosis was advanced maternal age or a family history of a single-gene disorder, currently most pregnant women receive an invasive prenatal diagnosis because of abnormal screening results. This chapter discusses the common methods of prenatal genetic diagnosis, the information they convey, and the implications for the newborn.

NONINVASIVE TECHNIQUES

MATERNAL SERUM SCREENING

Maternal serum screening is part of routine obstetric care worldwide. It is used to identify a high-risk pregnancy in a low-risk population of pregnant women. First-trimester maternal serum screening consists of measuring pregnancy-associated plasma protein A and the free beta subunit of human chorionic gonadotropin (hCG). Second-trimester maternal serum screening consists of measurement of alpha-fetoprotein (AFP), hCG, unconjugated estriol (uE$_3$), and inhibin A—proteins that are made by the fetus or placenta.

Biochemical Screening for Neural Tube Defects

AFP is one of the major proteins in fetal serum. Its precise physiologic role is unknown. It can be detected as early as 4 weeks' gestation when it is synthesized by the yolk sac (Bergstrand, 1986). Subsequently, it is produced in the fetal liver and peaks in the fetal serum between 10 and 13 weeks' gestation. AFP is then excreted into the fetal urine or leaks into the amniotic fluid through the skin before keratinization at 20 weeks' gestation. It is also present in cerebrospinal fluid. AFP in maternal serum is exclusively fetal in origin (Crandall, 1981). Maternal serum AFP peaks at 32 weeks' gestation because of greater placental permeability for the protein (Ferguson-Smith, 1983). For interpretation of results, accurate gestational dating and knowledge of maternal race, weight, and presence or absence of diabetes are critical.

Brock and Sutcliffe (1972) observed that there were markedly increased levels of AFP in the amniotic fluid of fetuses with anencephaly and open neural tube defects. Subsequently, it was shown that elevated amniotic fluid AFP levels were associated with increased maternal serum AFP (Ferguson-Smith, 1983). The possibility of a screening test for open neural tube defects became apparent. In the initial collaborative efforts aimed at studying maternal serum AFP, results were expressed as multiples of the median (MoM) to allow comparisons between laboratories. It has become a convention to describe results greater than 2.5 MoM as abnormally high and less than 0.6 MoM as abnormally low. Both findings require further investigation.

If the AFP is elevated, the patient is offered an ultrasonographic examination to verify gestational age, determine fetal viability, and diagnose many of the structural abnormalities that can be associated with an elevated AFP. Although the AFP test was developed to screen for neural tube defects, abnormally high results are not specific for this condition (Box 18-1). If the ultrasonographic examination is unrevealing, the patient undergoes amniocentesis to assay the amniotic fluid for the presence of AFP and acetylcholinesterase, which are elevated in open spina bifida (Crandall et al, 1983). Although an elevated AFP is compatible with a normal diagnosis, a study of 277 infants with elevations of maternal serum AFP and normal levels of amniotic fluid AFP revealed a higher incidence of intrauterine growth restriction and non–neural tube anomalies (Burton and Dillard, 1986).

Aneuploidy Screening

Maternal serum AFP screening has also been used to detect chromosomally abnormal fetuses since the observation was made that a low AFP value was more likely in a fetus with trisomy 18 or 21 than in a normal fetus (Merkatz et al, 1984). Several prospective studies have demonstrated that expressing risk for Down syndrome as a combined function of maternal age and AFP value, and offering amniocentesis to all women with a risk of 1 in 270 or greater (the equivalent risk in a 35-year-old woman based on age alone), makes it possible to detect approximately one third of otherwise unexpected cases of Down syndrome in fetuses (Dimaio et al, 1987; Palomaki and Haddow, 1987). Low AFP values are probably caused by decreased hepatic production in the affected fetus. Although it would make sense to ascribe this phenomenon to the small size of the liver, one study found no association between fetal weight and low AFP values in chromosomally abnormal fetuses (Librach et al, 1988). The differential diagnosis of a decreased AFP level is shown in Box 18-2. Because a low AFP value detects only one third of fetuses with Down syndrome, a normal AFP value does not rule out trisomy 21.

Experience with using low maternal AFP levels as a screen for fetal chromosome abnormalities has led to the evaluation of many other proteins produced by both the fetus and placenta. Three of these—uE$_3$, hCG, and inhibin A—were incorporated into second-trimester maternal serum screening panels (Wenstrom et al, 1999). Measurements of all four can be combined to improve the sensitivity and specificity of Down syndrome detection. AFP, uE$_3$, and hCG are only weakly correlated with one another, and their values are all independent of maternal age (Norton, 1994). Elevations of hCG are the most specific markers for fetal trisomy 21 (Bogart et al, 1987; Rose and Mennuti, 1993), whereas estriol levels are approximately 25% less than normal. Pregnancies affected by fetal trisomy 18 also have reduced levels of uE_3 and hCG. Each measurement is compared with population-specific normal values (i.e., MoM), which are then converted to a likelihood ratio that is expressed as a numeric risk for Down syndrome. Women whose serum screening results indicate a fetal Down syndrome risk of greater than 1 in 270 are offered amniocentesis. Approximately 5% of all serum screen values are calculated to be false-positive results to achieve a sensitivity of detection of at least 70% for cases of Down syndrome.

In 1996 the National Health Technology Assessment Program in the United Kingdom launched a study comparing the performance of first-trimester to second-trimester screening—the Serum, Urine, and Ultrasound Screening Study (SURUSS) (Wald et al, 2003). In addition to the well-validated second-trimester markers, the first-trimester serum markers (pregnancy-associated plasma protein A and free beta hCG) and an ultrasound marker, nuchal translucency (NT), were measured. The results suggested that combining all measurements in an integrated panel improved the sensitivity of detection of trisomy 21 to 93% at a fixed false-positive rate of 5%; this was followed by the largest obstetric clinical trial ever performed in the United Sates and funded by the National Institutes of Health—the First and Second Trimester Evaluation of Risk (FASTER) study (Malone

et al, 2005a). In this prospective study of 38,189 pregnant women, 117 had a fetus affected with Down syndrome. All study subjects were required to have a first-trimester NT measurement, as well as first- and second-trimester serum screening. The results of the study showed that first-trimester combined serum and sonographic screening was better than conventional second-trimester screening, and that the highest sensitivity was achieved by the integrated test that combined results from both trimesters. The excellent results achieved by both of these large-scale studies resulted in the American College of Obstetricians and Gynecologists recommendation that all pregnant women be offered screening for Down syndrome as part of their routine prenatal care (American College of Obstetricians and Gynecologists, 2007).

ULTRASONOGRAPHIC EXAMINATION OF THE FETUS

Ultrasonographic examination of the fetus is the best non-invasive method for gestational dating, definition of fetal anatomy, serial measurements of fetal growth, and evaluation of dynamic parameters such as cardiac contractility, fetal urine production, and fetal movement. In addition, it has been suggested that antenatal visualization of the fetus promotes maternal-infant bonding (Fletcher and Evans, 1983). The advent of antenatal ultrasonography has had a significant influence on the types of patients who are admitted to the neonatal intensive care unit.

First Trimester

With the advent of transvaginal scanning and improved imaging, coupled with advances in first-trimester biochemical screening, fetal ultrasonography during the first trimester has become routine. A major emphasis of first-trimester sonography is screening for aneuploidy, using the following markers: nuchal translucency measurement, absent nasal bone, cystic hygroma, and abnormal ductus venosus blood flow.

NUCHAL TRANSLUCENCY MEASUREMENT

Ultrasonographic visualization and quantification of the normal subcutaneous fluid-filled space at the back of the fetal neck is known as the *nuchal translucency measurement* (Said and Malone, 2008). This particular fluid-filled space is especially well seen in the first-trimester fetus (10 to 14 weeks' gestation; Figure 18-1). In normal fetuses, the maximal thickness of the subcutaneous translucency between the skin and soft tissue overlying the fetal spine increases as a function of crown-rump length. Normal standards have been established for each gestational week. An enlarged NT measurement is thought to be caused by abnormal or delayed development of the lymphatic system, fetal cardiovascular abnormalities, or defects in the intracellular matrix (Said and Malone, 2008). An increased NT thickness is associated with a higher risk of fetal trisomy 21 (Snijders et al, 1998), cardiac defects in chromosomally normal fetuses (Hyett et al, 1996), and anomalies such as diaphragmatic hernia, omphalocele, skeletal defects, Smith-Lemli-Opitz syndrome, and spinal

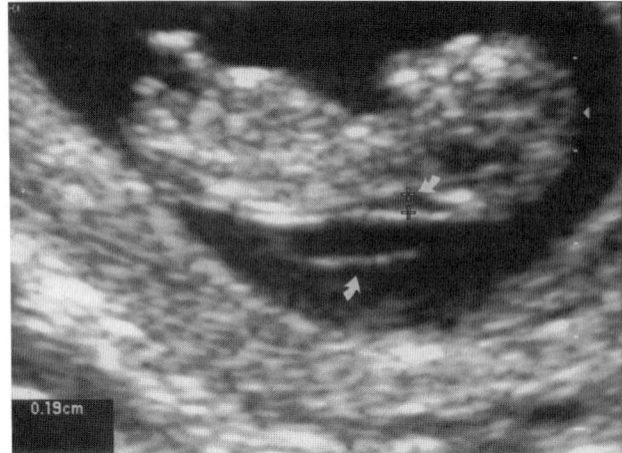

0.19cm

FIGURE 18-1 *(See also Color Plate 3.)* **Sagittal ultrasonographic image of a first-trimester fetus.** The nuchal translucency measurement is the distance between the two crosses. A measurement larger than normal standards for gestational age indicates that the fetus is at high risk for Down syndrome, congenital heart disease, or both. *(Courtesy Dr. Fergal Malone.)*

muscular atrophy (Sonek, 2007). In the largest prospective study (96,127 pregnant women) to examine the association of NT and aneuploidy, Snijders et al (1998) detected 82.2% of the cases of trisomy 21 at a false-positive rate of 8.3%. The implementation of large-scale, first-trimester sonographic screening protocols into clinical practice has emphasized the need for quality assessment, training, and standardized measurements. Assessment of the risk of fetal chromosomal abnormalities in the first trimester allows pregnant women the option of earlier (invasive) diagnostic testing. The disadvantage of this approach is that earlier diagnosis of aneuploidy may preferentially identify fetuses already destined for miscarriage.

CYSTIC HYGROMA

Cystic hygroma manifests sonographically in the first trimester as an enlarged echolucent space that extends along the entire fetal body (Said and Malone, 2008). What distinguished it from the NT is the presence of characteristic septations. Cystic hygroma in the first trimester is the single most powerful sonographic marker that is associated with aneuploidy (Malone et al, 2005b). In the FASTER trial there were 134 cases of cystic hygroma among 38,167 study subjects (incidence of 1 in 285). In the 134 cases, 67 were associated with chromosome abnormalities, (51%), 22 were associated with major structural anomalies (primarily skeletal and cardiac) (34%), and five were associated with fetal death (8%) (Malone et al, 2005b). Therefore pediatricians and neonatologists need to have a high level of suspicion for anomalies in live born infants with an in utero history of cystic hygroma.

ABSENT NASAL BONE

In the original description of his eponymous syndrome, Dr. Langdon Down noted that affected individuals had a small nose (Down, 1995). In one study, absence of the nasal bone in the fetal facial profile was noted in 43 of 59 (73%) fetuses with trisomy 21 and in 3 of 603 (0.5%) of chromosomally normal fetuses (Cicero et al, 2001). The prevalence of absence of the nasal bone is affected by ethnicity (most common in individuals of African ancestry), gestational age, and NT thickness. Using standardized imaging techniques, the nasal bone is absent in 70% of fetuses with trisomy 21, 55% of fetuses with trisomy 18, and 34% of fetuses with trisomy 13 (Cicero et al, 2004).

ABNORMAL DUCTUS VENOSUS BLOOD FLOW

The use of first-trimester Doppler assessment has identified abnormal blood flow velocity patterns across the ductus venosus (Said and Malone, 2008). Blood flows in the ductus during ventricular systole (the S wave) and diastole (the D wave) have characteristic forms with high velocity (Sonek, 2007). This velocity decreases during atrial contraction (the A wave), but in normal fetuses forward blood flow is maintained. When there is complete cessation or reversal of forward flow, the A wave is considered to be abnormal. Abnormal ductal flow is associated with chromosomal abnormalities, cardiac defects, and adverse pregnancy outcomes (Sonek, 2007).

Second Trimester

Within the context of prenatal genetic diagnosis, ultrasonography can be used to detect congenital anomalies. A malformation is present in 2% to 3% of live births (Nelson and Holmes, 1989). This risk is doubled in twins. Fetal structures that are normally filled with fluid are especially well visualized by ultrasonography. In approximately 10% of infants with anomalies, the central nervous system is involved (Hill et al, 1983). Ultrasonography is particularly useful in the diagnosis of anencephaly, microcephaly, encephalocele, and hydrocephalus. By 20 weeks' gestation, the fetal facial structures can be examined with this method for cyclopia, cleft lip, and micrognathia. Nuchal thickening is suggestive of Down syndrome, familial pterygium coli, and other chromosome abnormalities (Benacerraf et al, 1987; Chervenak et al, 1983). Fetal cardiovascular structures may be reliably examined at 20 weeks' gestation. The presence or absence of four cardiac chambers, the dynamic relationships between the cardiac valves and the locations of the vessels allow diagnoses such as hypoplastic left heart, double-outlet right ventricle, tricuspid atresia, tetralogy of Fallot, and Ebstein anomaly. Pericardial effusion and arrhythmias may be similarly observed.

Gastrointestinal anomalies occur in approximately 0.6% of live births, and one third of them are associated with chromosome abnormalities (Barss et al, 1985). The decrease in fetal swallowing seen in some cases of bowel obstruction (from atresia, stenosis, annular pancreas, or diaphragmatic hernia) may lead to polyhydramnios that results in a uterine size greater than expected for gestational dates. Although gastroschisis and omphalocele are readily diagnosed on ultrasonography, they may be confused with each other, and their differing prognoses may cause considerable parental anxiety (Griffiths and Gough, 1985). Gastroschisis usually occurs as an isolated anomaly; infants generally do well after surgical repair. The kidneys are identifiable by 14 weeks' gestation, but the presence of perirenal fat and large adrenal glands may obscure the diagnosis of renal agenesis (Hill et al, 1983). Renal cysts, hydronephrosis, and obstructive uropathy are easily visualized. Oligohydramnios is indicative of poor renal function.

Multiple standard curves have been developed for fetal anthropometric measurements (Elejalde and Elejalde, 1986; Saul et al, 1988). These instruments are particularly helpful in diagnosing skeletal dysplasias and evaluating growth restriction. Fetal genitalia may be determined reliably in the second trimester. In addition, ultrasonographic examination is of benefit in the diagnosis and management of multiple pregnancies.

Although there have been no documented adverse outcomes related to ultrasound exposure during human pregnancy, the reported experimental biologic effects—altered immune response, cell death, change in cell membrane functions, formation of free radicals, and reduced cell reproductive potential—necessitate judicious use of this technology. Another concern is the appropriate pediatric follow-up for prenatally observed conditions with unclear clinical significance, such as minimal hydronephrosis and echogenic bowel.

SECOND TRIMESTER GENETIC SONOGRAM

The *genetic sonogram* is a term that is used to describe the use of a second-trimester sonographic examination to adjust the risk of fetal aneuploidy (Breathnach et al, 2007). The genetic sonogram relies on the identification of major structural anomalies in association with soft markers—that is, findings that are normal variants that often resolve in the third trimester. An example of a soft marker for trisomy 18 is the presence of choroid plexus cysts. Therefore the presence of choroid plexus cysts, with other soft markers such as echogenic bowel, single umbilical artery, or both, in association with an omphalocele or a neural tube defect, would strongly increase the suspicion of fetal trisomy 18.

NEW IMAGING MODALITIES

New fetal imaging modalites include three-dimentional ultrasound examination and magnetic resonance imaging (Lee and Simpson, 2007). Three-dimensional sonography improves detection of cleft palate, and magnetic resonance imaging improves assessment of fetal brain anomalies.

CELL-FREE NUCLEIC ACIDS IN MATERNAL BLOOD

Lo et al (1997) first described the circulation of large amounts of cell-free DNA in maternal plasma and serum samples. Since then, knowledge regarding the biology of fetal cell-free DNA and mRNA in the maternal circulation has greatly expanded (Maron and Bianchi, 2007). The placenta is the predominant source of the circulating nucleic acids. To date, two main clinical applications have transitioned from bench to bedside: fetal rhesus D genotyping (Bianchi et al, 2005) and fetal gender determination (Rijnders et al, 2001). Both have been routinely available in the United Kingdom and Europe for a number of years and are just beginning to be available in the United States (Hill et al, 2010). Fetal gender determination is particularly useful in guiding maternal steroid administration in

patients at risk of congenital adrenal hyperplasia, as well as aiding further management of fetuses at risk for X-linked disorders. Extensive research is ongoing toward using circulating cell-free fetal nucleic acids for the noninvasive prenatal diagnosis of aneuploidy and in developing assays of normal fetal developmental gene expression at different gestational ages (Maron et al, 2007).

INVASIVE TECHNIQUES

AMNIOCENTESIS

Amniocentesis refers to the removal of up to 20 mL of amniotic fluid from the pregnant uterus. Contained within this fluid are cellular components (desquamated fetal epithelial and bladder cells) that serve as sources of chromosomes, DNA, or enzymes. Most of the cellular elements are nonviable; therefore amniocytes generally require tissue culture under specific conditions to provide enough material for diagnosis (Gosden, 1983). Herein lies one of the major disadvantages of the procedure, in that results are received late in the second trimester after fetal movement has been perceived by the pregnant woman. In contrast, the amniotic fluid itself may be assayed biochemically immediately after being removed for the presence of AFP, acetylcholinesterase, bilirubin, lecithin, sphingomyelin, or phosphatidylcholine.

The indications for genetic amniocentesis are (1) an abnormal maternal serum screen result indicating an increased risk of aneuploidy or neural tube defect, (2) maternal age of 35 years or older at the time of delivery, because there is an increased risk for fetal chromosome abnormalities, (3) a previous pregnancy that resulted in a fetus or an infant with chromosome abnormalities, (4) one parent with a balanced chromosome translocation, (5) a family history of a child with a neural tube defect, (6) a family history of a metabolic disorder for which the enzyme defect is known, (7) maternal history of an X-linked disorder, (8) a family history of a disorder for which DNA diagnosis is available, and (9) detection of a sonographic abnormality that is associated with aneuploidy.

Extensive clinical experience with amniocentesis has accrued over the past 30 years (Simpson et al, 1976; U.S. National Institutes of Health, 1976). Historically, institutions in the United States currently quoted a 1% to 2% incidence of minor complications, such as amniotic fluid leakage, uterine cramping, and vaginal spotting after the procedure. The incidence of more serious complications, such as chorioamnionitis and miscarriage, is 0.25% to 0.5% (Centers for Disease Control and Prevention, 1995). More recently, however, the rate of fetal loss after second-trimester amniocentesis was calculated using data from the FASTER trial (Eddleman et al, 2006). The spontaneous fetal loss rate at less than 24 weeks' gestation did not differ statistically significantly between those that did and did not undergo the procedure. The procedure-related loss rate after amniocentesis was 0.06%.

Because results of amniocentesis are received relatively late in the pregnancy, the Canadian early and Mid-Trimester Amniocentesis Trial focused on evaluation of the procedure when performed between 12 and 15 weeks' gestation. This study showed a higher fetal loss rate and a 1.3% risk of fetal clubfoot when amniocentesis was performed between 11 and 13 weeks' gestation (Canadian Early and Mid-Trimester Amniocentesis Trial Group, 1998). The rate of clubfoot in the early amniocentesis group was tenfold the risk in the general population. The cause of clubfoot is thought to be a disruption of normal foot development secondary to transient oligohydramnios (Farrell et al, 1999). For these reasons, early amniocentesis is not generally recommended.

CHORIONIC VILLUS SAMPLING

The increased use of first-trimester biochemical and ultrasound screening has increased uptake of chorionic villus sampling as the diagnostic follow-up procedure of choice. Chorionic villus sampling (CVS) involves the aspiration of the chorion frondosum between 10 and 11 weeks' gestation (Figure 18-2). The fact that the procedure is performed early is advantageous, because most women at this point do not have external manifestations of pregnancy and have not yet perceived fetal movement. The chorionic villi are composed of syncytiotrophoblast and mesenchymal core cells that are actively growing and dividing. In contrast to the dying epithelial cells shed into the amniotic fluid, chorionic villus cells do not require prolonged culture to provide enough mitoses for a cytogenetic diagnosis. Karyotype results are generally available within 1 week of the procedure. Initially, direct preparations derived from syncytiotrophoblast were used for analysis, but the number of apparently mosaic abnormal results proved unacceptable. Cultured preparations derived from the cell of the mesenchymal core are more closely related in embryonic origin to the actual fetus (Bianchi et al, 1993). It is currently recommended that both direct and cultured preparations be used for cytogenetic analysis. Mosaicism, defined as the presence of two or more cell lines carrying different chromosomal constitutions, is a true biologic (not technical) problem in CVS. In several large studies, 0.8% to 1.7% of 1000 cases demonstrated a chromosome abnormality that was present in the villus but not in the fetus (Hogge et al, 1986; Ledbetter et al, 1992) This finding has led to the observation that postzygotic nondisjunction is more common than was previously suggested.

The indications for CVS are the same as those for amniocentesis, with two exceptions. First, neural tube defects cannot be diagnosed by this procedure, and AFP or other serum screening is not routinely offered at this early point in gestation. Second, evidence shows that the fetomaternal hemorrhage associated with placental biopsy results in elevated maternal serum AFP immediately after the procedure (Brambati et al, 1988).

CVS is performed transcervically or transabdominally. With the transcervical technique, the inherent risks of fetal and maternal infection appear to be greater, because it is impossible to sterilize the cervix. Under ultrasonographic guidance, a flexible catheter is passed through the endocervix and placed into the chorion frondosum. A small segment of placenta is then aspirated into sterile tissue culture medium, and the catheter is withdrawn (Jackson, 1985). In contrast, the transabdominal technique uses a needle to obtain villus material; sterilization of the skin surface is straightforward (Brambati et al, 1988). With either

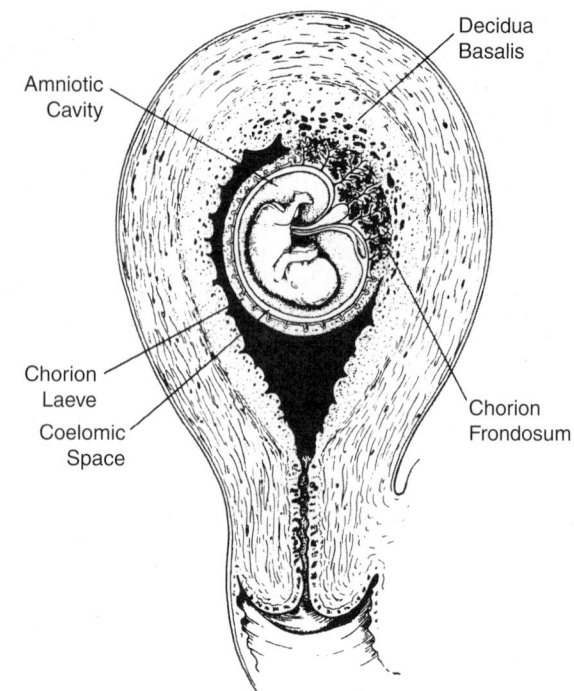

FIGURE 18-2 **A pregnant uterus containing a fetus at approximately 9 weeks' gestation.** The chorion frondosum, if sampled for biopsy, can provide fetal cells for chromosome, enzyme, or DNA analysis. (*From Jackson LG: First trimester diagnosis of fetal genetic disorders,* Hosp Pract (Off Ed) *20:40, 1985.*)

method, approximately 10 to 50 mg of tissue is obtained. Subsequently, the villi are dissected from maternal decidua and processed for tissue culture or DNA extraction.

The safety and accuracy of these techniques have been extensively monitored. A randomized National Institutes of Health clinical trial compared amniocentesis with CVS (Rhoads et al, 1989). The Centers for Disease Control and Prevention and the National Institutes of Health held a consensus conference to summarize worldwide experience. After adjustment for confounding factors such as gestational age, the risk of miscarriage after CVS was found to be on the order of 0.5% to 1.0% (Centers for Disease Control and Prevention, 1995).

The advantages and disadvantages of CVS are summarized in Box 18-3. For patients at high risk for single-gene disorders amenable to DNA diagnosis (e.g., cystic fibrosis, sickle cell anemia, Duchenne muscular dystrophy), CVS is probably the preferred prenatal diagnostic method. Alternatively, for patients with relatively low risk (e.g., a 35-year-old woman being tested for chromosome abnormalities), an amniocentesis may be more appropriate. There have been a few reports of serious maternal sepsis and transient bacteremia in association with transcervical CVS (Barela et al, 1986; Silverman et al, 1994).

The 1% incidence of mosaicism in villus samples may necessitate a further invasive technique, such as amniocentesis or cordocentesis, to confirm or refute diagnoses. However, the detection of mosaicism in a CVS sample may identify a fetus at risk for uniparental disomy. *Uniparental disomy* refers to the inheritance of both copies of a chromosome pair from a single parent. This inheritance occurs when a trisomic fetus undergoes rescue and loses

---

BOX 18-3 **Advantages and Disadvantages of Chorionic Villus Sampling**

ADVANTAGES

- Performed in first trimester; results available quickly
- Cells obtained are mitotically active
- Amount of tissue obtained is preferable for DNA analysis
- Placental mosaicism is detected

DISADVANTAGES

- Miscarriage rate slightly higher
- Increased fetomaternal hemorrhage after procedure
- Risk of serious maternal infection
- Risk of fetal limb and jaw malformations

BOX 18-4 **Indications for Fetal Blood Sampling**

- Thrombocytopenia
- Rapid third-trimester diagnosis of chromosome abnormalities*
- Immunodeficiency
- Congenital infection
- Acid-base abnormalities
- Metabolic disorders*
- Fetal blood type incompatibility*
- Hemoglobinopathy*

*Diagnosis can also be made by a DNA-based test performed on any nucleated fetal material, such as amniocytes.

---

the extra copy of the chromosome. One third of the time, the fetus will be left with two chromosomes that originated in a single parent. Uniparental disomy is an important mechanism in conditions such as Prader-Willi syndrome.

Initially, there was concern regarding the association between CVS and the risk of limb deficiencies in infants whose mothers underwent the procedure. The risk of limb malformations was first suggested by a number of studies describing an increased incidence of transverse limb anomalies and the hypoglossia-hypodactyly syndrome in infants whose mothers had undergone CVS (Burton et al, 1992; Firth et al, 1991; Firth et al, 1994; Hsieh et al, 1995). The overall rate of non–syndrome-related transverse limb deficiency from 65 centers performing CVS is 7.4 per 10,000 procedures (Centers for Disease Control and Prevention, 1995). This number is reasonably similar to that in population-based registries that monitor infants with all limb deficiencies, which give a rate of 5 to 6 per 10,000 live births (Centers for Disease Control and Prevention, 1995). Factors likely to influence the rate of limb malformations include gestational age (risk of limb deficiency is greatest at or before 9 weeks' gestation and decreased at or after 10 weeks' gestation), type of catheter used, and operator experience. The overall risk of limb deficiency appears to be on the order of 1 per 3000 procedures (Centers for Disease Control and Prevention, 1995). A higher incidence of hemangioma has also been suggested in infants born after CVS (Burton et al, 1995). The most important issue at present, however, is the fact that relatively few maternal-fetal medicine and obstetric clinics have personnel who are adequately trained to perform the procedure (Cleary-Goldman et al, 2006).

CORDOCENTESIS

Percutaneous umbilical blood sampling, or cordocentesis, was first described as a means of obtaining fetal immunoglobulin M (IgM) measurements in the prenatal diagnosis of congenital toxoplasmosis (Daffos et al, 1985). Under continuous ultrasonographic imaging, the insertion site of the umbilical cord into the placenta is identified. The umbilical vein is punctured with a 20-gauge needle, the sample is withdrawn, and the umbilical cord is observed for signs of hemorrhage. The technique has been used diagnostically in many clinical settings (Forestier et al,

1988) (Box 18-4). Regarding genetic diagnosis, the lymphocytes are a source of cells for a rapid karyotype; this is helpful in two situations: (1) when anomalies have been noted on ultrasonographic examination, but it is too late in gestation to perform an amniocentesis (antenatal diagnosis of trisomy 13 or 18 influences delivery room management), and (2) for confirmation of a fetal karyotype when amniocentesis or CVS has shown mosaicism (Gosden et al, 1988).

SUMMARY

There has been a major shift away from using maternal age as an indication for prenatal genetic diagnosis. Instead, the results of biochemical and sonographic screening tests, which are increasingly being performed in the first trimester, are used to guide the need for amniocentesis and CVS. Safety considerations and patient preferences have influenced the emphasis on noninvasive prenatal diagnosis. The results of large-scale clinical trials, such as the SURUSS and the FASTER study, have shown a high sensitivity and specificity for fetal Down syndrome detection using noninvasive techniques. Circulating cell-free fetal nucleic acids in maternal blood are already being used for noninvasive diagnosis of fetal gender and rhesus D genotype, and many potential opportunities exist to use this material for future clinical applications.

SUGGESTED READINGS

American College of Obstetrician and Gynecologists: Screening for fetal chromosomal abnormalities, ACOG Practice Bulletin No.77, *Obstet Gynecol* 109: 217-227, 2007.

Breathnach FM, Fleming A, Malone FD: The second trimester genetic sonogram, *Am J Med Genet C Semin Med Genet* 145C:62-72, 2007.

Eddleman KA, Malone FD, Sullivan L, et al: Pregnancy loss rates after midtrimester amniocentesis, *Obstet Gynecol* 108:1067-1072, 2006.

Malone FD, Canick JA, Ball RH, et al: First-trimester or second-trimester screening, or both, for Down's syndrome, *N Engl J Med* 353:2001-2011, 2005a.

Malone FD, Ball RH, Nyberg DA: First-trimester septated cystic hygroma: prevalence, natural history, and pediatric outcome, *Obstet Gynecol* 106:288-294, 2005b.

Maron JL, Bianchi DW: Prenatal diagnosis using cell-free nucleic acids in maternal body fluids: a decade of progress, *Am J Med Genet C Semin Med Genet* 145C: 5-17, 2007.

Said S, Malone FD: The use of nuchal translucency in contemporary obstetric practice, *Clin Obstet Gynecol* 51:37-47, 2008.

Complete references and supplemental color images used in this text can be found online at www.expertconsult.com

EVALUATION OF THE DYSMORPHIC INFANT

Chad R. Haldeman-Englert, Sulagna C. Saitta, and Elaine H. Zackai

Genetic disorders have a major impact on public health, as indicated by several large epidemiologic studies (Table 19-1) (Hall et al, 1978; McCandless et al, 2004; Scriver et al, 1973). The latest data indicate that genetic factors contribute to more than two thirds of the conditions prompting admission to a children's hospital (McCandless et al, 2004). Early identification of the genetic nature of a given condition may then help to appropriately focus resources for providing better care to these individuals. It is therefore critical to implement a systematic approach to evaluating a dysmorphic or malformed infant. This chapter outlines such a general approach.

The clinical geneticist incorporates the following five essential tools in the evaluation of a child suspected of having a primary genetic disorder:

- History: prenatal, birth, and medical
- Pedigree analysis or family history
- Specialized clinical evaluation that includes a detailed dysmorphology examination
- Comprehensive literature search
- Focused genetic laboratory analyses (e.g., chromosomes, fluorescence in situ hybridization, DNA microarray, sequencing)

HISTORY

PRENATAL

A complete gestational history should be generated, including results of prenatal testing such as maternal serum screening, ultrasonography, chorionic villus sampling (CVS), and amniocentesis (Box 19-1). The maternal age at conception should be documented, because the risk of chromosomal anomalies such as nondisjunction rises with maternal age. It is important to identify prenatal exposures to infection and medications, maternal habits such as alcohol and drug use, maternal chronic illnesses such as maternal diabetes, and pregnancy-related complications. An additional significant historical component involves the presence of abnormal levels of amniotic fluid. Oligohydramnios (decreased amniotic fluid volume) can be associated with either a fluid leak or a genitourinary abnormality, whereas polyhydramnios (excess amniotic fluid volume) can be seen in fetuses with neuromuscular disease or gastrointestinal malformations.

It is also important to identify exposure to environmental agents that might act as teratogens. Teratogens are environmental agents that may cause structural and functional diseases in an exposed fetus. Each teratogen may have a characteristic expression pattern, with a specific range of associated structural anomalies and dysmorphic features. Effects and the extent of the effects depend on the time of exposure, duration, and dosage as well as interactions

TABLE 19-1 Genetic Disorders in Pediatric Hospital Admissions

Genetic disorders	Montreal (1973)	Seattle (1978)	Cleveland (2004)
Chromosome, single gene (%)	7.3	4.5	11
Polygenic (%)	29	49	60
Nongenetic disorders (%)	64	47	29
Total number of admissions	12,801	4115	5747

Data from Hall JG, Powers EK, McIlvane RT, et al: The frequency and financial burden of genetic disease in a pediatric hospital, *Am J Med Genet* 1:417-436, 1978; McCandless SE, Brunger JW, Cassidy SB: The burden of genetic disease on inpatient care in a children's hospital, *Am J Hum Genet* 4:121-127, 2004; and Scriver CR, Neal JL, Saginur R, et al: The frequency of genetic disease and congenital malformation among patients in a pediatric hospital, *Can Med Assoc J* 108:1111-1115, 1973.

BOX 19-1 Elements of Prenatal History for the Dysmorphic Infant

MATERNAL HEALTH

Age
Disease: diabetes, hypertension, seizure disorder

MODE OF CONCEPTION

Natural
Assisted reproductive technologies
   Fertility medications
      In vitro fertilizatioin
      Intracytoplasmic sperm injection
      Gamete intrafallopian transfer
      Artificial insemination

EXPOSURES

Medications
Alcohol
Environmental agents
Infections (gestational age at exposure)

PRENATAL TESTING

Ultrasonography (gestational age performed)
Triple screen
Chorionic villus sampling, amniocentesis, and indications

---

with maternal and genetic susceptibility factors. In general, more severe effects are typically correlated with exposure early in the pregnancy and with more extensive (i.e., higher dose) exposure. The list of well-documented human teratogens is short and includes such substances as alcohol, thalidomide, warfarin, trimethadione, valproate, and hydantoin. If history of an exposure is documented, an effort should be made to identify the developmental time and level of exposure. This information is critical, because

TABLE 19-2 Dermatoglyphic Patterns Associated With Specific Dysmorphic Disorders

Dermatoglyphic Pattern	Associated Disorders
Excess arches	Trisomy 13, trisomy 18, Klinefelter syndrome (47,XXY), deletion 5p (cri du chat), fetal phenytoin exposure
Excess ulnar loops	Trisomy 21
Excess whorls	Smith-Lemli-Opitz syndrome, Turner syndrome (45,X), 18q deletion

---

BOX 19-2   Adjunct Studies in the Evaluation of the Dysmorphic Infant

- Investigation of internal malformation
- Assessment of neurologic function
- Identification of organ systems involved
- Ultrasonography magnetic resonance imaging
- Brain imaging
- Electroencephalography as indicated
- Electromyography as indicated
- Prognosis
- Treatment and intervention

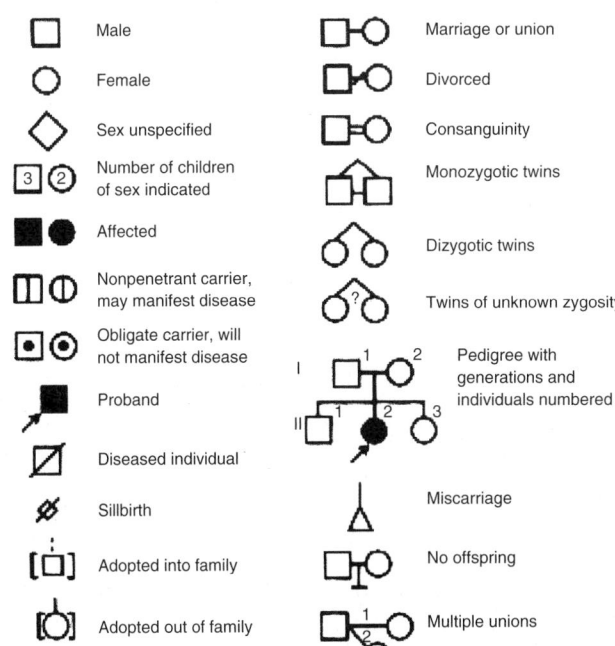

FIGURE 19-1 Symbols commonly used for pedigree notation. (*From Nussbaum RL, McInnes RR, Willard HF, eds:* Thompson and Thompson's genetics in medicine, *ed 7, Philadelphia, 2007, WB Saunders, p 117.*)

the counseling and calculation of recurrence risk for a given malformation are vastly different if environmental exposures are involved.

BIRTH

Another important component of the gestational history is obtaining information on fetal activity, size, and position. Often the mother's subjective impressions can be further confirmed by examining obstetric records of the perinatal period. A history of hypotonia may be further supplemented by reports of poor fetal movements and breech presentation. Perinatal information including gestational age, fetal position at delivery, the length of labor, type of delivery, and any evidence of fetal distress, such as passage of meconium, are all relevant data (Table 19-2). Apgar scores, the need for resuscitation, birth parameters (weight, length, and head circumference), any malformations seen at birth, and all abnormal test results should be noted.

MEDICAL

A full review of the medical issues of the child should include the baby's general health, test results, identification of any chronic medical issues, and need for hospitalization. Evaluation of growth, review of systems, developmental assessment, and notation of unusual behaviors can also provide important clues to a diagnosis.

PEDIGREE ANALYSIS AND FAMILY HISTORY

A critical part of any genetic evaluation is to obtain the family history (Box 19-2); this is best accomplished by creating a three-generation pedigree, which is a schematic

diagram depicting familial relationships using standard accepted symbols (Figure 19-1). This formal record can also be used to summarize positive responses elicited during the interview. Special attention should be paid to ethnic origins of both sides of the family, consanguinity, and any first-degree relatives with similar malformations to those of the patient being evaluated, also known as the *index case*, *proband*, or *propositus*. An extended family history should be used to identify relatives with congenital anomalies, developmental abnormalities, or physical differences. Often photographs can provide clear objective evidence of a descriptive history.

Reproductive histories, especially of the parents, should be elicited. Specifically, questions should be asked about infertility, miscarriages, and stillbirths. The occurrence of more than two first-trimester miscarriages increases the probability of finding a balanced translocation in one parent (Campana et al, 1986; Castle and Bernstein, 1988). A balanced translocation is a rearrangement of genetic material such that two chromosomes have an equal exchange without loss or gain of material. There are typically no associated clinical features with such a rearrangement. However, when chromosomes align to recombine for meiosis in the sperm or egg, this exchange produces a risk of unequal distribution and an unbalanced translocation in the resulting fetus. In this case, there would be aneuploidy for part of a chromosome. It has been estimated that 25% of stillbirths exhibit single or multiple malformations, and in at least half of these cases there is a genetic etiology for the malformations. Couples with two or more pregnancy losses should undergo routine chromosome analysis or karyotyping. When possible, such analysis should be performed on the stillborn fetus or on products of conception.

Obtaining a formal family history is helpful in discovering information that is often critical to making a diagnosis. Positive responses may help to discern a Mendelian pattern of inheritance for a given genetic disorder. For example, a disease affecting every generation, with both males and females involved, such as Marfan syndrome, would most likely be autosomal dominant. A pattern of X-linked recessive disease, such as hemophilia, would show affected males related through unaffected or minimally affected females; transmission in this pattern should not occur from father to son.

PHYSICAL EXAMINATION FOR DYSMORPHOLOGY

A congenital malformation can be described as a "morphologic defect of an organ, part of an organ, or larger region of the body resulting from an intrinsically abnormal developmental process" (Jones, 2006). The term *dysmorphology* was introduced by Dr. David Smith in the 1960s to describe the study of human congenital malformations (Aase, 1990). This study of "abnormal form" emphasizes a focus on structural errors in development with an attempt to identify the underlying genetic etiology and pathogenesis of the disorder.

In a landmark study, Feingold and Bossert (1974) examined more than 2000 children to define normal values for a number of physical features. These standards were devised as screening tools to objectively identify children with differences possibly attributable to a genetic disorder. Important measurements include head circumference, inner and outer canthal distances, interpupillary distances, ear length, ear placement, internipple distances, chest circumference, and hand and foot lengths. Other graphs and measurements using age-appropriate standards can be found in compendia such as the *Handbook of Physical Measurements* (Hall et al, 2007).

The assessment should begin with newborn growth parameters that can reflect the degree of any prenatal insult. Measurements such as height, weight (usually reflecting nutrition), and head circumference should be plotted on newborn graphs. Gestational age–appropriate graphs should be used for premature infants. It is often helpful to express values that are outside the normal range as 50th percentile for a different gestational age. For example, a full-term baby with microcephaly may have a head circumference of less than the 5th percentile for 38 weeks. This can be expressed as a measurement at the 50th percentile for 33 weeks, which imparts the degree of microcephaly more clearly.

A complete physical examination should include assessment of patient anatomy for features varying from usual or normal standards. This assessment can often provide clues to embryologic mechanisms. The data obtained should then be interpreted in regard to normal standards using comprehensive standard tables that are available for these purposes. Special attention to familial variants should be given.

The shape and size of the head and fontanels should be noted as well as the cranial sutures, with assessment for evidence of craniosynostosis or an underlying brain malformation. Any scalp defects should also be noted. The shape

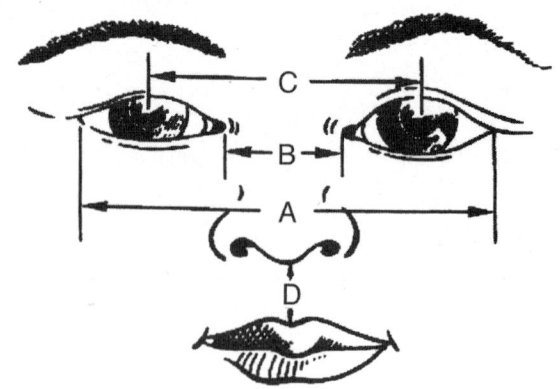

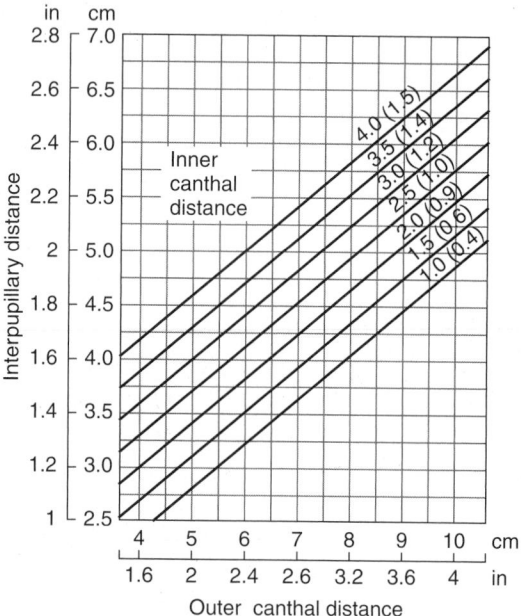

FIGURE 19-2 Various eye measurements are depicted (*top*). *A* indicates the outer canthal distance, *B* indicates the inner canthal distance, and *C* indicates the interpupillary distance (IPD), which is difficult to measure directly. The IPD can be determined using the graph at the *bottom* or with the Pryor formula: IPD = (A − B) 2 + B. (*From Feingold M, Bossert WH: Normal values for selected physical parameters: an aid to syndrome delineation, Birth Defects 10:1-16, 1974.*)

of the forehead, appearance of the eyebrows (noting synophrys), and the texture and distribution of hair should be noted. The spacing of the eyes, or canthal measurements (Figure 19-2), the interpupillary distances (Figure 19-3; see also Figure 19-2), palpebral fissure lengths (Figure 19-4), presence or absence of colobomata and epicanthal folds, and noting whether the palpebral fissures are turned upward or downward are components of the dysmorphology examination. Examination of the ears should include a search for preauricular and postauricular pits, tags, and assessment of the placement (Figure 19-5), length (Figure 19-6), and folding of the ear is important. Ear development occurs in a temporal frame similar to that of the kidneys, and external ear anomalies can be associated with renal anomalies. Evaluation of the nose should cover the shape of nasal tip, the alae nasi, presence of anteverted nares, the length of the columella, and patency of the choanae.

The mouth and throat are examined for the presence of a cleft lip or palate; the shape of the palate and uvula are noted, and the presence of unusual features, such as tongue deformities, lip pits, frenula, and natal teeth, are recorded. A small retrognathic or receding chin, which can be a part of several syndromes or an isolated finding, should be noted. The neck is inspected for excess nuchal folds or skin and evidence of webbing. Any bony abnormalities in the neck should prompt an evaluation of the cervical vertebrae to confirm cervical and airway stability.

Evaluation of the chest and thorax involves lung auscultation and cardiac examination. Abnormal findings should prompt a consultation with a cardiologist and appropriate echocardiographic or invasive studies as needed. External measurements include determining the internipple distance and its ratio in regard to the chest circumference (Figure 19-7). The abdominal examination is focused on

determining whether organomegaly is present, a finding typically associated with an inborn error of metabolism. The umbilicus should also be examined, with any hernias and the number of vessels present in the newborn cord being noted. A two-vessel cord, in which only a single artery is present, can be associated with renal anomalies. The genitourinary examination concentrates on determining whether anomalies such as hypospadias, chordee, cryptorchidism, microphallus, and ambiguous genitalia are present. These external anomalies may be associated with internal anomalies involving the upper urinary tract as

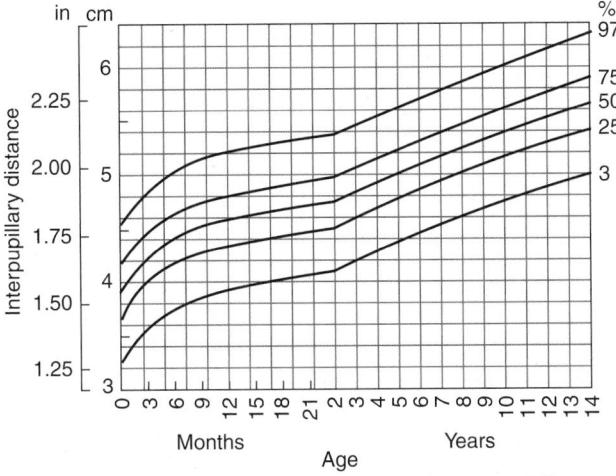

FIGURE 19-3 A nomogram for interpupillary distance at different ages for both sexes. (*From Feingold M, Bossert WH: Normal values for selected physical parameters: an aid to syndrome delineation,* Birth Defects 10:1-16, 1974.)

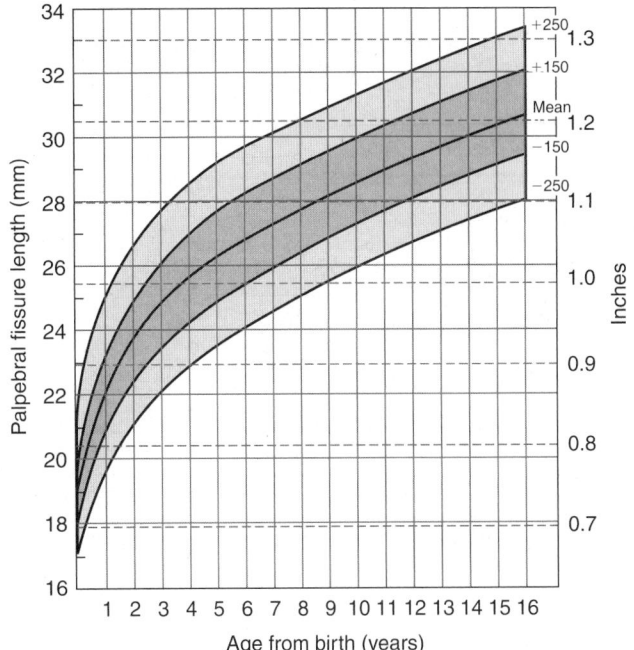

FIGURE 19-4 A graph of palpebral fissure length from birth to age 16 years for both sexes. (*From Hall JG, Allanson JE, Gripp KW, et al:* Handbook of physical measurements, *Oxford, 2007, Oxford University Press.*)

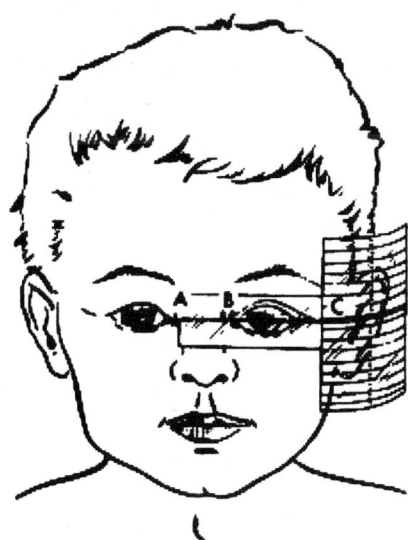
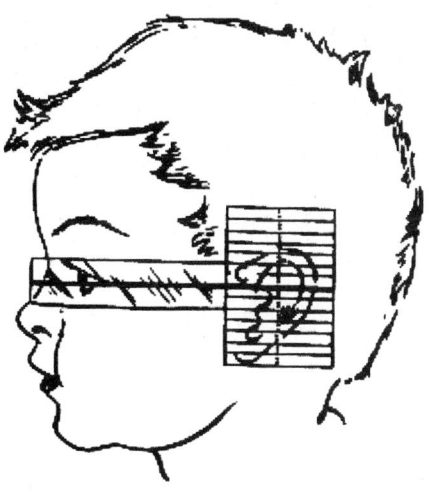

FIGURE 19-5 Ear placement. Using the medial canthi (*A* and *B*) as landmarks, one draws a central horizontal line and extends it to a point (*C*) on the side of the face. Ears attached below this line are considered low set.

well. The anus is examined for evidence of tags, its placement, and its patency.

The back should be assessed, especially for the shape of the spine and any associated defects, such as myelomeningocele. These defects prompt further radiologic evaluation to assess for potential functional limitations. In addition, a sacral dimple or hair tuft at the base of the spine should be noted, because either could signify developmental abnormalities in the underlying neural tissue.

Minor anomalies are often manifested in the extremities. Gross differences in the hands and feet include polydactyly (more than five digits), whether the extra digits are located in a preaxial or postaxial position should be noted, syndactyly (fusion of the digits), clinodactyly (incurving of the digits), and extremity length, which should be expressed as a percentile measured on age-appropriate

graphs (Figures 19-8 and 19-9). Often these data can provide important clues to a unifying syndrome.

Dermal ridge patterns, or dermatoglyphics, are formed on the palms and soles early in embryonic life, and they vary considerably among individuals. This variation can be inherited and can be influenced by disturbances to the development of the peripheral limb buds. Environmental exposures and chromosomal aberrations can greatly affect the formation of these structures and are reflected by the dermatoglyphic pattern of an individual. Each of the distal phalanges has one of three basic dermal ridge patterns: arches, whorls, or loops (Figure 19-10). The predominance of a single pattern can be an associated feature of a genetic disorder. For example, the occurrence of arches on eight or more digits is a rare event, but is frequently encountered in children with trisomy 18 (Box 19-3).

Deltas, or triradii, form at the convergence of three sets of ridges on the palm. This junction is where the hypothenar, thenar, and distal palmar patterns converge. There are typically no triradii in the hypothenar area of the palm, but when patterning is present or is large, a distal triradius arises, which is found in only 4% of normal Caucasian individuals but in 85% of patients with trisomy 21 (Down syndrome). A single transverse palmar crease is found in 4% of controls, but in more than half of patients with trisomy 21 (Figure 19-11) and in even greater proportions in patients with other trisomies. The hallucal area of the foot, located at the base of the big toe, also has a dermal ridge pattern, usually a loop or whorl. A simple pattern or open field in this region is found in less than 1% of controls but in more than 50% of patients with Down syndrome (Figure 19-12). This unusual dermal pattern is also associated with hypoplasia of the hallucal pad and a wide space between the great and second toes in these patients.

An examination of the skin is also important, to look for phakomatoses or skin manifestations that herald the presence of an underlying disorder. Examples are café-au-lait spots (associated with neurofibromatosis type I) and ash leaf spots (associated with tuberous sclerosis and detected

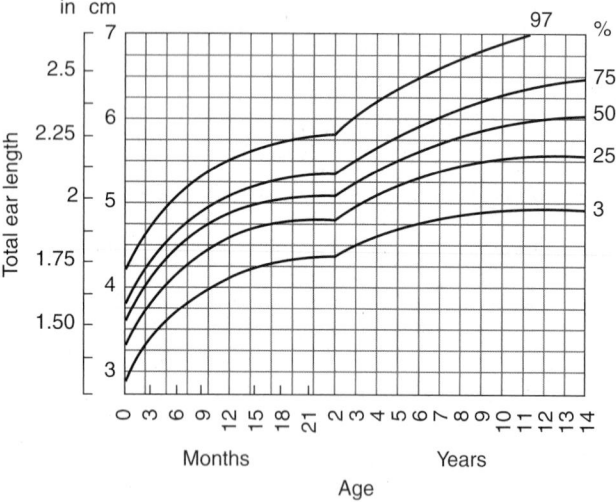

FIGURE 19-6 Graph showing various percentiles for ear length plotted against age. (*From Feingold M, Bossert WH: Normal values for selected physical parameters: an aid to syndrome delineation,* Birth Defects *10:1-16, 1974.*)

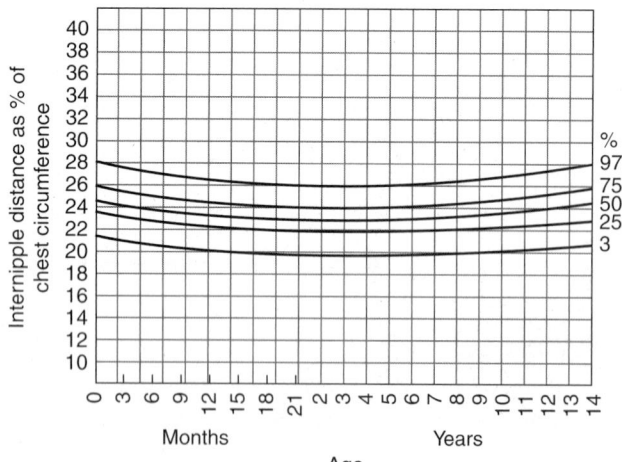

FIGURE 19-7 The internipple distance as a percentage of the chest circumference plotted against age for both sexes. (*From Feingold M, Bossert WH: Normal values for selected physical parameters: an aid to syndrome delineation,* Birth Defects *10:1-16, 1974.*)

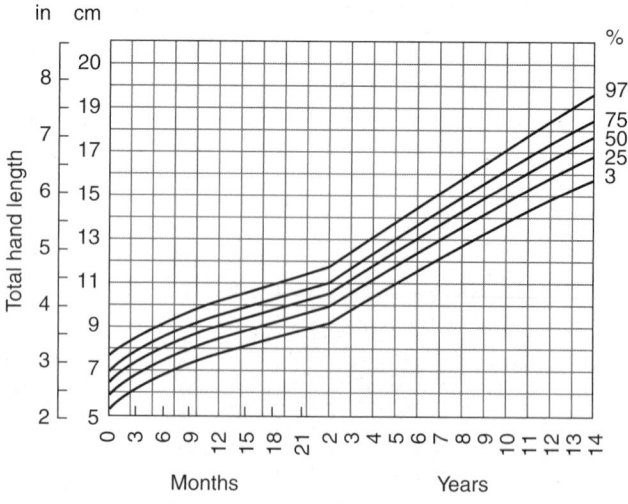

FIGURE 19-8 The total hand length plotted against age for both sexes. (*From Feingold M, Bossert WH: Normal values for selected physical parameters: an aid to syndrome delineation,* Birth Defects *10:1-16, 1974.*)

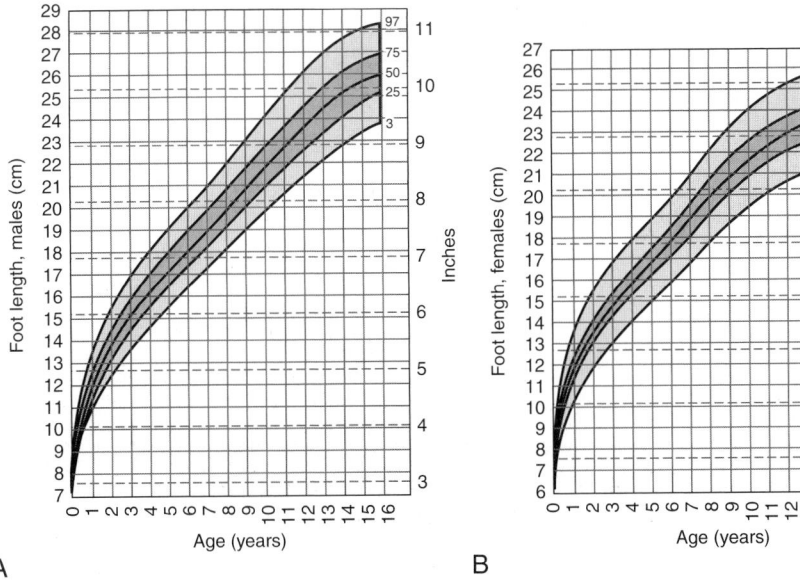

A

B

FIGURE 19-9 Total foot lengths plotted against age for boys **(A)** and girls **(B)**. (*From Hall JG, Allanson JE, Gripp KW, et al: Handbook of physical measurements, Oxford, 2007, Oxford University Press.*)

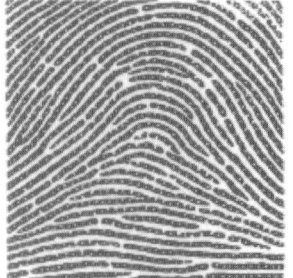

Simple Arch

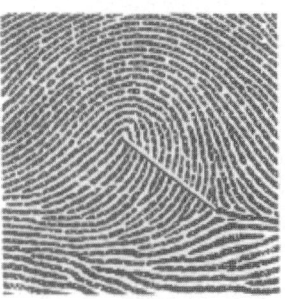

Loop

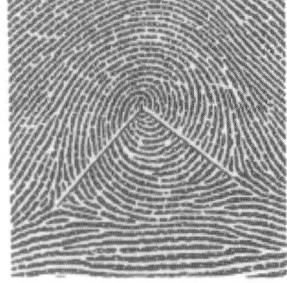

Whorl (Spiral)

FIGURE 19-10 Basic fingerprint patterns (dermatoglyphics). (*From Holt SB: The genetics of dermal ridges, Springfield, Ill, 1968, Charles C Thomas.*)

BOX 19-3 | **Underlying Mechanisms of Malformation**

SYNDROME
Pathogenetically related pattern of anomalies

SEQUENCE
Pattern of anomalies derived from a presumed or known prior anomaly or mechanical disturbance

ASSOCIATION
Nonrandom occurrence of multiple anomalies

FIELD DEFECT
Disturbance of a developmental field leading to a pattern of anomalies

---

with the use of a Wood's lamp). Irregular pigmentation, such as hypomelanosis of Ito, can be suggestive of chromosomal mosaicism, in which the different skin pigmentation patterns represent a different, mixed chromosomal composition. Hemangiomas and other skin diseases are also noteworthy.

Finally a careful neurologic examination with input from a specialist is often warranted in the child with multiple anomalies, because the neurologic status is often the most reliable prognostic indicator. Evaluation of tone, feeding, unusual movements, and the presence of seizure activity are critical pieces of diagnostic information.

ADJUNCT STUDIES

An exhaustive physical examination often reveals differences that require further evaluation for diagnostic, prognostic, and treatment purposes (Box 19-4). Poor feeding or cyanosis may lead to detection of internal organ malformations on echocardiogram or abdominal ultrasonography. Differences in head shape suggest the need for skull radiographs, three-dimensional computed tomography,

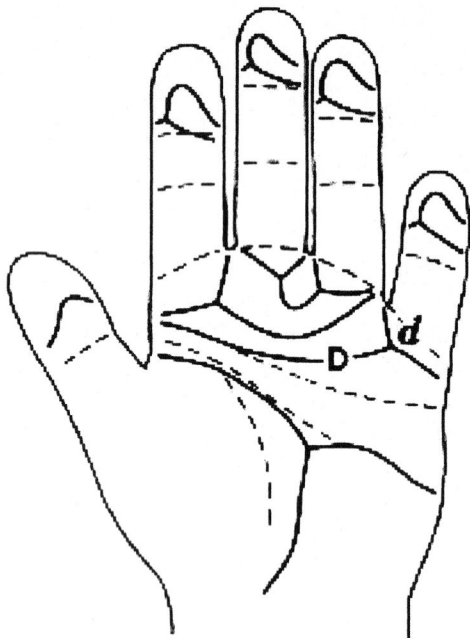

FIGURE 19-11 The patterns on the hand of a patient with Down syndrome depicting the palmar crease (*D*). (*From Holt SB:* The genetics of dermal ridges, *Springfield, Ill, 1968, Charles C Thomas.*)

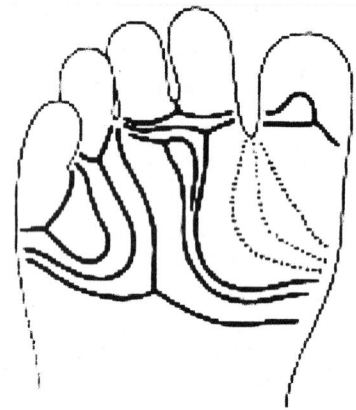

FIGURE 19-12 The distal sole of the foot of a patient with Down syndrome, depicting the characteristic "open field" pattern. (*From Holt SB:* The genetics of dermal ridges, *Springfield, Ill, 1968, Charles C Thomas.*)

> **BOX 19-4** **Processes Leading to Altered Form or Structure**
>
> **DEFORMATION**
>
> Abnormal form resulting from mechanical forces
>
> **DISRUPTION**
>
> Morphologic defect caused by interference with a previously normal developmental process
>
> **DYSPLASIA**
>
> Altered morphology because of abnormal organization of cells into a given tissue

> **BOX 19-5** **Examples of Morphologic Differences**
>
> - Malformation
> - Deformation
> - Disruption
> - Dysplasia
> - Cardiac septal defects, cleft lip
> - Club foot
> - Amniotic bands
> - Localized: hemangioma
> - Generalized (skeletal): achondroplasia

electroretinograms are needed to predict visual prognosis. Often there are well-characterized genetic disorders that have a specific pattern of abnormal findings in these highly specialized studies. Even when a unifying diagnosis is reached, there is often variation in the clinical phenotype, and determining the patient's prognosis on a system-by-system basis is typically the most appropriate and accurate way to proceed.

LITERATURE REVIEW

The occurrence of malformations can fit into one of several categories (Box 19-5). The next step toward reaching a diagnosis is to analyze the data generated from the evaluation and attempt to categorize the findings. A syndrome is a "collection of anomalies involving more than one developmental region or organ system," (Aase, 1990). The word itself means a "running together" or "pattern of multiple anomalies thought to be pathogenically related." Therefore a given congenital anomaly may be an isolated defect in an otherwise normal individual or part of a multiple malformation syndrome. Furthermore, the primary malformation itself can determine additional defects through an interrelated cascade of physical and functional processes; if ensuing malformations are related to one primary defect, factor, or event, a pathogenetic sequence has occurred. A classic example is the Pierre-Robin sequence or constellation, consisting of a small recessed jaw, midline U-shaped cleft palate, and relatively large and protruding tongue. The primary anomaly is the small jaw, which does not allow adequate room for the tongue and displaces it superiorly. The displaced tongue prevents closure of the palatine shelves, causing the cleft palate. The recurrence risk with this isolated occurrence is negligible. However,

or magnetic resonance imaging of the brain. A disproportionality of the limbs prompts a skeletal survey and bone age measurement.

It is prudent in children with anomalies involving multiple systems to obtain the input of relevant specialists. This step is often essential to medical decision making and the planning of interventions. Abnormal neurologic findings should prompt a consultation with a trained specialist and interpretation of studies such as head ultrasonography, brain magnetic resonance imaging, brainstem auditory evoked responses, and electroencephalogram for seizure activity. Muscle dysfunction might result in the ordering of electromyography, muscle ultrasound, or nerve conduction studies. Visual involvement requires a funduscopic examination by an experienced pediatric ophthalmologist, and sometimes studies of visual evoked responses or

---

BOX 19-6   Elements of Perinatal and Birth History for the Dysmorphic Infant

- Fetal activity
- Delivery
- Type (e.g., indication for cesarean section)
- Gestational age
- Fetal presentation
- Apgar scores, history of distress, or resuscitation
- Growth parameters
- Malformations noted

BOX 19-7   Elements of Pedigree Analysis and Family History for the Dysmorphic Infant

Identification of relatives with:
- Congenital anomalies (especially those similar to proband's)
- Mental retardation

Photographs (objective evidence)

Parental reproductive history
- Pregnancy losses (gestational ages)
- Infertility

Medical histories of primary relatives

Ethnic origin

Consanguinity

---

one should also remember that such sequences can also be part of a larger constellation of findings that does fit into a syndrome, as Pierre-Robin sequence can when it is part of velocardiofacial syndrome (caused by a deletion of chromosome 22q11) or Stickler syndrome (associated with mutations in the type II collagen gene). The recurrence risk for an affected individual passing on these particular syndromes to their children is 50%.

In addition, a cluster of several malformations that are not developmentally related can occur in a nonrandom fashion called an *association* that may appear without characteristic dysmorphic features. One such statistically nonrandom association of defects consists of vertebral defects, anal atresia, cardiac defects, tracheoesophageal fistula, esophageal atresia, renal dysplasia, and limb anomalies (VACTERL). It should be noted that not all features need to be present and that the extent of involvement of each system is widely variable. Recently, the CHARGE syndrome (coloboma, heart disease, atresia choanae, retarded growth and development, genital anomalies, and ear anomalies/deafness) was considered an association until the *CHD7* gene was identified to cause approximately 60% of the cases (Lalani et al, 2006).

These associations often manifest as sporadic rather than familial occurrences. Because they are not clearly related by a common etiology or pathogenesis, they are not considered syndromes and do not technically constitute a diagnosis. Instead, they are a recognition of a statistically significant association of features. It is important to remember that many of these same anomalies can occur as features of chromosomal aneuploidy or other syndromes. Syndromic malformations tend to occur in more than one developmental field. A field defect or complex is a set of primary malformations in a developmental field that originates from a single or primary abnormality in embryonic development (see Box 19-5).

When generating a differential diagnosis of malformations that might occur together, the evaluator must also consider structures that may appear abnormally formed, but in fact are structures that underwent normal development and then received some insult that distorted their true form (Box 19-6). For example, a *deformation* describes the abnormal form, shape, or position of a part of the body that was caused by mechanical forces. Examples are clubfoot, hip dislocation, and craniofacial asymmetry; they can result from intrinsic (embryonic) or extrinsic (intrauterine) mechanical forces that alter the shape or position of an organ or part that had already undergone normal differentiation. Deformations are estimated to occur in 2% of births,

and such factors as fetal crowding from the presence of multiple fetuses and uterine malformations, as well as oligohydramnios, and a face presentation during delivery can cause them.

Along similar lines, a *disruption* describes a "morphologic defect of an organ, part of an organ, or larger region of the body resulting from the extrinsic breakdown of, or an interference with, an originally normal developmental process," (Aase, 1990). The classic example of a disruption is entanglement of the fetus in amniotic bands. Amniotic bands are ribbons of amnion that have ruptured in utero and cause disruptions of normal developmental processes in the fetus, either through physical blockage or interruption of the blood supply or by entangling and tearing of developing structures. This effect is seen most often with digits and limbs, and remnants of the bands, or constriction marks, can frequently be seen at birth. If the fetus should swallow a band, a cleft palate might result; the etiology is a very different etiology from that of cleft palate occurring as a primary malformation. Recurrence risk counseling of the parent would be very different in these two scenarios.

Dysplasias occur when there is "an abnormal organization of cells into tissue(s) and its morphologic results," (Aase, 1990). Dysplasia tends to be tissue specific rather than organ specific (e.g., skeletal dysplasia) and can be localized or generalized.

In summary, structural or morphologic changes identified at birth can occur during intrauterine development as a result of malformations, deformations, disruptions, or dysplasia. However, approximately 90% of deformations undergo spontaneous correction. Malformations and disruptions often require surgical intervention when possible. Dysplasias are typically not correctable, and the affected individual experiences the clinical effects of the underlying cell or tissue abnormality for life (see Box 19-7). Examples of these entities are listed in Box 19-7.

After the history and physical evaluation are complete, a cross-reference of two or more anomalies is useful to generate a differential diagnosis. When the rest of the neonate's physical and history findings are added, the possibilities can often be narrowed down to a few entities that may be amenable to diagnostic testing. If multiple anomalies are present, it is usually best to start with the least common. As Aase (1990) has stated, "The best clues are the rarest. The physical features that will be the most helpful on differential diagnosis are those infrequently seen either in isolation or as part of syndromes. Quite often, these are not the most obvious anomalies or even the ones that have the greatest significance for the patient's health." Cross-referencing is usually best accomplished by using published compendia of malformation syndromes. These compendia have been supplemented by databases that are accessible online (i.e., GeneReviews, *Online Mendelian Inheritance in Man*, and PubMed). The availability of such tools allows the cross-referenced features to be compared easily with those of other described syndromes that may include similar malformations. This systematic review produces a differential diagnosis for the constellation of features described and identifies references to pertinent literature.

The recognition of patterns of genetic entities involves the comparison of the proband with the examiner's personal experience of known cases and a search of the literature. Multiple anomalies may be causally related, occur together in a statistically associated basis, or occur together merely by chance. Diagnosis of a genetic disorder relies heavily on the ability of the clinician to suspect, detect, and correctly interpret physical and developmental findings and to recognize specific patterns. Accurate diagnosis of a syndrome in a child is important to the identification of major complications and their treatment if possible. It is also crucial for long-term management of patients and for parental counseling about recurrence in future offspring.

SPECIALIZED LABORATORY TESTS

In sorting through the array of possibilities listed, the geneticist uses one other important tool—the availability of highly specialized cytogenetic and molecular genetic testing, including:

- Karyotype
- Fluorescence in situ hybridization
- DNA microarray (see Chapter 20)
  - Comparative genomic hybridization
  - Single nucleotide polymorphism or oligonucleotide arrays
- Molecular analysis

The standard karyotype, or analysis of stretched and stained chromosome preparations usually taken from a peripheral blood sample, can often confirm a suggested diagnosis or explain a set of major malformations not classically encountered together. Further description of specific chromosomal abnormalities is addressed in Chapter 20; it is sufficient to note that multiple malformation syndromes can result from large visible chromosome rearrangements that lead to deletion or addition of material (aneuploidy). These rearrangements can involve an entire arm of a chromosome or can be submicroscopic, requiring further special testing. Such small deletions can often be detected by fluorescence in situ hybridization analysis, which is performed using a probe specific for the deleted region.

It has become the standard of care in several centers to offer more specialized molecular testing, such as a DNA microarray or individual gene sequencing, as an adjunct to or instead of karyotype analysis. In general, microarray-based methods are currently focused on detecting copy number changes (smaller deletions or duplications not detectable by a karyotype) and can be performed in a targeted or genome-wide fashion (Emanuel and Saitta, 2007). As more information is made available about the role of individual gene mutations in newborns with congenital malformations, testing for these mutations is becoming available in diagnostic laboratories. It can be useful to check with a geneticist or genetics counselor for the availability of gene mutation testing that may be clinically available or performed on a research basis. GeneTests is an internet database of laboratories worldwide that provides such services.

DIAGNOSIS

There are cases in which, after a detailed examination, exhaustive literature search, and genetic testing, no unifying diagnosis is evident. Aase (1990), a dysmorphologist, advises, "Don't panic! The absence of a diagnosis may be distressing to the diagnostician and the family, but it is much less dangerous than the possibility of assigning the wrong diagnosis with the risk of erroneous genetic and prognostic counseling and possibly hazardous treatment." Therefore, in cases in which there is no clear diagnosis, prognosis and treatment should be determined according to the organ systems involved and the extent of their impairment. In addition, when the infant has a severe, untreatable impairment or the patient's condition is critical, it may be prudent to offer and obtain consent for a full postmortem examination by an experienced pathologist. A skin sample, and sometimes blood, can be taken from the expired fetus for establishing a cell line or for extracting DNA for future testing. Information gained from such investigations may often become relevant for family members, including the parents, allowing one to provide accurate recurrence risk counseling and perhaps offer prenatal testing of a new pregnancy. Such information can often help to provide closure for the family as well.

When should a genetics evaluation be considered? The following clinical situations prompt a further genetic evaluation and counseling by a specialist:

- Multiple anatomic anomalies
- History of maternal exposure to teratogens
- Familial disorders
- Increased carrier frequency or ethnic risk
- Multiple pregnancy losses

As described previously, if a birth defect is identified in the presenting patient or proband, especially if the defect is associated with other anatomic anomalies, short stature, or developmental delays, the features of a specific genetic syndrome may be present. A known history of maternal exposure to a potential teratogen would also be an indication for consultation. Conditions appearing to be familial, a family history of hereditary disorders involving malformation of a major organ, or major physical differences such as unusual body proportions, short stature, or irregular skin pigmentation, would warrant genetic investigation. Mental retardation, blindness, hearing loss, or neurologic deterioration in multiple family members suggests a genetic etiology. Likewise, a strong family history of cancer or a defined ethnic risk such as Ashkenazi Jewish heritage and its association with a higher carrier frequency for Tay-Sachs disease would be an indication for genetic evaluation. The occurrence of multiple pregnancy losses would also raise the suspicion of a genetically influenced cause and indicate the need for further investigation and counseling.

SUMMARY

Diseases with underlying genetic bases have significant effects on health care and its delivery. An appreciation of these entities, coupled with an organized, systematic evaluation, can help to define the nature of a given disorder and aid in the development of the optimal plan of treatment and care for the patient.

SUGGESTED READINGS

Aase JM: *Diagnostic dysmorphology*, New York, 1990, Plenum.

Carey JC, editor: Elements of morphology: standard terminology, *Am J Med Genet* 149A:1-127, 2009.

Gehlerter TD, Collins FS, Ginsburg D, editors: *Principles of medical genetics*, ed 2, Baltimore, Md, 1998, Williams & Wilkins.

GeneTests. Available online at www.ncbi.nlm.nih.gov/sites/GeneTests/?db=GeneTests.

Hall JG, Allanson JE, Gripp KW, et al: *Handbook of physical measurements*, Oxford, 2007, Oxford University Press.

Hennekam RCM, Krantz ID, Allanson JE, editors: *Gorlin's syndromes of the head and neck*, ed 5, New York, 2010, Oxford University Press.

Jones KL: *Smith's recognizable patterns of human malformation*, ed 6, Philadelphia, 2006, WB Saunders.

Nussbaum RL, McInnes RR, Willard HF, editors: *Thompson and Thompson's genetics in medicine*, ed 7, Philadelphia, 2007, WB Saunders.

Online Mendelian Inheritance in Man (OMIM). Available online at www.ncbi.nlm.nih.gov/omim/.

Rimoin DL, Connor JM, Pyeritz RE, et al: *Emery and Rimoin's principles and practice of medical genetics*, ed 5, New York, 2006, Churchill Livingstone.

Schinzel A: *Catalogue of unbalanced chromosome aberrations in man*, Berlin, 2001, Walter de Gruyter.

Spranger J, Benirschke K, Hall JG, et al: Errors of morphogenesis: concepts and terms, *J Pediatr* 100:160-165, 1982.

Stevenson RE, Hall JG, editors: *Human malformations and related anomalies*, ed 2, New York 2006, Oxford University Press.

Complete references used in this text can be found online at www.expertconsult.com

SPECIFIC CHROMOSOME DISORDERS IN NEWBORNS

Chad R. Haldeman-Englert, Sulagna C. Saitta, and Elaine H. Zackai

It has been estimated that 3% of newborns have a major structural anomaly that will affect their quality of life. Although most of these patients have a single malformation, 0.7% of infants have multiple major malformations. In an additional 2%, a major anomaly is discovered by the age of 5 years. Early identification of the genetic nature of a given condition can aid in treatment and help to identify resources for providing better health care to these individuals. This chapter will focus on genetic disorders and syndromes with underlying chromosomal abnormalities that typically manifest in the newborn period, in addition to the shift in genetic evaluation and diagnosis with the advent of newer array-based diagnostic techniques.

HUMAN KARYOTYPE

Chromosomes consist of tightly compacted DNA whose structure is maintained by association with histones and other proteins. When treated and stretched, chromosomes from dividing cells can be visualized under the light microscope as linear structures with two arms joined by a centromere. The short arm is designated p (petit) and the long arm is designated q. The ends of the p and q arms are known as *telomeres*. Human chromosomes were first visualized in 1956 (Lejeune and Turpin, 1960), and each pair shows a distinctive size, centromeric position, and staining or banding pattern after treatment with special dyes, allowing it to be identified and classified. Each chromosome is identified by a number, in general from largest to smallest, in standard international cytogenetic nomenclature. This presentation, or karyotype (Figure 20-1), normally consists of 46 chromosomes, with 22 pairs of autosomes and one set of sex chromosomes—two X chromosomes for females (46,XX), and an X and a Y for males (46,XY).

Karyotype analysis is performed in cells undergoing mitosis, or cell division, in which the chromosomes condense and can be stained and visualized. Thus, cells that can be stimulated to divide and grow in culture, such as peripheral blood lymphocytes, skin fibroblasts, and amniocytes, are typically used. Cells from bone marrow and chorionic villi are normally undergoing rapid cell division and can also be karyotyped successfully. Historically, several different staining methods have been described. However, G-banding (Giemsa staining) is the standard cytogenetic method used. This technique permits a resolution of at least 400 bands among all the chromosomes and can be adapted to allow for high-resolution analysis of up to 800 bands to analyze structural rearrangements as small as 5 to 10 million or megabase pairs (Mb).

Gamete formation, either spermatogenesis or oogenesis, is accomplished by a process known as *meiosis*. In the first part of meiosis (meiosis I), homologous chromosomes align as pairs and cross over, exchanging genetic material,

also known as *recombination*. In this stage, reduction division, the recombined pairs separate and the typical diploid content (46 chromosomes) of the cell is reduced by half to a haploid complement of 23 chromosomes. In the next stage, meiosis II, the chromosomes separate, similar to mitosis (Nussbaum et al, 2007). The full diploid state of the cell will be restored at the time of fertilization.

An imbalance of genetic material, or aneuploidy, occurs from a net loss or gain of genetic material during sperm or egg formation or, less commonly, during the initial divisions of the embryo. This missing or extra genetic material can be small pieces or parts of chromosomes or an entire chromosome itself. The classic recognizable aneuploidy syndromes involve trisomy (three copies of a given chromosome) such as those of chromosomes 13, 18, and 21, or monosomy (only a single copy) of a complete chromosome, such as X. Trisomies in particular can occur from nondisjunction, a failure of normal chromosome separation. In such cases, a pair of homologues does not separate in meiosis; one daughter cell receives both homologs of that pair, and the other cell receives none. This event can occur in either part of gamete division, meiosis I or meiosis II. Most human meiotic nondisjunction arises during oocyte formation, specifically in maternal meiosis I. Nondisjunction of meiosis I is especially pronounced in trisomies of the acrocentric chromosomes (13, 14, 15, 21, and 22) and in XXX trisomy (MacDonald et al, 1994; Zaragoza et al, 1994). The occurrence of meiotic nondisjunction increases significantly with maternal age. Therefore prenatal karyotyping from amniocentesis or chorionic villus sampling is offered to women aged 35 years and older (Hook and Cross, 1982).

Nondisjunction can also occur in mitosis, with uneven division of genetic material during early embryonic cell division. This can result in two cell lines, one trisomic lineage that is potentially viable and one monosomic line. If this event occurs after the first postzygotic division, cells with a normal chromosome complement may also exist with cells containing an aneuploid complement as a mosaic chromosome constitution.

Partial aneuploidy may result from several mechanisms, such as rearrangements of material between nonhomologous chromosomes that can occur in the gametes of a balanced translocation carrier. The carrier parent who has no net loss or gain of genetic material is usually phenotypically normal; however, the offspring are at increased risk for an unbalanced rearrangement and its phenotypic consequences. Attention has also been focused on deletion syndromes caused by the loss of genetic material from several chromosomes (e.g., 1p-, 4p-, 5p-), with a resulting, often recognizable phenotype. Other microdeletions have been associated with segmental duplications, or large blocks of DNA that contain chromosome-specific repetitive

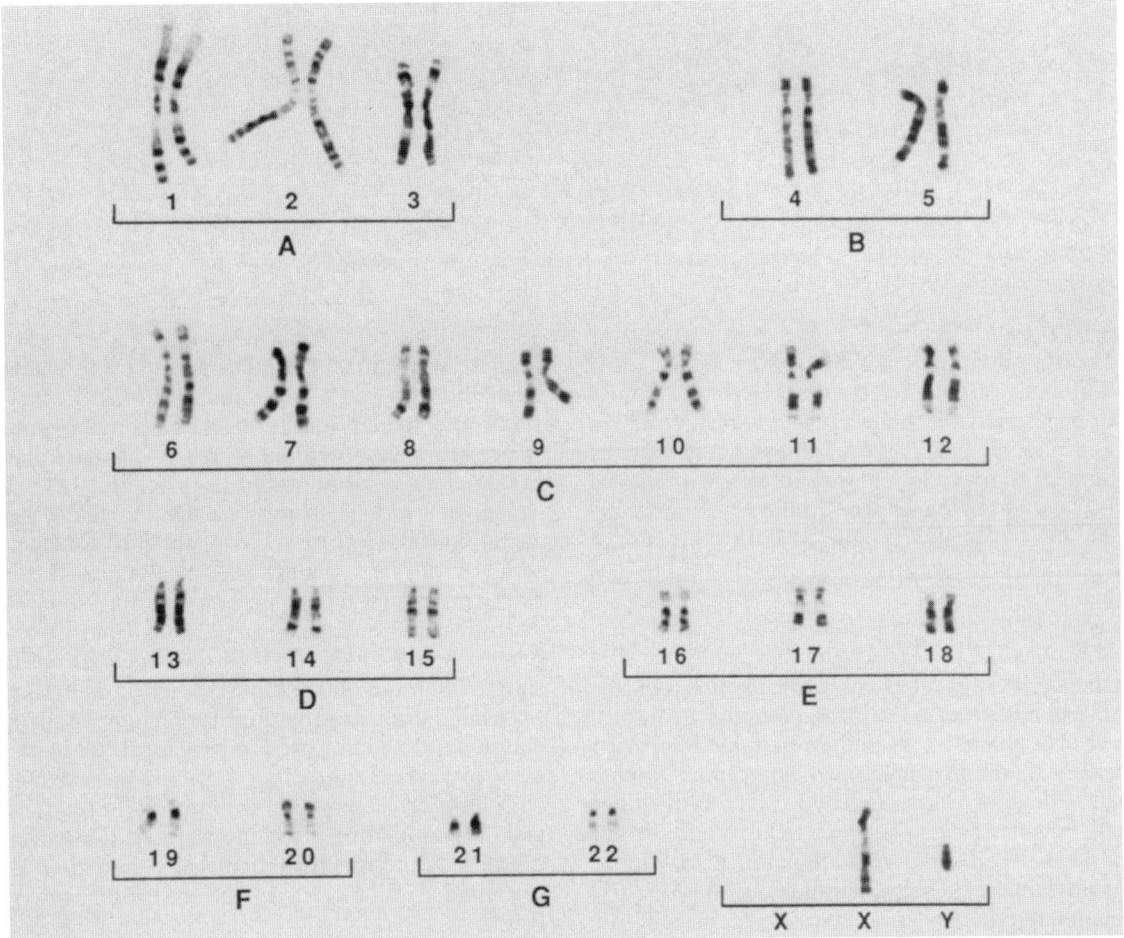

FIGURE 20-1 G-banded human male karyotype. The 46 chromosomes are arranged into 23 pairs, each with a specific banding pattern.

sequences (Emanuel and Saikh, 2001). It is thought that the repeats can mediate misalignment between two homologs and have been shown to be present in regions of the genome prone to instability, such as the pericentromeric regions of chromosomes 7q11, 15q11, 17q11, and 22q11, leading to the phenotypes seen in Williams-Beuren syndrome, Prader-Willi or Angelman syndrome, Charcot-Marie-Tooth disease or hereditary neuropathy with liability to pressure palsies, and DiGeorge or velo-cardiofacial syndrome, respectively (Emanuel and Saitta, 2007). The use of fluorescent in situ hybridization (FISH) and chromosome-specific subtelomeric FISH and the advent of DNA microarrays has allowed the identification of smaller chromosomal rearrangements that were largely unrecognized until recently. The use of high-resolution microarrays in infants with multiple congenital anomalies has in many cases led to the identification of a specific genotype, with clinical investigations then further defining the associated phenotype (Bejjani and Shaffer, 2008).

TRISOMIES

DOWN SYNDROME (TRISOMY 21)

Lejeune and Turpin (1960) demonstrated that trisomy of human chromosome 21 caused the constellation of findings recognized as Down syndrome (Figure 20-2). This chromosome disorder was the first to be described and is the most common viable autosomal trisomy, occurring in approximately 1 in 700 to 800 live births (Hook, 1992). The vast majority (>90%) occurs secondary to meiotic nondisjunction, and a pronounced maternal age effect is encountered. Approximately 3% to 5% of cases are caused by a translocation, that could be either de novo or passed from a balanced translocation-carrier parent, that becomes unbalanced and trisomic in the baby. Typically, the translocated chromosome 21 rearranges with another acrocentric chromosome, often chromosome 14, resulting in a Robertsonian translocation. Mitotic nondisjunction, or mosaic Down syndrome, has been demonstrated in approximately 3% of cases as well, with variable features ranging from normal to a typical Down syndrome phenotype.

Clinical Features

It is the more common occurrence of Down syndrome in babies of older mothers that led to the use of prenatal karyotyping for advanced maternal age (>35 years) at the time of conception, with samples typically obtained by amniocentesis after 15 weeks' gestation, or chorionic villus sampling at 10 to 12 weeks' gestation. Maternal serum analyte testing is used for prenatal screening purposes, with results showing low alpha-fetoprotein, low unconjugated estriol, and elevated total human chorionic gonadotropin.

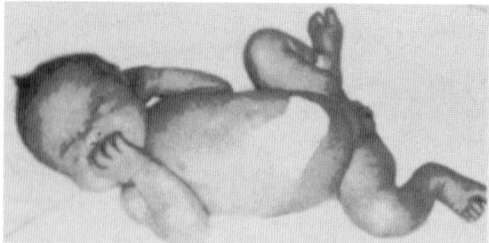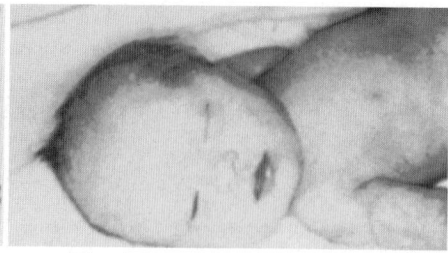

FIGURE 20-2 Newborn with Down syndrome (trisomy 21) illustrating some of the characteristic facial features, including upward-slanting palpebral fissures and a flat facial profile.

Associated ultrasonographic findings for Down syndrome, including a cardiac defect, shortened long bones, underdeveloped fetal nasal bone, nuchal translucency or thickening, echogenic small bowel, and duodenal atresia ("double-bubble" sign), may be seen in 50% to 60% of fetuses. Most patients with Down syndrome, if not diagnosed prenatally, are usually recognized at birth because of the typical phenotypic features, which then prompt karyotype analysis.

The constellation of physical findings associated with Down syndrome consists of brachycephaly, presence of a third fontanel, upward-slanted palpebral fissures, epicanthal folds, Brushfield spots in the irises, flattened nasal root, small posteriorly rotated ears with over-folded superior helices, prominent tongue, short neck with excess nuchal skin, single palmar creases, brachydactyly, fifth-finger clinodactyly, exaggerated gap between the first and second toes, open field hallucal pattern, and hypotonia (see Figure 20-2). Often the physical features conform to an easily distinguishable phenotype, but in some cases, prematurity or ethnic variations can make a clinical diagnosis less straightforward. An immediate karyotype is indicated to confirm the diagnosis and as preparation for counseling the family.

Malformations involving many organ systems have been described in Down syndrome, and whether the diagnosis is known prenatally or determined in the newborn period, several clinical investigations are warranted when this diagnosis is suggested. The most common malformation is congenital heart disease (seen in approximately 50% of cases), which may require surgical intervention. Atrioventricular canal defects are often encountered (mean of 40%), although ventricular septal defects (VSDs), atrial septal defects (ASDs), tetralogy of Fallot, and patent ductus arteriosus (PDA) are all described in the disorder. An echocardiogram is indicated in all cases, and medical and surgical interventions of cardiac lesions are routine. Gastrointestinal malformations, especially duodenal atresia (2% to 5%), in addition to Hirschsprung disease and less frequently encountered conditions, such as esophageal atresias, fistulas, and webs throughout the tract, have been described. It is critical to carefully monitor the baby's feeding and bowel function before considering discharge from the nursery.

Although growth parameters can be in the range of 10% to 25% at birth, significantly decreased postnatal growth velocity is encountered in these patients. Separate growth curves have been devised for patients with Down syndrome (Fernandes et al, 2001), because growth retardation involving height, weight, and head circumference has been well documented. An initial ophthalmologic evaluation is also indicated in the first few months of life and then annually, because strabismus, cataracts, myopia, and glaucoma have been shown to be more common in children with Down syndrome. In addition, hearing loss of heterogenous origin is present in approximately half of patients, with middle ear disease contributing to this problem.

Spinal cord compression caused by atlantoaxial subluxation from ligamentous laxity and subsequent neurologic sequelae can be a complication of the disorder. Screening radiographs are typically performed at approximately 3 years of age. Physicians should be vigilant in evaluating the cervical spine, especially before administration of anesthesia and before an older child's participation in sports. Other associated disorders that merit screening are hypothyroidism in approximately 5% of patients, often with the presence of thyroid autoantibodies. Initial evaluation occurs with newborn screening programs, followed by additional thyroid-stimulating hormone and free thyroxine levels at 6 months, 12 months, and then yearly thereafter. Bone marrow dyscrasias, such as neonatal thrombocytopenia, and transient self-resolving myeloproliferative disorders, such as leukemoid reaction, have been observed in the first year of life. An elevated rate of leukemia with a relative risk of 10 to 18 times normal up to age 16 years has been described. Acute nonlymphoblastic leukemia is seen at higher rates in congenital or newborn cases, but the distribution becomes similar to that of non–Down syndrome patients after age 3 years. Survival of patients with Down syndrome is shorter after a diagnosis of acute lymphoblastic leukemia than in diploid patients (Epstein, 2001).

Patients with Down syndrome demonstrate a wide range of developmental abilities, with highly variable personalities and behavioral phenotypes as well (Pueschel et al, 1991). Central hypotonia with concomitant motor delay is most pronounced in the first 3 years of life, as are language delays. Therefore immediate and intensive early intervention and developmental therapy are critical for maximizing the developmental outcome. A wide range of intelligence has been described, with conflicting data on genetic and environmental modifiers of outcome (Epstein, 2001). Seizure disorders occur in 5% to 10% of patients, often manifesting in infancy.

The most common causes of death in patients with Down syndrome are related to congenital heart disease, to infection (e.g., pneumonia) that is thought to be associated with defects in T-cell maturation and function, and to malignancy (Fong and Brodeur, 1987). Once medical and surgical interventions for the correction of associated congenital malformations are complete and successful, the long-term survival rate is good. However, fewer than half of patients survive to 60 years, and fewer than 15% survive past 68 years. Neurodegenerative disease with features of Alzheimer's disease is encountered in most patients who are older than 40 years, although frank dementia is not typical. Men with Down syndrome are almost always infertile, whereas small numbers of affected women have reproduced (Epstein, 2001).

In counseling the family of a newborn diagnosed with Down syndrome, it is important to include the organ systems affected in their baby and the severity of each malformation when defining a prognosis. Above all, the wide variability of the phenotype should be emphasized, with a care plan tailored to the needs of the individual patient.

Genetic Counseling

If a complete (full chromosome) or mosaic trisomy 21 is found, parental karyotypes are generally not analyzed, because the karyotypes are normal in virtually all cases. After having one child with Down syndrome, a mother's recurrence risk for another affected child is approximately 1% higher than her age-specific risk (Hook, 1992). This fact is especially significant in younger mothers, whose age-specific risks are low. If a de novo translocation resulting in Down syndrome is found, the recurrence risk is less than 1%. If the mother is found to carry a constitutional balanced Robertsonian translocation, the risk for another translocation Down syndrome fetus is approximately 15% at the gestational age when amniocentesis is offered, and 10% at birth. However, if the father is the translocation carrier, the recurrence risk is significantly smaller, approximately 1% to 2% (Epstein, 2001). Whereas newer array-based diagnostic techniques will identify the copy number change associated with the trisomy, structural rearrangements such as Robertsonian translocations are not readily detected. In this situation, a karyotype will provide information regarding the mechanism of the copy number change, which is needed for accurate recurrence risk counseling.

EDWARDS SYNDROME (TRISOMY 18)

Trisomy 18 is encountered in 1 in 6000 live births and is associated with a high rate of intrauterine demise. It is estimated that only 5% of conceptuses with trisomy 18 survive to birth and that 30% of fetuses diagnosed by second-trimester amniocentesis die before the end of the pregnancy (Hook, 1992). Findings on prenatal ultrasonography can raise suspicion for the disorder—growth retardation, oligohydramnios or polyhydramnios, heart defects, myelomeningocele, clenched fists, and limb anomalies. Maternal serum screening can show low values for alpha-fetoprotein, unconjugated estradiol, and total human chorionic gonadotropin, indicating the need for subsequent karyotype analysis and fetal ultrasonographic monitoring.

Clinical Features

Phenotypic features present at birth consist of intrauterine growth restriction (1500 to 2500 g at term), small narrow cranium with prominent occiput, open metopic suture, low-set posteriorly rotated ears, and micrognathia with small mouth. Characteristic clenched hands with

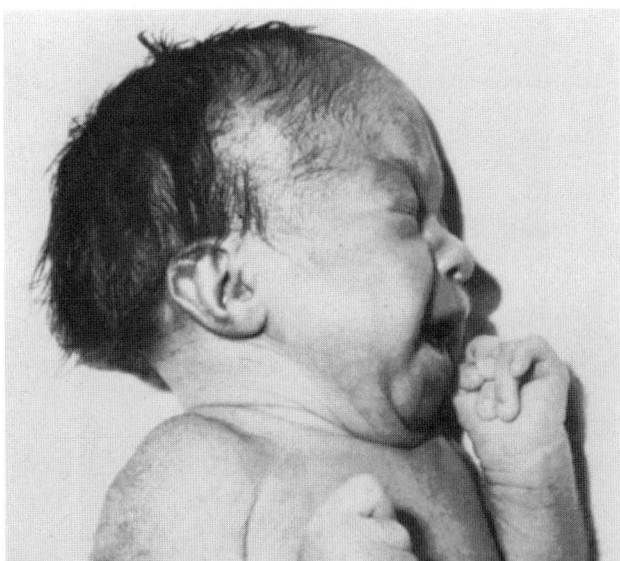

FIGURE 20-3 Newborn with trisomy 18, showing prominent occiput, characteristic facial appearance, and clenched hands.

overlapping digits, excess of arches on dermatoglyphic examination, hypoplastic nails, and "rocker-bottom" feet or prominent heels with convex soles (Figure 20-3) are also described. Additional malformations encountered in this syndrome are congenital heart disease (ASD, VSD, PDA, pulmonic stenosis, aortic coarctation), cleft palate, clubfoot deformity, renal malformations, brain anomalies, choanal atresia, eye malformations, vertebral anomalies, hypospadias, cryptorchidism, and limb defects, especially of the radial rays.

The prognosis in this disorder is extremely poor, with more than 90% of babies succumbing in the first 6 months of life and only 5% alive at 1 year old. Death is caused by central apnea, infection, and congestive heart failure. The newborn period is characterized by poor feeding and growth, typically requiring tube feedings. A few patients have been described who have survived into childhood and beyond. Universal poor growth and profound mental retardation with developmental progress stopping at that of a 6-month-old infant (Baty et al, 1994) have been documented. Malignant tumors such as hepatoblastoma and Wilms' tumor have been described in some of the survivors. In the few patients in whom cardiac surgery was performed, outcome was not shown to be improved.

Genetic Counseling

The typical estimate of a recurrence risk for trisomy 18 in a future pregnancy is a 1% risk over the maternal age–specific risk for any viable autosomal trisomy (Hook, 1992). Trisomy occurring from a structural rearrangement, such as a translocation, warrants parental karyotype analysis before the recurrence risk can be assessed.

PATAU SYNDROME (TRISOMY 13)

It has been estimated that approximately 2% to 3% of fetuses with trisomy 13 survive to birth, with a frequency of 1 in 12,500 to 21,000 live births (Hook, 1992). As with

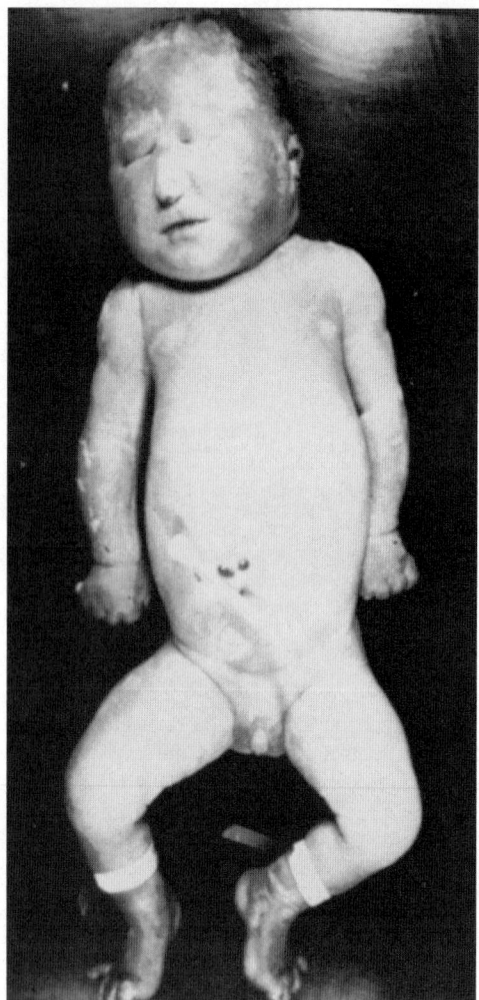

FIGURE 20-4 Stillborn with trisomy 13. The facial appearance is that of cebocephaly, which is associated with holoprosencephaly. There is an extra digit on the ulnar border of the right hand.

other trisomies, amniocentesis performed for advanced maternal age or indicated by fetal ultrasonographic findings may lead to a prenatal diagnosis of trisomy 13.

Clinical Features

Trisomy 13–associated malformations include congenital heart disease, cleft palate, holoprosencephaly, renal anomalies, and postaxial polydactyly (Figure 20-4). In addition, microcephaly, eye anomalies, and scalp defects can suggest the diagnosis. Brain malformations such as holoprosencephaly are found in more than half the patients, with concomitant seizure disorders. Microcephaly, split sutures, and open fontanels are encountered. A scalp defect (cutis aplasia) that can sometimes be mistakenly attributed to a fetal scalp monitor is specific to the disorder, being found in 50% of cases. Eye malformations, including iris colobomas and hamartomatous cartilage "islands," can be seen on funduscopic examination.

Congenital heart disease is present in approximately 80% of patients, usually VSD, ASD, PDA, or dextrocardia. Limb anomalies, such as postaxial polydactyly, single palmar creases, and hyperconvex narrow fingernails, are

also seen. The fingers can be flexed or overlapped and can show camptodactyly. An increased frequency of nuclear projections in neutrophils, giving a drumstick appearance similar to that of Barr bodies, can also be found. This finding would be especially striking in males, in whom Barr bodies would not be expected.

As with trisomy 18, prognosis for the fetus with trisomy 13 is extremely poor, with 80% mortality in the neonatal period, and less than 5% of patients surviving to 6 months old. Mental retardation is profound, and many patients are blind and deaf as well. Feeding difficulties are typical.

Genetic Counseling

Recurrence risk data suggest that, as with trisomy 18, the chance that a woman will have a child with any trisomy after a pregnancy affected by trisomy 13 is rare. The estimated risk is 1% higher than the maternal age–related risk for the recurrence of any viable autosomal trisomy in a subsequent pregnancy.

TURNER SYNDROME (45,X)

In early embryogenesis, two active X chromosomes are required for normal development. Turner syndrome, a phenotype associated with loss of all or part of one copy of the X chromosome in a female conceptus, occurs in approximately 1 in 2500 female newborns. The 45,X karyotype or loss of one entire X chromosome accounts for approximately half of the cases. A variety of X chromosome anomalies—including deletions, isochromosomes, ring chromosomes, and translocations—account for the remainder of the causes. It is important to note that approximately 0.1% of fetuses with a 45,X complement survive to term; the vast majority (>99%) is spontaneously aborted. This fact underscores the requirement for both X chromosomes during embryonic development. Additional studies indicate that in approximately 80% of cases, it is the paternally derived X chromosome that is lost (Willard, 2001).

Clinical Features

There is wide phenotypic variability in patients with Turner syndrome. Features present at birth include short stature, webbed neck, craniofacial differences (epicanthal folds and high arched palate), hearing loss, shield chest, renal anomalies, lymphedema of the hands and feet with nail hypoplasia, and congenital heart disease. Typical cardiac defects are bicuspid aortic valve, coarctation of the aorta, valvular aortic stenosis, and mitral valve prolapse.

Growth issues, especially short stature, are the predominant concern in childhood and adolescence; the mean adult height of patients with Turner syndrome is 135 to 150 cm without treatment. Growth hormone therapy, which is routinely offered starting at approximately 4 to 5 years old, can lead to an average gain of 6 cm or more in final adult height (Willard, 2001). Primary ovarian failure caused by gonadal dysplasia (streak gonads) can result in delay of secondary sexual characteristics and primary amenorrhea. Cyclic hormonal therapy is initiated at the age of puberty to aid the development of secondary sex characteristics and menses as well as to help bone mass. Infertility, related to gonadal dysplasia, is typical and has been successfully treated with assisted reproduction techniques and donor oocytes. It is important to evaluate for structural cardiovascular defects in the patient before pregnancy.

In terms of intellectual development, specific difficulties with spatial and perceptual thinking lead to a lower performance intelligence quotient; however, this syndrome is not characterized by mental retardation.

TRIPLOIDY (69,XXX OR 69,XXY)

As its name implies, triploidy is a karyotype containing three copies of each chromosome. Mechanisms that lead to this state include fertilization of the egg by two different sperm (dispermy) and complete failure of normal chromosome separation in maternal meiosis. The vast majority of triploid fetuses are spontaneously aborted, accounting for up to 15% of chromosomally abnormal pregnancy losses. Live births of affected fetuses are rare, and reports of survival beyond infancy are only anecdotal. Mosaicism with combinations of diploid and triploid cells (mixoploid) has also been documented. Malformations, including hydrocephalus, neural tube defects, ocular and auricular malformations, cardiac defects, and 3-4 syndactyly of the fingers, are associated findings. In addition, the placenta is often abnormal, typically large, and cystic.

DELETION SYNDROMES

In addition to the aneuploid conditions described previously, partial monosomy of a chromosome can lead to a recognizable pattern of malformations. Three known syndromes that are associated with the deletion or loss of genetic material from the short, or *p* arms of chromosomes 1, 4, and 5 are described. All these syndromes are associated with deletions that involve the loss of many genes located in a specific region.

CHROMOSOME 1p DELETION SYNDROME (1p-)

Monosomy for the distal short arm of chromosome 1, or deletion of 1p36, has been associated with a constellation of clinical findings. A characteristic facies consisting of frontal bossing, large anterior fontanel, flattened midface with deep set eyes, and developmental delay has been described (Figure 20-5). Orofacial clefting, hypotonia, seizures, deafness, and cardiomyopathy are also noted.

This deletion syndrome is estimated to occur in approximately 1 in 10,000 live births, and it is the most frequently occurring subtelomeric deletion. Greater recognition of the phenotype, the availability of a specific FISH test, and current widespread use of DNA microarrays will likely lead to improved diagnosis of this condition. The majority of deletions arise de novo in the patient, with approximately 3% being attributable to malsegregation of a balanced parental translocation. The size of the deletion varies, from submicroscopic (<5 Mb) to large, cytogenetically visible deletions greater than 30 Mb. A correlation between the size of the deletion and the severity of clinical features is suggested.

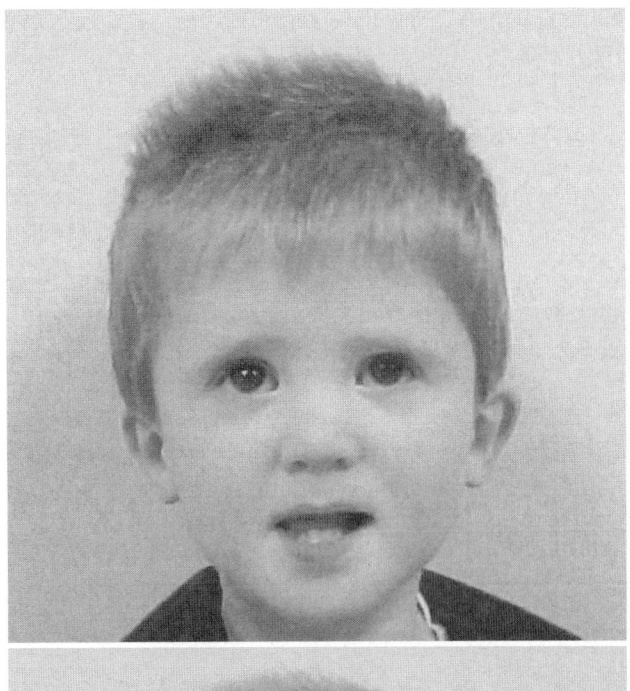
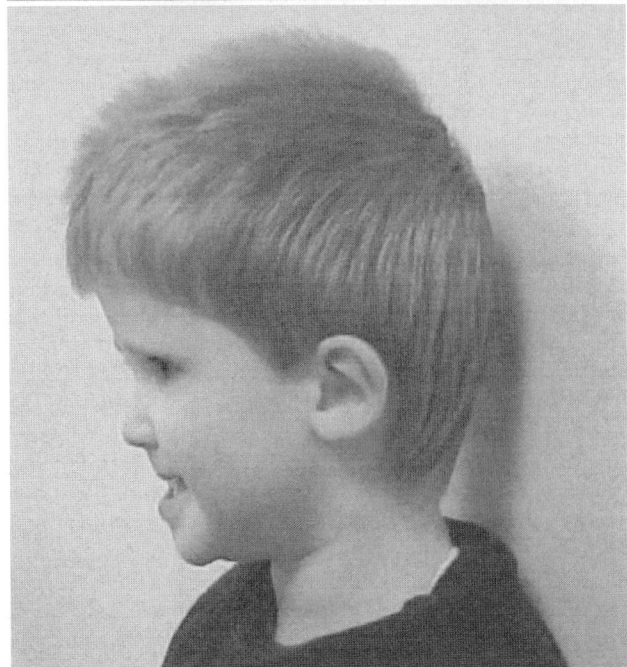

FIGURE 20-5 Child with deletion of chromosome 1p.

WOLF-HIRSCHHORN SYNDROME (4p-)

Distal deletions of the short arm of chromosome 4 are associated with a recognizable pattern of malformation. This syndrome is estimated to occur in 1 in 50,000 births and has features such as intrauterine growth restriction, microcephaly, midline structural defects such as cleft lip and cleft palate, cardiac septal defects, and hypospadias. The characteristic facial features are described as the Greek helmet facies, as evidenced by hypertelorism with epicanthi, a high forehead with a prominent glabella, and a beaked nose. Prominent, low-set ears are also seen. Hypotonia, failure to thrive, and developmental delay are common, with one third of infants dying in the first year of life.

Many patients have lived well into childhood and even into adulthood, although profound growth and mental retardation is typical and often accompanied by seizures.

Although most deletions are cytogenetically visible on karyotype analysis, small submicroscopic deletions have also been described. In cases in which the clinical features are suggestive but the karyotype is not revealing, further cytogenetic analysis using specific 4p telomere probes or a DNA microarray can be diagnostic. More than 80% of 4p deletions arise de novo in the patient, with minimal risk of recurrence. In the 10% to 15% of cases resulting from a translocation, analyzing parental samples is clinically indicated for appropriate recurrence risk counseling.

CRI DU CHAT SYNDROME (5p-)

Partial monosomy of chromosome 5p is seen in approximately 1 in 50,000 live births and is associated with a multiple congenital anomaly syndrome named for the unusual cry of the affected babies, described as similar to that of a cat, or *cri du chat*. The constellation of features associated with this disorder includes low birthweight, microcephaly, round face, hypertelorism or telecanthus, downward-slanting palpebral fissures, epicanthi, and broad nasal bridge. Hypotonia and cardiac defects are also seen, including ASD, VSD, and tetralogy of Fallot. Early issues include failure to thrive and pronounced developmental delay. The unusual cry usually resolves during infancy, and survival into adulthood is possible but is typically associated with severe mental retardation. Intensive therapy appears to provide some benefit, and more sensitive measures of cognition demonstrate clearly better receptive language skills than expressive language ability. Therefore children may understand more complex verbal language than their expressive skills might demonstrate (Cornish et al, 1999).

It is estimated that almost 100 genes are lost when the putative critical region from 5p15.2 to p15.33 is deleted (Shaffer et al, 2001; Zhang et al, 2005). Close to 90% of 5p deletions arise de novo in the affected child, incurring a minimal risk of recurrence (<1%). The remainder arise from malsegregation of a balanced translocation in a carrier parent, which would be associated with a 10% to 15% risk of recurrence of an unbalanced karyotype in a future live born infant. Parental chromosome analysis is indicated for proper recurrence risk counseling.

DNA MICROARRAYS

Recently, emphasis has been placed on characterizing variations of the genome that fall in the range between the single nucleotide and visible chromosomal changes—submicroscopic structural variants (less than 5 Mb) that cannot be seen by standard karyotype. An emerging technology rapidly gaining acceptance in various clinical settings involves the use of DNA microarrays (Bejjani and Shaffer, 2008; Miller et al, 2010). In general, microarray-based methods are focused on detecting copy number changes, and rearrangements such as balanced translocations or inversions are not detectable using this methodology. Microarray testing can be performed in either a targeted or genome-wide fashion. Two types of DNA microarray platforms are used currently: array comparative

genomic hybridization, which can utilize bacterial artificial chromosomes containing large DNA segments as probes, or small oligonucleotides as DNA probes. Other approaches use single nucleotide polymorphism arrays that include probes based on known polymorphisms present in the human genome. Single nucleotide polymorphism-based arrays or dense oligonucleotide arrays have the advantage of detecting gains or losses of shorter stretches of the genome, because the probes for a given region can be densely arrayed, and the sensitivity for detecting alterations of that region is greatly enhanced.

With a single test, microarrays can detect genomic errors associated with disorders that are usually identified by cytogenetic analysis and multiple FISH studies. Whereas microarray analysis is proving robust and providing an exceptional level of resolution from a diagnostic perspective, the major difficulty with the current interpretation of the results lies in assigning causality and clinical significance to the multiple alterations that are detected in each individual. Toward this end, the availability of databases with information on normal variation in multiple ethnic populations and testing of unaffected parents remain standard approaches to discerning whether a copy number change is likely to cause disease.

SEGMENTAL DUPLICATIONS AND MICRODELETION SYNDROMES

A greater appreciation of the complexity of the human genome and its structure has now been afforded with the completion of the human genome sequence. This work has focused attention on regions of the genome that are prone to rearrangement. The presence of such unstable regions appears to have a significant role in the etiology of several genetic disorders (Emanuel and Shaikh, 2001; Emanuel and Saitta, 2007). These disorders result from inappropriate dosage of crucial genes in a given genomic segment via either structural mechanisms (deletion or duplication) or functional mechanisms (imprinting or uniparental disomy). It has also been demonstrated that many of these regions of genomic instability have a common element: the presence of large, chromosome-specific low copy repeats that most likely mediate misalignment and unequal crossover during recombination, leading to rearrangements such as a deletion and duplication (Figure 20-6). Many of these large repeat structures are localized to a single chromosome or within a single chromosomal band. Examples of such genomic disorders are hemophilia A (inversion of Xq28), Sotos syndrome (in which a number of patients have a deletion of 5q35), Smith-Magenis syndrome (deletion of 17p11.2), Charcot-Marie-Tooth disease (interstitial duplication on 17p12), and the reciprocal deletion of this same region of 17p12, leading to hereditary neuropathy with liability to pressure palsies and a small percentage of patients with neurofibromatosis type I (deletion involving 17q11.2).

In this section, we focus on several deletion syndromes that occur on chromosomes whose underlying genomic structure contains segmental duplications such as Williams-Beuren syndrome (involving chromosome 7q11.2), Prader-Willi syndrome or Angelman syndrome (involving an imprinted region of chromosome 15q11

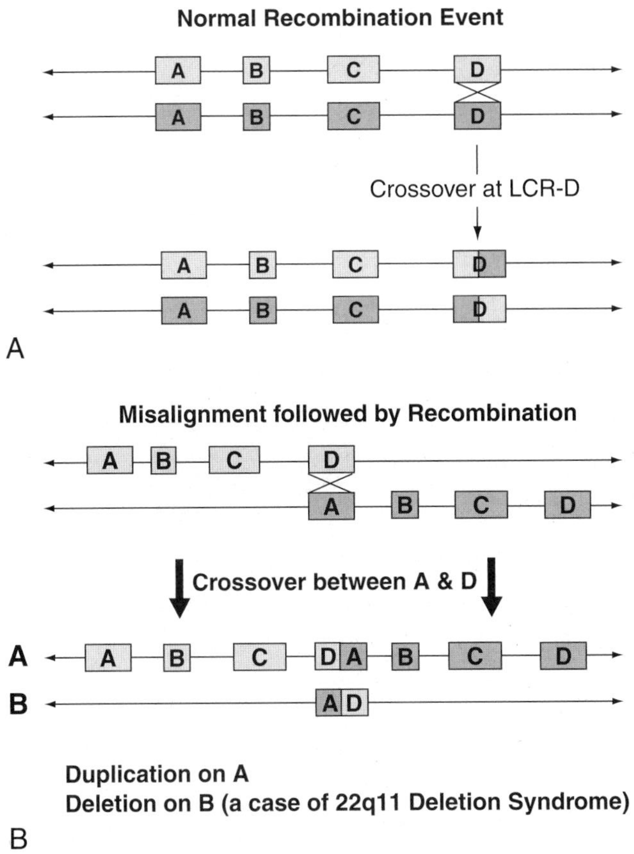

Normal Recombination Event

Crossover at LCR-D

A

Misalignment followed by Recombination

Crossover between A & D

A

B

Duplication on A
Deletion on B (a case of 22q11 Deletion Syndrome)

B

FIGURE 20-6 A, Alignment of low copy repeats (LCRs) before exchange. **B,** Misalignment of LCRs before exchange can result in rearrangement.

through 15q13), and DiGeorge or velocardiofacial syndrome (DGS/VCFS), the most commonly occurring microdeletion syndrome in humans, involving chromosome 22q11.2. It is important to note that in several of these microdeletion syndromes, there is the possibility that a reciprocal duplication of the exact same region may also occur (see Figure 20-6). Typically, the duplication syndromes cause fewer abnormalities and have wide phenotypic variability, but they are often characterized by developmental delays or behavioral abnormalities.

In addition, there are newly recognized microdeletion syndromes (e.g., 1q21.1, 3q29, 15q13.3, 16p11.2, and 17q21) that are rapidly being identified because of the increased use of DNA microarrays in the clinical and research settings. These regions are similarly flanked by segmental duplications, likely predisposing to their rearrangements. Many of the patients with these newly recognized rearrangements are not clinically diagnosed in the newborn period, because they may not have significant anatomic malformations or dysmorphic features that prompt a genetic evaluation; however, they can present during childhood with variable clinical findings. Typically there is developmental delay, often autistic spectrum disorder, or an intellectual disability. These syndromes are complicated because they have been reported in unaffected family members, which proves to be a challenge when ascribing causality to the rearrangement.

When an abnormality is identified by microarray analysis, the genes located in the affected region can be identified. It is then possible to decide what role, if any, the affected genes have in the observed phenotype. For example, deleted genes could be identified that may predispose a patient to cancer because of a germline loss of one copy of a tumor suppressor gene (Adams et al, 2009), resulting in careful surveillance for tumor formation. Therefore a new genetic paradigm is developing where patients are initially genotyped (genotype-first), followed by evaluation of the altered genes in a given region to determine their possible effect on the future phenotype.

WILLIAMS-BEUREN SYNDROME (7Q11.2 DELETION)

The estimated incidence of Williams-Beuren syndrome is 10,000 live births. The phenotype has a variable spectrum, but usually consists of distinctive facies, growth and developmental retardation, cardiovascular anomalies, and occasionally infantile hypercalcemia (Figure 20-7). Babies with Williams-Beuren syndrome usually show some degree of intrauterine growth restriction with mild microcephaly. Facial features include epicanthal folds with periorbital fullness of subcutaneous tissues, flat midface, anteverted nostrils, long philtrum, thick lips, large open mouth, and stellate irises that may not be discernible at birth. Most infants have a cardiovascular abnormality; supravalvular aortic stenosis (SVAS) is the most commonly associated defect, seen in more than 50% of cases. Pulmonary artery stenosis is also often encountered. It is interesting to note that isolated SVAS can also exist as a separate autosomal dominant trait and has been shown to occur from mutations of the elastin gene that is located within the deletion region on 7q11.2. Patients with Williams-Beuren syndrome are typically missing one copy of the elastin gene.

Hypercalcemia, which is manifested in approximately 10% of patients with this disorder, is severe and persists through infancy. Umbilical and inguinal hernias are also associated features. Issues in infancy include feeding and growth problems, with pronounced irritability and colicky behavior. Hoarse voice, strabismus, hypertension, and joint mobility restrictions may develop later in childhood. In terms of development, the typical mild to moderate mental retardation can be masked by advanced language skills, although gross motor and visual-motor integration skills are especially affected. Attention-deficit disorders are common, and a characteristic outgoing personality is often described in affected children.

Many of the classic features of Williams-Beuren syndrome are not clearly discernible in the newborn period, but the diagnosis should be suggested in any child with SVAS, hypercalcemia, and facial features consistent with the disorder. The diagnosis can be confirmed quickly by performing a DNA microarray or FISH using probes specific for the deleted region of chromosome 7q11.2. Because the condition is typically sporadic and most deletions arise de novo, the risk of recurrence in subsequent pregnancies is minimal. An affected adult, however, would pass on the condition in an autosomal dominant manner, with a 50% risk of the disorder in his or her child.

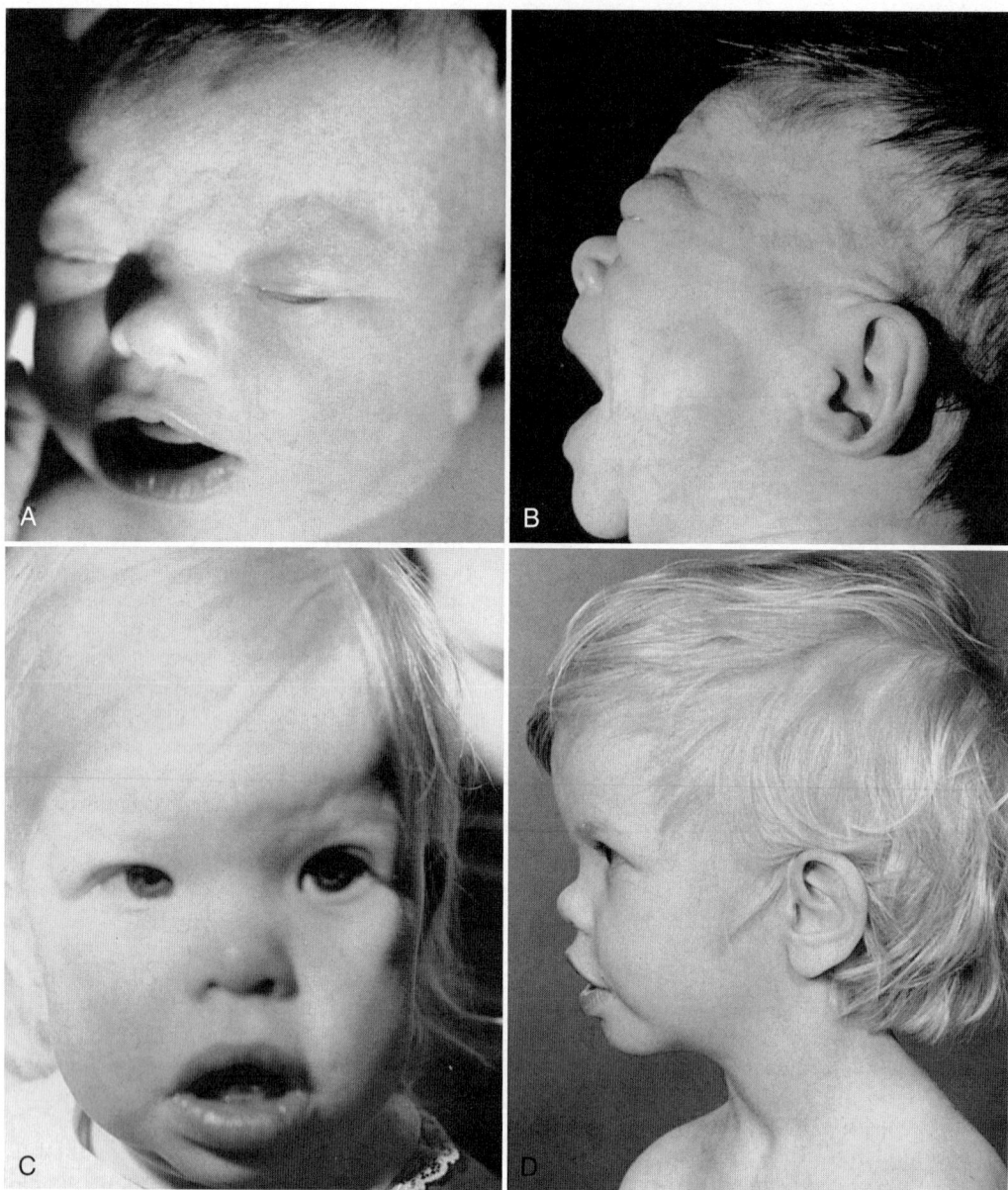

FIGURE 20-7 **Williams syndrome. A,** Neonate with a coarse face, periorbital fullness, wide mouth, and thick lips with decreased Cupid's bow. **B,** Neonate profile showing periorbital fullness, flat nasal bridge with full tip, and prominent cheeks. **C,** This infant has periorbital fullness, flat nasal bridge, thick lips with decreased Cupid's bow, pouty lower lip, and low-set, full cheeks. **D,** Infant profile showing dolichocephaly (increased antero-posterior diameter of head), a higher nasal bridge than in the neonate, full nasal tip, pouty lower lip, long neck, sloping shoulders, and part of pectus excavatum.

22q11.2 DELETION SYNDROME

A deletion of chromosome 22q11.2 has been identified in the majority of patients with DiGeorge syndrome, VCFS, and conotruncal anomaly face syndrome, leading to the realization that these clinical entities all reflect features of the same genomic disorder (McDonald-McGinn et al, 1997). The list of findings associated with 22q11.2 deletion is extensive and varies by patient. Estimates indicate that 22q11 deletion occurs in approximately 1 in 3000 live births (Burn and Goodship, 1996). This disorder is the most common microdeletion syndrome occurring in humans and is a significant health concern in the general population.

The phenotype is characterized by a conotruncal cardiac anomaly and often aplasia or hypoplasia of the thymus and parathyroid glands. The majority of patients with a deletion can receive a diagnosis as newborns or infants with significant cardiovascular malformations, including interrupted aortic arch type B, truncus arteriosus, or tetralogy of Fallot, along with functional T-cell abnormalities and hypocalcemia. In addition, facial dysmorphia may be present (Figure 20-8), including hooded eyelids, hypertelorism, overfolded ears, bulbous nasal tip, a small mouth, and micrognathia. Since the initial report by DiGeorge in 1968, the spectrum of associated clinical features has been expanded to include anomalies such as palatal anomalies,

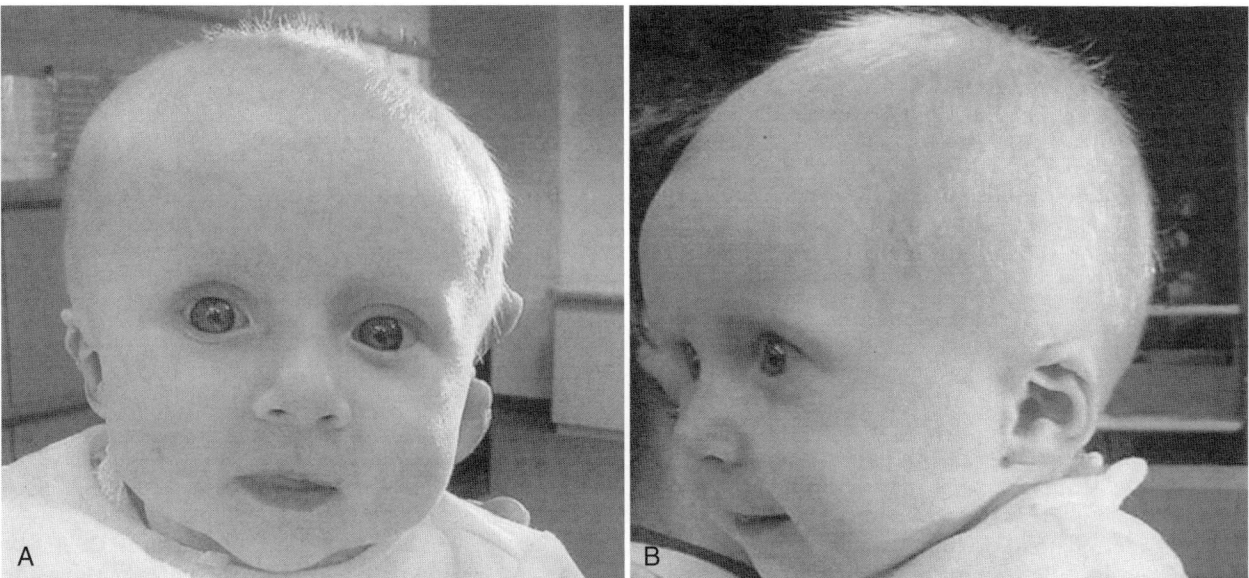

FIGURE 20-8 Facial differences associated with 22q deletion.

vascular rings, feeding and swallowing problems, gastroesophageal reflux, renal agenesis, and hypospadias (McDonald-McGinn et al, 1997). Before advances in the medical and surgical management of children with complex congenital cardiac disease and immune deficiencies, this disorder was associated with significant morbidity and mortality.

Developmental delays or learning disabilities have been reported in most patients with 22q11.2 deletion, and a wide range of developmental and behavioral findings have been observed in young children (Emanuel et al, 2001). In the preschool years, children with a 22q11.2 deletion were most commonly found to be hypotonic and developmentally delayed with language and speech difficulties. Severe or profound retardation was not seen, and one third of patients functioned within the average range.

The vast majority of patients (80% to 90%) have the same large deletion, approximately 2.4 to 3 Mb, that is detected by FISH (Figure 20-9) or DNA microarray. The deletion remains unchanged when inherited from an affected parent. However, the phenotype can be widely variable, even within a family. Although smaller recurrent deletions that are half the size of the common deletion occur (1.5 Mb), a smaller size does not indicate milder symptoms, making genotype-phenotype correlations difficult. To date, no explanation for the great phenotypic variability has been forthcoming, and it is currently an area of active investigation (Emanuel and Shaikh, 2001).

Most 22q11 deletions occur as de novo events, with less than 10% of them being inherited from an affected parent. The prevalence of these de novo 22q11.2 deletions indicates an extremely high mutation or rearrangement rate within this genomic region that is probably related to the presence of recombination-permissive duplicated DNA sequences, segmental duplications, or low copy chromosome 22–specific repeats in 22q11

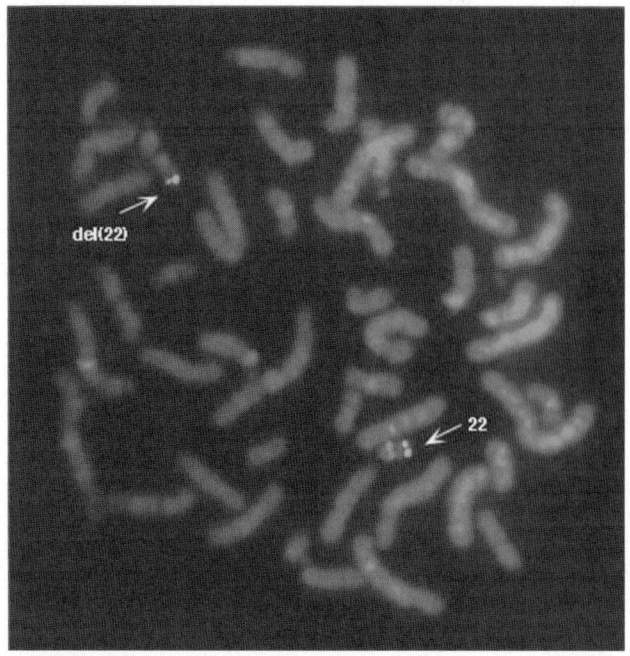

FIGURE 20-9 *(See also Color Plate 4.)* Fluorescence in situ hybridization study of a 22q deletion. *(Courtesy Beverly S. Emanuel.)*

(Emanuel and Shaikh, 2001; Emanuel and Saitta, 2007; Shaikh et al, 2007).

NEW MICRODELETION AND MICRODUPLICATION SYNDROMES

As mentioned previously, several newly identified genetic syndromes have been described with the increased use of DNA microarrays (Slavotinek, 2008). These regions are frequently flanked by segmental duplications, which is the likely reason for their prevalence in diverse patient populations, as well as the fact that there are reciprocal rearrangements (deletion or duplication). Almost all of the patients with these deletions or duplications were not initially recognized based on their clinical features, but were instead ascertained by microarray analysis.

Deletions of 1q21.1 of 1.35 Mb have been seen in patients with variable presentations including developmental and behavioral abnormalities, mild facial dysmorphia, and microcephaly (Brunetti-Pierri et al, 2008; Mefford et al, 2008). The 3q29 microdeletion syndrome is approximately 1.6 Mb and was initially discovered (Willatt et al, 2005) in patients with mild-to-moderate mental retardation, microcephaly, and nonspecific facial dysmorphia. Duplications of this region have also been described in patients with developmental delays, mental retardation, and microcephaly (Lisi et al, 2008). The 15q13.3 region is distal to the more commonly known 15q11-q13 locus associated with Prader-Willi and Angelman syndromes. Patients with the 1.5-Mb deletion of 15q13.3 have variable phenotypes, but typically manifest with seizures or abnormal electroencephalograms (Sharp et al, 2008). A smaller 680-kb deletion has also been described in a range of patients with neurobehavioral phenotypes (Shinawi et al, 2009). Interestingly, this deletion is often maternally inherited, suggesting that there might be an imprinting mechanism involved. A recurrent 550-kb deletion of 16p11.2 has been discovered in approximately 1% of patients with autism (Weiss et al, 2008), and the reciprocal duplication associated with attention deficit-hyperactivity disorder and schizophrenia (McCarthy et al, 2009; Shinawi et al, 2010). 17q21.31 deletions involving approximately 500 to 650 kb were also found in patients with developmental delays, learning disabilities, and variable facial dysmorphia (Koolen et al, 2008; Shaw-Smith et al, 2006).

DISORDERS OF IMPRINTED CHROMOSOMES

A growing recognition of mechanisms regulating gene expression has emerged in the last decade. Two of the most exciting concepts with important clinical correlates are imprinting and uniparental disomy. The term *genomic imprinting* implies that a whole region of a chromosome or a group of genes in a given region are subject to a difference in their expression that depends on whether they reside on the maternally inherited or paternally inherited chromosome. In these cases, a genetic disorder might manifest according to the parent from which the genomic region was inherited. The genes in an imprinted region are not necessarily mutated, but they are marked such that the cell can distinguish between the maternal and paternal copies and coordinate expression on the basis of that distinction. At the molecular level, it appears that differences in the methylation of the DNA, and its replication and regulation at the transcriptional level, appear to be involved in this mechanism. This mechanism has become an area of important research advancements, and there are now more than 100 known or predicted genes and chromosomal regions thought to be important in human disease (www.geneimprint.com/site/genes-by-species).

PRADER-WILLI SYNDROME

It has been demonstrated that occasionally, instead of inheriting one copy of each chromosome from each parent, both copies of a given chromosome can come from the same parent. This phenomenon, known as *uniparental disomy* (UPD), is associated with advanced maternal age. It becomes a significant issue when the involved chromosome is imprinted or has regions on it that are imprinted.

Prader-Willi syndrome (PWS) involves the loss of activity from the paternally derived proximal long arm of chromosome 15 (15q11). This loss can occur through deletion or disruption of this region or through maternal uniparental disomy such that no paternal chromosome 15 is present (Nicholls et al, 1989). Newborns have pronounced central hypotonia, hyporeflexia, and a weak cry. The poor tone manifests as sucking and swallowing difficulties that can lead to failure to thrive and the need for feeding tubes in infancy. Facial differences that have been described include bifrontal narrowing, almond-shaped eyes, and a small, downturned mouth. Genitalia are often hypoplastic, with cryptorchidism being common in boys with this syndrome. The commonly reported small hands and feet are not usually demonstrated in the newborn. Strabismus and hypopigmentation relative to the family are also common.

A history of poor fetal activity during the pregnancy can often be elicited, especially if the mother has had prior pregnancies. Consistent with the hypotonia, breech presentation and perinatal insults are found more frequently than usual. The extreme hypotonia begins to improve in the first year of life, as does motor development, although developmental delay is the rule, especially for gross motor skills and speech. The feeding improves in the first few years of life and gives way to often uncontrollable hyperphagia and obesity. This issue and other behavioral problems, including severe temper tantrums and obsessive-compulsive disorder, are encountered throughout life. The majority of patients manifests mild to moderate mental retardation. Early diagnosis and preemptive implementation of behavioral therapy are essential components of the optimal management of these issues.

Deletions of the region critical in Prader-Willi syndrome have been demonstrated in up to 70% of patients. The deletion can be detected by DNA microarray or FISH analysis using a probe specific for this region of chromosome 15. A small number of patients have a disruption of this area as the result of a chromosomal translocation. To date, no single gene in this region has been implicated as the cause, but expression of the genes in this region is under intense investigation. It has been noted, however, that patients who have Prader-Willi syndrome as a result of a deletion of the region are more likely to be hypopigmented. This feature has been attributed to deletion of a gene involved in pigmentation, the so-called P gene (Rinchik et al, 1993). Recurrence risks are negligible in cases in which de novo deletions are found and sporadic occurrence is usually encountered.

Approximately 20% to 25% of patients with Prader-Willi syndrome show maternal UPD that can be detected by means of a molecular assay designed to assess specific

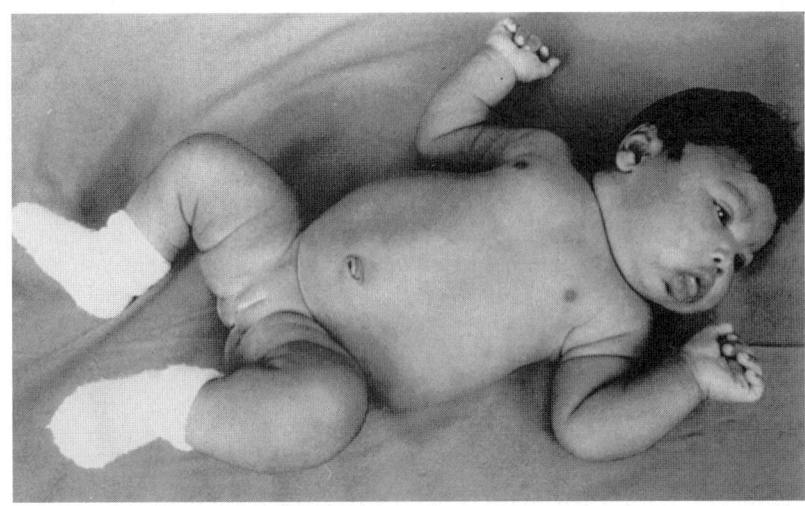

FIGURE 20-10 Macrosomic infant with macroglossia and lax abdominal musculature. These findings are typical of Beckwith-Wiedemann syndrome. *(From Viljoen DL, Jaquire Z, Woods DL: Prenatal diagnosis in autosomal dominant Beckwith-Wiedemann syndrome,* Prenat Diagn *11:167-175, 1991.)*

methylation differences between maternal and paternal alleles. Methylation analysis is abnormal in more than 99% of affected individuals, but will not determine whether the cause is attributed to a deletion or maternal UPD. Further study is required if an abnormal result is obtained. A maternal age effect has been demonstrated in UPD cases, and recurrence risks in families without deletions are estimated at 1 in 1000. In addition, this region of the genome is subject to regulation by imprinting. Large chromosome-specific segmental duplications are found in 15q11 and have been implicated in mediating the recurrent deletion of this genomic region (Emanuel and Shaikh, 2001; Emanuel and Saitta, 2007).

ANGELMAN SYNDROME

Loss of genetic material from the 15q11 region from the maternal copy of chromosome 15 is associated with Angelman syndrome. Clinical features are not evident in the newborn period and infancy, but include significant mental retardation, seizures, ataxic gait, tongue thrusting, inappropriate bursts of laughter, and facial differences including protruding jaw, wide mouth, thin upper lip, and widely spaced teeth. The mental retardation and hypopigmentation overlap with the features of Prader-Willi syndrome, but Angelman syndrome is a distinct entity.

Seventy percent to 75% of patients have a deletion of 15q11 that is detectable by FISH analysis. A small percentage (3% to 5%) have evidence of paternal isodisomy (two paternal copies) of the entire chromosome 15, with no apparent maternal chromosome. Unlike in Prader-Willi syndrome, Angelman syndrome has been associated with mutations in a single gene, *UBE3A*—an enzyme involved in the ubiquitin pathway of protein degradation, detected in up to 10% of patients. In addition, mutations of an imprinting center locus on chromosome 15 are thought to be associated with 1% to 2% of Angelman phenotypes (Shaffer et al, 2001). Methylation analysis can be performed and will detect abnormalities in approximately 75% to 80% of patients, because of a deletion or UPD. If methylation analysis is normal but Angelman syndrome is still suspected, *UBE3A* sequence analysis should be

considered. The vast majority of cases result from a sporadic event, and the risk of recurrence can be best evaluated once the genetic mechanism has been determined for a given patient.

BECKWITH-WIEDEMANN SYNDROME

Beckwith-Wiedemann syndrome affects approximately 1 in 14,000 newborns and manifests as an overgrowth syndrome in the neonatal period. The characteristic findings are macrosomia, abdominal wall defect, and macroglossia (Figure 20-10). Affected babies are large for gestational age with proportionate length and weight. Infants of mothers with diabetes also manifest with macrosomia, but are more likely to have a weight disproportionately greater than length. Advanced bone age is also noted in Beckwith-Wiedemann syndrome. Hemihypertrophy caused by asymmetric growth is common, as is visceromegaly of various organs, including the spleen, kidneys, liver, pancreas, and adrenal glands.

Other characteristic features of the syndrome are macroglossia, linear creases of the earlobe with indentations on the posterior helix, and severe hypoglycemia. Although the hypoglycemia responds quickly to therapy, it can be present for several months; therefore recognition of the condition and immediate therapeutic intervention are critical in these cases. The hypoglycemia resolves spontaneously with age, and the physical diagnostic features also become less prominent with age, making the diagnosis more difficult to ascertain.

Equally important is the establishment of routine ultrasonographic surveillance at regular intervals, because children with Beckwith-Wiedemann syndrome are at increased risk of malignant tumors, especially Wilms' tumor. The estimated risk is as high as 8% for patients with hemihypertrophy. Many centers currently perform ultrasonography at 3-month intervals until the school-age years (approximately 8 years old). Monitoring of serum alpha-fetoprotein levels at the same intervals until age 4 years has proved valuable, as several cases of hepatoblastoma have also been reported and detected with this adjunct study.

Although most cases of Beckwith-Wiedemann appear to arise de novo, up to 15% may be familial. In familial cases,

208 PART V Genetics

the transmission is autosomal dominant, because of mutations of the *CDKN1C* gene in 40% of familial cases, but only 5% to 10% of de novo cases. In addition, this region of the genome (11p15.5) appears to be imprinted such that the maternal allele is not usually expressed. The insulin-like growth factor type 2 (*IGF2*) gene is located in this region and encodes an important factor involved in fetal growth. Mutations causing overexpression of the paternal allele or underexpression of the maternal allele can result in an imbalance of expression leading to the overgrowth and tumor formation encountered in these patients. Paternal UPD has proved to be a mechanism involved in 10% to 20% of sporadic cases of Beckwith-Wiedemann syndrome. A method for detecting methylation abnormalities at two distinct genetic loci within 11p15 accounts for approximately 60% of patients and is related to the overexpression of the *IGF2* gene. Therefore all the available testing methods combined can detect the cause in approximately 85% of the patients with Beckwith-Weidemann syndrome. The recurrence risk for future affected siblings or offspring of the proband depends on the specific genetic abnormality causing the disorder and can range from low (UPD, methylation abnormality) to as high as 50% (*CDKN1C* mutation).

RUSSELL-SILVER SYNDROME

Russell-Silver syndrome presents in neonates with intrauterine growth retardation followed by postnatal growth deficiency. The head size is usually normal, causing a relative macrocephaly that may have the appearance of hydrocephalus. Facial features can include a broad and prominent forehead, triangular-shaped face with a small chin, and downturned corners of the mouth. The fingers can show brachydactyly, camptodactyly, or more commonly fifth-finger clinodactyly. Other concerns involve limb-length discrepancy, delayed bone age, café au lait macules, hypospadias in males, developmental delays, diaphoresis, and hypoglycemia during the first 3 years of life. These patients are often examined by a geneticist as a toddler with growth retardation, proportionate short stature, and normal head circumference. When evaluating patients with growth retardation, it becomes important to know the prenatal and postnatal growth parameters, because they might provide a clue to the diagnosis of Russell-Silver syndrome.

The molecular mechanisms underlying the pathogenesis show that Russell-Silver syndrome is likely caused by abnormalities of imprinted genes. Maternal UPD of chromosome 7 is present in 7% to 10% of patients, and

the symptoms are likely caused by overexpression of the maternal *GRB10* gene that suppresses activity of various growth factor receptors. In approximately 35% of the patients, imprinting abnormalities of 11p15.5 occur because of a loss of the paternally expressed *IGF2* gene, leading to decreased prenatal and postnatal growth. This finding contrasts with some patients with Beckwith-Wiedemann syndrome, in whom *IGF2* is overexpressed causing increased growth. To that end, patients with Russell-Silver syndrome do not have a significantly increased risk for neoplasia compared to patients with Beckwith-Wiedemann syndrome, and routine cancer surveillance protocols are typically not recommended.

SUMMARY

This chapter has summarized the rapidly expanding field of chromosomal and genomic disorders, concentrating on those that commonly manifest in the newborn. The widespread development and clinical implementation of molecular cytogenetic techniques have allowed the identification of subtle rearrangements that were previously undetectable. These advances now enable the discernment of new syndromes in which the chromosomal anomaly may be defined before a characteristic phenotype is recognized. In addition, a greater understanding of the role of segmental duplications and their effects on human genetic disorders as well as of the influence of mechanisms that regulate gene expression, such as imprinting, is emerging. The tremendous advances in genomics led by the completion of the Human Genome Project and the development of new molecular diagnostic tools present new challenges for clinicians to better diagnose, understand, and care for patients with genetic disorders and their families.

SUGGESTED READINGS

GeneReviews. Available on line at http://www.ncbi.nlm.nih.gov/sites/GeneTests/?db=GeneTests
Jones KL: *Smith's Recognizable Patterns of Human Malformation*, ed 6, Philadelphia, PA, 2006, WB Saunders.
Online Mendelian Inheritance in Man (OMIM): Available on line at http://www.ncbi.nlm.nih.gov/omim/
Rimoin DL, Connor JM, Pyeritz RE, Korf BR, editors: *Emery and Rimoin's Principles and Practice of Medical Genetics*, ed 5, New York, NY, 2006, Churchill Livingstone.
Schinzel A: *Catalogue of Unbalanced Chromosome Aberrations in Man*, Berlin, 2001, Walter de Gruyter.
Shaffer LG, Slovak ML, Campbell LJ, editors: *An International System for Human Cytogenetic Nomenclature (ISCN) 2009: Recommendations of the International Standing Committee on Human Cytogenetic Nomenclature*, Basel, 2009, S Karger.
Slavotinek AM: Novel microdeletion syndromes detected by chromosome microarrays, *Hum Genet* 124:1-17, 2008.

Complete references used in this text can be found online at www.expertconsult.com

CHAPTER
21

INTRODUCTION TO METABOLIC AND BIOCHEMICAL GENETIC DISEASE

Stephen Cederbaum

Inborn errors of metabolism or biochemical genetic disorders are one type of genetic disease that may be encountered in the neonatal period as an acute or more indolent illness. In these disorders, a mutation in a gene leads to an absent or defective gene product or enzyme and results in the accumulation of the precursor of the enzyme or a byproduct of it, a shortage of the product of the enzymatic reaction, or a combination of both. In reality the effects of many inborn errors on normal physiology are much more profound, causing many changes in gene expression and normal biochemical function. One example is a case of propionic acidemia in which interference with the mitochondrial respiratory apparatus is rarely measured except by the ascertainment of an elevated blood lactate level, but which may be much more frequent and represent only the most obvious and easily measured alteration.

Inborn errors of metabolism may be inherited by any genetic mechanism—autosomal dominant, autosomal recessive, sex-linked recessive, or through a mutation in the independently inherited mitochondrial genome (mtDNA), which leads to a circumstance in which the mother alone passes the abnormal DNA to all of her children, but the affected or carrier father to none of his offspring.

Most inborn errors are inherited as autosomal recessive conditions, with the carrier parents rarely expressing any obvious metabolic phenotype. A small minority is inherited in a sex-linked recessive or codominant manner, and they will be discussed in the context of their particular disease. Examples would be ornithine transcarbamylase deficiency (a urea cycle disorder) and Fabry disease (a lysosomal storage disorder), the latter not appearing in the neonatal period.

When viewed from the perspective of disease mechanism, most genetic disorders, whether single gene or involving imbalance of chromosomal materials, could be considered to be inborn errors of metabolism. One or more changes in the DNA result in either altered gene expression or expression of a mutated gene, which then lead secondary to an altered product of the reaction or reactions. We will not use this expansive and grandiose interpretation of inborn errors, but rather confine ourselves to the more traditional definition described in the first paragraph. Thus disorders such as cystic fibrosis and spinal muscle atrophy, considered inborn errors that require broader interpretation, will not be considered.

The advent of newborn screening in the early part of the 1960s for phenylketonuria (PKU) established a new paradigm for approaching inborn errors of metabolism and making the diagnosis and treatment prior to the symptomatic presentation, and hence preventing rather than treating the condition. This approach has proved to be remarkably successful for PKU and congenital hypothyroidism, with few patients becoming mentally retarded. In subsequent years the menu of tests expanded gradually, but it has greatly expanded in the last decade with the implementation of expanded newborn screening using tandem mass spectrometry (MS/MS) technology, which allows for ascertainment of a constellation of disorders and should alter the probability of, and the diagnostic testing for, inborn errors when incorporated into the diagnostic algorithms of the ill newborn. Moreover, the advancing technology permits some of the newborn dried blood spot to be used for a wider palette of tests, some of which may already be available. The consequences of this expansion have a downside for the neonatologist and the neonatal intensive care unit staff members. For a variety of reasons the sick and premature newborn, usually receiving intravenous alimentation and having immature or damaged organs, is far more likely to have a false-positive newborn screening test and require follow-up testing. It is important to recognize that a number of traditionally tested diseases are outside of this class of disorders, such as hypothyroidism, congenital adrenal hyperplasia, cystic fibrosis, and hemoglobinopathies.

When considering inborn errors of metabolism, it is important to consider the molecular basis of mutation. Large deletions of a gene are certain to eliminate enzymatic function and any residual gene product. Smaller deletions, especially if they remove one or more of the in-phase coding triplets, may permit a stable protein to be made and to function to some extent. Most small deletions, however, cause the synthesis of unstable and out-of-phase proteins that do not function and have a short half-life within the cell. Some single-based change mutations can introduce a stop codon, causing the synthesis of the polypeptide to halt abruptly and leave a nonfunctional enzyme. Single-base changes introducing a new amino acid vary in their effects from complete loss of activity to a lesser impact, and finally to having no effect whatsoever. When considering that the mutation test is then all modulated through the unique genetic background of the individual, there is no single final phenotype, severity, or time of onset for any genetic disorder. This variation must be considered when any diagnosis, genetic or not genetic, is considered.

CLASSIFICATION OF INBORN ERRORS OF METABOLISM

Each professional uses classification systems to permit effective reasoning as to possible causes of a symptom complex. A system for understanding inborn errors of metabolism is shown in Box 21-1. Each group has common characteristics, modes of presentation, types of molecules involved, and tests that would be applied. Because the demarcation between the groups is not sharp, other systems can see them differently. This discussion is restricted to those disorders that may be symptomatic in the newborn period or in early infancy, whereas many severe disorders would be unlikely to be associated with neonatal disease and will be given less emphasis. The disorders more commonly seen in the neonatal period are listed in Box 21-2.

The first group consists of newborns with progressive lethargy, poor suck, neurologic deterioration, and often death. They have inborn errors of amino acids, the urea cycle, organic acids, or sugar metabolism. This group of patients is the product of normal pregnancies and deliveries and becomes ill after 36 hours of life, when the maternal circulation no longer cleanses the accumulating small molecules from the fetal or infant blood and the offending metabolites accumulate in intoxicating amounts (Box 21-3). Examples include maple syrup urine disease, methylmalonic and propionic acidemias, galactosemia, and ornithine transcarbamylase deficiency. The general characteristics are given in Box 21-4; they are the disorders for which expanded newborn screening may lead to earlier detection and a more rapid diagnosis. These patients' condition is most likely to resemble sepsis, and they should be treated with antibiotics. Most disorders manifesting acutely in the newborn period will be detected by the newborn screen, with only some urea cycle disorders and lactic acidoses likely to be missed by this screening panel. When diagnosed, these conditions are

---

BOX 21-1   Classification of Inborn Errors of Metabolism, 2007

Small molecule disorders
- Amino acids
- Organic acids
- Sugars

Lysosomal storage disorders
- Mucopolysaccharides
- Sphingolipids
- glycolipids

Energy metabolism disorders
- Oxidation disorders
- Fatty acid mobilization and metabolism disorders
- Glycogen storage diseases

Peroxisomal and membrane biogenesis disorders
Carbohydrate-deficient glycoprotein disorders
Cholesterol biosynthetic disorders
Disorders of biogenic amines, folate, and pyridoxine
Transport disorders
Purine and pyrimidine metabolism disorders
Receptor disorders

BOX 21-2   Common Types of Inborn Errors of Metabolism With Newborn Presentation

- Amino acid disorders
- Organic acid disorders
- Disorders of ammonia metabolism
- Disorders of carbohydrate metabolism
- Disorders of gluconeogenesis or hypoglycemia
- Disorders of fatty acid oxidation
- Primary lactic acidoses (respiratory chain defects)
- Disorders of vitamin or metal metabolism
- Storage diseases (infrequently)
- Peroxisomal disorders
- Disorders of sterol metabolism
- Congenital defects in glycosylation

BOX 21-3   Metabolic Diseases With Newborn Coma Secondary to Toxic Metabolite Accumulation or Mitochondrial Failure

- Galactosemia
- Inborn errors of ammonia metabolism
- Maple syrup urine disease
- Nonketotic hyperglycinemia
- Methylmalonic acidemia with or without homocystinuria
- Propionic acidemia
- Isovaleric acidemia
- Multiple carboxylase deficiency
- Glutaric aciduria type 2
- Fatty acid oxidation defects
- Primary lactic acidosis
- Pyruvate dehydrogenase deficiency
- Pyruvate carboxylase deficiency
- Mitochondrial respiratory chain or electron transport chain defects

---

BOX 21-4   Characteristics of Small Molecule Disorders

- High levels of metabolites in body fluids
- Normal physical phenotype
- Neonatal presentation
- Periods of stability and instability
- Considered to be intoxication disorders
- Can often be treated by external manipulation

Lysosomal storage disorders (format)
- Usually born normally
- Course is progressive, relentless, and indolent
- Deposition of material seen clinically and microscopically
- May be deforming
- Cannot be addressed exogenously

Disorders of energy metabolism
- Mixed presentation between the first two categories
- Can be catastrophic at presentation
- May be present at birth or develop later
- Usually progressive
- May cause malformations
- May have episodes of deterioration
- Usually not treatable by exogenous means
- May be tissue specific or preferential

treated with dialysis, limitation of protein intake except for galactosemia, fluid, and caloric support, and some specific interventions. The association of identifying physical and laboratory characteristics and various disorders is listed in Tables 21-1 and 21-2. The individual disorders are discussed in Chapters 22 and 23. When a diagnosis of a metabolic disorder appears likely, plasma amino acids, urine organic acids, plasma acylcarnitine, and plasma carnitine tests should be repeated, and ammonia and lactate should be determined.

The second major category of inborn errors is the lysosomal storage diseases. This group of disorders results from defective function of a catabolic hydrolase located in the lysosome that is generally responsible for breaking down complex glycosaminoglycans and sphingolipids that are products of normal cellular turnover (see Box 21-4). Unlike the small molecule disorders in which the metabolites are found freely circulating in the body fluid compartments, these compounds accumulate intracellularly, are not removed by the maternal circulation, and are present in limited amounts in the body fluids. They most often cause no apparent symptoms in the newborn period or early infancy, because the pathologic metabolites accumulate slowly with time. Exceptions to this finding are the severe form of α-glucosidase deficiency or Pompe disease, the neonatal form of α-galactosidase deficiency, or Krabbe disease and galactosialidosis. These findings are discussed in Chapter 23, and some are listed in Table 21-1. The disorders of mucopolysaccharides and glycolipids lead to the characteristic features pejoratively and inappropriately referred to as *gargoylism*, which consist of an exaggerated eyebrow, coarse-appearing facies, thick skin, hirsutism, and multiple abnormalities of the bones and joints seen on a radiograph. Attention to the disorder is often drawn by the hepatosplenomegaly. The metabolites are synthesized in the body and are not influenced by dietary intake.

TABLE 21-1   Unique or Characteristic Physical Findings in Inborn Errors* (Major Examples)

Finding	Error	Finding	Error
Hepatomegaly	Galactosemia Glycogen storage diseases Gluconeogenic defects Disorders of fatty acid oxidation and transport Mitochondrial respiratory or electron transport chain defects Hereditary tyrosinemia type 1 Urea cycle defects Peroxisomal defects Niemann-Pick disease type C Congenital defects in glycosylation	Retinitis pigmentosa	Mitochondrial respiratory or electron transport chain defects Sjögren-Larsson syndrome Peroxisomal disorders Abetalipoproteinemia
Hepatosplenomegaly	Gangliosidoses Niemann-Pick disease type C Mucopolysaccharidoses Wolman disease Ceramidase deficiency	Optic atrophy or hypoplasia	Pyruvate dehydrogenase complex deficiency Mitochondrial disorders Leigh disease Peroxisomal disorders
		Corneal clouding or opacities	Mucolipidoses Mucopolysaccharidoses Steroid sulfatase deficiency
Macrocephaly	Glutaric acidemia type 1 Canavan disease	Cataracts	Galactosemia Lowe syndrome Mitochondrial respiratory or electron transport chain defects Peroxisomal disorders Congenital defects in glycosylation
Microcephaly	Mitochondrial respiratory or electron transport chain defects Leigh disease Methylmalonic acidemia with homocystinuria		
		Dislocated lens	Methionine synthetase deficiency Sulfite oxidase deficiency
Coarse facial features	Gangliosidosis Mucolipidoses Mucopolysaccharidosis type VII Sialidosis Galactosialidosis	Bone or limb deformities or contractures	Storage, peroxisomal, or connective tissue disorders Inborn errors of cholesterol biosynthesis
		Thick skin	Mucolipidoses Gangliosidoses Mucopolysaccharidoses
Macroglossia	Pompe disease Gangliosidoses Mucopolysaccharidoses Mucolipidoses	Desquamating, eczematous, or vesiculobullous skin lesions	Acrodermatitis enteropathica Organic acidemias Early-onset forms of porphyria
Dystonia or extrapyramidal signs	Gaucher disease type 2 Glutaric acidemia type 1 Krabbe disease Crigler-Najjar syndrome Biopterin defects	Ichthyosis	Gaucher disease type 2 Steroid sulfatase deficiency
		Alopecia	Multiple carboxylase deficiency
		Steely or kinky hair	Menkes disease
Macular "cherry red spot"	G_{M1} gangliosidosis Galactosialidosis Niemann-Pick disease type A Tay-Sachs disease (G_{M2} gangliosidosis)	Persistent diarrhea	Glucose galactose malabsorption Congenital lactase deficiency Congenital chloride diarrhea Sucrase isomaltase deficiency Acrodermatitis enteropathica Congenital folate malabsorption Wolman disease Galactosemia

*For discussion of specific disorders, see Chapters 22 and 23.

TABLE 21-2   Characteristic or Unique Laboratory or Diagnostic Testing Outcomes in Inborn Errors (Major Examples)

Outcome	Error	Outcome	Error
Metabolic acidosis with or without increased anion gap	Organic acidemias Maple syrup urine disease Fatty acid oxidation defects Ketothiolase deficiency Ketogenesis defects Disorders of pyruvate metabolism Mitochondrial respirator or electron transport chain defects, including Leigh disease Galactosemia Glycogen storage disease type 1 Gluconeogenesis defects	Thrombocytopenia	Organic acidemias Pearson syndrome
		Anemia	Organic acid disorders Wolman disease Pearson syndrome Severe liver failure Galactosemia
		Vacuolated lymphocytes or neutrophils	Lysosomal storage disorders
Respiratory alkalosis	Urea cycle disorders	Cardiomegaly	Pompe disease Barth syndrome Fatty acid oxidation defects Mitochondrial respiratory or electron transport chain defects Carbohydrate-deficient glycoprotein syndrome
Hyperammonemia	Urea cycle disorders Methylmalonic acidemia Organic acidemias Fatty acid oxidation disorders		
Ketosis	Organic acidemias Maple syrup urine disease Glutaric acidemia type 2 Ketogenesis defects Glycogen storage disease type 1 Gluconeogenesis disorders	Electrocardiographic abnormalities	Pompe disease (short PR interval, large QRS interval) Fatty acid oxidation disorders Mitochondrial respiratory or electron transport chain defects
Lactic acidosis	Mitochondrial respiratory or electron transport chain defects, including Leigh disease Pyruvate dehydrogenase complex deficiency Pyruvate carboxylase deficiency Organic acidemias Glutaric acidemia type 2 Fatty acid oxidation defects Ketogenesis defects Glycogen storage disease type 1 Gluconeogenesis disorders	Ventricular hypertrophy	Pompe disease Organic acidemias Glutaric acidemia type 2 Fatty acid oxidation defects Mitochondrial respiratory or electron transport chain defects, including Leigh disease
		Dysostosis multiplex	Gangliosidoses Mucopolysaccharidoses Mucolipidoses Sialidosis
Hypoglycemia	Hyperinsulinism Glycogen storage disease type 1 Gluconeogenesis disorders Maple syrup urine disease Glutaric acidemias Fatty acid oxidation defects Ketogenesis defects Galactosemia Severe liver failure Mitochondrial respiratory or electron transport chain defects	Stippled calcifications of patellae	Peroxisomal disorders Cholesterol biosynthetic defects
		Adrenal calcifications	Wolman disease
		Rhizomelica	Rhizomelic chondrodysplasia punctata
		Hair abnormalities	Menkes disease Argininosuccinicaciduria
Lipemia	Glycogen storage disease type 1 Lipoprotein lipase deficiency	Basal ganglia lesions on MRI	Organic acidemias (later in life) Pyruvate dehydrogenase complex deficiency Mitochondrial respiratory or electron transport chain defects, including Leigh disease
Positive urinary-reducing substances	Galactosemia Hereditary fructose intolerance Lowe syndrome		
Discolored urine	Alkaptonuria Tryptophan malabsorption	Cerebellar atrophy or hypoplasia	Pyruvate dehydrogenase complex deficiency Mitochondrial respiratory or electron transport chain defects, including Leigh disease Carbohydrate-deficient glycoprotein syndrome
Leukopenia	Organic acidemias Glycogen storage disease type 1B Barth syndrome Pearson syndrome	Agenesis of corpus callosum	Pyruvate dehydrogenase complex deficiency Pyruvate carboxylase deficiency Mitochondrial respiratory or electron transport chain defects

MRI, Magnetic resonance imaging.

The third important category of metabolic disorders is insufficient generation of energy by the mitochondrial machinery. These disorders can be caused by the inability to provide substrates such as glucose in glycogenoses; the inability to deliver substrate to the site of oxidation, such as the fatty acid and carnitine transport disorders; the inability to break down fatty acids in a stepwise fashion to provide reduced flavin adenine dinucleotide to be oxidized; or the deficient function of the mitochondrial respiratory pathway and energy-generating system itself. These disorders have characteristics in between those of the acute, small molecule disorders and the storage disorders

Box 21-5   Signs and Symptoms of Inborn Errors in the Newborn

- Neonatal catastrophe (life threatening)
- Poor suck and feeding
- Gastrointestinal problems, vomiting
- Respiratory distress
- Cardiac failure
- Neurologic abnormalities: alertness, tone, seizures
- Organomegaly
- Ocular abnormalities
- Cutaneous changes

Box 21-6   Metabolic Diseases With Congenital Malformations or Dysmorphic Features

- Cholesterol biosynthetic disorders
- Peroxisomal disorders
- Glutaric aciduria type 2
- Primary lactic acidoses
- Congenital defects in glycosylation
- Lysosomal storage disorders
- Menkes disease

(see Box 21-4). They differ from the small molecule disorders in the possible onset immediately at birth or before, and from storage disorders in the generally normal physical features with hepatomegaly alone, a regular feature of glycogen storage disorders. The small molecule and energy-generating disorders are discussed in Chapter 22 and the lysosomal storage disorders are discussed in Chapter 23.

Of the remaining groups that are encountered less frequently, the peroxisomal biogenesis disorders, carbohydrate-deficient glycoprotein disorders, and Smith-Lemli-Opitz syndrome (a cholesterol biosynthetic disorder) are discussed in Chapter 23. Other disorders are too infrequent to be considered in a general neonatology textbook. Disorders of biogenic amines are discussed in Chapter 22 and in greater depth in Chapter 63 on neonatal seizures, along with consideration of pyridoxine and folate disorders.

SIGNS AND SYMPTOMS OF INBORN ERRORS

The limited symptomatic repertoire of the sick newborn is well established, but it is worth repeating. For this reason, the first thought when confronting a newborn in deteriorating condition, with lethargy, poor suck, temperature instability, and neurologic abnormalities, is sepsis (Box 21-5). Most metabolic specialists have never confronted a sick newborn who has not had a "septic workup" and who is not receiving standard antibiotics. The issue then becomes when to perform a metabolic workup. The standard answer is that it should be performed when the neonatologist is concerned that the newborn in extremis does not fit the pattern that they expect from a child with sepsis or hypoxia. That threshold would vary by individual. Negative results of tests for infectious agents, a nonconfirmatory white count, hypoglycemia, unexpectedly severe acidosis, or hyperammonemia could be important triggers. Although dysmorphic features are not characteristic of inborn errors, there are some that may have subtle or occasionally pronounced abnormality on a physical examination; they are listed in Box 21-6 and in Table 21-2.

Modern neonatology has one tool that was previously unavailable: the expanded newborn screen. This screening will diminish the probability of many disorders, and the newborn screening follow-up hotline should be on the speed dial of every neonatal intensive care unit. The only acutely presenting disorders not ascertained by these studies are most hyperammonemias and lactic acidoses. These test results are available immediately in any tertiary or secondary care hospital. With a high level of concern and near normal levels of lactate and ammonia, the standard battery of metabolic studies should be performed only when the index of suspicion for a metabolic disorder is particularly high and no alternative explanation for the poor condition of the patient is likely. When deemed necessary, these studies should include plasma amino acids, plasma acylcarnitine levels, and urinary organic acids. The abnormalities associated with individual disorders are discussed in Chapter 22.

EMERGENCY TREATMENT

An acutely ill child with an inborn error of metabolism is an emergency, and rapid rescue treatment is mandatory. When considering a differential diagnosis, special emphasis should be placed on disorders for which there is treatment, as opposed to those for which there is no treatment. As with all acutely ill patients, supportive care, including cardiorespiratory, hemodynamic status, fluids, and electrolytes, is the mainstay of treatment. Transfer from institution to institution should not be performed unless the patient's condition is stable and there is adequate vascular access for emergency treatment. Transfer to a tertiary care center with experience in caring for these children is desirable and should be performed as quickly as possible.

Virtually all disorders require a maximum source of calories (150 calories/kg is desirable, but 120 calories/kg is a minimum target) to prevent or diminish catabolism, and glucose is the most important part of this, especially in the absence of primary lactic acidemia or acidosis. As much lipid as is safe should be added to compensate for the caloric deficit.

Hemodialysis, and especially extracorporeal membrane oxygenation, will remove most metabolites rapidly, but these are extreme interventions in a newborn. These interventions should be performed routinely in extreme and symptomatic hyperammonemia (ammonia levels of 400 mol/L or more), and many would consider dialysis in severe acidosis caused by acids other than lactate or ketones. Once a diagnosis is established, specific therapy can be initiated. It is important to emphasize that during this period of generic therapy, prolonged deprivation of exogenous protein or amino acids will cause endogenous protein breakdown and exacerbate the metabolic process. As a result, protein is added to the intravenous support fluids after 36 to 48 hours, beginning with 0.25 to 0.5 g/kg/day and increasing gradually to maintenance levels of 1.2 to 1.5 g/kg/day, pending a definitive diagnosis and assuming that it is tolerated.

SUGGESTED READINGS

Fernandes J, Saudubray J-M, van den Berghe G, et al, editors: *Inborn metabolic diseases: diagnosis and treatmented*, ed 4, Germany, 2006, Springer-Verlag.

Online Mendelian Inheritance in Man, OMIM: McKusick-Nathans Institute of Genetic Medicine, Johns Hopkins University (Baltimore, Md.) and National Center for Biotechnology Information, National Library of Medicine (Bethesda, Md.), Accessed {date of download}. Available at www.ncbi.nlm.nih.gov/omim/.

Saudubray JM, Charpentier C: Clinical phenotypes: diagnosis/algorithms. In Valle D, et al, editors: *The metabolic and molecular bases of inherited disease*. Available online at www.ommbid.com, see Chapter 66.

Saudubray J-M, Desguerre I, Sedel F, et al: Classification of inborn errors of metabolism. In Fernandes JM, Saudubray J-M, van den Berghe G, Walter JH, editors: *Inborn metabolic diseases: diagnosis and treatment*, Heidelberg, 2006, Springer-verlag, pp 1-47.

Valle D, et al, editors: *The metabolic and molecular bases of inherited disease*. Available online at www.ommbid.com.

INBORN ERRORS OF CARBOHYDRATE, AMMONIA, AMINO ACID, AND ORGANIC ACID METABOLISM

Stephen Cederbaum and Gerard T. Berry

The inborn errors of carbohydrate, ammonia, amino acid, and organic acid metabolism have one factor in common: all can be associated with acute, life-threatening disease during the newborn period. The most notable exception in this broad group of small-molecule disorders is phenylketonuria (PKU). There are often few signs secondary to classic PKU in the first 6 months of life, underscoring the importance of newborn screening in establishing the diagnosis of this disease. Although this chapter will present the most common phenotype for these disorders, special emphasis will be placed on the neonatal presentations. The fact that a number of the more mild forms can manifest later merely emphasizes the importance of newborn screening in their mitigation. The disorders that constitute each group are listed in Boxes 22-1 to 22-4. The interrelationships among the major metabolites, biochemical cycles, and organelle pathways in the most critical facets of intermediary metabolism are simplified and depicted in Figure 22-1. The primary lactic acidosis and mitochondrial respiratory chain disorders, as well as the defects in fatty acid oxidation, are included in the section on inborn errors of organic acid metabolism.

INBORN ERRORS OF CARBOHYDRATE METABOLISM

HEREDITARY GALACTOSEMIA

Galactose-1-Phosphate-Uridyltransferase Deficiency

The three enzymes of the galactose metabolic pathway that are responsible for the rapid conversion of galactose to glucose in the liver after ingestion of dietary lactose or the breakdown of endogenous galactose-containing compounds are galactokinase, galactose-1-phosphate uridyl transferase (GALT), and uridine diphosphate (UDP) galactose-4-epimerase (Figure 22-2). All three enzymes have been associated with inborn errors of galactose metabolism (Berry et al, 2006; Fridovich-Keil and Walter, 2008). Although a deficiency of any of the three enzymes can lead to galactose accumulation in plasma, the term *galactosemia* refers to GALT deficiency, the most common of the three enzyme deficiencies in the newborn period. The frequency of clinically significant galactosemia is estimated at 1 in 60,000 births in the United States, but would be higher if the more frequent partial deficiencies are considered. The clinical syndrome of transferase-deficiency galactosemia has changed since the advent of newborn screening. In instances of the rapid availability of newborn screening results (3 to 4 days of life) patients rarely require hospitalization. In the past, a severe multiorgan toxicity

syndrome was a much more common occurrence, associated with unlimited intake of lactose in the proprietary formula or breast milk. Because death from *Escherichia coli* sepsis can occur with only 1 to 2 weeks of exposure to galactose, the incidence of the disorder in the prescreening era was estimated to be less than 1 in 200,000 births. Today, even when picked up later after screening, the disorder is rarely fatal because the liver dysfunction is reversible and sepsis is largely prevented.

If patients survive the neonatal period and there is no diagnosis, the most common initial clinical signs of GALT deficiency is poor growth, irritability, lethargy, vomiting, and poor feeding. Jaundice may be present in the first few weeks of life and can persist. Initially the hyperbilirubinemia may be indirect and is only later associated with an elevation of the direct component as well. The current tendency to change formulas can mask the disease if a non–lactose-containing formula is substituted fortuitously. With continual lactose ingestion, multiorgan toxicity syndrome ensues, which is associated with liver disease that can progress to cirrhosis with portal hypertension, splenomegaly, ascites, renal tubular dysfunction, and sometimes full-blown renal Fanconi syndrome. Anemia, primarily caused by decreased red blood cell (RBC) survival, and lethargy; brain edema associated with a bulging fontanel

---

BOX 22-1   Inborn Errors of Carbohydrate Metabolism

- Hereditary galactosemia
- Glycogen storage diseases
- Hereditary fructose intolerance
- Fructose-1,6-bisphosphatase deficiency

BOX 22-2   Inborn Errors of Ammonia Metabolism

- Ornithine transcarbamylase deficiency
- Argininosuccinicaciduria
- Citrullinemia
- Carbamylphosphate synthetase deficiency
- Transient hyperammonemia of the newborn

BOX 22-3   Inborn Errors of Amino Acid Metabolism

- Maple syrup urine disease
- Hereditary tyrosinemia type 1
- Nonketotic hyperglycinemia
- Methionine synthetase deficiency
- Phenylketonuria

BOX 22-4   Inborn Errors of Organic Acid Metabolism

- Methylmalonic acidemia
- Propionic acidemia
- Isovaleric acidemia
- Multiple carboxylase deficiency
- Glutaric acidemia type 1
- Fatty acid oxidation disorders
  - Glutaric acidemia type 2
  - Very-long-chain acyl-CoA dehydrogenase deficiency
  - Medium-chain acyl-CoA dehydrogenase deficiency
  - Short-chain acyl-CoA dehydrogenase deficiency
  - Long-chain 3-hydroxy acyl-CoA dehydrogenase deficiency
  - Carnitine transporter defect
  - Carnitine palmitoyltransferase type I deficiency
  - Carnitine palmitoyltransferase type II deficiency
  - Acylcarnitine translocase deficiency
- Defects in ketone metabolism
  - Ketothiolase deficiency
  - Succinyl-CoA: 3-ketoacid-CoA transferase deficiency
  - 3-Hydroxy-3-methylglutaryl-CoA lyase deficiency
- Primary lactic acidoses
  - Pyruvate dehydrogenase complex deficiency
  - Pyruvate carboxylase deficiency
  - Phosphoenolpyruvate carboxykinase deficiency
  - Mitochondrial respiratory/electron transport chain defects
    - Barth syndrome
    - Pearson syndrome
    - Leigh disease

CoA, Coenzyme A.

can also occur. Cataracts may be evident in the first few weeks of life. However, some infants are born with congenital cataracts that are associated with abnormalities of the embryonal lens; they are central in nature and require slit-lamp examination for documentation.

After initiation of a lactose-free diet in the newborn period, the problems related to liver and kidney disease, anemia, and brain edema usually disappear, unless there has been severe organ damage such as hepatic cirrhosis. Most infants begin to grow and develop at a normal rate. However, patients treated prospectively can manifest long-term complications related to speech defects, delay in language acquisition, learning problems, frank mental retardation, autistic features, and hypergonadotropic hypogonadism in most of the females. The cause of these so-called diet-independent complications is unknown. Patients with galactosemia continue a lactose-restricted diet for their entire lives, although many lapse as they get older and may not suffer from detectable consequences. A minority of patients with GALT deficiency develop a neurodegenerative condition. One of the first abnormalities to be detected—albuminuria—reflects a poorly understood renal glomerular component. This component develops within 24 to 48 hours of ingestion of lactose and disappears as quickly after elimination of lactose from the diet. In addition to hyperbilirubinemia, there may be mild to severe elevations of serum alanine aminotransferase (ALT) and aspartate aminotransferase (AST) levels and various abnormalities related to renal tubular dysfunction, such as hyperchloremic metabolic acidosis, hypophosphatemia, glucosuria, and generalized aminoaciduria. Vitreous hemorrhages are newly recognized complications in the newborn period.

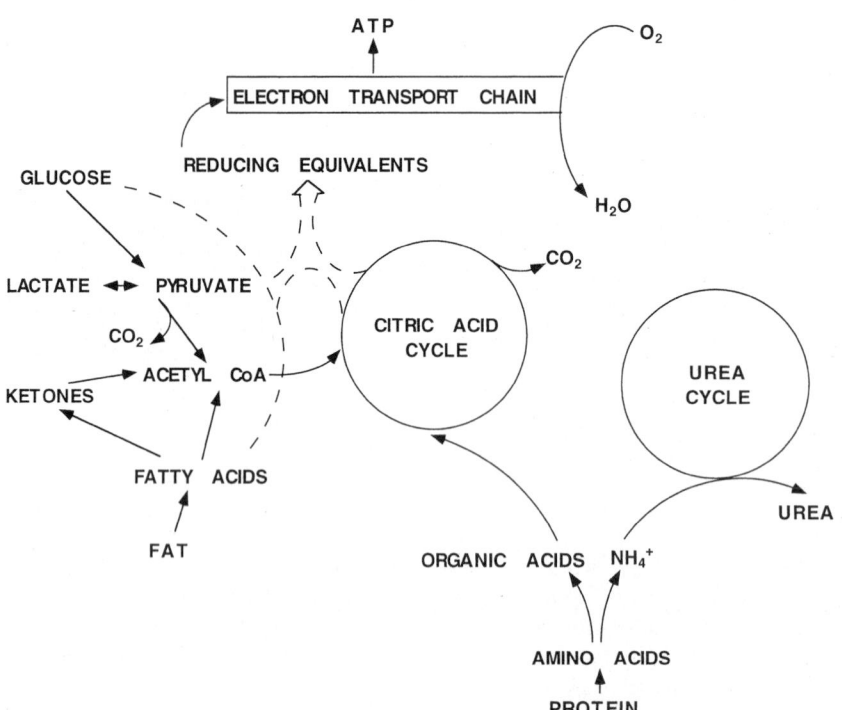

FIGURE 22-1   Intermediary metabolism interactions among the glycolytic, citric acid cycle, mitochondrial respiratory–electron transport chain, amino acid, organic acid, and urea cycle pathways. Defects in these primarily catabolic pathways are the chief source of inborn errors of metabolism that involve the small, simple—not the large—complex molecules. *ATP,* Adenosine triphosphate. (*Adapted from Cowett RM, editor:* Principles of perinatal-neonatal metabolism, *ed 2, New York, 1998, Springer-Verlag, p 800.*)

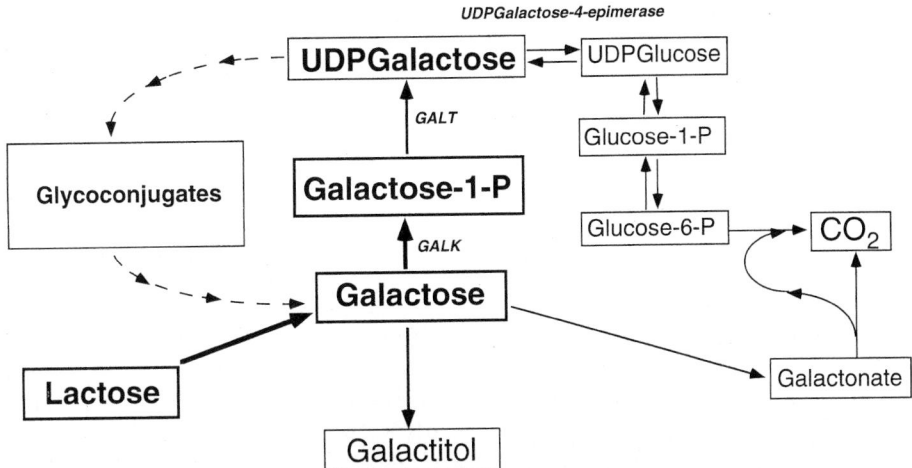

FIGURE 22-2 The important reactions in the galactose metabolic pathway are shown in relation to exogenous, via lactose primarily, and endogenous de novo synthesis of galactose. The reactions catalyzed by enzymes that have not been well delineated or are purported to exist are shown by *broken lines*. Carbon skeletons exit the galactose pool via galactokinase (GALK)–mediated conversion to galactose-1-phosphate (galactose-1-P), aldose reductase–mediated conversion to galactitol, and as galactonate. In patients with severe galactose-1-P-uridyltransferase (GALT) deficiency, there is little or no conversion of galactose-1-P to uridine diphosphate galactose (UDPgalactose). The epimerization of UDPglucose to UDPgalactose by UDPgalactose-4-epimerase, the utilization of UDPgalactose in the synthesis of glycoconjugates such as glycoproteins, and their subsequent degradation may constitute the pathways of de novo synthesis of galactose. *(Adapted from Berry GT, Nissim I, Gibson JB, et al: Quantitative assessment of whole body galactose metabolism in galactosemic patients,* Eur J Pediatr 156:S44, 1997.)

When an infant's condition is initially diagnosed, either through the newborn screening program or because of the recognition of clinical signs, blood galactose levels may be as high as 5 to 20 μmol/L, and the RBC galactose-1-phosphate level is significantly elevated, as are urine galactitol levels. During this phase of severe hypergalactosemia, positive reducing substances are present in the urine. After the patient starts a lactose-free diet, the RBC galactose-1-phosphate levels in patients with classic galactosemia fall, but they never return to the normal range, remaining mildly elevated for the lifetime of the patient.

As noted in the newborn screening chapter, a patient's condition can be ascertained by elevated plasma galactose levels, reduced levels of GALT, or both. Because newborn blood spots can be obtained before significant lactose ingestion occurs, screening by galactose in plasma alone is unsatisfactory. Many programs screen for GALT deficiency alone and sacrifice diagnosis of the far less frequent and less lethal kinase and epimerase deficiencies. Many modern screening follow-up programs eschew the measurement of RBC galactose-1-phosphate levels and instead confirm the enzymatic deficiency with a quantitative assay and perform mutation analysis. Mutation analysis can identify those with a poorer prognosis and those who are unlikely to exhibit clinical symptoms. The mutations also provide information for genetic counseling and prenatal diagnosis, with the latter also performed effectively by enzymatic means. A GALT variant labeled the *Duarte variant*, after its place of discovery, is far more frequent than the more severe mutations and gives approximately three fourths of the activity of the normal allele. Compound heterozygotes for this allele (*D2*) and a null allele (*G*) have approximately 25% of normal activity in red blood cells and are not associated with clinical symptoms.

GLYCOGEN STORAGE DISEASES

The glycogen storage diseases (GSDs) can be divided into those types that primarily affect the liver and those that affect striated muscle (Kishnani et al, 2001; Smit et al, 2006). With some forms, such as GSD type 3 or debrancher deficiency, both striated muscle and the liver may be affected. According to European prevalence data, the overall frequency of GSD is 1 in 20,000 to 25,000 (Kishnani et al, 2001). With the exceptions of GSD type 2 and or Pompe disease, a lysosomal defect, most of the patients with glycogenosis do not come to clinical attention in the newborn period. With the exception of a form of phosphorylase kinase deficiency, which is labeled as *type IX* and is inherited in a sex-linked recessive manner, all are inherited in an autosomal recessive manner. Patients with the three most common forms of GSD—types 1, 3, and 6—have a phenotype that mimics a small-molecule disorder, because glucose homeostasis is affected.

Glucose-6-Phosphatase Deficiency

GSD type 1 is caused by decreased activity of glucose-6-phosphatase, the enzyme that is perched at the terminus of both glycogenolysis and gluconeogenesis. Several different biochemical abnormalities can result in this phenotype, now classified as GSD types 1a, 1b, and 1c. The enzyme that resides on the anticytoplasmic side of internal membrane spaces of the hepatocyte catalyzes the hydrolysis of glucose-6-phosphate to glucose and phosphate. Impairments in the transport of either glucose-6-phosphate (type 1b–much less frequent than type 1a) or phosphate (type 1c–extremely rare) may cause decreased function of this enzyme. The frequency of GSD type 1 is estimated to be 1 in 100,000 births, with most cases being type 1a.

This condition infrequently manifests in the neonatal period, because "demand" feeding or feeding at short intervals prevent symptomatic hypoglycemia and hepatomegaly has usually not yet occurred. The major clinical findings are poor growth and enlarged abdominal girth as a result of hepatomegaly, and any of the signs that may be related to hypoglycemia. The major laboratory findings are fasting hypoglycemia, ketosis, lactic acidosis, hyperlipidemia (i.e., hypertriglyceridemia), and hyperuricemia. In patients with type 1b disease caused by a defect in the microsomal transporter of glucose-6-phosphate, there may be a history of recurrent infections because of neutropenia and defective neutrophil function and inflammatory bowel disease that may be present in the first year of life. Diagnosis used to be based on hepatic enzyme analyses, but molecular diagnostic testing is currently the first choice. The most important aspect of therapy is the prevention of brain damage from hypoglycemia and growth failure. The mainstay of therapy is frequent feedings and restriction of lactose and sucrose (Kishnani et al, 2001; Smit et al, 2006). The use of continuous nasogastric feedings or uncooked cornstarch, particularly during the night, has significantly improved the care of affected children, and although it does not correct all the biochemical perturbations, it does improve growth and can prevent hypoglycemic spells. Intercurrent illness with increased glucose utilization is particularly hazardous and a careful plan for emergencies is essential. The leukopenia of type 1b is helped by a regimen of granulocyte colony stimulating factor.

Lysosomal α-1,4-Glucosidase Deficiency

GSD type 2, or Pompe disease, is a deficiency of the lysosomal enzyme α-glucosidase. The clinical presentation of patients is most often in the newborn or early infancy period with symptoms of heart failure. The frequency is estimated at 1 in 100,000 births. There is usually marked cardiomegaly with massive biventricular cardiac wall thickening and a typical abnormal electrocardiogram, confirming biventricular hypertrophy and with a short PR interval. Decreased cardiac output can lead to heart failure and passive congestion. Infants may also have generalized hypotonia because of a skeletal myopathy. There is increased deposition of glycogen within the lysosomes of striated muscle. Except in the instance of passive congestion, the liver is not usually enlarged. Diagnosis is based on enzyme analysis in dried blood spots or leukocytes (Goldstein et al, 2009; Pompe Disease Diagnostic Working Group et al, 2008; Zhang et al, 2008). Cardiac transplantation has been performed to prevent death in infancy. Onset of symptoms as late as adulthood occurs when the mutations in one or both of the alleles cause less complete enzyme loss.

In the last several years enzyme replacement therapy for this disorder has been developed and has had a favorable effect on the outcome. More than half of the patients with infantile onset, for whom the disease had previously been fatal within the first year, can now be rescued with varying degrees of residual disability. Patients with adolescent and adult onset may do better depending on the speed with which the diagnosis was made, therapy initiated, and the degree of irreversible muscle damage that has occurred.

HEREDITARY FRUCTOSE INTOLERANCE

Fructose-1,6-Bisphosphate Aldolase B Deficiency

Hereditary fructose intolerance is a rare disorder caused by a deficiency of the enzyme fructose-1,6-bisphosphate aldolase in liver (Steinmann et al, 2001). The enzyme deficiency results in an impairment in the conversion of fructose-1-phosphate to glyceraldehyde and dihydroxyacetone phosphate and therefore in the effective metabolism of fructose. The disorder is inherited as an autosomal recessive trait. Symptoms are triggered by eating fructose or sucrose, which produces fructose. The signs begin when juices and fruit are added to the infant diet and are mitigated by the aversion that the infant develops to these foods and drinks. The major clinical findings are pallor, lethargy, poor feeding, vomiting, loose stools, poor growth, hepatomegaly, and any sign that could be related to hypoglycemia. The major laboratory findings consist of hypoglycemia; hypophosphatemia; elevations of serum ALT and AST, including any of the findings that may be associated with hepatocellular disease; and the presence of reducing substances in the urine. The liver disease may be severe. Patients may be jaundiced with hyperbilirubinemia. There may be bleeding diathesis. In addition to liver disease, renal tubular dysfunction can lead to the renal Fanconi syndrome. The intuition of the physician is crucial in establishing the diagnosis. Previously an intravenous fructose tolerance test was performed under controlled circumstances, to determine whether serum phosphate and glucose levels decrease and serum AST and ALT values rise after 15 to 30 minutes of fructose administration. In the past, confirmation depended on enzyme analysis, but molecular diagnostic testing is more widely available now and avoids both the risk of provocative testing and the laborious enzymatic analysis. The treatment consists of elimination of dietary fructose and sucrose. Many patients enter adulthood with excellent teeth and an aversion to foods containing sucrose or fructose.

FRUCTOSE-1,6-BISPHOSPHATASE DEFICIENCY

Deficiency of the enzyme fructose-1,6-bisphosphatase results in an inability to hydrolyze fructose-1,6-bisphosphate to fructose-6-phosphate (Steinmann et al, 2001). It is a rare disorder. This enzyme is indispensable in gluconeogenesis. The main clinical features are hypoglycemia and signs related to glucose deprivation in the central nervous system (CNS). The symptoms are due primarily to inadequate food intake and not fructose ingestion, although fructose may exacerbate the abnormalities induced by fasting adaptation. Enlargement of the liver because of diffuse steatosis may be present only during periods of fasting and enhanced gluconeogenesis. The laboratory findings consist of hypoglycemia, ketosis, and lactic acidosis. The acidosis caused by accumulation of lactic, 3-hydroxybutyric, and acetoacetic acids can be severe in this disease. Diagnosis depends on enzymatic or mutation analysis. The therapy consists primarily of avoidance of fasting and the need for gluconeogenesis.

Inborn Errors of Ammonia Metabolism

Inborn errors of the urea cycle, because they manifest in infancy, exemplify the small-molecule weight disorders in which symptoms occur episodically, are exacerbated by protein catabolism, and can be treated by the control of catabolic stimuli, dietary modification, and the enhanced removal of offending metabolites. Four disorders in particular cause the majority of cases that occur in the newborn period and in infancy; they are carbamyl phosphate synthetase I deficiency, ornithine transcarbamylase (OTC) deficiency, argininosuccinate (ASA) synthetase deficiency (citrullinemia), and ASA lyase deficiency (argininosuccinic acidemia). The other four genetic disorders of the urea cycle, *N*-acetylglutamate synthase deficiency, arginase deficiency, ornithine transporter deficiency, and citrin deficiency, are rare or do not manifest with neonatal hyperammonemia, or both. In aggregate, disorders of the urea cycle may be as frequent as 1 in 25,000 births or more. The entire cycle is outlined in Figure 22-3 and will be important in understanding the therapeutic modalities.

One round through the urea cycle condenses two molecules of toxic ammonia and one molecule of bicarbonate to form a molecule of urea that is nontoxic and is readily excreted in the urine. *N*-Acetylglutamate, the product of the first enzyme in the cycle, is an obligatory activator of carbamyl phosphate synthetase. These two reactions and OTC, which is responsible for citrulline synthesis, occur in the mitochondrion. The next three reactions occur in the cytoplasm after citrulline is transported out of the mitochondrion. The transport of ornithine back into the mitochondrion and the shuttling of aspartate to the cytoplasm are clearly imperative and account for the two other genes that cause urea cycle defects.

With the exception of arginase deficiency, each of these enzyme deficiencies has been associated with disease in the newborn period. Clinical presentation in the newborn period is similar for all these defects (Brusilow and Horwich, 1995; Leonard, 2006). Almost all the infants are well in the first 12 to 24 hours of life until they begin to feed poorly, vomit, hyperventilate, become irritable and lethargic, and become comatose, usually with seizures. When these diseases are not treated aggressively, they are almost always fatal. The treatment requires specific therapy to lower the waste nitrogen burden, including the toxic substance ammonia, and address the increased intracranial pressure. The severe encephalopathic and life-threatening features may be related in large part to brain edema. Chronic hepatomegaly has been reported in patients with argininosuccinic aciduria, whereas hepatomegaly is evident only during hyperammonemic episodes in the other urea cycle disorders. Acute hyperammonemia is associated with transaminase elevation and liver synthetic dysfunction, but these are rarely more than transient. Histologic examination of the liver shows modest fatty infiltration and fibrosis. Children with argininosuccinic aciduria can also manifest a specific abnormality of the hair known as *trichorrhexis nodosa*.

The main laboratory finding in the urea cycle defects (UCDs) is a plasma ammonium elevation. Plasma ammonium values may vary in different laboratories. In general, however, with automated chemistry testing for ammonia, the normal plasma values in older infants, children, and adults range between 10 and 35 µmol/L. However, the normal plasma ammonium value in newborns may occasionally be as high as 110 µmol/L but is usually somewhat lower. In patients with newborn-onset UCDs who are acutely ill, the plasma ammonium levels are often higher than 1000 or 2000 µmol/L. Patients with UCDs usually do not have metabolic acidosis unless they are in a terminal state with vascular collapse or respiratory failure. Instead, the characteristic acid-base abnormality associated with hyperammonemia is respiratory alkalosis caused by the effect of ammonia on the respiratory control centers in the brainstem.

The various UCDs can usually be distinguished on the basis of the pattern and levels of plasma amino acids. Because citrulline is the product of the carbamyl phosphate synthetase type 1 (CPS-I) and OTC reactions and the substrate for ASA synthetase, its value is critical. In newborn-onset *N*-acetylglutamate synthase (NAGS), CPS-I and OTC deficiencies, plasma citrulline concentrations may be undetectable and are always low. With OTC deficiency, there is increased urinary orotate excretion secondary to carbamyl phosphate accumulation and pyrimidine synthesis. With NAGS or CPS-I deficiency, carbamyl phosphate production is decreased or absent, and orotate excretion is decreased. In citrullinemia, the eponymous amino acid citrulline has markedly elevated concentrations. With argininosuccinic aciduria, plasma citrulline concentration is moderately elevated, in the range of 100 to 300 µmol/L, and can be readily detected during a study of plasma by amino acid analysis.

Because the ability of infants with these disorders to excrete waste nitrogen as urea is impaired, therapy is initially focused on the reduction of nitrogen intake by decreasing dietary protein and providing essential amino acids or the ketoacid analogues. This approach theoretically permits adequate growth without an excessive nitrogen load. Excessive protein leads to hyperammonemia, but too much restriction of protein during long-term therapy leads to poor growth and can provoke catabolism to maintain essential amino acid levels. Actually this approach fails when the patient is in a catabolic state and in negative nitrogen balance, as occurs in the catastrophically ill infant presenting in the first week of life with massive hyperammonemia. For such an infant with hyperammonemia and coma, the mainstay of therapy is dialysis treatment. Hemodialysis (or extracorporeal membrane oxygenation) is the most effective way of reducing plasma ammonium levels, because it affords the greatest clearance of ammonia (Rutledge et al, 1990). Continuous arteriovenous hemofiltration (CAVH) provides a lower clearance rate, but has the added benefit of continuous use and a lesser likelihood of major swings in intravascular volume that can exacerbate an already fragile state and cerebral edema. Ammonia clearance with peritoneal dialysis is only approximately one tenth that of CAVH and is not recommended for specific UCD therapy in the newborn period. Ammonia is not cleared effectively by exchange transfusion.

While the intensive care personnel are waiting for dialysis to be started, alternative waste nitrogen therapy using intravenous sodium benzoate, sodium phenylacetate (together as Ammonul), and, for patients with

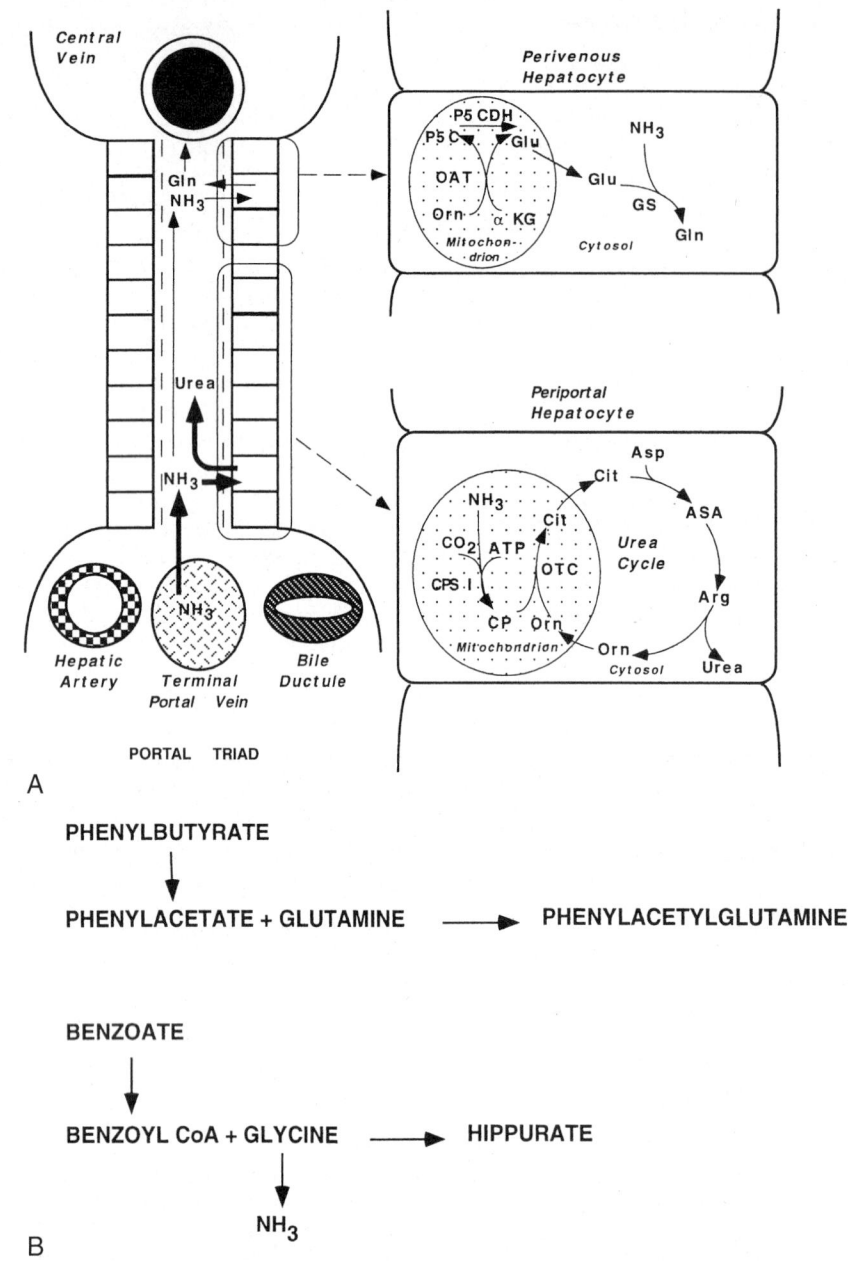

FIGURE 22-3 A, Depicted is the nonhomogeneous distribution of enzymes involved in ammonia metabolism in hepatocytes of an acinar sinusoid as they are linearly distributed from the portal triad to the region of the central vein or terminal hepatic venule. The specific enzymatic reactions are shown for an individual periportal and perivenous hepatocyte. The glutamine synthetase (GS) and ornithine aminotransferase (OAT) enzyme activities are expressed exclusively in the one- to three-cell layers surrounding the central vein—that is, the region of zone 3 of the liver lobule—whereas the urea cycle enzymes are concentrated within the periportal hepatocytes. However, the urea cycle enzyme activities are higher in zone 1 immediately surrounding the portal triad than in the middle zone 2. The hepatocytes are shown as *squares,* the hepatic mitochondria as *shaded circles,* and the lining of the space of Disse as the *broken lines* on either side of the linear array of hepatocytes. *Arg,* Arginine; *ASA,* argininosuccinate; *Asp,* aspartate; *ATP,* adenosine triphosphate; *Cit,* citrulline; *CP,* carbamylphosphate; *CPS-I,* carbamylphosphate synthetase type 1; *Gln,* glutamine; *Glu,* glutamate; α-KG, α-ketoglutarate; NH_3, ammonia; CO_2, CO_2 or bicarbonate; *Orn,* ornithine; *P5C,* pyrroline 5-carboxylate; *P5CDH,* pyrroline-5-carboxylate dehydrogenase. **B,** The medications sodium phenylacetate and phenylbutyrate and sodium benzoate promote alternative waste nitrogen disposal by participating in these two mitochondrial reactions. *(Adapted from Tuchman M, et al: Hepatic glutamine synthetase deficiency in fatal hyperammonemia after lung transplantation,* Ann Intern Med *127:447, 1997.)*

ASA synthetase and ASA lyase deficiencies especially, arginine hydrochloride should be given (Brusilow, 1991; Brusilow and Batshaw, 1979; Brusilow et al, 1979). The medications and the proper dose for a bolus and 24-hour sustaining infusions of Ammonul are available from Ucyclyd Pharma (Scottsdale, Arizona). This product is rarely stocked except in pharmacies of tertiary care metabolic centers. Arginine hydrochloride is thought to be helpful in NAGS, CPS-I, and OTC deficiencies and is given at a continuous dose of 250 mg/kg per 24 hours. A dose of 600 mg/kg/day is recommended for ASA lyase particularly and for citrullinemia. Arginine supplementation the body arginine pool, and in citrullinemia and argininosuccinic acidemia it increases ornithine to promote synthesis of citrulline and ASA. ASA contains both waste nitrogen atoms destined for excretion as urea and has a renal clearance rate equal to the glomerular filtration rate, provided that it is continuously synthesized and excreted. Accordingly, ASA should serve as an effective substitute for urea as a waste nitrogen product. The excretion of citrulline, which contains only one molecule of ammonia, also exceeds that of ammonia, although it does not appear to be eliminated as efficiently as ASA.

Sodium benzoate promotes ammonia excretion when it is conjugated with glycine to form hippurate, which is cleared by the kidney at fivefold the glomerular filtration rate (see Figure 22-3). Theoretically, 1 mole of waste nitrogen is synthesized and excreted as hippurate for each mole of benzoate administered. The hippurate synthetic mechanism resides primarily in the hepatic mitochondria and depends on an intact mitochondrial energy system for adenosine triphosphate (ATP) synthesis. The glycine consumed in this reaction can be replaced by either serine or the glycine cleavage pathway. Sodium phenylacetate, as well as sodium phenylbutyrate, which is used for long-term therapy in the absence of sodium benzoate, conjugates with glutamine to form phenylacetylglutamine, which is excreted by the kidney (see Figure 22-3). Sodium phenylbutyrate is converted to phenylacetate in the liver. Glutamine contains two nitrogen atoms, whereas glycine contains one. Two moles of waste nitrogen are removed for each mole of phenylacetate administered. This acetylation reaction occurs in the kidney and the liver.

The outcome for patients with severe newborn-onset CPS-I and OTC deficiencies is poor. Sometimes dialysis therapy cannot rescue severely affected boys with X-linked OTC deficiency in the first few days of life (Enns et al, 2008). Prospectively administered alternative pathway therapy in conjunction with high-calorie fluids usually prevents death and severe hyperammonemia in patients known from family studies or prenatal diagnosis to be at risk. This therapy is done best in collaboration with an expert in the treatment of urea cycle disorders. Even after institution of successful therapy, the morbidity and mortality rates are high in these severely affected patients and mental retardation is common in survivors (Brusilow and Horwich, 1995). There is a significant correlation between the duration of newborn hyperammonemic coma and the developmental quotient score at 12 months of age (Msall et al, 1984). Four of five reported children in whom duration of coma was 2 days or less had normal intelligence quotient scores, whereas all seven children in whom coma lasted 5 days or longer were severely mentally retarded. Currently liver transplantation is recommended for patients with CPS-I and OTC deficiencies in the newborn period. The patient should have almost no residual enzyme activity and grow to a sufficient size for the treatment to be feasible and safe. Early diagnosis and treatment is important because of the devastating effects of prolonged newborn hyperammonemic coma.

Mutational analysis of DNA is available for all of these disorders at www.genetests.org. If the lesion in a particular family is known, prenatal diagnosis by means of direct DNA analysis is also feasible. With the exception of OTC deficiency, all the UCDs are inherited as autosomal recessive traits.

TRANSIENT HYPERAMMONEMIA OF THE NEWBORN

Transient hyperammonemia of the newborn is a distinct clinical syndrome that was first identified by Ballard et al (1978). The disease usually develops in premature infants during the course of treatment for respiratory distress syndrome. The plasma ammonium level may be enormously elevated, as high as that found in any of the patients with the most severe type of UCD. Its onset is usually in the first 24 hours after birth, when the infant is undergoing mechanical ventilatory support. Affected babies can manifest all the signs associated with hyperammonemic coma. The diagnosis may not be obvious, however, because many of these same infants are receiving sedatives and muscle relaxants to optimize therapy of their life-threatening pulmonary disease and an ammonia level is not determined. Important clues are the absence of deep tendon reflexes, the absence of normal newborn reflexes, and a decrease or absence of response to painful stimuli. As with hyperammonemic coma in UCD, this medical emergency requires dialysis therapy.

The cause of this disease is unknown. The plasma amino acid levels are similar to those found in CPS-I or OTC deficiency. Investigators have hypothesized that the disorder may be caused by impairment of hepatic mitochondrial energy production or shunting of portal blood away from the liver, such as in patent ductus venosus. The mortality rate in transient hyperammonemia of the newborn is high. A patient who can be treated early and aggressively may survive the episode. There is no evidence that any of the survivors have suffered any further episodes of hyperammonemia, nor has there been any further evidence of impaired ammonia metabolism.

INBORN ERRORS OF AMINO ACID METABOLISM

MAPLE SYRUP URINE DISEASE

Branched-Chain 2-Keto Dehydrogenase Complex Deficiency

Maple syrup urine disease (MSUD) is a rare inborn error of amino acid metabolism (Chuang et al, 2001; Wendel and de Baulny, 2006). It is inherited as an autosomal recessive trait and is caused by a deficiency of the enzyme branched-chain 2-keto dehydrogenase (BCKAD) complex. This enzyme catalyzes the conversion of each of the 3-ketoacid derivatives of the branched-chain amino acids (BCAAs)—leucine, isoleucine, and valine—into their decarboxylated coenzyme metabolites within the mitochondria (Figure 22-4). The disease occurs in 1 in 200,000 newborn infants around the world, but in the Mennonite communities of the United States, the frequency is 1 in 358 because of a founder effect for a point mutation in the $E_1\alpha$ gene. The most common presentation of the disorder occurs in the newborn period. Other forms with later onset caused by less complete enzyme deficiencies occur, but they are not the subject of this chapter. The newborn

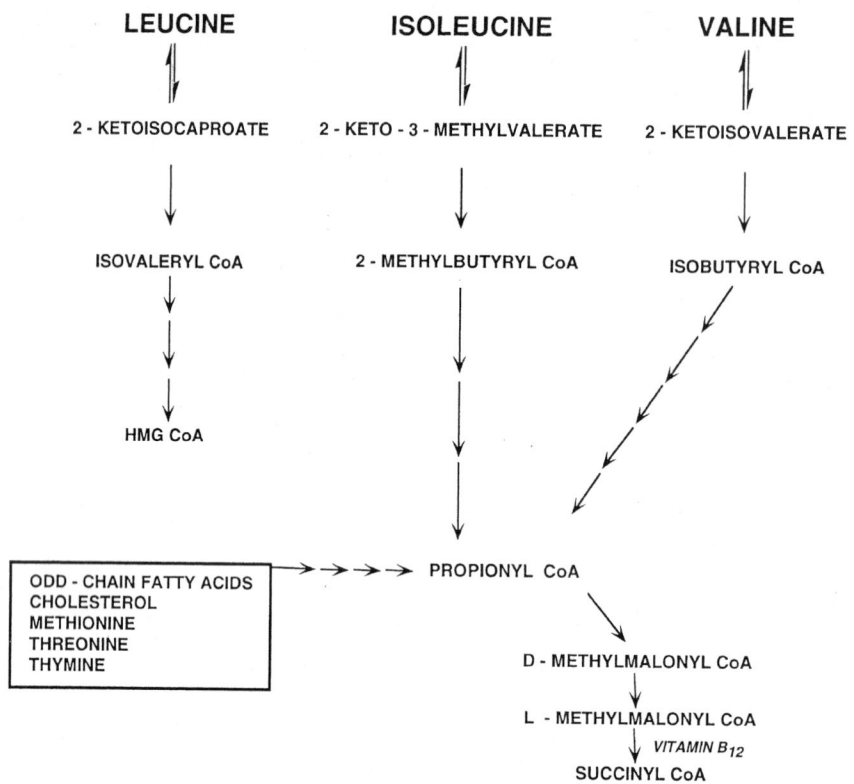

FIGURE 22-4 The branched-chain amino acids leucine, isoleucine, and valine are reversibly transaminated to their corresponding 2-keto analogues, which are substrates for the single decarboxylase (branched-chain 2-keto dehydrogenase) enzyme deficient in maple syrup urine disease. Reduced activity of isovaleryl coenzyme A (CoA) dehydrogenase, the next enzyme in the leucine degradative pathway, is the cause of isovaleric acidemia. The immediate precursor of ketones, 3-hydroxy-3-methylglutaryl CoA (HMG-CoA), is the final product of the leucine catabolic pathway. However, its production more strongly depends on the oxidation of fatty acids as in ketogenesis and in cholesterol biosynthesis. Propionyl CoA, which accumulates in both propionic and methylmalonic acidemia, can be synthesized from isoleucine, valine, odd-chain fatty acids, cholesterol, methionine, threonine, and thymine. The adenosyl form of vitamin B_{12} is the important cofactor in the L-methylmalonyl CoA mutase–catalyzed conversion of l-methylmalonyl-CoA to the citric acid cycle intermediate, succinyl CoA.

presentation is associated with a severe and catastrophic illness and usually results in death without specific medical intervention. Typically the infants are well at birth; only after 2 or 3 days of ingestion of breast milk or formula do they begin to manifest poor feeding and regurgitation. Lethargy becomes evident; the cry may be shrill and high pitched. There may be hypotonia alternating with hypertonia and opisthotonic posturing. The odor of maple syrup may be detected in saliva, on the breath, in urine and feces, and in cerumen obtained from the ear. The babies become more and more obtunded and eventually lapse into a deep coma. The anterior fontanel may be bulging. Seizures may develop. The life-threatening encephalopathic features may simply be related to brain edema (Chuang et al, 2001).

The clinical biochemical laboratory hallmark is metabolic acidosis. The anion gap may be raised, but not necessarily. There is almost always ketonuria. The plasma ammonium values are usually normal. The complete blood count is usually normal. The levels of the plasma BCAAs leucine, isoleucine, and valine are elevated, with striking elevation in leucine, the probable toxic metabolite. The normal ranges for plasma leucine, isoleucine, and valine in the newborn period are 29 to 152 μmol/L, 11 to 87 μmol/L, and 71 to 236 μmol/L, respectively. In patients who are critically ill, the leucine levels may range between 1900 and 6900 μmol/L. In the past, almost every newborn infant who was recognized to have MSUD and

was severely ill was treated with peritoneal dialysis in a tertiary care center. The treatment was clinically successful in most instances, but it did not allow for as rapid a rate of reduction in plasma BCAA levels as did hemodialysis or CAVH (Rutledge et al, 1990).

It is now clear that a nutritional approach works as well as peritoneal dialysis in newborns with MSUD (Berry et al, 1991; Chuang et al, 2001; Morton et al, 2002; Parini et al, 1993; Wendel and de Baulny, 2006). It is best performed with the use of a BCAA-free modified parenteral nutrition solution for infants and older children with acute metabolic decompensation, but this is rarely available in any center that does not have a larger Mennonite population. Protein-free intravenous alimentation augmented with a low-volume, enteral solution of the 17 nonbranched chain amino acids for 24 to 48 hours is satisfactory. An insulin drip may also be necessary to curtail the effects of the catabolic stimulus (Berry et al, 1991; Wendel et al, 1982). On the basis of the rate of plasma leucine decline, the staff at Children's Hospital of Philadelphia have found that this nutritional therapy is comparable to peritoneal dialysis when plasma leucine levels are as high as 1908 to 3053 μmol/L. However, CAVH or hemodialysis may achieve more rapid normalization of the plasma BCAAs and their corresponding branched-chain ketoacids when the levels of leucine are in the range of 4580 to 6870 μmol/L. Newborn infants with an odor of maple syrup, a metabolic acidosis, and ketonuria require immediate metabolic consultation assistance and a confirmatory plasma amino acid quantitation. This is truly a medical emergency with a high risk of death and permanent brain damage. Most patients who are successfully treated by 7 days of age do not have mental retardation. Patients whose diagnosis and therapy are delayed—and perhaps even in those whose disorder is diagnosed in the first week of life, but who have suffered such severe damage because of increased intracranial pressure—often have substantial decreases in developmental or intelligence quotient, as well as signs compatible with spastic diplegia or quadriplegia.

Expanded newborn screening is going to lead to a changed picture for this disorder. In jurisdictions in which the turnaround time for the program are as fast as 3 to 4 days of life, the patient will likely be less ill and the diagnosis will be known. The outcome will be better because less risk of permanent damage will have occured.

The mainstay of long-term therapy for patients with MSUD who survive the newborn period is a special formula devoid of the BCAAs. The amount of BCAAs necessary to sustain growth but maintain plasma leucine, isoleucine, and valine levels in the normal range is supplied with a regular proprietary formula in limited amounts. In the first week of life, this amount is approximately 100 mg of leucine per kilogram of body weight daily and 50 mg/kg daily of both isoleucine and valine. The BCAA requirements, and thus the rates of utilization of the BCAAs for protein accretion, drop rapidly in the first year of life in conjunction with the decline in growth velocity in young infants. As with PKU, it is imperative that the administration of the special amino acid formula be carefully monitored by means of frequent plasma amino acid quantitations. One of the most common errors made in the treatment of MSUD is the failure to administer adequate amounts of supplemental isoleucine and valine solutions to maintain normal plasma levels, because proprietary formulas alone do not always meet the needs of each growing baby (i.e., adequate amounts of each BCAA are not supplied by a formula alone). Deficiency of BCAAs can result in a severe exfoliative rash and anemia. The rash may mimic that of severe acrodermatitis enteropathica (Giacoia and Berry, 1993).

As with many of the inborn errors of amino acid, organic acid, and ammonia metabolism, protein administration in the infant whose disease is controlled and who is in metabolic balance with diet therapy must be discontinued during periods of intercurrent infections because catabolism, possibly driven by counterregulatory hormones or cytokines, triggers metabolic decompensation through the release of branched-chain ketoacid from skeletal muscle. Metabolic decompensation is further exacerbated by poor nutritional intake. It is imperative that during these times, adequate calories and fluids be given to prevent the crisis from escalating into a medical emergency.

In selected instances, a molecular diagnosis of MSUD may be undertaken; this diagnosis is especially useful in targeted populations such as the Mennonites. Rarely patients may have a defect in the enzyme 2(E_2) component (Danner et al, 1985) or, as discussed in the Primary Lactic Acidosis section, in the enzyme 3(E_3) component. The rare patient with MSUD may respond favorably to high-dose thiamine therapy with a reduction in BCAAs and a lower need for protein restriction.

HEREDITARY TYROSINEMIA TYPE 1 OR HEPATORENAL TYROSINEMIA

Fumarylacetoacetate Hydrolase Deficiency

Tyrosinemia type 1 is caused by a deficiency of the enzyme fumarylacetoacetate hydrolase (Tanguay et al, 1995). This enzymatic reaction is distal in the phenylalanine and tyrosine pathway, and the disorder is actually an inborn error of organic acid metabolism, with hypertyrosinemia being a secondary and variable biochemical effect. Tyrosinemia type 1 is a rare disease inherited in an autosomal recessive manner. The highest incidence is found in those of French-Canadian ancestry as a result of a founder effect (De Bracketeer and Larochelle, 1990).

The phenotype is variable. At one extreme, the patient is in early infancy and has severe, usually fatal disease in which liver disease dominates the clinical picture. At the other end of the spectrum is a more chronic phenotype, and patients exhibit hypophosphatemic rickets related to renal Fanconi syndrome. These patients usually also have evidence of liver disease, although milder. Most of the patients with severe liver disease phenotype do not come to clinical attention in the newborn period. Careful search, however, may reveal laboratory findings compatible with this disease, even in newborn infants. In the phenotype seen in early infancy, the clinical findings are hepatomegaly, a bleeding diathesis, and jaundice. Ascites is not uncommon. The laboratory findings consist of abnormal liver function and dysfunction tests with increases in serum AST, ALT, and direct and indirect bilirubin; prolongations of PT and PTT; and findings related to renal Fanconi syndrome, such as glycosuria, hypophosphatemia, hypouricemia, proteinuria caused by β_2-microglobulin hyperexcretion, and generalized amino aciduria and organic aciduria.

More specific laboratory abnormalities consist of an abnormally high serum alpha-fetoprotein level. There may be an elevation of plasma tyrosine; however, the hypertyrosinemia and a more prominent hypermethioninemia are caused by a secondary impairment in liver function. The most important metabolites are those related to the substrate, fumarylacetylacetic acid, the handling of which is defective. Increased levels of the diagnostic metabolite succinylacetone can be detected on urine organic acid quantitation by gas chromatography–mass spectrometry (GC-MS) in most instances and even more sensitively by an isotope dilution method, and in RBCs by the δ-aminolevulinic acid dehydratase inhibition assay. As in all metabolic disorders, the metabolite abnormalities may not be present or detectable at all times.

Newborn screening methods are likely to alter the phenotype of this disorder. Increasingly, analysis of blood spot succinylacetone is being added to the expanded newborn screening panels and will likely lead to preemptive diagnosis and treatment in the majority of cases. The false-negative rate for this analysis is not known at this time. Newborn screening by older methods has been performed in Quebec for many years.

In the past, most of the infants with the hepatic form of tyrosinemia type 1 died in early to late infancy. However, a medical therapy has been developed that uses the agent 2-(2-nitro-4-trifluoromethylbenzoyl)-1,3-cyclohexanedione

(NTBC), which inhibits *p*-hydroxyphenylpyruvate dioxygenase (Lindstedt et al, 1992), thus blocking the conversion of *p*-hydroxyphenylpyruvate, the transamination product of tyrosine, to fumarylacetoacetate and thereby retarding the synthesis and accumulation of succinyl acetate and succinyl acetone. This therapy has been used successfully to improve liver and renal function as well as to normalize or improve the various laboratory abnormalities. It is unclear, however, whether NTBC therapy will eliminate the need for liver transplantation, which has been the mainstay of long-term therapy until recently.

One of the most devastating complications for older infants with tyrosinemia type 1 who have been stabilized clinically and biochemically is the development of hepatocellular carcinoma. This development is prevalent in tyrosinemia treated with diet, and most patients who survive infancy or who have a chronic phenotype succumb to liver cancer. It is recommended that NTBC therapy be started in infants who are acutely ill while they are waiting for a liver transplantation, which may be deferred until the third year of life, while monitoring the liver for development of a hepatoma. Early treatment with NTBC surely retards the development of tumors, but patients receiving therapy develop hepatomas and preemptive transplantation, although at a later age. Liver transplantation is still a highly prevalent therapy. Most liver transplantations have been successful, and the patients have done well with immunosuppressive therapy with only minimal persistent evidence of renal tubular dysfunction while eating a normal diet.

Hepatorenal tyrosinemia has no direct effect on the nervous system, and most patients are free of neurologic findings and mental retardation. Because succinylacetone can inhibit delta-amino levulinic acid dehydratase, the enzyme deficient in a rare type of acute intermittent porphyria, porphyria symptoms have frequently occurred in the pre-NTBC era and have proved fatal in some instances.

Hepatorenal tyrosinemia is not to be confused with transient tyrosinemia of the newborn, which is prevalent in premature infants and is probably the most common disturbance of amino acid metabolism in man; it is secondary to a delayed maturation of *p*-hydroxyphenylpyruvate dioxygenase activity (Levine et al, 1939; Tanguay et al, 1995) or with the hypertyrosinemia secondary to liver disease. Current screening methods are unlikely to detect this condition that was found frequently in the past.

NONKETOTIC HYPERGLYCINEMIA

Glycine Cleavage Complex Deficiency

Nonketotic hyperglycinemia is a rare defect of glycine metabolism (Dulac and Rolland, 2006; Hamosh and Johnston, 1995.) and is inherited as an autosomal recessive trait. The disorder is caused by deficient activity of the glycine cleavage enzyme complex (GCC), which consists of the products of four genes. Its frequency is fewer than 1 in 200,000 newborn infants. Although several variant forms exist, most infants who come to clinical attention in the newborn period—presumably most patients with this disease—have a severe, catastrophic illness that mimics the most acute forms of ammonia, amino acids, or organic acid

metabolism. The infants may be healthy at birth but begin to show severe hypotonia and seizures after 12 to 36 hours. They quickly become comatose, and there is a loss of all the newborn and deep tendon reflexes.

The clinical findings are predominantly those of an acute encephalopathy. The electroencephalogram (EEG) usually shows a characteristic pattern of spike and slow waves. The babies may have hiccups from diaphragmatic spasms. The main laboratory finding is an elevation of plasma glycine and a proportionally higher elevation of glycine in the cerebrospinal fluid (CSF). Unfortunately, plasma glycine levels may be normal in the newborn period. The urine glycine is usually also elevated. The most common diagnostic criterion is the raised CSF–plasma glycine ratio. Values greater than 0.08 are considered to be diagnostic, whereas those between 0.04 and 0.08 are highly suspicious of the diagnosis. The amino acid serine, which is also a product of the defective enzyme reaction, is depressed in plasma, and there is a corresponding increase in the glycine-to-serine ratio in body fluids. Prenatal CNS lesions have been reported (Dobyns, 1989).

The pathophysiology of this brain disease is not well understood; it is believed that glycine, an active neurotransmitter, may interfere with the activity of specific chloride channels, thus perturbing the membrane potential and depolarization of neurons. There also appears to be an impairment in alpha-motor neuron outflow tract activity, producing a clinical state that mimics Werdnig-Hoffmann disease. No acidosis or ketosis is seen in this disease—thus the name, *nonketotic hyperglycinemia*. Many of the disorders of organic acid metabolism, such as methylmalonic acidemia and propionic acidemia, are also associated with elevations of plasma glycine, presumably because of a secondary impairment in the GCC, and have been referred to in the past as the *ketotic hyperglycinemia syndromes*.

Although many therapies have been tried in this disease—such as protein restriction, benzoate to trap glycine as the byproduct hippurate, strychnine to affect the lower motor neuron function, and dextromethorphan to block *N*-methyl-D-aspartate receptors—there is no generally effective treatment. The seizures are variably controlled and life may be prolonged, but no meaningful improvement occurs in most instances. Many affected babies die in the newborn period despite medical support with assisted ventilation, and most others die within 2 to 4 years. A transient form of nonketotic hyperglycinemia has also been reported in newborns (Luder et al, 1989; Schiffmann et al, 1989). Valproate may result in hyperglycinemia because of secondary inhibition of the GCC, as is postulated to explain secondary hyperglycinemia in disorders of organic acid metabolism, such as propionic acidemia. Milder forms exist and milder symptoms appear at a later age. This disorder cannot be diagnosed by newborn screening.

METHIONINE SYNTHETASE DEFICIENCY, OTHER DISORDERS OF HOMOCYSTEINE REMETHYLATION AND CYSTATHIONINE SYNTHASE DEFICIENCY

In humans, the essential amino acid methionine is converted to homocysteine, and in the process a methyl group is transferred to an acceptor molecule from

S-adenosylmethionine that serves as a donor for methyl groups in many different reactions (see Figure 22-5) (Mudd et al, 1995). Subsequently the homocysteine may either be completely metabolized through the cysteine pathway to sulfate or it may be remethylated back to methionine to maintain the critical levels of methionine. Defective methionine remethylation or a deficiency in methionine synthetase leads to a form of homocystinemia (the name *homocystinuria* is anachronistic and does not reflect the current reality of ascertainment or testing as well as does *homocystinemia*). Patients with classic homocystinemia, caused by a deficiency of the cystathionine beta-synthase enzyme, rarely manifest signs in early infancy (Mudd et al, 1995). In contrast, patients with methionine synthetase deficiency or methionine remethylation defect may come to clinical attention in the newborn period (Rosenblatt and Fenton, 2001). The patients may have either an abnormality in vitamin B_{12} metabolism, which can also produce methylmalonic acidemia and homocystinuria, or an isolated defect in folate metabolism or the methionine synthetase enzyme (Rosenblatt and Fenton, 2001). In this reaction the methyl group from 5-methyltetrahydrofolate, which is derived from 5,10-methylene tetrahydrofolate, is transferred to methylcobalamin and subsequently to homocysteine.

The clinical findings associated with the methionine synthetase deficiencies are poor growth and development. There may be severe cortical atrophy and possible brain lesions caused by thromboses of the arteries or veins, as in classic homocystinuria. Infrequently they can manifest as an acute intoxicating disorder in the newborn period. The laboratory findings consist of an elevation in plasma homocysteine values and a normal or decreased methionine value. Often the homocysteine values are not as elevated as in classic cystathionine β-synthetase deficiency. If there is a defect in folate or vitamin B_{12} metabolism that produces secondary impairment in methionine synthetase activity, there may also be megaloblastic anemia.

Some patients with a defect in cobalamin metabolism respond to treatment with high doses of intramuscular hydroxycobalamin. The treatment of methionine synthesis deficiency is a normal protein intake or methionine supplementation to restore methionine levels in plasma to normal and to restore CNS pools of methionine, which may be critical in one-carbon transfer reactions. It is also possible to retard homocysteine accumulation and restore methionine levels by administering betaine, which can enhance remethylation of homocysteine to methionine through the alternate betaine methyltransferase pathway. Some investigators have also used pharmacologic doses of cobalamin, folate, and pyridoxine to stimulate flux through either the methionine synthetase or the classic homocysteine pathway. Unfortunately, if infants with this type of disorder are not treated early, there is usually a permanent and devastating effect on cognitive and motor function. Milder and occasionally asymptomatic forms are known.

Classic homocystinemia caused by cystathionine synthase deficiency can be ascertained by expanded newborn screening in a minority of cases. The elevated methionine that is the critical detected metabolite may require several days to become apparent; that is unfortunate because cystathionine synthetase deficiency is a treatable disorder.

Expanded newborn screening has altered the landscape for several B_{12} processing defects. Ascertainment of elevated methylmalonic acid with the C3 acylcarnitine, the C4 dicarboxylacyl carnitine, or both usually allows for earlier diagnosis and treatment, with apparent mitigation of long-term effects. These disorders are more common than classical homocystinemia, the latter having a frequency in most populations of 1 in 200,000 births or less.

PHENYLKETONURIA

Phenylalanine Hydroxylase Deficiency

PKU is the most common inborn error of amino acid metabolism that can result in mental retardation (Scriver et al, 2001; Walter et al, 2006). Its frequency is between 1 in 10,000 to 1 in 25,000 births, depending on where in the United States it is studied. There are areas of the world such as Ireland, Turkey, and Iran in which it is more frequent, and others such as Finland, Japan, and among Ashkenazi Jews in which it is less prevalent. PKU is caused by a defect in the activity of the enzyme phenylalanine hydroxylase, which converts phenylalanine to tyrosine, a reaction that resides primarily in the liver. Thus in PKU it is the deficiency of this liver enzyme that results in brain disease. Because of the paucity of findings in the newborn period or early infancy, PKU usually was not diagnosed until late infancy or later until newborn screening was instituted. It is important for physicians caring for newborns to be aware of the pitfalls of screening, which are summarized in Chapter 27. This disease, inherited as an autosomal recessive trait, exemplifies the interaction of a gene and the manipulatable environment (i.e., diet) in the expression of a disease (Scriver et al, 2001).

After birth, the baby with PKU who is undergoing normal postnatal catabolism, or ingesting adequate amounts of breast milk or a proprietary formula, will experience a gradual and persistent increase in plasma phenylalanine levels. The cutoff value for newborn screening differs by jurisdiction, but both phenylalanine value and the phenylalanine:tyrosine ratio are considered when calling a presumptive positive. The diagnosis is rarely missed if testing occurs after 24 hours of age. By 5 to 7 days of age in the untreated patient, the eponymous phenylketone is found in urine, and another side product of phenylalanine accumulation, phenylacetic acid, may impart the characteristic "mousey" odor to urine and the patient. This odor may be detected when levels of phenylalanine exceed 600 to 900 μmol/L, but it is not detected in every patient. With modern newborn screening programs, the neonatologist will rarely see a case of PKU in the hospital and will usually be dealing with a patient who has a preemptive diagnosis and is treated as an outpatient. Greater detail about the disorder can be obtained in Scriver et al (2001), but a synopsis will be given here.

In the first 6 months of life, the affected babies may have difficulty with feeding and vomiting. In some instances, persistent vomiting has been associated with the diagnosis of pyloric stenosis, for which corrective surgery has been performed, perhaps inappropriately. Developmental delay is usually evident in the second 6 months of life. Patients may have seizures, sometimes infantile spasms in early infancy associated with a hypsarrhythmic EEG pattern. Persistent elevation of plasma phenylalanine levels greater than 600 μmol/L may be sufficient to result in mental retardation.

The mechanism of brain disease in PKU is still unknown. It may be related to the effect of high phenylalanine levels on the transport of amino acids across the blood-brain barrier and then into brain neurons or glial elements. The plasma levels of tyrosine may be decreased, especially in patients who are not receiving tyrosine supplementation in the special amino acid powder used as a daily nutrient. Investigators have speculated for many years that hypotyrosinemia has a role in the CNS deficits, because tyrosine (only a liver enzyme) cannot be synthesized within the CNS by phenylalanine hydroxylase (a liver enzyme). Older infants often exhibit long tract findings, such as spastic quadriparesis and spastic quadriplegia. The untreated infant demonstrates microcephaly acquired postnatally and may also have severe behavioral problems in addition to a diagnosis of autism. Typical findings consist of elevated serum plasma phenylalanine levels, normal or subnormal plasma tyrosine levels, and increased urinary excretion of phenylpyruvic acid, phenyllactic acid, and phenylacetic acid (rarely measured routinely, but easily seen if urine organic acids are studied).

The mainstay of therapy is a low-protein diet and the use of a special amino acid–containing formula that does not include phenylalanine. The patient must receive an adequate amount of phenylalanine from protein in proprietary formulas and later from table foods, which is tracked by means of a phenylalanine exchange system, to allow for the normal daily utilization of phenylalanine for protein synthesis while maintaining plasma phenylalanine levels in a range as close as possible to normal, but less than 360 μmol/L. As the patient ages, care-givers may have to be content with levels less than 600 μmol/L. Deviations from normal plasma levels are believed to be associated with chronic, perhaps acute, effects on brain function and testing performance; therefore the diet should be maintained for life. More recently, other forms of therapy have been used. Preparations of the large neutral amino acids that compete for the same transporter as phenylalanine may be given, especially to patients who cannot comply with the low–natural protein diet, and more importantly the mandatory daily ingestion of the medical food devoid of phenylalanine, but replete with unpalatable amino acids. Positive effects have been frequently claimed, but few carefully controlled studies are available. The positive effects of this supplement have variously been attributed to competition with phenylalanine absorption in the gastrointestinal tract, competition for transport into the brain, and repletion of neurotransmitters. A small fraction of patients with full-blown PKU respond favorably to high doses of tetrahydrobiopterin, the natural cofactor for phenylalanine hydroxylase, with a substantial fall in plasma phenylalanine levels and an increased tolerance for natural protein. The more mild forms of hyperphenylalaninemia are even more responsive. The therapy is expensive. Injections or implantations of a reservoir in which there is an enzyme that breaks down phenylalanine in the body are in the early phases of testing.

The phenylalanine hydroxylase gene has been cloned and sequenced, and the mutations responsible for most abnormalities in humans are known. DNA sequencing and mutational analysis can be used to identify carriers in families and to provide a scientific rationale during family counseling.

In rare cases, patients with hyperphenylalaninemia have severe disease not because of deficiency of the phenylalanine hydroxylase apoenzyme, but because of deficiency of the active cofactor of this enzyme, tetrahydrobiopterin. Several defects in the metabolism of biopterin can produce this type of hyperphenylalaninemia. Patients with these uncommon types of PKU usually come to attention in the newborn period because of severe seizure activity. Patients with biopterin deficiency can have evidence of severe brain damage despite treatment with a low-phenylalanine diet. Brain damage may be related to deficiencies of other neurotransmitters whose synthesis also depends on adequate levels of tetrahydrobiopterin. These various other defects, such as the dihydropteridine reductase, 6-pyruvoyl tetrahydropterin synthetase, and the guanosine triphosphate cyclohydrolase deficiencies, can be ascertained by urinary measurements of neopterin and biopterin in urine. They are responsive to therapy with neurotransmitter replacement and tetrahydrobiopterin.

If women with PKU are poorly treated during pregnancy, their children may be born with microcephaly and congenital heart defects. Mental retardation is common. Adequate treatment before 8 weeks' gestation is essential, and control of phenylalanine levels before pregnancy is most desirable.

INBORN ERRORS OF ORGANIC ACID METABOLISM

Defects in the catabolism of the BCAAs are responsible for most of the disorders of organic acid metabolism (Figure 22-5). Typical examples are methylmalonic, propionic, and isovaleric acidemias. An organic acid is any organic compound that contains a carboxy functional group but no α-amino group as in an amino acid. In this section, we consider the disorders of fatty acid oxidation, ketone body metabolism, and lactic acid metabolism as well as the more classic inherited defects in organic acid metabolism.

Until recently, these disorders were diagnosed only after symptoms have appeared. It is now more common to be confronted with an asymptomatic or early symptomatic patient and a good idea of the diagnosis. As discussed earlier, acidosis and encephalopathy are usually the hallmarks of these syndromes when they manifest in the newborn period.

METHYLMALONIC ACIDEMIA

L-Methylmalonyl–Coenzyme A Mutase Deficiency

Methylmalonic acidemia, along with propionic acidemia, is thought to be the most common of disorders of organic acid metabolism (Fenton et al, 2001; Wendel and de Baulny, 2006). Although more than one enzyme defect may result in methylmalonic acidemia, all are inherited as autosomal recessive traits. In California, defects in cobalamin metabolism are more frequent than apoenzyme deficiency, specifically L-methylmalonyl–coenzyme a (CoA)

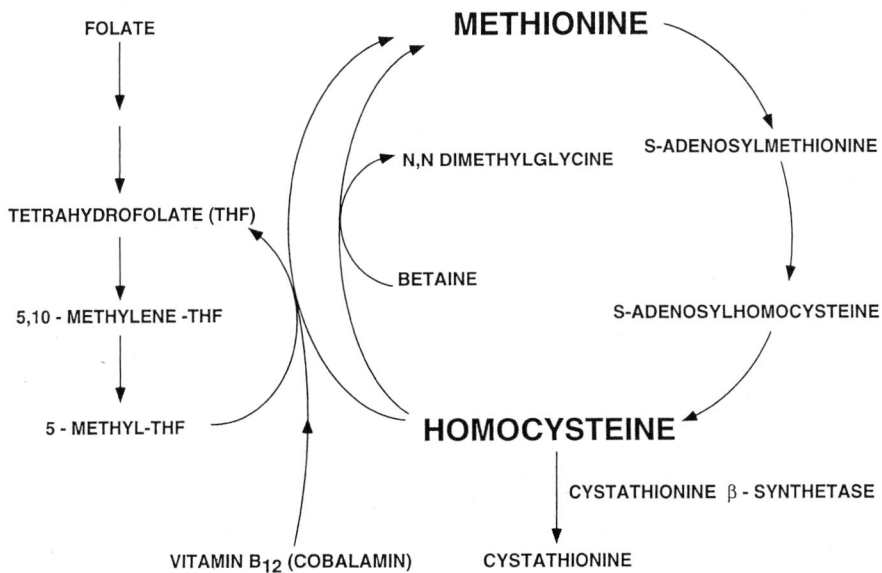

FIGURE 22-5 The pathways, metabolites, and vitamin cofactors important in the interconversion of methionine and homocysteine are shown in this abbreviated scheme of the trans-sulfuration pathway. In a methyl-transfer reaction, homocysteine is converted to methionine; the reaction is catalyzed by a cobalamin-containing enzyme, 5-methyl-tetrahydrofolate-homocysteine methyltransferase or methionine synthase. An alternate reaction involves betaine-homocysteine methyltransferase. Therefore vitamin B_{12} and folate are important vitamins in homocysteine and methionine metabolism. The 5,10-methylene tetrahydrofolate (THF) derived from dietary folate is converted to 5-methyl THF by the enzyme 5,10-methylene THF reductase. In classic homocystinuria, the deficient enzyme is the cystathionine β-synthetase, which catalyzes the conversion of homocysteine to cystathionase, a precursor of cysteine. This pathway is readily operative in the adult, so that cysteine is a nonessential amino acid. In newborn infants, however, synthesis of cysteine does not occur at the same rate as in adults. Adenosylmethionine-dependent methyl transfer may be extremely important in the central nervous system. Most of the patients who come to clinical attention in the newborn period have defects in the remethylation of homocysteine to methionine; therefore these patients may have a severe deficiency of adenosylmethionine in the brain and spinal cord.

mutase (see Figure 22-4). This enzyme is present in mitochondria, and it depends on adenosyl-cobalamin for activity. Impaired function can result from either a mutation of the L-methylmalonyl-CoA mutase apoenzyme or deficient availability of the adenosyl form of vitamin B_{12}. The latter may result from impaired cellular metabolism of vitamin B_{12}, including defective activity of the enzyme adenosylcobalamin synthetase. Some patients, but not usually newborn infants with methylmalonic acidemia caused by apoenzyme deficiency, are responsive to pharmacologic therapy with vitamin B_{12}. Methylmalonic acidemia, therefore, is one of the important disorders that can be considered a vitamin-responsive inborn error of metabolism. Because of deficient activity of L-methylmalonyl-CoA mutase, the substrate L-methylmalonyl-CoA accumulates in mitochondria and is subsequently hydrolyzed to methylmalonic acid. Methylmalonic acid is capable of diffusing out of cells in which it is being produced, so it may be detected in excess in blood, CSF, and urine of patients with these various forms of the disease. The precursors of L-methylmalonyl-CoA are the BCAAs isoleucine and valine, in addition to methionine, threonine, thymine, and odd-chain fatty acids (see Figure 22-4).

There are many different phenotypes of methylmalonic acidemia that range from severe, catastrophic newborn-onset disease in the first week of life to an almost benign form that has been detected in adults with partial L-methylmalonyl-CoA mutase deficiency. Most patients in the newborn period have a severe phenotype. Dialysis therapy is not effective in some of the patients in the first week of life with catastrophic illness, possibly because of a delay in diagnosis and treatment or the breakdown of other

systems, including the heart and circulation. The most striking presentation is in the second or third day of life. The baby is usually well at birth, as with UCDs, but then gradually begins to manifest problems with feeding, vomiting, lethargy, and perhaps seizures. There may be respiratory distress as a symptom of metabolic acidosis. The important laboratory findings include metabolic acidosis usually associated with an increased anion gap, ketosis, and hyperammonemia. The elevation of plasma ammonium may be as high as in severe newborn-onset hyperammonemic syndromes. Because ketonuria is relatively uncommon in newborn infants, even in stressed infants with hypoglycemia caused by poor feeding, and because diabetes mellitus is so uncommon in the newborn period, the physician caring for newborn infants must always consider an inborn error of organic acid metabolism when confronted with an acutely ill baby with ketosis. Other laboratory findings are thrombocytopenia, leukopenia, and anemia caused by effects of the metabolite on hematopoietic elements in bone marrow. Plasma amino acid analysis may reveal elevations of several amino acids, such as glycine and alanine. Secondary carnitine deficiency with elevations of carnitine esters is expected (Chalmers et al, 1984). Methylmalonic acid is detected at high levels in urine with GC-MS. Older patients with methylmalonic acidemia during crisis have suffered acute pancreatitis and devastating lesions to the basal ganglia.

The diagnosis can be confirmed with an assay of the activity of L-methylmalonyl-CoA mutase enzyme in cultured skin fibroblasts. In addition, various other disturbances in vitamin B_{12} metabolism can be studied by analyzing skin fibroblasts in culture. It is more common to dissect the condition clinically, ascertain the response to vitamin B_{12}, and use mutation analysis to confirm the exact site of the genetic lesion.

The treatment of acute disease consists of protein restriction, empirical therapy with vitamin B_{12} (1 mg/day intramuscularly), intravenous fluids with 10% glucose and sodium bicarbonate to correct dehydration, electrolyte imbalance and acidosis, high-calorie feeds via a nasogastric tube, and often dialysis. The use of carnitine (25 to 200 mg/kg/day intravenously or orally) is often recommended, but its usefulness as an acute treatment has not been proved. The treatment of chronic state centers on the judicious use of a low-protein diet, an amino acid supplement low in the MMA precursors, carnitine to alleviate free carnitine deficiency, and appropriate calories and fluid. Vitamin B_{12} is used only when a specific and reproducible response is noted.

Most diagnoses are ascertained by expanded newborn screening. If the results are rapidly available, the outlook for the neonatal period may be improved. Episodes of decompensation will still occur. Patients who are particularly brittle or who develop renal failure receive either liver, kidney, or combined liver-kidney transplants, but their efficacy at curing the primary disease process has not been proved.

PROPIONIC ACIDEMIA

Propionyl Coenzyme A Carboxylase Deficiency

Propionic acidemia was the first classic defect in organic acid metabolism to be described in humans (Fenton et al, 2001; Wendel and de Baulny, 2006). The first patient, described by Childs et al in 1961, was sick on the first day of life with severe metabolic acidosis and ketosis. He responded to massive alkali therapy and survived the newborn period. He subsequently suffered multiple episodes of metabolic decompensation with ketoacidosis, usually precipitated by infections or protein ingestion. He also had developmental delay, a seizure disorder, and episodic neutropenia and thrombocytopenia. He died at 7 years old. His sister also demonstrated ketosis and metabolic acidosis in the first week of life, but because of better control of her disease, there were few severe episodes of decompensation in the first and second decades of life.

Propionic acidemia, which is caused by a selective deficiency of propionyl-CoA carboxylase, is inherited as an autosomal recessive trait. This disorder was originally called *ketotic hyperglycinemia*, because of elevations in plasma glycine along with ketosis. The precursors of propionyl-CoA include the amino acids isoleucine, valine, methionine and threonine, thymine, and odd-chain fatty acids (see Figure 22-4). Of the several hundred patients described with this disease, most clinical presentations are in the newborn period with poor feeding, vomiting, lethargy, and hypotonia. The patients commonly have seizures and hepatomegaly. The metabolic acidosis may be severe with or without an increase in the anion gap. Ketosis is usually present, but not always. Patients who survive may often show choreoathetosis, because of persistent damage to the basal ganglia. Usually episodes of metabolic decompensation characterized by acidosis and ketosis can be precipitated by excessive protein intake or more commonly infection, with the attendant catabolism. Such episodes can result in permanent neurologic damage. Subsequent findings therefore include developmental delay, seizures, cerebral atrophy, and EEG abnormalities. During the acute attacks, leukopenia, thrombocytopenia, and less rarely anemia, probably caused by suppression of maturation of bone marrow hematopoietic precursors, may be exacerbated.

The diagnosis can be confirmed with GC-MS analysis. The urine has excess concentrations of various propionate metabolites, such as methyl citrate, propionylglycine, 2-methyl-3-hydroxybutyrate, 2-methylacetoacetate, and several other, rarer compounds. The plasma glycine value may be elevated, and during acute attacks the plasma ammonium value is frequently increased. The enzyme activity of propionyl-CoA carboxylase can be assayed in white blood cells or extracts of cultured skin fibroblasts for definitive diagnosis. Numerous mutations have been described in the two genes that encode the subunits of this multimeric enzyme.

Therapy consists of a low-protein diet and adequate calories. As in MMA, there is secondary carnitine deficiency with elevations of propionylcarnitine. The use of L-carnitine to relieve a deficiency of free carnitine and promote greater urinary excretion of propionylcarnitine to lower mitochondrial propionyl-CoA levels is not proved. Because intestinal bacteria can also contribute to propionate production, antimicrobial therapy with metronidazole has been used during an acute attack and for long-term therapy. In the acutely ill newborn, the immediate treatment consists of elimination of protein, total parenteral nutrition, administration of an adequate amount of calories (10% glucose intravenously or a nonprotein formula, or both, via nasogastric tube infusion), administration of alkali to eliminate metabolic acidosis, and platelet transfusion if warranted by thrombocytopenia. Patients frequently require hemodialysis, because of severe acidosis and coma. It is unclear whether administration of sodium benzoate and sodium phenylacetate, as in the treatment of hyperammonemia associated with UCDs, is of benefit to the patient with secondary hyperammonemia. Several patients with propionic acidemia have undergone liver transplantation with mixed success. Episodes of acidosis are often recurrent between 1 and 3 years of age, after which some ability to modulate the effects of catabolism occurs.

Most patients with this condition are now ascertained by expanded newborn screening. If the results are rapidly available, the outlook for the neonatal period may be improved. Episodes of decompensation will still occur.

ISOVALERIC ACIDEMIA

Isovaleryl–Coenzyme A Dehydrogenase Deficiency

Isovaleric acidemia is caused by a selective deficiency of the enzyme isovaleryl-CoA dehydrogenase (Sweetman and Williams, 2001; Wendel and de Baulny, 2006). It is inherited as an autosomal recessive trait. There are two major phenotypes; an acute form manifests as catastrophic disease in the newborn period, and the late-onset type is characterized by chronic, intermittent episodes of metabolic decompensation. The degree of enzyme deficiency and the mutations differ between the two extreme presentations. In the acute form, the infants become extremely sick in the first week of life. There is usually a history of poor feeding, vomiting, lethargy, and seizures. The characteristic sweaty feet or rancid cheese odor caused by isovaleric acid is noted on the body or in urine, especially if it is acidic. Metabolic acidosis is present, usually with an elevated anion gap and ketosis. There may be secondary hyperammonemia, thrombocytopenia, neutropenia, and sometimes anemia, resulting in pancytopenia. The babies usually lapse into a coma. Dialysis therapy may be necessary. As with other organic acid disorders for which an amino acid determines organic acid production (see Figure 22-4), treatment also consists of protein restriction, intravenous fluids with glucose, and perhaps sodium bicarbonate, protein-free formula with calories via nasogastric tube, glycine (250 mg/kg/day), and carnitine supplementation (Sweetman and Williams, 2001). Intravenous L-carnitine may be beneficial. The excretion of isovaleric acid as the glycine conjugate is highly efficient, and symptomatic relief can occur rapidly. Glycine is often available in compounding pharmacies that make their own IV alimentation solutions.

In the chronic, intermittent form of isovaleric acidemia, patients have repeated episodes of metabolic decompensation precipitated by infections, primarily or excessive protein intake. Some of these episodes may mimic Reye syndrome. The same therapeutic principles are applied as for the treatment of the neonatal disorder. The mainstay of long-term therapy is a diet with limited natural protein, a valine-free amino acid supplement, and long-term administration of glycine (Berry et al, 1988), which enhances the production of the nontoxic compound isovalerylglycine and serves to reduce the free levels of isovaleric acid in body fluids. In addition, carnitine administration can augment the excretion of isovaleryl carnitine (Berry et al, 1988; Mayatepek et al, 1991). The benefit of carnitine treatment in the chronic state, however, remains unproved. Some patients who remain largely asymptomatic are ascertained through the expanded newborn screening programs.

Newborn screening and the rapid treatment protocols can alter the outlook for this condition. In the prescreening era, many patients with neonatal onset could not be saved, and a number of those with the more indolent forms have been retarded. This situation should change with preemptive treatment.

The diagnosis can be made from marked elevations of isovalerylglycine in urine. There is usually also increased excretion of 3-hydroxyisovaleric acid. The enzyme isovaleryl-CoA dehydrogenase can be assayed in extracts of cultured skin fibroblasts. As with many other conditions, the typical metabolic profile should allow confirmation directly by mutation analysis bypassing the enzyme assay.

MULTIPLE CARBOXYLASE DEFICIENCY

There are two enzymatic defects leading to deficiency of the same suite of carboxylase enzymes, holocarboxylase synthetase deficiency and biotinidase deficiency (Wolf, 2001). All the carboxylase enzymes—propionyl-CoA carboxylase, pyruvate carboxylase, 3-methylcrotonyl-CoA

carboxylase, and acetyl-CoA carboxylase—require covalent linkage with biotin for normal activity. In holocarboxylase synthetase deficiency, the enzyme that catalyzes the covalent linkage of biotin to a lysine residue of these various carboxylases is deficient. In the second form of the disorder, the absence of the enzyme biotinidase does not allow for biotin recycling after a carboxylase enzyme is degraded, and hydrolyzed biotinidase deficiency does not usually manifest in the newborn period.

Patients with severe deficiency in holocarboxylase synthetase, however, characteristically are catastrophically ill in the newborn period. Patients have severe metabolic acidosis with lactic acidosis and become comatose. As with biotinidase deficiency, administration of biotin is life saving. Holocarboxylase synthetase deficiency is one of the few disorders of organic acid metabolism for which the administration of a vitamin in megadoses produces a dramatic turnabout in clinical and laboratory findings. Diagnosis depends on GC-MS analysis of urine and the demonstration of markedly increased levels of lactate, 3-methylcrotonylglycine, and propionate metabolites. In most patients the affinity of the holocarboxylase synthetase enzyme for biotin is diminished, and for the biochemical disturbances to normalize or improve, patients need between 10 and 60 mg of biotin daily. The enzyme deficiency can be confirmed in cultured skin fibroblasts or by mutation analysis. The disorder is inherited as an autosomal recessive trait.

Both biotinidase deficiency, ascertained by direct enzyme assay, and holocarboxylase synthetase deficiency are detected in the expanded newborn screening panels. The outcomes should alter because of this earlier diagnosis.

GLUTARIC ACIDEMIA TYPE 1

Glutaryl–Coenzyme A Dehydrogenase Deficiency

An isolated deficiency of glutaryl-CoA dehydrogenase causes glutaric acidemia type 1 (GA-1) (Goodman and Frerman, 2001). Multiple phenotypes are known. In the most dramatic presentation, which accounts for fewer than half of the known patients with GA-1, the illness develops acutely in the first year of life, usually after an infection or other catabolic event. Acute encephalopathy is followed by the development of what appears to be a severe form of extrapyramidal cerebral palsy (Hoffmann et al, 1991). The affected infants have incurred bilateral damage to the caudate and putamen in the basal ganglia, resulting in an incapacitating dystonic syndrome. Some patients have a slowly progressive course with developmental delay, hypotonia, dystonia, and dyskinesia in the first 2 years of life. Other patients are relatively asymptomatic.

In general, GA-1 is not a disorder that is associated with acute disease in the newborn period. However, macrocephaly at birth is common (Goodman and Frerman, 2001). The etiology of any of the CNS lesions is unknown, but toxicity caused by dicarboxylic acid accumulation has been postulated. Magnetic resonance imaging (MRI) of the head typically shows bilateral widening of the Sylvian fissures associated with hypoopercularization, resulting in the "bat-wing" appearance. Sometimes the fluid accumulation mimics subdural hygromas, and a few patients have been noted to have subdural hematomas. The congenital nature of these findings suggests that GA-1 has its onset in utero and affects CNS development. Usually infants do not demonstrate bilateral damage to the basal ganglia in the newborn period. Diagnosis depends on the demonstration of glutaric acid and 3-hydroxyglutaric acid in urine and is confirmed by the demonstration of deficiency of glutaryl-CoA dehydrogenase activity or protein levels on Western blot analysis in cultured fibroblasts, or more commonly by mutation analysis.

Newborn screening may be complicated in this disorder. Whereas the majority of patients have positive findings of elevated C5DC in the newborn acylcarnitine profile, a minority with severe disease may have normal or near normal results. These same patients might not show the characteristic elevation of 3-hydroxyglutarate in urine. For this reason an initial elevation of C5DC in urine can and should elicit the close attention of a metabolic specialist who then must help to interpret results of the follow-up testing.

A rare disorder, GA-1 is especially common in Saulteaux-Ojibway Indians of Canada (Greenberg et al, 1995) and in the Old-Order Amish of Lancaster County, Pennsylvania (Morton et al, 1991). A low-protein diet can help in the treatment of these patients; acute illnesses, usually viral in nature, should be treated vigorously with fluids containing glucose and adequate amounts of calories to prevent or diminish catabolism. Bicarbonate may be necessary to correct acid-base imbalance. Carnitine has also been used to reduce mitochondrial glutaryl-CoA levels.

FATTY ACID OXIDATION DISORDERS

Glutaric Acidemia Type 2 or Multiple Acyl Coenzyme A Dehydrogenase Deficiency

Glutaric acidemia type 2 (GA-2) is characterized by deficiency of multiple acyl-CoA dehydrogenase enzymes (Goodman and Frerman, 2001; Stanley et al, 2006). All these dehydrogenase proteins have in common the binding of a protein called *electron transfer flavoprotein* (ETF). This protein is responsible for accepting electrons in any of these oxidative dehydrogenation reactions from the flavin adenine dinucleotide (FAD) cofactor. A mutation in any of the three genes that encode the protein subunits of either ETF or the ETF dehydrogenase, which is responsible for further transferring the electrons from ETF to coenzyme Q_{10} within the mitochondria leads to this condition. Deficiency of riboflavin, a component of FAD, or its transport may also lead to this condition. Among the compounds accumulating in this condition are short-, medium-, and long-chain fatty acids, glutaric and isovaleric acids, dimethylglycine, and sarcosine.

The three major phenotypes of GA-2 are (1) a newborn-onset type with congenital anomalies, (2) a newborn-onset type without anomalies, and (3) a milder or later-onset type, sometimes called *mild acyl-CoA dehydrogenase deficiency* or *ethylmalonic adipic aciduria*.

Severely affected newborn patients with GA-2 often have multiple malformations, may be premature, and are usually ill within the first week of life (Frerman and Goodman, 2001). The patients demonstrate hypotonia,

encephalopathy, hepatomegaly, hypoglycemia, and metabolic acidosis; often the odor of isovaleric acid is present. There may be facial dysmorphism consisting of a high forehead, low-set ears, hypertelorism, and a hypoplastic midface. The kidneys may be palpably enlarged, associated with large renal cysts; they may also have rocker-bottom feet, muscular defects of the inferior abdominal wall, and anomalies of the external genitalia, including hypospadias and chordee. Most of the patients with GA-2 and multiple malformations do not survive the first weeks of life. In some, the malformations are not so noticeable, and only renal cysts are identified at autopsy. Some of these patients have cardiomyopathy. In contrast, some of these infants can survive the newborn period.

The phenotype in the third form of GA-2 is highly variable. Some patients are relatively free of disease and have intermittent episodes of vomiting, dehydration, hypoglycemia, and acidosis during childhood or adult life. In some, there may be hepatomegaly and muscle disease.

Laboratory studies in patients with the newborn-onset type usually show severe metabolic acidosis with lactate elevation and increased anion gap, mild to moderate hyperammonemia, and hypoglycemia without a moderate or large ketonuria. The liver function and dysfunction test results may be abnormal, with increases in serum transaminases and prolongations of PT and PTT. A chest radiograph may show heart enlargement because of hypertrophic cardiomyopathy. Abdominal ultrasonography or computed tomography may reveal renal cysts. The diagnosis is made from the characteristic pattern of organic acid metabolites on urine GC-MS analysis. It consists of glutarate; ethylmalonate; 3-hydroxyisovalerate; 2-hydroxyglutarate; 5-hydroxyhexanoate; adipic, suberic, sebacic, and dodecanedioic acids; isovalerylglycine; isobutyrylglycine; and 2-methylbutyrylglycine. The ketones, acetoacetic acid, and 3-hydroxybutyric acid are usually not present or are only minimally elevated if present, being inappropriate for the degree of fatty acid metabolites that indicate free fatty acid mobilization and the potential for enhanced ketogenesis. The renal cystic disease may also be associated with evidence of impaired renal tubular function. Generalized aminoaciduria may be present. The amino-containing compound sarcosine may be elevated in serum as well as in urine. There may be secondary carnitine deficiency, and abnormal carnitine esters such as isovalerylcarnitine and butyrylcarnitine can be detected in blood. The ETF and ETF dehydrogenase deficiency can be detected through the use of specific antibodies on Western blot analysis of cultured skin fibroblasts or of functional assays in skin cells. Mutation analysis in this condition as in others may be superseding the more cumbersome enzyme studies.

Prenatal diagnosis can be achieved by demonstration of glutarate in amniotic fluid, from results of dehydrogenase assays in cultured amniocytes, or by mutation analysis. Despite much debate, criteria for newborn screening have not been well established, and many false positive tests have occurred for this rare disorder.

Although treatment with intravenous glucose, riboflavin, carnitine, and diets low in protein and fat generally have not been successful for catastrophically ill newborns, there has been some success in patients with milder or later-onset disease. Riboflavin is suggested to be administered to the newborn with severe disease, but riboflavin at a dose of 100 to 300 mg/day has been effective in only a few older patients (Gregersen et al, 1982; Harpey et al, 1983). The rationale for this therapy is that riboflavin, being a precursor of FAD, increases the concentrations of FAD and allows for better interaction with mutated and defective ETF or ETF dehydrogenase proteins. Finally, some artificial electron acceptors such as methylene blue have been used in the newborn period without success.

VERY-LONG-CHAIN, MEDIUM-CHAIN, AND SHORT-CHAIN ACYLFATTY ACID OXIDATION DEFECTS

Fatty acids are oxidized in a complex process by which they are taken up into the cell and transported into the mitochondrion for beta oxidation and energy production. There are at least 31 enzymes involved in the process and defects in the majority have been described. Of these many disorders, the most frequent are those of carnitine metabolism and transport, and various steps in the beta oxidation pathways. The presentations are sufficiently different to bear independent description, but in general they all have hypoketotic hypoglycemia and energy deficits. Most spare the CNS.

When severe, the defects have been associated with coma, hypoglycemia, liver disease, cardiac, and skeletal myopathy (Roe and Ding, 2001; Stanley et al, 2006). All of these defects involve abnormalities in enzymes that participate in or facilitate the mitochondrial beta oxidation of fatty acids. In general the pathophysiology associated with these disorders has the potential to put the patient in a life-threatening condition in which there is a state of catabolism and enhanced liberation of free fatty acids by adipose stores. The most prevalent disorders will be discussed here.

Medium-Chain Acyl-Coenzyme A Dehydrogenase Deficiency

The most common of these disorders is the medium-chain acyl-CoA dehydrogenase (MCAD) deficiency, with a frequency of approximately 1 in 20,000 births in Northern European populations (Roe and Ding, 2001; Stanley et al, 2006). Most patients' disease does not manifest until late infancy, but some with the most severe enzyme deficiencies manifest in the first days of life and may die without explanation, something recently appreciated with the advent of expanded newborn screening. It is also a well-known cause of sudden infant death syndrome having been found in 2% to 3% of cases in which it has been investigated. The typical patient is an older infant who, after an infection, experiences anorexia, vomiting, dehydration, lethargy, and hypoglycemia that may be associated with seizures. Similarly, older patients have features that mimic those of Reye syndrome and can die because of brain edema.

In MCAD deficiency, the initial episode is associated with a high mortality rate. If not diagnosed by newborn screening, the laboratory studies usually show hypoglycemia and an absence of moderate to large ketones in urine that would be expected to accompany hypoglycemia. The plasma ammonium values may be mildly elevated, the liver

may be enlarged, and serum ALT and AST levels may be slightly increased. During an acute episode, urine GC-MS analysis of organic acids characteristically shows increased levels of adipic, suberic, and sebacic acids as well as their unsaturated and hydroxylated analogues. However, this result is not pathognomonic of a disorder of fat metabolism, because infants who are fed medium-chain triglyceride–enriched formulas also show dicarboxylic aciduria. Acylcarnitine studies of plasma from patients with MCAD deficiency demonstrates increased levels of C8, C6, and C10 species. Urine also contains glycine conjugates such as suberylglycine and hexanoylglycine. A secondary carnitine deficiency can be present. The MCAD enzyme can be assayed in cultured skin fibroblasts, but mutation analysis is the more common means of confirming the diagnosis.

After the MCAD gene was cloned and sequenced, a large number of more common and private mutations were identified. The most conspicuous gene is *R329E*, a highly prevalent mutation in people of Northern European ancestry and known to cause a severe enzyme deficiency. The major treatment is avoidance of fasting for more than 12 hours, especially in association with an intercurrent illness. Some practitioners are more conservative and advocate fasting of no more than 4 to 6 hours in the first year of life, whether sick or well. Although not of proven efficacy, many physicians recommend a moderately fat-restricted diet for these patients. It is thought that once the disease is diagnosed and preventive programs are instituted, the disease should not be life threatening or fatal.

With the advent of newborn screening, a larger group of patients has been found and some more common mutations in these patients have never been seen in a case ascertained because of symptoms. Finding these individuals has given rise to the notion that many patients found by newborn screening are destined never to become symptomatic. Whereas ascertainment of such mutations can be reassuring, too little is known about them to allow complete reassurance and full relaxation of preventive precautions. Newborn screening also finds individuals heterozygous for a severe mutation when no other mutation is found. These patients are considered to be biochemically manifesting heterozygotes and are thought to be at no medical risk from this condition.

Very-Long-Chain Acyl-Coenzyme A Dehydrogenase Deficiency

Most of the patients with a previous diagnosis of long-chain acyl-CoA dehydrogenase (LCAD) deficiency (Roe and Ding, 2001; Stanley et al, 2006) actually had very-long-chain acyl-CoA dehydrogenase (VLCAD) deficiency (Yamaguchi et al, 1993). Patients with this disease may be ill in the newborn period because of liver disease with hypoglycemia, cardiomyopathy, and skeletal myopathy. The membrane-bound VLCAD—as opposed to the soluble LCAD, whose specific metabolic role is unknown—is the main enzyme for initiating oxidation of free fatty acids that are derived from adipose stores, such as palmitic, stearic, and oleic acids. The fasting state may include coma. In its absence, however, the patients may exhibit hypotonia, hepatomegaly, and cardiomegaly. With an acute metabolic decompensation, urine organic acid analysis may demonstrate dicarboxylic aciduria. There may be a secondary carnitine deficiency with increased concentrations of long-chain fatty acids (LCFAs) bound to carnitine.

VLCAD deficiency can be fatal; sudden death in early infancy has been reported. Therapy is directed toward replenishment of glucose, calorie administration, and treatment of any potential brain edema. The myopathy and cardiomyopathy, however, may proceed even in the absence of fasting. Most investigators suggest a reduction in dietary fat intake, supplementation in medium-chain triglycerides, and maintenance of an adequate intake of essential fatty acids. Diagnosis can be made through enzyme assay in cultured skin fibroblasts, but commonly by mutation analysis.

Expanded newborn screening has expanded our horizons in this disorder as it has for MCAD deficiency. In addition to patients who may be homozygous for two mild mutations or compound heterozygous for a mild mutation, and who are at much reduced clinical risk, heterozygotes for a pathologic mutation and a wild type gene have been found and are presumably at no greater risk than others in the population.

Short-Chain Acyl-Coenzyme A Dehydrogenase Deficiency

The short-chain acyl-CoA dehydrogenase deficiency is a disorder mired in controversy (Roe and Ding, 2001; Stanley et al, 2006). Patients with a severe enzyme deficiency are infrequent, and the majority of them have no symptoms attributable to the disorder, as judged by the variability of symptoms in those ascertained symptomatically and the absence of obvious disease in similarly affected siblings. The situation is further complicated by extensive mutation analysis, especially in those ascertained through positive newborn screens. Because of the prevalence of common polymorphisms that impair but do not eliminate enzymatic activity, the majority of ascertained individuals have no symptoms and appear unlikely to develop them. This problem has led some people to declare the disorder harmless and to pay no attention to it. Other more sober voices accept it as a benign disease and disorder in the majority of patients, but recognize the possibility that a small minority may become symptomatic and treat them appropriately by warning the parents to react to unusual and unexpected symptoms. There tends to be some acrimony at meetings from members of the most extreme positions on either end of the spectrum.

Acylcarnitine analysis on either newborn screen or later shows elevated C4 carnitine. Organic acid analysis shows elevated levels of ethylmalonic and methylsuccinic acids, with higher levels tending to occur with greater enzyme deficiencies. Diagnosis can be made by assaying the short-chain acyl-CoA dehydrogenase enzyme in cultured skin fibroblasts and by a fatty acid oxidation profile in these same cells. Mutation analysis is now the norm for this condition.

Long-Chain 3-Hydroxy Acyl-Coenzyme A Dehydrogenase Deficiency

The long-chain 3-hydroxy acyl-CoA dehydrogenase deficiency is associated with acute illness, fasting-induced hypoglycemia, hypoketosis, cardiomegaly, and muscle weakness (Roe and Ding, 2001; Stanley et al, 2006).

As with VLCFA oxidative abnormalities, some older patients may have episodes of illness associated with elevated serum creatine phosphokinase levels and myoglobinuria. A few patients have had sensory motor neuropathy and pigmentary retinopathy. Half the patients do not survive. Some patients may have severe liver disease with fibrosis in addition to necrosis and steatosis. Women who are carriers for this disease may also manifest the HELLP syndrome when carrying an affected child.

The diagnosis was made in symptomatic individuals and was suggested by symptoms and demonstration of longer chain 3-hydroxydicarboxylic acids on urine organic acid analysis. Enzymatic diagnosis can be made in lymphocytes or in skin fibroblasts. More commonly the diagnosis is confirmed by a combination of clinical biochemical abnormalities and DNA mutation analysis. The majority of moderate to severe cases are diagnosed by expanded newborn screening and follow-up.

Treatment of this disorder has involved frequent high-carbohydrate feedings, dietary fat restriction, and supplementation with uncooked cornstarch. Administration of medium-chain triglycerides may be helpful. Carnitine and riboflavin have also been tried without benefit. A high level of parental vigilance is required to begin therapy quickly at signs of metabolic decompensation. Liver and neurologic disease can progress despite any intervention. The outcome of severely affected patients is guarded.

Carnitine Transporter Defect and Deficiencies of Carnitine Palmitoyltransferase I and II and Acylcarnitine Translocase

Carnitine is essential for fatty acid oxidation because transport of LCFAs into mitochondria depends on an adequate amount of carnitine and the presence of two enzymes that covalently link carnitine to fatty acid or remove the linkage and one transporter that carries it across the inner mitochondrial membrane (Roe and Ding, 2001; Stanley et al, 2006). These enzymes are carnitine palmitoyltransferase I and II and a carnitine translocase. Cellular levels of carnitine in turn depend on a sodium-dependent carnitine transporter.

Primary carnitine deficiency appears to be associated with a carnitine transporter defect (Roe and Ding, 2001; Stanley et al, 2006). Patients with the transporter defect may present with symptoms in infancy or in childhood, but rarely in the newborn period. Earliest reports concern the extended newborn period or early infancy. The disease is characterized by hypoketotic hypoglycemia, hyperammonemia, elevations of transaminases, cardiomyopathy, and skeletal muscle weakness. In some of the older patients, cardiomyopathy may be the presenting sign. The characteristic laboratory finding in this disease is extremely low plasma carnitine levels. The total carnitine levels are usually less than 10 μmol/L in plasma. A dicarboxylic aciduria is not usually evident on urine organic acid analysis.

Newborn screening has altered our view of this disorder. Most cases are ascertained with low carnitine on screening and are usually diagnosed with mutation analysis and the failure of carnitine levels to rise in the postnatal period. Most physicians treat the disorder with carnitine to raise plasma carnitine levels while the evaluation is in progress. Newborn screening has also ascertained asymptomatic and affected mothers and has altered our perception of this condition and its severity. In addition, largely asymptomatic mothers affected with an organic acidemia and low carnitine levels in the mother and fetus have been detected.

This disorder is the only one in which pharmacologic administration of carnitine has dramatic effects on the clinical and laboratory abnormalities. The treatment is 100 to 200 mg/kg/day of L-carnitine. Repletion of plasma carnitine levels is the benchmark by which the efficacy of treatment is judged, but the degree of repletion of tissue levels (skeletal muscle and heart) is inferred but rarely demonstrated. Treatment is successful in the short, intermediate, and longer terms, but no information on the lifespan of these patients who appear healthy is available.

Carnitine Palmitoyltransferase Type I Deficiency

Carnitine palmitoyltransferase type I (CPT-I) is responsible for covalently linking LCFAs such as palmitate to carnitine. Although one patient with deficiency of CPT-I came to attention in the newborn period, most come to attention in early to late infancy (Roe and Ding, 2001; Stanley et al, 2006). The clinical findings are hypoketotic hypoglycemia, encephalopathy, and hepatomegaly; there is usually no evidence of cardiomyopathy or skeletal myopathy in CPT-I deficiency. Renal tubular acidosis, which is caused by impaired distal hydrogen ion secretion, has rarely been reported. Characteristic laboratory findings are the absence of dicarboxylic aciduria and high plasma levels of total carnitine and free carnitine; however, the plasma acylcarnitine profile is not abnormal. The definitive diagnosis rests on measuring CPT-I enzyme activity in cultured skin fibroblasts or mutation analysis. Frequent feeding, reduction of dietary fat, supplementation with medium-chain triglycerides, and avoidance of fasting all have been beneficial in the long-term management of patients with CPT-I deficiency. These patients are now often found by expanded newborn screening because of an abnormal ratio of carnitine to the carnitylated long-chain fatty acids.

Acylcarnitine Translocase Deficiency

Acylcarnitine translocase deficiency is an exceedingly rare defect. It was initially reported in a male infant who suffered a cardiac arrest at 36 hours of age in association with fasting stress and ventricular dysrhythmias (Roe and Ding, 2001; Stanley et al, 2006). Because of the failure to transport long-chain acylcarnitines across the intermitochondrial membrane after the synthesis by CPT-I, the patient had very low total plasma levels of carnitine, most of which was long-chain esterified carnitine; he also had recurrent episodes of hypoglycemia, vomiting, gastroesophageal reflux, and mild chronic hyperammonemia as well as severe skeletal myopathy and mild hypertrophic cardiomyopathy. The continuous nasogastric feeding of a low-fat, high-carbohydrate formula failed to normalize clinical abnormalities, and the patient died at 3 years of age. At that time, liver failure had also developed. Pathophysiologic findings in this patient suggested that accumulation of long-chain acylcarnitine species may be toxic for several organs, including heart, liver, and skeletal muscle. In addition, the acute development of ventricular dysrhythmias may be related to accumulation of such species in cardiac tissue. It is often considered to be almost invariably fatal or very serious, but the probability is that more mild cases with reduced but not absent transporter activity have not been found.

Carnitine Palmitoyltransferase Type II Deficiency

There are two phenotypes of carnitine palmitoyltransferase type II (CPT-II) deficiency (Roe and Ding, 2001; Stanley et al, 2006). The enzyme is responsible for the hydrolysis of LCFA bound to carnitine after transport across the intermitochondrial membrane. Most of the patients reported with CPT-II deficiency have a mild deficiency of the enzyme and in adulthood exhibit episodes of muscle weakness and myoglobinuria brought on by prolonged exercise. The other phenotype is caused by a more serious enzyme defect and manifests in early infancy. The first detailed report was of a 3-month-old boy with hypoketotic hypoglycemia, coma, seizures, hepatomegaly, cardiomegaly, cardiac arrhythmias associated with an increase in long-chain acylcarnitine levels in tissues, and the absence of urinary dicarboxylic aciduria. The enzyme is also expressed in renal tissue and skeletal muscle. Renal dysgenesis has been noted in three patients (Zinn et al, 1991). Reports of onset in the newborn period associated with an abnormal physical appearance and MRI (Hug et al, 1991) and in later infancy have been recorded. Several mutations have been described. Decreased activity of the CPT-II enzyme may be demonstrated in cultured skin fibroblasts.

DEFECTS IN KETONE METABOLISM

After LCFAs are broken down first to medium-chain and finally to short-chain fatty acids such as acetoacetyl CoA, they must be converted in the liver to 3-hydroxy-3-methylglutaryl CoA (HMG-CoA) before hydrolysis to acetoacetate, the ketone body used by the body for energy. Depending on the mitochondrial redox potential—that is, the ratio of the reduced form of nicotinamide adenine dinucleotide (NAD) to its oxidized form (NADH/NAD$^+$)—some of the acetoacetate is converted to 3-hydroxybutyrate, and both ketone bodies are transported out of liver mitochondria and hepatocytes into blood, where they may be used by other tissues, especially brain. Acetoacetyl CoA derived from the last turn of the beta oxidation spiral together with acetyl CoA forms HMG-CoA in a reaction catalyzed by HMG-CoA synthetase. Normally, acetoacetyl CoA can also be hydrolyzed to acetyl CoA by the mitochondrial acetoacetyl-CoA thiolase. Patients with a deficiency of this thiolase do not have a defect in ketone body synthesis but, rather, metabolic acidosis associated with excess ketosis (Mitchell and Fukao, 2008; Stanley et al, 2006).

The clinical features of the thiolase deficiency are variable. Severe acute metabolic decompensation has been reported in infants, but there are also asymptomatic adults with the disorder. The episodes are heralded by fasting or increased protein intake, because isoleucine is a precursor of 2-methylacetoacetyl CoA, which is also a substrate for the mitochondrial acetoacetyl-CoA thiolase enzyme. Therefore this block leads to a defect in distal catabolism of isoleucine and in processing of the precursor of ketone body formation—namely, acetoacetyl-CoA. Cardiomyopathy has been identified in rare patients. The characteristic urinary metabolite pattern detected on urine organic acid analysis is the presence of isoleucine metabolites, such as 2-methylacetoacetate, 2-methyl-3-hydroxybutyrate, and triglylglycine. During acute decompensation, lactate and the traditional ketone bodies are detected in excess amounts in the urine. Some older children have been mistakenly identified as having ketotic hypoglycemia because glycine may be elevated in plasma. Deficiency in the mitochondrial acetoacetyl-CoA thiolase can be demonstrated in cultured skin fibroblasts and by mutation analysis. Treatment of acute episodes consists of intravenous glucose and administration of alkali to correct metabolic acidosis, which may be severe. Long-term therapy involves mild protein restriction, avoidance of fasting, and prompt attention to any intercurrent illness or development of ketonuria.

The synthesis of acetoacetate from HMG-CoA depends on the HMG-CoA lyase enzyme. A deficiency of this enzyme represents the most profound defect in ketone body synthesis (Roe and Ding, 2001; Stanley et al, 2006). Approximately one third of patients with this disease are in the first week of life. In this subgroup of patients, the onset is dramatic and the disease is catastrophic, being characterized by vomiting, lethargy, coma, seizures, hepatomegaly, hypoglycemia, little or no ketones in urine, and hyperammonemia. Most of the complications are related to severe effects of hypoglycemia on the CNS in addition to acidemia, which may be profound. The characteristic urine metabolites detected by GC-MS analysis are 3-hydroxy-3-methylglutaric acid, 3-methylglutaconic acid, and 3-hydroxyisovaleric acid. Only small, inappropriate amounts of acetoacetic acid and 3-hydroxybutyric acid may be detected. Lactate values may be elevated during the acute metabolic decompensation. Inherited as an autosomal recessive trait, the HMG-CoA lyase deficiency can be demonstrated in cultured skin fibroblasts or by mutation analysis. Treatment of the acute episode consists of administration of intravenous glucose and alkali to correct metabolic acidosis. Most long-term therapy consists of a high-carbohydrate diet. Some patients treated with protein-restricted diets, but the most important element in long-term care is the avoidance of fasting.

The last defect to be discussed in the area of disturbances in ketone body metabolism is the succinyl-CoA 3-ketoacid-CoA transferase deficiency (Mitchell and Fukao, 2008; Stanley et al, 2006). In this disease, the ketone bodies, acetoacetic acid, and 3-hydroxybutyric acid are synthesized adequately in the liver, but they cannot be metabolized in the extrahepatic tissues because of the failure of activation of acetoacetate to acetoacetyl CoA by the transferase enzyme. Conversion to a CoA derivative is required for hydrolysis to acetyl CoA for final metabolism in the Krebs citric acid cycle. This disorder is rare, and most of the affected patients in the newborn period do not survive. Such patients usually exhibit severe ketosis and lactic acidosis. The hallmark of the disease is persistent ketosis, even after correction of overt metabolic acidosis and the institution of frequent feedings with the avoidance of fasting.

Plasma values of acetoacetate and 3-hydroxybutyrate are always mildly to moderately elevated, resulting in intermittent ketonuria. The most important aspect of therapy is the avoidance of fasting, during which acidosis and ketosis can be overwhelming. The gene that encodes this enzyme has been cloned, and several mutations have been detected.

PRIMARY LACTIC ACIDOSIS

The term *congenital lactic acidosis* (CLA) refers to a group of diseases in which impaired lactate metabolism is caused by a defect in the mitochondrial respiratory or electron transport chain (ETC), or the tricarboxylic acid (TCA; Krebs) cycle, in which there is a primary defect in pyruvate metabolism that secondarily leads to impaired lactate handling (see Figure 22-1) (De Meirleir et al, 2006; Munnich, 2006; Munnich et al, 2001; Robinson, 2001). However, there are a limited number of reports on inborn errors of the TCA cycle. Most of the information on CLA focuses on mitochondrial ETC, pyruvate dehydrogenase (PDH) complex, and pyruvate carboxylase (PC) defects, all of which have been reviewed (De Meirleir et al, 2006; Munnich, 2006; Munnich et al, 2001; Robinson, 2001) with more detailed information on conditions that must be treated more superficially in this chapter.

Some patients with CLA present have overwhelming lactic acidosis in the neonatal period. In others, lactate may be elevated only in CSF, a "cerebral" lactic acidosis syndrome and present more indolently. Depending on the nature of the enzyme deficiency, lactate, pyruvate, and alanine levels can be elevated in the blood. The ratio of blood lactate to pyruvate (L:P ratio) can be helpful in distinguishing the different types of inborn errors. For example, the L:P ratio is often normal (10 to 20) in PDH complex and modestly elevated in PC deficiencies, but can be greatly elevated in an ETC defect. Unlike most of the disorders previously considered in this chapter, these conditions are not detectable by newborn screening and become apparent only when a patient's symptoms are recognized.

Pyruvate Dehydrogenase Deficiency
Pyruvate Dehydrogenase Complex Deficiency

PDH is a complex of three primary enzymes— plus a phosphatase, a kinase, and at least one other element of less known function—that combine as a multimer with a very large molecular weight and a number of copies of each enzyme. The first enzymatic step is a decarboxylation reaction catalyzed by a heterodimeric system consisting of the E-1α subunit, encoded by a gene on the X-chromosome, and E-1β, which is autosomally encoded as are all the other subunits in this complex. Defects in all the known genes have been reported, but mutations in the X-linked E-1α outnumber all others by far and may represent as much as 25% of known causes in patients with CLA.

Severe PDH deficiency sometimes manifests in the neonatal period with profound lactic acidosis, elevated blood lactate and pyruvate, elevated plasma alanine, and congenital anomalies of the brain noted on MRI, including absent or underdeveloped corpus callosum, heterotopic migration deficits, and a somewhat typical dysmorphic appearance. Typically, the L:P ratio is normal and distinguishes it from disorders of the mitochondrial respiratory chain.

The patients are hypotonic and respirator dependent and have a poor prognosis. The diagnosis is rarely known immediately, and the standard intravenous support of high glucose exacerbates the metabolic acidosis and worsens the outlook for the patient. The diagnosis is inferred when all the clinical biochemical data are collated and can be confirmed by an enzymatic deficiency in lymphocytes or cultured skin fibroblasts or by mutation analysis of the E-1α gene in particular. The enzyme assay is difficult in the most experienced hands, and it is difficult to understand the high residual activity that is often recorded.

The majority of patients are more indolent on clinical presentation, with developmental delay that may resemble Leigh syndrome, and they may have a modest elevation of lactate, with pyruvate being the most telling biochemical marker of the disease. This group of patients often respond well biochemically to a high-fat and low-carbohydrate diet. Fat, as acetyl CoA, enters the energy pathway after the block, whereas glucose must traverse the PDH reaction to provide all but minimal energy generation.

Other defects of the PDH complex including two other subunits, the activating and deactivating enzymes, and a subunit X of unknown function are rare and usually result in chronic psychomotor retardation syndrome in late infancy and childhood. The E₃ subunit defect causes a unique syndrome, because the subunit is important in the PDH complex, the BCKAD complex, and the α-ketoglutarate dehydrogenase complex. Therefore these patients have multiple deficiencies involving the BCAA as in MSUD, as well as Krebs cycle metabolites that are indicative of a block in the TCA cycle. Most of the patients are later than the newborn period and have severe progressive neurodegenerative disease. The key laboratory findings are elevations of lactic acid in blood, BCAAs in plasma, and detection of α-ketoglutarate in urine by urine organic acid analysis. PDH phosphatase deficiency is a rare cause of congenital lactic acidosis. Other than the E₃ deficiency, other defects in PDH are responsive, at least biochemically to the high-fat, low-carbohydrate diet.

Pyruvate Carboxylase Deficiency

Pyruvate carboxylase is an enzyme that is involved in gluconeogenesis and that adds bicarbonate to pyruvate to form oxaloacetate, a compound also involved in replenishing intermediates of the tricarboxylic acid cycle. There are two main types of PC deficiency (De Meirleir et al, 2006; Robinson, 2001). Type A is characterized by lactic acidosis in the newborn period and delayed development. However, the disease is of a chronic nature. In type B, the catastrophic form of the disorder, the infant is acutely ill, usually in the first week of life, with encephalopathy, severe metabolic acidosis with lactic acidosis, and hyperammonemia (De Meirleir et al, 2006; Munnich et al, 2001; Robinson, 2001). The mortality rate in this form is high.

As discussed earlier, PC is a biotin-containing enzyme. Most of the patients with a type B form of PC deficiency have been of French or English origin. Unlike patients with a type A defect, in whom the blood L:P ratio is normal because both lactate and pyruvate are comparably elevated, patients with the type B defect often have an elevated L:P ratio. Because of the importance of the PC product

oxaloacetate in providing adequate cellular levels of aspartate, citrulline metabolism in the urea cycle is defective, leading to elevations of plasma citrulline and plasma ammonium concentrations. Although PC is also an important enzyme in gluconeogenesis, hypoglycemia has not been commonly reported. The liver may be enlarged. There is no effective treatment for PC deficiency when it is associated with progressive neurodegeneration. The gene that encodes the PC subunits, of which four combine to make an active enzyme, has been cloned and sequenced. An expanding number of mutations have been identified and provide a basis for prenatal diagnosis. PC deficiency may be detected in cultured skin fibroblasts or in liver biopsy samples.

Phosphoenolpyruvate Carboxykinase Deficiency

Phosphoenolpyruvate carboxykinase enzyme also functions in gluconeogenesis, and there are two forms in liver, one in the cytosol and the other in the mitochondrial compartment. It is an exceedingly rare disorder. Patients do not usually come to attention until childhood with hypotonia, failure to thrive, hepatomegaly, lactic acidosis, and hypoglycemia. Although there is no adequate experience in identifying the optimal therapy for these patients, it is reasonable to assume that frequent feedings and avoidance of fasting are important in avoiding severe metabolic imbalance.

Mitochondrial Respiratory Chain or Electron Transport Chain Defects

Oxidative phosphorylation is the key process performed by the mitochondria of cells. Any inborn error of metabolism that involves the tightly coupled and regulated process of mitochondrial energy metabolism may have profound effects on health and disease, because oxidative phosphorylation is the process by which we convert nutrients into energy. The various derivatives of the nutrients, such as pyruvate and fatty acids, are converted to CO_2 in mitochondria. The energy derived from such controlled chemical combustion is harnessed by allowing the reducing equivalents (in the form of NADH or the reduced form of flavin adenine dinucleotide [FADH₂], which are derived from such metabolism) to combine with oxygen to form water, and in the process the synthesis of ATP is coupled to the orderly flow of electrons down the respiratory chain components.

The important components in the mitochondrial respiratory chain are complex 1 (NADH dehydrogenase), complex 2 (ETF dehydrogenase), complex 3 (cytochromes b, c_1) and the terminal complex in this chain, and complex 4, which is cytochrome c oxidase (COX) (Shoffner, 1995). In addition, there is a complex 5, or ATP synthetase, and an adenine nucleotide translocase, which permits transport of adenosine diphosphate into and ATP out of the mitochondria. Complex 2 is involved primarily in fatty acid oxidation and oxidation of succinate derived from the Krebs cycle, because the reducing equivalents extracted from fatty acids, glutaric acid, and succinate flow from ETF into complex 2. The polypeptides that compose these various complexes are derived from both the nuclear genes and the genes on mitochondrial DNA (mtDNA). Except for complex 2, mtDNA is important in production of the subunits of all the respiratory chain complexes. CLA involving the ETC components has been associated with both nuclear and mtDNA mutations. In addition to the actual complex components, there are many more genes responsible for the assembly of various subunits into the functional complexes, all of which are encoded in nuclear DNA (nDNA). There are estimates that defects in any one of more than 500 genes can result in an ETC deficiency.

On the basis of molecular diagnostic testing, the oxidative phosphorylation diseases can be divided into the following four genetic groups (Shoffner, 1995):

- Group 1: nDNA mutations
- Group 2: mtDNA point mutations
- Group 3: mtDNA deletions and duplications
- Group 4: unidentified genetic defects

The relationship between phenotype and mtDNA mutations is not straightforward, probably because of the phenomenon of heteroplasmy. Mitochondria with their unique mtDNA are inherited solely from the mother. Random segregation of mitochondria having mtDNA mutations leads to heteroplasmy and, ultimately, a variable concentration of defective mitochondria within cells and among tissues (Wallace et al, 1988). Much of our understanding of the detailed molecular mechanisms that contribute to or produce the ETC gene disturbances concern the mtDNA mutations, although the application of molecular methodology and increasingly inexpensive mass sequencing is allowing more definition of the nDNA disorders that compose the majority of the ETC disease seen in newborn and infancy periods. With the exceptions of the neurogenic muscle weakness, ataxia, and retinitis pigmentosa (NARP caused predominantly by mutations at position 8993 of the mitochondrial genome), only a minority of the mtDNA defects actually are known to manifest in the newborn period (Wong, 2007). Other examples of syndromes caused by mtDNA mutations are the MELAS (mitochondrial encephalopathy, lactic acidosis, and stroke-like—episodes position 3243), MERRF (myoclonic epilepsy with ragged-red—fiber position A8344G), Leber hereditary optic neuropathy (Wallace et al, 1988), and sporadic deletion–duplication syndromes such as Pearson syndrome (Di Donato, 2009). The diseases that affect young infants are benign infantile mitochondrial myopathy, cardiomyopathy, or both; lethal infantile mitochondrial disease; lethal infantile cardiomyopathy; subacute necrotizing encephalomyopathy (SNE) or Leigh disease; Pearson syndrome; Alpers' disease; and the most dramatic form, with presentation often in the first few days of life, during which an acid-base disturbance dominates the clinical picture (Carrozzo et al, 2007; Gibson et al, 2008). The hallmarks of mitochondrial disease are almost always multisystem involvement and unambiguous lactate acidemia or acidosis. Although some debate exists as to whether lactate elevation is present in all mitochondrial disorders that present in life, it is a virtual requirement for such a diagnosis in newborns and early infants.

The nuclear encoded mitochondrial DNA depletion syndromes, which may include fatal hepatopathy, are caused by mutations in the *SUCLG1*, *SUCLA2*, *MPV17*, *RRM2B*, *PEO1*, *TP*, *POLG1*, *DGUOK*, and *TK2* genes. The ribosomal translational defects (*EFG1* and *EFTμ* genes) are the relatively new groups of mitochondrial diseases (Di Donato, 2009; DiMauro and Schon, 2008). Both are part of the group I genetic disease types.

The diagnostic tools to unravel these disorders have proliferated recently. We assess lactate in the CSF after lumbar puncture, lactate (among other metabolites) in the brain by magnetic resonance spectroscopy (MRS) during an MRI, more readily obtained in a sick newborn than previously, and DNA technology that has become faster and less expensive and includes full sequencing of the mitochondrial genome. Older and still useful technologies such as muscle biopsy with histologic analysis by light and electron microscopy, mitochondrial complex assay on either fresh (preferred, but infrequently available) or flash-frozen tissue and skin fibroblast studies are still available. In fatal cases, a rapid autopsy and proper preservation of tissue specimens are essential. Finally, a newer and increasingly frequently diagnosed family of disorders includes mitochondrial depletion syndromes caused by a number of genetic defects in the mtDNA synthesis apparatus or the availability of nucleotides. A less frequent, newly recognized family of disorders are the coenzyme Q biosynthetic disorders, diagnosed reliably only by coenzyme Q_{10} levels in muscle, and not in plasma.

Although the subject of much debate, there is no credible evidence that mitochondrial disease is treatable, with the obvious exception of a small minority caused by coenzyme Q deficiency. Given the inability to identify these patients quickly, it is reasonable to treat acutely ill patients with presumed mitochondrial disorders with high doses of coenzyme Q. However, indiscriminant use of this cofactor is to be discouraged.

Benign Infantile Mitochondrial Myopathy, Cardiomyopathy, or Both

Benign infantile mitochondrial myopathy is associated with congenital hypotonia and weakness at birth, feeding difficulties, respiratory difficulties, and lactic acidosis. In this poorly understood, developmental-like disorder, only skeletal muscle appears to be affected, and histochemical analyses show a COX deficiency that returns to normal levels after 1 to 3 years of age. An nDNA mutation in a gene important in a fetal isoform of an ETC polypeptide specific for muscle oxidative phosphorylation was hypothesized to be the cause of this problem. A developmental switch from the defective fetal gene to the adult form may be responsible for the gradual improvement. It was thought to be the only example of a developmental defect in oxidative phosphorylation that is probably nuclear encoded and in which the treatment is only supportive during the early newborn period to prevent death from respiratory disease. However, a recent study suggests that the etiology may be a maternally inherited, homoplasmic m.14674T>C mt_tRNA^{Glu}: mutation (Horvath et al, 2009).

The form also associated with cardiomyopathy may be a variant of the benign isolated myopathy and involves striated muscle in both skeletal and cardiac muscle. It manifests in the newborn period with lactic acidosis and a cardiomyopathy that improves during the first year of life. The exact gene defect is unknown. More attention must be paid to these two disease entities, because with early optimal medical care, affected infants may have an excellent prognosis.

Lethal Infantile Mitochondrial Disease

Infants with lethal infantile mitochondrial disease are severely ill in the first few days or weeks of life or in the extended newborn period. They exhibit hypotonia,

CASE STUDY

A boy was born to nonconsanguinous, healthy parents after a full-term gestation. Biventricular hypertrophy with a predominant right-sided component had been observed on fetal ultrasonography at 24 weeks' gestation. He was delivered by cesarean section because of variable decelerations, and he emerged without meconium staining or passage. Respiratory distress developed shortly after birth. An echocardiogram showed concentric right ventricular hypertrophy with elevated right ventricular pressure (70 mm Hg). Initial laboratory studies showed acute metabolic acidosis (blood lactate >18 mmol/L; arterial pH, 6.91).

His weight was 2.36 kg (10th percentile), his length was 46 cm (5th percentile), and his head circumference was 31 cm (5th percentile). He had a right ventricular heave and an intermittent fourth heart sound. There was no liver enlargement. Muscle bulk was normal, and deep tendon reflexes were intact. Metabolic investigations showed persistent arterial lactic acidemia (range, 3 to 11 μmol/L) with increased pyruvate (range, 0.02 to 0.44 μmol/L). The L:P ratio ranged from 25 to 290. The activities of the respiratory chain complexes II, III, and IV were normal in cultured skin fibroblasts. A left quadriceps muscle biopsy was used for histochemical analysis and to prepare a 10% extract for respiratory chain studies. Histochemical analysis showed no ragged-red fibers with the modified Gomori trichrome stain, but a diffusely weak response to staining for cytochrome c oxidase (COX, ETC complex 4). Biochemical analysis showed markedly reduced COX activity, contrasting with normal activities of other complexes. Direct sequencing of the three COXs and all 22 transfer RNA genes of mtDNA, all the COX-assembly

nuclear genes known to harbor pathogenic mutations (*SURF1, SC01, SCO2, COX10,* and *COX15*), and the two other nuclear ancillary genes (*COX11* and *COX17*) showed no mutations. Southern blot analysis showed no deletions, but results were inconclusive regarding mtDNA depletion. However, sequencing of the two genes known to be associated with the myopathic (Saada et al, 2001) and the hepatocerebral (Mandel et al, 2001) mtDNA depletion syndromes (*TK2* and *dGK*) did not show any mutations.

A series of echocardiograms documented biventricular, hypertrophic, nonobstructive cardiomyopathy. The patient died on the seventh hospital day after a sudden episode of hemoglobin desaturation. An autopsy was performed 4 hours after death. The right ventricle was found to be thickened and enlarged, with relative sparing of the left side. The pulmonary vasculature of the lungs showed hypertrophy that extended to the most distal vessels. Routine microscopic findings in skeletal muscle were normal, and the CNS was without microscopic or macroscopic abnormalities.

This baby had a fatal syndrome defined clinically by prenatal cardiomyopathy and severe pulmonary hypertension in the newborn period. The syndrome was caused by isolated ETC complex 4 deficiency. The pathophysiology centered on the heart and lungs. How much disease was caused by the involvement of other organs remains unclear. This case is an example of a mitochondrial metabolic disorder, but without a specific molecular genetic cause. A more extensive evaluation by current methods might or might not have revealed a diagnosis.

---

muscle weakness, failure to thrive, and severe lactic acidosis. Death often occurs by 6 months of age and almost always is associated with overwhelming lactic acidosis. Skeletal muscle shows lipid and glycogen accumulation and abnormally shaped mitochondria on electron microscopic examination. Hepatic dysfunction may be a prominent finding in these patients. Generalized proximal renal tubular dysfunction may occur, leading to the renal Fanconi syndrome. The ETC defects reported in these patients include defects in complexes 1, 3, and 4. Original reports concerned infants with a phenotype resembling severe Werdnig-Hoffman disease with COX deficiency and renal Fanconi syndrome.

Lethal Infantile Cardiomyopathy

Defects of the mitochondrial respiratory chain have varied neonatal presentations and are commonly caused by isolated COX deficiency (Shoffner, 1995). Clinical features of COX deficiency reflect involvement of one or more tissues and include encephalopathy, myopathy, cardiomyopathy, liver disease, and nephropathy (Munnich et al, 2001). The heterogeneous clinical features are due, in part, to the dual genetic control of COX. The three catalytic subunits—COX I, COX II, COX III—are encoded by mtDNA, whereas the remaining subunits (COX IV to COX VIII) are encoded by nDNA. In addition, the proper assembly of COX requires several nDNA-encoded proteins. The various syndromes caused by COX deficiency are only partially understood at the genetic level. Most infants with isolated complex IV deficiency are likely to have nDNA gene defects in COX assembly genes, including *SURF1, SCO2, COX15, COX10, SC01,* and *LRPPRC* (Di Mauro and Schon, 2008).

Subacute Necrotizing Encephalomyelopathy or Leigh Disease

Probably because of a failure to recognize the clinical signs, infants with SNE or Leigh disease usually come to clinical attention after the newborn period. This disease is

characterized as a progressive neurodegenerative disorder with severe hypotonia, seizures, extrapyramidal movement disorders, optic atrophy, and defects in automatic ventilation or respiratory control (Finsterer, 2008; Leigh, 1951). It is clear that there are many causes of SNE. As discussed earlier, PDH complex deficiency (PDHE1 alpha-subunit and PDHX1) can lead to Leigh disease. Patients with defects in the ETC have also been reported to have findings compatible with SNE. The mtDNA mutation causing NARP is an example. Reported nuclear gene defects include ETC complex I (NDUFS1), complex II (SDHA), complex IV (SURF1, COX15), coenzyme Q_{10} biosynthetic defects, mitochondrial ribosomal translational defects, and SUCLA2. Many neuropathologists believe that the diagnosis of SNE depends on an analysis of CNS tissue at autopsy. However, MRI characteristically shows bilateral symmetrical lesions of the basal ganglia as occurs in other mitochondrial disorders.

There is no effective treatment for this disease, unless the cause is a specific inability to synthesize coenzyme Q_{10}. It is possible that most of the patients with Leigh disease have disturbances in nuclear-encoded genes. Although, as discussed later, the NARP lesion caused by a group 2 mtDNA mutation is one important cause in early infancy. Clearly, this is not one disease entity, because the specific neuropathologic findings for SNE have also been reported in a patient with Menkes' disease, in which there is a secondary ETC complex 4 deficiency, because copper is an important metal cofactor of COX.

The following clinical findings have been noted in infants with SNE: optic atrophy, ophthalmoplegia, nystagmus, respiratory abnormalities, ataxia, hypotonia, spasticity, seizures, developmental delay, psychomotor retardation, myopathy, and renal tubular dysfunction. Some patients may manifest hypertrophic cardiomyopathy, liver dysfunction, and microcephaly. The neuropathologic lesions include demyelination, gliosis, necrosis, relative neuronal sparing, and capillary proliferation in specific brain lesions.

There are lesions of the basal ganglia, which are bilaterally symmetrical, as well as of the brainstem, cerebellum, and the cerebral cortex to a lesser degree. Commonly, elevation in blood lactate is only slight to moderate, as well as intermittent, in this diverse group of patients. In some instances, lactate values may be elevated only in the CSF. The most commonly reported biochemical abnormalities are deficiencies in COX, complex 4 NADH dehydrogenase, or complex 1 and PDH. In a few rare patients, the abnormality in oxidative phosphorylation has been reported to be secondary to NARP mutation. This involves a T:C transition at base pair 8993 of the adenosine triphosphatase (ATPase) 6 gene, changing a leucine to a proline at position 156 in the ATPase 6 polypeptide. Investigators have speculated that defects such as those in COX and the NADH dehydrogenase, when associated with neuropathology of Leigh disease, are caused by nuclear gene mutations and not mtDNA gene defects such as the NARP point mutation in the ATPase 6 gene.

The diseases in group 3 (see earlier), exemplified by the Kearns-Sayre and chronic progressive external ophthalmoplegia syndromes, are genetic but not familial and are caused by mtDNA deletions or duplications that are spontaneous mutations. These disorders do not usually come to clinical attention in infancy. The only example of such a mutation manifesting in early infancy is the Pearson syndrome. This disorder is systemic and primarily affects the hematopoietic system and pancreas function. The characteristics are severe macrocytic anemia with varying degrees of neutropenia and thrombocytopenia. Bone marrow examination shows normal cellularity, but extensive vacuolization of erythroid and myeloid precursors, hemosiderosis, and ringed sideroblasts. This disease of the bone marrow can lead to death in infancy. However, patients who are able to recover or who benefit from aggressive therapy may demonstrate other signs of this systemic disorder in late infancy or childhood, such as poor growth, pancreas dysfunction, mitochondrial myopathy, lactic acidosis, and progressive neurologic damage.

Barth Syndrome

Barth syndrome is an X-linked disorder associated with cardiomyopathy, skeletal muscle disease, and neutropenia (Yen et al, 2008). Skeletal muscle shows abnormal mitochondrial morphology. Important laboratory findings include decreased plasma-free carnitine, increased urinary excretion of 3-methylglutaconate on GC-MS analysis of urine organic acids, and decreased levels of serum cholesterol in early infancy. Positional cloning identified a gene for this disorder on Xq28 that encodes for a phospholipid remodeling enzyme, cardiolipin acyl transferase. Several mutations have been identified. It has been hypothesized that the organic acid 3-methylglutaconate accumulates because of defective mitochondrial transport. Patients must be supported from birth to early infancy. It is possible that if severe cholesterol deficiency can be avoided, affected infants may survive and may be relatively free of cardiomyopathy during childhood. Of diagnostic importance, not all patients with 3-methylglutaconic aciduria have Barth syndrome. A few have isolated leucine-dependent 3-methylglutaconyl-CoA hydratase deficiency or Costeff syndrome, but most have ill-defined mitochondropathies.

Unidentified Genetic Defects

A number of diseases are believed to be caused by mitochondrial respiratory chain problems, but the specific mutations remain unknown. These disorders constitute the group 4 mutations, or the disorders of unknown inheritance (Shoffner, 1995). Alpers disease was once one such example. It has also been called *progressive infantile poliodystrophy*. Infants and children with this progressive disease experience progressive cerebral cortical damage, sometimes also involving the cerebellum, basal ganglia, and brainstem; in some, liver disease may progress to cirrhosis. The neuropathologic lesions consist of spongiform or microcystic cerebral degeneration, gliosis, necrosis, and capillary proliferation Seizures are prominent, including myoclonus. Laboratory abnormalities include abnormal NADH oxidation or complex 1 defects, impaired pyruvate handling, PDH complex deficiency, TCA cycle malfunction, and decreased mitochondrial cytochrome $a + a_3$ content. This disorder is caused by mutations in one or more gene defects associated with mtDNA depletion, such as the autosomal recessive disease caused by mutations in the DNA polymerase gamma 1 (*POLG1*) gene and can usually be defined by mutation analysis.

Early Lethal Lactic Acidosis

In an unknown fraction of patients with primary disturbances in mitochondrial oxidative phosphorylation or ETC defects, massive lactic acidosis develops within 24 to 72 hours after birth. Commonly the condition is untreatable, because it is relentless and unresponsive to alkali therapy. Dialysis is a remedy but not a cure. Often, affected infants have no obvious organ damage early in the course or evidence of malformations; this is also true for infants with the PDH complex deficiency, which is probably a more common cause of overwhelming acidosis in the first week of life. In addition, acidemia per se can easily cause the coma or impaired cardiac contractility that may be encountered. Some infants have survived with aggressive therapy.

The care of babies with these different forms of severe lactic acidosis almost always brings an ethical dilemma to the forefront for physicians and nurses of the neonatal intensive care unit as well as for the babies' families. To further complicate the issues, enzymatic and molecular analyses usually are not immediately available. The disease in most patients probably remains idiopathic, and no DNA mutation, nuclear or mitochondrial, will be identified without extensive, expensive, and extremely inconvenient and Herculean efforts. A rigid approach to care is impractical and unwise. Decisions regarding management must be individualized, because the mitochondrial dysfunction and resultant pathophysiology can vary among infants.

SUGGESTED READINGS

Blau N, Hoffmann GF, Leonard J, et al, editors: *Physicians guide to the treatment and follow-up of metabolic diseases*, Heidelberg, 2006, Springer.
Fernandes J, Saudubray JM, Van den Berghe G, et al: *Inborn Metabolic diseases: diagnosis and treatment*, Heidelberg, 2006, Springer.
Scriver CR, Beaudet AL, Sly WS, et al: *The metabolic and molecular bases of inherited disease*. ed 8, New York, 2001, McGraw-Hill. Updated material is available online at www.ommbid.com.

Complete references used in this text can be found online at www.expertconsult.com

LYSOSOMAL STORAGE, PEROXISOMAL, AND GLYCOSYLATION DISORDERS AND SMITH-LEMLI-OPITZ SYNDROME IN THE NEONATE

Janet A. Thomas, Carol L. Greene, and Gerard T. Berry

Lysosomal storage diseases (LSDs), peroxisomal disorders, congenital disorders of glycosylation (CDGs), and Smith-Lemli-Opitz (SLO) syndrome are single-gene disorders, most of which demonstrate autosomal recessive inheritance. The combined incidence of LSDs has been reported to be 1 in 1500 to 8000 live births in the United States, Europe, and Australia (Fletcher, 2006; Meikle et al, 2006; Staretz-Chacham et al, 2009; Stone and Sidransky, 1999; Wenger et al, 2003; Winchester et al, 2000). The incidence of peroxisomal disorders is estimated to be more than 1 in 20,000. The most current estimate for SLO syndrome is 1 in 20,000, and a similar frequency of 1 in 20,000 is estimated for the congenital disorders of glycosylation.

These four categories of metabolic diseases involve molecules important in cell membranes and share overlapping clinical presentations. Clinical presentations are heterogeneous, with a broad range of age at presentation and severity of symptoms. All are chronic and progressive. Age of onset varies from prenatal to adulthood, and severity can range from severe disability and early death to nearly normal lifestyle and life span. For each condition, interfamilial variability is greater than intrafamilial variability. The genetic and clinical characteristics of conditions in these categories that can manifest in the neonatal period (except Pompe disease, which is addressed in Chapter 22) are also summarized in Tables 23-1 to 23-3.

Important presentations that should lead the neonatologist to consider these disorders in the differential diagnosis are as follows:

1. In utero infection—hepatosplenomegaly and hepatopathy, possibly with extramedullary hematopoiesis
2. Nonimmune hydrops fetalis, ichthyotic or collodion skin, or both
3. Neurologic only—early and often difficult to control seizures, hypertonia or hypotonia, with or without altered head size and with or without eye findings
4. Coarse facial features with bone changes, dysostosis multiplex, or osteoporosis
5. Dysmorphic facial features with or without major malformations
6. Rarely, known family history or positive prenatal diagnosis

Only for the last three presentations are these conditions likely to be considered early in the differential diagnosis. Most babies with these conditions are born to healthy, nonconsanguineous couples with normal family histories, and these disorders are usually considered late, if at all, as in Case Study 1.

LYSOSOMAL STORAGE DISORDERS

Lysosomes are single-membrane–bound intracellular organelles that contain enzymes called *hydrolases*. These lysosomal enzymes are responsible for splitting large molecules into simple, low-molecular-weight compounds, which can be recycled. The materials digested by lysosomes and derived from endocytosis and phagocytosis, are separated from other intracellular materials by the process of autophagy, which is the main mechanism whereby endogenous molecules are delivered to lysosomes. The common element of all compounds digested by lysosomal enzymes is that they contain a carbohydrate portion attached to a protein or lipid. These glycoconjugates include glycoproteins, glycosaminoglycans, and glycolipids.

Glycolipids are large molecules with carbohydrates attached to a lipid moiety. Sphingolipids, globosides, gangliosides, cerebrosides, and lipid sulfates all are glycolipids. The different classes of glycolipids are distinguished from one another primarily by different polar groups at C1. Sphingolipids are complex membrane lipids composed of one molecule each of the amino alcohol sphingosine, a long-chain fatty acid, and various polar head groups attached by a β-glycosidic linkage. Sphingolipids occur in the blood and nearly all tissues of the body, the highest concentration being found in white matter of the central nervous system (CNS). In addition, various sphingolipids are components of the plasma membrane of practically all cells. The core structure of natural sphingolipids is ceramide, a long-chain fatty acid amide derivative of sphingosine. Free ceramide, an intermediate in the biosynthesis and catabolism of glycosphingolipids and sphingomyelin, composes 16% to 20% of normal lipid content of stratum corneum of the skin. Sphingomyelin, a ceramide phosphocholine, is one of the principal structural lipids of membranes of nervous tissue.

Cerebrosides are a group of ceramide monohexosides with a single sugar, either glucose or galactose, and an additional sulfate group on galactose. The two most common cerebrosides are galactocerebroside and glucocerebroside. The largest concentration of galactocerebroside is found in the brain. Glucocerebroside is an intermediate in the synthesis and degradation of more complex glycosphingolipids.

Gangliosides, the most complex class of glycolipids, contain several sugar units and one or more sialic acid residues. Gangliosides are normal components of cell membranes and are found in high concentrations in ganglion cells of the CNS, particularly in nerve endings and dendrites. G_{MI} is the major ganglioside in brain of vertebrates.

CASE STUDY 1

C.J. was a 2200-g girl, born to a 24-year-old mother (third pregnancy, second viable child) after a 32-week gestation, by cesarean section performed for fetal distress. Pregnancy was complicated by the finding on ultrasonography of fetal hydrops and ascites and possible hepatosplenomegaly at 24 weeks' gestation. Fetal blood sampling showed a hematocrit of 31% and elevations of γ-glutamyl-transferase and aspartate transaminase values. Results of viral studies were negative, and chromosomes were normal. At delivery, the infant was limp and blue with a heart rate of 60 beats/min. Physical examination and chest radiograph showed marked abdominal distention, hepatosplenomegaly, multiple petechiae and bruises, a bell-shaped thorax, generalized hypotonia, talipes equinovarus, contractures at the knees, a large heart, and hazy lung fields with low volumes. Disseminated intravascular coagulopathy and evidence of liver disease developed rapidly, with elevated aspartate transaminase, γ-glutamyl-transferase, and increasing hyperbilirubinemia. The patient's condition was maintained with a ventilator and treatment with antibiotics for possible sepsis.

Results of evaluations for bacterial and viral agents were negative. Metabolic studies, including ammonia, lactate, very long chain fatty acids (VLCFAs), and urine amino and organic acids, yielded unremarkable measurements. The white blood cells were noted to have marked toxic granularity consistent with overwhelming bacterial sepsis or metabolic storage disease.

The patient experienced continued cardiorespiratory deterioration, had bilateral pneumothoraces and pneumopericardium, and died on the third day of life. Consent for autopsy was obtained from the family. A standard autopsy was performed and showed the presence of large, membrane-bound vacuoles within hepatocytes, endothelial cells, pericytes, and bone marrow stromal cells, which are typical of a metabolic storage disorder. Similar cells were also found within the placenta. There was no evidence of an infectious cause. Unfortunately, because a lysosomal storage disorder was not considered as a possible cause at the time of death, no frozen tissue or cultured fibroblasts were available to pursue the diagnosis. As a result of efforts by a research laboratory and the recurrence of disease in the couple's subsequent pregnancy, a diagnosis of β-glucuronidase deficiency, or mucopolysaccharidosis type VII, was confirmed.

CASE STUDY 2

M.E. was born by normal spontaneous vaginal delivery, at full term according to dates based on early ultrasonography, with weight of 2.2 kg, length of 45 cm, and head circumference of 31.5 cm. On the basis of physical examination, gestational age was assessed as 36 weeks. A heart murmur was noted, and investigation showed the presence of a small ventricular septal defect with no hemodynamic significance. Submucous cleft palate was noted. Examination for dysmorphic features showed simple, posteriorly rotated ears, mild epicanthic folds, micrognathia, and unilateral simian crease. Tone was moderately decreased. Irritability and severe feeding problems were noted, and gavage feeding was required; growth was poor despite adequate calories. The results of a karyotype analysis were normal, and the results of studies for velocardiofacial syndrome were negative. Vomiting developed, and further evaluation showed no acidosis, hypoglycemia, or hyperammonemia. Liver-associated values and cholesterol level were normal, as were results of studies of amino acids, organic acids, and acylcarnitine profile. Vomiting became more severe and did not respond to elemental formula, and pyloric stenosis was detected. Feeding problems persisted after successful surgical correction. Delivery of more than 140 kcal/kg by gavage was poorly tolerated, but resulted in weight gain; however, length and head growth remained poor.

SLO syndrome was suggested despite the normal cholesterol value obtained on analysis in the hospital laboratory. Studies performed in a specialized laboratory showed the 7- and 8-dehydrocholesterol values to be elevated and the cholesterol value decreased. Cholesterol supplementation led to some improvement in behavior and feeding. A decrease to 110 kcal/kg/day was tolerated without worsening of growth, and weight for height gradually returned to normal. A review of records confirmed that the pregnancy had been accurately dated by ultrasonography at 10 weeks' gestation, confirming that M.E. was small for gestational age and microcephalic at birth, with subsequent growth typical for SLO syndrome. The incorrect assessment of gestational age as 36 weeks on examination was found to result from a failure to appreciate the effect of hypotonia on the findings for gestational age. The family was counseled about autosomal recessive inheritance, including the availability of prenatal diagnosis.

CASE STUDY 3

H.K. was born at term to healthy parents by cesarean section performed for breech presentation after an otherwise uncomplicated pregnancy. Hypotonia and dysmorphic features were noted in the delivery room, including inner epicanthic folds, flat occiput, large fontanels, shallow orbital ridges, low nasal bridge, micrognathia, redundant skin folds at the neck, and unilateral simian crease. Brushfield spots were present. Investigation of a heart murmur revealed patent ductus arteriosus and a small atrial septal defect. There was mild hepatomegaly but normal liver function, no acidosis, and no hypoglycemia. Suck was poor, and gavage feeding was required.

Karyotype was normal and there was no evidence of trisomy 21 in blood in 50 interphase cells examined. The option of skin biopsy to search further for evidence of mosaicism for trisomy 21 was considered. Thyroid function values were normal. Urine amino and organic acid values were normal, as was the acylcarnitine profile. Plasma VLCFA analysis showed elevation consistent with a diagnosis of Zellweger syndrome, along with a typical increase in pipecolic acid value and impaired capacity for fibroblast synthesis of plasmalogens. The baby died at 3 months of age, and autopsy showed polymicrogyria and small hepatic and renal cysts. The family was counseled about autosomal recessive inheritance, including the availability of prenatal diagnosis.

Gangliosides function as receptors for toxic agents, hormones, and certain viruses, are involved in cell differentiation, and they can also have a role in cell-cell interaction by providing specific recognition determinants on the surface of cells.

Ceramide oligosaccharides (i.e., globosides) are a family of cerebrosides that contain two or more sugar residues, usually galactose, glucose, or *N*-acetylgalactosamine. Glycosaminoglycans and oligosaccharides are essential constituents of connective tissue, parenchymal organs, cartilage, and the nervous system.

Glycosaminoglycans, also called *mucopolysaccharides*, are complex heterosaccharides consisting of long sugar chains rich in sulfate groups. The polymeric chains are bound to specific proteins (core proteins). Glycoproteins contain oligosaccharide chains (long sugar molecules) attached covalently to a peptide core. Glycosylation occurs in the endoplasmic reticulum and Golgi apparatus. Most glycoproteins are secreted from cells and include transport proteins, glycoprotein hormones, complement factors, enzymes, and enzyme inhibitors. There is extensive diversity in the composition and structure of oligosaccharides.

CASE STUDY 4

M.J. had hypotonia at birth after an uncomplicated pregnancy. Minor dysmorphic features were noted, including high nasal bridge, large ears, and inverted nipples. Feeding difficulties were significant, and growth was poor. Findings on head ultrasonography were unremarkable, as were those of head magnetic resonance imaging, although the radiologist questioned whether the cerebellum might be slightly small. Results of a karyotype analysis were normal. Hypothyroidism, discovered on newborn screening, was promptly treated and closely monitored. There was no acidosis or hypoglycemia, and liver enzyme values were normal; results of amino and organic acid analyses and acylcarnitine profile were all normal.

The baby was discharged on a diet providing 130 kcal/kg/day. On follow-up, growth remained poor, and development was severely delayed. At 6 months of age, she was admitted to the hospital for an episode of acutely altered mental status and low blood pressure. Mild acidosis, borderline elevations of lactate and ammonia, and significant elevation of liver enzymes all resolved over the course

of the hospital stay. Cardiac ultrasonography showed mild ventricular dysfunction, which also resolved. Amino and organic acid values were normal, as was the acylcarnitine profile. Urine oligosaccharide levels showed an unusual pattern, and urine mucopolysaccharide values were normal.

At 2 years of age, developmental delay remained marked, and hypotonia persisted with reflexes absent. The creatinine phosphokinase level was normal, but liver function values were again abnormal. Because mitochondrial disease was suspected, the patient was scheduled for liver biopsy, but clotting values were abnormal. A congenital disorder of glycosylation was suspected, and a transferrin assay confirmed the diagnosis. A review of neonatal records revealed a comment from a neurology consultant about the unusual distribution of fat on the buttocks and thighs of M.J. as a neonate. The family was counseled about autosomal recessive inheritance, including availability of prenatal diagnosis.

The degradation of glycolipids, glycosaminoglycans, and glycoproteins takes place especially within lysosomes of phagocytic cells, related to histiocytes and macrophages, in any tissue or organ. A series of hydrolytic enzymes cleaves specific bonds, resulting in sequential, stepwise removal of constituents such as sugars and sulfate, and degrading complex glycoconjugates to the level of their basic building blocks. Lysosomal storage diseases most commonly result when an inherited defect causes significantly decreased activity in one of these hydrolases. Other causes are failure of transport of an enzyme, substrate, or product. Whatever the specific cause, incompletely metabolized molecules accumulate, especially within the tissue responsible for catabolism of the glycoconjugate. Additional excess storage material may be excreted in urine. The mechanisms of cellular dysfunction and damage in the majority of LSDs remain unknown. Various hypotheses have been offered, such as a pivotal disturbance in the normal process of autophagy (Ballabio and Gieselmann, 2009; Kiselyov et al, 2007). In this pathophysiologic construct, endoplasmic reticulum membrane engulfment of cellular components, such as mitochondrial derivatives targeted for destruction, is perturbed. As a consequence, deleterious pathways become activated, leading to unwanted ubiquitination of targeted molecules and apoptosis.

Lysosomal storage diseases are classified according to the stored compound. Clinical phenotype depends partially on the type and amount of storage substance. There are more than 50 different LSDs and a significant fraction, approximately 20 LSDs, may have manifestations in the newborn infant (Staretz-Chocham et al, 2009). The disorders selected for discussion in this chapter are all known to manifest in the neonatal period.

CLINICAL PRESENTATIONS

Table 23-1 summarizes the clinical characteristics of the neonatal presentations of lysosomal storage disorders.

Niemann-Pick A Disease (Acute, Sphingomyelinase Deficient)
Etiology

Niemann-Pick A disease is caused by a deficiency of sphingomyelinase. Sphingomyelinase catalyzes the breakdown of sphingomyelin to ceramide and phosphocholine, and

its deficiency results in sphingomyelin storage within lysosomes. Cholesterol is also stored, suggesting that its metabolism is tied to that of sphingomyelin. Sphingomyelin normally composes 5% to 20% of phospholipid in liver, spleen, and brain, but in these disorders it can compose up to 70% of phospholipids. Patients with Niemann-Pick A disease usually have enzyme activity less than 5% of normal.

Clinical Features

Clinical features of this disorder may appear in utero or up to 1 year of age. Affected infants usually have massive hepatosplenomegaly (hepatomegaly greater than splenomegaly), constipation, feeding difficulties, and vomiting with consequent failure to thrive. Patients eventually appear strikingly emaciated with a protuberant abdomen and thin extremities. Neurologic disease is evident by 6 months of age, with hypotonia, decrease or absence of deep tendon reflexes, and weakness. Loss of motor skills, spasticity, rigidity, and loss of vision and hearing occur later. Seizures are rare. A retinal cherry-red spot is present in about half of cases, and the electroretinographic findings are abnormal. Respiratory infections are common. The skin may have an ochre or brownish yellow color, and xanthomas have been observed. Radiographic findings consist of widening of medullary cavities, cortical thinning of long bones, and osteoporosis. In the brain and spinal cord, neuronal storage is widespread, leading to cytoplasmic swelling together with atrophy of cerebellum. Bone marrow and tissue biopsy samples may show foam cells or sea-blue histiocytes, which represent lipid-laden cells of the monocyte-macrophage system. Similarly, vacuolated lymphocytes or monocytes may be present in peripheral blood. Tissue cholesterol levels may be threefold to tenfold of normal, and patients may have a microcytic anemia and thrombocytopenia. Death occurs by 2 to 3 years of age.

Niemann-Pick C Disease
Etiology

Niemann-Pick C disease is caused by an error in the intracellular transport of exogenous low-density lipoprotein (LDL)–derived cholesterol, which leads to impaired esterification of cholesterol and trapping of unesterified cholesterol in lysosomes. The incidence may be higher than

TABLE 23-1 Lysosomal Storage Disorders in the Newborn Period: Genetic and Clinical Characteristics of Neonatal Presentation

Disorder	Onset	Facies	Neurologic Findings	Distinctive Features	Eye Findings	Cardiovascular Findings	Dysostosis Multiplex	Hepatomegaly/ Splenomegaly	Defect	Gene Location Molecular Findings	Ethnic Predilection
Niemann-Pick A disease	Early infancy	Frontal bossing	Difficulty feeding, apathy, deafness, blindness, hypotonia	Brownish-yellow skin, xanthomas	Cherry-red spot (50%)	−	−	++/+	Sphingomyelinase deficiency	ASM gene at 11p15.1-p15.4 3 of 18 mutations account for approximately 92% of mutant alleles in the Ashkenazi population	1:40,000 in Ashkenazi Jews with carrier frequency of 1:60
Niemann-Pick C disease	Birth to 3 mo	Normal	Developmental delay, vertical gaze paralysis, hypotonia, later spasticity	−	−			+/++	Abnormal cholesterol esterification	$NPC1$ gene at 18q11 accounts for >95% of cases; $HE1$ gene mutations may account for remaining cases	Increased in French Canadians of Nova Scotia and Spanish Americans in the southwest United States
Gaucher disease type 2	In utero to 6 mo	Normal	Poor suck and swallow, weak cry, squint, trismus, strabismus, opsoclonus, hypertonic, later flaccidity	Congenital ichthyosis, collodion skin	−	−	−	+/++	Glucocerebrosidase deficiency	1q21; large number of mutations known; five mutations account for approximately 97% of mutant alleles in the Ashkenazi population, but approximately 75% in the non-Jewish population	Panethnic
Krabbe disease	3-6 mo	Normal	Irritability, tonic spasms with light or noise stimulation, seizures, hypertonia, later flaccidity	Increased CSF protein	Optic atrophy	−	−	−/−	Galactocerebrosidase deficiency	14q 24.3-q32.1; >60 mutations with some common mutations in specific populations	Increased in Scandinavian countries and in a large Druze kindred in Israel
G_{M1} gangliosidosis	Birth	Coarse	Poor suck, weak cry, lethargy, exaggerated startle, blindness, hypotonia, later spasticity	Gingival hypertrophy, edema, rashes	Cherry-red spot (50%)	−	+	+/+	β-Galactosidase deficiency	3 pter-3p21; heterogeneous mutations; common mutations in specific populations	Panethnic
Farber disease type I	2 wk to 4 mo	Normal	Progressive psychomotor impairment, seizures, decreased reflexes, hypotonia	Joint swelling with nodules, hoarseness, lung disease, contractures, fever, granulomas, dysphagia, vomiting, increased CSF protein	Grayish opacification surrounding retina in some patients, subtle cherry-red spot	Occasional	−	Hepatomegaly in 50%, splenomegaly less common	Lysosomal acid ceramidase	8p21.3-22; 9 disease-causing mutations identified	Panethnic

Disorder	Age at onset	Facial/somatic	Neurologic	Clinical findings	Eye	Cardiac		HSM	Defect	Gene/locus	Ethnicity
Farber disease types II and III	Birth to 9 mo (≤20 mo)	Normal		Joint swelling with nodules, hoarseness	Normal macula, corneal opacities	−	−	HSM less common than in type I		8p21.3-p22	Panethnic
Farber disease type IV (neonatal)	Birth	Normal		Nodules not consistent findings	Corneal opacities (1/3)	−	−	++/++		Unknown	Panethnic
Congenital sialidosis	In utero to birth	Coarse, edema	Mental retardation, hypotonia	Neonatal ascites, inguinal hernias, renal disease	Corneal clouding	−	+	+/+	Neuraminidase deficiency	*NEU 1* gene (sialidase) at 6p21	Panethnic
Galactosialidosis	In utero to birth	Coarse	Mental retardation, occasional deafness, hypotonia	Ascites, edema, inguinal hernias, renal disease, telangiectasias	Cherry-red spot, corneal clouding	Cardiomegaly progressing to failure	+	+/+	Absence of a protective protein that safeguards neuraminidase and beta-galactosidase from premature degradation	20q13.1	Panethnic
Wolman disease	First weeks of life	Normal	Mental deterioration	Vomiting, diarrhea, steatorrhea, abdominal distention, failure to thrive, anemia, adrenal calcifications	−	−	−	+/+	Lysosomal acid lipase deficiency	10q23.2-q23.3; variety of mutations identified	Increased in Iranian Jews and in non-Jewish and Arab populations of Galilee
Infantile sialic acid storage disease	In utero to birth	Coarse, dysmorphic	Mental retardation, hypotonia	Ascites, anemia, diarrhea, failure to thrive	−	Congestive heart failure	+	+/+	Defective transport of sialic acid out of the lysosome	*SLC17A5* gene at 6q	Panethnic
I-cell disease	In utero to birth	Coarse	Mental retardation, deafness	Gingival hyperplasia, restricted joint mobility, hernias	Corneal clouding	Valvular disease, congestive heart failure, cor pulmonale	++	+++/+++	Lysosomal enzymes lack mannose-6-PO$_4$ recognition marker and fail to enter the lysosome (phosphotransferase deficiency, 3-subunit complex $[\alpha_2\,\beta_2\,\gamma_2]$)	Enzyme encoded by two genes; α and β subunits encoded by gene at 12p; γ subunit encoded by gene at 16p	Panethnic
Mucolipidosis type IV	Birth to 3 mo	Normal	Mental retardation, hypotonia	—	Severe corneal clouding, retinal degeneration, blindness	−	−	−/−	Unknown; some patients with partial deficiency of ganglioside sialidase	*MCOLN1* gene at 19p13.2-13.3 encoding mucolipin; two founder mutations accounting for 95% of mutant alleles in Ashkenazi population	Increased in Ashkenazi Jews
Mucopolysaccharidosis type VII	In utero to childhood	Variable coarseness	Mild to severe mental retardation	Hernias	Variable corneal clouding	Variable	++	Variable	β-Glucuronidase deficiency	*GUSB* gene at 7q21.2-q22; heterogeneous mutations	Panethnic

−, Not seen; +, typically present, usually not severe; ++, usually present, and moderately severe; +++, always present, usually severe; *CSF*, cerebrospinal fluid; *HSM*, hepatosplenomegaly.

1 in 150,000 births (Wraith et al, 2009). Cell lines from patients can be divided into two complementation groups, NPC1 and NPC2, corresponding to different genes (Millat et al, 2001). In each group, the primary defect is abnormal cholesterol esterification, but the enzyme responsible for cholesterol esterification—acetyl coenzyme A (CoA) acetyltransferase (ACAT)—is not deficient. The storage of sphingomyelin is secondary. It has been suggested that the defect is in transport of cholesterol out of the lysosome, making cholesterol unavailable to ACAT (Natowicz et al, 1995). Sphingomyelinase activity appears normal or elevated in most tissues, but is partially deficient (60% to 70%) in fibroblasts from most patients with this disorder. Storage of sphingomyelin in tissues is much less than in Niemann-Pick A or B disease and is accompanied by additional storage of unesterified cholesterol, phospholipids, and glycolipids in the liver and spleen. Only glycolipids are increased in the brain.

Clinical Features

The age of onset, clinical features, and natural history of Niemann-Pick C disease are highly variable. Onset can occur from birth to 18 years of age. Fifty percent of children with onset in the neonatal period have conjugated hyperbilirubinemia, which usually resolves spontaneously but is followed by neurologic symptoms later in childhood. In the severe infantile form, hepatosplenomegaly is common, accompanied by hypotonia and delayed motor development. Further mental regression is usually evident by the age of 1 to 1.5 years, in association with behavior problems, vertical supranuclear ophthalmoplegia, progressive ataxia, dystonia, spasticity, dementia, drooling, dysphagia, and dysarthria. Seizures are rare. Foam cells and sea-blue histiocytes may be found in many tissues. Neuronal storage with cytoplasmic ballooning, inclusions, meganeurites, and axonal spheroids are also seen. Death may occur in infancy or as late as the third decade of life. Niemann-Pick C disease can also manifest as fatal neonatal liver disease, often misdiagnosed as fetal hepatitis. Patients with mutations in the *NPC2* gene (*HE1*) may have remarkable features consisting of pronounced pulmonary involvement leading to early death caused by respiratory failure (Millat et al, 2001).

Gaucher Disease Type 2 (Acute Neuropathic)
Etiology

Three types of Gaucher disease have been defined. Type 1, the nonneuropathic form, is the most common and is distinguished from types 2 and 3 by the lack of CNS involvement. Type 1 disease most commonly manifests in early childhood, but may do so in adulthood. Type 2 disease, the acute neuropathic form, is characterized by infantile onset of severe CNS involvement. Type 3 disease, the subacute neuropathic form, is also late in onset with slow neurologic progression. Almost all types of Gaucher disease are caused by a deficiency of lysosomal glucocerebrosidase and result in storage of glucocerebroside in visceral organs; the brain is affected in types 2 and 3. Although there is significant variability in clinical presentation among

individuals with the same mutations, there is a clear correlation between certain mutations and clinical symptoms involving the CNS (Beutler and Grabowski, 2001). The enzyme splits glucose from cerebroside, yielding ceramide and glucose. A few patients with Gaucher disease type 2 have a deficiency of saposin C, a cohydrolase required by glucocerebrosidase.

Clinical Features

Typically, the age of onset of Gaucher disease type 2 is approximately 3 months, consisting of hepatosplenomegaly (splenomegaly predominates) with subsequent neurologic deterioration. Hydrops fetalis, congenital ichthyosis, and collodion skin, however, are well-described presentations (Fujimoto et al, 1995; Ince et al, 1995; Lipson et al, 1991; Liu et al, 1988; Sherer et al, 1993; Sidransky et al, 1992). In a review of 18 cases of Gaucher disease manifesting in the newborn period, Sidransky et al (1992) found that eight of the patients had associated dermatologic findings and six patients had hydrops. The etiology of the association of such findings and Gaucher disease is unclear, although the enzyme deficiency appears to be directly responsible (Sidransky et al, 1992). Ceramides have been shown to be major components of intracellular bilayers in epidermal stratum corneum, and they have an important role in skin homeostasis (Fujimoto et al, 1995). Therefore Gaucher disease should be considered in the differential diagnosis for infants with hydrops fetalis and congenital ichthyosis. For the subset of patients in the prenatal period or at birth, death frequently occurs within hours to days, or at least within 2 to 3 months.

Krabbe Disease (Globoid Cell Leukodystrophy)
Etiology

The synonym for Krabbe disease, globoid cell leukodystrophy, is derived from the finding of large numbers of multinuclear macrophages in cerebral white matter that contain undigested galactocerebroside. Disease is caused by a deficiency of lysosomal galactocerebroside β-galactosidase, which normally degrades galactocerebroside to ceramide and galactose. Deficiency of the enzyme results in storage of galactocerebroside. Galactocerebroside is present almost exclusively in myelin sheaths. Accumulation of the toxic metabolite psychosine, also a substrate for the enzyme, has been postulated to lead to early destruction of oligodendroglia. Impaired catabolism of galactosylceramide is also important in pathogenesis of the disease.

Clinical Features

Age of onset ranges from the first weeks of life to adulthood. The typical age of onset of infantile Krabbe disease is between 3 and 6 months, but there are cases of early onset in which neurologic symptoms are evident within weeks after birth. Symptoms and signs are confined to the nervous system; no visceral involvement is present. The clinical course has been divided into three stages. In stage I, patients who appeared relatively normal after birth exhibit hyperirritability, vomiting, episodic fevers, hyperesthesia, tonic spasms with light or noise stimulation, stiffness, and seizures.

Peripheral neuropathy is present, but reflexes are increased. Stage II is marked by CNS deterioration and hypertonia that progresses to hypotonia and flaccidity. Deep tendon reflexes are eventually lost. Patients with stage III disease are decerebrate, deaf, and blind with hyperpyrexia, hypersalivation, and frequent seizures. Routine laboratory findings are unremarkable except for an elevation of cerebrospinal fluid protein. Cerebral atrophy and demyelination become evident in the CNS, and segmental demyelination, axonal degeneration, fibrosis, and macrophage infiltration are common in the peripheral nervous system. The segmental demyelination of peripheral nerves is demonstrated by the finding of decreased motor nerve conduction. The white matter is severely depleted of all lipids, especially glycolipids, and nerve and brain biopsies show globoid cells. Death from hyperpyrexia, respiratory complications, or aspiration occurs at a median age of 13 months.

G_{M1} Gangliosidosis
Etiology

Infantile G_{M1} gangliosidosis is caused by a deficiency in lysosomal β-galactosidase. The enzyme cleaves the terminal galactose in a β linkage from oligosaccharides, keratan sulfate, and G_{M1} ganglioside. Deficiency of the enzyme results in storage of G_{M1} ganglioside and oligosaccharides. Clinical severity correlates with the extent of substrate storage and residual enzyme activity. The same enzyme is deficient in Morquio disease type B.

Clinical Features

Age of onset ranges from prenatal to adult. Infantile or type 1 G_{M1} gangliosidosis may be evident at birth as coarse and thick skin, hirsutism on the forehead and neck, and coarse facial features consisting of a puffy face, frontal bossing, depressed nasal bridge, maxillary hyperplasia, large and low-set ears, wide upper lip, moderate macroglossia, and gingival hypertrophy. These dysmorphic features, however, are not always obvious in the neonate. A retinal cherry-red spot is seen in 50% of patients, and corneal clouding is often observed. Shortly after birth, or by 3 to 6 months of age, failure to thrive and hepatosplenomegaly become evident, as does neurologic involvement with poor development, hyperreflexia, hypotonia, and seizures. Cranial imaging shows diffuse atrophy of the brain, enlargement of the ventricular system, and evidence of myelin loss in white matter.

The neurologic deterioration is progressive, resulting in generalized rigidity and spasticity and sensorimotor and psychointellectual dysfunction. By 6 months of age, skeletal features are present, including kyphoscoliosis and stiff joints with generalized contractures, and striking bone changes are seen—vertebral beaking in the thoracolumbar region, broadening of shafts of the long bones with distal and proximal tapering, and widening of the metacarpal shafts with proximal pinching of four lateral metacarpals. Tissue biopsy samples demonstrate neurons filled with membranous cytoplasmic bodies and various types of inclusions as well as foam cells in the bone marrow. Death generally occurs before 2 years of age. A severe neonatal-onset type of G_{M1} gangliosidosis with cardiomyopathy has also been described (Kohlschütter et al, 1982).

Farber Lipogranulomatosis
Etiology

Farber lipogranulomatosis results from a deficiency of lysosomal acid ceramidase. Ceramidase catalyzes the degradation of ceramide to its long-chain base, sphingosine, and a fatty acid. Clinical disease is a consequence of storage of ceramide in various organs and body fluids.

Clinical Features

Four types of Farber lipogranulomatosis can manifest in the neonatal period. Type I, classic disease, is a unique disorder with onset from approximately 2 weeks to 4 months of age. Patients exhibit hoarseness progressing to aphonia, feeding and respiratory difficulties, poor weight gain, and intermittent fever caused by granuloma formation, and swelling of the epiglottis and larynx. Palpable nodules appear over joints and pressure points, and joints become painful and swollen. Later, joint contractures and pulmonary disease appear. Liver and cardiac involvement can occur, and patients can have a subtle retinal cherry-red spot. Severe and progressive psychomotor impairment can occur, as can seizures, decreased deep tendon reflexes, hypotonia, and muscle atrophy. Affected patients die in early infancy, usually from pulmonary disease.

Type 2, or intermediate, Farber lipogranulomatosis manifests from birth to 9 months of age as joint and laryngeal involvement and nodules. Death occurs in early childhood. Type 3 disease (mild) manifests slightly later, from approximately 2 months to 20 months of age, with survival into the third decade. Clinically types 2 and 3 are both dominated by subcutaneous nodules, joint deformity, and laryngeal involvement. Liver and pulmonary involvement may be absent. Two thirds of patients have a normal intelligence quotient. Type 4, or neonatal visceral, Farber lipogranulomatosis manifests at birth as hepatosplenomegaly caused by massive histiocyte infiltration of the liver and spleen, with infiltration also in the lungs, thymus, and lymphocytes. Subcutaneous nodules and laryngeal involvement may be subtle. Death occurs by 6 months of age.

In all types of Farber lipogranulomatosis, tissue biopsy samples show granulomatous infiltration, foam cells, and lysosomes with comma-shaped, curvilinear tubular structures called *Farber bodies*. Cerebrospinal fluid protein may be elevated in patients with type 1 disease.

Sialidosis
Etiology

Sialidosis is caused by a deficiency of neuraminidase, which is responsible for the cleavage of terminal sialyl linkages of several oligosaccharides and glycopeptides. The defect results in multisystem lysosomal accumulation of sugars rich in sialic acid.

Clinical Features

Type I sialidosis is characterized by retinal cherry-red spots and generalized myoclonus with onset generally in the second decade of life. Type II is distinguished from type I by the early onset of a progressive, severe phenotype with somatic features. Type II is often subdivided into juvenile, infantile, and congenital forms. Congenital sialidosis begins in utero and manifests at birth as coarse features, facial edema, hepatosplenomegaly, ascites, hernias, and hypotonia, and occasionally frank hydrops fetalis. Radiographs demonstrate dysostosis multiplex and epiphyseal stippling. Delayed mental development is quickly apparent. The patient may have recurrent infections. Severely dilated coronary arteries, excessive retinal vascular tortuosity, and an erythematous macular rash may also be features of this disease (Buchholz et al, 2001). Most patients are stillborn or die before 1 year of age. Age of onset for the infantile form of sialidosis ranges from birth to 12 months. Clinical features are coarse facial features, organomegaly, dysostosis multiplex, retinal cherry-red spot, and mental retardation. Death occurs by the second or third decade. In both types of sialidosis, vacuolated cells can be seen in almost all tissues, and bone marrow foam cells are present.

Galactosialidosis

Etiology

Galactosialidosis results from a deficiency of two lysosomal enzymes, neuraminidase and β-galactosidase. The primary defect in galactosialidosis has been found to be a defect in protective protein–cathepsin A, an intralysosomal protein that protects the two enzymes from premature proteolytic processing. The protective protein has catalytic and protective functions, and the two functions appear to be distinct. Deficiency of enzymes results in the accumulation of sialyloligosaccharides in tissue lysosomes and in excreted body fluids.

Clinical Features

Galactosialidosis has been divided into three phenotypic subtypes based on age at onset and severity of clinical manifestations. Most cases occur in adolescence and adulthood, but early infantile and late infantile presentations occur. Patients develop early infantile galactosialidosis between birth and 3 months of age with ascites, edema, coarse facial features, inguinal hernias, proteinuria, hypotonia, and telangiectasias, and, occasionally, frank hydrops fetalis. Patients subsequently demonstrate organomegaly, including cardiomegaly progressing to cardiac failure, psychomotor delay, and skeletal changes, particularly in the spine. Ocular abnormalities can occur, including corneal clouding and retinal cherry-red spots. Death occurs at an average age of 8 months, usually from cardiac and renal failure. Galactosialidosis can be a cause of recurrent fetal loss or recurrent hydrops fetalis.

Late infantile galactosialidosis manifests in the first months of life as coarse facial features, hepatosplenomegaly, and skeletal changes consistent with dysostosis multiplex. Cherry-red spots and corneal clouding may also be present. Neurologic involvement may be absent or mild. Valvular heart disease is a common feature, as is growth retardation, partially because of spinal involvement and often in association with muscular atrophy. Early death is not a feature of the late infantile form. Vacuolated cells in blood smears and foam cells in bone marrow are present in all forms of galactosialidosis.

Wolman Disease

Etiology

Wolman disease is caused by lysosomal acid lipase deficiency, which is an enzyme involved in cellular cholesterol homeostasis and responsible for hydrolysis of cholesterol esters and triglycerides. The result of enzyme deficiency is defective release of free cholesterol from lysosomes, which leads to upregulation of LDL receptors and 3-hydroxy-3-methylglutaryl-CoA reductase activity. De novo synthesis of cholesterol and activation of receptor-mediated endocytosis of LDL then occur, leading to further deposition of lipid in lysosomes. The result is the accumulation of cholesterol esters and triglycerides in most tissues of the body, including the liver, spleen, lymph nodes, heart, blood vessels, and brain. An extreme level of lipid storage occurs in cells of the small intestine, particularly in the mucosa. In addition, neurons of the myenteric plexus demonstrate a high level of storage, with evidence of neuronal cell death, which may account for prominence of gastrointestinal symptoms (Wolman, 1995).

Clinical Features

Clinical presentation of Wolman disease is within weeks of birth, with evidence of malnutrition and malabsorption, including symptoms of vomiting, diarrhea, steatorrhea, failure to thrive, abdominal distention, and hepatosplenomegaly. Adrenal calcifications may be seen on radiographs, and adrenal insufficiency appears. The presence of adrenal calcifications in association with hepatosplenomegaly and gastrointestinal symptoms is strongly suggestive of Wolman disease. Later, mental deterioration becomes apparent. Laboratory findings include anemia secondary to foam cell infiltration of the bone marrow and evidence of adrenal insufficiency. The serum cholesterol level is normal. Death usually occurs before 1 year of age.

Infantile Sialic Acid Storage Disease

Etiology

Infantile sialic acid storage disease is caused by a defective lysosomal sialic acid transporter that is responsible for efflux of sialic acid and other acidic monosaccharides from the lysosomal compartment. The defective transporter results in greater storage of free sialic acid and glucuronic acid within lysosomes and increased sialic acid excretion.

Clinical Features

Infantile sialic acid storage disease often manifests at birth as mildly coarse features, hepatosplenomegaly, ascites, hypopigmentation, and generalized hypotonia. Mild dysostosis multiplex may be seen on radiographs. Failure to thrive and severe mental and motor retardation soon appear. Cardiomegaly may be present. Corneas are clear, but albinoid fundi have been reported (Lemyre et al, 1999). Vacuolated cells are seen on a tissue biopsy sample, and electron microscopy demonstrates swollen lysosomes filled with finely granular material. CNS changes include myelin loss, axonal spheroids, gliosis, and neuronal storage. Death occurs in early childhood. Infantile sialic acid storage disease can also manifest as fetal ascites, nonimmune fetal hydrops, or infantile nephrotic syndrome (Lemyre et al, 1999).

I-Cell Disease (Mucolipidosis Type II)
Etiology

In normal cells, targeting of enzymes to lysosomes is mediated by receptors that bind a mannose-6-phosphate recognition marker on the enzyme. The recognition marker is synthesized in a two-step reaction in the Golgi complex. It is the enzyme that catalyzes the first step of this process, uridine diphosphate–N-acetylglucosamine: lysosomal enzyme N-acetylglucosaminyl-1-phosphotransferase, that is defective in I-cell disease. As a result, the enzymes lack the mannose-6-phosphate recognition signal, and the newly synthesized lysosomal enzymes are secreted into the extracellular matrix instead of being targeted to the lysosome. Consequently, multiple lysosomal enzymes are found in plasma in 10- to 20-fold their normal concentrations. Affected cells, especially fibroblasts, show dense inclusions of storage material that probably consists of oligosaccharides, glycosaminoglycans, and lipids; these are the inclusion bodies from which the disease name is derived. This disorder is found more frequently in Ashkenazi Jews, because of a putative founder effect.

Clinical Features

I-cell disease can manifest at birth as coarse features, corneal clouding, organomegaly, hypotonia, and gingival hyperplasia. Birthweight and length are often below normal. Kyphoscoliosis, lumbar gibbus, and restricted joint movement are often present, and there may be hip dislocation, fractures, hernias, or bilateral talipes equinovarus. Dysostosis multiplex may be seen on radiographs. Severe psychomotor retardation, evident by 6 months of age, and progressive failure to thrive occur. The facial features become progressively more coarse, with a high forehead, puffy eyelids, epicanthal folds, flat nasal bridge, anteverted nares, and macroglossia. Linear growth slows during the first year of life and halts completely thereafter. The skeletal involvement is also progressive, with development of increasing joint immobility and claw-hand deformities. Respiratory infections, otitis media, and cardiac involvement are common complications. Death usually occurs in the first decade of life because of cardiorespiratory complications.

Mucolipidosis Type IV
Etiology

Although mucolipidosis type IV is associated with a partial deficiency of the lysosomal enzyme ganglioside sialidase, a deficiency of mucolipin 1 (TRPML1), a member of the transient receptor potential TRMPL subfamily of channel proteins, is the cause of the disorder (Bargal et al, 2000; Sun et al, 2000). Mutations in the MCOLN1 gene result in lysosomal storage of lipids such as gangliosides, plus water-soluble materials such as glycosaminoglycans and glycoproteins in cells from almost all tissues.

Clinical Features

The age of onset for mucolipidosis type IV ranges from infancy to 5 years. Presenting features are corneal clouding (may be congenital), retinal degeneration, blindness, hypotonia, and mental retardation. Survival of affected patients into the fourth decade of life has been reported (Chitayat et al, 1991). Cytoplasmic inclusions are noted in many cells, including those in conjunctiva, liver, and spleen, as well as fibroblasts.

Mucopolysaccharidosis Type VII (Sly Disease)
Etiology

Sly disease is a member of a group of lysosomal storage disorders that are caused by a deficiency of enzymes catalyzing the stepwise degradation of glycosaminoglycans. Skeletal and neurologic involvement is variable. There is a wide spectrum of clinical severity among the mucopolysaccharidoses and even within a single enzyme deficiency. Most of these disorders manifest in childhood, but type VII is included in this chapter because of its well-recognized neonatal and infantile presentations. Sly disease is caused by β-glucuronidase deficiency and results in lysosomal accumulation of glycosaminoglycans, including dermatan sulfate, heparan sulfate, and chondroitin sulfate, causing cell, tissue, and organ dysfunction.

Clinical Features

Sly disease can manifest as a wide spectrum of severity. Patients with the early-onset or neonatal form may have coarse features, hepatosplenomegaly, moderate dysostosis multiplex, hernias, and nonprogressive mental retardation. Corneal clouding is variably present. Frequent episodes of pneumonia during the first year of life are common. Short stature becomes evident. Granulocytes have coarse metachromic granules. A severe neonatal form associated with hydrops fetalis, and early death has been recognized frequently. Milder forms of the disease with later onset are also known.

DIAGNOSIS, MANAGEMENT, AND PROGNOSIS

Growing recognition of lysosomal storage disorders in the neonate has led to expansion of the spectrum of possible clinical presentation in the newborn period. Diagnostic tools and options for treatment also continue to advance. For example, efforts are currently underway to develop newborn screening for mucopolysaccharidoses (Whitley et al, 2002), with the goal to offer treatment with enzyme infusion or bone marrow transplantation (BMT) to affected babies (Vogler et al, 1999). The state of New York has implemented newborn screening for Krabbe disease using dried blood spots. The test uses a tandem mass-spectrometry–based enzyme analysis (Li et al, 2004a). This test has resulted in a fairly large number of positive newborn screens for Krabbe disease, most of which appear to be false positives, including enzyme perturbations that are not linked with clinical disease (Duffner et al, 2009).

As a consequence, an expert advising panel, the Krabbe Consortium of New York State, has been generated to establish standardized clinical evaluation guidelines. The goal is to help physicians determine which infant with a positive newborn screen may express disease and require treatment, such as hematopoietic stem cell transplantation in early infancy. The neonatologist is urged to work closely with appropriate experts to explore diagnostic and treatment protocols on an individual basis. Larger panels of multiplex testing for various other LSDs are in the testing stages (Li et al, 2004b) and some states in the United States are poised to begin implementing LSD newborn screening. Currently a federal advisory committee actively reviews and makes recommendations to the U.S. Secretary of Health and Human Services about the introduction of new newborn screening tests in the United States, with the aim of vetting proposed tests for need, cost effectiveness, and availability of effective and timely therapy.

Recognizing lysosomal storage disorders in the newborn period can be difficult, because they often mimic more common causes of illness in newborns, such as respiratory distress, nonimmune hydrops fetalis, liver disease, and sepsis. The initial step in the diagnosis of these disorders is to consider them in the differential diagnosis of a sick or unusual-appearing newborn. At times the phenotype may suggest a specific diagnosis, such as respiratory distress and painful, swollen joints in Farber lipogranulomatosis or gastrointestinal symptoms, hepatosplenomegaly, and adrenal calcifications in Wolman disease. Subtle dysmorphic features, coarsening of features, and radiographic evidence of dysostosis multiplex are also strong indications that lysosomal storage disorders should be considered. Routine laboratory findings are often normal or nonspecific. Affected infants do not have episodes of acute metabolic decompensation. Anemia and thrombocytopenia may be seen because of bone marrow involvement. Vacuolated cells may be found in peripheral blood, but the absence of this finding does not exclude lysosomal storage disease. Elevated cerebrospinal fluid protein is seen in Krabbe disease and Farber lipogranulomatosis type I.

Nonimmune hydrops fetalis deserves special mention. The physician must consider LSDs as the cause of nonimmune hydrops fetalis or unexplained ascites in the affected newborn infant. The following LSDs are potential causes: sialidosis type II, MPS types VII and IV, ISSD, Salla disease, galactosialidosis, Gaucher disease type II, G_{M1} gangliosidosis, I-cell disease, Niemann-Pick disease types A and C, Wolman disease, and Farber's disease (Staretz-Chacham et al, 2009). The mechanisms of edema are unclear. Furthermore, not all of the 13 LSDs routinely appear in the neonatal period.

Directed analysis of urine is helpful for conditions in which characteristic metabolites are excreted in urine. One- or two-dimensional electrophoresis or thin-layer chromatography can detect excess excretion of urine glycosaminoglycans, oligosaccharides, or free sialic acid, but all urinary tests for the diagnosis of lysosomal storage disorders can have false-negative results. Examination of bone marrow or other tissues may demonstrate storage macrophages in Gaucher disease and in Niemann-Pick disease types A and C. Small skin or conjunctival biopsy specimens may demonstrate storage within lysosomes in most of these disorders.

Definitive diagnosis for all lysosomal storage disorders, except for Niemann-Pick C disease, is confirmed by enzymatic assays in serum, leukocytes, fibroblasts, or a combination of these. The diagnosis of Niemann-Pick C disease requires measurement of cellular cholesterol esterification and documentation of a characteristic pattern of filipin-cholesterol staining in cultured fibroblasts during LDL uptake. Analysis of DNA mutations may be helpful for the diagnosis of Niemann-Pick C disease, Gaucher disease, and some other conditions, and it will become increasingly available for other conditions. An imperfect genotype-phenotype correlation impedes the use of mutation analysis as a prognostic tool. In addition, prenatal diagnosis is available for most lysosomal storage disorders through the use of enzyme assays performed on amniocytes or chorionic villus cells or measurements of levels of stored substrate in cultured cells or amniotic fluid. As mutation analysis becomes more prevalent, it will increasingly substitute for biochemical and enzymatic methods.

These conditions must also be considered in the dying infant, and the neonatologist must be prepared to request the appropriate samples for diagnosis at the time of death. In surviving patients, treatment and management must be considered. All the lysosomal storage disorders are chronic and progressive conditions for which there is no curative treatment. Gene transfer therapy holds promise, but is not currently available for lysosomal storage disorders. With few exceptions, current standard medical management is supportive and palliative. Patients must be continually reassessed for evidence of disease progression and associated complications. These complications manifest at variable ages and can include hydrocephalus, valvular heart disease, joint limitation, and obstructive airway disease.

For several disorders, particularly neonatal Gaucher disease and Niemann-Pick C disease, splenectomy may be indicated to improve severe anemia and thrombocytopenia. This procedure enhances the risk of serious infections, and it can accelerate the progression of disease at other sites. Patients with Krabbe disease may have significant pain of radiculopathy and spasms, and alleviation of that pain is important for the patient's comfort. The administration of glutamic acid transaminase inhibitor, vigabatrin, has been used in a small number of patients with Krabbe disease, because part of the pathology may involve a secondary deficiency of γ-aminobutyric acid (Barth, 1995). Low-dose morphine has also been reported to improve the irritability associated with this disorder (Stewart et al, 2001).

Enzyme replacement therapy with imiglucerase (Cerezyme), a recombinant enzyme, is available for Gaucher disease. Although enzyme replacement therapy has successfully reversed many of the systemic manifestations of the disease, it has been suggested that enzyme replacement therapy should not be given to patients with Gaucher disease type 2 who already have severe neurologic signs, because no substantial improvement has been demonstrated to occur in the neurologic symptoms of patients treated (Erikson et al, 1993; Gaucher disease, 1996).

Bone marrow transplantation has been tried for a variety of lysosomal storage disorders. The rationale for the procedure is that circulating blood cells derived from the transplanted marrow become a source of the missing enzyme. Results of bone marrow transplantation in disorders of glycosaminoglycans show that after successful engraftment, leukocyte and liver tissue enzyme activity normalizes, organomegaly decreases, and joint mobility increases. Skeletal abnormalities stabilize but do not improve. Whether brain function can be improved in patients with CNS disease remains questionable. Some patients maintained their learning capability or intelligence quotient, but others continued to deteriorate. Clinical experience and studies in animal models indicate that BMT before the onset of neurologic symptoms can prevent or delay the occurrence of symptoms, whereas there is no clear benefit if transplantation is performed when symptoms are already present (Hoogerbrugge et al, 1995). BMT in patients with nonneuropathic Gaucher disease can result in complete disappearance of all symptoms; however, the procedure is associated with significant risks (Hoogerbrugge et al, 1995) that must be balanced against lifelong enzyme replacement therapy. Currently it is unclear to what extent patients with the neuropathic types of Gaucher disease (types 2 and 3) would benefit from transplantation; therefore it is generally not recommended.

BMT has also been attempted in a small number of patients with infantile Krabbe disease, Farber lipogranulomatosis, and Niemann-Pick A disease. The outcome after transplantation for these few patients has been poor, with continued disease progression and death. Krivit et al (2000) reported successful long-term bone marrow engraftment in a patient with Wolman disease that resulted in normalization of peripheral leukocyte lysosomal acid lipase enzyme activity. The patient's diarrhea resolved; cholesterol, triglyceride; and liver function values normalized; and the patient attained developmental milestones. Lysosomal storage diseases are not all equally amenable to BMT, and the use of BMT as a treatment modality for most lysosomal storage disorders remains uncertain. In a small number of cases, BMT has been performed in utero after prenatal diagnosis showing an affected infant, and experimental protocols are available for families who wish to pursue this option.

The goal of therapy for a dietary protocol proposed for the treatment of Wolman disease is reduced accumulation of storage material in intestine and phagocytes. The diet, which should be started as soon as the diagnosis of Wolman disease is suggested, consists of (1) discontinuing breastfeeding or feeding with a formula containing triglycerides and cholesterol esters and (2) keeping the infant on a fatty ester–free diet (Wolman, 1995). The diet should include all necessary vitamins, including fat-soluble vitamins. In addition, daily smearing of the skin of a different extremity with a small amount (10 to 50 μL) of sunflower or safflower oil or preferably soy, canola, flax, cod liver, or algal oil is required for preventing essential fatty acid deficiency, which complicates the restricted diet (Wolman, 1995). The absorption of fatty acids through skin spares the gastrointestinal tract from accumulation and is associated with the formation of phospholipids and triglycerides (Wolman, 1995). Preliminary results of this approach suggest that treatment appears to halt disease progression.

CONGENITAL DISORDERS OF GLYCOSYLATION

ETIOLOGY

Previously called *carbohydrate-deficient glycoprotein syndromes*, CDGs are a large and increasing family of genetic diseases resulting from deficient glycosylation of glycoconjugates, mainly glycoproteins and glycolipids. Most extracellular proteins, such as serum proteins (e.g., transferrin and clotting factors), most membrane proteins, and several intracellular proteins (e.g., lysosomal proteins), are glycosylated proteins. Glycosylation, the addition of sugar chains (glycans) to proteins, occurs in every human cell and serves a number of functions, including aiding in correct folding of the nascent protein, participating in cell adhesion phenomena, protecting against premature proteolytic destruction, and modifying biologic function (Grünewald, 2007). The glycans are defined by their linkage to the protein N-glycan or O-glycan. N-Glycosylation consists of the assembly of a glycan on and in the endoplasmic reticulum and its attachment to a particular asparagine of target proteins, followed by remodeling of this glycan mainly in Golgi (Jaeken and Matthijs, 2007); therefore it is a two-part process of assembly and processing. O-Glycosylation consists of assembly of a glycan and its attachment to a serine or threonine of a target protein, or the attachment of a monosaccharide (mannose, fructose, or xylose) to one of these amino acids. No processing pathway is present in O-glycosylation (Jaeken and Matthijs, 2007). Combined N- and O-glycosylation defects and lipid glycosylation defects have also been described (Jaeken and Matthijs, 2007).

Given the ubiquitous occurrence of glycoproteins and the number of apparent genes involved in glycosylation (more than 200; approximately 1% of the human genome), it is not surprising that the number of described CDG defects is increasing rapidly and clinical manifestations are diverse (Jaeken, 2006; Jaeken et al, 2008; Morava et al, 2008b). Currently, 21 disorders in protein N-glycosylation, 12 in protein O-glycosylation, five in both protein N- and O-glycosylation, and two in lipid glycosylation have been described (Jaeken, 2006; Jaeken and Matthijs, 2007; Marklová and Albahri, 2007). The number of described disorders is expected to continue to grow.

The disorders of N-glycosylation have been divided into two primary categories. CDG-I disorders result from defects in N-glycan assembly (designated CDG-Ia to -Im). On isoelectrofocusing of serum transferrin, the most widely used screening test for N-glycosylation disorders, a type I pattern is observed. This pattern is characterized by a decrease of anodal fractions and an increase of disialotransferrin and asialotransferrin. A type II pattern, showing an increase of trisialofractions, monosialofractions, or both is seen in CDG-II defects, which represent defects in N-glycan processing (designated CDG-IIa-IIf).

O-Glycosylation defects have been found to be causative in a number of muscular dystrophies with reduced glycosylation of α-dystroglycan. These disorders, collectively referred to as α-*dystroglycanopathies*, encompass previously described disorders, such as Walker-Warburg syndrome, muscle-eye-brain disease, Fukuyama congenital muscular dystrophy, and limb-girdle muscular dystrophy (Mercuri et al, 2009; Topaloglu, 2009). Six known or putative glycosyltransferase genes have been identified in these disorders (Godfrey et al, 2007). In general, this is a heterogeneous group of autosomal recessive disorders with a wide spectrum of clinical severity, and it shares the common pathologic feature of hypoglycosylated α-dystroglycan (Godfrey et al, 2007). α-Dystroglycan is a major component of the dystrophin-associated glycoprotein complex that forms a link between the actin-associated cytoskeleton and extracellular matrix. It is a highly glycosylated peripheral membrane protein that binds many of its extracellular matrix partners through its carbohydrate modifications (Godfrey et al, 2007). In the dystroglycanopathies, these modifications are either absent or reduced, resulting in decreased binding of ligands (Barresi and Campbell, 2006). O-Glycosylation defects have also been described in hereditary multiple exostoses syndrome, familial tumoral calcinosis, Schneckenbecken dysplasia, spondylocostal dysostosis type 3, Peters plus syndrome, and the progeria variant of Ehlers-Danlos syndrome (Grünewald, 2007; Jaeken et al, 2008; Jaeken and Matthijs, 2007).

Combined N- and O-glycosylation defects are important because they appear to affect trafficking in the glycosylation machinery (Grünewald, 2007). The disruption of multiple glycosylation pathways is caused by mutations of the conserved oligomeric Golgi (COG) complex. This large complex spanning eight subunits plays a key role in protein transport between the endoplasmic reticulum and Golgi and within the Golgi complex (Grünewald, 2007; Jaeken, 2006). COG7 deficiency, first described in two siblings with poor intrauterine growth, dysmorphic features, encephalopathy, cholestatic liver disease, and perinatal asphyxia, shows a partial combined N- and O-glycosylation defect caused by decreased transport of CMP-sialic acid and UDP-galactose into Golgi and reduced activity of two glycosyltransferases involved in the galactosylation and sialylation of O-glycans (Jaeken, 2006). An autosomal recessive cutis laxa syndrome has recently been found to be also associated with a combined glycosylation defect (Morava et al, 2008a).

Two disorders of lipid glycosylation have been described. Amish infantile epilepsy was the first identified and is caused by a defect of lactosylceramide α-2,3 sialyltransferase (GM3 synthase; Jaeken, 2006). This enzyme catalyzes the initial step in the biosynthesis of most complex gangliosides from lactosylceramide (Jaeken and Matthijs, 2007). The defect causes accumulation of lactosylceramide associated with decreased gangliosides of the GM3 and GD3 series (Jaeken, 2006). Glycosylphosphatidylinositol deficiency is the second disorder in glycolipid glycosylation described, but the first reported genetic defect in glycosylation of the glycosylphosphatidylinositol (GPI) anchor (Jaeken and Matthijs, 2007). Glycosylphosphatidylinositol-anchored proteins have heterogeneous functions as enzymes or adhesion molecules. Finally, the term *CDG-x* indicates syndromes with strong evidence for a glycosylation defect, but in which the defective gene has yet to be identified (Jaeken and Matthijs, 2007). This clinically heterogeneous group is also growing rapidly.

CLINICAL FEATURES

The phenotypic spectrum of CDG defects is extremely broad and ranges from mild to severe disease and from a single-organ system to multisystem disease. Clinical features alone are insufficient to define the CDG subtype. CDG should be considered a possible diagnosis in any unexplained clinical condition, but especially in multiorgan disease with neurologic involvement. Discussion of the clinical presentation of all forms of CDG is beyond the scope of this chapter (Table 23-2).

CDG-Ia is the classic and most common presentation. The basic defect in CDG-Ia is a deficiency of the enzyme phosphomannomutase, which is required for the early steps of protein glycosylation (Jaeken, 2006; Jaeken et al, 2001; van Schaftingen and Jaeken, 1995). Patients with CDG-Ia at birth exhibit dysmorphic features consisting of a high nasal bridge, prominent jaw, large ears, and inverted nipples, feeding difficulties, and subsequent growth failure, hypotonia, lipocutaneous abnormalities (including prominent fat pads on the buttocks), and mild to moderate hepatomegaly. The clinical progression of this disorder is divided into four stages. In stage I—the infantile, multisystem stage—patients show evidence of multisystem involvement, including variable strokelike episodes, thrombotic disease, liver dysfunction, pericardial effusions and cardiomyopathy, proteinuria, and retinal degeneration. The coagulopathy likely stems from the number of clotting and anticlotting proteins that are N-linked glycoproteins. Mental retardation, peripheral neuropathy, and decreased nerve conduction velocities are observed. Strabismus and alternating esotropia are present in almost all patients, and retinitis pigmentosa and abnormalities of the electroretinogram are present in most. Cranial imaging shows varying degrees of cerebral, cerebellar, and brainstem hypoplasia. Electroencephalogram results are usually normal. Liver biopsy samples typically show steatosis and fibrosis, and multicystic changes in kidneys have been noted.

Stage II, the childhood stage, is characterized by ataxia and mental retardation. Skeletal abnormalities may become more prominent, consisting of contractures, kyphoscoliosis, pectus carinatum, and short stature. Stage III, generally occurring in the teenage years, is characterized primarily by lower extremity atrophy. Adulthood, or stage IV, is characterized by hypogonadism. In general, patients have an extroverted disposition and happy appearance. Approximately 20% of patients die during the first year of life because of severe infection, liver failure, or cardiac insufficiency.

Patients with CDG-Ib are unique among patients with these disorders. They may have vomiting, diarrhea, hypoglycemia, and liver disease (coagulopathy, hepatomegaly, hepatic fibrosis). In addition, they often have a protein-losing enteropathy (also seen in CDG-Ih; Jaeken and Matthijs, 2007). Development is normal. The remaining forms of CDG-I and CDG-II are similar in presentation to type Ia. Additional features include seizures, normal cerebellar development, delayed myelination, optic atrophy, blindness, frequent infections, hypoventilation and apnea, and further dysmorphic features such as adducted thumbs, high-arched palate, coarse facies, widely spaced nipples, and low-set ears.

TABLE 23-2 Common Congenital Disorders of Glycoprotein

Findings	Types of CDG							
	Ia	Ib	Ic	Id	Ie	IIa	IIb	x
Enzyme defect	Phosphomannomutase	Phosphomannose isomerase	α1,3-Glucosyltransferase	α1,3-Mannosyl transferase	Dol-P-Man synthase	GlcNAc transferase 2	Glucosidase I	Unknown
Dysmorphic features	+	+/−	+/−	+/−	+	+	+	+
Psychomotor retardation	+	−	+	+	+	+		+
Hypotonia	+	+/−	+	+	+	+		+
Cerebellar hypoplasia	+	−	+/−	−	+/−	−	−	−
Seizures	+/−	+/−	+/−	+	+	+	+	−
Eye findings	Strabismus, esotropia	−	Strabismus	Optic atrophy	Cortical blindness	−	−	−
Liver disease	+	+	−	−	+	+	+	−
Coagulopathy	+	+	+	−	+	+	+	−
Other	Multiorgan involvement, peripheral neuropathy, subcutaneous fat distribution, inverted nipples, strokelike episodes, cardiomyopathy, ataxia, microcephaly, hypothyroidism	Protein-losing enteropathy, cyclic vomiting, diarrhea, hypoglycemia	Microcephaly, feeding difficulties, ataxia	Microcephaly, reduced responsiveness, adducted thumbs	Microcephaly, delayed myelination	Stereotype behavior, frequent infections, ventricular septal defect, widely spaced nipples, delayed myelination	Early death, generalized edema, hypoventilation, apnea, demyelinating polyneuropathy	Leukocyte adhesion deficiency syndrome type II (guanosine diphosphate–fucose transporter); phenotype: elevated peripheral leukocytes, absence of CD 15, Bombay blood group phenotype, failure to thrive, recurrent infections, short arms and legs, simian crease

Adapted from Westphal V, Srikrishna G, Freeze H: Congenital disorders of glycosylation: Have you encountered them? *Genet Med* 2:329-337, 2000.
+, Present; −, absent; +/−, occasionally present.

The phenotypic presentation of dystroglycanopathy is extremely variable. At the severe end of the spectrum are individuals with Walker-Warburg syndrome, muscle-eye-brain disease, and Fukuyama congenital muscular dystrophy. These conditions are characterized by congenital muscular dystrophy with severe structural brain and eye abnormalities and death typically before the age of 1 year (Godfrey et al, 2007; Jaeken, 2006; Jaeken and Matthijs, 2007). Toward the more mild end of the spectrum are individuals in adulthood with limb-girdle muscular dystrophy with no brain or eye involvement (Godfrey et al, 2007; Jaeken and Matthijs, 2007). Intermediate phenotypes lie between the two extremes.

The presence of carbohydrate-deficient transferrin in serum and cerebrospinal fluid is a distinctive biochemical feature of CDG. Laboratory findings are often nonspecific (e.g. elevated liver function studies or hypoalbuminemia), but concentrations of plasma glycoproteins such as α_1-antitrypsin, thyroxin-binding globulin, and transferrin are frequently abnormal (Marklová and Albahri, 2007). Clotting factors such as factors V, XI, II, X, antithrombin III, proteins C and S, and thyroid hormones (triiodothyronine, thyroxine, and reverse T3) are also frequently decreased (Marklová and Albahri, 2007; Morava et al, 2008b). Abnormal clotting is an important indicator of a glycosylation disorder (Morava et al, 2008b).

DIAGNOSIS

CDG should be considered in newborns with several of the following features:

- Neurologic signs, including hypotonia, hyporeflexia, or seizures
- Ophthalmic signs, including abnormal eye movements, cataracts, glaucoma, optic nerve atrophy, or retinitis pigmentosa
- Hepatic and gastrointestinal signs such as ascites or hydrops, hepatomegaly, diarrhea, and protein-losing enteropathy
- Endocrinologic signs, including hyperinsulinemic hypoglycemia and hypothyroidism
- Signs of renal or cardiac disease
- Congential muscular dystrophy
- Congenital joint contractures
- Dysmorphic features, microcephaly, structural brain anomalies, or abnormal skin findings

Isoelectrofocusing of serum transferrin is the screening method of choice, but only to detect defects of N-glycosylation. Confirmatory enzyme assays or molecular studies are required to pinpoint the specific defect. Urine oligosaccharide analysis, Bombay blood phenotype, serum apoC-III screening, or membrane bound sialyl-Lewis[X] antigen may be helpful in distinguishing subclasses of CDG II disease (Marklová and Albahri, 2007). If suspicion of CDG remains, further structural analysis of the lipid-linked oligosaccharide (LLO) and the peptide-protein N-linked oligosaccharide should follow, if available (Marklová and Albahri, 2007). Patients with CDG can often be identified through neonatal screening for congenital hypothyroidism, because of an associated thyroid-binding globulin deficiency and an increased thyroid-stimulating hormone level. Prenatal diagnosis by transferrin isoelectric focusing is not reliable. Prenatal diagnosis is possible in all types of CDG for which the molecular defect is known (Grünewald, 2007). The vast majority of CDG disorders are autosomal recessive disorders or presumed autosomal recessive disorders; hereditary multiple exostoses syndrome is autosomal dominant.

TREATMENT AND MANAGEMENT

The treatment and management for most types of CDGs are primarily supportive and palliative. There is no curative or corrective treatment. In infancy, evidence of multisystem involvement and the resulting complications must be treated promptly. There is substantial mortality in the first years of life because of severe infection or vital organ failure (Grünewald, 2007; Jaeken, 2006). The exception is treatment of CDG-Ib with oral mannose therapy. In this disorder, oral mannose effectively bypasses the impaired pathway and allows glycosylation to continue (Freeze, 1998; Jaeken, 2006; Jaeken and Matthijs, 2007). Therapy improves the protein-losing enteropathy and liver disease (Grünewald, 2007). Oral fucose therapy has also been used in patients with CDG-IIc, a GDP-fucose transporter defect (Grünewald, 2007). Therapy appears to improve the fucosylation of glycoproteins and to improve control of recurrent infections, but it has no effect on neurologic complications of the disorder (Grünewald, 2007).

PEROXISOMAL DISORDERS

DISORDERS OF PEROXISOME BIOGENESIS

Peroxisomes are single-membrane–bound cellular organelles that contain no internal structure or DNA and are characterized by an electron-dense core and a homogeneous matrix. Peroxisomes are found in all cells and tissues except mature erythrocytes, and they are in highest concentration in the liver and kidneys. They are formed by growth and division of preexisting peroxisomes and are randomly destroyed by autophagy. Their half-life is 1.5 to 2 days. Peroxisomal proteins are encoded by nuclear genes, synthesized in cytosol, and imported posttranslationally into the peroxisome. The import of proteins into the peroxisome is mediated by receptors and requires adenosine triphosphate hydrolysis.

Peroxisomes contain enzymes that use oxygen to oxidize a variety of substrates, thereby forming peroxide. The peroxide is decomposed within the organelle by the enzyme catalase to water and oxygen. This process protects the cell against peroxide damage through compartmentalization of peroxide metabolism within the organelle. Peroxisomes can also function to dispose of excess reducing equivalents and may contribute to thermogenesis, producing heat from cellular respiration (Gould et al, 2007).

More than 50 enzymes have been found within peroxisomes (Gould et al, 2001). The proteins have multiple functions, both synthetic and degradative (Wanders et al, 2001). The primary synthetic functions are plasmalogen synthesis and bile acid formation. Plasmalogens constitute 5% to 20% of phospholipids in cell membranes and 80% to 90% of phospholipids in myelin. They are involved in platelet activation and may also protect cells against oxidative stress. Degradative functions include (1) β-oxidation of VLCFA (≥C23), fatty acids (down to C8 to C6), long-chain dicarboxylic acids, prostaglandins, and polyunsaturated fatty acids; (2) oxidation of bile acid intermediates, pipecolic acid and glutaric acid (intermediates in lysine catabolism), and phytanic acid; (3) deamination of D- and L-amino acids, (4) metabolism of glycolate to glyoxylate; (5) polyamine degradation (spermine and spermidine); and (6) ethanol clearance. At least 16 conditions caused by single peroxisomal enzyme deficiencies have been confirmed (Wanders et al, 2007).

Peroxisomal disorders constitute a clinically and biochemically heterogeneous group of inherited diseases that result from the absence or dysfunction of one or more peroxisomal enzymes. Conditions in which multiple peroxisomal enzymes are affected can result from a disturbance of biogenesis or the organelle. Pathophysiology apparently involves either deficiency of necessary products of peroxisomal metabolism or excess of unmetabolized substrates. Disorders with similar biochemical defects may have markedly different clinical features, and disorders with similar clinical features may be associated with different biochemical findings. General features of peroxisomal disorders, each of which can manifest or be evident in the newborn period, are as follows:

- Dysmorphic craniofacial features
- Neurologic dysfunction, primarily consisting of severe hypotonia, possibly associated with hypertonia of the extremities and seizures
- Hepatodigestive dysfunction, including hepatomegaly, cholestasis, and prolonged hyperbilirubinemia

Rhizomelic shortening of the limbs, stippled calcifications of epiphyses, renal cysts, and abnormalities in neuronal migration may also be seen.

Peroxisomal biogenesis disorders are composed of at least 12 complementation groups (Matsumoto et al, 2001). All involve defects in proteins targeted to the organelle. Genes and proteins required for peroxisomal biosynthesis are referred to as *peroxins* and are encoded by *PEX* genes. The *PEX* genes responsible for disease in most human patients are known, and more than 50% of patients with peroxisomal biogenesis disorders have mutations in *PEX1* (Moser, 2000; Steinberg et al, 2006). This section We discusses the peroxisomal disorders that can manifest in the newborn period.

Zellweger syndrome is the prototype of neonatal peroxisomal disease. It is a disorder of peroxisome biogenesis caused by failure to import newly synthesized peroxisomal proteins into the peroxisome. The proteins remain in the cytosol, where they are rapidly degraded. In this condition, peroxisomes are absent from liver hepatocytes or exist as "ghosts." Neonatal adrenoleukodystrophy and infantile Refsum disease are also disorders of peroxisome biogenesis in which, as in Zellweger syndrome, disruption of function of more than one peroxisomal enzyme is demonstrable. A few residual peroxisomes, however, may be seen in the liver. These disorders represent a continuum of clinical severity. Rhizomelic chondrodysplasia punctata is caused by a defect in a subset of peroxisomal enzymes. In this disorder, liver peroxisomes are demonstrable and normal in number, but their distribution and structure are abnormal.

There is circumstantial evidence that in utero elevations of VLCFAs may be key to congenital CNS abnormalities. Powers and Moser (1998) proposed that VLCFAs and phytanic acid that accumulate in these peroxisomal disorders are incorporated into myelin and cell membranes, and that alteration of normal constituents of the membrane adversely affects membrane function. Specifically, these investigators suggest that abnormal constituents accelerate cell death and impede neuronal migration, accounting for the conspicuous CNS abnormalities in disorders of peroxisomal biogenesis.

To date, four disorders of peroxisomal fatty acid β-oxidation have been defined: acetyl-CoA oxidase deficiency, D-bifunctional protein deficiency, peroxisomal thiolase deficiency, and 2-methylacyl-CoA racemase deficiency (Wanders et al, 2007). The clinical presentation of the first three disorders resembles that of biogenesis disorders. Individuals with the fourth disorder have a late-onset neuropathy.

Clinical Presentations

Table 23-3 summarizes the clinical features of disorders of peroxisome biogenesis that can present in the neonate.

Zellweger Syndrome

Zellweger syndrome is most often evident at birth, with affected babies having dysmorphic facial features including large fontanels, high forehead, flat occiput, epicanthus, hypertelorism, upward-slanting palpebral fissures,

---

TABLE 23-3 Disorders of Peroxisomal Biogenesis in the Newborn Period

Feature	Zellweger Syndrome	Neonatal Adrenoleukodystrophy	Infantile Refsum Disease	Rhizomelic Chondrodysplasia Punctata
Onset	Birth	Birth to 3 mo	Birth to 6 mo	Birth
Facies	High forehead, large fontanels, upward-slanting palpebral fissures, hypoplastic supraorbital ridges, epicanthic folds, micrognathia, abnormal ears	Milder features of Zellweger syndrome	Epicanthic folds, midface hypoplasia, low-set ears	Depressed nasal bridge, hypertelorism, microcephaly
Neurologic findings	Weakness, hypotonia, seizures, psychomotor retardation, sensorineural hearing loss	Hypotonia, seizures, slow psychomotor development and neurodegeneration	Mild hypotonia, normal early development followed by degeneration, ataxia, sensorineural hearing loss	Severe psychomotor retardation
Ophthalmologic findings	Cataracts, glaucoma, corneal clouding, retinitis pigmentosa, optic nerve dysplasia, Brushfield spots	Retinopathy	Retinitis pigmentosa	Cataracts
Other findings	Hepatomegaly, multicystic kidneys, congenital heart disease, growth failure, chondrodysplasia punctata	Impaired adrenal function	Hepatomegaly, anosmia, diarrhea	Severe shortening of proximal limbs, joint contractures, ichthyosis
Diagnosis	↑ plasma VLCFA, phytanic acid, pipecolic acid, and bile acid intermediates, ↓ plasmalogens	Same as for Zellweger syndrome	Same as for Zellweger syndrome	↑ phytanic and pipecolic acids, ↓ plasmalogens, normal VLCFA and bile acid intermediates

VLCFA, Very-long-chain fatty acid; ↑, elevated; ↓, reduced.

hypoplastic supraorbital ridges, abnormal ears, severe weakness and hypotonia, hepatomegaly, multicystic kidneys, and congenital heart disease. Seizures, feeding difficulties, and postnatal growth failure soon manifest. Ophthalmologic examination may detect cataracts, corneal clouding, glaucoma, optic atrophy, retinitis pigmentosa, and Brushfield spots. Somatic sensory evoked responses and electroretinograms are abnormal. Hearing assessment often shows an abnormal brainstem auditory evoked response consistent with sensorineural hearing loss. Skeletal radiographs demonstrate epiphyseal stippling, and cranial imaging shows leukodystrophy and neuronal migration abnormalities. Hepatic cirrhosis and severe psychomotor retardation occur later. Laboratory analysis may demonstrate abnormal liver function values, hyperbilirubinemia, or hypoprothrombinemia. Death usually occurs within the first year of life, the average life span being 12.5 weeks.

Neonatal Adrenoleukodystrophy

Clinically, neonatal adrenoleukodystrophy is similar to, but less severe than, Zellweger syndrome. Differences include less dysmorphology, absence of chondrodysplasia punctata and renal cysts, and fewer neuronal and gray matter changes. Patients with neonatal adrenoleukodystrophy may have striking white matter disease, however, and often show degenerative changes in adrenal glands. They also have slow psychomotor development followed by neurodegeneration that usually begins before the end of the first year of life. Disease progression is slower than that observed in Zellweger syndrome, and longer survival is usual, to an average of approximately 15 months of age.

Infantile Refsum Disease

Patients with infantile Refsum disease also have relatively mild dysmorphic features, such as epicanthic folds, midface hypoplasia with low-set ears, and mild hypotonia. Early neurodevelopment is normal, possibly up to 6 months of age, but then slow deterioration begins. Later, sensorineural hearing loss (100%), anosmia, retinitis pigmentosa, hepatomegaly with impaired function, and severe mental retardation are evident. Patients learn to walk, although their gait may be ataxic and broad based. Diarrhea and failure to thrive may also be seen. Chondrodysplasia punctata and renal cysts are absent. Neuronal migration defects are minor, and adrenal hypoplasia occurs. The life span of patients with infantile Refsum disease ranges from 3 to 11 years.

Rhizomelic Chondrodysplasia Punctata

Patients with rhizomelic chondrodysplasia punctata at birth have facial dysmorphia, microcephaly, cataracts, rhizomelic shortening of extremities with prominent stippling, and coronal clefting of vertebral bodies. The chondrodysplasia punctata is more widespread than in Zellweger syndrome and may involve extraskeletal tissues. Infants with this disorder have severe psychomotor retardation from birth onward and severe failure to thrive. In addition, patients may have joint contractures, and 25% experience ichthyosis. Neuronal migration is normal. Life span is usually less than 1 year.

DISORDERS OF PEROXISOMAL β-OXIDATION

D-Bifunctional protein deficiency is more rare than peroxisomal biogenesis disorders and results in a phenotype similar to Zellweger syndrome. In general, children have severe CNS involvement consisting of profound hypotonia, uncontrolled seizures, and failure to acquire any significant developmental milestones. Children are usually born full term without evidence of intrauterine growth restriction. Dysmorphic features, similar to those seen in Zellweger syndrome, are notable in most children. In most cases, neuronal migration is disturbed with areas of polymicrogyria and heterotopic neurons in the cerebrum and cerebellum. Death generally occurs before 1 year of age, but survival to at least 3 years of age is possible.

Acetyl-CoA oxidase deficiency is less common. Patients exhibit global hypotonia, deafness, and delayed milestones with or without facial dysmorphic features. Patients may demonstrate early developmental gains, but then show regression of skills. Retinopathy with extinguished electroretinograms, failure to thrive, hepatomegaly, areflexia, and seizures have also been reported.

One patient with peroxisomal thiolase deficiency has been described (Goldfischer et al, 1986). The child had marked facial dysmorphia, muscle weakness, and hypotonia. She demonstrated no psychomotor development during her 11 months of life. Autopsy showed renal cysts, atrophic adrenal glands, minimal liver fibrosis, hypomyelination in cerebral white matter, foci of neuronal heterotopia, and a sudanophilic leukodystrophy (Goldfischer et al, 1986).

X-linked adrenoleukodystrophy is the most common peroxisomal disorder, because of altered function of a membrane transport protein ABCD1 that affects metabolism of VLCFAs, and does not usually present in the neonatal period. However, three patients with contiguous deletions involving the *ABCD1* gene have exhibited a phenotype similar to peroxisomal biogenesis disorders (Corzo et al, 2002).

DIAGNOSIS, MANAGEMENT, AND PROGNOSIS OF PEROXISOMAL DISORDERS

The key to diagnosing peroxisomal disease is a high index of suspicion. Peroxisomal disorders should be considered in newborns with dysmorphic facial features, skeletal abnormalities, shortened proximal limbs, neurologic abnormalities (including hypotonia or hypertonia), ocular abnormalities, and hepatic abnormalities. Babies with abnormal visual, hearing, or somatosensory evoked potentials should also be considered for these diagnoses.

Peroxisomal disorders are not associated with acute metabolic derangements or abnormal routine laboratory tests. Measurements of VLCFAs, phytanic acid, pipecolic acid, bile acid intermediates, and plasmalogens are required for diagnosis. Zellweger syndrome is associated with elevations of VLCFAs, phytanic acid, pipecolic acid, and bile acid intermediates, and a decrease in plasmalogen synthesis. Neonatal adrenoleukodystrophy and infantile Refsum disease have similar biochemical findings; however, the defect in plasmalogen synthesis and the degree of VLCFA accumulation are less severe. Laboratory findings in rhizomelic chondrodysplasia punctata are elevations of phytanic and pipecolic acids, a decrease in plasmalogen, and normal levels of VLCFAs and bile acid intermediates. Therefore screening that uses only levels of VLCFAs fails to detect rhizomelic chondrodysplasia punctata. D-Bifunctional protein deficiency is associated with deficient oxidation of C23:0 and pristanic acid, leading to elevations of pristanic acid and, to a lesser extent, phytanic acid. This deficiency results in an elevated pristanic acid-to-phytanic acid ratio, which is generally not elevated in peroxisomal biogenesis disorders. Abnormal VLCFA and elevation of varanic acid (an intermediate metabolite in β-oxidation) are also seen. Accumulation of bile acid intermediates is a variable finding. Abnormalities in phytanic acid and plasmalogens are age dependent. The elevation of phytanic acid might not be demonstrable in young infants, and reduction in red blood cell plasmalogen levels may not be evident in children older than 20 weeks (Gould et al, 2007). A liver biopsy may be a useful adjunct diagnostic tool to assess for the presence or absence and structure of peroxisomes. Definitive diagnoses for all types of peroxisomal disease require cultured skin fibroblasts for measurement of VLCFA levels and their β-oxidation and, as needed, assay of the peroxisomal steps of plasmalogen synthesis, phytanic acid oxidation, subcellular localization of catalase, enzyme assays, and immunocytochemistry studies. Prenatal diagnosis with a variety of methods is available (Steinberg et al, 2005). DNA diagnosis is possible for most patients, but is "challenging for the Zellweger syndromes spectrum since 12 *PEX* genes are known to be associated with this spectrum of peroxisomal biogenesis disorders" (Steinberg et al, 2006). DNA study for deletions also has a role in diagnostic evaluations in some cases before counseling for recurrence risk, as demonstrated by the neonatal presentation of cases with deletion of the *ABCD1* gene on the X chromosome (Corzo et al, 2002). The complexities of prenatal diagnosis emphasize the need for studies of tissue on the proband to determine the potential for and appropriate strategies to offer in prenatal diagnosis for any family.

One of the more interesting recent developments in peroxisomal disease is the preliminary work on combined liquid chromatography-tandem mass spectroscopy application for blood spot–based newborn screening. It is targeted at conditions with abnormal VLCFAs, especially X-linked adrenoleukodystrophy, that typically manifest in childhood and for which presymptomatic therapy may alter the course of the usual progressive disease. The method is promising, but still under investigation (Hubbard et al, 2006).

Treatment for all peroxisomal disorders in the newborn period remains supportive. These disorders are chronic, progressive diseases with no currently available curative therapy. Setchell et al (1992) described the effects of administration of primary bile acids on liver function in a 6-month-old infant with Zellweger syndrome. The effects included normalization of serum bilirubin and liver enzyme levels and a decrease in hepatic inflammation, bile duct proliferation, and canalicular plugs. The patient also showed an improvement in growth and neurologic function (Setchell et al, 1992).

Martinez (1992) reported the use of docosahexaenoic acid ethyl ester in two patients with neonatal adrenoleukodystrophy. Both patients had an increase in erythrocyte omega fatty acid levels and plasmalogens accompanied by significant improvement in clinical parameters, including alertness, motor performance, vocabulary, and visual evoked responses. Martinez et al (2000) also reported on the effects of docosahexaenoic acid supplementation in 13 patients with generalized peroxisomal disorders. The effects were normalization of blood docosahexaenoic acid levels, increased plasmalogen concentrations, decreased plasma VLCFAs, and improvement to near normal of liver enzymes. Although patients with severe neonatal Zellweger syndrome presentation did not benefit, patients with milder peroxisomal biogenesis disorders—in which clinical course is more variable—experienced improvement in vision, liver function, muscle tone, and social contact. Three patients showed normalization of brain myelin, and myelination improved in three others (Martinez et al, 2000).

In addition, a "triple" dietary approach consisting of oral administration of ether lipids, decreased phytanic acid intake, and the oral administration of glyceryl trioleate and glyceryl trierucate (Lorenzo's oil) leads to biochemical improvement and may have value in patients with mild forms of peroxisomal biogenesis defects (Gould et al, 2007). Although treatment protocols are available for infants affected with disorders of peroxisomal biogenesis, improvement in long-term outcome remains limited in all but the mildly affected patients. However, treatment involving diet and bone marrow transplant, when appropriate, has been demonstrated to significantly improve the outcome of some patients affected with adrenoleukodystrophy (Moser et al, 2001).

SMITH-LEMLI-OPITZ SYNDROME

ETIOLOGY

Smith-Lemli-Opitz syndrome is a well-recognized autosomal recessive malformation syndrome, with an estimated incidence ranging from 1 in 10,000 to 70,000 in various populations (Porter, 2008; Yu and Patel, 2005). Because of the identification of an underlying biochemical defect, SLO syndrome has been reclassified as an inborn error of metabolism. In 1993, it was discovered that SLO syndrome is caused by a defect in cholesterol biosynthesis that results in low levels of cholesterol and elevated levels of 7-dehydrocholesterol (7DHC) and its isomer, 8-dehydrocholesterol (8DHC). Patients have markedly reduced activity of the enzyme 7DHC reductase, the enzyme responsible for conversion of 7DHC to cholesterol (Porter, 2008; Salen et al, 1995; Waterham and Clayton, 2006), which is located on chromosome 11 (Kelley and Hennekam, 2000; Waterham and Clayton, 2006). Cholesterol is a major lipid component of cellular membranes such as myelin, and it is an important structural component of lipid rafts, which play a major role in signal transduction (Porter, 2008; Yu and Patel, 2005). In addition, bile acids, steroid hormones, neuroactive steroids, and oxysterols are all synthesized from cholesterol (Merkens et al, 2009; Porter, 2008). The possible role of these various pathways in the etiology of SLO syndrome is still being defined (Merkens et al, 2009; Porter, 2008).

The cause of the clinical phenotype of SLO syndrome may be related to deficient cholesterol, deficient total sterols, the toxic effects of either 7DHC or compounds derived from 7DHC, or a combination of these factors (Porter, 2008; Yu and Patel, 2005). A single underlying pathologic mechanism is unlikely (Porter, 2008).

The pivotal connection between cholesterol and SLO syndrome involves development and differentiation of the vertebrate body plan, although additional metabolic effects have not been ruled out. Among those proteins exerting decisive influence on patterning during embryogenesis are the Hedgehog proteins. One variant, Sonic hedgehog (Shh), becomes covalently linked to cholesterol at the protein's amino-terminal signaling domain. This linkage is needed to restrict the locus of action of Shh to the region of plasma membrane. Although it was originally suggested that failure to modify Shh could account for multiplicity of structural abnormalities in patients with SLO syndrome (Farese and Herz, 1998), the process is thought to be more complex and to involve other signaling proteins such as Patched (PTCH) and Smoothened (SMO) (Farese and Herz, 1998; Kelley and Hennekam, 2000; Porter, 2008).

CLINICAL FEATURES

Recognition of the biochemical defect in SLO syndrome provided the diagnostic test required to recognize the most mild and most severe cases, substantially expanding the clinical spectrum of the condition. Classic SLO syndrome is often evident at birth; affected patients have microcephaly and facial dysmorphism, including bitemporal narrowing, ptosis, epicanthic folds, anteverted nares, broad nasal tip, prominent lateral palatine ridges, micrognathia, and low-set ears. Other features are 2- to 3-syndactyly of toes (found in 95% of patients), small proximally placed thumbs, and occasionally postaxial polydactyly and cataracts. Males usually have hypospadias, cryptorchidism, and a hypoplastic scrotum, but may have ambiguous or female genitalia. Pyloric stenosis, cleft palate, pancreatic anomalies, Hirschsprung disease, and lung segmentation defects have also been reported. Hypotonia progressing to hypertonia and moderate to severe mental deficiencies are also present. Feeding difficulties and vomiting are common problems in infancy. Irritable behavior and shrill screaming may also pose problems during infancy. Older children frequently have hyperactivity, self-injurious behavior, sleep difficulties, and autistic characteristics. Cranial imaging studies show (and autopsy confirms) defects in brain morphogenesis, including hypoplasia of frontal lobes, cerebellum, and brainstem, dilated ventricles, irregular gyral patterns, and irregular neuronal organization.

Historically, approximately 20% of patients die within the first year of life, although others may survive for more than 30 years. Life expectancy appears to correlate inversely with the number and severity of organ defects and with the kinds and numbers of limb, facial, and genital abnormalities (Kelley and Hennekam, 2000; Tint et al, 1995). Developmental outcomes are also highly variable, ranging from severe mental retardation to normal intelligence. Development of treatment protocols for SLO syndrome may contribute to improvements in prognosis, but improved recognition of more mildly affected patients

may explain the increasing reports of SLO syndrome in patients with mild mental retardation or normal intelligence (Jezela-Stanek et al, 2008). Testing for SLO syndrome has been suggested for all patients with idiopathic intellectual impairment, behavioral anomalies, or both, when associated with nonfamilial two- and three-toe syndactyly and failure to thrive (Jezela-Stanek et al, 2008).

DIAGNOSIS

The diagnosis of SLO syndrome is based on findings of elevated levels of 7DHC and 8DHC. Plasma cholesterol levels are usually but not always low; as many as 10% of patients at all ages have normal cholesterol levels (Kelley and Hennekam, 2000). In addition, the standard method for analysis of cholesterol in most hospital laboratories identifies 7DHC and 8DHC as cholesterol. Therefore most laboratories report normal cholesterol levels in patients who have low cholesterol, but elevations of 7DHC and 8DHC sufficient to bring the total level into the "normal" range (Kelley and Hennekam, 2000; Porter, 2008). The difference between mild and more severe disease appears to be one of degree; the enzyme defect is more severe and the block is more complete in patients with severe disease (Kelley and Hennekam, 2000; Tint et al, 1995). Clinical severity in SLO syndrome correlates best with either reduction in absolute cholesterol levels or the sum of 7DHC plus 8DHC expressed as a fraction of total sterol (Waterham and Clayton, 2006). Recently, maternal apolipoprotein E (ApoE) genotype was implicated in phenotype heterogeneity (Witsch-Baumgartner et al, 2004). Maternal ApoE2 genotypes were associated with a severe SLO syndrome phenotype, whereas ApoE genotypes without the E2 allele were associated with a milder phenotype (Witsch-Baumgartner et al, 2004; Yu and Patel, 2005).

Confirmation of diagnosis via molecular analysis is available. Genotype-phenotype correlation, however, is relatively poor (Jezela-Stanek et al, 2008; Porter, 2008). Prenatal diagnosis is possible. A mother carrying an affected fetus may have an abnormally low unconjugated estriol value. Ultrasonography detects many but not all affected fetuses, and biochemical analysis of amniotic fluid and of chorionic villus samples is accurate and unambiguous in most cases (Kelley and Hennekam, 2000). A direct correlation between the level of 7DHC in amniotic fluid and clinical severity has been demonstrated; however, a similar correlation does not exist for the level of cholesterol (Yu and Patel, 2005). When molecular mutations are known, analysis may be useful.

TREATMENT

There are two goals of therapy for SLO syndrome: to increase the level of cholesterol in plasma and other body fluids and to lower the level of 7DHC. Treatment consists of providing exogenous cholesterol, in the form of either dietary cholesterol or cholesterol suspension, to replenish body stores of cholesterol and downregulate the patient's endogenous cholesterol synthesis, thus decreasing the amount of 7DHC produced. A goal of cholesterol supplementation of 20 to 60 mg/kg per day was initially advocated, but doses higher than 300 mg/kg per day have been used without adverse outcome (Irons et al, 1995; Kelley and Hennekam, 2000). In infants with SLO syndrome, the use of breast milk should be encouraged because it supplies approximately 133 mg/L of cholesterol (Irons et al, 1995).

Providing bile acids to facilitate adequate absorption of dietary cholesterol is controversial, especially because fat malabsorption is unusual and certain bile acids can decrease tissue uptake of cholesterol (Kelley and Hennekam, 2000). Dietary cholesterol supplementation appears to restore both adrenal and bile salt deficiencies (Yu and Patel, 2005). Steroid replacement therapy may still be needed during times of stress or illness. Use of 3-hydroxy-3-methyl-CoA (HMG-CoA) lyase inhibitors such as lovastatin has also been suggested as a mechanism to decrease levels of 7DHC. However, because the results of animal studies suggest that downregulation of cholesterol synthesis might not decrease 7DHC, and because of concern about a decrease in the synthesis of other essential isoprenoid compounds, HMG-CoA reductase inhibitors are not routinely used in therapy (Kelley and Hennekam, 2000). Furthermore, this treatment could be theoretically detrimental in patients with SLO syndrome with little or no enzyme activity (Yu and Patel, 2005). Statins may also impair dietary cholesterol absorption (Merkens et al, 2009). In addition, a retrospective study of simvastatin use in patients with SLO syndrome failed to demonstrate a positive effect on anthropometric measures or behavior (Haas et al, 2007).

Although many questions remain about optimal therapy and outcomes, therapeutic interventions appear to increase plasma cholesterol levels, decrease 7DHC levels, and improve irritability, behavior, and growth (Elias et al, 1997; Irons et al, 1995; Kelley and Hennekam, 2000; Waterham and Clayton, 2006). Parents reported children to be more alert, active, and happier during therapy. Therapy was well tolerated. Unfortunately, a study of 14 patients with SLO syndrome indicated that cholesterol supplementation had hardly any effect on developmental progress (Sikora et al, 2004). Treatment probably does not significantly change sterol levels in brain which are dependent on de novo cholesterol synthesis because of limited ability of cholesterol to cross the blood-brain barrier (Porter, 2008; Waterham and Clayton, 2006). Direct delivery of cholesterol to the CNS by low-pressure catheter infusions has been proposed, but not tested (Yu and Patel, 2005). Gene therapy, the use of neuroactive steroids, and inhibition of glycosphingolipids are also being investigated as possible therapeutic options in SLO syndrome (Merkens et al, 2009).

For maximal benefit, it has been suggested that treatment should begin prenatally, because SLO syndrome has many features that are consistent with in utero involvement of the disease process. Antenatal supplementation by fetal intravenous and intraperitoneal transfusions of fresh frozen plasma were shown to increase fetal cholesterol in one patient (Irons et al, 1999). Treatment should otherwise begin as soon as possible after birth or as soon as the diagnosis is confirmed. Patients with severe SLO syndrome may need gavage or gastrostomy feeding for management of reflux and gastrointestinal dysmotility, and many have protein allergies and require elemental formulas. Growth is often a problem, but the temptation to overfeed must be avoided because overfeeding would contribute to feeding problems and could not rescue intrauterine growth restriction in severe SLO syndrome (Kelley and Hennekam, 2000).

SUGGESTED READINGS

Barth PG: Sphingolipids. In Fernandes J, Saudubray J-M, van den Berghe G, editors: *Inborn Metabolic Diseases: Diagnosis and Treatment*, ed 2, Berlin, 1995, Springer-Verlag, pp 375-382.

Beutler E, Grabowski GA: Gaucher Disease. In Scriver CR, Beaudet AL, Sly WS, Valle D, et al, editors: *The Metabolic and Molecular Bases of Inherited Disease*, ed 8, New York, 2001, McGraw-Hill, pp 3635-3668.

Fletcher JM: Screening for lysosomal storage disorders: a clinical perspective, *J Inherit Metab Dis* 29:405-408, 2006.

Gould S, Raymond G, Valle D: The peroxisome biogenesis disorders. In Valle D, Beaudet AL, Vogelstein B, et al: *The Metabolic and Molecular Bases of Inherited Disease*, ed 8, New York, 2001, McGraw-Hill, pp 3181-3217.

Grünewald S: Congenital disorders of glycosylation: rapidly enlarging group of (neuro)metabolic disorders, *Early Hum Devel* 83:825-830, 2007.

Jaeken J: Congenital disorders of glycosylation. In Fenandes J, Saudubray JM, van den Berghe G, et al: *Inborn Metabolic Diseases: Diagnosis and Treatment*, ed 4, Heidelberg, 2006, Springer Medizin Verlag, pp 523-530.

Jaeken J, Matthijs G, Carchon H, et al: Defects of *N*-glycan synthesis. In Scriver CR, Beaudet AL, Sly WS, et al: *The Metabolic and Molecular Bases of Inherited Disease*, ed 8, New York, 2001, McGraw-Hill, pp 1601-1622.

Meikle PJ, Grasby DJ, Dean CJ, et al: Newborn screening for lysosomal storage disorders, *Mol Genet Metab* 88:307-314, 2006.

Moser HW, Smith KD, Watkins PA, et al: X-linked adrenoleukodystrophy. In Valle D, Beaudet AL, Vogelstein B, et al: *The Metabolic and Molecular Bases of Inherited Disease*, ed 8, New York, 2001, McGraw Hill, pp 3257-3301.

Porter FD: Smith-Lemli-Opitz syndrome: pathogenesis, diagnosis, and management, *Eur J Hum Genet* 16:535-541, 2008.

Staretz-Chacham O, Lang TC, LaMarca ME, et al: Lysosomal storage disorders in the newborn, *Pediatrics* 123:1191-1207, 2009.

Stone DL, Sidransky E: Hydrops fetalis: lysosomal storage disorders in extremis, *Adv Pediatr* 46:409-440, 1999.

Wanders R, Barth P, Heymans H: Single peroxisomal enzyme deficiencies. In Valle D, Beaudet AL, Vogelstein B, et al: *The Metabolic and Molecular Bases of Inherited Disease*, ed 8, New York, 2001, McGraw Hill, pp 3219-3256.

Waterham HR, Clayton PT: Disorders of cholesterol synthesis. In Fenandes J, Saudubray JM, van den Berghe G, Walters JH, editors: *Inborn Metabolic Diseases: Diagnosis and Treatment*, ed 4, Heidelberg, 2006, Springer Medizin Verlag, pp 414-415.

Complete references used in this text can be found online at www.expertconsult.com

SKELETAL DYSPLASIAS AND CONNECTIVE TISSUE DISORDERS

David L. Rimoin and George E. Tiller

The skeletal dysplasias, or osteochondrodysplasias, are disorders of the development and growth of cartilage and bone. The connective tissue disorders involve abnormalities of the cells' supporting and connecting structures in the matrix. In one series of 126,316 deliveries monitored over 15 years, the incidence of skeletal dysplasias was 2.14 in 10,000 (Rasmussen et al, 1996). With the growing use and accuracy of ultrasonography for prenatal care, a greater number of osteochondrodysplasias and connective tissue disorders are diagnosed prenatally.

The skeletal dysplasias have been classified into 37 groups on the basis of radiologic criteria (Superti-Furga and Unger, 2007). Other classifications vary according to molecular, clinical, pathologic, and radiologic criteria and may be confusing. For example, osteogenesis imperfecta (OI) can be classified as either a skeletal dysplasia or a connective tissue disorder. This chapter focuses on several of the more common skeletal dysplasias (see Table 24-1 for an expanded list) and connective tissue disorders that manifest prenatally or perinatally, but the discussion is not exhaustive. The osteochondrodysplasias have been reviewed extensively elsewhere (Cohen, 2006; Superti-Furga et al, 2001; Unger et al, 2007).

There are a large number of different connective tissue molecules, including collagens (over two dozen types), elastin, fibrillin (two types), and microfibril-associated glycoproteins. These molecules are components of tissues such as bone, cartilage, skin, vascular media, tendon, ligaments, and basement membrane in many organs. The heritable disorders of connective tissue are varied, may be very dissimilar clinically, and may manifest in utero or at any age postnatally. Those that may manifest at birth include the infantile (neonatal) form of Marfan syndrome, congenital contractural arachnodactyly (Beals syndrome), cutis laxa, Ehlers-Danlos syndrome, and Menkes disease.

CLINICAL SPECTRA OF DISORDERS WITH COMMON MOLECULAR BASES

The number of clinically distinguishable skeletal dysplasias and connective tissue disorders is extensive. With advances in molecular knowledge, several different dysplasias have been recognized to have mutations in the same genes. In some of these disorders, clinical similarities noted previously suggested a common etiology. One such clinical spectrum includes achondroplasia, hypochondroplasia, severe achondroplasia with developmental delay and acanthosis nigricans (SADDAN), and thanatophoric dysplasia, all of which are caused by mutations in the fibroblast growth factor receptor 3 (*FGFR3*) gene (Bellus et al, 1995; Shiang et al, 1994; Vajo et al, 2000; Wilcox et al, 1998). Another spectrum of disorders includes Stickler syndrome, Kniest dysplasia, spondyloepimetaphyseal dysplasia, spondyloepiphyseal dysplasias, hypochondrogenesis, achondrogenesis type II, and recessive multiple epiphyseal dysplasia, all of which are caused by mutations in the gene for collagen type II, *COL2A1* (Spranger et al, 1994; Winterpacht et al, 1993). With other disorders, the common etiology is not as obvious clinically: diastrophic dysplasia, atelosteogenesis type II, and achondrogenesis type 1B are all caused by mutations in the diastrophic dysplasia sulfate transporter (*DTDST*) gene (Bonafe and Superti-Furga, 2007; Hastbacka et al, 1994, 1996; Superti-Furga et al, 1996). The obverse is also evident, wherein a specific clinical entity (e.g., multiple epiphyseal dysplasias) may be caused by a mutation in one of several genes—a concept known as *genetic heterogeneity*.

APPROACH TO DIAGNOSIS

An early and precise diagnosis is important for prognosis, optimal immediate- and long-term management, accurate genetic counseling about recurrence risk, and identification of other possibly affected family members or disease carriers. An example is the group of disorders with punctate calcifications ("stippling") in epiphyses, called *chondrodysplasia punctata*. There are more than three types, each of which has a different cause and mode of inheritance: autosomal recessive, X-linked recessive, and X-linked dominant (see Table 24-1). As in any uncommon genetic condition, multiple factors may be required to arrive at the correct diagnosis: a complete physical examination, three-generation family history, radiologic studies, and biochemical or molecular tests.

Most skeletal dysplasias cause short stature, which can be proportionate or disproportionate. The disproportion may be evident as a short-limbed or short-trunk form of dwarfism. If the limbs are affected, there may be segmental shortening of the upper arms and thighs (rhizomelia), forearms and legs (mesomelia), or hands and feet (acromelia). Most skeletal dysplasias that manifest at birth involve short limbs. Accurate measurements of length (on a firm surface), arm span, and head and chest circumferences must be plotted on standard growth curves, with calculation of upper and lower body segment ratios to objectively assess disproportion.

Other skeletal characteristics can give important clues for specific disorders:

- Children with achondroplasia and thanatophoric dysplasia have large heads (macrocephaly). Cloverleaf skull deformity is present in some forms of thanatophoric dysplasia.
- A relatively long chest is seen in asphyxiating thoracic dystrophy.
- In achondroplasia the hand is short and the fingers form a trident configuration. In diastrophic dysplasia, there are distinctive "hitchhiker" thumbs.

TABLE 24-1 Skeletal Dysplasias Manifesting Prenatally or Perinatally

Dysplasia	Skeletal Features	Nonskeletal Features	Radiographic Features	Inheritance; Gene	Comments
Lethal					
Achondrogenesis type IB	Soft cranium; round face; short, round chest; very short limbs	Polyhydramnios	Poorly ossified calvarium; ribs short with fractures (beading); nonossified vertebrae; small pelvis; short broad femurs with metaphyseal spikes, short broad tibiae, and fibulae	AR; DTDST (diastrophic dysplasia sulfate transporter)	Same gene as diastrophic dysplasia and atelosteogenesis II
Achondrogenesis type II, hypo-chondrogenesis	Large head, flat face with cleft palate; short trunk; very short limbs (micromelia)	Fetal hydrops; distended abdomen;	Lack of vertebral mineralization; short limbs (all segments); enlarged cranium with normal ossification	AD; *COL2A1* (type II collagen)	Same gene as for spondyloepiphyseal dysplasia congenita, spondyloepimetaphyseal dysplasia, Stickler syndrome, Kniest syndrome
Asphyxiating thoracic dystrophy	Normal face; narrow, long chest; variable limb shortening	Lethal pulmonary insufficiency	Normal calvarium and vertebrae; very short ribs with anterior cupping; short limbs with wide proximal femoral metaphyses; premature ossification of proximal femoral epiphysis	AR	Survivors may have renal disease; possibly a variant of short-rib polydactyly III
Atelosteogenesis					
Type I	Flat face with cleft palate, micrognathia; very narrow chest; very short limbs (rhizomelic) with equinovalgus deformities; joint dislocations	Prematurity; stillbirth	Flat vertebrae with coronal and sagittal clefts, scoliosis, short ribs (11 pairs), small pelvis with enlarged sacrosciatic notch, short limbs, "drumstick" humeri and femurs, absent fibulas, short metacarpals triangular first metacarpals, dislocated knees	AD; filamin B	Filamin B mutations also seen in boomerang dysplasia, Larsen syndrome, and spondylocarpotarsal syndrome
Type II	Cleft palate, narrow chest, short limbs with dislocations, equinovarus deformities, gap between first and second digits	Laryngeal stenosis; patent foramen ovale	Occasional coronal and sagittal vertebral clefts; short ribs; normal sacrosciatic notch; short "dumbbell" humeri and femurs, small fibulas; large second and third metacarpals; small round midphalanges	AR; *DTDST* (diastrophic dysplasia sulfate transporter)	Same gene as for diastrophic dysplasia, achondrogenesis type IB, and some forms of multiple epiphyseal dysplasia (MED)
Campomelic dysplasia	Large cranium; small face with flat nose bridge, small chin (cleft soft palate); small, narrow chest; bowed thighs and legs, with dimple on leg	Polyhydramnios, congenital cardiac abnormalities, female external genitalia in XY males	Large dolichocephalic calvarium with shallow orbits; short and wavy ribs, often 11 pairs; hypoplastic scapula; small, flat vertebrae; tall, narrow pelvis; relatively long, thin limbs with bent femurs and short tibiae	AD (most are new mutations); *SOX9*	
Chondrodysplasia punctata, rhizomelic type 1 (*RCDP1*)	Face flat; very flat nasal bridge and tip; proximal shortening of limbs	Cataracts; joint contractures; ichthyosiform erythroderma	Wide coronal vertebral clefts; short humeri and femurs; stippled epiphyses of long bones, pelvis and periarticular areas; trapezoid ilia	AR; *PEX7* (peroxisome biogenesis factor 7)	Survivors may live a few years, with severe growth and mental retardation; biochemical abnormalities are decreased RBC plasmalogens and increased phytanic acid
Short-rib polydactyly					Heterogeneous ciliopathies

Continued

TABLE 24-1 Skeletal Dysplasias Manifesting Prenatally or Perinatally—cont'd

Dysplasia	Skeletal Features	Nonskeletal Features	Radiographic Features	Inheritance; Gene	Comments
Types I and III	Hydropic appearance, round flat face, micrognathia, extremely narrow chest, very short limbs, postaxial polydactyly	Cardiac, renal, anal malformations	Normal calvarium; very short, horizontal ribs; flat, wide intervertebral disc spaces; small pelvis; short limbs with lateral and medial metaphyseal spurs	AR; *DYNCH2H1* (dynein heavy chain 1B for type III only)	
Types II and IV	Hydropic; short face, flat nose, CLP; low-set ears; narrow chest, protuberant abdomen; moderately short limbs	Cardiac, renal, respiratory malformations	Very short, horizontal ribs; normal pelvis and vertebrae; short limbs with round metaphyses; premature epiphyseal ossification; polydactyly	AR; NEK1 (never in mitosis gene A-related kinase 1 for type II only)	
Thanatophoric dysplasia	Large cranium, proptosis, flat nasal bridge, narrow chest, very short limbs (all segments)	Polyhydramnios, hydrocephalus, brain anomalies, congenital cardiac abnormalities	Large calvarium, short base, small foramen magnum, cloverleaf skull (type 2); short, splayed, cupped ribs; small, very flat, U-shaped vertebrae; short, small, flat pelvis; short, bowed limbs; metaphyseal flare with spike	AD (most are new mutations); *FGFR3* (fibroblast growth factor receptor 3)	Same gene as for achondroplasia, hypochondroplasia, SADDAN
Nonlethal					
Achondroplasia	Large cranium; frontal bossing, flat nose bridge, short neck; slightly narrow chest; proximal limb shortening, short trident hands; short proximal and middle phalanges; joint laxity; thoracolumbar kyphosis	Hypotonia: delayed motor milestones; spinal stenosis causes spinal compression; small foramen magnum can cause hydrocephalus and apnea	Large calvarium, small foramen magnum, short base; diminished lumbosacral interpedicular space, short pedicles; short ribs with anterior cupping; short humeri and femurs; relatively long fibulas; metaphyseal flare; small iliac wings	AD (most are new mutations); *FGFR3*	Same gene as for hypochondroplasia, SADDAN, and thanatophoric dysplasia
Chondrodysplasia punctata, X-linked recessive	Hypoplasia of the distal phalanges; severe hypoplasia of nose; short stature	Cataracts; hearing loss; congenital ichthyosis, anosmia, and hypogonadism (in contiguous gene deletion patients)	Distal phalangeal hypoplasia; stippled epiphyses of long bones; paravertebral stippling	XLR; *ARSE* (arylsulfatase E)	Usually milder than X-linked dominant form; variable clinical severity, with neonatal death to longevity and diagnosis in adulthood
Chondrodysplasia punctata, X-linked dominant (Conradi-Hunermann syndrome)	Asymmetric rhizomesomelia	Congenital cataracts; ichthyosis; patchy alopecia	Stippled epiphyses of long bones; paravertebral stippling; tracheal calcifications	XLD; *ESP* (3β-hydroxy Δ8-Δ7 sterol isomerase)	Severe form of disease; usually lethal in males; females vary from stillborn to mild (diagnosis in adulthood); elevated 8(9)-cholestenol
Diastrophic dysplasia	Normal cranium; cleft palate; micrognathia; normal chest at birth; very short limbs; thumbs proximally placed and adducted (hitchhiker thumb); severe equinovarus of feet; limited movement of many joints	Cystic masses in auricles (cauliflower ears) during infancy; deafness caused by lack or fusion of ossicles; narrow external auditory canal	Premature ossification of rib cartilage; narrow L1-L5 interpedicular spaces; scoliosis; short limbs; disproportionately short ulna and fibula (mesomelia); broad flared metaphyses; ovoid first metacarpals; variable symphalangism of proximal interphalangeal joints	AR; *DTDST* (diastrophic dysplasia sulfate transporter)	Same gene as atelosteogenesis II, achondrogenesis type IB, and some forms of multiple epiphyseal dysplasia (MED); intrafamilial variability; normal life span if tracheomalacia or scoliosis do not impair respiratory function; normal intelligence

TABLE 24-1 Skeletal Dysplasias Manifesting Prenatally or Perinatally—cont'd

Dysplasia	Skeletal Features	Nonskeletal Features	Radiographic Features	Inheritance; Gene	Comments
Kniest syndrome	Large cranium; flat face with large eyes, flat nasal bridge, cleft palate; short limbs with proximal shortening (more severe in lower limbs), enlarged joints, flexion contractures	Infancy: tracheomalacia; childhood: myopia and retinal detachment, hearing loss, delayed motor development, normal intelligence	Frontal and maxillary hypoplasia with shallow orbits; slightly short ribs; flat vertebrae with coronal clefts; small pelvis with irregular acetabular roof; short limbs with broad, flared metaphyses (dumbbell), lateral bowing of femurs and tibiae; slightly short and broad tubular bones of hands and feet; epiphyses at knees not ossified	AD; *COL2A1* (type II collagen)	Same gene as for spondyloepiphyseal dysplasia congenita, spondyloepimetaphyseal dysplasia, Stickler syndrome, hypochondrogenesis, achondrogenesis type II
Spondyloepiphyseal dysplasia congenita	Flat face, cleft palate, short limbs	Infancy: tracheomalacia; childhood: myopia and retinal detachment, hearing loss, normal intelligence	Frontal and maxillary hypoplasia, flat vertebrae, small pelvis with irregular acetabular roof, short limbs, normal hands and feet	AD; *COL2A1* (type II collagen)	Same gene as for spondyloepimetaphyseal dysplasia, Stickler syndrome, hypochondrogenesis, achondrogenesis type II, Kniest syndrome

AR, Autosomal recessive; *AD*, autosomal dominant; *RBC*, red blood cell; *CLP*, cleft lip with or without cleft palate; *XLR*, X-linked recessive; *XLD*, X-linked dominant.

- Clubfeet may occur in diastrophic dysplasia, Kniest dysplasia, spondyloepiphyseal dysplasias, and OI type II.
- Postaxial polydactyly occurs in short-rib polydactyly and asphyxiating thoracic and chondroectodermal dysplasias. Occasionally, preaxial polydactyly can also occur in the short-rib dysplasias.
- Multiple joint dislocations can manifest at birth in Larsen syndrome, Ehlers-Danlos syndrome type VII, atelosteogenesis, and Desbuquois syndrome.

The presence of extraskeletal abnormalities may provide additional clues to diagnosis, as follows:

- Cleft palate may occur in campomelic, Kniest, spondyloepiphyseal, short-rib polydactyly (Majewski), atelosteogenesis types I and II, hypochondrogenesis, and diastrophic dysplasias.
- Congenital cataracts are frequent in some forms of chondrodysplasia punctata.
- Congenital cardiac defects occur in short-rib polydactyly dysplasias and Ellis van Creveld syndrome.

CLINICAL TESTING

Radiographs of the entire skeleton, including the skull, hands, feet, and lateral spine, are essential for accurate diagnosis. Atlases dedicated to skeletal dysplasias are essential for this purpose (Lachman, 2006; Spranger et al, 2002), even to the experienced radiologist or neonatologist. Ultrasound images of the brain, heart, and kidneys may be helpful if anomalies in those organs are suspected. Detailed family history and measurements of family members may be helpful; more mildly affected members might have gone without a diagnosis. Molecular investigations may be necessary to arrive at the proper diagnosis; given their complexity, such analyses should be considered after consultation with a clinical geneticist.

If the infant or fetus dies, specimens of cartilage and skin fibroblasts should be obtained for histochemical tests, biochemical assays, and molecular analysis; these can be used to make or confirm diagnoses and permit accurate future prenatal diagnosis. Even if the molecular or enzymatic basis of the condition is not understood at the time, the tissue may be useful in the future. If photographs and skeletal radiographs were not obtained premortem, they should be obtained postmortem.

DISORDERS OF BONE FRAGILITY

OSTEOGENESIS IMPERFECTA TYPES II AND III

OI is characterized by increased bone fragility. There are classically four major clinical types: types II and III are the most severe, manifesting prenatally and perinatally (Byers, 2002; Steiner et al, 2005). However, fractures at birth can occur in OI type I. Further heterogeneity in OI has recently been described.

Presentation

OI type II (perinatal lethal type) is estimated to affect 1 in 20,000 to 60,000 infants. Affected infants may be born prematurely, with low birthweight and disproportionately short stature. The limbs are short and bowed with extra, circular skin creases; the hips are abducted and flexed. The head is soft and boggy, and minimal calvarial bone can be felt. The sclerae are dark blue and the chest is narrow. The infant cries with handling because there are many fractures at different stages of healing. Sixty percent of affected babies are stillborn or die during the first day of life, and 80% die by 1 month. With the growing use of ultrasonography, affected fetuses may be detected in the early second trimester because of

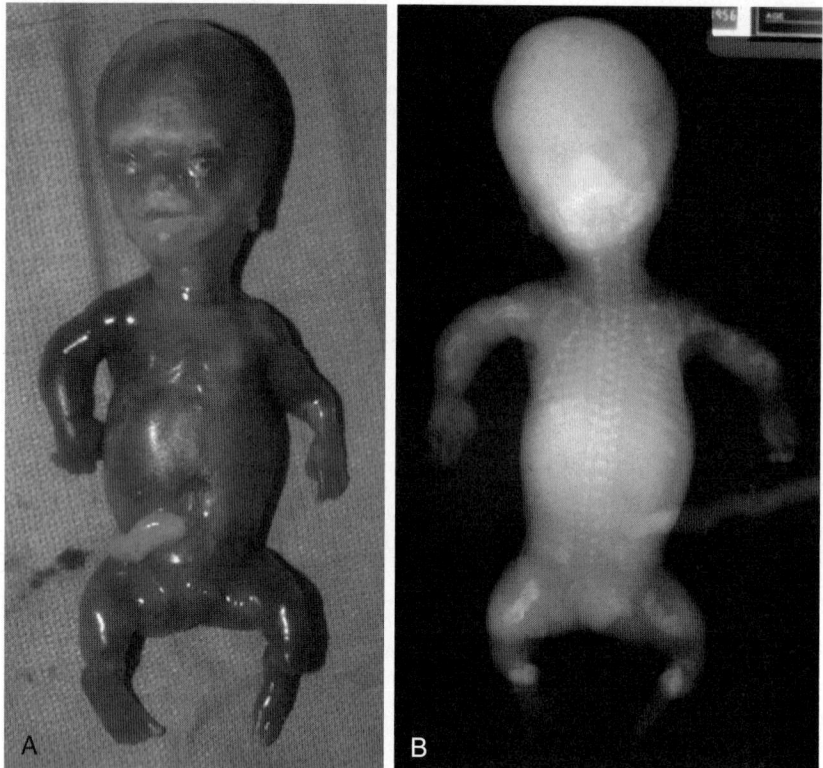

FIGURE 24-1 *(See also Color Plate 5.)* **Osteogenesis imperfecta type II. A,** A 20-week fetus. The limbs are angulated and deformed from multiple fractures. **B,** Radiograph of fetus (20 weeks' gestation) showing an absence of ossification in the calvarium, short telescoped or crumpled humeri and femurs, and short and wavy ribs with fractures.

short and bowed or angulated limbs and narrow thoraces (Figure 24-1).

OI type III (progressive deforming type) can manifest prenatally, perinatally, and in the first 2 years of life. Prenatal and perinatal clinical features resemble those in OI type II, but are less severe (Figure 24-2), and perinatal death is not uncommon. If not present at birth, fractures and deformations of the limbs develop in the first and second years. The highest prevalence of fractures in OI, up to 200, occur in type III. Extremely short stature, with adult heights of 92 to 108 cm, can result from microfractures in growth plates. The head may be large because the calvarium is soft with a large anterior fontanel. The sclerae may be blue initially, but are white by puberty. The head assumes a triangular shape, with a bossed, broad forehead and a tapered, pointed chin. Later in childhood, dentinogenesis imperfecta and hearing loss may develop. Severe kyphoscoliosis may occur, leading to cardiopulmonary compromise, which is the major cause of early death.

Radiolographic Features

Radiographs show the femurs in OI type II to be short, broad, and "telescoped" or "crumpled." The tibiae are short and bowed or angulated, and the fibulae may be thin (see Figure 24-1, *B*). There is minimal to no calvarial mineralization. The acetabulae and iliac wings may be somewhat flattened. The ribs are short, wavy, and thin or broad, with "beading" from callus formation at fetal fracture sites.

In OI type III, the femurs are short and deformed, but not crumpled as in OI type II (see Figure 24-2, *B* and *C*). The other long bones are thinner than usual, with healing fractures incurred in utero, bowing, and deformations. The calvarium is undermineralized with a large anterior fontanel, and there are many Wormian bones (small islands of bone in the suture spaces; see Figure 24-2, *D*). The ribs are thin and gracile.

Etiology

OI is most commonly caused by mutations in one of the two genes for type I collagen (*COL1A1* and *COL1A2*), the predominant protein building block of bone. More clinically severe forms of OI are the result of qualitatively abnormal collagen synthesis, rather than decreased production (Byers, 2002).

Inheritance

A fetus or infant with OI type II or III is usually the result of a spontaneous dominant-acting gene mutation, but there is a small risk of recurrence (approximately 6%) in subsequent siblings because of parental somatic or gonadal mosaicism. The parent is usually asymptomatic but may have minimal manifestations, such as short stature. Most cases of OI are inherited as autosomal dominant traits, although rare recessive forms have been shown to be caused by mutations in the cartilage-associated protein CRTAP (Barnes et al, 2006), prolyl 3-hydroxylase (LEPRE1), and cyclophylin B (van Dijk et al, 2009).

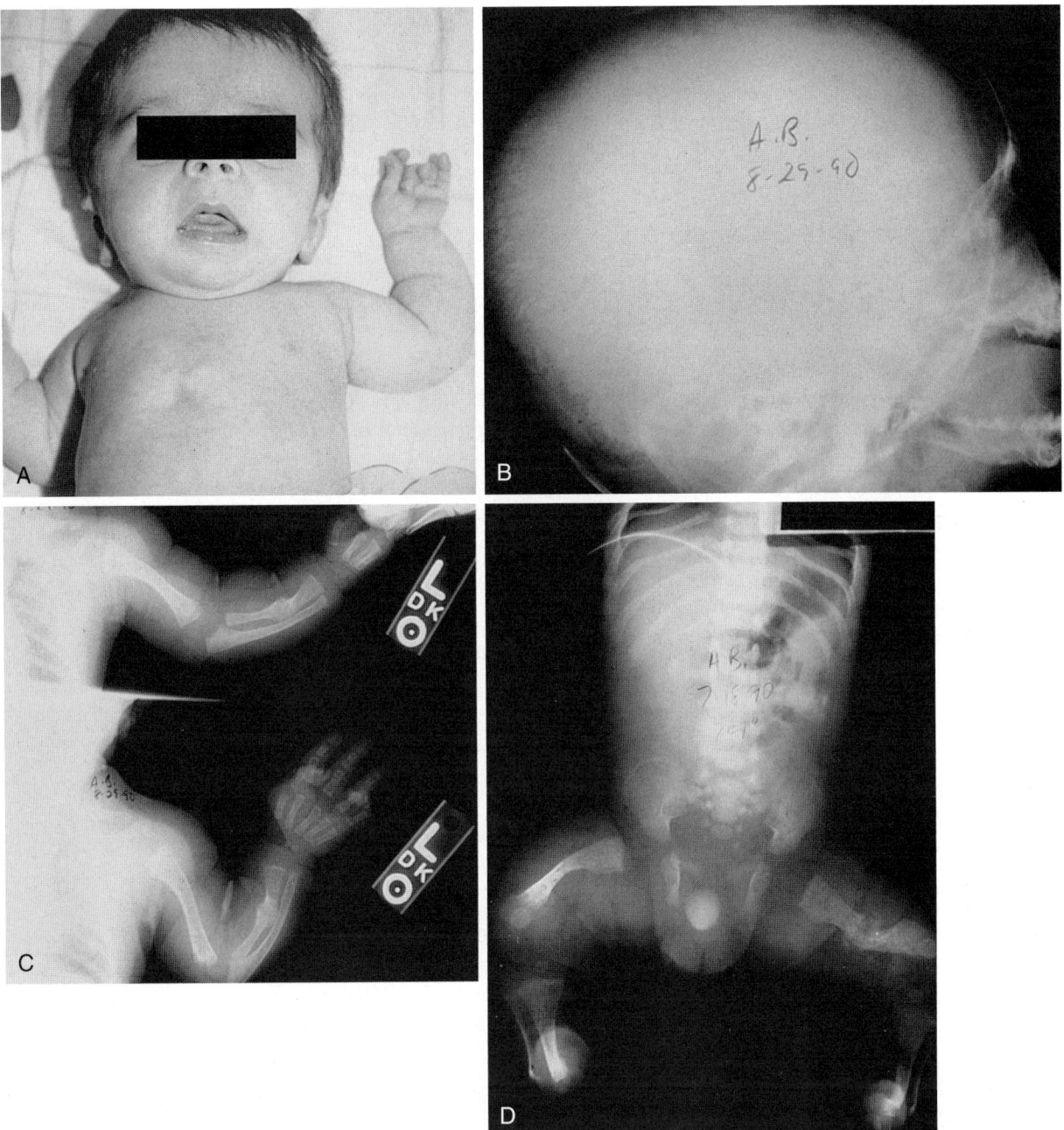

FIGURE 24-2 Osteogenesis imperfecta type III. **A,** Neonate with normal face, short neck, slightly short limbs. **B,** Radiograph shows that the calvarium is undermineralized with Wormian bones. **C,** Radiograph shows the upper limbs, which have bowed humeri and callus in the ulnae. **D,** Radiograph shows lower limbs with moderately short, thick femora, and angulated tibiae and fibulae. (*Courtesy Paige Kaplan, Children's Hospital of Philadelphia, Philadelphia, Penn.*)

Differential Diagnosis

Other lethal skeletal dysplasias may have similar abnormalities to those in OI type II and may be difficult to distinguish by prenatal ultrasonography; however, in experienced hands they can be differentiated based on several ultrasound findings. Krakow et al (2008) did a retrospective analysis of 1500 prenatally diagnosed cases of skeletal dysplasias. The three most common prenatal-onset skeletal dysplasias were osteogenesis imperfecta type 2, thanatophoric dysplasia, and achondrogenesis 2, accounting for almost 40% of cases. Postnatal radiographs clearly reveal distinctive differences among thanatophoric dysplasia,

campomelic dysplasia, achondrogenesis, and perinatal hypophosphatasia, among others.

Management

If the diagnosis of OI is made prenatally, cesarean delivery has not been shown to decrease fracture rate or improve survival rate of severely affected fetuses (Cubert et al, 2001). Those severely affected with OI II are not expected to survive the neonatal period. In OI type III, the neonate needs careful handling to minimize pain and prevent further fractures. Analgesia alleviates pain. Consideration can be given to treatment with bisphosphonates (using intravenous pamidronate), which increase bone density, reduce the frequency of fractures and pain, possibly prevent short stature and deformations, and permit ambulation (Aström et al, 2007). It is prudent to treat only severely affected children in whom the clinical benefits outweigh potential long-term effects.

Handling an Infant With Osteogenesis Imperfecta

When changing the diapers of an infant with OI, place a hand behind the buttocks with the forearm supporting the legs. Similarly, when the infant is lifted the buttocks, head, and neck must be supported. The infant can be laid on a pillow to be carried. To transport the infant, an infant seat that reclines as much as possible and allows easy placement or removal should be used. The seat can be padded with egg crating or 1-inch foam. A layer of foam can be placed between the seat's harnesses and the child for extra protection. The car seat must always be placed in the back seat. Sling carriers and "umbrella" strollers should not be used for infants with OI because they do not give sufficient leg, head, and neck support.

PERINATAL HYPOPHOSPHATASIA

Presentation

Perinatal hypophosphatasia is a lethal condition characterized by short, deformed limbs, a soft skull, blue sclerae, and undermineralization of the entire skeleton, so that many bones cannot be visualized and may seem absent on radiography. In the skull, only the base can be visualized radiologically. There may be rachitic changes and fractures. Seizures that are responsive to pyridoxine may occur. There is polyhydramnios during pregnancy, and death can occur in utero. The disorder affects approximately 1 in 100,000 live births; neonatal death is common (Whyte, 2000).

Radiographic Features

The radiologic features of perinatal hypophosphatasia include polyhydramnios (prenatal); underossification, especially of the calvarium and long bones (with marked variability); small thoracic cavity; short, bowed limbs; spurs in the middle portion of the forearms and lower legs; and dense vertebral bodies.

Etiology

Mutations in the *ALPL* gene are responsible for deficiency of the tissue-nonspecific isoenzyme of alkaline phosphatase (TNSALP), thus causing perinatal hypophosphatasia. The serum alkaline phosphatase (ALP) value is low. Serum values of inorganic pyrophosphate and pyridoxal 5′-phosphate (putative natural substrates for TNSALP) may be elevated, and urinary phosphoethanolamine is elevated (Mornet and Nunes, 2007).

TNSALP acts on multiple substrates: the essential function of TNSALP is in osteoblastic bone matrix mineralization. TNSALP hydrolyzes inorganic pyrophosphate to phosphate, thought to be critical in promoting osteoblastic mineralization. If TNSALP is deficient, there is extracellular accumulation of inorganic pyrophosphate, which inhibits hydroxyapatite crystal formation and mineralization of the skeleton. TNSALP is also needed for delivery of pyridoxal-5-phosphate into cells where it is a cofactor (vitamin B_6).

Inheritance

Perinatal hypophosphatasia is inherited as an autosomal recessive trait, with a 25% recurrence risk in future pregnancies. Prenatal diagnosis is optimized through the use of ultrasonography, assay of TNSALP activity in amniocytes, DNA mutation analysis if the previously affected infant's mutation was known, or a combination of these methods.

Differential Diagnosis

Differential diagnoses are osteogenesis imperfecta type II and achondrogenesis.

Management

Treatment is primarily supportive and directed toward minimizing pain and discomfort. Clinical trials with bone-targeted human recombinant enzyme replacement therapy are underway.

FGFR3 SPECTRUM

ACHONDROPLASIA

Presentation

Achondroplasia is the most common of the nonlethal chondrodysplasias; it affects 1 in 25,000 live births. It is characterized by short stature with short limbs, particularly rhizomelic (proximal) and acromelic (hands) shortening with trident hand configuration, large head with frontal prominence ("bossing"), flat nasal bridge and midface, long narrow trunk, joint laxity, and development of thoracolumbar kyphosis ("gibbus") in infancy (Figure 24-3).

The foramen magnum and cervical spinal canal may be narrow and can cause compression of the spinal cord. Standards have been published for foramen magnum size in achondroplasia (Hecht et al, 1985). Compression of the lower brainstem and cervical spinal cord can lead to hypotonia, central apnea, retardation, quadriparesis, and (rarely) sudden death (Pauli et al, 1984). Perinatal or infantile death can occur, but is unusual. Infants often sleep with their neck hyperextended, and symptoms can be exaggerated by neck flexion (Danielpour et al, 2007).

Radiographic Features

The calvarium is large with a relatively small foramen magnum and a short base. The lateral cerebral ventricles may be large, but hydrocephalus is not a common

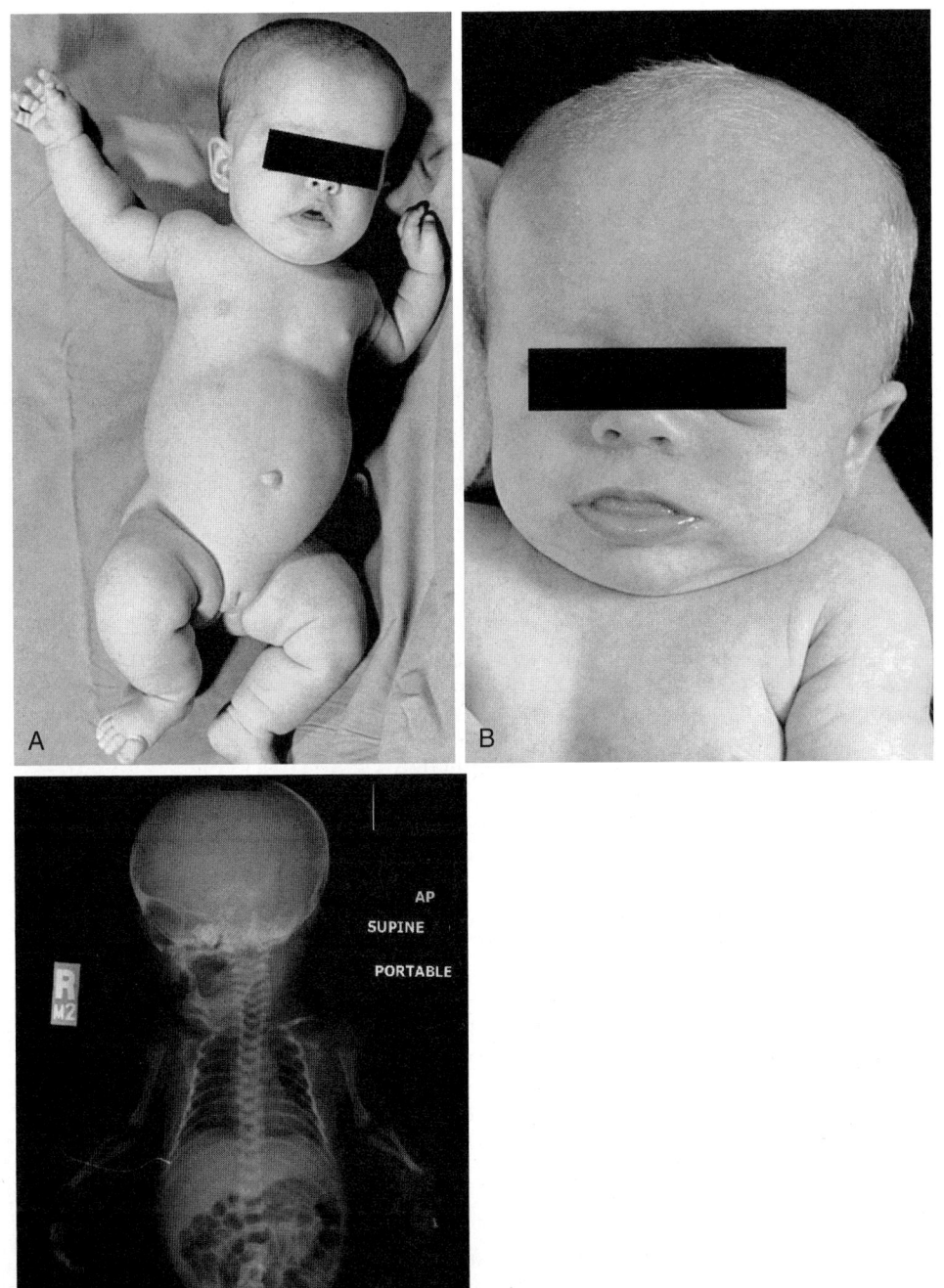

FIGURE 24-3 Achondroplasia. A, Infant with achondroplasia has macrocephaly and proximal limb shortening (rhizomelia). **B,** Infant with achondroplasia exhibits frontal bossing and flat nasal bridge. **C,** Neonatal film of achondroplasia illustrates a large skull, a somewhat narrow chest, short vertebral bodies with a lack of lumbar interpediculate flare, and rhizomelia. (**B,** *Courtesy Charles I. Scott, AI DuPont Institute, Wilmington, Del.*)

complication. The proximal long bones (humeri and femurs) are short, including the femoral neck. Fibulae are longer than tibiae. There is metaphyseal flaring. The hand is short with a trident configuration of the fingers, with short proximal and middle phalanges. Vertebrae are small and cuboid with short pedicles, and there may be anterior beaking of the first or second lumbar vertebrae; there is lack of flare of the interpedicular distance in the lumbar vertebrae. The pelvis has squared iliac wings ("elephant ear" appearance), a narrow greater sciatic notch, and flat acetabular roofs. Compression of the cervical cord, if present, can be ascertained with magnetic resonance imaging cerebrospinal fluid flow studies in flexion and extension.

Etiology

The cause of achondroplasia is a mutation of the gene for fibroblast growth factor receptor 3 (*FGFR3*). The FGFR3 protein is a membrane-spanning tyrosine kinase receptor, which may form dimers with other gene family members *FGFR1*, *FGFR2*, and *FGFR4*. The heterodimers serve as receptors for several fibroblast growth factors (Cohen, 2006). More than 97% of persons with achondroplasia have a mutation in the transmembrane domain of the *FGFR3* gene, in which glycine is substituted by arginine (Gly380Arg; Shiang et al, 1994). The same gene is mutated at different sites in hypochondroplasia, thanatophoric dysplasia, SADDAN, Muenke craniosynostosis, and Crouzon craniosynostosis syndrome with acanthosis nigricans (Vajo et al, 2000). Histopathologic examination demonstrates a defect in the organization and maturation of the cartilage growth plates of long bones because of differing degrees of constitutive activation of the receptor.

Inheritance

The inheritance pattern in achondroplasia is autosomal dominant. Approximately 80% of cases are sporadic occurrences in a family, representing new mutations. Cases may be associated with advanced paternal age, with molecular confirmation that the new mutations are of paternal origin. Affected individuals are fertile, and achondroplasia is transmitted as a fully penetrant autosomal dominant trait, meaning that each person who inherits the mutant gene will manifest the condition.

Differential Diagnosis

Differential diagnoses are SADDAN (Vajo et al, 2000) hypochondroplasia (Bellus et al, 1995).

Management

The infant with achondroplasia is often hypotonic; together with the large head, the hypotonia leads to delayed motor milestones. Development of thoracolumbar kyphosis may be exacerbated by unsupported sitting before truncal muscle strength is adequate; therefore infants should not be carried in flexed positions (including soft sling-carriers and umbrella strollers). Rear-facing car safety seats should always be used. Most infants lose their kyphosis and develop lumbar lordosis when they begin walking.

Hydrocephalus may occasionally develop during the first 2 years, so the head circumference and body length should be carefully measured and plotted on standard achondroplasia growth charts (Trotter et al, 2005). Routine imaging of the skull and brain is not recommended; however, development of hyperreflexia, hypotonia, or apnea may herald the development of clinically significant cord compression. Surgical decompression at the foramen magnum or the upper cervical spine may prevent neurologic damage, although most patients usually gain motor milestones late but spontaneously, because the foramen grows faster than the cord.

The upper airway in individuals with achondroplasia is small, often leading to obstructive apnea, snoring, and chronic serous otitis media beyond infancy. Treatment may consist of tonsillectomy, adenoidectomy, and placement of myringotomy tubes. Parents should be counseled about the clinical and hereditary aspects of the disorder and given a copy of the guidelines for health supervision of children with achondroplasia issued by the American Academy of Pediatrics (Trotter et al, 2005).

THANATOPHORIC DYSPLASIA

Presentation

Thanatophoric dysplasia is one of the most common lethal dysplasias (Unger et al, 2007), occurring in 1 in 45,000 births. It is characterized by extremely short limbs, long narrow trunk, large head with bulging forehead, prominent eyes, flat nasal bridge, wide fontanel, and occasionally cloverleaf skull deformity (Figure 24-4). It is differentiated into types I and II on the basis of radiologic features. Death occurs in the neonatal period from respiratory insufficiency. Polyhydramnios is common during pregnancy.

Radiographic Features

Femurs are short, flared at the metaphyses with a medial spike, and are bowed (type I) or straight (type II); other long bones are also short and bowed (see Figure 24-4). The calvarium is large with a short base and small foramen magnum; cloverleaf skull is sometimes present in type I and is severe in type II. Vertebrae are strikingly flat (platyspondyly) with a U- or H-shape in anteroposterior projection and uniform interpediculate narrowing. Ribs are short, cupped, and splayed anteriorly (Lachman, 2006).

Etiology

Thanatophoric dysplasia represents the severe end of the FGFR3 spectrum. In thanatophoric dysplasia type I, the most common mutation in the extracellular domain is a substitution of arginine at position 248 by cysteine (Arg248Cys), but other mutations have been described throughout the gene. In all studied cases of thanatophoric dysplasia type II, there is a substitution of lysine at position 650 by glutamate (Lys650Glu; Wilcox et al, 1998).

Inheritance

All cases of thanatophoric dysplasia, as with most cases of achondroplasia and hypochondroplasia, occur sporadically and result from new autosomal dominant mutations. Nevertheless, there may be a small risk of recurrence to siblings of a sporadic case, possibly caused by gonadal mosaicism.

Differential Diagnosis

Differential diagnoses are OI types II and III, achondroplasia (severe), achondrogenesis, and hypochondrogenesis.

Management

If the condition is diagnosed prenatally, the couple should receive genetic counseling and anticipate neonatal death. If the diagnosis is suggested after delivery and radiographically confirmed, management is solely supportive, with death from pulmonary insufficiency usually occurring within hours to days.

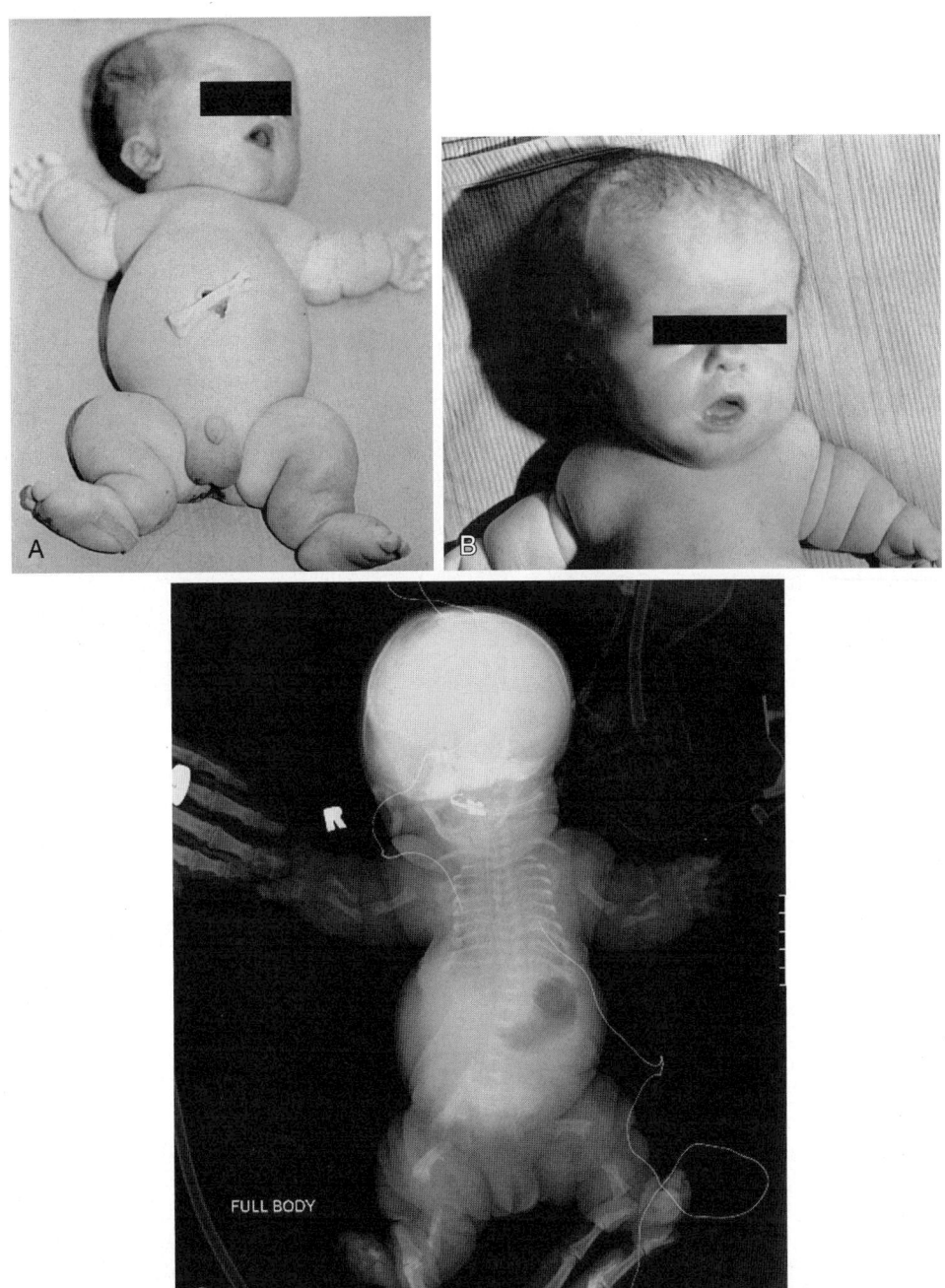

FIGURE 24-4 *(See also Color Plate 6.)* **Thanatophoric dysplasia. A,** Neonate with thanatophoric dysplasia has a large head, narrow chest, short limbs, extra creases on the limbs, short hands with trident fingers, and angulated abducted thighs. **B,** Neonate with thanatophoric dysplasia has a face with a bossed forehead, flat nose bridge, short neck, very short limbs with extra creases, and trident fingers. **C,** Radiograph of an infant with thanatophoric dysplasia demonstrates a large calvarium, short ribs with anterior splaying, flat vertebral bodies (platyspondyly), and short bowed femurs with medial metaphyseal spike. *(**B,** Courtesy Montreal Children's Hospital, Montreal, Quebec, Canada.)*

COL2A1 SPECTRUM

SPONDYLOEPIPHYSEAL DYSPLASIA CONGENITA

Presentation

Spondyloepiphyseal dysplasia congenita (SEDC) manifests with shortened neck, trunk and limbs, normal-sized hands and feet, flat facial profile, and occasional cleft palate and clubfoot (Unger et al, 2007). The name is derived from the spinal (spondylo-) and growth plate (epiphyseal) involvement. *Congenita* indicates that the condition is present from birth.

Radiographic Features

Radiographic features include ovoid or pear-shaped vertebral bodies in infancy, with platyspondyly more evident at a later age; odontoid hypoplasia evident in early childhood; midface hypoplasia; retrognathia; mild rhizomelia

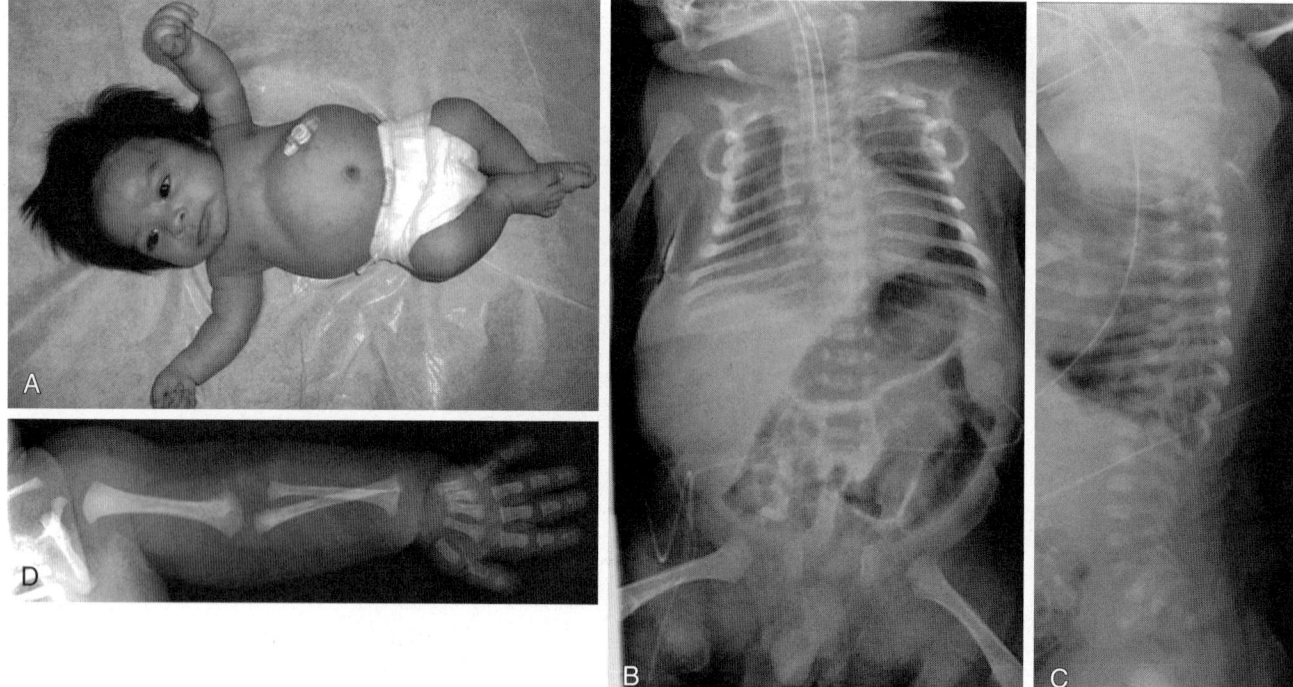

FIGURE 24-5 *(See also Color Plate 7.)* **Spondyloepiphyseal dysplasia congenita. A,** A 2-month-old infant demonstrating short neck, trunk, and limbs. Note the flat facial profile and normal size of hands and feet. **B,** Anteroposterior radiograph reveals platyspondyly and short chest. **C,** Lateral radiograph reveals platyspondyly. **D,** Upper limb radiograph reveals rhizomelia, mesomelia, and a normal-sized hand.

and mesomelia (Figure 24-5); absent ossification of the os pubis; apparent decreased bone age caused by epiphyseal involvement; and development of coxa vara, variable kyphosis, and scoliosis in childhood

Etiology

SEDC is caused by mutations in the gene for type II collagen (*COL2A1*), the predominant protein building block of cartilage. Mutations in *COL2A1* are also responsible for Kniest dysplasia, some forms of spondyloepimetaphyseal dysplasia and Stickler syndrome, and the perinatal lethal disorders achondrogenesis type II and hypochondrogenesis (Spranger et al, 1994; Tiller et al, 1995; Winterpacht et al, 1993).

Inheritance

SEDC is inherited in an autosomal dominant pattern. Offspring of affected individuals are at 50% risk for inheriting the disorder. Recurrence risk for unaffected parents is approximately 6%, because of parental gonadal mosaicism.

Differential Diagnosis

Differential diagnoses are the milder form of hypochondrogenesis and Morquio syndrome.

Management

Neonates may require intubation because of upper airway compromise. Care must be given when manipulating the cervical spine (as in endotracheal intubation), because

of odontoid hypoplasia. C1-C2 fusion may be required in early childhood to stabilize the cervical spine. Annual hearing screens are recommended during childhood. Regular ophthalmologic evaluation (semiannually before school age) is essential to detect early development of retinal detachment and to manage myopia. Osteoarthritis is a common feature in early adulthood, often requiring hip arthroplasty.

ACHONDROGENESIS II–HYPOCHONDROGENESIS

Presentation

The severe end of the COL2A1 spectrum manifests with fetal hydrops and maternal polyhydramnios, severe short trunk and limbs, and fetal or neonatal death caused by pulmonary hypoplasia.

Radiographic Features

Radiographic features include prenatal polyhydramnios, a large calvarium with normal ossification, midface hypoplasia, retrognathia, platyspondyly with underossification of the vertebral bodies (achondrogenesis II), short chest with a protuberant abdomen, marked shortening of all tubular bones (Figure 24-6), and small iliac wings.

Etiology

Achondrogenesis II–hypochondrogenesis is caused by mutations in the gene for type II collagen (*COL2A1*), the predominant protein building block of cartilage (Mortier et al, 2000).

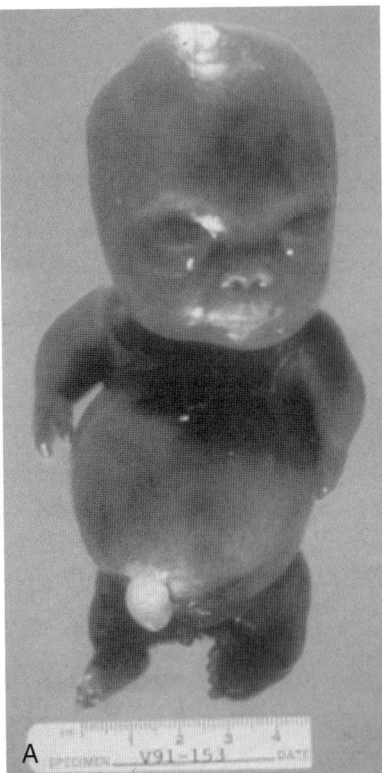 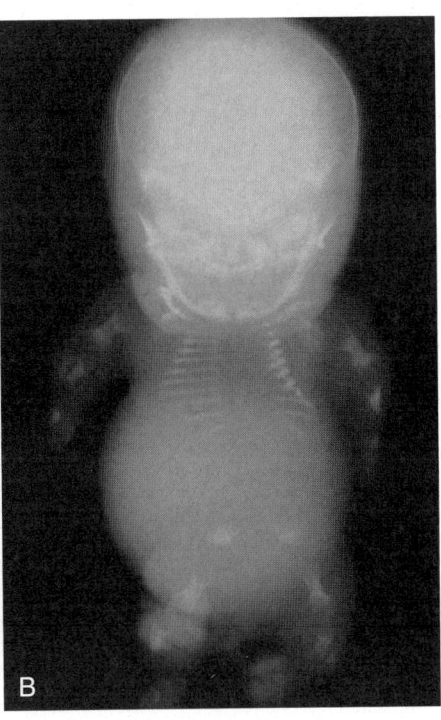

FIGURE 24-6 **Achondrogenesis type II. A,** This 20-week fetus demonstrates small chest and short limbs. **B,** This radiograph demonstrates poor ossification of vertebral bodies and short limbs.

Inheritance

All cases of achondrogenesis II–hypochondrogenesis are caused by spontaneous dominant-acting mutations in *COL2A1*. Recurrence risk has been reported as high as 6%, because of parental gonadal mosaicism (Forzano et al, 2007).

Differential Diagnosis

Differential diagnoses are achondrogenesis type I and osteogenesis imperfecta types II and III.

Management

If the condition is diagnosed prenatally, the couple should receive genetic counseling and anticipate neonatal death. If the diagnosis is suggested after delivery and radiographic confirmation is obtained, management is solely supportive, with death from pulmonary insufficiency usually occurring within hours to days.

DTDST SPECTRUM

DIASTROPHIC DYSPLASIA

Presentation

Newborns with diastrophic dysplasia exhibit limb shortening, cystic ear swelling, hitchhiker thumbs (developing several days after birth), spinal deformities (especially cervical kyphosis), and contractures of the large joints (Figure 24-7). Clubfoot and ulnar deviation

of the fingers may also be present. On occasion the disease can be lethal at birth, but most individuals survive the neonatal period (Bonafe and Superti-Furga, 2007).

Radiographic Features

The most characteristic clinical and radiologic feature is the proximally-placed hitchhiker thumb, with ulnar deviation of the fingers. Cervical kyphosis is a frequent finding. Long bones are moderately shortened and thick, with mild metaphyseal flaring, rounding of the distal femur, and bowing of the radius and tibia. Severe talipes equinovarus may be present. Iliac wings are hypoplastic, with flat acetabular roofs. The chest can be narrow, bell shaped, or both. Narrowing (lack of flare) of the interpedicular distance in the lumbar spine is reminiscent of achondroplasia.

Etiology

Diastrophic dysplasia is caused by mutations in the diastrophic dysplasia sulfate transporter gene (*DTDST*), which also cause the lethal disorders achondrogenesis type 1B and atelosteogenesis type 2, as well as a rare recessive form of multiple epiphyseal dysplasia. The gene product is a sulfate-chloride exchanger of the cell membrane (Superti-Furga et al, 1996); this affects incorporation of sulfate into proteoglycans (mucopolysaccharides), especially chondroitin sulfate B–containing proteoglycans, which are prevalent in cartilage.

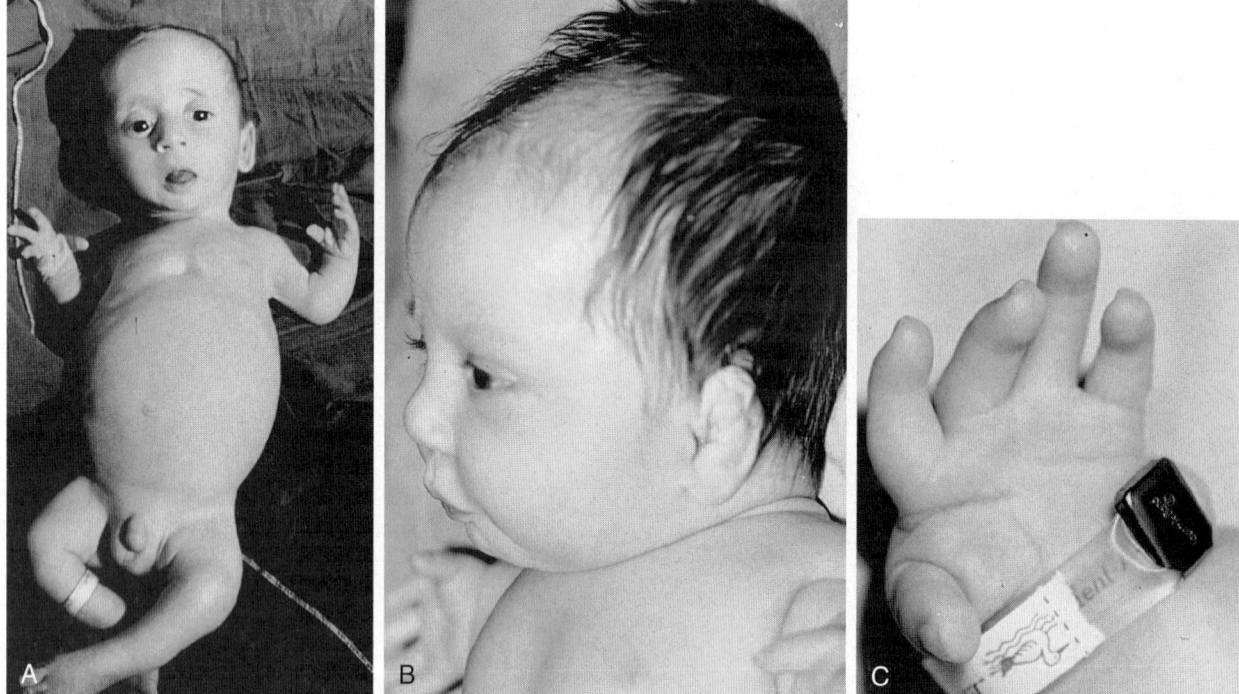

FIGURE 24-7 Diastrophic dysplasia. A, This infant has prominent eyes, small chin, slightly narrow chest, proximally placed angulated thumbs, and short limbs. **B,** Neonate profile showing small chin, swollen ears, and short neck. Note the proximally placed, angulated thumb. **C,** View of the neonate's hand shows the proximally placed angulated thumb and mild syndactyly. *(Courtesy Paige Kaplan, Children's Hospital of Philadelphia, Philadelphia, Penn.)*

Inheritance

Diastrophic dysplasia is inherited in an autosomal recessive pattern. Siblings of affected individuals are at 25% risk for inheriting an abnormal allele from both carrier parents.

Differential Diagnosis

Differential diagnoses are atelosteogenesis type II (part of the DTDST spectrum), spondyloepiphyseal dysplasia, and arthrogryposis.

Management

Mechanical ventilation may be required because of small chest circumference and a floppy airway. Maintenance of joint mobility and proper positioning through physical therapy is essential. Serial casting and or surgical correction of clubfeet may be required. Cervical kyphosis can impede endotracheal intubation and can result in cord compression, but may resolve spontaneously during infancy.

ACHONDROGENESIS 1B

Presentation

Achondrogenesis type IB is characterized by short stature, extremely short limbs, a relatively large head with a round face, short nose, small mouth, soft skull, and very short neck (Borochowitz et al, 1988). Polyhydramnios during pregnancy, premature delivery, and hydrops are common. The affected infant is stillborn or dies within hours of birth.

Radiographic Features

The long bones are extremely short, with square, globular, or triangular shapes and medial spikes in the metaphyses of the femurs (Figure 24-8). The calvarium and vertebrae are poorly ossified (type IB), and the ribs are short.

Etiology

Achondrogenesis type 1B is caused by mutations in the *DTDST* gene (see Diastrophic dysplasia, earlier).

Inheritance

Achondrogenesis 1B is inherited in an autosomal recessive pattern. Siblings of affected individuals are at 25% risk for inheriting an abnormal allele from both carrier parents.

Differential Diagnosis

Differential diagnoses are atelosteogenesis type II (part of DTDST spectrum), achondrogenesis type II, and hypochondrogenesis.

Management

If the condition is diagnosed prenatally, the couple should receive genetic counseling and anticipate neonatal death. If the diagnosis is suggested after delivery and radiographic confirmation is obtained, management is solely supportive, with death from pulmonary insufficiency usually occurring within hours to days.

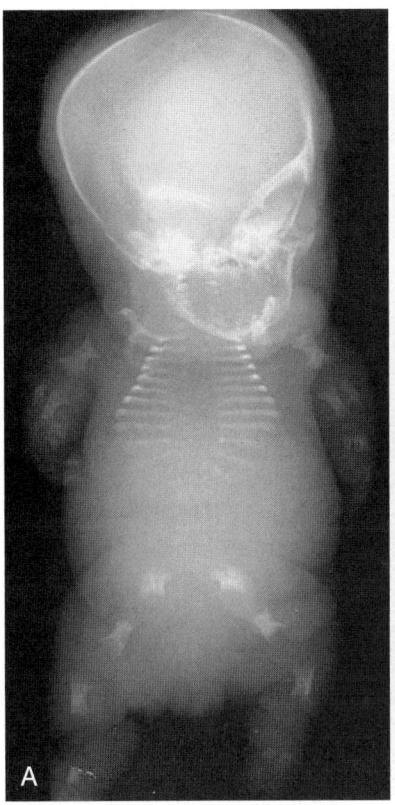
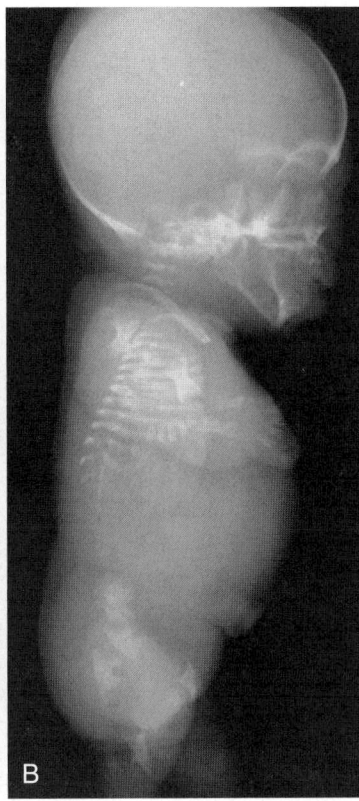

FIGURE 24-8 A and **B,** Achondrogenesis type IB. Cervical, thoracic, and lumbar vertebral bodies are not ossified, the sacrum is not ossified, the ribs are short, and the limbs are extremely short with medial femoral metaphyseal spikes. *(Courtesy Elaine Zackai, Children's Hospital of Philadelphia, Philadelphia, Penn.)*

OTHER SKELETAL DYSPLASIAS

CAMPOMELIC DYSPLASIA

Presentation

Campomelic dysplasia is characterized by short stature (birth length of 35 to 49 cm), large dolichocephalic skull, large anterior fontanel, high forehead, flat face, widely spaced eyes with short palpebral fissures, low-set ears, cleft soft palate, micrognathia, relatively long and slender thighs and upper arms, short bowed legs with dimples in the midshaft (in most cases), narrow chest, and kyphoscoliosis (Figure 24-9). Sex reversal or ambiguous genitalia affects 75% of the chromosomal males; there may be internal and external genital abnormalities (from mild anomalies to complete sex reversal) in XY males (Meyer et al, 1997; see Figure 24-9, *A* and *B*). Absence of the olfactory bulbs and tracts as well as heart and renal malformations may occur. Death, usually in infancy, results from pulmonary hypoplasia, tracheomalacia, or cervical spinal instability. Survivors are usually globally developmentally delayed. A few more mildly affected people without bowed limbs have been reported (Unger et al, 2008).

Radiographic Features

The most characteristic finding is midshaft angulation (campomelia) of the femurs, although it is not a constant finding. Other features include hypoplastic, undermineralized cervical vertebrae and thoracic pedicles; narrow iliac wings with dislocated hips; brachydactyly; clubfeet; anterior bowing of tibia; bell-shaped chest with thin, wavy ribs (with only 11 pairs); and scapular hypoplasia.

Etiology

Campomelic dysplasia is caused by mutations in or near the SRY-related HMG-Box gene 9 (*SOX9*; Tommerup, 1993). *SOX9*, with homology to the *SRY* gene, is a transcription factor involved in both bone formation and testis development.

Inheritance

Campomelic dysplasia is an autosomal dominant trait. Most cases are new sporadic occurrences in a family; recurrence caused by gonadal mosaicism has been reported (Smyk et al, 2007).

Differential Diagnosis

Differential diagnoses are osteogenesis imperfecta types II and III, diastrophic dysplasia, kyphomelic dysplasia, thanatophoric dysplasia, and spondyloepiphyseal dysplasia congenita (severe).

Management

Survival beyond the newborn period is rare; therefore support is primarily directed toward comfort measures. In survivors, care must be given to the cervical spine, which may be unstable. Chromosomal studies to determine gender and pelvic ultrasonography to examine internal genitalia

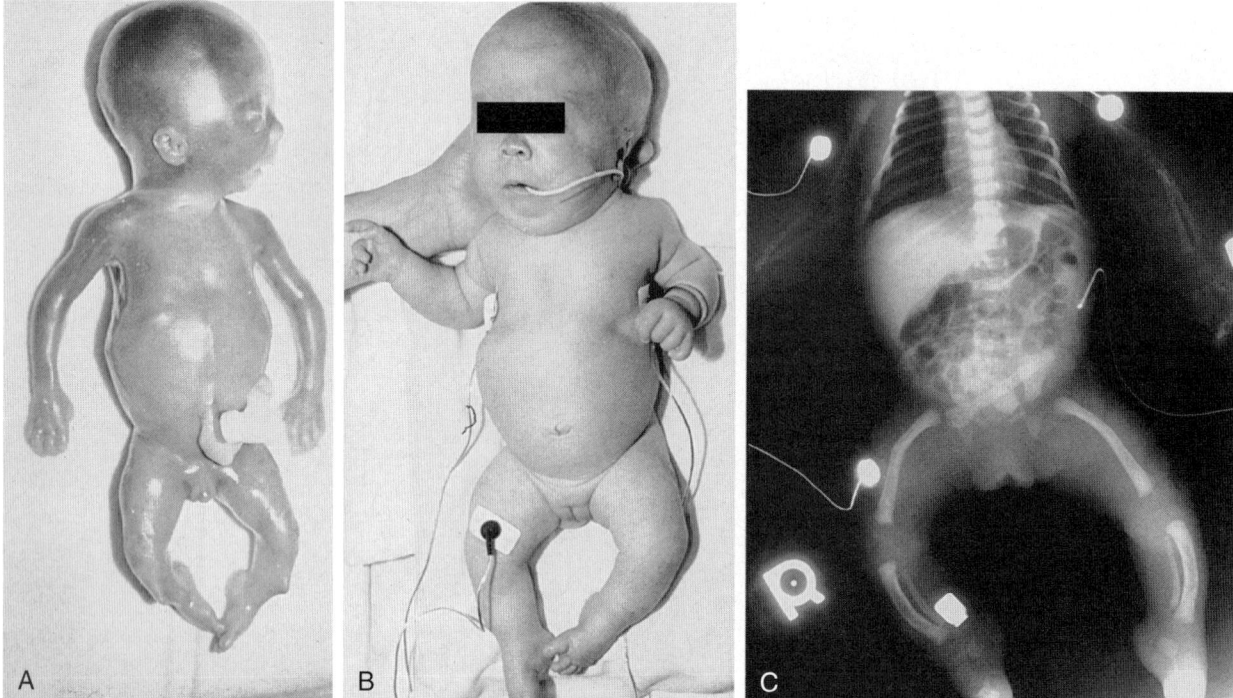

FIGURE 24-9 Campomelic dysplasia. **A,** 46,XY female 22-week-old fetus with normal head, long philtrum, micrognathia, low-set ears, mild narrowing of chest, proximally placed thumbs, and bowed or angulated lower limbs resembling those of osteogenesis imperfecta type II but less shortened. The external genitalia are female. **B,** Neonate with the long-limb form of the disorder has a relatively large head, micrognathia, narrow chest, and bowing of lower limbs with characteristic dimpling of lower leg. **C,** Radiograph shows the narrow chest, the relatively long, thin limb bones with bowing of the femurs and tibiae, and a long, narrow pelvis. *(Courtesy Paige Kaplan, Children's Hospital of Philadelphia, Philadelphia, Penn.)*

may be performed. Cleft palate may be repaired in those able to feed orally, and clubfeet may require casting or surgical correction.

CONNECTIVE TISSUE DISORDERS

CONGENITAL (NEONATAL, INFANTILE) MARFAN SYNDROME

Presentation

Infants with neonatal congenital Marfan syndrome (cMS) have a long, thin body and can have an aged appearance because of a lack of subcutaneous tissue and wrinkled, sagging skin (Morse et al, 1990; Figure 24-10). The craniofacial features include dolichocephaly, deep-set eyes with large or small corneas (and occasionally cataracts), high nasal bridge, high palate, small pointed chin with a horizontal skin crease, and large simple or crumpled ears. The fingers and toes are long and thin (arachnodactyly). Some joints are hyperextensible, and others have flexion contractures causing clubfoot, dislocated hips, or adducted thumbs. Infants tend to exhibit hypotonia with low muscle mass. Lenses are usually not subluxated at birth. The most important cause of morbidity and mortality is severe cardiovascular disease, which affects almost every neonate with cMS—namely, mitral and tricuspid valve prolapse and insufficiency and aortic root dilatation. The ascending aorta may be dilated and tortuous. Many infants die in the first year of life from congestive heart failure. Survivors have chronic hypotonia and contractures, are unable to walk, and require many surgical procedures.

Radiographic Features

Radiographic features include pectus deformity, spontaneous pneumothorax, dural ectasia, aortic root dilatation, and mitral valve prolapse. Many of these features may not be present in the newborn period.

Etiology

Congenital MS is caused by mutations in the gene encoding fibrillin 1 (*FBN1*; Dietz et al, 1991). Fibrillin is a glycoprotein associated with microfibrils, which form linear bundles in the matrices of many tissues, such as aorta, periosteum, perichondrium, cartilage, tendons, muscle, pleura, and meninges. There are two regions in *FBN1* in which many mutations causing cMS occur; these lie among exons 24 to 27 and exons 31 and 32 (Dietz, 2009). Molecular analysis does not yield mutations in all cases.

Inheritance

Marfan syndrome is an autosomal dominant disorder. Most neonates with cMS are sporadic occurrences within a family (Dietz et al, 1991; Morse et al, 1990). However, there is one well-documented neonate with cMS whose father had classic Marfan syndrome except for average height (Lopes et al, 1995).

Differential Diagnosis

Differential diagnoses are congenital contractural arachnodactyly (CCA), autosomal recessive cutis laxa, and Loeys-Dietz syndrome.

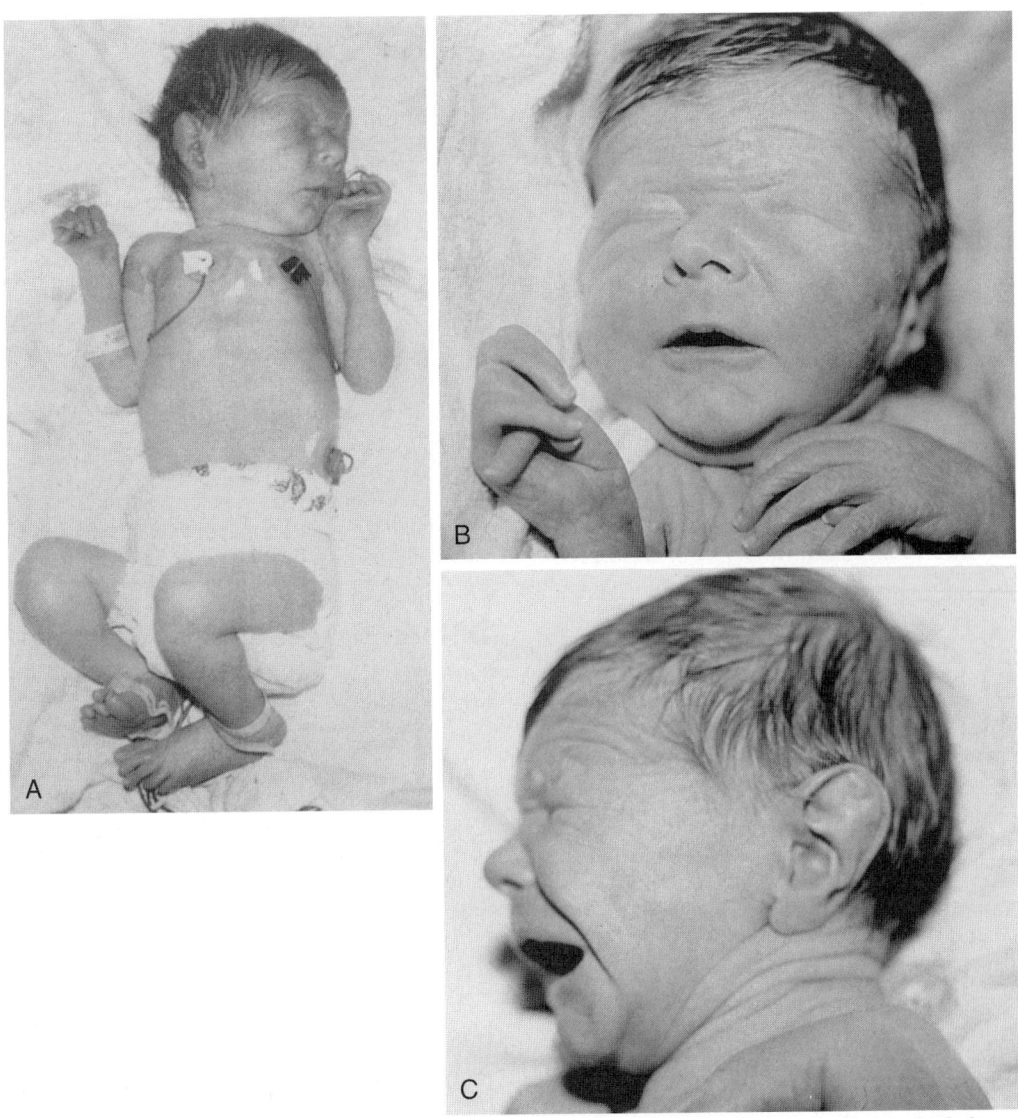

FIGURE 24-10 **Congenital Marfan syndrome. A,** Neonate with long, thin trunk and limbs (particularly the feet), lack of adipose tissue, and multiple skin creases giving an aged appearance. The ears are large and simple, and the chin is small with a horizontal crease. There are flexion contractures at the joints. **B,** The neonate's face shows laxity of skin, typical horizontal chin crease, and a pointed chin. The fingers are long with adduction contractures of the thumbs, which extend past the edge of the palm, and floppy wrists. **C,** Lateral view of the neonate's head showing simple, large ears and redundant skin on the neck. *(Courtesy Paige Kaplan, Children's Hospital of Philadelphia, Philadelphia, Penn.)*

Management

Patients require annual ophthalmologic and cardiac evaluation throughout childhood. Cardioselective beta-blockers, such as atenolol, are often implemented at the first signs of aortic root dilatation. The angiotensin II antagonist losartan has also shown promise in this regard (Brooke et al, 2008). Children should be screened for the development of scoliosis.

CONGENITAL CONTRACTURAL ARACHNODACTYLY (BEALS SYNDROME)

Presentation

CCA (Beals syndrome) is characterized by a thin, wasted appearance with minimal muscle and fat mass (similar to neonatal Marfan syndrome). Distinctive features include arachnodactyly with contractures of the large and small joints (Figure 24-11, *A*), as well as crumpled, overfolded helices of the external ear. Cardiovascular involvement is usually limited to mitral valve prolapse, but aortic root dilatation may occasionally develop (Godfrey, 2007).

Radiographic Features

Features are nonspecific and include elongated proximal phalanges; contractures of digits, ankles, knees, and hips; thin, gracile tubular bones; and gradual development of kyphoscoliosis.

Etiology

CCA is caused by mutations in the fibrillin 2 gene.

Inheritance

CCA is inherited in an autosomal dominant manner, with many patients representing the result of spontaneous mutations. Offspring of affected individuals are at 50% risk for inheriting the condition. Gonadal mosaicism has been described in CCA (Putnam et al, 1997).

Differential Diagnosis

Differential diagnoses are cMS, cutis laxa, and distal arthrogryposis.

Management

Proper nutrition is essential to ensure adequate weight gain. Joint contractures respond to physical therapy, but occasionally surgical release may be required. Surveillance for development of spinal curvature and aortic root dilatation, although rare, are essential throughout childhood.

EHLERS-DANLOS SYNDROMES

Presentation

The Ehlers-Danlos syndromes (EDSs) are a clinically and genetically heterogeneous group of connective tissue disorders, which are characterized by varying degrees of joint and skin hypermobility, excessive bruising, abnormal wound healing, and fragility of tissues (Steinmann et al, 2002; Wenstrup and de Paepe, 2008). This group of disorders was reclassified in 1997 (Beighton et al, 1998). The classic type (formerly type I) and the arthrochalasia type (formerly type VII) are the most likely to manifest in the newborn period. Type I is often characterized by premature delivery of an affected fetus as a result of a rupture of the fragile amniotic membranes. The infant may be floppy and in the breech position. There may be joint laxity and joint instability. In type VII, the major involvement is in the ligaments and joint capsules. Large and small joints are hypermobile and dislocatable; severe congenital dislocation of hips occurs.

In vascular (formerly type IV) EDS, the greatest danger is to the pregnant affected woman, for whom there is a high risk of uterine and arterial rupture. Although there is a 50% risk that the fetus will be affected, the problems of blood loss and prematurity are more important in the newborn period than the disorder itself.

Radiographic Features

Radiographic features are dependent on the particular type of EDS. Congenital hip dislocation may be evident on plain films. Hydronephrosis, bladder diverticula, and spontaneous pneumothorax may occur occasionally. Aortic dilatation and arterial aneurysms may be evident by echocardiography and other imaging modalities, but only occur in patients of school age or older.

Etiology

Mutations in two of the genes for type V collagen (*COL5A1* and *COL5A2*) are demonstrable in some cases of classic EDS (Malfait and de Paepe, 2005). The vascular type is caused by mutations in the gene for type III collagen, *COL3A1*. The arthrochalasia type is caused by mutations in either gene for type I collagen (*COL1A1* or *COL1A2*), which result in loss of the N-proteinase cleavage site of the protein.

Inheritance

Most types of EDS are inherited as autosomal dominant traits. Each child of an affected person has a 50% chance of inheriting and manifesting the disorder, although there can be marked intrafamilial variability (Malfait and de Paepe, 2005). One form of the arthrochalasia type, also referred to as *dermatosparaxis*, is inherited in an autosomal recessive pattern, and is caused by deficiency of procollagen N-peptidase. The kyphoscoliotic form (formerly type VI) is also inherited in an autosomal recessive pattern and is caused by a deficiency of lysyl hydroxylase, an enzyme that aids in crosslinking of collagen fibrils.

Differential Diagnosis

Differential diagnoses are cMS, congenital contractural arachnodactyly, and Larsen syndrome.

Management

Trauma should be avoided because of skin fragility. Effective closure of surgical wounds is challenging because of a tendency for dehiscence (Wenstrup and Hoechstetter, 2004).

CUTIS LAXA

Presentation

Cutis laxa is a genetically heterogeneous disorder, meaning that mutations in several different genes may be responsible for the phenotype. As such, the presentation can be highly varied. Infantile forms may exhibit loose, furrowed skin, a large anterior fontanelle, hypotonia, hernias, and congenital hip dislocation (see Figure 24-11, *B*) (Kaler, 2005; van Maldergem et al, 2011).

Radiographic Features

Radiographic features are in part dependent on the genetic form of the disorder. Nonspecific features include a large anterior fontanel, congenital hip dislocation, and hernias. The X-linked form may exhibit occipital horns. Arterial tortuosity, aortic root dilatation, and cortical and cerebellar anomalies may be seen in some forms, as well as gastrointestinal and urinary tract diverticula.

Etiology

The relatively mild, autosomal dominant form of cutis laxa is caused by mutations in the elastin gene, *ELN*. The X-linked recessive form (occipital horn syndrome) is caused by mutations in the *ATP7A* gene (allelic with Menkes syndrome). Autosomal recessive forms may be caused by mutations in the fibulin 4 (*FBLN4*) and fibulin

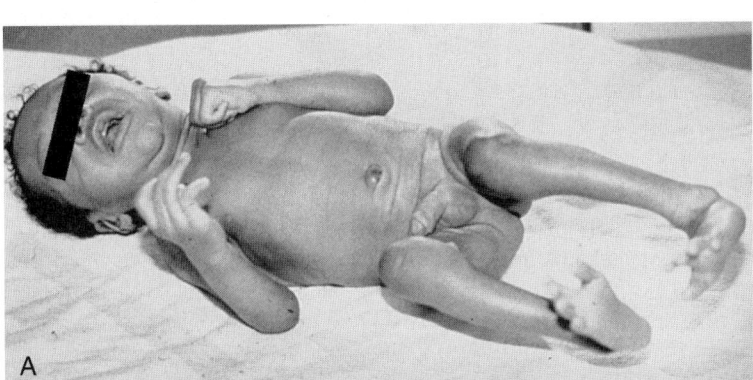

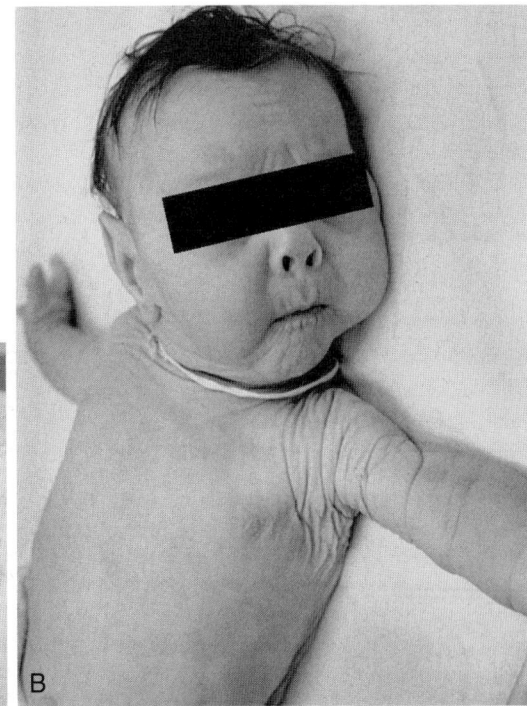

FIGURE 24-11 A, Congenital contractural arachnodactyly (Beals syndrome). This infant has a long, thin trunk and limbs, contractures of joints, and crumpled ears. **B,** Infant with cutis laxa. *(Courtesy Montreal Children's Hospital, Montreal, Quebec, Canada.)*

5 (*FBLN5*) genes or the A2 subunit of the V-ATPase gene (*ATP6V0A2*). Biochemical clues as to the etiology in a particular patient may include decreased serum copper and ceruloplasmin (X-linked form), and abnormal serum sialotransferrin isoelectric focusing in cases caused by ATP6V0A2 mutations.

Inheritance

Because cutis laxa is genetically heterogeneous, modes of inheritance include autosomal dominant, autosomal recessive, and X-linked recessive. The latter two modes are usually responsible for forms with neonatal and infantile presentation.

Differential Diagnosis

Differential diagnoses are EDS, Menkes syndrome, gerodermia osteodysplastica, and de Barsy syndrome.

Management

Serious childhood complications include developmental delay, pulmonary emphysema, aortic root dilatation, and arterial tortuosity. Annual ophthalmologic and cardiac examinations are essential, and referral to special education programs may be indicated.

MENKES SYNDROME

Presentation

Menkes syndrome often appears in the newborn period with nonspecific neurologic manifestations. Typically, developmental delay is evident in the first 2 to 3 months of life, with failure to thrive, seizures, and severe ocular manifestations.

Changes in the appearance of the hair include hypopigmentation, brittleness, patchy alopecia, and twisted shafts seen by light microscopy (i.e., pili torti; Figure 24-12). Early death is common and may occur in infancy (Kaler, 2010). Serum copper and ceruloplasmin concentrations are low, and the plasma dopamine-to-norepinephrine ratio may be elevated (Goldstein et al, 2009).

Radiographic Features

Features may evolve during infancy and may include bladder diverticula (seen on bladder ultrasound and voiding cystourethrogram [VCUG]), tortuous vessels (on echocardiogram, magnetic resonance imaging with contrast), gastric polyps (on upper GI), metaphyseal spurring, osteopenia, and Wormian bones on plain radiographs (Lachman, 2006; see Figure 24-12).

Etiology

Menkes syndrome is caused by mutations in a copper-transporting adenosine triphosphatase gene, *ATP7A* (Kaler et al, 1994). This enzyme takes part in the final processing of a number of copper-dependent enzymes, including dopamine beta-hydroxylase, tyrosinase, lysyl oxidase, superoxide dismutase, and cytochrome c oxidase. As a result, several physiologic processes and cellular functions are impaired, including collagen cross-linking, pigment production, and neurotransmission (Goldstein et al, 2009).

Inheritance

Menkes syndrome is an X-linked recessive disorder; therefore only males are affected. Female carriers may exhibit pili torti in some hair shafts because of lyonization (Moore

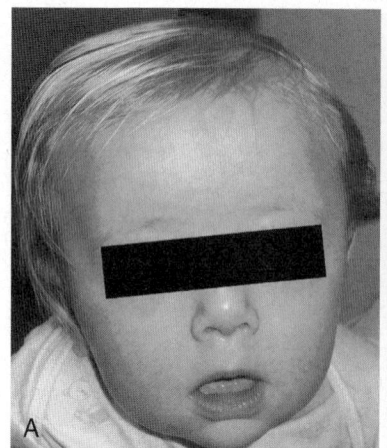
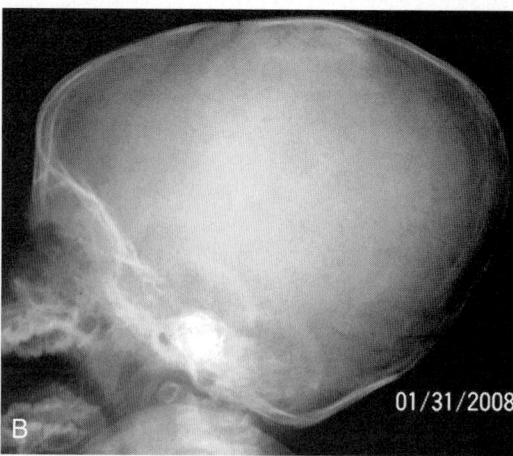

FIGURE 24-12 *(See also Color Plate 8.)* **Menkes syndrome. A,** Note blonde hair, fair complexion, and epicanthal folds in this 11-month-old Hispanic boy. **B,** Note multiple Wormian bones near the occiput.

and Howell, 1985). Sons born to carrier females have a 50% risk for manifesting the disease.

Differential Diagnosis

Differential diagnoses are cutis laxa (the occipital horn form is allelic), EDS, neonatal cMS, biotinidase deficiency, mitochondrial myopathies, nutritional copper deficiency, and organic aciduria.

Management

Early diagnosis allows for parenteral copper supplementation therapy (Kaler et al, 2008), but this is not effective in all patients. Patients should be monitored for the development of seizures, as well as a propensity for bone fragility, poor wound healing, and vascular fragility leading to excessive bleeding, hemorrhagic strokes, and subdural hematomas. Bladder diverticula may result in urinary retention and urinary tract infections and should be surgically corrected. Patients are at risk for moderate to severe developmental delay, and they should be referred to infant stimulation and early intervention programs.

SUGGESTED READINGS

Aström E, Jorulf H, Söderhäll S: Intravenous pamidronate treatment of infants with severe osteogenesis imperfecta, *Arch Dis Child* 92:332-338, 2007.

Brooke BS, Habashi JP, Judge DP, et al: Angiotensin II blockade and aortic-root dilation in Marfan's syndrome, *N Engl J Med* 358:2787-2795, 2008.

Kaler SG, Holmes CS, Goldstein DS, et al: Neonatal diagnosis and treatment of Menkes disease, *N Engl J Med* 358:605-614, 2008.

Trotter TL, Hall JG: The Committee on Genetics: Health supervision for children with achondroplasia, *Pediatrics* 116:771, 2005.

Wenstrup RJ, Hoechstetter LB: Ehlers-Danlos syndromes. In Cassidy SB, Allanson JE, editors: *Management of Genetic Syndromes*, ed 2, New York, 2004, Wiley-Liss, pp 211-224.

Complete references and supplemental color images used in this text can be found online at www.expertconsult.com

PART VII

CARE OF THE HEALTHY NEWBORN

INITIAL EVALUATION: HISTORY AND PHYSICAL EXAMINATION OF THE NEWBORN

Jeffrey B. Smith

The central focus of this chapter is the medical evaluation of the apparently well newborn in the first few days after birth in a hospital setting. Obtaining the history, performing the physical examination, and judging the significance of risk factors and findings all require skill and experience. For brevity, we mostly refer to the person evaluating the newborn as a *pediatrician*. In some institutions, the routine evaluation is performed by a general pediatrician, family practitioner, or pediatric nurse practitioner, and the neonatologist enters the well baby nursery only as a consultant. In other institutions, the neonatologist has direct responsibility for patients in the normal nursery in addition to the neonatal intensive care unit (NICU). In either setting, the neonatologist should develop and maintain proficiency in the evaluation of the normal newborn, a task that requires an approach and set of skills somewhat different than the evaluation of the NICU patient, who typically has a known symptom or high-risk condition. In the normal nursery, the vast majority of newborns are healthy and will not require medical intervention; therefore a primary goal is to identify the small minority with problems that have the potential to cause serious morbidity if not detected in a timely fashion. This goal includes identifying psychosocial and medical problems. For the healthy majority, the evaluation provides the basis for appropriate parental reassurance and education. For this reason, the emphasis of the discussion in this chapter is on common problems, variations of normal, and subtle abnormalities. Some symptoms and findings that suggest significant illness are also described, but the discussion in this chapter is not intended to provide a complete differential diagnosis or guide to management. Physical findings pertinent to specific diseases and organ systems are described with greater detail in other sections throughout the book. Evaluation of the dysmorphic infant is described in Chapter 19. Laboratory studies helpful in the routine care of the healthy newborn are discussed in Chapter 26.

HISTORY

The medical history of the newborn begins with pertinent information about the mother's past medical and pregnancy history, the current pregnancy, and the family. Information about the current pregnancy, labor, and delivery is central at the time of delivery, but the infant's postnatal history becomes progressively more important in the subsequent hours and days. An outline of basic components of the prenatal and newborn history is presented in Table 25-1. The history is potentially gathered from multiple sources, including records of prenatal outpatient visits and laboratory studies; the records of the mother's current and prior hospitalizations; the delivery record; newborn records created by nurses and other personnel; direct communications from the obstetrician, midwife, and nurses; and interviews with the mother and other family members. Most of the prenatal history is collected and recorded by members of the obstetric team. Systems should be in place to ensure that the pediatrician responsible for the newborn is directly informed about high-risk conditions in a timely manner, but the pediatrician has an independent responsibility to review the information available in the maternal record. From a potentially large amount of information, a key task for the pediatrician is to efficiently identify and highlight the portions that are relevant to the newborn's current situation and the task at hand.

To ensure that important information is not overlooked, a systematic approach to the collection and recording of the history is essential. Structured data systems, preferably electronic, can help to ensure that essential information is not missed. However, information gathering must be prioritized appropriately, because the relative importance of specific parts of the history depends on the clinical situation. For example, the physician paged to attend the emergency delivery of a fetus in distress should focus information gathering in the few minutes available on what is directly relevant to preparations for resuscitation. At that moment, it is not necessary to know the results of prenatal testing of the mother for hepatitis B. For the stable infant sent to room-in with the mother and for the critically ill infant admitted to the NICU, it becomes important to obtain this information in the next few hours, so that hepatitis B vaccine can be administered within the recommended 12 hours after birth if the mother does not have a documented negative test result for hepatitis B infection.

For the healthy newborn, history gathering at the time of the initial encounter after birth will emphasize the prenatal history (including maternal and family history), the delivery and neonatal transition, the initiation of feeding, and any symptoms or parental concerns that have manifested since birth. A major goal of the initial evaluation is

TABLE 25-1   Components of the Prenatal and Newborn History

Category	Typical Components of the History
Maternal identification	Name, medical record number, age, gravidity, parity, estimated gestational age
Maternal medical history	Allergies Significant past illnesses, hospitalizations, and surgeries Chronic illnesses, especially diabetes Chronic medications Psychiatric history
Previous pregnancies	Dates, routes of delivery, complications, and outcomes Breastfeeding history
Family history	General health status and history of family members Congenital anomalies, metabolic disorders, hearing impairment Food and other allergies of parents and siblings
Psychosocial history	Family structure, care of previous children Availability of support for parents (extended family, others) Living accommodations, access to transportation Language, racial or ethnic group, parental education level Smoking, alcohol, drugs of abuse Family strife, domestic violence
Current pregnancy	Estimated gestational age (and how determined) Singleton or multiple fetuses Fertilization history (e.g., assisted reproduction) Prenatal care (when started, number of visits, provider) Maternal blood type and screening for unusual isoimmune antibodies Screening for group B streptococcal colonization Other prenatal screening for infectious diseases* Glucose tolerance test results Results of maternal drug screening, if applicable Occupational or other exposure to teratogens Sexual contact with high-risk group Genetic screening tests Ultrasound studies and amniocentesis Complications, hospitalizations Prescription and nonprescription medications; herbal remedies Breastfeeding plans; plans for well-child care after discharge
Labor	Spontaneous, induced, augmented Duration of first and second stages Rupture of membranes: spontaneous versus artificial, duration Amniotic fluid: clear, meconium stained, bloody, foul smelling Signs of infection: fever, increased white blood cell count, uterine tenderness, tachycardia Antibiotics during labor and the indication Other medications during labor Fetal monitoring abnormalities
Delivery and delivery room stabilization	Route and presentation Indication for cesarean section, vacuum, or forceps, if applicable Stabilization and resuscitation measures; time to spontaneous breathing Apgar scores Placental abnormalities, if noted Cord blood gases, if obtained Ease versus difficulty of transition Medications administered (erythromycin eye drops, vitamin K) Abnormalities noted on initial examination
Postnatal history	Nursing or parental concerns Growth parameters (weight, length, head circumference, and percentiles) Vital signs, daily weights Glucose checks Activity and alertness Breastfeeding (frequency, duration, quality of latch) Bottle feeding (amount, frequency, reason) Voiding, wet diapers Meconium and transitional stools Procedures (lumbar puncture, circumcision) Results of laboratory tests and imaging studies

*Prenatal screening performed in accordance with medical recommendations and local regulations commonly include tests for group B *Streptococcus*, hepatitis B, syphilis, gonorrhea, and for immunity to rubella; it may also include tests for chlamydia, tuberculosis, HIV, and hepatitis C.

to identify risk factors for problems that may develop in the next few days, such as early-onset neonatal sepsis or exacerbated hyperbilirubinemia. Identification of psychosocial risk factors is also an important goal, and it remains important throughout the hospitalization. At the time of the predischarge evaluation, the key goal is to determine whether the infant can be discharged home safely. The prenatal and perinatal history will have already been documented and reviewed, so information-gathering for the predischarge evaluation will focus on the interval history, mostly collected from the nursing records and the parents.

Because of the frequency and potential morbidity of early onset neonatal sepsis, the presence or absence of risk factors for sepsis should be assessed as part of the initial evaluation of every newborn. Historical risk factors for early onset sepsis include prolonged rupture of the fetal membranes (18 hours or more), a maternal body temperature of 38° C or higher, uterine tenderness, foul-smelling or purulent amniotic fluid, an elevated maternal white blood cell count or left shift, and fetal or maternal tachycardia. Maternal colonization with group B streptococci is also considered a risk factor unless adequate intrapartum prophylaxis was administered or the fetal membranes were intact until delivery by cesarean section (American Academy of Pediatrics, 1997). Poor tolerance of labor, manifested by an unexplained need for resuscitation or a slow transition, can be a nonspecific symptom of sepsis.

Whereas gathering the history and performing the physical examination are distinct activities, described by convention in separate parts of a note, they are not performed in isolation. Knowledge of specific concerns, events, and risk factors in the history should prompt a more focused or detailed examination of the relevant body region or organ system than otherwise might be done. Conversely, specific questioning prompted by physical examination findings will often elicit information that was not volunteered in the earlier routine history gathering, such as a family history of a specific anomaly. When a note is written, the history, the physical examination, and laboratory studies are the data upon which the current assessment and plan of care are based. Once documented, the assessment and plan also become part of the patient's ongoing history.

PHYSICAL EXAMINATION

Physical examination requires skills whose refinement can continue to reward and challenge the pediatrician and neonatologist throughout a professional lifetime. No matter how experienced the practitioner, every examination represents an opportunity to add to or refine one's knowledge of significant abnormalities and of the wide range of variation of common, benign conditions. Nevertheless, the examiner knows that most newborns are in fact healthy; therefore one of the practical challenges of performing the routine newborn examination is to maintain a high level of vigilance and thoroughness throughout every examination.

The examination of the healthy newborn entails a complete physical examination in the sense that all parts of the body are examined. However, no actual examination or its write-up can be complete in the sense of exhaustively exploring and explicitly documenting all possible findings.

The degree of detail that is appropriate is a matter of judgment that will vary with the presenting situation and the findings discovered during the examination. Distinct subtypes of the newborn examination include examinations in the delivery room, at admission, and at discharge from the normal nursery, in addition to examinations initiated in response to specific concerns.

EVALUATION AT BIRTH

At the time of birth, attention focuses on the initiation of air breathing and cardiorespiratory stability. The assessment of successful adaptation or a need for resuscitation is described in Chapter 28. The infant whose condition remains unstable or who has major anomalies that are apparent on initial inspection will be transferred to an NICU for further evaluation and management.

DELIVERY ROOM DISPOSITION

The infant whose condition stabilizes after delivery, with or without intervention, is evaluated to determine whether the infant can remain with the mother. This examination centers on assessment of the adequacy of the cardiorespiratory transition, and it also includes a basic inspection for congenital anomalies such as imperforate anus or other problems that may indicate a need for admission to an NICU or observation nursery. Passage of a thin catheter through both nostrils and into the stomach can be done in the delivery room to rule out choanal and esophageal atresia. For routine deliveries, the delivery room discharge examination is often done by the obstetrician or nurse-midwife. If the pediatrician is present, the examination at this time can be expanded to serve as the nursery admission exam.

NURSERY ADMISSION EXAMINATION

For babies not requiring admission to an NICU or observation unit, this examination is done after the infant completes transition, and usually by 24 hours after birth. The purpose of a complete physical examination is to efficiently detect problems that, if present, are inapparent or may soon develop. This examination is the main focus of this chapter. The initial physical examination of the patient admitted to the NICU is similar, except that examination in the NICU should be initiated immediately after admission, and parts of the NICU examination may need to be modified or delayed because of physiologic instability or limited accessibility. Whether in the nursery or the NICU, the identification of historical risk factors or the detection of symptoms or abnormalities requires that the basic examination be expanded to focus additional attention on the areas relevant to the differential diagnosis.

TARGETED OR PROBLEM-DIRECTED EXAMINATION

When the physician is called to evaluate an infant because of specific symptoms or concerns, the examination will naturally focus on aspects relevant to those issues. Because the nonspecific nature of many symptoms in the infant often implies a large differential diagnosis, even the targeted examination will often need a wide focus. The daily follow-up examination can be regarded as a variety of targeted examination, guided by the infant's overall condition. For healthy infants remaining in the hospital for several days after birth, areas of active attention always include the infant's neurologic and cardiorespiratory stability, hydration status, feeding and elimination behavior, and jaundice.

NURSERY DISCHARGE EXAMINATION

The discharge examination is similar in scope to the well-baby admission examination, but with a slightly altered emphasis, based on the additional information provided by the period of observation in the hospital, and by the goal of determining whether the infant is ready for routine care at home. The discharge examination is still a complete physical examination that encompasses the entire body. However, it is not necessary for the discharge examination to duplicate all portions of the admission examination, provided that it was performed by the same person or specific aspects of the admission examination were sufficiently well documented by a trusted colleague. For example, it is unnecessary to repeat a search for physical anomalies that do not change with time, such as examination of the oral cavity for cleft palate, or to check again for red retinal reflexes if they were already found to be normal. Nevertheless, it is often more efficient to repeat the entire examination than to verify the completeness of an earlier examination by another. When the hospital stay is short, a combined admission-discharge examination is appropriate.

EVALUATION OF GESTATIONAL AGE

If the obstetric estimate of the gestational age is uncertain or appears unreliable, the gestational age of the newborn infant can be estimated based on physical examination criteria. No individual feature is a reliable guide to the gestational age, but scoring systems that use multiple features of physical and neuromuscular maturity have been evaluated extensively (Amiel-Tison, 1968; Dubowitz et al, 1970). The New Ballard Score is probably the most widely used in contemporary practice (Ballard et al, 1991). Detailed descriptions and a video demonstration of this examination are available at www.ballardscore.com.

ENVIRONMENT OF EXAMINATION

The environment in which the examination is performed can significantly affect the reliability of the examination via effects on the examiner or on the baby. The examiner must be aware of the limitations produced by a suboptimal environment and adjust the approach to the examination to compensate, arrange for the infant to be moved, or defer selected parts of the examination when appropriate. Important environmental considerations include lighting, room temperature, and the levels of background noise and other distractions. An often overlooked source of distraction is a situation that forces the examiner into a physically awkward or uncomfortable position, such as tall examiner bending over a low bed or examining table. If possible, the infant's clinical state and tolerance for handling can also have a major effect on the conduct of the examination. The wise examiner will postpone the examination of a hungry, crying infant if possible, and try to return when the infant is fed and calm.

The healthy infant is typically examined in a warmer bed in the delivery room or in a bassinet in the mother's room or in the nursery. An open warmer bed provides the best access to the patient, allowing the infant to be kept warm while completely undressed during the examination. The presence of a warmer bed in the delivery room adds to the advantages of performing the nursery admission examination soon after delivery, but often this is not practical. Most examinations of the healthy newborn are done with the infant in a bassinet, starting with the infant dressed in at least a shirt and hat, and wrapped in blankets. An adequate well-baby examination can be performed under these conditions, but the sequence of the examination should be modified to minimize the time the infant is fully undressed. The examiner must take extra care to ensure that the examination is complete and the entire skin surface is visualized at some point during the examination.

Performing the examination in the presence of the parents allows the examiner to show how the infant responds to handling, and to demonstrate immediately any findings that require explanation or reassurance. Watching the examination may stimulate the parents to ask questions that might otherwise not occur to them until later, and it provides the physician an immediate opportunity for further education. On the other hand, interruptions from parents and other family members can interfere with the examiner's train of thought, risking inadvertent distraction and omissions. In large, busy nurseries, it may be more practical for the pediatrician to examine a series of infants in the nursery and then report the results of the examination to each set of parents afterward. Specific findings should be demonstrated to the parents at that time, if appropriate. Regardless of whether the parents are present for the examination, the results of the examination should be communicated promptly. Parents may be anxious about findings that the pediatrician believes are of little consequence, and vice versa. Prompt and sensitive communication of the examination findings helps to build parents' trust, whereas delayed or poor communication can undermine the parents' relationship with the physician and the hospital.

CLINICAL APPROACH TO THE NEWBORN EXAMINATION

An important challenge of the newborn examination is the need to maintain a high level of vigilance and thoroughness, while projecting an attitude of comfortable reassurance appropriate to the reality that the overwhelming majority of newborns seen in the well-baby nursery are in fact healthy. Although the eyes and fingers of the experienced examiner will detect many abnormalities by pattern recognition alone, even the most expert examiner can miss important findings unless a disciplined, systematic approach is used. However, the desire to ensure that no essential aspect of the examination is missed or slighted needs to be balanced with the infant's limited tolerance for handling. It may seem easier to avoid omissions if the examiner always performs the examination in the same sequence, but a rigid approach that fails to adjust to the state and activity of the individual infant may yield a suboptimal examination that is inefficient and unnecessarily stressful for infant, parent, and examiner.

The physical examination of the newborn includes measurements of the weight, length, and head circumference, which must be compared with standardized growth data (Figure 25-1) to determine whether the infant is small (<10th percentile), appropriate, or large (>90th percentile) for gestational age (Battaglia and Lubchenco, 1967). The body temperature, heart rate, and respiratory rate are typically recorded at regular intervals by nurses, but the pediatrician should also consciously evaluate the heart and respiratory rate at the time of examination. The blood pressure is not routinely measured in healthy newborns, but the blood pressure should be checked in all four extremities if the history or examination suggest a problem with the circulation. Of the standard physical examination techniques, the most important in the examination of the newborn is observation. Palpation and auscultation are also important, whereas percussion is of relatively limited use. The routine examination also includes specific physical maneuvers for examining the hips and for eliciting a variety of reflex responses. A stethoscope, an ophthalmoscope, and a tape measure are the only pieces of equipment generally needed. A source of light for transillumination is helpful for specific purposes. Pulse oximetry can enhance early detection of critical congenital heart disease, but further study is needed to determine whether this procedure should become a standard of care in the routine assessment of the neonate (Mahle et al, 2009).

Sensitivity to the infant's state and responses can greatly facilitate the examination and make it less stressful for the infant and less time-consuming for the examiner. The newborn infant generally responds more slowly to a stimulus than does an older child or adult, and the response tends not to remain localized to the area of the stimulus. For example, a gentle touch to the face or extremity of a sleeping infant, or merely loosening a blanket, typically results in some limited initial movement of the area touched, followed with a slight delay by a wave of movement that spreads to involve the whole body, and which may be accompanied by partial arousal. If the examiner waits a few seconds for this wave of response to fully subside before proceeding to move or touch the infant again, the infant will often settle and remain asleep. With a series of such gentle, well-spaced interactions, the examiner can often complete important portions of the examination without waking the infant. If, however, the examiner provides a new stimulus soon after the first, before the secondary movements have finished spreading and while the infant is partially aroused, the new stimulus is likely to reinforce the initial stimulation and provoke full awakening and a crying.

The examination should begin with a deliberate pause to observe the infant in an undisturbed state. Before the infant is moved or undressed, the examiner should actively observe the infant and mentally note as much information as possible, including the state of alertness or sleep, color of visible portions of the skin and mucous membranes, respiratory rate and any audible sounds or signs of increased work of breathing, posture, spontaneous activity, and quality of cry. Throughout the examination, the examiner should alternate between focusing attention on specific elements of the examination (e.g., listen for a heart murmur, closely scrutinize a scalp lesion) and maintaining a global awareness of the infant's overall responses and activity. The experienced examiner's general impression of whether the patient is sick or healthy is an important part of the evaluation.

If the infant is sleeping or in a quiet alert state, the examiner will usually begin by gently uncovering the chest. Depending on the type of clothing the infant is wearing, it may be best at first to lift the shirt or gown just enough to slide the stethoscope underneath. Because the heart sounds and a soft murmur, if present, can be obscured easily by

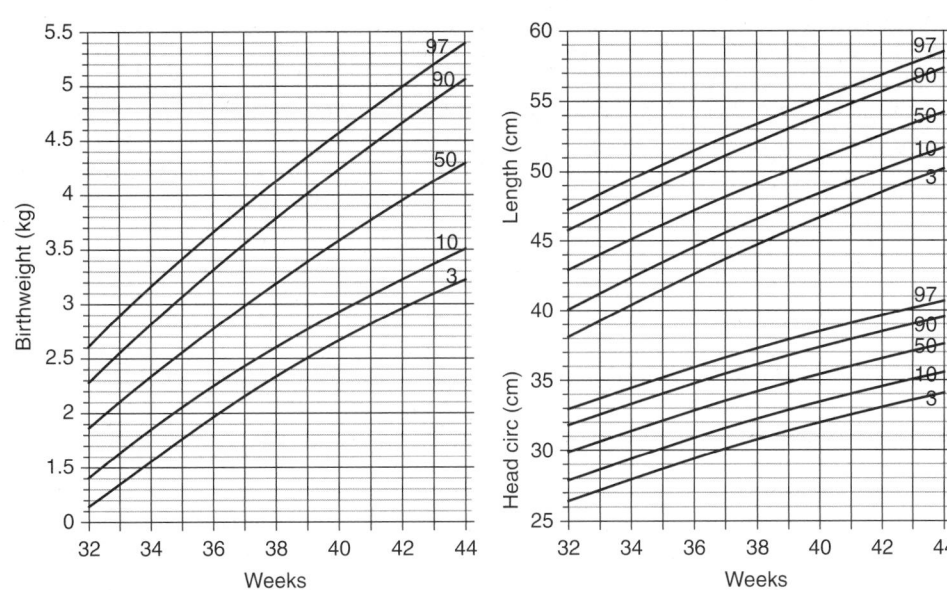

FIGURE 25-1 Fetal-infant growth chart for 32 to 44 weeks' gestation. *(Redrawn from Fenton TR: A new growth chart for preterm babies: Babson and Benda's chart updated with recent data and a new format.* BMC Pediatr 3:13, 2003. *The complete chart for 22 to 50 weeks' gestation can be downloaded from http://members.shaw.ca/ growthchart.)*

crying, the precordial area is usually auscultated first. If the infant remains quiet, the clothing can be removed further, and the stethoscope can be moved to other locations on the chest to expand the area of auscultation for breath and heart sounds, and then to the abdomen to listen for bowel sounds. If the infant is already crying or awakens and starts crying vigorously, auscultation can be deferred in favor of other parts of the examination. Auscultation of the chest can be performed later, after the infant has become quiet.

If the infant is lightly dressed and is being examined on an open warming bed, all clothing can be removed after the initial auscultation of the chest and abdomen; this allows the entire body to be easily observed throughout the examination with a systematic head-to-toe approach. If the infant is in an open crib, he or she may become cold and upset if undressed fully at the beginning of the examination. In this environment, it is preferable to allow the infant to remain at least partially clothed for as long as possible. For example, start by examining the head, and after replacing the infant's hat, open the shirt to finish examining the anterior chest and abdomen, closing but not buttoning or snapping the shirt while moving to examine the hips, genitalia, and lower extremities, and finally removing the shirt to examine the upper extremities and back. However, proceeding in this way requires extra attention on the part of the examiner to ensure that no parts of the examination are missed.

An experienced examiner can accomplish a thorough examination of the newborn more quickly than a novice, largely because of the acquired skill in handling the infant and minimizing wasted or redundant motions. Although there is no substitute for experience, the trainee's skill will develop more rapidly if close attention is paid to developing a fluid approach to the examination as a whole. The following paragraphs provide one example; each experienced examiner will develop his or her own preferred sequence. Further details of specific parts of the examination are described in subsequent sections.

After the initial moment of observation and auscultation of the anterior chest and abdomen, begin examining the head. Using both hands, gently encircle and palpate the entire scalp while inspecting parts of the scalp that are visible in this position (the back of the head and neck will be inspected later). Gently turn the head to one side (noting any limitation of range of motion), and inspect that side of the head, including the ear, and then the side of the neck. Roll the infant's head gently while working the fingers around the neck to the other side, palpating the neck and clavicular areas and applying gentle traction on the skin as needed to open the neck creases to allow full visualization. After reaching the other side of the neck, inspect the ear and side of the head. Next, proceed to the face, attending first to overall features of shape and symmetry and then focusing sequentially on the skin, eyes, nose, mouth, and oral cavity.

With the shirt open in front, inspect and palpate the anterior chest. Observe the respiratory pattern, noting the presence or absence of retractions. Additional auscultation of the chest may be done at this time, if not completed earlier. Open the diaper, and inspect and palpate the abdomen and umbilicus. Palpate the femoral pulses. One may examine the genitalia and perineum at this time, or wait

until after the examination of the hips and lower extremities, described next.

Inspect the lower extremities. Check the range of motion of the hips and perform the Barlow and Ortolani maneuvers. Palpate the legs, sliding the examiner's hands from the hips down to the ankles. The examiner should place the thumbs on the soles of the feet, with the fingers around the back of the ankles. From this position, the examiner can smoothly check the alignment of the feet, elicit the plantar grasp, and then slide the thumbs up along the outer edge of the soles to elicit Babinski's reflex. Next, lift and abduct the legs into a frog-leg position to provide a full view of the perineum and anus. Inspect the genitalia by gently retracting the labia majora in females, or depressing the skin at the base of the penis in males. Inspect and palpate the scrotum and testes. After this, the diaper can be refastened.

Attention next turns to the upper extremities. The shirt should be removed completely to allow unobstructed observation of the overall shape, symmetry, and movements of the arms and hands. With the infant supine, turn the head to elicit the asymmetric tonic neck reflex on each side. Palpate the whole arm gently, starting with one of the examiner's hands on each of the baby's shoulder's, and then slide down to the baby's hands, noting any swelling or discontinuities. Inspect the hands, fingers, nails, and palms. If the infant's hand is tightly fisted, do not attempt to pry the fingers open. Instead, gently flex the wrist to 90 degrees, which will cause the fingers to relax naturally. Inspect the palms, and then elicit the palmar grasp reflex. Without releasing the baby's hands, one can then perform the pull-to-sit maneuver. The examiner places his or her hand behind the infant's head and neck to provide support as the infant is gently lowered back toward the bed. When the infant's head and shoulders are a few inches from the bed, the examiner drops his or her hand rapidly to elicit the Moro reflex.

Next, place the hands on either side of the chest, under the arms at the shoulders, and raise the baby to an upright position, noting the strength and tone of the shoulder muscles. Lower the infant, still in an upright position, and try to elicit the supporting and stepping reflexes. Turn the infant to a prone position, suspended on the examiner's hand. Observe the infant's posture and tone, and elicit the incurvation response. Inspect the infant's back, from the vertex of the head down to the sacrum (pulling the diaper down, if needed). Gently place the infant back in the crib, and dress the infant. The red reflex examination can be performed at this time, or at any suitable moment when the eyes are open spontaneously.

The preceding description assumes routine findings throughout. The examiner should always be prepared to deviate from his or her preferred sequence in response to changes in the infant's state or if abnormalities are found that require a more extended examination of particular features. However, it remains important for the examiner to complete the entire examination and not become distracted by a prominent finding. On occasion, portions of an examination need to be deferred; this is more common in the NICU, because of patient instability, than in the well-baby nursery. In either environment, any limitations of the examination should be clearly documented, with the need for reexamination listed explicitly in the plan of care.

SKIN

The entire skin surface should be inspected during the course of the examination, with attention to the color, moisture, temperature, texture, and elasticity of the skin, the pattern and depth of skin creases, and the presence and character of any local alterations or lesions. The skin appendages—nails and hair—are inspected along with the skin, with attention to the color, size, shape, and any lesions of the nails, and to the growth pattern, color, texture, and distribution of scalp and body hair. Lighting must be adequate and consistent. Natural light is best, although not always available. Phototherapy lights must be turned off during the examination. Typically the skin in different regions of the body is examined sequentially during the course of the routine examination, but if abnormalities are seen, it can be helpful to reexamine the infant in a fully undressed state and in a warm environment, so that all parts of the body can be directly compared. The size, shape, location, distribution, and time course of lesions are all important for differential diagnosis.

Skin color is a composite of the infant's basic skin pigmentation, the adequacy of perfusion, the amounts of oxygenated and deoxygenated hemoglobin in the local circulation, and, at times, internal staining of skin by extravasated blood or pigmented molecules such as bilirubin. The skin can also be stained externally by in utero exposure to meconium or postnatally by foreign substances applied to the skin. The newborn is typically much more pink or red than the mother, because of the healthy infant's high hemoglobin level. With excessive hemoglobin levels, as in polycythemia or twin-twin transfusion, a deeply red or purple-red color (plethora) is evident. Pallor may be caused by anemia or poor perfusion. Central oxygenation is usually best evaluated by observing the color of the tongue and oral mucous membranes, because the color of lips can be misleading. Visual detection of central cyanosis requires approximately 5 g of desaturated Hb per 100 mL of blood, and may not be apparent in the presence of significant anemia (Snider, 1990). Cyanosis of the perioral area, hands, and feet (acrocyanosis), which is common in the first 24 hours after birth or if the infant is cold, is due to relatively poor perfusion of those areas, resulting in increased O_2 extraction by the tissues and an increase in the concentration of deoxyhemoglobin. Because skin color is dependent on perfusion, it can be a sensitive indicator of systemic perfusion. However, the infant's peripheral color can vary markedly and rapidly with activity and the local environmental temperature. Transient mottling of skin of the extremities and trunk (cutis marmorata) is common in newborn infants in response to cold. If mottling does not resolve with warming, other conditions should be considered, including hypertension and hypothyroidism. Harlequin color change is a striking but infrequently observed transient asymmetry of color and perfusion, in which one side of the body is vasodilated, with a clear line of demarcation at the midline.

The yellow-orange color of jaundice caused by unconjugated bilirubin becomes obvious if serum bilirubin levels are sufficiently high, but it can be difficult to detect at more moderate levels. Typically, jaundice first becomes apparent in the face and then progresses distally as bilirubin levels continue to rise. The detection of mild-to-moderate jaundice is easier if the infant's foot is lifted so that the face and foot can be seen side by side in the same visual field, with the foot providing a built-in control for the infant's basic skin pigmentation. This is particularly helpful in the black or brown infant, in whom mild jaundice is more difficult to detect than in the white infant, and in the Asian infant whose skin tones can exaggerate the appearance of mild jaundice.

A transient period of generalized erythema may be noted a few hours after birth, usually by the parents, often during a bath or with vigorous crying, resolving within minutes to an hour. Sometimes called *erythema neonatorum*, it appears to be associated with successful completion of neonatal transition of the circulation, and it rarely recurs with the same intensity after the first episode (Fletcher, 1998).

Skin creasing is affected by both development and movement. Creasing increases if movement is constrained, as in the fetus near term. An absence of creasing on the palms or soles of a term or near-term neonate can be caused by a prolonged lack of movement secondary to a neuromuscular disorder. Edema stretches the skin and obscures normal skin folds and creases. Edematous skin pits with gentle pressure. The distribution of edema is affected by gravity and thus changes with position. In contrast, lymphedema (as in Turner syndrome) tends to accentuate the creases, and is less affected by gravity (Fletcher, 1998).

Injuries caused by iatrogenic trauma in utero or at delivery are common; they include scars from injury by an amniocentesis needle, minor lacerations and abscesses from fetal scalp electrodes or fetal blood gas sampling, scalpel lacerations during cesarean section, and ecchymoses and abrasions from forceps or vacuum. Trauma can also occur from pressure on the fetus during labor, particularly over bony prominences. Such pressure may be involved in the development of subcutaneous fat necrosis, an uncommon condition hypothesized to be caused by hypoxic injury to fat and manifested by firm, subcutaneous nodules and plaques (Cohen, 2008). The lesions usually resolve spontaneously after several months, but can become inflamed and fluctuant and are occasionally associated with the late development of significant hypercalcemia. Aplasia cutis congenita is a focal lesion characterized by congenital absence of some or all layers of skin (Figure 25-2) and can

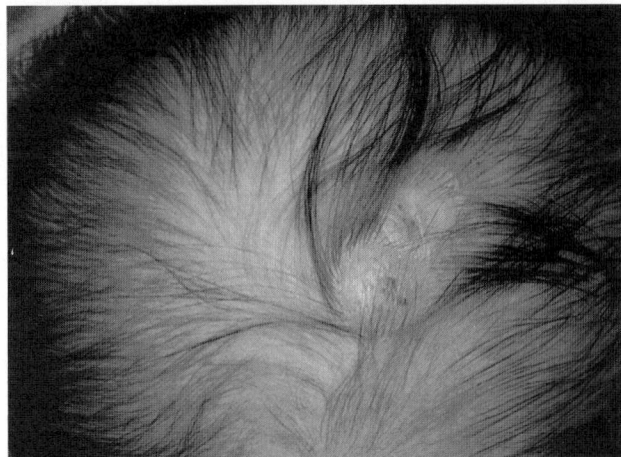

FIGURE 25-2 Aplasia cutis congenita. Lesions are usually single, but in this case there are two adjacent lesions near the vertex—one bullous and one membranous. (*Reprinted from Rudolph AJ:* Atlas of the newborn, vol 4, *Hamilton, Ont, Canada, 1997, BC Decker, p 30.*)

BOX 25-1 Common and Uncommon Causes of Skin Lesions in Neonates

PUSTULAR, VESICULOPUSTULAR, AND VESICULOBULLOUS LESIONS

- Common or benign: erythema toxicum neonatorum, transient neonatal pustular melanosis, miliaria crystallina, miliaria rubra, sucking blisters, neonatal acne (benign cephalic pustulosis)
- Infectious: herpes simplex, varicella, staphylococcal pustulosis, bullous impetigo, congenital candidiasis, syphilis, scabies
- Chronic or recurrent: epidermolysis bullosa, mastocytosis, epidermolytic hyperkeratosis, acropustulosis of infancy
- Positive Nikolsky's sign: epidermolysis bullosa, staphylococcal scalded skin syndrome
- Other: incontinentia pigmenti

NODULES AND PLAQUES

- Common or benign: milia, Ebstein's pearls, Bohn's nodules, sebaceous hyperplasia
- Yellow: sebaceous nevus, juvenile xanthogranuloma
- Brown or black: congenital pigmented nevus, epidermal nevus
- Other: subcutaneous fat necrosis, dermoid cyst, fibroma, infantile myofibromatosis, hamartomas, malignant tumors, leukemia

PAPULOSQUAMOUS AND SCALING LESIONS

- Common or benign: physiologic desquamation
- Healthy infant: atopic dermatitis, contact dermatitis, seborrheic dermatitis, local candida dermatitis, psoriasis
- Ill infant: acrodermatitis enteropathica, Langerhans cell histiocytosis, syphilis
- Other: ichthyosis syndromes, collodion baby, harlequin baby

EROSIONS AND ULCERATIONS

- Common or benign: sucking blisters, traumatic injury (e.g., scalp electrode, diaper erosions, reaction to adhesives)
- Other: aplasia cutis congenita, herpes simplex, epidermolysis bullosa, toxic epidermal necrolysis

ALTERED PIGMENTATION

- Common or benign: Mongolian spots, transient neonatal pustular melanosis, isolated café au lait macules
- Increased pigmentation: Mongolian spots, transient neonatal pustular melanosis, café au lait macules, lentigines, incontinentia pigmenti
- Decreased pigmentation: ash leaf macule, nevus depigmentosus, piebaldism, albinism
- Purpuric or erythematous: petechiae, dermal hematopoiesis ("blueberry muffin" lesions), neonatal lupus erythematosus

VASCULAR AND LYMPHATIC LESIONS

- Common or benign: Nevus simplex or salmon patch, petechiae on the presenting part, small hemangioma
- Other vascular: complicated hemangioma, vascular malformation, port-wine stain
- Lymphatic: cystic hygroma, lymphangioma, lymphedema

Data from Cohen B: *Pediatric dermatology*, ed 3, Philadelphia, 2005, Mosby; Eichenfield LF, Frieden IJ, Esterly NB, editors: *Neonatal dermatology*, (See also Color Plate 9.) *ed 2*, Philadelphia, 2008, Elsevier Saunders; and Fletcher MA: *Physical diagnosis in neonatology*, Philadelphia, 1998, Lippincott-Raven.

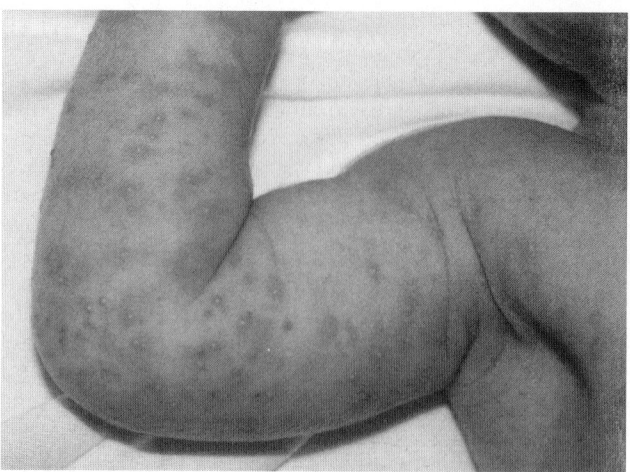

FIGURE 25-3 *(See also Color Plate 9.)* Erythema toxicum neonatorum with erythematous macules, wheals, and pustules. Pustules predominate in this example. At times, patchy or confluent areas of erythema occur without pustules. *(Reprinted from Eichenfield LF, Frieden IJ, Esterly NB, editors: Neonatal dermatology, ed 2, Philadelphia, 2008, Elsevier Saunders, p 88.)*

occur sporadically or in association with chromosomal defects or other malformations (Kos and Drolet, 2008). It occurs most often on the scalp near the vertex and can be mistaken for a traumatic injury.

Some common and uncommon skin conditions that may be seen in the newborn are outlined in Box 25-1. Fortunately, most of the skin findings encountered during the routine examination are due to a relatively few common conditions, mostly benign, that are described in the following paragraphs. If unusual or unfamiliar lesions that fall outside the examiner's "comfort zone" are observed, consultation with an appropriate subspecialist should be arranged.

Erythema toxicum neonatorum, or erythema toxicum, is the most common skin rash in the newborn, occurring in up to 70% of term infants (Howard and Frieden, 2008; Lucky, 2008). Lesions can be present at birth, but in most cases the lesions are first noted at 1 to 2 days. The lesions are seen predominately on the face and trunk, but can appear anywhere on the body except the palms and soles. New lesions may continue to appear for approximately 1 week while older lesions resolve. The typical lesion is an isolated elevated erythematous papule or pustule 1 to 2 mm in diameter, surrounded by an irregular area of erythema 1 to 3 cm in diameter (Figure 25-3). When extensive, the lesions can occur in clusters or become nearly confluent. Diagnosis can usually be made by appearance alone, but a scraping of the pustule will reveal an almost pure infiltrate of eosinophils if confirmation is needed in atypical cases.

Transient neonatal pustular melanosis is a self-limited process with lesions that evolve through three distinct phases (Howard and Frieden, 2008; Lucky, 2008; Figure 25-4). Initially, a superficial vesicopustule appears, which after rupturing leaves a fine collarette of scale around the unroofed pustule, which is without erythema. The final stage is a hyperpigmented macule that gradually disappears. The condition is most common in African American infants. In some cases, only the second or third stages are seen at birth, the initial stage presumably having occurred in utero.

Miliaria crystallina is the result of superficial obstruction of the sweat ducts, producing small, crystal-clear vesicles that resemble water droplets (Figure 25-5). It is mostly seen in warm climates or febrile infants. The vesicles are fragile and can be removed by wiping the skin with a soft damp cloth (Howard and Frieden, 2008; Lucky, 2008). Miliaria rubra, also called *heat rash* or *prickly heat*, results from sweat duct obstruction deeper in the epidermal layer, and is more

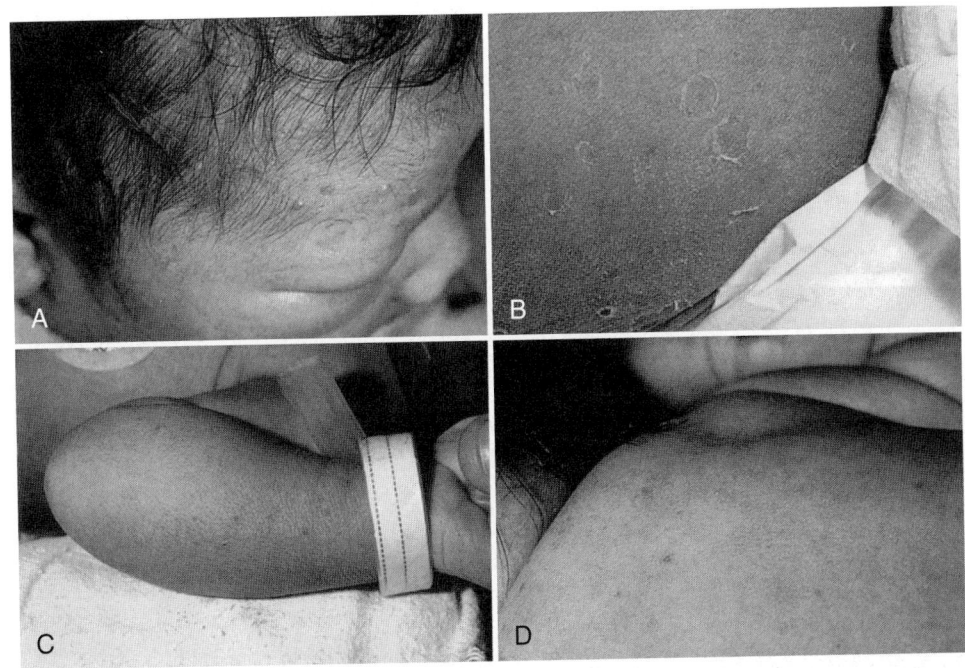

FIGURE 25-4 **Transient neonatal pustular melanosis.** The first stage consists of small superficial pustules, without inflammation **(A)**. Collarettes of scale, the second stage, may be seen at birth without evident pustules **(B)**, or may develop postnatally after pustules have ruptured **(C)**. Small hyperpigmented macules remain in the final stage **(D)**, gradually fading over weeks or months. *(Reprinted from Eichenfield LF, Frieden IJ, Esterly NB, editors:* Neonatal dermatology, *ed 2, Philadelphia, 2008, WB Saunders, p 89.)*

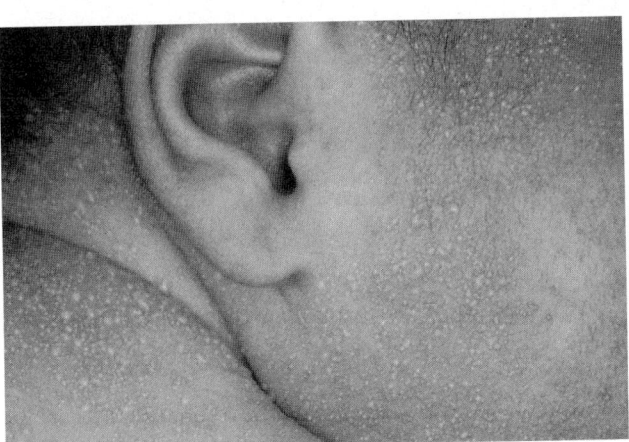

FIGURE 25-5 *(See also Color Plate 10.)* **Miliaria crystallina.** The tiny, clear vesicles resemble water droplets, with no signs of inflammation. *(Reprinted from Rudolph AJ:* Atlas of the newborn, vol 4, *Hamilton, Ont, Canada, 1997, BC Decker, p13.)*

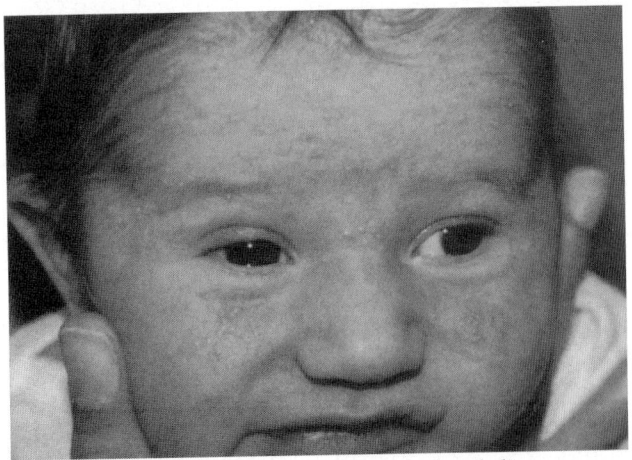

FIGURE 25-6 *(See also Color Plate 11.)* **Neonatal cephalic pustulosis (neonatal acne).** Small, red papules and pustules are seen on the cheeks and forehead, with some extension into the scalp. Comedones are absent. *(Reprinted from Eichenfield LF, Frieden IJ, Esterly NB, editors:* Neonatal dermatology, *ed 2, Philadelphia, 2008, WB Saunders, p 90.)*

common after the first week. Occasionally miliaria rubra will look sufficiently pustular as to mimic lesions caused by staphylococcal, candidal, or herpes simplex.

Sucking blisters and calluses result from vigorous sucking on a hand or forearm in utero, and they can cause a tense, fluid-filled blister, which when ruptured forms an erosion or a callus. The lesion is most often solitary, but may be bilateral, and is without inflammation. A sucking pad or callus may develop on the lips postnatally as a result of vigorous and frequent nursing.

Neonatal cephalic pustulosis, or neonatal acne may occasionally be seen at birth, but more typically appears later, with a mean age of onset of 2 to 3 weeks (Howard and Frieden, 2008; Lucky, 2008). It is characterized by inflammatory, erythematous papules and pustules located primarily on the cheeks with extension over the face and

into the scalp (Figure 25-6). It can be difficult to distinguish clinically from miliaria rubra, but both are benign conditions and biopsy is not warranted.

Infectious causes of skin lesions are relatively uncommon in the immediate newborn period, but often need to be considered in the differential diagnosis. Superficial skin infections of *Staphylococcus aureus* are rarely present at birth, but can develop within the first few days. Thrush and candidal diaper dermatitis, common later but not immediately after birth, usually pose no diagnostic difficulty. Congenital candidiasis, which is uncommon, typically manifests within the first day with a papulovesicular eruption that progresses to pustules, followed by crusting and desquamation (Figure 25-7). Lesions can be widespread and may appear on any part of the body, including the palms and soles (Carder,

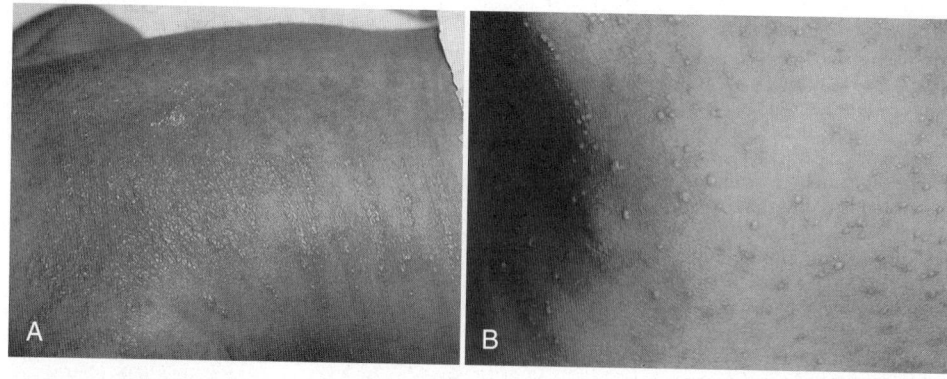

FIGURE 25-7 *(See also Color Plate 12.)* **Congenital candidiasis.** The rash may be a diffuse, erythematous pustular eruption **(A)** or have diffusely distributed but distinct pustules **(B).** In premature infants, a diffuse scaldlike erythematous dermatitis may be seen (not shown). *(Reprinted from Eichenfield LF, Frieden IJ, Esterly NB, editors:* Neonatal dermatology, *ed 2, Philadelphia, 2008, Elsevier Saunders, p 214.)*

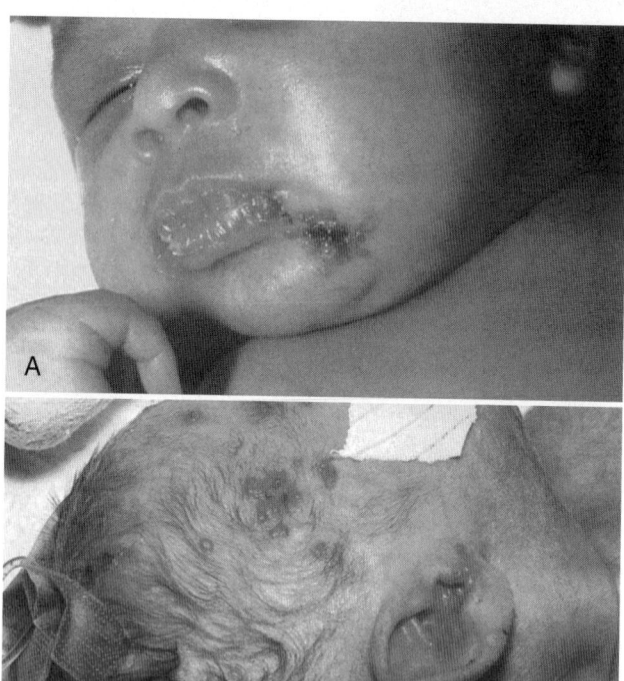

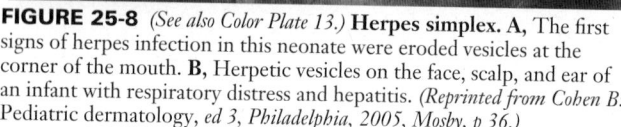

FIGURE 25-8 *(See also Color Plate 13.)* **Herpes simplex. A,** The first signs of herpes infection in this neonate were eroded vesicles at the corner of the mouth. **B,** Herpetic vesicles on the face, scalp, and ear of an infant with respiratory distress and hepatitis. *(Reprinted from Cohen B:* Pediatric dermatology, *ed 3, Philadelphia, 2005, Mosby, p 36.)*

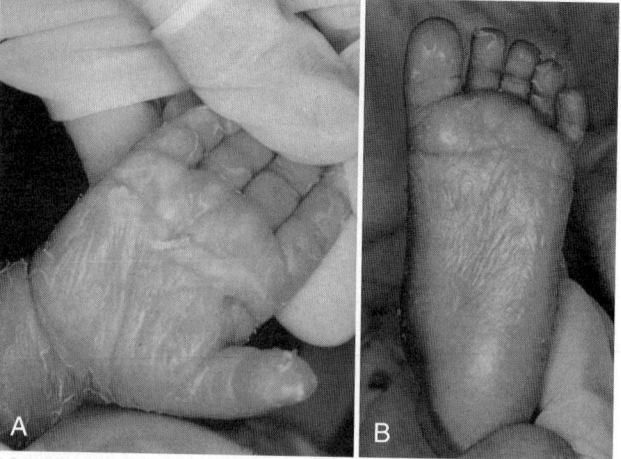

FIGURE 25-9 *(See also Color Plate 14.)* Desquamation on the palms **(A)** and soles **(B)** of an infant with congenital syphilis. *(Reprinted from Rudolph AJ:* Atlas of the newborn, vol 4, *Hamilton, Ont, Canada, 1997, BC Decker, p 108.)*

2008; Darmstadt et al, 2000). Neonatal herpes simplex is unlikely in the first few days after birth, unless the fetal membranes were ruptured for many days, but it must be considered whenever vesicles are seen in the newborn. The skin lesions of herpes simplex start as small, 2- to 4-mm vesicles on an erythematous base, become pustular after 1 to 3 days, and develop an eschar (Friedlander and Bradley, 2008; Figure 25-8). The mucosal lesions are usually shallow ulcerations. The "blueberry muffin" skin lesions of congenital rubella and cytomegalovirus, caused by dermal hematopoiesis, are unlikely to be seen as an isolated finding. Affected infants typically have multiple stigmata of congenital infection including growth retardation, microcephaly, and hepatosplenomegaly. Cutaneous findings of congenital syphilis are present in only a minority of infected infants, but they classically involve the palms, soles, and perioral

and anogenital areas (Dinulos and Pace, 2008; Howard and Frieden, 2008). The rash is highly variable, taking papulosquamous, vesiculobullous, macular erythematous, annular, and polymorphous forms. Desquamation limited to the palms and soles, with no rash or peeling elsewhere, is suggestive of congenital syphilis (Figure 25-9).

Milia, Ebstein's pearls, and Bohn's nodules are epidermal inclusion cysts (Lucky, 2008; Figure 25-10). Milia are tiny epidermal inclusion cysts seen primarily on the face and scalp in small numbers; they are smooth, firm, white papules with no associated erythema. They may be present at birth or appear somewhat later, and they generally resolve spontaneously within a few months. Larger inclusion cysts, which usually occur singly, are called *pearls;* the foreskin and the ventral surface of the penis and scrotum are common locations. Epidermal inclusion cysts located on the palate are called *Ebstein's pearls,* and those on the alveolar ridge are called *Bohn's nodules.*

Sebaceous hyperplasia occurs mostly on the face, especially on the nose and upper lip. It is due to hypertrophy of the sebaceous glands caused by androgenic hormonal stimulation in utero, and it gradually resolves over several weeks. It is characterized by sheets of smooth, yellow-white papules with the regular spacing of involved follicles and no surrounding erythema (Figure 25-11).

Physiologic desquamation occurs in many full-term infants. These infants will have some dry skin with fine

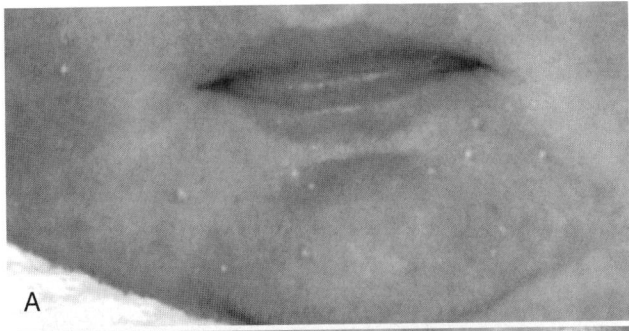

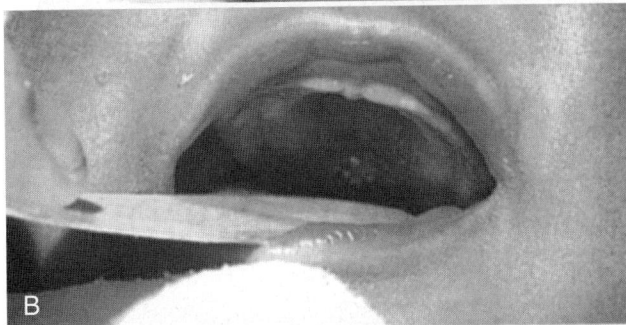

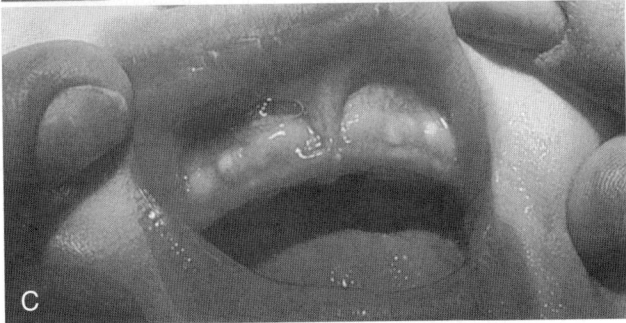

FIGURE 25-10 Epidermal inclusion cysts. Milia are most commonly seen on the face (**A**), but can occur anywhere on the body. Ebstein's pearls occur on the midline of the hard palate, most commonly near the junction with soft palate (**B**). Bohn's nodules are found along the gum margins and on the lateral palate (**C**). Dental lamina cysts (not shown) are similar inclusions located on the crest of the alveolar ridge. (*Reprinted from Fletcher MA:* Physical diagnosis in neonatology, *Philadelphia, 1998, Lippincott-Raven, p124* [**A**]; *and Eichenfield LF, Frieden IJ, Esterly NB, editors:* Neonatal dermatology, *ed 2, Philadelphia, 2008, Elsevier Saunders, pp 503-504* [**B** and **C**].)

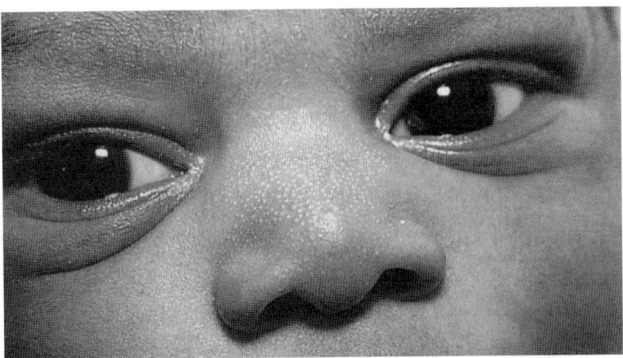

FIGURE 25-11 (*Supplemental color version of this figure is available online at www.expertconsult.com.*) **Sebaceous hyperplasia.** Sheets of tiny, white-yellow follicular papules, without inflammation, are seen on the nose. (*Reprinted from Eichenfield LF, Frieden IJ, Esterly NB, editors:* Neonatal dermatology, *ed 2, Philadelphia, 2008, Elsevier Saunders, p 87.*)

desquamation at 1 to 2 days of age, particularly on the hands and feet. A more exaggerated variety of physiological desquamation is common in postmature infant (born at greater than 41 ⁶⁄₇ weeks post-menstrualage). These infants are often born with dry, thickened skin that cracks and peels extensively and then normalizes spontaneously over the course of approximately 1 week. The condition is usually not difficult to distinguish from the rare inherited disorders of cornification (ichthyosis) that manifest in the neonatal period (Irvine and Paller, 2008). These disorders include Harlequin ichthyosis (caused by mutations in the *ABCA12* gene) and "collodion babies" who appear encased in a thickened, shiny skin that resembles collodion, a phenotype associated with a number of different ichthyotic conditions.

Mongolian spots (dermal melanocytosis) are macular areas of a slate grey, blue-grey, blue-black, or deep brown color. The distinctive appearance is due to the presence of melanocytes located in the dermis, instead of their typical site at the dermal-epidermal junction. The spots are most commonly located on the lower back and buttocks, but can occur elsewhere. Mongolian spots in this location—which are common in East Asian, East African, Native American, and Polynesian infants—tend to fade over several years, whereas similarly appearing lesions that occur elsewhere on the body may never resolve (Gibbs and Makkar, 2008; Lucky, 2008). Dermal melanocytosis in the area of the first and second divisions of the trigeminal nerve is called the *nevus of Ota*. The nevus of Ito is a similar lesion occurring on the neck, upper back, and shoulders in the area of the posterior supraclavicular and lateral brachial cutaneous nerves. Unlike Mongolian spots, these nevi do not become less pigmented with time, and malignant melanoma or malignant nevi can develop within them, though rarely.

Café au lait macules are tan-brown macules that can occur anywhere on the body. They are common as an isolated finding in the newborn and are generally benign, but can be markers of other conditions (Gibbs and Makkar, 2008). The presence of six or more café au lait macules greater than 5 mm in diameter is considered presumptive evidence of neurofibromatosis type 1. Multiple large café au lait macules with irregular borders may be a manifestation of the McCune-Albright syndrome.

The salmon patch (or nevus simplex) is a benign vascular lesion consisting of erythematous macules or patches frequently seen at the nape of the neck ("stork bite"), on the eyelids and glabella ("angel's kisses"), and somewhat less frequently on the nose and upper lip (Lucky, 2008; Figure 25-12). The lesions are caused by dilated capillaries in the upper dermis, with normal overlying skin. Those on the face usually fade or resolve completely within 1 to 2 years, but 25% to 50% of those on the neck persist throughout life (Lucky, 2008).

After vaginal delivery of a healthy infant, it is not unusual or concerning to see petechiae on the presenting part (i.e. the part of the fetus closest to the pelvic inlet of the birth canal at the onset of labor) or on other areas of the body subjected to localized pressure during delivery. A tight nuchal cord can cause extensive ecchymoses and petechiae on the entire head. Widespread petechiae are abnormal, however, and are suggestive of thrombocytopenia or platelet dysfunction.

Hemangiomas are soft, pink-red, compressible vascular tumors composed of proliferating endothelial cells. Small

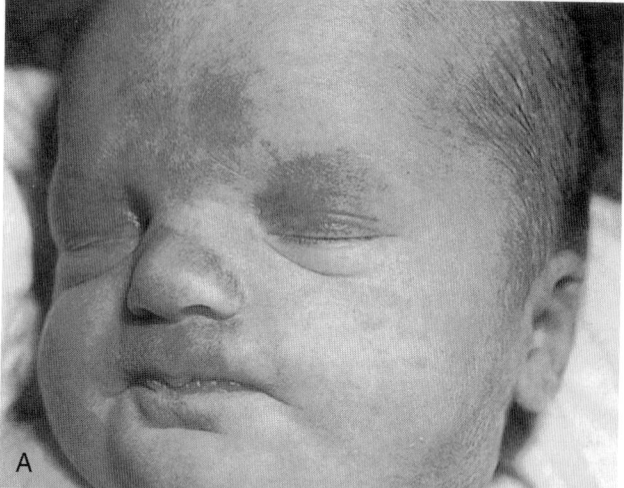

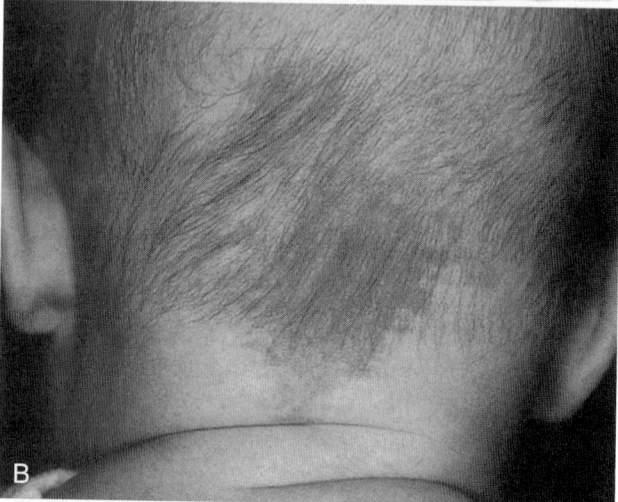

FIGURE 25-12 *(See also Color Plate 15.)* Salmon patches are commonly seen on the glabella, eyelids, nose, or upper lip, either singly or in all these locations **(A)**, and on the nape of the neck **(B)**. *(Reprinted from Eichenfield LF, Frieden IJ, Esterly NB, editors: Neonatal dermatology, ed 2, Philadelphia, 2008, Elsevier Saunders, p. 95.)*

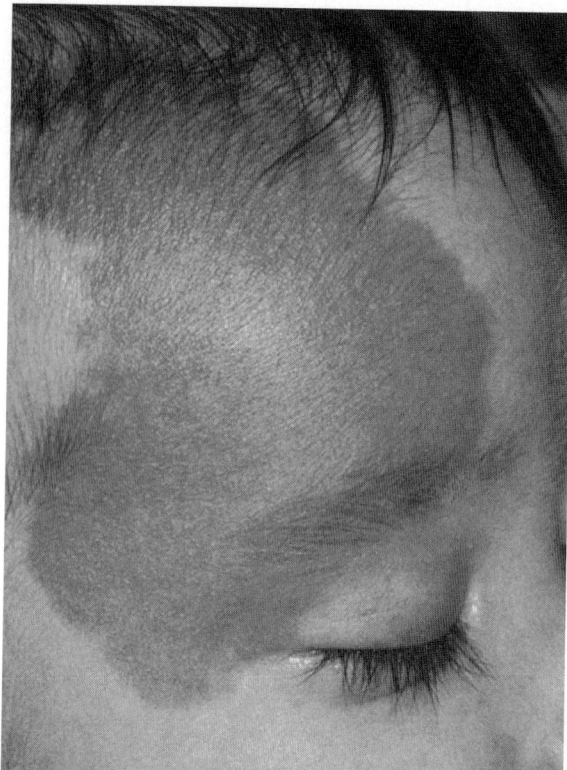

FIGURE 25-13 This infant with the Sturge-Weber syndrome has a port-wine stain in the distribution of the ophthalmic division of the facial nerve. *(Reprinted from Cohen B: Pediatric dermatology, ed 3, Philadelphia, 2005, Mosby, p 49.)*

hemangiomas are recognized at or shortly after birth in 1% to 3% of healthy term infants and become apparent in 10% of all infants by 1 month old (Cohen, 2005). Hemangiomas are more common in female infants by 2:1 to 9:1 as compared with males. The incidence is much higher (22% to 30%) in preterm infants weighing less than 1000 g, but only slightly higher (15%) in those weighing 1000 to 1500 g (Amir et al, 1986; Enjolras and Garzon, 2008). Infantile hemangiomas typically undergo a period of growth beyond that of surrounding tissues for 6 to 12 months, typically followed by spontaneous involution. Approximately 25% regress by 2 years of age, 40% to 50% regress by 4 years of age, 60% to 75% regress by 6 years of age, and 95% regress by adolescence (Cohen, 2005). Before the hemangioma becomes obvious, careful examination may reveal a precursor lesion manifesting as telangiectasias surrounded by an area of pallor or as pale, erythematous, or bruise-like macules and patches. In contrast, vascular malformations are nonproliferative lesions, usually present at birth. The Kasabach-Merritt phenomenon occurs in association with specific types of large vascular tumors that cause platelet trapping and severe thrombocytopenia, and is not associated with the true hemangioma of infancy (Enjolras and Garzon, 2008). In the rare Klippel-Trenaunay syndrome, capillary malformation and varicose veins are associated with overgrowth of an affected limb.

Port-wine stains are capillary malformations evident at birth as pink or red patches that grow proportionately with the child and persist throughout life (Enjolras and Garzon, 2008). The initial pink-red color typically changes to a deeper red or purple hue with age. Approximately 10% of port-wine stains that involve the area supplied by the ophthalmic (V1) branch of the trigeminal nerve (Figure 25-13) are associated with seizures, arterial brain malformations, and ocular abnormalities that constitute the Sturge-Weber syndrome (Enjolras et al, 1985).

HEAD

The head is mainly examined by inspection and palpation. The overall size, shape, and features of the skull should be noted. The head circumference (maximal occipital-frontal circumference) should be measured in every neonate and plotted on an appropriate growth chart (see Figure 25-1). The measurement of the head circumference is subject to error and can be significantly affected by molding of the skull during labor, so the head circumference should be measured again if the result appears discordant with the visual examination or with the infant's weight and length, and repeated after molding has resolved. The soft tissue of the scalp should be examined for swelling, ecchymoses, and other evidence of injury because of the forces of labor, and for iatrogenic injuries including those from application of a vacuum device, placement of scalp electrodes, fetal blood sampling, and lacerations with a scalpel during cesarean section.

The quantity of scalp hair present in the newborn is highly variable, but abnormalities in the distribution, texture, and patterning of the hair are potentially informative. The hair usually forms a single whorl near the vertex, but double whorls occur in approximately 5% of newborns. Abnormal placement or the presence of more than two whorls may be a marker of abnormal brain development (Smith and Gong, 1974).

The infant skull is composed of several bony plates, separated by sutures and fontanels. This structure allows the skull to deform during labor (Figure 25-14). The entire surface of the skull should be palpated to identify the location and size of the major fontanels and assess for discontinuities. The soft tissue over a fontanel should normally be flat; a raised or bulging fontanel suggests that intracranial pressure is increased. It is common to find a palpable discontinuity at a suture, because of vertical displacement of a skull bone relative to its neighbor as a result of molding. In some cases, one bone can truly override the other. Such discontinuities at a suture must be distinguished from the step-off of a displaced skull fracture. Premature fusion of one or more of the cranial sutures, or craniosynostosis, results in a variety of abnormal skull shapes, depending on which sutures are involved (Fletcher, 1998; Volpe, 2008). Fusion of the saggital suture produces a narrow skull elongated in the anterior-posterior dimension (scaphocephaly or dolichocephaly). Fusion of the coronal sutures causes a widened skull that is shortened in the anterior-posterior dimension (brachycephaly). Unilateral closure of either a coronal or lambdoid suture causes an oblique deformity (frontal or occipital plagiocephaly, respectively). Closure of a metopic suture produces a triangular skull with a prominent, narrow forehead (trigonocephaly). Depending on the timing of the fusion, the skull shape may be abnormal at birth or become visibly deformed later. The fused suture typically has a palpable elevation or ridge, which must be distinguished from displacement of a normal suture caused by molding. In the absence of craniosynostosis or overriding, normal mobility at a suture can be verified by gently applying alternating pressure to the bones on either side of the suture line.

Caput succedaneum is a diffuse edematous swelling of the scalp caused by pressure during delivery that results in fluid accumulation external to the periosteum. The caput is boggy, has diffuse edges, is not limited by suture lines,

and most commonly is located over the vertex. It is usually present at birth and resolves over several days. In contrast, a cephalohematoma is caused by hemorrhage under the periosteum; it forms a distinct, firm bump laterally that does not cross suture lines (Figure 25-15). The cephalohematoma may not appear until several hours after birth, and it often increases in size over the first 12 to 24 hours. It typically remains palpable for 2 to 3 weeks, during which time it may develop a calcified rim. Unlikely a cephalohematoma, a subgaleal hematoma is not confined by the

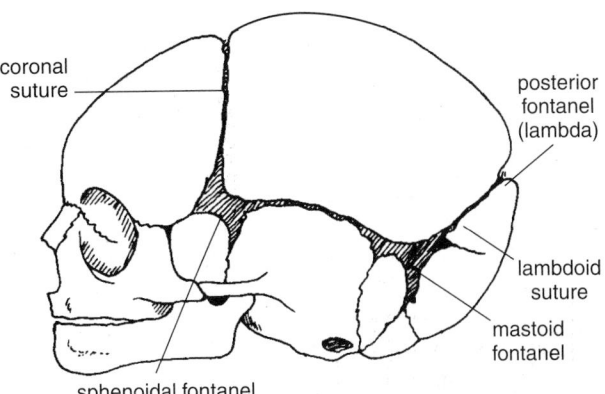

A

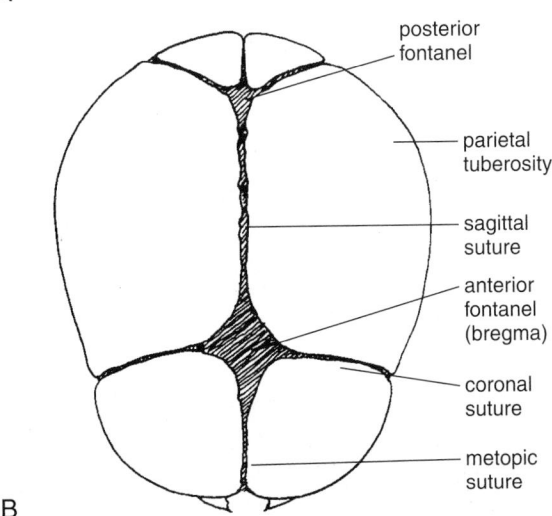

B

FIGURE 25-14 The major sutures and fontanels of the newborn skull. *(Reprinted from Fletcher MA: Physical diagnosis in neonatology, Philadelphia, 1998, Lippincott-Raven, p 175.)*

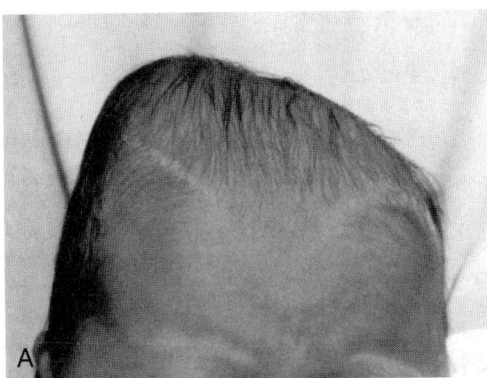

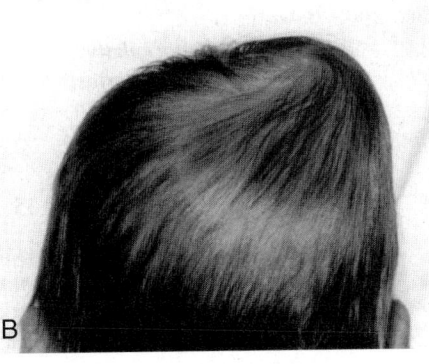

FIGURE 25-15 *(See also Color Plate 16.)* Anterior **(A)** and posterior **(B)** views of a large cephalohematoma under the periosteum of the right parietal bone. *(Reprinted from Fletcher MA: Physical diagnosis in neonatology, Philadelphia, 1998, Lippincott-Raven, p 185.)*

periosteum and can involve massive blood loss. Depending on the volume of blood that has accumulated, it can be palpated as a firm or fluctuant mass with poorly defined edges that may extend onto the neck or forehead. Large subgaleal hematomas are uncommon, but potentially life threatening.

Craniotabes (or craniomalacia) is a softening of the skull, most commonly involving the parietal bones near the vertex. Gentle pressure on the involved bone produces a sudden collapse, with recoil when the pressure is released, similar to the way a ping-pong ball collapses when squeezed. It has usually been attributed to localized bone resorption or interference with ossification caused by prolonged pressure on the fetal skull from the maternal pelvis, but it may be associated with maternal vitamin D deficiency in some populations (Yorifuji et al, 2008).

A localized defect in the skull can occur in association with aplasia cutis congenita. A small soft-tissue mass or bulge at the occiput or in the midline of the forehead near the bridge of the nose may be caused by an encephalocele protruding through a small defect in the skull. Large encephaloceles and major neural tube defects will be obvious if present. Hydranencephaly, if suspected, can be detected by transillumination of the skull.

FACE

The face and facial expressions should be observed throughout the course of the entire examination. In addition, there should be a moment when attention is directed to the overall arrangement and proportion of the features of the face as a whole. It is helpful to view the face from the front, in profile, and looking down from the top of the head. Important characteristics to note include the symmetry and expressiveness of the face, both at rest and during crying, and the relative sizes, spacing, and orientation of the features. After this overview, specific attention should be paid to the ears, eyes, eyebrows, eyelids, nose and nasal passages, lips, palate, and mouth. Suggested abnormalities should be described as precisely as possible. Measurements of the facial features are not part of the routine newborn examination, but comparison with reference nomograms can be helpful if dysmorphism is suspected (see Chapter 19).

EARS

The external ear is a relatively common site of minor anomalies. The external ear develops from the first and second branchial arches, from which the six hillocks of His grow, migrate, and fuse to form the pinna. Most of the pinna derives from the second branchial arch. The third arch contributes the tragus, antitragus, and anterior wall of the canal (Figure 25-16). The position and orientation of each ear should be noted, as well as the size, shape, and structure of the helix, and any signs of trauma. The ear is palpated to assess the firmness and recoil of the cartilage and to detect any masses or abnormalities of texture. The skin near the pinna is examined for skin tags, pits, and sinus tracts. Minor variations in the shape of the ear and ear lobe are common, and they usually have only cosmetic significance. A lop ear is characterized by downward folding of the superior helix caused by underdevelopment of

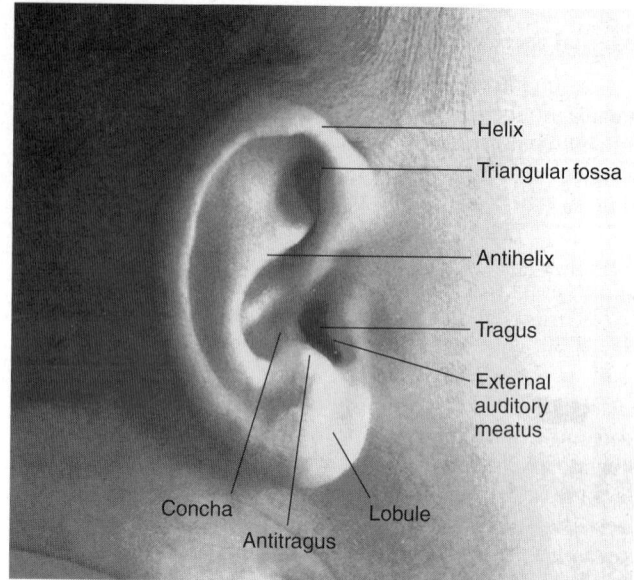

FIGURE 25-16 Anatomy of the external ear. *(Reprinted from Fletcher MA: Physical diagnosis in neonatology, Philadelphia, 1998, Lippincott-Raven, p 285.)*

the upper third of the pinna; this needs to be distinguished from folding caused by positioning in utero. A cup ear is a protruding ear with an excessively concave concha. Microtia implies a severely dysplastic and malformed ear, and it is often associated with abnormalities of the middle ear and other malformations.

Assessment of hearing by observation of behavioral responses has been essentially replaced in the routine examination by automated testing of hearing before hospital discharge (American Academy of Pediatrics, 2007; US Preventive Services Task Force, 2008). Otoscopy to inspect the eardrum is not part of the routine examination in the immediate newborn period. The eardrum is more horizontal in neonates than in adults, lying almost parallel to the external canal. Movement of the eardrum is more difficult to detect than in older infants, and visualization of the eardrum is often impeded by the presence of amniotic debris, vernix, or blood in the ear canal. Moreover, findings typical of otitis media in older infants (dullness of the tympanic membrane, decreased light reflex and translucence, and diminished mobility) may be present in healthy newborns.

EYES

As part of the inspection of the face, the size, spacing, and orientation of the eyes, lids, and eyebrows should be assessed. In microphthalmos the entire eye is small, whereas microcornea can be an isolated finding in an otherwise normal eye. Hypertelorism implies that the spacing between the bony orbits is excessively wide. In telecanthus, the inner canthi are displaced laterally, giving a false impression of hypertelorism. Hypotelorism is often associated with holoprosencephaly, Trisomy 13, and other genetic abnormalities. The palpebral fissures are downslanting if the medial canthi are higher than the lateral canthi, and upslanting if the lateral canthi are higher. Ptosis can be difficult to detect reliably in the neonate unless it is severe or unilateral. It may be congenital or caused by trauma or inflammation. Transient episodes of gaze disconjugation are common in otherwise healthy newborns, but persistent eye deviation requires follow-up. Obstruction at both ends of the lacrimal sac produces a mucocele (or dacryocele), which appears as a bluish subcutaneous mass that can be mistaken for a hemangioma or an encephalocele. Mucoceles can sometimes extend into the nasal passages and cause respiratory distress.

The routine examination of sclera, cornea, and internal portions of the newborn eye is often limited by the presence of significant eyelid edema in the first few days after birth. If the corneas and conjunctivae cannot be adequately visualized during spontaneous eye opening or with gentle lid retraction, it is normally preferable to defer further examination of the eyes until the swelling recedes, rather than to attempt to retract the lids forcibly. A coloboma is a congenital defect in the formation of the eye, which can affect any or all of the external or internal structures of the eye. Colobomas of the iris, most frequently located inferomedially and producing a keyhole-shaped pupil, are the most common type visible on external examination. As part of the routine examination, the lower lid of each eye should be retracted so that the entire pupil is visible, if not the entire cornea. If a coloboma of the lid or iris is seen, ophthalmologic evaluation of internal structures of the eye is advisable. Cloudy corneas represent glaucoma until proven otherwise and require prompt ophthalmologic evaluation even if obvious enlargement of the cornea and globe (buphthalmos) is not present. Small subconjunctival hemorrhages are common in newborns, particularly after vaginal delivery, and do not indicate trauma unless other findings are present.

An examination of the red reflex of the eyes should be performed in all neonates before discharge from the nursery and at subsequent health supervision visits (American Academy of Pediatrics, 2008). Anything that interferes with the transmission of light through the normally transparent parts of the eye on its path to the fundus and back to the examiner will result in an abnormality of the red reflex. Problems potentially detected by the red reflex examination include cataracts, aqueous and vitreous opacities, and retinal abnormalities including tumors and chorioretinal colobomas. High-refractive errors and strabismus may also produce abnormalities or asymmetry of the red reflex. Dark spots in the red reflex, a markedly diminished reflex, the presence of a white reflex, or asymmetry of the reflexes are indications for immediate referral to an ophthalmologist experienced in neonatal evaluation (American Academy of Pediatrics, 2008). The red reflex examination is to be rated as normal when the reflections of the two eyes viewed both individually and simultaneously are equivalent in color, intensity, and clarity, and there are no opacities or white spots within the area of either or both red reflexes (American Academy of Pediatrics, 2008). The red reflex examination is vital for early detection of vision-threatening and potentially life-threatening abnormalities, including retinoblastoma. Unfortunately, the sensitivity of the routine red reflex examination for retinoblastoma is low, and most retinoblastomas are first detected by family members rather than pediatricians, despite routine screening (Abramson et al, 2003).

NOSE

The nose should be inspected for deformities, with attention to the size, shape, and symmetry of the various components of the nose, including the nostrils, columella, alae nasi, and the bridge, root, and tip. Asymmetries of the nose caused by in utero compression are common and need to be distinguished from malformations. Passage of a catheter beyond the nasopharynx via each nare, usually done in the delivery room, rules out choanal atresia but does not ensure that the size of the nasal passages is adequate for normal breathing. The quality and volume of air flow through each nostril can be evaluated by listening with the bell of a stethoscope or by observing the deflection of a wisp of cotton placed under the nostril. With the mouth closed, the infant should be able to breath comfortably via each nostril separately; this can be assessed by briefly occluding each nostril with the examiner's fingertip. If unilateral atresia or stenosis is present, the infant will exhibit signs of distress when the patent nostril is occluded. Flaring of the alae nasi may occur as the sole or initial symptom of mild respiratory distress, or it may accompany grunting and retractions.

MOUTH AND ORAL CAVITY

The lips, perioral area, and oral cavity should be inspected both at rest and during crying. The shape of the philtrum should be evaluated when the mouth is relaxed, because stretching of the upper lip during crying can give a false impression of a flat philtrum, which is suggestive of fetal alcohol syndrome. Perioral cyanosis is common and benign in normal infants in the immediate newborn period, whereas cyanosis of the tongue and mucous membranes is always abnormal and requires immediate investigation. The mucous membranes will be moist and shiny with saliva if the infant is well hydrated. Excessive oral secretions can be caused by esophageal atresia or impaired swallowing. An excessively short frenulum that restricts protrusion of the tongue can be a cause of feeding difficulty.

In the routine examination, the oral cavity is usually inspected without the use of a tongue depressor or other instruments. Epstein's pearls, Bohn's nodules, and dental lamina cysts (Figure 25-10) are common findings that should be indicated to the parents as benign. With patience and some adjustment of the head position, the entire palate and much of the pharynx can often be visualized. The tonsils are normally inconspicuous in neonates. The uvula is short but highly mobile. The soft palate elevates during crying if cranial nerves (CNs) IX and X are intact.

Inspection of the oral cavity is supplemented by palpation with a gloved finger to assess the shape and integrity of the palate, and to feel for natal teeth and masses. Although clefting of the lip and anterior palate will be obvious at a glance, an isolated cleft of the posterior palate may be missed unless deliberately sought by palpation. Eliciting the sucking reflex allows the strength and coordination of sucking to be assessed. In the routine examination of a vigorous, alert infant, elicitation of a gag reflex is unnecessarily upsetting to the infant and is normally avoided. The gag reflex should be tested if the infant is neurologically depressed or has difficulty swallowing.

NECK

It is usually convenient to combine palpation of the neck for lymphadenopathy and masses with palpation of the clavicles. The entire skin surface of the neck should be visualized and palpated, while turning the head and retracting the skin to open the neck creases and folds. The range of motion of the head and neck is evaluated at the same time. Congenital muscular torticollis at birth is commonly but not invariably accompanied by a palpable fibrous tumor (fibromatosis colli) in the shortened sternocleidomastoid muscle. Nonmuscular causes of torticollis include tumors of the posterior fossa or cervical spine and malformations of the cervical spine. A short neck, low hairline at the back of the head, and restricted mobility of the upper spine are characteristic features of the Klippel-Feil syndrome. Redundant skin or a webbed neck may be seen in Trisomy 21 and in Turner and Noonan syndromes. Cystic hygromas are soft, fluctuant masses that transilluminate and are usually unilateral. Branchial cleft cysts or sinuses are also found laterally, from the level of the mastoid to the center of the sternocleidomastoid muscle. Thyroglossal duct cysts are located in the midline high in the neck or under the chin. Further investigation is needed if the larynx or trachea are displaced from the midline, or if enlargement of the thyroid gland is suspected.

CHEST WALL

Although evaluation of the heart and lungs is a central focus of the examination of the chest, the skin, soft tissue, and bony structures of the thorax should not be neglected. The position of the nipples and the presence of any accessory nipples should be noted. The definition and stippling of the areola and the size of the breast bud are developmental features helpful as part of scoring for gestational age estimation. Transient galactorrhea occurs in approximately 5% of term neonates (Madlon-Kay, 1986). Variations in the shape of the xiphoid process are common, and parents can be reassured that a prominent or bifid xiphoid is benign and will usually become much less apparent as the infant grows. A mildly depressed sternum (pectus excavatum) or protuberant one (pectus carinatum) is usually of no clinical consequence. A small, bell-shaped chest in an infant with respiratory distress may reflect lung hypoplasia or a disorder of skeletal growth. An increase in the anterior-posterior diameter of the chest (barrel chest) may reflect an increase in the intrathoracic volume caused by air trapping from meconium aspiration or pneumothorax. Palpation of the chest wall may reveal irregularities or tenderness, and crepitus may be felt at the site of a fractured clavicle or rib. Crepitus can also be caused by dissection of air into the subcutaneous tissue from a pneumothorax or pneumomediastinum, but this is an unlikely occurrence in an asymptomatic infant.

LUNGS AND RESPIRATION

The respiratory examination begins with observing the color of the tongue and mucous membranes, respiratory rate, breathing pattern, and work of breathing. Respiratory problems are unlikely to be found in an infant who is centrally pink and breathing comfortably at a relaxed rate.

In the normal newborn, the abdomen expands smoothly with each contraction of the diaphragm, while the chest moves inward slightly.

The respiratory rate of the newborn infant is highly variable when the infant is awake, changing with activity such as feeding and crying. Tachypnea during sleep is more clearly associated with respiratory problems than is tachypnea during awake states. During a routine examination of the healthy infant, it is not necessary to measure the exact respiratory rate, as long as it is clearly within a normal range in an asymptomatic infant, but the respiratory rate should be determined if tachypnea or an unusually slow rate is seen. Because short pauses and brief periods of rapid breathing are common in normal newborns, accurate measurement of the respiratory rate requires counting for a full minute, preferably when the infant is asleep or at least not crying. During crying, the quality and vigor of vocalization are assessed, and the infant is observed for changes in color and perfusion. Central cyanosis that only appears during crying may be caused by cardiac or respiratory disease and requires further evaluation. Cyanosis that resolves during crying may be due to choanal atresia or stenosis, apnea, or hypoventilation.

The classic symptoms of respiratory distress are nasal flaring, grunting, and retractions. Nasal flaring and mild grunting are common in the immediate postnatal period, but in the healthy newborn they should resolve within 15 to 20 minutes after birth. Increasing respiratory distress caused by decreasing lung compliance is typically reflected in a progression from nasal flaring, or mild tachypnea, or both; to nasal flaring plus mild or intermittent grunting; and then to flaring, grunting, and increasingly severe retractions. The respiratory rate generally decreases as the work or effort of breathing increases, as indicated by the development of grunting and increasing retractions. When respiratory distress is mild, intermittent grunting at a slower respiratory rate may alternate with periods of mild tachypnea. As grunting becomes more severe, the expiratory phase becomes increasingly prolonged. The length of the grunt, rather than its loudness, correlates with the severity of distress. Intermittent mild grunting can be misinterpreted by parents as crying. The rhythm of grunting and its occurrence at the end of expiration are key features that help to distinguish it from other vocalizations. Retractions require a forceful inspiratory effort and decreased lung compliance, and they may be absent or less prominent than expected in an infant with neuromuscular depression.

Nasal congestion, airway obstruction, and airway secretions can produce sounds that are audible without a stethoscope. Noisy or congested nasal breathing and intermittent sneezing not associated with upper respiratory infection is common in the first few days after birth. A hoarse cry suggests an abnormality affecting the vocal cords. Because intubation of vigorous infants born through meconium-stained amniotic fluid is no longer routine (Halliday and Sweet, 2001), hoarseness or stridor caused by vocal cord trauma in healthy term infants is less common than previously. Inspiratory stridor is due to narrowing or partial obstruction of the upper airway. The presence and loudness of the stridor depends on respiratory effort as well as the extent of airway narrowing, so that stridor worsens with forceful inspiration during crying. Stridor during crying in an infant with no respiratory distress when quiet is often due to tracheolaryngomalacia, and it is usually benign. Stridor that is present during quiet breathing or present during both inspiration and expiration suggests the presence of a more significant airway obstruction that requires further evaluation.

In the routine examination of the infant who is observed to be centrally pink and breathing comfortably in room air, brief auscultation of the chest of a sleeping or quiet infant is usually sufficient to ensure that the breath sounds are clear, and that air entry is adequate and equal bilaterally. Sounds are not well localized in the neonate, and the infant might not remain quiet for long, so attention to the quality of the breath sounds is usually more helpful than attempting to compare multiple sites. Detection of abnormal lung sounds including crackles, wheezes, and rhonchi requires further assessment. If more detailed examination is indicated, auscultate over the four major quadrants anteriorly, on the sides, and on the upper and lower back bilaterally. Diaphragmatic hernia manifesting in the neonatal period usually causes significant respiratory distress, but rarely a small diaphragmatic hernia is detected by the presence of bowel sounds in the chest in an asymptomatic infant. Spontaneous cough, which is abnormal in neonates, is most commonly caused by infection or aspiration.

Percussion of the chest, rarely done as part of routine examination of newborn, can be useful for estimating the position of the upper margin of the liver. Percussion can also be used to detect a large effusion or lung consolidation, but infants with these conditions will have other symptoms of respiratory distress, so the diagnosis will rely on imaging studies and not the physical examination. Transillumination can be useful for supporting a rapid diagnosis of pneumothorax in a distressed infant, but it is not reliable for detecting a small pneumothorax that produces minimal symptoms.

Respiratory symptoms are sensitive but nonspecific indicators of illness in the newborn, because alterations in respiration (including apnea) can accompany illness of many different etiologies. Common causes of subtle or mild respiratory distress detected in the routine evaluation include retained fetal lung fluid (transient tachypnea of the newborn), spontaneous pneumothorax, neonatal sepsis, pneumonia, meconium or amniotic fluid aspiration, and congenital heart disease. Any infant with respiratory distress should be transferred to an NICU or observation nursery for further evaluation, monitoring, and treatment.

CARDIOVASCULAR

The evaluation of the cardiovascular system during the routine examination has two major goals: to assess the current status of the circulation and to detect signs of congenital heart disease, particularly the critical, ductal-dependent forms that can produce rapid clinical deterioration in the newborn period. Although detection of heart disease is important, abnormal circulatory findings in the newborn are more often secondary to other problems, including sepsis, hypovolemia, anemia, and hypoglycemia. The cardiovascular system undergoes marked changes after birth involving the transition to air breathing, the progressive decrease of pulmonary vascular resistance, and the closure of the ductus arteriosus. These changes affect the physical examination of healthy infants and those with congenital heart disease; therefore the time after birth is always an important consideration in the interpretation of the examination.

Physical examination of the cardiovascular system is not limited to examination of the heart and pulses. It also requires attention to the infant's general behavior and activity, to respiratory symptoms, to the color of the tongue and oral mucosa, and to the temperature, color and perfusion of all regions of the body. These features will usually be inspected at different times during the course of the routine examination, but they should be reevaluated during the heart and chest examination if cardiovascular abnormalities are suspected.

Important features of the pulses are the rate, rhythm, volume and character. The heart rate of the resting well newborn averages 120 to 130 beats/min, with high variability. Transient sinus tachycardia during vigorous crying is common, but persistent tachycardia with a rate greater than 160 beats/min suggests a need for further investigation. A low resting heart rate caused by sinus bradycardia (80 to 100 beats/min) during sleep is common in healthy full-term infants. Isolated premature beats can be noted occasionally in otherwise healthy infants and are almost always benign. The femoral pulses in a normal neonate are not easy to palpate, and they are easily obliterated with pressure. They usually receive a grade of 2 on the traditional scale of 0 to 4. A patent ductus arterious will not cause bounding pulses until the pulmonary vascular resistance has dropped enough to allow significant left-to-right shunting. Uniformly weak pulses suggest a low output state, usually accompanied by signs of poor perfusion. If a decrease or delay of the femoral relative to the brachial pulses is detected, measurement of the blood pressure in all four extremities can reveal a gradient in the blood pressure caused by coarctation of the aorta. However, normal pulses and four-limb blood pressures do not rule out a coarctation if the ductus arteriosus remains open.

The precordial area and heart are examined by inspection, palpation, and auscultation. A precordial impulse can be visible in normal newborns, especially during activity, but visible prominence of the precordial area together with a palpably increased cardiac impulse suggest cardiomegaly or a hyperdynamic state. Displacement of the cardiac impulse to the right suggests dextrocardia or a shift in the mediastinum. Thrills are rarely palpable in the newborn.

Auscultation of the heart should be performed with specific questions in mind, with attention attuned sequentially for heart sounds, clicks, murmurs, and other abnormal sounds. Most sounds and murmurs in the newborn are relatively high-pitched, so the diaphragm is usually used initially. The bell can be used for further evaluation of low-pitched sounds, if needed. The first heart sound, produced by closure of the mitral and tricuspid valves, is usually single in newborns and best heard in the precordial area. The second sound, produced by closure of the aortic and pulmonary valves, is usually best heard at the left upper sternal border. With focused attention, slight splitting of the second sound and its variation with respiration can be appreciated. Third and fourth heart sounds are abnormal in the newborn. Systolic ejection clicks may be heard in some normal neonates in the first several hours after birth, but ejection clicks are abnormal after this period (Johnson, 1990).

The timing, location, intensity, radiation, quality, and pitch are important characteristics of heart murmurs that can help to distinguish physiologic from pathologic murmurs. With repeated examination, physiologic heart murmurs may be detected in as many as 60% of infants during the first 48 hours (Johnson, 1990). These murmurs are most commonly systolic ejection murmurs that are transient and soft (grade I or II), and they are usually attributed to flow through a closing ductus arteriosus or to increasing flow across the pulmonic valve as pulmonary vascular resistance drops. Vibratory systolic murmurs resembling Still's murmur can be heard in some newborns. A murmur detected on a routine newborn examination that is not clearly physiologic needs further evaluation.

Detection of a suspicious murmur is the most common reason for further evaluation in an otherwise asymptomatic newborn, but absence of a murmur does not rule out congenital heart disease. Examples include transposition of the great arteries and atrioventricular (AV) canal defect. A decrease or loss of a murmur can be an ominous sign that accompanies clinical deterioration associated with ductal closure in an infant with ductal-dependent pulmonary or systemic blood flow.

Pathologic murmurs detected in the first few hours of life are usually caused by obstruction of ventricular outflow such as aortic stenosis or pulmonic stenosis; they are crescendo-decrescendo murmurs, usually grade II or III. This type of murmur may also be caused by subaortic stenosis associated with hypertrophic cardiomyopathy in a macrosomic infant of a mother with diabetes. Murmurs associated with defects that produce left-to-right shunting usually appear after a few days, when the pulmonary vascular resistance has dropped sufficiently. Pansystolic murmurs (which include and obscure the first heart sound) that are heard soon after birth are most commonly caused by AV valve insufficiency, whereas left-to-right shunting through a ventricular septal defect produces a pansystolic murmur that typically appears only after 1 to 2 days. Diastolic murmurs are rare in newborns. A continuous murmur in a neonate usually represents an aortopulmonary communication or an arteriovenous fistula. The location of an extrathoracic arteriovenous fistula may be revealed by auscultation of a bruit, most commonly in the head or liver.

ABDOMEN

Examination of the abdomen begins with observation of the configuration, fullness, and movement with respiration of the abdominal wall. Major abdominal wall abnormalities such as omphalocele, gastroschisis, prune belly syndrome, and bladder extrophy will be obvious on initial inspection in the delivery room and may be diagnosed prenatally. Although a large omphalocele will never be missed, a small one may produce only a slight widening of the umbilicus and proximal umbilical cord (Figure 25-17). If such an omphalocele is not detected in the delivery room before the umbilical cord is clamped and cut, the intestine within it may be damaged. The abdomen of the neonate ranges from flat to moderately protuberant, with substantial variation depending on feeding and the passage of gas and meconium. A markedly distended abdomen suggests the possibility of significant ascites, a large mass, or

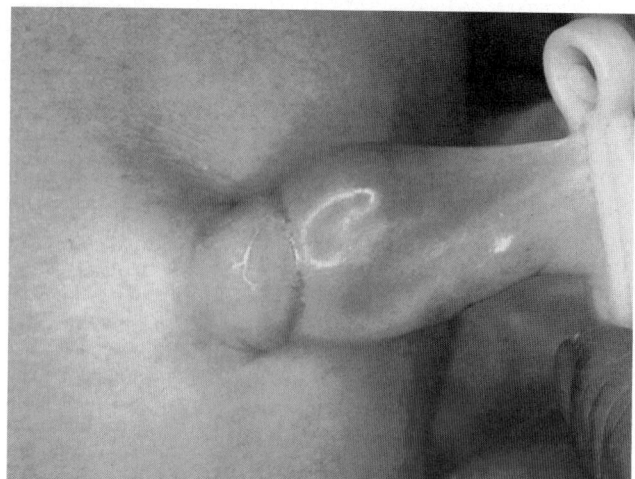

FIGURE 25-17 A small omphalocele that could be injured if the cord were to be clamped too close to its insertion. (*Reprinted from Rudolph AJ: Atlas of the newborn, vol 4, Hamilton, Ont, Canada, 1997, BC Decker, p 109.*)

an intestinal obstruction. A proximal obstruction such as esophageal or duodenal atresia does not cause abdominal distension, however. A sunken or scaphoid abdomen may be seen in the infant with respiratory distress caused by a diaphragmatic hernia. The umbilicus should be inspected for meconium staining, for signs of infection, and for the rare occurrence of pallor and edema or the visible discharge of urine caused by a patent urachus. At 1 or 2 days after birth, slight redness of the periumbilical skin is common, because of irritation from the cord clamp, and needs to be distinguished from an omphalitis or cellulitis. Counting of the umbilical vessels is best done in the delivery room, on the freshly cut cord.

If the infant is asleep or resting quietly, it is prudent to auscultate for bowel sounds before proceeding to palpate the abdomen. Palpation should be initially gentle and superficial, to detect any signs of tenderness and the presence of an enlarged liver or spleen. Tenderness must be distinguished from the tendency of the infant to stiffen the abdominal muscles in reaction to the touch of the examiner's fingers, which are usually colder than the infant's skin. If the examiner's fingers remain in gentle contact within the same spot, the temperature difference will disappear in a moment, and the baby will usually relax and allow the examiner to proceed without a struggle. In the healthy infant, the liver edge may be at or slightly above the right costal margin, or palpable 1 to 2 cm below. The spleen is rarely palpable unless it is enlarged. Gentle palpation of the lower abdomen can detect an enlarged bladder, which is the most common cause of a midline abdominal mass in neonates. Deep palpation to detect small masses or enlargement of the kidneys is most easily done soon after birth, before the infant has fed much, and when the infant is quiet. However, a satisfactory examination can be done even in a crying infant by keeping the fingers in position, and gradually increasing the depth of palpation each time the infant briefly relaxes the abdominal muscles while taking a breath between cries. It is helpful to support the flank with one hand while palpating for the kidney with the other, or to palpate with the thumb while supporting the flank with fingers of the same hand. Percussion of the abdomen is not particularly helpful in routine examination, but it can sometimes help to define the boundaries of an enlarged liver or bladder.

GENITALIA AND PERINEUM

Brief inspection after delivery is usually sufficient to identify the infant as male or female. The evaluation and management of the infant with ambiguous genitalia is discussed in Chapter 92. In both male and female infants, a soft swelling or bulge in the inguinal area may be due to an inguinal hernia. The bulge typically appears or increases in size during crying and is easily reduced with gentle pressure when the infant relaxes. The perineum is inspected to locate the anus and assess the tone of the anal sphincter. Absence of a normal anal opening should be detected as part of the initial evaluation in the delivery room. However, external observation of an apparently normal anus does not guarantee internal patency of the anus, which is best confirmed by the normal passage of meconium.

The genitalia are mainly examined by inspection, supplemented by palpation, with the infant in a supine, frog-leg position. In the newborn male, the foreskin normally covers the entire head of the penis, which is adherent to the glans. The urethral opening is usually hidden by the foreskin and need not be visualized if the foreskin is intact. The foreskin is typically incomplete if hypospadias is present, which allows the abnormal position of the urethral opening to be identified easily. Congenital chordee, a ventral angulation of the head of the penis, may accompany hypospadias or occur in isolation. Chordee can be missed unless the examiner straightens the penis by gently retracting the skin along the shaft towards the base of the penis. In infants who have a generous pad of subcutaneous fat at the base of the penis, this maneuver also helps to avoid a false impression that the penis is short. Dribbling of urine or a weak stream, if observed, is suspicious for bladder dysfunction or urethral obstruction. The scrotal sac and inguinal areas are palpated to locate the testes and assess their size. The scrotal rugae usually appear at approximately 36 weeks' gestation and cover the entire scrotum at term. Enlargement of the scrotal sac is most commonly caused by a hydrocele. Transillumination can help to distinguish a hydrocele from swelling because of congenital testicular torsion or other masses. Bowel sounds may be audible in a scrotum enlarged by an inguinal hernia.

During the inspection of the female genitalia, the examiner must gently retract the labia majora laterally to allow full visualization. The sizes and positions of the labia minora, clitoris, urethra, and vaginal opening should be noted. Relative prominence of the labia minora is normal in preterm infants. Partial labial fusion and an increase in the size of the clitoris may represent virilization caused by congenital adrenal hyperplasia or related endocrine abnormalities. The posterior fourchette should be at least 1 cm from the anal opening. Enlargement of the uterus because of hydrometrocolpos may produce a protruding perineal mass. Vaginal tags and mucoid vaginal discharge are common at birth, resulting from exposure to maternal estrogen. A slightly bloody vaginal discharge (pseudomenses) caused by hormonal withdrawal is common in healthy females during the first week after birth.

BACK

The back is inspected for asymmetry or abnormal positioning of the shoulders, ribs, and hips. Major neural tube defects and large masses such as a large sacrococcygeal teratoma will be detected prenatally or on initial inspection in the delivery room. In the routine examination, the lumbosacral area should be inspected carefully for the presence of deep or unusual dimpling of the skin over the sacrum, for sinus tracts, for unusual tufts of hair, and for small masses such as a lipoma or hemangioma, any of which may be associated with spina bifida occulta or tethering of the spinal cord. The spine is inspected for straightness and palpated for the integrity and alignment of the posterior spinous processes.

MUSCULOSKELETAL SYSTEM

Routine assessment of the musculoskeletal system begins with plotting the height, weight, and head circumference on appropriate growth charts. Detailed measurements of the limbs and trunk can be made if growth appears disproportionate, but they are not part of the routine examination. The infant's posture, muscle mass, and movements should be observed. As the different parts of the body are surveyed during the course of the examination, any limitation in the normal range of joint motion and any localized swelling or tenderness should be noted. Major limb or skeletal malformations will usually be appreciated on initial inspection in the delivery room, but minor anomalies such as supernumerary digits, syndactyly, or nail hypoplasia can be missed if a disciplined approach is not taken. Lack or restriction of normal movement of an extremity can be caused by trauma, most commonly a fractured humerus or clavicle, or by an intrinsic abnormality of the joint or limb. Although they generally require no treatment, fractures of the clavicle are sufficiently common that the clavicles should be specifically examined in every newborn. Crepitus and tenderness at the site of a clavicle fracture may be more easily detected if the examiner palpates a clavicle with one hand while using the other to elevate and rotate the ipsilateral shoulder.

Deformations caused by in utero positioning are not always easy to distinguish from malformations on an initial examination. Mild inward bowing of the lower legs and feet is common in newborns. If an inward-turning foot can be brought easily to a neutral position, a clubfoot deformity is unlikely, and the angulation of the foot can be expected to normalize spontaneously.

EXAMINATION OF THE HIPS

Assessment for developmental dysplasia of the hip (DDH) is an important component of the examination of every newborn (American Academy of Pediatrics, 2000; Sewell et al, 2009). Frank dislocations, partial dislocations, and instability of the humoral head in the socket can be detected by examination in the newborn period. Nevertheless, DDH is not always detectable at birth. Statistical risk factors for DDH include a positive family history, female sex, and breech presentation. In addition to the Ortolani and Barlow maneuvers, the examination also involves a focused inspection for indirect clues related to the possible presence of DDH.

During general inspection of the infant, attention should be paid to the resting posture and spontaneous movements; any asymmetry or unusual positioning of the legs should be noted. Asymmetry of the gluteal or femoral skin folds may be a sign of unilateral hip dislocation. A unilateral dislocation may also produce an apparent inequality of leg length, seen either with the legs in extension (Thomas' sign) or with the feet flat on the bed and the knees bent (Galeazzi's sign). A restricted range of motion, particularly abduction, is a clue that may detect either unilateral or bilateral dislocations.

The dislocation of the femoral head during a Barlow maneuver or its relocation during an Ortolani maneuver produces what is called a *clunk* that must be distinguished from high-pitched clicks of the hip that are common and benign. Clunks and clicks are perceived by palpation and are not actually audible. The key element defining the clunk is a distinct sensation of abrupt movement of the femoral head as it passes over the rim of acetabulum and drops into or out of the socket. A dislocated or dislocatable hip has the distinctive clunk, whereas a subluxable hip is characterized by a feeling of looseness or sliding without a distinct clunk (American Academy of Pediatrics, 2000). Both maneuvers are performed with the infant supine, starting with the legs held in neutral rotation and the hips flexed to 90 degrees but not more. Each hip is examined separately. For the Ortolani maneuver, the index and middle fingers of the examiner's hand are placed along the greater trochanter with the thumb placed along the inner thigh near the knee. The other hand stabilizes the pelvis. The examiner gently abducts the hip by rotating the thumb outward while lifting anteriorly with the fingers. A distinct sensation of movement is felt when a posteriorly dislocated hip relocates during abduction. For the Barlow maneuver, the index and middle fingers are also positioned along the greater trochanter, but the examiner's hand is rotated so that the base of the thumb is on top of the knee. The maneuver is performed by adducting the leg until the knee is in the midline, and then applying gentle pressure to the knee in a downward direction along the adducted femur. A clunk is felt if this maneuver induces the femoral head to exit the acetabulum posteriorly. Minimal force is used in either maneuver.

The examination is considered positive for DDH if a clunk of dislocation or reduction is elicited during the Barlow or Ortolani maneuvers, in which case prompt referral to an orthopedist is strongly recommended. The examination is considered equivocal if the Barlow and Ortolani test results are negative, but warning signs such as asymmetric creases, apparent or true leg length discrepancy, or limited abduction are found. In this case, the recommended next step in evaluation is a follow-up examination of the hips by a pediatrician at 2 weeks (American Academy of Pediatrics, 2000).

NEUROLOGIC EXAMINATION

The neurologic system is assessed during the course of the general newborn examination and by performing some specific maneuvers to elicit neonatal reflexes. Because the healthy infant's responses vary with the state of alertness, and because the infant's tolerance for prolonged examination is limited, eliciting a perfect response to each maneuver should not be expected. Fortunately, there is sufficient redundancy in the routine examination that it is not difficult in most cases for the examiner to be satisfied that the infant is neurologically normal. When the examination is not fully reassuring, repeating selected parts of the examination at a later time may be more helpful in clarifying findings than attempting an extended examination at one time. The newborn screening examination includes assessment of the infant's alertness, spontaneous activity, posture, muscle tone and strength, head control, and responses to manipulation and handling.

The overall assessment of alertness, tone, and activity is one of the most important components of the newborn examination. Diminished alertness, tone, or spontaneous activity are sensitive but nonspecific indicators of illness that are much more likely the result of other causes, such as neonatal sepsis, than a specific neurologic abnormality. The typical healthy newborn is easily awakened from sleep and remains alert through the remainder of the routine examination, shifting among states of quiet alertness, active alertness, and crying. The examiner's initial attempt to quietly auscultate the breath and heart sounds of a sleeping infant is often foiled by the infant's prompt arousal and crying. The healthy newborn demonstrates a vigorous cry when upset, but is able to self-console or to be consoled with holding, sucking, or feeding. An infant who is stuporous or difficult to arouse is clearly abnormal and needs further evaluation, as does an infant who is unusually irritable or inconsolable. The typical newborn will be rather alert for several hours after delivery, but may then provoke parental concern by becoming relatively sleepy and uninterested in feeding for the remainder of the first 24 hours. As long as the infant continues to be easily arousable and the examination result remains otherwise normal, parents can be reassured that the infant will likely begin feeding much more vigorously on the second day. Decreases in tone or alertness occurring 1 day or more after birth in a previously vigorous infant are not normal and require prompt investigation for sepsis or other problems, including inborn errors of metabolism that can cause progressive symptoms starting a few days after birth because of accumulation of toxic metabolites.

Because the newborn cannot respond to verbal questions or commands, assessment of the infant's sensory functions in the routine examination depends on observation of the strength and quality of the infant's movements in response to handling during the examination and to specific local stimulation, such as the elicitation of the palmar and plantar grasp reflexes and the rooting and sucking reflexes. Assessment of vision in the routine newborn examination is limited to observing pupillary constriction and a blink response to light, which are subcortical responses, and to observing the infant's visual attentiveness. The healthy term newborn is expected to be able to visually fixate on and follow the examiner's face, but failure to observe this response during the course of the routine examination is common, because it can take more time and patience to elicit than are available. Hearing can be evaluated behaviorally by observing the infant's responses to the ringing of a bell and other sounds. However, behavioral testing can only detect profound, bilateral hearing loss, and it has been effectively replaced in the routine newborn examination by automated hearing tests (American Academy of Pediatrics, 2007; US Preventive Services Task Force, 2008).

The assessment of motor function relies on the observation of the infant's posture and spontaneous movements, observation of the infant's general responses to stimulation and handling, and the elicitation of specific reflexes. The healthy term newborn normally maintains a resting posture with elbows, hips, and knees strongly flexed. The scarf sign, forearm recoil, square window of the wrist, the heal-to-ear maneuver, and popliteal angle are measures of tone and flexibility commonly scored in the gestational age assessment (Ballard et al, 1991; Dubowitz et al, 1970). The active tone and strength of upper extremity muscle groups are routinely assessed by eliciting the palmar grasp and by arm traction during the pull-to-sit maneuver. Lower extremity strength and tone are assessed during the general examination of hips and feet, and by testing for the supporting reaction, stepping reflex, Babinski's reflex, and ankle clonus. The neck flexors may be evaluated during the standard pull-to-sit maneuver, or by lifting the shoulders to pull the baby to a sitting position. The neck extensors can be evaluated by tilting the infant forward from a sitting position, or evaluated along with truncal tone by suspending the infant in a prone position with the examiner's hand under the chest (ventral suspension maneuver).

When observing the infant's movements, the examiner should note any asymmetry and pay attention to qualitative characteristics such as the relative smoothness versus jerkiness or tremulousness of movement. Unusual jitteriness may be a symptom of hypoglycemia or hypocalcemia, especially in infants of mothers with diabetes, infants that are small or large for gestational age, or infants who were exposed to opiates or other drugs in utero and are experiencing withdrawal. Passive restraint of an extremity should inhibit jittery movements, but will not stop the rhythmic contractions of clonic seizure activity. In addition to clonic movements, signs of neonatal seizures can include tonic posturing, repetitive stereotyped movements of the face or extremities, tonic horizontal eye deviation or nystagmoid jerking, staring or blinking, apnea, and unexplained changes in heart rate or blood pressure. Although it is uncommon to observe an actual seizure during the routine newborn examination, the pediatrician or neonatologist is frequently called to evaluate an infant because of concern about unusual movements seen by a parent or nurse. In the otherwise healthy newborn who is fully alert and responsive, jerky or abrupt movements that are evoked by stimulation (e.g., startles), that can be suppressed by passive restraint (e.g. jitteriness), and that are not accompanied by autonomic changes or changes in alertness are unlikely to be seizures. Transient episodes of disconjugate gaze are also not unusual in normal newborn infants, particularly when the infant is entering or awakening from sleep.

Neonatal Reflexes

The neonatal or primitive reflexes frequently tested during routine examination of the newborn include the Moro reflex, the asymmetrical tonic neck reflex, truncal incurvation (Galant reflex), the palmar and plantar grasp reflexes, the Babinski's reflex, and the placing and stepping reflexes. The Moro reflex can be elicited following the pull-to-sit maneuver, by lowering the infant until there is only a slight space between the neck and bed, and then allowing the infant to fall back suddenly. Alternatively, the Moro response can be elicited by the "drop" method: the examiner lifts the baby completely off the bed, supporting the head and trunk with both hands and keeping the baby supine, and then rapidly lowers the baby by approximately 4 to 8 inches. The complete Moro reflex involves a quick bilateral abduction of the arms and extension of the forearms with full opening of the hands, followed by smoother and slower return of the hands toward the midline, with curling of the fingers. The startle reflex is similar to the Moro reflex, but without full extension or hand opening, and may occur spontaneously or be evoked by a sudden noise or movement.

The position of the neck affects the tone of the extremities via the asymmetrical tonic neck reflex. This should be kept in mind during observation of the infant's spontaneous movements, because it can cause a false impression of asymmetry if the position of the neck is not taken into account. To test the asymmetric tonic neck reflex, turn the infant's head 90 degrees to one side for 15 seconds, keeping the infant lying on the back with the shoulders horizontal. In the complete response, the ipselateral arm and leg will extend and the contralateral arm and leg will flex, producing the "fencing" posture. The test is then repeated with the head turned to the other side. Observation of the complete response is reassuring, but its absence is not necessarily abnormal, because partial and unidirectional responses are common in normal newborns. However, an unusually sustained or exaggerated response is abnormal.

The truncal incurvation reflex is elicited with the infant held in ventral suspension by stroking lightly down the back on one side, and then the other. The normal response is for the infant to curve the spine strongly, concave toward the stimulated side.

The supporting, placing, and stepping reflexes are elicited with the infant held upright. The supporting reaction is elicited by lowering the infant vertically until both feet touch the surface of the bed or table. A positive response, usually seen after a slight delay, is partial extension at the hips and knees, as though the infant is attempting to stand and support his or her weight. The stepping reaction is tested by lowering the infant so that one foot touches the surface, with the infant tilted slightly forward. The infant should flex that leg and extend the other, as though taking a step. The response can sometimes be sustained for several alternating steps. The placing reaction is elicited by lifting the infant to bring the dorsum of one foot in contact with the underside of a table or bassinet edge. In a positive response, the infant lifts the foot up and places it on the top surface.

Babinski's reflex, which is normal in neonates, consists of dorsal flexion of the big toe and spreading of the other toes in response to stroking the foot laterally. Firm pressure on the sole of the foot, in contrast, will elicit a plantar grasp. The deep tendon reflexes are usually not elicited during routine examination of the well newborn, but they are helpful as part of a more complete examination if neurologic abnormalities are suspected. The pectoralis, biceps, brachioradialis, thigh adductor, crossed adductor, knee jerk, and ankle jerk reflexes are the most readily elicited (Volpe, 2008). Ankle clonus may be elicited by quickly dorsiflexing the foot, which in a healthy term infant should produce no more than approximately five beats of alternating extension and flexion with rapidly decaying intensity.

Brachial Plexus Injury

Although fortunately not common, brachial plexus injury is one of the more frequent neurologic abnormalities found in the otherwise healthy newborn, occurring in about 0.5 to 2 per 1000 live births. Often there is a history of difficult delivery because of shoulder dystocia. Brachial plexus injury can occur in isolation or in conjunction with fractures of the clavicle or humerus. Typical findings in Erb's palsy are an inability to abduct and externally rotate the shoulder, flex the elbow, and supinate the forearm because of injury to C5-C6 (Volpe, 2008). If C7 is involved, wrist and finger extension are also weak (Figure 25-18). A distal brachial plexus injury involving C8-T1 causes weakness of wrist and finger flexion.

Cranial Nerves

Observation and maneuvers during the routine examination provide at least partial assessment of all the cranial nerves (Volpe, 2008) except for the olfactory nerve (CN I), which is not routinely tested. Visual attentiveness, the ability to fix and follow, eyelid closing in response to light, and the pupillary light reflex require the optic nerve (CN II). The pupillary light reflex also tests the oculomotor nerve (CN III). Extraocular movements are controlled by CNs III, IV, and VI. Vertical gaze is difficult to assess in neonates, but horizontal gaze in both directions can usually be verified by observing spontaneous eye movements or by the rotation test. The examiner performs the rotation test by turning in place while holding the infant upright and supporting the back of the head. If vestibular functions (CN VIII) are intact, the infant will turn the head in the direction of rotation or, if the head is restrained, turn the eyes in that direction. Eliciting rooting or a facial grimace in response to touching the face tests the sensory portion of the trigeminal nerve (CN V). The corneal reflex can be tested by touching the cornea with a wisp of sterile cotton, but this is not part of the routine newborn examination. CNs V, VII, IX, X, and XII are all involved in normal sucking and swallowing. The motor portion of CN V controls the muscles of mastication, which are involved in the jaw-closing phase of the suck and are assessed during elicitation of the suck when the infant bites down on the examiner's finger. Although not part of the routine examination, the masseter or jaw-jerk reflex can be elicited by placing the forefinger of one hand on the infant's relaxed chin and tapping it with the forefinger of the other hand.

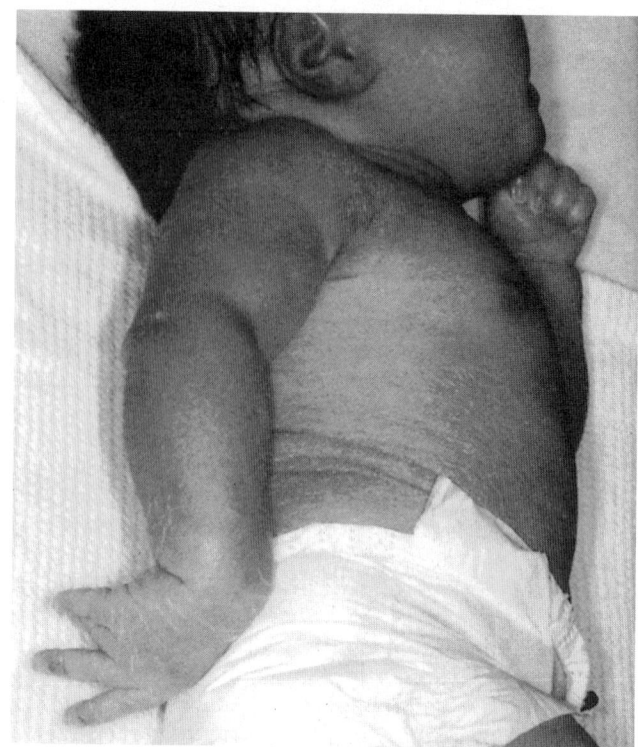

FIGURE 25-18 Hand and arm position in an infant with Erb's palsy involving C5, C6, and C7. *(Reprinted from Fletcher MA: Physical diagnosis in neonatology, Philadelphia, 1998, Lippincott-Raven, p 450.)*

The facial nerve (CN VII) is required for pursing of the lips in sucking, as well as normal facial expression and tone. Compression of the facial nerve by in utero positioning or by forceps injury are common causes of unilateral facial weakness in the newborn period (Figure 25-19). CNs IX and X are needed for normal swallowing and the gag reflex. CN XII is involved in the milking action of the tongue during sucking and swallowing. Taste, mediated by CN VII (anterior two thirds of the tongue) and IX (posterior third) is not evaluated in the routine examination. Sternocleidomastoid function (CN XI) is assessed by evaluating head flexion and lateral rotation. Because head control is often poor in normal newborns, it can be difficult to detect an abnormality unless it is unilateral. However, an asymmetric abnormality of a sternocleidomastoid is caused more commonly by torticollis than dysfunction of CN XI. The vestibular portion of CN VIII is assessed by the rotation test, as noted previously, or by the doll's eye maneuver. The auditory portion of CN VIII is best assessed using brainstem auditory evoked responses, rather than behavioral responses to auditory stimulation.

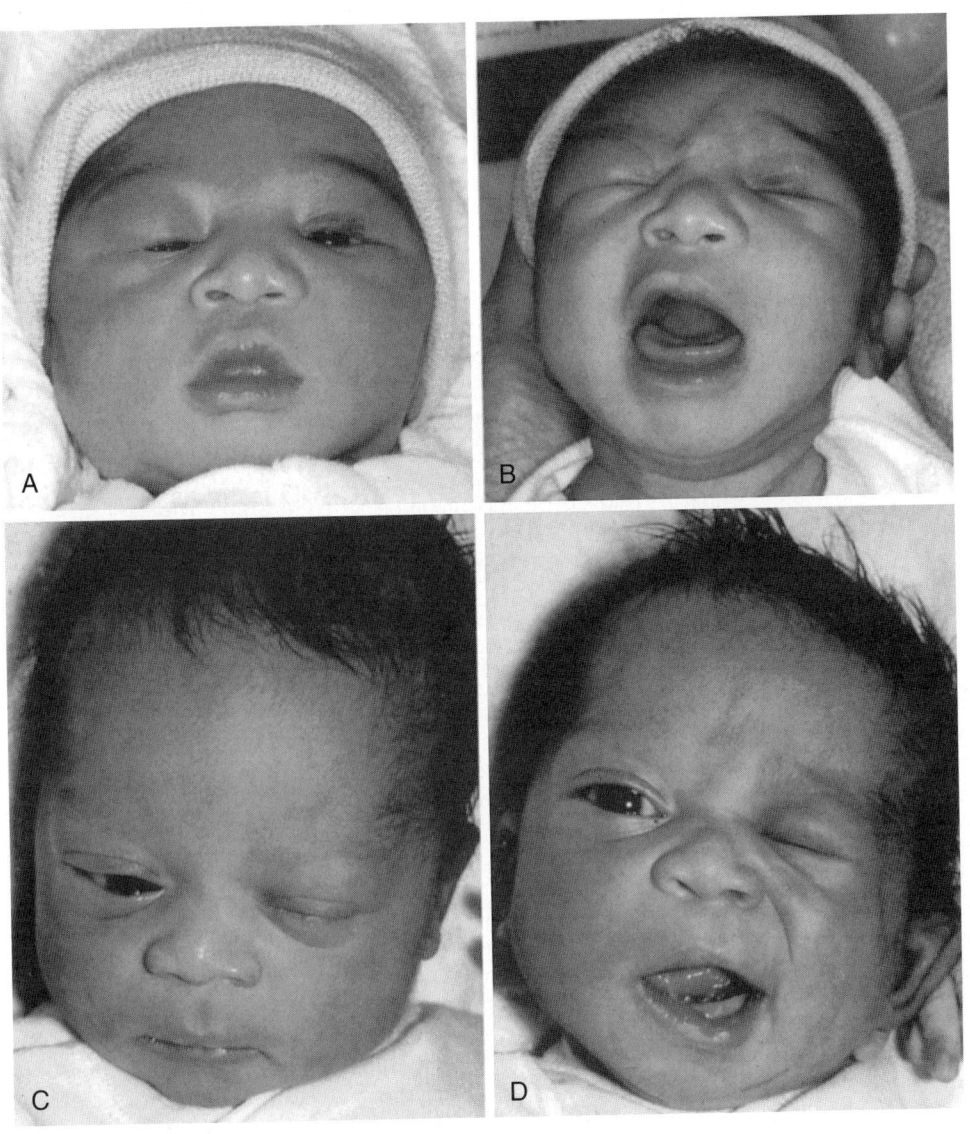

FIGURE 25-19 *(See also Color Plate 17.)* **Unilateral facial weakness in two infants.** There is mild facial asymmetry with flattening of the nasolabial folds at rest (**A** and **C**) and more obvious asymmetries of the grimace and eye closing during crying (**B** and **D**). The weakness is on the infant's left side in **A** and **B**, and on the infant's right side in **C** and **D**. *(Reprinted from Fletcher MA:* Physical diagnosis in neonatology, *Philadelphia, 1998, Lippincott-Raven, p 457.)*

SUGGESTED READINGS

Books

Cohen B: *Pediatric Dermatology*, ed 3, Philadelphia, 2005, Mosby.

Eichenfield LF, Frieden IJ, Esterly NB, editors: *Neonatal Dermatology*, ed 2, Philadelphia, 2008, Saunders.

Fletcher MA: *Physical Diagnosis in Neonatology*, Philadelphia, 1998, Lippincott-Raven.

Rudolph AJ: *Atlas of the Newborn*, Hamilton, Ontario, 1997, B.C. Decker.

Volpe JJ: *Neurology of the Newborn*, ed 5, Philadelphia, 2008, Saunders.

Guidelines and Policy Statements

Early detection of developmental dysplasia of the hip: clinical practice guideline. Committee on Quality Improvement, Subcommittee on Developmental Dysplasia of the Hip. American Academy of Pediatrics, *Pediatrics* 105:896-905, 2000.

Hospital stay for healthy term newborns: policy statement. American Academy of Pediatrics, *Pediatrics* 125:405-409, 2010.

Red reflex examination in neonates, infants, and children: Joint policy statement. American Academy of Pediatrics Section on Ophthalmology, American Association for Pediatric Ophthalmology and Strabismus, American Academy of Ophthalmology, American Association of Certified Orthoptists, *Pediatrics* 122:1401-1404, 2008.

Universal screening for hearing loss in newborns: US Preventive Services Task Force recommendation statement, *Pediatrics* 122:143-148, 2008.

Online Resources

Lehmann CU, Cohen BA: Dermatlas: an online collaborative education tool, *The Internet Journal of Dermatology* 1, 2002. Available at http://dermatlas.med.jhmi.edu/derm/.

Ballard JL, Khoury JC, Wedig K, Wang L, Eilers-Walsman BL, Lipp R: New Ballard Score, expanded to include extremely premature infants, *J Pediatr* 119:417-423, 1991. Descriptions and video demonstrations by JL Ballard. Available at www.ballardscore.com.

Pediatric NeuroLogic Exam, Available at http://library.med.utah.edu/pedineurologic-exam/html/home_exam.html. A tutorial with video demonstrations and descriptions by PD Larsen and SS Stensaas.

Complete references and supplemental color images used in this text can be found online at www.expertconsult.com

ROUTINE NEWBORN CARE

James A. Taylor, Jeffrey A. Wright, and David Woodrum

Two central paradoxes underlie the care of healthy newborn infants. First, although birth is perhaps the oldest and most natural of all human processes, the infant mortality rate has been extraordinarily high until recently. The second paradox in providing newborn care is that neonates are at once the healthiest and most vulnerable patients in medicine. Recent medical history is replete with examples of the pendulum swinging too far in each direction around these paradoxes. The promotion of scheduled feeding using infant formulas rather than breastfeeding is an example of the medicalization of neonatal care. Conversely, recent resistance to treatments that prevent uncommon but disastrous conditions represent a denial of the benefits provided by medical care.

Therefore optimal care of a normal neonate is an attempt to balance these competing forces. Systems of care should be designed to support the concept that newborn infants are extraordinarily healthy and require little intervention beyond promotion of breastfeeding. Interventions for which there is evidence that the benefits far outweigh the risks should be provided as unobtrusively as possible. Simultaneously, while promoting natural care for these newborns, health care providers need to be vigilant for the early identification of neonates who are at risk for conditions such as dehydration, sepsis, and severe hyperbilirubinemia.

The goal of this chapter is to provide an evidence base for the promotion of healthy newborn care by parents, the rationale for monitoring full-term neonates for various conditions, a risk-benefit analysis of common treatments, and the significance of common prenatal and postnatal findings. Rather than providing a comprehensive prescription for the care of these infants, it is hoped that the reader will integrate the information provided in this chapter with expert opinion and clinical experience to determine the proper care of healthy newborns.

INITIAL ASSESSMENT

Timing of the initial assessment of a full-term newborn is dependent on the condition of the infant and parental preference. In most instances a health care professional who is present at the birth will make a general appraisal of the infant and alert the child's provider if there is an acute problem necessitating an immediate evaluation. Usually the neonate will be healthy and the assessment can be timed so as not to interfere with breastfeeding, bonding with the family, and routine care.

Before examining a healthy newborn, the mother's medical history should be reviewed to identify issues that would affect the care or prognosis of the infant. For example, a history of diabetes in the mother would lead to glucose testing in the neonate. Maternal drug use should be assessed for possible teratogenic effects, possibility of

symptoms of withdrawal in the infant, and compatibility with breastfeeding. It is important to review the pregnancy history and focus on estimated gestational age, the results of screening for genetic conditions, and the results of prenatal ultrasound examinations. Perinatal events such as type of delivery, length of time that membranes were ruptured, and Apgar scores should also be reviewed. Finally, it is critical to review the mother's social history to insure that the newborn will be raised in a nurturing environment and to identify high-risk situations for which interventions are needed before or shortly after discharge from the newborn nursery.

The results of several laboratory tests commonly performed on pregnant women will determine the need for treatment or monitoring during the newborn nursery stay. These tests include maternal HIV, hepatitis B surface antigen status, and syphilis. The mother's blood type, Rh status, and antibody test results are useful in identifying newborns with an increased risk of hyperbilirubinemia. It is important to note the results of testing for maternal colonization with group B *Streptococcus* (GBS) and the type and timing of antenatal antibiotic prophylaxis in mothers with a positive test result for GBS.

The infant's weight, length, and head circumference should be measured shortly after birth and plotted on a standardized chart. Although the most common reason for a significant discrepancies among weight, height, and head circumference percentiles is an inaccurate measurement, a valid discrepancy warrants close clinical observation or testing. Glucose testing may be indicated for newborns found to be small or large for gestational age. If the estimated gestational age of the infant is inconsistent with the growth parameters a formal evaluation using a Dubowitz-Ballard assessment of gestational age may be helpful.

When examining a newborn infant for the first time, the initial focus is directed toward an overall assessment of the child's health. Observation and auscultation of the chest allows for detection of an irregular heart rate, murmur, or acute lung condition such as pneumothorax. The heart rate and respiratory rate can be measured. Normal values for heart and respiratory rate in a newborn infant are 100 to 160 beats/min and 35 to 60 breaths/min. Evaluation of skin color may be useful for identifying cyanotic congenital heart disease or pulmonary conditions in a neonate. If uncertainty exists about the presence of cyanosis, oxygen saturation can be measured quickly with a pulse oximeter. The newborn's tone, general posture, and movement should be assessed; abnormalities may be indicative of an acute or chronic central nervous system problem or sepsis.

There are several purposes for the rest of physical examination, including maternal reassurance and education about normal variations. Asymptomatic conditions can be

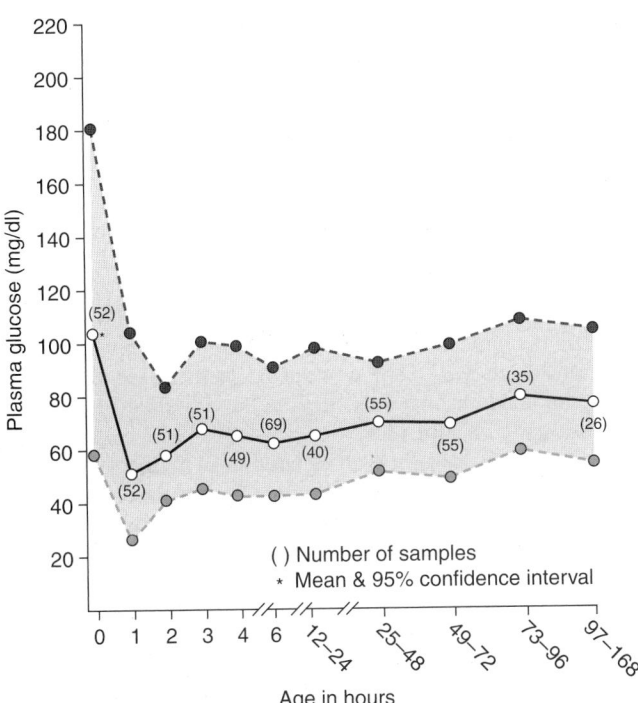

FIGURE 26-1 Predicted plasma glucose values during the first week of life in healthy term neonates appropriate for gestational age. (*Adapted from Srinivasan G et al: Plasma glucose values in normal neonates: a new look.* J Pediatr *109:114, 1986.*)

diagnosed, such as some types of congenital heart disease or developmental dysplasia of the hips. Finally, the examination is a useful screen for rare but serious conditions.

ROUTINE TESTING

GLUCOSE

The fetal blood glucose level is approximately 80% of the maternal level. After birth and separation of the infant from its major energy supply, the infant's glucose falls by an average factor of 0.5. Over the next several hours, it gradually increases to a level approaching that of older infants (Figure 26-1). Critical factors involved in this normal adaptive process include transient inhibition of the infant's insulin secretion and an increase in the counter regulatory hormones, including growth hormone, cortisol, epinephrine, and glucagon (Polin et al, 2004). The end result is the promotion of liver glycogen breakdown, gluconeogenesis, and tissue lipolysis. Given this normal sequence of events, there is no reason to routinely screen the blood glucose in infants who are products of uncomplicated pregnancies, labor, and delivery. Clinical scenarios that might be expected to alter the normal sequence of events and indicate the need for early glucose screening include:

- A pregnancy history of maternal treatment with β-agonists or intrapartum intravenous glucose
- Infants of diabetic mothers
- Infants demonstrating intrauterine growth restriction
- Premature infants
- Infants delivered after in utero or intrapartum fetal distress

> **BOX 26-1   Clinical Signs Compatible With Hypoglycemia**
>
> - Poor feeding
> - Lethargy
> - Hypotonia
> - Irritability
> - Tremor
> - Seizure-like activity
> - Apnea

- Infants with midline facial anomalies, which might be markers for pituitary deficiency
- Infants demonstrating hepatomegaly, suggesting glycogen storage disease
- Any infant showing clinical signs of hypoglycemia (Box 26-1)

The treatment approach to confirmed hypoglycemia depends on the glucose level, the presence of symptoms, or both (see Chapter 94).

NEWBORN METABOLIC SCREENING

Newborn screening for metabolic disorders began in 1962 when 29 states participated in a trial of testing for phenylketonuria. With the implementation of screening programs, criteria were proposed for determining which conditions should be screened. It was recommended that only disorders that were important health problems be included in screening programs. The condition should be detectable before the onset of significant symptoms. Importantly, a specific treatment to prevent adverse clinical consequences from the disorder should be available, and the screening program for the condition should be cost effective (Tarini, 2007). Based on these criteria, conditions such as congenital hypothyroidism and congenital adrenal hyperplasia were slowly added to newborn screening tests in many states, and subsequently conditions such as sickle cell disease were added. Although there is no specific treatment for sickle cell disease, there was evidence that the use of a newborn screening program to identify infants with the disorder led to early initiation of penicillin treatment, which resulted in fewer deaths from sepsis than when disease was identified at the onset of symptoms (Vichinsky et al, 1988). Given the demonstrable effectiveness of early identification, sickle cell disease met criteria for newborn screening.

The advent of tandem mass spectrometry in the 1990s revolutionized newborn metabolic screening. With this technology it is possible to test for a multitude of conditions using a small sample of blood. In 1995, the average number of conditions included in state-mandated screening programs was eight; by 2005 this had increased to 19, with some states testing for up to 46 conditions. Unfortunately, this increase in newborn screening has been controversial. Some of the conditions included do not meet the established criteria for screening, in that there are no known effective treatments, and in some cases it is not known whether the targeted condition always leads to disease. In addition, with increasing numbers of tests come increasing numbers of false-positive results, with the resulting parental anxiety and potential for the overuse of medical services (Tarini et al, 2006).

In an attempt to define a rational list of disorders for which newborn screening is appropriate, the American College of Medical Genetics used an iterative process to identify 29 "core conditions" that should be included in mandatory screening programs (Watson et al, 2006). As of 2009, approximately 25 of these conditions were included in the screening panels of at least 48 states (National Newborn Screening and Genetics Resource Center, 2009). The most common disorders included in newborn metabolic screens in the United States are congenital hypothyroidism (1 case per 3000 to 4000 infants) and sickle cell disease (American Academy of Pediatrics [AAP] Newborn Screening Task Force, 2000). The incidence of phenylketonuria is approximately 1 in 15,000. For many of the core conditions for which screening is recommended, incidence rates are in the range of 1 in 100,000 to 1 in 200,000 (Kaye et al, 2006). For some disorders, the incidence rate is unknown.

The expansion in newborn screening programs presents a challenge to health care providers. It is difficult to remain knowledgeable about all of the conditions that are screened, the incidence of the various conditions, and their natural histories and treatments. Fortunately, many states have informative Web sites providing up-to-date information for parents and health care professionals. In addition, the American College of Medical Genetics maintains online information for health care practitioners, including synopses of conditions commonly included in screening programs and appropriate management of infants with a positive result (accessible at http://www.acmg.net/resources/policies/ACT/condition-analyte-links.htm).

HEARING SCREEN

Newborn hearing screening has become nearly universal in the United States. Thirty states plus Guam, Puerto Rico, and the District of Columbia have established mandatory early hearing screening programs, and 17 states plus Guam, Puerto Rico, and the District of Columbia require all health insurers to cover the test (National Conference of State Legislatures, 2009). Newborn hearing screening and early intervention is endorsed by the AAP (AAP Joint Committee on Infant Hearing, 2007), and the U.S. Preventive Services Task Force (2008). Many nurseries now use a two-step screen, first using automated otoacoustic emissions screening followed by auditory brainstem response done in those who fail the otoacoustic emissions screening.

Before universal screening, there were questions about the utility of newborn hearing screening, including whether the false-positive rate creates more harm than the benefit of detecting a small number of infants with hearing loss (approximately 1 in 1000 newborns) and whether early intervention is effective (Keren et al, 2002). The specificity of a two-step screening program for hearing loss approaches 0.99. However, even with this high specificity, there at least six false-positive screens for every true positive screening result, because of the low rate of hearing loss (Nelson et al, 2008). The effect of false-positive screens has been minimally investigated. In one study, at 6 months of age, parents of newborns

with false-positive screens continued to express worries about their child's hearing after subsequent testing confirmed normal hearing. Fortunately, using standardized measures, there was no evidence of an increase in general anxiety these parents compared with parents of babies with normal newborn hearing screens (van der Ploeg et al, 2008).

False-negative screens are also a concern, because the equipment used is designed for screening and because most auditory brainstem response screening is designed to detect moderate or greater hearing loss. As a result, there is a chance that the screen will be falsely negative in approximately 2% of newborns (Johnson et al, 2005), and pediatricians should continue surveillance of hearing status during childhood.

The results of recent studies have shown improved reading and communication skills in hearing-impaired children identified during the period of universal newborn hearing screening. Furthermore, hearing-impaired children who enroll in treatment programs during the first 3 months of life have better language outcomes at school age (McCann et al, 2009; Vohr et al, 2008). Investigators in a Belgian study found that a cause for hearing loss can be determined in approximately half of children identified by newborn screening, of which 60% have genetic origins and 19% have cytomegalovirus infection (Declau et al, 2008).

It is challenging to ensure that all children with positive newborn screening test results have confirmatory audiologic testing and begin treatment by 3 to 6 months of age. The number of patients lost to follow-up remains problematic in many areas, and services such as amplification may take time to arrange. Efforts must be made to improve these problems for hearing screening programs to be maximally effective.

PRENATAL ULTRASOUND SCREENING FOR BIRTH DEFECTS

Second-trimester ultrasound screening for fetal anomalies has become increasingly routine. Major fetal organ system abnormalities can, for the most part, be identified and referred for appropriate fetal and neonatal management. There are, however, a number of ultrasound findings that have a variable natural history, may or may not be markers for serious conditions, and do not always result in a definitive prenatal workup. These findings often do not fit within the pediatric lexicon, and they can present a challenge to the pediatrician regarding parent counseling and determining management in the neonatal period.

Central Nervous System Findings

Choroid plexus cysts are found in 1% to 3% of second-trimester fetal ultrasound examinations. They are transient, functionally benign in nature, and resolve spontaneously before term. If one or more choroid plexus cysts are found in isolation on prenatal ultrasound examination, no adverse effect on fetal growth and development has been noted. Therefore, without other risk factors, no further evaluation is needed in an infant with this isolated finding and a benign prenatal course. Choroid plexus cysts are believed to be a "soft marker" for aneuploidy (particularly trisomy

18) when associated with other fetal anomalies or with maternal risk factors such as maternal age. In such situations, begin an appropriate prenatal evaluation, such as karyotyping (DiPietro et al, 2006; Lopez and Reich, 2006; Sohaey, 2008b).

Agenesis of the corpus callosum is reported to occur in 0.01% to 0.7% of unselected postnatal populations. Aneuploidy has been reported in 10% to 20% of children with this prenatal ultrasound finding. Major organ system abnormalities are reported to occur in up to 60% of such fetuses. Notably, when absence of the corpus callosum is an isolated fetal ultrasound finding, the reported rate of a relatively normal developmental outcome ranges from 50% to 75%. Well-conducted, long-term studies are lacking. Postnatal follow-up for infants with a history of a finding of agenesis of the corpus callosum on prenatal ultrasound examination should include, at a minimum, close long-term clinical assessment (Chadie et al, 2008; Fratelli et al, 2007; Woodward, 2008).

Mild ventriculomegaly is a relatively uncommon fetal ultrasound finding that may be a soft marker for aneuploidy, fetal infection, or other central nervous system abnormalities. As such, it is recommended that serial imaging studies be undertaken, in some cases including a more extensive workup. In the presence of a benign fetal assessment, most infants appear to do reasonably well after delivery. Close pediatric developmental followup and serial imaging studies are important to consider (Leitner et al, 2009; Melchiorre et al, 2009; Sohaey and Filipek, 2008).

Cardiac Findings

Echogenic cardiac focus is an incidental ultrasound finding in 3% to 4% of healthy fetuses. Notably, there is an increased incidence of twofold to threefold in Asian populations. It is said to be a soft marker for chromosomal abnormalities when associated with other screening abnormalities. If the results of a physical examination of a newborn are normal and there are no other ultrasound findings, no further evaluation is needed (Borgida et al, 2005; Koklanaris et al, 2005; Ouzounian et al, 2007; Sohaey, 2008b).

Gastrointestinal Findings

Echogenic bowel, when noted to be present during a second-trimester ultrasound examination and determined to be grade 0 or 1 (i.e., less echogenic than bone) is a normal variant. Density greater than that of bone (grade 2 to 3) is abnormal and is potentially a marker for cystic fibrosis, trisomy 21, gastrointestinal anomalies, or in utero infection. Isolated echogenic findings are considered benign with a good prognosis and require no special workup or postnatal management (Al-Kouatly et al, 2001; Patel et al, 2004; Sohaey, 2008a).

Cholelithiasis is an uncommon third-trimester fetal ultrasound finding that needs to be differentiated from hepatic calcification. Cholelithiasis is a benign condition requiring no special evaluation or treatment. An imaging examination at 1 year of age for a child with this prenatal finding may be helpful in documenting expected resolution (Agnifili et al, 1999; Sohaey, 2008b).

Hepatic calcifications are uncommon fetal ultrasound findings; they are often isolated, single and, in a low-risk pregnant patient, of no significance. When numerous, hepatic calcifications may be markers for fetal aneuploidy, infection, meconium peritonitis, hepatic tumor, or vascular insult. Twenty percent are associated with some form of fetal pathology. Neonatal management depends on the prenatal workup and the clinical presentation in the newborn period (Oh, 2008; Simchen et al, 2002).

Urinary Tract Findings

Mild fetal pelviectasis is one of the more common abnormalities detected by second-trimester ultrasound examination, with a reported incidence of 0.5% to 5% in unselected pregnant populations. Diagnostic criteria vary, but generally include a second-trimester renal pelvis diameter of 4 to 10 mm and 7 to 10 mm during the third trimester. Some authors consider mild fetal pelviectasis to be a soft marker for trisomy 21. When mild fetal pelviectasis is an isolated finding, the prognosis is good and the condition usually resolves either in utero or during early childhood. In a meta-analysis, it was reported that 11% of children with a history of mild fetal pelviectasis demonstrated postnatal pathology. Authors of a prospective cohort follow-up study reported uropathy in 18% of the patients. There is a lack of consensus as to postnatal management, with some authorities recommending close clinical assessment and others recommending follow-up renal ultrasound examinations at approximately 1 week and 1 month of life (Coelho et al, 2007; Lee et al, 2006; Sohaey and Arnold, 2008).

CAR SEAT TRIALS

The observation that preterm infants had episodes of hypoxia when monitored in car seats led the AAP to recommend in 1991 that preterm infants should be observed and monitored for apnea, bradycardia, or oxygen desaturation in their car safety seat before hospital discharge—the so-called car seat challenge (AAP Committee on Injury and Poison Prevention and Committee on Fetus and Newborn, 1991, 1996; Bull et al, 1999). In the United States, the car seat challenge expanded to include late preterm infants, most of whom did not have respiratory problems during their newborn hospital stay. It has been reported that 25% of late preterm infants do not fit securely into standard car safety seats, and 12% of healthy late preterm infants have apneic or bradycardic events in their car seats (Merchant et al, 2001).

The authors of a Cochrane Review questioned whether car seat trials actually prevent morbidity or mortality, and whether there are adverse effects of not passing this test, such as prolonging the hospital stay or creating parental anxiety. Their review did not disclose any randomized trials, and they concluded that "it is unclear whether undertaking a car seat challenge is beneficial or indeed whether it causes harm" (Pilley and McGuire, 2006). Since then, there has been one randomized trial in healthy term infants comparing car seats to car beds, and no differences were found in rates of oxygen desaturation or apneic events (Kinane et al, 2006). Further study is needed to determine whether car seat trials in late preterm neonates are warranted.

ROUTINE AND COMMON MEDICAL TREATMENTS

PREVENTION OF OPHTHALMIA NEONATORUM AND CONJUNCTIVITIS

Approximately15% to 20% of babies will develop conjunctivitis in the first few weeks of life. Conjunctivitis can be caused by a sexually transmitted bacteria, normal skin or nasopharyngeal flora, or chemical irritation (Krohn et al, 1993). In addition, eye discharge can be caused by obstruction of the nasolacrimal duct rather than from the conjunctivitis. The most worrisome infection is that from *Neisseria gonorrhea*, which can be invasive to the cornea in a matter of hours and lead to blindness. Despite effective preventive measures known since the 1880s, there are still thousands of children blinded by this infection worldwide each year.

Most states in the United States have laws or regulations that require administration of topical antibiotic ointment to the conjunctivae of babies within a few hours of birth. This practice has been effective in reducing the cases of blindness caused by gonococcal conjunctivitis. It is moderately effective in preventing conjunctivitis caused by chlamydia.

Parents may question the need to expose all babies to eye medication, especially if the mother has been tested and found to be without gonorrhea or chlamydia. Some countries have stopped routine administration of eye prophylaxis. In those countries, an increase in infection, primarily caused by chlamydia, has been noted. With informed consent, parents can opt out of eye prophylaxis for their newborn.

There is lay literature recommending the instillation of colostrum or breast milk into the eyes of babies to prevent or treat conjunctivitis. Although colostrum has antimicrobial action, its efficacy has not been adequately studied.

Povidone-iodine solution has been shown to be more effective and cause less irritation than erythromycin ointment. It is also less expensive, but is not yet approved for this use by the U.S. Food and Drug Administration (Isenberg et al, 1995). Whether instillation of povidone-iodine in the eyes may affect newborn thyroid screens—as has been reported with use of this solution on umbilical cord stumps—is not clear (Lin et al, 1994).

VITAMIN K

Vitamin K is necessary for biologic activation of several human proteins, most notably coagulation factors II, VII, IX, and X. Because placental transfer is limited, cord blood levels of vitamin K_1 (phylloquinone) are 30-fold lower than maternal levels. Intestinal bacteria synthesize menaquinone (vitamin K_2), which has 60% of the activity of phylloquinone. However, neonates have a decreased number of bacteria in their gut that manufacture vitamin K_2; levels of this form of vitamin K are not found in the livers of infants until they are 2 to 3 months old. Therefore newborn infants are deficient in vitamin K at birth and are at risk for significant bleeding. Fortunately intramuscular vitamin K rapidly activates clotting factors, greatly decreasing this risk.

Three presentations of vitamin K–deficient bleeding (VKDB) have been described. Early VKDB manifests in the first 24 hours after birth. It is not prevented by postnatal administration of vitamin K, and it usually occurs in infants born to mothers who are taking medications that inhibit vitamin K. Common medications that inhibit vitamin K include many anticonvulsants, isoniazid, rifampin, warfarin, and some antibiotics such as cephalosporins. Early VKDB is frequently serious because of intracranial and intraabdominal hemorrhage. It is estimated that in neonates at risk for early VKDB, the incidence is as high as 12% (Van Winckel et al, 2009). Classic VKDB occurs in infants during the first week of life. Although the clinical presentation is often mild, blood loss can be significant, and intracranial hemorrhages have been reported. Although estimates vary, the incidence of classic VKDB in the absence of vitamin K supplementation is likely 0.25% to 1.7% (AAP Committee on Fetus and Newborn, 2003). Late VKDB occurs in infants between the ages of 2 and 12 weeks and is usually severe. The mortality rate from late VKDB is approximately 20%, and 50% of children with this disorder have intracranial hemorrhages. Late VKDB is associated with exclusive breastfeeding. Human milk contains only 1 to 4 µg/L of vitamin K, whereas commercially available formula contains 50 µg/L or greater. In neonates who do not receive supplemental vitamin K, the incidence of late VKDB is estimated at 4.4 to 7.2 in 100,000 (or 1 in 15,000 to 1 in 20,000; Van Winckel et al, 2009). Vitamin K administered shortly after birth is effective in preventing classic and late VKDB. Since 1961 the recommended dose of vitamin K for term infants born in the United States has been 1 mg given intramuscularly. However, the results of a study suggesting an association between intramuscular vitamin K given at birth and childhood cancer created controversy regarding this practice (Golding et al, 1990, 1992). The results of subsequent studies have indicated conclusively that there is no increased risk for solid tumors in children given intramuscular vitamin K; however, the possibility that there is a slightly increased risk for leukemia cannot be excluded (Puckett and Offringa, 2000). Because of concerns regarding an increased risk of childhood cancers, a switch to oral vitamin K occurred in some countries, but not in the United States. It is apparent that a single oral dose of vitamin K has an efficacy similar to an intramuscular dose in preventing classic VKDB, but offers less protection against late VKDB. Repeated doses of an oral vitamin K preparation until an infant is 8 to 12 weeks old increases the efficacy of this route of administration. However, it is not clear that even multiple doses of an oral formulation of vitamin K are as effective as a single intramuscular dose, given at birth. In a multinational review, rates of late VKDB in infants receiving various regimens of oral vitamin K were mostly in the range of 1.2 to 1.8 in 100,000 compared with 0 cases in 325,000 children receiving an intramuscular dose (Cornelissen et al, 1997). The oral regimens assessed included a dose at birth of 1 mg. Reported rates of VKDB in infants who received

2 mg orally at birth, with doses repeated subsequently, are lower but still somewhat higher than in neonates treated with intramuscular vitamin K (Busfield et al, 2007; Von Kries et al, 2003). Early data from the Netherlands, where infants received 1 mg orally at birth and 25 mcg daily for up to 12 weeks, suggested that this regimen was as efficacious as an intramuscular dose (Cornelissen et al, 1997). However, in a subsequent study from the Netherlands, the rate of late VKDB was 3.2 in 100,000 in a group of infants with undiagnosed biliary atresia who had been treated with this dosing schedule (van Hasselt et al, 2008). Unrecognized cholestatic liver disease is a significant risk factor for VKDB. Finally, no cases of late VKDB were found among 396,000 Danish infants who received an oral dose of 2 mg of vitamin K at birth and 1 mg weekly until the age of 3 months (Hansen et al, 2003).

Risks from intramuscular vitamin K include pain at the injection site and the possibility of a serious medication error. The risks of a significant complication from the injection are probably negligible; in one study, zero significant complications were reported after 420,000 injections (Von Kries, 1992). In the United States, oral administration is complicated by the lack of an oral vitamin K preparation being licensed for newborns. In some settings, infants have received the intramuscular preparation orally; however, tolerance may be a problem, and the efficacy of this preparation when given orally might not be comparable to the oral formulations used in Europe. In addition, compliance with repeated doses of oral vitamin K in infants may be suboptimal. Finally, it is unknown whether the use of repeated administration of oral vitamin K in the dose range of 1 to 2 mg each week is associated with an increased risk of childhood cancers.

For parents who have questions regarding the best method to prevent classic and late VKDB, the clinician is advised to discuss the pros and cons of intramuscular versus oral vitamin K. If the parents choose oral administration, a dose of 2 mg of vitamin K should be given shortly after birth, with subsequent doses until the infant is at least 4 weeks old if he or she is breastfed. In a policy statement, the AAP suggests that, if an oral vitamin K formulation becomes licensed for use in the United States, a dose of 2 mg can be given at birth and repeated at 1 to 2 weeks of age and at 4 weeks of age for neonates whose parents decline intramuscular vitamin K (AAP Vitamin K Ad Hoc Task Force, 1993).

CIRCUMCISION

Neonatal circumcision is a polarizing issue for health care professionals and parents. Those who favor routine circumcision highlight health benefits such as decreased urinary tract infections (UTIs), reduced risk of penile cancer, and possibly lower rates of sexually transmitted diseases, including HIV (Schoen, 2008). Those who oppose the procedure indicate that the number of circumcisions needed to be performed to prevent one of these outcomes (i.e., the number needed to treat [NNT]) is large, the risks of the procedure balance out these benefits, circumcision leads to loss of sexual sensation, and subjecting a neonate to a painful procedure without clear benefits may be unethical (Andres, 2008).

It is clear that circumcision reduces the risk of UTI by approximately 10-fold; however, given the low incidence of UTI in male infants, 100 boys need to be circumcised to prevent one UTI. Similarly, although circumcision has been shown to prevent penile cancer, it is an extremely rare condition and the NNT is about 900 (Christakis et al, 2000). There has been recent interest in circumcision as a method for preventing HIV. The results of studies in three African countries indicate that circumcision reduces the risk of HIV infection by 56%. Because the incidence of HIV in these countries is high, the calculated NNT is approximately 72 (Mills et al, 2008). Given the same efficacy, the NNT to prevent one case of HIV infection in Canada, where the incidence is 13 in 100,000, or in the United States, where the incidence is 23 in 100,000, is greater than 5000 (Andres, 2008; Hall et al, 2008).

Circumcision is generally a safe procedure. Although some increased bleeding is reported after 1% of circumcisions, the rate of significant complications is approximately 0.2% (Christakis et al, 2000; Gee and Ansell, 1976; Wiswell and Geschke, 1989). Bleeding, sometimes requiring suturing of a vessel, is the most common significant complication, followed by penile injury and infection. Infection is more common after a circumcision using a Plastibell rather than a Gomco clamp; hemorrhage is reportedly similar after either technique (Gee and Ansell, 1976).

Circumcision is an uncomfortable experience for the neonate. Small amounts of sucrose solutions can be offered to the baby for soothing. Pain from the actual surgery can be significantly decreased with the use of a dorsal penile nerve block or ring block. In one study, 65% of infants who had received a dorsal nerve block had no or minimal response to the initial clamping of the foreskin (Taeusch et al, 2002).

A poor cosmetic outcome can be caused by removal of too little foreskin. It has been estimated that 1-9.5% of circumcisions are redone because of parental concern regarding the appearance. In a prospective study, among boys younger than 3 years who had been circumcised using either a Plastibell or with a Mogen clamp, the glans was fully exposed in only 35.6%. However, in older circumcised males the glans was fully exposed in more than 90% (Van Howe, 1997). This finding suggests that parents of a circumcised infant should be counseled that the vast majority of properly done circumcisions will lead to an acceptable cosmetic appearance over time.

In the United States, the Gomco clamp is the most commonly used apparatus for performing circumcisions, followed by the Plastibell and Mogen clamp (Stang and Snellman, 1998). The use of the Mogen clamp leads to shorter procedures and, reportedly, less pain and bleeding than the other techniques (Kurtis et al, 1999; Taeusch et al, 2002). However, less foreskin is removed with the Mogen clamp than with the other two techniques (Alanis and Lucidi, 2004).

HEPATITIS B VACCINE

The implementation of routine hepatitis B immunization during infancy has been associated with a dramatic decrease in the incidence of this infection. Between 1990 (before routine vaccination of infants) and 2004 the overall incidence of acute hepatitis B in the United States declined by 75%, and by 94% among children and adolescents (Centers for Disease Control and Prevention, 2005). The Centers for Disease Control and Prevention and the AAP recommend that the initial dose of the three-dose hepatitis B immunization series be given in the newborn nursery; however, this recommendation is far from being followed universally. In 1999, it was estimated that 54% of newborns in the United States received a dose of hepatitis B vaccine at birth. However, at that time a recommendation was made to suspend birth dosing until vaccines were made that did not contain thimerosal (a preservative containing mercury). Even after a thimerosal-free hepatitis B vaccine was produced, many newborn nurseries in the United States did not immediately resume newborn immunization programs. This issue, combined with the reluctance of some parents to have their newborns immunized, has led to continued suboptimal rates of administration of the birth dose of hepatitis B vaccine (Clark et al, 2001). Among infants born in the United States between 2003 and 2005, it was estimated that 50.1% received a dose of the vaccine by the age of 3 days (Centers for Disease Control and Prevention, 2008).

There are at least two advantages of providing the first dose of hepatitis B vaccine during the newborn nursery stay. First, newborns who receive a dose at birth are more likely to complete their hepatitis B immunization series on time than those who receive a first dose later (Yusuf et al, 2000). Second, because a dose of hepatitis B vaccine given within 12 hours of birth can prevent vertical transmission of hepatitis B infections in 75% to 90% of cases, early provision of immunization serves as a safety net in cases where there has been an error in identifying a mother who is positive for hepatitis B surface antigen (Centers for Disease Control and Prevention, 2005).

The main disadvantage of providing a dose of hepatitis B vaccine during the nursery stay is that it can complicate documentation of hepatitis B immunization status in a child by increasing the number of vaccination providers. There is no evidence that administration of a dose of hepatitis B vaccine at birth leads to more evaluations for sepsis because of adverse events related to the immunization.

ONGOING CARE

UMBILICAL CORD CARE AND SINGLE UMBILICAL ARTERY

Umbilical cord care recommendations vary from "dry cord care" to the use of dyes and cleansing with alcohol, soap and water, or antiseptics. Concern over the possible toxic effects of dye and antiseptics led many hospitals in the United States to adopt the dry cord care method of cord care. Unfortunately this method may be responsible for causing an increase in the risk for omphalitis (Janssen et al, 2003; Simon and Simon, 2004). In addition, the results of a randomized trial in Nepal indicate that cord care using topical chlorhexidine reduces the risk of developing omphalitis; however, that population may be at higher risk compared with those born in the United States (Mullany et al, 2006).

Because omphalitis is rare, and its more severe complication necrotizing fasciitis is even rarer, large trials are needed to determine which cord care regimen is best for preventing these complications. Until such trials are conducted, there is no clear advantage of one regimen over another. Providers caring for newborns need to keep these diagnoses in mind and encourage parents to report redness around the umbilical cord stump.

A single umbilical artery is detected in about 4 out of 1000 births. There is an association of the single umbilical artery with a number of congenital anomalies, including renal or genitourinary malformations, cardiac malformations, and chromosomal anomalies such as Down syndrome. In this era of near universal use of prenatal fetal ultrasonography, any associated anomalies are usually discovered (Deshpande et al, 2009; Johnson and Tennenbaum, 2003). Unless there are abnormalities noted on physical examination, there is no need to repeat diagnostic ultrasound examinations after birth in a child with a single umbilical artery.

BREASTFEEDING

There is voluminous evidence that the optimal feeding for normal neonates is human milk provided via the mother's breast. From this most preferred feeding there is a continuum to least preferred feeding that includes: maternal milk given by an artificial method, donor human milk (although this is rarely used by most health care facilities), and commercially available infant formula. It is incumbent on health care professionals and health care systems to vigorously promote the optimal feeding for normal newborns. This promotion includes education to prospective mothers, knowledge of the characteristics of human milk and the normal course of lactation, organization of health care facilities to optimize the initiation of breastfeeding after delivery, early recognition of suboptimal breastfeeding and interventions to correct problems, and adoption of a parsimonious list of contraindications to breastfeeding.

Nutritional Composition of Human Milk

Although the composition varies among mothers, by age of the child, and even within a feeding, the nutritional components of mature human milk can be summarized (Picciano, 2001). The caloric content of human milk is approximately 0.67 Kcal/mL (20 Kcal/ounce). Approximately 50% of these calories are provided by the lipid components. Importantly, human milk contains omega-3 fatty acids. Lactose is the principal carbohydrate, providing approximately 40% of the calories. The protein in human milk is divided into two categories, casein and whey, that are provided in a 40:60 ratio. The sodium content of human milk is low, averaging approximately 7 mEq/L. With the exception of vitamins D and K, the amounts of minerals and micronutrients available are all adequate for optimal infant growth. The evolutionary advantage afforded by the relatively low concentrations of vitamin D and vitamin K in human milk is unclear.

Healthy newborns receive surprisingly little breast milk in the first few days of life. Average intake of colostrum during the first day of life is approximately 10 mL/kg and

20 mL/kg during the second 24 hours of life (Casey et al, 1986; Evans et al, 2003). Maternal milk production dramatically increases during the period from 36 to 96 hours of life; this increase in quantity is accompanied by a change from colostrum to mature milk (Casey et al, 1986; Saint et al, 1984). The increase in milk production is perceived by the mother as breast fullness. In one study, mothers noted that their breasts were noticeably fuller when their infants were an average of 53 hours old. This finding was closely correlated with the mean age (58 hours) when infants transferred greater than 15 mL of milk from the breast (Dewey et al, 2003).

Given the low volume of milk provided initially, neonates have a decrease in weight and an increase in serum sodium during the first few days of life (Marchini and Stock, 1997). Average maximal weight loss in breastfed infants is 5% to 7% of birthweight and occurs between 48 and 72 hours of life (Macdonald et al, 2003; Marchini and Stock, 1997; Rodriguezet al, 2000). With the onset of copious production of mature milk, neonates begin to gain weight and their serum sodium levels fall (Marchini and Stock, 1997). Infants fed human milk regain their birthweight, on average, by the age of 8.3 days; 97.5% have regained their birthweight by 21 days of age (Macdonald et al, 2003).

Health Benefits of Human Milk

There is copious research on numerous health benefits for infants who are breastfed. The list of benefits that have been found include: decreased incidence of conditions such as gastrointestinal infections, lower respiratory tract disease, otitis media, hypertension, obesity, diabetes, allergies, and asthma; improved cognitive development; and reduced risk of sudden infant death syndrome (Hoddinott et al, 2008). Unfortunately, because it is unethical to conduct individual randomized controlled trials on breastfeeding, most of these benefits have been documented in observational studies. Such studies are subject to numerous problems that might bias the results toward the null hypothesis or an overestimation of the benefits (Kramer et al, 2009). Perhaps the biggest problem with observational studies on breastfeeding is that there is significant confounding by socioeconomic status, for which it is difficult to adequately account in analyses.

The best evidence of the health benefits of breastfeeding comes from a large trial conducted in Belarus. Health care professionals at participating hospitals were randomly assigned to receive training on promoting breastfeeding using the Baby-Friendly Hospital Initiative (BFHI) developed by the World Health Organization and the United Nations Children's Fund (BFHI is further described in a following section) or to continue to provide standard care. A total of 17,046 mother-infant dyads were enrolled in the study (Kramer et al, 2001). All participating infants were born at 37 weeks' gestation or later and weighed more than 2500 g; all the mothers intended to breastfeed their infants. The rate of any breastfeeding at 3 months old was significantly higher among infants born in BFHI hospitals than at control sites (43% and 6%, respectively). Rates of breastfeeding were also significantly higher at BFHI locations at 6 and 12 months of age. Most pertinent, rates of

BOX 26-2 Baby-Friendly Hospital Initiative: Ten Steps to Successful Breastfeeding

1. Maintain a written breastfeeding policy that is routinely communicated to all health care staff.
2. Train all health care staff in the skills necessary to implement this policy.
3. Inform all pregnant women about the benefits and management of breastfeeding.
4. Help mothers initiate breastfeeding within 1 hour of birth.
5. Show mothers how to breastfeed and how to maintain lactation, even if they are separated from their newborns.
6. Give infants no food or drink other than breast milk unless medically indicated.
7. Practice "rooming-in"—allow mothers and infants to remain together 24 hours a day.
8. Encourage unrestricted breastfeeding (i.e., on demand).
9. Give no pacifiers or artificial nipples to breastfeeding infants.
10. Foster the establishment of breastfeeding support groups and refer mothers to them on discharge from the hospital or clinic.

gastrointestinal infection and atopic dermatitis were significantly lower in babies who had been born at BFHI hospitals. These data provide strong evidence for a significant beneficial effect of breastfeeding.

Among children enrolled in the original study who were assessed at 6.5 years of age, the verbal intelligence quotient of those born at BFHI hospitals was 7.5 points higher than those born at control sites (Kramer et al, 2008). Whether this finding was related to the components in the breast milk or from the physical act of breastfeeding is unclear; regardless of the mechanism, the effect is profound. In other follow-up studies, no difference between the two groups of children were found in the rates of asthma, allergy, or obesity (Kramer et al, 2007); however, the design of the study provides a conservative estimate of the effects of breastfeeding.

Promotion of Breastfeeding

Given the demonstrable improvements in outcomes, health care providers should promote breastfeeding as the preferred method of feeding newborn infants and facilitate its initiation during the newborn nursery stay. As a comprehensive program, implementation of the 10 steps of the BFHI (Box 26-2) has been shown to significantly increase the rates of breastfeeding (Kramer et al, 2001). There is evidence to support the efficacy of each of the 10 separate steps, although for some of the steps, such as excluding pacifiers, the evidence is contradictory (Cramton et al, 2009; O'Connor et al, 2009).

From a practical standpoint there are several evidence-based interventions during the newborn nursery stay that increase the rate or prolongation of breastfeeding. These interventions include the use of frequent demand feedings as opposed to a rigid feeding schedule, early skin-to-skin contact between mother and infant, professional advice on breastfeeding techniques, and exclusion of commercial formula from discharge packs (Anderson et al, 2003; Britton et al, 2007; Donnelly et al, 2000; Renfrew et al, 2000).

Breastfeeding Problems

The vast majority of difficulties with breastfeeding are related to a delay in transfer of adequate quantities of human milk to the infant. Delayed lactogenesis occurs in 20% to 30% of mothers; however, in most instances the primary problem is related to infant breastfeeding behaviors in the first few days of life. Although the clinical correlate is not well defined, weight loss of greater than 10% of birthweight is considered excessive in breastfed infants. Studies on breastfed neonates indicate that approximately 10% of infants lose more than 10% of their birthweight during the first few days of life (Dewey et al, 2003).

It is important to identify mother-infant dyads who are at risk for breastfeeding problems, so that early interventions can prevent excessive weight loss. Mothers with previous breast surgery, particularly breast reduction, are at increased risk of primary insufficient lactation. Flat or inverted nipples can also make breastfeeding more difficult. Prolonged labor and cesarean delivery have been associated with delayed onset of milk production (Dewey et al, 2003).

The adequacy of breastfeeding behaviors can be assessed during the newborn nursery stay using scoring systems such as the Infant Breastfeeding Assessment Tool. Low scores on this measure during the first day of life are moderately predictive of excessive weight loss in the neonate (Dewey et al, 2003). Decreased numbers of voids and stools in the newborn are also helpful in identifying children with breastfeeding problems, but this information is most useful after day 3 of life.

Supplementation of Breastfeeding

It is usually unnecessary to provide any nutrition or fluid to full-term breastfed infants beyond human milk. Dextrose water or commercial formula may be needed in neonates with hypoglycemia who are not responsive to breastfeeding. Supplementation may also be indicated in newborns who have lost more than 10% of birthweight or have decreased urine and stool output. Supplementation should be considered a temporary intervention, and its provision should not interfere with the onset of successful breastfeeding.

Contraindications to Breastfeeding

The few absolute contraindications to breastfeeding include maternal HIV infection, untreated tuberculosis in the mother, evidence of current cocaine use or antimetabolite drugs in the mother, and galactosemia in the neonate (Gartner et al, 2005). There are a myriad of other drugs for which there is concern regarding long-term neurodevelopmental outcomes in the infant. Selective serotonin reuptake inhibitors are commonly used to treat depression and anxiety in young women. Among drugs in this category, sertraline and paroxetine are thought to be the safest for use in breastfeeding mothers, whereas fluoxetine and citalopram are believed to have the most potential for toxicity in the neonate (Field, 2008). Overall there have been few adverse effects noted with use of any of these drugs, and generally the potential risks associated with these medications are thought to be outweighed by the benefits of breastfeeding (Field, 2008). Similarly, although methadone is detectable in the breast milk of women receiving this medication, serum levels in neonates are low and unlikely to cause a significant effect (Jansson et al, 2008).

Hepatitis C virus RNA has been found in the milk of mothers infected with this virus. Despite this finding, transmission of infection via breastfeeding has not been documented. Maternal hepatitis C infection is not considered a contraindication to breastfeeding (Gartner et al, 2005).

BOTTLE FEEDING

Commercial formula that provides adequate nutrition, vitamins, and minerals is available for infants of mothers who do not wish to breastfeed their infants or when breastfeeding is contraindicated or impossible. There are three major categories of formula used in neonates: cow milk–based, soy, and hydrolyzed formula. Of these, cow milk–based formula is used most commonly. The main carbohydrate in cow milk–based formula is lactose. Soy formulas were developed for infants with a possible cow's milk allergy. Because the main carbohydrate in soy formulas is sucrose or corn syrup, soy formula can be used in neonates with possible galactosemia. Protein hydrolysate formulas were initially developed for use in infants who are highly intolerant to cow's milk protein (Kleinman, 2009). These formulas are purported to lead to fewer allergies in babies and children than does cow milk–based formula, but the evidence for this is limited (Osborn and Sinn, 2006). All extensively hydrolyzed formulas are lactose free (Kleinman, 2009). These formulas are indicated in infants with definitive evidence of cow's milk protein allergy because 10% to 14% of them also have a soy allergy (Bhatia and Greer, 2008).

Standard preparations of formulas available for use in healthy term neonates provide 0.67 Kcal/mL. Most formulas are fortified with 10 to 12 mg/L of iron; however, some low-iron cow milk–based formulas are available. It is recommended that all formula-fed newborns receive the iron-fortified products. Vitamin D at the concentration of approximately 400 IU/L is provided in all the commercially available formulas (Kleinman, 2009).

Mothers who elect to bottle-feed report feeling unsupported for their decision by health care professionals, and up to 50% feel pressured to breastfeed (Lakshman et al, 2009). Although the benefits of breastfeeding should be provided to mothers who have not decided how to feed their babies, the role of health care providers is to support the decision of those who have elected to bottle-feed. It is also important to provide practical education about bottle-feeding to these parents; this is frequently neglected in many newborn nurseries (Lakshman et al, 2009).

Newborns who are bottle-fed can feed ad libitum beginning shortly after birth. Average formula intake in term newborns during the first day of life is 15 to 20 mL/kg and 40 to 45 mL/kg during the second day. During the nursery stay, neonates who are formula fed typically lose less weight than breastfed infants (Dollberg et al, 2001).

ANTICIPATORY GUIDANCE

A primary duty of providers of newborn care is to ensure that parents of new infants have the knowledge and skills to provide for normal growth and development. Parents who are taught about normal newborn development and behavior have more realistic expectations about the work involved and look upon their child with more fondness. Conversely, before discharge from the newborn nursery, it is important to assess the parents' ability to provide a safe and nurturing environment for the neonate. Parents showing concerning behaviors, possibly leading to abuse or neglect, should have supervision and interventions to help them, possibly leading to termination of parental rights (Davidson-Arad et al, 2003; Wattenberg et al, 2001).

There are several major challenges for parents of normal newborns: sleep deprivation, learning to calm a crying infant, significant life changes, and the new worries that come with being responsible for a totally dependent being. Postpartum depression is more common and of longer duration than previously thought, and it occurs in at least 10% of mothers. This condition is related to sleep deprivation and has major and long-lasting effects on infant homeostasis and development (Chaudron, 2003).

Anticipatory guidance should be given to help prepare new parents for the common tasks of newborn care and to educate them about the many normal variations in newborn behavior. Learning how to soothe a baby is one of the first needed parenting tasks. Providers can help by giving suggestions to reduce crying and to better cope with infants who are more sensitive and harder to soothe (Barr et al, 2009).

Most parents have questions about feeding, elimination, bathing, cord care, genital care, jaundice, and common rashes. There are numerous checklists of educational topics that can be overwhelming to new parents. In addition, learning styles can vary, with some preferring written materials and while others preferring audio-visual materials or hands-on demonstration. Ideally, education should be targeted toward the topics of interest and with the appropriate materials for learning style (Dusing et al, 2008).

Mothers are often not in a good learning state in the immediate postpartum period because of pain, postpartum hormonal changes, and the stress of being in a hospital. However, there is heightened receptivity to change during this period, so attempts to teach or make lifestyle changes (e.g., smoking cessation) may be more effective. There is some evidence that providing parental education using tools such as interactive video and computers may be superior to traditional teaching (Snowdon et al, 2009; Trepka et al, 2008).

Given the obstacles to providing meaningful education during the nursery stay, it is probably better for practitioners to focus on a few key points of anticipatory guidance rather than reciting a litany of instructions. There is also a philosophical choice in deciding whether to emphasize the overall health of a newborn or to concentrate on prevention or identification of illness. There is little evidence for the efficacy of most anticipatory guidance provided to parents during the newborn nursery stay. A notable exception is the advice to put infants to sleep in the supine position (described in the following section). There is also emerging evidence that education about the normality of inconsolable crying in infants helps parents cope with this

stressful situation, and it could reduce the risk of shaken baby syndrome (Barr et al, 2009).

Sleep Position

With the exception of immunizations, no child health intervention in the past two decades has resulted in a larger decrease in postneonatal infant mortality than the "Back to Sleep" campaign. The remarkable change in the predominant sleep position of infants from prone to supine has led to a 30% to 50% reduction in the rate of sudden infant death syndrome (SIDS) in the United States (AAP Task Force on Sudden Infant Death Syndrome, 2005). A multipronged effort including brochures, public service announcements, and education provided by health care professionals was used to affect the change in sleep position (Willinger et al, 2000). Obviously education provided to parents during the newborn nursery stay is a crucial determinant of the sleep position of an infant. In addition to providing education, there is evidence that parents model sleep position for their babies after how they saw nurses and physicians place their neonate in the bassinet in the newborn nursery (AAP Task Force on Sudden Infant Death Syndrome, 2005; Colson and Joslin, 2002). Therefore it is crucial that neonates are placed on their backs to sleep in the newborn nursery. In addition, there is an additive effect of both physicians and nurses recommending the supine sleep position (Willinger et al, 2000).

In addition to supine position, there are other factors related to the sleep environment that can effect the risk of SIDS in a newborn infant. It is recommended that infants sleep on firm surfaces and without excessive bedding such as pillows. Many experts also recommend against co-sleeping between parents and infants; however, this topic is controversial and the evidence is somewhat contradictory. Similarly, although use of a pacifier has been found to reduce the risk of SIDS, there is a reluctance to recommend these devices because of concerns about reducing breastfeeding (AAP Task Force on Sudden Infant Death Syndrome, 2005; Willinger et al, 2000).

DISCHARGE AND FOLLOW-UP

For infants born in the United States at 35 weeks' gestation or later, the average length of the initial hospital stay is 48 to 52 hours (Datar and Sood, 2006; Kuzniewicz et al, 2009; Paul et al, 2009). Because approximately 50% of infants born by vaginal delivery are discharged before the age of 48 hours, and because up to 40% of those born by cesarean delivery are discharged before 72 hours of age, a large proportion of neonates are discharged before the age of 3 to 4 days, when bilirubin levels typically peak and breastfeeding is well established (Paul et al, 2006). It is recommended that infants discharged before 48 hours have a follow-up appointment with a provider within 48 hours (AAP Committee on Fetus and Newborn, 2004). This follow-up can be accomplished either by a visit to a health care provider or via a home nursing visit.

Risk factors for readmission after an initial hospital stay of less than 48 to 72 hours include gestational age less than 39 weeks (and especially less than 37 weeks), primiparous mother, and Asian race (presumably because of an increased risk of hyperbilirubinemia) (Burgos et al, 2008; Grupp-Phelan et al, 1999; Liu et al, 1997; Paul et al, 2006). Consideration of a longer nursery stay is suggested for infants with one or more of these risk factors. In addition, early discharge is not recommended for term newborns who have not voided, passed at least one stool, or demonstrated adequate breastfeeding (AAP Committee on Fetus and Newborn, 2004). However, there is little evidence to support these recommendations.

COMMON PROBLEMS DURING THE NURSERY STAY

HYPOTHERMIA AND HYPERTHERMIA

Upon leaving the womb, a newborn is immediately challenged with maintaining a normal body temperature. If a neonate is not quickly dried at birth, he or she may lose up to 1° C body temperature per minute. Healthy term babies are able to increase heat production through glycogenolysis and nonshivering thermogenesis for minutes to a few hours, depending on environmental conditions (Aylott, 2006). Babies typically have a decline in body temperature during the first hour of life with a gradual increase during the following 12 hours (Li et al, 2004). By the second day of life, the infant's body temperature becomes more stable, but heat loss can occur again with bathing or other stresses (Takayama et al, 2000).

Being too cold or too hot causes metabolic stress to the newborn, so efforts to maintain a steady and neutral thermal environment should be provided. The best practice is to dry the baby immediately after delivery and place the infant skin-to-skin with the mother. Although the AAP and the American College of Obstetricians and Gynecologists jointly recommend keeping infants' core temperatures within the narrow range of 36.5° to 37° C, in one study of healthy term newborns the average temperature was 36.5° C, with a normal range from 36.0° to 37.9° C (Takayama et al, 2000). Thin babies tend to have lower body temperatures, and heavier babies tend to have higher body temperatures. Hypothermia should be managed by placing the baby skin-to-skin with a parent or under a radiant warmer.

Standard practice at most nurseries is to measure axillary temperatures, probably because of reports in the 1960s and 1970s of perforations caused by rectal thermometers; however, axillary temperatures may not always accurately reflect core temperature (Hutton et al, 2009).

An elevated body temperature at birth generally reflects the intrauterine temperature and is not usually a sign of sepsis (Baumgart, 2008). Isolated hyperthermia during labor is associated with neonatal encephalopathy, occurring in approximately 1 in 2000 births (Blume et al, 2008). After the first 3 to 4 days of life, increased temperatures are most likely caused by dehydration from suboptimal breast milk supply (Maayan-Metzger et al, 2003). A single increased temperature in an otherwise normally behaving newborn is not a strong predictor of infection, but has been reported as a sign of intracranial hemorrhage (Fang et al, 2008).

ELIMINATION

Voiding

Approximately 15% of healthy newborns void at the time of delivery, and 95% void by 24 hours of age. The cause of delayed voiding is likely a consequence of stress on the infant during labor and delivery (Vuohelainen et al, 2007; 2008), which is a protective mechanism for the baby. Normally no intervention is needed once homeostatic adaption to extrauterine life is stable.

The differential diagnosis of delayed voiding (defined as no urine output by 24 to 48 hours of age) includes renal and postrenal causes. With the frequent use of prenatal ultrasound examination, it is unusual that a significant renal anomaly is discovered because of a delay in voiding. Most infants with bilateral renal agenesis have other findings, such as oligohydramnios or Potter sequence. Unilateral renal agenesis does not usually give symptoms of decreased urine output. Renal vascular thrombosis can also cause anuria, and babies with this condition are usually ill. Severe cystic kidney disease can involve urinary outflow obstruction. The diagnosis of cystic kidneys is usually made after the newborn period, or it is found incidental to evaluation of other anomalies and not because of delayed voiding.

Postrenal causes of delayed voiding include neuropathic bladder dysfunction and anatomic obstruction of urinary flow by anomalies in ureters, the bladder, or the urethra. Persistent or recurrent bladder distention after catheterization is found with occult lower spinal cord anomalies. Presacral teratoma or other tumors can cause compression and urinary blockage as well. In male infants, there is the possibility of posterior urethral valves. Physical findings of loose abdominal skin or musculature and a distended bladder suggest this diagnosis.

In a healthy-appearing newborn with a normal result on prenatal ultrasound examination, the absence of enlarged kidneys or palpable suprapubic mass, allowing up to 72 hours for a spontaneous first void, will avoid excessive testing. In fussy neonates, infants with other genitourinary abnormalities, enlarged kidneys, or distended bladder, testing should begin immediately. Ultrasound examination of bladder, kidneys, and posterior urethra is often diagnostic.

Normal newborns have decreased renal concentrating ability and excessive extracellular free water at birth. As a result, neonates will continue to void despite low intake of fluids. This process is normal, with excess fluid volumes being intrinsically protective against dehydration. Conversely, delayed voiding is not indicative of dehydration in the first 72 hours of life.

Defecation

Similar to the first void, the first passage of meconium occurs by an average of 7 hours of age. One third of newborns pass meconium before their first feeding. Late preterm newborns tend to pass meconium later than term infants, and 32% of preterm infants do not pass meconium in the first 2 days of life. In the first few days of life, intake is not well correlated with meconium output. However, the number of wet and soiled diapers reflects adequacy of breast milk production on day 4 of life. Fewer than four soiled diapers on day 4 correlates with inadequate milk production (Nommsen-Rivers et al, 2008). By 2 weeks of age, breastfed infants pass feces more frequently than bottle-fed infants; they also have larger variability in time between bowel movements (Sievers et al, 1993).

Because 99.7% of healthy newborns pass meconium by 34 hours of age, those who are delayed beyond that time deserve extra vigilance during examination to avoid missing obstructions, such as an imperforate anus (Metaj et al, 2003). A baby with abdominal distention or vomiting and delayed stooling deserves evaluation for a possible gastrointestinal tract obstruction.

JAUNDICE

There are few conditions in newborn infants that create as much controversy and clinician and parental angst as does hyperbilirubinemia. Since the discovery of phototherapy in 1956 and its integration into medical care in the 1960s, the standard management of neonatal jaundice in the United States has gone through three distinct phases. Until the early 1990s, clinicians visually monitored full-term neonates during their 2- to 5-day newborn nursery stay and obtained serum bilirubin levels on those with significant jaundice. Phototherapy was begun when the total bilirubin was 15 mg/dL, and an exchange transfusion was indicated if the level rose to 20 mg/dL (Watchko et al, 1983). The wisdom of this approach was challenged by several significant events. First, there was a growing awareness of the increase in costs associated with the prolonged hospitalization of a healthy infant for phototherapy to treat a relatively modest level of hyperbilirubinemia. Second, Kemper et al (1989, 1990) conducted a series of studies documenting that mothers of neonates who received phototherapy were at risk of overmedicalizing their children. Finally and most significantly, informal and formal reviews of data on jaundice in full-term newborns, without hemolytic disease, revealed that the risk of kernicterus in such infants was extraordinarily low (Newman and Maisels, 1992; Watchko et al, 1983).

Based on this evidence, a "kinder and gentler" approach to the management of hyperbilirubinemia in term infants was advocated, leading to the AAP practice parameter in 1994 (AAP Provisional Committee for Quality Improvement and Subcommittee on Hyperbilirubinemia, 1994). Under this guideline, phototherapy for a healthy, 72-hour-old, full-term newborn was not definitively recommended unless the serum bilirubin was 20 mg/dL or greater. Unfortunately, publication of this guideline corresponded to a shortening of the nursery stay by term infants to as little as 24 hours. Therefore infants were discharged home before their levels of bilirubin peaked at 3 to 4 days of life, and there were numerous reports of infants with extremely high bilirubin levels and a general impression that the incidence of kernicterus was increasing. In retrospect, it does not appear that the incidence of kernicterus increased, but case reports and anecdotal evidence led to significant consternation by clinicians, parents, and quality assurance organizations (Burke et al, 2009).

Because newborns are usually discharged well before bilirubin levels reach their peak, it is clear that predictive models were needed to assess risk in newborns who are discharged early. Bhutani et al (1999) developed a nomogram based on data from neonates in whom serum bilirubin levels were measured multiple times. Infants who had initial bilirubin levels above the 95th percentile for any time period were significantly more likely to have "significant hyperbilirubinemia" detected in subsequent bilirubin measurements. These data were used in the development of the 2004 AAP practice guideline (AAP Subcommittee on Hyperbilirubinemia, 2004b). With this iteration of the guideline, clinicians are provided hourly guidance on levels of bilirubin for which phototherapy or exchange transfusions are indicated. Separate curves for low-risk, medium-risk, and high-risk neonates have been developed. Internet-based tools are available that provide the appropriate management for an infant with a specific bilirubin at a specific hour of life.

Although the AAP bilirubin nomogram provides useful information, there are some caveats. First, in the study by Bhutani et al (1999), 39.5% of infants with an initial bilirubin level greater than the 95th percentile had significant hyperbilirubinemia at subsequent testing. Therefore more than 60% of such infants had less severe hyperbilirubinemia when retested. The nomograms for medium- and high-risk infants are based almost exclusively on expert opinion rather than actual data. Given these limitations, it is important for the clinician to determine management of a jaundiced neonate on an individual basis, remaining cognizant of the infant's medical condition, social situation, and parental preferences.

There are numerous neonatal conditions that increase the risk for hyperbilirubinemia (Dennery et al, 2001); chief among these is hemolysis secondary to maternal antibodies to red blood cell antigens. Thankfully, hemolysis secondary to antibodies to Rh factor is rare because of proper management of Rh-negative mothers. Because there is no way to prevent hemolysis from an ABO incompatibility, it may be useful to test cord blood from neonates born to mothers with blood type O for blood type and the presence of antibodies on their red cells (i.e., Coombs' test) at birth. The increase in bilirubin secondary to ABO compatibility is highly variable, even with a positive direct Coombs' test. Some infants will have an early and dramatic rise in serum bilirubin and evidence of hemolysis, whereas in others no effect can be detected clinically. In addition to ABO incompatibility, some women will have antibodies to minor red cell antigens that can usually be diagnosed prenatally. In most instances the increases in bilirubin associated with antibodies against minor antigens are mild.

Other neonatal conditions that are risk factors for hyperbilirubinemia include bruising secondary to birth trauma and polycythemia. Decreased intake of breast milk can lead to decreased passage of stool. Because intestinal bacteria break down conjugated bilirubin to the unconjugated form, a decrease in stooling can lead to increased reabsorption of this unconjugated bilirubin (enterohepatic circulation). Breastfeeding is a significant risk factor for hyperbilirubinemia particularly when intake is limited. The propensity for developing significant jaundice is variable in different racial groups. Asian and American Indian infants are at the highest risk for significant hyperbilirubinemia (Dennery et al, 2001). Finally, late preterm infants are at significantly increased risk for significant hyperbilirubinemia and kernicterus.

Traditionally, visual assessment has been used to judge whether a newborn infant has significant jaundice. This method of assessment is moderately accurate, but may be sufficient to rule out the need for serum bilirubin testing in many full-term newborns with no risk factors for jaundice (Moyer et al, 2000; Riskin et al, 2008). Transcutaneous bilirubinometers offer a noninvasive method for screening for hyperbilirubinemia. Depending on the technology and brand used, these instruments generally provide estimates of transcutaneous bilirubin (TcB) that correlate well with serum values. However, in practice it is not clear whether categorical estimates of the severity of neonatal jaundice using the transcutaneous meter are actually better than a visual assessment (Kaplan et al, 2008). Because the TcB may be lower or higher than the serum level in actual clinical practice, it should be considered as a screening tool only. Serum bilirubin testing remains the standard on which management decisions are based. Transcutaneous testing may be warranted for infants with risk factors for significant hyperbilirubinemia, even in the absence of significant jaundice.

Unless levels are high enough to require an exchange transfusion, phototherapy is effective for treating an infant with significant hyperbilirubinemia. Although repeated measurements of direct bilirubin are not cost effective, one assessment is helpful before or immediately after initiating phototherapy to rule out direct hyperbilirubinemia (Newman et al, 1991). An assessment of the potential for hemolysis as the etiology of the elevated bilirubin, possibly including a review of maternal and infant blood type, direct Coombs' test, hematocrit, reticulocyte count, and red cell morphology may also be useful.

There is no conclusive evidence as to whether continuous phototherapy leads to more rapid reduction in serum bilirubin levels than does intermittent treatment (AAP Subcommittee on Hyperbilirubinemia, 2004b; Lau and Fung, 1984). Unless bilirubin levels are approaching exchange transfusion levels, it is probably reasonable to discontinue treatment for several minutes to 1 hour at frequent intervals to allow parents to feed and hold their baby. Serial bilirubin measurements are needed to determine the adequacy of therapy and to determine when phototherapy can be discontinued. A rebound bilirubin level obtained 24 hours after discontinuation of phototherapy may be helpful in some clinical situations.

RESPIRATORY COMPLICATIONS

The term or late preterm fetus accomplishes the transition from dependency on the placenta to the newborn cardiorespiratory system, for the most part, without incident. After birth, pulmonary blood flow increases, fetal shunts reverse and begin to close, spontaneous breathing effort is initiated, and fetal lung fluid is cleared. Effective cardiorespiratory function, as represented by an absence of respiratory distress (nasal flaring, grunting, chest wall retractions, a respiratory rate of greater than 60 per minute) and an oxygen saturation in the middle 90s should be established by several hours of age (Levesque et al, 2000; O'Brien et al, 2000).

This normal sequence of events fails to occur in 2% to 8% of infants born at 34 weeks; gestation or later (Farchi et al, 2009; Hansen et al, 2008; Yoder et al, 2008). It is important to keep in mind that initial presenting symptoms are relatively nonspecific. Agrawal et al (2003) studied a large number of consecutive births in an attempt to determine the frequency and nature of different early-onset respiratory disorders and found that more than half did not meet specific diagnostic criteria. When confronted with a neonate with early onset respiratory symptoms, the most important diagnostic considerations include:

- Complex structural cardiac system anomalies; incidence estimated to be between 0.2% and 0.3%, often but not always identified by in utero imaging studies
- Diaphragmatic hernia, incidence estimated to be between 0.04% and 0.08%, commonly identified by second-trimester ultrasound (de Buys Roessingh and Dinh-Xuan, 2009)
- Respiratory distress syndrome (RDS); incidence estimated to vary between 0.45% and 2.4%, depending on the population studied; risk increased in the late preterm and infants delivered by cesarean section, particularly if accomplished before labor (Jain et al, 2009; Tita et al, 2009; Yoder et al, 2008)
- Persistent pulmonary hypertension of the newborn; incidence of 0.1% to 0.3%; often occurs in association with other acute respiratory conditions; questionable increased risk with maternal selective serotonin reuptake inhibitor treatment (Andrade et al, 2009; Chambers et al, 2006; Konduri and Kim, 2009)
- Meconium aspiration syndrome; incidence reported to vary between 2% and 9% of infants delivered through meconium-stained amniotic fluid (7% to 20% of all deliveries); risk increased in infants delivered after 40 weeks' gestation, intrapartum distress, or both (Bhutani, 2008; Liu and Harrington, 2002)
- Spontaneous pneumothorax; incidence between 0.1% and 0.8%; infants born by cesarean delivery may be at increased risk (Benterud et al, 2009; Zanardo et al, 2007)
- Transient tachypnea of the newborn (TTNB); incidence variable between 0.3% and 3.9%; risk factors include late prematurity and cesarean section; initial diagnosis sometimes difficult to differentiate from pneumonia and early RDS (Guglani et al, 2008; Jain et al, 2009; Tita et al, 2009; Yoder et al, 2008)
- Pneumonia; incidence difficult to determine, with one recent retrospective report estimated rate at 0.3%; risk factors include maternal chorioamnionitis and prolonged ruptured membranes; sometimes difficult to differentiate from RDS and/or TTNB (Yoder et al, 2008)

A review of the maternal history—particularly pregnancy, labor, and delivery—can provide useful diagnostic information. For example, the results of a second-trimester ultrasound examination could reveal the possibility of a cardiac defect or diaphragmatic hernia. A positive maternal GBS test result without adequate treatment, prolonged rupture of amniotic membranes, or evidence of chorioamnionitis suggests the possibility of pneumonia. For infants with respiratory distress born by cesarean section before the onset of labor, a diagnosis of RDS should be considered and assessment of gestational age should be performed. Finally, TTNB is a diagnosis of exclusion; it is prudent to rule out other causes before it is considered as the cause of respiratory distress in a term neonate.

In most cases minimal initial diagnostic efforts for a term newborn with unsuspected respiratory distress should include a chest radiograph and assessment of the arterial oxygen saturation. The results of these studies, in combination with maternal history, should provide information helpful to: (1) establish initial management, such as the need for supplemental oxygen, continuous monitoring, or both; (2) determine the need for further work-up or treatment, possibly including an echocardiogram, laboratory testing, and treatment for possible sepsis; or (3) give a referral for further specialty consultation, intensive care, or both (in severe cases).

CARDIOVASCULAR ISSUES

Congenital heart disease is a relatively common condition in newborns, with an estimated incidence of 81 cases per 10,000 live births (Reller et al, 2008). Ventricular septal defect (VSD) is by far the most common defect, accounting for more than 30% of all cases. The increasing accuracy of prenatal ultrasound examination has greatly improved the early diagnosis of complex congenital heart disease. The results of population-based reviews indicate that the sensitivity of routine prenatal ultrasound examination in identifying selected congenital defects is as high as 70% and ranges as high as 85% for hypoplastic left heart (Chew et al, 2007; Rasiah et al, 2006). For mothers at high risk of delivering a newborn with congenital heart disease, the use of fetal echocardiography is helpful for delineating the anatomy and significance of specific lesions. However, many of the most common defects, particularly VSD, are not typically detected prenatally.

In the absence of a prenatal diagnosis, detection of congenital heart disease is by physical examination. Sequential examinations are most helpful. At birth, many babies have loud murmurs that are thought to be from either a closing ductus arteriosus or tricuspid regurgitation (Silberbach and Hannon, 2007). These murmurs are transient and not indicative of disease. Conversely, murmurs associated with VSDs may not be heard for several days when the pressures on the right side of the heart have dropped enough to permit a significant shunting of blood from left to right. Although the ratio of pathologic to benign murmurs is higher in newborns than in older children, most of the murmurs heard during the newborn nursery stay in a healthy neonate are not clinically significant. Characteristics that increase the likelihood that a murmur signifies the presence of congenital heart disease include an intensity of 3/6 or greater, a harsh quality, occurrence during all of systole or into diastole, and being heard best at the lower sternal border or right upper border (Mackie et al, 2009). In a healthy newborn, the most common presentation of congenital heart disease is a somewhat harsh systolic murmur that is heard best at the lower left sternal border in an asymptomatic infant, indicative of a VSD.

In addition to auscultation, it is helpful to assess a newborn with a murmur for dysmorphic features and other anomalies, because these findings increase the likelihood that the murmur is indicative of congenital heart disease. It is important to evaluate the adequacy of femoral pulses to rule out coarctation of the aorta. Femoral pulses may be difficult to palpate in a neonate; if there is uncertainty, upper and lower extremity blood pressures can be measured. Although it is not a good screening tool, measurement of oxygen saturation may be helpful in diagnosing a cyanotic lesion in a child with a murmur or other signs of heart disease, particularly because hypoxia is frequently difficult to detect in newborns (Mahle et al, 2009). Chest radiographs and electrocardiograms are usually of limited value in evaluating healthy newborns with murmurs (Mackie et al, 2009; Oeppen et al, 2002).

Full-term neonates frequently have alterations in cardiac rhythm and rate. Heart rates in full-term infants can range as high as 200 beats/min or as low as 80 beats/min. These values are usually indicative of normal variation and are not clinically meaningful unless there are other signs of illness or if there is a lack of variability in rate with stimulation or attempts at calming the newborn. Arrhythmias are also not uncommon, occurring in approximately 1% of newborns (Oeppen et al, 2002). By far, the most common arrhythmia in a healthy-appearing, full-term newborn is from premature atrial contractions (Larmay and Strasburger, 2004; Southall et al, 1981). These contractions are almost always benign and are usually transient. If there is concern about an irregular rhythm in a newborn, an electrocardiogram can be obtained. With premature atrial contractions, the irregular beat is initiated by a P wave. Although the QRS complex may be widened, it is always be preceded by the P wave. In most cases no further work-up is needed. Cardiology consultation may be warranted if premature atrial contractions are persistent or if widened QRS complexes are seen on an electrocardiogram.

POSSIBLE NEONATAL SEPSIS

Group B *Streptococcus* Screening and Intrapartum Antibiotics

Since the 1970s, GBS has been a major cause of neonatal sepsis (Schuchat, 1998). The implementation of intrapartum antibiotic prophylaxis (IAP) to prevent early-onset GBS disease in neonates was associated with an 80% decrease in the rate of infection (Phares et al, 2008). The currently recommended strategy to prevent GBS disease is to obtain rectovaginal cultures on all pregnant women at 35 to 37 weeks' gestation and to administer penicillin or ampicillin during labor to those colonized with the bacteria. In situations where the mother's GBS status is unknown before the onset of labor, IAP is advised for those with certain risk factors for neonatal infection (Box 26-3; Schrag et al, 2002). A third strategy may become available with the development of rapid strep testing, which can be done intrapartum. Overall, it is estimated that IAP can reduce

BOX 26-3   Risk Factors for Group B *Streptococcus* Sepsis in Newborns

- Delivery before 37 weeks' gestation
- Maternal fever during labor (body temperature >38.5° C)
- Prolonged rupture of membranes (>18 hours)
- Chorioamnionitis (maternal fever >38.5° C, tender uterus, fetal tachycardia)
- Prior child with group B *Streptococcus* disease
- Group B *Streptococcus* infection during pregnancy (urinary tract infection or bacteremia)
- Young maternal age
- African American race
- Hispanic ethnicity
- Meconium-stained amniotic fluid
- Newborn low absolute neutrophil count (e.g., immature:total ratio >0.2)

the risk of early-onset GBS disease by 83% (Ohlsson and Shah, 2009). The overall rate of early-onset disease in the United States is approximately 0.3 to 0.4 cases per 1000 live births (Centers for Disease Control and Prevention, 2009; Van Dyke et al, 2009).

Unfortunately, despite an effective strategy to prevent the infection, the rate of GBS disease in the United States increased between 2003 and 2006 (Centers for Disease Control and Prevention, 2009). Much of this increase was seen in African American infants. Although the rate of infection was 2.8-fold higher in premature infants than term newborns, 72% of the cases of GBS disease during this period were in full-term neonates. In addition, although 93% of mothers of infants in this series with GBS had been screened, IAP was administered to only 20%. Finally, although GBS cultures are highly accurate, there is always the possibility of a false-negative screen. In one review, 61% of infants with GBS disease were born to mothers with a negative test result before delivery (Van Dyke et al, 2009). These statistics highlight the need for continued vigilance for signs of GBS infection in term newborns by health care providers, even in an era of surveillance and IAP.

Guidelines for prevention of GBS sepsis indicate that neonates are adequately treated only if IAP is administered at least 4 hours before delivery (Schrag et al, 2002). There is no clinical evidence to support this recommendation; it is based on expert opinion and is used to provide a margin of safety. However, there is evidence that penicillin given 2 hours before delivery is 90% effective in preventing GBS sepsis, and IAP provided less than 2 hours prior to delivery may be less effective (Illuzzi and Bracken, 2006). Blood levels are higher in the neonate than in the mother, even 30 minutes after a dose of penicillin, but the clinical importance of this has not been studied (Colombo et al, 2006).

Term infants whose mothers have received IAP for a positive GBS screen at least 4 hours before delivery can be safely discharged at 24 hours of age if there are no signs or symptoms of infection (Ohlsson and Shah, 2009). One area of consternation is how long to observe term newborns when antibiotics were not given more than 4 hours before delivery. In the current guidelines it is recommended that such infants be monitored in the hospital for

at least 48 hours after birth. The pressure for early newborn discharge has led some to compromise this period of observation. Most infants with sepsis manifest it early in life—many at birth, and nearly all by 12 hours of age (Escobar et al, 2000). Among a group of 172 term infants with documented early-onset GBS infection, 95% had presenting symptoms within 24 hours after delivery. More importantly, among the 33 neonates in this study that had GBS infection despite IAP, 31 had signs of infection before 24 hours of age (93.9%; 95% confidence interval, 79.8% to 99.3%; Bromberger et al, 2000). These data suggest, but do not definitively indicate, that some term newborns born to GBS positive mothers who received IAP less than 4 hours before delivery can be discharged by 48 hours of age. This decision is best made on an individual basis considering all risk factors, examination of the baby, vital sign stability, the results of any available laboratory tests, and parental wishes.

Assessment of Term Newborn for Possible Sepsis

The decision to remove a baby from the care of his or her parents during the period of initial homeostasis, and bonding should not be done without significant concern for the well-being of the infant. These decisions can have permanent effects on the parent-child relationship (Paxton and Nyington, 2001; Pearson and Boyce, 2004). Conversely, neonatal sepsis is such a dangerous and potentially rapidly progressive condition that any suggestive signs and symptoms cannot be ignored. It is between these extremes that the provider dwells and must make decisions often based on uncertainty and vague information.

The strongest predictor of sepsis is whether the baby is ill. This predictor can be somewhat challenging to determine given the limited repertoire of behaviors in newborns. Neonates typically have erratic temperature, poor feeding, periods of lethargy, and crying, all of which can also be symptoms of infection. Some of the earliest signs of infection include resting tachypnea or tachycardia, especially with reduced heart rate variability and transient decelerations (Griffin et al, 2005). This level of early identification requires continuous monitoring which, although routinely used on premature infants, is not routinely performed on term newborns. Because the infection entry portal is often the lungs, increased respiratory rate or increased work of breathing are the most common symptoms noted (Andersen et al, 2004). Fever is not a common symptom in an infected newborn, and usually babies with high temperatures are found to have other causes, especially after 24 hours of age (Maayan-Metzger et al, 2006). Decreased skin perfusion or mottling and decreased or increased tone are also worrisome signs.

GBS is not the only cause of sepsis in newborns. Coliforms were the dominant cause in the 1950s, and current causes may involve a natural cycle in the dominant bacteria causing sepsis. There are also sporadic cases of sepsis caused by enterococci, *Serratia* spp., and gram-negative bacteria such as *Escherichia coli*, *Proteus* spp., and *Klebsiella* spp. Although the decision of whether to evaluate or treat a neonate for possible sepsis cannot be informed only by the GBS status of the mother, and because other causes of infections are rare, most guidelines focus on GBS sepsis risk.

In general, the physical examination is as good as laboratory testing in identifying ill newborns (Escobar et al, 2000). Laboratory tests can aid in the prediction that a baby is ill, but testing is also viewed as invasive by parents, so it is often helpful to carefully explain the tests and how the results will be used to make decisions. There is no one single test that has shown superiority, and opinion on testing varies. Among the most useful tests are the absolute neutrophil count, immature-to-total neutrophil ratio, and the procalcitonin level (Carrol et al, 2002; van Rossum et al, 2004). The C-reactive protein or erythrocyte sedimentation rate may help, but have lower predictive values (Galetto-Lacour et al, 2003).

The decision to start testing or treating a term newborn for suspected sepsis should be multivariate and include: (1) risk factors during pregnancy, labor, and delivery (see preceding section); (2) current age in hours of the newborn; (3) presence of concerning signs and symptoms; and (4) physical examination. One single finding, such as an elevated temperature in an otherwise normally behaving newborn, is not usually sufficient evidence to start intravenous antibiotics. If the status of a term newborn is not rapidly changing, the use of close observation and periodic reassessment of risk factors and findings may prevent unnecessary testing or treatment.

SUGGESTED READING

Burke BL, Robbins JM, Bird TM, et al: Trends in hospitalizations for neonatal jaundice and kernicterus in the United States, 1988-2005, *Pediatrics* 123: 524-532, 2009.

Bhutani VK, Johnson L, Sivieri EM: Predictive ability of a predischarge hour-specific serum bilirubin for subsequent significant hyperbilirubinemia in healthy term and near-term newborns, *Pediatrics* 103:6-14, 1999.

Dewey KG, Nommsen-Rivers LA, Heinig MJ, et al: Risk factors for suboptimal infant breastfeeding behavior, delayed onset of lactation, and excess neonatal weight loss, *Pediatrics* 112:607-619, 2003.

Nommsen-Rivers LA, Heinig MJ, Cohen RJ, et al: Newborn wet and soiled diaper counts and timing of onset of lactation as indicators of breastfeeding inadequacy, *J Hum Lact* 24:27-33, 2008.

Escobar GJ, Li DK, Armstrong MA, et al: neonatal sepsis workups in infants >/=2000 grams at birth: a population-based study, *Pediatrics* 106:256-263, 2000.

Kramer MS, Aboud F, Mironova E, et al: Breastfeeding and child cognitive development: new evidence from a large randomized trial, *Arch Gen Psychiatry* 65:578-584, 2008.

Kramer MS, Chalmers B, Hodnett ED, et al: Promotion of Breastfeeding Intervention Trial (PROBIT): a randomized trial in the Republic of Belarus, *JAMA* 285:413-420, 2001.

Kuzniewicz MW, Escobar GJ, Newman TB: Impact of universal bilirubin screening on severe hyperbilirubinemia and phototherapy use, *Pediatrics* 124: 1031-1039, 2009.

Lee RS, Cendron M, Kinnamon DD, et al: Antenatal hydronephrosis as a predictor of postnatal outcome: a meta-analysis, *Pediatrics* 118:586-593, 2006.

Phares CR, Lynfield R, Farley MM, et al: Epidemiology of invasive group B streptococcal disease in the United States, 1999-2005, *JAMA* 299:2056-2065, 2008.

Van Dyke MK, Phares CR, Lynfield R, et al: Evaluation of universal antenatal screening for group B streptococcus, *N Engl J Med* 360:2626-2636, 2009.

Tarini BA, Christakis DA, Weich HG: State newborn screening in the tandem mass spectrometry era: more tests, more false-positive results, *Pediatrics* 118: 448-456, 2006.

Complete references and supplemental color images used in this text can be found online at www.expertconsult.com

NEWBORN SCREENING

Inderneel Sahai and Harvey L. Levy

Newborn screening is directed primarily at disorders in which the clinical complications develop postnatally. In metabolic diseases, these complications result from biochemical abnormalities that appear after birth, when the infant is no longer protected by fetal-maternal exchange. For example, the infant with phenylketonuria (PKU) has a normal blood phenylalanine level at birth, but within a few hours demonstrates hyperphenylalaninemia. The infant with congenital hypothyroidism (CH) is also protected in utero, most likely from placental transfer of maternal thyroxine (T_4). If the hyperphenylalanemia in PKU is not controlled by diet or the hypothyroidism in CH is not corrected by supplemental T_4, the infant begins to show signs of developmental delay and subsequently becomes mentally retarded. If therapy begins during the first weeks of life, mental retardation in both disorders is prevented.

PKU was the first metabolic disorder known to benefit from dietary therapy. This fact was established by the middle 1950s. By the late 1950s, it was evident that the diet could prevent mental retardation if initiated in the neonatal period. Detecting PKU in all affected infants at that early age, before irreversible brain damage occurred, then became the challenge. This challenge entailed neonatal screening for a biochemical marker of the disease. In 1962, Guthrie developed a simple bacterial assay for phenylalanine that required only a small amount of whole blood soaked into filter paper (Guthrie and Susi, 1963). Therefore infants in newborn nurseries could be routinely tested for PKU in blood specimens obtained by lancing the heel and blotting the drops of blood onto a filter paper card. This filter paper blood specimen (dried blood spot specimen) could be mailed to a central laboratory for PKU testing. An increased concentration of phenylalanine in the specimen indicated PKU in the infant.

By the middle 1960s, many states had established routine newborn screening programs for PKU using the Guthrie method. Infants with PKU were identified in larger numbers than anticipated and were showing normal development while receiving treatment (O'Flynn, 1992). The success of PKU screening led to the addition of tests for other metabolic diseases, including galactosemia, maple syrup urine disease (MSUD), and homocystinuria. These additional tests could be performed on the same blood specimen obtained for PKU screening. Over time, a test was added for the endocrine disorder congenital hypothyroidism, followed by screening tests for sickle cell disease, congenital adrenal hyperplasia (CAH), biotinidase deficiency, cystic fibrosis, and others.

In 1990, tandem mass spectrometry (MS/MS) was first applied to the Guthrie specimen, opening a new era in newborn screening (Levy, 1998; Millington et al, 1990). This technology allowed for the accurate detection of numerous biochemical markers with a single assay, thereby making redundant several assays traditionally used in screening

for metabolic disorders. Furthermore, it enabled analysis of biomarkers not detectable by previous methodologies, thus greatly expanding the spectrum of conditions identifiable in the neonate (Levy and Albers, 2000). By the early 1990s, Naylor (Chace and Naylor, 1999) and Rashed et al (1995) began using this technology to routinely screen neonates for more than 20 biochemical disorders with high specificity and an extremely low rate of false-positive results. Currently most programs in the United States and screening programs in Europe and elsewhere have integrated MS/MS into newborn screening, and many are screening for more than 50 individual conditions (http://genes-r-us.uthscsa.edu).

In order to standardize screening panels nationwide, the American College of Medical Genetics has recommended a panel of 29 core conditions for screening (Table 27-1). An additional 25 secondary conditions were listed for which test results could be reported (American College of Medical Genetics, 2006). These secondary conditions, revealed in the course of screening for the 29 core conditions, are not well known or documented treatment is unavailable.

Molecular diagnostic techniques (i.e., DNA analysis) are also commonly used in newborn screening, predominantly as secondary tests for diseases such as cystic fibrosis or medium-chain acyl-CoA dehydrogenase deficiency (MCADD). Molecular testing substantially improves the positive predictive value of a primary screening result that is based on metabolite testing only (Ranieri et al, 1994; Wilcken et al, 1995; Ziadeh et al, 1995). With the initiation of pilot screening for severe combined immunodeficiency syndrome wherein the markers measured are DNA molecules (i.e., T cell receptor excision circles), the role of molecular technology has extended into primary marker analysis (Baker et al, 2009; Vogt, 2008). The use of molecular testing in screening will most likely expand further with advances in DNA technology.

Screening for neuroblastoma, the most common solid tumor of childhood, was formerly being performed in Japan and some European programs measuring vanillylmandelic acid and homovanillic acid in urine collected from infants (Sawada, 1993). However, this screening was abandoned because it failed to identify individuals with poor-prognosis neuroblastoma, instead identifying infants who had a form of neuroblastoma that either spontaneously regressed or could be effectively treated after clinical detection (Woods et al, 2003).

SCREENING PROCEDURE

SPECIMEN

The blood specimen is generally obtained from the heel of the infant. This simple sampling method, conceived and introduced by Guthrie and Susi (1963), has had an

TABLE 27-1   Core Disorders Recommended for Screening by American College of Medical Genetics

Disorder	Acronym	Primary Marker
Metabolic Disorders Detected Using Tandem Mass Spectrometry		
Organic acid disorders		
Beta-ketothiolase deficiency (mitochondrial acetoacetyl CoA thiolase deficiency)	BKT	C5:1/C5OH
Cobalamin defects A, B	CBL (A,B)	C3
Isovaleric acidemia*	IVA	C5
Glutaric aciduria I	GA-I	C5DC
3-Hydroxy 3-methylglutaryl-CoA lyase deficiency*	HMG	C5OH/C5-3M-DC
Multiple carboxylase deficiency*	MCD	C3/C5OH
3-Methylcrotonyl-CoA carboxylase deficiency	3MCC	C5OH
Methylmalonic aciduria (mutase)*	MMA	C3
Propionic acidemia*	PA	C3
Fatty acid oxidation defects		
Carnitine uptake defect (carnitine transporter defect)	CUD	C0
Long-chain hydroxyacyl-CoA dehydrogenase deficiency*	LCHAD/D	C16OH/C18:1OH
Medium-chain acyl-CoA dehydrogenase deficiency	MCAD/D	C8
Trifunctional protein deficiency*	TFP	C16OH/C18:1OH
Very-long-chain acyl-CoA dehydrogenase deficiency	VLCAD/D	C14:1/C14
Amino acid disorders		
Argininosuccinic aciduria (argininosuccinate lyase deficiency)*	ASA	ASA
Citrullinemia I (argininosuccinate synthase deficiency)*	CIT-I	Citrulline
Phenylketonuria	PKU	Phenylalanine
Maple syrup urine disease*	MSUD	Leucine
Homocystinuria	HCY	Methionine
Tyrosinemia type I	TYR-I	Tyrosine
Other Metabolic Disorders		
Biotinidase deficiency	BIOT	Biotinidase activity
Galactosemia*	GALT	Total galactose, GALT activity
Endocrine Disorders		
Congenital adrenal hyperplasia*	CAH	17-Hydroxyprogesterone
Congenital hypothyroidism	CH	T4, TSH
Hemoglobin Disorders		
Sickle cell anemia	HbSS	Hb variants
Sickle cell disorder	HbS/C	Hb variants
Hemoglobin S/β-thalassemia	HbS/betaTh	Hb variants
Other Disorders		
Cystic fibrosis	CF	Immunoreactive trypsinogen
Hearing	HEAR	

GALT, Galactose-1-phosphate uridyl transferase; T_4, thyroxine; *TSH*, thyroid-stimulating hormone.
*Can manifest acutely in the first week of life.

enormous effect on newborn screening. The specimen is easily obtained and easily and inexpensively sent by mail to a central testing facility. There are no complications in obtaining the specimen from the newborn, contrary to early fears that its collection would lead to infection or result in excessive bleeding.

SPECIMEN COLLECTION PROCEDURE

The blood specimen should be obtained from the lateral or the medial side of the heel (Figure 27-1). Blood should be applied to only one side of the filter paper card, but it should saturate each circle on the card. Contamination of the filter paper specimen with iodine, alcohol, petroleum jelly, stool, urine, milk, or a substance such as oil from the fingers can adversely affect the results of the screening tests. In addition, exposure to heat and humidity can inactivate enzymes and produce false results. The specimen should be dried in air at room temperature for at least 3 hours before being placed in an envelope.

Specimens are sometimes collected in capillary tubes, by venipuncture of a dorsal vein or from a central line, and then spotted on filter paper. There is little or no substantial difference in analyte levels between blood collected

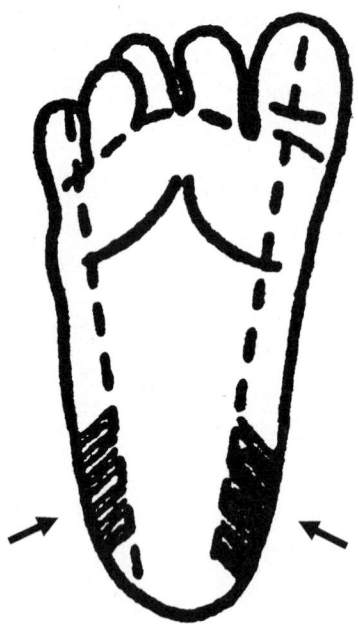

FIGURE 27-1 *Hatched areas* at medial and lateral sides of the heel in this drawing of the sole indicate the proper sites for a heel stick in the newborn.

directly from the heel and that collected by any of these other methods (Lorey and Cunningham, 1994). However, there is the danger of introducing amino acids from total parental nutrition solutions given through a central line into blood collected from this line, resulting in a false-positive increase in amino acids or interference in some molecular assays by the heparin from the line. In general, it is preferable that blood for screening be spotted on filter paper directly from the heel.

TIMING OF COLLECTION

Newborn screening encompasses a gamut of conditions, each with its own ideal screening period during which there is the greatest chance of diagnosing the disorder and before onset of symptoms. As a result, it is worth noting that recommendations on the timing of specimen collection, although appropriate for the majority, may not be ideal for all conditions on the screening panel. In congenital adrenal hyperplasia, in which the symptoms can manifest within the first week of life, the optimal time for collection of the specimen is within 24 to 48 hours after birth. Formerly there was concern that with the newborn screening specimen collected early, often during the first day of life, some infants with metabolic disorders or CH might not have a sufficient degree of abnormality for identification. However, MS/MS methodology with its improved sensitivity and specificity has considerably improved the reliability of screening for metabolic conditions in early specimens (Chace and Naylor, 1999) and using thyroid-stimulating hormone (TSH) as the primary marker for CH, or as a second-tier test when T_4 is the primary marker, has similarly allowed early screening for CH to be reliable.

Specimen collection timings vary around the world. In Europe and Australia, most screening specimens are collected within 48 to 72 hours, whereas specimens in

the United Kingdom are not collected until the infant is 5 to 8 days old (U.K. Newborn Screening Program Centre, 2008). In the United States, most screening specimens are collected within 24 to 72 hours after birth. The specimen should be obtained from every newborn infant before nursery discharge or by the third day of life, whichever is first. In infants whose initial specimen was obtained within the first 24 hours of life, as may happen with the practice of early nursery discharge, a second blood specimen should be obtained no later than 7 days of age to be certain that a diagnosis is not missed.

Special circumstances require specific attention to newborn blood specimen collection. Premature infants or those with very low birthweight, as well as infants who are sick and those in neonatal intensive care units (NICUs), are at a risk of unreliable screening owing to factors such as the unique physiology of the infant, therapeutic interventions, and a focus on critical activities in caring for the very sick neonate. Consequently, a single specimen is inadequate for screening in this subpopulation, and additional specimens should be collected for retesting. Serial screening with collection of three specimens—upon admission to the NICU, between 24 and 48 hours of life, and at discharge or at 28 days of life, whichever is sooner—has been proposed as an adequate and efficient protocol for this population (Clinical and Laboratory Standards Institute, 2009). In addition, some programs recommend screening every month until discharge for babies who continue to remain in the NICU.

A blood specimen should be collected from any infant who is being transferred to a different hospital or to a NICU, regardless of age. The first specimen should be collected before transfer, and a second specimen at the receiving hospital by 4 days of age. This dual collection policy covers the infant from whom a newborn specimen might not have been obtained in the turmoil that frequently accompanies the transfer of neonates.

In a newborn who is to receive a blood transfusion, a screening specimen should be collected before transfusion, and a second specimen should be collected 2 days after the transfusion. In addition, a third screening specimen should be obtained 2 months after the transfusion, when most of the donor red blood cells (RBCs) have been replaced. This practice ensures reliable testing for analytes present in RBCs, if a pretransfusion specimen has not been obtained.

Newborn screening tests are usually performed in a centralized state, provincial, or regional laboratory. In a regional program, the specimens may be received by the state program and then delivered to the regional state or private laboratory, or they may be sent directly to the regional laboratory. In either case, the individual state programs serve as the state data and follow-up centers.

SCREENING TESTS

The testing procedure begins with the punching of small discs (each usually 3 mm in diameter) from the screening specimen. These small discs are then analyzed by various methodologies for the individual markers being sought. Amino acids and acylcarnitines, the markers for the majority of screened metabolic conditions, are simultaneously measured by MS/MS (Rinaldo et al, 2004). MS/MS is superior in terms of accuracy of measurement of the individual analytes when compared with alternate methods originally used for screening amino acids, such as bacterial assays or fluorometric techniques.

Immunoassays, including fluoroimmunoassay and enzyme-linked immunosorbent assays, are used to test for endocrinopathies such as congenital hypothyroidism and CAH, for infectious diseases such as congenital toxoplasmosis and human immunodeficiency virus (HIV) seropositivity, and for cystic fibrosis. Hemoglobin electrophoresis of blood eluted from the filter paper disc is used for sickle cell disease screening. An enzyme assay is often used to screen for galactosemia and is always used to screen for biotinidase deficiency. Molecular assays are applied to quantify T cell receptor excision circles in dried blood to screen for severe combined immunodeficiency syndrome. More commonly, molecular assays are used to identify known mutations in certain disorders as a second-tier test. Several platforms, such as DNA microarrays and microsphere-based assays, can multiplex several molecular and immunological assays for high-throughput screening and are being used by screening programs (Dobrowolski et al, 1999; Green and Pass, 2005; McCabe and McCabe, 1999).

SECONDARY TESTS

An abnormal finding on a newborn screening test is not diagnostic of a disorder. Abnormalities in the newborn specimen can be transient or artifactual. Accordingly, when an abnormality is identified, the original specimen is retested for the analyte that was abnormal. Additional tests can be performed by the screening laboratory to substantiate the finding and improve the specificity of screening (Matern et al, 2007; Rinaldo et al, 2006).

In screening for congenital hypothyroidism, many programs initially measure T_4 in the original newborn blood specimen. Specimens in which a low T_4 level is found are further tested for an increased level of TSH, which would indicate congenital hypothyroidism. A normal TSH level would suggest transiently low T_4, a common finding in premature infants, or T_4-binding globulin deficiency. Some screening programs have adopted screening protocols in which the primary analysis is for TSH, and T_4 is measured as a second-tier test in specimens with high concentrations of TSH. Similarly, in screening for galactosemia an elevated galactose measurement in a specimen can trigger the analysis of galactose-1-phosphate uridyltransferase (GALT) enzyme activity as a second-tier test.

Second-tier molecular testing is also performed in some screening laboratories. For example, in screening for cystic fibrosis, an initial out-of-range primary marker prompts DNA analysis to identify several specific pathogenic mutations (Comeau et al, 2004; Rock et al, 2005; Wilcken et al, 1995). Screening programs following this two-tiered immunoreactive trypsinogen-DNA approach can identify up to 99% of patients with cystic fibrosis and report a positive predictive value ranging between 1/9.5 to 1/25 (Grosse et al, 2004). Molecular assays to detect disease-causing mutations are currently used as second-tier tests for several other disorders, and their use is likely to expand with advances in DNA technology. These uses include testing for the prevalent c.985A>G mutation in MCADD, the predominant E474Q mutation in long-chain 3-hydroxyacyl-CoA dehydrogenase deficiency (LCHADD; Dobrowolski et al, 1999), and a panel of several GALT mutations in galactosemia screening.

The final interpretation of the screening results is based on the primary analysis and, if available, the results of second-tier testing. However, it is important to realize that screening is not intended to be diagnostic; abnormal screening results must be supported by confirmatory investigations. These studies require additional specimens and are performed by clinical laboratories or sometimes by the screening laboratory.

PHYSICIAN CONTACT FOR ABNORMAL RESULTS

Table 27-2 indicates disorders or other reasons for abnormal screening results, sorted according to the primary analyte usually used to screen for the condition. For example, a low T_4 level together with an elevated TSH concentration indicates congenital hypothyroidism, and a marked elevation of 17-hydroxyprogesterone (17-OHP) indicates the likelihood of CAH. An elevation of an acylcarnitine could indicate an organic acid or fatty acid oxidation disorder.

Any infant for whom such a screening result is reported should be evaluated by the primary care provider as soon as possible to facilitate the next steps towards the confirmation and management of the disorder. However, several conditions screened for are extremely rare, and primary health care professionals might not have sufficient information available to be able to direct appropriate intervention in screen-positive infants. To overcome the challenge, readily accessible, one- to two-page explanations of the possible disorders represented by the abnormality and the recommended confirmatory tests, known as *ACT sheets* and *confirmatory algorithms* (Kaye et al, 2006), are available on the Web site of the American College of Medical Genetics (www.acmg.net/resources/policies/ACT/condition-analyte-links.htm).

Although all specimens with a metabolite concentration that crosses its threshold are considered screen-positive, all screen-positive results are not associated with the same likelihood of being associated with a disorder. Most infants with a positive screening result that is only mildly abnormal are less likely to have a disorder (see later discussion of false-positive results) than are infants with analyte concentrations that are several fold above the cutoff. Applying a uniform approach for all positive results in terms of urgency of intervention or battery of tests suggested can result in unnecessary parental anxiety and medical costs. However, if recommendations for further action and workup are customized in accordance with the potential significance of the abnormality, both parental anxiety and costs associated with false-positive results can be reduced. To achieve this goal, some programs subcategorize positive screening results. The New England Newborn Screening Program uses primary marker concentrations, second-tier analyses, biomarker profiles for markers analyzed by MS/MS, and acuity of the likely disorder to subcategorize out-of-range screening results (Sahai et al, 2007). The primary care providers are supplied with category-based, customized fact sheets when a positive screening result is reported

TABLE 27-2 Disorders or Other Reasons for Abnormal Screening Results Sorted by Primary Marker Analyzed

Marker			Disorders	Possible Causes of False Positives
Markers Analyzed Using Tandem Mass Spectrometry				
Free carnitine (C0)	Low		CUD	Poor feeding, maternal CUD
Free carnitine (C0)	High		CPT-I	Carnitine supplementation
Propionylcarnitine (C3)	High		MMA, PA, CBL (A,B)	Hemolysis,* maternal biotin deficiency, carrier of associated disorders
Butyrylcarnitine (C4)	High		SCADD/EE/IBDD	Hypoglycemia from other causes,* FIGLU elevation
Tigylcarnitine (5:1)	High		BKT deficiency	VLBW neonate
Isovalerylcarnitine (C5)	High		IVA	Antibiotics containing pivalic acid, IVA/MBCD carrier, VLBW neonate, neonate receiving total parental nutrition, FAS hemoglobin profile*
Glutarylcarnitine (C5DC)	High		GA-I	MCADD carrier, twin or multiple births*
3-Methylglutarylcarnitine (C5-3M-DC)	High		HMG	Severe respiratory distress, neonates receiving ECMO*
Hydroxyisovalerylcarnitine (C5OH)	High		3MCC	Maternal MCC, maternal biotin deficiency
Octanoylcarnitine (C8)	High		MCADD	MCADD carrier, MCT supplementation
Tetradecenenoylcarnitine (C14:1)	High		VLCADD	Carrier
Hydroxyhexadecanoylcarnitine (C16OH)	High		LCHADD/TFP	Carrier
Hexadecanoylcarnitine (C16)	High		CPT-II	Severe hemolysis*
Arginine (Arg)	High		ARG	Hyperalimentation
Argininosuccinic acid (ASA)	High		ASA	—
Citrulline (Cit)	Low		OTC/CPS/NAGS	Poor feeding*
Citrulline (Cit)	High		CIT-I	Hyperalimentation
Phenylalanine (Phe)	High		PKU	Hyperalimentation, specimen contaminated with artificial sweetener*
Leucine (Leu)	High		MSUD	Hyperalimentation, hydroxyprolinemia
Methionine (Met)	High		HCY	Hyperalimentation
Tyrosine (Tyr)	High		TYR-I	Prematurity, transient immaturity of enzyme
Markers analyzed by assays other than tandem mass spectrometry				
Biotinidase activity (Bio)	Low		BIOT	Exposure of specimen to heat, improper drying
Total galactose (T-Gal)	High		GALT	GALE deficiency, GALK deficiency, contamination with milk/cream
Activity GALT	Low		GALT	Exposure of specimen to heat
17-Hydroxyprogesterone (17-OHP)	High		CAH	Physiologic stress (seen commonly in NICU babies), VLBW, EDTA in specimen
T4/TSH	Low/High		CH	Neonates in NICU, maternal thyroid medications
Immunoreactive trypsinogen (IRT)	High		CF	VLBW neonate, NICU
T cell receptor excision circles (TREC)	Low		SCID	Other immunodeficiencies, Di George syndrome, heparin in specimen*

BIOT, biotinidase deficiency; *BKT*, beta-ketothiolase deficiency; *CAH*, congenital adrenal hyperplasia; *CBL*, cobalamin defect; *CF*, cystic fibrosis; *CH*, congenital hypothyroidism; *CIT-I*, citrullinemia I; *CPT*, carnitine palmitoyltransferase deficiency; *CUD*, carnitine uptake defect; *ECMO*, extracorporeal membrane oxygenation; *EDTA*, ethylenediamine tetraacetic acid; *EE*, ethylmalonic encephalopathy; *FIGLU*, formiminoglutamic; *GA-I*, glutaric aciduria I; *GALE*, uridine diphosphate galactose-4-epimerase; *GALK*, galactokinase; *GALT*, galactosemia; *HCY*, homocystinuria; *HMG*, 3-hydroxy 3-methylglutaryl-CoA lyase deficiency; *IBDD*, Isobut yryl-CoA dehydrogenase deficiency; *IVA*, isovaleric acidemia; *LCHADD*, long-chain 3-hydroxyacyl-CoA dehydrogenase deficiency; *MBCD*, 2-methylbutyryl-CoA dehydrogenase deficiency; *MCC*, methylcrotonyl-CoA carboxylase; *MCT*, medium-chain triglycerides; *MSUD*, maple syrup urine disease; *MMA*, methylmalonic aciduria; *MCADD*, medium-chain acyl-CoA dehydrogenase deficiency; *NICU*, neonatal intensive care unit; *PA*, propionic acidemia; *PKU*, phenylketonuria; *SCADD*, Short-chain acyl-CoA dehydrogenase; *SCID*, severe combined immune deficiency; *TFP*, trifunctional protein deficiency; *TYR-I*, tyrosinemia type I; *VLBW*, very low birthweight; *VLCADD*, very-long-chain acyl-CoA dehydrogenase deficiency.
*Associations observed in the New England Newborn Screening Program.

(Sahai and Eaton, 2008). These sheets include information on disorders associated with the marker, estimated likelihood of being affected, clinical presentations of likely disorders, factors contributing to false positives, and recommendations for further management. The follow-up recommendations can range from immediate admission to a hospital, where further evaluation and therapy for the illness can be initiated without delay, to simply repeating the filter paper analysis on a sample collected a few days later. Other programs approach this problem differently, but with the same goal in mind, providing the primary care providers with the information needed to put the result in the appropriate context for the family.

Any infant for whom an abnormal screening result is reported should be seen as soon as possible and evaluated with a careful history and physical examination. When specific guidelines based on the individual results are not provided by the screening program, and the infant is ill or the likely disorder manifests acutely within the first few days of life (see Table 27-1), a specialist should be contacted. The infant may need to be admitted to the hospital where further evaluation and therapy for the illness can be initiated without delay.

If the infant is active and alert with good feeding and shows no abnormal signs on initial evaluation, and the suspected disorder does not require immediate attention, a second filter paper blood specimen can be obtained and sent to the screening laboratory for repeated testing, or confirmatory testing can be performed on a less urgent basis. In many cases, confirmatory testing or referral to a specialist is required only if the second test indicates the presence of a disorder. However, the follow-up of an initial positive screening result can vary. In some programs, more specific confirmatory testing is the first response to a presumptive positive newborn screen, with a less intense time frame for individuals in whom the level of suspicion is lower.

The physician should contact the screening laboratory when an infant whose screen has been reported as normal or whose screening results have not yet been reported has symptoms that suggest a metabolic disorder. The screening laboratory can check the results in the infant's newborn specimen. If the testing has been completed and the newborn specimen is retained in storage, the laboratory may wish to recover the specimen and repeat the tests. The physician should also contact the screening laboratory for the results of repeated tests and inform the family of the results as soon as possible. If the second result is normal, the duration of the family's anxiety may be shortened.

SCREENED DISORDERS

Following are brief summaries of the categories of the most common disorders detected by newborn screening. There is no attempt to describe any of the disorders in detail or their rare variants.

METABOLIC DISORDERS

Amino Acid Disorders

The amino acid disorders are caused by an enzymatic defect in the catabolic pathway of amino acids, with consequent accumulation of specific amino acids above the block. Screening relies on the detection of these elevated amino acids in the newborn specimen. The clinical manifestations may be a result of the toxic effects of the accumulating amino acid and metabolites produced by alternate pathways, a deficiency of the products of the normal pathway, or both. PKU is the best-known example of an amino acid disorder and is the paradigm for screened disorders in the newborn.

In addition to PKU, MSUD and homocystinuria are historically significant in the context of screening, because they are among the original metabolic conditions for which screening was performed before the introduction of MS/MS and therefore the expansion of screening. Screening for other amino acid disorders, such as the urea cycle defects and tyrosinemia type I, became possible only with the advent of MS/MS technology.

In PKU, the cardinal screening feature is an increased level of phenylalanine. PKU should always be identified by newborn screening. If untreated, patients with PKU experience severe mental retardation and other neurologic abnormalities. The average incidence of the disorder is approximately 1 in 12,000 live births. With screening by MS/MS, PKU can reliably be identified as early as the first day of life (Chace et al, 1998). Not all infants with an elevation of phenylalanine have PKU. Mild elevations can indicate benign mild hyperphenylalaninemia. Liver disease, such as that associated with galactosemia, tyrosinemia type I or citrin deficiency, can also produce increased phenylalanine. Therefore treatment for PKU should never be started on the basis of a positive screening test result alone. The dietary therapy is complicated and can be hazardous to an infant who does not have PKU. If the screening test reveals a marked elevation of phenylalanine (≥6 mg/dL) and the metabolic profile (including reduced tyrosine) is supportive of PKU, the infant should be referred directly to a metabolic center for confirmatory testing and prompt consideration of dietary treatment. If the screening level of phenylalanine is only slightly increased, retesting a second specimen before initiating a complete diagnostic work-up may suffice.

The primary indicator for MSUD in the newborn blood specimen is an increase in leucine. To improve the specificity for MSUD of an abnormal leucine measurement, some screening programs also report the ratio between leucine and a reference amino acid or alloisoleucine analysis as a second-tier test (Matern et al, 2007). The average incidence of classic MSUD is 1 in 185,000. MSUD can be a fulminant disease associated with severe ketoacidosis, vomiting, and lethargy, and it can progress rapidly to coma and death. Consequently, the finding of a substantially increased leucine level in the newborn blood specimen should prompt an immediate telephone call from the screening program to the attending physician. If the infant is ill, he or she should be transported immediately to an NICU at a medical center with a metabolic specialist. Confirmatory plasma and urine specimens should be obtained, and emergency therapy should be initiated. Plasma amino acid analysis in an infant with MSUD will show marked increases in leucine, isoleucine, and valine as well as alloisoleucine (the branched-chain amino acids). The urine specimen will test strongly positive for ketones and will contain large quantities of the branched-chain ketoacids and amino acids. The characteristic odor reminiscent of maple syrup, which appears earliest in cerumen and only later in urine, will probably be detected on a cotton-tipped swab inserted in the infant's ear. Milder variants of MSUD can be missed by newborn screening (Bhattacharya et al, 2006). A newborn with the intermediate variant might not have a blood leucine elevation, or the increase may be so mild as to be below the cutoff value. In the intermittent variant, the blood leucine concentration is normal in the newborn period, becoming elevated only in later infancy or childhood during acute metabolic episodes precipitated by febrile illness or surgery.

Individuals with homocystinuria are clinically normal at birth but, if untreated, may develop ectopia lentis (dislocation of the lens), thromboembolism, osteoporosis, and mental retardation. The worldwide frequency of all forms of homocystinuria has been estimated at 1 in 344,000, but may be considerably higher (Skovby et al, in press). The newborn blood screening marker for detecting homocystinuria is an increased level of methionine. Homocysteine can be measured as a second-tier analysis to improve specificity (Matern et al, 2007). The diagnosis of homocystinuria may be missed if the blood methionine concentration is not elevated at the time the newborn specimen is collected (Whiteman et al, 1979). Reducing the cutoff value for methionine can substantially increase the frequency of identified infants (Peterschmitt et al, 1999), but may also result in an increased number of false-positive results. A high methionine level alone is not diagnostic of homocystinuria. Liver disease of a nonmetabolic nature can produce a strikingly high methionine level, as can isolated hypermethioninemia (methionine-S-adenosyltransferase [MAT] I/III deficiency), a metabolic disorder that may be benign. Two additional rare disorders also produce hypermethioninemia: glycine-N-methyltransferase deficiency associated with liver disease (Luka et al, 2002; Mudd et al, 2001) and S-adenosylhomocysteine hydrolase deficiency, which may result in developmental delay and hypotonia (Baric et al, 2004). Furthermore, transient hypermethioninemia may occur in newborn infants. Confirmation of the disorder requires quantitative amino acid analyses of plasma and urine. In the infant with homocystinuria, homocystine is usually detectable in plasma and urine, plasma total homocysteine is increased as is methionine, and cystine is reduced. In isolated hypermethioninemia, methionine is markedly increased in plasma, but there is no detectable homocystine in plasma or urine and the plasma cystine concentration is normal. Hypermethioninemia secondary to liver disease owing to tyrosinemia type I, or to nonspecific liver disease, is usually accompanied by increased tyrosine.

The three urea cycle disorders currently screened by MS/MS analysis are citrullinemia, argininosuccinic acidemia, and arginase deficiency. Citrullinemia and argininosuccinic acidemia produce hyperammonemia, often in the neonatal period, accompanied by poor feeding, tachypnea, lethargy, and vomiting. Respiratory alkalosis is characteristic. Severe hyperammonemia in the newborn is a medical emergency and should trigger prompt consultation with a metabolic specialist or referral to an NICU at a metabolic center. Discontinuation of protein and the provision of intravenous fluids with high caloric content are the first steps to take. L-Arginine or L-citrulline, as well as the "scavenger drugs" sodium phenylbutyrate and sodium benzoate, may be administered. Hemodialysis might be required to control the neurotoxic hyperammonemia, which can lead to irreversible brain damage, coma, and death. It is hoped that with early identification through newborn screening, patients with urea cycle disorders will be protected by presymptomatic therapy in the neonatal period. Arginase deficiency can also present acutely with hyperammonemia as described earlier, although more frequently it manifests as developmental delay and spastic diplegia in childhood with a milder degree of hyperammonemia (Crombez and Cederbaum, 2005).

Tyrosinemia type I is an amino acid disorder that can be diagnosed by finding an elevation of succinylacetone in MS/MS analysis (Allard et al, 2004). However, the preanalytic processing required for succinylacetone is more involved than that required for the amino acids and acylcarnitines. As a result, succinylacetone is not currently measured by all screening programs. These programs may rely on elevations of tyrosine for identification of this disorder. Unfortunately, moderate elevations of tyrosine that are transient occur frequently in neonates, especially those who have low birthweights and are sick, necessitating frequent requests for repeated screening with virtually no detection of tyrosinemia type I. Unfortunately moderate transient elevations of tyrosine occur frequently in neonates, especially those who have low birthweights and are sick, necessitating frequent requests for repeated screening. Virtually no cases of tyrosinemia type I have been detected based on elevated tyrosine because almost all infants with tyrosinemia type I have had normal tyrosine levels when screened (Frazier et al, 2006). Consequently, the newborn detection of tyrosinemia type I by a tyrosine marker alone is ineffective. Tyrosinemia type I leads to liver and renal tubular disease and can later result in hepatocellular carcinoma. It is treated with administration of 2-(2-nitro-4-trifluoromethylbenzoyl)-1,3-cyclohexanedione (NTBC; Orfadin) and a diet low in phenylalanine and tyrosine. Tyrosinemia types II and III are identified by an increased level of tyrosine in newborn screening. Tyrosinemia type II can result in mental retardation, painful hyperkeratoses, and keratoconjunctivitis, and it is treated by a low tyrosine-phenylalanine diet. Tyrosinemia type III seems to be benign, although developmental delay has been reported occasionally (Ellaway et al, 2001).

Medium-Chain Acyl-CoA Dehydrogenase Deficiency and Other Fatty Acid Oxidation Disorders

The fatty acid oxidation disorders include those in which the long-chain fatty acids cannot traverse the mitochondrial membranes to be oxidized within the mitochondrial matrix (i.e., the carnitine palmitoyltransferase disorders) and those that constitute defects in fatty acid oxidation per se. In either category, the problem is the inability to fully oxidize fatty acids. Fatty acid oxidation is essential to supply energy as adenosine triphosphate via the Krebs cycle and as ketones in the presence of a low supply of glucose. The disorders involving defective transport concern carnitine, whereas those with defective oxidation are named according to the enzyme that is deficient (see Table 27-1). The clinical consequence of these disorders is fasting intolerance resulting in hypoketotic hypoglycemia, lethargy, hyperammonemia, metabolic acidosis, hepatomegaly, and sometimes sudden death. Cardiomyopathy is an additional feature of very-long-chain acyl-CoA dehydrogenase deficiency (VLCADD) and long-chain hydroxyacyl CoA dehydrogenase deficiency (LCHADD). Each fatty acid disorder is associated with a specific or almost specific acylcarnitine pattern on MS/MS analysis.

The most common fatty acid oxidation disorder is MCADD. Tragically, before newborn screening was available, this disorder was often diagnosed only retrospectively after a sudden unexplained death, usually when postmortem examination revealed a fatty liver. This devastating outcome and a frequency of 1:15,000 to 1:20,000 (Zytkovicz et al, 2001), comparable with that of PKU, made MCADD the primary reason for the addition of MS/MS technology to newborn screening. To reduce the rate of false-positive results in screening for MCADD, some programs have added molecular testing of the c.985A>G MCAD mutation as second-tier screening. Because this mutation occurs in as many as 90% of persons with MCADD, this additional analysis of a newborn blood specimen with an elevation of the octanoylcarnitine marker for MCADD substantially improves the predictive value of the screening abnormality (Zytkovicz et al, 2001).

The treatment for fatty acid oxidation disorders is avoidance of fasting with high-carbohydrate, low-fat feedings and, of critical importance, prompt attention to acute illnesses in which vomiting occurs. Carnitine supplementation may be beneficial. Medium-chain triglycerides (i.e., MCT oil) is given for the long-chain disorders VLCADD and LCHADD. Any infant with a fatty acid oxidation disorder should be evaluated at a metabolic center. Most of these disorders are treatable, but screening enables early diagnosis and genetic counseling for the family even when early treatment may not be effective, such as in neonatal carnitine palmitoyltransferase II deficiency (CPT-II) (Albers et al, 2001a).

Organic Acid Disorders

Organic acid disorders are a heterogenous group of disorders with a combined frequency of approximately 1 in 50,000 (Zytkovicz et al, 2001). Many of them can be identified through MS/MS screening (see Table 27-1). The marker for this disease group, as for the fatty acid oxidation disorders, is an abnormal acylcarnitine pattern. If a screening result suggests an organic acidemia, a metabolic specialist should be consulted immediately. The major organic acid disorders identified in newborn screening are propionic acidemia, the methylmalonic acidemias, and isovaleric acidemia.

The organic acidemias can manifest in the neonatal period with a life-threatening, sepsis-like picture of feeding difficulties, lethargy, vomiting, and seizures. Metabolic acidosis virtually always accompanies this presentation, and hyperammonemia is common. In this situation, protein administration should be discontinued and replaced by administration of intravenous fluids with high caloric content and carnitine. The hyperammonemia rarely requires specific treatment. The effects of early diagnosis and treatment on the clinical and neurologic development of individuals affected by an organic acid disorder are currently under investigation (Albers et al, 2001b).

Galactosemia

Galactosemia typically manifests in the neonatal period as failure to thrive, vomiting, and liver disease (Hughes et al, 2009). Death from bacterial sepsis, usually caused by *Escherichia coli*, occurs in a high percentage of untreated neonates (Levy et al, 1977). The average incidence of the disorder is 1 in 62,000.

Some screening programs use a metabolite assay for total galactose (galactose and galactose-1-phosphate) to detect galactosemia. Other programs screen the newborn specimen with a specific enzyme assay for activity of GALT, undetectable in severe galactosemia. The enzyme assay identifies only galactosemia, whereas the metabolite assay also identifies other galactose metabolic disorders, such as deficiencies of galactokinase and epimerase. Severe neonatal liver disease and portosystemic shunting caused by anomalies in the portal system can also increase the galactose level.

The most rapid confirmatory test for a positive result in galactosemia screening is urine testing for reducing substance. In almost all cases of severe galactosemia, this test produces a strongly positive reaction. Galactosemia with residual GALT activity, however, may be accompanied by a negative or only slightly positive result for urine reducing substance. If the urine contains reducing substance and the infant has clinical signs of galactosemia (e.g., poor feeding, jaundice, hepatomegaly), a blood specimen for confirmatory testing should be collected, and milk feeding (breast or formula) should be discontinued with substitution of a nonlactose formula such as soy or elemental. The infant should then be referred immediately to a pediatric metabolic center, where confirmatory testing should include the measurement of RBC galactose-1-phosphate and an enzyme assay for RBC GALT activity (Levy and Hammersen, 1978). Molecular testing for GALT mutations may also be performed. Approximately 70% of the patients with galactosemia carry the Q188R mutation (Elsas and Lai, 1998). Variant galactosemia is produced by mutations such as S135L. The N314D mutation produces the benign Duarte variant.

If the urine test is negative for reducing substance, the newborn screening result is most likely to be false-positive or to indicate a benign GALT enzyme variant (e.g., Duarte variant). Nevertheless, urine-reducing substance may be absent in infants with clinically significant variants of galactosemia. Consequently, follow-up testing should be performed for all infants with an initial positive galactosemia screening result.

Biotinidase Deficiency

Biotin recycling is necessary for the maintenance of sufficient intracellular biotin to activate carboxylase enzymes. Biotinidase is a key enzyme in biotin recycling. Lack of biotinidase activity results in reduced carboxylase activities and an organic acid disorder known as *multiple carboxylase deficiency* (Wolf and Heard, 1991). The clinical features of the disorder are developmental delay, seizures, hearing loss, alopecia, and dermatitis. The developmental delay and seizures usually manifest at 3 to 4 months of age. Death during infancy has also been reported.

Initiating biotin therapy in early infancy, when the disorder is presymptomatic, seems to prevent all the features of biotinidase deficiency. For this reason, a screening test has been developed and added to newborn screening in a number of newborn screening programs throughout the world (Hart et al, 1992). The frequency of identified newborns in these programs has a wide range, from 1:30,000 to 1:235,000. The average frequency is approximately 1 in 70,000. Almost all identified infants have been asymptomatic and have remained normal with biotin treatment.

ENDOCRINE DISORDERS

Congenital Hypothyroidism

Congenital hypothyroidism is the most common disorder identified by routine newborn screening. It is found in 1:3000 to 1:5000 screened infants (Dussault, 1993). The major clinical features of untreated congenital hypothyroidism are growth retardation and delayed cognitive development leading to mental deficiency. If treatment with pharmacologic doses of T_4 is initiated early, growth and mental development are normal.

Two screening approaches are used (Pass and Neto, 2009). One method is primary screening for low T_4 with secondary screening for high TSH. The second method is primary screening for high TSH levels. Either procedure reliably identifies congenital hypothyroidism. Nevertheless, affected infants can be missed with either approach. This situation may be due to a lack of the identifying marker abnormality at the time of specimen collection. Specifically, the T_4 level during the first 24 hours of life in an affected infant might not yet be sufficiently decreased for identification because of persistence of maternally transmitted T_4. Moreover, in the premature infant with congenital hypothyroidism, it might take 2 weeks or more for a TSH elevation to develop (Larson et al, 2003).

The reported false-positive rates of screening for congenital hypothyroidism range from approximately 0.05% to as high as 4% (Pass and Neto, 2009). Infants with false-positive results have transiently low T_4 or elevated TSH levels. Many of those with low T_4 levels are premature infants with a normal TSH concentration or infants with perinatal stress and elevated TSH levels. To avoid missing congenital hypothyroidism, screening programs require a second blood specimen from each of these infants. In addition to false-positive results, a low T_4 level with a normal TSH value can result from benign T_4-binding globulin deficiency (Dussault, 1993; Mandel et al, 1993) or hypothyroidism secondary to pituitary deficiency.

Infants with a positive screening test result should not be labeled as having congenital hypothyroidism until diagnostic testing confirms the disorder. This is especially true if the TSH concentration reported by the screening program is normal. If congenital hypothyroidism is confirmed, however, administration of T_4 should be started without delay to prevent irreversible brain damage.

Congenital Adrenal Hyperplasia

CAH caused by steroid 21-hydroxylase deficiency occurs in 1:16,000 to 1:20,000 births (White, 2009). Infants with the salt-losing form of CAH can rapidly become hyperkalemic and die precipitously, often without a specific diagnosis. The clinical diagnosis may be suspected in the newborn girl because of ambiguous genitalia. However, the diagnosis is usually not suspected in boys and in girls with atypical forms of CAH in which ambiguous genitalia may not occur. Infant girls with ambiguous genitalia might not be recognized as having CAH if the ambiguity is not obvious, or they could be misassigned as boys if the ambiguity is advanced. Because accurate gender assignment and initiation of hormone therapy as soon as possible are critical to a favorable prognosis in CAH, newborn screening is important in leading to early diagnosis and prompt therapy with pharmacologic doses of hydrocortisone. Consequently, testing for CAH has been incorporated into routine newborn screening in most programs.

Screening is based on identifying elevated levels of 17-OHP, the preferred substrate for 21-hydroxylase, and is usually measured using an immunoassay. Unfortunately, compared with other neonatal screening assays, the specificity of the CAH assay is low and false-positive results in newborn screening for CAH are relatively common, with the rate often as high as 0.5%. The finding may be due to a truly increased 17-OHP, as in perinatal stress and early specimen collection (within the first 24 hours of life), or to cross-reacting steroids, such as in prematurity and low birthweight (al Saedi et al, 1996). Cross-reacting steroids are produced by residual fetal adrenal cortex or result from decreased metabolic clearance by an immature liver.

A decidedly increased level of 17-OHP suggests CAH, and the infant should be referred to a pediatric endocrinologist for management. A second blood specimen is usually requested from infants found to have slight to moderately increased 17-OHP. If the infant shows signs of illness or has ambiguous genitalia, serum electrolytes should be measured. If these results indicate hyponatremia and hyperkalemia, the infant should be hospitalized without delay, and the electrolyte imbalance should be corrected immediately. Pediatric endocrinology consultation should also be sought. It may be possible to improve the positive predictive value by second-tier screening using DNA-based methods or liquid chromatography followed by tandem mass spectrometry, but currently these methods are not widely used by newborn screening programs.

SICKLE CELL DISEASE

In most newborn screening programs in the United States, the blood specimen is routinely tested for hemoglobin abnormalities. The major goal of this testing is to identify infants with sickle cell disease so that they can be given penicillin prophylaxis to prevent pneumococcal septicemia. Additional benefits of early detection are early referral to a comprehensive sickle cell program and early education and genetic counseling for parents (Smith and Kinney, 1993). Unfortunately, the long-term complications are not yet preventable.

Sickle cell screening is usually performed by means of hemoglobin electrophoresis of blood eluted from a disc of the Guthrie specimen. This procedure identifies sickle cell disease, sickle cell trait, and several other abnormal hemoglobins. Other than sickle cell disease, most of these abnormalities are benign. It is especially critical to differentiate the common and benign sickle cell trait from the much rarer sickle cell disease (homozygosity for S hemoglobin). For example, sickle cell disease affects approximately 1 in 600 African American persons, whereas sickle cell trait (carrier status for S hemoglobin) is present in 1 in 12. Infants with sickle cell trait do not have complications and should not be stigmatized as having sickle cell disease.

When sickle cell disease is confirmed, penicillin prophylaxis should be initiated as soon as possible, and the infant should be referred to a sickle cell disease center or hematologist. The combination of screening and careful follow-up has been highly effective in preventing pneumococcal sepsis in infants with sickle cell disease.

CYSTIC FIBROSIS

The frequency (1:2000 to 1:3000) and severity of cystic fibrosis explain its inclusion in routine newborn screening. As with sickle cell disease, therapy that can prevent the ultimate complications of cystic fibrosis is not yet available. However, early and usually presymptomatic diagnosis through screening leads to early nutritional therapy, pancreatic enzyme replacement, and antibiotic prophylaxis for pulmonary infection. Data from newborn screening suggest better growth, prevention of vitamin deficiency in early infancy, and some advantage in terms of pulmonary status later in life in children identified by screening (Farrell et al, 2001; McKay and Wilcken, 2008; Southern et al, 2009). Other benefits of newborn screening are identifying the parents' genetic potential for producing additional children with cystic fibrosis and, through presymptomatic identification, allowing the family to avoid months or years of delay in the correct diagnosis of a child with chronic respiratory problems or poor growth (Farrell and Mischler, 1992).

The analyte marker in newborn screening for cystic fibrosis is increased immunoreactive trypsinogen (IRT). Transient increases in IRT are common in healthy newborns as a result of perinatal stress or for unknown reasons. Consequently, the rate of false-positive results in cystic fibrosis screening using only IRT is relatively high. To reduce this rate, screening programs have adopted a second-tier DNA analysis for a panel of cystic fibrosis mutations when the specimen has increased IRT (Ferec et al, 1995). Despite this two-tiered approach to screening, a substantial number of infants who do not have cystic fibrosis must undergo a sweat test or complete DNA sequencing of the cystic fibrosis gene before the diagnosis can be eliminated.

SPECIFIC ISSUES IN NEWBORN SCREENING

CRITERIA FOR NEWBORN SCREENING

Under the auspices of the World Health Organization, Wilson and Jungner (1968) published a set of criteria for screening for disease that have generally been accepted as required for population screening. The ten criteria state that (1) the condition be an important health problem, (2) there be accepted treatment, (3) facilities for diagnosis and treatment be available, (4) there be a recognizable latent or early symptomatic stage, (5) there should be a suitable test, (6) the test should be acceptable to the population, (7) the natural history of the condition should be understood, (8) there should be a policy prescribing whom to treat, (9) the cost of case finding should be economically balanced in relation to medical care as whole, and (10) case-finding should be a continuing process.

These criteria were developed at a time when newborn screening was in its beginning stages and with screening for adult disorders in mind. For example, regarding to the first criterion, Wilson and Jungner recognized that the term *important* is relative; whereas diabetes was prevalent, treatment might not influence outcome while PKU was rare, but it warranted screening because of the serious consequences that would be prevented by early discovery and treatment.

There is a question as to the current relevance of the Wilson-Jungner criteria for newborn screening. Ideally, all the criteria should be applied to newborn screening. However, advances in technology have caused this application to be questioned (Green and Pollitt, 1999; Levy, 1999). As an example, screening using MS/MS allows detection of serious disorders for which there may not be acceptable or agreed upon therapy, or in which the natural history is largely unknown, challenging the criterion that the disorder included in screening have acceptable treatment. How is this dilemma resolved? The answer is not yet available. It is hoped that the experience and findings from expanded newborn screening will be used to develop a new set of criteria that will apply to newborn screening. These criteria will likely retain the essence of the Wilson-Jungner compilation, but with important modifications that could be applied to any new screening venture.

FALSE-POSITIVE RESULTS

The majority of positive results in newborn screening, particularly when this result is only mildly or moderately abnormal, are not due to a disorder. Unfortunately, because screening is primarily based on a quantitative measure, false-positive results must be addressed. Metabolite concentrations vary among individuals, and the distribution curves of the markers from affected and unaffected populations are expected to be different (Figure 27-2). In screening, a value that separates the two distribution curves is established as a cutoff.

The cutoff values of the quantitative biomarkers are established by the individual screening laboratories, and they can vary among the different laboratories because of variations in the testing technology. In general, the cutoff value should be set such that it is greater than the 99th percentile of the concentration in normal neonates and less than the 5th percentile of the concentration in affected neonates (Rinaldo et al, 2006). However, for disorders that are extremely rare, the population of affected neonates may be so small that establishing an appropriate cutoff becomes a challenge. In such cases, the laboratory may empirically set a cutoff at 3 to 4 SD from the population mean and adjust the values with experience to minimize the false positives without compromising the sensitivity. Specimens in which the concentration crosses the established cut-off are considered screen-positive. The metabolite concentration in a majority of unaffected individuals is below the cutoff value, but in a small proportion it crosses this threshold. The positive screening results that are not caused by a disorder are considered false positives. Because of some degree of overlap in the distribution curves of the affected and unaffected populations, these false positives cannot be entirely eliminated without compromising the sensitivity of screening. Furthermore other physiologic factors, such as immaturity of enzymes or stress and therapeutic interventions, can skew

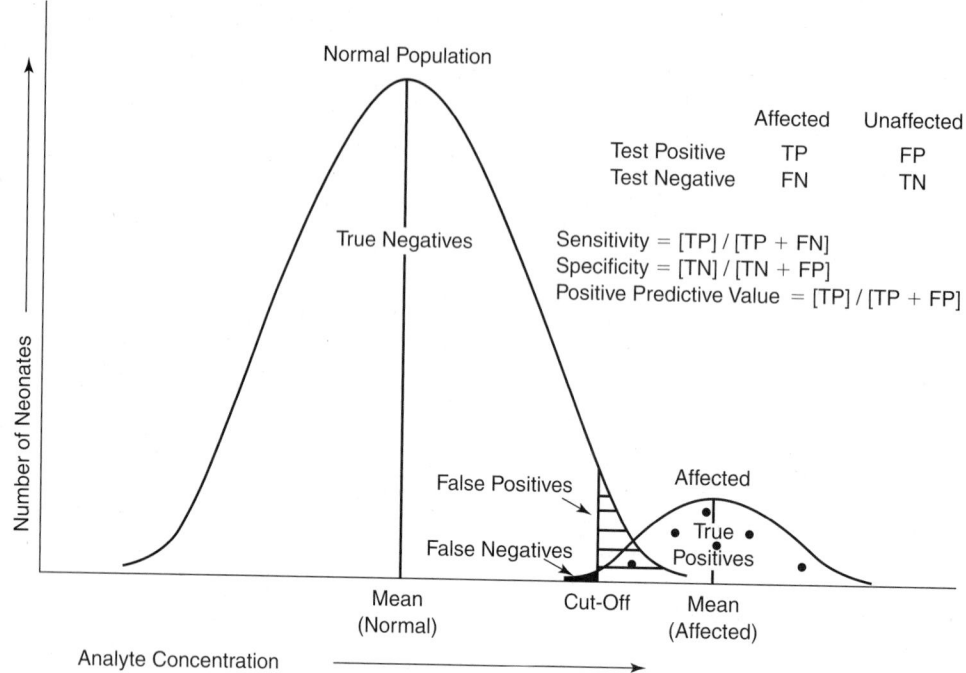

FIGURE 27-2 Distribution of quantitative markers measured in screening. For most conditions, the distribution in the unaffected or normal population overlaps that in the affected individuals. The number of false positives *(FP)*, false negatives *(FN)*, true positives *(TP)*, and true negatives *(TN)* depends on the established cutoff.

the concentrations of certain metabolites and lead to false-positive screening results. Currently, indicators measured using immunoassays (e.g.,17-OHP in CAH and T_4 in congenital hypothyroidism) or enzymatic activity (low GALT activity in galactosemia) are associated with the highest false-positive rates.

The false-positive results are more common in preterm and low-birthweight infants than in full-term infants. For example, up to 85% of preterm infants have transiently low T_4 levels (Paul et al, 1998). Transient increases in 17-OHP are another common abnormality in infants who are preterm or have low birthweights or have experienced perinatal stress (Pang and Shook, 1997). In addition, transient tyrosinemia is commonly observed in preterm and low-birthweight infants, although it can also occur in full-term infants (Levy et al, 1969).

Artifacts produced in the collection or transport of the Guthrie specimen account for some false-positive results. As mentioned in the discussion of the specimen collection procedure, collection of the specimen from a central line can result in mixing with amino acids in total parental nutrition solution and a false increase of amino acids in the specimen. Contamination with milk (or any drink containing milk) can result in a false elevation in galactose and the mistaken suspicion of galactosemia. Prolonged exposure to heat can reduce the activity of GALT in the specimen and produce a false impression of galactosemia when the enzyme assay is used to screen for this disorder. This error is common during the summer, especially when the specimens remain in a mailbox for a period of time. Some factors known to be associated with false positives are shown in Table 27-2 (Sahai et al, 2009).

With the substitution of MS/MS for the traditional bacterial or specific assays, such as those for PKU and MSUD, the number of false-positive results is distinctly lower. For

PKU screening, the false-positive rate is reported at 0.05% compared with 0.23% by earlier methods (Levy, 1998). In addition, with MS/MS the multiplexed approach allows for a profile of analytes rather than a single analyte level (e.g., phe/tyr ratio vs. only a phenylalanine level for PKU identification), further improving the specificity of screening (Chace et al, 1998; Schulze et al, 1999). Therefore the average positive predictive value for primary markers analyzed by MS/MS, previously reported to be 8% to 10% (Schulze et al, 2003; Wilken et al, 2003), can be improved substantially if the marker is evaluated in context with other metabolites that are screened or when a tiered approach is applied (Frazier et al, 2006; Sahai et al, 2007).

Second-tier assays, such as molecular assays for cystic fibrosis or secondary immunoassays for hypothyroidism, are commonly performed to reduce the false-positive rates for primary markers analyzed by immunoassays or enzymatic assays. Nevertheless, false-positive results cannot be entirely eliminated; therefore it is important to reassure the parents that not every abnormal result of newborn screening inevitably implies a disorder and that transient or nonspecific abnormalities are common. Although all infants with an abnormal screening result must undergo repeated testing, the families should be informed that an initial positive result might have no medical implications. This approach can alleviate excessive anxiety and prevent unnecessary diagnostic procedures and treatment.

INCREASED DETECTION BY SCREENING

For certain disorders screened by MS/MS, many more infants are identified than the expected numbers based on clinical identification. The greatest increases are in the fatty acid oxidation disorders, including short-chain acyl-CoA dehydrogenase deficiency SCADD, MCADD,

VLCADD, and carnitine deficiency, and in three organic acid disorders (glutaric acidemia type I, 3-methylcrotonyl-CoA carboxylase deficiency, and 3-ketothiolase deficiency; Wilken et al, 2003).

Although some of the excess detection by screening could represent cases that were symptomatic but not diagnosed clinically, it is likely that the greater part of the excess represents infants with benign or milder forms of the disorders who would not come to clinical attention. Notably, Spiekerkoetter et al (2003) identified a frequent mutation in asymptomatic patients with VLCADD detected by newborn screening, and Ensenauer et al (2004) found a common, mild, and perhaps asymptomatic mutation in patients with isovaleric acidemia identified by screening.

MISSED CASES

Infants with congenital hypothyroidism, PKU, intermittent MSUD, glutaric acidemia, tyrosinemia I, and other screened disorders have been undetected by newborn screening. Laboratory or program errors were reported as the most common cause of these missed cases (Holtzman et al, 1974). In some instances, a specimen was never collected, such as when infants were transferred to another hospital. However, in screening for a multitude of disorders, each with its own biomarker that varies with time and physiologic states, an occasional affected neonate may have normal biomarker concentrations in the newborn specimen simply because the timing of collection was not ideal for the particular condition. Therefore physicians must exercise clinical judgment and not fall into the trap of excluding a diagnosis because an infant has presumably been screened. Specific testing for metabolic and endocrine disorders should be performed in any infant or child with symptoms that suggest the presence of such a disorder, regardless of the assumed or actual newborn screening result.

THE FUTURE

Many factors are impinging on newborn screening, including rapidly advancing technology, new and increasingly available therapeutic approaches to previously untreatable disorders, and family support groups and influential citizens or legislators who are heavily invested in individual disorders that may or may not be ready for inclusion as screening tests. To address these pressures, a committee convened by the American College of Medical Genetics

and the Maternal and Child Health Division of the U.S. Department of Health and Human Services meets regularly to study newly proposed newborn screening tests (and those currently recommended) to judge their suitability for inclusion in the screening panels. One new candidate for screening severe combined immunodeficiency has passed through a careful vetting process and has been recommended for inclusion in the standard panel. Other candidate conditions being considered are the lysosomal storage disorders and adrenoleukodystrophy, for which enzyme or early bone marrow therapies are available and are being studied, Fragile X syndrome, and the Smith-Lemli-Opitz syndrome. These disorders will be judged on the basis of frequency, severity, availability of preemptive therapies, and the cost and robustness of the screening test itself. Some disorders have been included in isolated state panels on the basis of the political influences mentioned above.

Finally, there is the issue of retention of blood spots for future study. Despite multiple safeguards to protect the identity and anonymity of individuals, parents and civil libertarians are concerned that retention of these blood spots poses a threat to the privacy of individuals and that the specimens should be destroyed. If this view prevails, a resource of great value in the development of new and more effective tests, and one that is increasingly recognized as the avatar of personalized medicine, will be lost.

SUGGESTED READINGS

American College of Medical Genetics: Newborn Screening Expert Group. Newborn screening: toward a uniform panel and system, *Genet Med*, 2006.

Clinical and Laboratory Standards Institute: *Newborn screening for preterm, low birth weight and sick newborns: approved guideline. CLSI document I/LA31-A*, Wayne, Penn, 2009, Clinical and Laboratory Standards Institute.

Dobrowolski SF, Banas RA, Naylor EW, et al: DNA microarray technology for neonatal screening, *Acta Paediatr Suppl* 88:61-64, 1999.

Kaye CI, Accurso F, La Franchi S, et al: Newborn screening fact sheets, *Pediatrics* 118:e934-e963, 2006.

Matern D, Tortorelli S, Oglesbee D, et al: Reduction of the false-positive rate in newborn screening by implementation of MS/MS-based second-tier tests: the Mayo Clinic experience (2004-2007), *J Inherit Metab Dis* 30:585-592, 2007.

Pass KA, Neto EC: Update: newborn screening for endocrinopathies, *Endocrinol Metab Clin North Am* 38:827-837, 2009.

Rashed MS, Ozand PT, Bucknall MP, et al: Diagnosis of inborn errors of metabolism from blood spots by acylcarnitines and amino acids profiling using automated electrospray tandem mass spectrometry, *Pediatr Res* 38:324-331, 1995.

Sahai I, Marsden D: Newborn screening, *Crit Rev in Cli Lab Sci* 46:55-82, 2009.

Smith J, Kinney T: Clinical practice guidelines, quick reference guide for clinician: sickle cell disease: screening and management in newborns and infants, *Am Fam Physician* 48:95-102, 1993.

Wilken B, Wiley V, Hammond J, et al: Screening newborns for inborn errors of metabolism by tandem mass spectrometry, *N Engl J Med* 348:2304-2312, 2003.

Complete references used in this text can be found online at www.expertconsult.com

RESUSCITATION IN THE DELIVERY ROOM

Tina A. Leone and Neil N. Finer

The transition from fetal to neonatal life is a dramatic and complex process involving extensive physiologic changes that are most obvious at the time of birth. Individuals who care for newly born infants must monitor the progress of the transition and be prepared to intervene when necessary. In the majority of births this transition occurs without a requirement for any significant assistance. However, when the need for intervention arises, the presence of providers skilled in neonatal resuscitation can be life saving. Each year approximately 4 million children are born in the United States (Martin et al, 2008) and more 30-fold as many are born worldwide. It is estimated that approximately 5% to 10% of all births will require some form of resuscitation beyond basic care, making neonatal resuscitation the most frequently practiced form of resuscitation in medical care. Throughout the world approximately 1 million newborn deaths are associated with birth asphyxia (Lawn et al, 2005). Whereas early effective newborn resuscitation will not eliminate all early neonatal mortality, such intervention will save many lives and significantly reduce subsequent morbidities.

Attempts at reviving nonbreathing infants immediately after birth have occurred throughout recorded time with references in literature, religion, and early medicine. Although the organization and sophistication have changed, the basic principle and goal of initiating breathing have remained constant. During the last 20 years, attention has focused on the process of neonatal resuscitation. Resuscitation programs in other areas of medicine were initiated in the 1970s in an effort to improve knowledge about effective resuscitation and provide an action plan for early responders. The first such program was focused on adult cardiopulmonary resuscitation (Kattwinkel, 2006). These programs then began increasing in complexity and becoming more specific to different types of resuscitation needs. With the collaboration of the American Heart Association and the American Academy of Pediatrics, the Neonatal Resuscitation Program (NRP) was initiated in 1987 and was designed to address the specific needs of the newly born infant. The NRP textbook (Kattwinkel, 2006) now includes specific recommendations for the preterm infant. Various groups throughout the world also provide resuscitation recommendations that are more specific to the practices in certain regions. An international group of scientists, the International Liaison Committee on Resuscitation meets on a regular basis to review available resuscitation evidence for all the different areas of resuscitation and puts forth a summary of its review (Chamberlain, 2005).

The overall goal of the NRP is similar to other resuscitation programs, in that it intends to teach large groups of individuals of varying backgrounds the principles of resuscitation and provide an action plan for providers. Similarly, a satisfactory end result of resuscitation would be common to all forms of resuscitation, namely to provide adequate tissue oxygenation to prevent tissue injury and restore spontaneous cardiopulmonary function. However, when comparing neonatal resuscitation with other forms of resuscitation, several distinctions can be noted. First, the birth of an infant is a more predictable occurrence than most events that require resuscitation in an adult, such as an arrhythmia or a myocardial infarction. Although not every birth will require resuscitation, it is more reasonable to expect that skilled individuals can be present when the need for neonatal resuscitation arises. It is possible to anticipate with some accuracy which newborns will more likely require resuscitation based on perinatal factors and thus allow time for preparation. The second distinction of neonatal resuscitation compared with other forms of resuscitation involves the unique physiology involved in the normal fetal transition to neonatal life. The fetus exists in the protected environment of the uterus where temperature is closely controlled, the lungs are filled with fluid, continuous fetal breathing is not essential, and the gas exchange organ is the placenta. The transition that occurs at birth requires the newborn infant to increase heat production, initiate continuous breathing, replace the lung fluid with air, and significantly increase pulmonary blood flow so that gas exchange can occur in the lungs. The expectations for this transitional process and knowledge of how to effectively assist the process help to guide the current practice of newborn resuscitation.

FETAL TRANSITION TO EXTRAUTERINE LIFE

The complete transition from fetal to extrauterine life is complex and much more intricate than can be discussed in these few short paragraphs, but a basic knowledge of these processes will contribute to the understanding of the rationale for resuscitation practices. The key elements necessary for a successful transition to extrauterine life involve changes in thermoregulation, respiration, and circulation. In utero the fetal core temperature is approximately 0.5° C greater than the mother's temperature (Gunn and Gluckman, 1983). Heat is produced by metabolic processes and is lost over this small temperature gradient through the placenta and skin (Gilbert et al, 1985). After birth the temperature gradient between the infant and the environment becomes much greater and heat is lost through the skin by radiation, convection, conduction, and evaporation. The newborn infant must begin producing heat through other mechanisms such as lipolysis of brown adipose tissue (Dawkins and Scopes, 1965). If heat is lost at a pace greater than it is produced, the infant will develop hypothermia. Preterm infants are at particular risk because of increased heat loss through immature skin, a greater surface area–to–body weight ratio, and decreased brown adipose tissue stores.

The fetus lives in a fluid-filled environment, and the developing alveolar spaces are filled with lung fluid. Lung fluid production decreases in the days before delivery (Kitterman et al, 1979), and the remainder of lung fluid is reabsorbed into the pulmonary interstitial spaces after delivery (Bland, 1988). As the infant takes the first breaths after birth, a negative intrathoracic pressure of approximately 50 cm H_2O is generated (Vyas et al, 1986). The alveoli become filled with air, and with the help of pulmonary surfactant the lungs retain a small amount of air persisting at the end of exhalation, which is known as the *functional residual capacity* (FRC). Although the fetus makes breathing movements in utero, these efforts are intermittent and are not required for fetal gas exchange. Continuous spontaneous breathing is maintained after birth by several mechanisms, including the activation of chemoreceptors, the decrease in hormones that inhibit respirations, and the presence of natural environmental stimulation.

Spontaneous breathing can be suppressed at birth for several reasons, most critical of which is the presence of acidosis secondary to compromised fetal circulation. The natural history of the physiologic responses to asphyxia and acidosis has been described by researchers evaluating animal models. Geoffrey Dawes described the breathing response to acidosis in different animal species (Dawes, 1968). He noted that when pH was decreased, animals typically had a relatively short period of apnea followed by gasping. The gasping pattern then increased in rate until breathing ceased again for a second period of apnea. The physiologic effects that occur with worsening acidosis are noted in Figure 28-1. Dawes also noted that the first period of primary apnea could be reversed with stimulation, whereas the second period, secondary or terminal apnea, required assisted ventilation to ultimately establish spontaneous breathing. The first sign of improvement was noted to be an increase in heart rate. Further recovery was noted when the newborn begins gasping again. The secondary period of apnea varies in duration depending on the duration of asphyxia and degree of acidosis. In the clinical situation, the exact timing of onset of acidosis is generally unknown; therefore any observed apnea may be either primary or secondary. This finding is the basis of the resuscitation recommendation that stimulation may be attempted in the presence of apnea, but if not quickly successful, assisted ventilation should be initiated promptly. Without the presence of acidosis, a newborn may also develop apnea because of recent exposure to respiratory suppressing medications such as narcotics, anesthetics, and magnesium. These medications cross the placenta when given to the mother and may depress the newborn's respiratory drive, depending on the time of administration and dose.

Fetal circulation is unique because gas exchange takes place in the placenta. In the fetal heart, oxygenated blood returning via the umbilical vein is mixed with deoxygenated blood from the superior and inferior venae cavae, and it is distributed differentially throughout the body. The most oxygenated blood is directed toward the brain, and the most deoxygenated blood is directed toward the placenta. Thus blood returning from the placenta to the right atrium is preferentially streamed via the foramen ovale to the left atrium and ventricle and then to the ascending

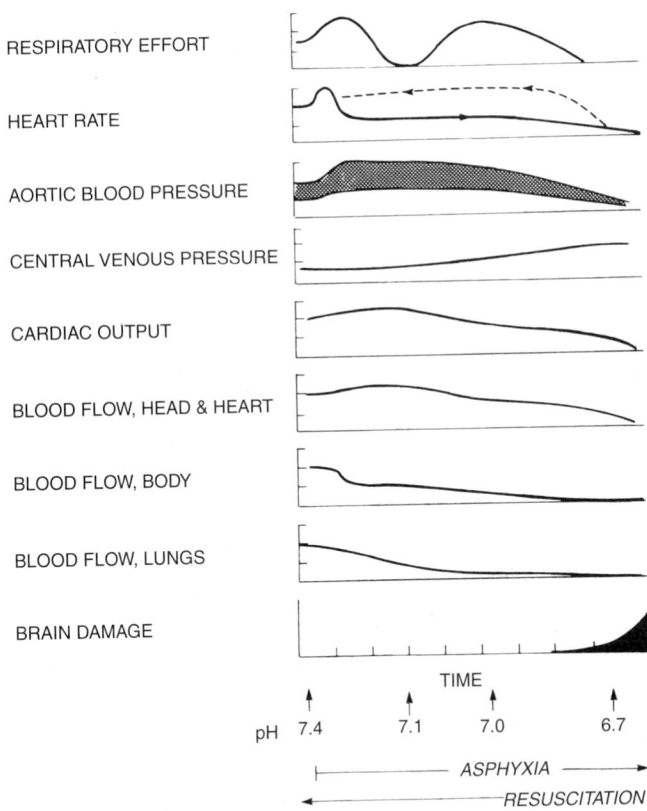

FIGURE 28-1 The sequence of cardiopulmonary changes with asphyxia and resuscitation. Time is on the horizontal axis. Asphyxia progresses from left to right; resuscitation proceeds from right to left. Units of time are not given. If there is complete interruption of respiratory gas exchange, the entire process of asphyxia from extreme left to right could occur in approximately 10 minutes. It could take much longer with an asphyxiating process that only partly interrupts gas exchange or does so completely, but only for repeated brief periods. With resuscitation, the process reverses, beginning at the point to which asphyxia has proceeded. (*Adapted from Dawes G: Foetal and neonatal physiology, Chicago, 1968, Year Book; and Avery GN: Neonatology, Philadelphia, 1987, JB Lippincott.*)

aorta, providing the brain with the most oxygenated blood. Fetal channels, including the ductus arteriosus and foramen ovale, allow most blood flow to bypass the lungs with their intrinsically high vascular resistance. As a result, pulmonary blood flow is approximately 8% of the total cardiac output. In the mature postnatal circulation, the lungs must receive 100% of the cardiac output. When the low-resistance placental circulation is removed after birth, the infant's systemic vascular resistance increases while the pulmonary vascular resistance begins to fall as a result of pulmonary expansion, increased arterial and alveolar oxygen tension, and local vasodilators. These changes result in a dramatic increase in pulmonary blood flow. The average fetal oxyhemoglobin saturation as measured in fetal lambs is approximately 50% (Nijland et al, 1995), but ranges in different sites within the fetal circulation between values of 20% and 80% (Teitel, 1988). The oxyhemoglobin saturation rises gradually over the first 5 to 15 minutes of life to 90% or greater as the air spaces are cleared of fluid. A diagram of the blood flow patterns in the fetus and normally transitioning newborn is shown in Figures 28-2 and 28-3. In the face of poor transition secondary to asphyxia,

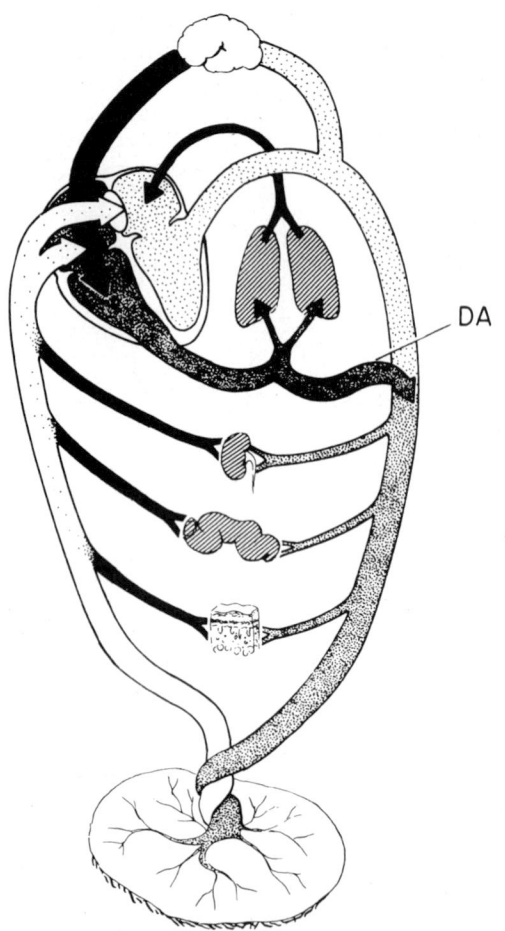

DA

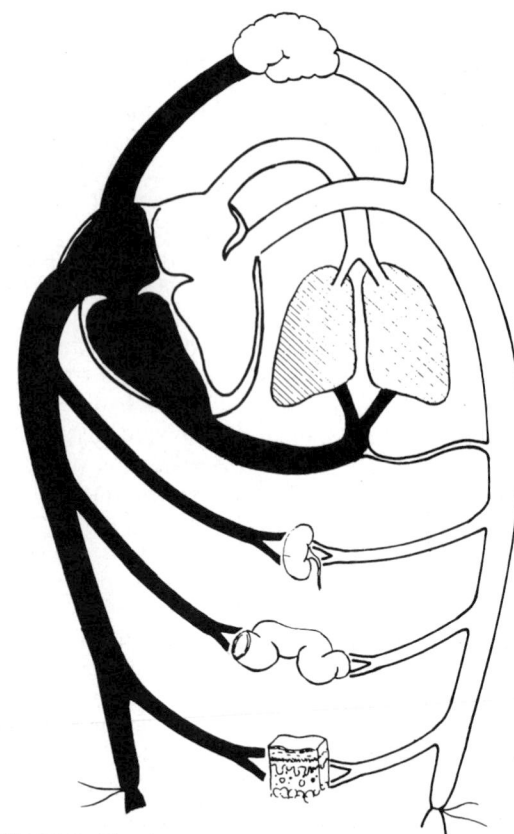

FIGURE 28-2 Fetal circulation. Oxygenated blood leaves the placenta by way of the umbilical vein (*vessel without stippling*). The blood flows into the portal sinus in the liver (not shown), and a variable portion of it perfuses the liver. The remainder passes from the portal sinus through the ductus venosus into the inferior vena cava, where it joins blood from the viscera (represented by the kidney, gut, and skin). Approximately half of the inferior vena cava flow passes through the foramen ovale to the left atrium, where it mixes with a small amount of pulmonary venous blood. This relatively well-oxygenated blood (*light stippling*) supplies the heart and brain by way of the ascending aorta. The other half of the inferior vena cava stream mixes with superior vena cava blood and enters the right ventricle (blood in the right atrium and ventricle has little oxygen, which is denoted by *heavy stippling*). Because the pulmonary arterioles are constricted, most of the blood in the main pulmonary artery flows through the ductus arteriosus (DA), so that the descending aorta's blood has less oxygen (*heavy stippling*) than blood in the ascending aorta (*light stippling*). (*From Avery GN: Neonatology, Philadelphia, 1987, JB Lippincott.*)

FIGURE 28-3 Circulation in the normal newborn. After expansion of the lungs and ligation of the umbilical cord, pulmonary blood flow increases and left atrial and systemic arterial pressures increase while pulmonary arterial and right heart pressures decrease. When the left atrial pressure exceeds right atrial pressure, the foramen ovale closes so that all of the inferior and superior vena cava blood leaves the right atrium, enters the right ventricle, and is pumped through the pulmonary artery toward the lung. With the increase in systemic arterial pressure and decrease in pulmonary arterial pressure, flow through the ductus arteriosus becomes left to right, and the ductus constricts and closes. The course of the circulation is the same as in the adult. (*From Avery GN:* Neonatology, *Philadelphia, 1987, JB Lippincott.*)

ENVIRONMENT AND PREPARATION

The environment in which the infant is born should facilitate the transition to neonatal life as much as possible and should be able to readily accommodate the needs of a resuscitation team when necessary. Hospitals vary in the approach to the details of how to prepare for resuscitation. For example, some hospitals have a separate room designated for resuscitation where the infant will be taken after birth, whereas others have the delivery room adjacent to the neonatal intensive care unit (NICU) and the infant is resuscitated in the NICU if necessary. Hospitals may bring all the necessary equipment into the delivery room when resuscitation is expected or have every delivery room equipped for any resuscitation. Wherever the resuscitation will take place, a few key elements must be considered. The room should be warm enough to prevent excessive newborn heat loss, bright enough to assess the infant's clinical status, and large enough to accommodate the necessary personnel and equipment to care for the baby.

When no added risks to the newborn are identified, the term birth frequently occurs without the attendance of a

meconium aspiration, pneumonia, or extreme prematurity, the lungs might not be able to develop efficient gas exchange; therefore the oxygen saturation might not increase as expected. In addition, in some situations the normal reduction in pulmonary vascular resistance does not fully occur, resulting in persistent pulmonary hypertension and decreased effective pulmonary blood flow with continued right-to-left shunting through the aforementioned fetal channels. Right-to-left shunting will lead to persistent hypoxemia and potentially to significant newborn illness requiring intensive care until the circulatory pattern adjusts to extrauterine life. The circulatory pattern associated with poor transition is noted in Figure 28-4.

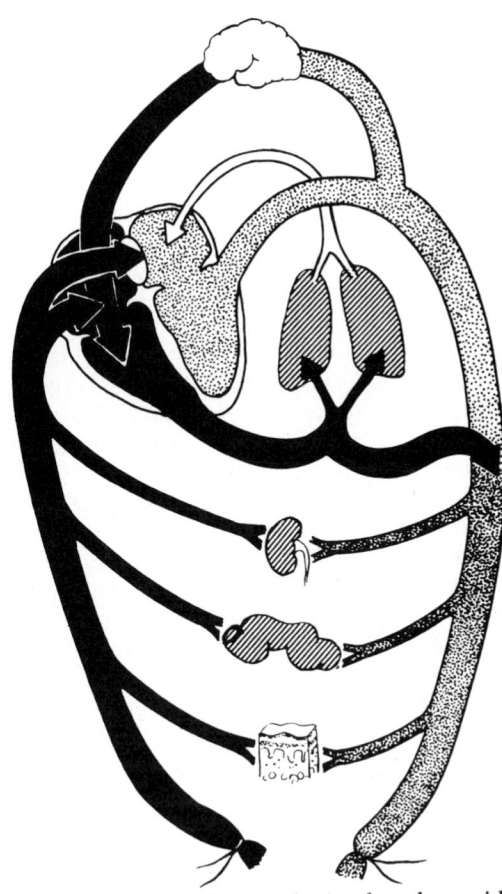

FIGURE 28-4 Circulation in an asphyxiated newborn with incomplete expansion of the lungs. Pulmonary vascular resistance is high, pulmonary blood flow is low (normal number of pulmonary veins), and flow through the ductus arteriosus is high. With little pulmonary arterial flow, left atrial pressure decreases below right atrial pressure, the foramen ovale opens, and vena cava blood flows through the foramen into the left atrium. Partially venous blood goes to the brain via the ascending aorta. The blood of the descending aorta that goes to the viscera has less oxygen than that of the ascending aorta (*heavy stippling*), because of the reverse flow through the ductus arteriosus. Therefore the circulation is the same as in the fetus, except that there is less well-oxygenated blood in the inferior vena cava and umbilical vein. (*From Avery GN: Neonatology, Philadelphia, 1987, JB Lippincott.*)

Maternal Factors	**Fetal Factors**	**Intrapartum Factors**
Maternal hypertension	Preterm delivery	Opiates in labor
Maternal infection	Breech presentation	Rupture of membranes >18 hours
Multiple gestation (preterm)	Shoulder dystocia	Meconium-stained amniotic fluid
		Nonreassuring fetal heart rate patterns
		Emergency cesarean section
		Prolapsed cord

TABLE 28-1 Risk Factors for Neonatal Resuscitation

Data from Aziz K et al: Ante- and intra-partum factors that predict increased need for neonatal resuscitation, *Resuscitation* 79:444-452, 2008.

specific neonatal resuscitation team. However, it is recommended that one individual be present who is responsible only for the infant and can quickly alert a neonatal resuscitation team if necessary. Even the best neonatal resuscitation triage systems will not anticipate the need for resuscitation in all cases. Using a retrospective risk assessment scoring system, 6% of newborns requiring resuscitation were not be identified based on risk factors (Smith et al, 1985). Similarly, a recent review found that when a risk-based determination of neonatal resuscitation team attendance at deliveries was used, 22% of infants at attended deliveries required at least assisted ventilation (Aziz et al, 2008). These investigators found that the most significant risk factors were preterm birth, emergency cesarean section, and meconium-stained amniotic fluid. Other significant risk factors for the need for resuscitation are listed in Table 28-1. Antenatal determination of risk allows the resuscitation team to be present for the delivery and to be more thoroughly prepared for the situation.

The composition of the neonatal resuscitation team will vary tremendously among institutions. Probably the most important factor in how well a team functions is how the group has prepared for the delivery. Preparation involves both the immediate tasks of readying equipment and personnel for an individual situation as well as the more broad institutional preparation of training team members and providing appropriate space and equipment. We believe that when there is a strong suspicion that the newborn infant will be born in a compromised state, a minimum of three team members should be present, including one member with significant previous experience leading neonatal resuscitations. Each team member is assigned tasks that are performed on a regular basis. The leader is expected to ensure that the appropriate interventions are performed and that they are performed well. All team members are encouraged and expected to speak up if a problem is noticed or if they believe an alternate course would be beneficial. It seems logical that teams that regularly work together and divide tasks in a routine manner will have a better chance of functioning smoothly during a critical situation. Institutions can facilitate team readiness with regular review of practices and mock codes or simulator training to practice uncommon scenarios. In our institution, University of California San Diego (UCSD), video-taped resuscitations are reviewed twice monthly with representatives from all disciplines involved in the resuscitation team (Carbine et al, 2000); this is done as a quality-assurance procedure and allows for ongoing identification of areas needing improvement. In addition, this practice provides an opportunity for education and discussion about potential solutions to repetitive problems of newborn resuscitation. UCSD also instituted a supplemental training program for pediatric trainees to obtain experience in a preclinical situation (Garey et al). These training sessions allow adequate time to review scenarios in detail, and trainees are given the opportunity to prepare and operate the equipment and practice procedures on an individualized basis. Others have used simulators to provide additional resuscitation training (Halamek, 2008). All of these training elements help to prepare teams for future resuscitations.

When preparing for a resuscitation that will occur in the immediate short-term period, additional aspects must be addressed. The most important element in preparing for the resuscitation is the discussion that occurs among the team members who will participate. This discussion, known as a *prebrief*, is an essential part of improving communication during resuscitation and involves reviewing the clinical information, reviewing the available resources and introducing the individuals who will participate, assigning tasks to individuals, and making equipment as readily available as possible. A discussion of the overall plan will help team members know what to expect and how to address problems that could occur. We have formalized this process by creating a prebrief checklist for the team to review while preparing for the delivery. Checklists are considered one of the most important methods of preventing medical errors. A briefing after the resuscitation (i.e., a postbrief) allows team members to address positive and negative aspects of the resuscitation. This briefing is an important element in the preparation for future resuscitations, because team members can immediately identify how to improve the care being provided. An example of our current checklist with prebrief and postbrief documentation is shown in Figure 28-5. To better train the staff in these techniques, UCSD instituted training in crew resource management, a methodology developed for training air crews from the late 1970s that evolved from a careful evaluation of the role of human error in air crashes (Cooper et al, 1980).

ASSESSMENT

Immediately after birth the infant's condition is evaluated by general observation and measurement of specific parameters. Typically a healthy newborn will cry vigorously and maintain adequate respirations. The color will transition from blue to pink over the first 2 to 5 minutes, the heart rate will remain in the range of 140 to 160 beats/min, and the infant will demonstrate adequate muscle tone with some flexion of the extremities. The overall assessment of an infant who is having difficulty with the transition to extrauterine life will often reveal apnea, bradycardia, hypotonia, and cyanosis or pallor. After the initial steps of resuscitation, interventions are based mainly on the evaluation of respiratory effort and heart rate, which need to be assessed continually throughout the resuscitation. Heart rate can be monitored by auscultation or palpation of the cord pulsations, with auscultation being the more reliable method (Owen and Wyllie, 2004). The continuous monitoring of this parameter gives providers an ongoing indication of the effectiveness of interventions.

The use of more sophisticated monitoring devices, such as a pulse oximeter or electrocardiographic leads, can be helpful during resuscitation. A pulse oximeter can provide the resuscitation team with a continuous audible and visual indication of the newborn's heart rate throughout the various steps of resuscitation while allowing all team members to perform other tasks. In addition, the pulse oximeter can be used as a more accurate measure of oxygenation than the evaluation of color alone, which is an unreliable measure of the infant's oxygen saturation (O'Donnell et al, 2007). Whenever interventions beyond brief positive-pressure ventilation by mask are required, a pulse oximeter should be considered. Electrocardiographic monitoring may be helpful, but at this point has been infrequently evaluated in the delivery room and does not provide information about oxygenation.

The overall assessment of a newborn was quantified by Virginia Apgar in the 1950s with the Apgar score (Apgar, 1953). The score describes the infant's condition at the time it is assigned and consists of a 10-point scale, with a maximum of 2 points assigned for each of the following categories: respirations, heart rate, color, tone, and reflex irritability. Table 28-2 shows the detailed components of the score. Although the components of the score include items that are assessed for determining interventions, the score itself is not used to determine the need for interventions. The score was initially intended to provide a uniform, objective assessment of the infant's condition and was used as a tool to compare different practices, especially obstetric anesthetic practices. Despite the intent of objectivity, there is often disagreement in score assignment among various practitioners (O'Donnell et al, 2006). Low scores are associated with increased risk of neonatal mortality (Casey et al, 2001), but have not been predictive of neurodevelopmental outcome (Nelson and Ellenberg, 1981). Interpreting the score when interventions are being provided may be difficult, and current recommendations suggest that clinicians should document the interventions used at the time the score is assigned (American Academy of Pediatrics Committee on Fetus and Newborn and American College of Obstetricians and Gynecologists and Committee on Obstetric Practice, 2006).

INITIAL STEPS: TEMPERATURE MANAGEMENT AND MAINTAINING THE AIRWAY

In the first few seconds after birth, all infants are evaluated for signs of life and a determination of the need for further assistance is made. This evaluation is done both formally as described in the NRP and informally as the initial care providers observe the infant in the first few moments of life. When the determination is made that further assistance and formal resuscitation are necessary, the infant is then placed on a radiant warmer and positioned appropriately for resuscitation to proceed. Appropriate positioning includes placing the infant supine on the warmer in such a way that care providers have easy access. In addition, the head should be in a neutral or "sniffing" position to facilitate maintenance of an open airway. Frequently the oropharynx contains fluid that can be removed by suctioning with a standard bulb syringe.

An infant born through meconium-stained amniotic fluid is at risk for aspirating meconium and developing significant pulmonary disease, known as *meconium aspiration syndrome*, which may also be accompanied by persistent pulmonary hypertension. For many years, routine management of all infants with meconium-stained amniotic fluid included suctioning of the mouth and pharynx once the head was delivered, but before the shoulders were delivered, and endotracheal intubation and tracheal suctioning in an attempt to remove any meconium from the trachea and prevent the development of meconium

DR Resuscitation Checklist Patient Label Here

Pre-Resuscitation Briefing

Leader ____________________________

MD(s) ____________________________

RN(s) ____________________________

RT(s) ____________________________

- ☐ Introductions/Roles
- ☐ Discuss Plan, communication expectations
    - o Special considerations?"
    - o Additional personnel/equipment?
    - o **"If any team member sees any developing problem or concern, I want to have it brought to my attention as soon as possible."**
    - o **Please call back all orders from Leader (e.g. "PIP is now 40")**

Pre-Resuscitation Checklist

Lead Resuscitator

- ❖ **Need urgent assistance, call x10770**
- ☐ Ensure briefing completed and introductions done
- ☐ Ensure RT checklist done
- ☐ Ensure RN checklist done
- ☐ Check status with resident receiving infant

Respiratory Therapy

- Brings RT bag (bring surfactant for < 28 weeks)
- Sets up Neopuff (30/5 and FiO2 .40, flow 8-10), appropriate masks
- Pedicap
- Sets up hand bag, checked (black bag if expecting difficult resus.)
- Intubation equipment checked, appropriate sized tubes
- Suction set at 80-100 mmHg, catheters, meconium aspirator if needed
- Pulse ox on and probe out
- NICO ET CO2 sensor
- Turn on video recorder

Nursing

- If crash C/section (call 2nd RN/MD) ensure line is set up, Epi drawn up.
- Barney bag
- Radiant warmer on MANUAL at 100%, probe and cover available, hat
- Stethescope
- Plastic wrap for < 28 weeks, Chemical mattress for <25 weeks
- ECG Leads

Debrief

Did we have all the information we need to admit this patient? Y/N

What did we do well? (Resident, Nurse, RT, Fellow, Attending in that order)

____

What can we improve upon? ____________________________

Do we need follow-up on any items: ____________________________

FIGURE 28-5 Delivery room resuscitation checklist form.

TABLE 28-2 The Apgar Score

Feature Evaluated	0 Points	1 Point	2 Points
Heart rate (beats/min)	0	<100	>100
Respiratory effort	Apnea	Irregular, shallow, or gasping respirations	Vigorous and crying
Color	Pale, blue	Pale or blue extremities	Pink
Muscle tone	Absent	Weak, passive tone	Active movement
Reflex irritability	Absent	Grimace	Active avoidance

aspiration syndrome. Routine suctioning of the mouth and nose before delivery of the shoulders has been shown to be of no benefit in decreasing the incidence of meconium aspiration syndrome, ventilation for meconium aspiration syndrome, or mortality (Vain et al, 2004). Recognizing that intubation may not be necessary for all infants and that the procedure may be associated with complications, a more selective approach was evaluated in randomized controlled trials (Wiswell et al, 2000). A metaanalysis of studies that have evaluated this question supported the notion that universal endotracheal suctioning does not result in a lower incidence of meconium aspiration syndrome or improve mortality compared with selective endotracheal suctioning (Halliday, 2000). The likelihood that an infant with meconium-stained amniotic fluid will develop meconium aspiration syndrome is increased in the presence of fetal distress. The selective approach to endotracheal suctioning requires a quick evaluation of the infant after delivery. If the infant is vigorous with good respiratory effort, normal heart rate, and normal tone, the steps of resuscitation proceed as usual. However, if the infant is not vigorous and has poor respiratory effort, a heart rate less than 100 beats/min, or decreased tone, rapid endotracheal intubation for suctioning is currently indicated, although this has not been evaluated in a standardized manner. When endotracheal intubation for suctioning is performed, the resuscitation team must continue to adequately monitor the infant and may need to proceed quickly to providing assisted ventilation if bradycardia is present.

Whereas temperature control is important for all newborn infants, it is particularly important for the extremely preterm infant. Preterm infants are commonly admitted to the NICU with core temperatures well below 37° C. In a population-based analysis of all infants younger than 26 weeks' gestation, more than one third of these preterm infants had an admission temperature of less than 35° C (Costeloe et al, 2000). More disturbing is the fact that these infants with hypothermia on admission survived less often than those with admission temperatures greater than 35° C. Admission temperatures can be improved in preterm infants by immediately covering the infant's body with polyethylene wrap before drying the infant (Vohra et al, 2004). With this approach the infant's head is left out of the wrap and is dried, but the body is not dried before wrap application. Other measures for maintaining infant temperatures include performing resuscitations in a room that is kept at an ambient temperature of approximately 27° to 30° C, using radiant warmers with servo-controlled temperature probes placed on the infant within minutes of delivery, and the use of accessory prewarmed mattress or heating pads for the tiniest infants. Hats are routinely used as a method of decreasing heat loss, but they have not been shown to be consistently effective (McCall et al, 2008). It is important to note that as a required safety feature, radiant warmers substantially decrease their power output after 15 minutes of continuous operation at full power. If this decrease in power is unrecognized, the infant will be exposed to much less radiant heat. By applying the temperature probe and using the warmer in servo-controlled mode, the temperature output will adjust as needed and the power will not automatically decrease.

ASSISTING VENTILATION

As the newborn infant begins breathing and replaces the lung fluid with air, the lungs become inflated and an FRC is established and maintained. With inadequate development of FRC, the infant will not be able to oxygenate and will develop bradycardia if inadequate FRC is prolonged. Providing assisted ventilation when the infant's spontaneous breathing is inadequate is probably the most important step in newborn resuscitation. The indications for providing assisted ventilation (positive-pressure ventilation) include apnea or bradycardia of less than 100 beats/min. Positive-pressure ventilation can be delivered noninvasively with a pressure delivery device and a face mask or invasively with the same pressure delivery device and an endotracheal tube. Pressure delivery devices can include self-inflating bags, flow-inflating or anesthesia bags, and t-piece resuscitators, each with its own advantages and disadvantages. The self-inflating bag is easy to use for inexperienced personnel and will work in the absence of a gas source. However, the self-inflating bag requires a reservoir to provide nearly 100% oxygen and does not consistently provide adequate positive end expiratory pressure (PEEP). These devices can deliver very high pressure if not used carefully. Although they have pressure blow-off valves, these valves do not always open at the target blow-off pressures (Finer et al, 1986). An anesthesia bag or flow-inflating bag requires a gas source for use, allows the operator to vary delivery pressures continuously based on the felt compliance, but requires significant practice to develop expertise. However, using a test lung and intermittent airway occlusion, experienced anesthesiologists were unable to recognize the increased resistance from an airway obstruction using only their hands (Spears et al, 1991). A t-piece resuscitator is easy to use, requires a gas source, and delivers the most consistent levels of pressure, but requires intentional effort to vary the pressure levels (Hoskyns et al, 1987). The flow-inflating bag and t-piece resuscitator allow the operator to deliver continuous positive airway pressure (CPAP) or PEEP relatively easily (Bennett et al, 2005; Finer et al, 2001).

A level of experience is required to perform assisted ventilation using a face mask and resuscitation device, and this is especially true for an infant with extremely low birthweight. It is important to maintain an open airway for pressure to be transmitted to the lungs. The procedure of obtaining and maintaining an open airway includes at minimum clearing fluid with a suction device, holding the head in a neutral position, and sometimes lifting the jaw slightly anteriorly. The face mask must make an adequate seal with the face in order for air to pass to the lungs effectively. No device will adequately inflate the lungs if there is a large leak present between the mask and the face. Wood et al (2008) measured face mask leaks of more than 55% when participants were evaluated, providing positive pressure to manikins at baseline. The amount of the leak was able to be decreased to approximately 30% with specific instruction (Wood et al, 2008). Until recently there were no masks that were small enough to provide an adequate seal over the mouth and nose for the smallest infants. Such masks are now readily available and facilitate bag-mask resuscitation of small infants. Signs that the airway is open and air is being delivered to the lungs include visual inspection of chest rise with each breath and improvement in the clinical condition, including heart rate and color. The use of a colorimetric carbon dioxide detector during bagging will allow confirmation that gas exchange is occurring by the observed color change of the device, or it will alert the operator of an obstructed airway by not changing color (Leone et al, 2006). Airway obstruction is common in the preterm infant during positive-pressure ventilation immediately after birth (Finer et al, 2009). It is important to remember that these devices will not change color in the absence of pulmonary blood flow, as occurs with inadequate cardiac output. At times, multiple maneuvers are required to achieve an open airway, such as readjusting the head and mask positions, choosing a mask of more appropriate size, and further suctioning of the pharynx. Alternate methods of providing an open airway include the use of a nasopharyngeal tube (Lindner et al, 1999), a laryngeal mask airway device (Grein and Weiner, 2005), or an endotracheal tube.

The amount of pressure provided with each breath during assisted ventilation is critical to establishing lung inflation and therefore adequate oxygenation. Although it is important to provide adequate pressure for ventilation, excessive pressure can contribute to lung injury. Achieving the correct balance of these goals is not simple and is an area of resuscitation that requires more study. A single specific level of inspiratory pressure will never be appropriate for every baby. Initial inflation pressures of 25 to 30 cm H_2O are probably adequate for most term infants. The NRP textbook (Kattwinkel, 2006) recommends initial pressures of 20 to 25 cm H_2O for preterm infants. The first few breaths may require increased pressure if lung fluid has not been cleared, as occurs when the infant does not initiate spontaneous breathing. Newborn infants with specific pulmonary disorders such as pneumonia or pulmonary hypoplasia also frequently require increased inspiratory pressure. It has been shown that using enough pressure to produce visible chest rise is associated with hypocarbia on admission blood gas evaluation (Tracy et al, 2004), and excessive pressure may decrease the effectiveness of surfactant therapy (Bjorklund et al, 1997). It may be possible to establish FRC without increasing peak inspiratory pressures by providing a few prolonged inflations (3 to 5 seconds of inspiration), although the use of prolonged inflations has not been associated with better outcomes than conventional breaths during resuscitation (Lindner et al, 2005). Choosing the actual initial inspiratory pressure is less important than continuously assessing the progress of the intervention. A manometer in the circuit during assisted ventilation provides the clinician with an indication of the administered pressure, although if the airway is blocked this pressure is not delivered to the lungs. The volume of air delivered to the lungs seems to be more important than the absolute pressure delivered in the development of lung injury. Tidal volume can be monitored with respiratory function monitors that are placed in the respiratory circuit (Schmolzer et al, 2010). The most critical component of continued assessment is evaluation of the infant's response to the intervention. If the condition of the infant does not improve after initiating ventilation, then the ventilation is most likely inadequate. In our experience the two most likely reasons for inadequate ventilation are a blocked airway and insufficient inspiratory pressure. The occluded airway can be noted using a colorimetric carbon dioxide device as described previously, and frequently it can be corrected with changes in position or suctioning while inadequate pressure is corrected by adjusting the ventilating device.

The use of continuous pressure throughout the breathing cycle seems to be beneficial for establishing FRC and improving surfactant function (Hartog et al, 2000; Michna et al, 1999; Siew et al, 2009); this is accomplished during assisted ventilation with the use of PEEP or with CPAP when

additional inspiratory pressure is not needed. In the absence of PEEP, a lung that has been inflated with assisted inspiratory pressure will lose on expiration most of the volume that had been delivered on inspiration. This pattern of repeated inflation and deflation is frequently thought to be associated with lung injury. In preterm infants, a general approach of using CPAP as a primary mode of respiratory support in NICUs has been associated with a low incidence of chronic lung disease (Ammari et al, 2005; Avery et al, 1987; Van Marter et al, 2000; Vanpee et al, 2007). Recently, te Pas and Walther (2007) evaluated a ventilation strategy that included the use of a I-piece resuscitator and a nasopharyngeal tube to deliver a prolonged breath followed by CPAP, compared with the use of a self-inflating bag to deliver positive pressure ventilation when needed without any CPAP provided until infants reached the NICU. Infants treated with the prolonged breath and CPAP required less endotracheal intubation and had lower rates of bronchopulmonary dysplasia. The use of CPAP compared with endotracheal intubation and mechanical ventilation as the initial mode of respiratory support was evaluated in the Continuous Positive Airway Pressure or Intubation at Birth (COIN) trial (Morley et al, 2008), but the intervention did not begin until after 5 minutes of life and therefore cannot inform the decision about the use of these therapies as immediate resuscitative interventions. The recently completed Surfactant Positive Airway Pressure and Pulse Oximetry Trial (SUPPORT Study Group 2010. Available at http://clinicaltrials.gov/ct2/show/NCT0023333 24?term=neonatal+respiratory+support&rank=15) evaluated the use of CPAP versus intubation and surfactant use in the first hour of life as the primary respiratory support for preterm infants. These trials suggest that CPAP is beneficial for improving some short-term outcomes associated with prematurtiy. Although these trials do not evaluate these therapies specifically in the resuscitation period, the respiratory support provided shortly after birth should probably mimic the support provided in the NICU after delivery.

If assisted ventilation is necessary for a prolonged period of time or if other resuscitative measures have been unsuccessful, ventilation must be provided by a more secure device such as an endotracheal tube. If it has been difficult to maintain an open airway while ventilating via a face mask, an appropriately placed endotracheal tube will provide a stable airway. This stability will allow more consistent delivery of gas to the lungs and therefore provide for the ability to establish and maintain FRC. At this time intubation is required for administering surfactant, and it can be used to administer other medications such as epinephrine if necessary for resuscitation. Finally, for non-vigorous infants born through meconium-stained amniotic fluid, intubation is performed for suctioning of the airway.

The intubation procedure is often critical for successful resuscitation, requires a significant amount of skill and experience to perform reliably, and may be associated with serious complications. The placement of a laryngoscope in the pharynx often produces vagal nerve stimulation, which leads to bradycardia. A photograph of the desired view of the larynx is shown in Figure 28-6. Assisted ventilation must be paused for the procedure, which if prolonged can lead to hypoxemia and bradycardia. Intubation has been shown to increase blood pressure

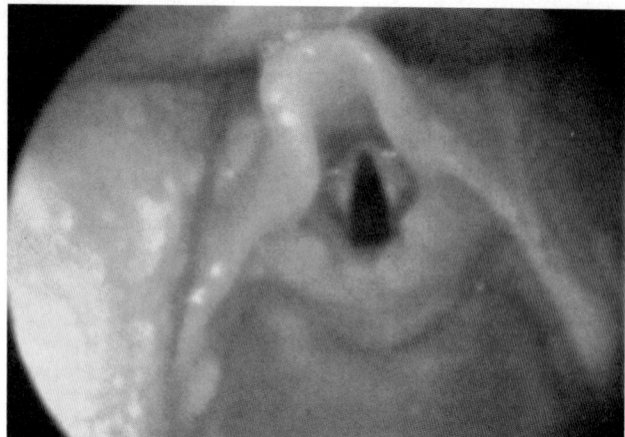

FIGURE 28-6 *(See also Color Plate 18.)* View of the glottis and vocal cords as the laryngoscope is gently lifted. *(From American Heart Association, American Academy of Pediatrics: Kattwinkel J, editor: Neonatal resuscitation textbook, ed 5, Elk Grove Village, Ill., 2006, American Academy of Pediatrics.)*

and intracranial pressure (Kelly and Finer, 1984). Trauma to the mouth, pharynx, vocal cords, and trachea are all possible complications of intubation. Performing the intubation procedure when the infant already has bradycardia and hypoxemia can lead to further decline in heart rate and oxygenation (O'Donnell et al, 2006). In addition, hypoxia and bradycardia are more likely when intubation attempts are prolonged beyond 30 seconds. Therefore it is most appropriate to make an attempt to stabilize the infant with noninvasive ventilation before performing the procedure, limiting each attempt to 30 seconds or less (Lane et al, 2004), and allow time for the infant to recover with noninvasive ventilation between attempts. If misplacement of the endotracheal tube in the esophagus goes unrecognized, the infant may experience further clinical deterioration. Clinical signs that the endotracheal tube has been correctly placed in the trachea include auscultation of breath sounds over the anterolateral aspects of the lungs (near the axilla), mist visible in the endotracheal tube, chest rise, and clinical improvement in heart rate and color or oxygen saturation. The use of a colorimetric carbon dioxide detector to confirm intubation significantly decreases the amount of time necessary to determine correct placement of the endotracheal tube from approximately 40 seconds to less than 10 seconds (Aziz et al, 1999; Repetto et al, 2001); this is the primary method of determining endotracheal tube placement.

Successful placement of the endotracheal tube is not always easy and is sometimes not possible. Airway anomalies may make alternate methods of airway management necessary. A laryngeal mask airway is one such alternative that has been described for use in patients with Pierre Robin sequence or other airway anomalies (Yao et al, 2004). Some practitioners have reported using the laryngeal mask airway for all positive-pressure delivery after birth, with success noted in infants as small as 1.2 kg (Gandini and Brimacombe, 1999). Administration of medications including surfactant and epinephrine through this device has undergone preliminary investigations (Chen et al, 2008; Trevisanuto et al, 2005).

TRANSITIONAL OXYGENATION AND OXYGEN USE

It is critical to remember that fetal arterial oxygen levels are much lower than newborn arterial oxygen levels. The transition from fetal to newborn levels does not take place instantaneously. Using pulse oximetry in the immediate newborn period, several investigators have established that this transition with an ultimate oxygen saturation level greater than 90% takes 5 to 15 minutes to occur in infants who do not otherwise require resuscitation. For term and preterm nonresuscitated infants, the median interquartile range (IQR) of oxygen saturation at 3 minutes was 76% (64% to 87%) and at 5 minutes was 90% (79% to 91%; Kamlin et al, 2006). Expected oxygen saturation levels are slightly lower for preterm compared with term and for infants delivered via cesarean section compared with those delivered vaginally (Rabi et al, 2006). Oxygen saturation levels measured in preductal sites are 5% to 10% higher than those measured from postductal sites for approximately 15 minutes of life (Mariani et al, 2007). A great deal of variability occurs in the saturation values among different healthy individuals during the first 5 minutes of life, but a resuscitation team can expect that there be a steady, albeit slow, increase in levels over several minutes. If values are below a threshold at different time points or not progressively increasing, intervention should be considered.

The use of pure oxygen for ventilation became routine practice in resuscitation simply because it seemed logical that oxygen would be beneficial. However, the recognition that oxygen could also be toxic led some investigators to question this previously well accepted practice. The toxicity of oxygen is anticipated when the cellular antioxidant capacity is impaired, as occurs during the reperfusion phase following an hypoxic-ischemic insult. After animal studies showed the potential harmful effects of oxygen (Poulsen et al, 1993; Rootwelt et al, 1992), clinical trials were conducted to evaluate the effects of oxygen use during resuscitation of depressed infants. Several worldwide trials have compared the use of pure (100%) oxygen with room (ambient) air (21% oxygen) as the initial ventilating gas for asphyxiated newborns. These trials found that air was as successful as oxygen in achieving resuscitation, and infants resuscitated with air had a shorter time to initiate spontaneous breathing and less evidence of oxidative stress (Ramji et al, 2003; Saugstad et al, 1998; Vento et al, 2001, 2003). Metaanalyses of several of the trials indicated that infants resuscitated with air had a lower risk of mortality than those resuscitated with pure oxygen (Rabi et al, 2007; Tan et al, 2005). These trials have been criticized because they were not all strictly randomized, and some sites were in developing countries; however, metaanalysis of the strictly randomized trials, which were mostly done in European centers, demonstrates significant benefit for survival with the use of air compared with pure oxygen (Saugstad et al, 2008).

The preterm infant may be more susceptible to any harmful effects of excessive oxygen exposure, because of decreased antioxidant enzyme capacity. Some of the infants in the previous oxygen trials were preterm, but few weighed less than 1000 g. Review of the outcomes for preterm infants (<37 weeks' gestation) demonstrated an even greater reduction in death for those initially resuscitated with room air compared with oxygen (Saugstad et al, 2005). NICUs generally attempt to reduce oxygen toxicity by limiting the amount of oxygen administered to newborns using an upper limit for oxygen saturation and adjusting supplemented oxygen levels to maintain saturation levels within that limit. The unlimited use of oxygen during resuscitation exposes the preterm infant to higher oxygen saturation levels than would routinely be accepted in the NICU. Several small trials of oxygen use during resuscitation of preterm infants have been performed in the last 3 years. Among 42 preterm infants younger than 32 weeks' gestation treated with either pure oxygen for 5 minutes or a targeted oxygen strategy beginning with 21% oxygen, all infants were provided some level of supplemental oxygen (Wang et al, 2008). Infants initiated on pure oxygen had higher pulse oximeter saturation (Spo_2) levels during transition, but did not have any differences in heart rate, need for intubation, or survival. The infants provided air from the start of resuscitation all required an increase in inspired oxygen to obtain the specified oxygen saturation targets. Using 30% versus 90% oxygen at the start of resuscitation and adjusting the concentration based on the clinical status of the infant, Escrig et al (2008) found that infants initially receiving 30% oxygen had lower overall exposure to oxygen without any adverse effects. The group receiving 30% oxygen received increased oxygen concentrations up to approximately 55% at 5 minutes, but both groups received similar oxygen concentrations after 4 minutes of life, with a level of approximately 35% by 15 minutes of life (Escrig et al, 2008). In a more recent study, these investigators also reported a decrease in the incidence of bronchopulmonary dysplasia in infants initially receiving 30% oxygen compared with 90% oxygen (Vento et al, 2009). Finally, the Room Air versus Oxygen Administration during Resuscitation (ROAR) study was a blinded, randomized controlled trial in 106 infants at 32 weeks' gestation or less comparing three oxygen strategies: one group received 100% throughout (HOB), one received 100% initially (MOB), and one received 21% (LOB) initially; the last two groups had the oxygen concentration titrated to keep Spo_2 at 85% to 92%. Spo_2 levels were below the specified target range 61% of the time in the LOB group and were above the target range 49% of the time in the HOB group (p <0.001; Rabi et al, 2008). Larger trials of preterm infants treated with different oxygen strategies are necessary to determine the long-term effects of resuscitation with different oxygen concentrations. Oxygen use in the first minutes of life could affect survival and common neonatal morbidities associated with prematurity and free radical disease, such as neurodevelopmental impairment, retinopathy of prematurity, bronchopulmonary dysplasia, and necrotizing enterocolitis.

The use of oxygen concentrations between 21% and 100% requires compressed air and a blender. Different organizations throughout the world have provided differing recommendations on the use of oxygen for newborn resuscitation. The most recent review of evidence for the updated NRP guidelines suggest that resuscitation could begin with either air or blended oxygen; if blended oxygen is unavailable, air is preferred to pure oxygen. The suggested goal for oxygen saturation values is the IQR at each minute (Kattwinkel et al, 2010). Our approach has been to begin with 40% oxygen and adjust slowly, attempting to mimic the gradual transition in Spo_2 values that occur in healthy newborns transitioning from fetal oxygenation levels with an expected increase in Spo_2 from the fetal level of approximately 50% to a target of 85% to 90% by 7 to 8 minutes, an increase of approximately 5% per minute. Figure 28-7 demonstrates continuous physiologic data during the first 10 minutes of life for an infant resuscitated using a targeted oxygen strategy.

ASSISTING CIRCULATION

In newborn infants, the need for resuscitative measures beyond assisted ventilation is extremely rare. Additional circulatory assistance can include chest compressions, administration of epinephrine, and volume infusion. In a large urban delivery center with a resuscitation registry, 0.12% of all infants delivered received chest compressions, epinephrine, or both during 1991 to 1993 (Perlman and Risser, 1995), and 0.06% of all infants delivered received epinephrine during 1999 to 2004 (Barber and Wyckoff, 2006). Ventilation remains the most critical priority in neonatal resuscitation; however, if adequate ventilation is provided for 30 seconds, and bradycardia with a heart rate less than 60 beats/min persists, chest compressions are initiated. Further attention to ventilation with the use of increased pressures or intubation may be required. Chest compressions are preferably provided with two thumbs on the sternum while both hands encircle the chest with (Menegazzi et al, 1993). The chest is then compressed in a 3:1 ratio coordinated with ventilation breaths.

Further circulatory support may be necessary if adequate chest compressions do not result in an increase in heart rate after 30 seconds. Epinephrine is then indicated as a vasoactive substance, which increases blood pressure by α-receptor agonism, improves coronary perfusion pressure, and increases heart rate by β-receptor agonism. Intravenous administration of epinephrine is more likely to be effective than endotracheal administration. The intravenous dose of 0.01 to 0.03 mg/kg (0.1 to 0.3 mL/kg of a 1:10,000 solution) is currently recommended. Early placement of an umbilical venous catheter is critical to delivering intravenous epinephrine quickly enough to be effective. In order to place an umbilical catheter as quickly as possible, it is necessary to have the equipment readily available and to begin the procedure as soon as possible. This could be accomplished by the lead resuscitator assigning the task of placing the catheter as soon as chest compressions are initiated. If there is any prenatal indication that substantial resuscitation will be required, the necessary equipment for umbilical venous catheter placement should be prepared before delivery as completely as possible. Epinephrine can be given by endotracheal tube, but the efficacy of this delivery method is not as certain; therefore an increased dose (0.05 to 0.1 mg/kg) is recommended. Epinephrine doses can be repeated every 3 minutes if heart rate does not increase. Excessive epinephrine can result in hypertension, which in preterm infants may be a factor in the development of intraventricular hemorrhage. However, the risks

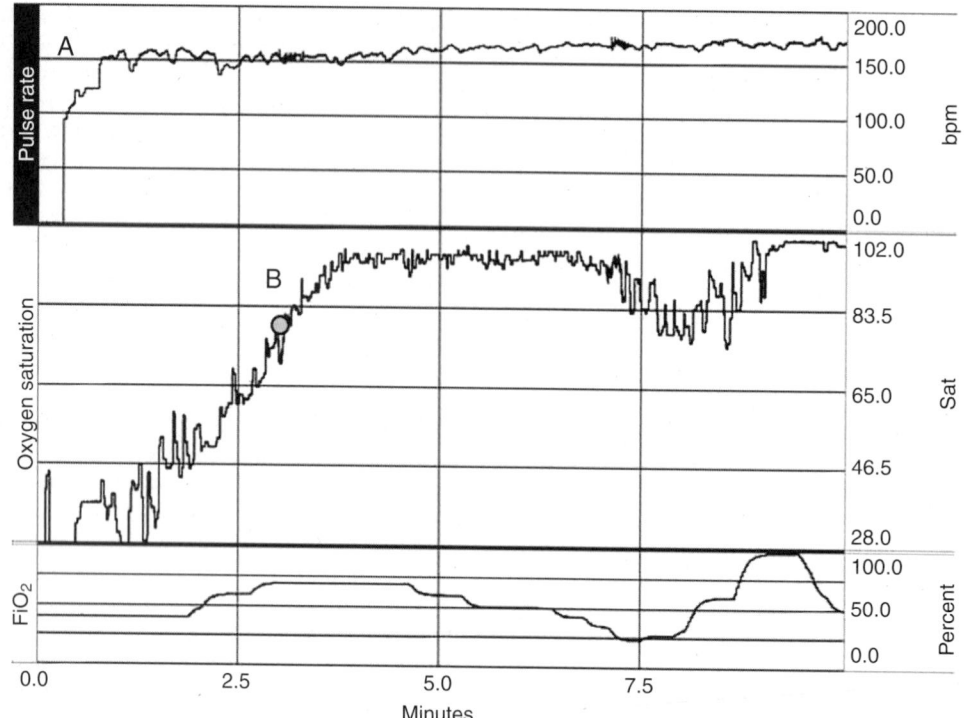

FIGURE 28-7 **Tracing of physiologic data during transition.** The pulse rate, oxygen saturation, and oxygen concentration (FiO$_2$) measured within 30 seconds of birth are displayed here. The pulse oximeter is placed on the infant's right hand as soon as possible. Point *A* shows when the pulse oximeter begins working. Point *B* shows the oxygen saturation (SpO$_2$) at 3 minutes (approximately 80%). This infant was initially treated with 40% oxygen, and the concentration was adjusted to achieve SpO$_2$ of 85% to 90% by 5 minutes of life. When the oxygen is weaned down to 21% at approximately 7.5 minutes of life, the SpO$_2$ decreases and oxygen concentration is increased again.

are balanced by the benefit of successful resuscitation in an infant who might not otherwise survive.

If the infant has not responded to all the prior measures, a trial of increasing intravascular volume should be considered, which involves administering crystalloid or blood. Situations associated with fetal blood loss are also frequently associated with the need for resuscitation. These situation include placental abruption, cord prolapse, and fetal maternal transfusion. Some of these clinical circumstances will have an obvious history associated with blood loss, whereas others might not be readily evident at the time of birth. Signs of hypovolemia in the newborn infant are nonspecific, but include pallor and weak pulses. Volume replacement requires intravenous access, for which emergent placement of an umbilical venous catheter is essential. Any infant who has signs of hypovolemia and has not responded quickly to other resuscitative measures should have an umbilical venous line placed and a volume infusion administered. The most common, and currently recommended, fluid for volume replacement is isotonic saline. A trial volume of 10 mL/kg is given initially and repeated if necessary. If a substantial blood loss has occurred, the infant may require infusion of red blood cells to provide adequate oxygen-carrying capacity. This infusion can be accomplished emergently with noncrossmatched, O-negative blood, with blood collected from the placenta or with blood drawn from the mother, who will have a compatible antibody profile with her infant at the time of birth. Because not all blood loss is obvious and resuscitation algorithms usually discuss volume replacement as a last resort of a difficult resuscitation, the

clinician needs to keep a high index of suspicion for significant hypovolemia so that action can be taken to correct the problem as promptly as possible. Therefore in situations where the possibility for hypovolemia is known before birth, it would be wise to prepare an umbilical catheter and an initial syringe of isotonic saline and discuss with the blood bank and the delivering physicians the possibility that non-crossmatched blood may be required.

SPECIFIC PROBLEMS ENCOUNTERED DURING RESUSCITATION

NEONATAL RESPONSE TO MATERNAL ANESTHESIA AND ANALGESIA

Medications administered to the mother during labor can affect the fetus by transfer across the placenta and direct action on the fetus or by adversely affecting the mother's condition, and therefore altering uteroplacental circulation and fetal oxygen delivery. The most commonly discussed complication of intrapartum medication exposure is perinatal respiratory depression after maternal opiate administration. The fetus can develop respiratory depression from the direct effect of the drug. Naloxone has been used during neonatal resuscitation as an opiate receptor antagonist to reverse the effects of fetal opiate exposure. Naloxone chloride (0.1 mg/kg per dose, intravenously, intramuscularly, or endotracheally) can be considered if the newly born infant does not develop spontaneous respirations after adequate resuscitation and the mother has received an opiate analgesic during labor, provided the opiate exposure is not chronic. Infants of mothers who have a chronic opiate exposure can potentially have a sudden withdrawal syndrome, including seizures if they receive a narcotic antagonist. It is also critical that assisted ventilation be provided as long as spontaneous respirations are inadequate. It should be noted that the administration of a narcotic antagonist is never an acutely required intervention during neonatal resuscitation, because these infants can be treated with assisted ventilation.

CONDITIONS COMPLICATING RESUSCITATION

When resuscitation has proceeded through the described steps without improvement in the infant's clinical condition, other problems should be considered. Some of these problems may be modifiable with interventions that could improve the course of the resuscitation. For example, an unrecognized pneumothorax could prevent adequate pulmonary inflation and if under tension could impair cardiac function. If the pneumothorax is recognized and drained, gas exchange and circulation can be improved. Some congenital anomalies that were not diagnosed antenatally make resuscitation more difficult. Congenital diaphragmatic hernia is difficult to recognize on initial inspection of the infant, but can cause significant problems with resuscitation. The abdominal organs are displaced into one hemithorax, and the lungs are unable to develop normally; this will cause ventilation to be difficult. If the intestines are displaced into the thorax and mask ventilation is provided, the intestines will become inflated, making ventilation more difficult. If the congenital diaphragmatic hernia is known before delivery or a presumptive diagnosis is made in the delivery room, the baby should be intubated early to prevent intestinal inflation. An orogastric suction tube should also be placed to decompress the inflated intestines.

Many other congenital anomalies that can lead to a difficult resuscitation will be more visibly obvious when the baby is born. For example, hydrops fetalis occurring for any reason can be associated with difficult resuscitation. Although most cases are diagnosed on fetal ultrasound examination before delivery, severe hydrops would be visible on examination with skin edema and abdominal distention. Frequently peritoneal and pleural fluid will need to be drained to achieve adequate ventilation. Abdominal wall defects such as gastroschisis require special attention in the delivery room to ensure that the exposed bowel is covered in plastic, to prevent excessive fluid loss, and is protected from twisting or trauma. An orogastric suction tube is also important to decompress the stomach and limit the chances of further vomiting. If assisted ventilation is necessary, early intubation as opposed to mask ventilation should be considered to prevent gastric distention. Infants with neural tube defects should also have any exposed tissues protected with a covering. In addition, all efforts should be made to avoid pressure on the defect.

Fetal congenital high airway obstruction can cause particularly difficult resuscitation. If a significant airway obstruction is diagnosed antenatally, an ex utero intrapartum treatment (i.e., EXIT) procedure can be planned. This procedure allows for establishing a stable airway before clamping the umbilical cord, which maintains placental function until the airway is secure. An airway obstruction may not necessarily be diagnosed before delivery and can cause difficult resuscitation. The therapy will vary depending on the cause of obstruction. An alternate airway (oral or nasopharyngeal) can be helpful if endotracheal intubation is not possible, as can occur with micrognathia. Tracheal suctioning can be attempted if a tracheal plug is suspected. In extreme situations of airway obstruction, an emergency cricothyroidotomy may be attempted.

Birth trauma of any kind has been documented to occur in approximately 2.6% of all deliveries in the United States (Moczygemba et al, 2010). The most serious injuries are the variety of head injuries that can occur, including subgaleal hemorrhage and intracranial hemorrhage. Subgaleal hemorrhage is more often associated with vacuum-assisted delivery; it and is important to recognize because of the rapid blood loss that can occur into this soft tissue space. Intracranial hemorrhages such as subdural hematomas can occur, although many such injuries are mild and can be found incidentally after uncomplicated vaginal delivery. Spinal cord injuries after birth are extremely rare, but can be severe with long-lasting functional limitations. Brachial plexus and other peripheral nerve injuries may be noticed in the delivery room and evaluated shortly after birth, but they should not interfere with the resuscitation efforts. Pressure injuries from forceps-assisted deliveries can be noted on examination and evaluated as necessary in accordance with the location of the injury. Fractures and lacerations can occur and need to be evaluated after the newborn infant has transitioned adequately.

LIMITS OF VIABILITY

Neonatal intensive care has increased survival at lower gestational ages, resulting in changes in the definition of viability over time. There is a variety of opinion among practitioners regarding the lower limit of gestational age when intensive care should be offered. The NRP states that not providing intensive care is appropriate at less than 23 weeks' gestation or 400 g birthweight. When the outcome is uncertain, parents of the infant are frequently included in the decision-making process. Making an informed decision about providing intensive care should be done with the best information available. One of the most useful resources to determine the likelihood of survival without severe disabilities has been provided by Tyson et al (2008) using the National Institute of Child Health and Human Development Neonatal Research Network data. Using information regarding the gestational age, birthweight, sex, number of fetuses, and antenatal steroid exposure, a calculation of the risk of mortality and neurodevelopmental impairment can be made. These predictive data that were compiled from the participating centers of the Neonatal Research Network, a group of mostly academic centers, may currently be the best national data available for predicting outcome, but they do not necessarily represent the outcome at any single unit or of any individual baby. When there is the possibility of delivery at a very preterm gestational age at a small, inexperienced center, all efforts should be made to transport the mother to an experienced inborn center.

CARE AFTER RESUSCITATION

Infants who survive a significant resuscitation require special attention in the hours to days that follow. Frequent complications immediately following resuscitation include hypoglycemia, hypotension, and persistent metabolic acidosis. In addition, infants with evidence of hypoxic ischemic encephalopathy may benefit from mild therapeutic hypothermia (Azzopardi et al, 2009; Jacobs et al, 2007; Shankaran et al, 2005). Mild therapeutic hypothermia, in which the core body temperature is kept at 33.5° C, has been extensively evaluated and has been effective at reducing death or impairment in infants with moderate to severe hypoxic ischemic encephalopathy. The decreased temperature is thought to decrease the secondary injury that occurs after an hypoxic-ischemic insult. Hypothermia can be accomplished with both whole-body and head cooling, although clinical trials of whole-body cooling more effectively achieved a reduction in adverse outcomes. The therapy is most beneficial when initiated as quickly as possible after an insult, with beneficial effects noted when treatment was initiated within 6 hours of birth. The timing of insult in relation to the time of birth is not always obvious, making it difficult to know the actual timing of initiating therapy after the insult.

Mild hypothermia therapy should be considered when an infant has required a significant resuscitation after birth, Apgar scores are low (especially a 5-minute score less than 5), fetal or neonatal acidosis are documented on cord or newborn blood gases, and signs of encephalopathy are apparent. In addition, the history of a significant event likely to cause a hypoxic-ischemic insult should trigger a thorough evaluation of the newborn to determine whether hypothermia therapy is indicated. Hypothermia therapy is not currently available at all institutions; however, all delivery services must be able to recognize the indications for therapy, so that a transfer can be initiated as quickly as possible, if necessary.

In infants born without a heart rate or any respiratory effort, if resuscitation is performed to the full extent without any response, discontinuation is recommended after 10 minutes. From a review of 13 years of data from a database including 81,603 deliveries, Haddad et al (2000) found that survival with an Apgar score of 0 at 1 minute occurred in 1.26 of 1000 delivered infants without major malformations. Of 33 infants assigned Apgar scores of 0 at both 1 and 5 minutes, 67% died before hospital discharge (Haddad et al, 2000). A recent review of the available literature for infants with Apgar scores of 0 at 10 minutes found that 94% of infants either died or were severely handicapped, whereas 3% were mild or moderately handicapped (Harrington et al, 2007).

The transition from fetal to neonatal life is a critical time in an individual's life and is an opportunity for care providers to have significant effect on the outcome of infants who need assistance. The need for neonatal resuscitation, even when no signs of encephalopathy are recognized, increases the risk that children will have lower scores on intelligence quotient tests at school age (Odd et al, 2009). This risk arises most likely because resuscitation is a marker for a prior insult. However, a well-performed resuscitation could be critical for a successful recovery. Neonatal care providers have an obligation to ensure that this process is performed as well as possible and that the techniques of resuscitation are evaluated in an objective manner to promote continued improvement.

SUGGESTED READINGS

Apgar V: A proposal for a new method of evaluation of the newborn infant, *Curr Res Anesth Analg* 32:260-267, 1953.

Carbine DN, Finer NN, Knodel E, et al: Video recording as a means of evaluating neonatal resuscitation performance, *Pediatrics* 106:654-658, 2000.

Costeloe K, Hennessy E, Gibson AT, et al: The EPICure study: outcomes to discharge from hospital for infants born at the threshold of viability, *Pediatrics* 106:659-671, 2000.

Kamlin CO, O'Donnell CP, Davis PG, et al: Oxygen saturation in healthy infants immediately after birth, *J Pediatr* 148:585-589, 2006.

Morley CJ, Davis PG, Doyle LW, et al: Nasal CPAP or intubation at birth for very preterm infants, *N Engl J Med* 358:700-708, 2008.

Saugstad OD, Ramji S, Soll RF, et al: Resuscitation of newborn infants with 21% or 100% oxygen: an updated systematic review and meta-analysis, *Neonatology* 94:176-182, 2008.

Shankaran S, Laptook AR, Ehrenkranz RA, et al: Whole-body hypothermia for neonates with hypoxic-ischemic encephalopathy, *N Engl J Med* 353:1574-1584, 2005.

Siew ML, te Pas AB, Wallace MJ, et al: Positive end-expiratory pressure enhances development of a functional residual capacity in preterm rabbits ventilated from birth, *J Appl Physiol* 106:1487-1493, 2009.

te Pas AB: Walther FJ. A randomized, controlled trial of delivery-room respiratory management in very preterm infants, *Pediatrics* 120:322-329, 2007.

Teitel DF: Circulatory adjustments to postnatal life, *Semin Perinatol* 12:96-103, 1988.

Tyson JE, Parikh NA, Langer J, et al: Intensive care for extreme prematurity: moving beyond gestational age, *N Engl J Med* 358:1672-1681, 2008.

Vohra S, Roberts RS, Zhang B, et al: Heat Loss Prevention (HeLP) in the delivery room: a randomized controlled trial of polyethylene occlusive skin wrapping in very preterm infants, *J Pediatr* 145:750-753, 2004.

Wiswell TE, Gannon CM, Jacob J, et al: Delivery room management of the apparently vigorous meconium-stained neonate: results of the multicenter, international collaborative trial, *Pediatrics* 105(1 Pt 1):1-7, 2000.

Complete references and supplemental color images used in this text can be found online at www.expertconsult.com

CHAPTER

29

STABILIZATION AND TRANSPORT OF THE HIGH-RISK INFANT

George A. Woodward, Roxanne Kirsch, Michael Stone Trautman, Monica E. Kleinman, Gil Wernovsky, and Bradley S. Marino

NEONATAL TRANSPORT MEDICINE

INTRODUCTION

Regionalization of medical care has improved the ability to centralize resources and improve patient outcomes. For optimal coordinated care, however, adequate medical transport needs to be developed and continually refined to enable delivery of patients to regional centers, and for specialized care to be available for and delivered to patients in distress. For centers that serve as a basic or specialized service, there will be times when subspecialty care is required. For those who deliver subspecialty care, there will also be times for most organizations when transfer to a similar level organization may be required for reasons such as capacity or extraordinary care. For hospitals that do not have birthing centers as part of their facility, the patient population, the acuity of the arriving patients, and potentially the ultimate morbidity and mortality of those patients depend on skilled, efficient, and quality neonatal transport. Although transfers to neonatal centers in the 1960s and early 1970s often occurred in an ad hoc manner, such as in a police car or an ambulance (i.e., a converted hearse) with variably skilled providers, transfer programs today offer a more sophisticated level of care. This level of care, however, is not consistent throughout cities, nationwide, and internationally. Many transport services and centers have grown around individual center needs, without clear attention to coordination and regionalization of services. Competitive systems, often located in similar areas or vying for similar patient populations, have resulted in the duplication of services at the ground and air levels, and at times increased risk and cost to patients and providers as part of the efforts to increase patient volume and revenue.

When considering transport of neonatal patients, several situations can occur. Intrafacility transport may be required for specialty services within a particular institution. Interfacility transport between lower and higher levels of service capability can also occur, as well as between relatively equivalent levels of service because of capacity or other issues. Transported patients may be of high acuity, relatively stable, or in various stages of convalescent care. Each type of transport requires anticipatory planning, appropriate staffing, adequate modalities (e.g., transport vehicles), and strong relationships between referring and receiving providers, in addition to skilled, qualified, and certified transport personnel. As noted in the next section, transfer agreements can help to minimize inefficiencies and enable rapid approval and eventually transport of patients.

This chapter will review considerations and requirements for neonatal transport; discuss issues involved in transport team operation, including equipment, personnel, mode of transport, and medical-legal issues; and present general and specific topics, including quality improvement opportunities, that might be encountered in a neonatal transport system (American Academy of Pediatrics et al, 2007; Cornette, 2004; Woodward et al, 2007).

REGIONALIZATION OF NEONATAL CARE, TRANSFER AGREEMENTS, AND BACK TRANSPORT

The concept of regionalization of neonatal care and transport developed from the formation of neonatal stations in the 1920s and 1940s (Oppenheimer, 1996). These stations were located within certain area hospitals, where additional resources were allocated to provide care for premature infants. One consequence of the formation of these stations was the development of equipment and protocols to transport premature infants from other area hospitals to those specialized areas to receive care.

In the 1960s and 1970s, as interest in neonatal care grew, so did the number of hospitals offering services for premature infants. To help optimize the care being delivered, the March of Dimes produced *Toward Improving the Outcome of Pregnancy* in a 1976 report (Committee on Perinatal Health, 1976). The report stratified maternal and neonatal care into levels based on their complexity, and it proposed the referral of high-risk patients to centers with sufficient personnel and resources to provide care. The goal was to create standard definitions so that comparisons of health outcomes, resource utilization, and costs among regional institutions could be made. High-risk maternity patients would be able to actively participate in selecting a delivery service, and businesses would be able to select appropriate health care resources for their employees. The subsequent March of Dimes publication in 1993 *Toward Improving the Outcome of Pregnancy: The 90s and Beyond* reiterated the importance of regionalized care and further delineated care levels (Committee on Perinatal Health, 1993). The concepts of regional care were adopted and incorporated into the Guidelines for Perinatal Care (American Academy of Pediatrics Committee on Fetus and Newborn and Bell, 2007; Woodward et al, 2007). Whereas the original driving forces for regionalization in the 1970s were the shortage of trained personnel to care for low birthweight (LBW) infants and the economic expense to maintain these skills, during the late 1980s and 1990s, technology and clinical expertise disseminated outside the regional tertiary centers, resulting in proliferation of the number of intermediate care neonatal intensive care units (NICUs). This proliferation has blurred many of the original distinctions between various care systems. Whether driven by third party payers or other factors, with various interpretations and applications of what "regional care" means, the results have been the creation of a variety of care options (Lainwala et al, 2007).

Limited space and cooperative longitudinal care planning in some tertiary care units have created the necessity for patient transport back to a unit with less acuity or fewer resources once their critical condition has resolved or stabilized (Attar et al, 2005; Donovan and Schmitt, 1991; Lynch et al, 1988). Regionalization guidelines should support the return to the community for patients who no longer need the highest care level. Patient selection for back transport (transport back to referring service, hospital, or a hospital closer to the patient's home) and care in another facility should match the capabilities and expertise of the community hospital (Stark and American Academy of Pediatrics Committee on Fetus and Newborn, 2004).

Although third-party payers often drive decision making, transport relationships develop between various institutions either by formalized transfer and preferred provider agreements or by historical and personal relationships (Attar et al, 2005). Transfer agreements can help to define the roles, understanding, and expectations between institutions and the transport service; they also help frequently to detail reimbursement issues. These agreements set the expectations for participating facilities, with the ultimate goal of the timely movement of patients from one facility to another 2007; Woodward et al, 2007). Whether optimal care can be provided in some smaller NICUs or outside of a tertiary unit is frequently debated. Nonetheless, there is a trend in the United States and elsewhere toward the centralization of perinatal care (Howell et al, 2002; Wall et al, 2004).

Several investigators have shown that mortality was lowest for deliveries of infants with very LBW that occurred in hospitals with tertiary care NICUs (Chien et al, 2001; Phibbs et al, 2007; Rautava et al, 2007; Robertson et al, 1994). Cifuentes et al (2003) supported the idea that whenever possible, women in early preterm labor should be moved to the regional hospital rather than transferring the infant after birth. The study was insufficiently powered, however, to make a recommendation regarding the difference between regional and large community NICUs (Cifuentes et al, 2003). In trying to discern which LBW infant might be better cared for in tertiary regional care centers, Vieux et al (2006) showed that the risk factors for requiring high levels of intensive care were low gestational age, twin pregnancy, maternal hypertension, antepartum hemorrhage, infection, and male gender, whereas antenatal steroid therapy and premature rupture of membranes were protective factors against requiring intensive care. Regional care concerns can apply to the neonates with extremely

LBW and to the late preterm population (Khashu et al, 2009). Investigators trying to describe the optimal neonatal unit caring for very preterm infants in Europe were unable to produce a consensus as to what the ideal neonatal unit size and patient volume should be (Van Reempts et al, 2007). Given the wide variability in levels of neonatal care and the inability to predict premature delivery, neonatal transport will continue to be a dynamic process.

TRANSPORT COMMUNICATIONS

When developing and maximizing transport capabilities, a key concept is the centralization of communication. Although a telephone call from a referring provider to a receiving provider might be the most efficient way to receive advice or notify a receiving provider of a potential transport, there are more centralized and effective means of communication. First, a centralized, easily recalled, advertised, and monitored (24 hours per day, 7 days per week) communication system should be available. Identifying and publishing a centralized access number for immediate access to the transport system or receiving center personnel are imperative for optimal communication and efficiency (Southard et al, 2005). Anyone who has transported or referred patients to systems without centralized access understands the challenges in working through operators, unit clerks, multiple providers, and often multiple services to enable a singular transport. This process is time consuming and often frustrating for the referring provider, and it is often time that could be better spent in direct assessment and care of the patient, rather than on the telephone with repetitive informational transfer. Ideally a centralized transport communication center would enable a referring provider to make a single call to a single number and immediately receive all the services that they might require. Those services include appreciation and recognition of the need for transfer, identification of appropriate hospital and facility, review of medical issues, and determination of required services (i.e., personnel, equipment, time of response) needed for transport. Also included would be simultaneous awareness of need for transport by the personnel responsible for arrangement of particular modes of transport, verification of bed capacity, and any other logistic items that may need to take place prior to the transport. A telephone call made to an individual provider requesting transport requires a sequential process from data gathering through acceptance for admission and eventual transport service or modality identification and dispatch. Centralized access to a communication center allows all those functions to occur simultaneously, enabling more rapid transport response and appropriate involvement of all those required for the management of the particular patient (American Academy of Pediatrics Committee on Fetus and Newborn and Bell, 2007; Woodward et al, 2007).

MEDICAL SUPERVISION

A key requirement for any system is to have appropriately skilled and immediately available medical command physicians (American Academy of Pediatrics Committee on Fetus and Newborn and Bell, 2007; Woodward et al, 2007). A medical command physician should be literate and expert in the medical area of concern. In most cases involving neonatal transport, this provider should be a neonatologist. There may be instances, however, when the referring or receiving physicians may request or desire additional medical expertise. For example, a cyanotic newborn with congenital heart disease may be temporarily improved or stabilized well by the referring neonatologist and have additional stabilization direction provided by the receiving medical command physician; however, invaluable additional management and planning might be added by a partnering cardiac intensive care physician. A communication or transfer center can allow for multiple providers to be linked together during an initial referral call to allow the highest level advice to be presented and discussed among the providers. These telephone calls should also include the transport personnel so that the providers have the background information and care plans delivered directly.

MODE OF TRANSPORT

Once the transport referral has been made, ideally through a communication center, and discussions have been started with the medical command physician, the transport can take place. Decision on mode of transport is an important component to consider at this juncture. In general, ground transport allows door-to-door service between facilities, enables a well-lighted environment, provides space for several providers as well as the patient and a family member, and is efficient in urban and short-range transfers. As the distance for transfer increases, and the need for decreased out-of-hospital time becomes more important, consideration of air transport becomes important depending on acuity and patient disease process. In general, air transport is most expeditious over approximately 50 miles, with helicopter being favored between 50 and 150 miles and airplane being effective for transports greater than 150 miles. The decision regarding mode of transport is influenced by several issues, which include available modes of transport, staffing and medical expertise of the providers involved in those particular modes, current and projected patient condition (which includes preliminary identification of the underlying disease process), consideration of stability or illness progression during the projected transport timeframe, capabilities of the referring facility and personnel, and the urgency of intervention and definitive placement of the patient. Other issues that influence the process include geographic and weather constraints, distance and duration of transport, and provider perception about the transport process. In addition to the potential risks of ground transport, which include traffic accidents, vibration, noise, and other issues, air transport creates concerns for accident, vibration, gravitational forces during acceleration and deceleration, excessive noise, temperature variations, and decreased humidity with altitude. Air transport also includes issues related to altitude physiology that can affect patients with respiratory issues or air trapping and their air-containing equipment (e.g., endotracheal tube cuffs, laryngeal mask airways; Wilson et al, 2008; Woodward et al, 2002, 2006). Dalton's Law recognizes that ambient oxygen decreases as altitude increases; therefore there may be a need for pressurization and augmentation with increased FiO_2. Boyle's Law states that as altitude increases, the volume of a gas also increases, and the barometric pressure is inversely related to the volume of the gas. This law is potentially a serious issue for patients with an enclosed gas collection, such as a simple or developing pneumothorax.

TRANSPORT PERSONNEL, EDUCATION, AND TEAM COMPOSITION

Awareness of the capabilities of the transport system and of the personnel involved in transport is imperative in decisions regarding mode of transport. Although it is ultimately the responsibility of the referring physician to identify the appropriate mode and personnel for transport, per Emergency medical Treatment and Active Labor Act (EMTALA), opportunities exist for tertiary care and referral centers to help to educate the referral providers regarding optimal transport planning and usage (Bolte, 1995; Woodward, 1995). In general, issues influencing transport decisions include current level of care, urgency for a different level of medical capability or equipment, current providers of care, stability of the patient, options available to the provider and patient, and efficiency and quality of the transport process. Ideally, these issues are the determinants of appropriate transfer; however, referring providers are often overwhelmed by the severity or acuity of the patient and their primary desire may be to have the patient removed from their facility as quickly as possible. The providers may decide on a transport or transfer process based solely on speed of transport process rather than quality of care. It is imperative for the receiving and tertiary care centers to educate the referring population on the importance of stabilization, initiation and quality of initial response, transport options, and definitive care to maximize potential patient outcome. When examining the transfer of patients, providers should ask a simple question: "Are we trying to deliver the patient to tertiary care, or are we trying to deliver tertiary care to the patient?" In most high-functioning transport and referral centers, the latter is true. The referring physician should expect to have tertiary care advice and direction delivered at the moment of the referral telephone call and continued throughout the transport process (American Academy of Pediatrics Committee on Fetus and Newborn and Bell, 2007; Woodward, 1995; Woodward et al, 2007). At no time should the care delivered to the patient decrease in sophistication after a referral call is made. If a transfer places the infant in a suboptimal environment or with providers who are not competent to address the infant's current or potential medical needs, the patient might receive suboptimal care and the referring provider is liable for arranging and providing inappropriate care.

When considering the team composition of the transport providers, it is important to consider the quality of the personnel, their expertise and experience, and their ability to work in the transport environment (King and Woodward, 2002a; King et al, 2001, 2007). There are many variations of transport teams in the United States and abroad. These teams can be composed of physicians, nurse practitioners, nurses, respiratory therapists, paramedics, and other health care providers. In the United States, medical (pediatric or specialty) trainees are often used as primary providers in the transport environment. Regardless of the formal educational background of an individual, there are several criteria that must be met to be optimally effective in the transport environment. First, the provider must have adequate certification, be licensed for the care they deliver, and be able to provide the assessments and interventions that the patient currently or potentially requires during the transport process. For example, a neonatal retrieval service must be able to manage acute and critical airways in the neonatal population, both at a referring hospital and during the transport. It is interesting that those same providers might not be credentialed to provide those skills within their home hospital; however, they have been certified to provide them in the ambulance environment. In general, this must be done under the auspices of a physician's care, which may be from an accompanying physician or via online medical control (real-time medical advice during the transport process). Transport care also often involves offline medical control, which involves the use of protocols developed by medical personnel. It is important to recognize that the transport timeframe is somewhat limited; therefore the personnel might not need to have the longitudinal or differential diagnosis expertise of a fully trained neonatologist. However, these personnel must have the acute care assessment abilities and intervention skills of an experienced neonatal expert. In addition to training the onsite personnel, it is imperative to have medical command physicians understand the opportunities and limitations of the transport services and environment and to understand the risks and challenges that referring personnel can potentially encounter with situations and patients who exceed their own personal or their facility's management abilities. The physicians must have significant awareness of the transport environment to understand the limitations of potential interventions. It is also imperative that medical command positions have superb communication skills, not only at the referring physician level but also within the transport team. Medical command physicians will need to be able to effectively and efficiently communicate with providers from different disciplines.

QUALITY IMPROVEMENT

Transport medicine offers an opportunity to identify areas for potential improvement within the inpatient arena, in the transport system, and at the referring facilities (Browning Carmo et al, 2008; Chen et al, 2005; Lim and Ratnavel, 2008; McPherson et al, 2008; Ramnarayan, 2009). This glimpse into medical sophistication and capability is one that is privileged and should be used to identify educational opportunities rather than prompt judgmental and critical review. Education by referring physicians and transport teams can have a significant effect on the quality and outcome of patient care and the volume of future referrals. Ideally, once a referral call is made, a receiving physician or medical command physician will direct the care so that the job of the transport team is to verify that an appropriate working diagnosis has been made and that adequate stabilization procedures have been performed. The team can verify that the interventions are secure and then transport the patient in a stable fashion. Systems that do not gather adequate information or offer appropriate

advice, or in which the referring facilities do not follow that advice or choose not to perform needed interventions, put the patient at risk by having a delay in care of initial interventions, prolonging the transport, and delaying delivery of definitive care. The transport team that has invested several hours at a bedside, stabilizing a newborn with medical or surgical issues, may be spending time in a facility that is not ideal, has a limited number of skilled personnel, and has minimal backup, thus prolonging the transport process and potentially putting that individual patient at risk (Chen et al, 2005; Haji-Michael, 2005). However, the patient and the system are at risk because the valuable resource of specialized neonatal transport personnel is not available for another patient.

Ideally, care delivery would be the same at referral and receiving centers; the development of practice guidelines can be helpful in that regard. Guidelines that are evidence based, developed by regional and local experts, and disseminated to referring locations and transport teams will help to standardize and enable consistent care across variable locations. It is necessary, however, to assess and reassess the quality of the guidelines and the competency of their use to ensure optimal results from this process. Even in the best of hands, near-miss or realized adverse events may happen. It is clear that identification of those events, discussion with families (where appropriate), and root cause analysis are imperative. Several studies have examined adverse events in transported patients. Ligtenberg et al (2005) noted that one third of patients had an adverse event, and 50% of those resulted from not following the advice of the medical command physician. Of that group, 70% of events were avoidable and 30% were logistical. In a review of the London Neonatal Transfer Service, Lim and Ratnavel (2008) noted that 36% of their patients had greater than or equal to one adverse event, and two thirds of those were due to human error; half of those occurred before the team arrived at the referral center, and their major etiologies included preparation and communication.

A neonatal transport service must determine if maternal transport is part of their purview. It is clear that preterm infants who are born at outside hospitals and require transfer to tertiary care centers or who are born at one tertiary care center and require transfer to another have worse outcomes that include increased mortality and morbidities such as intraventricular hemorrhage (IVH) and other medical issues (Baskett and O'Connell, 2009; Janse-Marec and Mairovitz, 2004; Jony and Baskett, 2007; O'Brien et al, 2004; Ohara et al, 2008). Developing appropriate criteria for transporting women in preterm labor may help to direct the optimal use of resources required with maternal transfer. Identifying the appropriate time to transport women in preterm labor, as well as those with other preterm medical issues, will help in developing appropriate criteria and limit resource utilization for maternal transfers. It is important to note that significant work regarding neonatal and maternal transport and regionalization of care in the United States, United Kingdom, Australia, Europe, and other areas has already been accomplished. There are, however, multiple opportunities to improve transport on an individual and regional basis in these developed countries and in other developing countries.

TRANSPORT ADMINISTRATION

As a hospital develops and optimizes a neonatal transport program, experts in transport medicine are integral to the success of this program (American Academy of Pediatrics Committee on Fetus and Newborn and Bell, 2007; Woodward et al, 2007). A quality medical director and program director, often a nurse or respiratory therapist, are essential to understand the potentially complicated and challenging environment of transport medicine. These leaders should be instrumental in identifying expectations, roles, and responsibilities for the process; this includes access through a communication center and developing and disseminating referral center expectations. These expectations include stabilization and preparation of the patient before transport, making an appropriate decision to transfer, choosing the appropriate transport process and destination, obtaining consent from the family for transport, discussing plans for stabilization and intervention with the medical command physician, and initiating that plan as able. Referral centers must be able to be direct when they believe that the suggested interventions are inappropriate or beyond their scope. The referring team also needs to be available to participate in transition care to the transport team and the receiving service. The receiving and transport team responsibilities include being immediately available for case discussion, having the ability to rapidly accept the patient if capacity is available, offering clear and concise expert recommendations, ensuring preparation of the environment and the staff both for the transport and arrival of the patient, organizing additional diagnostics and interventions, and providing available and accessible neonatal advice throughout the process. Most important, the team needs to ensure that appropriate skills and therapy are available and delivered throughout the process, from referral call through definitive placement, and ensure seamless transition at each point of care. The team needs to communicate well with referring and the patient's physicians and document their advice, interventions and activities in a clear, concise fashion to enable appropriate patient and provide protection for the transport service.

TRANSPORT EXPERTISE

As transport medicine has developed over the past 30 to 40 years, there has been an increase in the quality and volume of transport research, as well as organizations that are discipline and process specific. Multiple disciplines have organizations with transport focus and expertise, including the American Academy of Pediatrics Section on Transport Medicine, which includes executive committee representation from neonatology, pediatric critical care, and emergency medicine physicians, as well as a broad membership from other subspecialties and disciplines. The American Academy of Pediatrics Transport Section published its most recent Guidelines for Neonatal and Pediatric Transport in 2007; they also host a listserv at transmedaap@listserve.aap.org, which is a national repository of information and a conduit to others in the transport arena for transport-related issues.

There are many keys to success in transport medicine. These keys include integrity, professionalism, preparation, anticipation, education, competency, critical evaluation of current and new practices, the ability to critically assess the quality of care being delivered at every point along the way, and looking for opportunities to improve access, efficiency, and delivery of care. An area that is vital for appropriate transport care is the assurance of competency of the providers (American Academy of Pediatric Committee on Fetus and Newborn and Bell, 2007). As noted, providers can come from many different backgrounds and bring different skills from their clinical and training experience. It is imperative for the transport system and leadership to ensure that the skills required are present in their personnel. This responsibility includes initial education, continuing education, and competency assessment. A team may decide to have individuals who are experts in defined areas of care, such as a physician who manages airways and the pneumothorax, a nurse who manages intravenous access and medication delivery, and a respiratory therapist who is responsible for airway and ventilatory support, whereas another team may choose to have all team members competent in all skills. Specific procedures may be useful or needed in transport that are not as common in the hospital environment or to the hospital-based providers (e.g., laryngeal mask airway; Trevisanuto et al, 2005). However the team is structured, there must be clear and concise guidelines for ongoing training and assessment of the personnel. High-fidelity simulation models offer additional opportunities to assess and potentially improve technical and cognitive capabilities (LeFlore and Anderson, 2008). The American Academy of Pediatrics Guidelines for Air and Ground Transport of Neonatal and Pediatric Patients (available at www.aap.org) is an invaluable resource that outlines required education and competencies for each level and discipline.

The true quality of a transport service is sometimes difficult to determine, because many teams and services have been developed independently and are not part of larger regional systems. It is difficult to compare and contrast systems in different areas for which different patient populations are transported (Berge et al, 2005; Cornette and Miall, 2006; Craig, 2005; Doyle and Orr, 2002; Khilnani and Chhabra, 2008; Van Reempts et al, 2007).

One avenue for potential standardization of the transport environment is by assessment and accreditation by the Commission on Accreditation of Medical Transport Systems, which was initiated in 1990 as a direct response to the number of air medical accidents in the 1980s. This certification is voluntary in some areas and required in others, and it serves to assure providers, stakeholders, and the public of adherence to quality of care and transport safety standards. The Commission on Accreditation of Medical Transport Systems is an independent organization, supported by 16 member organizations, which publishes standards and arranges reviews of interested air and ground transport programs. Further information can be found at http:www.camts.org.

TRANSPORT SAFETY

Safety of the transport system and for its providers is paramount and must be assessed and ensured before transporting any patient. Vehicles must be safe and meet the standards for air or ground transport, the personnel must be appropriate, licensed, and competent, and the patients must be managed in the most appropriate and professional fashion. In addition, the logistics of travel must include a safe environment, including helmets and fire-retardant suits for those who fly in helicopters, three-point restraints, and appropriate ambulance seating arrangements. There should not be an occasion when providers put themselves at risk by being unrestrained or being in an area where unsecured debris or inappropriately placed equipment may damage a provider or a patient. Adherence to rules and regulations of air and ground transport is imperative as well (Clawson, 2002; Greene, 2009; King and Woodward, 2002b; Levick et al, 2006; National Highway Traffic Safety Administration, 2009).

It is imperative to recognize that there is risk with both air and ground transport. The air transport industry has seen an acute spike in tragic and fatal air accidents (Greene, 2009; National Transportation Safety Board Accident Database, 2009). This increase has caused the industry, and the U.S. government, to critically investigate these issues and offer suggestions to improve transport safety (Federal Aviation Administration Helicopter Safety Initiative, 2011; 10.5-year U.S. HEMS Safety, 2008). Requirements such as duty hours for pilots, weather restrictions, flight under instrument, flight rules with terrain avoidance equipment, and night vision goggles can to help minimize the risk for these transports. Although ground ambulances are used much more frequently, and the risk of injury and death is evident, the fatality rate is lower in ambulance accidents than it is in aircraft accidents (Becker, 2003; Becker et al, 2003; King and Woodward, 2002b). It is necessary, however, that the vehicles be maintained and operated in a safe manner. Many systems do not allow ambulances to exceed posted speed limits and use lights and sirens only as a way to identify an emergency response, not to enable the vehicle to circumvent or ignore standard traffic laws (Clawson, 2002). Appropriate equipment for ambulances is required as well, and the July 2009 statement by the American College of Surgeons Committee on Trauma regarding appropriate equipment for ambulances (also published as an American Academy of Pediatrics' policy statement) should be reviewed by all transport systems (American College of Surgeons Committee on Trauma, 2009; American College of Surgeons Committee on Trauma et al, 2009).

It is evident from the transport and pediatric literature that patient outcomes are improved with specialty providers. There have been multiple studies to examine this particular issue (Belway et al, 2006; Mullane et al, 2004). Perhaps the most compelling is the study by Orr et al (2009), which examined transports provided by variable providers within the same system. This study compared outcomes in patients whose care was delivered by specialized pediatric critical care teams with those whose care was delivered by general providers. Both teams had the same medical command oversight, equipment, and modalities. Patient outcomes were worse for those whose care was not delivered by specialty teams, and much improved for those who were. One challenge, however, with transport teams is that differentiation of medical resources, such as a neonatal specialty team, likely means that there may be a scarcity and potential need for rationing of those resources. It is possible to develop teams with a variety of personnel with complementary cognitive and procedural skill sets

and work toward appropriate triage of transport requests to ensure the proper level of onsite skill provision. There have been multiple attempts to develop triage tools for pediatric and neonatal care providers, including the Mortality Index for Neonatal Transport, the Modified Clinical Risk Index for Babies, and the Risk Score for Transported Patients, which are noted in the bibliography (Broughton et al, 2004a, 2004b; Markakis et al, 2006).

FAMILY-CENTERED CARE

Transport team research has shown that family-oriented care, as in other areas of the medical systems, is an important component of transport (Woodward and Fleegler, 2000, 2001). Families who have been formally surveyed appreciate the opportunity to participate in the care of their child. In neonatal transport, however, there are times when there are two patients who may require care in two disparate locations. A mother who has had a cesarean section and has delivered an acutely ill child in need of care in a higher facility is one such example. It is required that the mother be in one facility and the child be in another. The father may be conflicted regarding accompanying his new child on the transport or staying with the child's mother. Transport teams need to be sensitive to the challenges and opportunities for the family and include them in the process when possible. It is evident that when parents attend or accompany transport team members on critical care transports, they are not there to assess the medical skill set of the provider, but to provide support to their child. It is also a great opportunity for the transport team to demonstrate to the family that their patient is in focused, professional, caring, and capable hands.

MEDICAL LEGAL ISSUES

There are many medical legal issues in transport medicine, as elsewhere in the medical system (Hedges et al, 2006; Williams, 2001; Woodward, 2003). The Health Insurance Portability and Accountability Act (HIPAA) is a required component of transport planning and delivery. Discussion of patients should not take place in a public area or via public communication airways where non–patient-related personnel or bystanders could overhear information about a specific patient. As noted earlier, a requirement of EMTALA is that the referring physician chooses the appropriate mode of transport and ensures that the transport process and receiving hospital are appropriate for the particular patient. Patients cannot be transferred if they are unstable and the ability to further stabilize them is available at the initial site of care. If a patient must be transferred for care while in an unstable condition—a frequent scenario for critically ill patients who need care not available at the referring institution—consent must be obtained from the family, which acknowledges their understanding of the potential risks and benefits of the process. In practice, there are often patients in unstable condition who are transferred from lower to higher levels of care, because the level of care that can be provided at the referring or initial center is not optimal for the child. This reason is appropriate for transfer as compared with transferring patients because of financial or other economic drivers. The medical liability for transport is a shared process. Before the referring center calls regarding the patient and the center of referral has accepted care, the entire medical responsibility lies with the referring provider. Once the receiving team has accepted the patient and offered advice, medical liability is a shared process. The referring physician maintains the majority of the liability, as well as medical control of the patient, throughout the process until the transport team has left the referring hospital. It is important to recognize that most transport teams and personnel do not have privileges at referring hospitals and are working under the guidance and supervision of the referring physician team. Transport teams that act independently, or referring physicians who are not available when the transport team arrives, put both the referring provider and the transport team at risk if there is disagreement or inappropriate care delivered to the patient. There will be times, however, when there is disagreement regarding the optimal care to be delivered. For example, a child with a hypoplastic left heart syndrome and an open ductus arteriosus may be given a low-dose prostaglandin infusion and be in stable condition. A transport team can insist on intubation before a long air transport, whereas the referral physician might believe that intubation is not required and that it poses a risk to that particular patient. This situation can be challenging, and it must be handled appropriately. It is never appropriate to have obvious provider conflict occur at a patient's bedside, especially in front of family members. The appropriate way to handle a situation that cannot be easily mitigated is to involve the medical command physician with a telephone call to the referring physician in a discussion at a peer-to-peer level. Transport teams have been known to comply with the wishes of the referring providers to not perform advanced procedures at the referring hospital, only to perform those procedures in the ambulance, which is a much less desirable location. Ideally, all disagreements and considerations of different therapies are discussed in a collegial fashion in the appropriate environment to enable the safe care and transport of the child to the receiving center. As noted previously, documentation of all information received and advice offered is imperative. If there is future review or challenge to the care delivered during transport, as with any other care delivered in the hospital, clear and appropriate documentation should stand alone as an excellent defense. In addition, many centers use recorded (i.e., digital, tape, other retrievable recording process) for their intake and advice lines; this is another way to review, educate, and ensure that appropriate information is delivered in an effective communication style. The use of recorded lines with frequent review, for educational and quality assurance purposes, can be invaluable. Review with legal advisors can help to define the length of time the recorded materials should be maintained for quality improvement or patient record addendum.

PATIENT CARE DURING TRANSPORT

EXTREME PREMATURITY

The most effective method of transporting premature infants is within the mother as a maternal transport. By delivering at a referral hospital, the premature infant is exposed to all the variability of the extrauterine environment, with the added complexity of having to be transported to a facility capable of providing the level of care the infant needs. Most neonatal transport teams are regarded as extensions of the NICU. The team initiates and provides much of the same level of complex neonatal care as the receiving hospital, but in a changing environment. It is this changing environment that poses unique challenges for both patient and caregiver. These issues would be amplified in the case of a disaster with care and transfer required for premature infants (Gershanik, 2006).

Limit of Viability

The incidence of premature births has been increasing in the United States. Of the approximate 4.1 million live births occurring annually, 520,000 (12.7%) infants are born premature (Ananth et al, 2009; Martin et al, 2008). Although some premature infants require minimal care to survive, infants with very LBW often test the resources and skills of the most experienced care provider. The long-term outcome for many of these small infants is often unknown for months to years after leaving the hospital. In some instances, the long-term results have not been ideal (Donohue et al, 2009; Tyson and Saigal, 2005). Several studies of extremely premature infants born outside of tertiary care centers show increases in morbidity and mortality (Cifuentes et al, 2002; EXPRESS Group et al, 2009; Phibbs et al, 2007; Rautava et al, 2007). Human viability is currently limited by the physiology of pulmonary development and its ability to exchange gases. Currently this limit appears to be at approximately 22 to 24 weeks' gestation (Pignotti and Donzelli, 2008). Unfortunately, for transport teams and the care givers at referring hospitals, it is difficult to determine which infants born at the margins of viability should be resuscitated and provided with aggressive neonatal care and which should be allowed to die (American Academy of Pediatrics Committee on Fetus and Newborn and Bell, 2007; Buchanan, 2009). These decisions are best made collaboratively with the family, transport team members, and the referring and receiving physicians (Ahluwalia et al, 2008; Gunderman and Engle, 2005; Tyson et al, 1996) and may ultimately result in a patient transport, even when the likelihood for survival is minimal.

Thermoregulation

Problems in neonatal thermoregulation continue to be a major contributor to neonatal morbidity and mortality worldwide and can be especially problematic in neonatal transport (World Health Organization, 1996). During transport, neonates often cross into and out of multiple different environments with wide temperature and humidity variations. Although a normal term infant is capable of a significant homoeothermic response by using their sympathetic nervous system to vasoconstrict peripherally, thus placing their normal layer of insulating white fat between the body's core and the exposed skin, preterm infants lack the subcutaneous white fat insulation to protect their core temperature. Moreover, term infants use brown fat as a source for nonshivering thermogenesis. Preterm infants, although as sensitive to temperature as term infants, lack sufficient brown fat to sustain a response when exposed to a cold environment (Baumgart, 2008). The consequences of hypothermia can include hypoglycemia, metabolic acidosis, intraventricular hemorrhage, persistent pulmonary hypertension, and hypoxemia (Bartels et al, 2005). Silverman et al (1958) demonstrated that using a higher incubator temperature, even without additional humidity resulted in improved premature survival rates.

Additional measures such as chemical gel packs and polyethylene occlusive skin wrapping help in maintaining the temperature of an infant with very LBW (Vohra et al, 2004). For all newborns, an equally important condition to avoid is hyperthermia.

Although elevated temperatures in neonates occur with increased metabolic rates, prolonged seizures, dehydration, or infection, the most common cause of neonatal hyperthermia is high ambient air temperature and humidity (Baumgart, 2008). In a review of a subset of patients referred for a trial of hypothermia for hypoxic ischemic encephalopathy, patients with an elevated body temperature had poorer neurologic outcomes than those with normal body temperatures (Laptook et al, 2008; Yager et al, 2004). Humidity also has an extremely important role in temperature control of LBW infants, especially those receiving mechanical ventilator support. The importance of delivering humidified gas to neonates receiving mechanical ventilation is widely acknowledged (Sousulski et al, 1983). Ventilation with dry gases affects the airway epithelium in very LBW infants, and it can result in hypothermia secondary to their large surface area–to–body mass ratio and their relatively large respiratory minute volume (Fassassi et al, 2007). There is a linear correlation between incubator temperature and the humidity generated by heated humidity systems (Fassassi et al, 2007). Whereas ventilator complications can be reduced and thermoregulation can be improved by providing exogenous heat and humidity to the gases, active heated humidification systems are used infrequently during neonatal transport. Passive hygroscopic heat and moisture exchangers have been used for short-term conventional mechanical ventilation and with some types of high-frequency ventilation (Fassassi et al, 2007; Schiffmann, 1997; Schiffmann et al, 1999). Humidifying the incubator and the ventilator system helps in thermoregulation while transporting very LBW neonates.

Surfactant

Surfactant replacement has had a significant effect on newborn intensive care. Numerous systematic reviews have demonstrated the benefit of surfactant administration in reducing oxygen needs and ventilation requirements, as well as ventilator complications such as pneumothorax and pulmonary interstitial emphysema (Horbar et al, 1993; Liechty et al, 1991; Schwartz et al, 1994). Extremely LBW infants benefit from both prophylactic (defined as within 10 to 30 minutes of birth) and rescue surfactant administration (within 12 hours of birth) (Kendig et al, 1991; Soll, 2000). Infants given prophylactic surfactant appear to have fewer complications, including death, pneumothorax, and bronchopulmonary dysplasia (Soll and Morley, 2001), supporting its use during transport (Riek, 2004). Surfactant administration can be complicated by airway obstruction and right mainstem bronchus or esophageal instillation, justifying the American Academy of Pediatrics Committee on Fetus and

Newborn recommendations that "preterm and term neonates who are receiving surfactant should be managed by nursery and transport personnel with the technical and clinical expertise to administer surfactant safely and deal with multisystem illness" (Engle, 2008). While investigations are still ongoing as to the optimal manner of surfactant administration, future technology might eventually allow for surfactant to be delivered without airway intubation. Currently, aerosolized surfactant has yet to be shown to be superior to endotracheal tube administration (Berggren et al, 2000; Mazela et al, 2007). Although there are concerns about the composition variability of animal-derived surfactants, use of a synthetic surfactant such as Lucinactant creates other concerns. Lucinactant requires a special warming cradle to convert it from a gel to a liquid before administration, adding a level of difficulty to its administration during neonatal transport (Kattwinkel, 2005; Moya et al, 2005). Smaller community hospitals might not stock surfactant in their pharmacies, making it necessary for the transport team to carry it as part of their medical supplies. Earlier forms of surfactant came as lyophilized powder and could be reconstituted when needed. Currently, the most frequently used surfactant preparations in the United States are derived from either bovine or porcine lung extracts. These surfactants require refrigeration and are usually carried by transport teams in small containers cooled by gel packs. The same precautions used in the delivery room or the NICU apply to its use in transport. Checklists should be used to avoid inadvertently leaving this lifesaving therapy behind when the transport team is dispatched.

Before surfactant administration, proper endotracheal tube position must be confirmed either clinically or radiographically. Surfactant administration is generally done using transport team protocols, which usually mirror the package inserts. After administering surfactant, monitoring pulmonary compliance and adjusting the patient's ventilator support will occasionally extend the time of a transport to avoid clinical complications, such as pneumothorax or endotracheal tube occlusion, during the transfer process. Often by the time the transport team arrives at the receiving hospital, significant clinical improvement has occurred.

Surfactant has a role in other disease processes, such as meconium aspiration, sepsis, and pulmonary hemorrhage, during which a patient's endogenous surfactant is depleted or inactivated, thus creating a condition of secondary surfactant deficiency (Chinese Collaborative Study Group for Neonatal Respiratory Diseases, 2005; Finer, 2004; Wiswell et al, 2002).

HYPOXIC RESPIRATORY FAILURE

Meconium Aspiration Syndrome, Persistent Pulmonary Hypertension of the Newborn, Inhaled Nitric Oxide on Transport, and Extracorporeal Membrane Oxygenation Referrals

Hypoxic respiratory failure describes a heterogeneous group of neonatal disorders that have in common impaired oxygenation and the need for assisted ventilation. The most frequently observed conditions are respiratory distress syndrome, meconium aspiration syndrome, and persistent pulmonary hypertension of the newborn (PPHN), which can occur individually or in combination. Interfacility transport of the newborn with hypoxic respiratory failure is potentially hazardous, with a high risk for patient deterioration and complications of therapy, such as pneumothorax.

Assisted ventilation during neonatal transport can be accomplished with a variety of devices, although not all modes of mechanical ventilators have been modified for use in a mobile setting. Newborns with milder degrees of illness may be managed successfully with continuous positive airway pressure (Murray and Stewart, 2008). Infant transport ventilators range from simple time-cycled, pressure-limited machines to more sophisticated devices with flow sensitivity and the ability to synchronize. Certain high-frequency ventilators have been successfully adapted for the transport environment (see later).

Inhaled nitric oxide (iNO) is approved for use in term and near-term newborns with hypoxic respiratory failure with clinical or echocardiographic evidence of pulmonary hypertension. Persistent PPHN can exist in isolation or be secondary to another insult, such as sepsis or meconium aspiration syndrome. Administration of iNO to newborns with PPHN reduces the need for extracorporeal membrane oxygenation (ECMO; Clark et al, 2000; Lowe and Trautwein, 2007). With its availability to community NICUs, iNO is often initiated before transport to a tertiary care center. Once iNO is administered, abrupt cessation of therapy can result in rapid clinical deterioration from rebound pulmonary hypertension, so it is essential to continue iNO if already initiated (Kinsella et al, 1995). Transport teams may also consider initiation of iNO therapy for term and near-term newborns with hypoxic respiratory failure. If the referring facility does not have the capability to perform echocardiography, transport staff should carefully consider the possibility of congenital heart lesions that could be worsened by the use of iNO, including total anomalous venous return and lesions dependent on right-to-left ductal flow such as critical aortic stenosis.

The rationale for initiating iNO during transport is to reduce pulmonary vasoreactivity and improve stability during transport. However, there have been no prospective studies to determine whether this practice affects patient outcome. INO during transport has been delivered by a number of different systems, such as the aeroNOX (Aeronox Technology Corporation, Quezon City, Philippines) iNOvent, and INOmax DS (INO Therapeutics, New Jersey) transport systems (Kinsella et al, 1995, 2002; Lutman and Petros, 2008; Tung, 2001). The use of iNO in combination with high-frequency ventilation in non-ECMO centers can complicate the transfer process. If the transport team does not have the capability to provide mobile high-frequency ventilation, it is recommended that the referring hospital perform a trial of conventional mechanical ventilation before the arrival of the transport team to establish that the infant can tolerate the transition. Both high-frequency jet ventilation (Bunnell ventilators [Bunnell Inc., Utah]) and high-frequency flow interrupter ventilation (Bird ventilators [Viasys, California]) have been configured and used with nitric oxide during transport (Honey et al, 2007; Mainilli et al, 2007). The

high-frequency oscillator (SensorMedics 3100A [Viasys, California]) that is commonly used in many NICUs is impractical for ground transport and is not configured for helicopter or fixed wing transport. However, even with these technologies, 30% to 40% of critically ill neonates improve only temporarily with iNO therapy and will ultimately require higher care levels (Fakioglu et al, 2005; Kinsella et al, 2002).

In patients with pulmonary or cardiac failure that is unresponsive to maximal medical therapy, conventional ECMO is often used as a bridge therapy to allow either the lungs and heart to recover. Ideally, centers without ECMO capability have prospective criteria to guide the transfer of newborns before the need for ECMO cannulation. In some cases, the patient's condition is so unstable that conventional transport cannot be conducted safely. Selected programs have the capability to provide mobile ECMO, during which patients are cannulated for ECMO before transport to the referring institution. Mobile ECMO can also benefit patients already receiving ECMO at a tertiary facility who are in need of advanced quaternary therapies, such as heart or heart-lung transplants (Wagner et al, 2008; Wilson et al, 2002). The resources and skill set necessary to safely and consistently perform ECMO in the transport environment have, by their complexity, restricted the number of transport programs with mobile ECMO capabilities (Coppola et al, 2008).

NEUROLOGIC ISSUES

Perinatal Depression and Therapeutic Hypothermia

Hypoxic ischemic encephalopathy affects approximately 1 to 2 in 1000 term neonates (du Plessis and Volpe, 2002). Several early studies from the 1950s and 1960s suggested that hypothermia might be an effective therapy for the asphyxiated neonates, but there was no systemic long-term follow-up for these patients to confirm its effectiveness until a series of animal studies suggested that hypothermia was an effective neuroprotective therapy (Gunn et al, 1997, 1998). Several randomized trials of therapeutic hypothermia for term human infants have demonstrated a reduction in the combined outcome of death and neurodevelopmental disability when cooled, compared with a control population (Gluckman et al, 2005; Shankaran et al, 2005). However, the efficacy of hypothermia may diminish as the time from insult to cooling increases. Although clinical trials and current guidelines suggest that cooling should be initiated within 6 hours of insult, animal studies demonstrated that hypothermia is most effective if it is started as soon as possible (Gunn et al, 1997, 1998). For patients with a delay in referral or who are being transported from a distant center, waiting to start hypothermic therapy until arrival at the receiving center potentially places the patient at a significant disadvantage. The initial larger clinical trials did not address these issues in regard to critical care transport, but several case (Anderson et al, 2007), pilot (Eicher et al, 2005), and single-center studies have demonstrated the feasibility of controlled hypothermia during transport to significantly shorten the time to therapy initiation (Zanelli et al, 2008). Several new large-scale hypothermia trials that have been recently completed or are nearing completion include initiation of hypothermia before arrival at the referral center. The Total Body Hypothermia for Neonatal Encephalopathy Trial (the Toby Trial) compared standard intensive care plus total body cooling with standard intensive care for 72 hours. Recruited patients from referring hospital were assessed by the transport team, who performed amplitude integrated electroencephalograms and obtained consent if the patient was eligible and less than 6 hours of age. The patients randomized to cooling had gel packs applied if needed to cool the body to rectal temperature between 33° and 34° C (Azzopardi et al, 2009). The Australian Cooling Trial for Hypoxic-Ischemic Encephalopathy achieves the temperature range for referral study patients by turning off the normal heating systems and applying gel packs (at 10° C) around the infant's head and chest, until the rectal temperature is reduced to 33° to 34° C (Jacob et al, 2008). While hypothermia is still being evaluated as a therapeutic tool to manage hypoxic ischemic encephalopathy, the current management trend for term and near-term infants being considered for hypothermia is to delay actively warming the patient at a referral hospital until there is a consultation with a receiving hospital that offers therapeutic hypothermia. If criteria are met, further cooling could be achieved by placing wrapped disposable cooling packs next to the trunk and head with continuous monitoring of rectal temperature. Once the rectal temperature stabilizes, the infant is transferred to a transport incubator with the heater turned off, and the transport team applies cooling packs or a blanket as needed to maintain a rectal temperature of 33° to 34° C during transport. Just as careful temperature monitoring during hypothermia is necessary for the safe transport of these patients, observational studies suggest that the avoidance of hyperthermia is critically important. In an observational study, Laptook et al (2008) noted an increase in mortality or disability in asphyxiated neonates who had elevated skin or esophageal temperatures. As additional studies are completed, therapeutic hypothermia may enter common clinical and transport practices. When combined with other therapeutic interventions, hopefully therapeutic hypothermia will have a greater effect on the consequences of perinatal asphyxia.

Neonatal Seizures

The highest rate for seizures in pediatrics occurs during the neonatal period, with an incidence of 2 to 3.5 in 1000 live births (Cowan, 2002); however, there is considerable variability in treatment regimens among pediatric hospitals in the United States (Blume et al, 2009). Phenobarbital, phenytoin, or midazolam have not been shown to significantly improve seizure management or reduce morbidity and mortality (Booth and Evanse, 2004; Carmo and Barr, 2005; Painter et al, 1999). Despite the evidence of limited efficacy, phenobarbital remains the first line of therapy to treat neonatal seizures (Painter et al, 1999; Sankar and Painter, 2005). Before initiating therapy, the transport team needs to consider the diverse causes for neonatal seizures. Metabolic disorders such as hypoglycemia, hypocalcemia, and inborn errors of metabolism, cerebral vascular events including intraventricular hemorrhage and stroke,

bacterial and viral meningitis, infectious and developmental abnormalities can all manifest as or with neonatal seizures (Silverstein and Jensen, 2007). Having initiated treatment, the transport team needs to remain vigilant for potential changes in the patient's clinical status either as a response to therapy or from the primary disease process. Attention to the basics of airway, breathing, and circulation should continue throughout the transport, because the major anticonvulsants used to treat neonatal seizure all have potential side effects, most commonly respiratory depression and hypotension. Controversy remains as to whether to treat all forms of neonatal seizures, although treatment seems prudent in the transport environment (Bartha et al, 2007). In animal models, seizures create neural, biochemical, and structural changes that have long-term cognitive and behavioral consequences (Thibeault-Eybalin et al, 2009). Similar neurologic findings have been suggested in human neonates. Both of the large-scale clinical hypothermia trials for hypoxic ischemic encephalopathy noted poorer prognosis for children with hypoxic ischemic encephalopathy with seizures (Gluckman et al, 2005; Shankaran et al, 2005). Glass et al (2009) compared magnetic resonance imaging findings and the presence of seizures in a group of newborns with suggested hypoxic ischemic encephalopathy. Adjusting for the magnetic resonance imaging results, patients with seizures were more likely to have long-term neurologic issues than those without seizures (Glass et al, 2009). The ideal anticonvulsant agent would reliably stop clinical and electrographic seizures with minimal adverse effects (Thibeault-Eybalin et al, 2009). Several trials of new antiepileptic medications are underway. Topirmante, levetiracetam, bumetanide, and zonisamide have all been used to treat neonatal seizures, but there have been no randomized trial to demonstrate their effectiveness compared with current therapies. Trials with levetiracetam and bumetanide are reportedly ongoing. Further work is necessary to develop more effective and safer antiepileptic drugs so that, along with potentially neuroprotective strategies, the vulnerable and immature brain can be protected. Several trials and studies have been proposed to hopefully elucidate a better treatment strategy (Clancy, 2006).

STABILIZATION AND TRANSPORT OF THE NEONATE WITH CONGENITAL HEART DISEASE

Transport of the neonate with congenital heart disease (CHD) follows the general guidelines for the transport of any critically ill neonate. However, neonates with complex CHD often need therapeutic intervention, requiring the support of multiple subspecialty consultants, including the pediatric cardiothoracic surgeon and pediatric cardiologist (Allen et al, 2003; Stark et al, 2000). The care of the neonate with CHD generally necessitates transport to a specialized center (Castaneda et al, 1989; Penny and Shekerdemian, 2001). The preoperative care of the patient affects postoperative outcomes and mortality (Mahle and Wernovsky, 2000; Mahle et al, 2000; Robertson et al, 2004; Simsic et al, 2007; Wernovsky et al, 1995, 2000). With the increasing use of fetal ultrasound examination to diagnose CHD antenatally, the ability to intervene immediately at delivery has become increasingly expected. In a single tertiary care center, 53% of neonates with CHD had a prenatal diagnosis (Dorfman et al, 2008), with an additional 38% obtaining a diagnosis before discharge from the newborn nursery. The aspects of stabilization of the neonate with CHD either diagnosed by prenatal ultrasound or suggested by postnatal clinical examination include initial resuscitation, airway management, vascular access, a judicious use of supplemental oxygen, prostaglandin E1 (PGE1) therapy, inotropic support, and communication with cardiac specialty services for timely transport and intervention.

Neonates with Prenatally Diagnosed Congenital Heart Disease

Significant advances in the diagnosis and treatment of neonates with critical CHD across the last decade have altered the timing of intervention, the types of interventions available, and the way in which CHD is diagnosed. With increasing numbers of patients with prenatal diagnosis (Berkley et al, 2009; Friedman et al, 2002; Jone and Schowengerdt, 2009; Khoshnood et al, 2005), fewer neonates may have their initial presentation of CHD in the emergency department. In a single-center review, prenatal diagnosis accounted for 53% of presentations of CHD (Dorfman et al, 2008). Another European center reported that 51% of transports with CHD had a prenatal diagnosis (Bouchut, 2008). In addition, a single-center cohort of critical CHD showed 44.3% to have had a prenatal diagnosis (Schultz et al, 2008). Clearly, prenatal diagnosis of CHD has increased across the past decade.

Neonates with Suspected Congenital Heart Disease

In a single tertiary care center, Dorfman et al (2008) found that 38% of neonates received a diagnosis with CHD in the newborn nursery before discharge, and 8% of patients presented with CHD after initial hospital discharge at 4 to 27 days of life. The most common nursery findings prompting diagnosis of heart disease in the nursery were an isolated murmur, cyanosis, or both (Berkley et al, 2009; Table 29-1). In a single emergency department review of patients younger than 5 months with undiagnosed cardiac disease, the most common presentation was congestive

heart failure, shock, and cyanosis; if restricting the findings to a neonatal population, shock and profound cyanosis were the presenting symptoms (Savitsky et al, 2003). Another study showed that 45% of critical CHD cases (CHD with signs of shock, end organ dysfunction, or in cardiac arrest) were diagnosed postnatally, particularly left-sided obstructive lesions (Schultz et al, 2008). This finding is consistent with other centers showing a preponderance of left-sided obstructive lesions (excluding hypoplastic left heart syndrome) in those diagnosed postnatally (Friedberg et al, 2009).

The cyanotic neonate who fails the hyperoxia test without an obvious pulmonary etiology, who has an equivocal result on the hyperoxia test but has other signs or symptoms of CHD, or who is in shock within the first 3 weeks of life is highly likely to have complex CHD. Furthermore, pulse oximeter measurement of the postductal (probe on the foot) oxygen saturation has been found to be specific for the detection of CHD, particularly when combined with findings on the clinical examination (de-Wahl Granelli et al, 2009; Meberg et al, 2008, 2009; Reich et al, 2008; Sendelbach et al, 2008; Thangaratinam et al, 2007; Valmari, 2007). Although debate is ongoing as to the appropriateness of routine pulse oximetry as a screening tool (Sendelbach et al, 2008), the detection of saturations of less than 95% has a sensitivity of 72% to 77%, specificity rates over 99%, and false-positive rates of 0.2% to 0.6% in large-volume studies (Meberg et al, 2008; Valmari, 2007). These neonates are likely to have heart lesions that depend on blood flow through a patent ductus arteriosus to contribute to either systemic or pulmonary blood flow, or improvement of intercirculatory mixing. PGE1 given as continuous infusion will reopen the ductus arteriosus. In babies with ductal-dependent pulmonary blood flow, hypoxemia is lessened as the ductus opens, and the resultant metabolic acidosis will resolve. Babies with systemic flow that is dependent on the ductal connection to provide flow to the descending aorta will have congestive heart failure, low cardiac output, or shock, which is unlikely to be treatable by standard measures without reopening the ductus arteriosus. Patients with transposition of the great arteries will have improved intercirculatory mixing with a patent ductus arteriosus (Wernovsky, 2008; Wernovsky and Jonas, 1998). Interventions such as supplemental oxygen, airway management, volume resuscitation, inotropic therapy, and prostaglandin infusion require careful thought and consideration in the child with CHD.

Considerations of Therapies in the Neonate with Congenital Heart Disease

The neonatal resuscitation algorithm is still applicable in the presence of CHD (Johnson and Ades, 2005), but should be modified in certain circumstances. In presentations with hypoxemia that is unresponsive to supplemental oxygen, congestive heart failure, or shock, simultaneous attention is devoted to the basics of neonatal advanced life support and to assurance of a patent ductus arteriosus.

A stable airway must be maintained, allowing for adequate alveolar oxygenation and ventilation. In critically ill neonates with CHD presenting with severe cyanosis or circulatory collapse, intubation should be performed if

TABLE 29-1   Presenting Symptoms of Patients Diagnosed Postnatally

	Diagnosis in Nursery, n = 73 (%)	Diagnosis After Discharge, n = 16 (%)
Murmur	38	25
Cyanosis	32	0
Respiratory distress	7	19
Shock	4	38
Arrhythmia	3	0
Other	3	6
Multiple symptoms	14	13

Modified from Dorfman AT, Marino BS, Wernovsky G, et al: Critical heart disease in the neonate: presentation and outcome at a tertiary care center, *Pediatr Crit Care Med* 9:193-202, 2008.

possible after premedication with sedation and neuromuscular blockade (discussed subsequently). Reliable venous access is important, and arterial monitoring is helpful for ongoing assessment of blood pressure, acid-base status, and gas exchange. Volume resuscitation, inotropic support, and correction of metabolic acidosis may be required to maximize cardiac output and tissue perfusion. Blood glucose and ionized calcium should be checked and treated to achieve normal range for age. An evaluation for sepsis is typically performed simultaneously, and empiric antibiotic therapy is initiated while evaluation continues.

Supplemental Oxygen

Supplemental oxygen is a potent pulmonary vasodilator and systemic vasoconstrictor, and it can adversely affect the physiology in neonates with a single ventricle, as well as those with two ventricles with an unrestrictive ventricular septal defect or great vessel communication (see Chapter 55, Congenital Heart Disease). In these babies, the ratio of pulmonary vascular resistance to systemic vascular resistance will determine the proportion of blood flow to each vascular bed. The oxygen-induced pulmonary vasodilation can decrease pulmonary vascular resistance and increase pulmonary blood flow at the expense of systemic blood flow, thus reducing systemic output. Titrating oxygen via nasal cannula or face mask to a target peripheral saturation of 75% to 85% usually corresponds to adequate blood flow in both the pulmonary and systemic systems. In the setting of normal hemoglobin, cardiac output, and oxygen consumption, these oximetry values will provide adequate oxygen delivery. Higher oxygen saturations are typically not necessary and importantly may in fact ultimately result in decreased oxygen delivery to the peripheral tissues. Considerations for intubation and mechanical ventilation are discussed Intubation and Ventilation, later.

Prostaglandin E1 Therapy

In the instance of antenatally diagnosed CHD, ductal dependency (either for systemic or pulmonary blood flow) is often already determined. Whenever possible, PGE1 infusions should be prepared ahead of delivery and started promptly in a peripheral intravenous catheter. The dose of PGE1 varies according to the timing of the diagnosis and the degree of ductal closure that is present upon discovery (or suspicion) of the cardiac lesion. In most cases, PGE1 at 0.01 to 0.025 µg/kg/min via intravenous infusion is adequate for stabilization. PGE1 may be given via a central venous catheter or peripheral intravenous catheter, or in situations where intravenous access cannot be obtained, via an umbilical arterial catheter or intraosseous line. The dose is usually titrated down once the patent ductus arteriosus has been demonstrated echocardiographically. However, doses as high as 0.1 µg/kg/min may be required in the newborn with significant ductal constriction or in the neonate who at 1 to 2 weeks of life presents with a closing, closed, or severely restrictive ductus arteriosus. As in the prenatally diagnosed neonate, once therapeutic effect is achieved, the dose can generally be decreased without loss of therapeutic effect. Prostaglandin response is often immediate if ductal patency is important to the

hemodynamics of the infant. Failure to respond may mean that the initial diagnosis of ductal dependent CHD is incorrect, the ductus is unresponsive to PGE1 (which may occur in older infants), or that there is no ductus arteriosus present.

On rare occasion, the neonate may have progressive instability after initiating PGE1 therapy. This important diagnostic finding strongly suggests a congenital heart defect with obstructed blood flow out of the pulmonary veins or the left atrium. These lesions include (1) hypoplastic left heart syndrome with restrictive foramen ovale or intact atrial septum, (2) other variants of mitral atresia with a restrictive foramen ovale, (3) transposition of the great arteries with intact ventricular septum and restrictive foramen ovale, and (4) total anomalous pulmonary venous return with obstruction of the common pulmonary vein.

If the neonate clinically deteriorates despite PGE1 therapy, urgent echocardiography with plans for potential interventional cardiac catheterization or cardiac surgery need to be made. Early recognition of this deterioration despite PGE1 requires prompt transfer to a cardiac unit (Penny and Shekerdemian, 2001). Controversy exists as to whether PGE1 should be continued in these rare instances; it has generally been the authors' practice to continue the infusion at the usual dose. More important than the decision to continue or discontinue PGE1 is that the lack of response to PGE1 in a child with suspected CHD is a marker for rare forms of CHD that do not respond to medical management and require urgent surgical or catheter intervention.

Although PGE1 is critical in the management of most neonates with CHD, there are a number of potential adverse effects associated with PGE1 continuous infusion that must be anticipated, particularly in the premature or LBW infant, in which they occur more commonly. The most common adverse effects include hypotension (caused by vasodilation), apnea, rash, and fever (Kramer et al, 1995; Lewis et al, 1981). Other less common side effects include seizures, gastric outlet obstruction, cortical hyperostosis, and leukocytosis (Arav-Boger et al, 2001; Teixeira et al, 1984).

Although high-dose PGE1 infusions may occasionally be required, most often neonates are in stable condition receiving a low-dose infusion. The resultant vasodilation and hypotension is less common and usually treatable with fluid resuscitation rather than inotropic support (Kramer et al, 1995). A separate intravenous catheter is typically necessary for the purpose of volume administration and should be considered prior to transport. A 5 to 10 mL/kg bolus of normal saline, lactated Ringer's solution, or 5% albumin will generally normalize the blood pressure in cases of hypotension related to PGE1. Serum ionized calcium levels should be checked and normalized if low. If hypotension is refractory to fluid administration, an alternative cause of hypotension should be considered (e.g., a restrictive ductus, pericardial effusion, myocardial dysfunction, sepsis), and dopamine (3 to 5 µg/kg/min) may be given to offset the vasodilatory effects of PGE1.

If apnea and hypotension occur, they will usually manifest during the first hours of administration, but may occur at any time during the infusion. This occurrence mandates the need for ongoing cardiorespiratory monitoring even after stabilization on PGE1 infusion. Furthermore it has been shown that, although the side effect profile (particularly apnea) increases with increasing doses and lower weight, the clinical response is not dose dependent. In other words, infants can be maintained safely on a low-dose PGE1 infusion until definitive care is achieved and thereby potentially avoid the significant side effects of apnea and hypotension. Certainly, PGE1 therapy alone does not require mechanical ventilation without the presence of significant or recurrent apnea (Browning et al, 2007; Kramer et al, 1995) or other clinical states requiring mechanical ventilation. The use of low-dose PGE1 (<0.015 µg/kg/min) for duct-dependent lesions is unlikely to cause apnea requiring mechanical ventilation, and it is safe to transport the infant without establishing an artificial airway in most cases (Carmo and Barr, 2005).

When starting PGE1 infusion, it is prudent to remeasure arterial blood gases and reassess vital signs and perfusion within 15 to 30 minutes of initiation. Doing so allows effectiveness to be assessed and any adverse events to be addressed promptly.

Intubation and Ventilation

Although the initiation of PGE1 alone does not require the neonate to be intubated, the presence of profound hypoxemia, respiratory distress, or hemodynamic instability may demand airway intervention. In most cases, intubation should be performed after premedication with sedation (narcotic or benzodiazepine), preferably with neuromuscular blockade. Although intubation can be performed without sedation and neuromuscular blockade, there are physiologic reasons to use these agents for the intubation of a neonate with CHD. First, the catecholamine surge that will occur with a nonsedated intubation may result in significant dysrhythmias in the at-risk myocardium. Second, vagally mediated bradycardia from hypoxemia, hypercapnia, or laryngeal stimulation may lead to asystole in these neonates, who have little reserve. Finally, sedation and neuromuscular blockade will reduce total body oxygen consumption, raising the mixed venous oxygen saturation and improving oxygen delivery. Premedication with atropine (0.02 mg/kg) can blunt the vagal effects of laryngoscopy. Fentanyl (1 to 2 µg/kg) or midazolam (0.05 to 0.1 mg/kg) for sedation may be given, with titration of dose to effect. Chest wall rigidity may occur with low-dose fentanyl (more likely if given rapid push) and may require neuromuscular blockade for adequate ventilation.

In most cases, the neonate is preoxygenated with 100% FiO_2, which can be down-titrated to achieve an acceptable oxygen saturation given the underlying CHD after intubation. In an effort to maintain a balanced circulation, ventilation should attempt to achieve normocarbia (Pco_2, 35 to 40 mm Hg). In the single-ventricle patient (i.e., a patient in whom the systemic and pulmonary circulations are dependent on a single-ventricular pumping chamber) or the neonate with unrestrictive ventricular or great vessel communications, significant adjustments in ventilation will alter pulmonary vascular resistance, and therefore may have an effect on both pulmonary and systemic blood flow. Hyperventilation in the neonate decreases pulmonary vascular resistance, thereby increasing pulmonary blood flow potentially at the expense of systemic blood flow.

Although intubation and ventilation may be necessary interventions, it should be noted that preoperative mechanical ventilation is a risk factor for mortality or poor outcome after surgery for CHD in multiple studies (Gottlieb et al, 2008; Robertson et al, 2004; Simsic et al, 2007; Tabbutt et al, 2008).

Inotropic Therapy

The neonate with CHD discharged from the nursery before diagnosis may be experiencing congestive heart failure or circulatory collapse. These infants, while urgently requiring the opening of the ductus arteriosus to provide either systemic or pulmonary blood flow, may also require inotropic therapy to recover from the adverse effects of a myocardium that has decompensated in the face of high afterload (obstructive left-sided lesions requiring ductal patency for systemic blood flow) or hypoxemia (obstructive right-sided lesions requiring ductal patency for pulmonary blood flow). Appropriate volume status should be achieved in conjunction with the institution of inotropic therapy and secure access for its delivery. The choice of inotropic agent remains largely practitioner dependent.

Sympathomimetic amines are the most commonly used inotropic agents. They can be endogenous (dopamine and epinephrine) or synthetic (dobutamine and isoproterenol). Dopamine is a norepinephrine precursor and stimulates dopaminergic, β1-adrenergic, and α-adrenergic receptors in a dose-dependent manner. Dopamine improves myocardial contractility, which will increase stroke volume. This increase leads to improved cardiac output and higher mean arterial pressure, with resultant increased urine output. There is a low incidence of side effects at doses less than 10 µg/kg/min. Dobutamine is an analogue of dopamine; it stimulates β1-adrenergic receptors predominantly, with relatively weak β2-adrenergic receptor and α-adrenergic receptor activity. No definitive benefit has been found in the use of dopamine versus dobutamine, although dopamine is more likely to increase the systemic blood pressure in the short term. No differences in outcomes or mortality were found between the two inotropes (Subhedar and Shaw, 2003). Both drugs are generally initiated at 3 to 5 µg/kg/min. Epinephrine may also be used in neonates with hypotension and hemodynamic deterioration. Epinephrine has α1-, α2-, β1-, and β2-adrenergic effects. Few trials have been done to recommend epinephrine over other agents. A randomized controlled trial comparing epinephrine and dopamine in LBW infants found equal efficacy in treating hypotension (Valverde et al, 2006). The recommended starting dose is 0.03 to 0.05 µg/kg/min. Isoproterenol stimulates β1- and β2-adrenergic receptors. It has greater chronotropic effect and stronger vasodilatory effect because of the β2 stimulation. It needs to be started at low dose and titrated to effect, because of the strong chronotropic effect. Chronotropic effects will precede inotropic effects in a responsive heart and can produce tachyarrhythmias. Recommended starting dose is 0.01 to 0.05 µg/kg/min.

The adverse effects of the sympathomimetic amines include tachycardia, atrial and ventricular arrhythmias, and peripheral vasoconstriction causing increased afterload. Tachycardia will increase myocardial oxygen consumption, whereas arrhythmias and vasoconstriction decrease cardiac output.

Vascular Access

Umbilical venous catheters (UVCs) and umbilical arterial catheters (UACs) are useful in the stabilization, transport, and preoperative and postoperative management of the neonate with CHD. However, the placement of these lines is not without risk. Beyond the infectious risks, newborns with CHD are at a higher risk for thromboembolic events because of their underdeveloped clotting mechanisms, small vessel lumens, and low flow states. There is also an ongoing risk of systemic embolization of air and particulate matter in babies with an intracardiac right-to-left shunt. There has been much controversy surrounding the optimal placement of a UAC in premature infants, although there are scant data regarding full-term infants with CHD. A Cochrane Database review suggested that "high" catheters were associated with a decreased risk of vascular complications with no significant increase in adverse sequelae (Barrington, 2000; Hermansen et al, 2005). Although there is variation in definition, in general "high" catheters are above the level of the diaphragm and below the level of the left subclavian artery (approximately T6 to T10); "low" catheters are below the renal arteries but above the aortic bifurcation (approximately L3 to L5). Levels between high or low are associated with increased risks of complications, as are placements below the L5 level (Hermansen et al, 2005). Although transient placement of a UAC in this area will generally be well tolerated, long-term placement should be avoided if possible. The UVC should be placed, if possible, at the inferior vena cava/right atrial junction or in the atria. It might not be necessary to obtain ideal placement of either the UAC or UVC for stabilization and transport, and manipulation of lines and reconfirmation can delay transport and stabilization to the tertiary care center. The risk-benefit relation for the use of umbilical lines in the neonate with ductal dependent circulation has not been well delineated. The need for central access should be judged based on the clinical status of the neonate and stability for transport.

Transport of the Neonate With Congenital Heart Disease

Once the neonate with suspected or known CHD has been sufficiently resuscitated and stabilized, they should be transferred to an institution that provides subspecialty care in pediatric cardiology and pediatric cardiothoracic surgery. In a single tertiary center study of neonates presenting with CHD, 157 of 190 patients required at least one surgical or catheter intervention with a median of 3 days of life at time of surgery (Dorfman et al, 2008). To optimize management, early communication with the specialist center is vital. Successful transport involves two phases: referring hospital staff to the transport team and subspecialists, and transport staff to the accepting hospital staff. The need for this precise and thorough communication between respective teams cannot be overemphasized. Whenever possible, the pediatric cardiologist, neonatologist, or intensivist at the accepting hospital should be

included in formulating the transport management plan while the neonate is still at the referring hospital. This procedure will help to guide the timing and urgency of the transport, line placement, and recommendations for airway management and supplemental oxygen. Often the patient with a duct-dependent lesion will improve greatly with the institution of prostaglandin therapy and may not need to be rushed to the cardiac referral center as an emergent case.

Similar supports and treatments need to be put into place before transport of any critically ill neonate or infant. Secure vascular access should be obtained, with a port available for volume resuscitation that is not running the inotropic support or PGE1 infusion, to avoid interruption of this medication. Intubated patients should have the airway position recorded and secured and have a nasogastric or orogastric tube for decompression. The intubated infant should remain unfed, and medication administration and fluids should be given intravenously. Appropriate sedation should be used, as well as maintenance of normothermia and avoidance of hyperthermia, to minimize oxygen consumption.

Evaluation of acid-base status, oxygen delivery, temperature, serum glucose, and calcium should take place before transport and should be corrected when possible. Neonates with conotruncal anomalies are at particular risk for hypocalcemia, because they have an increased frequency of 22q11 deletion syndrome (Gallot et al, 1998), which may have associated thymic and parathyroid hypoplasia. Furthermore, the neonatal myocardium may be more dependent on calcium for inotropy than the adult. Ionized calcium levels less than 1 mg/dL may have a significant negative effect on contractility and should be considered for treatment with calcium gluconate (50 to 100 mg/kg) or calcium chloride (0.1 mEq/kg of elemental calcium or 0.01 g/kg) intravenously, via a central catheter if possible.

In patients with mixing lesions, single ventricle or in those with an unknown diagnosis, supplemental oxygen should be used and titrated to maintain pulse oximeter oxygen saturation of 75% to 85% for "balance" of circulation between pulmonary and systemic systems and to provide adequate oxygen delivery, because higher oxygen saturations may actually be deleterious, as noted previously. The accepting pediatric cardiologist can aid with lesion-specific advice and guidelines to optimize in-transport care.

Hypotension is a late finding of shock in neonates. Earlier, more sensitive signs, of impending decompensation include persistent tachycardia despite adequate intravascular volume and temperature control, poor tissue perfusion, and metabolic acidosis. Treatment of shock should occur before transport during the stabilization phase of management, although the patient in profound shock and with significant acidosis at presentation may require significant time for resolution of organ dysfunction and perfusion and clearance of acidosis. Finally, failure to respond to prostaglandin, assuming adequate dose and delivery, should promote prompt transfer to a cardiac unit able to care for lesions with obstruction to pulmonary venous outflow. Before leaving the referring hospital, hemodynamic status (capillary refill, heart rate, systemic blood pressure, and acid-base status) needs to be reassessed and communicated to the accepting hospital.

Summary of Cardiac Transport

Stabilization and transport of the neonate with known or suspected critical CHD affect their preoperative condition, potentially contributing to short-term mortality risk and long-term morbidity. One key to stabilization is the recognition of potential or confirmed CHD, appropriate resuscitation, airway management where indicated, stable vascular access, judicious oxygen utilization, PGE1, and inotropic support when necessary. Early consultation with a center specializing in pediatric cardiac care, for advice and timing of transport, will aid the initial care and stability of the infant on transport. Accurate, detailed information must be communicated among the referring hospital, the transport team, and the accepting hospital.

SURGICAL EMERGENCIES

Because most births occur in hospitals without an NICU or neonatal surgical abilities, the need for surgical evaluation or intervention is a common reason for interfacility transport. Whereas some surgical conditions are relatively not urgent in nature, there are several diagnoses that represent truly life-threatening conditions for which stabilization and transport require expertise and specialized resources.

Congenital Diaphragmatic Hernia

Advances in ultrasound technology have resulted in the prenatal diagnosis of up to 60% of fetuses affected by congenital diaphragmatic hernia (Gallot et al, 2007). A recent systematic review showed that outcome was improved for newborns with a prenatal diagnosis or born in a tertiary care center (Logan et al, 2007b). Newborns with undiagnosed CDH, especially those delivered at a community hospital, are at high risk for complications. Before transport, critically ill infants with suspected or known CDH should undergo tracheal intubation and placement of a large-bore nasogastric or orogastric tube to continuous suction, because many have received bag-mask ventilations and swallowed air can quickly travel beyond the pylorus and distend the intrathoracic intestinal contents (Grisaru-Granovsky et al, 2009; Logan et al, 2007b). Whenever possible, the same principles of management that are used in the tertiary care center should be used during transport: limitation of peak airway pressures and use of low tidal volumes to avoid ventilator-induced lung injury, judicious use of sedation, avoidance of chemical paralysis to permit spontaneous breathing, and maintenance of adequate systemic blood pressure with the use of fluid therapy and inotropes (Logan et al, 2007a). Although there is still controversy over the role of extracorporeal membrane oxygenation for newborns with CDH, transport to a high-volume center with ECMO capabilities should be strongly considered (Grushka et al, 2009; Morini et al, 2006).

Abdominal Wall Defects

The proper management of a newborn with gastroschisis or omphalocele is critical during the first several hours of life, and delivery in a tertiary care center has been associated with improved outcome (Quirk et al, 1996). In addition to the need for initial resuscitation and cardiorespiratory support, the correct treatment of the exposed bowel or sac may improve the infants' chances of a successful repair and long-term intestinal function.

The mean gestational age for newborns with gastroschisis is 36.6 weeks, and many affected infants are small for gestational age (Baerg et al, 2003; Lausman et al, 2007). As with other mildly premature and growth-restricted infants, patients with gastroschisis are at risk for hypothermia and hypoglycemia. Heat loss is exacerbated by the large surface area of the exposed intestines, which can also serve as a significant source of fluid loss. Prevention of heat and fluid losses can be accomplished by placing the lower part of the infant's body, including the intestines, into a transport bag (i.e., bowel bag or Lahey bag) before placement of the infant into the heated transport isolette. Significant fluid losses can occur through the exposed mucosa, and the patient may require aggressive fluid replacement (120 to 150 mL/kg/day). The use of antibiotics should be considered if risk factors for sepsis are present and reviewed with the pediatric surgeon.

Infants with gastroschisis are at risk for intestinal vascular compromise, because the vascular pedicle containing the arterial supply and venous drainage from the bowel must pass through the relatively small abdominal wall defect. Transport personnel must closely monitor the appearance of the bowel to detect signs of venous congestion or ischemia. Transporting the infant in the lateral position, with support of the exposed intestines to avoid tension or torque, is recommended. The use of intestinal pulse oximetry has been described for monitoring the bowel for ischemia through a transparent silo, but has not been studied as a tool during interfacility transport (Kim et al, 2006). Vascular compromise of the intestine is a surgical emergency, and communication with the receiving facility is essential to coordinate urgent intervention.

The transport of an infant with omphalocele has similar considerations, although unless the sac has ruptured there is significantly less risk of heat and fluid loss. Infants with an omphalocele are more likely than those with gastroschisis to have other birth defects (e.g., CHD). Furthermore, infants with giant omphaloceles often have respiratory insufficiency caused by diaphragmatic dysfunction, pulmonary hypoplasia, or both, and they may require ventilatory assistance.

All infants with gastroschisis or omphalocele require placement of a large-bore nasogastric or orogastric tube due to functional ileus or intestinal obstruction, as may occur with associated stenoses or atresias. In general, cannulation of the umbilical vessels is not recommended unless other methods for vascular access are not successful.

Esophageal Atresia and Tracheo Esophageal Fistula

Esophageal atresia, with or without tracheo esophageal fistula, is typically diagnosed within the first day of life because of increased secretions, poor feeding, and respiratory distress. General transport considerations include placement of a large-bore sump-type tube for continuous aspiration of the proximal esophageal pouch, positioning (prone with the head of bed elevated), and respiratory support as indicated. Direct aspiration of secretions into the trachea may occur with either a proximal or distal tracheo esophageal fistula. Transport providers should be aware that infants with a distal tracheo esophageal fistula (type C), characterized by the presence of air in the intestinal tract, are at risk for gastric and intestinal insufflation via the fistula when receiving positive-pressure ventilation. Bag-mask ventilation and continuous positive airway pressure should be avoided. If the infant requires endotracheal intubation, the endotracheal tube should be positioned as close to the carina as tolerated in an effort to position the distal tip beyond the fistula and minimize direct inflation of the distal esophageal segment with pressurized gas. In extreme cases, gastric rupture with pneumoperitoneum has been reported, requiring emergency paracentesis, laparotomy, or both (Maoate et al, 1999).

Midgut Volvulus

Malrotation with midgut volvulus can be a catastrophic event resulting in intestinal ischemia and shock, and it represents a surgical emergency in the neonate. The most common clinical presentation of midgut volvulus is bilious vomiting, which is a nonspecific sign of intestinal obstruction. Expeditious evaluation of the newborn with bilious vomiting is essential to facilitate prompt surgical intervention in the event that midgut volvulus is identified, to prevent progression of vascular insufficiency to actual intestinal necrosis. An upper gastrointestinal series is the radiologic test of choice to diagnose malrotation and midgut volvulus, although some practitioners have reported success with the use of ultrasound examination to identify the relationship of the superior mesenteric vessels (Lampl et al, 2009; Shew, 2009).

An infant with suspected midgut volvulus should be rapidly transported to a facility with pediatric radiology and surgical capabilities. Care of the infant with suspected midgut volvulus during interfacility transport is primarily supportive and includes circulatory support with intravenous fluid repletion, correction of metabolic abnormalities, and gastric decompression with a large-bore nasogastric or orogastric tube.

Necrotizing Enterocolitis

Necrotizing enterocolitis (NEC) is common in premature infants, and approximately 30% of newborns with NEC will require surgical intervention in the form of laparotomy or peritoneal drain placement (Guthrie et al, 2003). The clinical presentation of NEC is typically nonfocal and often mimics signs of systemic sepsis. Clinical and radiologic findings that are specific to NEC include abdominal distention and discoloration of the abdominal wall, dilated or thickened bowel loops, pneumatosis intestinalis, portal venous gas, and free intraperitoneal air.

Infants with suspected NEC should be transported to a facility with pediatric surgical capabilities. Care during transport is primarily supportive and includes intravenous fluids, administration of broad-spectrum antibiotics,

correction of metabolic abnormalities, and gastric decompression. Respiratory failure is common because of disordered control of breathing and elevation of the diaphragm from abdominal distension.

Meningomyelocele

Although most newborns with neural tube defects are diagnosed prenatally because of an elevated AFP and are therefore delivered in a tertiary care center, the unexpected birth of an infant with a meningomyelocele may be an indication for neonatal transport. For purposes of transport, the infant should be placed in the prone position and the spinal defect should be covered with moist sterile dressings as well as some form of plastic wrap to maintain moisture. The lesion can be covered with a moistened Telfa dressing and then loosely encircled with a Kerlix "donut," with the entire defect covered with a sterile drape. This dressing can be moistened as indicated during the transport process (Jason and Mayock, 1999). Avoid the use of latex gloves during care of these patients. If the skin covering the defect is disrupted, there is an increased risk of infection, and empiric antibiotics should be considered. Infants with meningomyelocele may or may not have accompanying hydrocephalus at birth; approximately 25% of affected patients will require shunting in the immediate newborn period, with up to 85% eventually undergoing shunt placement (Bowman et al, 2001).

SUGGESTED READINGS

Browning Carmo KA, Barr P, West M, et al: Transporting newborn infants with suspected duct dependent congenital heart disease on low-dose prostaglandin E1 without routine mechanical ventilation, *Arch Dis Child Fetal Neonatal Ed* 92:F117-F119, 2007.

Das UG, Leuthner SR: Preparing the neonate for transport, *Pediatr Clin N Am* 51:581-598, 2004.

Dorfman AT, Marino BS, Wernovsky G, et al: Critical heart disease in the neonate: presentation and outcome at a tertiary care center, *Pediatr Crit Care Med* 9: 193-202, 2008.

Engle WA: American Academy of Pediatrics Committee on Fetus and Newborn: Surfactant-replacement therapy for respiratory distress in the preterm and term neonate, *Pediatrics* 121:419-432, 2008.

King BR, Woodward GA: Procedural training for pediatric and neonatal transport nurses: Part I: - training methods and airway training, *Pediatr Emerg Care* 17:461-464, 2001.

Orr RA, Felmet KA, Han Y, et al: Pediatric specialized transport teams are associated with improved outcomes, *Pediatrics* 124:40-48, 2009.

Phibbs CS, Baker LC, Caughey AB, et al: Level and volume of neonatal intensive care and mortality in very-low-birth-weight infants, *N Engl J Med* 356: 2165-2175, 2007.

Polin RA, Randis TM, Sahni R: Systemic hypothermia to decrease morbidity of hypoxic-ischemic brain injury, *J Perinatol* 27:S47, 2007.

Silverstein FS, Jensen FE: Neurological progress: neonatal seizures, *Ann Neurol* 62:112, 2007.

Thangaratinam S, Daniels J, Ewer AK, et al: Accuracy of pulse oximetry in screening for congenital heart disease in asymptomatic newborns: a systematic review, *Arch Dis Child Fetal Neonatal Ed* 92:F176-F180, 2007.

Woodward GA, Insoft RM, Kleinman ME, editors: *Guidelines for air and ground transport of neonatal and pediatric patients,* Elk Grove Village, Ill, 2007, American Academy of Pediatrics.

Woodward GA, King BR, Garrett AL, et al: Prehospital care and transport medicine. In Fleisher G, Ludwig S, Henretig F, editors: *Textbook of pediatric emergency medicine,* ed 5, Philadelphia, 2006, Lippincott, Williams, and Wilkins, pp 93-134.

Complete references used in this text can be found online at www.expertconsult.com

TEMPERATURE REGULATION OF THE PREMATURE NEONATE

Stephen Baumgart and Sudhish Chandra

The human neonate is a homeothermic mammal. Even the smallest premature infants respond adaptively to changes in their environment. Response, however, may be insufficient to maintain core body temperature and can render preterm babies functionally poikilothermic, even in moderately temperate environments. Morbidity (e.g., poor brain and somatic growth) and mortality rates increase when core body temperature is permitted to decline much below 36° C (96.8° F), and moderate to severe hypothermia below 31° C (88.7° F) results in precipitous declines in heart rate and blood pressure.

COLD STRESS

Evaporative heat loss is widely as regarded the most stressful cooling event upon birth. Severe nonevaporative heat loss is also problematic for several reasons. First, a baby's exposed body surface area is much larger than an adult's, relative to metabolically active body mass (Table 30-1). Especially for the extremely low birthweight infant, the heat-dissipating area is fivefold to sixfold greater proportionate to that of the adult. Second, the baby's small size presents a much smaller heat sink to store thermal reserve. Finally, the radius of curvature of the body is less than in the adult, resulting in a thinner protective boundary layer of warm, still air.

Aside from these geometric considerations, characteristics of the premature infant's skin contribute to the problem of excessive heat loss. The skin and subcutaneous fascia provide little insulation against the flow of heat from the core to the surface. Moreover, the lack of a keratinized epidermal barrier exposes infants to vastly increased evaporative heat loss.

Finally, premature infants may not induce effective thermogenesis in response to cold stress. Shivering and nonshivering thermogenesis are compromised by low brown fat stores. Furthermore, the presence of hypoxia (common with preterm birth) seriously reduces nonshivering thermogenesis by reducing mitochondrial oxidative capacity.

PHYSICAL ROUTES OF HEAT LOSS

CONVECTION

Convective heat loss in newborns occurs when ambient air temperature is less than the infant's skin temperature. Convective heat loss includes natural convection (passage of heat from the skin to the ambient still air) and forced convection, in which mass movement of air over the infant conveys heat away from the skin. The quantity of heat lost is proportional to the difference between air and skin temperatures, and to air speed. The effect of forced convection in disrupting the microenvironment of warm, humid air layered near an infant's skin usually is not appreciated in the nursery, where drafts, air turbulence, and consequently heat loss can occur within the relatively protective environment of an incubator.

EVAPORATION

Passive transcutaneous evaporation of water from a newborn's skin (insensible water loss) results in the dissipation of 0.58 Kcal/mL of latent heat. As shown in Figure 30-1, transcutaneous water loss increases exponentially with decreasing body size and gestation. The tiniest premature baby, who is least able to tolerate cold stress, can incur evaporative heat loss in excess of 4 Kcal/kg/hr (water loss of approximately 7 mL/kg/hr). Evaporation is enhanced by low vapor pressure (i.e., high air temperature and low relative humidity) and air turbulence. The highest evaporative losses occur on the first day of life. During the first week of life in infants born at 25 to 27 weeks' gestation, evaporative heat losses may be higher than radiant losses (Hammarlund et al, 1986).

RADIATION

Radiant heat loss constitutes the transfer of heat from an infant's warm skin, via infrared electromagnetic waves, to the cooler surrounding walls that absorb heat. Radiant heat loss is proportional to the temperature gradient between the skin and surrounding walls. An infant's posture may affect radiant heat loss by increasing or reducing the exposed radiating surface area. In a moderately humid environment (relative humidity approximately 50%), babies experience an ambient temperature (termed *operant temperature*) determined 60% by wall temperature and 40% by air temperature.

CONDUCTION

Conductive heat loss to cooler surfaces in contact with an infant's skin depends on the conductivity of the surface material and its temperature. Usually babies are nursed on insulating mattresses and blankets that minimize conductive heat loss.

PHYSIOLOGY OF COLD RESPONSE

AFFERENTS

Homeothermic response to a cold environment begins with the sensation of temperature. Traditional physiology identifies two temperature-sensitive sites: the hypothalamus and the skin. Sensation of cold by neonatal skin triggers a cold-adaptive response long before core sensors

TABLE 30-1 Body Surface Area-to-Body Mass Ratio

	Body Weight (kg)	Surface Area (m²)	Ratio (cm²/kg)
Adult	70	1.73	250
Premature infant	1.5	0.13	870
Very premature infant	0.5	0.07	1400

in the hypothalamus become chilled. Some investigators conjecture that neonatal cold reception resides primarily in the skin, whereas warm reception resides in the hypothalamus. Both sensors are probably integrated, because cold sensory response is inhibited by core sensor hyperthermia and vice versa. Peripheral skin cold sensation is teleologically important, because early detection of heat loss from the skin aids in the infant's timely response for maintaining core temperature.

CENTRAL REGULATION

Integration of multiple skin temperature inputs probably occurs in the hypothalamus; however, no single control temperature seems to exist. Under different environmental conditions, temperature of the skin can fluctuate 8° to 10° C, and temperature of the hypothalamus may vary ±0.5° C. There are also diurnal temperature fluctuations, variations with general sympathetic tone, and blunted regulation with asphyxia, hypoxemia, and other central nervous system defects. Premature infants can regulate core temperature near 37.5° C (99.5° F), whereas term infants may respond by maintaining 36.5° C (97.7° F). Because important thermoregulatory processes are triggered by deviations of as little as 0.5° C at any temperature-sensitive site, environmental temperature homeothermy is important.

EFFERENTS

The effector limb of the neonatal thermal response is mediated primarily by the sympathetic nervous system, although infant behavior may also be involved. The earliest maturing response is vasoconstriction in deep dermal arterioles, resulting in reduced flow of warm blood from the infant's core into the exposed periphery. In addition, reducing blood flow effectively places a layer of insulating fat between the warm core tissue compartment and the cooler exposed skin surface in the term infant. Reduced fat content in babies with low birthweight diminishes this effective insulating property. Vasoconstriction nevertheless remains the newborn's first line of thermally insulating defense, and the response is present even in the most premature infant.

Brown fat constitutes a second sympathetic effector organ that provides a metabolic source of nonshivering thermogenesis. (Babies do not shiver like adults to generate heat, because muscle constriction-relaxation fibers are not yet myelinated.) Brown fat located in axillary, mediastinal, perinephric, and other regions of the newborn is particularly enervated and equipped with an abundance of mitochondria to hydrolyze and reesterify triglycerides

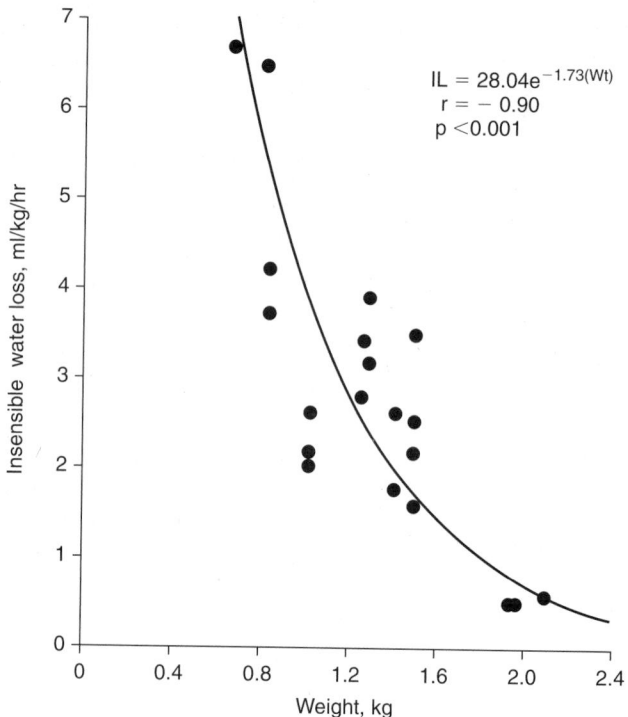

FIGURE 30-1 Exponential increase in evaporative water loss from skin of infants with very low birthweight who were nurtured under radiant warmers. (*Adapted from Baumgart S, et al: Fluid, electrolyte and glucose maintenance in the very low birthweight infant, Clin Pediatr 21:199-206, 1982.*)

and to oxidize free fatty acids. In the term infant, these reactions are exothermic and may increase metabolic rate by twofold or more. Preterm babies, however, have little brown fat and may not be capable of more than a 25% increase in metabolic rate despite the most severe cold stress (Hull, 1966).

Finally, recent evidence suggests that control of voluntary muscle tone, posture, and increased motor activity with agitation may serve to augment heat production in skeletal muscle via glycogenolysis and glucose oxidation. Clinical observations of infant posture, behavior, and skin perfusion and measurements of skin and core temperature gradient may ultimately provide the most useful guidelines for assessing infant comfort during incubation.

MODERN INCUBATION: INCUBATORS AND RADIANT WARMERS

The lifesaving requirement of an appropriate thermal environment was demonstrated conclusively by Day et al (1964) and further defined by Silverman et al (1966). Minor changes in heat balance create an oxygen and energy cost, inducing an increased metabolic rate that can be met only by increased ventilation or increased inspired oxygen and appropriate cardiovascular response to provide oxygen delivery to activated tissues.

THERMAL NEUTRAL ZONE

The thermal neutral zone is a narrow range of environmental temperatures within which an infant's metabolic rate is minimal and normal body temperature is maintained.

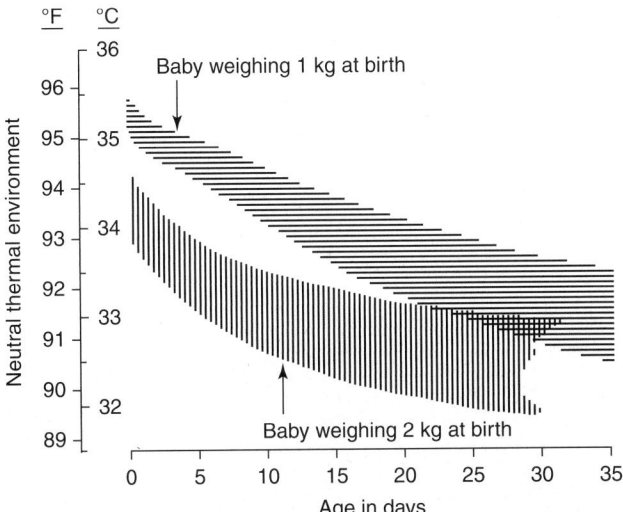

FIGURE 30-2 The range of temperature needed to provide neutral environmental conditions for a baby lying naked on a warm mattress in draft-free surroundings of moderate humidity (50% saturation) when mean radiant temperature is the same as air temperature. The *hatched areas* show the average neutral temperature range for a healthy baby weighing 1 or 2 kg at birth. Optimal temperature probably approximates the lower limit of neutral range as defined here. Approximately 1° C should be added to these operative temperatures to derive the appropriate neutral air temperature for a single-walled incubator when room temperature is less than 27° C (80° F), and more should be added if room temperature is significantly less. (*Adapted from Hey EN, Katz G: The optimum thermal environment for naked babies,* Arch Dis Child *45:328-334, 1970.*)

TABLE 30-2 Mean Temperature Needed to Provide Thermal Neutrality for a Healthy Baby Nursed Naked in Draft-Free Surroundings of Uniform Temperature and Moderate Humidity during the Days or Weeks after Birth

Birth-weight (kg)	Operative Environmental Temperature*			
	35° C	**34° C**	**33° C**	**32° C**
1.0	For 10 days	After 10 days	After 3 weeks	After 5 weeks
1.5		For 10 days	After 10 days	After 4 weeks
2.0		For 2 days	After 2 days	After 3 weeks
>2.5			For 2 days	After 2 days

Data from Hey E: Thermal neutrality, Br Med Bull 31:72, 1975.
*To estimate operative temperature in a single-walled incubator, subtract 1° C from incubator air temperature for every 7° C by which this temperature exceeds room temperature.

When thermally neutral, infants regulate temperature through vasomotor tone alone without regulatory changes in metabolic heat production. A range of critical environmental temperatures relevant to modern incubators was clearly articulated by Hey and Katz (1970; Figure 30-2, Table 30-2). Below this range, an increase in the infant's minimal metabolic rate was observed; therefore the thermal neutral temperature range was defined as the optimal incubator operating (operant) temperature. Several important considerations in regulating incubator temperature were included in these studies: (1) incubator wall temperature was maintained identical to air temperature, (2) relative humidity was controlled near 50%, and (3) the environment was maintained in a steady state, uninterrupted by turbulence or invasion of the incubator's enclosed perimeter.

Rigid application of older air temperature recommendations should be modified. Many modern incubators incorporate a double-walled design that results in lower radiant heat loss to colder incubator walls encountered in single-walled designs. As a result, slightly cooler air temperature may be required. In addition, many nurseries do not humidify incubators artificially, fearing the occurrence of condensation ("rain-out") resulting in bacterial colonization, particularly around door openings. Finally, it is important to recognize that the incubator's steady state temperature control is frequently interrupted for nursing and medical procedures that require opening doors to care for the infant. More than 1 hour may be required to recover prior steady state conditions after such procedures; therefore the thermal neutral zone must be redefined in practical terms. Silverman et al (1966) used a modified concept of the thermal neutral zone to simplify

clinical application. Reasoning that infants sense environmental temperature first on the skin, electronic negative-feedback (servo-controlled) regulation of the incubator heater in response to skin temperature was introduced. These authors demonstrated minimum metabolic expenditure near 36.5° C (97.7° F) abdominal skin temperature as measured by a shielded thermistor in a less rigidly defined incubator environment. The importance of frequently checking core temperatures (axillary or rectal) must be emphasized before delegating the infant's environment to thermostatic control. In addition, Chessex et al (1988) have demonstrated that incubator temperature can vary by more than 2° C when skin temperature servo control rather than air temperature control is used, obviating homeothermic environmental conditions.

Finally, with the modern use of open radiant warmer beds (improving access to the critically ill premature infant without interrupting heat delivery) skin temperature servo control is the only practical method for approximating the thermal neutral zone (Malin and Baumgart, 1987). The extension of infant warming to include extremely low birthweight, critically ill premature babies have generated new problems for determining a universally accepted optimal environment.

PARTITIONING INFANT HEAT LOSSES AND HEAT GAINS

Wheldon and Rutter (1982) demonstrated the special problems encountered in incubating infants with very low birthweight in a convection-warmed, closed-hood incubator environment (Figure 30-3). Figure 30-3, *A*, demonstrates the thermal balance achieved by a series of 12 infants (mean weight, 1.58 kg). Heat losses to radiation (R), convection (C), and evaporation (E) are modest, and their sum (Σ) is balanced by the infant's metabolic heat production (M). Used in this fashion, the incubator reduces physical heat losses such that the infant's minimal metabolism (larger than any single avenue of heat loss)

A

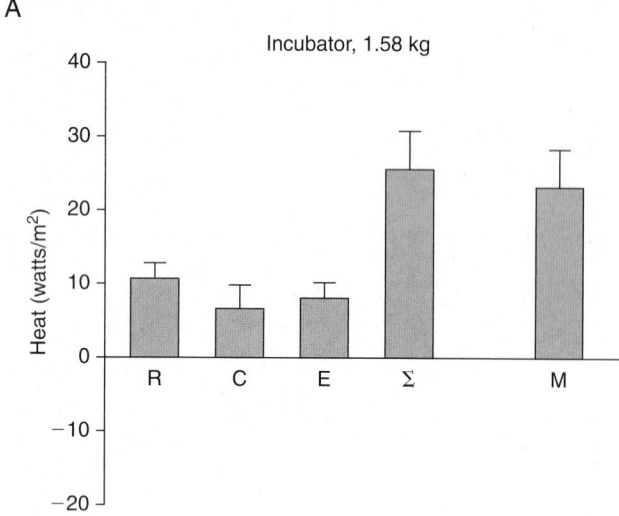

B

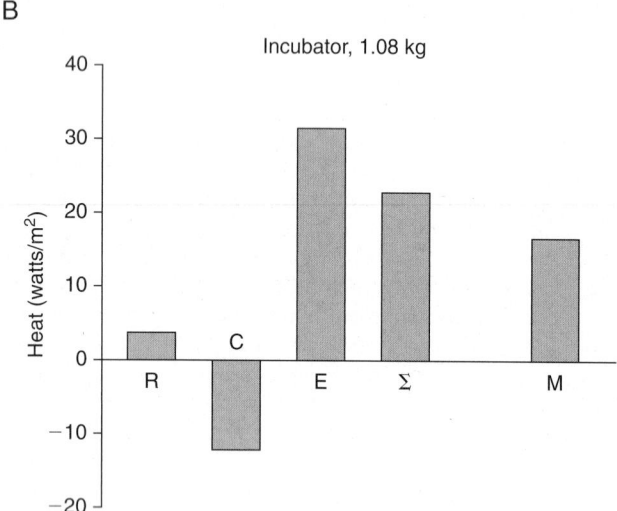

FIGURE 30-3 A, Partition of heat losses and gains in 12 premature infants nursed within incubators. **B,** Partition in an infant weighing 1.08 kg at birth. Heat losses to radiation (*R*), convection (*C*), and evaporation (*E*) are modest, and their sum (*Σ*) is balanced by the infant's metabolic heat production (*M*). (*Adapted from Wheldon AE, Rutter N: The heat balance of small babies nursed in incubators and under radiant warmers,* Early Hum Dev *6:131-143, 1982.*)

delicately balances minimal physical heat losses within the controlled thermal environment.

In contrast, a subject with very low birthweight (1.08 kg) is evaluated in Figure 30-3, *B*. As the incubator servo control increases warming power to accommodate massive evaporative heat loss, convective loss becomes a net gain (negative histogram bar). Radiant loss is diminished by warm walls inside the incubator. These conditions differ strikingly from those discussed previously: the incubator truly warms the infant rather than modestly attenuating convective heat loss, and evaporative heat loss vastly exceeds the infant's metabolism. The small infant's body temperature is balanced, therefore, between opposing physical parameters of evaporative and convective heat transfer. Metabolism plays a secondary role.

The modern use of radiant warmers that are servo controlled to maintain infant abdominal skin temperature

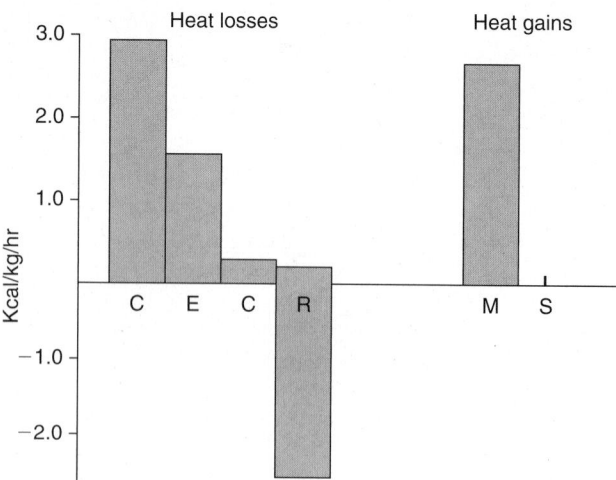

FIGURE 30-4 Partitional calorimetry in 10 critically ill premature newborns with low birthweight who were nursed under open radiant warmers. *C,* Convection; *E,* evaporation; *M,* infant's metabolic heat production; *R,* radiation. (*Adapted from Baumgart S: Radiant heat loss vs. radiant heat gain in premature neonates under radiant warmers,* Biol Neonate *57:10-20, 1990.*)

between 36.5° and 37° C (97.7° to 98.6° F) also demonstrates the opposition of physical forces described earlier. Figure 30-4 demonstrates the heat balance partition for 10 critically ill premature infants (mean weight, 1.39 kg) nursed on open radiant warmer beds (Baumgart, 1990). Because ambient room air temperature is 5° to 10° C cooler than air inside an incubator, convective heat loss is nearly double the infant's metabolic heat production. Evaporation adds to the net physical heat loss. In addition, small amounts of heat are lost to conduction and radiation (to cooler room walls). The infant's metabolism provides only one third of the energy required to maintain body temperature, with the majority of heat supplied by the servo-controlled radiant heat source injecting heat transdermally through skin blood flow. In this instance, radiant warming (not convection as in the incubator discussed earlier) delicately balances the infant's physical temperature environment. Wheldon and Rutter (1982) demonstrated similar results in their studies.

HYBRID INCUBATOR-RADIANT WARMER TECHNOLOGY

A more promising new development in commercially available incubators is a hybrid design, combining these two separate warming modes in one device. Manufacturers in the United States and Germany (Air-Shields [Hatboro, Pennsylvania], Hill-Rom [Batesville, Indiana], Drager [Lubeck, Germany], and General Electric, Ohmeda [Laurel, Maryland]) have launched such products. In the incubator mode, movable plastic walls enclose the tiny premature infant, providing servo-controlled air warming, while the overhead radiant warmer is incorporated into the roof of this design but remains off. In the radiant warmer mode, the plastic walls are dropped down, and the radiant warmer rises overhead on a motorized pylon and rapidly turns on to maintain servo-controlled skin temperature during infant care procedures. The infant is not moved, and no plastic barrier is placed between the infant and the radiant heat source when turned on in this mode. The servo control algorithms, and the integrity of the plastic enclosure in incubator mode, are critical to the performance of such devices, and the utility of these products (e.g., survival, quality of life) is still unproved. Published data are reviewed in the following sections.

VERSALET INCUWARMER

Greenspan et al (2001) tested nine premature lambs, randomized at delivery, to receive incubation from a conventional radiant warming bed (Resuscitaire) with subsequent transfer into an incubator C550 Isolette or from the hybrid Versalet 7700 Care System (Air-Shields, Hatboro, Pennsylvania) in both the warmer bed and the incubator modes. Deep central and surface temperatures, heart rate, blood pressure, and blood gas determinations were measured during warming in the radiant warmer bed mode (Versalet) or on the radiant warmer bed Resuscitaire and then during transition to the incubator mode (Versalet or Isolette), and then back to the warmer bed, and bed mode. The animals conditions all remained clinically stable throughout the entire transfer protocol on both arms of the study. Despite careful planning, loss of temperature probe data occurred when probes became unattached in the control group during transfers from one device to the other. There were no significant differences in recorded temperatures or in pH and blood gasses in either group. Compared with the standard warming techniques currently used in neonatal intensive care units (NICUs; separate warmer bed for resuscitation and stabilization with transfer as soon as possible into an incubator device), the Versalet provided similar thermal and cardiovascular stability without adverse physiologic events during transition to different modes of warming. The authors state that the contribution of this hybrid device to the ease of management and improved outcomes in humans needs to be evaluated in a clinical trial (Greenspan et al, 2001; Sherman et al, 2006). No such trial has yet been conducted, and the Versalet is currently not in production (Jay Greenspan, personal communication).

GIRAFFE OMNIBED

As a radiant warmer, the Giraffe OmniBed (General Electric, Ohmeda Division, Laurel, Maryland) evenly heats the infant's mattress with a curved reflector surface designed to distribute heat to the baby and its bed surface without overwarming bedside caregivers. Babies are warmed uniformly, regardless of their position on the bed platform surface, which can be rotated 360 degrees, accommodating intravenous and ventilator tubing and attached wire leads. The same platform tilts up to 12 degrees in Trendelenburg or reverse Trendelenburg positions. Three-sided access from drop-down walls in the radiant warmer mode facilitates procedures such as diaper and bedding changes, blood sampling, starting intravenous lines, performing tracheal intubation, administering medications, creating radiographs, and conducting ultrasound examinations without interrupting warming. A stable thermal environment in either the incubator or radiant warmer mode eliminates the stress of moving premature babies, such as when performing chest tube insertion or other surgical procedures

performed in the NICU and outside the operating room. In one of several industry sponsored studies, Leef et al (2001) reported that infants were handled significantly less with the Giraffe OmniBed, especially when converted to incubator mode (from 6.9 handling events per hour maximum on a standard radiant warmer bed device to 1.6 times per hour on an OmniBed-closed). These authors concluded that the OmniBed is conducive to providing developmentally appropriate care—that is, medically fragile newborns are not exposed to a variety of visual, auditory, and tactile stimuli that would not occur otherwise within the mother's womb. Consequences of such stimulation are unknown, although it seems reasonable to avoid excessive handling and inappropriate touches because of documented physiologic effects of procedural handling (Gressens et al, 2002).

In a second industry-sponsored study (Gaylord et al, 2001), there were no differences found in mean skin temperature among the four tested conditions in premature neonates (R = radiant warmer configuration of OmniBed; transition R to C = convection-warmed closed OmniBed and transition C to R). Mean heart rate, respiratory rate, blood pressure, and oxygen saturation were not statistically different among the four test conditions. These authors conclude that the Giraffe OmniBed provided thermal and physiologic stability across bed states, eliminating the risk of infant mishap as a result of bed transfer.

When transforming the Giraffe OmniBed from incubator to warmer bed and back, the closed-convection heat partition adapts to form a uniform open-radiant heating configuration with sequential alterations of air warming temperature, fan power, and radiant heat delivered while displaying all equipment and baby parameters in one control panel. For example, when returning to the closed-convection mode, the retracting radiant warmer pylon immediately disconnects electrical power to the warming element and opens a mechanical air vent to cool the reflector hood, avoiding overheating the infant upon descent. In closed-convection configuration, bidirectional airflow through a double wall construction provides a stably enclosed thermal environment. When either door port is opened, an air curtain minimizes infant heat loss.

Light and sound levels are carefully controlled within the OmniBed to promote infant health and development (Lynam, 2003). An alarm light easily visible to caregivers remains out of infant's view. The WhisperQuiet mode limits sound to create the most quiet and soothing environment possible. Alarm speakers are deflected to minimize any noise experienced by the baby. An in-bed scale further reduces infant handling.

In addition, servo-regulated humidification is supplied within the closed-incubator condition and can be set to a determined relative humidity between 70% and 80%, which is optimal to avoid excessive insensible water loss and electrolyte disturbances often experienced by premature neonates with extremely low birthweight in the first week of life when incubated dry. One recent non–industry-sponsored report of a clinical series compared the use of initial stabilization of babies with extremely low birthweight (<1000 g) under a radiant warmer followed by conventional incubation—dry versus use of humidity control in OmniBeds. The authors demonstrated that humidification improved care by decreasing fluid intake, with more stable electrolyte balance, and growth velocity (Kim et al, 2010). The authors did not address the risk-benefit issue of humidification and infection.

The Giraffe Humidifier immerses a heating element in a reservoir of sterile, distilled water. Water temperature at equilibrium ranges 52° to 58° C, which is bactericidal to most organisms thriving at temperatures of 20 to 45° C (most human pathogens). As an added safety measure against reservoir contamination, water is boiled off the immersion element as the humidified air is passed inside the infant's compartment. Sterile humidity is created in a vapor state, with no airborne droplets. In a third industry-sponsored study by Lynam and Biagotti (2002), humidified OmniBeds (in vitro, air control mode at 35° C, and humidified to 65% relative humidity) were cultured after investigator inoculation with reservoir contamination with four waterborne pathogens over a 4-week incubating period. No infant environment culture revealed growth of any pathogen. The authors concluded that there is no concern for an increased risk of infection to an infant when the reservoir is filled daily with sterile distilled water and the bed is routinely cleaned, according to their protocol.

LESS CONVENTIONAL TECHNIQUES

PLASTIC HOODS

Plastic hoods comprise rigid body shields sometimes used as miniature incubator hoods placed over infants on open radiant beds. Hoods are usually made of plastic (1 to 3 mm thick) and can obstruct the delivery of radiant heat to the baby's skin when placed between an infant and the radiant warming element. The plastic can form a heat sink, warming to 42° to 44° C, but disrupts the radiant warmer's servo control mechanism and is a poor strategy. In addition, such devices might not diminish insensible water loss, especially when used without humidity. Use with humidity—a technique often referred to as *swamping*, which has never been validated—encourages bacterial colonization with water born pathogens.

PLASTIC BLANKETS

Alternatively, a thin, flexible plastic wrap or polyethelene plastic "blanket" was introduced in 1968 for covering premature infants under radiant warmers (Baumgart, 1984; Baumgart et al, 1981, 1982a, 1982b). The blanket prevents convective heat loss and is thin enough to transmit almost completely radiant heat from the warmer. The flexible plastic molds closely around the infant's body (with care taken to avoid skin adhesion), conserves evaporation, and forms a microenvironment near the baby's body. The plastic acts as a mechanical barrier to prevent convective turbulence from disrupting this microenvironment. A two-thirds reduction in insensible water (and evaporative heat) loss under radiant warmers is prevented, resulting in less servo-controlled radiant heat delivery required to maintain body temperature in even the smallest infants. By moderating heat losses, oxygen consumption is reduced by approximately 10%. This reduction exactly matches the oxygen consumption cost of using radiant warmers reported by LeBlanc (1982). Risks of plastic blankets include sticking to immature skin, causing masceration

and accidental airway obstruction in patients without intubation. In rare cases, partial detachment of the skin thermistor probe can result in life-threatening hyperthermia. Diligence is required to avoid these complications. The risk for abnormal bacterial colonization has not been evaluated.

A polyethylene plastic bag was evaluated by Vohra et al (1999) to promote temperature maintenance during delivery room resuscitation under radiant warmers and during subsequent transport of infants to the NICU. A significantly higher admission rectal temperature and survival was reported for infants at less than 28 weeks' gestation. A larger, randomized trial of this technique was performed, confirming the prevention of heat loss with a polyethylene bag but not the improvement in mortality (Vohra et al, 2004). Recently another large, randomized trial was performed to compare polyethylene caps with polyethylene bags; it found that both methods were more effective than conventional treatment in improving NICU admission temperature for infants at less than 29 weeks' gestation (Trevisanuto et al, 2010).

SEMIPERMEABLE POLYURETHANE SKIN

A semipermeable, semiocclusive polyurethane dressing (Tegederm [3m Corporation, Maplewood, Minnesota] or Opsite [Smith & Nephew, London, United Kingdom]) can be applied like an artificial skin to shield premature infants with very low birthweight. These breathing polyurethane plastics do not cause skin breakdown and are often used to dress central venous catheter sites. Temperature probe detachment is less likely to occur because of skin adherence. These dressings can also be tailored to avoid airway obstruction. Insensible water loss may be reduced more than 30% with these dressings, and after carefully removing them the skin's naturally developing keratin moisture barrier may be preserved. Porat and Brodsky (1993) and Bhandari et al (2005) demonstrated that an adherent polyurethane layer over the torso and extremities of infants with very low birthweight improved fluid and electrolyte balance, reduced the occurrences of patent ductus arteriosus and intraventricular hemorrhage, and improved survival. Further study is required to demonstrate the safety of this technique.

PETROLEUM OINTMENTS

Another occlusive dressing for the skin of preterm infants with low birthweight during the first week of life is the application of Aquaphor (Biersdorf Co, Hamburg, Germany). Although early results were encouraging for preserving skin integrity and perhaps controlling excessive dehydration in dry incubators, the findings of a multicenter randomized trial were not so laudable (Edwards et al, 2004). Anecdotal reports suggest that bacterial infections may actually be more common with use of this technique. Clinicians should exercise critical judgment before adopting this practice.

KANGAROO CARE

Kangaroo care connotes warming by skin-to-skin contact with the mother or father, where premature infants are held naked between the axilla or the breasts, mimicking a kangaroo's pouch. First implemented in Bogota,

Columbia, this method was popularized for nonintubated premature infants in Scandinavian and European countries in the 1980s. Early studies suggested a significant reduction in early mortality and morbidity in premature infants weighing less than 1.5 kg and who are nursed by kangaroo care. Behavioral studies demonstrated more stable sleep patterns, less irritability at 6 months of age, and more eye contact with caregivers in infants nursed with kangaroo care. Kangaroo care has been shown to promote a thermal-neutral metabolic response and temperature stability in stably growing premature babies. Moreover during kangaroo care, infants with bronchopulmonary dysplasia have better oxygenation, and other infants show less periodic breathing and reduced apnea. In the modern nursery, kangaroo care be initiated during mechanical ventilation in uncomplicated patients. The infant should be placed between breasts with maximum skin contact and should be covered with a blanket to avoid outward convective and evaporative heat losses. After initial sessions of 30 minutes to 1 hour with careful intermittent temperature monitoring, periods up to 4 hours may be achieved successively. Kangaroo care integrates the family into the neonatal intensive care team. No adverse reports have been published, and use in many nurseries is on the rise.

SPECIAL CASES

EXTREMELY LOW-BIRTHWEIGHT INFANTS

Case Presentation

A baby boy ($23^{4/7}$ weeks' gestation, weighing 510 g) was born limp, cyanotic, with no respiratory effort, and a heart rate less than 100 beats/min. The baby was resuscitated under a radiant warmer and dried, and a stocking cap was placed over the head. The warmer's temperature probe recorded a low skin temperature because it did not attach well to skin. The radiant warmer was on full power to compensate for this low probe reading. After resuscitation, the baby was transported to the NICU in an incubator preheated to a temperature of 35° C. On arrival, the baby was weighed quickly and placed onto a preheated radiant warmer bed. Skin probe (servo control) temperature registered 33° C, with a rectal temperature of 35° C and axillary temperature of 34° C. The radiant warmer set point was targeted at 37° C, and temperatures were monitored every 15 minutes. A plastic blanket was used to minimize heat loss. Heated and 100% humidified air from a respiratory pack was run underneath the blanket. next, the baby was prepared with iodine solution and draped completely for umbilical catheterization (a 30-minute procedure). Over the first 2 hours of life, rectal temperature increased only to 34.5° C. The baby was transferred into a preheated and humidified incubator regulated by a skin probe set at 37° C. Two light bulbs (250 W) were positioned over the incubator hood for supplemental heat and for warming during any procedure requiring opening the incubator (e.g., serial weight determinations). Over the next 12 hours the baby had difficulty maintaining temperature despite incubator air temperature running near a set temperature of 37° C, and sometimes greater than 38.5° C.

Discussion

Temperature maintenance of an extremely premature infant should be part of resuscitation from the time of delivery. Despite radiant warming in the delivery room and convective incubation during transport, this baby had hypothermia on admission to the NICU. Low admission temperature correlates with increased mortality rates in these infants. They are born wet and prone to excessive transepidermal evaporative and convective heat losses. In addition, heat loss can be exacerbated by suboptimal radiant heating; blowing noncontrolled warm, humidified air under plastic blankets, which is probably not as effective as the still air envelope conserved by the blanket; and the pressure for performing procedures with surgical drapes that block radiant heat delivery.

Quick drying, proper placement directly under the radiant heater at birth, and covering the head are small but important steps of temperature resuscitation. Other techniques might be considered from birth, such a use of a plastic bag described by Vohra et al (1999) or a plastic blanket or polyurethane drape during umbilical catheterization. Finally, transferring infants into incubators before adequately rewarming them under a radiant warmer can prolong thermal recovery in hypoxic subjects who are incapable of generating enough metabolic heat to recover. The use of light bulbs to provide supplemental radiant heat in incubators attests to the incubator's intrinsic operating power deficiency (i.e., seeking to reduce heat loss, rather than rewarm cold babies). Moreover, such supplemental radiant heat sources are not controlled, produce more radiation in the visible light range, and are inefficient and potentially dangerous for promoting burns if placed too close to the infant's skin.

There are few data describing the best rate of rewarming. Cold-stressed babies should probably be nursed under a servo-controlled radiant heat source, and heat loss should be minimized. During rewarming the infants should be closely monitored, and heat delivery should be servo controlled. A rate of approximately 0.5° to 1° C per hour seems reasonable, but it might not be achievable. Profound cardiovascular and electrolyte disturbances characterize rewarming. Alternatively, a preheated and humidified incubator can be used to rewarm infants, although the rate may be slower. The incubator air or skin servo control temperature can be set 1° C higher than the baby's temperature and gradually increased until a normal core temperature is achieved. Hybrid incubators that can also be used as radiant warmer beds are available and are helpful in rewarming scenarios.

NEONATAL FEVER

Problem of Temperature Elevation

There is no universally accepted definition of neonatal fever. Craig (1963) defined *neonatal pyrexia* as a rectal (core body) temperature greater than 37.4° C; however, other investigators accept temperatures up to 37.8°C as normal. Between 1% and 2.5% of all newborns admitted to the nursery develop fever, judged by rectal or axillary temperatures and depending on the limits chosen. Fever is an inconsistent and infrequent sign of sepsis (fewer than 10%

of febrile neonates have culture-proven sepsis), and temperature elevation may be seen with several other clinical entities.

Mechanisms Producing Neonatal Fever

Mechanisms producing neonatal fever are understood incompletely and result from disturbances in the complex interactions between heat conservation and heat dissipation mechanisms. Fever can occur when immunogenic pyrogens (commonly prostagladin [PG E2]) leads to upward displacement of the normal thermal set-point in the hypothalamus, leading to activation of heat conservation and physiologic heat-generating responses. Generally heat conservation starts with peripheral vasoconstriction and is followed by thermogenesis (generally nonshivering in neonates) while the new set-point is achieved. It is important to note that newborn infants of different animal species react in peculiar ways to different known pyrogens. Human newborns can have severe bacterial infections without increased body temperature.

In addition to pyogenic mechanisms of febrile response in newborns, other phenomena can lead to elevated of body temperature. Newborn infants have poor heat dissipation mechanisms (absence of sweating); therefore exposure to excess heat or insulation (e.g., excessive swaddling) can quickly increase their core temperature. Such overheating commonly occurs when term babies are nursed in uncontrolled incubators or under radiant warmers. Temperature elevation can also occur with increased infant metabolic rate such as that seen with skeletal muscle rigidity and status epilepticus. Another cause of temperature elevation is occasionally observed in healthy, breast-feeding newborn infants on the third to fourth day of life, and it is believed to result from dehydration caused by insufficient milk production. Finally, there are more recent reports of an increased incidence of neonatal fever in infants of mothers receiving epidural analgesia. The mechanisms for temperature elevation in these latter instances are unknown.

Determining the Cause of Fever

Sepsis is an uncommon cause of fever. Paradoxically, neonates with sepsis more frequently have hypothermia as well. However, sepsis is probably the most treatable life-threatening illness occurring in febrile newborn infants, especially those with temperature elevations to greater than 38° to 39° C, who are more likely to have bacteremia, purulent menigitis, and pnemonia. Most neonatal febrile episodes are noted in first day of life (54% in one series); however, any fever occurring on the third day of life and body temperature greater than 39° C have both been correlated with a significantly higher chance of bacterial disease. Severe temperature elevation is also associated with viral disease, particularly herpes simplex encephalitis; therefore work-ups for sepsis in these infants should include lumbar puncture.

Hyperthermia has been reported in tiny premature infants as a complication of improper use of shielding devices under either convection-warmed incubator or radiant warmer conditions. When incubated, babies should always have a strictly monitored and controlled source of heat. Fever secondary to overheating, particularly associated with incubators, is more common in equatorial and tropical countries.

Dehydration is an infrequently recognized cause of fever in the newborn period. Dehydration occurring in healthy term infants between the third and fourth day of life was noted previously, and it is probably the result of inadequate milk intake. Dehydration fever is commonly seen in large breastfed babies whose milk intake is poor and who may be exposed to high environmental temperatures during the summertime or in tropical areas. Body temperature can range between 37.8° and 40° C. Rehydration leads to resolution of fever and is key to the diagnosis of dehydration fever.

In two reports (Lieberman et al, 1997; Pleasure and Stahl, 1990), fever was more common in neonates born to mothers receiving epidural analgesia during labor when compared with those without analgesia (7.5% versus 2.5% and 14.5% versus 1%, respectively). One of these reports (Lieberman et al, 1977) observed more frequent sepsis evaluations and antibiotic use in the offspring of women receiving epidural analgesia. With the increasing use of epidural analgesia during labor, recognizing epidural neonatal fever is an important consideration when evaluating a febrile neonate.

Unusual and uncommon causes of neonatal fever include neonatal typhoid fever and congenital malaria, which should be considered in immigrant populations or in third-world countries. An increase in unexplained neonatal fevers was associated with the introduction of routine hepatitis B vaccination versus historical controls (Lewis et al, 2001), but this was not confirmed in a subsequent, large prospective clinical study (Lewis et al, 2001). In addition, temperature elevations may be seen with hypothalamic or other central nervous system malformations or masses. Subarachnoid or other intracranial hemorrhages may also be associated with temperature elevation. On rare occasions, neonatal spinal neurenteric cyst can manifest with long-lasting neonatal fever and should be considered in the differential diagnosis of acute myelopathy with persistent fever in infancy (greater than 3 weeks' duration). The presence of myelopathy will help to establish this diagnosis.

Management

The clinical problem is that fever may be the only indication of severe bacterial disease. The relevant perinatal history should be evaluated for risk factors mitigating a laboratory evaluation, presumptive treatment for infection, or both. Furthermore, signs that are suggestive of sepsis (e.g., diminished activity, irritability, seizures) should be considered. All neonates with fever should be evaluated for hydration, weight loss, and foci of infection (i.e., cellulitis, septic arthritis or osteomyelitis, omphalitis, and the presence of colonized foreign bodies, such as a central venous line).

However, febrile neonates without clinical history or any signs of infection present a challenge with insufficient data in the literature regarding appropriate management. An infant's environment should be examined for overheating. In breastfeeding, infants with fever at 3 to 4 days of age and excessive weight loss, dehydration fever should be considered and treated to establish this diagnosis. Mothers receiving epidural analgesia often manifest shivering with their temperature rise, and they experience a rapid defervescence after discontinuing the epidural infusion. Recognition of this pattern may avoid unnecessary sepsis evaluations in neonates with early fever.

THERAPEUTIC HYPOTHERMIA FOR BRAIN PROTECTION FOLLOWING NEONATAL ASPHYXIA

Since 2005, therapeutic hypothermia has been considered the standard of care for a highly selected population of near-term and term infants suffering hypoxic-ischemic events after birth, or after medically witnessed cardiopulmonary arrest and resuscitation. Two randomized studies suggest that cerebral cooling with either whole body cooling to a core temperature of 33.5° C (considered moderate hypothermia) or selective head cooling to approxmately 10° C (with mild whole-body cooling to 34° C) reduces the risk for death or moderate to severe neurologic injury from approxiately two thirds, to less than half (Gluckman et al, 2005; Shankaran et al, 2005). In the United States, the National Institutes of Health Institute of Child Health and Human Development Experts Panel Workshop held in May 2005 emphasized using standardized protocols adapted from these randomized trials for hypothermia treatment, and it recommended continual follow-up until school age to develop and better refine therapy for treating moderate to severe clinical neonatal encephalopathy observed in term or near-term neonates (Higgins et al, 2006).

The Children's National Medical Center (CNMC) has adapted the Neonatal Network's whole-body hypothermia protocol (Shankaran et al, 2005). In addition, CNMC provides continuous electroencephalogram (EEG) neurologic monitoring as part of a protocol, without consideration of the EEG as a criteria for initiating cooling. A full montage video-EEG (using a modified International 10-20 system accepted for neonates) is recorded by computer for 120 hours after birth to include cooling and rewarming recovery. EEG data are displayed on a centralized monitoring station and reviewed at least daily for every patient treated for hypothermia. Amplitude-integrated EEG is also reviewed for characterization of background pattern and for detection of seizures that can contribute to evolving brain injury and are treated aggressively. Automated seizure detection software is confirmed on raw EEG signals by an electrophysiology neonatal neurologist who is integrated into the program. To receive cooling therapy, infants must be at 34 weeks' gestation or greater, arrive for treatment within 6 hours of birth, and have experienced a hypoxic-ischemic event. Evidence of hypoxic-ischemic injury includes: resuscitation being required at delivery, an umbilical vessel blood gas pH of 7.00 or less, or having a significant base deficit of at least –16. Also qualifying for therapy are blood gas disturbances within the first hour of life, with a pH of 7.01 to 7.15 and a base deficit of –10 to –15.9, along with an ominous perinatal history (e.g., fetal heart rate decelerations, umbilical cord prolapse or rupture, uterine rupture, severe maternal trauma preceding birth, abruption of the placenta, maternal life-threatening event requiring cardiopulmonary resuscitation). Signs of

moderate to severe neonatal encephalopathy must also be present to qualify for hypothermia intervention: lethargy, complete stupor, diminished or completely absent spontaneous activity and/or aberrant muscle tone, weak or absent sucking and Moro reflexes with pupils fixed and constricted or unresponsive and dilated, fixed flexion or extension posturing of extremities, or a clinically observed seizure. Infants with such symptoms persisting for several days have an approximately 60% risk for death before hospital discharge, whereas a majority of survivors experience moderate to severe life-long neurodevelopmental disabilities (e.g., cerebral palsy, deafness, blindness, mental retardation, or recurrent seizures as in epilepsy).

Infants meeting these criteria are quickly examined at admission and then placed supine onto a water-filled cooling blanket that is precooled to 5° C (41° F). CNMC uses a Blanketrol II device (Cincinnati Sub-Zero, Cincinnati, Ohio) that is used commonly in the emergency department to reduce high fevers and in the operating room to promote hypothermia before and during reconstructive heart surgery. An esophageal temperature probe is placed into the distal third of the esophagus to monitor the infant's core temperature, and the thermostatic controller in the water mattress' cooling unit is set to 33.5° C. A second, larger pediatric-size blanket is also attached in parallel to the cooling system and is suspended at the bedside as a "sail" heat capacitor. Water circulates through both blankets exposed to both the baby and the room air temperature to diminish continuously monitored temperature fluctuations in esophageal temperature (less than ±0.5° C). Although CNMC uses a warmer bed platform as a crib, the overhead warmer is not turned on during the cooling period. Abdominal wall skin temperature is monitored with a surface probe that is available with the warmer bed (in monitor-only mode). Temperatures of the esophagus, skin, and axilla are thus monitored and recorded every 15 minutes for the first 4 hours of cooling, every hour for the next 8 hours, and every 4 hours during the remaining 72-hour period of hypothermia. CNMC's electronic medical record (Cerner) provides hourly esophageal temperature recording. After 72 hours, the set-point of the controller on the cooling system is increased by 0.5° C increments per hour to promote gradual rewarming. The Neonatal Network reported febrile rebound and seizures during rewarming (Shankaran et al, 2005); however, CNMC has not experienced this with continuous EEG monitoring over 24 to 48 hours throughout rewarming and a subsequent recovery period. After 6 hours, the esophageal probe and cooling blankets are removed, and anterior abdominal wall skin temperature is then regulated using the radiant warmer's servomechanism set at 36° to 36.5° C (i.e., warmer is turned on). The purpose of rewarming slowly is to avoid rapid shifts in electrolytes (calcium and potassium in particular), cardiac arrhythmias, and in rewarming hyperthermia, because fever promotes further brain injury. Infants otherwise receive routine neonatal intensive care, with continuous monitoring of vital signs. Mild sinus bradycardia (80 to 90 beats/min) and small decreases in mean arterial blood pressure (less than 20 mm Hg) are commonly observed and treated easily with volume and pressor infusions, according to CNMC's standard institutional guidelines for babies developmentally.

Frequent blood samples are monitored for glucose regulation (infants are restricted to 4 to 6 mg/kg/min of dextrose infusion), coagulopathy (in particular treating fibrinogen levels less than 150 mg/dL and platelet levels less than 80,000 per millimeter), and major organ failure (e.g., electrolytes, blood urea nitrogen, creatinine, liver enzymes).

CNMC's clinical experience over the past 3 years in more than 98 babies meeting strict criteria for therapeutic hypothermia has been commensurate with that reported from the Neonatal Network (Shankaran et al, 2005). Target esophageal temperature was achieved at 33.5 ± 0.5° C (range 33° to 34° C) in 30 to 60 minutes without a major circulatory mishap at CNMC. Continuous EEG monitoring has been instructive for intervening seizure activity (observed on EEG in approximately one quarter of infants shortly after admission). CNMC electrophysiologists observed general improvements in background voltages and patterns on EEG recordings during and after hypothermia. Specifically, improvement of background activity, appearance of sleep wake cycling, and disappearance of seizures has been observed at the time of rewarming (El-Dib et al, 2007). The Neonatal Network observed seizures emerging frequently during rewarming, hence the precaution in re-warming more slowly. CNMC is presently acquiring and reviewing infant neurologic and neuron-developmental follow-up data on a 6-month schedule through the first 2 years of life. CNMC has also made the clinical observation that the water mattress felt warm to the touch (i.e., warmer than the examiner's hand) during most of the cooling period (Baumgart et al, 2007). Median ambient temperature in CNMC's NICU during October 2007 (23.1° C; range, 20.9° to 25.4° C) was usually less than both the blanket water and baby temperatures. No infant had acidemia during cooling. Temperature gradients suggest that whole-body cooling is achieved through surface cooling from skin exposed to the ambient environment, and not actually by heat loss into the water-blanket. CNMC observers believe that the water matress simply incubates infants at a lower temperature. Except during the first 30 minutes, the blanket more often provided warmth to maintain esophageal temperature at 33.5° C. Whole-body cooling might also be provided by regulating an incubator air temperature or a radiant heater to maintain esophageal temperature. It has been important to CNMC's outreach education program to emphasize that referring (i.e., resuscitating) institutions should perform cardio pulmonary resuscitation under warm conditions to facilitate cardiac response according to Neonatal Resuscitation Program guidelines. Cold resuscitation is not advocated until after careful clinical evaluation of a stabilized patient has been performed at CNMC to meet therapeutic cooling criteria.

SUMMARY

The premature newborn with very low birthweight is extremely vulnerable to harsh fluctuations in physical environment. These infants require frequent assessments of skin, core, and air temperature and relative humidity to design an optimal strategy for thermal regulation. In caring for smaller babies, heat replacement is often required, and refinement of techniques to accomplish replacement without inducing hyperthermia is needed. The use of therapeutic hypothermia in highly selective cases at risk for brain injury is no longer considered novel.

SUGGESTED READINGS

Baumgart S: Partitioning of heat losses and gains in premature newborn infants under radiant warmers, *Pediatrics* 75:89-99, 1985.

Bell EF, Rios GR: Air versus skin temperature servo control of infant incubators, *J Pediatr* 103:954, 1983.

Bell EF, Rios GR: A double-walled incubator alters the partition of body heat loss of premature infants, *Pediatr Res* 17:135-140, 1983.

Bell EF, Weinstein MR, Oh W: Heat balance in premature infants: Comparative effects of convectively heated incubator and radiant warmer, with and without plastic heat shield, *J Pediatr* 96:460-465, 1980.

Bruck K: Heat production and temperature regulation. In Stave U, editor: *Perinatal physiology*, New York, 1978, Plenum Publishing, pp 455-498.

Dawkins MJ, Hull D: The production of heat by fat, *Sci Am* 213:62-67, 1965.

Day RL, Caliguiri L, Kaminski C, et al: Body temperature and survival of premature infants, *Pediatrics* 34:171-181, 1964.

Knauth A, Gordin M, McNelis W, et al: Semipermeable polyurethane membrane as an artificial skin for the premature neonate, *Pediatrics* 83:945-950, 1988.

Marks KH, Lee CA, Bolan CD, et al: Oxygen consumption and temperature control of premature infants in a double-wall incubator, *Pediatrics* 68:93-98, 1981.

Mayfield SR, Bhatia J, Nakamura KT, et al: Temperature measurement in term and preterm neonates, *J Pediatr* 104:271-275, 1984.

Okken A, Blijham C, Franz W, et al: Effects of forced convection of heated air on insensible water loss and heat loss in preterm infants in incubators, *J Pediatr* 101:108-112, 1982.

Scopes JW: Thermoregulation in the newborn. In Avery CB, editor: *Neonatology, pathophysiology and management of the newborn*, ed 2, Philadelphia, 1981, JB Lippincott, pp 171-181.

Yager JY, Armstrong EA, Jaharus C, et al: Preventing hyperthermia decreases brain damage following neonatal hypoxic-ischemic seizures, *Brain Res* 1011:48-57, 2004.

Complete references used in this text can be found online at www.expertconsult.com

CHAPTER 31

ACID-BASE, FLUID, AND ELECTROLYTE MANAGEMENT

Michael A. Posencheg and Jacquelyn R. Evans

FLUID AND ELECTROLYTE BALANCE

Maintenance of fluid and electrolyte balance is essential for normal cell and organ function during intrauterine development and throughout extrauterine life. Pathologic conditions in the newborn often lead to disruption of the complex regulatory mechanisms of fluid and electrolyte homeostasis. Therefore a thorough understanding of the physiologic changes in neonatal fluid and electrolyte homeostasis and the provision of appropriate fluid and electrolyte therapy based on the principles of developmental fluid and electrolyte physiology are among the cornerstones of modern neonatal intensive care.

DEVELOPMENTAL CHANGES AFFECTING FLUID AND ELECTROLYTE BALANCE IN THE FETUS AND NEONATE

Developmental Changes in Body Composition and Fluid Compartments

Dynamic changes occur in body composition and fluid distribution during intrauterine life, labor and delivery, and the early postnatal period. Thereafter the rate of change in body composition and fluid distribution gradually decreases, with more subtle changes taking place especially after the first year of life (Friis-Hansen, 1961).

Changes during Intrauterine Development

In early gestation, body composition is characterized by a high proportion of total body water (TBW) and a large extracellular compartment (Brans, 1986; Friis-Hansen, 1983). As gestation advances, rapid cellular growth, accretion of body solids, and fat deposition result in gradual reductions in TBW content and extracellular fluid volume while the intracellular fluid compartment increases (Figure 31-1) (Friis-Hansen, 1983). In the 16-week-old fetus, TBW represents approximately 94% of total body weight, and approximately two thirds of the TBW is distributed in the extracellular and one third in the intracellular compartment. By term, TBW contributes only 75% of body weight, and almost half of this volume is located in the intracellular compartment. Therefore infants born prematurely have TBW excess and extracellular volume expansion compared with their term counterparts, with the majority of the expanded extracellular volume being distributed in the interstitium (Brace, 1992).

Changes during Labor and Delivery

Additional and more acute changes in TBW and its distribution occur during labor and delivery. Arterial blood pressure rises several days before delivery in response

to increases in catecholamine, vasopressin, and cortisol plasma concentrations and translocation of blood from the placenta into the fetus. This rise in arterial blood pressure, along with changes in the fetal hormonal milieu and an intrapartum hypoxia-induced increase in capillary permeability, results in a shift of fluid from the intravascular to the interstitial compartment. This fluid shift results in an approximately 25% reduction in circulating plasma volume in the human fetus during labor and delivery (Brace, 1992). The postnatal increase in oxygenation and changes in vasoactive hormone production then restore capillary membrane integrity and favor absorption of interstitial fluid into the intravascular compartment. The ensuing gradual movement of fluid from the expanded interstitial space into the bloodstream aids in maintaining intravascular volume during the first 24 to 48 hours postnatally, when oral fluid intake may be limited. However, prematurity, pathologic conditions, or both can disrupt this delicate process and interfere with the physiologic contraction of the extracellular fluid (ECF) compartment in the immediate postnatal period.

In the fetus, body composition and fluid balance depend on the electrolyte and water exchange between mother, fetus, and amniotic space (Brace, 1986). Antenatal events can have significant effects on postnatal fluid balance. Maternal indomethacin treatment or excessive administration of intravenous fluids during labor can result in neonatal hyponatremia with expanded extracellular water content (Rojas et al, 1984; vd Heijden et al, 1988). Placental insufficiency or maternal diuretic therapy can impair fetal hydration, leading to decreases in extracellular volume, urine output, and amniotic fluid volume (Van Otterlo et al, 1977). The timing of cord clamping after delivery is another important factor significantly affecting total circulating blood volume and extracellular volume in the neonate. Immediate cord clamping does not allow for placental transfusion, but if the cord clamping is delayed only 3 to 4 minutes after delivery with the newborn positioned at or below the level of the placenta, up to 25 to 50 mL/kg of blood is transfused into the neonate, representing an approximately 25% to 50% increase in the total blood volume (Linderkamp, 1982; Yao and Lind, 1974). The onset of infant respiratory effort after birth also increases placental transfusion regardless of the infant's position (Philip and Teng, 1977).

Changes in the Postnatal Period

In the first few days and weeks after birth, the most important effects on the pace of further changes in body composition, TBW content, and its distribution are exerted by gestational and postnatal ages, the presence or absence of pathologic conditions, the immediate environment, and the type of nutrition. In normal conditions in the first few

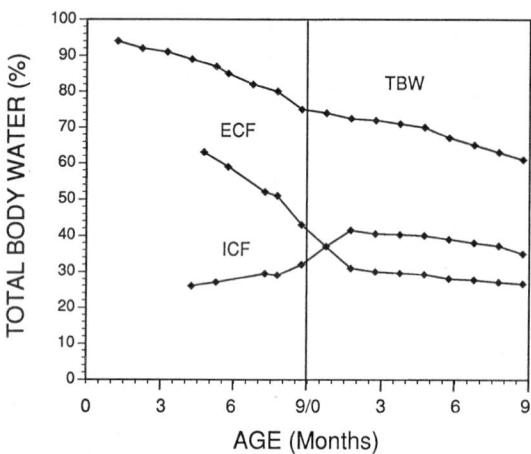

FIGURE 31-1 Total body water *(TBW)* content and its distribution between the extracellular fluid *(ECF)* and intracellular fluid *(ICF)* compartments in the human fetus, newborn, and infant from conception until 9 months of age. *(Data represent average values from Friis-Hansen B: Body water compartments in children: changes during growth and related changes in body composition, Pediatrics 28:169-181, 1961.)*

days after birth, the postnatal increase in capillary membrane integrity favors absorption of the interstitial fluid into the intravascular compartment. The ensuing rise in circulating blood volume stimulates the release of atrial natriuretic peptide from the heart, which in turn enhances renal sodium and water excretion (Sagnella and MacGregor, 1984) resulting in an abrupt decrease in TBW and attendant weight loss. Although it is generally accepted that this postnatal weight loss is primarily due to the contraction of the expanded ECF compartment (Cheek et al, 1961), some water loss from the intracellular compartment can also occur, particularly in infants with extremely low birthweight (ELBW) and increased transepidermal water losses (Costarino and Baumgart, 1991; Sedin, 1995).

Healthy term newborns lose an average of 5% to 10% of their birthweight during the first 4 to 7 days of life (Brace, 1992); thereafter they establish a pattern of steady weight gain. Because preterm infants have an increased TBW content and extracellular volume, they lose an average of 15% of their birthweight during transition (Shaffer and Meade, 1989) and, depending on the degree of prematurity and associated pathologic conditions, these neonates only regain their birthweight by 10 to 20 days after birth (Figure 31-2).

Physiology of the Regulation of Body Composition and Fluid Compartments

Although human cells have the ability to adjust their intracellular composition, ultimate regulation of the intracellular volume and osmolality relies on the control of the extracellular compartment. Therefore the human body must be able to monitor the volume and osmolality of the extracellular compartment and to correct the changes resulting from its interaction with the environment.

Regulation of the Intracellular Solute and Water Compartment

The major intracellular solutes are the cellular proteins necessary for cell function, the organic phosphates associated with cellular energy production and storage, and

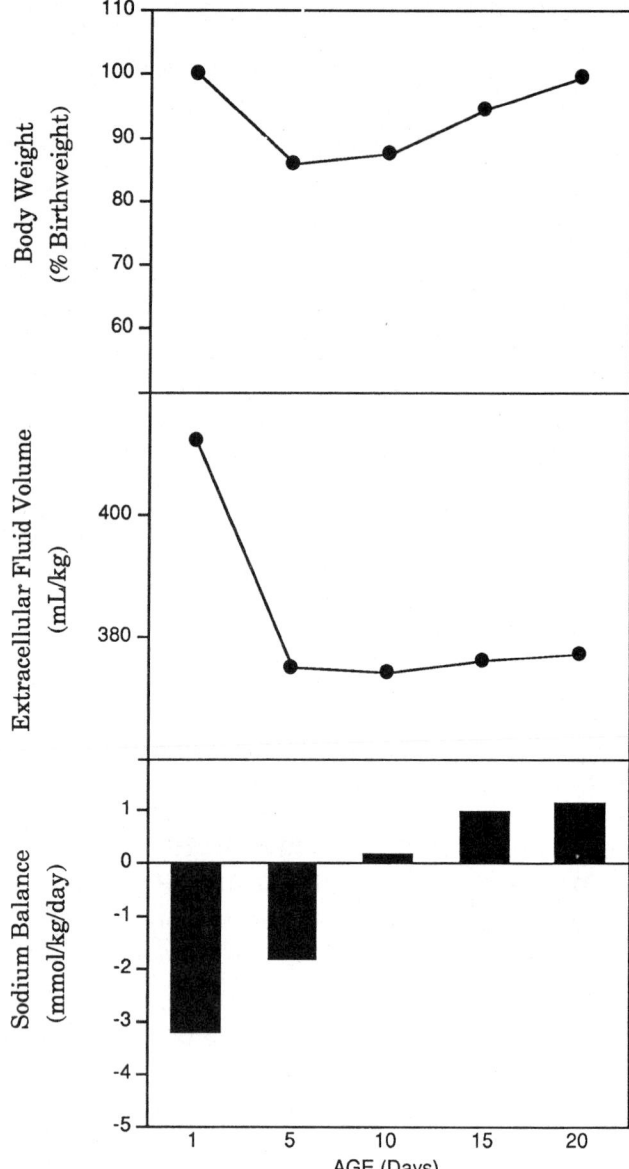

FIGURE 31-2 Postnatal changes in body weight (expressed in percent of birthweight), extracellular fluid volume (estimated by the bromide dilution method), and sodium balance (defined as the difference between sodium intake and urinary sodium excretion). *(From Shaffer SG, Weismann DN: Fluid requirements in the preterm infant, Clin Perinatol 19:233-250, 1992.)*

the equivalent cations balancing the phosphate and protein anions (MacKnight and Leaf, 1977). Potassium is the major intracellular cation, and sodium is the major extracellular cation. The energy derived from the concentration differences for sodium and potassium between the intracellular and extracellular compartments is used for cellular work. Because changes in osmolality of the extracellular compartment are reflected as net movements of water in or out of the cell, regulation of ECF concentration ultimately controls the osmolality and size of the intracellular compartment (MacKnight and Leaf, 1977). This physiologic principle must be kept in mind by the neonatologist managing sick term and preterm neonates with disturbances of sodium homeostasis. Rapid changes in serum sodium concentration and thus in extracellular osmolality directly affect the osmolality and size of the intracellular compartment and can lead to irreversible cell damage, especially in the central nervous system.

Regulation of the Intracellular-Extracellular Interface: The Interstitial Compartment

In the healthy term neonate, hydrostatic and oncotic pressures are well balanced, with both being approximately half those in the adult (Sola and Gregory, 1981). In normal physiologic conditions, movement of fluid across the capillary is determined by the direction of the net driving pressure $([P_C - P_T] - [\pi_P - \pi_T])$ and the water and protein permeability characteristics of the capillary wall (Figure 31-3). At the arterial end of the capillary, intracapillary hydrostatic pressure (P_C) is high, and plasma oncotic pressure (π_P) is relatively low, resulting in a net movement of fluid out of the capillary. As filtration of relatively protein-poor fluid continues along the capillary, plasma oncotic pressure rises and intracapillary hydrostatic pressure drops; therefore on the venous side, fluid moves from the interstitium into the capillary, so that much of the filtered fluid is reabsorbed at the end of the capillary bed. The fluid remaining in the interstitium (arterial-venous side of the capillary) is drained by the lymphatic system. Interstitial hydrostatic (P_T) and oncotic (π_T) pressures remain virtually unchanged along the capillary bed. However, pathologic conditions readily disturb the delicate balance between the hydrostatic and oncotic forces, leading to an expansion of the interstitial compartment at the expense of the intravascular compartment. The increased interstitial fluid volume (edema) then further affects tissue perfusion by altering the normal function of the extracellular-intracellular interface. Box 31-1 summarizes the mechanisms for conditions resulting in interstitial edema formation in the neonate. There are also some important developmentally regulated differences between the newborn and adult relating to the pathogenesis of edema formation. Capillary permeability to proteins is increased during the early stages of development (Brace, 1992; Gold and Brace, 1988). Because neonatal capillary permeability is further increased under pathologic conditions (see Box 31-1), protein concentration in the interstitial compartment may approach that of the intravascular space, favoring further intravascular volume depletion and interstitial volume expansion. When sick neonates are treated with frequent albumin boluses, much of the infused albumin leaks into the interstitium, creating a vicious cycle of intravascular volume depletion and edema formation. If the cycle is not interrupted, it can result in the formation of anasarca, which has an extremely poor prognosis. In summary, the sick neonate has a limited capacity to maintain appropriate intravascular volume and to regulate the volume and composition of the interstitium. The ensuing intravascular hypovolemia and edema formation result in vasoconstriction and disturbances in tissue perfusion and cellular function with further impairments in the regulation of extracellular volume distribution.

Regulation of the Extracellular Solute and Water Compartment

The regulation of the volume and osmolality of the extracellular compartment ensures the integrity of the circulation and maintains the osmolality of the extracellular

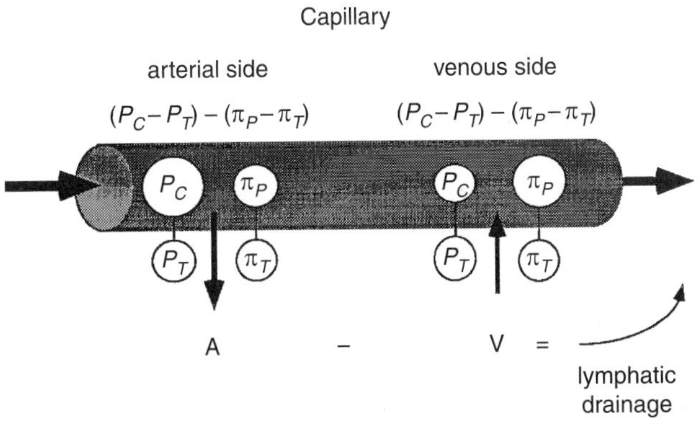

FIGURE 31-3 Filtration and reabsorption of fluid along the capillary under physiologic conditions.

BOX 31-1 Mechanisms for Conditions Causing Interstitial Edema in the Neonate

CONDTIONS FAVORING FLUID ACCUMULATION IN THE INTERSTITIAL SPACE BY CAUSING A DYSEQUILIBRIUM BETWEEN FILTRATION AND REABSORPTION OF FLUID BY THE CAPILLARIES

Increased hydrostatic pressure
　Elevated capillary hydrostatic pressure
　　Increased cardiac output
　　Venous obstruction
　Decreased tissue hydrostatic pressure
　Conditions associated with changes in the properties of the interstitial gel (edematous states, effects of hormones including prolactin)
Decreased oncotic pressure gradient
　Decreased capillary oncotic pressure
　　Prematurity, hyaline membrane disease
　　Malnutrition, liver dysfunction
　　Nephrotic syndrome
Increased interstitial oncotic pressure is usually the result of increased capillary permeability
Elevation of the filtration coefficient
　Increased capillary permeability
　　Organs with large-pore capillary endothelium (liver, spleen)
　　State of maturity (preterm infants > term newborns > adults)
　　Production of pro-inflammatory cytokines (sepsis, anaphylaxis, hypoxic tissue injury, tissue ischemia, ischemia-reperfusion, soft tissue trauma, extracorporeal membrane oxygenation)
　Increased capillary surface area
　Vasodilation

CONDITIONS ASSOCIATED WITH DECREASED LYMPHATIC DRAINAGE

Decreased muscle movement
　Neuromuscular blockade and/or heavy sedation
　Central and/or peripheral nervous system disease
Obstruction of lymphatic flow
　Increased central venous pressure
　Scar tissue formation (bronchopulmonary dysplasia)
　Mechanical obstruction (dressings, high mean airway pressure in mechanically ventilated newborns)

Modified from Costarino AT, Baumgard S: Neonatal water metabolism. In Cowett RM, editor: *Principles of perinatal/neonatal metabolism*, New York, 1991, Springer Verlag, pp 623-649.

compartment within 2% of the osmolar set point between 275 and 290 mOsm (Robertson and Berl, 1986). Blood pressure and serum sodium concentration (i.e., osmolality) are monitored by baroreceptors and osmoreceptors, respectively. The effector limb of the regulatory system consists of the heart, vascular bed, kidneys, and intake of fluid in response to thirst. The latter part of the effector system is inactive in critically ill term and preterm neonates whose fluid intake is completely controlled by caregivers. By regulating the function of the effector organs, several hormones have a role in the control of the extracellular compartment, including the renin-angiotensin-aldosterone system, vasopressin, atrial natriuretic peptide, brain (B-type) natriuretic peptide, bradykinin, prostaglandins, and catecholamines. Because volume changes in the extracellular compartment must be reflected by similar changes in the intravascular volume for effective operation of the regulatory mechanisms, regulation of the extracellular compartment relies on intact cardiovascular function and on the integrity of the capillary endothelium (Robertson and Berl, 1986). For example, under physiologic conditions, an increase in the extracellular volume is reflected by an increase in the circulating plasma volume, leading to rises in blood pressure and renal blood flow. The ensuing increase in glomerular filtration and urine output returns the extracellular volume to normal. In critically ill neonates, however, the capillary leak and reduced myocardial responsiveness resulting from immaturity and underlying pathologic conditions limit the increase in the circulating blood volume when extracellular volume expands. Thus, especially in sick preterm infants, blood pressure may rise only transiently, and renal blood flow may remain low after volume boluses as fluid rapidly leaks into the interstitium. Inappropriate central regulation of vascular tone results in vasodilatation, further decreasing effective circulating blood volume and compromising tissue perfusion; this leads to impaired gas exchange in the lungs, resulting in hypoxia with further increases in capillary leak. Unless interrupted by appropriate therapeutic measures, a vicious cycle with further deterioration readily occurs in the sick neonate.

Maturation of Organs Regulating Body Composition and Fluid Compartments

The heart, kidneys, skin, and endocrine system play the most important roles in the regulation of extracellular (and thus intracellular) fluid and electrolyte balance in the neonate. Immaturity of these organ systems, especially in infants with very low birthweight (VLBW), results in a compromised regulatory capacity, which must be noted when estimating daily fluid and electrolyte requirements in these patients.

Maturation of the Cardiovascular System

There is a direct relationship between gestational maturity and the ability of the neonatal heart to respond to acute volume loading (Baylen et al, 1986). The blunted Starling response of the immature myocardium results from its lower content of contractile elements and incomplete sympathetic innervations (Mahony, 1995). Because central vasoregulation and endothelial integrity are also developmentally regulated (Brace, 1992; Gold and Brace, 1988), an appropriate effective intravascular volume is seldom maintained in a critically ill preterm infant. Since regulation of the extracellular volume requires the maintenance of an adequate effective circulating blood volume, the immaturity of the cardiovascular system contributes to the limited capacity of sick preterm infants to effectively regulate the total volume of their extracellular compartment.

Maturation of Renal Function

The kidney has a crucial role in the physiologic control of fluid and electrolyte balance. It regulates extracellular volume and osmolality through the selective reabsorption of sodium and water, respectively. Immaturity of renal function renders preterm infants susceptible to both excessive sodium and bicarbonate losses (El-Dahr and Chevalier, 1990). In addition, the inability of the preterm infant to respond promptly to a sodium or volume load results in a tendency toward extracellular volume expansion with edema formation. Because prenatal steroid administration accelerates maturation of renal function (van den Anker et al, 1994), preterm infants treated with steroids in utero have a better capacity to regulate their postnatal ECF contractions. During the first few weeks of life, hemodynamically stable but extremely immature infants produce dilute urine and may develop polyuria because of their renal tubular immaturity. As tubular functions mature, their concentrating capacity gradually improves from the 2nd to 4th week of life. However, it takes years for the developing kidney to reach the concentrating capacity of the adult kidney.

Maturation of the Skin

Although term infants have a well-developed cornified layer of the epidermis, extremely immature neonates have only two or three cell layers in the epidermis (Cartridge-Patrick and Rutter, 1992). Because of the lack of an effective barrier to diffusion of water through the immature skin, transepidermal free water losses in the immature infant may be extremely high during the first few days postnatally. Gestational age, postnatal age, the pattern of intrauterine growth, and environmental factors have crucial roles in the magnitude of transepidermal free water losses (Figure 31-4). Although skin cornification rapidly increases, even in the extremely immature infant during the first few days after birth, full maturation of the epidermis does not occur for more than 28 days of age (Sedin, 1995). Chronic intrauterine stress (Hammarlund et al, 1983) and prenatal steroid treatment (Aszterbaum et al, 1993) also enhance maturation of the skin.

Increases in free water losses through the immature skin of the VLBW infant can result in early postnatal hypertonic dehydration with rapid changes in intracellular volume and osmolality. In many organs, especially the brain, these abrupt changes in intracellular volume and osmolality can lead to cellular dysfunction and ultimately cell death.

Maturation of End-Organ Responsiveness to Hormones Involved in the Regulation of Fluid and Electrolyte Balance

Several hormones, including but not limited to the renin-angiotensin-aldosterone system, vasopressin, atrial natriuretic peptide, and brain (B-type) natriuretic peptide, directly regulate the volume or composition of the extracellular compartment. These hormones exert their effects

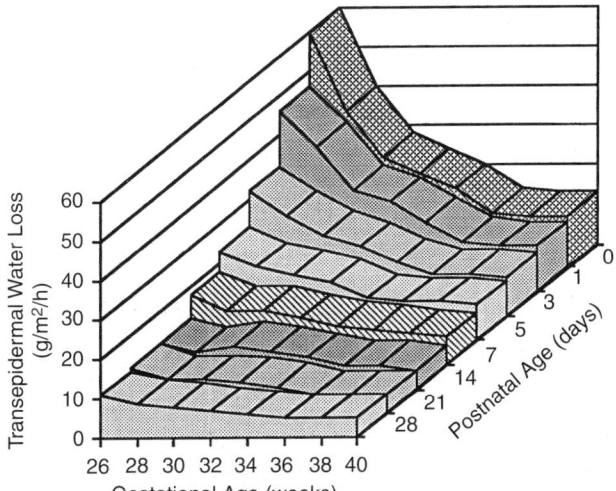

FIGURE 31-4 **Transepidermal water loss in relation to gestational age during the first 28 postnatal days in infants who are appropriate for gestational age.** There is an exponential relationship between transepidermal water loss and gestational age, the water loss being higher in preterm infants than in term infants. Transepidermal water loss is also significantly affected by postnatal age, especially in the immature preterm infant. The measurements were performed at an ambient air humidity of 50% and with the infants calm and quiet. (*From Hammarlund K, Sedin G, Stromberg B: Transepidermal water loss in newborn infants. VIII: Relation to gestational age and postnatal age in appropriate and small for gestational age infants,* Acta Paediatr Scand *72:721-728, 1983.*)

mainly by altering renal sodium and water excretion and by inducing changes in systemic vascular resistance and myocardial contractility. Other hormones, including the prostaglandins, bradykinin, and prolactin, modulate the actions of many of the regulatory hormones.

Renin-Angiotensin-Aldosterone System

Decreases in renal capillary blood flow stimulate renin secretion, which in turn initiates the production of angiotensin. Angiotensin induces vasoconstriction, increased tubular sodium and water reabsorption, and the release of aldosterone (Riordan, 1995). Aldosterone increases potassium secretion and further enhances sodium reabsorption in the distal tubule; therefore the primary function of this system is to protect the volume of the extracellular compartment and maintain adequate tissue perfusion (Bailie, 1992). However, its effectiveness in the neonate is somewhat limited by the decreased responsiveness of the immature kidney to the sodium- and water-retaining effects of these hormones (Sulyok et al, 1985). Vasodilatory and natriuretic prostaglandins generated in the kidney (Gleason, 1987) are the main counterregulatory hormones balancing the renal actions of the renin-angiotensin-aldosterone system. Therefore, when prostaglandin production is inhibited by indomethacin, the unopposed vasoconstrictive and sodium-retentive actions of the activated renin-angiotensin-aldosterone system contribute to the development of the drug-induced renal failure in the preterm infant (Gleason, 1987; Seri, 1995; Seri et al, 2002).

Vasopressin (Antidiuretic Hormone)

Vasopressin has its major effect in maintaining the osmolality of the extracellular compartment. Vasopressin selectively raises free water reabsorption in the kidneys and

results in blood pressure elevation (Elliot et al, 1996). Plasma levels of vasopressin are markedly elevated in the neonate, especially after vaginal delivery, and its cardiovascular actions facilitate neonatal adaptation (Pohjavuori and Raivio, 1985). The high vasopressin levels are in part also responsible for the diminished urine output of the healthy term neonate during the first day of life. Under certain pathologic conditions, the dysregulated release of, or the end-organ unresponsiveness to, vasopressin significantly affects renal and cardiovascular functions and electrolyte and fluid status in the sick preterm and term infant. In the syndrome of inappropriate secretion of antidiuretic hormone (SIADH), an uncontrolled release of vasopressin occurs in sick preterm and term infants, with resulting water retention, hyponatremia, and oliguria. In the syndrome of diabetes insipidus (DI), the lack of pituitary production of vasopressin or renal unresponsiveness to vasopressin results in polyuria, with increased thirst and hypernatremia.

Atrial Natriuretic Peptide

Via its direct vasodilatory and renal natriuretic actions, atrial natriuretic peptide (ANP) regulates the volume of the extracellular compartment in the fetus and neonate in a fashion opposite to that of the renin-angiotensin-aldosterone system (Iwamoto, 1992; Needleman and Greenwald, 1986; Seymour, 1985). ANP has a direct inhibitory effect on renin production and aldosterone release (Christensen, 1993).

The stretch of the atrial wall caused by an increase in the circulating blood volume is the most potent stimulus for the release of this hormone. Plasma levels of this hormone are high in the fetus (Claycomb, 1988). There are a few specific conditions in which the actions of atrial natriuretic peptide are directly relevant for the neonatologist. For example, the hormone is involved in the regulation of both the fluid shifts during labor (Brace, 1992) and the extracellular volume contraction during postnatal transition (Kojima et al, 1987; Ronconi et al, 1995; Rozycki and Baumgart, 1991; Tulassay et al, 1987). Furthermore, the oliguric effects of positive end-expiratory pressure ventilation are due in part to a decrease in atrial natriuretic peptide secretion (Christensen, 1993) along with the enhanced release of vasopressin (El-Dahr and Chevalier, 1990).

Brain (or B-type) Natriuretic Peptide

Similar to ANP, brain natriuretic peptide (BNP) is a hormone secreted by cardiac myocytes. Specifically, BNP is thought to be secreted by cardiac ventricular myocytes in response to increases in wall tension. Both of these peptides cause natriuresis, diuresis, and vasodilation while inhibiting the renin-angiotensin-aldosterone system (Gemelli et al, 1991; Holmes et al, 1993; Kojima et al, 1989). BNP levels increase rapidly after birth, with levels on the first day of life up to 20-fold higher than those at birth (Mir et al, 2003; Yoshibayashi et al, 1995), and correlate with the downward trend in pulmonary arterial pressure in the days after birth, unlike ANP (Ikemoto et al, 1996). BNP levels continue to fall during the first week of life (Koch and Singer, 2003; Mir et al, 2003). Infants and children with congestive heart failure have an elevated

BNP level, which is associated with decreased ejection fraction and increased heart failure score (Mir et al, 2002). In this way, BNP can be used as a surrogate for changes in ventricular volume from either pulmonary hypertension or ventricular overload. Clinical researchers have begun to investigate the utility of this peptide in diagnosing and managing cardiac disorders in neonates. The best-studied association to date is the relationship between BNP and a patent ductus arteriosus (PDA). Multiple studies have described a positive correlation between BNP level and a hemodynamically significant PDA (Choi et al, 2005; Czernik et al, 2008; Flynn et al, 2005; Sanjeev et al, 2005). BNP levels were associated with larger ductal size and degree of shunting, especially in infants older than 2 days (Flynn et al, 2005). Furthermore, significant correlations have been seen between BNP level and left atrial to aortic root diameter (Choi et al, 2005; Czernik et al, 2008) and diastolic flow velocity in the left pulmonary artery (Choi et al, 2005). BNP levels decline significantly with either medical or surgical therapy of a hemodynamically significant PDA (Choi et al, 2005; Sanjeev et al, 2005). The biologically inactive fragment N-terminal pro-B-type natriuretic peptide (NT-proBNP) has also been studied regarding its association with PDA with similar results (Farombi et al, 2008). NT-proBNP has a longer half-life (60 versus 20 minutes) than BNP and has also been associated with sepsis (Farombi et al, 2008). BNP has also been associated with other forms of cardiac dysfunction in neonates. Increases in BNP levels have been described in infants with persistent pulmonary hypertension of the newborn over the first 4 days of life, correlating with the degree of tricuspid regurgitation on an echocardiogram (Reynolds et al, 2004). BNP measurements can also be useful in differentiating infants in respiratory distress who have a cardiac etiology for their disease from those who do not (Ko et al, 2008; Reynolds et al, 2004). The usefulness of this test is limited by the variability of levels in the first few days of life as well as the variety of assays available to measure BNP levels. Its utility may ultimately lie in repeated measures in the same patient over time using the same assay and following trends.

Prostaglandins

Prostaglandins have a well-documented, counterregulatory role for the renal vascular and tubular effects of renin-angiotensin-aldosterone and vasopressin (Bonvalet et al, 1987). The inhibition of these actions of prostaglandins by indomethacin results in clinically important and sometimes detrimental renal vascular and tubular effects in the preterm infant. The actions of prostaglandins modulating the effects of the other regulatory hormones of neonatal fluid and electrolyte homeostasis are less well studied.

Prolactin

Prolactin plays a permissive role in the regulation of fetal and neonatal water homeostasis (Coulter, 1983; Pullano et al, 1989). High fetal plasma prolactin levels contribute to the increased tissue water content of the fetus. Interestingly, postnatal prolactin levels remain high in the preterm neonate until approximately the 40th postconceptional week (Perlman et al, 1978).

MANAGEMENT OF FLUID AND ELECTROLYTE HOMEOSTASIS

General Principles of Fluid and Electrolyte Management

Fluid and electrolyte management is the cornerstone of neonatal intensive care, and appropriate management requires an understanding of the previously outlined physiologic principles and careful monitoring of key clinical data. Requirements vary substantially from infant to infant and in the same infant over time; therefore intakes must be individualized and frequently reassessed. The primary goals are to maintain the appropriate ECF volume, ECF and intracellular fluid osmolality, and ionic concentrations.

Assessment of Fluid and Electrolyte Status

Maternal conditions during pregnancy, drugs and fluids administered to the mother during labor and delivery, and specific fetal and neonatal conditions all affect early fluid and electrolyte balance. Excessive administration of free water or oxytocin use in the mother can result in hyponatremia in the neonate. Maternal therapy with indomethacin, angiotensin-converting enzyme inhibitors, furosemide, and aminoglycosides can all adversely affect neonatal renal function. A newborn's history of oligohydramnios or birth asphyxia may also alert the clinician to the possibility of abnormal renal function. In young infants, altered skin turgor, sunken anterior fontanel, and dry mucous membrane are not sensitive indicators of dehydration, but tachycardia, hypotension, and metabolic acidosis may be seen when intravascular volume is moderately to severely affected. In addition, edema usually occurs early when there is volume overload. Serial measurements of body weight, intake and output, and serum electrolytes will usually provide the most precise and accurate information regarding overall fluid status. Appropriate fluid balance in the first few days after birth is associated with a urine output of 1 to 3 mL/kg per hour and a weight loss of 5% to 10% in term infants and 10% to 15% in preterm infants. In critically ill infants and in situations of altered homeostasis, additional clinical data that may help in diagnosis and management include blood urea nitrogen, serum and urine osmolarity or specific gravity, urine electrolytes and serum bicarbonate, along with close monitoring of blood pressure and heart rate. The frequency of monitoring depends on the extent of immaturity and the severity of the fluid and electrolyte disturbance and of the underlying pathologic condition.

Water Homeostasis and Management

Water Losses

Free water losses occurring through the skin and the respiratory tract are considered insensible losses, whereas the sensible water losses are composed of the amounts lost through urine and feces. Urine output is the most important source of sensible water loss. Extremely preterm infants without systemic hypotension or renal failure usually lose 30 to 40 mL/kg/day of water in the urine on the first postnatal day and approximately 120 mL/kg/day by the third day. In stable, more mature preterm infants born after the 28 weeks' gestation, urinary water loss is approximately 90 mL/kg/day on the first postnatal day and 150 mL/kg/day by the third day (Coulthard and Hey, 1985). Because of their renal immaturity, preterm neonates have a tendency to produce dilute urine, thereby increasing their obligatory free water losses.

Normal water losses in the stool are less significant, amounting to approximately 10 mL/kg/day in term infants and 7 mL/kg/day in preterm infants during the first postnatal week (Sedin, 1995). Water losses in the stool increase thereafter and are influenced by the type of feeding and the frequency of stooling.

Gestational age, postnatal age, and environmental factors determine the amount of daily insensible water losses through the skin (see Figure 31-4). During the first few postnatal days, transepidermal water losses may be 15-fold higher in extremely premature infants born at 23 to 26 weeks' gestation than in term neonates (Sedin, 1995). Although the skin matures rapidly after birth, even in extremely immature infants, insensible losses are still somewhat higher at the end of the first month than in the term counterparts. Prenatal steroid exposure is associated with substantially less insensible water loss (IWL) in premature infants (Aszterbaum et al, 1993; Omar et al, 1999; Sedin, 1995).

Among environmental factors, ambient humidity has the greatest effect on transepidermal water loss. In extremely immature neonates, a rise in the ambient humidity of the incubator from 20% to 80% decreases the transepidermal water loss by approximately 75% (Sedin, 1995). However, the use of an open radiant warmer more than doubles transepidermal water losses (Flenady and Woodgate, 2003). Applying a plastic heat shield while the infant is under the warmer can decrease transepidermal water loss by 30% to 50% (Costarino et al, 1992). At low ambient humidity, phototherapy increases transepidermal water losses by approximately 30%. However, one study showed that if the ambient humidity is at least 50% in the incubator, regular phototherapy lamps will not increase the transepidermal water loss in infants older than 28 weeks' gestation (Sedin, 1995). On the other hand, halogen spotlight phototherapy increases transepidermal water loss in premature infants by 20% despite constant skin temperature and relative humidity (Grunhagen et al, 2002). Newer light-emitting diode phototherapy devices are not associated with significant transepidermal water loss or changes in cerebral hemodynamics (Bertini et al, 2008). Other factors that increase IWL include activity, airflow, elevated body, and environmental temperature as well as skin breakdown and skin or mucosal defects (e.g., gastroschisis, epidermolysis bullosa).

Insensible water losses from the respiratory tract depend mainly on the temperature and humidity of the inspired gas mixture and on the respiratory rate, tidal volume, and dead space ventilation. In a healthy term newborn, the water loss through the respiratory tract is approximately half the total IWL if the ambient air temperature is 32.5°C and the humidity is 50% (Sedin, 1995). However, in infants undergoing mechanical ventilation there will be no insensible losses through the respiratory tract if the ventilator gas mixture is humidified at body temperature.

Extraordinary losses are also seen in the neonate requiring intensive care. The most commonly encountered extraordinary water losses occur when a nasogastric tube is placed under continuous suction (to be discussed later in this chapter). Large losses may also occur in association with chest tubes, other drains, ostomies, and fistulas as well as with emesis or diarrhea.

Management of Water Requirements

Appropriate management requires estimating any existing deficits or surpluses, calculating ongoing maintenance needs because of usual sensible and insensible losses and growth and additional needs as a result of extraordinary losses. The infant's prenatal history, birthweight, gestational age, and need for mechanical ventilation and the environment in which the infant is to be cared for should be considered when determining initial fluid and electrolyte needs. Frequent reevaluations are necessary. The most useful parameter for monitoring fluid balance is the weight of the baby, as rapid changes in weight will reflect changes in water balance. Serial weights can be used to estimate the IWL using the following formula:

$$IWL = Fluid\ intake - Urine\ output + Weight\ loss\ or$$

$$IWL = Fluid\ intake - Urine\ output - Weight\ gain$$

It is reasonable to initiate fluid volume based on the sum of an allowance for sensible water loss of 30 to 60 mL/kg/day and the estimated IWL. Figure 31-4 shows usual IWL ranges by gestational and postnatal age. Factors previously outlined that predictably affect IWL should be considered when prescribing fluids. Prevention of excessive IWL rather than replacement of increased IWL is associated with fewer complications in the preterm neonate and usually can be achieved by modifying the infant's environment. See Table 31-1 for usual maintenance fluid administration based on birthweight. These numbers are guidelines for initial management only; the approach must subsequently be individualized based on laboratory values and other clinical data.

It is important to remember that the TBW excess and extracellular volume expansion of preterm infants implies that their negative water and sodium balance during the first 5 to 10 postnatal days (see Figure 31-2; Shaffer and Meade, 1989) represents an appropriate adaptation to extrauterine life and should not be compensated for by increased fluid administration and sodium supplementation. If this principle is not followed and a positive fluid balance (i.e., weight gain) is achieved during the transitional period, preterm infants are at higher risk of a more severe course of respiratory distress syndrome (Shaffer and Weismann, 1992) and a higher incidence of patent ductus arteriosus (Bell et al, 1980), congestive heart failure (Bell et al, 1980),

TABLE 31-1 Estimated Maintenance Fluid Requirements

Birth-weight (g)	Fluid Requirements (mL/kg/day)			
	Day 1	Day 2	Day 3-6	≥ Day 7
<750	100-140	120-160	140-200	140-160
750-1000	100-120	100-140	130-180	140-160
1000-1500	80-100	100-120	120-160	150
>1500	60-80	80-120	120-160	150

pulmonary edema (Shaffer and Weismann, 1992), necrotizing enterocolitis (Bell et al, 1979), and bronchopulmonary dysplasia (Oh et al, 2005; Van Marter et al, 1990).

Infants with ELBW and others with anticipated fluid problems should be weighed daily or twice daily. Serum sodium levels should be measured every 4 to 8 hours until stabilized, usually by 3 to 4 days after birth, and urine output should be recorded and reviewed every 6 to 8 hours. Once data are available, fluids should be increased if weight loss is greater than 1% to 2% per day in term infants and 2% to 3% per day in preterm infants, if urine output is low, if urine specific gravity is rising, or if serum sodium concentration is rising. Overall, expected and appropriate weight loss in the first week of life is up to 10% in term infants and up to 20% in preterm infants. Conversely, fluids should be decreased if weight is not falling appropriately and serum sodium is decreasing. The goal is to reach 140 to 160 mL/kg/day of fluids by 7 to 10 days to allow for adequate caloric intake.

Treatment of Fluid Overload

Fluid overload commonly occurs in sick neonates, often because of the use of fluid bolus administration for hypotension. The diagnosis is based on weight gain, edema, and often hyponatremia. Overhydration can sometimes be prevented by the use of blood transfusions or dopamine instead of colloid or crystalloid, if appropriate, for blood pressure support. In addition to reducing the need for volume boluses, dopamine may facilitate the process of extracellular volume contraction via its renal and hormonal effects (Seri, 1995). Once overhydration has occurred, management is usually effected by 10% to 20% decrements of total daily fluid intake while carefully monitoring clinical and laboratory signs to ensure maintenance of adequate intravascular volume as well as normal glucose and electrolyte status while the ECF contraction occurs.

Treatment of Dehydration

Dehydration may be suspected based on clinical signs. The total water deficit may be estimated by using weight changes, calculating total inputs and outputs, and following serial sodium levels. Free water deficit (or excess) can be calculated as:

$$H_2O \text{ deficit (or excess) } (L) = [0.7 \times BW (kg)] \times \left\{ \frac{[Na (mEq/L)]_{current}}{[Na (mEq/L)]_{desired}} - 1 \right\}$$

In this formula, $0.7 \times BW$ is the estimation of TBW.

When dehydration is diagnosed, correction should generally occur over 24 hours, with half correction over 8 hours and the remainder over the next 16 hours. Longer correction times are indicated when dehydration is accompanied by moderate to severe hypernatremia. Treatment is best approached by considering separately the fluid resuscitation requirements, fluid to replace current deficits and ongoing losses, and maintenance requirements, because the volume of the fluid, the composition, and the rate of replacement differ for each. Resuscitation of the intravascular volume to restore blood pressure and perfusion should be provided with boluses of isotonic saline (0.9% saline), and this volume is included in the initial half correction. The remaining deficit replacement volume should

TABLE 31-2 Free Water Content (as Volume %) of Common Intravenous Solutions at Normal and High Serum Sodium Concentrations*

Intravenous Fluid	Serum Sodium Concentration			
	145 mEq/L		195 mEq/L	
	Isotonic (%)	Water (%)	Isotonic (%)	Water (%)
D₅W	0	100	0	100
0.2% saline	22	78	17	83
0.45% saline	50	50	39	61
0.9% saline	100	0	79	21
Lactated Ringer's solution	86	14	68	32

Modified from Molteni KH: Initial management of hypernatremic dehydration in the breastfed infant, *Clin Pediatr* 33:731-740, 1994.

*Note that isotonic saline provides 21% free water when given to a patient with a serum sodium concentration of 195 mEq/L and therefore will induce undesirable decreases in serum sodium concentration when used for volume resuscitation in the severely dehydrated hypernatremic neonate.

TABLE 31-3 Approximate Electrolyte Composition of Body Fluids (mEq/L)

Body Fluid	Sodium	Potassium	Chloride
Gastric	20-80	5-20	100-150
Small intestine	100-140	5-15	90-130
Bile	120-140	5-15	80-120
Ileostomy	45-135	3-15	20-115
Diarrhea	10-90	10-80	10-110

be with fluid of appropriate sodium content based on the serum sodium (see Sodium and Potassium Homeostasis and Management, later), usually 0.2% or 0.45% saline. Free water contents of the common intravenous fluids are listed in Table 31-2. Usual maintenance fluids and electrolytes must also be provided. Ongoing urine losses should be replaced volume for volume every 4 to 6 hours with a solution tailored to the urine's electrolyte concentration (usually 0.45% normal saline). Extraordinary losses caused by tubes, drains, emesis, diarrhea, and ostomies should always be sought in the dehydrated infant and also accounted for in fluid management. The composition of this latter replacement solution depends on the electrolyte concentration of the fluid loss. The most common extraordinary loss, gastric fluid, contains significant sodium and chloride. See Table 31-3 for approximate electrolyte compositions of body fluids.

Potassium replacement (usually by adding 20 to 40 mEq potassium per liter of replacement fluid) should not begin until adequate urine output is established. For additional details of fluid correction and sodium management, see the discussion under Management of Hypernatremia later in this chapter.

Sodium and Potassium Homeostasis and Management

Serum sodium values should be kept between 135 and 145 mEq/L. Sodium chloride supplementation at 1 to 2 mEq/kg/day should be started in preterm and sick term neonates only after completion of the postnatal extracellular volume contraction, usually after the first few days of life or after more than 5% of birthweight is lost (Hartnoll et al, 2001). In general, as long as the infant's fluid balance is stable, maintenance sodium requirements do not exceed 3 to 4 mEq/kg/day, and providing this amount usually ensures the positive sodium balance necessary for adequate growth. Extreme prematurity and pathologic conditions associated with delayed transition or disturbance of fluid and electrolyte balance may significantly alter the infant's daily sodium requirement. For example, although the preterm infant has a limited ability to excrete a sodium load (Hartnoll, 2003), some of the most immature infants may have sodium requirements of as much as 6 to 8 mEq/kg/day because of the decreased capacity of their kidneys to retain sodium. Neonates recovering from an acute renal insult and preterm infants with immature proximal tubule functions who are in a state of extracellular volume expansion (Ramiro-Tolentino et al, 1996) may need daily sodium bicarbonate supplementation to compensate for their greater renal bicarbonate losses.

Hyponatremia

Hyponatremia (serum sodium <130 mEq/L) represents a deficit of sodium in relation to body water content and may be caused by either total body sodium deficit or free water excess. In both situations, total body water may be decreased (hyponatremia with volume contraction), normal, or increased (hyponatremia with volume expansion). Hyponatremia may be hypotonic, isotonic, or hypertonic. To initiate effective treatment, it is important to attempt to determine the primary cause of the hyponatremia and whether there is associated volume expansion or contraction. The most common cause of hyponatremia in the sick neonate is excessive administration or retention of free water. In these situations the total body sodium content is normal, and the appropriate treatment is restriction of free water intake and not administration of sodium. In situations of true sodium deficit, the deficits can be estimated by assuming 70% of total body weight as the distribution space of sodium. The formula for calculating sodium deficit is:

$$Na^+ \text{deficit (or excess) (mEq)} \approx 0.7 \times kg \times [(Na^+)_{desired} - (Na^+)_{actual}]$$

In most situations of depletional hyponatremia, the sodium deficit should be replaced on a schedule that provides two thirds replacement in the first 24 hours and the remainder in the next 24 hours. Frequent measurements of serum electrolytes are needed to ensure that the correction is occurring appropriately. If the serum sodium concentration is less than 120 mEq/L, regardless of whether the hyponatremia is due to free water overload or total body sodium deficit, then correction of the serum sodium concentration up to 120 mEq/L is recommended with administration of 3% saline solution (513 mEq of sodium per liter). This correction should be done over 4 to 6 hours, depending on the severity of hyponatremia (Avner, 1995) and using the above formula. Although rapid intravenous bolus administration of 4 to 6 mL/kg of 3% saline solution has been effective in children with seizures or

coma (Sarnaik et al, 1991), rapid and complete correction of low serum sodium concentration in adults with chronic hyponatremia has been shown to be associated with pontine and extrapontine myelinolysis. Once the risk of acute central nervous system symptoms has been minimized and serum sodium concentration has reached 120 mEq/L, complete correction of hyponatremia should be performed more slowly over the next 48 hours. In patients with asymptomatic hyponatremia whose serum sodium concentration exceeds 120 mEq/L, hypertonic infusions are not indicated. Additional therapy should be directed at fluid restriction if the hyponatremia is dilutional or sodium repletion if the hyponatremia is depletional. The use of 5% dextrose in water with 0.45% to 0.9% saline is a reasonable replacement fluid for depletional hyponatremia once the sodium is above 120 mEq/L. More stable infants with chronic sodium losses can also be corrected with enteral sodium chloride. Figure 31-5 summarizes the clinical evaluation and therapy of neonates with hyponatremia.

Hypernatremia

Hypernatremia (serum sodium >145 mEq/L) reflects a deficiency of water relative to total body sodium and is most often a disorder of water rather than sodium homeostasis. Hypernatremia does not reflect the total body sodium content, which can be high, normal, or low depending on the cause of the condition. Hypernatremia can also be associated with hypovolemia, normovolemia, or hypervolemia (Box 31-2). If hypernatremia is primarily due to changes in sodium balance, it can result from pure sodium gain or, more commonly, sodium gain coupled with a lesser degree of water accumulation or, rarely, water loss. The hypernatremia-induced hypertonicity causes water to shift from the intracellular to the extracellular compartment, resulting in intracellular dehydration and the relative preservation of the extracellular compartment. This shift is the main reason that neonates with chronic hypernatremic dehydration often do not demonstrate overt clinical signs of intravascular depletion and dehydration until late in the course of the condition.

Compared with other organs, the central nervous system has a unique adaptive capacity to respond to the hypernatremia-induced hypertonicity, leading to a relative preservation of neuronal cell volume. The shrinkage of the brain stimulates the uptake of electrolytes such as sodium, potassium, and chloride (immediate effect) as well as the synthesis of osmoprotective amino acids and organic solutes (more delayed response). These idiogenic osmols aid in maintaining normal brain cell volume during longer periods of hyperosmolar stress (Trachtman, 1991). As long as hypernatremia develops rapidly (within hours), as in accidental sodium loading, a relatively rapid correction of the condition improves the prognosis without raising the risk of cerebral edema formation. Intracellular fluid accumulation does not occur because the accumulated electrolytes (sodium, potassium, and chloride) are rapidly extruded from the brain cells, and cerebral edema is unlikely. In these cases, reducing serum sodium concentration by 1 mEq/L per hour (24 mEq/L per day) is appropriate (Adrogue and Madias, 2000).

However, because of the slow dissipation of idiogenic osmols over a period of several days (Adrogue and Madias,

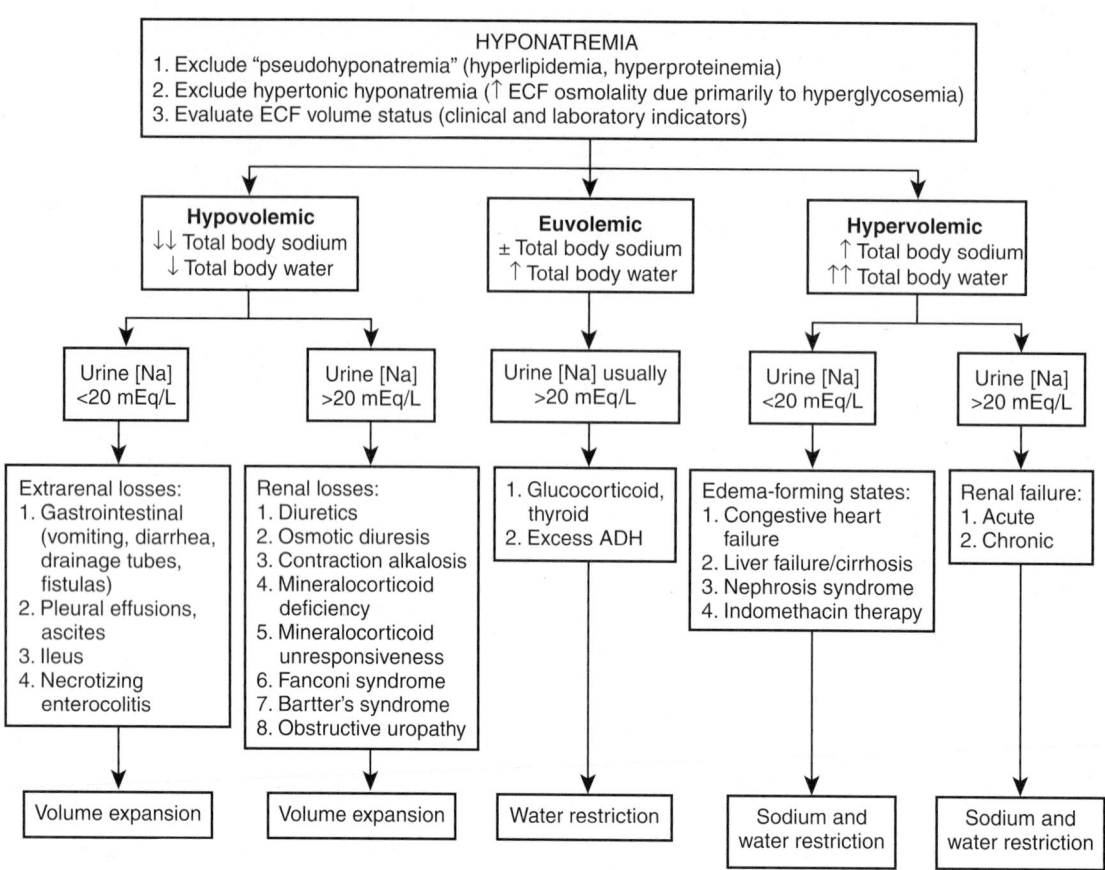

FIGURE 31-5 Flow diagram for the clinical evaluation and therapy of neonates with hyponatremia. *ADH*, Antidiuretic hormone; *ECF*, extracellular fluid. (*Modified from Avner ED: Clinical disorders of water metabolism: hyponatremia and hypernatremia*, Pediatr Ann *24:23-30, 1995.*)

2000), in cases of chronic hypernatremia or in cases in which the time frame is unknown, the hypernatremia should be corrected more slowly, at a maximum rate of 0.5 mEq/L per hour (12 mEq/L per day). If correction is performed more rapidly in these cases, the abrupt fall in the extracellular tonicity results in the movement of water into the brain cells, which have a relatively fixed hypertonicity because of the presence of the osmoprotective molecules. The result is the development of brain edema with deleterious consequences (Adrogue and Madias, 2000; Molteni, 1994).

In the breastfed term neonate, hypernatremia most commonly develops because of dehydration caused by inadequate breast milk intake (Molteni, 1994), but may also be caused by high sodium levels in maternal breast milk. Reduction in breastfeeding frequency has been shown to be associated with a marked rise in the sodium concentration of breast milk (Neville et al, 1991). A vicious cycle can ensue in which the infant sucks poorly, breast milk production drops, sodium concentration rises, and the infant becomes increasingly dehydrated, hypernatremic, and lethargic. Recognition may be delayed because these infants may appear quiet and content initially. Because this process is chronic, usually occurring over 7 to 14 days, signs of extracellular volume contraction are less prominent until the development of the full clinical presentation consisting of lethargy, irritability, abnormal muscle tone with or without seizures, and cardiovascular collapse

---

BOX 31-2 Conditions Causing Hypernatremia

HYPOVOLEMIC HYPERNATREMIA

Inadequate breast milk intake
Diarrhea
Radiant warmers
Excessive sweating
Renal dysplasia
Osmotic diuresis

EUVOLEMIC HYPERNATREMIA
Decreased Production of Antidiuretic Hormone
Central diabetes insipidus, head trauma, central nervous system tumors (craniopharyngioma), meningitis, or encephalitis

Decrease or Absence of Renal Responsiveness
Nephrogenic diabetes insipidus, extreme immaturity, renal insult, and medications such as amphotericin, hydantoin, aminoglycosides

HYPERVOLEMIC HYPERNATREMIA
Improperly mixed formula
$NaHCO_3$ administration
NaCl administration
Primary hyperaldosteronism

with renal failure. This presentation can be associated with serious central nervous system morbidity from both the hypertonicity (sagital or other venous sinus thrombosis, subdural capillary hemorrhage, white matter injury) and inappropriately rapid rehydration therapy (brain edema, myelinolysis).

In the extremely immature neonate, hypernatremia most commonly occurs from excessive transepidermal free water losses. The condition usually develops rapidly, within 24 to 48 hours after birth. The diagnosis is based on the attendant decrease in body weight and clinical signs of extracellular volume contraction. Prevention of this condition has been successful in the majority of immature neonates by frequent monitoring of serum electrolyte levels, appropriate adjustments of free water intake, and the use of humidified incubators (Modi, 2004).

The central and nephrogenic forms of diabetes insipidus are much less commonly encountered and result in hypernatremia because of the lack of production of and renal responsiveness to ADH, respectively. Hypernatremia can also develop in response to excessive sodium supplementation, mainly in the sick neonate receiving repeated volume boluses for cardiovascular support. In these cases, clinical signs of edema, increased body weight, and the history of volume boluses help to establish the diagnosis.

Treatment of Hypernatremia

Thorough analysis of the medical history and the changes in clinical signs, laboratory findings, and body weight usually aid in determining the major etiologic factor in hypernatremia and thus the appropriate treatment. In the critically ill infant, the cause of the serum sodium abnormality may be multifactorial however, and the treatment less straightforward. Although some cases of hypernatremia are a result of sodium excess with normal or high TBW, most cases in neonates are due to hypernatremic dehydration. Treatment of this condition is generally divided into two phases: the emergent phase where the intravascular volume is restored, usually by administration of 10 to 20 mL/kg of isotonic saline, and the rehydration phase, where the sum of the remaining free water deficit and usual maintenance needs are administered evenly over at least 48 hours.

The free water deficit can be calculated as:

$$H_2O \text{ deficit (or excess) (L)} = [0.7 \times BW\ (kg)] \times \{1 - [NA^+ (mEq/L)]_{current} / [NA^+ (mEq/L)]_{desired}\}$$

In this formula, $(0.7 \times BW)$ is the estimation of TBW.

It is important to note that the amount of free water required to decrease the serum sodium by 1 mEq/L is 4 mL/kg with moderate hypernatremia, but only 3 mL/kg when the hypernatremia is as high as 195 mEq/L (Molteni, 1994). Therefore the amount of free water required to decrease serum sodium by 12 mEq/L over a 24-hour period when hypernatremia is moderate is calculated as:

$$\text{Free water required} = \text{Current weight (kg)} \times 4mL/kg \times 12mEq/L \text{ or}$$
$$\text{Free water required} = \text{Current weight} \times 48\ mL/kg/day$$

And the amount of free water required to decrease serum sodium by 12 mEq/L over a 24-hour period when hypernatremia is severe is calculated as:

$$\text{Free water required} = \text{Current weight} \times 36\ mL/kg/day$$

The free water contents of the common intravenous fluids are listed in Table 31-2. In most mild to moderate hypernatremic states, during the rehydration phase, replacement fluids of 5% dextrose in 0.2% normal saline (31 mEq/L) or 0.45% normal saline (77 mEq/L) are appropriate. Infants with serum sodium levels greater than 165 mEq/L should initially be given 0.9% saline to avoid sudden drops in serum sodium concentration. When the serum sodium is greater than 175 mEq/L, however, normal saline will be hypotonic compared with the patient's serum. In these instances of severe hypernatremia, an appropriate amount of 3% saline (513 mEq/L) should be added to the intravenous (IV) fluid so that the sodium concentration is approximately 10 to 15 mEq/L less than the serum sodium level (Rand and Kolberg, 2001). The relative free water content of an IV solution for a specific patient with sodium perturbations can be calculated using the formula:

$$\text{Percentage of free water content} = 1 - (\text{IV fluid sodium} / \text{Serum sodium})$$

Serum electrolytes should be monitored every 2 to 4 hours until the desired rate of decline in serum sodium concentration is established. At this point, the frequency of the laboratory measurements can be relaxed to every 4 to 6 hours until the serum sodium concentration is less than 150 mEq/L. The speed of correction of hypernatremia depends on the rate of its development. This approach provides a reasonable chance that the serum sodium concentration will gradually decrease to the normal range over 2 to 4 days. Except in cases of acute massive sodium overload, the goal should be to drop the serum sodium concentration at a rate no greater than 1 mEq/L/h. A slower pace of correction of 0.5 mEq/L/h is prudent in patients with hypernatremia of chronic or unknown duration to avoid iatrogenic central nervous system sequelae.

Once serum sodium concentration, urine output, and renal function are normal, the patient should receive standard maintenance fluids, either intravenously or orally, depending on his or her condition. At this time, electrolyte status must still be monitored for an additional 24 hours to ensure that complete recovery has occurred. Hyperglycemia and hypocalcemia commonly accompany hypernatremia. The use of insulin to treat the hyperglycemia is not recommended, because it can increase brain idiogenic osmol content. Hypocalcemia should be corrected with appropriate calcium supplementation.

Potassium Homeostasis and Management

Serum potassium should be kept between 3.5 and 5 mEq/L. In the early postnatal period, neonates, especially immature preterm infants, have higher serum potassium concentrations than older persons. The etiology of the relative hyperkalemia of the newborn is multifactorial and involves developmentally regulated differences in renal function, Na$^+$,K$^+$-ATPase activity (Vasarhelyi et al, 2000), and hormonal milieu. Exposure to prenatal steroids in premature infants is associated with a decreased incidence of hyperkalemia, believed to be due to improved renal function (Omar et al, 2000).

In general, potassium supplementation should be started only after urine output has been well established, usually by the third postnatal day. Supplementation should be started at 1 to 2 mEq/kg/day and increased over 1 to 2 days to the usual maintenance requirement of 2 to 3 mEq/kg/day. Some preterm infants may need more potassium supplementation after the completion of their postnatal volume contraction, because of their increased plasma aldosterone concentrations, prostaglandin excretion, and disproportionately high urine flow rates. Most term and preterm neonates will require potassium supplementation if they are receiving diuretics.

Hypokalemia

Hypokalemia in the neonate is usually defined as a serum potassium level of less than 3.5 mEq/L. Hypokalemia can occur from potassium loss due to diuretics, diarrhea, renal dysfunction, or nasogastric drainage from inadequate potassium intake or from intracellular movement of potassium in the presence of alkalosis. Except in patients receiving digoxin, hypokalemia is rarely symptomatic until the serum potassium concentration is less than 2.5 mEq/L. Electrocardiogram (ECG) manifestations of hypokalemia include flattened T waves, prolongation of the QT interval, or the appearance of U waves. Severe hypokalemia can result in cardiac arrhythmias, ileus, and lethargy.

Treatment of Hypokalemia

Hypokalemia is treated by slowly replacing potassium either intravenously or orally, usually in the daily fluids. Rapid administration of potassium chloride is not recommended, because it is associated with life-threatening cardiac dysfunction. In extreme emergencies, potassium can be given as an infusion over 30 to 60 minutes of not more than 0.3 mEq/kg potassium chloride. If hypokalemia is secondary to alkalosis, the alkalosis should be corrected before considering increasing the potassium intake.

Hyperkalemia

Hyperkalemia in the neonate is defined as a serum potassium level greater than 6 mEq/L in a nonhemolyzed specimen. It is important to understand that most of the body's potassium is contained within cells; therefore serum potassium levels do not accurately reflect total body stores. However, a serum potassium greater than 6.5 to 7 mEq/L can be life threatening, even if stores are normal or low, because of its effect on cardiac rhythm. ECG manifestations of hyperkalemia include peaked T waves (the earliest sign), a widened QRS configuration, bradycardia, tachycardia, supraventricular tachycardia, ventricular tachycardia, and ventricular fibrillation. Because pH affects the distribution of potassium between the intracellular and the extracellular space, serum potassium levels rise during acidosis, which may occur acutely. The clinician should be aware of the potential for life-threatening arrhythmias to occur in infants with chronic lung disease on diuretics

and potassium supplements who develop a sudden respiratory deterioration with acidosis. Another common cause of hyperkalemia is renal dysfunction, of particular concern in very preterm and asphyxiated infants. In addition, infants who have suffered intraventricular hemorrhage or tissue trauma and those with intravascular hemolysis often have hyperkalemia caused by the release of potassium during breakdown of red blood cells. Finally, hyperkalemia may be one of the earliest manifestations of congenital adrenal hyperplasia.

Treatment of Hyperkalemia

When hyperkalemia is diagnosed, all potassium intake should be discontinued and the ECG should be monitored. Table 31-4 presents medications used in management of significant hyperkalemia. Calcium gluconate stabilizes cardiac membranes and alkali therapy, insulin, and inhaled albuterol (Singh et al, 2002) all rapidly enhance cellular uptake of potassium and can acutely drop serum potassium levels, but not decrease total body potassium. Intravenous furosemide and rectally administered sodium polystyrene sulfonate (Kayexalate) enhance potassium excretion and will lower total body stores, but they require several hours to take effect. Dialysis or exchange transfusion may be used when the hyperkalemia is life threatening and these measures do not result in improvement.

CLINICAL CONDITIONS ASSOCIATED WITH FLUID AND ELECTROLYTE DISTURBANCES

Extreme Prematurity

Infants born between 23 and 27 weeks' gestation, or with a birthweight of <1000 g (i.e., ELBW), are at particular risk for acute abnormalities of both fluid and electrolyte status in the immediate postnatal period. Their transepidermal water loss is much higher than that in more mature preterm neonates (see Figure 31-4), and it is difficult for their water balance to be maintained unless the excessive losses are prevented. It should be kept in mind that such an infant, when cared for in an open warmer without the use of a plastic heat shield, may lose up to 150 to 300 mL/kg/day of free water through the skin during the first 3 to 5 days of life. Infants whose mothers received antenatal glucocorticoids often have fewer problems because prenatal glucocorticoids enhance maturation of the epidermis and result in increases in urine output and fractional excretion of sodium (Ali et al, 2000; Omar et al, 1999).

Although the IWL primarily affects the extracellular volume, the intracellular compartment ultimately shares the loss of free water as osmotic pressure in the extracellular compartment rises. As water leaves the cells, intracellular osmolality rises and cell volume diminishes. In the central nervous system, as described earlier, these changes stimulate the generation of idiogenic osmols, resulting in selective increases in intracellular osmolality and a tendency toward normalization of neuronal cell volumes. This protective mechanism has significant clinical implications for the rate at which hypernatremia should be corrected, and the decrease in serum sodium concentration should not exceed 12 mEq/L/day, especially in the infant in whom the hypernatremia has been chronic (>12 hours).

TABLE 31-4 Medications Used for Treatment of Hyperkalemia

Medication	Dosage	Onset	Length of Effects	Mechanism of Action	Comments and Cautions
Calcium gluconate	100 mg/kg IV over 2-5 min	Immediate	30 min	Protects the myocardium from toxic effects of potassium; no effect on total body potassium	Can worsen digoxin toxicity
Sodium bicarbonate	1-2 mEq/kg	Immediate	Variable	Shifts potassium intracellularly; no effect on total body potassium	Maximum infusion: mEq/min in emergency situations
Tromethamine	3-5 mL/kg	Immediate	Variable	Shifts potassium intracellularly; no effect on total body potassium	—
Insulin plus dextrose	Insulin 0.1-0.15 U/kg IV plus dextrose 0.5 g/kg IV	15 to 30 min	2 to 6 h	Shifts potassium intracellularly; no effect on total body potassium	Monitor for hypoglycemia
Albuterol*	0.15 mg/kg every 20 min for three doses then 0.15-0.3 mg/kg	15 to 30 min	2 to 3 h	Shifts potassium intracellularly; no effect on total body potassium	Minimum dose, 2.5 mg
Furosemide	PO: 1-4 mg/kg/dose 1-2 times/day IV: 1-2 mg/kg/dose given every 12-24 hours	15 min to 1 h	4 h	Increases renal excretion of potassium	—
Kayexalate	1 g/kg PR every 6 hours	1 to 2 h (rectal route faster)	4 to 6 h	Removes potassium from the gut in exchange for sodium	Use with extreme caution in neonates, especially preterm; contains sorbital; may be associated with bowel necrosis and sodium retention

IV, Intravenous; *PO*, by mouth or gastric tube; *PR*, per rectum.
*From Singh BS, Sadiq HF, Noguchi A, et al: Efficacy of albuterol inhalation in treatment of hyperkalemia in premature neonates, *J Pediatr* 141:16, 2002.

Because serum sodium concentration is a reliable clinical indicator of extracellular tonicity, monitoring of this parameter every 6 to 12 hours during the first 2 to 3 postnatal days coupled with daily (or twice daily) measurements of body weight provide valuable information and appropriate guidance for the fluid and electrolyte management of the extremely immature preterm neonate. This is especially true in the absence of prenatal steroid exposure and if the infant is not cared for in a humidified incubator. Serum osmolality should be directly measured in patients in whom calculated serum osmolality is more than 300 to 320 mOsm/L.

Table 31-1 shows suggested maintenance fluid requirements by birthweight and postnatal day of life. Because immature neonates in an incubator with an ambient air humidity of 50% to 80% require significantly less free water and less frequent measurements of serum electrolyte and osmolality (Sedin, 1995), open radiant warmers should be used only for critically ill, extremely labile preterm infants requiring frequent hands-on medical management. In these cases, the use of a protective plastic heat shield can help decrease excessive evaporative losses, and total daily fluid intake, similar to that used for infants in incubators, may be started at approximately 100 mL/kg/day containing 5% to 10% dextrose in water with close monitoring for dehydration. Daily fluid intake is then increased by 10 to 30 mL/kg/day every 6 to 12 hours if the serum sodium concentration rises from the baseline, the goal being to keep serum sodium concentration below 145 to 150 mEq/L. As skin integrity improves during the course of

the 2nd to 3rd days, serum sodium concentration starts to fall. At this time, a significant stepwise limitation of total fluid intake is obligatory to allow a complete contraction of the extracellular volume to occur and to minimize the possibility of free water overload with its attendant risks for the development of ductal patency, pulmonary edema, and worsening lung disease.

Potassium chloride supplementation may be started as soon as urine output has been established and the serum potassium concentration is less than 5 mEq/L. Extremely premature infants are at risk for the development of both oliguric and nonoliguric hyperkalemia, so the serum potassium concentration should be monitored closely, and supplementation should be discontinued if warranted by changes in serum potassium values or in renal function. Critically ill, extremely immature neonates often receive excess sodium with volume boluses, medications, and the maintenance infusion of their arterial lines (Costarino et al, 1992). Therefore extra sodium supplementation usually should not be started during the first few postnatal days, to prevent a rise in total body sodium concentration and thus in extracellular volume, which will hinder the appropriate postnatal diuresis.

Many critically ill preterm infants retain their originally high extracellular volumes, even when sodium and water intakes are restricted, and such neonates also tend to lose more bicarbonate in the urine. Interestingly, proximal tubular bicarbonate reabsorption may be appropriate even in the VLBW infant despite the immaturity of their renal functions, as long as extracellular volume contraction takes place (Ramiro-Tolentino et al, 1996). Therefore the presence of the extracellular volume expansion appears to be an important factor in the renal bicarbonate wasting in these infants. The diagnosis of functional proximal tubular acidosis in such cases should not rely solely on the finding of an alkaline urine pH, because the distal tubular function is usually mature enough to acidify the urine once serum bicarbonate has decreased to its new threshold. Provided that liver function is normal, daily supplementation of bicarbonate in the form of sodium acetate, potassium acetate, or both normalizes blood pH and serum bicarbonate in these infants and also increases urine pH, aiding in the diagnosis. Once extracellular volume contraction occurs, these neonates generally achieve a positive bicarbonate balance (Ramiro-Tolentino et al, 1996), and supplementation becomes unnecessary.

Other general guidelines in the fluid and electrolyte management of the immature preterm infant during the 1st week of life are (1) daily calculation of fluid balance and estimation of sodium balance; (2) daily measurements of body weight, serum electrolytes, blood urea nitrogen, creatinine, and plasma glucose; and (3) testing of urine samples for glucose, and osmolality or specific gravity. The frequency of testing and the addition of other tests, including the measurement of serum albumin concentration and osmolality, depend on the clinical status, severity of underlying disease, and fluid and electrolyte disturbance of the individual patient.

Respiratory Distress Syndrome

There is a well-established relationship between fluid and electrolyte imbalance and respiratory distress syndrome. Surfactant deficiency results in pulmonary atelectasis, elevated pulmonary vascular resistance, poor lung compliance, and decreased lymphatic drainage. In addition, preterm infants have low plasma oncotic and critical pulmonary capillary pressures and suffer pulmonary capillary endothelial injury from mechanical ventilation, oxygen administration, and perinatal hypoxia (Dudek and Garcia, 2001; Sola and Gregory, 1981). These abnormalities alter the balance of the Starling forces in the pulmonary microcirculation, leading to interstitial edema formation with further impairment in pulmonary functions.

In the presurfactant era, an improvement in pulmonary function occurred only during the 3rd to 4th postnatal day. This improvement was usually preceded by a period of brisk diuresis characterized by small increases in glomerular filtration rate and sodium clearance and a larger rise in free water clearance (Costarino and Baumgart, 1991). Although the exact mechanism for this diuresis is not known, it is likely that improving endogenous surfactant production and capillary integrity promoted the recovery of the pulmonary capillary endothelium and lymphatic drainage. The ensuing changes in Starling forces then favored reabsorption of the hypotonic interstitial lung fluid into the circulation, and a delayed physiologic diuresis took place.

Currently, with the routine use of surfactant and antenatal steroids, the pulmonary compromise and its consequences are less severe. However, because significant improvements in lung function take place only after the

majority of the excess free water is excreted (Costarino and Baumgart, 1991), daily fluid intake should still be restricted to allow the extracellular volume contraction to take place. If this principle is not followed and a positive fluid balance occurs, preterm infants with respiratory distress syndrome are at higher risk for a more severe course of acute lung disease and have a higher incidence of patent ductus arteriosus, congestive heart failure, and necrotizing enterocolitis as well as a greater severity of the ensuing bronchopulmonary dysplasia.

Antenatal administration of steroids and postnatal use of surfactants have clearly altered the course and clinical presentation of respiratory distress syndrome (Ballard and Ballard, 1995; Kari et al, 1994). Antenatal steroid administration accelerates maturation of organs including those involved in the regulation of fluid and electrolyte balance (Ballard and Ballard, 1995), whereas the use of exogenous surfactant decreases pulmonary capillary leak and edema formation (Carlton et al, 1995). Furthermore, surfactant administration does not alter the rate and timing of ductal closure (Reller et al, 1993), although it may affect the pattern of shunting through the ductus arteriosus in the acute period (Kaapa et al, 1993; Kluckow and Evans, 2000). Thus, these interventions generally enhance extracellular volume contraction and aid in the stabilization of fluid and electrolyte homeostasis in preterm neonates with respiratory distress syndrome. However, maintenance of a negative water and sodium balance during the first few days of life remains the cornerstone of fluid and electrolyte management in these infants (Tammela, 1995; Van Marter et al, 1990).

On the basis of the events in the pathophysiology of pulmonary edema formation in these infants, the use of furosemide has long been suggested to promote a negative fluid balance and to directly inhibit pulmonary epithelial transport processes involved in edema formation in the lungs (Green et al, 1988; Yeh et al, 1984). However, furosemide induces only short-term improvements in pulmonary function in these patients, and no beneficial effects on long-term morbidity or mortality have been documented. Moreover, prophylactic use of the drug during the first postnatal days can lead to intravascular volume depletion with hypotension, tachycardia, and decreased peripheral perfusion as well as to acute and chronic disturbances in serum electrolytes and thus osmolality (Green et al, 1988; Shaffer and Weismann, 1992; Yeh et al, 1984). Furthermore, continued administration may be associated with an increased incidence of patent ductus arteriosus (Green et al, 1983). Therefore the use of furosemide during this period should be restricted to patients with oliguria of renal origin whose intravascular volume appears to be adequate.

Chronic Lung Disease or Bronchopulmonary Dysplasia

Low gestational age and birthweight, lack of antenatal steroid administration, severe respiratory distress syndrome with oxygen toxicity, volutrauma and barotrauma, air leak, inflammation, patent ductus arteriosus, and insufficient nutrition are among the known etiologic factors for the development of bronchopulmonary dysplasia. In addition, a high fluid and salt intake during the first weeks of life has been shown to increase the incidence and severity of chronic lung disease. Specifically, higher fluid intake and lack of appropriate weight loss in the first 10 days of life are associated with significantly higher risk for bronchopulmonary dysplasia, even after controlling for other known risk factors such as those listed previously (Oh et al, 2005). Therefore careful fluid and electrolyte management during the first weeks of life, allowing for the appropriate degree of weight loss, is of great importance in decreasing the incidence and severity of this condition (see Chapter 48).

Patent Ductus Arteriosus

A PDA has been associated with an increase in morbidity and mortality in epidemiological studies, especially in the infant with ELBW. However, trials aimed at prophylactic or therapeutic closure of the ductus have not demonstrated improvements in these outcomes. Several conditions, including hypoxemia, unstable cardiovascular status, metabolic acidosis, increases in extracellular volume, inflammatory mediators, and ductal prostaglandin synthesis, have been recognized to prolong patency of the ductus arteriosus (Hammerman, 1995; see Chapter 54). Accordingly, clinical management aimed at preventing the occurrence of ductal patency involves interventions that keep the cardiovascular status and oxygenation stable, minimize inflammation, restrict fluid intake, and maintain low levels of local prostaglandin synthesis by the administration of indomethacin (Clyman, 1996). Pharmacologic ductal closure with indomethacin is normally indicated during the first 2 postnatal weeks, because ductal sensitivity to prostaglandins rapidly diminishes thereafter (Clyman, 1996; Van Overmeire et al, 2000). Ibuprofen has been offered as an alternative inhibitor of cyclooxygenase, the enzyme responsible for prostaglandin synthesis, because of its equivalent efficacy in closing the symptomatic PDA with fewer adverse effects (Ohlsson et al, 2008). Specifically, ibuprofen may cause less renal dysfunction (Van Overmeire et al, 2000) and cerebral vasoconstriction (Mosca et al, 1997; Patel et al, 2000) when used in this manner. However, ibuprofen is not recommended for prophylactic use because it has an adverse effect on renal function in this setting and does not reduce grade III and IV IVH as indomethacin has been proven to do (Shah and Ohlssen, 2006). For more details, see Chapter 61.

Under physiologic circumstances in the immediate postnatal period, renal prostaglandin production is increased to counterbalance the renal actions of vasoconstrictor and sodium- and water-retaining hormones released during labor and delivery (Bonvalet et al, 1987; Gleason, 1987). Compared with the renal function of the adult kidney in euvolemia, the neonatal kidney is more dependent on the increased production of vasodilatory and natriuretic prostaglandins, rendering it more sensitive to the vasoconstrictive and sodium- and water-retaining actions of cyclooxygenase inhibition. In the preterm infant, indomethacin administration has been shown to have clinically significant, although mostly transient, renal side effects because of decreased prostaglandin production through inhibition of cyclooxygenase. In the indomethacin-treated neonate, the unopposed renal vasoconstriction and sodium

and water reabsorption leads to decreases in renal blood flow and glomerular filtration rate and to increases in sodium and free water reabsorption. These side effects occur despite the diminishing left-to-right shunt through the closing ductus. Characteristic clinical findings include a rise in serum creatinine level, oliguria, and hyponatremia (Cifuentes et al, 1979). Hyponatremia occurs because the free water retention caused by the unopposed renal actions of high plasma vasopressin levels is out of proportion to the sodium retention induced by angiotensin and noradrenaline. This pattern of renal response can most likely be explained by the fact that in a preterm infant, the function of the distal tubule is more mature than that of the proximal tubule (Lumbers et al, 1988), leading to an expanded but somewhat hypotonic extracellular space. Therefore fluid management of the preterm infant receiving indomethacin must focus on maintaining an appropriately restricted fluid intake and avoiding extra sodium supplementation. As the prostaglandin inhibitory effects of indomethacin diminish following the last dose, renal prostaglandin production returns to normal, and the retained sodium and excess free water are usually rapidly excreted, especially with the improvement in the cardiovascular status as the ductal shunt decreases.

Because furosemide increases prostaglandin production, the drug has been hypothesized to attenuate the renal side effects of indomethacin if the intravascular volume is judged to be adequate (Yeh et al, 1982). However, furosemide administration can increase the incidence of ductal patency (Green et al, 1983), so routine use of the drug might not be prudent in preterm infants treated with indomethacin, because of the theoretical risk of reopening the ductus arteriosus (Seri, 1995). Furthermore, the concomitant use of furosemide and indomethacin has been shown to worsen renal function, as evidenced by increases in serum creatinine and worsening hyponatremia without increasing overall urine output (Andriessen et al, 2009). As a result, furosemide should not be used early in life when the PDA is also being actively managed. In cases of hemodynamic instability or to avoid the potential effect of furosemide on ductal closure, dopamine infusion can be used to support the cardiovascular status and attenuate the indomethacin-induced oliguria (Cochran et al, 1989; Seri et al, 1984, 1993). However, there is controversy regarding the efficacy and clinical significance of this intervention (Baenziger et al, 1999; Fajardo et al, 1992; Seri, 1995).

Growing Premature Infant With Negative Sodium Balance

The 2- to 6-week-old growing preterm neonate who does not have significant chronic lung disease and is not undergoing diuretic treatment may have hyponatremia (serum sodium concentration 125 to 129 mEq/L) because of a relative sodium deficiency (Sulyok et al, 1979, 1985). Despite the low total body sodium and high activity of sodium retaining hormones, these infants continue to lose sodium in the urine mainly because of immature renal function. Although the infant is usually in a positive sodium balance, it is insufficient to compete with the increased sodium demand because of growth. The treatment of this condition is to provide extra sodium supplementation in the form of sodium chloride (usually 2 to 4 mEq/kg/day) to keep serum sodium values greater than 130 mEq/L.

Shock and Edema

In the uncompensated phase of shock, blood pressure is low; cardiac output may be low, normal, or high; effective circulating blood volume is usually decreased; transcapillary hydrostatic pressure is elevated; and capillary integrity and lymphatic drainage are impaired, resulting in edema formation and increased interstitial compliance. The latter condition further enhances fluid accumulation in the interstitium. The changes in the effective circulating blood volume also trigger the release of antidiuretic hormones, including catecholamines, renin-angiotensin-aldosterone, and vasopressin, resulting in the retention of sodium and free water. The specific cause of shock (e.g., infection, asphyxia, myocardial insufficiency, hypovolemia) may independently contribute to this chain of events, further compromising fluid and electrolyte balance. In affected infants, treatment is directed at normalizing tissue perfusion and oxygen delivery by restoring effective intravascular volume, cardiac output, and renal function with the use of vasopressor and inotropic support, as well as with the judicious use of volume expanders while monitoring blood pressure, cardiac output, and changes in organ blood flow (see Chapter 51). In shock refractory to these therapies, early initiation of low-dose glucocorticoid and mineralocorticoid replacement may help to break the vicious cycle by improving capillary integrity and thus effective circulating blood volume, and by potentiating the cardiovascular response to vasopressors and inotropic agents (Seri et al, 2000).

Syndrome of Inappropriate Anti-Diuretic Hormone Secretion

SIADH may be associated with birth asphyxia, intracerebral hemorrhage, respiratory distress syndrome, pneumothorax, and the use of continuous positive-pressure ventilation (El-Dahr and Chevalier, 1990; Leake, 1992). The syndrome is characterized by oliguria, free water retention, decreased serum sodium concentration and serum osmolality, increased urine concentration, and weight gain caused by edema formation. However, because the urinary concentrating capacity of the newborn is limited, a less than maximally diluted urine satisfies the diagnosis of SIADH in the presence of the other symptoms. The treatment is based on fluid and sodium restriction despite the oliguria and hyponatremia, as well as on appropriate circulatory and ventilatory support. The clinician must remember that total body sodium is normal, but TBW is elevated in such an infant, and that it is particularly dangerous to treat the hyponatremia caused by free water retention with large amounts of sodium. Because of their more immature renal functions, infants with extreme LBW during the first few weeks of life usually do not exhibit the full-blown syndrome despite their sometimes excessively high plasma vasopressin levels (Aperia et al, 1983).

Diminished vasopressin secretion or complete unresponsiveness of the renal tubules to vasopressin results in polyuria, dilute urine production, and increased serum osmolality (Leake, 1992), otherwise known as diabetes insipidus (DI). This condition is not common in neonates, but can occur in association with central nervous system injury or disease, such as in meningitis or cerebral hemorrhage affecting the pituitary gland (central DI) or in an inherited form (nephrogenic DI). The treatment of neonates with this condition consists of allowing for adequate free water intake and the use of desmopressin.

Surgical Conditions

Surgery has a major effect on metabolism, fluid balance, and electrolyte balance in the newborn. Preterm infants with acute or chronic lung disease are especially sensitive and respond to the procedure with significant catabolic responses, increases in capillary permeability with the attendant shift of fluid into the interstitial space, and retention of sodium and free water (John et al, 1989). The retention of sodium and free water is secondary to the decrease in effective circulating blood volume and to the increased plasma levels of sodium- and water-retaining hormones, including catecholamines, renin-angiotensin-aldosterone, and vasopressin.

Preoperative management has a significant effect on outcome and should be aimed at maintaining adequate effective circulating blood volume as well as cardiovascular and renal function. In preterm infants who have evidence of absolute or relative adrenal insufficiency (Watterberg, 2002), the provision of stress doses of steroids may be necessary. In the postoperative period, maintenance of the integrity of the cardiovascular system through the judicious use of volume expanders and pressor support, meticulous replacement of ongoing surgical and nonsurgical fluid and electrolyte losses, close monitoring, and intense and effective communication between the neonatal and surgical teams are essential to ensure a successful outcome. As capillary integrity improves, reabsorption and excretion of the expanded interstitial fluid volume occurs, with normalization in the secretion of hormones regulating fluid and electrolyte balance. At this time, the provision of maximized nutritional support becomes essential to restore the anabolic state and growth of the infant.

The most commonly encountered surgical water losses occur when a nasogastric tube is placed under continuous suction to provide relief for the gastrointestinal tract in conditions such as necrotizing enterocolitis and postoperative management after abdominal surgery. Because these losses may be substantial, they should be monitored and a portion of it should be replaced every 6 to 12 hours to maintain appropriate water and electrolyte balance. However, free water retention often develops after surgery; therefore full replacement of the nasogastric free water loss is not usually recommended. The composition of the replacement solution depends on the electrolyte concentration of the fluid loss. Gastric fluid usually contains 50 to 60 mEq/L of sodium chloride, and therefore, 0.45% sodium chloride with potassium is normally used as the fluid of choice for replacement. See Table 31-3 for estimated electrolyte compositions of body fluids.

ACID-BASE BALANCE

PHYSIOLOGY OF ACID-BASE BALANCE REGULATION

Like adults, newborns must maintain their extracellular pH, or hydrogen ion concentration, within a narrow range. A normal pH is essential for intact functioning of all enzymatic processes and, therefore, the intact functioning of all organ systems of the body. Newborns are subjected to many stresses that can affect their acid-base balance. In addition, neonates, especially if they are premature, have a limited ability to compensate for acid-base alterations; therefore acid-base disturbances are common in the neonatal period. An understanding of the principles of acid-base regulation is essential for proper diagnosis and treatment of these disturbances.

In healthy humans, the normal range of ECF hydrogen ion concentration is 35 to 45 mEq/L. Because pH is defined as the negative logarithm of hydrogen ion concentration (pH = $-log$[H$^+$]), these values of hydrogen ion concentration correspond to a pH range of 7.35 to 7.45. Acidosis is a downward shift in pH to less than 7.35, and alkalosis is an upward shift in pH to more than 7.45. Alterations in normal pH are resisted by complex physiologic regulatory mechanisms. The main systems that maintain pH are the body's buffer systems, the respiratory system, and the kidneys. Some of these systems respond immediately to sudden alterations in hydrogen ion concentration, whereas others respond more slowly to changes but maintain the overall balance between acid and base production, intake, metabolism, and excretion over the long term.

The physiologic regulatory systems that respond immediately to changes in acid-base balance include the various intracellular and extracellular buffers as well as the lungs. A buffer is a substance that can minimize changes in pH when acid or base is added to the system. The extracellular buffers, which include the bicarbonate-carbonic acid system, phosphates, and plasma proteins, act rapidly to return the extracellular pH toward normal. The intracellular buffers, which include hemoglobin, organic phosphates, and bone apatite, act more slowly and require several hours to reach maximal capacity.

The most important extracellular buffer is the plasma bicarbonate–carbonic acid buffer system, in which the acid component (carbonic acid [H_2CO_3]) is regulated by the lungs, and the base component (bicarbonate [HCO_3^-]) is regulated by the kidneys. The buffer equation is:

$$H^+ + HCO_3^- \leftrightarrow H_2CO_3 \leftrightarrow H_2O + (CO_2)_d$$

where $(CO_2)_d$ represents the dissolved carbon dioxide. At equilibrium, the amount of $(CO_2)_d$ exceeds that of H_2CO_3 by a factor of 800:1; therefore for practical purposes, $(CO_2)_d$ and H_2CO_3 can be treated interchangeably. The fact that CO_2 excretion can be controlled by the respiratory system markedly improves the efficiency of this buffer system at physiologic pH. The enzyme carbonic anhydrase allows rapid interconversion of H_2CO_3 to H_2O and CO_2. If the hydrogen ion (H$^+$) concentration increases for any reason, hydrogen combines with HCO_3^-, driving the buffer reaction toward greater production of H_2CO_3 and

CO_2. Carbon dioxide crosses the blood-brain barrier and stimulates central nervous system chemoreceptors, leading to increased alveolar ventilation and decreased concentration of extracellular CO_2. This respiratory compensation begins within minutes after a pH change and is complete within 12 to 24 hours. A similar compensation occurs in response to a decrease in H$^+$ concentration, leading to decreased alveolar ventilation and a resultant increase in extracellular CO_2.

The relationship of the two components of the bicarbonate–carbonic acid buffer system to pH is expressed by the Henderson-Hasselbalch equation:

$$pH = pK + log\frac{[HCO_3^-]}{[H_2CO_3]}$$

Because H_2CO_3 is in equilibrium with the dissolved CO_2 in the plasma, and because the amount of dissolved CO_2 depends on the partial pressure of CO_2, the equation can be modified as:

$$pH = pK + log\frac{[HCO_3^-]}{0.03} \times Pa_{CO_2}$$

Both the original equation and the modified equation are clinically difficult to use; therefore the modified Henderson-Hasselbalch equation can be rewritten as the Henderson equation without logarithms for easier clinical use.

$$[H^+] = 24 \times \frac{Pa_{CO_2}}{[HCO_3^-]}$$

This last equation clearly indicates the clinically most important aspect of acid-base regulation by the bicarbonate-carbonic acid buffer system, that the change in the ratio of Pa_{CO_2} to HCO_3^- concentration, and not in their absolute values, determines the direction of change in H$^+$ concentration and thus in pH. The status of the plasma bicarbonate-carbonic acid buffer system can be monitored easily by serial blood gas measurements, making understanding of this buffer system important in clinical care.

The physiologic regulation system that responds more slowly to changes in acid-base balance is the renal system. There must be a long-term balance between net acid increase caused by intake and production and net acid decrease caused by excretion and metabolism. Although infant formula and protein-containing intravenous fluids have small amounts of preformed acid, most of the daily acid load is derived from metabolism. A large amount of the acid produced is in the form of the volatile H_2CO_3 that can be excreted in the lungs. Nonvolatile or fixed acids are also produced, which must be excreted through the kidneys. Nonvolatile acids normally are sulfuric acid produced in the metabolism of the amino acids methionine and cysteine as well as smaller contributions from phosphoric acid, lactic acid, hydrochloric acid, and incompletely oxidized organic acids. In addition to the excretion of nonvolatile acids, however, the kidneys have a role in long-term acid-base regulation by controlling renal HCO_3^- excretion.

Two regions of the kidney act to achieve urinary acidification—the proximal tubule and the collecting tubule. The proximal tubule acidifies the urine by two mechanisms. The first mechanism is by the reabsorption of any HCO_3^- already present in the blood that is being constantly filtered through the glomeruli. The proximal tubule reabsorbs 60% to 80% of all filtered HCO_3^- and performs this role through an exchange of Na^+ for H^+ across the luminal membrane of the proximal tubular cells via the Na^+/H^+ exchanger. The excreted H^+ combines with filtered HCO_3^-, producing H_2CO_3 through the activity of carbonic anhydrase in the cellular brush border. The H_2CO_3 is then quickly converted to CO_2, which crosses into the tubular cell, where HCO_3^- is regenerated and reabsorbed back into the blood stream, probably in exchange for chloride (Cl^-). The regenerated H^+ ion reenters the cycle at the Na^+/H^+ exchanger.

The second mechanism by which the proximal tubule acidifies urine is by the production of ammonia (NH_3). Inside the tubular cell, NH_3 is produced by the deamination of glutamine. The NH_3 is secreted into the tubular lumen, where it combines with and traps free H^+ to form ammonium (NH_4^+).

The remaining urinary acidification occurs mostly in the collecting tubule. H^+ secretion in this region of the kidney is sufficient to combine with or titrate any remaining filtered HCO_3^- or any filtered anions, such as phosphate and sulfate. Hydrogenated phosphate and sulfate anions produce the titratable acid of the urine. The collecting tubule also takes up NH_3 from the medullary interstitium and secretes it into the urine, where again it can combine with and trap H^+ as NH_4^+. This urinary NH_4^+ can act as a cation and be excreted with urinary anions such as Cl^-, PO_4^-, and SO_4^-, thereby preventing loss of cations such as Na^+, Ca^{++}, and K^+. Total acid secretion in the kidney can be represented by

$$\text{Titratable acid} + NH_4^+ - HCO_3^-$$

and under normal conditions should equal the net production of acid from diet and metabolism that is not excreted in the form of CO_2 through the lungs.

In adults, the steady state for renal compensation for respiratory alkalosis is reached within 1 to 2 days and for respiratory acidosis within 3 to 5 days. Newborns are able to compensate for acidemia through the previously described renal mechanisms, although the renal response to acid loads is limited, especially in premature infants born before 34 weeks' gestation. Reabsorption of HCO_3^- in the proximal tubule and distal tubular acidification are also decreased, with a fairly rapid gestational age-dependent maturation of these functions after birth (Jones and Chesney, 1992).

To accomplish the tight regulation of pH necessary for survival, H^+ ions generated in the form of the volatile acid H_2CO_3 are excreted by the lungs as CO_2. H^+ ions generated in the form of nonvolatile acids are buffered rapidly by extracellular HCO_3^- and more slowly by intracellular buffers. HCO_3^- is then replenished by the kidneys via the reabsorption of much of the filtered HCO_3^- and by the excretion of H^+ in the urine as NH_4^+ and titratable acids.

DISTURBANCES OF ACID-BASE BALANCE IN THE NEWBORN

General Principles

The evaluation of the acid-base status in a newborn is one of the most common laboratory assessments made in the neonatal intensive care unit. The status of this system can be monitored with blood gas measurements and should be the starting point for the evaluation of any acid-base disorder. In the blood gas measurement, the pH and $Paco_2$ levels are directly measured; from these, the HCO_3^- level and base excess or deficit are calculated.

The whole blood buffer base, defined as the sum of the HCO_3^- and non-HCO_3^- buffer systems, is another important blood gas value used in evaluating acid-base disturbances. The difference between the observed whole blood buffer base of any blood gas sample and the expected normal buffer base of that sample is called the base excess or base deficit. The base excess and base deficit give an accurate measure of the amount of strong acid or base, respectively, that would be needed to titrate the pH back to normal once the respiratory contribution of the acid-base disturbance is also corrected. For example, a base excess of 10 mEq/L indicates that there is an additional 10 mEq of base per liter (or loss of 10 mEq of H^+ per liter) that is contributing to the acid-base abnormality. Conversely, a base deficit of 10 mEq/L indicates there is relatively more acid (or less base) in the ECF than expected after accounting for the effect of Pco_2 on pH.

Acid-base disorders are classified according to their cause as being either metabolic or respiratory. Metabolic acidosis occurs as a result of the accumulation of increased amounts of nonvolatile acid or decreased amounts of HCO_3^- in the ECF. Metabolic alkalosis occurs as a result of increased amounts of HCO_3^- in the ECF. Respiratory acidosis is caused by hypoventilation and decreased excretion of volatile acid (CO_2), whereas respiratory alkalosis is caused by hyperventilation and increased excretion of volatile acid (CO_2).

Acid-base disorders are also classified according to the number of conditions causing the disorder. When only one primary acid-base abnormality and its compensatory mechanisms occur, the disorder is classified as a *simple acid-base disorder*. When a combination of simple acid-base disturbances occurs, the patient has a mixed (or complex) acid-base disorder. Because secondary physiologic regulatory mechanisms often compensate for the alteration in pH caused by primary disturbances, it is sometimes difficult to differentiate simple from mixed disorders or even a simple disorder from its resulting compensation. One important principle that allows the determination of primary acid-base disturbance is that the compensatory regulatory mechanisms do not completely normalize the pH.

Nomograms, such as the one shown in Figure 31-6, can help in the diagnosis of the primary disturbance. The nomogram describes the 95% confidence limits of the expected compensatory response to a primary abnormality in either $Paco_2$ or HCO_3^-. Table 31-5 summarizes the expected respiratory and metabolic compensatory mechanisms for primary acid-base disorders (Brewer, 1990). If the compensation in a given patient differs from that predicted in Figure 31-6 or Table 31-5, the patient either has not had enough time to compensate for a simple acid-base disturbance or has a mixed acid-base disorder. Furthermore, the complete correction of an acid-base disturbance occurs only when the underlying process responsible for the abnormality has been treated effectively.

For identification of the primary disturbance, the analysis of blood gas values must be considered in light of the patient's history and physical findings and with an understanding of expected compensatory responses. Further laboratory evaluation is indicated if the problem is not immediately obvious or if the response to therapy is not as expected. The evaluation of the acid-base disturbance should always involve efforts to determine the underlying cause of the disturbance, because adequate treatment requires correction of the underlying disorder, if possible.

Transitional Physiology after Birth

As part of a discussion of normal physiology, it is important to understand the in utero environment just before delivery of the newborn and its effects on neonatal

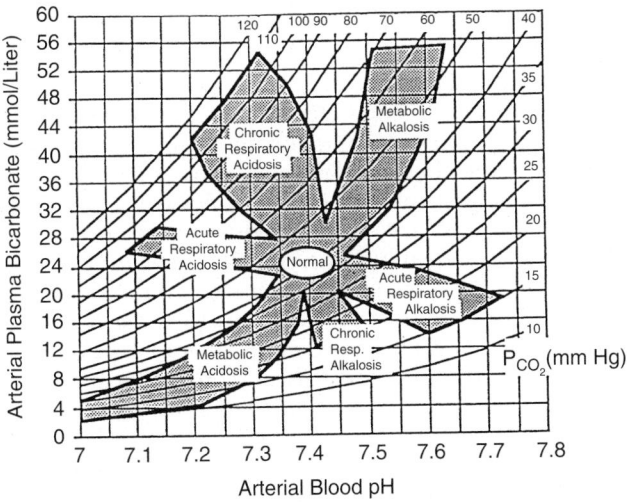

FIGURE 31-6 Acid-base nomogram illustrating the 95% confidence limits for compensatory responses to primary acid-base disorders. *(From Cogan MG, Rector FC Jr: Acid-base disorders. In Brenner BM, Rector FC Jr, editors:* The kidney, *Philadelphia, 1986, WB Saunders.)*

acid-base analysis shortly after birth. Hyperventilation of pregnancy is a known phenomenon with corresponding maternal PCO_2 levels of approximately 31 to 34 mm Hg (Thorp and Rushing, 1999). This relative respiratory alkalosis in the mother is compensated for by a corresponding metabolic acidosis in the mother and, therefore, fetus. As a result, umbilical arterial blood gases have a normal pH range of 7.20 to 7.28 with a corresponding base deficit ranging from 2.7 ± 2.8 mEq/L (SD) to 8.3 ± 4.0 mEq/L (SD) (Riley and Johnson, 1993; Sykes et al, 1982). In other words, a mild metabolic acidosis in the newborn shortly after birth can be expected and explained by normal physiology.

Metabolic Acidosis

Metabolic acidosis is a common problem, particularly in the critically ill newborn. Metabolic acidosis occurs when the drop in pH is caused by the accumulation of acid other than H_2CO_3 by the ECF, resulting in loss of available HCO_3^-, or by the direct loss of HCO_3^- from body fluids. Patients who have metabolic acidosis are divided into those with an elevated anion gap and those with a normal anion gap.

The anion gap reflects the unaccounted acidic anions and certain cations in the ECF. The unmeasured anions normally include the serum proteins, phosphates, sulfates, and organic acids, whereas the unaccounted cations are the serum potassium, calcium, and magnesium. Thus, in clinical practice, the anion gap is estimated using the formula

$$\text{Anion gap} = [Na^+]_{serum} - ([Cl^-]_{serum} + [HCO_3^-]_{serum})$$

The normal range of the serum anion gap in newborns is 8 to 16 mEq/L, with slightly higher values in very premature newborns. Accumulation of strong acids because of increased intake, increased production, or decreased excretion results in an increased anion gap acidosis, whereas loss of HCO_3^- or accumulation of H^+ results in a normal anion gap acidosis. A decrease in serum potassium, calcium, and magnesium concentrations, an increase in serum protein concentration, or a falsely elevated serum sodium concentration can also result in an increased anion gap in the absence of metabolic acidosis. In clinical practice, although

TABLE 31-5   Expected Compensatory Mechanisms Operating in Primary Acid-Base Disorders

Acid-Base Disorder	Primary Event	Compensation	Rate of Compensation
Metabolic acidosis			
Normal anion gap	↓ $[HCO_3^-]$	↓ Pco_2	For 1 mEq/L ↓ $[HCO_3^-]$, Pco_2 ↓ by 1-1.5 mm Hg
Increased anion gap	↑ Acid production ↑ Acid intake	↓ Pco_2	For 1 mEq/L ↓ $[HCO_3^-]$, Pco_2 ↓ by 1-1.5 mm Hg
Metabolic alkalosis	↑ $[HCO_3^-]$	↑ Pco_2	For 1 mEq/L ↑ $[HCO_3^-]$, Pco_2 ↑ by 0.5-1 mm Hg
Respiratory acidosis	↑ Pco_2	↑ $[HCO_3^-]$	For 10 mm Hg ↑ Pco_2, $[HCO_3^-]$ ↑ by 1 mEq/L
Acute (<12-24 h) Chronic (3-5 days)	↑ Pco_2	↑ $[HCO_3^-]$	For 10 mm Hg ↑ Pco_2, $[HCO_3^-]$ ↑ by 4 mEq/L
Respiratory alkalosis	↓ Pco_2	↓ $[HCO_3^-]$	For 10 mm Hg ↓ Pco_2, $[HCO_3^-]$ ↓ by 1-3 mEq/L
Acute (<12 h) Chronic (1-2 days)	↓ Pco_2	↓ $[HCO_3^-]$	For 10 mm Hg ↓ Pco_2, $[HCO_3^-]$ ↓ by 2-5 mEq/L

Modified from Brewer ED: Disorders of acid-base balance, *Pediatr Clin North Am* 37:430-447, 1990.

BOX 31-3   Common Causes of Metabolic Acidosis

INCREASED ANION GAP

- Lactic acidosis caused by tissue hypoxia
  - Asphyxia, hypothermia, shock
  - Sepsis, respiratory distress syndrome
- Inborn errors of metabolism
  - Congenital lactic acidosis
  - Organic acidosis
- Renal failure
- Late metabolic acidosis
- Toxins (e.g., benzyl alcohol)

NORMAL ANION GAP

- Renal bicarbonate loss
  - Bicarbonate wasting caused by immaturity
  - Renal tubular acidosis
  - Carbonic anhydrase inhibitors
- Gastrointestinal bicarbonate loss
  - Small bowel drainage: ileostomy, fistula
  - Diarrhea
- Extracellular volume expansion with bicarbonate dilution
- Aldosterone deficiency
- Excessive chloride in intravenous fluids

BOX 31-4   Inborn Errors of Metabolism Associated With Metabolic Acidosis

- Primary lactic acidosis
- Organic acidemias
- Pyruvate carboxylase deficiency
- Pyruvate hydroxylase deficiency
- Galactosemia
- Hereditary fructose intolerance
- Type I glycogen storage disease

a serum anion gap value greater than 16 mEq/L is highly predictive of the presence of lactic acidosis and a value less than 8 mEq/L is highly predictive of the absence of lactic acidosis, an anion gap value between 8 and 16 mEq/L cannot be used to differentiate between lactic and nonlactic acidosis in the critically ill newborn (Lorenz et al, 1999). Therefore if the anion gap is within this high normal range and lactic acidosis is suggested, measuring serum lactate is indicated.

An increased anion gap metabolic acidosis in the newborn is most commonly caused by lactic acidosis secondary to tissue hypoxia, as seen in asphyxia, hypothermia, severe respiratory distress, sepsis, and other severe neonatal illnesses. Other important but much less common causes of an increased anion gap metabolic acidosis in the neonatal period are inborn errors of metabolism, renal failure, and intake of toxins (Box 31-3). Box 31-4 lists inborn errors of metabolism that can manifest as increased anion gap metabolic acidosis in the newborn period.

In the syndrome of late metabolic acidosis of prematurity, first described in the 1960s, otherwise healthy premature infants at several weeks of age demonstrated mild to moderate increased anion gap acidosis and decreased growth. All the infants were receiving high-protein cow's milk formula, and they demonstrated higher net acid excretion compared with controls. This type of late metabolic acidosis is rarely seen, probably because of the use of special premature infant formulas and changes in regular formulas with decreased casein-to-whey ratios and lower fixed acid loads.

A normal anion gap metabolic acidosis most commonly occurs in the newborn as a result of HCO_3^- loss from the extracellular space through the kidneys or the gastrointestinal tract. Hyperchloremia develops with the HCO_3^- loss because a proportionate rise in serum chloride concentration must occur to maintain the ionic balance or to correct the volume depletion in the extracellular compartment. The most common cause of normal anion gap metabolic acidosis in the preterm newborn is a mild, developmentally regulated, proximal renal tubular acidosis with renal HCO_3^- wasting. In infants with this disorder, the serum HCO_3^- usually stabilizes at 14 to 18 mEq/L in the early postnatal period. The urinary pH is normal once the serum HCO_3^- falls to this level, because the impairment in proximal tubular HCO_3^- reabsorption is not associated with an impaired distal tubular acidification of similar magnitude (Jones and Chesney, 1992). The diagnosis of this temporary cause of acidosis can be established by the recurrence of a urinary alkaline pH when serum HCO_3^- is raised above the threshold after HCO_3^- or acetate supplementation. Even term newborns have a lower renal threshold for HCO_3^-, with normal plasma HCO_3^- levels in the range of 17 to 21 mEq/L. In most infants, plasma HCO_3^- increases to adult levels over the first year as the proximal tubule matures. Other common causes of normal anion gap metabolic acidosis seen in neonatal intensive care units are gastrointestinal HCO_3^- losses, often caused by increased ileostomy drainage, diuretic treatment with carbonic anhydrase inhibitors, and dilutional acidosis with rapid expansion of the extracellular space through the use of non-HCO_3^- solutions in the hypovolemic newborn.

The presence of metabolic acidosis in the newborn should be suggested by the clinical presentation and the history of predisposing conditions, including perinatal depression, respiratory distress, blood or volume loss, sepsis, and congenital heart disease associated with poor systemic perfusion or cyanosis. Metabolic acidosis is confirmed by blood gas measurements. The cause of metabolic acidosis is often readily discernible from the history and physical examination. Specific laboratory evaluation of electrolytes, renal function, lactate, and serum and urine amino acids may be undertaken, depending on the diagnosis that is suggested clinically. Figure 31-7 shows a simple flow diagram outlining an approach to diagnosis of metabolic acidosis in the newborn. It is important to remember that infants might not manifest an increased anion gap in the setting of lactic acidosis and thus require the direct measurement of lactate when a lactic acidosis is suspected (Lorenz et al, 1999).

The morbidity and mortality of metabolic acidosis depend on the underlying pathologic process, the severity of the acidosis, and the responsiveness of the process to clinical management. By far, the most important intervention for an infant with a metabolic acidosis is to identify the pathologic process contributing to the acidosis and to take measures to correct it. The administration of base, such as sodium bicarbonate, as supportive therapy for metabolic acidosis is unproven in its efficacy (Aschner and Poland, 2008).

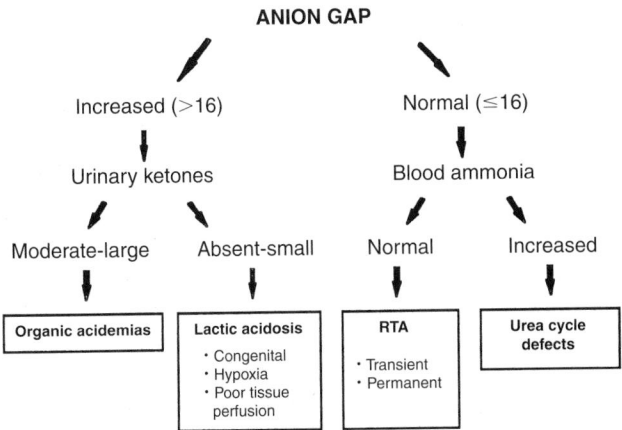

ANION GAP

FIGURE 31-7 **Diagnostic approach of increased anion gap and normal anion gap metabolic acidosis in the newborn.** Infants with lactic acidosis may not have an increased anion gap and lactate should be measured directly if suspected by the history and physical examination. *RTA,* Renal tubular acidosis. (*Adapted from Lorenz JM, Kleinman LI, Markarian K, et al: Serum anion gap in the differential diagnosis of metabolic acidosis in critically ill newborns,* J Pediatr *135:751-755, 1999.*)

The use of base administration is supported by findings on the beneficial cardiovascular effects of sodium bicarbonate in preterm newborns with an arterial pH of less than 7.25 and term newborns with an arterial pH of less than 7.30 (Fanconi et al, 1993). The use of sodium bicarbonate in this study was associated with an increase in myocardial contractility and a reduction in afterload, albeit transient. However, there is concern for harm associated with the administration of base, including increased mortality and intraventricular hemorrhage (Papile et al, 1978; Simmons et al, 1974; Usher, 1967), increased cerebral blood volume regardless of rate of administration (van Alfen-van der Velden et al, 2006), and decreased intracellular pH with cellular injury (Lipshultz et al, 2003).

If therapy with base is warranted, the clinician has three options: sodium bicarbonate, sodium (or potassium) acetate, and tromethamine. Sodium bicarbonate is the most widely used buffer in the treatment of metabolic acidosis in the neonatal period. Bicarbonate should not be given if ventilation is inadequate, because its administration results in an increase in P_aco_2 with no improvement in pH and an increase in intracellular acidosis. Therefore sodium bicarbonate should be administered slowly and in diluted form only to newborns with documented metabolic acidosis and adequate alveolar ventilation. Once a blood gas measurement has been obtained, the dose of sodium bicarbonate required to fully correct the pH can be estimated with the use of the following formula:

$$\text{Dose of NaHCO}_3 \text{ (mEq)} = \text{Base deficit (mEq/L)} \times \text{Body weight (kg)} \times 0.3$$

Sodium bicarbonate is thought to be confined mostly to the ECF compartment. Although there are controversies regarding the actual bicarbonate space in humans, the 30% of total body weight in the formula represents its estimated volume of distribution in the neonate. Most clinicians would use half of the calculated total correction dose for initial therapy to avoid overcorrection of

metabolic acidosis. Subsequent doses of sodium bicarbonate are then based on the results of additional blood gas measurements.

When clinicians are faced with a chronic metabolic acidosis caused by a prematurity-related proximal renal tubular acidosis with bicarbonate wasting, many choose to replace these losses over time. In this instance, either sodium or potassium acetate can be used as an alternative to sodium bicarbonate. Sodium acetate is a conjugate base of a weak acid (acetic acid) with a pKb of 9.25. pKb is a measure of the strength of a base, which depends on its base dissociation constant. It has been shown in one study to be an effective alternative to sodium bicarbonate in correcting this type of acid-base abnormality when added to parenteral nutrition (Peters et al, 1997). The median doses of acetate used in this randomized controlled trial were 2.6 mmol/kg/day on day 4 of life and 4.1 mmol/kg/day on day 8 of life. Infants randomized to acetate had an increased base excess and pH and increased Pco_2, and they received less bicarbonate boluses compared with control infants.

In certain clinical situations, tromethamine can be used as an alternative buffer to sodium bicarbonate. The theoretical advantages of tromethamine over sodium bicarbonate in the treatment of metabolic acidosis of the newborn include its more rapid intracellular buffering capability, its ability to lower $Paco_2$ levels directly, and the lack of an increase in the sodium load (Schneiderman et al, 1993). Tromethamine lowers P_aco_2 by covalently binding H^+ and thus shifting the equilibrium of the reaction

$$H^+ + HCO_3^- \leftrightarrow H_2CO_3 \leftrightarrow H_2O + CO_2$$

to the left, resulting in a decrease in CO_2 and an increase in HCO_3^-. Because the end-product (chelated tromethamine) is a cation that is excreted by the kidneys, oliguria is a relative contraindication to the repeated use of this buffer. Tromethamine administration also has been associated with the development of acute respiratory depression, most likely secondary to an abrupt decrease in P_aco_2 levels as well as from rapid intracellular correction of acidosis in the cells of the respiratory center (Robertson, 1970). Furthermore, because hypocapnia is associated with decreases in brain blood flow and a higher incidence of white matter damage, especially in the immature preterm neonate, close monitoring of $Paco_2$ is of paramount importance when tromethamine is being used. Finally, when large doses of tromethamine are administered, hyponatremia (Seri et al, 1998b), hypoglycemia, hyperkalemia, an increase in hemoglobin oxygen affinity, and diuresis followed by oliguria can occur. Because the tromethamine solution is hyperosmolar, and because rapid infusion of tromethamine can also lower blood pressure and intracranial pressure (Duthie et al, 1994), slow infusion is recommended. The suggested initial dose is 1 to 2 mEq/kg or 3.5 to 6 mL/kg given intravenously using the 0.3 M solution, with the rate of administration not exceeding 1 mL/kg/min. Once a blood gas measurement has been obtained, the dose of tromethamine required to raise the pH can be estimated using the formula

$$\text{Dose of tromethamine (mL)} = \text{Base deficit (mEq/L)} \times \text{Body weight (kg)}$$

Finally, during the correction of metabolic acidosis, particular attention should be paid to ensuring an appropriate potassium balance. Because potassium moves from the intracellular to the extracellular space in exchange for H^+ when acidosis occurs, the presence of a total body potassium deficit might not be appreciated during metabolic acidosis. Hypokalemia may become evident only as the pH increases and potassium returns to the intracellular space. Furthermore, intracellular acidosis cannot be completely corrected until the potassium stores are restored. Therefore close monitoring of serum electrolytes and potassium supplementation are important during the correction of metabolic acidosis in the sick newborn.

Respiratory Acidosis

Respiratory acidosis occurs when a primary increase in $Paco_2$ develops secondary to impairments in alveolar ventilation that result in an arterial pH of less than 7.35. Primary respiratory acidosis is a common problem in newborns, and causes include hyaline membrane disease, pneumonia owing to infection or aspiration, patent ductus arteriosus with pulmonary edema, chronic lung disease, pleural effusion, pneumothorax, and pulmonary hypoplasia. The initial increase in P_aco_2 is buffered by the non-HCO_3^- intracellular buffers without noticeable renal compensation for at least 12 to 24 hours (see Table 31-5). Renal metabolic compensation reaches its maximum levels within 3 to 5 days, and its effectiveness in the newborn is influenced mainly by the functional maturity of proximal tubular HCO_3^- transport.

Management of respiratory acidosis is directed toward improving alveolar ventilation and treating the underlying disorder. For sick newborns, adequate ventilation must often be provided by mechanical ventilation. In severe respiratory acidosis, tromethamine can be used to raise pH, because it lowers CO_2 levels. Tromethamine, however, produces only a transient decrease in P_aco_2, and toxic doses would quickly be reached if it were used to buffer all the CO_2 produced by metabolism over a sustained period. Therefore tromethamine should be used only as a temporizing measure in severe respiratory acidosis until alveolar ventilation can be improved.

Metabolic Alkalosis

Metabolic alkalosis is characterized by a primary increase in the extracellular HCO_3^- concentration sufficient to raise the arterial pH above 7.45. In the newborn, metabolic alkalosis occurs when there is a loss of H^+, a gain of HCO_3^-, or a depletion of the extracellular volume with the loss of more chloride than HCO_3^-. It is important to understand that metabolic alkalosis generated by any of these mechanisms can be maintained only when factors limiting the renal excretion of HCO_3^- are also present.

Metabolic alkalosis can result from a loss of H^+ from the body, from either the gastrointestinal tract or the kidneys, that induces an equivalent rise in the extracellular HCO_3^- concentration. The most common causes of this type of metabolic alkalosis in the newborn period are continuous nasogastric aspiration, persistent vomiting, and diuretic treatment. Less common causes of H^+ losses are congenital

chloride-wasting diarrhea, certain forms of congenital adrenal hyperplasia, hyperaldosteronism, posthypercapnia, and Bartter syndrome.

Metabolic alkalosis can also result from a gain of HCO_3^-, such as occurs during the administration of buffer solutions to the newborn. In the past, a metabolic alkalosis was intentionally created when sodium bicarbonate or tromethamine was used to maintain an alkaline pH to decrease pulmonary vasoreactivity in infants with persistent pulmonary hypertension, a practice not recommended anymore. Currently, iatrogenically produced metabolic alkalosis is primarily unintentional and due to chronic excessive administration of HCO_3^-, lactate, citrate, or acetate in intravenous fluids and blood products. Because excretion of HCO_3^- is normally not limited in the newborn, metabolic alkalosis resulting from HCO_3^- gain alone should rapidly resolve after administration of HCO_3^- is discontinued. However, if the alkalosis is severe and urine output is limited, inhibition of the carbonic anhydrase enzyme by the administration of acetazolamide may enhance elimination of HCO_3^-.

Metabolic alkalosis can also result from a loss of ECF containing disproportionately more chloride than HCO_3^-—the so-called contraction alkalosis. During the diuretic phase of normal postnatal adaptation, preterm and term newborns retain relatively more HCO_3^- than chloride (Ramiro-Tolentino et al, 1996). The obvious clinical benefits of allowing this physiologic extracellular volume contraction to occur, especially in the critically ill newborn, clearly outweigh the clinical importance of a mild contraction alkalosis that develops after recovery. No specific treatment is needed in such cases, because with the stabilization of the extracellular volume and renal function after recovery, acid-base balance rapidly returns to normal. Contraction alkalosis due to other causes, however, may require treatment.

For metabolic alkalosis to persist, factors limiting the renal excretion of HCO_3^- must be present. The kidneys are usually effective in excreting excess HCO_3^-, but this ability can be limited under certain conditions, such as decreased glomerular filtration rate, increased aldosterone production, and the more common clinical situation of volume contraction–triggered metabolic alkalosis with potassium deficiency. In the last condition, there is a direct stimulation of Na^+ reabsorption coupled with H^+ loss in the proximal tubule, and an indirect stimulation of H^+ loss in the distal nephron by the increased activity of the renin-angiotensin-aldosterone system. Contraction alkalosis responds to administration of saline to replace the intravascular volume in conjunction with additional potassium supplementation to account for renal potassium wasting. In the other disorders, however, the primary problem of reduced glomerular filtration rate or elevated aldosterone must be treated for the alkalosis to resolve.

One of the most commonly encountered clinical scenarios of chronic metabolic alkalosis actually occurs in the form of a mixed acid-base disorder in a preterm infant with chronic lung disease on long-term diuretic treatment. Such a newborn initially has a chronic respiratory acidosis that is partially compensated for by renal HCO_3^- retention. Prolonged or aggressive use of diuretics can lead to total-body potassium depletion and contraction of the extracellular volume, thus exacerbating the metabolic alkalosis. By stimulating proximal tubular Na⁺ reabsorption and thus H⁺ loss, distal tubular H⁺ secretion, and renal ammonium production, the diuretic-induced hypokalemia contributes to the severity and maintenance of the metabolic alkalosis. Furthermore, metabolic alkalosis per se worsens hypokalemia, because potassium moves intracellularly to replace hydrogen as the latter shifts into the extracellular space. Although the serum potassium concentration may be decreased, the serum levels in the newborn do not accurately reflect the extent of total-body potassium deficit because potassium is primarily an intracellular ion, with approximately 98% of the total body potassium being in the intracellular compartment. In addition, the condition is often accompanied by marked hypochloremia and hyponatremia. Hyponatremia occurs in part because sodium shifts into the intracellular space to compensate for the depleted intracellular potassium. If the alkalosis is severe, alkalemia (pH >7.45) can supervene and result in hypoventilation. In this situation, potassium chloride, and not sodium chloride supplementation, reverses hyponatremia and hypochloremia, corrects hypokalemia and metabolic alkalosis, and increases the effectiveness of diuretic therapy. Because chloride deficiency is the predominant cause of the increased pH, ammonium chloride or arginine chloride also corrects the alkalosis. These agents do not affect the other electrolyte imbalances such as the hypokalemia, so they should not be the only therapy given.

It is important to keep ahead of the potassium losses in infants receiving long-term diuretic therapy, rather than to attempt to replace potassium after intracellular depletion has occurred. Because the rate of potassium repletion is limited by the rate at which potassium moves intracellularly, correction of total body potassium deficits can require days to weeks. In addition, there is also a risk of acute hyperkalemia if serum potassium levels are driven too high during repletion, particularly in newborns in whom an acute respiratory deterioration may occur, with worsened respiratory acidosis and the subsequent movement of potassium from the intracellular to the extracellular space. The routine use of potassium chloride supplementation and close monitoring of serum sodium, chloride, and potassium levels are therefore recommended during long-term diuretic therapy to prevent these common iatrogenic problems.

Respiratory Alkalosis

When a primary decrease in Paco₂ results in an increase in the arterial pH beyond 7.45, respiratory alkalosis develops. The initial hypocapnia is acutely titrated by the intracellular buffers, and metabolic compensation by the kidneys returns pH toward normal within 1 to 2 days (see Table 31-5). Interestingly, respiratory alkalosis is the only simple acid-base disorder in which, at least in adults, the pH can completely be normalized by the compensatory mechanisms (Brewer, 1990). The cause of respiratory alkalosis is hyperventilation, which in the spontaneously breathing newborn is most often caused by fever, sepsis, retained fetal lung fluid, mild aspiration pneumonia, or central nervous system disorders. In the neonatal intensive care unit, the most common cause of respiratory alkalosis is iatrogenic secondary to hyperventilation of the intubated newborn. Because findings suggest an association between hypocapnia and the development of periventricular leukomalacia (Okumura et al, 2001; Wiswell et al, 1996) and chronic lung disease (Garland et al, 1995) in ventilated preterm infants, avoidance of hyperventilation during resuscitation and mechanical ventilation is of utmost importance in the management of sick preterm newborns. The treatment of neonatal respiratory alkalosis consists of the specific management of the underlying process causing hyperventilation.

SUGGESTED READINGS

Aschner JL, Poland RL: Sodium bicarbonate: basically useless therapy, *Pediatrics* 122:831, 2008.
Avner ED: Clinical disorders of water metabolism: hyponatremia and hypernatremia, *Pediatr Ann* 24:23, 1995.
Brewer ED: Disorders of acid-base balance, *Pediatr Clin North Am* 37:430, 1990.
El-Dahr SS, Chevalier RL: Special needs of the newborn infant in fluid therapy, *Pediatr Clin North Am* 37:323, 1990.
Hartnoll G: Basic principles and practical steps in the management of fluid balance in the newborn, *Semin Neonatol* 8:307, 2003.
Lorenz J: Fluid and electrolyte therapy in the very low-birthweight neonate, *Neoreviews* 9:e02, 2008.
Modi N: Management of fluid balance in the very immature neonate, *Arch Dis Child Fetal Neonatal Ed* 89:F108, 2004.
Oh W, Poindexter BB, Perritt R, et al: Association between fluid intake and weight loss during the first ten days of life and the risk of bronchopulmonary dysplasia in extremely low birthweight infants, *J Pediatr* 147:786, 2005.
Sedin G: Fluid management in the extremely preterm infant, In Hansen TN, McIntosh N, editors: *Current topics in neonatology*, London, 1995, WB Saunders, pp 50-66.

Complete references used in this text can be found online at www.expertconsult.com

CARE OF THE EXTREMELY LOW-BIRTHWEIGHT INFANT

Eric C. Eichenwald

In the past two decades, the field of neonatology has experienced significant progress in medical care and improvement in overall patient survival. Advancement in technology, greater use of prenatal glucocorticoids and neonatal surfactant replacement therapy, better regionalization of perinatal and high-risk neonatal care, and a more comprehensive understanding of the physiology of the immature infant have all contributed to dramatic increases in survival of very preterm infants. Care of premature infants with birthweights between 1000 and 1500 g has become almost routine in most neonatal intensive care units (NICUs) in the United States.

The most recent challenge in neonatology is the care of extremely low-birthweight (ELBW) infants (birthweight <1000 g), sometimes referred to colloquially as *micropremies*. These infants present one of the greatest medical and ethical challenges to the field. Although they represent a small percentage of overall births and NICU admissions, ELBW infants are often the most critically ill and at the highest risk for mortality and long-term morbidity of any NICU patient. They also contribute disproportionately to overall hospital days and consume a large percentage of NICU personnel time, effort, and costs of care. Care of these infants is in constant evolution, as a result of new discoveries in both basic and clinical research as well as to growing clinical experience. This chapter will review some of the special challenges in and practical aspects of the management of the ELBW infant. The reader is referred to specific chapters throughout the text for a more comprehensive review of specific problems and conditions.

EPIDEMIOLOGY

The percentage of babies born preterm in the United States has risen slowly over the past two decades (Behrman and Stith Butler, 2007). In the year 2007, preterm births (<37 weeks' gestation) accounted for 12.7% of all births, with approximately 1% of births occurring before 28 weeks' gestation. There is a significant racial disparity in the incidence of extreme preterm birth, with the African American ELBW birth rate being nearly double that of the Hispanic and non-Hispanic white populations. Associated with this increase in frequency of preterm births is the greater availability of assisted reproductive technologies. These technologies result in a higher incidence of LBW infants, because of the higher frequency of multiple gestations (Schieve et al, 2002). Twins, triplets, and higher-order multiple gestations currently represent almost a quarter all LBW deliveries in the United States (Martin et al, 2002) and contribute to the ELBW population. Multiple gestations add to the potential morbidity of extremely premature birth because of a higher frequency of intrauterine growth restriction and other medical complications of pregnancy.

Several studies have shown increased survival in the smallest and most premature infants over the past decade (Figures 32-1 and 32-2) (Fanaroff et al, 2007; Horbar et al, 2002; Lemons et al, 2001). See Chapter 1 for a complete discussion of these changes.

Improved survival has not been accompanied by a change in the incidence of several major morbidities among survivors (Tables 32-1 and 32-2). Little to no change in the frequency of severe intracranial hemorrhage, periventricular white matter injury, necrotizing enterocolitis, or bronchopulmonary dysplasia was observed in the Eunice Kennedy Shriver National Institute of Child Health and Human Development cohort of infants born in institutions participating in the Neonatal Research Network in 1995-1996 compared with and 1997-2002 (Fanaroff et al, 2007). Although the Vermont–Oxford NICUs reported a reduction in the incidence of severe intracranial hemorrhage in the early part of the 1990s, the incidence has remained static into the late 1990s (Horbar et al, 2002). With the current trends in survival and in hospital morbidity, the absolute number of extremely premature infants who survive to NICU discharge and are diagnosed with a major morbidity in the neonatal period is increasing. A significant percentage of these infants continues to suffer from neurodevelopmental and neurosensory disability into childhood (Hack et al, 2005; Marlow et al, 2005; Wood et al, 2000).

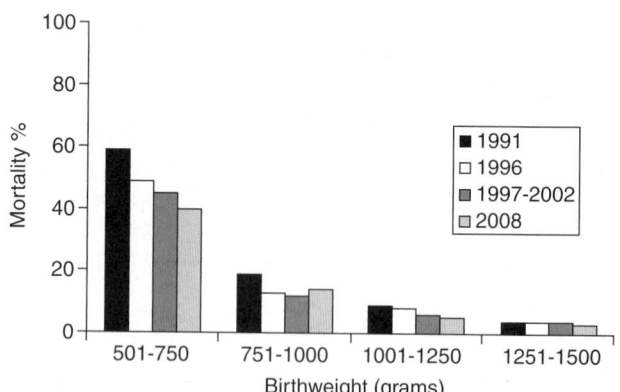

FIGURE 32-1 Mortality in very low birthweight infants receiving care in the National Institute of Child Health and Human Development Eunice Kennedy Shriver Neonatal Research Network Centers from 1991 to 2002 and the Vermont-Oxford Network in 2008. *(From Eichenwald EC, Stark AR: Management and outcomes of very low birth weight, N Engl J Med 358:1700-1711, 2008. Data from Lemons J, Bauer C, Oh W, et al: Very low birth weight outcomes of the National Institute of Child Health and Human Development Neonatal Research Network, January 1995 through December 1996, Pediatrics 107:1-8, 211, 2001; Fanaroff AA, Stoll BJ, Wright LL, et al: Trends in neonatal morbidity and mortality for very low birthweight infants, Am J Obstet Gynecol 196:147.e1-147.e8, 2007; and Horbar JD, Carpenter J, Kenny M, et al, editors: Vermont Network 2008 very low birth weight database summary, Burlington, Vt, 2009, Vermont Oxford Network.)*

PERINATAL MANAGEMENT

Extremely premature infants born in perinatal centers for high-risk infants, especially those with a high volume of such infants, have better short-term outcomes than infants transferred to such centers after birth (Arad et al, 1999; Bartels et al, 2006; Chien et al, 2001; Cifuentes et al, 2002; Phibbs et al, 2007; Shah et al, 2005; Towers et al, 2000). Therefore, if clinically feasible, the pregnant woman who seems likely to deliver an extremely premature infant should be transferred to a high-risk perinatal center for the expertise in both obstetric and neonatal management. Upon arrival, the expectant mother should be evaluated for factors that may have predisposed to preterm labor and assessed for the status of the fetal membranes and the presence or absence of chorioamnionitis. In addition, best obstetric estimate of gestational age (by date of last menstrual period and early ultrasonographic dating, if available), ultrasonographic assessment of fetal size and position, and the presence of other medical or obstetric complications (preeclampsia, placenta previa, abruptio placentae) should be documented. Specimens for rectovaginal cultures to detect the presence of group B streptococci should also be obtained on admission (Schrag et al, 2002), and treatment with penicillin or ampicillin (or vancomycin for the patient with a severe penicillin allergy) should be initiated until culture results are available. There is widespread agreement that prenatal glucocorticoids should be offered to any woman in whom delivery at 24 to 34 weeks' gestation threatens; treatment at earlier gestational ages is controversial and of unclear benefit. Although unlikely to arrest labor for an extended period, tocolytic agents should be considered for women with preterm uterine contractions without evidence of chorioamnionitis.

Premature rupture of the fetal membranes (PROM) occurs in 30% to 40% of women who deliver prematurely (Mazor et al, 1998). If PROM is diagnosed without evidence of chorioamnionitis, consideration should be given

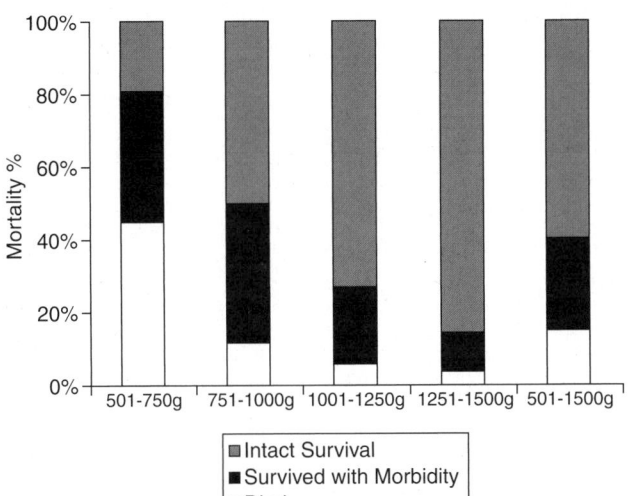

FIGURE 32-2 Proportion of very low birthweight infants who died, and the proportion who survived with short-term complications (bronchopulmonary dysplasia, severe intraventricular hemorrhage, necrotizing enterocolitis, or a combination of these disorders, or with no complications from 1997 to 2002 at the Eunice Kennedy Shriver National Institute of Child Health and Human Development Neonatal Research Network sites. *(From Eichenwald EC, Stark AR: Management and outcomes of very low birth weight, N Engl J Med 358:1700-1711, 2008. Data from Fanaroff AA, Stoll BJ, Wright LL, et al: Trends in neonatal morbidity and mortality for very low birth weight infants, Am J Obstet Gynecol 196:147.e1-147.e8, 2007.)*

TABLE 32-1 Survival and Selected Morbidities for Very Low Birthweight (501-1500 g) Infants Born in NICHD Neonatal Research Network Sites (1995-1996 Compared with 1997-2002)

Survival	1995-1996* n = 4438%	1997-2002† n = 18,153%
Survival without morbidity	84	85
Bronchopulmonary dysplasia	70	70
Home in supplemental oxygen	23	22
Necrotizing enterocolitis	15	11
Severe intraventricular hemorrhage	7	7
Periventricular white matter injury	12	12
Late-onset sepsis	5	3

NICHHD, National Institute of Child Health and Human Development.
*Lemons J, Bauer C, Oh W, et al: Very low birth weight outcomes from the National Institute of Child Health and Development Neonatal Research Network, January 1995 through December 1996, *Pediatrics* 107:1-18, 2001.
†Fanaroff AA, Stoll BJ, Wright LL, et al: Trends in neonatal morbidity and mortality for very low birth weight infants, *Am J Obstet Gynecol* 196:147, 2007.

TABLE 32-2 Survival With Selected Morbidities for Very Low Birthweight Infants: NICHD Neonatal Research Network, 1997-2002*

Birthweight	501-750 g n = 4046%	751-1000 g n = 4266%	1021-1250 g n = 4557%	1251-1500 g n = 5284%
Overall survival	55	88	94	96
Survived With Morbidity				
Overall	65	43	22	11
BPD alone	42	25	11	4
Severe IVH	5	6	5	4
NEC alone	3	3	3	2
BPD and severe IVH	10	4	2	<1

BPD, Bronchopulmonary dysplasia; *IVH*, intraventricular hemorrhage.
*Data from Fanaroff AA, Stoll BJ, Wright LL, et al: Trends in neonatal morbidity and mortality for very low birth weight infants, *Am J Obstet Gynecol* 196:147, 2007.

to the use of prophylactic antibiotic therapy (ampicillin or erythromycin) for the mother. Several studies have shown that such therapy prolongs the latency period, reduces the incidence of chorioamnionitis and endometritis, and improves neonatal outcome (Gibbs and Eschenbach, 1997; Mazor et al, 1998; Mercer et al, 1997). Tocolytic and antibiotic therapy in the setting of PROM may prolong latency by 48 to 72 hours in many extremely preterm pregnancies in which delivery threatens, allowing the administration of a complete course of glucocorticoids to the mother.

PRENATAL CONSULTATION

If possible, all parents who are at risk for delivery of an extremely premature infant should meet in consultation with a neonatologist before the infant's birth, preferably jointly with a perinatologist caring for the mother (Finer and Barrington, 1998). There are several goals of this consultation. First, the neonatologist and perinatologist should inform the parents about the proposed management of the pregnancy and delivery of the infant, including a discussion of the advantages of administration of glucocorticoids to the mother, the possible need for cesarean delivery, and delivery room care and resuscitation of the baby. Second,

the parents should be informed about the potential risks of both the extent of prematurity and the proposed therapeutic interventions (Tables 32-3 and 32-4). Third, the neonatologist should investigate the parents' beliefs and attitudes about delivery of an extremely premature infant and the potential for long-term morbidity. This outline for prenatal consultation is especially important if delivery is expected at the borderline of viability (23 to 24 weeks' gestation).

Data are sparse about the process and results of prenatal consultation with parents of an extremely preterm infant. Some studies suggest that significant incongruity exists among the attitudes of obstetricians, nurses, neonatologists, and parents about active delivery room resuscitation and treatment of extremely premature infants (Streiner et al, 2001; Zupancic et al, 2002). Reuss and Gordon (1995) have shown that the obstetric judgment of fetal viability was associated with an 18-fold increase in survival for infants with a birthweight less than 750 g, indicating that obstetric attitudes and decisions influence outcome. Obstetricians and nurses tend to overestimate, and parents tend to underestimate, mortality and morbidity in premature infants

TABLE 32-3 Major Problems of Extremely Low Birthweight Infants

System	Short-Term Problems	Long-Term Problems
Respiratory	Respiratory distress syndrome Air leaks Bronchopulmonary dysplasia Apnea of prematurity	Chronic lung disease Reactive airway disease
Gastrointestinal, nutritional	Feeding intolerance Necrotizing enterocolitis Growth failure	Growth failure Failure to thrive Inguinal hernias
Immunologic, infection	Immune deficiency Perinatal infection Nosocomial infection	Respiratory syncytial virus
Central nervous system	Intraventricular hemorrhage Periventricular white matter disease	Cerebral palsy Neurodevelopmental delay Hearing loss
Ophthalmologic	Retinopathy of prematurity	Blindness, retinal detachment Myopia Strabismus
Cardiovascular	Hypotension Patent ductus arteriosus	? Hypertension in adulthood Pulmonary hypertension
Renal	Water, electrolyte imbalance Acid-base disturbances	
Hematologic	Iatrogenic anemia Frequent transfusions Anemia of prematurity	
Endocrine	Transient hypothyroxinemia ?Cortisol deficiency	? Impaired glucose regulation ? Increased insulin resistance

TABLE 32-4 Incidence of Specific Interventions and Outcomes of Extremely Low Birthweight Infants (<1000 g) in the Vermont–Oxford Network, 2008

Outcome	Birthweight Category	
	501 to 750 g n = 9963	751 to 1000 g n = 12,341
Survival (%)	58	85
Respiratory Morbidity		
Chronic lung disease at 36 weeks (%)	66	39
Discharge home in oxygen (%)	38	20
Retinopathy of Prematurity		
Eye examination performed (%)	66	82
None (%)	25	51
Stages 1-2 disease (%)	47	40
≥Stage 3 disease (%)	27	8
Laser, cryotherapy (% treated)	15	5
Intraventricular Hemorrhage		
Cranial ultrasound examination	91	95
No intraventricular hemorrhage (%)	54	69
Grade 1-2 (%)	23	19
≥Grade 3 (%)	23	12
Patent ductus arteriosus (%)	63	53
Indomethacin, ibuprofen treatment (%)	61	52
Surgical ligation (%)	23	12
Nosocomial infection (%)	39	26
Necrotizing enterocolitis (%)	13	10
Survival without major morbidity (%)	12	38

Data from Horbar JD, Carpenter J, Kenny M, Michelle J, editors: *Vermont Oxford Network 2008 very low birth weight database summary*, Burlington, Vt, 2009, Vermont Oxford Network.

(Doron et al, 1998; Haywood et al, 1994). Parents report being more in favor of intervening regardless of gestational age or condition at birth compared with health care professionals (Streiner et al, 2001). In a survey by Ballard et al (2002), the majority of neonatologists responded that they would respect parents' wishes about resuscitation of a borderline viable infant. In practice, when parental preferences about active resuscitation are known before delivery of an extremely preterm infant, neonatologists report that they would alter their management of the infant in the delivery room accordingly after assessment of the baby after birth (Doron et al, 1998), indicating the important role for prenatal consultation. However, parental attitudes likely are strongly influenced by physician recommendations about aggressive resuscitation conveyed during the prenatal consultation. This consultation is further complicated by significant variability in physician's opinions about the benefits and burdens of providing intensive care at the borders of viability (De Leeuw et al, 2000). Physician attitudes may be influenced by fear of litigation for not actively resuscitating an extremely premature infant even if parental choices are made clear, as well as local, regional, and national norms (Partridge et al, 2009).

The earliest gestational age at which resuscitation should be initiated remains controversial among neonatologists (Finer et al, 1999), making firm recommendations for the actual content of prenatal consultation difficult (Kaempf et al, 2006). Most studies that describe the outcome of premature infants are based on birthweight rather than gestational age and thus confound the effects of extremely preterm birth with those of intrauterine growth restriction, but both parents and physicians are usually faced with making decisions based on the anticipated gestational age at delivery. However, the likelihood of survival without serious sequelae may be influenced by factors other than gestational age. Using prospectively collected data from the Eunice Kennedy Shriver National Institute of Child Health and Human Development Neonatal Research Network on infants born at 22 to 25 weeks' gestation between 1998 and 2003, Tyson et al (2008) presented an analysis of some of these factors. In a multivariate analysis, exposure to antenatal glucocorticoids, female sex, singleton gestation, and higher birthweight (in 100-g increments) were each associated with a decrease in the risk of death or of survival with neurodevelopmental impairment. The reduced risk was similar to the risk for infants with an additional week of gestational age. Other data from several studies suggest that in terms of survival and potential for long-term disability, encouragement of active management is appropriate for pregnancies expected to deliver at 25 weeks' gestation or later (Piecuch et al, 1997; Wood et al, 2000). The risk of death and severe morbidity is significantly higher before 25 weeks' gestation (El-Metwally et al, 2002). Mortality approaches 80% for infants delivered at 23 weeks' gestation, with the majority of survivors suffering from neurodevelopmental sequelae (Vohr et al, 2000; Wood et al, 2000). These data should be shared with parents during prenatal consultation, and appropriate guidance should be given for decision making about the pregnancy, delivery, and resuscitation of the infant. Some have argued that, because of the risk of long-term disability associated with extreme preterm birth and the difficulty of making an informed

decision immediately before delivery, parents should be given the opportunity to have these issues discussed during routine prenatal care (Harrison, 2008).

GENERAL PRINCIPLES OF CARE SPECIFIC TO EXTREMELY LOW-BIRTHWEIGHT INFANTS

FIRST HOURS

The first few hours after admission to the NICU are critical for the ELBW infant, although there are significant variations in practice among hospitals and practitioners. Careful adherence to details in the delivery room and during the first few hours after birth is essential to help avoid some of the immediate and long-term complications of the ELBW infant. All NICUs should have a consistent approach to the initial care of these fragile infants in the delivery room and upon admission to the NICU. A suggested treatment guideline for the first few hours after birth is presented in Table 32-5, and screening guidelines for common complications are shown in Table 32-6.

DELIVERY ROOM

At delivery, strict attention to maintenance of body temperature by means of rapid, gentle drying of the infant and the use of adequate heat sources is paramount to avoid cold stress. Use of a polyethylene occlusive skin wrap or bag immediately after delivery may also help to prevent initial evaporative heat losses (Vohra et al, 1999). Many ELBW infants need some form of assisted ventilation immediately after birth. If positive-pressure ventilation is required, it should be provided with low inspiratory pressure to prevent overdistention of the lungs, which can result in air leak and other lung injury, and adequate positive end-expiratory pressure (PEEP) to maintain lung volume by use of a flow-inflating bag, or optimally, a T-piece resuscitator that allows for more consistent delivery of inspiratory pressure and PEEP. Hyperventilation and hyperoxia also should be avoided; many units use continuous oxygen saturation monitoring in the delivery room, with supplemental oxygen titrated to maintain oxygen saturations in the range of 85% to 93%. The use of room air for resuscitation of these infants has been proposed to protect them from hyperoxia and damage to the lungs by oxygen free radicals. This issue is under active investigation (Lefkowitz, 2002), but most centers use blended oxygen for initial resuscitation, with an initial starting FIO_2 between 0.4 and 0.6 (see also Chapter 28.)

Considerable practice variation exists in the use and type of ventilatory support and timing of surfactant administration for the ELBW infant after birth. Some centers routinely intubate all ELBW infants in the delivery room for respiratory support and prophylactic surfactant administration (Egberts et al, 1997; Kendig et al, 1998). Soll (2009) has reported on a metaanalysis of eight randomized trials of the use of natural surfactant as prophylaxis versus as a rescue strategy for established respiratory distress syndrome (RDS) in the ELBW infant. Administration of exogenous surfactant before 15 minutes of age resulted in a reduction in the rates of neonatal mortality, air leak, and

TABLE 32-5 Treatment Guidelines for Initial Management of Extremely Low-Birthweight Infants

Time after Birth	Guideline	Time after Birth	Guideline
		First 24 to 48 Hours	
Delivery room	Ensure good thermoregulation "Gentle" ventilation as required Avoid hyperventilation and hyperoxia Administer surfactant (if prophylaxis approach) Initiate NCPAP (if early CPAP approach)	Cardiovascular	Monitor blood pressure, give vasopressors as required Maintain vigilance for presence of patent ductus arteriosus Obtain echocardiogram as indicated

NICU admission	Obtain weight measurement
	Administer surfactant within first hour (if rescue approach)
	Establish vascular access:
	    Peripheral intravenous catheter
	    Umbilical arterial catheter
	    Umbilical venous catheter (central, double-lumen)
	Start intravenous fluids as soon as possible with dextrose and amino acid solution
	Limit evaporative water losses (humidified incubator)
	Minimize stimulation
	Avoid hyperventilation and hyperoxia
	Maintain target oxygen saturations between 88% and 93%
	Obtain specimens for complete blood count with differential, blood culture, blood glucose measurement
	Give antibiotics as indicated
	Give parents information about their child
		Respiratory	Give additional surfactant doses as indicated
			Maintain low tidal volume ventilation
			Avoid hyperventilation and hyperoxia
			Extubate infant and start on continuous positive airway pressure when possible

		Fluid management	Obtain weight every 12 to 24 hours Monitor serum electrolyte, blood glucose, and calcium concentrations every 4 to 8 hours Limit evaporative water losses Administer skin care
		Hematologic	Obtain second blood count Administer transfusion support as indicated Monitor bilirubin, give phototherapy as indicated
		Infection	Consider discontinuing antibiotics if blood culture results are negative at 48 hours
		Nutrition	Start amino acid solution, parenteral nutrition
		Neurologic	Minimize stimulation Perform screening head ultrasonography
		Social	Arrange to meet with family

CPAP, Continuous positive airway pressure; *NCPAP*, nasal continuous positive airway pressure; *NICU*, neonatal intensive care unit.

the combined outcome of bronchopulmonary dysplasia (BPD) or death compared with a selective rescue approach. However, no trials comparing prophylactic administration with early rescue administration of exogenous surfactant (within the first 30 to 60 minutes) have been performed (see Chapter 46). In some centers, ELBW infants are observed briefly after birth, and if respiratory distress develops, they are intubated and ventilated for transfer to the NICU. Exogenous surfactant is given within 1 hour of birth, after endotracheal tube position and the presence of RDS are confirmed on chest radiograph. This strategy assures uniform distribution of surfactant to both lungs and allows initial stabilization and more intensive monitoring of the infant during its administration. Recent data suggest that many spontaneously breathing, extremely premature infants can be managed successfully with continuous positive airway pressure (CPAP) started in the delivery room (Aly et al, 2005b; Lindner et al, 1999; Morley et al, 2008; SUPPORT Study Group, 2010). Routine use of CPAP immediately after delivery may obviate the need for intubation in infants with a gestational age of 24 weeks or more, and increasing experience with this approach has been shown to improve its success (Aly et al, 2005b; Finer, 2006). According to one report, mechanical ventilation was avoided in approximately one third of infants with a gestational age of 25 weeks or less, and in nearly 80% of infants with a gestational age of 28 weeks or more using this approach (Aly et al, 2005b). Whereas aggressive use of early CPAP in the delivery room avoids intubation in some

ELBW infants, it remains unclear whether it improves longer term respiratory outcomes (Morley et al, 2008; SUPPORT Study Group, 2010).

If intubation is required, both oral and nasal routes for endotracheal tube placement are equally effective and have similar complication rates (Spence and Barr, 2002). Preference is usually institution specific, although successful placement of a nasal endotracheal tube requires more time.

ADMISSION TO THE NEONATAL INTENSIVE CARE UNIT

All infants should be weighed upon admission; frequent determination of subsequent weights is a valuable tool in managing fluid and electrolyte balance. In many centers, ELBW infants are initially placed under a radiant warmer for easier access (i.e., for surfactant administration and catheter placement). Because of the high transepidermal fluid losses in these infants, intravenous solutions containing 5% to 10% dextrose should be started as quickly as possible after admission, and efforts should be made to ameliorate evaporative water losses by increasing the relative humidity surrounding the infant. A plastic heat shield used in concert with the radiant warmer may decrease transepidermal water losses; alternatively, a polyethylene tent with an infusion of warmed humidified air may be used. Several studies suggest that fluid management is improved by using a humidified incubator instead of a radiant warmer, because of lower water losses (Gaylord et al, 2001;

TABLE 32-6   Recommended Screening for Common Complications of Extremely Low-Birthweight Infants

Complication	Screening
IVH	HUS on days 1-3; repeat on days 7-10
Germinal matrix hemorrhage	Repeat HUS weekly until findings normal
Intraventricular hemorrhage	Repeat HUS every 3 to 7 days until stable or resolved
IVH with ventricular dilation or intraparenchymal bleeding	Repeat HUS every 3 to 7 days until stable or resolved Consider measurement of resistive indices for progressive ventricular dilatation
Periventricular white matter disease	HUS at day 30; repeat at 36 weeks of postmenstrual age or at discharge Consider magnetic resonance imaging if HUS findings are equivocal
ROP	Perform OE examination at 4 to 6 weeks of postnatal age Repeat every 2 weeks if no ROP Repeat weekly if ROP present Repeat twice weekly for prethreshold disease or rapidly progressive ROP
Audiology screening	Hearing screen no earlier than 34 weeks of postmenstrual age, but before discharge home

HUS, Head ultrasonography; *IVH,* intraventricular hemorrhage; *OE,* ophthalmologic examination; *ROP,* retinopathy of prematurity.

Meyer et al, 2001). Exposure to high humidity may raise the rate of skin colonization with gram-negative organisms, although no increase in the rate of nosocomial infections was observed in several randomized trials comparing incubators with radiant warmers (Flenady and Woodgate, 2002). However, temperature regulation for the smallest infants in the first few days may be more difficult in an incubator than in a servo-controlled radiant warmer, because of rapid drops in air temperature as the incubator doors are opened to care for the infant (Meyer et al, 2001; see also Chapter 30).

VASCULAR ACCESS

Close monitoring of blood pressure, arterial blood gases, and serum chemistries during the first few days after birth is required in most sick ELBW infants; therefore it is advantageous to insert an umbilical arterial catheter for reliable access in infants who require assisted ventilation. Infusion of half-normal saline with 0.5 unit of heparin per milliliter at a low rate (0.5 to 1 mL/h) is usually enough to maintain catheter patency. Although using a saline solution rather than a dextrose-water solution in the umbilical arterial line may complicate fluid and electrolyte management, this disadvantage is offset by the advantage of reliable measurement of blood glucose levels, which are frequently required, without disturbing the infant. Placement of a central umbilical venous catheter (tip at the inferior vena cava–right atrial junction) at the same time the umbilical arterial catheter is placed also provides the clinician with reliable venous access for infusion of fluids, medications,

and blood products. Use of a double-lumen umbilical venous catheter often obviates insertion of a peripheral intravenous line over the first few days after birth and helps to preserve intravenous sites and skin integrity.

The length of time that umbilical catheters are left in place varies by hospital. In most centers, umbilical lines are generally discontinued after 7 to 10 days because of the potential for catheter-related infection and vascular complications, although it is unusual for arterial access to be needed beyond a few days after birth. Before the umbilical venous catheter is removed, it is advisable to insert a percutaneous central venous catheter with its tip at the junction of the superior or inferior vena cava and the right atrium, dedicated to infusion of parenteral nutrition (see Nutritional Management, later). This catheter helps to maintain intravenous access for nutritional purposes without raising the risk of catheter-related infections and reduces the need to establish and maintain peripheral intravenous lines (Janes et al, 2000; Parellada et al, 1999). The incidence of complications of percutaneous central catheters, including catheter-related infections, is lower if a limited number of NICU personnel insert and maintain the lines.

SKIN CARE

The skin of an infant born at 23 to 26 weeks' gestation is extremely immature and is ineffective as an epidermal barrier. Poor epidermal barrier function in the extremely preterm infant leads to disturbances in temperature regulation and water balance as well as breakdown in skin integrity, which can increase the risk of infection. The stratum corneum, which is responsible for epidermal barrier function, does not become functionally mature in the fetus until approximately 32 weeks' gestation (Rutter, 2000). However, acceleration of the maturation process occurs after birth, so most extremely premature infants have a mature epidermal barrier by approximately 2 weeks of postnatal age. Until that time, full-thickness skin injury can occur in the ELBW infant from seemingly innocuous causes, such as local pressure from body positioning, removal of adhesives, and prolonged exposure to products containing alcohol or iodine. Such injury can lead to larger transepidermal water losses, an even greater risk of nosocomial infection, and significant scarring.

Because of these risks, preservation of skin integrity should be incorporated into the care of the extremely preterm infant (Table 32-7). Limited use of adhesives and extreme care upon their removal, frequent repositioning of the infant to avoid pressure points on the skin, and use of soft bedding or a water mattress are the minimum requirements. Hydrocolloids (e.g., DuoDerm, ConvaTech, U.S.) applied to the baby in areas where adhesive tape may come in prolonged contact with the skin (i.e., umbilical catheter or endotracheal tube fixation) to prevent the direct application of tape to the baby may be useful, because it is more easily removed than standard adhesive tape. Polyurethane adhesive dressings (Tegaderm 3m, St. Paul, Minnesota) or hydrogels (Vigilon, Bard Medical, Covington, Georgia) may also be used to protect areas of skin friction and superficial wounds.

Prophylactic application of preservative-free emollient ointments (Aquaphor, Beiersdorf AG, Hamburg, Germany) to protect the skin of the ELBW infant has been studied

Data from Hoath S, Narendran V: Adhesives and emollients in the preterm infant, *Semin Neonataol* 5:289-296, 2000.

TABLE 32-7 Practical Guidelines for Skin Care of Extremely Low-Birthweight Infants

Interventions	Guidelines
Adhesive application	Increase adhesive tack by applying to dry, clean skin surface Avoid alcohol for skin cleansing Use smallest amount of tape possible Use a hydrocolloid or pectin-based layer on the skin, before application of heavy adhesive Avoid using adhesive over areas of skin breakdown Avoid adhesive bonding agents (e.g., benzoin) Use hydrophilic gel or pectin-based adhesives preferentially
Adhesive removal	Avoid adhesive removers and solvents Use a warm, wet cotton ball to periodically saturate hydrogel adhesives (avoid overdrying and oversaturation) Facilitate removal of adhesive with mineral oil, petrolatum, and emollients if reapplication is not necessary
Emollient application	Infants born at <27 weeks' gestation may benefit from emollient use Avoid multidose containers (e.g., large jars) Use nonperfumed, nonirritating hydrophilic emollients Recognize potential for emollients to interfere with adhesive and conductive properties of monitoring devices
Emollient removal	Wipe off gently with a soft cloth or gauze if site is contaminated Avoid repeated attempts to thoroughly cleanse the skin (undesired friction effect) Remove emollients before attaching thermistors or other monitoring devices

(Edwards et al, 2004; Lane and Drost, 1993; Nopper et al, 1996). Several small studies demonstrated smaller transepidermal water losses, improved skin condition, and lower risk of suspected or proven nosocomial infection with prophylactic application of emollient ointments. However, one report documented an increase in the rate of systemic yeast infections in a single NICU coincident with a change to use of prophylactic emollients in ELBW infants, who returned to baseline after such use was discontinued (Campbell et al, 2000). In the largest study to date, infants randomized to prophylactic emollient had better skin integrity during the first month after birth, but had a higher rate of nosocomial bacterial infection compared with a control group with no emollient use (Edwards et al, 2004). Given these concerns, routine use of prophylactic emollients is not recommended; however, selective use in ELBW infants at risk for significant skin breakdown may be effective as an adjunct to other types of local skin care already described.

MECHANICAL VENTILATION AND NASAL CONTINUOUS AIRWAY PRESSURE

A high percentage of ELBW infants require some level of assisted ventilation to survive. Data from animal models of RDS indicate that positive-pressure ventilation with large tidal volumes damages pulmonary capillary endothelium, alveolar and airway epithelium, and basement membranes. This mechanical damage results in leakage of fluid, protein, and blood into the airways, alveoli, and interstitial spaces, leading to inhibition of surfactant activity and further damage to the lungs. These data suggest that a ventilator strategy that avoids large changes in tidal volume may reduce ventilator-induced lung injury in ELBW infants, an important management goal. The optimal mode, timing, and application of ventilatory support used in the initial management of the ELBW infant to meet this goal remain controversial. However, the objectives of all strategies of assisted ventilation in the ELBW infant should be similar—(1) to provide the lowest level of ventilatory support possible that will both support adequate oxygenation and ventilation and prevent atelectasis and (2) to try to reduce acute and chronic lung injury secondary to barotrauma, volutrauma, and oxygen toxicity (Clark et al, 2000). Data also suggest that targeting oxygen saturations (88% to 93%) lower than those used historically in ELBW infants who are receiving supplemental oxygen may protect the lung from oxidative injury and result in better outcomes (Askie et al, 2003).

CONTINUOUS POSITIVE AIRWAY PRESSURE

In a classic study comparing the incidence of BPD between NICUs, Avery et al (1987) reported that the NICU with the lowest incidence used CPAP more frequently and more aggressively than the other units. Van Marter et al (2000) confirmed these observations.

Theoretically, early CPAP protects the immature lung from injury caused by positive-pressure tidal breaths, by preserving surfactant function, increasing alveolar volume and functional residual capacity, enhancing alveolar stability, and improving ventilation-perfusion matching. It also may stimulate the growth of the immature lung. Some NICUs now use CPAP (delivered via nasal prongs or nasopharyngeal tube at 5 to 7 cm H_2O) as the initial mode of assisted ventilation for ELBW infants, starting almost immediately in the delivery room (Lindner et al, 1999). CPAP used this way has been reported in retrospective studies to decrease the need for mechanical ventilation (Gittermann et al, 1997; Poets and Sens, 1996), the need for surfactant treatment, and the incidence of BPD (Aly, 2001; Aly et al, 2005b; de Klerk and de Klerk, 2001; Lindner et al, 1999). In one prospective study (Morley et al, 2008), infants with a gestational age of 25 to 28 weeks who were breathing spontaneously, but required ventilatory assistance at 5 minutes after birth, were randomly assigned to treatment with nasal CPAP or intubation and mechanical ventilation. In the infants assigned to CPAP, 56% did not require intubation, and surfactant use was halved. Although respiratory outcomes at 36 weeks postmenstrual age were equivalent in the two study groups, a greater number of infants who were assigned to initial treatment with CPAP had pneumothorax (9% versus 3%). Alternatively, CPAP may be used after prophylactic or rescue surfactant therapy is given during a brief period of intubation and positive-pressure ventilation (Booth et al, 2006; Verder et al, 1999). Observational studies of this approach show that approximately one fourth of infants born before

27 weeks' gestation do not require a subsequent course of mechanical ventilation and are less likely to develop BPD (Booth et al, 2006; Dani et al, 2004).

CPAP can be delivered by a conventional mechanical ventilator with continuous flow, a variable flow device that adjusts flow through the respiratory cycle, or via "bubble" CPAP, in which a tube is immersed in water to the desired depth to generate CPAP with continuous gas flow bubbling through the immersed tube. Animal data suggest that bubble CPAP improves lung volume and gas exchange compared with conventional CPAP (Pillow et al, 2007), perhaps secondary to effects of the higher intranasal pressures generated by the bubbling water (Kahn et al, 2008). Other data suggest that work of breathing and thoracoabdominal asynchrony may be lessened with variable flow devices (Liptsen et al, 2005). Whether these differences are clinically relevant remains to be elucidated.

CONVENTIONAL MECHANICAL VENTILATION

Most NICUs continue to use pressure-limited, time-cycled conventional ventilators for the initial respiratory management of the ELBW infant requiring mechanical ventilation. Synchronized intermittent mandatory ventilation (SIMV) remains the preferred mode of conventional ventilation for the ELBW infant. In the premature infant, SIMV, in which the inspiratory cycle is synchronized with the patient's own effort, is better than conventional IMV in terms of oxygenation, ventilation, work of breathing, and blood pressure variability (Cleary et al, 1995; Hummler et al, 1996; Jarreau et al, 1996). Technologic limitations in the ability of some ventilators to synchronize breaths with very weak inspiratory efforts may prevent use of SIMV in the smallest infants. With further advancement in ventilator design, other modes of patient-triggered ventilation, including volume guarantee, assist control, and pressure support, have become available to clinicians. These designs generally allow ventilation at lower pressures than conventional SIMV. These modes of ventilation are under investigation but have not been proved to produce better pulmonary outcomes than SIMV in ELBW infants (Donn and Sinha, 1998; Herrera et al, 2002), although one report suggested a shorter time to extubation in infants babies managed with pressure-support ventilation (Reyes et al, 2006).

Currently accepted conventional ventilatory strategies in the ELBW infant stress the avoidance of excessive tidal volumes by limiting peak inspiratory pressures and provision of adequate PEEP to maintain lung volume (Thome et al, 1998). This strategy helps to prevent repeated cycles of atelectasis and lung overdistention, a risk factor for ventilator-induced lung injury (Dreyfuss and Saumon, 1998). Hyperventilation ($Paco_2$ <35 mm Hg) has been associated with a higher risk for the development of BPD (Garland et al, 1995; Van Marter et al, 2000) and neurodevelopmental sequelae in ELBW infants (Wiswell et al, 1996).

In response to this suggestion of worse pulmonary outcome in hyperventilated infants, a strategy of minimal ventilation, or permissive hypercapnia, has been proposed for conventional ventilation in ELBW infants. In the largest study to date of this ventilatory strategy, Carlo et al (2002) randomly assigned 220 infants with birthweights between 501 and 1000 g to receive either minimal ventilation (target $Paco_2$ >52 mm Hg) or routine ventilation (target $Paco_2$ <48 mm Hg). No difference in the rate of BPD, death, or other major short-term morbidities was seen between the two groups. Potential risks of a high $Paco_2$ include increases in both cerebral perfusion and pulmonary vascular resistance and lower pH. Without clear data to support the benefit and safety of higher levels of hypercapnia, most centers target their conventional ventilatory strategy to maintain $Paco_2$ between 45 and 55 mm Hg in the first several days of mechanical ventilation in the ELBW infant.

In infants whose lung disease prevents extubation in the first several days after birth, changes in lung dynamics over the first 1 to 2 weeks often necessitate a change in ventilatory strategy. In the early stages of chronic lung disease, increased airway resistance and decreased lung compliance may require higher values for mean airway pressure, peak inspiratory pressure, PEEP, and inspiratory time than are usually used in initial ventilatory management. Once the need for more prolonged mechanical ventilation is established, many centers tolerate higher target $Paco_2$ values in an attempt to limit further ventilator-induced lung injury.

HIGH-FREQUENCY VENTILATION

Considerable interest has been generated over the past 15 years in the application of high-frequency ventilation (HFV) in newborns who have respiratory failure, because this technique allows ventilation with small tidal volumes. Results of studies using HFV in animal models of RDS have been promising in the prevention of lung injury, but results of clinical studies of this ventilatory technique have not. Despite many clinical trials, controversy continues to surround the indications for HFV in ELBW infants, whether HFV is more effective than other modes of ventilation for RDS, whether HFV reduces adverse outcomes (specifically BPD), and whether HFV is more likely to have significant long-term complications than conventional mechanical ventilation.

Early trials of HFV before surfactant replacement therapy demonstrated no pulmonary advantage of HFV over conventional mechanical ventilation and suggested an increase in rates of air leak and intracranial abnormalities in the HFV-treated infants (HIFI Study Group, 1989). Later trials in ELBW infants who were treated with surfactant also failed to demonstrate any reduction in the incidence of BPD in the HFV-treated infants (Johnson et al, 2002; Rettitz-Volk et al, 1998; Thome et al, 1999).

A rigorously controlled trial of HFV as the primary mode of assisted ventilation compared with conventional mechanical ventilation was the first to suggest a small advantage to the early use of HFV in reduction of BPD or death without an increase in the incidence of short-term complications in ELBW infants. Courtney et al (2002) compared high-frequency oscillatory ventilation (HFOV) with synchronized IMV in a randomized trial that enrolled 500 ELBW infants. These investigators found a small but significant decrease in the incidence of BPD in survivors, requirement of fewer doses of exogenous surfactant, and shorter time to successful extubation in the HFOV-treated group. No differences in other complications of prematurity were observed between the two groups.

These results suggest that, when used in experienced hands according to strict protocol, HFV confers some protection from lung injury in ELBW infants. It remains unclear whether this same advantage is gained when HFV is used in usual clinical circumstances in less experienced centers and whether the incidence of other complications may be affected by mode of ventilation. Some NICUs with the most experience with HFV use it routinely as the initial mode of ventilation for ELBW infants. Most centers continue to use conventional ventilation with low tidal volumes and reasonable ventilation goals as the initial mode of ventilation for ELBW infants, reserving HFV for infants in whom conventional ventilation and surfactant fail. This latter practice seems advisable, given the potential risks of HFV, including inadvertent lung overdistention, impaired cardiac output, and increased central venous pressure that may lead to intracranial hemorrhage.

POST-EXTUBATION CPAP FOR RESPIRATORY DISTRESS SYNDROME AND APNEA

CPAP is commonly used in ELBW infants after extubation to stabilize functional residual capacity and reduce the frequency of apneic spells after the lung disease has improved. All ELBW infants should be extubated as soon as they have recovered from acute RDS and should be given a trial of CPAP to protect them from further ventilator induced lung injury. When used in combination with methylxanthine therapy, CPAP decreases the need for reintubation because of progressive respiratory distress or apnea (Davis et al, 2003). Methylxanthine (aminophylline or caffeine) treatment before extubation has also been shown to lower the incidence of apnea and the need for reintubation in premature infants. Many ELBW infants benefit from prolonged use of CPAP by nasal prongs after extubation, especially those with frequent or severe episodes of apnea and bradycardia resistant to methylxanthine. Some centers currently provide assisted ventilation through nasal prongs (nasal intermittent positive pressure ventilation) to avoid intubation (Khalaf et al, 2001); this method may be more successful than conventional CPAP in avoiding postextubation failure in some infants (Bhandari et al, 2009). However, the smallest and least mature infants may need prolonged mechanical ventilation because of frequent, severe apneic spells that are unresponsive to other therapies.

ADJUNCTIVE THERAPIES TO PREVENT BRONCHOPULMONARY DYSPLASIA

Vitamin A Supplementation

ELBW infants have low stores of vitamin A. Because of the role of vitamin A in promoting lung healing, its deficiency has been linked to a higher risk for development of BPD. In a large multicenter trial, vitamin A supplementation (5000 IU given intramuscularly three times

per week for 4 weeks) reduced biochemical evidence of vitamin A deficiency and decreased the incidence of BPD by 12% without adverse effects in ELBW infants who required mechanical ventilation or supplemental oxygen at 24 hours of age (Tyson et al, 1999). Given these efficacy data and apparent safety, many NICUs choose to administer vitamin A supplementation as described previously to all ELBW infants starting at 24 hours after birth. However, widespread acceptance of this therapy has been limited by concerns over the need for thrice weekly intramuscular injections and its associated pain and stress to the infant.

Caffeine

In a prospective, masked, randomized trial involving infants with a birthweight of 500 to 1250 grams, the initiation of treatment with caffeine citrate (20 mg/kg loading dose, followed by 5 mg/kg/day) in the first 10 days after birth decreased the rate of BPD (a secondary outcome), as compared with placebo (36% versus 47%) without adverse effects (Schmidt et al, 2006). The composite primary outcome of death, cerebral palsy, cognitive delay, deafness or blindness at 18 to 22 months of age was also reduced in the subjects randomized to caffeine (Schmidt et al, 2007). The effect of caffeine on the incidence of bronchopulmonary dysplasia may be secondary to less ventilator-induced lung injury in the caffeine-treated infants, because shorter duration of positive pressure ventilation and supplemental oxygen therapy was associated with its use (Schmidt et al, 2006). These results suggest that caffeine should be administered routinely in ELBW infants in the first 10 days after birth, even if they continue to require mechanical ventilation.

Inhaled Nitric Oxide

Inhaled nitric oxide (iNO) may improve the pulmonary outcome in some VLBW infants, through mechanisms that are thought to involve decreased pulmonary vascular resistance or improved ventilation-perfusion matching, bronchodilatation, antiinflammatory effects, promotion of lung remodeling in response to injury, or normalized surfactant function. iNO used as rescue therapy for ELBW infants with severe hypoxic respiratory failure does not improve the pulmonary outcome or survival, and it may be associated with increased mortality or an increased incidence of intraventricular hemorrhage (Van Meurs et al, 2005). Results of trials of iNO involving premature infants with less severe lung disease who were at risk for BPD are mixed. In the Nitric Oxide for the Prevention of Chronic Lung Disease Trial (NO-CLD) study, a multicenter trial involving ventilator-dependent infants with a birthweight of 500 to 1250 g, treatment with iNO started at 7 to 14 days and continued for an average of 23 days of increased survival without BPD as compared with placebo (Ballard et al, 2006). In contrast, in a multicenter trial of iNO, treatment started before 48 hours of age and continued for 21 days (20 ppm for 3 to 4 days, then weaned to 10 ppm, 5 ppm, and 2 ppm for 7 days each) in infants with a birthweight of 500 to 1250 g who continued to require mechanical ventilation, only iNO-treated infants with a birthweight greater than 1000 g had a pulmonary benefit (Kinsella et al, 2006). Treated infants in this latter study were also less likely to have ultrasonic evidence of brain injury than were control infants. Long-term follow-up from the latter two studies suggests that iNO is safe and may improve long term pulmonary outcomes (Hibbs et al, 2008; Watson et al, 2009). iNO use for the prevention of BPD is not currently approved by the United States Food and Drug Administration. Routine use of iNO for the prevention of BPD should be discouraged until additional studies are available to define dosing and duration of therapy.

Systemic Corticosteroids

Inflammation also plays an important role in the pathogenesis of BPD; therefore pharmacologic doses of systemic corticosteroids have been widely used for prevention and treatment of BPD in ELBW infants. Several studies have examined early (<96 hours of age) administration of corticosteroids, usually dexamethasone, to prevent the development of BPD in infants at risk (Garland et al, 1999; Rastogi et al, 1996; Stark et al, 2001). A meta-analysis of studies in which corticosteroids were used to prevent rather than treat established BPD suggested that early corticosteroid treatment in ELBW infants results in more rapid extubation and a lower incidence of BPD (Halliday et al, 2002), although no effect on mortality was observed. However, a higher incidence of short-term complications, including hyperglycemia, hypertension, poor growth, and intestinal perforations and bleeding, was observed in the corticosteroid-treated infants (Garland et al, 1999; Stark et al, 2001; Watterberg et al, 2004). More importantly, long-term follow-up data suggest that exposure to corticosteroid for prevention or treatment of BPD raises the risk of neurological sequelae in treated infants, including poor head growth, cerebral palsy, and developmental impairment (American Academy of Pediatrics, 2010).

The apparently higher risk of long-term sequelae without an effect on overall mortality has tempered enthusiasm for systemic corticosteroid treatment to prevent or treat BPD in ELBW infants. The possible role of postnatal corticosteroids in the prevention of BPD in selected infants, such as those exposed to chorioamnionitis, was suggested by a trial of early treatment with hydrocortisone (Watterberg et al, 2004). The risk of impaired neurodevelopment may be lower with hydrocortisone than dexamethasone (Rademaker et al, 2007; Watterberg et al, 2007), and some centers are substituting hydrocortisone for dexamethasone if postnatal corticosteroids are used. However, it seems prudent to avoid routine use of systemic corticosteroids in ELBW infants for the prevention or treatment of BPD until further data are available (American Academy of Pediatrics, 2010).

NUTRITIONAL MANAGEMENT

Provision of adequate nutrition is central to effective care of ELBW infants (see Chapters 66 and 67). These infants are born with limited nutrient reserves, immature pathways for nutrient absorption and metabolism, and higher nutrient demands. In addition, medical conditions associated with extreme prematurity both alter requirements for and complicate the adequate delivery of nutrients. The goals of nutritional management of the ELBW infant are preservation of endogenous body stores, achievement of postnatal growth similar to intrauterine weight accretion and body composition, and maintenance of normal physiologic and metabolic processes concomitant with minimizing complications and side effects. However, few ELBW infants are able to meet these goals despite the use of central parenteral nutrition and caloric supplementation of enteral feedings. As a result, significant growth failure is commonplace (Berry et al, 1997; Ehrenkranz et al, 1999; Martin et al, 2009).

Enteral Nutrition

Medical problems of ELBW infants sometimes preclude initiation of enteral feedings for several days to weeks. However, the structural and functional integrity of the gastrointestinal tract depends on the provision of enteral feedings. Withholding enteral feedings at birth imposes risks for all the complications of luminal starvation, including mucosal thinning, flattening of the villi, and bacterial translocation. Early initiation (within the first few days after birth) of low volumes of milk (10 to 20 mL/kg/day, preferably with expressed breast milk; trophic feedings, or "gut priming") has been studied in several small trials in premature infants (McClure and Newell, 2000; Schanler et al, 1999a). Trophic feedings are not meant to give the infant significant nutrition, rather to promote continued functional maturation of the gastrointestinal tract. Documented benefits of trophic feedings include higher plasma concentrations of gastrointestinal hormones, a more mature gut motility pattern, lower incidence of cholestasis, increased calcium and phosphorus absorption, and improved and earlier tolerance of enteral feedings. Trophic feedings have not been associated with a higher risk of necrotizing enterocolitis or other adverse outcomes; therefore there is no clinical advantage to delaying initiation of feedings in the medically stable ELBW infant. (See also Chapter 66.)

Feeding intolerance, indicated by gastric residuals that exceed 25% to 50% of the volume fed, abdominal distention, or microscopic blood in the stool, is common in ELBW infants and may be difficult to differentiate from early stages of necrotizing enterocolitis. Feeding intolerance may preclude the advance of enteral nutrition for days to weeks, complicating nutritional management and prolonging the need for parenteral nutrition. Numerous feeding strategies to avoid episodes of feeding intolerance have been used in ELBW infants, including slow increase in enteral volume (<10 mL/kg/day), use of dilute rather than full-strength milk, continuous versus bolus tube-feeding, and use of prokinetic agents. None of these feeding strategies has been found to be clearly superior, although bolus feedings may decrease episodes of gastric residuals compared with continuous tube feedings and may allow a more rapid advance to full enteral volumes as well as promote better growth.

Episodes of feeding intolerance also are reduced in ELBW infants fed human milk rather than specialized formulas for premature infants (Schanler et al, 1999b). Other benefits of giving human milk in ELBW infants are a more rapid advance to full enteral volumes and its positive immunologic effects, with an associated reduction in the risk of necrotizing enterocolitis and late-onset sepsis. Data also suggest that neurodevelopmental outcome may be improved in ELBW infants fed expressed breast milk (Vohr et al, 2006). Human milk must be fortified with calcium, phosphorus, sodium, protein, and other minerals to provide adequate nutrition in the ELBW infant. In addition to commercially available human milk fortifiers, which increase the caloric density to approximately 24 calories per ounce, human milk can be fortified further to higher caloric densities with medium chain triglycerides, glucose polymers, and added protein.

Premature infants who are fed fortified human milk may grow more slowly than infants fed premature formulas (Schanler et al, 1999b), perhaps because of the variability in fat and caloric content of pumped breast milk or changes in the nutrient composition of human milk with fortification that affect fat absorption. Despite the potential for slower growth in infants fed human milk, its use should be strongly encouraged in ELBW infants because of the immunologic and other nutritional benefits. Further research on how best to fortify human milk is necessary to promote the best rate of growth in ELBW infants. (See also Chapters 65 and 66.) In addition, even after recommended enteral dietary intakes are reached, many ELBW infants continue to have a cumulative energy and protein deficit, which in part explains their later growth failure (Ehrenkranz et al, 1999; Embleton et al, 2001; Martin et al, 2009).

Early Parenteral Nutrition

Protein losses in ELBW infants receiving a glucose infusion alone begin immediately after birth and can approach 1.5 g/kg/day in the first 24 to 72 hours. Fortunately, these losses can be offset by early administration of an amino acid solution, even at low caloric intakes. Several studies have demonstrated the safety of early administration (within 24 hours after birth) of an amino acid solution, with no abnormal elevations of ammonia or blood urea nitrogen even in the most immature infants (Rivera et al, 1993; Van Goudoever et al, 1995). To prevent early protein deficit, ELBW infants should be given a source of parenteral protein as soon as possible after birth (see also Chapter 67). In one study, ELBW infants who received 3 g or more of protein per day at 5 days of age or less were less likely to have a weight below the 10th percentile at 36 weeks postmenstrual age and suboptimal head growth at 18 months of age when compared with ELBW infants who received less protein supplementation after birth (Poindexter et al, 2006).

In most centers, parenteral nutrition is used exclusively during the first few days after birth and then gradually reduced as enteral feedings are introduced. Longer duration of parenteral nutrition is associated with the development of a number of complications, including cholestasis, osteopenia, and sepsis. For example, the risk of an episode of late-onset sepsis in premature infants is 22-fold higher if parenteral nutrition is continued for

more than 3 weeks compared with 1 week or less (Stoll et al, 2002b).

MANAGEMENT AND PREVENTION OF INFECTION

Bacterial and fungal infections are an important cause of illness and death among ELBW infants. In addition to the immediate morbidity and mortality, local and systemic inflammation caused by infections may increase the risk for development of other complications of prematurity, including BPD and brain injury. ELBW infants are frequently exposed to perinatal and delivery complications that raise their risk of early-onset (<72 hours) infections. The need for prolonged intravenous access, exposure to parenteral nutrition, and mechanical ventilation also subject the ELBW infant to a high risk of late-onset (>72 hours) nosocomial infections. The frequent infections seen in the ELBW population are related to immaturity of both humoral and cellular immunity (see Chapter 36). In addition to the judicious use of antimicrobial therapy, environmental controls, nursery surveillance, and modulation of the immature immune response have been proposed as possible interventions to prevent infections in extremely premature infants.

Early-Onset Infections

The incidence of early-onset bacterial infections in very LBW (VLBW) infants is approximately 1% to 2%, with a mortality of approximately 40% to 50% (Stoll et al, 2002a; see also Chapter 39). The major risk factor for the development of perinatally acquired bacterial infections is PROM with chorioamnionitis, which frequently complicates premature deliveries. However, a significant percentage of extremely premature births may be associated with intrauterine infection before membrane rupture (Goldenberg et al, 2000). In one study, 41% of premature infants with early-onset sepsis were born less than 6 hours after membrane rupture (Stoll et al, 2002a).

Because the clinical signs of perinatally acquired infection are nonspecific, the index of suspicion and the concern about the possibility of intrauterine infection should always be high in the presence of premature birth. All ELBW infants, except for those delivered for maternal indications with no labor, should be evaluated for infection at birth by means of a complete blood count with differential and blood culture, and empiric antibiotic therapy with ampicillin and an aminoglycoside should be initiated. A white blood cell count less than 5000 cells/μL, a ratio of immature to total neutrophils ratio greater than 0.2 to 0.3, and neutropenia (absolute neutrophil count less than 1000 cells/μL) are all suggestive of infection, but may also be seen in infants with other conditions, including maternal preeclampsia and hypertension. The duration of initial antibiotic therapy depends on the results of the blood culture, blood counts, the clinical course, and the perinatal history. If the blood culture is negative for bacterial growth at 48 hours and the infant has improved clinically, consideration should be given to discontinuing antibiotics. Prolonged exposure to antibiotic therapy increases the likelihood of colonization with multiple antibiotic-resistant organisms, the development of fungemia, and necrotizing enterocolitis (Cotten et al, 2009); therefore it should be reserved for infants with documented infection or a very high index of suspicion of infection based on clinical or historical factors.

The distribution of pathogens causing early-onset sepsis in VLBW infants has changed, likely because of increased use of intrapartum antibiotics for prevention of group B streptococcal infections and treatment of preterm PROM (Puopolo and Eichenwald, 2010). As the rate of infections from group B streptococci has diminished with intrapartum antibiotic prophylaxis, the proportion of documented infections from gram-negative organisms has risen (Table 32-8; Stoll et al, 2002a). In an additional change of the epidemiology of early-onset infections in premature infants, possibly related to increased use of intrapartum antibiotics, the frequency of infections owing to ampicillin-resistant *Escherichia coli* strains has increased in some centers (Bizzarro et al, 2008; Joseph et al, 1998; Stoll et al, 2002a). Current recommendations for empiric antibiotic therapy for ELBW infants at risk of early-onset sepsis have not changed, but continued surveillance of the epidemiology and antibiotic resistance patterns of isolates within individual units is warranted. In infants with severe illness that may be caused by sepsis, broadening initial antibiotic coverage to include a third-generation cephalosporin should be considered.

LATE-ONSET INFECTIONS

Nosocomial infection is a common though preventable complication of intensive care of the ELBW infant. The incidence of late-onset sepsis in ELBW infants who survive beyond 3 days of age is 25% to 50%, depending on gestational age and birthweight, with the median age at onset of the first episode approximately 2 weeks (Fanaroff et al, 1998; Stoll et al, 2002b). The overall mortality rate is approximately 20% but may be as high as 80%, depending on the organism causing sepsis. The risk of neurodevelopmental impairment is increased by approximately 1.5-fold in ELBW survivors of nosocomial bloodstream infections (Stoll et al, 2004). Risk factors for the development of late-onset sepsis include prolonged hyperalimentation and lipid use, the presence of a central venous catheter, longer duration of mechanical ventilation, and delay in initiation of enteral feedings (Stoll et al, 2002b). These practices and procedures are common events that may be unavoidable in the care of ELBW infants. However, large variations have been observed among NICUs in the rate of late-onset infections in premature infants (Brodie et al, 2000; Stoll et al, 2002b), suggesting that individual NICU practices may affect the incidence of nosocomial infections.

The most common cause of late-onset infections in ELBW infants is coagulase-negative *Staphylococcus* (CoNS). The most significant risk factor for the development of CoNS infection is the use of a fat emulsion (e.g., Intralipid) infusion (Freeman et al, 1990). Infection with CoNS is almost never fatal but is associated with significant morbidity, such as prolonged ventilator use and hospital stay (Gray et al, 1995). Other organisms that cause late-onset infections in ELBW infants are associated with a much higher morbidity and mortality. The distribution

TABLE 32-8 Distribution of Pathogens among 84 Cases of Early-Onset Sepsis*

Organism	No.	%
Gram-negative:	51	60.7
Escherichia coli	37	44.0
Haemophilus influenzae	7	8.3
Citrobacter	2	2.4
Other	5	6.0
Gram-positive:	31	36.9
Group B streptococci	9	10.7
Viridans streptococci	3	3.6
Other streptococci	4	4.8
Listeria monocytogenes	2	2.4
Coagulase-negative staphylococci	9	10.7
Other	4	4.8
Fungi: *Candida albicans*	2	2.4
TOTAL	84	100

Data from Stoll B, Hansen N, Fanaroff A, et al: Changes in pathogens causing early onset sepsis in very low birth weight infants, *N Engl J Med* 347:240-247, 2002.
*Occurring in 5447 infants born between September 1, 1998, and August 31, 2000.

TABLE 32-9 Distribution of Pathogens Associated With the First Episode of Late-Onset Sepsis*

Organism	No.	%
Gram-positive:	922	70.2
Coagulase-negative staphylococci	629	47.9
Staphylococcus aureus	103	7.8
Enterococcus spp.	43	3.3
Group B streptococci	30	2.3
Other	117	8.9
Gram-negative:	231	17.6
Escherichia coli	64	4.9
Klebsiella spp.	52	4.0
Pseudomonas spp.	35	27
Enterobacter spp.	33	2.5
Serratia spp.	29	2.2
Other	18	1.4
Fungi:	160	12.2
Candida albicans	76	5.8
Candida parapsilosis	54	4.1
Other	30	2.3
TOTAL	1313	100

Data from Stoll B, Hansen N, Fanaroff A, et al: Late-onset sepsis in very low birth weight neonates: experience of the NICDH Neonatal Research Network, *Pediatrics* 110:285-291, 2002.
*In National Institute of Child Health and Development Neonatal Research Network institutions, September 1, 1998, through August 31, 2000.

of pathogens associated with the first episode of late-onset sepsis among 1313 infants in a cohort of VLBW babies over a 2-year period is shown in Table 32-9.

Presenting features of late-onset sepsis include increased apnea, feeding intolerance, abdominal distention, guaiac-positive stools, increased respiratory support, and lethargy and hypotonia (Fanaroff et al, 1998). Because these symptoms are nonspecific, ELBW infants are frequently evaluated for infection and treated with empiric antibiotic therapy. In one study, use of both vancomycin and antifungal therapy was inversely related to birthweight; approximately three fourth of infants with a birthweight less than 750 g was treated with vancomycin during their hospital stay, and approximately one third was treated with antifungals (Stoll et al, 2002b). Central catheters should be removed immediately to ensure adequate treatment of infants in whom sepsis is diagnosed, except for that caused by CoNS (Benjamin et al, 2001).

Endotracheal tube colonization with multiple organisms is common in infants who require prolonged mechanical ventilation. In general, such colonization should not be treated with antibiotics unless there is evidence of pneumonia or significant inflammation indicative of tracheitis. Prospective surveillance of common isolates and antimicrobial resistance patterns within individual NICUs can help to guide empiric antibiotic therapy in ELBW infants being evaluated and treated for presumed sepsis. However, indiscriminate use of broad-spectrum antibiotics in the absence of true infection can alter antimicrobial resistance patterns (Goldmann et al, 1996), raising the risk of late-onset infections and complicating therapy.

Prevention of Nosocomial Infection

Because of the frequency and potential severity of late-onset sepsis in ELBW infants, several strategies to prevent infection have been proposed. Using these practices as a guideline, Horbar et al (2001) observed a decrease in the CoNS infection rate from 22% to 16.6% over a 2-year period in VLBW infants in six study NICUs. Other investigators have confirmed that changes in practice, primarily surrounding the use and care of central venous catheters, can reduce the overall burden of late onset infections in individual units (Aly et al, 2005a; Kilbride et al, 2003). Some NICUs routinely screen ELBW infants by stool or respiratory secretion cultures for the presence of multiple antibiotic-resistant organisms, which would necessitate isolation (Gregory et al, 2009). Clusters of infections with unusual organisms should prompt surveillance cultures of infants, potential NICU environmental sources, and NICU staff (Foca et al, 2000). Restriction of broad-spectrum antibiotic use by hospital policy or treatment guidelines may limit the local spread of resistant organisms (Goldmann et al, 1996). Strict adherence to hand hygiene before and after every patient contact and avoidance of overcrowding within NICUs also help to decrease the incidence of infection. The use of alcohol-based hand gels at the bedside may improve compliance with hand hygiene (Harbarth et al, 2002).

In addition to practice and environmental controls, prophylactic use of antibiotics and modulation of the immune response of ELBW infants have been studied as methods to reduce the incidence of late-onset sepsis. Low-dose vancomycin given continuously via hyperalimentation solutions (Baier et al, 1998; Spafford et al, 1994), intermittently via peripheral vein (Cooke et al, 1997), or vancomycin lock of the central venous catheter (Garland et al, 2005) has been shown to reduce the incidence of CoNS in premature infants at risk. Concern about the emergence

of vancomycin-resistant organisms and the low mortality associated with CoNS infections has prevented widespread use of this approach. Prophylactic fluconazole given for 6 weeks lowered the incidence of fungal colonization and invasive disease in ELBW infants without associated complications or the emergence of resistant organisms (Kaufman et al, 2001, 2005; Manzoni et al, 2007). Such an approach might be advisable for NICUs with a high incidence of fungal infections in their ELBW population, but more study is needed to define any potential short- and long-term risks. Approaches that have been used with success in immunocompromised adult patients, such as antiseptic-impregnated central catheters, are promising but have not yet been studied adequately in premature infants.

Prophylactic intravenous administration of polyclonal immunoglobulin (IVIG) to prevent late-onset sepsis has been studied extensively in premature infants. Several trials have shown a decrease in the incidence of documented sepsis by a small but significant amount in premature infants treated with prophylactic IVIG and no effect on mortality or other complications of prematurity (Lacy and Ohlsson, 1995). The costs associated with this therapy to achieve the small decrease in infection rates, as well as the increased exposure to blood products, have limited its use; it is unclear whether selective prophylactic IVIG treatment of ELBW infants at highest risk for sepsis is warranted. However, IVIG therapy in addition to antibiotic therapy may be of benefit in reducing mortality in infants with established sepsis (Jenson and Pollock, 1997). Development of more targeted polyclonal or monoclonal γ-globulin preparations for specific organisms that cause sepsis in premature newborns may alter the use of IVIG in the future (Lamari et al, 2000; Weisman et al, 2009).

Another promising strategy under investigation for modulation of the immature immune response to help prevent infections in premature infants is treatment with hemopoietic colony-stimulating factors, including granulocyte colony-stimulating factor and granulocyte-macrophage colony-stimulating factor (Modi and Carr, 2000). Most studies of these factors have been conducted in neutropenic, small-for-gestational-age infants or infants delivered to women with preeclampsia. Treatment with granulocyte colony-stimulating factor in neutropenic infants resulted in an increase in neutrophil counts and reduced the incidence of sepsis (Kocherlakota and La Gamma, 1998). Prophylactic treatment with granulocyte-macrophage colony-stimulating factor in premature infants with normal neutrophil counts prevented the development of neutropenia in episodes of sepsis, but it remains unclear whether this type of therapy to address cellular immune deficiency in ELBW infants will reduce the incidence of infection without additional complications (Miura et al, 2001; Modi and Carr, 2000).

NEUROSENSORY COMPLICATIONS

The major neurosensory complications associated with extreme premature birth are intraventricular hemorrhage, periventricular white matter injury, and retinopathy of prematurity. Although the incidence of severe intraventricular hemorrhage has fallen with improvements in management and increased antenatal steroid use, it remains a major cause of brain injury with consequent abnormal neurodevelopment. Pharmacologic approaches to its prevention after birth have been generally unsuccessful. Prophylactic indomethacin reduces the incidence of severe intraventricular hemorrhage, but does not improve long-term neurodevelopment (Schmidt et al, 2001).

Periventricular white matter injury is the predominant form of brain injury in extremely preterm infants and correlates strongly with the development of cerebral palsy. Its pathogenesis is poorly understood, and no specific neuroprotective strategy is known. In some infants, cerebral blood flow and oxygen delivery measured with near infrared spectroscopy varies during variations of blood pressure considered to be in the normal range, and this lack of autoregulation of cerebral blood flow may lead to ischemic white matter injury (Evans, 2006). Whether aggressive treatment of hypotension in ELBW infants prevents or may lead to subsequent brain injury is uncertain, probably because blood pressure, which is easily measured, does not correlate well with systemic or cerebral blood flow (Fanaroff et al, 2006; Limperopoulos et al, 2007). A higher rate of white matter injury occurs in the setting of maternal or neonatal infection, or with elevated proinflammatory cytokines in amniotic fluid or cord blood, suggesting that inflammation has a role in the pathogenesis (Viscardi et al, 2004). Advanced magnetic resonance imaging techniques in infants with white matter injury show disturbances in cerebral growth, with reduced volume of both gray and white matter (Inder et al, 2005). These observations might serve to explain the motor and cognitive dysfunction often seen in infants with white matter injury.

Retinopathy of prematurity, a vascular proliferative disorder that affects the incompletely vascularized retina of preterm infants, is a major cause of blindness in these children. Severe retinopathy is 18-fold more likely to develop in infants delivered at less than 25 weeks' gestation compared with 28 weeks' gestation (Fanaroff et al, 2007). Periods of hyperoxia owing to exposure to excessive inspired oxygen concentration contribute to the development of retinopathy (Saugstad, 2006); however, the optimal target range of oxygen saturation is not known. Because fetal hemoglobin shifts the hemoglobin oxygen saturation curve to the left, oxygen saturations greater than 95% may be associated with arterial oxygen tension greater than 80 mm Hg, possibly excessive for the ELBW infant. Conversely, oxygen saturation that is too low can increase the risk of injury to the brain or other end organs (Deulofuet et al, 2006).

Adjusting inspired oxygen concentration to target lower oxygen saturations in extremely preterm infants may decrease the rate of severe retinopathy. In a prospective observational study, ELBW infants treated in centers with a restrictive approach to oxygen delivery (i.e., saturation alarm limits of 70% to 90%) had less retinopathy requiring cryotherapy (6.3 versus 27.7 %) than did those in units with a liberal approach (i.e., alarm limits of 88% to 98%), and neurodevelopmental outcome at 1 year of age was similar (Tin et al, 2001). In two other studies with historical controls, the incidence of severe retinopathy decreased after oxygen saturation alarm limits were lowered from 87%-97% to 85%-93% for infants born at 28 weeks' gestation and less until they reached 32 weeks postmenstrual age (Chow et al, 2003; Vanderveen et al, 2006). In a masked randomized trial comparing two different target oxygen saturation ranges (85% to 89% compared with 91% to 95%) in infants born between 24 and 27 weeks, ROP occurred less frequently in survivors assigned to the lower oxygen saturation group. However, death before discharge occurred more frequently in the lower oxygen saturation group, suggesting that the best target range for oxygen saturation remains unclear (SUPPORT Study Group, 2010).

DEVELOPMENTAL AND PARENTAL CARE

ELBW infants are particularly vulnerable to the potentially noxious stimuli of the NICU environment, including light, noise, frequent disturbances, and painful procedures. The ELBW infant reacts to the noisy and well-lit environment of many NICUs with greater variability of blood pressure, ventilatory requirements, and oxygen saturation as well as behavioral disorganization, which may have both short- and long-term effects on outcome (Jacobs et al, 2002). Modification of the NICU environment to limit exposure of ELBW infants to such stresses—by lowering ambient light and reducing noise, clustering caregiving periods and procedures to allow periods of uninterrupted sleep, and using positioning aids to promote containment—is an intuitive part of their care. Newer NICU designs, transitioning from open common rooms to private room settings, may also facilitate a better environment for vulnerable infants and enhance parental involvement. These environmental and developmental interventions in the NICU can improve physiologic stability and some short-term outcomes in preterm infants, including decreased severity of BPD and shorter length of hospital stay. It remains unclear whether individualized, developmentally supportive care or other developmental interventions started in the NICU improve long-term outcome in ELBW infants (Symington et al, 2009).

In addition to environmental modifications, NICUs should promote parental involvement with infants, even when they are critically ill. Open family presence guidelines and encouragement of parental caregiving when appropriate may help parents to bond with their baby. Many NICUs have embraced a philosophy of family-centered care, in which a stronger bond is forged with the families of NICU patients by encouraging collaboration among family members and care providers in policy and program development, professional education, and aspects of the delivery of care (Dunn et al, 2006). Skin-to-skin (kangaroo) care, in which the infant is placed unclothed on the mother or father's bare chest, was originally developed in nonindustrialized countries to maintain temperature regulation in premature infants. It is now used in many NICUs to promote parental attachment. Skin-to-skin care may have a positive effect on infant state organization and respiratory patterns, increase the rate of infant weight gain, improve maternal milk production, and have long-term benefits in infant development and parents' perceptions of their babies (Feldman et al, 2002). Skin-to-skin care can be initiated in ELBW infants within the first 2 weeks after birth, when they are more medically stable.

FUTURE DIRECTIONS

This chapter presents some of the special needs of the ELBW infant. The medical care of the ELBW infant is a complex combination of knowledge of developmental physiology, evidenced-based interventions, and clinical experience. Wide variability in approaches to care of these infants exists among practitioners and NICUs, as does variability in outcomes. Nevertheless, NICUs involved in treating ELBW infants should develop a coherent approach to the medical and ethical aspects of their care.

Future research should focus on identifying best practices to narrow the variability in approach to care and with the goal to prevent long-term disability. As more of these tiny infants survive, it is the responsibility of neonatologists to stay abreast of clinical improvements and the short- and long-term consequences of established and newly proposed medical interventions to provide the best care for these vulnerable infants and to keep parents informed and involved.

Complete references used in this text can be found online at www.expertconsult.com

CARE OF THE LATE PRETERM INFANT

Sowmya S. Mohan and Lucky Jain

Had he been alive today, Patrick Bouvier Kennedy would have been hailed as a triumph of neonatal care—after all, he was the son of the former United States President, John F. Kennedy and former First Lady Jacqueline B. Kennedy. Born prematurely at 34 weeks gestation, he would have been aptly labeled as a late preterm neonate; however, based on his birth weight (2.1 kg) and gestational age, few would have predicted the outcome he had then, were he born in 2009. But then, in 1963, little was available to the clinician for the management of hyaline membrane disease—no routine use of neonatal ventilators, no device to provide airway positive pressure, no surfactant, and no antenatal steroids. He died two days after his birth; the New York Times obituary said that "the battle for the Kennedy baby was lost because medical science has not advanced far enough."

(Jain and Carlton, 2009)

With more than 4 million live births per year (Martin et al, 2007), the United States has one of the highest birth rates among industrialized countries; it also has the stigma of having a disproportionately high prematurity rate. Decades of efforts to reduce preterm births have not affected this formidable problem. In recent years the problem has been highlighted by the rise in births between 34 and 36⁶/₇ weeks' gestation, a group referred to as *late preterm infants* (Figure 33-1). Late preterm infants have a checkered history, having been passed off as nothing more than "near term" infants, yet being feared as the "quick to spiral down group" when they develop respiratory distress syndrome or other complications. As the number of late preterm infants has grown, so has the awareness of their unique set of problems, such as delayed neonatal transition, wet lung syndrome, hypothermia, hypoglycemia, and hyperbilirubinemia (Figure 33-2). Although not unique to this population, these complications have sufficient differences in their manifestations and management, prompting the editors to add an entirely new chapter to this textbook devoted to the health issues of late preterm infants. In Chapter 14, the obstetric issues and epidemiology related to prematurity are addressed. This chapter focuses on the special considerations applicable to the clinical course and management of late preterm infants.

There has been a shift in the distribution of births away from term and post term and toward earlier gestational ages (Davidoff et al, 2006). This shift has resulted in a disproportionately high rate of premature births with estimates of up to 12.7% of live births being premature (Martin et al, 2007)—defined as <37 completed weeks' gestation or <260 days, counting from the first day of the last menstrual period (Raju, 2006). Within this group of premature babies, up to 75% are classified as late preterm infants (Adamkin, 2009). Although the reasons for such a high number of late preterm births are multifactorial,

higher rates of induced deliveries, cesarean births, and efforts to reduce stillbirths may have contributed to the increase.

Late preterm babies currently account for up to one third of all neonatal intensive care unit (NICU) admissions in the United States (Angus et al, 2001), adding strain to the overburdened system of health care delivery, particularly in community hospitals and rural areas. These admissions range from short stays, for problems such as transient tachypnea of the newborn (TTNB), to more complicated or extended NICU stays for problems such as persistent pulmonary hypertension of the newborn (PPHN). With the average NICU stay costing up to $3500 per day, the economic impact of caring for the late preterm baby can be significant. For example, in 1996 the State of California alone could have saved $49.9 million in health care costs by preventing non–medically indicated deliveries between 34 and 37 weeks' gestation (Gilbert et al, 2003). In addition to the expense of the initial hospitalization, the cost of caring for a late preterm baby can also be compounded by the increased incidence of hospital readmissions and the long-term care issues related to persistent problems. The effects of the increasing number of late preterm births create a societal burden in lost productivity, as parents take extended leave from work to be with their fragile newborns. More importantly, there may be lasting effects with neurodevelopmental delays extending into early school age. Because a significant proportion of brain growth occurs during the last 6 weeks of gestation (Adams-Chapman, 2006), late preterm infants are vulnerable to neuronal injury and disruption of normal brain development. Whereas more longitudinal studies are needed, preliminary studies show that late preterm infants are more likely to have a diagnosis of developmental delay within the first 3 years of life, require special needs preschool resources, and have more problems with school readiness (Morse et al, 2009).

Given their large numbers, the overall socioeconomic effects of the late preterm births can be significant. Strategies are required that can reduce the preventable fraction of late preterm births and work toward reducing the morbidity in others, when continuation of the pregnancy is deemed harmful to the fetus or the mother. This chapter explores the pathophysiology of the major morbidities that affect late preterm infants and discusses the unique challenges faced by clinicians in the management of these conditions.

DEFINITION

Late preterm birth is an accepted term used for infants born between 34 and 36⁶/₇ weeks' gestation (see Figure 33-1) (Raju et al, 2006). This group of infants was initially referred to as *near term*, but the misleading implication of

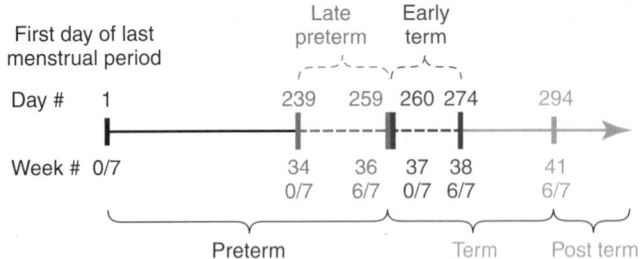

FIGURE 33-1 Definitions of late preterm and early term. *(Adapted from Engle WA, Kominiarek MA: Late preterm infants, early term infants, and timing of elective deliveries,* Clin Perinatol *35:325-341, 2008.)*

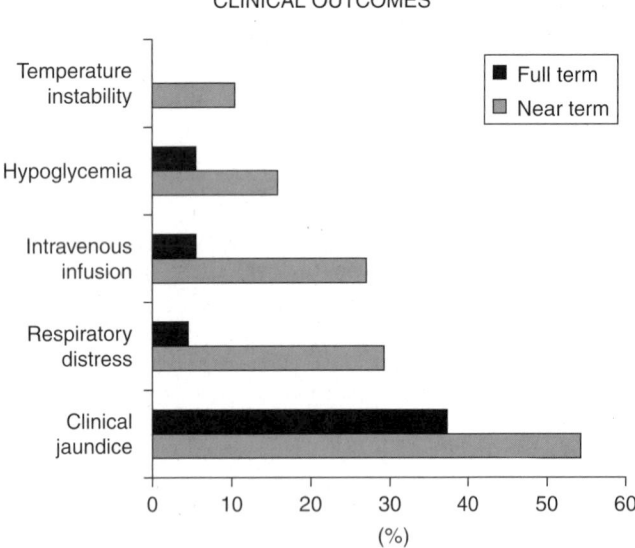

CLINICAL OUTCOMES

FIGURE 33-2 Graph of clinical outcomes in near-term (35 to 36⅚ weeks) and full-term infants as percentage of patients studied. *(Adapted from Wang ML, Dorer DJ, Fleming MP, et al: Clinical outcomes of near-term infants,* Pediatrics *114:372-376, 2004.)*

maturity has prompted the name change to *late preterm* (Box 33-1). This notion is further validated by recent studies showing that term infants born at 37 to 38 weeks' gestation have higher morbidity and mortality than those born at 39 weeks' gestation (Hansen et al, 2008; Madar et al, 1999; McIntire and Leveno, 2008; Shapiro-Mendoza et al, 2008); this has prompted the use of *early term* to describe births at 37 to 38 weeks' gestation.

The term *late preterm* and the gestational age limits were established by a panel of experts convened by the National Institutes of Health and the National Institute of Child Health and Human Development in 2005. While developing these criteria, the group considered many factors, including the obstetric guidelines that consider 34 weeks to be a maturational milestone. Beyond 34 weeks' gestation, surfactant is generally considered to be adequate and antenatal steroids are not offered to mothers with anticipated delivery (Raju et al, 2006). Unlike the smaller, more typical premature infant, late preterm infants appear mature because of their larger size, but have a higher incidence of transient tachypnea of the newborn (McIntire and Leveno, 2008; Wang et al, 2004), respiratory distress syndrome (RDS) (Clark, 2005; Wang et al, 2004), PPHN (Roth-Kleiner et al, 2003), respiratory failure, prolonged

---

- Late preterm infants—defined as born at 34 to 36⅚ weeks' gestation
- Physiologically immature with limited compensatory responses to extrauterine environment compared to term infants
- Greater risk than term infants for mortality and morbidities such as:
  - Temperature instability
  - Hypoglycemia
  - Respiratory distress
  - Apnea
  - Jaundice
  - Feeding difficulties
  - Dehydration
  - Suspected sepsis

Adapted from Engle WA, Tomashek KM, Wallman C: "Late preterm" infants: a population at risk, *Pediatrics* 120:1390-1401, 2007.

physiological jaundice, late neonatal sepsis (Raju, 2006), thermoregulation issues, hypoglycemia, feeding difficulties (Dudell and Jain, 2006; Escobar et al, 2006; Fuchs and Wapner, 2006), and risk of injury to the developing brain, which can lead to neurodevelopmental problems. These problems account for a substantially higher number of NICU admissions (see Figures 33-2 and 33-3).

PATHOPHYSIOLOGY AND CLINICAL COURSE

Although many of the diseases discussed in this section are not specific or unique to late preterm infants and are being covered in other chapters in this book, it is important to understand and recognize them as part of the unique challenge of caring for late preterm newborns.

RESPIRATORY

Several studies have consistently shown that late preterm infants have higher respiratory morbidity and mortality compared with full-term infants. Many late preterm infants develop respiratory distress soon after birth (sustained distress for more than 2 hours after birth accompanied by grunting, flaring, tachypnea, retractions, or supplemental oxygen requirement), which studies show occurs more often in late preterm infants than in term newborns (28.9% versus 4.2%, respectively) (Wang et al, 2004). In addition, within the early term and late preterm groups, infants born at 37 weeks' gestation are fivefold more likely, and babies born at 35 weeks' gestation are ninefold more likely, to have respiratory distress compared with babies born at 38 to 40 weeks' gestation (Escobar et al, 2006). For each gestational week of age, infants delivered by elective cesarean section tend to do worse (Figure 33-4). In fact, Madar et al (1999) found that the incidence of respiratory distress was significantly increased with every week of gestation less than 39 weeks: 30 in 1000 infants born at 34 weeks' gestation developed respiratory distress, 14 in 1000 born at 35 weeks' gestation, and 7.1 in 1000 born at 36 weeks' gestation. The etiology of respiratory distress is diverse and includes transient tachypnea of the newborn, RDS, persistent pulmonary hypertension, and apnea. Not surprisingly, of the affected babies, the incidence of respiratory

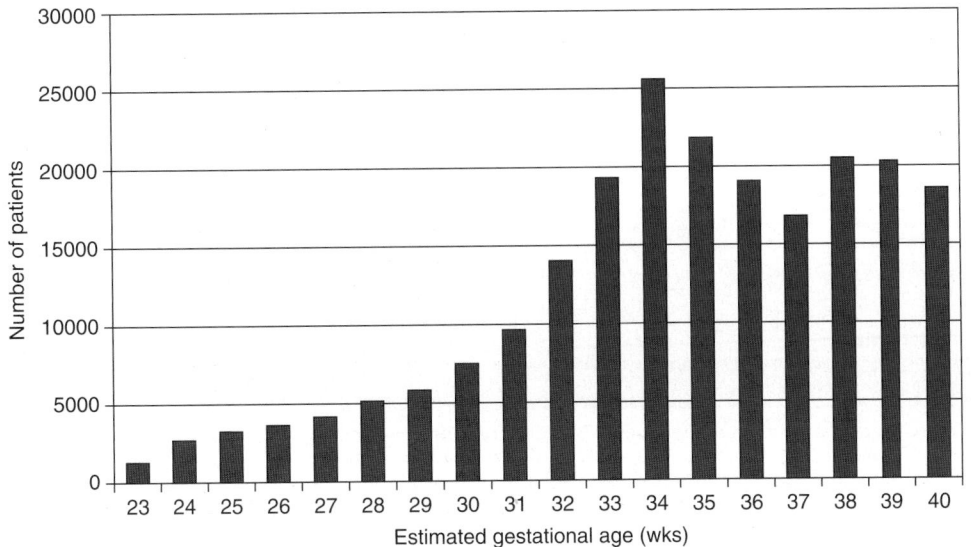

FIGURE 33-3 Distribution of neonatal intensive care unit (NICU) admissions by gestational age, highlighting the contribution made by late preterm and early preterm infants. Data were obtained from a large consortium of NICUs under a common management. (*Adapted from Clark RH: The epidemiology of respiratory failure in neonates born at an estimated gestational age of 34 weeks or more, J Perinatol 25:251-257, 2005.*)

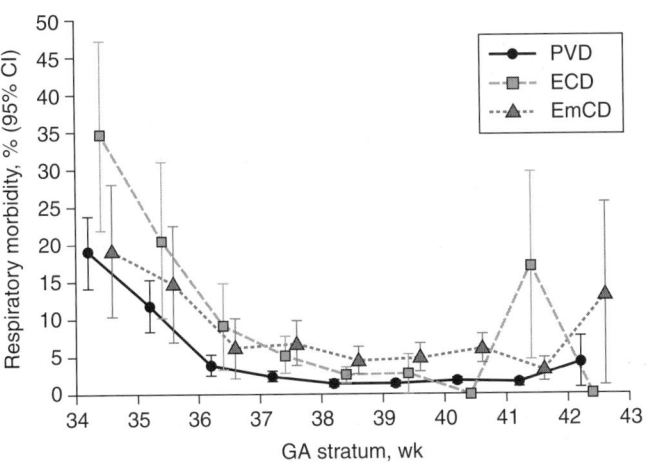

FIGURE 33-4 Respiratory morbidity in late preterm and early term infants and the impact of mode of delivery. *ECD*, Elective cesarean delivery; *EmCD*, emergency cesarean delivery; *PVD*, planned vaginal delivery. (*Adapted from De Luca R, Boulvain M, Irion O, et al: Incidence of early neonatal mortality and morbidity after late-preterm and tern cesarean section, Pediatrics 123:e1064-e1071, 2009.*)

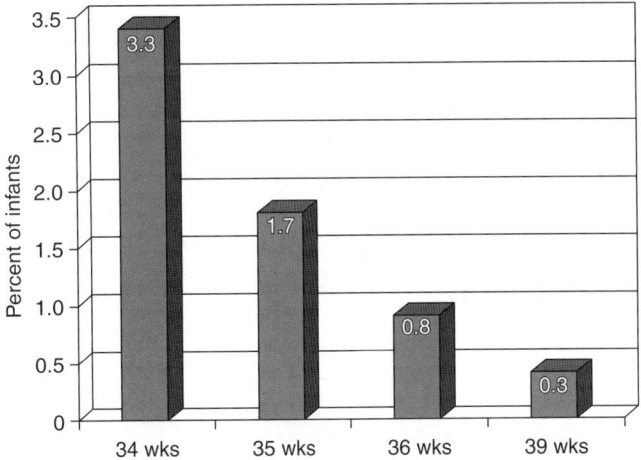

FIGURE 33-5 Percentage of infants born at late preterm gestations who require mechanical ventilation. (*Adapted from McIntire DD, Leveno KJ: Neonatal mortality and morbidity rates in late preterm births compared with births at term, Obstet Gynecol 111:35-41, 2008.*)

distress requiring mechanical ventilation corresponded to the degree of prematurity: 3.3% of late preterm infants born at 34 weeks' gestation, 1.7% at 35 weeks' gestation, and 0.8% at 36 weeks' gestation (Figure 33-5) (McIntire and Leveno, 2008).

Whereas respiratory issues often tend to be transient in a vast majority of these neonates, some develop into PPHN or severe hypoxic respiratory failure requiring additional therapies such as nitric oxide, high frequency ventilation, and extracorporeal membrane oxygenation (ECMO; Heritage and Cunningham, 1985; Keszler et al, 1992). Studies have shown that pulmonary hypertension is more likely in preterm infants (born at 34 to 37 weeks' gestation) who develop RDS than in similar infants born at 32 weeks' gestation. Such predisposition is attributed to a developmental increase in smooth muscle in the walls of pulmonary blood

vessels. PPHN is associated with increased pulmonary vascular resistance that eventually leads to right-to-left shunting by means of fetal pathways and ventilation-perfusion mismatching (Dudell and Jain, 2006). Management of neonates who develop significant pulmonary hypertension can be challenging, given the self propagated nature of hypoxia-induced pulmonary vasoconstriction. Treatment options include exogenous surfactant (shown to be effective if used earlier in the disease course; Dudell and Jain, 2006), inhaled nitric oxide (selectively lowers pulmonary vascular resistance and decreases extrapulmonary right-to-left shunting) (Kinsella et al, 1992, 1993), high-frequency ventilation, and ECMO.

A review of the Extracorporeal Life Support Organization Neonatal Registry from 1989 to 2006 by Dudell and Jain (2006) found that 14.5% of the ECMO patients during that time period were late preterm infants and had a mean gestational age of 35.3 weeks. Interestingly, affected

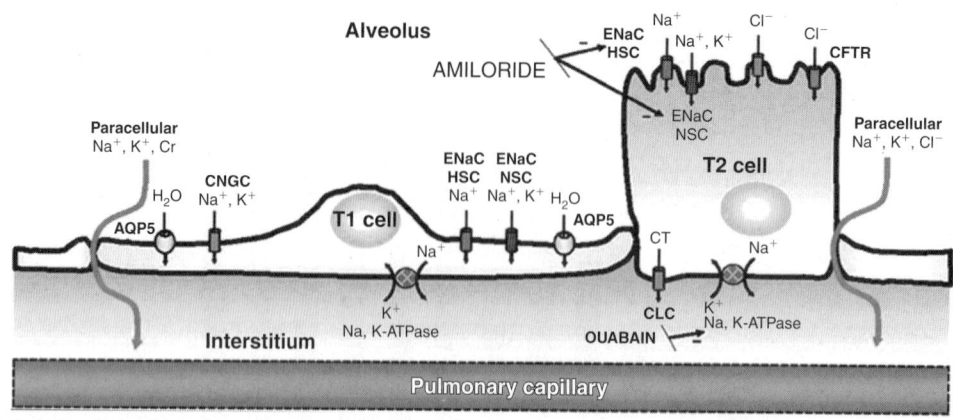

FIGURE 33-6 **Epithelial sodium (Na) absorption in the fetal lung near birth.** Na enters the cell through the apical surface of both ATI and ATII cells via amiloride-sensitive epithelial Na channels (*ENaC*), both highly selective channels (*HSC*) and nonselective channels (*NSC*), and cyclic nucleotide gated channels (seen only in ATI cells). Electroneutrality is conserved with chloride movement through cystic fibrosis transmembrane conductance regulator (*CFTR*) or through chloride channels (*CLC*) in ATI and ATII cells, and/or paracellularly through tight junctions. The increase in cell Na stimulates Na-K-ATPase activity on the basolateral aspect of the cell membrane, which drives out three Na ions in exchange for two K ions, a process that can be blocked by the cardiac glycoside ouabain. If the net ion movement is from the apical surface to the interstitium, an osmotic gradient would be created, which would in turn direct water transport in the same direction, either through aquaporins or by diffusion. (*From Jain L: Respiratory morbidity in late-preterm infants: prevention is better than cure! Am J Perinatol 25:75-78, 2008.*)

infants were more likely to require ECMO secondary to hypoxic respiratory failure or RDS instead of aspiration syndromes, which is the primary insult for term infants requiring ECMO (Dudell and Jain, 2006). In addition, late preterm infants were older at cannulation (likely because most of these infants are asymptomatic at birth, but gradually develop an increasing oxygen requirement with subsequent development of PPHN), had a longer duration of ECMO support, and were more likely to have intraventricular hemorrhage and other neurologic complications than term infants. Overall survival rate was significantly lower (74%) for late preterm infants compared with term infants (87%) (Dudell and Jain, 2006).

Why is it that, even in situations in which amniotic fluid testing shows a mature surfactant profile, late preterm infants are at risk for developing respiratory distress? Part of the answer lies in the delay in clearing fetal lung fluid. Throughout much of gestation, fetal lungs actively secrete fluid into alveolar spaces via a chloride secretory mechanism. This process can be blocked by inhibitors of Na-K-2Cl co-transport. The fluid that accumulates in the developing lung plays a critical role by providing a structural template that prevents the collapse of the developing lung and promotes its growth. At the time of delivery, the lung epithelium becomes integral in the process of switching from placental to pulmonary gas exchange (Bland, 2001; Jain, 1999). For effective gas exchange to occur in the lungs, alveolar spaces must be cleared of excess fluid, and pulmonary blood flow must be increased to match ventilation with the perfusion that is taking place. If either the ventilation or perfusion is inadequate, the infant will have a difficult time transitioning and will develop respiratory distress. In addition, during fetal development, many abnormalities can occur and interfere with the normal production of this lung fluid. Some problems during development include pulmonary artery occlusion, diaphragmatic hernia, and uterine compression of the fetal thorax from chronic leak of amniotic fluid. All these conditions inhibit normal lung development and growth (Jain and Eaton, 2006).

Although a small role in the clearance of this fluid can be attributed to Starling forces and "vaginal squeeze" (Bland, 2001; Jain, 1999), amiloride-sensitive sodium transport by lung epithelial cells through epithelial sodium channels (ENaCs) has emerged as a key event in the transepithelial movement of alveolar fluid (Figure 33-6) (Bland, 2001; Jain et al, 2001). Research has shown that these ENaCs orchestrate the clearing of fluid from the fetal lungs, and disruption of their function has been implicated in several disease processes affecting the newborn, including transient tachypnea of the newborn and hyaline membrane disease. The late preterm infant is more susceptible to these problems, in part because ENaC expression is developmentally regulated and peak expression in the alveolar epithelium is achieved only at term gestation, which leaves the preterm infant with lower expression of these channels, thus reducing their ability to clear fetal lung fluid after birth (Smith et al, 2000).

High doses of glucocorticoids have been shown to stimulate transcription of ENaCs in several sodium transporting epithelia and in the lung (Tomashek et al, 2007). In the alveolar epithelia, glucocorticoids were found to induce lung sodium reabsorption in the late gestation fetal lung (Tomashek et al, 2007). In addition to increasing transcription of sodium channel subunits, steroids increase the number of available channels, by decreasing the rate at which membrane-associated channels are degraded, and increase the activity of existing channels. Glucocorticoids have also been shown to enhance the responsiveness of lungs to β-adrenergic agents and thyroid hormones (Venkatesh and Katzberg, 1997).

In addition to problems with lung fluid clearance, several other factors may contribute to the overall burden of respiratory morbidity (Hansen et al, 2008; Kolas et al, 2006; Levine et al, 2001; Morrison et al, 1995; Roth-Kleiner et al, 2003; Villar et al, 2007). Given the shortcomings clinicians face in accurate estimation of gestational age, elective induction and cesarean section may have increased the burden of iatrogenic prematurity. In an attempt to minimize the occurrence of iatrogenic RDS in light of the increasing frequency of elective cesarean sections—commonly performed between 37 and 40 weeks' gestation (Hales et al, 1993)—fetal lung maturity testing was recommended before elective cesarean sections. Because of the risks and complications associated with amniocentesis, this testing is done infrequently (Dudell and Jain, 2006), especially in light of recent studies showing that even late preterm infants and some early term infants born by cesarean section before the onset of labor have respiratory distress despite having mature surfactant profiles. This finding prompted the American College of Obstetrics and Gynecologists (2002) to recommend scheduling elective cesarean section at 39 weeks or later or waiting for the onset of spontaneous labor, but unfortunately factors related to the convenience of scheduled elective cesarean section deliveries for both families and providers will continue to influence the timing of elective cesarean section (Dudell and Jain, 2006).

GASTROINTESTINAL

Nutrition

Feeding problems are one of the primary reasons for delay in the discharge of late preterm infants (Adamkin, 2006). Late preterm infants often have poor coordination of sucking and swallowing because of neuronal immaturity, decreased oromotor tone, and inability to generate adequate intraoral pressures during sucking (Engle et al, 2007; Kinney, 2006; Polin et al, 2003; Raju et al, 2006). Breastfeeding has also been shown to be more difficult for early term or late preterm infants compared with term infants (Raju, 2006). These problems can lead to poor caloric intake and dehydration.

These problems are compounded by the variations in practice and nutritional management of these infants, given the paucity of published studies in this regard. Recent studies have shown that issues such as hypoglycemia and poor feeding contributed to 27% of all late preterm babies requiring intravenous fluids, compared with only 5% of their term counterparts (Wang et al, 2004). In the face of poor enteral intake, TPN is indicated and can become an important therapy in the care of the late preterm infant, but is often delayed in anticipation of a quick recovery (Adamkin, 2006). The challenge then becomes providing adequate nutrition to support growth and equate the energy expenditure that can occur when the infant faces issues such as hypothermia, sepsis, and respiratory distress, which are often seen in late preterm infants. Studies show that the energy expenditure of nongrowing low-birth-weight infants (birthweight less than 2500 g) is 45 to 55 cal/kg/day (Adamkin, 2006). These calories come from several sources in the TPN including amino acids and lipids.

Late preterm infants are more adept at handling amino acids, allowing the protein content in TPN to be started at 2 g/kg/day. With a protein intake of 2.5 to 3 g/kg/day (with adequate caloric intake), a late preterm infant can achieve weight gain similar to a term infant fed human milk (Adamkin, 2006). More controversial is the use of intravenous lipids in late preterm infants. Of the late

preterm infants with respiratory distress or disease, there are two subgroups: infants with parenchymal lung disease without increased pulmonary vascular resistance (PVR) and those with signs of PPHN or increased PVR (Adamkin, 2006). The concern over the use of lipids in the late preterm infant with lung disease stems from adult studies showing that failure to clear infused lipids has an adverse effect on gas exchange in the lungs (Greene et al, 1976). Contrary to those findings, preterm neonates randomized to different lipid infusion rates did not demonstrate any effect on alveolar-arterial oxygen gradient, arterial blood pH, or oxygenation when randomly assigned to modest doses of lipids (0.6 to 1.4 g/kg/day) over the first week of life (Adamkin, 2006). The other argument for restricted use of lipids in late preterm infants specifically addresses the infants with increased PVR and respiratory disease. The concern is that the high polyunsaturated fatty acid content of lipid emulsions (with excess omega 6-linoleic acid) feeds into the arachidonic acid pathways, leading to synthesis of prostaglandins and leukotrienes, which can increase vasomotor tone and result in hypoxemia (Adamkin, 2006). Despite the lack of firm evidence for the effects of lipid emulsions in infants with severe respiratory failure with or without pulmonary hypertension, the recommendation is that infants with respiratory disease, but not increased PVR, should receive adequate lipids to prevent essential fatty acid deficiency; in infants with elements of PPHN, lipids should be avoided during the critical stages of their illness (Adamkin, 2006). Because of these issues and other concerns about parenteral nutrition (e.g., difficult in optimizing nutrition, the need for intravenous access and the potential for infiltrates or infection, risk of cholestatic jaundice with prolonged use of parenteral nutrition) enteral feeds should be started as soon as clinically possible while the infant is slowly weaned from the parenteral nutrition.

In general, nutritional experts recommend that 34- and 35-week late preterm infants receive nutrient-enriched (22 kcal/oz) milk, whereas older 36- and 37-week late preterm infants with an uncomplicated neonatal course be fed unfortified milk after discharge (Adamkin, 2006). These nutrient-enriched formulas have a higher protein content (1.9 versus 1.4 g/dL), increased energy (22 versus 20 kcal/oz), additional calcium, phosphorous, zinc, trace elements, and vitamins compared with standard formulas (Adamkin, 2006). This enrichment becomes essential to the late preterm infant who was born at 34 to 35 weeks' gestation or the older group of late preterm infants who had a difficult NICU course, where the goal is to compensate for earlier deprivation of adequate nutrition and allow for somatic and brain growth during the first year of life. These issues notwithstanding, these nutritional guidelines are not always followed, leading to variability in nutritional practices by providers. One study showed that, although nearly 46% of late preterm infants were discharged home with recommendations to use formula that contained more than 20 kcal/oz, this practice recommendation had a broad range of followers (4% to 72%) (Adamkin, 2006). The issue becomes more pressing in the late preterm infant with chronic conditions, such as bronchopulmonary dysplasia, that are often associated with growth failure caused by inadequate nutrient intake.

BOX 33-2   Causes of Hypoglycemia in the Late Preterm Infant

TRANSIENT HYPOGLYCEMIA IN THE LATE PRETERM INFANT

Maternal Conditions
- Glucose infusion in the mother
- Preeclampsia
- Drugs: tocolytic therapy, sympathomimetics
- Infant of diabetic mother

Neonatal Conditions
- Prematurity
- Respiratory distress syndrome
- Twin gestation
- Neonatal sepsis
- Perinatal hypoxia-ischemia
- Temperature instability: hypothermia
- Polycythemia
- Specific glucose transporter deficiency
- Isoimmune thrombocytopenia, Rh incompatibility

PERSISTENT HYPOGLYCEMIA IN THE LATE PRETERM INFANT

Endocrine Disorders
- Pituitary insufficiency
- Cortisol deficiency
- Congenital glucagon deficiency

Inborn Errors of Metabolism
- Carbohydrate metabolism: glycogen storage disease, galactosemia, fructose-1,6-diphoshatase deficiency
- Amino acid metabolism: maple syrup urine disease, propionic academia, methylmalonic academia hereditary tyrosinemia
- Fatty acid metabolism: acyl-coenzyme dehydrogenase defect, defects in carnitine metabolism, beta-oxidation defects
- Defective glucose transport

From Garg M, Devaskar SU: Glucose metabolism in the late preterm infant, *Clin Perinatol* 33:853-870, 2006. Reprinted with permission.

For mothers who choose to breastfeed their late preterm infant, it can often be more challenging compared with nursing a full-term infant. The challenge often lies in initiating and establishing breastfeeding because these infants are sleepier; have less stamina; have more difficulty maintaining body temperature; have problems with latching, sucking, and swallowing; and have more respiratory instability than full-term infants (Adamkin, 2006). Despite these obstacles, mothers should still be encouraged to provide breast milk given the numerous proven benefits of breast milk. In fact, recent studies have shown that the advantages of breast milk feeding for premature infants might be even greater than those for term infants (Adamkin, 2006).

Hypoglycemia

Hypoglycemia is defined as low circulating glucose concentrations, but the actual neonatal threshold value is still debated. A physiologic definition was established, based on abnormal electroencephalograms at glucose levels that were lower, with a glucose level less than 45 mg/dL being considered hypoglycemia (Koh et al, 1988). Hypoglycemia is often missed in late preterm infants, mainly because of the early transition of these infants to the well baby nursery or the mother's room in an effort to triage the limited number of acute care beds in the NICU and to allow the mother to bond with her new baby (Garg and Devaskar, 2006). However, developmental immaturity is associated with multiple problems, including decreased glycogen stores and feeding difficulties, both of which can lead to hypoglycemia (Box 33-2). Not surprisingly, the incidence of hypoglycemia in preterm infants is threefold greater than in full-term infants (Wang et al, 2004). In addition, severe hypoglycemia is a well-known risk factor for neuronal cell death and adverse neurodevelopmental outcomes (Garg and Devaskar, 2006). Therefore, if the hypoglycemia is not recognized and treated in a timely manner with intravenous fluids or feedings, the infant can develop neurodevelopmental abnormalities because the compensatory mechanisms for protecting the brain from hypoglycemia are not

fully developed (Cornblath and Ichord, 2000; Cornblath et al, 2000; Rozance and Hay, 2006; Vannucci and Vannucci, 2001). Therefore early recognition, diagnosis, and treatment of hypoglycemia are crucial to the late preterm infant's long-term outcome. It is recommended that institutions develop protocols for routine testing of blood sugars in late preterm infants. One can use existing serum glucose screening protocols for infants at high risk for hypoglycemia (i.e., small for gestational age, large for gestational age, infant of a diabetic mother). If none are available, the following is recommended: glucose checks between 1 and 2 hours after birth, followed by testing before the next three consecutive feeds and then before alternate feedings for the remainder of the first 24 hours. If the blood sugar is less than 40 to 45 mg/dL, the hypoglycemia protocol should be followed for management.

Hypoglycemia is not a problem in utero, because the fetus receives a steady supply of glucose primarily by maternal transfer through the placenta. Once the baby is delivered, this constant supply of glucose is abruptly stopped and the infant has to rely on glucose production primarily via hepatic glycogenolysis and gluconeogenesis (Halamek et al, 1997). After birth, the baby experiences a surge in catecholamines, glucagon, and corticosteroids, which play a key role in maintaining a euglycemic state. The increase in catecholamines leads to a surge in glucagon concentration and a decline in circulating insulin concentrations, which both contribute to maintaining a normal serum glucose level. Glucose levels are also affected by the unregulated insulin production by the immature pancreatic β cells (Garg and Devaskar, 2006). As a result, the late preterm newborn can experience significant hypoglycemia secondary to developmentally immature hepatic enzyme systems for gluconeogenesis, glycogenolysis, and hormonal dysregulation (Engle et al, 2007; Garg and Devaskar, 2006; Raju et al, 2006).

The neonatal glucose requirement is 6 to 8 mg/kg/min, which is a higher value than that observed in adults (3 mg/kg/min) (Bier et al, 1977). This demand for glucose increases if the late preterm infant has coexisting conditions such as sepsis, birth asphyxia, or cold stress (Greisen and Pryds, 1989; Halamek et al, 1997; Halamek and

Stevenson, 1998). Treatment options for hypoglycemia in the late preterm infant include establishing early feeds (supplementing with formula if quantity of breast milk is insufficient), glucose infusion through intravenous fluids, hydrocortisone, glucagon, epinephrine, diazoxide, and octreotide (Garg and Devaskar, 2006). The treatment choice for the late preterm infant is based on the underlying cause of the hypoglycemia. Regardless of the etiology of the hypoglycemia, it is important to have constant monitoring of the glucose levels until they stabilize and the baby is tolerating adequate nutrition.

Hyperbilirubinemia

Hyperbilirubinemia is the most common clinical condition requiring evaluation and treatment in the late preterm newborn and the most common cause for readmission during the first postnatal week of life (Bhutani et al, 2004; Brown et al, 1999; Escobar et al, 2005; Maisels and Kring, 1998). Studies show that late preterm infants are more likely than term infants to be rehospitalized for jaundice (4.5% versus 1.2% in term infants) (Escobar et al, 2005).

In general, neonatal hyperbilirubinemia in late preterm infants is more prevalent, more pronounced, and more protracted than in their term counterparts. Important risk factors for severe jaundice are summarized in Figure 33-7, *A*. A study by Newman et al (1999) showed that infants born at 36 weeks' gestation have an eightfold increase in the risk of developing a total serum bilirubin concentration greater than 20 mg/dL (343 μmol/L) when compared with those born at 41 weeks' gestation or later. Part of the reason for this increased risk is the immature hepatic metabolic pathways for bilirubin and the overall immaturity of gastrointestinal function and motility. The decreased ability for hepatic uptake and conjugation puts the late preterm infant at increased risk of elevated serum bilirubin levels, and the jaundice then becomes more prolonged, prevalent, and severe (Bhutani and Johnson, 2006). In addition, late preterm infants are at increased risk of kernicterus at bilirubin levels equal to or lower than that of term infants (Bhutani and Johnson, 2006). Kernicterus is a devastating, chronic, and disabling condition characterized by the tetrad of choreoathetoid cerebral palsy, neural hearing loss, palsy of vertical gaze, and dental enamel hypoplasia (Watchko, 2006).

Whereas the need for universal predischarge bilirubin testing in neonates is debated, it is generally accepted that late preterm infants are at higher risk and should not be included with term infants. The current recommendation from the American Academy of Pediatrics from 2004 for the management of hyperbilirubinemia recommends that all newborns be assessed for their risk of developing hyperbilirubinemia by using predischarge total serum bilirubin or transcutaneous bilirubin measurements (Kuzniewicz et al, 2009). The effectiveness of this policy was studied by Kuzniewicz et al (2009), and they concluded that universal bilirubin screening, whether using transcutaneous bilirubin or total serum bilirubin for measurements, was associated with increased identification of newborns needing phototherapy and a significantly lower incidence of severe hyperbilirubinemia (see Figure 33-7, *B* and *C*).

This finding underscores the need for close monitoring of late preterm infants, particularly breastfed infants whose mothers may not have a proper milk supply before being discharge home. Early discharges should be avoided until proper feeding has been established, and early follow-up should be arranged.

INFECTIOUS DISEASES

Late preterm infants are also more susceptible to infections because of their immunologic immaturity. The timing of the infection categorizes them as congenital (acquired before delivery), early onset (usually acquired during delivery and presenting within the first 72 hours), or late onset (often acquired in the hospital and presents after 72 hours of life). Congenital infections are commonly attributed to rubella, cytomegalovirus, herpes simplex virus, and HIV (Benjamin and Stoll, 2006). The severity of the infection and its effect on the late preterm infant depends on the stage of pregnancy at which the maternal infection occurred. With both herpes simplex virus and HIV, maternal-infant transmission is more frequent if a mother has a primary infection at the time of delivery, whereas maternal viral load is the main risk factor for HIV transmission from mother to newborn (Benjamin and Stoll, 2006).

Early-onset sepsis is almost always caused by perinatally acquired infections. In most cases, the late preterm infant is initially colonized by exposure to various organisms in the maternal genital tract including group B *Streptococcus* (GBS), *Escherichia coli*, and *Candida* spp. Additional risk factors for developing sepsis are prolonged rupture of membranes (greater than 18 hours), maternal fever, and chorioamnionitis (Centers for Disease Control and Prevention, 2002).

The third group—the late-onset sepsis—may be caused by perinatally or postnatally acquired organisms, but usually is a consequence of nosocomial transmission. The most common organisms are gram-negative rods, but sepsis could be caused by *Staphylococcus aureus*, *Enterobacter* spp., or *Candida* spp. Although the mortality rate is low for late preterm infants, infections increase the risk of complications and often involve longer hospital stays (Benjamin and Stoll, 2006).

In addition, research shows that late preterm infants undergo testing for sepsis more often than term infants (36.7% versus 12.6%; odds ratio, 3.97; 95% confidence interval, 1.82 to 9.21; $p = 0.00015$) and receive antibiotics more often and for a longer duration (7-day course 30% versus 17% in term infants) (Wang et al, 2004). Other studies show that the need for a sepsis evaluation increases with decreasing gestational age; 33% were evaluated for possible sepsis at 34 weeks' gestation compared with 12% at 39 weeks' gestation ($p < 0.01$), of which only 0.4% of infants had culture-proven sepsis (McIntire and Leveno, 2008). This higher frequency of screening late preterm newborns for sepsis compared with term infants may be multifactorial. First, records show that one third of all preterm deliveries occur after prolonged premature rupture of membranes, which can put the newborn at a significantly higher risk of infection. In addition, this higher rate of sepsis workups in the late preterm baby may be

A

IMPORTANT RISK FACTORS FOR SEVERE HYPERBILIRUBINEMIA

- Predischarge total serum bilirubin (TSB) or transcutaneous bilirubin (TcB) measurement in the high-risk or high-intermediate-risk zone
- Lower gestational age
- Exclusive breastfeeding, particularly if nursing is not going well and weight loss is excessive
- Jaundice observed in the first 24 h
- Isoimmune or other hemolytic disease (e.g., G6PD deficiency)
- Previous sibling with jaundice
- Cephalohematoma or significant bruising
- East Asian race

B   HOURLY PROGRESSION OF TOTAL SERUM BILIRUBIN (TSB) LEVELS:
RISK CATEGORIES

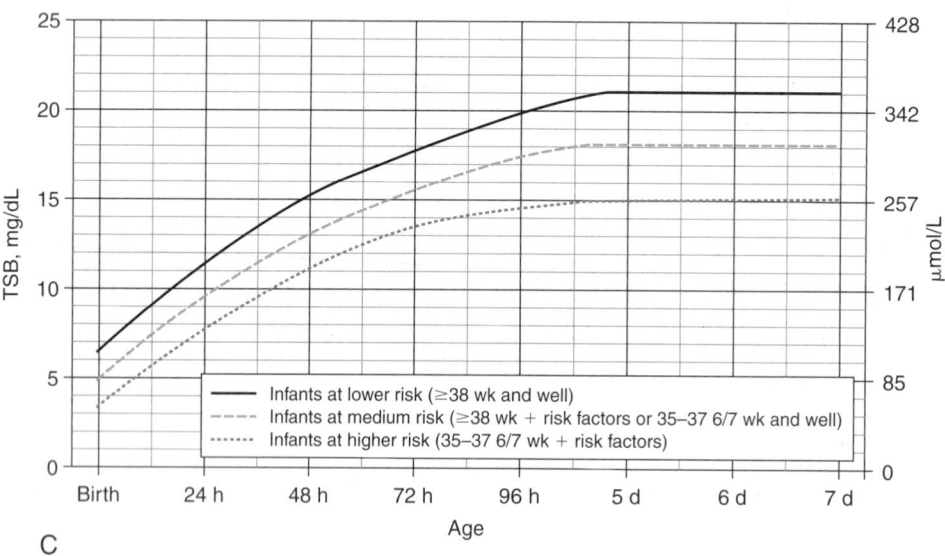

C

GUIDELINES FOR PHOTOTHERAPY IN HOSPITALIZED INFANTS ≥35 WEEKS' GESTATION

Note that these guidelines are based on limited evidence and that the levels shown are approximations. The guidelines refer to the use of intensive phototherapy, which should be used when the TSB level exceeds the line indicated for each category.

- Use total bilirubin. Do not subtract direct-reacting or conjugated bilirubin.
- Risk factors are isoimmune hemolytic disease, G6PD deficiency, asphyxia, significant lethargy, temperature instability, sepsis, acidosis, or an albumin level of <3.0 g/dL (if measured).
- For well infants at 35 to 37 6/7 weeks' gestation, on can adjust TSB levels for intervention around the medium-risk line. It is an option to intervene at lower TSB levels for infants closer to 35 weeks' gestation and at higher TSB levels for those closer to 37 6/7 weeks' gestation.
- It is an option to provide conventional phototherapy in the hospital or at home at TSB levels of 2 to 3 mg/dL (35–50 μmol/L) below those shown, but home phototherapy should not be used in any infant with risk factors.

FIGURE 33-7 Hyperbilirubinemia. **A,** Risk factors. **B,** Hourly progression of total serum bilirubin levels. **C,** Management guidelines. *(Adapted from Maisels MJ, Bhutani VK, Bogen D et al: Hyperbilirubinemia in the newborn infant > or = 35 weeks' gestation: an update with clarifications, Pediatrics 124:1193-1198, 2009.)*

a reflection of a standard protocol used for admissions to the NICU or due to their clinical presentation (e.g., respiratory distress, hypothermia, hypoglycemia), which could be a sign of sepsis or a reflection of the infants' immaturity.

THERMOREGULATION

Because of their relatively smaller size, the late preterm infant is susceptible to periods of hypothermia or cold stress. Unfortunately, as for other problems discussed earlier, this may be difficult to assess if the late preterm newborn has been sent to the mother's room or is not closely observed. Usually cold stress will manifest as tachypnea or apnea, poor feeding, poor color caused by peripheral vasoconstriction, and metabolic acidosis. Hypothermia and its related consequences can delay the respiratory transition and exacerbate hypoglycemia; these signs and symptoms may also be misinterpreted as possible sepsis, which then leads to unnecessary interventions and workups.

The reason that late preterm infants are particularly more susceptible to temperature instability is because of their physiologic immaturity of thermoregulation, which in turn is dependent on three main things: the amount of brown adipose tissue, white adipose tissue, and body surface area (Engle et al, 2007; Martin et al, 2006; Polin et al, 2003). Nonshivering thermogenesis is controlled by the hypothalamic ventromedial nucleus through the sympathetic nervous system, which releases the neurotransmitter norepinephrine. The norepinephrine then causes the brown adipose tissue to liberate free fatty acids, which are eventually oxidized and produce heat (Engle et al, 2007; Martin et al, 2006; Polin et al, 2003). Late preterm infants have decreased stores of brown adipose tissue and the hormones responsible for brown fat metabolism (i.e., prolactin, norepinephrine, triiodothyronine, and cortisol). These hormones peak at term gestation and the late preterm infant misses those last few weeks of in utero development (Engle et al, 2007; Polin et al, 2003). In addition to the decreased stores of hormones leading to thermogenesis, late preterm infants also have problems with hypothermia because of a decreased amount of white adipose tissue, which leads to less insulation, and their smaller size. The late preterm infant's relatively smaller size, compared with term infants, leads to an increased ratio of surface area to body weight, which allows for greater heat loss to the environment (Engle et al, 2007; Martin et al, 2006; Polin et al, 2003). Appropriate monitoring and triaging of the late preterm infant who is susceptible to temperature instability can avoid unnecessary morbidity, workups, interventions, and prolonged hospitalizations.

NEURODEVELOPMENTAL

During pregnancy, the infant's lungs and brain are among the last organs to mature and are therefore more prone to injury. Not surprisingly, research has shown that even healthy near-term or late preterm infants are at risk for developmental delays through the first 5 years of life (Raju, 2006). During the final few weeks of gestation, many aspects of brain maturity are still in progress. These aspects include maturing oligodendroglia, increasing neuronal arborization and connectivity, maturation of neurotransmitter systems, and continued brain growth that accounts for a 30% increase in brain size during the last few weeks of gestation (Figure 33-8) (Jain and Raju, 2006). At 34 weeks' gestation, the brain weighs only 65% of the weight of a 40-week term infant (Billiards et al, 2006; Kinney, 2006). Researchers have shown that the brain of a late preterm infant is still immature and continues to grow until 2 years of age, when it reaches 80% of adult brain volume. In addition, the cerebral cortex is still smooth and the gyri and sulci are not fully formed, and myelination and interneuronal connectivity is still

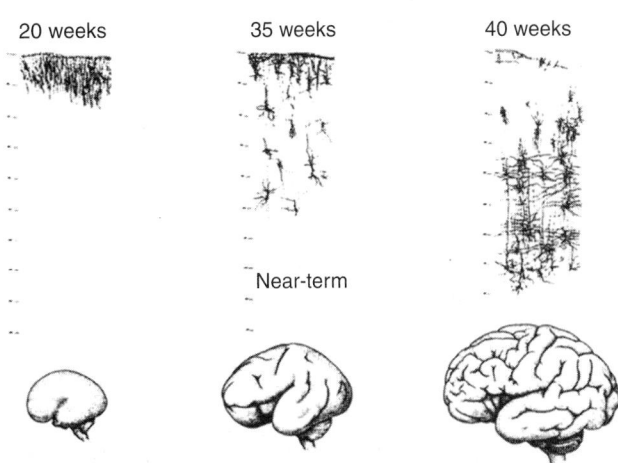

FIGURE 33-8 The immaturity of the laminar position and dendritic arborization of neurons, as demonstrated by Golgi drawings, in the cerebral cortex in the late preterm infant at 35 weeks' gestation is striking in comparison with neurons at mid-gestation (20 weeks) and at term (40 weeks). *(From Kinney HC, Armstrong DD: Perinatal neuropathology. In Graham DI, Lantos PE, editors:* Greenfield's neuropathology, *ed 7, London, 2002, Arnold, pp 557-559.)*

incomplete. Multiple insults during this critical phase of neuronal and glial maturation cause white and grey matter injury, especially in the thalamic region and the periventricular white matter (Kinney, 2006). These events can be correlated subsequently to delayed development and special education needs; therefore it is important to start early developmental follow-up, anticipatory guidance, and interventions for infants born at 32 to 36 weeks' gestation (Chyi et al, 2008).

HOSPITALIZATION OF THE LATE PRETERM INFANT

Based on the need for close monitoring and management of the various medical problems identified in late preterm infants, they are more likely than a full-term infant to require admission to an intensive care unit. Despite this finding, individual hospitals and nurseries follow different criteria regarding which infants to admit to the NICU, an intermediate care unit, or an observation area. Some routinely admit all infants <35 weeks, gestation to the NICU, whereas others do so on an individual basis. The most common reasons for admission include temperature instability, jaundice, respiratory distress, dehydration, poor feeding, and hypoglycemia (Vachharajani and Dawson, 2009; Wang et al, 2004). Studies have shown that 88% of infants born at 34 weeks' gestation, 12% born at 37 weeks' gestation, and 2.6% born at 38 to 40 weeks' gestation were admitted to the NICU (Engle and Kominiarek, 2008). Other studies have shown similar rates, and the overall trend was that the late preterm infant had significantly higher rates of NICU admission than the 39-week infants (McIntire and Leveno, 2008). In addition, the duration of hospitalization for the late preterm infant is inversely proportional to the baby's gestational age, which means that late preterm infants require longer hospitalization after birth than their term counterparts. On average, infants are hospitalized for 6 to 11 days at 34 weeks', 4 to 6 days at 35 weeks', and 3 to 4 days at 36 weeks' gestation (Escobar

TABLE 33-1 Mortality (rate per 1000 live births) in Infants Born at Late Preterm and Early Term Gestations

Gestational Age (weeks)	Early Neonatal Mortality (1-7 days)		Infant Mortality (1-365 days)	
	Mortality Rate	Risk Ratio	Mortality Rate	Risk Ratio
34	7.2	25.5	12.5	10.5
35	4.5	16.1	8.7	7.2
36	2.8	9.8	6.3	5.3
37	0.8	2.7	3.4	2.8
38	0.5	1.7	2.4	2.0
39	0.2	0.8	1.2	1.2

From Young PC, Glasgow TS, Li X, et al: Mortality of late-preterm (near-term) newborns in Utah, *Pediatrics* 119:e659-e665, 2007.

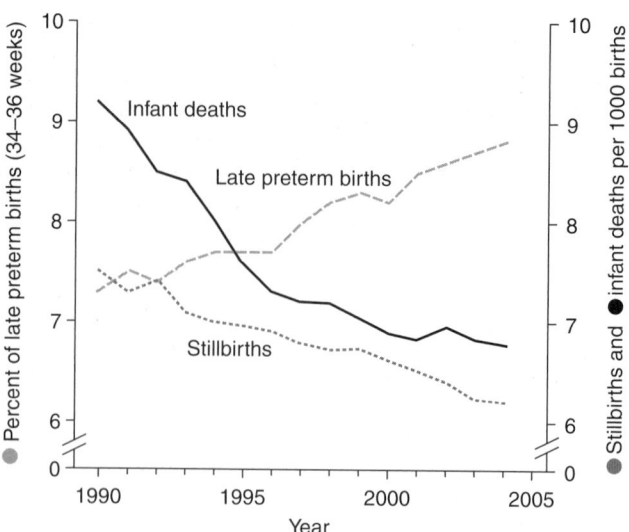

FIGURE 33-9 **Trends in late preterm birth, stillbirth, and infant mortality in the United States, 1990 to 2004.** The left axis shows trends in stillbirth and infant mortality rates; the right axis shows trends in late preterm births (34 to 36 weeks). Late preterm birth rates are shown per 100 live births; stillbirth rates per 1000 total births, and infant death rates per 1000 live births. (*Adapted from Ananth CV, Gyamfi C, Jain L: Characterizing risk profiles of infants who are delivered at late preterm gestations: does it matter?* Am J Obstet Gynecol *199:329-331, 2008.*)

et al, 2005; Gilbert et al, 2003; Khashu et al, 2009; McIntire and Leveno, 2008; Phibbs and Schmitt, 2006; Vachharajani and Dawson, 2009).

MORTALITY

Preterm birth is consistently recognized as the most pressing public health problem in perinatology by both clinicians and researchers, given its overall contribution to infant mortality. It also contributes substantially to neurocognitive, pulmonary, and ophthalmologic morbidity (Kramer et al, 2000). On review of infant birth and death files from 1995 to 2002 in the United States, Tomashek et al (2007) compared the overall and cause-specific mortality rates between singleton late preterm infants and term infants. They found that, despite significant declines since 1995 in mortality rates for late preterm and term infants, the infant mortality rate in 2002 was threefold higher in late preterm infants than in term infants (7.9 versus 2.4 deaths per 1000 live births); early, late, and postneonatal mortality rates were sixfold, threefold, and twofold higher, respectively. Another study by Young et al (2007) found that in a large cohort from Utah, the relative risk of death increased for every decreasing week in gestational age less than 40 weeks (Table 33-1). In addition, a large study involving 133,022 infants born at 34 to 40 weeks' gestation found that neonatal mortality rates were significantly higher for late preterm infants (1.1, 1.5, and 0.5 per 1000 live births at 34, 35, and 36 weeks, respectively, compared with 0.2 per 1000 live births at 39 weeks' gestation p <0.001) (McIntire and Leveno, 2008). In 2005, the U.S. infant mortality rate for late preterm infants was 7.3 versus 2.43 per 1000 live births in term neonates. Surprisingly, the mortality rate is 30% higher even for infants born between 37 and 39 weeks' gestation (early term) (Mathews and MacDorman, 2008). These studies and statistics again emphasize the fact that infants born just a few weeks early are at a much greater risk of morbidity and mortality than those born at term gestation. However, perinatal data collected over similar periods also reveal a remarkable decline in stillbirth rate (Figure 33-9). Perinatologists argue that this reduction in fetal demise is directly related to close monitoring of the fetus and early intervention (delivery) when needed.

RECOMMENDATIONS

ADMISSION CRITERIA

With more than 80% of all deliveries occurring in community hospitals (Jain and Raju, 2006), many of which have a relatively small number of deliveries, and health care teams that might not always be equipped to assess and manage the needs of a late preterm infant, it becomes increasingly important to establish safeguards for the screening, identification, and appropriate triage of these patients. A subcommittee on the American Academy of Pediatrics Committee on the Fetus and Newborn (Engle et al, 2007) outlined recommendations for the care of the late preterm newborn. Based on these guidelines and the potential complications associated with late preterm infants, we recommend that all infants born before 35 weeks' gestation weighing less than 2300 g should be admitted to a transitional nursery where the infant can be monitored closely until there has been adequate time to assess the baby's vital signs, feeding abilities, and thermoregulation, among other issues, before sending the baby to the mother's room. Sicker neonates who require intensive care obviously will need to be admitted to higher levels of care. In addition, each nursery should establish guidelines for frequency of monitoring vital signs, assessment for sepsis and use of antibiotics, and the use of supplemental oxygen. It is also important to determine a threshold (based on comfort level, staff training, and available resources) for transferring the newborn to a tertiary care center when the disease process associated with the late preterm infant continues to progress or worsen. Box 33-3 shows the recommendations for admission, management, and discharge of the late preterm infant. This list is not all-inclusive and was designed to be used as a guideline, and not as a replacement for good clinical judgment.

BOX 33-3   Admission and Discharge Criteria and Management of Late Preterm Infants

ADMISSION CRITERIA

- Admit all infants born before 35 weeks' gestation or weighing less than 2300 g at birth
- They should not to be sent to their mother's rooms in the first 24 hours until stable, unless arrangements can be made to provide transitional care and close monitoring in the mother's room.

HOSPITAL MANAGEMENT

- Physical examination on admission and discharge
- Determination of accurate gestation age on admission examination
- Vital signs and pulse oximeter check on admission, followed by vital signs every 3 to 4 hours in the first 24 hours, and every shift thereafter
- Caution against use of oxyhoods with high FiO₂; consider transfer to NICU or tertiary care center if FiO₂ exceeds 0.4
- A feeding plan should be developed. Formal evaluation of breastfeeding and documentation in the record by care givers trained in breastfeeding at least twice daily after birth
- Serum glucose screening per existing protocols for infants at high risk of hypoglycemia

DISCHARGE CRITERIA

- Discharge should not be considered before 48 hours after birth
- Vital signs should be within normal range for the 12 hours preceding discharge
  - Respiratory rate less than 60 breaths/min
  - Heart rate of 100 to 160 beats/min
  - Axillary temperature of 36.5° to 37.4° C measured in an open crib with appropriate clothing
- Passage of one stool spontaneously
- Adequate urine output
- Twenty-four hours of successful feeding: ability to coordinate sucking, swallowing, and breathing while feeding
- If weight loss is greater than 7% in 48 hours, consider further assessment before discharge
- Risk assessment plan for jaundice for infants discharged within 72 hours of birth
- No evidence of active bleeding at circumcision site for at least 2 hours
- Initial hepatitis B vaccine has been given or an appointment scheduled for its administration
- Metabolic and genetic screening tests have been performed in accordance with local or hospital requirements
- The late preterm infant has passed a car seat safety test
- Hearing assessment is performed and results documented in the medical record; follow-up if necessary has been arranged
- Parents have been trained and demonstrate competency in caring for the infant
- Family, environmental, and social risk factors have been assessed; when risk factors are present, discharge should be delayed until a plan for future care has been generated
- Identification of a physician with a follow-up visit arranged for 24 to 48 hours after discharge with a possibility of additional visits initially until the infant can demonstrate a consistent pattern of weight gain

Adapted from Engle WA, Tomashek KM, Wallman C: "Late Preterm" Infants: a population at risk, *Pediatrics* 120: 1390-1401, 2007.
FiO₂, Fractional concentration of oxygen in inspired gas; *NICU*, neonatal intensive care unit.

DISCHARGE CRITERIA

Because of the morbidities and risk factors associated with late preterm babies, they should not be discharged before 48 hours after birth. Before discharge,

while the baby is still in the NICU, the following are recommended:

1. Vital signs should be within normal range for at least 12 hours preceding discharge; this includes respiratory rate less than 60 breaths/min, heart rate of 100 to 160 beats/min, and axillary temperature 36.5 to 37.5° C in an open crib with appropriate clothing.
2. There should be documentation of passage of at least one stool spontaneously.
3. Adequate urine output should be accompanied by educating the parents about ways to assess the adequacy of output and appropriate interventions if the urine output appears to decrease, with at least 24 hours of successful feeding with adequate coordination of sucking, swallowing, and breathing during feedings.
4. Weight loss should not exceed 7% of birthweight in the first 48 hours of life.
5. Serum or transcutaneous bilirubin check—a transcutaneous bilirubin higher than 12 mg/dL should warrant a serum bilirubin check, which will then be stratified into risk category by using a bilirubin nomogram. Parents should also be educated on what to look for and what to do if their baby appears jaundiced.
6. Hearing screen, a car seat test, and metabolic and genetic screening tests should have been performed in accordance with state, local, and hospital protocols; if the baby is circumcised, there should be no bleeding at the site for at least 2 hours.
7. Hepatitis B vaccine should be given or an appointment should be made for its administration.
8. Parents should be educated about umbilical cord and skin care, identification of common signs and symptoms of illness, sleeping patterns and positions, instructions on using the thermometer and parameters for normal measurements, and instructions regarding responses to an emergency (i.e., CPR training before discharge).

If these guidelines (or other criteria outlined as standard of care) are not met, we recommend considering postponing discharge until the baby has been observed for a longer period of time and the issues have been resolved.

When additional risk factors are present (e.g., twin or multiple gestation, teenage mother), discharge should be delayed until an appropriate care plan has been generated. In addition, when indicated, it may be appropriate to arrange a nursing home health visit for closer monitoring, but this should not be used to replace the due diligence that must be done while the baby is in the hospital and the appropriate and timely follow-up with a pediatrician.

Follow-up after Discharge

After discharge from the hospital, the majority of the medical care a newborn baby receives occurs in two main settings: the primary care physician's office and the emergency department. To avoid fragmented care by multiple emergency department visits and to allow for an early assessment of the baby, it is recommended that the late preterm baby should be brought for a checkup by their pediatrician within 24 to 48 hours after discharge from the hospital.

In addition, because of their increased risk for developmental delays, these infants should be monitored closely to ensure that all milestones are achieved appropriately and that early intervention (e.g., physical therapy, occupational therapy, speech therapy) is in place if needed. Early developmental testing can also be useful in determining any cognitive delays, which can then be addressed with individualized educational programs.

Readmission to the Hospital

The late preterm infant is susceptible to many of the problems of smaller preterm infants. Because of the multiple factors discussed throughout this chapter, the close observation and intensity of management provided to smaller premature infants is often lacking. In addition, there are often more lenient criteria for discharge, which sets them (and their parents) up for failure and eventual readmission to the hospital. Tomashek et al (2007) looked at late preterm infants who were discharged early (<2 days after birth) from the hospital and found that 4.3% of late preterm and 2.7% of term infants were either readmitted or had an observational hospital stay.

Recent data suggest that the most frequent causes of emergency department visits by this subgroup of premature infants after being discharged home are dehydration, feeding problems, respiratory distress, apnea, fever, infection, and jaundice (Jain and Cheng, 2006). Whether they are evaluated in the emergency department or a pediatrician's office, it is important to have a lower threshold for readmitting these infants because of their vulnerability to serious complications. Their fragility is evidenced by their higher rate (4.4%) of rehospitalization than term infants (2%; Escobar et al, 2005). In addition, studies show that 34- to 36-week infants who were never admitted to the NICU (or if admitted, their NICU stay lasted less than 24 hours) had nearly a threefold and 1.3-fold higher risk of readmission compared with term infants, respectively (Escobar et al, 1999, 2005, 2006). Because late preterm infants are at a much higher risk for rehospitalization, they need close follow-up after discharge to assess breastfeeding and nutrition and to monitor for jaundice.

FUTURE RESEARCH

Since 1981, the number of premature births in the United States has increased by 30%. The majority of this increase is attributable to the increased number of late preterm infants (Pulver et al, 2009)—a unique and high-risk subgroup of premature infants. The identification and care of this group and their unique challenges have only recently been recognized as a high-priority area of research in the field of neonatology. There are many questions still to be answered regarding the care and outcomes associated with late preterm infants (Box 33-4). Topping this list of priorities is the need to know which babies are better off being delivered early, and for the rest, what can be done to take pregnancy as close to term as possible. Because answers to many issues related to preterm birth still remain elusive, clinicians have, rightly so, focused on ways to improve the postnatal management of these premature babies. New studies, albeit mostly retrospective, have added to

> **BOX 33-4** Unanswered Questions and Future Directions
>
> **EPIDEMIOLOGY, TRENDS, ETIOLOGY, AND PREVENTION OF LATE PRETERM BIRTHS**
> - Is there a subset of preventable late preterm births?
> - What is the effect of continuing such pregnancies (preterm rupture of membranes, preterm labor, medically indicated birth) on perinatal outcomes?
> - Is there a role for antenatal steroids in late preterm gestation pregnancies threatened with preterm delivery?
> - Should singleton and multiple gestation late preterm deliveries be treated differently?
>
> **CLINICAL MANAGEMENT AND OUTCOMES OF LATE PRETERM INFANTS**
> - Can standardized "care paths" for late preterm infants improve outcomes?
> - Optimal discharge strategies that minimize readmissions and other problems after discharge
> - Strategies for management of rapidly progressive and/or severe morbidities in late preterm infants
> - Standardized approach to central nervous system imaging and post-discharge follow-up
>
> **LONGTERM OUTCOMES**
> - Prospective studies of long-term outcomes of symptomatic and asymptomatic late preterm births to determine which infants should have long-term follow-up

the understanding of the spectrum of morbidities in late preterm infants; they have also formed the basis for current strategies to standardize management and optimize outcomes.

SUGGESTED READINGS

Definition, Epidemiology, and Background
Davidoff MJ, Dias T, Damus K, et al: Changes in the gestational age distribution among U.S. singleton births: impact on rates of late preterm birth, 1992 to 2002, *Semin Perinatol* 30:8-15, 2006.
Engle WA, Tomashek KM, Wallman C: Late-preterm" infants: a population at risk, *Pediatrics* 120:1390-1401, 2007.
Raju TN, Higgins RD, Stark AR, et al: Optimizing care and outcome for late-preterm (near-term) infants: a summary of the workshop sponsored by the National Institute of Child Health and Human Development, *Pediatrics* 118:1207-1214, 2006.

Pathophysiology and Clinical Course
Jain L: Alveolar fluid clearance in developing lungs and its role in neonatal transition, *Clin Perinatol* 26:585-599, 1999.
McIntire DD, Leveno KJ: Neonatal mortality and morbidity rates in late preterm births compared with births at term, *Obstet Gynecol* 111:35-41, 2008.
Wang ML, Dorer DJ, Fleming MP, et al: Clinical outcomes of near-term infants, *Pediatrics* 114:372-376, 2004.

Mortality
Kramer MS, Demissie K, Yang H, et al: The contribution of mild and moderate preterm birth to infant mortality. Fetal and Infant Health Study Group of the Canadian Perinatal Surveillance System, *J Am Med Assoc* 284:843-849, 2000.
Tomashek KM, Shapiro-Mendoza CK, Davidoff MJ, et al: Differences in mortality between late-preterm and term singleton infants in the United States, 1995-2002, *J Pediatr* 151:450-456, 2007.

Longterm Outcome
Chyi LJ, Lee HC, Hintz SR, et al: School outcomes of late preterm infants: special needs and challenges for infants born at 32 to 36 weeks gestation, *J Pediatr* 153:25-31, 2008.
Kinney HC: The near-term (late preterm) human brain and risk for periventricular leukomalacia: a review, *Semin Perinatol* 30:81-88, 2006.

Complete references and supplemental color images used in this text can be found online at www.expertconsult.com

PHARMACOKINETICS, PHARMACODYNAMICS, AND PHARMACOGENETICS

Robert M. Ward, Steven E. Kern, and Ralph A. Lugo

Dynamic changes in growth and physiologic maturation in newborns create unique complexities in drug therapy that affect absorption, distribution, metabolism, and elimination. Pharmacologic studies during this period of rapid growth and physiologic maturation reveal different patterns of change in kinetics, some related to postnatal age and others to postmenstrual age. These differences also provide information about varied patterns of maturation in drug metabolizing enzymes and pathways of elimination during early infancy. Therapeutic drug monitoring is used for a few drugs in neonatology, such as phenobarbital and gentamicin, when concentrations correlate with desired effects as well as adverse effects. Dosage adjustments to reach desired concentrations can be estimated at the bedside using simple calculations. Pharmacogenetics and pharmacogenomics of enzymes and receptors explain many variations among individuals in their responses to drugs. The immature, preterm newborn adds another level of complexity to drug metabolism, because of variability in the timing of the expression of these enzymes.

PRINCIPLES OF NEONATAL THERAPEUTICS

A thorough understanding of factors that affect drug concentrations helps to provide accurate, effective drug therapy and to identify the causes of therapeutic failure in neonates. Many important factors are not chosen consciously in a therapeutic plan, but have tremendous impact on its effectiveness. Because pharmacokinetics and pharmacodynamics in newborns follow the same general principles that govern drug actions in patients of any age, the diagnosis, drug selection, and administration needed to achieve a therapeutic goal must consider the effects of absorption, distribution, metabolism, and excretion on the dose-exposure relationship. When applied to the newborn, these principles should adjust for several unique physiologic and pharmacologic features of these immature patients, as outlined in Box 34-1 and discussed in detail here.

DIAGNOSIS

Effective treatment begins with an accurate diagnosis and assessment of clinical signs and symptoms. Although this principle applies to all areas of therapeutics, treatment in newborns presents special diagnostic challenges because the small size and fragility of such nonverbal patients may preclude useful, but inordinately invasive, diagnostic procedures. For example, many small immature newborns with chronic lung disease are treated for bronchospasm based on the findings of decreased air entry associated with desaturation and abnormal breath sounds. Relief of these symptoms with aerosolized bronchodilators may be interpreted as confirmation of the diagnosis. Although this interpretation may be correct, increased humidity or movement of the endotracheal tube bevel away from a pliable tracheal wall during an aerosol treatment may also produce the improvement. Therefore evaluation of any ineffective therapy should include reconsideration of the original diagnosis, just as conclusions about why a therapy succeeded should be made with a degree of skepticism.

ABSORPTION

Although most drug therapy for acute problems in the intensive care setting involves intravenous administration to ensure drug delivery to the site of action, this route is not always reliable in newborns (Gould and Roberts, 1979; Roberts, 1984). In a critical care setting, drugs should be infused toward the patient as close as possible to the site of vascular access. If a drug is injected away from the infant into a catheter with a slow infusion rate, the drug may reach the patient too slowly to achieve effective concentrations. Infusion solution filters may also prevent effective drug delivery by blocking large molecules, such as amphotericin, by direct adsorption of the drug to the filter, or by allowing a heavier drug to settle in the filtration chamber and mix slowly with the infusion solution. For drug therapy in which the driving force for tissue penetration is a concentration gradient between the circulation and the tissue (e.g., in meningitis), sustained low drug concentrations might be therapeutically suboptimal.

Intramuscular administration of drugs to newborns is generally suboptimal, but might be used when there is difficulty establishing intravenous access. Absorption of drugs from an intramuscular injection site is directly related to muscle blood flow, which is usually reduced in patients experiencing hypothermia or shock, when intravenous access can be difficult, but intramuscular doses are unlikely to be absorbed effectively. Furthermore, intramuscular administration of drugs can sclerose tissue and cause sterile abscesses or create large intramuscular collections of the drugs, which are then absorbed slowly, producing a "depot effect" in which serum concentrations rise slowly over a prolonged period. Intramuscular administration of drugs, especially for multiple doses, should be avoided in newborns. Although oral administration of drugs is preferred for treatment of chronic illnesses in newborns, this route is not well studied, particularly in acutely ill premature infants. Studies in adults show that less drug is usually absorbed from the stomach than from the intestinal tract because of the smaller surface area and differences in pH. Many newborns experience gastroesophageal reflux associated with delayed gastric emptying, which might also alter drug bioavailability. Delayed gastric emptying postpones

BOX 34-1   Pharmacologic Principles and Pitfalls in Management of the Very Low-Birthweight Infant

I. Diagnosis
  A. Limited diagnostic procedures
II. Absorption
  A. Intravenous
    1. Drug injection away from patient
    2. Uneven mixing of drugs and intravenous fluids
    3. Delayed administration because of low flow
    4. Part of the dose discarded with tubing changes
  B. Intramuscular
    1. Poor perfusion limits absorption
    2. Danger of sclerosis or abscess formation
    3. Depot effect
  C. Oral
    1. Poorly studied
    2. Affected by delayed gastric emptying
    3. Potentially affected by reflux
    4. Passive venous congestion may occur with chronic lung disease, decreasing absorption
III. Distribution, affected by
  A. Higher (85%) total body water (versus 65% in adults)
  B. Lower body fat—that is, approximately 1% body weight (versus 15% in term infants)
  C. Low protein concentration
  D. Decreased protein affinity for drugs
IV. Metabolism
  A. Half-life prolonged and unpredictable
  B. Total body clearance decreased
  C. Affected by nutrition, illness, and drug interaction
  D. Affected by maturational changes
V. Excretion: decreased renal function, both glomerular filtration rate and tubular secretion

reaching peak serum drug concentrations and prolongs the absorption phase, which reduces the peak concentration. If the total absorbed dose is reduced, the area under the concentration time curve (AUC) will decrease along with drug exposure. Passive venous congestion of the intestinal tract from elevated right atrial pressures decreases drug absorption in adults and may do so in premature infants with severe bronchopulmonary dysplasia complicated by cor pulmonale (Peterson et al, 1980). The administration of medications to newborns in small volumes of formula or during continuous gastric feedings may also alter drug absorption by binding to proteins, lipids, carbohydrates, or minerals in the feeding. When enteral drug therapy fails, possible effects of feeding patterns on drug absorption and action should be considered.

DISTRIBUTION

In pharmacokinetics, distribution is the partitioning of drugs among various body fluids, organs, and tissues. The distribution of a drug within the body is determined by several factors, including organ blood flow, pH and composition of body fluids and tissues, physical and chemical properties of the drug (e.g., lipid solubility, molecular weight, ionization constant), and the extent of drug binding to plasma proteins and other macromolecules (Plonait and Nau, 2004; Ward and Lugo, 2005).

Important differences among premature infants, children, and adults affect the distribution of drugs. Total body water varies from 85% in premature newborns to 75% in term newborns to 65% in adults (Friis-Hansen, 1961, 1971). Conversely, body fat content varies from 0.7% or less in extremely premature newborns to approximately 12% in term newborns (Friis-Hansen, 1971; Ziegler et al, 1976). These differences change the distribution of many drugs, especially polar, water-soluble drugs such as the aminoglycosides. Protein binding of drugs in the circulation is decreased in the premature newborn because of a smaller total amount of circulating protein and lower binding affinity of the protein itself (Aranda et al, 1976). With rare exceptions, only the free (not bound to protein) drug molecules cross membranes, exert pharmacologic actions, and undergo metabolism and excretion. Clinical measurements of serum or plasma drug concentrations usually reflect total circulating drug concentrations, which consist of both free and protein-bound drug. Thus, even when total circulating drug concentrations in the newborn may be low by adult standards, the free drug concentrations may be equivalent or even higher than those in the adult because of decreased protein binding in the newborn.

METABOLISM

Many drugs require metabolic conversion before elimination from the body. Biotransformation of a drug usually produces a more polar, less lipid-soluble molecule that can then be eliminated rapidly by renal, biliary, or other routes of excretion. Drug biotransformation is classified into two broad categories: nonsynthetic (phase I) reactions, which include oxidation, reduction, and hydrolysis; and synthetic or conjugation (phase II) reactions, which include glucuronidation, sulfation, and acetylation. Multiple forms of phase I and phase II enzymes exist to perform these metabolic functions. Although the liver is considered the major organ responsible for drug biotransformation, many other organs also contribute to drug metabolism.

For many drugs in the newborn, the half-life is prolonged and total body clearance is decreased compared with older children and adults. Important variations occur, however, among drug classes and among individuals that prevent broad generalizations. Glucuronide conjugation of bilirubin by uridine 5′-diphospho-glucuronosyltransferase (UGT) 1A1 is usually low at birth unless this enzyme has been induced in utero through maternal exposure to drugs, cigarette smoke, or other inducing agents (Maurer et al, 1968). In contrast, conjugation through sulfation is usually active at birth. Various factors after birth, such as nutrition, illness, and drug interactions, may hasten or retard the maturation of enzymes and organs responsible for drug metabolism in the newborn. Maturational changes in hepatic blood flow, drug transport into hepatocytes, synthesis of serum proteins, protein binding of drugs, and biliary secretion—alone and in combination—confound accurate predictions about drug metabolism after birth, leading to empiric dose adjustments (Morselli et al, 1980). Because smaller and more immature newborns are now surviving, many of these factors that were studied in larger, more mature neonates must be reassessed in this less mature population.

The primary types of enzymes involved in phase I reactions are cytochromes P450 (CYPs). CYPs are microsomal, mixed-function oxidases that catalyze chemical changes within a molecule, such as hydroxylation, methylation, demethylation, addition of oxygen, or removal of hydrogen (Leeder and Kearns, 1997). There are thousands of different CYP450 enzymes found in plants and animals on land and in water. CYPs with more than 40% of the same amino acid sequence are grouped as a numbered family (e.g., CYP3). Those with greater than 67% polypeptide homology belong to the same subfamily (e.g., CYP3A), and specific genes are denoted with a number (e.g., CYP3A5). The amino acid sequence of these enzymes determines the tertiary structure that creates a hydrophobic pocket with selective binding for chemicals and drugs. This substrate specificity creates groups of drugs, often with similar structure and function that are metabolized by the same CYP. In the preterm newborn, CYPs develop at different rates and in different patterns. Maturation correlates best with postmenstrual age for some CYPs and with postnatal age for others. Some CYPs do not reach adult activity until several years of age, whereas others develop activities twice that of the adult during childhood; therefore generalizations about patterns of maturation for CYPs are seldom valid. In addition, single nucleotide polymorphisms (SNPs) or substitutions in the DNA sequence for a CYP may reduce its metabolizing activity or completely eliminate it if the polypeptide cannot be formed.

The phase II conjugation enzymes, such as the UGTs, have several forms with different substrate specificity (e.g., UGT1A1 for bilirubin, UGT2B7 for morphine), although they are not as absolutely selective as the CYPs (Leeder and Kearns, 1997). Some phase II enzymes complement each other at birth for conjugation of specific drugs, such as acetaminophen that is conjugated primarily by sulfotransferases at birth and less so by UGT. Moreover, by adolescence, UGT has become the predominant conjugation pathway for acetaminophen.

EXCRETION

Drug elimination from the body can occur through several mechanisms, including renal excretion, biliary excretion, transcutaneous loss, gastrointestinal loss, and pulmonary exhalation. Renal excretion is one of the most important pathways for elimination of metabolized and unchanged drug. Neonatal renal function is diminished in absolute terms and when normalized to body weight or surface area. The neonatal glomerular filtration rate averages 30% of the adult rate per unit surface area. Glomerular function rises steadily after birth, whereas tubular function matures more slowly, causing a glomerular and tubular imbalance (Aperia et al, 1981). The postnatal increase in glomerular function reflects greater cardiac output, reduced renal vascular resistance, redistribution of intrarenal blood flow, and changes in intrinsic glomerular basement membrane permeability (Morselli et al, 1980). The dynamics of neonatal renal function markedly influence drug excretion. The rate of change of renal function and its susceptibility to hypoxemia, nephrotoxic drugs, and underperfusion prevent accurate predictions of drug elimination rates in newborns, which often must be measured empirically.

Some drugs, such as nafcillin and spironolactone, have metabolites that must be eliminated through biliary excretion. Drugs that are conjugated within the liver may also be excreted through bile, enter the intestinal tract, and undergo deconjugation and enterohepatic recirculation, similar to bilirubin. Although biliary excretion is not well studied in newborns, clinical conditions such as parenteral nutrition–associated cholestasis suggest that it may be highly variable among specific patients and conditions.

Transporters play important roles in removing drugs and preventing drug absorption. Organic anion transporter polypeptides provide facilitated transport of anions in many tissues, including the kidney and liver. Permeability glycoprotein is an efflux transporter that belongs to the adenosine triphosphate–binding cassette–multiple drug resistance family of transporters. Permeability glycoprotein prevents the absorption of many compounds across the intestinal wall or into the brain, where it functions as a significant portion of the blood brain barrier.

PHARMACOGENETICS AND PHARMACOGENOMICS

The human genome project described the protein structures of many enzymes involved in drug metabolism and identified genetic variants in the proteins that alter activity, many of which are produced by a change in a single nucleotide to create SNPs. As discussed in the previous sections, genetic variation in drug metabolizing enzymes and in drug transporters can have a significant influence on the relative activity of these systems within a particular individual. Knowledge of pharmacogenetic and pharmacogenomic factors that can effect pharmacokinetics, particularly with a relationship to drug metabolism and elimination, has been important for understanding ways to avoid unanticipated drug effects in adults and to some extent older children. In neonates, however, this knowledge is only beginning to develop. Moreover, because many of these drug-metabolizing systems that are subject to pharmacogenetic variation continue to mature during the first few years of life, it can be difficult to determine whether genetic variability or physiologic maturation are contributing to differences in drug metabolism by neonates. What should be appreciated from this limited knowledge, however, is that drug metabolism is often reduced in neonates, and scaling of drug dosage by simple body weight or allometrically with an exponent will not fully compensate for differences in clearance that exist in this newborn population. Clearance often varies several-fold among adults, and the same degree of variation is emerging among neonates whether caused by maturation of the expression of these enzymes by gestational age or induction of protein synthesis after birth.

One of the most prominent phase 1 metabolizing enzymes, CYP3A4, illustrates several important aspects of CYPs. CYP3A4 exists as a fetal form at birth (CYP3A7) that decreases over the first months of life as it is replaced by the adult form, CYP3A4, by 1 year of age (Lacroix et al, 1997). However, these changes are not linear, which confounds making accurate dosing adjustments by age. The maturation of metabolic activity of phase I enzymes to adult activity varies among the specific enzymes, requiring months for some and years for others (Kearns et al, 2003). During the fetal–neonatal period some CYPs increase in activity, but the most rapid increase in activity usually occurs after birth, regardless of the gestational age at birth (Koukouritaki et al, 2004). Drug-drug interactions influence activity of CYPs as well. Macrolide antibiotics, such as erythromycin and clarithromycin, and the azole antifungal drugs, such as fluconazole, inhibit the activity of CYP3A4 (Leeder and Kearns, 1997). These drugs can reduce clearance for drugs that are a substrate for CYP3A4, such as fentanyl or midazolam, and lead to toxicity without dosage adjustments. Conversely, inducers of CYP3A4 activity, such as rifampin and phenobarbital, can increase clearance of drugs that are substrates and reduce the concentration and effectiveness.

Large interindividual variation occurs for most of these enzymes and is complicated by inherited differences in activity. An SNP in the DNA for one of these enzymes is designated with an asterisk, such as CYP2C9*1, and can alter the protein structure enough to reduce or even inactivate its enzymatic activity. SNPs have been identified for most CYPs, especially CYP2D6, one of the first recognized inherited variations in activity for debrisoquine (Leeder and Kearns, 1997). Ethnic variations in these SNPs help to predict when activity is likely to be reduced or increased. For example, several inactivating SNPs of CYP2D6 have been recognized, indicating that 50% or more of Asians lack enough active CYP2D6 to metabolize codeine to morphine for a more potent analgesic effect (Ingelman-Sundberg, 2005). Study of the maturational changes in the pharmacokinetics of drugs metabolized by specific CYPs expands current knowledge of how these enzymes mature. A better understanding of the rates and patterns of maturation of different CYPs will help to guide appropriate dosage adjustments to improve drug therapy for newborns.

PHARMACOKINETIC PRINCIPLES

Pharmacokinetics describes the time course of changes in drug concentrations within the body. Although rates of change are often described with differential equations, useful concepts at the bedside are emphasized in this section. More detailed mathematical discussions of pharmacokinetics can be found elsewhere (Buxton, 2006; Rowland and Tozer, 2010).

COMPARTMENT

In pharmacokinetics, *compartment* refers to fluid and tissue spaces into which drugs penetrate. These compartments may or may not be equivalent to anatomic or physiologic fluid volumes. In the simplest case, the compartment may correspond to the vascular space and equal the volume of a real body fluid (i.e., blood). Large or highly polar molecules can be confined to this central compartment until they are eliminated by excretion or metabolism. Many drugs, however, diffuse reversibly out of the central compartment into tissues or other fluid spaces, generically referred to as *peripheral* or *tissue compartments*. Such compartments are seldom sampled directly, but their involvement in kinetic processes may be recognized from

the graphic or mathematical description of the kinetics of a drug. The number of exponential terms necessary to adequately describe the kinetic profile of a drug designates the number of compartments involved, recognizing that many more compartments may exist. For appropriate clinical application, rarely are more than three compartments required to describe a drug's pharmacokinetics.

APPARENT VOLUME OF DISTRIBUTION

The apparent volume of distribution might be better termed *volume of dilution*, because it is a mathematical description of the volume (L or L/kg) that dilutes a dose (mg or mg/kg) to produce the observed circulating drug concentration (mg/L or μg/mL). (To simplify cancellation of units, concentrations are expressed as mg/L, which is the same as μg/mL, the more conventional unit for drug concentrations.)

$$\text{Concentration (mg/L)} = \frac{\text{Dose (mg/kg)}}{\text{Apparent volume of distribution (L/kg)}}$$

For many drugs, the volume of distribution does not correspond to a specific physiologic body fluid or tissue—hence the term *apparent*. In fact, the volume of distribution for drugs that are bound extensively in tissues may exceed 1.0 L/kg, a physiologic impossibility that emphasizes the arithmetic, nonphysiologic nature of the apparent volume of distribution. The determination of distribution volume is described later.

FIRST-ORDER KINETICS

Removal of most drugs from the body can be described by first-order (exponential or proportional) kinetics, in which a constant proportion or percentage of a drug is removed per unit of time (e.g., 50% in one half-life interval), rather than a constant amount per unit of time. For drugs exhibiting first-order kinetics, the higher the concentration, the greater the amount removed during an interval of time. The following equations describe the concentration (C) of a drug whose first-order kinetics have a constant rate k (hour^{-1}), at time t, and an initial concentration of C_0 achieved after administration of a dose.

In differential equation form, the change in C with time is

$$\frac{dC}{dt} = -kC$$

The solution to this differential equation gives the exponential form, which describes C at time t:

$$C_t = C_0 e^{-kt}$$

If this equation is transformed using the natural logarithm (ln), it results in:

$$\ln C_t = \ln C_0 - kt$$

The last equation fits the equation of a straight line, so that a graph that plots *ln* C_t versus t has an intercept of *ln* C_0 at $t = 0$ and a slope of $-k$, the rate constant for the change in concentration; this can be used to calculate the half-life and to estimate appropriate dosages. Multiple rate constants in

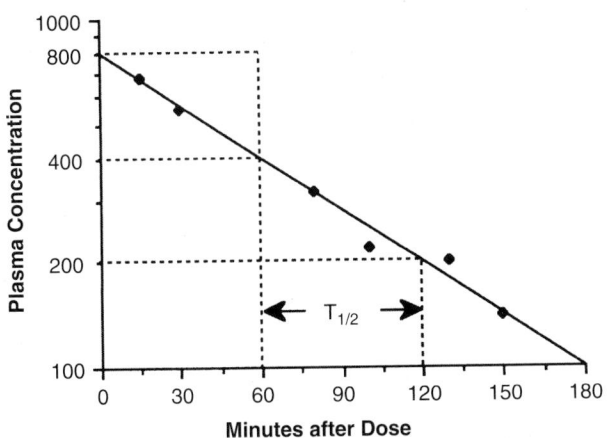

FIGURE 34-1 Apparent single-compartment, first-order plasma drug disappearance curve illustrating graphic determination of half-life from best-fit line of serial plasma concentrations.

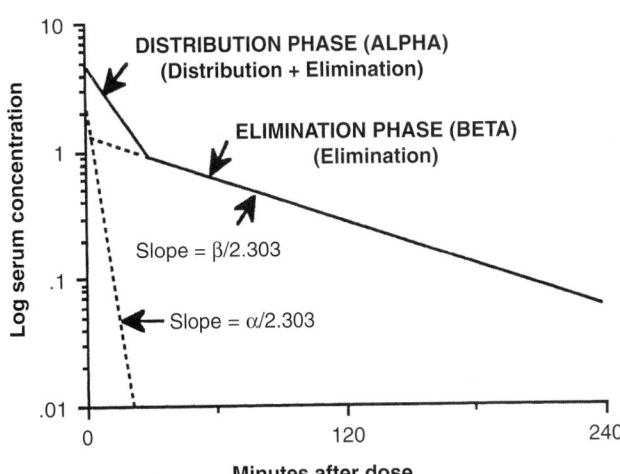

FIGURE 34-2 Multicompartment serum drug disappearance curve.

more complex equations are distinguished with the letter k and numbered subscripts or with Greek letters.

HALF-LIFE

The drug half-life ($t_{1/2}$) is the time required for a drug concentration to decrease by 50%. Half-life is a first-order kinetic process because the same proportion, 50%, of the drug is removed during equal periods. Half-life can be determined mathematically from the elimination rate constant k as:

$$t_{1/2} = \frac{\text{Natural logarithm 2}}{k} = \frac{0.693}{k}$$

Figure 34-1 illustrates a graphical method for determination of half-life. Drug concentrations measured serially are graphed on semilogarithmic axes, and the best-fit line is determined either visually or by linear regression analysis. In this illustration of first-order kinetics, the concentration decreases 50% (from 800 to 400) during the first hour and decreases another 50% (from 400 to 200) during the second hour. Thus the half-life is 1 hour. More drug is removed during one half-life at higher concentrations, although the proportion removed remains constant. The exponential equation for this graph is:

$$C = 800e^{-0.693t}$$

where $k = 0.693/h$ and $C_0 = 800$, allowing a mathematical calculation of half-life using the equation described previously:

$$t_{1/2} = \frac{0.693}{k\,(\text{hour}^{-1})} = \frac{0.693}{0.693/h} = 1\text{ hour}$$

MULTICOMPARTMENT, FIRST-ORDER KINETICS

The rate of removal of many drugs from the circulation is often biphasic. An initial rapid decrease in concentration is the distribution (α) phase, often lasting 15 to 45 minutes, which is followed by a sustained slower rate of removal, the elimination (β) phase. Such biphasic processes are best visualized from semilogarithmic graphs of concentration versus time. When such semilogarithmic graphs show

kinetics that best fit two straight lines, the kinetics are described as *biexponential*, or reflective of a drug that shows two-compartment first order pharmacokinetics (Figure 34-2). Two exponential terms are needed to describe the change in concentration over time, as:

$$C = Ae^{-\alpha t} + Be^{-\beta t}$$

In this equation, the rate constant for distribution is designated α to discriminate it from the rate constant for terminal elimination (β), where A and B are the *time* = 0 intercepts for the lines describing distribution and elimination, respectively. Division by 2.303 converts logarithms to natural logarithms.

After an intravenous dose, drug loss from the vascular space during the distribution phase occurs through both distribution and elimination (see Figure 34-2). The rate constant of distribution (α) can be determined by plotting the difference between the total amount of drug lost initially and the amount of drug lost through elimination (Greenblatt and Koch-Weser, 1975). This determination produces the line with the steeper slope (equal to $\alpha/2.303$) below the serum concentration graph in Figure 34-2. The single slope of the distribution phase and of the terminal elimination phase does not imply that distribution or elimination occurs through a single process. The observed rates usually represent the summation of several simultaneous processes, each with differing rates, occurring in various tissues.

When the time course of drug elimination is observed for prolonged periods, a third rate of elimination, or γ phase, may also be observed and is usually attributed to elimination of drug that has reequilibrated from deep tissue compartments back into the plasma. Such kinetics are designated *three-compartment first-order pharmacokinetics*. The kinetics of a drug are expressed with the smallest number of compartments that accurately describe its concentration changes over time.

APPARENT SINGLE-COMPARTMENT, FIRST-ORDER KINETICS

When a semilogarithmic graph of concentration versus time reveals a single slope with no distribution phase, the kinetics are characterized as *apparent one-compartment*,

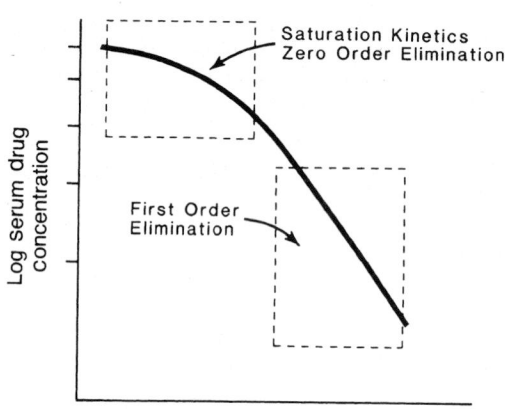

FIGURE 34-3 Representation of saturation, or zero-order (serum concentration–dependent), and first-order (serum concentration–independent) pharmacokinetics.

first-order (see Figure 34-1). Such kinetics can occur when a drug remains entirely within the vascular space or central compartment or when a drug passes rapidly back and forth between the circulation and peripheral sites until it is metabolized or excreted by first-order kinetics. The adjective *apparent* is used because careful study often shows that distribution occurs even though the kinetic curve has only a single slope. Single-compartment kinetics implies that the drug rapidly and completely distributes homogeneously throughout the body, which rarely occurs clinically.

In many pharmacokinetic studies in newborns, blood samples are not obtained early enough to allow calculation of the distribution phase, and the kinetics are described as single-compartment. If sampling begins after the distribution phase, the concentration time points may fit a single-compartment, first-order model, which determines the elimination rate constant (β). The kinetics cannot be assumed, however, to fit a single-compartment model from such a limited study. The more clinically limited but accurate approach to kinetic analysis, noncompartmental analysis, makes no assumptions about the number of compartments (Rowland and Tozer, 2010).

ZERO-ORDER KINETICS

Some drugs demonstrate zero-order kinetics, in which a constant amount of drug, rather than a constant proportion or percentage, is removed per unit of time. This relationship can be expressed as:

$$\frac{dC}{dt} = -k$$

It is important to understand when zero-order kinetics occurs, how to recognize it, and how it affects drug concentrations. Zero-order kinetics is sometimes referred to as *saturation kinetics*, because it can occur when excess amounts of drug completely saturate enzymes or transport systems so that they metabolize or transport only a constant amount of drug over time. Zero-order processes produce a curvilinear shape in a semilogarithmic graph of concentrations versus time (Figure 34-3). When drug concentrations are high from a drug overdose or the pathway for elimination is impaired as in renal dysfunction, kinetics

may become zero-order initially and be followed by first-order kinetics at lower concentrations. For drugs exhibiting zero-order kinetics, small increments in dose can cause disproportionately large increments in serum concentration. Certain drugs administered to newborns exhibit zero-order kinetics at therapeutic doses, and concentrations and must be recognized for their potential accumulation (Box 34-2).

NONCOMPARTMENTAL ANALYSIS

Noncompartmental analysis is based on describing drug exposure measured by the AUC without any assumptions about the pattern of elimination or number of compartments. Central to this analysis is the determination of drug clearance from the dose and the AUC:

$$Cl = Dose / AUC$$

If the dose is administered intravenously, then noncompartmental analysis allows the direct determination of drug clearance using this relationship. Estimation of the elimination half-life is generally done using the slope of the log transformed concentration measurements made during the end of a pharmacokinetic study. With an estimation of clearance and elimination rate, the apparent distribution volume can also be estimated from:

$$Cl = V \times K$$

Thus noncompartmental pharmacokinetics provides a simple means to assess fundamental pharmacokinetic parameters, which may be useful for dosing patients when detailed knowledge of the complete pharmacokinetic profile is not needed.

POPULATION PHARMACOKINETICS

Most pharmacokinetic studies in newborns are limited by the amount of blood that can be removed safely for sampling. To determine the kinetics safely, population pharmacokinetic approaches are valuable, particularly because they can accommodate unbalanced study designs for drug sampling. The population approach describes the concentration-versus-time profile for all the patients enrolled in a given study simultaneously, estimating population parameters that describe the general pharmacokinetic profile of the complete study group and patient specific parameters that define the individual patients in the study. The population approach can use fewer samples taken from each patient, if the samples are taken at different specified times over the complete time profile of interest for the study analysis. For example, one group of 28- to 32-week premature infants might have samples drawn at 1, 4, and 12 hours, whereas another group of 28- to 32-week premature infants might be sampled at 0.5, 2, and 8 hours. The concentrations from these two groups of similar patients are then analyzed in aggregate to provide information during both distribution and elimination phases, thus describing the kinetics with a limited volume of blood sampled from each patient.

Furthermore, the population approach allows for the investigation of patient covariates of interest that might explain differences seen within the population of patients enrolled in the trial. Typical covariates such as gestational age, gender, and disease conditions can also be assessed for their contribution to differences seen between subjects in a clinical study. These covariates can be helpful for gaining a better understanding of factors that may alter the pharmacokinetics of infants that might otherwise be considered similar.

TARGET DRUG CONCENTRATION STRATEGY

Drug treatment of newborns commonly uses the target drug concentration strategy (Box 34-3), in which drug therapy corrects a specific problem by producing an effective concentration of free drug at a specific site of action (Rowland and Tozer, 2010). The target site of drug action is usually inaccessible for monitoring concentrations. A specific concentration or range of circulating concentrations is correlated with the effective concentration at the site of action, which provides a "therapeutic" concentration range.

The requirements for effective and accurate application of the target drug concentration treatment strategy in adults have been discussed by Spector et al (1988). When applied to newborns, these requirements highlight the special problems of drug therapy in these patients and the special circumstances in which clinical drug concentration monitoring is appropriate. Some of these requirements are as follows:

- An available analytic procedure for accurate measurement of drug concentrations in small volumes of blood
- A wide variation in pharmacokinetics among individuals with the knowledge that population-based kinetics do not accurately predict individual kinetics
- Drug effects are proportional to plasma drug concentrations
- A narrow concentration range between efficacy and toxicity (narrow therapeutic index)
- Constant pharmacologic effect over time, in which tolerance does not develop
- Clinical studies that have determined the therapeutic and toxic drug concentration ranges

THERAPEUTIC DRUG MONITORING

Box 34-3 illustrates the basic assumptions of therapeutic drug monitoring—that total plasma drug concentrations correlate with dose, circulating unbound drug concentrations, unbound drug concentration at the site of action. Clinical measurements of drug concentrations usually include both bound and unbound drug, and the active portion is the portion that is unbound (see Distribution, earlier). The two broad indications for monitoring drug

BOX 34-3 Target Drug Concentration Strategy

Drug dose ↔ Plasma total drug concentration ↔ Plasma unbound drug concentration ↔ Target site unbound drug concentration ↔ Desired pharmacologic effect

Data from Shenier LB, Tozer TN: Clinical pharmacokinetics: the use of plasma concentrations of drugs. In Melmon KL, Morrelli HF, editors: *Clinical pharmacology: basic principles in therapeutics,* ed 2, New York, 1978, Macmillan, p 71.

concentrations are attainment of effective concentrations and avoidance of toxic concentrations. As Kauffman (1981) has indicated, drug concentration ranges are not absolute reflections of effective therapy. Patient response, not a specific drug concentration range, is the endpoint of therapy.

Although concentrations of aminoglycoside antibiotics, such as gentamicin, are monitored frequently in newborns, toxicity is rare (McCracken, 1986). Because of the limited evidence of toxicity in newborns, it is more important to measure aminoglycoside concentrations to achieve effective concentrations for treatment of culture-proven infections than to avoid toxicity. In newborns with serious therapeutic problems, measurement of serum drug concentrations should be used to achieve effective concentrations and to avoid toxicity. When the desired concentration range and kinetic parameters are known, doses may be estimated to reach that concentration with single bolus doses or bolus doses followed by continuous infusions.

PHARMACOKINETIC-BASED DOSING

The following equations can be used both to guide dosing and to derive kinetic parameters for individual patients.

$$\text{Dose} = \Delta C \times Vd = (C_{desired} - C_{initial}) \times Vd$$
$$mg/kg = (mg/L) \times (L/kg) = (mg/L) \times (L/kg)$$

where C = concentration, and Vd = volume of distribution.

This equation may be used to estimate dosage changes needed to increase or decrease concentration. For the first dose, the starting concentration is zero; afterward, the calculation of distribution volume should use the change (Δ) in concentration from the preceding trough to the peak associated with that dose. To reach a desired concentration rapidly, a loading dose can be administered followed by a sustaining infusion. The equation for calculation of infusion doses to maintain a constant concentration is shown:

$$\text{Infusion rate} = k \times Vd \times C$$
$$(mg/kg) \ (min^{-1}) = min^{-1} \times (L/kg) \times (mg/L)$$

where C = concentration, Vd = volume of distribution, and k = rate constant of elimination.

Steady state is reached when tissue concentrations are in equilibrium and the amount of drug removed equals the amount of drug infused. The time needed to reach a steady state depends on the elimination half-life. Whereas the time is not shortened by the administration of a loading dose, a loading dose can allow the patient to achieve

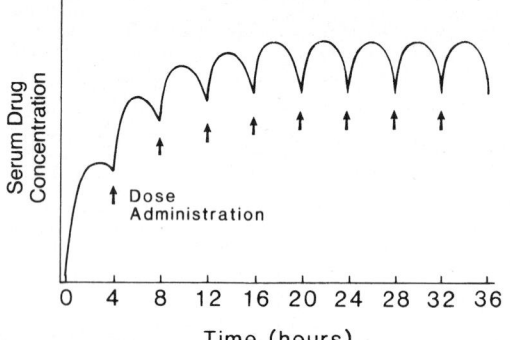

FIGURE 34-4 Representation of multiple dosing with accumulation of serum drug levels to steady-state concentration.

therapeutic concentrations rapidly that can be maintained with an infusion during steady state.

It is important to consider that if drug clearance decreases, the steady state concentration during an infusion will increase proportionally. In addition, the half-life increases and the rate constant decreases. Because concentrations are not measured for most of the drugs administered by continuous infusion in the neonatal intensive care unit (NICU), it is important to adjust dosages for factors that reduce clearance, such as kidney or liver dysfunction or reduced kidney or liver blood flow, to avoid high and toxic concentrations.

REPETITIVE DOSING AND THE "PLATEAU PRINCIPLE"

During the typical course of drug therapy, drug doses are administered before complete elimination of previous doses, and the drug accumulates in the body (Rowland and Tozer, 2010). During repeated administration, the peak and trough levels after each dose increase for a time. Steady-state, or plateau, concentrations are reached when the amount of drug eliminated equals the amount of drug administered during each dosing interval. During repetitive dosing, the steady-state concentrations achieved are related to the half-life, dose, and dosing interval relative to the half-life (Buxton, 2006; Rowland and Tozer, 2010). Figure 34-4 illustrates a hypothetical concentration-time curve for a drug with a half-life of 4 hours administered orally every 4 hours, so that the dosing interval corresponds to one half-life. Several important principles of pharmacokinetics are illustrated in this figure; the mathematics are described in detail elsewhere (Buxton, 2006). Drug concentrations rise and fall with drug administration (absorption) and elimination. For dosing intervals of one half-life, accumulation is 88% complete after the third dose, 94% complete after the fourth dose, and 97% complete after the fifth dose. At steady state, the peak and trough concentrations between doses are the same after each dose. If a drug is administered with a dosing interval equal to one half-life, the steady-state peak and trough concentrations are twofold those reached after the first dose. If the dosing interval is shortened to half of a half-life, the concentration decreases less before the next dose, more total drug is administered per day, and the steady-state peak and trough concentrations are considerably higher (3.4-fold the peak

and trough concentrations after the first dose); therefore the shorter the dosing interval–to–half-life ratio, the higher the drug accumulation. As noted during infusions, the length of time required to reach steady-state concentrations depends primarily on the elimination half-life, not the dosing interval.

CLEARANCE

Clearance of drugs, as for creatinine, describes the volume of blood from which all the drug is removed per unit of time. Clearance is proportional to organ blood flow and the intrinsic capacity of organs to metabolize or remove drug from the circulation. In its simplest form, clearance is proportional to the flow to a single organ (Q) and to the arterial-venous difference in drug concentrations compared with the amount of drug in the arterial circulation, expressed as

$$CL = Q \times \frac{C_{arterial} - C_{venous}}{C_{arterial}}$$

Total body clearance usually reflects the combined clearance of multiple organs with different enzyme activities and different rates of blood flow. Clearance can be measured by the rate of appearance of drug outside the body (similar to urinary creatinine clearance) or by the rate of disappearance of drug from the circulation compared with the circulating concentration. For calculations, clearance (CL) is defined as the dose divided by the area under the plasmaconcentration versus AUC and by the rate of drug input per Css average, where rate of input is the dosing interval (τ) and Css is the steady-state concentration. For a drug administered by continuous infusion, this is simply the infusion rate (mg/kg)hr^{-1} divided by *Css* as follows:

$$CL = \frac{Dose}{AUC} = \frac{Dose/\tau}{Css} = \frac{Infusion\ rate}{Css}$$

Once clearance is known, this equation can be rearranged to solve for the dose necessary to achieve any desired steady state concentration:

$$Infusion\ rate = Css \times CL$$
$$(mg/kg)\,h^{-1} = (mg/L) \times (mL/kg)\,h^{-1}$$

Clearance changes significantly for some drugs during fetal and infant development because the activity of metabolic enzymes increases with advancing gestational and postnatal age. Values for clearance and volume of distribution at different stages of preterm development are available for a few drugs and can be used to estimate the doses needed to achieve and maintain therapeutic concentrations associated with desired clinical responses.

Studies of the analgesic fentanyl illustrate the developmental changes in its kinetics and how they can be used to calculate dosages to reach and maintain concentrations associated with effective analgesia. Analgesia has been associated with a serum fentanyl concentration of 1 to 2 ng/mL (Santeiro et al, 1997). If analgesic treatment is initiated with a continuous infusion of fentanyl, five half-lives are needed to reach a steady state. The fentanyl half-life ranges from 3 hours in term newborns to 12.7 hours in premature newborns (Koehntop et al, 1986; Santeiro et al, 1997). Because of this prolonged half-life, the patient may be inadequately

TABLE 34-1   Fentanyl Development Kinetics

Gestational Age (wk)	Clearance at 0-47 Hours after Birth (mL/[min·kg])
29	9.6
33	11.4
37	13.2
41	15.0

Data from Saarenmaa E, Neuvonen PJ, Fellman V: Gestational age and birth weight defects of plasma clearance of fentanyl in newborn infants, *J Pediatr* 136:767-770, 2000.

treated for a long time, unless a loading dose is administered to reach an effective concentration more rapidly. In general, the initiation of analgesic treatment and increases in infusion doses of analgesics should begin with a loading dose based on the estimated volume of distribution in the central compartment (circulation) and desired concentration. The use of a loading dose shortens the time to reach higher effective analgesic concentrations, but also increases the likelihood of toxicity, as has been reported with digoxin.

Limited data are available regarding the gestational age–related changes in fentanyl clearance, but two studies show that it increases with advancing gestational age (Koehntop et al, 1986; Santeiro et al, 1997) and with increasing age after birth (Gauntlett et al, 1988; Santeiro et al, 1997). The linear graph of clearance versus gestational age from 38 neonates who began treatment within 47 hours after birth was used to derive mean rates of clearance at different gestational ages, as shown in Table 34-1.

Other investigators studied single-dose fentanyl kinetics during anesthesia and found an apparent central volume of distribution of fentanyl in neonates of 1.45 L/kg (Koehntop et al, 1986). Note that this distribution volume is smaller than the steady-state volume of distribution of 5.1 L/kg, also calculated after a single dose of fentanyl (Koehntop et al, 1986). In turn, the apparent steady-state volume of distribution after a single bolus dose of a lipophilic drug is usually smaller than that associated with continuous drug infusions, during which tissues throughout the body become saturated with drug. The steady-state distribution volume for fentanyl during continuous infusions was calculated as 17 L/kg (Santeiro et al, 1997). It should be noted that because fentanyl is highly lipid soluble, it distributes rapidly from the central compartment into the peripheral tissue compartment. This large distribution volume likely reflects the period during the infusion when the drug is leaving the circulation to penetrate peripheral tissues, such as fat. Because it may take 15 to 60 hours to achieve a steady-state concentration (five half-lives) after a fentanyl infusion is begun or the infusion rate is increased, a patient may need repeated bolus doses to maintain effective plasma concentrations in the central compartment. The best approach is to repeat the calculated loading dose until the desired clinical effect is achieved. This also illustrates why, for sedation specifically, dosing should be adjusted to achieve the desired clinical effect. Clearance calculations, however, can guide the starting doses to achieve effective sedation, as illustrated later.

The kinetic parameters for fentanyl in premature infants reported by Koehntop et al (1986) can be used to calculate a loading and infusion dose to reach a fentanyl concentration

of 2 ng/mL, which is considered an analgesic concentration (Saarenmaa et al, 2000). Fentanyl analgesic concentration is estimated for a premature newborn at a gestational age of 33 weeks (note that ng/mL is equivalent to µg/L) as follows:

$$C\ (\mu g/L) = \frac{Loading\ dose\ (\mu g/kg)}{Vd_{central}\ (L/kg)} \qquad [1]$$

$$Loading\ dose = 2\ \mu g/L \times 1.45\ L/kg = 2.9\ \mu g/kg \qquad [2]$$

$$\begin{aligned} Infusion\ rate\ (\mu g/kg \times h) &= C\ (\mu g/L) \times CL\ (mL/kg \times h) \\ &= 2\ \mu g/L \times 11.4\ mL/kg/min \times \\ &\quad 1\ L/1000\ mL \times 60\ min/h \\ &= 1.4\ \mu g/kg \times h \qquad [3] \end{aligned}$$

Two studies have observed rises in fentanyl clearance with increasing postnatal age (Gauntlett et al, 1988; Santeiro et al, 1997). This postnatal rise in clearance of fentanyl likely relates either to maturation of cytochrome P450 3A4 (the enzyme responsible for fentanyl metabolism) activity or to increased hepatic blood flow after birth, because fentanyl has a high hepatic extraction rate. For drugs like fentanyl with a high hepatic extraction ratio, the rate-limiting factor in clearance is the flow of blood to the liver (Saarenmaa et al, 2000). Some researchers have observed that increased intraabdominal pressure reduces fentanyl clearance, which is likely caused by reduced hepatic blood flow (Gauntlett et al, 1988; Koehntop et al, 1986). Clinical changes known to increase or decrease fentanyl clearance should be used to adjust starting dosages, but dosing should be adjusted primarily for the desired clinical effect.

MODELING AND SIMULATIONS

Pharmacokinetic modeling and simulations can be used to evaluate the effects of important developmental changes and disease processes upon pharmacokinetic parameters for distribution volume, elimination rate, and clearance. These models can identify clinical situations and conditions when doses are likely to require modification. Mathematical simulations create theoretical pharmacokinetic profiles for patients after a dose using the range of pharmacokinetic parameters determined from a patient population. These can then be calculated for 100 to 1000 hypothetical patients to define the expected range of concentrations that are likely after a dose. For drugs, such as antiinfectives with which serum concentrations have been correlated with effectiveness, this provides estimates of how large a dose is needed to reach effective concentrations. A recent study of fluconazole kinetics in newborns illustrates the application of this process (Wade et al, 2008).

PHARMACOKINETIC PRACTICAL EXAMPLES

ESTIMATED DOSE ADJUSTMENTS

Gentamicin and phenobarbital can be used to illustrate the practical application of the principles of pharmacokinetics and therapeutic drug monitoring already discussed.

The calculations can be performed with standard arithmetic calculators and provide close enough estimates of the kinetics for drugs with a long half-life to adjust dosages at the bedside.

GENTAMICIN

Assume that optimal gentamicin concentrations are

$$Peak = 6 \text{ to } 10 \ \mu g/mL$$
$$Trough = 0.5 \text{ to } 2 \ \mu g/mL$$

After the fourth dose (2.5 mg/kg) of gentamicin to an edematous premature newborn, the peak concentration was 5.0 μg/mL; 18 hours later, the trough was 2.5 μg/mL. It appears that the distribution volume is greater than anticipated, because the peak concentration is lower than expected, and the half-life is longer than anticipated because the trough is higher than expected. The time of drug administration and blood sampling were confirmed (an important step), so the half-life is 18 hours, because the concentration decreases 50% from 5.0 to 2.5 μg/mL in 18 hours, assuming that the kinetics are linear and first-order.

$$Vd \ (mL/kg) = \frac{Dose \ (mg/kg)}{\Delta C \ (\mu g/mL) \times 1 \ mg/1000 \ \mu g}$$

$$= \frac{2.5 \ mg/kg \times 1000 \ \mu g/mg}{(5.0 - 2.5) \ (\mu g/mL)}$$

$$= 1000 \ mL/kg$$

To ensure a trough concentration of 2.0 μg/mL or less, doses are administered every two half-lives or every 36 hours. When two half-lives have passed after the fourth dose, the gentamicin concentration should be approximately 1.25 μg/mL (50% of 2.5 μg/mL). Increasing the concentration from the 1.25 μg/mL (trough) to greater than 6 μg/mL (peak) requires a concentration difference of 4.75 μg/mL or greater. With a distribution volume of 1000 mL/kg, a dose of 4.75 mg/kg should raise the concentration from a trough of 1.25 μg/mL to a peak of 6.00 μg/mL. In one half-life, this concentration will decrease to 3.0 μg/mL, and in two half-lives or 36 hours to 1.5 μg/mL. An additional 4.75-mg/kg dose will raise the peak concentration to 6.25 μg/mL, which will fall to 3.12 μg/mL in one half-life and 1.6 μg/mL in two half-lives. The variation between the peak and trough concentrations after the last dose is within the measurement error for gentamicin and should achieve the optimum concentrations defined previously.

PHENOBARBITAL

Seizures that were difficult to control developed in a 3.6-kg asphyxiated newborn. Seizures continued after two 20-mg/kg phenobarbital doses until an additional 10-mg/kg dose was administered. A maintenance dose of 7 mg/kg per day was started 24 hours after the loading doses were administered. At 10 days, the child was increasingly somnolent. The phenobarbital level measured in a blood specimen taken 2 hours after administration of the oral maintenance dose was 50 μg/mL. Additional doses were withheld, and the phenobarbital concentration was checked daily. The results were as follows:

- 24 hours: 40 μg/mL
- 48 hours: 31 μg/mL
- 72 hours: 25 μg/mL
- 96 hours: 21 μg/mL

The maintenance dose (7 mg/kg) was resumed immediately after the 21 μg/mL concentration was measured and produced a peak concentration of 30 μg/mL after administration of the dose. These concentrations and doses can be used to calculate the volume of distribution and a dose to maintain the phenobarbital concentration between 20 and 30 μg/mL as follows:

$$Vd \ (L/kg) = \frac{Dose \ (mg/kg)}{\Delta C \ (\mu g/mL = mg/L)}$$

$$= \frac{7.0 \ (mg/kg)}{(30 - 21) \ (mg/L)}$$

$$= \frac{7 \ mg/kg}{9 \ mg/L}$$

$$= 0.78 \ L/kg$$

Half-life can be determined from inspection, because the concentration decreased from 50 to 25 μg/mL in 72 hours; therefore it should take 72 hours for the concentration to decrease by one half-life from 30 to 15 μg/mL. The concentration will decrease approximately 5 μg/mL every 24 hours, or one third of a half-life. Dividing the half-life into fractions is an approximation because it estimates the change in concentration as linear rather than exponential. To be more accurate, the concentration decreases 59% in half of one half-life. Although this approximation violates certain principles of pharmacokinetics, it allows estimation of the change in concentration for each one third of a half-life as one third of the change during one half-life. Therefore the concentration decreases approximately 5 μg/mL in 24 hours. The following approach can be used to estimate the daily phenobarbital dose needed to return the concentration to 30 μg/mL, a change in concentration of 5 μg/mL:

$$\Delta C \ (mg/L) = \frac{Dose \ (mg/kg)}{Vd \ (L/kg)}$$

$$5 \ mg/L = \frac{Dose \ (mg/kg)}{0.78 \ L/kg}$$

$$3.6 \ mg/kg = Dose \ (mg/kg)$$

DRUG-INDUCED ILLNESS

The extensive exposure of newborns to drugs in the NICU is not benign. Neonates in the NICU have higher rates of medication errors and potential adverse error rates (91 in 100 admissions) than do neonates in other areas of the hospital, and physician orders are responsible for 74% of errors and 79% of potential errors (Kaushal et al, 2001). Physician reviewers judged more than 90% of these errors to be preventable, and 16% were potentially life-threatening or fatal (e.g., heparin and digoxin overdoses).

Similar problems have been observed worldwide (Kunac et al, 2009). The causes of this drug-related morbidity and mortality are complex. Pharmacologic studies in pediatric patients are difficult because of a variety of problems ranging from ethics to study design (Ward and Green, 1988). The difficulty of studying therapeutics in the newborn has created a situation in which a plethora of drugs is administered with a paucity of pharmacologic data. For the smaller and more immature newborns who are now surviving, gestational age–appropriate pharmacologic data for efficacy, dose-response, and kinetics for most drugs remain limited and need further study (Ward and Kern, 2009).

Furthermore, drug-induced illness is seldom considered in newborns. Failure to recognize drug-induced illness in the newborn often leads to further pharmacologic treatment as the first approach to correct unrecognized drug-induced problems. This fact may reflect an expectation that drug therapy is usually effective and safe. Prudent management of newborns must recognize and weigh the potential benefits of unstudied drug therapy against potential drug-induced adverse effects, morbidity, and mortality. Some examples from the history of drug-induced mortality and morbidity in newborns should serve as a reminder of how more harm than good may accrue from uncontrolled or unstudied drug therapy in the NICU.

LESSONS FROM CHLORAMPHENICOL

Chloramphenicol was released for use in the 1940s, and reports of its efficacy for treatment of *Salmonella* spp. infections included pediatric patients. The manufacturer recommended doses of 50 to 100 mg/kg per day for patients weighing 15 kg or less. When Sutherland (1959) reported three cases of sudden death in newborns treated with high doses of chloramphenicol (up to 230 mg/kg per day), the drug was considered "well tolerated and nontoxic." Later the same year, Burns et al (1959) reported the disturbing results of a controlled trial of the following four prophylactic treatment regimens for newborn sepsis: (1) no treatment, (2) chloramphenicol alone, (3) penicillin and streptomycin, and (4) penicillin, streptomycin, and chloramphenicol. The groups that received chloramphenicol (100 to 165 mg/kg per day), in regimens 2 and 4, had overall mortality rates of 60% and 68%, respectively, whereas groups receiving regimens 1 and 3 had mortality rates of 19% and 18%, respectively. The deaths of these newborns demonstrated the stereotyped sequence of symptoms and signs caused by chloramphenicol, designated the *gray syndrome*, which consisted of abdominal distention with or without emesis, poor peripheral perfusion and cyanosis, vasomotor collapse, irregular respirations, and death within hours of the onset of these symptoms. Weiss et al (1960) attributed the gray syndrome in newborns to high concentrations of chloramphenicol secondary to its prolonged half-life in newborns who received dosages of more than 100 mg/kg per day, which are usually used in older children. They recommended maximum doses of 50 mg/kg per day in term infants younger than 1 month, half that dose for premature infants, and careful monitoring of chloramphenicol blood concentrations.

The discovery and explanation of chloramphenicol toxicity in newborns illustrate several important aspects of neonatal pharmacology. Because chloramphenicol was considered well tolerated in older children and adults, it was regarded as nontoxic for newborns. Chloramphenicol was so effective in newborns that higher doses were used without pharmacokinetic study. Higher doses were administered to newborns despite recognition that its clearance required glucuronide conjugation, which was known to be immature in newborns. The unexpected finding that chloramphenicol in doses of 100 to 165 mg/kg per day could be lethal to newborns was demonstrated because the study conducted by Burns et al (1959) included appropriate control groups. Because the mortality rate from the most effective antibiotic treatment regimen was equivalent to that of no antibiotic treatment, these investigators discontinued prophylactic use of antibiotics in the nursery.

Similar pharmacologic comparisons are needed for other drugs used in newborns. Additional thoughtful consideration should be given to clinicians' response to therapeutic failure. Fewer drugs and lower doses may be safer and more effective than additional drugs in higher dosages.

REDUCTION AND PREVENTION OF MEDICATION ERRORS IN NEWBORN CARE

Drug treatment is one of the most common approaches used in the care of sick newborns. At Primary Children's Medical Center 35-bed NICU in Salt Lake City, Utah, with an average of 785 patient-days per month, patients receive an average of 8700 (range 6990 to 11,290) doses of medications, pharmacy-formulated intravenous solutions, and aerosols each month (unpublished observations, 1994). These doses are usually prepared by pharmacists and administered by nurses, respiratory therapists, and (rarely) physicians. In such a large and complex system that produces so many drug treatments per month, errors are virtually inevitable despite several levels of prospective and redundant reviews by nurses, pharmacists, and NICU unit secretaries involved in the drug treatment process. At Primary Children's NICU, the medication error rate averages 0.04% for nurses and pharmacists and 0.07% for physicians (unpublished observations, 1994). Many errors are inconsequential, whereas others have serious adverse effects. Medication errors incur significant costs, ranging from the obvious ones such as direct patient injury, prolonged hospital stays, and additional corrective treatments to the more subtle costs associated with monitoring and regulation of medication use within hospitals (ASHP, 1995).

In a study of 393 malpractice claims reported to the Physician Insurers Association of America, the second-most common cause of malpractice claims was drug errors (Physician Insurers Association of America, 1993). Among 16 medical specialties with two or more claims, pediatric practice ranked sixth in the number of claims, yet it had the third highest average cost per indemnity. The medications most frequently involved in all claims were antibiotics, glucocorticoids, narcotic or non-narcotic analgesics, and narcotic antagonists. In pediatric practice, the medications most frequently involved were vaccines (diphtheria-pertussis-tetanus) and bronchodilators (theophylline). In the Physician Insurers Association of America review

(Physician Insurers Association of America, 1993), the five most common causes of drug errors were as follows:

- Incorrect doses
- Medications that were inappropriate for the medical condition
- Failure to monitor for drug side effects
- Failure of communication between physician and patient
- Failure to monitor drug levels

The primary opportunity for prevention of these five most common errors rests with the prescribing physician. Additional information and time for communication and documentation may be needed.

Prescriptions and drug orders are a means of communicating, but clinicians often devote too little attention to making them legible, clear, and unambiguous (ASHP guidelines on preventing medication errors in hospitals, 1993). Physicians should keep the following recommendations in mind to ensure that their medication orders communicate more effectively:

- Write instructions in full rather than with abbreviations.
- Avoid vague instructions (e.g., "take as directed").
- Specify exact dose strengths.
- Avoid abbreviations of drug names (e.g., *MS* could mean morphine sulfate or magnesium sulfate).
- Avoid *U* as an abbreviation for units, because the *U* may be mistaken for a 0 (zero).
- Avoid trailing zeroes (e.g., 5.0 mg).
- Use leading zeroes (e.g., 0.5 mg).
- Minimize the use of verbal orders.
- Ensure that prescriptions and signatures are legible, even if it means printing the name that corresponds to the signature.

The process for ordering, preparing, dispensing, and administering medications in an ICU with acutely ill patients is often complicated and may contribute directly to errors. The frequency of those errors, however, may be reduced in almost every NICU. Although complex and expensive computerized systems may help reduce medication errors, caregivers can take steps that are completely within their control to reduce medication errors without waiting for changes in the entire pharmacy process within the hospital (ASHP guidelines on preventing medication errors in hospitals, 1993).

DRUG EXCRETION IN BREAST MILK

The excretion of drugs in breast milk remains a source of confusion and concern for many physicians and families. Newer analytic techniques and more thorough pharmacokinetic studies have improved the available data in this area of neonatal pharmacology. The available data regarding drug exposure of the newborn through human milk have been organized, in decreasing levels of concern, from drugs that are associated with adverse effects on the infant during nursing to those that are of concern pharmacologically to those that have not been associated with problems during nursing. The list of drugs clearly contraindicated during nursing is surprisingly short (American Academy of Pediatrics, Committee on Drugs, 2001). On average, the breastfeeding infant receives approximately 2% to 3% of a maternal dose through milk. Drugs that are organic bases or are lipid soluble may reach higher concentrations in milk than in maternal serum.

SUMMARY

The extensive drug exposure of the sick newborn in the NICU is dangerous because of the frequency of adverse, sometimes fatal, drug reactions. Unfortunately, in the rapidly changing fetus and newborn, drug therapy is often empiric because of a lack of gestational age–appropriate kinetic data. Methods appropriate for the study of therapeutics in newborns present unique difficulties, but a review by Ward and Green (1988) may provide assistance for investigators. Drug therapy of newborns requires practical application of the principles of pharmacokinetics and pharmacodynamics—which describe the processes of drug absorption, distribution, metabolism, and excretion—to the estimation and individualization of dosages.

SUGGESTED READINGS

American Academy of Pediatrics: Committee on Drugs: The transfer of drugs and other chemicals into human breast milk, *Pediatrics* 108:776-789, 2001.

ASHP guidelines on preventing medication errors in hospitals: *Am J Hosp Pharm* 50:305-314, 1993.

Buxton ILO: Pharmacokinetics and pharmacodynamics: the dynamics of drug absorption, distribution, action, and elimination, In Brunton LL, Lazo JS, Parker KL, editors: *Goodman and Gilman's the pharmacological basis of therapeutics*, ed 11, New York, 2006, McGraw-Hill, pp 1-39.

Ingelman-Sundberg M: Genetic polymorphisms of cytochrome P450 2D6 (CYP2D6): clinical consequences, evolutionary aspects and functional diversity, *Pharmacogenomics J* 5:6-13, 2005.

Kaushal R, Bates DW, Landrigan C, et al: Medication errors and adverse drug events in pediatric inpatients, *J Am Med Assoc* 285:2114-2120, 2001.

Kearns GL, Abdel-Rahman SM, Alander SW, et al: Developmental pharmacology—drug disposition, action, and therapy in infants and children, *N Engl J Med* 349:1157-1167, 2003.

Kunac DL, Kennedy J, Austin N, et al: Incidence, preventability, and impact of Adverse Drug Events (ADEs) and potential ADEs in hospitalized children in New Zealand: a prospective observational cohort study, *Paediatr Drugs* 11:153-160, 2009.

Lacroix D, Sonnier M, Moncion A, et al: Expression of CYP3A in the human liver—evidence that the shift between CYP3A7 and CYP3A4 occurs immediately after birth, *Eur J Biochem* 247:625-634, 1997.

Leeder JS, Kearns GL: Pharmacogenetics in pediatrics. Implications for practice, *Pediatr Clin North Am* 44:55-77, 1997.

McCracken GH: Aminoglycoside toxicity in infants and children, *Am J Med* 80(Suppl 6B):172-178, 1986.

Rowland M, Tozer TN: *Clinical pharmacokinetics and pharmacodynamics: concepts and applications*, Baltimore, 2010, Williams and Wilkins.

Spector R, Park GD, Johnson GF, et al: Therapeutic drug monitoring, *Clin Pharmacol Ther* 43:345-353, 1988.

Wade KC, Wu D, Kaufman DA, et al: Population pharmacokinetics of fluconazole in young infants, *Antimicrob Ag Chemo* 52:4043-4049, 2008.

Ward RM, Lugo RA: Drug therapy in the newborn, In MacDonald MG, Seshia MMK, Mullett MD, editors: *Avery's neonatology: pathophysiology and management of the newborn*, ed 6, Philadelphia, 2005, Lippincott Williams and Wilkins, pp 1507-1556.

Complete references used in this text can be found online at www.expertconsult.com

NEONATAL PAIN AND STRESS: ASSESSMENT AND MANAGEMENT

Dennis E. Mayock and Christine A. Gleason

Relief of human suffering is one of the most important goals of all health care providers. Advances in neonatology have significantly improved neonatal morbidity and mortality, but pain, discomfort, and stress remain sad realities for babies in the neonatal intensive care unit (NICU). Assessing, managing, and trying to limit these clinical realities, particularly while caring for critically ill neonates, are challenging and increasingly controversial. Fortunately there has been considerable clinical and laboratory research and much clinical dialogue aimed at developing the best clinical practices in this problematic arena. This chapter describes the developmental biology, history, and public policies that have informed and shaped current clinical practices; it also summarizes relevant clinical and basic research regarding clinical assessment tools and both pharmacologic and nonpharmacologic management approaches. Finally, future directions in this field are discussed.

HISTORY AND DEVELOPMENT OF PUBLIC POLICIES

HISTORICAL TIMELINE: NEONATAL PAIN MANAGEMENT

Like all challenging medical issues, it is important to know the history and current practice of neonatal pain management to understand what direction research should take in the future. Management of neonatal pain and stress serves as an excellent example of this philosophy; therefore a brief history of neonatal pain management follows, beginning with the isolation of morphine from the opium poppy, which has been used to treat pain since approximately 3500 BC.

- 1806: Morphine (named for Morpheus, god of dreams) isolated from opium poppy by Friedrich Serturner (a pharmacist) and used to treat pain
- 1960s to 1980s: Infants believed to be too immature to feel pain; adverse effects of anesthetics feared; Liverpool method (pancuronium only, no anesthesia) used widely for patent ductus arteriosus (PDA) ligation in premature infants
- 1985: Landmark paper published by Anand et al (1985) describing adverse physiologic effects of Liverpool method and improved outcomes using anesthesia for PDA ligation; anesthesia and postoperative pain medication begin to become more widely used in neonatal care
- 1987: Joint statement issued by the American Academy of Pediatrics (AAP) and American Society of Anesthesiologists (ASA) regarding safety of (and necessity for) operative anesthesia and postoperative analgesia for neonates, regardless of their age or maturity
- 1990s: Use of morphine infusions in the NICU expands from operative and postoperative pain relief to include

preemptive sedation, particularly during mechanical ventilation
- 1999: Pilot study (NOPAIN) suggesting that neurologic outcome is improved if preemptive morphine infusions are used in a neonate receiving mechanical ventilation
  2000: AAP and Canadian Pediatric Society issue joint statement regarding neonatal pain management; primarily directed at surgical anesthesia and postoperative and procedural pain assessment and relief (American Academy of Pediatrics Committees on Fetus and Newborn and on Drugs, Sections on Anesthesiology and on Surgery et al, 2000)
- 2001: International evidence-based group develops consensus guidelines for prevention and management of neonatal pain, most of which are pharmacologically based
- 2003: The Joint Commission issues mandate regarding pain assessment and management in all hospitalized patients, including neonates
- 2004: Cochrane Review (Stevens et al, 2004) supports use of oral sucrose for procedural analgesia
- 2004: NEOPAIN trial results published (*Neurologic Outcomes and Pre-emptive Analgesia in Neonates*), concluding that preemptive morphine infusion did not improve outcomes in neonates receiving ventilation and did not relieve procedural pain
- 2005: Cochrane Review (Bellù et al, 2005) states "There is insufficient evidence to recommend routine use of opioids in mechanically-ventilated newborns."
- 2005: Lee et al (2005) conclude that "fetal perception of pain is unlikely before the 3rd trimester" and "little or no evidence addresses the effectiveness of direct fetal anesthetic or analgesic techniques."
- 2006: Cochrane Review (Shah et al, 2006) recommends breastfeeding or oral breast milk for neonatal procedural pain
- 2009: More than 40 infant pain assessment tools available around the world; most were developed for research and have not been validated for clinical use
- 2009: First national practice guidelines developed in Italy for procedural pain management for NICU patients

DEVELOPMENT OF PUBLIC POLICY

Since the late 1980s, in response to a public outcry regarding the recognition and management of pain in hospitalized patients, mandates have been promulgated by the U.S. Department of Health and Human Services, The Joint Commission, and other professional organizations. The initial public policy statement regarding pain management for neonates undergoing surgical interventions was issued as a joint communication by the AAP and the ASA

(American Academy of Pediatrics Committees on Fetus and Newborn and on Drugs, Sections on Anesthesiology and on Surgery, 1987; American Society of Anesthesiologists, 1987). This statement made it clear that anesthesia and analgesia could be given relatively safely to neonates despite their age or cortical immaturity. A second influential document was issued by the Acute Pain Management Guideline Panel of the U.S. Agency for Health Care Policy and Research (Acute Pain Management Guideline Panel, 1992; Agency for Health Care Policy and Research Pain Management Guideline Panel, 1992). This statement unequivocally endorsed the need for pain management in neonates. The result of the publication of these two documents was the initiation of research studies into the prevention and amelioration of neonatal pain.

The most influential of these documents came from The Joint Commission. The 2003 accreditation standards required health care providers to look across the continuum of life, including the neonatal period, at the complex nature of the pain experience so as to create new foundations for care (Joint Commission International Accreditation Standards for the Care Continuum, 2003). However, these guidelines do not provide specific instructions for assessing or managing pain in neonates. Neonatal caregivers needed to assess and treat perceived neonatal pain and discomfort, but had little research-based evidence on which to base their assessment and therapy. Organizations have commissioned interdisciplinary teams to incorporate regulatory directives and results of scientific investigation into institutional practice guidelines and standards for care (Anand, 2001; Howard et al, 2008a, 2008b; Lago et al, 2009). These guidelines include a patient's right to regular and systematic assessments of pain, interventions to relieve pain, evaluation of effectiveness of interventions, attention to long-term pain management needs, deleterious effects of unmanaged pain, and educational needs of families and staff members who provide care (American Pain Society, 2006; Bell, 1994; Carrier and Walden, 2001; Howard et al, 2008a, 2008b; Joint Commission on Accreditation of Healthcare Organizations, 2004; Lago et al, 2009).

As a result of these public policy initiatives and regulations, new tools for pain assessment and innovative methods to treat pain have been developed and evaluated. However, many old questions remain unanswered and new concerns have been raised. Neonates can suffer both acute and chronic pain. Treatment protocols for acute pain may not be appropriate for chronic pain, because the origin and resultant physiologic status can be quite different. Long-term use of narcotics and other drugs leads to drug tolerance and the need to wean slowly to avoid drug withdrawal. The drugs themselves, as well as drug tolerance and drug withdrawal, may all contribute to adverse effects on brain development and neurodevelopmental outcomes.

RECENT SURVEYS OF CLINICAL PRACTICE

Surveys of clinical practice have shown that attention to neonatal pain management has improved over the last decade, but they also demonstrate that much more needs to be done. This concern is evidenced by three recent surveys from NICUs. Prestes et al (2005) surveyed four Brazilian units in October 2001 prospectively. They found that, of 91 neonates

admitted to the NICU, there was documentation of systemic analgesia in only 25% of 1025 patient days. No specific drug was administered during arterial, venous, and capillary sticks, lumbar punctures, or intubation. Only 9 of 17 surgical patients received any postoperative analgesia (Prestes et al, 2005). Taylor et al (2006) surveyed 10 NICUs in North America to determine their use of postoperative analgesia. Data were collected for 25 consecutive postoperative admissions. Nurses documented pain assessments for 88% of the infants, whereas physicians documented pain assessments for only 9%. The study concluded that "documentation of postoperative pain assessment and management in neonates was extremely variable" and called for development of evidence-based guidelines for postoperative care and education of professional staff. Carbajal et al (2008) prospectively studied 430 infants admitted to tertiary NICUs in Paris between September 2005 and January 2006. Each neonate averaged 115 total procedures (75 of which were considered to be painful) and 16 procedures per day (10 of which were considered to be painful). Of a total of 42,413 painful procedures, 2.1% were performed with pharmacologic therapy; 18.2% with nonpharmacologic therapy; 20.8% with pharmacologic, nonpharmacologic, or both; and 79.2% without specific analgesia. All three of these recent survey studies found that despite current knowledge of pain assessment and treatment methods, most infants still are not provided any specific treatment to alleviate pain and discomfort

ONTOGENY AND DEVELOPMENT OF PAIN AND STRESS RESPONSES

The sensory system of the neonate, especially the preterm infant, is immature (Figure 35-1). Afferent input from both noxious and non-noxious stimuli terminate in the dorsal horn of the spinal cord in a diffuse manner on multiple cells; this results in the inability to distinguish between noxious and non-noxious stimuli and limits the care provider's ability to correctly interpret the infants' behavioral response. In the neonatal rat, separation of sensory input is not completed until 3 to 4 weeks after birth (approximately 1 to 2 years in humans; Beggs et al, 2002); this prevents the newborn from differentiating touch from painful sensory input. The responses of the infant are therefore nonspecific. With repeated painful exposures, infants may lose any discriminatory ability and develop hypersensitive states for long periods of time. This hypersensitivity persists even if non-noxious stimuli are introduced (Evans, 2001; Jennings and Fitzgerald, 1998). The responses are less synchronized in the immature central nervous system are also noted in the immature central nervous system because of underdeveloped myelination and slower synaptic transmission as manifested in longer and more variable latencies (Fitzgerald, 2005; Jennings and Fitzgerald, 1998).

Neuronal connections within the cortex appear to form at approximately 22 weeks' gestation (Kostovic and Jovanov-Milosevic, 2006), suggesting that higher cortical level pain processing may be limited despite the presence of a behavioral response (Fitzgerald and Walker, 2009). In addition, the neonate lacks sufficient descending modulatory control, thereby limiting their ability to benefit from endogenous control over noxious stimuli compared with adults (Fitzgerald and Koltzenburg, 1986; Hathway et al, 2006).

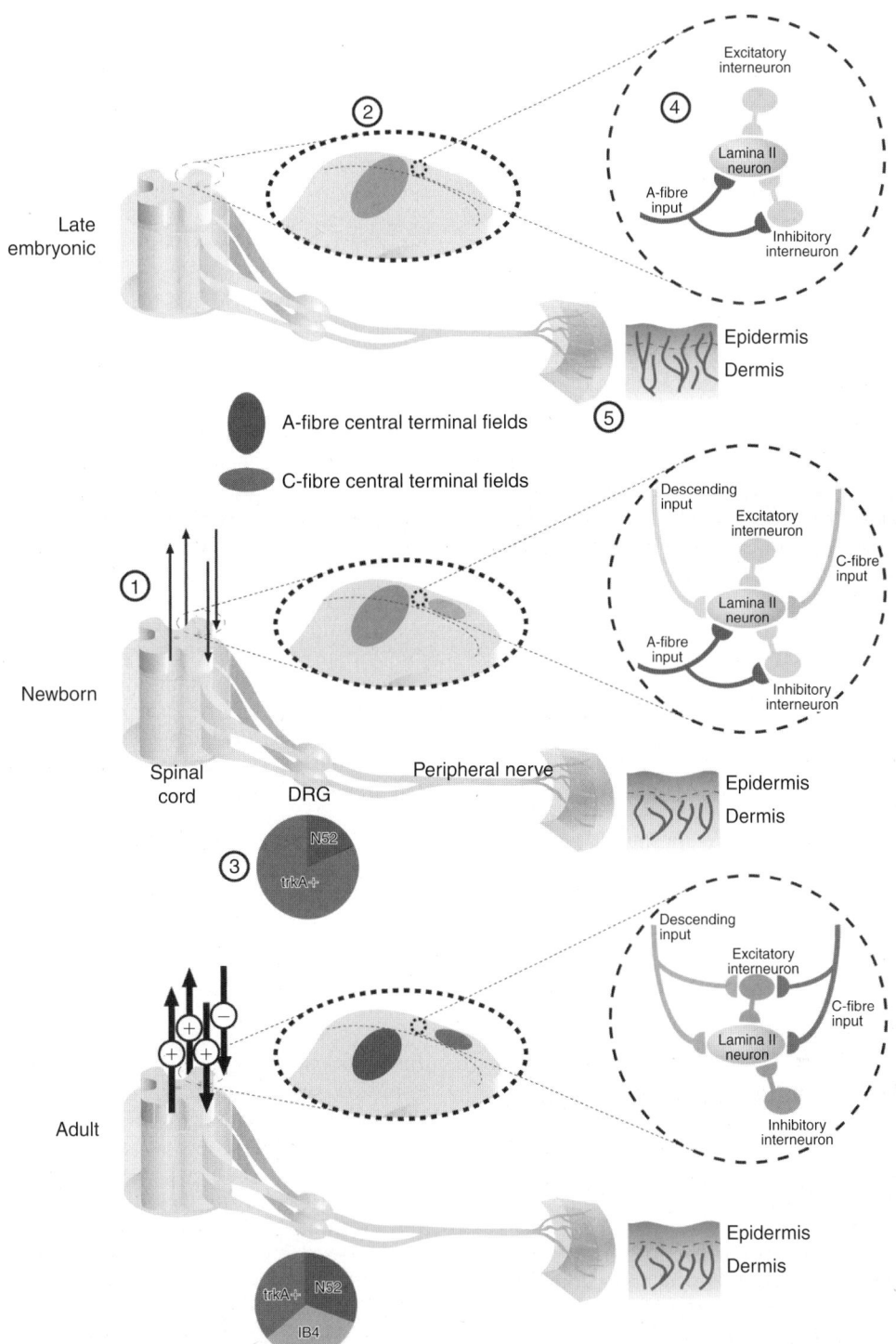

FIGURE 35-1 *1,* In early postnatal life, descending fibres are present, but inhibitory and excitatory influences are weak or absent. The connections gradually strengthen, becoming fully functional at the end of the third postnatal week. *2,* A-fibres are the first primary afferents to enter the dorsal horn gray matter and are present during the last few embryonic days. Their distribution is diffuse with exuberant, more superficial projections gradually retracting over the first 3 postnatal weeks. C-fibres are present in the dorsal horn during late embryonic stages, but only enter the gray matter 2 to 3 days before birth. Unlike A-fibres, they project to topographically appropriate regions in lamina II of the spinal cord as soon as they enter. C-fibre synaptic connectivity is present, although weak at the time of birth, with connections strengthening over the first 2 postnatal weeks. *3,* At birth the majority (approximately 80%) of dorsal root ganglion (DRG) neurons express the nerve growth factor (NGF) receptor trkA. Over the first postnatal week, this population reduces, with approximately half of these neurons losing their trkA expression and beginning to express receptors for glial cell line-derived neurotrophic factor (GDNF) (identifiable as the IB4-binding population). *4,* The balance of excitation and inhibition in the superficial dorsal horn develops postnatally, through changes in both local interneuron circuitry and descending fibres. A-fibre input is stronger in the neonate and weakens as the influence of C-fibre input increases. *5,* Primary afferent innervations of the skin occurs earlier than central projections. By late embryonic stages, primary afferents of all classes have reached the skin and innervate through the dermis into the epidermis. These projections die back during the immediate perinatal period to leave the full adult situation of dermal innervations present soon after birth. *(From Beggs S, Fitzgerald M: Development of peripheral and spinal nociceptive systems. In Anand KJ, Stevens BJ, McGrath PJ, editors:* Pain in neonates and infants, *ed 3, Philadelphia, 2007, Elsevier, p 15.)*

Noxious stimuli in adults result in the release of inflammatory and trophic factors that activate and sensitize nociceptors in the injured tissue. Such noxious stimuli lead to nociceptive afferent input to the central nervous system, exciting nociceptive circuits in the spinal cord, brainstem, thalamus, somatosensory cortex, cingulate cortex, and amygdale (Tracey and Mantyh, 2007; Woolf and Ma, 2007). However, noxious stimuli in infants do not evoke similar patterns of central nervous system activity as noted in adults (Fitzgerald, 2005). The response to noxious stimuli is more diffuse and less spatially focused in infants. Studies in rats have demonstrated major alterations in neuronal circuitry with maturation, appearing to mirror that seen in humans but in a compressed time period. These animal data may parallel developmental changes that have been noted in humans (Fitzgerald, 2005). Local tissue injury resulting from repeated heel sticks and invasive procedures triggers increased proliferation of nerve endings in surrounding tissues, particularly when this damage occurs early in gestation. As a result, scars (e.g., from heel sticks, old intravenous sites) and surrounding tissues can remain hypersensitive well beyond the neonatal period (Jennings and Fitzgerald, 1998; Reynolds and Fitzgerald, 1995). Pain assessment and management are thus most challenging in preterm infants who are exposed to the stressful NICU environment for long periods (Johnston and Stevens, 1996).

In summary, the immature nervous system in preterm infants lacks the ability to discriminate consistently between noxious and non-noxious stimuli, reacts often with similar behavior to a variety of stimuli, lacks the ability to modulate pain responses, and does not consistently manifest signs or symptoms that allow care providers to accurately assess the infant's level of pain and discomfort. Furthermore, infants cannot verbally report their level of pain. This later challenge remains a significant obstacle to accurate assessment of pain in the newborn and determination appropriate treatment.

ASSESSMENT OF NEONATAL PAIN AND STRESS

DEVELOPMENT OF BEHAVIORAL RESPONSES TO PAIN

Tools for assessment of neonatal pain and stress must be based on an understanding of the normal development of behavioral responses to pain and stress—an infant is not a small adult. Behavioral responses to noxious stimuli in infants are not always predictable because of immaturity of the central nervous system; therefore assessment of pain and response to therapeutic intervention can be similarly unpredictable. Significant structural and functional changes occur in pain pathways during development, many of which continue to take place after birth (see later discussion of ontogeny and development of pain and stress responses). When assessing pain and discomfort in infants, especially those born prematurely, it is important to remember that the patients are nonverbal and cannot say where and how badly they hurt. Indeed, even if they could verbalize such information, their ability to accurately localize and describe the pain would be limited as

discrimination between inputs (tactile or nociceptive) is immature. Moreover, their behavioral response repertoire is also limited and is not always predictable. These limitations make the use of assessment tools problematic, especially when trying to determine whether there has been a response to a drug or other intervention.

INFANT PAIN SCORES

Over the past two decades, more than 40 infant pain scales have been developed (Ranger et al, 2007). Most of these scales were developed for use in clinical trials to assess efficacy of various pharmacologic therapies and have not been validated for general clinical use. However, the use of these scales in clinical practice has led to better health care provider recognition that procedural pain and stress are common. Moreover, it is assumed that this pain and distress can be ameliorated by appropriate use of pharmacologic and nonpharmacologic approaches. However, assessment and treatment of chronic pain and discomfort in infants remains problematic. The pain instruments developed for assessment of acute pain were not designed or validated for the chronic pain and discomfort associated with mechanical ventilatory support, or for use in paralyzed or neurologically compromised infants (Anand, 1998). Furthermore, painful stimuli may be processed at the cortical level in infants without producing detectable behavioral changes (Slater et al, 2008). Therefore the clinician is left to decide whether the touted benefits of opiate sedation during mechanical ventilation in newborns outweigh the possible adverse effects, both acute and long term. The importance of selecting a valid, reliable, and practical pain assessment tool is evident from the current literature. These tools assess the response to noxious stimuli by categorizing the behavioral or physiologic reactions of the infant, or a combination of both (Grunau and Craig, 1987). The behavioral responses can include limb movements, muscle tone, crying, and characteristic facial expressions. The physiologic measures can include heart rate, oxygen saturation, and respiratory rate. Of note, specific facial expression changes have been determined to be the most reliable indicators of pain (brow bulge, eye squeeze, nasolabial furrow, taut lips, and open mouth) whereas crying is the least reliable indicator (Grunau and Craig, 1987; Guinsburg et al, 1997; Stevens et al, 1993). Use of facial expression changes can be challenging when the infant's face is partially covered with adhesives to secure tubes and lines, or with a phototherapy mask in place.

A recent publication lists the current available pain assessment tools that can be used in neonates (Stevens et al, 2007). The most commonly used tools are listed in Table 35-1.

Many pain assessment tools are available; however, they have not been systematically reviewed, and there is no specific gold standard for comparison. Because each instrument requires training and practice for optimal use, care providers should choose one that best fits the infant population being assessed to allow for consistency. The optimal approach to pain management should include reducing the frequency of painful procedures, reducing environmental stressors, facilitating neurologic developmental, determining the best technique to minimize the pain and stress

TABLE 35-1   Infant Pain Scales

Measure	Age Level	Indicators	Pain Type	Psychometric Properties
Unidimensional Behavioral Measures of Infant Pain				
Baby facial action coding system (Rosenstein and Öster, 1988)	Term infants	Facial actions based on adaptation from adult work	Procedural	Interrater reliability (r = 0.65-0.85)
Infant body coding system (Craig et al, 1993)	Preterm infants (32 wk GA) to term infants	Movement of hand, foot, arm, leg, head, torso	Procedural	Interrater reliability (r = 0.83), face validity, content validity
Neonatal facial coding system (Grunau and Craig, 1987)	Preterm infants (>25 wk GA) to term infants	Brow bulge, eye squeeze, naso-labial furrow, open lips, horizontal mouth, vertical mouth, lips pursed, taut tongue, chin quiver, tongue protrusion	Procedural	Interrater reliability (r = 0.88), content validity, face validity, construct validity, convergent validity, feasibility
Multidimensional Pain Measures in Infants				
Children's and infants' postoperative pain scale (Büttner and Finke, 2000)	Birth to 4 years	Crying, facial expression, posture of the trunk, posture of the legs, motor restlessness	Prolonged (postoperative)	Interrater reliability (<3 yr old subsample; r = 0.64-0.77), internal consistency (<1 yr old subsample; r = 0.96), content validity, construct and concurrent validity demonstrated in older subsample
Modified behavioral pain scale (Taddio et al, 1995a)	2-6 months	Facial expression, cry, body movement	Procedural	Interrater reliability (ICC = 0.95), internal consistency (r = 0.55-0.66), test-rest reliability (r = 0.95), content validity, construct validity (p <0.01), concurrent validity (r = 0.68-0.74)
Composite Pain Measures in Infants				
Clinical scoring system (Barrier et al, 1989)	1-7 months	Infant sleep during the preceding hour, facial expression, cry, motor activity, excitability, flexion, sucking, tone, consolability	Prolonged (postoperative)	Interrater reliability (r = 0.79-0.88), content validity, discriminant validity (p <0.0001)
Modified postoperative comfort score (Guinsburg et al, 1998)	<32 wk GA (postnatal age of 12-48 h)	Sleep, facial expression, sucking, hyperreactivity, agitation, hypertonicity, toe or finger flexion, consolability	Prolonged (mechanical ventilation)	Convergent validity in bedside (p <0.0001) and laboratory video coding (p = 0.02), content validity, divergent validity shown between placebo and analgesic samples (p <0.05)
Echelle Douleur Inconfort Nouveau-né (Debillon et al, 2001)	26-36 wk GA	Facial expression, movement, sleep, consolability	Prolonged (postoperative)	Interrater reliability (r = 0.59-0.74), content validity, construct validity (p <0.000)
Modified postoperative comfort score (Guinsburg et al, 1998)	Preterm infants	Sleep, facial expression, activity, tone, consolability, cry, sociability	Prolonged (postoperative)	Content validity, discriminant validity (p <0.0001)
Neonatal pain, agitation and sedation scale (Hummel et al, 2008)	<28-35 wk GA (age correction for prematurity)	Crying, irritability, behavior state, facial expression, extremities, tone, vital signs (heart rate, respiratory rate, blood pressure, oxygen saturation)	Prolonged (mechanical ventilation or postoperative)	Preliminary reliability and validity testing in progress
Pain assessment tool (Hodgkinson et al, 1994)	27 wk GA to full term	Posture, tone, sleep pattern, expression, color, cry, respirations, heart rate, oxygen saturations, blood pressure, nurse perception	Prolonged (postoperative)	Interrater reliability (r = 0.85), content validity, convergent validity (r = 0.38), concurrent validity (r = 0.76)
Scale for use in newborns (Blauer and Gerstmann, 1998)	24-40 wk GA	Central nervous system state, breathing, movement, tone, face, heart rate, mean blood pressure	Procedural (excluded postoperative)	Beginning indications of reliability, content validity, discriminant validity (p <0.05-0.01)
Distress scale for ventilated newborn infants (Sparshott, 1996)	—	Facial expression, body movement, color, heart rate, blood pressure, oxygenation, temperature	—	Face validity, content validity (Duhn and Medves, 2004)
Crying, requires increased oxygen, increased vital signs, expression, sleeplessness (Krechel and Bildner, 1995)	Neonates 32-60 wk GA	Crying, requires increased oxygen, increased vital signs, expression, sleeplessness	Prolonged (postoperative)	Interrater reliability (r = 0.72), content validity, concurrent validity (r = 0.49-0.73), discriminant validity (p <0.0001), concurrent validity for first 24 h (ICC = 0.34-0.65; McNair et al, 2004)

Continued

TABLE 35-1   Infant Pain Scales—cont'd

Measure	Age Level	Indicators	Pain Type	Psychometric Properties
Neonatal infant pain scale (Lawrence et al, 1993)	Preterm and full term	Facial expression, cry, breathing patterns, arm movement, leg movement, state of arousal	Procedural	Interrater reliability (*r* = 0.92-0.97), internal consistency (0.87-0.95), content validity, concurrent validity (*r* = 0.53-0.83)
Pain assessment in neonates scale GA (Hudson-Barr et al, 2002)	26-47 wk GA	Facial expression, cry, breathing patterns, extremity movement, state of arousal, oxygen saturation, increased heart rate	Procedural	Content validity, concurrent validity (*r* = 0.93)
Modified infant pain scale (Bucholz et al, 1998)	4-30 wk old	Sleep during evaluation, facial expression, quality of cry, spontaneous motor activity, excitability and responsiveness to stimulation, finger and toe flexion, sucking, overall tone, consolability, sociability, change in heart rate, change in blood pressure, fall in oxygen saturation	Prolonged preceding hour	Interrater reliability (postoperative; *r* = 0.85), content validity, convergent validity in dichotomous rating (*p* <0.0001)
Premature infant pain profile (Stevens et al, 1996)	Term and preterm neonates	GA, behavioral state, heart rate, oxygen saturation, brow bulge, eye squeeze, nasolabial furrow	Procedural	Interrater reliability (ICC = 0.93-0.96), intrarater reliability (ICC = 0.94-0.98), internal consistency (alpha = 0.59-0.76), content validity, construct validity (in preterm neonates, *p* = 0.0001-0.02; in term neonates, *p* <0.02), construct validity in clinical setting (*p* <0.0001), interrater reliability (*r* = 0.94-0.98; Ballantyn et al 1999), concurrent validity with cry duration (Johnston et al, 1999)

Modified from Stevens BJ et al: Assessment of pain in neonates and infants. In Anand KJ, Stevens BJ, MaGrath PJ, editors: *Pain in neonates and infants*, ed 3, Philadelphia, 2007, Elsevier, pp 70-75.
GA, Gestational age.

associated with procedures, delegating responsibility for pain assessment and treatment to the bedside nurse staff, and using a balanced multimodal approach to pain control (Allegaert et al, 2009).

BEDSIDE NONINVASIVE NEUROIMAGING TO EVALUATE PAIN AND STRESS

Several new modalities are being evaluated for their capability to help health care providers recognize pain in neonates. Near infrared spectroscopy might be a helpful technology. In a study of 29 infants between 26 and 36 weeks' gestation at birth, cortical activation occurred over both somatosensory cortices during unilateral tactile and painful stimuli (Bartocci et al, 2006). Amplitude-integrated electroencephalography also can be used to detect cortical activation in neonates (Toet and Lemmers, 2009). These and other new technologies will be needed to first recognize and then continually assess and manage pain and discomfort in our fragile patients.

LONG-TERM CONSEQUENCES OF NEONATAL PAIN AND STRESS

Untreated pain and stress has been linked to adverse long-term outcomes. Acute effects include elevations of cortisol, catecholamines, and lactate, hypertension, tachycardia, respiratory instability, glucose instability, and changes in cerebral blood flow. Chronic pain can affect growth, immune function, recovery, and length of hospitalization. In addition, a growing body of evidence has drawn attention to the potential deleterious effects of repeated handling, stress, and pain on long-term memory, social and cognitive development, and neural plasticity (Anand, 1998; Anand et al, 1987, 1989; Evans, 2001; Jennings and Fitzgerald, 1998; Pokela, 1994; Porter et al, 1999; Taddio et al, 1995a). Extrapolation of information from older children and adults can be inappropriate for our most vulnerable infants (Berde et al, 2005; Howard, 2003; Walker, 2008).

Pain and stress may alter neurodevelopment (Abdulkader et al, 2008; Anand et al, 1987, 2000). Pain suffered during neonatal intensive care has been associated with adverse long-term outcomes, such as altered pain perception to subsequent immunizations after circumcisions without anesthesia (Taddio et al, 1997), abnormal cortisol responses to stress in later infancy (Grunau et al, 2007), and altered pain responses in childhood (Grunau et al, 1998). There is concern that such hormonal changes might lead to the development of cardiovascular disease and type 2 diabetes in adulthood (Kajantie et al, 2002; Rosmond and Björntorp, 2000). As a result, appropriate use of sedation and analgesia might be beneficial to infants requiring intensive care support; however, a clear delineation of the benefits still requires further study.

CLINICAL PAIN AND STRESS MANAGEMENT STRATEGIES

SURGICAL ANESTHESIA

The recognition that surgical intervention in infants results in dramatic physiologic and metabolic changes similar to those noted in adults with significant pain has changed current practice. It is well recognized that infants perceive pain, and surgical intervention without anesthesia and analgesia leads to increased morbidity and excess mortality; however, experience obtained in older children and adults cannot be extrapolated to immature patients. Providing general anesthesia in infants requires an intimate knowledge of the developmental status and function of each organ system. A complete review of this subject is beyond the scope of this chapter. Interested readers are referred to *A Practice of Anesthesia for Infants and Children* by Spaeth and Kurth (2009) or *Anesthesia for Infants and Children* by Brett et al (2006).

FETAL SURGERY

The fetus has increasingly become a candidate for surgical intervention to repair fetal anomalies such as congenital cystic adenomatoid malformation of the lung, sacrococcygeal teratoma, and myelomeningocele, and to treat fetal disorders such as severe anemia secondary to hemolytic diseases. Many fetal interventions are accomplished using general maternal anesthesia, and therefore fetal anesthesia, but certain procedures are attempted with maternal analgesia and local anesthesia. Thus, during such fetal surgical interventions, the fetus requires consideration for pain management to attenuate fetal physiologic and hormonal stress responses (Fisk et al, 2001; Giannakoulopoulos et al, 1999). Anand et al (1987) summarized the available evidence regarding fetal and neonatal nociceptive activity in 1987 and put all care providers on notice that late gestation fetuses and newborns have intact cortical and subcortical centers necessary for pain perception and demonstrate physiologic responses to painful stimuli similar to evidence in adult subjects. A recent review of the literature supports the contention that the fetus perceives pain (Lee et al, 2005). The International Association for the Study of Pain supported the view that the human fetus is capable of reacting to nociceptive stimuli during the second trimester (Anand, 2006).

NEONATAL SURGERY

Selection of anesthetic agents to be used in neonates must account for the developmental status and function of each organ system and the potential adverse and toxic effects of specific anesthetic agents. Animal models have demonstrated that anesthetic agents can be both neuroprotective and neurotoxic in the immature brain. Frequently used anesthetics act by two principal mechanisms, either by decreasing excitation via *N*-methyl-D-aspartate (NMDA) receptors (e.g., ketamine, nitrous oxide) or by increasing inhibition via gamma-aminobutyric acid receptors (e.g., benzodiazepines, barbiturates, propofol, etomidate, isoflurane, enflurane, halothane). In the immature rat brain,

drugs that act by either of these two mechanisms can induce widespread neuronal apoptosis when given during the period of synaptogenesis (Ikonomidou et al, 1999; Ishimaru et al, 1999). The applicability of these findings to the human infant has been questioned (Soriano and Anand, 2005); however, recent data suggest that some toxicity may occur in human infants (Wilder et al, 2009).

Regional anesthesia for neonatal surgery is commonly used for minor interventions. As more experience with regional anesthesia for major surgical procedures is gained, such practice is expanding. Bösenberg (1998) presented results of the use of epidural analgesia for major neonatal surgical interventions in 240 infants weighing between 900 and 5800 g and reported that all infants had effective intraoperative analgesia with only two complications. Advantages of regional anesthesia may include less postoperative apnea, lees need for intubation, and better postoperative pain control. Sethna and Suresh (2007) reviewed this subject in depth recently.

POSTOPERATIVE PAIN MANAGEMENT STRATEGIES

Pain management after surgical intervention, like acute pain management, requires knowledge of the developmental status and function of each organ system and the potential adverse and toxic effects of specific analgesic agents. Many neonates remain intubated for mechanical ventilation after major surgery. Analgesia can be provided via intravenous administration of an analgesic agent, either by intermittent bolus dosing or by continuous infusion. Another option is continuation of regional analgesia (Bösenberg, 1998). Regional analgesia appears to be effective for pain control, but sedation may also be required in active or vigorous infants (Frumeinto et al, 2000). Regional anesthesia, when used alone, may also reduce the incidence of postoperative apnea in preterm infants (Craven et al, 2003).

Research-based evidence of appropriate postoperative pain management in neonates is limited. Taylor et al (2006) surveyed 10 NICUs regarding their postoperative pain assessment and management practices; they found that pain assessment documentation was extremely variable. Nursing documentation was done for most infants, whereas few physicians documented any assessment. Most infants were treated with opioids, benzodiazepines, or both, and some infants (7%) received no analgesia despite recent major surgery (Taylor et al, 2006). Van der Marel et al (2007) evaluated the use of rectal acetaminophen as an adjuvant treatment to continuous morphine infusion in postoperative neonates and could not demonstrate any additional analgesia effect. Recent evidence suggests that neonates require significantly less morphine to control pain and discomfort than older infants do, based on monitoring of pain scale data. Bouwmeester et al (2003a, 2003b) determined that neonates required less morphine for postoperative pain control and that the dose requirement increased with age. Both studies found that morphine, given by bolus or continuous infusion, was equally effective. The later study (2003b) found that mechanical ventilation decreased morphine metabolism and clearance.

The Association of Pediatric Anesthetists of Great Britain and Ireland commissioned guideline development for pain management after surgery and painful medical procedures (Howard et al, 2008a, 2008b). The level of evidence from the literature was determined and the recommendations were graded, allowing for better interpretation. These guidelines provided evidence-based recommendations and listed best clinical practice points when published evidence was insufficient to make formal recommendations.

MECHANICAL VENTILATION

The use of mechanical ventilation in neonates with respiratory failure is a fairly common practice in the United States, although decreasingly less than in the 1980s and 1990s. In older children and adults who require mechanical ventilation, sedation is routinely provided—most often with opiates (Gélinas et al, 2004). However, pharmacologic sedation is used less frequently in the adult intensive care unit because of concern regarding adverse cognitive outcomes and longer duration of ventilator support (Izurieta and Rabatin, 2002; Oderda et al, 2007). Extrapolation of evidence from past studies in adult patients led to the routine use of opiate sedation in neonates during mechanical ventilation (Kahn et al, 1998), with limited information regarding safety and efficacy (Anand et al, 2004; Simons et al, 2003b). As noted previously, the ability to assess and treat discomfort and pain is limited, and preemptive use of pharmacologic sedation during mechanical ventilation in newborns, especially preterm infants, remains controversial (Anand and Hall, 2007).

Mechanical ventilation in neonates is associated with an increase in hormonal stress responses, including increased cortisol and catecholamine levels (Guinsburg et al, 1998; Quinn et al, 1998). In the past, infants who appeared uncomfortable while receiving ventilatory support demonstrated asynchronous respiratory effort (i.e., "fighting" the ventilator), compromised gas exchange, and altered stress responses (Dyke et al, 1995). Furthermore, pain and stress in newborns receiving mechanical ventilation have been associated with decreased pulmonary compliance, atelectasis, and intrapulmonary shunting (Bolivar et al, 1995). More recently, with the introduction and use of surfactant replacement therapy and synchronized ventilatory technology, some of the problems with fighting the ventilator have been eliminated (Claure and Bancalari, 2009; Keszler, 2009).

Clinical studies from the 1990s demonstrated that opiate treatment prevented these adverse effects on neonatal ventilation and reversed the previously described hormonal stress changes (Quinn et al, 1993; Saarenmaa et al, 1999). Opiate sedation has been demonstrated to decrease stress scores in newborns who receive mechanical ventilation (Orsini et al, 1996; Quinn et al, 1993, 1998). In full-term infants receiving mechanical ventilation, the severity of respiratory failure as assessed by the oxygenation index directly correlated with the need for analgesia and sedation (Aretz et al, 2004).

A small randomized trial of routine morphine infusion in preterm infants receiving mechanical ventilation concluded that morphine lacked a "measurable analgesic effect" and there was "absence of a beneficial effect on poor neurological outcome" (Orsini et al, 1996). The larger clinical trial that followed (i.e., NEOPAIN) reported no beneficial effect of preemptive morphine infusions in ventilated preterm infants and an increased incidence of severe intraventricular hemorrhage in preterm infants born at 27 to 29 weeks' gestation and receiving morphine (Anand et al, 2004). Bhandari et al (2005) found that morphine infusions had no beneficial effects in preterm infants receiving mechanical ventilation. Additional bolus doses of morphine resulted in worse respiratory outcomes and longer requirement for ventilatory support. None of these controlled clinical trials provide evidence that routine narcotic sedation during mechanical ventilatory support in neonates is beneficial. In addition, the well-recognized and common adverse effects of narcotic exposure (e.g., hypotension, feeding intolerance, respiratory depression) are mentioned infrequently in sedation and pain treatment protocols in neonates receiving mechanical ventilation. Future trials have been deemed unethical if they involve withholding sedation from a group of infants. One approach to this dilemma would be to minimize the use of ventilatory support as much as possible.

A recent Cochrane Review evaluated the effects of opioid analgesics on pain, duration of mechanical ventilation, mortality, growth, and development in neonates requiring mechanical ventilation (Bellù et al, 2008). The authors found no differences in mortality, duration of mechanical ventilation, and short- and long-term neurodevelopmental outcomes. Preterm infants given morphine took longer to achieve full enteral feeding. If morphine sedation prolongs ventilatory support needs and time to full enteral feeds, then an increase in the risk of complications related to the use of venous lines (bloodstream infections) and parenteral nutrition (cholestasis) should be expected (Menon et al, 2008). Hällström et al (2003) studied risk factors for necrotizing enterocolitis in premature infants and found that the duration of morphine use was the strongest predictor for development of severe necrotizing enterocolitis. The Cochrane Review's overall conclusion regarding the use of sedation during mechanical ventilation was that "there is insufficient evidence to recommend routine use of opioids in mechanically ventilated newborns" (Bellù et al, 2008). Menon and McIntosh (2008) came to a similar conclusion in their recent review.

PROCEDURES

Infants undergoing intensive care suffer through many painful procedures, often several times each day. Although new pharmacologic and nonpharmacologic treatment strategies to decrease or eliminate some of this pain and stress have been developed, there is still a need to develop better management techniques. An article by D'Apolito (2006) reviews this issue in detail and outlines where knowledge remains limited.

BLOOD SAMPLING AND MONITORING

Heel sticks are routinely performed to obtain blood samples in neonates. The most appropriate method for relieving pain from a heel stick is yet to be determined. The heel should be warmed to aid blood sampling. Eutectic mixture of local anesthetics (EMLA) cream does not relieve the pain of a heel lance (Stevens et al, 1999b; Taddio et al, 1998). Shah et al (1997) and Larsson et al (1998a, 1998b) demonstrated that neonates experiencing venipuncture had lower pain scores than those who underwent heel stick for blood sampling. In selected neonates, venipuncture should be used preferentially over heel stick.

The pain of arterial puncture can be decreased by infiltrating the site with 0.1 to 0.2 mL of 0.5% or 1% lidocaine using the smallest-gauge needle possible (Franck and Gregory, 1993). Buffering the lidocaine with sodium bicarbonate is recommended to decrease the burning caused by lidocaine. In addition, EMLA may reduce the pain of arterial puncture.

TRACHEAL INTUBATION

The use of premedication to minimize the pain and stress of intubation has been demonstrated to benefit neonates (Simons et al, 2003a). However, concerns about rapid medication availability, ability to maintain the airway, and the ability to provide ongoing ventilatory support continue to cause controversy (Carbajal et al, 2007). Premedications typically include atropine, narcotics for sedation, and muscle relaxants. Atropine abolishes vagal bradycardia. Narcotics attenuate the increases in arterial blood pressure. Muscle relaxants attenuate the increases in intracranial pressure. Combinations decrease the time and number of attempts needed to intubate the infant.

When considering the use of medications for intubation, several questions need to be asked:
- Does the infant have adequate vascular assess?
- What is the urgency of intubation need?
- Is the infant known to have a difficult airway?
- When was the last feeding?
- Can the infant be preoxygenated while avoiding gastric distension?

If the decision is made to use medications for intubation, typical doses include:
- Atropine 0.02 mg/kg fast intravenous (IV) push
- Fentanyl 2 µg/kg slow IV push
- Vecuronium 0.1 mg/kg IV push

Alternative medications may include succinylcholine (1 to 2 mg/kg IV push) or rocuronium (1 mg/kg IV push).

The investigational agent sugammadex can reverse rocuronium-induced neuromuscular blockade in less than under 2 minutes. Sugammadex forms a 1:1 complex with steroidal nondepolarizing neuromuscular blockers in the plasma. Although approved for use in Europe, sugammadex is not currently available in the United States; it might render succinylcholine unnecessary. Rocuronium could be administered and if intubation is unsuccessful, paralysis could be immediately reversed with sugammadex (de Boer et al, 2007).

Propofol has been used as a premedication for intubation. Being a single agent, it is easier and faster to prepare than three separate drugs. Propofol is a hypnotic agent without anesthetic properties. If combined with remifentanil, there is no need for paralysis in older children (Batra et al, 2004); however, propofol is painful when injected in small veins, and extremely painful if it extravasates.

A major advantage is continued spontaneous breathing during the intubation procedure. The dose is 2.5 mg/kg IV; this dose might need to be repeated. Concerns over the use of propofol for intubation in neonates include minimal experience in neonates, uncertain pharmacokinetics and duration of action, and compatibility with precutaneously inserted central catheters lines.

Because intubation can raise both blood pressure and intracranial pressure, a short-acting benzodiazepine, such as midazolam, can be beneficial for infants with stable cardiovascular function. Fentanyl can be used as an alternative for infants with compromised cardiovascular function (McClain and Anand, 1996). Any infant who is pharmacologically paralyzed during mechanical ventilation should receive adequate sedation. In addition, the infant should receive pain medication if pain is suggested by the infant's condition or because of the procedures being performed.

CIRCUMCISION

The AAP Circumcision Policy Statement (American Academy of Pediatrics Task Force on Circumcision, 1999) states that analgesia must be provided to infants undergoing circumcisions. EMLA cream, dorsal penile nerve block, and subcutaneous ring block are all possible options. The AAP reports that subcutaneous ring block may provide the best analgesia (American Academy of Pediatrics Task Force on Circumcision, 1999). Subcutaneous ring block has been found to be more effective than EMLA or dorsal penile nerve block in other studies (Lander et al, 1997). Dorsal penile nerve block has been found to be more effective than EMLA, but this method is not always available (Lee and Forrester, 1992).

EMLA has been established as superior to placebo for pain relief during circumcision (Benini, 1993; Taddio et al, 1997). An effective method for applying EMLA in preparation for circumcision is to apply one third of the dose to the lower abdomen, extend the penis upward gently, pressing it against the abdomen, and then apply the remainder of the dose to an occlusive dressing placed over the penis. This dressing is then taped to the abdomen so that the cream surrounds the penis. Another method is to apply the cream and then place plastic wrap around the penis in a tubelike fashion to direct the urine stream out and away from the cream.

Acetaminophen is ineffective for the management of severe pain associated with the circumcision procedure, but it provides some analgesia in the postoperative period. Acetaminophen has been found to decrease pain 6 hours after circumcision (Howard et al, 1994).

OTHER INVASIVE PROCEDURES

Placement of a central venous catheter requires topical anesthesia with EMLA or infiltration of the skin with lidocaine. In addition, a parenteral opioid, such as morphine or fentanyl, is typically required. Consideration should also be given to regional blocks for central line placement.

The pain of a lumbar puncture is compounded by both the needle puncture and the distress caused by the body position required for the procedure. EMLA has been shown to decrease the pain of lumbar puncture in children (Halperin et al, 1989). Chest tube insertion requires an intravenous opioid, adequate local analgesia (lidocaine), or both.

PHARMACOLOGIC ANALGESIA INTERVENTIONS

The severity of the pain, etiology, available administration routes, and consideration of potential side effects should all be evaluated during selection of an analgesic. Once medication administration has begun, careful monitoring for side effects can decrease potential adverse events related to administration of pain medications to infants. A key component of effective pain management is reassessment after a painful intervention, although this is difficult to do with limited pain assessment tools.

NONOPIOID ANALGESICS

Nonsteroidal Antiinflammatory Drugs (Indomethacin, Ibuprofen)

Nonsteroidal antiinflammatory drugs (NSAIDs) inhibit prostaglandin synthesis by inhibiting the action of cyclooxygenase enzymes. Cyclooxygenase enzymes are responsible for the breakdown of arachidonic acid to prostaglandins. NSAIDs have many physiologic effects, including sleep cycle disruption, increased risk of pulmonary hypertension, cerebral blood flow alterations, decreased renal function by decreasing glomerular filtration rate, alteration in thermoregulatory control, and changes in platelet function. Moreover, development of the central nervous, cardiovascular, and renal systems is dependent on prostaglandins. These adverse effects are particularly worrisome for neonates and infants; however, these drugs are used frequently in the NICU for pharmacologic closure of the PDA. Aside from effects on renal and perhaps mesenteric circulation, which are difficult to separate from the PDA, no clear side effects have been reported.

Acetaminophen

Acetaminophen is the most widely administered analgesic in patients of all ages. Acetaminophen inhibits the activity of cyclooxygenase in the central nervous system, decreasing the production of prostaglandins, and peripherally blocks pain impulse generation (Arana et al, 2001). Neonates are able to form the metabolite that results in hepatocellular damage (Arana et al, 2001); however, it is inappropriate to withhold acetaminophen in newborns because of concerns of liver toxicity. The immaturity of the newborn's cytochrome P-450 system may actually decrease the potential for toxicity by reducing production of toxic metabolites (Collins, 1981).

Current recommendations are for less frequent oral dosing (every 8 to 12 hours in preterm and term neonates), because of slower clearance times, and higher rectal dosing because of decreased absorption (Arana et al, 2001; van Lingen et al, 1999). Typical oral doses for acetaminophen are 10 to 15 mg/kg every 6 to 8 hours for term neonates and 10 to 15 mg/kg every 4 to 6 hours for infants.

Administering 10 mg/kg may be inadequate for pain control, because this dose is based on antipyretic dose-response studies. The maximum recommended daily dose is 75 to 90 mg/kg for infants, 45 to 60 mg/kg for term and preterm neonates more than 32 to 34 weeks of postconceptual age, and 25 to 40 mg/kg/day for preterm neonates 28 to 32 weeks of postconceptual age (Berde and Sethna, 2002; Morris et al, 2003).

Rectally administered acetaminophen has a longer half-life, but absorption is highly variable because it depends on the individual infant and placement of the suppository. It should also be noted that the suppository may contain all of the drug in its tip and should be divided lengthwise if a partial dose is desired. The analgesic effect of acetaminophen may be additive when the agent is administered with opioids. This coadministration may enable a decrease in the opioid dose and therefore in corresponding opioid side effects; however, demonstration of this potential benefit awaits further study (van der Marel et al, 2007).

OPIOID ANALGESICS

Opioids are believed to provide the most effective treatment for moderate to severe pain in patients of all ages. There is a wide range of interpatient pharmacokinetic variability. Opioid dosing depends on the severity of the pain as well as the age and clinical condition of the infant. Opioids should be used in infants younger than 2 months only in a monitored setting such as an intensive or intermediate care unit (Yaster et al, 2003). Some clinicians propose a more conservative recommendation, restricting the use of opioids to monitored settings for any infant younger than 6 months.

Morphine

Morphine remains the standard for pain management in neonates, although not necessarily because it has been shown to be the most effective analgesic. Morphine is metabolized in the liver by uridine diphosphate glucuronyltransferase into two active metabolites: (1) morphine-6-glucuronide (M6G), a potent opiate receptor agonist, and (2) morphine-3-glucuronide (M3G), a potent opiate receptor antagonist. Both metabolites and some unchanged morphine are excreted in the urine. The predominant metabolite in preterm and full-term neonates is M3G. Because of slow renal excretion, the metabolites can accumulate substantially over time (Bouwmeester et al, 2003a, 2003b; Saarenmaa et al, 2000). There is a potential for late respiratory depression because of a delayed release of morphine from less well-perfused tissues and the sedating properties of the M6G metabolite (Anand et al, 2000).

Because the predominant metabolite of morphine in infants is M3G, a potent opiate receptor antagonist, using the lowest dose possible to achieve the needed analgesia should be considered. Escalating morphine doses will also increase the levels of M3G in the infant, interfering with the goal of adequate analgesia. Doses as low as 1 to 5 µg/kg/h can provide adequate analgesia, minimizing the risk of accumulation of high M3G levels with the metabolite's prolonged half-life (Bouwmeester et al, 2003a, 2003b).

Clearance or elimination of morphine and other opioids is prolonged in infants, because of the immaturity of the cytochrome P-450 system at birth. The rate of elimination and clearance of morphine in infants 6 months and older approaches that in adults. Chronologic age seems a better indicator than gestational age of how an infant metabolizes opioids (Scott et al, 1999; Yaster et al, 2003).

Infants are at greater risk for opioid-associated respiratory depression because of their immature responses to hypoxia and hypercarbia. There is an increase in unbound or free morphine and M6G available to reach the brain as a result of the reduced concentration of albumin and alpha$_1$ acid glycoproteins (Houck, 1998).

Hypotension, bradycardia, and flushing constitute the response to the histamine release and rapid intravenous administration of morphine. Histamine release may cause bronchospasm in infants with chronic lung disease, although this is not commonly seen (Anand et al, 2000). Morphine sedation may result in extended need for ventilatory support in neonates (Anand et al, 1999; Bhandari et al, 2005).

Dosing recommendations currently reflect the wide range of interpatient pharmacokinetic variability. In the past, 0.03 mg/kg of morphine IV was suggested as a starting dose in infants not receiving ventilation (Acute Pain Management Guideline Panel, 1992), whereas 0.05 to 0.1 mg/kg of morphine IV was recommended as an appropriate starting dose in infants receiving ventilation. Recently, much lower doses have been recommended (Anand et al, 2008; Bouwmeester et al, 2003b, 2004; Lynn et al, 2000; Saarenmaa et al, 2000). Titration to the desired clinical effect is required in adjusting both the dose and the frequency of administration. Furthermore, it is important to continually assess need and responses so that dosing can be adjusted both up and down (Allegaert et al, 2009). As the use of morphine for analgesia and sedation in neonates is explored further, it is becoming clear that some of the risks may outweigh the potential benefits (Allegaert et al, 2009; Anand et al, 2008; Black et al, 2008; Carbajal et al, 2005; Nandi et al, 2004; Ng et al, 2003; Ranger et al, 2007).

Fentanyl

Fentanyl is 80- to 100-fold more potent than morphine and causes less histamine release, making it a more appropriate choice for infants with hypovolemia, hemodynamic instability, or congenital heart disease. Another potential clinical advantage of fentanyl is its ability to reduce pulmonary vascular resistance, which can be of benefit for infants who have undergone cardiac surgery, have persistent pulmonary hypertension, or need extracorporeal membrane oxygenation (Anand et al, 2000). Bolus doses of fentanyl must be administered over a minimum of 3 to 5 minutes to avoid chest wall rigidity, a serious side effect observed after rapid infusion. Chest wall rigidity, which can result in difficulty or inability to ventilate, can be treated with naloxone or a muscle relaxant such as pancuronium or vecuronium.

Fentanyl is highly lipophilic. It has a quick onset and relatively short duration of action. Because of fentanyl's short duration of action, it is typically used as a continuous infusion for postoperative pain. In infants 3 to 12 months of age, total body clearance of fentanyl is greater than that of older children, and the elimination half-life is longer because of its increased volume of distribution (Singleton et al, 1987). Fentanyl has been demonstrated to have a prolonged elimination half-life in infants with increased abdominal pressure (Gauntlett et al, 1988; Koehntop et al, 1986). Because of tachyphylaxis, continuous infusions of fentanyl are often increased to maintain constant levels of sedation and pain management. Infusion dosing can reach substantial levels requiring prolonged withdrawal.

A rebound transient increase in plasma fentanyl levels is a phenomenon known to occur after discontinuation of therapy in neonates. It is a result of the accumulation of fentanyl in fatty tissues, which can prolong its effects after continued use; therefore caution must be exercised in the use of repeated doses or a continuous infusion.

Oral Opioids

Oral methadone can be used to wean infants from long-term opioid use. Methadone is widely used in neonates and children, although there are limited data regarding its efficacy and pharmacokinetics in this population (Chana and Anand, 2001; Suresh and Anand, 1998). The respiratory depressant effect of methadone is longer than its analgesic effect. Methadone is metabolized slowly, and it has a long half-life.

Codeine is prescribed at 0.5 mg to 1 mg/kg orally every 4 hours as needed. Scarce data are available to recommend use of codeine in neonates. Most pharmacies supply acetaminophen and codeine in a set formula, consisting of acetaminophen (120 mg) and codeine phosphate (12 mg per 5 mL) with alcohol (7%). The dose prescribed is limited by both the appropriate dose of codeine and the safe dose of acetaminophen. This combination is not recommended in neonates.

Oxycodone dosing is 0.05 mg/kg to 0.15 mg/kg orally every 4 to 6 hours as needed. No data are available to recommend oxycodone in neonates. The liquid form is not universally available.

MIXED OPIOID AGONIST-ANTAGONIST DRUGS

Nalbuphine is a mixed agonist-antagonist opioid receptor drug; therefore its administration in infants of opioid-addicted mothers may precipitate withdrawal. This agent is equianalgesic with morphine. Nalbuphine has a ceiling effect for analgesia. Additional studies are needed regarding the safety and efficacy of nalbuphine use in infants. It is not recommended for use in neonates, although it may be useful during opioid drug withdrawal (Jang et al, 2006).

LONG-TERM CONSEQUENCES OF NEONATAL OPIOID EXPOSURE

Experimental Animal Studies

Perinatal and neonatal opioid exposure in experimental animals is associated with both short- and long-term adverse neurologic effects that should make clinicians ask whether the use of such medications with questionable benefits should be used at all. Data from previous studies suggested that perinatal narcotic exposure restricts brain growth, induces neuronal apoptosis, and alters behavioral pain responses later in life (Handelmann and Dow-Edwards, 1985; Hu et al, 2002; Kirby et al, 1982; Seatriz and Hammer, 1993). One area of particular concern to clinicians is the developing cerebral circulation, which is extremely vulnerable to physiologic perturbations and the effects of drugs (Volpe, 1998). Cerebrovascular effects of drug exposure early in development can have lifelong consequences, including increased risk for stroke (Barker, 2000; Craft et al, 2006; Hanson et al, 2004). The acute effects of exogenous narcotics, including morphine, on the developing cerebral circulation have been described in piglets and include modulation of prostaglandin-induced pial artery dilation during hypoxia, alteration in endothelin production, and increases in endothelin A receptor mRNA expression (Armstead et al, 1990, 1996; Van Woerkom et al, 2004). Endogenous opioids are important regulators of cerebrovascular tone and angiogenesis (Blebea et al, 2000; Gupta et al, 2002; Pasi et al, 1991; Poonawala et al, 2005). Exposure to morphine in fetal sheep and neonatal rats permanently alters cerebrovascular control mechanisms (Mayock et al, 2005, 2006). We have also shown permanent neurobehavioral and neuropathologic changes in a rodent model of neonatal stress and morphine exposure (Boasen et al, 2009; McPherson et al, 2007; Vien et al, 2009). These and other animal studies demonstrate short- and long-term effects of neonatal morphine exposure, which is not surprising because opioid receptor-mediated signaling likely has a role in several aspects of early brain development (Durrmeyer et al, 2010). However, the clinical relevance of these animal studies regarding the long-term effects of neonatal opioids is difficult because of species differences in the timing of brain development, the development of opiate receptors and major neurotransmitter systems, and the pharmacokinetics of administered opioids. Overall, it is difficult but necessary to simulate the premature infant's NICU experience in an animal model (Durrmeyer et al, 2010).

Clinical Studies

Clinical studies addressing the short- and long-term effects of prolonged opiate use in neonates are limited. The few that exist are contradictory and confounded by illness severity. Bergman et al (1991) described reversible encephalopathic changes in neonates receiving long-term sedative and narcotic infusions. MacGregor et al (1998) demonstrated no adverse neurodevelopmental outcomes in a small group of newborns who received morphine for a median of 5 days. Roźe et al (2008) presented 5-year neurodevelopmental outcomes in very low-birthweight (VLBW) infants exposed to prolonged sedation or analgesia (defined as greater than 7 days of sedative or opioid drugs). They found that exposed VLBW infants had more severe or moderate disability at 5 years (42%) compared with those not exposed (26%), but after adjusting for gestational age and propensity score (as a way to ensure that treatment effects are only compared between infants who

are equally likely to receive that treatment), the association was no longer significant. Preterm infants (23 to 32 weeks' gestation at birth) evaluated at 36 weeks postconceptual age in the NEOPAIN study already demonstrated neurobehavioral abnormalities if exposed to morphine during ventilatory support (Rao et al, 2007).

TOPICAL AND LOCAL ANESTHETICS

Lidocaine reduces the pain and stress of venipuncture and IV catheter placement (Larsson et al, 1998a, 1998b; Long et al, 2003). EMLA cream has been demonstrated to reduce the pain of circumcision. Place the cream on the area where anesthesia is desired and then cover it with an occlusive dressing for 1 hour before the procedure. Longer application times provide deeper local anesthetic penetration, but can lead to toxicity. There is a slight risk of methemoglobinemia with the use of EMLA cream in infants and patients who are G6PD deficient. A rare occurrence, methemoglobinemia can occur when hemoglobin is oxidized by exposure to prilocaine. EMLA should not be used in patients with methemoglobinemia or in infants younger than 12 months who are also receiving methemoglobinemia-inducing drugs, such as acetaminophen, sulfonamides, nitrates, phenytoin, and class I antiarrhythmics. (Refer to Table 35-2 for recommended maximum doses of EMLA cream by age and weight.) A study of 30 preterm infants found that a single 0.5-g dose of EMLA applied for 1 hour did not lead to a measurable change in methemoglobin levels (Taddio et al, 1995b). A systematic review concluded that EMLA diminishes the pain during circumcision. Limited efficacy was noted with pain from venipuncture, arterial puncture, and percutaneous venous line placement. EMLA was not found to diminish pain from heel lancing (Taddio et al, 1998). Oral sucrose or glucose may be as effective as EMLA for venipuncture (Abad et al, 2001; Gradin et al, 2002).

SEDATIVES

Benzodiazepines

Benzodiazepines such as lorazepam and midazolam are sedatives which activate gamma-aminobutyric acid receptors and should not be used in place of an appropriate

TABLE 35-2 EMLA Cream: Recommended Maximum Dose by Age and Weight

Age	Body Weight (kg)	Maximum Total EMLA Dose (g)	Maximum Application Area (cm²)	Maximum Application Time (h)
Birth to 3 mo	or <5	1	10	1
3-12 mo	and >5 kg	2	20	4

Data from Taketomo CK, Hodding JH, Kraus DM, editors: *Pediatric dosage handbook*, 2001-2002, ed 8, Hudson, Ohio, Lexi-Comp Inc, p 595.
EMLA, Eutectic mixture of local anesthetics.

pain medication, because this class of medication has no analgesic effect. For painful procedures, an analgesic must be used in conjunction with the benzodiazepine. Benzodiazepines are administered to decrease irritability and agitation in infants and to provide sedation for procedures. In ventilated infants, benzodiazepines can help to avoid hypoxia and hypercarbia from breathing out of sync with the ventilator although, as noted for opioids, new synchronized infant ventilators make this clinical problem less likely. When given as continuous infusions, dosing often escalates rapidly to maintain apparent sedation resulting in need for prolonged weaning. Use of such medications has been associated with abnormal neurologic movements in both preterm (Lee et al, 1994) and term infants (Chess and D'Angio, 1998). In rats, prenatal exposure to diazepam results in long-term functional deficits and atypical behaviors (Kellogg et al, 1985); exposure of 7-day-old mice to diazepam induces widespread cortical and subcortical apoptosis (Bittigau et al, 2002); and midazolam potentiates pain behavior, sensitizes cutaneous reflexes, and has no sedative effect in newborn rats (Koch et al, 2008). Whether these data can be extrapolated to human infants is unknown, but clinicians have reason to be concerned and should use these drugs with caution in the NICU.

Dexmedetomidine

Dexmedetomidine is a potent and relatively selective α_2 adrenergic receptor agonist indicated for the short-term sedation of patients in intensive care settings, especially those receiving mechanical ventilatory support. The drug is administered by either bolus doses for short procedural sedation (1 to 3 µg/kg) or continuous intravenous infusion (0.25 to 0.6 µg/kg/h). Because dexmedetomidine does not produce significant respiratory depression, it has been used for procedural interventions in spontaneously breathing infants (Barton et al, 2008; Chrysostomou et al, 2009). As neonatologists become more familiar with dexmedetomidine, its use may increase (O'Mara et al, 2009); however, short- and long-term safety and effectiveness information needs to be assessed in infants, as has been initiated in adults (Pandharipande et al, 2007; Riker et al, 2009).

NONPHARMACOLOGIC ANALGESIC INTERVENTIONS

Nonpharmacologic interventions for prevention or relief of neonatal pain and stress are numerous and widely publicized in the medical literature. These interventions have been used either as the sole method of pain control or in combination with pharmacologic interventions. No one would argue with the statement that neonatal intensive care is associated with stress, pain, and discomfort. Because opioid analgesia and sedation have not been proved to be efficacious and may possibly be harmful, alternative methods of pain and stress relief need to be evaluated for efficacy and safety. A variety of approaches have been investigated. As stated clearly by Golianu et al (2007), "These therapies may optimize the homeostatic mechanisms of the infant, thereby mitigating some of the adverse consequences of untreated pain, as well as facilitating healthy physiologic adaptions to stress." However, widespread adoption of specific techniques is not consistent.

Nonnutritive sucking with pacifiers reduces pain responses to heel prick, injections, venipuncture, and circumcision procedures (Sexton and Natale, 2009; Shiao et al, 1997; South et al, 2005). Infant massage has been demonstrated to decrease plasma cortisol and catecholamine levels in preterm infants (Acolet et al, 1993; Kuhn et al, 1991).

Maternal skin-to-skin contact (also termed *kangaroo care*) is associated with greater physiologic stability and reduced responses to acute pain (Bergman et al, 2004; Fohe et al, 2000; Gray et al, 2000; Johnston et al, 2003; Ludington-Hoe and Swinth, 1996). Kangaroo care can decrease Neonatal Infant Pain Scale scores after vitamin K injections (Kashaninia et al, 2008). Maternal rocking has been shown to diminish neonatal distress (Jahromi et al, 2004). Breastfeeding reduces the physiologic and behavioral responses to acute pain and stress in neonates and has been recommended as the first line of treatment (Osinaike et al, 2007; Shah et al, 2006).

The Neonatal Individualized Developmental Care and Assessment Program (NIDCAP) systematically changes a protocol-based model of nursing care to a relationship-based approach (Als et al, 1994). There is a significant body of empiric evidence that use of the NIDCAP approach improves the clinical and neurodevelopmental outcomes of preterm infants (Als and Gilkerson, 1997; Brown and Heermann, 1997; Kleberg et al, 2002; Westrup et al, 2000; Wielenga et al, 2007), but recent metaanalyses of published studies could not demonstrate any improvement in long-term outcomes (Jacobs et al, 2002; Symington and Pinelli, 2006).

Another approach is multisensory stimulation of preterm infants undergoing painful procedures. This approach entails simultaneous gentle massage, soothing vocalizations, eye contact, smelling a perfume, and sucking on a pacifier. This technique was associated with analgesia and calming of the infants in several reports from one unit (Bellieni et al, 2001, 2002, 2007).

Music therapy may reduce the behavioral and physiologic responses to acute procedural pain (Hartling et al, 2009).

Oral sucrose (versus intragastric) reduces pain behavior in preterm and term infants and is used widely (Stevens et al, 1997, 2004). The mechanism of oral sucrose analgesia is believed to be the sweet taste stimulation of endogenous opioid release (Shide and Blass, 1989). Of all methods and techniques discussed, oral sucrose has been the most widely used. As more data regarding the limitations of pharmacologic treatment are published, consideration of nonpharmacologic interventions will likely become more important and commonplace.

IATROGENIC DRUG DEPENDENCE, TOLERANCE, WITHDRAWAL

A clear distinction must be made between opioid or benzodiazepine dependence, tolerance, and addiction. Physical dependence is demonstrated by the need to continue the administration of the drug to prevent signs or symptoms of physical withdrawal. Tolerance is a reduction in the drug effects after repeated administration, or the need to increase the dose to achieve the same clinical effect. Addiction is compulsive drug-taking behavior (Gutstein and Akil, 2001). Infants are not capable of becoming psychologically addicted, but they clearly develop tolerance and dependence.

DRUG WEANING CONSIDERATIONS

Baseline pain and withdrawal scores should be obtained before beginning the drug weaning process, and infants should be reassessed every 2 to 4 hours for signs of withdrawal. In addition, when an opioid dosage is being tapered, the infant should be assessed for the presence of pain a minimum of every 4 hours. If an infant is receiving both an opioid and a benzodiazepine, it is prudent to taper and stop only one class of medication at a time. Typically, a weaning schedule is 10% of the total initial dose every other day. Many patients can tolerate a relatively large initial decrease in dose, but subsequent decreases may need to be smaller. Environmental stressors should be eliminated or reduced whenever possible. It should be noted that the potential onset of withdrawal symptoms varies according to the half-life of the opioid or benzodiazepine and the half-life of active metabolites, which may be much longer than that of the parent compound (Tobias, 2000).

PALLIATIVE CARE

Palliation, as defined in the *New Oxford American Dictionary*, is "making a disease (or its symptoms) less severe or unpleasant without removing the cause." Most deaths in neonatal intensive care units occur after withdrawal of supportive measures, when the burden of care is extreme and the likelihood of recovery is remote (Cook and Watchko, 1996; Wall and Partridge, 1997). Traditionally, initiation of palliative care occurs when further medical interventions are no longer curative and death of the infant is expected. However, the AAP and the World Health Organization both support palliative care that starts early in the course of an illness and works with other therapies to prolong life. "The goal of palliative care is the achievement of the best quality of life for the patients and their families, consistent with their values, regardless of the location of the patient" (World Health Organization, 1998). Both the AAP (American Academy of Pediatrics Committee of Bioethics and Committee on Hospital Care, 2000) and the World Health Organization (1998) have provided guidelines for palliative care for infants that emphasize optimizing quality of life until death occurs and eliminating of the notion of euthanasia. Such care is an active process that includes family-centered care with attention to physical, emotional, and spiritual issues (Papadatou, 1997). Several good reviews of neonatal end-of-life care have been published (De Lisle-Porter and Podruchny, 2009; Institute of Medicine of the National Academies, 2003; Moro et al, 2006). Box 35-1 provides a comprehensive listing of the many aspects of end-of-life care that should be considered for the dying neonate.

Parents and other family members should be actively involved in palliative care. Palliative treatments focus on relief from clinical symptoms such as dyspnea, pain, agitation, vomiting, and seizures, in addition to maintaining dignity and providing warmth. Palliative care should also include attention relieving psychological stress in caregivers such as loneliness, depression, anxiety, grief, and separation from family and loved ones. Family members should be prepared for the end of life. They need to be provided with a description of the dying process that includes mention of the potential for gasping respiratory efforts and an estimate of the length of the dying process. Opportunities to create memories for the family should be offered, such as pictures, footprints, locks of hair, hats, or blankets.

Consideration of to the place of death is important. Should it occur in the hospital or at home with hospice care? Unfortunately, many deaths occur in busy NICUs with little privacy. Placement of the infant and the family on a postpartum ward with other parents and their healthy infants is also suboptimal. Ideally, for deaths likely to occur in the hospital, the infant and family should be placed in a private room with enough space for all family members to be present to support the parents in their grieving process.

Bereavement and follow-up discussions should be planned with the family. Care providers should discuss autopsy, discuss follow-up discussion times, and provide ongoing bereavement support to the family for as long as needed.

SUMMARY

Recognition and treatment of pain and discomfort in the neonate remain challenging issues. Despite significant progress in the understanding of human neurodevelopment, pharmacology, and more careful attention to the care of sick infants, there is still have much to learn. Because protecting and comforting these patients are important, and because external regulatory forces have required intervention to minimize distress, what is known about adult patients must be applied to infants. Some good has come from these endeavors, but errors have been made along the way.

It is important to minimize pain and distress in these patients to avoid more aggressive interventions. Such care will minimize the risks of adverse effects on neurodevelopment. Learning to provide good care without doing harm should be the goal. Nonpharmacologic methods of pain and distress control should be explored further. When pharmacologic intervention is necessary for pain control, use the least amount of drug that controls the pain. Escalation of drug doses may, in fact, be adding to the problem.

As newer techniques and medications are introduced to clinical practice, it must be demonstrates that such additions achieve the goal of pain control. It must also be demonstrates that neonatal interventions are safe over the lives of the patients. Better tools are needed to help optimize the outcomes for infants.

BOX 35-1   Guideline for End-of-Life Care of the Neonate

I. Patient population

Any infant in the NICU diagnosed with a medical condition incompatible with life.

II. Purpose

The guideline is for use by the bedside nurse in the NICU when faced with caring for an infant at the end of life. It provides the bedside nurse with alternative ways to encourage parents to perform normal parenting activities, such as bathing, holding, and picture taking with their infant, in the time surrounding his death. These activities may be the only, and sometimes last, opportunity the mother and father will have to parent their infant.

III. Background and rationale

Many NICUs have policies in place relating to bereavement and postmortem care of the neonate, but few have policies or guidelines on palliative care (Sudia-Robinson, 2003). Many nurses have not received sufficient training to support families or themselves through this bereavement process. Many nursing programs lack or have only recently added curricula regarding end-of-life care (Romesberg, 2004). This lack of protocols, along with the limited education available to professionals, serves to decrease the chance that infants and their families will receive the end-of-life care they deserve. Palliative care consists of three components: (1) pain and comfort management, (2) assistance with end-of-life decision making, and (3) bereavement support (March of Dimes, 2010).

IV. Procedure

  A. Inclusion criteria: any infant in the NICU with a diagnosis of nonviability or a fatal condition should be considered for inclusion in this guideline. These medical conditions may fall into three categories: (1) newborns born at the edge of viability with extremely low birthweight (<500 g) and <24 weeks' gestational, (2) newborns with complex or multiple congenital anomalies, and (3) newborns not responding to intensive care interventions and experiencing deterioration despite medical efforts to save them (Catlin and Carter, 2002). For these infants, the focus of care should change from curative to palliative.

  B. Predeath: any intervention should focus on supporting the parents during their infant's end-of-life care. Some nurses may be uncomfortable with their own feelings and have trouble communicating with parents at this time. Communication, however, is vital, and the words spoken should serve to validate the infant's life and death (Capitulo, 2005). Communication also helps the parents understand their infant's condition and offers them the opportunity to make choices concerning the extent of their participation in his end-of-life care (Workman, 2001).

    1. Communication

      a. The following are suggestions for successful communication techniques to use with parents:

        (1) Active listening

        (2) Open communication

        (3) Total presence

        (4) Uninterrupted time for parents to express their wishes

        (5) Nonverbal gestures such as touch

      b. Refer to the infant by name

      c. Inform parents of what to expect while their infant is dying (see, hear, smell, feel)

      d. Inform parents of their options for disposition of their infant's remains

        (1) Transfer to morgue

        (2) Pick up by mortuary

      e. Use language that does not confuse the parents.

        (1) Use definite words such as *death, die,* and *dying* instead of euphemisms such as *not doing well* or *passing away*

        (2) Words such as *good, stable,* or *better* could be misinterpreted to mean the infant could improve or survive

    2. Environment

      a. Do not restrict the number of visitors

      b. Provide privacy and comfort

        (1) Low lights

        (2) Decreased noise and activity

    3. Religion

      a. Ask parents about any religious preference

      b. Notify clergy of the parents' choice

      c. Offer baptism, blessing, anointing, or prayer

    4. Parental activity

      a. Provide a stuffed animal

      b. Keep the family involved

        (1) Decisions (medical and physical care)

        (2) Handprints, footprints

        (3) Kangaroo care, holding

        (4) Bathing

        (5) Dressing

        (6) Changing diaper

        (7) Any other parenting acts

        (8) Taking pictures of the infant and family members at any time during this process

  C. Active dying: the time period when the infant is dying offers special challenges for both the nurse caring for the dying infant and his family members. Pain management for the infant during the extubation and dying process is of extreme importance. Parents must be informed of what they may see, hear, and experience during this time. The family and infant should be offered a comfortable, private area for this process.

    1. Pain management

      a. Maintain intravenous access

      b. Medicate the infant appropriately

      c. Assess pain routinely and frequently after the withdrawal of life support

    2. Communication

      a. Inform the parents what to expect (see, hear, smell, feel)

      b. Inform the parents that their baby may not die immediately after removal of the endotracheal tube

      c. Be available for any questions or concerns the parents may have

    3. Environment

      a. Do not restrict the number of visitors

      b. Provide privacy and comfort

        (1) Low lights

        (2) Decreased noise and activity

    4. Religion

      a. If ceremonies or rituals have not been performed before now, offer any of the following:

        (1) Clergy of choice

        (2) Blessing, baptism, anointing, orprayer

      b. Parental activity

        (1) Offer the opportunity to hold the baby during extubation

        (2) Encourage the parents to notify the nurse if they believe their baby is in pain and needs assistance

Continued

BOX 35-1 Guideline for End-of-Life Care of the Neonate—cont'd

D. After death: once the infant has died, creating lasting memories is integral to the healing of the family. Regardless of whether the family participates in their infant's death care, no steps should be eliminated. When an infant dies, there are few, if any, memories of their time together, and parents will cherish any memento of their infant's life (Jansen, 2003). It is the nurse's responsibility to help ensure that as many memories as possible are created (Capitulo, 2005).

1. Communication
   a. Offer the parents opportunities to be involved with all aspects of after-death care.
   b. If parents decline, respect their decision, but gently remind them that this will be their only chance to perform these tasks.
   c. If parents decline, offer them the opportunity to help the nurse with the infant's care.
   d. Reassure the family that the nurse is available at any moment if assistance is required.

2. Environment
   a. A room with a bed and chairs for family and friends to be alone with their infant should be provided.
   b. Complimentary snacks and beverages should be made available.
   c. Family time with the infant should be unrushed and unlimited.

3. Parental activities
   a. Encourage the parents to hold and dress their infant.
   b. Offer the parents the opportunity to bathe their infant if this has not already been done.
   c. Offer the parents the opportunity to have family pictures taken at this time.

4. Memory makers: memory boxes should contain items that have meaning and have been a part of the infant's hospitalization. Objects that seem trivial to others will have profound significance for the family. They will be the only concrete evidence to the parents and family that their infant was alive. The nurse needs to be creative. There is no second chance to create memories for the family (Catlin and Carter, 2002).
   a. Identification band
   b. Name card
   c. Blood pressure cuff
   d. Oxygen saturation probe
   e. Thermometer
   f. Respiratory paraphernalia
   g. Measuring tape with infant's length marked and name and date written on it
   h. Polaroid or digital photographs pictures
   i. Stuffed animal
   j. Pacifier
   k. Diaper
   l. Lock of hair
   m. Handprints, footprints
   n. Swaddling blanket (do not discard blanket if soiled)
   o. Clothing (include postmortem gown, hat, socks, T-shirt; do not wash if soiled)
   p. Ring
   q. Mold of hand, foot, or both
   r. Cord clamp
   s. Phototherapy mask
   t. Dried washcloth and soap from bath, placed in a small plastic bag to preserve soap fragrance
   u. Black mourning (remembrance) pin

5. Final departure of parents: ensure that the parents do not leave with "empty arms"
   a. Memory box
   b. Stuffed animal
   c. Baby's blanket
   d. Pictures
   e. Baby's belongings

V. Nursing responsibilities
   A. Prepare the infant's body for transportation to the hospital morgue per hospital protocol.
   B. Complete the necessary paperwork.
   C. Ensure that all tasks are completed per hospital policy.

Adapted from De Lisle-Porter M, Podruchny AM: The dying neonate: family-centered end-of-life care, *Neonatal Netw* 28:75-83, 2009.
NICU, Neonatal intensive care unit.

SUGGESTED READINGS

Allegaert K, Veyckemans F, Tibboel D: Clinical practice: analgesia in neonates, *Eur J Pediatr* 168:765-770, 2009.

American Academy of Pediatrics Committees on Fetus and Newborn and on Drugs, Sections on Anesthesiology and on Surgery; Canadian Paediatric Society Fetus and Newborn Committee: Prevention and management of pain and stress in the neonate, *Pediatrics* 105:454-461, 2000.

Anand KJ, Anderson BJ, Holford NH, et al: Morphine pharmacokinetics and pharmacodynamics in preterm and term neonates: secondary results from the NEOPAIN trial, *Br J Anaesth* 101:680-689, 2008.

Anand KJ, Hall RW, Desai N, et al: Effects of morphine analgesia in ventilated preterm neonates: primary outcomes from the NEOPAIN randomised trial, *Lancet* 363:1673-1682, 2004.

Carbajal R, Lenclen R, Jugie M, et al: Morphine does not provide adequate analgesia for acute procedural pain among preterm neonates, *Pediatrics* 115:1494-1500, 2005.

Carbajal R, Roussit A, Danan C, et al: Epidemiology and treatment of painful procedures in neonates in intensive care units, *J Am Med Assoc* 300:60-70, 2008.

De Lisle-Porter M, Podruchny AM: The dying neonate; family-centered end-of-life care, *Neonatal Netw* 28:75-83, 2009.

Durrmeyer X, Vutskits L, Anand KJ, et al: Use of analgesic and sedative drugs in the NICU: Integrating clinical trials and laboratory data, *Pediatr Res* 67:117-127, 2010.

Fitzgerald M: The development of nociceptive circuits, *Nature Rev Neurosci* 6:507-520, 2005.

Howard R, Carter B, Curry J, et al: Quick reference summary of recommendations and good practice points, *Pediatr Anesth* 18(Suppl 1):4-13, 2008b.

Lago P, Garetti E, Merazzi D, et al: Guidelines for procedural pain in the newborn. For the Pain Study Group of the Italian Society of Neonatology, *Acta Paediatr* 98:932-939, 2009.

Stevens BJ, Riddell RR, Oberlander TE, et al: Assessment of pain in neonates and infants, In Anand KJ, Stevens BJ, McGrath PJ, editors: *Pain in neonates and infants,* ed 3, Philadelphia, 2007, Elsevier, pp 67-90.

Complete references used in this text can be found online at www.expertconsult.com

PART IX

IMMUNOLOGY AND INFECTIONS

IMMUNOLOGY OF THE FETUS AND NEWBORN

Calvin B. Williams, Eli M. Eisenstein, and F. Sessions Cole

Understanding the contribution of the newborn infant's immunologic response to neonatal disease requires a review of the complex immunologic environment of pregnancy and the developmentally regulated changes in fetal and neonatal immunity. The contrasting functions of the fetal, neonatal, and maternal immunologic responses (i.e., preservation of fetal well-being as an allogenic graft versus adequate immunologic protection in a nonsterile extrauterine environment) are regulated by a host of incompletely understood developmental and genetic mechanisms. The diversity and importance of these mechanisms are suggested by the heterogeneity and frequency of the infectious problems encountered in newborns. Differences in immunologic responsiveness between adults and newborns should not be considered defects or abnormalities. Just as the ductus arteriosus, a cardiopulmonary necessity in the intrauterine environment, closes at different rates in different infants, human fetal and newborn infant immunologic response mechanisms are developmentally and genetically programmed to change from graft preservation to identification and destruction of invading pathogens at different rates.

MATERNAL AND PLACENTAL IMMUNOLOGY

Although pregnancy is a natural process that is essential for the propagation of all mammalian species, from an immunologic perspective it poses a great dilemma. The fetus represents a hemiallogenic graft that expresses paternal antigens, which under ordinary circumstances would be rejected as foreign tissue. The fact that such rejection ordinarily does not occur cannot be explained by systemic suppression of the maternal immune system. Most studies of maternal immune function during pregnancy have not shown significant abnormalities (Aagaard-Tillery et al, 2006) and are consistent with the clinical observation that pregnant women are not at increased risk for opportunistic infection. Furthermore, maternal acceptance of the fetus does not occur exclusively as a result of physical separation between immunogenic fetal and maternal tissues. Trophoblastic tissue expressing paternal antigens comes into direct contact with maternal immune cells, and fetal cells can readily be detected in maternal peripheral blood (Price et al, 1991). Conversely, maternal leukocytes and somatic cells are present in significant numbers in the fetus and may persist into adult

life in a phenomenon known as *microchimerism* (Bianchi et al, 1996; Lo et al, 1996; Maloney et al, 1999). As a result, mechanisms must exist whereby antigen-specific responses against paternal antigens either are not initiated or are specifically suppressed. Beginning with the seminal studies of Peter Medawar more than 50 years ago, significant progress has been made in unraveling the immunologic mechanisms underlying maternal-fetal tolerance (Seavey and Mosmann, 2008; Trowsdale and Betz, 2006). Currently it appears that no single factor can explain the commensal immunologic relationship that exists between mother and fetus throughout pregnancy. Rather, several distinct but complementary innate and adaptive immune mechanisms contribute to this process.

Before fertilization, both systemic and local immunologic changes occur in the endometrium to favor acceptance of the fetal allograft. For example, progesterone induced by ovulation can reduce the proliferation of T cells and inhibit antigen-presenting cells (Ehring et al, 1998; Miyaura and Iwata, 2002). In addition, as discussed later, T cells with immunosuppressive properties accumulate cyclically in the endometrium during normal menses.

Semen has contrasting immunomodulatory effects on the female reproductive tract and immune system, respectively; however, seminal plasma induces expression of proinflammatory cytokines, including granulocyte-monocyte colony-stimulating factor (GM-CSF), interleukin (IL) 6, IL-8, and the chemokine monocyte chemotactic protein 1 by the uterine endometrium (Sharkey et al, 2007). These molecules help to induce a local inflammatory cell infiltrate containing macrophages, neutrophils, and dendritic cells, which may help to break down endometrial mucin and thereby facilitate adherence of the blastocyst to the endometrium (Dekel et al, 2010). GM-CSF also has embryotrophic effects that promote fetal growth and viability. Knockout mice lacking GM-CSF have normal implantation rates, but have 15% to 25% smaller litters (Robertson et al, 1999). However, semen contains immunosuppressive factors that teleologically are necessary to inhibit initiation of an immunologic reaction against sperm antigens. Therefore seminal plasma can induce secretion of the immunosuppressive cytokine IL-10 by monocytic cell lines (Denison et al, 1999) and is rich in transforming growth factor (TGF) β-family cytokines (Tremellen et al, 1998). TGF-β1 is essential for inducing local differentiation of certain forms of immunoregulatory T cells (Chen et al, 2003; Keskin et al, 2007).

Inflammatory mediators and cytokines produced by uterine tissues have a key role in embryonic implantation. Prostacyclin is expressed by uterine tissues by day 5 of gestation and is required for blastocyst adherence and subsequent placental decidualization (Lim et al, 1999). The IL-6 family of cytokines, which includes leukemia inhibitory factor (LIF), IL-11, and IL-6 itself, is also essential for placental implantation. This family of cytokines is defined by their receptors, which share a common signaling component, GP130, in addition to a cytokine-specific alpha chain. LIF is expressed by uterine endometrium, beginning during the mid-secretory phase of the menstrual cycle (Cullinan et al, 1996), probably in response to progesterone (Eijkemans et al, 2005). Implantation does not occur in LIF-deficient mice (Stewart, 1992). Interleukin-11, a cytokine that possesses hematopotic and antiinflammatory properties, has also been shown to be essential for implantation, albeit at a later stage than LIF. Placenta of mice deficient in the alpha chain of the IL-11 receptor fail to undergo decidualization, resulting in infertility (Robb et al, 1998). IL-6 itself is expressed by endometrial epithelial and stromal cells, mainly during the secretory phase of menses (Perrier d'Hauterive et al, 2004). Reduced expression of IL-6 mRNA has been noted in secretory-phase endometrium of women with recurrent miscarriages (Jasper et al, 2007). This finding was attributed to a possible role of IL-6 in facilitating placental decidualization and trophoblast development. In summary, an orchestrated series of specific proinflammatory and tolerogenic mechanisms support implantation and early fetal allograft survival.

TABLE 36-1 Selected Molecules of Immunologic Significance at the Fetal-Maternal Interface

Molecule	Expression Pattern	Functional Consequence
MHC class II	Not expressed by trophoblast, either constitutively or inducibly	Impaired CD4+ T cell activiation
MHC Class I Molecules		
HLA-A, HLA-B	Not expressed by trophoblast	Impaired CD8+ T cell activation
HLA-C	Expressed by trophoblast during 1st trimester	Modulation of NK cell function
HLA-G	Expressed by trophoblast	Inhibition of T cell and dendritic cell function; modulation of T cell and dendritic cell function
Fas ligand (CD178)	Expressed by placental decidual and glandular epithelium and by fetal trophoblast	Induces leukocyte apoptosis
PDL-1	Expressed on placental deciduas basalis	Immune inhibition Cofactor for induction of regulatory T cells
Galectins	Expressed by trophoblast early in pregnancy	Induction of T cell apoptosis

HLA, Histocompatibility leukocyte antigen; *MHC,* major histocompatibility complex; *NK,* natural killer; *PDL,* programmed cell death ligand.

STRATEGIES FOR IMMUNOLOGIC EVASION AT THE MATERNAL-FETAL INTERFACE

One possible way in which the hemiallogeneic fetus might avoid rejection is to evade detection by the maternal immune system. This approach clearly is not the entire explanation for tolerance of the fetal allograft. Indeed, fetal antigenic maturity in eliciting a maternal immunologic response has been well documented (Beer and Billingham, 1976; Billington, 1987). The view that maternal tolerance is an active process is further supported by observations that, at least in mice, maternal T lymphocytes specific for paternal antigens in particular are activated during pregnancy. In addition, the fact that paternally derived tumor cells are not rejected by pregnant female mice supports a central role for antigen-specific systemic immune inhibition (Tefuri et al, 1995); therefore, tolerance appears to be at least in part a metabolically active process. Nevertheless, several unique features of the maternal-fetal interface undoubtedly contribute to attenuation of antifetal immunity (Table 36-1).

One such mechanism is altered expression of major histocompatibility complex (MHC) proteins. MHC class II molecules are necessary for CD4+ T cell responses, which contribute both effector and regulatory functions needed for graft rejection. MHC class II molecules are not ordinarily constitutively expressed, except by certain antigen-presenting cells; however, proinflammatory stimuli such as interferon (IFN)-γ are capable of inducing MHC class II expression on most cell types. In contrast, fetal trophoblastic tissues do not express MHC class II

proteins, either in the resting state or in response to IFN-γ (Peyman et al, 1992). MHC class II gene silencing in trophoblasts is at least partially the result of the transcriptional repression of class II transactivator, a necessary transcription factor for class II gene expression (Murphy and Tomasi, 1998; Peyman et al, 1992).

More importantly, human trophoblasts also do not express conventional MHC class I human leukocyte antigen (HLA) A or HLA-B molecules. This fact undoubtedly contributes to reduced alloantigenic recognition at the fetal-maternal interface. Human trophoblasts express HLA-C, principally during the first trimester of pregnancy (King et al, 1996) and two nonclassic HLA molecules—HLA-E and HLA-G. The role of the latter in pregnancy has been studied extensively. HLA-G is a nonpolymorphic molecule encoded by a single gene that encodes seven alternatively spliced transcripts and exists as a protein in both membrane-bound and soluble forms. Its expression is primarily limited to fetal tissue, but it can be detected on some adult tissues, and its expression can be induced on other cells in response to infection, inflammation, or malignant transformation (Carosella et al, 2008). Unlike classical MHC molecules, HLA-G does not have a significant role in stimulating CD8+ T cells via the T cell receptor complex. Rather, the principal function of HLA-G molecules expressed by the trophoblast appears to be modulating the activity of natural killer (NK) cells. HLA-G has also been shown to have other immunomodulatory properties, including inhibition of cytotoxic T cell activity, inhibition of alloproliferative responses by CD4+ T cells, and modulation of dendritic cell maturation and function (Carosella et al, 2008). These data reveal that the unique MHC class I molecule expression pattern on fetal trophoblast constitutes an intricate mechanism for orchestrating the activity of immune cells.

Several additional interesting molecules expressed at the maternal-fetal interface confer unique immunologic properties to this environment. Fas ligand (FasL) is expressed in both maternal and fetal components of the uteroplacental unit throughout gestation. Activated T cells express the Fas receptor, which delivers an apoptotic (death) signal when bound by FasL. Implicit in these observations is the hypothesis that expression of FasL limits the reciprocal migration of activated fetal and maternal T cells. This idea is strengthened further by experiments examining the homozygous matings between generalized lymphoproliferative disease (gld) mice, which make a nonfunctional FasL. Pregnant generalized lymphoproliferative disease (gld) mice demonstrate leukocyte infiltration and necrosis at the decidual-placental border, with many resorption sites and small litters (Hunt et al, 1997). Progesterone-induced blocking factor is an immunomodulatory molecule released in response to progesterone by trophoblastic cells (Anderle et al, 2008). Its properties include indirectly suppressing NK cell function and inducing bias of CD4+ T cells toward Th2-type cytokine secretion (Szekeres-Bartho and Wegmann, 1996). The galectins represent a family of molecules expressed at the maternal-fetal interface with immunoregulatory properties. These glycoproteins regulate the immune response by recognition of cell surface glycans on immune cells. Galectins are expressed in human placenta primarily by the syntrophoblast early in pregnancy (Than et al, 2009). Upon cell surface contact, galectins downregulate the cellular immune response, in part by inducing programmed cell death (apoptosis) of T lymphocytes (Liu and Rabinovich, 2010).

A series of murine investigations points to a role for local metabolic factors in suppressing maternal T cell alloresponses in preventing spontaneous fetal loss. When monocytes are induced to differentiate into macrophages in vitro using macrophage colony-stimulating factor, they become inhibitors of T cell proliferation rather than activators. This inhibition was shown to be the result of selective degradation of tryptophan by the inducible enzyme indoleamine 2,3-dioxygenase (IDO). Serum tryptophan levels fall during pregnancy, possibly in response to IDO expression by syncytiotrophoblast cells, which make the enzyme as early as 7.5 days after coitus. Given the localization of IDO to the maternal-fetal interface and the immunosuppressive effects of tryptophan depletion, it seemed plausible to investigators that this pathway had a role in survival of the fetal allograft. This hypothesis was supported by experime nts with either normal or recombinase activating gene knockout mice, which lack T and B cells, together with the IDO inhibitor 1-methyl tryptophan. Normal mice carrying allogenic fetuses lose all their concepti by 11.5 days after coitus when they are treated with the inhibitor. In contrast, the delivery of healthy litters in RAG-deficient mice treated with 1-methyl-tryptophan demonstrates an immunologic basis for the observation (Munn et al, 1998). More

recently, an additional tolerogenic mechanism influenced by tryptophan metabolism has been suggested by studies of the indirect influence of the IDO pathway on differentiation and activation of regulatory T lymphocytes (Baban et al, 2009; Chen et al, 2008). However, the lack of fetal rejection observed in female, genetically deficient IDO mice suggests that IDO may be necessary, but not sufficient, in maintaining tolerance during pregnancy (Baban et al, 2004).

Another possible mechanism through which the maternal immune system might be rendered relatively indifferent to the presence of fetal alloantigens concerns antigen presentation within the uterine environment. Dendritic cells (DCs) are a type of antigen-presenting cell that is critical for cellular and humoral immune responses. Collins et al (2009) recently reported that the migration of DCs from decidual tissue to draining uterine lymph nodes is impaired compared with myometrial DCs. Therefore placental entrapment of DCs might represent a way by which presentation of fetal antigens to the maternal immune system is retarded, thereby potentially inhibiting initiation of allogenic immune responses.

NK cells found in the placental decidua are referred to as *decidual NK cells* (dNK cells) to distinguish them from NK cells found in maternal blood and those found in the nonpregnant uterine endometrium (Yagel, 2009). These cells comprise 70% of decidual lymphocytes, express a CD56+CD16− phenotype (Manaster et al, 2008), and have a unique gene expression profile which indicates that dNK cells are a unique cell population (Koopman et al, 2003). Furthermore, despite expressing high amounts of granzyme and other molecules necessary for mounting a cytotoxic response, these cells exhibit reduced cytotoxicity compared with peripheral blood NK cells (Kopcow et al, 2005) and were noncytotoxic to trophoblastic cells. In contrast to NK cells found in peripheral blood and tissues that have important innate immune functions, including surveillance against infection and tumor cells, it is not certain whether dNK cells have any role in immunity during pregnancy. Rather, they have been shown to have an essential role in promoting trophoblast invasion into the decidua and placental vascularization. These cells accomplish these tasks by secreting cytokines with effects on the placental vasculature including IFN-γ, chemokines that affect trophoblastic growth, and angiogenic factors including vascular endothelial growth factor, placental growth factor, angiopoietin-2, and NKG5 (Hanna et al, 2006).

To facilitate activation of dNK cells to perform their essential tissue remodeling functions, while at the same time avoiding overactivation that could possibly lead to cytotoxic damage to the trophoblast, their activity must be tightly modulated by a series of interactions between several activating and inhibitory receptors and their respective ligands (Manaster and Mandelboim, 2010). The nonclassic class I MHC molecules are among these dNK cell receptor ligands. For example, a principal physiologic ligand of β2-microglobulin–associated HLA-G is the inhibitory receptor leukocyte immunoglobulin (Ig)-like receptor 1 (Ponte et al, 1999). Free heavy chain HLA-G also binds to this receptor in a noninhibitory fashion, and this interaction could represent a feedback mechanism to avoid overinhibition (Gonen-Gross, 2010).

HLA-C is a major ligand for the different killer immuno-globulin-like receptors (KIRs), some of which are activating and others which are inhibitory. Amino acid allotypes at position 80 of HLA-C confer preferential binding to different forms of KIR, which in turn may result in clinically significant differences in dNK cell activation. Various combinations of maternal KIR and fetal HLA-C genes have been shown to confer differential risk for preeclampsia, as a result of differences in dNK cell-mediated placental vascular changes (Hiby et al, 2004).

A final innate immune condition necessary for successful completion of pregnancy is the absence of placental activation of complement. Fetal death occurs in mice that are genetically deficient in the complement regulatory protein Crry, accompanied by placental complement deposition and inflammation (Xu et al, 2000). Although there is no direct homolog of Crry in humans, complement inhibition has been shown to be essential for normal pregnancy in a murine model of the antiphospholipid syndrome, an autoimmune condition characterized by thrombosis, thrombocytopenia, and recurrent fetal loss. In this model, fetal injury occurs as a result of placental inflammation initiated by local dysregulation of complement proteins. Both complement activation and fetal loss can be prevented administering anticoagulants with complement-inhibitory properties such as heparin, but not by anticoagulants lacking complement-binding properties (Girardi et al, 2003, 2004). Some but not all human clinical interventional studies using anticoagulants with complement-binding properties to prevent fetal loss in the antiphospholipid syndrome have shown positive results (Di Nisio et al, 2005).

CYTOKINE SECRETION BY T CELLS DURING PREGNANCY

Bias in T cell cytokine secretion toward Th2-type cytokines and away from Th1-type cytokines has been proposed as an immunologic condition necessary for maintaining healthy pregnancy. Excessive exposure to Th1-type cytokines is clearly detrimental to the fetus. The Th1 cytokines IFN-γ and tumor necrosis factor-α have been shown to inhibit the growth of trophoblasts and to inhibit embryonic and fetal development (Haimovici et al, 1991). Th1 cytokines terminate normal pregnancy when injected into pregnant mice (Chaouat et al, 1990). Th2-type cytokines contribute to implantation as discussed previously, and to maintenance of pregnancy as suggested by LIF expression throughout pregnancy by placental leukocytes, decidua, and chorionic villous cells (Sharkey et al, 1999). LIF production by maternal T cells from healthy pregnancies is also positively associated with IL-4 production and inversely with IFN-γ (Piccinni et al, 1998). These studies have been interpreted to support the notion that the balance between Th1 and Th2 cytokines is important in maintaining pregnancy. However, it has been indicated that mice lacking all Th2-type cytokines (deleted by multiple genetic mutations) undergo normal allogenic pregnancies with normal litter sizes (Fallon et al, 2002). Based on this result, some investigators have concluded that Th1/Th2 cytokine shifts is an epiphenomenon that is irrelevant to maternal-fetal tolerance (Trowsdale and Betz, 2006).

ROLE OF REGULATORY T CELLS IN PREGNANCY

The mechanism whereby adaptive allogenic responses against paternal antigens are actively suppressed during pregnancy was largely unexplained until the discovery of a distinct lineage of T lymphocytes with dominant immunosuppressive properties (Brunkow et al, 2001). This type of regulatory T (Treg) cell is characterized by expression of a lineage-specific transcription factor, Foxp3. Upon activation via their antigen-specific T cell receptor, Treg cells are capable of suppressing immune effector cells, including dendritic cells and T effector cells through a variety of mechanisms (Tang and Bluestone, 2008), thereby preventing a fatal form of autoimmune disease throughout life (Kim et al, 2007). The ontogeny of Treg cells is discussed more fully in the section on adaptive immunity.

The possible role of Treg cells during pregnancy was first investigated in mice. These experiments disclosed that Treg cell numbers are expanded in peripheral lymphoid tissues, and this expansion is not dependent on the presence of alloantigen. Particularly high numbers of Treg cells are found at the maternal-fetal interface, where they comprise 30% of all CD4+ T cells. Treg cells are not required for pregnancy in syngeneic mice, in which the fetus does not display any foreign paternal antigens. In contrast, in allogenic pregnancy in which the fetus expresses paternal antigens, Treg cell depletion resulted in pregnancy failure (Aluvihare et al, 2004). In another series of experiments examining an abortion-prone strain of mice, allogeneic pregnancy loss could be prevented by adoptive transfer of Treg cells from healthy mice (Zenclussen et al, 2005). These data provide a plausible mechanism whereby the adaptive immune system can actively suppress cellular immune responses directed against paternal alloantigens.

Another line of evidence from studies performed in mice provides additional indirect support for an essential role of Treg cells in maintaining fetal tolerance in mice. Programmed death-1 (PD-1) is an inhibitory receptor expressed on activated lymphocytes. There are two programmed death ligands (PDLs) for the PD-1 receptor, PDL-1 and PDL-2. PDL-1 is expressed on the decidua basalis, the portion of the placenta abutting the fetal trophoblast, and by Treg cells. Blockade of PDL-1 using antibodies in allogenic pregnancy results in T cell–mediated fetal loss, indicating an essential role for this molecule in preventing rejection of the fetal allograft (Wang et al, 2008). This effect of anti–PDL-1 antibody is abrogated when Treg cells are depleted. Furthermore, in PDL-1–deficient mice, suppressive activity of Treg cells was found to be impaired (Habicht et al, 2007). Finally, an independent series of experiments has demonstrated an important role for PD-1–PDL-1 interaction in Treg cells (Krupnick et al, 2005). These data support a critical role for PD-1–PDL-1 interactions in generating functional Treg cell populations necessary for successful allogenic pregnancy.

Studies of Treg cells in humans further support an essential role for this cell type in initiating and maintaining healthy pregnancy. Treg cells are increased in the peripheral blood of women during the late follicular and luteal phases of the menstrual cycle. This increase is believed to occur in response to estradiol (Polanczyk et al, 2004; Tai et al, 2008). Soluble factors in seminal fluid may contribute to further local expansion of these cells at the time of copulation (Robertson et al, 2009). Human Treg cells selectively migrate to the placental decidua under the influence of soluble factors including human chorionic gonadotropin (Schumacher et al, 2009). Most but not all studies have shown that Treg cell numbers are increased in peripheral blood throughout pregnancy (Mjosberg et al, 2009; Somerset et al, 2004).

Alterations in Treg cells have been associated with certain pathologic conditions during pregnancy. Although preeclampsia does not appear to be associated with reduced numbers of Treg cells in peripheral blood, the ratio of Treg cells relative to CD4+ T cells bearing proinflammatory phenotypic markers, such as Th17 cells, is abnormal in preeclamptic women (Santner-Nanan et al, 2009). In addition, toxoplasma infection in pregnant mice is associated with reduced numbers of Treg cells in peripheral lymphoid tissues (Ge et al, 2008). This observation raises the possibility that embryopathy associated with prenatal infection is caused in part by the maternal immune system, because of the breakdown of maternal-fetal tolerance as a result of altered Treg cell differentiation.

A fascinating permutation of the role of Treg cells during pregnancy concerns the effects of these cells on the developing fetal immune system. As already noted, fetal lymphoid tissues are microchimeric—that is, they contain small but significant numbers of maternally derived cells. Because not all maternal antigens are inherited, it would be expected that the fetal immune system would reject these cells. Recently it was demonstrated that maternal cells expressing noninherited maternal antigens (NIMAs) are tolerated by the fetal immune system as a result of active suppression by fetal Treg cells (Mold et al, 2008). In this study, Treg cell numbers were not found to be increased in the fetal thymus, but were markedly increased in number in fetal lymphoid tissues. It is therefore likely that these cells represent an induced rather than a natural Treg cell population, which differentiates in peripheral lymphoid tissues under the influence of TGF-β. It was also shown in this study that small numbers of these NIMA-specific Treg cells persist into childhood, but can be reactivated using appropriate stimuli.

This property of Treg cells has important clinical implications in the transplantation setting. Bone marrow and solid organ transplants are known to be more successful when either the donor or recipient expresses NIMA (Burlingham, 2009; Dutta et al, 2009; van Rood et al, 2009). This finding is explained by restimulation of dormant, NIMA-specific T_{reg} cells by transplanted cells expressing these antigens, thereby contributing to active tolerance of the graft. In addition to their potential relevance for developing future clinical strategies for improving transplantation outcomes while reducing the need for pharmacologic immune suppression (Burlingham, 2009), these findings also show that some of what is learned by the fetal immune system in utero is retained into childhood, and perhaps throughout life.

DEVELOPMENTAL FETAL-NEONATAL IMMUNOLOGY

The newborn infant, especially the preterm infant, is at increased risk for developing a considerable spectrum of opportunistic infections, including *Candida* spp., herpes simplex, and cytomegalovirus. Developmental and genetic differences between adults and infants in immunologic responsiveness account for much of this enhanced susceptibility (Adkins et al, 2004; Levy, 2007), although under certain circumstances neonates can mount adult-level responses (Marchant et al, 2003; Sarzotti et al, 1996). Research has focused on the molecular, cellular, and functional definitions of these differences. This discussion focuses on those developmental aspects of innate and adaptive immunity known to be important for fetal or neonatal responsiveness to infection.

INNATE IMMUNITY

During fetal adaptation from the sterile intrauterine environment to neonatal colonization of mucosal surfaces, the innate immune system shields the newborn from infection while helping to orchestrate the acquisition of protective adaptive immune responses (Levy, 2007). These innate mechanisms include protective barriers like the vernix caseoa, which contains antimicrobial peptides and fatty acids (Tollin et al, 2005), developmentally controlled regulation of toll-like receptor signaling (Fusunyan et al, 2001; Lotz et al, 2006), expression of acute phase reactants (Jokic et al, 2000; Levy 2007) and complement proteins, and alterations in neutrophil and monocyte function (Forster-Waldl et al, 2005; Levy et al, 2004, 2006a, 2006b). Importantly, functional maturation of innate immunity allows for colonization with commensal organisms while reducing potentially dangerous inflammatory responses.

Complement

The complement system, a principal component of the innate immune response, consists of more than 40 plasma, cell surface, and regulatory proteins that interact dynamically to regulate multiple physiologic functions, including resistance to pyogenic infections, interaction between adaptive and innate immunity, and elimination of immune complexes, products of inflammatory injury, and apoptotic self cells (Carroll, 2004; Walport, 2001a; Zipfel and Skerka, 2009). Components of the complement system recognize and lyse bacteria, opsonize microorganisms nonspecifically, release anaphylatoxins, solubilize immune complexes, and induce B-cell proliferation and differentiation.

Activation of the complement cascade can occur via three pathways—classic, lectin, or alternative. The activation steps in these pathways have been reviewed recently (Thiel, 2007; Zipfel and Skerka, 2009). Several characteristics of the complement cascade are important for the fetal–neonatal immunologic response. First, whereas the specificity of classic pathway activation results from interaction of antigens with antibodies of several isotypes, activation of the alternative and lectin pathways is antibody-independent and can be initiated by structures such as endotoxin and polysaccharides frequently expressed by pathogenic organisms. For the fetus or infant who has not yet produced antigen-specific IgG for immunologic recognition, the alternative and lectin pathways may be critical for triggering the effector functions of the complement cascade (Kielgast et al, 2003; Simister, 2003; Stossel et al, 1973; Zilow et al, 1997). Second, the enzymatic activation of the complement cascade permits rapid amplification of its functions: deposition of a single immunoglobulin molecule or C3b fragment can generate enzymatic cleavage of thousands of later-acting components and thus multiple complement activities (Carroll, 2004; Walport, 2001a, 2001b; Zipfel and Skerka, 2009). In addition, the alternative pathway can be amplified via a positive feedback activation mechanism, because C3b, an activation product of the alternative pathway C3 convertase, is a component of this convertase (Janssen et al, 2006). Because of the importance of antibody-independent recognition for the immunologic responsiveness of the fetus and infant, the positive amplification loop of the alternative pathway is critical for rapid generation of complement effector functions without specific immunologic recognition. Third, the continuous activation of the alternative pathway requires rigorous regulation in the fetus to avoid tissue damage during organ remodeling (Zipfel et al, 2007). Finally, the contributions of the lectin pathway to fetal–neonatal complement activation and fetal well-being are still under investigation.

Complement activation via any of the three pathways occurs in four main steps: initiation of complement activation, C3 convertase activation and amplification, C5 convertase activation, and terminal pathway activity or the assembly of the membrane attack complex (Zipfel and Skerka, 2009) (Figure 36-1). Although the classic and lectin pathways may be triggered by recognition of ligands via complement activating soluble pattern recognition molecules (e.g., IgG or IgM antibodies, mannan-binding lectin [MBL], or the ficolins), the alternative pathway is spontaneously and constantly activated on biological surfaces in plasma and in most or all other body fluids (Pangburn and Muller-Ederhard, 1984). The spontaneous activation of the alternative pathway readily initiates amplification and requires rigorous regulation (Zipfel et al, 2007). Complement activation results in assembly of the

first enzyme in the cascade, C3 convertase, via early-acting components of the classical (C1, C4, and C2), alternative (factor B, factor D, and C3), or lectin (MBL, L-ficolin, M-ficolin, H-ficolin, MBL-associated serine proteases [MASP-1, -2, -3]), and a smaller MBL-associated protein (MAp19) pathway. C3 convertase is assembled via highly specific and limited proteolysis. Proteolytically activated components form specific enzymatic complexes composed of classical (C2b and C4b), alternative (C3bBb), or lectin (C2b and C4b) pathway components, which proteolytically cleave C3 into C3a and C3b (see Figure 36-1). These two endopeptidases (C3bBb and C4bC2b) have identical substrate specificities; each cleaves the single peptide bond $Argine_{77}$–$Serine_{78}$ of the alpha chain of C3 (Janssen et al, 2006). The rates of formation and dissociation of both C3 convertases are regulated by multiple soluble (e.g., factor H, factor I, C4b-binding protein) and membrane-associated proteins (e.g., membrane cofactor protein, delay accelerating factor) (Zipfel and Skerka, 2009). During the first phase of complement activation, small (8 to 10 kD) peptides are released by proteolytic cleavage from the second (C2a), third (C3a), and fourth (C4a) components of complement. These fragments have anaphylatoxin and antimicrobial activities and can establish chemotactic gradients for effector cells (Nordahl et al, 2004). If C3b is deposited close to the site of generation and surface-bound convertases are formed, complement cascade activation can be amplified (Gros et al, 2008). If C3b fragments coat microbial or apoptotic surfaces, they opsonize the particles for phagocytosis. Although C3b deposition on the surface membrane of intact self cells can be prevented by regulators that block further complement activation, C3b deposition on microbial surfaces or on modified self cells that lack such regulators amplifies complement activation (Zipfel and Skerka, 2009). The role of non–inflammation-inducing, C3b-mediated removal of

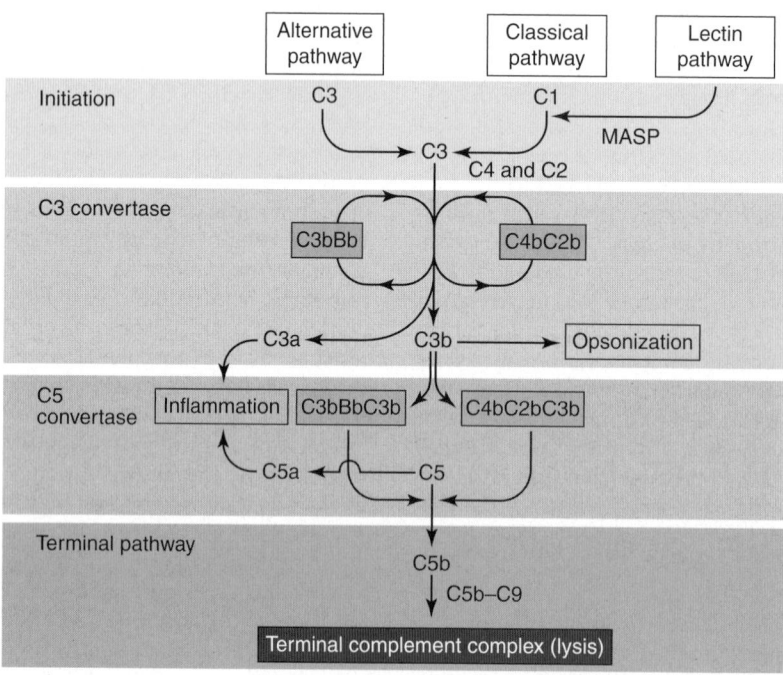

FIGURE 36-1 Summary of complement activation via the classic, alternative, and lectin pathways. *(From Zipfel PF, Skerka C: Complement regulators and inhibitory proteins,* Nat Rev Immunol *9:729-740, 2009.)*

cells during fetal organ remodeling has not been explored in detail.

If complement pathway activation continues beyond C3 cleavage, the binding of a second C3b molecule to either C3 convertase generates the alternative (C3bBbC3b) or classical or lectin (C4bC2bC3b) C5 convertases (see Figure 36-1). Both enzymes proteolytically cleave C5 to C5a and C5b. C5a is a powerful anaphylatoxin, and the C5b fragment can initiate activation of the terminal pathway (Ward, 2009). The C5a-induced inflammation and the C5b-initiated terminal pathway seem to be separately regulated (Zipfel and Skerka, 2009).

Binding of C5b to either of the active C5 convertases initiates directed, nonenzymatic assembly of the terminal pathway components C5, C6, C7, C8, and C9 to form the membrane attack complex (see Figure 36-1). The assembly and conformational changes of these soluble, hydrophilic proteins generate pores composed of lipophilic, membrane-inserting complexes (the membrane attack complex) that ultimately cause cell lysis by disrupting the osmotic gradient between the intracellular and extracellular environments (Morgan, 1999).

Studies of fetal and neonatal complement have focused on quantification of serum concentrations of individual components, examining maternal–fetal transport of these proteins, assessing specific effector functions of the classical and alternative pathways, and investigating contributions of complement activation to common neonatal diseases. In humans, Gitlin and Biasucci (1969) reported detectable concentrations of C3 (1% of adult levels) and C1 inhibitor (20% of adult levels) by immunochemical methods as early as 5 to 6 weeks' gestation. By 26 to 28 weeks' gestation, both C3 and C1 inhibitor concentrations increased to 66% of adult levels. Since these studies, multiple investigators have demonstrated that functionally and immunochemically measured classical and alternative pathway protein concentrations in cord blood increase with advancing gestational age and that they are only 50% to 75% of adult concentrations at full-term gestation (Sonntag et al, 1998; Wolach et al, 1997). Although cord blood lectin pathway component concentrations are lower than those in older children and adults, the correlation between MBL and gestational age has not been consistently observed (Hilgendorff et al, 2005; Kielgast et al, 2003; Kilpatrick et al, 1996; Lau et al, 1995; Swierzko et al, 2009; Thiel et al, 1995). The important roles of complement regulatory proteins, decay-accelerating factor, membrane cofactor protein, and CD59 have also prompted examination of the ontogeny of these proteins in the human fetus (Simpson et al, 1993).

On the basis of studies of genetically determined, structurally distinct complement variants in maternal and cord serum, no transplacental passage from mother to fetus of C3, C4, factor B, or C6 has been observed (Colten et al, 1981; Propp and Alper, 1968). The presence of detectable amounts of C2 and C1 inhibitor in cord blood, but not in the sera of mothers with genetic deficiencies of these proteins, suggests that fetal–maternal transport of these components does not occur.

Regulation of complement effector functions in the fetus and newborn infant has not been as extensively examined. Opsonization of invading microorganisms without specific immunoglobulin recognition requires activation of the alternative or lectin pathways. For infants born prematurely or without organism-specific maternal IgG, alternative or lectin pathway activation provides a critical mechanism for triggering complement effector functions (Maruvada et al, 2008; Super et al, 1989; Swierzko et al, 2009). For example, Stossel et al (1973) demonstrated opsonic deficiency in 6 of 40 cord sera examined because of decreased factor B concentrations, despite normal C3 and IgG levels. The functional contribution of the classic pathway to neonatal effector functions has been assessed through the use of cord blood–mediated opsonophagocytosis by adult polymorphonuclear leukocytes of group B streptococci type Ia (Edwards et al, 1983). This serotype may be opsonized by classical pathway components in the absence of specific antibodies and thus permits evaluation of the function of classical pathway activation. In 8 of 20 neonatal sera examined, decreased bactericidal activity was detected and correlated with significantly lower functional activity of C1q and C4. These studies did not determine whether this decrease was mediated by an inhibitor of function or by an intrinsic change in functional activity of these components in neonatal sera. The contribution of the lectin pathway to immunosusceptibility of the newborn infant has been suggested by studies of both MBL concentrations and pathway activity (Kielgast et al, 2003; Kilpatrick et al, 1996; Sumiya et al, 1991; Super et al, 1989; Swierzko et al, 2009; Thiel et al, 1995). Complement regulatory proteins (e.g., C4b-binding protein and factor H) also contribute to neonatal immunosusceptibility as suggested by the failure of neonatal serum to stop invasion by group B streptococci and *Escherichia coli* into human brain microvascular endothelial cells (Maruvada et al, 2008). The importance of the terminal complement component C9 for cytolysis of multiple isolates of *E. coli* was suggested by in vitro experiments in which killing of *E. coli* by neonatal serum samples was limited by C9, but not by other classical pathway components (Lassiter et al, 1992, 1994).

Although lower serum concentrations of classical, alternative, and lectin pathway complement proteins can contribute to enhanced susceptibility of infants to systemic infection, other complement functions important for fetal and neonatal well-being, but not related to antimicrobial response, can contribute to reduced capacity to activate the classical and alternative pathways. For example, reduced serum concentration of C4b-binding protein (8% to 35% of pooled adult plasma levels), which is a critical regulator of classical pathway C3 convertase activity, has been noted in fetal and neonatal sera (Fernandez et al, 1989; Malm et al, 1988; Melissari et al, 1988; Moalic et al, 1988). Lower C4b-binding protein concentration increases the functional anticoagulant activity of protein S, with which it complexes and thereby contributes to decreased coagulation function of the fetus and newborn. Consideration of functions besides immunologic effector functions may be important in furthering the current understanding of the developmental regulation of complement component production.

The contribution of complement activation to tissue injury has been investigated in several common neonatal diseases, including neonatal hypoxic ischemic encephalopathy, necrotizing enterocolitis, meconium aspiration syndrome, and intrauterine growth restriction and fetal loss (Girardi and Salmon, 2003; Girardi et al, 2006; Lassiter, 2004; Mollnes et al, 2008; Schlapbach et al, 2008; Schultz et al, 2005). Concern has also been raised that unregulated complement activation can occur in selected infants who undergo extracorporeal membrane oxygenation therapy (Johnson, 1994; Kozik and Tweddell, 2006).

Complement activation is an important regulator of multiple functions of the host immunologic response. Further study of the fetus and newborn infant will be aimed at understanding the developmental and genetic regulation of immunologic and nonimmunologic functions of this important group of plasma and cell surface proteins.

Natural Killer Cells

NK cells are a component of the innate immune response and represent approximately 10% to 15% of all peripheral blood lymphocytes. NK cells are present in the spleen, lungs, and liver, but rarely are found in lymph nodes and thoracic duct lymph (Cerwenka and Lanier, 2001). Interestingly, NK cells are the major type of lymphocyte found in the maternal decidual tissue, where they represent up to 70% of all lymphocytes (King et al, 1996). NK cells are distinguished from other lymphocytes by their morphology, function, and expression of distinct surface molecules. Expression of the cell surface markers CD16 (FγRIII) and CD56 (nerve cell adhesion molecule-1) can be used to identify the NK population by analytical flow cytometry. Mature NK cells appear larger and more granular than T or B cells (Cooper et al, 2001) Mature NK cells are also distinguished by the presence of both activating and inhibitory receptors that are used to selectively identify and kill virally infected cells and tumors (Biassoni et al, 2001). NK receptors recognize MHC class I molecules on target cells, resulting in signals that suppress NK cell function. Target cells that are deficient in or lack MHC class I activate NK cell function, resulting in the release of lysosomal granules. These granules contain serine proteases, perforin, and TGF-β, which disrupt the target cell membrane and induce an inflammatory response. Studies show significantly lower NK cell activity in fetuses and neonates compared with adults (Georgeson et al, 2001; Kadowaki et al, 2001).

NK cells are derived from a common hematopoietic progenitor that retains T and B cell developmental potential (Boos et al, 2008). NK cells first make their appearance in fetal liver as early as 6 weeks' gestation. Committed CD34+CD56- NK progenitors have been identified in the fetal thymus, bone marrow, and liver. In humans, there are several subsets of NK cells with distinct cell surface markers and function. For example, the CD56high CD16- subset is activated by IL-2 and also expresses CCR7 and CD62L, which allows these cells to traffic through lymph nodes (Di Santo, 2006). This subset is similar to NK cells that develop in the mouse thymus through an IL-7- and GATA3-dependent pathway and, in both species, is characterized by low cytotoxicity and enhanced cytokine production (Boos et al, 2008; Vosshenrich et al, 2006). In the human neonate, the NK population is immature; only half of all NK cells express CD56, and the NK cytolytic activity is lower (Dominguez et al, 1993). This functional reduction in NK activity has been proposed as a factor that contributes

to the severity of neonatal herpes simplex virus infections. Profound defects in NK cell activity result in familial hemophagocytic lymphohistiocytosis, a disease characterized by fever, hepatosplenomegaly, cytopenia, hyperferritinemia, and hemophagocytosis. Familial hemophagocytic lymphohistiocytosis arises from mutations in genes that encode proteins involved in the granule-exocytosis pathway and is a fatal disorder without bone marrow transplantation (Jordan and Filipovich, 2008; Orange, 2006).

NK cell receptors are fundamentally different from the T cell receptor (TCR) and B cell receptor (BCR). NK receptor gene expression does not require gene segment rearrangement, and the receptors are not clonally distributed. Instead, NK cells use an array of stimulatory and inhibitory receptors to regulate their cytolytic functions (Lanier, 2008). A cluster of 10 or more genes encoding KIRs was located on human chromosome 19q13.4 (Biassoni et al, 2001; Lanier, 1998). Each of these type I glycoproteins recognizes a different allelic group of HLA-A–, HLA-B–, HLA-C–, or HLA-G– encoded proteins, and each KIR is expressed by only a subset of NK cells. Another family of immunoglobulin-like receptor genes termed ILT is present near the KIR locus at 19q13.3. These receptors are not as restricted as the KIRs and bind multiple HLA class I molecules. A third inhibitory receptor gene locus has been identified on chromosome 12p12-p13. These genes encode a C-type lectin inhibitory heterodimeric receptor called CD94/NKG2 that binds HLA-E. Importantly, those KIRs, ILT receptors, and CD94/NGK2 molecules with long cytoplasmic tails and two immunoreceptor tyrosine-based inhibitory motifs (ITIMs) function as inhibitory receptors. Upon phosphorylation, the two ITIMs recruit and activate the Src homology domain 2 (SH2)-containing phosphatases, which turn off the kinase-driven activation cascade (Ravetch and Lanier, 2000). The KIR family member KIR2DL4 is distinct from other KIRs in structure and distribution. KIR2DL4 binds HLA-G, has a single ITIM in the cytoplasmic tail and a lysine in the transmembrane region, which allows association with adaptor proteins. This inhibitory receptor was found on all dNK cells in the placenta at term, but not on circulating maternal NK cells. This observation suggests that expression of KIR2DL4 is induced during pregnancy (Rajagopalan and Long, 1999).

Other KIR or members of the C-type lectin superfamily serve as activating receptors (Moretta et al, 2001). These receptors lack the long cytoplasmic tail of the inhibitory receptors and therefore do not contain ITIMs. Instead, they have a charged amino acid in the transmembrane region that allows the receptor to associate with the adaptor molecule DAP12 (Lanier et al, 1998). This adaptor contains an immunoreceptor tyrosine-based activation motif (ITAM) that allows these receptors to activate NK cells. The physiologic role of these HLA class I–specific activating receptors remains unknown. Another group of NK cell–activating receptors has been identified and termed natural cytotoxicity receptors (Moretta et al, 2001). These proteins (NKp46, NKp30, NKp44) are immunoglobulin superfamily members with little similarity to one another or to other NK receptors. They are highly specific for NK cells and appear to interact with non-HLA molecules.

CD244 (2B4) is a member of the signaling lymphocyte activation molecule family of receptors expressed on all human NK cells (Ma, 2007). Upon interaction with the ligand CD48 on target cells, NK signaling proceeds via interactions between the ITSM (switch motif) in the cytoplasmic tail of CD244 and one of two SH2 domain-containing adaptor proteins, SAP and EAT-2. SAP interactions result in activation, as evidenced in humans with X-linked lymphoproliferative disease, which is caused by loss-of-function mutations in the SAP linker. In the absence of SAP, interactions with EAT-2 may be inhibitory (Lanier, 2008).

Polymorphonuclear Neutrophils

As observed for T and B lymphocytes, neonatal polymorphonuclear neutrophils (PMNs) are present at early stages of gestation, but their functional capacities are different from those of adult PMNs. Progenitor cells that are committed to maturation along granulocyte or macrophage cell lineages (granulocyte-macrophage colony-forming units) are detectable in the human fetal liver between 6 and 12 weeks' gestation in proportions comparable to those observed in adult bone marrow (Christensen, 1989). Human fetal blood has detectable granulocyte-macrophage colony-forming units from 12 weeks' gestation to term (Christensen, 1989; Liang et al, 1988). Although these progenitor cells are detectable in the fetus and newborn infant, developmental differences between adult and mature neonatal PMNs have been demonstrated—in signal transduction, cell surface protein expression, cytoskeletal rigidity, rolling adhesion, microfilament contraction, transmigration oxygen metabolism, intracellular antioxidant mechanisms, and extracellular trap formation (Carr, 2000; Henneke and Berner, 2006; Hill, 1987; Levy, 2007; Ricevuti and Mazzone, 1987; Yost et al, 2009). The severity of functional differences correlates with the maturity of the infant and begins to decrease within the first few weeks after birth (Carr, 2000).

Besides intrinsic differences in PMN function, induction of specific functions and maturation of these cells are developmentally regulated by the availability in the microenvironment of specific inflammatory mediators and growth factors (Christensen, 1989; Vercellotti et al, 1987). For example, an activation product of the fifth component of complement, C5a, is a chemoattractant at sites of inflammation. Low concentrations of C5 in neonatal sera might not permit establishment of chemoattractant gradients at sites of inflammation in newborns comparable to those in adults. Differences between adult and fetal–neonatal PMN functions may thus reflect intrinsic cellular differences required for fetal well-being and differences in the availability or activity of substances that regulate PMN function.

The recognition that systemic bacterial infection in newborns is frequently accompanied by profound neutropenia prompted the investigation of neutrophil kinetics in infected infants (Christensen et al, 1980, 1982; Santos, 1980). These studies have suggested diverse, developmentally specific regulatory mechanisms required for mobilization of the neutrophil response to infection. The lack of neutrophil precursors in bone marrow aspirates of infected infants and systemic neutropenia motivated several investigators to give neutrophil replacement therapy to neutropenic, infected infants (Christensen et al, 1980). Although this approach has been successful in some cases, the results have not been uniformly beneficial (Cairo, 1987; Cairo et al, 1984; Menitove and Abrams, 1987; Stegagno et al, 1985). Similarly, the use of granulocyte CSF or GM-CSF to treat infants with suspected infection has generally not shown a reduction in mortality (Carr et al, 2003). This heterogeneity emphasizes the importance of individualizing immunologic interventions for the developmental stage of the infant and the invading microorganism being treated.

Monocytes and Macrophages

Cells committed to phagocyte maturation (granulocyte or monocyte-macrophage) are detectable in the human fetal liver by 6 weeks' gestation and in peripheral fetal blood by 15 weeks' gestation. Unlike granulocytes, whose tissue half-life is hours to days, macrophages migrate into tissues and reside for weeks to months. In a tissue-specific fashion, these cells regulate availability of multiple factors, including proteases, antiproteases, prostaglandins, growth factors, reactive oxygen intermediates, and a considerable repertoire of cytokines.

The importance of macrophages in the neonatal response to infectious agents has been documented in multiple studies. For example, increased antibody response and protection from lethal doses of *Listeria monocytogenes* were induced in newborn mice by administration of adult macrophages (Lu et al, 1979). Functional differences in chemotaxis, phagocytosis, and toll-like receptor signaling between adult and neonatal cells have been observed and most likely result from both intrinsic fetal–neonatal monocyte-macrophage characteristics, such as reduced IL-12p70 production, and from nonmacrophage factors (e.g., decreased production of the lymphokine IFN-γ) (English et al, 1988; Kollmann et al, 2009; Levy, 2007; Stiehm et al, 1984; van Tol et al, 1984). Inducible expression of individual complement proteins by lipopolysaccharide (LPS), a constituent of gram-negative cell walls, has also been shown to differ between adult and neonatal monocyte–macrophages (Strunk et al, 1994; Sutton et al, 1986). This difference suggests that, although signal transduction mediated by LPS, LPS-induced transcription, and accumulation of mRNAs, which direct the synthesis of the third component of complement and factor B, are comparable in adult and neonatal cells, a translational regulatory mechanism does not permit these important inflammatory proteins to be synthesized by LPS-induced neonatal cells. This observation emphasizes the fact that fetal–neonatal monocytes–macrophages can have functions developmentally distinct from those of adult cells. For example, in utero production of growth factors and removal of senescent cells during tissue remodeling may be critical to fetal development (Kannourakis et al, 1988). Concurrent induction of these functions and immunologic effector functions in fetal monocyte–macrophages would potentially elicit nonspecific inflammation in actively remodeling tissues.

Besides having antibacterial functions, neonatal monocyte–macrophages contribute to tissue-specific regulation of the microenvironment in individual organs. For example, considerable attention has focused on the contributions of these cells to antioxidant defenses and to regulation of protease-antiprotease balance. Because of the importance in tissue injury and repair, tissue and injury-specific treatment by appropriately targeted and primed monocyte–macrophages may provide therapeutic options for treating a spectrum of problems, from oxygen toxicity in the lung to hemorrhage in the brain.

ADAPTIVE IMMUNITY

Lymphocytes play multiple critical roles in the adaptive immune responses. Major lymphocyte lineages identified by cell surface and functional criteria include T, B, and NK cells (Kawamoto and Katsura, 2009). All three types develop from $CD34^+CD38^{dim}$ hematopoietic stem cells found in the fetal liver and bone marrow (see Figure 36-1). CD34 is also expressed on early committed progenitors, which differentially express other markers usefully in lineage determination. Some early T cell progenitors retain myeloid potential, suggesting a revision of the classic model base on the presence of a common lymphoid progenitor (Bell and Bhandoola, 2008; Wada et al, 2008). The process of lymphocyte differentiation is best viewed as a progressive narrowing of differentiation potential based on the sequential expression of specific transcriptional regulators (Mansson et al, 2010).

T Lymphocytes

T lymphocytes or T cells develop in the thymus, which is formed from the third branchial cleft and the third or fourth brachial pouch. Thymic lobes are generated when tissue from these sites moves caudally to fuse in the midline. Each lobe can be divided into three regions based on structure and function: the cortex, the corticomedullary junction, and the medulla. The thymic cortex is composed of specialized epithelial cells that express MHC class I and class II molecules and mediate the early stages of T cell maturation. This complex developmental process (Figure 36-2) begins when multipotent $CD1a^-$, $CD5^-$, $CD34^+$, and

$CD38^{low}$ stem cells enter the thymus at the corticomedullary junction and migrate into the outer cortex (Awong et al, 2009; Res et al, 1996). Maturation continues as cells migrate back through the cortex toward the corticomedullary junction. The first committed T cells express low levels of CD4 and show DNA rearrangement at the TCR δ gene locus. These events are followed by low levels of CD8 expression and by rearrangement at the TCR-β locus, which generates a pre-TCR on the cell surface (Spits et al, 1998). The pre-TCR is composed of several polypeptides, including a TCR-β chain and the invariant pre-Tα chain. Expression of the pre-TCR serves as an important developmental checkpoint (beta selection; von Boehmer and Fehling, 1997). Cells that do not successfully rearrange their TCR-β chain cannot express the pre-TCR and die by apoptosis (Falk et al, 2001). The remaining cells generate antigen-specific receptors when the TCR-α chain replaces pre-Tα. These intermediate- to late-stage progenitors also express both the CD4 and CD8 coreceptors and are called *double positives*. The minor population of δγT cells follows a similar developmental pattern.

Small double-positive cells ($CD4^+$, $CD8^+$, TCR^{low}) constitute approximately three fourths of all thymocytes, reflecting the critical and rate-limiting developmental stage that follows. Further maturation requires that the unique TCR on each thymocyte interact with self-peptide–MHC complexes expressed on the surface of thymic epithelial cells. Several factors control the outcome of this interaction, including the strength and timing of the TCR signal generated and the nature of the antigen-presenting cell (Hogquist et al, 2005). The TCR and associated CD3 signaling complex translate subtle differences in the affinity of ligand binding into cell fate decisions through induced conformational changes in the CD3 signaling complex (Dave, 2009; Gil et al, 2005; Hayes, 2005), differential utilization of mitogen-activated protein kinase signaling pathways (Sohn et al, 2008; Sugawara et al, 1998), and subcellular compartmentalization of mitogen-activated protein kinase proteins (Daniels et al, 2006). Heterogeneity among thymic epithelial cells and the peptides that they

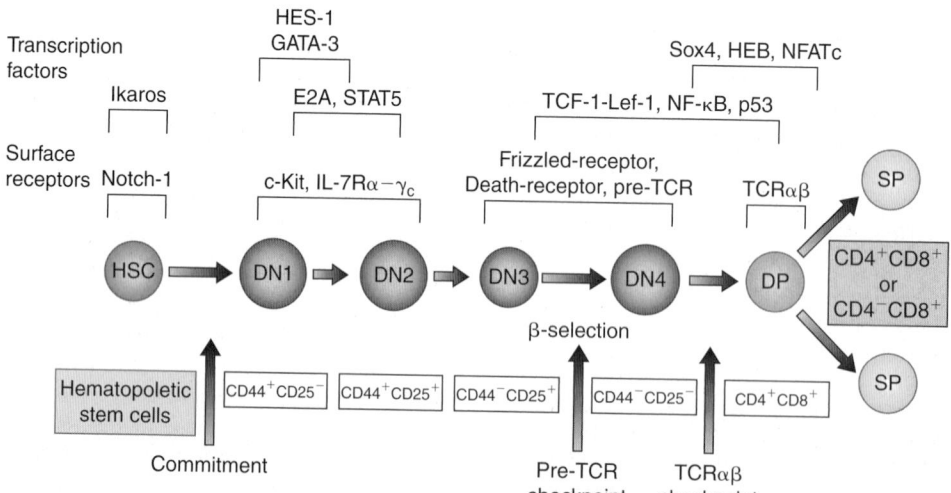

FIGURE 36-2 Transcription factors and checkpoints in thymic selection. *TCR*, T cell receptor. *(From Wu L, Strasser A: "Decisions, decisions": beta-catenin-mediated activation of TCF-1 and Lef-1 influences the fate of developing T cells, Nat Immunol 2:823-824, 2001.)*

present also contributes to the complexity of the selection process (Klein et al, 2009).

In the affinity-based model of thymic selection (see Figure 36-2), thymocytes that are unable to interact with thymic cortical epithelial cells fail to generate a survival signal and die by apoptosis, the default pathway for most developing cells. Weak interactions generate survival signals and continued development of positive selection. Studies in mice show that the result of positive selection is a thymocyte population containing a high frequency of cells that are broadly cross-reactive for multiple MHC alleles (alloreactivity) and for multiple peptides (Huseby et al, 2005). For many positively selected cells, subsequent high-avidity interactions with bone marrow–derived antigen-presenting cells in the thymic medulla result in activation-induced apoptosis or negative selection (Gong et al, 2001). Negative selection effectively culls from the positively selected pool of cells with cross-reactive TCR and is the primary mechanism for the elimination of self-reactive T cells (Huseby et al, 2003). For a small subset of thymocytes, high-affinity interactions with an agonist ligand can also induce a transcription factor, Foxp3, that is associated with regulatory T cell development rather than cell death (Jordan et al, 2001; Relland et al, 2009). Following avidity-based selection, mature T cells that express either the CD4 or CD8 coreceptor and a single TCR heterodimer are found in the thymic medulla just before the egress into the peripheral circulation. In the human embryo, the first naive, mature T cells appear at approximately 11 to 12 weeks of embryonic development. Thymopoiesis continues for many years thereafter, and integrity of this process is essential for a healthy immune system. Thymectomy early in life results in a substantial loss of naive T cells and in an oligoclonal memory T cell compartment (Prelog et al, 2009; Sauce et al, 2009). The decay process is accelerated by chronic CMV infection, resulting in an immunosenescent T cell phenotype similar to that seen in elderly individuals and associated with increased morbidity and mortality (Wikby et al, 2006).

The final phase of T cell development is independent of the thymus and involves peripheral (lymph nodes, spleen- and gut-associated lymphoid tissue) homeostatic mechanisms. These poorly understood events control the expansion of clones recognizing specific antigens and the development of T cell memory. Peripheral repertoire selection begins with migration of lymphocytes from the blood into lymphatic tissue. Naive T cells express the adhesion molecule L-selectin (CD62L) that interacts with peripheral-node addressins, a group of sialomucins present on high endothelial venules. Lymphocyte attachment, coupled with the shear forces produced by blood flow, results in rolling of the lymphocytes along the endothelial cell surface. Signals mediated by CC-chemokine receptor 7 (CCR7) molecules on the surface of rolling lymphocytes result in their tight binding to endothelial cells via integrins and in transendothelial migration (Forster et al, 2008). After entering the lymph nodes, movement of lymphocytes is also controlled by chemokines and their receptors (Worbs et al, 2007). CCR7 signaling directs cells to the T cell areas, whereas CXCR5-mediated signaling controls movement to B cell follicles (Reif et al, 2002). After activation, changes in chemokine receptor expression control

the mobilization and function of lymphocytes within the lymph nodes.

T cell activation requires a complex molecular cascade that results in reorganization of signaling molecules in the membrane into an "immunological synapse" and in signal transduction (Bromley et al, 2001). Many of the important biochemical events in this process have been described. TCR engagement by an appropriate MHC–peptide ligand results in phosphorylation of components of the CD3 complex. The CD3 complex is composed of the αβTCR and γ, δ, ε and ζ chains. These later molecules all contain specific amino acid sequences called *ITAMs*, which serve as molecular targets for the tyrosine kinases fyn and lck. The ζ chain is thought to be the most critical component and is found as a homodimer. Each ζ chain contains three ITAMs, which will bind the tyrosine kinase Zap-70 when sequentially phosphorylated. Appropriate phosphorylation of ζ results in a downstream cascade that involves the tyrosine phosphorylation of multiple cellular substrates including phospholipase Cγ1, the guanine nucleotide exchange factor Vav, and the adaptor protein Shc. Ultimately the genetic program of the cells is altered, leading to the transcription of genes for cytokines, cytokine receptors, and transcription factors (Cantrell, 2002).

After activation, CD4⁺ T cells differentiate into Th1, Th2, or Th17 effector cells or become induced Treg cells (Figure 36-3) (Murphy and Reiner, 2002; Zhu et al, 2010). Each of these CD4⁺ T cell types is defined by prototypical transcription factors and by secretion of a characteristic profile of cytokines in response to antigenic stimulation. The cytokine milieu in the local environment during antigen presentation is a primary factor influencing the developmental fate of a naive T cell following activation. IL-12 promotes Th1 cell development by a signal transducer and activator of transcription 4–dependent mechanism and

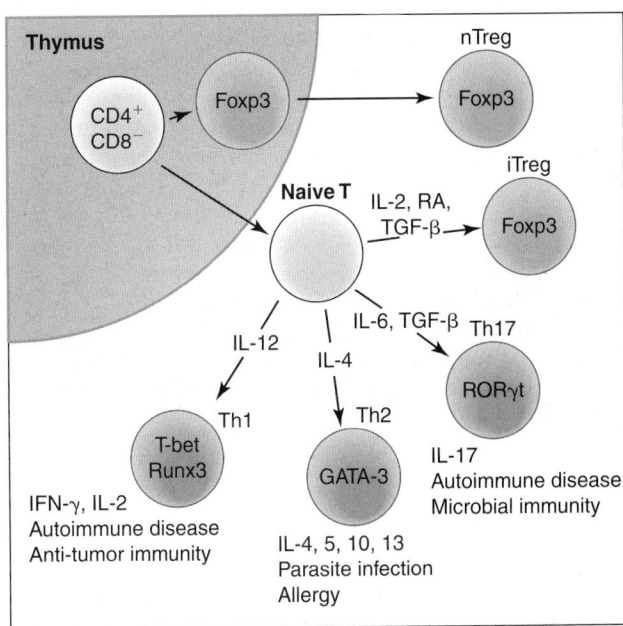

FIGURE 36-3 Cytokines and transcription factors associated with T cell differentiation. *IFN*, Interferon; *IL*, interleukin; *iTreg*, inducible regulatory T cell; *nTreg*, natural regulatory T cell; *TGF*, transforming growth factor. (*From Sakaguchi S, Yamaguchi T, Nomura T, et al: Regulatory T cells and immune tolerance*, Cell 133:775-787, 2008.)

results in expression of the transcription factor T-bet. Th1 cells secrete IL-2, IFN-γ, lymphotoxin alpha, and tumor necrosis factor-α. Th1 responses are generally proinflammatory. Th1 cytokines act synergistically to lyse virally infected cells and activate antigen-presenting cells as well as granulocytes. In addition to being the signature cytokine of Th1 cells, IFN-γ also promotes the development of the Th1 phenotype and inhibits the development of Th2 cells (Lighvani et al, 2001). Human neonatal T cells are biased against Th1 polarization relative to adult T cells (Levy, 2007). This bias has been linked to reduced IL-12(p35) gene expression by dendritic cells (Goriely et al, 2001, 2004) and IL-4–dependent apoptosis of Th1 cells after reexposure to antigen (Li et al, 2004). Poor Th1 function is associated with impaired killing of intracellular pathogens and a reduction in vaccine responsiveness (Levy, 2007).

IL-4–mediated activation of the transcription factor STAT6 is required for Th2 cell development (Kaplan et al, 1996). STAT6 activation drives expression of another transcription factor, GATA3, which promotes Th2 cell differentiation. Th2 cells produce IL-4, IL-5, IL-10, and IL-13. IL-4 induces immunoglobulin heavy-chain class switching to the IgE isotype and promotes the development of the Th2 phenotype. IL-5 is an eosinophil growth factor. Thus, Th2 cells are thought to promote antibody production and the allergic response by multiple mechanisms (Ouyang et al, 2001). Human fetal T cells are biased toward Th2 polarization (Prescott et al, 1998), and their abundant representation in the neonate contributes to the Th2 skewing of neonatal responses (Adkins et al, 2004).

The cytokines TGF-β and IL-6 activate STAT3, which induces the expression of the transcription factor RORγt and Th17 cell differentiation (Littman and Rudensky, 2010). Th17 cells, which are named for their secretion of the cytokine IL-17A and related family members, are proinflammatory cells associated with the clearance of intracellular pathogens and protection from infection by a number of bacterial and fungal species (Weaver et al, 2007). Abnormalities in Th17 cell development and function are also linked to immunodeficiency and autoimmunity. For example, humans with mutations in molecules affecting Th17 cell differentiation have the hyper-IgE syndrome (Al Khatib et al, 2009; de Beaucoudrey et al, 2008), and genes associated with Th17 cell differentiation are associated with increased susceptibility to Crohn's disease (Brand, 2009).

Activation of naive T cells requires a second signal, and the most potent costimulatory molecule is CD28. The ligands for CD28 are B7-1 and B7-2, which are present on the surface of antigen-presenting cells. Cyotoxic T-lymphocyte antigen 4 (CTLA-4), a molecule expressed only on activated T cells, also binds B7-1 and B7-2 and functions as a negative regulator of T cell activation. Experiments with knockout mice demonstrate that CD28 is the major costimulatory receptor and that signaling through CTLA-4 attenuates CD28-dependent responses (Alegre and Thompson, 2001; Subudhi et al, 2005). A maturational delay in the development of costimulatory function that contributes to reduced T cell responses in the neonatal period has been suggested (Orlikowsky et al, 2003), and the expression of costimulatory molecules is further suppressed by treatment with dexamethasone (Orlikowsky et al, 2005).

Control of the clonal proliferation seen in a primary immune response involves a number of inhibitory mechanisms, including Fas/FasL–mediated cell death, ligation of the cell surface molecule PD-1, and regulatory T cell–mediated suppression (Haribhai et al, 2007; Lettau et al, 2009; Riley, 2009; Sakaguchi et al, 2008). These mechanisms reset the peripheral immune system and thereby maintain adequate clonal diversity. A small number of activated T cells survives, and these cells differentiate into memory cells (Wakim and Bevan, 2010). Memory cells are defined by function (i.e., more rapid response) and by expression of certain cell surface markers. The transcription factors T-bet and eomesodermin influence memory development, probably by controlling expression of IL-7R and IL-15R (Intlekofer et al, 2005; Pearce et al, 2003). These receptors are linked to cell survival. Early memory T cells are L-selectin^{low}, CD45RO^{high}, and CD44^{high}. Late memory cells can become L-selectin^{high}, which is a surface marker seen in naive T cells. The ultimate number of memory cells has been shown in mice to reflect the initial antigenic load and clonal burst size. Memory T cells allow the secondary response to be more rapid and more potent, characteristics that form the basis for vaccinations. The memory phenotype is not seen early in life, but increases with age. The precise mechanisms that generate and maintain memory T cells have not been determined, although it is known that the persistence of CD8$^+$ memory T cells in mice does not depend on the persistence of specific antigen (Surh and Sprent, 2002; Williams and Brady, 2001). In one study, preterm and term infants developed comparable memory T cell responses after vaccination (Klein et al, 2010).

Immunocompetent T cells capable of responding to foreign lymphocytes in the mixed lymphocyte reaction are found in the fetal liver at 5 weeks' gestation. Before 8 weeks' gestation, lymphocytes are not detectable in the fetal thymus. After 8 weeks, lymphoid follicles, T lymphocytes, and Hassall's corpuscles can be identified. By 12 to 14 weeks' gestation, T lymphocytes can be found in the fetal spleen (Timens et al, 1987). By 15 to 20 weeks' gestation, the fetus has readily detectable numbers of peripheral T lymphocytes. The first T cell proliferative responses that occur are to mitogens and can be measured at approximately 12 weeks' gestation. By 15 to 20 weeks' gestation, antigen-specific responses can be detected (Adkins, 1999; Garcia et al, 2001). Fetal growth has been shown to influence T, B, and NK lymphocyte counts by 3% to 6% per week increase of gestational age (Duijts et al, 2009). Maturation of immune responses continues throughout the first year of life, a fact that affects vaccination schedules (Gans et al, 1998). A low level of thymopoiesis has been shown to continue into adulthood (Kennedy et al, 2001).

Regulatory T Cells

Natural regulatory T cells develop as a distinct lineage in the thymus dedicated to maintaining self tolerance (Sakaguchi et al, 2008). Induced Treg cells arise in the periphery from conventional CD4$^+$ T cells activated in the presence of TGF-β (Curotto de Lafaille and Lafaille,

2009). Expression of the forkhead-winged helix transcription factor Foxp3 ultimately identifies these cell types and is essential for the acquisition of suppressive effector function (Zheng and Rudensky, 2007). Treg cells are required for the maintenance of immunologic tolerance, as illustrated by the autoimmunity that arises after neonatal thymectomy and by the fatal autoimmune lymphoproliferative disease that develops shortly after birth in mice and humans deficient in Foxp3 (Bennett et al, 2001; Brunkow et al, 2001; Chatila et al, 2000; Sakaguchi et al, 1995; Wildin et al, 2001).

Treg cells have risen to the forefront of research in immunology because of their essential role in maintaining immunologic tolerance. Preclinical animal models have demonstrated that adoptive transfer of Treg cells can prevent or cure diabetes, experimental allergic encephalomyelitis (multiple sclerosis), inflammatory bowel disease, lupus, arthritis, and graft-versus-host disease (Hori et al, 2002; Kohm et al, 2002; Morgan et al, 2005; Mottet et al, 2003; Scalapino et al, 2006; Tang et al, 2004; Tarbell et al, 2004; Taylor et al, 2002). In humans, removal of Treg cells in vitro enhances the proliferation of T cells in response to self-antigens (Danke et al, 2004). Defects in Treg cell function and number have been described in a number of different human autoimmune diseases, including diabetes, multiple sclerosis, rheumatoid arthritis, and juvenile idiopathic arthritis (Baecher-Allan and Hafler, 2006). Clinical trials using the adoptive transfer of Treg cells after allogenic hematopoietic stem cell transplantation as therapy for graft-versus-host disease have begun in Germany and are planned in the United States (Roncarolo and Battaglia, 2007).

B Lymphocytes

B cells are lymphocytes that upon activation give rise to terminally differentiated, immunoglobulin-secreting plasma cells. Immunoglobulins form the humoral arm of the immune system and provide the main form of protection against many pathogens. B cell development can be divided into embryonic and adult phases. The embryonic phase begins in the fetal liver at the same gestational age as T cell development, follows a similar time course, and uses similar developmental strategies. The adult phase occurs in the bone marrow and continues throughout life. In both phases, B cell progenitors are selected at key developmental checkpoints for the presence of a functional BCR rearrangement and for the absence of BCR self-reactivity. Those progenitors with self-reactive receptors are either eliminated or generate new antigen receptors by continued gene segment rearrangements that are not self-reactive. Both B cell development and peripheral B cell homeostasis require signal transduction through the BCR. Although the B cell compartment is well formed before birth, diversification of the antibody repertoire and several important antibody responses are not developed until long after the neonatal period (Hardy and Hayakawa, 2001; Rohrer et al, 2000; Rolink et al, 2001; Yankee and Clark, 2000).

B cell development begins before 7 weeks' gestation in the human fetal liver, and pre-B cells in various stages of maturation are seen by 8 weeks' gestation. By 8 to 10 weeks' gestation, CD34+ hematopoietic stem cells are also found in the bone marrow. The early phase of B cell development, like T cell development, is antigen independent. The first committed progenitors (pro/pre-B-I) express CD34, terminal deoxynucleotidyl transferase (TdT), recombinase-activating genes (RAG) and CD19 (Li et al, 1993). They lack immunoglobulin gene rearrangement (Allman et al, 1999). The next lineage is marked by heavy chain (H) diversity to joining (D_H to J_H) gene segment rearrangements followed by variable to diversity/joining segment rearrangement. Terminal deoxynucleotidyl transferase is used during this process to insert nucleotides between the segments to create additional diversity at a region that encodes the V_H portion of the antibody-binding site. Late cells in this stage express an invariant surrogate light chain (Kitamura et al, 1992). The normal light chain genes remain in germline configuration.

The first developmental checkpoint in B cell development requires expression of surrogate light chain together with Ig-α and Ig-β on the cell surface as the pre-BCR, marking the transition to the pre–BII stage. Expression of the pre-BCR is essential for positive selection of cells that have a functional μH chain rearrangement and for expansion of the pre–B cell lineage (Gong and Nussenzweig, 1996). Cells with a nonfunctional H chain rearrangement or with H chains that assemble poorly with surrogate light chain are unable to progress. V_L to J_L rearrangement takes place next, and the newly expressed polymorphic L chain protein replaces the surrogate light chain. The completed BCR is antigen-specific and contains the mIgM molecule. A second developmental checkpoint occurs here, and those B cells with self-reactive receptors are eliminated or edited (Hartley et al, 1991). Only 10% to 20% of the immature B cells survive this negative selection and migrate to the spleen, which they enter through the terminal branches of the central arterioles. Once in the spleen, they rapidly differentiate into mIgM+, mIgD+, B220+ mature B cells that enter the recirculating pool of B lymphocytes (Hardy and Hayakawa, 2001).

When mature B cells contact antigen through the BCR, a signal is transduced that promotes further growth and differentiation into surface Ig+ memory cells and plasma cells (Calame, 2001). BCR signaling involves activation of the tyrosine kinases Syk and Btk, which are also involved in pre-BCR signal transduction. Certain mutations in Btk result in a failure of pre-BCR signaling and lead to X-linked agammaglobulinemia. Many B cell responses use the ability of B cells to capture antigen at vanishingly low concentrations, process the antigen into small peptide fragments, and then present the antigen to Th cells in the context of MHC class II molecules. Antigen-specific T cells then form conjugates with antigen-presenting B cells. The T cell membrane protein gp39 interacts with CD40 on B cells and triggers B clonal expansion, cytokine responsiveness, and isotype switching.

B lymphocytes with surface IgM are first found in the human fetal liver at 9 weeks' gestation and in the fetal spleen at 11 weeks' gestation (Owen et al, 1977; Timens et al, 1987). Antigen-specific antibody production can be detected in the human fetus by 20 weeks' gestation. Fetal spleen cells can synthesize in vitro IgM and IgG by 11 and 13 weeks' gestation, respectively.

TABLE 36-2   Characteristics and Functions of Immunoglobulins

	Molecular Weight (kD)	Serum Concentration (g/L)	Serum Half-life (Days)	Neutralization	Opsonization
IgG1	150	10	21	++	+++
IgG2	150	5	21	++	(+)
IgG3	170	1	7	++	++
IgG4	150	0.5	21	++	+
IgA1	160	3	7	++	+
IgA2	160	0.5	7	++	+
IgM	900	2	5	++	+
IgD	180	0.03	3	+	+
IgE	190	0.00003	3	−	−

Adapted from Mix E, Goertsches R, Zett UKL: Immunoglobulins: basic considerations, *J Neurol* 253:V9-V17, 2006.
Ig, Immunoglobulin; *NK,* natural killer.

Immunoglobulins

Immunoglobulins are a heterogeneous group of proteins that are detectable in plasma and body fluids and on the surfaces of mucosal barriers and B lymphocytes. Although these proteins have multiple, diverse functions, they are classified as a family of proteins because of their capacity to act as antibodies—that is, to recognize and bind specifically to antigens. The rapid advances in understanding molecular structure and regulation, genetic diversity, and differences in functions of immunoglobulins have been reviewed recently (Bengten et al, 2000; Mix et al, 2006). The functions of immunoglobulins relevant to fetal and neonatal immunity are summarized in Table 36-2.

There are five known classes of immunoglobulins: IgG, IgM, IgA, IgE, and IgD. Human IgM circulates as a pentamer or hexamer and IgA as a dimer. Multimers are formed in association with an additional J-chain (or join-chain). Functions of individual immunoglobulin classes are different but overlapping (see Table 36-2) (Mix et al, 2006). The prototype immunoglobulin molecule consists of a pair of identical heavy (H) chains that determine the immunoglobulin class in combination with a pair of identical light (L) chains (Figure 36-4). Disulfide bonds and electrostatic forces link the chains. Each immunoglobulin molecule contains two N-terminal, identical domains with antigen-binding activity (Fab). The Fab fragment consists of variable (V_H and V_L) and constant (C_H and C_L) regions on both the H and L chains. The Fab domains function to bind antigenic epitopes via complementarity determining regions. A third fragment (i.e., F crystalline [Fc]) is devoid of antibody activity, but mediates immunoglobulin effector functions (Table 36-3). The principal functions of the Fc fragment include: receptor-mediated phagocytosis (IgG1/3 and IgA), cytotoxicity (IgG1/3), release of inflammatory mediators (IgE), receptor-mediated transport through mucosa (IgA and IgM) and placenta (IgG1/3), and complement activation (IgG1/3 and IgM). The five different isotype classes of human immunoglobulins (IgG, IgM, IgA, IgD, and IgE) are defined structurally by differences in the Fc fragments. Within isotypes, there are four IgG subclasses (IgG1, IgG2, IgG3, and IgG4) and two IgA subclasses (IgA1 and IgA2).

Immunoglobulin G

IgG is the most abundant immunoglobulin class in human serum and accounts for more than 75% of all antibody activity in this compartment. Its monomeric form circulates in plasma, has a molecular mass of approximately 155 kD, and in adults constitutes approximately 45% of total body IgG in the extravascular compartment. The human conceptus is able to produce IgG by 11 weeks' gestation (Gitlin and Biasucci, 1969; Martensson and Fudenberg, 1965). The importance of the contribution of IgG to immunologic function is illustrated by the clinical problems encountered in individuals with genetically disrupted IgG production (hypogammaglobulinemia). These patients have recurrent infections if they do not receive treatment with immunoglobulin replacement therapy (Yong et al, 2008).

Several investigators have observed that infants in whom group B streptococcal sepsis develops have low concentrations of type-specific IgG, which has prompted attempts at acute or prophylactic treatment with immunoglobulin replacement therapy (Stiehm et al, 1987). Although successful in some trials, replacement therapy in newborns has not proved as efficacious as in individuals with genetically determined hypogammaglobulinemia (Cohen-Wolkowiez et al, 2009; Noya and Baker, 1989). This difference might be caused in part by fetal and neonatal IgG synthesis being regulated by both developmental and genetic mechanisms (Cates et al, 1988; Lewis et al, 2006).

The kinetics of IgG placental transport suggest both passive and active transport mechanisms (Saji et al, 1999; Simister, 2003). Because IgG transport begins at approximately 20 weeks' gestation, preterm infants are born with lower IgG concentrations than are their mothers or infants born at term. The full-term infant has a complete repertoire of adult, maternal IgG antibodies. Thus, provided that relevant maternal IgG has been transported to the fetus, newborns are generally immune to many viral and bacterial infections (e.g., measles, rubella, varicella, group B streptococcus, and *E. coli*) until transplacentally acquired antibody titers decrease to biologically nonprotective concentrations at 3 to 6 months of age (Pentsuk and van der Laan, 2009). The regulation of IgG production in

Complement Activation	Epithelial Transport	Placental Transport	Sensitization for Killing by NK Cells	Sensitization of Mast Cells and Basophils
Strong classic, alternative	−	+++	++	+
Classical, alternative	−	+	−	−
Strong classical, alternative	−	++	++	+
Alternative	−	(+)	−	−
Alternative	+++	−	−	−
Alternative	+++	−	−	−
Strong classical	+	−	−	−
Alternative	−	−	−	+++
−	−	−	−	

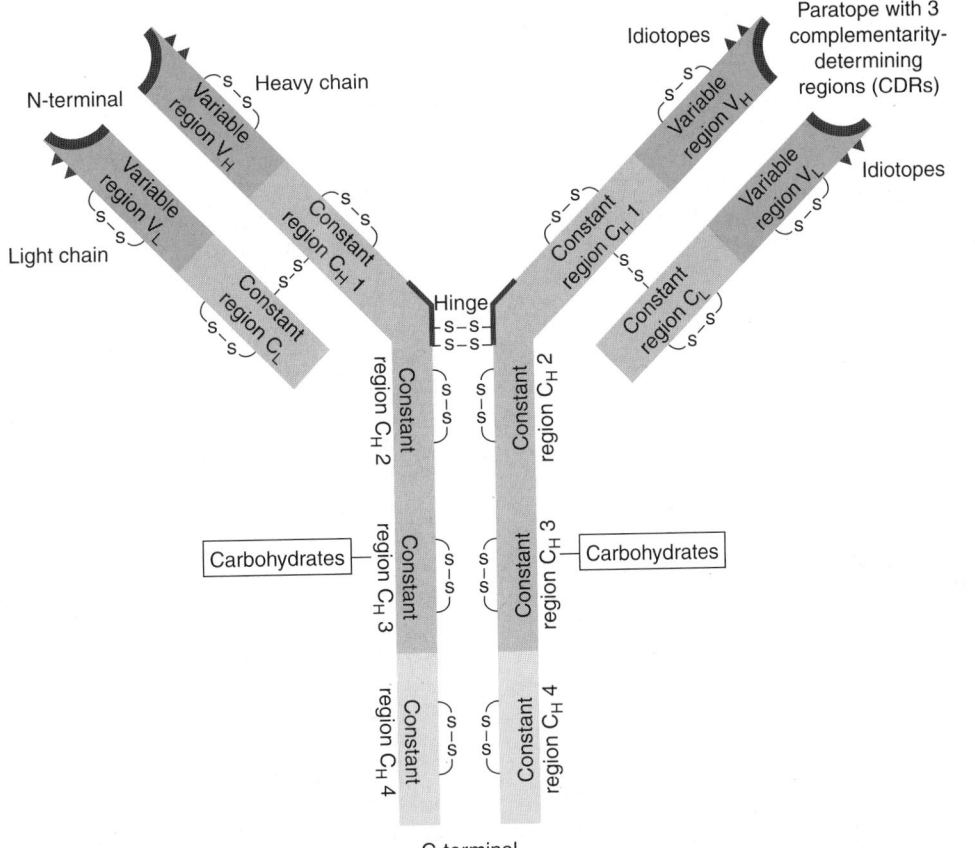

FIGURE 36-4 Structure of monomeric immunoglobulin. *(From Mix E, Goertsches R, Zett UK: Immunoglobulins: basic considerations, J Neurol 253(Suppl 5):V9-V17, 2006.)*

preterm infants has been a topic of study for more than 60 years (Ballow et al, 1986; Bauer et al, 2002; Bonhoeffer et al, 2006; Dancis et al, 1953; Meffre and Salmon, 2007; Schroeder et al, 1995). Although adults with antibody deficiency syndromes have a higher rate of infections when IgG concentrations are less than 300 mg/dL, the serum IgG concentrations of many preterm infants decrease to less than 100 mg/dL apparently without consequences. These observations suggest that preterm infants have additional immunologic protective mechanisms or that the protective capacity of humoral immunity is not accurately assessed by serum IgG concentrations alone in preterm infants. Studies also suggest that reduced endogenous secretion of IgG by newborns may result from reduced ability of neonatal B cells to undergo immunoglobulin isotype switching, because of decreased or ineffective expression of the ligand for the B cell surface protein CD40 on activated cord blood T cells (Brugnoni et al, 1994; Fuleihan et al, 1994).

TABLE 36-3 Severe Combined Immunodeficiency Classification

Mechanisms	Mutated Genes	Inheritance	Affected Cells
Premature cell death	*ADA*	AR	T, B, NK
Defective cytokine-dependent survival signaling	γc	X-L	T, NK
	JAK3	AR	T, NK
	IL7RA	AR	T
Defective VDJ rearrangement	*RAG1* or *RAG2*	AR	T, B
	Artemis	AR	T, B
Defective pre-TCR and TCR signaling	*CD3* δ, ξ, ε	AR	T
	CD45	AR	T

Adapted from Cavazzana-Calvo et al: Gene therapy for severe combined immunodeficiency: are we there yet? *J Clin Invest* 117:1456-65, 2007.
AR, Autosomal recessive; *NK,* natural killer; *TCR,* T cell receptor; *X-L,* X-linked.

IgG functions in host defenses in several ways. It can neutralize a variety of toxins in plasma by direct binding. As described previously in the section on complement, after antigen binding IgG can activate the complement cascade via interaction with early-acting, classical pathway complement components. The Fc portion of IgG can interact with cell surface receptors on mononuclear phagocytes and polymorphonuclear leukocytes and thereby promote clearance of immune complexes and phagocytosis of particles or microorganisms—a process known as *opsonization.* Finally, the presence of IgG on specific target cell antigens (e.g., tumors or allogeneic transplant tissues) can mediate antibody-dependent cellular cytotoxicity, a mechanism through which lymphocyte subpopulations bearing Fc receptors can acquire the capacity to recognize non–self-antigens.

Immunoglobulin M

IgM represents approximately 15% of normal adult immunoglobulin. IgM circulates in serum as a pentamer of disulfide-linked immunoglobulin molecules joined by a single cross-linking peptide (J-chain). The size of IgM (molecular mass >900 kD) restricts its distribution to the vascular compartment. Although the antibody-binding affinity of monomeric IgM is low, the multivalent structure of the molecule provides high pentameric antibody avidity. IgM synthesis has been detected in the human conceptus at 10.5 weeks' gestation (Rosen and Janeway, 1964). Because maternal-fetal transport of IgM does not occur, elevated (>20 mg/dL) concentrations of IgM in the fetus or newborn may be suggestive of intrauterine infection or immunologic stimulation (Alford et al, 1969; Stiehm et al, 1966). However, because it is technically difficult to distinguish IgM molecules with specificity for individual organisms, diagnosis of infections by analysis for specific IgM antibody remains of limited usefulness.

IgM is important for fetal and neonatal host defenses for several reasons. First, the IgM molecule is the most efficient of any immunoglobulin isotype in activation of the classical pathway of complement. As a result, it can trigger multiple effector functions of this cascade. Second, its pentameric structure provides conformational flexibility to accommodate multivalent ligand binding. Third, because of its localization in the vascular compartment and its high efficiency in complement activation, IgM has a prominent role in clearance from serum of invading microorganisms.

Immunoglobulin A

Although IgA accounts for approximately 10% of serum immunoglobulins, it is detectable in abundance in all external secretions (Brandtzaeg, 2010). In serum, IgA is present as a monomer (molecular weight, 160 kD), whereas in secretions it exists as a dimer (molecular weight, 500 kD) attached to a J chain identical to that found in IgM. In addition to this structural difference, mucosal IgA is attached to an additional protein called the *secretory component.* This protein is a proteolytic cleavage fragment of the receptor involved in the secretion of polymeric IgA onto mucosal surfaces and into bile. Secretory IgA produced locally on mucosal surfaces by plasma cells is thus readily distinguishable from serum IgA. Although the amount of IgA produced daily is not rigorously quantified, it is estimated to exceed immunoglobulin production of all isotypes combined. Despite its relative abundance, unlike IgM and IgG, IgA cannot activate the classical pathway of complement nor effectively opsonize for phagocytosis particles or microorganisms.

Although IgA is detectable on the surface of human fetal B cells at 12 weeks' gestation, adult concentrations of serum and secretory IgA are not achieved until approximately 10 years of age. Because serum IgA is not transplacentally transferred in significant amounts, IgA is almost undetectable in cord blood. Colostrum-derived secretory IgA can provide a source of IgA in both gastrointestinal tract and other secretions for the newborn infant (Brandtzaeg, 2010). Unlike other immunoglobulin isotypes, amino acid sequences of the hinge region of the IgA-2 subclass confer partial resistance to bacterial proteases. IgA is thus more resistant than other immunoglobulin isotypes to proteolytic effects of gastric acidity. Although considerable investigation suggests that passive immunization with IgA occurs with breastfeeding in humans, the overall importance of IgA in host defenses is currently not well characterized (Bailey et al, 2005).

Immunoglobulin E

The serum concentration of IgE is undetectable by standard immunochemical techniques and accounts for approximately 1/10,000 of the immunoglobulin in adult serum. It circulates in the monomeric form (molecular weight, 190 kD). Structurally, IgE lacks a hinge region. It is produced by most lymphoid tissues in the body, but in greatest amounts in the lung and gastrointestinal tract. It is not secreted, and its appearance in body fluids generally occurs only with induction of inflammation. IgE cannot activate complement or act as an effective opsonin. Its best-known role is as a mediator of immediate hypersensitivity reactions. Specifically, antigen-specific IgE triggers mast cell degranulation with resultant bronchoconstriction, tissue edema, and urticaria via interactions with IgE receptors on the mast cell surface. Because of the presence of IgE in lung secretions and its potential importance in mediating allergic pulmonary and gastrointestinal reactions, considerable interest has been recently focused on the use of serum IgE concentrations to identify premature infants at risk for developing reactive airways disease or in the diagnosis of gastrointestinal hypersensitivity reactions (Bazaral et al, 1971; Herz, 2008; Jarrett, 1984; Kagan, 2003).

Immunoglobulin D

Although IgD is found in trace quantities in adult human serum and has neither complement-activating activity nor the capacity to opsonize particles or microorganisms, approximately 50% of cord blood lymphocytes exhibit IgD on their cell surface (Colten and Gitlin, 1995; Haraldsson et al, 2000; Preud'homme et al, 2000). These pre–B lymphocytes express surface IgM and IgD simultaneously. Because of its wide distribution on B cells, IgD may have an important role in primary antigen recognition for the fetus and newborn infant.

Immunoglobulin Therapy

Because of low serum immunoglobulin concentrations, a concurrent greater susceptibility to infection in preterm infants, and successful use of immunoglobulin replacement in patients with genetically based hypogammaglobulinemia, several investigators have proposed prophylactic, intravenous administration of immunoglobulin (IVIG) to prevent antibody deficiency and nosocomial infection (Baker et al, 1992; Clapp et al, 1989; Cohen-Wolkowiez et al, 2009; Fanaroff et al, 1994; Kinney et al, 1991; Lewis et al, 2006; Magny et al, 1991; Weisman et al, 1994). Immunoglobulin therapy in very low-birthweight neutropenic infants with bacterial sepsis and shock has been tried with some success, when the potential benefits might outweigh the immunomodulatory properties of IVIG (Christensen et al, 2006). However, well-designed, placebo-controlled studies have failed to show consistent benefit of this strategy using different preparations of immunoglobulin, different treatment groups, and different dosage regimens (Ohlsson and Lacy, 2004a). These results suggest that serum immunoglobulin concentrations do not predict immunoglobulin function and immunologic response as accurately in the newborn infant as in the older child or adult.

In infants with sepsis, the results of immunoglobulin therapy have been difficult to interpret because of the complexities in study design associated with enrolling acutely ill infants and the small numbers of enrolled infants (Ohlsson and Lacy, 2004b). A recent metaanalysis of randomized, controlled studies that examined the effects of polyvalent immunoglobulin for treatment of sepsis or septic shock in newborn infants (12 trials, 710 newborn infants) suggested a reduction in mortality (Kreymann et al, 2007). However, heterogeneous study quality led the Cochrane reviews to suggest that there is still insufficient evidence to recommend routine use of this strategy. The availability of results from the large cohort recruited for the International Neonatal Immunotherapy Study (www.npeu.ox.ac.uk/inis) should provide a more definitive recommendation (INIS Study Collaborative Group, 2008). Other interventions including administration of colony-stimulating factors, antistaphylococcal antibodies, probiotics, glutamine supplementation,

recombinant human protein C, and lactoferrin have been reviewed recently (Cohen-Wolkowiez et al, 2009).

Besides prophylactic or acute treatment of systemic bacterial infection, the therapeutic scope of monoclonal and polyclonal immunoglobulin therapy has expanded over the last 10 years. For example, although controversy still exists concerning specific populations of infants for whom prophylaxis is appropriate, administration of anti–respiratory syncytial virus monoclonal antibody has become standard of care for prevention of respiratory syncytial virus (RSV) infection in high-risk infants and for management of nosocomial outbreaks of RSV (Fitzgerald, 2009; Halasa et al, 2005; Kurz et al, 2008; Wu et al, 2004). In addition, administration of intravenous IgG is a safe and effective immunomodulatory strategy for reducing the need for exchange transfusion in hemolytic disease of the newborn if the total serum bilirubin is rising despite intensive phototherapy (American Academy of Pediatrics Subcommittee on Hyperbilirubinemia, 2004; Smits-Wintjens et al, 2008; Walsh and Molloy, 2009). Intravenous immunoglobulin is also indicated for treatment of immune thrombocytopenia (Bussel and Sola-Visner, 2009). The administration directly into the ocular vitreous of antibody against vascular endothelial growth factor to bind and inactivate vascular endothelial growth factor has been shown in early studies to reduce the need for laser therapy for retinopathy of prematurity (Mintz-Hittner and Best, 2009). The historically promising use of oral immunoglobulin for preventing necrotizing enterocolitis has not proved effective in a recent Cochrane review of three trials ($n = 2095$ infants) (Foster and Cole, 2004). In view of the continued expansion of neonatal diseases that are potentially treatable with immunoglobulin, the use of immunoglobulin therapy must continue to be evaluated not only in terms of immediate benefits, but also in terms of long-term effects on immunologic function.

SPECIFIC IMMUNOLOGIC DEFICIENCIES

The most common reason for increased immunologic susceptibility to infection in newborns, besides prematurity, is iatrogenic immunosuppression caused by administration of corticosteroids for treatment or prevention of bronchopulmonary dysplasia. Although pulmonary and neurodevelopmental benefits have been attributed to this therapy (Abman and Groothius, 1994; Cummings et al, 1989), caution has developed concerning possible long-term, adverse neurodevelopmental effects of steroid administration (Bancalari, 2001; Barrington, 2002; Committee on the Fetus and Newborn, 2002). Although the mechanisms that lead to steroid-induced amelioration of pulmonary disease have not been elucidated completely, the pulmonary inflammatory response as measured by the concentrations of the anaphylatoxin C5a, leukotriene B4, IL-1, elastase-α1-proteinase inhibitor, and the number of neutrophils has been shown to be attenuated in infants receiving steroid treatment (Groneck et al, 1993). Whereas shorter courses of steroids can reduce side effects, including immunosusceptibility, the availability of nebulized steroids may provide effective antiinflammatory therapy with minimum toxicity (Cole et al, 1999).

There are more than 130 recognized primary immunodeficiency diseases (Notarangelo, 2010). The physician should attempt to differentiate infants with specific genetically regulated immunologic deficiencies from those with developmentally regulated, environmentally induced, or infection-related susceptibility to microbial invasion (Rosen, 1986; Rosen et al, 1984). Documenting a full family history during an antenatal visit can be helpful in identifying relatives removed by as many as two to four generations with histories suggestive of primary immunodeficiency disease, as most arise from single-gene defects. Genetic testing is widely available for many primary immunodeficiency diseases, although de novo mutations are common (Notarangelo, 2010). Several single-gene defects resulting in blocks in T and B cell development are shown in Figure 36-5. Several disorders arising from these defects can manifest in the first months of life.

SEVERE COMBINED IMMUNODEFICIENCY

Severe combined immunodeficiencyt (SCID) is a rare category of diseases that affect development of both B cells and T cells. The estimated frequency is between 1 per 70,000 and 1 per 100,000 live births (Buckley et al, 1997; Stephan et al, 1993). Before identifying the genes involved in producing the SCID phenotype, investigators classified patients with the disorder by analyzing the number, cell surface proteins, and function of circulating lymphocytes. The most common subgroups are T⁻B⁻ SCID, T⁻B⁺SCID, and adenosine deaminase deficiency.

T⁻B⁺ SCID accounts for more than half of all SCID cases, and both X-linked and autosomal recessive forms exist (Fischer, 2000). Approximately 80% of T⁻B⁺ SCID cases involve males with the X-linked form, which results from deleterious mutations in the common gamma chain (γc) shared by the IL-2, IL-4, IL-7, IL-9, and IL-15 cytokine receptors (see Figure 36-5) (Noguhi et al, 1993). Defects in the γc protein abrogate the development of T cells and NK cells and lead to B cell dysfunction despite normal B cell numbers. IL-7 receptor signaling is essential for T cell development within the thymus, and the deficiency of this cytokine accounts for the absence of T cells (Cao et al, 1995; DiSanto et al, 1995; Peschon et al, 1994). IL-15 is implicated in NK cell development, and reductions in IL-4 receptor signaling are thought to contribute to poor B cell function seen in γc deficient patients (Mrozek et al, 1996). Nevertheless, the precise mechanisms involved in the NK cell developmental defect and the B cell functional defect are largely unknown.

The less common autosomal recessive form of T⁻B⁺SCID is primarily due to mutations in the Janus-associated tyrosine kinase JAK3 (Macchi et al, 1995; Russell et al, 1995). This kinase is expressed in cells of hematopoietic lineage and associates with γc as part of the cytokine receptor signaling cascade. The T⁻B⁺NK⁻ immunophenotype of these patients is identical to that seen in γc deficiency. Rarely, patients with autosomal recessive T⁻B⁺ SCID have NK cells. In two such patients, a defect was found in the IL-7Rα chain (Puel et al, 1998). This finding was predicted by the phenotype of the IL7R knockout mouse, and the data imply that the IL-7 receptor is not essential for NK cell development.

Clinically, the X-linked and autosomal recessive forms of T⁻B⁺ SCID are indistinguishable. Affected infants often appear healthy at birth. In the neonatal period a morbilliform rash, probably the result of attenuated

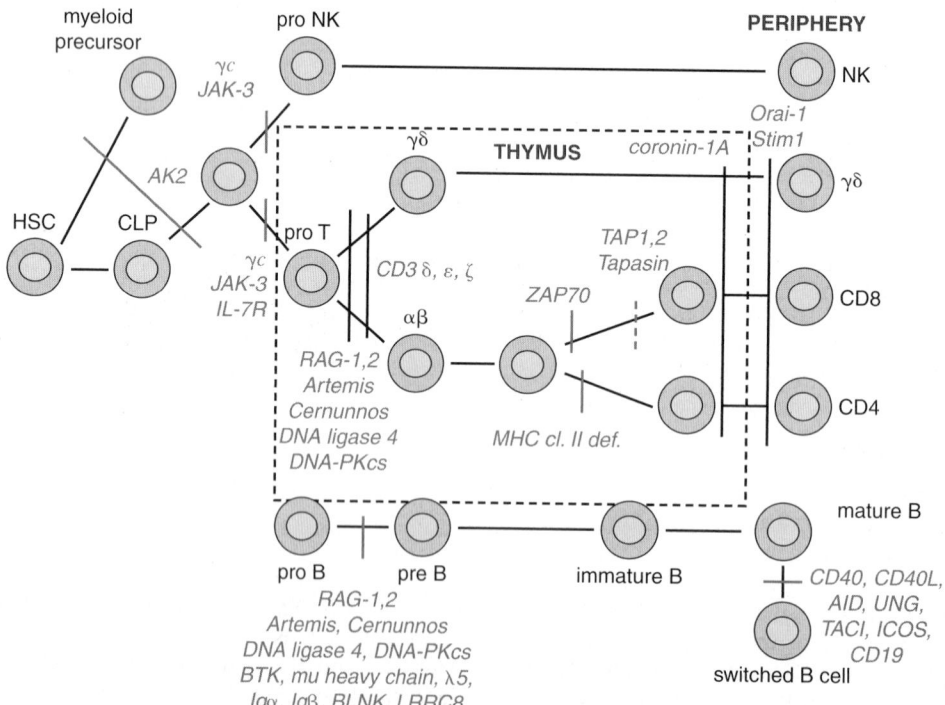

FIGURE 36-5 Blocks in T and B cell development associated with severe combined immunodeficiency and other primary immunodeficiencies. *NK*, Natural killer. (*From Notarangelo LD: Primary immunodeficiencies*, J Allergy Clin Immunol *125:S182-S194, 2010.*)

graft-versus-host disease from transplacental passage of maternal lymphocytes, may be the only symptom of SCID (Rosen, 1986). Over the first several months of life, as acquired maternal antibody levels drop, failure to thrive and undue susceptibility to infection become universal features. Intractable diarrhea, pneumonia, and persistent thrush, especially oral thrush, constitute the triad of findings most frequently seen in infants with this disease (Stephan et al, 1993).

Mutations in the gene encoding adenosine deaminase (ADA), an enzyme in the purine salvage pathway, account for approximately 20% of all cases of SCID. Mutations in another enzyme in the purine salvage pathway, purine nucleoside phosphorylase, are found in approximately 4% of patients with SCID (Fischer, 2000; Fischer et al, 1997). The ADA-deficient phenotype is variable, and neonatal onset, delayed onset, and partial forms have been described (Santisteban et al, 1993). In neonatal-onset ADA deficiency, patients have a profound T, B, and NK cell lymphopenia, with a clinical presentation similar to T⁻B⁺ SCID (Hirschhorn, 1990). Although ADA is normally present in all mammalian cells, life-threatening disease in ADA deficiency is limited to the immune system. Less severe manifestations include flaring of the costochondral junction as seen on the lateral chest radiograph (termed *rachitic rosary*) and pelvic dysplasia. Other findings associated with ADA deficiency include hepatic and renal dysfunction, deafness, and cognitive problems (Fischer, 2000; Rogers et al, 2001). Patients who lack ADA accumulate deoxy-adenosine triphosphate in red blood cells and lymphocytes, and the concentration correlates with disease severity. The ADA substrates, adenosine and deoxy-adenosine, are found at increased levels in the serum and urine. Studies in ADA-deficient mice suggest that developing thymocytes are particularly sensitive to these metabolic derangements and that the few T cells that mature have signaling defects (Blackburn et al, 2001). The precise mechanism by which the accumulation of ADA substrates results in the immunologic pathology seen in humans remains unclear (Yamashita et al, 1998).

The remaining 20% of SCID patients lack mature T and B cells, but have functional NK cells (T⁻B⁻NK⁺). These patients exhibit an autosomal recessive pattern of inheritance and have defects in the VDJ recombination machinery (Schwarz et al, 1996). Somatic recombination of variable, diversity, and joining DNA segments is a critical step in the development of B and T cells. A rearranged IgM heavy chain and TCR-β chain form components of the pre–B and pre–T receptors, which provide essential survival signals for developing lymphocytes. In the absence of recombination, these lymphocyte precursors do not receive a survival signal, die, and produce the T⁻B⁻ SCID phenotype. NK cells do not require somatic cell recombination and survive. In the recombination process, DNA cleavage is mediated by RAG1 and RAG2, which are the recombination-activating proteins that recognize specific sequences flanking V, D, and J segments. The two proteins act in concert to introduce a double-strand DNA break and leave hairpin-sealed coding ends. Recruitment of a DNA-dependent protein kinase and other components of the general DNA repair machinery completes the process.

Mutations in the genes encoding both RAG1 and RAG2 have been identified in patients with T-B-NK+ SCID (Cornero et al, 2000) and in some patients with Omenn's syndrome (Cornero et al, 2001). Omenn's syndrome is clinically characterized by failure to thrive, diarrhea, erythroderma, alopecia, hepatosplenomegaly, and lymphadenopathy. This concurrence of RAG mutations implies that factors other than RAG mutations also contribute to the Omenn's syndrome phenotype. Finally, a small subset of T-B-NK+ SCID patients also have increased sensitivity to ionizing radiation, which suggests mutations that affect the DNA repair mechanism (Fischer, 2000). This supposition is strengthened by murine and equine SCID in which specific defects in the DNA-dependent protein kinase involved in VDJ recombination and DNA repair have been identified.

The diagnosis of SCID is often suggested by an opportunistic or unusually severe infection in the setting of profound lymphopenia (<1000 lymphocytes per mm³) (Gennery and Cant, 2001). Only 10% of patients with SCID have lymphocyte counts in the normal range. T cells detectable in peripheral blood of affected infants shortly after birth may be either maternal T cells or circulating thymocytes. The thymus gland is not seen on chest radiographs. Histologically, the gland is composed of islands of endodermal cells that have not become lymphoid and contain no identifiable Hassall's corpuscles. Lymphocyte subpopulation analysis using monoclonal antibodies to cell surface markers and analytical flow cytometry is the most important confirmatory test. As noted previously, each phenotypic pattern suggests a specific diagnosis and molecular defect. Other useful tests include measurements of ADA and purine nucleoside phosphorylase activity in red blood cells and isohemagglutinins as a marker of specific IgM production. Quantitative immunoglobulin levels are not particularly helpful in the diagnosis of neonatal SCID, because most IgG is maternal in origin and IgA and IgM levels are often low in the neonatal period. Once the immunophenotype has been established, a precise molecular diagnosis should be obtained and genetic counseling should be provided. Females carrying deleterious mutations in the *IL2RG* gene (X-linked SCID) can be identified by nonrandom inactivation of the X chromosome in lymphocytes. Prenatal diagnosis is available by gene identification from a chorionic villous biopsy. In the absence of definitive prenatal genetic testing, all newborn siblings of patients with known SCID, and infant male first cousins of patients with known or suspected X-linked SCID, should be considered at high risk for this disorder and investigated promptly after birth.

An effective strategy for detecting newborn infants with SCID with statewide newborn screening was first implemented in Wisconsin (Routes et al, 2009). The test is based on the detection of T cell recombination excision circles by PCR and also identifies patients with lymphopenia resulting from other causes (Baker et al, 2009; Chan and Puck, 2005). When a fetus at risk for a genetic form of SCID is identified, treatment should begin in the delivery room and should be coordinated with antenatal diagnostic interventions. Specifically, cord blood samples should be obtained for white blood cell count and differential, lymphocyte subset determinations, karyotype (if not performed antenatally), mitogen stimulation studies, and immunoglobulin measurements. Because the majority of children with genetic SCID do not become ill within the 1st week of life, care in an incubator should be provided, and staff members should observe strict handwashing technique.

SCID is a pediatric emergency and is invariably fatal if untreated. Most untreated patients die in the 1st year of life. Treatment of SCID begins with aggressive antibiotic and antiviral therapy for infections, intravenous immunoglobulin replacement, and prophylaxis for *Pneumocystis carinii* infection. Besides greater susceptibility to opportunistic infections, these infants are also susceptible to development of graft-versus-host disease, either before birth as a result of engraftment of maternal T lymphocytes or after birth as a result of the engraftment of T lymphocytes present in transfused blood products (Pollack et al, 1982; Thompson et al, 1984). Therefore infants in whom SCID is suspected should receive only irradiated blood products and should not be given live viral vaccines.

Good and colleagues performed the first successful bone marrow transplantation (BMT) in a SCID patient (Gatti et al, 1968). Allogeneic BMT, preferably from an HLA-matched sibling, is now the standard treatment for most types of SCID (Buckley, 2000). In these transplants, conditioning regimens are not required for engraftment. Recipients usually become chimeric, with only T and NK cells of donor origin. B cell function is frequently deficient and many patients continue to require monthly therapy with IVIG. Survival rates for this type of BMT exceed 90%. When no HLA-identical donor is available, haploidentical transplants have been used successfully, although overall survival is lower with such transplants (Fischer, 2000). The rates of engraftment after haploidentical transplantation of T−B−NK+ SCID patients are low; this is likely due to host NK cell function, and some form of preconditioning may be indicated in this subset of patients. In addition to BMT, ADA deficiency can be treated with enzyme replacement. This treatment involves weekly injections of ADA coupled to polyethylene glycol. Response, consisting of decreasing deoxyadenosine triphosphate levels and increasing T cell numbers, is seen in most patients within weeks. Finally, gene therapy based on vector-mediated transfer of therapeutic gene into autologous hematopoietic stem cells has been used to treat patients with ADA and γc SCID and patients with chronic granulomatous disease. Results in more than 30 patients showed engraftment and clinical benefit, but were limited by transient expression and by insertional mutagenesis (Aiuti and Roncarolo, 2009).

WISKOTT-ALDRICH SYNDROME

Wiskott-Aldrich syndrome (WAS), another form of primary immunodeficiency, is characterized by severe eczema, thrombocytopenia, increased risk of malignancy, and susceptibility to opportunistic infection. Other manifestations, which may be present in the newborn period, include petechiae and bruises, bloody diarrhea, and hemorrhage after procedures. In infants with any of these clinical findings, abnormal low mean platelet volume in a complete blood count report is an important clue to possible WAS. WAS is inherited as a sex-linked

recessive trait (Rosen, 1986). In untreated cases, children survive longer than infants with SCID (median survival, 5.7 years). T lymphocytes in affected patients are decreased in number and diminished in function. Reductions in platelet size and thrombopoiesis are also noted. Affected children can be treated with BMT, and the 5-year survival rate after HLA-identical sibling BMT is approximately 90% (Filipovich et al, 2001). Although transplantation corrects the T cell defects, thrombocytopenia persists. As for children with SCID, all blood products given to children with WAS should be irradiated before administration to avoid T cell engraftment and graft-versus-host disease.

The gene responsible for the WAS was cloned in 1994 (Derry et al, 1994). It is composed of 12 exons and encodes a 502 amino acid cytoplasmic protein (WAS) expressed in all hematopoietic cells. Evaluation by flow cytometry for expression of this protein by lymphocytes can be used to diagnose WAS. Other mammalian WAS family members include a more widely expressed N-WAS and three WAVE/Scar isoforms. These proteins have multiple domains and are important regulators of actin polymerization (Symons et al, 1996); they have a common carboxy-terminal region through which they activate Arp2/3, an actin-nucleating complex involved in actin assembly and cytoskeletal structure. The amino termini are distinct and allow the proteins to couple Arp2/3 activation to a wide variety of different intracellular signals. More than 340 mutations in WAS have been described, which have profound effects on cell motility, signaling, and apoptosis (Rengan and Ochs, 2000).

DiGEORGE SYNDROME

The embryologic anlage of the thymus gland and the parathyroid gland is the endodermal epithelium of the third and fourth pharyngeal pouches. When normal development of these structures is disturbed, thymic and parathyroid hypoplasia can occur (Rosen, 1986). Infants with this disorder, DiGeorge syndrome, can exhibit abnormalities of calcium homeostasis during the neonatal period (hypocalcemia and tetany) and variable T cell deficits, which appear to depend on the presence and number of small, normal-appearing ectopic thymic lobes. In addition, these infants have congenital, conotruncal cardiac defects, low-set ears, midline facial clefts, hypomandibular abnormalities, and hypertelorism.

The availability of methodology for performing gene dosage studies and more refined cytogenetic techniques (fluorescence in situ hybridization) has permitted the description of a contiguous gene syndrome that includes the DiGeorge phenotype (Hall, 1993). The DiGeorge syndrome is known to result from varying sized deletions on chromosome 22q11 in more than 90% of patients (Markert, 1998; Shprintzen, 2008). This deletion has been linked to several other diagnostic labels, including velocardiofacial (Shprintzen) syndrome, Cayler syndrome, and Opitz G/BBB syndrome. Collectively, these are referred to as the *22q11 deletion syndromes*. The cardiac anomalies associated with the 22q11 deletion syndrome are variable, but usually involve the outflow tract and the derivatives of the branchial arch arteries. These defects include interrupted aortic arch type B, truncus arteriosus, and tetralogy of Fallot (Carotti et al, 2008).

Children with the 22q11 deletion syndrome also exhibit a higher incidence of receptive-expressive language difficulties, cognitive impairment, and behavioral problems including psychotic illness (Jolin et al, 2009; Scambler, 2000). The cardiovascular defects have been shown to be the result of haploinsufficiency of TBX1 (Merscher et al, 2001).

In the nursery, identification of infants with congenital conotruncal abnormalities or unexplained, persistent hypocalcemia should prompt consideration of this syndrome. Thymic implants can partially correct the immunologic deficits (Markert et al, 2007).

IMMUNIZATION

MATERNAL IMMUNIZATION

Immunization before or during pregnancy has been effective in preventing several specific neonatal infections including diphtheria, pertussis, tetanus, hepatitis B, and rabies (ACOG Technical Bulletin Number 160, 1993; Hackley, 1999; Immunization Practices Advisory Committee, 1991; Stevenson, 1999). For example, in developing countries, immunization during pregnancy with tetanus toxoid is a cost-effective method for preventing neonatal tetanus and for providing up to 10 years of protection for infants (Gill, 1991; Schofield, 1986; Vandelaer, 2003). The benefits are substantial for both mother and infant from induction before or during pregnancy of maternal IgG antibody that can be transferred to the fetus and protect both the fetus and mother against postpartum morbidity and mortality (Healy and Baker, 2006; Insel et al, 1994; Linder and Ohel, 1994). However, immunization during pregnancy is biologically distinct from immunization of nonpregnant individuals. Vaccine epitopes can be shared with vital fetal or placental tissues; therefore vaccination can lead to unanticipated maternal or fetal morbidity. Maternal immunization can induce an antibody response in the fetus, as has been demonstrated with tetanus toxoid (Gill et al, 1983) and thereby induce potentially undesirable immunologic side effects (e.g., immunologic unresponsiveness or tolerance) in the infant.

Nevertheless, the increase in availability of potentially protective, transplacentally transferred IgG through active maternal vaccination prompted the Institute of Medicine to recommend the establishment of a program of active immunization to control early-onset and late-onset group B streptococcal disease in both infants and mothers (Institute of Medicine and National Academy of Sciences, 1985). Efforts to develop safe, effective vaccines for protection from group B streptococcal infections have encountered the same difficulties with immunogenicity and safety observed in the development of other vaccines that induce protection from polysaccharide-encapsulated organisms (Baker et al, 1988; Noya and Baker, 1992). The availability of conjugate vaccines, which include group B streptococcal polysaccharide antigens covalently linked either to tetanus toxoid or to a protein in the membrane of group B streptococci (beta C protein) (Madoff et al, 1994; Wessels et al, 1993; Yang et al, 2007) have shown some promise.

The indications for active vaccination during pregnancy rest on assessment of maternal risk of exposure, the maternal-fetal-neonatal risk of disease, and the risk from the immunizing agents. (ACOG Technical Bulletin Number 160, 1993; Hackley, 1999; Stevenson, 1999). In general, immunization with live viral vaccines during pregnancy is not recommended (Box 36-1). Preferably, immunizations with live viral vaccines are performed before pregnancy occurs. However, rare instances may occur in which live viral vaccine administration is indicated. For example, if a pregnant woman travels to an area of high risk for yellow fever, administration of that vaccine might be indicated because of the susceptibility of the mother and the fetus, the probability of exposure, and the risk of the mother and fetus from the disease. More common examples in the United States include influenza and polio virus vaccination. If a chronic maternal medical condition would be adversely affected by influenza, active immunization may be indicated during pregnancy. Similarly, if imminent exposure to live polio virus in an unprotected woman is anticipated, live oral polio virus vaccine may be used during pregnancy. If immunization can be completed before the anticipated exposure, inactivated polio virus vaccine can be given. A summary of recommendations for immunizations during pregnancy is provided in Box 36-1.

For the pediatrician, maternal immunization represents an important preventive intervention. Breastfeeding does not adversely affect immunization, and inactivated or killed vaccines pose no special risk for mothers who are breastfeeding or for their infants. Maternal immunizations with vaccines against polysaccharide-encapsulated

---

BOX 36-1 Summary of Recommendations for Immunization during Pregnancy

LIVE VIRUS VACCINES

- Influenza (LAIV)—contraindicated
- Measles—contraindicated
- Mumps—contraindicated
- Rubella—contraindicated
- Yellow fever—safety not established (travel to high-risk areas only)
- Varicella—contraindicated

INACTIVATED VIRUS VACCINES

- Hepatitis A—consider if high risk of exposure
- Influenza—recommended
- Rabies—consider if indicated

INACTIVATED AND RECOMBINANT BACTERIAL VACCINES

- Cholera—to meet international travel requirements
- Meningococcal polysaccharide vaccine—consider if indicated
- Plague—selective vaccination of exposed persons
- Typhoid—safety not established
- Pneumococcal polysaccharide vaccine—consider if indicated
- Tetanus-diphtheria—consider if indicated
- Hepatitis B—consider if indicated
- Meningococcal conjugate vaccine—safety not established

POOLED IMMUNE SERUM GLOBULINS

- Hepatitis A—postexposure prophylaxis
- Measles—postexposure prophylaxis

Adapted from Centers for Disease Control and Prevention: *Guidelines for Vaccinating Pregnant Women* (May, 2007). Available at www.cdc.gov/vaccines/pubs/preg-guide.htm. *LAIV,* Live attenuated influenza vaccine.

organisms (e.g., *Haemophilus influenzae* type b and group B streptococci) can decrease morbidity and mortality from these diseases during the first 3 to 6 months of the infant's life (Amstey et al, 1985; Baker et al, 1988; Colbourn et al, 2007; Walsh and Hutchins, 1989). The benefit of decreasing the risks of development of hepatocellular carcinoma, cirrhosis, and chronic active hepatitis from perinatal transmission of hepatitis B through prenatal screening and active and passive immunization of the infant is substantial (Arevalo and Washington, 1998). The implications of maternal vaccination during pregnancy for preterm infants have not been studied.

The anthrax attacks of September 2001 have raised the possibility of the need for preexposure or postexposure immunization programs that may include pregnant women. Currently available data tend to suggest that the anthrax vaccine licensed since 1970 in the United States has no detrimental effects on pregnancy and does not increase adverse birth outcomes, although caution is advised when administering this vaccine during the first trimester (Inglesby, 2002; Ryan et al, 2008; Wiesen and Littell, 2002). A second infectious agent that might be used in a bioterrorist attack is variola virus (smallpox). Although eradicated in 1977, this virus remains a concern because of its lethality, especially in pregnancy (Enserink, 2002; Suarez and Hankins, 2002). Pregnancy is a contraindication to smallpox immunization (Wharton et al, 2003); however, if an intentional release of smallpox virus should occur, pregnant women should be immunized because of their high risk of mortality if unprotected (Suarez and Hankins, 2002).

INFANT IMMUNIZATION

Advances in understanding the developmental regulation of immunity have suggested that immunization during the neonatal period offers important advantages (Lawton, 1994). The recommendations of the American Academy of Pediatrics for immunization of infants can be found at http://aapredbook.aappublications.org/resources/IZ Schedule0-6yrs.pdf (Anonymous, 2002; Committee on Infectious Diseases et al, 2002). Immunization against *H. influenzae* type b should be considered for infants who are discharged from intensive care nurseries at or after 2 months of age. For the preterm infant, different clinical approaches to immunization are used by practitioners, including decreasing the dose of immunogen, postponing the first immunization until a corrected age of 2 months, or waiting for an arbitrary weight to be achieved by the infant (e.g., 4.5 kg). However, the American Academy of Pediatrics recommends administering full-dose diphtheria, tetanus, and pertussis immunization beginning at 2 months of age. These recommendations (i.e., that no correction needs to be made for prematurity when initiating routine immunization in preterm infants) have been supported by longitudinal evaluation of serum antibody response in preterm infants (Bernbaum et al, 1989; Conway et al, 1993).

The Advisory Committee on Immunization Practices (ACIP) of the United States Public Health Service recommends universal immunization of infants to protect against perinatal transmission of the hepatitis B virus (HBV) and chronic HBV infection (Mast et al, 2005). This recommendation has been endorsed by the Committee on Infectious Diseases of the American Academy of Pediatrics. Chronic HBV infection occurs in approximately 90% of infected infants and is associated with hepatocellular carcinoma and cirrhosis leading to end-stage liver disease. All medically stable infants born to women with a negative test result for hepatitis B surface antigen (HBsAg) and weighing more than 2000 g at birth should begin a hepatitis immunization schedule in the newborn period before hospital discharge. Only single-antigen hepatitis B vaccines should be used for the birth dose (Mast et al, 2005).

All infants regardless of gestational age at the time of birth, and whose mothers have a positive test result for HBsAg, should receive passive immunization with hepatitis B immunoglobulin and active immunization with a single-antigen HBV vaccine within 12 hours of birth. Repeated vaccinations are given at 1 to 2 months and again at 6 months of age. For premature infants weighing less than 2000 g and born to HBsAg-positive mothers, the birth dose is not counted as part of the vaccine series. Special efforts should be made to complete the hepatitis B vaccination schedule within 6 to 9 months in populations of infants with high rates of childhood hepatitis B infection (Peter, 1994). For premature infants with birthweights of less than 2000 g born to HBsAg-negative women, vaccination can be delayed until just before discharge. These infants do not need routine serologic testing for anti-HBsAg after the third dose of vaccine. The infant whose mother has a negative test result for HBsAg, but has received active or passive immunization during pregnancy because of exposure to hepatitis B, should receive no treatment as long as the mother was HBsAg-negative at the time of birth. For current HBV vaccinations recommendations, the reader is directed to the Centers for Disease Control and Prevention Web site: www.cdc.gov/hepatitis/HBV/VaccChildren.htm.

In 1999, the U.S. Agency for Toxic Substances and Disease Registry raised concern about the possibility that administration of thimerosal-containing vaccines, including the hepatitis B vaccines, might lead to exposure to mercury that exceeded federal guidelines (Clark et al, 2001). Since March 2000, HBV vaccines used in the United States have not contained thimerosal. These yeast-derived recombinant HBV vaccines contain 10 to 40 µg/mL of HBsAg protein, have excellent safety records, induce minimum adverse reactions, and are highly immunogenic (Greenberg, 1993). Multivalent vaccines are available, but are not recommended for the birth dose. Guidelines for hepatitis immunization of infants have been developed for implementation for term and preterm infants. However, vaccine responses in the extremely preterm infant whose mother is HBsAg-positive, a population seen with increasing frequency because of the coincidence of intravenous drug abuse and carriage of HBsAg, have not been studied.

Short-term and long-term neonatal immunologic protection after fetal exposure to maternally administered vaccines against anthrax or smallpox, the mass use of which might be prompted by a bioterrorist attack, has not been studied. Similarly, guidelines for neonatal immunization against these agents are not currently available. Before the eradication of smallpox, smallpox vaccine was routinely administered to older infants and children. No data or experience is available on immunization of newborn infants with anthrax vaccine. For postexposure prophylaxis in newborn infants, both chemotherapy (amoxicillin, ciprofloxacin, or doxycycline) and immunization should be considered. Clinicians faced with decisions concerning immunization strategies for pregnant women and newborn infants after a bioterrorist attack should consult the Web site for the Centers for Disease Control and Prevention (www.cdc.gov).

SUGGESTED READINGS

Chase NM, Verbsky JW, Routes JM: Newborn screening for T-cell deficiency, *Curr Opin Allergy Clin Immunol* 10:521-525, 2010.

D'Argenio DA, Wilson CB: A decade of vaccines: Integrating immunology and vaccinology for rational vaccine design, *Immunity* 33:437-440, 2010.

Koga K, Mor G: Toll-like receptors at the maternal-fetal interface in normal pregnancy and pregnancy disorders, *Am J Reprod Immunol* 63:587-600, 2010.

Leber A, Teles A, Zenclussen AC: Regulatory T cells and their role in pregnancy, *Am J Reprod Immunol* 63:445-459, 2010.

Levy O: Innate immunity of the newborn: basic mechanisms and clinical correlates, *Nat Rev Immunol* 7:379-390, 2007.

M'Rabet L, Vos AP, Boehm G, et al: Breast-feeding and its role in early development of the immune system in infants: consequences for health later in life, *J Nutr* 138:782S-1790S, 2008.

Mor G, Cardenas I: The immune system in pregnancy: a unique complexity, *Am J Reprod Immunol* 63:425-433, 2010.

PrabhuDas M, Adkins B, Gans H, et al: Challenges in infant immunity: implications for responses to infection and vaccines, *Nat Immunol* 12:189-194, 2011.

Trowsdale J, Betz AG: Mother's little helpers: mechanisms of maternal-fetal tolerance, *Nat Immunol* 7:241-246, 2006.

Willems F, Vollstedt S, Suter M: Phenotype and function of neonatal DC, *Eur J Immunol* 39:26-35, 2009.

Zaghouani H, Hoeman CM, Adkins B: Neonatal immunity: faulty T-helpers and the shortcomings of dendritic cells, *Trends Immunol* 30:585-591, 2009.

Zhu J, Yamane H, Paul WE: Differentiation of effector CD4 T cell populations, *Annu Rev Immunol* 28:445-489, 2010.

Complete references and supplemental color images used in this text can be found online at www.expertconsult.com

VIRAL INFECTIONS OF THE FETUS AND NEWBORN AND HUMAN IMMUNODEFICIENCY VIRUS INFECTION DURING PREGNANCY*

Mark R. Schleiss and Janna C. Patterson

VIRAL INFECTIONS OF THE FETUS AND NEWBORN

Viral infections of the fetus and newborn infant are common and underrecognized. Given the urgency of identifying invasive bacterial disease in the neonate, the identification of viral infections is often relegated to a matter of secondary importance. However, identifying viral infections can also be a matter of great urgency, because antiviral agents are available for many of the most common infections. Accordingly, an appropriately high index of clinical suspicion of a neonatal viral infection can be lifesaving. Moreover, identification of viral disease in the newborn period may be of great prognostic significance, particularly for neurodevelopmental issues. Making a diagnosis of a neonatal viral infection can help to direct and focus the anticipatory management of the child's pediatrician during the course of well-child care. This chapter reviews the epidemiology, pathogenesis, diagnosis, and short- and long-term clinical management of many of the more common viral infections encountered in neonates.

One of the great challenges in the evaluation of viral disease in the newborn is the ascertainment of the timing of acquisition of infection. Some infections can be acquired either in utero or in the early postnatal period. In this chapter, *congenital infection* is defined as any infection acquired in utero. *Perinatal infections* are defined as those acquired intrapartum, typically during the labor and delivery process. *Postnatal infections* are acquired in the post-partum period and are defined as infections acquired after delivery through the first month of life. In some situations, correctly identifying the timing of acquisition of infection can have substantial consequences, not only for the management of the infant, but for the long-term prognosis. Figure 37-1 outlines the most common timing of acquisition of neonatal viral infections with an emphasis on the relative importance of the many viruses that can be acquired congenitally, perinatally, or postnatally. There is considerable overlap across categories for some viral infections that can be transmitted at any of these time points, and this will be considered on a pathogen-by-pathogen basis.

GENERAL DIAGNOSTIC APPROACH

Clinicians caring for newborns have long recognized that there are some common clinical manifestations that suggest the presence of a congenital or perinatal viral infection. These manifestations include evidence of intra-uterine growth restriction, hydrops fetalis, hepatomegaly, splenomegaly, pneumonitis, bone lesions, rashes, and hematologic abnormalities (Box 37-1). Because the incidence of congenital viral infections is high (Alpert and Plotkin, 1986), it is appropriate for clinicians to have a high index of suspicion in any newborn with signs or symptoms. However, caution should be taken in efforts to lump all neonatal viral infections into a single diagnostic category. An unfortunate example of this manner of thinking is the continued use of the terminology *TORCH titers* in the diagnostic approach to a symptomatic neonate. The *TORCH* acronym, first coined by Nahmias et al (1971), stands for toxoplasmosis, other infections, rubella, cytomegalovirus (CMV), and herpes simplex virus (HSV). Numerous variants of this acronym have been suggested over the past four decades (Ford-Jones and Kellner, 1995; Kinney and Kumar, 1988; Ronel et al, 1995; Tolan, 2008). Unfortunately numerous clinical laboratories continue to offer the "TORCH panel," typically consisting of serologic tests for toxoplasmosis, HSV, CMV, and rubella. This acronym has outlived its usefulness (Lim and Wong, 1994), and should be discarded from clinical parlance, based on the following considerations:

- Measurements of immunoglobulin G antibody titers virtually always simply reflect transplacental maternal antibody and provide little information of relevance to the infant's infection status. With the exception of the identification of antibodies to *Treponema pallidum*, which is always of interest and significance, antibodies against the other members of the TORCH panel are of little diagnostic significance.
- Congenital and perinatal infection can occur with HSV and CMV, even in the face of preconception maternal immunity. Thus the finding of antibody in a TORCH titer is neither diagnostic of infection nor reassuring in regard to protection against that infection.
- Highly sensitive virologic and molecular tools are available to identify virtually all pathogenic viruses. These tools include standard culture and nucleic acid identification techniques, typically based on polymerase chain reaction (PCR) amplification of viral nucleic acids. Such studies can facilitate rapid pathogen-specific diagnosis; therefore the diagnosis of neonatal viral disease should depend on diagnostic virology, not serology.
- Most importantly, the use of the TORCH acronym vastly underemphasizes the great diversity of viral pathogens that have been associated with infection in the newborn. A list of the myriad of viral pathogens that have been reported to cause congenital infection and disease is included in Box 37-2. A discussion of

---

*In writing this chapter, the authors excerpted portions of the chapters *Identification, Evaluation, and Care of the Human Immunodeficiency Virus–Exposed Neonate* by Karen P. Beckerman and *Viral Infections of the Fetus and Newborn* by Erica S. Pan, F. Sessions Cole, and Peggy Sue Weintrub from the previous edition of this book.

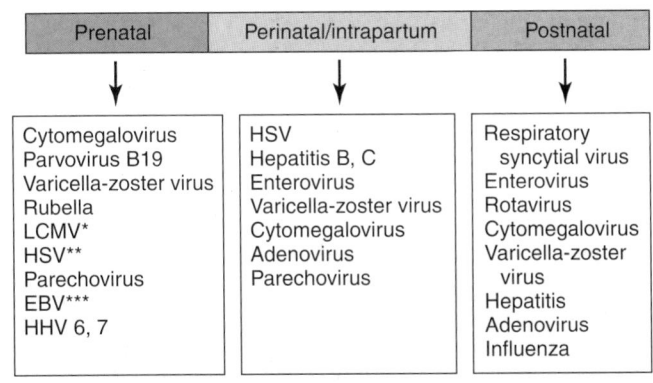

Prenatal	Perinatal/intrapartum	Postnatal
Cytomegalovirus Parvovirus B19 Varicella-zoster virus Rubella LCMV* HSV** Parechovirus EBV*** HHV 6, 7	HSV Hepatitis B, C Enterovirus Varicella-zoster virus Cytomegalovirus Adenovirus Parechovirus	Respiratory syncytial virus Enterovirus Rotavirus Cytomegalovirus Varicella-zoster virus Hepatitis Adenovirus Influenza

* Lymphocytic choriomeningitis virus
** Herpes simplex virus
*** Epstein Barr virus

FIGURE 37-1 **Relative importance of neonatal viral infections related to timing of acquisition of infection.** Viruses listed in declining relative order of importance relative to prenatal, perinatal (intrapartum), and postnatal timing of typical infection. Some neonatal virus infections (e.g., cytomegalovirus) can be substantial causes of disease whether acquired during gestation or postpartum, whereas others (e.g., respiratory syncytial virus) are typically acquired in the postnatal period. *EBV*, Epsteinn–Barr virus; *HSV*, herpes simplex virus; *HHV*, human herpes virus; *LCMV*, Lymphocytic choriomeningitis virus

---

BOX 37-1   Clinical Features Commonly Associated With Congenital Viral Infections in Neonates

- Intrauterine growth restriction
- Nonimmune hydrops fetalis
- Echogenic bowel (prenatal ultrasound)
- Hepatosplenomegaly
- Jaundice (>20% direct-reacting bilirubin)
- Hemolytic anemia
- Purpura, ecchymoses and petechiae
- Skeletal defects ("celery-stalking")
- Microcephaly and hydrocephaly
- Intracranial calcification
- Neuronal migration defects
- Pneumonitis
- Myocarditis
- Cardiac abnormalities
- Chorioretinitis
- Keratoconjunctivitis
- Cataracts
- Glaucoma

BOX 37-2   Viral Pathogens Reported to Cause Congenital Infections

Adenoviridae
- Adenovirus serogroup 3

Arenaviridae
- Lymphocytic choriomeningitis virus
- Lassa fever virus

Bunyaviridae
- Bunyamwera serogroup (Cache Valley virus)
- La Crosse encephalitis virus

Flaviviridae
- Hepatitis C virus
- Japanese encephalitis virus
- West Nile virus
- St. Louis encephalitis virus
- Yellow fever virus
- Dengue virus

Hepadenoviridae
- Hepatitis B virus

Herpesvirinae
- Herpes simplex viruses 1 and 2
- Varicella zoster virus
- Cytomegalovirus
- Epstein–Barr virus
- Human herpesviruses 6 and 7

Orthomyxoviruses and paramyxoviruses
- Influenza
- Measles

Parvoviridae
- Human parvovirus B19

Picornaviridae
- Poliovirus
- Coxsackievirus
- Enteric cytopathic human orphan virus
- Parechovirus
- Hepatitis A virus

Retroviridae
- Human T-lymphotropic viruses 1 and 2
- HIV

Togavirinae
- Mumps
- Western equine encephalitis virus
- Venezuelan equine encephalitis virus

---

many of the more unusual viral causes of congenital infection is beyond the scope of this chapter, but this table underscores the diversity of agents associated with fetal infection. A recent travel history or recent emigration might suggest consideration of some of these more unusual agents.

Rather than rely on a large battery of serologic tests, the clinician can usually narrow the differential diagnosis of a suspect neonatal or congenital viral infection with the history and physical examination, followed by the use of focused, specific diagnostic studies. Important questions include: What was the overall health of the mother during her pregnancy? What is her age and marital status (e.g., young, unmarried women have a higher risk of acquiring primary genital HSV infection). What is her immunization history? Has she had chickenpox? Did she have other common childhood viral infections? What part of the world is she from? Are there potential animal exposures (e.g., exposure to cat litter or consumption of undercooked meat might suggest toxoplasmosis; exposure to rodents might suggest lymphocytic choriomeningitis virus)? Does she have other children and, if so, what are their ages, overall health status, and histories of group day care attendance? Have there been recent illnesses in the household? What time of year is it? (For example, respiratory syncytial virus and enterovirus infections have characteristic seasonality in temperate zones.) What are her occupational exposures? Did she have any symptomatic infectious illnesses during pregnancy? The answers to these types of questions, considered in the context of the infant's physical examination, can direct the next steps in establishing a definitive etiologic diagnosis.

TABLE 37-1   Clinical Findings in Selected Congenital and Perinatal Infections That Suggest a Specific Diagnosis

Congenital Infection	Findings
Rubella	Cataracts, cloudy cornea, pigmented retina; petechiae with "blueberry muffin" rash; bone defects with longitudinal bands of demineralization ("celery stalking"); cardiovascular malformations (patent ductus arteriosus, pulmonary artery stenosis); sensorineural hearing loss; hydrops
Cytomegalovirus	Microcephaly with periventricular calcifications; chorioretinitis; petechiae with thrombocytopenia; jaundice; sensorineural hearing loss; bone abnormalities; abnormal dentition, hypocalcified enamel
Herpes simplex virus	Skin vesicles, keratoconjunctivitis, acute central nervous system findings (seizures), hepatitis, pneumonitis
Parvovirus B19	Hydrops, ascites, hepatomegaly, ventriculomegaly, hypertrophic myocardiopathy, anemia
Varicella zoster virus	Limb hypoplasia, dermatomal scarring in cicatricial pattern, gastrointestinal tract atresia
Lymphocytic choriomeningitis virus	Hydrocephalus, chorioretinitis, intracranial calcifications

Some of the classic presentations of the more common perinatal viral infections are reviewed in Table 37-1. It should be noted that there can be considerable overlap of these clinical features across the different infectious categories listed; for example, the "blueberry muffin" rash of congenital rubella syndrome may be indistinguishable from that of congenital CMV, and both syndromes can include sensorineural deafness. The presence of brain calcifications is similarly nonspecific, and this finding should always suggest a differential diagnosis that includes CMV, toxoplasmosis, lymphocytic choriomeningitis virus, and the recently described parechoviruses. Because neuroradiologic studies cannot reliably distinguish these entities, definitive diagnostic virology is necessary. Specific viral pathogens, their basic virology, the clinical manifestations of diseases they cause in the newborn, management strategies, and prospects for prevention are considered on a pathogen-specific basis in the remainder of this chapter.

HERPESVIRIDAE

Currently there are eight recognized human herpesviruses, which are subdivided into three categories based on aspects of viral biology, pathogenesis, and clinical presentations. These categories are the α-herpesviruses, consisting of HSV-1, HSV-2, and varicella-zoster virus (VZV); the β-herpesviruses, which include CMV and the roseola viruses HHV-6 and HHV-7; and the γ-herpesviruses, which include Epstein–Barr virus (EBV) and Kaposi's sarcoma herpesvirus (KSHV), reviewed in Schleiss (2009). Remarkably, all of these agents have been implicated in varying degrees as causes of clinically important congenital

and perinatal infections, although these associations are less well studied for the γ-herpesviruses.

HERPES SIMPLEX VIRUS INFECTIONS

HSV-1 and HSV-2 are highly related viruses. Although classically HSV-1 has been identified as a cause of oral infections (gingivostomatitis and pharyngitis), and HSV-2 has been implicated as the most common virus associated with genital herpes, in recent years these distinctions have become blurred. The greatest risk for the newborn is in the context of a first-time episode of maternal genital HSV infection occurring during pregnancy. The entity of neonatal herpes is reviewed in the following section, along with current management approaches for this infection.

VIROLOGY, EPIDEMIOLOGY, AND CLINICAL MANIFESTATIONS OF HSV DISEASE

HSV-1 and HSV-2 demonstrate a high degree of similarity, both at the molecular level and in their clinical manifestations. The degree of genetic relatedness of these two viruses is approximately 45%, and the genome structures and morphology of the virion (virus particle) are virtually identical (Kieff et al, 1972). HSV-1 and HSV-2 are both acquired predominantly at mucosal surfaces and require intimate contact for transmission. After primary infection in epithelial cells, intraaxonal trafficking of viral DNA to the dorsal route ganglia results in the establishment of latency. The latent state is characterized by the cessation of virtually all gene transcription, except for the latency-associated transcript (LAT), which is expressed in the dorsal route ganglia even as the virus maintains a quiescent state (Steiner et al, 2007; Taylor et al, 2002). The function of the latency-associated transcript is unknown, but it might involve a novel RNA-mediated mechanism, because there does not appear to be a protein product associated with the transcript (Umbach et al, 2008). After a number of triggers, including ultraviolet radiation, stress, and immunosuppression, the virus reactivates at the level of the dorsal route ganglia and initiates a cascade of viral transcription that leads to the production of infectious virus, which can traffic via the axon to the cutaneous surface or ocular surface, producing lesions (Toma et al, 2008). The recrudescence of HSV lesions, usually manifest as vesicular or ulcerative lesions at the site of primary infection, can in turn lead to person-to-person transmission, including maternal-fetal and maternal-infant transmission. Importantly, clinically evident lesions need not be present for person-to-person transmission of infection to susceptible individuals, because asymptomatic or subclinical shedding of virus is well documented, particularly in the setting of genital herpes.

A wide variety of disease syndromes are associated with primary and recurrent HSV infection. Classically HSV-1 has been described as causing disease "above the belt," whereas HSV-2 is associated with disease "below the belt." The finding of HSV-2 antibodies in seroprevalence studies is generally viewed as indicative of genital herpes, and in the pregnant patient it can be considered to be diagnostic of genital herpes. The most common disease associated with HSV infection is herpetic gingivostomatitis, characterized typically by perioral and intraoral lesions involving the pharyngeal mucosa. HSV infection of the oropharynx may present in adolescence as herpetic pharyngitis (McMillan et al, 1993); it can be indistinguishable from other causes of pharyngitis. Other common manifestations of HSV infection include primary cutaneous infection, which can manifest as herpes gladiatorum or as a herpetic whitlow (Johnson, 2004; Wu and Schwartz, 2009). In children with atopic dermatitis, cutaneous HSV infection can be associated with eczema herpeticum, a serious illness that can be associated with systemic symptom (Bussman et al, 2008). All of these cutaneous manifestations of HSV could put a newborn at risk for acquisition of infection if care is not taken to protect the infant. HSV encephalitis is unlikely to be transmitted person-to-person; it is the most common sporadic cause of viral encephalitis in North America, and it can be associated with primary infection or reactivation of latent infection. It is most commonly associated with HSV-1 (Baringer, 2008).

The most important manifestation of HSV disease is maternal genital herpes. Genital herpes can be associated with either HSV-1 or HSV-2. HSV is the most common cause of genital ulcerative disease in the developed world, and the prevalence has increased steadily in recent year (Fleming et al, 1997). Genital herpes is characterized by blisters, ulcers, or crusts on the genital area, buttocks, or both. Typically, symptomatic disease manifests with a mixture of vesicles, ruptured vesicles with resulting ulcers, and crusted lesions. Systemic flulike symptoms such as headache, fever, and swollen glands can accompany an outbreak of genital herpes, particularly during primary infection. Other symptoms include dysuria, urinary retention, vaginal or penile discharge, genital itching, burning or tingling, and groin sensitivity. Genital lesions vary in number, are painful in nature, and if untreated persist for up to 21 days (Whitley et al, 1998). It has been recognized in recent years that many individuals with genital herpes are asymptomatic and unaware of their status (Wald et al, 2000). Therefore a negative maternal history of HSV should not dissuade the clinician from considering the possibility of neonatal herpes in an infant with compatible signs and symptoms. Patients with recurrent symptomatic episodes continue to shed virus in between episodes, even after lesions have healed and crusted over (Leone, 2005). This information has important implications for the continued evolution of the HSV epidemic in the United States. Because individuals with asymptomatic genital herpes shed virus frequently in the absence of lesions, all HSV-2 seropositive individuals are probably at risk for transmitting infection in setting of sexual activity, labor and delivery, and intimate contact.

NEONATAL HERPES

For the neonatologist, the most important category of HSV-associated disease is that of neonatal herpes. In the United States, the reported range of neonatal herpes ranges from 1 in 2500 births to 1 in 8000 births (Corey and Wald, 2009; Kimberlin, 2005; Whitley, 2004). Approximately 70% to 85% of neonatal herpes simplex infections are caused by HSV-2 (Kimberlin et al, 2001). The majority of cases occur in infants born to women who were recently

infected, rather than to women with histories of recurrent genital herpes. Primary infection late in pregnancy poses a higher risk of transmission to the infant than do primary infections occurring before or early in pregnancy, suggesting that the evolution of a maternal antibody response confers some measure of protection for the infant (Brown et al, 2003; Caviness et al, 2008a). Primary genital herpes infection in a pregnant mother results in an attack rate of 33% to 50% for her infant, whereas recurrent maternal infection results in a 1% to 3% attack rate (Arvin, 1991; Brown et al, 1997; Prober et al, 1987). Overall, it is estimated that approximately 22% of pregnant women have genital herpes (HSV-2 seropositivity), and 2% of women will acquire HSV during pregnancy (Brown et al, 2005). Approximately 90% of these women are undiagnosed, because they are asymptomatic or have other subtle symptoms that are incorrectly attributed to other vulvovaginal disorders.

Strategies for preventing neonatal HSV infection can be optimized by identifying women with genital lesions at the time of labor for cesarean delivery, prescribing antiviral suppressive therapy as appropriate (see Treatment and Outcomes, later), and minimizing invasive intrapartum procedures for women in whom the diagnosis of genital herpes cannot be excluded. Rarely, cases of intrauterine infection have been described; these are often associated with overwhelming primary maternal infection and usually result in fetal demise. On occasion, placentitis is also observed (Baldwin and Whitley, 1989; Chatterjee et al, 2001; Florman et al, 1973; Hutto et al, 1987; Vasileiadis et al, 2003). Although intrauterine transmission is possible, the vast majority of HSV infections in newborns are acquired intrapartum, related to the presence of virus in the maternal genital track. Neonatal acquisition of HSV from an individual other than the mother, such as from a recurrent oropharyngeal lesion, is unusual (Light, 1979; Linnemann et al, 1978; Yeager et al, 1983). Neonatal HSV has been described as a complication of ritual circumcision (Rubin and Lanzkowsky, 2000). Approximately 85% of infants with neonatal HSV acquire infection from the maternal genital tract at the time of delivery, but only 15% to 30% of mothers who give birth to infants with neonatal HSV infection have a known history of genital HSV (Whitley, 1988). Intrapartum interventions that have the risk of penetrating fetal skin, such as scalp electrode monitoring, increase the risk of transmission to the infant (Golden et al, 1977; Parvey and Ch'ien, 1980).

Neonatal herpes can have devastating long-term consequences, making early recognition of paramount importance. Most infants with perinatal or postnatal HSV infection are normal at birth. Illness typically develops after 3 days of age; therefore the presence of skin lesions, oral ulcers, and other signs and symptoms in the first 72 hours of life should suggest diagnoses other than HSV. Premature infants appear to be at greater risk, possibly because of reduced transplacental transfer of protective antibody. Approximately 40% to 50% of affected infants are less than 36 weeks in gestational age (Whitley, 1988). Although a history of maternal cervical, vaginal, or labial lesions should be sought when neonatal HSV is being considered in the differential diagnosis, overt herpetic disease in the maternal genital tract is evident in approximately

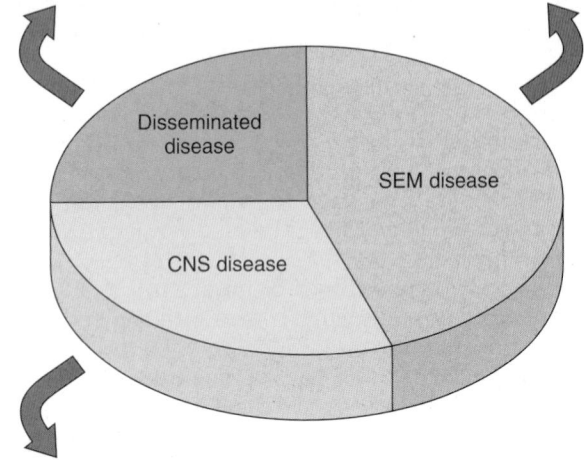

• Disease limited to skin, eyes, mucous membranes
• May progress to CNS or disseminated disease
• Frequent cutaneous recurrence in first year of life – increased risk of poor neurodevelopmental outcome

• Sepsis syndrome
• Hepatitis, DIC, pneumoia
• Skin vesicles may be absent
• High mortality even with therapy
• Survivors may be free of CNS disease

• Skin vesicles are absent in ~⅓ of cases
• Severe seizures common
• High incidence of CNS imaging abnormalities and neurologic sequelae

FIGURE 37-2 Characteristic presentations of neonatal herpes simplex virus (HSV) infection. Approximately 45% of neonatal HSV manifests as skin, eye, or mucous membrane disease (SEM disease); 25% as disseminated disease; and 30%, central nervous systems (CNS) disease. Characteristic features of each subtype of neonatal HSV are listed (*arrows*). Disease may span categories; for example, infants with SEM disease may progress to disseminated or CNS disease, and infants with CNS disease may develop skin vesicles later in hospital course, although up to one-third of infants with CNS disease never have cutaneous manifestations.

one third of patients (Overall, 1994). In the remaining two thirds, infection is presumably via asymptomatic maternal genital tract shedding of virus.

Infection can manifest in newborns in one of three forms: disease limited to the skin, eye, or mucous membrane disease (SEM); disease involving the central nervous system (CNS); or disseminated HSV infection, frequently manifesting as a sepsislike syndrome, with pneumonia, hepatitis, and viremia (Figure 37-2) (Kimberlin, 2005; Whitley, 2004). There can be overlap in these syndromes; for example, an infant with disseminated disease may initially have only skin lesions. The relative proportion of infants with disseminated disease has been declining in recent years, probably because earlier recognition and treatment of SEM disease have resulted in more timely intervention with antiviral therapy. Disseminated disease usually begins toward the end of the 1st week of life. Skin vesicles may be an early sign, but they are entirely absent in almost half of patients. The scalp should be inspected carefully, particularly near the site of insertion of fetal scalp electrodes, because such lesions are easy to overlook.

Systemic symptoms, although initially insidious in onset, progress rapidly. Poor feeding, lethargy, and fever may be accompanied by irritability or seizures if the CNS is involved. These symptoms are followed rapidly by jaundice, hypotension, disseminated intravascular coagulation, apnea, and shock. This form of disease is indistinguishable at its onset from both neonatal enterovirus infection and bacterial sepsis. HSV infection should be considered in the differential diagnosis of infants who have fever during the first 2 weeks of life, because fever can herald the onset of systemic disease. Localized disease may begin somewhat later, with most cases appearing in the 2nd to 3rd weeks of life. When the CNS is the primary site of infection, the skin or eyes may be involved: up to one third of infants with neonatal CNS disease will never have skin lesions during their clinical course. The infants are lethargic, irritable, and tremulous, and seizures are common and difficult to control.

Other less common but potentially localized or disseminated findings are keratoconjunctivitis, chorioretinitis, and pneumonitis, which can manifest as a focal infiltrate or as diffuse bilateral disease. Supraglottitis, intracranial hemorrhage, aseptic meningitis, and fulminant liver failure have been described (Abzug and Johnson, 2000; Erdem et al, 2002; Greenes et al, 1995; Kohl, 1994, 1999; Schlesinger and Storch, 1994). Less common presentations of neonatal herpes include hydrops fetalis (Anderson and Abzug, 1999) and laryngitis (Vitale et al, 1993).

Diagnosis

The cornerstone of the diagnosis of neonatal HSV is virologic detection; HSV serology is of little use. HSV-1 and HSV-2 are both easily recovered by culture of clinical samples. In disseminated disease, virus is present in blood, conjunctivae, respiratory secretions, and urine; it is also present in the central nervous system in approximately half of patients. In SEM disease, the virus can usually be found at the site of disease (i.e., within a vesicle). Definitive microbiologic diagnosis requires growth of the virus in tissue culture, or detection of viral nucleic acid by PCR. HSV can also be presumptively identified by immunofluorescence of infected cells using HSV-specific antibodies; such tests are commercially available and should be used in lieu of the outdated and insensitive Tzanck smear. Viral culture has the added advantage of allowing detection in the clinical virology laboratory of other agents that can mimic HSV disease in neonates, such as enteroviruses (see Enteroviruses later), because most diagnostic viral culture systems will support the growth of a variety of pathogens. When neonatal herpes is suggested, viral cultures of the throat, conjunctiva, blood, stool or rectum, and urine should be obtained, as should scrapings of vesicular, pustular, and ulcerative skin lesions. Of these sites, skin and conjunctival HSV cultures have the highest yield (Kimberlin et al, 2001).

All infants with presumed neonatal HSV disease should undergo lumbar puncture, even if SEM disease is the only observed clinical manifestation. In some infants, CNS infection may be present but subclinical, and the finding of HSV DNA in the cerebrospinal fluid (CSF) has important therapeutic and prognostic implications. Blood should be sent for viral blood culture or PCR, because viremia is a common finding in neonatal HSV infection (Diamond et al, 1999; Stanberry et al, 1994). Usually if the CNS is involved in the setting of neonatal HSV disease, evaluation of the CSF reveals a lymphocytosis, red blood cells, normal or high protein level, and low or normal glucose level. In addition to viral culture, CSF, blood, skin lesions, and other specimens should be analyzed by PCR for the presence of HSV genome (Ryan and Kinghorn, 2006). Caution should be taken with interpretation of a negative CSF PCR result: many infants with neonatal HSV disease will not have CNS involvement, so a negative CSF PCR considered in isolation does not exclude the diagnosis of neonatal HSV. PCR of DNA extracted from the dried newborn blood spot has been reported as a way to retrospectively identify HSV infection in young infants (Lewensohn-Fuchs et al, 2003). Some experts recommend obtaining a second CSF specimen for evaluation at the end of antiviral therapy, and it has been reported that persistence of HSV DNA may be a poor prognostic factor and an indication for continuing antiviral therapy (Kimberlin et al, 1996b; Malm and Forsgren, 1999; Mejías et al, 2009). In disseminated disease, transaminase elevations consistent with hepatocellular injury are typically present; in severe disease, fulminant hepatitis with hepatic necrosis may be observed. Infants with CNS disease should undergo neuroradiographic imaging with computed tomography (CT) or magnetic resonance imaging (MRI). Early in the course of illness, imaging may demonstrate nonspecific lack of gray-white matter junction differentiation and general signs of encephalitis. Later CT findings include dilated ventricles, parenchymal echogenicity, cystic degeneration, and intracranial calcifications (O'Reilly et al, 1995), whereas MRI images demonstrate a variable appearance (Vossough et al, 2008). Neonatal HSV-2 encephalitis can be multifocal or limited to only the temporal lobes, brainstem, or cerebellum. Deep gray matter structures are involved and hemorrhage is observed in more than half of patients. In approximately 20% of patients, lesions are seen only by diffusion-weighted imaging. In 40% of patients, watershed distribution ischemic changes are also observed in addition to areas of presumed direct herpetic necrosis. In contrast to the classical description in older patients, neonatal HSV encephalitis is not usually confined to the temporal lobes. Electroencephalography should also be considered in all infants with CNS involvement or with disseminated disease, to evaluate for seizures. Electroencephalography findings will be abnormal in approximately 80% of such patients (Kimberlin et al, 2001).

Treatment and Outcomes

The cornerstone of the treatment of neonatal HSV disease is the nucleoside analog known as *acyclovir*. The development of acyclovir in the 1980s was a watershed event in the management of HSV infection. The use of acyclovir and other antivirals is summarized in Table 37-2. Although acyclovir had an efficacy similar to a previously used antiviral agent (vidarabine) in a controlled trial, acyclovir has emerged as the drug of choice because of its greater ease of administration and its highly favorable toxicity profile. The current recommendation of the American Academy of Pediatrics (AAP) Committee on Infectious Diseases is that

neonatal HSV infections should be treated with high-dose acyclovir at a dose of 60 mg/kg/day intravenously, divided into three doses given every 8 hours, for either 14 days for infants with SEM disease or 21 days for infants with disseminated or CNS disease. Support for this recommendation was derived from a comparison of the results from an earlier study using standard-dose acyclovir (30 mg/kg/day) for 10 days (Kimberlin et al, 2001). There is no role for oral acyclovir in the management of neonatal HSV, and no role for topical acyclovir in neonatal SEM disease. Herpetic keratoconjunctivitis should receive topical ophthalmic antiviral therapy along with parenteral treatment. In addition to antiviral therapy, appropriate supportive care is essential, with anticipatory management targeting complications of neonatal HSV disease such as seizures, pneumonitis, and hepatic insufficiency. A beneficial role of intravenous immunoglobulin (IVIG) has been inferred from animal models of neonatal HSV disease, in which passive antibody is clearly beneficial (Bravo et al, 1996), but the absence of controlled studies precludes any recommendations in infants.

Even with timely institution of antiviral therapy, the prognosis following neonatal HSV infection is guarded. The mortality rates in infants with localized CNS disease range from 4% to 14% with antiviral therapy, and most survivors have long-term neurologic sequelae. Risk factors for increased morbidity and mortality from CNS infection include prematurity and seizures upon initiation of therapy (Kimberlin et al, 2001; Kohl, 1999). Infants with disseminated disease have a high mortality rate without antiviral therapy; 80% die, and most survivors have serious neurologic sequelae (Whitley, 1988). Intravenous antiviral therapy has decreased mortality of disseminated disease to approximately 30%, and approximately 80% of surviving infants have a normal neurologic outcome (Corey and Wald, 2009). Antiviral therapy has decreased the mortality of neonatal CNS infection from approximately 50% to 6%, but more than 70% of survivors have sequelae (Corey and Wald, 2009; Engman et al, 2008; Freij and Sever, 1988). Lethargy at initiation of therapy has been associated with a higher mortality rate in neonates with disseminated HSV infection (Kimberlin et al, 2001). Infants with skin involvement often have recurrent crops of skin vesicles for several years. In an infant younger than 6 months, readmission to the hospital for diagnostic evaluation and administration of intravenous acyclovir is appropriate when cutaneous recurrences are observed. It is postulated that recurrent cutaneous lesions may be associated with subclinical CNS reactivation, and it has been proposed that treatment of these recurrences with acyclovir will improve long-term outcome.

Management of asymptomatic neonates potentially exposed to HSV in the birth canal is controversial. This situation sometimes arises when a maternal perineal lesion is discovered after vaginal delivery. Some experts recommend neonatal surface cultures and administration of prophylactic antivirals, but there is little evidence to support this approach. The most important variable informing clinical management is probably the maternal history. Term infants exposed to HSV in the birth canal and born to women with long-standing histories of recurrent genital herpes are at low risk (<1%) of infection and, if the infant is

TABLE 37-2 Commonly Used Antiviral Agents in Neonatology Practice

Antiviral Agent	Indication	Dose, Route of Administration, Duration of Therapy	Comments
Acyclovir	Neonatal HSV	60 mg/kg/day, dosing every 8 h IV; 21 days for disseminated infection or CNS disease; 14 days for SEM disease	Monitor CBC twice weekly; adjust dosage for renal insufficiency
	Oral suppression following neonatal HSV	Efficacy for improving neurodevelopmental outcomes unproven; 10 to 20 mg/kg/dose twice daily; duration of therapy, 12 months	Neutropenia observed in ½ to ⅔ of infants; lesions while receiving suppressive therapy should suggest acyclovir-resistant strain
	VZV infection	15 mg/kg every 8 h for minimum of 5 to 7 days; longer courses may be needed for severe end-organ disease (pneumonia, hepatitis)	
	VZV postexposure prophylaxis	10 mg/kg PO four times per day; treat for at least 7 days (from 7 days after the earliest exposure until 14 days after the last exposure)	Use in conjunction with VariZIG
Trifluridine 1%	HSV ophthalmic disease	Apply as eye drops; 1 drop every 2 h to affected cornea while awake; maximum 9 drops per day	Manage in consultation with ophthalmologist
Ganciclovir	Congenital CMV; acquired CMV	12 mg/kg/day, dosing every 12 h IV; duration of therapy is 6 weeks for prevention of hearing loss; shorter courses of therapy (14 to 21 days) are reasonable for serious end-organ disease	Efficacy against CMV associated hearing loss in controlled trial; benefits of shorter courses of therapy unknown; neutropenia observed in 63% of patients in controlled trial; adjust dose for renal insufficiency; consider G-CSF if continued therapy desired in setting of neutropenia
Valganciclovir	Congenital CMV	32 mg/kg/day divided twice daily; no data available for duration or efficacy of oral formulation; CASG is currently performing a controlled clinical trial of 6 months oral suppression	Valine ester (prodrug) of ganciclovir; similar toxicity profile as GCV; long-term suppressive therapy not well studied in infants; theoretical concerns of carcinogenesis, gonadal toxicity
Lamivudine	Hepatitis B, HIV	For children 3 months to 16 years of age, recommended dose is 4 mg/kg, up to 150 mg per dose, twice daily	Chronic hepatitis B infection; also used for HIV therapy
Interferon α2b	Hepatitis B, hepatitis C	3 to 6 million international units/m² 3 times weekly; up to 24 months duration; combined with oral ribavirin for hepatitis C	Chronic hepatitis B infection; no data in neonates; chronic hepatitis C infection when administered with ribavirin; systemic side effects (fever, flu-like symptoms, anorexia); leucopenia; thyroid autoantibodies
Pegylated interferon α2b	Hepatitis B, hepatitis C	1.5 μg/kg once per week; no information on dosing in children <2 yr old	Chronic hepatitis B; administer in conjunction with ribavirin for hepatitis C; systemic side effects (fever, flulike symptoms, anorexia); leucopenia; thyroid autoantibodies; side effects less common with pegylated formulations
Adefovir	Hepatitis B	Not recommended in children <10 years of age; 0.3 mg/kg once daily PO in children 2 to 6 yr old has favorable pharmacokinetics	Chronic hepatitis B infection; no safety or efficacy data in infants or young children
Ribavirin (oral)	Hepatitis C	15 mg/kg/day PO; no information on dosing in children <2 years of age	Hemolytic anemia; teratogenic in animal models
Ribavirin (aerosol)	Respiratory syncytial virus	Standard ribavirin aerosol therapy is 6 g per 300 mL water for 18 h daily; short-duration therapy, 6 g per 100 mL water given for a period of 2 h 3 times per day	Not indicated for use with mechanical ventilator; conjunctivitis; bronchospasm
Amantadine	Influenza A	FDA-approved dosage for children 1 to 9 yr old for treatment and prophylaxis is 4.4 to 8.8 mg/kg/day, not to exceed 150 mg/day in children <9 yr old	Not approved for use in children <1 yr old; influenza B resistant; influenza A; H1N1 resistant
Rimantidine	Influenza A	Administered in one or two divided doses at a dosage of 5 mg/kg/day, not to exceed 150 mg/day in children <9 yr old	Not approved for use in children <1 yr old; influenza B resistant; influenza A H1N1 resistant
Oseltamivir	Influenza A, influenza B	For children <15 kg, recommended dose is 30 mg PO twice daily for 5 days (treatment) or 10 days (prophylaxis)	Not typically recommended in children <1 yr old; FDA-approved guidelines for emergency use of oseltamivir in pediatric patients younger than 1 year in 2009 in response to H1N1 influenza pandemic
Zanamivir	Influenza A, influenza B	Recommended dose of zanamivir for treatment of influenza is two inhalations (one 5-mg blister per inhalation for a total dose of 10 mg) twice daily (approximately 12 h apart)	Not recommended in children <5 yr old

CASG, Collaborative Antiviral Study Group; *CBC*, complete blood cell count; *CNS*, central nervous system; *FDA*, U.S. Food and Drug Administration; *G-CSF*, granulocyte colony-stimulating factor; *HSV*, herpes simplex virus; *IV*, intravenous; *PO*, by mouth; *SEM*, skin, eye, or mucous membranes; *VariZIG*, varicella-zoster immunoglobulin; *VZV*, varicella-zoster virus.

asymptomatic, observation without antiviral therapy is sufficient. If the maternal HSV history is unclear, the infant is premature, or other obstetric complications or risk factors are present (e.g., prolonged rupture of membranes, maternal fever, signs or symptoms of chorioamnionitis, fetal scalp electrode monitoring), then empiric antiviral therapy is warranted. After the appropriate specimens are collected and sent for viral culture and PCR analysis, the infant should receive parenteral acyclovir (60 mg/kg/day) pending the results of diagnostic virology studies. There is no role for topical or oral formulations of acyclovir in this setting.

Similarly controversial is the question of whether empiric acyclovir therapy should be administered to neonates who are readmitted for evaluation of febrile illness in the first 30 days of life. Standard practice in most children's hospitals is to rule out sepsis in this setting by administering broad-spectrum antibiotics pending the result of diagnostic cultures of blood, urine, and spinal fluid. Some experts recommend the use of empiric acyclovir in this setting (Long, 2008), citing data that indicate that the prevalence of neonatal HSV infection is similar to that of invasive bacterial infection in this setting, and that infants may exhibit fever and sepsis-like syndrome as the only manifestations of HSV infection (Caviness et al, 2008b). Other experts recommend a more selective approach, based on analysis of history, risk factors, and laboratory and radiographic analyses, such as liver function tests and chest radiograph (Kimberlin, 2008). Additional studies will be required to ascertain whether acyclovir should be included in the empiric antimicrobial regimen of all neonates who are evaluated for fever in the first few weeks of life.

In addition to its critical role in the management of the acute clinical syndromes of neonatal HSV infection, acyclovir may be of benefit when administered as long-term suppressive therapy in the first 6 months of life. The Collaborative Antiviral Study Group (CASG) has reported results of controlled studies evaluating long-term oral suppressive acyclovir therapy after neonatal HSV aimed at both prevention of recurrent skin lesions and neurologic sequelae. The observation driving this study is that recurrent skin lesions (more than three episodes) within the first 6 months of life predict an adverse neurologic prognosis, possibly because recurrent skin lesions are a surrogate marker for subclinical reactivation events in the CNS (Whitley, 1991). Phase I and II trials demonstrated fewer cutaneous recurrences in the treatment group, but did not have enough subjects to analyze the effect on neurologic outcomes (Kimberlin et al, 1996a). Whether reducing cutaneous recurrences in the 1st year of life will result in improved neurodevelopmental outcome remains unknown (Gutierrez and Arvin, 2003). Given the favorable safety profile of acyclovir, the use of long-term suppression after an episode of neonatal herpes is probably an appropriate management strategy, and it is likely to reduce the need for repeat hospitalization when lesions reappear. Any theoretical benefit of acyclovir must be considered against the potential risk of neutropenia, which has been reported in 20% to 50% of neonates receiving long-term acyclovir therapy. Although readily reversible with discontinuation of drug, this concern necessitates frequent monitoring of the absolute neutrophil count. The emergence of

acyclovir-resistant HSV strains is also a potential concern (Kimberlin et al, 1996a; Oram et al, 2000). That long-term oral suppressive therapy may be beneficial for improving long-term neurodevelopmental outcomes owing to neonatal HSV infection was suggested by a 2-year pilot study of oral suppressive therapy in a cohort of 16 infants (Tiffany et al, 2005). In this uncontrolled study, all children were independently mobile, free of seizures, and had normal vision and speech development at the time of final neurodevelopmental assessment.

Prospects for Prevention

Even with prompt recognition and therapy, the risk of long-term morbidity with neonatal HSV infection, particularly neurodevelopmental morbidity, remains significant. Ideally, prevention of neonatal HSV infection would be the best approach to solving the problem of HSV-induced long-term neurologic injury. Recent developments in the approach to HSV infections among women of childbearing age include consideration of maternal screening programs and the use of antiviral agents in women at risk for transmission of infection. The availability of reliable kits that allow specific serodiagnosis of HSV-1 and HSV-2 infections has enabled the identification of asymptomatic women with genital herpes who can be counseled appropriately during pregnancy (Sauerbrei and Wutzler, 2007). Although routine seroscreening of pregnant women is not currently considered a standard of care, screening in some instances, including situations where high maternal anxiety exists, seems justified. There is no evidence that routine administration of suppressive antivirals during pregnancy can improve outcomes or reduce disease in newborns (Sheffield et al, 2006), although this approach has become common in many obstetric practices (Hollier and Wendel, 2008). One benefit of suppressive antiviral therapy during pregnancy for a woman with a history of genital herpes may be a reduced likelihood of cesarean section, predicated on the assumption that suppressive therapy will prevent reactivation of HSV (Brown et al, 2003; Hollier and Wendel, 2008). Strategies for preventing neonatal herpes can also target prevention of intrapartum transmission by caesarean section. If a mother has active genital herpes simplex infection at the time of delivery, and if the membranes are either intact or have been ruptured for less than 4 hours, both the AAP and the American College of Obstetricians and Gynecologists (ACOG) recommend cesarean delivery. The role of intrapartum antivirals or immunoglobulin has not been studied in this setting.

Even with careful histories and meticulous physical examination during labor and delivery, many at-risk deliveries cannot be predicted or identified, because so many HSV-2–seropositive women are asymptomatic, do not know that they have genital herpes, and may unknowingly shed virus at the time of delivery. Infants in whom HSV infection is known or highly suspected should be put in isolation with contact precautions, and skin lesions should be covered. Finally, any health care provider with active herpetic whitlow or other skin lesions should not have direct patient care responsibilities for neonates.

Ultimately, prevention of neonatal HSV infection could be conferred by the development of a vaccine. Several phase I, II, and III clinical trials are ongoing to investigate the utility of various HSV vaccines to prevent genital infections (Stanberry and Rosenthal, 2005). A double-blind, randomized trial of an HSV-2 glycoprotein-D-subunit vaccine given with alum adjuvant and 3-O-deacylated-monophosphoryl lipid A, was reported in a study of individuals whose regular sexual partners had a history of genital herpes. The primary end point was the occurrence of genital herpes disease. The vaccine was efficacious in women who were seronegative for both HSV-1 and HSV-2, but it was not efficacious in women who were seropositive for HSV-1 and seronegative for HSV-2 at base line. The vaccine had no efficacy in men, regardless of serostatus (Stanberry et al, 2002). The basis for this discrepancy remains unexplained, but may relate to anatomic differences in how primary infections are established in men and women, or sex-related differences in immune response. It remains to be studied what effect widespread HSV-2 vaccination might have on the incidence or severity of neonatal HSV infection.

VARICELLA-ZOSTER VIRUS

Varicella-zoster virus (VZV) is a member of the α-herpesvirus subfamily of the *Herpesviridae*. Like the related HSV-1 and HSV-2, VZV can infect neurons where it can establish latent infection. Primary varicella infection, commonly known as *chickenpox*, usually results in a fever and a characteristic vesicular exanthem. The illness often includes other systemic symptoms, such as headache and malaise. Reactivation from latency, which can occur decades after the primary VZV infection, is usually referred to as *zoster* or *shingles*. Zoster is characterized by a painful vesicular rash in a dermatomal distribution, and in older patients can lead to postherpetic neuralgia.

The neonatologist may encounter consequences of maternal VZV infection in two different clinical presentations. In congenital varicella, VZV is transmitted to the fetus in the first or second trimester of pregnancy, where it can produce a number of teratogenic consequences (Auriti et al, 2009; Laforet and Lynch, 1947; Smith and Arvin, 2009; Srabstein et al, 1974). In contrast, neonatal varicella occurs in the setting of primary maternal varicella acquired late in the third trimester, and the affected infant can exhibit symptoms and signs in the neonatal period. This section reviews both of these presentations of VZV-related disease in infants.

Epidemiology of Maternal and Perinatal Varicella-Zoster Virus

Before the advent of routine childhood vaccination against chickenpox, it was estimated that the VZV seroprevalence in women of childbearing age was greater than 95%, because of the formerly ubiquitous nature of this infection. In this era, primary VZV infections during pregnancy occurred with a frequency of 5 to 7 per 10,000 pregnancies in the United States (Balducci et al, 1992; Brunell, 1992). The major concern in the setting of primary maternal VZV infection is the risk for congenital varicella syndrome (CVS). It is not yet clear whether the risk for CVS has been ameliorated by the widespread use of VZV vaccine.

For pregnant women with primary varicella infection, the transmission rate to the fetus is estimated to be approximately 25%. Only a subset of infected fetuses exhibit symptomatic disease. Approximately 100 cases of CVS have been reported in the literature (Sauerbrei and Wutzler, 2000). The risk of symptomatic intrauterine VZV infection after maternal varicella occurring during the first 20 weeks of pregnancy is approximately 1% to 2% (Enders et al, 1994; Paryani and Arvin, 1986; Pastuszak et al, 1994; Siegel, 1973). Symptomatic disease appears to be more common in female infants (Sauerbrei and Wutzler, 2000). CVS does not appear to occur in the setting of maternal zoster. A prospective study of infants born to 366 mothers with a clinical history of zoster during pregnancy found no infants with CVS (Enders et al, 1994).

Maternal infection in the third trimester is not associated with CVS, presumably because this falls outside the time frame when teratogenicity can occur. Maternal infection just before or after delivery poses a high risk for neonatal varicella. Before the advent of VZV vaccination, neonatal varicella was encountered much more commonly that CVS. For infants in which maternal illness begins 5 days or less before delivery or up to 2 days after delivery, the infant attack rate is 17% to 31% (Brunell, 1992; Feldman, 1986; Meyers, 1974). Because the incubation period for varicella is between 10 and 21 days, cases beginning in the first 10 days of life are considered to have been acquired in utero.

Pathogenesis and Clinical Manifestations

As noted, CVS is acquired from a maternal primary varicella infection that occurs during the first or second trimester. The virus is thought to be transmitted transplacentally during the viremia that precedes or accompanies the rash of chickenpox. Ascending infection from cervical infection has been proposed as a potential mechanism of transmission, but is probably much less common (Sauerbrei and Wutzler, 2000). Some of the congenital malformations associated with CVS may be a consequence of zosterlike virus reactivation events in the infected fetus rather than the direct effects of the primary viral infection. This explanation is supported by the common finding of unusual cicatricial rashes in dermatomal distributions in the newborn with CVS. Other clinical manifestations include asymmetric muscular atrophy with limb hypoplasia, low birthweight, neurologic abnormalities (cortical or spinal cord atrophy, seizures, microcephaly, encephalitis, Horner syndrome), and ophthalmologic abnormalities (chorioretinitis, microphthalmia, atrophy, and cataracts; Brunell, 1992; Feldman, 1986; Sauerbrei and Wutzler, 2000). Gastrointestinal abnormalities are reported in 15% to 23% of cases; findings include duodenal stenosis, dilated jejunum, small left colon, intestinal atresia or bands, and hepatic calcifications (Alkalay et al, 1987; Jones et al, 1994). Immature fetal cell–mediated immune response may explain the short latency period and the inadequate protection from the consequences of episodes of reactivation in utero (Higa et al, 1987; Kustermann et al, 1996). Pathology reports have noted destruction of neural tissue with residual dystrophic calcifications, chronic active inflammation in nonneural tissues surrounding viral inclusions, and evidence of chronic placental villitis (Bruder et al, 2000; Petignat et al, 2001; Qureshi and Jacques, 1996).

Maternal varicella near term or immediately postpartum can lead to neonatal varicella. Neonatal varicella is usually caused by maternal chickenpox acquired during the last 3 weeks of pregnancy. Infection may be transmitted perinatally by transplacental viremia (most cases) or by ascending infection from the birth canal; it can also be treated postnatally by the aerosol route or direct contact with infectious lesions. Serious postnatal infection acquired from maternal varicella via breastfeeding has not been reported. Neonatal varicella may develop despite the administration of varicella-zoster immunoglobulin (VariZIG) to the infant at birth. Transplacentally transmitted infections occur in the first 10 to 12 days of life, whereas chickenpox after that time is most likely acquired by postnatal infection. The clinical presentation differs markedly for cases in which maternal rash began 5 days or more before delivery from those in which maternal illness occurred from 5 days before to 2 days after delivery. When maternal varicella is noted more than 5 days before delivery, neonatal disease usually begins within the first 4 days of life and is typically mild. In contrast, neonatal varicella in an infant whose mother develops varicella from 5 days before until 2 days after delivery has a high risk of morbidity and mortality (Isaacs, 2000; Tan and Koren, 2006). In this second group, neonatal disease typically begins between 5 and 10 days after delivery, and a fatal outcome has been reported in 23% to 30% of cases (Brunell, 1966; Sauerbrei and Wutzler, 2001). When the disease appears in this setting, it closely resembles varicella in the immunodeficient or immunosuppressed host. Recurrent crops of skin vesicles develop over a prolonged period. Typical presenting signs are fever, hemorrhagic rash, and visceral dissemination with involvement of the liver, lung, and brain. Secondary bacterial infection may occur.

Prospective studies of the long-term outcomes of CVS have not been performed, and there is probably a wide continuum of disease. Among the 96 infants reviewed by Sauerbrei and Wutzler (2000), 14 (15%) had clinical signs of zoster during early infancy; these infants had been exposed to varicella between 8 and 24 weeks' gestation. Some experts consider early zoster infections as one criterion for diagnosis of CVS. Between 1% and 2% of infants without clinical evidence of CVS, but whose mothers had chickenpox in the second and third trimesters, develop zoster in the first few weeks of life; if this occurs, consideration should be given to ophthalmologic evaluations to rule out the possibility of CVS (Enders et al, 2004; Sauerbrei and Wutzler, 2000). Overall mortality rates for CVS are estimated at 30%. Deaths occur in the first few months of life, usually secondary to severe pulmonary disease (Pastuszak et al, 1994; Sauerbrei and Wutzler, 2000).

Diagnostic Studies

Prenatal diagnosis—by means of quantification of varicella-specific IgM on fetal blood obtained by cordocentesis or through PCR analysis of chorionic villi, fetal blood, and amniotic fluid—has been attempted (Cuthbertson et al, 1987; Kustermann et al, 1996; Mouly et al, 1997). Although the yield of PCR on amniotic fluid or fetal blood is higher than that of serologic analysis of fetal IgM or viral cultures, large prospective studies of the correlation of such findings with clinical outcomes have not been performed. Reported prenatal ultrasonographic findings include polyhydramnios, hydrops, progressive intrauterine growth restriction, microcephaly, limb hypoplasia, and liver hyperechogenicities (Petignat, 2001; Pretorius et al, 1992). Abnormal ultrasonographic findings might not develop in a fetus for at least 5 weeks after maternal infection (Kerkering, 2001).

Serologic studies can be performed postnatally on infants (Paryani and Arvin, 1986). Suspected congenital infection with varicella can be confirmed by the finding of persistent VZV IgG beyond the presumed duration of passive transfer of maternal antibodies (at least 6 to 7 months). Detection of fetal IgM can also confirm infection, but it is less useful because approximately one fourth of infants reported with classic CVS have positive VZV IgM titer values (Enders et al, 1994; Sauerbrei and Wutzler, 2000). Scrapings of skin lesions, as with herpes simplex infections, can show large multinucleated cells when stained with Wright or Giemsa stain (Tzanck smears), but this procedure is no longer recommended, because highly sensitive direct fluorescent antibody (DFA) tests are readily available and are more sensitive and specific (Chan et al, 2001; Coffin and Hodinka, 1995). VZV can also be detected from skin lesions by PCR (Leung et al, 2010). Although VZV can be detected by DFA staining of cells or PCR of DNA extracted from skin and visceral lesions, these tests in infants with suspected congenital infection are often extremely low yield compared with infants and children who have acquired varicella infection. Neuroradiographic demonstration of intracranial calcifications has been reported with CVS, but this is not a common finding (Kerkering, 2001).

Treatment

No controlled studies examining the effect of antiviral therapy to prevent or treat congenital varicella syndrome have been conducted. Some experts have recommended oral acyclovir for pregnant women with varicella, especially during the second and third trimesters (AAP Committee on Infectious Diseases, 2010a). Intravenous treatment with acyclovir for the infected pregnant woman is recommended for patients with serious complications of varicella, particularly pneumonia. Anecdotal observations suggest a potential effect of acyclovir on the progression of eye disease in CVS (Sauerbrei and Wutzler, 2000). However, there are no recommendations for the use of acyclovir or immunoglobulin for treatment or prevention of CVS. For neonatal varicella, treatment with intravenous acyclovir, 60 mg/kg/day divided into doses every 8 hours, is recommended, particularly for infants at the highest risk of adverse outcomes (i.e., the infant born to a woman who develops varicella from 5 days before until 2 days after delivery; see Table 37-2).

Prevention

If a susceptible pregnant woman has a significant exposure to varicella, administration of VariZIG to her and her newborn infant should be considered seriously. These recommendations are summarized in Box 37-3. Infants of mothers in whom varicella develops from 5 days before to 2 days after delivery should receive VZIG as soon as possible (AAP Committee on Infectious Diseases, 2010a). VariZIG is given intramuscularly at a recommended dose of 125 units per 10 kg bodyweight, up to a maximum of 625 units. If VariZIG is unavailable, IVIG (400 mg/kg) can be substituted. Passive immunoprophylaxis has been shown to prevent chickenpox in exposed older children (Brunell et al, 1969), but does not always prevent neonatal disease (Reynolds et al, 1999). Approximately 50% of exposed infants treated with immunoglobulin can still develop varicella, but the disease is often attenuated, and approximately 10% have severe disease (Hanngren et al, 1985). For healthy term infants exposed postnatally to varicella, including infants whose mother's rash began more than 48 hours after delivery, VariZIG is not generally indicated. VariZIG is not indicated for an infant whose mother has zoster. Breastfeeding is not contraindicated.

Follow-up of infants exposed to VZV and treated with VariZIG can include consideration of serologic testing (enzyme immunoassay, latex agglutination, or indirect fluorescent antibody staining for IgG) to determine whether asymptomatic infection has elicited immune protection. Some experts recommend repeated administration of VariZIG after a repeated exposure of an infant in whom varicella did not develop more than 3 weeks after administration of the initial dose of VariZIG, although the risk to these infants is less well defined. Infants receiving VariZIG should also be placed in respiratory isolation for 28 days or until discharge, because administration of VariZIG can prolong the incubation period.

In the event of a significant varicella exposure in a nursery situation, infants whose mothers have no history of chickenpox and who have undetectable antivaricella antibody titers should be considered candidates for VariZIG. All exposed infants less than 28 weeks of gestational age or birthweight less than 1000 g, regardless of maternal history, should receive VariZIG (see Box 37-3) (AAP Committee on Infectious Diseases, 2010a). The decision to use VariZIG in the premature infant greater than 28 weeks' gestation should be predicated on maternal

history of chickenpox or serologic evidence of protection. As of late 2010, VariZIG is available under an investigational new drug protocol and can be obtained by calling FFF Enterprises (800-843-7477; www.fffenterprises.com/Products/VariZIG.aspx).

Acyclovir has also been recommended by some experts for postexposure prophylaxis in the setting of a nursery outbreak of VZV (Hayakawa et al, 2003; Shinjoh and Takahashi, 2009). A suggested dose is 10 mg/kg by mouth, four times per day for 7 days. All exposed health care professionals without evidence of immunity should be excused from patient contact from day 8 to 21 after exposure to an infectious patient, or to day 28 if the individual has received VariZIG (AAP Committee on Infectious Diseases, 2010a).

The best means of prevention is to follow current recommendations for universal varicella immunization of all children at 12 to 15 months of age, as well as vaccinating all susceptible adolescents and adults at high risk of exposure to varicella. VZV vaccine is available in three formulations: a monovalent formulation for children and young adults, a combination vaccine given with the measles-mumps-rubella vaccine in children and young adults, and a monovalent formulation for adults older than 60 years for prevention of herpes zoster (shingles). There is no evidence that CVS occurs after exposure to varicella vaccine during pregnancy. From March 17, 1995, through March 16, 2005, 981 women were enrolled in a pregnancy registry for women exposed to varicella vaccine (Shields et al, 2001; Wilson et al, 2008). Pregnancy outcomes were available for 629 prospectively enrolled women. Among the 131 live births to VZV-seronegative women, there was no evidence of congenital varicella syndrome. Nonetheless it is recommended that adolescents and women of childbearing age should avoid pregnancy for at least 1 month after immunization.

CYTOMEGALOVIRUS

CMV infection is ubiquitous in the general population and generally produces few if any symptoms in the immunocompetent infant, child, or adult. The mild nature of primary infection in most persons belies the severe nature of CMV-induced illness in those with impaired, suppressed, or immature immune systems, including infected newborns. Among the perinatally acquired viral infections in the developed world, CMV imposes the largest economic burden and produces the greatest long-term neurodevelopmental morbidity. This section focuses on the epidemiology, pathogenesis, diagnosis, and therapeutic management of maternal, congenital, and perinatal CMV infections.

Epidemiology

In retrospect, the first description of congenital CMV disease was in 1904, when Ribbert observed the large inclusion-bearing cells that represent the typical histopathologic finding of CMV end-organ disease in a stillborn infant. In 1920 a viral cause was proposed for the "cytomegaly" seen in tissue sections of these inclusion-bearing cells (Goodpasture and Talbot, 1921), and it would be several more decades before the ubiquitous nature of this virus

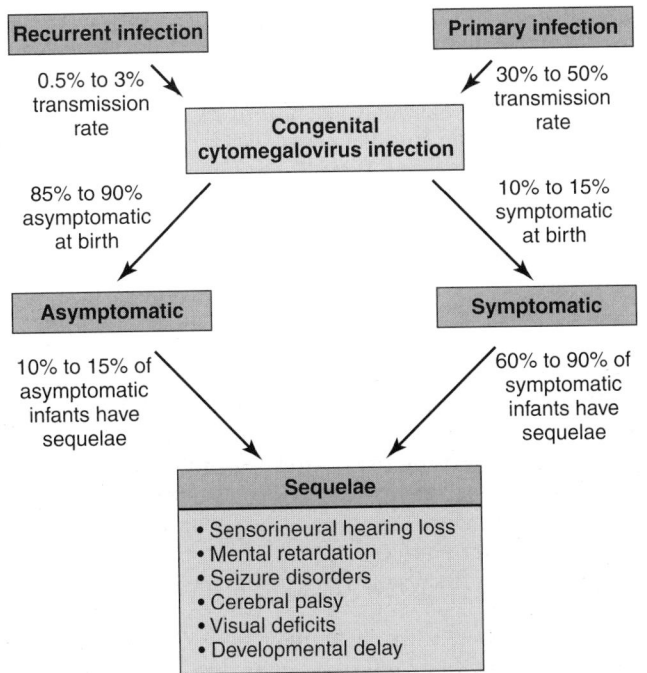

FIGURE 37-3 Profiles of congenital cytomegalovirus epidemiology, infection, and outcome. Transmission rates to the fetus are highest in the setting of primary maternal infection (up to 50%), although 0.5% to 3% of women with preconception immunity may nonetheless transmit cytomegalovirus (CMV) because of reinfection or reactivation of latent infection. Among all infants with congenital CMV infection, regardless of maternal immune status during pregnancy, approximately 10% to 15% have symptoms or signs at birth (e.g., microcephaly, chorioretinitis, hepatosplenomegaly, petechiae, purpura, thrombocytopenia, hepatitis, seizures, pneumonitis). Symptomatic infants have the highest risk of neurodevelopmental sequelae, although any infant with congenital CMV is potentially at risk for sequelae. Among asymptomatic congenitally infected infants with sequelae, the most common manifestation is sensorineural hearing loss, which may not be present at birth.

and the depth and breadth of the pathology it produces would be elucidated. In the developed world, CMV transmission occurs in 0.5% to 2% of all live births, making it the most common congenital viral infection (Demmler, 1991). Approximately 40,000 infants are born with CMV infection every year in the United States. Consequently, congenital CMV has a much greater impact than other more commonly recognized causes of birth defects in newborns. More than 8000 children per year will be permanently disabled by congenital CMV infection (Figure 37-3). This number is higher than those affected by other, better known childhood conditions such as Down syndrome, fetal alcohol syndrome, and spina bifida (Ross et al, 2006). Rates of congenital CMV infection tend to parallel those of maternal seropositivity and vary substantially across populations (Mustakangas et al, 2000). Although the lifetime risk of acquiring CMV infection is high, approaching 90% by the eighth decade of life (Staras et al, 2006), seroprevalence is substantially lower among women of childbearing age. Seronegative women are therefore at risk for acquiring primary infections during pregnancy. Primary infections pose an increased risk of transmission to the fetus, and possibly a higher risk of sequelae. Every year in the United States, approximately 27,000 seronegative women acquire a primary CMV infection (Colugnati et al, 2007).

Seroprevalence rates for CMV vary significantly globally and are generally inversely correlated with socioeconomic status. CMV seroprevalence is greater in childhood in developing countries. In developed countries, seroprevalence tends to be higher in blacks and Hispanics, low-income groups, and persons without higher education. Young maternal age, single marital status, and non-Caucasian race are associated with higher rates of congenital CMV infection. Women with increased occupational exposure to young children (including daycare providers) appear to be at elevated risk for primary CMV infections (Adler, 1989; Pass et al, 1986, 1990; Stagno and Britt, 2006; Stagno and Cloud, 1994). Health care providers in contrast are not at increased risk for acquisition of a primary CMV infection (Dworsky et al, 1983).

Pathogenesis

Morphologically and at the genome level, CMV is the largest pathogen (Schleiss, in press). There are approximately 160 known CMV genes; although based on its coding potential, CMV has the potential to encode more than 250 open reading frames. The mechanisms by which CMV injures the fetus are complex and involve a complex interplay of viral gene products, maternal immune response, and placental biology. CMV encodes genes modifying the cell cycle, cellular apoptosis mechanisms, inflammatory responses, and evasion of host immune responses. The pathogenesis of fetal injury in the setting of congenital CMV infection is incompletely understood. The pathogenesis of disease associated with acute CMV infection has been attributed to lytic virus replication, with end-organ damage occurring either secondary to virus-mediated cell death or from pathologic host immune responses targeting virus-infected cells (Britt, 2008; Schleiss, in press). Factors that contribute to fetal injury include the timing of infection relative to the gestational age of the fetus (Pass et al, 2006), the maternal immune status (Fowler et al, 1992), the extent of associated placental injury (Fisher et al, 2000), the magnitude of the viral load in the amniotic fluid (Lazzarotto et al, 2000), the induction of host genes occurring in response to infection (Challacombe et al, 2004), and possibly the genotype of the particular strain of CMV infecting the fetus (Arav-Boger et al, 2006). The relative contribution of maternal, placental, and fetal compartments in the pathogenesis of disease remains incompletely defined. Much of the injury that CMV produces in the newborn may be caused by placental insufficiency and not by viral infection of the fetus (Schleiss, 2006a). Delivery of oxygen, substrate, and nutritional factors to the fetus is impaired for a CMV-infected placenta. Moreover, CMV infection of the placenta might contribute to intrauterine growth restriction and fetal injury via induction of proinflammatory cytokines and modulation of normal trophoblast gene expression (Chan and Guilbert, 2005; Chou et al, 2006; La Torre et al, 2006; Maidji et al, 2007; Yamamoto-Tabata et al, 2004). Identified as a site for major pathogenic virus-induced injury, the placenta is increasingly considered to be a target for novel therapeutic interventions, such as CMV hyperimmune globulin for women with primary CMV infection during pregnancy (La Torre et al, 2006).

Congenital CMV infection appears to be pathologically more severe in the setting of primary maternal infection, which confers a 40% to 50% risk of intrauterine transmission during gestation, versus the 0.5% to 2% transmission risk in women with preconceptional immunity (Fowler et al, 2003). Congenital CMV infection in previously immune mothers appears to be related to reinfection with new strains of virus, with variations in epitopes of virally encoded proteins that may correlate with decreased maternal immune (Boppana et al, 1999, 2001). Many of the pathologic manifestations of congenital CMV infection that reflect visceral organ involvement (hepatitis and pneumonitis) are also observed in immunocompromised adults with disseminated CMV disease. The developing fetal brain is also highly susceptible to CMV-induced injury. CNS injury may be attributable to interference with important cellular functions of the stem and progenitor cells in the brain. The pathogenesis of CMV infection in the CNS seems to be strongly related to perturbations in neural migration, neural death, cellular compositions, and the immune system of the brain (Cheeran et al, 2009). In infants with severe symptomatic congenital CMV infection, histopathologic evidence of viral dissemination is commonly found in the brain, ear structures, retina, liver, lung, kidney, and endocrine glands (Bissinger et al, 2002). Distinctive features include large cells with large nuclei containing oval inclusions separated from the nuclear membrane by a clear zone, which gives them a characteristic "owl's eye" appearance. Inclusion-bearing epithelial cells have been described in the semicircular canals, vestibular membrane, cochlea, and other structures of the ear. In addition, temporal bone anomalies with cochlear, vestibular, and auditory canal defects have been noted in association with hearing loss in affected infants (Davis, 1969; Myers and Stool, 1968).

Clinical Presentation, Sequelae, and Prognosis

Prenatal ultrasonography provides clues to the possible diagnosis of fetal CMV infection. Findings include intrauterine growth restriction, microcephaly, ventriculomegaly, periventricular calcifications, echogenic bowel, polyhydramnios, pleural effusion, pericardial effusion, hepatosplenomegaly, intrahepatic calcifications, pseudomeconium ileus, and placental enlargement (Guerra et al, 2008; Nelson and Demmler, 1997). Fetal hydrops is also a common finding (Sampath et al, 2005). However, the sensitivity of ultrasound to detect congenital CMV infection is poor given that the majority of congenitally infected infants are asymptomatic. In a study of 600 pregnant women with primary CMV infection, abnormal ultrasound findings were detected in 51 of 600 (8.5%) pregnancies and in 23 of 154 (14.9%) fetuses in which congenital infection was documented. The positive predictive value of an abnormal ultrasound finding that predicted symptomatic congenital infection in women with primary CMV infection was only 35.3% when fetal infection status was unknown, compared with 78.3% when congenital CMV infection was confirmed (Guerra et al, 2000, 2008).

Signs and symptoms are apparent at birth in 10% to 15% of all children with congenital CMV infection. Table 37-1 outlines the clinical manifestations of symptomatic CMV infection. Each year in the United States, approximately 40,000 babies are born with congenital infection; of these, 4000 to 6000 have symptomatic disease (see Figure 37-3) (Sharon and Schleiss, 2007). Infection in the symptomatic infant can involve any organ and manifests along a spectrum from mild illness to severe disseminated multiorgan system disease. The mortality rate of symptomatic congenital CMV disease in the 1st year of life is estimated to be greater than 10% (Boppana et al, 1992). Clinical features include jaundice, hepatosplenomegaly, lethargy, respiratory distress, seizures, and petechial rash. Infants with symptomatic disease are often premature and small for gestational age. A wide spectrum of disease can be observed, including hemolysis, bone marrow suppression, hepatitis, pneumonitis, enteritis, and nephritis. Bone abnormalities have been described (Alessandri et al, 1995). Common laboratory abnormalities include thrombocytopenia, anemia, abnormal levels of liver enzymes (particularly elevated transaminases), and elevated conjugated bilirubin levels. End-organ involvement is often inferred on a clinical basis; it can be confirmed by isolation of the virus or viral DNA from tissue or by the histopathologic demonstration of characteristic inclusion bodies, positive in situ hybridization with CMV gene probes, or immunofluorescence using appropriate CMV-specific antibodies from tissue biopsies.

Of particular concern are the CNS pathologies observed with symptomatic congenital CMV infection. These pathologies include meningoencephalitis, calcifications, microcephaly, neuronal migration disturbances, germinal matrix cysts, ventriculomegaly, and cerebellar hypoplasia (Cheeran et al, 2009). CNS disease is usually characterized by at least one of the following signs and symptoms: lethargy, microcephaly, intracranial calcifications, hypotonia, seizures, hearing deficit, or an abnormal eye examination finding, such as chorioretinitis or optic atrophy. The clinical finding of microcephaly implicates the CNS as a site of infection with CMV, and abnormal findings on cranial imaging studies corroborate its involvement (Figure 37-4). Long-term neurodevelopmental disabilities are observed in 50% to 90% of children who are symptomatic at birth. In contrast, long-term neurodevelopment injury is strikingly less likely in congenitally infected infants who are asymptomatic at birth: when it does occur, it is typically limited to hearing deficits. If there is a control for sensorineural hearing loss (SNHL), the intellectual development of asymptomatic congenitally infected infants appears to be normal (Conboy et al, 1986, 1987; Stagno et al, 1982b). Among symptomatic congenitally infected infants, long-term sequelae can include microcephaly, hearing loss, motor deficits (paresis or paralysis), cerebral palsy, mental retardation, seizures, ocular abnormalities (chorioretinitis, optic atrophy), and learning disabilities (Cheeran et al, 2009; Sharon and Schleiss, 2007).

The incidence of hearing loss among children with congenital CMV infection ranges from 10% to 15% of those who are asymptomatic at birth to up to 60% of those who are symptomatic as newborns (Pass, 2005). SNHL can be progressive and fluctuating in both asymptomatic and symptomatically congenitally infected infants (Rosenthal et al, 2009). Among asymptomatic congenitally infected

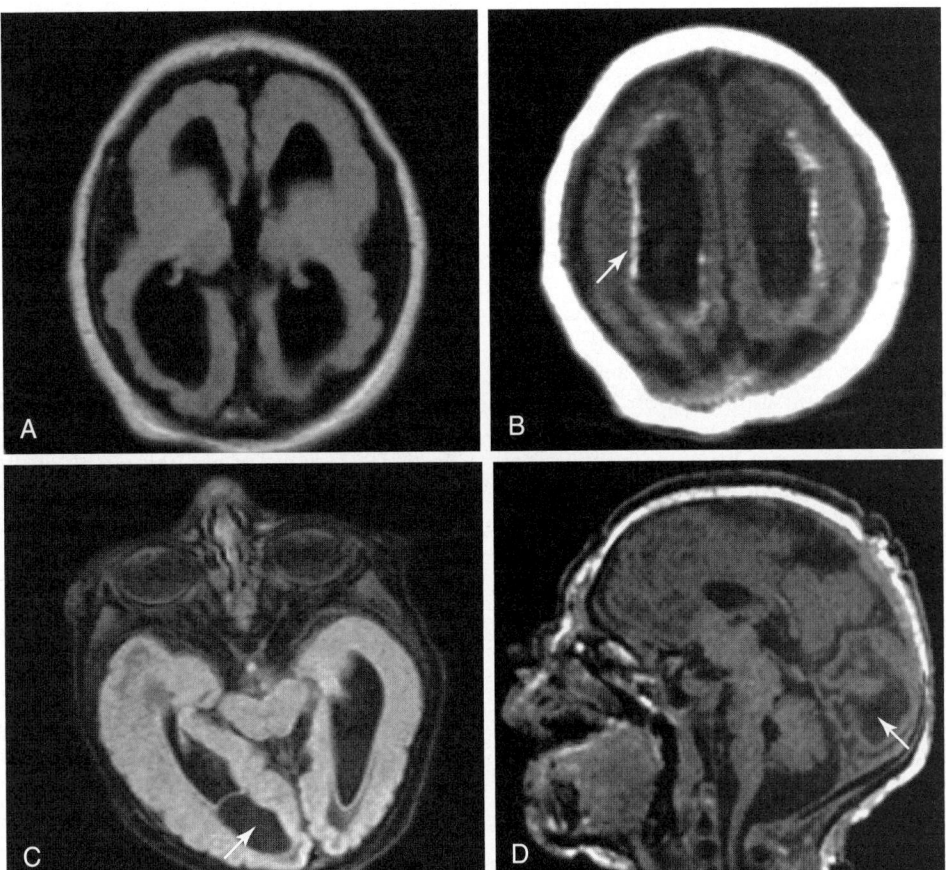

FIGURE 37-4 Magnetic resonance image abnormalities in infants with congenital cytomegalovirus (CMV) infection with neurologic manifestations. A, T1 axial flair image of neonate with congenital CMV diagnosed with CNS malformation in utero by prenatal ultrasound, demonstrating severe hydrocephalus and cortical dysplasia and polymicrogyria. **B,** Axial T1 image of infant with symptomatic congenital CMV infection demonstrating ventriculomegaly and periventricular enhancement *(arrow).* **C** and **D,** T1 flash axial **(C)** and sagittal **(D)** images of a symptomatic, congenitally infected infant demonstrating ventriculomegaly, polymicrogyria, and porencephalic cyst *(arrow).*

infants, SNHL tends to be high frequency in nature; it ranges in severity from a unilateral, mild hearing deficit to severe, bilateral, profound deafness. CMV-induced SNHL is a dynamic, evolving lesion; it may be present at birth or can appear later in childhood. Delayed-onset hearing loss usually occurs before 4 years of age (Dahle et al, 2000; Fowler et al, 1997; Rivera et al, 2002; Williamson et al, 1992), but has been reported to evolve and progress through 6 years of age and beyond. The pathogenesis of the SNHL is incompletely understood. SNHL appears to be related to an inflammatory labyrinthitis, possibly potentiated by the fact that the labyrinth is a site of immune privilege, allowing virus to persist in this compartment long after it has been cleared from the systemic compartment (Schleiss and Choo, 2006). Although some temporal bone and cochlear abnormalities have been described in a small case series of hearing-impaired infants with congenital CMV infection (Bauman et al, 1994), a more comprehensive analysis indicated that CMV-associated SNHL was not associated with structural abnormalities, such as enlarged vestibular aqueduct syndrome (Pryor et al, 2005). Logistic regression analysis of the clinical and laboratory parameters observed in 180 children with symptomatic congenital CMV infection showed that the presence of petechiae and intrauterine growth restriction were independently associated with the development of hearing loss

(Rivera et al, 2002). A retrospective review of symptomatic congenitally infected infants identified neurologic and radiologic sequelae in 81% of affected patients. There was a significant correlation between the severity of the initial pure-tone audiometry and the development of progressive hearing loss, in addition to a significant correlation between a less severe final pure-tone audiometry and the presence of cerebral palsy (Madden et al, 2005). All congenitally infected infants, regardless of the results of functional hearing assessment at birth, should be monitored prospectively for SNHL by an audiologist using age-appropriate diagnostic tools. For severe SNHL, cochlear implantation has been used with success (Lee et al, 2005; Yoshida et al, 2009).

Diagnosis and Infant Assessment

Congenital CMV infection is best diagnosed by detection of virus, either through culture techniques or via PCR, in samples collected within the first 2 to 3 weeks of life. The timing of these samples is important because subsequent viral isolation may represent neonatal infection acquired in the birth canal or after exposure to breast milk (Schleiss, 2006b). Urine and saliva are the clinical samples of choice for viral culture. Specimens are typically inoculated onto a monolayer of human fibroblasts. The high viral titer in these samples usually allows virus detection by cytopathic effect within 1 to 3 days; however, 2 to 4 weeks may be required (Revello and Gerna, 2002). Rapid virus isolation can be achieved using monoclonal antibodies to CMV-specific early protein with low-speed centrifugation of the clinical isolate onto the monolayer of fibroblasts growing on cover slips inside shell vials. This "shell vial" assay has a high sensitivity and specificity, and it allows the confirmation of diagnosis within 24 hours of inoculation (Gleaves et al, 1984; Rabella and Drew, 1990).

PCR can readily amplify CMV DNA from various clinical samples, including urine, cerebrospinal fluid, blood, plasma, saliva, and biopsy material (Revello and Gerna, 2002). If primer selection and amplification conditions are carefully chosen, PCR can yield results comparable to a standard tissue culture test. Obvious advantages of PCR over culture are the small sample requirement, the short time requirement for test results, and the ability to use frozen specimens for diagnosis. The magnitude of the systemic viral load in the congenitally infected infant can be a predictor of neurodevelopmental prognosis. In some studies, the magnitude of viral DNA in blood (DNAemia) assessed by quantitative PCR correlated with an increased risk of long-term sequelae, including SNHL (Lanari et al, 2006). Quantitative PCR assays, particularly of blood, should be ordered in the evaluation of congenitally infected infants and may be useful in making decisions about which infants to treat with antiviral therapy.

Serodiagnosis of congenital CMV is problematic. In congenital CMV infection, antibody production by the infected fetus begins in utero; however, serodiagnosis of congenital infection is complicated by the presence of maternal IgG antibodies that cross the placenta. Although a negative antibody titer in infant and maternal sera provides sufficient evidence to exclude the diagnosis of congenital CMV infection, positive titers in the newborn by no means confirm congenital infection. The presence of IgM antibodies to CMV in cord or neonatal blood is highly specific and in principle represents fetal antibody response, but many IgM commercial detection assays cross-react with IgG antibodies. Therefore a positive IgM titer has limited sensitivity in diagnosing congenital CMV infection and should not take the place of viral culture or PCR (Revello et al, 1999b).

A recent development in molecular diagnostics for congenital CMV infection has been the use of dried blood spots (DBSs) as a source of CMV DNA for PCR-based detection (Barbi et al, 2006; Scanga et al, 2006; Yamagishi et al, 2006). DBS screening is amenable to long-term storage, so diagnosis can be made retrospectively, even after several years. The test might be useful in the future for implementation of widespread population-based newborn screening for congenital CMV infection (Dollard et al, in press; Kharrazi et al, 2010). However, recent evidence from a large multicenter study suggests that DBS is not sufficiently sensitive for diagnosis of congenital CMV compared with detection in other bodily fluids such as saliva and urine (Boppana et al, 2010). An alternative approach would be to analyze the DBSs obtained from infants with failed newborn hearing screens, because congenital CMV infection can be identified in approximately 3% of such cases (Choi et al, 2009). This approach would allow early

detection and more timely intervention; however, it would fail to identify those congenitally infected infants who pass the newborn hearing screening but later develop SNHL.

Cranial ultrasonography, head CT, and brain MRI are used to detect brain lesions associated with congenital CMV infection. CNS anomalies can be detected in some infants in utero. Fetal MRI can also detect abnormalities, including microcephaly and cortical anomalies, even when the ultrasound is normal; this appears to be the preferred modality for diagnosis of fetal CNS involvement (see Figure 37-4; Benoist et al, 2008; Doneda et al, 2010). Because the finding of CNS disease is a potential harbinger of permanent sequelae, diagnostic CNS imaging is warranted in all suspected cases of congenital infection (Ancora et al, 2007; Boesch et al, 1989; Boppana et al, 1997; Kylat et al, 2006). Any of the standard imaging modalities is valuable in assessing CNS involvement. Ultrasound, because of its convenience, is an appropriate initial study and is particularly valuable and sensitive in detecting periventricular calcifications and lenticulostriate vasculopathy associated with mild to moderate ventricular dilatation. MRI provides important additional information, particularly the presence of associated polymicrogyria, hippocampal dysplasia, and cerebellar hypoplasia (de Vries et al, 2004); therefore the staged sequential use of ultrasound and MRI is probably the preferred approach to CNS imaging in this setting.

Careful initial hearing evaluation and longitudinal monitoring for SNHL is required in all infants with documented congenital CMV infection, given that this complication is the most common late sequela of congenital CMV infection. Early recognition of SNHL and institution of appropriate interventions (speech–language therapy, centers for deafness education, and cochlear implants) can markedly improve the developmental, social, and language skills of a child with hearing impairment. Any child born with congenital CMV infection, whether symptomatic or not, deserves careful and recurring evaluation for cognitive delays, visual impairment, or motor disabilities. Follow-up evaluation should include a multidisciplinary team approach involving a pediatric infectious diseases specialist, pediatric otolaryngologist, and child behavioral-developmental specialist, in addition to a physical therapist, ophthalmologist, and neurologist as needed.

Treatment: Antiviral Intervention in the Newborn and the Pregnant Patient

Experience with the use of antiviral therapies against CMV in immunosuppressed patients, particularly solid organ and hematopoietic stem cell recipients and patients with HIV infection, is considerable (Boeckh and Ljungman, 2009; Razonable, 2005). Several studies in recent years have extended this experience to infants and children and have clearly indicated a benefit of antiviral therapy against CMV infection in several settings. In a phase 3, randomized, nonblinded controlled trial of ganciclovir for newborns with congenital CMV disease (Kimberlin et al, 2003), a group of infants with virologically confirmed congenital CMV received a 6-week course of ganciclovir (6 mg/kg every 12 hours). The primary endpoint was improved hearing or retention of normal hearing. Significant differences between treated and untreated groups were noted, including a statistically higher likelihood of normal or improved hearing at 6 months of age in treated infants compared to controls. Although almost two thirds of the treated infants had neutropenia, it was reversible when antiviral therapy was halted. In a follow-up assessment, infants with symptomatic congenital CMV involving the CNS who received intravenous ganciclovir therapy had fewer developmental delays at 6 and 12 months, using the Denver Developmental Screening test, compared with untreated infants (Oliver et al, 2009). Because the use of ganciclovir can promote improved hearing and neurodevelopmental outcomes, antiviral therapy should be considered for all infants with congenital CMV infection with any evidence of CNS involvement (microcephaly, abnormal CNS imaging study, positive CSF for CMV DNA, chorioretinitis, or evidence of SNHL).

Ganciclovir should also be used in any infant with severe or life-threatening end-organ CMV disease, whether acquired via congenital infection or via a postnatal route (see Table 37-2) (Schleiss and McVoy, 2004). CMV retinitis in the congenitally infected infant can represent a particularly problematic management issue; it has been reported that up to 6 months of antiviral therapy may be required to control chorioretinitis in the symptomatic congenitally infected infant (Shoji et al, 2010). All infants with documented congenital infection should have an ophthalmologic evaluation. If chorioretinitis is present, it should be managed in consultation with an ophthalmologist and infectious diseases expert. Although ganciclovir improves neurodevelopmental outcomes for symptomatic infants, it is not clear whether ganciclovir holds the promise of improving outcomes in infants with asymptomatic congenital CMV infection. Because some of these infants are at risk to progress to SNHL, clinical trials are warranted to explore whether antiviral therapy could prevent development of hearing loss. Other investigational studies including the assessment of the therapeutic potential in infants of the prodrug of ganciclovir, valganciclovir, are needed. The potential role of valganciclovir in long-term (suppressive) therapy of CMV in congenitally infected infants is currently under investigation. The CASG is currently conducting a clinical trial of 6 weeks versus 6 months of valganciclovir (www.casg.uab.edu; Nassetta et al, 2009). A number of case reports and small case series have reported the safety, tolerability, and possibly efficacy of long-term oral therapy with valganciclovir in the setting of congenital CMV infection (Amir et al, 2010; Hilgendorff et al, 2009; Lombardi et al, 2009; Yilmaz Çiftdogan and Vardar, 2011), but the uncontrolled nature of these reports precludes any recommendations for oral therapy at this time.

The prospect of treating the pregnant patient to prevent transmission of CMV to the fetus is an area of active investigation. Ganciclovir has demonstrated teratogenic risk in some studies (Schleiss and McVoy, 2004); although this has never been demonstrated in humans, it has limited research in this area. A case report of the use of oral ganciclovir in a pregnant liver transplant patient did not show any evidence of teratogenicity (Pescovitz, 1999). Ganciclovir has been demonstrated to cross the placenta, and therefore could theoretically be used to treat CMV infection in utero (Brady et al, 2002). An observational study of 20

women with 21 fetuses, with confirmed congenital CMV infection treated with oral valacyclovir, demonstrated placental transfer of valacyclovir with measurable concentrations in the amniotic fluid and a subsequent reduced viral load in the fetal blood (Jacquemard et al, 2007). There have been several case reports of treatment of congenital CMV infection in utero with oral, parenteral, or intraamniotic ganciclovir with varying degrees of success (Miguelez et al, 1998; Puliyanda et al, 2005; Revello et al, 1993, 1999a). Although it is probably safe, prenatal treatment of fetal CMV infection with ganciclovir is currently not supported by the available data; further study with a randomized controlled trial is needed.

Passive immunization with CMV human immunoglobulin (HIG) has been studied for the in utero treatment and prevention of congenital CMV infection. CMV HIG is a pooled, high-titer immunoglobulin preparation derived from donors with high levels of CMV antibody. Nigro et al (2005) completed a prospective study of CMV HIG for the treatment of pregnant women with primary CMV infection, including some women with confirmed fetal CMV (Nigro et al, 2005). The women were enrolled in the therapy group if they had an amniocentesis and confirmed congenital CMV infection, as evidenced by a positive PCR in the amniotic fluid; they were enrolled in prevention group if they did not have an amniocentesis. In the therapy group, only 1 in 31 of the treated mothers delivered an infant with congenital CMV disease, compared to 7 in 14 mothers who were not treated with HIG. In the prevention group 6 of 37 mothers receiving HIG delivered infants with congenital CMV, compared to 19 of 7 mothers who did not receive treatment. Overall, there was a statistically significant reduction of risk for congenital CMV infection with HIG therapy. In a subsequent study, three fetuses treated with HIG had resolution of their ultrasonographically detected cerebral abnormalities; in contrast the two untreated fetuses had persistence of their cerebral abnormalities (Nigro et al, 2008). In addition to fetal effects, CMV HIG has been demonstrated to affect the placenta. In pregnancies treated with HIG, significant reductions in placental thickness have been demonstrated (La Torre et al, 2006). The reduction in placental thickness with HIG treatment suggests that at least part of the beneficial effect of treatment is mediated at the level of the placenta (Schleiss, 2006a). Randomized controlled trials of HIG for the treatment and prevention of congenital CMV infection are needed. Until such data are available, clinicians could consider treatment with CMV HIG in pregnant patients with confirmed fetal CMV infection.

Natal Acquisition of CMV Infection: Implications for the Premature Infant

In addition to congenital infection, CMV can produce disease in the newborn infant after natal acquisition; this can occur via one of three mechanisms: (1) transmission in the birth canal during vaginal delivery after exposure to infectious cervicovaginal secretions, (2) through ingestion of breast milk, and (3) via blood transfusion. Of these potential mechanisms, the most common is via breast milk (Schleiss, 2006c), with transmission in the birth canal occurring less commonly. It has long been recognized that

CMV is shed by the cervix (Montgomery et al, 1972) and excreted in the breast milk of seropositive women (Hayes et al, 1972; Stagno, 1982a). The risk of CMV transmission in infants who are breastfed by seropositive women shedding virus in their breast milk has been reported to be between 58% and 69% (Dworsky et al, 1983; Stagno et al, 1980). CMV infection acquired in the postnatal period in healthy term infants by this route typically is asymptomatic, only rarely producing any morbidity. There is no convincing evidence that acquisition of CMV via breast milk leads to any adverse neurodevelopmental sequelae (Kurath et al, 2010). In a study of CMV transmission through breastfeeding, all the infants who acquired CMV infection had normal neurodevelopment at a mean follow-up of 51 months of age (Vollmer et al, 2004).

Although the safety of breastfeeding has been established in term infants in CMV-seropositive women, controversy exists regarding the safety of breastfeeding low-birthweight, premature infants. Studies in low-birthweight and very low-birthweight (VLBW) preterm infants yield conflicting results regarding to the risk of developing symptomatic infection after breast milk acquisition of CMV (Schleiss, 2006c). In one study of VLBW premature infants (<32 weeks' gestation, <1500 g) exposed to CMV via breast milk, virus transmission occurred in 33 of the 87 exposed infants (Maschmann et al, 2001). Approximately half of these infants were ill and exhibited symptoms such as hepatopathy, neutropenia, thrombocytopenia, and sepsislike deterioration. Conflicting reports of early postnatal CMV infection in preterm infants in highly immune populations have suggested that symptomatic CMV infection acquired by breast milk is rare (Mussi-Pinhata et al, 2004; Kurath et al, 2010). Proposed efforts to reduce the infectivity of breast milk from seropositive mothers have included freezing breast milk at –20°C, Holder pasteurization, and short-term pasteurization (Hamprecht et al, 2004). Of these methods, freezing is the most studied and most likely to maintain the salutary immunologic properties of breast milk. Some experts recommend freeze-thawing all breast milk before feeding the VLBW premature infant if the mother is known to be CMV seropositive, or if her CMV serostatus is unknown. Although freezing breast milk may lower the incidence of postnatally acquired CMV infection, it does not entirely eliminate the risk (Maschmann et al, 2006). It is presumed that VLBW premature infants are at increased risk because they possess fewer transplacentally acquired antibodies against CMV than do term babies, and thus are more likely to develop disease upon infection. It has recently been shown that treating the VLBW infant with IVIG appeared to reduce the likelihood of transmission of CMV by breast milk (Capretti et al, 2009), although this is not currently considered to be an indication for the use of IVIG in the premature infant. Further evidence is necessary to make recommendations regarding what, if any, interventions are appropriate in low-birthweight, preterm infants receiving breast milk from CMV-seropositive mothers.

CMV can be transmitted through blood transfusion, and transfusion-associated infections were at one time a major problem in the neonatal intensive care setting (Adler, 1986; Adler et al, 1983, 1984; Prober et al, 1981). Two approaches are currently used to decrease the risks of transfusion-associated CMV, leukocyte reduction, and directed transfusion of CMV-negative blood products (Lamberson et al, 1988). Although leukocyte reduction has had a dramatic effect on the risk of transfusion-associated CMV, reports are conflicting in the literature regarding the question of whether this intervention is completely effective at eliminating the risk of transfusion-transmitted CMV (Allain et al, 2009; Fergusson et al, 2002; Vamvakas, 2005). A recent survey of the American Association of Blood Banks physician membership revealed that 65% of those responding believed that leukocyte-reduced and CMV-negative blood components were equivalent in their ability to prevent transfusion-associated transmission of CMV (Smith et al, 2010). Leukoreduction should be adequate for preventing the overwhelming majority of transfusion-associated CMV infections in the newborn intensive care unit. However, despite the American Association of Blood Banks survey results on attitudes toward leukocyte-reduced blood products, fetuses and neonates are more likely to receive CMV-negative products compared with other groups receiving transfusions, and additional studies are warranted to ascertain what risk may exist for premature infants receiving leukocyte-reduced products from CMV-seropositive donors.

Prevention

One important strategy for addressing the problem of congenital CMV is the education of women of childbearing age about the risks of transmission and strategies for prevention. Child care providers (including daycare workers, special education teachers, and therapists) appear to have a higher risk of occupational exposure to CMV, because of extensive contact with infants and young children (Adler, 1989; Pass et al, 1986, 1990). Education of the potential occupational risk in this group is essential. In contrast to these child care providers, health care workers who appropriately use routine infection control practices are not at increased risk of CMV acquisition. CMV infections in pregnant women are typically clinically "silent." Like most healthy individuals, more than 90% of pregnant women with primary CMV infections have no symptoms. When symptoms occur, they are nonspecific and vague, often described as a flulike syndrome. Potential manifestations include fever, fatigue, headache, myalgia, lymphadenitis, and pharyngitis, but these are the exception and not the rule. Because most maternal CMV infections are asymptomatic, a major goal is education of all women of childbearing age on hygienic practices (ACOG Practice Bulletin, 2002; Jeon et al, 2006; Ross et al, 2006). Hygienic strategies are important because the saliva and urine of infected children are significant sources of CMV infection among pregnant women. Strategies include washing hands whenever there is contact with a child's saliva or urine, not sharing food, utensils, or cups, and not kissing a child on the mouth or cheek (Anderson et al, 2007; Cannon and Davis, 2005). It is also essential that women become better educated on the importance of CMV infection. A survey of women in 2005 showed that only 14% of women knew what CMV was, but most believed that preventative measures for an infection that could harm an unborn baby would generally be acceptable (Ross et al, 2008). The effectiveness of educating pregnant women on methods to prevent CMV transmission has been demonstrated (Adler et al, 1996). In a study in which seronegative mothers with a child in group day care were instructed on measures to prevent CMV transmission, pregnant mothers had a significantly lower rate of CMV infection when compared with nonpregnant mothers attempting conception (Adler et al, 2004). In addition, a study in France recently demonstrated a lower CMV seroconversion rate after counseling pregnant women on hygienic measures (Vauloup-Fellous et al, 2009).

Prenatal maternal screening for CMV antibodies is controversial. Because women who are CMV-immune can be reinfected with new strains that can then be transmitted to the fetus, with subsequent sequelae (Boppana et al, 1999, 2001), the finding of a positive preconception titer for CMV IgG antibody may provide a false sense of reassurance and decrease a pregnant patient's motivation to engage in careful hygienic practices. A recent study evaluated three screening strategies and suggested that universal maternal screening for CMV could be a cost-effective strategy if a treatment were available that could achieve a 47% reduction in disease (Cahill et al, 2009).

Ultimately the control of congenital CMV could be realized by the development of an effective vaccine. No CMV vaccines are currently licensed; however, because of the enormous economic impact of congenital CMV, the Institute of Medicine has identified a CMV vaccine as the highest-level priority for new vaccine development (excluding HIV vaccines) for the United States (Stratton et al, 2001). The CMV envelope glycoprotein B has been the most studied subunit vaccine candidate for this purpose, because it is a target of neutralizing antibody in all CMV-seropositive individuals. Results of a phase II, placebo-controlled, randomized, double-blind trial of the recombinant CMV envelope glycoprotein B with MF59 adjuvant were published recently (Pass et al, 2009). In this study, three doses of the CMV vaccine or placebo were administered at 0, 1, and 6 months to healthy women within 12 months postpartum. Women in the vaccine group were less likely than the placebo group to become infected with CMV ($p = 0.02$) with 18 of 225 women becoming infected with CMV in the vaccine group, compared to 31 o 216 in the placebo group. This report is the first to document efficacy of any CMV vaccine in a clinical trial and should help to accelerate the pace of future vaccine development and testing. Other clinical trials include evaluation of live, attenuated CMV vaccines and the testing of subunit vaccines targeting other key proteins involved in the humoral and cellular immune responses to CMV infection (Schleiss, 2008).

HUMAN HERPESVIRUS 6 AND 7

Human herpesvirus (HHV) 6 was isolated in tissue culture in 1986 from peripheral blood leukocytes of patients with both lymphoproliferative disorders and HIV infection (Bernstein and Schleiss, 1996; Schleiss, 2009). The virus was eventually shown to have a tropism for T cells, and molecular studies revealed homology with CMV. These findings suggested that the virus belonged to the family Herpesviridae. For several years after discovery, its role in disease was unclear, but it is now known to be the

major etiologic agent of roseola infantum (exanthem subitum) and has been implicated in other clinical syndromes. HHV-6 is a prototypical β-herpesvirus, with a double-stranded DNA genome contained within an icosahedral capsid, surrounded by an outer envelope. HHV-6 is subclassified as either variant A or B, based on differences in nucleotide sequence, restriction enzyme profile, and reactivity with monoclonal antibodies. HHV-6B is the subtype typically associated with exanthem subitum (Yamanishi et al, 1988). HHV-6 and HHV-7 are ubiquitous in nature, and typically cause infection in the first 2 years of life.

HHV-7 is highly related to HHV-6 and, like HHV-6, is responsible for roseola infantum (Tanaka et al, 1994). HHV-7 is a β-herpesvirus, structurally and molecularly similar to CMV and HHV-6. It was first isolated from CD4+ T cells of a healthy individual. The high degree of homology with HHV-6 creates difficulty in interpretation of serologic assays, which are largely investigational in nature and not generally useful for clinical practice, because there is considerable cross-reactivity of antibodies between HHV-6 and HHV-7 proteins. As with HHV-6, infection with HHV-7 appears to be ubiquitous, although infection appears to be acquired somewhat later in life than is HHV-6 (Caserta et al, 1998; Suga et al, 1997). Approximately 40% to 45% of children have antibodies to HHV-7 by 2 years of age, and 70% of children are seropositive by 6 years of age. Like other β-herpesviruses, HHV-7 can be found in the saliva, suggesting a route for person-to-person transmission. Based on its identification in cervical secretions, HHV-7 also has the potential for perinatal transmission (Okuno et al, 1995).

It is of interest to examine the evidence that suggests that HHV-6, like CMV, can cross the placenta and infect the fetus in utero, given the extensive molecular similarities between these two viruses. In one early study, HHV-6 DNA was detected by PCR in approximately 25% of pregnant seropositive women at the time of delivery, and in approximately 1% of cord blood samples, suggesting the possibility of congenital transmission (Dahl et al, 1999). Examination of 305 cord blood samples in another study identified HHV-6 DNA by PCR in 1.6% of infants (Adams et al, 1998). Interestingly, this potential vertical transmission rate of 1% to 2% is similar to congenital infection rates commonly reported for CMV. Congenital HHV-6 transmission was first definitively reported in a study of 5638 cord bloods; 57 samples (1%) had HHV-6 DNA by PCR, but none had HHV-7 (Hall et al, 2004). Of note, these infections were all asymptomatic, and the HHV-6 genome variant in one third of congenital infections was HHV6A, in contrast to the more common variant HHV6B, which is encountered in virtually all postnatal infections. Although the rate of congenital HHV-6 transmission at approximately 1% is highly similar to that observed for congenital CMV, the mechanisms of transmission are different. It has been shown that vertical transmission of HHV-6 most often occurs (90% of cases) because of the germline passage of chromosomally integrated HHV-6 (Hall et al, 2008). The mode of inheritance of HHV-6 genome in this form of vertical transmission appears to be exclusively maternal (Hall et al, 2010). HHV-6 is unique among the human Herpesviridae regarding its capacity to integrate into the host chromosome and mediate germline transmission of viral genome from mother to fetus. Remarkably, HHV-6 is the first functional virus of any type reported to be passed through the human germline. The clinical consequences of such transmission, and the differences in germline transmission of viral genome and the more common postnatal acquisition of HHV-6 in early childhood, remain unknown. That HHV-6 genome appears to integrate into the telomere—a chromosomal component important in cellular aging and in cancer—suggests that there may be interesting long-term consequences associated with vertical germline transmission of this virus (Arbuckle et al, 2010; Nacheva et al, 2008) that remain to be elucidated.

HHV-6 and HHV-7 DNA has been found to be present in cervical secretions, placenta, and peripheral blood mononuclear cells of pregnant women (Caserta et al, 2007). Whether intrapartum transmission of these viruses can occur in the birth canal during delivery remains unknown. HHV-6 DNA can also be found in breast milk. Perinatal transmission via this mechanism has been postulated (Joshi et al, 2000), but has not been demonstrated.

KAPOSI'S SARCOMA HERPESVIRUS AND EPSTEIN–BARR VIRUS

In 1994 a novel herpesvirus, HHV-8 or KSHV, was identified in patients with AIDS-associated Kaposi's sarcoma (KS; Chang et al, 1994). This virus was assigned to the γ-herpesvirus family of the Herpesviridae, based on its molecular and sequence similarity to the other prototypical γ-herpesvirus, Epstein–Barr virus. Subsequent studies have linked KSHV to both AIDS-associated KS and the endemic forms of KS that are prevalent in elderly Mediterranean men. Little is known about routes of transmission of KSHV in nonpregnant patients, let alone whether it can be transmitted perinatally. The clinical significance of acquiring primary KSHV infection outside of the HIV setting is also unclear. Serologic evidence from sexually transmitted disease clinics suggests that sexual contact is a risk factor for acquiring KSHV. The epidemiology of primary HHV-8 infection appears to vary considerably worldwide. Indeed, the routes of acquisition of infection and mechanisms responsible for person-to-person transmission remain uncertain. After the virus was initially discovered, the unique role it seemed to play in inducing malignant disease in HIV-infected patients suggested that the primary route of transmission of HHV-8 was through sexual contact, particularly among gay men. However, more recent evidence suggests that other routes of infection exist, including transmission by saliva (Pica and Volpi, 2007).

A recent cross-sectional study of the seroprevalence of HHV-8 in children and adolescents in the United States indicated a prevalence of approximately 1% (Anderson et al, 2008). There appears to be considerable regional variation in prevalence in the United States. In a population of children in south Texas, the seroprevalence was 26%, strongly suggesting that nonsexual modes of transmission predominate (Baillargeon et al, 2002). In Sub-Saharan Africa, prevalence in children is even higher, approaching 60% in some studies (Sarmati, 2004). There are reports of infections in infants that suggest possible vertical transmission, but congenital infection has not been demonstrable

by PCR techniques (Sarmati et al, 2004). HHV-8 can also be transmitted by blood transfusion (Hladik et al, 2006); this observation would suggest that transplacental transmission is at least theoretically feasible. In a study of 89 KSHV-seropositive women, 13 mothers (14.6%) had KSHV DNA detected in their peripheral blood mononuclear cells; 2 of 89 samples drawn at birth from infants born to these mothers had KSHV DNA detectable within their peripheral blood mononuclear cells. These findings suggest that KSHV can be transmitted perinatally, but infrequently (Mantina et al, 2001). As serologic and nucleic acid–based diagnostics tests become more widely available, a better assessment of the worldwide seroepidemiology of HHV-8 infection and an increased understanding of its modes of transmission will be achievable.

Most primary infections with HHV-8 are probably asymptomatic, although the clinical course of primary symptomatic HHV-8 infection in immunocompetent children has been described (Andreoni et al, 2002). In this study, fever and rash were noted with primary infection. The rash first appeared on the face and gradually spread to the trunk, arms, and legs. It initially consisted of discrete red macules that blanched with pressure and eventually became papular. An upper respiratory tract infection appeared as a secondary symptom in most children, and a lower respiratory tract infection appeared as a secondary symptom in one third of symptomatic children. Additional information on the epidemiology and modes of transmission of this pathogen, particularly in the prenatal and intrapartum period, is needed.

There is a minimal amount of information available about prenatal and perinatal modes of transmission of EBV. EBV is the causative agent of infectious mononucleosis and is associated with nasopharyngeal carcinoma, Burkitt's lymphoma, and lymphoproliferative disease in immunocompromised patients (Schleiss, 2009). Primary EBV infection during pregnancy appears to be rare. In a prospective study, susceptibility to EBV infection in 1729 pregnant women was evaluated by screening for EBV antibodies. Fifty-eight subjects (3.4%) had no detectable EBV antibody and were presumably susceptible. Of the 54 women who agreed to participate in this study, none acquired EBV antibody during pregnancy (Le et al, 1983). It is not clear whether transplacental passage of EBV in seropositive pregnant women occurs. Because EBV can be acquired by blood transfusion, such a mode of transmission is feasible. It has been postulated that high-titer antibodies cross the placenta and protect the fetus from hematogenous transmission of virus in women who reactivate EBV during pregnancy (Purtilo and Sakamoto, 1982). A solitary case report describes the occurrence of severe EBV disease in a premature infant, born at 28 weeks' gestation, who was examined on the 42nd day of life with hepatosplenomegaly, hemolytic anemia, thrombocytopenia, and atypical lymphocytosis (Andronikou et al, 1999). In another study, the potential for EBV vertical transmission from a seropositive mother to her child was evaluated in 67 pregnant women by nested PCR (Meyohas et al, 1996). Two of 67 neonates were positive for EBV DNA, suggesting that mother-to-child transmission of free EBV or of maternal EBV-infected cells can occur during pregnancy in the setting of latent EBV infection, but no clinical consequences of these putative congenital infections were reported. In a study of six pregnant women with evidence of primary EBV infection, four pathologic births were observed: one spontaneous abortion, two premature babies, one of whom died, and one stillborn with multiple malformations (Icart et al, 1981). However, the assessment of primary infection was drawn solely from the serologic profile (including the presence of anti–early antigen antibodies) and the relationship of EBV infection to adverse pregnancy outcome was undefined, and it was unclear whether intrauterine EBV infection was present. In another study, placentas and some fetuses were studied in five cases of pregnancy interruption caused by maternal infectious mononucleosis in early gestation (Ornoy et al, 1982). Decidual lesions, consisting of perivasculitis and necrotizing deciduitis, were noted, and endovasculitis, perivasculitis, and occasional vascular obliteration were found in villi, as well as mononuclear and plasma cell infiltrates. Two fetal hearts exhibited evidence of myocarditis. These observations suggested a pathogenic role for placental and fetal EBV infection, but no direct virologic evidence of EBV was obtained, and these observations have not been duplicated. Accordingly a recent review concluded that maternal EBV infection did not impose a serious threat to pregnancy outcome (Avgil and Ornoy, 2006) and that no strong evidence for teratogenicity or fetal injury existed.

HUMAN PARVOVIRUS B19

Parvovirus B19, a small, single-stranded DNA virus, is the only member of the parvovirus family that causes human disease. The virus was identified in 1975 (Cossart et al, 1975) and was first linked to a disease in 1981—aplastic crisis in children with sickle cell anemia (Pattison et al, 1981). Primary infection with parvovirus B19 is commonly known as *fifth disease* or *erythema infectiosum;* it is classically described as a childhood exanthem with a "slapped cheek" appearance (Anderson et al, 1984). The agent is less ubiquitous than other common childhood exanthematous illnesses, such as HHV-6; therefore many individuals reach adulthood with no prior evidence of infection, placing women of childbearing age at potential risk. Considerable interest in the role of this virus in hydrops fetalis (nonimmune) and fetal aplastic crisis has evolved since the first cases of fetal death associated with maternal parvovirus B19 infection were reported in the 1980s (Brown et al, 1984; Kinney et al, 1988).

Epidemiology

Parvovirus B19 infection is global in nature. It is common in childhood and continues at a low rate throughout adult life. One study identified an annual seroconversion of 1.5% in women of childbearing age unrelated to their occupation (Koch and Adler, 1989). The peak incidence of erythema infectiosum is in the late winter and early spring. Periodic epidemics at intervals of a few years are typical. The virus is spread by respiratory droplet (Anderson and Cohen, 1987), by blood products (especially pooled clotting factor concentrates; Jordan et al, 1998), and transplacentally (Ergaz and Ornoy, 2006). Approximately 50% to 80% of adults in the United States are seropositive

for human parvovirus B19 (Anderson, 1987; Vyse et al, 2007). A significant proportion of childbearing women are thus susceptible to infection (Markenson and Yancey, 1998; Yaegashi et al, 1998). Preconception seroprevalence to parvovirus B19 ranges from 24% to 84% (Ergaz and Ornoy, 2006). During pregnancy the risk of acquiring parvovirus B19 infection is low, ranging from 0% to 16.5% in different studies (Ergaz and Ornoy, 2006). The risk of primary maternal infection is higher during epidemics, with reported seroconversion rates ranging between 3% (Kerr et al, 1994) and 34% (Woernle et al, 1987).

It is estimated that one fourth to half of maternal parvovirus infections result in transmission of infection to the fetus (Alger, 1997; Gratacos et al, 1995; Koch et al, 1998). The vast majority of pregnancies are unaffected (Berry et al, 1992; Sheikh et al, 1992). The risk of adverse fetal outcome is increased if maternal infection occurs during the first two trimesters of pregnancy (Skjoldebrand-Sparre et al, 2000), particularly before 20 weeks' gestation. There are conflicting reports regarding the prognosis once fetal infection has been established. A longitudinal study of fetal morbidity and mortality in more than 1000 women with primary parvovirus B19 infection in pregnancy demonstrated a risk of fetal hydrops of 3.9% and a risk of fetal death of 6.3%; fetal death was observed only if maternal infection occurred before the 20th week of gestation (Enders et al, 2004). A recent retrospective analysis of intrauterine parvovirus B19 infection at a single site suggested that the rate of adverse fetal outcome is much higher than previously appreciated, with fetal hydrops and demise occurring in greater than 10% of pregnancies (Beigi et al, 2008), although the total number of cases reported in this series was low; this primarily represented a referral population to a tertiary care center.

Pathogenesis

The most common mode of transmission of parvovirus B19 is via a respiratory route. Typically, once the virus establishes infection, viremia occurs, followed by mild systemic symptoms such as fever and malaise. Viremia is short-lived, lasting only 1 to 3 days, and the characteristic immune-mediated rash develops 1 to 2 weeks later. Once the rash appears, an individual is no longer infectious. Arthropathy caused by parvovirus B19 is common; it is observed more frequently in adults with primary infection than in children. It typically manifests late in the course of illness with acute onset of arthralgias or frank arthritis involving the hands, knees, wrists, and ankles. The symptoms usually subside within 1 to 3 weeks, although approximately 20% of affected women have persistent or recurring arthropathy for months to years (Woolf et al, 1989).

Potential pathogenic mechanisms involve the recognized affinity of parvovirus B19 for progenitor erythroid cells of bone marrow. The blood group P antigen is a main cellular receptor for parvovirus B19, and it is found on red blood cells and on placental trophoblast cells (Jordan et al, 2001). The P antigen is also expressed on fetal cardiac myocytes, enabling parvovirus B19 to infect myocardial cells (Rouger et al, 1987) leading to myocarditis (von Kaisenberg et al, 2001). Myocarditis induced by parvovirus B19 can contribute to high-output cardiac failure, and the myocardial inflammation and subendocardial fibroelastosis may also contribute to fetal hydrops (Morey et al, 1992). Fetal infection most likely occurs hematogenously via the placenta during maternal viremia. Parvovirus B19 infection in utero causes a pronormoblast arrest, which leads to fetal anemia, nonimmune hydrops, and sometimes progressive congestive heart failure (Ergaz and Ornoy, 2006; Kinney et al, 1988). The fetus is especially susceptible to adverse consequences of red blood cell infection, secondary to the intrinsic short fetal erythrocyte life span and rapidly expanding blood volume, especially during the second trimester. It has also been postulated that parvovirus B19 infection leads to cytotoxicity and subsequent anemia by inducing apoptosis of infected red blood cells (Yaegashi et al, 1999, 2000). The NS1 protein of parvovirus B19 induces cell death by apoptosis in erythroid-lineage cells by a pathway that involves caspase 3, whose activation may be a key event during parvovirus-induced cell death (Moffatt et al, 1998). The NS1 protein also has a key role in the arrest of infected cells at the G1 phase of the cell cycle prior to apoptosis induction (Chisaka et al, 2003). In addition to erythroid precursors and myocytes, other organs appear to be involved in fetal parvovirus B19 infection. Fetal brain infection has been reported. Neuropathologic findings in the infected hydropic fetus include perivascular calcifications, primarily in the cerebral white matter, as well as multinucleated giant cells. Viral DNA has been demonstrated in the brain and liver (Isumi et al, 1999). Data also suggest that the maternal cell–mediated immune response at the placental level contributes to the pathogenesis of congenital infection. In one study, placentas from women whose pregnancies were complicated by parvovirus B19 infection had increased infiltration of CD3 T cells and elevated levels of interleukin 2 (Jordan et al, 2001).

Clinical Spectrum

Parvovirus B19 infection causes erythema infectiosum, or fifth disease, in normal hosts, aplastic crisis in patients with hemolytic disorders, and chronic anemia in immunocompromised hosts. A substantial proportion of infected adult women may also have arthropathy in association with parvovirus B19 infection (Woolf et al, 1989). Maternal symptoms have been present in up to two thirds of documented cases of nonimmune hydrops fetalis associated with parvovirus B19 infection (Yaegashi et al, 1998).

The major clinical presentation of parvovirus B19 infection in the fetus is hydrops fetalis. Various estimates suggest that human parvovirus B19 infection contributes from 10% to 27% of cases of nonimmune hydrops fetalis (Essary et al, 1998; Markenson and Yancey, 1998; Yaegashi et al, 1994). Nonimmune hydrops fetalis was the main complication in 0.9% to 23% of pregnancies among proven maternal infections with parvovirus B19 (Ergaz and Ornoy, 2006). A risk of 7.1% for hydrops fetalis has been described for pregnant women who acquire parvovirus B19 infection between 13 and 20 weeks' gestation (Enders et al, 2004). Parvovirus B19 does not appear to have a major role in intrauterine fetal demise in the absence of hydrops fetalis (Riipinen et al, 2008). In addition to hydrops fetalis, in recent years there have been increasing numbers of case reports of neurologic and ophthalmologic anomalies associated with fetal parvovirus B19 infections. Although some studies undertaken to examine the association between fetal infection and congenital anomalies failed to reveal any associations (Kinney et al, 1988; Mortimer et al, 1985), parvovirus B19 has increasingly been recognized as a cause of neuronal migration defects (Pistorius et al, 2008). The role of parvovirus B19 in neurodevelopmental injury has not been fully explored. There have been at least three case reports of fetal encephalopathy associated with in utero infection with parvovirus B19 (Alger, 1997). Parvovirus B19 has recently been recognized as a cause of CNS injury in older children, including encephalitis, meningitis, stroke, and peripheral neuropathy (Douvoyiannis et al, 2009). Consideration should be given to performing brain imaging studies in infants with symptomatic in utero parvovirus B19 infection. Such infants need careful neurodevelopmental follow-up. Few data are available regarding long-term outcomes of infants infected in utero. Two prospective studies in the United Kingdom of approximately 300 congenitally exposed infants found the risk of major congenital or developmental abnormality to be less than 1% (Miller et al, 1998).

Parvovirus B19 has been implicated in some cases of congenital anemia (Heegaard and Brown, 2002). In one series of 11 children with a diagnosis of Diamond-Blackfan syndrome, 3 of 11 bone marrow aspirates revealed evidence of parvovirus B19 DNA. All three of these children, but none of the parvovirus B19 PCR-negative cases, underwent spontaneous remission (Heegaard et al, 1996). In light of these data, all infants undergoing evaluation for congenital anemias should be evaluated for the possibility of parvovirus B19 infection.

Laboratory Evaluation

In primary care, the diagnosis of human parvovirus B19 infection is most commonly made clinically through recognition of the characteristic rash. Serologic confirmation is necessary in high-risk situations, such as after a significant exposure of a pregnant woman to a child with erythema infectiosum. Both radioimmunoassays and enzyme-linked immunosorbent assays are available for detection of human parvovirus B19–specific IgG and IgM antibodies (Kinney and Kumar, 1988). Presence of anti–parvovirus B19 IgM in fetal blood or amniotic fluid may confirm fetal infection, but may be detected in only one fifth of infected fetuses (Torok et al, 1992). False-positive results of parvovirus B19 IgM testing have been reported, including cross-reactions with anti-rubella IgM (Dieck et al, 1999).

Monitoring of the pregnant patient with a primary parvovirus B19 infection is an important clinical problem. In the context of a human parvovirus B19 infection in a symptomatic, pregnant woman, elevated or rising weekly measurements of maternal alpha-fetoprotein suggest fetal infection, and rising concentrations may be a marker for an increased risk for hydrops fetalis (Carrington et al, 1987). However, some studies have failed to demonstrate any association between the magnitude of the elevation of the α-fetoprotein and the severity of fetal anemia (Simms et al, 2009). Serial fetal ultrasonographic evaluations of infected pregnant women are recommended to evaluate and follow for fetal hydrops or intrauterine demise. The findings of echogenic bowel, ascites, pleural or pericardial effusion, or scalp edema are considered to be important markers of fetal infection and pathology. Middle cerebral artery Doppler to evaluate for fetal anemia may be another useful prospective surveillance tool, because fetal anemia can be detected using this technique before fetal hydrops is evident (Feldman et al, 2010). Other techniques to diagnose fetal parvovirus B19 infection have been studied and used, but most are not readily available. Virus can be cultured from tissue in suspension cultures of bone marrow cells from persons with hemolytic anemias, but it is difficult to isolate; therefore this method is not feasible for prenatal or postnatal diagnosis. Electron microscopy and histology have permitted visualization of parvovirus in fetal blood, ascitic fluid, tissue, and amniotic fluid, but the utility and sensitivity of these evaluations have not been well studied (Markenson and Yancey, 1998). A number of commercial PCR assays are available, and these can be performed on serum, amniotic fluid, or fetal tissue. Presumptive diagnosis can also be made based on finding IgM antibody in the maternal and fetal blood. PCR for parvovirus B19 DNA or in situ hybridization studies can be performed using maternal blood, amniotic fluid, cord blood, or fetal tissues. The detection of B19 DNA in maternal blood appears to have the best diagnostic sensitivity for identifying maternal B19 infection, and new-generation EIA and IgG avidity assays appear to hold promise for improved serodiagnosis during pregnancy (Enders et al, 2006, 2008).

Treatment

Spontaneous resolution of fetal hydrops with normal neonatal outcome has been reported in approximately one third of cases (Humphrey et al, 1991; Rodis et al, 1998a; Sheikh et al, 1992). Because two thirds of fetuses do not recover without intervention, fetal transfusion is usually recommended (Boley and Popek, 1993; Brown et al, 1994). The earlier fetal transfusion is attempted, the more likely it is to be successful. Cordocentesis allows precise assessment of the magnitude of fetal anemia, which can then be corrected by blood transfusion, typically using packed red blood cells. Using this approach, outcomes have been favorable in most reported series, even among severely anemic fetuses. In one report, packed red cell transfusion was performed in 30 patients with fetal anemia (hemoglobin values ranging from 2.1 to 9.6 g/dL). The overall survival rate was 83.8% (Schild et al, 1999). In a report of 13 cases with severe hydrops fetalis who received intrauterine transfusion, 11 of 13 survived (84.6%), whereas all the nontransfused fetuses with severe hydrops fetalis died (Enders et al, 2004).

Prognosis

Mortality rates for fetal hydrops resulting from all nonimmune causes continue to exceed 50%, even with current aggressive therapies and intensive care (Huang et al, 2007; Wy et al, 1999). Hydrops secondary to parvovirus B19 seems to have a better outcome than that from other causes (Enders et al, 2004; Ismail et al, 2001). Although

few long-term prospective studies of infants born to mothers with documented primary parvovirus B19 infection have been conducted, most report normal developmental outcome. One case-control study involving approximately 200 mother–infant pairs found no differences in frequency of developmental delay between infants born to women with confirmed primary parvovirus B19 infection during pregnancy and infants born to mothers with evidence of preconceptional immunity (Rodis et al, 1998b). Other studies have also suggested a favorable long prognosis in children born to women with primary parvovirus B19 infections during pregnancy (Miller et al, 1998).

Prevention

If a pregnant woman has a significant exposure to an infectious case of parvovirus B19, counseling should be provided regarding the potential risk of infection. Anti–parvovirus IgM and IgG serologic analyses and serum PCR should be performed; if they show evidence of primary infection, then serial fetal ultrasonographic evaluations should be performed. Postexposure passive immunization with immunoglobulin is not currently recommended because the period of maternal viremia has passed by the time the diagnosis of acute parvovirus B19 infection is made (Boley and Popek, 1993). Although high-dose IVIG has been used to attempt to prevent hydrops fetalis during pregnancy in the setting of acute infection (Selbing et al, 1995), treatment with this modality in the pregnant woman or the neonate has not been shown to improve fetal outcomes; therefore it is not routinely recommended. Human IgG monoclonal antibodies with potent neutralizing activity have been generated, and these are suggested as candidates for the development of immunotherapeutic approaches for individuals chronically infected with parvovirus B19 virus or for acutely infected pregnant women (Gigler et al, 1999), but these interventions are not commercially available. There has been limited progress in the development of a candidate parvovirus B19 vaccine. Phase 1 studies of a recombinant vaccine based on baculovirus-produced capsids have been conducted, and this vaccine was found to have a favorable safety and immunogenicity profile (Bansal et al, 1993). Efforts are under way to research and develop vaccines to prevent parvovirus B19 infections using other expression systems (Lowin et al, 2005).

Pregnant health care providers should be counseled about the potential risks to their fetus from parvovirus B19 infections and should, at a minimum, wear masks and use standard droplet precautions when caring for immunocompromised patients with chronic parvovirus B19 infection or patients with parvovirus B19–induced aplastic crises. Some hospitals exclude pregnant health care providers from caring for these high-risk patients, but this issue remains controversial.

RUBELLA

Rubella virus is an enveloped, single-stranded, positive sense RNA virus belonging to the family Togaviridae. Although togaviruses are typically vector-borne infections, rubella is the notable exception, being transmitted instead by respiratory droplet. Humans are the only known natural host for rubella virus. Rubella infection, commonly known as the *German measles*, usually results in a mild illness with an accompanying exanthem in adults and children; however, rubella produces serious consequences in pregnant patients, in whom fetal infection can lead to serious anomalies. An ophthalmologist named Norman Gregg offered the first description of congenital rubella syndrome (CRS) in 1941 while investigating an epidemic of neonatal cataracts (Gregg, 1941). Not until the global pandemic of 1964 to 1965, however, were the multiple teratogenic manifestations of CRS fully appreciated and the permanent neurodevelopmental consequences for newborns fully recognized. The capacity to grow the virus in tissue culture led rapidly to the development of a vaccine and subsequent a reduction in the incidence of CRS in the United States and other developed countries. However, CRS is still encountered in the developing world, and unfounded concerns about the safety of measles-mumps-rubella vaccine have set the stage for potential reemergence of these diseases (Omer et al, 2009). Therefore a working knowledge of CRS remains highly relevant to the care of newborns.

EPIDEMIOLOGY

Since the development of rubella vaccine in 1969, the incidence of rubella in the United States has decreased dramatically. The annual incidence of rubella cases has dropped 99%, from 58 per 100,000 population in 1969 to less than 0.5 per 100,000 population in 1997 to 1999 (Danovaro-Holliday et al, 2001). CRS cases in the United States have demonstrated a similar dramatic decline, and in 2004 the Centers for Disease Control and Prevention (CDC) concluded, against the background of few or no reports of rubella activity from the 50 states and the virtual absence of reported CRS, that endemic rubella had been eliminated from the United States (Centers for Disease Control and Prevention, 2005; Plotkin, 2006; Reef et al, 2006). The persistence of rubella in Latin America serves as the source for a small number of importation cases of rubella that are recognized in the United States annually (Castillo-Solórzano et al, 2003). In parts of the world where routine rubella immunization is unavailable or not used, rubella and CRS continue to be common. Rubella is still an important and potentially preventable cause of birth defects globally, with more than 100,000 cases of CRS occurring annually in developing countries.

Maternal rubella infection that occurs in the period of time from 1 month before conception through the second trimester of pregnancy may be associated with transmission of infection and, depending on the timing of infection, disease in the infant. The frequency of congenital infection after maternal rubella with a rash is 70% to 85% if infection occurs during the first 12 weeks of gestation, 30% to 54% during the first 13 to 16 weeks of gestation, and 10% to 25% at the end of the second trimester (Miller et al, 1982; South and Sever, 1985). The classic findings of congenital rubella are most typically associated with the onset of maternal infection during the first 8 weeks of gestation (Miller et al, 1982). Both the risk of fetal infection and severity of disease decline after the first trimester, and the risk of any teratogenic effect is extremely low after 17 weeks' gestation (Lee and Bowden, 2000).

PATHOGENESIS

Rubella virus is transmitted via respiratory droplets. Once the oral or nasopharyngeal mucosae are infected, viral replication occurs in the upper respiratory tract and nasopharyngeal lymphoid tissue. The virus then spreads contiguously to regional lymph nodes and hematogenously to distant sites. Fetal infection is believed to occur as a consequence of maternal viremia. The mechanism by which rubella infection of the fetus leads to teratogenesis has not been fully determined, but the cytopathology in infected fetal tissues suggests necrosis, apoptosis, or both, as well as inhibition of cell division of precursor cells involved in organogenesis (Atreya et al, 2004; Lee and Bowden, 2000). The rubella replicase protein p90 interacts with a cellular cytokinesis-regulatory component (i.e., the citron-K kinase) in the process leading to tetraploidy and cell cycle arrest. In tissue culture, a number of unusual manifestations of rubella replication have been observed, including mitochondrial abnormalities and disruption of the cytoskeleton. Characteristic markers of apoptosis such as DNA fragmentation, nuclear chromatin condensation, and annexin V staining can be observed following rubella infection in cell culture. Cytoplasmic inclusions have also been reported in some cell lines. Microarray analysis following rubella infection in cell culture demonstrated upregulation of cytokines and interferon, suggesting that the induction of inflammatory responses may serve as another possible mechanism of injury induced by rubella (Adamo et al, 2008). Fetuses infected with rubella demonstrate cellular damage in multiple sites and a noninflammatory necrosis in target organs, including eyes, heart, brain, and ears (Lee and Bowden, 2000).

CLINICAL SPECTRUM

The peak incidence of endemic rubella is in the late winter and early spring months. Up to 50% of primary infections are asymptomatic. The period of maximal communicability extends from a few days before until 7 days after onset of the rash. Often a prodrome of mild systemic symptoms precedes the rash by 1 to 5 days. Viremia can be detected as early as 9 days before the onset of rash. Lymphadenopathy, which can precede a rash, often is present in the posterior auricular or suboccipital region. The rash classically begins on the face and spreads caudally to the trunk and extremities. Symptoms generally last up to 3 days, and the incubation period ranges from 14 to 21 days. Transmission by breastfeeding in a case of postpartum acquisition of infection has been described (Klein et al, 1980). Typical illness in adults and children with acquired rubella infection consists of an acute generalized maculopapular rash, fever, and arthralgias, arthritis, or lymphadenopathy. Conjunctivitis is also common. Encephalitis (1:5000 cases) and thrombocytopenia (1:3000 cases) are complications.

Infants with congenital rubella are usually born at term, but often are small for gestational age. The most common isolated sequela is hearing loss (Miller et al, 1982; Ueda et al, 1979). The next most common findings are heart defects, cataracts, low birthweight, hepatosplenomegaly, and microcephaly. The triad of deafness, cataracts, and congenital heart disease constitutes the classic syndrome.

In addition, systemic illness can occur and be characterized by purpura, hepatosplenomegaly, jaundice, pneumonia, and meningoencephalitis; 45% to 70% of infants have cardiac lesions, including patent ductus arteriosus, peripheral pulmonic stenosis, and valve abnormalities (Reef et al, 2000; Schluter et al, 1998). Recently, an extensive review of published reports of cardiovascular disease in the setting of congenital rubella syndrome demonstrated that branch pulmonary artery stenosis is the most commonly identified isolated lesion (Oster et al, 2010). A variety of other signs may be present. Additional ocular findings are pigmentary retinopathy, microphthalmia, and strabismus. The skin lesions have been described as resembling a blueberry muffin and represent extramedullary dermal hematopoiesis; an identical rash can be observed in congenital CMV infection (Avram et al, 2007; Bowden et al, 1989; Brough et al, 1967; Mehta et al, 2008).

The clinical manifestations of CRS vary to some extent depending on the timing of fetal infection. In a prospective study following pregnant women with confirmed rubella infection by trimester, a full range of rubella-associated defects (including congenital heart disease and deafness) were observed in nine infants infected before the 11th week. Thirty-five percent of infants (9 of 26) infected between 13 and 16 weeks' gestation had deafness alone (Miller et al, 1982). Cataracts typically occur secondary to maternal rubella infection occurring before day 60 of pregnancy; heart disease is found almost exclusively when maternal infection is before the 80th day (i.e., first trimester). Disease manifestations that may have their onset after birth (late-onset disease) include: a generalized rash with seborrheic features that may persist for weeks, acute or chronic interstitial pneumonia, abnormal hearing resulting from presumed labyrinthitis, central auditory imperception, and progressive rubella panencephalitis (Franklin and Kelley, 2001; Phelan and Campbell, 1969; Reef et al, 2000; Sever et al, 1985).

A higher than expected incidence of autoimmune diseases, such as thyroid disorders and diabetes mellitus, have also been reported years after the diagnosis of congenital rubella (Forrest et al, 2002; Gale, 2008; McEvoy et al, 1988; Reef et al, 2000). Infants with late-onset disease have demonstrated immunologic abnormalities, including dysgammaglobulinemia or hypogammaglobulinemia (Hancock et al, 1968; Hayes et al, 1967; Soothill et al, 1966). Hyper-IgM syndrome has also been described in association with autoimmune disease in a child with CRS (Palacin et al, 2007). Other studies have demonstrated dysfunction of cellular immune responses in children with CRS (Fuccillo et al, 1974; South et al, 1975; Verder et al, 1986). The pathogenesis of these rubella-related syndromes is poorly understood. Psychiatric disturbances, including some with features of autism spectrum disorders, have been observed decades after CRS (Hwang and Chen, 2010).

LABORATORY EVALUATION

It is common obstetric practice to screen all pregnant women for rubella antibodies, and because of the devastating consequences of CRS, this is a reasonable policy to continue, even in the setting of eradication of endemic rubella in the United States. Women who are exposed to rubella should be screened for evidence of previous immunity; if none is found, they should be tested for rubella IgG and IgM antibodies. A positive IgM titer or a rise in paired IgG titers is indicative of recent infection. Women with such findings should also be evaluated to try to determine the likely gestational age at time of infection in order to assess the potential risk to the fetus.

The laboratory diagnosis of congenital rubella can be made definitively only during the 1st year of life, unless the virus can be recovered later from an affected site, such as the lens. Diagnosis can be made with any one of the following four criteria:
1. Positive anti-rubella IgM titer, preferably determined with enzyme immunoassays, but indirect assays are acceptable
2. A significant rise in rubella IgG titer between acute and convalescent measurements 2 to 3 weeks apart or the persistence of high titers longer than expected from passive maternal antibody transfer
3. Isolation of rubella virus cultured from nasal, blood, throat, urine, or CSF specimens (throat swabs have the best yield)
4. Detection of virus by reverse transcriptase PCR in specimens from throat swabs, CSF, or cataracts obtained from surgery (Centers for Disease Control and Prevention, 2001)

An infected infant can excrete the virus for many months after birth despite the presence of neutralizing antibody and, thus, may pose a hazard to susceptible individuals. In rare cases the virus can be recovered after 1 year of age. An exception to this rule is the cataract, in which the virus can remain for as long as 3 years. In late-onset disease, the virus can also be found in affected skin and lung.

Other laboratory findings are thrombocytopenia, hyperbilirubinemia, and leukopenia. Radiographic findings include large anterior fontanel, linear areas of radiolucency in the long bones (i.e., celery stalking), increased densities in the metaphyses, and irregular provisional zones of calcification (Chapman, 1991; Reed, 1969). The radiographic changes seen in rubella are not pathognomonic of the disease, but resemble those seen in other congenital viral infections, including congenital cytomegalovirus infection (Alessandri et al, 1995).

TREATMENT AND PROGNOSIS

There is no specific therapy for congenital rubella. Initially the infant may need general supportive care, such as administration of blood transfusion for anemia or active bleeding, seizure control, and phototherapy for hyperbilirubinemia. Long-term care requires a multidisciplinary approach consisting of occupational and physical therapy, close neurologic and audiologic monitoring, and surgical interventions as needed for cardiac malformations and cataracts.

The consequences of fetal rubella infection may not be evident at birth. In one study of 123 infants with documented congenital rubella, 85% of cases were not diagnosed until after discharge from the nursery (Hardy, 1973). Communication disorders, hearing defects, some mental or motor retardation, and microcephaly by 1 to 3 years of age were among the major problems that were discovered after the newborn period. A predisposition to inguinal hernias was also noted. Longitudinal studies of somatic growth show that most infants with congenital rubella remain smaller than average throughout infancy, but grow at a normal rate. Stunting of growth was more common after rubella infection in the first 8 weeks of pregnancy than after later infection. Even in the absence of mental retardation, neuromuscular development is commonly abnormal. A study of neurodevelopmental outcomes in 29 affected children without mental retardation found that 25 had other abnormalities; hearing loss, difficulties with balance and gait, learning deficits, and behavioral disturbances were found in more than half of the affected children (Desmond et al, 1978).

PREVENTION

There is no effective antiviral therapy against congenital rubella infection, so the most useful practice is to ensure that women who are considering pregnancy are immune. The Advisory Committee on Immunization Practices recommends screening of all pregnant women for rubella immunity and postpartum vaccination of those who are susceptible (Centers for Disease Control and Prevention, 2001). Immunity to rubella appears to confer almost complete protection against CRS. Rare cases of documented subclinical maternal reinfection with rubella have been reported (Morgan-Capner et al, 1991; Saule et al, 1988). In rare cases, maternal reinfection can lead to CRS (Banerji et al, 2005). Approximately 20 cases of CRS after maternal reinfection have been reported in the literature, and none have caused symptomatic CRS when the known reinfection occurred after 12 weeks' gestation (Bullens et al, 2000).

Live attenuated rubella virus vaccine is safe and effective, although the duration of immunity is uncertain. It is typically administered in the United States in a trivalent formulation in combination with measles-mumps-rubella vaccine or in a quadrivalent combination with measles-mumps-rubella-varicella vaccine. The vaccine is recommended for children at 12 to 15 months of age and at 4 to 5 years of age. It is also recommended for women of childbearing age in whom results of both a hemagglutination inhibition antibody test and a pregnancy test are negative. Although no cases of symptomatic congenital rubella infection have been reported as a consequence of vaccination during pregnancy in the more than 500 cases monitored, vaccination is not recommended during pregnancy because of the theoretical hazard to the fetus (Josefson, 2001; Nasiri et al, 2009; Tookey, 2001). A mild rubella-like illness is sometimes seen after immunization, with arthralgia occurring 10 days to 3 weeks after injection. If a woman is found to be susceptible, vaccine should be administered during the immediate postpartum period before discharge. Breastfeeding is not a contraindication to postpartum immunization. Immunization in the postpartum period has rarely produced polyarticular arthritis, neurologic symptoms, and chronic rubella viremia (Tingle et al, 1985).

The problem of management of the pregnant woman who is exposed to rubella or who contracts the disease should be resolved after the known risks are weighed. If serum antibody is detectable at the time of exposure, the fetus is probably protected. If no antibody is detectable, additional serum samples at 2 to 3 weeks after exposure and again at 4 to 6 weeks after exposure should be obtained. These samples can be run concurrently with the first serum to ascertain whether infection has occurred (i.e., seroconversion). There is no evidence that administration of immunoglobulin prevents rubella infection or viremia. Moreover, administering immunoglobulin may provide an unwarranted sense of security, because infants with congenital rubella have been born to women who received immunoglobulin shortly after exposure. Regardless of these limitations, administration of immunoglobulin may be considered if the pregnancy is not terminated. Immunoglobulin can reduce the likelihood of fetal infection, but will not eliminate the risk; therefore the CDC does not routinely recommend the use of immunoglobulin in a pregnant woman for postexposure prophylaxis unless she does not wish to terminate the pregnancy under any circumstances (Centers for Disease Control and Prevention, 2001). Decisions about the termination of pregnancy should be made only after maternal infection has been proved and should also account for the risk of rubella-associated damage to the fetus, which is highest when maternal infection occurs during the first 8 weeks of pregnancy.

LYMPHOCYTIC CHORIOMENINGITIS VIRUS

Lymphocytic choriomeningitis virus (LCMV) is a member of the family Arenaviridae. Rodents are the primary reservoir, particularly mice and hamsters. Like other arenaviruses, LCMV has a bisegmented negative-strand RNA genome. The S segment encodes for the virus nucleoprotein and glycoprotein, whereas the L segment encodes for the virus polymerase (L) and Z protein. Susceptible rodents are infected asymptomatically in utero, can harbor chronic infection, and excrete virus in urine, feces, saliva, nasal secretions, milk, and semen for life. Typically mice remain asymptomatic, although hamsters may demonstrate viremia and viruria with variable symptoms (Jahrling and Peters, 1992). Sequelae of human exposure to LCMV range from asymptomatic infection to nonspecific, flulike symptoms; a proportion of infections have neurologic manifestations. LCMV was first described as a cause of congenital infection in England in 1955 in a 12-day-old infant (Komrower et al, 1955) and later in the United States (Barton and Mets, 2001; Barton et al, 1993, 2001; Larsen et al, 1993). Because LCMV has only recently been recognized as a source of congenital infection, it is likely underdiagnosed (Jamieson et al, 2006).

EPIDEMIOLOGY

Human seroprevalence ranges between less than 1% and 10% worldwide and varies extensively with geographic region (Ambrosio et al, 1994; Childs et al, 1991; Marrie and Saron, 1998; Stephensen et al, 1992). One study noted a higher prevalence in women (Marrie and Saron, 1998). Lower socioeconomic status and older age are associated with higher seroprevalence. Studies conducted in the 1940s through the 1970s found that approximately 8% to 11% of cases of aseptic meningitis and encephalitis were associated with LCMV infection (Meyer et al, 1960; Park et al, 1997b). In temperate climates, human exposure is more common during the fall and winter, when rodents move indoors. Outbreaks have been reported in laboratory personnel working with hamsters and mice (Dykewicz et al, 1992; Hinman et al, 1975; Vanzee et al, 1975). Multiple outbreaks associated with pet hamsters have also been reported in the United States (Biggar et al, 1975; Maetz et al, 1976) and Europe (Brouqui et al, 1995; Deibel et al, 1975); however, congenital infection is relatively rare. A total of 54 cases have been diagnosed worldwide since the first case in 1955, and 27 of those occurred in the United States (Barton and Mets, 2001; Greenhow and Weintrub, 2003). There has been an increased recognition of congenital LCMV in recent years; 34 of the cases described in a review were reported since 1993 (Jamieson et al, 2006). The true frequency of congenital LCMV infection is unknown, because there is no active surveillance. As with other congenital infections, there may be a wide spectrum of disease, including asymptomatic and subclinical or nonspecific infections.

PATHOGENESIS

Humans acquire LCMV infection from aerosolized particles, bites, or fomite contact with virus excreted from rodents (Jahrling and Peters, 1992). Human-to-human horizontal transmission by organ transplantation has been documented (Fischer et al, 2006). In this report, abdominal pain, altered mental status, thrombocytopenia, elevated aminotransferase levels, coagulopathy, graft dysfunction, renal failure, seizures, and either fever or leukocytosis were variably present within 3 weeks after transplantation. Seven of the eight recipients died, 9 to 76 days after transplantation. The pathogenesis of LCMV infection is poorly understood, although it is likely an immunopathologic process mediated by the host CD8+ T-cell response (Craighead, 2000). It is also postulated that the high rate of spontaneous mutations that arise during LCMV replication allows both variability in pathogenicity and a mechanism of escape from humoral response during the initial phase of infection (Ciurea et al, 2001).

Like other arenaviruses, LCMV replicates either at the site of infection or in corresponding lymph nodes; this localized replication is followed by viremia. It is thought that during the viremic stage, the virus travels to parenchymal organs and the CNS. Pathologic findings include lymphocytic infiltration and extramedullary hematopoiesis. In two congenitally infected infants for whom neuropathology results were available, cerebromalacia, glial proliferation, and perivascular edema were reported (Barton et al, 1993). In adult mice inoculated intracranially with LCMV, subsequent viral proliferation in the ependyma, meninges, or both have been described, with injury mediated by CD8+ T cells (Doherty et al, 1990). This viral infiltration, along with the host inflammatory response, can lead to aqueductal stenosis and subsequent hydrocephalus. Studies in a murine model suggest that cytokine-chemokine cascades mediate much of the neuropathology observed in the setting of CNS infection (Christensen et al, 2009).

CLINICAL SPECTRUM

It is estimated that asymptomatic or mild LCMV infections occur in approximately one third of patients infected; however, the classic presentation of LCMV infection is a nonspecific, flulike, or mononucleosis-like illness that is often biphasic. Symptoms are fever, malaise, nausea, vomiting, myalgias, headache, photophobia, pharyngitis, cough, and adenopathy. After defervescence and resolution of these constitutional symptoms, a second phase of CNS disease may develop. Neurologic manifestations occur in approximately one fourth of infectious episodes and vary from aseptic meningitis to meningoencephalitis. Transverse myelitis, Guillain-Barré syndrome, and deafness have also been reported. Other manifestations are pneumonitis, arthritis, myocarditis, parotitis, and dermatitis. Recovery may take months, but usually occurs without sequelae (Craighead, 2000).

When LCMV infection occurs during pregnancy, maternal symptoms typically appear during the first and second trimesters, but only 50% to 60% of mothers of infants diagnosed with LCMV congenital infection recall having symptoms (Wright et al, 1997). Known maternal exposure to rodents is reported in approximately one fourth to one half of cases (Barton and Mets, 2001). Usually, exposed women are from rural settings, come from lower socioeconomic settings with substandard housing conditions, or have pet rodents in the home (i.e., hamsters).

The complete spectrum of disease secondary to congenital LCMV infection is still uncertain, although chorioretinitis and hydrocephalus are the predominant characteristics reported among children diagnosed with congenital LCMV infection. Chorioretinitis is present in more than 90% of cases. Other ocular findings are chorioretinal scars, optic atrophy (usually bilateral), nystagmus, esotropia, exotropia, leukocoria, cataracts, and microphthalmia (Barton and Mets, 2001; Brezin et al, 2000; Enders et al, 1999). Some ophthalmologic findings resemble those described in the lacunar retinopathy of Aicardi syndrome (Wright et al, 1997), a finding of interest insofar as Aicardi syndrome can, like congenital CMV or LCMV infection, produce intracranial calcifications. A wide range of neurologic defects are described, including microencephaly, encephalomalacia, chorioretinitis, porencephalic cysts, neuronal migration disturbances, periventricular infection, and cerebellar hypoplasia (Bonthius et al, 2007). Congenital LCMV should be considered in the differential diagnosis of neonatal hydrocephalus (Schulte et al, 2006).

Most infants are born at term, and birthweights are generally appropriate or large for gestational age. Thirty-five percent to 40% of infants reported with congenital LCMV have had microcephaly or macrocephaly at birth (Barton and Mets, 2001). Systemic symptoms are rare, although hepatosplenomegaly and jaundice have been noted. Other individual case report findings are pes valgus, dermatologic findings consistent with staphylococcal scalded-skin syndrome (Wright et al, 1997), spontaneous abortion (Biggar et al, 1975), and intrauterine demise secondary to hydrops fetalis (Enders et al, 1999; Meritet et al, 2009). It is important to note that, because systemic symptoms are typically minimal at birth, the diagnosis of congenital LCMV infection often is not considered until an affected infant is a few months of age, when microcephaly, macrocephaly, visual loss, or developmental delay may be noted.

LABORATORY EVALUATION

Serology is the most reliable and feasible method to diagnose LCMV. In most reports, the diagnosis was established by testing of the infant's serum, CSF, or both; in some, maternal serum testing was the key. Testing all three fluids provides the most information. Because of the low baseline population seroprevalence, positive titers for LCMV are much more useful for diagnosis than detection of antibodies to microbes such as CMV and toxoplasmosis. There is a commercially available immunofluorescent antibody test that detects both IgM and IgG for LCMV. It has better sensitivity than the complement fixation and neutralizing antibody tests that also have been used (Lehmann-Grube et al, 1979; Lewis et al, 1975). Complement fixation titers generally do not rise until more than 10 days after onset of infection, but immunofluorescent antibody results may be positive within the first few days of illness (Deibel et al, 1975). The CDC also has an enzyme-linked immunosorbent assay test for IgM and IgG; it may be more useful for diagnosis in an older child because it can detect increased IgG later than and persistent IgG for longer than the immunofluorescent antibody test. Some studies have found antibody as late as 30 years after suspected exposure. Virus can be cultured in Vero cell lines or inoculated into newborn mice, but use of these methods is uncommon. Reverse transcriptase–PCR has been used in serum and CSF to diagnosis LCMV and as a surveillance tool; it may become more available in the future (Enders et al, 1999; McCausland and Crotty, 2008; Park et al, 1997a).

Information about routine laboratory data in patients with a diagnosis of congenital LCMV infection is minimal, but thrombocytopenia and hyperbilirubinemia have been reported. CSF findings are variable. Up to one half of cases demonstrate a mild increase in white blood cell count (up to 64 cells/μL in one case series of 18 infants), the serum protein concentration may be normal or mildly elevated, and the serum glucose concentration may be normal or mildly decreased (Wright et al, 1997). Among infants reported in whom neuroradiographic imaging was performed, 89% (17 of 19) had hydrocephalus or periventricular calcifications. Flattened gyri, lissencephaly, and schizencephaly have been reported (Barton and Mets, 2001), compatible with a role for LCMV in fetal neuronal migration defects (Bonthius et al, 2007).

TREATMENT

Ribavirin has been used for management of other arenavirus infections and inhibits LCMV growth in vitro (Géssner and Lother, 1989). Although novel approaches are being used to develop antivirals against LCMV and other pathogenic arenaviruses (de la Torre, 2008), there are currently no recommendations for the use of antiviral agents against these viruses. In the outbreak associated with solid organ transplantation, one affected recipient received ribavirin and reduced levels of immunosuppressive therapy and survived (Fischer et al, 2006).

PROGNOSIS

Because congenital LCMV infections have been recognized relatively recently and the existing data come from case reports, there may be a wider spectrum of disease than is currently appreciated. The proportion of asymptomatic infected infants is unknown. For the 25 infant cases reported, estimated mortality rates are 16% to 35% between birth and 21 months of age (Barton and Mets, 2001; Wright et al, 1997). Among infants who survived, 84% (32 of 38) have neurologic sequelae, including spastic quadriparesis, mental retardation, developmental delay, seizures, and visual loss (Barton and Mets, 2001). Sensorineural hearing loss is less common and has been reported in only two infants (Barton and Mets, 2001; Wright et al, 1997). Some ophthalmologists suggest that among patients with developmental delay and visual loss consistent with chorioretinitis, LCMV congenital infection may be underdiagnosed. A study in Chicago of prospectively diagnosed patients with chorioretinitis and patients in a home for severely mentally retarded children with chorioretinal scars found six children with elevated LCMV titers and normal toxoplasmosis, CMV, rubella, and HSV titers (Mets et al, 2000). Two children with chorioretinal scars and elevated LCMV titers have been reported in France (Brezin et al, 2000).

PREVENTION

Public health officials and clinicians should be aware that (1) wild, laboratory, and pet rodent exposure can lead to intrauterine infection with LCMV virus and (2) congenital infection has been associated with potentially devastating ophthalmologic and neurologic sequelae. Pregnant women need to be educated about the potential risks of exposure to infected rodent excreta and instructed to avoid rodents and rodent droppings whenever possible. Obstetricians and neonatologists should seek a history of pet or wild rodent exposure for counseling purposes and to aid in the evaluation of infants with unexplained CNS pathologies. The diagnosis of LCMV should be considered in all unexplained cases of infant hydrocephalus. There are currently no vaccines approved by the U.S. Food and Drug Administration (FDA) for the prevention of arenavirus disease, although candidate multivalent arenavirus vaccines capable of providing T cell–mediated protection against a variety of pathogenic arenaviruses are currently in development (Botten et al, 2010).

ENTEROVIRUSES

Enteroviruses are single-stranded, positive-sense RNA viruses. These viruses belong to the family Picornaviridae (*pico* means very small in Spanish). The enteroviruses of humans include polioviruses 1, 2, and 3, coxsackieviruses A and B (named after Coxsackie, New York the city where these viruses were first identified and characterized), and the echoviruses (*echo* is an acronym for enteric cytopathic human orphan). Of these, poliovirus infection has historically been responsible for the greatest morbidity in infants. Severe, often fatal poliovirus disease used to occur with great frequency in infants infected in the perinatal period, with a high incidence of residual paralysis in survivors (Bates, 1955; Cherry, 2005). Fortunately, poliovirus infections have become rare in the developed world, because of the widespread implementation of effective immunizations. However, neonatal diseases associated with coxsackieviruses and echoviruses, for which there are no vaccines, remain common and can be associated with serious morbidity and occasional mortality. Typically acquired from a maternal source, these agents are associated with a wide range of clinical syndromes in the neonatal intensive care unit, including CNS infection, myocarditis, and a sepsis-like syndrome. Enteroviruses are also responsible for a large number of hospital readmissions for evaluation of febrile syndromes in infants younger than 2 months.

EPIDEMIOLOGY

Enterovirus infections are seasonal, occurring most commonly during the summer and autumn in temperate climates. The incidence varies from year to year, with outbreaks sometimes caused by a single coxsackievirus or echovirus serotype and sometimes by several (Sawyer et al, 1994). In older children, enteroviruses are transmitted by the fecal-oral route and are typically associated with a variety of febrile syndromes, including febrile exanthematous syndromes, aseptic meningitis, pneumonia with or without pleural effusion, and myocarditis. Disease in newborn infants is relatively uncommon, but reflects the frequency of infection in the general population (Krajden and Middleton, 1983). Enteroviruses may also be associated with nosocomial outbreaks. Nursery and obstetric clinic outbreaks of both coxsackievirus B (Bhambhani et al, 2007; Brightman et al, 1966; Rantakallio et al, 1970) and echovirus infections (Chen et al, 2005; Jankovic et al, 1999; Nagington et al, 1978) have been reported and associated with severe, and sometimes fatal, illnesses.

Enteroviral infections account for at least one third of neonatal febrile admissions for suspected sepsis and for between half and two thirds of all admissions during peak enteroviral season (Byington et al, 1999; Dagan, 1996). Neonatal aseptic meningitis is also frequently caused by enteroviral infections. In a review of neonatal meningitis seen over a 15-year period in Galveston, Texas, enterovirus was the most common cause of meningitis in newborn infants older than 7 days of age (Shattuck and Chonmaitree, 1992). Enteroviruses, along with other viruses, have been implicated as a potential cause of sudden infant death syndrome (SIDS), possibly from myocarditis or pulmonary infection (Grangeot-Keros et al, 1996; Shimizu et al, 1995), but this association has been controversial. In one study of SIDS victims, a comprehensive assessment was undertaken to attempt to identify potential viral infection of the myocardium. Overall, 62 SIDS victims and 11 controls were studied. Enteroviruses were detected in 14 (22.5%), adenoviruses in 2 (3.2%), Epstein–Barr viruses in 3 (4.8%), and parvovirus B19 in 7 (11.2%) cases, whereas control group samples were completely negative for viral nucleic acid (Dettmeyer et al, 2004). However, an evaluation of histopathologic features and PCR analysis from 24 SIDS cases failed to demonstrate any association with viral infection (Krous et al, 2009), leaving this putative association unclear.

ETIOLOGY AND PATHOGENESIS

Neonates can acquire enteroviral infections secondary to in utero transmission, intrapartum transmission during labor and delivery, or postnatally. Intrauterine infections appear to occur via transplacental spread, secondary to maternal viremia, and this mode of transmission appears to be responsible for up to 22% of cases of neonatal enteroviral infection (Kaplan et al, 1983; Modlin, 1986). Enteroviruses have been implicated as a cause of fetal demise (Johansson et al, 1992; Konstantinidou et al, 2007; Nielsen et al, 1988). Intrapartum or postnatal transmission is more common than transplacental transmission. The dominant mode of transmission of serious neonatal infection is through contact with maternal blood, fecal material, or vaginal or cervical secretions, most likely during or shortly after delivery (Hawkes and Vaudry, 2005; Jenista et al, 1984). After acquisition of infection, viremia ensues in the infant, leading to a variety of end-organ diseases. Virus strain or serotype appears to be a factor in predicting the severity of illness, as does the quantity of the inoculum. The presence or absence of transplacental maternally derived antibody also dictates the severity of disease in the infected infant. Severe disease occurs in the absence of type-specific antibody, a scenario that is more likely if the maternal infection is acquired near the time of delivery. Breastfeeding appears to provide a relative degree of protection against acquisition of infection in neonates (Sadeharju et al, 2007).

One of the most comprehensive analyses of the incidence of neonatal enterovirus disease came from a prospective study in Rochester, N.Y. This study demonstrated that approximately 13% of all newborns tested positive for enterovirus from throat or stool cultures during a typical season (June to October; Jenista et al, 1984). Although this result represented a remarkably high incidence, 79% of these infections were asymptomatic. The most common clinical findings in the 21% of symptomatic infections were lethargy and fever. These infants were typically admitted to hospital for an evaluation to rule out sepsis, making enterovirus infection a more common reason for hospitalization owing to an infectious disease than group B streptococcus, herpes simplex virus, and cytomegalovirus infections combined.

It appears that any of the non–polio enteroviruses can cause disease in the newborn infant. A variety of clinical syndromes are associated with certain enteroviruses. A retrospective chart review of 24 neonatal enteroviral infections in Toronto, Canada, found that 10 infants died, 12 had aseptic meningitis, and 5 had myocarditis (Krajden and Middleton, 1983). Of the 24 isolates, 7 were echovirus, 15 were coxsackievirus B, one was coxsackievirus A, and one was nontypable. In infants requiring hospitalization with acute enterovirus disease, coxsackievirus B is associated primarily with myocarditis and aseptic meningitis (Kibrick and Benirschke, 1958). Recent reports have identified coxsackievirus B1 as an emerging cause of life-threatening myocarditis and other severe, fatal syndromes in neonates (Verma et al, 2009; Wikswo et al, 2009). Echoviruses are associated with severe nonspecific febrile illnesses with disseminated intravascular coagulation (Nagington et al, 1978), aseptic meningitis (Cramblett et al, 1973), or hepatitis (Modlin, 1980). With both coxsackievirus and echovirus, nonspecific febrile illnesses, with or without an exanthem, are commonly observed. Enterovirus 71 is particularly notable for its etiologic role in epidemics of severe neurologic diseases in children (Chen et al, 2010). Nursery-based outbreaks of this neurovirulent enterovirus have also been described (Huang et al, 2010).

Except for transplacental infections, the portal of entry for enterovirus is via the oral or respiratory route. After replication in the pharynx and the gastrointestinal tract, virus seeds the tonsils, cervical and mesenteric nodes, and Peyer's patches. The pathogenesis of enterovirus disease stems from the ensuing viremia, which can lead to infection of the heart, CNS, liver, pancreas, adrenal glands, skin, mucous membranes, and respiratory tract. This feature of enterovirus replication and dissemination helps to explain the diverse disease manifestations that may be observed following infection. The humoral immune response is associated with recovery from systemic and end-organ infection, although virus may continue to be shed in the stool for several weeks. Failure to clear enteroviral infection, particularly from the CNS, should suggest an underlying humoral immunodeficiency, although this would not typically be observed in the neonatal period, when maternally derived Ig is present in the newborn (McKinney et al, 1987; Misbah et al, 1992). Depending on the extent of disease, extensive end-organ pathology may be observed. In coxsackievirus B infections, myocardial necrosis, and inflammation may be seen that are patchy or diffuse, with extensive infiltration by lymphocytes, mononuclear cells, histiocytes, and polymorphonuclear leukocytes. Similar infiltrates are seen in the meninges in both coxsackievirus and echovirus aseptic meningitis. Brainstem encephalitis can be observed with enterovirus 71 infection, often in association with pulmonary edema (Wang and Liu, 2009). When liver or adrenal glands are involved, there is usually extensive hemorrhage as well as inflammation and necrosis; such fatal fulminant infections are often associated with echovirus 11 (Mostoufizadeh et al, 1983).

CLINICAL SPECTRUM

When neonatal disease is acquired vertically from the mother, the infant is typically asymptomatic at birth, although premature delivery is more common. The mother may be febrile at this time or may have a history of recent high fevers and gastrointestinal symptoms. Fever, anorexia, and vomiting develop in the baby after an incubation period of 1 to 5 days. The onset of illness occurs in the first week of life in more than 50% of affected infants (Krajden and Middleton, 1983). At that point, the clinical evolution depends on the infecting virus and the extent of end-organ involvement. In most instances, the disease is mild and self-limited. Symptomatic infections may be characterized by rash, aseptic meningitis, hepatitis, and pneumonia. A review of 29 infants younger than 2 weeks with enteroviral infections reported that 5 of 29 infants had severe multisystem disease, and all survived (Abzug et al, 1993). In another study in Salt Lake City, 1779 febrile infants younger than 90 days and undergoing evaluation for sepsis were enrolled; 1061 had enterovirus testing, and 214 (20%) were enterovirus positive (57% from blood, and

74% from CSF). The mean age of infants with enterovirus infection was 33 days; 91% were admitted, and 2% required intensive care (Rittichier et al, 2005).

These observations underscore the generally benign and self-limited nature of neonatal enterovirus disease; however, morbidity can be substantial in severe disseminated disease. A viral sepsis syndrome—characterized by disseminated intravascular coagulation, refractory hypotension, and death—may occur in the setting of severe disease. Typically these severe infections are acquired in the immediate perinatal period. The mother is commonly symptomatic and may have been empirically treated with broad-spectrum antibiotics for possible chorioamnionitis. A maternal history of suspected chorioamnionitis in the absence of positive bacterial cultures should suggest this association, particularly during the typical "enterovirus season" observed in temperate climates. If myocarditis is present, congestive heart failure is often severe. Some infections, particularly those with echoviruses, are characterized by a rampant and overwhelming hepatitis (Modlin, 1980). Others exhibit primarily pulmonary disease or gastrointestinal involvement including diarrhea and necrotizing enterocolitis (Lake et al, 1976). Intracranial bleeding ranging from small to massive, severe hemorrhage has also been reported as a complication of neonatal enteroviral infection (Abzug, 2001; Abzug and Johnson, 2000; Swiatek, 1997). Other rarely associated findings include disseminated vesicular rash, dermal hematopoiesis, and hemophagocytic syndrome (Barre et al, 1998; Bowden et al, 1989; Sauerbrei et al, 2000). The severity of CNS infection is similarly variable. Enteroviruses, particularly enterovirus 71, can produce overwhelming meningoencephalitis, sometimes with cranial nerve signs. It is more common, however, to see moderate or mild meningitis characterized by temporary irritability, lethargy, fever, and feeding difficulty.

Acquired postnatal enteroviral disease in infants is characterized primarily by high fever, irritability, lethargy, or poor feeding. One fourth of infected infants develop diarrhea or vomiting with or without an erythematous maculopapular rash. Conjunctivitis has also been observed. Respiratory tract symptoms are less common (Dagan, 1996). As noted, there is significant overlap between enteroviral and bacterial neonatal infections, and the two syndromes are difficult to distinguish; therefore many febrile infants will be admitted to the hospital and treated with broad-spectrum antibiotics and, if the CNS is involved, with acyclovir for possible bacterial sepsis and neonatal HSV infection. Such treatment seems unavoidable, except in circumstances in which enterovirus infection can be diagnosed rapidly and definitively. Duration of illness varies from less than 24 hours to longer than 7 days, but generally lasts 3 to 4 days.

LABORATORY EVALUATION

Viral culture from stool or rectal swab, nasopharyngeal swab, blood, buffy coat, urine, or CSF represents the gold standard diagnosis. Stool or rectal swab cultures can remain positive for several weeks following the initial infection, underscoring the importance of fecal-oral transmission in the epidemiology of these infections. Recently, reverse transcriptase PCR assays have become standardized and are available from many commercial and reference laboratories. Serologic tests for enteroviruses have been reported, but are less useful than culture and PCR (Swanink et al, 1993).

Laboratory evaluation is predicated on the clinical syndrome and the end organs involved. Infants with aseptic meningitis typically have moderate CSF pleocytosis, which can be either lymphocytic or polymorphonuclear, but may lack pleocytosis even in the setting of documented CNS infection (Seiden et al, 2010). Accordingly, during periods of active enterovirus infection in the community, CSF should be sent for PCR even if a pleocytosis is absent. Thrombocytopenia, elevated transaminase levels, hyperbilirubinemia, hyperammonemia, hematologic abnormalities consistent with disseminated intravascular coagulation, anemia, peripheral leukocytosis, and abnormal chest radiographs are among other potential laboratory findings. When myocarditis is a diagnostic possibility, echocardiogram and electrocardiogram are indicated and may reveal diminished LV function, or dysrhythmias. Liver biopsy may be warranted in cases of fulminant hepatic failure (Abzug, 2001).

TREATMENT

The cornerstone of treatment of neonatal enteroviral disease is supportive care. Myocarditis and heart failure can be treated with inotropic support, diuretics, aggressive fluid management, and other supportive measures. Disseminated intravascular coagulation should be treated with blood products and other supportive measures as indicated. There is no evidence that steroids are of benefit. IVIG has been reported anecdotally to treat neonatal enteroviral infections with varying degrees of success (Kimura et al, 1999; Valduss et al, 1993). Only one randomized trial has systematically studied its use in 16 neonates with severe enteroviral infection; nine of these infants were randomized to receive IVIG, at a dose of 750 mg/kg. Decreased viremia and viruria along with faster resolution of irritability, jaundice, and diarrhea was demonstrated in patients administered IVIG with high titers of neutralizing enteroviral-specific antibodies. However, there were no significant differences in other major clinical outcomes, such as duration of hospitalization, fever, and symptoms of acute illness between treatment and control groups (Abzug et al, 1995). To attempt to augment the enterovirus type–specific antibody level in the setting of symptomatic neonatal disease, maternal plasma transfusion has been attempted (Jantausch et al, 1995; Rentz et al, 2006), based on the rationale that neonates typically acquire infection from their mothers in the peripartum period. Although reports of success using IVIG for treatment of neonatal enterovirus infections is largely based on anecdotal reports in limited numbers of patients, its use should be considered for severely symptomatic infections with life-threatening end-organ disease.

The antiviral drug pleconaril has been developed specifically to treat picornavirus infections (enteroviruses and rhinoviruses). A small case series of infants with severe enteroviral hepatitis suggested a beneficial effect (Aradottir et al, 2001). Another small case series indicated that five of six neonates with severe enteroviral infection who were treated with pleconaril survived, with minimal or no sequelae (Rotbart and Webster, 2001). However, a multicenter study of pleconaril treatment for enteroviral meningitis in children younger than 12 months conducted by the CASG and sponsored by the National Institutes of Health demonstrated no significant differences in duration of positivity by culture or PCR, hospitalization, or symptoms comparing the treatment and placebo groups (Abzug et al, 2003). Pleconaril did appear to have an effect on enteroviral meningitis in adults, promoting more rapid resolution of illness (Desmond et al, 2006), but the role of this drug in infants and children remains undefined. The drug continues to be investigational and is only available through the CASG, which is currently comparing pleconaril with placebo in severe symptomatic neonatal enteroviral infections (www.clinicaltrials.gov).

SHORT- AND LONG-TERM PROGNOSIS

Prognostic factors for severe neonatal disease include peripartum maternal illness, earlier age of onset of neonatal disease, absence of serotype-specific antibody, and absence of fever and irritability (Abzug et al, 1993). All these risk factors are most consistent with vertical intrauterine enteroviral infection rather than postnatally acquired infection. The highest mortality rates are associated with the combination of severe hepatitis, coagulopathy, and myocarditis. Severe hepatitis caused by enteroviral infection is associated with mortality rates ranging from 30% to 80% (Abzug, 2001; Modlin, 1986). By the time disseminated intravascular coagulation has developed, the prognosis is grave. Prothrombin time longer than 30 seconds was a risk factor for death in one retrospective case review (Abzug, 2001).

Few long-term follow-up studies have been published, but the available information suggests that infants who survive severe enteroviral neonatal disease have a complete recovery in most instances. Outcomes of 6 of 11 survivors with follow-up ranging from 9 to 48 months reported normal growth and no residual medical problems or liver dysfunction (Abzug, 2001). The long-term prognosis following CNS infection is unclear. A number of early studies of infants younger than 3 months with aseptic meningitis suggested that there may be some impairment of intellectual development in comparison with carefully selected control groups (Farmer et al, 1975; Sells et al, 1975). However, in a series of nine children with enteroviral meningitis and nine matched controls evaluated for sequelae at approximately 4 years of age, no differences in mean intelligence quotient, head circumference, detectable sensorineural hearing loss, or intellectual functioning were detected. Receptive language functioning of the meningitis group was significantly less than that in control subjects (Wilfert et al, 1981). A similar case-control follow-up study of 33 subjects, who were compared with siblings used as controls, reported no neurodevelopmental sequelae (Bergman et al, 1987). Older children with enterovirus 71 infection involving the CNS are at risk for significant neurodevelopmental sequelae (Chang et al, 2007).

PREVENTION

Anecdotal reports of the use of IVIG in nursery outbreaks to prevent further horizontal transmission of enteroviral infection produce conflicting results (Carolane et al, 1985; Kinney et al, 1986; Nagington et al, 1983). Because there are multiple non–polio enteroviral serotypes that cause clinical disease, development of anti-enteroviral immunization is conceptually difficult, although vaccines are in development for enterovirus 71 (Zhang et al, 2010). Standard contact precautions should be used for the treatment of hospitalized infants with known or suspected enteroviral infections.

HUMAN PARECHOVIRUS

Recently two viruses formerly classified with the echoviruses, echovirus 22 and 23, were shown to comprise a separate genus within the Picornaviridae family, the genus *Parechovirus*; these viruses are now referred to as *human parechoviruses types 1* and *2*. A total of 10 distinct parechoviruses have now been recognized (Drexler et al, 2009; Harvala et al, 2010; Pajkrt et al, 2009). These viruses have been recognized recently as significant neonatal pathogens (Harvala et al, 2010). The primary site of parechovirus replication is believed to be the respiratory and gastrointestinal tract. Replication in the gastrointestinal tract is associated with prolonged shedding of infectious virus in the feces. As a result, fecal-oral transmission, as with enteroviruses, appears to be the predominant route of infection. Parechovirus infections may also be acquired via a respiratory route, with subsequent virus shedding detectable in respiratory secretions. Viremia leads to secondary seeding of other organs and systemic symptoms. Neonates with parechovirus infection, particularly parechovirus 3, have a clinical presentation similar to infants with severe enteroviral disease, with a sepsislike illness in severe cases (Verboon-Maciolek et al, 2008a; Wolthers et al, 2008). Hepatitis is also a prominent feature of neonatal infection. The most frequent signs are fever, seizures, irritability, rash, and feeding problems. It has been postulated that parechovirus 3 is a newly emerging infection, and the relative lack of maternal antibody may predispose the neonate to more severe disease (Harvala et al, 2010). Parechovirus can also cause aseptic meningitis and encephalitis in the neonate, with the predominate site of injury being the periventricular white matter (Gupta et al, 2010; Levorson et al, 2009; Verboon-Maciolek et al, 2008b). Parechovirus RNA has also been found at autopsy in children younger than 2 years (Sedmak et al, 2010), including from infants with otherwise unexplained deaths. Management is similar to that for neonatal enterovirus disease—namely, supportive care.

The other virus classified in the *Parechovirus* genus is Ljungan virus (Tolf et al, 2009). This virus was first described in 1998 and was found to cause type 1 diabetes–like symptoms and myocarditis in bank voles; it also appears to be endemic in other wild rodent populations. The virus does not appear to have a role in the development of diabetes in humans (Tapia et al, 2010). This zoonotic virus has recently emerged as a recognized cause of fetal infection (Niklasson et al, 2007, 2009b). Ljungan virus infection appears in particular to be associated with severe CNS abnormalities, including hydrancephaly and hydrocephalus (Niklasson et al, 2009a). A study from Sweden identified a strong epidemiologic association between small rodent abundance and the incidence of intrauterine fetal death in humans. Ljungan virus antigen was detected in this study in half of the intrauterine fetal death cases tested (Niklasson et al, 2009).

HEPATITIS VIRUSES

There are six distinct viruses known to cause viral hepatitis—hepatitis A, B, C, D (delta agent), E, and G. Hepatitis G is of importance for the pregnant patient, although only B and C are of major importance in the newborn. The main features of each virus type are listed in Table 37-3 (Jonas, 2000; Koff, 2007; Krugman, 1992). Hepatitis A virus (HAV) is passed by fecal-oral transmission and is a rare cause of neonatal disease, although it has been nosocomially transmitted in the setting of a neonatal intensive care unit. Hepatitis E virus is similar to hepatitis A in its mode of transmission and clinical manifestations, except for an increased mortality in pregnant women infected with hepatitis E (Aggarwal et al, 2009; Teshale et al, 2010). There are no data regarding perinatal transmission of hepatitis E. Hepatitis D virus may cause only coinfection or super-infection with hepatitis B virus. Its only clinical significance is that hepatitis B infection may become more severe when hepatitis D virus is present. Perinatal transmission has been described (Ramia and Bahakim, 1998), but is uncommon.

Hepatitis G virus (HGV), also known as *GB virus type C*, has been associated with acute and chronic hepatitis and usually is noted as a coinfection with hepatitis B or C. This virus has a tropism for lymphocytes and may influence the course and prognosis in HIV-seropositive patients (Reshetnyak et al, 2008). Perinatal transmission can occur in 60% to 80% of infants born to HGV-viremic mothers, but there has not been any report of clinical hepatitis attributed to the HGV infection in this setting (Ohto et al, 2000; Wejstal et al, 1999; Zanetti et al, 1998; Zuin et al, 1999). The clinical significance and effects of HGV infection are still poorly understood. Hepatitis B and C viruses are both transmitted vertically and among the viral hepatitis are of the greatest important to the care of newborns.

HEPATITIS B

The issues that are most important to neonatologists are the frequency with which hepatitis B virus (HBV) is transmitted to infants at the time of birth, the short-term and long-term consequences of these infections, the importance of greater surveillance for maternal carriage of HBV, the role of antiviral therapy to prevent transmission and disease progression, and the availability of effective HBV immunoprophylaxis (Arfaoui et al, 2010; Krugman, 1988).

Incidence

In certain parts of the world and among certain ethnic groups, as many as 7% to 10% of all infants acquire hepatitis B infections at the time of birth, and almost all of these infections become chronic. In the United States, it has been estimated that approximately 20,000 infants are

TABLE 37-3   Viral Hepatitis Types A, B, C, D, E, and G: Comparison of Clinical, Epidemiologic, Immunologic, and Therapeutic Features

Feature	Hepatitis A	Hepatitis B	Hepatitis C	Hepatitis D (Delta)	Hepatitis E	Hepatitis G/GBVC
Virus	Hepatitis A virus (HAV)	Hepatitis B virus (HBV)	Hepatitis C virus (HCV)	Hepatitis D virus (HDV)	Hepatitis E virus (HEV)	Hepatitis G virus (HGC), (GB virus type C [GBV-C])
Family	Picornavirus	Hepadnavirus	Flavivirus	Satellite	Calicivirus	Flavivirus
Genome	RNA	DNA	RNA	RNA	RNA	RNA
Incubation period	15-40 days	50-180 days	1-5 months	2-8 weeks	2-9 weeks	Unknown
Mode of transmission						
Oral (fecal)	Usual	No	No	No	Usual	No
Parenteral	Rare	Usual	Usual	Usual	No	Usual
Perinatal	Rare	Yes	Yes	Only with HBV	Unknown	Yes
Other	Food- or water-borne	Sexual contact	Sexual contact less common	Sexual contact less common	Water-borne transmission in developing countries	Sexual contact; probably less common
Sequelae						
Carrier state	No	Yes	Yes	Yes	No	Yes
Chronic disease	No cases reported	Yes	Yes	Yes	No cases reported	Yes; controversial
Interventions						
Immunoglobulin	Yes	Yes	No	No	No	No
Vaccine	Yes	Yes	No	No	No	No
Antiviral therapy	No	Yes	Yes	No	No	No

Modified from Krugman S: Viral hepatitis: A, B, C, D, and E: prevention, *Pediatr Rev* 13:245-247, 1992.

born annually to mothers who are chronic HBV carriers (Mast et al, 1998). Since 1990 the incidence of acute hepatitis B in the United States has declined dramatically, with the largest declines occurring in children younger than 15 years (98%) and in young adults 15 through 24 years of age (90%). The frequency of transmission depends primarily on the prevalence of the hepatitis B carrier state among women of childbearing age. Hepatitis B is a carcinogenic virus; perinatal acquired infection can lead to chronic liver failure and hepatic carcinoma in adult life (Balistreri, 1988; Beasley and Hwang, 1984; Chan and Sung, 2006).

The incidence of neonatal hepatitis B infection depends on the timing of infection and the overall prevalence of the disease in the population under study. Women with acute hepatitis B infection during the first or second trimester rarely transmit the virus to their infants (Krugman, 1988; Stevens, 1994). Transplacental transfer has been described, but appears to be rare. The carriage rate for hepatitis B surface antigen (HBsAg) varies from 0.1% in the United States and Europe to 15% in Taiwan and parts of Africa, with intermediate rates in Japan, South America, and Southeast Asia. Transmission rates among immigrant women in Western countries appear to parallel the rates in their countries of origin (Krugman, 1988).

The most important route of transmission is transmission that occurs during labor and delivery. The likelihood of transmission is great if symptomatic acute disease is present (60% to 70% transmission; Gerety and Schweitzer, 1977). Infants of hepatitis B e antigen (HBeAg)–positive mothers have an 80% to 90% chance of becoming HBsAg carriers (Lee et al, 1978; Okada et al, 1976). The risk of an infant acquiring hepatitis B if born to an HBsAg-positive but HBeAg-negative mother is 5% to 20%. Chronic

neonatal infection occurs in less than 10% of infants of HBeAg antigen–negative mothers (Krugman, 1988). Although HBsAg has been found in breast milk, breast-feeding does not appear to have any influence on the rate of transmission (Beasley et al, 1975). The World Health Organization currently recommends that all mothers who are hepatitis B positive breastfeed their infants, and that their infants be immunized at birth.

Etiology and Pathogenesis

HBV is a DNA virus that localizes primarily in hepatic parenchymal cells but circulates in the bloodstream, along with several subviral antigens, for periods ranging from a few days to many years. Several distinct genotypes have been identified, and these subtypes show biologic variability in transmission and disease progression (Magnius and Norder, 1995; Schaefer et al, 2009). Transplacental leakage of HBeAg-positive maternal blood is a potential source of intrauterine infection (Lin et al, 1987). During either acute or persistent viremia in the mother, the virus itself or viral antigens may rarely cross the placenta and cause intrauterine infection, but more commonly infection occurs perinatally during labor or delivery (Chisari and Ferrari, 1995; Xu et al, 2001). The finding of hepatitis antigens in the newborn might not indicate the presence of infection, but rather the passive transfer of antigen only; therefore antigen tests should be interpreted cautiously in this setting. Hepatitis B infection of placental trophoblast has been documented and is compatible with a transplacental route of infection in some circumstances (Bai et al, 2007). Most infants born to mothers infected with HBV have a negative test result for HBsAg at birth, but in the absence of prophylaxis are at risk for becoming

TABLE 37-4 Licensed Monovalent and Combination Hepatitis B Vaccines

Clinical Scenario	Monovalent Vaccines		Combination Vaccines		
	Recombivax Hepatitis B Dose, µg (mL)	Enginerix-B Dose, µg (mL)	Twinrix*	Comvax†	Pediatrix‡
Newborns born to HBsAg-negative mothers	5 (0.5)	10 (0.5)	NA	NA	NA
Newborns born to HBsAg-positive mothers§	5 (0.5)	10 (0.5)	NA	NA	NA
Infants, children, and adolescents <20 yr old	5 (0.5)	10 (0.5)	NA	5 (0.5)	10 (0.5)
Adults >20 yr old	10 (1.0)	20 (1.0)	20 (1.0)	NA	NA

*Twinrix is a combination of Engerix-B (20 mg) and hepatitis A vaccine, licensed for use in people 18 years of age and older in a three-dose series at a 0-, 1-, and 6-month schedule.
†Comvax is a combination of Recombivax HB (5 µg) and *Haemophilus influenzae* type b (PRP-OMP) recommended for use at 2, 4, and 12 to 15 months of age. This vaccine should not be administered at birth.
‡Pediatrix is a combination of diptheria and tetanus toxoids and acellular pertussis (i.e., DTaP), inactivated poliovirus, and hepatitis B (Engerix B, 10 mg). It is recommended for use at 2, 4, and 6 months of age, but should not be administered at birth, before 6 weeks of age, or after 7 years of age.
§Hepatitis B immunoglobulin (0.5 mL) should be adminstered simultaneously with vaccination.

HBsAg-positive during the first 3 months of life, suggesting that transmission is primarily peripartum (Krugman, 1988, 1992; Mulligan and Stiehm, 1994; Shapiro, 1993).

Clinical Spectrum and Laboratory Evaluation

Infants with hepatitis B infection do not show clinical or chemical signs of disease at birth. Without immunoprophylaxis, the usual pattern is the development of chronic antigenemia with mild and often persistent enzyme elevations, beginning at 2 to 6 months of age (Mulligan and Stiehm, 1994). Less commonly the infection becomes clinically manifest, with jaundice, fever, hepatomegaly, and anorexia, followed by either recovery or chronic active hepatitis. Rarely, fulminant hepatitis is seen and can be fatal (Delaplane et al, 1983).

Laboratory tests are essential in the diagnosis of hepatitis B infection. Evaluations of serum enzymes and of bilirubin reflect the extent of liver damage. Several helpful serologic tests identify the virus involved (Krugman, 1988). HBsAg appears early, usually before liver disease is found; it persists in those who become chronic carriers or disappears in the 5% of infants who resolve the infection. HBeAg and anti-HBe testing can be used to assess infectivity; although they are not as frequently used for serodiagnosis, they are useful markers of the likelihood of perinatal transmission. PCR and other nucleic acid detection techniques are important in confirming diagnosis, assessing viral load, and monitoring the response to therapy.

Prevention

The primary goal of prevention strategies for hepatitis B is to prevent chronic infection and chronic liver disease. In the United States over the past two decades, a comprehensive immunization strategy has been implemented consisting of four components:

1. Universal immunization of all infants beginning at birth
2. Prevention of perinatal infection through routine screening of all pregnant women and appropriate immunoprophylaxis of infants born to HBsAg-positive women (or women whose HBsAg status is unknown)

3. Routine immunization of children and adolescents who have not been immunized previously
4. Immunization of nonimmunized adults at increased risk of infection

For infants, the three-dose vaccination schedule should be initiated in the neonatal period or by 2 months of age (Table 37-4). Four doses can be given if a birth dose is given and a combination vaccine is used to complete the series. Vaccination can be delayed until just before hospital discharge in preterm (birthweight less than 2000 g) infants born to HBsAg-negative mothers.

All infants born to HBsAg-positive women should receive both active and passive immunization within 12 hours of birth. The doses and recommended options for administration of the hepatitis B vaccines that are currently licensed in the United States are provided in Table 37-4. If maternal HBsAg status is unknown, it should be checked immediately, and the infant should receive the first dose of HBV vaccine immediately. Infants born to women who test positive, or to women in whom the HBsAg is unknown, should be given hepatitis B immunoglobulin as soon as possible within 1 week after birth. The highest immunization failure rates have been observed in infants of HBeAg-positive women and those infected in utero (Farmer et al, 1987; Tang et al, 1998). It is recommended that infants born to HbsAg-positive mothers undergo postimmunization testing for anti-HBS and HbsAg 3 to 9 months after completion of the series, for identification of breakthrough carriers and of infants who may benefit from revaccination (AAP Committee on Infectious Diseases, 2010a).

Treatment

There is no therapy for acute hepatitis B infection. Interferon (IFN) α and antiretroviral drugs such as lamivudine, an antiretroviral drug that blocks HBV polymerase, and adefovir, a reverse transcriptase inhibitor, have been approved for treatment of chronic hepatitis B in children, but success is widely variable (Giacchino and Cappelli, 2010). Three therapeutic agents for chronic HBV infection in children have been approved in the United States, including standard IFN-α, lamivudine, and adefovir (Kurbegov and Sokol, 2009). These antiviral therapies are summarized in Table 37-2. IFN-α appears to be the most effective (approximately 30% HBeAg seroconversion; 10% HBsAg seroconversion), although benefits are primarily observed in children with alanine aminotransferase levels more than twofold the upper limit of normal. The virologic response rates for lamivudine mirror those of IFN-α (23% to 31% HBeAg seroconversion) with easier administration and a more favorable safety profile, but lower HBsAg seroconversion (2% to 3%) and high rates of drug resistance. Adefovir demonstrates a favorable safety profile and is less likely to select for resistance than lamivudine, but virologic response was limited to adolescent patients and was lower than that of lamivudine (16% HBeAg seroconversion; <1% HBsAg seroconversion). Entecavir and tenofovir, both approved therapies for adults with chronic HBV infection, are in trials for use in children. Some experts recommend "watchful waiting" of children, because current therapies are only 30% effective at best. Young children are often believed to be immune tolerant of hepatitis B infection (i.e., they have viral DNA present in serum, but normal transaminase levels and no evidence of active hepatitis). These children should have transaminases and viral load monitored, but are not typically considered to be candidates for antiviral therapy.

Prognosis

Most long-term follow-up studies have shown that children vaccinated at birth have high levels of protection until at least 5 years of age. Approximately 5% to 10% of infants born to HbeAg-positive mothers become chronic HBV carriers despite combined active and passive immunoprophylaxis with hepatitis B immunoglobulin and HBV vaccine (Kato et al, 1999). Failure of immunoprophylaxis may be associated with the level of maternal viremia and specific HBV genetic variants (Ngui et al, 1998). Infants who become infected with HBV perinatally have a 90% risk of chronic infection, and 15% to 25% of those with chronic infection die of HBV-related liver disease (primarily hepatocellular carcinoma) as adults. There is some evidence that the risk of carcinoma correlates with specific hepatitis B genotypes (Sherman, 2010).

HEPATITIS C

In 1989, hepatitis C virus (HCV) was found to be the main cause of non-A, non-B, parenterally transmitted hepatitis; subsequently, HCV has been found to account for a significant portion of the cases of sporadic acute and chronic hepatitis (Choo et al, 1989; Reyes et al, 1990; Weiss and Persing, 1995). Hepatitis C virus is a small, single-stranded RNA virus that is a member of the family Flavivirus; this family consists primarily of vector-borne infections, such as St. Louis encephalitis virus and West Nile virus. Hepatitis C virus is an exception in this family because it is not transmitted by insect vectors. Seven genotypes are described, with significant biologic differences in regard to disease progression and responsiveness to therapy (Klenerman et al, 2009). Vertically transmitted hepatitis C infection in infants is associated with a higher rate of chronic hepatitis, but less liver injury compared with adult HCV infections (Tovo et al, 2000).

Incidence

The seroprevalence for anti-HCV antibody in pregnant women ranges from 0.7% to 4.4% worldwide (Conte et al, 2000). In the United States, seroprevalence of hepatitis C decreased during the 1990s and has remained low and stable since then. The overall seroprevalence is estimated to be 1.3%, with a seroprevalence in pregnant women ranging from 1% to 2% (AAP Committee on Infectious Diseases, 2010a). Forty percent to 50% of women with HCV have no identified known risk factors for infection (Bortolotti et al, 1998). Estimates from the 1990s suggested that the vertical transmission rate of HCV is approximately 5% to 11% in HIV-negative mothers, and ranges from 10% to 20% from mothers coinfected with HIV (Hillemanns et al, 2000; Palomba et al, 1996; Polywka et al, 1997; Tajiri et al, 2001). More recent studies, however, suggest a lower rate of vertical transmission, ranging from 2.7% to 3.6% (Ferrero et al, 2003; Syriopoulou et al, 2005). One study has shown, in a multivariate analysis, that higher risk of vertical transmission is related more to maternal use of injection drugs than to HIV infection itself, although the mechanism for this finding is still unclear (Resti et al, 2002). The risk of transmission correlates with maternal viremia, and transmission appears to be rare in the absence of viremia. The risk of HCV infection from transfused blood after the advent of HCV screening is estimated to be less than 1 in 1 million units transfused.

Etiology and Pathogenesis

HCV is transmitted less efficiently than HBV by sexual contact. Risk factors for HCV infection include transfusion, intravenous drug use, frequent occupational exposure to blood products, and household or sexual contact with an infected person (Weiss and Persing, 1995). In children, perinatal transmission is the most common route of infection (Mohan et al, 2010). Preparations of IVIG contaminated with HCV were reported between April 1993 and February 1994, but since that time, routine screening for HCV with PCR and application of a viral inactivation process during manufacturing have been implemented to reduce the risk of transmission (Schiff, 1994).

Perinatal transmission is the leading cause of childhood HCV infection (Mohan et al, 2010). Transmission of HCV from mother to child is thought to occur either in utero or at the time of delivery. Viral genotypes and infection and replication in maternal peripheral blood monocytes can also affect the ability of the virus to infect the fetus or newborn (Azzari et al, 2000; Zuccotti et al, 1995). Perinatal transmission is confined almost always to women with detectable HCV ribonucleic acid (RNA) in the peripheral blood by the PCR, but all children born to women with anti-HCV antibodies should be tested for HCV. Data regarding the correlation of HCV RNA titer in the mother with the risk of vertical transmission are conflicting, although most studies have reported an association (Conte et al, 2000; Lynch-Salomon and Combs, 1992; Ohto et al, 1994; Resti et al, 1998; Tajiri et al, 2001). Maternal peripheral blood mononuclear cell infection by HCV, membrane rupture of longer than 6 hours before delivery, and procedures exposing the infant to maternal blood infected with HCV during vaginal delivery are associated with an increased risk of transmission. Internal fetal monitoring is also a risk factor for transmission (Mast et al, 2005). Maternal coinfection with HCV and human immunodeficiency virus, maternal history of intravenous drug use and of HCV infection of the sexual partner of the mother are also risk factors for transmission (Fiore and Savasi, 2009; Indolfi and Resti, 2009). Transmission rates as high as 25% have been reported in HCV-infected, HIV-positive women. The effect of vaginal delivery versus cesarean section on transmission rates is unclear (Gibb et al, 2000; Paccagnini et al, 1995); current recommendations do not support the practice of cesarean delivery in women with HCV infection.

Transmission of HCV via breast milk has not been demonstrated conclusively, although HCV can be found in breast milk and colostrum (Gurakan et al, 1994; Zimmermann et al, 1995). Studies comparing breastfed and bottle-fed infants born to HCV-infected mothers have not shown a statistically significant difference in vertical transmission (Lin et al, 1995; Resti et al, 1998). Accordingly, maternal HCV infection is not a contraindication to breastfeeding (Mast, 2004); however, it may be prudent for mothers who are HCV-infected and who choose to breastfeed to consider abstaining from breastfeeding if their nipples are cracked and bleeding.

Clinical Spectrum and Laboratory Evaluation

Acquired HCV infection typically causes jaundice in one third of cases and significant increases in alanine aminotransferase (ALT) in almost all persons infected. Most neonates perinatally infected with HCV demonstrate little in the way of clinical symptomatology; they may have elevated liver ALT either transiently or intermittently. The increases in ALT values, when tested, are most commonly noted between 3 and 6 months of age. HCV-RNA PCR results may be negative initially at birth or within the first few days of life, but typically become positive by 1 to 2 weeks of age and remain so until at least 5 years of age. The highest sensitivity of PCR is reported after 1 month of age (Polywka et al, 2006; Thomas et al, 1997). Confirmatory anti-HCV IgG serology should be delayed until exposed infants are at least 15 to 18 months old, when at least 99% will have cleared maternal antibody (Dunn et al, 2001). Before 18 months of age, only a positive HCV PCR result can confirm diagnosis of neonatal infection; positive anti-HCV IgG results simply reflect passively acquired maternal antibody. IgM assays are not available or reliable for perinatal diagnosis of HCV. Liver ultrasonographic findings are usually normal or may consist of a mild diffuse increase in echogenicity. Liver biopsies, when performed, typically demonstrate mild to moderate chronic persistent hepatitis (Palomba et al, 1996; Tovo et al, 2000).

Treatment

Interferon and ribavirin are both approved by the FDA to treat adults and children with chronic hepatitis C. Antiviral agents are summarized in Table 37-2. Only 10% to 25% of adults treated with interferon have a sustained remission of disease (Bonkovsky and Woolley, 1999). Treatment with a combination of interferon and ribavirin achieves remission in closer to half of treated adults (Cornberg et al, 2002). Randomized controlled trials indicate that patients treated with pegylated interferons (so called because they are formulated and stabilized with polyethylene glycol), both as dual therapy with ribavirin and as monotherapy, experience higher sustained viral response rates than do those treated with nonpegylated interferon (Shepherd et al, 2004). Data on the use of these agents in infants and children are limited, although the use of IFN-α2b in combination with ribavirin was recently approved by the FDA (Palumbo, 2009). In a case series of four pediatric patients treated with interferon for 1 year, viremia decreased to undetectable levels during treatment in all four patients, but two patients became viremic again once the treatment was stopped (Tovo et al, 2000). There are significant genotype-dependent differences in responsiveness to antiviral therapy; patients with genotype 1 had the lowest levels of sustained virologic response, and patients with genotype 2 or 3 had the highest (Palumbo, 2009; Shepherd et al, 2004). The use of IFN-α2b in combination with ribavirin provides a much more favorable sustained virologic response in children with HCV genotype 2/3 (84%) than in those with HCV genotype 1 (36%; González-Peralta et al, 2005). For genotype 1 hepatitis C treated with pegylated interferons combined with ribavirin, it has been shown that genetic polymorphisms near the human *IL28B* gene, encoding interferon lambda 3, are associated with significant differences in response to the treatment (Ge et al, 2009; Thomas et al, 2009). Interferon therapies are available only in parenteral formulations and are associated with significant side effects; therefore further research into its utility in pediatric HCV infection is needed.

Infants and children with persistent elevations in liver transaminases should be referred to a pediatric gastroenterologist for evaluation and management. The necessity for, as well as the frequency of, screening tests of liver function has not been established.

Prognosis

In 60% to 80% of HCV-infected adults, chronic hepatitis occurs, and in one third of HCV-infected adults, chronic HCV infection leads to cirrhosis or liver failure within 20 to 30 years after infection (Iwarson et al, 1995; Leone and Rizzetto, 2010). In patients with cirrhosis, the incidence of hepatocellular carcinoma is 2% to 5% per year. There are limited data regarding long-term follow-up in HCV-infected infants, but existing knowledge indicates that most children remain viremic until at least 5 to 6 years of age, and most develop chronic, persistent hepatitis. Studies monitoring infected children beyond 6 years of age have not been completed, but they are at risk for cirrhosis and hepatocellular carcinoma. Transient hepatitis C viremia with subsequent resolution has been reported (Padula et al, 1999; Ruiz-Extremera et al, 2000; Zanetti et al, 1995). All the infants who have been followed for an average of 3 to 4 years have been reported to have normal growth and development (Tovo et al, 2000).

Prevention

Although development of an HCV vaccine is a major public health priority (Houghton and Abrignani, 2005), there is currently no vaccine available. Like all other infants, infants with HCV should receive routine hepatitis B immunization. In addition, they should receive hepatitis A vaccination at 2 years of age. Parents should be advised to avoid unnecessary administration of medicines known to be hepatotoxic. Standard precautions are recommended for the hospitalized infant.

ADENOVIRUS

Adenoviruses are so named because they were originally recovered from human adenoidal tissue; they are medium-sized (90 to 100 nm), nonenveloped icosahedral viruses composed of a nucleocapsid and a double-stranded linear DNA genome. They are the largest of the nonenveloped viruses. There are 53 described adenovirus serotypes in humans.

EPIDEMIOLOGY AND CLINICAL MANIFESTATIONS

Adenoviruses are responsible for a wide variety of clinical syndromes, including conjunctivitis, respiratory track disease, and gastroenteritis. Adenovirus causes 5% to 10% of upper respiratory infections in children, and many infections in adults as well. No clear seasonality has been described for adenovirus infections.

ADENOVIRUS INFECTIONS IN NEWBORNS

There are a limited number of reports of adenovirus infection in young infants, but published case series indicate that adenovirus can cause serious, life-threatening disease in the neonate. A review of neonatal adenovirus infection (Abzug and Levin, 1991) identified several characteristic historical features, including prolonged rupture of membranes, history of maternal illness, vaginal mode of delivery, and onset of illness within the first 10 days of life. Serotypes 2, 3, 7, 11, 13, 19, 21, 30, and 35 have been implicated (Abzug and Levin, 1991; Andiman et al, 1977; Matsuoka et al, 1990; Osamura et al, 1993; Pinto et al, 1992; Sun and Duara, 1985). Clinical findings in various case reports and case series have included lethargy, fever or hypothermia, anorexia, apnea, hepatomegaly, bleeding, and progressive pneumonia (Figure 37-5). Laboratory abnormalities include thrombocytopenia, coagulopathy, and hepatitis. Acquisition of infection from the mother via vaginal delivery is the presumed mode of transmission in most cases, although transplacental spread has also been implicated.

Although most neonatal adenovirus infection is believe to be acquired in the birth canal, congenital infections have been described, presumably because of transplacental transmission. A wide range of fetal pathologies including pleural effusion, hepatitis, myocarditis, meningitis, and CNS abnormalities have been described (Baschat et al, 2003; Meyer et al, 1985; Rieger-Fackeldey et al, 2000). Adenovirus has been implicated as a potential cause

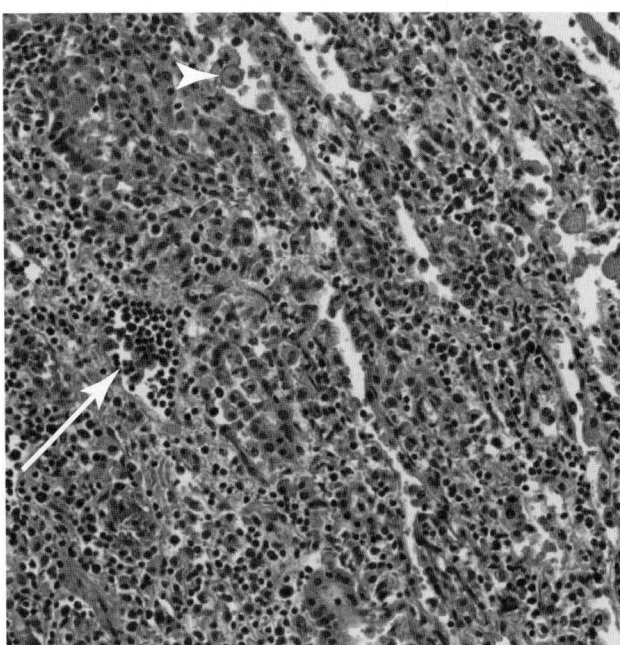

FIGURE 37-5 *(See also Color Plate 19.)* Postmortem histologic analysis from an infant who died from disseminated adenovirus infection at 2 weeks of age. Hematoxylin and eosin stain of lung demonstrating inflammatory infiltrates *(arrow)* and intranuclear inclusions *(arrowhead)*. This infant had a viral sepsis syndrome characterized by hepatic failure, disseminated intravascular coagulation, and pneumonitis from adenovirus infection presumed to have been acquired intrapartum.

of chorioamnionitis and premature birth (Tsekoura et al, 2010; Van den Veyver et al, 1998).

PREVENTION AND INTERVENTION

Intravenous ribavirin has been administered to a neonate with disseminated adenovirus infection undergoing extracorporeal membrane oxygenation, with evidence of viral clearance within 48 hours of initiating therapy (Aebi et al, 1997). Adenovirus vaccines were at one time available for use in military personnel (Gaydos and Gaydos, 1995; Tucker et al, 2008), but are not currently in production. Adenoviruses are hardy and resistant to inactivation by physical and chemical methods that kill most viruses, adding to the challenge of hospital infection control during outbreaks of infection.

RESPIRATORY VIRUSES

Although relatively uncommon, any one of the respiratory viruses can cause symptomatic respiratory disease in newborn infants. The association has been described for rhinoviruses, adenoviruses, parainfluenza viruses, influenza virus, and respiratory syncytial virus. Adenovirus, rhinovirus, and parainfluenza virus infections are generally characterized by mild rhinorrhea in neonates. All of these viruses, however, can cause clinical symptoms indistinguishable from those of bacterial infection, leading to increased diagnostic testing and empiric antibiotic treatment. Influenza virus infections are usually mild, but in the absence of maternally transmitted antibody, they can be life threatening, with severe pneumonia, hypoxia, and a prolonged course. During the H1N1 influenza pandemic of 2009 to 2010, pregnant women were at uniquely high risk for severe influenza (Jamieson et al, 2009), and infections were described in neonates (Sert et al, 2010).

The most extensive nursery outbreaks, however, have been caused by respiratory syncytial virus (RSV; Hall et al, 1979; Wilson et al, 1989). Because of the importance that RSV plays in the newborn nursery, this virus is considered in greater detail in the following section.

RESPIRATORY SYNCYTIAL VIRUS

RSV is the major cause of viral pneumonia and bronchiolitis in infants and children. In temperate climates, it causes large annual epidemics during the winter and early spring months (typically ranging from November through April). During these months, RSV appears to be responsible for up to 20% of all pediatric hospital admissions (Hall et al, 2009). Nosocomial infections are frequent during these times, and illness among hospital staff members is a major factor in its spread from infant to infant. Several nursery outbreaks have been described. In one of these outbreaks, cultures were obtained prospectively so that a full picture of the virus's pathogenicity and epidemiology could be drawn (Hall et al, 1979). Twenty-three of 66 infants hospitalized for 6 days or more were infected. Virtually all infants were symptomatic. Clinical manifestations included pneumonia, upper respiratory infection, apneic spells, and nonspecific signs. Pneumonia and apnea were seen almost exclusively in infants older than 3 weeks, and nonspecific signs were most commonly observed in younger infants. Four (17%) infants died, two unexpectedly, during the course of infection. The spread of infection in the unit was difficult to interrupt; infants in isolettes did not seem to be protected against acquisition of the infection. Eighteen of the 53 nursery personnel were infected during the outbreak; 83% of the infected nursery providers were symptomatic. Of particular importance is the observation that RSV infection, both in term and in preterm infants, is commonly associated with a new onset of apnea (Bruhn et al, 1977). Boys are at greater risk than girls for serious RSV disease. RSV-associated apnea has been the probable explanation for some case reports of deaths attributed to SIDS (Eisenhut, 2006). RSV lower respiratory track disease can be slow to resolve. After discharge from initial hospitalization, risk factors for infant rehospitalization secondary to RSV infection include premature gestational age, chronic lung disease, siblings in daycare or school, chronologic age of less than 3 months, and exposure to tobacco smoke (Carbonell-Estrany and Quero, 2001).

Diagnosis can be confirmed by DFA staining of nasopharyngeal or tracheal aspirate, nasopharyngeal swab, or other respiratory secretions. Culture of RSV can require 3 to 5 days and can be used if DFA staining is not available. PCR is also available for the rapid diagnosis of infection.

Treatment and prevention of RSV infection in infants attracted considerable attention during the 1990s because of the clinical and economic impacts of these infections (Groothuis, 1994; Kinney et al, 1995; Levin, 1994; Meissner, 1994). Considerable debate has ensued concerning the efficacy, safety, and potential effect on health care workers of ribavirin therapy, so its use remains controversial

---

BOX 37-4   Guidelines for Prophylaxis in Preterm Infants at Start of RSV Season

PROPHYLAXIS RECOMMENDED

- Infants born at ≤28 weeks, 6 days of gestation during first RSV season*
- Infants born at 29 weeks, 0 days through 31 weeks, 6 days of gestation if less than 6 months of age at beginning of RSV season
- Infants and children less that 24 months of age with chronic lung disease requiring medical therapy (e.g., supplmental oxygen, bronchodilators, diuretics, corticosteroids) within the 6 months before RSV season
- Infants born at 32 weeks, 0 days through 34 weeks, 6 days of gestation if one of the following two risk factors are present:
  - Attending child care
  - Sibling younger than 5 years of age

PROPHYLAXIS CONSIDERED

- Infants with congenital anomalies of the airways
- Infants younger than 24 months of age with hemodynamically significant congenital heart disease, as manifest by congestive heart failure, pulmonary hypertension, and cyanosis
- Infants with severe neuromuscular disease
- Infants with immune deficiencies
- Infants with cystic fibrosis

RSV, Respiratory syncytial virus.
*Earliest date to consider initiation of prophylaxis depends upon geographic location: July 1 for southeast Florida, September 15 for north central and southwest Florida, November 1 for most other areas of the United States.

(Meissner, 2001; Ventre and Randolph, 2004; Wald and Dashefsky, 1994). Treatment consists of nebulization of ribavirin by a small-particle aerosol generator supplied by the manufacturer into an oxygen hood, tent, or mask from a solution containing 20 mg of ribavirin per milliliter of water (see Table 37-2). The aerosol has been administered on various schedules for 3 to 5 days (e.g., 12 to 20 h/day). The efficacy of ribavirin in this setting remains unclear. Some long-term benefit on recurrent wheezing may be realized (Ventre and Randolph, 2004). Corticosteroids are not effective in the treatment of RSV.

Prevention efforts have focused on passive and active immunization. Standard immunoglobulin has not been shown to be efficacious for prevention of RSV infection in high-risk infants (Meissner et al, 1993). The efficacy of monthly prophylactic administration of RSV-specific immunoglobulin (750 mg/kg or 150 mg/kg) in 249 infants with cardiac disease or bronchopulmonary dysplasia was examined in a multicenter trial (Groothuis, 1994). In the high-dose (750 mg/kg) group, there were fewer lower respiratory tract infections, hospitalizations, days in hospital, and days in the intensive care unit as well as less use of ribavirin. Subsequently a mouse monoclonal antibody was developed, which provides similar protection against RSV (i.e., palivizumab). Unlike anti-RSV immunoglobulin, which is a pooled human blood product, the monoclonal antibody does not confer the theoretical risk of acquiring blood-borne pathogens. Palivizumab is also substantially easier to administer because it is an intramuscular injection. Recommendations by the AAP for the use of palivizumab are summarized in Box 37-4. Additional preventive measures for high-risk infants include eliminating or minimizing exposure to tobacco smoke, avoiding crowds and situations in which exposure to infected individuals cannot be controlled, careful hand hygiene education of parents, vaccinating against influenza beginning at 6 months of age, and restricting participation in child care during the RSV season whenever feasible. The prospects for infant or maternal immunization with live attenuated and protein subunit vaccines are under active investigation and development (Crowe, 2001; Fretzayas and Moustaki, 2010; Piedra, 2000).

Nosocomial spread of RSV and other respiratory viruses can be minimized by emphasis on hand washing by care providers between contacts with patients. Without additional special precautions, an attack rate of approximately 26% has been observed (Madge et al, 1992). Use of standard contact precautions, such as cohort nursing and the use of gowns and gloves for all contacts with RSV-infected children, can reduce the risk of nosocomial RSV infection to 9.5% (Madge et al, 1992).

GASTROINTESTINAL VIRUSES

The most important of the viruses that cause diarrhea from the perspective of the neonatal nursery are the rotaviruses. This important group of viruses, with at least four serotypes, is responsible for a large proportion of significant and sometimes severe diarrhea in infants 6 to 24 months of age (Cohen, 1991; Greenberg et al, 1994; Haffejee, 1991; Taylor and Echeverria, 1993). Recent evidence suggests that rotavirus extracts an unexpectedly significant burden of disease on infants as young as 2 to 3 months of age (Clark et al, 2010). Nursery-acquired infections are common; surprisingly, such infections appear to be benign in most infants. Two studies performed in nurseries in Sydney, Australia, and in London found that 30% to 50% of 5-day-old babies shed the virus (Chrystie et al, 1978; Murphy et al, 1977). However, more than 90% of the infected infants were asymptomatic. The remaining symptomatic infants had loose stools and vomiting, but this figure was only slightly higher than the proportion of uninfected infants with the same symptoms. The full scope of rotavirus disease in the newborn and in the premature infant remains to be fully defined. The recent advent and licensure of several rotavirus vaccines should have a significant effect on both nosocomial and community-acquired rotavirus disease (Bernstein, 2009).

HUMAN IMMUNODEFICIENCY VIRUS INFECTION DURING PREGNANCY

CHANGING EPIDEMIOLOGY OF THE HIV/AIDS PANDEMIC

From 1980, when previously healthy, young, gay men first began to have complaints of fever, malaise, weight loss, lymphadenopathy, and malaise, to the identification in 1983 of 36 cases in Kinshasa, Zaire (Congo) of acquired immunodeficiency syndrome (AIDS) by a team of representatives from the CDC and National Institutes of Health, the scope of HIV infection has evolved into a global pandemic. The Joint United Nations Program on

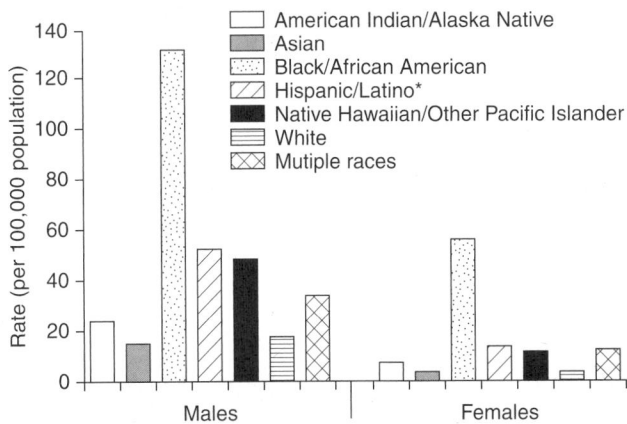

FIGURE 37-6 Estimated rates of diagnoses of HIV infection among adults and adolescents, by sex and race/ethnicity, in 2008 for 37 states with confidential name-based HIV infection reporting. Estimated rates resulted from statistical adjustment that accounted for reporting delays, but not for incomplete reporting. *(From Centers for Disease Control and Prevention:* HIV Surveillance Report 20, 200, *June 2010. Available at www.cdc.gov/hiv/topics/surveillance/resources/reports. Accessed November 24, 2010.)*

HIV/AIDS estimated that, as of the end of 2008, up to 35 million individuals were living with HIV/AIDS globally. Relevant to this chapter, women accounted for 60% of all adults living with HIV (Christie et al, 2008).

Currently, national and international surveillance for HIV infection and the resulting illness of AIDS is routine. In the United States, CDC surveillance data for 2005 to 2008 revealed an 8% increase in the absolute number of newly diagnosed HIV infections, whereas the overall rate of new infections was stable. Women currently account for 25% of the HIV-infected U.S. population, with African American women having the highest rate of diagnosed infection among women (Figure 37-6). In Florida, an HIV prevalence study among pregnant women from 1998 to 2007 found that black women were 11-fold more likely than white women to have HIV infection (Salihu et al, 2010). The incidence of HIV infection is challenging to measure and has not been measured directly. Based on a relatively new antibody test that can distinguish recent (median, 156 days) seroconversion from longstanding infection, it is estimated that there were 13,000 to 15,000 HIV infections among U.S. women in 2006 (Hall et al, 2008).

Estimates of HIV prevalence in pregnant women worldwide are challenging to obtain and may be underestimated, because those who consent to testing and counseling are more likely to be HIV negative. For example, in an urban antenatal clinic in Zambia, 25% of women accepting HIV testing were found to be HIV positive, whereas anonymous sampling of infants' cord blood demonstrated a prevalence of 29% among women who refused testing ($p < 0.0001$ for a difference in HIV prevalence between the two groups; Stringer et al, 2005). In Zimbabwe, HIV prevalence among antenatal clinic attendees has been declining, although rates remain high: 32.1% in 2000 and 23.9% in 2004 (Mahomva et al, 2006). Infection rates in antenatal clinics in KwaZulu-Natal, South Africa, reached 37.5% (Ramogale et al, 2007). In the country of South Africa alone, there are an estimated 220,000 pregnant women living with HIV infection. Most African cities exhibit an HIV prevalence rate in the 20% to 40% range, whereas estimates in India are markedly lower—closer to 1% to 2% (Dandona et al, 2008; Lionel et al, 2008).

A markedly disproportionate burden of disease is spread among a few countries as evidenced by this summary statement in a 2008 World Health Organization report: "Close to 90% of all pregnant women living with HIV in low and middle-income countries live in 20 countries and 75% are concentrated in 12 countries" (World Health Organization, 2008). The high prevalence of HIV infection among women living in settings where antiretroviral medications are not universally available results in many cases of pediatric HIV infection. Mother-to-child transmission accounts for 90% of HIV infections in children. A recent estimate is that a staggering 2.1 million children younger than 15 years are infected with HIV (World Health Organization, 2008).

In addition to the expansive societal and economic cost directly resulting from maternal HIV infection, there is a ripple effect of HIV infection on prevalence and morbidity of other infections. Tuberculosis and malaria are now common opportunistic infections of HIV in low-income countries. Herpes and HIV are considered "overlapping epidemics" (Corey et al, 2004), and the interplay is complex. Reactivation of HSV increases HIV RNA levels in plasma, and mucocutaneous shedding of HIV-1 is greater during mucocutaneous replication of HSV-2. Less publicized but more morbid effects are seen on the risk for puerperal sepsis, which is increased in HIV-infected women. A study in Zimbabwe demonstrated an 11-fold increase in risk for puerperal sepsis among HIV-infected women compared with HIV-negative women (Zvandasara et al, 2006). The same trend is exhibited in European settings; the European Collaborative Study found a fourfold increased risk for puerperal sepsis among HIV-infected women in 14 HIV reference centers across five countries (Fiore et al, 2004). Clearly the effect of HIV is multidimensional, and interdisciplinary cooperation is essential to effect change.

PATHOGENESIS OF HIV DISEASE

Transmission of the Virus

Transmission of HIV infection requires the exchange of bodily fluids. Numerous studies have demonstrated that casual household or community contacts are not associated with transmission or acquisition of HIV/AIDS. The three general mechanisms by which the virus can be passed from one individual to another are sexual, parenteral, and perinatal.

Different types of exposure to infection are associated with different risks of infection (Royce et al, 1997). One sexual transmission occurs for every 100 to 1000 exposures. Male-to-female transmission risk is about 10-times greater than female-to-male transmission risk. Needle-stick injury from an infected source carries a transmission risk of approximately 0.3% (Panlilio et al, 2005), with the risk from needle sharing being significantly greater. The risk of transmission through blood transfusion is greater than 90%, although this rarely occurs in the United States because of current screening methods used by blood banks.

Mother-to-Child Transmission

Transfer of virus from maternal to fetal or neonatal tissues is thought to occur during one of three discrete periods—antepartum (before the onset of labor), peripartum (during labor and delivery), and during breastfeeding. Studies of early viral dynamics in infected neonates suggest that the peripartum period is the time of highest risk (Mofenson, 1997). The risk of vertical transmission is heightened by premature rupture of membranes, high maternal viral load, and low maternal CD4 counts (Ioannidis and Contopoulos-Ioannidis, 1999; Mofenson et al, 1999). Without antiretroviral treatment, the risk of vertical transmission is estimated to be 15% to 20% in Europe, 15% to 30% in the United States, and 25% to 35% in Africa (Volmink et al, 2007). With highly active antiretroviral therapy, the risk of vertical transmission in the United States has been reduced to 1% to 5% (Coovadia, 2009).

Transmission through breast milk carries a 5% to 20% risk of transmission, largely dependent on the viral load and CD4 count of the mother (World Health Organization, 2008). A Kenyan study that randomized infants of HIV-infected mothers to breast versus formula feeding found that breastfeeding increased the risk of HIV transmission by 16% (Nduati et al, 2000b).

Prevention of Mother-to-Child Transmission

The cornerstone of preventing mother-to-child transmission of HIV is knowledge of the mother's HIV status. Updated recommendations from the CDC in 2006 (Branson et al, 2006) reinforced the importance of antenatal testing by stating that:
1. HIV screening should be included in the routine panel of prenatal screening tests for all pregnant women.
2. HIV screening is recommended after the patient is notified that testing will be performed, unless the patient declines (i.e., opt-out screening).
3. Separate written consent for HIV testing should not be required; general consent for medical care should be considered sufficient to encompass consent for HIV testing.
4. Repeated screening in the third trimester is recommended in certain jurisdictions with elevated rates of HIV infection among pregnant women (described as one diagnosed HIV case per 1000 pregnant women per year).

Research has shown that HIV testing rates are highest when included in standard testing for pregnant women both in high-income and low-income countries. A study done in Birmingham, Alabama, found that HIV testing rates increased from 75% to 88% (p <0.001) subsequent to the 1999 Institute of Medicine recommendation to make HIV testing a routine part of antenatal care (Stringer et al, 2001). Similarly, in Zimbabwe, testing rates increased from 65% to 99.9% (p <0.001) after implementation of an opt-out HIV testing approach in antenatal clinics (Chandisarewa et al, 2007).

HIV testing rates in most low-income countries are lower than those seen in Zimbabwe, but modest gains are being made. Globally, HIV testing in low- and middle-income countries rose from 10% of pregnant women attending antenatal clinics in 2004 to 18% in 2007 (World

Health Organization, 2008). As antiretroviral therapy becomes more readily available and the effects of this therapy on vertical transmission become more widely known, the incentive to perform HIV testing among pregnant women should increase.

Maternal Therapy

The introduction of potent antiretroviral therapies in the middle 1990s markedly reduced deaths caused by AIDS in most regions of the developed world. Antiretroviral therapies have not only reversed AIDS mortality trends in the developed world; they have also dramatically altered patterns of HIV transmission from mothers to children. The results of the Pediatric AIDS Clinical Trial Group Study 076 lead to a profound change in the approach to medical care for HIV-positive pregnant women (Connor et al, 1994). This prospective, placebo-controlled, randomized trial demonstrated that zidovudine prophylaxis during pregnancy, delivery, and early infancy reduced the rate of vertical HIV transmission from 25% to 8%. Less than 2 years later, additional antiretroviral agents became available for treatment of HIV infection. It also became possible to monitor viral load via plasma HIV-1 RNA assays. These monitoring and treatment tools created the potential for the well-controlled management of HIV infection in pregnant women seen today, where it is common to see viral loads of less than 1000 copies per milliliter and vertical transmission risk as low as 1%. Numerous studies have been conducted in low- and middle-income countries as well, demonstrating the benefit of antiretroviral therapy during pregnancy for prevention of vertical transmission of HIV (Dorenbaum et al, 2002; Ioannidis et al, 2001; Namukwaya et al, 2010).

Current guidelines exist for antiretroviral therapy in pregnant women (Panel on Treatment of HIV-Infected Pregnant Women and Prevention of Perinatal Transmission, 2010; available at http://aidsinfo.nih.gov/Content Files/PerinatalGL.pdf). Antiretroviral therapy is recommended for all HIV positive pregnant women during the latter trimesters of their pregnancy, with reassessment of the need to continue antiretroviral therapy after birth of the infant. If a woman is already receiving antiretroviral therapy that successfully suppresses viremia, it is recommended to continue the same regimen but find substitutes for any teratogenic drug (e.g., efavirenz). If the woman has a new HIV diagnosis, is antiretroviral therapy–naïve, and does not require antiretroviral therapy for her own health, therapy should be initiated for prophylaxis against vertical transmission based on the parameters in Box 37-5. If the mother is symptomatic from her infection or has a history of antiretroviral therapy use, the Perinatal Guidelines should be referenced for additional recommendations (Panel on Treatment of HIV-Infected Pregnant Women and Prevention of Perinatal Transmission, 2010).

Internationally, women in countries with the highest HIV prevalence often have less 25% intrapartum antiretroviral therapy coverage (Figure 37-7). United Nations goals target an 80% coverage rate of antiretroviral therapy in pregnant women, but drug availability still varies widely between countries. Rapid increases in antiretroviral availability in some African countries during 2004 to 2007 prove that such services can be provided quickly and

---

BOX 37-5   Treatment Recommendations for HIV-Infected, Antiretroviral-Naive Asymptomatic Pregnant Women

- Perform HIV antiretroviral drug resistance testing before initiating combination antiretroviral drug therapy and repeat after initiation of therapy if viral suppression is suboptimal.
- Prescribe a combination antiretroviral drug prophylaxis regimen (i.e., at least three drugs) for prophylaxis of perinatal transmission.
  - Consider delaying initiation of antiretroviral prophylaxis until after first trimester is completed.
  - Avoid use of efavirenz or other potentially teratogenic drugs in the first trimester and drugs with known adverse potential for the mother (e.g., combination stavudine/didanosine).
  - Use zidovudine as a component of the antiretroviral regimen when feasible.
  - If the woman has CD4 count >250 cells/mm^3, use nevirapine as a component of therapy only if the benefit clearly outweighs the risk, because of an increased risk of severe hepatic toxicity.
- Although the use of zidovudine prophylaxis alone is controversial, consider it if the woman has plasma HIV RNA level <1000 copies/mL on no therapy.
- Continue antiretroviral prophylaxis regimen during intrapartum period (zidovudine given as continuous infusion during labor while other antiretroviral agents are continued orally).
- Evaluate the need for continuing the combination regimen postpartum; discontinue the combination regimen unless the woman has indications for continued therapy. If regimen includes a drug with a long half-life, such as NNRTI, consider stopping NRTIs at least 7 days after stopping NNRTI.

Adapted from Panel on Treatment of HIV-Infected Pregnant Women and Prevention of Perinatal Transmission: [Perinatal Guidelines] *Recommendations for use of antiretroviral drugs in pregnant HIV-1-infected women for maternal health and interventions to reduce perinatal HIV transmission in the United States,* May 24, 2010, pp 1-117. http://aidsinfo.nih.gov/ContentFiles/PerinatalGL.pdf. Accessed November 22, 2010.

---

effectively in low-income countries given adequate political and financial support (Figure 37-8) (World Health Organization, 2008).

Antiretroviral Drug Resistance

Resistance to available antiretroviral drug therapy has become an increasingly important problem requiring continual reevaluation of antiretroviral therapy regimens for women and prophylactic regimens against perinatal transmission in both mother and infant. Drug resistance in the context of longitudinal maternal antiretroviral therapy is beyond the scope of this chapter, but current recommendations for appropriate drug regimens can be accessed in the Perinatal Guidelines (Panel on Treatment of HIV-Infected Pregnant Women and Prevention of Perinatal Transmission, 2010). It is important to conduct resistance testing before antiretroviral therapy initiation in women or infants, with the exception of the recommended 6 weeks of postnatal zidovudine for infants described in the following section). Selection of an appropriate combination drug regimen is best undertaken with the advice of a clinician specializing in the care of HIV-infected pediatric or adult patients.

In low- and middle-income countries, a single dose of nevirapine is often used to prevent vertical transmission of HIV (Guay et al, 1999). Whereas single-dose nevirapine is the most widespread approach to prophylaxis against perinatal transmission of HIV because of cost, limited availability of other drugs, and ease of administration, issues of

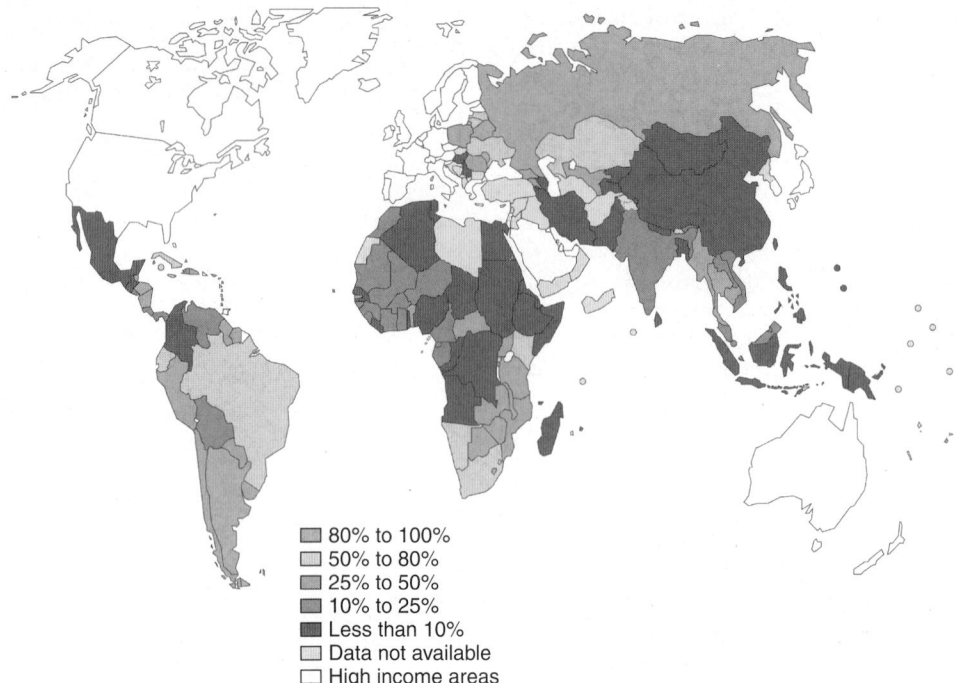

80% to 100%
50% to 80%
25% to 50%
10% to 25%
Less than 10%
Data not available
High income areas

FIGURE 37-7 Coverage of antiretroviral agents to prevent mother-to-child transmission of HIV in low- and middle-income countries: 2007. *(From World Health Organization:* Towards universal access: scaling up priority HIV/AIDS interventions in the health sector. Progress Report 2008. *Available at www.who.int/hiv/pub/2008progressreport/en. Accessed November 22, 2010.)*

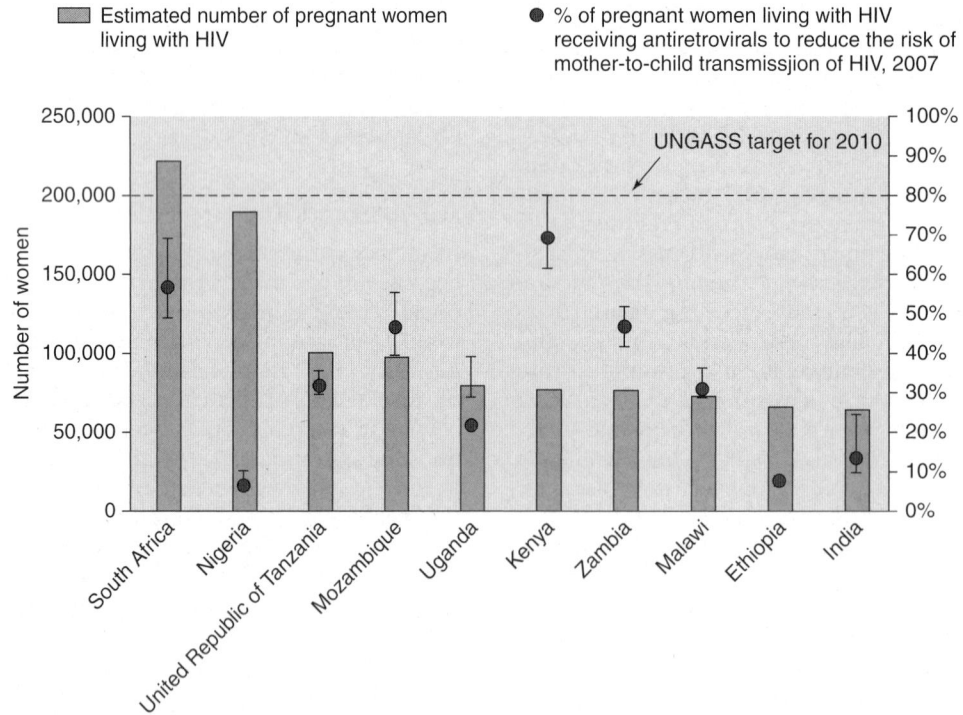

UNGASS: United Nations General Assembly Special Session on HIV/AIDS in 2001

⊢——⊣ The bar indicates the uncertainty range around the estimate.

FIGURE 37-8 Percentage of pregnant women living with HIV receiving antiretroviral agents for preventing mother-to-child transmission of HIV in the 10 countries with the highest estimated number of pregnant women living with HIV: 2007. *(From World Health Organization:* Towards universal access: scaling up priority HIV/AIDS interventions in the health sector. *Progress Report 2008. Available at www.who.int/hiv/ pub/2008progressreport/en. Accessed November 22, 2010.)*

nevirapine resistance are paramount. One study published in 2010 was terminated early because of the significant difference in nevirapine resistance and associated treatment failure in infants exposed to single-dose perinatal nevirapine prophylaxis (Palumbo et al, 2010). Another study from Uganda found 100% resistance to nevirapine in 6-month-old HIV-infected infants who had received 6 weeks of daily nevirapine in addition to single-dose nevirapine prophylaxis perinatally. Resistance patterns were less prevalent in infants who had received only the single-dose perinatal prophylaxis (16% at 6 months; $p=0.005$; Church et al, 2008). Appropriate drug regimens for prophylaxis against perinatal transmission in the face of viral mutation and resistance patterns will likely remain a moving target in high-, middle- and low-income countries.

Delivery Method

In 1999, two studies (one randomized clinical trial and one metaanalysis) showed a decreased risk of vertical transmission of HIV with cesarean section before rupture of membranes or onset of labor (European Mode of Delivery Collaboration, 1999; International Perinatal HIV Group, 1999). This evidence was compelling enough for the ACOG to issue new guidelines in August 1999 recommending that all HIV positive pregnant women be offered elective cesarean at 38 completed weeks of gestation. The current ACOG recommendations, updated in 2000 and again in December 2010, recommend that all HIV-positive pregnant women with plasma viral loads greater than 1000 copies per milliliter be "counseled regarding the benefits of an elective cesarean delivery" in addition to a zidovudine infusion 3 hours before the operation (Jamieson et al, 2007). Currently, no study has answered whether elective cesarean delivery further decreases the risk of transmission in women with undetectable viral loads or in those receiving antiretroviral therapy.

Infant Feeding

In the United States, where replacement feeding (i.e., infant formula) is affordable and safe, it is recommended that HIV-positive mothers avoid breastfeeding entirely to minimize the estimated risk of 9% to 14% of postnatal HIV transmission through breast milk. Cell-associated HIV has been detected in human breast milk even among women receiving highly active antiretroviral therapy.

Globally, there is less clarity on best practices for infant feeding. When formula feeding is not affordable, feasible, acceptable, sustainable, and safe, then breastfeeding appears to be best for all infants of HIV-infected mothers. Current World Health Organization guidelines updated in 2010 recommend that mothers known to be HIV-infected either breastfeed and receive antiretroviral interventions or avoid all breastfeeding. The guidelines further clarify that feeding recommendations should be formulated at a national or subnational level based on local epidemiology and socioeconomic and infrastructure realities rather than trying to modify feeding recommendations for each individual mother (World Health Organization, 2010).

Data from a randomized controlled trial in Zambia showed that abrupt weaning at 4 months after birth versus

gradual weaning at the mother's time of choice (median, 16 months) yielded no difference in HIV-free survival at 24 months of age (Kuhn et al, 2008). Among children who became infected, early weaning increased mortality. This finding contrasts with data from Kenya that showed an increased risk of HIV transmission in breastfed infants at 24 months of age (37% risk of HIV infection in breastfed versus 21% risk in formula-fed infants; Nduati et al, 2000a). Most vertical transmission occurred during the first 6 months of breastfeeding, and the overall risk of transmission from breastfeeding was 16%. The 2-year all-cause mortality was similar between the two groups in this study.

Safety of breastfeeding in low-resource settings can be enhanced further by antiretroviral therapy for mothers, breastfeeding infants, or both. A synthesis of related studies was reviewed by Coovadia (2009). The mild-borne transmission of HIV-1C (MASHI) study in Botswana (Thior et al, 2006), the Six Week Extended-Dose Nevirapine study in India, Ethiopia, and Uganda (Six Week Extended-Dose Nevirapine Study Team et al, 2008), the post-exposure prophylaxis of infants (PEPI) study in Malawi (Kumwenda et al, 2008), and the Mitra study in Tanzania (Kilewo et al, 2008) have all assessed the utility of prophylactic antiretroviral agents in breastfeeding infants. There was variation in drug choice and duration, but most of these studies showed decreased vertical transmission in breastfeeding infants on some form of antiretroviral drug. A larger effect on vertical transmission, however, is observed from continuation of maternal antiretroviral therapy throughout the breastfeeding period. Maternal antiretroviral therapy in low-resource settings has decreased the vertical transmission rates during breastfeeding to 1% to 5% (Coovadia, 2009).

Evaluation and Treatment of HIV-Exposed Infants

Infant Testing

Infants born to HIV-infected mothers should have an initial serum evaluation by HIV-DNA or RNA PCR assay. This test is most sensitive if performed initially at 2 weeks of age; however, some physicians also do this testing in the first few days after birth to rule out in utero infection, particularly when the situation is high risk. High-risk situations would include unknown maternal HIV status with concerning history or known maternal HIV infection without prophylactic antiretroviral treatment. A negative test result in the first few days after birth requires confirmatory testing at a later time. Table 37-5 shows the recommended testing and evaluation schedule for an HIV-exposed infant (Havens et al, 2009).

If a mother's HIV status is unknown at the time of delivery, a rapid antibody test should be performed on mother or baby. Test results should be available within a few hours. If this test result is positive, prophylactic antiretroviral therapy should be initiated in the infant within 12 hours of birth, even in the absence of a confirmatory test.

Presumptive HIV-negative status of the infant is achieved with two negative tests results, one at 2 weeks old or later and the other at 4 weeks old or later. These are nucleic acid amplification tests (NAATs) and can be either DNA or RNA PCR. A definitive HIV-negative status is achieved

TABLE 37-5 Evaluation and Treatment of the Infant Exposed to HIV-1 (Birth to 18 Months of Age), in Addition to Routine Pediatric Care and Immunization

Action*	Birth	14 days	4 wk	6 wk	8 wk	4 mo	12-18 mo
History and physical examination†	X		X				
Assess risk of other infections	X						
Antiretroviral prophylaxis‡	X	X	X	X			
Recommend against breastfeeding	X	X	X	X	X	X	X
Hemoglobin or complete blood cell count	X		X§		X§		
HIV-1 DNA PCR or RNA assay¶	‖	X**	X		††	X	
Initiate PCP prophylaxis‡‡							
Enzyme immunoassay for antibody to HIV-1§§							X

From Havens PL et al: Evaluation and management of the infant exposed to HIV-1 in the United States, *Pediatrics* 123:175, 2009.

PCR, polymerase chain reaction; *PCP, Pneumocystis jirovechii* pneumonia;

*See text (in Havens et al, 2009) for detailed discussion of each action. If the infant has a diagnosis of HIV-1 infection during this period, laboratory monitoring and immunizations should follow guidelines for treatment of pediatric HIV infection.

†Review maternal health information for possible exposure to coinfections. Frequency of examinations is determined, in part, by frequency of visits for immunizations in infancy.

‡Antiretroviral prophylaxis is initiated as soon as possible after birth, but certainly within 12 hours. Zidovudine prophylaxis is continued for 6 weeks.

§Checked at 4 weeks by some experts and rechecked at 8 weeks if the week 4 hemoglobin level is significantly low.

¶All HIV-1–exposed infants should undergo virologic testing for HIV-1 with HIV-1 DNA PCR or RNA assays at 14 to 21 days of age and, if results are negative, repeated at 1 to 2 and 4 to 6 months of age to identify or exclude HIV-1 infection as early as possible. Any positive test result at any age is promptly repeated to confirm the diagnosis of HIV-1 infection.

‖HIV-1 DNA PCR or RNA assay testing in the first few days of life allows identification of in utero infection and might be considered if maternal antiretroviral agents were not administered during pregnancy or in other high-risk situations. A negative test result at this age requires repeated testing to exclude HIV-1 infection.

**If HIV-1 RNA or DNA testing of the newborn infant was not performed shortly after birth, or if such test results were negative, diagnostic testing with HIV-1 NAAT is delayed until 14 to 21 days of age, because the diagnostic sensitivity of virologic assays increases rapidly by the age of 2 weeks. A negative test result at this age requires repeated testing to exclude HIV-1 infection. *Presumptive uninfected* indicates negative nucleic acid amplification test (NAAT) result at ≥14 days and ≥4 weeks (1 month) of age; *definitive uninfected* indicates negative NAAT result at ≥1 and ≥4 months of age.

††No NAAT is needed at 8 weeks of age if previous test results at 2 and 4 weeks of age were negative. A single negative NAAT result at 8 weeks identifies a presumptively uninfected infant.

‡‡Infants with HIV-1 infection should be given PCP prophylaxis until 1 year of age, at which time infants are reassessed on the basis of age-specific CD4+ T-lymphocyte count and percentage thresholds. Infants with indeterminate HIV-1 infection status should receive prophylaxis starting at 4 to 6 weeks of age until they are deemed to be presumptively or definitively uninfected with HIV-1. Prophylaxis is not recommended for infants who meet criteria for presumptive or definitive lack of HIV-1 infection; therefore an NAAT at 2 and 4 weeks of age allows avoidance of PCP prophylaxis if both results are negative.

§§Many experts confirm the absence of HIV-1 infection with a negative HIV-1 antibody assay result at 12 to 18 months of age.

when a negative NAAT test obtained at 4 weeks old or later is added to a negative NAAT results from 4 months old or later (AAP Committee on Infectious Diseases, 2010b). Many clinicians will also obtain an antibody test at 12 to 18 months after birth. By this time, an HIV-negative infant should have cleared any passively acquired maternal antibodies and have a negative antibody test result, a process referred to as *seroreversion*. If the infant's antibody test is positive at this time, an NAAT test should be repeated in addition to close clinical evaluation for signs of infection.

Infant Treatment

Infants exposed to HIV should receive 6 weeks of prophylactic zidovudine (Table 37-6). It is important that families be given the entire quantity of medication at the time of hospital discharge to avoid challenges for compliance resulting from difficulty in filling a prescription (e.g., limited availability of the proper drug formulation, insurance coverage issues).

If the mother has a positive antibody test and received no intrapartum prophylactic zidovudine, some experts would consider early initiation of additional infant antiretroviral medication. However, a careful analysis of the pros and cons of potential toxicity versus decreased transmission risk is imperative. As stated by the Committee on Pediatric AIDS, "If infant prophylaxis with antiretroviral drugs in addition to ZDV is being considered, decisions

and choice of antiretroviral drugs should be determined in consultation with a practitioner who is experienced in care of infants with HIV infection," (American Academy of Pediatrics Committee on Pediatric AIDS, 2008).

If the infant has a positive NAAT test result before 6 weeks of age, antiretroviral treatment should be initiated immediately. As stated in *Red Book Online* (AAP Committee on Infectious Diseases, 2010b), "Initiation of antiretroviral therapy is recommended for all HIV-1-infected infants as soon as infection is confirmed, regardless of clinical, immunologic, or virologic parameters." Before initiation, however, it is recommended that infants have resistance testing, because infants can acquire resistant virus from their mothers. Extensive guidelines exist for selecting an appropriate combination drug regimen (available at: http://aidsinfo.nih.gov/ContentFiles/PediatricGuidelines.pdf). A specialist in the treatment of pediatric HIV infection should also be consulted. Although it was once thought that treatment with antiretroviral therapy should be delayed until an infant had signs of illness, it is now known that infected infants have a decreased mortality when treatment is started early. Several studies in South Africa have found that early antiretroviral therapy slowed disease progression, and one study found a 76% reduction in early infant mortality and a 75% reduction in HIV disease progression when antiretroviral therapy was initiated early (Violari et al, 2008).

TABLE 37-6 Intrapartum Maternal and Neonatal Zidovudine Dosing for Prevention of Mother-to-Child Transmission of HIV

Dosing	Duration
Maternal Intrapartum	
2 mg/kg IV over 1 hour, followed by continuous infusion of 1 mg/kg/h	Onset of labor until delivery
Neonatal	
>35 weeks' gestation: 2 mg/kg by mouth[*],[†] (or 1.5 mg/kg IV) started within 6-12 h of delivery, then every 6 h	Birth to 6 wk
30-35 weeks' gestation: 2 mg/kg by mouth (or 1.5 mg/kg IV) started within 6-12 h of delivery, then every 12 h, advanced to every 8 h at 2 weeks of age	Birth to 6 wk
<30 weeks' gestation: 2 mg/kg by mouth (or 1.5 mg/kg IV) started within 6-12 h of delivery, then every 12 h, advanced to every 8 h at 4 weeks of age	Birth to 6 wk

From Panel on Treatment of HIV-Infected Pregnant Women and Prevention of Perinatal Transmission: [Perinatal Guidelines] *Recommendations for use of antiretroviral drugs in pregnant HIV-1-infected women for maternal health and interventions to reduce perinatal HIV transmission in the United States*, May 24, 2010; pp 1-117. http://aidsinfo.nih.gov/ContentFiles/PerinatalGL.pdf. Accessed November 22, 2010.

IV, Intravenous.

*Zidovudine dosing of 4 mg/kg given every 12 h has been used for infant prophylaxis in some international perinatal studies. Although there are no definitive data to show equivalent pharmacokinetic parameters or efficacy in preventing transmission, a regimen of zidovudine 4 mg/kg by mouth twice daily instead of 2 mg/kg by mouth four times daily may be considered when there are concerns about adherence to drug administration to the infant.

†A simplified zidovudine dosing regimen has been developed for use in low resource settings. This regimen consists of 10 mg by mouth twice daily for infants weighing less than 2.5 kg at birth and 15 mg twice daily for infants weighing more than 2.5 kg at birth. This regimen could be considered for infants in higher resource settings born after 35 weeks' gestation if simplicity in zidovudine dosing and administration is of prime importance.

Prophylaxis with trimethoprim-sulfamethoxazole against opportunistic infections should also be initiated in any infant with possible HIV infection at 6 weeks of age and continued until at least 1 year of age. With a presumptive HIV-negative diagnosis, prophylaxis can be deferred. Although the occurrence of opportunistic infections has declined with more widespread access to testing and antiretroviral therapy, *Pneumocystis jirovechii* pneumonia remains a common serious opportunistic infection in HIV-1–infected infants, responsible for one third of pediatric AIDS diagnoses (AAP Committee on Infectious Diseases, 2010b). A Cochrane review that evaluated a study in HIV-positive Zambian children found a 33% reduction in mortality among children receiving cotrimoxazole prophylaxis versus placebo (Grimwade and Swingler, 2006).

Side Effects of Antiretroviral Therapy Exposure in Infants

Antiretroviral therapy has been overwhelmingly successful in the prevention of vertical transmission of HIV, but few human studies have assessed drug safety and toxicity in infants (Thorne and Newell, 2007). Most antiretroviral drugs are pregnancy category B or C; however, efavirenz was changed to a D classification in 2005 when an association with infants with neural tube defects was seen (De Santis et al, 2002; Fundarò et al, 2002).

A few case reports of mitochondrial toxicity (hyperlactatemia, some with additional motor or cognitive symptoms) in HIV-uninfected, antiretroviral therapy–exposed infants have come from Europe (Blanche et al, 1999; Noguera et al, 2004; Tovo et al, 2005). Some of the symptoms resolved or improved with time. However, large cohort studies in the United States have not shown excess death owing to mitochondrial dysfunction, although they might be underpowered to detect mild dysfunction.

One study done in Malawi showed a hypersensitivity reaction, primarily consisting of a rash, in 16 of 852 (1.9%) infants treated with nevirapine for 28 weeks. This reaction was not seen in the control group, which received only 1 week of zidovudine and lamivudine (Chasela et al, 2010).

Studies are inconsistent regarding the risk of prematurity in antiretroviral therapy–exposed infants. European studies have shown an increased risk of prematurity in infants born to mothers receiving antiretroviral therapy regimens containing a protease-inhibitor drug (European Collaborative Study and Swiss Mother and Child HIV Cohort Study, 2000; Thorne et al, 2004). Some U.S. studies have not confirmed this association; however, a U.S. study confirmed a significantly increased risk of very low birthweight in infants born to women receiving protease-inhibitor–containing antiretroviral therapy versus other combination antiretroviral therapy (adjusted odds ratio, 3.56) (Tuomala et al, 2002).

Several studies have identified anemia in infants exposed to prophylactic zidovudine; typically it is mild and transient, but occasionally severe anemia develops (Connor et al, 1994; Taha et al, 2002; Wiktor et al, 1999). Slightly longer term effects were seen in a French study in which decreased levels of platelets, lymphocytes, and neutrophils were persistent in the treatment group after adjusting for several factors, including maternal CD4+ count and prematurity (Le Chenadec et al, 2003). Two European studies have found neutropenia in children exposed to antiretroviral therapy up to 8 years of age (Bunders et al, 2005; European Collaborative Study, 2004). These effects are of uncertain clinical significance, but as prenatal and postnatal antiretroviral therapy exposure increases in duration and number of drugs, studies to assess both subtle and significant sequelae in exposed infants will be crucial.

Special Case of HIV-Exposed Uninfected Infants

An increasing area of research is focused on HIV-exposed, uninfected (HIV-EU) infants. HIV-EU infants may be at increased risk of death and morbidity. One study demonstrated a fivefold increased risk of death to the infant after the death of an HIV-infected mother (Newell et al, 2004). Other studies have found no increase in morbidity among HIV-EU infants when compared with unexposed infants (Taha et al, 2000). Whereas these findings may simply reflect different levels of background disease burden among vulnerable children when their mother is ill or dead, there may be an additional immunologic effect on the infant from the mother's HIV infection. In rural Kenya, a study of tetanus antibody levels found a 22% reduction in cord:maternal ratio of tetanus antibodies after adjusting for maternal vaccination and other factors in infants born to HIV-positive mothers. An even greater reduction in infant antibody titers was seen with maternal HIV and malaria coinfection (Cumberland et al, 2007). A large study in Zambia found that HIV-EU infants had twice the risk of death or severe morbidity when the mother's CD4+ T-cell counts were low even when controlling for maternal mortality, separation due to maternal hospitalization, lower birthweight, and other factors (Kuhn et al, 2005). Another study documented an increase in mortality and morbidity (e.g., respiratory infections) in HIV-EU infants over community baseline in Latin America and the Carribean (Mussi-Pinhata et al, 2007). All these studies are, however, limited by lack of a control group of unexposed infants in the same study setting. Early evidence supporting the possibility of impaired neonatal immunity in HIV-EU infants needs further investigation.

CONCLUSION

Pediatric HIV infection has become a disease of the developing world, where more than 90% of HIV-exposed and more than 98% of HIV-infected children live. Without therapy, morbidity and mortality are high for all HIV-infected individuals and are worse for children. Exposed, uninfected children face the virtual certainty of becoming orphans by their tenth birthdays and a 50% chance of some day becoming infected.

HIV transmission is preventable, whether sexual, vertical, or parenteral. Progression to AIDS and death is also preventable. Although the arrest of all HIV transmission remains an unfulfilled goal, potent antiretroviral combination therapy has dramatically decreased AIDS deaths and virtually eliminated vertical transmission of the virus in the United States and other high-income countries. Vigilance in researching sustainable prevention measures and continued advocacy at national and international levels can arrest HIV transmission worldwide.

SUGGESTED READINGS

Branson BM, Handsfield HH, Lampe MA, et al: Revised recommendations for HIV testing of adults, adolescents, and pregnant women in health-care settings, *MMWR Recomm Rep* 55:1, 2006.

Centers for Disease Control and Prevention: *HIV Surveillance Report 20, 2008.* Available at www.cdc.gov/hiv/topics/surveillance/resources/reports/. Accessed November 24, 2010.

Cheeran MC, Lokensgard JR, Schleiss MR: Neuropathogenesis of congenital cytomegalovirus infection: disease mechanisms and prospects for intervention, *Clin Microbiol Rev* 22:99-126, 2009.

Coovadia H: Current issues in prevention of mother-to-child transmission of HIV-1, *Curr Opin HIV AIDS* 4:319, 2009.

Corey L, Wald A: Maternal and neonatal HSV infections, *N Engl J Med* 361:1376-1385, 2009.

Corey L, Wald A, Celum CL, et al: The effects of herpes simplex virus-2 on HIV-1 acquisition and transmission: a review of two overlapping epidemics, *J Acquir Immune Defic Syndr* 35:435, 2004.

Ergaz Z, Ornoy A: Parovirus B19 in pregnancy, *Reprod Toxicol* 21:421-435, 2006.

Fiore S, Savasi V: Treatment of viral hepatitis in pregnancy, *Expert Opin Pharmacother* 10:2801-2809, 2009.

Hall CB, Weinberg GA, Iwane MK, et al: The burden of respiratory syncytial virus infection in young children, *N Engl J Med* 360:588-598, 2009.

Hall CB, Caserta MT, Schnabel KC, et al: Transplacental congenital human herpesvirus 6 infection caused by maternal chromosomally integrated virus, *J Infect Dis* 201:505-507, 2010.

Hawkes MT, Vaudry W: Nonpolio enterovirus infection in the neonate and young infant, *Paediatr Child Health* 10:383-388, 2005.

Kimberlin DW: Advances in the treatment of neonatal herpes simplex infections, *Rev Med Virol* 11:157-163, 2001.

Lee JY, Bowden DS: Rubella virus replication and links to teratogenicity, *Clin Microbiol Rev* 13:571-587, 2000.

Nassetta L, Kimberlin D, Whitley R: Treatment of congenital cytomegalovirus infection: implications for future therapeutic strategies, *J Antimicrob Chemother* 63:862-867, 2009.

Palumbo P, Lindsey JC, Hughes MD, et al: Antiretroviral treatment for children with peripartum nevirapine exposure, *N Engl J Med* 363:1510, 2010.

Panel on Antiretroviral Therapy and Medical Management of HIV-Infected Children: *Guidelines for the use of antiretroviral agents in pediatric HIV infection,* 2010, pp 1-219. Available at http://aidsinfo.nih.gov/ContentFiles/PediatricGuidelines.pdf. Accessed November 22, 2010.

Panel on Treatment of HIV-Infected Pregnant Women and Prevention of Perinatal Transmission: *Recommendations for use of antiretroviral drugs in pregnant HIV-1-infected women for maternal health and interventions to reduce perinatal HIV transmission in the United States,* 2010, pp 1-117. Available at http://aidsinfo.nih.gov/ContentFiles/PerinatalGL.pdf. Accessed November 22, 2010.

Plotkin SA: The history of rubella and rubella vaccination leading to elimination, *Clin Infect Dis* 43(Suppl 3):S164-S168, 2006.

Prevention of respiratory syncytial virus infections: Indications for the use of palivizumab and update on the use of RSV-IGIV. Committee on Infectious Diseases and Committee of Fetus and Newborn, *Pediatrics* 102:1211-1216, 1998.

Smith CK, Arvin AM: Varicella in the fetus and newborn, *Semin Fetal Neonatal Med* 14:209-217, 2009.

Stagno S: Breastfeeding and the transmission of cytomegalovirus infections, *Ital J Pediatr* 28:275-280, 2002.

Thorne C, Newell ML: Safety of agents used to prevent mother-to-child transmission of HIV: is there any cause for concern? *Drug Saf* 30:203, 2007.

Violari A, Coton MF, Gibb DM, et al: CHER Study Team: Early antiretroviral therapy and mortality among HIV-infected infants, *N Engl J Med* 359:2233, 2008.

Volmink J, Siegfried NL, van der Merwe L, et al: Antiretrovirals for reducing the risk of mother-to-child transmission of HIV infection, *Cochrane Database Syst Rev* 1:CD003510, 2007.

World Health Organization: *Towards universal access: scaling up priority HIV/AIDS interventions in the health sector. Progress Report 2008.* Available at www.who.int/hiv/pub/2008progressreport/en/. Accessed November 22, 2010.

World Health Organization: *Guidelines on HIV and infant feeding 2010. Principles and recommendations for infant feeding in the context of HIV and a summary of evidence.* 2010. Available at www.who.int/child_adolescent_health/documents/9789241599535/en/index.html.

Complete references and supplemental color images used in this text can be found online at www.expertconsult.com

TOXOPLASMOSIS, SYPHILIS, MALARIA, AND TUBERCULOSIS

Pablo J. Sánchez, Janna C. Patterson, and Amina Ahmed

TOXOPLASMOSIS

Toxoplasmosis is the disease state that results from infection with the obligate protozoan parasite *Toxoplasma gondii*. *T. gondii* is a coccidian that is ubiquitous in nature, and the cat is the definitive host. The organism exists in the following three forms:

1. An oocyst that is shed in cat feces from sporozoites formed within the cat's intestinal tract
2. A tachyzoite or endozoite that is the proliferative form and was formerly referred to as a *trophozoite*
3. A tissue cyst that has an intracystic form termed *cystozoite* or *bradyzoite*.

Nonfeline mammals or birds ingest infective oocysts from contaminated soil. Tissue cysts then accumulate in the organs and skeletal muscle of these animals. The possible routes of transmission from animal to human are direct contact with cat feces, ingestion of undercooked meat containing infective cysts, and ingestion of fruits or vegetables that have been in contaminated soil. Congenital infection results from placental infection and subsequent hematogenous spread to the fetus.

EPIDEMIOLOGY

Toxoplasmosis is a worldwide medical problem. High prevalence of infection has been documented in Europe, Central and Latin America, and parts of Africa. However, seroprevalence rates differ considerably from one country to another, from one region of a country to another, and even from one ethnic group to another in the same region. These widely disparate seroprevalence rates among different adult populations throughout the world have been explained by differences in eating and sanitation practices that contribute to acquisition of infection. Eating undercooked or raw meat or unwashed raw fruits and vegetables, drinking unpasteurized goat's milk, working with meat, having three or more kittens, and even certain climactic conditions have been associated with higher risks of infection (Jones et al, 2009).

Among women of childbearing age in the United States, the prevalence of antibody to *T. gondii* varies from approximately 3% to 30%, depending on the region of the country (Boyer and McAuley, 1994; Remington et al, 2001). The lowest seroprevalence rates have been found in the Mountain and Pacific states, and the highest rates have been seen in the Northeastern and Southeastern United States. Seroprevalence rates for pregnant women seem to be decreasing, although regional and ethnic differences persist.

The prevalence of congenital infection in Massachusetts and New Hampshire has been documented to be 0.08 per 1000 births through immunoglobulin (Ig) M screening of newborn blood specimens collected on filter paper (Guerina et al, 1994). This finding compares with a rate of 3 to 10 per 1000 live births in Paris and Vienna, where maternal seroprevalence rates of approximately 70% and 40%, respectively, are observed. In Massachusetts, a case-control study involving 14 years of newborn screening for congenital toxoplasmosis found that the mother's birth outside the United States, particularly in Cambodia and Laos, as well as the mother's educational level and higher gravidity were strongly predictive of congenital infection (Jara et al, 2001). With approximately 4 million live births annually in the United States, there are an estimated 400 to 4000 babies born each year with congenital toxoplasmosis (Feldman et al, 2010).

NATURAL HISTORY

Infection of the fetus occurs as a consequence of maternal primary infection during pregnancy or, rarely, just before conception (Villena et al, 1998b). Reactivation of latent *T. gondii* infection during pregnancy does not lead to fetal infection, except among immunocompromised women such as those infected with the human immunodeficiency virus (HIV) or those undergoing chemotherapy (Bachmeyer et al, 2006; Dunn et al, 1997; European Collaborative Study, 1996; Langer, 1983; Mitchell et al, 1990; O'Donohoe et al, 1991; Remington et al, 2001). Under these circumstances, however, the risk is low. In addition, maternal reinfection can result in congenital toxoplasmosis (Gavinet et al, 1997; Hennequin et al, 1997). Acute maternal infection, which is usually acquired early in pregnancy, can lead to fulminant fetal infection resulting in stillbirth, nonimmune fetal hydrops, preterm birth, and perinatal death (Wong and Remington, 1994); however, chronic *T. gondii* infection rarely has been associated with sporadic abortion (Remington et al, 1964).

Infection of the fetus occurs transplacentally during maternal parasitemia. Placental infection is an important intermediary step, and up to 16 weeks may elapse between placental infection and subsequent infection of the fetus. This time delay has been termed the *prenatal incubation period* (Remington et al, 2001). Congenital toxoplasmosis has occurred in twins and triplets (Couvreur et al, 1991; Sibalic et al, 1986; Wiswell et al, 1984). The clinical manifestations are usually similar in monozygotic twins, whereas discrepancies in clinical findings are common in dizygotic twins.

Approximately 40% of infants born to mothers who acquired toxoplasmosis during pregnancy are infected with *T. gondii*. The rate of vertical transmission varies according to the trimester in which the mother became infected, with fetal infection rates increasing as pregnancy advances (Dunn et al, 1999; Remington et al, 2001; Wong and Remington, 1994). Specifically, when maternal infection occurs in the first trimester, 15% of infants are infected, whereas maternal infection in the second and third trimesters results in transmission rates of 30% and 60%, respectively. The severity of clinical manifestations is greatest, however, when maternal infection is acquired early in pregnancy. Maternal infection in the first trimester results in severe disease in as many as 40% of infected fetuses, and in still birth or perinatal death in an additional 35% of infants. Approximately 15% of newborns have subclinical disease; however, maternal infection in the third trimester is rarely if ever associated with severe fetal disease or still birth, and approximately 90% of infants in such situations have subclinical infection.

Postnatally, transmission of *T. gondii* can occur from transfusion of blood or blood products or from transplantation of organ or bone marrow from a seropositive donor with latent infection. Although the organism has been detected in human milk, transmission by breastfeeding has not been documented.

The majority of newborns with congenital toxoplasmosis lack clinical signs of infection, although thorough evaluation may demonstrate eye or neurologic abnormalities in approximately 20% of cases. Clinically apparent disease is present in approximately 10% to 25% of infected infants (Alford et al, 1969, 1974; Guerina et al, 1994). The clinical manifestations of toxoplasmosis are often indistinguishable from those seen with other congenital infections, such as cytomegalic inclusion disease and congenital syphilis. Approximately one third of infants have a generalized form of the disease that principally involves organs of the reticuloendothelial system. The abnormalities include temperature instability, hepatosplenomegaly, jaundice, pneumonitis, generalized lymphadenopathy, rash, chorioretinitis, anemia, thrombocytopenia, eosinophilia, and abnormal cerebrospinal fluid (CSF) indices (Table 38-1; Boyer and McAuley, 1994; Eichenwald, 1960). The other two thirds of infected infants principally manifest neurologic disease.

Central nervous system involvement is the hallmark of congenital *T. gondii* infection (Diebler et al, 1985; McAuley et al, 1994; Remington et al, 2001). Chorioretinitis, intracranial calcifications, and hydrocephalus are the most characteristic findings, occurring in approximately 86%, 37%, and 20% of symptomatic infants, respectively (see Table 38-1) (Boyer and McAuley, 1994; Eichenwald, 1960; Remington et al, 2001). This constellation of findings has been referred to as the *classic triad of congenital toxoplasmosis;* its presence should alert the clinician to the diagnosis. Intracranial calcifications may be single or multiple, but typically are generalized and located in the caudate nucleus, choroid plexus, meninges, and subependyma (Müssbichler, 1968); they also may occur periventricularly, as in cytomegalovirus infection. They are visualized best by computed tomography (CT), but are often detected on ultrasonography as well. Intracranial calcifications may resolve with appropriate antimicrobial therapy (McAuley et al, 1994). Hydrocephalus may be the only manifestation of disease; it results from the extensive periaqueductal and periventricular vasculitis with necrosis that causes obstruction of the ventricular system. Ventriculoperitoneal shunting is often required (Martinovic et al, 1982; McAuley et al, 1994). Abnormalities of the CSF are common; characteristically, they consist of lymphocytic pleocytosis

TABLE 38-1 Clinical Findings Among Infants With Congenital Toxoplasmosis

Finding	Infants with Findings (%)	
	Neurologic Disease* (108 Cases)	Generalized Disease† (44 Cases)
Chorioretinitis	94	66
Abnormal cerebrospinal fluid	55	84
Anemia	51	77
Convulsions	50	18
Intracranial calcification	50	4
Jaundice	29	80
Hydrocephalus	28	0
Fever	25	77
Splenomegaly	21	90
Lymphadenopathy	17	68
Hepatomegaly	17	77
Vomiting	16	48
Microcephaly	13	0
Diarrhea	6	25
Cataracts	5	0
Eosinophilia	4	18
Abnormal bleeding	3	18
Hypothermia	2	20
Glaucoma	2	0
Optic atrophy	2	0
Microphthalmia	2	0
Rash	1	25
Pneumonitis	0	41

Adapted from Remington JS, McLeod R, Thulliez P, Desmonts G: Toxoplasmosis. In Remington JS, Klein JO, editors: *Infectious diseases of the fetus and newborn infant,* ed 5, Philadelphia, 2001, WB Saunders, p 246.
*Infants with otherwise undiagnosed central nervous system diseases in the first year of life.
†Infants with otherwise undiagnosed non-neurologic diseases during the first 2 months of life.

and a markedly elevated protein content. Microcephaly, when present, indicates severe brain injury. Hypothermia and hyperthermia may occur secondary to hypothalamic involvement. *T. gondii* has been detected in the inner ear and mastoid, with the associated inflammation resulting in deafness. An ascending flaccid paralysis with myelitis has also been reported (Campbell et al, 2001).

Chorioretinitis secondary to congenital toxoplasmosis can manifest at any age. It usually manifests as strabismus in infants. Defects in visual acuity are more common in older children. Typically the eye lesion consists of a focal necrotizing retinitis that is often bilateral with involvement of the macula and even the optic nerve. Complications include blindness, iridocyclitis, and cataracts (Arun et al, 2007; Phan et al, 2008).

Other less common manifestations of congenital toxoplasmosis are nonimmune hydrops fetalis, myocarditis, nephrotic syndrome, and immunoglobulin abnormalities with both hypergammaglobulinemia and hypogammaglobulinemia described. Bony abnormalities consisting of metaphyseal lucencies similar to those seen in congenital syphilis have also been reported (Milgram, 1974). A variety of endocrine abnormalities may occur, including hypothyroidism, diabetes insipidus (Oygur et al, 1998; Yamakawa et al, 1996), precocious puberty, and growth hormone deficiency.

DIAGNOSIS

Isolation of *T. gondii* from body fluids and tissues provides definitive evidence of infection. The organism can be isolated from placenta, amniotic fluid, fetal blood obtained by cordocentesis, umbilical cord blood, infant peripheral blood, and CSF by means of intraperitoneal and subcutaneous inoculation into laboratory mice (Foulon et al, 1999a; Remington et al, 2001; Wong and Remington, 1994). Mouse inoculation may require as long as 4 to 6 weeks for demonstration of the parasite. Although it is not a practical method, isolation of the organism should be attempted whenever possible. It is available at the *Toxoplasma* Serology Laboratory, Palo Alto Medical Foundation (860 Bryant Street, Palo Alto, California 94301; telephone: 415-326-8120). In addition, tissue culture has been used to isolate *T. gondii* from amniotic fluid.

Histopathologic examination of the placenta and tissues obtained at postmortem examination or by biopsy from stillborns or infants should be performed because the specimens may demonstrate the presence of tachyzoites. In addition, tachyzoites have been demonstrated in CSF, ventricular fluid, and aqueous humor by specialized staining techniques.

Polymerase chain reaction (PCR) analysis has been used successfully to detect *T. gondii* DNA in amniotic fluid, placenta, CSF, brain, urine, and fetal and infant blood (Foulon et al, 1999a; Fricker-Hidalgo et al, 1998; Grover et al, 1990; Guy et al, 1996; Hohlfeld et al, 1994; Jenum et al, 1998; Romand et al, 2001). PCR performed on amniotic fluid obtained by amniocentesis has become the preferred method of confirming in utero infection (Kasper et al, 2009). False-negative results have been reported, however, and interlaboratory variability in performance of PCR assays has been documented (Guy et al, 1996; Romand et al, 2001). PCR performed on neonatal CSF is recommended for the evaluation of possible central nervous system involvement.

Serologic assays for measurement of antibodies to *T. gondii* in serum and body fluids are the most widely used methods of diagnosing congenital toxoplasmosis (Boyer, 2001; Boyer and McAuley, 1994; Dannemann et al, 1990; Foudrinier et al, 1995; Guerina et al, 1994; Lappalainen et al, 1993; Madi et al, 2010; Naessens et al, 1999; Naot et al, 1991; Pinon et al, 2001; Rabilloud et al, 2010; Remington et al, 1985; Robert-Gangneux, 2001; Robert-Gangneux, 1999a, 1999b; Villena et al, 1999; Wong and Remington, 1994). These tests are commercially available at the *Toxoplasma* Serology Laboratory. The more commonly used tests that detect *T. gondii*-specific IgG antibodies are the Sabin-Feldman dye test, which is considered the gold standard but requires live organisms, indirect immunofluorescent antibody test, IgG enzyme-linked immunosorbent assay (ELISA), direct agglutination, and IgG avidity test.

In addition, a differential agglutination test has been developed as a confirmatory test to differentiate acute from chronic maternal infection. This test compares the IgG serologic titer obtained with the use of formalin-fixed tachyzoites (HS antigen) with those obtained with acetone- or methanol-fixed tachyzoites (AC antigen). The latter preparation contains stage-specific *T. gondii* antigens that are recognized by IgG antibodies only during early infection. An additional assay to assist in ruling out maternal infection acquired in the first 3 months of pregnancy is the IgG avidity test performed by the ELISA technique. This test is based on the principle that, although the antibody-binding avidity or affinity for an antigen is initially low after primary antigenic stimulation, IgG antibodies that are present from previous antigenic stimulation are usually of high avidity. Therefore a high-avidity result in the first trimester would exclude an infection acquired in the previous 12 weeks. Finally, an enzyme-linked immunofiltration assay has been developed that allows discrimination between IgG antibodies of maternal origin and IgG synthesized by the fetus as well as identification of antibody subtypes in infected neonates (Zufferey et al, 1999).

Tests that detect *T. gondii*-specific IgM are (1) the double-sandwich IgM ELISA, which has a sensitivity of 75% to 80% and a specificity of 100% (Guerina et al, 1994); (2) the IgM immunosorbent agglutination assay, which is the most sensitive test but should not be performed on umbilical cord blood, because even small quantities of maternal IgM antibodies contaminating the specimen will yield a false-positive result (Boyer and McAuley, 1994); and (3) the IgM immunofluorescent antibody test. The last test is not recommended because it has a much lower sensitivity than either the IgM ELISA or IgM immunosorbent agglutination assay and it has poor specificity secondary to rheumatoid factors and antinuclear antibodies, contributing to false-positive results. Other tests that are still being investigated include a *T. gondii*-specific IgA ELISA and IgA immunofiltration assay; a *T. gondii*-specific IgE immunofiltration assay; and IgG, IgM, and IgA immunoblotting tests.

Because the majority of adults with acquired *T. gondii* infection are asymptomatic, evaluation of the pregnant woman and fetus is usually prompted by either seroconversion or an elevated maternal *Toxoplasma* spp. IgG titer (Couvreur et al, 1988; Daffos et al, 1988; Montoya et al, 2008). The latter may reflect chronic or past infection; therefore the acuity of the maternal infection is determined serologically with the HS-AC differential agglutination test where agglutination titers to formalin-fixed tachyzoites (HS antigen) are compared with titers against acetone- or methanol-fixed tachyzoites (AC antigen). In general, an acute pattern demonstrates high AC and HS titers, while a nonacute pattern demonstrates high AC titers and low HS titers. This method can differentiate an acute from a remote infection in pregnant women, whereas IgM and IgA antibodies detectable by ELISA or ISAGA are elevated for prolonged periods. If recent maternal infection is documented by an acute pattern on the HS-AC test, seroconversion, or rising IgG antibody titers, the fetus should be evaluated by ultrasonography, and amniotic fluid should be tested for specific *Toxoplasma* spp. DNA with PCR. PCR has supplanted the need for cordocentesis, and a positive result confirms fetal infection (Hohlfeld et al, 1994). Postnatally, serologic testing of paired maternal and infant sera should be performed at a reliable laboratory that will include assays for *Toxoplasma* spp. IgG and IgM antibodies.

Neonatal serum for *Toxoplasma* spp. IgA determination by ELISA also should be considered, because it may yield the only positive result in some infants.

Subinoculation of placental tissue, amniotic fluid, and umbilical cord blood into mice should be considered. If results of these tests suggest possible infection, the newborn should be evaluated fully with complete blood cell count and platelet determination, liver function tests, CSF evaluation (including tests for IgG and IgM antibodies and PCR;) (Wallon et al, 1998), cranial ultrasound or CT imaging of the head, ophthalmologic examination, and hearing evaluation. The presence of neonatal IgM antibody in serum or CSF, or a positive PCR result for blood or CSF, indicates congenital infection. In addition, at-risk infants should undergo serologic follow-up to detect rising serum IgG titers during the 1st year of age or persistence of IgG antibody beyond 12 to 15 months of age, when maternal IgG antibody has disappeared (Robert-Gangneux et al, 1999a, 1999b). Uninfected infants show a continuous decline in *T. gondii* IgG titer with no detectable IgM or IgA antibodies.

Low IgG titers and an HS-AC differential agglutination test that indicate remote maternal infection do not require further evaluation of the mother or infant unless the mother is infected with HIV. Because fetal infection has occurred during chronic *T. gondii* infection in HIV-infected pregnant women, their infants should be evaluated serologically at birth for evidence of congenital infection. It has been suggested that HIV-infected pregnant women who have low CD4+ T lymphocyte counts and who are seropositive for *T. gondii* antibody receive prophylaxis to prevent fetal infection (Beaman et al, 1992; Wong and Remington, 1994). However, insufficient data currently are available to recommend that such therapy be given routinely for this indication. Nevertheless, if such women previously have had toxoplasmic encephalitis, prophylaxis with pyrimethamine, sulfadiazine, and leucovorin (folinic acid) should be considered (Masur et al, 2002).

THERAPY

It is currently recommended that fetuses and infants younger than 1 year who are infected with *T. gondii* receive specific therapy effective against this congenital pathogen, even if they have no clinical signs of disease (Couvreur et al, 1988; Daffos et al, 1988; Foulon et al, 1999b; Friedman et al, 1999; Gilbert et al, 2001; Hohlfeld et al, 1989; Koppe et al, 1986; McAuley et al, 1994; McGee et al, 1992; McLeod et al, 2009; Peyron and Wallon, 2001; Roizen et al, 1995; Vergani et al, 1998; Wallon et al, 1999; Wong and Remington, 1994). On the basis of comparison with untreated historical controls, outcome is improved substantially by neonatal treatment. The effectiveness of maternal and fetal treatment is less clear. Spiramycin has been used in pregnant women with acute toxoplasmosis to reduce transplacental transmission of *T. gondii*. If fetal infection is confirmed after the 17th week of pregnancy, however, treatment with pyrimethamine, sulfadiazine, and folinic acid is recommended. Prenatal treatment of congenital toxoplasmosis is believed to reduce the clinical severity of infection in the newborn while shifting the disease to a more subclinical form. This effect in turn may ameliorate the long-term neurologic complications that

are commonly seen among infants who have clinical manifestations in the neonatal period. A recent metaanalysis of the effectiveness of prenatal treatment of toxoplasmosis infection found no evidence that such treatment significantly decreased clinical manifestations of disease in infected infants (Thiebaut et al, 2007).

Neonatal treatment has also resulted in reductions in sensorineural hearing loss and neurodevelopmental and visual handicaps. Table 38-2 shows the recommended guidelines for the treatment of congenital toxoplasmosis. In infants with congenital toxoplasmosis, the treatment consists of pyrimethamine, sulfadiazine, and folinic acids (Boyer and McAuley, 1994; McAuley et al, 1994; McLeod et al, 1992; Remington et al, 2001). The actual duration of therapy is not known, although prolonged courses of at least 1 year are preferred. Currently most experts recommend combined treatment until the patient is 1 year old (Remington et al, 2001; Villena et al, 1998a, 1998b).

Complete blood cell counts and platelet determination must be monitored closely while the patient is receiving therapy, because granulocytopenia, thrombocytopenia, and megaloblastic anemia can occur. These parameters usually improve once a higher dose of folinic acid is administered or pyrimethamine and sulfadiazine are discontinued temporarily. The indications for adjunctive therapy with corticosteroids such as prednisone (0.5 mg/kg twice per day) are CSF protein concentration 1 g/dL or higher and chorioretinitis that threatens vision; corticosteroid treatment is continued until either condition resolves. Current therapies are not effective against encysted bradyzoites and therefore might not prevent reactivation of chorioretinitis and neurologic disease.

PROGNOSIS

Maternal toxoplasmosis acquired during the first and second trimesters has been associated with still birth and perinatal death secondary to severe fetal infection in approximately 35% and 7% of cases, respectively. Among infants born with congenital toxoplasmosis, the mortality rate has been reported to be as high as 12%. In addition, infants with congenital toxoplasmosis are at high risk for ophthalmologic, neurodevelopmental, and audiologic impairments, including mental retardation (87%), seizures (82%), spasticity and palsies (71%), and deafness (15%) (Eichenwald, 1960; Hohlfeld et al, 1989; Koppe et al, 1986; McAuley et al, 1994). Of neonates with subclinical infection, long-term follow-up reveals eye or neurologic disease in as many as 80% to 90% by the time they reach adulthood (Couvreur and Desmonts, 1962; Couvreur et al, 1984; McLeod et al, 2000; Saxon et al, 1973; Wilson et al, 1980). Data from the United States National Collaborative Treatment Trial show that treatment of neonates with congenital toxoplasmosis early and for 1 year resulted in more favorable outcomes than were reported for untreated infants or infants who were treated for only 1 month.

PREVENTION

Pregnant women whose serologic status for *T. gondii* is negative or unknown, as well as women who are attempting to conceive, should be educated on the prevention

TABLE 38-2 Treatment Guidelines for Toxoplasmosis

Condition	Therapy	Dose (Oral Unless Specified)	Duration
Pregnant woman with acute toxoplasmosis	Spiramycin for first 21 wk of gestation or until term if fetus not infected*	1 g every 8 h without food	Until fetal infection documented or excluded at 21 wks; if fetal infection documented, replaced with pyrimethamine, leucovorin, and sulfadiazine (see below)
	Pyrimethamine (if fetal infection confirmed after 18th week of gestation or if infection acquired in last few weeks of gestation) *and*	Loading dose: 100 mg/day in two divided doses for 2 days followed by 50 mg/day	Until delivery
	Sulfadiazine* *and*	Loading dose: 75 mg/kg/day in two divided doses (maximum, 4 g/d) for 2 days; then 100 mg/kg/day in two divided doses (maximum, 4 g/day)	Until delivery
	Leucovorin†	10-20 mg/d	Until delivery
Congenital *Toxoplasma gondii* infection in infant	Pyrimethamine *and*	Loading dose: 2 mg/kg/day for 2 days; then 1 mg/kg/day for 2 or 6 months; then 1 mg/kg/day on Mon, Wed, and Fri each week	≥1 yr
	Sulfadiazine* *and*	100 mg/kg/day in 2 daily divided doses	≥1 yr
	Leucovorin (folinic acid)†	10 mg 3 times weekly	≥1 yr
	Corticosteroids (prednisone)‡	1 mg/kg/daily in 2 daily divided doses	Until resolution of elevated (≥1 g/dL) CSF protein or active chorioretinitis that threatens vision

Data from Boyer KM, McAuley B: Congenital toxoplasmosis, *Semin Pediatr Dis* 5:42, 1994; and Remington JS, McLeod R, Thulliez P, Desmonts G: Toxoplasmosis. In Remington JS, Klein JO, editors: *Infectious diseases of the fetus and newborn infant*, ed 5, Philadelphia, 2001, WB Saunders, p 293.
CSF, Cerebrospinal fluid.
*Available only on request from the U.S. Food and Drug Administration (301-827-2127; fax, 301-927-2475).
†Monitor blood and platelet counts weekly; adjust dosage for megaloblastic anemia, granulocytopenia, or thrombocytopenia.
‡When signs of inflammation or active chorioretinitis have subsided, dose can be tapered and eventually discontinued; use only in conjunction with pyrimethamine, sulfadiazine, and leucovorin.

of congenital toxoplasmosis through avoidance of at-risk behaviors that may expose them to cat feces or encysted bradyzoites in raw meat (Centers for Disease Control and Prevention, 2000; Eskild et al, 1996; Foulon et al, 2000; Jones et al, 2001; Wilson and Remington, 1980). Such women should be taught to wear gloves when changing cat litter boxes or gardening and to wash hands after such activities. Daily changing of cat litter will also decrease the chance of infection, because oocysts are not infective during the first 1 to 2 days after passage. In addition, feeding cats commercially prepared foods rather than undercooked meats or wild rodents reduces the likelihood of their becoming infected and capable of transmitting the infection to a pregnant woman. Oral ingestion of *T. gondii* can be prevented by either cooking meat to well done, smoking it, or curing it in brine, and by washing kitchen surfaces that come into contact with raw meat. Vegetables and fruits should be washed, and hands and kitchen surfaces should be cleaned after handling fruits, vegetables, and raw meat. Flies and cockroaches may serve as transport hosts for *T. gondii*, so their access to food must be prevented.

Routine serologic screening of women during pregnancy has been an effective means of prevention in such countries as France and Austria, where the incidence of congenital toxoplasmosis is high. No such screening is currently recommended in the United States. However, high-risk women, including those who are immunocompromised, should be screened early in pregnancy.

Neonatal screening for IgM antibody has also been advocated so that asymptomatic infants can be detected and treated before neurologic symptoms develop (Peterson and Eaton, 1999). This strategy, however, has been hampered by the lack of readily available and reliable IgM test kits. Moreover, such screening will not detect the approximately 25% of infected infants who lack anti-*Toxoplasma* spp. IgM antibody. Further study involving cost analyses is needed to define the best preventive strategy for congenital toxoplasmosis in specific populations, regions, and countries.

SYPHILIS

Syphilis is caused by infection with the spirochete *Treponema pallidum*. In adults, this spirochete is transmitted through sexual contact, but infants acquire the infection from their mothers, either in utero or during delivery. The history of syphilis epidemics is one of intermittent peaks. During the 1930s and 1940s in the congenital syphilis clinic of the Harriet Lane Home (Baltimore, Md.), 60 to 80 infants and children attended each week for arsenic therapy. Many more were lost to follow-up before completing their 2- to 3-year course of treatment. It was unusual if fewer than three or four new examples were discovered in the general outpatient department in the course of 1 week. Then, for several decades, the frequency of new cases of congenital syphilis declined.

INCIDENCE AND EPIDEMIOLOGY

After years of declining incidence, congenital syphilis is again on the rise. Recent Centers for Disease Control and Prevention (CDC) surveillance data show a 23% increase in congenital syphilis cases from 2005 to 2008 as shown in Figure 38-1 (Centers for Disease Control and Prevention, 2010a). This increase is directly linked to a rise in primary and secondary syphilis in women from 2004 to 2007. In 2008, there was a total of 431 congenital syphilis cases in the U.S. Half of these cases were in infants born to black mothers, primarily in the South. Approximately 30% of the mothers of these infected infants did not receive prenatal care. When mothers did receive prenatal care and their infants still became infected, 27% were screened <30 days before delivery (likely resulting in a false negative test) and 24% screened positive but were not treated (Centers for Disease Control and Prevention, 2010a). An outbreak was also reported among Pima Indians in Arizona in 2007-2009 in which a total of 106 cases were identified, including six congenital cases, two of which resulted in stillbirth (Centers for Disease Control and Prevention, 2010b). A similar epidemic was seen in Alabama with a peak of 238 cases in 2006 with the largest increase seen in heterosexual women (Centers for Disease Control and Prevention, 2009).

Worldwide more newborns are affected by congenital syphilis than by any other neonatal infection (Schmid, 2004). Countries such as Ethiopia, Swaziland, and Mozambique have prevalence rates of maternal syphilis as high as 12% to 13% (World Health Organization, 2007). There are an estimated 2 million pregnancies affected annually, and most women infected with syphilis within 1 year of their pregnancy will transmit the infection to their infant.

Adverse outcomes in these pregnancies are severe: 17% to 40% result in stillbirth, 10% to 23% in neonatal death, and 10% to 30% result in congenital syphilis infection (World Health Organization, 2007).

The global problem of congenital syphilis is further confounded by the high prevalence of HIV, which reaches 25% to 40% in some African cities. Mothers who are coinfected with syphilis and HIV may be less likely to respond to penicillin treatment, which increases the risk of congenital syphilis in the fetus (Lukehart et al, 1988). In addition, HIV-infected mothers with untreated syphilis may be at increased risk of transmitting HIV to their fetus secondary to a placentitis that allows the virus to pass from maternal to fetal circulation (Pollack et al, 1990). In one study of HIV-infected women from Tanzania, coinfection with syphilis doubled the risk of still birth (Kupka et al, 2009). The extent of negative synergy between these two infections will become increasingly clear as research progresses.

PREVENTION

Screening for syphilis in pregnancy is the primary method of preventing congenital syphilis. The American Academy of Pediatrics and the American Congress of Obstetricians and Gynecologists in *Guidelines for Perinatal Care* (2002) recommend screening all pregnant women at the first prenatal visit, after exposure to an infected partner, and at delivery. Reinforcing this recommendation is the Reaffirmation Recommendation Statement by the U.S. Preventive Services Task Force (2009) that "Grade A evidence" is present for screening all pregnant women for syphilis infection.

As summarized by Miller and Karras (2010) in reference to the latest CDC surveillance data, "the increase in the

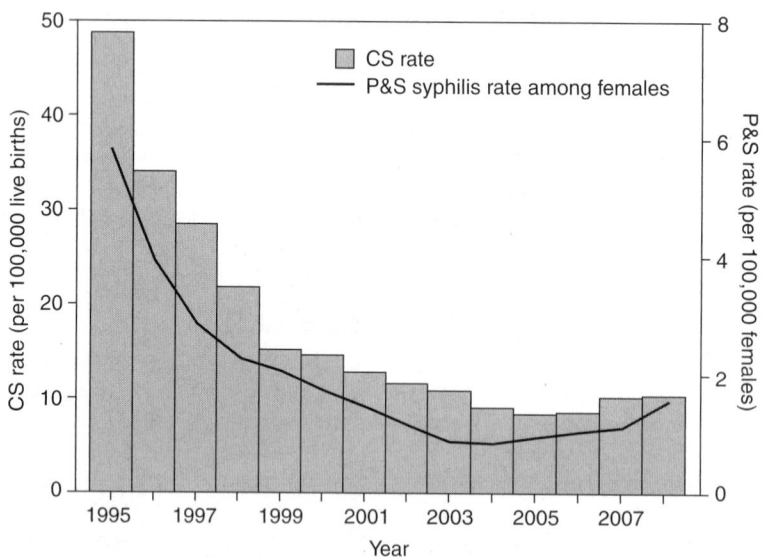

* CS rates from 1995 to 2006 were calculated using yearly live birth data as denominators. Rates for 2007 and 2008 were calculated using live birth data for 2006. Available at http://www.cdc.gov/nchs/births.htm.
† P&S syphilis rates were calculated using bridged race population estimates for 2000-2007 based on 2000 U.S. Census counts. Available at hhtp://wonder.cdc.gov/wonder/help/bridged-race.html.

FIGURE 38-1 Congenital syphilis (CS) rate among infants less than 1 year old and the rate of primary and secondary syphilis (P&S) among females 10 years or older. National Electronic Telecommunication System for Surveillance, United States, 1995-2008. (*Data from Centers for Disease Control and Prevention: Congenital syphilis: United States, 2003-2008,* MMWR Morb Mortal Wkly Rep *59:413, 2010.*)

congenital syphilis rate, the substantial burden of primary and secondary syphilis among black women in the south, and the high case/fatality ratio associated with congenital syphilis require that congenital syphilis prevention be given high priority in areas with high syphilis morbidity and evidence of heterosexual syphilis transmission."

ETIOLOGY AND PATHOGENESIS

The organism responsible for syphilis is *Treponema pallidum*. This delicate, corkscrew-shaped, flagellated, highly motile spirochete is almost identical in appearance to *Treponema pertenue*, which causes yaws. Because *Treponema* spp. enter the fetal bloodstream directly, the primary stage of infection is completely bypassed. There is no chancre and no local lymphadenopathy. Instead, the liver, the immediate target of the invasion, is flooded with organisms that then penetrate all the other organs and tissues of the body to a lesser degree. Other sites of invasion include skin, mucous membranes of the lips and anus, bones, and the central nervous system. If fetal invasion has taken place early, the lungs may be heavily involved in a characteristic pneumonia alba, but this condition is usually life threatening. *Treponema* spp. may be found in almost any other organ or tissue of the body, but seldom cause inflammatory and destructive changes in loci other than the ones named previously.

Under the microscope, the tissue alterations consist of nonspecific interstitial fibrosis with or without evidence of low-grade inflammatory response in the form of round cell inflammation. Necrosis follows fairly regularly in bone, but only rarely in other tissues. Localization and gumma formation are not common in the neonate; however, extramedullary hematopoiesis in the liver, spleen, kidneys, and other organs can be seen.

Syphilis in infants is acquired primarily by transplacental transmission, which can occur at any time during pregnancy but ordinarily occurs during 16 to 28 weeks' gestation. Fetuses infected early may die in utero or are at high risk for significant neurodevelopmental morbidity. The usual outcome of a third-trimester infection is the birth of an apparently normal infant who becomes ill within the first few weeks of life. Virtually all infants born to women with primary or secondary infection have congenital infection, but approximately half are clinically symptomatic. As hospitals and insurers strive to cut costs, early discharge of new mothers has hindered identification of congenitally infected, asymptomatic infants whose mother's infections occurred late in the third trimester and whose syphilis serologic test results are not yet positive at the time of delivery (Dorfman and Glaser, 1990). It is critical that at-risk infants have a source of primary health care capable of tracking both maternal and infant syphilis status (Chhabra et al, 1993; Zenker and Berman, 1991). Early latent infection results in a 40% infant infection rate, and late latent infection results in a 6% to 14% infant infection rate (Wendel, 1988).

CLINICAL PRESENTATION

Congenital syphilis is challenging to diagnose in neonates because 60% of infected infants are asymptomatic. Early presentation is typically within the first 4 weeks after birth and is characterized by the signs and symptoms

summarized in Table 38-3. Persistent rhinitis ("snuffles") was estimated to occur in two thirds of patients in the early literature, but is now less prevalent (Ingall et al, 2006). Prematurity and low birthweight is seen in 10% to 40% of infants (Saloojee et al, 2004). Additional diagnoses associated with congenital syphilis include nonimmune hydrops, nephrotic syndrome, and myocarditis.

Cutaneous lesions can appear at any time from the 2nd week after birth and onward. These copper-colored lesions can be either sparse or numerous; round, oval, or iris-shaped; and circinate or desquamative (Figure 38-2). Even more characteristic than their appearance is their distribution, which most frequently includes the perioral, perinasal, and diaper regions. Palms and soles are also involved, but the rash is soon replaced there by diffuse reddening, thickening, and wrinkling. In heavily infected infants, the rash may become generalized. Mucocutaneous junctions become involved in typical fashion. The lips become thickened and roughened and tend to weep.

TABLE 38-3 Clinical Features of Congenital Syphilis in the Neonatal Period

Feature	Prevalence (%)
Hepatomegaly with or without splenomegaly	33-100
Radiographic bone changes	75-100
Lymphadenopathy	50
Blistering skin rash	40
Respiratory distress	34
Jaundice	33
Pseudoparalysis of Parrot	12
Fever	16
Bleeding	10

Adapted from Remington JS, Klein JO, Wilson CB, et al, editors: *Infectious diseases of the fetus and newborn infant*, ed 6, Philadelphia, 2006, Saunders, p 572 and Saloojee H, Velaphi S, Goga Y, et al: The prevention and management of congenital syphilis: an overview and recommendations, *Bulletin of the World Health Organization* 82, 2004.

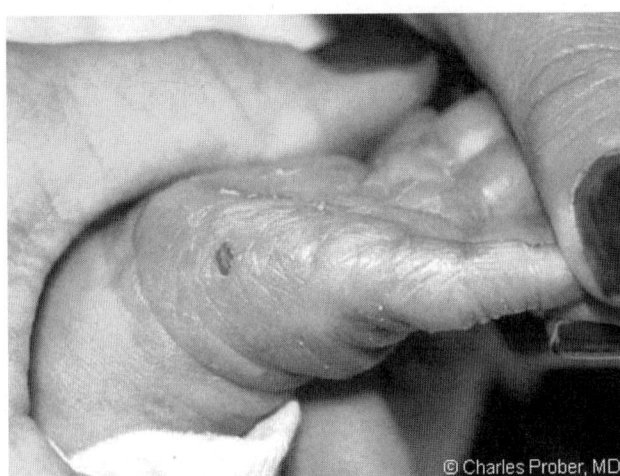

FIGURE 38-2 Congenital syphilis with desquamation over the hand. *(From American Academy of Pediatrics Committee on Infectious Diseases: Syphilis: clinical manifestations images. Red Book Online Visual Library, 2009, American Academy of Pediatrics. Available at http:// aapredbook.aappublications.org/cgi/content/figsonly/2009/1/3.129. Accessed November 19, 2010.)*

Radial cracks appear that traverse the vermillion zone up to and a bit beyond the mucocutaneous margins of the lips. These cracks are the beginnings of the radiating scars that may persist for many years as rhagades. Similar mucocutaneous lesions involve the anus and vulva, but in these locations, the white, flat, moist, raised plaques known as *condylomata* are also encountered, although less frequently.

Radiographs of the bones show characteristic osteochondritis and periostitis in 80% to 90% of infants with symptomatic congenital syphilis (Figure 38-3). In most cases, the bone lesions are asymptomatic, but in a few they are severe enough to lead to subepiphyseal fracture and epiphyseal dislocation with an extremely painful pseudoparalysis of one or more extremities. Approximately 20% of asymptomatic, congenitally infected infants have metaphyseal changes consistent with congenital syphilis. Radiographic alterations include an unusually dense band at the epiphyseal ends, below which is a band of translucency whose margins are at first sharp but that later become serrated, jagged, and irregular. The shafts become generally more opaque, but spotty areas of translucency throughout may give them a moth-eaten look. The periosteum of the long bones becomes more thickened. Epiphyses separate because the dense end plate breaks away from the shaft by fracture through the subepiphyseal zone of decalcification. Pseudoparalysis of Parrot can occur because of bone pain from these changes.

Signs of visceral involvement include hepatomegaly, splenomegaly, and general glandular enlargement. Palpable epitrochlear nodes are not pathognomonic, but are highly suggestive of congenital syphilis. The liver may be greatly enlarged, firm, and nontender. Associated with this finding may be jaundice, which appears in the 2nd or 3rd weeks of life, is seldom intense, and does not persist for many days. Anemia, probably indicative of bone marrow infection and hematopoietic suppression, may become severe. Lesions in the gastrointestinal tract and pancreas can occur and produce distention and delay in the passage of meconium.

Clinical signs of central nervous system involvement seldom appear in the newborn infant, although one third to

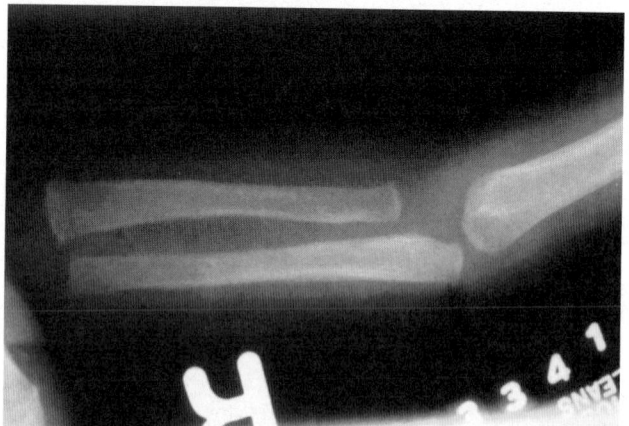

FIGURE 38-3 The radiograph displays the characteristic "celery stalking" and widening of the metaphases in long bones found in untreated congenital syphilis. *(From American Academy of Pediatrics Committee on Infectious Diseases: Syphilis: clinical manifestations images. Red Book Online Visual Library, 2009, American Academy of Pediatrics. Available at http://aapredbook.aappublications.org/cgi/content/figsonly/2009/1/3.129.)*

half of those infected suffer such involvement. One study by Beeram et al (1996) found no difference in leukocyte values or protein between the CSF of symptom-free infants born to syphilis-seropositive mothers (positive rapid plasmin reagin [RPR] test result confirmed by positive fluorescent treponemal antibody-absorbent [FTA-ABS]) and symptom-free control infants for whom sepsis for associated sepsis risk factors had been ruled out. In addition, only 2 of the 329 infants born to syphilis-infected mothers with no or inadequate treatment had a positive venereal disease research laboratory (VDRL) test result on their CSF specimen. Another study of neonatal CNS invasion by *T. pallidum* found the sensitivity and specificity of CSF VDRL to be 71% and 92%, respectively (Sanchez et al, 1993). Overall, the added value of CSF evaluation in asymptomatic infants appears marginal, because few cases of congenital syphilis are diagnosed based on CSF abnormalities in the absence of other laboratory or clinical findings. However, the CDC and the European International Union against Sexually Transmitted Infections guidelines still recommend that infants with confirmed disease (e.g., those with increasing quantitative titers) or infants who have a normal physical examination result but with an inadequately treated, syphilis-infected mother have a CSF evaluation for VDRL, cell count, and protein (Centers for Disease Control and Prevention, 2006; French et al, 2009). Further research may inform future guideline development.

DIAGNOSIS

The suggestion of congenital syphilis infection should be spurred by a positive maternal antibody test (RPR or VDRL). If the mother's treponemal test (treponema pallidum particle agglutination assay [TP-PA] or FTA-ABS) is also positive, a RPR or VDRL test should be performed on the infant's serum per current *Red Book* recommendations by the American Academy of Pediatrics (2009). Cord blood is not a reliable testing source for neonatal infection as false-positive RPR rates of 10% and false-negative RPR rates of 5% have been reported (Rawstron and Bromberg, 1991). However, a serum-positive antibody test alone does not confer a diagnosis of congenital syphilis, because of transplacental transfer of maternal nontreponemal and treponemal IgG antibodies. Because IgG is transferred across the placenta, its finding in the baby's serum simply means that the mother either currently has or has had syphilis. She may have been successfully treated during pregnancy and yet still has antibodies in her blood, or she may not have received treatment at all and still has not passed the disease on to her fetus. Conversely, if an antibody test is done on the infant's serum because of clinical suspicion in the absence of a positive maternal antibody test, the infant's antibody test can also be falsely negative if the mother acquired infection late in pregnancy, because she may not have had time to form antibodies herself or has not passed them to her fetus.

IgM does not cross the placenta, so the presence of specific IgM antibodies in the infant is generally diagnostic. Whereas the IgM immunoblot appears to be the best available method to detect *T. pallidum*-specific IgM in neonates, the CDC (2006) does not identify this as a commercially available and recommended test (Herremans et al, 2010). Treponemal tests on infant serum are not necessary. Comparison of maternal and infant nontreponemal serologic titers at delivery and followed over time are most informative for infant diagnosis. These titers should be accessed via the same test and in the same laboratory to ensure valid comparisons. If the infant titer is fourfold higher than the mother's titer, it is considered highly suggestive of congenital infection. Additional criteria for treatment in the neonate include inadequate maternal treatment in a mother with syphilis and the presence of clinical, laboratory, or radiographic evidence in the infant.

Evaluation of an infant with a concerning physical examination result and maternal profile should include darkfield or fluorescent antibody test of skin lesions or mucous discharge. In addition, a complete blood cell count with differential should be obtained, and CSF studies for cell count, protein and VDRL are recommended. If clinically indicated, long-bone radiographs can be diagnostic.

Clearly the evaluation for congenital syphilis is complex, and serial investigations may be necessary for definitive diagnosis. An algorithm for evaluation is shown in Figure 38-4.

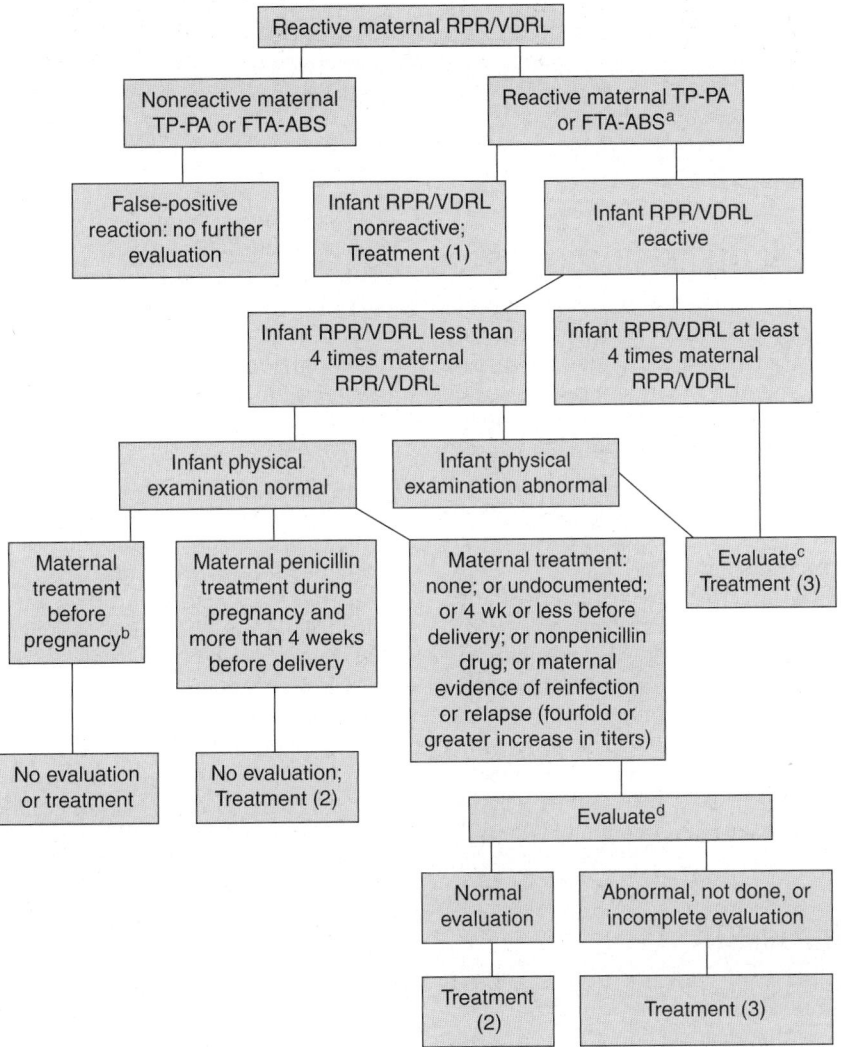

RPR indicates rapid plasma reagin (test); VDRL, Venereal Disease Research Laboratory (test); TP-PA, *Treponema pallidum* particle agglutination (test); FTA-ABS, fluorescent treponema antibody absorption (test).

[a] Test for human immunodeficiency virus (HIV) antibody. Infants of HIV-infected mothers do not require different evaluation or treatment.

[b] Women who maintain a VDRL titer 1:2 or less (RPR 1:4 or less) beyond 1 year after successful treatment are considered serofast.

[c] Evaluation consists of complete blood cell (CBC) and platelet count; cerebrospinal fluid (CSF) examination for cell count, protein, and quantitative VDRL. Other tests as clinically indicated: long-bone and chest radiographs, neuroimaging, auditory brainstem response, eye examination, liver function tests.

[d] CBC, platelet count; CSF examination for cell count, protein, and quantitative VDRL; long-bone radiography.

TREATMENT:

(1) If the mother has had no treatment, undocumented treatment, treatment 4 weeks or less before delivery or evidence of reinfection or relapse (fourfold or greater increase in titers) AND the infant's physical examination is normal, THE treat infant with a single intramuscular (IM) injection of benzathine penicillin (50 000 U/kg). If these criteria are not met, no treatment is required. In both scenarios, no additional evaluation is needed.

(2) Benzathine penicillin G, 50 000 U/kg, IM, × 1 dose.

(3) Aqueous penicillin G, 50 000 U/kg, IV, every 12 hours (1 week of age or younger), every 8 hours (older than 1 week), or procaine penicillin G, 50 000 U/kg, IM, single daily dose, × 10 days.

FIGURE 38-4 Algorithm for evaluation and treatment of infants born to mothers with reactive serologic tests for syphilis. (*From American Academy of Pediatrics Committee on Infectious Diseases:* Syphilis, Red Book Online, *2009, American Academy of Pediatrics. Available at http://aapredbook.aappublication s.org/cgi/content/full/2009/1/3.129. Accessed November 19, 2010.)*

TABLE 38-4   Recommended Treatment of Pregnant Patients With Syphilis

Stages of Syphilis	Drug (Penicillin)	Route	Dose (Units)
Early (<1 yr duration)			
Primary, secondary, or early latent			
HIV antibody-negative	Recommended: benzathine	IM	2.4 million single dose; possibly repeat in 1 wk
HIV antibody-positive*	Recommended: benzathine	IM	2.4 million single dose; possibly repeated weekly for 3 wk
	Alternative: penicillin desensitization		
Latent (>1 yr duration)†	Recommended: benzathine	IM	2.4 million weekly for 3 wk
	Alternative: penicillin desensitization		
Neurosyphilis	Recommended: aqueous	IV	3-4 million every 4 hr for 10-14 days
	Alternative: procaine‡	IM	2.4 million daily for 10-14 days

From Remington JS, Klein JO, Wilson CB, et al, editors: *Infectious diseases of the fetus and newborn infant*, ed 6, Philadelphia, 2006, WB Saunders, p 567.
IM, Intramuscular; *IV*, intravenous.
*With normal cerebrospinal fluid findings, if performed.
†Lumbar puncture to exclude neurosyphilis is recommended for HIV-antibody–positive patients.
‡Probenecid, 500 mg orally, four times per day for 10 to 14 days, should also be prescribed.

TREATMENT AND LONG-TERM OUTCOMES

Treatment of all pregnant women infected with syphilis is recommended. Guidelines for maternal treatment are found in Table 38-4 and are tailored to the stage of disease (e.g., primary, secondary, latent). Treatment of an infected infant requires 10 days of intravenous or intramuscular penicillin. Specific dosing and treatment regimens are outlined in Table 38-5, followed by long-term follow-up recommendations in Table 38-6. Notably, if a single dose is missed during the treatment of an infected infant, restarting the entire series is recommended.

Late manifestations of infection in untreated infants, even if initially asymptomatic, can occur years after birth. Pathognomonic presentations include the Hutchinson triad (interstitial keratitis, eight cranial nerve deafness and Hutchinson's [peg-shaped] teeth), mulberry molars (first lower molar with many small cusps), and Clutton's joints (synovitis with hydrarthrosis, tenderness, and limited range of motion) (Fiumara et al, 1970). Mental retardation can also be a feature of late, untreated congenital syphilis (Brosco et al, 2006).

CONGENITAL MALARIA

Malaria is a parasitic disease of epidemic proportion. An estimated 200 to 500 million cases occur worldwide each year, resulting in 2 to 3 million deaths. The greatest burden of disease occurs in Sub-Saharan Africa, although malaria is increasingly recognized as a significant public health problem in Asia and Oceania. In areas of high transmission, mortality is concentrated largely among young children and pregnant women. Malaria is caused by four *Plasmodium* species: *P. falciparum*, *P. vivax*, *P. ovale*, and *P. malariae*. Of these, *P. falciparum* is the major cause of morbidity and mortality. Humans typically acquire infection through the bite of the *Anopheles* spp. mosquito. Transmission may also occur through blood transfusion or vertically from the mother to fetus, resulting in congenital malaria.

Despite the prevalence of malaria in the developing world, it has historically been believed that congenital malaria occurs infrequently in areas of high transmission (Bruce-Chwatt, 1952; Covell, 1950; McGregor, 1984). As of 1995, only 300 cases of congenital malaria had been reported in the literature (Balatbat et al, 1995), largely from outside of malarious areas. The rarity of vertical transmission has been attributed to the effectiveness of the placenta as a barrier against passage of maternal parasitized red blood cells as well as the protective effect of maternally derived antibodies in the fetus and newborn. Recent reports, however, suggest that congenital malaria is no longer a rare occurrence in endemic areas and has likely been underrecognized and underreported (Akindele et al, 1993; Falade et al, 2007; Fischer, 1997, Ibhanesebhor, 1995; Menendez and Mayor, 2007; Uneke, 2007a, 2007b).

Although endemic malaria has been eliminated from the United States, approximately 1200 cases of malaria are reported to the CDC annually, almost exclusively in travelers and immigrants from endemic countries. From 1966 to 2005, 81 cases of congenital malaria were reported to the National Malaria Surveillance System of the CDC (Lesko et al, 2007). The majority of infants were born to foreign-born women. As an increasing number of people travel to and emigrate from malarious areas, the number of cases of malaria (and consequently congenital malaria) will continue to increase. The lack of familiarity with this disease in the United States renders it a diagnostic and therapeutic challenge for clinicians, with delays in diagnosis potentially leading to significant morbidity and mortality (Griffith et al, 2007). It is therefore critical to maintain a high index of suspicion for congenital malaria in the evaluation of infants born to women from endemic countries.

DEFINITION

Congenital malaria is defined as malaria acquired by the fetus or newborn from the mother, either in utero or at parturition, but there exists no consensus on the application of this definition. Most commonly, *congenital malaria* is defined as the presence of *Plasmodium* spp. parasites

TABLE 38-5 Recommended Treatment of the Newborn With Syphilis

Penicillin	Dosage
Aqueous penicillin G	50,000 units/kg every 12 hours during first 7 days of life and every 8 hours thereafter for a total of 10 days
or	
Penicillin G, procaine	50,000 units/kg/day, intramuscular, in a single dose every day for 10 days

From Centers for Disease Controls and Prevention: *Sexually transmitted diseases treatment guidelines, 2006.* Available at www.cdc.gov/std/treatment/2006/congenital-syphilis.htm. Accessed November 17, 2010.

TABLE 38-6 Follow-up after Treatment or Prophylaxis for Congenital Syphilis

Patient Category	Follow-up Procedures
Infants with diagnosis of congenital syphilis	RPR testing every 2-3 mo until negative or decreased fourfold; if RPR titer is stable or increasing after 6-12 mo after treatment, reevaluate and treat again; perform treponemal antibody test after age of 15 mo; if initial CSF analysis is abnormal or infant shows signs of CNS disease, repeat CSF evaluation every 6 mo until normal; with abnormal CSF not due to intercurrent illness on retesting, treat again; careful developmental evaluation, vision testing, and hearing testing are indicated
Infants who received treatment in utero or at birth because of maternal syphilis	RPR testing at birth and then every 3 mo until result is negative; treponemal antibody test after age of 15 mo
Women who received treatment for syphilis during pregnancy	RPR testing as often monthly until delivery, then every 6 mo until negative result obtained or titer decreased fourfold; repeated treatment any time there is a fourfold rise in RPR titer

From Remington JS, Klein JC, Wilson CB, et al, editors: *Infectious diseases of the fetus and newborn infant,* ed 6, Philadelphia, 2006, Saunders, 2006, p 572. *CSF,* Cerebrospinal fluid; *RPR,* rapid plasmin reagin.

in the peripheral blood in the first 7 days of life (Covell, 1950; Menendez and Mayor, 2007; Moran and Couper, 1999; Sotimehin et al, 2008; Uneke, 2007a). This definition is applicable in areas of high malaria transmission where, among older infants, it would be difficult to distinguish congenitally acquired from mosquito-acquired disease. Outside endemic areas, where postnatal transmission can be reasonably excluded, clinical onset of disease often does not occur until after the 1st week of life, and age-specific criteria are not useful for the diagnosis of congenital malaria. It is likely that because of the delay in clinical presentation, many cases of congenital malaria in endemic areas are misclassified as being acquired from mosquitoes.

Alternate applications of the definition of congenital malaria include the detection of parasites in peripheral blood or in umbilical cord blood (Fischer, 1997) within the first 24 hours of life (Larkin and Thuma, 1991). It has been argued that congenital malaria should be distinguished

from cord blood parasitemia, which is not uncommon in some endemic areas and frequently clears without involving the peripheral circulation. Reinhardt (1978) found parasites in thick smears of umbilical cord blood in 22% of 19 infants born to women in the Ivory Coast, but the peripheral blood smears were negative for all of the infants. Similarly, 4% of 1009 infants born to Tanzanian women had parasites in cord blood, but parasitemia was detected on peripheral smear in only 2 of 11 infants (McGregor, 1984). Parasitemia detected shortly after birth may also resolve without evolving into clinically symptomatic disease. In a recent multicenter study, the correlation between maternal, placental, umbilical cord, and peripheral parasitemia was evaluated in 1875 mother-baby pairs in Nigeria. Thick and thin blood smears were obtained within 4 hours of birth, and smear-positive (cord or peripheral) neonates were retested on days 2, 3, and 7 of life, with treatment for those with symptoms or persistent parasitemia. The overall prevalence of congenital malaria was 5.1%, with parasitemia detected in 19% of infants born to mothers with peripheral parasitemia, 21% of those born to mothers with placental malaria, and 45% of those with positive cord smears. Spontaneous clearance of parasitemia occurred in 62% of infants before day 2, whereas 33% were symptomatic within 3 days of birth (Falade et al, 2007). It has now been well established that (1) maternal and placental parasitemia are important risk factors for congenital malaria, (2) a correlation between umbilical cord parasitemia and neonatal parasitemia exists, and (3) congenital malaria can occur in the absence of symptoms (Mukhtar et al, 2006; Sotimehin et al, 2008; Uneke, 2007a). However, the definition of *congenital malaria* has yet to be standardized to facilitate a better understanding of the epidemiology of this disease and the outcomes of prevention measures.

EPIDEMIOLOGY

Congenital malaria has traditionally been considered a rare consequence of malaria in pregnant women living in endemic areas. Covell (1950) published a review of cases of congenital malaria reported in areas with rates of placental parasitemia ranging from 5% to 74%, and rates of maternal malaria ranging from 1% o 68%. The prevalence of congenital malaria—defined as parasitemia detected in the first 7 days of life—was estimated to be 0.3% (16 of 5324 births) among immune mothers. Subsequent reports supported the observed low frequency of congenital malaria—defined as umbilical cord parasitemia or parasitemia in the first 24 hours of life—among indigenous populations (Bruce-Chwatt, 1952; Cannon, 1958; MacGregor, 1984; Williams and McFarlane, 1970). These observations have been cited repeatedly in the literature to support the notion that congenital malaria is an uncommon occurrence in endemic areas despite the high prevalence of maternal and placental malaria. More recent reports, however, suggest that the prevalence of congenital malaria was underestimated, with rates from endemic and nonendemic areas ranging from 8% to 33% (Desai et al, 2007; Menendez and Mayor, 2007). In Zambia during a season of heavy malaria transmission, incidence rates for congenital malaria ranged from 4% to 15% (Nyirjesy et al, 1993). A survey of seven sites in

Sub-Saharan Africa indicated a prevalence of congenital malaria—defined as umbilical cord blood parasitemia—ranging from 0% to 23% (Fischer, 1995). Congenital malaria, defined as neonatal parasitemia, was detected in 15.3% and 17.4% of neonates born in two sites in Nigeria (Mukhtar et al, 2006; Runsewe-Abiodun et al, 2006). The apparent increase in the frequency of congenital malaria has been attributed to increasing resistance of *P. falciparum* to antimalarial drugs resulting in increased maternal parasitemia, increased virulence of the parasite, and reduced transmission of antibody from mother to newborn because of malaria chemoprophylaxis administered to pregnant women. It is equally likely that congenital malaria was previously underreported because of the difficulty in differentiating congenital malaria from postnatally acquired malaria in neonates, or it was underdetected because of low parasite densities in newborns. It is evident that congenital malaria is not an uncommon occurrence in areas of high transmission. The variability in prevalence of disease may be attributed to differences in the definition of congenital malaria or the methods used for parasite detection. The inconsistency may also represent true environmental differences with differences in levels of maternal immunity.

In contrast to the rarity of congenital malaria in indigenous populations, Covell (1950) found the prevalence of congenital malaria among nonimmune populations (i.e., Europeans residing in or visiting endemic areas) to be approximately 7%. It was postulated that congenital malaria is more common in infants born to these women because of lower levels of malaria-specific maternal antibodies being transmitted to the fetus. Most published reports of congenital malaria describe infants born in nonendemic countries whose mothers emigrated from malarious areas to areas free of malaria. These women presumably developed a recrudescence of disease because of waning immunity from lack of continued exposure

In the United States, the occurrence of congenital malaria is well documented because the country has been free of indigenous disease since the 1950s. From 1950 to 1991, 49 cases of congenital malaria were reported in the literature (Hulbert, 1992), and additional cases were reported during the next 15 years (Balatbat et al, 1995; Baspinar et al, 2006; D'Avanzo et al, 2002; Gereige and Cimino, 1995; Starr and Wheeler, 1998; Viraraghavan and Jantausch, 2000). In an updated review, Lesko et al (2007) tabulated 81 cases reported to the CDC between 1966 and 2005. Almost all the cases were among infants whose mothers were foreign born, suggesting that congenital malaria is primarily a health problem of recent immigrants rather than of U.S.-born travelers to malaria-endemic countries. Forty-four women (54%) had emigrated from Asia, 27 (33%) from South or Central America, and 7 (9%) from Africa. Until 1979, one to two cases were reported annually (Malviya and Shurin, 1984). An abrupt rise to 16 cases around 1981 (Figure 38-5) correlated with an increase in the total number cases of malaria that occurred as a result of a large influx of refugees and immigrants from Southeast Asia, with 15 of the 16 infants being born to mothers from that region (Quinn et al, 1982).

Congenital malaria occurs with all *Plasmodium* species. Among the 107 cases of congenital malaria reported by Covell (1950), mostly from Africa, 64% were infected with *P. falciparum*, 32% by *P. vivax*, and 2% by *P. malariae*. Although *P. falciparum* remains the predominant pathogen in Sub-Saharan Africa, *P. vivax* may account for a larger proportion of cases in Asia. Among 27 cases reported in Thailand between 1981 and 2005, 82% of were cause by *P. vivax* (Wiwanitkit, 2006). *P. malariae* is less frequently a causative agent, with fewer than 10 cases reported worldwide since 1950 (de Pontual et al, 2006). Concurrent infection with *P. malariae* and *P. vivax* has been documented (MacLeod et al, 1982). In the United States, the predominant *Plasmodium* species causing congenital malaria

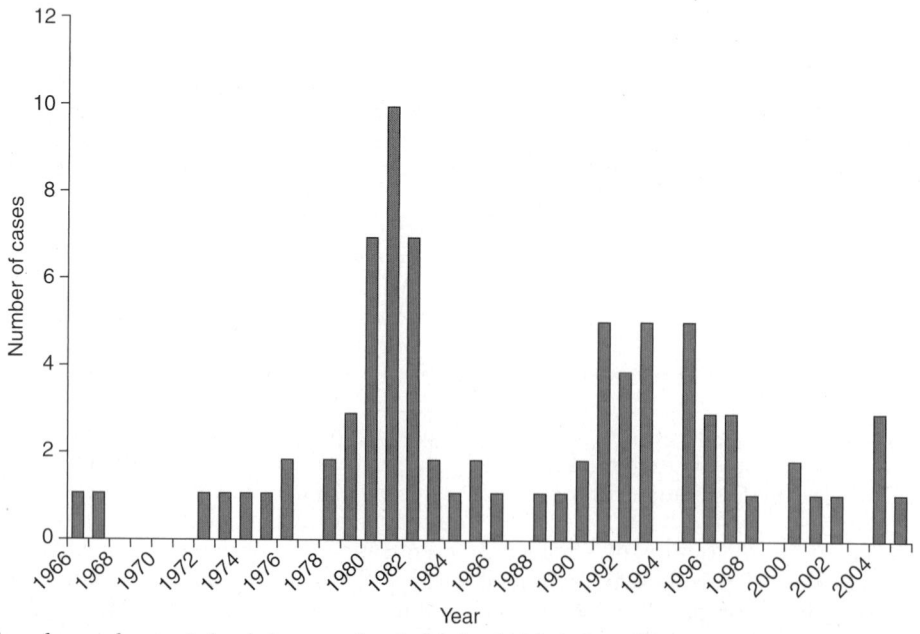

FIGURE 38-5 Number of cases of congenital malaria reported to the National Malaria Surveillance System per year, 1966-2005. *(From Lesko CR, Arguin PM, Newman RD: Congenital malaria in the United States: a review of cases from 1966 to 2005,* Arch Pediatr Adolesc Med *161:1062-1067, 2007.)*

reflects the countries of origin of the mothers, as noted previously. In Hulbert's (1992) review of 49 cases, 82% of infections were caused by *P. vivax*. In the updated review by Lesko et al (2007), the predominant infecting species remained *P. vivax* (81%), although all four species were represented.

PREGNANCY AND MALARIA

Malaria in pregnancy is an immense public health problem in the developing world, with substantial effects on maternal, fetal, and infant health. It is well established that both the frequency of disease and density of parasitemia are higher in pregnant women compared with nonpregnant women (Coll et al, 2008; Desai et al, 2007; Rogerson et al, 2007). In Sub-Saharan Africa, 25 million pregnant women are at risk for *P. falciparum* infection every year (Desai et al, 2007). Among 20 studies conducted between 1985 and 2000, the median prevalence of maternal malaria infection (defined as peripheral or placental infection) in all was 28% (Steketee et al, 2001). Thus, one in four pregnant women in areas of stable transmission in Africa have evidence of malaria infection at the time of delivery. The increased susceptibility likely represents a combination of immunologic and hormonal changes combined with the unique ability of infected erythrocytes to sequester in the placenta (Rogerson et al, 2007). The risk is indisputably greater for primigravidae, with primigravidae having a twofold to fourfold increased risk of placental malaria compared with multigravidae (Desai et al, 2007; McGregor, 1984; Uneke, 2008).

The clinical features of *P. falciparum* malaria in a pregnant woman depend to a large degree on her immune status, which in turn is determined by her prior exposure to malaria. In pregnant women with little or no preexisting immunity, such as women from nonendemic countries or travelers to malarious areas, infection is associated with high risks of severe disease with significant maternal and perinatal mortality. In contrast, women residing in areas of stable malaria transmission usually have a high level of immunity to malaria. Infection may be frequently asymptomatic and therefore unsuspected or undetected, but it is associated with placental parasitization, with consequent effects on maternal and fetal outcomes. The most significant consequence of pregnancy-associated malaria is maternal anemia. It is estimated that in Sub-Saharan Africa between 200,000 and 500,000 pregnant women develop anemia as a result of malaria, and that up to 10,000 maternal anemia-related deaths are a consequence of *P. falciparum* parasitemia (Uneke, 2008). Malaria in pregnancy also has potentially devastating effects on the fetus and newborn, including spontaneous abortion, still birth, premature delivery, congenital infection, and neonatal death (Coll et al, 2008; Fischer, 2003). The most notable consequence is low birthweight (LBW), likely because of fetal growth restriction. In areas of high transmission in Africa, the risk of LBW approximately doubles if women have placental malaria, with the greatest effect in primigravidae (Desai et al, 2007). Pregnancy-associated malaria is believed to be responsible for 30% to 35% of LBW infants and for 75,000 to 200,000 infant deaths each year (Coll et al, 2008).

TRANSMISSION

The timing and mechanism of transmission of *Plasmodium* spp. parasites from the mother to the fetus is not well understood. Postulated mechanisms include maternal transfusion into fetal circulation either during pregnancy or at delivery, or direct penetration of parasitized red blood cells through the chorionic villi or through premature separation of the placenta. In utero transmission is supported by the finding of malarial parasites in fetal tissues at autopsy (Mertz et al, 1981), by umbilical cord blood parasitemia (McGregor, 1984) and the onset of clinical signs of malaria within hours of birth (Brandenburg and Kenny, 1982; Covell, 1950; Gereige and Cimino, 1995). Antenatal transmission is also suggested by findings from Malawi, where approximately 50% of newborns with cord blood parasitemia were infected with parasites of a different genotype than their mothers at the time of delivery (Fischer, 2003). Alternatively, clinical findings in infants with congenital malaria may be delayed for several weeks after birth, suggesting infection at parturition. It is generally understood that the placenta acts as an effective barrier to prevent the transfer of malaria parasites from maternal into fetal circulation, supporting transmission at parturition as the most likely mechanism. Vertical transmission of malaria probably does not occur as a result of transplacental passage of exoerythrocytic parasites. More likely, transmission occurs by transfusion of parasitized maternal erythrocytes through a breach in the placental barrier that may occur either prematurely during pregnancy or during labor. Transmission of malaria by breastfeeding is not known to occur. The fate of the *Plasmodium* spp. parasite is unclear after it is transmitted to the fetus. As discussed previously, parasites detected in umbilical cord blood or shortly after birth may be cleared spontaneously, resulting in no disease manifestation. Alternatively, parasitemia may be maintained and proliferate until multiplication permits the development of clinical disease.

CLINICAL PRESENTATION

The clinical picture of overt congenital malaria is detailed in cases reported outside of endemic areas (Harvey et al, 1969; Hindi and Azimi, 1980; Hulbert, 1992; Lesko et al, 2007). The manifestation of disease, although occasionally noted within hours of birth (Brandenburg and Kenny, 1982; Gereige and Cimino, 1995), is typically delayed until the infant is several weeks old. In the classic review of 49 infants with congenital malaria reported in the United States between 1950 and 1992, the mean age at onset of symptoms was 5.5 weeks, with 96% of infants presenting between 2 and 8 weeks of age (Hulbert, 1992). Among cases reported to the CDC from 1966 to 2005 (Lesko et al, 2007), the median age of symptom onset for 81 infants was 21.5 days for all species combined (Figure 38-6). Infants infected with *P. malariae* were significantly older at symptom onset (mean, 53 days) compared with those infected with *P. vivax* or *P. falciparum*.

The prolonged interval between birth and onset of clinical manifestations may be explained by transmission late in pregnancy or at delivery, such that multiple erythrocytic

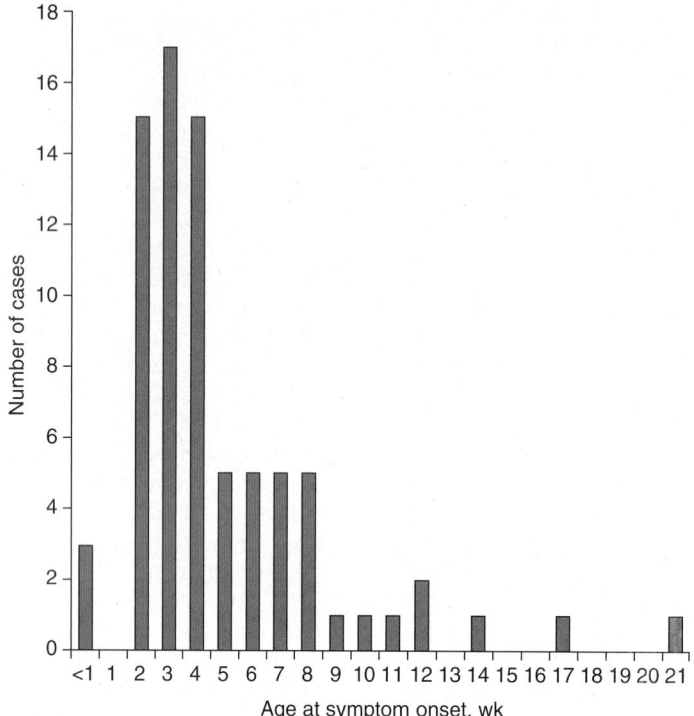

FIGURE 38-6 Age in weeks at symptom onset of infants with reported congenital malaria, United States, 1966-2005. *(From Lesko CR, Arguin PM, Newman RD: Congenital malaria in the United States: a review of cases from 1966 to 2005, Arch Pediatr Adolesc Med 161:1062-1067, 2007.)*

life cycles are required to produce clinically evident disease. Alternatively, the delay may be attributed to the presence of transplacentally acquired maternal antimalarial antibodies. When such antibodies are present in sufficient concentrations, as in infants born to immune mothers, parasitic replication can be prevented or attenuated, and clinical signs can be mild, delayed, or even absent. The presence of a high concentration of fetal hemoglobin in newborns may also promote resistance to multiplication of parasites. Among infants born to mothers with low or nonexistent immunity, parasitic replication is more likely uninhibited, and clinical signs of malaria may supervene. Preterm infants, who do not benefit from passive immunity, can manifest clinical signs earlier than full-term infants. In a review of premature neonates with congenital malaria, 4 of 5 infants received a diagnosis in the 1st week of life (Ahmed et al, 1998), although the prompt medical evaluation afforded these infants may have facilitated earlier detection.

The clinical features of congenital malaria are nonspecific and often resemble those of bacterial or viral sepsis and other congenital infections. Fever is almost uniformly present, although without the classic paroxysmal pattern described for malaria beyond the neonatal period. Hulbert (1992) noted fever in all 44 infants for whom clinical information was available. In the cases reported from 1966 to 2005, fever was reported in 70 of 81 cases (86%) (Lesko et al, 2007). Hepatomegaly and splenomegaly suggestive of a transplacentally acquired infection are found in a substantial portion of infants (Table 38-7). Anemia (often hemolytic), thrombocytopenia, and hyperbilirubinemia are the most commonly reported laboratory findings. Additional signs, symptoms, and laboratory findings are listed in Table 38-7.

TABLE 38-7 Frequency of Symptoms, Signs, and Laboratory Findings Among 81 Infants With a Diagnosis of Congenital Malaria (United States, 1966-2005)

Symptoms, Signs, and Laboratory Findings	Infants, No. (%)*
Fever	70 (86)
Anemia	28 (36)
Splenomegaly	25 (31)
Hepatomegaly	16 (20)
Thrombocytopenia	12 (15)
Jaundice	11 (14)
Irritability	8 (10)
Anorexia	8 (10)
Vomiting	8 (10)
Cough	6 (7)
Diarrhea	3 (4)
Lethargy	3 (4)
Hemolysis	3 (4)
Pallor	3 (4)
Hyperbilirubinemia	2 (3)
Failure to thrive	2 (3)
Seizures	2 (3)
Dyspnea	1 (1)
Purpura	1 (1)
Tachycardia	1 (1)
Monocytosis	1 (1)

From Lesko CR, Arguin PM, Newman RD: Congenital malaria in the United States: a review of cases from 1966 to 2005, *Arch Pediatr Adolesc Med* 161:1062-1067, 2007.
*Percentages do not total 100% because each case can have more than one symptom, sign, or laboratory finding.

In endemic areas, the traditional belief has been that congenital malaria is rare and that when it occurs the infant is typically asymptomatic and develops no clinical features. The lack of symptoms has been attributed to transplacentally acquired antibodies from the mother as well as the protective effects of high levels of fetal hemoglobin. Depending on the region, spontaneous clearance of peripheral parasitemia has been documented in 87% to 100% of neonates (Lesko et al, 2007; Mukhtar et al, 2006). Larkin and Thuma (1991) found peripheral parasitemia within 24 hours of age in 19 of 51 newborns (65%), but only 7 had clinical signs of disease. Because all 19 newborns received antimalarial therapy, it is unknown how many would have manifested disease if untreated. More recently, Falade et al (2007) noted spontaneous clearance of parasitemia in 62% of 95 neonates before day 2 of life. Of the remaining infants, 34% were symptomatic within 3 days of birth, with fever and refusal to eat being the most common signs of disease. When active surveillance for malaria was conducted in newborns being evaluated for possible bacterial sepsis in Nigeria, 16 of 203 (8%) neonates had parasitemia, and 10 (5%) met the definition of congenital malaria (Ibhanesebhor, 1995). Predominant features of disease included fever, respiratory distress, anemia, and hepatomegaly. In another area in Nigeria, of 202 neonates less younger than 1 week who were admitted for evaluation of sepsis, 71 (35%) were diagnosed with congenital malaria (Ekanem et al, 2008). Fever was the most common symptom and was present in 93% of infants. Refusal to feed and jaundice were reported in approximately 33%. These observations suggest that, as in infants diagnosed outside endemic areas, the clinical presentation of congenital malaria in endemic areas does not differ significantly from bacterial sepsis. Because the clinical symptoms of congenital malaria may be indistinguishable from that of neonatal sepsis, it is suggested that screening for malaria be included as part of routine investigation of newborns with fever in areas of high malaria transmission (Ekanem et al, 2008; Runsewe-Abiodun et al, 2006).

DIAGNOSIS

Diagnostic tests for malaria include blood smears, rapid antigen detection tests (RDTs) and PCR. Definitive diagnosis of congenital malaria is based on the microscopic demonstration of parasites on stained thick and thin blood films. Thick blood smears test for the presence of parasites by concentration of red blood cells, whereas thin blood smears allow species identification and quantification of parasitemia. In cases of suggested congenital malaria, specimens for smears should be obtained from both the infant and the mother. If test results from the initial set of smears are negative, additional sets should be obtained every 12 to 24 hours; three sets are generally considered sufficient for diagnostic evaluation. Response to therapy may also be measured by clearance of parasitemia on blood films.

RDTs are based on the immunochromatographic detection of parasite-specific antigens circulating in the bloodstream. Many RDTs are commercially available outside the United States, and, depending on the antigens targeted, the tests may detect only *P. falciparum* or all *Plasmodium* species. RDTs are simple to use, do not require specialized training or facilities, and offer a useful alternative to microscopy in situations where reliable microscopic diagnostics are not readily available. However, the tests have

demonstrated mixed results in multiple trials, and sensitivity remains a problem, especially at low parasite densities. Information regarding the sensitivity of these tests is limited for neonatal or congenital malaria. In the evaluation of an RDT for the diagnosis of congenital malaria in Nigeria, parasitemia was detected by microscopy in 21 of 192 newborns (10.9%) at 0 to 3 days of age, whereas the RDT result (OptiMAL [Flow Inc, Portland, Oregon]) was negative in all infants, including those diagnosed by microscopy. Whether the poor performance of the test was due to low-level parasitemia or suboptimal state of the parasites, the RDT was determined not to be useful for the diagnosis of congenital malaria (Sotimehin et al, 2007). It is recommended that microscopy be conducted in parallel with RDTs because low level parasitemia may not be detected or, if parasitemia is detected, for species identification and determination of parasite density.

The major advantage of PCR for the diagnosis of malaria is its ability to detect low level parasitemia and identify parasites to a species level. Currently PCR is used mainly to confirm positive blood smears, particularly when the results of the smear are not definitive or there is a mixed species infection. PCR may detect DNA from circulating nonviable parasites after treatment, resulting in difficulty differentiating an active infection from a recently cleared infection. Although PCR is a highly sensitive alternative to microscopy, the infrastructure and expertise required preclude its use in malaria-endemic areas and many health care settings in the United States.

As with malaria in general, the diagnosis of congenital malaria outside of endemic areas is often delayed because of nonspecific features and lack of clinical suspicion. Among the 81 cases reviewed by Lesko et al (2007), a median length of delay of 8.5 days was noted for 15% of the infants. Occasionally the diagnosis is made incidentally. In all four cases of congenital malaria reported by Quinn et al (1982), *Plasmodium* spp. parasites were noted by hematology technicians on routine smears performed for blood cell counts. Maternal history of recent travel to or emigration from an endemic area may suggest the diagnosis, but is often obscured by the lack of clinical or laboratory findings in the mother. Lesko et al (2007) found that, of the mothers for whom a history was available, 67% reported having fever during pregnancy, and 26% reported a diagnosis of malaria during pregnancy. Maternal blood films were performed after either symptomatic illness or malaria diagnosis in the infant. Overall only 42% of women had parasitemia detected, although it is not clear whether an adequate number of smears were conducted for each patient. As a result, lack of peripheral parasitemia in the mother of an infant with suspected congenital malaria does not exclude the diagnosis.

Further confounding the early recognition of disease in the infant is the potentially prolonged lapse between malaria exposure in the mother and transmission of infection to the infant. *P. vivax* and *P. ovale* may remain dormant in the liver, especially if the infected individual did not receive therapy for the exoerythrocytic stage, which can cause a delayed relapse of malaria in travelers or immigrants. *P. malariae* can persist for 20 to 40 years before clinical symptoms or demonstrable parasitemia appear (D'Avanzo et al, 2002). Congenital malaria has been reported in an infant whose mother lived in the United States for 5 years before delivery and had no signs or symptoms or malaria for more than 20 years (Harvey et al, 1969). In North Carolina, congenital *P. malariae* infection was reported in a 10-week-old infant who was born to a mother who had emigrated from the Democratic Republic of Congo 4 years before delivery (D'Avanzo et al, 2002). In a review by Lesko et al (2007), the median duration from the mother's last exposure to delivery was 9.5 months. The time elapsed since exposure was longest for those with *P. malariae* infection, ranging from 2 to 12 years.

Recognizing that congenital malaria is an exceptional occurrence in the United States, it is still important to include malaria in the differential diagnosis of fever in infants born to mothers who have been exposed to malaria, even if the exposure is remote and even if the woman is asymptomatic. Of 11 infants with congenital malaria in the United States born to women known to have parasitemia at or shortly after delivery, only five underwent testing by blood smears, and all five had negative test results at the time of delivery (Lesko et al, 2007). Data are insufficient to determine the overall risk of an infant developing congenital malaria when born to a woman at risk for parasitemia or identified with parasitemia at birth. Consequently, the evaluation of infants born outside endemic areas to women with epidemiologic risk factors for parasitemia should be individualized. In malaria endemic areas, and as a public health measure, it has been recommended that blood smears should be checked as part of the evaluation of neonates with fever born to mothers who have had fever within a few weeks of delivery (Uneke, 2007a).

TREATMENT

The management of malaria consists of supportive care and antimalarial therapy. Information regarding treatment of congenital malaria is limited, and recommended chemotherapy is similar to that of noncongenital infections. The treatment regimen is based on the infecting species, the possibility of drug resistance, and the severity of disease. For mild infections caused by *P. vivax*, *P. ovale*, and *P. malariae* or chloroquine-sensitive *P. falciparum*, chloroquine orally (10 mg base/kg initially followed by 5 mg base/kg 6, 24, and 48 hours later) is recommended. Treatment with primaquine is not necessary for congenitally acquired *P. vivax* or *P. ovale* infection because, like transfusion-associated malaria, congenital infection does not involve the exoerythrocytic phase.

The treatment of congenital malaria due to chloroquine-resistant *P. falciparum* is poorly defined. In older children, three treatment options currently recommended are: (1) oral quinine plus either tetracycline, doxycycline, or clindamycin; (2) atovaquone-proguanil; or (3) mefloquine. For the treatment of congenital malaria, oral quinine sulfate and trimethoprim-sulfamethoxazole for 5 days was recommended by Quinn et al (1982), who used the regimen to treat a 1-month-old infant. Ahmed et al (1998) used a similar regimen for the treatment of an infant born at 28 weeks' gestation to a mother from Zaire. Other regimens used successfully in neonates include oral quinine sulfate and pyrimethamine-sulfadoxine (Gereige

and Cimino, 1995) and intravenous quinine hydrochloride followed by oral quinine (Airede, 1991). Intravenous quinine is no longer available in the United States. Because of the rarity of congenital malaria in the United States, the changing pattern of resistance, and the potential toxicity associated with drugs used for therapy, current treatment recommendations should be sought from the Malaria Branch of the CDC (www.cdc.gov/malaria). For health care professionals, assistance with management of malaria is also available 24 hours a day through the CDC Malaria Hotline (770-448-7788).

Severe malaria occurs most commonly with *P. falciparum* infection and is characterized by one or more of the following: (1) parasitemia greater than 5% of red blood cells, (2) central nervous system or other end-organ involvement, (3) shock, (4) acidosis, (5) severe anemia, or (6) hypoglycemia. Management of severe malaria involves parenteral treatment in an intensive care setting. Until recently, the only parenteral therapy available in the United States was quinidine gluconate. Quinidine is more cardiotoxic than quinine and should be administered with continuous cardiac monitoring. Exchange transfusion may be warranted when parasitemia exceeds 10% or if there are complications at lower parasite densities.

The efficacy of treatment should be monitored by examining blood smears (i.e., malaria smears) every 12 hours until negative for malaria parasites. Response to therapy with chloroquine for non-*P. falciparum* malaria is usually favorable (Brandenburg and Kenny, 1982; Dowell and Musher, 1991; Hindi and Azimi, 1980). It has been suggested that infants born to mothers with parasitemia at delivery should be treated presumptively for congenital malaria (Lesko et al, 2007). Data are insufficient to determine the risk of an infant developing congenital malaria when born to a mother with parasitemia. Although there is evidence from endemic areas that parasitemia detected at or shortly after delivery may clear spontaneously, the clinical relevance of this observation in nonendemic areas is unclear. It is recommended that physicians judge each case individually, considering factors such as access to medical care and reliability of follow up in deciding whether to treat infants presumptively.

PROGNOSIS

Malaria during pregnancy is likely an underappreciated risk factor for increased infant morbidity and mortality in endemic areas. In a review of studies published between 1985 and 2000, Steketee et al (2001) determined population-attributable risks for maternal malaria of 3% to 8% for infant mortality. It was estimated that 75,000 to 200,000 infant deaths annually are associated with malaria during pregnancy, although what proportion of these are related to congenital malaria is unknown. Outside endemic areas, the short-term outcome of congenital malaria has been favorable. Most infants respond rapidly to therapy with clearance of parasitemia. There were no reports of death or adverse outcomes in the 49 cases reported from 1950 to 1992 or in the 81 cases reported to the CDC from 1966 to 2005 (Hulbert, 1992; Lesko et al, 2007). It is unclear, however, whether the outcomes are due to an overall favorable prognosis or reporting bias.

PREVENTION

The prevention of congenital malaria is based on a pregnant woman's avoidance of exposure and use of chemoprophylaxis. Malaria infection in pregnant women is more common and more severe than in nonpregnant women. Malaria also increases the risk for adverse pregnancy outcomes, including prematurity, abortion, and still birth. Nonimmune pregnant women are at the highest risk for these adverse outcomes. Based on these observations, the CDC advises women who are pregnant or likely to become pregnant to avoid travel to areas with malaria transmission. If such travel is unavoidable, consultation with an infectious disease or malaria expert is advised. The use of mosquito netting, mesh screens on windows, insecticides, and mosquito repellents can decrease potential exposure to malaria parasites. For pregnant women traveling to areas where there is no chloroquine-resistant *P. falciparum* malaria, prophylaxis with chloroquine is advised. The safety of chloroquine for the fetus when used at the recommended doses for malaria prophylaxis is well established (MacLeod et al, 1982). For travel to areas where chloroquine resistance has been reported, mefloquine is the only medication that is currently recommended for prophylaxis during pregnancy. Atovaquone-proguanil is not recommended during pregnancy because of insufficient information on potential adverse effects. Doxycycline is contraindicated because of adverse effects on the fetus caused by a related drug, tetracycline, which include dysplasia and discoloration of teeth and inhibition of bone growth. Health care professionals caring for women who cannot take the recommended antimalarial agent should contact the CDC Malaria Hotline (770-488-7788).

Pregnant women originally from areas where malaria is endemic but who are now living in nonendemic areas may be only partially immune. When traveling to their countries of origin, they should be considered nonimmune and thus should receive the same recommendations as nonimmune women.

The burden of malaria among pregnant women in endemic areas is well recognized, and prevention and control strategies for areas of high *P. falciparum* transmission are aimed at reducing maternal and infant mortality. The World Health Organization has proposed a three-pronged approach: (1) intermittent preventative treatment with an effective antimalarial agent at scheduled antenatal visits, (2) insecticide-treated nets, and (3) effective case management of clinical infection. A metaanalysis of more recent intervention trials suggests that successful prevention of these infections reduces the risk of severe maternal anemia by 38%, LBW by 43%, and perinatal mortality by 27% among paucigravidae women (Desai et al, 2007). Unfortunately, the full implementation of antenatal malaria prevention efforts is burdened by the challenges associated with health care delivery in the developing world.

CONGENITAL TUBERCULOSIS

Tuberculosis remains one of the deadliest communicable diseases worldwide. More than 2 billion people, equivalent to one third of the world's population, are infected with *Mycobacterium tuberculosis*. Each year, an estimated 9 million new tuberculosis cases are identified, and 2 million people die from the disease. The greatest burden of disease is in developing countries, where tuberculosis remains a major public health threat. While case rates have declined steadily in the United States and Europe, the corresponding numbers have increased dramatically in the former Soviet Union and Sub-Saharan Africa, in part fueled by the epidemic of human immunodeficiency virus (HIV).

Despite the prevalence of tuberculosis worldwide, congenital tuberculosis occurs rarely, with fewer than 400 cases reported in the English-language literature. The majority of reports describe infants born in low-burden countries to mothers who have emigrated from high-burden countries. Although some reports originate from countries where tuberculosis is endemic, it is likely that congenital tuberculosis is underrecognized and underreported in these areas, largely because of the nonspecific clinical features of disease and the limited diagnostic capability.

In the United States, 10,000 to 15,000 cases of tuberculosis are reported annually. Although the overall rate of tuberculosis infection has been declining steadily since 1992, the proportion of cases in foreign-born populations has increased. More than 50% of cases reported in 2008 occurring among the foreign born. With increased global mobility and the epidemiologic trends of tuberculosis, it is likely that tuberculosis and congenital tuberculosis will continue to be observed in developed countries. The nonspecific features of congenital tuberculosis and the mortality associated with untreated disease underscore the importance of maintaining a high index of suspicion for tuberculosis in pregnant women and young infants.

DEFINITION

Transmission of *M. tuberculosis* from the mother to the neonate can occur in utero, intrapartum, or postpartum. Although congenital infection is classically considered the result of in utero infection of the fetus, the term *congenital tuberculosis* has historically referred to infection acquired either in utero or intrapartum. The infection can be transmitted by direct spread to the fetus from the placenta via the umbilical vein or by aspiration or ingestion of infected amniotic fluid, either in utero or intrapartum.

Beitzke (1935) proposed diagnostic criteria to distinguish congenital tuberculosis from postnatally acquired tuberculosis. The criteria required that the infant have proven tuberculosis lesions and one of the following: (1) a primary hepatic complex as evidence of dissemination of the tubercle bacilli via the umbilical vein or (2) in the absence of a primary complex, the presence of tuberculous lesions in the first few days of life or the exclusion of postnatal infection by separation of the infant at birth from the mother and other potential sources of infection. These criteria were developed before the introduction of chemotherapy, when infant mortality with congenital tuberculosis was high and diagnosis was largely based on autopsy findings. It is difficult and no longer practical to apply Beitzke's criteria. The demonstration of a primary hepatic complex with liver and regional node involvement requires an open surgical procedure; a percutaneous liver biopsy may demonstrate caseating granulomas, but the primary complex will seldom be identified. Cantwell et al (1994) proposed revised criteria that are more applicable to current practice and improve diagnostic sensitivity. To meet the criteria, the infant must have proven tuberculous lesions and at least one of the following: (1) lesions in the first week of age, (2) a primary hepatic complex or caseating hepatic granulomas, (3) tuberculous infection of the placenta or maternal genital tract, or (4) exclusion or postnatal transmission by thorough investigation of contacts. Whereas the distinction between congenital tuberculosis and postnatally acquired disease may be relevant for academic or epidemiologic purposes, it does not affect the management, treatment, or prognosis of disease.

EPIDEMIOLOGY

From 1953 through 1984, the incidence of tuberculosis in the United States declined steadily, reaching a nadir of 9.4 cases per 100,000 population. From 1985 through 1992, there was a 20% increase in the total number of cases. The resurgence of disease was attributed to multiple factors, including the HIV epidemic, increased immigration, and a decline in public health funding for tuberculosis control. With the availability of antiretroviral therapy for HIV and fortification of public health measures, the epidemiologic trend was reversed. Since 1992, the case rates for tuberculosis have decreased annually to a case rate of 4.2 per 100,000 in 2008. Despite the decrease in the total burden of disease, tuberculosis continues to disproportionately affect the foreign-born and racial and ethnic minorities. In 2008, 59% of all cases of tuberculosis in the United States occurred in foreign-born persons (CDC, 2008).

The current epidemiology of tuberculosis in pregnancy is not well delineated. With the resurgence of tuberculosis in the 1980s, the largest increase in the incidence of disease occurred in the 25- to 44-year age group, and the number of cases among women of childbearing age rose by 40% (Cantwell et al, 1994). In 1991, almost 40% of tuberculosis cases in minority women occurred in those between 15 and 35 years of age (Smith and Teele, 1995). These trends persist through the present time, thus placing women of childbearing age, especially those who are foreign born, and their newborns at continued risk.

The risk of congenital tuberculosis in infants born to women with tuberculosis is unknown. Blackall (1969) reported only three cases among infants born to 100 mothers with tuberculosis. Ratner et al (1951) identified no cases among infants born to 260 mothers with the disease. In a study of 1369 infants separated at birth from their tuberculous mothers and placed in foster care, only 12 became tuberculin-positive during 4 years of observation, and in all 12 cases there was a source of infection in the postnatal environment (Smith and Teele, 1995). The low incidence of congenital tuberculosis is in part attributable to the high likelihood of infertility in women who have endometrial tuberculosis (Balasubramanian et al, 1999). However, in areas with high rates of tuberculosis transmission, neonates may be undiagnosed or underreported, and the incidence of congenital infection or vertical transmission remains unknown.

Fewer than 400 cases of congenital tuberculosis have been reported in the literature, with the majority being in the prechemotherapy era (Laartz et al, 2002). Hageman et al (1980) reported two cases of congenital tuberculosis and reviewed another 24 reported in the English-language literature since the introduction of isoniazid (INH) in 1952. In the subsequent 30 years, more than 30 additional cases of neonates with congenital tuberculosis have been described (Abughali et al, 1994; Cantwell et al, 1994; Chen and Shih, 2004; Doudier et al, 2008; Grover et al, 2003; Hatzistamatiou et al, 2003; Laartz et al, 2002; Manji et al, 2001; Mazade et al, 2001; Nicolaidou et al, 2005; Pejham et al, 2002; Saitoh et al, 2001). The more recent reviews are cited in Table 38-8. Not surprisingly, the majority of infants were born to foreign-born mothers living in nonendemic areas.

PATHOPHYSIOLOGY

In pregnant women, tuberculous bacillemia can result in dissemination of infection to the placenta, the endometrium, or the genital tract. Genital tuberculosis that occurred before pregnancy may be asymptomatic, but often results in sterility, thus likely accounting for the low overall frequency of congenital infection. Vertical transmission may occur in one of three ways: (1) hematogenous spread from the infected placenta via the umbilical vein, (2) in utero aspiration or ingestion of amniotic fluid infected from the placenta or endometrium, or (3) ingestion of infected amniotic fluid or secretions from maternal genital lesions during delivery. The hematogenous route and in

TABLE 38-8   Reviews of Cases of Congenital Tuberculosis Cases Reported in the English-Language Literature in the Era of Chemotherapy

Reference	Years Cases Reported	No. of Cases	Age at Clinical Presentation (d)	No. of Infants With Reactive TST	Common Symptoms	Mortality (%) (With Treatment)
Hageman et al, 1980	1952-1980	26	NR	2 of 14	Respiratory distress, fever, hepatomegaly	46 (12)
Cantwell et al, 1994	1980-1994	31	Median 24 (range 1 to 84)	0 of 9	Hepatosplenomegaly, respiratory distress, fever	38 (22)
Abughali et al, 1994	1952-1994	58	NR	1 of 19?	Respiratory distress, hepatomegaly, fever	45 (14)
Laartz et al, 2002	1994-2002	16	Mean 17.4 (range, 1 to 60)	1 of 4	Respiratory distress, hepatomegaly, fever	20

NR, Not reported; *TST,* tuberculin skin test.

utero aspiration each probably account for approximately half of the cases of congenital tuberculosis.

Tuberculous bacilli have been demonstrated in the decidua, amnion, and chorionic villi of the placenta. It is unlikely that the fetus can be infected directly from the mother without the presence of a caseous lesion in the placenta, although massive involvement of the placenta does not always result in congenital tuberculosis. When a tubercle ruptures into the fetal circulation, bacilli in the umbilical vein can infect the liver, forming a primary focus with involvement of periportal lymph nodes. The bacilli also may pass through the liver and right ventricle and into the lung, or they can enter the left ventricle via the foramen ovale and pass into the systemic circulation. The organisms in the lung remain dormant until after birth, when oxygenation and circulation result in their multiplication and the subsequent development of a primary pulmonary focus. Alternatively, if the caseous lesion in the placenta ruptures directly into the uterine cavity and infects the amniotic fluid, the fetus can inhale or ingest the bacilli, leading to primary foci in the lung, intestine, or middle ear. Pathologic examination of tuberculosis in the fetus and newborn usually demonstrates disseminated disease, with the liver and lungs being principally involved. In Siegel's study (1934) of 38 postmortem cases, the lungs were involved in 97%, the liver in 82%, and the spleen in 76% of the infants. Other sites described are the gastrointestinal tract, kidneys, adrenal glands, and skin (Agrawal and Rehman, 1995; Hageman et al, 1980; Sood et al, 2000). It is not always possible to determine whether sites represent multiple primary foci or are secondary to primary lesions in the lung or liver. The only lesion in the neonate that is unquestionably associated with congenital infection is a primary complex in the liver; all others may be acquired congenitally or postnatally.

M. tuberculosis infection acquired in utero or perinatally may be indistinguishable from postpartum infection. Postnatal acquisition of *M. tuberculosis* acquired by airborne inoculation, either from the mother or another contagious adult in the infant's environment, is the most common route of infection of the neonate. In addition, postnatal infection can occur from ingestion of infected breast milk from a mother with a tuberculous breast abscess. In the absence of a breast abscess, transmission of tuberculosis via breast milk has not been documented. The distinction between congenital tuberculosis and postnatally acquired disease may be important for academic or epidemiologic purposes, but the management, treatment, and prognosis of the disease processes are the same.

CLINICAL PRESENTATION

The clinical presentation of congenital tuberculosis is neither distinctive nor specific. Manifestations of disease resemble those of neonatal sepsis or other congenital infections. The affected infant is commonly born prematurely (Amodio et al, 2005; Davis et al, 1960; Foo et al, 1993; Katumba-Luenya et al, 2005; Premkumar et al, 2008; Wanjari et al, 2008). A retrospective cohort study from Mexico of infants born to 35 mothers with pregnancies complicated by tuberculosis demonstrated an approximately twofold risk of prematurity compared with newborns of mothers without tuberculosis (Figueroa-Damian and

Arredondo-Garcia, 2001). Clinical signs may be evident shortly after birth, but typically do not appear until 2 to 4 weeks of age (see Table 38-8). Among the 29 cases reviewed by Cantwell et al (1994), the median age of presentation was 24 days. In an updated review of 16 cases reported since 1994, the mean age at presentation was slightly younger at 17.4 days (Laartz et al, 2002).

Before the availability of INH, congenital tuberculosis was almost uniformly fatal. Notable signs included failure to thrive, jaundice, and central nervous system involvement. In the post-INH era, the most commonly described features of disease are respiratory distress, hepatomegaly with or without splenomegaly, and fever (Abughali et al, 1994; Cantwell et al, 1994; Hageman et al, 1980). Additional findings are listed in Table 38-9. Although it is important to evaluate for meningitis in an infant with suspected congenital tuberculosis, central nervous involvement occurs in fewer than 50% of cases (Hageman et al, 1980; Starke, 1997). Otitis media with aural discharge has been described as the presenting sign of congenital tuberculosis (Ng et al, 1996; Senbil et al, 1997), accompanied by regional lymphadenopathy (Gordon-Nesbitt and Rajan, 1973; Hatzistamatiou et al, 2003; Figure 38-7) or facial palsy (Pejham et al, 2002). It is presumed that the infection is due to the accumulation of infected amniotic fluid in the eustachian tube, either in utero or at birth. Cutaneous manifestations of congenital tuberculosis include papular, pustular, or vesicular lesions often surrounded by erythema (Al-Katawee et al, 2007; Azimi and Grossman, 1996; Hageman et al, 1980; Loeffler et al, 1996; Sood et al, 2000). Biopsy of the lesions is often confirmatory, demonstrating granulomatous inflammation and the presence of acid fast bacilli (AFB) on tissue stain (Hageman et al, 1980; Loeffler et al, 1996). A unique case of congenital tuberculosis involving the spine was recently reported in India (Grover et al, 2003).

TABLE 38-9   Clinical Signs of Congenital Tuberculosis in 58 Infants

Sign	No. of Patients	% of Patients
Respiratory distress	44	76
Hepatomegaly with or without splenomegaly	38	65
Fever	33	57
Lymphadenopathy	19	33
Poor feeding	18	31
Lethargy, irritability	16	30
Abdominal distention	15	26
Failure to thrive	9	15
Ear discharge	9	15
Rash	5	9
Abnormal funduscopic findings	4	7
Jaundice	4	7
Seizure	3	5
Bloody diarrhea	3	5
Ascites	3	5

Adapted from Abughali N, Van Der Kuyp F, Annable W, et al: Congenital tuberculosis, *Pediatr Infect Dis J* 13:738-741, 1994.

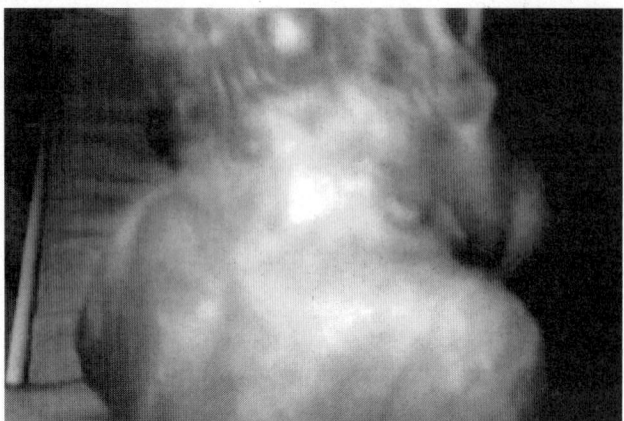

FIGURE 38-7 Cervical and suboccipital tuberculous lymphadenitis in a 6-day-old premature infant. *(From Hatzistamatiou Z, Kaleyias J, Ikonomidou U, et al: Congenital tuberculous lymphadenitis in a preterm infant in Greece,* Acta Paediatr *92:392-394, 2003.)*

DIAGNOSIS

The timely diagnosis of congenital tuberculosis requires a high index of suspicion. Clinical signs of disease in the neonate are nonspecific, and disease in the mother may be unsuspected, contributing to further delay in diagnosis. The diagnosis of congenital tuberculosis should be considered in any neonate with suspected infection who is unresponsive to conventional antimicrobial therapy. Evaluation for suspected disease should include a tuberculin skin test (TST), chest radiography, lumbar puncture, and mycobacterial culture of appropriate specimens. Biopsy specimens of affected tissue, either from the infant or the mother, and the placenta have been confirmatory in several case reports (Abughali et al, 1994; Cantwell et al, 1994; Chou, 2002; Hageman et al, 1980; Laartz et al, 2002; Loeffler et al, 1996).

The TST is the most commonly used diagnostic test for tuberculosis. The test uses 5 tuberculin units of purified protein derivative injected intradermally on the volar surface of the forearm. The reaction is measured 48 to 72 hours later as millimeters of induration. As many as 10% to 40% of immunocompetent children with culture-proven tuberculosis do not initially react to a TST. Host factors such as young age and immunocompromised state can also decrease the sensitivity of the TST. Specificity may be compromised by cross reactivity with bacille-Calmette-Guérin vaccine or with environmental nontuberculous mycobacteria. The TST result is usually negative in neonates with congenital or perinatal tuberculosis, either secondary to immature cell-mediated immunity or because of overwhelming disease (see Table 38-8). Hageman et al (1980) found that only 2 of 14 infants who underwent skin testing had positive test results; on repeated testing, seven infants subsequently demonstrated positive tuberculin skin tests, the earliest being at 6 weeks of age, almost 4 weeks after presentation with clinical signs. Similarly, results of TSTs performed in 9 of 29 patients described by Cantwell et al (1994) were all negative, with results of subsequent testing being positive in 2 of the 9 infants. Among the 16 infants with congenital tuberculosis recently reviewed by Laartz (2002), three of four infants tested had nonreactive TST results.

Recent advances in diagnostic tools for tuberculosis include whole-blood interferon γ release assays (IGRAs), which are immunologically based tests that measure interferon γ production from lymphocytes in response to antigens that are fairly specific to *M. tuberculosis*. The two types of assays currently available include the Quantiferon Gold (Cellestis, Valencia, California) and the enzyme-linked immunosorbent spot assay. Advantages of these tests include lack of cross-reactivity with bacille-Calmette-Guérin vaccine and most nontuberculous mycobacteria. The correlation between IGRAs and TSTs is variable, and negative results do not definitively exclude tuberculosis. Published experience with the use of IGRAs in children is limited, and the negative predictive value of these tests in this population is unclear. Although IGRAs are endorsed by the CDC for use in circumstances in which a TST is indicated (Mazurek et al, 2010), the tests are not recommend for use in children younger than 5 years of age (American Academy of Pediatrics, 2009). Data on the use of IGRAs in newborns is limited to case reports, and these assays should not be substituted for TSTs in the evaluation of congenital tuberculosis.

Given the frequency of respiratory distress in infants with congenital tuberculosis, it is not surprising that chest radiograph findings are frequently abnormal at first examination. Typically, a nonspecific parenchymal infiltrate is noted, although a miliary pattern representative of disseminated disease is occasionally observed (Agrawal and Rehman, 1995; Airede, 1990; Nemir and O'Hare, 1985; Pal and Ghosh, 2008; Polansky et al, 1978; Singh et al, 2006; Figure 38-8). Sixteen of 26 patients (62%) reviewed by Hageman et al (1980) had abnormal radiographic findings on presentation; seven had a miliary pattern and nine had nonspecific changes. Radiographic abnormalities developed subsequently in four additional infants. Among the 29 cases reviewed by Cantwell et al (1994), 23 infants (79%) had chest radiographic abnormalities, the majority being nonspecific infiltrates. Cavitation secondary to progressive pulmonary involvement has been reported (Cunningham et al, 1982). CT imaging of the chest may demonstrate adenopathy suggestive of tuberculosis or confirm miliary disease (Das et al, 2008; Singh et al, 2006). An ultrasound or CT image of the abdomen may reveal enlargement of the liver, spleen, or both, possibly with areas of abscesses (Amodio et al, 2005; Berk and Sylvester, 2004; Grover et al, 2003; Senbil et al, 1997). Congenital tuberculosis involving the spine was identified by radiographs and confirmed by magnetic resonance imaging in India (Grover et al, 2003) (Figure 38-9).

Microbiologic confirmation of disease in the neonate should be sought using specimens from multiple sites. For infants and children unable to expectorate sputum, gastric aspirates are considered the specimens of choice. Additional sources for culture include endotracheal aspirate, bronchial washing, middle-ear discharge, and lymph node tissue. CSF should be analyzed and cultured, although isolation of *M. tuberculosis* from CSF is uncommon (Abughali et al, 1994; Hageman et al, 1980). Traditionally the detection of mycobacterial organisms by smear or culture has been considered difficult, because children have paucibacillary disease relative to adults. With three morning gastric aspirates collected appropriately in hospitalized

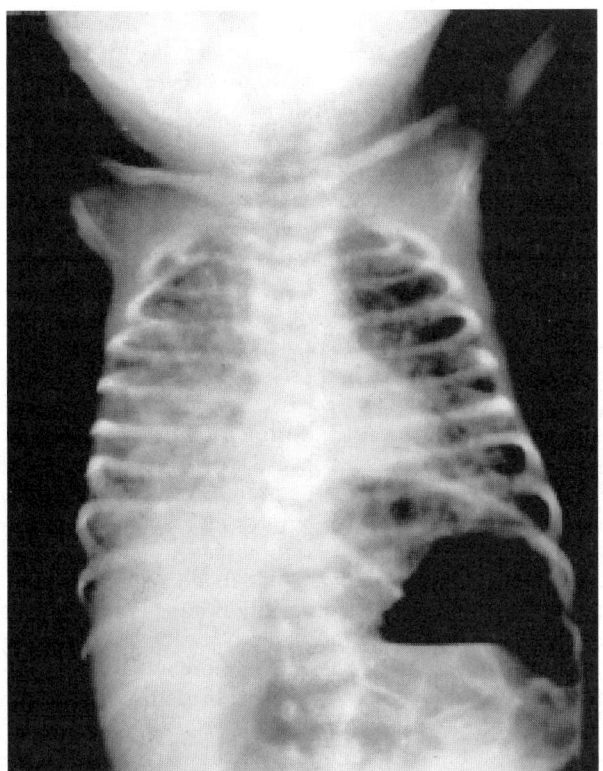

FIGURE 38-8 Miliary tuberculosis in a neonate with congenital tuberculosis. *(From Singh M, Kothur K, Dayal D, et al: Perinatal tuberculosis a case series,* J Trop Pediatr *53:135-138, 2006.)*

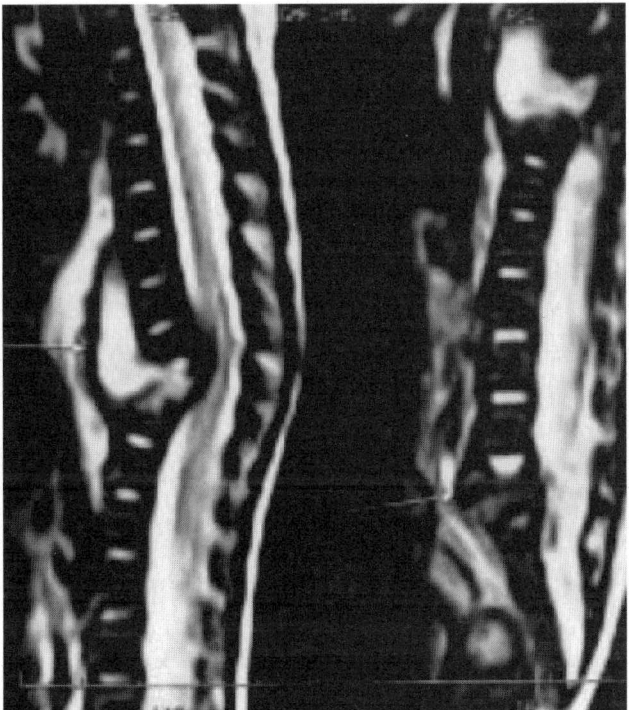

FIGURE 38-9 Saggital magnetic resonance image on the *left* demonstrates destruction of T9 to T11 vertebral bodies with the collapse of T10, leading to a kyphotic deformity causing cord compression. A large prevertebral collection is also seen. The image on the *right* demonstrates destruction with collapse of L5 and S1 vertebral bodies. *(From Grover SB, Pati NK, Mehta R, et al: Congenital spine tuberculosis: early diagnosis by imaging studies,* Am J Perinatol *20:150, 2003.)*

children with a clinical diagnosis of tuberculosis, only 40% of children had positive cultures (Starke and Taylor-Watts, 1989). In comparison, cultures of aspirates from infants evaluated at the same institution had a 75% yield (Starke and Taylor-Watts, 1989; Vallejo et al, 1994).

The improved diagnostic yield in infants likely reflects more widely disseminated and progressive disease, with higher bacillary loads. Hageman et al (1980) found positive cultures of *M. tuberculosis* in 10 of 12 gastric aspirates, 3 of 3 liver biopsy specimens, 3 of 3 lymph node specimens, and 2 of 4 bone marrow biopsy specimens. Among the 31 cases reviewed by Cantwell et al (1994), noninvasive procedures and biopsy were useful for the diagnosis of congenital malaria in the majority infants (Table 38-10). More recent reports confirm the high yield of cultures from a variety of specimens in neonates (Berk and Sylvester, 2004; Chou, 2002; Mazade et al, 2001; Premkumar et al, 2008; Wanjari et al, 2008). Histologic examination of tissue may suggest the diagnosis before culture results are available. Biopsy of skin lesions, lymph nodes, and the liver have suggested the diagnosis in several cases by demonstration of granulomas or acid-fast bacilli on staining before culture results are available (Berk and Sylvester, 2004; Davis et al, 1960; Hageman et al, 1980).

Whereas *M. tuberculosis* can require 7 to 21 days for growth by standard culture technique, results from techniques such as PCR may be available within 48 hours. A comparison of PCR, AFB smear, and culture with clinical diagnosis in children found a sensitivity of 60% and a specificity of 97% (Smith, 2002). Although PCR has been useful for diagnosing congenital tuberculosis in a few case reports, it is not sensitive enough to preclude obtaining specimens for culture. Isolation of *M. tuberculosis* is still important to determine susceptibilities and to optimize treatment.

The mother of a newborn in whom congenital tuberculosis is suspected is often asymptomatic or has subclinical disease. In the series of congenitally infected infants reported by Hageman et al (1980), the majority of mothers did not have a diagnosis until after the disease became apparent in their infants. Cantwell et al (1994) found that 50% of the mothers of infected infants were not ill at the time their newborns exhibited clinical signs of disease. Evaluation of the mother should include a TST, a chest radiograph, and, if the radiograph is consistent with tuberculosis disease, collection of sputum for microbiological confirmation. It is not unusual for the mother to have extrapulmonary disease such as meningitis or peritonitis (Laartz et al, 2002; Naouri, 2005), and evaluation may need to be extended to identify such sites if pulmonary disease is not discovered. In mothers with no clinical evidence of disease, endometritis should be considered. Pathologic examination and culture of the placenta (if available) or endometrial biopsy can confirm the diagnosis of genital transmission (Asensi et al, 1990; Balasubramanian et al, 1999; Cantwell et al, 1994; Cooper et al, 1985; Niles, 1982; Surve et al, 2006). In several case reports, the diagnosis of maternal tuberculosis was solely and ultimately made by endometrial biopsy and culture (Pejham et al, 2002). In addition, culture of amniotic fluid should be performed. All mothers with tuberculosis should be tested for HIV infection and, if the mother is seropositive, the infant should be evaluated for perinatally acquired HIV infection.

TREATMENT AND MANAGEMENT

The successful management of congenital tuberculosis depends on early recognition and treatment of disease. In suspected cases, treatment should not be delayed until results of cultures or other diagnostic tests are available.

TABLE 38-10 Results of Diagnostic Procedures Performed on 29 Infants With Congenital Tuberculosis Reported from 1980 to 1994

Type of Specimen	Acid-Fast Smear*	Mycobacterial Culture	Smear or Culture
Gastric aspirate	8/9	8/9	9/11
Endotracheal aspirate	7/7	7/7	7/7
Ear discharge	2/2	1/1	2/2
Cerebrospinal fluid	1/2	1/2	1/2
Urine	0/2	0/2	0/2
Peritoneal fluid	1/1	1/1	1/1
Bronchoscopic specimen	1/1	1/1	1/1
Biopsy specimen	14/19	11/12	16/21
Lymph node	7/8	6/6	7/8†
Liver	4/6	1/2	4/6†
Skin	1/3	1/1	1/3
Lung	1/1	1/1	2/2
Bone marrow	—	1/1	1/1
Ear	1/1	1/1	1/1

Adapted from Cantwell MF, Shehab ZM, Costello AM, et al: Brief report: congenital tuberculosis, *N Engl J Med* 330:1051, 1994.
*Results expressed as number of positive results per number of patients tested.
†All biopsy specimens of lymph node and liver that tested negative on smear and culture showed histopathologic changes consistent with tuberculosis (i.e., giant cell transformation of granulomas, with or without caseation).

Multiple drug therapy for an extended duration has long been recognized as the standard of care for tuberculosis. Because of the rarity of the condition, clinical trials have not been conducted to establish the optimal treatment regimen for congenital tuberculosis. It is assumed that the regimens used for older infants and children are safe and effective for the treatment of neonates with congenital tuberculosis. Consultation with a pediatric infectious disease specialist or tuberculosis expert is advised.

Until susceptibility results are known, infants with proven or suspected tuberculosis should be treated with a four-drug regimen consisting of INH rifampin (RIF), pyrazinamide (PZA), and ethambutol (Table 38-11). Some experts would recommend administration of three drugs (INH, RIF, PZA) if antimicrobial resistance is not suspected in the mother, because either she or the source case are known to have a susceptible strain or she has no risk factors for resistant *M. tuberculosis*. The adjunctive use of corticosteroids is recommended for the treatment of tuberculosis meningitis based on decreased mortality and morbidity demonstrated in adults and children (Girgis et al, 1991). Supplementation with pyridoxine, although not routinely recommended for otherwise healthy older children, should be provided to breastfeeding infants receiving INH. If the *M. tuberculosis* isolate is determined to be susceptible, the regimen can be narrowed to three drugs (INH, RIF, PZA) for the first 2 months of initial treatment, and subsequently to 2 drugs (INH, RIF) to complete the continuation phase of treatment. Once the infant is discharged to home, directly observed therapy is recommended to ensure adherence and to prevent relapse.

The optimal duration of treatment for infants with congenital tuberculosis is unknown. The typical duration of treatment for susceptible *M. tuberculosis* is 6 months for pulmonary disease, pulmonary disease with hilar adenopathy, or hilar adenopathy alone (American Academy of

TABLE 38-11 Commonly Used Drugs for Treatment of Tuberculosis in Infants, Children, and Adolescents

Drugs	Dose Forms	Daily Dose (mg/kg)	Twice per Week Dose (mg/kg)	Maximum Dose	Adverse Reactions
Ethambutol	Tablets (100,400 mg)	20-25	50	2.5 g	Optic neuritis (usually reversible), decreased red-green color discrimination, gastrointestinal tract disturbances, hypersensitivity
Isoniazid	Scored tablets (100, 300 mg) Syrup 10 mg/mL	10-15†	20-30	300 mg daily	Mild hepatic enzyme elevation, hepatitis,† peripheral neuritis, hypersensitivity
				900 mg twice per week	Diarrhea and gastric irritation caused by vehicle in the syrup
Pyrazinamide	Scored tablets (500 mg)	30-40	50	2 g	Hepatotoxic effects, hyperuricemia, arthralgia, gastrointestinal tract upset
Rifampin	Capsules (150, 300 mg) Syrup formulated capsules	10-20	10-20	600 mg	Orange discoloration of secretions or urine, staining of contact lenses, vomiting, hepatitis, influenza-like reaction, thrombocytopenia, pruritus; oral contraceptives may be ineffective

From American Academy of Pediatrics Committee on Infectious Diseases: Section 3. Summaries of Infectious Diseases. Tuberculosis. In Pickering LK, editor: *2009 red book: report of the committee on infectious diseases*, ed 28, Elk Grove Village, Ill, 2009, American Academy of Pediatrics, p 688.
†When isoniazid in a dose exceeding 10 mg/kg/d is used in combination with rifampin, the incidence of hepatotoxic effects may be increased.

Pediatrics, 2009). For extrapulmonary disease, the duration is extended to 9 to 12 months, and for drug-resistant *M. tuberculosis* the duration may be extended even further to prevent failure or relapse. Most experts would treat infants with congenital tuberculosis for 9 to 12 months because of the decreased immunocompetence of neonates (Starke, 1997).

Although there is a fair amount of data to support the safety of INH, data on the safety and pharmacokinetics of other agents are limited. Careful monitoring for signs and symptoms of hepatitis and other adverse effects of drug therapy is recommended. Routine determination of serum transaminases in children is indicated with severe tuberculosis (e.g., military or meningitis), for those with concurrent liver or biliary disease, or for those receiving other potentially hepatotoxic drugs. Routine monitoring of liver function also should be considered for neonates with congenital tuberculosis given the paucity of data on adverse effects of anti-tuberculosis agents in this age group (Patel et al, 2008). The risks of optic neuritis with ethambutol should be considered when this agent is used, and vision should be monitored periodically.

The management of infants born to mothers who have latent tuberculosis infection (LTBI) or tuberculosis disease is outlined in Figure 38-10. Recommendations are based on the categorization of infection in the mother and the potential risk of transmission of tuberculosis to the infant (American Academy of Pediatrics, 2009). Infants born to mothers with potentially contagious tuberculosis should be evaluated for congenital tuberculosis. Separation of the infant and mother is necessary only in cases in which the mother is highly infectious at the time of delivery. The mother with latent tuberculosis infection is not contagious. To prevent reactivation disease in the mother and subsequent exposure of the infant, the mother should receive treatment with INH for LTBI. In addition, latent tuberculosis infection in the mother may be a marker for contagious tuberculosis within the household, and it is recommended that all household members and close contacts of the mother be evaluated for tuberculosis.

Breastfeeding is not contraindicated in women with LTBI. The breast milk of a woman with tuberculosis does not contain tubercle bacilli. For women with tuberculosis who are potentially infectious and separated from the newborn, breast milk may be manually expressed and fed to the infant. Once the mother is noninfectious or the infant is receiving therapy, breastfeeding can be resumed. The exception, however, is the mother with an active tuberculous breast lesion. In this situation the breast milk may be pumped and discarded until resolution of the lesion (Efferen, 2007).

PROGNOSIS

The prognosis for congenital tuberculosis was dismal in the prechemotherapy era, the diagnosis often being only made at autopsy. Although the survival rate subsequently improved, mortality remained approximately 50% secondary to delayed diagnosis. In a review of 26 cases reported between 1952 and 1980, 12 (46%) patients died, 9 of whom were untreated but with a diagnosis made at autopsy. The subsequent reviews demonstrate a decrease in case fatality (see Table 38-8), with earlier diagnosis and treatment. Timely diagnosis and initiation of anti-tuberculosis therapy are critical for a favorable outcome.

PREVENTION

Prevention of congenital tuberculosis requires the treatment and prevention of disease in women of childbearing age. Risk factors for acquiring tuberculosis infection or progressing to disease should be assessed at prenatal visits, and women identified as being high risk for LTBI or progression to disease should undergo tuberculin skin testing as recommended by the CDC (Centers for Disease Control, 2000). Women who are TST positive should undergo evaluation for active disease. The treatment of active tuberculosis during pregnancy is considered standard, and early treatment has been shown to improve maternal and neonatal outcome (Figueroa-Damian and Arredonondo-Garcia, 1998). While not without potential complications, treatment during pregnancy is less of a hazard to a pregnant woman and her fetus than tuberculosis itself. The treatment of LTBI during pregnancy is somewhat more controversial. Some experts advocate treatment during pregnancy, whereas others support a delay in therapy until weeks to months after delivery. Although there is no demonstrated teratogenic potential for the use of INH, there is concern that pregnant and postpartum women are more vulnerable to INH-related hepatotoxicity (Franks et al, 1989).

Most children with pulmonary tuberculosis, especially those younger than 10 years, have paucibacillary disease and often have little to no cough. Isolation of the hospitalized pediatric patient is directed at accompanying adult contacts who may be source cases and potentially contagious. Visitation of the hospitalized pediatric patient should be restricted to adults in whom contagious tuberculosis has been excluded. Hospitalized children with negative sputum AFB smears (if obtained) require standard precautions, assuming that contagious tuberculosis has been excluded in the visitors. Airborne precautions are recommended for the following pediatric patients: (1) children and adolescents with adult-type cavitary disease, (2) extensive pulmonary infection, (3) those with smears positive for AFB, and (4) congenitally infected neonates undergoing endotracheal intubation (American Academy of Pediatrics, 2009).

Compared with older children, neonates likely have a higher concentration of bacilli in their sputum. As noted previously, AFB smears on tracheal aspirates and other specimens are frequently positive in this population compared with older children. Transmission of tuberculosis from congenitally infected neonates to health care workers and other hospitalized infants has been reported and is likely related to aerosolization of bacilli during respiratory manipulation (Crockett et al, 2004; Laartz et al, 2002; Lee et al, 1998; Mouchet et al, 2004). Neonates suspected of having congenital tuberculosis should be placed in respiratory isolation if intubated or if undergoing any procedure with the potential for aerosolization of infected sputum. Exposed infants, visitors, and health care workers should undergo evaluation for tuberculosis infection or disease.

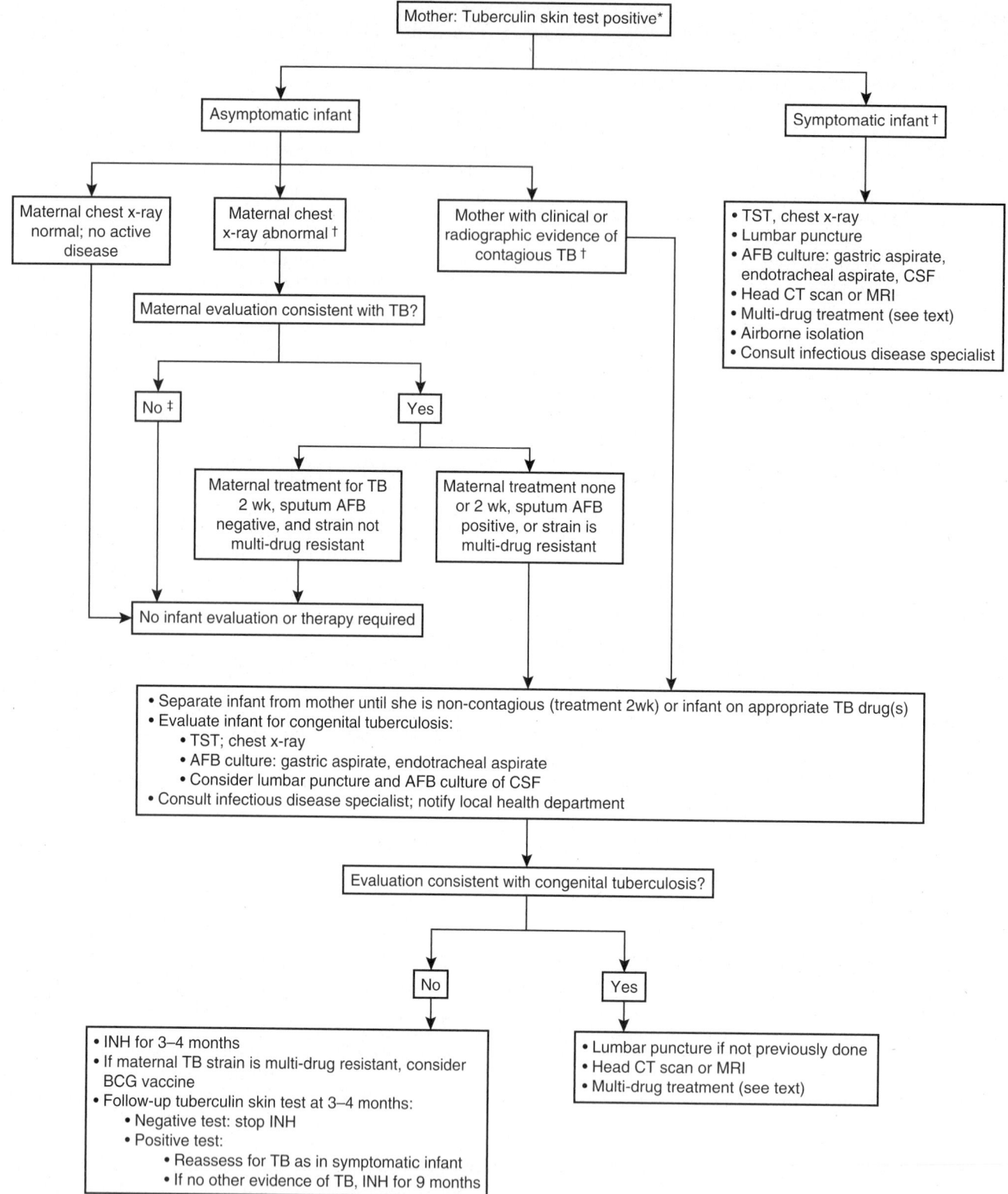

FIGURE 38-10 Management of infants born to mothers with a positive tuberculin skin test (TST) result. *BCG,* Bacille Calmette-Guérin; *CSF,* cerebrospinal fluid; *CT,* computed tomography; *INH,* isoniazid; *MRI,* magnetic resonance imaging. (*Adapted from American Academy of Pediatrics: Tuberculosis. In Pickering LK, editor:* 2003 Red book: report of the committee on infectious diseases, *ed 26, Elk Grove Village, Ill, 2003, American Academy of Pediatrics, p 642.*)
*Household contacts should have a TST and further evaluation for contagious tuberculosis (TB). Consult local health department. The mother should receive treatment for latent tuberculosis infections. All persons with TB should be tested for human immunodeficiency virus (HIV) infection.
†Acid-fast bacillus (AFB) culture of amniotic flid and placenta, if available; placenta for histopathologic examination.
‡Includes mother with chest radiographic findings consistent with old, healed TB.

SUGGESTED READINGS

Toxoplasmosis

Beaman MH, Luft BJ, Remington JS: Prophylaxis for toxoplasmosis in AIDS, *Ann Intern Med* 117:163-164, 1992.

Boyer K: Diagnostic testing for congenital toxoplasmosis, *Pediatr Infect Dis J* 20:59-60, 2001.

Centers for Disease Control and Prevention: CDC recommendations regarding selected conditions affecting women's health: Preventing congenital toxoplasmosis, *MMWR Morb Mortal Wkly Rep* 49(RR-2):59-68, 2000.

Feldman DM, Timms D, Borgida AF: Toxoplasmosis, parvovirus and cytomegalovirus in pregnancy, *Clin Lab Med* 30:709-720, 2010.

Jones JL, Dargelas V, Roberts J, et al: Risk factors for Toxoplasma gondii infection in the United States, *Clin Infect Dis* 49:878-884, 2009.

Kasper DC, Sadeghi K, Prusa AR, et al: Quantitative real-time polymerase chain reaction for the accurate detection of *Toxoplasma gondii* in amniotic fluid, *Diagn Microbiol Infect Dis* 63:10-15, 2009.

Koppe JG, Loewer-Sieger DH, DeRoever-Bonnet H: Result of 20-year follow-up of congenital toxoplasmosis, *Lancet* 1:254-256, 1986.

Masur H, Kaplan JE, Holmes KK, et al: Guidelines for preventing opportunistic infections among HIV-infected persons: 2002 recommendations of the U.S. Public Health Service and the Infectious Diseases Society of America, *MMWR Morb Mortal Wkly Rep* 51(RR-8):5, 2002.

McLeod R, Kieffer F, Sautter M, et al: Why prevent, diagnose and treat congenital toxoplasmosis?, *Mem Inst Oswaldo Cruz* 104:320-344, 2009.

Rabilloud M, Wallon M, Peyron F: In utero and at birth diagnosis of congenital toxoplasmosis: use of likelihood ratios for clinical management, *Pediatr Infect Dis J* 29:421-425, 2010.

Syphilis

American Academy of Pediatrics Committee on Infectious Diseases: Syphilis, Red Book Online: 2009. Available at http://aapredbook.aappublications.org/cgi/content/full/2009/1/3.129. Accessed November 17, 2010.

Beeram MR, Chopde N, Dawood Y, et al: Lumbar puncture in the evaluation of possible asymptomatic congenital syphilis in neonates, *J Pediatr* 128:125-129, 1996.

Centers for Disease Control and Prevention: Sexually Transmitted Diseases Treatment Guidelines, 2010. *MMWR* 59:1-110, 2010. Accessed

Centers for Disease Control and Prevention: Congenital syphilis: United States, 2003-2008, *MMWR* 59:413-417, 2010.

Herremans T, Kortbeek L, Notermans DW: A review of diagnostic tests for congenital syphilis in newborns, *Eur J Clin Microbiol Infect Dis* 29:495-501, 2010.

Ingall J, Sanchez P, Baker C: Syphilis, In Remington JS, Klein JO, Baker C, et al: *Infectious diseases of the fetus and newborn infant*, ed 6, Philadelphia, 2006, WB Saunders, pp 545-580.

World Health Organization Department of Reproductive Health and Research: The global elimination of congenital syphilis: rationale and strategy for action: 2007. Available at www.who.int/reproductivehealth/publications/rtis/9789241595858/en/index.html. Accessed November 17, 2010.

Malaria

Desai M, ter Kuile FO, Nosten F, et al: Epidemiology and burden of malaria in pregnancy, *Lancet Infect Dis* 7:93-104, 2007.

Hulbert TV: Congenital malaria in the United States: report of a case and review, *Clin Infect Dis* 14:922-926, 1992.

Lesko CR, Arguin PM, Neman RD: Congenital malaria in the United States: a review of cases from 1966 to 2005, *Arch Pediatr Adolesc Med* 161:1062-1067, 2007.

Menendez C, Mayor A: Congenital malaria: the least known consequence of malaria in pregnancy, *Semin Fetal Neonatal Med* 12:207-213, 2007.

Tuberculosis

Abughali N, Van Der Kuyp F, Annable W: Kumar ML: Congenital tuberculosis, *Pediatr Infect Dis J* 13:738-741, 1994.

Cantwell MF, Shehab ZM, Costello AM, et al: Brief report: congenital tuberculosis, *N Engl J Med* 330:1051-1054, 1994.

Hageman J, Shulman S, Schreiber M, et al: Congenital tuberculosis: critical reappraisal of clinical findings and diagnostic procedures, *Pediatrics* 66:980-984, 1980.

Laartz BW, Narvarte HJ, Hold D, et al: Congenital tuberculosis and management of exposures in a neonatal intensive care unit, *Infect Control Hosp Epidemiol* 23:573-579, 2002.

Complete references and supplemental color images used in this text can be found online at www.expertconsult.com

NEONATAL BACTERIAL SEPSIS

Patricia Ferrieri and Linda D. Wallen

NEONATAL BACTERIAL SEPSIS

Throughout pregnancy, the fetus is protected from bacterial and viral infections by the chorioamniotic membranes, the placenta, and various antibacterial factors, that are poorly described in amniotic fluid. It is thought that some subclinical infections of the fetus, amniotic fluid, membranes, or placenta may contribute to the onset of preterm labor and the delivery of preterm infants. There are several mechanisms by which bacteria can reach the fetus or newborn and initiate infection. Maternal blood stream infections, caused by bacteria such as *Listeria monocytogenes* and *Mycobacterium tuberculosis*, can reach the fetus and cause infection. Bacteria such as group B streptococcus (GBS) can be acquired from the vagina, cervix, or fecal contamination of the birth canal through either ruptured or intact membranes, leading to amnionitis, intrauterine pneumonitis, and premature delivery (Ancona et al, 1980; Ferrieri, 1990; Larsen and Sever, 2008; Payne et al, 1988). Finally, infection can occur via aspiration of birth canal contents or colonization of mucosal surfaces during passage through the birth canal, leading to pneumonia, followed by bacteremia and sepsis after 1 day or later; this may be the mode by which *Neisseria gonorrhoeae*, *Escherichia coli*, and GBS are acquired.

Early-onset bacterial sepsis remains a major cause of neonatal morbidity and mortality, although the sepsis-associated death rates per 100,000 live births have declined significantly from 2001-2011. Much of this decline in mortality is because of the introduction of intrapartum antibiotic prophylaxis in pregnant women during labor and delivery (Centers for Disease Control and Prevention, 2007, 2009; Schrag et al, 2002; Schrag and Stoll, 2006). Mortality rates in infected premature infants and very immature infants are significantly higher than in term infants. Major improvements in neonatal intensive care and early identification and recognition of infected infants have all contributed to reduced mortality rates in the newborn period.

PATHOGENESIS OF EARLY-ONSET NEONATAL BACTERIAL INFECTIONS

There are multiple portals through which bacteria can enter and infect the newborn. The primary portals of entry appear to be the respiratory tract, as suggested by the high frequency of acute respiratory distress and pneumonia, which occurs in infants with early-onset disease. Acquisition via the placenta is suggested in some instances by the presentation of high-grade bacteremia and severe sepsis clinically apparent at the time of birth in the presence of intact membranes in infants born via cesarean section. The primary maternal event in this sequence, leading to infection of the fetus and newborn infant, is colonization of the maternal genital tract with organisms such as the GBS.

Bacteria that reside in the cervix, vagina, or rectum can ascend into the amniotic cavity through intact or ruptured membranes and lead to chorioamnionitis. Bacteria can initially spread into the choriodecidual space and can occasionally cross intact chorioamniotic membranes. Although organisms recovered from the amniotic sac in the mother are usually polymicrobial and include such organisms as the GBS, group D enterococcus, aerobic gram-negative bacteria, and anaerobes such as *Bacteroides* spp. (Gibbs et al, 1980), a single organism causing bacterial sepsis is the rule in de novo sepsis of the newborn infant. Genital microplasmas are at times recovered from women as well as *Chlamydia* spp., but the precise pathogenic role is unclear (Krohn et al, 1995; Pankuch et al, 1984). *Ureaplasma* spp., and *Chlamydia* spp. can be isolated from infants' respiratory tract after birth; these two plus *Mycoplasma hominis* can be recovered from the respiratory tract after birth, but they are not associated with sepsis syndrome.

Although many microorganisms recovered from the amniotic cavity are thought to induce spontaneous preterm labor, and possibly premature rupture of membranes, the exact mechanisms by which this may occur are debatable. Clinical or subclinical chorioamnionitis can incite a marked inflammatory response with the release of cytokines that can contribute to the onset of preterm labor and premature rupture of membranes. Other risk factors for clinical intraamniotic infection include young maternal age, prolonged labor, prolonged rupture of membranes (≥18 hours), internal scalp fetal monitoring, the presence of urinary tract infections, and a history of bacterial vaginosis (Newton et al, 1989; Soper et al, 1989). Despite inherent antibacterial properties in amniotic fluid, these may not be sufficient to overcome a large bacterial inoculum, because of rapid multiplication of bacteria during a prolonged labor or the absence of type-specific maternal antibodies for various pathogens (Ferrieri, 1990).

Infants who immediately display signs of respiratory distress and after birth undoubtedly have onset of infection before or during labor and delivery. Particularly with hypoxia in utero, the infant may gasp and inhale contaminated amniotic fluid, leading to pneumonia, blood stream infection, sepsis, and a severe systemic response syndrome. Infants who display such signs at birth or within a short time after birth have the highest mortality rates. Infants who have an initial asymptomatic period after birth may display symptoms gradually as the organisms multiply in the lung and in the blood. An example of another invasive site of entry is the scalp lesion created by a monitoring device, which becomes contaminated in the setting of amniotic fluid infected with the GBS. An overarching mechanism for continued bacteremia is the absence of sufficient local and systemic host defenses, such as adequate complement levels or type-specific immunity against the invading microorganism (Ferrieri, 1990).

The inflammatory cascade is initiated by activation of macrophages by bacterial cell wall constituents, toxins, or enzymes. A number of proinflammatory cytokines can be released, such as interleukin (IL) 6, IL-8, and tumor necrosis factor-α (TNF-α). These cytokines can alter vascular permeability and vascular tone, decrease myocardial contractility, activate clotting systems, increase pulmonary vascular resistance, and activate other phagocytic cells, such as polymorphonuclear leukocytes (PMNs). Ideally, proinflammatory and antiinflammatory cytokines would be balanced; however, this is usually not the case and the bacteria persist with subsequent consequences. It is common in newborn infants and, particularly in preterm infants, to have dissemination of bacteria to other organs such as the meninges, kidneys, and bone.

EPIDEMIOLOGY OF EARLY-ONSET BACTERIAL INFECTIONS

Before the availability and use of antibiotics in the late 1940s and 1950s, there were few survivors of neonatal bacterial sepsis, contributing to the high perinatal mortality rate of that period. There have been changes in the types of bacteria responsible for neonatal infection over the years. In the 1930s and 1940s, the group A streptococcus was a prominent cause of neonatal sepsis; this organism is now rather rare (Bizzarro et al, 2005). In the 1950s, nursery outbreaks of *Staphylococcus aureus* infections appeared across North America and Europe, prompting changes in techniques of hygiene and encouraging the development and use of penicillinase-resistant antibiotics (Bizzarro et al, 2005). In the 1960s, *Escherichia coli* became the most common cause of bacterial sepsis, followed in the 1970s by the GBS. Even in an era of intrapartum antibiotic prophylaxis of GBS colonized mothers, the GBS remains the most common bacterial pathogen in neonatal centers of North American and Europe, followed by *E. coli* (Schrag et al, 2006). An update on neonatal sepsis at Yale, between 1989 to 2003, revealed an overall decrease in sepsis caused by both GBS and *E. coli* (Bizzarro et al, 2005). Regional differences exist, however, and must be considered before attempting to apply epidemiologic data to individual perinatal units. For example, *Listeria monocytogenes* is a frequent isolate in some western European countries, and *S. aureus* is found commonly in Germany and Scandinavia (Posfay-Barbe and Wald, 2009).

The incidence of early-onset bacterial infection is variable and ranges from one to five per 1,000 live births; however, it is clear that the incidence has declined as a result of intrapartum antibiotic therapy (Centers for Disease Control and Prevention, 2007, 2009). Recent data from the CDC revealed a downward trend from 2000 to 2003 (from 0.52 to 0.31 case per 1000 live births), followed by an increase from 2003 to 2006 (from 0.31 to 0.40 case per 1000 live births) (Centers for Disease Control and Prevention, 2009). Stratified by race, the incidence increased significantly among black infants from 2003 to 2006 (from 0.53 to 0.86 case per 1000 live births), whereas the incidence among white infants did not change significantly (from 0.26 to 0.29 case per 1000 live births). When stratified by gestational age, the average incidence of early-onset GBS disease among preterm infants during 2003 to 2006

was 2.8-fold higher among black infants compared with white infants (1.79 case versus 0.67 case per 1000 live births). It is of interest that both preterm black and white infants had increases in early-onset disease from 2003 to 2006 that were not statistically significant. Early-onset disease among full-term white infants was stable during 2003 to 2006, whereas term black infants had a significant increase of the incidence during this period, from 0.33 to 0.7 case per 1000 live births.

The overall rates of late-onset GBS disease remained stable from 2000 to 2006 (0.36 case versus 0.30 case per 1000 live births) (Centers for Disease Control and Prevention, 2009). No overall incidence trend was observed from 2003 to 2006. When stratified by race, late-onset disease incidence among black infants decreased significantly by 42% from 2005 to 2006 (0.95 case versus 0.55 case per 1000 live births). Between 2003 and 2006 there were no significant trends among black or white infants.

Infants described with early-onset sepsis frequently have one or more identifiable risk factors (Dutta et al, 2010). Prematurity is considered the single greatest risk factor for early-onset bacterial infections. Because it is accepted that ELBW infants have impairment of host defenses, and since preterm birth may be associated with low-grade chorioamnionitis, it is not surprising that the attack rates for infection by pathogens such as GBS are 26- to 30-fold higher in preterm infants, compared to term newborn infants, with an associated high mortality. Other risk factors for early-onset sepsis are maternal age, health and nutrition, colonization with well-known pathogens (e.g., GBS), and rupture of membranes for longer than 18 hours (Schuchat et al, 2000). Neonatal susceptibility to GBS infection is increased with deficiencies in circulating levels of GBS type-specific antibody and complement, which is further heightened by any element of neutrophil dysfunction, as may be seen in the more premature infants (Ferrieri, 1990; Foxman, 2007; Makhoul et al, 2009; Nandyal, 2008).

BACTERIAL PATHOGENS IN EARLY-ONSET INFECTIONS

GROUP B STREPTOCOCCAL INFECTIONS

Since the early 1930s when Rebecca Lancefield reported her grouping system for hemolytic streptococci, group A streptococcus (*Streptococcus pyogenes*) was widely acknowledged as the major pathogen associated with puerperal sepsis. GBS was initially thought to be a commensal until 1938, when Frye reported seven cases of GBS-associated puerperal fever with three deaths (Eickhoff et al, 1964). Before the 1960s, GBS was not recognized frequently as a cause of human disease. However, in the late 1960s GBS emerged as the leading cause of neonatal sepsis in newborn infants (Bizzarro et al, 2005; Zaleznik et al, 2000). Before the era of maternal intrapartum prophylaxis, GBS had a reported national incidence of approximately two per 1000 live births and was associated with approximately 50% mortality in the newborn infant. As mentioned previously, over the past decade with the introduction of antibiotic maternal prophylaxis, there has been a significant decrease in the incidence of GBS to its current rate of approximately 0.32 per 1000 live births for early-onset disease.

Transmission of GBS from Mothers to Infants

In the United States, approximately 20% to 35% of pregnant women are asymptomatic carriers of GBS in the genital and gastrointestinal tract during pregnancy and at the time of delivery (Ferrieri, 1990; Ferrieri et al, 2004b; Zaleznik et al, 2000). The prevalence of GBS colonization during pregnancy varies. Among women who were positive for GBS between 26 and 28 weeks' gestation, only 65% remain colonized at term, whereas 8% of those with negative prenatal cultures were positive for GBS at term (Ancona et al, 1980; Zaleznik et al, 2000). Treatment of GBS-colonized women during pregnancy only temporarily eradicates the organism, and most women are recolonized within several weeks. At birth, 50% to 65% of infants who were born to GBS-colonized mothers have positive GBS cultures from mucous membranes and skin (external ear canal, throat, umbilicus, and anal or rectal sites) (Shet and Ferrieri, 2004). Before the introduction of intrapartum antibiotic prophylaxis, approximately 1% to 2% of colonized infants developed GBS infection, and the overall incidence of neonatal GBS infection was approximately two per 1000 live births in the United States. With intrapartum prophylaxis, approximately 60% to 80% of GBS cases occur in infants born to women with negative antenatal GBS screens (Verani and Schrag, 2010).

A small number of GBS-infected infants acquired their bacteremia because of hematogenous transmission through the placenta. In these situations, the mother commonly displays signs and symptoms of chorioamnionitis, although it may occur in the absence of maternal symptoms (Baker and Edwards, 1995).

Detection of GBS colonization has been emphasized since approximately 1996; studies to determine the optimal sites of sampling have been key to the effectiveness of intrapartum prophylaxis. GBS resides in the genitourinary and gastrointestinal tracts, where large numbers of gram-negative bacteria are also present. The majority of colonization studies have revealed high rates of both rectal and vaginal colonization with GBS (Ancona et al, 1980; Hickman et al, 1999; Zaleznik et al, 2000). The use of the selective broth enrichment medium that inhibits the growth of gram-negative enteric bacilli and other normal flora can increase culture sensitivity for GBS to greater than 90%. The most widely used selective medium is Todd-Hewitt broth with either gentamicin or colistin and nalidixic acid. As recommended in a 2002 publication from the Centers for Disease Control and Prevention, the optimal time for performing antenatal cultures is between 35 and 37 weeks' gestation, and the highest culture yield is obtained when both the lower vaginal area and anal or rectal sites are sampled (Schrag et al, 2002).

Epidemiologic studies of GBS-colonized women have shown that those with heavy colonization (3+ to 4+) are more likely to transmit GBS to their infants (Ancona et al, 1980). The colonization of GBS in pregnant women may be long standing, intermittent, or transient. There is a definite association between GBS colonization and other risk factors for neonatal sepsis; these include preterm labor, preterm delivery, premature rupture of membranes, prolonged rupture of membranes, and maternal fever.

In the past few years, rapid diagnostic tests to detect GBS colonization in pregnant women have included real-time polymerase chain reaction (PCR); compared with broth enrichment cultures, there is an approximately 10% to 15% increased sensitivity (P. Ferrieri, unpublished data). The advantages of PCR detection of maternal vaginal or rectal colonization are the rapid turnaround time, as well as the increased sensitivity. Although more expensive than traditional culture-based detection assays, the results are available 1 to 2 days sooner. The argument that this does not provide semiquantitative data on the degree of GBS colonization in the mother is moot, because even low grade colonization in pregnant women is a risk factor for neonatal GBS sepsis. However, women with heavy (3+ to 4+) colonization, determined by semiquantitative assessment of vaginal or rectal cultures, are more likely to pass the microorganism to their infants (Ancona et al, 1980).

Chemoprophylaxis and Intrapartum Antibiotics

Prevention is of key importance in decreasing invasive GBS disease. The challenge has been to widely promulgate screening cultures in pregnant women. Revised guidelines from the CDC were published in 2002 and presented only the culture screening based approach for prevention and chemoprophylaxis, rather than the two preventive approaches published in 1996: a culture screening-based and a risk-based approach (Schrag et al, 2002). The risk-based approach involved the use of antibiotics based solely on the presence of antenatal or intrapartum risk factors such as maternal fever, preterm labor or premature rupture of membranes (<37 weeks' gestation); prolonged rupture of membranes (≥18 hours); history of a previous newborn infant with GBS disease; and GBS bacteruria during pregnancy. Challenges to the implementation of the CDC guidelines, such as failure to seek prenatal care and the use of suboptimal laboratory culture techniques continue in certain populations. Data for the United States as a whole show a decrease in the incidence of early-onset GBS concurrent with the implementation of maternal GBS screen and intrapartum antibiotic prophylaxis guidelines. The current estimate for the overall United States population for early-onset GBS disease is 0.32 per 1000 live births (Van Dyke et al, 2009).

Intrapartum Antibiotic Prophylaxis

GBS is sensitive to penicillin, which is the drug of choice because of its narrow spectrum; the alternative is ampicillin. If a mother is allergic to penicillin but not at high risk for anaphylaxis, the use of cefazolin has been proposed (Schrag et al, 2002). When patients are at high risk for anaphylaxis in which the GBS is known to be susceptible to clindamycin and erythromycin, they can receive either of these drugs intravenously (IV) until delivery. When GBS is resistant to clindamycin or erythromycin or the antibiotic susceptibility is unknown, vancomycin given every 12 hours IV until delivery is the current recommendation (Schrag et al, 2002). In the United States, GBS exhibits considerable resistance against erythromycin (5% to 32%) and clindamycin (3% to 21%) (Castor et al, 2008). It is therefore important to have antibiotic testing done on the group B streptococcal isolates from pregnant women. For laboratories performing PCR on maternal vaginal or rectal cultures, it is recommended that the swabs be placed in a selective enrichment broth containing inhibitory antibiotics (either colistin and nalidixic acid or gentamicin and nalidixic acid) against gram-negative bacteria. If the PCR result is positive, the broth culture can be subcultured and antibiotic testing can be pursued. Because of the higher sensitivity of PCR, compared with the selective broth-enrichment culture, the organism will not grow in 10% to 15% of occasions.

Group B Streptococcal Sepsis in Neonates

The majority of infections in newborn infants occur within the first week of life and are designated as early-onset disease (Table 39-1). Late-onset infections occur in infants 7 days or older, with the majority of these infections appearing in the first 3 months of life. Although chemoprophylaxis has led to a significant decrease in the incidence of early-onset GBS disease, there is no evidence that chemoprophylaxis prevents late-onset disease (Cohen-Wolkowiez et al, 2009; Hamada et al, 2008; Jordan et al, 2008). Young infants with early-onset invasive GBS disease usually have pneumonia, sepsis, often; less often they have meningitis, osteomyelitis, or septic arthritis (Koenig and Keenan, 2009). The frequency of meningitis, osteomyelitis, or septic arthritis is higher among infants with late-onset disease.

There are nine antigenically distinct GBS serotypes, based on their capsular polysaccharide analysis (types Ia, Ib, II to VIII) and a proposed new type, IX (Diedrick et al, 2010; Henrichsen et al, 1984; Slotved et al, 2007). In the United States and Western Europe, types Ia, II, and III account for the majority of isolates from infants

with early-onset disease (Diedrick et al, 2010; Zaleznik et al, 2000). However, recent studies in the United States have demonstrated that serotypes Ia, III, and V, the latter emerging in recent years (Diedrick et al, 2010; Elliott et al, 1998; Harrison et al, 1998), account for the majority (70-75%) of early-onset invasive disease in newborn infants and parturient women (Diedrick et al, 2010; Zaleznik et al, 2000). Late-onset GBS disease in infants is dominated by serotype III followed by serotypes Ia and V (Shet and Ferrieri, 2004). A polysaccharide capsule is considered the most important virulence factor (Cieslewicz et al, 2005; Kasper et al, 1996; Paoletti et al, 1997, 2001); however, the role of surface localized GBS proteins (Ferrieri et al, 2004a; Johnson and Ferrieri, 1984; Lindahl et al, 2005; Smith et al, 2004) in pathogenesis and immune protection has gained favor (Maione et al, 2005; Tettelin et al, 2005).

The remaining GBS isolates from invasive disease consist primarily of types Ib and II, but types IV, VI, VII, and VIII compose a small fraction. Type IV GBS represented between 0.4% and 0.6% of colonizing GBS isolates (Diedrick et al, 2010), but it was relatively uncommon for type IV isolates to be found in invasive GBS (Ferrieri et al, 2008; Puopolo and Madoff, 2007). Recent studies in the United Arab Emirates, Turkey, and Zimbabwe showed large proportions of type IV GBS among their isolates (Amin et al, 2002; Diedrick et al, 2010; Ekin and Gurturk, 2006; Moyo et al, 2002). In Zimbabwe it was the fourth most common serotype, comprising 4.6% of the colonizing and invasive isolates (Moyo et al, 2002). Serotypes VII and VIII are uncommon in Western countries.

Infected infants have low levels of type-specific antibody to the infecting GBS serotype (Baker and Edwards, 2003). Vaccines against the common GBS serotypes have been shown to elicit a specific antibody response in humans (Baker and Edwards, 2003; Kasper et al, 1996; Paoletti et al, 1997, 2001). Sera from these vaccinated individuals protected against GBS challenge in neonatal mice, thereby showing the potential of vaccines to prevent invasive neonatal GBS disease in infants (Paoletti et al, 1997). The prospect of a multivalent GBS vaccine, with or without conjugated GBS surface localized proteins, makes the study of the common GBS serotypes important because of the possibility of serotype replacement or capsular switch (Cieslewicz et al, 2005; Lipsitch, 1999; Maione et al, 2005; Tettelin et al, 2005).

ESCHERICHIA COLI INFECTIONS

Historically, *E. coli* has been the second-most common pathogen causing sepsis and meningitis in newborn infants. The antigenic structure of *E. coli* is complex, composed of approximately 150 somatic or cell wall O antigens, 50 flagellar H antigens, and approximately 80 capsular K antigens. However, a limited number of K antigen *E. coli* strains cause meningitis, and approximately 80% of the strains causing meningitis and 40% of the strains causing bacteremia or sepsis express K1 (Mulder et al, 1984). The capsular K1 polysaccharide antigen is highly homologous to the capsular antigen of group B *Neisseria meningitidis*. Because a high percentage of women may have bacteriuria with strains of *E. coli* that express the K1 antigen or are

TABLE 39-1 Manifestations of Early-Onset and Late-Onset Group B Streptococcal Disease

Characteristic	Early-Onset Disease	Late-Onset Disease
Age at onset	Birth through day 6 of life	Day 7 to 3 months
Symptoms	Respiratory distress, apnea	Irritability, fever, poor feeding
Findings	Pneumonia, sepsis	Sepsis, meningitis, osteoarthritis
Maternal obstetrical complications	Frequent	Uncommon
Mode of transmission	Vertical, in utero, or intrapartum	Nosocomial, horizontal
Predominant serotypes	Ia, III, V[*]	III, Ia, V[*]
Effect of intrapartum antibiotic prophylaxis recommended by the Centers for Disease Control and Prevention	Reduces incidence by 85%-90%	No effect

[*]In decreasing order of frequency

colonized with it at the time of delivery, it is surprising that *E. coli* sepsis or meningitis is not more common. It has been estimated that disease occurs in 1 in 100 to 200 infants colonized by K1 *E. coli*. Surveillance data from the National Institute of Child Health and Human Development Neonatal Research Network, a consortium of 16 U.S. academic neonatal centers, revealed that in the era of widespread implementation of antibiotic prophylaxis, *E. coli* sepsis increased from 3.2 to 6.8 cases per 1000 live births. This increase was observed in the 1998-2000 era and persisted in 2002 to 2003. Approximately 85% of *E. coli* infections in very low-birthweight (VLBW) infants were ampicillin resistant (Stoll et al, 2002). However, most evidence suggests that intrapartum antibiotic prophylaxis has not been associated with a concomitant adverse impact of increasing *E. coli* or other non-GBS bacterial causes. Among preterm infants, however, the incidence of *E. coli* and ampicillin-resistant *E. coli* infections increased significantly (Bizzarro et al, 2005). A recent retrospective case-control study between 1997 and 2001 concluded that exposure to intrapartum antibiotic prophylaxis therapy in mothers did not increase the odds of invasive, early-onset *E. coli* infection. In fact, among full term infants, exposure to 4 hours or greater of intrapartum antibiotic therapy was associated with decreased odds of early-onset *E. coli* infection (Schrag et al, 2006).

LISTERIA MONOCYTOGENES INFECTIONS

Listeria monocytogenes is a small, facultatively anaerobic, gram-positive motile bacillus that produces a narrow zone of beta hemolysis on blood agar plates, and can be confused with GBS unless a careful Gram stain, a catalase reaction, and other tests are performed. Most disease is due to three primary serotypes: 1a, 1b, and 4b. The last serotype has been described in most outbreaks of listeriosis (Posfay-Barbe and Wald, 2009). Most cases of listeriosis appear to be food borne, including those acquired by pregnant women.

Foods that can be contaminated by *L. monocytogenes* include raw vegetables such as cabbage, raw milk, fish, poultry, processed chicken, beef, and hot dogs (Schlech, 2000). Transmission to the fetus occurs through either a hematogenous (transplacental) route or via an ascending infection through the birth canal. Frequently, infections with *Listeria* spp. early in gestation result in abortion; later in pregnancy, infection with *Listeria* spp. can result in premature delivery of a stillborn or infected newborn. Approximately 70% of *Listeria*-infected women deliver before 35 weeks' gestation. Illness in the mother may be undetected because of vague influenza-like illnesses that may not come to medical attention. In approximately half of perinatal cases, illness in the mother has preceded delivery by 2 days to 2 weeks. At autopsy of stillborn infants or of those who die in the perinatal period, granulomas may be found throughout such organs as the liver and lungs, and infection is widely disseminated, including involvement of the meninges. Treatment of *Listeria* spp. infection or bacteremia during pregnancy can prevent infection in the fetus (Kalstone, 1991). Like GBS infection, *Listeria* spp. infection may have either an early-onset or late-onset presentation. Epidemics of neonatal *Listeria* spp. infection have been described after ingestion of contaminated foods such as cheese or coleslaw. The first clearly documented food borne (coleslaw) outbreak of listeriosis was in 1981 from the Eastern Maritimes in Canada (Schlech, 2000); it was associated with a fatality rate of 27%. There are reports of repeated abortions in women with colonization in the gastrointestinal tract, and cold-enrichment cultures can be performed to try to detect fecal carriage in such women. However, cold enrichment cultures are inferior to selective media for *Listeria* spp. in isolating the organism from various foods or stool specimens. Rapid antigen tests based on nucleic acid amplification are not in common use in clinical diagnostic laboratories. There is no current vaccine for *Listeria* spp. infection, but preventive measures have included the surveillance programs from the U.S. Department of Agriculture, prohibiting the sale of contaminated meats. Between 1996 and 2006, the incidence of *Listeria* spp. infections declined by 36%; however, an outbreak of disease in 2002 related to contaminated turkey meat led to 54 illnesses, eight deaths, and three fetal deaths in nine states (Posfay-Barbe and Wald, 2009).

MISCELLANEOUS BACTERIAL PATHOGENS

Bacteria responsible for early-onset neonatal sepsis have changed dramatically over time. There are regional differences in the organisms commonly responsible for early-onset sepsis. In addition to the organisms mentioned previously, other bacterial pathogens associated with early-onset bacteremia or sepsis in newborn infants are *Enterococcus* spp., viridans group *Streptococcus* spp., *Klebsiella* spp., *Enterobacter* spp., *Haemophilus influenzae* (typeable and nontypeable), *S. aureus*, *Streptococcus pneumoniae*, group A streptococcus and other beta-hemolytic streptococci, and coagulase-negative staphylococci.

CLINICAL SIGNS OF BACTERIAL SEPSIS

There is great variability in the clinical presentations of infants with early-onset bacterial sepsis (Box 39-1). Most infants exhibit respiratory distress in the first 12 hours of life, frequently immediately after birth. In these infants, the progression may be rapid with cardiovascular instability, shock, and death. Presentation within the first 12 hours of life suggests that the infection with pneumonia and bacteremia occurred at or near the time of birth

---

BOX 39-1   Common Clinical Signs of Neonatal Sepsis

- Abnormal neurologic status: irritability, lethargy, poor feeding
- Abnormal temperature: hyperthermia or hypothermia
- Apnea
- Bleeding problems: petechiae, purpura, oozing
- Cardiovascular compromise: tachycardia, hypotension, poor perfusion
- Cyanosis
- Gastrointestinal symptoms: abdominal distention, emesis, diarrhea
- Jaundice
- Respiratory distress: tachypnea, increased work of breathing, hypoxemia
- Seizures

		Bacterial Infection Present		
		YES	NO	
Laboratory Test Result	POSITIVE	True Positive TP	False Positive FP	Positive Predictive Value = (TP)/(TP+FP)
	NEGATIVE	False Negative FN	True Negative TN	Negative Predictive Value = (TN)/(FN+TN)
		Sensitivity = (TP)/(TP+FN)	Specificity = (TN)/(FP+TN)	

FIGURE 39-1 Diagram of the relationships among sensitivity, specificity, positive predictive value, and negative predictive value. *FN,* Number with infection incorrectly diagnosed as healthy by the test. *FP,* number of healthy infants incorrectly diagnosed as infected by the test; *TN,* number of healthy infants correctly diagnosed as not infected by the test; *TP,* number of infants with infection correctly diagnosed by the test.

or during the immediate postnatal period. Infants with hypoxia in utero may gasp, inhaling contaminated amniotic fluid and setting the stage for early-onset pneumonia, bacteremia, and sepsis.

The signs of early-onset infection may be subtle, with tachypnea suggesting "wet lung disease" or may be more overt with grunting, flaring, and subcostal and intercostal retractions. Because the signs of sepsis can be relatively nonspecific, such as poor feeding and increased sleepiness, they can be overlooked. In newborn or intermediate or intensive care nurseries, one must be attuned to subtle abnormal findings in newborn infants. The clinical signs of neonatal sepsis include hyperthermia or hypothermia, respiratory distress, apnea, cyanosis, jaundice, hepatomegaly, abdominal distention, feeding abnormalities, and neurologic abnormalities. Autopsy findings in preterm infants with fatal early-onset GBS infection suggested that surfactant deficiency respiratory distress syndrome was common (Payne et al, 1988).

LABORATORY TESTING

There are many laboratory tests that have been evaluated for infants with possible sepsis, and the results must be interpreted with caution, assessing the sensitivity and specificity of a particular test as well its positive and negative predictive accuracy (Figure 39-1). The sensitivity of a test is defined as the proportion of individuals with proven or probable sepsis in whom the result is abnormal; the specificity is the proportion of healthy or noninfected infants in whom the result is normal. Ideally, a test would have a high sensitivity and a high specificity, but this is rarely achievable. High sensitivity is the most desirable characteristic when dealing with serious and treatable diseases such as neonatal sepsis. Because sepsis is generally treated with antibiotic agents that have a low toxicity, diagnostic tests do not need to have a high specificity, but should have a high sensitivity, which will allow sepsis to be excluded. A positive predictive accuracy is the probability that an infant with an abnormal laboratory result is infected; a negative predictive value is the probability that infection with a normal or negative result is free of infection. The more sensitive the test, the greater its negative predictive value; the more specific a test, the higher its positive predictive value.

MICROBIOLOGIC CULTURES

Previously, cultures of superficial body sites in newborn infants (external auditory canal, gastric aspirate, umbilicus, and nasopharynx) were used to identify bacterial pathogens when more specific blood culture results were negative. Most centers no longer use surface cultures to make clinical decisions regarding either the institution or the discontinuation of antibiotic therapy, because surface cultures are of limited value in predicting the etiology of bacterial sepsis in newborn infants (Evans et al, 1988; Shenoy et al, 2000). Examination of gastric aspirates by Gram stain as a screening mechanism has also lost favor, as has examination for PMNs. Although the presence of increased numbers of PMNs may represent amnionitis and an inflammatory response, these cells may reflect a maternal origin and have no specificity in predicting bacterial sepsis for the infants (Vasan et al, 1977).

Blood Cultures

The gold standard for detection of bacteremia in newborn infants with suspected sepsis is a positive blood culture. With the introduction of newer blood culture detection instruments that are semiautomated and examined for the presence of growth by CO_2 production by the internal computer of the instrument every minute, the sensitivity of detecting positive blood cultures has increased. Another variable that influences the sensitivity of detection of bacteremia is the volume of blood obtained and placed in the culture bottles. Ideally 1 to 3 mL of blood from infants should be obtained, but this not always possible in very small infants. Most positive blood cultures are detected within 24 to 48 hours using the new technology (Garcia-Prats et al, 2000). However, the use of intrapartum antibiotics for prophylaxis in mothers with either GBS colonization or suspected amnionitis on account of any cause can reduce the ability to detect bacteremia in newborn infants. In a term infant who was asymptomatic at the initiation of antibiotic therapy, it may be reasonable to stop antibiotic administration if the blood cultures remain negative after 48 hours. However, the decision to discontinue treatment with antibiotics should include the assessment of results of other laboratory tests used for sepsis screens, and should not solely rely on a negative blood culture. When

TABLE 39-2 Predictive Values of Components of the White Blood Cell Count and of C-Reactive Protein

Laboratory Result	Sensitivity (%)	Specificity (%)	Predictive Value (%)	
			Positive	Negative
ANC <1750 cells/mm³	38-96	61-92	20-77	96-99
ANC <10% (≈5580 cells/mm³ for term)	48	73	4	98
I/T ratio ≥0.2	90-100	30-78	11-51	98
I/T ratio ≥0.3	35	89	7	98
CRP > 1mg/dL	70-93	78-94	27	100

Adapted from Gerdes JS: Diagnosis and management of bacterial infections in the neonate, *Pediatr Clin North Am* 51:939-959, 2004.
ANC, Absolute neutrophil count; *CRP,* C-reactive protein; *I/T,* immature to total neutrophils (ratio), calculated by the number of immature neutrophils (bands, metamyelocytes, and myelocytes) divided by the total number of neutrophils (immature plus mature).

the suspicion of sepsis is high, clinicians should consider continuing antibiotic therapy for a complete course despite negative blood cultures (Ottolini et al, 2003).

Urine Cultures

The frequency of positive urine cultures in infants with early-onset sepsis is relatively low, and it is rare to find bacteriuria in infants with negative blood culture results (DiGeronimo, 1992). Infants with late-onset sepsis tend to have a higher rate of positive urine cultures (Visser and Hall, 1979). In the era of widespread intrapartum antibiotic prophylaxis in the mother, positive urine cultures may be obscured because of excretion of antibiotics in the urine of newborn infants. When pyelonephritis is found in newborn infants, it likely represents metastatic seeding of the kidney during a bout of bacteremia. In the first 72 hours of life, because the yield from urine cultures is low, it is not generally recommended to obtain these specimens. However, in the older newborn infant, a urine sample collected by an aseptic technique (urinary catheter or suprapubic bladder aspiration) is an important part of the sepsis workup.

Cerebrospinal Fluid

Lumbar punctures are deferred in infants with any instability or uncorrected bleeding disorders. The details of examination of cerebrospinal fluid and the diagnostic approach for examining cerebrospinal fluid will be discussed under the section on bacterial meningitis.

WHITE BLOOD CELL COUNT AND NEUTROPHIL INDICES

Normal white blood cell (WBC) counts range from 9000 to 30,000 cells/mm³ at the time of birth, and differences in the site of sampling can affect these values. The absolute neutrophil count (ANC), the absolute band count of immature neutrophils, and the ratio of immature neutrophils to total neutrophils (I/T) are regarded as more useful than total leukocyte counts in the diagnosis of neonatal sepsis.

The lower limit or total neutrophil count rises to 7200 cells/mm³ by 12 hours of age, and then declines to approximately 1720 cells/mm³ by 72 hours of age (Manroe et al, 1979; Schmutz et al, 2008). Postnatally the absolute band

count also undergoes similar changes, with peak values of 1400 cells/mm³ at 12 hours of age, and then declines. In contrast, the I/T ratio is maximum at birth and then declines to a value of 0.12 beyond 72 hours of age (Manroe et al, 1979; Schelonka et al, 1994). However, in VLBW infants there is a greater reference range for the total neutrophil counts (Manroe et al, 1979; Mouzinho et al, 1994). There are no significant differences in I/T ratio or absolute immature neutrophil counts in VLBW infants. There is considerable overlap of the cutoff values of the ANC, absolute band count, and I/T ratio between healthy and infected newborns.

There are a number of clinical conditions that affect the total neutrophil count. Prolonged crying, meconium aspiration syndrome, maternal fever, and asphyxia are all associated with an increase in the total neutrophil count, and there may be an increase in the total immature neutrophil forms, as well as an increased I/T ratio. Maternal hypertension is associated with a decrease in total neutrophils. At high altitudes, a higher upper limit of neutrophil values occurs (Schmutz et al, 2008).

In approximately two thirds of infants with sepsis, the total neutrophil count is abnormal. Neutropenia is the best predictor of sepsis, whereas neutrophilia does not correlate well. The absolute neutrophil band count is not a sensitive marker of sepsis, but has a relatively good predictive value and specificity. The I/T ratio is considered to have the best sensitivity of all of the neutrophil indices (Table 39-2) (Gerdes, 2004).

PLATELET COUNTS

Approximately 25% to 30% of infants exhibit thrombocytopenia at the time of diagnosis of sepsis, and this frequency increases during the course of infection. Accelerated platelet destruction and possibly depressed production caused by bacterial products on the bone marrow are the underlying mechanisms for thrombocytopenia in infected infants. Disseminated intravascular coagulation may be seen in some infants with severe sepsis.

ACUTE PHASE REACTANTS AND ERYTHROCYTE SEDIMENTATION RATE

A number of acute phase reactants have been studied to help identify infants with likely sepsis. Most biochemical markers currently in use are derived from components of the complex inflammatory response to an invading pathogen. These markers have been studied during the past 20 years and continue to be under investigation. Of issue is the availability of tests for these inflammatory mediators when investigating an infant with possible sepsis, and the value of these tests in assisting with the early diagnosis of sepsis. It is known that some proinflammatory cytokines peak rapidly, within 1 to 4 hours after a sepsis stimulus (Lam and Ng, 2008). C-reactive protein (CRP) rises to a maximum at 12 to 24 hours, and procalcitonin (PCT) rises at 4 hours, peaks at 6 hours, and plateaus 8 to 24 hours after a stimulus. CRP is induced by proinflammatory cytokines. Among the early markers are the proinflammatory mediators, such as IL-1β, IL-6, the chemokine IL-8, TNF-α, and interferon gamma; these activate host defenses against bacterial and other infecting agents, whereas antiinflammatory mediators such as IL-4, IL-10, and transforming growth factor β$_1$ (TGF-β$_1$) are important in regulating and limiting the inflammatory response, thus preventing an excessive reaction that could lead to organ damage and tissue cell death (Mehr and Doyle, 2000). Survival should be considered a fine balance between the proinflammatory cytokines and the antiinflammatory mediators. Because of the limitations of other assessment markers of potentially infected neonates, such as WBC counts and band counts, the advantages of having a surrogate marker readily available are apparent.

CRP is probably the most studied acute phase reactant in neonatal sepsis (Benitz et al, 1998; Jaye and Waites, 1997; Lam and Ng, 2008; Weitkamp and Aschner, 2005). Monitoring of CRP levels has been widely promulgated as a way to diagnose neonatal infection and to adjust the duration of antibiotic therapy in infants with suspected versus proven sepsis (Benitz et al, 1998; Ehl et al, 1997; Gerdes, 2004; Philip and Mills, 2000). Depending on the laboratory, a CRP value of 1 to 8 mg/dL is considered the upper limit of normal; it is important to know the different cutoff values in the laboratory supporting one's neonatal units. Theoretically, results can be available within 30 minutes. CRP is produced by the liver in response to stimulation by the proinflammatory cytokine IL-6, which is produced by both T and B cells (Lam and Ng, 2008; Weitkamp and Aschner, 2005). Because exposure of the host to bacterial products results in a substantial and rapid increase in IL-6 concentrations, it appears that IL-6 is potentially a more useful marker than CRP during the early phase of an infection. In one study, the IL-6 concentration had a sensitivity of 89% versus 60% for CRP at the onset of clinical suspicion of a neonatal infection (Lam and Ng, 2008). The negative predictive values of IL-6 are much higher than those for CRP (Lam and Ng, 2008), and this was also found in cord blood IL-6 levels, where the sensitivity of detection was high. This finding can be useful in deciding which infants do not require antibiotic therapy and those in whom antibiotics can be discontinued after a relatively short course.

In a recent study, the high-sensitivity CRP (hsCRP) measurement has been shown to provide increased sensitivity for detecting neonatal infection (Edgar et al, 2010). Not all diagnostic laboratories can provide hsCRP in a timely fashion. In addition, the optimum diagnostic cutoff levels for CRP and hsCRP are debatable.

A recent study examined the combination of hsCRP, serum soluble intercellular adhesion molecule 1 (sISAM-1), soluble E-selectin (sE-selectin), and serum amyloid A, individually and in combination, for the diagnosis of sepsis in a neonatal intensive care unit (Edgar et al, 2010). In this study, all four measurements had some diagnostic value for neonatal infection; however, s1SAM-1, hsCRP, and sE-selectin demonstrated the highest negative predictive value individually (sISAM, 84%; hsCRP, 79%; and sE-selectin, 74%) (Edgar et al, 2010). Use of a combination of these measurements enhanced the diagnostic value, with sensitivities of 90.3% and a negative predictive value of 91.3% (Edgar et al, 2010). However, the application of this set of diagnostic markers is not available for most facilities, and more investigative work is needed to confirm their role in excluding early-onset infection.

In another study, early markers (IL-6, TNF-α, IL-8, interferon gamma, CRP, IL-18, the antiinflammatory cytokine IL-10, the I/T ratio, and PCT, a later marker of infection) were studied for use in detection of early-onset sepsis in 123 newborn infants (Bender et al, 2008). This study concluded that IL-6 combined with PCT was a fair measure of evaluating early-onset infection, and that the traditional I/T ratio was almost as efficient as IL-6. Combining an early marker such as IL-6 and an I/T ratio may reduce the number of diagnostic tests and nonconclusive values. The combined value of IL-6 and PCT at the first blood drawing had a sensitivity of 71% and specificity of 88% (Bender et al, 2008).

There are many studies of procalcitonin in the literature, and most have concluded that procalcitonin is superior to CRP levels in the early diagnosis of neonatal sepsis (Lam and Ng, 2008). PCT is the precursor of calcitonin, normally synthesized in the C-cells of the thyroid gland. PCT is induced by systemic inflammation and bacterial sepsis and is produced by such cells as hepatocytes, nephrons, and monocytes. The physiologic function of PCT is unknown. In bacterial infections, plasma PCT concentrations increase from 0.001 to 0.01 ng/mL (baseline range) to values ranging from 1 to 1000 ng/mL. PCT concentrations rise much faster than CRP (6 to 8 hours versus 48 hours for maximum levels). In healthy newborn infants, plasma PCT concentrations increase gradually after birth, reaching peak levels at approximately 24 hours of age (range, 0.1 to 20 ng/mL) and then decrease to normal values less than 0.5 ng/mL by 48 to 72 hours of age (Stocker et al, 2010). Various studies on the use of PCT as a marker of neonatal sepsis have yielded contradictory results regarding its application to clinical decision making for both diagnosis and adjustment of the length of antibiotic therapy. In a recent study of 121 newborn infants with suspected early-onset sepsis, serial PCT determinations allowed shortening of the duration of antibiotic therapy (Stocker et al, 2010). However, there are currently few institutions or intensive care units that are applying PCT as a regular measurement for diagnosis or for adjustment of length of antibiotic therapy. Larger studies are needed to determine the true value of PCT in diagnosis and therapy.

To date, studies on the role of various cytokine determinations in assisting with diagnosis and treatment of early-onset sepsis are intriguing, but have not translated to widespread use. Other molecular technologies are also being studied to diagnose neonatal sepsis by the rapid identification and differentiation of gram-negative and gram-positive bacterial bloodstream infections. PCR, using universal bacterial primers, targets conserved regions of the 16SrRNA gene common to all bacteria, but not found in other organisms (Dutta et al, 2009). In one study, universal primer PCR was performed in newborn infants with clinically suspected sepsis. PCR was performed before starting antibiotic therapy, and repeated at 12, 24, and 48 hours after starting drug therapy (Dutta et al, 2009). The sensitivity, specificity, and positive and negative predictive values of universal primer PCR were 96.2%, 96.3%, 87.7%, and 98.8% respectively. Results of testing in two patients were blood culture positive, but 0-hour PCR negative, and results in 7 patients were 0-hour PCR positive, but blood culture result was negative. Of the patients with a result of 0-hour PCR positive, 7 remained positive at 12 hours but none remained positive at 24 and 48 hours after starting antibiotic therapy. Although universal bacterial primer PCR may be a useful test for diagnosing an early episode of culture-proven sepsis, it cannot be used for diagnosis if the patient has been exposed to 12 hours or more of antibiotic therapy (Dutta et al, 2009). Much larger studies are certainly required before this assay can be recommended for routine clinical use in newborn infants suspected of sepsis.

PREVENTION

INTRAPARTUM ANTIBIOTIC PROPHYLAXIS

There were initial concerns about adverse effects of implementing the CDC consensus strategies, but these have proved unwarranted. The primary risks considered were maternal anaphylaxis from administered antibiotics, and these were unfounded. The possibility of the emergence of infections in mothers and infants caused by antibiotic resistant organisms (e.g., *E. coli*) was addressed in part by studies conducted by the Neonatal Network of the National Institute of Child Health and Human Development. In 2002, they reported a change in the pathogens causing early-onset sepsis, with an increase in sepsis caused by *E. coli* from 3.2 to 6.8 per 1000 live births (Stoll et al, 2002). Most of the *E. coli* isolates were resistant to ampicillin. Mothers of infants with ampicillin-resistant *E. coli* infections were more likely to have received intrapartum antibiotic prophylaxis than were those with ampicillin-sensitive strains (Stoll et al, 2002). In another study comparing a period of no prophylaxis to periods of risk-based and universal screening-based prophylaxis, no change in the incidence of infection with ampicillin-resistant organisms was observed overall or among VLBW infants (Puopolo and Eichenwald, 2010). However, an increased proportion of infections was caused by ampicillin-resistant organisms. Mothers of infants with ampicillin-resistant infections were also more likely to have been treated with ampicillin (Chen et al, 2005). A 10-year study of the effect of intrapartum antibiotic prophylaxis on GBS and *E. coli* sepsis in Australasia revealed a steady decline in early-onset GBS infection, but also a trend to decreasing early-onset *E. coli* sepsis in all infants and a stable rate for this infection in VLBW infants (Daley et al, 2004).

INTRAPARTUM MANAGEMENT OF PARTURIENTS

The universal GBS screening strategy recommended by the CDC is done at 35 to 37 weeks' gestation. Antepartum antibiotic therapy is recommended for women with a previous infant with invasive GBS disease, a positive GBS screening culture result during pregnancy, unknown GBS status (culture either not performed or incomplete or results unknown), and any of the following features: delivery before 37 weeks' gestation, rupture of chorioamniotic membranes for greater than 18 hours, intrapartum temperature of 100.4° F (38° C) or higher, and GBS bacteriuria during pregnancy.

Women who are not allergic to penicillin can be given penicillin G (5,000,000 units as a loading IV dose followed by 2.5 million units every 4 hours until delivery) or ampicillin (2g IV as a loading dose followed by 1g every 4 hours until delivery). For women who are allergic to penicillin, the recommendation is to determine, ideally during prenatal care, whether the patient is at high risk for anaphylaxis (i.e., history of immediate hypersensitivity reactions). Women who are not at high risk for anaphylaxis can receive cefazolin (2g IV and 1g IV every 8 hours until delivery). Women who are at high risk for anaphylaxis whose GBS isolate is not resistant to clindamycin or erythromycin can receive clindamycin (900 mg IV every 8 hours until delivery) or erythromycin (500 mg IV every 6 hours until delivery) (Schrag et al, 2002). Women with clindamycin-erythromycin–resistant GBS isolates can receive vancomycin (1g IV every 12 hours until delivery).

INTRAVENOUS IMMUNE GLOBULIN FOR PREVENTION OF EARLY-ONSET SEPSIS

Premature infants are susceptible to early-onset sepsis because of diminished transplacental transfer of immunoglobulins and decreased synthesis of immunoglobulin (Ig) G. An intravenous infusion of immunoglobulin (IVIg) will increase the typically low levels of serum immunoglobulin in preterm infants, and it has been proposed to improve immune function that may lead to improved clinical outcome (Wynn et al, 2009). Clinical trials examining the possible benefit of IV-Ig began over 15 years ago (Chirico et al, 1987; Conway et al, 1990; Haque et al, 1986). The very premature infants are the group most likely to receive and potentially benefit from these adjuvant treatments and preventative interventions. A Cochrane metaanalysis showed a reduction in mortality of newborn infants treated with IV-Ig for what were subsequently proved to be bacterial infections (relative risk, 0.55; 95% confidence interval, 0.31 to 0.98) (Ohlsson and Lacy, 2010). However, a review of the studies included in the metaanalysis revealed the inclusion of few very premature infants. A large international, placebo-controlled, double-blind, randomized clinical trial has recently been undertaken in approximately 5000 newborn infants to examine the benefit of polyclonal IV-Ig treatment for proven or suspected sepsis (Wynn et al, 2010). However, because randomization will allow the inclusion of neonates of all gestational and postnatal ages with suspected or proven infection, the subgroup sample sizes may leave the issue of clinical efficacy for early- and late-onset sepsis in the different gestational age groups unanswered. A metaanalysis that included almost 4000 preterm (<37 weeks' gestation) or low birthweight (<2500 g) infants showed a modest reduction in the development of sepsis after IV-Ig prophylaxis in preterm neonates (Wynn et al, 2010). Currently available data do not support the suggested immunologic enhancements expected for IV-Ig in very premature neonates. There is continued interest in the potential of IV-Ig as treatment or prophylaxis for infection in very premature infants, but large trials are needed to provide convincing data.

Other immunomodulating factors such as granulocyte colony-stimulating factor (G-CSF) have been studied to both prevent and treat neonatal sepsis. An earlier metaanalysis showed that G-CSF administration improved mortality in all neonates and in the subgroups of neutropenic and preterm infants (Bernstein et al, 2001). A recent Cochrane metaanalysis concluded that prophylaxis with G-CSF does not significantly reduce mortality in all infants, although in premature infants with neutropenia (ANC < 1750) mortality may be improved (Carr et al, 2009). It is possible that combination therapies using IV-Ig and other immunomodulating factors, such as granulocyte-macrophage colony-stimulating factor (GM-CSF), G-CSF, and complement-containing blood products, may lead to improved immune function in these highly susceptible infants; however, these studies are not currently being conducted.

DIAGNOSTIC APPROACH TO NEONATES WITH SUSPECTED SEPSIS

Obviously, all symptomatic newborn infants must be carefully evaluated for the possibility of bacterial sepsis and treated with antibiotics, if necessary. Although the presence of various risk factors should increase the suspicion of sepsis, the absence of risk factors in a symptomatic infant cannot be dismissed. In adjusting to postnatal life, some infants exhibit abnormal signs transiently, such as tachypnea, before becoming asymptomatic. However, any infant who has other findings or is still symptomatic with only one finding by 6 hours of life should have a diagnostic evaluation performed with a complete blood cell count (CBC) and differential, a blood culture, and as appropriate, a lumbar puncture and a chest radiograph. Antibiotic therapy can be stopped when the physical findings are normal, the clinical suspicion of sepsis is low, and the screening results for sepsis, including the blood culture, remain negative. If the blood culture result is positive, the lumbar puncture findings abnormal, or there are clinical signs of sepsis, then the infant should be treated with an appropriate course of antibiotics (Figure 39-2).

Management of the asymptomatic infant with risk factors for sepsis is more controversial. Escobar et al (2000) retrospectively reviewed 2785 newborns with birthweight greater than 2000 g and who were evaluated for sepsis after birth. Asymptomatic status was associated with a significantly decreased odds ratio for infection. Low absolute neutrophil count and meconium-stained amniotic fluid were associated with an increased risk of infection. The highest infection rates occurred in infants whose mother had a clinical diagnosis of "definite" chorioamnionitis, but chorioamnionitis was significantly associated with an increased risk of neonatal infection only in infants whose mothers had not received intrapartum antibiotics (Escobar et al, 2000).

Current practice management for the infant with no signs or symptoms of sepsis, but with risk factors such as maternal chorioamnionitis or incomplete GBS maternal prophylaxis, includes performing a limited sepsis evaluation (CBC with differential and blood culture). If the WBC count, absolute neutrophil count, and the I/T ratio are all normal, then the infant is usually observed in the hospital and discharged at approximately 48 hours. If the screening tests are abnormal, the infant undergoes a complete sepsis evaluation with subsequent antibiotic therapy initiated.

Recent CDC and American Academy of Pediatrics guidelines for the prevention of early-onset neonatal GBS sepsis have a slightly different approach to management of the at-risk asymptomatic infant (see Figure 39-2; Verani and Schrag, 2010). If there are signs of sepsis in the newborn, then a full sepsis workup and antibiotic therapy are recommended. If there is maternal chorioamnionitis, a limited sepsis evaluation and antibiotic are recommended. For infants whose mother received greater than 4 hours of antibiotic therapy, it is recommended that the infant be observed in the hospital for approximately 48 hours. For infants whose mother did not receive more than 4 hours of antibiotic prophylaxis, a 48 hour in-hospital observation is recommended. If the infant is less than 37 weeks' gestation, or the duration of rupture of membranes is greater than or equal to 18 hours, then a limited evaluation and observation in the hospital for approximately 48 hours are recommended.

TREATMENT

ANTIMICROBIAL THERAPY

The choice of antibiotic administration for an infant with suspected early-onset sepsis depends on the predominant bacterial pathogens and the antibiotic susceptibility profiles for the microorganisms causing early-onset disease in a particular geographic region. Any decision to discontinue antimicrobial therapy should be based on the level of suspicion for sepsis at the time treatment was begun, the culture results, laboratory test results, and the clinical behavior and course of the infant. If sepsis is highly suspected in an infant, antibiotics should be considered for a full course even if the culture results are negative.

Empiric therapy for early-onset sepsis generally consists of combinations of antibiotics effective against gram-positive (e.g., GBS, *L. monocytogenes*) and gram-negative pathogens (e.g., *E. coli*). The two most commonly used combinations are (1) ampicillin with an aminoglycoside, usually gentamicin, and (2) ampicillin with a third-generation cephalosporin, usually cefotaxime. Cefotaxime has minimal toxicity and is well tolerated by newborn infants. However, the third-generation cephalosporins, as well as vancomycin, a glycopeptide antibiotic, have been associated with the development of vancomycin-resistant enterococci and, in the case of cephalosporins, with the induction of various β-lactamase producing gram-negative bacteria, including extended-spectrum β-lactamase producing organisms (Bryan et al, 1985). These latter bacteria

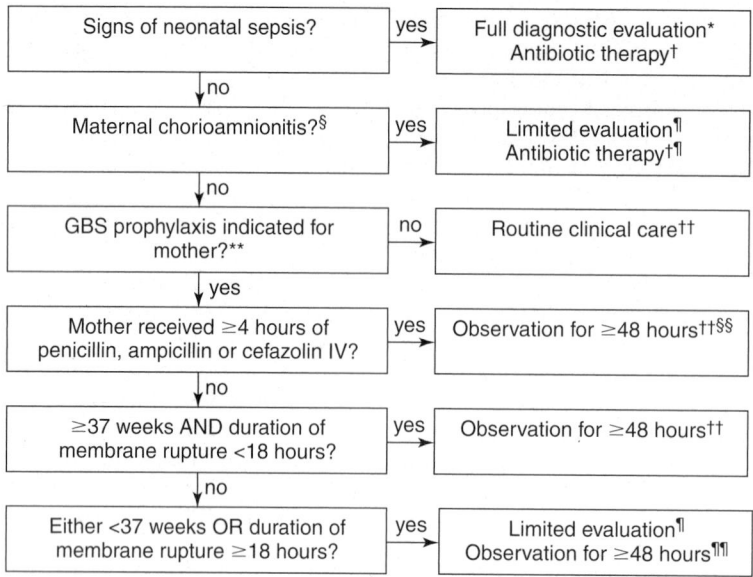

Signs of neonatal sepsis? → yes → Full diagnostic evaluation*
Antibiotic therapy†

↓ no

Maternal chorioamnionitis?§ → yes → Limited evaluation¶
Antibiotic therapy†¶

↓ no

GBS prophylaxis indicated for mother?** → no → Routine clinical care††

↓ yes

Mother received ≥4 hours of penicillin, ampicillin or cefazolin IV? → yes → Observation for ≥48 hours††§§

↓ no

≥37 weeks AND duration of membrane rupture <18 hours? → yes → Observation for ≥48 hours††

↓ no

Either <37 weeks OR duration of membrane rupture ≥18 hours? → yes → Limited evaluation¶
Observation for ≥48 hours¶¶

* Includes CBC with differential, platelets, blood culture, chest radiograph (if respiratory abnormalities are present), and LP (if patient stable enough to tolerate procedure and sepsis is suspected).

† Antibiotic therapy should be directed towards the most common causes of neonatal sepsis including GBS and other organisms (including gram negative pathgoens), and should take into account local antibiotic resistance patterns.

§ Consultation with obstetric providers is important to determine the level of clinical suspicion for chorioamnionitis. Chorioamnionitis is diagnosed clinically and some of the signs are non-specific.

¶ Includes blood culture (at birth), and CBC with differential and platelets. Some experts recommend a CBC with differential and platelets at 6-12 hours of age.

** GBS prophylaxis indicated if one or more of the following: (1) mother GBS positive at 35-37 weeks' gestation, (2) GBS status unknown with one or more intrapartum risk factors including <37 weeks' gestation, ROM ≥18 hours or T ≥100.4°F (38.0°C), (3) GBS bacteriuria during current pregnancy, (4) history of a previous infant with GBS disease.

†† If signs of sepsis develop, a full diagnostic evaluation should be done and antibiotic therapy initiated.

§§ If ≥37 weeks' gestation, observation may occur at home after 24 hours if there is a knowledgeable observer and ready access to medical care.

¶¶ Some experts recommend a CBC with differential and platelets at 6-12 hours of age.

FIGURE 39-2 Algorithm for recommended management of newborns at risk for group B streptococcal disease. (*Adapted from Verani JR, Schrag SS: Group B streptococcal disease in infants: progress in prevention and continued challenges,* Clin Perinatol 37:375-392, 2010.)

are resistant to all β-lactam antibiotics and frequently are resistant to other antibiotics, but not to meropenem. Another disadvantage of the cephalosporin antibiotics is the lack of effectiveness against enterococci or *L. monocytogenes*. *L. monocytogenes* is usually treated with ampicillin and an aminoglycoside until the blood culture result is negative and the infant has shown an improved outcome. In infants with bacteremia and sepsis caused by GBS, gentamicin is frequently combined with ampicillin or penicillin, although there are no data to suggest that the addition of the aminoglycoside improves outcome. However, it is common practice to use the combination of these two drugs during the first few days of therapy and then to continue the full course of therapy with ampicillin or penicillin alone.

When the likelihood of infection is very low, the antibiotic therapy should be stopped. In most hospitals using modern blood culture instrumentation, 48 hours should be considered sufficient to determine whether a blood culture result is negative, assuming that no antibiotics were being given when the culture was obtained (Garcia-Prats et al, 2000). Blood culture bottles with antimicrobial binding resins are in common use in microbiology laboratories,

enhancing the ability to demonstrate positive blood cultures. Infants with proven bacteremia, but without meningitis, are commonly treated for 7 to 10 days. The use of antibiotics with nephrotoxicity (i.e., aminoglycosides) should be monitored using appropriate drug levels.

IMMUNOLOGICAL THERAPIES FOR TREATMENT OF EARLY-ONSET SEPSIS

Various adjunctive therapies have been proposed to improve the immune status of the infant in an attempt to mitigate the mortality of neonatal sepsis. These included IV-Ig, granulocyte transfusions and G-CSF or GM-CSF treatment. Overall, there are insufficient data to recommend the routine use of any of these therapies for the treatment of sepsis in newborn infants. However, mortality in cases of subsequently proven infection was reduced in the IV-Ig–treated infants, and a large randomized controlled trial of IV-Ig use was recently completed (Ohlsson and Lacy, 2010). Clinical studies also did not show that granulocyte transfusions provided a significant benefit to neonates with culture-proven early-onset infections (Vamvakas and Pineda, 1996). However, in infants with overwhelming sepsis, severe neutropenia, and depletion of bone marrow neutrophil stores, treatment with granulocyte transfusions improved survival (Cairo et al, 1992).

Using GM-CSF and G-CSF to enhance the quantity and quality of neutrophils has also been studied in human neonates (Carr et al, 2009). Although these agents have induced circulating numbers of neutrophils and appeared to be relatively safe, they have not significantly reduced neonatal sepsis mortality (Wynn et al, 2009). In two meta-analyses, subgroup analysis showed a significant reduction in mortality in the group of infants with systemic infection and neutropenia (Bernstein et al, 2001; Carr et al, 2009). Future studies may prove that selective use of these therapies is beneficial in specific subgroups of septic infants.

NEONATAL BACTERIAL MENINGITIS

Neonatal bacterial meningitis is ominous because of its mortality and morbidity, and it is associated with the same pathogens that cause bacterial sepsis, with GBS and *E. coli* accounting for approximately 70% of all cases, and *L. monocytogenes* accounting for an additional 5% in the first week of life. On occasion, it is possible to isolate *Streptococcus pneumoniae* and *Haemophilus influenzae*, and in infants who are older than 1 week residing in neonatal intensive care units, coagulase-negative staphylococci are the most common isolates. The underlying pathogenesis of bacterial meningitis is a seeding of the meninges during a bacteremic phase in the infant. Studies in neonatal rats have shown that high-grade bacteremia is more likely to lead to bacterial meningitis than lower grade bacteremia.

GBS meningitis (with a mortality approaching 30% and a morbidity of 50%) usually presents as late-onset disease, and the most common GBS serotype identified is III (Levent et al, 2010). In a recent paper by Ansong et al (2009), GBS meningitis complicated 22 in 145 (15%) episodes of early-onset GBS sepsis and 13 in 23 (57%) of episodes of late-onset GBS sepsis. GBS meningitis can occur in the presence of negative blood cultures, and 20% of infants in this study had negative blood cultures (Ansong et al, 2009).

Approximately 80% of all serotypes of *E. coli* that cause meningitis in newborn infants possess the K1 or capsular antigen. The K1 capsular polysaccharide antigen is considered one of the primary virulence factors of this capsular type of *E. coli*, because antibody against K1 antigen has been shown to be protective in neonatal rat models of infection. Mortality rates for neonatal *E. coli* meningitis vary from 20% to 30% in some centers and 50% to 60% in others (Dodge, 1994).

PATHOLOGY AND CLINICAL MANIFESTATIONS

At autopsy, infants who die of meningitis have purulent exudates of the meninges and the surfaces of the ventricles associated with inflammation. Historically, hydrocephalus and a noninfectious encephalopathy were demonstrated in approximately 50% of infants who died of bacterial meningitis.

The signs and symptoms of neonatal meningitis are not easy to distinguish from those of sepsis. The most common presenting symptoms are lethargy, feeding problems, instability of temperature regulation, vomiting, respiratory distress, and apnea. A bulging fontanel may be seen, but this is usually a late manifestation. Seizures are frequently observed and can be caused by either direct central nervous system inflammation or by metabolic abnormalities such as hypoglycemia or hyponatremia.

DIAGNOSIS

The gold standard for diagnosis of meningitis is the analysis of the cerebrospinal fluid, including the WBC count, glucose and protein levels, Gram stain, and culture. The interpretation of cerebrospinal fluid cell counts in newborn infants may be difficult (Garges et al, 2006; Greenberg et al, 2008; Polk and Steele, 1987; Unhanand et al, 1993). During the first week of life, the cerebrospinal fluid WBC count slowly decreases in full-term infants, but may remain high or even increase in premature infants. There is no change in cerebrospinal fluid WBC counts or protein content with gestational age, but there is a significant decrease with postnatal age (Mhanna et al, 2008). The cerebrospinal fluid cell counts, protein, and glucose concentrations from healthy infants may overlap with those from infants with meningitis, and from 1% to 10% of infants with proven meningitis have normal results on a cerebrospinal fluid analysis (Hristeva et al, 1993; Garges et al, 2006; Greenberg et al, 2008). Finally, approximately 30% of all infants with positive results of cerebrospinal fluid cultures for bacteria have negative blood culture results (Garges et al, 2006; Wiswell et al, 1995).

A Gram stain of cerebrospinal fluid must be examined carefully for every infant with suspected meningitis. The stains for approximately 20% of newborns with proven meningitis are reported as showing "no bacteria seen." Although an increase is expected in neutrophils with bacterial meningitis, one may see a predominance of lymphocytes within a conversion to PMNs. With *L. monocytogenes*, a mononuclear cellular response is found in examination of the cerebrospinal fluid. In clinical care units, it is routine to repeat the cerebrospinal fluid examination and culture 2 to 3 days after the initiation of antibiotic therapy. This examination is especially important if the patient has not responded clinically and is experiencing seizures or continued fever. At times it is difficult to eradicate the organism from the cerebrospinal fluid, and consideration can be given to examining the inhibitory and bactericidal concentrations in cerebrospinal fluid. It is especially important to repeat the cerebrospinal fluid examination before stopping antibiotics in patients with more complicated courses, and for enteric gram-negative bacterial meningitis.

THERAPY

Infants with bacterial meningitis are frequently ill and should be monitored in intensive care units when the critical needs can be met with aggressive management. These patients may require mechanical ventilation, complex fluid management to attenuate the effects of cerebral edema and effects of secretion of inappropriate anti-diuretic hormone (ADH), seizure control, vasopressor support, and cardiopulmonary monitoring. The choice of appropriate antibiotic therapy is based on several factors, including the achievable cerebrospinal fluid levels of drugs that have in vitro efficacy against the microorganism. In the case of gram-positive bacteria, the use of penicillin and ampicillin will achieve 10- to 100-fold higher concentrations than the minimal inhibitory concentrations needed to inhibit the bacteria, and there is rapid sterilization of the cerebrospinal fluid. In contrast, aminoglycosides, such as gentamicin and tobramycin, achieve only 40% of peak serum levels and may not achieve minimal inhibitory concentrations more than those equal to or slightly greater than found in vitro for gram-negative bacteria.

In many intensive care units, ampicillin and gentamicin are recommended for the initial therapy for neonatal meningitis. An alternative regimen of ampicillin and cefotaxime can also be used, recognizing the potential for the introduction of cephalosporin-resistant gram-negative isolates in the unit. Although used in the past, neither intrathecal nor intraventricular administration of antibiotics has been found to improve the morbidity or mortality of gram-negative meningitis (Shah et al, 2008). Once the microorganism has been identified and the antibiotic susceptibility results are available, either a single drug or a combination of drugs found to be effective in vitro should be used. Usually penicillin or ampicillin is used for GBS meningitis; in the first few days of therapy, dual therapy with an aminoglycoside may be used. For *L. monocytogenes*, it is common to treat with ampicillin with or without gentamicin. Ampicillin or cefotaxime with or without an aminoglycoside can be used for infection with gram-negative enteric bacteria. The precise length of antibiotic therapy depends on the rapidity of response and sterilization of cerebrospinal fluid. In general, continue therapy for approximately 2 weeks after sterilization of the cerebrospinal fluid, or a minimum of 2 weeks for gram-positive meningitis and a minimum of 3 weeks for gram-negative meningitis. In difficult situations, therapy may be required for as long as 4 to 6 weeks.

It may be prudent to repeat a cerebrospinal fluid examination and culture after initiation of therapy, especially if the clinical response is less than satisfactory. If organisms are seen on gram-stained smears of the fluid, modification of the therapeutic regimen should be considered. In general, approximately 3 days or more are required for an antibiotic regimen to sterilize the cerebrospinal fluid in infants with gram-negative meningitis. In infants with gram-positive meningitis, sterilization is usually seen within 36 to 48 hours. Neuroimaging should be considered to exclude parameningeal foci and abscess formation and to assist in assessing the infant's prognosis.

PROGNOSIS

Complications from neonatal meningitis include brain abscess, communicating or noncommunicating hydrocephalus, subdural effusions, ventriculitis, deafness, and blindness. Generally the severity of complications is related to severity of the disease during the early neonatal period. It is imperative to follow hearing competency and to examine these infants for prolonged periods after recovery. The infant who has experienced meningitis may appear relatively healthy at the time of discharge, and only after careful follow-up do perceptual difficulties, reading problems, or signs of brain damage become apparent. Approximately 40% to 50% of survivors have some evidence of neurologic damage, with severe damage being obvious in 11%. Infants who survive neonatal meningitis should have regular audiology, language, and neurologic evaluations until they enter school (Edwards et al, 1985; Stevens et al, 2003).

SUGGESTED READINGS

Ansong AK, Smith PB, Benjamin DK, et al: Group B streptococcal meningitis: cerebrospinal fluid parameters in the era of intrapartum antibiotic prophylaxis, *Early Hum Dev* 85:S5-S7, 2009.

Bender L, Thaarup J, Varming K, et al: Early and late markers for the detection of early-onset neonatal sepsis, *Dan Med Bull* 55:219-223, 2008.

Castor ML, Whitney CG, Como-Sabetti K, et al: Antibiotic resistance patterns in invasive group B streptococcal isolates, *Infect Dis Obstet Gynecol* 727505:2008, 2008.

Centers for Disease Control and Prevention: Trends in perinatal group B streptococcal disease: United States, 2000-2006, *MMWR Morb Mort Wkly Rep* 58:109-112, 2009.

Diedrick MJ, Flores AE, Hillier SL, et al: Clonal analysis of colonizing group B Streptococcus, serotype IV, an emerging pathogen in the United States, *J Clin Microbiol* 48:3100-3104, 2010.

Edgar JD, Gabriel V, Gallimore JR, et al: A prospective study of the sensitivity, specificity and diagnostic performance of soluble intercellular adhesion molecule 1, highly sensitive C-reactive protein, soluble E-selectin and serum amyloid A in the diagnosis of neonatal infection, *BMC Pediatr* 10:22, 2010.

Ferrieri P, Baker SJ, Hillier SL, et al: Diversity of surface protein expression in group B streptococcal colonizing and invasive isolates, *Indian J Med Res* 119:191-196, 2004a.

Garges HP, Mood MA, Cotton CM, et al: Neonatal meningitis: what is the correlation among cerebrospinal fluid cultures, blood cultures, and cerebrospinal fluid parameters? *Pediatrics* 117:1094-1100, 2006.

Jordan HT, Farley MM, Craig A, et al: Revisiting the need for vaccine prevention of late-onset neonatal group B streptococcal disease: a multistate, population based analysis, *Pediatr Infect Dis J* 27:1057-1064, 2008.

Koenig JM, Keenan WJ: Group B streptococcus and early-onset sepsis in the era of maternal prophylaxis, *Pediatr Clin North Am* 56:689-708, 2009.

Lam HS, Ng PC: Biochemical markers of neonatal sepsis, *Pathology* 40:141-148, 2008.

Levent F, Baker CJ, Rench MA, et al: Early outcomes of group B Streptococcal meningitis in the 21st century, *Pediatr Infect Dis J* 29:1009-1012, 2010.

Puopolo KM, Eichenwald EC: No change in the incidence of ampicillin-resistant, neonatal, early-onset sepsis over 18 years, *Pediatrics* 125:e1031-1038, 2010.

Verani JR, Schrag SJ: Group B streptococcal disease in infants: progress in prevention and continued challenges, *Clin Perinatol* 37:375-392, 2010.

Wynn JL, Neu J, Moldawer LL, et al: Potential of immunomodulatory agents for prevention and treatment of neonatal sepsis, *J Perinatol* 29:79-88, 2009.

Wynn JL, Seed PC, Cotton CM: Does IVIg administration yield improved immune function in very premature neonates? *J Perinatol* 30:635-642, 2010.

Complete references used in this text can be found online at www.expertconsult.com

HEALTH CARE–ACQUIRED INFECTIONS IN THE NURSERY

David A. Munson and Jacquelyn R. Evans*

For decades, nosocomial or health care–acquired infection (HAI) has been considered by many as an unavoidable problem associated with prolonged stays in an intensive care nursery. Immature skin and immune systems, pathologic skin flora, and necessary invasive interventions all put the premature neonate at high risk for HAI. But some centers have clearly shown that, despite these risk factors, HAIs ranging from catheter-associated infections to acquisition of respiratory viruses can largely be prevented (Andersen, 2005; Bloom et al, 2003; Kilbride et al, 2003). There is a direct financial cost to the health care system associated with infections acquired while in the hospital, but more importantly there is growing evidence that the deleterious effects of the inflammatory response to infection may adversely affect long-term outcomes, including increased rates and severity of bronchopulmonary dysplasia and neurodevelopmental impairment (Adams-Chapman and Stoll, 2001, 2006; Gonzalez et al, 1996; Hintz et al, 2005; Jobe and Ikegami, 1996; Leviton et al, 1999; Rojas et al, 1995; Shah et al, 2008; Stoll et al, 2004).

The growing numbers of surviving very low-birth-weight (VLBW) infants magnifies the impact of this problem. Clinicians must make efforts to minimize the exposure of newborns to known risk factors for infection. Continuous surveillance and monitoring of endemic HAI rates and patterns of responsible pathogens are necessary to establish a reference point in each nursery and facilitate early identification of epidemics. Prevention of infections in the neonatal patient requires an expanding skill set in addition to organized hospital-wide initiatives. Familiarity with quality improvement concepts, standardization of practice, and hospital programs such as antimicrobial stewardship are all essential to preventing harm in the smallest patients.

DEFINITIONS

The Centers for Disease Control and Prevention (CDC) provides the following surveillance definition for an HAI: illness associated with a pathogen or its toxins that is not present or incubating at the time of admission to the intensive care unit (Horan et al, 2008). As simple as this definition seems, it does leave some room for confusion for the clinician caring for the neonatal population. Infections that manifest early in the 1st week of life are typically related to perinatal risk factors and vertical transmission from the mother. HAIs are more often related to patient colonization and environmental risk factors. Unfortunately, there

is no specific postnatal age that distinguishes maternally transmitted infections from HAIs (Baltimore, 1998), and it may be difficult to differentiate a late-onset, perinatally acquired infection from an HAI. Most sources define HAIs as infections occurring after 3 days of age (Baltimore, 1998; Stoll et al, 2002a). The CDC defines HAI as any infection that occurs after admission to the neonatal intensive care unit (NICU) and that was not transplacentally acquired (Garner et al, 1988). Other authorities suggest that HAI be defined as any infection occurring more than 5 to 7 days after birth (Baltimore, 1998).

The majority of HAIs in the neonatal population are bloodstream infections associated with an intravascular device. Criteria for central line–associated bloodstream infections (CLABSIs), as defined by the CDC, are (1) isolation of a recognized pathogen from one blood culture specimen or of a skin commensal from two blood culture specimens; (2) one or more clinical signs of infection, such as temperature instability, apnea, and bradycardia; and (3) the presence of an intravascular device at the time the culture specimen is collected (Horan and Gaynes, 2004). Ventilator-associated pneumonias are difficult to diagnose in the NICU, but can contribute to morbidity, especially in patients with evolving lung disease. Although the use of Foley catheters is low in the NICU compared with other intensive care units, the acquisition of urinary tract infections while in the NICU is still a problem.

A summary of definitions of important HAIs in infants is provided in Box 40-1. The prevention of the spread of respiratory viruses is another area that demands attention, especially in a unit caring for infants with significant bronchopulmonary dysplasia. The NICU, as with other intensive care units, must remain vigilant in the control of bacteria resistant to antibiotics such as methicillin-resistant *Staphylococcus aureus* (MRSA) and vancomycin-resistant enterococcus (VRE). As community-acquired MRSA is becoming more prevalent, it is becoming more difficult to determine the origin of MRSA in a neonatal patient.

INCIDENCE

WELL BABY (HEALTHY NEWBORN) NURSERY

Accurate rates of HAI in the well baby nursery are difficult to ascertain because there is no systematic reporting or surveillance network for this issue; however, the incidence appears to be low. Some researchers estimate rates of less than 1 per 100 patients discharged (Baltimore, 1998). Typical risk factors for acquiring a HAI, such as invasive procedures and presence of an intravascular device, are uncommon in the healthy newborn population. Discharge

*Acknowledgment: In writing this chapter, the authors excerpted significant portions of the chapter *Nosocomial Infections in the Nursery* by Ira Adams-Chapman and Barbara Stoll from the previous edition of this book.

from the hospital within 48 hours of birth and rooming-in practices have helped further to decrease the risk of exposure in modern mother-baby units. Early discharge may also limit surveillance efforts, because patients may be discharged home before they become symptomatic from HAIs (Goldmann, 1989).

NEONATAL INTENSIVE CARE UNIT

The majority of neonatal HAIs occur in term and preterm infants hospitalized in special care nurseries. It is difficult to determine and compare reports of endemic HAI rates in different NICU populations. Any comparison of surveillance data between institutions is limited by differences in patient demographics (e.g., birthweight,

---

BOX 40-1   Definitions of Nosocomial Bacteremia and Pneumonia for Patients Younger than 12 Months, from the Centers for Disease Control and Prevention

NOSOCOMIAL BLOODSTREAM INFECTIONS

- Recognized pathogen isolated from blood culture and pathogen is not related to infection at another site
- Must have at least one of the following clinical symptoms: fever (body temperature >38°C, rectal), hypothermia (body temperature <37°C, rectal), apnea, bradycardia, and a skin commensal isolated from two blood culture specimens on separate occasions.

PNEUMONIA

- Chest radiograph with new or progressive infiltrate, cavitation, consolidation, or pneumatoceles
- Worsening gas exchange and three of the following:
  - Temperature instability
  - White blood cell count <4000 or >15,000 with ≥10% bands
  - New-onset purulent sputum, change in character of sputum, increased respiratory secretions, or increased suctioning requirements
  - Physical examination findings consistent with increased work of breathing or apnea
  - Wheezing, rales, or rhonchi
  - Cough
  - Bradycardia or tachycardia

URINARY TRACT INFECTION

- Clinical symptoms (fever [body temperature >38°C, rectal], hypothermia [body temperature <37°C, rectal], apnea or bradycardia, dysuria, lethargy or vomiting) and positive urine culture (≥100,000 microorganisms/mL) with no more than two species identified
- May also qualify as a UTI if the above symptoms are present without another cause and has at least one of the following
  - Positive dipstick for leukocyte esterase, nitrate, or both
  - Pyuria
  - Organisms seen on Gram stain of unspun urine
  - At least two urine cultures with the same uropathogen with ≥100 colonies/mL
  - ≤100,000 colonies/mL of a single uropathogen if the patient is receiving an effective antimicrobial agent
  - Physician diagnosis of UTI
  - Physician institutes appropriate therapy for a UTI

Modified from Horan TC, Andrus M, Dudeck MA: CDC/NHSN surveillance definition of health care-associated infection and criteria for specific types of infections in the acute care setting, *Am J Infect Control* 36:3091-332, 2008.
UTI, Urinary tract infection.

---

gestational age distribution, underlying severity of disease, birth in the hospital versus elsewhere), back transport policies, and the use of different definitions for HAI.

Among a cohort of 6215 VLBW infants (weight <1500 g) who were monitored by the National Institute of Child Health and Human Development (NICHD) Neonatal Research Network, 21% of those who survived beyond 3 days of age had at least one episode of late-onset sepsis (Stoll et al, 2002b). There was significant variability among the participating centers, with rates ranging from 10.6% to 31.7% at individual sites (Stoll et al, 2002b). Moreover, rates were inversely related to birthweight and gestational age, ranging from 43% for infants weighing 401 to 750 g at birth to 7% for infants weighing 1251 to 1500 g at birth. These data are similar to those reported by Brodie et al (2000). In their study, 19% of 1354 infants weighing less than 1500 g at birth had HAIs, and the rates were highest for infants at the lowest birthweights (39%, <750 g; 27%, 750 to 999 g; 10%, 1000 to 1499 g). A point prevalence survey conducted by the 29 level II to level IV nurseries participating in the Pediatric Prevention Network revealed a prevalence of 11.4% for HAI (Sohn, 2001).

The CDC National Healthcare Safety Network (NHSN) was developed in 2005 and replaced the National Nosocomial Infections Surveillance system that reported national data before that time. Some investigators believe that reporting overall incidence rates may be misleading, because of the wide variations in practice and patient populations in different units; therefore the NHSN system monitors device-associated HAI rates by using an approach that accounts for variability in device use and length of hospital stay (Edwards et al, 2008; Emori et al, 1991; Gaynes et al, 1996). These data are also stratified by birthweight categories and expressed as incidence density per 100 or 1000 patient-days. These two adjustments modify the relative risk on the basis of the severity of the illness and the duration of exposure to the risk factor. A number of states in the United States have mandatory reporting of HAIs through the NHSN, and the number of participating medical centers is growing. The NHSN data are similar to institutional and collaborative epidemiologic data reported elsewhere. Rates of device-associated infections are presented in Table 40-1. These rates remained constant in the 1990s (Gaynes et al, 1996; National Nosocomial Infections Surveillance System Report, 2000), but appear to have dropped considerably in the 2007 report (Edwards et al, 2008), suggesting that preventive strategies for CLABSIs may be having an effect.

ANATOMIC SITES OF INFECTION

WELL BABY NURSERY

HAIs in the well baby nursery are most commonly superficial, involving the skin, mouth, or eyes. These infections include omphalitis, pustules, abscesses, and bullous impetigo (Goldmann, 1989). Nursery epidemics of diarrhea caused by bacterial and viral enteropathogens have been reported, but they occur infrequently (Goldmann, 1989).

NEONATAL INTENSIVE CARE UNIT

National and institutional surveillance data demonstrate that bloodstream infections are responsible for the majority of HAIs among NICU patients (Gaynes et al, 1996; National Nosocomial Infections Surveillance System Report, 2000; Sohn et al, 2001). The remaining cases involve the respiratory tract, eye, ear, nose, throat, or gastrointestinal tract (Figure 40-1). Surveillance data for meningitis are limited. Reports suggest that late-onset meningitis may be underdiagnosed in the high-risk population of VLBW infants (Stoll et al, 2002b). There are widespread differences in clinical practice regarding the inclusion of a lumbar puncture with cerebrospinal fluid

analysis in the evaluation of a neonate with possible sepsis. This variation in practice has been challenged by recent data suggesting that generally accepted cerebrospinal fluid parameters are not sensitive or specific for meningitis in the neonate (Smith et al, 2008). Although early onset meningitis remains a rare event, clinicians need to consider including a lumbar puncture in the initial evaluation of a neonate with signs and symptoms of infection.

RISK FACTORS

Some risk factors for acquiring an HAI are reflections of the patient population and are difficult or impossible to modify. Other risk factors are directly related to the level of supportive care associated with intensive care medicine and may be difficult yet possible to modify. Risk factors for HAI include lower gestational age and low birthweight; invasive procedures; invasive devices, especially intravascular catheters and endotracheal tubes; parenteral nutrition and intravenous lipids; colonization of skin, gastrointestinal tract, and airway with invasive organisms; selected drugs administered to the neonate; and issues surrounding nursery staffing, nursery crowding, and hand washing (Box 40-2) (Gaynes et al, 1996; Kawogoe et al, 2001; Perlman et al, 2007; Stoll et al, 1996, 2002a; Stover et al, 2001; Suara et al, 2000). Minimizing exposure to known risk factors for infection is important to reduce the rate of HAIs in the nursery.

The risk of developing an HAI is inversely related to gestational age and birthweight (Gaynes et al, 1996, Kawogoe et al, 2001; National Nosocomial Infections Surveillance System Report, 2000; Stoll et al, 1996, 2002a; Stover

TABLE 40-1   Rate of Device-Associated HAIs

Birthweight (g)	NHSN 2008 CLABSI per 1000 catheter days	NHSN 2008 VAP per 1000 ventilator days
<750	3.7	2.6
751-1000	3.3	2.1
1001-1500	2.6	1.5
1501-2500	2.4	1.0
>2500	2.0	0.9

Modified from Edwards JR, Peterson KD, Andrus ML, et al: National Healthcare Safety Network (NHSN) Report, data summary for 2006 through 2007, issued November 2008. National Healthcare Safety Network Facilities, *Am J Infect Control* 36:609-626, 2008. Level III NICU pooled data.
CLABSI, Central line–associated bloodstream infection; *HAI*, health care–acquired infection *NHSN*, National Healthcare Safety Network; *VAP*, ventilator-associated pneumonia.

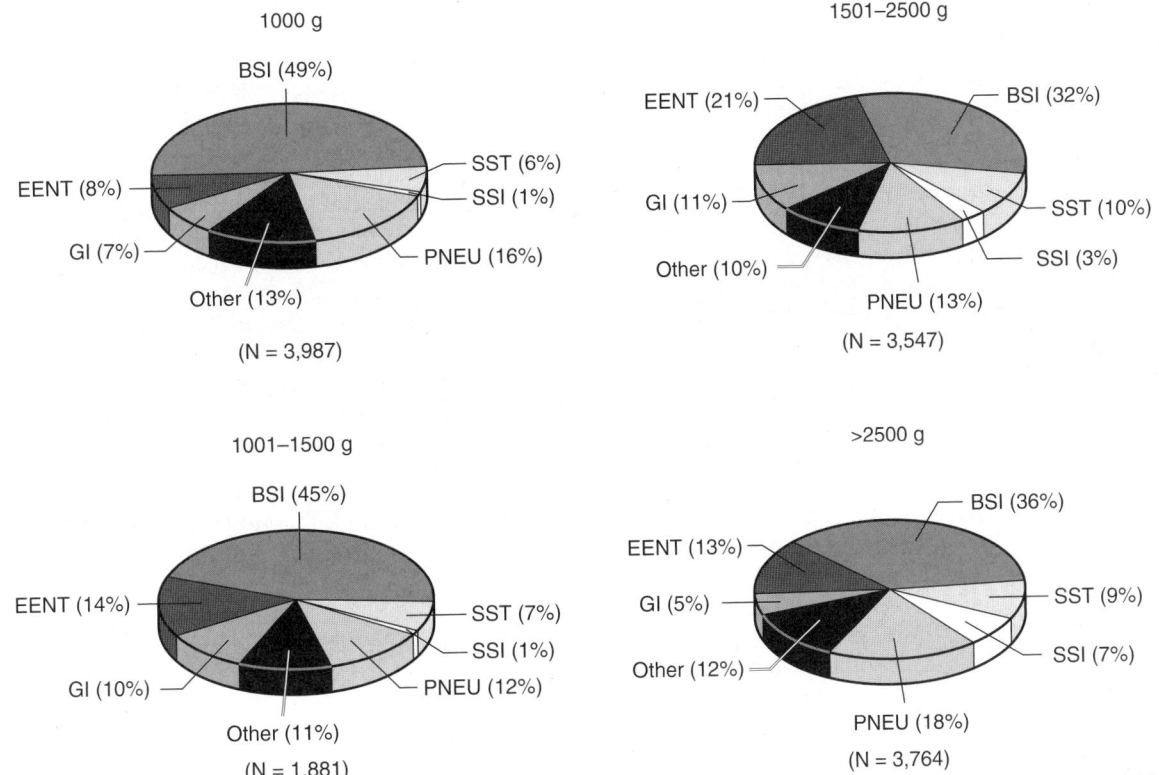

FIGURE 40-1 Distribution of health care–acquired infections by site of infection. (*Data from Gaynes RP, Edwards JR, Jarvis WR, et al: Nosocomial infections among neonates in high-risk nurseries in the United States,* Pediatrics 98:357-361, 1996.)

BOX 40-2   Risk Factors for Acquiring Health Care–Acquired Infections in the Neonatal Intensive Care Unit

- Prematurity
- Low birthweight
- Invasive device
- Intravascular device (CVC, PAL, PICC, PIVC, umbilical catheter)
- Mechanical ventilator
- Urinary catheter
- Ventriculoperitoneal shunt
- Medications
- Histamine$_2$-blocking agents
- Steroids
- Others
- Prolonged administration of hyperalimentation
- Intralipid administration
- Delayed enteral feedings
- Feeding with formula rather than human milk
- Inadequate nursery staffing and overcrowding
- Poor compliance with handwashing

CVC, Central versus catheter; *PAL,* percutaneous arterial line; *PICC,* peripherally inserted central catheter; *PIVC,* percutaneous intravenous catheter.

et al, 2001; Suara et al, 2000). Previous reports estimate that there is a 3% lower risk of acquiring an HAI with each 500-g increment in birthweight (Goldmann, 1989). Infants with birthweights less than 1000 g have twice the rate of nosocomial bloodstream infections than do infants with birthweights greater than 1000 g (Brodie et al, 2000; Geffers et al, 2008; Gaynes et al, 1996; National Nosocomial Infections Surveillance System Report, 2000; Stoll et al, 2002a; Stover et al, 2001). Severity of illness scores may be more predictive than birthweight alone, because they reflect physiologic stability and the cumulative need for intervention and invasive therapies (Goldmann, 1989; Gray et al, 1995).

The use of any type of invasive device increases the risk for infection. The most common invasive devices used in the nursery are intravascular catheters, mechanical ventilators, ventriculoperitoneal shunts, and urinary catheters. In general, the risk rises as the duration of exposure lengthens. Compared with adult patients, neonates are at higher risk for catheter-related bloodstream infections and at lower risk for ventilator-associated pneumonia and urinary tract infections (Langley et al, 2001; National Nosocomial Infections Surveillance System Report, 2000). These patterns correlate with the frequency with which these invasive devices are used in the neonatal patient population.

Prolonged duration of mechanical ventilation is the primary risk factor for development of hospital-acquired pneumonia. Contamination of respiratory equipment—especially with gram-negative organisms that thrive in moist environments, such as *Acinetobacter, Pseudomonas,* and *Flavobacterium* spp.—frequently leads to colonization of the respiratory tract. There is some evidence that aspiration of gastric and oropharyngeal secretions around the uncuffed endotracheal tube may occur, and this could be a mechanism for ventilator-associated pneumonia (Farhath et al, 2008). The various closed-system suctioning devices may decrease the risk of iatrogenic contamination during suctioning. Defining a ventilator-associated pneumonia in the neonatal population remains a challenge. Patients in the NICU do not often meet all of the parameters defined by the CDC (see Box 40-1), but acute worsening of pulmonary function in an infant with a ventilator could represent a new-onset pneumonia. Collaboration among the largest NICUs is needed to better define this entity in the neonatal population.

Intravascular devices commonly used in the neonatal population are peripheral intravenous catheters (PIVs), umbilical catheters, peripherally inserted central catheters (PICCs), surgically placed central venous catheters (CVCs) and percutaneous arterial catheters. Regardless of the type of device used, the rate of catheter-related bloodstream infections is directly related to the number of days the catheters are in place and inversely related to the gestational age and birthweight of the patients (Gaynes et al, 1996; Kawogoe et al, 2001; National Nosocomial Infections Surveillance System Report, 2000; Stoll et al, 2000a; Suara et al, 2000). Coagulase-negative *Staphylococcus* (CONS) remains the primary pathogen associated with catheter-related bloodstream infections (Garland et al, 2001).

PIVs are the most commonly used device for vascular access in neonates. In adults, the removal of such catheters after 72 hours is recommended. Data in neonates are insufficient to recommend elective removal of PIVs after 72 hours, because studies have not shown a clear correlation between the higher colonization rate noted after 72 hours and an increased rate of catheter-related bloodstream infection (Oishi, 2001; Pearson, 1996). Further study is needed to answer this question.

Data comparing the infection rates of the various types of intravascular catheters are limited. Theoretically the risk should be lower for tunneled catheters, because the Dacron cuff proximal to the exit site of a surgically placed catheter can inhibit the migration of organisms into the catheter tract (Mermel et al, 2001). Adult data suggest that tunneled catheters have lower infection rates than nontunneled catheters; however, a report of 79 surgical neonates requiring tunneled lines showed a rate of infection of 9.9 per 1000 catheter days (Klein et al, 2003), comparable to or worse than reported rates of PICC line infections in other NICU populations. This issue needs further study in the neonatal population, especially because PICCs are being used with greater frequency for long-term vascular access in neonates (Stoll et al, 2002a). Some recent trials comparing PIVs to PICC lines for the provision of parenteral nutrition have challenged the notion that the presence of a central line increases the risk of infection above the risk that exists simply with the use of peripheral catheters. It appears that the use of a PICC line decreases the risk of complications associated with PIVs without increasing the rate of infection, at least in the initial weeks of life (Ainsworth et al, 2007). There is certainly much work to be done to determine the ideal access for the different populations cared for in the NICU.

The use of intravenous lipid emulsions increases the risk for infection (Freeman et al, 1990). Lipid emulsions decrease the flow rate through the intravenous catheter and potentiate the growth and proliferation of some microorganisms. Lipid emulsions can interfere with host defense mechanisms by impairing the function of neutrophils and reticuloendothelial macrophages (Freeman et al, 1990; Langevin et al, 1999; Nugent, 1984). Extrinsic contamination has been reported but rarely occurs in the United States (Hernandez-Ramos et al, 2000). Freeman et al (1990) reported that the use of a lipid emulsion was positively and independently predictive for the development of CONS bacteremia. Infants who demonstrated CONS sepsis were 5.8-fold more likely to have been exposed to lipid emulsions. Administration of such emulsions has also been linked to a higher risk for HAI with *Candida* and *Malassezia* spp. in neonates (Long and Keyserling, 1985; Redline et al, 1985; Saiman et al, 2000).

Histamine-blocking agents and postnatally administered corticosteroids are the medications most commonly associated with an increased risk of HAIs among newborns. It is hypothesized that the reduced gastric pH associated with the use of histamine$_2$-blocking agents promotes bacterial overgrowth and invasion of pathogenic bacteria (Beck-Sague et al, 1994; Stoll et al, 1999). Dexamethasone has been used in ventilator-dependent preterm infants to facilitate weaning from the ventilator and to minimize the risk of chronic lung disease. The use of dexamethasone has decreased in the last decade in VLBW infants secondary to concerns of spontaneous bowel perforation and adverse effects on growth and neurodevelopmental outcome (O'Shea et al, 1999; Stark et al, 2001, Vohr et al, 2000). However, there is renewed interest in a role for steroids after the first week of life, especially in infants who have demonstrated a high risk for developing chronic lung disease (Doyle et al, 2005, 2006, 2007). Because the use of dexamethasone has been associated with an increased risk of infection in VLBW infants (Stoll et al, 1999; Yeh et al, 1997), neonatologists will need to include this concern in any risk-benefit analysis of the use of steroids in their patients.

Nursery design and staffing influence the risk of infection. Overcrowding and larger workloads decrease compliance with hand washing and raise the risk of HAI (Archibald et al, 1997; Fridkin et al, 1996; Harbarth et al, 1999; Robert et al, 2000; Vicca, 1999). Inadequate numbers of staff and the use of temporary or inexperienced staff members both adversely affect the rate of infection. The adverse effects of inadequate staffing and overcrowding were demonstrated by Hayley and Bregman (1982), who showed a relationship between nurse-to-patient ratio and colonization of patients with MRSA. Fridkin et al (1996) found that patient-to-nurse ratio was an independent predictor of development of a catheter-related bloodstream infection. Furthermore, strategic nursery design and improvement in nursing staffing correlate with lower rates of HAIs (Gladstone et al, 1990).

DISTRIBUTION BY PATHOGEN

The predominant pathogens responsible for nosocomial bloodstream infections have changed over time. Goldmann (1989) proposed that these trends are explained by changes in the neonatal intensive care patient population and advancing technology. *S. aureus* was the most common nosocomial pathogen in the 1950s and 1960s. In the 1960s and 1970s, gram-negative organisms emerged

TABLE 40-2 Distribution of Pathogens Responsible for Bloodstream Infections

Pathogen	No.	%
Coagulase-negative staphylococci	3833	51.0
Staphylococcus aureus	563	7.5
Group B streptococci	597	7.9
Enterococcus spp.	467	6.2
Candida spp.	518	6.9
Escherichia coli	326	4.3
Other *Streptococcus* spp.	205	2.7
Enterobacter spp.	219	2.9
Klebsiella pneumoniae	188	2.5

Data from Gaynes RP, Edwards JR, Jarvis WR, et al: Nosocomial infections among neonates in high-risk nurseries in the United States, *Pediatrics* 98:357-361, 1996.

as the predominant pathogens; globally, these organisms remain the most important pathogens responsible for HAIs in the nursery (Stoll, 2001). National surveillance data in the United States indicate that CONS is currently the most common nosocomial pathogen (Gaynes et al, 1996; National Nosocomial Infections Surveillance System Report, 2000) (Table 40-2). In the United States, the distribution of pathogens has not changed significantly over the past decade (Gaynes et al, 1996; Stoll et al, 1996, 2002a) (Box 40-3). Among a cohort of infants with birthweights less than 1500 g with late-onset infections, the NICHD Neonatal Research Network reported that gram-positive organisms were responsible for 70% of cases, gram-negative organisms for 18%, and fungi for 12% (Stoll et al, 2002a). These findings are similar to those of a 10-year retrospective analysis of pathogens in a single center, in which gram-positive organisms caused 57% of late-onset infections (Karlowicz et al, 2000). The distribution of infecting pathogens did not differ with birthweight or timing of infection (Stoll et al, 2002a). More recent articles evaluating interventions and mechanisms of infection confirm the continued predominance of CONS in neonatal line infections in the United States (Garland et al, 2008) as do review articles (Curtis and Shetty, 2008).

For the clinician, understanding the specific colonization and resistance patterns in the individual NICU is perhaps more important than being aware of national trends. The emergence of nosocomial pathogens with antimicrobial resistance is a concern. In patients of all ages, reports estimate that 50% to 60% of HAIs are caused by resistant organisms (Jones, 2001; Weinstein, 1998). Organisms showing patterns of increasing antibiotic resistance of importance to NICU patients are VRE, MRSA, and multidrug-resistant gram-negative organisms (Bizzarro and Gallagher, 2007).

GRAM-POSITIVE BACTERIA

CONS is the most common endemic nosocomial pathogen in neonates (Brodie et al, 2000; Garland et al, 1996, 2008; Gray et al, 1995; National Nosocomial Infections Surveillance system report, 2000; Stoll et al, 2002a). The majority of CONS infections are bloodstream infections. Reported incidence ranges from 51% to 78% among VLBW infants (Gray et al, 1995; Isaacs et al, 1996; Stoll, 1996, 2002a). Gray et al (1995) reported a cumulative incidence of 17.5 episodes of CONS sepsis per 100 patient-days and an incidence density of 6.9 episodes of CONS sepsis per 1000 patient-days.

Known risk factors for CONS infection are low birthweight, lower gestational age, use of central venous catheters, prolonged administration of hyperalimentation, use of intravenous lipid emulsions, postnatal administration of corticosteroids, and prolonged hospital stay (Brodie et al, 2000; Freeman et al, 1990; Goldmann, 1989; Johnson-Robbins et al, 1996). CONS is the pathogen most commonly associated with catheter-related infections, partially because it produces a capsular polysaccharide adhesin (poly-*N*-succinyl glucosamine), which enhances its ability to adhere to intravascular devices. Although some studies suggest that prophylactic use of vancomycin reduces the risk of CONS catheter-related infections, this practice is not recommended because of the serious risk of encouraging antibiotic-resistant organisms, especially VRE and staphylococci. The use of a vancomycin lock, where vancomycin is instilled into the catheter and then removed after a specified dwell time, has more promise in terms of balancing the risk of systemic exposure and prophylaxis against contamination of the catheter lumen. Garland et al (2005) demonstrated a reduction in the rate of CLABSI from 17.8 to 2.4 per 1000 catheter days using this technique. Although promising, several units have achieved comparable reductions without the use of this kind of intervention. Consequently, the role of an antibiotic lock will likely find its place in certain circumstances or in populations that have demonstrated persistently elevated risks for infection.

Enterococci are responsible for both endemic and epidemic HAIs in the NICU. Use of central venous catheters, prolonged hospital stay, and prior antibiotic use are recognized risk factors for colonization with these organisms. The gastrointestinal tract is often the primary source of infection; however, the pathogens are typically spread via the hands of health care workers or through environmental contamination. The widespread use of antibiotics has led to the emergence of VRE. There are published guidelines to prevent the spread of VRE, which include hand washing, isolation, barrier precautions, and cohorting of infected patients (Gross and Pujat, 2001; Hospital Infection Control Practices Advisory Committee, 1995). Educational programs to limit the indiscriminate use of antibiotics have been effective in decreasing the spread of VRE (Goldmann et al, 1996; Isaacs, 2000).

S. aureus has caused epidemics in well baby nurseries and in NICUs. In the nursery, the major reservoirs for staphylococci are colonized or infected infants. These infants transmit the organism to health care workers, who subsequently infect other infants. The skin, nares, and umbilicus are the most common sites of colonization. Unfortunately, routine surveillance cultures are not useful because colonization rates correlate poorly with infection rates. Studies in adult patients have shown that many patients who demonstrate *S. aureus* bacteremia were colonized with the identical strain at the time of admission to the hospital, suggesting that some of the infections with *S. aureus* are community acquired rather than hospital acquired (von Eiff et al, 2001). Similarly, health care workers can be colonized with a community-acquired strain of *S. aureus*, which they then transfer to vulnerable infants. Importantly, there has been a significant increase in methicillin-resistant strains of *S. aureus* causing infections in the NICU. A review of the National Nosocomial Infections Surveillance data from 1995 to 2004 indicated a 308% increase in the incidence of MRSA over that 10-year time frame. As of the 2004, MRSA accounted for 34% of *S. aureus* infections in the reported data (Lessa et al, 2009). Consequently, when covering for a possible *S. aureus* infection, it is critical to select an antibiotic that is effective against methicillin-resistant strains.

Group B *streptococcus* (GBS) remains an important cause of late-onset infection in neonates, but do not have a clear role as an HAI. Intrapartum antibiotic treatment to prevent vertical transmission of GBS from a colonized mother to her infant has led to a decrease in early-onset GBS disease. In contrast, the incidence of late-onset GBS disease has remained unchanged, presumably because prophylaxis does not eradicate colonization of the genital tract or the environment.

GRAM-NEGATIVE ORGANISMS

Gram-negative organisms are a particularly important cause of nosocomial bloodstream infections, pneumonia, and meningitis because they generally cause severe disease.

Escherichia coli is the most common gram-negative pathogen. Other gram-negative organisms responsible for HAI are *Klebsiella*, *Pseudomonas*, *Enterobacter*, *Acinetobacter*, *Serratia*, *Haemophilus*, and *Salmonella* spp. (see Box 40-3).

The attributable mortality is much higher for gram-negative infections than for gram-positive infections. Stoll et al (2002a) reported that infants with gram-negative infections had a 3.5-fold higher risk of death. Karlowicz et al (2000) found that gram-negative infections were associated with fulminant death within 48 hours of a positive blood culture result in 69% of cases. *Pseudomonas* spp. appear to be particularly virulent, causing death in 42% to 75% of infected neonates (Karlowicz et al, 2000; Leigh et al, 1995; Stoll et al, 2002a). A more recent study by Makhoul et al (2005) and colleagues in Israel confirms that gram-negative infections are associated with a substantially higher mortality.

FUNGAL ORGANISMS

Fungal infections are discussed in detail in Chapter 41. Invasive fungal infection is estimated to occur in 1% to 4% of VLBW infants and the incidence in extremely low-birthweight (ELBW) infants has been reported to be significantly higher. The risk may even approach 20% in infants with a birthweight less than 750 g (Bartels et al, 2007; Benjamin et al, 2006; Clerihew et al, 2006; Fridkin et al, 2006; Makhoul et al, 2002, 2007; Rodriguez et al, 2006; Stoll et al, 2002a). Rates and predominant fungal species vary among clinical centers. The smallest and most premature infants appear to be at the highest risk, particularly when they are exposed to broad-spectrum antibiotics or long courses of antibiotics. Other identified risk factors are prolonged mechanical ventilation, prolonged use of central venous catheters, prior use of lipid emulsions, and the use of histamine type 2 antagonists (Benjamin et al, 2001; Long and Keyserling, 1985; Makhoul et al, 2002; Saiman et al, 2000).

Efforts at preventing nosocomial fungal infection have focused on the use of prophylactic fluconazole for VLBW infants. This strategy has been shown to decrease the rate of invasive disease in randomized trials, but the baseline rates in the control arms in some studies have been high (Kaufman et al, 2001). Consequently it has been difficult to determine how generalizable the findings are. Furthermore, metaanalysis has not demonstrated an associated improvement in mortality (Clerihew et al, 2007). A number of retrospective studies describing the implementation of fluconazole prophylaxis in individual units have also suggested a reduction in invasive fungal disease (Aghai et al, 2006; Bertini et al, 2005; Dutta et al, 2005; Healy et al, 2005; Manzoni et al, 2006; Uko et al, 2006). Although no study has found an increase in fluconazole-resistant fungus, resistance remains a concern with any prophylactic strategy. Limiting a prophylactic strategy to units with a high rate of invasive candidal disease and to patients with the highest risk will likely ultimately provide the greatest benefit with the lowest risk.

VIRAL ORGANISMS

Viral organisms that cause HAI in the NICU include respiratory syncytial virus (RSV), rhinovirus, metapneumovirus, influenza, varicella, rotavirus, and enterovirus.

Isolated infections generally result from contact with infected caregivers or family members. Nursery epidemics may occur in addition to isolated individual cases.

Respiratory Syncytial Virus

Careful hand washing is the most effective measure to prevent RSV infection. Recommendations for preventing RSV epidemics in the inpatient setting include cohorting of patients, barrier precautions, and careful hand washing (Goldmann, 2001; Hall, 2000; Karanfil et al, 1999; Mlinarić-Galinović and Varda-Brkić, 2000; Snydman et al, 1988). Rapid testing to detect the virus in nasal washings facilitates efforts to cohort infected patients, which has been shown to be an effective control measure (Madge et al, 1992; Snydman et al, 1988). RSV is a fastidious organism capable of surviving on inanimate objects for prolonged periods; therefore some authorities advocate the use of gowns and gloves, because of the increased risk of contamination through casual contact between the patient and the environment (Goldmann, 2001; Hall, 2000; Karanfil et al, 1999; Mlinarić-Galinović and Varda-Brkić, 2000). Several case reports have described the use of palivizumab, an RSV monoclonal antibody, to control nosocomial outbreaks; however, the efficacy of administering monthly injections to hospitalized patients has not been critically or systematically evaluated (Cox et al, 2001; Macartney et al, 2000). Preterm infants born before 32 weeks' gestation and those with chronic lung disease remain at high risk for RSV infection after hospital discharge; therefore the American Academy of Pediatrics (AAP) recommends that all high-risk infants (<32 weeks' gestation, chronic lung disease, or asymptomatic acyanotic congenital heart disease, such as a patent ductus arteriosus or ventricular septal defect) receive up to five doses of palivizumab during the RSV season (American Academy of Pediatrics, 1998, 2009a; Meissner et al, 1999). These guidelines were updated in 2003 to also include patients with cyanotic congenital heart disease. They have been modified again in 2009 to clarify the risk factors for the 32- to 35-week gestational age group (American Academy of Pediatrics, 2009a).

Influenza

Influenza is spread primarily via airborne transmission. Hand washing and immunization of health care workers are the primary tools to prevent nosocomial spread of this virus (Nichol and Hauge, 1997). Most infection control guidelines recommend that every health care worker wear a mask during contact with infected patients. Although several drugs are available for the prophylaxis and treatment of influenza, they have not been studied in newborns and cannot be recommended at this time (Meissner, 2001). At-risk infants should receive the influenza vaccine during the winter months once they reach the age of 6 months.

With the appearance of the novel H1N1 influenza strain, the season for possible flu exposure has increased substantially. In addition, newborns are thought to be in a high-risk population if they are born to mothers who are actively infected. Guidelines for minimizing risk to the infant have been offered by the CDC. Pregnant women with symptoms that are consistent with H1N1 influenza should receive treatment as soon as possible. If tolerated, the mother should wear a mask during labor and delivery. After the delivery, the infant should be cared for away from the mother until he or she has received 48 hours of treatment and has become afebrile and able to control cough and secretions. The infant should be assisted in lactation if she intends to breastfeed, because the breast milk itself is not thought to be a means of viral transmission (CDC, 2009).

Varicella

Potential exposures and epidemics of nosocomial varicella have been reported, but true nosocomial infection in the NICU is rare. The index case is typically an asymptomatic infected health care worker or family member who has had contact with a susceptible infant before the onset of clinical disease in the health care worker or family member. The incubation period lasts 14 to 16 days, and infected persons are contagious 24 to 48 hours before the appearance of the rash. The relative risk of infection varies according to the intensity of the exposure and the presence of maternal antibody in the infant. The majority of transplacental antibody transfer occurs during the third trimester; therefore most extremely preterm infants are born before this process is complete. ELBW infants may be at risk even if their mothers have a documented titer of varicella antibodies. The AAP recommends administration of varicella zoster immunoglobulin (VZIG) to any newborn whose mother shows signs of varicella infection within 5 days before delivery or within 2 days after delivery. If the exposure is postnatal, whether via a family member or a health care worker, an exposed preterm infant born before 28 weeks' gestation or weighing less than 1000 g birthweight should receive immunoprophylaxis regardless of the mother's varicella history or serologic status. A postnatally exposed preterm infant born after 28 weeks' gestation should receive VZIG only if the mother lacks clinical or serologic evidence of prior disease (American Academy of Pediatrics, 2009b).

Airborne and contact precautions are recommended for all infants with active varicella disease for at least 5 days after vesicles appear and until all lesions have crusted. Airborne and contact precautions should be used for any exposed susceptible patient from 8 to 21 days after the exposure. Administration of VZIG potentially prolongs the incubation period; therefore all exposed infants who receive this product should be isolated for up to 28 days after the exposure. An infant born to a mother with active varicella should be isolated for 21 days, or for 28 days if the infant received VZIG. The infants should also be isolated from the mother until all of her lesions have crusted.

Rotavirus

Although rare, epidemics of rotavirus diarrhea may occur in the nursery (Herruzo et al, 2009; Jain and Glass, 2001; Lee et al, 2001; Widdowson et al, 2000); they are primarily caused by inadequate hand washing and cross-contamination between patients. Standard and contact precautions should be followed throughout the duration of the illness. Some patients have prolonged fecal shedding of low concentrations of the virus; therefore some infection control

experts recommend contact precautions for the duration of the hospitalization of such patients. Rotavirus is an important cause of diarrhea in older infants and should be suspected with any apparent epidemic of diarrhea. There are now two live virus vaccines available for the prevention of rotavirus infection, but their use in the NICU remains controversial because of concerns about the possibility of illness occurring in immunocompromised infants via spread of the vaccine related virus. Currently the AAP recommends the administration of rotavirus vaccine at the time of discharge or after discharge (American Academy of Pediatrics, 2009c).

Enterovirus

There are numerous serotypes of enteroviruses, including polioviruses, Coxsackie viruses A and B, echovirus, and nonassigned subtypes (Chambon et al, 1999). Enterovirus infections have been described among neonates in the well baby nursery and the neonatal intensive care setting (Chambon et al, 1999; Isaacs et al, 1989; Sizun et al, 2000; Takami et al, 2000, Wreghitt et al, 1989). Both individual cases and epidemics can occur. The seasonal distribution of enterovirus infections in neonates mirrors what is seen in the community.

The clinical presentation associated with enteroviral infection is variable. Many patients are asymptomatic; however, several case reports describe overwhelming infection with multisystem organ dysfunction and death (Jankovic et al, 1999; Keyserling, 1997). Clinical manifestations of severe disease include meningoencephalitis, hepatic dysfunction, disseminated intravascular coagulation, myocarditis, pneumonitis, gastroenteritis, and muscle weakness (Abzug et al, 1993; Isaacs et al, 1989; Keyserling, 1997; Wreghitt et al, 1989). The severity of disease and the likelihood of death are often more pronounced in perinatally acquired cases than in nosocomially acquired cases, presumably related to the lack of maternal antibody present in the neonate (Isaacs et al, 1989; Modlin et al, 1981).

Infection control measures during an enteroviral epidemic include hand washing with alcohol-based preparations or antimicrobial soaps and cohorting of infected patients. Surveillance cultures of specimens from the throat and rectum may be helpful in identifying asymptomatic colonized infants. Blood and cerebrospinal fluid cultures should be obtained from any patient with clinical symptoms of disease. Polymerase chain reaction analysis is helpful in making a rapid diagnosis (Nigrovic, 2001). No antiviral agents are currently available to treat enteroviral infections in newborns (Nigrovic, 2001). Although commercially available intravenous immunoglobulin preparations have high levels of neutralizing antibodies to common enterovirus serotypes, there is no clear evidence that administration of immunoglobulin alters the process or outcome of enteroviral infection (Abzug et al, 1993; Dagan et al, 1983; Keyserling, 1997); therefore the use of these products remains controversial in patients with enteroviral infection.

EPIDEMICS

Numerous nursery epidemics have been reported. Common sources for infection are contaminated equipment (i.e., breast pump, thermometer, ventilator), environmental reservoirs, soaps, and lapses in hand hygiene practices (Focca et al, 2000; Hervas et al, 2001; Hoque et al, 2001; Jeong et al, 2001; Jones et al, 2000; McNeil et al, 2001; Reiss et al, 2000; van den Berg et al, 2000; Wisplinghoff et al, 2000; Yu et al, 2000). Clinicians must have a high index of suspicion to detect nursery outbreaks, especially when clusters of infections with unusual pathogens occur in a nursery. Continuous surveillance and monitoring of the endemic infection rates are crucial for determining when there has been a significant change in the baseline pattern of infection for a given nursery. Modern molecular technology facilitates identification and tracking of specific strains of bacteria to help determine the common source of infection (Chambon et al, 1999; Jeong et al, 2001; Jones et al, 2000; Takami et al, 2000).

Epidemics must be identified promptly, and immediate control measures must be instituted. Efforts should be made to identify the causal agent and the mode of transmission. Surveillance of staff members may be necessary, even if they are asymptomatic. Reinforcement of hand-washing policies is of utmost importance. Cohorting infected patients may be helpful in limiting the spread of organisms in the nursery. In an effort to minimize the risk of cross-contamination between patients, staff members caring for colonized or infected infants should not care for infants who are not infected or colonized.

INFECTION CONTROL

The CDC has developed a two-tiered approach to infection control. Standard precautions should be used with all patient contact regardless of the underlying diagnosis or infectious status. These precautions consist of universal precautions (designed to prevent blood and body fluid contamination) and body substance precautions (designed to prevent contamination with moist substances). Transmission-based precautions are necessary when a patient is infected with a known or suspected pathogen that is associated with a high risk of contamination via airborne or droplet transmission or contact with the skin or contaminated surfaces (Garner, 1996).

The routine use of gowns is not an effective measure to decrease the endemic HAI rate in the nursery (Garner, 1996; Goldmann, 1989, 1991). Gowns should be used in specific circumstances in which the risk for contamination is high or the infant is being held. Gowns should be changed after each patient encounter.

Visitation policies are not restrictive in most modern nurseries. Various regulatory agencies have developed guidelines for sibling visitation (Box 40-4) (American Academy of Pediatrics, 1985). Infection and colonization rates have not risen with use of the current standards. Siblings should be screened for infection or recent exposures before visiting.

PREVENTION OF HEALTH CARE–ACQUIRED INFECTIONS

Several intensive care nurseries have described their success in decreasing the rate of central line–associated infections (Andersen et al, 2005; Bloom et al, 2003; Kilbride et al, 2003). Until recently it was considered implausible

---

BOX 40-4	**Guidelines for Sibling Visitation in the Nursery**

- Siblings should not have been exposed to known communicable diseases (e.g., varicella).
- Siblings should not have fever or symptoms of acute illness (i.e., upper respiratory infection or gastroenteritis).
- Children should be supervised by their parents or a responsible adult during the entire visit.
- Children should be prepared in advance for the visit.

Adapted from the American Academy of Pediatrics Committee on the Fetus and Newborn: Postpartum (neonatal) sibling visitation, *Pediatrics* 76:650, 1985.

---

by many that HAIs could be eliminated completely. But the challenge that faces neonatologists, nurses, respiratory therapists, physical therapists, clerks, environmental service staff, and anyone else who affects the care of the neonate now must be framed by the following question: can we get to zero? Much is known about the mechanisms of catheter-related infections and the factors that increase risk. Effective prevention strategies focus on modifying the known risks, such as standardization of procedures that relate to central line care, strategic nursery design, adequate staffing, hand-washing compliance, minimization of catheter days, and promotion of enteral nutrition, especially with human milk (Adams-Chapman and Stoll, 2002; Goldmann, 1989; Horbar et al, 2001). Care "bundles" incorporating a group of interventions aimed at standardizing central line care can be effective if a particular intensive care unit is committed to implementing them. One hundred percent compliance with adequate hand hygiene is required to eliminate the spread of viruses and bacteria, particularly those that are drug resistant. Monitoring, surveillance, and benchmarking of the HAI rates in the nursery are also critical components of any prevention program (Box 40-5). There is power in simply knowing how an individual unit compares to others, and there is empowerment in knowing that preventing HAIs is possible (Schulman et al, 2009).

HAND HYGIENE

Historic Perspective

Hand washing has clearly been shown to be the most effective and least expensive means of preventing the spread of HAI; however, compliance with this simple practice is poor (Jarvis, 1994; Larson, 1999; Pittet, 2000; Pittet et al, 2000). Historically, the benefits of hand washing have been known since the early nineteenth century. Labarraque, a French pharmacist, was one of the first to demonstrate that cleansing the hands with solutions containing lime or soda could be used as disinfectants and antiseptics (Boyce et al, 2002). The issue was further elucidated by Ignaz Semmelweis in the 1850s, who noted that the mortality and puerperal infection rates were higher among women receiving care from physicians than in those receiving care from midwives. He postulated that the puerperal fever in these patients was caused by "cadaverous particles" transmitted from the autopsy suite on the hands of the students and physicians. After

---

BOX 40-5   Principles for the Prevention of Health Care–Acquired Infections in the NICU

- Observe recommendations for standard precautions with all patient contact.
- Observe recommendations for transmission-based precautions as indicated.
  - Gowns
  - Gloves
  - Masks
  - Isolation
- Use good nursery design and engineering.
  - Appropriate nurse-to-patient ratio
  - Avoidance of overcrowding and excessive workload
  - Readily accessible sinks, antiseptic solutions, soaps, and paper towels
  - Maintain hand-washing practices.
  - Improving hand-washing compliance
  - Washing of hands before and after each patient encounter
  - Appropriate use of soap, alcohol-based preparations, or antiseptic solutions
  - Alcohol-based antiseptic solution at each patient's bedside
  - Emollients provided for nursery staff
  - Education and feedback for nursery staff
- Minimize risk of contamination of CVCs.
  - Maximal sterile barrier precautions during CVC insertion
  - Local antisepsis with chlorhexidine gluconate
  - Minimal entries into the line for laboratory tests
  - Aseptic technique when entering the line
  - Minimal CVC days
  - Sterile preparation of all fluids to be administered via a CVC
- Provide meticulous skin care.
- Encourage early and appropriate advancement of enteral feedings.
- Provide education and feedback for nursery personnel.
- Perform continuous monitoring and surveillance of HAI rates in the NICU.

CVC, Central venous catheter; *HAI,* health care–acquired infection; *NICU,* neonatal intensive care unit.

BOX 40-6   Recommendations for Hand Hygiene Practices in the NICU

INDICATIONS FOR HAND HYGIENE

- Wash hands with a nonantimicrobial soap or an antimicrobial soap and water when hands are visibly soiled or contaminated with proteinaceous material.
- If the hands are not visibly soiled, then alcohol-based, waterless antiseptic agents are strongly preferred for routine decontamination of hands in all other clinical situations.
- Alcohol-based, waterless antiseptic agents should be available at each patient area and other convenient locations, and in individual pocket-sized containers for health care providers.
- Antimicrobial soaps can be considered in settings with few time constraints and easy access to hand hygiene facilities.
- Decontaminate hands after contact with intact patient skin (i.e., checking pulse or lifting).
- Decontaminate hands after contact with body fluids or excretions, mucous membranes, nonintact skin, or wounds.
- Decontaminate hands before applying sterile gloves or inserting a central intravascular catheter.
- Decontaminate hands before inserting indwelling urinary catheters or other invasive devices not requiring surgical procedures.
- Decontaminate hands after removing gloves.
- Decontaminate hands before caring for patients with severe neutropenia or severe immunosuppression.
- Decontaminate hands after contact with inanimate objects in the immediate vicinity of the patient.

RECOMMENDED TECHNIQUES FOR HAND HYGIENE

- When using a waterless antiseptic agent, apply enough of the product to cover all surfaces of the hands and fingers, and rub hands together until they are dry. Each manufacturer has guidelines for the volume to be used; in general, enough should be applied so that it takes 15 to 25 seconds to dry.
- When using a nonantimicrobial or antimicrobial soap, wet hands, apply 3 to 5 mL of solution to the hands, and rub for at least 15 seconds. Be sure to cover all surfaces of the hands and fingers. Rinse hands with warm water, and dry thoroughly. Foot pedals, automatic faucets, or towel barriers should be used to turn off the water.

Adapted from Boyce JM, Pittet D, et al: Guidelines for hand hygiene in health-care settings: recommendations of the Healthcare Infection Control Practices Advisory Committee and the HICPAC/SHEA/APIC/IDSA Hand Hygiene Task Force, *Infect Control Hosp Epidemiol* 23(Suppl 12):S33-S40, 2002.
NICU, Neonatal intensive care unit.

---

he instructed physicians to cleanse their hands with a chlorine solution between patients, the maternal infection and mortality rates dropped dramatically (Boyce et al, 2002; Semmelweis, 1983). This intervention represents the first clinical evidence suggesting that cleansing contaminated hands with an antiseptic agent was more effective than washing them with plain soap and water and that hand antisepsis could reduce the spread of contagious disease via the hands of health care workers (Boyce et al, 2002).

Guidelines for Hand Hygiene Practices in the Neonatal Intensive Care Unit

Clinical Indications for Hand Hygiene

Hand hygiene techniques are effective in decreasing the colonization rate of resident and transient flora and have been shown to reduce cross-contamination among patients. Several studies have shown that the hands of health care workers become contaminated during routine patient care activities, including "clean" procedures such as lifting patients and checking vital signs, as well as during contact with intact skin (Casewell and Phillips, 1977; Pittet et al, 1999). Attempts have been made to stratify the type of activity with the likelihood of contamination, but they have not been validated by quantitative bacterial contamination analysis. Direct patient contact and respiratory tract care seem to be particularly associated with contamination (Pittet et al, 1999). Organisms such as RSV, *S. aureus,* and gram-negative bacilli are able to survive on inanimate objects, so changing diapers or holding an infant infected with one of these organisms, and even touching items in the infant's environment, may result in contamination (Boyce et al, 2002; Goldmann, 1989; Hall, 2000).

Recommendations concerning indications and techniques for hand hygiene are summarized in Box 40-6 (Boyce et al, 2002; Garner and Favero, 1986; Larson, 1995). Current recommendations strongly support the use of waterless alcohol-based preparations as the primary agents for hand hygiene, except when the hands are soiled with organic material (Boyce et al, 2002). The bottom line is that hands need to be cleaned before and after every patient contact. Until there is 100% compliance with this simple intervention, HAIs will continue to be a problem.

TABLE 40-3   Antimicrobial Spectrum and Characteristics of Hand Hygiene Antiseptic Agents

Group*	Gram-Positive Bacteria	Gram-Negative Bacteria	Mycobacteria	Fungi	Viruses	Speed of Action	Comments
Alcohols	+++	+++	+++	+++	+++	Fast	Optimum concentration 60%-90%, no persistent activity
Chlorhexidine (2% and 4% aqueous)	+++	+++	+	+	+++	Intermediate	Persistent activity, rare allergic reactions
Iodine compounds	+++	+++	+++	++	+++	Intermediate	Causes skin burns, usually too irritating for hand hygiene
Iodophors	+++	+++	+	++	++	Intermediate	Less irritating than iodine
Phenol derivatives	+++	+	+	+	+	Intermediate	Activity neutralized by nonionic surfactants
Triclosan	+++	++	+	−	+++	Intermediate	Acceptability varies
Quaternary ammonium compounds	+	++	−	−	+	Slow	Used only in combination with alcohols, ecologic concerns

Reprinted with permission from Boyce JM, Pittet D, et al: Guidelines for hand hygiene in health-care settings: recommendations of the Healthcare Infection Control Practices Advisory Committee and the HICPAC/SHEA/APIC/IDSA Hand Hygiene Task Force, *Infect Control Hosp Epidemiol* 23(Suppl 12):S33-S40, 2002.
+++, Excellent; ++, good, but does not include the entire bacterial spectrum; +, fair; −, no activity or not sufficient.
*Hexachlorophene is not included because it is no longer an accepted ingredient of hand disinfection.

Preparations for Hand Hygiene

Washing the hands with soap causes suspension and mechanical removal of microorganisms and dirt from the hands. *Hand disinfection* refers to the same process, but with the use of an antimicrobial product to kill or inhibit microorganisms. Table 40-3 compares properties of the various hand hygiene agents.

The cleansing activity of plain soap results from its detergent properties (Boyce et al, 2002). Hand washing with soap alone reduces bacterial colonization of the hands, but has no significant antimicrobial activity and is ineffective at removing pathogenic flora. Soaps containing antimicrobial agents are typically used in the NICU environment.

The antimicrobial activity of alcohol stems from its ability to denature proteins (Boyce et al, 2002). Because proteins are not readily denatured in the absence of water, solutions containing 50% to 80% alcohol are most effective (Boyce, 2000; Boyce et al, 2002). Alcohol has a rapid onset of action and reduces bacterial colonization, but has no residual activity. The efficacy of alcohol-based products is influenced by the type of alcohol used, concentration, contact time, volume used, and whether the hands are wet when the product is applied (Boyce et al, 2002; Mackintosh and Hoffman, 1984). When used in adequate amounts, alcohol is usually more effective than other hand hygiene products (Boyce, 2000; Boyce et al, 2002).

Chlorhexidine gluconate is a cationic bis-biguanide whose antimicrobial activity is caused by attachment and disruption of cytoplasmic membranes (Boyce et al, 2002). The onset of action is slower than the alcohol-based preparations; however, its major benefit is the persistent antimicrobial activity, which may last up to 6 hours after application (Boyce et al, 2002; Larson, 1995). Varying percentages of this product have been added to other hand hygiene preparations, especially the alcohol-based preparations, to confer greater residual activity.

Hexachlorophene is a bisphenol compound with bacteriostatic properties. Its activity is due to its ability to inactivate essential enzymes systems. It has good activity against *S. aureus*, but weak activity against gram-negative bacteria, fungi, and *Mycobacterium tuberculosis*. Hexachlorophene also has residual activity. Hexachlorophene was used for routine bathing of newborn infants until 1972, when the U.S. Food and Drug Administration (FDA) warned against its use because of an increased occurrence of cystic degeneration of the cerebral white matter in infants who had been bathed in the 3% solution (Shuman et al, 1975). This product should be considered only in term infants during a severe outbreak of *S. aureus*. Most experts recommend diluting the material 1:4 with water to decrease the risk of systemic absorption.

Iodine and iodophors penetrate the cell walls of organisms, impairing protein synthesis and altering the cellular membranes (Boyce et al, 2002). The amount of iodine present determines the level of antimicrobial activity. Combining iodine with polymers (i.e., povidone or poloxamer) increases the solubility, promotes sustained release of iodine, and decreases skin irritation. The activity of this product is affected by pH, exposure time, temperature, the presence of organic (blood or sputum) or inorganic material, and the concentration of iodine.

Compliance

Despite the fact that the benefits of hand washing have been reported since the nineteenth century, compliance with hand-washing protocols remains unacceptably low. The overall compliance rate is approximately 40% (Pittet, 2000). Reported barriers to compliance with hand hygiene recommendations include skin irritation, poor accessibility of sinks or cleansing agents, greater priority for patient needs, insufficient time, heavy workload and understaffing, and lack of information (Box 40-7). A common misconception is that using gloves obviates the need for adequate hand hygiene.

BOX 40-7 Factors Influencing Compliance With Hand Hygiene Practices

OBSERVED RISK FACTORS FOR POOR ADHERENCE TO RECOMMENDED PRACTICES

- Physician status (rather than a nurse)
- Nursing assistant status (rather than a nurse)
- Working in an intensive care unit
- Working during the week compared with the weekend
- Wearing gowns and gloves
- Automated sink faucet
- Activities with high risk of contamination
- High numbers of indications for hand hygiene per hour of patient care

SELF-REPORTED FACTORS FOR POOR ADHERENCE TO RECOMMENDED PRACTICES

- Agents are irritating or drying
- Inconvenient location of sinks and supplies
- Inadequate supplies (e.g., soap, paper)
- Too busy
- Patient needs take priority
- Perceived low risk of acquiring infection
- Gloves obviate the need for hand hygiene
- Lack of knowledge of guidelines and recommendations
- Disagreement with recommendations

Data from Pittet D: Improving compliance with hand hygiene in hospitals, *Infect Control Hosp Epidemiol* 21:381-386, 2000; and Boyce JM: Using alcohol for hand antiseptics: dispelling old myths, *Infect Control Hosp Epidemiol* 21:438-441, 2000.

Leakage and contamination of gloves have been reported (Boyce et al, 2002; Larson, 1995). Disposable single-use gloves should be removed after each patient encounter, and hands should be washed before and after their use.

Hand hygiene is extremely cost effective. The additional hospital charges associated with a single HAI almost equal the yearly hand hygiene budget. Pittet et al (2000) estimated the cost of a hand hygiene intervention program to be less than $57,000 per year. Assuming that only 25% of the observed decrease in infections was attributable to improved hand hygiene practices, they estimated a savings of $2,100 for every infection averted.

PREVENTION OF CENTRAL LINE–ASSOCIATED BLOODSTREAM INFECTIONS

The care and maintenance of central venous catheters may affect the risk of catheter-related bloodstream infection. Before insertion of an intravascular device, attempted sterilization of the skin insertion site is of utmost importance. The recommended technique for skin antisepsis is to use two consecutive 10-second applications or a single 30-second application of the selected antibacterial agent. Sterile water rather than alcohol should be used to remove antiseptics from the skin. Povidone-iodine (10%) solution is commonly used for skin antisepsis; however, data suggest that chlorhexidine gluconate is more effective at decreasing skin colonization and subsequent CLABSIs in adults, as well as colonization of peripheral intravenous catheters in neonates (Darmstadt and Dinulos, 2000; Garland et al, 1995).

Hub colonization and repeated entry into the line for administration of medications or collection of specimens for laboratory studies are both associated with an increased risk for infection. Salzman et al (1993) conducted a prospective study in which surveillance cultures of catheter hubs were performed three times per week, and blood cultures and hub cultures were conducted for any suspected episode of sepsis. These investigators found that 54% of 28 episodes of CLABSI were preceded by or coincided with colonization of the catheter hub with the same pathogen. This mechanism has been confirmed in the neonatal population by Garland et al (2008). Mahieu et al (2001b) reported that catheter manipulation for blood sampling and fluid or tubing changes raised the risk of colonization. Despite the lack of large randomized controlled trials, the available data suggest that the use of heparin in intravenous fluids is associated with a lower risk of bacterial colonization and thrombosis (Appelgren et al, 1996; Mahieu et al, 2001b). It is hypothesized that heparin prevents bacteria from adhering to the catheter and that the preservatives in heparin preparations have some limited antibacterial properties.

Various products have been designed to decrease the risk of catheter-related infection in adult patients. Although data on their use are promising, many of the currently available products are not specifically designed for the neonate, and their safety and efficacy have not been tested in this patient population. Antiseptic- or antibiotic-impregnated catheters have been shown to significantly decrease the risk of CLABSI in adults (Elliott, 2000; Marin et al, 2000; Pai et al, 2000; Tennenberg et al, 1997; Veenstra et al, 1999). Pierce et al (2000) reported that pediatric patients randomly assigned to the use of a heparin-bonded device had a lower incidence of CLABSI than controls (4% versus 33%; $p < 0.005$). Studies are in progress to evaluate the efficacy of antibiotic lock therapy in neonates. Johnson et al (1994) treated a small group of pediatric patients with CLABSIs with antibiotic lock therapy for 10 days. They reported that 10 of 12 catheters were salvaged. There are limited data describing the use of antibiotic lock therapy in neonates. Garland et al (2002) randomly assigned 82 VLBW infants to saline control or vancomycin antibiotic lock therapy of catheters in an effort to prevent CLABSI. These researchers found a significantly lower incidence density of catheter-related infections, no evidence of toxicity, and no cases of VRE in the neonates receiving antibiotic lock therapy.

UMBILICAL CORD CARE

Umbilical cord infections remain a significant cause of neonatal mortality in developing nations, although not in the United States (Zupan and Garner, 2000). In clinical practice, there are numerous approaches to umbilical cord care in the healthy term infant because the available data are insufficient to recommend the use of a specific agent or regimen (Zupan and Garner, 2000). Most authorities agree that the umbilical cord should be separated from the placenta with the use of good aseptic technique. Subsequently, some experts recommend "natural drying," but others support the use of an antiseptic agent such as alcohol, silver sulfadiazine, chlorhexidine, triple dye, or gentian violet (Darmstadt and Dinulos, 2000; Hsu et al, 1999; Pezzati et al, 2002; Zupan and Garner, 2000). Hexachlorophene and iodine are used sparingly because of concerns about their systemic absorption and toxicity. Studies have shown that antiseptic products decrease umbilical cord colonization. Unfortunately, this decrease has not clearly resulted in a lower incidence of umbilical cord infections. In a meta-analysis that included "no intervention" as an alternative, Zupan and Garner (2000) were unable to determine which regimen was superior. In general, they found that time to cord separation was prolonged when antiseptics were used, but there were no significant differences in the incidence of infection or death with the use of a particular agent for cord care.

SKIN CARE

The skin of VLBW preterm infants is immature and functions as an ineffective barrier to prevent transepidermal loss of water and invasion of bacteria. The stratum corneum (the outermost layer of skin) has both mechanical and chemical properties that decrease the risk of infection (Darmstadt and Dinulos, 2000). This layer of skin matures at approximately 32 weeks' gestation. In a prematurely born neonate, the maturation process is accelerated and is usually complete by 2 to 4 weeks after birth (Darmstadt and Dinulos, 2000).

Unfortunately, there is no consensus on the most effective skin care practices for VLBW infants (Baker et al, 1999; Munson et al, 1999). Neonatologists had hoped that the application of a topical emollient would protect the developing epidermal layer, reduce the risk of infection, and prevent transepidermal water loss. Several studies have documented that such a practice decreases water loss; however, there was no significant reduction in HAI in VLBW infants randomly assigned to receive routine application of one emollient product (Aquaphor) in a study performed by Edwards et al (2001). Infants randomly assigned to emollient therapy had more nosocomial bloodstream infections, particularly with CONS. This difference was most evident in infants with birthweights of 501 to 750 g.

The efficacy of other topical agents warrants further study. Efforts to prevent traumatic injury to the skin of VLBW infants include the use of transparent dressing over bony prominences, semipermeable barriers between the skin and adhesive tape, and water-activated electrodes and the avoidance of agents such as tincture of benzoin, Mastisol, and adhesive removers (Adams-Chapman and Stoll, 2002; Darmstadt and Dinulos, 2000; Hoath and Narendran, 2000).

MANAGEMENT OF HEALTH CARE–ACQUIRED INFECTIONS

CATHETER-RELATED BLOODSTREAM INFECTIONS

Management of neonates with CLABSIs is problematic because of the limited intravenous access in most patients, as well as the lack of consensus among clinicians. Current recommendations for adults regarding catheter removal

with associated CLABSI suggest the removal of nontunneled central venous catheters associated with bacteremia or fungemia, unless the pathogen is CONS (Mermel et al, 2001). A patient with a catheter-related infection caused by CONS should undergo catheter removal if culture results are persistently positive or if the patient's condition is unstable (Benjamin et al, 2001; Karlowicz et al, 2000).

Benjamin et al (2001) retrospectively reviewed data on infants with CLABSIs and compared outcomes in patients in whom catheters were removed at the onset of infection with those in whom catheters remained in place. Forty-six percent (59 of 128) of infants in whom catheter sterilization was attempted had complications, compared with 8% (2 of 25) of those in whom catheters were removed. In particular, infants with gram-negative infections were more likely to have complications if their catheters remained in place. A study of infants with CLABSIs caused by CONS found no difference in the complication or mortality rate in patients in whom removal of the catheter was delayed (Karlowicz et al, 2000). However, patients with a CONS infection related to their central line were more likely to have persistently positive culture results when their lines were not removed with the first positive culture (43% versus 13% for immediate catheter removal). The attempt to retain the catheter was never successful if culture results remained positive for more than 4 days. Additional prospective randomized trials are needed to validate these observational data.

ANTIBIOTIC AND ADJUNCTIVE THERAPIES

Antibiotic therapy that is effective against a culture-proven or suspected pathogen is the primary treatment for HAIs. As a general rule, antibiotic choice should initially cover a broad spectrum of pathogens and should then be narrowed as soon as possible to cover the specific bacteria identified once sensitivities are known, or it should be discontinued if infection is not proved and is not likely. One should consider coverage for *Pseudomonas* spp. or other resistant gram-negative organisms in patients with a rapid clinical deterioration (Karlowicz et al, 2000; Stoll et al, 2002a). However, empiric broad-spectrum antibiotic use should be limited as much as possible to avoid complications of resistant bacterial and fungal infections.

A metaanalysis of the prophylactic use of intravenous immunoglobulin (IVIG) in preterm neonates found only a 3% reduction in HAI and no reduction in mortality (Modi and Carr, 2000; Ohlsson and Lacy, 2001a). The benefit in patients with culture-proven sepsis remains unclear, and IVIG is therefore not recommended for routine use in such patients (Modi and Carr, 2000). Some authorities speculate that the benefit of IVIG would be greater if products containing high concentrations of specific antibodies against pathogens frequently responsible for neonatal infections were developed (Hill, 2000; Ohlsson and Lacy, 2001b; Weisman et al, 1994). Hemopoietic colony-stimulating factors (granulocyte and granulocyte-macrophage) are effective in raising the neutrophil count, but have not consistently decreased HAI rates or mortality

(Carr et al, 2003; Modi and Carr, 2000). Studies are being conducted in adults to evaluate the efficacy of administering various cytokine preparations known to modulate the inflammatory response.

CONCLUSION

Interventions to reduce HAI are urgently needed. Infants with HAIs have significantly longer hospital stays (79 versus 60 days; $p < 0.001$) and higher hospital costs (Gray et al, 1995; Mahieu et al, 2001a; Pittet et al, 1994; Stoll et al, 2002a). The higher costs are primarily caused by daily hospital charges and pharmaceutical fees (Mahieu et al, 2001a). The attributable cost of a nosocomial infection has been estimated to be approximately $40,000 per adult case and $1200 per neonatal case (Mahieu et al, 2001a; Pittet et al, 1994). The magnitude of these costs is significant, especially when considering the growing number of surviving VLBW infants, who are at the highest risk for acquiring an HAI. Moreover, infants who experience an HAI are significantly more likely to die than are those who remain uninfected (Stoll et al, 1996, 2002a).

A variety of new therapeutic alternatives is currently being investigated. Clinicians must continue to focus on developing effective prevention strategies, including strict hand-washing policies, minimal use of invasive devices, promotion of enteral nutrition surveillance of infection patterns, and education for the nursery staff members. Quality improvement approaches can be effective in implementing the necessary practices within a given unit.

SUGGESTED READINGS

Bloom BT, Craddock A, Delmore PM, et al: Reducing acquired infections in the NICU: observing and implementing meaningful differences in process between high and low acquired infection rate centers, *J Perinatol* 23:489-492, 2003.

Clerihew L, Austin N, McGuire: Prophylactic systemic antifungal agents to prevent mortality and morbidity in very low birth weight infants, *Cochrane Database Syst Rev* 4:CD003850, 2007.

Curtis C, Shetty N: Recent trends and prevention of infection in the neonatal intensive care unit, *Curr Opin Infect Dis* 21:350-356, 2008.

Kilbride HW, Wirtschafter DD, Powers RJ, et al: Implementation of evidence-based potentially better practices to decrease nosocomial infections, *Pediatrics* 111(4 Pt 2):e519-e533, 2003.

Meissner HC, Long SS: American Academy of Pediatrics Committee on Infectious Diseases and Committee on Fetus and Newborn: revised indications for the use of palivizumab and respiratory syncytial virus immune globulin intravenous for the prevention of respiratory syncytial virus infections, *Pediatrics* 112:1447-1452, 2003.

Perlman SE, Saiman L, Larson EL: Risk factors for late-onset health care-associated bloodstream infections in patients in neonatal intensive care units, *Am J Infect Control* 35:177-182, 2007.

Parellada JA, Moise AA, Hegemier S, et al: Percutaneous central catheters and peripheral intravenous catheters have similar infection rates in very low birth weight infants, *J Perinatol* 19:251-254, 1999.

Schulman J, Wirtschafter DD, Kurtin P: Neonatal intensive care unit collaboration to decrease hospital acquired bloodstream infections: from comparative performance reports to improvement networks, *Pediatr Clin N Am* 56:865-892, 2009.

Stoll BJ, Adams-Chapman I, et al: Abnormal neurodevelopmental outcome of ELBW infants with infection, *Pediatr Res Suppl* 53:2212, 2003.

Stoll BJ, Hansen NI, Adams-Chapman I, et al: National Institute of Child Health and Human Development Neonatal Research Network: neurodevelopmental and growth impairment among extremely low-birth-weight infants with neonatal infection, *J Am Med Assoc* 292:2357-2365, 2004.

Complete references used in this text can be found online at www.expertconsult.com

FUNGAL INFECTIONS IN THE NEONATAL INTENSIVE CARE UNIT

Margaret K. Hostetter

EPIDEMIOLOGY

Invasive fungal infection occurs in approximately 1% to 2% of all infants admitted to U.S. neonatal intensive care units (NICUs) (Stoll et al, 1996), and the incidence rises dramatically with decreasing gestational age. Among the fungi, *Candida* spp. is the dominant pathogen, with infections evenly distributed among *C. albicans* and non–*C. albicans* species (*C. parapsilosis, C. orthopsilosis, C. metapsilosis, C. glabrata, C. guilliermondii, C. krusei,* and *C. lusitaniae*). *Candida* spp. are the third most common cause of late-onset sepsis in the NICU, with a fatality rate more than sevenfold greater than that of *Staphylococcus epidermidis*, the most common pathogen (Benjamin et al, 2000; Saiman et al, 2001). Other fungi encountered include *Aspergillus fumigatus, A. flavus, Malassezia furfur, M. pachydermatis.* The yeast *Cryptococcus neoformans* and the fungi *Histoplasma capsulatum, Blastomyces dermatitidis,* and *Coccidioides immitis* are rarely if ever seen in the NICU.

The most important risk factor for fungal infection is gestational age. In a survey of 2847 infants from six different nurseries, the incidence of candidemia in infants weighing less than 800 g (7.55%) was 25-fold that of the infant weighing more than 1500 g (Figure 41-1) (Saiman et al, 2000). This latter group acquires blood-borne candidal infection in association with congenital anomalies, especially those of the gastrointestinal tract (Rabalais et al, 1996). Candidemia carries a mortality rate exceeding 25% in most studies (Chapman and Faix 2000; Weese-Mayer et al, 1987).

Colonization with ubiquitous fungal species occurs in at least 25% of very low-birthweight infants (Baley et al, 1986), and both the amount of *Candida* spp. in the gastrointestinal tract (Pappu-Katikaneni et al, 1990) and colonization at sites such as endotracheal tubes (Rowen et al, 1994) have been correlated with increased risk of invasive disease caused by *Candida* spp. Prospective studies correlating colonization by other fungal genera (e.g., *Aspergillus, Malassezia* spp.) with risk of invasive disease have not been done.

Apart from colonization and gestational age, other host factors that contribute to the susceptibility of the infant in the NICU to fungal infection include 5-minute Apgar scores less than 5, and an age-dependent immunocompromised state ascribable to reduced numbers of T cells, impaired phagocyte number and function, and reduced levels of complement (Marodi et al, 1994; Rebuck et al, 1995; Witek-Janusek et al, 2002; Zach and Hostetter, 1989). Concomitants of nursery care that are thought to increase the risk of fungal infections include length of stay greater than 1 week, indwelling central venous catheters, abdominal surgery, parenteral nutrition, intralipids, H_2 (histamine) receptor antagonists, endotracheal intubation, and prolonged use of broad-spectrum antimicrobials, especially third-generation cephalosporins (Cotten et al, 2006; Saiman et al, 2001; Saiman et al, 2000). Other centers have identified associations with systemic steroids and catecholamine infusions in retrospective studies and with topical petrolatum in a prospective case-control study (Benjamin et al, 2000; Botas et al, 1995; Campbell et al, 2000).

Interestingly, a number of variables appear not to associate with candidal colonization, including the use of antibiotics in the mother, premature rupture of the membranes, the infant's gender, the use of antimicrobial agents other than third-generation cephalosporins in the infant, surgical procedures, or frequency of intubation (Saiman et al, 2001). Although ≈5% of NICU staff members carry *C. albicans* on the hands and 19% carry *C. parapsilosis*, there is no correlation with site-specific rates of infant colonization (Saiman et al, 2001).

This chapter will place major emphasis on infections caused by *Candida* spp. and other fungi, as well as the approach to diagnosis, treatment, and management of infants with fungal infection.

INFECTIONS CAUSED BY *CANDIDA* SPECIES

CONGENITAL CANDIDIASIS

Appearing within the first 24 hours of life in both full-term and premature infants, congenital candidiasis, a very rare entity, manifests as a deeply erythematous skin rash in the setting of pronounced neutrophilia, with white blood cell counts often rising to 50,000 or more, and infrequently *Candida* spp. funisitis (see Local Infections, later). In the full-term infant, there are no invasive consequences, and desquamation typically ensues within 2 to 3 days. In contrast, the condition is life threatening in the premature infant (Dvorak and Gavaller, 1966; Johnson et al, 1981) and is distinguished by a pustular rash, hazy infiltrates reminiscent of respiratory distress syndrome on chest radiograph, and frequently positive blood cultures. The premature infant is thought to acquire the organism from inhaling infected amniotic fluid.

Diagnosis in both premature and full-term infants requires the visualization of the organism on Gram stain from a bullous lesion or an opened pustule. On rare occasions, the placenta has yielded the diagnosis. Treatment for the full-term infant requires only the full-body application of topical antifungal creams containing either nystatin or azoles, such as miconazole or clotrimazole. In the premature infant, initiating parenteral amphotericin B deoxycholate at a dose of 1 to 1.5 mg/kg is mandatory, but respiratory involvement typically heralds death despite anti-fungal therapy.

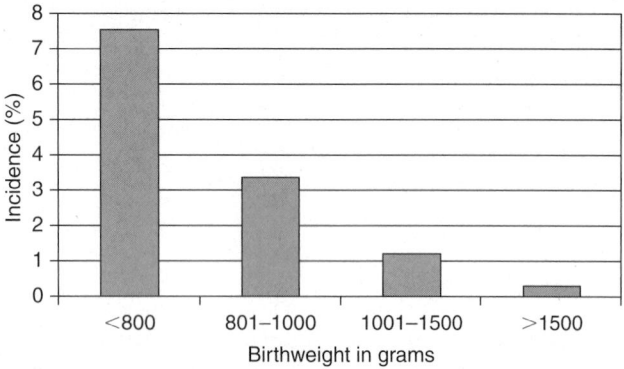

FIGURE 41-1 Incidence of candidemia related to birthweight in grams. *(Data from Saiman L et al: Risk factors for candidemia in Neonatal Intensive Care Unit patients. The National Epidemiology of Mycosis Survey study group,* Pediatr Infect Dis J *19:319-324, 2000.)*

LOCAL INFECTIONS WITH *CANDIDA* SPECIES

Diaper Dermatitis

Diaper dermatitis manifests as an erythematous, erosive dermatitis of the perineal region, typically with pustular satellite lesions beyond the borders of the rash. Predisposing factors include systemic antibiotics, glucosuria, and wet diapers. Care must be taken to differentiate this tractable condition from invasive fungal dermatitis (see Invasive Fungal Dermatitis, later). The infection responds well to topical antifungal ointments.

Funisitis

Infection of the umbilical cord with *Candida* spp., although rare, is an indicator of chorioamniotitis and carries a poor prognosis, especially in the premature infant (Qureshi et al, 1998). A minority (16%) of infants in one study had associated congenital candidiasis. Intrauterine contraceptive devices or cervical cerclage were reported in 16% of the mothers.

Urinary Tract Infection

Isolation of *Candida* spp. from a catheterized specimen or suprapubic aspiration, as opposed to a bagged sample, is a reliable indicator of infection, although asymptomatic colonization of urinary catheters, stents, or nephrostomy tubes can be difficult to distinguish from true infection (Lundstrom and Sobel, 2001).

The presence of candiduria in infants in the NICU is associated with renal candidiasis—the latter manifested by cortical abscesses or fungal mycelia in the collecting system ("fungus balls")—almost half the time and may be a cause of frank obstruction (Bryant et al, 1999). Therefore, in contrast to older children or adults, the finding of candiduria in an infant in the NICU should at least prompt blood cultures and renal imaging. If blood cultures prove to be positive, a full evaluation for disseminated candidiasis should be undertaken (see Systemic Infection, later).

Because of the high prevalence of associated upper tract disease, imaging of the kidneys by ultrasonography should occur after isolation of the organism from a sterile urine specimen. Approximately one half of the patients who eventually develop upper tract manifestations will display them on the first ultrasound (Bryant et al, 1999). Therefore follow-up imaging is recommended both to ensure the clearance of fungal mycelia, if present, and to monitor for later development of this complication. Unfortunately, no standard interval for monitoring has been proposed; however, in the infant with persistent funguria or candiduria, a single negative ultrasound should not be considered definitive.

Removal of a colonized urinary catheter may suffice for treatment in a patient without pyuria or systemic symptoms. Disease confined to the lower tract is best addressed with azoles (e.g., fluconazole, 4 to 6 mg/kg/day). Upper tract disease requires parenteral amphotericin B in systemic doses (1 to 1.5 mg/kg/day). Liposomal amphotericin B may not be an acceptable alternative. The particles in at least one liposomal preparation (Abelcet) appear to be too large to penetrate the adult kidney (Hell et al, 1999), and this author has seen a premature newborn whose persistent candiduria failed to resolve until treatment was changed to amphotericin B deoxycholate.

PERITONITIS

Candida spp. peritonitis typically develops as a consequence of bowel perforation or rarely as a complication of peritoneal dialysis. In the former situation, multiple organisms such as gram-negative rods and enterococci may also be involved, and the neonate is at risk for sepsis with any one of them (Johnson et al, 1980). Peritonitis associated with a peritoneal dialysis catheter usually occurs as an isolated process, and the outcome is much better.

Spontaneous intestinal perforation associated with *Candida* spp. peritonitis with or without sepsis has been described within 7 to 10 days of birth in infants weighing less than 1000 g, typically in the absence of necrotizing enterocolitis (Adderson et al, 1998; Holland et al, 2003; Meyer et al, 1991; Mintz and Applebaum, 1993). Hallmark clinical findings include bluish discoloration of the abdomen and a gasless pattern on abdominal film. A substantial proportion of these infants will have systemic candidiasis, although *Staphylococcus epidermidis* can also be seen. In a small study of seven patients (Holland et al, 2003), deficiency of the muscularis propria was found in six.

Diagnosis requires visualization of the organism on a Gram stain of peritoneal fluid sterilely obtained or culture of the organism from the same source. Isolation of *Candida* spp. from the peritoneal fluid should always prompt a search for bowel perforation, by either radiology or surgical exploration, depending upon the clinical circumstances.

Treatment of *Candida* spp. peritonitis caused by necrotizing enterocolitis or bowel perforation requires surgical evaluation, supportive therapy, and direct address of all contaminating microorganisms in the peritoneal fluid and the bloodstream. The typical regimen may include ampicillin and an aminoglycoside for enterococci and gram-negative rods, clindamycin for anaerobes, and systemic antifungal therapy, most likely with amphotericin B. The isolation of *Candida* spp. from peritoneal dialysate can be treated with removal of the catheter and a short course (7 to 10 days) of amphotericin B therapy in a dose of

0.3 to 0.5 mg/kg/day. The catheter can typically be reinserted within 24 to 48 hours, once the Gram stain is free of yeast cells.

SYSTEMIC INFECTION

CANDIDEMIA ASSOCIATED WITH CENTRAL VENOUS CATHETERS

The association between prematurity and blood-borne candidal infections has been recognized for 25 years (Baley et al, 1984; Johnson et al, 1984). Over this same period of time, the incidence of candidemia has escalated from 25 to 123 cases per 10,000 NICU admissions (Kossoff et al, 1998; Saiman et al, 2000). The median time of onset is approximately 30 days of age (Baley et al, 1984). In a large multicenter study, colonization of the gastrointestinal tract preceded candidemia in 43% of cases (Saiman et al, 2000).

A variety of nonspecific clinical findings may be associated with this presentation of candidal disease, including respiratory decompensation, feeding intolerance, temperature instability, or mild thrombocytopenia. It is unclear whether the latter manifestation relates more to the use of heparin in vascular catheters or to the presence of *Candida* spp. in the blood stream.

Isolation of *Candida* spp. from a blood culture should never be regarded as a contaminant and should prompt an immediate search for evidence of dissemination, which occurs in approximately 10% of premature newborns with candidemia (Noyola et al, 2001; Patriquin et al, 1980). A thorough evaluation includes ophthalmologic examination and ultrasonography of the heart, venous system, and abdomen. When lumbar puncture is performed, 10% to 50% of infants with candidemia may have associated meningitis (Benjamin et al, 2006; Faix, 1984); in one prospective study, almost 50% of extremely low-birthweight (ELBW) infants with *Candida* spp. meningitis (13/27) had negative blood cultures (Benjamin et al, 2006).

Numerous studies have shown that central venous catheters should be removed within 24 hours after identification of yeasts in the blood culture (Karlowicz et al, 2000); in particular, removal of the central venous catheter within 3 days is associated with a significantly shorter median duration of candidemia (3 versus 6 days) and a reduced mortality rate (0% versus 39%). In at least one study of candidemia, delayed removal of central venous catheters was associated with neurodevelopmental impairment at 18 to 22 months (Benjamin et al, 2006). Many experts recommend routine echocardiograms for patients with catheter-associated candidemia to look for thrombi before removal of the catheter. However, even with the prompt removal of the catheter and the institution of appropriate antifungal therapy, a substantial proportion of infants may exhibit prolonged candidemia lasting 1 to 3 weeks (Chapman and Faix, 2000).

DISSEMINATED CANDIDIASIS

Mortality rates approach 30% for this dreaded complication of candidal infection. *C. albicans* is the leading pathogen. Organ involvement is most common in the vascular tree at catheter sites (15.2%), followed by the

kidneys (7.7%) (Noyola et al, 2001; Patriquin et al, 1980). Eye involvement occurs in approximately 6% of infants. Thrombi within the vascular bed may be particularly difficult to eradicate with antifungal therapy; infants with right atrial thrombi may benefit from atriotomy (Foker et al, 1984). Other sites less frequently involved include the liver, spleen, and skeletal system. In infection of the bones and joints in premature newborns, *Candida* spp. are typically the second most likely pathogen, preceded by *Staphylococcus aureus* (Ho et al, 1989).

ANTI-FUNGAL THERAPY FOR SYSTEMIC INFECTION

As is true of most medications used in the neonatal ICU, dosing recommendations for antifungal therapies have not undergone rigorous testing in this patient population. With that caveat in mind, it is important to discuss practice guidelines for this difficult clinical problem. Amphotericin B is the standard antifungal therapy for treatment of systemic neonatal fungal infection. The drug binds to ergosterol in the membrane of fungi, facilitating membrane leakage. Rapid institution of parenteral amphotericin B deoxycholate in doses of 1.0 to 1.5 mg/kg/day, given by intravenous infusion over 2 to 6 hours, is the therapy of choice for systemic infection, including catheter-associated candidemia and disseminated candidiasis. No more than 24 hours should elapse before the infant is receiving a dose of 0.7 to 1.0 mg/kg/day. Some experts recommend instituting empiric antifungal therapy in acutely thrombocytopenic ELBW infants (Benjamin et al, 2003). Dose adjustment for renal dysfunction is necessary only if serum creatinine increases significantly during therapy. Amphotericin B has poor cerebrospinal fluid penetration; therefore accompanying meningitis should prompt the addition of 5-flucytosine in doses of approximately 12.5 to 37.5 mg/kg per dose given by mouth every 6 hours (in patients with normal renal function). Peak serum concentrations of this drug should be kept between 40 and 60 µg/mL to avoid bone marrow suppression or hepatotoxicity. Fluconazole may also be added to amphotericin B for meningeal penetration, if 5-flucytosine is unavailable or cannot be used.

Infants being treated with amphotericin B who experience a twofold rise in creatinine, which is evidence of renal tubular compromise or renal tubular acidosis, may benefit from use treatment with one of the liposomal amphotericin preparations. AmBisome has been used in neonates at well-tolerated doses of 5 to 7 mg/kg per dose every 24 hours intravenously, infused over 2 hours (Juster-Reicher et al, 2003; Weitkamp et al, 1998), although the failure of many liposomal preparations to penetrate renal parenchyma can militate against fungal clearance from this organ.

With prompt removal of an offending central venous catheter, and no evidence of dissemination, the duration of therapy for catheter-associated candidemia is typically 10 to 14 days after the blood culture becomes negative (Donowitz and Hendley, 1995). Disseminated candidiasis, including *Candida* spp. meningitis, requires at least 3 weeks or more of parenteral therapy; the course is typically completed when all foci have been eradicated. Most infectious disease experts will use fungicidal doses of parenteral amphotericin B or a liposomal preparation for the entire course. Azoles (such as fluconazole at 6 mg/kg intravenously at varying dosing intervals) are antifungal agents that interfere with ergosterol synthesis by inhibiting C-14 alpha demethylase, a cytochrome P450 enzyme. Use of an azole to complete the latter part of an antifungal course must account for the inability of the infant's immune system to compensate for the fungistatic activity of the azoles. Azoles such as itraconazole and posaconazole are preferable to fluconazole for aspergillus and zygomycetes, but no studies have been done to recommend neonatal dosing guidelines.

Although not a first-line antifungal medication, echinocandins such as caspofungin, which interrupt biosynthesis of β-(1,3)-D-glucan, an integral part of the fungal cell wall, have also been used in doses of 1 to 2 mg/kg/day to treat invasive candidal disease in the newborn in several case reports; this drug is particularly helpful for species such as *Candida glabrata*, *Candida krusei* or *Candida lusitaniae*, which may have decreased susceptibility or de novo resistance to amphotericin B (Odio et al, 2004; Saez-Llorens et al, 2009).

ANTI-FUNGAL PROPHYLAXIS

Five randomized, controlled trials comparing intravenous fluconazole (3 mg/kg/day) with placebo or no treatment in very low-birthweight (VLBW) or ELBW infants for 4 to 6 weeks (Cabrera et al, 2002; Kaufman et al, 2001; Kicklighter et al, 2001; Manzoni et al, 2007; Parikh et al, 2007) met criteria for analysis in Cochrane reviews (Clerihew et al, 2007). Kaufman and Manzoni reported significantly lower incidence of invasive fungal infection, whereas there was no difference in treated versus untreated infants in other studies (Cabrera et al, 2002; Kicklighter et al, 2001; Parikh et al, 2007). The only study to evaluate neurologic outcomes found no difference in neurologic impairment at 16 months (Kaufman et al, 2001). Fluconazole prophylaxis did not create a significant difference in the risk of death before discharge in any of the five studies or in a metaanalysis (Clerihew et al, 2007). No study documented clinically significant adverse effects of fluconazole or the emergence of fluconazole resistance.

One study from a single center compared nonrandomized fluconazole prophylaxis in 2002 to 2006 with an untreated, retrospective cohort (2000 to 2001) and reported that invasive candidiasis decreased from 0.6% to 0.3%, although the proportion of invasive disease caused by non–*C. albicans* species increased from 26% to 41% after the introduction of fluconazole prophylaxis (Healy et al, 2008). Interestingly, fluconazole prophylaxis in this study was extended to several infants with birthweights greater than 1000 g, if risk factors (e.g., maternal HIV infection, intestinal abnormalities) were present.

The finding that prophylactic fluconazole reduces the incidence of invasive fungal infection must be interpreted with caution (Clerihew et al, 2007, 2008):

1. The incidence of invasive fungal infection in the placebo groups (Kaufman et al, 2001; Manzoni et al, 2007; Parikh et al, 2007) was significantly higher (13% to 16%) than in other large cohort studies of

VLBW or ELBW infants in the United States (6% to 7%) or the United Kingdom (1% to 2%).
2. Fluconazole prophylaxis may have impaired the microbiologic isolation of some fungal species and led to underdiagnosis of infection in the treatment group.
3. Six years after the introduction of fluconazole prophylaxis, one study reported that non–*C. albicans* species with relatively reduced susceptibility to the azoles were the most common causes of invasive fungal infection (Parikh et al, 2007). This study did not detect a significant effect of fluconazole prophylaxis in reducing invasive candidal disease.

Based on these results and cautionary notes, infants weighing less than 1000 g who receive third-generation cephalosporins and central venous catheters may be the best group to be evaluated for a statistically significant benefit of fluconazole prophylaxis in preventing invasive fungal infection, neurologic complications, and death before hospital discharge. Study durations less than 6 years may be insufficient to detect the emergence of fluconazole resistance.

INFECTIONS ASCRIBABLE TO OTHER FUNGI

INVASIVE FUNGAL DERMATITIS

Invasive fungal dermatitis typically manifests in the infant weighing less than 1000 g who displays macerated or bruised lesions that are contaminated with fungal species. In the initial report, three of seven confirmed cases had *C. albicans*, *C. parapsilosis*, *C. tropicalis*, *Trichosporon beigelii*, *Curvularia* spp., or *Aspergillus niger* and *A. fumigatus* were cultured from the remainder (Rowen et al, 1995). Among cases considered "probable," seven of eight had *C. albicans*. Systemic complications including fungemia, meningitis, or infection of the urinary tract occurred in four of seven confirmed cases and seven of eight probable cases. More cases than controls had postnatal steroids and prolonged hyperglycemia. Disseminated infection occurred in 69%, all ascribable to *Candida* spp.

Diagnosis requires a skin biopsy specimen demonstrating fungal invasion beyond the stratum corneum or a positive potassium hydroxide preparation of skin scrapings; growth of the identical organism from an otherwise sterile site (blood, cerebrospinal fluid, or urine obtained via supra pubic aspiration) is confirmatory. Treatment requires systemic doses of amphotericin B in the range of 0.7 to 1.0 mg/kg/day; in infants who do not develop systemic infection, oral therapy with fluconazole or topical antifungal creams may suffice. Oral therapy is not advisable for pathogens like *Aspergillus* spp., and repeated skin biopsies may be necessary to define duration of therapy.

LINE INFECTIONS CAUSED BY LIPOPHILIC ORGANISMS

The species *Malassezia furfur* and *Malassezia pachydermatis* are lipophilic organisms commonly carried on the skin, even in patients without tinea versicolor (Marcon and

Powell, 1992). Cutaneous colonization can infect hyperalimentation fluids or parenteral lipid formulations. Infants typically exhibit mild but nonspecific signs: respiratory decompensation, glucose intolerance, or thrombocytopenia (Dankner et al, 1987; Stuart and Lane, 1992). Diagnosis requires isolation of the organism from blood by growth on fungal medium overlaid with olive oil, because *Malassezia* spp. will not grow in the absence of lipids (Marcon et al, 1986). Removal of the intravascular catheter usually suffices for therapy, although some experts recommend the addition of amphotericin B in dosages of 0.5 mg/kg/day for 7 days.

MISCELLANEOUS FUNGAL INFECTIONS

Aspergillus species

Although rarely seen in neonates, systemic infection with *Aspergillus* spp. suggests severe immune system compromise, such as DiGeorge Syndrome or myeloperoxidase deficiency (Chiang et al, 2000; Marcinkowski et al, 2000). Disseminated disease has occurred in premature newborns without additional immunologic abnormalities (Rowen et al, 1992). Diagnosis requires isolation of the fungus from a normally sterile tissue site or visualization by Gomori-methenamine silver stain on a biopsy specimen of infected tissue. Of note, a commercially available enzyme-linked immunosorbent assay for diagnosis of aspergillosis on serum specimens had an 83% rate of false positive results in premature newborns (Siemann et al, 1998). Treatment requires systemic amphotericin B in doses of 1.0 to 1.5 mg/kg/day. Fungistatic therapies such as the triazoles are not recommended for aspergillosis.

Trichosporon beigelii

In a cluster of five neonatal cases of infection caused by *T. beigelii*, a yeast found ubiquitously in soil, no common source was identified (Fisher et al, 1993). Two of three premature infants infected with this organism died. Resistance to achievable concentrations of amphotericin B complicates therapy.

SUGGESTED READINGS

Benjamin DK Jr, Stoll BJ, Fanaroff AA, et al: Neonatal candidiasis among extremely low birth weight infants: risk factors, mortality rates, and neurodevelopmental outcomes at 18 to 22 months, *Pediatrics* 117:84-92, 2006.

Clerihew L, Austin N, McGuire W: Prophylactic systemic antifungal agents to prevent mortality and morbidity in very low birth weight infants, *Cochrane Database Syst Rev* 4:CD003850, 2007.

Cotten CM, McDonald S, Stoll B, et al: The association of third-generation cephalosporin use and invasive candidiasis in extremely low birth-weight infants, *Pediatrics* 118:717-722, 2006.

Faix RG: Systemic Candida infections in infants in intensive care nurseries: high incidence of central nervous system involvement, *J Pediatr* 105:616-622, 1984.

Juster-Reicher A, Flidel-Rimon O, Amitay M, et al: High-dose liposomal amphotericin B in the therapy of systemic candidiasis in neonates, *Eur J Clin Microbiol Infect Dis* 22:603-607, 2003.

Karlowicz MG, Hashimoto LN, Kelly RE Jr, et al: Should central venous catheters be removed as soon as candidemia is detected in neonates? *Pediatrics* 106:E63, 2000.

Noyola DE, Fernandez M, Moylett EH, et al: Ophthalmologic, visceral, and cardiac involvement in neonates with candidemia, *Clin Infect Dis* 32:1018-1023, 2001.

Odio CM, Araya R, Pinto LE, et al: Caspofungin therapy of neonates with invasive candidiasis, *Pediatr Infect Dis J* 23:1093-1097, 2004.

Rowen JL, Atkins JT, Levy ML, et al: Invasive fungal dermatitis in the < or = 1000-gram neonate, *Pediatrics* 95:682-687, 1995.

Saiman L, Ludington E, Pfaller M, et al: Risk factors for candidemia in Neonatal Intensive Care Unit patients. The National Epidemiology of Mycosis Survey study group, *Pediatr Infect Dis J* 19:319-324, 2000.

Saiman L, Ludington E, Dawson JD, et al: Risk factors for Candida species colonization of neonatal intensive care unit patients, *Pediatr Infect Dis J* 20:1119-1124, 2001.

Complete references and supplemental color images used in this text can be found online at www.expertconsult.com

PART X

RESPIRATORY SYSTEM

CHAPTER
42
LUNG DEVELOPMENT: EMBRYOLOGY, GROWTH, MATURATION, AND DEVELOPMENTAL BIOLOGY

Maria Victoria Fraga and Susan Guttentag

The primary function of the lung is to accomplish exchange of oxygen and carbon dioxide to accommodate the needs of aerobic cellular respiration. The oxygen consumption of the adult human ranges from 250 mL/min at rest to 5500 mL/min at peak exercise (Warburton et al, 2000). To accommodate these metabolic needs, a large surface area, and a thin alveolar-capillary membrane are required to enable efficient diffusion of oxygen more so than carbon dioxide. Ultimately the zone of gas exchange will attain a surface area of 50 to 100 m² and a volume of 2.5 to 3.0 L in the adult human; therefore a primary goal of lung organogenesis is to expand the lung surface area to meet these needs. A second goal of lung organogenesis is to minimize the diffusing distance from alveolus to red blood cell, coordinating the development of an extensive capillary network with a thin, expansive alveolar epithelial surface. A third goal of lung development is production of a protective aqueous barrier overlying the delicate alveolar epithelium while mitigating the effects of the surface tension generated by this barrier, specifically alveolar collapse, through the production of a surface active agent or surfactant.

The trachea, airways, and alveoli are in constant contact with the external environment. Consequently with every inhalation, epithelial surfaces encounter large numbers of microorganisms and potentially toxic particles and gases. Lung organogenesis must also incorporate mechanisms for clearance of microorganisms and allergens that may result in epithelial infection or injury. Similarly the lung must defend against nonparticulate gases that are potentially harmful. Oxygen, although critical to cellular function, can be the source of harmful reactive oxygen species and inhaled pollutants similarly require detoxification. The appropriate development and maintenance of these lung functions are critical to the health and survival of newborn infants. This chapter focuses on developmental aspects of each function that place the premature neonate at increased risk for lung injury and disease.

KEY EVENTS IN LUNG DEVELOPMENT

Lung formation begins early in human gestation (by day 25), and growth extends well into childhood (Burri, 2006; Kumar et al, 2005). Lung development can be organized into stages (embryonic, pseudoglandular, canalicular, saccular, and alveolar), although the timing of these stages is somewhat imprecise and considerable overlap can occur.

Figure 42-1 shows a timeline of fetal and postnatal lung development.

DEVELOPMENT OF AIRWAYS AND GAS EXCHANGE SURFACES

The initial phase of lung development, the embryonic phase, is marked by the formation of the lung bud and initial branching of presumptive airways. The lung bud is first recognizable as a laryngotracheal groove of the ventral foregut at 25 days' gestation. Within a few days the groove closes so that the only remaining lumenal attachment to the foregut is in the region of the developing hypopharynx and larynx. The lung bud, consisting of epithelium and surrounding mesenchyme, then begins the first of a series of dichotomous divisions that give rise to the conducting airways and five primordial lung lobes (two left and three right). Tracheoesophageal fistulas, tracheal atresia, and tracheal stenosis result from errors in separation of the laryngotracheal groove, whereas failure of partitioning of the lung bud can result in pulmonary agenesis, most typically of the right lung.

Branching continues into the pseudoglandular stage of lung development. By 7 weeks' gestation, the trachea and the segmental and subsegmental bronchi are evident. By the end of 16 weeks' gestation, all bronchial divisions are completed. It is important to remember that, although the conducting airways will certainly enlarge as the fetus and newborn grow (airway diameter and length increase twofold to threefold between birth and adulthood), large airway branching ceases after 16 weeks' gestation.

Closure of the pleuroperitoneal folds is a critical event of the pseudoglandular phase, reaching completion by 7 weeks' gestation and resulting in separation of the thoracic cavity from the peritoneal cavity. Failure of pleuroperitoneal closure results in a diaphragmatic defect and continuity between these cavities. At 10 weeks' gestation, when the midgut returns to the peritoneal cavity from the umbilical cord, abdominal contents are free to pass into the thoracic cavity and restrict the space into which the lung grows. The resulting congenital diaphragmatic hernia leads to pulmonary hypoplasia of the lung ipsilateral to the diaphragmatic defect as bowel and solid viscera migrate into the thorax. Pulmonary hypoplasia can also extend to the contralateral lung as the mediastinum shifts because of accumulating abdominal viscera in the thorax.

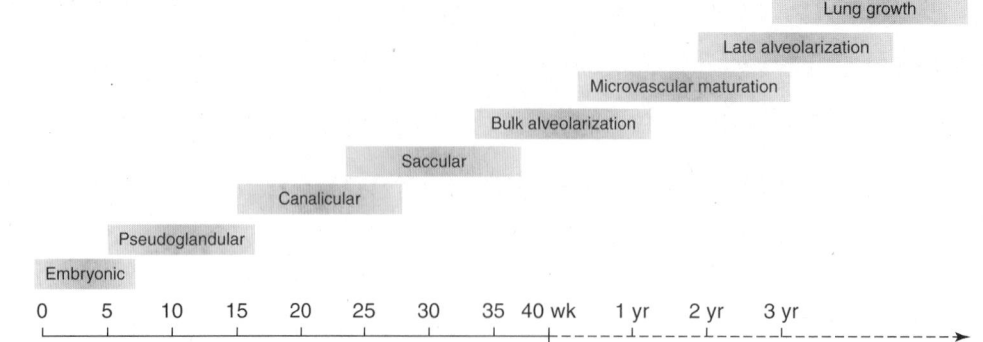

FIGURE 42-1   Human lung development. Timeline of major events in human fetal and postnatal lung development.

The canalicular phase is marked by completion of the conducting airways through the level of the terminal bronchioles, and the development of the rudimentary gas exchange units that are no longer invested with cartilaginous support. The acinus is the gas exchange unit of the lung and encompasses a respiratory bronchiole and all of its associated alveolar ducts and alveoli. A terminal bronchiole with all its associated acinar structures constitutes a lobule. Branching of these distal airspaces continues on a more limited basis during the canalicular phase, finally achieving a total of 23 airway subdivisions.

Evolution of the relationships between the airspaces, capillaries, and mesenchyme acquires greater significance during the saccular phase of lung development (24 to 38 weeks' gestation), enabling an alveolocapillary membrane sufficient to participate in gas exchange (0.6 μm) by approximately 24 weeks. Beyond this point, the efficiency of gas exchange is determined by the available surface area. Lengthening and widening of the terminal sacs expands the gas exchange surface area. Each saccule consists of smooth-walled airspaces with thickened interstitial spaces containing a double capillary network. These will give rise to two to three alveolar ducts, further expanding the available surface area. Expansion of these rudimentary gas exchange units continues well into the 3rd trimester of human gestation; therefore the human lung is not fully mature structurally, even at term delivery.

Postnatal lung development can be subdivided into additional stages (Burri, 2006). True alveoli become evident as early as 36 weeks' gestation, initiating the alveolar phase of lung development. The development of primary alveoli is followed by a further expansion of the gas-exchange surface area through the formation of septae or secondary crests (see Alveolarization, later). Postnatal alveolarization extends from term through 1 to 2 years of age. An initial phase of bulk alveolarization occurs within the first 6 months postnatally, with a more modest addition of secondary alveoli through the remainder of this period. The alveoli of the infant lungs are different from adult alveoli. These immature secondary alveoli contain a double capillary bed, whereas adult alveoli are invested by a single capillary bed. Microvascular maturation, the next phase of postnatal lung development, occurs between the first few postnatal months of life through 3 years of age (see Development of the Pulmonary Vasculature, later).

There is considerable controversy regarding when the lung ceases to add alveoli. Estimates have ranged from as early as 2 years to as late as 20 years old in humans; this is further complicated by the observation that alveolar expansion can occur in response to pneumonectomy in adult animals and humans. The acquisition of alveoli after the maturation of the microvasculature has been termed *late alveolarization*. This activity has been most often demonstrated in subpleural regions of the lung and likely invokes mechanisms similar to secondary crest formation.

The addition of alveoli is not the only means for expanding the surface area of the lung. While alveolarization wanes over the first 3 years of life in the human, growth of the lung continues to expand the gas exchange surface. Between 2 years of age and adulthood, lung tissue expands with lung volume roughly proportionately to the increase in bodyweight of the child. Thus, because of the combined processes of prenatal lung development, postnatal lung development, and lung growth, there is tremendous potential for expansion of the gas exchange surface area that is developmentally programmed into the fetal lung to account for the growing needs of the infant, child, and adult for aerobic cellular respiration. The extent to which these developmental mechanisms can be harnessed after premature birth, with or without superimposed lung injury, is a topic of active investigation.

COMPOSITION OF AIRWAYS AND ALVEOLI

As branching morphogenesis proceeds, the epithelium lining the successive generations of airways and alveoli gives rise to specialized cells that participate in gas exchange, surfactant production, mucociliary clearance, detoxification, and host defense. Differentiation proceeds in a centrifugal fashion from proximal to distal airspaces, lagging behind branching. Temporal and contextual signals foster the regionalization of epithelial cell types.

Proximal Airways

The airway epithelium is tall and columnar, decreasing to a more cuboidal appearance more distally (Jeffrey, 1998; Snyder et al, 2009). The endodermal epithelial lining cells of the trachea and bronchi partition into four cell types: undifferentiated columnar, ciliated, secretory-goblet, and basal cells. Ciliated cells critical to the process of mucus clearance are first apparent between 11 and 16 weeks' gestation and become less prevalent in more distal airways. Three types of secretory cells—those with largely mucous granules, those with serous granules, and some with both types of granules—can be seen as early as 13 weeks' gestation. The number of mucin-producing goblet cells in airways peaks at mid-gestation in the fetus and declines into adulthood. Finally, immature basal cells expressing epidermal keratin have been noted as early as 12 weeks' gestation. Basal cells have a critical role in regenerating injured large airway epithelium (see Stem and Progenitor Cells in the Lung, later).

Cartilaginous support of the tracheobronchial tree begins and proceeds in a centrifugal fashion beginning in the primitive trachea at 4 weeks, reaching the main bronchi by 10 weeks, and proceeding to the most distal terminal bronchioles by approximately 25 weeks' gestation. Cartilaginous investment of airways is complete by the 2nd month postnatally. Submucosal glands are found in the interstitium between the cartilaginous tissue and surface epithelium, and they have a major role in airway host defense. Submucosal gland development can be characterized by five stages: (1) epithelial budding and invasion of the lamina propria, (2) development of a lumen, (3) initiation of tube branching, (4) dichotomous branching, and (5) repeated dichotomous branching. By comparison, the airways of infants and children contain relatively more submucous glands than do adults. The glands are lined by mucous cells proximally and serous cells more distally, the latter comprising 60% of the total epithelial cell content of the glands. Serous cells secrete water, electrolytes, and proteins with antimicrobial, antiinflammatory, and antioxidant properties, whereas the mucous cells produce primarily mucins. In addition to this host defense role, submucosal glands also contain a population of basal cells that respond to injury of the airway by replenishing the airway epithelium.

Muscular investment of the airways begins as early as 6 to 8 weeks gestation as smooth muscle cells are identifiable around the trachea and large airways. Fetal airway smooth muscle is innervated and able to contract during the first trimester. It is also responsive to methacholine challenge that is reversible with β-adrenergic agonists. Muscularization increases through fetal life and childhood such that there is an increase in the amount of smooth muscle relative to airway size compared with adults. Furthermore, there is a rapid increase in bronchial smooth muscle immediately after birth, whether born at term or prematurely.

An additional airway cell deserves mention because of its role in a wide variety of pediatric diseases. Pulmonary neuroendocrine cells (PNECs) are found throughout the airways, often in innervated clusters known as pulmonary neuroendocrine bodies (NEBs) located at branch points in the bronchial tree (Cutz et al, 2007). Although they arise from foregut endoderm, the cell of origin is distinct from other epithelial components of the lung. Solitary PNECs are sensitive to stretch- and hypoxia-mediated secretion, producing both amines (i.e., serotonin) and peptides (i.e., bombesin) that are important in regulating bronchial tone. Pathologic conditions recently associated with PNECs and NEBs, most often characterized by hyperplasia, include bronchopulmonary dysplasia, disorders of respiratory control (congenital central hypoventilation syndrome and sudden infant death syndrome), cystic fibrosis, and pulmonary hypertension. Neuroendocrine hyperplasia of infancy is a rare form of interstitial lung disease of infancy associated with expansion of the number of PNECs and NEBs, yet little is known about the mechanism of disease.

Distal Airways

The bronchiolar epithelium differs from the more proximal airway epithelium. In addition to being more cuboid in appearance, the epithelium contains progressively fewer ciliated cells and goblet cells, which are ultimately absent from the terminal bronchioles. Instead, the nonciliated, secretory Clara cell is found in increasing numbers and density down the conducting airways, such that the Clara cell is the most abundant cell of the terminal bronchiole (Jeffrey, 1998). Clara cells are first evident by 16 to 17 weeks' gestation, initially exhibiting large glycogen stores that are replaced by secretory granules. Between 23 and 34 weeks' gestation, there is a dramatic increase in Clara cell numbers in distal bronchioles. Clara cells are critical to the host defense and detoxification functions of the lung. This specialized cell produces the highest levels of cytochrome P-450 and flavin monooxygenases in the lung. While critically important in detoxification, these enzymes participate in the bioactivation of procarcinogens as well, placing the Clara cell in a precarious position as a primary target of toxic metabolites. The Clara cell also has an important role in immunoregulation in the distal airways. Important host defense products of the Clara cell include Clara cell secretory protein (CCSP or CC10), surfactant proteins A, and D, leukocyte protease inhibitor, and a trypsinlike protease. The function of Clara cell SP-B in airways is less certain, especially because Clara cells do not produce a mature 8-kDa SP-B protein, but may also contribute to host defense. The secretion of antiproteases from Clara cells suggests that they modulate the protease-antiprotease balance in the distal lung.

Alveolar Epithelium

During the 4th through 6th months of gestation, the epithelial cells lining the acini begin to differentiate further (Mallampalli et al, 1997). The cuboidal epithelial cells accumulate large glycogen stores and develop small vesicles containing loose lamellae. The large glycogen pools provide a ready source of substrate required for the production of increasing amounts of surfactant phospholipids, and they decrease in size as surfactant production advances in the fetal lung. In cells destined to become type 2 cells, lamellar bodies become larger, more numerous, and more densely packed with surfactant phospholipids and proteins, whereas those cells destined to become type 1 cells, upon losing their relationship to mesenchymal fibroblasts, lose the prelamellar vesicles and become progressively thinner, thereby adopting a phenotype more suitable for gas exchange. Alveolar type 1 and 2 cells are readily identified early in the saccular stage of fetal lung development. There remains considerable controversy regarding the origin of type 1 cells. In culture, these cells demonstrate slow turnover, with a doubling time estimated to be between 40 and 120 days, suggesting that they are functionally terminally differentiated in vivo. Furthermore, in response to epithelial denudation occurring with lung injury, type 2 cells proliferate to reestablish epithelial continuity, and then lose

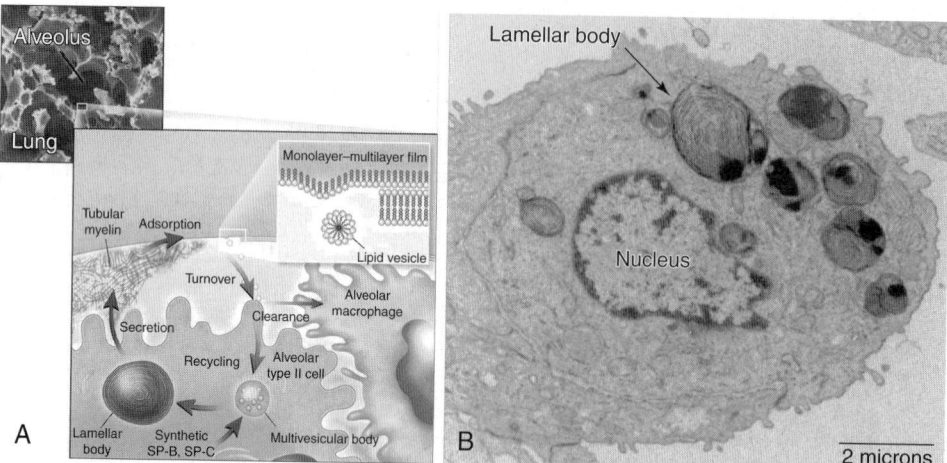

FIGURE 42-2 Surfactant life cycle. A, Schematic diagram depicting the life cycle of surfactant. **B,** Electron micrograph of a type II alveolar epithelial cell showing the prominent lamellar bodies near the apical surface. (*A, Reprinted with permission from Whitsett J, Weaver T: Hydrophobic surfactant proteins in lung function and disease,* N Engl J Med 347:2141–2148, 2002. Copyright 2002 Massachusetts Medical Society. All rights reserved.)

phenotypic features such as lamellar bodies and acquire markers of type 1 cells, suggesting that rapid repopulation of type 1 cells requires a type 2 cell intermediary.

There is increasing appreciation for the alveolar type 1 cell as more than a passive membrane for gas exchange (Williams, 2003). The large surface area and small cytoplasm/nucleus ratio provides for a thin alveolocapillary membrane to facilitate gas exchange. However, this large surface area also provides a large absorptive surface in the lung. The presence of water and ion channels, some distinct from those in type 2 cells, facilitates the maintenance of a relatively dry alveolus. Type 1 cells may also regulate cell proliferation locally, signal macrophage accumulation, and modulate the functions of local peptides, proteases and growth factors.

Although most notable for its role in surfactant production, the alveolar type 2 cell provides additional important functions in the alveolus (Fehrenbach, 2001). Alveolar type 2 cells are local progenitor cells, as mentioned previously. Like type 1 cells, alveolar type 2 cells contain specialized ion and water channels as well as ion pumps in both the apical and basal membranes that contribute to the movement of water and ions across the epithelium (see Static Stretch: Fetal Lung Fluid Protection, later). Type 2 cells contain and secrete important antioxidants (superoxide dismutases 1, 2, and 3, glutathione) and molecules of innate host defense (SP-A, SP-D, lysozyme) to participate in detoxification and sterilization of the alveolar microenvironment.

More recently, it is becoming clear that alveolar type 2 cells may also play a part in exacerbating alveolar pathology. The type 2 cell participates in the coagulation-fibrinolysis cascade through the production of fibrinogen, urokinase-type plasminogen activator, and tissue factor, especially under pathologic circumstances. Type 2 cells are increasingly recognized as a source of cytokine and chemokine production in the lung, as well as growth factors that can promote fibrosis. Finally, cross-talk between epithelial cells, cell matrix, interstitial cells, and local inflammatory cells can foster the resolution of injury and inflammation or prolong lung remodeling after injury with detrimental effects, such as lung destruction and fibrosis. Although previously heralded as the defender of the alveolus, the

alveolar type 2 cell have a much more complex role in alveolar health and disease.

SURFACTANT

Pulmonary surfactant is essential to alveolar health. A thin layer of liquid is constantly secreted into the alveolar lumen to protect the delicate alveolar epithelium. The surface tension generated by this aqueous layer opposes alveolar inflation and promotes alveolar collapse at the end of expiration, because of Laplace's law, which states that the collapsing pressure on the alveolus is directly proportional to the surface tension while inversely proportional to the radius of the alveolus. The film of pulmonary surfactant at the air-liquid interface lowers surface tension as alveolar surface area decreases, thereby preventing end-expiratory atelectasis, maintaining functional residual capacity, and lowering the force required for subsequent alveolar inflations.

Pulmonary surfactant is a complex mixture of phospholipids, neutral lipids, and proteins that is synthesized, packaged, and secreted by alveolar type 2 cells (Zuo et al, 2008). The life cycle of surfactant is depicted in Figure 42-2. Storage of surfactant occurs in the lamellar body, a lysosome-derived membrane-bound organelle that undergoes regulated secretion in response to a variety of stimuli, including stretching. In the alveolus, surfactant phospholipids transition through an extracellular storage form—tubular myelin. Phospholipid and protein components are recycled out of the surfactant monolayer at the air-liquid interface and taken back into the alveolar type 2 cell, where they can be repackaged into lamellar bodies. Alternatively, alveolar macrophages are able to engulf and degrade surfactant components.

The predominant surfactant phospholipid is saturated dipalmitoylphosphatidylcholine, with the remaining phospholipids consisting of monounsaturated phosphatidylcholine, phosphatidylglycerol and other phospholipids (Table 42-1). Dipalmitoylphosphatidylcholine is the only surface active component of lung surfactant capable of lowering surface pressure to nearly zero. The presence of unsaturated phospholipids and other lipid components like

TABLE 42-1 Composition of Pulmonary Surfactant

Component	Percentage (by Weight)
Lipid	90
Saturated phosphatidylcholine	45
Unsaturated phosphatidylcholine	25
Phosphatidylglycerol	5
Other phospholipids	5
Neutral lipids	10
Protein	10
Surfactant proteins	5
Serum proteins	5

cholesterol enables the monolayer to remain fluid at body temperature during the respiratory cycle. Phospholipid content in the fetal lung increases with advancing gestation because of increased activity of enzymes responsible for phospholipid synthesis within alveolar type 2 cells. The expression and activity of enzymes of the choline incorporation pathway, the predominant pathway for surfactant phospholipid synthesis, are developmentally regulated and induced by hormones. The inductive hormones that have direct clinical relevance are glucocorticoids and agents that increase intracellular cyclic adenosine monophosphate (cAMP) such as the β-adrenergic agonist (and tocolytic) terbutaline.

Surfactant contains a group of specific proteins with importance to surfactant function and host defense. The four surfactant proteins SP-A, -B, -C, and -D are subdivided based on their physical characteristics into either hydrophobic (SP-B and -C) or hydrophilic (SP-A and -D) proteins. The hydrophobic surfactant proteins play a major role in the surface-active properties of surfactant, whereas the primary roles of the hydrophilic surfactant proteins are in host defense, immunomodulation, and surfactant clearance and metabolism (see Surfactant, earlier).

Together, the hydrophobic proteins facilitate the mobilization of surfactant phospholipid from tubular myelin to the surface monolayer, promote spreading of phospholipids in the surfactant film, and assist in film stability at end-expiration (Zuo, 2008). SP-B plays a central role in alveolar health because of its critical function in surfactant homeostasis. It is a secretory protein that exhibits strong association with membranes, unlike SP-C, which contains a membrane-spanning domain and covalently attached fatty acids (palmitate) that render it integral to phospholipid membranes (Conkright et al, 2001). Both SP-B and SP-C are synthesized as large precursor proproteins that undergo extensive posttranslational processing as they pass through the secretory pathway, ultimately reaching the lamellar body. SP-B is essential for the process of lamellar body formation, and the alveolar type 2 cells of infants with inherited deficiency of SP-B are devoid of lamellar bodies. Because the lamellar body is where SP-C processing is completed, infants with inherited deficiency of SP-B are also deficient in mature SP-C, instead accumulating a larger, nonfunctional precursor of SP-C. Therefore patients with inherited deficiency of SP-B, despite having relatively normal surfactant phospholipid profiles, make a

pulmonary surfactant with poor surface tension properties because of the combined defects in SP-B and SP-C. Conversely, because SP-C does not have either a direct nor indirect role in SP-B protein processing, animals with SP-C deficiency have normal SP-B, normal lamellar bodies, and relatively normal surfactant function, and they exhibit no perinatal lethality because of surfactant dysfunction.

Like the enzymes of surfactant phospholipid production, SP-B and SP-C exhibit developmental and hormonal regulation of expression (Mendelson, 2000). In human fetuses, SP-C mRNA is detected as early as 12 weeks' gestation and SP-B mRNA by 14 weeks' gestation, but the mature proteins are not detectable in fetal lung tissue until after 24 weeks' gestation. SP-B protein is not detectable in amniotic fluid until after 30 weeks' gestation, increasing toward term (Pryhuber et al, 1991), because of developmental regulation of posttranslational events in the proteolytic processing of proSP-B and proSP-C (Guttentag, 2008). Consequently, infants delivered prematurely have reduced levels of both surface active components of surfactant, phospholipid, and hydrophobic surfactant proteins, because of the developmental regulation of surfactant proteins and the enzymes of phospholipid production in alveolar type 2 cells. The rate of type 2 cell differentiation, and secondarily surfactant production by the fetal lung, is modulated by levels of endogenous corticosteroids and is accelerated by administering antenatal glucocorticoid to women in preterm labor. The response of the surfactant system to glucocorticoid involves all the lipid and protein components, and it occurs primarily through increased gene expression, thus representing precocious maturation mimicking the normal developmental pattern. Endogenous thyroid hormones, prostaglandins, and catecholamines also have stimulatory effects on type 2 cell maturation and clearance of lung fluid at birth. Certain proinflammatory cytokines (e.g., tumor necrosis factor [TNF]-α and transforming growth factor [TGF-β]) inhibit surfactant production in experimental systems and may downregulate surfactant in conditions such as sepsis and inflammation. A partial list of hormones capable of inducing or inhibiting lung maturation is presented in Table 42-2.

DEVELOPMENT OF THE PULMONARY VASCULATURE

The pulmonary vasculature consists of the vascular supply to the acini and the bronchial circulation (Hislop, 2005). During early fetal life, the airways act as a template for pulmonary blood vessel development. The earliest pulmonary vessels form de novo in the tissue that surrounds the lung bud by differentiation of mesenchymal cells into endothelial cells and then capillaries, a process known as *vasculogenesis*. Mesodermal cells within the mesenchyme investing the developing lung tube differentiate into endothelial cells, proliferate, organize into chords, and develop a central lumen. As each new airway buds into the mesenchyme, a new plexus forms and adds to the pulmonary circulation, thereby extending the arteries and veins. By 5 weeks' gestation, a capillary network surrounds each bronchus and circulation of blood between the right ventricle and the left atrium via this network is evident.

TABLE 42-2 Hormonal Regulators of Lung Maturation

Inducers	Glucocorticoids (cortisol)	Major endogenous modulator of alveolar development and surfactant production
	β-Adrenergic agonists (epinephrine), cAMP	Increase surfactant production and secretion, especially during labor and delivery
	Thyroid hormones (T_3, T_4)	Enhance glucocorticoid effects on lipid synthesis
	Retinoic acid	May interact with glucocorticoids to regulate surfactant phospholipid and protein production
	Bombesin-related peptides, parathyroid hormone–related protein	May contribute to surfactant lipid synthesis
Inhibitors	Protein kinase C activators (proinflammatory cytokines)	Inhibit surfactant protein gene transcription during infection, inflammation
	TGF-β family	Inhibit type 2 cell maturation during early gestation and with inflammation
	TNF-α	Inhibit SP-B and SP-C gene transcription during infection
	Insulin	Inhibit surfactant protein gene transcription in infants of poorly controlled diabetic women
	Dihydrotestosterone	Delayed type 2 cell maturation in males

By the canalicular stage of lung development, continued branching of the airways is accompanied by thinning of the epithelium. At this stage, new blood vessels form from preexisting vessels, a process known as *angiogenesis*. By comparison, angiogenesis is initiated by endothelial cell proliferation and sprouting from established vessels, resulting in the extension of a vascular network into undervascularized regions. Vasculogenesis is the primary mode of pulmonary vascular development until 17 weeks' gestation, when all preacinar airways and their accompanying vessels are present, whereas angiogenesis becomes the predominant mode of vascular development in the later stages of lung development. Although originally thought to be sequential processes, it is generally accepted that vasculogenesis occurring in the periphery and more central angiogenesis occur concurrently during lung development (deMello et al, 1997). Interconnections between vascular networks arising from both angiogenesis and vasculogenesis increase in the saccular phase of lung development.

In the human lung, a second circulatory system, the bronchial circulation, arises from the dorsal aorta supplying systemic blood. The bronchial vasculature develops after the pulmonary circulation, with bronchial vessels first apparent by 8 weeks' gestation. The network of bronchial vessels is extensive, with bronchial arteries demonstrated as distal as the alveolar ducts in the adult respiratory tree.

The inappropriate branching of bronchial vessels from the dorsal aorta is implicated in the formation of bronchopulmonary sequestration, a space-occupying lung malformation that can result in hypoplasia of the ipsilateral lung.

Vasculogenesis and angiogenesis are the primary mechanisms of vascular development throughout intrauterine life. The human lung at term contains only a small portion of the adult number of alveoli, and the airspaces walls are represented by a thick primary septum consisting of a central layer of connective tissue surrounded by two capillary beds, each of them facing one alveolar surface (Burri, 2006). As alveolar architecture changes with the appearance of secondary septa, or secondary crests, folding of one of the two capillary layers occurs within the secondary septa. This double capillary network is not present in the adult lung. Microvascular maturation involves fusion of the double capillary network into a single capillary system. The expansion of surface area and lumenal volume compresses the interstitium, bringing the capillary networks in close proximity to potential air spaces and thereby promoting both alveolar surface area expansion and capillary bed fusion. Interestingly, by the third postnatal week during which lung volume increases by 25%, there is a concomitant 27% decrease of the interstitial tissue volume that is believed to promote focal microvascular fusions. Subsequently, there is preferential growth of fused areas that continues until 3 years of age.

Lastly, it is well known that lung volume increases approximately 23-fold between birth and young adulthood, and capillary volume expands 35-fold. It has been recently shown that this increase in capillary volume occurs by insertion of new capillary meshes in the absence of capillary sprouting. This new concept in capillary network growth has been named *intussusceptive microvascular growth*, and involves the formation of transluminal tissue pillars that then expand, resulting in increased capillary surface area (Burri, 2006).

Muscularization can be detected early in development of the pulmonary arteries (Hislop, 2005). Initially the muscular investment of the vasculature is derived from the migration of bronchial smooth muscle cells from adjacent airways. Muscularization of preacinar and resistance arteries of the pulmonary vasculature begins in the canalicular stage and continues through the remainder of gestation. This second phase of smooth muscle cells investing pulmonary vessels develops from the surrounding mesenchyme. Fibroblasts in close proximity to developing arteries alter their cellular shape and begin to express α-smooth muscle actin, a marker of smooth muscle cells. A third phase of vascular muscularization has been described, largely in the distal lung, in which capillary endothelial cells undergo a process of endothelial-mesenchymal transition that encompasses endothelial cell division, separation, and migration from the endothelial layer and expression of smooth muscle cell markers.

Muscularization of pulmonary arteries normally extends to the level of the terminal bronchiole and is minimal to absent in blood vessels surrounding respiratory bronchioles. Abnormal extension of smooth muscle along arterioles supplying acinar structures occurs in infants dying from persistent pulmonary hypertension of the newborn and in severe bronchopulmonary dysplasia.

TABLE 42-3 Composition of Human Fetal Lung Fluid Compared With Other Body Fluids

Component	Lung Fluid	Interstitial Fluid	Plasma	Amniotic Fluid
Sodium (mEq/L)	150	147	150	113
Potassium (mEq/L)	6.3	4.8	4.8	7.6
Chloride (mEq/L)	157	107	107	87
Bicarbonate (mEq/L)	3	25	24	19
pH	6.27	7.31	7.34	7.02
Protein (g/dL)	0.03	3.27	4.09	0.10

MECHANISMS OF LUNG DEVELOPMENT

Fetal and postnatal lung development depend on several key developmental processes: branching morphogenesis to promote branching of the lung bud into the surrounding mesenchyme, static and cyclic stretching of the lung that assist in promoting lung branching, alveolarization to enhance the expansion of the gas exchange surface area, and vasculogenesis and angiogenesis to ensure that the developing epithelial surface area is invested with a similarly extensive vascular supply.

BRANCHING MORPHOGENESIS

Branching morphogenesis is the fundamental mechanism of lung development. Branching is mediated by the accelerated growth of epithelial cells lateral to branch points with concomitant growth arrest at the branch point (Affolter et al, 2009). This process requires extensive communication between the cells lining the tubular lung bud and cells contained within the invested mesenchyme. Classic tissue recombination experiments in which mesenchyme from proximal airways was transplanted to distal airways (and vice versa) indicate that the mesenchyme has an important inductive role in dictating the branching pattern and cell fate of the expanding epithelium. More recently, studies of mouse lung development indicate that three modes of branching—domain branching, planar bifurcation, and orthogonal bifurcation—are the basic mechanisms that characterize the complex three-dimensional development of the respiratory tree through the pseudoglandular phase (Metzger and Krasnow, 1999). These routines occur repetitively during lung development and appear to be set by a genetic clock dictating when side branches form, a bifurcation program determining when a branch bifurcates, and a rotator function controlling the planar orientation of the bifurcation.

STRETCH AND MECHANOTRANSDUCTION

The role of physical factors in modulating lung size is well established; normal lung growth requires adequate space in the chest cavity and appropriate tonic and cyclic distending forces. Genetic defects that compromise the thoracic skeleton and space-occupying lung masses like congenital cystic adenomatoid malformations are associated with pulmonary hypoplasia because of the restriction of intrathoracic space. Denervation of the diaphragm to eliminate fetal breathing movements is also associated with pulmonary hypoplasia, as is the manipulation of fetal lung fluid volume.

Static Stretch: Fetal Lung Fluid Production

Fetal lung fluid is a product of the epithelial lining of the developing lung (Wilson et al, 2007), averaging 4 to 6 mL/kg/h. Because of the resistance imparted by laryngeal abduction, fluid accumulates to a total volume of 20 to 30 mL/kg during gestation, providing end-expiratory pressure of approximately 2.5 cm H_2O pressure (Kitterman, 1996). The composition of fetal lung fluid is distinct from both amniotic fluid and plasma, as shown in Table 42-3. The increased chloride content of fetal lung fluid compared with serum is the result of active chloride secretion by the tracheal and distal pulmonary epithelium, largely because of the chloride channel CLC-2/CLCN2. Fetal lung fluid secretion can be enhanced by prolactin, KGF, PGE2 and PGF2, whereas it is inhibited by a variety of mediators, including β-adrenergic agonists, vasopressin, serotonin, and glucagon.

Fetal lung fluid is an essential component of lung development, but it presents a significant obstacle to the transition to air breathing upon delivery. Three important events must occur to decrease the amount of fetal lung fluid and its potential effect on alveolar surface tension: absorption, bulk removal, and maturation of pulmonary surfactant. The transition to air breathing must be coupled with a conversion from a secretory pulmonary epithelium to one that is absorptive. Enhanced sodium transport across the alveolar epithelium is in part responsible for this change. Much evidence suggests that induction of components of the epithelial sodium channels (ENaC) around the time of birth is a major factor in promoting sodium transport with water passively following the movement of sodium. Absence of the α-subunit of ENaC in transgenic mice is perinatal lethal because of the failure of fetal lung fluid clearance. Induction of ENaC components occurs at a transcriptional level in response to changes in extracellular matrix components, glucocorticoids, aldosterone, and oxygen. By comparison, agents that increase intracellular cAMP levels (i.e., β-agonists, phosphodiesterase inhibitors, and cAMP analogues), while not increasing the number of sodium channels, increase the probability of a channel being open to sodium transport. In addition, glucocorticoid and thyroid hormones have important roles in priming the lung epithelium to be responsive to the actions of β-adrenergic agonists on sodium transport across lung epithelia near term. Water channels consisting of aquaporins are also induced during the late fetal period to facilitate fluid movement, but their contribution is unclear because of the perinatal survival of mice in which aquaporin 5 or both aquaporins 5 and 1 were absent.

Conversion to an absorptive surface is not sufficient to minimize the fetal lung fluid at the time of term delivery. The absence of uterine contractions is associated with an increased incidence of retained fetal lung fluid in infants delivered by cesarean section without the benefit of labor. On delivery of the head and neck, continued uterine contractions on the fetal thorax promote expulsion of bulk fluid from the fetal lung. However, animal studies have shown that the magnitude of the benefit of thoracic compression during labor is modest (Bland, 2001). The primary mechanism by which labor facilitates clearance of lung fluid is through hormonal effects on fluid clearance, especially through catecholamine-induced changes in the ENaC opening. The onset of air breathing, associated with increased intrathoracic negative pressure, assists in the clearance of residual fetal lung fluid into the loose interstitial tissues surrounding alveoli. Fluid is then reabsorbed via lymphatics and pulmonary blood vessels. It is generally accepted that the amount of residual liquid in the lung after complete transition is approximately 0.37 mL/kg body weight.

Cyclic Stretch: Fetal Breathing Movements

Fetal breathing is an essential stimulus for lung growth (Kitterman, 1996). Fetal breathing is readily detectable as early as 10 weeks' gestation. Fetal breathing occurs for 10% to 20% of the time at 24 to 28 weeks' gestation, increasing to 30% to 40% after 30 weeks' gestation. Originating from the diaphragm, fetal breathing is erratic in frequency and amplitude, and it changes throughout gestation. The volume of fluid moved is small and insufficient to be cleared from the trachea. Respiratory rates range from 30 to 70 breaths/min, and periods of apnea of up to 2 hours have been recorded. Sustained periods of fetal breathing increase in duration with advancing gestation. The frequency of fetal breathing varies with sleep state (inhibited during quiet sleep) and exhibits diurnal variation, with the lowest rates recorded early in the morning. Fetal breathing is hormonally responsive and the inhibition of fetal breathing with the onset of labor is attributed to the action of increased circulating prostaglandins. Maternal medications can influence the frequency of fetal breathing movements. Central nervous system stimulants are associated with increased fetal breathing (i.e., caffeine, amphetamines), whereas depressants are associated with decreased fetal breathing (i.e., anesthetics, narcotics, ethanol). Maternal smoking is associated with reduced fetal breathing, largely because of increased fetal hypoxemia. Animal studies have shown that permanent cessation of fetal breathing, regardless of the insult, is associated with impaired fetal lung growth. However, the effects of short-term alterations in fetal breathing frequency and amplitude on fetal lung development are unknown. Together, constant distention from the production and retention of fetal lung fluid, and episodic cyclic fetal breathing, are important mechanisms for lung growth during fetal life.

ALVEOLARIZATION

Branching morphogenesis is the primary developmental program that establishes the conducting airways of the lung, but it is important to remember that alveolarization is the developmental program that will establish the large surface area involved in gas exchange (Galambos and Demello, 2008). This process will result in a 20-fold increase in surface area between birth (with between 0 and 50 million alveoli) and adulthood (>300 million alveoli). Primitive saccules develop low ridges (primary septa) that subdivide the saccule into an alveolar duct containing primary alveoli and outpouchings between the ridges (secondary septa/crests) that establish secondary alveoli (Figure 42-3). Regions destined for secondary septation exhibit increased elastin deposition (Mariani et al, 1997), and elastin localizes to the tips of the secondary crests as they form. Septae contain a connective tissue core separating two capillary membranes, suggesting that the septum is formed by the folding of a capillary on itself, as mentioned previously. Septation also leads to the development of the pores of Kohn, allowing gaseous continuity between acini. The process of alveolarization is poorly understood, but is receiving much attention because of observations that infants who die after severe bronchopulmonary dysplasia exhibit alveolar simplification with little evidence of secondary septation. It remains unclear to what extent the process of alveolarization is disrupted by preterm birth and whether this developmental program can be resurrected after preterm birth in the absence or presence of lung injury.

INTERDEPENDENCE OF ALVEOLAR AND VASCULAR DEVELOPMENT

Recent evidence suggests that the pulmonary capillary bed actively promotes normal alveolar development and contributes to the maintenance of alveolar structures throughout life (Thebaud and Abman, 2007). The observation that combined abnormalities in the airways and vasculature occur in bronchopulmonary dysplasia supports this hypothesis. Intraacinar arteries and veins continue to develop after birth by angiogenesis as long as alveoli continue to increase in number and size. This process may be reciprocal because vascular growth around the distal airspaces suggests an inductive influence from the alveolar epithelial cells as well.

MOLECULAR BASIS FOR LUNG DEVELOPMENT

The developmental processes that contribute to lung organogenesis are under the regulation of interdependent signaling pathways mediated by secreted growth factors that are themselves under the control of large networks of transcription factors controlling gene expression. Gene regulatory networks common to other organs that depend on branching morphogenesis during development, most notably in the kidney and mammary gland, are also found in the lung. Selected regulatory networks are highlighted in the following sections to illustrate these systems. For more detailed reading, additional references are provided (Kaplan, 2000; Kumar et al, 2005; van Tuyl and Post, 2000; Warburton et al, 2000;).

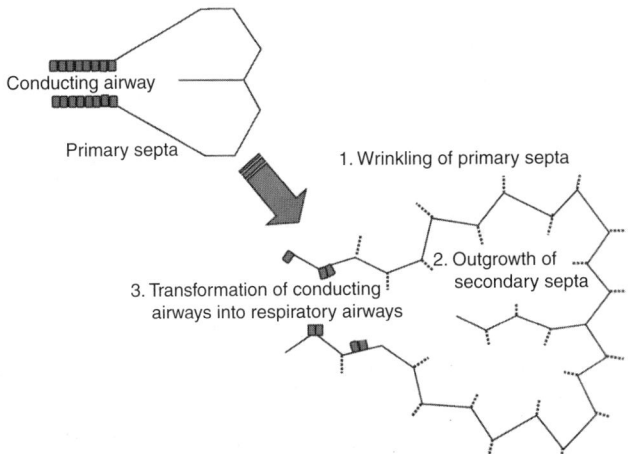

FIGURE 42-3 Development of primary versus secondary alveoli. The development of secondary alveoli from primary alveoli allows for expansion of the total surface area available for gas exchange. Continued growth of primary septa results in a wrinkled appearance that is followed by elastin deposition at points where secondary septae, also known as secondary crests, will form by an in-folding of the epithelium that pulls underlying capillaries into the septum. Finally the more proximal epithelium becomes differentiated into alveolar epithelial cells capable of participating in gas exchange. Shaded cells represent bronchiolar epithelial cells.

GROWTH FACTORS IN LUNG DEVELOPMENT

The initiation of branching morphogenesis is the result of the interplay of signals between the developing lung epithelial tube and its surrounding mesenchyme. Central to this process is the family of fibroblast growth factors (FGFs) that are produced and secreted by mesenchymal cells, and bind to receptors on the plasma membrane of epithelial cells, establishing a system of mesenchymal-epithelial cross talk. In particular, the growth factor FGF10 secreted by mesenchymal cells binds to the receptor FGFR2b on nearby epithelial cells. This signal will be strongest in the closest epithelial cells because of a gradient that develops with diffusion of the secreted FGF10. Binding of ligand to receptor results in signal transduction within the epithelial cell that induces expression of a group of genes via the mitogen-activated protein kinase pathway. One of the genes induced by FGF10/FGFR2b signaling, Sprouty 2 (*Spry2*), inhibits the mitogen-activated protein kinase pathway, resulting in inhibition further FGF10/FGFR2b signaling. Therefore a signal propagated by the mesenchyme has an effect that is subsequently dampened within the epithelial cell. Examination of genes expressed early in the formation of a branch point in response to FGF10 revealed a large number of genes that regulate cell adhesion, cytoskeleton, and cell polarity—all essential elements of cell migration (Lu et al, 2005). Surprisingly, bud initiation was not associated with the expression of genes that promote proliferation, which appears to be more important for branch elongation. Still, animals expressing reduced FGF10 develop pulmonary hypoplasia with reduced numbers of large airways (Abler et al, 2009; Ramasamy et al, 2007). Furthermore, increased FGF10 signaling during fetal lung development in mice by intrapulmonary injections of recombinant FGF10 produced cystic structures with epithelial characteristics dependent

on the location of the injection: proximally with Clara cells, distally with alveolar type 2 cells (Gonzaga et al, 2008). These data provide strong evidence that FGF10 signaling has diverse responses—from initiation of branching to differentiation of epithelial cells—depending on the temporal or spatial context of signaling.

Like branching morphogenesis, lung vascular development is a complex and highly organized process that requires multiple vascular signaling molecules to interact in a specific temporospatial sequence. Vascular endothelial growth factor (VEGF) is a critical growth factor in angiogenesis and vasculogenesis. The expression of the VEGF ligand by epithelial cells and VEGF receptors by endothelial cells of the developing human fetal lung reinforces the interdependence of the airspace and vascular development. The expression of VEGF mRNA and protein is localized to the epithelial cells at the distal tips of developing lung branches, and expression levels increase with time (Galambos and Demello, 2007; Hislop, 2005). VEGF gene expression is induced in epithelial cells by the hypoxic environment of the growing fetal lung through the actions of the oxygen-sensing hypoxia-inducible factor (HIF) family of transcription factors. From the single VEGF gene, five different VEGF protein isoforms can be produced, although VEGFA (VEGF165) is the most studied. Each isoform has different affinities for each of the three VEGF receptors (Flt-1/VEGFR1, Flk-1/KDR/VEGFR2, and Flt-4/VEGFR3). Vascular endothelial cells express primarily VEGFR-1 and VEGFR-2, whereas VEGFR-3 is on the plasma membrane of the lymphatic endothelium. VEGF receptors are expressed on the plasma membrane endothelial cells surrounding the developing airways from very early in gestation, and expression of VEGFR2/Flk1 is considered the earliest marker of an endothelial progenitor cell. In vitro and in vivo experiments have shown that VEGFA induces endothelial cell proliferation and migration, both key elements of vascular sprouting, as well as tube formation through interactions with VEGFR2. VEGFR1 appears to have more importance in transforming primitive endothelial tubes into more stable vascular networks, in part by reducing endothelial proliferation through downregulation of VEGF production. The embryonic lethality of animals with reduced VEGF expression attests to the critical importance of VEGF and VEGFR signaling to vascular development in the fetus, though not limited to the developing pulmonary vasculature.

TRANSCRIPTION FACTORS IN LUNG DEVELOPMENT

The ligand-receptor interactions important to branching morphogenesis and pulmonary vascular development are in part determined by the actions of transcription factors on facilitating or reducing gene expression. Transcription factors are also critical in the differentiation of the lung epithelium from the most rudimentary lung bud out to the type 1 and 2 alveolar epithelial cells. The more important transcription factors in epithelial cell determination in the lung include the Gli, hepatocyte nuclear factor (HNF), GATA, and Hox families of transcription factors (Kumar et al, 2005; Warburton et al, 2000).

The most important transcription factor in the lung is thyroid transcription factor-1 (TTF-1), a product of the *Nkx2.1* gene. TTF-1 is considered a master regulator of lung development, as transgenic mice null for *Nkx2.1* exhibit complete absence of lung branching. However, *Nkx2.1* also has a prominent role in establishing cell fate proximally to distally along the branching lung epithelium. TTF-1 expression is detected as early as 11 weeks' gestation in humans, and continues to be expressed by epithelial cells at the distal tips of the branching lung epithelium, ultimately becoming more restricted to Clara cells and alveolar type 2 cells. TTF-1 is critical for the expression of genes that are unique to differentiated epithelium, such as CC10 expression in Clara cells and surfactant proteins in alveolar type 2 cells. DNA binding sites for TTF-1 are found in the promoter regions of all four surfactant proteins, CC10, and *Nkx2.1* itself, creating a positive feedback loop for sustained TTF-1 expression. TTF-1 function is highly dependent on phosphorylation of critical amino acids, although it remains unclear which kinase is involved in this process (DeFelice et al, 2003). Interestingly, VEGFA expression is reduced in animals unable to phosphorylate TTF-1, providing another important link between epithelial and vascular development. TTF-1 is itself regulated by other transcription factors that bind to the promoter region of the *Nkx2.1* gene, specifically HNF-3β and GATA-6. Therefore the ability of networks of transcription factors to bind to gene regulatory elements of DNA in a coordinated fashion during fetal lung development enables the temporospatial expression of growth factor networks that foster branching morphogenesis, the process of differentiation that ultimately gives rise to the approximately 40 cell types that constitute the human lung, as well as critical coordination of both epithelial and vascular development.

OTHER TOPICS IN LUNG DEVELOPMENT

DEVELOPMENT OF PULMONARY HOST DEFENSE

The adult human lung takes in approximately 7 L/min of air contaminated with a variety potential pathogens that can cause epithelial injury. The continuous exposure of the epithelial surface of the conducting airway to inhaled pathogens requires the presence of an efficient innate immune response system to prevent infections. The proximal and distal airway epithelia have a major role in clearing pathogens by secreting antimicrobial as well as antiinflammatory molecules. Components of mucociliary clearance appear as early as 11 weeks' gestation with the differentiation of ciliated epithelial cells and the expression of mucus in mucus-secreting goblet cells within the epithelium and submucosal glands, as discussed previously. The number of goblet cells peaks in mid-gestation (30% to 35% of total airway epithelial cells), decreasing toward term to levels lower than in adults, and then increasing after birth. The postnatal increase in goblet cells occurs after preterm birth as well, giving premature infants a greater number of goblet cells than in term infants. Therefore premature

infants are prone to more mucus production in smaller airways than are term infants, and premature infants have relatively fewer ciliated cells to assist in mobilization of secretions.

A number of microbial defense molecules are produced and secreted by epithelial cells into the airways (Bartlett et al, 2008). They include lysozyme, C-reactive protein, lactoferrin, collectins, β-defensins, and the only human member of the cathelicidin family, hCAP-18/LL-37 (Hiemstra, 2007). Two lung collectins were originally identified as surfactant-related proteins—the hydrophilic surfactant proteins SP-A and SP-D. Although originally identified as products secreted by epithelial cells lining airways (Clara cells) and alveoli (type 2 cells), SP-A and SP-D have been found in other sites associated with epithelial surfaces exposed to the external environment (Haagsman et al, 2008). They interact with microorganisms, inflammatory cells, and leukocytes to facilitate clearance of microorganisms from the airspace, and they modulate allergic responses.

The basis for the interactions of the lung collectins with microbes and antigens centers on the binding of sugars by the carbohydrate recognition domains of these proteins (Wright, 2005). Both collectins bind a variety of fungi and *Pneumocystis carinii*, and they have an important role in inhibiting a variety of respiratory viruses, including influenza A and respiratory syncytial virus. Differences in the structure of the carbohydrate recognition domain provide SP-A and SP-D with altered affinities for different sugar molecules, allowing complementary functions and improving the diversity of microbial interactions. Interactions with gram-negative organisms frequently depends on the ability of SP-A and SP-D to bind lipopolysaccharide, whereas the mechanism of SP-A interactions with gram-positive organisms, including group B beta-hemolytic streptococci, are not as clear.

The lung collectins also modulate the functions of a variety of immune cells, including macrophages, neutrophils, eosinophils, and lymphocytes (Wright, 2005). In addition to opsonizing microorganisms, functions of the lung collectins include stimulating chemotaxis of macrophages and neutrophils, enhancing cytokine production by macrophages and eosinophils, attenuating lymphocyte responses by inhibiting T cell proliferation, and modulating the production of reactive oxygen and nitrogen species used in killing microorganisms.

Like the hydrophobic surfactant proteins, SP-A and SP-D exhibit both developmental and hormonal regulation of expression (Mendelson, 2000). In human fetuses, SP-A mRNA is undetectable before 20 weeks' gestation, and SP-A protein is first detectable in amniotic fluid by 30 weeks' gestation, increasing toward term (Pryhuber et al, 1991). In humans, SP-A gene expression is induced by cAMP and glucocorticoids, although the response to glucocorticoids in biphasic, showing attenuation at higher doses. Retinoids, insulin, and growth factors such as TGF-β and TNF-α inhibit SP-A gene expression. Like SP-A, SP-D levels in human lung are low during the second trimester (Dulkerian et al, 1996), are detectable in amniotic fluid, and increase toward term (Whitsett, 2005). Levels of both SP-A and SP-D increase markedly in the first days after preterm birth.

DEVELOPMENT OF DETOXIFICATION SYSTEMS

Although essential to cellular processes, oxygen concentrations beyond the physiologic limits may be hazardous to cells. The lung is particularly susceptible to reactive forms of oxygen and free radicals, because it is the organ with the highest exposure to atmospheric oxygen. The fetal lung is exposed to oxygen tensions of 20 to 25 mm Hg in utero, and the transition to air breathing is associated with a fourfold to sevenfold increase in oxygen tension, presenting a significant oxidant stress. Oxygen free radicals arise from endogenous production through metabolic reactions, or by exogenous exposure, from air pollutants and cigarette smoke, and they can result in lung injury from oxidation of proteins, DNA, and lipids. Therefore it is imperative for the lung to develop an antioxidant detoxification system, and for this system to be functional upon the fetal transition to air-breathing.

Oxygen free radicals are highly toxic substances. Superoxide, produced by the reduction of molecular oxygen by the addition of an electron, is formed by all cells and occurs in particularly high concentrations in phagocytic cells to facilitate the killing of microorganisms. Hydrogen peroxide is generated from the transfer of a single electron to superoxide, and hydroxyl radicals are generated from the interaction of hydrogen peroxide with superoxide. The free electrons of free radicals interact with membrane lipids, resulting in lipid peroxidation, with sulfhydryl and other groups on exposed amino acids in proteins and with DNA causing direct damage. These lipid, protein, and nucleic acid modifications damage airway and alveolar epithelial cells as well as capillary endothelial cells, leading to altered epithelial integrity, interstitial and airspace edema, and infiltration of inflammatory cells. Increased reactive oxygen species levels have also been implicated in initiating inflammatory responses through the activation of transcription factors such as NFκB and AP-1, signal transduction pathways, and chromatin remodeling that foster the expression of proinflammatory mediators (Rahman et al, 2006).

Oxygen can have additional effects beyond the direct toxicity of free radicals. Oxygen levels regulate the activity of plasminogen activator inhibitor-1 and other protease-antiprotease systems within the airspaces, thereby modulating the destructive effects of proteases elaborated from inflammatory cells. Oxygen can also regulate cellular growth responses by altering the secretion of growth factors and DNA synthesis, generally through oxygen-sensing transcription factors, such as the HIF family.

Antioxidants attenuate the effects of oxygen free radicals in the lungs, and in the lung there are both nonenzymatic and enzymatic antioxidants. The major nonenzymatic antioxidants are glutathione (GSH), vitamins C (ascorbate) and E (primarily α-tocopherol), β-carotene, and uric acid. Enzymatic antioxidants include superoxide dismutases 1, 2, and 3, catalase, and a variety of peroxidases. Animal studies indicate that many of the antioxidant enzymes are induced before term delivery, and limited data suggest that the same is true of human fetuses (Weinberger et al, 2002). Premature animals fail to induce antioxidant enzymes in response to oxidative lung injury (Thibeault, 2000). Therefore preterm infants are significantly more compromised in antioxidant defenses and, because of the need for oxygen in the treatment of respiratory distress syndrome, they are more susceptible to oxygen toxicity.

NOVEL CONCEPTS IN LUNG DEVELOPMENT

STEM AND PROGENITOR CELLS IN THE LUNG

The ability of lung epithelium to replace cells damaged from normal aging or injury has become the focus of recent attention (Rawlins et al, 2008; Warburton et al, 2008). Stem cells are undifferentiated and have an unlimited capacity for self-renewal. Asymmetric divisions allow for self-renewal through one daughter cell while enabling the other daughter cell to become more terminally differentiated. Progenitor cells are more committed, and although capable of self-renewal, they have more restricted cell fates. Thus far, three cell types in the lung have been identified as progenitor cells, having the capacity for self-renewal and for replacement of a variety of specialized lung epithelial cells. Basal cells in large airways and submucosal glands, identified by the expression of Trp63/p63 and cytokeratin 5, are able to self-renew and give rise to ciliated and secretory cells. Clara cells in smaller airways, identified by the expression of CC10/Scgb1a1, seem to be more committed progenitor cells because they are able to self-renew or differentiate into ciliated cells. A subset of Clara cells at the bronchoalveolar duct junction are both CC10/Scgb1a1 and SP-C positive, and thus have the potential to produce either Clara cells or alveolar type 2 cells. The most limited lung epithelial progenitor cell is the alveolar type 2 cell, which divides rapidly to reestablish epithelial continuity in damaged alveoli and then transdifferentiates into alveolar type 1 cells. The mesenchymal progenitor cells that provide for vascular and muscular components of the developing lung have been studied less. Candidate cells have been identified that give rise to endothelial cells in the process of vasculogenesis and airway smooth muscle cells along the branching lung epithelial tubes.

Evidence for the existence of stem-progenitor cells in the lung is strong, but limited largely to mouse models of lung development and lung repair; therefore extrapolation to humans should be done with caution. The capacity for self-renewal is tantalizing, but it means that such cells have a risk for autonomous growth such as cancer. Controversy exists around the potential to harness these populations of cells as a means for correcting errors in lung development (pulmonary hypoplasia), genetic diseases of the lung (cystic fibrosis), and abnormal repair of injured lungs (bronchopulmonary dysplasia).

EPITHELIAL TO MESENCHYMAL TRANSITION

Fibrosis often occurs as the result of severe injury to the lung and has historically been a component of bronchopulmonary dysplasia (BPD). Emerging evidence suggests that expansion of fibroblast populations in fibrotic lesions is not simply the result of increased proliferation of local fibroblast populations, rather the transformation of epithelial cells into mesenchymal components, a process known as *epithelial-mesenchymal transition* (EMT) (Guarino

TABLE 42-4   Potential Effects of Premature Birth on Lung Development and Maturation

Event	Effect of Preterm Birth	Potential Consequences
Development of conducting airways	Branching: no effect; completed to the level of the respiratory bronchi by 24 wk gestation Tone: increased secondary to lung disease in part reflecting developmental deficiency of nitric oxide	None Increased airways resistance
Alveolarization	Variable depending on timing of delivery and severity of lung disease; may also be compromised by excess glucocorticoids	Reduced lung growth and lung surface area with increased alveolar size; impaired pulmonary function
Development of alveolocapillary membrane	Minimal, reaches adult diameter by 24 wk gestation; glucocorticoids induce precocious thinning	Gas exchange largely dependent upon surface area, not alveolocapillary diameter
Type II cell differentiation	Variable immaturity and deficient surfactant production depending on timing of delivery; improved with antenatal glucocorticoids	Developmental deficiency of surfactant content and composition results in RDS
Type I cell differentiation	Variable depending on timing of delivery; cells develop from type II cells	Gas exchange largely dependant upon surface area
Hydrophobic surfactant proteins (SP-B, SP-C)	Variable depending on timing of delivery and other factors, such as infection, that can impair gene transcription	High alveolar surface tension; RDS
Hydrophilic surfactant proteins (SP-A, SP-D)	Variable depending on timing of delivery; both proteins appear relatively late in third trimester	Comprised host defense: ability to clear microorganisms from airways, alveolar space, or both; impaired ability to modulate inflammatory responses
Clara cell differentiation	Variable depending on timing of delivery; these cells appear in middle 2nd trimester, but antioxidant products appear late in 3rd trimester	Impaired antioxidant and antimicrobial defenses; may contribute to chronic lung disease and pneumonia
Induction of antioxidant systems	Variable depending on timing of delivery; expression of antioxidants occurs late in third trimester	Lung injury from oxidant stress exacerbated by need for increased oxygen; may contribute to chronic lung disease
Mucociliary clearance	Variable depending on timing of delivery; goblet cells decrease in number toward term	Increased mucous production may obstruct small airways
Development of the pulmonary capillary bed	Variable depending on timing of delivery in parallel to alveolar development	Variable degrees of impaired gas exchange commensurate with impaired alveologenesis and any superimposed lung injury; pulmonary hypertension
Pulmonary arteries	Variable depending on presence and severity of associated lung disease	Pulmonary hypertension associated with chronic lung disease
Fetal lung liquid	Fluid loss: variable effects depending on magnitude and duration of fluid loss (i.e., prolonged premature rupture of membranes) as well as timing of delivery Fluid retention: variable effects depending on timing of delivery, because hormone surges near term and in labor promote reabsorption before delivery	Pulmonary hypoplasia Transient tachypnea of the newborn
Fetal breathing movements	Variable depending on timing of delivery, but also depending on maternal exposure to substances that reduce fetal breathing movements	Unlikely to have effects in preterm infants unless coexisting conditions severely limit fetal breathing
Respiratory drive	Variable depending on timing of delivery	Apnea of prematurity

RDS, Respiratory distress syndrome.

et al, 2009; Thiery and Sleeman, 2006). EMT is an essential part of gastrulation and the development of cardiac valves. Neural crest cells are the best model system for EMT, because these epithelial cells must lose their local attachments and travel long distances before locating their final niche and differentiating accordingly. The evidence is clear that the changes in cell phenotype characteristic of EMT—from sedentary, interconnected epithelial cell expressing epithelial marker proteins to mobile, proliferative mesenchymal cell expression markers of fibroblasts and secreting collagen and other components of extracellular matrix—are under the control of local growth factors. In the lung, the most prominent growth factor in EMT associated with pulmonary fibrosis is TGF-β, a growth factor essential for normal branching morphogenesis during early lung development.

It remains uncertain whether EMT has a similarly important role in lung development as it does in cardiac development, and whether EMT alone is important to the abnormal repair response to lung injury. EMT has the potential to reduce epithelial populations, resulting in lung destruction, while expanding mesenchymal fibroblast pools and enhancing local matrix deposition that reduces lung elasticity. Many of the models of EMT are derived from lung cancer cell lines or mouse models, limiting their applicability to humans. However, improved understanding of the processes controlling EMT could lead to novel therapies for limiting or reversing pulmonary fibrosis after lung injury. Furthermore, given the potential for EMT to contribute to lung destruction, a more common feature of the "new BPD," early events in EMT may be particularly important targets of preventive therapy in premature infants.

ROLE OF miRNA IN LUNG DEVELOPMENT AND MATURATION

Regulation of normal development and consequences of abnormal development are at the heart of understanding the implications of preterm birth and developing potential protective lung therapies. The central tenet of DNA to RNA to protein is being challenged by new epigenetic mechanisms—histone modifications, modification of DNA and RNA, silencing RNA, and micro RNA (miRNA)—for regulating gene expression. The evidence that miRNA has an important role in normal fetal development is strong (Nana-Sinkam et al, 2009). miRNAs are small, noncoding RNAs (generally 19 to 25 nucleotides long) found within cells that target genes for RNA degradation or inhibition of protein synthesis. There are more than 500 recognized miRNA, some of which are particularly enriched in lung cell populations. MiRNAs are generated from a process that begins in the nucleus. Long primary miRNA are transcribed, processed, and exported from the nucleus, followed by further cytoplasmic maturation before the final miRNA is able to interact with regions of messenger RNA, usually in the 3' untranslated region of RNA that extends beyond the RNA sequence used for protein translation.

Emerging evidence indicates that miRNA is essential for normal lung development, because targeted deletion of Dicer, a key enzyme in miRNA processing, results in abnormal airway development and excessive apoptosis in the lungs. The miR-17-92 cluster of miRNA is highly expressed in embryonic mouse lung, decreasing into adulthood as lung development progresses. Altered expression of the miRNA cluster miR-17-92 suggests a primary role for these miRNA in maintaining a population of undifferentiated lung epithelium during lung development. Because of their role in regulating developmental and pathologic processes, miRNAs are increasingly seen as targets for therapeutic interventions. Obstacles to miRNAs as therapeutic agents are similar to obstacles encountered in other gene therapies, including mode of delivery, cell and tissue specificity, and the potential for off-target effects.

SUMMARY

Lung branching morphogenesis is coordinated with pulmonary vascular development to provide a large surface area and thin alveolocapillary membrane for adequate gas exchange in the transition to air breathing and to meet the needs of a growing infant and child. Although maturation occurs late in fetal lung development, it is similarly critical in the transition to air breathing. Although the fetal lung developmental program requires an array of transcription factors, hormones, and growth factors promoting branching morphogenesis, lung growth is equally dependent on intact neural input to modulate fetal breathing, stability of an appropriately sized thorax, and the presence of adequate lung and amniotic fluid. Furthermore the maturation of the host defense and detoxification systems minimize the effects of increased oxygen tension and exposure to potential pathogens accompanying the transition to air breathing. Premature birth affects all these functions as illustrated in Table 42-4. Bronchopulmonary dysplasia is the net result of multiple injuries to the underdeveloped lungs of premature newborns that compromise postnatal growth and development, and thus impairing function. Integrated approaches to therapy that reflect the interdependency of these lung functions have the most promise for minimizing the effects of premature birth on childhood and, ultimately, adult lung function.

SUGGESTED READINGS

Burri PH: Structural aspects of postnatal lung development: alveolar formation and growth, *Biol Neonate* 89:313-322, 2006.

Galambos C, Demello DE: Regulation of alveologenesis: clinical implications of impaired growth, *Pathology* 40:124-140, 2008.

Hislop A: Developmental biology of the pulmonary circulation, *Paediatr Respir Rev* 6:35-43, 2005.

Jeffrey PK: The development of large and small airways, *Am J Respir Crit Care Med* 157:S174-S180, 1998.

Kaplan F: Molecular determinants of fetal lung organogenesis, *Mol Genet Metab* 71:321-341, 2000.

Kitterman JA: The effects of mechanical forces on fetal lung growth,, *Clin Perinatol* 23:727-740, 1996.

Kumar VH, Lakshminrusimha S, El Abiad MT, et al: Growth factors in lung development, *Adv Clin Chem* 40:261-316, 2005.

Mallampalli RK, Acarregui MJ, Snyder JM: Differentiation of the alveolar epithelium in the fetal lung. In McDonald JA, editor: *Lung growth and development*, vol 100, New York, 1997, Marcel Dekker, pp 119-162.

Mendelson CR: Role of transcription factors in fetal lung development and surfactant protein gene expression, *Annu Rev Physiol* 62:875-915, 2000.

Thibeault DW: The precarious antioxidant defenses of the preterm infant, *Am J Perinatol* 17:167-181, 2000.

Warburton D, Schwarz M, Tefft D, et al: The molecular basis of lung morphogenesis, *Mech Dev* 92:55-81, 2000.

Zuo YY, Veldhuizen RA, Neumann AW, et al: Current perspectives in pulmonary surfactant–inhibition, enhancement and evaluation, *Biochim Biophys Acta* 1778:1947-1977, 2008.

Complete references used in this text can be found online at www.expertconsult.com

CONTROL OF BREATHING

Estelle B. Gauda and Richard J. Martin

The developmental aspects of respiratory control are of considerable interest to physiologists and clinicians for a multitude of reasons. The transition from fetal to neonatal life requires a rapid conversion from intermittent fetal respiratory activity not associated with gas exchange to continuous breathing upon which gas exchange is dependent. In addition, the circuitry that regulates respiratory control serves as a unique link between the maturing lung and brain. The term infant has the repertoire of respiratory and cardiovascular responses that meets his or her metabolic demands during wakefulness, sleeping, crying, and feeding even though the breathing pattern may be punctuated with apneic pauses and sighs (augmented breaths), and the neurocircuitry that controls breathing is not completely developed. In some term infants who appear well, developmental abnormalities in the neurocircuitry and neurochemistry that regulate respiratory rhythmogenesis can lead to profound disorders of breathing, placing them at increased risk for sudden death. Infants who have died of sudden infant death syndrome (SIDS), and those infants with central congenital hypoventilation and Rett syndrome, have provided a window of opportunity for careful epidemiologic, genetic, neurochemical, and anatomic study that has allowed researchers to better understand which genes regulate the development of the respiratory system and how environmental factors in fetal and early neonatal life may adversely affect normal development.

The infant who is born prematurely has also provided a unique opportunity to observe the natural developmental trajectory of respiratory control. Breathing in the most premature infants is akin to fetal breathing, which is episodic, punctuated by periods of disturbingly long apneic pauses interspersed with frequent periods of hyperventilation and sighs (augmented breaths). The purpose of fetal breathing movements is not gas exchange, rather it is lung development by inducing sufficient stretch of the chest wall. For the infant who is born prematurely, the frequent apneic events and hypoventilation associated with oxygen desaturations and bradycardia are of significant concern. The purpose of this chapter is to present what is currently known about the neuroanatomy, neurocircuitry, and neurochemistry that controls breathing during development to better understand how infants breathe, why premature infants have apnea of prematurity, why term infants have apnea of infancy, and how genetic errors and environmental influences modify mechanisms that control breathing during fetal and early neonatal life.

ANIMAL MODELS OF CONTROL OF BREATHING

Much of our understanding of basic mechanisms that lead to a stable respiratory pattern is derived from animal studies, both adult and newborn. Earlier studies used the newborn pig, dog, and cat, as well as fetal and newborn sheep models, to better understand developmental physiology, and much has been gained from these models. However, a more detailed understanding of the neuroanatomy, neurocircuitry, and neurochemistry has been obtained using in vitro models from newborn rats and mice. Of particular relevance, the stage of respiratory development of the rat born at term is similar to that of the human infant born at 25 to 29 weeks' gestation; therefore the newborn rodent model is applicable to breathing in the premature infant. Studies using either of two in vitro models (brainstem slices that include the area that contains the "pacemaker cells mediating rhythmogenesis" and the isolated brainstem spinal cord preparation from fetal and newborn rodents) have led to an explosion of information about all aspects of maturation of respiratory control within the last decade (Richter and Spyer, 2001). Because the stability and viability of the in vitro preparations are best when tissues are used from late embryonic or early postnatal rodents (within first week of postnatal life), data from these in vitro models are relevant to respiratory control during early development.

OVERVIEW OF RESPIRATORY CONTROL

The leading hypothesis regarding autonomic control of breathing is that respiratory rhythm is generated from a core group of synaptically coupled excitatory neurons in the brainstem located in the pre-Bötzinger complex (PBC). These neurons depolarize during the three phases of respiration: inspiration, postinspiration, and expiration. The timing of the respiratory cycle is controlled by inhibitory interneurons that discharge during specific phases of the respiratory cycle. Collectively this complex network of neurons is called the *central pattern generator* (Duffin, 2004; Smith et al, 2009).

Inspiratory, postinspiratory, and expiratory neurons depolarize with each phase of the respiratory cycle coincident with activity motoneurons innervating the muscles of respiration (Figure 43-1). Whereas inspiration is always associated with phrenic nerve activity and contraction of the diaphragm, the first phase of expiration (E1), known as *postinspiratory activity*, can be associated with phrenic nerve activity, and the second phase of expiration (E2) is not (see Figure 43-1).

With development, the intrinsic properties and neurotransmitter profiles of respiratory-related neurons and synaptic inputs from (1) higher brain centers (frontal and insular cortex, hypothalamus, reticular activating system and amygdala, (2) mechanoreceptors in the lungs and upper airways, (3) peripheral chemoreceptors in the carotid body, and (4) central chemoreceptors on the ventral medullary surface modify the excitability of respiratory-related

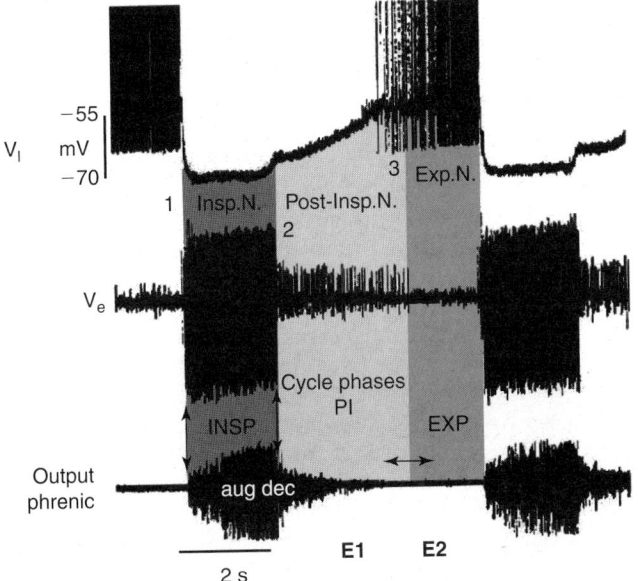

FIGURE 43-1 Simultaneous triple recordings of electrical activities of the main populations of respiratory neurons: *1*, an inspiratory neuron (large spikes, middle tracing); *2*, a postinspiratory neuron (small spikes, middle tracing); *3*, an expiratory neuron (top tracing) and the phrenic nerve (bottom tracing). Note the augmenting (aug) activity of the phrenic nerve during inspiration and the decrementing (dec) activity of the phrenic nerve during the postinspiratory (PI) phase of the respiratory cycle. The postinspiratory phase is the first phase of expiration (E1) and is associated with phrenic nerve activity. In the second phase of expiration (E2), the phrenic nerve is silent. *(Reproduced from Richter DW, Spyer KM: Studying rhythmogenesis of breathing: comparison of in vivo and in vitro models, Trends Neurosci 24:464-472, 2001.)*

neurons. In addition, the intrinsic "sensing" properties of mechanoreceptors and chemoreceptors are also changing. Last, the integrated respiratory output is also dependent on the strength of the synapse between the premotor respiratory neurons and the respiratory motoneurons innervating the diaphragm, intercostals and muscles of the upper airway, and the corresponding neuromuscular junctions (Figure 43-2). The effect of development on respiratory motoneurons and the neuromuscular junction will not be discussed in depth in this chapter; for further discussion of this topic the reader is referred to two excellent reviews (Greer and Funk, 2005; Mantilla and Sieck, 2008).

MUSCLES OF RESPIRATION

The muscles of respiration include the pump muscles (diaphragm, intercostal muscles, and abdominal muscles) and muscles of the upper airway (alae nares, pharyngeal muscles, and laryngeal muscles). Upper airway muscles modulate the rate of inspiratory and expiratory airflow. During the inspiratory phase of the respiratory cycle the diaphragm, external intercostals (in infants), and posterior cricoarytenoid (laryngeal dilator) contract. During the postinspiratory phase, the diaphragm and the thyroarytenoid (laryngeal constrictor) contract. Diaphragmatic and thyroarytenoid postinspiratory activity is common in newborns, both human (Eichenwald et al, 1993) and animals (England et al, 1985). Because the chest wall of newborn infants, particularly premature infants, is highly compliant, diaphragmatic and laryngeal postinspiratory activity retards expiration to maintain functional residual

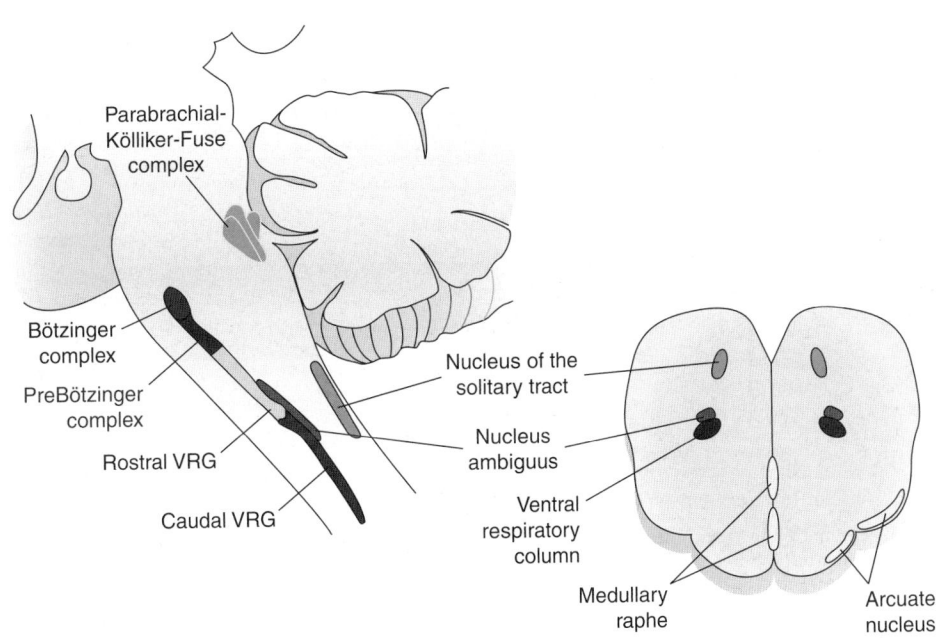

FIGURE 43-2 Schematic illustrating the anatomic relationship between the regions in the human brainstem that compose the respiratory network. These regions include specialized neurons in the dorsolateral pons (parabrachial and Kölliker–Fuse nuclei) nucleus of the solitary tract (nTS), and ventral respiratory column. The ventral respiratory column is organized rostrocaudally extending from the level just below the facial nucleus to the C1 level of cervical cord. The ventral respiratory column consists of the Bötzinger complex, pre-Bötzinger complex, and the rostral and caudal ventral respiratory groups (VRGs). Vagal motor neurons of the nucleus ambiguus innervate the laryngeal muscles. The medullary raphe, arcuate nucleus, located just underneath the ventral medullary surface, contains neurons that depolarize in response to hypercapnia and hypoxia. The retrotrapazoid nucleus (not shown) are CO_2/H^+ chemosensors, and is located rostrally below the facial nucleus on the ventral medullary surface. *(Modified with permission from Benarroch EE: Brainstem respiratory control: substrates of respiratory failure of multiple system atrophy, Mov Disord 22:155-161, 2007.)*

capacity. This postinspiratory activity is often audible, known as *grunting*, and is heard in infants with low lung-volume disease states, such as surfactant deficiency and atelectasis. As outlined previously, the second phase of expiration (E2) is often quiescent regarding muscle activity; the diaphragm relaxes and the lungs recoil. During forced expiration often seen during exercise and significant hypercapnia, the internal intercostals and abdominal muscles may contract during E2. Brainstem nuclei that are involved in the control of upper airway muscles include the upper airway motoneurons of the nucleus ambiguous, the dorsal motor nucleus of the vagus, and the hypoglossal nucleus (Jordan, 2001; Nunez-Abades et al, 1992). Projections from respiratory-related neurons synapse onto these upper airway motoneurons, thereby regulating the activity of these nerves and muscles during the respiratory cycle.

RESPIRATORY CENTER NEUROANATOMY

As shown in the anatomic illustration (see Figure 43-2) and the schematic (Figure 43-3), the respiratory-related neurons are located in three main areas in the brainstem: (1) the dorsal respiratory group within the nucleus tractus solitarii, (2) the ventral respiratory column (VRC) that extends from the facial nucleus to the ventrolateral medulla at the spinal-medullary junction, and (3) the pontine respiratory group within the dorsolateral pons (Alheid and McCrimmon, 2008). The VRC can be subdivided into a rostral part, involved in rhythmogenesis, and a caudal part involved in pattern formation. The rostral VRC contains both the rostral ventral respiratory group (VRG), which contains a large proportion of bulbospinal inspiratory neurons that project directly to the phrenic and external intercostal motoneurons, and the caudal VRG, which contains bulbospinal expiratory neurons that project to abdominal and internal intercostal motoneurons. Bulbospinal neurons are neurons that originate in the medulla and synapse onto motoneurons in the spinal column. Of importance, within the rostral VRC are two areas that are essential to formation of respiratory rhythm: the Bötzinger complex, and PBC. The Bötzinger complex contains propriobulbar expiratory neurons that provide strong inhibitory inputs onto inspiratory and expiratory bulbospinal neurons in the VRC. Propriobulbar neurons are neurons originating in the brainstem that send projections to other neurons in the brainstem. The PBC contains a core group of synaptically coupled excitatory neurons that have pacemaker properties, similar to the pacemaker cells in the AV node of the heart. These pacemaker cells are rostral to the nucleus

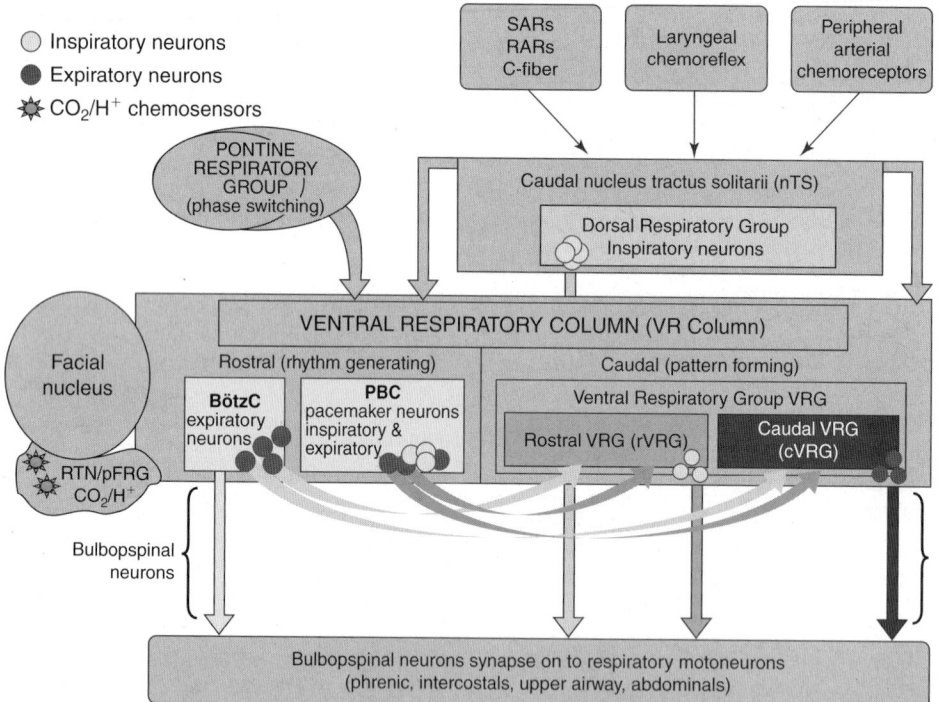

FIGURE 43-3 Simplified schematic illustrating the major pontine-medullary brainstem network controlling respiration and afferent and efferent projections. The pontine respiratory group contains two nuclei that send neuronal connections to respiratory-related neurons in the ventral respiratory column (VRC). The pontine respiratory group mediates phase switching between inspiration and expiration. Within the nucleus tractus solitarii (nTS) are the inspiratory neurons of the dorsal respiratory group with projections to motoneurons in the spinal column. The nTS also receive monosynaptic inputs from vagally mediated reflexes in the lung and upper airways (including slowly adapting receptors [SARs], rapidly adapting receptors [RARs], and C-fibers receptors), laryngeal chemoreceptors, and peripheral arterial chemoreceptors. Projections from second-order neurons in the nTS then synapse on to neurons in the rostral and caudal VRC. The VRC extends from the level of the facial nucleus to C1 in the cervical spinal cord. The rostral VRC is involved in respiratory rhythmogenesis and contains the expiratory neurons of the Bötzinger complex (BötzC) and the pacemakers cells of the pre-Bötzinger complex (PBC). The BötzC and PBC contain propriobulbar neurons that project to inspiratory neurons in the rostral ventral respiratory group (VRG) and expiratory neurons in the caudal VRG. The BötzC also contains bulbospinal neurons that synapse on to phrenic motoneurons in the spinal cord, whereas the PBC only contains propriobulbar neurons. Neurons in the VRG are responsible for shaping the respiratory pattern and receive inputs from second-order neurons in the nTS and from rhythm-generating neurons in the BötzC and PBC. Bulbospinal neurons from the DRG, BötzC, rVRG, and cVRG synapse onto motoneurons that control the activity of the muscles of respiration.

ambiguous, have both intrinsic inspiratory and expiratory bursting properties, and are essential to maintaining respiratory rhythm (Smith et al, 1991). Progressive destruction of the PBC disrupts rhythmogenesis, leading to death in an animal model (Ramirez et al, 1998).

Another important group of neurons are those within the retrotrapezoid nucleus (RTN) located along the ventral medullary surface beneath the facial nucleus (see Figure 43-3). These neurons have chemosensitive properties and depolarize in response to increasing CO_2 and decreasing pH, and they are presumed to synapse on rhythm and pattern generating neurons in the VRC (Guyenet et al, 2008). All these neuronal groups and networks for rhythmogenesis are present in newborn animals born at term (e.g., sheep, cats, pigs) or born prematurely (e.g., rodents) in which rhythmogenesis is well established before birth. Episodic spontaneous fetal breathing movements occur in human fetuses as early as 10 weeks' gestation (de Vries et al, 1985). In rodents, respiratory rhythmogenesis is first detected at embryonic day 15 in rats and day 17 in mice (Thoby-Brisson and Greer, 2008). The emergence of this respiratory related activity in rats is coincident with the characteristic expression of neurokinin 1 receptors of the PBC (Thoby-Brisson and Greer, 2008).

In summary, respiratory rhythm and inspiratory-expiratory patterns emerge from dynamic interactions between: (1) excitatory neuron populations in the PBC and rostral VRG, which are active during inspiration and form the inspiratory motor output; (2) inhibitory neuron populations in the PBC that provide inspiratory inhibition within the network; and (3) inhibitory neuron populations in the Bötzinger complex, which are active during expiration and provide expiratory inhibition within the network and to phrenic motor neurons (see Figure 43-3) (Smith et al, 2009).

NEUROCHEMISTRY MEDIATING RESPIRATORY CONTROL

Glutamate is the major neurotransmitter mediating excitatory synaptic input to brainstem respiratory neurons and respiratory premotor and motor neurons through binding to the α-amino-3-hydroxy-5-methylisoxazole-4-propionic acid kainite (Bonham, 1995) and metabotropic glutamate receptors (Pierrefiche et al, 1994). GABA (gamma-aminobutyric acid) and glycine are the two major inhibitory neurotransmitters mediating inhibitory synaptic input in the respiratory network; they have a key role in pattern generation and termination of inspiratory activity (Haji et al, 2000). GABA (via $GABA_A$ receptors) and glycine (via glycine receptors) mediate fast synaptic inhibition via activation of chloride channels (Bianchi et al, 1995). $GABA_B$ receptors, which are metabotropic G-protein coupled receptors, have a greater role in inhibiting respiratory rhythm in adult mammals (Kerr and Ong, 1995). Throughout development, glutamate always functions as an excitatory neurotransmitter; however, it is not the case that GABA and glycine are always inhibitory neurotransmitters. During early development, GABA and glycine mediate excitatory neurotransmission in many neuronal networks, including the respiratory network (Putnam et al, 2005). The expression of $K^{\pm}$ chloride cotransporters (KCC2 and NKCC2) reduces the intracellular chloride concentrations that

change the effect of GABA binding to $GABA_A$ receptors from depolarizing during late embryonic and early postnatal to hyperpolarizing with maturation (Rivera et al, 1999).

NEUROMODULATION OF RESPIRATORY PATTERN AND RHYTHM

The baseline excitatory and inhibitory influences mediated by glutamate and GABA–glycine, respectively, on major neuronal networks are further altered by many endogenously released neuromodulators that shape and fine tune respiratory pattern and rhythm throughout development, as outlined in Table 43-1. For example, acetylcholine, substance P, cholecystokinin, cholecystokinin (CCK) and thyrotropin-releasing hormone all exert an excitatory drive, whereas opioids and somatostatin exert an inhibitory drive on respiratory-related neurons. Dopamine, adenosine, serotonin, and norepinephrine can have excitatory and inhibitory influences depending on the specific receptors that the neuromodulator binds. Neurons within the PBC that are the kernel of rhythmogenesis are also distinctly identified by being immunopositive for the glutamate transporter, NK1, μ-opioid, and $GABA_B$-receptors. Although these cells are primarily excitatory and release glutamate, they can be modulated by synaptic inputs that release substance P, opioids, and GABA (Doi and Ramirez, 2008). Recently these rhythmogenic neurons have been found to produce, and be excited by, brain-derived neurotrophic factor (Bouvier et al, 2008).

GENETIC MUTATIONS AFFECTING BIOGENIC AMINES

Some neuromodulators may be more critical for supporting respiratory rhythmogenesis than others. By identifying the genetic mutations that are associated with marked abnormalities in respiratory control, a better understanding of the key role of several neuromodulator systems has been elucidated. For example, serotonergic neurons in the caudal medullary raphe nuclei have extensive projections to phrenic and hypoglossal motoneurons, the nucleus tractus solitarii (nTS), the RTN, and the PBC (Pilowsky et al, 1990; Voss et al, 1990). Thus, as reviewed by Kinney et al (2009), the serotonergic system has a significant influence on the modulation and integration of diverse homeostatic functions. Medullary serotonergic neurons are also CO_2 sensitive (Richerson et al, 2001). In genetically modified mice that do not develop medullary serotonergic neurons, CO_2 sensitivity is reduced by 50% (Hodges et al, 2008). Individuals with Prader–Willi syndrome, who may exhibit breathing abnormalities at birth) have mutations in the *Necdin* gene associated with abnormalities in the brainstem serotonergic system (Zanella et al, 2008a). Mice lacking the *Necdin* gene also have abnormal brainstem serotonergic neurochemistry (Zanella et al, 2008b). In some infants who have died of SIDS, disruptions of the brainstem serotonergic system have been identified (Kinney et al, 2009; Paterson et al, 2006b). Abnormalities in norepinephrine production also disrupt normal breathing. Rett syndrome is an X-linked disorder with mutations in the methyl CpG binding protein 2 (*MECP2*) gene. Affected individuals have severe respiratory disturbances that can be fatal. Genetically

TABLE 43-1 Neurotransmitters and Neuromodulators That Mediate Respiratory Rhythm

Neuromodulator	Receptor Subtype	Source of the Endogenous Ligand	Excitatory or Inhibitory on Respiratory Rhythm	Comment
Glutamate	NMDA, AMPA GluR		Excitatory	Major excitatory neurotransmitter
Ach	M3	PAG, LC, X	Excitatory	
NE	α_1-adrenergic	LC	Excitatory	
Serotonin	5-HT_{2A2B}, 5-HT_3, 5-HT_4	Raphe	Excitatory	
Dopamine	Likely D1	PVN, hypothalamus	Excitatory	
ATP	$P2X_2$	Ventral medulla; CO_2/H^+ cells in the RTN	Excitatory	
Adenosine	$P2Y_1$	Ventral medulla	Excitatory	
Substance P	NK1	nTS, NA	Excitatory	
CCK	CCK_1	nTS, raphe	Excitatory	
TRH	TRH-R, R2	raphe	Excitatory	
GABA	$GABA_A$ $GABA_B$		Inhibitory	Major inhibitory neurotransmitter (can be excitatory during fetal life)
Glycine	GlyR		Inhibitory	Can be excitatory during fetal life
NE	α_2-adrenergic	Pons	Inhibitory	
Dopamine	D_4	PVN, hypothalamus		
Adenosine	A1, A2	Ubiquitous from metabolism of ATP that increases during hypoxia	Inhibitory	Contributes to respiratory depression at baseline (A1), and mediates HVD
Opioid	μ, δ, κ	nTS, PBN, PVN, raphe	Inhibitory	Prominent inhibitory effect during early development
PDGF	PDGF-β	nTS,	Inhibitory	Contributes to HVD

Data combined from Doi A, Ramirez JM: Neuromodulation and the orchestration of the respiratory rhythm, *Respir Physiol Neurobiol* 164:96, 2008; and Simakajornboon N, Kuptanon T: Maturational changes in neuromodulation of central pathways underlying hypoxic ventilatory response, *Respir Physiol Neurobiol* 149:273, 2005.
Ach, Acetylcholine; *ATP*, Adenosine triphosphate; *CCK*, cholecystokinin; *GABA*, gamma-aminobutyric acid; *HVD*, hypoxic ventilatory depression; *LC* locus ceruleus; *NA*, nucleus ambiguus; *NE*, norepinephrine; *nTS*, nucleus tractus solitarii; *PAG*, periaqueductal gray; *PBN*, parabrachial nucleus; *PDGF*, platelet-derived growth factor; *PVN*, paraventricular nucleus; *RTN*, retrotrapezoid nucleus; *TRH*, thyrotropin-releasing hormone; *X*, vagal nucleus.

modified mice that lack the *Mecp2* gene have reduced levels of norepinephrine and serotonin in the medulla and have breathing patterns similar to humans with Rett syndrome (Roux et al, 2008). Pharmacologic treatment to increase brain norepinephrine and serotonin levels stabilizes breathing and prolongs the life of these mice (Roux et al, 2007).

PERIPHERAL MECHANORECEPTOR INPUTS THAT MODULATE RESPIRATORY PATTERN AND RHYTHM

The nTS in the brainstem (see Figure 43-3) is where sensory afferents that are transmitting pressure signals from the upper airway, volume signals from the lung, and chemical signals from the blood and cerebrospinal fluid, synapse onto second-order neurons that send projections either monosynaptically or polysynaptically to phrenic motor neurons via respiratory-related bulbospinal neurons.

VAGALLY MEDIATED REFLEXES

Essentially all bronchopulmonary reflexes that modify depth and duration of inspiration and expiration are mediated through the vagal nerve. The vagal nerve has both myelinated and unmyelinated fibers. Myelinated vagal

afferent fibers are activated via (1) slowly adapting stretch receptors (SARs), which are activated by volume and stretch of the lung (mediating the Breuer-Hering Reflex), or (2) rapidly adapting receptors (RARs), which are activated in response to inhaled irritants (e.g., ammonia, cigarette smoke) and large inflations or deflations of the lung (Kubin et al, 2006). Changes in respiratory timing of inspiration and expiration are the respiratory response to activation of SARs, whereas sighing (i.e., augmented breaths) and coughing are the characteristic ventilatory responses to activation of RARs. Unmyelinated vagal afferents, specifically C fibers, are activated by a multitude of chemical stimuli, including CO_2 and capsaicin, in addition to lung edema and elevated temperature. Rapid shallow breathing and apnea are the characteristic ventilatory responses to the activation of C-fibers in the airways.

BREUER–HERING REFLEX DURING DEVELOPMENT

The duration of inspiration and expiration is greatly influenced by lung inflation, and the most well-characterized bronchopulmonary reflex is the pulmonary stretch reflex mediated through SARs, discovered by Josef Breuer in 1868. In adult cats, Breuer showed that expansion of the lungs reflexively inhibits inspiration and promotes expiration, and that deflation of the lungs promotes inspiration and inhibits expiration (Widdicombe, 2006). In the nTS, these afferents monosynaptically synapse on to second-order neurons called *pump cells* and *inspiratory-β neurons*. These second-order neurons then send projections to respiratory-related bulbospinal neurons in the VRC. Bulbospinal neurons synapse on the phrenic motoneurons in the cervical spinal cord. SARs also influence the activity of a subset of propriobulbar VRC neurons that are involved in rhythmogenesis (for review, see Kubin et al, 2006).

The Breuer–Hering (B-H) reflex does not appear to be important in regulating fetal breathing movements, because vagotomy performed in fetal sheep has little effect on the incidence, frequency, or amplitude of these breathing movements (Hasan and Rigaux, 1992). However, the B-H reflex is important in establishing continuous breathing and adequate gas exchange at birth (Wong et al, 1998). The reflex maintains functional residual capacity in newborns and infants, because vagotomy within 48 hours of birth results in respiratory failure associated with marked atelectasis in newborn sheep (Lalani et al, 2001; Wong et al, 1998). Vagal innervation in utero was initially thought to be necessary for the development of surfactant (Alcorn et al, 1980), but this belief has recently been challenged by new findings from Gahlot et al (2009). These studies showed that vagal denervation performed at 110 to 113 days' gestation (term gestation, 147 days) in fetal sheep had no effect on alveolar architecture, number of type II cells, morphology of lamellar bodies, or the level of surfactant proteins A and B and total phospholipids in lung tissue (Gahlot et al, 2009).

In humans, the contribution of the B-H to tidal breathing is determined by occluding the airway at either end expiration, where the next occluded inspiratory effort is prolonged and expiratory effort is shortened, or end inspiration, where the next occluded expiratory effort is prolonged and inspiratory effort is shortened. The inspiratory and expiratory time of the occluded effort is compared to the inspiratory and expiratory time of the preceding nonoccluded breath to determine the percentage increase or decrease of the inspiratory or expiratory times. With this technique, the B-H reflex has been shown to contribute significantly to tidal breathing in infants, which is strongest at birth and then decreases during the 1st year of life (Rabbette et al, 1994). It is reasoned that the strength of the B-H reflex is inversely related to gestational and postnatal age because of the excessively compliant chest wall in newborns, which collapses at lung volumes less than functional residual capacity. With decreasing lung volumes during expiration, the B-H deflation reflex will become activated and thereby shorten expiratory time and prolong inspiratory time. Several factors increase the strength of the B-H reflex, including premature birth (De Winter et al, 1995; Kirkpatrick et al, 1976), prone sleeping position (Landolfo et al, 2008) and active sleep (Hand et al, 2004) and respiratory distress syndrome (RDS) (Rabbette et al, 1994).

RAPIDLY ADAPTING RECEPTORS DURING DEVELOPMENT

Lung deflation, mechanical stimulation, and chemical irritants also stimulate vagal afferents of RARs causing augmented breaths and increased mucous production

(Widdicombe, 2006). RAR afferents synapse on RAR cells and inspiratory Iγ neurons throughout the nTS (Kubin et al, 2006). RAR cells receive monosynaptic excitatory inputs from vagal afferents, which are excited by irritants, particularly ammonia. RAR cells then send projections to the pons respiratory group and bulbospinal inspiratory and expiratory neurons. Stimulation of RARs as a result of lung deflation monosynaptically activates inspiratory Iγ neurons in the nTS, which then send axonal projections to bulbospinal neurons (Kubin et al, 2006).

RARs are particularly important in restoring lung inflation in premature and term infants, because the excessive compliance of the chest wall in newborn infants causes low lung volumes during tidal breathing. RARs become active at low lung volumes, leading to threshold activation of vagal afferents that results in augmented breaths, restoring lung volume. The frequency of augmented breaths is inversely related to gestational age, with premature infants having the greatest number (Alvarez et al, 1993), and the characteristic pattern of the augmented breath differs between newborns and adults. Augmented breaths in infants have a biphasic pattern with two large inspiratory efforts in succession, whereas in adults only one large inspiratory effort is seen. Augmented breaths in preterm and term infants are also relatively larger than those in adults; immediately after the augmented breath, preterm and term infants often hypoventilate or have apnea. In contrast, ventilation often increases after the augmented breath in adults (Qureshi et al, 2009). The increased frequency of augmented breaths and the hypoventilation and apnea after augmented breaths in premature infants suggest that peripheral arterial chemoreceptor inputs may have a greater influence on respiration in infants than in adults. Peripheral arterial chemoreceptors reflexively alter ventilation in response to acute changes in arterial CO_2 and O_2 tensions (discussed later). In response to an augmented breath, Pa_{O_2} rapidly increases and $PaCO_2$ rapidly decreases, which reduces the excitatory input from peripheral arterial chemoreceptors, leading to hypoventilation or apnea. Peripheral arterial chemoreceptors are also key in inducing augmented breaths, because carotid sinus nerve denervation in animals is associated with decreased frequency of augmented breaths (Matsumoto et al, 1997). As a result, increased activity of RARs during lung deflation and increased sensitivity of peripheral arterial chemoreceptors in early development both likely contribute to the increased frequency and ventilatory consequences of augmented breaths in premature infants.

C-FIBER RECEPTORS AND RESPONSES DURING DEVELOPMENT

Pulmonary and bronchial C-fiber receptors are unmyelinated vagal fibers located throughout the respiratory tract, extending from the nose to the lung parenchyma. Pulmonary C-fibers are accessible from the pulmonary circulation, whereas bronchial C-fibers are accessible from the bronchial circulation and have similar sensitivity to various stimuli (Coleridge and Coleridge, 1984). C-fibers are activated by a variety of substances: inflammatory mediators, capsaicin, lobeline, and phenylbiguanidine. Capsaicin and phenylbiguanidine are often used experimentally to identify vagal afferents as C-fibers and characterize stimulus-response profiles. C-fiber simulation induces central and local effects: cough, apnea, and laryngospasm, followed by rapid shallow breathing, bradycardia, and hypotension mediated by the central reflex pathways. Bronchoconstriction, increased mucous secretion, and bronchial and nasal vasodilation are mediated by local or axon reflexes (Carr and Undem, 2003). The central effects involve transmission of impulses to interneurons in the central nervous system, which influences the activity of autonomic or somatic efferent nerves. The local, direct effects are mediated by the release of neuropeptides, particularly substance P, from C-fiber endings. By far the most common respiratory response from C-fiber stimulation is reflex apnea characterized by prolongation of expiratory time from excitation of postinspiratory neurons and continuous firing of central expiratory neurons (Coleridge and Coleridge, 1984). Central integration of pulmonary C-fiber afferent information also occurs in the subnucleus of the nTS. Unlike the relay pathways that have been carefully delineated for the SARs, and to a lesser extent for the RARs, the specific second-order neurons in the nTS that are activated in response to bronchopulmonary C-fiber stimulation have not been completely identified. It is likely, however, that the central integration of pulmonary C-fiber stimulation occurs within the nTS, because the interruption of synaptic transmission within the subnucleus of the nTS ablates reflex response of pulmonary C-fibers from intraatrial injections of phenylbiguanidine (Bonham and Joad, 1991).

In newborns, the stimulation of pulmonary C-fibers by chemical stimulants causes bronchoconstriction and apnea (Frappell and MacFarlane, 2005). Capsaicin-induced apneic response and the sensitivity of the reflex was greatest in newborn rat pups younger than 10 postnatal days (Wang and Xu, 2006). Bronchopulmonary C-fibers are also stimulated by acidosis, adenosine, reactive oxygen species, hyperosmotic solutions, and lung edema. Furthermore, inflammatory mediators in the local environment sensitize C-fibers to other stimuli (Lee and Pisarri, 2001). Pulmonary C-fiber–mediated respiratory inhibition may be causing persistent apnea beyond term postconceptional age in infants born at the limit of viability who have significant lung disease (Eichenwald et al, 1997). As proposed by Lee and Pisarri (2001), C-fiber activation may also account for the increased frequency of apnea observed in infants with viral infections, especially caused by respiratory syncytial virus (Pickens et al, 1989).

LARYNGEAL REFLEXES

Receptors that respond to changes in upper airway pressure and chemical compounds are abundantly distributed throughout the laryngeal mucosa. These receptors can be slowly adapting, rapidly adapting irritant receptors, or C-fibers. Water receptors that are simulated by hyposmolarity and low chloride content may also be involved. Stimulation of upper airway mechanoreceptors and chemoreceptors modifies activity of upper airway muscles as well as the pattern and timing of diaphragmatic activity. The upper airway reflex that mediates significant cardiorespiratory effects that occur in newborns is the laryngeal chemoreflex (LCR). The LCR is one of the most potent defensive reflexes protecting the respiratory tract from inadvertent aspiration (Harding et al, 1978). These receptors are stimulated by liquid in the airway, which induces coughing, swallowing, and arousal in mature models. However, the response in immature models is apnea followed by hypoventilation, laryngeal constriction, and swallowing. In addition to respiratory inhibition, bradycardia, peripheral vasoconstriction, and redistribution of blood flow also occurs. Of importance, the associated apnea and bradycardia can be life threatening in newborns (Boggs and Bartlett, 1982; Sasaki et al, 1977; Thach, 2001; Wetmore, 1993), and in newborn infants baseline hypoxemia enhances the severity of the apnea and bradycardia induced by the LCR (Wennergren et al, 1989). Afferent fibers for this reflex travel in the superior laryngeal nerve, a branch of the vagus. These afferents synapse onto neurons in the nTS which then send (1) excitatory projections to motoneurons of the recurrent laryngeal nerve in the nucleus ambiguous, causing constriction of the thyroarytenoid muscle (laryngeal constrictor) resulting in laryngospasm; (2) inhibitory projections to phrenic motoneurons in the cervical spinal cord, inhibiting diaphragmatic contraction resulting in apnea; and (3) an excitatory pathway to cardiac vagal neurons in the nucleus ambiguous causing bradycardia. However, the circuitry from second-order neurons in the nTS to cardiac vagal afferent neurons has not been demonstrated clearly. The LCR occurs in the fetus and likely functions to prevent aspiration of amniotic fluid, which contains approximately half the chloride content of pulmonary fluid (Bland, 1990; Reix et al, 2007). With premature birth, the reflex may be involved in the apnea and bradycardic responses associated with feeds and gastroesophageal reflux that reaches the larynx or nasopharynx. Whether the immature response is still present in term infants or how the maturation of the reflex is affected by premature birth has not been determined. Because of its profound inhibitory cardiorespiratory effects, stimulation of the LCR may be an important reflex that is operative in some SIDS cases and infants with acute life-threatening events (Duke et al, 2001; Gauda et al, 2007; Richardson and Adams, 2005; Thach, 2001).

CHEMICAL CONTROL OF BREATHING (CO_2/H^+ AND O_2)

In air-breathing animals, respiratory rhythmogenesis is primarily driven by the level of P_{CO_2} in the blood and cerebrospinal fluid and, to a lesser extent, by oxygen tension. In fact, for every increase of 1mm Hg in P_{CO_2}, ventilation will increase by 20% to 30%. Specialized chemosensitive cells in the brainstem depolarize in response to changes in CO_2/H^+; they drive breathing through synaptic inputs to respiratory-related neurons (Spyer and Gourine, 2009). Although peripheral arterial chemoreceptors in the carotid body also depolarize in response to increasing CO_2/H^+, these receptors are primarily responsible for modifying breathing in response to changes in oxygen tension (reviewed later). As a result of careful anatomic, physiologic, neurochemical, and genetic studies, the location and the development of central chemoreceptors and some of the genetic factors that drive the development of these receptors in health and disease have been determined. Several groups of neurons in the brainstem, specifically in the medullary raphe, RTN, nTS, locus ceruleus, and the fastigial nucleus are responsive to CO_2/H^+ in vitro and in vivo; therefore they are characterized as chemosensitive. The demonstration that (1) focal acidification either with acetazolamide (inhibits carbonic anhydrase) or local elevations of CO_2 in these regions in either nonanesthetized or anesthetized adult animals increases ventilation, and (2) focal ablation or disruption of the region inhibits the ventilatory response, is essential for a region to be identified as chemosensitive (Feldman et al, 2003). Although several regions are CO_2/H^+ sensitive, there appears to be some specificity in the contribution of each of the regions in chemical control of breathing wakefulness and sleep (Feldman et al, 2003). The greatest density of CO_2/H^+–sensitive neurons in the brainstem is in serotonergic cells of the raphe of the caudal medulla and glutamatergic neurons of the RTN, located just below the ventral medullary surface. The serotonergic neurons in the caudal raphe project to phrenic motoneurons, where they modulate neuronal plasticity in response to hypoxia (Feldman et al, 2003). The RTN receives afferent polysynaptic excitatory inputs from peripheral arterial chemoreceptors cartoid body (Takakura et al, 2006) and sends projections to neurons in the VRC, including the PBC (Guyenet et al, 2008). In animals older than 7 postnatal days, the activity of the RTN depends on intrinsic pH sensitivity and synaptic drive. The parafacial respiratory group may be the precursor to the RTN, and these neurons have intrinsic bursting properties starting at embryonic day 19 (Guyenet et al, 2008). In humans the arcuate nucleus in the medulla (not to be confused with the arcuate nucleus in the hypothalamus) is believed to be the homologous chemosensitive region, as described in animals based on the following findings: (1) the arcuate nucleus is located along the ventral medullary surface, (2) it contains a large population of glutamatergic neurons and a smaller population of serotonergic neurons (Paterson et al, 2006a), (3) it depolarizes in response to hypercapnia (Gozal et al, 1994), and (4) the absence of the arcuate nucleus in a human infant was associated with lack of CO_2 sensitivity during life (Folgering et al, 1979).

DEVELOPMENT OF CENTRAL CO_2/H^+ SENSITIVITY

In fetal sheep, hypercapnia causes an increase in the depth of fetal breathing movements, with no change in inspiratory or expiratory time. In humans, maternal exposure to CO_2 also increases fetal breathing (Ritchie and Lakhani, 1980). Ventilatory responses to CO_2 are present immediately after birth in most mammalian species, and CO_2 sensitivity increases with maturation. However, in the newborn rat, CO_2 sensitivity is robust during the first several days of postnatal life; it declines markedly in the next 2 weeks of life and then gradually increases to reach adult levels by the end of the 3rd week (Stunden et al, 2001). Premature and term infants tested at 2 days of postnatal age have modest ventilatory responses to 2% and 4% CO_2, although the strength of the ventilatory response is less in the more immature infants (Frantz et al, 1976). In premature and late preterm infants, CO_2 sensitivity increases with postnatal age, reaching a mature response within 4 weeks of postnatal development (Figure 43-4) (Frantz et al, 1976;

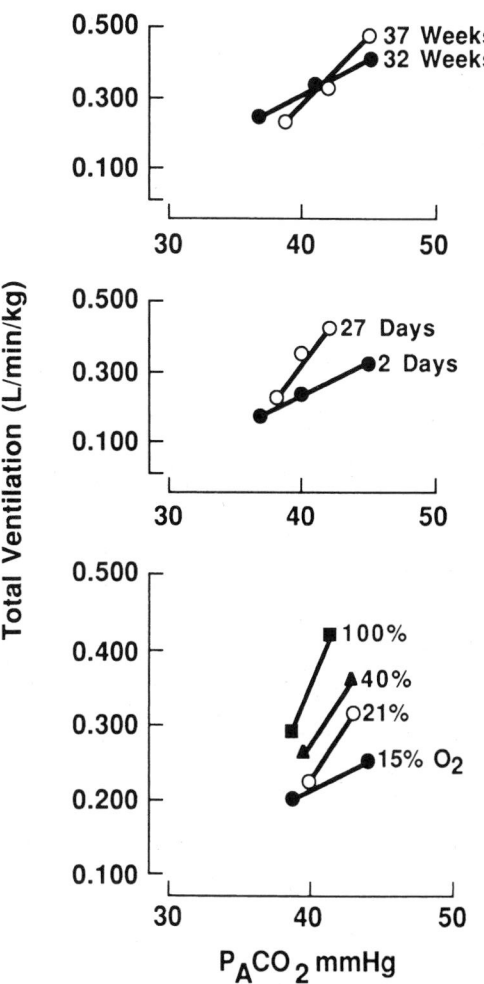

FIGURE 43-4 The relationship between ventilatory sensitivity to carbon dioxide and gestational age *(top panel)*, postnatal age *(middle panel)*, and the concentration of inspired oxygen *(bottom panel)*. *(From Rigatto H, Brady J, Verduzco RT: Chemoreceptor reflexes in preterm infants: the effect of gestational and postnatal age on the ventilatory response to inhaled carbon dioxide,* Pediatrics *55:614-620, 1975; and Rigatto H, Verduzco RT, Cates DB: Effects of O_2 on the ventilatory response to CO_2 in preterm infants,* J Appl Physiol *39:896-899, 1975.)*

Rigatto et al, 1975a, 1975c). Similar to the response in the fetus, the increase in ventilation is predominately due to an increase in tidal volume and not respiratory rate. Using the increase in inspiratory effort against an occluded airway as an indicator of central respiratory drive, when exposed to 2% and 4% CO_2, the increase in CO_2 sensitivity with postnatal development is due to an increase in central respiratory drive in human infants (Frantz et al, 1976). Premature infants with apnea of prematurity have reduced ventilatory responses to CO_2 compared with control infants at the same postconceptional age (Durand et al, 1985; Gerhardt and Bancalari, 1984). This finding suggests that infants with apnea of prematurity have reduced central respiratory drive to breathe when compared with infants who do not have apnea of prematurity at the same postconceptional age.

It is unknown whether maturation of synaptic inputs from chemosensitive neurons to respiratory related neurons in the brainstem, or maturation of intrinsic properties of chemosensitive neurons, accounts for the increase in CO_2 sensitivity with early postnatal development. Although such studies of human infants are impossible, data from studies performed in neonatal rats show that intrinsic responses of chemosensitive neurons in the nTS and locus ceruleus are already mature at birth. It is less clear whether there is a developmental increase in the sensitivity of chemosensitive neurons in the medullary raphe, an increase in the number of chemosensitive neurons in the RTN, or both (Putnam et al, 2005). However, within the first several weeks of postnatal development in the rat, the size of brainstem neurons changes, and both dendritic arborization in the nTS and astrocyte proliferation increase. Astrocytes contribute substantially to the pH of the extracellular milieu surrounding chemosensitive neurons (Putnam et al, 2005). It is likely that all these morphologic and neurochemical changes within and between neurons and astrocytes in the brainstem contribute to maturation of CO_2 sensitivity within the early weeks of postnatal development.

MATURATION OF PERIPHERAL CO_2/H^+ CHEMOSENSITIVITY IN THE CAROTID BODY

The arterial chemoreceptors in the carotid body, located at the bifurcation of the carotid artery, are primarily responsible for reflex control of ventilation in response to changes in arterial oxygen tension. Specialized cells within the carotid body also depolarize in response to changes in blood CO_2/H^+, reflexively increasing ventilation in response to acidosis and hypercapnia and reflexively decreasing ventilation in response to hypocapnia. Histologically, the carotid body chemoreceptors consist of (1) type I or glomus cells, similar to presynaptic neurons, that are chemosensitive and contain neurotransmitters and autoreceptors; (2) postsynaptic afferent nerve fibers from the carotid sinus nerve, which oppose glomus cells (Gonzalez et al, 1994), contain neurotransmitters and postsynaptic receptors, and have cell bodies in the petrosal ganglion; (3) type II cells similar to glial cells, which are not chemosensitive; (4) microganglion cells that express cholinergic traits (Gauda et al, 2004); and (5) blood vessels and sympathetic fibers innervating these vessels. The commissural nucleus of the nTS is the primary target for afferents from peripheral arterial chemoreceptors. Although these afferent processes contain glutamate, dopamine, and substance P, it is glutamate, binding to both NMDA and non-NMDA receptors on second-order neurons in the nTS, that is responsible for chemical transmission of excitatory inputs from the peripheral arterial chemoreceptors (Vardhan et al, 1993). These second-order neurons then send tonic excitatory projections to CO_2 sensitivity neurons in the RTN (see Development of Central CO_2/H^+ Sensitivity, earlier), bulbospinal neurons in the dorsal respiratory group, and VRG that synapse onto respiratory motoneurons.

In order to separate the contribution of peripheral arterial chemoreceptors from that of central chemoreceptors on ventilatory control, studies performed in animals have either perfused the carotid body separately from the systemic circulation or directly measured the neuronal output from the carotid body (in vivo or in vitro) in response to changes in arterial gas tension. With these approaches, it has been determined that peripheral chemoreceptors sense changes in arterial CO_2/H^+ more rapidly than do central chemoreceptors (Smith et al, 2006).

Sensitivity of the peripheral arterial chemoreceptors to CO_2 increases with postnatal development in newborn animals (Carroll et al, 1993); however, in human infants, the contribution of peripheral arterial chemoreceptors to ventilatory response to CO_2 is difficult to delineate. Inferences can be made from the ventilatory response that is seen within a few seconds of exposure to a particular concentration of CO_2, O_2, or both, because the response time of the peripheral arterial chemoreceptors is faster than that of the central chemoreceptors. What is inferred is that, after the first 2 days after birth, peripheral arterial chemoreceptors in newborns are highly responsive to changes in Pco_2. Hypoventilation and apnea are frequently seen in newborn infants after a sigh or augmented breath, in which the Pco_2 is rapidly reduced. This response is secondary to a high-gain system that is regulated at the level of the peripheral arterial chemoreceptors. In premature infants, the Pco_2 apneic threshold is close to the Pco_2 that mediates regular breathing (Khan et al, 2005). The level of Pco_2, however, increases the response of the peripheral arterial chemoreceptors to any level of arterial O_2 tension (Pao_2), and this O_2-CO_2 interaction at the carotid body increases with development (Carroll et al, 1993).

MATURATION OF HYPOXIC CHEMOSENSITIVITY

The contribution of afferent inputs from peripheral arterial chemoreceptors during maturation is more easily accessed by determining the acute change in ventilation in response to changes in oxygen tension. This determination is often made according to hypoxic gas exposure in newborn animals; an acute increase in ventilation within 30 seconds of hypoxic exposure is a measure of the strength of the peripheral arterial chemoreceptors. Whereas hypoxic gas exposure is occasionally used in human infants to test peripheral arterial chemoreceptor function, the reduction in ventilation in response to short acute exposure to hyperoxia (Dejours test) is more frequently performed to assess the strength of the reflex during postnatal development. Although the peripheral arterial chemoreceptors can respond to lower than baseline Pao_2 in the fetus, peripheral arterial chemoreceptors do not contribute significantly to fetal breathing, and functioning peripheral arterial chemoreceptors are not necessary for continuous breathing to occur at birth (for a historical overview, see Walker, 1984). However, studies using newborn animals (e.g., cats, dogs, rats, sheep, pigs) show that carotid body denervation shortly after birth destabilizes breathing, often leading to persistent apneic periods and death of the animal within days to weeks (Gauda and Lawson, 2000). Therefore it is believed that trophic factors from peripheral arterial chemoreceptors acting on central mechanisms that control breathing during early postnatal development are the key to stable rhythmogenesis throughout life. The critical period for these trophic influences appears to be within the first 2 weeks of postnatal development (Gauda et al, 2007). Exposures during this critical period of development that can lead to lifelong alterations in chemoreceptor function include environmental exposure to the extremes of oxygen tension (chronic hypoxia and hyperoxia), intermittent hypoxia (associated with apnea of prematurity) (Carroll,

2003; Gauda et al, 2007), nicotine exposure (Gauda et al, 2001; Hafstrom et al, 2005), and maternal separation in male rats (Genest et al, 2004).

Acute insensitivity to changes in oxygen tension associated with birth and then a gradual increase in hypoxic chemosensitivity during the first 2 to 3 weeks of postnatal development are two phases that affect the contribution of peripheral arterial chemoreceptors on breathing. Although oxygen tension less than 25 mm Hg stimulates the carotid body in exteriorized fetal sheep, peripheral arterial chemoreceptors are not functional at any level of hypoxic exposure for the first several days after birth in most mammalian species, including human infants (term and preterm). It is speculated that the resetting of peripheral arterial chemoreceptors occurs at birth because of the increase in arterial oxygen tension during the transition from fetal to neonatal life. After birth, there is a gradual increase in hypoxic chemosensitivity that occurs during the first 2 weeks of postnatal life (Rigatto et al, 1975b). Mechanisms accounting for the increase in hypoxic chemosensitivity of peripheral arterial chemoreceptors with maturation in most mammalian species have been reviewed recently by Gauda et al (2009). Although premature infants may have reduced peripheral chemoreceptor responses soon after birth, by 2 weeks of postnatal age they often have enhanced peripheral arterial chemoreceptor influences on eupneic breathing. Furthermore, premature infants who have a greater frequency of apnea and periodic breathing have a greater reduction in ventilation when exposed to short bouts of hyperoxia (Dejours test) (Rigatto and Brady, 1972), suggesting a greater influence of peripheral arterial chemoreceptors on eupneic breathing in this infant population (Al Matary et al, 2004; Nock et al, 2004).

GENETIC REGULATION OF CENTRAL AND PERIPHERAL CHEMORECEPTOR DEVELOPMENT

Development of central and peripheral chemoreceptors is genetically regulated by the expression of the transcription factor *PHOX2B*. *PHOX2B* is a homeobox gene located on chromosome 4 that is specifically expressed in limited types of neurons involved in autonomic processes (Dauger et al, 2003). Its expression is required for the development of the carotid body, nTS, and catecholaminergic neurons, and it is expressed in chemosensitive glutamatergic neurons in the RTN that receive polysynaptic inputs from peripheral arterial chemoreceptors (Guyenet et al, 2008). Mutations in the *PHOX2B* gene affect the development of key structures that regulate chemical control of breathing. Congenital central hypoventilation syndrome (CCHS) is characterized by impaired ventilatory responses to CO_2 and hypoxia and other abnormalities of autonomic control (Berry-Kravis et al, 2006). More than 90% of individuals with CCHS have mutations in the *PHOX2B* gene (for a review, see Amiel et al, 2009; Dubreuil et al, 2009.

NEONATAL HYPOXIC VENTILATORY DEPRESSION

Although the peripheral arterial chemoreceptors function to increase ventilation in response to hypoxia, minute ventilation significantly declines after 2 to 3 minutes of hypoxic exposure. This decline is commonly referred to as *hypoxic roll-off*, *hypoxic ventilatory decline*, or *hypoxic ventilatory depression*. Hypoxic ventilatory depression occurs in individuals at all ages, but it is most pronounced in the fetus and newborn (Bissonnette, 2000). Whereas the hypoxic ventilatory decline is usually still above baseline ventilation in mature models, the hypoventilatory response in newborns is usually below baseline ventilation and is often associated with apnea. Mechanisms accounting for hypoxic respiratory depression are most well characterized in the fetal animals in which the central brainstem nuclei mediating this response are located in the pons. Transverse section of the upper pons results in a sustained hyperventilatory response to hypoxia in fetal and newborn sheep (Gluckman and Johnston, 1987). Hypoxia activates expiratory neurons in the ventrolateral pons, and chemical blockade of this area blocks the hypoxic respiratory depression in newborn rats (Dick and Coles, 2000).

Several neuromodulators have been implicated in mediating hypoxic ventilatory decline, including norepinephrine, adenosine, GABA, serotonin, opioids, and platelet-derived growth factor (see Table 43-1) (Simakajornboon and Kuptanon, 2005). All these neuromodulators have been shown to contribute to the ventilatory depression in newborns, but particular attention has been given to adenosine. Degradation of intracellular and extracellular ATP is the main source of extracellular adenosine, which then mediates its cellular effects by binding to A1, A2a, A2b, and A3 adenosine receptors. In response to hypoxia, brain adenosine levels can increase 2.3-fold in fetal sheep (Koos et al, 1994), and 100-fold in rats in response to ischemia (Winn et al, 1981). Nonspecific adenosine receptor blockers, particularly caffeine and methylxanthine, are commonly administered to premature infants to increase central respiratory drive, and aminophylline inhibits hypoxic ventilatory depression in newborn infants (Darnall, 1985). A_1-adenosine inhibitory receptors are found on respiratory related neurons (Bissonnette and Reddington, 1991). Specific A_1-adenosine receptor agonists depress phrenic output in a reduced brainstem spinal cord preparation, whereas A_1-adenosine receptor blockers reverse this inhibitory effect (Dong and Feldman, 1995). In fetal sheep, the hypoxic respiratory depression appears to be mediated by excitatory A_{2a} receptors, because blockade of A_{2a} receptors eliminates hypoxic ventilatory roll-off in conscious newborn sheep. Xanthine (e.g., caffeine, aminophylline) blocks both A_1 and A_{2a} adenosine receptors; therefore the effectiveness of methylxanthine in stabilizing ventilation and decreasing the frequency of apnea in premature infants may be directly altering the ventilatory response to hypoxia as well as nonspecifically increasing respiratory drive (see Apnea of Prematurity, later).

SLEEP STATE AND BREATHING

Sleep state has a profound influence on breathing in the fetus and newborn, and most disorders of breathing that affect the young and old are worse during sleep. Active sleep (AS) and quiet sleep (QS) in infants is equivalent to rapid eye movement (REM) and non-REM sleep, respectively in older children and adults. Breathing during AS is mostly driven by inputs from the reticular activating system with less influence from Pco_2, whereas breathing during QS is driven by chemical control. Similar to REM sleep in adults, AS is associated with paralysis of striated muscles. Although this paralysis may be necessary to prevent acting out dreams, paralysis of striated muscles that are involved in breathing can be problematic for the newborn. AS and REM sleep are characterized by rapid eye movements, increase in cerebral blood flow and metabolic rate, and irregular breathing because of inhibition of the intercostals and upper airway dilating muscles. The discoordination between chest wall muscles and the diaphragm during active sleep causes paradoxic breathing: the chest wall moves in during inspiration with the abdomen moving outward. The more compliant the chest wall, the greater propensity for paradoxic breathing, which is common in the most immature infants. In addition, during inspiration, intrathoracic pressure becomes more negative, and this "suction pressure" causes narrowing or collapse of the compliant upper airway, particularly pharyngeal structures, leading to upper airway obstruction. Paradoxic breathing movements seen on physical examination or detected on inductive plethysmography are often interpreted as a sign of upper airway obstruction. During QS, breathing is characterized by smooth, regular breaths of consistent frequency and depth associated with tonic and phasic activity of the muscles of respiration that are in phase with each other. The chest wall and the abdomen move outward during inspiration, whereas they move inward during expiration. AS and QS can be reliably assessed at 30 to 32 weeks' gestation (Curzi-Dascalova et al, 1993). At this gestation, premature infants spend 80% of their sleep time in SA. This time decreases to 50% by term, and in adulthood REM sleep accounts for only 20% of sleep time. Sleep state in normal infants also modifies the time to arousal and the ventilatory responses. The time to arousal upon exposure to a hypoxic, somatosensory or auditory stimuli is greater in AS compared with QS in infants during the first 6 months of life (Horne et al, 2005). Of interest, the arousal latency in response to hypoxic stimulus in AS is longer in preterm infants at 2 to 5 weeks postnatal age than that of term infants at the same postnatal age (Verbeek et al, 2008). The level of oxygen desaturation at the time hypoxic arousal occurs is similar in the two sleep states (Richardson et al, 2007). Respiratory pauses and periodic breathing are more common during AS in both term and premature infants, but the ventilatory response to CO_2 is greater during QS (Cohen et al, 1991). Because of the complexity of the ventilatory response to hypoxia and the frequent occurrence of arousals induced by hypoxic exposure, assessing the affect of sleep state on the ventilatory response to hypoxia in newborns is more difficult. Other than the clear difference in arousal in response to hypoxic stimulus between the two sleep states, differences between sleep states on other respiratory parameters are more variable (Richardson et al, 2007).

Although most disorders of breathing, such as obstructive sleep apnea, become more severe during sleep, the breathing disorder that is most significantly influenced by sleep state in the newborn is CCHS. As noted previously, CCHS is characterized by abnormalities in central chemoreception and chemical control of breathing; therefore, with maturation, as the frequency of QS increases, so does

the severity of the disorder. During QS, CO_2 sensitivity is markedly impaired in affected individuals, and exposure to hypercapnia does not significantly increase minute ventilation (Paton et al, 1989). In infants who died of SIDS, their sleep state during their terminal event cannot be known. However, adequate arousal mechanisms are key in preventing respiratory failure and death, and impaired arousal mechanisms are hypothesized to be causative in SIDS. Prone sleeping position increases the percent of QS (Horne et al, 2002), and QS is associated with increased time to hypoxic arousal in human infants (Richardson et al, 2007). A hypoxic microenvironment from rebreathing with defected arousal and autoresuscitative mechanisms is hypothesized to have occurred in infants who have died of SIDS in the face-down (i.e., prone) sleeping position (Patel et al, 2001). Therefore sleep state can have a significant influence on control of breathing during health and disease, especially in the newborn infant.

This chapter has outlined the neurocircuitry and neurochemistry of the respiratory network along with its synaptic inputs that undergo significant maturation during the newborn period. Because these pathways are less developed in premature infants, premature infants have apnea of prematurity, which often requires active therapeutic intervention and can delay hospital discharge. At preterm gestational ages, the components of the respiratory network, similar to other developing organ systems, are plastic and uniquely vulnerable to pathologic processes. Therefore the episodes of intermittent hypoxemia and bradycardia that accompany apnea of prematurity may be a cause of acute and chronic morbidities in this high-risk population. What follows is a discussion of the clinical presentation of physiology and pathophysiology of breathing seen in premature infants and therapeutic interventions.

APNEA OF PREMATURITY

Respiratory pauses are universal features of preterm birth and are most prominent in infants of the lowest gestational age. There is no consensus as to when a respiratory pause can be defined as an apneic episode. It has been proposed that apnea be defined by its duration (e.g., longer than 15 seconds) or accompanying bradycardia and desaturations. However, even the 5- to 10-second pauses that occur in periodic breathing can be associated with bradycardia or desaturation. It should be emphasized that periodic breathing—ventilatory cycles of 10 to 15 seconds with pauses of 5 to 10 second—is a normal breathing pattern that should not require therapeutic intervention. It is thought to be the result of dominant peripheral chemoreceptor activity responding to fluctuations in arterial oxygen tension. Episodic bradycardia and desaturation in preterm infants is almost invariably secondary to apnea or hypoventilation (Figure 43-5) (Martin and Abu-Shaweesh, 2005). The rapidity of the fall in oxygen saturation after a respiratory pause is directly proportional to baseline oxygenation, which is related to lung volume and severity of lung disease.

Apnea is classified traditionally into three categories based on the absence or presence of upper airway obstruction: central, obstructive, and mixed. Central apnea is characterized by total cessation of inspiratory efforts with no

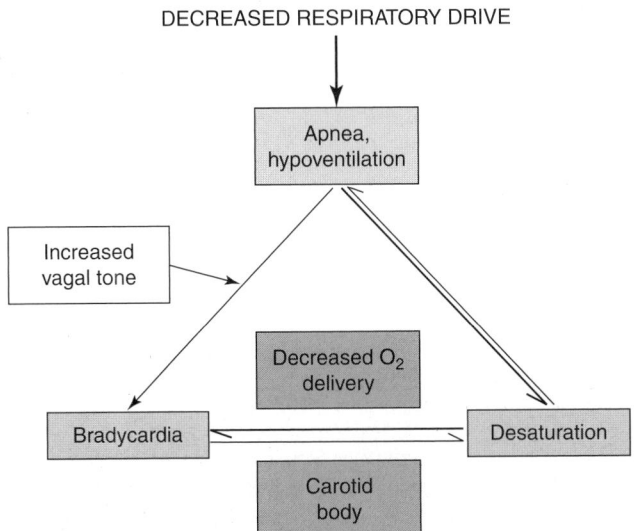

DECREASED RESPIRATORY DRIVE

FIGURE 43-5 Schematic representation of the sequence of the events whereby apnea results in various combinations of desaturation and bradycardia. *(From Martin RJ, Abu-Shaweesh JM: Control of breathing and neonatal apnea,* Biol Neonate *87:288-295, 2005.)*

evidence of obstruction. In obstructive apnea, the infant tries to breathe against an obstructed upper airway, resulting in chest wall motion without airflow through the entire apneic episode. Mixed apnea consists of obstructed respiratory efforts, usually following central pauses. The site of obstruction in the upper airways is primarily in the pharynx, although it also may occur at the larynx and possibly at both sites. It is assumed that there is an initial loss of central respiratory drive, and its recovery is accompanied by a delay in activation of upper airway muscles superimposed on a closed upper airway (Gauda et al, 1987). Mixed apnea typically accounts for more than 50% of long apneic episodes, followed in decreasing frequency by central and obstructive apnea. Purely obstructive spontaneous apnea in the absence of a positional problem is probably uncommon. Because standard impedance monitoring of respiratory efforts via chest wall motion cannot recognize obstructed respiratory efforts, mixed versus obstructive apnea is frequently identified by the accompanying bradycardia or denaturation.

THERAPEUTIC APPROACHES FOR APNEA OF PREMATURITY

Presentation of apnea can reflect a nonspecific alteration in either the environment (e.g., thermal) or general well being of preterm infants. For example, neonatal sepsis can manifest as an increase in frequency or severity of apnea, and the underlying cause must be treated. Studies using a rat pup model suggest that the systemically released cytokine interleukin-1β binds to its receptor on vascular endothelial cells at the blood-brain barrier. This binding induces synthesis of prostaglandin E2, which induces respiratory depression in the brainstem (Hofstetter et al, 2007). These studies provide new insight into mechanisms whereby sepsis often manifests as apnea of prematurity. Anemia, presumably via decreased oxygen delivery, is also frequently implicated as a cause of apnea, although transfusion of packed red cells is of variable benefit for apnea of prematurity.

CONTINUOUS POSITIVE AIRWAY PRESSURE

Continuous positive airway pressure (CPAP) at 4 to 6 cm H_2O is a relatively safe and effective therapy. Because longer episodes of apnea frequently involve an obstructive component, CPAP appears to be effective by splinting the upper airway with positive pressure and decreasing the risk of pharyngeal or laryngeal obstruction (Miller et al, 1985). CPAP also benefits apnea by increasing functional residual capacity, thereby improving oxygenation status. At a higher functional residual capacity, time from cessation of breathing to desaturation and resultant bradycardia is prolonged. High-flow nasal cannula therapy has been suggested as an equivalent treatment modality to allow CPAP delivery while enhancing infant mobility. Although this approach is used widely, its efficacy for apnea of prematurity has not been studied in depth. Noninvasive ventilatory strategies, using a nasal mask to deliver intermittent positive pressure, avoid the need for full ventilatory support in some infants. For severe or refractory episodes, endotracheal intubation and mechanical ventilation may be needed. Minimal ventilator settings should be used to allow for spontaneous ventilatory efforts and to minimize the risk of barotrauma.

XANTHINE

Methylxanthine has been the mainstay of pharmacologic treatment of apnea of prematurity for several decades. Both theophylline and caffeine are used and have multiple physiologic and pharmacologic mechanisms of action. Xanthine therapy appears to increase minute ventilation, improve CO_2 sensitivity, decrease hypoxic depression of breathing, enhance diaphragmatic activity, and decrease periodic breathing. The likely major mechanism of action is through competitive antagonism of adenosine receptors. Adenosine acts as an inhibitory neuroregulator in the central nervous system via activation of adenosine A_1 receptors (Herlenius et al, 1997). In addition, activation of adenosine A_{2A} receptors appears to excite GABAergic interneurons, and released GABA may contribute to the respiratory inhibition induced by adenosine (Mayer et al, 2006).

Methylxanthine has some well-documented acute adverse effects. Toxic levels can produce tachycardia, cardiac dysrhythmias, feeding intolerance, and seizures (infrequently), although these effects are seen less commonly with caffeine at the usual therapeutic doses. Mild diuresis is caused by all methylxanthines. The observation that xanthine therapy causes an increase in metabolic rate and oxygen consumption of approximately 20% suggests that caloric demands can be increased with this therapy at a time when nutritional intake already is compromised.

A recent large, international, multicenter clinical trial was designed to test short- and long-term safety of caffeine therapy for apnea of prematurity. In the neonatal period, caffeine treatment was associated with a significant reduction in the postmenstrual ages at which both supplemental oxygen and endotracheal intubation were needed (Schmidt et al, 2007). Of even greater interest was the significant decrease in cerebral palsy and cognitive delay in the caffeine-treated group (Schmidt et al, 2007). This finding raises interesting questions regarding possible mechanisms underlying this beneficial effect of caffeine on

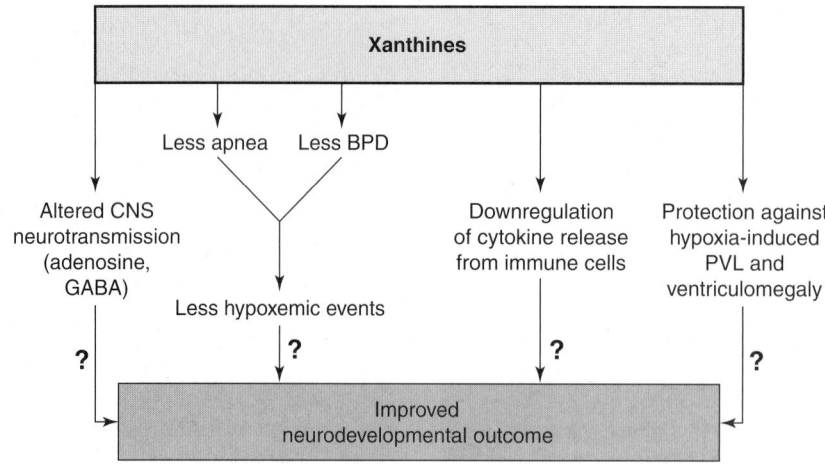

FIGURE 43-6 Multiple proposed mechanisms are demonstrated whereby xanthine therapy for apnea of prematurity improves neurodevelopmental outcome. These outcomes include functional changes in neurotransmitters in the brain, a decrease in hypoxemic episodes that accompany apnea, especially in the presence of BPD, a proposed protective effect of adenosine receptor inhibition on hypoxia induced white matter injury, and the benefit of adenosine receptor blockade on cytokine mediated lung or brain injury. *(Modified from: Abu-Shaweesh JM, Martin RJ: Neonatal apnea: what's new?* Pediatr Pulmonol *43:937-944, 2008.)*

neurodevelopmental outcome (Figure 43-6). These beneficial effects include the observation in animal models that loss of the adenosine A_1 receptor gene is protective against hypoxia-induced loss of brain matter (Back et al, 2006) and a potential benefit of caffeine on immune mechanisms that mediate lung and brain injury (Chavez-Valdez et al, 2009).

RELATIONSHIP TO GASTROESOPHAGEAL REFLUX [GER]

GER is often incriminated as a cause for neonatal apnea. Despite the frequent coexistence of apnea and GER in preterm infants, investigations of the timing of reflux in relation to apneic events indicate that they are rarely related temporally. When these events coincide, there is no evidence that GER prolongs the concurrent apnea (Di Fiore et al, 2005). Although physiologic experiments in animal models reveal that reflux of gastric contents to the larynx induces reflex apnea, there is no clear evidence that treatment of reflux affects the frequency of apnea in most preterm infants. Therefore pharmacologic management of reflux with agents that decrease gastric acidity or enhance gastrointestinal motility generally should be reserved for preterm infants who exhibit signs of emesis or regurgitation of feedings, regardless of whether apnea is present. Therapy for such infants should begin with nonpharmacologic approaches, such as thickened feeds, because acid suppression therapy has been shown to increase the risk of lower respiratory infection in infants (Orenstein et al, 2009). Recent data indicate considerable differences of opinion among neonatologists, pediatric gastroenterologists, and pediatric pulmonologists regarding diagnosis and management of this problem (Golski, 2010).

RESOLUTION AND CONSEQUENCES OF NEONATAL APNEA

Apnea of prematurity generally resolves by 36 to 40 weeks' postconceptional age; however, apnea frequently persists beyond this time in more immature infants. Available data indicate that cardiorespiratory events in such infants return to the baseline normal level at 43 to 44 weeks' postconceptional age (Ramanathan et al, 2001). In other words, beyond 43 to 44 weeks' postconceptional age, the incidence of cardiorespiratory events in preterm infants does not significantly exceed that in term infants. The persistence of cardiorespiratory events may delay hospital discharge for a subset of infants. In these infants, apnea longer than 20 seconds is rare; rather they exhibit frequent bradycardia to less than 70 to 80 beats/min with short respiratory pauses (Di Fiore et al, 2001). The reason that some infants exhibit marked bradycardia with short pauses is unclear, but available data suggest a vagal phenomenon and benign outcome. For a few of these infants home cardiorespiratory monitoring, until 43 to 44 weeks' postconceptional age, is offered in the United States as an alternative to a prolonged hospital stay. The apparent lack of a relationship between persistent apnea of prematurity and SIDS has significantly decreased the practice of home monitoring, with no increase in the SIDS rate. Infants born prematurely experience multiple problems during their time in the neonatal intensive care unit, and many of these conditions can contribute to poor neurodevelopmental outcomes. For example, a history of prior hyperbilirubinemia has been associated with persistent apnea of prematurity in preterm infants and animal models (Amin et al, 2005; Mesner et al, 2008). The problem of correlating apnea with outcome is compounded by the fact that nursing reports of apnea severity may be unreliable, and impedance monitoring techniques will fail to identify mixed and obstructive events. Despite these reservations, available data suggest a link between the number of days that apnea and assisted ventilation were recorded during hospitalization and impaired neurodevelopmental outcome (Janvier et al, 2004). A relationship has also been shown between delay in resolution of apnea and bradycardia beyond 36 weeks' corrected age and a higher incidence of unfavorable neurodevelopmental outcome (Pillekamp et al, 2007). Finally, a high number of cardiorespiratory events recorded after discharge via home cardiorespiratory

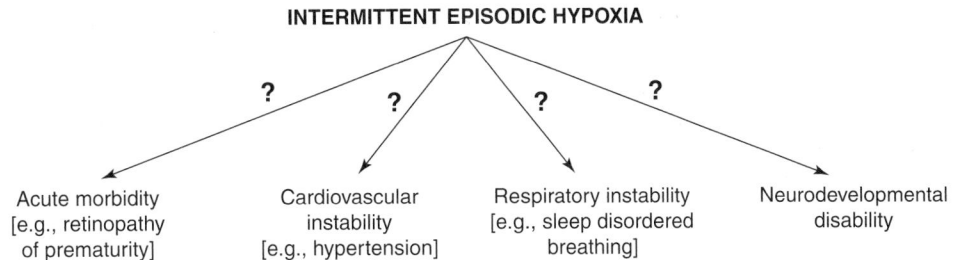

FIGURE 43-7 Proposed acute and longer-term morbidities that might be a consequence of intermittent hypoxic episodes in early postnatal life. *(Modified from Martin RJ, Wilson CG: What to do about apnea of prematurity,* J Appl Physiol *107:1015-1016, 2009.)*

monitoring appear to correlate with less favorable neurodevelopmental outcome (Hunt et al, 2004). Future studies might focus more on the incidence and severity of desaturation events, because techniques for long-term collection of pulse oximeter data are now more advanced. Furthermore, it is likely that recurrent hypoxia is the detrimental feature of the breathing abnormalities exhibited by preterm infants. Figure 43-7 summarizes proposed morbidities that might be attributable to intermittent hypoxic episodes in early life. Recurrent episodes of desaturation during early life and resultant effects on neuronal plasticity related to peripheral and central respiratory control mechanisms may serve as an important future direction for study. Ongoing investigation into the genetic background of infants with CCHS may also serve to enhance our understanding of the problem of apnea in preterm infants (Berry-Kravis et al, 2006).

SUGGESTED READINGS

Abu-Shaweesh JM, Martin RJ: Neonatal apnea: what's new? *Pediatr Pulmonol* 43:937-944, 2008.
Alheid GF, McCrimmon DR: The chemical neuroanatomy of breathing, *Respir Physiol Neurobiol* 164:3-11, 2008.

Bianchi AL, Denavit-Saubie M, Champagnat J: Central control of breathing in mammals: neuronal circuitry, membrane properties, and neurotransmitters, *Physiol Rev* 75:1-45, 1995.
Gauda EB, Carroll JL, Donnelly DF: Developmental maturation of chemosensitivity to hypoxia of peripheral arterial chemoreceptors: invited article, *Adv Exp Med Biol* 648:243-255, 2009.
Kinney HC, Richerson GB, Dymecki SM, et al: The brainstem and serotonin in the sudden infant death syndrome, *Annu Rev Pathol* 4:517-550, 2009.
Martin RJ, Wilson CG: What to do about apnea of prematurity, *J Appl Physiol* 107:1015-1016, 2009.
Nock ML, DiFiore JM, Arko MK, et al: Relationship of the ventilatory response to hypoxia with neonatal apnea in preterm infants, *J Pediatr* 144:291-295, 2004.
Richter DW, Spyer KM: Studying rhythmogenesis of breathing: comparison of in vivo and in vitro models, *In TRENDS in Neurosciences* 24:464-472, 2001.
Schmidt B, Roberts RS, Davis P, et al: Long-term effects of caffeine therapy for apnea of prematurity, *N Engl J Med* 357:1893-1902, 2007.
Thach BT: Maturation and transformation of reflexes that protect the laryngeal airway from liquid aspiration from fetal to adult life, *Am J Med* 111:69S-77S, 2001.

Complete references and supplemental color images used in this text can be found online at www.expertconsult.com

PULMONARY PHYSIOLOGY OF THE NEWBORN

Robert M. DiBlasi, C. Peter Richardson, and Thomas Hansen

LUNG MECHANICS AND LUNG VOLUMES

The lungs possess physical, or mechanical, properties that resist inflation, such as elastic recoil, resistance, and inertance. The dynamic interaction between these properties determines the effort that must be exerted during spontaneous breathing and the resting and extreme values for the volume of gas in the lung.

ELASTIC RECOIL

The lung contains elastic tissues that must be stretched for lung inflation to occur. Hooke's law requires that the pressure needed to inflate the lung must be proportional to the volume of inflation (Figure 44-1). Conventionally, volume of inflation is plotted on the *y*-axis, and the distending pressure is plotted on the *x*-axis. In this way, the constant of proportionality is volume divided by pressure, or lung compliance. Throughout the range of tidal ventilation, the relationship between pressure and volume is linear. At higher lung volumes, as the lung reaches its elastic limit (i.e., total lung capacity), this relationship plateaus, making the pressure-volume relationship nonlinear.

The lungs and the chest wall function as a unit (the respiratory system) coupled by the interface between the parietal and visceral pleura. Therefore, respiratory system compliance (CRS) can be partitioned into lung compliance (CL) and chest wall compliance (CCW), where CRS = 1/CL + 1/CCW. The tendency for the lung to collapse inward at end-exhalation is balanced by the outward recoil of the chest wall resulting in a negative (subatmospheric) intrapleural pressure. The functional residual capacity (FRC) is the volume of gas in the lungs when the elastic forces of these two structures reach equilibrium (Greenspan et al, 2005). Inflation of the respiratory system above FRC requires a positive distending pressure that must overcome the elastic recoil of both the lung (transpulmonary pressure; alveolar-intrapleural pressure) and the chest wall (transthoracic pressure; intrapleural pressure-atmospheric pressure) (Gappa et al, 2006). Deflation below FRC requires an active expiratory maneuver. Residual volume (RV) is defined as the volume of air that cannot be expired with a forced deflation.

As depicted in Figure 44-1, the relative compliance of the lung of the newborn is similar to that of the adult (Krieger, 1963). However, the infant's chest wall is composed primarily of cartilage, whereas in adults the chest wall is completely ossified and therefore, CCW is greater in infants than adult (see Figure 44-1) and pleural pressure is only slightly subatmospheric. Measurements of lung and chest wall compliance suggest that the newborn should have a lower percent RV and a lower percent FRC

than the adult. In fact, the percent FRC in the newborn is equal to the adult's, and the infant's percent RV is slightly greater. This seeming paradox exists because FRC and RV are measured while the infant is breathing, and predictions from the pressure volume curves assume that there is no air movement and passive relaxation of all respiratory muscles (Bryan and England, 1984).

Establishment of the FRC is vital to the role of maintaining adequate lung mechanics and gas exchange. The highly compliant newborn chest wall exerts very little outward distending pressure, and thus the lung is more prone to collapse at end-exhalation (Hülskamp et al, 2005. Data suggest three mechanisms by which the newborn can limit expiratory flow and increase the intrapulmonary pressure to maintain a normal FRC during spontaneous breathing: (1) by increasing expiratory resistance through laryngeal adduction (glottic narrowing), (2) by maintaining inspiratory muscle activity throughout expiration, and (3) by initiating high breathing frequencies to limit the expiratory time (Magnenant et al, 2004; te Pas et al, 2008).

RESISTANCE

Resistance to gas flow arises because of friction between gas molecules and the walls of airways (i.e., airway resistance) and because of friction between the tissues of the lung and the chest wall (i.e., viscous tissue resistance). Airway resistance represents approximately 80% of the total resistance of the respiratory system, and tissue resistance and inertial forces account for the remaining 20% (Polgar and String, 1966). In the newborn, nasal resistance represents nearly half the total airway resistance; in the adult, it accounts for about 65% of the airway resistance (Polgar and Kong, 1965).

Gas flows only in response to a pressure gradient (Figure 44-2). During laminar flow, the pressure difference needed to move gas through the airway is directly related to the flow rate times a constant—airway resistance. During turbulent flow, however, this pressure is directly proportional to a constant times the flow rate squared. Gas flow becomes turbulent at branch points in airways, at sites of obstruction, and at high flow rates. Turbulence occurs whenever flow increases to a point that Reynolds' number exceeds 2000. This dimensionless number is directly proportional to the volumetric flow rate and gas density, and it is inversely proportional to the radius of the tube and gas viscosity. Obviously, turbulent flow is most likely to occur in the central airways where volumetric flow is high, rather than in lung periphery where flow is distributed across a large number of airways. Both types of flow exist in the lung, so the net pressure drop is calculated as follows (Pedley et al, 1977):

$$\Delta P = (K_1 \times \dot{V}) + (K_2 \times \dot{V}^2) \tag{1}$$

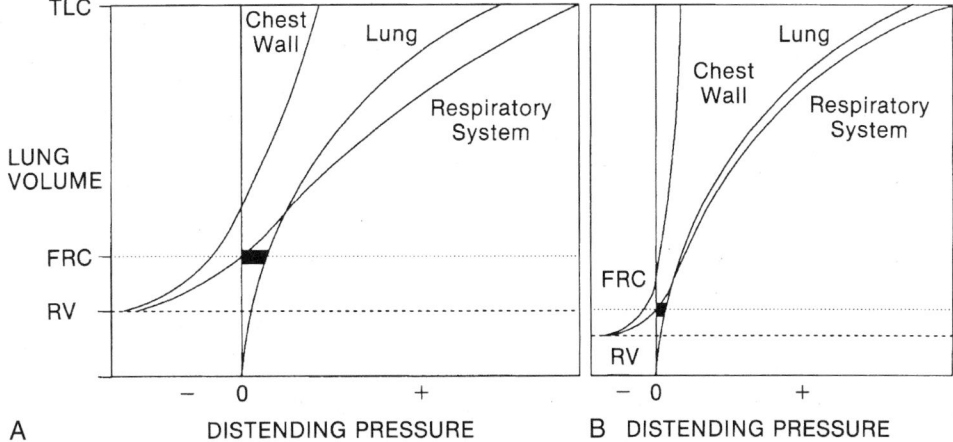

FIGURE 44-1 This is an idealized plot of volume as a function of distending pressure for the lung, chest wall, and respiratory system (lung plus chest wall) of an adult **(A)** and an infant **(B)**. These curves are derived by instilling or removing a measured volume of gas from the lung and allowing the respiratory system to come to rest against a shuttered airway. At this point only elastic forces are acting on the respiratory system, and airway pressure is equal to alveolar pressure. Intrapleural pressure can be measured using an esophageal balloon. Because airway pressure is equal to alveolar pressure, the distending pressure for the lung can be measured as *airway pressure – intrapleural pressure*. The distending pressure for the chest wall is *intrapleural pressure – atmospheric pressure*, and the distending pressure for the respiratory system is *airway pressure – atmospheric pressure*. Compliance is the change in volume divided by the change in distending pressure. The shaded area is the resting intrapleural pressure at functional residual capacity. Lung volumes depicted include residual volume *(RV)*, functional residual capacity *(FRC)*, and total lung capacity *(TLC)*.

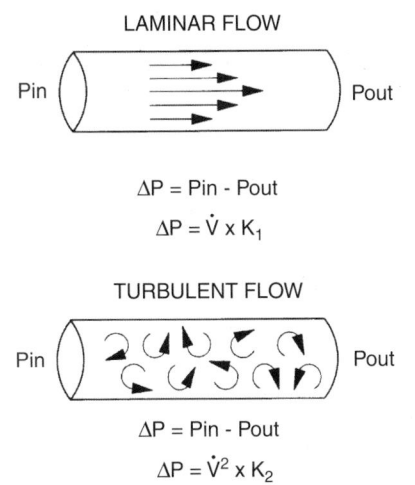

$$\Delta P = \dot{V} \times K_1$$

$$\Delta P = \dot{V}^2 \times K_2$$

FIGURE 44-2 Gas flow ($\dot{V}$) through tubular structures occurs only in the presence of a pressure gradient (Pin > Pout). For laminar flow, P is directly proportional to $\dot{V}$.

$$\Delta P = \dot{V} \times \frac{8 \times L \times \mu}{\pi \times r^4}$$

In this case, the constant of proportionality (K_1) is directly related to the length of the airway (L) and the viscosity of the gas (μ) and indirectly proportional to the fourth power of the radius of the airway (r). For turbulent flow, ΔP is proportional to $\dot{V}$. The constant of proportionality (K_2) is directly proportional to the length of the airway and the density of the gas and inversely proportional to the fifth power of the radius of the airway.

It is possible to take advantage of the differences between laminar and turbulent flow to determine the site of airway obstruction in the lung. If obstruction to gas flow is in the central airways, turbulent flow is affected the most. Because turbulent gas flow is density dependent, allowing the patient to breathe a less dense gas (such as helium mixed with oxygen) reduces the resistance to gas flow. If the site of obstruction is peripheral, the mixture of helium and oxygen does not appreciably affect resistance.

Inflation of the lung increases the length of airways and might therefore be expected to increase airway resistance; however, lung inflation also increases airway diameter. Because airway resistance varies with the fourth to fifth power of the radius of the airway, the effects of changes in airway diameter dominate, and resistance is inversely proportional to lung volume (Rodarte and Rehder, 1986). Similarly, airway resistance is lower during inspiration than during expiration because of the effects of changes in intrapleural pressure on airway diameter. During inspiration, pleural pressure becomes negative, and a distending pressure is applied across the lung. This distending pressure increases airway diameter as well as alveolar diameter and decreases the resistance to gas flow. During expiration, pleural pressure increases and airways are compressed. Collapse of airways is opposed by their cartilaginous support and by the pressure exerted by gas in their lumina. During passive expiration, these defenses are sufficient to prevent airway closure. When intrapleural pressure is high, during active expiration, airways may collapse, and gas may be trapped in the lung. This problem may be accentuated in the small preterm infant with poorly supported central airways.

INERTANCE

Gas and tissues in the respiratory system also resist accelerations in flow. Inertance is a property that is negligible during quiet breathing and physiologically significant only at rapid respiratory rates.

DYNAMIC INTERACTION

Compliance, resistance, and inertance all interact during spontaneous breathing (Figure 44-3). This interaction is described by the equation of motion for the respiratory system:

$$P(t) = \left(V[t] \times \frac{1}{C} \right) + (\dot{V}[t] \times R) + (\dot{V}[t] \times I) \qquad (2)$$

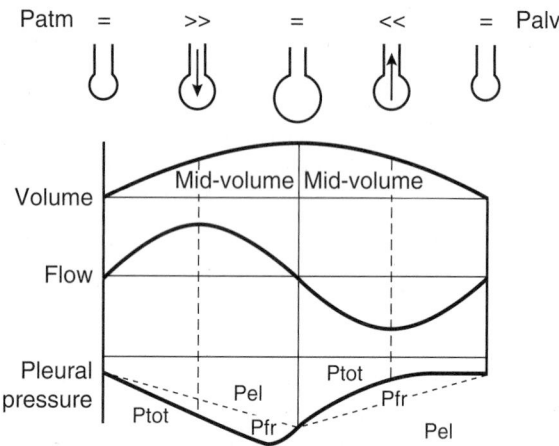

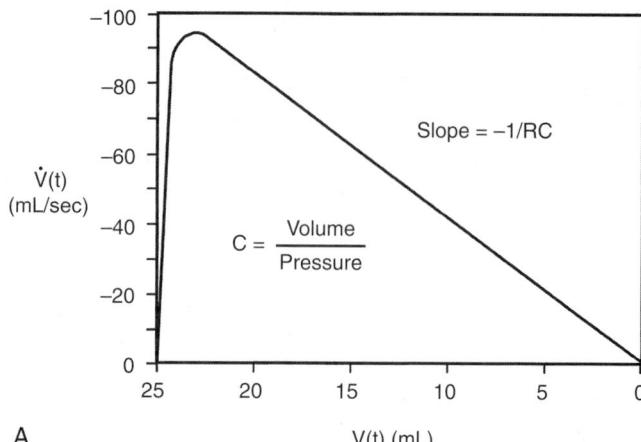

A

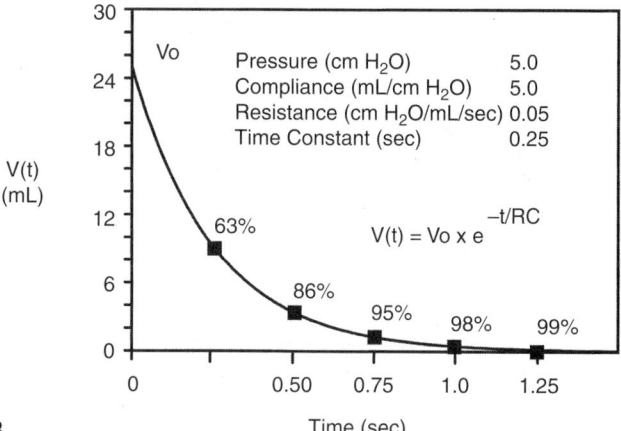

B

FIGURE 44-3 Gas flows from the atmosphere into the lung only if atmospheric pressure *(Patm)* is greater than alveolar pressure *(Palv)*. At end exhalation, when Patm equals Palv, there is no gas movement in or out of the lung. During a spontaneous inspiration, the diaphragm contracts, the chest wall expands, and the volume in the intrathoracic space increases. As a result, pleural pressure *(Ppl)* decreases relative to Patm, and a gradient is created between Ppl and Palv, distending the lung, increasing alveolar volume, and decreasing Palv. A gradient is also created between Patm and Palv, and gas flows from the atmosphere into the alveolar space. The rate of gas flow increases rapidly, reaches a maximum (peak flow), then decreases as the alveolus fills with gas and Palv approaches Patm. At peak inspiration, Palv equals Patm, and lung volume is at its maximum, as is Ppl. The *curved solid line* connecting end expiration to end inspiration is the total driving pressure for inspiration *(Ptot)*. The *dotted line* represents the pressure needed to overcome elastic forces alone *(Pel)*. The difference between the two lines is the pressure dissipated overcoming flow resistive forces *(Pfr)*. During exhalation, this cycle is reversed.

FIGURE 44-4 **A,** Plot of flow of gas out of the lung versus volume of gas remaining in the lung V(t) for a passive exhalation. Flow of gas out of the lung is negative by convention. After an initial sharp increase, flow decreases linearly as the lung empties. Static compliance of the respiratory system is obtained by dividing the exhaled volume by the airway pressure at the beginning of the passive exhalation. Resistance is calculated from the slope of the flow-volume plot $-(1/RC)$ and the compliance. This technique has the advantage of not requiring measurements of pleural pressure and being relatively unaffected by chest wall distortion. **B,** V(t) is plotted as a function of time for a passive exhalation. The graph is an exponential with the equation

$$V(t) = Vo \times e^{-t/RC}$$

V_0 is the starting volume, and *e* is mathematical constant (roughly 2.72). For this example, the time constant of the respiratory system (Trs) is roughly 0.25 second. Calculations show that when exhalation persists for a time equal to one time constant (t = 0.25 sec = 1 × Trs), 63% of the gas in the lung is exhaled. For t = 2 Trs, 86% of the gas is exhaled; for 3 Trs, 95%; for 4 Trs, 98%; and for 5 Trs, 99%. If expiration is interrupted before a time t = 3 Trs, gas is trapped in the lung.

where P(t) is the driving pressure at time, t, V[t] is the lung volume above FRC, C is the respiratory system compliance, $\dot{V}$[t] is the rate of gas flow, R is the resistance of the respiratory system, $\ddot{V}$[t] is the rate of acceleration of gas in the airways, and I is the inertance of the respiratory system. If I is neglected, the equation simplifies to:

$$P(t) = \left(V[t] \times \frac{1}{C}\right) + (\dot{V}[t] \times R) \quad (3)$$

At times of zero gas flow (end expiration and end inspiration), the equation further simplifies to:

$$P(t) = (V[t] \times 1/C) \text{ and } C = V(t)/P(t) \quad (4)$$

This series of equations and Figure 44-3 demonstrate that at points of no gas flow (end expiration and end inspiration), only elastic forces are operating on the lung. During inflation or deflation of the lung, however, both elastic and resistive forces are important.

Although the solution to the equation of motion for the respiratory system is beyond the scope of this discussion, the behavior of the respiratory system during passive exhalation is a special situation for which a solution can be obtained relatively easily using the occlusion technique (Lesouef et al, 1984; McIlroy et al, 1963). Before a passive exhalation maneuver, the infant is given a positive pressure breath, and the airway is occluded—invoking the Hering-Breuer reflex and a brief apnea. Airway pressure is measured, and the occlusion is released. Expired gas flow is measured using a pneumotachometer and integrated to volume; flow is then plotted as a function of volume (Figure 44-4, *A*). During a passive exhalation, there are no external forces acting on

the respiratory system (P[t] = 0), so the equation of motion simplifies to a first-order differential equation:

$$\left(V[t] \times \frac{1}{C}\right) + (\dot{V}[t] \times R) = 0$$

Rearranging yields the linear equation

$$\dot{V}(t) = -\left(\frac{1}{[RC]}\right) \times V(t) \quad (5)$$

where the slope is $-1/RC$, which can be determined using a linear regression of $\dot{V}(t)$ versus V(t).

This equation states that during passive exhalation, flow plotted against volume is a straight line with slope –1/(RC). The quantity RC has the units of time and is termed the *respiratory system time constant (Trs)*. Trs defines the rate at which the lung deflates during a passive exhalation (see Figure 44-4). Time constants affect the rate of lung inflation in the same manner in which they affect lung deflation (see Chapter 45).

WORK OF BREATHING

The work of breathing is a reflection of the amount of energy required to overcome the elastic and resistive elements of the respiratory system and move gas into and out of the lung during spontaneous breathing. Work of breathing is defined as the cumulative product of distending pressure and the given volume displaced during inhalation or exhalation (Figure 44-5):

$$WOB = \int PdV$$

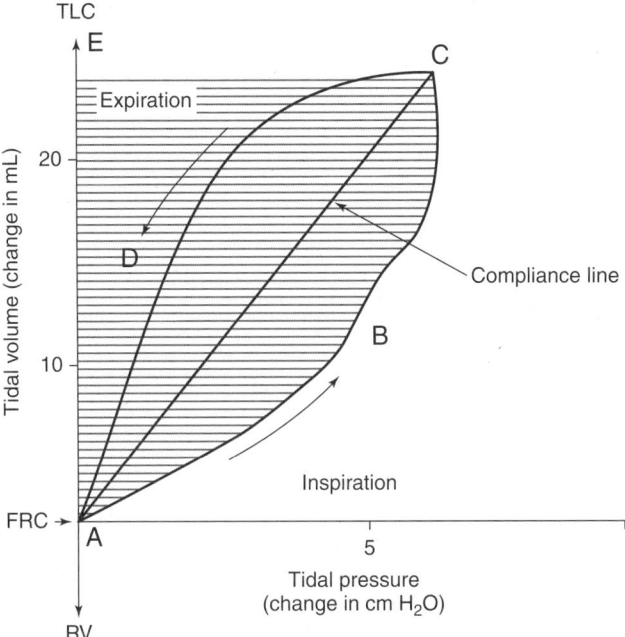

FIGURE 44-5 Pressure-volume loop showing the compliance line (*AC*, joining points of no flow); work done in overcoming elastic resistance (*ACEA*), which incorporates the frictional resistance encountered during expiration (*ACDA*); work done in overcoming frictional resistance during inspiration (*ABCA*); and total work done during the respiratory cycle (*ABCEA*), or the entire shaded area. *(Figure and legend taken from Wood BR: Physiologic principles, In Goldsmith JP, Karotkin EH, editors: Assisted ventilation of the neonate, ed 4, Philadelphia, 2003, WB Saunders, pp 15-30.)*

where P is pleural pressure in time relative to pleural pressure at end exhalation and V is the volume in time relative to the volume at end exhalation.

The work of breathing required to ventilate the lungs of normal newborns is approximately 10% of that required in adults (McIlroy and Tomlinson, 1955). However, infants have been shown to have a higher oxygen cost and lower mechanical efficiency associated with the work of breathing than adults (Thibeault et al, 1966). In healthy infants, the majority of the work of breathing is being done by the diaphragm during inhalation. Approximately one third of the total inspiratory work of breathing is related to overcoming the resistance to gas flow in the airways (Mortola et al, 1982). Exhalation is usually passive due to potential energy stored in the lung and the chest wall at end-inhalation but may become active as expiratory resistance increases or lung volumes decrease below FRC.

MEASUREMENTS OF RESPIRATORY SYSTEM MECHANICS

Respiratory system mechanics are objective measurements used to determine the severity of lung disease, changes in pathophysiology, response to therapeutic interventions, and progression of lung growth and development. Table 44-1 shows mechanics values for well and sick newborn infants. Lung mechanics in infants are typically measured during spontaneous breathing (dynamic) and by applying maneuvers during passive breathing conditions (static).

As mentioned previously, the mechanical behavior of the respiratory system (chest wall and lung) can be decoupled effectively by measuring pleural pressure. Because measuring pleural pressure is not feasible, esophageal pressure measured in the distal third of the esophagus, using an air-filled catheter attached to a pressure transducer, can be used to estimate pleural pressure. Thus, transpulmonary pressure is estimated by the difference between airway pressure and esophageal pressure and is useful in measuring lung and chest wall mechanics.

Dynamic compliance takes advantage of gas flow transiently being equal to zero at end inspiration and end expiration (see Figure 44-3). Dynamic compliance is calculated by dividing the change in volume between these two points in time by the concomitant change in distending pressure. Static compliance is the compliance measured when the infant is completely passive and can be estimated using an inspiratory hold at end inhalation during assisted ventilation (McCann et al, 1987).

TABLE 44-1 Lung Volumes and Mechanics of Well and Sick Neonates

Measurements	Units	Normal	RDS	BPD
Tidal volume	mL/kg	5-7	4-6	4-7
FRC	mL/kg	25-30	20-33	20-30
Compliance	mL/cm H₂O	1-2	0.3-0.6	0.2-0.8
Resistance	cm H₂O/L/sec	25-50	60-160	30-170

FRC, Functional residual capacity.
Data from Choukroun et al, 2003; Cook et al, 1957; Gerhardt and Bancalari, 1980; McCann et al, 1987; Polgar and Promadhat, 1971; Polgar and String, 1966; Reynolds and Etsten, 1966.

Another estimate of static respiratory system compliance requires instilling a known volume of gas into the lung, then measuring airway pressure at equilibrium in the absence of airflow and respiratory muscle activity (see Figure 44-1). This single occlusion technique is used to measure compliance during the passive exhalation maneuver described previously (see Figure 44-4). In the normal infant, it is generally assumed that dynamic compliance is equal to static compliance. However, in infants that are tachypneic or who have elevated airway resistance, the dynamic compliance may underestimate the static compliance of the lung (Katier et al, 2006).

As was mentioned earlier, measurements of compliance are affected by lung size. For example, if a 5 cm H_2O distending pressure results in a 25-mL increase in lung volume in a newborn, calculated lung compliance is 5 mL/cm H_2O. In an adult, the same 5 cm H_2O distending pressure increases the lung volume by roughly 500 mL, and calculated compliance is 100 mL/cm H_2O. Although the calculated lung compliances are different, the forces needed to carry out tidal ventilation are similar (i.e., lung function is normal in both circumstances). This example points out that if lung compliances are to be compared, they must be corrected for size. This is usually performed by dividing compliance by resting lung volume to get specific compliance. For the newborn, resting lung volume is roughly 100 mL, so specific compliance is 0.05 mL/cm H_2O/mL lung volume. For the adult, resting lung volume is nearly 2000 mL, so specific compliance is 0.05 mL/cm H_2O/mL lung volume—identical to that of the newborn. Thus, one might expect an infant born small for gestational age to have low lung compliance and normal specific compliance.

Lung compliance changes with volume history, meaning that it decreases with fixed tidal volumes and increases after deep breaths that recruit air spaces that may have been poorly ventilated or collapsed. The periodic sigh in spontaneous breathing is typically associated with an increase in lung compliance and in oxygenation (Frappell and MacFarlane, 2005). However, sighs in premature infants are often followed by apnea and hypoventilation that could lead to destabilization in infants affected with lung disease (Qureshi et al, 2009).

Many respiratory disorders result in nonhomogeneous increases in small airway resistance in the lung (see Table 44-1). Therefore, if lung compliance remains relatively uniform, the product of resistance and compliance (Trs) varies throughout the lung. During lung inflation, units with normal resistance have the lowest Trs and fill rapidly. Units with high resistance have a longer Trs and fill more slowly. At rapid respiratory rates when the duration of inspiration is short, only those lung units with a short Trs are ventilated. In effect, the ventilated lung becomes smaller. As discussed earlier, as the lung becomes smaller, its measured compliance decreases. Therefore, in infants with ventilation inhomogeneities, dynamic lung compliance decreases as respiratory rate increases. This decrease in lung compliance with increasing respiratory rate is termed *frequency dependence of compliance*, and it is suggestive of inhomogeneous small airway obstruction.

Resistance of the total respiratory system can be measured using the passive exhalation technique described previously (see Figure 44-4), or it can be calculated from measurements of distending pressure, volume, and flow (see Figure 44-3). Points of equal volume are chosen during inspiration and expiration. The gas flow and the distending pressure are measured at each point. The pressure needed to overcome elastic forces should be the same for inspiration and expiration and therefore cancel out. Total resistance, consequently, is equal to distending pressure at the inspiratory point minus distending pressure at the expiratory point, divided by the sum of the respective inspiratory and expiratory point gas flows. Investigators have calculated compliance and resistance by measuring distending pressure, gas flow, and volume (see Figure 44-3), then fitting these measurements to the equation of motion (see Equation 3), using multiple linear regression techniques, and solving for the coefficients 1/C and R (Bhutani et al, 1988).

The forced oscillation technique is used to estimate R_{RS} in spontaneously breathing subjects (Goldman et al, 1970). A loudspeaker is used to generate a sinusoidal pressure wave (P_{RS}) to the infant's nose via a face mask, with the mouth occluded, and the resulting gas flow is measured using a pneumotachograph. The $P_{RS}/\dot{V}$ relationship, called impedance (Z), is expressed as an amplitude ratio, called modulus ($|Z|$), and a phase shift (Φ) of both signals (Desager et al, 1996). Applying the simple RLC lung model described earlier in Equation 2 yields:

$$Z_{RS} = R_{RS} + j[\omega I_{RS} - 1/\omega C_{RS}]$$

where $j = \sqrt{-1}$ and $\Phi = 2\pi$ (frequency). The imaginary term on the right in the equation is termed reactance. At low frequencies, $1/\omega C_{RS} \gg \omega I_{RS}$, and Φ is negative. At high frequencies, the inertance term predominates, and Φ is positive. At an intermediate frequency, called resonant frequency, the effects of compliance and inertance are equal and cancel each other. The forced oscillations can be superimposed on spontaneous breaths (Jackson et al, 1996), making this technique suitable for infants. Forced oscillations methods can also be used with more complex lung models separating airway impedance from tissue impedance (Peslin et al, 1972).

FRC is measured by inert gas dilution techniques (helium dilution) or inert gas displacement (nitrogen washout) (Figure 44-6). Both of these techniques measure gas that communicates with the airways. The total volume of gas in the thorax at end expiration (thoracic gas volume [TGV]) can be measured using a body plethysmograph and applying Boyle's law. This technique measures all gas in the thorax—even trapped gas that is not in contact with the airways. Obviously, FRC measured by inert gas dilution is less than TGV if significant volumes of trapped gas are present.

ALVEOLAR VENTILATION

The tissues of the body continuously consume O_2 and produce CO_2 (Figure 44-7). The primary function of the circulation is to pick up O_2 from the lungs and deliver it to the tissues, then to pick up CO_2 from the tissues and deliver it to the lungs. The exchange of O_2 and CO_2 with the blood occurs within the alveolar volume of the lungs. The alveolar volume acts as a "large sink" from which O_2 is continuously extracted by the blood and to which CO_2 is continuously added. This mechanism for acquiring O_2 from

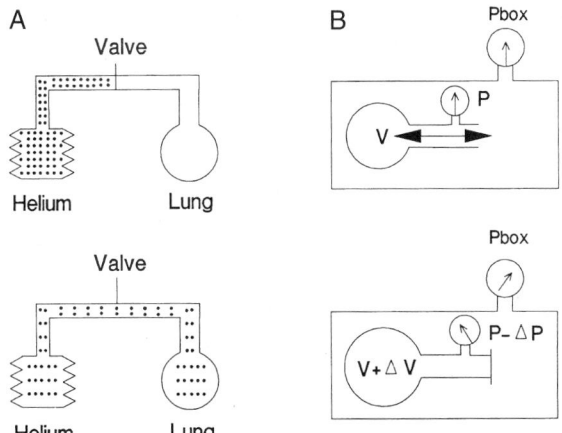

FIGURE 44-6 A, Measurement of functional residual capacity (FRC) by helium dilution. At end exhalation, the infant breathes from a bag containing a known volume (V_{bag}) and concentration of helium (He_i) in oxygen. The gas in the infant's lungs dilutes the helium oxygen mixture to a new concentration (He_f): FRC = Bag volume × (He_I – He_f)/ He_f. **B,** Measurement of thoracic gas volume (TGV) using a plethysmograph. The infant breathes spontaneously in a sealed body plethysmograph. At end exhalation, the airway is closed with a shutter. As the infant attempts to inspire against the shutter, the volume of the thorax increases and airway pressure decreases. The increase in volume of the thorax can be measured from the change in the pressure inside of the plethysmograph (Pbox). By Boyle's law: P × TGV = (P – ΔP) × (TGV + ΔV), where P is atmospheric pressure, (P – ΔP) is airway pressure during occlusion, and (TGV + ΔV) is thoracic volume during occlusion. Therefore, TGV = (P – ΔP) × ΔV/ΔP. Because ΔP is small compared with P, this can be simplified to TGV = P × ΔV/ΔP.

the atmosphere and excreting CO_2 into the atmosphere is the alveolar ventilation (Slonim and Hamilton, 1987).

The alveolar volume of the lung includes all lung units capable of exchanging gas with mixed venous blood: respiratory bronchioles, alveolar ducts, and alveoli. Because the conducting airways do not participate in gas exchange, they constitute the anatomic dead space (V_D). At end exhalation, the FRC is the sum of the volume of gas in the alveolar volume and in the anatomic dead space. During normal breathing, the amount of gas entering and leaving the lung with each breath is the tidal volume (V_T):

$$V_T \times \text{respiratory rate (RR)} = \text{minute ventilation} (\dot{V})$$

Part of each V_T is wasted ventilation because it moves gas in and out of the V_D. Therefore, alveolar ventilation ($\dot{V}_A$) can be expressed as:

$$\dot{V}_A = (V_T - V_D) \times RR \qquad (6)$$

Alveolar ventilation is an intermittent process, whereas gas exchange between the alveolar space and the blood occurs continuously. Because arterial O_2 and CO_2 tensions (Pao_2 and $Paco_2$) are roughly equal to the O_2 and CO_2 tensions within the alveolar space, these fluctuations in breathing could result in intermittent hypoxemia and hypercarbia. Fortunately the lung has a large buffer—the FRC. The FRC is four to five times as large as the V_T; therefore, only a fraction of the total gas in the lung is exchanged during normal breathing. This large buffer continues to supply O_2 to the blood during expiration and acts as a sump to accept CO_2 from the blood, so alveolar O_2 and CO_2 tensions (Pao_2 and $Paco_2$) change little throughout the ventilatory cycle.

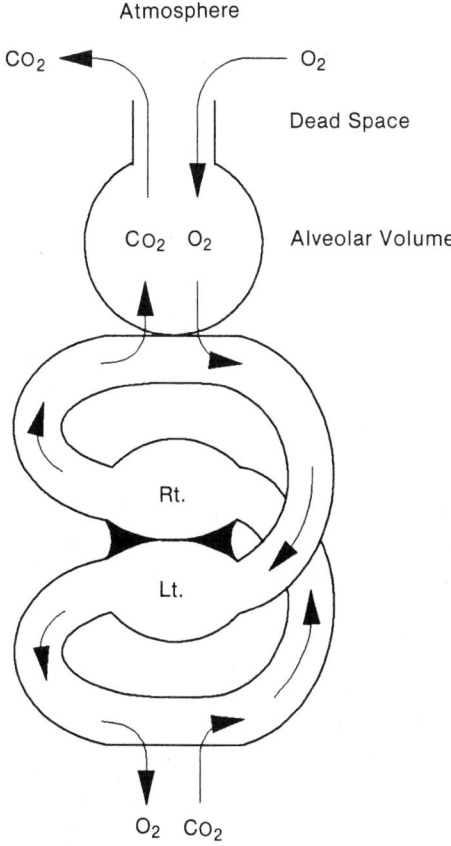

FIGURE 44-7 Schematic showing coupling of alveolar ventilation to tissue oxygen consumption.

Alveolar ventilation is linked tightly to metabolism. When alveolar ventilation is uncoupled from the body's metabolic rate, hypoventilation or hyperventilation results. During hypoventilation, less O_2 is added to the alveolar space than is removed by the blood, and less CO_2 is removed from the alveolar space than is added by the blood. As a result, Pao_2 decreases and $Paco_2$ increases. The net result of hypoventilation is hypoxemia and hypercapnia. Administering supplemental O_2 increases the quantity of O_2 in each breath delivered to the alveolar space, and it may prevent arterial hypoxemia. For example, suppose a 1-kg male infant has a V_T of 6 mL, an anatomic V_D of 2 mL, and a respiratory rate of 40 breaths/min. His alveolar ventilation is 160 mL per minute ([6 mL – 2 mL] × 40/ min). If he breathes room air (21% O_2), he delivers 33.6 mL of O_2 to the alveolar space every minute (160 mL/min × 0.21). If he maintains the same V_T but breathes only 20 times per minute, his alveolar ventilation decreases to 80 mL per minute, only 16.8 mL of O_2 (80 mL/min × 0.21) is delivered to the alveolar space each minute, and his Pao_2 and Pao_2 decrease. If he is allowed to breathe 50% O_2, O_2 delivery to the alveolar space increases to 40 mL per minute (80 mL/min × 0.50), and both his Pao_2 and Pao_2 increase. Because O_2 administration has no effect on the accumulation of CO_2, it does not prevent hypercapnia.

Hyperventilation delivers more O_2 to the alveolar space than can be removed by the blood and removes more CO_2 than can be added by the blood. As a result, Pao_2 increases and $Paco_2$ decreases.

Measurements of alveolar ventilation and anatomic V_D in the infant rely on the relationship between CO_2 production (VCO_2), $\dot{V}_A$, and $PaCO_2$. The mathematical expression of this relationship states (Cook et al, 1955):

$$F_ACO_2 = \frac{\dot{V}CO_2}{\dot{V}_A} \tag{7}$$

F_ACO_2 is the fraction of CO_2 in total alveolar gas, or

$$F_ACO_2 = PaCO_2/(P_B - 47) \tag{8}$$

P_B is the barometric pressure, and 47 mm Hg is the vapor pressure of water at body temperature.

Therefore,

$$\dot{V}_A = \frac{[\dot{V}CO_2 \times (P_B - 47)]}{P_ACO_2} \tag{9}$$

If minute ventilation ($\dot{V}$) is measured, dead space ventilation ($\dot{V}_D$) is calculated as:

$$\dot{V}_D = \dot{V} - \dot{V}_A \tag{10}$$

and V_D is calculated by dividing by the respiratory rate.

This method measures the anatomic V_D in the lung. As seen in the next section, portions of some gas exchanging units in the lung can also function as V_D; therefore, the total V_D, or the physiologic V_D, may be greater than the anatomic V_D. Physiologic V_D is calculated by substituting $PaCO_2$ into Equation 9 for P_ACO_2. When $PaCO_2 = P_ACO_2$, all the V_D is anatomic V_D, and the gas-exchanging units are all functioning normally. As physiologic V_D increases, however, $PaCO_2$ increases relative to P_ACO_2. Therefore, the difference between $PaCO_2$ and P_ACO_2 (the aA.DCO$_2$) is a measure of efficiency of gas exchange in the lung.

For clinical purposes, $\dot{V}CO_2$ in Equation 9 is assumed to be a constant so that $\dot{V}_A$ is proportional to $1/PaCO_2$. Thus, increased $PaCO_2$ means that alveolar ventilation has decreased; decreased $PaCO_2$ means that alveolar ventilation has increased.

VENTILATION-PERFUSION RELATIONSHIPS

Under ideal circumstances, ventilation and perfusion of the lung are evenly matched ($\dot{V}/\dot{Q} = 1$), both in the lung as a whole and in each individual air space. The air spaces receive O_2 from the inspired gas and CO_2 from the blood. O_2 is transported into the blood, while CO_2 is transported to the atmosphere. Even though $\dot{V}/\dot{Q}$ is 1, CO_2 and O_2 are exchanged in the lung at the same ratio at which they are exchanged in the tissues: A little less CO_2 is transported out than O_2 is transported in, so the respiratory exchange ratio R equals 0.8. If there is no diffusion defect, the gas composition of the air spaces and the blood comes into equilibrium. N_2 makes up the balance of dry gas. The sum of partial pressures of all gases in the air spaces must equal atmospheric pressure. The ideal alveolar gas composition is $PO_2 = 100$, $PCO_2 = 40$, $PN_2 = 573$, and $PH_2O = 47$ (all in mm Hg) at an atmospheric pressure of 760 mm Hg. The ideal arterial blood composition is the same. Therefore, differences between alveolar and arterial gas composition under ideal circumstances are all zero. Knowing the values for $PaCO_2$ and inspired gas, ideal alveolar gas

composition can be calculated from the alveolar gas equations (Farhi, 1966):

$$P_AO_2 = P_IO_2 - P_ACO_2 \times [F_IO_2 + (1 - F_IO_2)/R] \tag{11}$$

$$\text{where } P_IO_2 = F_IO_2 \times (P_B - PH_2O) \tag{12}$$

$$P_AN_2 = F_IN_2 \times [P_ACO_2 \times (1 - R)/R + (P_B - PH_2O)] \tag{13}$$

Under normal circumstances, and certainly in the presence of lung disease, this ideal situation is not the case; some air spaces receive more ventilation than perfusion, and others receive more perfusion than ventilation. A reduction of ventilation may occur because of atelectasis, alveolar fluid, or airway narrowing. Reduced ventilation in one part of the lung may cause increased ventilation elsewhere. A reduction of perfusion may occur if air spaces are collapsed or overdistended or because of gravitational effects, and increased perfusion may occur in congenital heart disease. As with ventilation, reduced perfusion in one part of the lung may cause increased perfusion in other regions. If an air space is relatively overventilated (high $\dot{V}/\dot{Q}$), its gas composition trends toward that of inspired gas, which in the case of room air is $PO_2 = 150$ mm Hg and $PCO_2 = 0$ mm Hg. If an air space is relatively underventilated (low $\dot{V}/\dot{Q}$), its gas composition tends toward that of mixed venous blood, which is $PO_2 = 40$ mm Hg and $PCO_2 = 46$ mm Hg. What counts is the $\dot{V}/\dot{Q}$ ratio, not absolute values of $\dot{V}$ or $\dot{Q}$ (West, 1986).

To understand $\dot{V}/\dot{Q}$ imbalance, it is common to view the lung as a three-compartment model (Figure 44-8): $\dot{V}/\dot{Q} = 0$ (Figure 44-8, *A*); $\dot{V}/\dot{Q} = 1$ (Figure 44-8, *B*); and $\dot{V}/\dot{Q} = $ infinity (Figure 44-8, *C*). The O_2 saturation of blood in each compartment depends on the PO_2 and the O_2 dissociation curve. For illustrative purposes, in a badly diseased lung, 50% of ventilation goes to $\dot{V}/\dot{Q} = 1$ and 50% to $\dot{V}/\dot{Q} = $ infinity, whereas 50% of perfusion goes to $\dot{V}/\dot{Q} = 1$ and 50% to $\dot{V}/\dot{Q} = 0$. Perfusion of $\dot{V}/\dot{Q} = 0$ causes venous admixture, whereas ventilation of $\dot{V}/\dot{Q} = $ infinity causes alveolar V_D. The mixed alveolar gas composition is easily calculated as the mean. For mixed arterial blood, the PO_2 must be read from the O_2 dissociation curve, but because the CO_2 dissociation curve is fairly linear, the values for CO_2 are easily calculated as the mean. The abnormalities in distribution of $\dot{V}$ and $\dot{Q}$ have created an Aa.DO$_2$ = 70, aA.DCO$_2$ = 23, and aA.DN$_2$ = 32 mm Hg (see Figure 44-8). The Aa.DO$_2$ is greater than the sum of the other two because the O_2 dissociation curve is not linear. Of course, the situation in most lungs is not as extreme as the one illustrated. From this illustration, however, it can be seen that:

1. Open low $\dot{V}/\dot{Q}$ units produce increased Aa.DO$_2$, significant hypoxemia, and increased aA.DN$_2$, but because they are poorly ventilated and have a PCO_2 close to the ideal value, they do not change the aA.DCO$_2$ significantly.
2. High $\dot{V}/\dot{Q}$ units produce increased Aa.DO$_2$ without hypoxemia and increased aA.DCO$_2$, but because they are poorly perfused and have a PN_2 close to the ideal value, they do not change the aA.DN$_2$ significantly.

For the calculation of Aa.DO$_2$ and aA.DN$_2$, it is customary to calculate the ideal alveolar gas composition for O_2 and N_2 from the alveolar gas equations and use these values with those measured for arterial PO_2 and PN_2. This

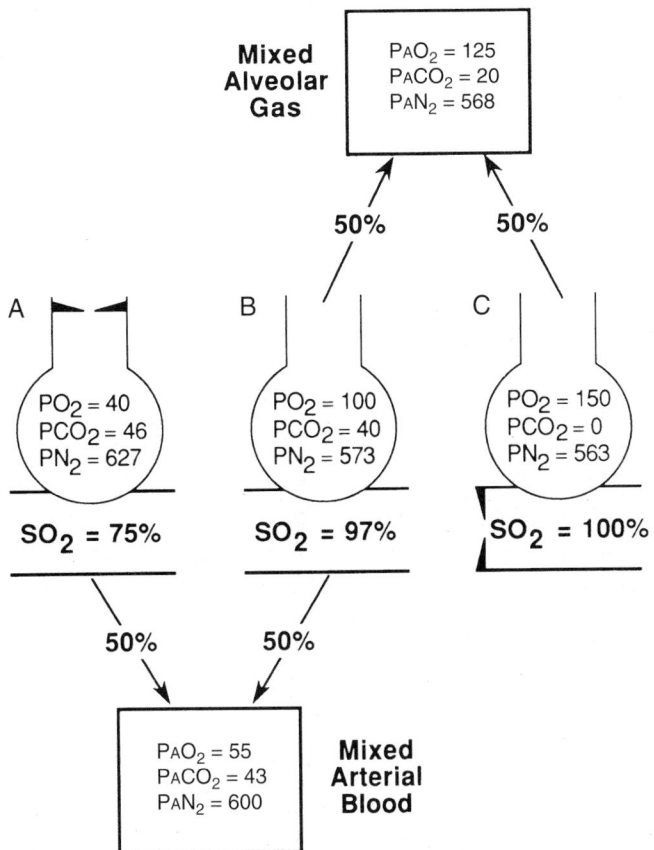

FIGURE 44-8 Three-compartment model of the lung with

$$\frac{\dot{V}}{\dot{Q}} = 0 \ (A), \quad \frac{\dot{V}}{\dot{Q}} = 1 \ (B), \quad \frac{\dot{V}}{\dot{Q}} = \text{infinity} \ (C)$$

The inspired gas is room air, and *B* is the ideal compartment. The sum of alveolar gas partial pressures is always 713 mm Hg. SO_2 is oxygen saturation in capillary blood. PaO_2 is read from the oxygen dissociation curve for a saturation of 86%. By calculated differences, $Aa.DO_2$ is 70 mm Hg, $aA.DCO_2$ is 23 mm Hg, and $aA.DN_2$ is 32 mm Hg.

emphasizes that part of the $Aa.DO_2$ and $aA.DN_2$ responsible for hypoxemia. For $aA.DCO_2$, both an arterial and mixed alveolar sample are required.

In the newborn, a fourth compartment in the model is important. A significant part of the venous return may be shunted from right to left at the foramen ovale, ductus arteriosus, pulmonary arteriovenous vessels, or lung mesenchyme without airway development, thus adding mixed venous to mixed arterial blood. This substantially increases the $Aa.DO_2$ but has little effect on $aA.DCO_2$ and no effect on $aA.DN_2$. The last mentioned is because there is no significant exchange of N_2 in the body, so venous and arterial PN_2 are the same. The effect on $aA.DCO_2$ is small because venous PCO_2 is only slightly higher than arterial. From this analysis, it can be seen that hypoxemia is produced by a true right-to-left shunt and open low $\dot{V}/\dot{Q}$ units. Diffusional problems are not thought to be important in the newborn. Hypoxemia may be modeled as a venous admixture, the part of mixed venous blood, expressed as a fraction of cardiac output, that when added to blood equilibrated with an ideal lung would produce the measured arterial oxygen saturation. It is calculated as follows:

$$\frac{\dot{Q}va}{\dot{Q}t} = \frac{C_cO_2 - C_aO_2}{C_cO_2 - C_{\bar{v}}O_2} \tag{14}$$

where $\dot{Q}va/\dot{Q}t$ = venous admixture, CO_2 = oxygen content, $\dot{c}$ = pulmonary capillary, a = arterial, and $\bar{v}$ = mixed venous blood. For practical application, $C_{\bar{v}}O_2$ is calculated from a constant a $\bar{v}.O_2$ difference, which does introduce an error.

If an infant breathes 100% O_2 for 15 minutes, most N_2 is washed out of the lung, and the PO_2 in open low $\dot{V}/\dot{Q}$ Q units becomes so high that associated blood is 100% saturated with O_2. The remaining venous admixture is attributed to true right-to-left shunt ($\dot{Q}s/\dot{Q}t$). If an infant has the total venous admixture $\dot{Q}va/\dot{Q}t$ measured while breathing room air, then true shunt ($\dot{Q}s/\dot{Q}t$) measured while breathing 100% O_2, the venous admixture caused by open low $\dot{V}/\dot{Q}$ units ($\dot{Q}o/\dot{Q}t$) can be calculated as the difference. The venous admixture caused by open low $\dot{V}/\dot{Q}$ units can also be calculated from the $aA.DN_2$ (Markello et al, 1972):

$$\frac{\dot{Q}o}{\dot{Q}t} = \frac{PaN_2 - PAN_2}{PoN_2 - PAN_2} \tag{15}$$

where P_oN_2 is the PN_2 in the units (see Figure 44-8), PaN_2 is measured, and PAN_2 is the ideal value calculated from the alveolar gas equation. In newborns with a significant value for true shunt, this value really represents venous admixture as a fraction of effective pulmonary blood flow ($\dot{Q}o/\dot{Q}c$.). A better estimate for $\dot{Q}o/\dot{Q}t$ can be obtained from simple arithmetic (Corbet et al, 1974):

$$\frac{\dot{Q}o}{\dot{Q}t} = \left(\frac{\dot{Q}o}{\dot{Q}\dot{c}}\right) \times \frac{\left(1 - \dfrac{\dot{Q}Va}{\dot{Q}t}\right)}{\left(1 - \dfrac{\dot{Q}o}{\dot{Q}\dot{c}}\right)} \tag{16}$$

The true right-to-left shunt can then be estimated without 100% O_2 breathing using the equation:

$$\frac{\dot{Q}s}{\dot{Q}t} = \frac{\dot{Q}va}{\dot{Q}t} - \frac{\dot{Q}o}{\dot{Q}t} \tag{17}$$

The normal values for the various indices of ventilation-perfusion imbalance in normal newborn infants are shown in Table 44-2.

HEART-LUNG INTERACTION

EFFECTS OF THE LUNG ON THE HEART

There exists considerable potential for the lung to affect the heart. Because they share the thoracic cavity, changes in intrathoracic pressure accompanying lung inflation are transmitted directly to the heart. In addition, all of the blood leaving the right ventricle must traverse the pulmonary vascular bed, so changes in pulmonary vascular resistance may greatly affect right ventricular function.

EFFECTS OF CHANGES IN INTRATHORACIC PRESSURE ON THE HEART

Negative Intrathoracic Pressure

During spontaneous inspiratory efforts, the chest wall and diaphragm move outward, intrathoracic volume increases, and intrathoracic pressure decreases (Figure 44-9, *A*). The

TABLE 44-2 Indices of Ventilation-Perfusion Imbalance in the Normal Newborn Breathing Room Air

	Aa.DO$_2$ mm Hg	$\frac{\dot{Q}va}{\dot{Q}t}$	aA.DN$_2$ mm Hg	$\frac{\dot{Q}o}{\dot{Q}t}$	$\frac{\dot{Q}s}{\dot{Q}t}$	aA.DCO$_2$ mm Hg
Newborn	25	0.25	10	0.10	0.15	1
Adult	10	0.07	7	0.05	0.02	1

Adapted from Nelson NM: Respiration and circulation after birth. In Smith CA, Nelson NM, editors: *The physiology of the newborn infant.* Springfield, Ill, 1976, Charles C Thomas.

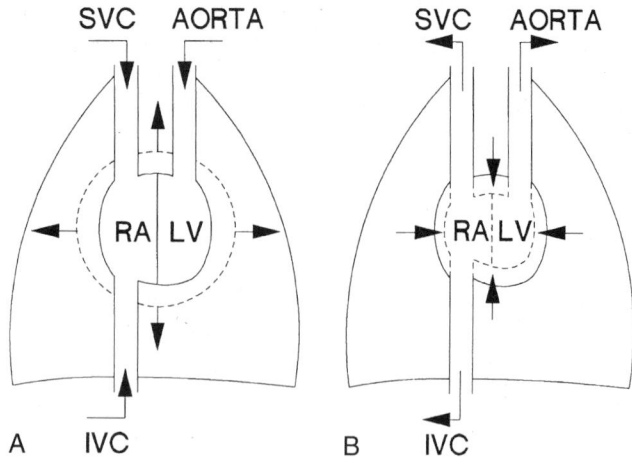

FIGURE 44-9 A, Negative intrathoracic pressure increases the volume of the heart and decreases the pressure within the chambers. This facilitates return of blood from the superior vena cava *(SVC)* and inferior vena cava *(IVC)* to the right atrium *(RA)* and impedes ejection of blood from the left ventricle *(LV)* into the extrathoracic aorta. **B,** Positive intrathoracic pressure decreases the volume of the heart and increases pressure within its chambers. This impedes blood return to the right atrium and augments ejection of blood from the left ventricle.

heart also resides within the thoracic cavity and is subject to the same negative intrathoracic pressure during inspiration. With a decrease in intrathoracic pressure, the heart increases in volume, and the pressure within its chambers decreases relative to atmospheric pressure. Analogous to the lung, when the pressure within the heart decreases, blood is literally sucked back into the heart from systemic veins and arteries. On the right side of the heart, the phenomenon serves to increase the flow of blood from systemic veins into the right atrium, increasing right ventricular preload and ventricular output. On the left side of the heart, ventricular ejection is impaired. During systole, the left ventricle must overcome not only the load imposed by the systemic vascular resistance, but also the additional load imposed by the negative intrathoracic pressure (McGregor, 1979).

In infants with normal lungs, spontaneous respiratory efforts result in relatively small swings in pleural pressure (2 to 3 mm Hg) that have little effect on the pressure within the heart. With airway obstruction or parenchymal lung disease, however, swings in pleural pressure can be much greater (5 to 20 mm Hg), and systemic arterial pressure may fluctuate as much as 5 to 20 mm Hg depending on where in the respiratory cycle ventricular systole occurs. In older children with asthma or some other form of airway obstruction, these fluctuations in blood pressure constitute pulsus paradoxus and are indicative of severe airway obstruction.

Positive Intrathoracic Pressure

During positive-pressure ventilation, the lung inflates and pushes the chest wall and diaphragm outward (Figure 44-9, *B*). This outward push generates a pressure in the thoracic space that is greater than atmospheric pressure. The magnitude of the increase (relative transmission of airway pressure to the pleural space) is determined by the volume of lung inflation (which, in turn, is determined by the airway pressure and lung compliance) and by the compliance of the chest wall and diaphragm. If the lung is compliant and the chest wall rigid, little airway pressure is lost inflating the lung, but considerable pressure is generated in the thoracic cavity as the lung attempts to push the rigid chest wall outward. In this instance, intrathoracic pressure (intrapleural pressure) is much greater than atmospheric and in fact nearly equal to airway pressure. If the lung is poorly compliant and the chest wall highly compliant, most of the airway pressure is dissipated trying to inflate the lungs, and little is transmitted to the thoracic cavity.

The effects of positive intrathoracic pressure on the heart are opposite to those of negative intrathoracic pressure.

The heart is compressed by the lungs and chest wall, and blood is squeezed out of the heart and the thoracic cavity. Return of blood from systemic veins is impaired, and right ventricular preload and output decrease. If the increase in intrathoracic pressure coincides with ventricular systole, the effect is to augment left ventricular ejection and reduce the load on the left ventricle.

In the infant undergoing positive-pressure ventilation, the degree to which lung inflation compromises venous return is related to the relative compliances of the lung and chest wall. If the infant's lung is poorly compliant and the chest wall is compliant, as in hyaline membrane disease, there is little effect of lung inflation on venous return. If the infant's lung is normally compliant but tight abdominal distention prevents descent of the diaphragm, intrathoracic pressure increases dramatically during positive pressure ventilation, and venous return and cardiac output can be impaired. This mechanism may help explain the circulatory instability of infants after repair of gastroschisis or omphalocele. A similar situation may arise in the preterm infant with pulmonary interstitial emphysema and massive lung overinflation. In these infants, the heart is tightly compressed between the hyperinflated lungs, the other structures of the mediastinum, and the diaphragm. Venous return may be severely limited and venous pressures so increased that massive peripheral edema often accompanies the reduction in cardiac output.

Although the effects of increased pleural pressure on the right atrium are detrimental, the effects on the left ventricle may be extremely beneficial (Niemann et al, 1980). During cardiopulmonary resuscitation, the chest wall is compressed against the lung, and intrathoracic pressure increases. Because the left ventricle is in the thorax, left ventricular pressure increases as well. A gradient is created, favoring flow of blood out of the ventricle and thorax and into the extrathoracic systemic circulation. Between chest compressions, elastic recoil causes the chest wall to pull

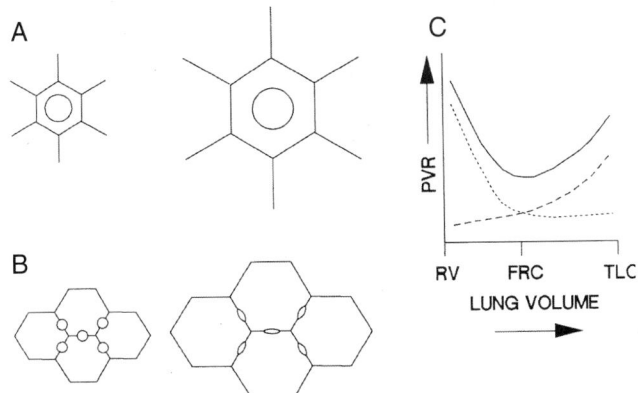

FIGURE 44-10 **A**, Effects of lung inflation on extra-alveolar vessels. **B**, Effects of lung inflation on alveolar vessels. **C**, Effect of lung volume on pulmonary vascular resistance *(PVR; solid line)*. Inflation is from residual volume *(RV)* to functional residual capacity *(FRC)* to total lung capacity *(TLC)*. *Dashed line* represents alveolar vessels; *dotted line* represents extraalveolar vessels.

away from the lung and heart, decreasing pleural pressure, favoring return of venous blood, and priming the heart for the next chest compression. A similar phenomenon may result in augmentation of systemic pressure when ventilator breaths coincide with ventricular systole.

EFFECT OF LUNG INFLATION ON PULMONARY VASCULAR RESISTANCE

The pulmonary interstitium comprises three different interconnected connective tissue compartments, each containing a different element of the pulmonary circulation (Fishman, 1986). The first—the perivascular cuffs—consists of a sheath of fibers that contain the preacinar pulmonary arteries, lymphatics, and bronchi. The second consists of the intersegmental and interlobular septa and contains pulmonary veins and additional lymphatics. The third connects these two within the alveolar septa and contains the majority of the pulmonary capillaries. The first and second compartments represent the extra-alveolar interstitium, whereas the third represents the alveolar interstitium. The perivascular cuffs are surrounded by alveoli and expand during lung inflation (Figure 44-10, *A*). As a result, pressure within each cuff decreases, distending extra-alveolar blood vessels and decreasing their resistance to blood flow. The alveolar interstitium lies between adjacent alveoli and contains the majority of gas-exchanging vessels in the lung. These vessels are exposed to alveolar pressure on both sides and during lung inflation (Figure 44-10, *B*) are compressed so that their resistance to blood flow increases.

Therefore, during lung inflation (Figure 44-10, *C*), the resistance in extra-alveolar vessels decreases, whereas resistance in alveolar vessels increases. As a result, the overall pulmonary vascular resistance decreases initially, with lung inflation reaching its nadir at FRC, and then increases with further inflation.

If transition from intrauterine life to extrauterine life is to be successful, after birth all of the right ventricular output must traverse the pulmonary vascular bed. To some extent, this adaptation is facilitated by a reduction in pulmonary vascular resistance that occurs with inflation

of the lungs (see Figure 44-10) to a stable FRC. Inflation of the lung beyond FRC increases pulmonary vascular resistance. If care is not taken during positive pressure ventilation, it is possible to inflate the lung to the point that alveolar vessels close and blood flow through the lung is impaired. When this occurs, either cardiac output decreases or the blood bypasses the lung via the foramen ovale or ductus arteriosus. Clinically, this is manifest as circulatory insufficiency from impaired right ventricular output or hypoxemia from right-to-left shunting of blood, or both.

EFFECTS OF THE HEART ON THE LUNG

Pulmonary Edema

Pulmonary edema is the abnormal accumulation of water and solute in the interstitial and alveolar spaces of the lung (Bland and Hansen, 1985; Staub, 1974). In the lung, fluid is filtered from capillaries in the alveolar septa into the alveolar interstitium (Figure 44-11, *A*) and then siphoned into the lower pressure extra-alveolar interstitium. The extra-alveolar interstitium contains the pulmonary lymphatics, and under normal conditions, they remove fluid from the lung so that there is no net accumulation in the interstitium. Pulmonary edema results only when the rate of fluid filtration exceeds the rate of lymphatic removal. There are only three mechanisms by which this can occur (Figure 44-11, *B*): (1) the driving pressure for fluid filtration (filtration pressure) increases, (2) the permeability of the vascular bed (hence, the filtration coefficient K_f) increases, or (3) lymphatic drainage decreases.

Increased Driving Pressure

Filtration pressure can be increased by increased intravascular hydrostatic pressure, decreased interstitial hydrostatic pressure, decreased intravascular oncotic pressure, or increased interstitial oncotic pressure (Figure 44-11, *C* and *D*). By far the most common cause of increased filtration pressure is increased intravascular hydrostatic pressure (Box 44-1). In the newborn, intravascular hydrostatic pressure increases with increased left atrial pressure from volume overload or a number of congenital and acquired heart defects. In the preterm and term newborn, evidence suggests that alterations in pulmonary blood flow that are independent of any change in left atrial pressure may also influence fluid filtration in the lung. Preterm infants with patent ductus arteriosus and left-to-right shunts exhibit signs of respiratory insufficiency before they develop any evidence of heart failure, and experiments performed in newborn lambs show that fluid filtration in the lung can be increased by increasing pulmonary blood flow without increasing left atrial pressure (Feltes and Hansen, 1986). In the newborn with a reduced pulmonary vascular bed, either from lung injury or from hypoplasia, cardiac output appropriate for body size may represent a relative overperfusion to the lung and can result in increased fluid filtration. This phenomenon has been invoked to explain the lung edema that often complicates the course of the infant with bronchopulmonary dysplasia.

The exact cause of pulmonary edema that accompanies severe hypoxia or asphyxia in the newborn is still a

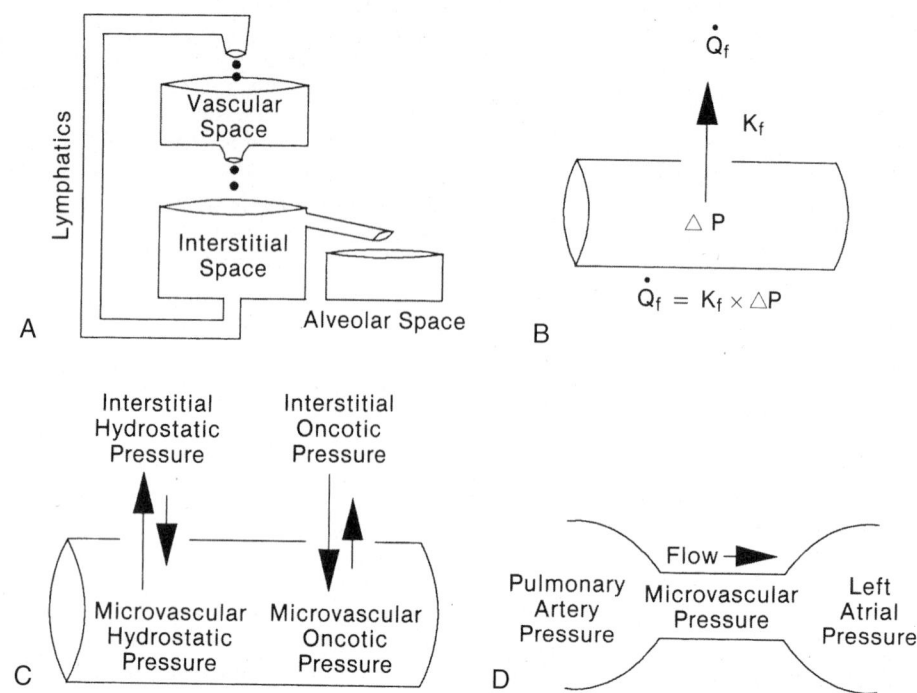

FIGURE 44-11 **A,** In the lung, fluid is continuously filtered out of vessels in the microcirculation into the interstitium and then returned to the intravascular compartment by the lymphatics. Only when the rate of filtration exceeds the rate of lymphatic removal can fluid accumulate in the interstitium. Spillover of fluid into the alveolar space occurs only when the interstitial space fills or when the alveolar membrane is damaged. **B,** Fluid flows out of vessels at a flow rate ($\dot{Q}_f$) that is equal to the driving pressure for fluid flow (ΔP) times the filtration coefficient (K_f): ($\dot{Q}_f$) = $K_f \times \Delta P$. K_f can be thought of as the relative permeability of the vascular bed to fluid flux. K_f in the normal lung is a small number so that despite a driving pressure of roughly 5 mm Hg, the net rate of fluid filtration is approximately 1 to 2 mL/kg per hour. **C,** The driving pressure for fluid flow out of the microvascular bed represents a balance of two sets of pressures. Within the blood vessel, hydrostatic pressure tends to push fluid out of the vessel into the interstitium. This pressure is partially opposed by a smaller hydrostatic pressure within the interstitium pushing fluid back into the blood vessel. Within the blood vessel, there also exists a discrete oncotic pressure that results predominantly from intravascular albumin that tends to draw fluid from the interstitium back into the blood vessel. This pressure is partially opposed by an interstitial oncotic pressure tending to draw fluid from the blood vessel into the interstitium. **D,** The intravascular hydrostatic pressure must be less than pulmonary artery pressure (Ppa) for blood to flow into the microvascular bed and greater than left atrial pressure (Pla) for blood to flow out. Intravascular pressure within the microvascular bed is roughly equal to 0.4 (Ppa − Pla) + Pla. The interstitial hydrostatic pressure is roughly equal to alveolar pressure. The intravascular oncotic pressure can be calculated from the plasma albumin concentration. The interstitial oncotic pressure is roughly two thirds of the intravascular oncotic pressure. The balance of these pressures favors filtration out of the vessel (in the normal lamb, this pressure is roughly 5 mm Hg).

BOX 44-1   Increased Intravascular Hydrostatic Pressure

INCREASED LEFT ATRIAL PRESSURE
Intravascular volume overload
 Overzealous fluid administration
 Overtransfusion
 Renal insufficiency
Heart failure
 Left-sided obstructive lesions
 Left-to-right shunts
 Myocardiopathies

INCREASED PULMONARY BLOOD FLOW
Normal pulmonary vascular bed
 Patent ductus arteriosus
 Increased cardiac output
Reduced pulmonary vascular bed
 Bronchopulmonary dysplasia
 Pulmonary hypoplasia

In addition, there may be some element of pulmonary venous constriction. Finally, there is evidence that hypoxia and acidosis may redistribute pulmonary blood flow to a smaller portion of the lung and result in relative overperfusion and edema, similar to that seen with anatomic loss of vascular bed (Hansen et al, 1984).

Several investigators have suggested that upper airway obstruction may cause pulmonary edema by decreasing interstitial hydrostatic pressure relative to intravascular hydrostatic pressure. Other data suggest, however, that with airway obstruction, vascular pressures decrease with intrapleural pressure in such a way that filtration pressure remains unchanged (Hansen et al, 1985).

Hypoproteinemia in infants results in a decrease in intravascular oncotic pressure. Its effects on filtration pressure, however, are blunted by the simultaneous decrease in protein concentration in the interstitial space of the lung. As a result, edema is unlikely to occur unless hydrostatic pressure also increases (Hazinski et al, 1986).

Increased Permeability

Another possible mechanism for increased fluid filtration in the lung is a change in the permeability of the microvascular membrane to protein—high-permeability

controversial issue. Data suggest that it is the result of increased filtration pressure and not the result of any alteration in permeability. Heart failure accounts for some of the increased filtration pressure following severe asphyxia.

pulmonary edema. In this form of edema, the sieving properties of the microvascular endothelium are altered so that K_f increases and patients may develop pulmonary edema despite relatively normal vascular pressures (Albertine, 1985). Furthermore, even small changes in vascular pressures can result in a dramatic worsening of pulmonary status. High-permeability pulmonary edema usually implies either direct or indirect injury to the capillary endothelium of the lung. Direct injuries result from local effects of an inhaled toxin such as oxygen. Indirect injuries imply that the initial insult occurs elsewhere in the body and that the lung injury occurs secondarily. An example of indirect lung injury is sepsis: Neutrophils activated by bacterial toxins attack endothelial cells in the lung and increase permeability to water and protein (Brigham et al, 1974). Indirect injuries usually involve bloodborne mediators, such as leukocytes, leukotrienes, histamine, or bradykinin. Alveolar overdistention can also cause high-permeability pulmonary edema, presumably by direct injury of the pulmonary vascular bed. This type of vascular injury probably accounts for some of the edema that accompanies diseases such as hyaline membrane disease and bronchopulmonary dysplasia, in which maldistribution of ventilation results in areas of alveolar overdistention (Carlton et al, 1990).

Decreased Lymphatic Drainage

In the normal lung, the rate of lung lymph flow is equal to the net rate of fluid filtration, and as long as lymphatic function can keep up with the rate of fluid filtration, water does not accumulate in the lung. Although lymphatics can actively pump fluid against a pressure gradient, studies show that this ability is limited and that lung lymph flow varies inversely with the outflow pressure (pressure in the superior vena cava). Several groups of investigators have demonstrated that, in the presence of an increased rate of transvascular fluid filtration, the rate of fluid accumulation in the lung is substantially greater if systemic venous pressure is increased (Drake et al, 1985). Recent data suggest that the ability of the lymphatics to pump against an outflow pressure is impaired in the fetus and newborn. In fact, in fetal lambs, lymph flow ceases at an outflow pressure of roughly 15 mm Hg (Johnson et al, 1996). This explains why pulmonary edema often complicates the course of infants with bronchopulmonary dysplasia and cor pulmonale and explains the particular problem of edema with pleural effusions complicating the postoperative course of patients following cavopulmonary shunts.

More recently, investigators have shown that the ability of the lymphatics to pump can be affected by other mediators with pumping increased by α-adrenergics and certain leukotrienes and impaired by nitric oxide, β-adrenergics (Von Der Weid, 2001), and products of hemolysis (Elias et al, 1990).

CONGENITAL PULMONARY LYMPHANGIECTASIS

Congenital pulmonary lymphangiectasis is a rare form of pulmonary lymphatic dysfunction that can be characterized into two groups: (1) cases associated with congenital heart disease and (2) cases not associated with congenital heart disease. The cardiac anomalies may include hypoplastic left heart syndrome, total anomalous pulmonary venous drainage, and pulmonary stenosis, including Noonan syndrome (France and Brown, 1971). The group that does not include associated cardiac anomalies may be of early or late onset and has a wide spectrum of severity. In some individuals, the lesion is asymptomatic, whereas in others it can lead to severe respiratory failure, usually in the first hours after birth but sometimes during the first weeks or months of life. Most infants with this condition die early in the neonatal period. Pulmonary lymphangiectasis has been reported twice as often in males and has been seen in families (Scott Emaukpor et al, 1981).

Usually the radiologist is the first to suggest the diagnosis after observing dilated lymphatic vessels and sometimes small accumulations of pleural fluid on the chest radiograph. The older infant may have no symptoms or mild to moderate tachypnea with various degrees of hypoxemia. If pleural fluid has accumulated, examination of the fluid is important. If the infant has received milk feedings, pleural fluid is chylous, and if not, there is an elevation in mononuclear cells and moderate protein of up to about 4%. These findings in the absence of fever or other signs of systemic illness are diagnostic of impaired lymphatic drainage.

Lung biopsy is probably not indicated and can be hazardous because once the distended lymphatic channels are severed, they can leak fluid for weeks. Only if the diagnosis is in doubt is open lung biopsy appropriate.

In noncardiac associated diffuse lymphangiectasis, only supportive treatment is available. The long-term prognosis depends on the severity of the lesion, but this form of pulmonary lymphangiectasis is compatible with asymptomatic life as an adult (Wohl, 1989).

SYMPTOMS OF PULMONARY EDEMA

As discussed previously, fluid filtered into the alveolar interstitium ordinarily moves rapidly along pressure gradients into the extra-alveolar interstitium where it is removed by the lymphatics. A delay in this process at birth can result in clinical transient respiratory distress (see Chapter 47). The extra-alveolar interstitium has a large storage capacity. Fluid does not begin to spill over into the alveoli and airways until total lung water is increased more than 50%, unless the alveolar membrane is damaged. Therefore, the first signs and symptoms of pulmonary edema are related to the presence of extra fluid in the interstitial cuffs of tissue that surround airways. As fluid builds up in these cuffs, airways are compressed, and the infants develop signs of obstructive lung disease. The chest may appear hyperinflated, and auscultation reveals rales, rhonchi, and a prolonged expiration. Early in the course, chest radiographs reveal lung overinflation and an accumulation of fluid in the extra-alveolar interstitium—linear densities of fluid that extend from the hilum to the periphery of the lung (the so-called sunburst appearance) and fluid in the fissures. With more severe edema, fluffy densities appear throughout the lung as alveoli fill with fluid (Figure 44-12). Heart size may be increased in infants with edema from increased intravascular pressure. Initially, infants present with increased $PaCO_2$ secondary to impaired ventilation. Later PaO_2 decreases secondary to ventilation-perfusion mismatching and alveolar flooding. In adults, a ratio of protein concentration in tracheal aspirate to that in plasma greater than 0.5 may help to differentiate permeability pulmonary edema from high-pressure pulmonary edema (Fein et al, 1979).

TREATMENT OF PULMONARY EDEMA

Treatment of pulmonary edema is directed at relieving hypoxemia and lowering vascular pressures. Hypoxemia should be treated with the administration of oxygen and, if necessary, positive pressure ventilation. Positive end expiratory pressure frequently improves oxygenation in individuals with pulmonary edema by improving ventilation-perfusion matching within the lung. Available evidence suggests that positive pressure ventilation does not reduce the rate of transvascular fluid filtration in the lung (Woolverton et al, 1978). Optimal treatment of pulmonary edema requires correction of the underlying cause. In infants with patent ductus arteriosus (see Figure 44-12) or other heart disease amenable to surgery, this is often easily accomplished. In cases of permeability edema or edema from nonsurgical heart defects, correction of the underlying cause may not be possible. In these instances, the only remaining option is to lower vascular pressures (even in permeability edema, lowering vascular pressures lowers the rate of fluid filtration and may also improve lymphatic function). This can be accomplished by lowering circulating blood volume by use of diuretics and fluid restriction, by improving myocardial function with the use of digitalis or other inotropic agents, or in severe cases by using a systemic vasodilator to reduce afterload and lower vascular pressures directly.

More recent data suggest that clearance of fluid from the alveolar space may be accelerated by β-adrenergic agents (Frank et al, 2000) and by dopamine (Saldias et al, 1999). Whether these agents will have any clinical efficacy remains to be determined.

PULMONARY HEMORRHAGE

Landing (1957) described pulmonary hemorrhage in 68% of lungs of 125 consecutive infants who died in the 1st week of life; massive pulmonary hemorrhage was found in 17.8% of neonatal autopsies at the Johns Hopkins Hospital (Rowe and Avery, 1966). Fedrick and Butler (1971) judged massive pulmonary hemorrhage to be the principal cause of death in about 9% of neonatal autopsies.

Etiology and Pathogenesis

Pulmonary hemorrhage usually occurs between the 2nd and 4th days of life in infants who are being treated with mechanical ventilation. It has been associated with a wide variety of predisposing factors, including prematurity, asphyxia, overwhelming sepsis, intrauterine growth retardation, massive aspiration, severe hypothermia, severe Rh hemolytic disease, congenital heart disease, and coagulopathies. It is often associated with central nervous system injury, such as asphyxia or intracranial hemorrhage. Cole et al (1973) studied a group of infants with pulmonary hemorrhage to determine the clinical circumstances under which the illness occurred as well as the hematocrit and protein composition of fluid obtained from lung effluent and arterial or venous blood. Their results indicated that the lung effluent was, in most cases, hemorrhagic edema fluid and not whole blood (i.e., as indicated by hematocrit values significantly lower than those of whole blood). In addition, they did not find that coagulation disorders initiated the condition but probably served to exacerbate it in some cases. They postulated that the important precipitating factor was acute left ventricular failure caused by asphyxia or other events that might increase the filtration pressure and so injure the capillary endothelium of the lung. Thus, pulmonary hemorrhage may be considered as the extreme form of high-permeability pulmonary edema.

Pulmonary edema following central nervous system injury probably results from increased hydrostatic pressure and some increase in vascular permeability (Malik, 1985). With the massive sympathetic discharge that accompanies central nervous system injury, left atrial pressure increases, and pulmonary arteries and veins constrict. As a result, microvascular pressure increases dramatically and causes dramatic damage to the microvascular endothelium, increasing its permeability to proteins and red blood cells. In infants with overwhelming sepsis and endotoxin production, increased microvascular permeability is apparent in the pulmonary circulation as well, undoubtedly contributing to the massive pulmonary hemorrhage sometimes seen in this group of infants. Pulmonary hemorrhage also has

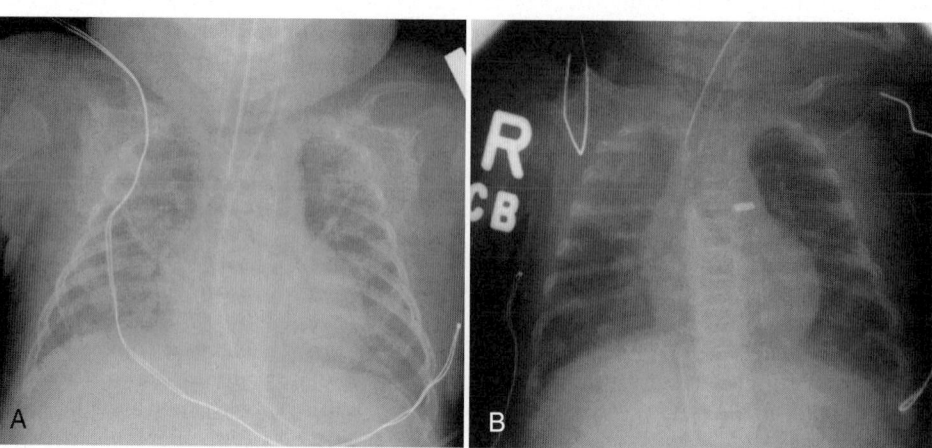

FIGURE 44-12 A, Preterm infant with a large patent ductus arteriosus and pulmonary edema. **B**, The same infant 24 hours after the ductus arteriosus was closed by surgical ligation.

been described occasionally in the presence of a large patent ductus arteriosus, with a left-to-right shunt that results in high flow and high pressure injurious to the vascular bed.

Pulmonary hemorrhage is also associated with surfactant replacement therapy. Presumably the hemorrhage results from the rapid increase in pulmonary blood flow that accompanies improved lung function after surfactant therapy. The contribution of the patent ductus arteriosus to this increased blood flow remains to be determined. A meta-analysis suggests that surfactant replacement may be associated with an increased risk of pulmonary hemorrhage. This risk, however, is still extremely small compared to the known benefits of surfactant replacement (Pappin et al, 1994; Raju and Langenberg, 1993).

Diagnosis

Infants with any of the conditions mentioned previously should be observed carefully for possible pulmonary hemorrhage. Particular note should be made of any occurrence of blood-stained fluid from endotracheal tube aspirates, especially if repeated suctioning shows an increase in the amount of hemorrhagic fluid. The infant's chest radiograph may show the fluffy appearance of pulmonary edema in addition to the underlying pathology, and the infant may have increased respiratory distress. Frank pulmonary hemorrhage, when it occurs, is an acute emergency, and the fluid has the appearance of fresh blood being pumped directly from the vascular system, although hematocrit values of the fluid are at least 15 to 20 points lower than the hematocrit of circulating blood, in keeping with hemorrhagic pulmonary edema.

Treatment

Effective treatment of pulmonary hemorrhage requires (1) clearing the airway of blood to allow ventilation; (2) use of adequate mean airway pressure, particularly end expiratory pressure; (3) resisting the temptation to administer large volumes of blood because in most cases the infant has not had a large loss of volume, and thus, administration of excessive volume exacerbates the increase in left atrial pressure and hemorrhagic pulmonary edema; rather, red cell replacement should be done as a slow administration of packed cells after the infant's pulmonary status has been stabilized; and (4) evaluation of the possibility of coagulopathy and administration of vitamin K and platelets, if appropriate.

SUGGESTED READINGS

Choukroun ML, Tayara N, Fayon M, Demarquez JL: Early respiratory system mechanics and the prediction of chronic lung disease in ventilated preterm neonates requiring surfactant treatment, *Biol Neonate* 83:30-35, 2003.

Cook CD, Cherry RB, O'Brien D, et al: Studies of respiratory physiology in the newborn infant: I. Observations on normal premature and full term infants, *J Clin Invest* 34:975-982, 1955.

Corbet AJ, Ross JA, Beaudry PH, et al: Ventilation-perfusion relationships as assessed by aADN$_2$ in hyaline membrane disease, *J Appl Physiol* 36:74-81, 1974.

Frappell PB, MacFarlane PM: Development of mechanics and pulmonary reflexes, *Respir Physiol Neurobiol* 149:143-154, 2005.

Gappa M, Pillow JJ, Allen J, et al: Lung function tests in neonates and infants with chronic lung disease: lung and chest-wall mechanics, *Pediatr Pulmonol* 41:291-317, 2006.

Greenspan JS, Miller TL, Shaffer TH: The neonatal respiratory pump: a developmental challenge with physiologic limitations, *Neonatal Netw* 24:15-22, 2005.

Hülskamp G, Pillow JJ, Stocks J: Lung function testing in acute neonatal respiratory disorders and chronic lung disease of infancy: a review series, *Pediatr Pulmonol* 40:467-470, 2005.

Katier N, Uiterwaal CS, de Jong BM, et al: Passive respiratory mechanics measured during natural sleep in healthy term neonates and infants up to 8 weeks of life, *Pediatr Pulmonol* 41:1058-1064, 2006.

Lesouef PN, England SJ, Bryan AC: Passive respiratory mechanics in newborns and children, *Am Rev Respir Dis* 129:552-556, 1984.

McCann EM, Goldman SL, Brady JP: Pulmonary function in the sick newborn infant, *Pediatr Res* 21:313-325, 1987.

McIlroy MB, Tomlinson ES: The mechanics of breathing in newly born babies, *Thorax* 10:58-61, 1955.

Qureshi M, Khalil M, Kwiatkowski K, Alvaro RE: Morphology of sighs and their role in the control of breathing in preterm infants, term infants and adults, *Neonatology* 96:43-49, 2009.

Complete references and supplemental color images used in this text can be found online at www.expertconsult.com

PRINCIPLES OF RESPIRATORY MONITORING AND THERAPY

Eduardo Bancalari and Nelson Claure

RESPIRATORY MONITORING

One of the most important aspects of newborn intensive care is monitoring of cardiorespiratory function, ventilation, and oxygenation. This can be accomplished by bedside monitoring devices and laboratory analysis. The information provided by these monitoring techniques is an essential tool in the diagnosis and treatment of respiratory problems in the newborn.

BREATHING FREQUENCY, APNEA, AND HEART RATE MONITORING

Transthoracic impedance is the standard method used to monitor neonatal respiration. This technique is based on changes in the thorax's electrical impedance caused by changes in gas volume during respiration measured by surface electrodes. Transthoracic impedance is mainly used to monitor breathing frequency and to detect apnea (Olsson and Victorin, 1970).

Breathing is detected when the change in impedance exceeds a set threshold. A low threshold decreases sensitivity for apnea, and small disturbances such as cardiogenic oscillations can be falsely considered as breathing. Conversely, a high threshold may lead to false apnea alarms during shallow breathing. Monitors can automatically adjust this threshold or the impedance amplitude, or use sophisticated methods for detecting breathing or apnea. Transthoracic impedance is not reliable in assessing absolute tidal volume, but it can be used to assess relative changes.

This technique is more effective in detecting apneas of central origin than obstructive apnea because the latter can produce internal displacement of gas volumes that still change impedance. More specific techniques are used for diagnosis and classification of apnea, including thermistors and CO_2 monitors to detect gas exhalation and respiratory inductance plethysmography that measures expansion of the chest and abdomen. Transthoracic impedance monitors can also measure heart rate and are used to detect brady- and tachycardia. More sophisticated devices or built-in algorithms are utilized to detect cardiac rhythm anomalies.

VENTILATION MONITORING

The basic clinical determination of the adequacy of ventilation in the mechanically ventilated neonate consists of assessment of chest expansion, breathing frequency and auscultation. This can be complemented by monitoring tidal volume (V_T) and minute ventilation utilizing flow sensors available in most neonatal ventilators. This allows for monitoring of spontaneous breathing, assessment of respiratory system mechanics and detection of excessive or insufficient V_T, hypoventilation, and gas trapping (Becker and Donn, 2007).

These flow sensors are either mainstream (connected between the endotracheal tube and the ventilator circuit) or built into the ventilator. In small infants, mainstream flow sensors have better accuracy than those built into the ventilator because V_T and flow are only a fraction of the gas volumes compressed in the circuit and the circulating bias flow (Cannon et al, 2000; Chow et al, 2002). Although mainstream flow sensors are usually small and typically have a dead space volume <1 mL, they can induce rebreathing of exhaled gases and affect CO_2 elimination in small preterm infants (Claure et al, 2003; Figueras et al, 1997).

BLOOD GAS MONITORING

Determination of arterial blood gas status is key to the management of respiratory failure and lung disease in the neonate. Measurements of oxygen (Pao_2) and carbon dioxide ($Paco_2$) tension in arterial blood are considered the reference standard by which the efficacy and adequacy of ventilation and oxygenation are assessed.

In order to obtain repeated arterial blood samples, placement of invasive catheters is required. In neonates, umbilical artery catheters (UACs) are commonly used during the acute phases of respiratory failure. Samples obtained from a UAC are the most accurate when proper sample handling and laboratory procedures are followed. However, there are important issues that must be considered before their placement and during their use to ensure that the risk-to-benefit ratio remains favorable. UAC have risks during placement and use, including perforation of the vessels, formation of thrombi and emboli, vasospasm and infection. UAC lines with the tip above the celiac plexus are associated with fewer complications than those below the renal or mesenteric artery (Barrington, 2000).

Alternatively, percutaneous lines in the radial, ulnar, or dorsalis pedis artery are used when placement of a UAC is not possible. When an invasive line is not available, arterial punctures to the radial, ulnar, temporal, posterior tibialis, or dorsalis pedis artery are done to obtain blood samples. These latter results should be interpreted carefully because the procedure frequently disturbs the infant and alters blood gases. An alternative is to obtain blood samples from the peripheral capillary bed of the medial or lateral plantar surface. These are obtained after warming of the area, which produces hyperemia or "arterialization." These samples provide a gross estimate of arterial blood gases, and they should also be interpreted cautiously (Courtney et al, 1990). Erroneous estimation usually occurs due to contamination by venous blood or air. This procedure can also disturb the infant and alter the basal status. Errors in blood gas measurement are often technique related. Contamination by an air bubble can reduce Pco_2 and alter the Po_2 in the direction of the air's oxygen tension. Contamination by fluids can reduce Po_2 and Pco_2 while also affecting pH. Because blood cell metabolism continues, reducing the time from sampling to analysis and cold temperature storage and transport attenuate its effects.

During conditions such as transport or when the turn-around time is important, bedside portable blood analysis devices have proven to be most effective (Murthy et al, 1997). Another alternative measurement method is that of indwelling electrodes inserted through a UAC that provide a continuous stream of blood gas information (Rais-Bahrami et al, 2002).

TRANSCUTANEOUS BLOOD GAS MONITORING

Transcutaneous measurement of O_2 ($TcPo_2$) and CO_2 ($TcPco_2$) tensions provide a noninvasive estimate of Pao_2 and $Paco_2$, respectively. Local hyperperfusion of the skin induced by heating creates a skin-electrode unit under the transcutaneous sensor, and electrochemical measurements in an electrolyte solution within this unit determine the partial pressure of O_2 and CO_2.

During measurement of $TcPo_2$, oxygen diffusing from the capillaries to the skin is reduced by the electrode, and the resulting electrical current is proportional to the Po_2 of the capillary bed. Because skin metabolism continues, local hyperemia is needed to maintain skin perfusion sufficiently high that the measured $TcPo_2$ is not affected by the skin's O_2 consumption. For this reason, accuracy of $TcPo_2$ depends on electrode temperature with improved accuracy at or above 43° C (Huch et al, 1976). Under adequate conditions, $TcPo_2$ correlates with Pao_2 (Peabody et al, 1978). However, conditions such as arterial hypotension and acidosis often result in underestimation due to insufficient skin perfusion (Versmold et al, 1979).

During $TcPco_2$ measurement, CO_2 molecules diffusing from the capillary bed change the pH of the electrolyte solution in the skin-electrode unit. This changes the electric potential between a reference and the electrode that is then translated into $TcPco_2$. Metabolism in the skin produces CO_2, and if the local perfusion is not adequate, the measured values can exceed those of $Paco_2$. $TcPco_2$ measurements can also be affected by conditions affecting peripheral perfusion (Peabody and Emery, 1985) and tend to overestimate $Paco_2$ in hypercapnia as local perfusion decreases (Martin et al, 1988).

Recent reports have demonstrated improved $TcPco_2$ measurement accuracy in preterm infants of <29 weeks' gestation, but inconsistent precision due to large between-patient variability (Aliwalas et al 2005; Bernet-Buettiker et al, 2005; Tingay et al, 2005). $TcPco_2$ measurements have also been shown to be tightly correlated to capillary Pco_2. Although capillary blood gases may not be the optimal reference, these are often the only available method for long-term monitoring because indwelling lines are available only during the acute phase of respiratory failure. In preterm infants, $TcPco_2$ may reduce the need for blood sampling and the number of painful punctures, but the main benefit is the ability to monitor continuously. For this reason, $TcPco_2$ is commonly used as an adjunct to standard blood gas sampling to provide information on trends and respiratory stability. This is particularly useful in the management of invasive ventilatory support where close tracking of the effects of ventilator changes is required.

The thin epidermal skin layer of the neonate has a relatively low metabolism. Nonetheless, some transcutaneous monitors include a metabolic correction factor. Measurements of $TcPo_2$ and $TcPco_2$ require a period of stabilization after sensor application until skin perfusion increases. A tight seal around the skin-electrode unit is required for accuracy. Similar to blood gas sampling, an air bubble transiently lowers $TcPco_2$ and shifts $TcPo_2$ toward the partial pressure of O_2 in room air until the O_2 is reduced.

The transcutaneous electrode is usually applied on the thorax or the thigh. The need for high electrode temperature combined with the premature infant's skin sensitivity requires frequent change of the application site to avoid thermal injury. Transcutaneous measurements have an intrinsic delay with respect to changes occurring in the arterial blood.

END-TIDAL CARBON DIOXIDE MONITORING

Monitoring of the partial pressure of CO_2 in end-tidal gases ($PetCo_2$) is based on the assumption that gases measured at the airway opening at the end of exhalation represent alveolar gases and that these match the arterial levels. $PetCo_2$ is obtained by infrared sensors placed mainstream or by side-stream gas sampling. $PetCo_2$ measurements are dependent on tidal volume size because the exhaled gas has to carry alveolar gas. The accuracy of $PetCo_2$ is affected by lung disease with an increased arterial to alveolar CO_2 gradient that results in underestimation of $Paco_2$ (Sivan et al, 1992). For this reason, $PetCo_2$ is more often used in term or near-term neonates and pediatric patients who require CO_2 monitoring for reasons other than lung disease.

ARTERIAL OXYGEN SATURATION BY PULSE OXIMETRY

Estimation of the oxygen saturation in arterial blood (Sao_2) by pulse oximetry (Spo_2) is based on the differences in the rates of light absorption between oxygenated and deoxygenated or reduced hemoglobin (Hb) in the red and infrared regions of light. Deoxygenated Hb absorbs more red light and less infrared light than oxygenated Hb. As Sao_2 increases, the ratio of the absorption of red light to that of infrared light decreases. It is assumed that in the circulation, changes in this ratio can only be produced by pulsating arterial blood. In neonates, Spo_2 has been shown to correlate well with measured saturation in arterial samples (Hay et al, 1989).

The absorption by pulsatile blood is only a small fraction of the light absorbed by tissue and venous blood. Thus, changes in pulse amplitude or patient movement that disrupt the optical pathway from transmitter to receiver side of the probe, or produce venous blood fluctuations, can affect Spo_2 accuracy, although newer techniques have reduced the effect of the latter (Hay et al, 2002). The accuracy of Spo_2 is also affected by conditions such as low perfusion or by inappropriate placement such as excessive tightening of the probe (Bucher et al, 1994).

Data indicate reliable detection of hypoxemia spells by pulse oximetry (Bohnhorst et al, 2000; Hay et al, 2002). Nonetheless, some hypoxemia episodes detected by pulse oximetry are considered artifactual because of their temporal association with infant movement. However, increased infant activity leading to heart rate, lung volume, and ventilation changes has been shown to trigger hypoxemia (Bolivar et al, 1995; Dimaguila et al, 1997) with increased frequency during periods when the infants are awake compared to periods of active or quiet sleep (Lehtonen et al, 2002).

OXYGEN THERAPY

PRINCIPLES

Neonates presenting with acute respiratory failure or with some degree of respiratory distress suffer abnormalities of gas exchange that almost invariably result in hypoxemia. Depending on the severity and duration of hypoxemia and the metabolic demands for oxygen, this can lead to reduced O_2 availability and tissue hypoxia. Hypoxemia in the neonate can result from reduced alveolar oxygen content, low ventilation-perfusion ratio, reduced diffusion capacity, and extrapulmonary right-to-left shunts.

The most common form of respiratory therapy for the neonate with hypoxemia consists of oxygen supplementation. The increased fraction of inspired oxygen (Fio_2) increases the alveolar O_2 tension (PAo_2) in both well- and partially ventilated areas of the lung. The resulting increase in the alveolar-arterial O_2 gradient (A-aDo_2) in part compensates for the conditions producing hypoxemia mentioned earlier. The proportion of neonates requiring supplemental O_2 increases with lower gestational ages because premature birth is associated with many of the factors that contribute to hypoxemia.

The primary goal of oxygen therapy is to maintain adequate O_2 availability to the tissues, especially to the central nervous system and the heart, and to improve an incomplete hemodynamic adaptation to extrauterine life evident by persistently elevated pulmonary vascular resistance and patency of the ductus arteriosus. These goals, however, need to be attained without inducing the side effects of O_2 toxicity on the eye, brain, and other organs that are common in the premature infant.

Normal Sao_2 for room-air-breathing term or healthy preterm infants is reportedly greater than 93%, with Pao_2 levels above 70 mm Hg (Fenner et al, 1975; O'Brien et al, 2000; Richard et al, 1993). Maintenance of such oxygenation levels in premature infants with lung disease and immaturity would almost invariably require high inspired O_2 levels. Earlier strategies to "normalize" oxygenation with use of high Fio_2 in this population resulted in high rates of retinopathy of prematurity (ROP) and blindness (Campbell, 1951; Cross, 1973; Crosse and Evans, 1952). Conversely, strict curtailment of supplemental O_2 regardless of the oxygenation level was associated with increased rates of neurologic damage and death (Avery, 1960; Bolton and Cross, 1974; Patz et al, 1952).

The preterm infant is at risk for O_2-induced injury because of an immature antioxidant system that is unable to balance the oxidative effects of O_2 radicals. In the past, severe neonatal lung injury was only partly attributed to exposure to high Fio_2. However, animal experiments have showed that lung damage was caused by high alveolar O_2 independent of Pao_2 (Miller et al, 1970; Northway et al, 1967; Taghizadeh and Reynolds, 1976). In preterm infants, hyperoxia has been linked to neurologic damage and impairment (Ahdab-Barmada et al, 1980; Collins et al, 2001; Haynes et al, 2003). For this reason, when supplemental O_2 is administered to hypoxemic neonates, oxygenation is continuously monitored to avoid hyperoxemia.

METHODS OF ADMINISTRATION

In neonates, supplemental O_2 is usually administered by means of a head box, mask, nasal cannula, nasal continuous positive airway pressure (CPAP), or a mechanical ventilator. In mechanically ventilated infants or in infants receiving nasal CPAP, supplemental O_2 is administered by the mixture of air and O_2 in the ventilator or CPAP device. In all four methods, verifying that correct mixing in the air-O_2 blender produces the desired Fio_2 (by means of an O_2 analyzer) is recommended.

A head box, the least invasive of these methods, is generally used for infants who only need supplemental O_2. Depending on the size of the infant, a minimum flow is required to flush exhaled gases and to minimize entrainment of ambient air. Gas warming and humidification is recommended to avoid drying of the airways and secretions as well as to avoid convective heat losses.

Nasal cannulas deliver a constant flow of the air-O_2 mixture to the nostrils. The actual Fio_2 is determined by the delivered flow and the infant's inspiratory flow. With increasing flows the actual inspired O_2 concentration approaches the mixture delivered by the cannula, whereas higher inspiratory flows, in larger infants or during periods of increased demands, reduce the actual inspired O_2 by entraining more room air (Walsh et al, 2005). The actual Fio_2 during oral breathing has not been determined. Cannula flows >1 lpm can produce positive pressure at the nose at levels similar or above typical CPAP levels (Locke et al, 2003), which can become very high if the prongs fit tightly in the nostrils. Gas conditioning is recommended to avert drying of the nose and the risk of mucosal damage (Kopelman and Holbert, 2003). Nasal cannulas have gained popularity because they are flexible and facilitate access to and mobility of the infant.

TREATMENT STRATEGIES

The effects of the introduction of continuous monitoring of oxygenation in the care of preterm infants in relation to ROP have been inconsistent (Bancalari et al, 1987; Grylack, 1987; Yamanouchi et al, 1987). Data showing that ROP severity was associated with duration of hyperoxemia emphasized the importance of monitoring and curtailing hyperoxemia (Flynn et al, 1987). However, infants with severe ROP were also found to spend considerable periods of time in hypoxemia.

Continuous monitoring of arterial oxygen saturation by pulse oximetry (Spo_2) has become an important and standard component of neonatal intensive care. The use of Spo_2 has recently been extended to the delivery room for titration of Fio_2 during resuscitation (Dawson et al, 2009; Escrig et al, 2008). Although the optimal range of Spo_2 in premature infants has not been fully defined, existing data suggest deleterious effects of hyperoxemia, with higher rates of ROP and worse respiratory course in neonatal centers that have tolerant policies toward high Spo_2 levels (Anderson et al, 2004; Tin et al, 2001). Observational data indicate that more restrictive policies toward high Spo_2 can reduce rates of ROP (Chow et al, 2003; Wright et al, 2006). Tolerance of high Spo_2 levels in convalescent infants beyond the neonatal period has been proposed to improve growth and neurologic outcome, as well as to stop the progression of threshold ROP. However, clinical trials showed minimal benefits that were outweighed by deterioration in lung function caused by the additional O_2 required to maintain higher Spo_2 (Askie et al, 2003; STOP-ROP Study Group, 2000).

Implementation of policies to curb hyperoxemia should also consider the potential deleterious effects of insufficient oxygenation. Hypoxemia can increase patency of the ductus arteriosus (Noori et al, 2009; Skinner et al, 1999) as well as increase the resistance of the pulmonary vasculature and airways, particularly in infants with established lung disease (Abman et al, 1985; Cassin et al, 1964; Halliday et al, 1980; Tay-Uyboco et al, 1989; Teague et al, 1988).

Observational data showed that policies targeting lower Spo_2 ranges were associated with better outcomes (Chow et al, 2003; Wright et al, 2006). However, it is unknown how closely such ranges were actually maintained and is possible that the side effects of lower Spo_2 levels were not detected because infants were maintained above those ranges most of the time. Those findings should be interpreted with caution in face of recent evidence from a large blinded randomized-controlled trial showing increased mortality when targeting a lower Spo_2 range (Carlo et al, 2010).

The use of pulse oximetry to avoid hyperoxemia and hypoxemia must be done in the context of the sigmoid-shaped oxygen dissociation curve between Pao_2 and Spo_2. Although Spo_2 levels in the upper range can be associated with a wide range of Pao_2 levels (Brockway and Hay, 1998), data indicate that a Spo_2 threshold of 93% or 94% can avoid most Pao_2 values >80 mm Hg (Bohnhorst et al, 2002; Castillo et al, 2008; Hay et al, 1989; Poets et al, 1993). On the other end, most Spo_2 values <80% or 85% are associated with Pao_2 <40 mm Hg. Thus, a moderate and stepwise increase in Fio_2 when Spo_2 decreases below this threshold can adequately correct hypoxemia and is unlikely to produce hyperoxemia unless the additional oxygen is excessive or prolonged unnecessarily. When Fio_2 is increased in response to a hypoxemia spell, Spo_2 should be continuously observed, and Fio_2 should be weaned as the spell ends.

Policies of oxygenation monitoring should clearly identify both intended range and the alarm limits of Spo_2. Although in many centers they coincide, these ranges serve different purposes. The intended range usually defines a prescribed basal level of oxygenation to be maintained by the staff, whereas the alarm limits usually define specific conditions that require immediate intervention.

In practice, the use of the low and high Spo_2 alarms differs. The low Spo_2 alarm, typically set between 85% and 88%, is generally used to detect acute hypoxemia. Setting Spo_2 alarms below these levels is often aimed at ensuring that the caregiver will respond only to the most severe events, thereby indirectly avoiding overuse of supplemental O_2. The high Spo_2 alarm is primarily used to avoid hyperoxemia and is typically set between 93% and 95%. The high Spo_2 alarm level is quite important because it has been shown to be closely linked to the actual mean Spo_2 observed in preterm infants receiving supplemental O_2 (Hagadorn et al, 2006).

Observational data have shown that preterm infants spend only half the time within the intended range of Spo_2, with the remaining 30% of the time above and 20% of the time below this range (Hagadorn et al, 2006; Laptook et al, 2006). Setting Spo_2 alarm limits within 2% of the intended range produces some improvement, but not strikingly so. Staff compliance to Spo_2 alarms plays an important role, with the prescribed high Spo_2 alarm level being frequently altered by the staff (Clucas et al, 2007). Insufficient staff education and communication can also influence the maintenance of Spo_2 within the intended range. However, a recent survey showed that only a third of the caregivers were aware of and could identify their center's oxygenation policies (Nghiem et al, 2008).

Policies for oxygen supplementation for preterm infants who reach term-corrected postmenstrual ages (e.g., 36 weeks) vary significantly between centers (Ellsbury et al, 2002). Centers with policies that target higher Spo_2 have greater proportions of infants on supplemental O_2, and many of those infants could be off O_2 if lower Spo_2 levels are tolerated or if their actual needs are frequently evaluated (Walsh et al, 2004). This is also the case during the discharge period as well as during home oxygen therapy.

Many preterm infants present with hypoxemia spells, and these are more frequent in infants with evolving chronic lung disease (Bolivar et al, 1995; Dimaguila et al, 1997; Garg et al, 1988). These spells often require a transient increase in Fio_2, but a delayed response can prolong the hypoxemia spell, whereas a delayed weaning of Fio_2 after hypoxemia ends can induce hyperoxemia. It is also evident that caregivers often tolerate or maintain high Spo_2 levels with the purpose of reducing the frequency of the spells or attenuating their severity (Claure et al, 2009, 2011). However, this is not truly effective and may actually increase the risk of ROP (McColm et al, 2004). Neonatal center policies should clearly define the response of the caregiver to these events to minimize both excessive and inadequate oxygenation.

Currently, automated systems to adjust the inspired oxygen for maintenance of Spo_2 within a set range are being developed and tested (Claure et al, 2001, 2009, 2011; Urschitz et al, 2004). Reports indicate improvements in terms of maintenance of an oxygenation range as well as reductions in hyperoxemia, exposure to supplemental O_2, and staff workload with these automated systems. Large trials are necessary to determine the effects of this form of Fio_2 control on short- and long-term neonatal outcomes. At the present time, most clinical effort is focused on avoiding the extreme high and low ranges of Spo_2. Forthcoming are the findings of multicenter trials being conducted to compare the effects of maintaining Spo_2 within different ranges in terms of ophthalmic, neurologic, and respiratory outcome. The information obtained from these trials will further refine the oxygen management strategies.

NONINVASIVE RESPIRATORY SUPPORT

Because of the severe complications associated with invasive mechanical ventilation, there has been a persistent search for less invasive alternatives to support infants with respiratory failure. This is especially relevant in the small preterm infant, who is more susceptible to acute complications and chronic pulmonary sequelae. Alternatives have ranged from transdermal oxygenation to lung volume maintenance by sternal traction. The strategies that have shown to be most clinically effective are nasal continuous positive airway pressure and, more recently, nasal intermittent positive pressure ventilation. These strategies can be used to support infants with respiratory failure in lieu of invasive mechanical ventilation.

NASAL CONTINUOUS POSITIVE AIRWAY PRESSURE

CPAP was introduced in 1971 by George Gregory to stabilize lung volume in preterm infants with respiratory distress syndrome (RDS) (Gregory et al, 1971). Initially, the constant pressure was delivered through a mask or head box and later was applied through nasal prongs. With the introduction of surfactant therapy, more infants were intubated and treated with mechanical ventilation, and the use of nasal CPAP declined for a period of several years; in the past decade, however, it has been reintroduced as a safer alternative to mechanical ventilation.

Physiologic Effects

Nasal CPAP (N-CPAP) prevents alveolar collapse and stabilizes functional residual capacity, thereby reducing pulmonary shunts and resulting in improved oxygenation.

N-CPAP also stabilizes large and small airways and can decrease the work of breathing and obstructive apnea episodes. By preventing alveolar closure and reopening with each breath, N-CPAP can also preserve surfactant.

Indications

Nasal CPAP is used primarily in infants with RDS who because of surfactant deficiency have decreased functional residual capacity (FRC). N-CPAP is also effective in the transition period immediately after birth while reabsorption of fetal lung fluid and establishment of FRC is occurring. N-CPAP is also effective in reducing apneic episodes and in stabilizing respiratory function after extubation (Locke et al, 1991; Martin et al, 1977; Miller et al, 1985). Nasal CPAP is also used in infants with increased pulmonary blood flow and pulmonary edema secondary to heart lesions with left-to-right shunting such as patent ductus arteriosus (PDA). Nasal CPAP can also be used effectively in infants with airway obstruction.

Devices for Nasal CPAP

Nasal CPAP has been applied using a variety of systems and devices. Most of the evidence suggests that best results are obtained using double short nasal prongs (De Paoli et al, 2002). The devices used to generate the pressure can be a water column such as the one used for "bubble CPAP" or an adjustable valve at the end of a continuous-flow system or a variable-flow system. Although there are data suggesting that some of these systems are superior to others, in clinical practice the stability and permeability of the nasal interface is probably the most important factor determining the success or failure of this form of respiratory support. Recently, nasal cannulas have been used as a method for generating nasal CPAP. The limitation of this method is that it is difficult to control and measure the actual pressures and inspired oxygen concentrations that are delivered to the infant because both depend on the gas flow and the leaks around the cannulas and through the mouth.

Clinical Application

As mentioned earlier, the major indication for N-CPAP use in preterm infants is RDS. There is considerable debate as to the ideal time to start N-CPAP and about the population of infants in which it should be used. In recent years most centers have used N-CPAP soon after birth in infants who have sufficient respiratory drive. The exceptions are infants who are depressed at birth or those who have severe respiratory failure and are intubated to administer surfactant. The success rate with this strategy depends on the maturity of the infant and the severity of the respiratory failure, but more than 50% of preterm infants who are not depressed at birth can be managed successfully with N-CPAP, avoiding the use of invasive ventilation (Ammari et al, 2005; Dani et al, 2004; Kamper and Ringsted, 1990; Reininger et al, 2005). The sooner N-CPAP is started, the better the results are in infants with RDS (Gittermann et al, 1997; Hegyi and Hiatt, 1981; Jonsson et al, 1997; Verder et al, 1999). It has been suggested that the early use of N-CPAP instead of invasive ventilation could lead to a reduction in the incidence of bronchopulmonary dysplasia (BPD). However, two large prospective randomized trials addressing this question did not show that early use of N-CPAP reduces BPD (Finer et al, 2010; Morley et al, 2008).

The other frequent indication for N-CPAP is to stabilize respiratory functions after weaning from mechanical ventilation and extubation (Andreasson et al, 1988; Engelke et al, 1982; Higgins et al, 1991). Although it is not clear whether the use of N-CPAP in this situation reduces the need for reintubation, it clearly prevents a deterioration of respiratory function (Davis and Henderson-Smart, 1999; Peake et al, 2005).

The other indication for N-CPAP is to reduce the incidence of apneic episodes in preterm infants, in which it has been shown to be very effective (Martin et al, 1977; Miller et al, 1985).

The levels of N-CPAP that are used in clinical practice range from 3 to 8 cm H_2O, but there are few data to justify a specific level. In practice, the level of N-CPAP used is determined by the severity of the lung disease, reflected by the inspired oxygen concentration and the degree of lung expansion in the chest radiograph. The more severe the disease is, the higher the level of N-CPAP that is used. As the respiratory condition improves and the oxygen requirement decreases the level of N-CPAP is reduced to 3 to 4 cm H_2O before removing the prongs.

Complications

The complications of N-CPAP can be related to the pressure that is applied or to the interface with the nose. The application of excessive pressure can cause overdistention and alveolar rupture with pulmonary interstitial emphysema and pneumothorax. It can also reduce venous return, increase pulmonary vascular resistance, and reduce cardiac output. Overdistention of the lung can also reduce compliance and induce hypoventilation.

When the nasal prongs are too large or are applied with too much pressure over the nasal septum, they can produce erosions or pressure necrosis that sometimes makes it impossible to continue the N-CPAP. Avoiding these complications and keeping the nasal prongs in place is a task that requires considerable time and skill. During N-CPAP there is a risk of gas being pushed into the stomach. A nasogastric catheter is often used to avoid accumulation of gas and gastric distention.

NONINVASIVE VENTILATION

Noninvasive forms of respiratory support have been introduced with the aim of avoiding the use of invasive ventilation in infants in respiratory failure. N-CPAP is effective in improving gas exchange by stabilizing lung volume and the airways. However, it is not fully effective in maintaining ventilation in infants with weak inspiratory effort and inconsistent respiratory drive.

Intermittent positive pressure ventilation via nasal devices was among the original forms of support used in preterm infants in respiratory failure (Llewellyn et al, 1970). Recently, it has been reintroduced in neonatal care for indications including respiratory distress and apnea and to facilitate weaning from invasive mechanical ventilation.

Devices for Noninvasive Ventilation

The devices used for neonatal noninvasive positive pressure ventilation consist of conventional time-cycled pressure-limited ventilators that utilize the same circuits and gas conditioning devices used for invasive ventilation, with the main difference being that in lieu of the endotracheal tube, positive pressure is applied through the same interfaces used for N-CPAP.

Noninvasive positive pressure can be delivered in the intermittent mandatory ventilation mode (N-IMV) where the positive pressure cycles are delivered at fixed intervals. In some ventilators, ventilator cycles can be synchronized to the neonate's inspiration to provide nasal synchronized IMV (N-SIMV). Synchronized noninvasive ventilation can also be provided in the assist/control (N-A/C) and pressure support (N-PSV) modes to assist every spontaneous inspiration.

The most commonly reported method for synchronization in noninvasive ventilation is the Graseby pressure capsule placed on the abdomen (Barrington et al, 2001; Bhandari et al, 2007; Friedlich et al, 1999; Khalaf et al, 2001). Mainstream flow sensors have been used for synchronization in noninvasive ventilation, but they are likely to require frequent sensitivity adjustments to avoid autocycling due to variable gas leaks around the interface and the mouth. This is particularly important during noninvasive

A/C or PSV. Internal flow sensors are available in many new ventilators. However, data on their use in neonatal noninvasive ventilation are lacking, and it is unlikely that small infants are able to produce flows large enough to be detected by the internal sensors.

Devices that alternate between two levels of positive airway pressure (Bi-PAP) are also available. In these devices the increase in pressure is achieved by an increase in circulating flow instead of a valve. For this reason, in Bi-PAP the increase in pressure is small compared to that in conventional ventilators, and it is achieved over a relatively long time. Synchronization of the increase in airway pressure with the infant's inspiration using the Graseby capsule is available in some countries.

Another approach has been that of applying high-frequency ventilation nasally, but it is unclear what proportion of the oscillating pressure is transmitted to the infant's airways.

Clinical Application

In infants with apnea, the cycling positive pressure at the upper airway may produce an intermittent stimulus that prevents or attenuates the duration of breathing pauses of central origin. In infants with central apnea, resumption of breathing following ventilator cycles has been described, and the reduction of apnea in comparison to N-CPAP is more striking among infants with more frequent apnea spells (Bisceglia et al, 2007; Lin et al, 1998; Ryan et al, 1989).

Noninvasive ventilation can improve gas exchange and ventilation compared to N-CPAP in infants with respiratory insufficiency during the first hours after birth as well as during weaning from mechanical ventilation (Bisceglia et al, 2007; Moretti et al, 1999). In contrast, infants with mild respiratory distress who are stable on N-CPAP and are able to maintain adequate gas exchange only reduced their spontaneous breathing effort when receiving noninvasive ventilation (Aghai et al, 2006; Ali et al, 2007; Chang et al, 2011). In the preterm infant, the chest wall is excessively compliant, and the breathing effort is in part dissipated by an inward motion of the chest. Hence, the reduced breathing effort with noninvasive ventilation can also be explained by a reduction in chest distortion (Ali et al, 2007; Kiciman et al, 1998).

In spite of applying cycles of relatively small positive pressure, Bi-PAP can improve CO_2 elimination and oxygenation (Migliori et al, 2005) compared to N-CPAP. Noninvasive application of high-frequency ventilation was also shown to be useful as a rescue for avoidance of intubation in a group of infants failing N-CPAP (van der Hoeven et al, 1998).

In addition to the effects on apnea, ventilation, and breathing effort, it is possible that the increase in mean airway pressure during noninvasive ventilation can better maintain lung volume than N-CPAP alone. It is also possible that CO_2 removal is improved during noninvasive ventilation by clearance of exhaled gases from the upper airway.

The use of noninvasive ventilation to achieve a reduction in the need for intubation or the duration of invasive mechanical ventilation is aimed at reducing the associated risks of lung injury. This is obviously more relevant in the smaller and more immature infants in whom N-CPAP more frequently fails. In infants with RDS, nasally delivered IMV has not consistently reduced the rate of intubation compared to N-CPAP (Kugelman et al, 2007; Meneses et al, 2011), but it has been shown to facilitate early extubation after surfactant administration (Bhandari et al, 2007). In some of these trials, noninvasive ventilation reduced BPD appreciably, but this was not a consistent finding. The possible beneficial effects of nasal ventilation during the initial respiratory failure still need to be confirmed.

During weaning from mechanical ventilation, adequate maintenance of lung volume is often achieved by N-CPAP. However, many infants fail because of insufficient ventilation resulting from central apnea, a weak respiratory pump, or poor lung mechanics due to the underlying lung disease. Noninvasive ventilation has consistently been shown to be an effective way to reduce extubation failure (Barrington et al, 2001; Friedlich et al, 1999; Khalaf et al, 2001; Moretti et al, 2008), mainly by reducing apnea and improving gas exchange. Smaller infants and those with poor lung function at extubation were more likely to benefit from nasal ventilation than larger infants or infants with better lung function (Khalaf et al, 2001).

Ventilator cycles delivered at fixed intervals can fall toward the end of spontaneous inspiration or during exhalation and disturb the infant's breathing pattern, whereas delivery of the ventilator cycle when the upper airway is patent may improve transmission of the pressure and reduce the risk of gas being pushed into the esophagus. Both nonsynchronized and synchronized modes of nasal ventilation have been shown to be more effective than N-CPAP, but data are lacking on the superiority of synchronization in terms of efficacy or safety. Data on the most effective mode, frequency, and duration of the cycle and, most importantly, peak pressures during noninvasive ventilation are also lacking. Until more data are available, a conservative approach with relatively low ventilator settings and in ranges near those used for intubated infants recovering from RDS or near extubation is recommended. This is particularly important in setting peak pressures, because V_T monitoring is not available during noninvasive ventilation.

Potential Drawbacks

The risks for gastrointestinal complications observed with N-CPAP may be greater during noninvasive ventilation because of the additional positive pressure. An earlier report indicated an increased rate of gastrointestinal complications (Garland et al, 1985), but more recent clinical trials have not confirmed this.

Because of the additional pressures, the risks for pneumothorax and pulmonary interstitial emphysema may also be increased. Although there are no data on these side effects, caution should be exercised and high peak pressures or ventilator rates should be avoided. The risks for nasal damage and obstruction often observed during N-CPAP are also present in noninvasive ventilation. Proper application and maintenance of the nasal interface and avoidance of excessive force on the nasal septum are important to avoid these complications.

INVASIVE MECHANICAL VENTILATION

Because of the high incidence of respiratory failure in the neonate, mechanical ventilation has been one of the main therapies responsible for the progress in neonatal critical care. This is especially relevant in the small preterm infant who, besides lung immaturity, has a soft chest wall and poor central respiratory drive, making the need for mechanical ventilation very common.

INDICATIONS

The decision to initiate invasive mechanical ventilation in the newborn is very important because of the serious complications associated with this mode of therapy and because in smaller infants, it is often difficult to wean them from respiratory support. There is considerable variation between different centers in the criteria used to initiate mechanical ventilation. Most often, this decision is based on the gestational age of the infant, the severity of the respiratory failure, and the disease process that is underlying the respiratory failure. This is also done considering the alternatives available to support the infant's respiratory function. The experience of the team and the outcomes of infants exposed to mechanical ventilation in each institution should also be an important consideration. In units with vast experience and good outcomes, ventilation may be used more liberally, whereas in units with limited experience and high rates of complications, other alternatives should be considered before embarking on invasive ventilation.

The initiation of mechanical ventilation is usually based on the clinical condition of the infant and the evaluation of arterial blood gases. In the preterm infant, mechanical ventilation is frequently started because of recurrent episodes of apnea and hypoxemia that require some intervention to recover. In more immature infants, ventilation is often begun in the delivery room because of severe respiratory depression and bradycardia not responsive to stimulation. The other common indication for mechanical ventilation is when levels of $Paco_2$ rise rapidly, indicating alveolar hypoventilation. Although there are no specific levels of $Paco_2$, most centers initiate mechanical ventilation when $Paco_2$ rises acutely above 55 to 65 mm Hg and the pH decreases below 7.25 to 7.20.

The introduction of positive pressure ventilation is associated with complications and seldom results in improved lung function. In fact, intermittent positive pressure ventilation (IPPV) frequently results in further deterioration in pulmonary function due to the negative effects of high inspired oxygen concentrations, ventilation-associated infections, and overdistention of the lung. The effectiveness of mechanical ventilation is primarily due to the support of the infant's failing respiratory pump and the reduction in the work of breathing. One exception to this is the infant with RDS in whom the positive airway pressure produces recruitment of distal air spaces with improvement in ventilation-perfusion matching and gas exchange.

In other instances, mechanical ventilation is started because of hypoxemia not responsive to continuous positive airway pressure. Although there are no set levels of Pao_2 or Fio_2 to start ventilation in preterm infants with

RDS, the initiation of mechanical ventilation is frequently associated with the decision to administer exogenous surfactant. The indications for surfactant vary between institutions, but there is good evidence that early administration of surfactant results in better outcomes, and therefore, in an infant with RDS, surfactant is usually given when the inspired oxygen concentration required to maintain acceptable O_2 saturation levels increases above 30% to 40%. If the infant has hypercapnia or clinical signs of significant distress and impending failure, ventilation may be started earlier. In many centers surfactant is given as prophylaxis to all infants below certain gestational age, usually 26 to 28 weeks. After the infant becomes more stable, he or she is extubated to nasal CPAP.

In full-term infants, the indication for mechanical ventilation is usually more conservative because these infants are better able to cope with increased work of breathing. The indication also varies depending on the underlying cause of the respiratory failure. For example, in an infant with respiratory failure due to a congenital diaphragmatic hernia, ventilation is usually started immediately after birth, whereas in an infant with a congenital pneumonia or meconium aspiration, a more conservative approach can be taken, and ventilation may not be started until there is evidence of rising $Paco_2$ and hypoxemia requiring inspired oxygen concentrations up to 40% to 60%. The clinical evaluation of the infant is critical in deciding whether invasive ventilation should be started.

INSPIRED GAS CONDITIONING

During normal breathing, inspired gas is heated and humidified in the nasal passages and airways. By the time it reaches the distal airways, it is fully saturated with water vapor at core body temperature, that is, 100% relative humidity at 37° C for an absolute humidity of 44 mg H_2O per liter of gas. The isothermal saturation point region in the respiratory tract, where inspired gas equilibrates with core body temperature and is fully saturated, is near the main bronchi. As inspiratory flow increases, this point moves distally into the airways.

The nose and airways function as heat and moisture exchangers. There, a portion of heat and water added to the inspired gas is recovered during exhalation, with the net loss depending on the temperature and relative humidity of the gas. This requires continuous replenishment of water to the aqueous mucosal layer by the airway epithelium and loss of heat. In contrast to ambient air at 22° C and 50% saturated (absolute humidity of 9.7 mg H_2O per liter of gas) medical gases are typically colder (15° C or less) and dry (<2% relative humidity) and therefore require more heat energy and humidity. Hence, all forms of respiratory support where medical gases are used require conditioning of the inspired gas. This is a key component of mechanical ventilation because the endotracheal tube (ETT) bypasses the nose and upper airway.

Inadequate conditioning of the inspired gas can increase water and heat loss (Fonkalsrud et al, 1980). Exposure to dry and cold inspired gas can also produce inflammation of the airway epithelium and increase the risk of airway damage (Marfatia et al, 1975; Todd et al, 1991). Insufficient humidification can also affect the mucociliary transport system, reducing clearance of secretions, pathogens, and foreign particles as well as increase the risk of airway blockage by mucus plugs (Fonkalsrud et al, 1975). These effects are likely to be more striking in small infants, infants with impaired thermoregulation, and those who are fluid and energy limited. In small preterm infants, a few minutes of mechanical ventilation with inadequately conditioned gases can increase airway resistance and reduce lung compliance (Greenspan et al, 1991). Inadequate gas conditioning has also been associated with increased risk for air leaks and augmented need for O_2 (Tarnow-Mordi et al, 1989).

The standard method for conditioning of the inspired gases consists of a heater/humidifier (H/H) device and heated breathing circuits. Dry and cold medical gases are heated in the H/H chamber to 37° C to increase the water carrying capacity to 44 mg per liter of gas at 100% relative humidity. The gas travels through the ventilator circuit, where it is heated to 39° C to prevent condensation. The gas temperature decreases as it travels through the ETT, and gas is delivered at approximately 37° C and near 100% saturated at the distal end.

Many conditions can affect gas conditioning. Air temperature in an incubator or radiant warmer above the 39° C set point can inadvertently reduce heating at the ventilator circuit and result in condensation. To avoid this, the temperature probe can be insulated or place outside the incubator or radiant warmer. If gas heating at the ventilator circuit is not adequate, low ambient temperatures and low circulating gas flows can also produce condensation. In general, presence of water condensate in ventilator circuit and minimal consumption of the humidifier water indicate inadequate conditioning of the gas. Water condensation can occur in the ETT and connector when incubator temperature is low and result in water droplets being pushed into the airway.

Humidity of the inspired gas can also be increased by water nebulization. In contrast to the size of the water vapor molecules (0.0001 μm), the size of aerosolized water particles ranges between 0.5 and 5 μm, which can potentially transport virus or bacteria. Thus, water nebulization is not an efficient or safe method, particularly for prolonged use.

Gas conditioning is also recommended during nasal CPAP or nasal ventilation and oxygen head box or nasal cannula use because the nasal passages and airways may not achieve adequate conditioning of the cold and dry medical gases. These gases are typically heated to 32° C, but heating at or above room temperature may be sufficient. On the other hand, passing the gas through a water bath may not produce a sufficient gain in humidity because of the low water carrying capacity of cold gas. Thick and dry nasal mucus and airway secretions are observed when gas conditioning is insufficient. Lack of conditioning may also affect body temperature and water losses.

CONVENTIONAL POSITIVE PRESSURE VENTILATION

Principles

Neonatal positive pressure ventilation can be described in its basic form as the cycled application of two distinct levels of positive pressure at the infant's airway via an ETT.

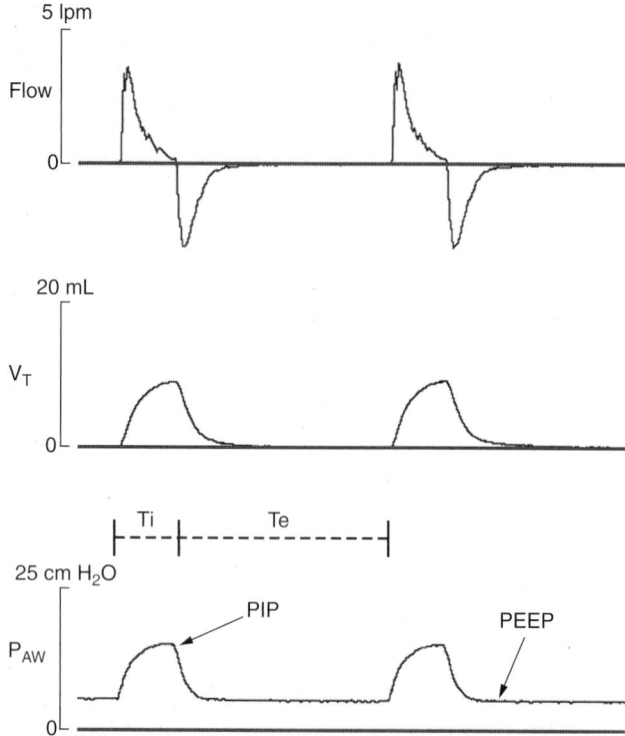

FIGURE 45-1 **Time-cycled pressure-limited ventilation.** In this example, recordings of flow, tidal volume (V_T), and airway pressure (P_{AW}) show that ventilator cycles, occurring at intervals determined by Te, increase P_{AW} from the PEEP level to PIP during the set Ti. The increase in pressure with respect to the alveolar pressure drives gas into the lung to achieve V_T. The inspiratory flow, which determines the rate of lung inflation, peaks initially and subsequently declines to zero as the lung is inflated.

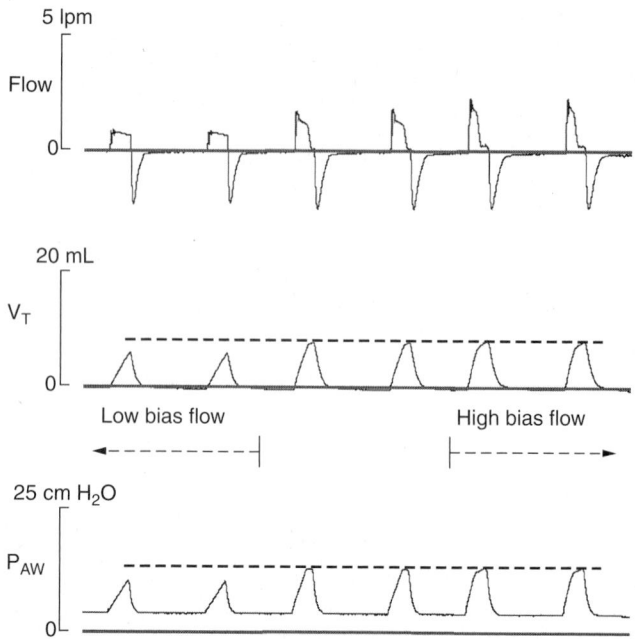

FIGURE 45-2 **Effect of circulating bias flow.** Recordings of flow, tidal volume (V_T) and airway pressure (P_{AW}) show how increasing bias flow rates in the ventilator circuit change the profile of P_{AW} with a more rapid rise toward the peak pressure. This produces a higher peak flow that indicates faster lung inflation. An insufficient bias flow rate does not permit generating the desired peak pressure with each ventilator cycle and results in a smaller V_T.

The positive end-expiratory pressure (PEEP) provides a continuous distending pressure to the lung and is aimed at maintaining lung volume. This is important because the ETT bypasses the upper airway mechanism that normally prevents lung volume loss by active closure of the glottis. The positive pressure applied at the airway opening is intermittently increased to a predetermined peak inspiratory pressure (PIP) during a set inspiratory time (Ti). The rise in airway pressure produces a gradient with respect to the alveolar pressure that drives a tidal volume (V_T) of gas into the lung. This form of ventilation is known as time-cycled pressure-limited ventilation.

Neonatal ventilators utilize a constant flow of conditioned gas, also known as bias flow, through the breathing circuit to produce positive pressure. A controlled obstruction by a valve at the expiratory port of the ventilator produces PEEP, and the intermittent increase to PIP at intervals determined by the set expiratory time (Te) as shown in Figure 45-1.

The circulating gas flow determines the profile of the airway pressure by modulating the rise to the set PIP. The airway pressure rise is faster and PIP is reached earlier at higher circulating flow rates. A fraction of this bias flow is driven into the infant's airways during tidal inflation. The infant's inspiratory flow, which indicates how fast is the lung being inflated, is in part determined by the profile of the airway pressure. The rapid rise in airway pressure produces a rapid increase in the infant's inspiratory flow

to a high peak inspiratory flow that decays as the lung is inflated. In this pattern of rapid lung inflation, most of the V_T is delivered early in the inspiratory phase, as shown in Figure 45-2. In contrast, a slow rising airway pressure produces a slower inflation and a smaller peak inspiratory flow. A low bias flow may not be sufficient to reach the set PIP within a fixed Ti and in consequence produce a smaller V_T, also shown in Figure 45-2. In most neonatal ventilators, the bias flow is constant during both the inspiratory and expiratory phases, whereas other ventilators self-adjust the flow necessary to produce a desired profile. In other ventilators, the caregiver can set a maximal flow to be delivered by the ventilator to the circuit during the cycle, which also modifies the airway pressure profile.

The bias flow should be sufficient to sustain the PEEP level when the infant's spontaneous respiratory flow demands increase. Otherwise, it may create an inspiratory load that the infant has to overcome with each breath. This is noted as a decline in PEEP during spontaneous inspiration toward zero pressure, or it can even become negative. The bias flow is also responsible for removal of exhaled gases, and an insufficient bias flow may cause rebreathing. On the other hand, a very high bias flow produces an almost square inspiratory airway pressure waveform that increases the velocity of lung inflation. This may have undesirable consequences because the lung will be expanded much faster than during a normal physiologic inflation. In general, circulating bias flow rates for ventilated preterm infants are set between 5 and 8 liters per minute, with higher circulating flow rate settings to accommodate gas leaks around the airway or the demands of larger neonates.

Respiratory System Mechanics during Positive Pressure Ventilation

The neonate's respiratory system mechanical properties (i.e., compliance and airway resistance) determine its time constant as their product. The respiratory time constant, which is a measure of the time to achieve equilibrium between the applied pressure and the alveolar pressure, varies with different lung diseases and their severity.

The compliance of the respiratory system (C_{RS}) is a measure of the recoil pressure that opposes expansion volume and is determined by the compliance of lung (C_L) and the chest wall. In the neonate, and most particularly in the preterm infant, C_{RS} is mainly determined by the compliance of lung because the chest wall is highly distensible. Lung diseases characterized by lung restriction, such as respiratory distress syndrome, where the increased lung recoil is indicated by a low C_{RS} and a short time constant, are quite prevalent in preterm infants. In addition, they have a respiratory pump that is often too weak to produce the pressure required to achieve an adequate V_T, and thus they require mechanical ventilation.

During positive pressure ventilation, a decreased C_{RS} is characterized by a smaller V_T for a given peak pressure and a relatively brief duration of inflation. As shown in Figure 45-3, the shorter time constant is illustrated by a shorter duration of inflation with an earlier return of the inspiratory flow to zero. This marks the point when the airway and alveolar pressures are at equilibrium. At this point, the PIP equals the lung's recoil pressure, with C_{RS} as the ratio between V_T and the applied pressure. When C_{RS} decreases, prolonging Ti is ineffective, and a higher PIP is required to maintain V_T constant.

The resistance of the airways opposes the flow of gas, which dissipates part of the driving pressure during lung inflation. In diseases characterized by increased airway resistance, this attenuates the infant's inspiratory flow and results in a slower inflation rate. The longer time constant indicates the increased time required for alveolar pressure to rise and equilibrate with the applied pressure. When airway resistance increases, the set Ti may not be long enough to achieve V_T, as shown in Figure 45-4. Although setting a longer Ti may be reasonable, this should be done cautiously because the increased airway resistance also attenuates the expiratory flow and prolongs the time required to achieve complete exhalation. A long Ti combined with a Te that does not allow complete exhalation will result in gas trapping.

Modes of Conventional Ventilation

Modes of conventional neonatal ventilation are generally classified according to the parameter controlled by the ventilator in each cycle as well as by the timing and duration of the cycle. Ventilator cycles can be pressure or volume controlled depending on whether the ventilator targets a set peak pressure or volume, respectively. Ventilator cycles can be delivered at fixed intervals regardless of the timing with respect to the infant's spontaneous breathing or they can be delivered in synchrony with the spontaneous inspiration. The duration of the inspiratory phase of each ventilator cycle can be constant or it can adapt to the time

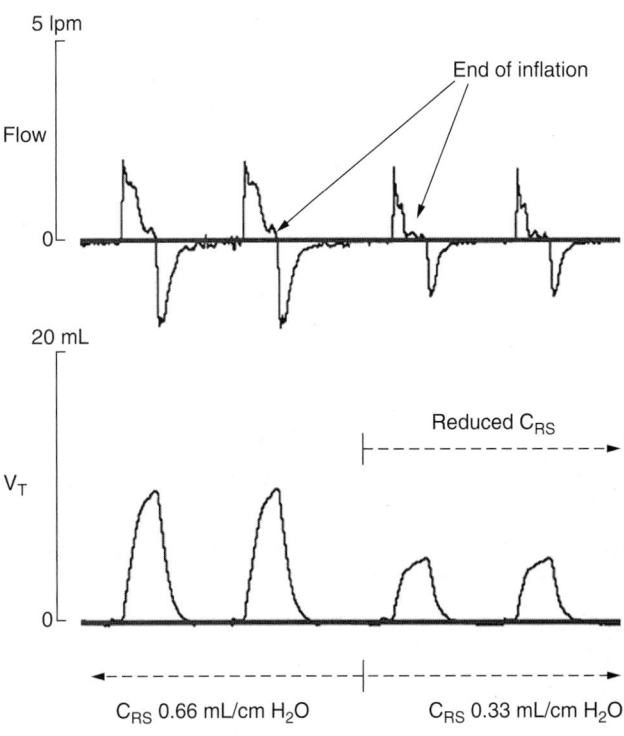

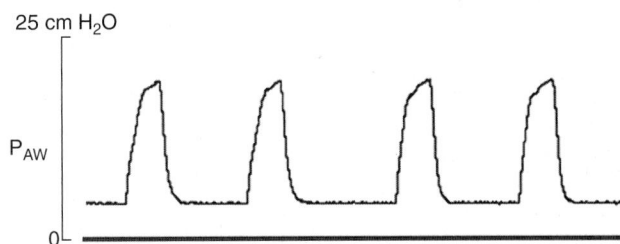

FIGURE 45-3 **Effect of lung compliance.** In this example, recordings of flow, tidal volume (V_T), and airway pressure (P_{AW}) show the effects of a decrease in lung compliance (C_L). A reduction in C_L results in a proportional decrease in V_T for the same driving P_{AW}. The effect is also noted by a shorter time constant indicated by an earlier return of the inspiratory flow to zero marking the end of lung inflation.

required to complete lung inflation, deliver the set volume, or to reach the end of spontaneous inspiration.

Intermittent Mandatory Ventilation

The time-cycled pressure-limited (TCPL) ventilation mode described earlier and illustrated in Figure 45-1 has been most commonly known as intermittent mandatory ventilation (IMV). This mode can be classified as pressure controlled because ventilator cycles deliver the PIP set by the caregiver. These cycles are of constant inspiratory duration, that is, Ti, and are delivered at fixed intervals, that is, Te is determined by the set ventilator frequency. For many years IMV has been one of the most commonly used modes of neonatal ventilation during the acute as well as the more chronic phases of neonatal respiratory disease.

In IMV, the increase in airway pressure due to PIP in each ventilator cycle produces a given lung inflation during the set Ti. If Ti is too short, complete lung inflation may not be achieved, whereas a long Ti that maintains a pressure plateau does not achieve a larger V_T and instead

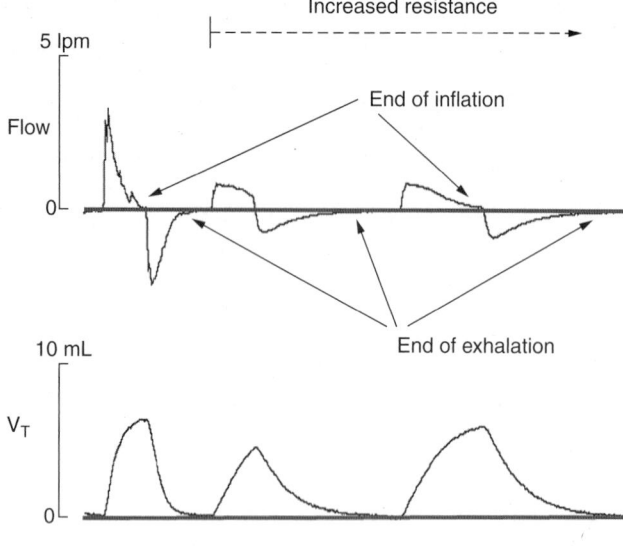

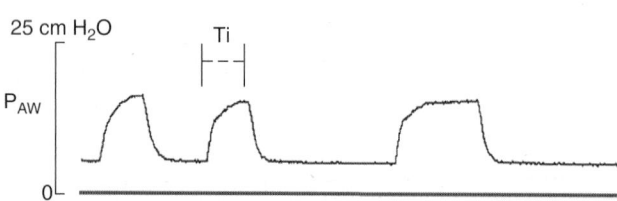

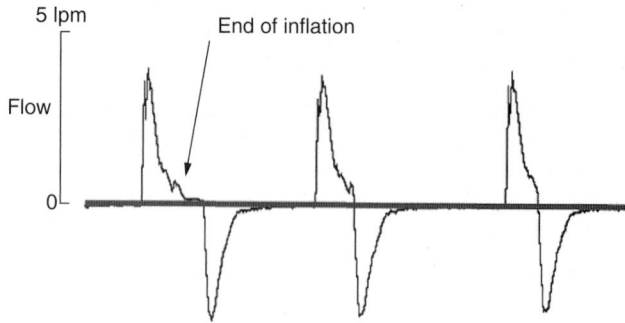

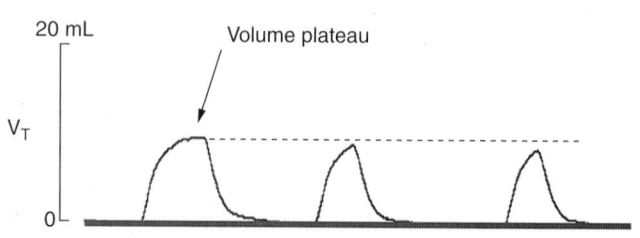

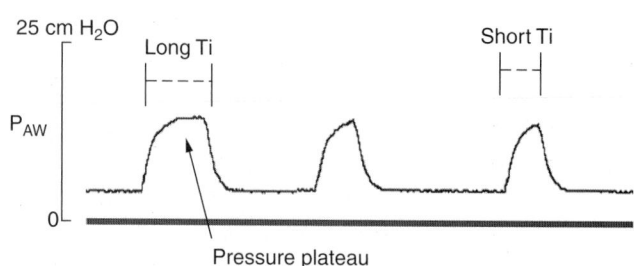

FIGURE 45-4 Effect of airway resistance. In this example, recordings of flow, tidal volume (V_T), and airway pressure (P_{AW}) show the effects of an increase in airway resistance. The increase in resistance results in a decrease in inspiratory flow that does not permit delivery of V_T in the set Ti. The prolonged time constant is noted by the increased time required to achieve full inflation and to complete exhalation.

FIGURE 45-5 Inspiratory duration. Recordings of flow, tidal volume (V_T), and airway pressure (P_{AW}) illustrate the effects of inspiratory time (Ti). A Ti that prolongs the inspiratory phase beyond the time needed to achieve inflation does not increase V_T and only keeps the lung expanded. A Ti of insufficient duration does not permit achieving full inflation, as indicated by an inspiratory flow that does not return to zero and leads to a decrease in V_T.

produces an inspiratory hold while the lung is kept inflated as illustrated in Figure 45-5. In infants with respiratory failure Ti is usually set in the range of 0.25 and 0.4 second. Caution should be exercised when setting ventilator cycles of longer Ti or high ventilator frequencies that could result in gas trapping due to an insufficient Te to allow full exhalation as shown in Figure 45-6. This is particularly important when the infant's time constant is long because of a high airway resistance or when the ventilator frequency results in Te <0. 5 seconds.

During IMV, total minute ventilation results from the ventilation produced by the ventilator and the contribution of the infant's spontaneous breathing effort. During clinical use, PIP is usually adjusted to maintain V_T between 3 and 5 mL/kg of body weight which is considered adequate for infants with lung disease. Ventilator frequency is adjusted depending on the infant's ability to contribute to minute ventilation and maintain sufficient gas exchange. $PaCO_2$ levels between 40 and 50 mm Hg are considered adequate, but higher levels are often accepted in infants with chronic ventilator dependency.

Although the management of IMV is relatively simple, there are some important limitations. With IMV, cycles are often delivered out of synchrony with the infant's inspiration (Greenough et al, 1983a, 1983b). Asynchronous ventilator cycles delivered toward the end of the infant's inspiration can prolong or increase lung inflation. IMV cycles delivered during the infant's exhalation can prolong its duration and in some cases elicit active exhalation against the positive pressure. Reports suggest associations between asynchrony and the occurrence of air leaks and intraventricular bleeding (Greenough and Morley, 1984; Greenough et al, 1984; Perlman et al, 1983, 1985; Stark et al, 1979). In older IMV ventilators, V_T cannot be measured, and PIP is adjusted based on the expansion of the chest, which does not permit determination of hypoventilation and gas trapping and assessment of spontaneous ventilation.

Synchronized Intermittent Mandatory Ventilation

Synchronized intermittent mandatory ventilation (SIMV) is for the most part similar to IMV except that ventilator cycles are delivered in synchrony with the onset of spontaneous inspiration. In SIMV, ventilator management is similar to that of IMV during the different phases of respiratory failure. SIMV was rapidly accepted and has become

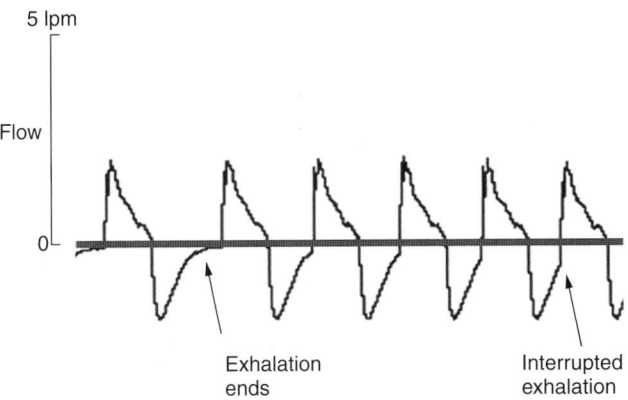

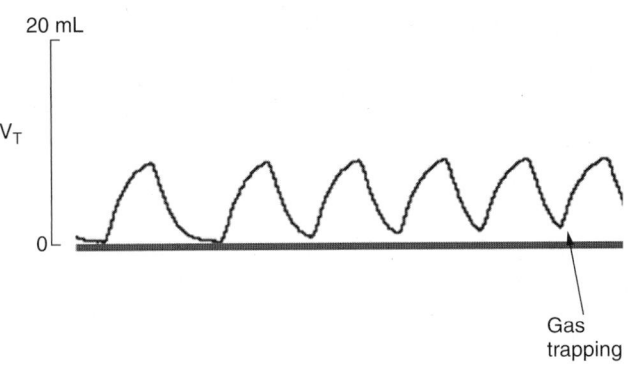

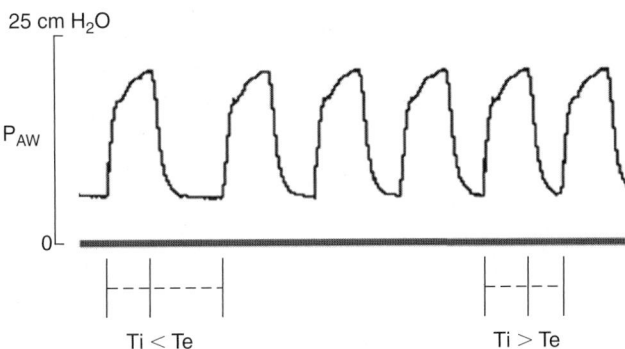

FIGURE 45-6 Gas trapping. Recordings of flow, tidal volume (V_T), and airway pressure (P_{AW}) illustrate the potential for gas trapping at high ventilator rates. As the ventilator rate increases, Te becomes insufficient to complete exhalation where every exhalation is interrupted by a new ventilator cycle. This produces a volume of gas trapped in the airways and alveoli and a reduction in V_T.

one of the most common modes of neonatal ventilation. During SIMV, spontaneous breathing is continuously monitored by the ventilator, and the first spontaneous inspiration during a time window of constant duration triggers a ventilator cycle. These time windows are opened consecutively, and their duration is similar to the interval between cycles in IMV. If no spontaneous inspiration is detected by the time the window elapses, a backup ventilator cycle is delivered. In this manner the number of ventilator cycles the infant receives every minute is the same as in IMV, but the interval between them is not constant.

Different techniques have been incorporated into neonatal ventilators to achieve synchronization, including the Graseby abdominal pressure capsule, esophageal balloons, transthoracic impedance, airway pressure changes, and

flow sensors. The last are used by most neonatal ventilators for synchronization and V_T monitoring.

SIMV produces a greater and more consistent V_T in comparison to IMV because of the increased transpulmonary pressure in ventilator cycles that are in synchrony with spontaneous inspiration (Bernstein et al, 1994; Hummler et al, 1996). Thus, lower PIP and slightly shorter Ti are often sufficient because the infant's inspiratory effort contributes to generating the V_T. As lung disease subsides, the infant's lung mechanics improve, and spontaneous breathing effort becomes more consistent, PIP is gradually adjusted to maintain a V_T between 3 and 5 mL/Kg. During acute respiratory failure, a ventilator SIMV frequency ranging between 40 and 60 b/m is usually required to maintain $Paco_2$ between 40 and 50 mm Hg. At this frequency, SIMV is likely to assist almost all spontaneous breaths. During weaning, SIMV frequency is gradually reduced as spontaneous unassisted breathing can better maintain acceptable $Paco_2$ levels. In infants with chronic lung disease, $Paco_2$ levels between 50 and 65 mm Hg are often tolerated for weaning of the ventilator settings as long as respiratory acidosis is not observed. The relative advantages of SIMV in comparison to IMV include faster weaning and a shorter ventilator dependency with improved respiratory outcome in the smaller infants (Chen et al, 1997; Bernstein et al, 1996).

As the SIMV frequency is weaned, the spontaneous breathing effort must be able to sustain most of the ventilation, thus requiring a greater breathing effort. It has been suggested that the work of breathing in unassisted spontaneous breaths between SIMV cycles is counterproductive and can potentially lead to diaphragmatic fatigue. Conversely, it has also been suggested that exposure to fewer ventilator cycles may reduce the risk of lung injury and improve diaphragmatic fitness toward an eventual extubation. Failure to synchronize leads the ventilator to cycle at the backup IMV rate. Delayed cycling prolongs the duration of inspiration and can disrupt the breathing pattern (Beck et al, 2004), whereas autocycling produce asynchrony between ventilator and infant.

Assist-Control Ventilation

In A/C, every spontaneous inspiration is assisted by a synchronous ventilator cycle. If the ventilator does not detect spontaneous breaths because of either apnea or very shallow breathing, it provides an IMV rate with the same PIP as the assisted breaths. A/C can also be used during the acute and weaning phases of respiratory failure.

A/C is primarily managed by adjustment of PIP to maintain V_T within an adequate range. As the respiratory failure resolves with improving lung mechanics and stronger spontaneous breathing effort, PIP is gradually weaned as V_T remains within an acceptable range. In the more immature infants, the respiratory drive is not consistent, and such infants have frequent apnea. Thus, the "controlled" or backup IMV rate becomes more relevant in the maintenance of ventilation during apnea.

In infants with respiratory failure, the Ti required to achieve lung inflation usually ranges between 0.25 and 0.4 seconds. Longer Ti is not recommended because of the potential for gas trapping with ventilator cycles delivered at the infant's often high breathing frequency. A long Ti can also disrupt spontaneous breathing (Beck et al, 2004; Dimitriou et al, 1998; Upton et al, 1990). Some ventilators provide flow cycling where Ti terminates at the end of the spontaneous inspiration or at the end of lung inflation. The advantages of A/C include a reduction in spontaneous breathing effort relative to IMV or SIMV because in contrast to these modes, A/C assists every inspiration (Bernstein et al, 1994; Kapasi et al, 2001). It has been suggested that assisting every spontaneous inspiration in A/C prevents diaphragmatic fatigue and can reduce the duration of weaning and ventilator dependency compared to IMV (Baumer, 2000; Beresford et al, 2000; Chan and Greenough, 1993; Donn et al, 1994). However, A/C has not been shown to be more effective than SIMV (Chan and Greenough, 1994; Dimitriou et al, 1995).

In A/C, PIP should be adjusted to avoid a large V_T that can produce hyperventilation, whereas the backup rate should be just sufficient to prevent hypoventilation during apnea. Autocycling is a problem in A/C because neonatal ventilators do not have a limit on cycling frequency and therefore can produce hyperventilation or gas trapping.

Pressure Support Ventilation

In PSV, the ventilator also provides a positive pressure breath with every spontaneous inspiratory effort. The start of the support pressure is in synchrony with the onset of the infant's inspiration and termination of the support pressure occurs toward the end of spontaneous inspiration or when lung inflation is completed, that is, flow cycling. The use of PSV is aimed at unloading the respiratory pump with support pressure that helps overcome the elastic and resistive loads imposed by the preterm infant's underlying lung disease. PSV can be used as a stand-alone mode with an IMV backup rate for apnea or in some ventilators as an adjunct to SIMV to assist the spontaneous breaths, whereas the SIMV cycles with a higher peak pressure are used to maintain lung volume.

Although PSV can be used during both the acute and weaning phases of respiratory failure, it is most commonly used during weaning. A consistent respiratory drive is required for the use of PSV as a stand-alone mode. For this reason, a backup IMV rate is recommended particularly in preterm infants to prevent hypoventilation. During PSV, gas leaks around the ETT can produce autocycling and extend the duration of the cycle. To avoid the risk of hyperventilation or gas trapping, trigger and termination sensitivity levels must be adjusted and limits on cycle duration must be set.

When PSV is used as an adjunct to SIMV, PSV can reduce the spontaneous breathing effort compared to SIMV alone even with support pressures set at a fraction of the peak pressures of the SIMV cycles (Gupta et al, 2009; Osorio et al, 2005; Patel et al, 2009). More importantly, by reducing the need for high SIMV rates, PSV can facilitate weaning in comparison to SIMV alone in preterm infants of birthweight (BW) less than 1000 g (Reyes et al, 2006). In that study PSV set at 30% to 50% of the peak pressure

of the SIMV cycles were sufficient to maintain acceptable $Paco_2$ levels with significantly lower SIMV rates.

Volume-Targeted Ventilation

In volume-targeted ventilation, automatic adjustments to the peak positive pressure or the duration of ventilator cycle are done to maintain a target V_T. Volume targeted ventilation modes have been proposed as means to reduce ventilator-associated lung injury caused by ventilation with excessive or insufficient tidal volumes during conventional pressure-controlled ventilation. A number of volume-targeted modes are available in neonatal ventilators. These differ in the timing of the adjustment or in the duration of the mechanical cycle, that is, whether it occurs as the cycle is delivered to the infant or in the subsequent cycle. These modes also differ in the volume parameter that is controlled—whether it is the tidal volume received by the infant or the volume delivered by the ventilator to the circuit, and whether this is measured during the inspiratory phase or during exhalation.

Volume-Controlled Ventilation

In volume-controlled ventilation (VC), the ventilator delivers a set volume of gas into the ventilator circuit in each cycle. VC cycles are delivered in the IMV, SIMV, or A/C modes described earlier. The time required to deliver the set volume depends on the ventilator flow rate, which can be constant during the cycle or variable with an initial peak followed by a gradual decline. The flow continues until the set volume is delivered. The cycle ends before the set volume is delivered if its duration exceeds the set Ti or the airway pressure exceeds the set PIP. In small infants, most of the volume delivered by the ventilator is compressed in the circuit, and the actual V_T delivered to the infant is only a fraction. Some ventilators use algorithms to correct the measured volume by the compressed volume to estimate true V_T.

VC has been proposed as a strategy to facilitate weaning and reduce the complications of positive pressure ventilation. Clinical trials showed that compared to pressure limited ventilation in the A/C mode, VC reduced the weaning time and the duration of mechanical ventilation in infants weighing at least 1200 g at birth (Sinha et al, 1997). Weaning was also faster with VC in infants of birthweight <1000 g, but the total duration of mechanical ventilation did not change and respiratory outcome did not differ significantly (Singh et al, 2006).

Pressure-Regulated Volume-Controlled Ventilation

In pressure-regulated volume-controlled ventilation (PRVC), the peak pressure of pressure-controlled ventilator cycles is adjusted from one cycle to the next to maintain a target volume. The targeted volume can be that delivered by the ventilator or the actual estimated or measured V_T. During PRVC, gas leaks around the ETT can produce overestimation of volume during the inspiratory phase and consequently lead to inappropriate reductions in peak inspiratory pressure.

Compared to conventional IMV, PRVC in A/C mode was effective in reducing the duration of mechanical ventilation and the incidence of intraventricular hemorrhage (IVH) in infants with RDS of BW <1000 g (Piotrowski et al, 1997). These advantages can be attributed, in addition to volume targeting, to synchronized delivery of PRVC cycles. These advantages were not evident when PRVC was compared to SIMV (D'Angio et al, 2005).

Volume Guarantee Ventilation

In volume guarantee ventilation (VG), the peak pressure of each ventilator cycle is adjusted to maintain a target V_T based on exhaled V_T measured in previous cycles. Measurement of exhaled V_T is aimed at circumventing the effects of gas leaks around the ETT during the inspiratory phase. VG can be used in combination with A/C, PSV, SIMV, or IMV modes.

VG was proposed as a potential alternative to avoid both extremes of V_T and to achieve a consistent weaning of peak pressure. The stability of V_T and gas exchange in infants with RDS can be improved by VG when combined with A/C or PSV as noted by fewer breaths with too small or large V_T and less hypocapnia (Abubakar and Keszler, 2001; Cheema et al, 2007; Herrera et al, 2002; Keszler and Abubakar, 2004). In infants with RDS or who had received surfactant, VG achieved the proper reduction in PIP, but this was dependent on setting a lower target V_T than the V_T attained with the pressure-controlled modes (Abd El-Moneim et al, 2005; Abubakar and Keszler, 2001; Cheema and Ahluwalia, 2001; Herrera et al, 2002; Nafday et al, 2005; Olsen et al, 2002). However, it must be noted that the smaller target V_T was in some cases not sufficient, resulting in increased Pco_2 and spontaneous breathing effort (Herrera et al, 2002).

VG was proposed as a means to attenuate hypoxemia spells triggered by hypoventilation during periods of agitation and decreased compliance in preterm infants. VG reduced the duration of the hypoxemia spells compared to SIMV, but only when the target V_T was increased which resulted in a considerable increase in airway pressure (Polimeni et al, 2006).

New and Experimental Modes

Proportional Assist Ventilation

In proportional assist ventilation (PAV), the ventilator pressure is increased in proportion to the measured volume, flow, or both generated by the infant's inspiratory effort. This achieves a perceived reduction of the elastic and resistive loads imposed by lung disease that commonly prevent the infant from producing an adequate V_T. The proportionality factors by which the positive pressure increases in relation to volume or flow are the elastic (volume proportional) and resistive (flow proportional) gains. The elastic and resistive gain factors must be individualized to each infant's lung compliance and airway resistance. Elastic gain factors that exceed the lung elastance (inverse of compliance) can lead to a runaway increase in pressure, whereas excessive resistive gain factors can produce oscillations in airway pressure. For this reason, PAV devices provide peak pressure and volume limits. Because PAV amplifies only the spontaneous breathing effort, a backup IMV rate is needed to prevent hypoventilation during apnea.

By compensating for the loads induced by lung disease, PAV reduced the breathing effort in infants recovering from RDS (Musante et al, 2001). Compared to conventional modes that deliver a constant pressure during inspiration, PAV produced similar ventilation with lower ventilator and transpulmonary pressures (Schulze et al, 1999, 2007).

Neurally Adjusted Ventilatory Assist

Neurally adjusted ventilatory assist (NAVA) is a mode where the ventilator pressure is adjusted in proportion to the electrical activity of the crural diaphragm measured by esophageal electrodes. NAVA was developed to improve the coupling of the infant's inspiration and the ventilator by overcoming conditions that delay or limit pneumatic triggering of the ventilator cycle. A study in preterm infants approaching extubation showed NAVA can produce comparable gas exchange with lower pressures than PSV, but no physiologic effects of the better synchrony, including breathing effort, were noted. This study showed the feasibility of noninvasive NAVA after extubation (Beck et al, 2009).

Data are lacking on the effects of different NAVA proportionality factors between diaphragmatic electrical activity and ventilator pressure within the same infant or between infants, because electrical activity of the diaphragm cannot be normalized. A backup ventilator rate is needed to prevent hypoventilation during apnea.

Targeted Minute Ventilation

Targeted minute ventilation (TMV) is an experimental mode where the ventilator rate is adjusted to maintain minute ventilation at a target level. If minute ventilation exceeds or decreases below the target level, the ventilator rate is reduced or increased, respectively. If spontaneous breathing can maintain a normal minute ventilation, the ventilator rate is reduced. In preterm infants recovering from RDS, TMV reduced the ventilator rate to half without impairing gas exchange compared to SIMV. Although these infants were able to sustain their ventilation for long periods, at times they required increased ventilator rates (Claure et al, 1997).

Mandatory minute ventilation (MMV) is a form of targeted minute ventilation where the ventilator rate is turned off when spontaneous breathing maintains ventilation. If minute ventilation falls below the target level, a constant ventilator rate of VC cycles is provided. In near-term infants ventilated for reasons other than lung disease, MMV weaned the rate and reduced the mean airway pressure compared to SIMV (Guthrie et al, 2005).

Adaptive backup ventilation is a form of backup support. In this mode, a ventilator rate is provided during apnea as well as during the occurrence of hypoxemia detected by Spo_2. In preterm infants recovering from RDS, this hybrid backup mode reduced the incidence and duration of hypoxemia spells compared to a backup ventilator rate for apnea alone (Herber-Jonat et al, 2006).

HIGH-FREQUENCY VENTILATION

Because of the association between pulmonary overdistention, lung injury, and the development of BPD, the possibility of achieving gas exchange with very small tidal volumes has been of great interest to neonatologists for many years. This led to the development of instruments that can generate changes in airway pressure at rates in excess of 10 Hertz (600/min) with the aim of producing ventilation with very small tidal volumes, usually much smaller than the dead space.

Gas Transport during High-Frequency Ventilation

During conventional ventilation, gas exchange occurs by introducing of fresh gas into the distal airspaces with each inspiration. In contrast, during high-frequency ventilation (HFV), the volume of fresh gas delivered by each cycle is very small and does not reach the most distal portions of the lung. Therefore, different mechanisms must explain alveolar ventilation and gas exchange. These include bulk flow into the more proximal portions of the lung, enhanced mixing of gas within the conducting airways, and out-of-phase movement between different regions of the lung that have different time constants. There is also enhanced diffusion of gas in large and medium-sized airways due to asymmetrical velocity profiles during inspiration and expiration. Finally, there is molecular diffusion in the more distal air spaces that moves the different gas molecules from areas of higher to lower concentrations. These mechanisms have been mostly explored in adult lung models, and therefore it is not clear how well they apply to the immature or sick neonatal lung.

Devices for HFV

Several types of high-frequency (HF) ventilators have been used in the neonate, including jet ventilators, oscillators, and flow interrupters.

Jet ventilators generate a high-velocity gas flow that is injected through a small-diameter tube that opens into the airway connector. Expiration is passive, and the cycling rate is determined by an electrically operated valve that opens and closes the jet at a predetermined rate and timing. The high velocity of the gas injected into the airway produces a Venturi effect that pulls additional gas from the ventilator circuit. This is known as "gas entrainment." Tidal volume is determined primarily by the driving pressure of the gas, the inspiratory time, and the resistance of the injection port. Because expiration is passive during high-frequency jet ventilation (HFJV), there is a risk of gas trapping and lung overdistention (Bancalari et al, 1987). This risk is higher when the time constant of the respiratory system is increased by airway obstruction and when large tidal volumes are delivered. Because of this, jet ventilators are used at lower rates (4 to 10 Hz). Jet ventilators are used in combination with conventional ventilators that provide PEEP and may also provide conventional positive pressure cycles.

Oscillatory ventilators use a piston or a membrane driven by an electromagnetic force and connected to the ventilator circuit. The mean airway pressure is determined by the gas flow through the circuit and a variable resistance, whereas the tidal volume is generated by the size of the excursion of the piston or membrane. With these devices, the expiratory phase is active because during expiration, airway pressure falls below baseline. This reduces the risk of gas trapping. Flow interrupters are a hybrid between jets and oscillators. They produce airway pressure changes by interrupting the gas source at very high rates using a standard ventilator circuit rather than an injection cannula. They are relatively simple and are usually offered as an additional mode in conventional ventilators. Most do not have enough power to generate sufficient tidal volumes to effectively ventilate large infants or infants with very stiff lungs.

Clinical Experience

The indications for HFV vary widely among different centers. Although some use HFV routinely as a primary mode of support, most centers use HFV as rescue when conventional ventilation has failed. This includes preterm infants who require increasing ventilator settings to maintain CO_2 elimination and oxygenation within acceptable limits and those with evidence of pulmonary interstitial emphysema. In larger infants, HFV is also indicated in situations where conventional ventilation is not sufficient to maintain acceptable CO_2 elimination or oxygenation, and especially in infants with persistent pulmonary hypertension secondary to hypoplastic lungs due to congenital diaphragmatic hernia or oligohydramnios or to severe lung disease due to meconium aspiration or pneumonia.

HFV in RDS

The clinical results with the use of HFV in infants with RDS have been inconsistent. Whereas some studies have shown better outcomes such as increased survival with no BPD (Courtney et al, 2002), others have not shown differences (Johnson et al, 2002). Some studies have suggested a higher risk of air leaks (Thome et al, 1999), and others higher incidence of intracranial hemorrhage with HFV (HIFI Study Group, 1989; Moriette et al, 2001).

Many of the earlier studies were performed before exogenous surfactant was available, and therefore the results are not applicable to the present situation where most preterm infants are exposed to antenatal steroids and, when indicated, receive exogenous surfactant. A meta-analysis of the most recent trials suggests a possible advantage for HFV in the outcomes "BPD at 36 weeks" or "death or BPD" at 36 weeks corrected age. However, when the results were analyzed using adjustments for heterogeneity between trials, the beneficial effect disappeared (Thome et al, 2005). The results of this meta-analysis revealed a significant increase in the risk of air leaks and a trend for higher risk of IVH grades III and IV with HFV. When the results of HFV were compared with conventional ventilation, including only studies where HFV was used with high-volume strategies and conventional ventilation with an optimized low positive pressure and tidal volume strategy, there were no significant differences in any of the outcomes (Bollen et al, 2007; Thome et al, 2005). Because of the inconsistency of the results and the lack of solid evidence of benefits of HFV over conventional ventilation in infants with RDS, the selection of one modality over the other is mostly based on individual preference.

HFV in PPHN

The clinical evidence with the use of HFV in infants with PPHN is not solid and comes from a few, relatively small trials. Some of these studies suggested a decreased need for extracorporeal membrane oxygenation (ECMO) in infants with PPHN treated with HFV compared to those managed with IPPV (Clark et al, 1994). However, other studies have not shown clear advantage of HFV over conventional management (Kinsella et al, 1997; Rojas et al, 2005). HFV may offer some advantage over conventional ventilation in infants with hypoplastic lungs secondary to congenital diaphragmatic hernia (Desfrere et al, 2000).

Other Indications

HFV has also been used in infants with bronchopleural fistulas in an attempt to reduce the amount of gas leak into the pleural space (Gonzalez et al, 1987; Walsh and Carlo, 1989). It can also be used during bronchoscopy or during airway surgery because in contrast to conventional ventilation, it can produce adequate gas exchange with a partially open airway and large gas leaks (Nutman et al, 1989).

Side Effects of HFV

Because during HFV the tidal volumes are extremely small, when HFV is used in unstable lungs there is a possibility of progressive loss of lung volume and atelectasis. For this reason it is necessary to use mean airway pressures that are usually higher than those used during conventional IPPV. In fact there is evidence that during HFV the use of an open lung strategy utilizing recruiting maneuvers and high mean airway pressures produces better outcomes than utilizing lower pressures (Thome et al, 2005). As a result of these higher pressures, it is likely that HFV may negatively influence cardiovascular function (Osborn and Evans, 2003; Trindade et al, 1985; Truog and Standaert, 1985; Weiner et al, 1987) and may also explain the higher incidence of pneumothorax reported in some studies with HFV (Thome et al, 2005).

Because of the effectiveness of HFV in enhancing alveolar ventilation it is easy to drive $Paco_2$ to very low values within a very short period of time. For this reason it is important to monitor $Paco_2$ values closely, especially when HFV is initiated or when settings are changed. Because of the very short inspiratory and expiratory times, it is extremely important to maintain the airway as patent as possible, ensuring a correct position of the endotracheal tube. Any obstruction will produce a decrease in pressure transmission and in tidal volume and can lead to gas trapping. This is even more important with jet ventilation. During jet ventilation, it is also critical to ensure proper humidification of the inspired gas to prevent airway damage that can be produced by the high velocity of gas injected into the airway.

Ventilator Settings during HFV

The ventilator settings during HFV are simpler to adjust than with conventional ventilation. The mean airway pressure determines the lung volume and is adjusted to achieve better ventilation-perfusion ratio and oxygenation. This is done considering the severity and type of lung disease. Most infants with RDS are managed with mean airway pressures between 8 and 15 cm H_2O. Higher levels may be necessary in some cases with severe lung disease and poorly compliant lungs.

The tidal volume is determined by the delta pressure, and this, in combination with the frequency, determines the Co_2 elimination. In contrast to conventional ventilation, during HFV the tidal volume is reduced as the frequency increases because the shorter times for inspiration and expiration prevent the equilibration of pressures between the ventilator circuit and the distal portions of the lung. Therefore, during HFV a reduction in rate may result in larger tidal volumes, more Co_2 elimination, and lower $Paco_2$ levels.

During HF oscillation or with flow interrupters the frequencies used range from 8 to 15 Hz, whereas during jet ventilation lower frequencies between 4 and 10 Hz are used.

The pressure transmission to the distal airways is greatly influenced by the resistance of the tube and the airway, so only a small fraction of the delta pressure generated by the ventilator is transmitted to the terminal airspaces. For this reason, the delta pressure during HFV represents more of a relative value used to adjust the ventilator than the real pressure change in the distal airways.

WEANING FROM MECHANICAL VENTILATION

Weaning from IPPV is extremely difficult in very immature infants who have poor inconsistent respiratory drive, a weak respiratory pump, and immature and many times damaged lungs. This combination of factors explains why they frequently become ventilator dependent for long periods of time.

For many years, infants who were ventilated received most of their minute ventilation from the ventilator and were not allowed to have effective spontaneous ventilation. In recent years this has changed, and ventilators are used as an assist support, preserving the patient's respiratory drive and effort. This has been possible by the introduction of synchronized patient-triggered ventilation (PTV) and has resulted in better outcomes and shorter times on mechanical ventilation.

Because of the high rate of complications associated with prolonged mechanical ventilation, weaning should start as soon as respiratory function is stabilized. The order in which the different ventilator parameters are decreased is determined by the relative risk of complications associated with each of them. With the possibility of measuring V_T, it has become much simpler to define the appropriate PIP that is required to generate an adequate V_T of 3 to 5 mL/kg body weight. As lung compliance improves PIP can be reduced to keep V_T within this range.

The level of PEEP is usually kept between 4 and 8 cm H_2O depending on the type of underlying lung disease and the level of oxygenation and Fio_2 requirement. The PEEP level is decreased gradually as the oxygenation improves until a level of 4 to 5 cm H_2O is reached, and this level is maintained until extubation. The inspired oxygen concentration is adjusted according to the level of arterial oxygen tension or O_2 saturation measured by pulse oximetry. The ideal ranges of oxygenation have not been defined, but most clinicians accept saturations between 88% and 95% in preterm infants and up to 98% in term infants. In infants with evidence of pulmonary hypertension, higher levels are targeted to prevent pulmonary vasoconstriction.

If V_T measurement is not available, the reduction in PIP is based on the observation of chest movement, the degree of aeration on chest radiograph, and $Paco_2$ levels. The ventilator rate is adjusted depending on the type of ventilation strategy being used. When the infant is ventilated with synchronized modes such as A/C or pressure support (PS), the infant determines the rate of the mechanical breaths so that the set rate is only the backup that the ventilator will provide when the infant's own rate falls below that level. Therefore, this rate is only relevant when the infant becomes apneic or hypoventilates. When the infant is controlled, the rate in the ventilator is not determined by the infant, and the adjustment in mechanical rate is based on the arterial Pco_2 level.

During weaning, it is advisable to do gradual changes and adjust one parameter at a time to evaluate the response of the infant to each change. With the availability of continuous oxygen and Co_2 monitoring, it is not always necessary to wait for results of arterial gas measurement to change ventilator settings, and the weaning can proceed faster.

Synchronized Patient-Triggered Ventilation

The use of patient-triggered synchronized ventilation has become common practice in neonatal units. Most randomized trials comparing PTV with nonsynchronized ventilation have shown reduction in the duration of mechanical ventilation in infants treated with synchronized modes (Greenough, 2001). This may be because, during PTV, the infant retains more control of ventilation, and the effectiveness of the mechanical and spontaneous breaths is enhanced by the summation of the ventilator positive pressure and the negative pressure generated by the respiratory muscles.

A/C and SIMV are the most common modes of synchronized ventilation in the neonate. It has been suggested that assisting each spontaneous inspiration in A/C may avoid respiratory muscle fatigue and facilitate weaning. However, the duration of weaning has not been consistently shorter with A/C than with SIMV (Beresford et al, 2000; Chan and Greenough, 1994). On the other hand, a randomized trial comparing the use of pressure support ventilation as an adjunct to SIMV to assist every spontaneous inspiration revealed a faster weaning and shorter duration of ventilation compared with SIMV alone in preterm infants (Reyes et al, 2006).

Volume Monitoring and Targeting

The continuous monitoring of V_T allows rapid weaning of PIP as the mechanical conditions of the lung improve. This can be achieved by a manual decrease of PIP as V_T increases, or automatically by using volume-targeted ventilation where weaning is achieved automatically independent of the clinician, who only sets the V_T targeted by the ventilator. Evidence from randomized trials using volume-targeting strategies suggest that faster weaning from mechanical ventilation can be achieved, although the results have not been entirely consistent (Singh et al, 2006; Sinha et al, 1997).

Nasal CPAP and Nasal Ventilation

After extubation, the infant is exposed to a number of mechanical impediments that explain the frequent need for reintubation in the smaller preterm infants. These include upper airway damage and retained secretions leading to obstruction and atelectasis, loss in lung volume due to poor respiratory effort, and a highly compliant chest wall. For these reasons, the use of continuous positive airway pressure applied through the nose can significantly reduce the deterioration that occurs frequently after extubation. Surprisingly, despite this improvement in respiratory function, the need for reintubation has not been consistently shown to be reduced by the use of N-CPAP after extubation (Davis and Henderson-Smart, 2003).

In contrast with N-CPAP, the use of nasal ventilation after extubation has been shown to significantly reduce extubation failure (Davis et al, 2001; De Paoli et al, 2003). Although these studies have included small numbers of infants, the effects have been consistent. This is a promising therapeutic alternative that needs further evaluation and the development of suitable equipment to provide synchronized noninvasive support.

Respiratory Stimulants

Respiratory stimulants such as aminophylline and caffeine have been shown to be effective to increase respiratory center activity in preterm infants and to decrease the incidence of severe apneic episodes. These drugs have also been shown to facilitate successful weaning from mechanical ventilation and decrease the need for reintubation. For this reason most preterm infants receive a loading dose of caffeine or aminophylline before extubation, and they are maintained on these stimulants at least during the first days after extubation while they are also maintained on N-CPAP or nasal ventilation (Henderson-Smart and Davis, 2003).

Permissive Hypercapnia

Tolerance of higher carbon dioxide levels may reduce the need for support and reduce the duration of ventilation. However, the results of clinical trials have been inconsistent. Whereas initial trials suggested faster weaning from mechanical ventilation in the group with higher Co_2 levels (Carlo et al, 2002; Mariani et al, 1999), a more recent study showed no benefit in duration of ventilation and a possible increase in mortality and central nervous system (CNS) impairment in infants with higher $Paco_2$ (Thome et al, 2006). Although these results shed doubt on the benefits of high Co_2 levels in premature infants during the acute stages of their clinical course, in infants with chronic lung disease it is necessary to tolerate high Co_2 levels to wean them from mechanical ventilation.

Dead Space Reduction

The large anatomical dead space in preterm infants in addition to the instrumental dead space can also delay weaning from mechanical ventilation (Figueras et al, 1997).

Continuous tracheal gas insufflations (CTGI) pumped through small capillaries to the distal end of the endotracheal tube to produce a continuous washout can reduce arterial CO_2 and shorten the weaning process (Dassieu et al, 2000). This method is limited by the need for special ventilators and endotracheal tube. Continuous washout of the flow sensor by a controlled gas leak can also improve CO_2 elimination and facilitate weaning (Claure et al, 2003; Estay et al, 2010).

Extubation from IMV versus Endotracheal CPAP

For many years infants on mechanical ventilation were extubated only after they had tolerated some time on CPAP via endotracheal tube. This practice was changed after a small, simple trial demonstrated that infants extubated from a low IMV rate had better success rates than those kept on CPAP for 6 hours before extubation (Kim and Boutwell, 1987).

Weaning from High-Frequency Ventilation

Infants ventilated with HFV are frequently switched to conventional ventilation before extubation. However, infants can be extubated directly from HFV following similar steps to those used to wean from conventional ventilation. The reduction in mean airway pressure (MAP) is done after oxygenation and lung expansion is estimated by chest radiographs while the FIO_2 is adjusted to maintain the desired oxygenation levels.

The oscillatory amplitude is gradually reduced in response to the levels of $PaCO_2$. If the MAP is weaned to low levels before the infant has spontaneous respiratory effort, this can lead to hypoventilation, loss in lung volume, and atelectasis. For this reason, it is advisable to lower the delta pressure and allow the CO_2 to rise and stimulate spontaneous respiration before the MAP is lowered below 10 or 8 cm H_2O.

Prediction of Successful Extubation

It is difficult to decide the best time for extubation in ventilated infants. It is obvious that many infants remain intubated for longer than necessary. This is evidenced by the fact that many infants who are accidentally extubated tolerate it well without needing further respiratory support. Various tools have been evaluated to predict successful extubation. These include measurement of lung mechanics, minute ventilation, inspiratory effort strength and ability to cope with mechanical loads, and stability of respiratory pattern during periods when the ventilator cycling is stopped (Kamlin et al, 2006). Some of the tools have been shown to predict with some accuracy successful extubation, but these tests have not been widely accepted in neonatal clinical practice.

The decision to extubate an infant is usually based on the level of inspired oxygen and ventilator support that the infant is requiring to maintain acceptable arterial blood gas levels. In general terms, if an infant needs less than 30% to 40% oxygen, a ventilator rate less than 15 per minute, and peak airway pressures below 15 cm H_2O and keeps acceptable blood gases, most clinicians attempt extubation. The lower the gestational age, the more likely it is that the infant will not tolerate extubation and will require reintubation. In most cases this failure is because of poor respiratory effort or severe apneic episodes.

Automated and Computer-Assisted Weaning

In the targeted minute ventilation mode described earlier, the ventilator rate is automatically reduced during periods of consistent spontaneous breathing where minute ventilation is maintained at or above the target level. In a study of preterm infants recovering from RDS, this experimental mode reduced the ventilator SIMV rate set by the clinical team by half while arterial blood gases remained unchanged (Claure et al, 1997). A similar reduction in rate was observed in near-term infants without lung disease when supported by mandatory minute ventilation, a mode where the ventilator rate is turned off if minute ventilation exceeds a set level or delivers a set rate of volume-controlled breaths when minute ventilation decreases below this level (Guthrie et al, 2005).

Preterm infants often need supplemental O_2, which increases their risk for eye and lung injury, particularly when exposure to oxygen is prolonged. In these infants, hyperoxemia is induced by an excessive FIO_2, and therefore it is modifiable by appropriate weaning. Automated weaning of supplemental oxygen was achieved by systems developed to adjust FIO_2 in a continuous manner. Systems of automated FIO_2 control have been shown to be as or more effective than routine or dedicated manual control in maintaining oxygenation within a desired range, with most of the improvement due to significant reductions in hyperoxemia (Claure et al, 2009, 2011).

Ventilator management involves adjustments of several parameters that affect the infant's ventilation and gas exchange. Computerized algorithms for ventilator management have been proposed to achieve efficient and consistent weaning. In infants with RDS, ventilator management assisted by one of these algorithms led to improvements in gas exchange and avoided unnecessary increases in ventilator settings (Carlo et al, 1986). Data indicated that during routine care, hypoxemia and hypercapnia were more diligently corrected than hyperoxia and hypocapnia, whereas computer-assisted management was similarly effective in correcting both extremes. The potential benefits of computer-assisted weaning on long-term outcome have not been explored.

ACUTE COMPLICATIONS OF RESPIRATORY SUPPORT

PULMONARY GAS LEAKS

Some of the most serious complications of mechanical ventilation are pulmonary gas leaks. These include pulmonary interstitial emphysema (PIE), pneumothorax, pneumomediastinum, pneumopericardium, pneumoperitoneum, and intravascular gas.

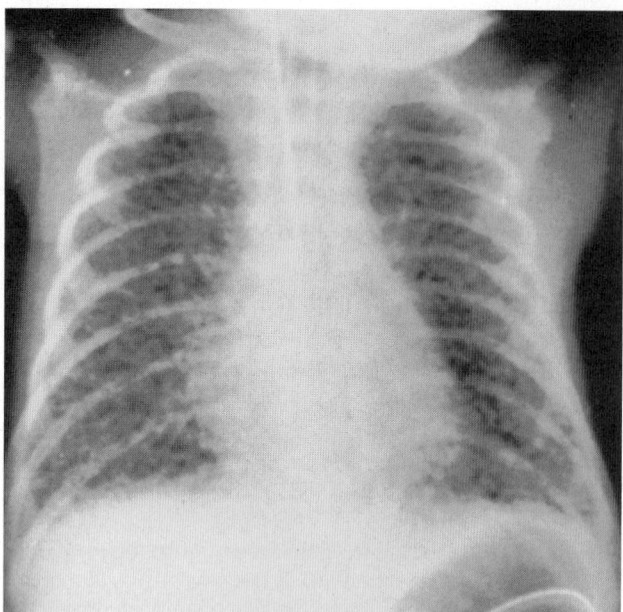

FIGURE 45-7 Pulmonary interstitial emphysema. A grossly hyper-inflated lung with coarse radiolucencies extending from the pleura to the hilum. These radiolucencies represent gas bubbles in the perivascular and peribronchial interstitial cuffs.

Pulmonary Interstitial Emphysema

PIE is the result of rupture of air spaces from overdistention. Although it may be seen in infants breathing spontaneously it is much more common in preterm infants undergoing mechanical ventilation and in infants with evidence of pulmonary infection. Once alveolar rupture occurs, gas is forced from the air spaces into the connective tissue sheaths surrounding airways and vessels and into the interlobular septa containing pulmonary veins. The air follows a track along these sheaths to the hilum of the lung, producing the characteristic radiographic appearance of PIE (Figure 45-7). The PIE occupies space within the lung parenchyma, decreasing lung compliance. Gas trapped within the interstitial cuffs compresses airways and increases airway resistance. In addition, gas in the interstitial space impairs lymphatic drainage, increasing interstitial fluid. This leads to significant deterioration in gas exchange with increase in $Paco_2$ and decrease in Pao_2.

The main cause of PIE is airspace overdistention and rupture. Therefore, minimizing pulmonary overdistention should reduce the risk of PIE. Shorter inspiratory times also decrease the incidence of PIE by reducing overdistention and avoiding an inspiratory hold (Heicher et al, 1981; OCTAVE Study Group, 1991).

PIE is a serious complication of mechanical ventilation. Infants with PIE have a significantly increased risk of developing chronic lung disease as well as higher mortality rates (Gaylord et al, 1985; Powers and Clemens, 1993).

Management

Because the gas leak can behave like a check valve, gas trapping occurs, resulting in further alveolar overdistention and rupture. Therefore, the first step in treatment must be to interrupt this cycle by putting to rest the more severely involved areas in the lung. If PIE is unilateral, this can be accomplished by positioning the infant with the involved side down (Swingle et al, 1984). Mechanical ventilation using short inspiratory times (0.1 to 0.2 seconds), low inflation pressures, and small tidal volumes can reduce the gas leak (Meadow and Cheromcha, 1985). Unfortunately, it is difficult to maintain oxygenation and ventilation while using low volumes. A multicenter controlled trial found that HFJV allowed the use of lower peak and mean airway pressures in infants with PIE than did rapid-rate conventional ventilation and led to more rapid improvement in PIE (Keszler et al, 1991).

Pneumothorax

Pneumothorax can occur spontaneously in healthy infants because of the very high transpulmonary pressures produced at birth. However, the incidence is much higher in the presence of underlying lung disease and in infants exposed to mechanical ventilation. Pneumothorax develops in 5% to 10% of spontaneously breathing infants with hyaline membrane disease. Although positive pressure ventilation increases the risk dramatically, treatment with surfactant has markedly lowered this risk.

Pneumomediastinum occurs when gas tracks through the perivascular and peribronchial cuffs to the hilum and then ruptures into the mediastinum. From there, gas can rupture into the pleural space, producing a pneumothorax. If the leak is large, it produces a tension pneumothorax that collapses the lung and results in severe hypoxia and hypercapnia. In addition, by compressing mediastinal structures, venous return to the heart may be impeded, resulting in circulatory collapse.

Diagnosis

Because of the severe consequences of a tension pneumothorax, it is important to diagnose it as early as possible. In the spontaneous breathing infant, pneumothorax usually produces tachypnea, grunting, pallor, and cyanosis. The cardiac sounds may be shifted away from the side of the pneumothorax, and the affected hemithorax and abdomen may appear to be bulging. In the infant on positive pressure ventilation, signs are frequently more dramatic, with sudden onset of hypoxemia and cardiovascular collapse (Ogata et al, 1976). Transillumination of the chest is positive over the affected side, and the pneumothorax is confirmed by chest radiograph that shows gas in the pleural space and partial collapse of the lung with shift of the mediastinum to the opposite side (Figure 45-8).

Management

A small pneumothorax in a spontaneously breathing infant may be observed closely until spontaneous resolution occurs. Infants with larger symptomatic pneumothoraces and all infants receiving positive pressure ventilation require thoracostomy and pleural tube placement. The tube may be inserted at the midaxillary line and directed anteriorly, or placed in the second intercostal space in the midclavicular line and directed toward the diaphragm so that the tip lies between the lung and the anterior chest

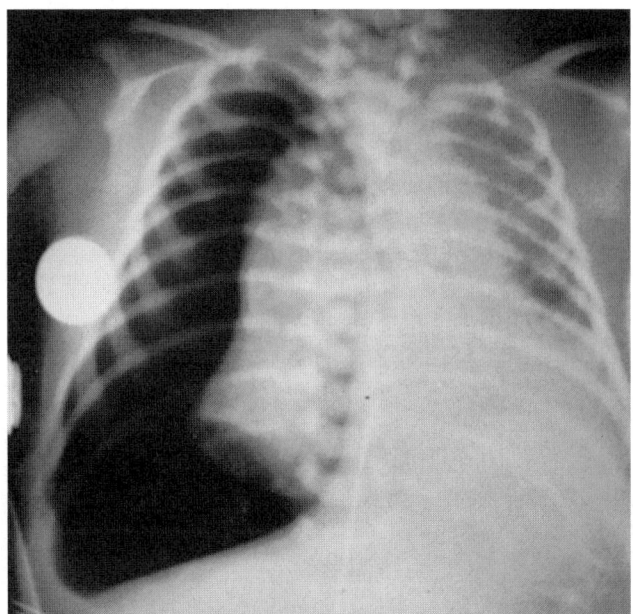

FIGURE 45-8 Tension pneumothorax. The lung on the involved side is collapsed, and the mediastinum is shifted to the opposite side, with bulging of the pleura into the intercostals spaces.

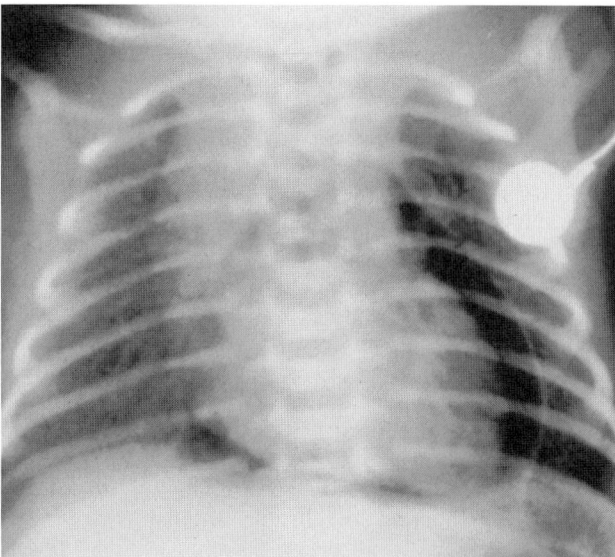

FIGURE 45-9 Pneumopericardium. A thin rim of pericardium is visible and clearly separated from the heart by gas within the pericardial sac.

wall. When placing the tube, the operator must avoid puncturing the lung, especially when a trocar, rather than a curved hemostat, is used to direct the tube. It also is possible to drain pneumothoraces using pigtail catheters that are placed percutaneously into the pleural space. This technique produces less trauma but may not be effective when large gas leaks are present. The thoracostomy tube is connected to a water seal with 10 to 20 cm H_2O negative pressure and is left in place until it ceases to drain. The negative pressure should be discontinued, and the tube should be left under the water seal for 12 to 24 hours before removal.

Pneumopericardium

Pneumopericardium results from direct tracking of interstitial gas along the great vessels into the pericardial sac. Gas under tension in the pericardium impairs atrial and ventricular filling, decreases stroke volume, and ultimately decreases cardiac output and systemic blood pressure. Infants present with increasing cyanosis, decreased heart sounds, and decreased systemic blood pressure and pulse pressure. The chest radiograph is diagnostic, showing gas surrounding the cardiac silhouette (Figure 45-9). Needle aspiration alleviates the acute symptoms, but because recurrence rate is high, continuous tube drainage is necessary in most cases.

Pneumoperitoneum

Pneumoperitoneum results from dissection of air from the mediastinum along the sheaths of the aorta and vena cava into the peritoneal cavity. Infants with this condition present sudden abdominal distention and a typical abdominal radiograph. Occasionally, the pneumoperitoneum may be large enough to cause respiratory embarrassment by compromising descent of the diaphragm and may require

drainage. This cause of peritoneal free gas must be distinguished from a primary gastrointestinal perforation.

Intravascular Gas

It has been suggested that the intravascular gas is pumped under high pressure through the pulmonary lymphatics into the systemic venous circulation (Booth et al, 1995). The intravascular gas results in immediate cardiovascular collapse and is often diagnosed when gas is seen in vessels or in the heart chambers when a chest radiograph is taken to determine the cause of cardiovascular collapse. Intravascular gas is usually a fatal complication.

AIRWAY COMPLICATIONS

Prolonged endotracheal intubation can produce airway damage and subglottic stenosis. The risk is increased by a too snugly fitting endotracheal tube, prolonged duration of intubation, and traumatic intubation. Some infants may require tracheostomy and even surgery to repair the stenosis. Inadequate humidification of the inspired gas can produce necrotizing tracheobronchitis, a necrotic inflammatory process involving the trachea and main bronchi. Infants present with acute respiratory deterioration due to airway obstruction, hyperexpansion on chest radiograph, and poor chest movement. Emergency bronchoscopy may be necessary to relieve airway obstruction.

Atelectasis frequently occurs during prolonged ventilation and after extubation from mechanical ventilation. This can also be secondary to airway injury due to trauma produced by suction catheters and by inadequate conditioning of the inspired gas.

VENTILATOR-ASSOCIATED PNEUMONIA

Ventilator-associated pneumonia is a very common complication of mechanical ventilation at any age, and it is likely to occur even more frequently in the immune-compromised premature infant. Unfortunately, it is not commonly diagnosed in this population because of the lack of specific criteria and the difficulty of differentiating pneumonia from other acute and chronic pulmonary pathologies observed previously in infants requiring prolonged mechanical ventilation. Despite these limitations, it should be suspected any time there is deterioration in lung function with radiographic changes suggestive of pneumonia. Changes in the amount and quality of the secretions obtained from the airway and colonization with pathogens is another indication of possible pulmonary infection that may require antibiotic therapy. Some evidence indicates that a large proportion of ventilated premature infants have aspiration of gastric contents into their airways. This is more common in fed infants and those receiving methylxanthines (Farhath et al, 2006). The consequences of this are not clear, but this could further contribute to the risk of pulmonary infection and chronic lung damage.

SUGGESTED READINGS

Avery ME: Recent increase in mortality from hyaline membrane disease, *J Pediatr* 57:553-559, 1960.

Bancalari A, Gerhardt T, Bancalari E, et al: Gas trapping with high-frequency ventilation: jet versus oscillatory ventilation, *J Pediatr* 110:617-22, 1987.

Bancalari E, Flynn J, Goldberg RN, et al: Influence of transcutaneous oxygen monitoring on the incidence of retinopathy of prematurity, *Pediatrics* 79:663-669, 1987.

Beck J, Reilly M, Grasselli G, et al: Patient-ventilator interaction during neurally adjusted ventilatory assist in low birth weight infants, *Pediatr Res* 65:663-668, 2009.

Becker MA, Donn SM: Real-time pulmonary graphic monitoring, *Clin Perinatol* 34:1-17, 2007.

Bollen CW, Uiterwaal CS, van Vught AJ: Meta-regression analysis of high-frequency ventilation vs conventional ventilation in infant respiratory distress syndrome, *Intensive Care Med* 33:680-688, 2007.

Carlo WA, Finer NN, Walsh MC, et al: Target ranges of oxygen saturation in extremely preterm infants. SUPPORT Study Group of the Eunice Kennedy Shriver NICHD Neonatal Research Network, *N Engl J Med* 362:1959-1969, 2010a.

Chang HY, Claure N, D'ugard C, et al: Effects of synchronization during nasal ventilation in clinically stable preterm infants, *Pediatr Res* 69:84-89, 2011.

Chow LC, Vanderhal A, Raber J, et al: Are tidal volume measurements in neonatal pressure-controlled ventilation accurate, *Pediatr Pulmonol* 34:196-202, 2002.

De Paoli AG, Davis PG, Lemyre B: Nasal continuous positive airway pressure versus nasal intermittent positive pressure ventilation for preterm neonates: a systematic review and meta-analysis, *Acta Paediatr* 92:70-75, 2003.

Finer NN, Carlo WA, Walsh MC, et al: Early CPAP versus surfactant in extremely preterm infants, *N Engl J Med* 362:1970-1979, 2010.

Gregory GA, Kitterman JA, Phibbs RH, et al: Treatment of the idiopathic respiratory-distress syndrome with continuous positive airway pressure, *N Engl J Med* 284:1333-1340, 1971.

Hay WW Jr, Rodden DJ, Collins SM, et al: Reliability of conventional and new pulse oximetry in neonatal patients, *J Perinatol* 22:360-366, 2002.

Keszler M, Abubakar K: Volume guarantee stability of tidal volume and incidence of hypocarbia, *Pediatr Pulmonol* 38:240-245, 2004.

Moretti C, Giannini L, Fassi C, et al: Nasal flow-synchronized intermittent positive pressure ventilation to facilitate weaning in very low-birthweight infants: unmasked randomized controlled trial, *Pediatr Int* 50:85-91, 2008.

Morley CJ, Davis PG, Doyle LW, et al: Nasal CPAP or intubation at birth for very preterm infants, *N Engl J Med* 358:700-708, 2008.

Reyes ZC, Claure N, Tauscher MK, et al: Randomized, controlled trial comparing synchronized intermittent mandatory ventilation and synchronized intermittent mandatory ventilation plus pressure support in preterm infants, *Pediatrics* 118:1409-1417, 2006.

Walsh M, Engle W, Laptook A, et al: Oxygen delivery through nasal cannulae to preterm infants: Can practice be improved? National Institute of Child Health and Human Development Neonatal Research Network, *Pediatrics* 116:857-861, 2005.

Complete references used in this text can be found online at www.expertconsult.com

RESPIRATORY DISTRESS IN THE PRETERM INFANT

J. Craig Jackson

INTRODUCTION

This chapter on the causes of respiratory distress in the preterm infant will focus primarily on respiratory distress syndrome (RDS) also known as hyaline membrane disease and on surfactant replacement therapy. However, the chapter also includes discussion of two less frequent causes - pneumonia/sepsis and pulmonary hypoplasia. Other causes of respiratory distress that are more commonly seen in term infants, such as transient tachypnea of the newborn (TTNB), are discussed in Chapter 47. Table 46-1 lists causes of respiratory distress in newborns of all gestational ages and demonstrates the relative frequency of each diagnosis. This table provides a useful differential diagnosis for respiratory distress in preterm neonates, particularly if polycythemia and hypoglycemia are included. More than half of extremely low birthweight newborns will have some type of respiratory distress (Figure 46-1). In that population respiratory distress syndrome is by far the most common diagnosis (50.8%), followed by transient tachypnea of the newborn (4.3%) and pneumonia/sepsis (1.9%). In higher birthweight preterm newborns, the incidence of any type of respiratory distress is much lower, but in symptomatic babies, the incidence of RDS and pneumonia/sepsis is lower, whereas TTNB is more common. Compared to the three diagnoses featured in Figure 46-1, the incidence of other causes of respiratory distress (see Table 46-1) is very low in preterm infants. However, these less common diagnoses should be considered in preterm infants with respiratory distress who follow an atypical clinical course.

RESPIRATORY DISTRESS SYNDROME

RISK FACTORS

The main risk factor for RDS, by far, is prematurity (see Figure 46-1). Other factors that increase the risk of RDS include perinatal asphyxia, maternal diabetes, lack of labor, absence of antenatal steroid administration to the mother, male gender, and White race. The central feature of RDS is surfactant deficiency due to lung immaturity, commonly a result of premature birth or delayed lung maturation associated with maternal diabetes or male gender. Surfactant dysfunction can also be caused by perinatal asphyxia, pulmonary infection, or excessive fetal lung liquid due to delivery without labor.

PATHOPHYSIOLOGY OF RDS

Because alveoli with insufficient (or dysfunctional) surfactant are unstable and tend to collapse, patients with RDS develop generalized atelectasis, ventilation-perfusion mismatching, and subsequent hypoxemia and respiratory acidosis.

During breathing (either spontaneous or assisted), shear stresses in the alveoli and terminal bronchioles occur due to the repetitive reopening of collapsed alveoli and the overdistention of open alveoli (Nilsson et al, 1978). These forces can quickly damage the fragile lung architecture, leading to leakage of proteinaceous debris into the airways (i.e., hyaline membranes). This debris (Figure 46-2) may impair the function of what little surfactant is present, leading to a downward spiral that may end in respiratory failure and death if not interrupted.

If supportive therapy is successful, the repair phase begins during the 2nd day after birth with the appearance of macrophages and polymorphonuclear cells. Debris is phagocytosed and the damaged epithelium is regenerated. Edema fluid in the interstitium is mobilized into lymphatics, leading to the "diuretic" phase of RDS characterized by high urine output.

With uncomplicated RDS, the patient improves by the end of the first week after birth. However, infants born at <1250 g and larger newborns needing high concentrations of oxygen and positive-pressure ventilation for severe RDS may develop inflammation and inappropriate repair of the growing lung, leading to emphysema and fibrosis (see Chapter 48).

PURPOSE OF SURFACTANT

Surface tension is generated from molecular attractive forces within a liquid that oppose spreading; it is the reason that water 'beads up' on a clean surface. If you try to inflate a bubble under water with a straw (Figure 46-3, *A*), the

TABLE 46-1 Causes of Respiratory Distress

Respiratory distress syndrome	46%
Transient tachypnea of newborn	37%
Pneumonia/sepsis	5%
Meconium aspiration syndrome	2%
Congenital cardiac malformation	2%
Chromosomal disorder/multiple congenital anomalies	1.4%
Spontaneous pneumothorax	1.2%
Perinatal asphyxia	1.1%
Pulmonary hemorrhage	1.0%
Persistent pulmonary hypertension	0.8%
Diaphragmatic hernia	0.8%
Apnea of prematurity	0.6%
Pulmonary hypoplasia	0.3%
Pulmonary dysplasia	0.2%
Hydrothorax	0.2%
Postsurgical diaphragmatic palsy	0.2%
	100%

Data from Rubaltelli FF, Dani C, Reali MF, et al: Acute neonatal respiratory distress in Italy: a one-year prospective study, *Acta Paediatr* 87:1261-1268, 1998.

spreading of the water's surface and enlargement of its surface area will be opposed by its surface tension (T). According to Laplace's law, the pressure (P) required to inflate the bubble is proportional to T divided by the radius of the bubble (r). If you simultaneously try to inflate two interconnected bubbles, the smaller one will deflate into the larger one, because of its smaller radius (Figure 46-3, *B*).

Surfactants are surface active materials that lower surface tension; a detergent is a type of surfactant which causes water to spread out on a surface rather than beading up. The surface tension of clean water resists the creation of bubbles, but the addition of detergent allows bubbles to form. Because the surfactant properties of detergents do not persist, all of the small bubbles eventually collapse into the large ones, and finally even the large ones collapse.

Lung surfactant has the miraculous property of reducing surface tension as the size of the bubble decreases. In clean water with high surface tension, the pressure required to keep open a bubble as the radius decreased would be greater than the pressure keeping open a larger bubble, so the smaller bubbles would eventually collapse into larger ones (or small alveoli would collapse into larger

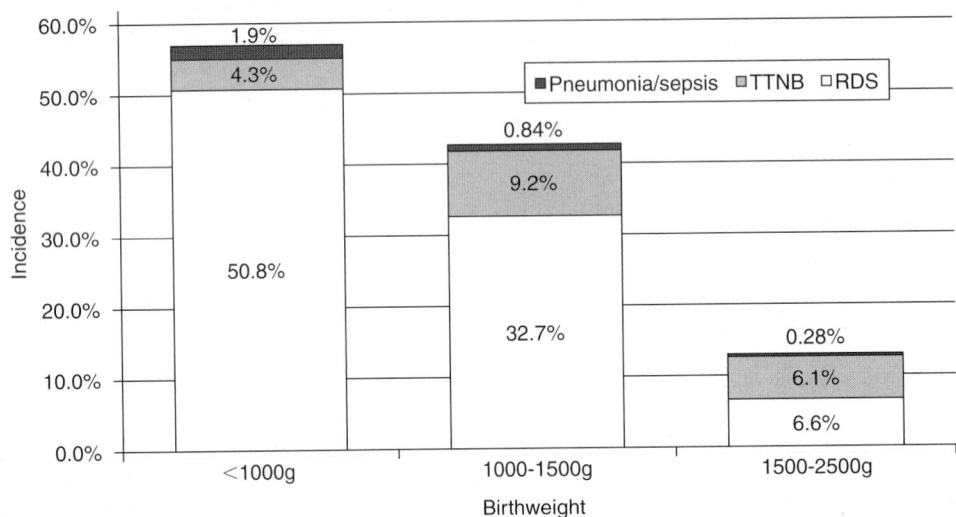

FIGURE 46-1 Incidence of respiratory problems in preterm newborns. (*Data from Rubaltelli FF, Dani C, Reali MF, et al: Acute neonatal respiratory distress in Italy: a one-year prospective study,* Acta Paediatr *87:1261-1268, 1998.*)

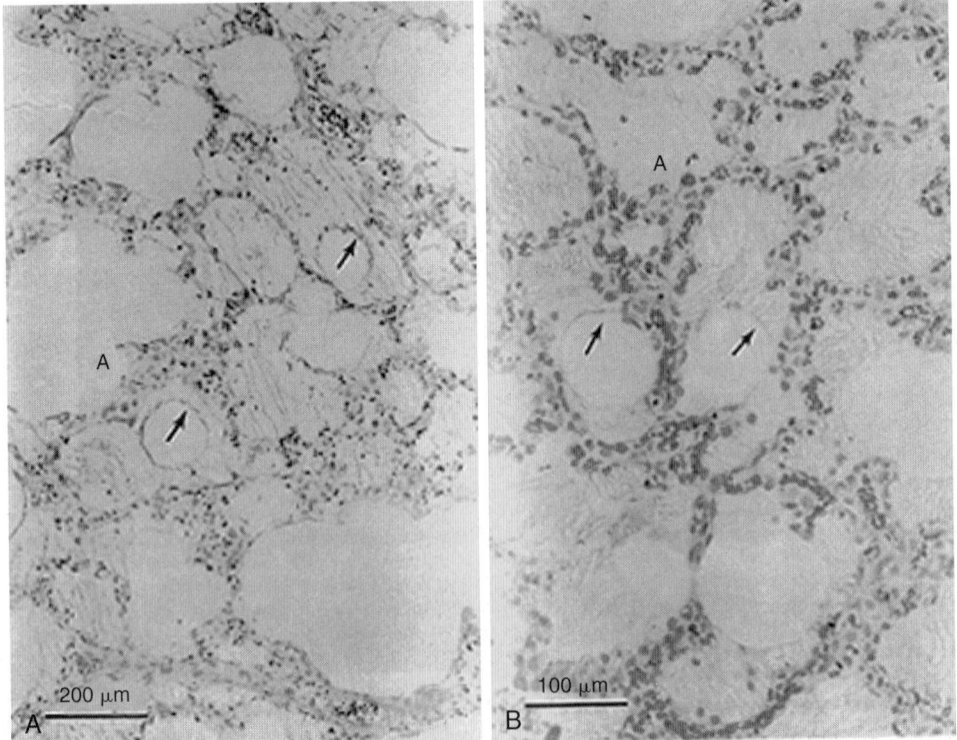

FIGURE 46-2 **Photomicrographs of lung tissue from experimental animal with RDS, flash frozen during inflation.** Note liquid-air interface (*arrows*). The alveolar debris forms hyaline membranes. **A,** Low power. **B,** Higher power. (*From Jackson JC, MacKenzie AP, Chi EY, et al: Mechanisms for reduced total lung capacity at birth during hyaline membrane disease in premature newborn monkeys,* Am Rev Respir Dis *142:413-419, 1990. American Thoracic Society.*)

ones), as shown in Figure 46-3, *B*. However, if the bubbles are lined with good-quality surfactant, the surface tension falls quickly as the radius gets smaller because the surfactant molecules become crowded during deflation (Figure 46-4). When the radius is very small, the surface tension

falls almost to zero, and the pressure required to keep the smaller bubble open is negligible. Thus, it does not collapse.

During inflation, as the radius of the bubble increases, surface tension increases even faster. This means that the amount of pressure in the larger bubbles will be higher than in smaller ones; in the lung where bubbles are interconnected, this pressure difference will cause flow *to* the smaller alveoli, thus keeping all the alveoli about the same size.

The cumulative result of the alveoli remaining open during deflation is a nonlinear pressure-volume relationship. The lung with sufficient surfactant retains gas during expiration, compared to rapid and almost complete loss of gas in the surfactant-deficient lung (Figure 46-5, *A*). During inflation, more pressure is required to achieve similar tidal volume (Figure 46-5, *B*), because of poor compliance ($\Delta V/\Delta P$) from having to reopen collapsed alveoli. For instance, to achieve a tidal volume of 5 mL/kg, an infant with RDS may require a pressure increase of 25 cm H_2O; dividing the volume change, ΔV, by pressure change, ΔP, we calculate that the compliance is only 0.25 mL/kg/cm H_2O, which is about one third of normal.

In the absence of adequate amounts of functional surfactant in the newborn lung, there is widespread alveolar collapse with overdistention of open alveoli (Figure 46-6). Because reopening collapsed alveoli requires high pressure, the spontaneously breathing newborn with surfactant deficiency must generate highly negative intrathoracic pressure. Clinically, this is manifested by retractions of the respiratory muscles during inspiration. Newborns may also attempt to prevent alveolar collapse by grunting. This partial closure of the glottis during expiration helps maintain an end-expiratory pressure that may keep unstable alveoli open.

A consequence of widespread alveolar collapse is intrapulmonary shunting of blood past atelectatic lung, without the opportunity for blood in pulmonary capillaries to pick up oxygen from, or deliver carbon dioxide to, the alveoli. In addition, lungs that are poorly inflated have widespread collapse of pulmonary vessels, leading to pulmonary hypertension. The elevated pulmonary artery pressures lead to right-to-left shunting of unoxygenated

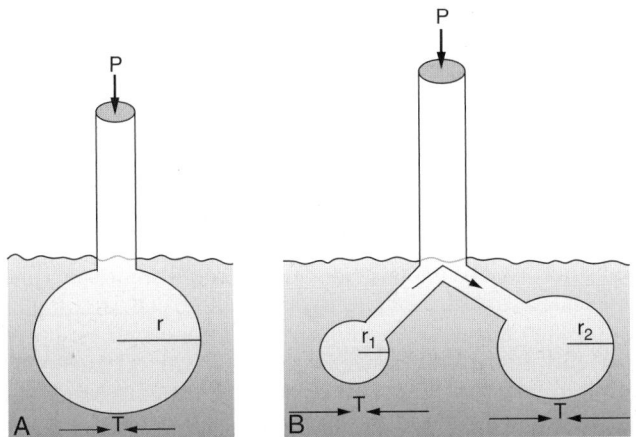

FIGURE 46-3 **Effect of surface forces generated by inflating bubbles under water. A,** Single bubble of radius *(r)* resists inflation and thus requires pressure *(P)* to overcome the surface tension *(T)*. **B,** If the surface tension is the same in two bubbles of unequal size, the smaller one will collapse into the larger one, because of the Laplace relationship, P = T/r (small r requires larger pressure to stay inflated).

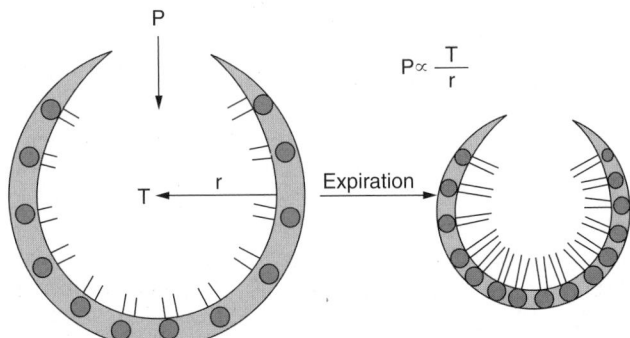

FIGURE 46-4 Surfactant molecules on surface crowding during deflation. *(From Jackson JC: Respiratory distress syndrome (figure 212–1). In: Osborn LM, DeWitt TG, First LR, Zenel JA, editors:* Pediatrics, *Philadelphia, 2005, Elsevier Mosby.)*

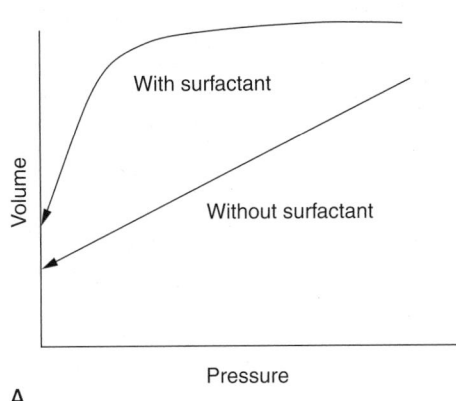

A

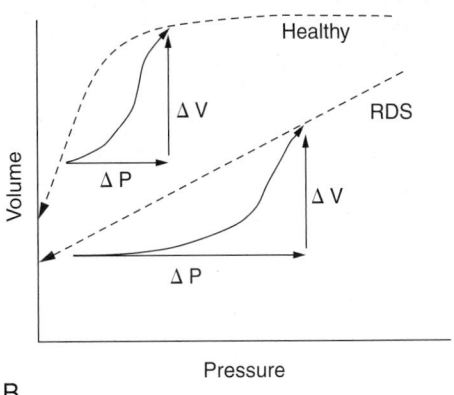

B

FIGURE 46-5 **Effect of surface forces on pressure-volume relationships.** During deflation **(A)**, the lungs with surfactant retain gas even at very low pressures, because of falling surface tension as the alveoli get smaller. The alveoli without surfactant collapse as the alveoli get smaller. During inflation of RDS lungs **(B)**, the starting lung volume (functional residual capacity) is lower, and much more pressure is required during inflation, compared to healthy lungs.

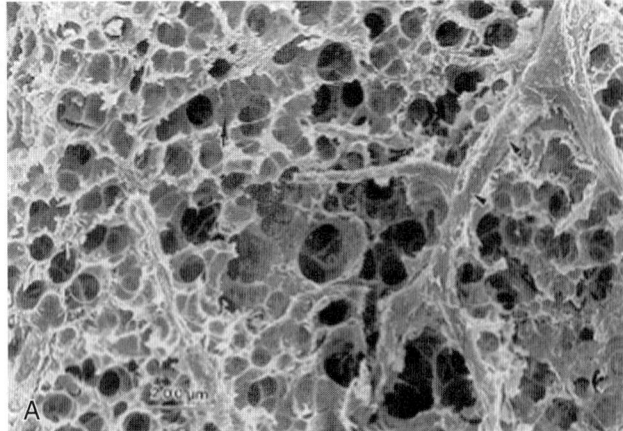

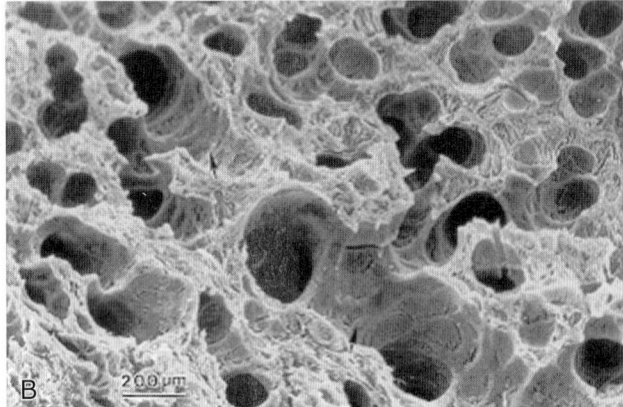

FIGURE 46-6 Histology of RDS. Scanning electron micrograph of lung frozen during inflation with air, in premature monkey healthy premature monkey **(A)** compared to one with RDS **(B).** Lungs affected by RDS have collapsed alveoli full of liquid and proteinaceous debris, with overdistended terminal airways. (*From Jackson JC, Truog WE, Standaert TA, et al: Effect of high-frequency ventilation on the development of alveolar edema in premature monkeys at risk for hyaline membrane disease,* Am Rev Respir Dis *143:865-871, 1991. American Thoracic Society.*)

blood across the patent ductus arteriosus to the descending aorta (see Chapter 52).

ORIGIN AND COMPOSITION OF SURFACTANT

Pulmonary surfactant is composed of approximately 90% lipids and 10% proteins. The main phospholipid in surfactant is dipalmitoylphosphatidylcholine (DPPC), also known as lecithin. It is surface active because of its hydrophilic head and hydrophobic tails (Figure 46-7). However, DPPC by itself does not adsorb efficiently at the air-liquid interface and is in the form of a gel at body temperature. The presence of some unsaturated phospholipids and cholesterol helps to make it more fluid (Mingarro et al, 2008).

The remainder of surfactant's ingredients is shown in Figure 46-8. One of them, phosphatidylglycerol (PG), is sometimes used as a marker of lung maturation; it interacts with the hydrophobic surfactant proteins to improve biophysical activity. Even minor components of pulmonary surfactant play important roles; for instance, free fatty acids improve the stability of the interfacial film, especially after repeated compression. The composition of surfactant is complex because it has evolved to balance the need

FIGURE 46-7 The main ingredient of lung surfactant, dipalmitoylphosphatidylcholine (DPPC).

for low viscosity for optimal spreading and redistribution along the smallest airways with the need for a stable and low surface tension.

Surfactant phospholipids are assembled in the type II pneumocytes of the lung epithelium into lamellar bodies in the form of bilayered membranes (Figure 46-9). Surfactant-associated proteins SP-B and SP-C are essential for the transition to a monolayer at the air-liquid interface. The molecular structure of the hydrophobic SP-B is complex and it interacts with the phospholipid monolayer as shown in Figure 46-10. Its absence is associated with fatal neonatal respiratory failure. Surfactant-associated proteins SP-A and SP-D are hydrophilic and have roles in immune defense. SP-A is involved in reuptake and reuse of secreted surfactant (see Chapter 42).

CLINICAL SIGNS OF RDS

The cardinal clinical signs of RDS are tachypnea, grunting, and increased work of breathing (Box 46-1). The newborn respiratory rate is elevated in an attempt to increase the exchange of oxygen and carbon dioxide, but with exhaustion, the rate may decline or even stop. Grunting is used to create positive pressure in the lungs to reduce the collapse of air sacs. Signs of increased work of breathing include nasal flaring and retraction of respiratory muscles, especially the intercostal and subcostal muscles. Because the ribcage in premature infants is so flexible, the sternum may deeply retract during inspiration. Cyanosis results from inadequate oxygenation, and pallor from acidosis due to poor elimination of carbon dioxide. The combination of increased work of breathing, cyanosis, and acidosis causes lethargy and disinterest in feeding, and eventually apnea. Rather than progressing through these signs during the first hours of life, newborns with intrapartum asphyxia or extreme prematurity may present with apnea immediately following birth.

On auscultation, breath sounds may be distant or shallow from the fast inspiratory rate and low tidal volume, and fine inspiratory rales may be heard due to reopening of moist, collapsed air sacs. The onset of symptoms is always within hours after birth and, in severe cases, may occur with the first few breaths after delivery. In general, the respiratory distress from RDS tends to get worse over the first 1 to 3 days after birth, and then usually improves gradually over a few days (although the natural course may be interrupted by exogenous surfactant therapy).

Differential Diagnosis

Clinical improvement during first 12 hours after birth suggests TTNB, and onset after the first 24 hours suggests pneumonia and sepsis. Tachypnea without increased work of breathing suggests cyanotic heart disease; the diagnosis of obstructed pulmonary veins from total

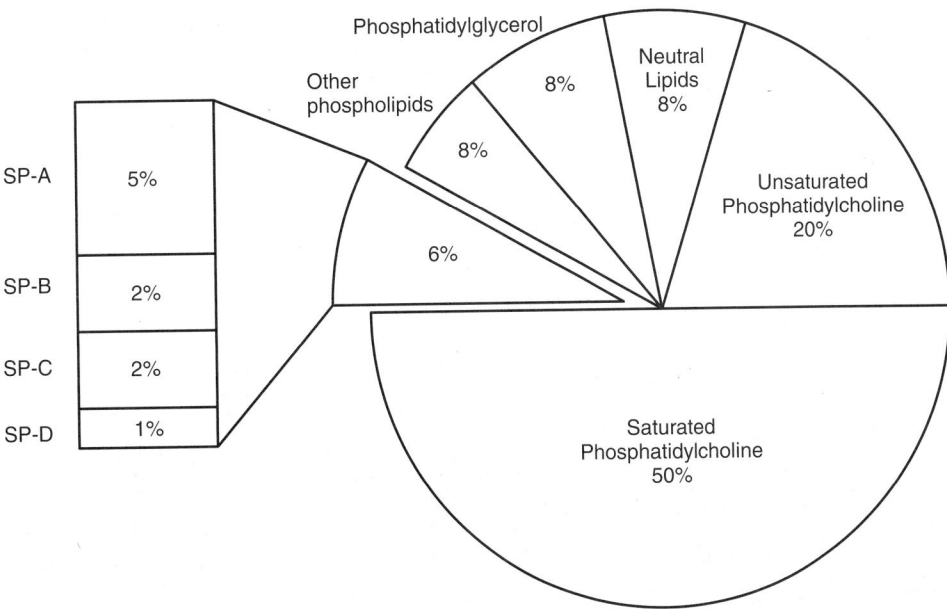

FIGURE 46-8 Composition of surfactant. (*From Jobe AH, Ikegami M: Biology of surfactant*, Clin Perinatol 28:655-669, 2001, WB Saunders.)

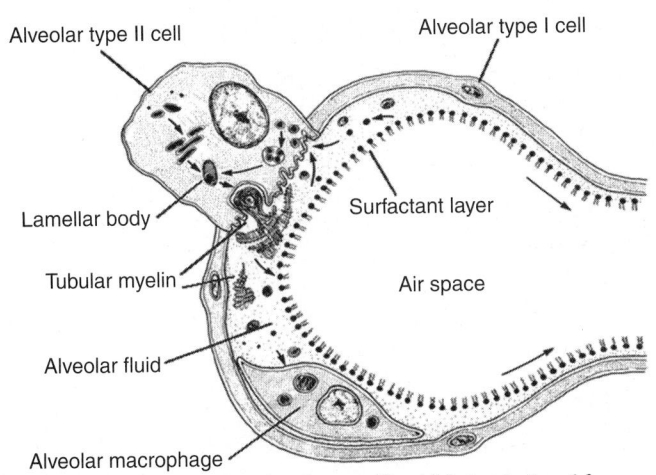

FIGURE 46-9 Assembly of surfactant. (*Republished and adapted from Hawgood S, Clements JA: Pulmonary surfactant and its apoproteins*, J Clin Invest 86:1-6, 1990. The American Society for Clinical Investigation.)

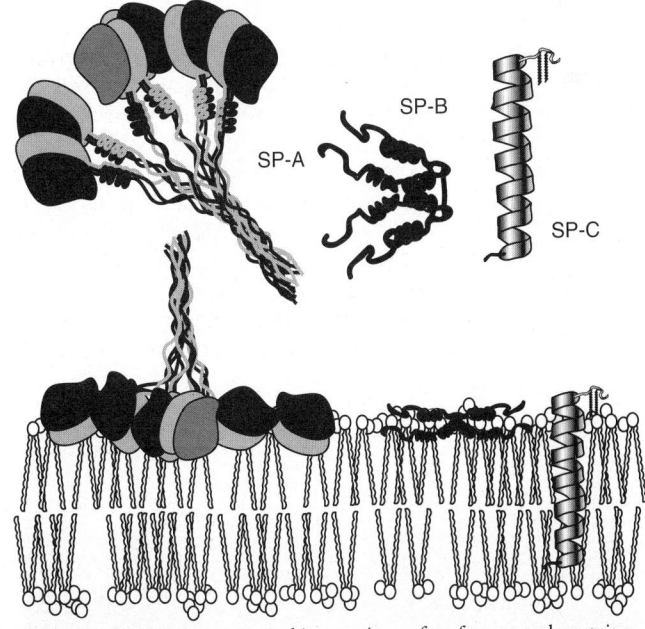

FIGURE 46-10 Structure and interactions of surfactant and proteins. (*From Pérez-Gil J: Molecular interactions in pulmonary surfactant films*, Biol Neonate 81:6-15, 2002. Karger AG Basel.)

anomalous venous return is occasionally confused with RDS. Hypoventilation without increased work of breathing suggests a central nervous system problem such as intracranial hemorrhage or asphyxia. Asymmetric breath sounds may be due to pneumothorax (which is a complication of RDS), congenital diaphragmatic hernia, or unilateral pleural effusion. Meconium staining of amniotic fluid suggests the possibility of meconium aspiration syndrome, but this is rare in premature infants—green-stained amniotic fluid in this population is more likely to be due to infection or to bile refluxed into the esophagus because of intestinal obstruction, rather than meconium.

LABORATORY FEATURES OF RDS

Initially, the arterial blood gases or oxygen saturation monitor may show only hypoxemia or desaturation. The $Paco_2$ may be normal because of tachypnea, but is almost

---

BOX 46-1   Clinical Signs of RDS

Tachypnea
Grunting
Increased work of breathing
  Nasal flaring
  Retraction of respiratory muscles (intercostal, subcostal, sternal)
Cyanosis
Pallor
Lethargy
Disinterest in feeding
Apnea

always elevated. Later, as the infant tires, the $Paco_2$ will rise further and cause respiratory acidosis. With imminent respiratory failure, there may be metabolic acidosis due to inadequate oxygen delivery to tissues, and from poor peripheral perfusion due to respiratory acidosis.

Differential diagnosis: Extremely elevated $Paco_2$ within minutes of birth suggests pulmonary hypoplasia, tension pneumothorax, congenital diaphragmatic hernia, or obstruction of the airways due to debris or an anatomic cause. The tachypneic, cyanotic newborn with low $Paco_2$ may have transient tachypnea of the newborn or cyanotic congenital heart disease. A positive blood culture suggests pneumonia and sepsis. Low blood glucose (<40) suggests symptomatic hypoglycemia, and high hematocrit (>65) suggests symptomatic polycythemia.

RADIOGRAPHIC FEATURES OF RDS

The classic radiographic findings of RDS include a reticulogranular (i.e., ground-glass) pattern and air bronchograms (Figure 46-11). The lungs are diffusely and homogeneously dense because of widespread collapse of alveoli. The appearance is reticular (i.e., netlike) because the small airways are open (black) and surrounded by interstitial and alveolar fluid (white); in severe cases, the lungs may appear complete white on the film. Air bronchograms are commonly seen because the large airways beyond the second or third generation are more visible than usual as a result of radiodensity from engorged peribronchial lymphatics and fluid-filled or collapsed alveoli. Another cardinal feature is low lung volume (e.g., the diaphragms are at the eighth rib level or higher) due to widespread alveolar collapse and low functional residual capacity.

Differential diagnosis: Normal or high lung volumes, especially with prominent interstitial fluid pattern, suggest TTNB. In this case, there are coarse white lines (engorged lymphatics and interstitial water) radiating from the hilum rather than the crisp black lines (air bronchograms) of RDS. Other causes of a coarse (rather than diffuse) fluid pattern include pneumonia with sepsis, and obstructed pulmonary venous drainage due to total anomalous pulmonary venous return. An abnormal cardiac silhouette or size should suggest congenital heart disease, and asymmetry of the lungs suggests pneumothorax, congenital diaphragmatic hernia, or lung anomaly. Very low lung volumes, especially with pneumothorax, may indicate pulmonary hypoplasia.

INITIAL DIAGNOSTIC EVALUATION FOR POSSIBLE RDS

The initial diagnostic evaluation (Box 46-2) is shaped by the differential diagnoses listed in Table 46-1, and by the urgency to intervene quickly for serious but infrequent conditions such as bacterial pneumonia and sepsis, hypoglycemia, and polycythemia. It is often helpful to obtain both anteroposterior and lateral radiographs for the initial evaluation. If congenital heart disease is suspected on clinical grounds, an echocardiogram is indicated.

TREATMENT OF PATIENTS WITH RDS

The treatment of patients with RDS is outlined in Box 46-3. All patients with RDS need the basics of warmth, hydration, and nutrition appropriate for the degree of prematurity, as described in other chapters. Because pulmonary edema contributes to surfactant dysfunction in RDS, it is important to avoid excessive intravenous (IV) fluid administration.

Newborns with significant tachypnea (e.g., more than 60 breaths per minute) or increased work of breathing

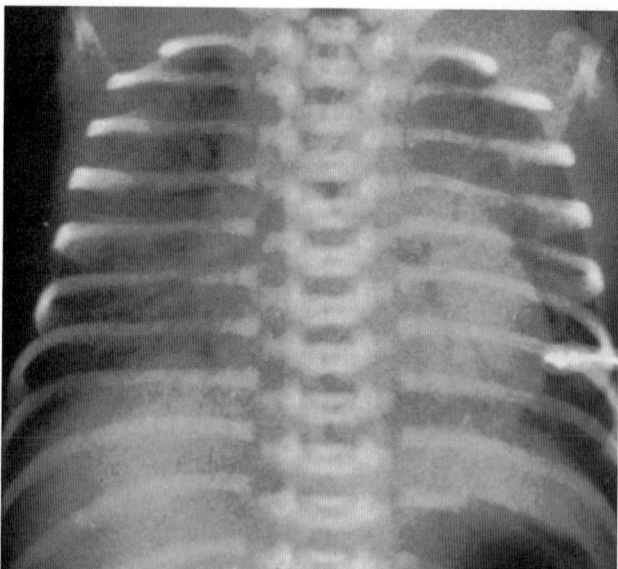

FIGURE 46-11 Radiograph of RDS. Note low lung volumes and reticulogranular pattern. (*From Welty S, Hansen TN, Corbet A: Respiratory distress in the preterm infant. In Taeusch HW, Ballard RA, Gleason CA, editors: Avery's diseases of the newborn, ed 8, Philadelphia, 2005, Elsevier.*)

> **BOX 46-2   Initial Diagnostic Evaluation for Possible RDS**
>
> Arterial or capillary blood gas
> Blood glucose
> Complete blood count
> Blood culture
> AP and lateral chest radiograph
> Echocardiogram (if clinically indicated)

> **BOX 46-3   Treatment of Established RDS**
>
> Warmth by radiant warmer or incubator
> Hydration at approximately 60–80 mL/kg/d
> Nutrition
>   Initially D5W or D10W (with protein, if possible)
>   NPO if respiratory rate over 60 or moderate/severe work of breathing
>   Gavage feeds if stable
>   Consider parenteral nutrition if enteral feeds are delayed
> Antibiotics if at risk for pneumonia and sepsis
> Supplemental oxygen
>   Oxygen saturation monitoring, with appropriate target for infants at risk for retinopathy of prematurity
> Exogenous surfactant
> CPAP or mechanical ventilation, as needed
>
> *CPAP,* Continuous positive airway pressure.

(moderate or severe) often do not have the energy required for oral feeding, and there is some risk of aspiration if nipple feeding is attempted. Initially, IV fluids and nothing by mouth (NPO) status may be appropriate, with consideration of small gavage tube gastric feedings if the baby is otherwise stable. Parenteral nutrition may be indicated because of the increased caloric expenditures associated with work of breathing. Antibiotics should be considered unless the risk of pneumonia and sepsis is negligible.

The techniques of respiratory support are described in other chapters. See Chapter 45 regarding risks and benefits of different modes of respiratory therapy.

RESPIRATORY COMPLICATIONS OF RDS

Air leak complications occur in patients with RDS because of the asymmetry of alveolar inflation and the sheer stresses in terminal bronchioles, leading to dissection of air into the interstitium (causing pulmonary interstitial emphysema) and through the visceral pleura (causing pneumothorax). The former can be seen in up to 50% of patients with RDS, and the latter in 5% to 10%, even in those treated with exogenous surfactant.

Hemorrhagic pulmonary edema (i.e., pulmonary hemorrhage) occurs more frequently in the most premature infants, probably due to left ventricular failure and excessive left-to-right flow through a patent ductus arteriosus, with resultant disruption of the pulmonary capillaries (Cole et al, 1973). It may also be related to insufficient attention to reducing mechanical ventilator settings after lung compliance improves following exogenous surfactant treatment. Onset is typically at 1 to 3 days of age, with sudden respiratory deterioration associated with pink or red frothy fluid in the ET tube, and widespread white-out on chest radiograph. Treatment considerations include increased positive end-expiratory pressure (PEEP); there is also evidence that exogenous surfactant may be beneficial (Pandit et al, 1995).

Bronchopulmonary dysplasia (BPD), also known as chronic lung disease, is probably due to abnormal lung repair following lung injury from RDS (see Chapter 48).

PREVENTION OF RDS

Box 46-4 outlines the key measures for prevention and treatment of RDS.

Antenatal Steroids

Antenatal steroids were shown in 1972 to be effective in reducing the risk of RDS (Liggins and Howie, 1972). A consensus panel convened by the National Institutes of

---

BOX 46-4 Prevention of RDS

Antenatal steroids
Prevention of asphyxia
Continuous positive airway pressure
Exogenous surfactant
Surfactant, then CPAP

CPAP, Continuous positive airway pressure.

Health concluded that "antenatal corticosteroid therapy is indicated for women at risk of premature delivery with few exceptions and will result in a substantial decrease in neonatal morbidity and mortality, as well as substantial savings in health costs" (NIH Consensus Panel, 1995). They recommended that the treatment be used from 24 to 34 weeks' gestation without limitation by gender or race, and whether or not surfactant therapy was available. Although the beneficial effects were found to be greatest if treatment was begun more than 24 hours before delivery, there was also a benefit when given for less than 24 hours.

A metaanalysis in 2006 (Roberts and Dalziel, 2006) reviewed 21 published trials and concluded that antenatal corticosteroids did not increase a mother's risk of death, chorioamnionitis, or puerperal sepsis. Treatment was associated with a 31% reduction in neonatal death, 34% reduction in RDS, 46% reduction in cerebroventricular hemorrhage, and 54% reduction in necrotizing enterocolitis (all significant at p <0.05 or less).

Although there is now widespread consensus on use of antenatal steroids, many issues remain controversial, including the type of corticosteroid to use; the dose, frequency, and timing of use; and the route of administration. A metaanalysis in 2008 (Brownfoot et al, 2008) reviewed 10 trials and found that antenatal dexamethasone appears to decrease the incidence of intraventricular hemorrhage but possibly increases the rate of NICU admissions, compared with betamethasone. Oral antenatal dexamethasone was found in one study to increase the incidence of neonatal sepsis compared to intramuscular drug (Egerman et al, 1998). More research is needed to optimize antenatal steroid administration.

Because the effectiveness appears to wane if antenatal steroids are given more than 1 week before premature delivery, several trials have been conducted to determine whether one or more repeat doses at weekly intervals was beneficial. Although a metaanalysis (Crowther and Harding, 2007) found modest improvements in occurrence and severity of RDS, there were concerning findings of smaller birthweight and head circumference, indicating that there is insufficient evidence to recommend repeated doses (Bonanno and Wapner, 2009).

Prevention of Asphyxia

Prevention of asphyxia may decrease the incidence and severity of RDS, because asphyxia leads to hypoxemia and acidosis, which reduce surfactant synthesis. Leakage of fluids from capillaries into alveoli may also impair surfactant function. Thus, delivery by cesarean section should be considered for signs of fetal distress if the fetus is deemed to be viable, or if the fetus is in the breech presentation during labor. Compliance with consensus neonatal resuscitation techniques outlined by the American Academy of Pediatrics and American Heart Association (Kattwinkel, 2006) is critical, especially because premature infants are at much higher risk for needing intervention at birth. Maternal transfer to a center experienced in management of premature infants, if it can be accomplished safely, is associated with improved neonatal outcome.

Continuous Positive Airway Pressure

Gregory et al (1971) first introduced continuous positive airway pressure (CPAP) for newborns with RDS, primarily by endotracheal tube. Since then, a variety of devices have been developed, including short nasal prongs that do not add much to the work of breathing (De Paoli et al, 2002). Avery et al (1987) reported that centers that used early nasal CPAP for RDS had a lower incidence of chronic lung disease.

The goals of CPAP are to prevent end-expiratory alveolar collapse, reduce the work of breathing, and better match ventilation to perfusion. If started in the delivery room, it may help the newborn establish functional residual capacity, in addition to stabilizing the chest wall and reducing airway resistance. Furthermore, adequate expansion of the lungs at birth improves pulmonary blood flow. Some have speculated that prophylactic use of CPAP in the delivery room might make intubation for exogenous surfactant unnecessary (De Klerk and De Klerk, 2001), and that avoidance of intubation and mechanical ventilation may lower the risk of BPD (see Chapter 48).

The COIN Trial randomized 25- to 28-weeks' gestation newborns who were breathing spontaneously at 5 minutes of age either to CPAP or to prophylactic intubation with early extubation to CPAP if possible. The investigators found that 46% of the CPAP group eventually required intubation anyway during the first 5 days, and the rate of pneumothorax was 9% compared to only 3% in those intubated routinely (p <0.001) (Morley et al, 2008). This suggests that routine intubation may be safer than immediate CPAP in the extremely premature infant, but it also demonstrated that some patients in this extremely high-risk population do well with early CPAP. Success with CPAP, especially in this population, requires considerable experience and skill (Bohlin et al, 2008).

Recently, some centers have begun using humidified high-flow nasal cannulas in infants with RDS (Lampland, 2009) to achieve the benefits of positive airway pressure with fewer of the perceived disadvantages of CPAP (challenges in keeping the nasal prongs in the nares, easier handling of the patient, and less risk of pressure necrosis of the nasal septum). However, the pressure generated from this therapy, although proven to produce clinical effect, is variable, unpredictable, and unregulated, and the commercially available systems are not approved by the U.S. Food and Drug Administration (FDA) for this indication. It should only be used by practitioners aware of the balance of risks and benefits, and those prepared to recognize and treat pneumothorax and respiratory failure.

The use of CPAP following tracheal administration of exogenous surfactant is discussed later in the section on timing of surfactant administration.

Exogenous Surfactant

Historical Summary

The development of exogenous surfactant for treatment of RDS is one of the most important advances in the history of newborn medicine. This history is well told elsewhere (e.g., Halliday, 2008). The key milestones include von Neergaard's discovery in 1929 that surface tension contributes to lung recoil, Gruenwald's demonstration in 1947 that lungs of stillborn infants have high surface tension, Prattle's speculation in 1955 that absence of surfactant active material contributes to RDS, Clement's description in 1957 of surfactant dysfunction in experimental animals, and Avery and Mead's demonstration in 1959 that RDS in human infants is due to surfactant deficiency. There was an increase in research interest and funding for RDS treatment after U.S. President Kennedy's son, born at 34 weeks' gestation, died of RDS in 1963. In 1972, Enhorning and Robertson used natural surfactant to delay the progression of RDS in preterm rabbits, and in 1980 Fujiwara et al demonstrated the first successful use of exogenous surfactant in human infants. By 1990, exogenous surfactant was widely used throughout the developed world, and many large clinical trials have been conducted since then to refine and improve surfactant treatment and prevention of RDS. Compared to standard therapy without surfactant, a metaanalysis of 13 randomized controlled trials suggests that animal-derived exogenous surfactant reduces the risk of pneumothorax by 58%, pulmonary interstitial emphysema by 55%, mortality by 32%, and the combined outcome of BPD or death by 17% (Seger and Soll, 2009).

Types of Surfactant Available

A list of commonly used surfactant preparations can be found in Table 46-2. The first generation of commercially available artificial surfactants (e.g. Exosurf [colfosceril]) was composed mainly of DPPC and did not have SP-B or SP-C. However, a metaanalysis of 11 randomized controlled trials showed that natural surfactants were faster acting than artificial surfactants with lower incidence of pneumothorax and mortality (Soll and Blanco, 2001).

TABLE 46-2 Surfactant Preparations and Their Sources

Brand Name	Generic Name	Constituents
Nonprotein Synthetic Surfactants		
Adsurf	Pumactant (ALEC)	DPPC, PG
Exosurf	Colfosceril palmitate	DPPC
Protein-Containing Animal Surfactants		
Curosurf	Poractant α	Porcine lung tissue
Alveofact	SF-RI 1	Bovine lung lavage
BLES	Bovine lipid extract surfactant	Bovine lung lavage
Infasurf	Calactant CLSE	Bovine (calf) lung lavage
Surfacten	Surfactant-TA	Bovine lung homogenate
Survanta	Beractant	Bovine lung tissue
Peptide-Containing Synthetic Surfactants		
Venticute	rSP-C surfactant	DPPC, POPG, PA, rSP-C
Surfaxin	Lucinactant	DPPC, POPG, PA, KL4

Adapted from Sinha S, Moya F, Donn SM: Surfactant for respiratory distress syndrome: are there important clinical differences among preparations? *Curr Opin Pediatr* 19:150-154, 2007.
ALEC, Artificial lung-expanding compound; *DPPC*, dipalmitoylphosphatidylcholine; *PG*, phosphatidylglycerol; *rSP-C*, recombinant human SP-C; *POPG*, palmitoyl-oleoyl phosphatidylglycerol; *PA*, palmitic acid.

Clinical trials comparing the available natural surfactants have been inconclusive. Speer et al (1995) showed no differences in a small study, whereas Baroutis et al (2003) showed differences in days of intubation, oxygen use, and duration of hospitalization, but not survival. A comparison of Infasurf and Survanta by Bloom and Clark (2005) was stopped because of lack of statistical significance in the primary outcome variable. Ramanathan et al (2004) compared Curosurf and Survanta, finding that the former was less costly because of fewer doses, but there were no important clinical differences in outcome.

A new generation of synthetic surfactants is under development to lower cost and because of theoretical concerns about immunologic or infectious complications from animal-derived surfactant. These new products have synthetic peptides or proteins, such as KL4 in lucinactant, which mimics the actions of natural surfactant-associated proteins SP-B and SP-C. Lucinactant has been shown to be superior to older synthetic surfactants (Sinha et al, 2005), but its superiority to animal surfactants has not been conclusively proven (Moya et al, 2005). In addition, there are uncertainties regarding the metabolic fate of lucinactant and its component chemicals, and there may be risks from the requirement to convert the lucinactant gel into liquid by using a special warming cradle immediately before instillation (Engle et al, 2008); the authors added that "efforts to develop more effective and safer surfactant formulations continue to be warranted because of concerns with animal-derived surfactants for transmission of microbes, exposure to animal proteins and inflammatory mediators, susceptibility to inactivation, and inconsistent content."

Surfactant Selection

The important issue for clinical providers and managers is which surfactant to stock in their pharmacy, because of the expense of the preparations and the need to standardize dosing guidelines. Compared to first-generation synthetic surfactants, current studies strongly support use of natural surfactants because of reduced risk of air leak and more rapid response to treatment. Among natural surfactants that are commercially available, no differences in long-term outcomes have been conclusively proven. However, poractant alfa (Curosurf) when given as prophylaxis with an initial dose of 200 mg/kg appears to have some advantages when compared to beractant (Survanta) and calfactant (Infasurf), such as fewer repeat doses, quicker oxygen weaning, and potentially less cost. The benefit may be related to the larger amount of phospholipid in each dose. For hospitals currently using beractant and calfactant, the advantages of poractant alfa must be considered in light of the logistical issues and potential drug errors when a hospital changes from one preparation to another, especially when there may be better products on the horizon.

Timing of Surfactant Administration

In theory, surfactant would ideally be given with the first breath. This concept was evaluated by Kattwinkel et al (2004) by delivering the head of the infant, suctioning the nasopharynx, and then instilling calfactant into the airway before delivery of the shoulders. CPAP was initiated immediately after delivery, but the trachea was not routinely intubated. The treatment appeared feasible and safe, but the sample size (23) was too small to prove that the approach was beneficial compared to surfactant instillation via endotracheal tube during the first minutes after delivery.

Prophylactic surfactant generally refers to the administration of doses within the first 15 minutes after birth. To avoid giving an unnecessary, expensive medication and subjecting a newborn to the risks of tracheal intubation, prophylactic endotracheal surfactant should ideally be given only to patients who would have eventually developed RDS and met treatment criteria for surfactant anyway. However, in practice, the clinician can only select those patients at highest risk and for whom clinical trials indicate that the benefits of prophylactic surfactant outweigh the risks. One such population is the baby born at <30 weeks' gestation whose mother was not given antenatal steroids (Table 46-3). In the highest risk populations, a metaanalysis of eight clinical trials suggests that prophylactic surfactant reduces mortality (by 39%), frequency and severity of RDS, pneumothorax (by 38%), and the combined outcome of BPD and death, compared to infants who received placebo or rescue surfactant (Soll and Morley, 2001). However, the criteria for selecting the high risk infants remain controversial. Table 46-3 provides one practical approach for the clinician who must make a decision in the delivery room as to whether to begin surfactant immediately or to wait. However, some centers manage even 25-week gestational newborns with initial CPAP, with only one third eventually needing surfactant (Aly et al, 2004). A randomized study of 27 to 31 weeks' gestation newborns with signs of early RDS demonstrated that infants intubated for surfactant during the first hour of life followed immediately by extubation and CPAP had a lower rate of subsequent ventilation, incidence of pneumothorax, and chronic lung disease compared to newborns treated with early CPAP alone (Rojas, 2009). This observation may be especially important for hospitals not equipped to provide mechanical ventilation for this population.

Early rescue surfactant (usually defined as treatment at 1 to 2 hours after birth) may be indicated for infants of <30 weeks' gestation at the first signs of RDS. The clinical trials showing superiority of prophylactic surfactant over rescue (Soll and Morley, 2001) compared prophylaxis to *late* rescue (needing mechanical ventilation and >40% Fio_2 and typically treated 4 to 6 hours after birth).

TABLE 46-3   Sample Algorithm for When to Begin Exogenous Surfactant

When to Give First Dose of Surfactant	Populations to Consider
Prophylactically, within 15 minutes after birth	<26 weeks' gestation *and* 26 to 30 weeks if (a) no antenatal steroids *or* (b) needs intubation anyway
Early rescue, preferably in first 60 minutes after birth	<30 weeks' gestation at first signs of RDS
Treatment of established RDS, preferably started within 12 hours after birth	All newborns with established RDS, regardless of gestational age, if they need ventilator and at least 30–40% O_2

One clinical trial showed clinical advantages of prophylactic compared to early-rescue surfactant (Kattwinkel et al, 1993) but a historically controlled study showed that aggressive use of CPAP led to a large reduction in the need for any surfactant at all and was associated with lower rates of BPD and other morbidity (De Klerk and De Klerk, 2001). Furthermore, immediate intubation in the delivery room may be associated with significant procedure morbidity, including apnea and bradycardia. Thus, there is no compelling evidence favoring prophylactic over early rescue surfactant for preterm infants at the time of this writing, except in those patients at highest risk (see Table 46-3) such as extremely preterm infants whose mothers did not receive antenatal steroids (Sweet and Halliday, 2009).

Late rescue surfactant: Clinical trials have firmly established the benefits of surfactant compared to no surfactant in preterm infants with established RDS (Engle et al, 2008). However, as noted previously, prophylactic or early rescue surfactant is more beneficial than late rescue in the highest-risk populations. In lower-risk populations (e.g., near-term infants) it is likely that the late rescue approach offers a better balance of benefit, risk of intubation, and cost efficiency than treatment before or at the earliest onset of RDS. Entry criteria in clinical trials of rescue surfactant compared to no surfactant usually required that RDS be severe enough to require mechanical ventilation and at least 30 to 40% supplemental oxygen. Many of the trials were conducted before nasal CPAP was widely used, so the indications for intubating and administering surfactant in infants tolerating CPAP are unknown. However, those with a requirement for very high concentration of supplemental oxygen (e.g., >80%) or with sustained severe hypercarbia (e.g., $Paco_2$ >60 torr) will likely benefit.

Combining surfactant therapy with CPAP: Because of advances in use of CPAP since the first clinical trials of surfactant, some have advocated immediate extubation to CPAP after surfactant dosing (Verder et al, 1999) to avoid complications from the endotracheal tube (including excessive tidal volumes and airway inflammation that may lead to BPD). Stevens et al (2007) reviewed six randomized controlled clinical trials of this treatment approach in infants with clinical signs of RDS. The "early rescue/CPAP" group was intubated for early surfactant therapy followed by immediate extubation to nasal CPAP. In comparison to the late rescue group, early rescue/CPAP was associated with a 33% reduction in need for mechanical ventilation, 48% reduction in air leak syndrome, and 49% reduction in incidence of BPD. They also noted that initiation of surfactant treatment at an Fio_2 of less than 0.45 was associated with lower incidence of air leak, compared to waiting until the Fio_2 was higher.

Methods of Surfactant Dosing

Animal studies suggest that surfactant distribution is better distributed when administered as a bolus rather than by infusing it slowly over several minutes (Fernandez et al, 1998). The package inserts of many surfactant preparations recommend moving the infant into multiple positions for better distribution of surfactant, but there are no clinical trials supporting one particular method. Therefore, surfactant should be given as quickly as tolerated, and with the least disruptive infant positioning.

Exogenous surfactant is generally given via an endotracheal tube. However, tracheal intubation is potentially risky, and sometimes difficult to accomplish, so administration through a laryngeal mask airway (LMA) may be considered. In a pilot study of 8 preterm infants (body weight range 880 to 2520 g) receiving nasal CPAP for RDS, the LMA administration approach appeared to be safe and potentially effective (Trevisanuto et al, 2005).

Number of Surfactant Doses and Dosing Intervals

A metaanalysis of two clinical trials that compared one versus multiple doses of animal-derived surfactant suggests a 49% reduction in incidence of pneumothorax and a trend toward a 37% reduction in mortality when multiple doses are used (Soll and Ozek, 2009). There are no data to suggest that dosing should continue once the patient's ventilator and oxygen requirement are at minimal levels, or beyond four doses. The interval between doses is usually at least 6 hours, and most protocols recommend discontinuation of dosing after 48 hours. In an attempt to reduce the incidence of BPD, clinical trials of surfactant administration at several days of age are underway.

Clinical Care after Dosing

Because natural surfactants may work quickly, the clinician must be prepared after dosing to immediately lower the Fio_2 while carefully monitoring the pulse oximeter. The tidal volume, as measured by the ventilator and/or by careful observation of chest wall movement, may gradually increase, resulting in a need to lower inspiratory pressures to avoid air leak syndrome, lung injury, and possibly pulmonary hemorrhage. Blood gases should be monitored by transcutaneous monitors and/or intermittent sampling. PEEP should be maintained but may be reduced if the starting levels at dosing were high, given that functional residual capacity increases shortly after surfactant administration.

A poor response to exogenous surfactant may occur because the patient does not have surfactant deficiency but rather, lung hypoplasia, pneumonia, or congenital heart disease. Other causes for a lack of response may be poor distribution of the surfactant, such as administration down the right stem bronchus due to malposition of the endotracheal tube, plugging of the tube, or malposition of the tube in the esophagus. A less likely reason is an inadequate dose of surfactant.

The rapid improvement in lung compliance after exogenous surfactant therapy may lead to excessive pulmonary blood flow from left-to-right shunting from a patent ductus arteriosus (Raju and Langerberg, 1993). It is uncertain whether early and aggressive intervention to close the ductus with medication or surgery will reduce the risk of pulmonary hemorrhage.

PULMONARY HYPOPLASIA

DEFINITION AND INCIDENCE

One or both lungs of newborns with pulmonary hypoplasia are smaller than normal, including reduced numbers of lung cells, airways, blood vessels, and alveoli.

Pulmonary hypoplasia is the cause of respiratory distress at birth in only 0.3% of newborns with respiratory symptoms (Rubaltelli et al, 1998), but it is commonly fatal, especially in preterm infants. The incidence is about 1 per 1000 live births, and 90% are associated with congenital anomalies or pregnancy complications (Churg et al, 2005). There is a continuum of severity of pulmonary hypoplasia—from negligible to severe—and therefore all but the most severe cases are difficult to diagnose. This is especially true when attempting to diagnose prenatally by imaging studies, but is also true during clinical assessment of the newborn, and even after postmortem examination of the lungs.

When considering the causes of pulmonary hypoplasia, it is useful to categorize them into associated conditions, each with representative diagnoses, as in Table 46-4. This chapter on respiratory distress in preterm infants focuses on the problem of pulmonary hypoplasia associated with oligohydramnios from preterm premature rupture of membranes (PPROM) because this cause of pulmonary hypoplasia occurs almost exclusively in preterm infants. When PPROM occurs at 15 weeks' gestation, the incidence

of pulmonary hypoplasia is 80% and at 19 weeks it is 50%, whereas after 26 weeks it is near zero (Rothschild et al, 1990). Other conditions associated with pulmonary hypoplasia are covered in other chapters.

PATHOLOGY

The easiest method of defining pulmonary hypoplasia during postmortem exam is to calculate the ratio of lung weight to body weight. At 28 weeks' gestation, a ratio of 0.015 is at the 5th percentile, whereas at 35 weeks', the 5th percentile is at a ratio of 0.012. The lung-to-body weight ratio may be artificially elevated if the lungs are wetter than usual from edema, hemorrhage, inflammation, or lymphangiectasia—this may lead to the false conclusion that the patient does not have pulmonary hypoplasia. Conversely, the ratio may be artificially low if the body is heavier than usual because of renal cystic disease, hydrops, ascites, tumors, hydrocephaly, and so forth. Therefore, a better method for postmortem diagnosis of pulmonary hypoplasia is to measure the lung volume by inflating the lung with fixative at physiologic pressure and then measuring the displacement of fluid when the lung is immersed. Pulmonary hypoplasia assessed by this method is defined as lung volume less than the 5th percentile of standards for each gestational age (Churg et al, 2005). This method facilitates comparison of postmortem to in utero estimates of lung volume made during antenatal imaging. However, low lung volume does not necessarily correlate with deficiency of lung structure and function. A postmortem technique more physiologically relevant than lung volume is the radial alveolar count, which is proportional to alveolar surface complexity (Churg et al, 2005) and thus gas exchange surface area; however, this procedure is complex and time-consuming.

Impairment of lung development before 16 weeks causes reduced airway branching, reduced cartilage development, reduced acinar complexity and maturation, delayed vascularization, and delayed thinning of the air-blood barrier. Impairment after 16 weeks typically causes reduced acinar complexity and maturation. These outcomes are predictable, given the time in gestation when these structures are developing (Figure 46-12, *A*).

Because the growth of lung blood vessels parallels the development of the airways, pulmonary hypoplasia causes decreased total size of the pulmonary vascular bed, decreased number of vessels per unit of lung tissue, and increased pulmonary arterial smooth muscle. This last phenomenon accounts for persistent pulmonary hypertension after birth.

CLINICAL SIGNS

The preterm newborn with pulmonary hypoplasia often presents with immediate signs of respiratory distress and cyanosis indistinguishable from those in the newborn with severe respiratory distress syndrome (see earlier section on clinical signs of RDS). However, respiratory failure from severe pulmonary hypoplasia often becomes apparent within minutes of birth, whereas respiratory failure from RDS usually progresses over the first few hours after birth. The thorax may appear small or bell-shaped

TABLE 46-4 Categories of Conditions Associated With Pulmonary Hypoplasia

Category	Representative Diagnoses

Restriction of thoracic space	Diaphragmatic hernia or eventration
	Intrathoracic mass
	   Congenital cystic adenomatoid malformation
	   Bronchogenic cyst
	   Extralobar sequestration
	   Thoracic neuroblastoma
	Pleural effusions
	   Chylothorax
	   Hydrothorax

Oligohydramnios	Renal
	   Bilateral renal agenesis or dysplasia
	   Bladder outlet obstruction (posterior urethral valves)
	Nonrenal
	   Prolonged preterm rupture of membranes

Skeletal anomalies	Chondroectodermal dysplasia Osteogenesis imperfecta Thanatophoric dwarfism
Hydrops fetalis	Rh isoimmunization
Neuromuscular and central nervous system anomalies	Fetal akinesia Anencephaly Arnold-Chiari malformation
Cardiac anomalies	Hypoplastic right or left heart Pulmonary stenosis Ebstein's anomaly
Abdominal wall defects	Omphalocele Gastroschisis
Syndromes	Trisomy 13, 18, 21 Larsen's Cerebrocostomandibular Jarcho-Levin Roberts Lethal multiple pterygium

Adapted from Churg AM, Myers JL, Tazelaar H, Wright J, editors: *Thurlbeck's pathology of the lung*, ed 3, New York, 2005, Thieme.

and, if oligohydramnios was severe, there may be flattening of the face and deformation (such as contractures of the extremities). Hypercarbia may be severe on the earliest blood gas measurement, despite aggressive mechanical ventilation. The hypoxemia from surfactant deficiency and lung immaturity may be compounded by right-to-left shunting of deoxygenated blood due to pulmonary hypertension, leading to severe desaturation. If there is also a tension pneumothorax, there may be asymmetry of breath sounds or malposition of heart sounds, as well as impaired cardiac output from impaired venous return to the thorax.

RADIOGRAPHIC SIGNS

Because lung immaturity and surfactant deficiency accompany pulmonary hypoplasia, particularly in preterm infants, the lungs may be radiographically dense with air

bronchograms, as with RDS, but the lung volumes may be smaller and the diaphragms higher than in RDS. With severe pulmonary hypoplasia, the thorax may appear bell-shaped, and early pneumothorax is common.

TREATMENT

After birth, treatment for pulmonary hypoplasia is similar to that provided to patients with RDS, including assisted ventilation and exogenous surfactant. Even with cautious ventilation, however, tension pneumothoraces are common and are often the proximate cause of death, so the neonatal team should be prepared for urgent needle decompression of the chest and insertion of a chest tube. Permissive hypercapnia is appropriate, and high-frequency ventilation may be necessary for adequate ventilation and removal of very high arterial Pco_2 levels. If pulmonary

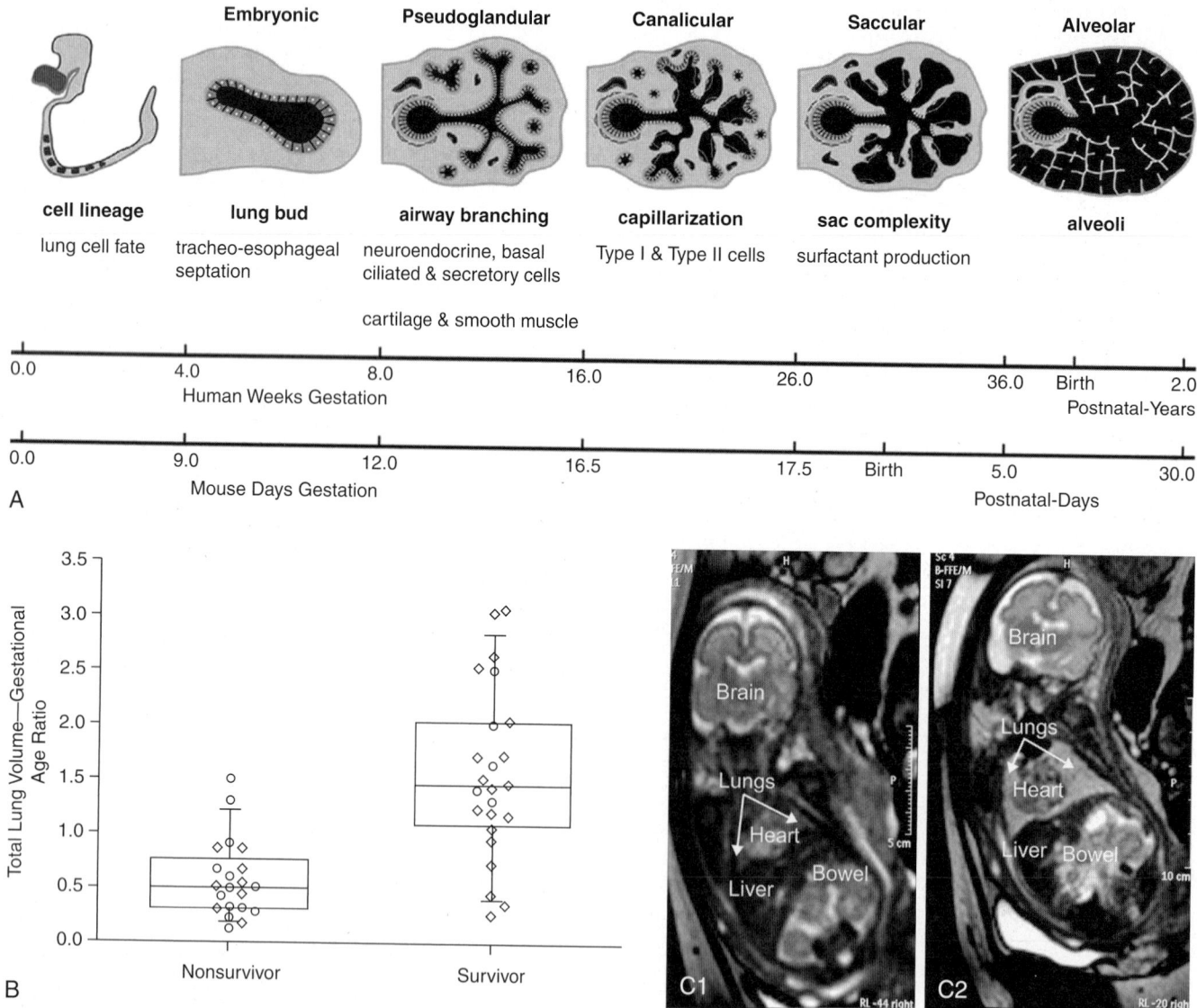

FIGURE 46-12 **A,** Stages of lung development. **B,** Measurement of fetal lung volume by magnetic resonance imaging and outcomes after delivery. **C,** Lung growth after occlusion of the fetal trachea for 6 days: (*C1*) before tracheal occlusion and (*C2*) after tracheal occlusion. (*A from Kimura J, Deutsch GH: Key mechanisms of early lung development,* Pediatr Dev Pathol *10:335-347, 2007. Allen Press, Inc.* **C** *from Kohl T, Geipel A, Tchatcheva K, et al: Life-saving effects of fetal tracheal occlusion on pulmonary hypoplasia from preterm premature rupture of membranes,* Obstet Gynecol *113:480-483, 2009, Lippincott Williams and Wilkins.*)

hypertension is present, as it commonly is, inhaled nitric oxide for pulmonary vasodilation is logical, but clinical trials with sufficient sample size to prove better survival are lacking (Chock et al, 2009). Extracorporeal membrane oxygenation may be appropriate for larger preterm infants if the pulmonary hypoplasia, surfactant deficiency, and pulmonary hypertension are expected to improve within a few days. However, it is very difficult to select appropriate candidates with pulmonary hypoplasia for extracorporeal membrane oxygenation, and it is often unsuccessful with severe disease or in combination with other major life-threatening malformations.

PRENATAL DIAGNOSIS

An accurate prenatal test for pulmonary hypoplasia is important because it may affect the obstetric management. It would be particularly helpful to be able to discriminate lethal from nonlethal pulmonary hypoplasia, especially before 24 weeks' gestation when termination of the pregnancy may be an option. This is an easier task than quantifying the degree of fetal pulmonary hypoplasia, which—as noted previously—is challenging even for the pathologist.

A metaanalysis of clinical parameters for prediction of fatal pulmonary hypoplasia following prelabor rupture of membranes before 28 weeks' gestation concluded that gestational age at rupture was a better predictor of pulmonary hypoplasia than latency or oligohydramnios (van Teeffelen et al, 2010).

In 1992, ultrasound measurement of the fetal chest circumference was shown to be helpful in predicting fatal pulmonary hypoplasia (Ohlsson et al, 1992), whereas in 2002 the best prediction was achieved by combining clinical, biometric, and Doppler parameters (Laudy et al, 2002). These parameters included thoracic, cardiac, and abdominal circumference, the largest vertical amniotic fluid pocket, and pulsed Doppler measurements of the arterial pulmonary branches. Nonsurvivors with pulmonary hypoplasia due to fetal urinary anomalies were noted to have lower in utero lung volumes as determined by fetal MRI, adjusted for gestational age (Zaretsky et al, 2005), but there was no clear separation between the survivors and nonsurvivors (Figure 46-12, B). Furthermore, there was considerable overlap of the confidence intervals before 26 weeks' gestation, which limits the usefulness of MRI assessment of fetal volume for prenatal counseling. Three-dimensional ultrasound measurements of lung volume had better diagnostic accuracy for predicting pulmonary hypoplasia, compared to two-dimensional measurements of thoracic/heart area ratio (Gerards et al, 2008). Although there will continue to be advances in fetal imaging to assess lung volume, it will likely remain difficult to differentiate lethal from nonlethal pulmonary hypoplasia.

The management of the preterm pregnancy with premature rupture of membranes near the limit of fetal viability is beyond the scope of this chapter. However, a recent review article by Waters and Mercer (2009) offers a management algorithm that illustrates the areas of controversy. For the patient who desires conservative management of premature rupture before the limit of viability, the algorithm recommends serial assessments for signs of infection or labor, as well as interval ultrasound examinations to

watch for the development of pulmonary hypoplasia. If this occurs, antenatal antibiotics and corticosteroids should be considered if more aggressive management is desired.

PRENATAL TREATMENT

Treatment of oligohydramnios with amnioinfusion with saline has been proposed to improve fetal survival by increasing the latency period (the interval between PROM and delivery) and thus the gestational age at delivery. In a small study, it appeared to reduce the incidence of pulmonary hypertension from about 50% to 10% with PPROM in the 20th week of gestation (De Carolis et al, 2004). However, the procedure restores adequate amniotic fluid volume in only a minority of patients in which it is performed, and there are procedure-related complications such as chorioamnionitis and placental abruption (Tan et al, 2003). When it is successful, the benefit may come from restoration of back-pressure from the amniotic sac fluid to the lungs, stimulating fetal lung growth and development during the critical canalicular stage between 16 and 26 weeks' gestation.

Based on this same logic, there have been efforts to reverse pulmonary hypoplasia in utero by fetal tracheal occlusion. In a case report of PPROM at 16 weeks' gestation, fetoscopic tracheal balloon occlusion was performed at 27 4/7 weeks (Kohl et al, 2009). Within 6 days, the fetal lung volume as measured by MRI increased from 13 to 70 mL (Figure 46-12, C) and the lung blood flow normalized. The fetus was delivered at 28 4/7 weeks using the EXIT procedure (ex utero–intrapartum treatment), had no signs of pulmonary hypertension, and was discharged home at 8 weeks of age. This approach has been used for fetuses with congenital diaphragmatic hernia (Done et al, 2008), but with mixed results. Whether this technique proves to be valuable for PPROM is uncertain, but the restoration of lung size in only 6 days suggests that pulmonary hypoplasia may be more reversible than previously assumed.

PNEUMONIA

INCIDENCE

The incidence of pneumonia/sepsis in preterm infants with birthweight 1500 to 2500 g is only 0.28%, whereas in patients with birthweight <1000 g the incidence is several-fold higher at 1.9% (see Figure 46-1) (Rubaltelli et al, 1998). If only newborns with respiratory distress are considered, the overall incidence (in mostly term infants) is 5% (see Table 46-1)—the third most likely cause after RDS (46%) and TTNB (37%). The data in Figure 46-1 indicate that the incidence of pneumonia in newborns with respiratory distress who are <1000 g, 1000 to 1500 g, and 1500 to 2500 g is 4%, 2%, and 1%, respectively. The NICHD Neonatal Research Network reported an incidence of blood culture–proven early-onset sepsis (<72 hours after birth) in newborns of birthweight <1500 g of 1.9% during 1991–1993 (Stoll et al, 1996) and 1.5% during 1998–2000 (Stoll et al, 2003). In the earlier period, group B streptococcus was the most frequent pathogen (31%) followed by *Escherichia coli* (16%) and *Haemophilus influenzae* (12%). In the more recent period, the most common pathogens were *E. coli*

(44%), group B streptococcus (11%), coagulase-negative staphylococcus (11%), *viridans* streptococci and other streptococci (8%), *H. influenzae* (8%), *Citrobacter* (2%), *Listeria monocytogenes* (2%), and *Candida albicans* (2%).

CLINICAL SIGNS

The clinical signs of pneumonia after preterm birth are often indistinguishable from the more common problem of RDS. Bacterial pneumonia is usually accompanied by sepsis because newborns are frequently unable to confine bacteria to the lung, and therefore some infants will exhibit clinical signs of sepsis or shock, including poor perfusion and hypotension, in addition to respiratory failure. Many premature infants with pneumonia also have surfactant deficiency from RDS, further obscuring the diagnosis of pneumonia.

LABORATORY AND RADIOGRAPHIC SIGNS

Blood cultures will be positive in some premature newborns with pneumonia, but the presence of maternal antibiotics in the blood of the newborn reduces confidence in a negative result. Leukopenia, increased percentage of immature granulocytes, and elevated inflammatory markers such as C-reactive protein increase the likelihood of sepsis/pneumonia, but with poor positive predictive value. Tracheal aspirate culture (but not Gram stain) obtained immediately after placement of an endotracheal tube may help with diagnosis and guide therapy, especially when the blood culture is negative (Booth et al, 2009).

Premature newborns with pneumonia will have pulmonary infiltrates on chest radiograph, but the radiographic appearance is difficult to distinguish from RDS (although classically in term newborns it has a more coarse and wet appearance). Because newborns are unable to localize pulmonary infection, lobar infiltrates are rarely an indication of pneumonia—plugging of airways with secretions is more likely.

TREATMENT

Antibiotics directed at the most common organisms (see earlier discussion) should be started immediately when pneumonia in the preterm infant is suspected. Ampicillin and gentamicin are reasonable choices, to be administered for 48 hours pending culture results. Empiric vancomycin has the disadvantage of promoting the emergence of vancomycin-resistant organisms, and a delay in treating coagulase-negative staphylococcal bacteremia until cultures

are positive is rarely of consequence to the patient. If the blood culture is negative, and the mother has been pretreated with antibiotics, a longer course of antibiotics (e.g., 5 to 7 days) may be prudent, especially if there are laboratory abnormalities such as elevated C-reactive protein and a clinical course suggestive of sepsis or pneumonia.

Because it is so difficult to tell which preterm infants with respiratory distress have pneumonia and which have the more common problems of RDS or TTNB, one approach is to empirically treat with antibiotics all premature newborns with respiratory symptoms. The likelihood of infection in newborns <1000 g with respiratory distress is about 4% (see Incidence, earlier), and so 24 extremely premature newborns will be needlessly treated for every one who will benefit. This number can be reduced by avoiding empiric antibiotics at birth for newborns who are prematurely delivered for maternal indications, such as hypertension. Both PROM and premature labor increase the risk of infection.

Among the possible adverse consequences of unnecessary empiric antibiotics are interference with the colonization of the intestinal tract with nonpathogenic bacteria, selection of antibiotic-resistant bacteria, and fungal infection. On the other hand, the development of bronchopulmonary dysplasia is associated with inflammation from chorioamnionitis (Speer, 2009), and so antibiotics even in the absence of frank pneumonia may be beneficial.

SUGGESTED READINGS

Engle WA: American Academy of Pediatrics Committee of Fetus and Newborn: Surfactant-replacement therapy for respiratory distress in the preterm and term neonate, *Pediatrics* 121:419-432, 2008.

Halliday HL: Surfactants: past present and future, *J Perinatol* 28:S47-S56, 2008.

Lampland AL, Plumm B, Meyers PA, et al: Observational study of humidified highflow nasal cannula compared with nasal continuous positive airway pressure, *J Pediatr* 154:177-182, 2009.

Rojas MA, Lozano JM, Rojas MX, et al: Colombian Neonatal Research Network: Very early surfactant without mandatory ventilation in premature infants treated with early continuous positive airway pressure: a randomized, controlled trial, *Pediatrics* 123:137-142, 2009:2009.

Seger N, Soll R: Animal derived surfactant extract for treatment of respiratory distress syndrome, *Cochrane Database Syst Rev* 2:CD007836, 2009.

Sinha S, Moya F, Donn SM: Surfactant for respiratory distress syndrome: are there important clinical differences among preparations, *Curr Opin Pediatr* 19:150-154, 2007.

Soll R, Ozek E: Multiple versus single doses of exogenous surfactant for the prevention and treatment of neonatal respiratory distress syndrome, *Cochrane Database Syst Rev* 1:CD000141, 2009.

Sweet DG, Halliday HL: The use of surfactants in 2009, *Arch Dis Child Educ Pract Ed* 94:78-83, 2009.

Waters TP, Mercer BM: The management of preterm premature rupture of the membranes near the limit of fetal viability, *Am J Obstet Gynecol* 201:230-240, 2009.

Complete references used in this text can be found online at www.expertconsult.com

RESPIRATORY FAILURE IN THE TERM NEWBORN

Thomas A. Parker and John P. Kinsella

The evaluation and management of respiratory failure in the term newborn poses unique challenges and remains one of the most vexing problems facing clinicians in the newborn intensive care unit. Although some of the pathophysiologic features of respiratory failure in the term infant are similar to the premature newborn condition, several disorders occur more commonly in the term newborn (e.g., meconium aspiration) and are often made more difficult to evaluate and manage because of cardiac and pulmonary vascular abnormalities that complicate the clinical course. Indeed, the traditional perspective of categorizing hypoxemia and respiratory failure in the term newborn as cardiac, pulmonary vascular, or due to air-space (lung) disease is insufficient. For example, the syndrome of persistent pulmonary hypertension of the newborn (PPHN) is defined by severe pulmonary vasoconstriction leading to suprasystemic pulmonary artery pressure with extrapulmonary right-to-left venoarterial admixture across the fetal channels of the oval foramen and the arterial duct. However, PPHN rarely occurs without concomitant parenchymal lung disease and disturbances in cardiac performance.

In this chapter we present an algorithm for evaluation of the term newborn with hypoxemia and respiratory failure, review the syndrome of PPHN, and discuss common causes of respiratory failure in the term newborn.

EVALUATION OF THE TERM NEWBORN WITH HYPOXEMIA/ RESPIRATORY DISTRESS

One of the most anxiety-provoking experiences for many clinicians (particularly those in training) is the initial evaluation and management of a term newborn with hypoxemia/respiratory distress. Traditional textbooks provided a wealth of information about individual conditions once identified. However, there are few sources designed to guide the clinician in an ordered fashion through a comprehensive diagnostic evaluation. In this section, we propose an approach to the evaluation of the hypoxemic newborn that may be useful in clarifying the etiology of hypoxemia/respiratory distress and in determining the proper sequence of diagnostic and therapeutic interventions.

HISTORY

Marked hypoxemia in the newborn can be caused by parenchymal lung disease with V/Q mismatch or intrapulmonary shunting, pulmonary vascular disease causing extrapulmonary right-to-left shunting (PPHN), or anatomic right-to-left shunting associated with congenital heart disease. Evaluation should begin with the history and assessment of risk factors for hypoxemic respiratory failure. Relevant history may include the results of prenatal

ultrasound studies. Lesions such as congenital diaphragmatic hernia (CDH) and congenital cystic adenomatoid malformation are diagnosed prenatally with increasing frequency. Although many anatomic congenital heart defects can be diagnosed prenatally, vascular abnormalities (e.g., coarctation of the aorta, total anomalous pulmonary venous return) are more difficult to diagnose with prenatal ultrasound. A history of a structurally normal heart by fetal ultrasonography should be confirmed by echocardiography in the newborn with cyanosis (see later).

Other historical information that may be important in the evaluation of the cyanotic newborn includes a history of severe and prolonged oligohydramnios causing pulmonary hypoplasia. Also important is a history of prolonged fetal bradyarrhythmia and/or tachyarrhythmia and marked anemia (caused by hemolysis, twin-twin transfusion, or chronic hemorrhage) that may cause congestive heart failure, pulmonary edema, and respiratory distress. Maternal illness (e.g., diabetes mellitus), medication use (e.g., aspirin or medications containing nonsteroidal antiinflammatory drugs causing premature constriction of the ductus arteriosus, association of Ebstein's malformation with maternal lithium use), and illicit drug use may contribute to acute cardiopulmonary distress in the newborn. Risk factors for infection that cause sepsis/pneumonia should be considered, including premature or prolonged rupture of membranes, fetal tachycardia, maternal leukocytosis, uterine tenderness, and other signs of intraamniotic infection.

Events at delivery may provide clues to the etiology of hypoxemic respiratory failure in the newborn. For example, if positive-pressure ventilation is required in the delivery room, the risk of pneumothorax increases. A history of meconium-stained amniotic fluid, particularly if meconium is present below the cords, is the sine qua non of meconium aspiration syndrome. Birth trauma (e.g., clavicular fracture, phrenic nerve injury) or acute fetomaternal or fetoplacental hemorrhage may cause respiratory distress in the newborn (Box 47-1).

PHYSICAL EXAMINATION

The initial physical examination provides important clues to the etiology of cyanosis. Marked respiratory distress in the newborn (retractions, grunting, nasal flaring) suggests the presence of pulmonary parenchymal disease with decreased lung compliance. However, it is important to recognize that upper airway obstruction (e.g., Pierre Robin sequence or choanal atresia) and metabolic acidemia also can cause severe respiratory distress. In contrast, the newborn with cyanosis alone or cyanosis plus tachypnea (i.e., nondistressed tachypnea) typically has cyanotic congenital heart disease, most commonly transposition of the great vessels (TGV) or idiopathic PPHN.

BOX 47-1   Neonatal Respiratory Failure: History and Risk Factor Assessment

PRENATAL

Prenatal ultrasound study results
History of oligohydramnios and duration
History of fetal brady/tachyarrhythmia
Maternal illnesses, drugs , medications
History of fetal distress
Risk factors for infection

DELIVERY

History of positive pressure ventilation in DR
Meconium stained amniotic fluid
Hemorrhage
Birth trauma
Low Apgar score

BOX 47-2   Physical Examination

RESPIRATORY DISTRESS (RETRACTIONS, GRUNTING, NASAL FLARING)

Suggests lung parenchymal disease (compliance), upper airway disease or metabolic acidemia

NO SIGNIFICANT RESPIRATORY DISTRESS (TACHYPNEA ALONE)

Suggests hypoxemia caused by cyanotic heart disease without lung disease

---

BOX 47-3   Acute Response to Supplemental Oxygen (High Fio_2 by Hood, Mask)

MINIMAL OR TRANSIENT CHANGE IN SA_{O2}

Cyanotic heart disease, PPHN

MARKED IMPROVEMENT IN SA_{O2}

Parenchymal lung disease, CHD with ductal-dependent systemic blood flow

---

The presence of a heart murmur in the first hours of life is an important sign in the newborn with cyanosis or respiratory distress. In this setting, it is unusual for the common left-to-right shunt lesions (patent ductus arteriosus, atrial septal defect, ventricular septal defect) to produce an audible murmur because pulmonary vascular resistance (PVR) remains high and little turbulence is created across the defect. A murmur that sounds like a ventricular septal defect in the first hours of life is most commonly caused by tricuspid regurgitation (associated with PPHN or an ischemic myocardium).

The response to supplemental oxygen can also provide important clues to the pathophysiology of hypoxemic respiratory failure in the term newborn (Boxes 47-2 and 47-3).

INTERPRETATION OF PULSE OXIMETRY MEASUREMENTS

The interpretation of preductal (right hand) and postductal (lower extremity) saturation by pulse oximetry provides important clues to the etiology of hypoxemia in the newborn. Right-to-left shunting across the ductus arteriosus (but not the patent foramen ovale) causes postductal desaturation (with a >5% preductal/postductal saturation difference). However, it is important to recognize that variability in oximetry readings may be related to differences in available devices and affected by local perfusion.

If the measurements of preductal and postductal Sao_2 are equivalent, this suggests either that the ductus arteriosus is patent and PVR is subsystemic (i.e., the hypoxemia is caused by parenchymal lung disease with intrapulmonary shunting or cyanotic heart disease with ductal-dependent pulmonary blood flow) or that the ductus arteriosus is closed (precluding any interpretation of pulmonary artery pressure without echocardiography). It is uncommon for the ductus arteriosus to close in the first hours of life in the presence of systemic or suprasystemic pulmonary artery pressures.

The most common cause of preductal-postductal gradients in oxygenation is suprasystemic PVR in PPHN causing right-to-left shunting across the ductus arteriosus (associated with meconium aspiration syndrome,

---

TABLE 47-1   Role of Pulse Oximetry in Evaluation of Neonatal Hypoxemic Respiratory Failure

Preductal Sao_2 = postductal Sao_2	1. Intrapulmonary shunt: PVR < SVR 2. Cyanotic congenital heart disease with L→R PDA: Ductal-dependent Qp: pulmonary atresia/stenosis, tricuspid atresia, Ebstein's anomaly 3. PPHN:R→L shunt at PFO: PVR > SVR, ductus closed
Preductal Sao_2 > postductal Sao_2	1. PVR > SVR with R→L PDA: PPHN: MAS, RDS, CDH 2. Ductal-dependent Qs: HLHS, IAA, coarctation 3. Anatomic PV disease: alveolar-capillary dysplasia, pulmonary vein stenosis, TAPVR with obstruction
Preductal Sao_2 ≤ postductal Sao_2	1. TGV with pulmonary hypertension 2. TGV with coarctation of aorta

HLHS, Hypoplastic left heart syndrome; *IAA,* interrupted aortic arch; *L→R PDA,* left-to-right shunting across the patent ductus arteriosus; *PV,* pulmonary vein; *PVR,* pulmonary vascular resistance; *Qp,* pulmonary blood flow; *Qs,* systemic blood flow; *SVR,* systemic vascular resistance; *TAPVR,* total anomalous pulmonary venous return; *TGV,* transposition of the great vessels.

---

surfactant deficiency/dysfunction, CDH, non-CDH pulmonary hypoplasia, or idiopathic). However, ductal-dependent systemic blood flow lesions (hypoplastic left heart syndrome, critical aortic stenosis, interrupted aortic arch, coarctation) may also present with postductal desaturation. Moreover, anatomic pulmonary vascular disease (alveolar-capillary dysplasia, pulmonary venous stenosis, anomalous venous return with obstruction) can cause suprasystemic PVR with right-to-left shunting across the ductus arteriosus and postductal desaturation.

Finally, the unusual occurrence of markedly lower preductal Sao_2 compared to postductal measurements suggests one of two diagnoses: TGV with pulmonary hypertension or TGV with coarctation of the aorta (Table 47-1).

BOX 47-4   CXR and Laboratory Evaluation

CHEST RADIOGRAPH

Hypoxemia out of proportion to radiographic changes suggests congenital heart disease with ductal-dependent pulmonary blood flow or extrapulmonary right-to-left shunting with PPHN

ARTERIAL BLOOD GAS, COMPLETE BLOOD COUNT, BLOOD PRESSURE

ABG: Assess respiratory and metabolic acidemia
CBC: For evidence of infection
BP: Ductal-dependent systemic blood flow and closing PDA (e.g., coarctation)

BOX 47-5   Role of Echocardiography in Evaluation of PPHN and the Use of Inhaled NO

EXTRAPULMONARY SHUNT

Right-to-left shunting at the arterial duct and/or oval foramen is observed in infants with suprasystemic pulmonary hypertension.
If echocardiography demonstrates adequate left ventricular performance, consider iNO use after effective lung recruitment (see functional measurements below)

ANATOMY

Inhaled NO may be contraindicated in the presence of duct-dependent systemic blood flow: e.g., hypoplastic left heart syndrome

LEFT VENTRICULAR PERFORMANCE

Inhaled NO may be contraindicated in the presence of left ventricular systolic/diastolic dysfunction (e.g., mitral insufficiency with L→R atrial shunting with R→L ductal shunting suggesting possible right-ventricle-dependent systemic blood flow

---

LABORATORY AND RADIOLOGIC EVALUATION

One of the most important tests to perform in the evaluation of the newborn with cyanosis is the chest radiograph (CXR). The CXR can demonstrate the classic findings of respiratory distress syndrome (air bronchograms, diffuse granularity, underinflation), diffuse parenchymal lung disease in pneumonia, meconium aspiration syndrome, and CDH. Perhaps the most important question to ask when viewing the CXR is whether the severity of hypoxemia is out of proportion to the radiographic changes. In other words, marked hypoxemia despite supplemental oxygen in the absence of severe pulmonary parenchymal disease radiographically suggests the presence of an extrapulmonary right-to-left shunt (idiopathic PPHN or cyanotic heart disease; Boxes 47-3 and 47-4).

Other essential measurements include an arterial blood gas to determine the blood gas tensions and pH, a complete blood count to evaluate for signs of infection, and blood pressure measurements in the right arm and a lower extremity to identify aortic obstruction (interrupted aortic arch, coarctation).

RESPONSE TO SUPPLEMENTAL OXYGEN

Marked improvement in SaO_2 (increase to 100%) with supplemental oxygen (by hood, mask, or endotracheal tube) suggests the presence of intrapulmonary shunt or V/Q mismatch due to lung disease or reactive PPHN. The response to mask continuous positive airway pressure is also a useful discriminator between severe lung disease and other causes of hypoxemia. Most patients with PPHN have at least a transient improvement in oxygenation in response to interventions such as high inspired oxygen and/or mechanical ventilation. If the preductal SaO_2 never reaches 100%, the likelihood of cyanotic heart disease is high.

ECHOCARDIOGRAPHY

Echocardiography has become a vital tool in the clinical management of newborns with hypoxemic respiratory failure (Box 47-5). The initial echocardiographic evaluation is important to rule out structural heart disease causing hypoxemia (e.g., coarctation of the aorta, total anomalous pulmonary venous return). Moreover, it is critically important to diagnose congenital heart lesions for which inhaled nitric oxide (iNO) treatment would be contraindicated. In addition to the lesions mentioned earlier,

congenital heart diseases that can present with hypoxemia unresponsive to high inspired oxygen concentrations (i.e., dependent on right-to-left shunting across the ductus arteriosus) include critical aortic stenosis, interrupted aortic arch, and hypoplastic left heart syndrome. Decreasing PVR with iNO in these conditions could lead to systemic hypoperfusion, worsening the clinical course and delaying definitive diagnosis.

Echocardiographic evaluation is an essential component in the initial evaluation and ongoing management of the hypoxemic newborn. Not all hypoxemic term newborns have echocardiographic signs of PPHN. As noted earlier, hypoxemia can be caused by intrapulmonary right-to-left shunting or V/Q disturbances associated with severe lung disease. In unusual circumstances, right-to-left shunting can occur across pulmonary-to-systemic collaterals. However, extrapulmonary right-to-left shunting at the foramen ovale and/or ductus arteriosus (PPHN) also complicates hypoxemic respiratory failure and must be assessed in order to determine initial treatments and evaluate the response to those therapies.

PPHN is defined by the echocardiographic determination of extrapulmonary venoarterial admixture (right-to-left shunting at the foramen ovale and/or ductus arteriosus), not simply evidence of increased PVR (i.e., elevated PVR without extrapulmonary shunting does not directly cause hypoxemia). Echocardiographic signs suggestive of pulmonary hypertension (e.g., increased right ventricular systolic time intervals, septal flattening) are less helpful.

Doppler measurements of atrial- and ductal-level shunts provide essential information when managing a newborn with hypoxemic respiratory failure. For example, left-to-right shunting at the foramen ovale and ductus arteriosus with marked hypoxemia suggests predominant intrapulmonary shunting, and interventions should be directed at optimizing lung inflation.

Finally, the measurements made with echocardiography can be used to predict or interpret the response or lack of response to various treatments. For example, in the presence of severe left ventricular dysfunction with pulmonary hypertension, pulmonary vasodilation alone may be ineffective in improving oxygenation. The echocardiographic findings in this setting include right-to-left ductal shunting (caused by suprasystemic PVR) and mitral insufficiency with left-to-right atrial shunting. In this setting, efforts to reduce PVR should be accompanied by targeted therapies to increase cardiac performance and decrease left ventricular afterload.

This constellation of findings suggests that left ventricular dysfunction may contribute to pulmonary venous hypertension, such as occurs in congestive heart failure. In this setting, pulmonary vasodilation alone (without improving cardiac performance) will not cause sustained improvement in oxygenation. Careful echocardiographic assessment will provide invaluable information about the underlying pathophysiology and help guide the course of treatment.

The initial echocardiographic evaluation determines both structural and functional (i.e., extrapulmonary right-to-left shunting in PPHN, left ventricular performance) causes of hypoxemia. Serial echocardiography is important to determine the response to interventions (e.g., pulmonary vasodilators) and to reevaluate cases where specific interventions have not resulted in improvement or with progressive clinical deterioration. For example, in a patient with extrapulmonary right-to-left shunting and severe lung disease, pulmonary vasodilation might reverse the right-to-left venous admixture with little improvement in systemic oxygenation. These observations unmask the critically important contribution of intrapulmonary shunting to hypoxemia.

PERSISTENT PULMONARY HYPERTENSION OF THE NEWBORN

As described previously, PPHN is a syndrome associated with diverse neonatal cardiac and pulmonary disorders that are characterized by high PVR causing extrapulmonary right-to-left shunting of blood across the ductus arteriosus and/or foramen ovale. The syndrome of PPHN and the role of iNO are discussed in more detail in other chapters. However, because its relationship to respiratory failure in term newborns is so vital to understanding the clinical pathophysiology and approaches to treatment, we address some historical perspectives in this section. Indeed, in order to understand the acronym PPHN, it is important to consider its historical evolution in term newborns with respiratory failure and critical hypoxemia, and the advances that led to current management strategies.

In the early 1960s, the association of respiratory distress syndrome with pulmonary hypertension and right-to-left ductal shunting was described in the landmark studies of Rudolph et al (1961) and the clinical observations of Stahlman (1964). Although it is now recognized that pulmonary hypertension with right-to-left venoarterial admixture often complicates the course of newborns with diverse diseases, its first recognition in term infants who were hypoxemic (but without significant lung disease) was likely by Roberton et al in 1967. These authors described 13 infants born at or near term who had marked hypoxemia but without other clinical signs of idiopathic respiratory distress syndrome (i.e., decreased lung compliance). They speculated that the cause of hypoxemia was right-to-left shunting,

but did not specifically implicate suprasystemic levels of pulmonary vascular resistance as the cause of the hypoxemia. The first clear description of the pathophysiology of PPHN (associated with right-to-left shunting across patent fetal channels) is attributed to Gersony et al, who, in 1969, coined the phrase "persistence of the fetal circulation" (PFC) in describing two newborns with clear lung fields who had critical hypoxemia associated with severe pulmonary hypertension and right-to-left shunting across the foramen ovale and ductus arteriosus. One infant was treated with tolazoline with only transient improvement in oxygenation. In 1970, Lees used the term *primary pulmonary hypertension* to describe this group of newborns. In 1971, Siassi et al described five infants with persistent pulmonary vascular obstruction associated with right-to-left shunting across the ductus arteriosus, and in one case marked medial hypertrophy of the muscular pulmonary arteries demonstrated on autopsy. This observation of a structural abnormality of the pulmonary circulation was further elucidated by Haworth and Reid (1976) in three infants who died with persistent fetal circulation and had extension of smooth muscle into the walls of smaller intra-acinar arteries. The phrase "persistent pulmonary hypertension of the newborn" was first used by Levin et al (1976) to describe a group of newborns with severe pulmonary hypertension, clear chest radiographs, and right-to-left shunting across the ductus arteriosus demonstrated both by simultaneous temporal arterial and umbilical arterial sampling (i.e., postductal desaturation) and by cardiac catheterization.

These initial descriptions of PFC focused on a discreet subset of newborns who had adequate cardiac performance without structural heart disease, absence of significant parenchymal lung disease, and suprasystemic pulmonary vascular resistance causing hypoxemia through right-to-left shunting of blood across the oval foramen and/or the arterial duct. However, it soon became clear that PFC could complicate the course of other diseases of the newborn, including meconium aspiration (initially described by Stahlman in 1964 and later by Fox et al, 1977), and pulmonary hypoplasia/congenital diaphragmatic hernia (Harrison and de Lorimier, 1981).

Nomenclature for this syndrome was clearly quite varied. Although there was initial appeal of the term persistent fetal circulation (PFC) (Behrman, 1976), this description is not quite accurate because of the absence of the placenta and onset of air breathing after delivery. Over time, most authors have embraced PPHN as the proper name for this syndrome, with the classic PFC subtype (idiopathic PPHN) representing a relatively small percentage of the cases now commonly encountered. Pathophysiologic mechanisms and etiologic classifications of PPHN described by Rudolph (1980) and further characterized by Geggel and Reid (1984) and Gersony (1984) provided an important framework for understanding the complex nature of this syndrome as management strategies evolved over the past two decades.

Because of the role of pulmonary hypertension in newborns with hypoxemic respiratory failure (initially severe hyaline membrane disease [HMD] and subsequently PFC, as described earlier), early approaches to management included a focus on pulmonary vasodilation using one of the few pharmacologic agents available at the time (tolazoline). Its use was first described by Cotton in 1965 in newborns with HMD, and later in infants with PPHN by Gersony et al (1969), Korones and Eyal (1975), and Levin et al (1976). However, its efficacy was limited by variable responsiveness and significant complications including systemic hypotension and gastrointestinal hemorrhage (Goetzman et al, 1976; Stevenson et al, 1979).

Multiple approaches to the treatment of PPHN evolved after its first recognition as a disease marked by severe pulmonary hypertension. However, discovery of the elusive selective pulmonary vasodilator would markedly change our understanding and clinical management of this syndrome. Indeed, the most striking change in the management of PPHN in the past decade has evolved from improved understanding of the role of endogenous NO production and exogenous NO delivery on pulmonary vasoregulation. Because the successful transition from fetal placental dependence to survival at birth requires that PVR rapidly decline and pulmonary blood flow increase, the role of NO in the transitional circulation has been intensively investigated to understand its relationship to the pathophysiology and treatment of PPHN.

NO was recognized as a potent vasodilator by Gruetter et al, as early as 1979, and in 1980, Furchgott and Zawadzki reported that acetylcholine-induced vasorelaxation was dependent on an intact endothelium through the elaboration of an endothelium-derived relaxing factor (EDRF) that diffused to the subjacent vascular smooth muscle. In 1987, investigators from two separate laboratories reported that the biologic activity of EDRF was identical to NO or an NO-containing substance. Palmer et al (1987) induced the release of EDRF from porcine aortic endothelial cells in culture and compared the effects on superfused aortic strips with that of NO in solution. They found that the effects of EDRF were indistinguishable from those of NO. Ignarro et al (1987) used a bioassay cascade superfusion technique with intrapulmonary arteries and veins, identified EDRF pharmacologically and chemically as NO, and found that EDRF and NO produced similar vasorelaxation and were inhibited by common antagonists. Ignarro et al also recognized that NO was inactivated by combining with hemoproteins and speculated that hemoglobin could trap endogenously produced NO that diffused into the vascular lumen, thus preventing any downstream vasorelaxation by this paracrine mediator.

The recognition that the endogenous production of this EDRF/NO mediator could be competitively blocked by modified L-arginine analogues prompted early experiments into the effects of NO in the fetal and transitional pulmonary circulation. Abman et al performed the first experiments on the role of EDRF in the ovine fetal circulation, demonstrating that endogenous EDRF/NO production modulates basal pulmonary vascular tone in the late-gestation fetus, and that pharmacologic NO blockade inhibits endothelium-dependent pulmonary vasodilation (Abman et al, 1990). These investigators also showed that pharmacologic NO blockade attenuates the rise in pulmonary blood flow at delivery, thus implicating endogenous NO formation in postnatal adaptation after birth and linking this laboratory observation to the life-threatening clinical condition of PPHN. In addition, experiments

using this ovine model showed that increased fetal oxygen tension augments endogenous NO release (McQueston et al, 1993; Tiktinsky and Morin, 1993), and the increase in pulmonary blood flow in response to rhythmic distention of the lung and high inspired oxygen concentrations are mediated in part by endogenous NO elaboration (Cornfield et al, 1992).

The observation that dilute NO gas could be therapeutically delivered by inhalation was first described by Higgenbottam et al (1988), who reported that brief (10-minute) inhalational NO treatment caused potent and selective pulmonary vasodilation in adults with severe pulmonary hypertension (Pepke-Zaba et al, 1991). Frostell et al (1991) demonstrated the selectivity of iNO in an adult animal model of hypoxic pulmonary vasoconstriction, and the first description of the potent, sustained, and selective vasodilator effect of iNO in newborn lambs was reported by Kinsella et al in 1992.

Clinical approaches to PPHN and the role of iNO are discussed in separate chapters, and in relationship to specific diseases of the term newborn in the following sections.

SPECIFIC PULMONARY CONDITIONS CAUSING RESPIRATORY DISTRESS IN THE TERM NEWBORN

TRANSIENT TACHYPNEA OF THE NEWBORN

Transient tachypnea of the newborn (TTNB) is among the most common causes of respiratory distress in the newborn period, affecting 0.5% to 4% of all late preterm and term neonates. Symptoms of respiratory distress typically start within the first several hours after birth and result from failure of adequate absorption of fetal lung fluid. Studies have consistently shown that risk factors for TTNB include prematurity, delivery by cesarean section (particularly without preceding labor), and male sex (Jain et al, 2009; Riskin et al, 2005).

Early theories of lung fluid clearance focused on the role of thoracic compression during vaginal delivery and were supported by the observation that TTNB is more common among babies born by cesarean section (Milner et al, 1978). However, more recent studies have demonstrated that the complex process of lung liquid clearance likely begins well before term birth (Brown et al, 1983). During fetal life, the lung epithelium is responsible for the production of a substantial volume of alveolar fluid, a process that is essential for normal fetal lung growth (Olver and Strang, 1974). With parturition, increased levels of epinephrine, glucocorticoids, and other hormones effectively cause the lung epithelia to transition from a secretory to a resorptive phenotype (Baines et al, 2000; Barker et al, 1990). Activated endothelial sodium channels (ENaC) at the apical surface of lung type II epithelial cells transport sodium and water from the alveolar space into the type II cells (Olver et al, 1986). Sodium is then actively moved from the type II cell into the interstitium by Na/K ATPase, causing passive movement of water, which is then resorbed into the pulmonary circulation and lymphatics. Supporting a possible role for abnormal activity of ENaC and Na/K ATPase in TTNB, a recent study found that genetic polymorphisms in β-adrenergic receptor encoding genes (which regulate expression of these channels) are more common in babies with TTNB (Aslan et al, 2008).

The diagnosis of TTNB remains problematic for clinicians. The most typical presenting symptoms, tachypnea/respiratory distress and the need for supplemental oxygen, are common among most neonatal respiratory disorders, and unfortunately, there exist no reliable diagnostic tests for TTNB (Guglani et al, 2008). For those reasons, the diagnosis remains one of exclusion, and vigilance for other, more severe disorders is imperative. Typically, symptoms of TTNB develop within the first several hours after birth. The degree of respiratory impairment, including the respiratory rate, use of accessory respiratory muscles, and impairment in gas exchange, varies widely. Chest radiographs should be considered in any baby presumed to have TTNB. Although radiographs commonly show prominent perihilar markings and fluid in the fissures, clinicians and radiologists often disagree in their interpretation of these findings in TTNB (Kurl et al, 1997).

Once a presumptive diagnosis of TTNB is made, treatment is largely supportive. Oxygen should be provided to maintain normal arterial oxygen saturations. The degree of tachypnea and respiratory distress should determine whether a baby is allowed to feed by mouth. If there is a suspicion of pneumonia or sepsis, empiric antibiotic therapy should be considered. A controlled trial of furosemide administration to accelerate clearance of lung fluid showed no benefit in attenuating the course of TTNB (Wiswell et al, 1985). Alternative or additional diagnoses should be considered in any infant who is deteriorating or requires mechanical ventilation. With supportive care, full recovery is to be expected after TTNB. However, compared with well infants of a similar gestational age, the diagnosis of TTNB is associated with a significantly prolonged hospital course (Riskin et al, 2005). Moreover, recent epidemiologic studies have suggested that newborns with TTNB are at a mildly increased risk for the later development of asthma (Birnkrant et al, 1996; Liem et al, 2007; Schaubel et al, 2006).

MECONIUM ASPIRATION SYNDROME

Meconium aspiration syndrome (MAS) is among the most common causes of hypoxemic respiratory failure in term newborns who require intensive care (Figure 47-1). Recent studies estimate that the incidence of MAS in babies greater than 37 weeks' gestation ranges from 0.4% to 1.8% (Dargaville and Copnell, 2006; Singh et al, 2009). Among babies born after 39 weeks' gestation with lung disease requiring mechanical ventilation, more than half suffer from MAS (Gouyon et al, 2008).

Moreover, MAS is the primary diagnosis for a significant proportion of those newborns who require extracorporeal membrane oxygenation (ECMO) in the United States (26%) and the United Kingdom (51%) (Brown et al, 2010).

Although a significant percentage of term births are complicated by the passage of meconium before or at delivery, fewer than 10% of those exposed to meconium develop MAS. Among those 10%, fetal acidemia is believed to result in increased intestinal peristaltic activity, passage of meconium, and fetal gasping, which draws particulate meconium deep into the lung. Supporting this theory, autopsy studies of babies who died of MAS demonstrate distal

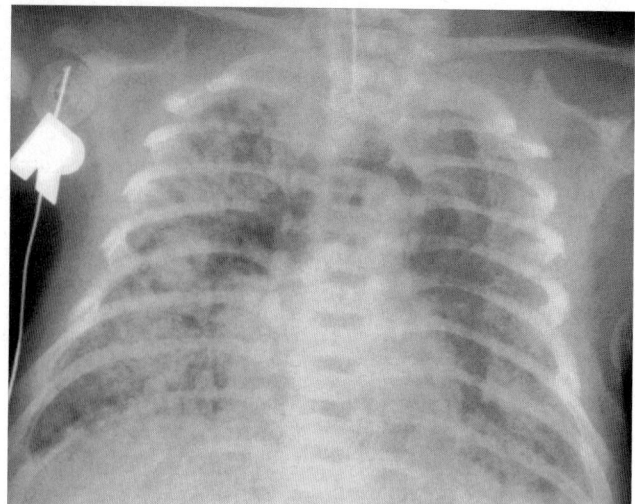

FIGURE 47-1 **Chest radiograph of MAS.** Term newborn with severe MAS. Note anterior pneumomediastinum and small left anteromedial pneumothorax.

muscularization of small pulmonary arterioles, suggesting long-standing hypoxemia (Murphy et al, 1984). Particulate meconium in the distal lung causes check-valve obstruction of air passages and leads to regional hyperinflation and atelectasis. In addition, meconium inactivates surfactant, leading to secondary surfactant deficiency (Moses et al, 1991). Moreover, babies with MAS are at high risk for persistent pulmonary hypertension, which significantly increases their morbidity and complicates their management.

Historically, prevention of MAS has focused on decreasing exposure of the fetal and newborn lung to the noxious effects of intrapulmonary meconium-contaminated amniotic fluid. Infusion of saline into the amniotic cavity (i.e., amnioinfusion) during labor has been studied as a means for diluting meconium and relieving pressure on the umbilical cord, a potential cause for fetal acidemia. In the largest trial investigating this practice, Fraser et al (2005) found no reduction in the risk of MAS. An alternative strategy to decreasing lung exposure to meconium is intrapartum oro- and nasopharyngeal suction of fetuses born through meconium-stained amniotic fluid. Although this practice was widely adopted in the 1970s, more recent studies have failed to demonstrated benefit (Vain et al, 2004), and the practice is no longer endorsed by the American College of Obstetricians and Gynecologists (ACOG) (Committee on Obstetric Practice, 2007). Whether the routine practice of tracheal suction of depressed, meconium-exposed infants immediately after birth is efficacious has not been adequately studied. In recent reports, surfactant lung lavage has demonstrated some promise in improving lung function in animal models of MAS (Dargaville et al, 2003), but a small clinical trial of this practice demonstrated no benefit (Gadzinowski et al, 2008). The lack of clear efficacy among any of these preventative strategies intended to remove meconium likely speaks to the complex and multifactorial nature of the pathophysiology of MAS.

The clinical signs of MAS vary widely among babies and may relate to the degree of antenatal compromise; the timing, volume, and consistency of aspirated meconium; and the presence of associated problems. Clinical signs of MAS typically present immediately after birth with tachypnea, increased work of breathing, and cyanosis. Other common associated findings are metabolic acidosis, cardiac dysfunction and hypotension, and postductal desaturation indicative of right-to-left shunting of blood at the ductus arteriosus caused by pulmonary hypertension. Because of the potential for ball-valve obstruction of small airways and failure to empty distal lung segments, pneumothorax can complicate the clinical picture. In recent series, the risk of pneumothorax among ventilated babies with MAS ranged between 10% and 24% (Dargaville and Copnell, 2006; Velaphi and Van Kwawegen, 2008). Like the degree of clinical signs, findings on chest radiograph vary widely. The classic chest x-ray shows diffuse, fluffy infiltrates. However, some babies have milder initial radiographic findings, and there is often progression of visible parenchymal disease over time, likely related to secondary surfactant dysfunction.

Approximately half the babies with MAS require mechanical ventilation. Ventilator strategy should be individualized to each baby and to the pathology evident on the chest radiograph. In general, because of the likelihood of increased airway resistance, a conventional strategy utilizing slower rates with long inspiratory and expiratory times allows for better gas dispersion and more adequate emptying during expiration. Gas trapping and regional or generalized hyperinflation can occur, particularly when rapid rates are used with a conventional mode of ventilation. Some babies respond better to ventilation with a high-frequency device, though there is also a high risk of hyperinflation. When severe, hyperinflation causes impaired gas exchange and hypercarbia, limits systemic venous return (adversely affecting cardiac performance), increases the risk of pneumothorax, and may exacerbate pulmonary hypertension.

In addition to management of parenchymal lung disease in MAS, special consideration must be paid to other problems, particularly pulmonary hypertension. The risk for PPHN is quite high, exceeding 50% in some series. Studies demonstrate that iNO improves oxygenation in MAS and is particularly efficacious when combined with a ventilator strategy that focuses on improving lung recruitment such as high-frequency oscillatory ventilation (HFOV) (Kinsella et al, 1997). Treatment with systemic antibiotics should be strongly considered in babies with PPHN for a number of reasons. These include the fact that intrauterine infection might be a precipitating factor in the initial passage of meconium and that in vitro studies suggest that presence of meconium might facilitate the growth of bacteria in the lung.

In spite of the availability of iNO and high-frequency modes of ventilation, some babies do not respond to medical therapy and require treatment with ECMO. Among babies with MAS treated with ECMO, reported survival ranges between 94% and 97%, markedly higher than for newborns treated for other respiratory conditions (Brown et al, 2010; Gill et al, 2002).

SURFACTANT PROTEIN DEFICIENCY

The details of surfactant biology and of respiratory distress syndrome in premature newborns are presented elsewhere in this textbook. However, term newborns may rarely present with a clinical syndrome dominated by respiratory failure that may be indistinguishable from surfactant deficiency in preterm infants. In the setting of unexplained and protracted respiratory failure in term infants, genetic alterations of surfactant-associated proteins, particularly the surfactant proteins B and C (SP-B and SP-C) and the ABC Binding Cassette A3 protein (ABCA3), must be considered and ruled out. As described later, there is considerable overlap in the clinical presentation of babies with mutations of SP-B, SP-C, and ABCA3. Though onset, severity of clinical signs, and a family history of lung disease may offer clues to the underlying disorder, a full histologic and genetic evaluation should be considered. Genetic analysis of blood or buccal swab for mutations of the genes responsible for SP-B, SP-C, and ABCA3 are the definitive tests for each disease, but analysis is both costly and time-consuming. Moreover, analysis is not routinely available, necessitating transport of specimens to a small number of labs specializing in these analyses. In addition, bronchoalveolar lavage (BAL) aspirate should be analyzed by ELISA for the presence of SP-B and pro-SP-C. Lung biopsy, evaluated by both standard and electron microscopy, can also provide important clues to the underlying diagnosis.

Surfactant Protein B (SP-B) Deficiency

Mature SP-B is a small 79-amino-acid hydrophobic protein that plays several key roles in the processing and function of normal pulmonary surfactant (Nogee et al, 2000). Transgenic mouse models suggest that SP-B is critical for phospholipid packaging into lamellar bodies, the formation of tubular myelin, and spreading/function of the surfactant monolayer. In addition, normal SP-B appears to be essential for normal processing of surfactant protein C (Vorbroker et al, 1995). In all babies described to date with SP-B deficiency, the genetic mutation has been inherited from the parents (autosomal recessive) rather than occurring as a spontaneous mutation (Hamvas et al, 1994). Although multiple genetic mutations have been described, approximately 70% of affected babies carry the 121ins2 mutation (Dargaville and Copnell, 2006). In a recent series of term babies referred for genetic evaluation of unexplained respiratory failure, 2 of 17 had detectable mutations of the surfactant protein B sequence (Somaschini et al, 2007).

Almost all babies with recognized deficiency of SP-B develop clinical signs of severe respiratory distress, including tachypnea, grunting, and retractions, within the first several hours of life. Similar to preterm newborns with HMD, chest radiographs classically reveal diffuse, hazy airspace disease with visible air bronchograms. Severe pulmonary hypertension may be a prominent feature of the disease. Treatment with surfactant is either ineffective or unsustained, and progressive respiratory failure is the rule (Hamvas, 2006). Lung transplantation is currently the only effective long-term treatment, with both short- and long-term outcomes similar to those for other infants undergoing lung transplantation (Palomar et al, 2006).

Analysis of fluid obtained by BAL/tracheal aspirate from babies with SP-B deficiency should fail to detect any immunoreactive SP-B. The presence of proSP-C increases suspicion of SP-B deficiency because intact SP-B is necessary for normal posttranslational processing of the protein to mature SP-C. Histologic findings include alveolar cell hyperplasia, interstitial thickening, and variable degrees of fibrosis and alveolar proteinosis. Staining of lung tissue for pro-SP-B is variable, but staining for mature SP-B should be minimal (because of cross-reactivity with epitopes on pro-SP-B) or absent. Initial DNA analysis focuses on the 121ins2 mutation. More exhaustive testing for other known mutations is warranted if initial testing is negative.

Surfactant Protein C (SP-C) Deficiency

Mature SP-C is a 35-amino-acid hydrophobic protein. SP-C is believed to enhance spreading of surfactant and to participate in normal surfactant catabolism (Whitsett et al, 2005). As with SP-B, multiple mutations of SP-C have been described; however, the majority of these mutations arise spontaneously and result in sporadic disease. Whether the abnormal phenotype associated with SP-C deficiency arises from dysfunction of the alveolar surfactant or from accumulation of abnormal cellular SP-C and consequent type II cell injury is not known.

In contrast to SP-B deficiency, babies with SP-C deficiency have a wide range of clinical presentations. Some may develop symptoms within the first several hours of life, similar to SP-B deficiency, whereas others present later in child- or adulthood with interstitial lung disease. The reasons that underlie the variable onset, presentation, and severity of individuals with SP-C deficiency are not currently understood.

In common with SP-B deficiency, the lung histopathology of patients with SP-C deficiency is nonspecific and widely variable. Common findings include accumulation of alveolar protein and macrophages and epithelial cell hyperplasia. Ultrastructural examination may reveal disorganized lamellar bodies with aggregates of small vesicles with electron-dense cores in the type II cells (Nogee et al, 2001). Allele-specific testing using PCR for the most common 173T mutation provides an initial screen for SP-C deficiency. If negative, direct sequencing of the entire SP-C gene should be undertaken.

ATP-Binding Cassette A3 Gene (ABCA3) Deficiency

The ATP-binding cassette (ABC) transporter proteins are essential for normal transport of compounds in numerous biologic systems (Mulugeta et al, 2002). Deficiencies of individual ATP-binding cassettes have been associated with clinical diseases in a number of different organ systems. The ABCA3 protein is highly expressed in the lung and is involved in the transport of lipids. Individuals lacking the gene for ABCA3 have abnormal accumulation of surfactant-rich lamellar bodies within their type II alveolar cells, with apparent inability to transport surfactant into the alveolar space. A study by Shulenin et al (2004) details a variety of mutations within the ABCA3 gene in a substantial portion of term infants with unexplained respiratory failure and suspected surfactant protein deficiency.

Age at presentation for individuals with ABCA3 deficiency is highly variable, ranging from the immediate newborn period to later in childhood. There may be a family history of consanguinity. Clinical manifestations of disease in the neonate may be indistinguishable from those with SP-B deficiency, with onset of respiratory failure within hours of birth. The disease may be progressive and fatal. In addition, ABCA3 deficiency may also manifest as severe persistent pulmonary hypertension of the newborn (Kunig et al, 2007). A recent report suggests that more mild, transient neonatal symptoms may not prompt a diagnostic evaluation in the newborn period, though recurrent pulmonary symptoms may lead to later investigation (Doan et al, 2007). These reports raise the possibility that deficiency of ABCA3 may be underrecognized in infants or children with a mild or normal phenotype.

The predominant pathologic findings of neonates with ABCA3 deficiency presenting with neonatal respiratory failure include alveolar proteinosis (Bullard et al, 2006), type II cell hyperplasia with dense lamellar bodies, and accumulation of alveolar macrophages in the distal airspace. Inheritance is believed to be autosomal recessive. Unlike SP-B deficiency, a single predominant mutation has not been described; rather, multiple distinct mutations affecting different protein domains have been identified (Brash et al, 2006).

Surfactant Proteins A and D

Although lung structural abnormalities have been described in mice lacking SP-A and SP-D, no phenotype attributable to abnormalities of either of these surfactant-associated proteins has been described in human infants.

CONGENITAL DIAPHRAGMATIC HERNIA

CDH is a complex clinical syndrome caused by a developmental defect in the diaphragm, resulting in a spectrum of potentially severe cardiopulmonary abnormalities (Figure 47-2). The estimated incidence of CDH ranges from approximately 1:2500 to 1:7000 live-born babies

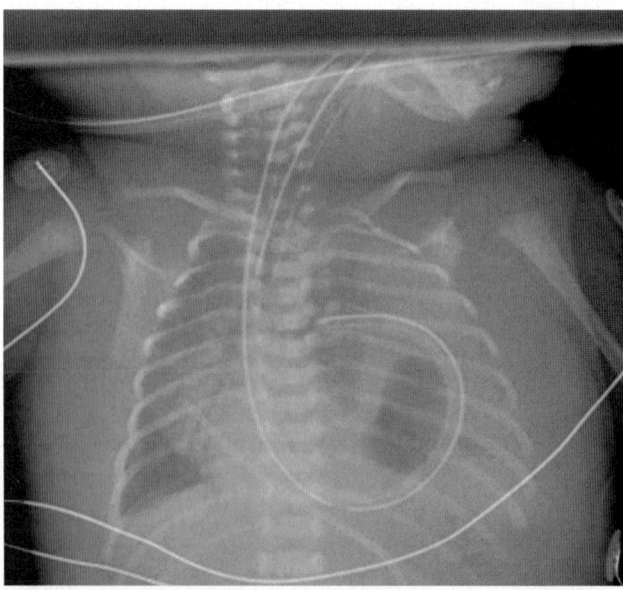

FIGURE 47-2 Chest radiograph of CDH. Note proper position of orogastric tube and UVC (*arrow*) in an infant with left-sided congenital diaphragmatic hernia.

(Prober, 2007). Approximately 80% to 85% of diaphragmatic hernias occur on the left side. In rare circumstances, they may be bilateral. Anatomically, CDH is classically divided by location into posterolateral (Bochdalek) defects, retrosternal anterior (Morgagni) defects, and other anterior or central defects. The vast majority, 90% to 95%, are of the Bochdalek type. However, recent work has suggested that the classical anatomic distinctions cannot always be clearly differentiated (Prober, 2008). Moreover, the implications of hernia location on severity of illness or mortality are not clearly defined.

As many as 30% to 40% of babies with CDH have additional congenital anomalies, most commonly of the heart, central nervous system, and genitourinary system. The remaining 60% to 70% of babies have isolated CDH without other identifiable major anatomic malformations. CDH may occur as an element of several well-recognized syndromes or of a chromosomal abnormality (particularly trisomy 18). A recent study suggests that, in babies with CDH but without a recognized genetic syndrome, 10% to 15% have heart defects, most commonly septal defects, conotruncal malformations, and obstruction of the left ventricular outflow tract (Lin et al, 2007). Coexisting cardiac disease complicates the management of babies with CDH and likely increases mortality.

Medical management of the newborn with a CDH remains one of the most complex and challenging situations for a neonatologist. A host of interrelated issues must be considered, including optimal mechanical ventilation strategies, presence and treatment of pulmonary hypertension, evaluation of cardiac performance, and consideration of support with ECMO. Unfortunately, owing to the relative infrequency of CDH, definitive studies guiding clinical decisions in the management these babies are lacking.

The optimal mode and strategy of mechanical ventilation in CDH has not been definitively established. Previously, aggressive hyperventilation and alkalinization as a means to lower pulmonary vascular resistance was advocated (Bohn et al, 1987). More recently, with the recognition that aggressive mechanical ventilation to the point of hyperventilation may cause significant iatrogenic lung injury and worsen outcome, this approach has generally been abandoned (Sakurai et al, 1999). However, prospective trials to clearly guide ventilator strategy are lacking. Many experts now advocate a gentle ventilation strategy that minimizes peak inspiratory pressure, targets $PaCO_2$ levels between 40 and 60 torr, and tolerates postductal desaturation if preductal saturations are adequate. If a conventional ventilator strategy is used and peak inspiratory pressures needed to achieve these goals are unacceptably high (generally 25 to 30 cm H_2O), transition to HFOV is undertaken (Bohn 2002; Boloker et al, 2002; Finer et al, 1998). As an alternative, some advocate earlier or initial use of HFOV (Bagolan et al, 2004; Frenckner et al, 1997; Reyes et al, 1998). Though definitive evidence in support of this gentle ventilation strategy is lacking owing to the retrospective nature of the cited reports, mortality in several centers has fallen coincident with adoption of this approach.

Pulmonary hypertension (PH) is a well-recognized complication of CDH. Decreased cross-sectional area of the pulmonary circulation, structural remodeling of the pulmonary vessels, and diminished size and function of the left ventricle have all been implicated in the PH associated with CDH. Newborns with CDH should all undergo early echocardiography to ascertain the presence of associated heart defects, to assess the degree of pulmonary hypertension, and to evaluate the function of the left and right ventricles. Treatment of early PH in babies with CDH is controversial. Inhaled nitric oxide did not reduce mortality among a group of infants with CDH failing aggressive medical therapy (Neonatal Inhaled Nitric Oxide Study Group, 1997). Moreover, newborns treated with iNO in that study more frequently required ECMO than the control group, likely related to the adverse effects of pulmonary vasodilation in the presence of severe left ventricular dysfunction, potentially worsening systemic hemodynamics. Current evidence does not support the routine use of iNO in the first 24 hours after birth in infants with CDH. Consideration of its use should be limited to those babies with optimized lung inflation and well-defined PH who do not have evidence of impaired left ventricular performance and right ventricle–dependent systemic blood flow (Kinsella et al, 2005). Other pharmacologic pulmonary vasodilators to treat acute PH in babies with CDH have not been carefully evaluated. In babies with severe PH and a closed ductus arteriosus, consideration should be given to restoration of ductal patency with prostaglandin infusion, to allow the right ventricle to serve as a source of systemic blood flow (Kinsella et al, 2005).

Animal models of CDH demonstrate biochemical and physiologic evidence of surfactant deficiency (Glick et al, 1992). In these models, surfactant replacement lowers PVR and improves gas exchange and lung mechanics (O'Toole et al, 1996; Wilcox et al, 1994). Studies of human babies with CDH also suggest a delay in surfactant maturation, and postmortem studies of babies with CDH commonly demonstrate the presence of hyaline membranes (Hisanaga et al, 1984; Moya et al, 1995). Taken together, these studies raise the possibility that surfactant replacement therapy might have a role in the management of babies with CDH. Although initial anecdotal evidence supported this possibility, a more recent retrospective study of more than 500 term babies with CDH suggested that surfactant treatment was associated with greater ECMO use, increased chronic lung disease, and reduced overall survival (Van Meurs et al, 2004). These findings strongly argue against the routine use of surfactant replacement in babies with CDH.

Owing to the infrequency of CDH and the wide variability in therapeutic approaches (both among centers and over time at individual centers), few studies of long-term outcome have been published. Moreover, almost all represent the experience of single centers. That said, several small recent studies suggest that babies born with CDH are at risk for a number of serious long-term morbidities, including impaired neurodevelopmental outcome, wheezing/asthma, protracted pulmonary hypertension, sensorineural hearing loss, gastroesophageal reflux (GER), scoliosis, and pectus excavatum (Peetsold et al, 2009). One recent study reports lower than anticipated scores on tests of intelligence and adaptive behavior among 11 CDH survivors who were not treated with ECMO (Bouman et al, 2000).

Stolar et al (1995) report that among 51 babies treated with ECMO, the subset of those with CDH had worse cognitive outcome than those with alternative underlying diagnoses. Neurologic (physical) testing was similar between the two groups. Though concerning, these findings must be interpreted with caution, because mean age at evaluation was only 31 months. CDH is also associated with a high rate of sensorineural hearing loss (SNHL), nearly 50% in a recent study (Morini et al, 2008). The causes that underlie the high incidence of SNHL in this population, and whether it represents a genetic/anatomic predisposition or is a result of treatment-related risk factors, have yet to be clarified.

As might be expected, several cardiopulmonary sequelae of CDH have been reported. In a follow-up study of adolescents born with CDH, Trachsel et al (2005) report several abnormalities elicited by pulmonary function testing. Compared with normal controls, CDH survivors demonstrated mild to moderate airway obstruction, and nearly half were responsive to bronchodilators. CDH patients also had decreased inspiratory muscle strength and maximum minute ventilation. In spite of these findings, these adolescents generally had minimal compromise of daily activities. The persistence of pulmonary hypertension in some patients with CDH remains a major concern. After CDH repair and with readiness for extubation from mechanical ventilation, some infants with underlying pulmonary hypertension develop suprasystemic pulmonary artery pressures with discontinuation of iNO. Kinsella et al (2003) has reported successful ongoing treatment of these babies with delivery of noninvasive iNO via nasal cannula. Schwartz et al (1999) report that 38% of their CDH patients who required ECMO had echocardiographic evidence of PH well beyond the newborn period, with a mean follow-up age of over 3 years. Importantly, most of those children had no apparent physical signs or symptoms of PH, supporting the need for proactive, ongoing surveillance. Although recent studies focused on the long-term follow-up of pulmonary vascular disease in these patients are lacking, the American Academy of Pediatrics recommends serial echocardiographic evaluation of children with CDH who have persistent pulmonary hypertension after repair (Lally and Engle, 2008). Newer pharmacologic agents for PH, such as phosphodiesterase inhibitors (sildenafil) or endothelin antagonists such as bosentan may offer effective longer-term therapy for PH, but have not been investigated in this population.

Postnatal nutrition presents a major challenge for many survivors of CDH. Among 121 CDH survivors, Muratore et al (2001) reported that one third had failure to thrive requiring the placement of a gastrotomy tube for the provision of adequate calories, and 25% demonstrated evidence of oral aversion. Many reports have documented the high incidence of GER after repair of CDH, and recent studies report that 12% to 28% require fundoplication for severe GER (Diamond et al, 2007; Fasching et al, 2000; Su et al, 2007).

PULMONARY HYPOPLASIA

In the absence of a diaphragmatic hernia, pulmonary hypoplasia and respiratory failure can develop in association with a number of other conditions. An extensive list of conditions associated with pulmonary hypoplasia has been generated, but most cause either restriction of normal fetal breathing motion or compression of the developing lung. Thus, among the most common causes of pulmonary hypoplasia are low amniotic fluid volumes, neuromuscular disorders, pleural effusions/chylothoraces, and space-occupying lung lesions.

Inadequate amniotic fluid volume to allow for normal fetal breathing can result from a number of circumstances. Because fetal urine is a primary contributor to amniotic fluid volume, any abnormality of renal development that limits fetal urine production or urine flow can result in pulmonary hypoplasia. In addition, preterm premature rupture of membranes (PPROM), particularly with persistent leak of amniotic fluid, can result in pulmonary hypoplasia. Estimates of the risk of pulmonary hypoplasia with PPROM vary widely, and multiple studies have attempted to define the variables related to oligohydramnios sufficient to result in pulmonary hypoplasia (Hadi et al, 1994; Kurkinen-Raty et al, 1998; Vergani et al, 1994). Though absolute criteria are not adequately defined, most authors agree that gestational age at onset of oligohydramnios is a critical determinant of risk (Kurkinen-Raty et al, 1998; Nimrod et al, 1984). In some studies, longer latency from rupture of membranes to delivery (particularly in excess of 4 weeks) and the severity of resulting oligohydramnios (median amniotic fluid pocket ≤2 cm) also increase the risk of pulmonary hypoplasia (Kurkinen-Raty et al, 1998; McIntosh and Harrison, 1994). Vergani et al (2004) found that, among babies born to mothers with prolonged premature rupture of membranes before 28 weeks' gestation, mortality was approximately 50%, and nearly half of those who died had pulmonary hypoplasia. Amnioinfusion to reestablish amniotic fluid volume may decrease the incidence of pulmonary hypoplasia (Vergani et al, 2004).

Definitive diagnosis of pulmonary hypoplasia can only be made at autopsy. Norms have been established for both the gestational age–corrected ratio of lung weight to body weight and for histologic evaluation of radial alveolar counts (Askenazi and Perlman, 1979; Lauria et al, 1995). Clinical criteria for pulmonary hypoplasia are less well defined. Neonates may present with a bell-shaped chest and elevated diaphragms on chest radiograph. Management of pulmonary hypoplasia should focus on maximizing lung inflation while avoiding pneumothorax, the incidence of which ranges widely, depending on the study (Klaassen et al, 2007; Leonidas et al, 1982). Ventilator strategies include permissive hypercapnia to minimize lung injury and use of HFOV. If pulmonary hypertension is defined echocardiographically, use of iNO should be considered. With sustained postnatal ventilatory support, the pulmonary hypertension associated with pulmonary hypoplasia may resolve over time. For additional discussion of pulmonary hypoplasia in preterm infants, see Chapter 46.

SUMMARY

The initial evaluation of respiratory distress/hypoxemia in the term newborn presents one of the most difficult challenges faced by pediatricians and neonatologists. An ordered approach using information derived from the history, physical examination, pulse oximetry measurements, radiographic and laboratory measurements, and echocardiography can help elucidate the cause of hypoxemia and respiratory failure and direct each step of clinical management. Recognizing the important contributions of parenchymal lung disease, pulmonary vasoconstriction, and cardiac performance is critical to successful clinical management of the term newborn with respiratory failure.

SUGGESTED READINGS

Bohn D: Congenital diaphragmatic hernia, *Am J Respir Crit Care Med* 166:911-915, 2002.

Bullard JE, Wert SE, Nogee LM: ABCA3 deficiency: neonatal respiratory failure and interstitial lung disease, *Semin Perinatol* 30:327-334, 2006.

Committee on Obstetric Practice, American College of Obstetricians and Gynecologists: ACOG Committee Opinion No. 379: Management of delivery of a newborn with meconium-stained amniotic fluid, *Obstet Gynecol* 110:739, 2007.

Dargaville PA, Copnell B: The epidemiology of meconium aspiration syndrome: incidence, risk factors, therapies, and outcome, *Pediatrics* 117:1712-1721, 2006.

Hamvas A: Inherited surfactant protein-B deficiency and surfactant protein-C associated disease: clinical features and evaluation, *Semin Perinatol* 30:316-326, 2006.

Kinsella JP, Ivy DD, Abman SH: Pulmonary vasodilator therapy in congenital diaphragmatic hernia: acute, late, and chronic pulmonary hypertension, *Semin Perinatol* 29:123-128, 2005.

Lally KP, Engle W: for the AAP Section on Surgery and the Committee on Fetus and Newborn: Postdischarge follow-up of infants with congenital diaphragmatic hernia, *Pediatrics* 121:627-632, 2008.

Prober BR: Overview of epidemiology, genetics, birth defects, and chromosome abnormalities associated with CDH, *Am J Med Genet Part C Semin Med Genet* 145C:158-171, 2007.

Vain NE, Szyld EG, Prudent LM, et al: Oropharyngeal and nasopharyngeal suctioning of meconium-stained neonates before delivery of their shoulders: multicentre, randomised controlled trial, *Lancet* 364:597-602, 2004.

Whitsett JA, Wert SE, Xu Y: Genetic disorders of surfactant homeostasis, *Biol Neonate* 87:283-287, 2005.

Complete references used in this text can be found online at www.expertconsult.com

BRONCHOPULMONARY DYSPLASIA

Roberta L. Keller and Roberta A. Ballard

HISTORICAL OVERVIEW

Bronchopulmonary dysplasia (BPD), also referred to as *chronic lung disease of prematurity*, is the most common chronic lung disease of childhood. BPD was first described by Northway et al in 1967 as a severe chronic lung injury in premature infants who survived hyaline membrane disease after treatment with mechanical ventilation and oxygen. Four distinct clinical stages were described radiographically and pathologically, progressing from typical respiratory distress syndrome (RDS), with alveolar interstitial edema as well as atelectasis, to massive fibrosis and consolidation of the lung with areas of cystic emphysema and overinflation.

BPD as originally described occurred predominantly in larger preterm infants born at 30 to 34 weeks' gestation with a history of severe respiratory distress necessitating high levels of ventilatory support and oxygen exposure for a prolonged period of time. These infants were born before the introduction of antenatal corticosteroids or postnatal surfactant replacement therapy and at a time when ventilators were first being adapted for use in the newborn.

Since that time, much has been learned about BPD, and the disorder as originally described has become rare. The infants who are more commonly affected with BPD today are those of extremely low birthweight and born at less than 26 weeks' gestation. After exposure to antenatal corticosteroids, combined with postnatal exogenous surfactant for treatment of RDS, these infants frequently do remarkably well initially, requiring low levels of supplemental oxygen and ventilatory support. They often have a subsequent period of several days during which there is minimal or no requirement for ventilatory support, before entering into a more chronic phase of variable requirements for assisted ventilation and supplemental oxygen. The form of BPD seen in the contemporary tiny preterm infant who has had minimal initial respiratory distress has been termed the *new* BPD, with arrested lung development affecting both alveologenesis and the pulmonary vascular bed (Abman, 2001, 2008; Bancalari, 2001; Jobe, 1999). Although the initial definition of BPD was a persistent requirement for supplemental oxygen 28 days after birth, in a subsequent attempt to define the functional implications of abnormal postnatal lung development, the need for oxygen at 36 weeks postmenstrual age (PMA) was found to be a better predictor of later pulmonary illness in extremely premature infants (Shennan et al, 1988). The definition of BPD was reviewed most recently at a National Institutes of Health–sponsored workshop (Jobe and Bancalari, 2001). This group specified diagnostic criteria including the need for oxygen, positive pressure ventilation, and/or continuous positive airway pressure (CPAP) at 36 weeks' PMA to better characterize the severity of BPD, with an oxygen reduction challenge test (to room air) performed in infants who are receiving supplemental oxygen only (Table 48-1). Using similar criteria, data from the NICHD Neonatal Network demonstrated increasing frequency of respiratory morbidity and neurodevelopmental impairment at follow-up with increasing severity of BPD (Ehrenkranz et al, 2005). Further, the definition of BPD using the need for supplemental oxygen alone was equally predictive of later pulmonary morbidity as was the need for oxygen plus an abnormal chest radiograph.

In the presurfactant era, there was remarkable consistency in the postmenstrual age at which infants surviving without later pulmonary morbidity were weaned off supplemental oxygen (Shennan et al, 1988). Subsequent studies have shown substantial proportions of infants with no BPD who do have later respiratory morbidity and even higher proportions of infants with BPD who have no respiratory morbidity (Ehrenkranz et al, 2005). Because survival for the most immature newborns has improved since the introduction of surfactant replacement therapy and the broadening use of antenatal corticosteroids, it may be that later assessments of pulmonary status, at 40 weeks PMA, for example, will prove better measures of later lung function and respiratory morbidity (Keller et al, 2009).

BRONCHOPULMONARY DYSPLASIA

EPIDEMIOLOGY

BPD is now relatively rare in infants born beyond 32 to 34 weeks' gestation, but it may be increasing in the smallest, most immature infants born at less than 26 weeks' gestation or less than 1000 g as survival has improved. In the NICHD Neonatal Network, the incidence of BPD at 36 weeks postmenstrual age in all infants weighing 501 to 1500 g at birth increased from 19% in 1990 to 22% in 2000, with another increase to 27% in 2003. Increased survival has been associated with these trends. As a result, survival without morbidity was unchanged from 1990 to 2002, with BPD now a greater chronic health burden in former premature infants than it was previously (Fanaroff et al, 2007). Comparable infants from the larger Vermont Oxford Network had an incidence of BPD of 29% in 2003 and 26% in 2007. The highest rates of BPD are in the smallest infants, 66% for those 501 to 750 g and 40% for those 751 to 1000 g birthweight (from 2007), but both networks report wide variability in the incidence of BPD at different centers. For infants less than or equal to 1000 g at birth, the incidence of BPD was 44% in infants in the NICHD Neonatal Network (from 1995 to 1999) (Ehrenkranz et al, 2005). Increasing severity of BPD was associated with decreasing gestational age, male sex, and race (relatively higher incidence for white infants and lower incidence for black infants).

TABLE 48-1   Diagnostic Criteria for Bronchopulmonary Dysplasia

Treatment with F_{IO_2} greater than 0.21 for at least 28 days	
PLUS	
Failure of room air challenge test at 36 weeks' postmenstrual age	
CLASSIFICATION OF SEVERITY	
Mild	Requires up to 0.30 effective F_{IO_2}*
Moderate	Requires greater than 0.30 effective F_{IO_2}*
Severe	Requires ventilatory support, usually with oxygen

Data from Jobe AH, Bancalari E: Bronchopulmonary dysplasia, *Am J Respir Crit Care Med* 163:1723-1729, 2001.
F_{IO_2}, Fraction of inspired oxygen.
*Effective F_{IO_2} is based on infant's weight and the concentration and flow of oxygen through a nasal cannula or in a hood.

The level of respiratory support after the initial recovery from RDS may be the best indicator of the risk of subsequent BPD in very immature infants. In the Extremely Low Gestational Age Newborn (ELGAN) study, three patterns of respiratory support in infants <28 weeks' gestation 3 to 14 days of age were described (Laughon et al, 2009b). The overall incidence of BPD was 51%. Infants with a persistently low level of oxygen supplementation had the lowest rate of BPD (17%), infants with a deterioration in their pulmonary status (initially low level of oxygen supplementation increasing in the 2nd week) had an intermediate incidence of BPD (51%), and infants with persistently higher oxygen requirements had the highest rate of BPD (67%). Mechanical ventilation was also closely associated with these patterns of oxygen supplementation. At postnatal day 7, fewer than 5% of infants in the low-oxygen group were receiving mechanical ventilation, almost 40% of the pulmonary deterioration group were intubated, and 50% of the higher oxygen group were intubated. Consistent with these data, infants enrolled in the placebo arm of the Nitric Oxide Chronic Lung Disease (NO CLD) Trial had an incidence of BPD or death of 75% if they were requiring mechanical ventilation at 7 days (Ballard, 2007; Ballard et al, 2006).

PATHOBIOLOGY

The etiology of BPD is clearly multifactorial and involves derangements in multiple aspects of lung function (e.g., surfactant production), repair from injury (e.g., elastin deposition) and growth and development (e.g., alveologenesis). Various factors contribute to this process, including a susceptible host with immature lung structure, and developmental deficiencies of factors crucial to lung development and function such as surfactant, nitric oxide, innate immune defense, and antioxidant capability (Figure 48-1). Inadequate nutrition, resulting in postnatal growth failure, may further exacerbate structural lung abnormalities and impair the ability of these infants to recover.

Pathologic Findings in the "New" Form of the Disease

In the chronic stage of BPD as originally described, the lung had extensive alveolar fibrosis, airway abnormalities and pulmonary vascular remodeling (Bonikos et al, 1976,

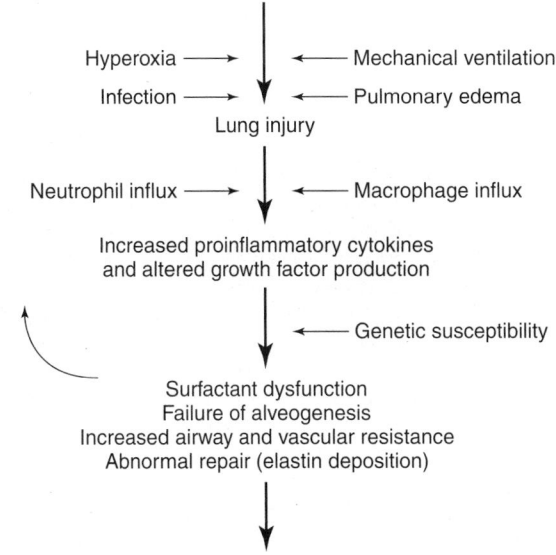

FIGURE 48-1   The pathogenesis of BPD. Lung injury in the immature lung secondary to hyperoxia, mechanical ventilation, and infection initiates an inflammatory response with an altered milieu of growth and inflammatory factors. Continuing insults contribute to the long-term changes in lung structure that characterize BPD. *BPD,* Bronchopulmonary dysplasia.

Northway et al, 1967). In contrast in the "new" BPD, the lungs are more uniformly inflated with minimal airway injury and less prominent fibrosis. The major abnormalities are a decrease in alveolar number (referred to as *alveolar hypoplasia*) and dysregulated microvascular growth (Bhatt et al, 2001; Burri, 1997; Coalson et al, 1999; De Paepe et al, 2006, 2008; Husain et al, 1998; Maniscalco et al, 2002). In the very preterm infants in whom this new BPD is seen (Figure 48-2), the lung is completing the canalicular stage of development at the time of birth; some investigators have noted an arrest of the lung at the saccular stage of development (De Paepe et al, 2006). There are a number of factors that interfere with the progress of postnatal alveologenesis which may contribute to the disordered lung development seen in contemporary premature newborns.

ETIOLOGIC FACTORS

We currently understand BPD to have a multifactorial etiology with many contributing factors.

Host Susceptibility and Genetic Predisposition

By far the most important factor in the pathogenesis of BPD is prematurity, although infants with intrauterine growth restriction are at increased risk (Bose et al, 2009; Lal et al, 2003). In addition, it has been known for some time that infants born to certain families are more likely to have RDS at any given gestational age than those in other families. Twin studies have supported this clinical impression, revealing that 50% to 80% of the variance in the

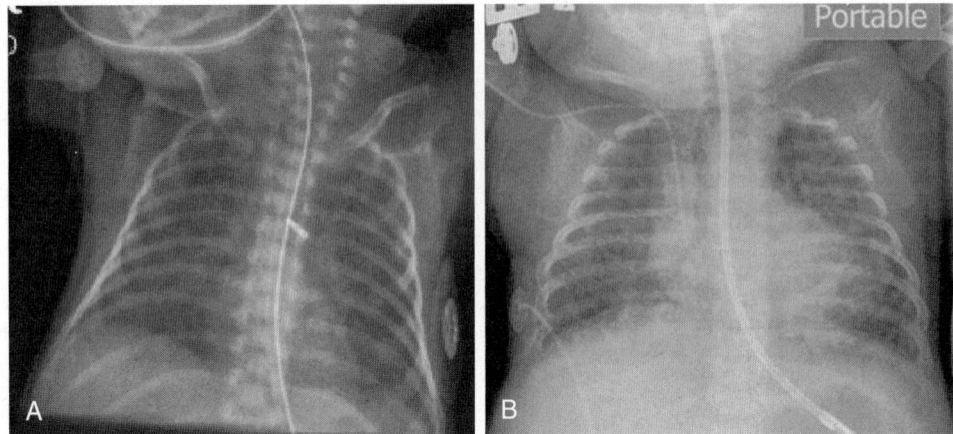

FIGURE 48-2 Radiographs of bronchopulmonary dysplasia characteristic of the new and old forms of the disease. **A,** Bilateral fine granular opacification consistent with atelectasis or edema in an infant with moderate disease. **B,** Bilateral coarse interstitial opacification consistent with fibrosis or edema and areas of hyperinflation in an infant with severe disease.

occurrence of BPD is due to genetic factors (Bhandari et al, 2006; Lavoie et al, 2008). In addition, a family history of asthma and reactive airway disease may increase the risk of BPD (Hagan et al, 1995; Nickerson and Taussig, 1980). Several studies have described the association of BPD with single nucleotide polymorphisms (SNPs) for genes involved in the inflammatory response, innate immunity, surfactant function and the extracellular matrix such as interleukins, collectins, surfactant-associated proteins, and proteases. Other pathways that are candidates for altering an infant's risk of BPD include (1) factors affecting alveologenesis and vascular growth and remodeling, such as those involved in vascular endothelial growth factor (VEGF), nitric oxide (NO), and transforming growth factor-β_1 (TGF-β_1) production and signal transduction; and (2) factors affecting the response to oxidative stress. In addition to further evaluations of these and other candidate gene relationships in larger and confirmatory patient populations, genome-wide association studies, wherein the entire genome is sequenced, could yield more information about the genes responsible for the familial associations that have been seen. These investigations may ultimately lead to more directed therapies for high-risk, susceptible infants.

Inflammation

A complex inflammatory response clearly plays a major role in the development of BPD (Yoon et al, 1999). This response may be triggered by a number of other factors thought to be a part of the pathobiology of BPD. These triggers include a fetal inflammatory response and increased concentrations of inflammatory cytokines in amniotic fluid, cytokines produced as a result of neonatal infection, and other neonatal inflammatory insults such as oxidant damage due to oxygen toxicity and volutrauma associated with mechanical ventilation.

The inflammatory response is reflected in increased numbers of neutrophils in tracheal aspirate samples as early as the 2nd day of life (Arnon et al, 1993). Although alveolar macrophages are essential for recognition, ingestion, and elimination of lung pathogens, they also produce fibroblast, epithelial, and endothelial cell growth factors, leading to lung tissue repair. In addition, they can have deleterious effects through release of oxygen radicals and can release fibronectin, a large glycoprotein that is a growth factor for fibroblasts, as well as releasing the growth factor TGF-β, which stimulates the growth of mesenchymal cells and inhibits proliferation of epithelial cells. Selected cytokines, chemokines, and other inflammatory factors are found to be elevated in lung lavage fluid of infants in whom BPD develops, while levels of IL-10, CC10, and VEGF are reported to be decreased in infants with BPD (see Box 48-1) (Bose et al, 2008; Ryan et al, 2008). A recent study of blood cytokine levels in preterm infants found that higher concentrations of IL-1β, IL-6, and interferon-γ were associated with BPD or death (Ambalavanan et al, 2009). Studies of mediators in lung fluid, compared to plasma, may have the advantage of reflecting the milieu adjacent to the epithelium and therefore lung inflammation rather than the systemic fetal or neonatal inflammatory response. Box 48-1 lists the factors found in tracheal aspirate or lavage samples that are associated with the development of BPD in the preterm infant.

Neonatal Infection

Airway microbial colonization with a variety of organisms, including *Ureaplasma urealyticum*, is associated with a diagnosis of chorioamnionitis, evidence of lung inflammation and an increased risk of BPD (Bhandari et al, 1998; Cordero et al, 2001; Groneck et al, 1996; Young et al, 2005). Recovery of *Ureaplasma* spp. or *Mycoplasma hominis* from cord blood in preterm infants has also been associated with an increased neonatal inflammatory response (Goldenberg et al, 2008), and postnatal bacterial sepsis with gram-positive, gram-negative, or fungal organisms is associated with an increased risk of BPD (Gagliardi et al, 2007; Stoll et al, 2002). There has been a lot of interest in the relationship of fastidious organisms to preterm lung disease. *Ureaplasma urealyticum* infection has been associated with precocious pulmonary interstitial fibrosis on postmortem evaluation (Viscardi et al, 2002), and a recent systematic review demonstrated a significant association between recovery of *Ureaplasma* from the respiratory tract and BPD at 36 weeks (OR 1.6; 95% confidence interval [CI] 1.1, 2.3), although studies with smaller sample sizes were more likely to report a significant association than those with larger ones (Schelonka et al, 2005). Despite these data, in small randomized studies, early appropriate antibiotic (macrolide) therapy does not alter recovery of the organism from tracheal aspirate samples or the incidence of BPD, regardless of colonization status (Baier et al, 2003; Ballard et al, 2009a, 2009b). Thus, if the new BPD in the tiny preterm infant is a syndrome of arrested lung development, it may be that even short-term exposure to microbial organisms and the resultant inflammatory response (increasing with prolonged ventilation) contribute to the arrest of normal alveolarization and microvascular growth.

Oxygen Toxicity and Oxidative Stress

In the initial cases of BPD reported by Northway et al (1967), it was clear that exposure to high oxygen concentration was a factor in development of the disease. Subsequent reports have continued to show an association between high levels of supplemental oxygen or prolonged oxygen exposure and lung damage in ventilated preterm infants. More recent evidence (STOP-ROP, 2000) suggests that even a slight increase in inhaled oxygen concentration over a prolonged time increases respiratory morbidity. In experimental animals, prolonged hyperoxic exposure recapitulates the clinical and morphometric findings of the older and newer forms of BPD (Coalson et al, 1995; Warner et al, 1998), and oxidative stress has been implicated in the pathogenesis of the morphometric changes in these models (Chang et al, 2003; Ratner et al, 2009). The damage to the lung caused by oxygen toxicity appears to be mediated by reactive oxygen species that are produced during univalent reduction of molecular oxygen. These species include superoxide anion (O_2^-), hydrogen peroxide (H_2O_2), and hydroxyl radical (OH^-). Evidence suggests the presence of an oxidant-antioxidant imbalance in lungs that are at risk for BPD. Vento et al (2009) found that even short exposure to hyperoxia during resuscitation increased the duration of mechanical ventilation and the incidence of BPD in extremely premature newborns. The infants resuscitated with high oxygen in that study had higher ratios of oxidized-to-reduced glutathione levels in blood as well as increased urine levels of oxidized proteins and DNA in the 1st week of life. Similarly, preterm infants exposed to higher inspired oxygen concentrations during resuscitation in another small randomized study had increased total blood hydroperoxides (Ezaki et al, 2009). Other observational studies have found higher concentrations

of lipid peroxidation metabolites, as well as excess carbonylated proteins, in preterm infants later developing BPD, compared to preterm controls without BPD, further supporting the concept of oxidant-antioxidant imbalance (reviewed in Saugstad, 2003). Antioxidant defenses are decreased in preterm infants, and critical nutrients such as retinoic acid (shown to suppress both superoxide and hydrogen peroxide formation in stimulated neutrophils and macrophages) are deficient (reviewed in Shenai, 1999). Nitric oxide, either endogenous or exogenous in origin, may function as either a pro- or antioxidant. However, no significant differences were seen in plasma carbonylated or nitrosylated protein levels in infants treated with inhaled nitric oxide (iNO) versus placebo in the randomized NO CLD Trial over the first 10 days of gas administration, when iNO dose was 10 to 20 ppm (Ballard et al, 2008). An early randomized trial of allopurinol, a xanthine oxidase inhibitor studied for its potential neuroprotective effects, demonstrated no differences in the incidence of BPD at 28 days (Russell et al, 1995). In a more recent trial, intratracheal recombinant human superoxide dismutase did not affect the incidence of BPD at 36 weeks, but treated infants had less pulmonary morbidity than control infants at 1-year follow-up (Davis et al, 2003). The effect of lower target oxygen saturation parameters on the incidence of BPD was studied in the NICHD Neonatal Network Surfactant Positive Airway Pressure and Pulse Oximetry Trial (SUPPORT) Trial (Carlo et al, 2010). Although the incidence of BPD and BPO or death was decreased in infants managed with lower oxygen saturations, these differences were small in magnitude and not statistically significant. In addition, infants tended to be maintained at the higher end of the target range with substantial overlap between the two groups.

Ventilation With Volutrauma

As is the case with exposure to high oxygen, the association between overdistention of the preterm lung and the development of BPD is well established. It is clear that overinflation produces stress fractures of the capillary endothelium, epithelium, and basement membrane. This mechanical injury causes leakage of fluid into the alveolar spaces, with additional inflammatory response and the release of additional proinflammatory cytokines. The relative contribution of high peak inspiratory pressures (*barotrauma*) versus overdistention of the lung (*volutrauma*) to lung injury previously was a source of some controversy. Hernandez et al (1989) compared the respective roles of high tidal volume with high peak inspiratory pressure (PIP) in immature New Zealand White rabbits to look at the effect on microvascular permeability in animals that were treated with chest wall restriction with a full-body plaster cast. Preventing overdistention also prevented any significant increase in microvascular permeability, even with manometer-indicated pressures up to 45 cm H_2O. In contrast, when isolated excised lungs were ventilated with peak inspiratory pressures of only 15 cm H_2O for 1 hour (with overdistention), there was an 850% increase in microvascular permeability. This finding suggests that preterm infants with relatively healthy lungs and highly compliant chest walls may experience significant lung injury even at apparently low ventilator pressures. In addition, in the preterm lamb model, manual ventilation with as few as six very large breaths at birth may compromise the therapeutic effect of subsequent surfactant administration, leading to significant lung damage (Bjorklund et al, 1997; Dreyfuss et al, 1998). Evidence that exposure to high tidal volumes in preterm human infants contributes to BPD comes from several sources. In particular, there is an association between hypocarbia and an increased incidence of BPD (Garland et al, 1995; Kraybill et al, 1989), as well as a known strong association between the occurrence of pneumothorax and pulmonary interstitial emphysema with lung overdistension.

Multiple attempts have been made to decrease the incidence of BPD through improved ventilatory strategies (see also Chapter 45 on the principles of respiratory care). The use of high-frequency oscillatory ventilation (HFOV) as a primary mode of ventilation is one such strategy (Courtney et al, 2002; Johnson et al, 2002; Moriette et al, 2001). Although a statistically significant decrease in the incidence of BPD has been described in some studies, none of the studies using HFOV achieved large clinically relevant differences in outcome. A recent (2009) Cochrane Collaboration metaanalysis of randomized clinical trials of HFOV (with 10 of 17 trials published since 2000) found that there was not a significant overall effect of ventilation mode on the incidence of BPD (RR 0.90; 95% CI 0.78, 1.03) (Cools et al, 2009). In addition, over time, as lung protection strategies on conventional ventilation have become more standard, any benefit of high frequency ventilation on the incidence of BPD has decreased (Bollen et al, 2003). On the other hand, a randomized trial to evaluate a minimal ventilation strategy (higher $PaCO_2$ and lower pH targets compared to more standard $PaCO_2$ and pH targets) demonstrated no differences in the incidence of BPD or death (63% vs. 68%), other major morbidities, and long-term outcomes (Carlo et al, 2002). However, the need for ventilatory support at 36 weeks PMA was significantly lower in the minimal ventilation group compared to the routine conventional ventilation treatment group (1% vs. 16%). Thus, the more permissive approach to assisted ventilation appears to influence the severity of BPD, although this approach alone may be insufficient to prevent the disorder.

In 1987, Avery and associates published a descriptive review of treatment center differences in the incidence of BPD. At one neonatal center, use of nasal CPAP immediately after delivery was associated with a much lower incidence of BPD than that reported by the other centers. Van Marter et al (2000) compared the practices and outcomes for neonatal units in Boston and at Columbia University and found that the incidence of BPD at Columbia overall was much lower, as was the use of interventions, including mechanical ventilation, surfactant administration, indomethacin treatment, and sedation. The use of nasal CPAP was higher and infants at Columbia were intubated less frequently than at the other centers. These investigators found that the best predictor of subsequent BPD at any time point from day 1 to 7 was the requirement for mechanical ventilation at that time, regardless of which institution the infant was in.

The need for early ventilation identifies the sickest infants who would usually die without intervention. In a report from Columbia University, mortality was 66% among infants ≤1250 g birthweight who received mechanical ventilation (after initial resuscitation) (Ammari et al, 2005). These infants generally were more depressed at delivery, with lower Apgar scores. Among infants who received nasal CPAP after resuscitation, 55% of those <26 weeks were intubated by 72 hours of age. Gestational age <26 weeks, birthweight ≤750 g, severe RDS by radiograph, and poor initial oxygenation had positive predictive values of 50% to 55% for failure of CPAP, and infants who required intubation were more likely to have a diagnosis of pneumothorax, severe intracranial hemorrhage, and BPD. This group of infants was supported with "bubble" CPAP, where the end expiratory pressure is created by an underwater seal. Bubble CPAP has been shown to deliver consistently higher intraprong pressures than ventilator-delivered CPAP set to the same end-expiratory pressure (Kahn et al, 2008). Nasal CPAP, in general, and bubble CPAP, in particular, have been successful in maintaining a greater proportion of premature infants extubated after mechanical ventilation, a strategy that may be particularly indicated in the most premature babies (Gupta et al, 2009; Ho et al, 2002). Other advances in the delivery of nasal CPAP since the initial description of its use in preterm infants include the use of a dedicated variable-flow nasal CPAP system, with nasal prongs or a nasal mask, which appears to significantly decrease the work of breathing in comparison to ventilator-delivered nasal CPAP (DeKlerk and DeKlerk, 2001; Pandit et al, 2001).

The preferential application of nasal CPAP to prevent BPD was studied in the Continuous Positive Airway Pressure or Intubation at Birth (COIN) Trial. Infants from 25 to 28 weeks' gestation needing assisted ventilation at 5 minutes of age were randomized to receive nasal CPAP or mechanical ventilation (Morley et al, 2008). There was a significant decrease in the need for oxygen supplementation at 28 days of age (65% vs. 54%), but no difference at 36 weeks PMA (39% vs. 34%). More infants in the mechanical ventilation group received surfactant, and significantly more infants in the CPAP group had pneumothoraces (9% vs. 3%). In addition, 46% of the infants in the CPAP group still required intubation in the first 5 days of life, with many of these babies in the lowest gestational age group (25 to 26 weeks). The NICHD Neonatal Network SUPPORT Trial also evaluated the strategy of preferential application of nasal CPAP to extremely premature infants (Finer et al, 2010). Of the infants in the CPAP group, 83% were ultimately intubated, and there was no significant difference in the incidence of BPD or BPD or death at 36 weeks' PMA. Thus, it appears that the most premature infants are very likely to be intubated, regardless of the strategy used, even at the most experienced centers.

It is clear that loss of functional residual capacity (FRC) with onset of generalized atelectasis can also be a major contributor to the development of BPD. In infants who are being ventilated below a normal FRC, repetitive opening and closing of lung units occurs in the presence of maldistribution. This then leads to areas of significant overdistension. There is accumulating evidence from both

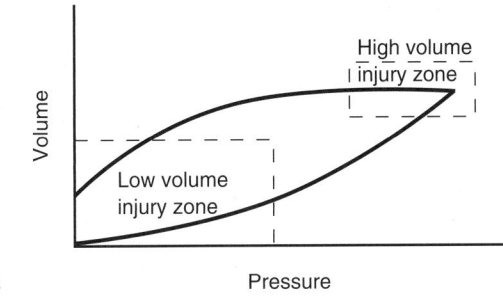

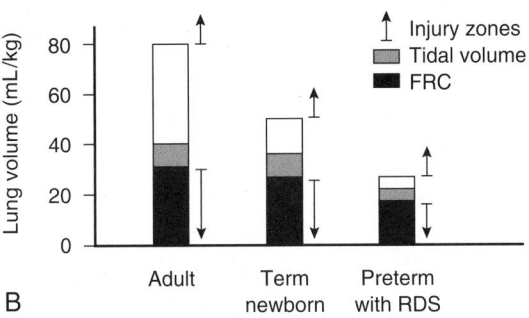

FIGURE 48-3 **A,** Static pressure-volume curve indicating areas of lung injury from either high-volume ventilation or low-volume ventilation with atelectasis. **B,** Lung volumes for a normal adult, a term newborn, and a preterm with RDS. The low- and high-volume injury zones are indicated by *arrows*. The preterm lung is susceptible to injury with ventilation because of the small volume/kg between the two injury zones. *FRC,* Functional residual capacity; *RDS,* respiratory distress syndrome.

animal and human newborn studies that the optimal use of PEEP is associated with a lower risk for BPD. Figure 48-3 demonstrates the appearance of static pressure-volume curves for infants either with normal lungs or with RDS and also depicts the potential areas of lung injury from either high-volume ventilation or low-volume ventilation with atelectasis. There is general agreement that the least injurious approach to supporting ventilation in the preterm infant would be to avoid intubation and stabilize FRC with CPAP. However, many preterm infants are too small or too sick to tolerate the use of nasal CPAP alone and therefore will require intubation and mechanical ventilation. At this time, the approach that would seem most likely to contribute to prevention of BPD is the use of an optimal PEEP to support a normal FRC combined with low-tidal-volume ventilation.

Pulmonary Edema and Patent Ductus Arteriosus

It is clear from animal studies (Bland et al, 2000) that abnormalities of lung fluid balance contribute to BPD. Persistent patency of the ductus arteriosus is thought to contribute to development of BPD through this mechanism. A recent retrospective study from the NICHD Neonatal Network found that a patent ductus arteriosus (PDA) was an independent risk factor associated with the development of BPD, as were higher fluid intake and lesser weight loss in the first 10 days of life (Oh et al, 2005).

Post-hoc analyses of infants enrolled in the Trial of Indomethacin Prophylaxis in Preterms (TIPP) suggest that the relationship of the diagnosis of PDA to BPD is complex (Kabra et al, 2007; Schmidt et al, 2006a). Although prophylactic indomethacin decreased the risk of PDA among these preterm infants, it increased the risk of BPD among infants who did not have a PDA, an effect that seemed to be explained by increased oxygen requirements and decreased weight loss in the 1st week in indomethacin-treated infants. Further, there was an independent association between surgical ligation and the development of BPD among infants who subsequently received treatment for PDA. A post-hoc analysis of a small randomized trial of prophylactic surgical PDA ligation conducted when the use of antenatal steroids was limited, demonstrated increased BPD among surviving infants who underwent prophylactic ligation, but no difference in the combined outcome of death or BPD at 36 weeks (70% vs. 66%) (Clyman et al, 2009). Antenatal glucocorticoids remain an important modulating factor in the pathophysiology of both PDA and BPD, and although these diagnoses are strongly associated with each other, there is currently no definitive evidence to determine whether treatment of PDA reduces the incidence of BPD (see Chapter 54 for full discussion of PDA) (Bose and Laughon, 2006).

Poor Nutrition

All of the aforementioned etiologic factors are intensified by the inadequate nutritional status that is virtually always present in sick preterm infants. These infants have delayed feeding, inadequate parenteral nutrition due to restricted fluid intake, and a catabolic state secondary to increased work of breathing. A recent publication described growth failure in 75% of extremely low-gestational–age newborns at 28 days of age (Martin et al, 2009). Inadequate nutrition decreases alveolar number, a state that can be reversed by normalizing nutritional intake (Massaro et al, 2004). In addition, there are vitamin deficiencies, particularly of vitamin A; the latter condition has been associated with disruption of epithelial cell integrity in an animal model. They also have diminished amounts of antioxidant agents including vitamin E, which probably leads to potentiation of oxygen free radical injury. Each of these factors leads to increased susceptibility to infection, which leads in turn to a further cycle of impaired defense against injury.

Surfactant Dysfunction

Surfactant dysfunction is common among extremely low birthweight infants who remain intubated beyond the 1st week of life (Figure 48-4) (Merrill et al, 2004). In addition, episodes of infection or respiratory deterioration (sustained increase in inspired oxygen concentration or mean airway pressure), have been associated with worsening surfactant function. Surfactant content of surfactant proteins (SP) B and C is tightly correlated with surfactant function in preterm infants, with lower SP levels correlated with higher surface tension. This is particularly true of SP-B, which is down-regulated by TGF-β (McDevitt et al, 2007); other studies in animals and humans have demonstrated

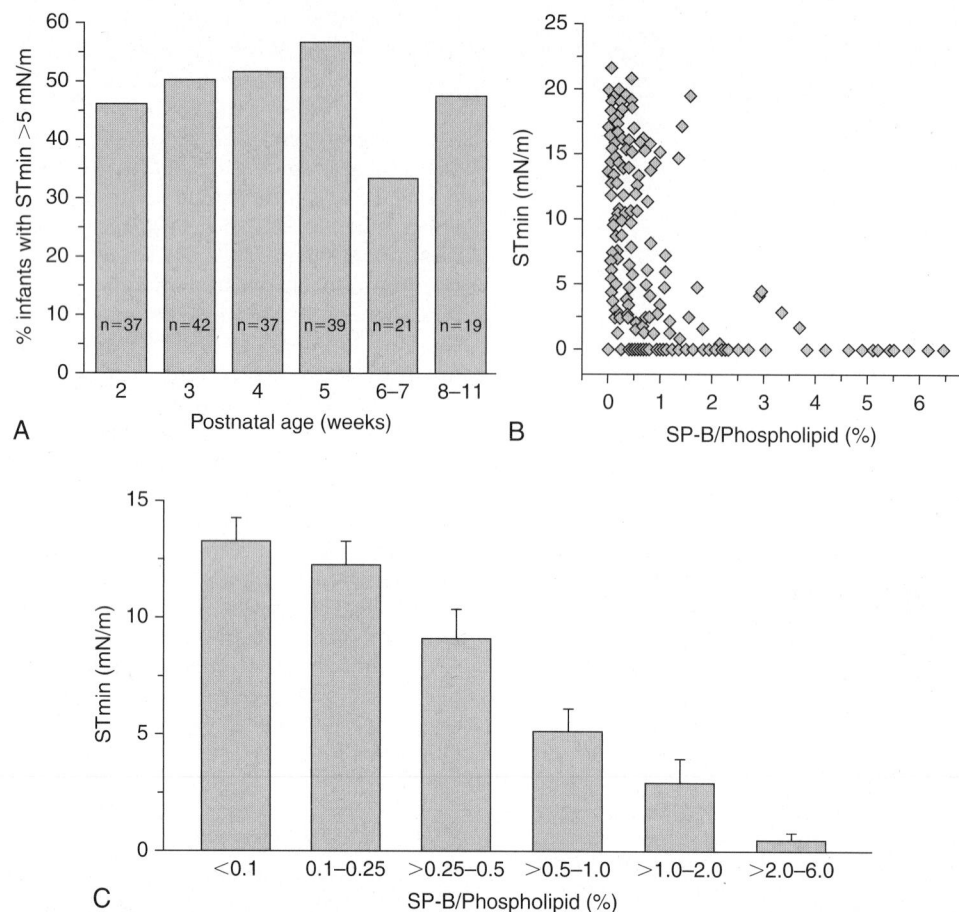

FIGURE 48-4 **Surfactant dysfunction in ventilated preterm infants. A,** Prevalence of surfactant dysfunction (STmin >5 mN/m) during weeks 2 to 11 of life in ventilated preterm infants. **B** and **C,** Inverse relationship of SP-B content (normalized to phospholipid content) to STmin in ventilated preterm infants; low surface tension is associated with higher SP-B content. *SP-B,* Surfactant protein-B; *STmin,* minimum surface tension. (*Adapted from Merrill JD, Ballard RA, Cnaan A, et al: Dysfunction of pulmonary surfactant in chronically ventilated premature infants,* Pediatr Res *56:918-926, 2004.*)

decreased surfactant protein content or expression after exposure to oxygen and cytokines.

Later administration of animal-based surfactants as rescue for clinical decompensation in preterm newborns has been evaluated, with a short-term decrease in ventilator settings after surfactant administration (Bissinger et al, 2008; Katz and Klein 2006; Pandit et al, 1995). A pilot randomized study of lucinacant (Surfaxin, Discovery Labs, Warrington, PA), a synthetic surfactant containing an SP-B-like polypeptide, from days 3 to 10 at two different doses versus placebo, had no effect on the prevention of BPD or death at 36 weeks (Laughon et al, 2009a). There is a large multicenter trial in progress to study the prevention of BPD or death by an animal-derived SP-B containing a surfactant, calfactant (Infasurf, Ony Inc, Amherst, NY) in combination with inhaled NO, administered to high-risk preterm infants who are requiring mechanical ventilation at 7 to 14 days (Trial of Late Surfactant, TOLSURF).

Adrenal Insufficiency

It has been suggested (Watterberg and Scott, 1995; Watterberg et al, 1996) that preterm infants may have developmental immaturity of the hypothalamic-pituitary-adrenal axis and that the risk of BPD is increased secondary to inadequate response to inflammatory lung injury. Banks

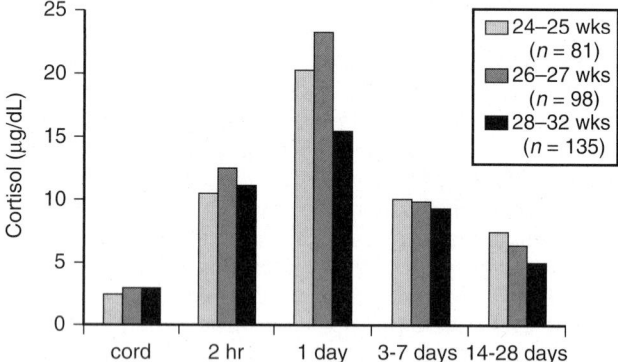

FIGURE 48-5 **Plasma cortisol concentrations in premature infants during the first 4 weeks of life.** Data are mean levels stratified by gestational age: 24 to 25 weeks (*n* = 81), 26 to 27 weeks (*n* = 98), and 28 to 32 weeks (*n* = 135).

et al (2001), reported, however, in a study of cortisol levels in 314 preterm infants, that even the earliest gestation infants (24 to 25 weeks) have an increase in cortisol after delivery and that levels were not associated with gestational age (Figure 48-5). More important, there was only a weak association with severity of illness. Using the CRIB (Clinical Risk Index for Babies) score to adjust for clinical risk factors, low cortisol at 3 to 7 days of life contributed only very minimally to increasing the risk for BPD, and there was no correlation at 14 to 28 days. A subsequent cohort of infants from the PROPHET (Prophylaxis of Early Adrenal Insufficiency to Prevent Bronchopulmonary Dysplasia) study demonstrated no relationship between cortisol levels in the 1st week of life and BPD, although increasing cortisol levels were associated with increasing incidence of other acute and chronic morbidities (Aucott et al, 2008). The PROPHET study, and a concurrent study in Finland, were designed to investigate lower dose "replacement" hydrocortisone dosing (0.5 to 2.0 mg/kg/d) for the prevention of BPD (Peltoniemi et al, 2005; Watterberg et al, 2004). Both studies were terminated prematurely, because of concern for increased gastrointestinal perforation in the hydrocortisone-treated group, and no beneficial effect on the primary outcomes of death or BPD was seen. Hydrocortisone was intended as an anti-inflammatory in these trials, and there was a significant interaction between exposure to chorioamnionitis and hydrocortisone treatment in the PROPHET study, with the exposed, treated infants more likely to survive without BPD. There was also a differential beneficial effect of treatment in the subset of infants with chorioamnionitis who also had evidence of fetal inflammation. Infants with lower baseline and ACTH-stimulated cortisol levels were more likely to respond to hydrocortisone in the Finnish study, but not in the larger PROPHET trial. Of interest is the fact that formation of alveolar septae in animals, a critical step in alveologenesis, occurs during a period of low serum glucocorticoid levels. Further, dexamethasone administered to newborn rodents results in persistent impaired septation and alveologenesis (Massaro and Massaro, 2000). Thus, there is not consistent evidence that adrenal insufficiency contributes to BPD in the general population of at-risk premature infants.

Inhibition of Normal Lung Development and Vascular Development

Some of the contributing factors described previously directly impair normal formation of secondary septae and therefore, microvascular development and alveolarization. Others arrest alveolarization by as yet unknown processes that also involve structural differences in the extracellular matrix. These insults, occurring during the saccular stage of lung development, include inflammation and cytokine overexpression, dexamethasone exposure, hyperoxia, hypoxia, and inadequate nutrition (Albertine et al, 1999; Jobe, 1999; Massaro and Massaro, 2000; Massaro et al, 2004).

PREVENTIVE FACTORS

The Bronchopulmonary Dysplasia Group, convened to identify strategies for investigation of therapies to prevent or treat BPD, proposed classes of drugs to prevent or treat evolving BPD (at 7 to 14 days) (Walsh et al, 2006a). These included anti-inflammatory agents such as antenatal and postnatal corticosteroids (PNCS) and other small molecules, antioxidants, inhaled nitric oxide, late surfactant replacement, and improved vitamin A preparations. Additional approaches that have been proposed and evaluated include alternative ventilation strategies and the primary use of nasal CPAP.

Antenatal Steroids

Numerous clinical studies and several large meta-analyses have demonstrated that a single course of antenatal glucocorticoids administered to women at high risk for premature delivery results in a significant decrease in the mortality rate and in the morbidity associated with prematurity, including RDS, intraventricular hemorrhage (IVH), PDA, and necrotizing enterocolitis (NEC). However, the effect of antenatal glucocorticoids on the incidence of BPD among survivors has been inconsistent, although some studies have demonstrated a benefit (Gagliardi et al, 2007; Van Marter et al, 1990). The inconsistent effect of antenatal steroids on BPD may be due to increased survival of higher risk, less mature preterm infants (see also Chapter 46 on RDS).

Surfactant Replacement Therapy

Surfactant replacement therapy is clearly associated with decreased severity of RDS and its associated mortality. Although there is not substantial evidence that survivors have a decreased incidence of BPD, survival without BPD appears to be improved in some of the meta-analyses that have been undertaken (Engle and the Committee on Fetus and Newborn, 2008). In addition, it is possible that later replacement surfactant, during a period of secondary surfactant dysfunction (Merrill et al, 2004), could be an effective way to prevent BPD in those infants who continue to require mechanical ventilation after the 1st week of life.

Gentle Ventilation and Nasal Continuous Positive Airway Pressure

As described previously, there is evidence that volutrauma as well as atelectasis contribute directly to lung damage as well as releasing cytokines, which further the cycle of damage. Numerous trials of ventilatory modes, including patient-triggered ventilation, high-frequency ventilation, and minimal ventilation (with the goal of keeping the $Paco_2$ above 55 mm Hg), have been attempted (see also Chapter 45 on the principles of respiratory care) (Carlo et al, 2002; Stark, 2002). Some of these trials have demonstrated decreased duration of mechanical ventilation; however, none has demonstrated a substantial clinical benefit in prevention of BPD (Greenough et al, 2008).

Although the primary use of nasal CPAP delivered with the bubble CPAP system (as practiced at Columbia University) is associated with lower rates of BPD (Aly et al, 2004; Van Marter et al, 2000), the multicenter COIN Trial did not show a significant benefit on the incidence of BPD at 36 weeks. The failure to show an effect on BPD in the COIN Trial may be related to differences in Pco_2, pH, and Fio_2 limits (65 mm Hg, 7.20, and 0.60, respectively) between the trial centers and Columbia (Ammari et al, 2005), and tolerance for an extended period of transition after delivery of these preterm infants, wherein these limits may be even more permissive. Additional studies are ongoing; however, given that the pathogenesis of BPD is complex, it may be that other differences in practice, combined with the early initiation of nasal CPAP, preserve lung growth and development and prevent BPD in extremely low gestational age newborns. Regardless, the effects of the more permissive respiratory care limits on neurodevelopmental outcome are still largely unknown. A single study comparing oxygen saturation limits of 91% to 94% versus 95% to 98% from 32 weeks PMA on showed no difference in neurodevelopmental outcomes at 1 year corrected age, although infants in the higher target saturation group had more prolonged oxygen supplementation, a higher incidence of BPD at 36 weeks, and increased need for oxygen supplementation at neonatal discharge (Askie et al, 2003).

Fluid Restriction

Multiple studies suggest that fluid overload contributes to an increased risk of BPD (Oh et al, 2005). In addition, some clinical trial data suggest that excessive fluid administration increases the risk of PDA, NEC, and death (Tammela, 1995). However, extremely restrictive fluid administration contributes to the problem of undernutrition, thereby contributing to failure of alveologenesis.

Vitamin A

Vitamin A is an essential nutrient for maintaining respiratory tract epithelial cells and also is stored in the septal cells of the alveoli involved in alveolar septation. Compelling animal data (Albertine et al, 1999) support the need for vitamin A (Figure 48-6). Because vitamin A is accumulated predominantly in the third trimester, preterm infants have deficient liver stores of this vitamin (Zachman, 1989). These infants, who often are unable to tolerate enteral feedings, are at particular risk for vitamin A deficiency because vitamin A added to parenteral nutrition solutions is degraded by light and can adhere to the intravenous tubing, making it largely inaccessible. A number of clinical trials have investigated whether supplementation with vitamin A, typically by intramuscular injections,

would result in a decrease in BPD. The largest study to date, by the NICHD Neonatal Network, also used one of the higher doses that has been studied and demonstrated a significant decrease in BPD or death at 36 weeks following treatment with vitamin A (55% vs. 62%) (Tyson et al, 1999). A recent metaanalysis of all published trials revealed that vitamin A supplementation was associated with a modest reduction in death or BPD at 36 weeks, which was of borderline statistical significance (RR 0.91, 95% confidence interval 0.82, 1.00, NNT 17) (Darlow and Graham, 2007). Vitamin A is well tolerated and relatively inexpensive, although it does involve repeated intramuscular injections. However, a recent survey found that ≤20% of centers routinely administer vitamin A supplementation to at-risk infants, with inadequate evidence or lack of substantial effect cited as the rationale for lack of supplementation at these centers (Ambalavanan et al, 2004). In addition, there was no treatment effect on pulmonary morbidity or neurodevelopmental impairment at 18 to 22 months corrected age in the NICHD trial participants (Ambalavanan et al, 2005).

Postnatal Corticosteroids

Preterm infants who are given PNCS demonstrate some decreased inflammatory markers and suppression of cytokine-mediated inflammatory reactions in their tracheal aspirates (Groneck et al, 1993). Numerous theoretical reasons have been advanced regarding why postnatal administration of steroids might decrease the incidence of BPD, including the potential for increased surfactant synthesis, enhanced β-adrenergic activity, increased antioxidant production, stabilization of cell and lysosomal membranes, and inhibition of prostaglandin and leukotriene synthesis (Watterberg et al, 1999). These potential benefits are balanced against the knowledge that dexamethasone results in persistent decreases in alveolar numbers in animal models (Massaro and Massaro, 2000). Clinical trials have demonstrated acute improvements in dynamic compliance and pulmonary resistance after treatment with PNCS, although small follow-up studies have demonstrated no differences in respiratory morbidity despite fewer children with abnormal pulmonary function at >5 years of age

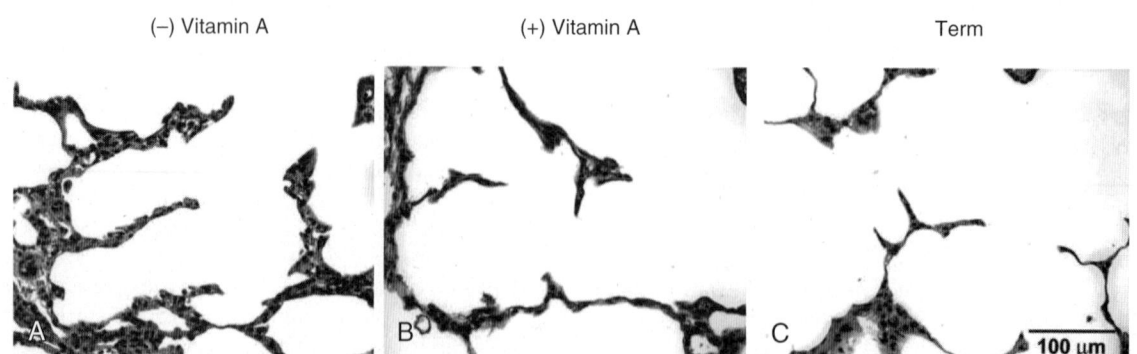

(−) Vitamin A   (+) Vitamin A   Term

FIGURE 48-6 Histopathology of evolving chronic lung disease (CLD) of prematurity in lambs that were mechanically ventilated for 3 weeks at 20 breaths/minute (approximately 15 mL/kg tidal volume). **A,** Preterm lamb ventilated for 3 weeks, treated daily with saline (the vehicle for vitamin A) given intramuscularly. **B,** Preterm lamb ventilated for 3 weeks, treated daily with vitamin A (5000 U/day) given intramuscularly. **C,** Term lamb ventilated for 3 weeks (control). The most simplified distal air spaces and most thickened alveolar walls are in the lung tissue of the preterm lamb that was not treated with vitamin A (seen in **A**). Secondary septa also are least evident in the preterm lamb that was not treated with vitamin A. All panels are of the same magnification (scale bar = 100 μm).

(Nixon et al, 2007). Based on two recent meta-analyses of treatment before and after 7 days of age (Halliday et al, 2009a, 2009b), postnatal dexamethasone has similar beneficial effects on death or BPD at 36 weeks (RR 0.72 to 0.73; 95% CIs within 0.61, 0.85 for both treatment intervals) and decreased need for mechanical ventilation, with no significant impact on survival to hospital discharge. The aggregation of studies comparing hydrocortisone administered in the 1st week of life to placebo demonstrates no effects on mortality or BPD.

Major concerns exist regarding both short- and long-term side effects of PNCS, including hypertension, hyperglycemia, hypertrophic cardiomyopathy, adrenal suppression, and decreased growth. With administration of PNCS in the 1st week of life, the risk of gastrointestinal perforation is significantly increased, regardless of which steroid is administered (RR 1.81; 95% CI 1.33, 2.48). This effect may be associated with concurrent administration of indomethacin. Individual studies have reported an increased risk of later cerebral palsy (CP) in children treated with dexamethasone in infancy (Shinwell et al, 2000; Yeh et al, 1998). The metaanalyses support this concern with dexamethasone initiated in the 1st week of life (with no effect seen with hydrocortisone), although the relationship was not statistically significant when treatment is initiated after 7 days of age (Halliday et al, 2009a, 2009b). The lack of substantial beneficial effects and the concern regarding adverse effects led the American Academy of Pediatrics and Canadian Pediatric Society to recommend against any routine use of postnatal dexamethasone in 2002 (Committee on the Fetus and Newborn, 2002). A more recent assessment, while acknowledging the uncertainty around specific outcomes, does illustrate the overlap between the number needed to treat (prevent BPD) and the number needed to harm (cause CP) for early dexamethasone treatment (Schmidt et al, 2008). This is further supported by an independent metaanalysis (Shinwell and Eventov-Friedman, 2009), demonstrating significantly increased risk of neurodevelopmental impairment (NDI) and CP with any dexamethasone exposure, and a large cohort study demonstrating a dose-dependent increased risk of death or NDI at 18 to 22 months corrected age, regardless of postmenstrual age at the time of dexamethasone exposure (Wilson-Costello et al, 2009). Thus, the avoidance of postnatal dexamethasone is prudent, given what is known about the risks and benefits, and there are insufficient data to support the use of any other systemic steroid at this point in time. At minimum, infants who might be candidates for dexamethasone therapy would be those with severe, persistent disease, treated under a protocol with a short exposure (3 days), with dosing initiated at <0.25 mg/kg/day, and after informing the family of the short- and long-term effects. Potential criteria for treatment would be Fio_2 >0.60, mean airway pressure >12 to 14 cm H_2O, and age >7 days. Interestingly, Walsh et al (2006b) reported decreasing PNCS rates in three major North American neonatal networks from 2001 to 2003, following the societies' statement, with no concurrent change in the rate of BPD.

Although inhaled steroids initiated in the first 2 weeks of life have been studied for prevention of BPD, there are no data suggesting either immediate or later clinical improvement with this intervention, although there is a trend toward decreased systemic steroid use in these infants (Shah et al, 2007). A pilot study of budesonide with beractant (Survanta, Abbot, Columbus, Ohio) compared to beractant alone for treatment of RDS resulted in a significantly lower rate of death or BPD at 36 weeks (32% vs. 61%), without evidence of substantial adverse effects (Yeh et al, 2008). These findings are somewhat surprising, given that the majority of infants received only a single dose of the study medication. In addition, the incidence of BPD was very high in this study. Thus these findings would need to be confirmed in a larger study to ensure safety and efficacy before adopting this approach.

Antioxidant Therapy

Some evidence in the baboon model of BPD indicates that a catalytic antioxidant metalloporphyrin can protect against hyperoxia-induced lung injury (Chang et al, 2003; Tanswell and Jankov, 2003). Superoxide dismutase is a naturally occurring enzyme that protects against oxygen free radical injury. Human studies have suggested that administration of intratracheal recombinant human superoxide dismutase (rhSOD) is well tolerated and might have beneficial effects on the lung (Davis, 2002; Davis et al, 2003). The large randomized trial of rhSOD, which was stopped prematurely because of lack of efficacy for prevention of BPD, did demonstrate an improvement in respiratory morbidity at 1 year corrected age. Some investigators have raised concern regarding antioxidant therapies in the newborn (Jankov et al, 2001). Further trials of this intervention are needed before it can be recommended as useful in preventing BPD.

Inhaled Nitric Oxide

Prolonged inhaled nitric oxide (iNO) from birth in preterm animal models of BPD improves endogenous surfactant function as well as lung growth, angiogenesis, and alveologenesis (Ballard et al, 2006; Bland et al, 2005; McCurnin et al, 2005). In addition, recovery with iNO attenuates the impaired alveolar and microvascular development associated with prolonged hyperoxia exposure in the rodent (Lin et al, 2005). Prematurity in the baboon, and presumably in the human, is associated with developmentally deficient endogenous NO production (Shaul et al, 2002). Accordingly, iNO in this situation is viewed as replacement therapy. Multiple studies of iNO initiated in the first 72 hours of life for prevention of BPD in ventilated, preterm infants have been conducted, with variable efficacy (Kinsella et al, 1999, 2006; Schreiber et al, 2003; van Meurs et al, 2005). Safety concerns were raised because of increased severe intracranial hemorrhage in a single study that enrolled sicker infants with a higher baseline oxygenation index (van Meurs et al, 2005). However, improved neurologic outcomes have been found in studies that enrolled less ill newborns (Kinsella et al, 2006; Mestan et al, 2005). These studies treated infants for variable duration, up to 21 days, with a dose of 5 to 10 ppm. A large European study enrolled infants at <24 hours of age on CPAP or mechanical ventilation and treated them with 5 ppm for 21 days, but failed to find an effect on BPD (Mercier

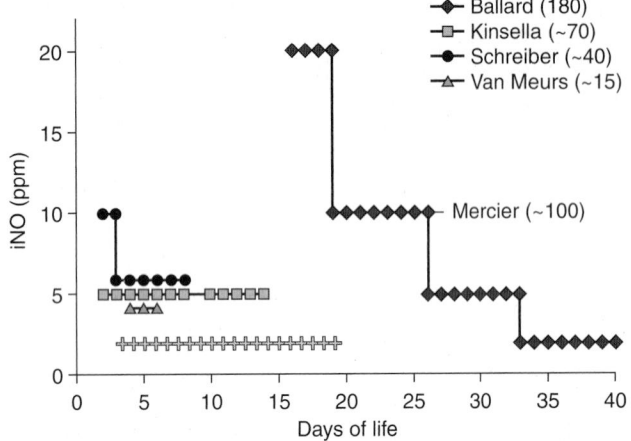

FIGURE 48-7 Summary of large trials of inhaled nitric oxide for prevention of bronchopulmonary dysplasia by day of life versus inhaled nitric oxide dose *(ppm)*. Duration of treatment and total nitric oxide dose is depicted. *INO,* Inhaled nitric oxide. *(Adapted from Truog WE: Inhaled nitric oxide for the prevention of bronchopulmonary dysplasia,* Expert Opin Pharmacother 8:1505-1513, 2007.)*

et al, 2009). In the NO CLD Trial, which enrolled ventilated infants 500 to 1250 g at 7 to 21 days with evolving BPD, infants received at least 24 days of iNO therapy, with a dose of 10 to 20 ppm for at least 10 days (Ballard, 2007; Ballard et al, 2006) (see Figure 48-7 for comparison of dosing and duration of trials). In this study, the rate of survival without BPD at 36 weeks significantly increased from 37% to 44%. Treated infants were also ventilated for fewer days, resulting in a relative cost savings with iNO (Zupancic et al, 2009). There was a significant interaction of treatment with the age at study entry, with infants who entered earlier (at 7 to 14 days), more likely to benefit (increase in survival without BPD from 27% to 49%; NNT = 4). The benefit of treatment persisted at 40 weeks' PMA, with iNO-treated infants more likely to be discharged or hospitalized off all respiratory support, and both the earlier and later (15 to 21 days) treated groups had evidence of benefit at that point in time (Keller et al, 2009). In addition, the smallest infants (500 to 799 g) could be enrolled while receiving nasal CPAP (8.4% of total enrollment), and even with this subset of infants, there was a trend toward a differential benefit of iNO therapy. Pulmonary morbidity at 1 year was decreased in the iNO-treated group (fewer infants requiring supplemental oxygen and decreased use of bronchodilators, diuretics, and inhaled and systemic steroids) (Hibbs et al, 2008). At that point, all subgroups of treated infants appeared to have a benefit from treatment. iNO therapy initiated at 7 to 21 days also was safe; there was no difference in the rate of any comorbidities of prematurity between the treatment and control groups, and at 2 years, there was no difference in the rate of NDI by treatment group (Walsh et al, 2009).

Caffeine

Recently, Schmidt et al (2006b) reported that the administration of caffeine, initiated in the 1st week of life for prevention or treatment of apnea of prematurity, decreased the risk of BPD at 36 weeks from 47% to 36% in infants 500 to 1250 g. The primary intervention for persistent

apnea was continuous positive airway pressure, and infants treated with caffeine were permanently weaned off of mechanical ventilation, positive airway pressure, and oxygen earlier (average 0.9 to 1.5 weeks) and had less exposure to PNCS (14% vs. 20%). Caffeine was discontinued at a median of 34 weeks PMA, once apnea episodes had resolved. There was a transient decrease in weight gain in treated infants, but no other substantial adverse effects were seen. In addition, the caffeine-treated group had a significantly lower rate of survival without NDI (40% vs. 46%; OR 0.79; 95% CI 0.65, 0.96) at 18 to 21 months corrected age (Schmidt et al, 2007). For use of caffeine for prevention of BPD, the NNT is 10, and for NDI it is 34 (Schmidt et al, 2008). Although this trial enrolled relatively larger preterm infants who had otherwise met criteria for extubation in the 1st week of life, and the mechanism of the effect of caffeine on BPD is unknown (Bancalari, 2006), caffeine to facilitate extubation or treat apnea of prematurity appears to be a safe and effective therapy for prevention of BPD.

CLINICAL COURSE AND TREATMENT

As mentioned earlier, the classic BPD described by Northway et al is now extremely rare with the advent of antenatal steroids, postnatal surfactant, and ventilators and ventilator strategies better suited for preterm newborn infants. Thus, here we address only the clinical course of the new BPD. As pointed out by Bancalari (2001) and others, a majority of infants who have BPD currently are extremely low-birthweight infants (usually under 1000 g and 28 weeks' gestation) who require prolonged ventilator support, often for management of apnea or poor respiratory effort. Because of exposure to antenatal steroids and treatment with postnatal surfactant, these infants often initially require relatively low concentrations of oxygen and have fairly mild respiratory disease. They are extremely susceptible to infection, however, and in the first weeks of life, they may develop sepsis and/or tracheitis and pneumonia. Infection contributes to the deterioration of respiratory status that occurs during this period in many of these infants; infectious episodes are associated with secondary surfactant dysfunction, as are other episodes of respiratory deterioration (Merrill et al, 2004). A number of other factors are involved in the development of BPD, including high-level oxygen and ventilator support administered during periods of clinical decompensation, which sets up the cycle of ongoing ventilator support and further lung injury.

Management of infants at risk for or with established BPD should be directed at (1) minimizing ventilatory support and overdistention while (2) supporting and maintaining adequate FRC with end-expiratory pressure. These goals can best be achieved with the use of nasal CPAP systems (variable-flow or bubble CPAP delivery) (Courtney et al, 2001; Pandit et al, 2001). Successful use of nasal CPAP requires tolerance of permissive hypercapnia during the transition immediately after birth (the recommendation of the group at Columbia is to tolerate levels as high as 70 mm Hg), as well as subsequent tolerance of Paco₂ values in the 60s. This recommendation has led to the need for further investigation of the appropriate level of Pco_2 in these preterm infants. There has been concern that elevated levels might be associated with IVH or other adverse neurodevelopmental effects. However, recent studies in the human suggest that both *hypo*capnia (not hypercapnia) and hyperoxia place infants at increased risk for disabling cerebral palsy (Collins et al, 2001). In addition, there is some evidence that high $Paco_2$ levels may actually be neuroprotective (Vanucci et al, 1995, 1997). In fact, some data (Laffey et al, 2000) indicate that Pco_2 values up to 100 mm Hg actually protect the lung from reperfusion injury and that buffering the low pH that results from high Pco_2 negates the protective effect of the high Pco_2.

Another management issue that is crucial for maintaining infants on nasal CPAP is the expected level of oxygen saturation to be achieved. Again, there is enormous controversy regarding the appropriate oxygen status of these infants. It should be emphasized that in utero, the fetus is exposed to a Pao_2 of only 25 to 27 mm Hg and arterial oxygen saturations below 80%. Yet, without sufficient data, keeping the preterm infant's oxygen saturation (Sao_2) in a range of 90% to 95% is commonplace. In some institutions, levels have routinely been kept above 95%. The data from the STOP-ROP trial did not demonstrate significant benefit against progression of retinopathy of prematurity with exposure to Sao_2 ranges that were greater than 96%, compared with 89% to 94%, although there was a low likelihood of ophthalmologic harm (STOP-ROP, 2000). Further, Askie et al (2003) reported no effect of lower oxygen saturation targets on subsequent neurodevelopmental outcomes or growth at 1 year corrected age. Finally, both of these trials demonstrated increased adverse pulmonary outcomes in the higher target saturation groups, despite the older gestational age at initiation of additional oxygen supplementation. The SUPPORT Trial and others should report whether keeping oxygen saturation at lower levels (routine Sao_2 in the 80s) might result in improvement in long-term pulmonary and neurodevelopmental outcomes, a strategy that has been advocated by developmental biologists for prevention of later morbidity, in recognition of the normally low oxygen tensions in the intrauterine environment (Maltepe and Saugstad, 2009).

Additional questions that are as yet unresolved relate to specific levels of Fio_2 that are directly toxic to the developing human lung (which affects the threshold at which an infant on NCPAP might be placed on mechanical ventilation) and whether maintenance of chronic oxygen saturations above a certain level might minimize secondary vascular changes associated with pulmonary hypertension in infants with established BPD. However, many practitioners do not feel comfortable discharging infants with BPD without supplemental oxygen unless Sao_2 is consistently ≥92%.

Ventilation

In spite of the development of numerous sophisticated ventilators for the newborn, there is still no clear advantage to any one approach to ventilating the preterm infant (see also Chapter 45). The general approach should be one of preventing atelectasis, sustaining FRC, using a minimal tidal volume (usually 4 to 6 mL/kg), and allowing the

infant to trigger his or her own ventilation as much as possible (Carlo et al, 2002). It is also clear that infants can be extubated more successfully if they are extubated directly to nasal CPAP, with either variable-flow or "bubble" CPAP delivery systems (Gupta et al 2009; Ho et al, 2002).

Nutrition

Optimizing both enteral and parenteral nutrition is essential to growth and recovery of preterm infants with BPD. Beginning parenteral nutrition in the first days after birth, as well as the use of aggressive feeding regimens, is crucial to success in these infants. In addition, appropriate vitamin supplementation should be considered, although, as noted previously, vitamin A supplementation is of marginal benefit and is infrequent in North American centers.

Caffeine

Caffeine therapy was initiated in The Caffeine of Prematurity (CAP) Trial in premature infants (500 to 1250 g) for treatment or prevention of apnea. The caffeine was administered as a loading dose of 20 mg/kg followed by a maintenance dose of 5 mg/kg/d, with the dose advanced up to 10 mg/kg/d as needed for ongoing apnea (Schmidt et al, 2006b). Caffeine was demonstrated to be safe and effective for prevention of BPD.

Inhaled Nitric Oxide

Infants treated with inhaled nitric oxide in The NO CLD Trial received a minimum of 24 days of therapy, with iNO continued when infants were extubated, while on nasal CPAP or nasal cannula support (Ballard 2007; Ballard et al, 2006). The dose schedule was 20 ppm × 3 days ± 24 hours (almost all infants received 4 days of therapy) followed by 7 days each of 10 ppm, 5 ppm, and 2 ppm. There was no difficulty in weaning off the gas, and infants did not have acute changes in lung function with iNO initiation (DiFiore et al, 2007). This protocol is becoming accepted practice in a number of institutions, given the favorable risk: benefit profile of the drug, particularly when initiated at 7 to 14 days. Although some have expressed concerns regarding cost of this therapy, it is cost effective and likely to be cost saving, because of the decreased duration of assisted ventilation and neonatal hospitalization, even without considering the longer term effects of preventing BPD (Zupancic et al, 2009).

Diuretics

In infants with well-developed BPD, pulmonary edema is a major component of the illness. Diuretics, therefore, have been used for some time (Hazinski, 2000). There is clear evidence that either daily or alternate-day therapy with furosemide improves lung mechanics and gas exchange in infants with established BPD (Rush et al, 1990). Thiazide-type diuretics alone or in combination with spironolactone also have improved lung function in some studies. There is no evidence for long-term benefits of diuretic therapy; nevertheless, most centers use diuretics at some point in the management of infants with BPD. There are metabolic effects of diuretic use, some of which are attenuated by every-other-day dosing. If long-term diuretics are administered, it is important that supplemental KCl also be administered to prevent the diuretic-induced metabolic alkalosis associated with hypochloremia as well as hypokalemia. In chronic BPD, an infant who has become hypercarbic will, over time, have a compensatory metabolic alkalosis (pH of 7.30 to 7.35 in the presence of a modestly elevated serum bicarbonate). However, if the infant is receiving diuretics and is not receiving adequate supplements of KCl, the infant's loss of potassium and chloride can lead to a primary metabolic alkalosis. The infant then might hypoventilate to reduce blood pH. Additional potential complications of long-term therapy with loop diuretics include hypercalciuria with nephrocalcinosis and its sequelae, and osteopenia, which can occur in these former premature infants as a result of decreased intrauterine mineral accretion, insufficient postnatal mineral supplementation, and the metabolic effects of the drugs. Ototoxicity is also of concern in this vulnerable population, although it is not known if permanent hearing loss is a direct result of diuretic therapy or an association with more severe neonatal illness.

Bronchodilator Therapy

With established BPD, there is a significant increase in airway resistance, and there may also be persistent or intermittent wheezing. Several studies of short-term, inhaled, or parenteral β_2-adrenergic agonist therapy have demonstrated some improvement in ventilation with such therapy. Inhaled albuterol has been the most widely used agent. Systemic use of bronchodilators has been more restricted because of a high incidence of side effects and a very narrow therapeutic index (DeBoeck et al, 1998). Hazinski (2000) pointed out that there are two pitfalls to the use of β_2 agonist drugs: (1) there can be β agonist–induced vasodilatation, which may lead to hypoxia; and (2) β agonist–induced augmentation of airway instability in an infant with both BPD and tracheomalacia may occur. Both of these pitfalls may lead to complex ventilation-perfusion ($\dot{V}/\dot{Q}$) relations (Hazinski 2000). Baraldi and Fillipone (2007) have reviewed reports of lung function in BPD. In studies of children >6 years of age with the new BPD, obstructive lung disease was present. Subsequently, Hilgendorff et al (2008) evaluated former premature infants at term-corrected age and found bronchodilator-responsive airway disease in 18 of 27 infants despite no clinical evidence of airway obstruction. However, an additional four infants had a paradoxical response to the medication, consistent with airway malacia. Thus, further evaluation of routine bronchodilator therapy in infants with established BPD should be studied, to identify if this use of bronchodilators could, in fact, attenuate later respiratory morbidity (see later discussion).

Postnatal Corticosteroids

As discussed earlier, there has been a widespread effort to prevent chronic lung disease with the use of postnatal dexamethasone. Currently, recommendations of the American Academy of Pediatrics and the Canadian Pediatric Society are that the use of postnatal steroids be restricted to randomized, controlled trials and, when these agents are given outside such trials, they be used only under exceptional circumstances of severity and after fully informing the parents of the potential problems with neurodevelopmental outcome.

Pulmonary Hypertension

Although it is known that infants dying with BPD have dysmorphic pulmonary vascular development (Abman, 2008), the prevalence of pulmonary hypertension in the disease is unknown. The diagnosis is challenging, with some practitioners recommending periodic screening echocardiograms (Bancalari et al, 2005), but the sensitivity and specificity of this technique is not adequate, even in an experienced center (Mourani et al, 2008). Pulmonary hypertension does not universally portend a poor prognosis, with 89% of former premature newborns demonstrating improvement over time (Khemani et al, 2007). Although therapies for chronic treatment of pulmonary hypertension have shown efficacy in older patient populations, the risk-benefit profile for infants and young children is unknown.

Future Directions

Given the pathobiology of BPD, there are multiple potential targets for prevention of the disease. The rationale for late treatment (beginning in the 2nd week of life) with an SP-B containing surfactant is sound, and a Trial of Late Surfactant (TOLSURF) in infants receiving inhaled nitric oxide has been initiated. A recent publication described antioxidant activity in multiple animal-derived surfactant preparations (Dani et al, 2009), and antioxidant supplementation remains promising for the prevention of BPD. Another promising therapy that has not been further pursued is α-1 antitrypsin therapy, to modify the protease-antiprotease imbalance that affects extracellular matrix development (Stiskal et al, 1998), and there is good rationale to target antagonism of TGF-β signaling (Nakanishi et al, 2007). In addition, bone marrow–derived mesenchymal stem cells offer some promise for repair in the rat hyperoxia-injured lung (van Haaften et al, 2009). Budesonide delivered by inhalation with surfactant as an anti-inflammatory agent also deserves further evaluation, possibly given after 7 days of age in combination with iNO.

OUTCOME

The mortality rate among infants with BPD who are discharged on therapy from the hospital is roughly 10%. Mortality was 38% in a recent report of children with BPD and pulmonary hypertension (Khemani et al, 2007). As anticipated, children with severe pulmonary hypertension (systemic-to-suprasystemic) were more likely to die. In long-term follow-up assessments of preterm infants, BPD clearly is one of the major conditions associated with poor neurodevelopmental outcome (along with IVH and periventricular leukomalacia), and exposure to PNCS increases the risk of NDI that is associated with BPD (Wilson-Costello et al, 2009). Poor nutrition, impaired growth, and prolonged and recurrent hospitalization likely also contribute to these poor outcomes. Children with BPD have increased rates of pulmonary hospitalization and medication use in the first 1 to 2 years of life, and data from the EPICURE study of former preterm infants at ≤25 weeks' gestation show that this pattern persists at 30 months and 6 years of age (Hennessy et al, 2008). Additional long-term morbidity associated with BPD may include upper airway damage secondary to endotracheal intubation (Statement on the care of the child with chronic lung disease, 2003), and systemic hypertension has also been described in severe cases (Alagappan and Malloy, 1998). Given the multiple systems involved, it is likely that these infants would benefit from multidisciplinary follow-up care, including neurodevelopmental screening and intervention, appropriate nutritional and feeding support, and cardiopulmonary care, provided in a coordinated and collaborative environment.

SUMMARY

BPD remains the most common form of chronic lung disease in children. It is estimated that there are between 25,000 and 30,000 infants with BPD at any one time in the United States. The morbidity of the disease is high, with chronic illness and long-term neurodevelopmental impairment, and is accompanied by financial costs to families and society. The American Thoracic Society published a well-referenced position paper on the care of the child with chronic lung disease of infancy and childhood that addresses many of the important ongoing issues in the care of these children (Statement on the care of the child with chronic lung disease, 2003).

It is hoped that combining treatment with caffeine with new approaches to ventilation, including the aggressive early use of nasal CPAP, treatment of high-risk infants with iNO and potentially with late doses of surfactant, further development of anti-inflammatory and antioxidant approaches, and possible stem cell therapy will ameliorate the impact of BPD. Ultimately, therapies tailored to specific biomarkers or genetic susceptibility should be possible.

SUGGESTED READINGS

Abman SH, editor: *Bronchopulmonary dysplasia*, 2010, Informa Healthcare. London.

Ballard RA, Truog WE, Cnaan A, et al: for the NO CLD Study Group: Inhaled nitric oxide in preterm infants undergoing mechanical ventilation, *N Engl J Med* 355:343-353, 2006:Correction, *N Engl J Med* 357:1444, 2007.

Baraldi E, Filippone M: Chronic lung disease after premature birth, *N Engl J Med* 357:1946-1955, 2007.

Bland RD, Coalson JJ, editors: *Chronic lung disease in early infancy*, New York, 2000, Marcel Dekker.

Hibbs AM, Walsh MC, Martin RJ, et al: One-year respiratory outcomes of preterm infants enrolled in the Nitric Oxide (to prevent) Chronic Lung Disease trial, *J Pediatr* 153:525-529, 2008.

Jobe AH, Bancalari E: Bronchopulmonary dysplasia, *Am J Respir Crit Care Med* 163:1723-1729, 2001.

Merrill JD, Ballard RA, Cnaan A, et al: Dysfunction of pulmonary surfactant in chronically ventilated premature infants, *Pediatr Res* 56:918-926, 2004.

Mestan KK, Marks JD, Hecox K, et al: Developmental outcomes of premature infants treated with inhaled nitric oxide, *N Engl J Med* 353:23-32, 2005.

Schmidt B, Roberts RS, Davis P, et al: Caffeine for Apnea of Prematurity Trial Group: Caffeine therapy for apnea of prematurity, *N Engl J Med* 354:2112-2121, 2006.

Schmidt B, Roberts RS, Davis P, et al: Caffeine for Apnea of Prematurity Trial Group: Long-term effects of caffeine therapy for apnea of prematurity, *N Engl J Med* 357:1893-1902, 2007.

Statement on the care of the child with chronic lung disease of infancy and childhood: American Thoracic Society documents, *Am J Respir Crit Care Med* 168:356-396, 2003.

Wilson-Costello D, Walsh MC, Langer JCEunice Kennedy Shriver National Institute of Child Health and Human Development Neonatal Research Network, et al: Eunice Kennedy Shriver National Institute of Child Health and Human Development Neonatal Research Network, Impact of postnatal corticosteroid use on neurodevelopment at 18 to 22 months' adjusted age: effects of dose, timing, and risk of bronchopulmonary dysplasia in extremely low birthweight infants, *Pediatrics* 123:E430-E437, 2009.

Complete references and supplemental color images used in this text can be found online at www.expertconsult.com

CHAPTER
49

SURGICAL DISORDERS OF THE CHEST AND AIRWAYS

Roberta L. Keller, Salvador Guevara-Gallardo, and Diana L. Farmer

ANOMALIES OF THE AIRWAYS

NASOPHARYNGEAL OBSTRUCTIVE DISORDERS

Respiratory distress due to nasal obstruction may manifest as a serious, life-threatening event shortly after birth. Because newborns are preferential nasal breathers for the first 2 to 3 weeks of life, nasal obstruction may cause severe cyanosis, particularly during oral feedings, with airway obstruction relieved only when the mouth is open to cry (Ramsden et al, 2009). There are several causes of neonatal nasal obstruction, including congenital choanal atresia, nasal pyriform aperture stenosis, nasolacrimal duct cyst, and nasal hypoplasia. Buckling or, less commonly, dislocation of the nasal septum due to birth trauma can also cause breathing problems; most cases respond to decongestant and steroid nasal drops, but dislocations require surgical manipulation (Prescott, 1995).

Congenital Choanal Atresia

Caused by persistence of the buccopharyngeal membrane, congenital choanal atresia occurs in between 1 per 5000 and 1 per 9000 births and has a significant female preponderance. In the majority of choanal atresia cases, the obstructing membrane is of mixed bony and membranous composition (Brown et al, 1996). Choanal atresia is more frequently unilateral; bilateral malformations are more serious and constitute an emergency at birth (Ramsden et al, 2009). Over half of all cases are associated with other congenital anomalies, bilateral cases more so than unilateral (Burrow et al, 2009; Hall, 1979). The most common collection of anomalies was originally termed the *CHARGE association*, consisting of some combination of *c*olobomas of the eyes, *h*eart defects, *a*tresia of the choanae, *r*etardation of growth or development, *g*enitourinary defects, and *e*ar anomalies associated with deafness (Pagon et al, 1981). The association was officially named *CHARGE syndrome* in 2004, when a common mutation in the *CHD*7 gene on chromosome 8 was identified in 60% of cases (Vissers et al, 2004).

Because the newborn is a preferential nasal breather, there may be serious difficulties soon after birth, especially in cases of bilateral atresia. Unilateral atresia may present simply with unilateral discharge and possibly feeding difficulties, but may not present until later in childhood. The inability to pass a catheter through the nose may suggest the diagnosis. Computed tomographic (CT) scan of the nasopharynx is the method of choice for making a definitive diagnosis and for evaluating the nature and severity of nasal obstruction (Benjamin, 1985; Crockett et al, 1987).

Emergent management of choanal atresia is focused on ensuring the oropharyngeal airway is patent and may necessitate endotracheal intubation. A McGovern nipple, an orogastric tube, or a modified endotracheal tube can be used to overcome the seal between the palate and the tongue (Fulton et al, 2007). Tracheostomy is rarely necessary and typically only required when associated with other anomalies (Asher et al, 1990). Surgical repair is the mainstay of treatment and can be performed within a few days of birth. Patency can be established by various methods according to surgeon preference. Correction can be accomplished using the transnasal approach under endoscopic visualization and relieving the obstruction by using dilators (Stahl and Jurkiewicz, 1985) followed by placement of temporary stents to prevent subsequent closure. The transnasal approach works best with thin buccopharyngeal membranes and tends to have higher recurrence and reoperation rates (Hengerer et al, 2008; Samadi et al, 2003). The transpalatal approach entails surgical correction of the offending defect and is typically performed for thick bony membranes. However, despite the minimal rate of reoperation, this approach is associated with a higher rate of palate growth deformities. In an attempt to avoid altering palate growth, modern endoscopic biting and drilling instruments were introduced to improve the transnasal technique (Josephson et al, 1998; Stankiewicz, 1990), and studies continue to demonstrate increasing support for the endoscopic repair of choanal atresia (Ramsden et al, 2009).

Congenital Nasal Pyriform Aperture Stenosis

Nasal pyriform aperture stenosis is a rare cause of nasal obstruction and should be suspected when encountering difficulty in passing a nasal catheter. Characterized by excessive bone formation in the medial nasal processes of the maxillary bone, the condition may be isolated or associated with other anomalies, such as a solitary maxillary central incisor tooth or, more seriously, midline defects such as pituitary hypoplasia with endocrine insufficiency (Beregszaszi et al, 1996), diabetes insipidus (Godil et al, 2000), other manifestations of holoprosencephaly, and craniosynostosis (Van Den Abbeele et al, 2001). Similar to choanal atresia, an oral airway may be necessary to relieve the breathing difficulty. Although the obstruction can be suitably demonstrated by CT scan of the nasopharynx (Truong and Oudjhane, 1994), because of its high association with holoprosencephaly, a karyotype analysis and brain CT and/or magnetic resonance imaging (MRI) may be required if brain abnormalities are suspected (Devambez et al, 2009). In most cases, nasal obstruction is mild and

672

may respond to nasal decongestants. In refractory cases of obstruction, sublabial surgery is necessary to remove excessive bone, and nasal stenting is required (Tate and Sykes, 2009).

Pierre Robin Syndrome (Robin Sequence)

Although this suite of upper airway problems was first described by Pierre Robin in 1923, characterization of Pierre Robin syndrome remains difficult and controversial. A constellation of anomalies within the spectrum of cleft palate, micrognathia, and glossoptosis, the Pierre Robin syndrome has recently been linked to mutations in the *SOX9* gene (Benko et al, 2009; Jakobsen et al, 2007). Given the varying definitions published, the incidence of Pierre Robin syndrome is difficult to pinpoint; it has been reported to occur in anywhere from 1 in 8500 to 1 in 20,000 births (Breugem and Mink van der Molen, 2009). It is the abnormal development of the mandible that is of clinical significance, as the micrognathia can lead to airway obstruction and cyanosis (Cozzi and Pierro, 1985). Obstruction is common when the infant is in the supine position, during feeding, and in active sleep, when pharyngeal muscle tone is absent. Excessive air swallowing, followed by gastric distention, vomiting, and tracheal aspiration, are frequent problems. The pharyngeal obstruction is maintained by the generation of large negative pressures in the lower pharynx during inspiration and swallowing (Fletcher et al, 1969). Chronic obstruction leads to carbon dioxide retention, failure to thrive, and development of pulmonary hypertension with right ventricular failure (Johnson and Todd, 1980).

As with the imprecise diagnosis of Pierre Robin syndrome, the severity of respiratory obstruction and the management indicated is varied. Mild cases may present with only mild glossoptosis, and because oral feeds are tolerated without respiratory obstruction, these cases can be managed by side-to-side nursing (Caouette-Laberge et al, 1994; Cole et al, 2008). In the event of respiratory symptoms with feedings or failure to thrive, a nasogastric tube for feedings may be required (Cole et al, 2008). In severe cases of respiratory distress, nasopharyngeal intubation should be performed, typically by passing a 3.5-mm tube through the nose and into the hypopharynx (Heaf et al, 1982; Stern et al, 1972). This prevents the generation of negative pressure and greatly relieves the respiratory difficulty. The nasopharyngeal tube may be left in place for weeks or even months with adequate lavage and suctioning. Other treatments include tongue-lip adhesion surgery to hold the tongue forward and tracheostomy if a nasopharyngeal tube does not adequately relieve the obstruction (Gilhooly et al, 1993). Recent reports of mandibular distraction and velar extension appliances have been introduced in attempts to avoid tracheostomy (Buchenau et al, 2007; Denny and Kalantarian, 2002). Nutrition can be maintained with a hypercaloric formula fed by nasogastric or gastrostomy tube. With adequate airway management and the passage of time, the problem becomes less threatening, especially after a few months, when the infant gains better control of the tongue (Mallory and Paradise, 1979). Oral feedings can then be introduced, usually with a long lamb's

nipple to help hold the tongue forward. With adequate nutrition and growth of the mandible, the problem usually resolves by 6 to 12 months of age, when cleft palate repair can safely take place.

Glossoptosis-Apnea Syndrome

Pierre Robin syndrome is not the only condition characterized by mechanical obstruction by the tongue. Infants with Beckwith-Wiedemann syndrome may have considerable breathing difficulties and apnea due to the associated macroglossia. Infants with a normal-sized tongue who also have conditions such as unilateral choanal atresia, choanal stenosis, or swelling of the nasal mucosa may generate considerable negative pressure in the pharynx; this, combined with inadequate muscular control over the tongue, may lead to pharyngeal obstruction with respiratory distress, cyanosis, and severe episodes of apnea (Cozzi and Pierro, 1985).

Pharyngeal Incoordination

Pharyngeal incoordination causes choking and cyanosis with feedings and may be complicated by aspiration pneumonia (Avery and Fletcher, 1974). Affected infants have difficulties in swallowing their own secretions. The condition may be seen in infants with severe hypoxic-ischemic encephalopathy and pseudobulbar palsy, Arnold-Chiari malformation, and Möbius syndrome. Drugs with antimuscarinic effects, such as atropine, can decrease secretions and may produce some relief. Although some infants may gradually improve, long-term management may require initiation of tube feedings or even gastrostomy.

LARYNGEAL DEFORMITIES

Congenital Laryngeal Stridor

A relatively common condition, congenital laryngeal stridor or laryngomalacia is the most frequent cause of stridor in infants (Zoumalan et al, 2007). Laryngomalacia is characterized by the prolapse of poorly supported supraglottic structures—the arytenoids, the aryepiglottic folds, and the epiglottis—into the airway during inspiration, causing respiratory obstruction and difficulty with feeding (Olney et al, 1999). Despite loud, high-pitched inspiratory stridor and significant chest retractions that typically present during the first month of life, the infant seldom has cyanosis, hypercarbia, notable feeding difficulty or growth failure, or an abnormal cry (Richardson and Cotton, 1984). Laryngomalacia is worse in the supine position with the neck flexed and subsides in the prone position with the neck extended (Cotton and Richardson, 1981). Obstruction is worse during episodes of agitation and lessens when the infant is calmed. Severe forms of laryngomalacia may cause apneic events, pulmonary hypertension, or difficulties with feeding and/or weight gain. Although CT scan is effective at demonstrating the abnormal prolapse of the aryepiglottic folds supporting the diagnosis (Galvin et al, 1994), confirmation should be obtained at laryngoscopy (Friedman et al, 1990; Wiatrak, 2000), with specific care to avoid fixating the supraglottic tissues with the instrument. Some practitioners prefer to pass a flexible fiberoptic bronchoscope through the nose (Berkowitz, 1998), which does not disturb the supraglottic tissues. In some cases, gastroesophageal reflux or episodes of obstructive apnea may be associated with this condition (Belmont and Grundfast, 1984). About 18% of infants with a congenital lesion of the airway have a second lesion of some kind. Thus, the evaluation of stridor must include the examination of the entire upper airway and upper digestive tract (Friedman et al, 1984). Most cases will resolve with conservative management within 12 to 24 months (Thompson, 2007). Conservative therapy entails positioning the infant prone as much as possible, and most demonstrate improvement over roughly 18 months (Smith and Catlin, 1984). However, approximately 20% will require surgical intervention. A very few patients may have severe obstructive apnea, cor pulmonale, and/or failure to thrive. In these cases supraglottoplasty may be indicated. Tracheostomy is reserved for supraglottoplasty failures (Richter and Thompson, 2008).

Vocal Cord Paralysis

Unilateral cord paralysis is usually left-sided and typically presents without marked stridor or retractions manifesting as aspiration. The infant may cough and choke during feedings, as laryngeal closure with swallowing is impaired. The condition is due to a lesion involving the recurrent laryngeal nerve, perhaps caused by excessive stretching of the neck during delivery. Another possible cause is trauma from ligation of a patent ductus arteriosus (Davis et al, 1988). Right-sided vocal cord paralysis has been reported as a complication of extracorporeal membrane oxygenation (ECMO) (Schumacher et al, 1989), presumably as a result of the surgical dissection for insertion of the catheters. Stridor may be less if the infant lies on the paralyzed side, when the affected cord can fall away from the midline (Cotton and Richardson, 1981). The condition tends to improve over a period of several weeks or months. Generally, medialization of the vocal cord is not recommended in neonates under 6 months of age, with tracheostomy preferred in severe cases of respiratory obstruction (Parikh, 2004).

Bilateral cord paralysis is a much more serious condition, accompanied by high-pitched inspiratory stridor; frequently, however, the cry is normal. Usually, severe central nervous system problems are to blame, such as hypoxic-ischemic encephalopathy, cerebral hemorrhage, Arnold-Chiari malformation, hydrocephalus, or brainstem dysgenesis. Associated problems may include pharyngeal incoordination with swallowing difficulty and esophageal dysfunction, recurrent apnea episodes, and tracheal aspiration of mucous secretions and formula. The stridor may resolve slowly if brain swelling subsides after birth, as is the case with ventriculoperitoneal shunt placement. The diagnosis may be suspected at laryngoscopy but should be confirmed by flexible fiberoptic bronchoscopy, rigid bronchoscopy, or ultrafast cine CT scan. Tracheostomy frequently is required (Smith and Catlin, 1984), and the prognosis usually is poor secondary to the underlying problems.

Laryngeal Atresia

Laryngeal atresia is the result of failed recanalization of the larynx during embryologic development, resulting in a newborn with complete laryngeal obstruction presenting with severe respiratory distress. In some cases the larynx may be completely obstructed by a laryngeal web, seen in the delivery room during attempts to intubate the cyanotic infant. An endotracheal tube sometimes can be forced beyond the obstruction into the trachea. Otherwise, a large-bore needle should be inserted percutaneously into the trachea to maintain marginal gas exchange while preparations for emergency tracheostomy are made. Most infants with laryngeal atresia have other lethal malformations (Smith and Catlin, 1984). Most cases are now diagnosed prenatally from ultrasound findings consistent with congenital high airway obstruction syndrome (CHAOS), such as polyhydramnios and enlarged hyperechoic lungs with an associated flattened or inverted diaphragm (Hedrick et al, 1994; Kalache et al, 1997). The mother may be evaluated for ascites or hydrops fetalis due to impaired venous return to the heart; the amniotic fluid lecithin may be very low in such cases. In the absence of other lethal malformations, the characteristic ultrasound diagnosis may permit preparations for emergency tracheostomy after delivery of the infant or an ex-utero intrapartum treatment (EXIT)-to-airway procedure, discussed later. Survivors of fetal intervention for CHAOS have now been seen (Hirose et al, 2004).

CONGENITAL SUBGLOTTIC STENOSIS

Congenital subglottic stenosis, manifesting as inspiratory stridor from birth, is caused by partial obstruction of the cricoid. In a full-term infant the normal subglottic lumen is 4.5 to 5.5 mm in diameter, whereas that of a preterm neonate is 3.5 mm in diameter. A subglottic diameter of 4 mm or less in a full-term infant or 3 mm or less in a premature infant is consistent with a diagnosis of subglottic stenosis. Subglottic stenosis is diagnosed by direct laryngoscopy supplemented with rigid bronchoscopy and chest radiography to evaluate other airway lesions and/or concomitant lung disease, as the latter may be common in the premature infant. Treatment consists of dilation or endoscopic lysis with a carbon dioxide laser in cases of membranous stenosis. However, most cases severe enough to require intervention are cartilaginous and require an anterior cricoid split, obviating the need for and complications of tracheostomy in most cases (Cotton and Seid, 1980; Schroeder and Holinger, 2008; Smith and Catlin, 1984).

Congenital Subglottic Hemangioma

Subglottic hemangioma, often occurring in association with cutaneous hemangioma, may cause inspiratory stridor and expiratory wheezing that progress with enlargement of the tumor (Cotton and Richardson, 1981). The presence of a cutaneous hemangioma in the facial beard distribution is often associated with a subglottic hemangioma (Orlow et al, 1997). This diagnosis is suspected when asymmetric subglottic narrowing is seen on plain radiographs and is confirmed by flexible and rigid endoscopy demonstrating a sessile vascular lesion, most commonly in the posterolateral subglottis (Ahmad and Soliman, 2007; Rahbar et al, 2004). Although some practitioners have advocated high-dose corticosteroid therapy (Brown et al, 1972) and others have tried intralesional injections of steroids, in many cases intubation or tracheostomy is eventually required. Results of removal by carbon dioxide or potassium-titanyl-phosphate laser have been encouraging, enabling treatment without tracheostomy; however, associated complications such as subglottic stenosis have been reported (Ahmad and Soliman, 2007; Healy et al, 1984; Kacker et al, 2001).

Laryngotracheoesophageal Cleft (Congenital Laryngeal Cleft)

In laryngotracheoesophageal cleft, a longitudinal communication is present between the airway and the esophagus, stretching from the larynx into the upper trachea or sometimes as far as the carina. This rare condition is reported in 1 in 10,000 to 1 in 20,000 births and is caused by an interruption in the cephalic advancement of the tracheoesophageal septum, which prevents the proper fusion of the posterior cricoid lamina (Pezzettigotta et al, 2008). Affected infants have respiratory distress with inspiratory stridor and cyanosis, associated with tracheal aspiration of saliva and feedings. The chest radiograph may show evidence of aspiration pneumonia, and the cine esophagogram shows contrast material spilling into the trachea. The diagnosis can be established with direct laryngoscopy and bronchoscopy. Given the high association with other congenital anomalies and syndromes, such as tracheal atresia, tracheoesophageal fistula, and Opitz-Frias syndrome, a thorough evaluation of all organ systems and genetic karyotype are recommended.

Laryngotracheoesophageal clefts are classified by severity of symptoms into four groups (types I–IV), which are used to determine the management strategy and the need for surgical intervention. For all types, initial management involves adequately securing the airway with an endotracheal tube or tracheostomy (Richardson and Cotton, 1984). Mild cases can sometimes be managed by conservative therapy, including swallow rehabilitation and antireflux medication; otherwise, endoscopic surgery may be necessary for refractory type I and type II clefts (Pezzettigotta et al, 2008). More severe cases requiring extensive reconstruction may require employing an anterior translaryngotracheal approach or even a partial upper sternotomy. Despite these reconstruction attempts, mortality remains high, at nearly 50% among all types of clefts and higher in cases with associated congenital anomalies and type IV clefts (Myer et al, 1990; Roth et al, 1983; Simpson et al, 1996).

TRACHEAL DEFORMITIES AND OTHER TRACHEAL DISORDERS

Tracheal Agenesis

In the rare condition of tracheal agenesis, the trachea is either atretic just below the vocal cords or absent all the way down to the carina (Altman et al, 1972). Clinical manifestations include severe distress, absence of vocal sound, and severe cyanosis. Prenatal presentation may manifest as

CHAOS, and EXIT may allow survival in severe cases (Vaikunth et al, 2009). Affected infants usually have a tracheoesophageal fistula as well as severe cardiac malformations, lung lobation defects, and sometimes renal and anal anomalies. Despite the presence of a larynx, intubation cannot be accomplished at delivery; however, if the tracheal tube is positioned in the esophagus and connected to a mechanical ventilator, reasonable gas exchange can be obtained via the tracheoesophageal fistula (Sandu and Monnier, 2007). When the tracheal atresia is high, a tracheostomy can be done. If survival seems possible, gastric division and a gastrostomy for feeding should be performed. Reconstructive surgery is not likely to be successful, however, and the prognosis is extremely poor, if not because of poor ventilation, then because of the underlying malformations.

Congenital Tracheal Stenosis

In congenital tracheal stenosis, a segment of the trachea is narrowed, usually starting in the subglottic region. The affected segment may be short or long; occasionally, the entire trachea is hypoplastic, and the bronchi may be involved. The narrowing is caused by complete or nearly complete tracheal cartilage rings. The patient may have inspiratory stridor, expiratory wheezing, and often cyanotic episodes. Mild inflammation and small mucous plugs may cause life-threatening deterioration. In many cases, other congenital malformations are also present, such as vascular ring anomalies, congenital heart defects, tracheoesophageal fistula (especially the H type), and hemivertebrae (Benjamin et al, 1981); there also is an association with pulmonary agenesis (Voland et al, 1986). A series of cases without accompanying defects has been reported in premature infants who presented with difficulties at tracheal intubation (Hauft et al, 1988).

Patients with this deformity usually can be intubated, but the endotracheal tube cannot be advanced and should not be forced. Mechanical ventilation with generous levels of positive end-expiratory pressure (PEEP) may help stabilize the infant. Tracheostomy is not indicated and interferes with making the diagnosis (Nakayama et al, 1982). Sometimes the diagnosis can be made by chest radiographs, using air as the contrast medium, with inspiration and expiration films. Investigators have described a high-kilovoltage technique, the so-called lateral airways xeroradiogram (Benjamin, 1980). Fluoroscopy often is useful (Lobe et al, 1987). Either flexible fiberoptic bronchoscopy in the NICU or rigid bronchoscopy in the operating room is usually required. Because it is important to examine the lower limits of the stenosis, it may be necessary to proceed with tracheobronchography, but this may sometimes cause acute decompensation (Loeff et al, 1988). Today, ultrafast cine CT scan has become a useful diagnostic technique to define the lower limits of the stenosis (Galvin et al, 1994).

In most cases, the stenosis requires treatment of some kind in the operating room. Balloon dilation alone is not likely to be successful in the case of a complete tracheal cartilage ring, because cartilage cannot be stretched. For short-segment stenosis, balloon dilation with laser may be used: at rigid bronchoscopy, the cartilage ring is split at the midline posterior aspect using the KTP laser, and the bronchoscope is advanced with the aid of serial balloon dilations

(Othersen et al 2000). For longer-segment stenosis, Longaker et al (1990) described segmental resection of the stenosis with end-to-end anastomosis to shorten the trachea, followed by serial balloon dilations through a rigid bronchoscope. Backer et al, described the successful use of free autografts of resected trachea for this type of tracheoplasty. However, for long-segment stenosis, slide tracheoplasty has become the standard treatment (Lipshutz et al, 2000). In this procedure, the stenosis is transected in the middle, the upper segment is incised longitudinally along the anterior aspect, the lower segment is incised longitudinally at the posterior aspect, the incised segments are slid over one another, and the edges are anastomosed, effectively shortening the trachea while widening the narrowed lumen.

The use of cardiopulmonary bypass has improved treatment and is advocated by some as averting the need for complex anesthesiology techniques (Loeff et al, 1988). After midline sternotomy, tracheal resection, and tracheoplasty with shortening of the trachea, the patient may need fixation in a brace for at least 6 weeks to maintain neck flexion and prevent excessive stretching of the anastomosis (Nakayama et al, 1982). Premature infants with congenital tracheal stenosis cannot undergo tracheal resection and tracheoplasty with cardiopulmonary bypass procedures. For these patients, aggressive balloon dilations are recommended, with splitting of the weaker posterior aspect of the tracheal rings (Messineo et al, 1992).

Tracheobronchomalacia (Tracheomalacia)

Tracheobronchomalacia, or the delayed development of tracheal cartilage, is rare and results in an excessively compliant trachea. This condition may be primary or associated with tracheoesophageal fistula, bronchopulmonary dysplasia, extrinsic tracheal compression, or prolonged intubation (Sotomayor et al, 1986). Tracheobronchomalacia should be suspected in infants presenting with respiratory distress, cyanotic spells, or persistent respiratory symptoms including expiratory stridor, persistent or recurrent wet cough, or recurrent respiratory infections (Masters, 2009). Chest radiograph shows diffuse overinflation, and the abnormalities of the trachea can be well demonstrated with ultrafast cine-CT scan (Galvin et al, 1994; Kimura et al, 1990), which provides a particularly good assessment of the peripheral extent of the lesion. At bronchoscopy, the anterior and posterior walls of the trachea are approximated during expiration (Saltzberg, 1983). The bronchoscope may support the walls of the trachea, alleviating the respiratory distress by passage of the bronchoscope to the carina, but potentially disguising the extent of the abnormalities.

Downing and Kilbride (1995) found that the factors associated with the development of tracheomalacia were immaturity, higher mean airway pressure, and prolonged mechanical ventilation. Affected infants may have significant dynamic compression of the trachea. Because the trachea of premature infants is very compliant and may be excessively stretched and injured during mechanical ventilation, very immature infants are particularly prone to tracheomalacia. Some premature infants have greatly enlarged tracheas or tracheomegaly after mechanical ventilation (Bhutani et al, 1986).

Many infants with tracheomalacia spontaneously improve by 1 to 2 years of age, when the cartilage has become strong enough to support tracheal patency (Sandu and Monnier, 2007). Severe cases typically necessitate tracheostomy with an elongated tracheostomy tube. However, current treatments for milder cases include tracheal intubation with continuous positive airway pressure (CPAP) or PEEP, which prevents tracheal collapse, and aortopexy (fixation of the aorta to the sternum), which has the effect of supporting the attached trachea (Bullard et al, 1997; Filler et al, 1992; Jacobs et al, 1994; Wiseman et al, 1985). Many of the most severely affected patients respond well to aortopexy (McCoy et al, 1992).

Tracheal Compression by Vascular Rings

Tracheal compression can be caused by several factors: (1) a double aortic arch, (2) a right aortic arch, (3) a left-sided origin of the (right) innominate artery, (4) a right-sided origin of the left common carotid artery, or (5) an anomalous origin of the left pulmonary artery from the right pulmonary artery (Hendren and Kim, 1978). With a right aortic arch, the trachea is compressed by the main pulmonary trunk, aortic arch, and ligamentum arteriosus. The anomalous innominate or common carotid arteries form a tight crotch, which impinges on the anterior trachea. The anomalous left pulmonary artery returns to the left by passing between the esophagus and the trachea, compressing the trachea between the right and the left pulmonary arteries. Infants with tracheal compression have inspiratory stridor and expiratory wheezing with symptoms usually appearing later in the neonatal period. Affected infants often lie with the head and neck hyperextended to stretch the trachea and make it less compressible. If the esophagus is compressed, feeding is associated with regurgitation.

There are several methods of diagnosis. The chest radiograph may show mild overinflation, a right-sided aorta, and, with appropriate technique, evidence of tracheal narrowing. A barium swallow examination may show indentation of the esophagus. Bronchoscopy should reveal a pulsatile mass at the carina. MRI has proved to be accurate in defining most vascular malformations compressing the airway (Simoneaux et al, 1995), with echocardiography regarded as less reliable in this situation (Rimell, 1997). Recently, it was demonstrated that prenatal diagnosis by ultrasound avoided unnecessary delays in the repair of symptomatic vascular rings and that repair on identification of symptoms prevented the development of secondary tracheobronchomalacia (Tuo et al, 2009). After surgical division of the vascular ring, the respiratory distress may persist for weeks or longer because of localized tracheal deformity (either stenosis or tracheomalacia), emphasizing the need for immediate repair on diagnosis. In cases of isolated vascular rings, repair provides cure with minimal postoperative complications (Ruzmetov et al, 2009).

Tracheal Compression by Extrinsic Masses

The trachea may also be compressed by a bronchogenic cyst, an enteric duplication cyst, a thoracic neurogenic tumor, or a mediastinal teratoma (Benjamin, 1980). These may be demonstrated by anteroposterior and lateral chest

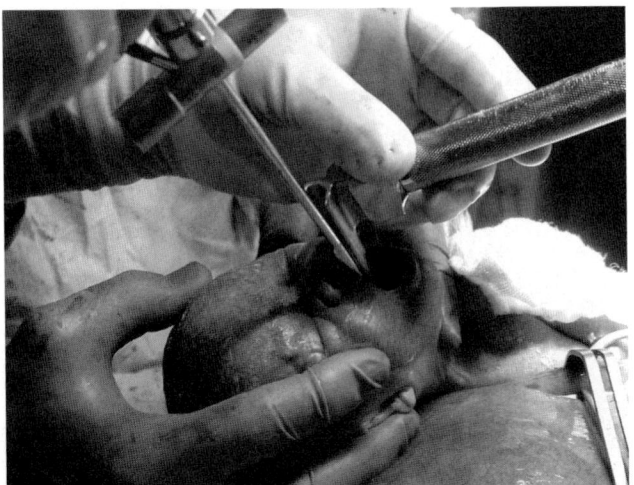

FIGURE 49-1 Direct laryngoscopy, bronchoscopy, and esophagoscopy are performed during an EXIT procedure. Using these methods, airway obstruction can be overcome and endotracheal intubation can be performed. *(From Hirose S, Farmer DL, Lee H, et al: The ex utero intrapartum treatment procedure: looking back at the EXIT, J Pediatr Surg 39:375-380; discussion 375-380, 2004.)*

films and are especially apparent on CT scan. Such masses may also compress the esophagus and can be demonstrated with a barium swallow.

Congenital High Airway Obstruction Syndrome and the Ex-Utero Intrapartum Treatment Procedure

CHAOS actually describes a spectrum of rare anomalies, including laryngeal web, laryngeal atresia, laryngeal cyst, and tracheal atresia or stenosis. Most cases are sporadic with the true incidence unknown, and thus the natural history of this disease is not well known. CHAOS is characterized by enlarged lungs, dilated distal airway, everted diaphragm, ascites, and, ultimately, nonimmune hydrops fetalis. Prenatal diagnosis is becoming more common with the progress of ultrasound and MRI techniques. The exact nature of the airway obstruction may not be entirely clear, however, and the time required to establish a safe airway soon enough after delivery carries various risks, including anoxic brain injury.

As with any anomaly that causes either direct respiratory airway obstruction or airway compression by means of mass effect, CHAOS poses a difficult problem for the clinical team during delivery. The EXIT procedure was developed as a solution to this problem: By preserving fetoplacental circulation throughout a scheduled cesarean section delivery, a safe fetal airway can be established before umbilical cord ligation (Figure 49-1) (Harrison et al, 1996; Hirose et al, 2004). Infants with CHAOS still require postnatal airway reconstruction after delivery, but once a tracheostomy is in place, laryngeal or tracheal reconstruction is essentially an elective procedure and can be performed once the patient's overall status is optimized (Hirose et al, 2004). The rate of live births seen with the EXIT procedure has been promising, although long-term outcomes have yet to be assessed (Abraham et al, 2010).

DISORDERS OF THE MEDIASTINUM

In the posterior mediastinal space, thoracic neuroblastomas and neurenteric duplication cysts are most commonly encountered in the newborn. Bronchogenic cysts occur in the middle mediastinal space. An enlarged thymus and a mediastinal teratoma are the masses most often seen in the anterior mediastinum.

Thymus

The thymus occupies the upper anterior mediastinum, and it is more prominent in the newborn period than at any other time of life. It may be so large as to reach the diaphragm or obscure both cardiac borders on radiographs. The normal thymus can be distinguished from an abnormal mass by the absence of tracheal deviation or compression. The thymus changes in position with respiration and is less prominent with deep inspiration. It also involutes with stress as well as with corticosteroid therapy. Absence of the thymic shadow in an infant should alert the clinician to the possibility of severe combined immune deficiency syndrome (SCIDS) or DiGeorge syndrome with hypocalcemia and cardiac anomalies.

The cardiothymic-to-thoracic ratio provides an index of thymic size. The shadow of the enlarged thymus is the most common radiopaque mass visualized in the anterior mediastinum of the newborn. The enlarged thymus causes little if any trouble in the neonatal period. Fletcher and associates, as well as Gewolb et al, (1979) noted that a large thymus is present on the first day of life in infants at risk for hyaline membrane disease, presumably because of less-than-normal levels of glucocorticoids before birth (Fletcher et al, 1979).

Congenital Mediastinal Teratoma

Mediastinal teratomas rarely cause symptoms in the newborn infant. However, when an anterior mediastinal mass is associated with respiratory distress in the newborn, the strong likelihood is that the lesion is a mediastinal teratoma. These teratomas are invariably not malignant, and surgical resection is sufficient treatment. Mogilner et al (1992) described a newborn with severe respiratory distress and tracheal compression who underwent emergency thoracotomy and mediastinal teratoma resection. Another infant had emergency resection for respiratory distress but died with poor cardiac function; as in that case, the tumor may be large enough to cause underdevelopment of the heart with severe circulatory insufficiency (Thambi Dorai et al, 1998). In other cases, the tumor may cause mild lung hypoplasia.

Congenital Bronchogenic Cysts

Bronchogenic cysts arise from the foregut and are usually extrapulmonary, located in the mediastinum (just above the tracheal bifurcation), pericardium, abdomen and neck (Langston and Thurlbeck, 1986; Winters and Effmann, 2001; Winters et al, 1997). The minority of bronchogenic cysts are found within the lung, and some pathologists believe that these may not be distinct from

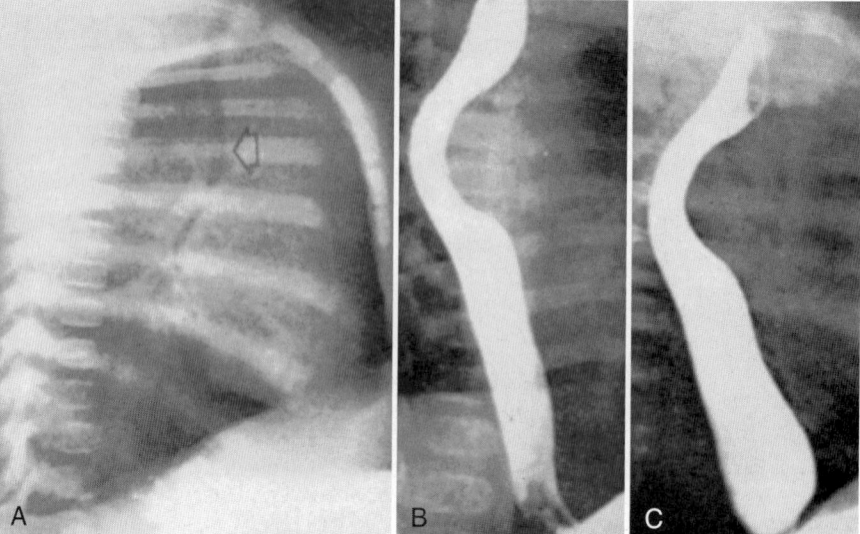

FIGURE 49-2 A, The lateral film shows the trachea displaced anteriorly. **B,** The anteroposterior film shows the barium-filled esophagus displaced to the right. **C,** Another lateral film shows the barium-filled esophagus displaced posteriorly. *(From Hope JW, Koop CE: Differential diagnosis of mediastinal masses,* Pediatr Clin North Am *3:379, 1959.)*

intralobar sequestrations or CCAM Type 1 (Stocker, 2009). Bronchogenic cysts can be seen on prenatal ultrasound, although they are more likely to present later as they increase in size over time, with airway compression, recurrent infection, hemoptysis, or pneumothorax (Langston, 2003). Intrauterine airway compression can result in congenital lobar emphysema (CLE; see later discussion). Lesions are filled with fluid and debris, and they can be appreciated by esophagram if external compression is present, or CT scan, with criteria developed to distinguish these cysts from other mediastinal masses (Winters and Effmann, 2001). The diagnosis is made histologically, after resection, with the cyst wall lined by respiratory epithelium and a fibromuscular layer that may contain glands, resembling a bronchus (Stocker, 2009).

In the newborn, bronchogenic cysts are encountered infrequently; most do not come to the attention of the practitioner until later in infancy or childhood. Bronchogenic cysts seldom attain a large size. They contain clear fluid, they are lined with columnar or cuboidal epithelium, and their walls generally contain smooth muscle and cartilage, the latter indicating their bronchial origin. These cysts lie near the carina in the middle mediastinal space. They produce lung overdistention or atelectasis, depending on whether airway obstruction is complete or partial, and this is accompanied by respiratory distress in the newborn infant. Opsahl and Berman reported a case that showed overinflation on the left followed by clearing and then similar overinflation on the right (Opsahl and Berman, 1962). Radiographic examination often shows a mass lesion at or just above the carina, and displacing the lower trachea forward (Figure 49-2, *A*). Ultrasonography may help localize the lesion more accurately. The barium swallow examination may reveal indentation of the esophagus, the cyst pushing it backward at the level of the carina (Figure 49-2, *B* and *C*). Bronchoscopy reveals compression of the trachea and sometimes of one major bronchus, usually from the posterior aspect. Sometimes the bronchogenic cyst may communicate with the airway and contain air. In the immediate newborn period, there may be retention

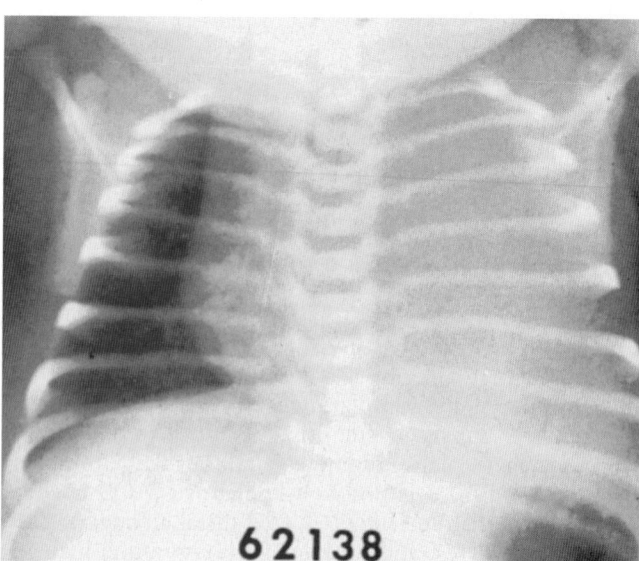

62138

FIGURE 49-3 The left lung shows delayed clearance of lung liquid, associated with bronchial obstruction by a bronchogenic cyst. *(From Griscom NT, Harris GBC, Wohl MEB, et al: Fluid filled lung due to airway obstruction in the newborn,* Pediatrics *43:383, 1969.)*

of fetal lung fluid in the lung compromised by the bronchogenic cyst; the fluid may take days to be cleared. This phenomenon produces a characteristic appearance on the chest radiograph (Figure 49-3). Treatment for bronchogenic cyst consists of early surgical excision, with uniformly good results.

Neurenteric Duplication Cysts

These mediastinal cysts may be derived from the esophagus, stomach, or small bowel, so they may also be called enterogenous cysts. Although they are not encountered frequently, they are far from uncommon in the newborn. They are duplicated segments of the foregut that have become partially or completely detached from the parent viscus. They lie in the posterior mediastinum but with

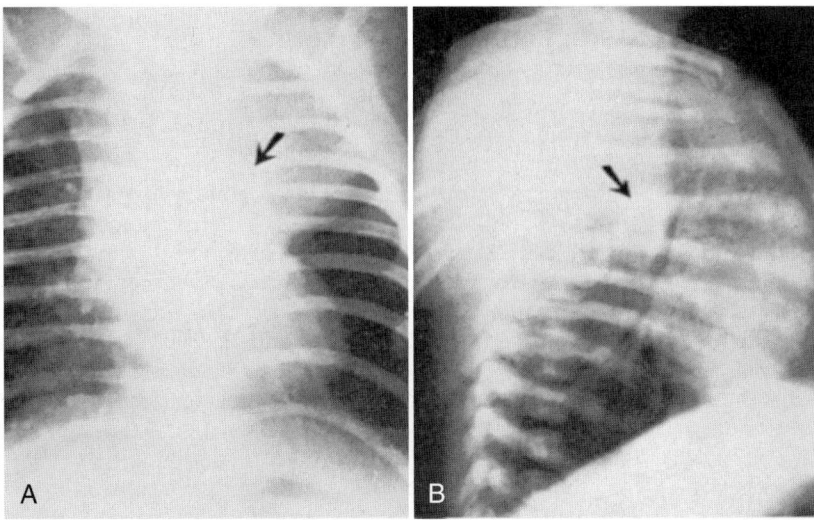

FIGURE 49-4 Congenital thoracic neuroblastoma. The mass is in the left upper hemithorax **(A)** and in the posterior mediastinum **(B)**. *(From Hope JW, Koop CE: Differential diagnosis of mediastinal masses,* Pediatr Clin North Am *6:379, 1959.)*

increasing size may project far into one or the other hemithorax. Their walls are composed of a mucosal layer, characteristic of their site of origin, and one or more muscular layers. They contain secreted fluid that is the same as that of their parent viscus; the fluid in a gastrogenic cyst contains pepsin and hydrochloric acid in the same concentration as in gastric juice.

The foregut becomes duplicated in the course of embryonic development by failure of complete resorption of primitive occluding epithelium, resulting in the formation of a supernumerary wall and eventually a separate lumen and cyst. The high percentage of vertebral anomalies associated with neurenteric duplication cysts led Veeneklaas to suggest that the primary embryonic defect lies in abnormal persistence of the primitive foregut adherence to the notochord (Veeneklaas, 1952). When the foregut descends from its early position in the neck, this adhesion causes anomalies of the vertebral bodies derived from the notochord. This adhesion also breaks off the duplicated portion of the foregut and prevents its complete descent into the thorax and abdomen along with the mature foregut.

Clinical signs depend on the size and location of the duplication cyst. Because all of these cysts are posterior and lie close to the trachea, esophagus, and great vessels, they are seldom present without signs of abnormality. Cyanosis, tachypnea, and dyspnea often are present from birth. Swallowing difficulty and vomiting are less frequent. Recurrent lower respiratory tract infections are findings in a few older infants with such cysts. Frank hemorrhage from the lungs or stomach, or in the form of melena, is not at all uncommon. In most instances, hemorrhage indicates that the cyst is of gastrogenic origin, with peptic acid erosion into the trachea or esophagus. Technetium scans are useful for delineating cysts lined with gastric mucosa. Radiographs of the chest show abnormal densities that are often difficult to distinguish from unusual cardiac contours. The barium swallow examination commonly shows displacement of the esophagus, usually forward because the mass is in the posterior mediastinum. The cyst may partially or totally compress the bronchus, with consequent lung overdistention or atelectasis. Sometimes the symptoms are intermittent as the cyst enlarges or empties. Bronchoscopy

may show compression of the trachea or bronchus from without, usually from the posterior aspect. Superina et al (1984) reviewed 25 years of experience with neurenteric duplication cysts; they noted that a spinal component may accompany the mediastinal cyst in as much as 20% of the children. They recommended careful radiographic evaluation of the spinal canal with CT scan and then excision of the intraspinal cyst, if possible, before the onset of neurologic signs in later childhood. The MRI scan may give improved delineation of intraspinal cysts (Azzie and Beasley, 2003). Operative resection is indicated as soon as the diagnosis of mediastinal mass is made. It is neither necessary nor wise to delay exploration, because all intrathoracic masses will eventually become symptomatic.

Congenital Thoracic Neuroblastoma

Neuroblastoma, the most common solid tumor in the mediastinum of infants, arises from sympathetic neural tissue along the vertebral column and is therefore located in the posterior mediastinum. It may extend into both lungs, causing respiratory distress, and it may extend into the spinal canal, later causing neurologic signs. The chest mass may be obvious on routine radiographs obtained for unrelated reasons in the newborn (Figure 49-4), or on chest radiographs taken to evaluate significant respiratory distress (Li et al, 2001). In older infants the diagnosis may follow chest radiography for lower respiratory tract infection, or radiographs may be taken to investigate dyspnea with physical signs of a solid intrathoracic mass. In some cases the tumor mass shows calcification, well visualized with the CT scan. A thoracic neuroblastoma may sometimes be found on fetal ultrasound examination (Moppett et al, 1999).

Differentiation from other posterior mediastinal masses may be impossible before exploration; neuroblastoma is not likely to be so sharply demarcated as a neurenteric duplication cyst. Invasion of neighboring lung parenchyma strongly supports a diagnosis of neuroblastoma. The MRI scan is superior to the CT scan for discerning spread to lymph nodes, spinal canal, and chest wall (Slovis et al, 1997), and also for discerning liver metastases. Elevations of urinary vanillylmandelic acid and homovanillylic acid may be present, but this finding is less common in the newborn, and its absence does not rule out neuroblastoma. If the patient has systemic hypertension, plasma levels of epinephrine, norepinephrine, and dopamine may be elevated, but this has not been reported in a thoracic neuroblastoma. Also, results of assays for various clinical biologic markers may be positive; for example, serum ferritin and serum lactate dehydrogenase may be elevated, but this is not usual in the newborn. A bone marrow aspirate should be obtained for cytologic evaluation, and a nuclear bone scan should be performed to exclude the possible remote spread of metastases. A number of cytogenetic biologic markers may be detected in the excised tumor tissue (e.g., cellular DNA ditetraploidy, increased N-*myc* oncogene copy number); these usually indicate malignancy in older children (Ladenstein et al, 2001), but again, they are commonly negative in the newborn.

Surgical exploration is indicated for any intrathoracic mass. If the tumor proves to be a neuroblastoma, as much of it should be excised as is feasible. The tumor should be staged by histologic examination according to the system of Evans et al (1971) and subsequent therapy should be dictated by the stage. In general, chemotherapy is not indicated unless distant metastases are present.

The outlook for neuroblastomas in extra-adrenal locations is better than that for their adrenal counterparts (Young et al, 1970). The outlook for neuroblastomas manifesting in the first year of life also is good. Many of these tumors are cystic in nature, and the histologic examination suggests that the neuroblasts are arranged in clumps rather than in sheets; this "neuroblastoma in situ" feature carries a high likelihood of spontaneous regression and therefore a good prognosis. Most neuroblastomas in the newborn are Evans stage A, with a good outlook. So-called stage D (S) also is quite common (Moppett et al, 1999); although there are metastases to the liver, marrow, or skin, the prognosis is still good because metastases to the bone are rare. The clinical markers are seldom elevated, and results of assays for the cytogenetic markers are seldom positive, all of which indicate a reasonable outlook. If the lesion can be completely removed and no bone metastases are found, then most infants survive. Some clinicians suggested that the chance of spontaneous regression is so high in the newborn that even surgery may not be necessary (Li et al, 2001; Morgan, 1995). However, intraspinal spread may occur, in which case the later clinical course is more troublesome, with paraparesis and neurogenic bladder (Moppett et al, 1999); most authors consider surgery to be advisable.

DISORDERS OF THE CHEST WALL

Abnormalities of the bone and muscle of the chest wall may be a mechanical hindrance to ventilation.

SKELETAL DISORDERS

Although abnormalities involving bone are rare, they may be recognized immediately and are sometimes amenable to operative correction.

Defects of Sternal Fusion

Defects in fusion of the sternum are uncommon. Complete separation of the two halves of the sternum allows protrusion of cardiovascular structures, a condition known as *ectopia cordis* (Maier and Bortone, 1949). Lethal malformations of the heart are commonly associated with this condition. Upper sternal clefts are more common. Early operation is advised to shield the underlying structures from injury, and because of the greater ease of approximating the separated parts in the first days of life compared with later (Sabiston, 1958). A lower sternal cleft and ectopia cordis with a congenital heart defect may be associated with congenital apertures in the upper abdominal wall, in the pericardium, and in the anterior diaphragm, with a Morgagni-type diaphragmatic hernia, the so-called pentalogy of Cantrell (Cantrell et al, 1958).

Pectus Excavatum

The most common of the sternal defects is pectus excavatum, sometimes associated with Pierre Robin syndrome or Marfan syndrome. Rarely is it a fixed or severe deformity until several months of postnatal age. A family history of some type of anterior thoracic deformity was found in 37% to 43% of patients (Nuss et al, 1998; Shamberger et al, 1988). The heart may be compressed between the sternum and the vertebral column and displaced to the left, impinging on the space of the left lung. There is usually no respiratory or cardiac distress. Only later in childhood may there be cosmetic and psychological distress sufficient to warrant intervention. Although routine chest radiographs may suffice in evaluating the severity of chest wall deformity, chest CT is typically preferred because this modality provides the bony and cartilaginous anatomic details as well as any information regarding cardiac compression necessary when considering surgical intervention. Using chest CT allows one to calculate the Haller index (HI), or the ratio of the transverse distance to the anteroposterior distance. A normal HI is about 2.5, and most cases of pectus excavatum that qualify for operative correction are greater than 3.25 (Haller et al, 1987). However, the indications for operative correction are debatable. Those with severe cardiac or pulmonary compression, abnormal cardiac or pulmonary function studies, or failed previous repairs are candidates for repair. Periodic evaluation of cardiovascular status with echocardiogram and electrocardiography in addition to assessment of pulmonary function are appropriate in the presence of progressive deformity. In our opinion, correction should not be undertaken until the child is several years of age and then only in those few children in whom the deformity appears to be progressing. Serial photographs are the best way to document changes in pectus excavatum. Results of both minimally invasive and open operative correction are excellent in the majority of patients; surgery is almost always associated with improved self-image and perceived functional activity (Fonkalsrud, 2009; Kelly et al, 2008; Nuss, 2008). Recurrences are possible during later active growth.

Poland Syndrome

Hypoplasia or absence of the pectoral muscles, typically only on one side, is termed Poland syndrome and may be associated with cartilage agenesis of the second through fifth ribs on the ipsilateral side—the ribs of attachment for the pectoralis major muscle. There may be associated syndactyly, hemivertebrae, scoliosis, and hypoplasia of the breast and nipple (Urschel, 2009). Breathing may be paradoxical and the cardiac impulse easily observed through the soft tissues, but there is rarely any severe respiratory distress that would necessitate emergent intervention. Later in childhood, and uncommonly, there may be increasing respiratory symptoms with scoliosis-related lung disease and/or heart failure. No operative intervention is required in infancy, although mammoplasty may be desirable later on in affected girls after puberty.

Thoracic Dystrophies
Asphyxiating Thoracic Dystrophy (Jeune's Syndrome)

A rare deformity of the thoracic cage in approximately 1 in 100,000 to 130,000 live births, asphyxiating thoracic dystrophy is an autosomal recessive chondrodystrophy, associated with short-limbed dwarfism and often polydactyly (Figure 49-5). It was first described by Jeune et al (1955). The ribs are horizontal, hypoplastic, and short, with flared costochondral junctions. The thorax is small, bell-shaped, and rigid; this results in displacement of the liver and spleen well into the abdominal cavity. Some degree of lung hypoplasia may be present, and if present is often severe and lethal (Phillips and van Aalst, 2008). The pelvis shows flaring of the iliac wings and acetabular abnormalities (Kohler and Babbitt, 1970). Prenatal diagnosis with ultrasonography is possible. Renal cystic dysplasia may be present, resulting in hypertension and renal failure. In the past, most patients with this condition did not survive the first month. Oberklaid et al (1977) studied 10 cases and noted that only two patients were alive at the time of the report. One of the two was in excellent health at 15 years of age. The more severely affected infants had respiratory distress from birth. Three patients have been described in one family; because it is an autosomal recessive trait, the expectation would be for an occurrence in one of four siblings, so mutations must be common. No parent-child occurrence has been described. Davis et al (2001) reported an operative technique for lateral thoracic expansion in 10 patients with chest wall deformities limiting thoracic capacity—including 8 patients with classic Jeune syndrome. Three were younger than 1 year of age at the time of surgery, and 6 were ventilator dependent. All of the infants older than 1 year of age at the time of surgery improved, with measured lung volumes increasing in 2 of 3 studied, and thoracic volumes by computed tomography increasing in 4 of 5 studied. The only deaths were in 2 infants younger than 1 year of age at the time of surgery, suggesting that lateral thoracic expansion is a safe and effective procedure for patients beyond the first year

of age. A vertical expandable prosthetic titanium rib (VEPTR) procedure has also been introduced for the purpose of progressive expansion of the chest cavity in thoracic insufficiency patients. However, long-term improvements in lung function specifically in patients with Jeune's syndrome have yet to be reported (Phillips and van Aalst, 2008).

Other Thoracic Dystrophies

Severe underdevelopment of the thoracic rib cage, accompanied usually by lethal pulmonary hypoplasia, may be seen in other conditions, such as the thanatophoric dwarfism syndrome, the short rib–polydactyly syndrome, and the camptomelic dwarfism syndrome. Affected infants do not survive for long after birth.

NEUROMUSCULAR DISORDERS

Other causes of thoracic dysfunction are diseases of the nerves and muscles, including congenital myasthenia gravis, congenital spinal muscular atrophy (Werdnig-Hoffmann disease), congenital myotonic dystrophy, glycogen storage disease, and congenital spinal injury. Such conditions are usually recognized in the context of the associated systemic muscular weakness. Newborns with myasthenia gravis have episodes of muscle weakness, poor feeding, weak cry, hypoventilation, and apnea with a positive response to an anticholinesterase medication. In congenital spinal muscular atrophy, there is lung hypoplasia associated with absent fetal breathing, and as a result the thorax is small. Other features include severe hypotonia, muscle fasciculation, respiratory failure, and early death; the inheritance is autosomal recessive. In congenital myotonic dystrophy, there is lung hypoplasia from absent fetal breathing; affected infants have respiratory distress at birth, rapidly need mechanical ventilation, and are soon ventilator dependent. Mothers of these infants have myotonia, difficulty in relaxing muscle contractions; the inheritance is autosomal dominant.

DISORDERS OF THE PLEURAL CAVITY

The pleural cavity lies between the parietal pleura, lining the chest wall, and the visceral pleura, lining the lung and other structures. The blood supply to both pleural surfaces is systemic. Venous drainage of the parietal pleura is to the systemic system and the visceral pleura to the pulmonary system. The pleural surfaces filter fluid into the pleural space and the pleural lymphatics then resorb fluid from the pleural cavity (Wiener-Kronish et al, 1985). This process is hindered in the setting of abnormal lymphatic development or abnormal systemic venous pressures (because the thoracic lymphatic system drains directly to the systemic veins), resulting in chylothorax. Chylothorax can also occur as a result of surgical disruption of the thoracic duct or in the setting of lymphatic malformations. Other causes of hydrothorax in the newborn include hydrops fetalis, transudate associated with congenital lung lesions or group B streptococcal pneumonia, empyema (usually associated with nosocomial pneumonia), or fluid extravasation from a displaced central venous catheter.

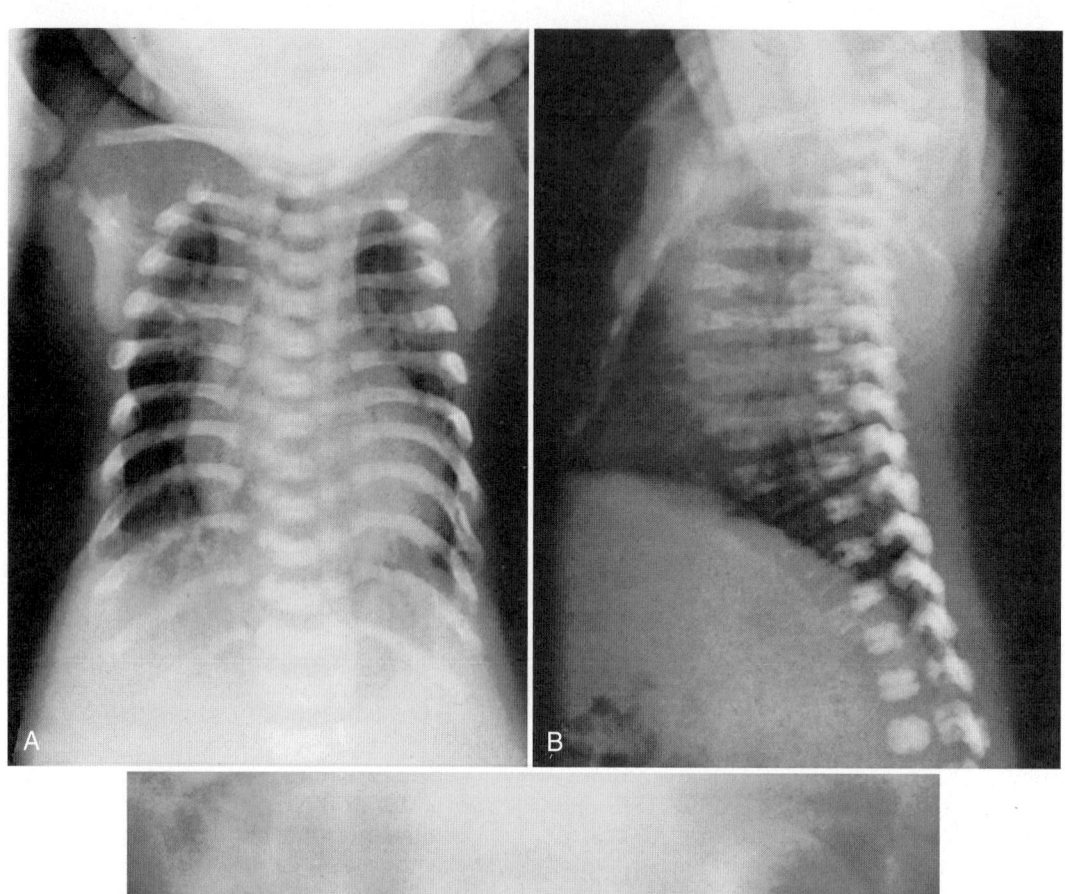

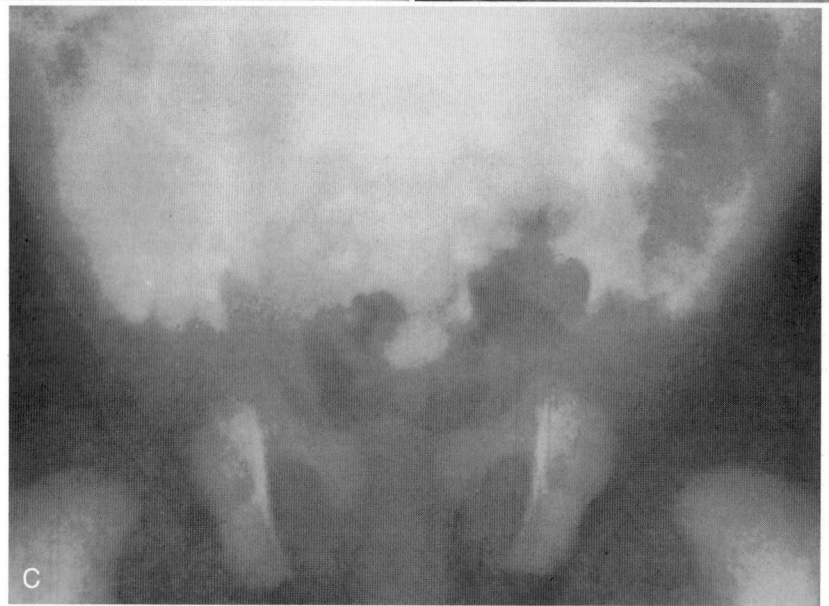

FIGURE 49-5 Radiographs from an infant with asphyxiating thoracic dystrophy. A and **B,** On anteroposterior and lateral views of the chest, the thoracic dimension is seen to be reduced in comparison with the abdominal dimension. **C,** Radiograph of the pelvis shows flaring of the iliac crests and bony protrusions of the acetabulae. *(A and **B,** Courtesy of Dr John Kirkpatrick; **C,** from Avery ME, Fletcher BD, Williams RG: The lung and its disorders in the newborn infant, ed 4, Philadelphia, 1981, WB Saunders.)*

CONGENITAL CHYLOTHORAX

The prenatal diagnosis of an isolated pleural effusion without an associated thoracic malformation or hydrops fetalis is most likely to be a chylothorax (or lymphatic effusion, because chyle cannot be present in the absence of fat-containing enteral feeds). A large fetal chylothorax may evert the diaphragm and can be the cause of hydrops fetalis, likely due to hypoproteinemia or impaired venous return in the setting of increased intrathoracic pressure. Fetal chylothorax portends a worse prognosis for survival

if it is bilateral or associated with hydrops, and prognosis is better if the effusion resolves without reaccumulation (Longaker et al, 1989). Large fetal chylothoraces can result in pulmonary hypoplasia. In utero intervention may be undertaken in cases of large or bilateral effusions, or hydrops, and may improve the chances of survival. These interventions include transabdominal thoracentesis (with ongoing ultrasound monitoring for fluid reaccumulation) and placement of an indwelling thoracoamniotic shunt (if the effusion reaccumulates), to allow continued drainage of fluid. Fetuses diagnosed with chylothorax should be evaluated for associated conditions that may affect their prognosis, including Down, Noonan, and Turner syndromes.

Newborns with congenital chylothorax often present with severe respiratory distress, requiring immediate respiratory support and urgent drainage of pleural fluid. Characteristics of chylous fluid include a high cell count with a lymphocytic predominance, a high triglyceride level (usually above serum levels, but not present unless enteral feeds initiated), and high protein content (Table 49-1). The introduction of small-volume fat-containing feeds with resultant elevated fluid triglyceride levels can confirm the diagnosis if biochemical indices are otherwise not confirmatory. A review of 39 cases of pediatric chylothorax revealed that the composition was consistent with previously described classic characteristics (Buttiker et al, 1999). Total cell counts were >1000/mm^3 in 92% of cases, and 85% of effusions had >90% lymphocytes (range 57% to 89% in 6 additional children). Fluid triglyceride levels were >1.1 mmol/L (98 mg/dL) in all but one case, with values ranging from 0.56 to 26.6 mmol/L (50 to 2358 mg/dL).

Management of Chylothorax

Neonatal management of chylothorax includes replacement of protein, clotting factors, and immunoglobulins as needed. Ongoing respiratory support may be needed, and often a chronic chest drain is required to decrease respiratory compromise. Feeds are usually restricted, either providing medium-chain triglycerides (MCT) only (because MCT are generally absorbed directly from the intestine without processing to chylomicrons) or a nonfat diet. If these measures fail, a period of total enteric rest is undertaken, with parenteral nutrition administered, until resolution of the chylous effusion. Some practitioners believe that a period of enteric rest is necessary to decrease strain on the lymphatic system, because lymphatic efflux from the intestine is an important component of thoracic lymph fluid. Once chest drainage has resolved, feeds are reintroduced with an MCT-only formula for 3 to 6 weeks before transitioning to a normal diet.

There are no controlled studies demonstrating that one strategy is superior to others to hasten resolution of chylothorax, and in one series, 50% of pediatric chylothoraces resolved with MCT-only diets (Le Coultre et al, 1991). A later series from the same institution had 80% (41 of 51)

resolution with conservative, nonoperative management (MCT-only diet or enteric rest) up to 4 weeks' duration (Beghetti et al, 2000). The primary risk of this approach is infection, because these children have prolonged hospitalizations with central venous access, chest drains, no enteral feeds, and protein and immunoglobulin losses. Eight of 51 children had severe infections in this series. Children who were less likely to have spontaneous resolution of chest drainage included patients with elevated central venous pressure who had more prolonged effusions and higher output than those with surgical injury. There were more frequent operative interventions in this group (6 of 14 children), which were undertaken only if 4 weeks of conservative therapy failed to decrease drainage to <10 mL/kg/d (Beghetti et al, 2000). In one series, 4 of 11 children with drainage after 4 weeks resolved their chylothorax by 6 weeks, with 2 of the remaining children too unstable to undergo surgical intervention (Buttiker et al, 1999). Operative interventions include thoracic duct ligation, pleurodesis, and/or placement of a pleuroperitoneal shunt. Most practitioners recommend about 4 weeks of conservative management, awaiting resolution of chylous drainage, because all interventions other than shunt placement require a thoracotomy. Effusions are unlikely to resolve after 6 weeks, and waiting too long for operative intervention may result in significant compromise to the child.

An adjunctive medical approach is the administration of somatostatin or its analogue, octreotide, to decrease pleural drainage. Somatostatin is delivered only via continuous infusion, whereas octreotide can also be given via intermittent subcutaneous injection, because of its longer half-life. The mechanism of effect is thought to be via decreased intestinal secretions and absorption, and therefore intestinal efflux and abdominal lymphatic return (Kalomenidis, 2006). Some practitioners proceed quickly to the use of these medications, believing they decrease the volume and duration of chest drainage compared to conservative management; however, this has not been studied in a controlled setting, so the efficacy and risks of this approach are unknown. Others use these medications once conservative measures have failed. Potential risks of therapy include hormonal effects of glucose instability and hypothyroidism and gastrointestinal effects such as cholelithiasis, hepatocellular injury, nausea, diarrhea, abdominal distention, and decreased intestinal perfusion. In this regard, a case of necrotizing enterocolitis in a newborn post repair of aortic coarctation was reported (Mohseni-Bod et al, 2004), as was a case of strangulation-ileus in an 18-month-old with asplenia syndrome (Matsuo et al, 2003). These serious side effects raise concerns, particularly regarding concomitant feeding during administration of the medications. Octreotide has been reported more commonly in newborns in case reports in the literature, in doses ranging from 7 to 240 µg/kg/d (Helin et al, 2006; Roehr et al, 2006). Dosing is either titrated up until chest drainage is minimal (typically starting at 3.5 µg/kg/h and advancing in several steps to 10 µg/kg/h), or started at the higher dose and titrated down once drainage has abated. The infusion is usually continued for several days after chest drainage is controlled, and then weaned off over several days. There are reports of recurrence after discontinuation of the medication

TABLE 49-1 Characteristics of Chylous Effusions

Characteristic	Description
Appearance	Clear yellow (milky with fat-containing feeds)
Cell count	>1000 cells/mm^3
Lymphocyte proportion	>80%
pH	7.4–7.8
Triglycerides	>110 mg/dL
Cholesterol	65–220 mg/dL
Albumin	1.2–4.1 g/dL
Total protein	2.2–5.9 g/dL

Adapted from Rocha G: Pleural effusions in the neonate, *Curr Opin Pulm Med* 13:305-311, 2007.

(Roehr et al, 2006). Octreotide has also been used in treatment of congenital chylothorax (Bulbul et al, 2009; Paget-Brown et al, 2006; Roehr et al, 2006). Monitoring of serum glucose, thyroid function, liver enzymes and indicators of cholestasis during therapy is recommended.

CONGENITAL THORACIC MASSES AND CYSTS

Fetal lung masses vary in the degree of abnormality of parenchyma and vasculature and likely represent a spectrum of developmental abnormalities, which may be difficult to distinguish antenatally (Ankermann et al, 2004; Langston 2003). In fact, some investigators have suggested classifying these lesions solely on the basis of the vascular supply (systemic vs. pulmonary) and whether or not lung structure is normal (Achiron et al, 2004), because the histology and likely the developmental pathways leading to the individual lesions are overlapping. Some level and degree of fetal airway obstruction has been implicated as the etiology of many of these lesions (Langston, 2003). In antenatal series, congenital cystic adenomatoid malformation of the lung (CCAM) is frequently the most common lesion reported (Achiron et al, 2004). However, in postnatal series, CCAM is often less common (with various imaging modalities and pathology available to clarify the diagnosis after birth), particularly when only cystic lesions are considered (Langston, 2003; Stocker, 2009; Winters and Effmann, 2001). There are multiple reports of "hybrid" lesions, with features of both CCAM and bronchopulmonary sequestration (BPS), emphasizing that these lesions constitute a spectrum of anomalies (Langston, 2003; Winters and Effmann, 2001).

Congenital Cystic Adenomatoid Malformation of the Lung

CCAMs develop from an overgrowth of lung tissue, extending from different levels of the airway. In general, they are unilateral. The lesions may communicate with the airways, allowing them to transition from being fluid-filled in utero to air-filled postnatally, but they do not contain normal alveoli. Stocker et al (1977) originally classified the lesions based on their cystic components, with lesions containing larger cysts demonstrating features consistent with a more proximal airway origin, microcystic lesions demonstrating features consistent with an intraacinar origin, and intermediate cysts demonstrating features consistent with origin from the bronchiole. Subsequent revisions of this classification have included less common proximal and distal lesions and have suggested new nomenclature based on the fact that not all lesions are either adenomatoid or cystic. The term congenital pulmonary airway malformation (CPAM) has been proposed by Stocker (2002), and others have suggested variable, more descriptive terminology which includes both the pulmonary airway malformations and other congenital chest lesions (Achiron et al, 2004; Bush, 2001; Langston, 2003). This chapter uses the terms CCAM and BPS, because much of the literature evaluating surgical approaches, natural history, and follow-up employs these terms. Table 49-2 shows the stages of lung development with the corresponding airway malformation and CCAM/CPAM type. Consistent with this classification, persistent epithelial expression of the nuclear regulatory protein TTF-1 has been found in CCAM types 1 to 3 (see later discussion), indicating developmental arrest in the pseudoglandular stage (Morotti et al, 2000), and targeted fetal airway overexpression of the growth factor FGF-10 in rats produces CCAM-like lesions (Gonzaga et al, 2008).

CCAM Types

Type 0 CCAM originates from the tracheobronchial tree. There is normal lung lobulation, but no formation of alveoli (Stocker, 2002). There are only bronchial-like structures present, indicating an arrest of development in the pseudoglandular stage (Davidson et al, 1998). Lungs may be normal weight or small, but regardless, this lesion is rapidly lethal because of severe, intractable respiratory failure. The lesion has been termed *acinar dysplasia* (Rutledge and Jensen, 1986). It is diffuse and bilateral, recurs in families, and can be associated with other anomalies, suggesting a genetic etiology (Gillespie et al, 2004; Moerman et al, 1998). In a large pathology series, fewer than 2% of the pulmonary airway malformations were characterized as acinar dysplasia (Stocker, 2002).

TABLE 49-2   Stages of Airway Branching and Lung Development With Corresponding Congenital Airway Malformation

Developmental Stage	Developmental Events	CCAM Type	
		Stocker	Adzick
Embryonic 0–7 weeks	Formation of tracheal bud and growth and branching to segmental bronchi	Type 0 Tracheobronchial Type 1 Bronchial/bronchiolar	Macrocystic
Pseudoglandular 7–17 weeks	Completion of airway branching to terminal bronchioles (preacinar); gland formation	Type 2 Bronchiolar	
Canalicular 17–27 weeks	Formation of respiratory bronchioles to prealveolar structures	Type 3 Bronchiolar/alveolar duct	Microcystic
Saccular 28–36 weeks	Formation of secondary septae	Type 4 Distal acinar	
Alveolar 36 weeks–2 years	Formation of alveoli		

From Cha I, Adzick NS, Harrison MR, Finkbeiner WE: Fetal congenital cystic adenomatoid malformations of the lung: a clinicopathologic study of eleven cases, *Am J Surg Pathol* 21:537-544, 1997; Hislop AA: Airway and blood vessel interaction during lung development, *J Anat* 201:325-334, 2002.

In contrast, type 1 CCAM is the most common lesion in postnatal series of airway malformations, identified in 60% to 65% of cases (Stocker, 2002, 2009). Cysts are large, usually greater than 2 cm, and usually limited in number, often with a dominant cyst present. The cysts usually communicate with each other, and they may decrease in size as they drain progressively during advancing gestation. Postnatally, they are aerated, with fluid also present in some lesions. Type 1 CCAMs are restricted to a single lobe in 95% of the cases, with bilateral lesions rare. The lesions are lined by a spectrum of respiratory epithelial cells, ranging from cuboidal to ciliated pseudostratified columnar epithelium, and mucus-producing cells may occur in gland-type tissue. The walls of the lesions may resemble walls of bronchi. Respiratory distress depends on the size of the lesion, with some lesions detected only by incidental imaging, or after infection or malignant transformation. There does appear to be a risk of malignant transformation in nonresected or residual CCAM tissue, which occurs sometimes in patients with evidence of chronic inflammation or a history of recurrent lower respiratory tract infections. The specific link to neoplasm has not been elucidated, though the diagnosis of bronchoalvolar carcinoma (BAC) is made in relatively young patients (10 to 42 years) and a spectrum of malignancy has been described (MacSweeney et al, 2003; Mani et al, 2007). This is the only CCAM type that is associated with malignancy, and the young age of affected patients suggests that the CCAM lesion is the etiology of the malignancy (MacSweeney et al, 2003).

Type 2 CCAMs are characterized by multiple, smaller macroscopic cysts, 0.5 to 2 cm diameter, which may not be evident by chest radiograph. These lesions account for 15% to 20% of congenital pulmonary airway malformations. The lesions are lined by respiratory epithelial cells, ranging from cuboidal to columnar in morphology, and appear as multiple bronchiole-type structures, although intraacinar structures may also be interspersed (Rosado-de-Christenson and Stocker, 1991). These lesions are most commonly associated with other anomalies, in 50% of cases, which include severe bilateral renal dysplasia or agenesis, agenesis of other genitourinary structures, sirenomelia, extrapulmonary sequestration, and diaphragmatic hernia (Stocker, 1977, 2009). Conotruncal cardiac malformations have been described in association with type 1 and type 2 CCAM (Hüsler et al, 2007; Stocker et al, 1977), and ventricular septal defects have been diagnosed in fetuses and infants with all CCAM types.

Type 3 CCAMs are uncommon lesions, occurring in 5% to 10% of CCAM cases (Stocker, 2002). These lesions are generally solid, with microscopic cysts (although single larger cysts can be present), and involve an entire lobe or the entire lung. There is often a mass effect in the thorax, and the lesions can cause lung hypoplasia through compression of adjacent structures. The lesions themselves contain bronchiolar and alveolar duct-type morphology with cuboidal epithelium, and there are alveoli-like structures.

Type 4 lesions have been more recently described, and account for 10% of CCAM (Stocker, 2002). With large cysts present, some of these lesions may be mistaken for type 1 CCAM. They are usually confined to one lobe and tend to be peripheral in location. Infants and children may present with mild respiratory distress, or more severe symptoms if pneumonia occurs, or if the lesion ruptures, causing pneumothorax. CCAM type 4 can also be detected by incidental imaging. The lesions are lined with alveolar type I (flat) and type II (rounded) epithelial cells. The presence of substantial portions of cells representing the more proximal areas of the lung should raise suspicion for pleuropulmonary blastoma (PPB), a distinction that is important (because of malignancy associated with PPB; see later discussion), but one that can be difficult.

Other classification systems for CCAM have included the type 3 CCAM with hyperplastic lung disorders implicating airway obstruction, including polyalveolar lobe and laryngeal atresia, and types 1 and 2 with other bronchopulmonary malformations (Langston, 2003). The approach to CCAM diagnosed in utero has led to a different classification system, based on the natural history of these fetal lesions (see later discussion). Macrocystic CCAM is defined when a lesion contains cysts that are greater than or equal to 5 mm (types 1 and 2 CCAM), and microcystic CCAM is defined as a solid lesion, with cysts less than 5 mm (type 3 CCAM) (Adzick et al, 1985). Some lesions categorized by these criteria on fetal ultrasound have been diagnosed as BPS after postnatal resection (Davenport et al, 2004).

Fetal Diagnosis and Natural History

Fetal diagnosis of CCAM is often made when mediastinal shift due to mass effect from the lesion is identified and a cystic, intermediate, or solid mass is detected. This may occur during routine fetal survey, or when the mother is referred for evaluation of polyhydramnios (thought to occur when the mass compresses the esophagus) (Adzick, 2009). A systemic vascular supply is more consistent with a diagnosis of BPS (Winters and Effmann, 2001). In a recent population-based study from the United Kingdom, confirmed CCAM (postnatal or postmortem) occurred in 9 per 100,000 births, without accounting for lesions that were not further investigated secondary to prenatal resolution (Gornall et al, 2003). In this study, 57% (21 of 37) of fetal CCAMs were confirmed, and 5 cases were missed (prenatal detection rate 21 of 26 [81%]). Generally, growth of CCAM lesions increases until about 28 weeks' gestation, after which time it plateaus and the lesion regresses in size while the fetus continues to grow (Adzick, 2009; Kunisaki et al, 2007). Fetal and neonatal problems that arise as the result of CCAM include the development of nonimmune hydrops, and lung hypoplasia, which may be due to compression of the otherwise normally developing lung. Factors associated with the development of nonimmune hydrops include an everted ipsilateral hemidiaphragm, a predominantly cystic lesion, and a mass-to-thorax ratio (MTR) ≥0.56 (Vu et al, 2007). The MTR is the transverse diameter of the mass divided by the transverse diameter of the thorax in an axial image containing the four-chamber view of the heart. An earlier publication from Crombleholme et al (2002) evaluated factors associated with the development of excessive fluid in a single compartment, which they termed nonimmune hydrops. In this study, the CAM volume ratio (CVR) was evaluated retrospectively and applied prospectively. The CVR calculates the volume of the mass (length × weight × height × 0.52) divided by the head circumference. With CVR >1.6, 75% (12 of 16) fetuses developed hydrops, and with CVR ≤1.6, only 17% (7 of 42) fetuses developed hydrops. In a series evaluating fetal macrocystic and microcystic lesions, generally the fetuses with microcystic lesions had poorer outcomes, with intrauterine demise or early neonatal death (Adzick et al, 1985). Compared to normal lung, CCAM lesions have unregulated growth, with increased proliferation and decreased apoptosis (Cass et al, 1998), although they are relatively hypovascular (Cangiarella et al, 1995). In fetal CCAM tissue, increased PDGF-B and decreased fatty acid binding protein-7 (FABP-7) expression have been detected (Liechty et al, 1999; Wagner et al, 2008).

Prenatal Management

Initial ultrasound evaluation of the fetus with possible CCAM should include assessment of lesion size with relevant indices, vascular supply, degree of mediastinal shift, ipsilateral diaphragmatic conformation (normal, flat, or everted), polyhydramnios, placentomegaly, and the presence of any other fluid collections (ascites, integumentary edema, pleural or pericardial effusion) indicating the development of hydrops fetalis. Additional prenatal evaluation of the fetus with CCAM should include a full fetal survey to identify other anomalies, a karyotype, and an echocardiogram, to evaluate for congenital heart disease and to assess cardiac inflow patterns and outputs. These cardiac indices may help identify impending hydrops, mandating closer ultrasound follow-up and repeated echocardiographic measurements. Most referral centers recommend at least weekly follow-up ultrasound examinations evaluating lesion size and monitoring for development of hydrops until 28 to 29 weeks' gestation, at which point regression of the lesion should be occurring. Thereafter, ultrasound evaluations can be spread out to every 2 weeks. Some referral centers have advocated twice-weekly surveillance if the CVR is greater than 1.6, until 28 weeks' gestation (Adzick, 2009). In a recent series, 21 of 54 fetal lung masses decreased in size or resolved by delivery (Davenport, 2004; Davenport et al, 2004), and a similar proportion of fetal CCAM cases were not detectable at birth in a population-based study (13 of 37, 35%) (Gornall et al, 2003).

The diagnosis of hydrops in a fetus with CCAM portends a poor prognosis, with either fetal demise or preterm delivery of a compromised infant (Gornall et al, 2003; Grethel et al, 2007; Kunisaki et al, 2007). Thus, impending or definite hydrops is an indication for fetal intervention. The specific intervention depends on the type of lesion. In fetuses with a macrocystic CCAM, a growing, dominant cyst, and impending or definite hydrops, placement of a thoracoamniotic shunt results in a decrease in cyst size and hemodynamic improvement, with relatively good neonatal survival (12 of 16 in two series) (Adzick et al, 1998; Wilson et al, 2004). However, shunt placement at <21 weeks gestation may be associated with chest wall deformity, which can compromise later respiratory function, so other interventions may need to be taken at that early gestation (Merchant et al, 2007). Fetal thoracentesis is rarely effective as definitive treatment, because cyst fluid invariably reaccumulates, but it might serve as a temporizing measure until further treatment can be undertaken. For fetuses with impending hydrops and a microcystic CCAM (or failed decompression of a large cyst), open fetal resection (lobectomy or pneumonectomy) likely improves the chances of survival, although mortality remains high (10 of 23 in one series), and nonsurvivors tended to be more premature (Grethel et al, 2007). This selected approach to fetal resection has resulted in resolution of hydrops and mediastinal shift in survivors (Adzick, 2009). For fetuses at 28 to 30 weeks' gestation, or in the case where fetal surgery is contraindicated because of preterm labor, an EXIT-to-resection procedure may provide a chance for survival (Adzick, 2009; Grethel et al, 2007). EXIT procedures have also been undertaken in later-gestation fetuses with persistent large lesions (mean CVR 2.2) despite other fetal interventions, although the impact of this strategy on survival and other outcomes is unknown (Adzick, 2009; Hedrick et al, 2005). Antenatal glucocorticoid therapy to enhance fetal lung maturation should be administered before undertaking any of these procedures. This practice, utilizing betamethasone (12 mg IM every 24 h × 2 doses), led to the observation that fetuses with microcystic CCAM (type 3) and hydrops resolved their hydrops after betamethasone exposure (Tsao et al, 2003). In this series, three fetuses with mild-to-moderate hydrops treated at 21 to 26 weeks' gestation avoided further fetal interventions, were delivered at term, and survived. Glucocorticoid administration may temporarily arrest cell proliferation and/or push maturation of different cell types in these more distal lung lesions, consistent with known effects of glucocorticoids on the developing lung. However, more severe hydrops, particularly in the case of maternal mirror syndrome, may represent irreversible physiologic changes that compromise the pregnancy regardless of the intervention (Adzick, 2009). There is an ongoing multicenter placebo-controlled trial enrolling mothers carrying nonhydropic fetuses with CVR >1.4 at <26 weeks' gestation, wherein women are randomized to betamethasone versus placebo. The primary outcome is the development of hydrops fetalis, with secondary outcomes of CCAM growth and neonatal survival. This trial should be able to clarify the role of antenatal glucocorticoids in the prenatal management of microcystic/type 3 CCAM.

Postnatal Management

In fetuses that do not develop hydrops fetalis, the prognosis is good and likely depends on the type of lesion and the presence of other anomalies. Generally, the prognosis of type 1 CCAM is good, particularly if fetal intervention is not required. There is resolution of any symptoms after resection, which usually can be accomplished by lobectomy. Type 2 CCAM has a worse prognosis, because of the association with additional serious malformations. Type 3 CCAM was thought to be uniformly lethal from its earliest descriptions (Stocker et al, 1977), and it can be associated with lung hypoplasia. For fetuses with large microcystic CCAM, fetal resection, if indicated, may mitigate hypoplasia. However, more recent series have described substantial spontaneous regression of microcystic CCAM, with an increased rate of in utero resolution compared to macrocystic lesions (Davenport et al, 2004). In a large series from a single referral center, neonatal survival was 98% (118 of 121) (Grethel et al, 2007). Five infants underwent fetal procedures, with 1 death, and there were 2 neonatal deaths. In a population-based series, there were no postnatal deaths following 20 live births, with a single IUFD and 5 terminations (Gornall et al, 2003). Three fetal interventions (thoracentesis or thoracoamniotic shunt placement) were undertaken in these patients.

Newborns with CCAM may be asymptomatic, or they may present with respiratory distress with or without pulmonary hypertension, which can be severe enough to require ECMO support (Adzick, 2009; Kunisaki et al, 2007). However, even in a series of large fetal CCAM (at least 3 cm × 3 cm), only 4 of 9 infants had respiratory distress requiring resection in the first week of life. For newborns with antenatally diagnosed CCAM, lesions may be detected on chest radiograph, as solid masses, or fluid or air-filled cysts (Figure 49-6). Mediastinal shift, mass effect, or areas of air trapping due to airway obstruction may be appreciated. Some centers use ultrasound as an adjunctive modality in the neonatal period, but many surgeons prefer CT scan as the definitive imaging study, which also can detect lesions that are no longer present on fetal ultrasound (Winters and Effmann, 2001). CT scans can also determine if there are multiple bronchopulmonary malformations, which may also require resection, and the use of intravenous contrast allows for definition of the vascular supply, helping to differentiate CCAM from BPS (Johnson and Hubbard, 2004). For asymptomatic newborns, surgeons will often defer this study until several months of age, because surgical resection is also deferred. The usual surgical approach is lobectomy, for the majority of lesions confined to a single lobe. More diffuse lesions might require bilobectomy or pneumonectomy. These surgical approaches are likely to result in the removal of normal lung, but it also may decrease the risk of air leak and infection after resection (Shanmugam, 2005), and compensatory lung growth does occur after lobectomy (Nakajima et al, 1998). Additional postoperative complications may include prolonged pleural effusion, pneumothorax, pneumonia, and wound infection (Kim et al, 2008; Waszak et al, 1999).

The need for resection in asymptomatic newborns remains controversial, and there is no consensus on this topic. In a national survey of Canadian pediatric surgeons, there was not even consensus between different surgeons within individual centers (Lo and Jones, 2008). The majority of respondents in this survey (67%) endorsed resecting asymptomatic lesions present on CT, with 78% selecting 2 to 12 months as the age for operation. The concerns with not resecting a lesion is that it remains a persistent nidus for lower respiratory tract infection, and there is the potential for malignant transformation. However, the latter concern is confined to type I CCAM. Twenty-nine children with fetal CCAM that were asymptomatic at birth were followed expectantly to >6 months of age (Aziz et al, 2004). Three (10%) developed recurrent pneumonias and underwent surgery at a median of 8 months; 17 children were followed for a median of 3 years without any complications. Although there was no difference in postoperative complications in children undergoing elective resection versus those with recurrent infections, symptomatic children had a significantly longer length of stay.

Generally, children who have undergone resection for CCAM are healthy. Pulmonary function data demonstrate normal vital capacity, residual volume, and expiratory flows between 1 and 2 years postlobectomy (Nakajima et al, 1998). There are some reports of reactive airway disease and lower respiratory tract infection (Kunisaki et al, 2007) and, in more severely affected children, chronic lung disease and pulmonary hypertension (Keller et al, 2006; Kunisaki et al, 2007).

Bronchopulmonary Sequestration

Bronchopulmonary sequestrations do not have a connection to the normal tracheobronchial tree (Rosado-de-Christenson et al, 1993). The lesions have a systemic arterial supply. Sequestrations are categorized into *extralobar* sequestrations, which are lesions that have their own pleural investment and systemic (80% of the time) venous drainage (and are therefore separate from the lung), and *intralobar* sequestrations, which are integral to the lung pleura and drain via the pulmonary venous system. These lesions usually require lobectomy for removal, because they are invested within the lung. The origin of intralobar sequestration is somewhat controversial. Some experts believe it is not a congenital lung lesion, but is rather always acquired after lung infection and injury, because inflammation, fibrosis, and cystic degeneration are its primary pathologic features (Frazie et al, 1997). In this large

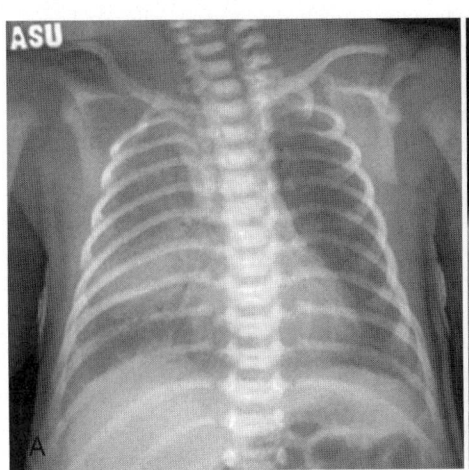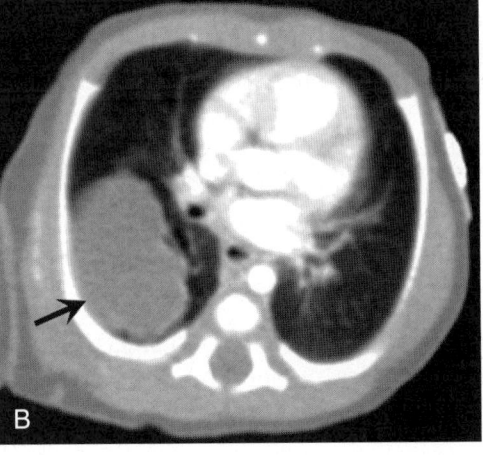

FIGURE 49-6 Chest radiograph **(A)** and thoracic CT with contrast **(B)** from newborn with fetal diagnosis of microcystic CCAM. Right chest mass (*arrow*) measured 2.3 × 3.3 cm at its largest aspect. The infant was asymptomatic.

pathologic series, intralobar lesions, usually diagnosed in adulthood and presenting as lower respiratory tract infection, account for about 75% of BPS. Others believe that intralobar sequestration can be congenital in origin, but is relatively rare in that setting when compared to extrapulmonary sequestration (Winters and Effmann, 2001). Thus, the remainder of this discussion focuses on extralobar sequestration.

Extralobar sequestrations likely originate as an independent bud from the foregut that derives its blood supply from splanchnic vessels (Rosado-de-Christenson et al, 1993). Usually the connection to the foregut is lost during development, although some lesions have persistent connections to the esophagus or the stomach (also referred to as bronchopulmonary foregut malformations). As accessory lobes, they occur within both the thorax and abdomen. As noted, hybrid lesions with features of CCAM and sequestration can occur (Lopoo et al, 1999; Winters and Effmann, 2001). The lesions are usually situated on the left side (65% to 90%), with the most common location between the lower lobe and the hemidiaphragm (approximately 70% of cases). Extrapulmonary BPS can also occur in the abdomen, the mediastinum, the pericardium, and the diaphragm itself. It is more common in males than females (3 to 4:1 ratio), and it also commonly occurs in association with other anomalies, particularly congenital diaphragmatic hernia. Additional associated anomalies include foregut duplication cysts, bronchogenic cysts, CCAM, pericardial defects, and ectopic pancreas. Histologically, these lesions appear as normal lung, except with dilated airway structures and, commonly, lymphangiectasia. A normal-appearing bronchus is present about 50% of the time. Associated pleural effusions are not uncommon (up to 10% of fetal BPS) (Johnson and Hubbard, 2004) and may be secondary to torsion of the vascular pedicle with resultant venous obstruction and elevated pressure or lymphatic abnormalities (Hernanz-Schulman et al, 1991).

Fetal diagnosis of intrathoracic BPS is suspected when there is an echogenic mass, which may also contain cysts. Depending on its size, the mass may be associated with some degree of mediastinal shift (Lopoo et al, 1999). It can be difficult to distinguish BPS from CCAM, but when a systemic arterial supply is identified, the diagnosis of BPS is highly likely. If there is also an associated ipsilateral pleural effusion, the diagnosis is almost certainly BPS (Johnson and Hubbard, 2004). Infradiaphragmatic masses also need to be distinguished from neuroblastoma, other tumors (such as lymphangioma) and adrenal hemorrhage (Curros and Brunelle, 2001; Winters and Effmann, 2001). As with CCAM, BPS often regress spontaneously over time, and if there are no associated anomalies, the outcome of these fetuses is good (Adzick et al, 1998; Lopoo et al, 1999). Close ultrasound follow-up is prudent, however, until regression is documented. When pleural effusion occurs, there is a risk of development of tension hydrothorax. In these cases, repeated fetal thoracentesis or placement of a thoracoamniotic shunt can avert or resolve hydrops fetalis, which may improve the chances for survival (Lopoo et al, 1999).

On postnatal imaging, BPS may be present as a radiographic density on plain film. The presence of linear or cystic lucencies within the radiopaque density suggests a persistent communication between an extralobar sequestration and the gastrointestinal tract (Leithiser et al, 1986; Laberge et al, 2005). An upper gastrointestinal study can demonstrate communication with the GI tract and is indicated for surgical planning if feeding difficulties are present. Ultrasound can also be useful in demonstrating the lesion (most easily seen if it is located at the lung base), and Doppler studies can identify a systemic feeding vessel. The use of contrast-enhanced CT has variable sensitivity for delineation of the vascular supply, although the lesion itself can often be demonstrated even when it has resolved by fetal imaging. MR with angiography can also be useful in demonstrating the lesion and its blood supply. Conventional angiography can also identify the vasculature and may be useful if the child requires cardiac catheterization to delineate additional pathology or physiology (Winters and Effmann, 2001).

Symptomatic BPS is usually identified in the first 6 months of life, with respiratory distress or feeding difficulties. Less commonly, recurrent infection, congestive heart failure (due to a high output state), or pulmonary hemorrhage are present. Distress at birth can be severe, particularly with large lesions complicated by a pleural effusion, or hydrops fetalis. For infants that present with symptoms in the first week of life, early resection is indicated (Azizkhan and Crombleholme, 2008). Because the lesion is delimited, sequestrectomy is not a complex operation. However, the feeding vessels can be very large in more severe cases, mandating a thoracotomy. The primary risk associated with an unresected BPS is recurrent infection, although this risk is not well quantified as there are likely adults with persistent, small, asymptomatic lesions. Thus, as with CCAM, there is controversy as to whether fetal lesions that are not identified on plain film should be further investigated in asymptomatic infants, and in general, whether asymptomatic lesions should be resected. Sequestrectomy can be accomplished thoracoscopically at 3 to 15 months, with rapid recovery and short hospitalization (Albanese et al, 2003). This approach may preserve rib architecture and limit later chest wall deformity (Rothenberg and Pokorny, 1992). Early resection, before infectious complications (the primary risk associated with an unresected lesion) may limit complications, because secondary changes such as emphysema might be averted (Rosado-de-Christenson et al, 1993). Some have attempted coil embolization of the feeding vessel(s), with hope of complete or partial involution of the lesion (Chien et al, 2009; Curros et al, 2000). In some cases, only partial occlusion can be achieved and a second procedure is necessary. Acute complications associated with the procedure include transient lower limb ischemia (due to distal migration of embolic material) and pain, fever, and pleural effusion. These complications are self-limited or treatable. Recanalization can also occur, and children who subsequently develop infection due to a persistent lesion do require surgery.

OTHER CYSTIC LESIONS

Additional cystic lung lesions include congenital lobar emphysema, pleuropulmonary blastoma, and acquired cysts (pneumatoceles or emphysema, in association with infection or bronchopulmonary dysplasia, respectively). Extra pulmonary cystic lesions include foregut cysts (bronchogenic or enteric duplication cysts) and neuroenteric cysts, which are less common than the other lesions and usually present later in infancy or childhood (Langston, 2003).

Congenital Lobar Emphysema

Because there is no evidence of lung destruction, the common term *congenital lobar emphysema* (CLE) is a misnomer, with this lesion as known as *congenital lobar overinflation* (Langston, 2003). The upper lobes are most commonly affected, with the left upper lobe the single most commonly affected lobe. Lesions occupying multiple lobes are infrequent (Mani et al, 2004). CLE is thought to arise from an obstructed lobar bronchus, which can either be intrinsic (including malacia) or extrinsic in origin. Although the affected lobe is larger than usual, the number of alveoli in the involved area is within normal limits. The exception to this is the subset of these lesions with *polyalveolar lobe*, which was present in 9 of 33 cases of CLE in one series and has an overlapping clinical presentation with CLE (Mani et al, 2004). This form of lung hyperplasia is consistent with pathophysiology associated with fetal airway obstruction (Langston, 2003).

CLE can be detected on fetal ultrasound, although it is difficult to make the correct diagnosis (Babu et al, 2001; Olutoye et al, 2000). Clinical reports have described the appearance of the lesion by ultrasound as cystic and/or echogenic, with mediastinal shift present, and subsequent regression with advancing gestation. As expected, these lesions are suspected to be CCAM or BPS, based on these findings. Fetal MRI can be helpful in characterizing the lesion, although it is not diagnostic (Olutoye et al, 2000). The postnatal clinical presentation and histology (after resection) distinguish CLE from the other lesions. The majority of children with CLE present with respiratory distress, cyanosis or recurrent pulmonary infections in the first 6 months of life, with 13 of 33 (39%) symptomatic on the first day of life in one series (Mani et al, 2004). Chest radiograph demonstrates a hyperinflated lung (transitioning from fluid-filled to air-filled over the initial postnatal days), with compression of other areas of the lung and mediastinal shift. These findings are generally diagnostic. In children with less severe presentation, bronchoscopy or CT scan can be helpful in management decisions, because some surgeons will elect to manage these patients expectantly, with resolution of symptoms in some cases (Stigers et al, 1992). After resection, prognosis is generally good, with compensatory lung growth present on the affected side (McBride et al, 1980). Airway obstruction continues to be a feature of the disease on pulmonary function tests, although these findings could be consistent with either compensatory lung growth exceeding airway growth (dysanapsis) or intrinsic, diffuse airway abnormality.

Pleuropulmonary Blastoma

PPB is a rare but malignant lesion arising from the lung or the pleura. Lesions can be predominantly cystic, predominantly solid, or mixed type and can occur in association with other congenital lung lesions (Priest et al, 1996). The diagnosis and resection of this lesion is important, because

of the risk of metastasis, recurrence, and associated malignancies (Priest et al, 1996). Although these lesions tend to present later in childhood than CCAM lesions, there is overlap in the timing of presentation (Stocker, 2002), and PPB can be detected on fetal ultrasound (Miniati et al, 2006); thus, the consideration of this diagnosis in the perinatal period is relevant for counseling and surveillance, even if a newborn is not symptomatic.

Symptomatic infants usually present with respiratory distress. Before resection, most lesions are thought to be CCAM, based on their appearance on fetal ultrasound or postnatal CT scan (Miniati, et al, 2006). Resected lesions contain cuboidal or columnar epithelial cells with underlying rhabdomyosarcoma cells (or other sarcomas). The malignant cells may not be widespread in the lesion, making the diagnosis of PPB challenging even by histology (Hill and Dehner, 2004; Stocker, 2002, 2009). Because of the difficulty in distinguishing CCAM from PPB, careful histologic evaluation of prophylactically resected CCAM is recommended, as those with stellate and spindle cells should be followed closely (Papagiannopoulos et al, 2001). Furthermore, PPB may require a more extensive resection than CCAM, so this distinction is important in determining surgical approach as well (MacSweeney et al, 2003). Tumor cells often have complex chromosomal rearrangements, and affected children can exhibit other neoplastic diseases: medulloblastoma, nephroblastoma, thyroid dysplasia and malignancy, and brain sarcoma (Priest et al, 1996; Stocker, 2002). Kindreds also demonstrate multiple malignancies, suggesting that familial surveillance for disease might be indicated (Priest et al, 1996).

Postinfectious Pneumatoceles

A number of infectious agents are more commonly associated with pneumatoceles. In our experience, the most common infection associated with pneumatocele in the newborn (maybe because of its higher frequency of infection) is *Staphylococcus aureus* pneumonia. Other infections seen in the neonatal intensive care unit that are associated with development of pneumatocele include pneumonia due to *Actinomyces* and *Candida* species, *Pseudomonas aeruginosa* and *Klebsiella pneumonia* (Stocker, 2009). Pneumatocele is often present on initial chest radiograph documenting the infiltrate, although they can also occur later in the process. These pneumatoceles can rupture, resulting in pneumothorax, which may be under tension, or they can compress lung tissue through mass effect, resulting in worsening respiratory status. Acutely, urgent interventions may be needed to improve ventilation and oxygenation, and chronically, long-term ventilator support may be necessary, particularly in former premature infants with bronchopulmonary dysplasia (BPD). Both of these scenarios raise the possibility of benefit from surgical intervention to allow functioning lung to expand. Placement of chest drains into the pneumatocele(s), either percutaneously or under direct visualization via video-assisted thoracoscopic surgery (VATS) procedure, can be definitive, because the usual course for these cysts is regression and resolution (Fujii and Moulton, 2008; Kunyoshi et al, 2006) (Figure 49-7). For patients with chronic ventilator dependence, a resection of the affected lobe could be considered, but

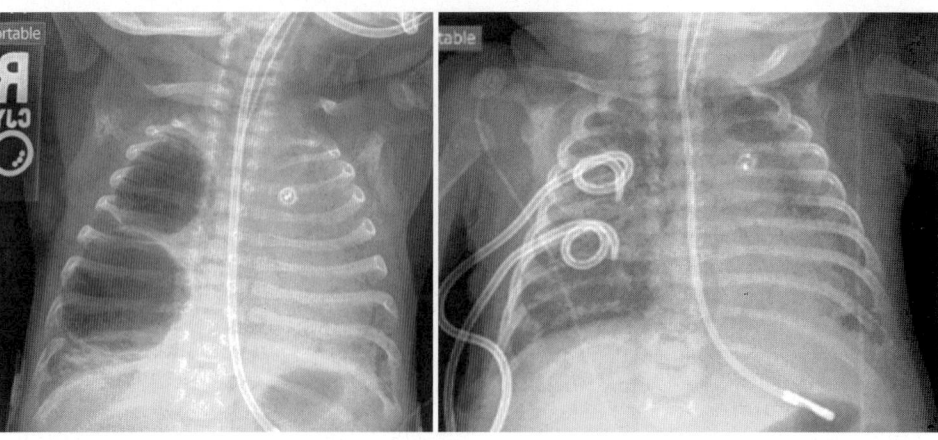

FIGURE 49-7 Chest radiographs from former preterm infant with pneumatoceles secondary to *Staphylococcus aureus* pneumonia. Cysts are compressing lung and causing mediastinal shift (*left*). Placement of draining thoracostomy tubes decompressed the cysts and decreased mediastinal shift, but infant ultimately succumbed to respiratory failure secondary to bronchopulmonary dysplasia.

any potential benefit from the procedure would need to be weighed against the need for thoracotomy (Al-Saleh et al, 2008).

Hyperinflation and Emphysema in Chronic Lung Disease

Similar to postinfectious pneumatoceles, frank cysts or hyperinflated lung in association with chronic lung disease (BPD following prematurity or developmental lung abnormalities) can cause compression on more functional areas of the lung and respiratory compromise (Moylan and Shannon, 1979; Stocker, 2009). In some cases, these infants are acutely decompensated, or they remain ventilator dependent despite maximal medical therapy. Evaluation of six infants with BPD and decompensated lobar hyperinflation in one series revealed extensive lobar bronchomalacia, with almost complete collapse of the affected airway through the expiratory phase or the entire respiratory cycle (Azizkhan et al, 1992). Lobectomy resulted in acute improvement, although ultimately only half of the infants survived.

Miscellaneous Cysts

Lymphatic, lymphangiomatous, mesothelial, and parenchymal cysts can be detected in the thorax, so these lesions may need to be included in the differential diagnosis of cystic lesions (Langston, 2003).

DISORDERS OF THE DIAPHRAGM

CONGENITAL DIAPHRAGMATIC HERNIA

Congenital diaphragmatic hernia (CDH) is a disorder of lung and pulmonary vascular hypoplasia which results from failure of formation of the diaphragm (Areechon and Eid, 1963; Hislop and Reid, 1973; Kitagawa et al, 1971). This may be due to primary deficiency of the embryonic pleuroperitoneal fold, which is one of the critical primordial diaphragmatic structures that must fuse at 6 to 8 weeks' gestation to form an intact diaphragm (Clugston et al, 2006). Failure of this event results in herniation of abdominal contents into the hemithorax, and the subsequent arrest of preacinar airway branching at 10 to 14

weeks' gestation is consistent with this early developmental defect. Hypoplasia is bilateral, although the lung ipsilateral to the hernia is most affected. Airway diameter is substantially decreased, but increase in airway muscle occurs as a later postnatal event (Broughton et al, 1998). Although acinar alveolar counts are normal, overall alveolar hypoplasia is present due to the branching defect ($<10 \times 10^6$ vs. 50×10^6 alveoli at term). Because of the interdependence of lung and vascular growth, both alveolar and capillary surface areas are decreased (Hislop and Reid, 1973; Joshi and Kotecha, 2007; Kitagawa et al, 1971). Vascular branching is impaired, with a decreased diameter of the vessels and increased muscle mass that is inversely related to the degree of lung hypoplasia (Kitagawa et al, 1971; Naeye et al, 1976). Some morphometric reports have demonstrated abnormal distal extension of the muscular media to the intraacinar arteries, whereas others have not demonstrated abnormal distal muscularization (Geggel et al, 1985; Kitagawa et al, 1971). The mechanism of developmental lung and vascular hypoplasia is unknown but may include decreased static transthoracic pressure (secondary to open communication with the peritoneal cavity) and decreased phasic pressure alterations (secondary to impaired fetal breathing movements). Compensatory alveolar growth does occur in survivors, although it is more pronounced in the contralateral lung, and relative perfusion to the ipsilateral lung can be persistently diminished (Okuyama et al, 2006; Thurlbeck et al, 1979; Wohl et al, 1977). These findings are consistent with evidence of greater injury present in the more hypoplastic and vulnerable ipsilateral lung, compared to the contralateral lung in survivors of CDH, with consequent impairment of lung growth (Hislop and Reid, 1973; Thurlbeck et al, 1979; Wohl et al, 1977).

The most common form of CDH is the posterolateral Bochdalek hernia. CDH is more common on the left side (75% to 80% of cases) than the right, likely because of slightly later fusion of the left-sided structures. Bilateral hernias account for 1% to 2% of cases. Morgagni (anterior and medial) hernias are much less frequent in occurrence and usually are not associated with substantial lung hypoplasia, although they may be associated with pericardial, sternal, and abdominal wall defects as part of the pentalogy of Cantrell spectrum. There is a predominance of males to females in CDH (1.4 to 1.6:1 ratio) ,and the occurrence of CDH (including stillbirths) is about 1:4000 births (Gallot et al, 2007; Levison et al, 2006; Yang et al, 2006). Additional anomalies occur in about 40% of affected infants and fetuses (Gallot et al, 2007; Yang et al, 2006). Musculoskeletal (including ribs, vertebrae and digits) and cardiac anomalies are most common, although the patterns of malformation differ in association with right-sided CDH compared to left-sided CDH (Slavotinek et al, 2007). CDH can be associated with aneuploidy (most frequently trisomy 18), and it can present in autosomal recessive (e.g., Fryns syndrome), sex-linked (e.g., Simpson-Golabi-Behmel syndrome) and autosomal dominant (e.g., Cornelia De Lange syndrome) disorders (Slavotinek 2007; Slavotinek, Warmerdam et al, 2007). With the exception of these disorders, recurrence rate is quoted at 1% to 2%, and more recent genetic studies have identified microdeletions in affected infants through use of microarray technology (Kantarci et al, 2006; Slavotinek, 2005). It is unclear whether or not infants with isolated CDH (no other anomalies found by antenatal and postnatal investigation) are at increased risk for these minor chromosomal aberrations, because large-scale investigations have taken place with very limited positive findings. Single gene mutations have been identified in animal models and some humans as causal in CDH, and certain areas of the genome may be critical regions wherein other causal genes might be found (Ackerman and Pober, 2007; Clugston et al, 2006).

In recent population-based studies, overall survival among live-born affected infants ranged from 52% to 61% (Colvin et al, 2005; Gallot et al, 2007; Stege et al, 2003; Yang et al, 2006). Data from the California Birth Defects Monitoring Program (1989–1997) demonstrated improved survival over time (Levison et al, 2006), with overall survival in 1997 up to 72% (Yang et al, 2006). Data from France (1986–2003) also showed modest improvements in survival over time, although other population-based studies have shown no change over a similar era (1991–2001) (Gallot et al, 2007; Stege et al, 2003). Survival of live-born infants with isolated (no additional anomalies) CDH has been higher (63% to 77%) than survival in live-born infants with other anomalies or chromosomal aberrations (19% to 43%) (Gallot et al, 2007; Stege et al, 2003; Yang et al, 2006). Survival is low (<10%) in affected infants with chromosomal abnormalities, and there is a risk of intrauterine fetal demise in both isolated (2%) and non-isolated (11%) CDH. Although individual referral centers have reported survival rates ranging from 75% to 93% (Bohn, 2002; Boloker et al, 2002; Downard and Wilson, 2003), there have been studies documenting a hidden mortality, demonstrating that a proportion of live-born infants die within hours of birth and before arrival at a surgical center (Harrison et al, 1994; Mah et al, 2009). In a recent study from Ontario, Canada, survival decreased from 67% to 58% (133 of 229) for multicenter compared to population-based data, after accounting for infants who never reached a referral center (Mah et al, 2009).

Both population-based and center-based studies have identified some risk factors for mortality for live-born infants undergoing full resuscitative measures and ongoing neonatal care. All of these likely are related to the severity of the CDH, with respect to the degree of lung and vascular hypoplasia. For instance, prenatal diagnosis has been associated with increased mortality and may be due to the identification of more severe CDH (because mediastinal shift will be more pronounced and present earlier in gestation; see later discussion) (Colvin et al, 2005; Gallot et al, 2007; Stege et al, 2003; Stevens et al, 2009). A low 5-minute Apgar score has also been associated with decreased survival in population-based and multicenter studies and may reflect initial cardiorespiratory compromise due to severity of lung hypoplasia (Colvin et al, 2005; Congenital Diaphragmatic Study Group, 2001; Levison et al, 2006; Wilson et al, 1997). Other postnatal factors that are associated with increased mortality include prematurity (<37 weeks) and air leak (Boloker et al, 2002; Colvin et al, 2005; Levison et al, 2006), which are associations with decreased lung development or increased lung injury. Interestingly, two studies have shown somewhat conflicting data around the timing of term delivery and survival. For infants receiving extracorporeal membrane oxygenation (ECMO) support, late term (40 to 41 weeks' gestation) infants had somewhat better survival compared to early term (38 to 39 weeks' gestation) infants, although the relationship was not statistically significant, and fewer ECMO-related complications were seen in the late-term group (Stevens, 2002). However, overall survival was slightly better for early term (37 to 38 weeks' gestation) versus late term (39 to 41 weeks' gestation) in another study that included infants not receiving ECMO support (Stevens et al, 2009). Other data show that infants not born at a tertiary center (outborn), but subsequently transferred to the tertiary center, have higher survival rates than those that are born at a tertiary center (inborn), which may reflect the hidden mortality associated with more severe CDH (Boloker et al, 2002; Levison et al, 2006). For those infants who do undergo surgical repair, the need for a prosthetic patch is associated with subsequent mortality, indicating a larger diaphragmatic defect and likely more severe lung hypoplasia (Bryner et al, 2009; Lally et al, 2006; Wilson et al, 1997).

Prenatal Diagnosis and Management

CDH is usually suspected on prenatal ultrasound when mediastinal shift away from the hernia side is appreciated. Prenatal detection rates are higher with left-sided than right-sided hernias, and bilateral hernias can be difficult to discern because of the distorted anatomy. CDH in fetuses with additional anomalies are also detected at a higher rate than CDH in isolated cases (Gallot et al, 2007). Fetal MRI can be helpful in determining the diagnosis, if the anatomy is difficult to identify. A prenatal diagnosis of CDH mandates careful evaluation for other anomalies, including a fetal echocardiogram, because of the high rate of additional anomalies and the lower survival rates. Some of this evaluation may be limited by the anatomic distortion due to the hernia. A karyotype and other genetic analysis (as indicated) are also recommended. Additional prognostic information regarding the severity of the hernia can be gathered during antenatal evaluation by ultrasound and MRI, although the prognostic ability of these measures is likely center dependent, as survival varies to some extent across centers. The most useful discriminator of CDH severity is herniation of the liver into the hemithorax (Jani et al, 2006; Metkus et al, 1996). Liver herniation can occur with both right-sided and left-sided CDH. In left CDH, the left lobe of the liver develops in the thorax. Thus, the course of the hepatic vasculature is distorted and indicative of liver herniation. Bowel-only right-sided hernias are very uncommon. Other antenatal discriminators of severity that have been used include stomach herniation and polyhydramnios (a later finding, secondary to GI obstruction or esophageal dysmotility). A number of ultrasound measures have been developed as intrauterine measures of lung size (Keller, 2007). The lung-to-head ratio (LHR) is widely used for this purpose (Metkus et al, 1996). It is the perpendicular area of the lung contralateral to the hernia at the level of the cardiac atria divided by the biparietal diameter. It has been used predominantly in mid-gestation (22 to 27 weeks), with an LHR ≤1.0 combined with liver herniation accepted as the most severe group of CDH. LHR has been studied in left CDH, although it has also been extrapolated to right CDH and likely has prognostic ability, although LHR thresholds for severity could be lower in right CDH since the normal right lung is larger than the left lung (Hedrick et al, 2004; Peralta et al, 2005). Investigators have developed nomograms for normal LHR over 12 to 32 weeks, which has led to an observed-to-expected (O/E) LHR measurement, employing the mean LHR at any gestational age as the "expected LHR," which increases with advancing gestational age because of a more rapid increase in lung area compared to head circumference (Peralta et al, 2005). It follows that the LHR ≤1.0 will represent a higher O/E LHR earlier in gestation than it does later in gestation and the O/E LHR will be higher with right CDH than left CDH for a given LHR and gestational age (Jani et al, 2009). In a large database of 354 fetuses with isolated CDH (including 25 fetuses with right CDH), the O/E LHR was predictive of survival independent of liver herniation (Jani et al, 2007). Subsequent analyses of this data have stratified fetuses with and without liver herniation, because survival does differ between these groups for a given O/E LHR range (Deprest et al, 2009). In these analyses, survival was <20% for fetuses with isolated left CDH and O/E LHR ≤25%. Fetuses with a higher O/E LHR of 26% to 35% survived in greater numbers: 30% if liver was herniated and almost 60% if liver was not herniated. The lower bound of the 95% confidence interval for O/E LHR in unaffected fetuses is 60% (Jani et al, 2007). Decreasing O/E LHR was also related to increasing time on assisted ventilation, prolonged hospitalization and an increased risk for prosthetic patch repair (Jani et al, 2009).

Fetal MRI techniques have also been pursued for prognostic information in CDH. Liver herniation can be determined by fetal MRI, and at some centers it is the preferred technique for this determination. A number of different nomograms to determine lung volume as a percent of normal (based on estimated fetal size or gestational age) have been developed. Recently, Büsing et al (2008) evaluated seven published nomograms for estimation of relative fetal lung volume in 68 fetuses with isolated left CDH evaluated at their center. They generated receiver operating characteristic curves for each of the seven equations and found high (0.800 to 0.900) area under the curve (AUC) for prediction of survival, regardless of technique used. In this dataset, prediction of need for ECMO was not as strong (AUC 0.653 to 0.739), although individual centers have found that relative fetal lung volume is a very

useful predictor of the need for subsequent ECMO support (Barnewolt et al, 2007).

Fetal intervention to enhance intrauterine lung growth has evolved to the current technique of endoscopic temporary balloon tracheal occlusion. Only fetuses likely to be the most severely affected newborns are candidates, if additional anomalies are not found after careful investigation. A randomized controlled trial evaluating this technique was terminated prematurely because of unexpectedly high survival in the control group, with no difference in survival between tracheal occlusion and standard care infants (Harrison et al, 2003). The tracheal occlusion procedure was complicated by premature delivery (mean gestational age 30.8 weeks), often stemming from premature rupture of the membranes, and this may have compromised survival in the intervention group. With development of smaller instruments, this technique can now be accomplished as a fully endoscopic procedure (Jani et al, 2009). Incorporation of a second procedure to remove the intratracheal balloon (i.e., plug-unplug) has also decreased the need for delivery by EXIT procedure, allowing for vaginal delivery in the majority of cases, if otherwise indicated. This technique has been accomplished for fetuses with LHR ≤1.0, in an uncontrolled experience in Europe, although the survival rate is promising compared to fetuses that did not undergo intervention with similar prognostic features. At last report, 210 cases were accomplished at 23 to 33 weeks' gestation. Median gestational age at delivery utilizing this technique has increased to 35 weeks, although premature rupture of the membranes occurred in almost half of the affected pregnancies. With operator experience, the procedure has been accomplished more rapidly, and shorter procedures were associated with lower rates of premature membrane rupture. Elective prenatal removal of the intratracheal balloon (i.e., unplug) was accomplished at a median of 34 weeks in 70% of the cases. Survival to neonatal discharge was 47% (98 of 210); 6 deaths were fetal and 10 deaths occurred secondary to difficulty with removal of the intratracheal balloon. From their historical experience, the investigators cite an expected survival of only 24%. In a subset of these fetuses, and some expectantly managed with CDH, Cannie et al (2009) evaluated changes in relative lung volume over gestation by fetal MR. They found that relative lung volume was largely unchanged in fetuses without intervention, and it tended to increase more consistently in fetuses with CDH when tracheal occlusion was undertaken at ≥29 weeks' gestation (n=8). There are several ongoing nonrandomized trials of this minimally invasive technique in the United States. In Europe, investigators are currently undertaking a randomized trial of the technique for fetuses with moderate lung hypoplasia (O/E LHR 25% to 34.9% or 35% to 44.9% with liver herniation) and plan to undertake tracheal occlusion at 30 to 32 weeks' gestation (trial registration number: NCT00763737).

Postnatal Diagnosis and Management

Most newborns with CDH will present immediately or within several hours of birth with respiratory distress, cyanosis, decreased or bronchial breath sounds on the hernia side, and a scaphoid abdomen. An occasional infant will

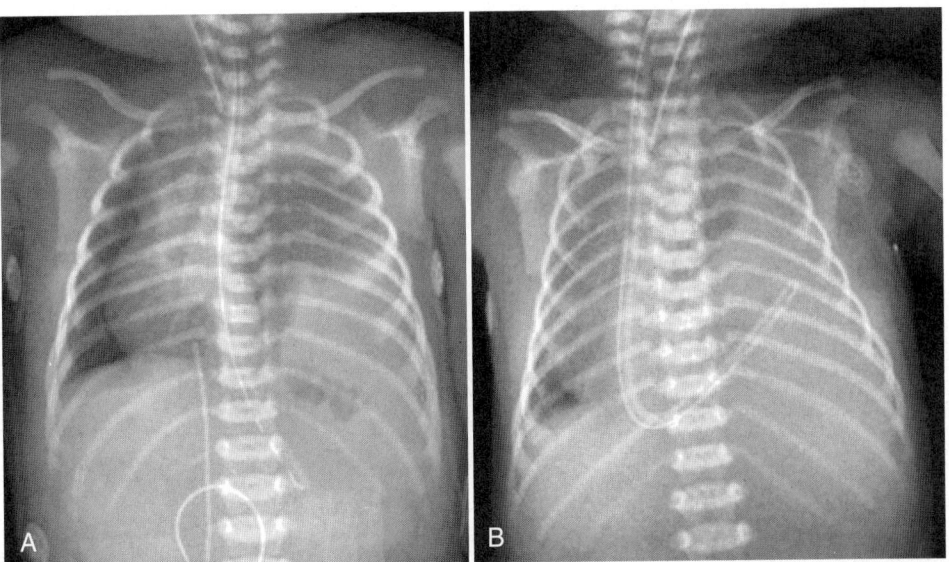

FIGURE 49-8 **Chest radiographs in two infants with left congenital diaphragmatic hernia before surgical repair. A,** Infant has CDH without liver herniated or stomach herniated into thorax. He subsequently underwent primary repair of the diaphragmatic defect, was extubated within several days of surgery, and was discharged to home without supplemental oxygen. **B,** Infant has severe CDH with liver and stomach herniated into thorax. He subsequently required ECMO support, underwent prosthetic patch repair for diaphragmatic aplasia, and succumbed to respiratory failure and pulmonary hypertension after decannulation from ECMO support.

not have symptoms until several days or months of age and often will have feeding intolerance and mild respiratory distress (Kitano et al, 2005). An initial chest radiograph will show a smaller lung on the hernia side, with bowel gas in the chest and shift of mediastinal structures (Figures 49-8 and 49-9). The findings of a small lung, with no mediastinal shift and usually without concern for herniated bowel, should raise suspicion for other diagnoses, which may require an alternate surgical approach or may not require surgery at all (see later discussion). Newborns with a fetal diagnosis of CDH or those presenting soon after birth are usually endotracheally intubated with a Replogle placed to continuous gastric suction to minimize accumulation of thoracic intraintestinal air. Some centers also routinely use pharmacologic paralysis until surgical repair of the diaphragmatic defect is accomplished and the hernia contents are reduced. Other centers use paralysis only in the most severe cases. Hypoplastic lungs with small alveoli have poor compliance, and thus ventilation is severely reduced (Keller, 2007). Because of the decreased alveolar surface area for gas exchange and the restrictive pulmonary vascular bed, oxygenation is severely impaired. Because these physiologic challenges cannot be overcome without lung growth, most high-volume centers use a gentle ventilation strategy. This strategy attempts to achieve adequate oxygen delivery while minimizing oxygen toxicity and ventilator-induced lung injury and preserving the potential for lung growth. Actual targets for ventilation and oxygenation vary somewhat, but consistency in care within a center is important (Logan et al, 2007). Ventilation target is often Pco_2 45 to 65 mm Hg (permissive hypercapnia). For oxygenation, a more liberal strategy allows for a preductal (right upper extremity) and postductal (descending aorta or lower extremity) arterial saturation (Sao_2) differential, with oxygenation targets based on preductal Sao_2 (permissive oxygenation).

Oxygenation targets are generally preductal Sao_2 ≥95% in less severely affected infants and Sao_2 ≥85% in more severely affected infants. Ventilator pressures are limited, with either positive inspiratory pressure (PIP) targeted at ≤25 to 28 cm H_2O or mean airway pressure (Paw) on high-frequency ventilation at ≤15 cm H_2O. Aggressive weaning strategies are used to achieve gentle ventilation goals and to minimize lung injury. Lung recruitment is not an effective strategy to achieve persistent improvements in oxygenation in CDH (Kinsella et al, 1997), and increases in PIP to achieve transient improvements in oxygenation lead to further increases in ventilator support, with worsening compliance due to lung injury and edema (Kays et al, 1999). There are also some centers that advocate low PEEP and high ventilator rates (which are physiologic in lung hypoplasia). With high ventilator rates, gas trapping and auto-PEEP may be an important factor, so limitation of the PEEP set on the ventilator is important (Boloker et al, 2002). In addition, low PEEP (2 to 3 cm H_2O) is associated with higher lung compliance in infants with CDH than PEEP of 4 to 6 cm H_2O (Dinger et al, 2000).

Employment of gentle ventilation strategies has been associated with improved survival at individual centers (Kays et al, 1999; Wilson et al, 1997); however, regardless of actual targets for ventilation and oxygenation and preferential mode of ventilation, it is likely that other aspects of care, such as infant stimulation and positioning and sedation and feeding practices, affect survival and other outcomes. Although there are a number of ancillary treatments employed in infants with CDH (antenatal glucocorticoids, surfactant replacement therapy, inhaled nitric oxide, and other pulmonary vasodilator therapies), there are no studies documenting broad efficacy of these treatments in term infants with CDH. Some have advocated the primary use of high-frequency ventilation in these infants, but there is no evidence of benefit to survival or other

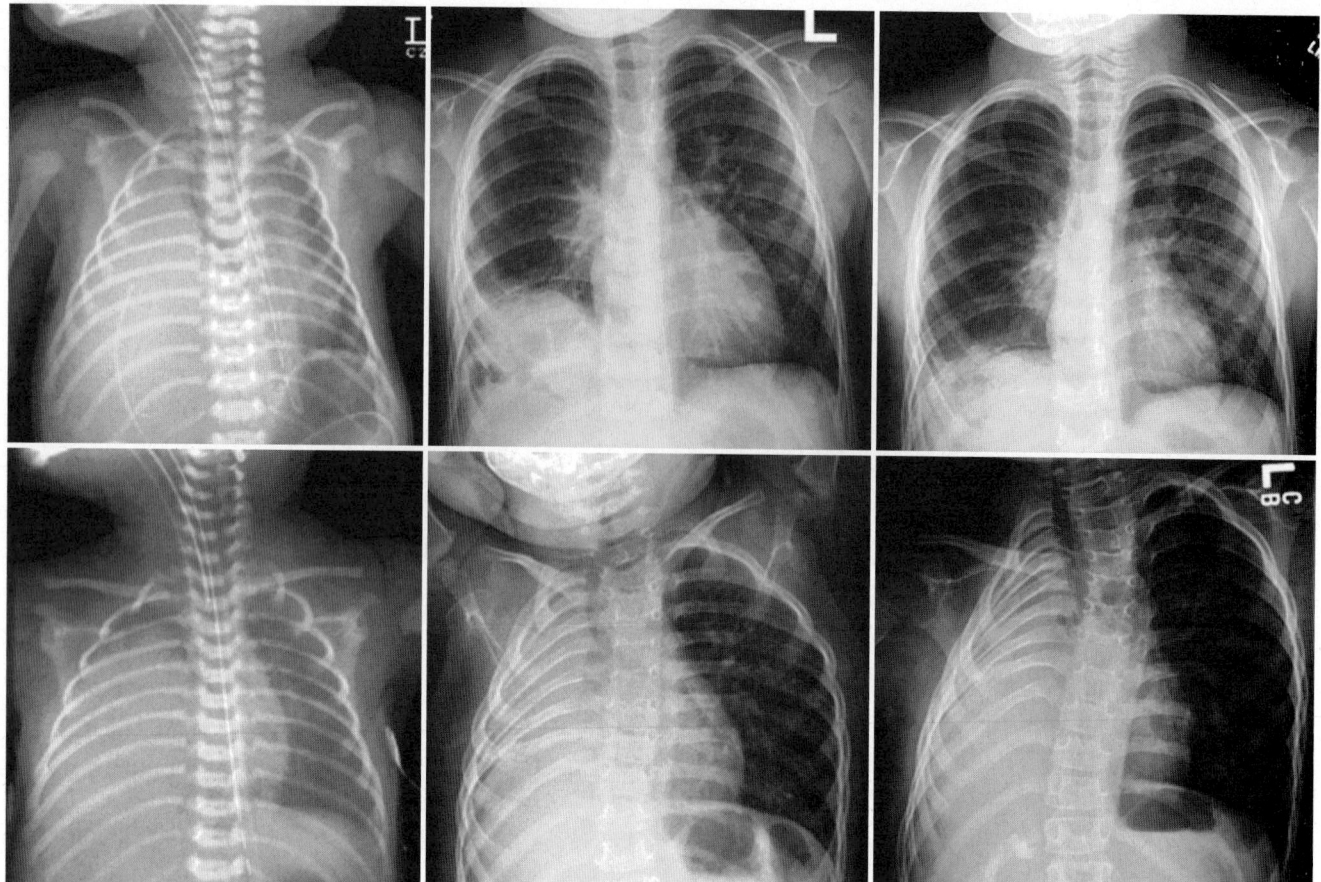

FIGURE 49-9 Chest radiographs in two infants with respiratory distress at admission to the intensive care nursery, and at 3 and 5 years of age (*left to right*). *Upper panel* shows infant with right congenital diaphragmatic hernia with liver herniated into thorax and diaphragmatic aplasia. Note mediastinal shift into left hemithorax, with subsequent improvement in aeration and then normalization of right lung volume. *Lower panel* shows infant with hepatopulmonary fusion. Surgical repair required resection of hypoplastic nubbin of lung. Note lack of mediastinal shift at presentation, compensatory growth of left lung with trachea deviated to the right, and scoliosis.

outcomes based on the mechanical ventilation technique alone (when similar permissive targets are used), although a clinical trial to study this question has been proposed in Europe (trial registration number: NTR1310). In addition, the use of prostaglandin infusion to maintain ductal patency and improve right heart function in cases of prolonged pulmonary hypertension has been advocated (Bohn, 2002). The one ancillary treatment that has shown benefit is the use of extracorporeal membrane oxygenation (ECMO), which improved survival to hospital discharge in the United Kingdom Collaborative study, although the effect dissipated at follow-up with later deaths among initial survivors (Mugford et al, 2008).

ECMO can be used to rescue newborns with CDH, particularly those with lung injury evident by pneumothorax (Sebald et al, 2004), and it may be used in the setting of gentle ventilation (where pneumothorax is a less frequent occurrence), to avoid prolonged high ventilator pressures or Fio_2. Although CDH has become the most common indication for neonatal respiratory ECMO, survival to discharge for these infants in 2003 declined to 40% (Rais-Bahrami, 2005). Because ECMO is a temporary therapy designed to allow for resolution of a reversible process, it is unlikely that all infants with CDH will benefit from ECMO support; some will have lethal pulmonary

hypoplasia (Antunes et al, 1995). Thibault and Haney described persistent pulmonary hypertensive changes in vessels of infants with CDH dying after ECMO support, and others have described recurrent pulmonary hypertension (Payne et al, 1991; Thibault and Haney, 1998). However, there is a challenge in determining which infants are very unlikely to benefit from ECMO. In our center, the University of California San Francisco (UCSF) Children's Hospital, there is an active inborn service for fetuses with antenatal diagnoses of anomalies such as CDH. Since 1991, no infants with CDH have survived to discharge and remained on ECMO support for >9 days (Table 49-3), despite an overall ECMO survival for infants with CDH that is similar to international data (Rais-Bahrami, 2005). More recently, in infants with CDH, the primary inclusion criterion for ECMO support has been imminent or actual inadequate oxygen delivery (persistent preductal $Sao_2 \leq$ low 80s or worsening metabolic acidosis) within gentle ventilation parameters. Families of infants with severe CDH are given the option to not pursue ECMO support, and ECMO is rarely offered late in the clinical course for infants who have never been weaned from mechanical ventilation. From 2003–2009 (since the full complement of care practices with gentle ventilation and pressure limitation have been formally implemented in our

TABLE 49-3 Infant Survival to Hospital Discharge by Duration of ECMO Support: 1991–2009*

ECMO Duration (days)	2003–2009 (n = 10)	1991–2002 (n = 33)	Survival (%)
1	0	0/2	0/2 (0)
2	0	0/1	0/1 (0)
3	0	2/2	2/2 (100)
4	0/1	1/1	1/2 (50)
5	0/1	5/6	5/7 (71)
6	1/1	5/6	6/7 (86)
7	0	1/1	1/1 (100)
8	1/1	1/2	2/3 (66)
9	0	2/2	2/2 (100)
10–14	0/4	0/8	0/12 (0)
15–23	0/2	0/2	0/4 (0)
Total	2/10 (20)	17/33 (52)	19/43 (44)

*Overall survival from 2003 to 2009 was 78/104 (75%), compared to 2/10 (20%) with ECMO support.

patients), utilization of ECMO support for CDH has been low (10%) in our center, and only 20% (2 of 10) of infants survived with ECMO, all with a duration of ECMO ≤8 days (no infant had pneumothorax). In contrast, survival to discharge during this period for all infants with Bochdalek hernias who had a full attempt of resuscitation and ongoing care (regardless of whether or not there were associated anomalies) was 78 of 104 (75%). Findings from the United Kingdom are consistent with our experience with prolonged ECMO support. The two independent predictors of mortality among infants with CDH were duration of ECMO support >2 weeks and use of renal replacement therapy for renal insufficiency. Survival among both of these groups was approximately 20% (2 of 11 for prolonged ECMO and 4 of 18 for renal insufficiency) (Tiruvoipati et al, 2007). Longer ECMO runs, renal complications, and multiple complications were also independently associated with mortality in infants with CDH in an analysis from the Extracorporeal Life Support Organization (ELSO) database (Stevens et al, 2002). Thus, failure to decannulate an infant at <10 to 14 days of support is likely an indicator of severe lung and vascular hypoplasia. In these severely affected infants, it often takes longer than 4 weeks to resolve pulmonary hypertension (Dillon et al, 2004; Keller et al, 2006), and therefore awaiting resolution of pulmonary hypertension in these cases before decannulation would require prolonged ECMO support. Prolonged ECMO runs are prone to mechanical complications, which may further prolong the ECMO run or be irrecoverable. Thus, it is unclear to what degree prolonging ECMO support could increase survival in CDH, unless there is still evidence of reversibility in the infant's condition. In the case of availability of a specific therapy, such as perfluorocarbon partial liquid ventilation, wherein lung growth might be induced, the benefits of continuing ECMO support might become evident (Hirschl et al, 2003). Although there has been difficulty obtaining this drug in the United States, a larger randomized trial in infants with CDH

requiring ECMO support could be indicated. Otherwise, strategies to limit the duration of ECMO support in CDH could be employed, accepting ventilator settings at decannulation that are significantly higher than what might otherwise be acceptable for newborns coming off ECMO support. These strategies could include prevention of complete lung collapse with aggressive pulmonary toilet, because re-recruitment of lung volume can be difficult in these infants (which may be related to small-caliber airways that have been damaged by pre-ECMO support regimens). Also, for infants cannulated prerepair, performance of the CDH repair post-ECMO decannulation could further limit time on ECMO support. Surgical repair of the diaphragmatic defect while on ECMO is associated with higher mortality, even after adjusting for other markers of CDH severity (Bryner et al, 2009). This phenomenon may be related to hematologic complications related to the repair (which are independently associated with decreased survival) (Stevens et al, 2002). However, some centers advocate CDH repair as soon as possible after stabilization on ECMO support (Bryner et al, 2009). In addition, some centers utilize an "EXIT-to-ECMO" approach for fetuses with high risk criteria based on fetal evaluation (low relative lung volume) (Kunisaki et al, 2007). These fetuses are intubated and ventilated during an EXIT procedure. If they meet certain criteria for adequate gas exchange, they are delivered for conventional management. If they do not meet these criteria, they are cannulated and placed on ECMO support. Using this strategy, Kunisaki et al reported a 71% (10 of 14) survival with 11 infants going directly to ECMO support and 7 of 11 surviving. Most infants required prolonged mechanical ventilation and hospitalization.

Repair of the diaphragmatic defect usually occurs after some degree of stabilization of cardiopulmonary status, either with conventional therapy or ECMO support. Two small studies randomizing infants to immediate (<24 hours of age) versus delayed surgery have showed no difference in survival (Moyer et al, 2002). However, Nakayama et al (1991) demonstrated that lung compliance improves before surgery after a short period (several days) of stabilization in infants with CDH, and Sakai et al (1987) demonstrated that compliance worsens with early surgery in almost all infants. We studied infants with severe CDH (liver herniation and LHR <1.4) and found that, although compliance did not improve before surgery after a period of stabilization, compliance did improve within 24 hours after surgery (Keller et al, 2004). Thus, the rationale for delayed surgery is sound with respect to lung function. Some centers advocate very delayed surgery, while awaiting complete resolution of pulmonary hypertension (Wung et al, 1995). However, this approach can be problematic, because pulmonary hypertension may require weeks for resolution (Dillon et al, 2004; Keller et al, 2010). Subsequent failure to reduce the hernia contents is likely to delay establishment of enteral nutrition, with a consequent increased risk of infection and complications from parenteral nutrition. The achievement of even modest reduction in Fio_2 before surgery allows for a transient increase, if needed, after surgery, and even in cases where Fio_2 remains high, the modest improvement in lung function that occurs with surgery may help with further recovery for the infant in the most severe cases. Another issue with respect to timing of surgery arises when an infant also has congenital heart disease that requires neonatal surgery. Most centers will undertake CDH repair and then proceed to the cardiac surgery once the infant meets reasonable hemodynamic criteria for the surgical intervention (Cohen et al, 2002). In newborns who might require urgent cardiac surgery, survival is unlikely except if the lung hypoplasia is very mild. In a large series of 280 infants with CDH and congenital heart disease, overall survival was 41%, but only 5% for infants with single ventricle physiology and 18% (2 of 11) for infants with TAPVR (Graziano, 2005).

Surgical repair of CDH involves reduction of the hernia contents and closure of the diaphragmatic defect. The surgical approach is usually via laparotomy, to abrogate the detrimental effect of thoracotomy on lung function. Some surgeons will preferentially do a thoracotomy for a right CDH repair. For selected patients, thoracoscopic repair of the diaphragmatic defect is becoming more common (Kim et al, 2009; Yang et al, 2005). Infants who have achieved low ventilator settings and Fio$_2$ before surgery are likely candidates for this approach, because operative instability or the need for prosthetic patch repair of the diaphragm can result in conversion to an open procedure. A prosthetic patch is placed when a diaphragmatic defect cannot be closed primarily. There is significant variability among surgeons in the need for patch repair, however. Clinical series have demonstrated that it is more common in the case of liver herniation and right CDH (which may also be an association with herniated liver) (Fisher et al, 2008; Kunisaki et al, 2008). Patch repair can be accomplished with use of a polytetrafluoroethylene (PTFE, Gore-Tex) or a bioabsorbable intestinal mucosa (SurgiSIS) material. Polypropylene (Marlex) and other materials have been used sporadically (Riehle et al, 2007). Use of an abdominal silo and/or prosthesis to close the abdominal wall is sometimes necessary and may decrease the need for a prosthetic diaphragm (Bryner et al, 2009; Rana et al, 2008). Some surgeons advocate construction of a latissimus dorsi flap for initial CDH repair when primary closure of the diaphragmatic defect cannot be accomplished (Barbosa et al, 2008). This technique allows for some potential for diaphragmatic function in the innervated flap, which usually remains abnormal at late follow-up even with primary repair (Arena et al, 2005). However, the technique is time-consuming and may not be tolerated in patients during the acute neonatal period, so others have reserved this technique only for hernia recurrence (Sydorak et al, 2003). Generally, use of a prosthetic patch for diaphragmatic closure is associated with increased risk of hernia recurrence, although the actual risk varies widely and may be dependent on multiple factors, including surgical technique (Jancelewicz et al, 2010). Recurrent herniation may be associated with small bowel obstruction. It is also associated with persistent chest wall deformity, which might be due to the severity of the underlying disease or the complication of reherniation (requiring multiple surgical procedures). Some surgeons have moved toward use of composite patches (more than one material), which may decrease the risk of recurrence by allowing for both durability and accommodation of rapid growth in infancy

(Jancelewicz et al, 2010; Riehle et al, 2007). Another area of variable practice is related to the intraoperative placement of a thoracostomy tube. Some of this controversy is related to the application of negative pressure, because that creates additional transpulmonary pressure and potential for barotrauma and lowers lung compliance (Dinger et al, 2000). However, negative pressure drainage is not necessary. Because the ipsilateral thorax will fill with fluid after reduction of the hernia contents as a result of the hypoplastic lung, placement of an anterior thoracostomy tube in a supine infant will prevent the accumulation of excess pleural fluid (which can occur with chylothorax). Chylous pleural effusion will cause respiratory compromise. However, it may be difficult to ascertain the cause of this deterioration because mediastinal structures remain shifted for some period of time postoperatively and may be modestly more exaggerated with tension hydrothorax. Chylothorax is not uncommon after CDH repair. In a recent series, it occurred in 7% of infants (10 of 152), and it was more common in infants who required prosthetic patch repair (8 of 10) (Gonzalez et al, 2009). Both surgical trauma and underlying hemodynamics due to right heart failure may contribute to the etiology of this problem in infants with CDH (see Chylothorax earlier, for diagnosis and management).

Long-Term Morbidity

Survivors of CDH have substantial pulmonary and gastrointestinal morbidity at follow-up (Muratore et al, 2001a, 2001b). Gastroesophageal reflux, failure to thrive, and need for tube feedings are common. Although low lung volumes and restrictive lung disease may be seen in the first months of life, obstructive lung disease is the most common finding in early childhood and at later follow-up (Koumbourlis et al, 2006; Vanamo et al, 1996). Children requiring prosthetic patch repair and prolonged mechanical ventilation are most likely to have later morbidity, but the relative contribution of anatomic abnormalities, physiologic derangements, and secondary injury to these outcomes is unknown. Developmental delay and hearing loss also occur and require careful follow-up for early identification and intervention (Cortes et al, 2005; Friedman et al, 2008; Jaillard et al, 2003; Keller et al, 2008).

Hepatopulmonary Fusion

Hepatopulmonary fusion likely represents a severe form of CDH. It has been described variably in the literature as both CDH and severe eventration (Keller et al, 2003; Rais-Bahrami et al, 1996; Robertson et al, 2006). All reported cases have occurred on the right side, although there is a report of a late-presenting left CDH with fusion of liver and lung tissue (Baeza-Herrera et al, 2000). It is not clear if this is the same entity that other authors have described, because these infants usually present in extremis, with respiratory failure and pulmonary hypertension (Keller et al, 2003; Rais-Bahrami et al, 1996; Robertson et al, 2006). The embryology of this defect is speculative, and the distinction between severe CDH versus eventration is probably not critical. However, the diaphragm is not intact, it is usually moderately to severely hypoplastic, and there is fusion of hepatic and pulmonary tissue without pleura or liver capsule present, no dissectable plane, and a fibrous membrane adherent to the liver and the lung (Slovis et al, 2000). In cases where hepatopulmonary fusion is determined or suspected, there is a lack of mediastinal shift, consistent with severe right lung hypoplasia rather than a mass effect from a large right CDH with herniated liver (Keller et al, 2003; Slovis et al, 2000). The suspicion of this diagnosis is important, because the surgical approach may differ. The need to separate the liver and the lung (usually requiring ligation or resection of part of the hypoplastic lung due to risk of air leak and hemorrhage) will require a thoracotomy. We have utilized contrast MR imaging preoperatively to help make this distinction and found enhanced lung tissue adherent and conforming to the dome of the liver in a case of hepatopulmonary fusion, suggestive of the anatomy subsequently encountered at the time of surgical repair (Keller et al, 2003). The goal of surgery is to separate the thoracic and abdominal cavities, often requiring placement of a prosthetic patch. In our experience, if these children survive, later growth of the right lung is much more restricted than it is in children with severe right CDH (see Figure 49-9). Whether this is due to more pronounced ipsilateral lung hypoplasia, less pronounced contralateral lung hypoplasia, or the need for resection at the time of surgical repair is unclear. However, chest wall deformity and scoliosis are significant problems in these children.

CONGENITAL EVENTRATION OF THE DIAPHRAGM

Congenital eventration of the diaphragm occurs when the hemidiaphragm is partially or completely nonmuscular. The intact diaphragm is elevated with a normal insertion. Thus, intraabdominal organs are present in the thorax, but still confined below the diaphragm. The right and left hemidiaphragms are equally affected, and 13% (6 of 48) of affected infants had bilateral eventration in an early series (Tsugawa et al, 1997; Wayne et al, 1974). With diaphragmatic eventration, movement of the hemidiaphragm is paradoxical, leading to respiratory distress, atelectasis, and recurrent pulmonary infections. Infants presenting later may have gastrointestinal symptoms. Surgical intervention involves plication of the diaphragm to eliminate the paradoxical movement. Results are generally good, with severe lung hypoplasia uncommon and improvement in symptoms without recurrence. However, infants with associated conditions, particularly neuromuscular disorders, may not survive. Some surgeons advocate plication even when symptoms are not present, to preserve potential for lung growth (Tsugawa et al, 1997).

DIAPHRAGMATIC PARESIS

Phrenic nerve injury due to birth trauma or surgical trauma can result in temporary paresis of the diaphragm, with an elevated hemidiaphragm and paradoxical movement evident by ultrasound or fluoroscopy. If infants are persistently symptomatic, diaphragmatic plication may allow for weaning from mechanical ventilation or lesser levels of respiratory support, but these injuries should also recover on their own over time (Tsugawa et al, 1997; Wayne et al, 1974).

NEONATAL SCIMITAR SYNDROME

Scimitar syndrome consists of three findings of right lung hypoplasia, partial anomalous pulmonary venous return, and unilateral pulmonary sequestration. These features may not all be present, and additional cardiac anomalies may also be detected. Scimitar syndrome can be suspected on fetal ultrasound, because of findings of cardiac dextroposition with a small right pulmonary artery (Abdullah et al, 2000). The presentation of scimitar syndrome in the first days of life is usually severe, with tachypnea and pulmonary hypertension (Gao et al, 1993; Huddleston et al, 1999). Some infants will present later with failure to thrive. Chest radiograph reveals an elevated right hemidiaphragm with the mediastinum shifted to the right, consistent with primary lung hypoplasia. The classic finding of the scimitar vein is often not appreciated. The associated cardiac anomalies include left-sided obstructive lesions and atrial and ventricular septal defects. Because these infants have a normally developed diaphragm, the surgical approach will depend on hemodynamic effects of the anomalous venous return and the sequestration (if present). Thus, careful hemodynamic and vascular assessment is critical and may be accomplished through cardiac catheterization and angiography or, in some cases, by MR angiography. Some infants will undergo pneumonectomy, others ligation or coil embolization of systemic feeding vessels, and others no intervention because the hypoplastic lung may have very little blood flow. Pulmonary vein stenosis can also complicate the hemodynamic status, and medical or surgical treatment for additional cardiac lesions may need to be addressed.

SUGGESTED READINGS

Azizkhan RG, Crombleholme TM: Congenital cystic lung disease: contemporary antenatal and postnatal management, *Pediatr Surg Int* 24:643-657, 2008.

Büsing KA, Kilian AK, Schaible T, et al: MR relative fetal lung volume in congenital diaphragmatic hernia: survival and need for extracorporeal membrane oxygenation, *Radiology* 248:240-246, 2008.

Gallot D, Boda C, Ughetto S, et al: Prenatal detection and outcome of congenital diaphragmatic hernia: a French registry-based study, *Ultrasound Obstet Gynecol* 29:276-283, 2007.

Harrison MR, Adzick NS, Flake AW, et al: Correction of congenital diaphragmatic hernia in utero VIII: Response of the hypoplastic lung to tracheal occlusion, *J Pediatr Surg* 31:1339-1348, 1996.

Hirose S, Farmer DL, Lee H, et al: The ex utero intrapartum treatment procedure: looking back at the EXIT, *J Pediatr Surg* 39:375-380, 2004:discussion 375-380.

Jani J, Keller RL, Benachi A, et al: Prenatal prediction of survival in isolated left-sided diaphragmatic hernia, *Ultrasound Obstet Gynecol* 27:18-22, 2006.

Keller RL: Antenatal and postnatal lung and vascular anatomic and functional studies in congenital diaphragmatic hernia: implications for clinical management, *Am J Med Genet C Semin Med Genet* 145C:184-200, 2007.

Nuss D: Minimally invasive surgical repair of pectus excavatum, *Semin Pediatr Surg* 17(3):209-217, 2008.

Richter GT, Thompson DM: The surgical management of laryngomalacia, *Otolaryngol Clin North Am* 41:837-864, 2008:vii.

Rocha G: Pleural effusions in the neonate, *Curr Opin Pulm Med* 13(4):305-311, 2007.

Wiatrak BJ: Congenital anomalies of the larynx and trachea, *Otolaryngol Clin North Am* 33:91-110, 2000.

Zoumalan R, Maddalozzo J, Holinger LD: Etiology of stridor in infants, *Ann Otol Rhinol Laryngol* 116:329-334, 2007.

Complete references used in this text can be found online at www.expertconsult.com

PART XI

CARDIOVASCULAR SYSTEM

EMBRYOLOGY AND PHYSIOLOGY OF THE CARDIOVASCULAR SYSTEM

H. Scott Baldwin and Ellen Dees

This chapter begins with a review of cardiac anatomy and of the cell types that make up the heart, and then discusses in detail the morphology and physiology of the developing heart. Although we mention certain genes that are important in cardiac development, this is not a comprehensive review of the genetic regulation of heart development, because several reviews have recently become available (Bruneau, 2008; Moon, 2008). Rather, we focus on aspects of heart development of particular interest to clinical neonatologists. These include the creation of inflow and outflow poles of the heart, alignment of these structures with the cardiac chambers, septation of the cardiac chambers, and the physiology of blood flow in the embryo, fetus, and newborn.

The heart begins as a field of cells that move ventrally and midline within the embryo, fusing into a tube. This primitive heart tube is formed in the human embryo by 3 weeks gestation (Figure 50-1, 21 days). At the posterior (dorsal) end of the tube is the venous pole, or sinus venosus. In mammals, this includes connections to the yolk sac (vitelline veins), placenta (umbilical veins), and embryo proper (cardinal veins). At the anterior (ventral) end of the tube is the arterial pole, or bulbus cordis, which will pass flow from the heart tube back into the body. In the primitive heart, this connection is to the aortic sac, which is connected to paired dorsal aortae. The tube itself is divided into an atrial segment, adjacent to the venous pole, an atrioventricular canal, and a ventricular segment adjacent to the arterial pole. Within the primitive heart tube, faint constrictions can be seen between these segments. Each of these segments is histologically and functionally distinct from the beginning—atrial and ventricular myocytes have distinct characteristics even when isolated from the primitive mesoderm. Thus, as the heart tube is being formed it already has primitive compartments. Furthermore, the differentiating cardiomyocytes are forming functional contractile units mature enough to begin spontaneous contractions by the time the heart tube is formed. These are initially peristaltic in nature, moving blood from venous inlet to arterial outlet.

Thus, as soon as the heart forms into an organized tubular structure, its primitive connections to the body are formed and its contractile function is operational, such that it begins to pump fluid to the rapidly growing embryo. Red blood cells begin to enter the circulation from blood islands in the yolk sac by the time the heart starts to beat at 22 days' gestation (Carlson, 2004). For the first 6 weeks, the yolk sac remains the exclusive source of hematopoietic cells, until the liver (and to a lesser extent spleen) take over. The bone marrow gradually becomes populated with hematopoietic cells beginning in the second trimester of pregnancy, and by birth is the major source of blood cells (Carlson, 2004). Development of a circulatory system early is critical to maintaining nutrition and oxygen delivery to developing tissues, which at this point are beyond depending on simple diffusion of nutrients.

From the primitive heart tube state, the heart undergoes significant growth and morphologic alterations. These include establishing laterality, such that the symmetry of the heart tube is lost, and there are well-defined left and right structures within the heart and vessels. As laterality is being established, the heart undergoes a dramatic change in shape, via a process known as cardiac looping. This occurs in the human embryo during week 4 of gestation (see Figure 50-1, 25 to 28 days). From this stage, the heart realigns its inflow and outflow segments, septates, and forms valves in processes that are detailed in this chapter. The final product will be a mature heart (Figure 50-1, bottom panel: human heart at 9 weeks' gestation) with the following structures:

1. A venous pole that is now connected to systemic veins from the upper body (superior vena cava), lower body (inferior vena cava), liver (hepatic veins), and coronary circulation (coronary sinus), all of which pass into the right atrium.
2. A separate left atrium, connected to the venous system separately by ingrowth of pulmonary veins from the lungs.
3. An atrioventricular canal that begins as a single unrestricted opening and septates into two atrioventricular valves. The tricuspid valve opens from right atrium into right ventricle, and the mitral valve opens from left atrium to left ventricle.
4. A primitive ventricular segment that has grown in cell number and by cell hypertrophy into two distinct and separate chambers, a right and left ventricle. By processes known as compaction and trabeculation, the working myocardium of each ventricle has become highly organized and adapted to the unique requirement of a pulmonary (right) or systemic (left) ventricle.
5. An arterial pole that has separated in a spiral fashion to create two separate outflow tracts of the heart. The right ventricle retains the proximal part of the original bulbus cordis connection as the conus; thus its structure differs from that of the left ventricle.

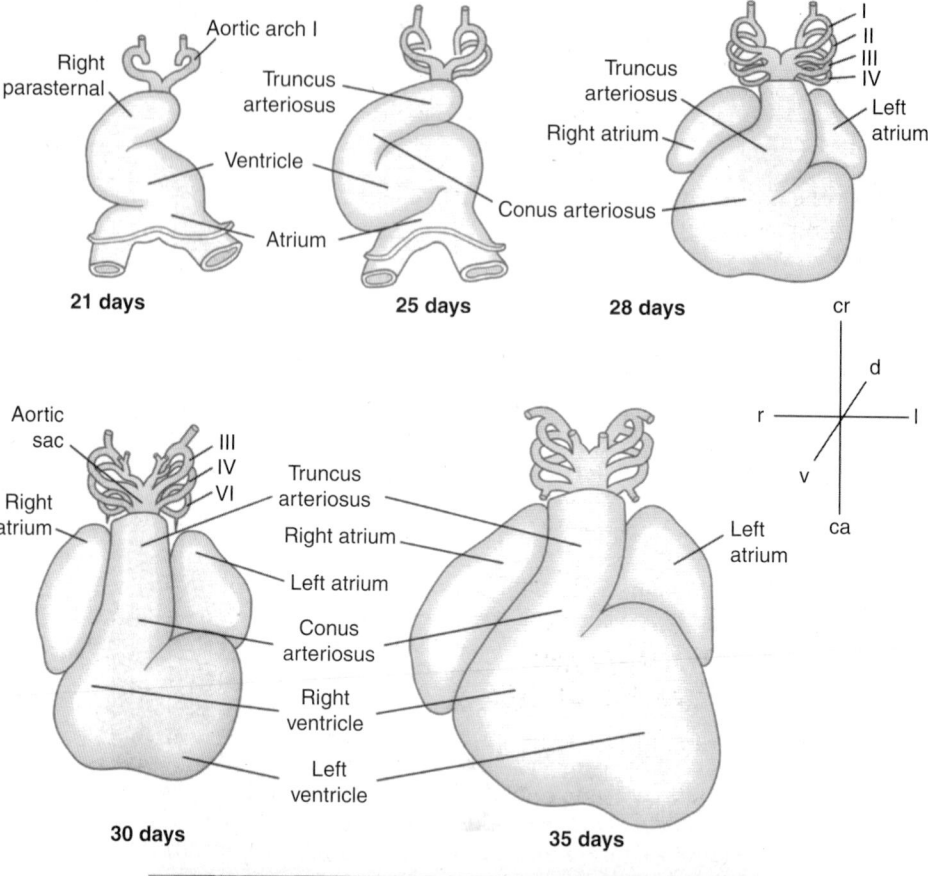

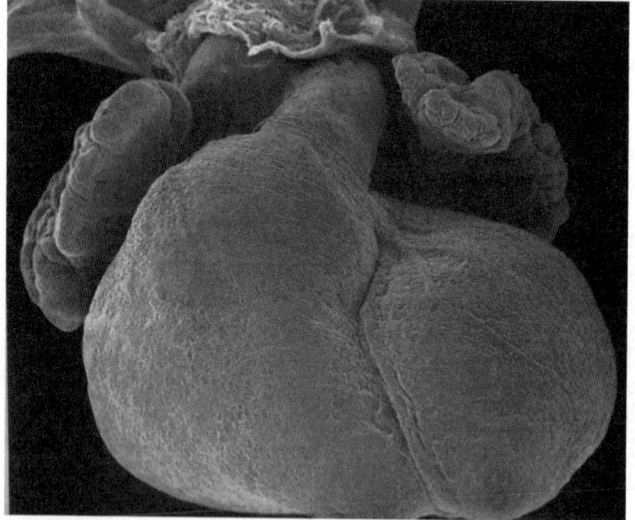

FIGURE 50-1 Morphology of the human heart, 3 to 5 weeks' gestation. Orientation in the body as shown, with cranial-caudal (cr, ca); dorsal-ventral (d, v); and left-right (l, r) planes. The heart tube is initially linear, with the inflow region dorsal/caudal and the outflow ventral/cranial. During week 4, the heart undergoes looping, realigning the segments such that the inflow is shifted dorsal/leftward, and the outflow ventral/rightward. After looping, the atrial and ventricular segments are approximately on the same plane in the cranial/caudal axis. (*Top from Carlson BM:* Human embryology and developmental biology, *ed 4, Philadelphia, 2009, Mosby, p 457.*) Below is a SEM of a human heart at 9 weeks' gestation, after looping, and after septation of the atria, ventricles, and great arteries. (*Bottom from Steding G:* The anatomy of the human embryo, *Basel, 2009, Karger, p 215.*)

The right ventricle is referred to as a tripartite ventricle, with inflow, outflow, and conal segments. The pulmonary valve forms between the conus and the pulmonary artery, and the pulmonary arteries send blood to both lungs. The left ventricle is more conical in shape and is structured as a highly efficient pump. It connects to the aorta, with an aortic valve in between. Because of the spiral septation, the great arteries cross as they arise from the ventricles, with the pulmonary artery coursing anterior to the aorta.

6. Paired dorsal aortae connected to the aortic sac that have extensively remodeled into a single leftward aortic arch and descending aorta. This connects proximally to the coronary arteries, the head and neck arteries, and to a temporary structure important in fetal life, the ductus arteriosus.

7. Networks of coronary arteries have formed within the myocardium of the heart. These grow toward and connect to the aorta as right and left coronary arteries.

8. Networks of myocytes have differentiated into the conduction system of the heart, including the sinoatrial node, the atrioventricular node, and the His-Purkinje system of the ventricles.

CELL TYPES WITHIN THE HEART AND THEIR ORIGINS

The mature heart has three cell layers: the endocardium, an epithelial lining one cell layer thick; the myocardium, a precisely oriented network of myocytes that perform the contractile work of the heart; and the epicardium, an epithelium that covers the external surface of the heart. Beyond this, the heart resides within a pericardial sac, similar in composition and function to the pleura, which covers the lungs.

Much, but not all, of the heart has its embryonic origin from a field of lateral plate mesodermal cells referred to as the cardiogenic mesoderm (Figure 50-2). The primitive heart tube forms as a two-layer structure, with an endocardium and a myocardium, both cell types coming from cardiac mesoderm. The endocardium remains as an epithelium, but a subset of cells delaminate and invade the proteinaceous matrix between the endocardium and myocardium to form the endocardial cushions. These cells will be vital to proper valve development and to complete septation of the atria and ventricles. The myocardium primarily remains muscle, but a subpopulation of these cells also change course and differentiate into Purkinje fibers of the conduction system.

There is a recently appreciated secondary field of cardiac mesoderm that enters the heart after formation of the primitive heart tube and contributes primarily to the ventricles and outflow region of the heart (Kelly and Buckingham, 2002; Mjaatvedt et al, 2001; Waldo et al, 2001). Also termed the anterior heart field, this is a population of cardiac mesoderm anterior and medial to the original heart field, surrounding the aortic sac (Mjaatvedt et al, 2001). Discovery of the anterior heart field was primarily accomplished using cell lineage tracing studies. In chick hearts marked just after fusion of the heart tube, a population of unmarked cells interposed themselves between marked cells of the distal and middle heart tube one day later (Mjaatvedt et al, 2001). Interestingly, if the paired heart fields are completely excised in the chick, a small beating mass of cells resembling an outflow tract still forms, lending further confirmation to the existence of this second population of cardiomyocytes (Mjaatvedt et al, 2001). Studies in mouse compared to chick suggest that the anterior heart field in mouse may extend further into the right ventricle (Kelly and Buckingham, 2002; Zaffran et al, 2004). What differences there are in humans remain unknown. However, the notion that there is a population of cells forming the outflow tract and right ventricle that is distinct from those that form the inflow tract and left ventricle may at least partially explain why heart defects often affect the outflow tract without affecting the inflow tract region of the heart.

Although most of the heart comes from cardiac mesoderm, there are a few critical populations of cells that migrate into the developing heart from outside (see Figure 50-2). One such population is neural crest cells, which migrate in from the developing branchial arches and innervate the heart as well as forming much of the smooth muscle of the proximal aorta. Proper neural crest migration is important to the developing aortic arch system, pulmonary arteries, and ductus arteriosus. Another external population of cell forms that make important contributions to the mature heart is a cluster of cells that forms dorsal and inferior to the heart tube known as the proepicardial organ (Ishii et al, 2007; Nahirney et al, 2003). The origin of these cells is a subject of debate; one leading theory is that they are derived from liver primordium (Ishii et al, 2007). These cells expand

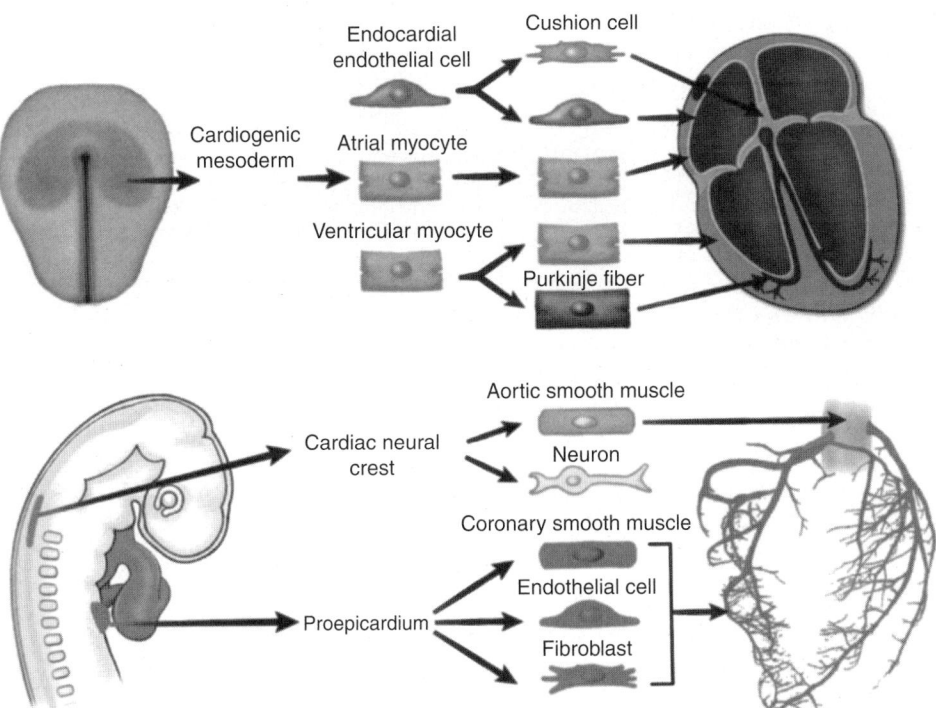

FIGURE 50-2 The cell types of the heart. Most of the heart myocardium and endocardium comes from cardiogenic mesoderm, but there are important cell types that migrate into the developing heart, including cardiac neural crest and proepicardium. (*From Mikawa T: Cardiac lineages. In Harvey RP, Rosenthal N, editors:* Heart development, *San Diego, Calif., 1999, Academic Press, p 31.*)

as an epithelial sheet covering the surface of the heart to form the epicardium. Subgroups of cells delaminate from the sheet and migrate into the myocardium beneath. In the chicken, these cells differentiate into vascular smooth muscle and vascular endothelial cells to form the coronary arteries. They also differentiate into cardiac fibroblasts, which make up a sizable population of cells residing within the myocardium, between myofibers. In the mouse and human, the origin of the coronary endothelial cells is unknown.

Thus, in addition to cardiomyocytes, the heart is composed of cells from epithelial and neural crest origins that migrate in with spatial and temporal precision during cardiac development. The next several sections highlight the steps of this process.

FORMATION OF THE EMBRYONIC CARDIAC CRESCENT AND HEART TUBE

It is important to point out that most of what is known about the early stages of embryonic development come from extensive studies of avian and mouse models (Abu-Issa and Kirby, 2007; Baldwin, 1996, 1999; Combs and Yutzey, 2009; Cui et al, 2009; de Lange et al, 2004; Dyer and Kirby, 2009; Fishman and Chien, 1997; Garcia-Martinez and Schoenwolf, 1992, 1993; Melnik et al, 1995; Redkar et al, 2001; Yutzey and Bader, 1995). This is extended, with some acknowledged gaps, to human development. In its earliest stages, the embryo exists as a bilayer disk of two epithelial sheets of cells suspended between two fluid-filled cavities, the yolk sac and the amniotic cavity. The ventral layer (facing the yolk sac) is the hypoblast, which will eventually be relegated to extraembryonic structures. The dorsal layer (facing the amniotic cavity) is the epiblast, which will actually form all 3 embryonic germ layers: the ectoderm (nervous system and skin), mesoderm (heart, skeleton, muscle and connective tissue), and endoderm (gut). Mesoderm and embryonic endoderm separate from the primitive ectoderm by a process known as gastrulation (Figure 50-3, *A*). Gastrulation begins as a groove form in the epiblast starting at the tail end (caudal) and gradually extending cranially to an endpoint known as the prechordal plate. The groove is known as the primitive streak, and its leading edge the primitive node. Along the primitive streak, epiblast cells delaminate from the epithelial sheet and invade the potential space between the epiblast and hypoblast. The heart forms as a crescent of cells cranial to the prechordal plate and extending along both sides. Fate mapping studies suggest that many cell fate decisions may be set during gastrulation or even before (Fishman and Chien, 1997; Garcia-Martinez and Schoenwolf, 1993). For example, within the cardiac crescent, the apex of the crescent is formed from cells that have migrated through the primitive streak closest to the primitive node and contains precursors of the outflow-tract myocardium. The cells on either side of this region have migrated through the mid-portion of the streak and are ventricular myocyte precursors. Finally, the most lateral and caudal cells are those that have migrated through the most posterior part of the streak and will become atrial myocytes. The exact details of when and how this occurs are still under debate and refinement as better techniques become available (Abu-Issa and Kirby,

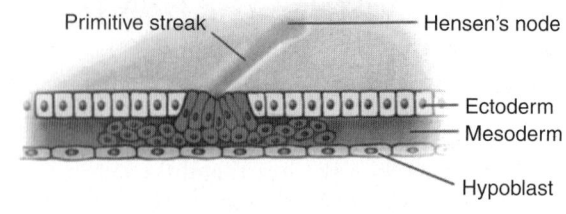

A

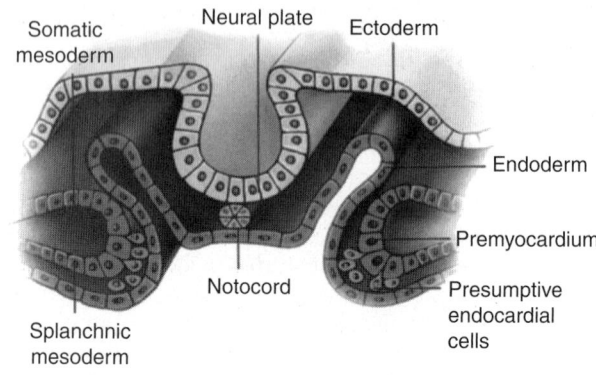

B

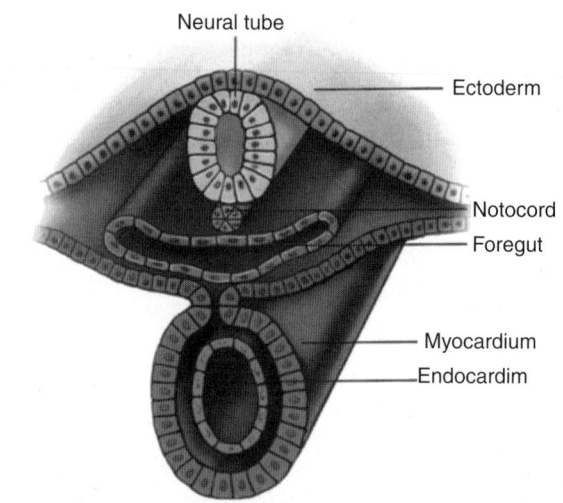

C

FIGURE 50-3 **Gastrulation and the formation of the three germ layers. A,** Both mesoderm and endoderm are formed during gastrulation. **B,** As the Mesoderm forms the paired premyocardium, endoderm folds into the gut tube. **C,** The heart tube, now composed of myocardium and endocardium, is pushed ventrally as it forms. (*From Mikawa T: Cardiac lineages. In Harvey RP, Rosenthal N, editors:* Heart development, *San Diego, Calif., 1999, Academic Press, p 20.*)

2007; Cui et al, 2009; Ehrman and Yutzey, 1999). One concept coming from recent fate-mapping studies using live-cell tracking and time-lapse imaging is that of cells moving as a cohort (tissue motion) rather than individually migrating; this is a way to maintain cells' relative positions within a tissue and, eventually, an organ (Cui et al, 2009).

LOOPING AND LATERALITY OF THE HEART TUBE

The cardiac crescent is a symmetric structure and fuses into an initially symmetric-appearing heart tube. This occurs as the ectoderm dorsal to the crescent is folding to

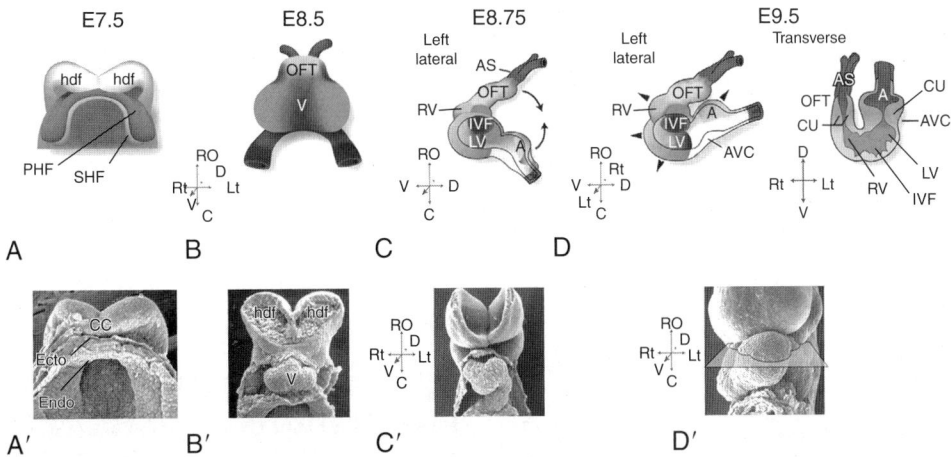

FIGURE 50-4 Diagrams **(A to D)** and corresponding scanning electron micrographs **(A′ to D′)** of embryos during the stages of looping. Shown are mouse embryos, at embryonic days as labeled. Orientation in three dimensions is depicted by the arrows, rostral-caudal *(RO, C)*; dorsal-ventral *(D, V)*; and right-left *(Rt, Lt)*. In **A**, note the primary and secondary heart fields *(PHF and SHF)* beneath the headfold *(hdf)*. In **A′**, the cardiac crescent *(cc)* is between the ectodermal *(ecto)* and endodermal *(endo)* germ layers. Labeled in **B** and **B′** are the outflow tract *(OFT)*, primitive ventricle *(V)*, and sinus venosus *(SV)*. The heart begins to loop, as shown by *arrows* in **C**; note the alignment of inflow region *(atrium; A)* and SV with the left ventricle *(LV)*, and of the outflow region (aortic sac *[AS]* and *OFT)* with the right ventricle *(RV)*. The interventricular foramen has begun to septate the ventricles *(IVF)*. By the completion of looping, the ventricular chambers have significantly enlarged, as indicated by the *arrowheads* in **D**. The atria and ventricles are on the same rostral-caudal plane, as shown by the *rectangle* in **D′**, corresponding to the transverse section diagram above. The endocardial cushions *(CU)* begin to form after completion of looping; see next section. (*Adapted from Moon A: Mouse models of congenital cardiovascular disease,* Curr Top Dev Biol *84:174, 176, 2008.*)

create the neural canal, and the endoderm initially ventral to the crescent is folding to create the foregut (Figure 50-3, *B*). As the foregut forms, it moves dorsally, pushing the cardiac crescent ventrally and medially, such that the two arms of the crescent fuse into a tube sitting directly in front of the foregut (Figure 50-3, *C*). As fusion of the heart fields occurs, the heart is already beating. In a human fetus this happens at approximately 22 days' gestation. Over the next week, there is tremendous growth of the head, such that the heart goes from being the most "cranial" structure in the embryo to a position tucked underneath the developing head of the embryo.

As the head grows up and over the heart tube, the heart tube itself begins to undergo a dramatic change in shape known as looping. Here the heart tube loses its symmetry, and distinct left and right morphology can be identified (Steding, 2009). Much is known about the molecular signaling and gene expression patterns involved in looping. The basic left-right asymmetry of the embryo is set during gastrulation by concentration gradients of the factors sonic hedgehog (shh) and fibroblast growth factor 8 (fgf-8). This gradient is created by ciliary motion at the primitive node and causes a cascade of downstream genes to be activated, including nodal, lefty, and pitx-2 (Capdevila et al, 2000; Rodriguez-Esteban et al, 2001; Tsukui et al, 1999). Within the heart tube, several cardiac transcription factors have been shown to be important to looping, including Nkx2-5, MEF2, and Hand2 (Christoffels et al, 2006; Cui et al, 2009; Han and Olson, 2005; Han et al, 2006; Hiroi et al, 2001; Jamali et al, 2001a,b; Karamboulas et al, 2006; McFadden et al, 2005; Srivastava et al, 1997; Tsukui et al, 1999; Yamagishi et al, 2001). Disruption of any of these factors in mice by gene knockout causes embryonic lethality, with a block in heart development at the looping stage. Morphologically, cardiac looping involves differential growth, with higher proliferation of myocytes along the

outer curvature than inner (Moorman and Christoffels, 2003), including those being added from the secondary heart field (Kioussi et al, 2002). All of this serves to elongate the outflow tract and enlarge the ventricles relative to the atria (Moorman and Christoffels, 2003). In addition, there are mechanical forces literally pulling, twisting, and realigning structures of the primitive heart tube. This is thought to involve the cytoskeleton, including nonmuscle myosin (Brueckner, 2001; Linask and Vanauker 2008; Supp et al, 1997), microtubules (Icardo and Ojeda, 1984), and nonmuscle actin bundles (Itasaki et al, 1991).

Normal looping occurs to the right (D-looping), that is, the sinus venosus and atria move toward the left and posterior, and the ventricles and bulbus cordis move to the right and anterior. Importantly, the venous pole also moves cranially such that it lines up with the arterial pole along the horizontal body axis. This is seen from several different angles in Figure 50-4. The bulbus cordis remains to the right of the primitive ventricle. This repositioning is critical for proper atrioventricular and ventriculo-arterial connections. Also with looping, an outer and an inner curvature of the heart is established. The anterior outer curvature is an area of rapid myocardial growth and expansion to form the ventricular chambers. The posterior inner curvature undergoes slower growth and acts rather like a fulcrum for the looping process. The inner curvature myocardium contributes to the atrioventricular canal and is critical to the formation of the endocardial cushions.

ABNORMALITIES IN CARDIAC LOOPING

Sometimes, looping can occur to the left, with the venous pole and atria moving rightward and the ventricles and arterial pole moving leftward. This is referred to as L-looping and most commonly occurs as an entity termed congenitally corrected transposition. Here the ventricles loop to the left, and the bulbus cordis ends up to the left of the primitive ventricle. When the great arteries septate, there is L malposition of the great arteries, so the aorta is to the left of the pulmonary artery (parallel, not crossed). The resulting circulation is right atrium to left ventricle to pulmonary artery; left atrium to right ventricle to aorta. In isolation, then, this defect allows for normal circulation— although with the right ventricle, which is structured to pump to the low-pressure pulmonary circulation, as the systemic ventricle. In addition, however, there are often other cardiac defects ranging from a ventricular septal defect with pulmonary valve stenosis to more complex defects involving hypoplasia of one of the ventricles or hypoplasia, aplasia, or malformation of one or more valves.

L-looping may also be associated with more global defects known as heterotaxy syndromes. Heterotaxy syndromes are a heterogeneous group of congenital defects, with the commonality being abnormal left-right asymmetry of the embryo (Ghosh et al, 2009). In heterotaxy, left-right assignments along the body axis are randomized. Thus, it is possible to have mirror-image asymmetry, or bilateral symmetry, with either two right sides or two left sides. This is often termed right or left isomerism. This can affect the abdomen, lungs, and heart. In the abdomen the gut, liver and spleen may be reversed from normal (abdominal situs inversus). There may be malrotation of the bowel and anomalies of the biliary tree. The spleen, being a normally left-sided structure, can be duplicated in left isomerism (polysplenia), and absent in right isomerism (asplenia). Asplenic patients require antibiotic prophylaxis in childhood to protect against bacterial infections. Asplenic patients usually have left-isomerization of the lungs and heart as described later; polysplenic patients have right-isomerization of the lungs and heart as well. Lung abnormalities in heterotaxy manifest in the bronchial and lung anatomy. The normal left lung is bilobed and the left main bronchus travels beneath the left pulmonary artery (hyparterial). The normal right lung is trilobed and the main bronchus travels above the right pulmonary artery (eparterial). Thus, careful examination of a chest x-ray in left isomerism reveals bilateral hyparterial bronchi, and in right isomerism shows bilateral eparterial bronchi.

In the heart, the atrial sidedness is randomized in heterotaxy. Here the atria may be normal (situs solitus), left-right reversed (situs inversus), or unclear (situs ambiguus; including bilateral right or bilateral left atria). The atria are most practically defined by their venous return, systemic to the right atrium and pulmonary to the left. But in heterotaxy this is not always possible, as the pulmonary or systemic veins may return to both atria. The pulmonary veins grow in from the developing lungs normally joining the back wall of the left atrium. When the left-right cues are scrambled, the pulmonary veins often return ipsilaterally: left-sided veins to left-sided atrium and right-sided veins to right-sided atrium. Likewise, the systemic veins may return to either or both atria in heterotaxy—for example, a right superior vena cava to right atrium and left superior vena cava to left atrium. This is because the systemic veins start out as paired symmetric structures (see section on systemic veins), with involution of certain structures occurring as part of the establishment of left-right asymmetry in the embryo. Finally, certain patterns of additional cardiac defects often accompany asplenia/right isomerism. These include failure of septation if the ventricles resulting in a single ventricle, pulmonary underdevelopment (stenosis or atresia of the pulmonary valve), bilateral superior vena cava, and anomalous pulmonary venous return. For polysplenia/left isomerism, commonly associated defects include endocardial cushion defects (see later discussion), left-sided obstructive lesions such as coarctation of the aorta, and interruption of the inferior vena cava (IVC) with azygous continuation to the superior vena cava.

VENTRICULAR INLET SEPTATION: ENDOCARDIAL CUSHIONS

After cardiac looping has occurred, the orientation of the heart tube has changed drastically, but the progression of blood flow through it remains in essentially the same sequence: into the heart from the venous pole, through the common atrium into the common ventricle, and out the conotruncus to the aorta. Inflow and atrial segments are leftward, and the ventricle and outflow are to their right. If the process arrests near this point, a heart may form with its entire inlet portion aligned over the leftward ventricle (a double inlet left ventricle), or its entire outlet portion aligned over the rightward ventricle (a double outlet right ventricle). Both of these entities are seen in humans. What are very rarely seen are a double inlet right ventricle, or a double outlet left ventricle—even if there is L-looping and/or dextrocardia, this basic sequence is maintained.

During the next phase of heart development, the atrioventricular (inlet) and ventriculoarterial (outlet) structures will realign and septate, such that there is a valved inlet and a valved outlet for each ventricle. In human embryos, this occurs during week 7 of gestation (Dhanantwari et al, 2009; Steding, 2009). These valves are formed primarily from the endocardial cushions. The endocardial cushions are also critical to complete ventricular and atrial septation, completing the portions of septum adjacent to the AV valves. This is detailed further in sections on atrial and ventricular septation. Thus, the endocardial cushions form the crux of the heart: a point in the center of the heart at which separate AV canals are to the left and right, and atrial and ventricular septa are aligned above and below.

Within the primitive heart tube, even before looping, there are faint constrictions at the atrioventricular groove and in the forming conotruncus (see Figure 50-4). The endocardial cushions initially appear as swellings in the atrioventricular and conotruncal segments of the primitive heart, by six weeks gestation (Figure 50-5, *A* and *B*). The swellings are caused as cells from the inner lining of the heart (endocardium) delaminate and migrate into the extracellular matrix in between the endocardium and the myocardium. Signaling involving the TGF-β family between the myocardium and endocardium play a crucial role in initiating and maintaining this process (Brown et al, 1996, 1999; Jiao et al, 2006). The delaminating cells change phenotype in a process known as epithelial-to-mesenchymal transformation. The cells lose their epithelial, or sheetlike, characteristics and acquire a mesenchymal

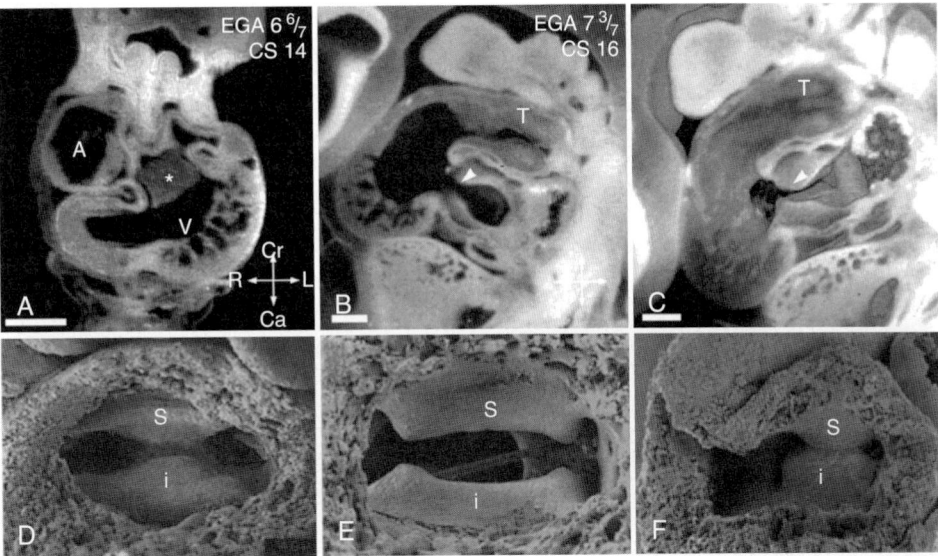

FIGURE 50-5 **Formation of the endocardial cushions.** **A** to **C,** Episcopic fluorescence image capture(EFIC) images of sectioned paraffin-embedded human embryos at 6⁶⁄₇ weeks (**A**) and 7³⁄₇ weeks (**B** and **C**) gestation. **C** is a three-dimensional volume reconstruction of the same embryo as **B.** Seen are atria (*A*), ventricles (*V*), AV cushions (* and *arrowhead*) and truncus and semilunar valve cushions (*T*). Scale bar = 0.515 mm in **A** and 0.389 mm in **B** and **C.** (*From Dhanantwari P, Lee E, Krishnan A, et al: Human cardiac development in the first trimester: a high-resolution magnetic resonance imaging and episcopic fluorescence image capture atlas,* Circulation *120:347, 2009.*) **D** to **F** are different views of scanning electron micrographs of human embryos at week 6 gestation, showing the superior (s) and inferior (i) atrioventricular cushions, with the tricuspid (left) and mitral (right) orifices. (*From Steding G:* The anatomy of the human embryo, *Basel, 2009, Karger, p 221.*)

phenotype, losing junctions with neighboring cells, invading the matrix, and proliferating faster (Combs and Yutzey, 2009; Kim et al, 2001; Lincoln et al, 2004; Shelton and Yutzey, 2007). Why some cells respond to such signals and undergo epithelial-to-mesenchymal transformation while neighboring cells remain epithelial is unclear.

In both the AV canal and conotruncus, four distinct cushions form, named by their anatomic locations. For the AV canal these are superior, inferior, left lateral, and right lateral. In the conotruncus they are right superior, right dorsal, left inferior, and left ventral. The AV and conotruncal cushions are separate with one important exception: The left ventral conal cushion and the superior AV cushion are in continuity along the inner curvature of the heart. This proximity will persist in the fully septated heart as aortic-mitral valve continuity. The atrioventricular canal septates as the superior and inferior cushions grow and extend (see Figure 50-5, *D* to *F*), finally fusing in the midline. This results in complete separation of the AV canal into left (mitral) and right (tricuspid) sides. The AV valves form from remnants of the cushions: a leftward mitral valve with two leaflets, and a rightward tricuspid valve with three leaflets.

Failure of complete fusion between the superior and inferior cushions in the midline results in a cleft within the anterior leaflet of the mitral valve. This is a mild form of an endocardial cushion defect, often associated with a primum atrial septal defect (see section on atrial septation) and known as a partial atrioventricular canal. The septal leaflet of the tricuspid valve also forms from this superior and inferior cushions and can be abnormal as well, although this is less often clinically significant. More profound failure of proper AV cushion expansion and fusion results in a complete atrioventricular canal. Here the crux

of the heart is unformed. There remains a common orifice overlying both ventricles, with defects in the adjacent atrial and ventricular septa. The common atrioventricular valve has leaflet structure based on the unseptated AV canal, with four or sometimes five separate leaflets corresponding to the two lateral, the superior (referred to as anterior bridging) and inferior leaflets.

The AV canal myocardium, part of the primitive heart tube, does not persist in the adult heart. There is no muscular connection between the mature atrial and ventricles. The process for isolation of the atrial and ventricular muscle appears to occur as the epicardium of the AV sulcus establishes continuity with the developing endocardial cushions beneath; this occurs all along the ventricular margin of the AV canal (Wessels et al, 1996). The only remaining connection between atria and ventricles is within the conduction system, the AV node (Anderson and Ho, 1998, 2003; Anderson et al, 2000). Occasional muscular bridges of tissue remain as accessory muscle connections, which can be clinically important as substrate for arrhythmias (specifically AV reciprocating tachycardias, a common form of supraventricular tachycardia).

VENTRICULAR OUTFLOW TRACT SEPTATION: CONTRIBUTION OF ENDOCARDIAL CUSHIONS

While the AV cushions form a three-dimensional crux of the heart, the conotruncal cushions form a three-dimensional spiral, completing an almost 180-degree rotation (Carlson, 2004; Ya et al, 1998). During septation of the outflow tracts, the primitive bulbus cordis is separable into two segments, the truncus adjacent to the aortic sac, and the conus adjacent to the ventricular myocardium (Figure 50-6, *A*).

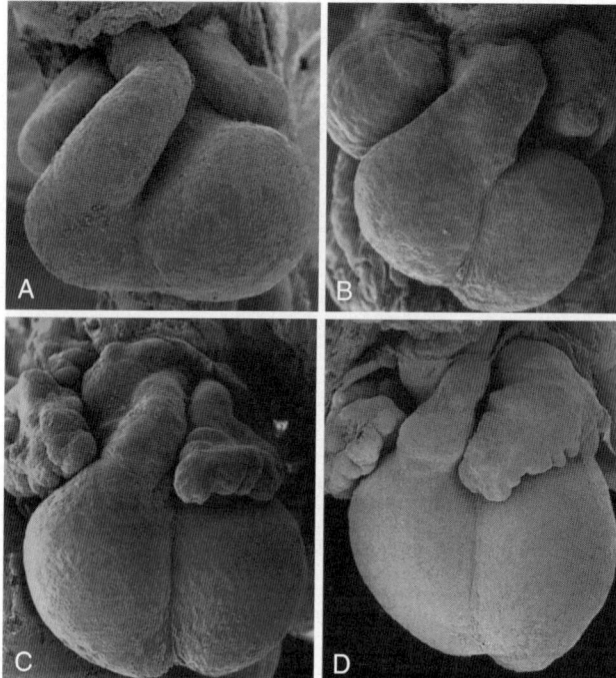

FIGURE 50-6 Septation of the outflow tracts, as viewed externally by scanning electron microscopy. **A** is a human embryo at 5 weeks' gestation; the conus and truncus of the common outflow tract are labeled. **B** is an embryo at 6 weeks' gestation. **C** and **D** are 7 and 8 weeks' gestation, respectively. Now completely separate pulmonary and aortic outflow tracts are identified. (*Adapted from Steding G: The anatomy of the human embryo, Basel, 2009, Karger, pp 211, 213, 214, 215.*)

The right superior and left inferior cushions are within the truncal region and will contribute to the aorticopulmonary septum. The right dorsal and left ventral cushions are within the conus region and are important for pulmonary and aortic valve formation, and for completion of septation between the ventricles at the level of the pulmonary and aortic valves.

Again, for this process to occur correctly, the continuity of the superior AV cushion and left ventral conus cushion is critical. To align the septated great arteries directly over the ventricles, the arterial trunk must shift to the left. There is evidence from mouse models that failure to achieve continuity of the superior AV cushion and left ventral conus cushion results in malalignment of both great arteries over the right ventricle, along with a ventricular septal defect (van den Hoff et al, 1999; Waller et al, 2000). Clinically, this is an entity known as double-outlet right ventricle (DORV). Part of the clinical definition of a DORV is presence of a conus segment of both ventricles (bilateral conus). Anatomically, the normal conus is a muscular "neck" within the right ventricle between the tricuspid and pulmonary valves. Embryologically, this is a remnant of the conus of the primitive heart tube that is retained by the right ventricle. In the left ventricle, the fusion of the superior AV and left ventral conal cushions results in mitral aortic continuity and lack of a conal segment. If this fusion of cushions and leftward shifting of the truncus do not occur, then a conus is retained in the left ventricular outflow tract, which is malpositioned to the right.

VENTRICULAR OUTFLOW TRACT SEPTATION: ROLE OF NEURAL CREST

As discussed in the section on cell types making up the heart, the developing outflow tract has the added complexity of contributions from outside the primitive heart tube. These include two important populations of cells, neural crest and anterior heart field cells. The cell movement of the anterior heart field was discussed in the section on cardiac looping. Recent data regarding gene expression in the secondary heart field have demonstrated newly appreciated roles for several genes already studied in the primary heart field, including *Hand1*, *Nkx2-5*, *Gata4*, and *Mef2* (Dodou et al, 2004; Dyer and Kirby, 2009; Verzi et al, 2005; Ward et al, 2005a, 2005b; Zeisberg et al, 2005). Gene expression defects here can lead to right ventricular hypoplasia and outflow tract abnormalities, including tetralogy of Fallot (Ward et al, 2005; Zeisberg et al, 2005).

The second population of cells that migrate into the developing outflow tracts is the cardiac neural crest. Neural cells originate in the anterior rhombencephalon, and migrate as a sheet through the pharyngeal region and into the aortic arches. The third, fourth, and sixth arches are the primary sites of neural crest migration and activity (see section on arch development and Figure 50-10 for detail). The neural crest cells surround the epithelia of the arch arteries and extend into the truncus and proximal conus. Here they interact with endocardial cushion cells to separate the great arteries and close the conal septum. These neural crest cells are also important for development of the nearby parathyroid, thyroid, and thymus glands. In human DiGeorge syndrome, cardiac conotruncal and arch defects are associated with developmental defects in each of these three glands as well. Extensive work has been done in chick models using neural crest ablation, and these studies show a very high prevalence of persistent truncus arteriosus, interrupted aortic arch, tetralogy of Fallot, DORV, and ventricular septal defects, along with abnormal parathyroid, thyroid, and thymus development (Creazzo et al, 1998; Harvey and Rosenthal, 1999; Kirby and Waldo, 1995; Nishibatake et al, 1987; Waldo and Kirby, 1993; Waldo et al, 1996, 2005).

The genetic defects underlying DiGeorge syndrome have been elusive, but knowledge is advancing. A deletion of up to 3 megabases in chromosome 22 (22q11) has long been known to be associated with DiGeorge, based on kindred studies in families with the syndrome. In humans, the defect is autosomal dominant, with variable penetration, meaning that one copy of the gene deletion is sufficient to cause disease and that the disease severity varied from family member to family member. A similar deletion generated experimentally in mice yielded a model of the cardiovascular features of DiGeorge syndrome (Lindsay et al, 1999). Recently, three independent investigators narrowed in on TBX1 as the responsible gene in these mice (Jerome and Papaioannou, 2001; Lindsay et al, 2001; Merscher et al, 2001). TBX1 is a transcription factor in a family known to be important in embryonic patterning. Homozygous mutations of TBX1 caused obliteration of the third, fourth, and sixth pharyngeal arches with embryonic lethality and caused most of the extracardiac defects as well, along with an abnormal ear, jaw, and pharynx

(Jerome and Papaioannou, 2001). Heterozygous mutants, which are analogous to the human disease state, showed more variable disease. The cardiac defects primarily affected the fourth pharyngeal arch and caused abnormal patterning of the great arteries in 50% of embryos in one study (Lindsay et al, 2001). This group had 1 heterozygous mouse mutant out of 14 that also exhibited parathyroid and thymic insufficiency. Possibly, humans are more sensitive to gene dosage and exhibit the full range of defects in the haploinsufficient state. There may be other modifying genes as well, because there seems to be an important contribution of genetic background to the phenotype in mice, with more severe arch anomalies presenting in more inbred strains (Jerome and Papaioannou, 2001). This is a confounding factor of many gene targeting strategies and perhaps a clue as to why significant phenotypic variation can occur in humans with identical mutations. Interestingly, isolated TBX1 mutations appear to be very rare as causes of clinical DiGeorge syndrome (Beaujard et al, 2009; Portnoi, 2009; Rauch et al, 2010); most patients having a larger megabase deletion.

SEPARATION OF AORTA AND PULMONARY ARTERY: NORMAL DEXTROPOSITION

Within the truncus segment, septation is also occurring during remodeling of the conus. This normally occurs as the truncal cushions fuse in a spiral fashion. Starting at the level of the AV valves, the newly forming pulmonary artery is directly anterior to the aorta. Further along the outflow tract, the pulmonary artery and aorta are more left-right to one another, as the spiral extends. As the aorta arches to the left, the proximal transverse arch passes anterior to the pulmonary artery, completing a 180-degree turn of the spiral (see Figure 50-6). This rotation involves not only the truncal cushions but the rotation of the myocardial tube as well (Bajolle et al, 2006; Lomonico et al, 1986). If this 180-degree twist does not occur or is incomplete, the result is transposed great arteries. This is defined by the aortic valve being anterior to the pulmonary valve. The left-right orientation of the valves is most commonly preserved (aortic rightward), although can vary within a 90-degree range from directly anterior-posterior to directly side by side. L-transposition, aortic leftward, is most often associated with L-looped ventricles or heterotaxy syndromes and is rare in isolated transposition.

CARDIAC VALVE FORMATION

Cardiac valve development begins with the endocardial cushions during week 7 of gestation, but formation of mature atrioventricular (mitral and tricuspid) and semilunar valves (aortic and pulmonic) takes several weeks for completion (Combs and Yutzey, 2009; de Lange et al, 2004; Dhanantwari et al, 2009; Hinton et al, 2006; Kanani et al, 2005; Lincoln et al, 2004; Steding, 2009). As the endocardial cushions enlarge, they protrude into the lumen of the heart. Here, subject to constant flow of blood, the protrusions condense and elongate. Endocardial cells overlying the cushions proliferate slowly, and there is programmed cell death (apoptosis) of mesenchymal cells underneath.

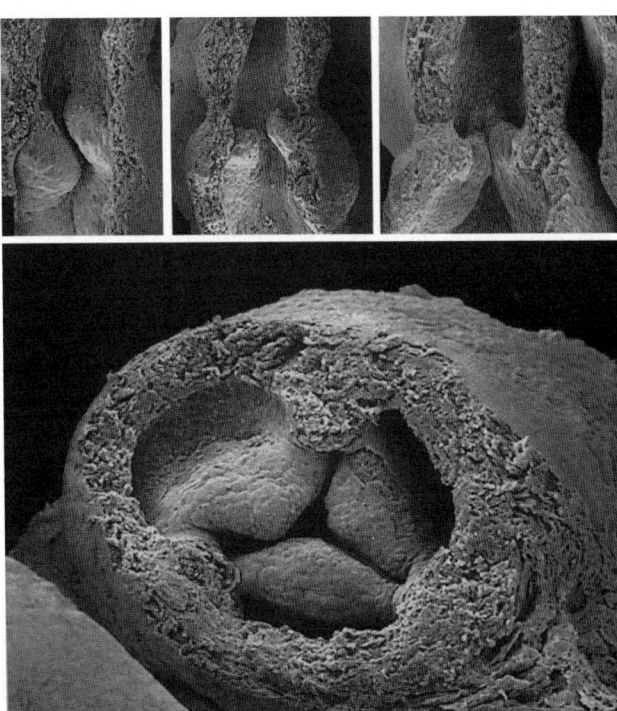

FIGURE 50-7 Semilunar valve formation, as seen by scanning electron microscopy. Human embryos at weeks 7 and 8 above, and week 9 below. The views *above* are coronal sections through the pulmonary trunk, viewed from the ventral side. The embryo *below* is shown from a transverse section through the pulmonary trunk, revealing the pulmonary valve leaflets. (*From Steding G:* The anatomy of the human embryo, *Basel, 2009, Karger, p 239.*)

The valves undergo extensive remodeling of the extracellular matrix; in the case of the semilunar valves, this results in a fibrous layer (primarily collagen) on the arterial side, a spongiosa layer (glycosaminoglycans) in the middle, and an elastic layer (elastin) on the ventricular side (Combs and Yutzey, 2009; Hinton et al, 2006; Shelton and Yutzey, 2007). In the case of the semilunar valves, this remodeling process of the endocardial cushions continues through the last trimester of pregnancy and into the neonatal period (Aikawa et al, 2006; Hinton et al, 2006). The morphology of this process is shown in Figure 50-7.

Recent studies have shed some light on the genetics of cardiac valve disease. For example, Noonan's syndrome is characterized by cardiac malformations including a dysplastic pulmonary valve. Linkage studies of families with Noonan's syndrome uncovered a candidate gene on chromosome 12, the PTPN11 gene (Tartaglia et al, 2001). The PTPN11 encodes for SHP-2, a signaling molecule important for growth factors, cytokines, and hormones (Tartaglia et al, 2001). A specific role in mediating growth factors during semilunar valve formation had been proposed (Chen et al, 2000), and several human mutations in the gene have been shown to cause overactivation of the SHP-2 protein (Tartaglia et al, 2002). This suggests a gain-of-function mechanism for the pathogenesis of Noonan's syndrome, an interesting distinction from the more familiar concept of loss of functioning protein causing disease. Likewise, mutations in the Notch1 receptor and various components of the Notch signaling pathway, have been associated with the formation of aortic valves and with multiple stages of cardiac development (Garg et al, 2005; High and Epstein, 2008).

DEVELOPMENT OF THE VENTRICLES AND VENTRICULAR SEPTUM

The majority of the ventricular septum is muscular and made up of a protrusion of ventricular myocardium that starts at the apex of the primitive ventricle and extends into the ventricular cavity. The early septating ventricle, then, appears as a bilobed structure (Dhanantwari et al, 2009; Steding, 2009) (Figure 50-8). As the septum extends upward, the separation becomes nearly complete. There is controversy as to how the septum extends so quickly to form a wall between the left and right ventricles. Part of the answer seems to be rapid proliferation of these myocytes, which retain the ability to divide even as a working myocardium. This property is lost soon after birth, as the mature myocardium is for the most part incapable of proliferation. Small muscular ventricular septal defects (VSDs) are very common in newborns. One study screening asymptomatic newborns found an incidence of 53 per 1000 neonates with small muscular VSDs; only one tenth of these infants had physical exam signs of their VSD. Nearly 90% of these small defects were closed by 10 months of age (Roguin et al, 1995). These data and others suggest continued low-level proliferation in human ventricles after birth.

We have said that as the muscular septum grows and extends from the ventricular apex, the separation between the left and right ventricles becomes nearly complete. There are two important regions of the entire ventricular septum that are completed by endocardial cushions, as discussed in the preceding sections. First, the AV endocardial cushions form the posterior septum adjacent to the AV valves. Second, the conal cushions form the conal septum below the great arteries. An important feature of this process not discussed earlier is the fact that these regions of septum contain muscle as well as cushion tissue. The muscle gets there via a process called myocardialization, during which the muscle cells of the inner curvature of the heart invade the conal cushion and superior AV cushions as they

form the septum (Harvey and Rosenthal, 1999). These migrating myocytes are nonproliferative, and the entire inner curvature is involved. Thus, the mitral-aortic continuity discussed earlier is completely fibrous and devoid of muscle. Yet the posterior AV septum and the conal septum are muscular structures, because of the process of muscularization. This process is considered by some investigators to complete the looping process; a DORV could then be considered a failure of the final stages of looping.

The left and right ventricles differ not only by their relative positions to one another, but also in their basic muscular structure and in their function. Each ventricle can functionally be subdivided into inflow and outflow regions. The RV, as we have discussed, has a conal segment as well and is therefore referred to as a tripartite ventricle. In the mature heart, the LV is a high-pressure system, connected to systemic pressures, whereas the RV is connected to the lower-pressure pulmonary circulation. The LV form follows its function, with concentric rings of myofibrils that contract with a slight twisting motion, which allows for an efficient ejection of blood. In the embryo, the myocardium thickens and arranges itself in processes known as trabeculation and compaction. Trabeculation refers to projections of muscular tissue into the lumen of the ventricle, such that the inner surface is no longer smooth-walled, but ridged. Compaction refers to the alignment of myocytes from random and loosely packed, as they are in the immature myocardium, into bundles of tightly packed and well-coordinated myocytes working as a unit in the mature myocardium (Harvey and Rosenthal, 1999).

DEVELOPMENT OF THE ATRIA AND ATRIAL SEPTUM

Like the ventricular septum, the atrial septum begins as a ridge of muscular tissue, superior and midline, which expands to divide the right side of the atrium containing the orifice of the sinus venosus from the left side of the atrium containing the orifice of the common pulmonary vein. This structure is known as the septum primum, and it grows inferiorly toward the fusing AV cushions. As discussed previously, the fusing AV cushions will form the

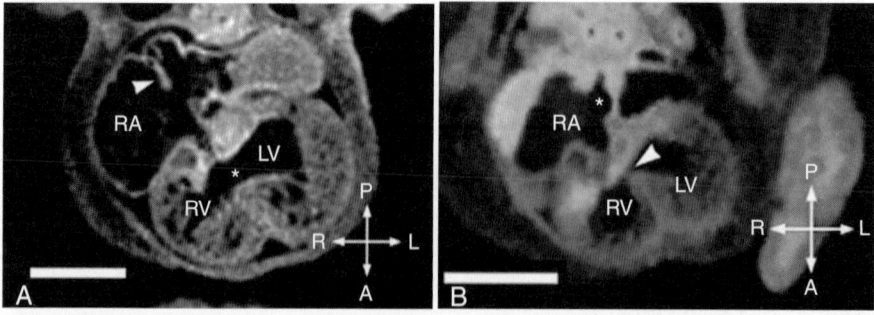

FIGURE 50-8 Atrial and ventricular septation. Human fetal MRI images in transverse plane, showing four chambers of the heart (*LV*, left ventricle; *RA*, Right atrium; *RV*, right ventricle). Orientation as shown by the *arrows*: P (posterior), A (anterior), R (right), and L (left). **A,** Fetus at 7⅚ weeks' gestation. The atrial septum primum is marked by the *arrowhead*, with the foramen primum below allowing shunting of blood from RA to LA. Between the ventricles, the muscular intraventricular septum is forming but is not yet complete (*). Scale bar is 1.25 mm. **B,** Fetus at 8 weeks' gestation. Here the atrial septum primum (*) is fused with the endocardial cushions inferiorly; not seen is the foramen ovale that allows continuous right-to-left atrial shunting in the fetus. The *arrowhead* shows a small residual ventricular septal defect in the inlet (posterior) septum, not yet closed by endocardial cushion tissue. Scale bar is 1.5 mm. (*Adapted from Dhanantwari P, Lee E, Krishnan A, et al: Human cardiac development in the first trimester: a high-resolution magnetic resonance imaging and episcopic fluorescence image capture atlas,* Circulation *120:345-346, 2009.*)

inferior portion of the atrial septum. Before septum primum and the cushions completing atrial septation, however, small perforations appear, enlarge, and coalesce within the primum septum (see Figure 50-8). The impetus for this is not known. Soon afterward, a new crescent of atrial septum forms on the right atrial side of the septum primum and begins extending alongside the septum primum. During fetal life, blood flow from the right atrium into the left prevents fusion of these two septae. The septum secundum is significantly more rigid than the septum primum, which flaps open to allow continued right-to-left flow (see Figure 50-8). After birth and separation from the low-resistance placenta, the left atrial pressure rises significantly and the atrial shunt reverses. This causes the septum primum to effect a seal against the septum secundum, often leaving a small opening known as the foramen ovale. A patent foramen ovale, generally 3 mm or less with a trivial degree of left-to-right flow, is a normal finding in a newborn and even in many older children and adults. A defect larger than 5 mm may constitute a secundum atrial septal defect (ASD), a true deficiency in atrial septal tissue in the region of the foramen ovale.

Failure of the cushions to form the inferiormost part of the atrial septum results in a primum atrial septal defect. Such defects do not close spontaneously and may be associated with other endocardial cushion defects, most commonly a cleft mitral valve. Finally, there is a small contribution to the atrial septum near the junctions of the superior and inferior vena cavae (see later discussion). Defects in this process result in a sinus venosus ASD, and there are superior or inferior types. Such defects again result from deficiency of atrial septal tissue and do not close spontaneously.

SYSTEMIC AND PULMONARY VEIN DEVELOPMENT

The sinus venosus of the primitive heart tube is a symmetric structure and receives three sets of paired (left and right) systemic veins: the vitelline, umbilical, and common cardinal (Figure 50-9, A). This is the situation at 4 to 5 weeks' gestation (Minniti et al, 2002).

The vitelline veins return from the yolk sac, a structure that communicates with the primitive gut via the vitelline duct. The duct normally regresses completely, but an occasional remnant can be seen as a Meckel's diverticulum (Carlson, 2004). Distally, the vitelline veins regress along with the duct and proximally lose their connection to the sinus venosus by 6 weeks. The midportions of these vessels, however, expand within the liver to contribute toward the hepatic and portal veins, and a small segment to the IVC (see Figure 50-9, A and later discussion) as well.

The umbilical veins return from the placenta carrying oxygenated blood. These are the first to develop, by 3 weeks' gestation. As the liver develops, the umbilical veins develop connections to the liver venous plexus, and the connection to the sinus venosus involutes. Outside the embryo within the umbilical cord, the left and right umbilical veins fuse into one; thus there is a single umbilical vein in the newborn. Within the embryo, the left and right segments remain separate, and the left umbilical vein becomes connected to the right hepatic veins via a new channel that forms, the ductus venosus (see Figure 50-9, A). This circulation is formed by the 7th week of gestation. Again the umbilical veins are carrying oxygenated blood to the right atrium. This flow is primarily directed toward the atrial septum, and therefore primarily through the foramen ovale into the left atrium and systemic circulation.

The cardinal veins carry the venous return from the embryo proper. The left and right common cardinal veins are relatively short segments that connect to the sinus venosus. On each side, anterior and posterior cardinal veins join to form the common cardinal vein, the anterior carrying the venous return from the upper body and the posterior from the lower body. The right anterior and right common cardinal vein will form the superior vena cava in the mature circulation. The left common cardinal vein and left segment of the sinus venosus form the coronary sinus, which receives venous return from the coronary system. These structures are pulled rightward as the IVC forms, such that the opening (os) of the coronary sinus ends up in the right atrium once atrial septation is complete. The IVC is more complex and is made up of five segments, coming from urogenital, mesenteric, and hepatic venous channels fusing together to the right of the spine as their leftward paired counterparts involute. Because numerous vessels go into making the IVC, interruption of the IVC can sometimes occur at various segments. This is most often in the setting of heterotaxy, but can occur in isolation. When the IVC is interrupted, one of two major vessels that connect the lower and upper body venous systems generally enlarges to receive the flow and shunt it into the SVC. These are the rightward azygous vein, which runs from the suprarenal segment of the IVC to the SVC, and the leftward hemiazygous vein, which takes a more tortuous course from the leftward lumbar and renal veins up into the thoracic cavity, where it turns rightward to join the azygous vein. Thus, an interrupted IVC generally has either azygous or hemiazygous continuation to the SVC.

The pulmonary veins grow in progressively from the developing lung vasculature, first as a common pulmonary vein from both lungs. This vein fuses into the back of the left atrium (Wessels et al, 2000). As the atrium expands, the common pulmonary vein becomes increasingly absorbed into the back wall, such that first 2, then 4 of its distal branches eventually enter independently into the left atrium, 2 from the left and 2 from the right lung (see Figure 50-9, B). The original atrial segment of the heart tube is not part of the functioning atria in the mature heart, instead relegated to the right and left atrial appendages.

AORTIC ARCH DEVELOPMENT

The primitive heart tube connects to the aortic sac, the precursor to the ascending aorta, and begins pumping to the developing systemic circulation of the embryo as soon as it is formed. The aortic sac connects to paired dorsal aortae posteriorly via an aortic root, which gives rise to a series of arches, the branchial arches (Figure 50-10, top). It is along these arches that the neural crest migrates into the conotruncus and supports development of the arch arteries. Again these are paired structures, and there are a total of six pairs, although not all are patent at the same time. Arches 1 to 4 carry the blood flow in the 4-week embryo.

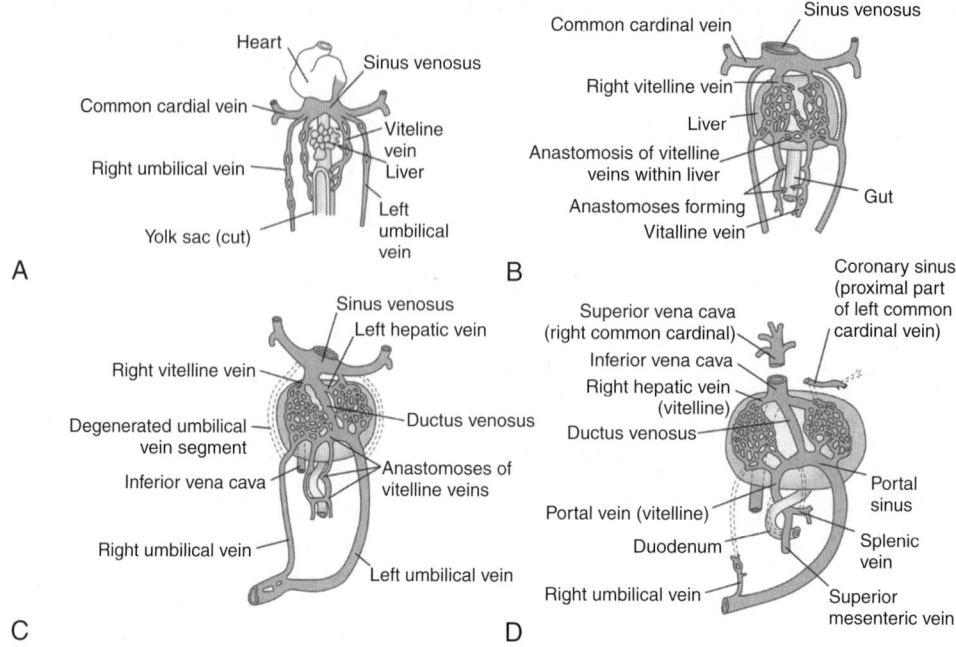

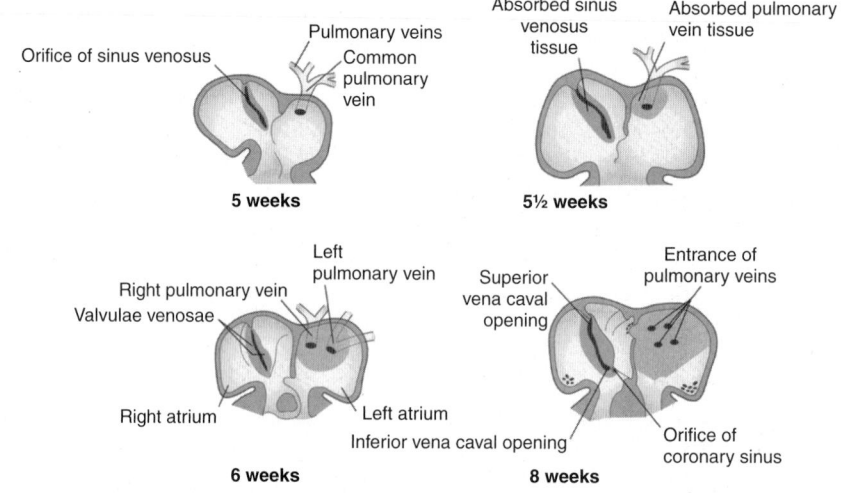

FIGURE 50-9 Stages of development of the systemic veins (*top*) and pulmonary veins (*bottom*). Stages of systemic vein development are shown in **A** to **D**, during which the paired umbilical, vitelline, and cardinal veins give rise to the single umbilical vein, liver vasculature including the portal system, and the inferior and superior vena cavae. Stages of pulmonary vein development are shown by week gestation as labeled; the common pulmonary vein progressively absorbs into the back wall of the left atrium. (*From Carlson BM: Human embryology and developmental biology, ed 4, Philadelphia, 2009, Mosby, pp 452-453.*)

Arches 1 and 2 mostly regress completely, although parts contribute to some of the arteries of the face. Arch 3 does not persist as an arch, but contributes to the formation of the carotid arteries, both left and right. The left limb of arch 4 remains in continuity with the aortic root, together making up the true aortic arch and its first branch, the brachiocephalic (innominate) artery. The right limb of arch 4 becomes part of the right subclavian artery, which retains its proximal connection with the brachiocephalic artery (Waldo et al, 1996). This arch remodeling has occurred by 7 weeks' gestation; see Figure 50-10, *bottom*. In some cases, either independently or as part of another developmental cardiac defect, the right limb of arch 4 remains patent and the left forms the left subclavian artery—this forms a right aortic arch with mirror-image branching. Arch 5 is small and never fully develops. Arch 6 forms with the developing pulmonary artery vasculature and makes up the proximal left and right pulmonary arteries and the ductus arteriosus (Waldo and Kirby, 1993). The ductal arch persists throughout fetal life as another means of right-to-left shunt, allowing blood from the right ventricle to bypass the pulmonary circulation and cross over into the descending aorta.

CORONARY ARTERIES

The coronary arteries were for many years assumed to sprout from the ascending aorta and grow over the surface of the heart. This is now known to be incorrect. The coronary arteries derive from the epicardium of the heart. Early in development, bilateral clusters of cells appear near the septum transversum, where the liver bud approaches the heart. These cells spread out over the surface of the heart as an epithelium, forming the epicardium. Some of

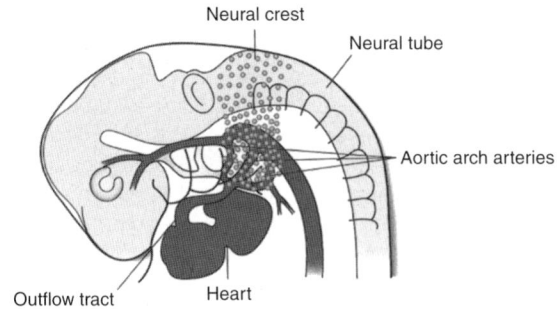

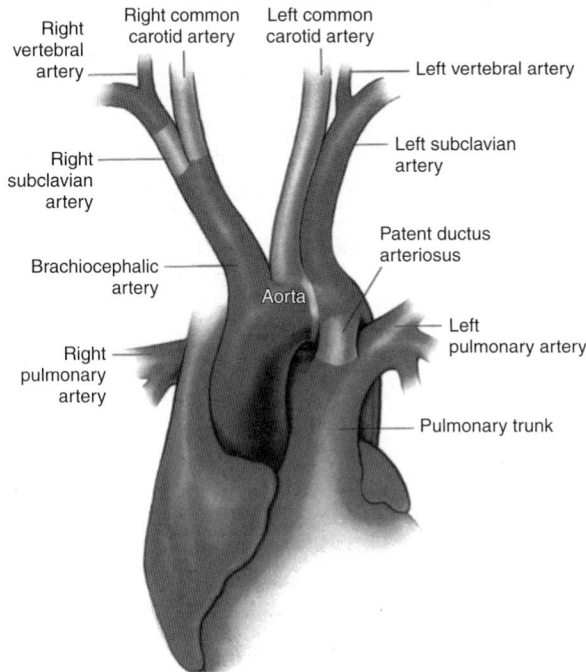

FIGURE 50-10 *Top,* Migration pattern of neural crest cells into pharyngeal arches 3, 4, and 6. *Bottom,* Normal aortic arch at term. Most of the pharyngeal arch segments have regressed. The third arch persists in part as the left and right common carotid arteries. The left fourth arch persists as the true aortic arch, while a portion of the right fourth arch makes up the proximal right subclavian artery. The sixth arch persists as the ductus arteriosus (ductal arch). *(From Kirby ML: Contribution of neural crest to heart and vessel morphology. In Harvey RP, Rosenthal N, editors: Heart development, San Diego, Calif., 1999, Academic Press, pp 180-181.)*

the epicardial cells delaminate from the epithelium and migrate into the myocardium below. Lineage tracing studies in the chicken have shown these cells to form the coronary vasculature, both endothelial cells and arterial smooth muscle, and cardiac fibroblasts (Cheng et al, 1999; Mikawa and Fischman, 1992; Mikawa and Gourdie, 1996; Reese et al, 1999). The coronary vessels form, grow, and fuse with one another to form a working vasculature. This corresponds with the process of growth and trabeculation of the ventricles. With increasing complexity and thickness of the myocardium, simple diffusion of nutrients from the blood inside the heart is no longer adequate. The coronary vasculature, then, provides the necessary blood supply to a working myocardium by extending its surface vessels on the right and left to plug into the aorta just above the aortic valve. It is likely that neural crest signaling plays an important guiding role here; this has been suggested in

mammals by the presence of neural crest cells in the proximal coronary arteries (Carlson, 2004). Detailed studies in chick have not supported the presence of neural crest in the coronary arteries, however (Waldo et al, 1994). Occasionally this process can go awry, and a coronary artery (usually the left) can join the pulmonary artery instead of the aorta. This does not damage the fetal myocardium given the low oxygen state of the fetus, with little difference in oxygen tension between the aorta and pulmonary artery. After birth, however, ischemia sets in rapidly, often causing a significant myocardial infarction early in life.

CONDUCTION SYSTEM

There has been controversy regarding the origin of the conduction system, and again this controversy was recently resolved. The conduction system was suspected to originate from neural crest by many investigators, thus migrating in from outside the heart. Lineage tracing studies show conclusively that the cells of the conduction system actually differentiate in situ from myocytes (Cheng et al, 1999; Gourdie et al, 1998; Hyer et al, 1999; Moorman et al, 1997; Waldo et al, 1994). There is evidence that the developing coronary vasculature is a source of signaling for this transdifferentiation to occur; the conduction system tends to develop alongside coronary vessels (Hyer et al, 1999). Conduction system myocytes express different markers, junctions, and have different action potential profiles that allow for automaticity (Alyonycheva et al, 1997; Hoogaars et al, 2007; Moorman et al, 1997; Takebayashi-Suzuki et al, 2001; Wessels et al, 1992). Under normal conditions, the automaticity of the remaining conduction system is suppressed as the dominant pacemaker of the heart forms, the sinoatrial (SA) node. The SA node tends to have the fastest depolarization and to set the pace for the heart rate starting at about 1 month's gestation (Phoon, 2001). If the SA node slows down for any reason, other "pacemakers" will substitute. Atrial myocytes tend to have the next most rapid automatic rates, followed by the His bundles, then by ventricular myocytes. The heart rate in a 5-week fetus is 100 beats per minute (Phoon, 2001). This increases gradually to a rate of 160 beats per minute by 8 weeks' gestation, then declines slightly during gestation to the 120s to 130s (Phoon, 2001).

PHYSIOLOGY OF TRANSITION

The fetal heart and circulation at the end of 9 weeks are completely formed (Phoon, 2001). As depicted in Figure 50-11, there are four chambers of the heart, two atria in communication via a patent foramen ovale, and two ventricles with complete septation. The left ventricular myocardium is configured differently from the right such that it is capable of working under higher pressure (afterload). There are fully competent atrioventricular valves (the mitral and tricuspid) and fully competent semilunar valves (the aortic and pulmonary) that ensure one-way flow through the heart. The venous blood from the systemic and pulmonary circulations return fully to the atria. The arterial blood is pumped to the body and to the lungs via the great arteries, with a communication between the two via the patent ductus arteriosus.

Before birth, the placenta is a critical component of the fetal circulation, with a single umbilical vein and two umbilical arteries (see Figure 50-11). A full 50% of the fetal blood volume is in the placenta, and 50% in the body. In the fetus, the systemic cardiac output is combined from left and right ventricles, with the right ventricle actually contributing more than the left to the total (approximately 65% vs. 35%) (Teitel, 1992). This is via the "ductal arch" connecting the main pulmonary artery to the ductus arteriosus and descending aorta. The aortic arch contributes about 60% of its flow to the head and neck vessels, and the rest combines with the ductal flow to reach the lower body and return to the placenta. Blood returning from the placenta (oxygenated) returns via the umbilical veins through the ductus venosus to the IVC and right atrium. This blood is under higher pressure than the systemic return from the fetus and is streamed such that at least 25% is directed across the foramen ovale into the left atrium and systemic circulation. The remainder combines the SVC return to cross the tricuspid valve into the right ventricle. Only about 10% of the right ventricular output actually goes to the lungs; this small amount of blood returns to the heart via the pulmonary veins into the left atrium, mixes with the oxygenated blood that has crossed the foramen ovale from the right atrium, and passes on to the systemic circulation (Teitel, 1992).

After birth, two major factors trigger changes in circulation. These are the initiation of respirations with lung expansion and alveolar gas exchange, and cutting of the umbilical cord. The result is a drastic reduction in IVC return to the right side of the heart as the placental flow ceases; at the same time there is a drastic increase in capacity of the pulmonary circulation. Thus, return to the right atrium decreases and return to the left atrium increases, as does left atrial pressure. This forces the flap of the foramen ovale up against the atrial wall, reducing the volume and reversing the direction of atrial level shunting. Thus the fetus has a large patent foramen ovale with right-to-left flow, which after birth becomes a smaller orifice with left-to-right flow. Approximately 20% of older children and adults retain a small patent foramen ovale, with a trivial left-to-right shunt. Also immediately after birth, the increased oxygen tension of the blood that occurs with breathing causes the ductus arteriosus to begin constricting (functional closure). This is a function of smooth muscle within the wall of the ductus arteriosus and is prostaglandin sensitive. After functional closure, the permanent process of anatomic closure, involving apoptosis of smooth muscle and proliferation of connective tissue, converts the ductus arteriosus into a fibrous ligament (the ligamentum arteriosus). A similar but slower process occurs in the ductus venosus, also causing it to be closed by fibrosis.

SUMMARY

We have reviewed heart development, with attention to the morphology, cell biology, genetics, and physiology of the heart as it forms and remodels. The field of developmental biology of the heart continues to advance rapidly on all of these fronts. New technologies allow earlier and earlier visualization of the developing human heart, recently as early as week 6 of gestation by cardiac MRI (Dhanantwari et al, 2009), and week 10 to 11 by cardiac ultrasound (Becker and Wegner, 2006; Bennasar et al, 2009; Cook et al, 2004; Gembruch et al, 2000; Marques Carvalho et al, 2008; Neuman and Huhta, 2006; Vimpelli et al, 2006; Weiner et al, 2002). Early ultrasound has the additional benefit of assessment of cardiac physiology in the embryo, using Doppler technology Phoon, 2001. Novel genetic techniques allow us to apply what is learned from animal models to humans, and to recreate human disease in animal models with greater specificity. The common goals to be applied to human disease are early recognition of congenital heart malformations, prevention where feasible, and state-of-the-art intervention to allow an abnormal heart to function as normally as possible. Currently such intervention is surgical and cardiac catheterization–based and continues to evolve. In the future, gene therapy, cardiac stem cell grafting, and in vitro tissue engineering will likely be added to the therapeutic potentials for patients with congenital heart malformations.

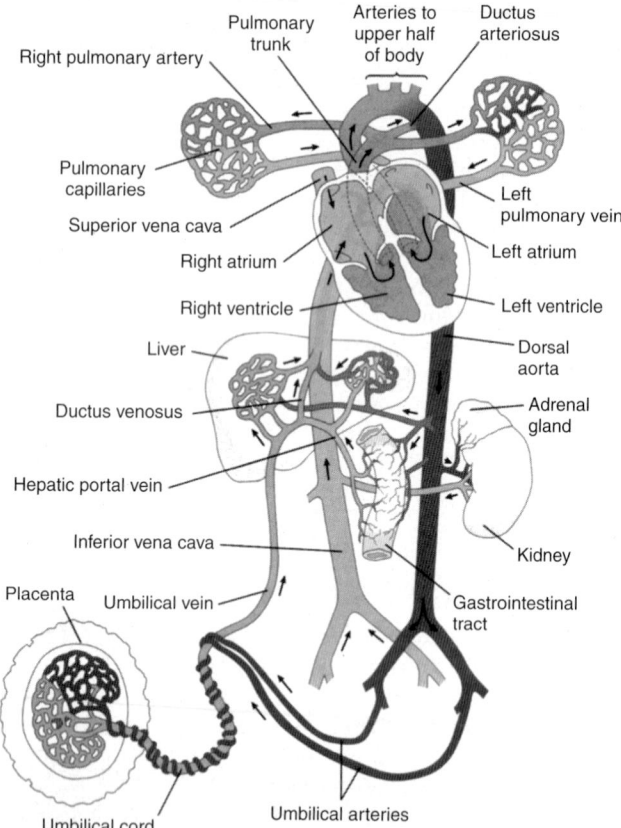

FIGURE 50-11 (*See also Color Plate 20.*) **The fetal circulation at term.** Deoxygenated blood is indicated in *dark gray* and oxygenated in *light gray*, with *shades in between* indicating mixing of blood. Oxygenated blood returns from the placenta to the heart and mixes with deoxygenated blood from the fetal systemic veins. Note that the upper body receives higher oxygen content than the lower body, as deoxygenated blood enters the descending aorta via right to left flow at the ductus arteriosus. (*From Carlson BM:* Human embryology and developmental biology, *ed 4, Philadelphia, 2009, Mosby, p 466.*)

SUGGESTED READINGS

Bruneau BG: The developmental genetics of congenital heart disease, *Nature* 451:943-948, 2008.
Combs MD, Yutzey KE: Heart valve development: regulatory networks in development and disease, *Circ Res* 105:408-421, 2009.
Cook AC, Yates RW, Anderson RH: Normal and abnormal fetal cardiac anatomy, *Prenat Diagn* 24:1032-1048, 2004.

Dhanantwari P, Lee E, Krishnan A, et al: Human cardiac development in the first trimester: a high-resolution magnetic resonance imaging and episcopic fluorescence image capture atlas, *Circulation* 120:343-351, 2009.

Dyer LA, Kirby ML: The role of secondary heart field in cardiac development, *Dev Biol* 336:137-144, 2009.

Ghosh S, Yarmish G, Godelman A, et al: Anomalies of visceroatrial situs, *AJR Am J Roentgenol* 193:1107-1117, 2009.

High FA, Epstein JA: The multifaceted role of Notch in cardiac development and disease, *Nat Rev Genet* 9:49-61, 2008.

Lindsay EA, Vitelli F, Su H, et al: Tbx1 haploinsufficiency in the DiGeorge syndrome region causes aortic arch defects in mice, *Nature* 410:97-101, 2001.

Phoon CK: Circulatory physiology in the developing embryo, *Curr Opin Pediatr* 13:456-464, 2001.

Steding G: *The anatomy of the human embryo*, Basel, 2009, Karger.

Tartaglia M, Mehler EL, Goldberg R, et al: Mutations in PTPN11, encoding the protein tyrosine phosphatase SHP-2, cause Noonan syndrome, *Nat Genet* 29:465-468, 2001.

Ward C, Stadt H, Hutson M, Kirby ML: Ablation of the secondary heart field leads to tetralogy of Fallot and pulmonary atresia, *Dev Biol* 284:72-83, 2005.

Complete references and supplemental color images used in this text can be found online at www.expertconsult.com

CARDIOVASCULAR COMPROMISE IN THE NEWBORN INFANT

Istvan Seri and Barry Markovitz

Although the prevalence of hypotension in the neonates admitted for intensive care is unclear, up to 50% of very low birthweight (VLBW) neonates present with blood pressure values considered to be low in the immediate transitional period (McLean et al, 2008). However, VLBW neonates account for only around 25% of all neonates diagnosed with hypotension in neonatal intensive care units. The lack of clear data on the prevalence of neonatal hypotension is primarily due to the uncertainty about the lower limit of the gestational- and postnatal-age dependent normal blood pressure range in neonates (Engle, 2008). This is illustrated, among others, by the significant differences in the prevalence of the use of vasopressor/inotropes in preterm neonates during the transitional period among different intensive care units across the nation (Al-Aweel et al, 2001).

Shock is a "state of cellular energy failure resulting from an inability of tissue oxygen delivery to satisfy tissue oxygen demand" (Singer, 2008). As long as pulmonary gas exchange is adequate, shock is caused by hypovolemia, cardiac or vasoregulatory failure, or a combination of these etiologies. According to this definition, when oxygen delivery is inadequate to meet oxygen demand, the organs will fail. This situation, if not corrected, will result in irreversible damage and ultimately death. Oxygen delivery to the organs is dependent on many factors, but fundamentally on the oxygen content of the blood and the volume of blood flowing to those organs. Because oxygen content is primarily determined by the hemoglobin concentration and oxygen saturation, with less contribution from the dissolved oxygen (see later discussion), it is relatively easily evaluated and monitored in the newborn intensive care unit. However, reliably assessing systemic and organ blood flow and tissue oxygen delivery and consumption at the bedside is difficult. These parameters need to be continuously measured in absolute numbers to provide adequate information on the rapidly changing hemodynamic status in sick preterm and term infants. Recent advances in our ability to monitor systemic and organ blood flow and tissue oxygenation as well as vital organ (brain) function at the bedside will likely lead to a better understanding of the complex hemodynamic changes associated with neonatal cardiovascular compromise (Cayabyab et al, 2009). These advances should lead to the development of treatment modalities more appropriately based on the etiology, pathophysiology, and phases of shock, thereby improving clinically relevant outcomes.

At present in clinical practice, tissue perfusion is routinely assessed by monitoring heart rate, blood pressure, capillary refilling time, acid-base status, serum lactate levels, and urine output. However, recent Doppler ultrasound and near infrared spectroscopy (NIRS) data have highlighted that these parameters are relatively poor, although at present are the only routinely available, indicators of acute changes in organ blood flow and tissue oxygen delivery in critically ill neonates (Kluckow and Evans, 1996, 2000; Lopez et al, 1997; Pladys et al, 2001; Tyszczuk et al, 1998). These observations and the lack of evidence that treatment of neonatal cardiovascular compromise improves outcomes (Barrington et al, 2006; Seri and Noori, 2005) call for a paradigm shift in our thinking about pathophysiology, diagnosis, and treatment of neonatal shock. This suggests that the assessment of the hemodynamic status in critically ill neonates should include the complex interactions among blood flow and blood pressure as well as tissue oxygen delivery and consumption (Cayabyab et al, 2009; Noori and Seri, 2008).

PATHOPHYSIOLOGY, PHASES, AND ETIOLOGY OF NEONATAL SHOCK

PRINCIPLES OF OXYGEN DELIVERY

Oxygen is the most vital substrate necessary for mitochondrial respiration and is not stored in the body. As mentioned earlier, interruption of oxygen supply to cells can result in irreversible damage (sometimes within minutes), particularly in vital organs such as the brain and myocardium.

Oxygen delivery ($\dot{D}O_2$) to the tissues is the "raison d'être" of the cardiorespiratory system, and shock is therefore defined as inadequate systemic tissue oxygen delivery (see earlier). Oxygen delivery can be expressed as

$$\dot{D}O_2 = \text{cardiac output (CO)} \times \text{arterial oxygen content } (CaO_2)$$

where

$$CO = \text{heart rate (HR)} \times \text{stroke volume (SV)}$$

and

$$CaO_2 = [1.34 \times \text{hemoglobin concentration [Hb]} \times \text{arterial oxygen saturation } (SaO_2)] + [0.003 \times \text{arterial partial pressure of oxygen } (PaO_2)]$$

Stroke volume is the result of complex interplay among preload, afterload, and contractility (Figure 51-1), all three of which are, at present, impossible to monitor reliably and continuously in real time at the bedside. Preload is the end-diastolic volume of the ventricle (a three dimensional reflection of pre-contractile myocardial cell fiber-length), and, up to a point, the greater the preload, the larger the stroke volume (the Frank-Starling relationship). Afterload is the force the ventricle must generate against the systemic or pulmonary vascular resistance. As long as appropriate perfusion pressure is ensured, the lower the afterload, the better the cardiac output. Contractility (the

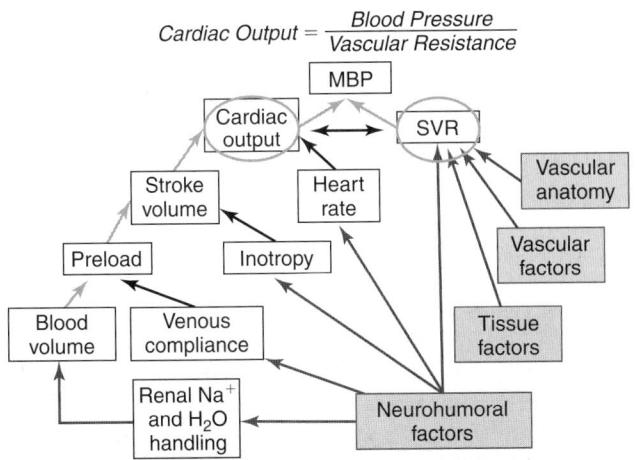

$$Cardiac\ Output = \frac{Blood\ Pressure}{Vascular\ Resistance}$$

FIGURE 51-1 Factors regulating cardiac output, blood pressure, and systemic vascular resistance. From a physiologic standpoint, SVR and cardiac output are the regulated (independent) variables and MBP is the dependent variable. *MBP,* Mean blood pressure; *Na⁺,* sodium; *SVR,* systemic vascular resistance. *(Modified from Klabunde RE, www. cvphysiology.com.)*

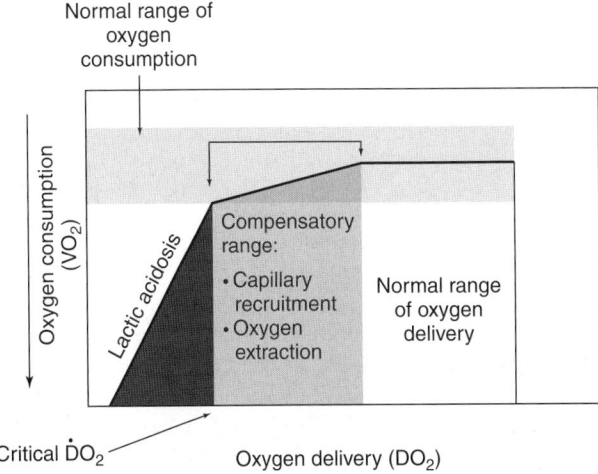

FIGURE 51-2 Relationship between oxygen consumption and delivery. In the normal range of oxygen delivery, oxygen consumption is unaffected by changes in the delivery rate of oxygen to the tissues. As oxygen delivery decreases below the normal range, tissue oxygen consumption remains in the normal range for a while because of activation of local compensatory mechanisms such as capillary recruitment and increased oxygen extraction. However, when oxygen delivery decreases to the "critical" point, compensatory mechanisms can no longer satisfy tissue oxygen demand, and anaerobic metabolism commences, resulting in significantly decreased ATP and increased lactate production.

intrinsic ability to generate force per unit time) may be assessed noninvasively but not continuously by echocardiogram. However, at present most of the measures of cardiac contractility are both preload and afterload dependent. Hence, contractility is not truly an independent variable. Typically, cardiac output in neonates is considered heart rate–dependent, because the neonate's ability to augment stroke volume is somewhat limited compared to children or adults.

From this simple model, it is easily appreciated that if there is an acute decline in CaO_2, by a decrease in either the [Hb] or SaO_2 or both, the cardiac output will increase in response to maintain $\dot{DO}_2$. On the other hand, because neither [Hb] nor SaO_2 can be physiologically increased rapidly, there is no acute compensation for a low cardiac output due to decreases in myocardial contractility and/or preload.

Oxygen consumption can be similarly readily expressed as

$$\dot{V}O_2 = CO \times (CaO_2 - C\bar{v}O_2)$$

where $C\bar{v}O_2$ is the mixed venous oxygen content.

This relationship is based on the Fick principle, from which, knowing flow rate and arterial-venous content difference of a trace element (in this case, oxygen), one can calculate the uptake or removal rate of the tracer.

Normally $\dot{DO}_2$ and $\dot{V}O_2$ are well matched, and O_2 extraction is usually approximately 25%. If the SaO_2 is 100%, SvO_2 would be expected to be 75%. If cardiac output falls, $\dot{V}O_2$ may be maintained constant by capillary bed vasodilation and recruitment and/or by increased O_2 extraction by the tissues. Increased O_2 extraction is manifested as a lower $C\bar{v}O_2$ and therefore greater $CaO_2 - C\bar{v}O_2$ difference. The relationship between $\dot{DO}_2$ and $\dot{V}O_2$ may be graphically displayed as in Figure 51-2. Once oxygen extraction is maximal, at the critical $\dot{DO}_2$ threshold, anaerobic metabolism ensues, resulting in lactic acidosis. If not reversed, the oxygen debt accumulates, and organ failure and death will ensue. In general, during aerobic metabolism 38 mol ATP is produced per 1 mol glucose, whereas during anaerobic metabolic conditions, 2 mol ATP and 2 mol lactate are produced per mol glucose.

Before reaching the stage of delivery-dependent $\dot{V}O_2$, the SvO_2 can be used as a proxy for $\dot{DO}_2$. Assuming $\dot{V}O_2$, [Hb], and SaO_2 are constant over a short period of time, a decline in SvO_2 represents a decreasing cardiac output. SvO_2 may be measured intermittently via a catheter—ideally placed in the pulmonary artery in a patient without intracardiac shunts to obtain a true mixed venous sample. In practice, central venous oxygen saturation is used ($ScvO_2$), measured with a catheter placed at the superior vena cava–right atrial junction. A catheter too low in the right atrium may measure very desaturated blood streaming from the coronary sinus or hepatic veins. Catheters with an oximetric probe at the tip may be used for continuous $ScvO_2$ monitoring in real time. However, for several reasons, measurement of $ScvO_2$ is not done routinely in neonates in neonatal intensive care units except for some neonates with congenital heart disease in the postoperative period following surgical correction of the cardiac condition.

In general, these principles are valuable guides to understanding and managing global $\dot{DO}_2$ and $\dot{V}O_2$, but they do not help us readily when evaluating individual organ $\dot{DO}_2$. Furthermore, the limitations of measuring $\dot{V}O_2$, $\dot{DO}_2$, and even just $ScvO_2$ are often daunting. However, regional tissue oxygen saturation (rSO_2) can be assessed noninvasively with NIRS in different tissues including the brain, kidneys, intestine, and muscle (see later discussion).

Finally, there is a class of neonates where calculations using the Fick principle can be critical in directing therapy. Newborns with congenital heart disease and intracardiac shunts may have perturbations in the usual pulmonary to systemic blood flow ratio (Qp:Qs). Normally, of course, in patients with parallel circulations and no shunts, Qp:Qs = 1. By comparing the oxygen utilized by the body with that taken up by the lung, Qp:Qs can be estimated.

$$Qs = \dot{V}O_2/(CaO_2 - C\bar{v}O_2)$$

and

$$Qp = O_2 \text{ uptake}/(CpvO_2 - CpaO_2)$$

where pa is pulmonary artery and pv is pulmonary vein.

After substituting and eliminating common terms,

$$Qp:Qs = (SaO_2 - SvO_2)/(SpvO_2 - SpaO_2)$$

This formula usually requires two assumptions (unless being measured directly as in the cardiac catheterization laboratory); first, that $SpvO_2$ is 95% to 100%, and second, that SvO_2 measured through a central venous line reflects a mixed venous sample (see also Chapter 55).

The value of this calculation can be easily illustrated with an example. A newborn infant with hypoplastic left heart syndrome is found to have an SaO_2 of 95% and SvO_2 of 80%. Using the formula just given, assuming a $SpvO_2$ of 100% and recognizing that SaO_2 and $SpaO_2$ are the same in this patient, we arrive at a Qp:Qs of 3:1. Such an imbalance may result in congestive heart failure from pulmonary overcirculation (the single right ventricle is now doing 4 cardiac outputs/minute), or there will be inadequate systemic blood flow resulting in shock, or both. This explains why we "aim" for an SaO_2 of 75% in such infants (ideally), because this would represent a Qp:Qs of 1:1.

PHASES OF NEONATAL SHOCK

From a pathophysiologic standpoint, three phases of shock depicting advancing severity have been identified (McLean et al, 2008; Zaritsky and Chernow, 1984).

In the "compensated phase," complex neuroendocrine and autonomic compensatory mechanisms maintain perfusion and oxygen delivery in the normal range to the vital organs (brain, heart, and adrenal glands) at the expense of decreased perfusion to the remaining organs (nonvital organs). This is achieved by vasodilation and vasoconstriction of the vessels to vital and nonvital organs, respectively, in response to a fall in perfusion pressure and/or oxygen delivery (Iwamoto, 1993; Sheldon et al, 1979). Blood pressure is maintained within the normal range, and heart rate increases. As perfusion of nonvital organs is decreased because of the compensatory vasoconstriction of their vascular beds, there often are clinical signs of compromised nonvital organ function such as decreased urine output. In addition, signs of poor peripheral perfusion can often be detected, such as cold extremities and prolonged capillary refill time.

If adequate treatment is not commenced, the infant will most likely develop hypotension due to failure of the neuroendocrine and autonomic mechanisms, and shock enters its "uncompensated phase." Systemic perfusion (cardiac output) will decrease, perfusion of all organs including the vital organs becomes compromised, and lactic acidosis develops (Zaritsky and Chernow, 1984).

If treatment is ineffective in the uncompensated phase of shock, multiorgan failure develops and shock may enter its "irreversible phase," where permanent damage to the

various organ systems occurs and further interventions will be ineffective in reversing the patient's condition.

DEVELOPMENTAL REGULATION OF CARDIAC OUTPUT AND ITS DETERMINANTS

Cardiac output is the product of stroke volume and heart rate and is determined by the amount of blood returning to the heart (preload), the strength of myocardial contractility, and the resistance against which the heart must pump (afterload). However, it is important to note that afterload and vascular resistance should not be used interchangeably. Rather, afterload is the load or force the heart faces during contraction and is affected by the impedance of the central vasculature, the resistance of the peripheral vascular beds, the ventricular mass, and the inertia of the blood. If myocardial function is intact, cardiac output depends solely on preload and afterload according to the relationships described by the Starling curve.

Therefore, low cardiac output and thus low systemic blood flow can result from various combinations of the three determinants of cardiac output: low cardiac preload, poor myocardial contractility, or high cardiac afterload. Decreases in preload lead to diminished stroke volume and cardiac output, and it is most often caused by low effective circulating blood volume. This can be due to loss of circulating blood volume following hemorrhage (absolute hypovolemia), or the circulating volume may be inadequate for the vascular space as in vasodilatory shock or as a side effect of administration of lusitropes (relative hypovolemia). Because approximately 75% of the circulating blood volume is on the venous side of the circulation at any given point in time, the increases in venous capacitance caused by venodilation significantly contribute to relative hypovolemia under these circumstances. Because preload is also augmented by the negative intrathoracic pressure generated at each spontaneous inspiration, the positive intrathoracic pressure associated with positive pressure mechanical ventilation reduces venous return and hence preload and cardiac output (Biondi et al, 1988; Henning, 1986).

The strength of myocardial contractility depends on the filling volume and pressure, and the maturity (Friedman, 1972) and integrity of the myocardium. Thus, decreases in preload (hypovolemia, cardiac arrhythmia) as well as prematurity (especially extreme immaturity), hypoxic insults, and infectious (viral or bacterial) agents (Walther et al, 1985) all negatively affect the ability of the myocardium to contract with resultant decreases in cardiac output.

If cardiac afterload is too high, the ability of the myocardium to pump against the increased resistance may become compromised, and cardiac output may fall (Osborn et al, 2002; Roze et al, 1993). Such increases in afterload are associated with enhanced endogenous catecholamine release during the period of immediate postnatal adaptation along with loss of the low-resistance placental circulation. Similar increases in afterload are seen in hypovolemia, hypothermia, or when inappropriately high doses of vasopressor-inotropes are being administered to a patient with intact cardiovascular adrenoreceptor responsiveness (Seri, 2006). High afterload can affect either ventricle, and if the output of one of the ventricles is reduced, this will affect the function of the other ventricle, especially when the fetal channels are closed. For instance, if the right ventricular output is low because of high pulmonary vascular resistance, the amount of blood traversing the lungs to the left ventricle will be reduced, leading to low systemic blood flow with blood pooling in the systemic venous system.

Hemodynamic changes during transition to extrauterine life have special implications, especially for the preterm neonate. With delivery and the separation of the placenta, the fetal circulation is replaced so that the systemic and pulmonary circuits separate and the cardiovascular system functions as a circulation in series (Kiserud and Acharya, 2004). However, when this process is compromised by ductal patency, the increase in SVR and blood pressure combined with the decrease in pulmonary vascular resistance (PVR) results in left-to-right shunting across the ductus arteriosus (Evans et al, 2004; Noori and Seri, 2008). In the healthy term neonate, the rapidly constricting ductus arteriosus prevents the development of hemodynamically significant left-to-right shunting across the ductus. However, in the preterm neonate, shunts through the persistently patent ductus arteriosus (PDA) and/or foramen ovale may compromise circulation (Kluckow and Evans, 2000a). Indeed, in 50% to 70% of VLBW neonates, the ductus remains open (Noori and Seri, 2008; Reller et al, 1993) and, as the right-sided pressures fall, blood will shunt left to right from the systemic circulation back into the pulmonary circulation. In most VLBW neonates, pulmonary vascular resistance initially decreases relatively rapidly for physiologic and nonphysiologic reasons (Noori and Seri, 2008). Physiologic mechanisms most important in the postnatal decrease of PVR include the mechanical effects of initiation of air breathing on PVR and the increased postnatal oxygenation-associated direct, paracrine, and endocrine vasodilation (Faro et al, 2007). Iatrogenic causes include surfactant administration or the inappropriate targeting of higher arterial oxygen saturations (Kluckow and Evans, 2000a; Noori and Seri, 2008). With the left-to-right ductal shunting, pulmonary overcirculation develops and left ventricular output, the gold standard of bedside assessment of systemic perfusion, cannot be used as a measure of systemic perfusion (Figure 51-3) (Kluckow and Seri, 2008). Indeed, under these circumstances, left ventricular output measures systemic perfusion and ductal blood flow. In earlier studies investigating the posttransitional changes in systemic perfusion and/or the effects of vasoactive agents on cardiovascular function, this fact has often not been acknowledged (Lundstrom et al, 2000; Roze et al, 1993). Therefore, the conclusions drawn from some of these studies (Roze et al, 1993) need to be reevaluated. More recent studies have acknowledged this hemodynamic paradigm and used right ventricular output to assess systemic perfusion in the VLBW neonate during the transitional period (Abdel-Hady et al, 2008; Bouissou et al, 2008; Kluckow and Evans, 2000b; West et al, 2006). However, right ventricular output only represents systemic perfusion as long as left-to-right shunting across the foramen ovale does not become significant. In many preterm neonates, however, as left-to-right shunting across a nonconstricting PDA increases during the first 12 to 36 hours, left atrial volume and pressure increase, often leading to the development of a significant left-to-right shunt across the foramen ovale (Evans and Iyer, 1994b). The left-to-right shunt

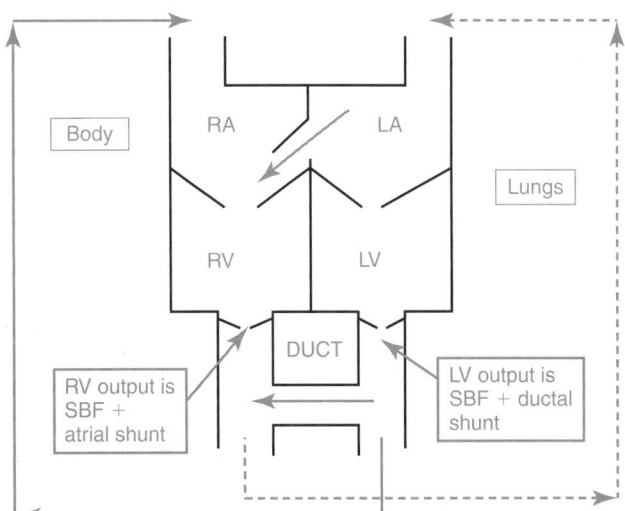

FIGURE 51-3 **The impact of left-to-right shunting across the PDA and PFO on LVO and RVO measurements.** Effect of left-to-right shunting across the PDA and foramen ovale on LVO and RVO. Under these circumstances, LVO represents the sum of total pulmonary venous return and ductal blood flow, whereas RVO measures the sum of systemic venous return and left-to-right shunting across the PFO. *LVO,* Left ventricular output; *PDA,* patent ductus arteriosus; *PFO,* patent foramen ovale; *RVO,* right ventricular output; *SBF,* systemic blood flow. (*From Kluckow M, Seri I: Clinical presentations of neonatal shock: the VLBW infant during the first postnatal day. In Kleinman CS, Seri I, editors:* Hemodynamics and cardiology. Neonatal questions and controversies, *Philadelphia, 2008, Saunders, pp 147-177.*)

through the patent foramen ovale (PFO) will then render the use of right ventricular output as a measure of systemic blood flow inaccurate, because right ventricular output now represents systemic inflow and PFO flow (Kluckow and Seri, 2008). This hemodynamic scenario results in the lack of an acceptable conventional measure of systemic blood flow in these neonates. To circumvent this problem, superior vena cava (SVC) flow has been used as a measure of upper body blood flow in preterm neonates with the fetal channels open (Kluckow and Evans, 2000b; Kluckow, 2005). The use of SVC flow has provided novel insights into the mechanisms of transitional hemodynamics, such as the observation that intraventricular hemorrhage (IVH) develops in many VLBW neonates as systemic blood flow improves, resulting in reperfusion of the brain (Kluckow and Evans, 2000c). These observations are supported by the findings of studies using NIRS to assess cerebral oxygen delivery in VLBW neonates during the transitional period (Victor et al, 2006a, 2006b). Although there is an association between low SVC flow during the first postnatal days and poor neurodevelopmental outcome at 3 years of age in VLBW neonates (Hunt et al, 2004), the vulnerability of SVC flow measurements to error and the technical difficulties associated with its use as a surrogate measure of systemic blood flow have forced these measurements to remain a research rather than a clinical tool (Evans, 2008).

DEVELOPMENTAL REGULATION OF SYSTEMIC BLOOD PRESSURE

Systemic blood pressure is the product of systemic blood flow and systemic vascular resistance. There is an association between low blood pressure and central nervous system injury in the preterm neonate (Bada et al, 1990; Goldstein et al, 1995; Miall-Allen et al, 1987; Watkins et al, 1999). Yet, blood pressure correlates only weakly with blood flow in this patient population during the period of immediate postnatal adaptation when the fetal channels are open (Kluckow and Evans, 2000b). Thus, in preterm infants during the first postnatal day, blood pressure may be low because resistance is low in the presence of normal or high blood flow. Alternatively, blood pressure may be normal or high because resistance is high in the presence of normal or low blood flow (Evans and Kluckow, 1996, 2000). The uncertainty surrounding the nature of the relationship between blood pressure and systemic blood flow during the transitional period results from our inability to appropriately define the normal blood pressure range (Engle, 2008) and systemic blood flow (see earlier), and to characterize the developmental regulation of organ blood flow and vital organ assignment (see later discussion) in the preterm neonate.

DEVELOPMENTAL REGULATION OF ORGAN BLOOD FLOW AND ITS AUTOREGULATION AND VITAL ORGAN ASSIGNMENT

Even very immature preterm neonates autoregulate their cerebral blood flow (CBF) (Seri et al, 1998; Tsuji et al, 2000; Tyszczuk et al, 1998). However, the autoregulatory blood pressure range in this patient population is believed to be narrow, and the "normal" blood pressure is very close to the lower elbow of the autoregulatory curve (Greisen, 2005, 2008). Organ blood flow autoregulation is impaired in preterm neonates who are more immature and sicker (McLean et al, 2008; Tsuji et al, 2000; Wong et al, 2008). In these patients, changes in blood pressure are mirrored by changes in CBF with a high coherence, and these babies are at higher risk for cerebral injury (O'Leary et al, 2009; Pryds et al, 1989; Tsuji et al, 2000; Wong et al, 2008). Factors that impair cerebral and other organ blood flow autoregulation include birth asphyxia, acidosis, infection, hypoglycemia, tissue hypoxia and ischemia, and sudden alterations in arterial carbon dioxide tension ($PaCO_2$) (Greisen, 2008). It is of clinical importance that the CO_2-CBF reactivity is more robust than the pressure-flow reactivity, as 1 mm Hg change in $PaCO_2$ results in 4% change in CBF, whereas 1 mm Hg change in blood pressure is associated with a 1% change in CBF only (Greisen, 2005; Müller et al, 2002). The impairment of CBF autoregulation in the preterm neonate during the immediate postnatal period has been proposed to contribute to cerebral injury with loss of vascular reactivity to both blood pressure and CO_2 (O'Leary et al, 2009; Pryds et al, 1989). However, the finding that impaired autoregulation may also be a consequence of a preceding ischemic insult (Greisen, 2008) makes clarification of this question particularly difficult.

The vessels of the vital organs respond to decreased perfusion pressure and/or oxygen delivery with vasodilation (i.e., high-priority vascular beds), whereas the vessels of the nonvital organs, with low-priority vascular beds, vasoconstrict. Several lines of evidence in human neonates and developing animals suggest that the assignment of the forebrain circulation to a high-priority vascular bed may not

be complete at birth (Ashwal et al, 1984; Hernandez et al, 1982; Victor et al, 2006b). For instance, the vessels of the forebrain of dog pups vasoconstrict like those of a nonvital organ whereas the vessels of the hindbrain vasodilate in response to hypoxic exposure (Hernandez et al, 1982). The finding that CBF autoregulation also appears in the brainstem first and in the forebrain only later in gestation (Ashwal et al, 1984) supports the notion that there are developmentally regulated differences in the timing of the blood flow autoregulatory functions and vital organ assignment characteristics between the forebrain and the hindbrain. The cellular mechanisms responsible for the assignment of vital and nonvital organ status from a blood flow regulatory standpoint are poorly understood. Based on these findings, it is tempting to speculate that the diminished capacity of the forebrain vessels to vasodilate in the very preterm neonate during the complex process of cardiovascular transition after delivery may contribute to hypoperfusion of the forebrain. These neonates may present with blood pressure values in the perceived normal range while being in the compensated phase of shock. Because this early phase of shock is difficult to recognize immediately after delivery, forebrain hypoperfusion and, on adaptation to the extrauterine environment, the ensuing reperfusion can go unnoticed. This proposed vital organ assignment-associated reperfusion cycle might contribute to cerebral injury in the very preterm neonate (Noori et al, 2009).

To summarize the pathogenesis of the abnormal circulatory adaptation in the very preterm neonate, there is indirect evidence that the sudden increase in systemic vascular resistance after separation from the placenta combined with myocardial immaturity plays a role in the development of the low flow state (Kluckow and Evans, 2000b). Because the preterm myocardium is adapted to a low-resistance intrauterine environment, characterized by reduced contractile elements, and has a limited ability to respond to increased afterload (Hawkins et al, 1989; Takahashi et al, 1997), it likely struggles to cope with the sudden increase in vascular resistance immediately after birth. This is compounded by shunts out of the systemic circulation through the fetal channels and the negative circulatory effects of positive pressure ventilation. In addition, the vessels of the forebrain initially vasoconstrict as the compensated phase of shock develops. As the final outcome of these hemodynamic events, critically low systemic and forebrain blood flow develops in many of these patients even with blood pressure values in the suspected normal range. Then, as treatment, endocrine, neuroendocrine and other compensatory responses to stress are initiated, the cardiovascular system adapts, and systemic blood flow improves, with reperfusion of the organs including the forebrain. However, if the low flow state is severe, a reperfusion injury may occur during the period of cardiovascular stabilization, especially in the extremely vulnerable immature central nervous system. Thus, hemodynamic compensation of shock in the very preterm neonate during the immediate postnatal period may not protect against central nervous system injury. Finally, patients in the uncompensated phase of shock with recognized circulatory compromise face the very same hemodynamic scenario, as by definition reperfusion of all organs including the brain will take place.

DEVELOPMENTAL REGULATION OF CEREBRAL OXYGEN DEMAND-DELIVERY COUPLING

Very little is known about the regulation of oxygen demand–oxygen delivery coupling in neonates, especially in the transitional period. Yet, several lines of evidence indicate that the very preterm neonate is unable to couple cerebral oxygen demand with blood flow, and instead increases oxygen extraction when oxygen demand is increased (Victor et al, 2006a, 2006b). This phenomenon may be linked to the developmental delay in the vital organ assignment of the forebrain immediately after delivery (see earlier discussion).

PATHOGENESIS OF NEONATAL SHOCK

Etiologic Factors

The etiologic factors leading to the development of neonatal shock include hypovolemia, myocardial dysfunction, abnormal peripheral vasoregulation, or a combination of two or all three of these factors.

Hypovolemia

Hypovolemia may be absolute (loss of intravascular volume), relative (increased venous capacitance), or combined such as is often seen in septic shock. Hypovolemia results in cardiovascular compromise primarily by the decrease in cardiac output (systemic blood flow) caused by the decrease in preload. In addition, if blood loss is the primary cause of hypovolemia, the associated decrease in oxygen carrying capacity contributes to the development of the circulatory compromise. Hypovolemia is probably overdiagnosed in neonatology, because it is a relatively uncommon primary cause of circulatory compromise, especially during the first postnatal day. In the preterm newborn there is no evidence that hypotensive neonates as a group are hypovolemic (Barr et al, 1977; Wright and Goodhall, 1994). However, when hypovolemia occurs, it can be difficult to detect clinically.

Absolute hypovolemia in the newborn can be due to several conditions. Intrapartum fetal blood loss is usually caused by an open bleed from the fetal side of the placenta, and therefore it is likely to be detected. More difficult to diagnose is the closed bleeding of an acute fetomaternal hemorrhage or an acute fetoplacental hemorrhage. The latter can occur during delivery where the umbilical cord comes under some pressure (breech presentation or nuchal cord). Because the umbilical vein is occluded before the artery, blood continues to be pumped into the placenta, and if the cord is clamped early, this blood remains trapped in the placenta. This probably happens to some degree in all babies with tight nuchal cords who, as a group, have lower hemoglobin levels (Shepherd et al, 1985). However, in some neonates, a tight nuchal cord may also cause severe circulatory compromise (Vanhaesebrouck et al, 1987). Postnatal hemorrhage may occur from any site and is frequently associated with perinatal infections or severe asphyxia-induced endothelial damage and the ensuing disseminated intravascular coagulation. Finally, acute abdominal surgical problems and conditions associated with the nonspecific inflammatory response syndrome and subsequent increased capillary leak with loss of fluid into the interstitium can lead to significant decreases in

the circulating blood volume. Iatrogenic causes of absolute hypovolemia include inadequate fluid replacement in conditions of increased insensible losses in the very preterm neonate and gastroschisis before closure of the defect, or the inappropriate use of diuretics.

Relative hypovolemia, that is, a decrease in the effective circulating blood volume, may occur in pathologic conditions leading to vasodilation such as in conditions associated with the nonspecific inflammatory response syndrome (sepsis, necrotizing enterocolitis [NEC], asphyxia, major surgical procedures, use of extracorporeal membrane oxygenation [ECMO]). In addition, the use of afterload-reducing agents (e.g., milrinone, PGE_2) may cause significant vasodilation (especially venodilation), thereby decreasing the effective circulating blood volume.

Finally, absolute and relative hypovolemia most frequently occurs in conditions associated with the nonspecific inflammatory response syndrome such as sepsis, asphyxia, and major surgical procedures.

Myocardial Dysfunction

Decreased myocardial contractility results in decreased cardiac output (primarily in stroke volume) and thus decrease in oxygen delivery to the tissues.

Acquired heart disease presenting as circulatory compromise includes primary cardiomyopathies, postasphyxial myocardial dysfunction due to hypoxic-ischemic injury, viral myocarditis, and myocardial dysfunction in the late stages of septic shock. Studies have shown a high incidence of ischemic electrocardiographic changes, elevated blood cardiac enzyme levels, and low cardiac output in neonates after intrapartum asphyxia (Primhak et al, 1985; Tapia-Rombo et al, 2000). For more detail on structural heart disease and cardiomyopathies, see Chapter 55.

Among the different types of congenital heart disease, structural heart defects that produce a ductus-dependent systemic circulation such as the hypoplastic left heart syndrome, critical coarctation, and critical aortic stenosis, if not diagnosed prenatally or immediately after delivery, classically present as acute circulatory compromise with pallor, tachypnea, impalpable pulses, and hepatomegaly as the duct starts closing. The presentation may be initially misdiagnosed as sepsis.

Abnormal Peripheral Vasoregulation

Peripheral vasodilation causes circulatory compromise by resultant decrease in cardiac output and blood pressure and the associated diminution in preload related to the venous return decrease. If myocardial function is intact, compensatory increase in the heart rate may maintain appropriate levels of tissue oxygen delivery for a period of time. Pathologic peripheral vasodilation in neonates occurs primarily in conditions associated with the nonspecific inflammatory response syndrome such as sepsis, NEC, asphyxia, major surgical procedures, use of ECMO, or respiratory distress syndrome of prematurity. It is of clinical importance that preterm neonates born to mothers with chorioamnionitis, especially if they have evidence of funisitis (fetal vessel inflammation), frequently present with hypotension and hyperdynamic, vasodilatory cardiovascular compromise at birth or shortly after delivery (Yanowitz et al, 2002, 2004, 2006).

Clinical Presentations of Shock in Neonates Associated With Multiple Etiologic Factors

Transitional Circulatory Compromise of the Very Preterm Neonate

The transitional circulatory changes in the first 12 to 24 hours after birth denote a period of unique circulatory vulnerability for the extremely preterm infant. During normal postnatal adaptation, pulmonary vascular resistance falls, systemic vascular resistance rises with removal of the placenta from the circulation, the ductus arteriosus closes, and the foramen ovale is closed by the reversal of the atrial pressure gradient. During this time frame, the left ventricle has to double its output. Given that the very preterm infant's cardiovascular system is adapted to the low-resistance intrauterine environment and its myocardium is immature, it is not surprising that these patients have difficulties during this critical period. In addition, as discussed earlier, developmentally regulated factors such as the state of vital organ assignment of the forebrain and cerebral oxygen demand-flow coupling make cardiovascular adaptation of the very preterm neonate an even more complex process (Ashwal et al, 1984; Hernandez et al, 1982; Noori et al, 2009; Victor et al, 2006b). It is important to note that there is much more to understand about the complex interactions between immediate postnatal cardiovascular adaptation and immaturity, organ development, myocardial and vasoregulatory function, and vital organ assignment.

Various studies have revealed an association between low blood pressure and central nervous system morbidities such as IVH (Bada et al, 1990; Miall-Allen et al, 1987; O'Leary et al, 2009; Watkins et al, 1999), white matter damage (Limperopoulos et al, 2007; Tsuji et al, 2000), and poor long-term neurodevelopmental outcome (Batton et al, 2009; Dempsey et al, 2009; Fanaroff et al, 2006; Goldstein et al, 1995; Martens et al, 2003; Soul et al, 2007). However, because blood pressure alone is not an accurate reflection of systemic and organ blood flow in this patient population during the immediate postnatal period (Kluckow and Evans, 1996, 2000; Lopez et al, 1997; Pladys et al, 2001; Tyszczuk et al, 1998), it is important to recognize that successful treatment of hypotension may not necessarily ensure normalization of organ blood flow. Furthermore, blood pressure in the normal range does not necessarily translate into normal cerebral blood flow and tissue perfusion in these patients, because their forebrain may initially function as a nonvital organ from a blood flow regulatory standpoint. This translates to the clinical situation discussed earlier, especially in very preterm neonates immediately after delivery. These patients are suspected to present with the compensated phase of shock with normal blood pressure and decreased "nonvital" organ blood flow, which in their case includes the forebrain. Because the compensated phase of shock is difficult if not impossible to diagnose in very preterm neonates in the transitional period, the clinician may not be aware of the ongoing hemodynamic compromise. Indeed, if only blood pressure is being followed to diagnose cardiovascular compromise, systemic blood flow can only be assumed normal if mean blood pressure is over 40 mm Hg during the first postnatal day in the preterm neonate born before 30 weeks' gestation (Osborn et al, 2001). However, when blood pressure and capillary refill time (CRT) are considered together, a mean blood pressure of ≥30 mm Hg and a CRT of ≤3 s have an 86% positive predictive value for a normal SVC flow used as a surrogate of systemic blood flow in these patients with the fetal channels open (Osborn et al, 2001).

Another special characteristic of the process of cardiovascular adaptation in this patient population is that early shunts through the preterm ductus arteriosus and foramen are not balanced and thus can produce left-to-right shunts of significant clinical importance (Evans and Kluckow, 1996; Kluckow and Evans, 2000a; Kluckow, 2005). Although the immediate postnatal physical constriction of the ductus is characterized by great variation (Kluckow and Evans, 2000a), in those cases in which constriction fails, very large shunts can occur within a few hours of birth, leading to high and not low pulmonary blood flow as previously thought. These abnormal hemodynamic changes may be further augmented by surfactant administration.

As discussed earlier in detail and depicted in Figure 51-3, in the transitional circulation of the preterm infant, neither ventricular output will consistently reflect systemic blood flow because of the shunts across the ductus arteriosus and foramen ovale (Evans and Iyer, 1994b; Evans and Kluckow, 1996). Consequently, measurement of either ventricular output can overestimate systemic blood flow by more than 100% in some cases (Evans and Kluckow, 1996; Noori et al, 2006). As mentioned earlier, SVC flow can be used as a marker of total systemic blood flow (Kluckow and Evans, 2000b), and serial measurements of SVC flow have been used to describe the natural history of systemic blood flow changes in preterm neonates in the early postnatal period (see Figure 51-1) (Kluckow and Evans, 2000c, 2001). These initial studies have found that around 30% of preterm neonates born before 30 weeks have a period of low systemic blood flow, mostly during the first 12 hours of life (Kluckow and Evans, 2000b). Gestational age was the dominant predictor of the low flow state with 70% of neonates born before 26 weeks' gestation having a period of low systemic flow compared to around 10% at 29 weeks. However, a more recent study (Paradisis et al, 2009) found only a <20% incidence of low systemic blood flow in neonates born before 26 weeks' gestation, suggesting that factors other than gestational age may also be important in the developmental low flow state after delivery. Advances in obstetrical, perinatal, and delivery room care, the mode of ventilatory support, and the diameter of the ductus arteriosus (Evans and Iyer, 1994a) are suspected additional factors associated with the decrease in incidence of low SVC flow of the very preterm neonatal population (Noori et al, 2009; Paradisis et al, 2009). The low-flow state can persist for up to 24 hours but usually improves thereafter. As discussed earlier, there is a strong relationship between recovery from the low-flow state and subsequent IVH (Kluckow and Evans, 2000c). The finding that IVH occurs after systemic blood flow has improved indicates the involvement of a hypoperfusion-reperfusion cycle in the pathogenesis of this injury. Follow-up to 3 years identified the low-flow state as a significant risk factor for poor neurodevelopmental outcome (Hunt et al, 2001). In addition to low SVC flow, hypotension and pressure-passive CBF have also been implicated in the development of IVH (Limperopoulos et al; 2007; Pryds et al, 1989). As mentioned earlier, PaCO₂ is even a more potent regulator of CBF than blood pressure (Greisen, 2005; Müller et al, 2002). Hence, hypocapnia and hypercapnia in very preterm neonates during the immediate postnatal period are associated with periventricular leukomalacia (Khwaya and Volpe, 2008; Wiswell et al, 1996) and IVH (Fabres et al, 2007; Kaiser et al, 2006; McKee et al, 2009), respectively. In summary, abnormal circulatory adaptation during the early postnatal transition is one of the causative factors in adverse outcomes of preterm infants born before 30 weeks' gestation (also see earlier discussion).

Vasopressor-Resistant Hypotension

Although the just-described transitional problems may or may not present with low blood pressure (compensated or uncompensated phase of shock), there is a group of preterm neonates in whom persistent hypotension that is resistant to conventional vasopressor-inotropic support develops (Ng et al, 2001, 2006; Noori et al, 2006b; Seri et al, 2001; Watterberg, 2002). Although a well-recognized entity, the underlying systemic hemodynamic changes in this condition only recently have been characterized (Noori et al, 2006). These babies are more likely to be extremely preterm (<27 weeks) and/or have been critically ill or suffered a degree of perinatal asphyxia. The problem may be apparent on the first postnatal day (Ng et al, 2006) but may persist beyond and represent a state of vasodilatory shock with normal to high systemic blood flow and possibly supranormal cardiac output (Lopez et al, 1997). There are striking analogous features of this presentation in preterm neonates to those of vasodilatory shock described in adults, particularly the lack of responsiveness to vasopressor-inotropes (Landry and Oliver, 2001). Potential mechanisms for the uncontrolled vasodilation include dysregulated cytokine release, excess nitric oxide synthesis, overactivation of the K$_{ATP}$ channels in the vascular smooth muscle cell membrane in response to tissue hypoxia, and downregulation of the cardiovascular adrenergic receptors (Hausdorff et al, 1990; Seri et al, 2001). In the preterm infant, the foregoing mechanisms are exacerbated by the immaturity-associated relative adrenal insufficiency (Cole, 2009; Watterberg et al, 1999; Watterberg, 2002) preceding asphyxia or may be secondary to the transitional circulatory failure as described earlier. In the term neonate, an association between congenital diaphragmatic hernia and relative adrenal insufficiency has also been reported (Pittinger and Sawin, 2000).

Sepsis

Although clinical evidence of circulatory compromise is a leading feature of many infectious processes in the newborn, the hemodynamics in neonatal septic shock have not been systematically studied. In older subjects, two distinct hemodynamic patterns occur: warm shock, characterized by loss of vascular tone, increased systemic blood flow, and low blood pressure, and cold shock, characterized by increased vascular tone, low systemic blood flow, and eventually falling blood pressure. Cold shock has been well described in the newborn (Meadow and Rudinsky, 1995),

whereas the warm shock phase is more difficult to recognize clinically unless the blood pressure and the cardiovascular status in general are being closely monitored. The mediators of neonatal warm septic shock remain unclear, but in adult sepsis, dysregulated cytokine release and upregulated nitric oxide production as well as deficiency of vasopressin production play an important role (Landry and Oliver, 2001). The significance of this to newborn sepsis remains unclear, but it may have relevance to the vasopressor-resistant hypotension seen in preterm babies (Ng et al, 2001, 2006; Noori et al, 2006; Noori and Seri, 2008; Seri et al, 2001).

Pulmonary Hypertension With or Without Meconium Aspiration Syndrome

Term neonates with severe respiratory failure and pulmonary hypertension have a high incidence of low ventricular outputs (Evans et al, 1998). The low-output state is commonest in the early course of the disease, resolving spontaneously with time and/or clinical improvement. The causes of such circulatory compromise are probably multifactorial but include abnormal postnatal cardiovascular adaptation secondary to perinatal hypoxic-ischemic insult, the negative effects of positive pressure ventilation, and the systemic effect of raised pulmonary vascular resistance. In one study, low left ventricular output was a significant predictor of the need for ECMO in this patient population (Kinsella et al, 1992).

DIAGNOSIS OF CIRCULATORY COMPROMISE

There is no agreement regarding what constitutes the gold standard in diagnosing circulatory compromise. Conventionally, blood pressure has been and still is used as a gold standard. As mentioned earlier, recent data suggest that sole reliance on blood pressure can lead to inaccurate and sometimes significantly delayed diagnosis of circulatory compromise, especially in the very preterm infant during the immediate postnatal period. On the other hand, it is clear from the observations about vasodilatory shock that continuous blood pressure monitoring is imperative. The other commonly used clinical signs of circulatory compromise, such as increased heart rate, slow skin CRT, increased core-peripheral temperature difference, low urine output, and acidosis due to increased lactate production, aid in establishing the diagnosis of circulatory compromise in the preterm or term infant but have significant limitations.

Heart Rate and Blood Pressure

Heart rate is continuously, accurately, and routinely monitored in neonates requiring admission to neonatal intensive care units (NICUs). Because many factors other than those regulating the cardiovascular system affect heart rate, it has a limited yet widely utilized role in the diagnosis of circulatory compromise. As for the blood pressure, in babies with invasive intraarterial access, continuous and accurate measurement of this parameter is routinely done. The accuracy of the noninvasive oscillometric method is less certain, especially when severe hypotension develops. Normal ranges for blood pressure in babies of different gestations have been defined in the literature (epidemiologic

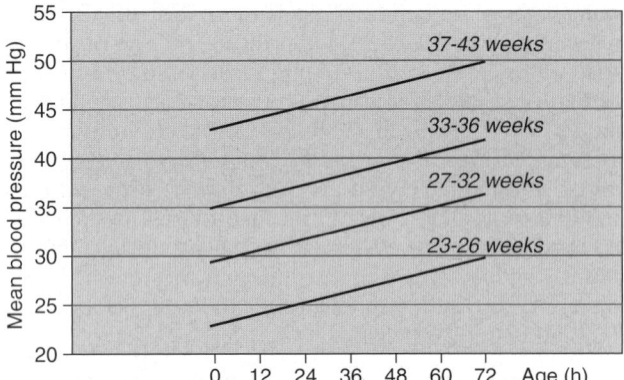

FIGURE 51-4 **Gestational and postnatal age-dependent nomogram for mean blood pressure values in neonates during the first 3 days of life.** The nomogram is derived from continuous arterial blood pressure measurements obtained from 103 neonates with gestational ages between 23 and 43 weeks. Each line represents the lower limit of 80% confidence interval of mean blood pressure for each gestational age group. Thus, 90% of infants for each gestational age group are expected to have a mean blood pressure equal to or greater than the value indicated by the corresponding line (the lower limit of confidence interval). (*From Nuntnarumit P, Yang W, Bada-Ellzey HS: Blood pressure measurements in the newborn,* Clin Perinatol 26:981-996, 1999.)

definition of hypotension) and it is clear that gestation and postnatal age are the dominant influences on blood pressure (Lee et al, 1999, Nuntnarumit et al, 1999; for a comprehensive review, see Engle, 2008). The nomogram from the data of Nuntnarumit et al in Figure 51-4 shows the 10th percentile for mean blood pressure of babies from different gestations at different postnatal ages.

The normal gestational- and postnatal-age dependent blood pressure range is not known, primarily because it is affected by additional factors such as disease severity, history of perinatal insult, presence of infection or ductal shunting, and interindividual variations (Engle, 2008; McLean et al, 2008). In addition to the epidemiologic definition of hypotension, increasing severity of hypotension can be defined from a pathophysiologic standpoint as the blood pressure value at which CBF becomes pressure-passive (autoregulatory blood pressure threshold; the definition used for the pediatric and adult patient population), brain function is affected (functional blood pressure threshold), and tissue ischemia develops (ischemic blood pressure threshold) (McLean et al, 2008). Preliminary data are available for the autoregulatory and functional blood pressure threshold in very preterm neonates during the first few postnatal days (Munro et al, 2004; Victor et al, 2006b). However, there is no information on the ischemic threshold in very preterm neonates, and very little is known about these pathophysiologic measures of hypotension in the term neonate or in any neonate beyond the transitional period. Perhaps the best method to define hypotension would be the demonstration of causation between gestational- and postnatal-age dependent blood pressure values and clinically relevant outcome measures such as mortality or long-term neurodevelopmental disability. However, because there are no data available on this interaction, there is uncertainty about the normative values. Besides, treatment may have its own side effects; hence there is controversy about when to intervene in

the critically ill neonate with suspected hypotension and circulatory compromise (Barrington and Dempsey, 2006; Noori and Seri, 2008).

In clinical practice, hypotension during the first postnatal day is usually defined in one of three ways: as a mean blood pressure <30 mm Hg, a mean blood pressure below the patient's gestational age in weeks at the time of birth (Lee et al, 1999), or, more recently, a blood pressure value that is accompanied by clinically detectable evidence of circulatory compromise (decreased urine output, poor peripheral perfusion, and/or lactic acidosis) (Dempsey et al, 2009). As mentioned earlier, there is only a weak relationship between mean blood pressure and SVC flow, a surrogate measure of systemic blood flow in preterm neonates with the fetal channels open in the immediate postnatal period (Kluckow and Evans, 1996, 2000; Lopez et al, 1997; Pladys et al, 2001). Thus, if blood pressure alone is used to guide treatment, patients in the unrecognized compensated phase of shock may not be treated appropriately. For instance, in the extremely preterm neonate with mean blood pressure between 20 and 40 mm Hg in the immediate postnatal period, the state of systemic blood flow and CBF is unclear based on the blood pressure values alone. Recent advances in our ability to apply complex, continuous cardiovascular monitoring providing data in absolute numbers using impedance-based electrical cardiometry, NIRS, and amplitude-integrated EEG combined with the intermittent use of Doppler flow measures hold the promise of gaining a better understanding of the hemodynamic changes occurring during transition and beyond in the neonatal patient population (Noori et al, 2009). However, at present only preliminary research data are available with the use of this complex approach.

Capillary Refill

Several recent studies have attempted to validate this widely used clinical tool for accuracy. However, there is no validated standard for assessing decreased peripheral perfusion and its relationship to systemic flow in the newborn. Further, in the different types of shock (warm vs. cold shock) the state of peripheral perfusion is different (vasodilation vs. vasoconstriction). Hence it is impossible to objectively assess the practical utility of this clinical tool in neonates. Accordingly, in VLBW neonates, a poor correlation was recently found between the capillary refill time, assessed on the forehead, sternum, and toe, and mean blood pressure, urine output, and SVC flow (Miletin et al, 2009). An earlier study documented a similar lack of tight relationship in VLBW neonates; only when capillary refill was >5 seconds did CRT have any clinically relevant degree of specificity (Osborn, 2001). Although a CRT of ≤3 seconds is traditionally accepted as normal, a CRT of 4.23 ± 1.47 seconds with a range of 1.63 to 8.78 seconds was reported in a large population of healthy newborns during the first 72 postnatal hours. CRT does not appear to change during the first 72 postnatal hours in healthy term newborns (Raju et al, 1999). Environmental, axillary, hand, and foot temperatures have been reported to indirectly relate to CRT (Raju et al, 1999). Interestingly, the duration of the pressure applied when eliciting CRT affects the measurement in term neonates <4 hours after delivery (LeFlore and Engle, 2005). This study also found an unanticipated moderate, direct correlation between blood pressure and CRT with a prolongation of CRT at higher blood pressures in this patient population (LeFlore and Engle, 2005). In general, interobserver variability has been reported to be fair, but a variation in the measurement among the different sites (sternum, forehead, hand, and feet) may be significant, although this issue needs to be more systematically studied.

Core-Peripheral Temperature Difference

There are few data to support the accuracy of this test in older infants (Tibby et al, 1999). As for preterm neonates less than 30 weeks' gestational age, there was also no relationship between this measure and SVC flow in the immediate postnatal period (Osborn, 2001). However, because SVC flow measurements have their limitations, these studies need to be repeated when a more accurate and continuous measure of systemic blood flow assessment becomes available for neonates with fetal channels open.

Low Urine Output and Hyperkalemia

Urine output is a frequently utilized clinical measure to assess renal perfusion and function. However, because urine output is low during the first postnatal day as a result of delivery-associated increases in stress hormones (catecholamines, vasopressin, renin-angiotensin) causing renal vasoconstriction and increased tubular reabsorption of sodium and water, its value in assessing compensated shock during the transitional period is limited. After the first 2 to 3 days, however, a decrease in urine output may be the earliest clinical sign of compensated shock in neonates of all gestational ages. In addition, a strong relationship has been documented in very preterm infants between low SVC flow and subsequent low urine output and hyperkalemia (Kluckow and Evans, 2001). However, because hyperkalemia may occur in the very preterm neonate without oliguria (i.e., nonoliguric hyperkalemia of the extremely preterm neonate) (Vemgal and Ohlsson, 2007), and because there could be other causes of hyperkalemia (acidosis), hyperkalemia alone should not be used as a measure of poor systemic perfusion.

Lactic Acid, pH, and Base Excess

In a large series, pH and base excess were found to have little relationship with low SVC flow in preterm babies in the immediate postnatal period (Kluckow and Evans, 1999). This finding is likely explained by lack of a strong relationship between pH, base excess, and lactic acid levels in neonates (Deshpande and Platt, 1997). However, because serum lactate levels can now be sequentially followed routinely on blood gases, and because changes in serum lactate are informative of changes in the cardiovascular status, this indirect measure of cellular oxygen delivery and consumption has been used in clinical practice. Interestingly, combining a CRT of >4 seconds with an elevated serum lactate concentration of >4 mmol/L has a specificity of 97% for detecting a low SVC flow state in VLBW neonates during the first postnatal day (Miletin et al, 2009). One needs to keep in mind, though, that a given serum lactate level primarily represents past hemodynamic events and not necessarily the present state of cardiovascular function. Thus, as with urine output, by the time lactic acidosis develops and

is detected, the initiating event may or may not be present anymore. It is not a surprise, therefore, that rising lactate levels are more predictive of adverse outcome than a high value early on followed by a subsequent decline (Deshpande and Platt, 1978).

Organ Blood Flow

With the use of Doppler ultrasonography and, more recently NIRS, blood flow to various organs can be assessed at the bedside. As for CBF, several methodologies have been studied in both preterm and term neonates including Doppler ultrasonography, xenon clearance, and NIRS (Greisen et al, 1984; Lemmers et al, 2006; Seri et al, 1998; Toet et al, 2005, 2006; Tsuji et al, 2000; Tyszczuk et al, 1998). Because peripheral arteries tend to be too small for size measurement, Doppler studies in such vessels are limited to parameters of velocity from which it is not possible to derive blood flow. Consequently, peripheral artery Doppler tends to be more useful for assessing changes over a time frame in which it is unlikely that the vessel size will have changed (Seri et al, 1998). Xenon clearance is not practical outside a research setting. However, recent advances in NIRS technology have introduced the potential of continuous assessment of brain, renal, mesenteric, and muscle oxygenation (i.e., blood flow) at the bedside in the critically ill neonate (Fortune et al, 2001; Lemmers et al, 2008; van Bel et al, 2008) (see next section).

Near-Infrared Spectroscopy

NIRS uses changes in oxygenation over time or the difference between oxygenated and deoxygenated hemoglobin to assess flow. The technology has been very useful as a research tool (Fortune et al, 2001; Lemmers et al, 2008; Meek et al, 1999a; Tsuji et al, 2000; Tyszczuk et al, 1998; van Bel et al, 2008). In addition, with better understanding of biophysical principles that govern light behavior in tissues, and the associated advances in software algorithms and sophisticated NIRS probe development, continuous assessment of regional tissue oxygenation (rSO_2) has become available and gained evidence-based application in neonatal intensive care (Adcock et al, 1999; Andropoulus et al, 2004; Lemmers et al, 2008; Nagdyman et al, 2008; van Bel et al, 2008).

Indeed, commercially available monitors with up to four channels can be now applied to infants, typically on the forehead to gauge cerebral rSO_2 and over the flank, felt to be measuring renal rSO_2. Although more validation is needed with invasive measurements (Nagdyman et al, 2008), it is evident that when cardiac output falls, the renal rSO_2 declines. First, cerebral rSO_2 may be preserved, but any interference with global cerebral blood flow can also be readily detected with this monitor. These monitors are very useful during cardiac surgical procedures on infants (Andropoulus et al, 2004; Azakie et al, 2005; Farouk et al, 2008), where precipitous drops in cerebral rSO_2 may be the only warning of a malpositioned venous or arterial cannula while on cardiopulmonary bypass. In addition, emerging findings suggest that monitoring rSO_2 in critically ill term and preterm neonates without congenital heart disease during transition to extrauterine life (van Bel et al, 2008) and treatment for various conditions such as preterm neonates with a PDA (Cayabyab et al, 2008; Lemmers et al,

2008), asphyxiated infants with or without cooling (Ancora et al, 2009; Meek et al, 1999b; Toet et al, 2006), or term neonates receiving ECMO (Fenik and Rais-Bahrami, 2009; van Heijst et al, 2004) provides clinically useful information (van Bel et al, 2008). Whether titration of therapy based on rSO_2 measurements in neonates with critical conditions other than congenital heart disease requiring surgery (Andropoulus et al, 2004) improves patients' outcomes remains unknown. In our experience, however, renal rSO_2 reliably declines well before signs of uncompensated shock such as hypotension or acidosis develop (see later discussion), enabling earlier intervention.

Echocardiographic Systemic Blood Flow Measures

In the mature circulation, systemic blood flow is the cardiac output. Although the output of both ventricles will be the same, cardiac output is traditionally measured from the left ventricular output. In clinical practice, Doppler ultrasound offers a noninvasive but noncontinuous method to measure cardiac output. Measuring blood flow directly in the pulmonary artery and ascending aorta enables us to evaluate outputs from the right and left ventricles, respectively (Alverson et al, 1982; Evans and Kluckow, 1996; Walther et al, 1985). However, as discussed earlier, in transitional circulation of the newborn infant, neither ventricular output will consistently reflect systemic blood flow because of the shunts across fetal channels (Evans and Iyer, 1994b; Evans and Kluckow, 1996; Kluckow and Seri, 2008). Use of SVC flow as a surrogate for systemic blood flow has been a valuable research tool offering insights into hemodynamic events unfolding during the immediate postnatal period when shunting across fetal channels precludes the use of traditional measures of systemic blood flow assessment (see earlier discussion) (Evans, 2008).

Doppler measures of left ventricular output have been validated against more invasive measures in neonates and older subjects (Mellander et al, 1987). Right ventricular output and SVC flow are less well validated but correlate well with left ventricular output in neonates with no confounding shunts (Evans and Iyer, 1994b; Kluckow and Evans, 2000; Tsai-Goodman et al, 2001). Despite this, the validity of these measures has been questioned based on comparison to cardiac output thermodilution measures in critical care patients (Notterman et al, 1989). However, thermodilution itself has an intrinsic error in that the volume of the required cold saline injection influences cardiac output (Tournadre et al, 1997). Thus, the quest for an ideal gold standard method continues.

There are significant intrinsic errors to Doppler flow measures as well. Intraobserver variability rates of around 10% and interobserver variability rates up to 20% are common (Hudson et al, 1990; Kluckow and Evans, 2000). Most of the error relates to vessel size measurement that is derived from a diameter. Thus, small differences are magnified in the conversion to a cross-sectional area. The other major problem of Doppler flow measurements is that there is reliance on ultrasound technology and echocardiographic skill that may not often be available 24 hours a day in many neonatal intensive care units.

In neonates, most studies quote a normal range for left and right ventricular output between 150 and 300 mL/kg/min

(Alverson et al, 1982; Evans and Kluckow, 1996; Walther et al, 1985; West et al, 2006). It is important to note that, in the transitional neonatal circulation, left ventricular output can be affected by ductal shunting to a greater extent than the right ventricular output is affected by atrial shunting. Therefore, right ventricular output is a better measure of low flow than left ventricular output during the first 1 to 2 postnatal days. Accordingly, a relationship has been documented between indirect measurements of systemic (and thus cerebral) perfusion such as right ventricular output and blood pressure (and cerebral function) in preterm infants during the first 2 postnatal days. This is a period when ductal shunting significantly decreases the accuracy of left ventricular output measurements reflecting systemic blood flow (West et al, 2006). SVC flow may also be used to estimate systemic flow in the early postnatal period. The normal range in well preterm babies is between 40 and 120 mL/kg/min, with the median rising from 70 mL/kg/min at 5 hours of age to 90 mL/kg/min at 48 hours (Kluckow and Evans, 2000).

In summary, the mainstay of diagnosing neonatal circulatory compromise has been a combination of blood pressure measurement and evaluation of the previously described clinical parameters. However, none of these parameters has a sufficient degree of accuracy to allow it to be relied on as the sole evaluator of systemic blood flow and tissue perfusion. Therefore, the addition of echocardiographic and NIRS hemodynamic assessment to blood pressure monitoring and thorough continuous clinical evaluation of the patient are necessary to better understand changes in organ blood flow and tissue perfusion, especially in preterm neonates during the vulnerable period of immediate transition to extrauterine life. The goal should be to maintain normal systemic blood flow in the presence of an acceptable blood pressure using the normal range for blood pressure that controls for gestation and postnatal age and following the indirect clinical and laboratory signs of tissue perfusion (urine output, serum lactate levels, CRT). If there is no immediate access to echocardiography or NIRS technology, the clinician will have to rely on blood pressure monitoring while recognizing the limitations of this approach. Over the past few years, training in functional echocardiography for neonatologists has become available in a structured format in several programs in the United States and abroad (Kluckow et al, 2008), although the medicolegal implications of such training remain unknown.

TREATMENT

Selection of the most appropriate treatment strategy requires identification of the pathogenesis for neonatal shock (Kluckow, 2005; Kluckow and Seri, 2008; Seri, 2001; Seri and Noori, 2005). As described earlier, the most frequent etiologic factors responsible for neonatal cardiovascular compromise are inappropriate peripheral vasoregulation, resulting in vasodilation or vasoconstriction, and dysfunction of the immature myocardium (Gill and Weindling, 1993; Kluckow and Seri, 2008; Noori and Seri, 2005; Seri, 1995; Osborn et al, 2002). Absolute hypovolemia is a much less frequent primary cause of neonatal hypotension, especially in preterm infants in the immediate postnatal period (Barr et al, 1977; Wright and Goodhall, 1994).

ASSOCIATION BETWEEN SYSTEMIC HYPOTENSION, HYPOPERFUSION, AND THEIR TREATMENT AND MORTALITY OR NEURODEVELOPMENTAL IMPAIRMENT

The impact of hypotension and/or its treatment on mortality, brain injury, or neurodevelopmental impairment is unclear, primarily because it is assumed that treatment will improve outcomes, and therefore the common practice has been to treat hypotension (Noori et al, 2009). Therefore, there are no prospective studies evaluating the impact of untreated hypotension on clinically relevant short- and long-term outcomes. In addition, the gestational- and postnatal-age dependent definition of hypotension based on physiology, pathophysiology, and clinically relevant outcome measures is lacking (Engle, 2008). Finally, the finding that hypotension as currently defined is unlikely to be predictive of brain injury (McLean et al, 2008; Limperopoulos et al, 2007) is important in examining the association between hypotension and its treatment and neurodevelopmental impairment.

VOLUME ADMINISTRATION

Observations that hypotensive neonates as a group are not hypovolemic (Barr et al, 1977; Wright and Goodhall, 1994), low blood pressure is frequently associated with normal or even high ventricular output and low index of resistance (Pladys et al, 1999) and dopamine is more effective in normalizing blood pressure than volume administration (Lundstrom et al, 2000) support indirectly that absolute hypovolemia is an infrequent primary cause of neonatal hypotension in the transitional period. Therefore, particularly in the preterm infant during the immediate postnatal period, fluid resuscitation is recommended to be minimized. Furthermore, because myocardial dysfunction frequently contributes to the development of neonatal hypotension (Gill and Weindling, 1993) and aggressive volume administration in this patient population increases pulmonary, cardiovascular, gastrointestinal, and central nervous system morbidity and mortality (Kavvadia et al, 2000; Lundstrom et al, 2000; Van Marter et al, 1990), judicious use of fluid administration is highly warranted. However, absolute hypovolemia is a major contributing etiologic factor to neonatal shock in neonates with sepsis and/or in the postoperative period in patients undergoing major surgery. Indeed, early and aggressive resuscitation of children and neonates with sepsis has been documented to decrease mortality (Han et al, 2003) and has been recommended by the American College of Critical Care Medicine (Bierley et al, 2009).

Controversy has recently emerged concerning the type of fluid administration to preterm neonates with cardiovascular compromise. Most studies have shown that isotonic saline is as effective as 5% albumin in increasing the blood pressure (Oca et al, 2003; So et al, 1997). In addition, albumin may impair gas exchange and induce fluid shift from the intracellular compartment (Ernest et al, 1999) and is associated with increased mortality (Nadel et al, 1998). Therefore, given comparable efficacy of isotonic saline and albumin in the face of differences in cost and the suggested increased mortality and morbidity

associated with albumin administration (Kavvadia et al, 2000; Lundstrom et al, 2000; Van Marter et al, 1990), isotonic saline has been the initial choice of treatment in the neonatal patient population. However, a recent randomized controlled trial found that in hypotensive, mostly preterm neonates, albumin administration resulted in a greater likelihood of achieving normotension and decreased the subsequent use of vasopressors when compared to isotonic saline (Lynch et al, 2008). The findings of this study need to be replicated before the routine use of albumin can be recommended as the initial treatment for neonatal cardiovascular compromise. Therefore, unless evidence of serum or blood loss or hypoalbuminemia is present, volume support in hypotensive preterm and term infants is provided in the form of 10 to 20 mL/kg of isotonic saline (Noori and Seri, 2008b; Seri, 2001). It is also important to note that, because of the unbalanced nature of normal saline, caution should be exercised with administration in large amounts over a short period of time, as this may worsen the metabolic acidosis (Mirza et al, 1999; Prough and Bidani, 1999). Should the limited-volume administration be ineffective, pharmacologic cardiovascular support with a vasopressor-inotrope or an inotrope is recommended (Kluckow, 2005; Noori and Seri, 2008; Osborn et al, 2002; Seri and Noori, 2005; Seri, 1995, 2001) and should be initiated.

If there is an identifiable volume loss, the type of fluid lost should be replaced. In cases of blood loss, transfusion with packed red blood cells after the initial crystalloid or colloid bolus or packed red blood cells suspended in fresh frozen plasma with a hematocrit around 55% may be used. In cases of increased transepidermal water losses, higher free water administration without an increase in sodium supplementation is indicated. When polyuria is present, the composition and volume of the replacement fluid may be adjusted to the urinary sodium and free water losses. However, replacement of half of the excessive urinary losses with 0.45% saline will usually suffice.

DOPAMINE AND DOBUTAMINE

Dopamine and dobutamine treatment was introduced in the management of neonatal hypotension in the early and mid-1980s, respectively, without appropriately designed randomized and blinded clinical trials. Thus, as mentioned earlier, we have no clear evidence that the use of these sympathomimetic amines (or any other sympathomimetic amine) improves neonatal mortality or morbidity. A number of studies have recently extended their focus beyond the dopamine- and dobutamine-induced heart rate and blood pressure changes by examining the drugs' effect on neonatal myocardial contractility, systemic and organ blood flow (Bouissou et al, 2008; Lundstrom et al, 2000; Noori et al, 2006; Osborn et al, 2002; Pellicer et al, 2005; Roze et al, 1993; Seri et al, 1998, 2002; Zhang et al, 1999; 2009). Some of the earlier studies, however, used left ventricular output to assess the impact of these medications on systemic blood flow even when shunting across fetal channels occurred (Lundstrom et al, 2000; Roze et al, 1993; Zhang et al, 1999). Therefore, the conclusions drawn in these studies need to be carefully reevaluated (Kluckow and Seri, 2008).

Hemodynamic Effects

Dopamine, an endogenous catecholamine, is the sympathomimetic amine most frequently used in the treatment of hypotension in preterm infants (Seri, 1995). It exerts its cardiovascular actions via the dose-dependent stimulation of the cardiovascular dopaminergic, α- and β-adrenergic, and serotoninergic receptors. In addition, by stimulating epithelial and peripheral neuronal dopaminergic and adrenergic receptors, the drug exerts significant renal and endocrine effects independent of its cardiovascular actions (Seri, 1995). Although dopamine affects all three major determinants of cardiovascular function (preload, myocardial contractility, and afterload), the drug-induced increases in myocardial contractility (Lundstrom et al, 2000; Zhang et al, 1999) and peripheral vascular resistance (afterload) (Lundstrom et al, 2000; Roze et al, 1993; Zhang et al, 1999) are the most important factors in increasing systemic blood pressure and improving the cardiovascular status.

The original dose-range recommendation of 2 to 20 µg/kg/min of dopamine was based on pharmacodynamic data obtained in adults without cardiovascular compromise. However, changes in cardiovascular adrenergic receptor expression caused by critical illness (Hausdorff et al, 1990) and relative or absolute adrenal insufficiency and immaturity (Watterberg and Scott, 1995; Watterberg 2002), as well as the dysregulated production of local vasodilators during severe illness, decrease the sensitivity of the cardiovascular system to dopamine, resulting in the emergence of hypotension resistant to conventional doses of the drug (Ng et al, 2001, 2006; Noori et al, 2006; Seri et al, 2001). Thus, with the advancement of the disease process, increased doses of dopamine and other sympathomimetic amines may be needed to exert the same magnitude of cardiovascular response. Therefore, dopamine administration should be tailored to the drug's pharmacodynamic effects in a given patient at the bedside rather than driven by the conventional dose recommendations based on data obtained in healthy adults. Indeed, although many neonatologists do not advance the dose of dopamine beyond 20 µg/kg/min, there is no evidence that, when required to normalize blood pressure, high-dose dopamine treatment with or without additional epinephrine administration has detrimental vasoconstrictive effects (Perez et al, 1986; Seri et al, 2001). However, there are no data available on changes in cardiac output and organ blood flow in response to high-dose catecholamine treatment in vasopressor-resistant neonatal shock, and close attention should be paid to signs of inappropriate vasoconstriction when this therapy is applied. More recently, administration of low-dose hydrocortisone has been shown to ameliorate the need for high-dose vasopressor administration in most patients (Cole, 2008; Ng et al, 2001; Noori et al, 2006; Seri et al, 2001; 2006).

Unlike dopamine, dobutamine is a relatively cardioselective sympathomimetic amine with significant α- and β-adrenoreceptor–mediated direct inotropic effects and limited chronotropic actions (Ruffolo, 1987). Dobutamine administration is usually also associated with a variable decrease in total peripheral vascular resistance and, at least in adults, with improved coronary blood flow and myocardial oxygen delivery (Ruffolo, 1987). Furthermore, unlike dopamine, dobutamine increases myocardial contractility exclusively through the direct stimulation of myocardial adrenergic receptors. Because myocardial norepinephrine stores are immature and rapidly depleted in the newborn, and because dobutamine may decrease afterload, newborns with primary myocardial dysfunction and elevated peripheral vascular resistance are most likely to benefit from dobutamine treatment (Martinez et al, 1992; Osborn et al, 2002). Interestingly, though addition of dobutamine to dopamine in preterm infants with RDS was effective in increasing blood pressure, it was associated with supranormal cardiac output states and low systemic vascular resistance (Lopez et al, 1997). Whether the benefits of supranormal cardiac output by providing adequate tissue oxygen delivery throughout the body outweigh the risks of sustained hypercontractility, potentially resulting in myocardial injury, remains to be investigated.

Randomized studies have uniformly demonstrated that dopamine is more effective than dobutamine in increasing blood pressure in the preterm infant, and a recent metaanalysis of the findings confirmed that dopamine was more successful than dobutamine in treating hypotension, with fewer infants in the dopamine group facing treatment failure (Subdehar and Shaw, 2000). However, there was no difference in short-term adverse neurologic outcome between the two groups. In the absence of long-term outcome data, no firm recommendations can be made regarding the choice of drug in treating hypotension of preterm infants in the immediate postnatal period. In addition, no information was forthcoming on changes in systemic blood flow. However, when carefully titrated to the optimum hemodynamic effect, dopamine (and epinephrine) increased blood pressure and CBF in hypotensive VLBW neonates during the first postnatal day (Pellicer et al, 2004). Neurodevelopmental follow-up of patients enrolled in this study at 2 to 3 years of age did not reveal evidence of an independent vasopressor-inotrope–associated increase in morbidity (Pellicer et al, 2009). Although the findings of this study provide some reassurance concerning the possibility of a dopamine (or epinephrine) associated increase in neurodevelopmental morbidity in VLBW neonates during the first postnatal day, the original study (Pellicer et al, 2005) was not sufficiently powered to put these concerns to rest.

As discussed earlier, because of the weak relationship between blood pressure and systemic blood flow in very preterm neonates during the immediate postnatal period, an increase in blood pressure does not necessarily guarantee that tissue perfusion has improved along with the blood pressure (Kluckow and Evans, 1996, 2000; Kluckow and Seri, 2008; Lopez et al, 1997; Pladys et al, 2001). Therefore, if there is evidence of peripheral vasoconstriction, especially in VLBW neonates during the first postnatal day, high-dose dopamine treatment should only be attempted if systemic blood flow can be monitored by functional echocardiography and/or NIRS. This treatment approach may result in further impairment in systemic blood flow despite improvements in blood pressure (Osborn et al, 2002). However, in present clinical practice these measures of blood flow monitoring are not routinely available, and the neonatologist has to rely on monitoring blood pressure and the indirect measures of cardiovascular function. If evidence of vasoconstriction is present with higher doses of dopamine (or epinephrine), the neonatologist should consider accepting lower-end blood pressure values for gestational and postnatal age and decrease the dose of vasopressor-inotrope to levels where significant α-adrenoreceptor stimulation is less likely (Kluckow and Seri, 2008; Seri, 1995). In these cases, addition of dobutamine should be considered and the blood pressure maintained at least in the low-normal range because systemic hypotension has been linked to poor long-term neurodevelopmental outcome in the VLBW neonatal patient population (Bada et al, 1990; Miall-Allen et al, 1987). A combination of dobutamine and low-dose dopamine may achieve the most important goals of treatment by maintaining blood pressure and systemic blood flow in acceptable ranges if monitoring of both cardiovascular parameters is possible. In most of these patients, physiologic glucocorticoid and mineralocorticoid replacement with hydrocortisone is likely to be effective, although the potential side effects of early hydrocortisone exposure in preterm neonates should be kept in mind (see later discussion) (Cole, 2008; Kluckow and Seri, 2008; Seri et al, 2001; Seri and Noori, 2005). In summary, because both hypotension and low systemic blood flow have been associated with impaired neurodevelopmental outcome, the primary goal of management of the hypotensive very preterm neonate should be the correction of both measures of cardiovascular function.

A recent study demonstrated that in hypotensive preterm neonates with a significant left-to-right shunting across the PDA, dopamine administration increases systemic blood pressure, pulmonary pressure, and SVC flow, used as a surrogate of systemic blood flow in these patients (Bouissou et al, 2008). Dopamine administration has not been associated with evidence of increased pulmonary vascular resistance and decreased right ventricular output in neonates without a significant left-to-right shunting across the PDA (Clark et al, 2002; Wardle et al, 1999). This finding suggests that when pulmonary blood flow is increased, vasoconstrictive mechanisms may be upregulated in the pulmonary circulation, resulting in more pronounced α-receptor–mediated dopamine-induced pulmonary vasoconstriction. The findings of an earlier study demonstrating a variable pulmonary resistance response to dopamine in preterm neonates with a hemodynamically significant PDA support this notion (Liet et al, 2002).

In hypotensive term and preterm neonates beyond the immediate postnatal period, where vasodilatory shock is the more likely presentation, dopamine administration in doses tailored to the cardiovascular response is warranted and appears to be beneficial (DiSessa et al, 1981; Martinez et al, 1992; Seri and Noori, 2005) unless evidence of primary myocardial dysfunction is present (Seri, 1995, 2001).

The vasodilatory dopamine receptors are primarily expressed in renal, mesenteric, and coronary circulations (Seri, 1995). Dopamine has been shown to selectively decrease renal vascular resistance (Seri et al, 1998, 2002) and increase glomerular filtration rate (Seri et al, 1993) in preterm infants as early as the 23rd week of gestation. However, dopamine appears to decrease mesenteric vascular resistance in preterm infants only beyond the first

postnatal day (Hentschel et al, 1995; Robel-Tillig et al, 2007; Seri et al, 1998, 2000), and the effect may be variable (Zhang et al, 1999). Similarly, there are some differences in the reported magnitude of drug-induced increases in ventricular function, cardiac output, and systemic vascular resistance (Clark et al, 2002; Lundstrom et al, 2000; Roze et al, 1993; Zhang et al, 1999). These findings may be best explained by differences in intravascular volume status, postnatal age, developmentally regulated expression of cardiovascular adrenergic and dopaminergic receptors, and severity of adrenergic receptor downregulation among different populations of critically ill infants studied. It is important to note that none of the studies found evidence for a direct effect of dopamine on cerebral blood flow as long as blood pressure was in the autoregulatory range (Lundstrom et al, 2000; Seri et al, 1998, 2000; Zhang et al, 1999). Thus, dopamine administration appears to be devoid of potentially harmful selective hemodynamic effects in the brain. As expected, in hypotensive neonates dopamine (and epinephrine) increase both blood pressure and CBF (Pellicer et al, 2004).

There are very few data available on direct renal, cerebral, or pulmonary hemodynamic effects of dobutamine in the newborn. A nonrandomized study comparing the effects of dopamine and dobutamine on blood pressure and mesenteric blood flow in preterm infants found that both drugs increased blood pressure and were equally effective in decreasing mesenteric vascular resistance (Hentschel et al, 1995). Because dobutamine does not stimulate the dopaminergic receptors, β-adrenoreceptor–induced selective vasodilation may be responsible for the observed mesenteric vasodilation in dobutamine-treated patients.

Epithelial and Neuroendocrine Effects

Independent of the just-described cardiovascular effects, dopamine exerts direct renal (Seri, 1995) and endocrine (Seri, 1995) actions in the newborn. Via its direct effects on sodium, phosphorous and water transport processes and Na/K ATPase activity in renal tubules, dopamine increases sodium, phosphrus, and free water excretion and may increase the hypoxic threshold of renal tubular cells during episodes of hypoperfusion and hypoxemia (Seri, 1995). Via its renal vascular and epithelial actions, dopamine also potentiates the diuretic effects of furosemide (Tulassay and Seri, 1986) and theophylline (Bell et al, 1998). Although dopamine has the theoretical potential to attenuate renal side effects of indomethacin, the data in the literature are contradictory (Seri, 1995). Differences in the level of maturity, disease severity, ductal shunting, intravascular volume status, and indomethacin dose may be responsible for such conflicting results. Among its endocrine actions, the dopamine-induced decreases in plasma prolactin, thyrotropin, and growth hormone levels (Seri, 1995) may be of clinical importance. The decrease in plasma prolactin may attenuate the preterm infant's propensity to edema formation but may also have an immune function (Seri, 1995). The inhibition of thyrotropin release necessitates the postponement of routine neonatal thyroid screening until after dopamine administration has been discontinued (Seri, 1995). The potential impact on long-term neurodevelopmental outcome and immunologic function of drug-induced alterations in neuroendocrine function has not been investigated in the preterm or term neonate. Because dobutamine does not directly stimulate dopaminergic receptors, its administration is thought to be devoid of neuroendocrine effects.

EPINEPHRINE, NOREPINEPHRINE, AND OTHER CARDIOVASCULAR AGENTS AND HORMONES

In a randomized controlled trial, low to medium doses of epinephrine, when titrated to optimal hemodynamic response, have been shown to increase blood pressure and CBF in hypotensive VLBW neonates (see earlier discussion) (Pellicer et al, 2004). Because of epinephrine's significant effect on glycogenolysis, its administration is associated with an increase in serum lactate levels independent of the drug's cardiovascular actions (Valverde et al, 2005). This effect should be kept in mind when following serum lactate levels to assess the changes in cardiovascular status due to epinephrine administration. Therefore, the epinephrine-induced improvement in perfusion cannot be ascertained by following serum lactate levels alone, because these levels will likely increase independent of drug-induced improvement in the cardiovascular status.

Until very recently, findings on the cardiovascular effects of norepinephrine in neonates were only published in abstract form (Derleth, 1997). However, a recent observational study in late preterm and term neonates with persistent pulmonary hypertension of the newborn (PPHN) treated with inhaled nitric oxide (iNO) and signs of circulatory failure found that medium doses of norepinephrine improve systemic and pulmonary cardiovascular function in these neonates by decreasing the pulmonary artery–to–aortic pressure gradient and improving cardiac performance (Tourneux et al, 2008). Although these findings are encouraging, the routine use of norepinephrine in the treatment of neonates with PPHN and cardiovascular compromise requires further confirmation.

It is not known whether there is a difference in the cardiovascular response and/or side effects of sympathomimetic amines with the combined use of epinephrine and dopamine compared to the use of increasing doses of dopamine beyond 20 µg/kg/min with or without dobutamine. There have been no detrimental vasoconstrictive effects reported using either high doses of epinephrine with or without dopamine, or norepinephrine in preliminary publications (Campbell and Byrne, 1998; Derleth, 1997; Seri and Evans, 1998). These findings are best explained by the decreased cardiovascular sensitivity of these critically ill preterm infants to catecholamines, necessitating the high sympathomimetic support in the first place. However, one must be extremely careful when escalating treatment with these potent vasopressor-inotropes to avoid causing significant vasoconstriction and decreased tissue perfusion. In addition to sympathomimetic amines, arginine-vasopressin has been reported to improve cardiovascular function in a small number of newborns with vasodilatory shock after cardiac surgery (Rosenzweig et al, 1999).

There are very few data available on the cardiovascular effects of milrinone, a phosphodiesterase-III (PDE-III) inhibitor in the neonatal patient population. It has been more widely used to reduce afterload in neonates with congenital heart disease with low cardiac output syndrome after surgery (Hoffman et al, 2003). As for its use in term infants without congenital heart disease, milrinone administration has been shown in a small case series to improve the oxygenation index without compromising systemic blood pressure when given to term neonates with PPHN treated with iNO during the first 2 postnatal days (McNamara et al, 2006). The preferential effect of milrinone on the pulmonary circulation in neonates with PPHN treated with iNO may be due to the upregulation of PDE-III in pulmonary vessels in response to iNO administration. It is unclear if milrinone has a positive inotropic effect in neonates (Barrington and Dempsey, 2006).

Recently, a randomized placebo-controlled blinded clinical trial investigated whether the use of milrinone would minimize or prevent the suspected increase in systemic vascular resistance and the associated systemic hypoperfusion in VLBW infants during the first postnatal day (Paradisis et al, 2009). However, there was no improvement in the incidence of low SVC flow used as a surrogate of systemic blood flow in patients treated with milrinone compared to the placebo group. These findings may be explained, at least in part, by the little-appreciated complexity of the pathophysiology of cardiovascular compromise in the very preterm neonate after delivery. They further suggest that systemic and cerebral hypoperfusion and reperfusion in this patient population may not solely occur because of the inability of the immature myocardium to pump against the sudden postnatal increase in systemic vascular resistance (Noori et al, 2009).

STEROID ADMINISTRATION

There is now overwhelming evidence provided by descriptive studies (Heckmann and Pohlandt, 2002; Helbock et al, 1993; Ng et al, 2001; Noori et al, 2006a; Seri et al, 2001) and confirmed by randomized blinded prospective trials (Bouchier and Weston, 1997; Effird et al, 2005; Gaissmaier and Pohlandt, 1999; Ng et al, 2006; Watterberg et al, 1999) that brief steroid treatment stabilizes the cardiovascular status and decreases the need for vasopressor-inotropic support in the critically ill preterm and term newborn with vasopressor-resistant hypotension. Because there is overwhelming evidence that early and/or medium-to-high cumulative doses of dexamethasone have detrimental effects on the developing brain (Baud et al, 2004; Halliday et al, 2003; O'Shea et al, 1999; Shinwell et al, 2000; Yeh et al, 2004), and because in addition to glucocorticoids, mineralocorticoids also have significant effects on the cardiovascular system (Wehling, 1997; Wehling et al, 1995), even low-dose dexamethasone administration to treat vasopressor-resistant hypotension has fallen by the wayside in recent years. This section therefore addresses only the actions, side effects, recommended doses, and remaining clinically relevant concerns of hydrocortisone administration to treat vasopressor-resistant hypotension in the critically ill neonate. It is of note that the available evidence for the effectiveness of low-dose hydrocortisone to increase blood pressure and decrease vasopressor-inotrope requirement in the preterm neonate is so strong that it would take 74 and 188 future studies demonstrating no effect of hydrocortisone on blood pressure increase and the decrease in vasopressor requirement, respectively, to eliminate the statistical power of the present findings (Higgins et al, 2010).

Because in most patients and after some time, cardiovascular stability will be achieved by the use of vasopressors-inotropes and/or inotropes alone, it is important to understand the rationale of hydrocortisone administration, especially because the drug has its own side effects (see later discussion). First, it is widely accepted that the sooner one normalizes blood pressure, especially in the VLBW neonate during the immediate postnatal period, the better the outcome. However, because normal blood pressure in the first 24 hours may not guarantee normal cerebral perfusion (see earlier discussion) and because an association but not causation has been documented between hypotension and adverse outcomes, stabilization of the cardiovascular status with little blood pressure fluctuation remains an intuitively desirable goal but one without much direct evidence to support it. More importantly, hydrocortisone specifically addresses the underlying etiology of the cardiovascular instability in most critically ill neonates and thus is the logical choice of treatment. Indeed, findings of developmental endocrinology and cardiovascular physiology as well as recent clinical data support a role for hydrocortisone use in critically ill hypotensive neonates, especially in VLBW neonates. In critical illness, desensitization of the cardiovascular system to catecholamines takes place through the downregulation of cardiovascular adrenergic receptors and second messenger systems (Hausdorff et al, 1990). This process is attenuated or prevented by the regulatory actions of glucocorticoids on the expression of cardiovascular adrenergic receptors and second messenger systems (Hausdorff et al, 1990). In addition, the direct increase in myocardial and vascular smooth muscle cell contractility induced by mineralocorticoids plays an effective role (Wehling, 1997; Wehling et al, 1995). In addition, corticosteroids contribute to the maintenance of capillary integrity, inhibit catecholamine metabolism and reuptake of norepinephrine into sympathetic nerve endings, increase the expression of angiotensin type 2 receptors in the myocardium, and inhibit prostacyclin production and the induction of inducible nitric oxide synthase. Each of these actions of corticosteroids aids in maintaining the sensitivity of the cardiovascular system to catecholamines in response to acute stress or critical illness. In addition, because of the role of glucocorticoids in the physiologic regulation of adrenergic receptor expression (Hausdorff et al, 1990), the emergence of vasopressor resistance in itself may indicate a state of relative adrenal insufficiency. Indeed, the findings of several recent studies indicate that critically ill preterm and term infants are likely to develop relative adrenal insufficiency because of their immature adrenal function (Ng et al, 2004; Watterberg, 2002; Watterberg and Scott, 1995) and hypothalamopituitary axis (Fernandez et al, 2008; Fernandez and Watterberg, 2009), respectively. It is important to emphasize that, based on these findings, it appears that in the VLBW neonate, adrenal unresponsiveness to endogenous or exogenous ACTH (Ng et al, 2004; Watterberg, 2002) and in the late preterm and term neonate, unresponsiveness of the hypothalamopituitary axis to stress (Fernandez and Watterberg,

2009; Fernandez et al, 2008) are the primary causes for the development of relative adrenal insufficiency. Thus, these patients have limited capacity to produce sufficient adaptive increases in endogenous steroid production to prevent the development of cardiovascular adrenergic receptor downregulation and desensitization of the cardiovascular system to catecholamines during their illness. Therefore, in critically ill preterm and term infants with vasopressor-resistant hypotension, steroid administration also serves as hormone substitution therapy.

As for the clinical application and effects of hydrocortisone, available evidence indicates that hydrocortisone in preterm and term infants with vasopressor-resistant hypotension increases blood pressure within 2 hours of the initiation of treatment (nongenomic effects) and decreases vasopressor requirement within 8 to 12 hours of the first dose of the drug (genomic effects) (Figure 51-5) (Ng et al, 2006; Noori et al, 2006; Seri et al, 2001). A recent study in preterm infants without a PDA also documented that the hydrocortisone-induced improvement in blood pressure is associated with improvements in all aspects of cardiovascular function including stroke volume and tissue perfusion (Figure 51-6) (Noori et al, 2006b).

As for the side effects of early or late low-dose hydrocortisone administration, the potential occurrence of short- and long-term sequelae is of great interest. As for the short-term side effects, it has been repeatedly documented that coexposure of preterm neonates to indomethacin and hydrocortisone during the first postnatal week significantly increases the risk of spontaneous gastrointestinal (mostly ileal) perforations (Peltoniemi et al, 2005; Watterberg et al, 2004). This serious untoward effect significantly curtails the use of hydrocortisone in the VLBW neonate during the first postnatal week; the very patient population in whom vasopressor-resistant hypotension and relative adrenal insufficiency are most prevalent during the immediate postnatal period. It is interesting to note that findings of one of these studies suggest that VLBW neonates with low baseline serum cortisol levels may be at less risk for developing ileal perforations when treated with low-dose hydrocortisone and a cyclooxygenase inhibitor during the first postnatal days (Peltoniemi et al, 2005). However, this observation needs to be confirmed before it can be used to predict the likelihood of spontaneous intestinal perforation based on the basal serum cortisol level alone. As for the other short-term side effects of hydrocortisone, one earlier study found an increase in the incidence of systemic fungal infections (Botas et al, 1995). However, none of the other studies have documented a significant increase in bacterial or fungal infections in neonates. Finally, hydrocortisone administration–associated transient hyperglycemia and hypertension have been reported in a few cases in the literature.

As for the potential long-term side effects, the most pressing question is whether low to moderate doses of hydrocortisone interfere with neurodevelopment, especially in preterm neonates. The findings of a recent study indicate that early, low-dose hydrocortisone treatment is not associated with an increased incidence of cerebral palsy and that infants exposed to hydrocortisone in the original placebo-controlled blinded clinical trial during the first 10 postnatal days to prevent the development

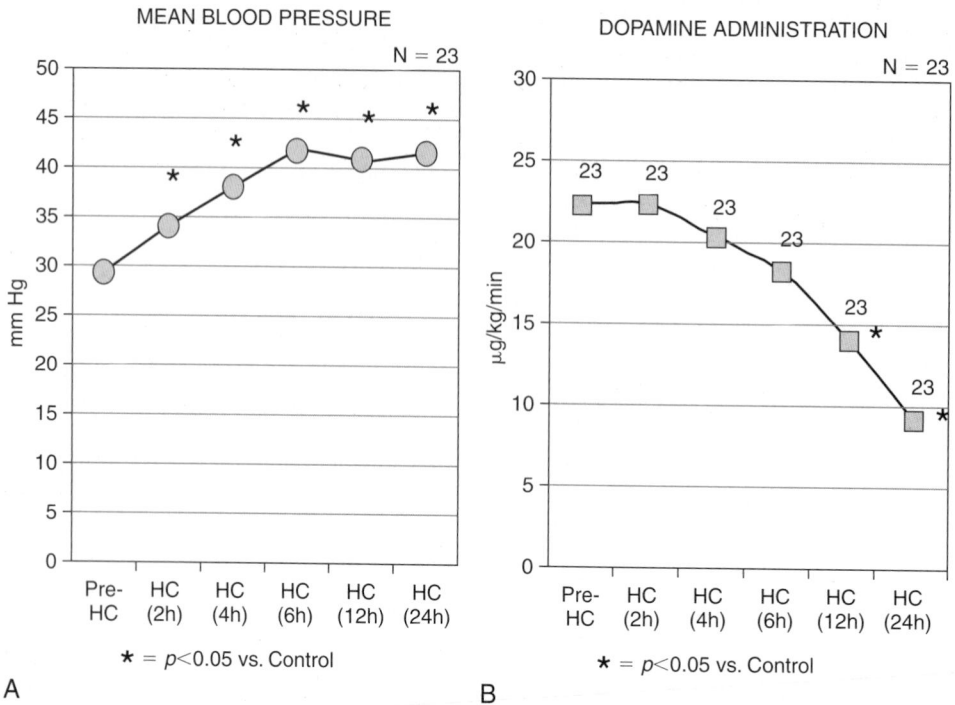

FIGURE 51-5 Effect of hydrocortisone on mean blood pressure and the dose of dopamine during the first 24 hours of hydrocortisone treatment in 23 preterm neonates with vasopressor-resistant shock. **A,** Mean blood pressure (mean ± SD) and **(B)** dopamine requirement (mean ± SD) during the 12 hours before and the first 24 hours after the first dose of hydrocortisone. Before hydrocortisone administration, blood pressure remained low **(A),** despite significantly increased dopamine doses **(B,** * = $p < 0.05$ vs. baseline [0 h]). However, mean blood pressure increased significantly by 2 hours after the first dose of hydrocortisone **(A,** * = P < 0.05 vs. baseline [0 h]) and continued to rise until 6 hours of hydrocortisone therapy, remaining stable thereafter **(A,** * = $p < 0.05$ vs. baseline [0 h]; * = $p < 0.05$ vs. HC [2 h]). In addition, the dose of dopamine significantly decreased by 12 and 24 hours of hydrocortisone therapy **(B,** * = $p < 0.05$ vs. baseline [0 h]). (*From Seri I, Tan R, Evans J: Cardiovascular effects of hydrocortisone in preterm neonates with pressor resistant hypotension,* Pediatrics *107:1070-1074, 2001.*)

of bronchopulmonary dysplasia (Watterberg et al, 2004) actually showed some evidence of improved developmental outcome at 18 to 22 months corrected age compared to controls (Watterberg et al, 2007). As for the use of higher cumulative doses of hydrocortisone outside the immediate transitional period, the results of a study examining structural and functional brain development at an age of 8 years suggest that hydrocortisone, used for the treatment of bronchopulmonary dysplasia in ventilator-dependent preterm neonates at a median age of 18 days and at cumulative doses over 50 mg, does not interfere with brain development (Lodygensky et al, 2005). Although these findings are reassuring, lack of power (Watterberg et al, 2007) and the retrospective nature of the study design (Lodygensky et al, 2005) warrant caution before the use of early or late and low- to medium-dose hydrocortisone could be declared safe in preterm neonates, at least from a neurodevelopmental standpoint.

SUPPORTIVE MEASURES

Maintenance of a normal intravascular volume, arterial pH, and serum ionized calcium concentrations is necessary for the optimum cardiovascular response to catecholamines. Because a metabolic acidosis of <7.25 may compromise myocardial function in the preterm infant (Fanconi et al, 1993), it is recommended that the arterial pH be maintained above this range in cases of acidosis with a significant metabolic component. However, more

data are needed in support of this recommendation in the neonatal patient population. Administration of sodium bicarbonate (Fanconi et al, 1993) or, in cases with severe combined respiratory and metabolic acidosis, the administration of tromethamine rapidly improves arterial pH. However, the efficacy and potential short- and long-term adverse effects of such supportive treatment measures have not been studied in the neonatal patient population, and there is indeed very little evidence that bicarbonate administration in metabolic acidosis caused by tissue hypoperfusion is beneficial (Aschner and Poland, 2008). Finally, although positive pressure ventilation may raise pleural pressure and has the potential to reduce venous return, it may also reduce left ventricular afterload by reducing transmural pressure and decreasing or eliminating the work of breathing. Decreasing or eliminating the work of breathing will also decrease or eliminate the concomitant cardiac output diverted to respiratory muscles. Therefore, the net hemodynamic effect of positive pressure ventilation is improved systemic oxygen delivery independent of any potential improvement in pulmonary gas exchange.

In summary, sustained stabilization of the cardiovascular status with provision of appropriate blood pressure, cardiac output, and tissue perfusion and oxygenation remains a difficult task in most of the critically ill hypotensive newborns. Treatment of these patients requires the ability to preferably continuously monitor the most important measures of cardiovascular function (blood pressure, systemic blood flow, and tissue oxygenation); a thorough

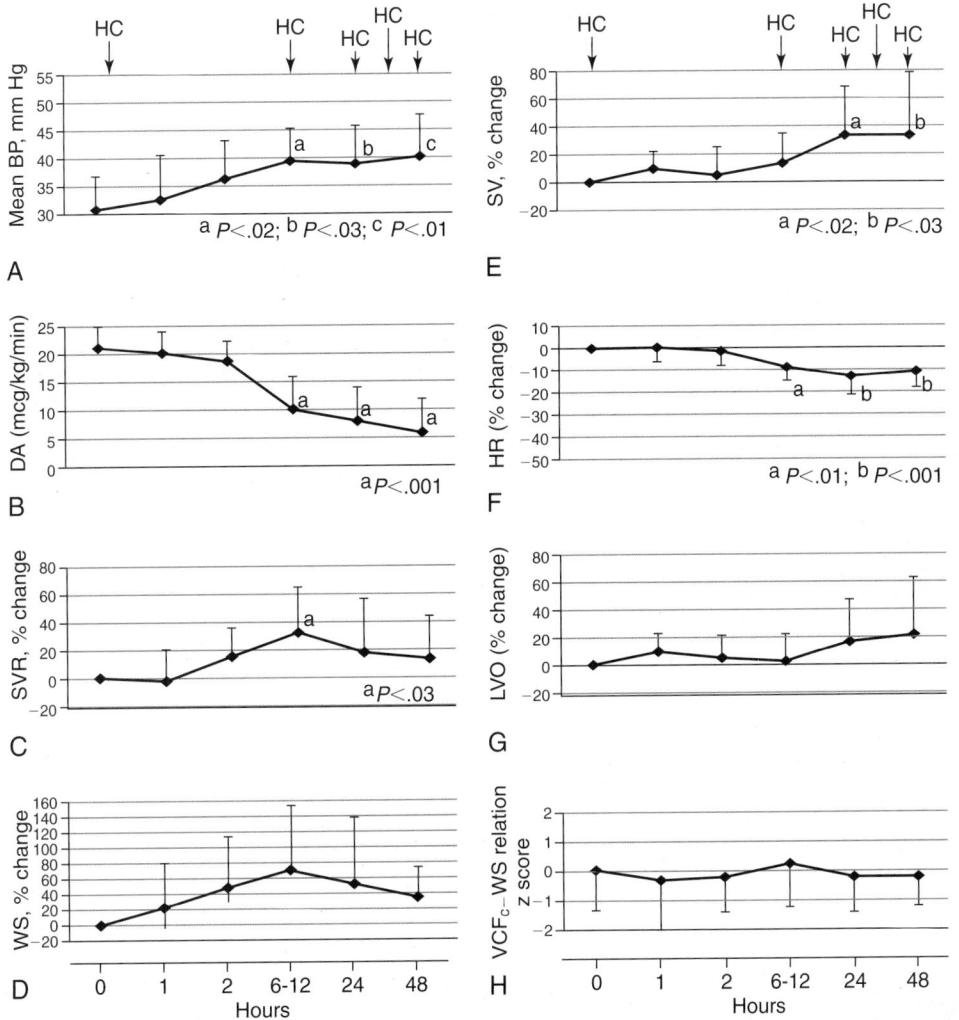

FIGURE 51-6 **Effect of hydrocortisone on mean blood pressure and the dose of dopamine during the first 24 hours of hydrocortisone treatment in 23 preterm neonates with vasopressor-resistant shock.** Changes in preterm neonates (n=15) in mean BP (**A,** [a]P < .02, [b]P < .03, [c]P < .01) and dopamine dosage (DA) (**B,** [a]P < .001) and percentage changes relative to baseline (0 hour) in SVR (**C,** [a]P < .03), WS (**D**), stroke volume (SV) (**E,** [a]P < .02, [b]P < .03), heart rate (HR) (**F,** [a]P < .01, [b]P < .001), and left ventricular output (LVO) (**G**) are shown at 1, 2, 6 to 12, 24, and 48 hours after the first dose of hydrocortisone. In addition, **H** depicts the changes in load-independent contractility as assessed by the VCFc-WS relation. *HC* with arrows indicate approximate timing of hydrocortisone doses. Significant P values for pairwise comparisons versus the baseline (0 hour) with adjustment for multiple comparisons (Bonferroni) are shown. See text for details. (*From Noori S, Friedlich P, Wong P, et al: Hemodynamic changes following low-dose hydrocortisone administration in vasopressor-treated neonates, Pediatrics 118:1456-1466, 2006b.*)

understanding of the pathogenesis and pathophysiology of neonatal shock; and the mechanisms of action, pharmacodynamics, and potential side effects of sympathomimetic amines and other medications used in the management of neonatal shock.

SUGGESTED READINGS

Brierley J, Carcillo JA, Choong K, et al: Clinical practice parameters for hemodynamic support of pediatric and neonatal septic shock: 2007 update from the American College of Critical Care Medicine, *Crit Care Med* 37:666-688, 2009.

Di Sessa TG, Leitner M, Ti CC, et al: The cardiovascular effects of dopamine in the severely asphyxiated neonate, *J Pediatr* 99:772-776, 1981.

Efird MM, Heerens AT, Gordon PV, et al: A randomized-controlled trial of prophylactic hydrocortisone supplementation for the prevention of hypotension in extremely low birth weight infants, *J Perinatol* 25:119-124, 2005.

Engle WD: Definition of normal blood pressure range: the elusive target. In Kleinman CS, Seri I, editors: *Hemodynamics and cardiology: neonatal questions and controversies*, Philadelphia, 2008, Saunders, pp 39-65.

Garland JS, Alex CP, Pauly TH, et al: A three-day course of dexamethasone therapy to prevent chronic lung disease in ventilated neonates: a randomized trial, *Pediatrics* 104:91-99, 1999.

Khwaja O, Volpe JJ: Pathogenesis of cerebral white matter injury of prematurity, *Arch Dis Child Fetal Neonatal Ed* 93:F153-F161, 2008.

Kluckow M, Evans N: Hypoperfusion, hyperkalaemia and serum lactate levels in the preterm infant, *Pediatr Res* 43:179A, 1998.

Kluckow M, Seri I, Evans N: Functional echocardiography: an emerging clinical tool for the neonatologist, *J Pediatr* 150:125-130, 2007.

Noori S, Friedlich P, Seri I, Wong P: Cardiac function following PDA ligation in the ELBW neonate, *J Pediatr* 150:597-602, 2007.

Noori S, Stavroudis TA, Seri I: Systemic and cerebral hemodynamics during the transitional period after premature birth, *Clin Perinatol* 36:726-736.

Paradisis M, Evans N, Kluckow M, et al: Pilot study of milrinone for low systemic blood flow in very preterm infants, *J Pediatr* 148:306-313, 2006.

Complete references used in this text can be found online at www.expertconsult.com

PERSISTENT PULMONARY HYPERTENSION

Robin H. Steinhorn and Steven H. Abman

Neonatal respiratory failure affects 2% of all live births and is responsible for more than one third of all neonatal deaths (Angus et al, 2001). Persistent pulmonary hypertension of the newborn (PPHN) is a frequent complication of respiratory disease in neonates and is defined as the failure to achieve or sustain the normal decrease in pulmonary vascular resistance at birth. PPHN complicates the course of approximately 10% of infants with respiratory failure and can lead to severe respiratory distress and hypoxemia associated with considerable mortality and morbidity (Kinsella and Abman, 1995; Walsh-Sukys et al, 2000). Newborns with PPHN are at risk for severe asphyxia and its complications, including death, chronic lung disease, neurodevelopmental sequelae, and other problems. This chapter reviews the pathophysiology of PPHN and clinical strategies that utilize a physiologic approach to the treatment of newborns with severe PPHN.

NORMAL FETAL PULMONARY VASCULAR DEVELOPMENT AND TRANSITION

Pulmonary hypertension is necessary to support gas exchange during fetal life. Because the placenta, not the lung, serves as the organ of gas exchange, most of the right ventricular output must cross the ductus arteriosus to the aorta, and only 5% to 10% of the combined ventricular output is directed to the pulmonary vascular bed. Even though the surface area of the pulmonary vasculature increases as the fetal lung grows, pulmonary vascular resistance increases with gestational age when corrected for lung or body weight, suggesting that active pulmonary vascular constriction is prominent during late gestation. Multiple pathways appear to be involved in maintaining high pulmonary vascular tone before birth. Pulmonary vasoconstrictors in the normal fetus include low oxygen tension, endothelin-1, leukotrienes, and Rho kinase. Vasoconstriction is also promoted by low basal production of vasodilators such as prostacyclin and nitric oxide (NO).

At birth, a rapid and dramatic decrease in pulmonary vascular resistance redirects half of the combined ventricular output to the lung, leading to an 8- to 10-fold increase in pulmonary blood flow. Increased pulmonary blood flow increases pulmonary venous return and left atrial pressure, promoting functional closure of the one-way valve of the foramen ovale. Systemic vascular resistance increases at birth, at least in part because of removal of the low-resistance vascular bed of the placenta. The largest drop in pulmonary vascular resistance occurs shortly after birth, although resistance continues to drop over the first several months of life until it reaches the low levels normally found in the adult circulation. As pulmonary vascular resistance falls below systemic levels, blood flow through the patent ductus

arteriosus (PDA) reverses. In the first several hours of life, the ductus arteriosus functionally closes, largely in response to the increased oxygen tension of the newborn. This effectively separates the pulmonary and systemic circulations and establishes the normal postnatal circulatory pattern.

The most critical signals for these transitional changes in the pulmonary vasculature are mechanical distention of the lung, a decrease in carbon dioxide tension, and an increase in oxygen tension in the lungs. The fetus prepares for this transition late in gestation by increasing pulmonary vascular expression of nitric oxide synthases and soluble guanylate cyclase (Figure 52-1). The importance of the NO–cyclic guanosine monophosphate (cGMP) pathway in facilitating normal transition has been demonstrated by acute or chronic inhibition of nitric oxide synthase (NOS) in fetal lambs, which produces pulmonary hypertension after delivery (Abman et al, 1990; Fineman et al, 1994). The prostacyclin pathway is another important vasodilatory pathway (see Figure 52-1). Cyclooxygenase is the rate-limiting enzyme that generates prostacyclin from arachidonic acid. Although both cyclooxygenase-1 and cyclooxygenase-2 are found in the lung, cyclooxygenase-1 in particular is upregulated during late gestation (Brannon et al, 1998). This upregulation leads to increased prostacyclin production in late gestation and early postnatal life (Brannon et al, 1994; Leffler et al, 1984). In turn, prostacyclin stimulates adenylate cyclase to increase intracellular cyclic adenosine monophosphate (cAMP) levels, which, as with cGMP, lead to vasorelaxation through a decrease in intracellular calcium concentrations.

PATHOPHYSIOLOGY OF PPHN

When the normal cardiopulmonary transition fails to occur, the result is PPHN. The first reports of PPHN described term newborns with profound hypoxemia who lacked radiographic evidence of parenchymal lung disease and echocardiographic evidence of structural cardiac disease (Gersony et al, 1969; Levin et al, 1976). In these patients, hypoxemia was caused by marked elevations of pulmonary vascular resistance leading to right-to-left extrapulmonary shunting of blood across the PDA or patent foramen ovale (PFO) during the early postnatal period. Because of the persistence of high PVR and blood flow through these "fetal shunts," the term *persistent fetal circulation* was originally used to describe these findings.

Subsequently, it was recognized that these physiologic patterns may complicate the clinical course of neonates with diverse causes of hypoxemic respiratory failure. As a result, the term *PPHN* is now commonly used to describe a syndrome characterized by common pathophysiologic features including sustained elevation of pulmonary vascular

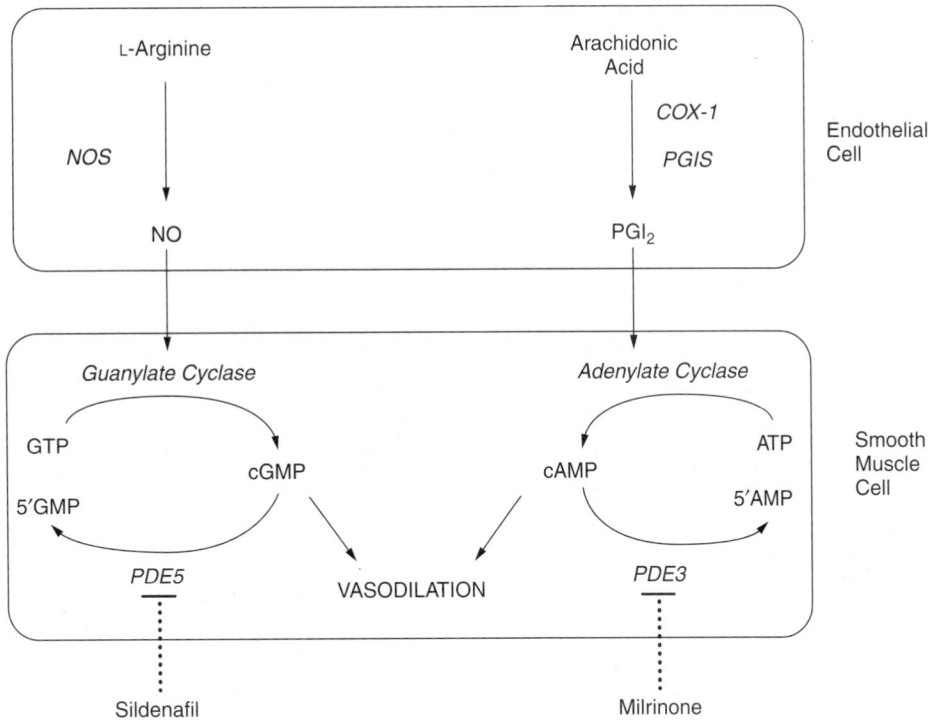

FIGURE 52-1 Nitric oxide *(NO)* and prostacyclin (i.e., prostaglandin I₂ *[PGI₂]*) signaling pathways that regulate pulmonary vascular tone in the developing lung.

resistance and hypoxemia due to right-to-left extrapulmonary shunting of blood flow across the ductus arteriosus or foramen ovale. These physiologic findings may be associated with a wide range of cardiopulmonary disorders such as meconium aspiration, sepsis, pneumonia, asphyxia, congenital diaphragmatic hernia, respiratory distress syndrome (RDS), and others. However, although hypoxemic respiratory failure in term newborns is often presumed to be associated with PPHN-type physiology, many hypoxemic term newborns will lack evidence for extrapulmonary shunting across the PDA or PFO. Thus, the term *PPHN* should generally be reserved to describe neonates in whom extrapulmonary shunting contributes to hypoxemia and impaired cardiopulmonary function. Recent estimates suggest an incidence for PPHN of 1.9/1000 live births, or an estimated 7400 cases/year in the United States (Walsh-Sukys et al, 2000).

PPHN is often characterized as one of three types: (1) maladaptation: the structurally normal but abnormally constricted pulmonary vasculature due to lung parenchymal diseases such as meconium aspiration syndrome, respiratory distress syndrome, or pneumonia; (2) excessive muscularization: the lung with normal parenchyma but remodeled pulmonary vasculature characterized by increased smooth muscle cell thickness and distal extension of muscle to vessels that are usually nonmuscular (Figure 52-2); or (3) the hypoplastic vasculature, associated with underdevelopment of the pulmonary vasculature, as seen in congenital diaphragmatic hernia. This designation is imprecise, however, and high PVR in most patients likely involves overlapping changes among these categories. For example, neonates with meconium aspiration often have clinical evidence of altered vasoreactivity, but excessive muscularization is often found at autopsy. Neonates with

congenital diaphragmatic hernia are primarily classified as having vascular hypoplasia, yet lung histology of fatal cases typically shows marked muscularization of pulmonary arteries, and clinically, these patients can respond to vasodilator therapy.

Autopsy studies of fatal PPHN demonstrate severe hypertensive structural remodeling even in newborns who die shortly after birth (Figure 52-3), suggesting that many cases of severe disease are associated with chronic intrauterine stress (Geggel and Reid, 1984). However, the exact intrauterine events that alter pulmonary vascular reactivity and structure remain poorly understood. Epidemiologic studies have demonstrated strong associations between PPHN and maternal smoking and ingestion of cold remedies that include aspirin or other nonsteroidal antiinflammatory products (Alano et al, 2001; Van Marter et al, 1996). Exposure to nonsteroidal antiinflammatory drugs (NSAIDs) during the third trimester can cause constriction of the fetal ductus arteriosus in utero, a finding that has been associated with idiopathic PPHN (Alano et al, 2001; Levin et al, 1979). In experimental models, surgical ductal constriction or ligation performed in fetal lambs produces very rapid antenatal remodeling of the pulmonary vasculature. The physiologic and anatomic findings in these lambs after birth are similar to those observed in human infants, including increased fetal pulmonary artery pressure, pulmonary vascular remodeling, and profound hypoxemia after birth (Wild et al, 1989).

New data suggest that exposure to selective serotonin reuptake inhibitors (SSRIs) during late gestation may increase the likelihood of PPHN (Chambers et al, 2006), although it is not clear how many infants will develop severe disease. In support of this association, newborn rats exposed in utero to fluoxetine develop pulmonary

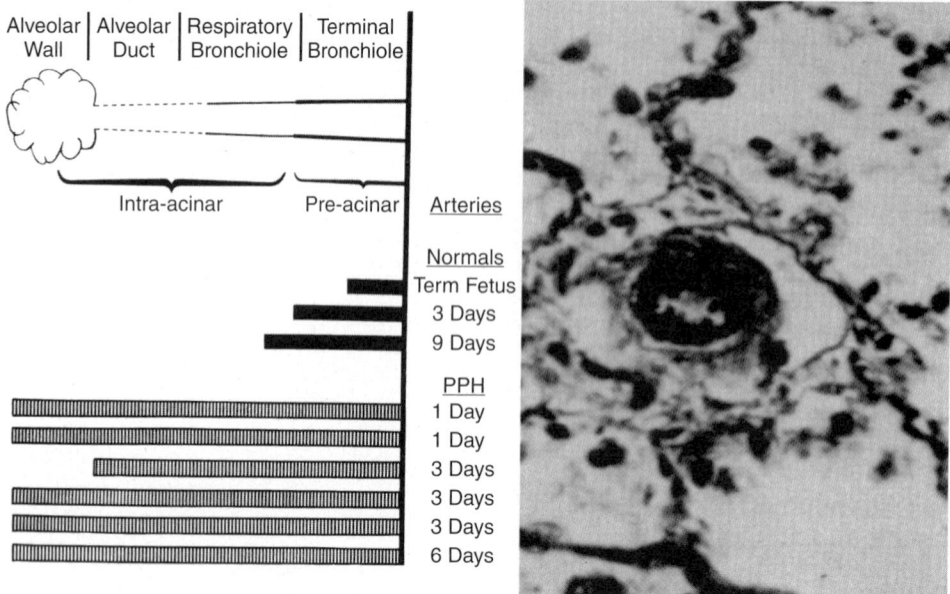

FIGURE 52-2 Vascular maldevelopment of PPHN, showing smooth muscle hyperplasia and extension of smooth muscle to the level of the intraacinar arteries, which does not normally occur until much later in the postnatal period. (*From Murphy JD, Rabinovitch M, Goldstein JD, et al: The structural basis of persistent pulmonary hypertension of the newborn infant*, J Pediatr 98:962-967, 1981.)

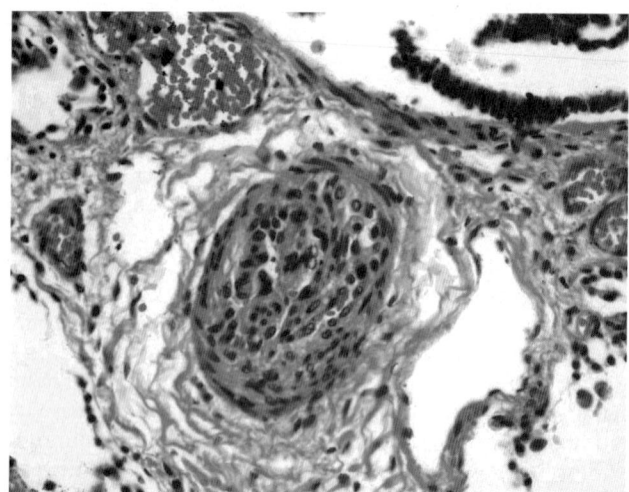

FIGURE 52-3 *(See also Color Plate 21.)* Histology of a pulmonary vessel from an infant with fatal PPHN illustrating the dramatic remodeling that can be associated with severe PPHN.

vascular remodeling, abnormal oxygenation, and higher mortality when compared with vehicle-treated controls (Fornaro et al, 2007). Because SSRIs have been reported to reduce pulmonary vascular remodeling in adult models of pulmonary hypertension, these findings may also serve to highlight the unique nature of fetal pulmonary vascular development.

It is not yet clear whether genetic factors increase susceptibility for neonatal pulmonary hypertension. Studies of adults with idiopathic and familial primary pulmonary hypertension have identified germline mutations in the bone morphogenetic protein receptor type 2 gene (BMPR2), a member of the transforming growth factor-β signaling family. However, whether polymorphisms of genes for the BMP or other transforming growth factor-β receptors, other critical growth factors, vasoactive

substances, or other products increase the risk for the neonatal PPHN syndrome is unknown.

Based on work from animal models, there is strong evidence that disruptions of the NO-cGMP, prostacyclin-cAMP, and endothelin signaling pathways play an important role in the vascular abnormalities associated with PPHN. The NO-cGMP pathway has been a topic of particularly intense investigation in the past two decades. Decreased expression and activity of endothelial nitric oxide synthase (eNOS) have been documented in the PPHN lamb model (Shaul et al, 1997; Villamor et al, 1997), and decreased eNOS expression has also been reported in umbilical venous endothelial cell cultures from human infants with meconium staining who develop PPHN (Villaneuva et al, 1998). These important findings were rapidly followed by clinical testing of inhaled nitric oxide (iNO) as a therapy for hypoxemic respiratory failure and PPHN, as described later.

Although prostacyclin appears to be important in the normal pulmonary vascular transition, less is known of the role of abnormal prostacyclin-cAMP signaling in PPHN. Some data suggest that abnormalities in prostacyclin synthesis and downstream adenylate cyclase responses exist, analogous to the abnormalities reported for NO-cGMP signaling (Lakshminrusimha et al, 2009a; Shaul et al, 1991). In addition, production of the vasoconstrictor arachidonic acid metabolite, thromboxane, plays a role in pulmonary hypertension produced by chronic hypoxia (Fike et al, 2005). Circulating levels of the potent vasoconstrictor endothelin (ET-1) are elevated in lambs and newborn infants with PPHN (Kumar et al, 1996; Rosenberg et al, 1993). Endothelin effects are mediated through two receptors: ET-A receptors on smooth muscle cells that mediate vasoconstriction, and ET-B receptors on endothelial cells that mediate vasodilation. There is evidence that in pulmonary hypertension, the balance of ET receptors is shifted to the vasoconstrictor (ET-A) pathways (Ivy et al,

1998). In addition, endothelin may affect vascular tone by increasing production of reactive oxygen species such as superoxide and hydrogen peroxide, which also act as vasoconstrictors (Wedgwood et al, 2001).

OTHER CAUSES OF NEONATAL PULMONARY HYPERTENSION

Neonatal pulmonary hypertension differs from pediatric and adult pulmonary hypertension in that it resolves in the majority of patients and has not been associated with genetic factors. A notable exception is alveolar capillary dysplasia with misalignment of lung vessels (ACD/MPV), a rare but universally lethal cause of pulmonary hypertension in the newborn (Boggs et al, 1994; Sen et al, 2004). Affected infants typically present shortly after birth with cyanosis and respiratory distress refractory to all known therapies including extracorporeal support, although later presentations (at several weeks or months of life) are increasingly recognized. Currently, the diagnosis can only be made by direct examination of lung tissue. Characteristic findings include simplification of lung architecture, widened and poorly developed cellular septa with a paucity of capillaries, and strikingly muscularized small arterioles accompanied by pulmonary veins within the same connective tissue sheath. Approximately 10% of alveolar capillary dysplasia cases have been reported to have a familial association, indicating a potential genetic component. Although the search for a candidate gene has proven difficult, a recent report showed an association with haploinsufficiency for the forkhead (FOX) transcription factor gene cluster and ACD/MPV associated with additional congenital heart defects and/or gastrointestinal anomalies (Stankiewicz et al, 2009).

Recently, mutations in the gene encoding the transporter ABCA3 have been reported as a cause of severe neonatal lung disease. Infants with ABCA3 mutations lack typical lamellar bodies, indicating that ABCA3 is critical for surfactant function at birth (Wert et al, 2009). Although ABCA3 deficiency is typically associated with parenchymal lung disease, a recent report of an infant with severe pulmonary hypertension due to ABCA3 deficiency described a presentation with relatively clear lung fields on chest radiographs (Kunig et al, 2007). Infants with prolonged, severe pulmonary hypertension out of proportion to the degree of lung disease may therefore benefit from a lung biopsy and/or targeted genetic evaluations to determine the etiology of their respiratory failure.

In preterm infants, there is increasing recognition that chronic lung disease may be associated with significant pulmonary hypertension. In the United States alone, it is estimated that up to 10,000 babies develop bronchopulmonary dysplasia (BPD) each year, a disease characterized by developmental abnormalities of lung structure, including impaired alveolarization and vascularization. Although the incidence of pulmonary hypertension associated with BPD is not known, it is clear that altered pulmonary vascular growth and significant pulmonary hypertension frequently complicate the course of BPD (Kinsella et al, 2006; Mourani et al, 2009). Moreover, severe or prolonged pulmonary hypertension increases the risk of late morbidity and death (Khemani et al, 2007). The pathogenesis of pulmonary hypertension associated with BPD is complex:

antenatal factors such as growth restriction, oligohydramnios, or fetal inflammation appear to play a role, and postnatal injury due to ventilator-induced lung injury and/or oxidant stress is also important. Similar to the reduction in alveolarization associated with BPD, work in animal models indicates that impaired angiogenesis is a component of abnormal lung development, which leads to decreased vascular growth and abnormal vascular structure. Identifying pulmonary hypertension in infants with BPD requires a high index of suspicion and careful longitudinal evaluation. Echocardiography is currently the most practical screening tool and should be considered in infants who continue to require oxygen supplementation at 36 weeks' corrected gestational age. In infants with evidence for significant pulmonary hypertension by echocardiogram, cardiac catheterization will allow for more accurate quantification of the severity of disease, as well as allow for vasoreactivity testing (Mourani et al, 2008).

CLINICAL EVALUATION OF INFANTS WITH PPHN

Clinically, PPHN is most often recognized in the term or near-term neonate, but may infrequently occur in premature neonates as well. PPHN typically manifests as respiratory distress and cyanosis within hours of birth and may be associated with a variety of lung and/or cardiac disorders (Box 52-1). Although PPHN is often associated with signs of perinatal distress, such as asphyxia, low Apgar scores, or meconium staining, idiopathic PPHN can present without signs of acute perinatal distress.

PPHN is characterized by hypoxemia that is poorly responsive to supplemental oxygen. An important goal for the initial clinical evaluation is to determine whether a hypoxemic infant has PPHN-type physiology (Abman and Kinsella, 1995). Because a PFO and PDA are normally present early in life, elevated pulmonary vascular resistance in the newborn will produce extrapulmonary shunting of blood through these fetal channels, leading to severe and potentially unresponsive hypoxemia. In the presence of right-to-left shunting across the patent ductus arteriosus, "differential cyanosis" is often present, which is difficult to observe by physical exam but may be detected by a gradient in the PaO_2 and/or oxygen saturation between the right radial artery and descending aorta sites. Because the left subclavian artery may have either a preductal or postductal origin from the aorta, it is best to apply the oximeter probe to one of the feet for postductal pulse oximetry monitoring. It is also important to remember that a similar pattern of postductal desaturation may be observed in ductus-dependent cardiac diseases, including hypoplastic left heart syndrome, coarctation of the aorta, and interrupted aortic arch.

In many infants, intrapulmonary shunt or ventilation-perfusion mismatch resulting from parenchymal lung disease is the predominant abnormality, rather than shunting of blood flow across the PDA and PFO. In this setting, hypoxemia is related to the amount of pulmonary arterial blood perfusing the nonaerated lung regions. Although PVR is often elevated in hypoxemic newborns without PPHN, high PVR does not contribute significantly to hypoxemia in these cases. Rapid improvement in response to supplemental oxygen suggests ventilation/perfusion

BOX 52-1   Disorders Associated With Neonatal Pulmonary Hypertension

PULMONARY

Meconium aspiration syndrome
Respiratory distress syndrome (term and preterm newborns)
Lung hypoplasia—primary
Congenital diaphragmatic hernia
Pneumonia/sepsis
Idiopathic
Transient tachypnea of the newborn
Alveolar-capillary dysplasia
Associated abnormalities in lung development:
- Congenital lobar emphysema (rare association)
- Cystic adenomatoid malformation (rare association)
- Idiopathic, with impaired distal alveolarization
- Others

CARDIOVASCULAR

Myocardial dysfunction (asphyxia; infection; stress)
Structural cardiac diseases:
- Mitral stenosis, cor triatriatum
- Endocardial fibroelastosis
- Pompe's disease
- Aortic atresia, coarctation of the aorta, interrupted aortic arch
- Transposition of the great vessels
- Ebstein's anomaly, tricuspid atresia
Hepatic arteriovenous malformations (AVMs)
Cerebral AVMs
Total anomalous pulmonary venous return
Pulmonary vein stenosis (isolated)
Pulmonary atresia

ASSOCIATIONS WITH OTHER DISEASES

Neuromuscular disease
Metabolic disease
Polycythemia
Thrombocytopenia
Maternal drug use or smoking

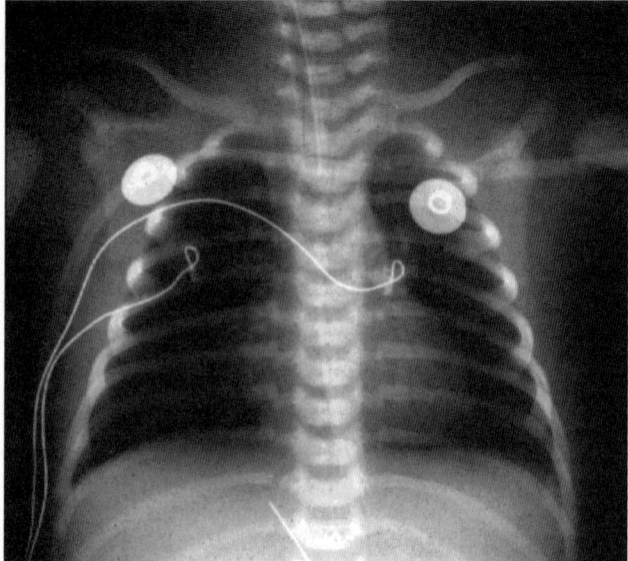

FIGURE 52-4 Typical chest radiograph of an infant with persistent pulmonary hypertension, showing mild hyperexpansion and oligemic lung fields.

mismatch due to primary lung disease, although this may not be obvious with severe parenchymal lung disease. Further, most infants with PPHN have at least a transient improvement in oxygenation in response to interventions such as high inspired oxygen and/or mechanical ventilation. Therefore, these clinical findings can only suggest, and not confirm, the diagnosis.

Radiographic findings are variable, depending on the primary disease associated with PPHN. Classically, the chest x-ray in idiopathic PPHN is oligemic, normally or slightly hyperinflated, and lacks parenchymal infiltrates (Figure 52-4). In general, the degree of hypoxemia is disproportionate to the severity of radiographic lung disease. Laboratory findings may include hypoglycemia, hypocalcemia, polycythemia, or thrombocytopenia.

The echocardiogram plays an essential diagnostic role and is an important tool for managing newborns with PPHN. The initial echocardiographic evaluation rules out structural heart disease causing hypoxemia or ductal shunting (e.g., coarctation of the aorta or total anomalous pulmonary venous return), determines the predominant direction of shunting at the PFO and PDA, and assesses ventricular function. As stated earlier, not all term newborns with hypoxemia have true PPHN physiology. Although

elevated pulmonary artery pressure is commonly found in association with neonatal lung disease, the diagnosis of PPHN is not certain without evidence of bidirectional or predominantly right-to-left shunting across the foramen ovale or ductus arteriosus. Echocardiographic signs such as increased right ventricular systolic time intervals and septal flattening are suggestive, but less definitive in making a diagnosis. In addition to demonstrating the presence of PPHN physiology, the echocardiogram is critical for the evaluation of left ventricular function. Although right-to-left shunting at the ductus arteriosus and foramen ovale is typical for PPHN, in some infants predominant right-to-left shunting at the ductus associated with left-to-right shunt at the foramen ovale may reveal that left ventricular dysfunction is contributing significantly to the underlying pathophysiology. High pulmonary venous pressure due to left ventricular dysfunction will elevate pulmonary arterial pressure, causing right-to-left shunting with little vasoconstriction. When severe left ventricular dysfunction accompanies pulmonary hypertension, pulmonary vasodilation alone may be ineffective in improving oxygenation and must be accompanied by targeted therapies to increase cardiac performance and decrease left ventricular afterload. Thus, careful echocardiographic assessment provides invaluable information about the underlying pathophysiology and will help guide the course of treatment.

At present, there is no single biochemical marker that has emerged with sufficient sensitivity and specificity for the diagnosis and management of PPHN. However, brain-type natriuretic peptide (BNP), an endogenous peptide hormone secreted by the cardiac ventricles in response to increased wall stress, may have some utility. A recent report suggests that high BNP levels (particularly those >850 pg/mL) may help differentiate infants with PPHN physiology from those with pulmonary causes of respiratory failure (Reynolds et al, 2004). Because BNP levels are widely used for rapid assessment of cardiac failure in adults, they can be easily and rapidly measured in most hospitals. However, the correlation between BNP levels and hypoxemia was weak, indicating that this test should not be used alone to gauge the severity of PPHN, but rather in combination with other clinical and echocardiographic data.

GENERAL MANAGEMENT FOR PPHN

General management principles for the newborn with PPHN include maintenance of normal temperature, electrolytes (particularly calcium), glucose, hemoglobin, and intravascular volume. Mechanical ventilation is almost always required to improve oxygenation, to achieve normal lung volumes, and to avoid the adverse effects of high or low lung volumes on pulmonary vascular resistance. The goal of mechanical ventilation should be to optimize lung volumes, and care should be taken to avoid settings that may induce ventilator-induced lung injury, which can lead to inflammatory changes, pulmonary edema, and decreased lung compliance. Some newborns with parenchymal lung disease associated with PPHN physiology demonstrate marked improvements in oxygenation as well as decreased right-to-left extrapulmonary shunting after lung recruitment during high-frequency ventilation (Kinsella and Abman, 2000).

The use of surfactant therapy to recruit the lung remains variable between centers (Fliman et al, 2006). Single-center trials have shown that surfactant improves oxygenation, reduces airleak, and reduces need for ECMO in infants with meconium aspiration (Findlay et al, 1996). A multicenter trial showed benefit in infants with parenchymal lung diseases such as meconium aspiration syndrome and sepsis, and also demonstrated that the benefit was greatest for infants with relatively mild disease (Lotze et al, 1998). However, this trial also failed to show a reduction in ECMO utilization in the subset of newborns with idiopathic PPHN. Therefore, the use of surfactant should only be considered for infants with parenchymal lung disease.

Acidosis can act as a pulmonary vasoconstrictor and should be avoided. However, variability exists between centers regarding the use of hyperventilation to achieve alkalosis in order to improve oxygenation. The use of alkalosis was frequent before the approval of inhaled nitric oxide (iNO) based on studies that found transient improvements in PaO_2 after acute hyperventilation (Drummond et al, 1981). However, no studies have demonstrated long-term or safety benefit. The pulmonary vascular response to alkalosis is transient, and prolonged alkalosis may paradoxically worsen pulmonary vascular tone, reactivity, and permeability edema (Laffey et al, 2000). Further, alkalosis produces cerebral constriction, reduces cerebral blood flow and oxygen delivery to the brain, and may be associated with worse neurodevelopmental outcomes (Ferrara et al, 1984). Similarly, there is currently no evidence to suggest that the use of sodium bicarbonate infusions to induce alkalosis provides any short-term or long-term benefit (Walsh-Sukys et al, 2000).

Systemic hemodynamics should be optimized with volume and cardiotonic therapy (dobutamine, dopamine, and milrinone), to enhance cardiac output and systemic O_2 transport. Systemic hypotension may worsen right-to-left shunting, impair oxygen delivery, and worsen gas exchange in patients with parenchymal lung disease.

However, the goal is more complex than simply increasing blood pressure, and careful attention should also be paid to right and left ventricular function. For instance, the level of systemic arterial pressure is the major component of afterload for the left ventricle, and marked increases in systemic pressure have the potential to worsen left ventricular dysfunction. Some clinicians advocate increasing systemic blood pressure to prevent right-to-left shunting across the ductus arteriosus. Although this strategy may improve oxygenation, if it is not accompanied by a reduction in pulmonary vascular resistance, the right ventricle will also be presented with substantial increases in afterload. Because the right ventricle of the fetus and young neonate exhibits a high degree of sensitivity to afterload (Reller et al, 1987), this approach should be used with caution and accompanied by careful longitudinal assessment of biventricular function.

Infants who fail to respond to medical management, as evidenced by failure to sustain improvement in oxygenation with good hemodynamic function, may require treatment with extracorporeal membrane oxygenation or ECMO (UK Collaborative ECMO Trial Group, 1996). The oxygenation index (OI; calculated as [mean airway pressure × FiO_2 × 100]/PaO_2) is often used to gauge the severity of disease, with OI >40 used as an indication for evaluation for ECMO. ECMO remains an effective and potentially life-saving rescue modality for severe PPHN, although it is also costly, labor intensive, and associated with potential adverse effects, such as intracranial hemorrhage and ligation of the right common carotid artery.

Even with all available therapies, the mortality rate for PPHN remains between 5% and 10%. In addition, approximately 25% of infants with moderate or severe PPHN will exhibit significant neurodevelopmental impairment at 12–24 months (Clark et al, 2003; Konduri et al, 2007; Neonatal Inhaled Nitric Oxide Study Group, 2000). This important observation may indicate that the underlying disease, antenatal factors, and/or early therapeutic approaches are associated with early neurological injury.

INHALED NITRIC OXIDE FOR PPHN

The primary goal of PPHN therapy is selective pulmonary vasodilation. iNO therapy (5 to 20 ppm) improves oxygenation and decreases the need for ECMO therapy in patients with diverse causes of PPHN (Clark et al, 2000; Davidson et al, 1998; Kinsella et al, 1997; Neonatal Inhaled Nitric Oxide Study Group, 1997; Roberts et al, 1997). Inhaled NO is well suited for the treatment of PPHN: it is a rapid and potent vasodilator, and because nitric oxide is a small gas molecule, it can be delivered as inhalation therapy to airspaces approximating the pulmonary vascular bed. In contrast, intravenous dilators such as prostacyclin, tolazoline, and sodium nitroprusside may produce nonselective effects on the systemic circulation, leading to hypotension as well as increased right-to-left shunting and impaired oxygenation. Large placebo-controlled trials enrolled infants with an oxygenation index of >25 and provided clear evidence that iNO significantly decreases the need for extracorporeal life support in newborns with diverse causes of hypoxemic respiratory failure and PPHN,

TABLE 52-1   Summary of the Large, Multicenter Randomized Trials of Inhaled NO in Term Newborns With Hypoxemic Respiratory Failure and/or PPHN, Showing the Effect of iNO on ECMO Utilization and Mortality

	n	OI	% ECMO		% Mortality	
			Control	iNO	Control	iNO
NINOS	235	44	55	39*	17	14
Roberts	58	44.4	71	40*	7	7
Clark	248	39	65	48*	8	7
Davidson	155	24.7	34	22	2	8
Konduri	299	19.2	12	10	9	7

Table adapted from Konduri (2004); data from Clark et al, 2000, Davidson et al, 1998, Konduri et al, 2004, Neonatal Inhaled Nitric Oxide Study Group, 1997 and Roberts et al, 1997.
*Indicates significantly different than control group

as shown in Table 52-1 (Clark et al, 2000; Neonatal Inhaled Nitric Oxide Study Group, 1997). These studies also showed that doses of 5 to 20 ppm were effective, and that increasing the dose beyond 20 ppm in nonresponders did not improve outcomes (Neonatal Inhaled Nitric Oxide Study Group, 1997). Further, sustained treatment with 80 ppm NO increased the risk of methemoglobinemia (Davidson et al, 1998). Weaning can generally be accomplished in 4 to 5 days, and prolonged need for inhaled NO therapy without resolution of disease should lead to a more extensive evaluation to determine whether other underlying anatomic lung or cardiovascular disease is present, such as pulmonary venous stenosis, alveolar capillary dysplasia, or severe lung hypoplasia (Goldman et al, 1996).

Although well-controlled trials led to the U.S. Food and Drug Administration (FDA) approval of iNO for therapy of PPHN, it is important to note that iNO did not reduce the mortality, length of hospitalization, or risk of neurodevelopmental impairment associated with PPHN (see Table 52-1) (Clark et al, 2003; Neonatal Inhaled Nitric Oxide Study Group, 2000). Moreover, beginning iNO at a milder or earlier point in the disease course (for an oxygenation index of 15 to 25) did not decrease the incidence of ECMO and/or death, or improve other patient outcomes, including the incidence of neurodevelopmental impairment (Konduri et al, 2004, 2007). Finally, although preterm infants (<34 weeks' gestation) may exhibit pulmonary hypertension as a component of their respiratory failure, there is less evidence to indicate whether iNO benefits this population.

These clinical trials have also revealed that as many as 40% of infants will not respond or sustain a response to iNO. The reasons for an inadequate response are diverse and require the clinician to carefully analyze the relative roles of parenchymal lung disease, pulmonary vascular disease, and cardiac dysfunction for each infant. For instance, if severe airspace disease is associated with PPHN, strategies such as high-frequency ventilation that optimize lung expansion are likely to be effective, and the two therapies used together are more effective than either used individually (Kinsella et al, 1997). Cardiac function should also be carefully assessed longitudinally. In particular, infants with severe left ventricular dysfunction are likely

to have pulmonary venous hypertension and are unlikely to respond to pulmonary vasodilation unless there is also optimization of cardiac performance.

Because iNO is usually delivered with high concentrations of oxygen, these therapies could interact and lead to enhanced production of reactive oxygen and reactive nitrogen metabolites, both of which may contribute to vasoconstriction and/or inadequate responses to iNO. Although hyperoxic ventilation is used to promote pulmonary vasodilation in PPHN, we know surprisingly little about what oxygen concentrations will maximize benefits and minimize risk, and there is little to indicate that increasing oxygen concentrations beyond 50% to 60% further enhances pulmonary vasodilation in the normal or remodeled pulmonary circulation (Lakshminrusimha et al, 2007, 2009b; Rudolph and Yuan, 1966). Furthermore, studies in newborn lambs with pharmacologic or anatomic pulmonary hypertension indicate that even brief (30-minute) exposures to 100% O_2 blunt subsequent responsiveness to NO (Farrow et al, 2008a; Lakshminrusimha et al, 2006a, 2007, 2009b). High concentrations of oxygen may be toxic to the developing lung through formation of reactive oxygen species, such as superoxide anions (Lakshminrusimha et al, 2006a). Superoxide may react with arachidonic acid to increase concentrations of isoprostanes and may also combine with NO to form peroxynitrite (Lakshminrusimha et al, 2006b). Both are potent oxidants with the potential to produce vasoconstriction, cytotoxicity, and damage to surfactant proteins and lipids.

NEW INSIGHTS INTO PPHN PATHOPHYSIOLOGY AND TREATMENT

Alterations in downstream signaling mechanisms in pulmonary vascular smooth muscle cells may also lead to inadequate vascular responses to iNO. NO mediates vasodilation by stimulating soluble guanylate cyclase (GC) in vascular smooth muscle cells, which then converts guanosine triphosphate to cGMP (see Figure 52-1). cGMP is the central and critical second messenger that regulates contractility of the smooth muscle cell by modulating the activity of cGMP-dependent kinases, phosphodiesterases, and ion channels. Therefore, there are multiple critical points in the pathway downstream from NO production that serves as attractive targets for manipulating cellular cGMP concentrations. For example, expression and activity of soluble guanylate cyclase are decreased in the abnormally remodeled pulmonary vessels of the PPHN lamb model, which could potentially diminish responses to both endogenous and exogenous NO. This finding would indicate that new compounds that directly stimulate sGC at a NO-independent but heme-dependent site may be helpful, a hypothesis that appears to be promising in pre-clinical testing (Deruelle et al, 2006).

Recent evidence indicates that the low cGMP concentrations associated with PPHN may also be due in part to increased activity of cGMP-specific phosphodiesterases (PDE5). Inhibition of PDE5 activity would thus be expected to increase cGMP concentrations (see Figure 52-1), dilate the pulmonary vasculature, and/or increase the efficacy of iNO. Recently approved by the FDA for the treatment of adult pulmonary hypertension, sildenafil is a potent and highly specific PDE5 inhibitor that has been used in several preclinical studies of animal models of pulmonary hypertension. For example, in lambs with experimental pulmonary hypertension, both enteral and aerosolized sildenafil dilated the pulmonary vasculature and augmented the pulmonary vascular response to iNO (Ichinose et al, 2001; Weimann et al, 2000). Intravenous sildenafil was found to be a selective pulmonary vasodilator with efficacy equivalent to inhaled nitric oxide in a piglet model of meconium aspiration, although hypotension and worsening oxygenation resulted when sildenafil was used in combination with iNO (Shekerdemian et al, 2002, 2004). Data have now begun to emerge on the use of sildenafil in human infants with PPHN. A recent report of a small cohort of human infants with PPHN demonstrated that enteral sildenafil improved oxygenation and survival compared to placebo (Baquero et al, 2006). More recent findings from a multicenter, dose-range study of intravenous sildenafil for infants with severe pulmonary hypertension indicate that the drug was generally well tolerated, with improvements in oxygenation noted in the cohorts that received higher infusion doses (Steinhorn et al, 2009). It is interesting to note that systemic administration of sildenafil improved oxygenation, but had little effect on systemic blood pressure. Seven infants received sildenafil before initiation of iNO and showed similar improvements in oxygenation. Of these, six survived to discharge without need for additional therapy with iNO or ECMO. These data suggest that sildenafil has the potential to independently decrease pulmonary vascular resistance and improve oxygenation in human infants with PPHN.

Similar to cGMP, cAMP also stimulates the cascade that leads to smooth muscle relaxation, and amplification of the cAMP signaling pathway could therefore enhance pulmonary vasodilation. Prostacyclin is a second central vasodilator that is upregulated after birth, primarily in response to ventilation of the lung. Prostacyclin stimulates adenylate cyclase to increase intracellular cAMP levels, which, similar to cGMP, produce vasorelaxation through a decrease in intracellular calcium concentrations. Intravenous PGI_2 is standard therapy for older children with pulmonary hypertension, but the use of systemic infusions of PGI_2 may be limited by systemic hypotension and/or ventilation-perfusion mismatch in neonatal PPHN populations. Inhaled PGI_2 has been shown to have vasodilator effects limited to the pulmonary circulation, and its efficacy has been reported to be similar to that of iNO (Khan et al, 2009). The actions of inhaled PGI_2 and iNO appear to be additive in humans and even synergistic in some studies. Reports of inhaled PGI_2 use in neonates with PPHN are limited, but case reports indicate it may enhance oxygenation in infants who are poorly responsive to iNO (Kelly et al, 2002). New agents are being developed specifically for inhalation (e.g., iloprost), and it will be interesting to learn if they also promote pulmonary vasodilation in neonatal populations (Ivy et al, 2008). Inhibition of phosphodiesterase type 3 (PDE3), which metabolizes cAMP, might also enhance cAMP signaling in PPHN (Chen et al, 2009). Milrinone, a PDE3 inhibitor, has been shown to decrease pulmonary artery pressure and resistance and to act additively with iNO in animal studies (Thelitz et al, 2004). A recent report indicates that the addition of intravenous milrinone to neonates with severe PPHN and poor iNO responsiveness was associated with improvements in oxygenation without compromising hemodynamic status (McNamara et al, 2006).

There is mounting evidence that oxidant stress plays an important role in the pathogenesis of PPHN. An increase in reactive oxygen species such as superoxide and hydrogen peroxide in the smooth muscle and adventitia of pulmonary arteries has been demonstrated in the PPHN lamb model (Brennan et al, 2003; Lakshminrusimha et al, 2006b; Wedgwood et al, 2005), as well as in postnatal models induced by chronic hypoxia (Fike et al, 2008). Possible sources for elevated concentrations of reactive oxygen species include increased expression and activity of NADPH oxidase and "uncoupled" nitric oxide synthase activity (Aschner et al, 2007; Konduri et al, 2003), as well as a reduction in endogenous superoxide dismutase activity (Brennan et al, 2003). Elevated concentrations of reactive oxygen species promote vascular smooth muscle cell proliferation in PPHN and produce abnormal vascular reactivity through mechanisms that blunt cGMP accumulation. Interestingly, one of the mechanisms may be through oxidant-mediated activation of cGMP-specific phosphodiesterases (Farrow et al, 2008a).

If reactive oxygen species promote vasoconstriction, it is possible that scavengers of reactive oxygen species will augment responsiveness to both endogenous and exogenous NO and promote pulmonary vasodilation. Superoxide dismutase scavenges and dismutates the superoxide radical to hydrogen peroxide, which is subsequently converted to water by catalase and glutathione peroxidase. Administration of recombinant human superoxide dismutase (rhSOD) has been tested in preterm infants without adverse effects and with trends toward decreased pulmonary morbidity (Davis et al, 2003). In lambs with pulmonary hypertension, rhSOD was found to dilate the pulmonary circulation and enhance responsiveness to inhaled NO (Steinhorn et al, 2001). A recent study examined the effects of rhSOD on oxygenation over a 24-hour period in ventilated PPHN lambs (Lakshminrusimha et al, 2006b). A single dose of rhSOD improved oxygenation to a degree similar to that observed for iNO. Further, rhSOD treatment appeared to block formation of oxidants such as peroxynitrite and isoprostanes and restore activity of endogenous nitric oxide synthase (Farrow et al, 2008b). Thus, an antioxidant therapeutic approach may have multiple beneficial effects: Scavenging superoxide may increase the availability of both endogenous and inhaled NO and may also reduce oxidative stress and limit lung injury (Firth and Yuan, 2008).

SUMMARY

Persistent pulmonary hypertension complicates the course of up to 10% of neonates with respiratory failure. It is associated with a diverse set of cardiopulmonary conditions, and its pathophysiologic mechanisms are characterized by vascular dysfunction, injury, and remodeling that occurs before and after birth. In the past 20 years, experimental work on basic mechanisms of vascular regulation of the developing pulmonary circulation has improved the range of therapeutic approaches to neonates with PPHN.

In particular, inhaled NO has proved to be a selective and effective pulmonary vasodilator for infants with PPHN, although successful clinical management requires meticulous care of all aspects of the associated lung and cardiac disease. Current research is focused on developing a better understanding of cellular responses in the remodeled vasculature that will likely elucidate additional signaling pathways and lead to new therapeutic strategies. More work is needed to further improve the survival and neurodevelopmental outcomes of sick newborns with pulmonary hypertension, especially in patients with lung hypoplasia and advanced structural vascular disease.

SUGGESTED READINGS

Angus DC, Linde-Swirble WT, Clermont G, et al: Epidemiology of neonatal respiratory failure in the United States, *Am J Respir Crit Care Med* 164:1154-1160, 2001.

Chambers CD, Hernandez-Diaz S, Van Marter LJ, et al: Selective serotonin-reuptake inhibitors and risk of persistent pulmonary hypertension of the newborn, *N Engl J Med* 354:579-587, 2006.

Fineman JR, Wong J, Morin FC III, et al: Chronic nitric oxide inhibition in utero produces persistent pulmonary hypertension in newborn lambs, *J Clin Invest* 93:2675-2683, 1994.

Kinsella JP, Abman SH: Clinical approach to inhaled NO therapy in the newborn, *J Pediatr* 136:717-726, 2000.

Lakshminrusimha S, Swartz DD, Gugino SF, et al: Oxygen concentration and pulmonary hemodynamics in newborn lambs with pulmonary hypertension, *Pediatr Res* 66:539-544, 2009b.

McNamara PJ, Laique F, Muang-In S, et al: Milrinone improves oxygenation in neonates with severe persistent pulmonary hypertension of the newborn, *J Crit Care* 21:217-222, 2006.

Mourani PM, Mullen M, Abman SH: Pulmonary hypertension in bronchopulmonary dysplasia, *Progr Pediatr Cardiol* 27:43-48, 2009.

Mourani PM, Sontag MK, Younoszai A, et al: Clinical utility of echocardiography for the diagnosis and management of pulmonary vascular disease in young children with chronic lung disease, *Pediatrics* 121:317-325, 2008.

Rudolph AM, Yuan S: Response of the pulmonary vasculature to hypoxia and H+ ion concentration changes, *J Clin Invest* 45:399-411, 1966.

Steinhorn RH, Kinsella JP, Pierce C, et al: Intravenous sildenafil in the treatment of neonates with persistent pulmonary hypertension, *J Pediatr* 155:841-847, 2009.

UK Collaborative ECMO Trial Group: UK collaborative randomised trial of neonatal extracorporeal membrane oxygenation, *Lancet* 348:75-82, 1996.

Walsh-Sukys MC, Tyson JE, Wright LL, et al: Persistent pulmonary hypertension of the newborn in the era before nitric oxide: practice variation and outcomes, *Pediatrics* 105:14-20, 2000.

Complete references and supplemental color images used in this text can be found online at www.expertconsult.com

FETAL AND NEONATAL ECHOCARDIOGRAPHY

Margaret M. Vernon and Mark Lewin

Echocardiography is the application of ultrasound to the evaluation of the cardiovascular system. Over the past several decades, echocardiography has become the gold standard for the determination of congenital and acquired cardiac malformations. Echocardiography provides reliable and reproducible information on cardiovascular form and function. Detailed cardiac structures can be identified, with differentiation of abnormal from normal anatomy, using high-resolution two-dimensional echocardiography. Accurate measures of myocardial thickness and cavity dimensions can be obtained via M-mode echocardiography. Components of hemodynamics, such as blood flow velocity and spatial direction, can be used to derive pressure measurements by the use of Doppler echocardiography.

Echocardiography is important not only in the diagnostic evaluation of congenital heart disease but also in the overall assessment of the cardiovascular system in disorders unique to the fetus and newborn infant. The information obtained is real-time, noninvasive, and acquired at the patient's bedside. Physiologic data points can be measured in a serial manner, which can be of great value in managing the fetus or sick neonate as conditions are explored and responses to management strategies are gauged. This chapter reviews the basic principles of echocardiography and their applications in the prenatal and newborn setting.

APPLICATION OF ULTRASOUND TO CARDIAC IMAGING

PHYSICS OF ULTRASOUND

Ultrasound energy is generated by the stimulation of piezoelectric crystals housed in a unit called a transducer. When ultrasound energy is transmitted into biologic tissue, the majority is absorbed; however, a small amount is reflected back to the transducer. Reflected energy is processed and an image created on a screen. Ultrasound scatter is greatest at the interfaces between biologic tissues of disparate densities. Hence, bone and air, when adjacent to soft tissues such as the heart, create poor acoustic windows for ultrasound transmission. Soft tissue and fluid are excellent media for ultrasound transmission and provide clear windows for cardiac imaging (Weyman, 1994).

The range of frequencies used for diagnostic assessment of biologic tissue is 2 to 12 MHz (1 MHz = 1 million cycles per second). Low-frequency ultrasound energy penetrates tissue better than high-frequency ultrasound; however, higher-frequency ultrasound provides for greater spatial resolution of fine structures. This principle is dictated by a fundamental law of physics that defines the relation between ultrasound frequency and wavelength:

velocity of sound in biologic tissue
$$= \text{ultrasound frequency} \times \text{wavelength}$$

An ultrasound wavelength distance is the physical limit beyond which two structures in space cannot be distinguished. Hence, the smaller the wavelength (i.e., the higher the frequency), the greater the ability to distinguish two points in space that are very close to each other.

Let us look at the following example. Two structures exist in space 0.5 mm apart. The velocity of sound in biologic tissue is a constant at approximately 1540 meters/second. Applying a frequency of 2 MHz of ultrasound energy will result in a wavelength of 0.77 mm, whereas applying a frequency of 8 MHz of ultrasound energy will result in a wavelength of 0.19 mm. Hence, to the operator using the 2-MHz transducer, the two structures will not be distinguishable from each other and will appear as one (in that the distance between them is less than the ultrasound wavelength), whereas the operator using the 8-MHz transducer will be able to differentiate between the structures with ease. Accordingly, higher frequencies, at a minimum 5 MHz and more typically 8 to 12 MHz, are used in the neonatal setting because penetration is less important in the small subject and the objective is to maximize fine structure resolution.

BASIC IMAGING COMPONENTS

Two-Dimensional Imaging

Development of phased-array transducers has allowed for sector scanning and the display of two-dimensional (2D) images. This is the most commonly applied modality of echocardiography and is used primarily for determination of anatomic structure.

M-Mode

The earliest form of echocardiographic imaging, M-mode echocardiography, displays fine detail of cardiac structure along a time line. A single thin plane of ultrasound energy is focused onto a targeted region of the heart. All structures within the targeted plane of insonation are then displayed in real time as they change during various portions of the cardiac cycle.

M-mode echocardiography is commonly used for measurement of myocardial wall thickness and cavity dimensions and is useful in estimating ventricular cavity size for calculation of the ventricular *shortening fraction*—an estimate of ventricular function. By angling the plane of insonation through the short axis of the left ventricle at the level of the tips of the papillary muscles, one can obtain an M-mode display of the change in ventricular cavity dimension over time (Figure 53-1). The ratio of the difference between left ventricle end-diastolic dimension (LVEDD) and left ventricle end-systolic dimension (LVESD) to the left ventricle end-diastolic dimension is

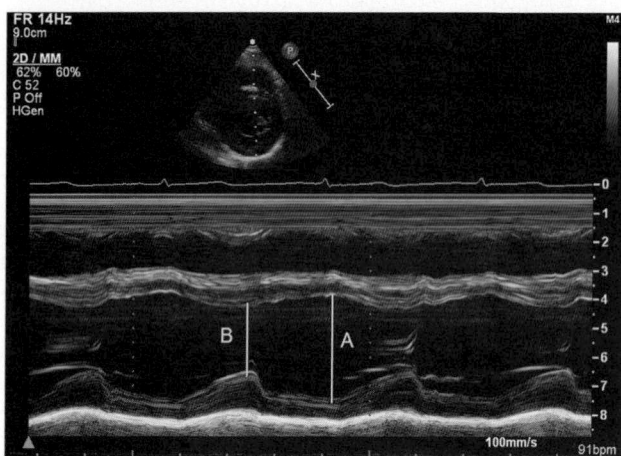

FIGURE 53-1 M-mode tracing of the left ventricular dimensions over time obtained in the short-axis view. The electrocardio-graphic tracing helps identify the timing of the cardiac cycle as systolic or diastolic. Measurement A demonstrates the left ventricle end-diastolic dimension, and measurement B, the left ventricle end-systolic measurement. The shortening fraction is calculated at 35%.

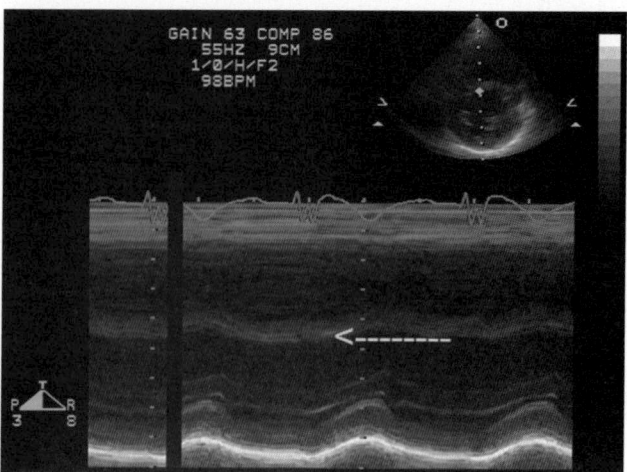

FIGURE 53-2 M-mode tracing of the left ventricular dimensions over time obtained in the short-axis view. The electrocardio-graphic tracing helps identify the timing of the cardiac cycle as systolic or diastolic. The interventricular septum moves paradoxically (*arrow*) because of elevated right ventricular pressure. Therefore, a shortening fraction cannot be calculated accurately.

the shortening fraction [(LVEDD – LVESD)/LVEDD × 100 = %SF]. The normal range is 28% to 38%, which correlates with a ventricular volumetric ejection fraction ratio of 55% to 65%, suggesting normal ventricular function. Interpretation of the %SF must also take into account the overall dimensions of the left ventricle. For example, an infant with a volume load due to mitral regurgitation or a large patent ductus arteriosus (PDA) may have a normal %SF but may have a dilated, enlarged left ventricle when normalized for body surface area. The %SF also can be helpful in investigating the cause of hypotension in infants. With hypotension due to myocardial dysfunction, the infant will have a dilated left ventricle and diminished %SF. With hypotension due to vasodilatation, such as is seen in various conditions of sepsis, the infant may have a normal or hyperdynamic %SF, often exceeding 40%. Volume-depleted infants will exhibit a normal %SF but a small left ventricular cavity size.

Although it is the most commonly used technique for determination of ventricular function, the M-mode measurement of %SF has a number of limitations. It provides for only a single-plane assessment of ventricular contraction and is invalid in conditions in which there is wall motion abnormality. Paradoxical movement of the ventricular septum away from the posterior wall during systole may create a spuriously low %SF value. Hence, %SF measures may be difficult to interpret in the presence of right bundle branch block, right ventricle dilatation due to atrial septal defect, or right ventricular hypertension due to either a congenital cardiac lesion (for example, tetralogy of Fallot) or pulmonary hypertension (Figure 53-2).

Doppler

Application of the Doppler principle allows for determination of the velocity and direction of moving objects. Because blood and myocardial tissue both are in motion throughout the cardiac cycle, either can be assessed by Doppler echocardiography. Doppler imaging can be performed in a number of ways. In pulsed-wave Doppler echocardiography, transducer crystals alternately fire pulses of energy and then "listen" for reflected signal return. This mode allows for determination of spatial signal position but limits the ability to measure blood traveling at higher velocities. In continuous-wave Doppler echocardiography, half of the transducer crystals fire continuously while the other half "listen" continuously. This mode allows for unambiguous assessment of increased velocities but limits the ability to pinpoint the precise location at which the velocity is obtained. In combination, pulsed-wave and continuous-wave Doppler modes provide a complete picture of blood flow direction and velocity.

Color Doppler echocardiography uses pulsed-wave principles to create a 2D sector display of all velocities within a given region of interest. A sector within a 2D image is identified and pixels of color are displayed overlying the area of interrogation. Each color pixel reflects the direction of motion; the shade of color reflects the velocity. By convention, "warm" colors such as red and orange designate direction of flow toward the transducer, and "cold" colors such as blue and white designate flow away from the transducer (Figure 53-3). When flow velocities exceed the characteristics of the transducer, the smooth, laminar color pattern changes to a speckled color pattern, suggesting a region of more turbulent flow. Whether this represents a pathologic velocity change requires pulsed Doppler interrogation. Doppler techniques are also applied to tissue motion of the myocardium, yielding information helpful in ascertaining parameters of myocardial function. Although tissue signals move at much lower velocities than blood signals, determination of Doppler-derived tissue velocities can aid in understanding complex states of systolic and diastolic dysfunction (Mertens and Friedberg, 2009). Distinct patterns of normal and abnormal motion of various myocardial segments have been described.

Data derived from Doppler echocardiography are used to provide physiologic information. Using the principles of flow hydraulics across a tubular system with

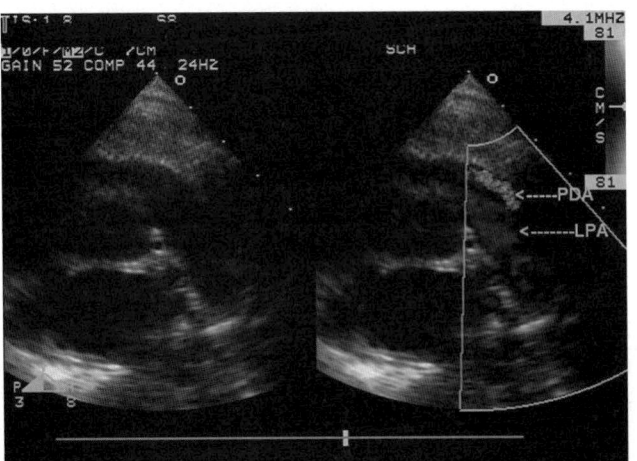

FIGURE 53-3 *(Supplemental color version of this figure is available online at www.expertconsult.com.)* **Side-by-side two-dimensional and color Doppler echocardiographic images of a ductus arteriosus.** Flow in the PDA is red, indicating flow toward the transducer (in this case left-to-right) and is directed toward the MPA from the aorta. The PDA color signal is speckled, indicating a more turbulent region of flow. High velocity in the PDA is the normal state, indicating appropriately elevated pressures in the aorta as compared to the lower pressures in the pulmonary artery. The flow in the LPA is blue, indicating flow away from the transducer. The LPA color flow signal is laminar (smooth), indicating a lower velocity of flow. Turbulent flow at this portion of the LPA in a neonate is most commonly associated with physiologic branch pulmonary artery stenosis, a transient phenomenon associated with neonatal transitional physiology. *PDA,* Patent ductus arteriosus; *LPA,* left pulmonary artery.

discrete narrowing, velocity data can be translated into pressure data via modification of the Bernoulli equation (Figure 53-4):

$$P_1 - P_2 = 4 \times (V_2 - V_1)^2$$

Normal velocities in the heart are rarely greater than 1 meter/second. Velocities proximal to areas of narrowing are typically less than 1 meter/second and can often be ignored. Hence, the equation can be simplified to:

$$\text{pressure change} = 4 \times V\text{max}^2$$

This principle can be applied in a variety of clinical settings. For example, in the presence of tricuspid regurgitation (TR), the peak right ventricle pressure (which will equal the pulmonary artery pressure in the absence of pulmonary outflow obstruction) can be estimated by measuring the regurgitant jet peak velocity. A TR peak velocity of 2 meters/second suggests a pressure difference between the right atrium and the right ventricle of 16 mm Hg ($4 \times (2)^2$). We express this as a right ventricular pressure of 16 mm Hg + right atrial (or central venous) pressure. In infants and children, right atrial pressure is estimated to be between 3 and 10 mm Hg, with 5 mm Hg typically chosen as an estimated guess. Hence, in the preceding example, the patient would have a right ventricle pressure of 21 mm Hg, which is within normal limits. Alternatively, an infant with severe chronic lung disease may have a TR peak jet of 4.1 meters/second (Figure 53-5). This would translate to a pressure estimate of 64 mm Hg ($4 \times (4.1)^2$); 68 mm Hg added to the estimated right atrial pressure of 5 mm Hg gives a right ventricle pressure of 73 mm Hg, which suggests pulmonary hypertension. The Bernoulli equation also is commonly used to assess pressure gradients across stenotic valves or vessels, for example valvular aortic stenosis or coarctation of

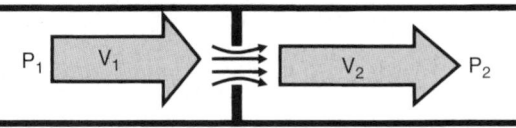

FIGURE 53-4 Bernoulli equation of flow dynamics describes the relationship between pressure differences and velocity differences across an area of narrowing in a closed fluid system. P_1, proximal pressure; P_2, downstream distal pressure; V_1, proximal velocity; V_2, distal downstream velocity.

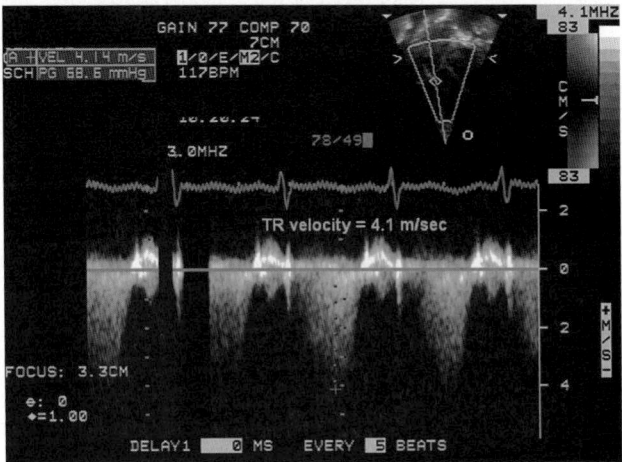

FIGURE 53-5 **Example of a Doppler signal.** Time is on the *x*-axis, and velocity is in meters/second on the *y*-axis. The Doppler signal is obtained by positioning a marker just proximal to the tricuspid valve annulus in order to sample the tricuspid regurgitant *(TR)* jet flow. In this example the TR peak velocity measures 4.1 m/sec. Using the modified Bernoulli equation, the predicted right ventricular pressure is $4 \times (4.1)^2 = 68$ mm Hg + right atrial pressure. This predicts elevated right ventricular pressure (normal is typically in the range of 20 mm Hg). In the absence of obstruction to flow through the pulmonary artery, the right ventricular pressure is equivalent to pulmonary artery pressure. We can therefore quantify pulmonary artery pressure based on the velocity of the TR jet.

the aorta. Using the maximum velocity, we derive the "peak instantaneous" gradient across the site of obstruction.

FETAL IMAGING TECHNIQUES

Fetal echocardiography is the ultrasonic evaluation of the fetal cardiovascular system. Echocardiography is the main diagnostic modality used to evaluate the fetal heart. Cardiac formation is complete by 8 weeks after conception, and ventricular contraction can be detected by ultrasound imaging at that time. The optimal timing for performance of a comprehensive transabdominal fetal echocardiogram is 18 to 20 weeks' gestation; however, as resolution has improved, earlier diagnosis and reassurance may be possible late in the first trimester (Smrcek et al, 2006).

Similar to a pediatric transthoracic echocardiogram, a fetal echocardiogram involves assessing cardiac anatomy in a sequential fashion. Initial imaging establishes fetal position in utero (vertex, breech, or transverse). Once fetal

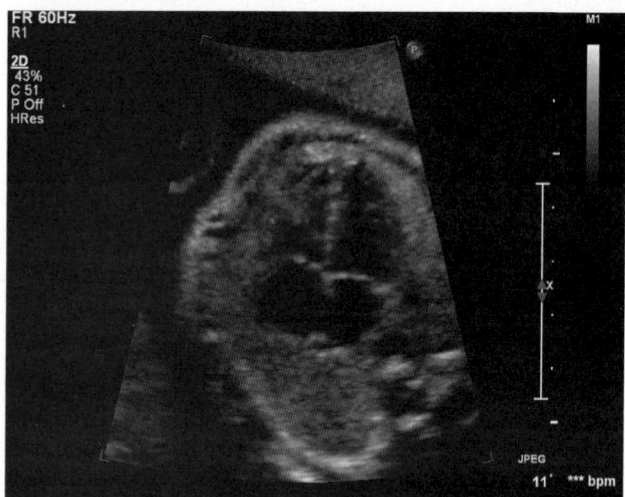

FIGURE 53-6 Four-chamber view of a normal fetal heart. All four chambers are visible with relative symmetry in size between the ventricles and atria. The right ventricle is identified by the presence of the moderator band and increased myocardial trabeculations in comparison with the left ventricle. The descending aorta is seen directly behind the left atrium.

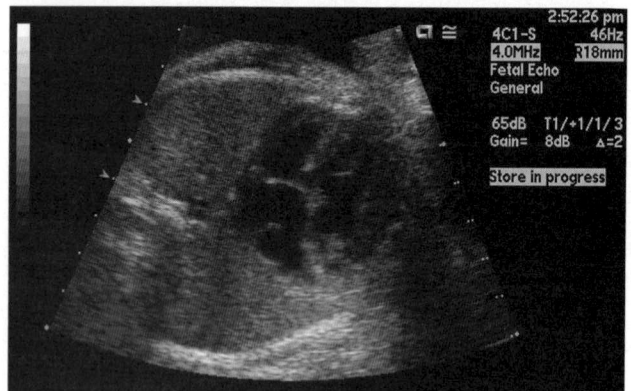

FIGURE 53-7 Four-chamber view of the fetal heart with complex congenital heart disease. There is a large ventricular septal defect as well as a large primum atrial septal defect. There is size discrepancy between the two ventricular chambers. This fetus was diagnosed with an unbalanced complete atrioventricular canal defect (CAVC).

left and right are established, the fetal abdominal situs is confirmed as well as the position of the heart within the thorax. Although uncommon as a whole, congenital heart disease and abnormalities of laterality (heterotaxy syndrome) are commonly found together. The cardiovascular system is then evaluated beginning below the diaphragm in the abdomen and ending at the thoracic inlet as a series of imaging planes. The four-chamber view (Figure 53-6) is the most important in a comprehensive examination of the fetal heart. In this view, cardiac position, size, rate and rhythm, and qualitative contractility can all be assessed. Additionally many congenital heart defects can be detected (Figure 53-7). After a four-chamber view is obtained, attention turns to visualization of the left and right ventricular outflow tracts and an assessment of ventriculoarterial concordance. Establishing the origin of the main pulmonary artery from the right ventricle and the aorta from the left ventricle is mandatory. Finally, the systemic and pulmonary venous return is evaluated.

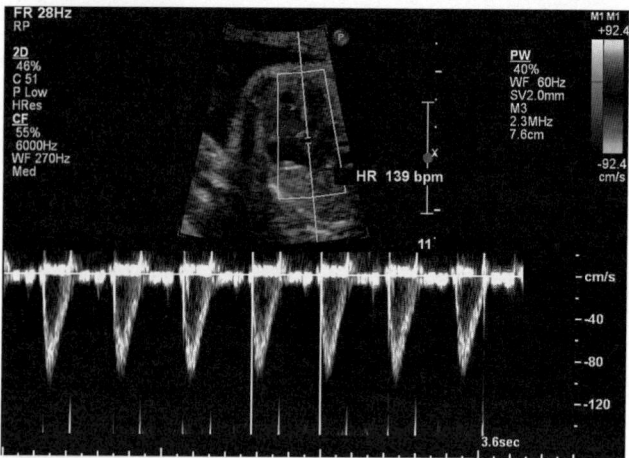

FIGURE 53-8 The fetal heart rate is documented using aortic valve Doppler. The time between successive beats is measured and a heart rate per minute calculated.

Structures are evaluated in orthogonal imaging planes in order to form a composite picture of the heart including any identified malformation. In addition to obtaining clear pictures of each structure, flow is evaluated with color Doppler and pulsed Doppler. Valve regurgitation and/or stenosis can be detected and valve leaflet motion observed. From 2D images, structures can be measured and compared with established normals for varying gestation ages.

Once a comprehensive assessment of the cardiac anatomy is complete, the heart rate is documented (Figure 53-8). The rate and rhythm of the fetal heart are evaluated by mechanical surrogate events, specifically the movement of atria and ventricles or blood flow across valves.

NEONATAL IMAGING TECHNIQUES

A systematic and standardized approach is important in performing the echocardiogram in the neonate. Follow-up echocardiographic studies may be curtailed and limited in scope; however, initial evaluation should be complete and include investigation of all aspects of the heart and great vessels using 2D, Doppler, color Doppler, and M-mode imaging. Standard imaging locations are used to create a complete picture of the heart and great vessels (Figure 53-9). These include images obtained mid-chest (parasternal imaging plane), four-chamber views (apical imaging), and abdominal views through the liver and diaphragm (subcostal imaging) and between the clavicles (suprasternal notch views). 2D imaging "sweeps" result in acquisition of tomographic cuts of the heart as the transducer is fanned through an imaging plane. This allows for "mental reconstruction" in the development of a three-dimensional understanding of cardiac structure, function, and structural relationships. Subcostal imaging is unique to neonates and pediatric patients: The liver acts to enhance acoustic transmission, and the proximity of the transducer to the heart optimizes image resolution.

Although echocardiography is considered a noninvasive diagnostic test, care should be taken during the performance of the echocardiogram, particularly in small, premature infants. In the older, less cooperative child, sedation is

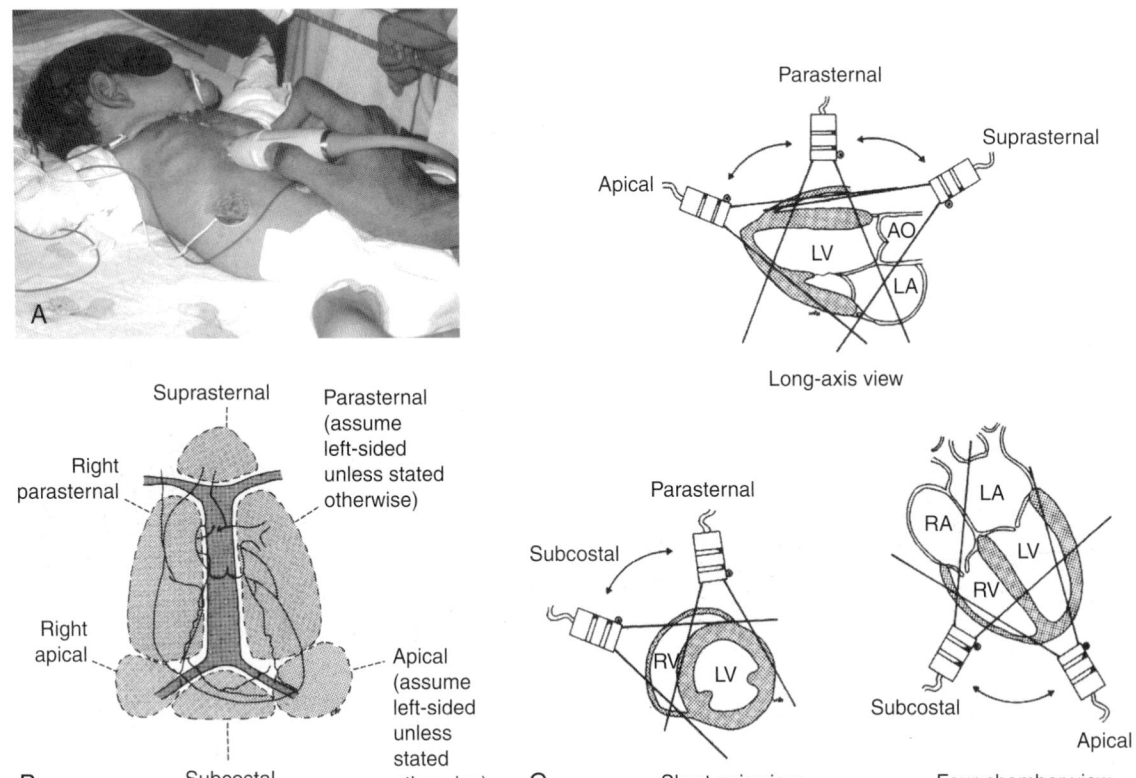

FIGURE 53-9 A, Demonstration of position of ultrasound transducer using the subcostal approach in a neonate. **B,** By moving the transducer to multiple windows surrounding the heart, echocardiographic two-dimensional tomographic imaging provides for a three-dimensional look at the heart via "mental reconstruction" once each of the corresponding windows has been examined. **C,** Long-axis, short-axis, and four-chamber views of the heart contribute to visualization of the overall detail of complex cardiac anatomy. (**B** and **C,** *Courtesy American Society of Echocardiography.*)

necessary to obtain patient compliance, and therefore continuous assessment during the procedure and monitoring thereafter are essential. Application of cold ultrasound gel and environmental exposure may cause temperature instability. Applying pressure on the abdomen during subcostal imaging or extending the neck during suprasternal imaging may cause destabilization of the patient due to either cardiac or pulmonary compromise. Either the person performing the echocardiogram or another assigned person should monitor heart rate, blood pressure, and ventilatory parameters during the procedure in unstable, ill infants.

FETAL ECHOCARDIOGRAPHY: GOALS OF IMAGING

Congenital heart disease, which refers mainly to anatomic malformations of the heart, constitutes one of the most common congenital anomalies. The reported incidence rate per 100 liveborn infants is 0.3 at birth and nearly 1 by the end of the first year of life (Botto et al, 2001).

Technical advances in ultrasound imaging have improved the antenatal detection of congenital heart disease (CHD); however, cardiac anomalies continue to be one of the most frequently overlooked lesions during prenatal obstetrical ultrasound examination.

The ultimate goal of fetal echocardiography is the accurate definition of any anatomic abnormality of the heart during the prenatal time period. Although a variety of maternal or fetal disorders may result in abnormality of the fetal cardiovascular system (Table 53-1), a majority of

TABLE 53-1 Indications for Fetal Echocardiography

Maternal Indications	Fetal Indications
Family history of CHD including prior child or pregnancy with CHD	Abnormal obstetrical screening ultrasound
Metabolic disorders (e.g., diabetes)	Extracardiac abnormality
Exposure to teratogens	Chromosomal abnormality
Exposure to prostaglandin synthetase inhibitors (ibuprofen)	Arrhythmia
	Hydrops
Infection (rubella, Coxsackie, parvovirus B19)	Increased first-trimester nuchal translucency
Autoimmune diagnosis (e.g., Sjögren's, SLE)	Multiple gestation and suspected twin-twin transfusion syndrome
Familial inherited disorder (Marfan, Noonan syndromes)	
In vitro fertilization	

CHD, Congenital heart disease; *SLE,* systemic lupus erythematosus.

children diagnosed with congenital heart disease are born with no known risk factors. Currently, however, a comprehensive cardiovascular evaluation is recommended only in those with identified risk factors.

Fetal diagnosis depends on the ability to obtain standard views. The components of a comprehensive evaluation are listed in Table 53-2, although not all may be visualized in every fetus at every examination. In addition, some lesions can evolve in utero.

Once a diagnosis is established, the secondary goal of fetal echocardiography, parental counseling, can begin. Complete parental counseling includes not only a discussion of

TABLE 53-2   Components of the Fetal Echocardiogram

Overview	Fetal number and position
	Stomach position and abdominal situs
	Cardiac position
Biometric examination	Cardiothoracic ratio
	Biparietal diameter and head circumference
	Femur length
	Abdominal circumference
Cardiac imaging	Four-color view
	LVOT
	RVOT
	Great arteries
	Three-vessel view
	Bicaval view
	Ductal arch
	Aortic arch
Doppler examination	Inferior and superior vene cavae
	Pulmonary veins
	Ductus venosus
	Foramen ovale
	Atrioventricular valves
	Semilunar valves
	Ductus arteriosus
	Transverse aortic arch
	Umbilical artery
	Umbilical vein
Measurement data	Atrioventricular valve diameter
	Semilunar valve diameter
	Main pulmonary artery
	Ascending aorta
	Branch pulmonary arteries
	Transverse aortic arch
	Ventricular length
	Ventricular short-axis dimensions
Examination of rate and rhythm	M-mode study of atrial and ventricular wall motion
	Doppler examination of atrial and ventricular flow patterns

LVOT, Left ventricular outflow tract; *RVOT,* right ventricular outflow tract.

TABLE 53-3   Indications for Echocardiographic Evaluation in the Neonate

Conditions Associated With Congenital Heart Defects	
Syndromes	**Nonsyndromes**
Trisomies 13, 18, 21	Congenital diaphragmatic
22q11 microdeletion syndromes:	hernia
DiGeorge	Gastroschisis
Velocardiofacial	Omphalocele
VACTER association	Tracheoesophageal fistula
CHARGE association	
Holt-Oram syndrome	
Goldenhar's syndrome	
De Lange's syndrome	
Turner's syndrome	
Noonan's syndrome	
Williams syndrome	
Infantile Marfan syndrome	

Conditions Associated With Impact on Cardiovascular System
Congenital diaphragmatic hernia
Chronic lung disease
Gestational diabetes mellitus
Sacrococcygeal teratoma
Twin-twin transfusion syndrome
Arteriovenous malformation
Perinatal asphyxia
Severe anemia

CHARGE, Coloboma, heart disease, retarded growth/development and/or central nervous system anomalies, genital hypoplasia, ear anomalies and/or deafness; *VACTER,* vertebral abnormalities, anal atresia, cardiac abnormalities, tracheoesophageal fistula and/or esophageal atresia, renal agenesis/dysplasia.

the abnormality identified, but also the frequently increased risk for extracardiac anomalies and chromosomal abnormalities and long-term outcome. Prenatal management plans need to be discussed, including local laws regarding termination of a pregnancy. Finally, perinatal management plans can be created to smooth the transition to the postnatal time period. Prenatal detection of CHD has been shown to improve outcome by reducing postnatal acidosis and mortality (Tworetzky et al, 2001; Verheijen et al, 2001).

NEONATAL ECHOCARDIOGRAPHY: GOALS OF IMAGING

Echocardiography is considered the gold standard in the diagnosis of congenital heart lesions. In addition, noninvasive cardiac imaging provides diagnostic support for the management of a variety of neonatal conditions. The indications for the performance of an echocardiogram in the nursery or newborn intensive care unit include the assessment of the neonate with a presumed syndromic or genetic condition that is at high risk for cardiac disease (e.g., trisomy 21), the infant with a noncardiac lesion where there is an increased risk of associated congenital

heart disease (e.g., omphalocele), and the neonate with a condition that may adversely affect hemodynamics (e.g., arteriovenous malformations). These are summarized in Table 53-3. The goals of neonatal cardiac imaging are similar to that of the fetal echocardiogram. Cardiac and abdominal situs are assessed, a complete evaluation is made of the anatomic structure of the heart and proximal vasculature, and a determination is made as to the functional (systolic and diastolic) properties of the myocardium.

For an accurate determination to be made as to the dimensions of chambers, valves, and vessels, a normative data set is required. The most common methodology involves normalizing measurements to body surface area. A number of data sets are available for comparison; in order to achieve consistency, each pediatric echocardiography laboratory must decide which of these data sets will be used. Various normative (Z-score) calculators are also available online (www.parameterz.com) with references and descriptors included for ease of use. The identification of a pathologically large or small structure is especially troublesome when the patient is markedly premature. Comparative data for such children are scant and are often based on data collected from a very small number of "normal" patients. Determination of dimensions (e.g., left ventricle, aortic valve, or pulmonary artery) in such premature patients is therefore subject to a fair bit of interpretation; in these cases, consultation with the pediatric cardiologist is imperative in order to make appropriate management decisions.

Serial echocardiographic evaluations are often necessary in order to care for the neonate. This is particularly the case when changes are occurring in the patient's clinical condition. We follow left atrial and left ventricular chamber dimensions as pulmonary vascular resistance drops in order to determine the left-to-right shunt impact in the face of a patent ductus arteriosus. We follow interventricular thickness and left ventricular outflow tract obstruction in the infant of a diabetic mother to determine if serial improvement occurs over time. The neonatal cardiopulmonary system is a highly fluid system, subject to perturbation from numerous outside influences and thus requires close monitoring in the labile child. Echocardiography is but one tool in the armamentarium of the neonatologist and cardiologist to assist with this monitoring.

FETAL-TO-NEONATAL TRANSITION PHYSIOLOGY: ECHOCARDIOGRAPHY-DERIVED ASSESSMENT

During fetal life, the placenta serves as the organ of gas exchange. This fundamental difference between the fetal and neonatal circulations is behind the complex physiological transition that occurs following birth and the clamping of the umbilical cord. With the initiation of respiration and expansion of the lungs, oxygen is brought to the alveoli. This results in a dramatic fall in pulmonary vascular resistance (PVR) and increase in pulmonary blood flow. Simultaneously, the umbilical cord is clamped, resulting in a sudden increase in systemic vascular resistance (SVR). The combination of this sudden increase in SVR and decrease in PVR leads to a reversal of flow through the ductus arteriosus. In utero flow was from right to left (pulmonary artery to descending aorta) and now flow reverses, becoming left to right (from descending aorta to pulmonary artery). Finally, because of the marked increase in pulmonary blood flow, venous return to the left atrium increases and left atrial pressure exceeds right atrial pressure. The redundant flap of tissue of the foramen ovale is pressed against the septum and closes the foramen.

Echocardiography is a very useful tool in the evaluation of a newborn. The information obtained is real-time, noninvasive, and acquired at the bedside. It is the primary imaging modality used when clinical events such as tachypnea, tachycardia, or persistent cyanosis suggest an abnormality in transitional physiology. Anything increasing the pulmonary vascular resistance or delaying the fall in pulmonary vascular resistance, such as acidosis, hypoxemia, polycythemia, lung disease, or immaturity, may impair the normal neonatal transition. Additionally, it is the uniqueness of the fetal circulation that allows many complex lesions to be tolerated silently in utero only to unmask themselves during the transitional period. Alterations from normal are most frequently associated with persistent patency of the ductus arteriosus, persistently elevated pulmonary vascular resistance, or the presence of congenital heart disease.

SUSPECTED CONGENITAL HEART DISEASE

Confirmation of the absence of structural heart disease or alternatively the identification of a significant congenital heart defect can be extremely helpful to the team caring for an ill neonate, particularly one with a recognized extracardiac anomaly. In those in whom congenital heart disease is confirmed, high-quality 2D images combined with color and pulsed- and continuous-wave Doppler are frequently sufficient for development of a comprehensive management strategy, including a surgical plan if necessary (Tworetzky et al, 1999).

ASSESSMENT OF THE DUCTUS ARTERIOSUS

Before the routine use of echocardiography, a hemodynamically significant PDA was diagnosed clinically by the presence of a murmur, hyperdynamic precordium, bounding and palmar pulses, increased ventilatory support, and radiographic evidence of cardiomegaly with increased pulmonary vascular markings. In the present era, a complete transthoracic echocardiogram is recommended before medical treatment of a presumed PDA.

The echocardiographic assessment of a PDA documents not only the size of the ductus but also the direction of flow across the ductus. Additionally, pulsed- and continuous-wave Doppler can be used to establish flow velocity and predict the pressure difference between the aorta and pulmonary artery. It is important not only to confirm the presence of a PDA, but also to ensure the absence of structural heart defects. In addition, the determination of aortic arch sidedness or branching pattern is important should surgical ligation be required (Murdison et al, 1990). Typically the aortic arch is a left aortic arch with a left-sided ductus, but a right aortic arch with a right-sided ductus can occur and alters the surgical approach to ductal ligation.

EVALUATION OF PERSISTENT PULMONARY HYPERTENSION

Persistent pulmonary hypertension of the newborn (PPHN), occasionally referred to as persistent fetal circulation, results when there is severe vasoconstriction of the pulmonary vasculature resulting in elevation of pulmonary arterial pressure and right ventricular pressure. Blood continues to bypass the lungs by shunting across the foramen ovale and ductus arteriosus. Several factors may disrupt the normal decrease in pulmonary vascular resistance and increase in pulmonary blood flow at birth, including apnea and parenchymal lung disease, both of which interfere with ventilation. Meconium aspiration and severe respiratory distress syndrome are the major parenchymal lung diseases. Pneumonia and asphyxia can cause PPHN as well.

In infants with PPHN, transthoracic echocardiography confirms the absence of structural heart disease, demonstrates atrial- and ductal-level shunting, and provides an estimate of pulmonary arterial pressure by measuring the velocity of the tricuspid regurgitation jet, if present. The Doppler pattern of flow in the ductus establishes flow direction as well as velocity. From flow velocity a pressure gradient (or lack thereof) between the aorta and pulmonary artery can be estimated by applying the Bernoulli equation (Musewe et al, 1990). The appearance of the Doppler pattern sampled in the branch pulmonary arteries may also provide information about the pulmonary vascular resistance and response to therapy.

In addition, echocardiography may be used to assess ventricular function in an infant with PPHN (Figure 53-10).

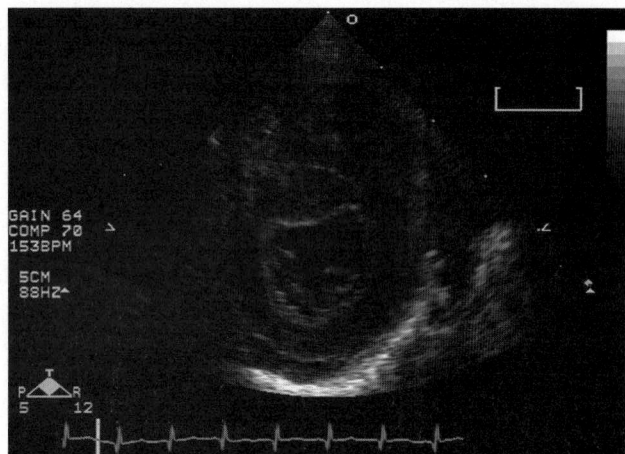

FIGURE 53-10 Short axis imaging of the ventricles. Normally the left ventricular pressure exceeds the right resulting in bowing of the ventricular septum into the right ventricular cavity. In PPHN, the right ventricular pressure (RVp) may be equivalent or even exceed the left ventricular pressure (LVp), altering the ventricular septal position, as seen in this image where the septum bows abnormally into the left ventricle. This septal position suggests the RVp exceeds the LVp.

Neonates with PPHN typically have right ventricular dysfunction (Valdes-Cruz et al, 1981). Although the etiology of cardiac dysfunction in PPHN is unclear, prenatal constriction of the ductus arteriosus has been suggested as a possible mechanism (Morin, 1989).

Extracorporeal membrane oxygenation (ECMO) is frequently used in infants with severe PPHN whose hypoxemia does not respond to mechanical ventilatory support and pulmonary vasodilators such as oxygen and nitric oxide. Echocardiography can be used to document improvement or causes of difficulties in circuit flow. Additionally, an echocardiogram is often crucial to rule out congenital heart defects that may mimic PPHN, including total anomalous pulmonary venous return with obstruction.

LIMITATIONS OF ECHOCARDIOGRAPHY

Although an extremely useful tool that has revolutionized the approach to diagnostic evaluation of the cardiovascular system in the neonate, echocardiography has a number of limitations:

- *Discrepancy between "echo-derived" and "catheter-derived" gradients.* Doppler echocardiography measures the "peak instantaneous" pressure difference at any point in time during flow across a stenotic valve. In the case of a stenotic aortic valve, this may occur during the upstroke of systole, not at the peak of systole. Catheter-based measures of pressure are taken at the peak of systole; hence, echo-derived pressure gradients do not equal, and usually exceed, catheter-derived measures. This discrepancy does not invalidate the measures of either modality but rather highlights the point that they are measures of gradients occurring during two different points in systole. Historically, clinical decision making has been based on catheter-derived information; therefore, echocardiographically derived data should be interpreted in this light. Other factors that may have an impact on differences in echocardiographic versus catheter-based gradients are level of sedation, hydration status, medications (inotropes), and ventilatory strategy.
- *Stress of the test.* Lengthy environmental exposure, temperature instability, and pressure application on the chest or abdomen during transducer contact may result in stress for the premature or hemodynamically unstable infant, often necessitating termination of the procedure or limiting the scope of the ultrasound evaluation.
- *Inadequate visualization of structures.* Lung disease can cause acoustic impedance, limiting the ability to visualize structures. Air within the thorax due to air trapping, pneumothorax, or pneumopericardium can result in a dramatic deterioration in image clarity.
- *Inadequate Doppler signal for velocity measurement.* Small blood volumes traveling at low velocity may be difficult to identify with echocardiography. Examples are coronary arteries in the very small, premature infant and pulmonary vein flow in patients with severe lung disease in whom pulmonary blood flow may be limited. Identification of pulmonary venous anatomy and flow in infants on extracorporeal membrane oxygenation also may be difficult as a result of reduced pulmonary circulation. Transesophageal echocardiography may be indicated in these patients because of the enhanced imaging resolution of this modality.

OTHER CARDIOVASCULAR IMAGING MODALITIES

TRANSESOPHAGEAL ECHOCARDIOGRAPHY

Technologic advancements in miniaturization have allowed for the development of tiny transducer housings and small footprints for the performance of surface echocardiography in the neonate. Similar technology has allowed for the development of transesophageal echocardiography (TEE), in which a small transducer can be introduced into the esophagus of an infant typically weighing as little as 2.5 to 3.0 kg. Newer technology has become available that expands the size range for TEE such that premature infants as small as approximately 1 kg can be safely imaged. TEE is helpful in elucidating structures in the posterior mediastinum, such as pulmonary veins, and in overcoming acoustic impediments at the surface such as air and bone (Randolph et al, 2002). Most important, TEE has allowed for imaging to take place during interventional procedures in the operating room or catheterization laboratory (Figure 53-11). This eliminates the need to place a transducer directly on the chest or abdomen, thereby avoiding potential contamination of the operative field. Interventional procedures can be guided by TEE imaging, yielding immediate feedback to the proceduralist that has been well validated as a means of improving overall outcomes.

INTRACARDIAC ECHOCARDIOGRAPHY

Recently, ultrasound transducer technology has been incorporated into the tips of catheters, allowing for intracardiac imaging (Hijazi et al, 2009). This is primarily of use in the cardiac catheterization laboratory for the imaging of

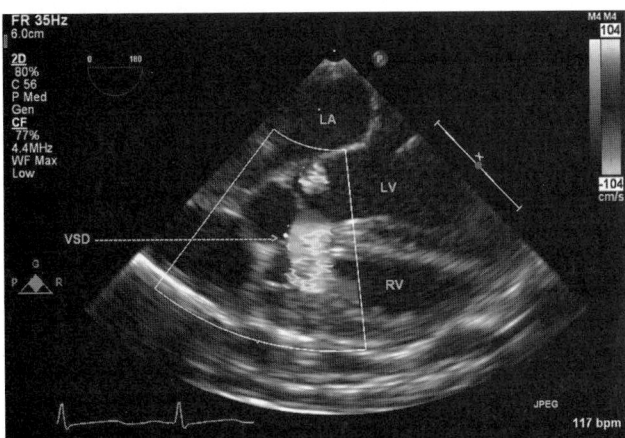

FIGURE 53-11 *(Supplemental color version of this figure is available online at www.expertconsult.com.)* Color Doppler image obtained during transesophageal imaging in the operating room preceding surgical closure of a moderate sized membranous ventricular septal defect. The color signal is blue, indicating flow away from the transducer, in this case left-to-right. *LA,* Left atrium; *LV,* left ventricle; *RV,* right ventricle; *VSD,* ventricular septal defect.

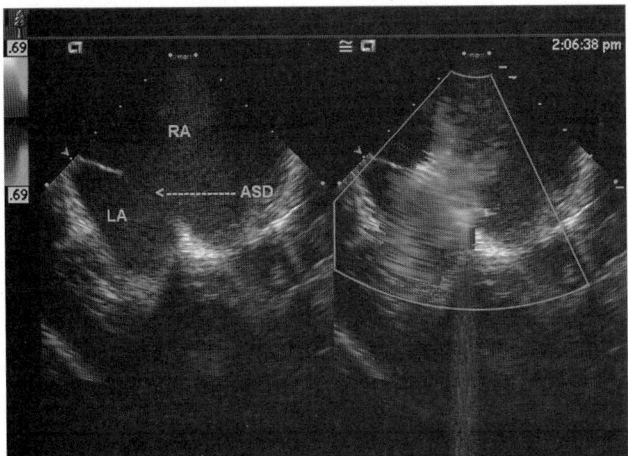

FIGURE 53-12 *(Supplemental color version of this figure is available online at www.expertconsult.com.)* Side-by-side two-dimensional and color Doppler imaging of a large secundum atrial septal defect *(ASD)* obtained by intracardiac echocardiographic (ICE) imaging. The color signal is red and laminar, indicating low velocity, left-to-right flow through the ASD. The right atrium *(RA)* is dilated in comparison with the left atrium *(LA)* because of the volume load on the right heart caused by this shunt lesion.

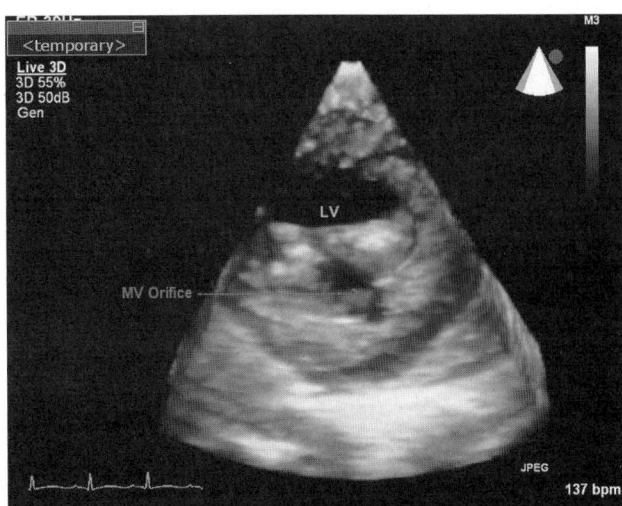

FIGURE 53-13 Three-dimensional echocardiographic image of a pathologic mitral valve. Using this imaging technique, a view of the mitral valve position within the left ventricular cavity is obtained that allows for a more thorough understanding of the nature of the anomaly. In this case the mitral valve is seen in a cross-sectional, short-axis view peering into the left ventricular cavity. The mitral orifice is hypoplastic, resulting in obstruction to inflow. *LV,* Left ventricle; *MV,* mitral valve.

structures and devices during interventional procedures. In the pediatric interventional laboratory, the primary use is for the percutaneous device closure of atrial septal defects (Figure 53-12). Although these catheters provide an additional imaging modality, because of the currently available technology the size of these catheters (8F) precludes their use in the femoral veins of younger children (less than approximately 10 kg). Additionally, in most cases small children yield excellent transthoracic images, thus obviating the need for direct intracardiac assessment.

THREE-DIMENSIONAL ECHOCARDIOGRAPHY

Integration of multiplanar image data into a real-time three-dimensional (3D) display has been a goal of echocardiography. The earliest methods required acquisition of data that then required offline 3D image rendering. Over the past several years systems have been made available that are capable of displaying "live" 3D echocardiographic images (Figure 53-13). This has resulted in our ability to interpret data as it is being obtained, making possible real-time bedside feedback. 3D echocardiography allows for enhanced identification of spatial relationships and structural malformations (Marx and Su, 2007). 3D echocardiographic technology has been miniaturized such that it is now available in an adult-sized TEE transducer. This allows for the benefits of TEE (improved image resolution and ease of image acquisition during procedures) to be combined with the enhanced data available from 3D imaging. In the foreseeable future, 3D TEE should be available in small transducers amenable to imaging the newborn and small child. 3D echocardiography will continue to evolve and promises to become an important modality as technologic advances continue.

SUMMARY

Echocardiographic assessment has become inseparable from effective management of the ill neonate. The ability to use noninvasive cardiac evaluation not only aids in the identification of congenital cardiac lesions but, just as important allows for a thorough understanding of the newborn physiologic state. Pharmacologic, ventilatory, and surgical decision making are by necessity based on clarity surrounding how these management strategies affect, and are affected by, cardiac status. In addition, the understanding of prenatal cardiac issues (e.g., anatomic anomalies, rhythm disturbances, myocardial function) can only be performed via fetal echocardiographic imaging. Neonatal outcomes are therefore dependent on both accurate fetal and postnatal echocardiographic diagnosis and the application of these data to overall multidisciplinary newborn care.

ACKNOWLEDGMENTS

We thank Drs. Jack Rychik and Meryl S. Cohen for those portions of this chapter extracted from "Echocardiography in the Neonatal Intensive Care Unit" in *Avery's Diseases of the Newborn*, 8th edition.

Complete references and supplemental color images used in this text can be found online at www.expertconsult.com

PATENT DUCTUS ARTERIOSUS IN THE PRETERM INFANT

Ronald I. Clyman

The ductus arteriosus represents a persistence of the terminal portion of the sixth branchial arch. During fetal life, the ductus arteriosus serves to divert blood away from the fluid-filled lungs toward the descending aorta and placenta. After birth, constriction of the ductus arteriosus and obliteration of its lumen results in separation of the pulmonary and systemic circulations. In full-term infants, obliteration of the ductus arteriosus takes place through a process of vasoconstriction and anatomic remodeling. In the preterm, the ductus arteriosus frequently fails to close. The clinical consequences of a patent ductus arteriosus (PDA) are related to the degree of left-to-right shunt through the PDA with its associated change in blood flow to the lungs, kidneys, and intestines. Although the magnitude of shunt flow plays a significant role in creating neonatal morbidity, equally important factors are the duration of exposure to the shunt and the infant's ability to compensate for the shunt.

DIAGNOSIS

Two-dimensional echocardiography and color Doppler flow mapping are the gold standards for assessing the magnitude and direction of PDA shunting. Ductus diameter ≥1.5 mm, left atrial-to-aortic root (LA:Ao) ratio ≥1.5, reversal of forward blood flow in the descending aorta during diastole, and end-diastolic flow velocity in the left pulmonary artery ≥0.20 m/s are signs consistent with a moderate-to-large PDA shunt (Table 54-1) (El Hajjar et al, 2005).

Clinical signs of a PDA (systolic murmur, hyperdynamic precordial impulse, full pulses, widened pulse pressure, and/or worsening respiratory status) usually appear later than echocardiographic signs and are less sensitive in determining the degree of left-to-right shunt. Certain signs such as continuous murmur or hyperactive left ventricular impulse are relatively specific for a PDA but lack sensitivity; conversely, worsening respiratory status, although a sensitive indicator, is relatively nonspecific for a PDA. Tachycardia is not a useful or reliable indicator of a PDA in preterm infants. Infants with large left-to-right shunts may have evidence of cardiomegaly and increased pulmonary arterial markings on their chest radiographs; however, in general, the chest radiograph and electrocardiogram are not useful in diagnosing a PDA. Although elevated plasma concentrations of brain natriuretic peptide (BNP) correlate with the presence of a moderate sized left-to-right PDA shunt (El-Khuffash and Molloy, 2007), changes in BNP concentrations have poor sensitivity and specificity in predicting increases or decreases in PDA shunt magnitude (Chen et al, 2010).

INCIDENCE

Pulsed Doppler echocardiographic assessments of full-term infants indicate that functional closure of the ductus has occurred in almost 50% by 24 hours, in 90% by 48 hours, and in all by 72 hours. The rate of ductus closure is delayed in preterm infants; however, essentially all healthy preterm infants (and 90% of those with respiratory distress syndrome) who are ≥30 weeks' gestation will close their ductus by the 4th day after birth. Preterm infants of <30 weeks' gestation, with severe respiratory distress, have a 65% incidence of persistent ductus patency beyond the 4th day of life. Even among these infants, spontaneous closure can occur during the neonatal period. Sixty-seven percent of very low-birthweight (VLBW) infants (weighing between 1000 and 1500 g at birth) will spontaneously close their ductus by 7 days after birth (94% will close before hospital discharge) (Nemerofsky et al, 2008). On the other hand, spontaneous, ductus closure only occurs in 30% to 35% of infants weighing <1000 g at birth during the neonatal period (Koch et al, 2006; Nemerofsky et al, 2008). Among VLBW infants who are discharged from the hospital with a persistent PDA, 14% will still have a persistent PDA or have had coil occlusion of their PDA at 1 year of age (Herrman et al, 2009).

Infants who are small for gestational age (Cotton et al, 1981; Del Moral et al, 2007; Rakza et al, 2007), develop late-onset septicemia (Gonzalez et al, 1996), or receive excessive fluid administration during the first days of life also are more likely to develop a clinically symptomatic PDA (Bell and Acarregui, 2001). On the other hand, nonwhite infants and infants who receive antenatal glucocorticoids have a reduced risk of PDA (Chorne et al, 2007a; Clyman et al, 1981a; Furzan et al, 1985). Administration of exogenous surfactant can alter both the incidence and presentation of a PDA. Although surfactant has no effect on the contractile behavior of the ductus, its effects on pulmonary vascular resistance lead to an earlier clinical presentation of the left-to-right shunt in preterm animals (Clyman et al, 1982; Shimada et al, 1989) and humans (Alpan et al, 1995; Kaapa et al, 1993; Reller et al, 1991, 1993). Similarly, lowering the "tolerable" range of oxygen saturations in preterm infants has led to an increased incidence of PDA (see later discussion of effects of oxygen on the ductus) (Noori et al, 2009).

REGULATION OF DUCTUS ARTERIOSUS PATENCY

In the full-term infant, closure of the ductus arteriosus occurs in two phases: (1) "functional" closure of the lumen within the first hours after birth by smooth muscle constriction, and (2) "anatomic" occlusion of the lumen over the next several days due to extensive neointimal thickening and loss of smooth muscle cells from the inner muscle media.

TABLE 54-1   Echocardiographic Characteristics Associated With Different Degrees of PDA Left-to-Right Shunts

PDA Shunt	Ductus Diameter (mm)		LA:Ao Ratio		LPA Diastolic Velocity (m/s)		DAo Flow Reversal	
	>1.5 (%)	<1.5 (%)	>1.5 (%)	<1.5 (%)	>0.2 (%)	≤0.2 (%)	Yes (%)	No (%)
Closed	0	100	0	100	0	100	0	100
Small	33	67	26	74	12	88	8	92
Moderate	86	14	56	44	53	47	60	40
Large	98	2	74	26	93	7	95	5

Data modified from Chen S, Tacy T, Clyman RI: Utility of B-type natriuretic peptide measurements for monitoring changes in patent ductus arteriosus shunt magnitude, *E-PAS* 2010. *DAo flow reversal*, Holodiastolic flow reversal in the descending aorta; *LA:Ao ratio*, left atrial:aortic root ratio; *LPA diastolic velocity*, left pulmonary artery end-diastolic velocity.

BALANCE BETWEEN VASOCONSTRICTION AND VASORELAXATION

Ductus arteriosus patency, therefore, is determined by the balance between dilating and constricting forces. The factors known to play a prominent role in ductus arteriosus regulation involve those that promote constriction (oxygen, endothelin, calcium channels, catecholamines, and Rho kinase) and those that oppose it (intraluminal pressure, prostaglandins, nitric oxide, carbon monoxide, potassium channels, cyclic adenosine monophosphate [cAMP] and cyclic guanosine monophosphate [cGMP]). The relative importance of each of these factors depends on the intrauterine and extrauterine environment, the degree of ductus maturation, and the genetic background and species being studied.

In Utero Regulation

The fetal ductus normally has a high level of intrinsic tone (Kajino et al, 2001). The intrinsic tone is due to mechanisms that both depend on and are independent of extracellular calcium (Kajino et al, 2001). The contractile proteins (smooth muscle myosin, calponin, and caldesmon) are more differentiated in the ductus than they are in adjacent fetal arteries (Colbert et al, 1996; Sakurai et al, 1996; Slomp et al, 1997). In addition, the fetal ductus arteriosus is more sensitive to the contractile effects of calcium than are the aorta and the pulmonary artery (Crichton et al, 1997). This may be due in part to increased Rho kinase activity in the ductus (Clyman et al, 2007). Endothelin-1 also appears to play a role in producing the elevated basal tone of the fetal ductus arteriosus (Coceani et al, 1999). Although catecholamines can constrict the ductus arteriosus (Tomita et al, 1996), there is little information about their role or the role of ductus innervation in regulating ductus tone. The presence of catecholamine-containing nerves varies with the species being studied (Bergwerff et al, 1999). The presence of high circulating catecholamine concentrations during the transition to extrauterine life suggests a role for catecholamines in ductus closure (Padbury et al, 1985).

The factors that oppose ductus arteriosus constriction in utero are better understood. The elevated vascular pressure within the ductus lumen (due to the constricted pulmonary vascular bed) plays an important role in opposing ductus constriction (Clyman et al, 1989a). The fetal ductus also produces several vasodilators that maintain its patency. Vasodilator prostaglandins (PGs) appear to be the dominant vasodilators that oppose ductus constriction in the later part of gestation (Momma et al, 1999). Inhibitors of prostaglandin synthesis constrict the fetal ductus both in vitro and in vivo. PGE_2 is the most potent prostaglandin produced by the ductus (Clyman et al, 1978; Coceani et al, 1978) and appears to be the most important prostanoid to regulate ductus patency. The response of the ductus to PGE_2 is unique among blood vessels because it is extraordinarily sensitive to this vasodilating substance. Prostaglandin E_2 produces ductus relaxation by interacting with several of the prostaglandin E receptors (EP_2, EP_3, and EP_4) (Bouayad et al, 2001). In contrast with other blood vessels, all of the EP receptors in the ductus can activate adenylate cyclase and relax the vessel (Bouayad et al, 2001). The increased cAMP concentrations inhibit the sensitivity of the contractile proteins to calcium (Crichton et al, 1997). Inhibitors of phosphodiesterase (the enzyme that degrades cAMP) relax the ductus in utero (Toyoshima et al, 2006). Low phosphodiesterase levels in the fetal ductus account for its increased sensitivity to PGE_2 (Liu et al, 2008). In addition, one of the EP receptors (EP_3) also relaxes the ductus by opening K_{ATP} channels and hyperpolarizing the smooth muscle cells (Bouayad et al, 2001).

Both isoforms of the enzyme responsible for synthesizing prostaglandins (cyclooxygenase [COX]-1 and COX-2) are expressed in the fetal ductus (Takahashi et al, 2000). Depending on the species, both nonselective (e.g., indomethacin and ibuprofen) and selective cyclooxygenase inhibitors constrict the ductus. In the fetal mouse, COX-2 appears to be the COX isoform responsible for producing the prostaglandins that regulate the ductus (Loftin et al, 2001), whereas in the fetal sheep, both COX-1 and COX-2 play a role in ductus patency (Takahashi et al, 2000).

In addition to the prostaglandins that are made within the ductus wall, circulating PGE_2 concentrations also regulate fetal ductus tone. Circulating concentrations of PGE_2 appear to be of placental origin (Thorburn, 1992). In the late-gestation fetal lamb, the circulating concentrations of PGE_2 (approximately 1 nM) are close to those that produce maximal relaxation of the ductus (Clyman et al, 1980). Circulating PGE_2 is cleared primarily by the pulmonary endothelium. Decreased pulmonary blood flow in the fetus results in reduced pulmonary clearance and contributes to the elevated fetal plasma PGE_2 concentrations (Clyman et al, 1981b).

Nitric oxide (NO), formed mainly by endothelial nitric oxide synthase (eNOS), is made by the fetal ductus arteriosus. NO appears to play an important role, early in gestation, in maintaining ductus patency in rodent fetuses (Momma et al, 1999). PGE_2 and NO appear to be preferentially coupled for reciprocal compensation because cyclooxygenase inhibition upregulates NO (Sodini et al, 2008). Although NO is also made in the ductus of larger species, its importance in maintaining ductus patency under normal in utero conditions has not been conclusively demonstrated (see later discussion of the role of NO in fetuses exposed to indomethacin tocolysis and in premature newborns) (Fox et al, 1996).

Carbon monoxide relaxes the ductus arteriosus, and both hemoxygenase-1 and -2 (the enzymes that make carbon monoxide) are found within the endothelial and smooth muscle cells of the ductus. Under physiologic conditions, the amount of carbon monoxide made by the ductus does not seem to affect ductus tone; however, in circumstances where its synthesis is upregulated, such as in endotoxemia, it may exert a relaxing influence on the ductus (Coceani et al, 1997). There is little evidence to suggest that adenosine or β-adrenergic stimulation play a significant role in ductus patency (Friedman et al, 1983).

Although the initial response to, pharmacologic inhibition of prostaglandin synthesis and signaling is to constrict the ductus in utero (Momma et al, 2005), chronic inhibition of prostaglandin synthesis (Loftin et al, 2001; Reese et al, 2006) and signaling (Nguyen et al, 1997) produces the opposite effect: namely, a persistent patent ductus in utero and a newborn mouse that fails to close its ductus after birth (Loftin et al, 2001; Nguyen et al, 1997). The exact mechanisms responsible for the persistent ductus patency that follows chronic inhibition of prostaglandin signaling have yet to be elucidated. Inhibition of prostaglandin production leads to increased nitric oxide production (Baragatti et al, 2003, 2007); however, inhibition of nitric oxide production does not appear to increase the rate of ductus closure in the COX-null mice (Reese et al, 2006). Inhibition of prostaglandin signaling may also contribute to delayed closure by inhibiting hyaluronic acid production and intimal cushion formation in the ductus (Yokoyama et al, 2006a). Intimal cushions play an important role in permanent ductus closure after birth (see later discussion). In addition to its function as a vasodilator, PGE_2 also plays a significant role in the development of ductus contractility (Reese et al, 2009). PGE_2 is necessary for the expression of several genes that control postnatal oxygen-induced ductus constriction (see later discussion). Specifically, PGE_2 increases the expression of CaL- and K^+-channel genes (CaLalpha1c, CaLbeta2, Kir6.1, and Kv1.5), which regulate calcium entry, without affecting genes that regulate calcium sensitization (Rho kinase–associated genes). Chronic inhibition of prostaglandin synthesis decreases the expression of CaL- and K^+-channel genes. Phosphodiesterase expression, which decreases the ductus's sensitivity to cAMP- or cGMP-dependent vasodilators, is also decreased by chronic COX inhibition (Reese et al, 2009).

It is interesting to note that pharmacologic inhibition of prostaglandin synthesis in human pregnancy also is associated with an increased incidence of patent ductus arteriosus after birth (Norton et al, 1993). However, this appears to be due to indomethacin's ability to produce ductus constriction in utero. In utero constriction produces ischemic hypoxia, increased nitric oxide production, and smooth muscle cell death within the ductus wall. These factors prevent the ductus from constricting after birth and make it resistant to the constrictive effects of postnatal indomethacin (Clyman et al, 2001; Goldbarg et al, 2002).

Postnatal Regulation

There are several events that promote ductus constriction in the full-term newborn after delivery: (1) an increase in arterial PO_2, (2) a decrease in blood pressure within the ductus lumen (due to the postnatal decrease in pulmonary vascular resistance), (3) a decrease in circulating PGE_2 (due to the loss of placental prostaglandin production and the increase in prostaglandin removal by the lung), and (4) a decrease in the number of PGE_2 receptors in the ductus wall (Bouayad et al, 2001). Although the newborn ductus continues to be sensitive to the vasodilating effects of NO, it loses its ability to respond to PGE_2 (Abrams et al, 1995; Clyman et al, 1983). All of these factors promote ductus constriction after birth.

The postnatal increase in arterial PaO_2 plays an important role in ductus constriction. Normoxic contraction can be demonstrated in the absence of the ductus endothelium (Fay, 1971), and in the presence of inhibitors of prostaglandin, nitric oxide, and endothelin signaling. This suggests that these vasoactive substances are not essential for normoxic constriction. In most species, oxygen appears to constrict the ductus arteriosus (1) through a mechanism that involves smooth muscle depolarization and (2) through a mechanism that is independent of changes in membrane potential (Roulet and Coburn, 1981). Oxygen depolarizes the ductus smooth muscle cells by inhibiting K^+ channels (Michelakis et al, 2000; Reeve et al, 2001). Following the depolarization of the membrane, calcium enters the ductus smooth muscle through L-type (Clyman et al, 2007; Nakanishi et al, 1993) and T-type (Akaike et al, 2009; Yokoyama et al, 2006b) voltage-dependent calcium channels. Several O_2-sensitive K^+ channels have been found in the fetal ductus (including Kv1.5 and Kv2.1). These vary with species and gestational age and may account for the differing sensitivity of the ductus to oxygen (Hayama et al, 2006; Wu et al, 2007). Oxygen also appears to have a direct effect on the CaL-channels themselves (Thebaud et al, 2008) and on the store-operated calcium channels (Hong et al, 2006). In addition, oxygen may increase smooth muscle sensitivity to calcium by activating Rho kinase–mediated pathways (Hong et al, 2006; Kajimoto et al, 2007; Keck et al, 2005; Roulet and Coburn, 1981).

The unique oxygen sensors within the ductus wall are still not clearly elucidated and may vary by species. The mitochondrial electron transport chain may act as an oxygen sensor by generating reactive oxygen species that constrict the avian, rabbit, and human ductus (Cogolludo et al, 2009; Michelakis et al, 2002; Reeve et al, 2001). This does not appear to be the mechanism in the ovine ductus (Clyman et al, 1989b), where reactive oxygen species dilate the ductus, and where the oxygen-induced events appear to involve a cytochrome P450 hemoprotein (Coceani et al, 1989a, 1994). Preterm infants treated with cytochrome P450 inhibitors have an increased incidence of PDA (Cotton et al, 2009).

Elevated oxygen tensions can also increase the formation of the potent vasoconstrictor endothelin-1 (Coceani et al, 1989b). The exact role of endothelin-1 in postnatal ductus closure is still unclear (Coceani et al, 1999; Fineman et al, 1998; Michelakis et al, 2000; Shen et al, 2002; Taniguchi and Muramatsu, 2003). This is due, in large part, to the marked species variation in its contribution to ductus constriction. Endothelin receptor stimulation accounts for 44% of the oxygen-induced constriction in the rat, but only 13% in the rabbit (Shen et al, 2002). In the human ductus, inhibition of endothelin production does not inhibit oxygen-induced constriction (Michelakis et al, 2000).

Although the contractile effects of oxygen play an important role in postnatal ductus constriction, they may not be essential for postnatal ductus closure. Mice lacking the endothelin A receptor have diminished oxygen-induced ductus constriction; however, their ductus closes normally after birth (Coceani et al, 1999). The postnatal increase in PaO_2 also has profound modulatory effects on other vasoactive systems (Smith, 1998). Elevated oxygen tensions can increase the ductus's contractile response to neural mediators (Ikeda et al, 1973) and can decrease the formation of vasodilator prostaglandins (Kajino et al, 2001). Although neural and hormonal factors contribute to ductus closure, they do not appear to mediate the oxygen-induced constriction itself.

Developmental Regulation

Gestational age has a marked effect on the rate of ductus closure after birth. In contrast with the full-term ductus, the premature ductus is less likely to constrict after birth. This is due to several mechanisms. The intrinsic tone of the extremely immature ductus (<70% of gestation) is decreased compared to the ductus at term (Kajino et al, 2001). This may be due to the presence of immature smooth muscle myosin isoforms, with a weaker contractile capacity (Brown et al, 2002; Colbert et al, 1996; Reeve et al, 1997; Sakurai et al, 1996) and to decreased Rho kinase expression and activity (Clyman et al, 2007; Cogolludo et al, 2009; Kajimoto et al, 2007). Calcium entry through L-type calcium channels appears to be impaired in the immature ductus (especially under hypoxic conditions) (Clyman et al, 2007; Cogolludo et al, 2009; Thebaud et al, 2008). The potassium channels that promote ductus relaxation also change during gestation (switching from K_{Ca} channels, which are not regulated by oxygen tension, to K_V channels, which can be inhibited by increased oxygen concentrations) (Thebaud et al, 2004; Waleh et al, 2009; Wu et al, 2007). Reduced expression and function of the putative oxygen-sensing K_V channels appear to contribute to ductus patency in the preterm rabbit, sheep, baboon, mouse, and chicken (Cogolludo et al, 2009; Thebaud et al, 2004; Waleh et al, 2009). In contrast, a decrease in K_V channel expression occurs with advancing gestation in the rat, which suggests that in that species DA closure may occur by eliminating K_V channels (Wu et al, 2007).

Although circulating catecholamine concentrations are elevated during the transition to extrauterine life (Padbury et al, 1985), immature animals are less responsive to circulating catecholamines than are animals near term (Agren et al, 2007; Padbury et al, 1985).

Premature infants have elevated circulating concentrations of PGE_2, which may play a significant role in maintaining ductus patency during the first days after birth. This is due to the decreased ability of the premature lung to clear circulating PGE_2 (Clyman et al, 1981b). In the preterm newborn, circulating concentrations of PGE_2 can reach the pharmacologic range during episodes of bacteremia and necrotizing enterocolitis and are often associated with reopening of a previously constricted ductus arteriosus (Gonzalez et al, 1996).

In most mammalian species, the major factor that prevents the preterm ductus from constricting after birth is its increased sensitivity to the vasodilating effects of PGE_2 and NO (Clyman et al, 1998). The preterm ductus's increased sensitivity to PGE_2 is due to increased cAMP signaling. There is both increased cAMP production, due to enhanced prostaglandin receptor coupling with adenyl cyclase, and decreased cyclic AMP degradation by phosphodiesterase in the preterm ductus (Liu et al, 2008; Waleh et al, 2004). As a result, inhibitors of prostaglandin production (e.g., indomethacin, ibuprofen, and mefenamic acid) are usually effective agents in promoting ductus closure in the premature infant. It follows that drugs interfering with NO synthesis or function also could become useful adjuncts, especially in situations where indomethacin has proven to be ineffective (Keller et al, 2005; Seidner et al, 2001).

Increased prostaglandin sensitivity can also contribute to delayed ductus closure in some late gestation newborns. Among infants ≥37 weeks' gestation with a persistent PDA, approximately 30% will close their PDA after indomethacin treatment and another 30% will develop partial ductus constriction (Takami et al, 2007).

The factors responsible for the changes that occur with advancing gestation are currently unknown. Prenatal administration of vitamin A has been shown to increase both the intracellular calcium response and the contractile response of the preterm ductus to oxygen (Wu et al, 2001). However, vitamin A administration does not improve the rate of ductus closure in preterm infants (Ravishankar et al, 2003). Thyroid hormones may play a role in ductus arteriosus maturation because full-term infants with congenital hypothyroidism have an increased incidence of PDA that appears to respond to thyroid hormone replacement therapy (Guarnieri et al, 2008). Similarly, a lower occurrence of PDA has been found in thyroid hormone–treated preterm infants (Osborn and Hunt, 2007; van Wassemaer and Kok, 2008). Elevated cortisol concentrations in the fetus also foster ductus maturation by decreasing the sensitivity of the ductus to the vasodilating effects of PGE_2 (Clyman et al, 1981c). Prenatal administration of glucocorticoids significantly reduces the incidence of PDA in premature humans and animals (Clyman et al, 1981a, 1981c; Collaborative Group on Antenatal Steroid Therapy, 1985; Momma et al, 1981; Thibeault et al, 1978; Waffarn et al, 1983). Postnatal glucocorticoid administration also reduces the incidence of PDA (Group VONSS, 2001). However, postnatal glucocorticoid treatment also increases the incidence of several other neonatal morbidities (Watterberg et al, 2004).

Genetic Regulation

Both species and genetic background play a significant role in determining the relative importance of ductus regulatory pathways. There is a marked species difference among several of these pathways: Although endothelin receptor stimulation may account for 44% of the oxygen-induced contraction in the rat, it contributes to only 13% of the contraction in the rabbit (Shen et al, 2002) and plays a negligible role in the human ductus (Michelakis et al, 2000). Oxygen depolarizes the ductus smooth muscle cells by inhibiting K channels (Michelakis et al, 2000; Reeve et al, 2001). In the rabbit, an increase in the expression of K_V channels appears to be responsible for the developmental increase in the oxygen-induced contraction (Thebaud et al, 2004). In contrast, in the rat, K_V channel expression decreases with advancing gestation (Wu et al, 2007). Ductus patency is critically dependent on vasodilator prostaglandins in most species; however, notable exceptions exist in the guinea pig, chicken, and emu ductus, where locally derived prostaglandins do not appear to play a role in patency (Agren et al, 2007; Bodach et al, 1980; Dzialowski and Greyner, 2008).

Several genes have been identified (from mouse mutation models and from human genetic syndromes) that are associated with PDA in the full-term neonate. These include homeobox genes (Prx1 and Prx2) (Bergwerff et al, 2000); chromosomal region 12q24, designated PDA1 (Mani et al, 2002); the Noonan's syndrome gene, PTPN11 (Ko et al, 2008); and genes that regulate myosin heavy chains (Morano et al, 2000; Zhu et al, 2006), filamin 1 (Anderson et al, 2009), prostaglandin signaling (COX2 and EP4) (Loftin et al, 2001; Segi et al, 1998), gap junctions (connexin 43) (Huang et al, 1998), and neural crest transcription factors (TFAP2B and myocardin) (Huang et al, 2008; Zhao et al, 2001).

Although Bhandari et al (2009) found that familial factors accounted for 76% of the variance in risk for persistent PDA in preterm twins, they attributed most of the effect to shared environmental rather than genetic factors. On the other hand, several single nucleotide polymorphisms (SNPs) in candidate genes have been identified that are associated with PDA in preterm infants: ATR type 1 (Treszl et al, 2003), interferon (IFN)-γ (Bokodi et al, 2007), estrogen receptor-alpha PvuII (Derzbach et al, 2005), TFAP2B, PGI synthase, and TRAF1 (Dagle et al, 2009). Recent studies suggest that an interaction between preterm birth and TFAP2B may be responsible for some of the PDAs that occur in preterm infants: TFAP2B is uniquely expressed in ductus smooth muscle (Ivey et al, 2008); it regulates other genes that are important in ductus smooth muscle development (Ivey et al, 2008); mutations in TFAP2B produce PDA in mice and humans (Zhao et al, 2001); and TFAP2B polymorphisms are associated with preterm PDAs (especially those that are unresponsive to indomethacin) (Dagle et al, 2009).

ANATOMIC CLOSURE: HISTOLOGIC CHANGES

In the full-term newborn there is progressive intimal thickening and fragmentation of the internal elastic lamina after delivery. As the intima increases in size, it ultimately forms mounds that occlude the already constricted lumen. The increase in intimal thickening is due (1) to migration of smooth muscle cells from the muscle media into the intima and (2) to proliferation of luminal endothelial cells. The process of intimal cushion formation starts with the accumulation of hyalurona (HA) below the luminal endothelial cells. This is accompanied by the loss of laminin and collagen IV from the basement membrane of the endothelial cells and their subsequent separation from the internal elastic lamina. Laminin and collagen IV ultimately reform under the detached endothelial cells, but HA continues to accumulate in the subendothelial space. The hygroscopic properties of HA cause an influx of water and widening of the subendothelial space; this creates an environment well suited for cell migration. Accompanying the increase in HA is an increase in fibronectin (FN) and chondroitin sulfate (CS) in the neointimal space (de Reeder et al, 1988). The endothelial and smooth muscle cells of the ductus arteriosus differ from those of the adjacent vessels in their ability to form neointimal cushions. Isolated endothelial cells of the ductus arteriosus have an increased rate of HA, FN, and CS accumulation compared with those of the aorta or pulmonary artery (Boudreau et al, 1992). Hyaluron makes ductus smooth muscle cells migrate faster. The potentiating effect of HA on ductus smooth muscle cells is mediated through a hyaluron-binding protein (RHAMM). After delivery, there is a marked increase in ductus arteriosus transforming growth factor (TGF)-β expression, which accentuates the accumulation of HA within the neointima. Prostaglandins, acting through the EP4 receptor, also appear to play a critical role in HA production in the ductus (Yokoyama et al, 2006a). Fibronectin plays an important role in facilitating ductus smooth muscle cell migration. When fibronectin production in the ductus is inhibited, intimal cushion formation is blocked (Mason et al, 1999). CS appears to have no direct effect on ductus smooth muscle cell migration (Boudreau et al, 1990).

Ductus arteriosus smooth muscle cells use a family of cell surface receptors, called integrins, to interact with, adhere to, and migrate through the extracellular matrix that surrounds them. When ductus smooth muscle cells of the inner muscle media begin to migrate into the subendothelial space, two new integrin complexes appear on their cell surface: the αvβ3 and the α5β1 receptors. The αvβ3 integrin is essential for migration of ductus smooth muscle cells in vitro. The α5β1 integrin binds exclusively to fibronectin and mediates the potentiating effects of fibronectin on ductus smooth muscle cell migration. During the process of migration, ductus smooth muscle cells secrete laminin, which also has an important promigratory role.

Intimal cushion formation in the ductus is also associated with striking alterations in elastin fiber assembly. In contrast to the aorta, where formation of well-developed elastic laminae is seen between layers of muscle cells, smooth muscle cells of the ductus muscle media are surrounded by thin and fragmented elastin fibers. Smooth muscle cells in the neointima are surrounded by even fewer elastin fibers (de Reeder et al, 1990). The disruption of normal elastin fiber assembly in the ductus does not appear to be due to increased elastase activity or decreased tropoelastin production. Rather, it appears to be due to a developmental mechanism that reduces insolubilization of elastin and prevents formation of intact elastic laminae (Hinek et al, 1991; Hinek and Rabinovitch, 1993; Zhu et al, 1993). The exact relationship between impaired elastin assembly and smooth muscle migration into the neointima is still open for speculation. Impaired assembly of thick elastic laminae might facilitate smooth muscle cell migration by removing a physical barrier to which they might attach. The elastic laminae of the ductus appear abnormally well developed and similar to those in the aorta in some genetic forms of PDA; when this occurs, intimal cushions fail to develop (de Reeder et al, 1990).

RELATIONSHIP BETWEEN VASOCONSTRICTION AND ANATOMIC CLOSURE

In full-term animals, loss of responsiveness to PGE$_2$ shortly after birth prevents the ductus arteriosus from reopening once it has constricted (Abrams et al, 1995; Clyman et al, 1983). This is due, in part, to decreased synthesis of PGE$_2$ receptors in the ductus after birth. Both the loss of vasodilator regulation and the anatomic events that lead to permanent closure appear to be controlled by the degree of ductus smooth muscle constriction. Experimental models that alter the ability of the ductus to constrict at term also prevent the normal histologic changes that occur after birth (Clyman et al, 1989a; Fay and Cooke, 1972; Jarkovska et al, 1992; Loftin et al, 2001; Mason et al, 1999; Nguyen et al, 1997). Constriction produces ischemic hypoxia of the vessel wall (Clyman et al, 1999). In the full-term newborn ductus, the ischemic hypoxia that accompanies constriction is due to loss of intramural vasa vasorum blood flow, which occurs even before luminal blood flow has been eliminated (Kajino et al, 2002). With advancing gestation, the thickness of the ductus wall increases to a dimension that requires the presence of intramural vasa vasorum to provide nutrients to its outer half. These collapsible, intramural vasa vasorum provide the ductus with a unique mechanism for controlling the maximal diffusion distance for oxygen and nutrients across its wall. In the full-term newborn, the intramural tissue pressure that develops during ductus constriction obliterates vasa vasorum flow to its muscle media; this turns the entire thickness of the muscle media into a virtual avascular zone. The profound ischemic hypoxia that follows the compression of the vasa vasorum inhibits local production of PGE$_2$ and NO, induces local production of hypoxia inducible factors such as HIF1α and vascular endothelial growth factor (VEGF), and produces smooth muscle apoptosis in the ductus wall. VEGF plays a critical role in the migration of the ductus smooth muscle cells into the neointima and in the proliferation of intramural vasa vasorum (Clyman et al, 2002). After postnatal ductus constriction, several genes known to be essential for vascular remodeling (TGF-β, VCAM-1, E-selectin, IL-8, MCSF-1, CD154, IFN-γ, IL-6, and TNF-α) are increased in the ductus wall. In addition, VLA4-positive monocytes/macrophages (CD68- and CD14-positive) adhere to the ductus wall. The inflammatory response that follows postnatal ductus constriction may be as necessary for ductus remodeling, because the extent of neointimal remodeling is significantly correlated with the degree of mononuclear cell adhesion (Waleh et al, 2005).

In preterm infants, the ductus frequently remains open for many days after birth, preventing it from developing profound hypoxic ischemia. Although alterations in prostaglandin signaling appear to be responsible for as many as 60% to 70% of the delayed ductus closures, cyclooxygenase inhibitors (such as indomethacin and ibuprofen) become less effective in closing the ductus with increasing postnatal age. A number of factors conspire to make the postnatal preterm ductus increasingly resistant to indomethacin- and ibuprofen-induced closure. After delivery, COX-2 expression and PGE$_2$ production increase in the ductus wall (Guerguerian et al, 1998). However, in contrast to the full-term ductus, where all of the PGE$_2$ EP receptors are downregulated after birth, in the preterm ductus, the dominant PGE$_2$ receptor, EP$_4$, continues to be synthesized after birth and the ductus continues to relax with prostaglandin stimulation. In addition, despite the presence of persistent ductus luminal blood flow, there is a progressive decrease in ATP concentrations within the preterm newborn ductus smooth muscle cells. The decreased ATP concentrations limit the preterm newborn ductus's ability to constrict (Levin et al, 2005). Similarly, the mild degrees of hypoxia that develop within the postnatal preterm ductus induce the production of other vasodilators within its wall that do not depend on prostaglandin signaling to affect contractility (e.g., nitric oxide, TNF-α, and IL-6) (Clyman et al, 2002; Waleh et al, 2005). These "other" vasodilators produce a change in the vasodilator-balance that maintains ductus patency. Ductus patency becomes less dependent on prostaglandin generation and more dependent on other vasodilators during the first weeks after birth. These postnatal changes may explain why the effectiveness of indomethacin wanes with increasing postnatal age (Clyman, 1996; Schmidt et al, 2001). In premature animals and humans, the combined use of a nitric oxide synthase inhibitor and indomethacin produces a much greater degree of ductus constriction than indomethacin alone (Keller et al, 2005; Seidner et al, 2001). It follows that drugs that interfere with NO synthesis could become a useful adjunct, especially in situations where indomethacin has been found to be ineffective.

Even when it does constrict, the premature ductus frequently fails to develop the same degree of profound hypoxia and anatomic remodeling that occurs in the full-term newborn ductus. The preterm ductus requires a greater degree of constriction, and a more complete degree of luminal closure, than the full-term ductus in order to develop a comparable degree of hypoxia. This is due to the thinness of the preterm ductus wall. In contrast with the full-term ductus, the thin-walled preterm ductus can extract all of the oxygen and nutrients it needs from its luminal blood flow. The preterm ductus does not need intramural vasa vasorum to provide oxygen and nutrients to its wall, and, as a result, before 26 weeks' gestation, intramural vasa vasorum are absent from the ductus wall. The absence of intramural vasa vasorum leaves the preterm ductus without a mechanism to rapidly increase the diffusion distance across its wall during postnatal constriction. As long as there is any degree of luminal patency and flow, the thin-walled preterm ductus fails to become profoundly hypoxic and fails to undergo anatomic remodeling. The preterm ductus requires that the lumen be completely obliterated before it can develop the same degree of hypoxia found at term. Once the preterm ductus develops profound ischemic hypoxia, it will undergo most of the anatomic changes seen at term (Kajino et al, 2001; Seidner et al, 2001). However, if the premature ductus does not develop the degree of ischemic hypoxia needed to induce cell death and anatomic remodeling, it will continue to be responsive to vasodilators and continue to be susceptible to vessel reopening.

HEMODYNAMIC AND PULMONARY ALTERATIONS

The pathophysiologic features of a PDA depend both on the magnitude of the left-to-right shunt and on the cardiac and pulmonary responses to the shunt. There are important differences between immature and mature infants in the heart's ability to handle a volume load. Immature infants have less cardiac sympathetic innervation. Before term, the myocardium has more water and less contractile mass. Therefore, the immature fetal ventricles are less distensible than at term and generate less force per gram of myocardium (even though they have the same ability to generate force per sarcomere) (Friedman, 1972). The relative lack of left ventricular distensibility in immature infants is more a function of the ventricle's tissue constituents than of poor muscle function. As a result, left ventricular distention secondary to a large left-to-right PDA shunt may produce a higher left ventricular end-diastolic pressure at smaller ventricular volumes. The increase in left ventricular pressure increases pulmonary venous pressure and causes pulmonary congestion.

Studies in preterm animal and human newborns (Clyman et al, 1987; Shimada et al, 1994) have shown that despite these limitations, preterm newborns are able to increase left ventricular output, and maintain their "effective" systemic blood flow, even with left-to-right PDA shunts equal to 50% of left ventricular output. With shunts >50% of left ventricular output, "effective" systemic blood flow falls, despite a continued increase in left ventricular output. The increase in left ventricular output associated with a PDA is accomplished not by an increase in heart rate, but by an increase in stroke volume (Clyman et al, 1987; Shimada et al, 1994). Stroke volume increases primarily as a result of the simultaneous decrease in afterload resistance on the heart and the increase in left ventricular preload. Despite the ability of the left ventricle to increase its output in the face of a left-to-right ductus shunt, blood flow distribution is significantly rearranged. This redistribution of systemic blood flow occurs even with small shunts (Clyman et al, 1987). Blood flow to the skin, bone, and skeletal muscle is most likely to be affected by the left-to-right ductus shunt. The next most likely organs to be affected are the gastrointestinal tract and kidneys because of a combination of decreased perfusion pressure and localized vasoconstriction. Mesenteric blood flow is decreased in both fasting and fed states in the presence of a PDA (McCurnin and Clyman, 2008). Significant decreases in organ blood flow may occur before there are signs of left ventricular compromise (Meyers et al, 1990; Shimada et al, 1994) and may contribute to

the decreased feeding tolerance and decreased glomerular filtration rate (Cassady et al, 1989; Clyman, 1996; Patole et al, 2007) that have been observed with ductus patency.

The decreased ability of the preterm infant to maintain active pulmonary vasoconstriction (Lewis et al, 1976) may be responsible in part for the earlier presentation of a "large" left-to-right PDA shunt (Gersony et al, 1983; Jacob et al, 1980). Dopamine can increase systemic blood pressure and systemic blood flow in preterm infants with hypotension and a PDA, by increasing pulmonary vascular resistance and decreasing the left-to-right shunt across the ductus (Bouissou et al, 2008). Therapeutic maneuvers, such as surfactant replacement, or prenatal conditions, such as intrauterine growth retardation, that lead to a rapid drop in pulmonary vascular resistance can exacerbate the amount of left-to-right shunt and lead to pulmonary hemorrhage (Alpan et al, 1995; Raju and Langenberg, 1993; Rakza et al, 2007). Randomized, controlled trials have shown that early ductus closure decreases the incidence of significant pulmonary hemorrhage (Al Faleh et al, 2008; Clyman and Chorne, 2008; Domanico et al, 1994). Although phototherapy has been associated with the persistence of a PDA, a recent randomized controlled trial found that chest shielding did not alter the incidence or severity of PDA (Travadi et al, 2006).

The factors responsible for preventing plasma fluid and protein from moving into the lung interstitium and from the interstitium into the air spaces have been described elsewhere. In premature animals, a wide-open PDA increases hydraulic pressures in the pulmonary vasculature; this, in turn, increases the rate of fluid transudation into the pulmonary interstitium (Alpan et al, 1991). Any increase in microvascular perfusion pressure in premature infants with respiratory distress syndrome may increase interstitial and alveolar lung fluid because of their low plasma oncotic pressures and increased capillary permeability. Leakage of plasma proteins into the alveolar space inhibits surfactant function and increases surface tension in the immature air sacs (Ikegami et al, 1983), which are already compromised by surfactant deficiency. The increased FiO_2 and mean airway pressures required to overcome these early changes in compliance may be important factors in the development of chronic lung disease (Brown, 1979; Clyman, 1996; Cotton et al, 1978). Depending on the gestational age and the species examined, changes in pulmonary mechanics may occur as early as 1 day after birth or not before several days of exposure to a PDA left-to-right shunt (McCurnin et al, 2008; Perez Fontan et al, 1987). Although it is true that preterm animals with a PDA have increased fluid and protein clearance into the lung interstitium, because of an increase in pulmonary microvascular filtration pressure, a simultaneous increase in lung lymph flow appears to eliminate the excess fluid and protein from the lung (Alpan et al, 1991). This compensatory increase in lung lymph acts as an "edema safety factor," inhibiting fluid accumulation in the lungs. As a result, there is no net increase in water or protein accumulation in the lung and there is no change in pulmonary mechanics (Alpan et al, 1989; Clyman, 1996; Krauss et al, 1989; Perez Fontan et al, 1987; Shimada et al, 1989). This delicate balance between the PDA-induced fluid filtration and lymphatic reabsorption is consistent with the observation, made in human infants, that closure of the ductus arteriosus within the first 24 hours after birth has no effect on the course of the newborn's hyaline membrane disease. However, if lung lymphatic drainage is impaired, as it is in the presence of pulmonary interstitial emphysema or fibrosis, the likelihood of edema increases dramatically. After several days of lung disease and mechanical ventilation, the residual functioning lymphatics are more easily overwhelmed by the same size ductus shunt that could be accommodated on the 1st day after delivery. As a result, it is not uncommon for infants with a persistent PDA to develop pulmonary edema and alterations in pulmonary mechanics at 7 to 10 days after birth. In these infants, improvement in lung compliance occurs after closure of the PDA (Clyman, 1996; Gerhardt and Bancalari, 1980; Johnson et al, 1978; Naulty et al, 1978; Stefano et al, 1991; Szymankiewicz et al, 2004; Yeh et al, 1981a).

Recently, a premature baboon model of PDA has been used to examine the factors responsible for the alteration in pulmonary mechanics that occur in the presence of a PDA (McCurnin et al, 2008). Animals delivered at 67% term gestation (equivalent to 26 weeks' human gestation) were given surfactant and mechanically ventilated for 2 weeks. One group was treated with a cyclooxygenase inhibitor to close the ductus; the other group had a persistent PDA. Exposure to a persistent PDA for 2 weeks did not appear to alter surfactant secretion, pulmonary epithelial protein permeability, or presence of surfactant inhibitory proteins. Nor did it alter the expression of genes that regulate inflammation and tissue remodeling. The animals with an open ductus had an increased amount and altered distribution of water in their lungs. In contrast with the full-term lung, which mobilized fluid rapidly after birth, the preterm lung mobilized lung fluid much more slowly. A persistent PDA led to a small but significant increase in lung water at 2 weeks after delivery. In addition, closure of the PDA with a cyclooxygenase inhibitor, such as indomethacin or ibuprofen, produced increased expression of alveolar epithelial sodium channels, which facilitate fluid removal from the alveolar compartment. This finding may account for the decreased incidence of significant pulmonary hemorrhage in infants who are treated with prophylactic indomethacin after birth (Al Faleh et al, 2008; Clyman and Chorne, 2008; Domanico et al, 1994).

Pharmacologic closure of the PDA was also associated with improved lung development in the preterm baboons. In contrast to the animals with an open ductus, where an arrest in alveolar development (the hallmark of the new "BPD") was noticeable by 2 weeks after birth, pharmacologic closure of the PDA led to improved alveolarization (McCurnin et al, 2008).

Not all of the changes associated with a PDA are necessarily detrimental to the immature infant with respiratory distress syndrome. The recirculation of oxygenated arterial blood through lungs that are not fully expanded can lead to improved arterial PaO_2 (Clyman et al, 1987; Dawes et al, 1955). Decreases in systemic arterial O_2 content have been observed after PDA closure, despite the absence of any alterations in pulmonary mechanics.

TREATMENT

TREATMENT OPTIONS FOR CLOSING A PDA

Surgical ligation produces definitive ductus arteriosus closure; however, it is associated with its own set of morbidities: thoracotomy, pneumothorax, chylothorax, scoliosis, and infection (Roclawski et al, 2009). The incidence of unilateral vocal cord paralysis (which increases the requirements for tube feedings, respiratory support, and hospital stay) has been reported to be as high as 67% in extremely low birthweight (ELBW) infants, after PDA ligation (Clement et al, 2008; Smith et al, 2009). Between 30% and 50% of infants with birthweights ≤1000 g will require inotropic support for profound hypotension during the postoperative period (Moin et al, 2003). In addition, neonatal transport to another facility may be required if surgical expertise is not readily available. Early surgical ligation of the PDA has recently been shown to be an independent risk factor for the development of bronchopulmonary dysplasia (Chorne et al, 2007b; Clyman et al, 2009). Studies in premature baboons support the concept that surgical ligation may produce detrimental effects on lung function and growth. Although pharmacologic ductus closure minimizes the postnatal arrest in alveolar development that occurs in preterm infants (see earlier discussion) (McCurnin et al, 2008), no benefit for alveolar growth has been observed after surgical ligation (Chang et al, 2008; McCurnin et al, 2005). This raises the possibility that ductus ligation, while eliminating the detrimental effects of a PDA on lung development, may create its own set of problems that counteract any of the benefits derived from ductus closure (Chorne et al, 2007b; Clyman et al, 2009).

Inhibition of prostaglandin synthesis with nonselective inhibitors of COX-1 and COX-2 (e.g., indomethacin and ibuprofen) appears to be an effective alternative to surgical ligation (Gersony et al, 1983). In most intensive care nurseries, indomethacin and ibuprofen have replaced surgery as the preferred therapy for closing a persistent PDA. However, both have been associated with several potential adverse effects in the newborn. Indomethacin produces significant reductions in renal (Pezzati et al, 1999; Rennie et al, 1986), mesenteric (Coombs et al, 1990; Van Bel et al, 1990), and cerebral blood flow (Austin et al, 1992; Edwards et al, 1990; Laudignon et al, 1988; Patel et al, 2000; Pryds et al, 1988; Van Bel et al, 1989). Indomethacin also reduces cerebral oxygenation (McCormick et al, 1993; Patel et al, 2000). Alterations in creatinine clearance and oliguria (that are minimally responsive to dopamine or furosemide therapy [Barrington and Brion, 2002; Brion and Campbell, 2001]) are common problems with the initial doses of indomethacin. Renal function returns toward normal after the initial doses of indomethacin or after drug discontinuation (Seyberth et al, 1983). Indomethacin's action on these organ systems may not be due entirely to its inhibition of prostaglandin synthesis (Chemtob et al, 1991; Malcolm et al, 1993; Speziale et al, 1999). Indomethacin also has effects on lipoxygenase activity and histamine and endothelin release (Docherty and Wilson, 1987; Konig et al, 1987; Therkelsen et al, 1994), although the relevance of these effects to any neonatal morbidity is still unknown.

Although indomethacin produces significant physiologic alterations, none of the controlled, randomized trials that have examined the relationship between indomethacin and neonatal morbidity have found an increase in the incidence of necrotizing enterocolitis, gastrointestinal perforation, retinopathy of prematurity (ROP), chronic lung disease, or cerebral white matter injury after indomethacin treatment (Fowlie and Davis, 2002). Although indomethacin, by itself, has not been shown to increase the incidence of gastrointestinal perforations, the combination of indomethacin *and* postnatal steroids, administered simultaneously, has been shown to increase the incidence of gastrointestinal perforations/necrotizing enterocolitis (Peltoniemi et al, 2005; Watterberg et al, 2004).

Indomethacin's cerebral vasoconstrictive effects are frequently cited as a concern for neonatologists (Edwards et al, 1990; Leffler et al, 1985); however, a Cochrane systematic review found that indomethacin prophylaxis is more likely to decrease rather than increase the incidence of periventricular leukomalacia (Fowlie and Davis, 2002). There is no evidence that prophylactic indomethacin has any adverse effect on neurodevelopmental outcome at 18 months (Schmidt et al, 2001); in fact, there is evidence that it may have long-term benefits at 4.5 and 8 years (Ment et al, 2000, 2004; Vohr et al, 2003).

Although there may be general consensus on the efficacy of indomethacin for treatment of a PDA, questions about proper dosage, treatment duration, and optimal timing of treatment remain quite controversial. Indomethacin's plasma clearance depends on postnatal age (Brash et al, 1981; Smith et al, 1984; Thalji et al, 1980; Yaffe et al, 1980; Yeh et al, 1989). Therefore, a dosage regime recommended for infants at the end of the 1st week (when the half-life of the drug is 21 hours) (Yaffe et al, 1980; Yeh et al, 1989) may lead to elevated and prolonged plasma concentrations when used in infants on day 1 (when the half-life is 71 hours) (Smith et al, 1984). Conversely, a single loading dose of indomethacin (0.2 mg/kg), without subsequent maintenance doses, can be effective in closing a PDA when administered within the first 24 hours after delivery (Krueger et al, 1987).

Many variations in dosage regimens have been evaluated (Gork et al, 2008; Herrera et al, 2007). A prolonged low-dose course of indomethacin (0.1 mg/kg every 24 hours for 5 to 7 days) may increase the rate of permanent closure, especially in infants who still have residual ductus flow after completing the standard short course (2 to 3 doses over 24 hours) (Hammerman and Aranburo, 1990; Quinn et al, 2002; Rennie and Cooke, 1991; Rhodes et al, 1988). This dosage regimen still needs further evaluation because in some reports (Rennie and Cooke, 1991; Rhodes et al, 1988) a higher mortality rate was observed in the infants receiving prolonged maintenance indomethacin. Although some have suggested that the dose of indomethacin be increased when conventional dosing fails to produce ductus closure (Gal et al, 1990; Shaffer et al, 2002; Sperandio et al; 2005), a randomized controlled trial examining this issue found that the rate of ductus closure was not substantially improved despite a nearly threefold increase in serum indomethacin concentrations. More worrisome was the fact that the higher indomethacin concentrations produced

significant increases in the incidence of moderate to severe ROP and late renal dysfunction (Jegatheesan et al, 2008).

The postnatal age at which indomethacin is administered plays an important role in determining its effectiveness. Even when indomethacin concentrations have been maintained in the "desired" range, the drug's ability to produce ductus closure remains inversely proportional to the postnatal age at the time of treatment (Achanti et al, 1986; Brash et al, 1981; Rennie et al, 1986; Rheuban et al, 1987; Thalji et al, 1980). With advancing postnatal age, dilator prostaglandins play less of a role in maintaining ductus patency (see earlier discussion). As a result, indomethacin becomes less effective in producing PDA closure (Achanti et al, 1986). It appears that in some situations, prostaglandins may not be the dominant factor maintaining ductus patency (Chorne et al, 2007a; Cotton et al, 1991).

Recurrence of a symptomatic PDA can occur after initial successful treatment. The rate of reopening, which is greatest among the most immature infants, appears to be related to the timing and completeness of ductus closure after the treatment course (Clyman, 1996; Narayanan et al, 2000). Permanent anatomic closure requires tight constriction of the ductus lumen and the development of ductus wall hypoxia (see earlier discussion). Of infants delivered at <28 weeks' gestation in whom clinical ductus closure was achieved after indomethacin treatment, 80% will reopen their ductus and develop clinical symptoms if there is any evidence of luminal patency on the Doppler examination performed at the end of indomethacin treatment (Narayanan et al, 2000). Unfortunately, there are limitations in the Doppler's ability to detect complete luminal closure. Even when there is no evidence of ductus patency on the Doppler/echocardiogram, a significant number of preterm infants will still have a tiny patent ductus lumen. The more immature the ductus (i.e., the thinner the ductus wall), the greater the likelihood that profound hypoxia and anatomic remodeling will not occur. These vessels will reopen at a later date: 23% of those born before 26 weeks reopen in spite of echocardiographic evidence of closure; in contrast, only 9% of those born between 26 and 27 weeks will reopen if the ductus is found to be closed by echocardiography. Early treatment produces a tighter degree of ductus constriction and, as a result, higher rates of ductus wall hypoxia and permanent closure (Narayanan et al, 2000).

Ibuprofen, another nonselective cyclooxygenase inhibitor, has been shown to close the ductus in animals (Coceani et al, 1979) and preterm infants. It appears to be as effective as indomethacin in producing PDA closure in VLBW infants (at least in infants with a mean gestational age of 28 weeks) (Van Overmeire et al, 2000). In contrast with indomethacin, ibuprofen does not appear to affect mesenteric blood flow (Malcolm et al, 1993; Pezzati et al, 1999; Speziale et al, 1999) and has less of an effect on renal perfusion, oliguria (Malcolm et al, 1993; Pezzati et al, 1999; Speziale et al, 1999), and cerebral blood flow (Chemtob et al, 1990; Mosca et al, 1997; Patel et al, 2000; Speziale et al, 1999). Animal studies suggest that ibuprofen may have some cytoprotective effects in the intestinal tract (Grosfeld et al, 1983). However, aside from its renal sparing effects, comparison trials have not found ibuprofen to be superior to indomethacin in the prevention of other neonatal morbidities (necrotizing enterocolitis, gastrointestinal perforation, and bronchopulmonary dysplasia) (Ohlsson et al, 2008). In addition, ibuprofen does not appear to have the same intracranial hemorrhage sparing effects that are seen with indomethacin (see later discussion). The optimal age-appropriate dosing schedule for ibuprofen is still under consideration (Hirt et al, 2008). Ibuprofen's effects on total and free serum bilirubin concentrations (Ahlfors, 2004; Zecca et al, 2009) raise concerns about the safety of some of the higher dose options.

INDOMETHACIN AND INTRACRANIAL HEMORRHAGE

Previous studies have shown that indomethacin can decrease the incidence of intracranial hemorrhage (ICH) in preterm infants and experimental animals (this has not been the case with ibuprofen). The effects of indomethacin on ICH do not appear to be due to its effects on ductus patency (Ment et al, 1985, 1988). Indomethacin decreases cerebral blood flow, decreases reactive postasphyxial cerebral hyperemia, and accelerates maturation of the germinal matrix microvasculature (Dahlgren et al, 1981; Ment et al, 1983, 1992). Because most intracranial hemorrhages occur within the first 3 days after birth, one would expect to see beneficial effects only when indomethacin is given in a prophylactic strategy (within the first 18 hours after birth). When prophylactic indomethacin is given to infants with normal echoencephalograms, there is a significant reduction in both the incidence of all grades (I–IV) as well as the most severe grades (III, IV) of ICH. Because 30% to 50% of infants who develop an ICH have evidence of an ICH on their screening preindomethacin echoencephalogram, the beneficial effects of prophylactic indomethacin are less dramatic when it is administered to populations where the prior ICH status is unknown. When indomethacin is administered prophylactically, without knowledge of prior ICH status, there is no longer a difference in the overall incidence of ICH; however, there is still a significant reduction in the incidence of severe (grade III, IV) ICH (Clyman, 1996). Although randomized controlled trials have not shown an effect of prophylactic indomethacin on neurodevelopmental outcome at 18 months (Schmidt et al, 2001), there is evidence for long-term benefits at 4.5 and 8 years (Ment et al, 2000, 2004; Vohr et al, 2003).

PDA AND NEONATAL MORBIDITY: TO TREAT OR NOT TO TREAT

A persistent PDA increases pulmonary hyperemia and pulmonary edema and decreases renal, mesenteric, and cerebral perfusion; however, clear evidence is lacking for or against many of the approaches to PDA treatment (Bose and Laughon, 2006; Clyman and Chorne, 2007; Laughon et al, 2004). Although a prolonged, persistent left-to-right shunt through a PDA shortens the life span of animals and humans (Brooks et al, 2005; Campbell, 1968; Loftin et al, 2001; Van Israel et al, 2003), there has been growing debate in recent years about whether or not to treat a persistent PDA during the neonatal period (Laughon et al, 2004). Preterm infants have a high rate of spontaneous PDA closure during the first 2 years. Therefore, early

treatment runs the risk of exposing infants to drugs or procedures they might not need.

Published randomized controlled trials (RCTs) provide only a limited amount of information to help guide current PDA treatment choices. Most of these have focused on the timing of treatment and the risks and benefits of prophylactic versus early indomethacin treatment. Numerous RCTs (and their metaanalyses) have shown that indomethacin prophylaxis decreases (1) the incidence of severe early pulmonary hemorrhages, (2) the occurrence of severe grades of intraventricular hemorrhage, (3) the risk of developing a symptomatic PDA, and (4) the need for surgical PDA ligation (Al Faleh et al, 2008; Bandstra et al, 1988; Clyman and Chorne, 2008; Domanico et al, 1994; Fowlie and Davis, 2002; Ment et al, 1994; Schmidt et al, 2001). On the other hand, indomethacin prophylaxis results in overtreatment of infants who would normally close their ductus spontaneously (Koch et al, 2006).

Even less information exists about the consequences of a persistent, symptomatic, moderate-to-large PDA shunt on neonatal morbidity. To date, only two small RCTs, performed about 30 years ago, have specifically examined the role of a persistent untreated symptomatic PDA on neonatal morbidity (Cotton et al, 1978; Kaapa et al, 1983). Both studies found that a persistent PDA increased pulmonary morbidity and prolonged the need for respiratory support. Whether these findings are still applicable in the setting of modern neonatal treatment is a matter for controversy among neonatologists.

The role of a PDA in the development of necrotizing enterocolitis is even more controversial. Although some retrospective, population-based studies have reported an association between PDA and NEC (Cassady et al, 1989; Dollberg et al, 2005; Sankaran et al, 2004), there is little evidence from RCTs to either support or refute the idea that a PDA plays a role in the development of necrotizing enterocolitis. At this time, there are no RCTs in the medical literature that address this issue. Nor is there information about the advisability of continuing or stopping enteral feeding in the presence of a PDA.

Although indomethacin has been shown to be effective in producing ductus closure (Gersony et al, 1983), its long-term benefits on chronic lung disease, necrotizing enterocolitis, or survival have yet to be established (Clyman and Chorne, 2007; Cooke et al, 2003; Knight, 2001; Yeh et al, 1981a, 1981b). These uncertainties have resulted in several areas of controversy regarding PDA management: (1) whether or not to use indomethacin prophylaxis, (2) when to treat a moderate-to-large PDA, and (3) whether or not enteral feeding should be stopped in the presence of a PDA or during treatment of a PDA (Amin et al, 2007; Bose and Laughon, 2006; Clyman and Chorne, 2007; Knight, 2001; Laughon et al, 2004). At this time, 95% of U.S. neonatologists believe that a moderate-to-large PDA should be treated if it persists in ELBW infants who still require mechanical ventilation; in contrast, only 30% use indomethacin prophylactically (Jhaveri et al, 2009). The number of neonatologists who treat a persistent PDA when it occurs in infants who do not require mechanical ventilation varies significantly by geographic region. Marked differences in neonatologists' willingness to feed infants in the presence of a PDA appears to account for the large geographic variations in indomethacin use and rates of PDA ligation. Of interest, 70% of U.S. neonatologists believe that enteral feedings need to be stopped in the presence of a PDA. In contrast, non-U.S. neonatologists have exactly the opposite opinion: 70% believe that enteral feedings should continue in the presence of a PDA (Jhaveri et al, 2009).

A PERSONALIZED APPROACH

Prolonged exposure to the left-to-right shunt can ultimately lead to congestive failure, pulmonary hypertension, and death. Therefore, our recommended approach has been to use early pharmacologic treatment of a PDA in the newborn period, because pharmacotherapy has not been shown to produce increased morbidity and early treatment is more likely to result in successful ductus closure. In certain settings (where ICH, pulmonary hemorrhage, and PDA ligations are frequent occurrences), indomethacin prophylaxis may even be a preferred alternative. On the other hand, ductus ligation, while eliminating one potential cause for neonatal morbidity, may introduce its own set of problems. Further investigations will be needed to determine which infants are most likely to benefit from surgical ligation and which infants might best be left untreated when pharmacologic approaches are no longer an option.

SUGGESTED READINGS

Clyman R, Cassady G, Kirklin JK, et al: The role of patent ductus arteriosus ligation in bronchopulmonary dysplasia: reexamining a randomized controlled trial, *J Pediatr* 154:873-876, 2009.

Dagle JM, Lepp NT, Cooper ME, et al: Determination of genetic predisposition to patent ductus arteriosus in preterm infants, *Pediatrics* 123:1116-1123, 2009.

El Hajjar M, Vaksmann G, Rakza T, et al: Severity of the ductal shunt: a comparison of different markers, *Arch Dis Child Fetal Neonatal Ed* 90:F419-422, 2005.

Fowlie PW, Davis PG: Prophylactic intravenous indomethacin for preventing mortality and morbidity in preterm infants. *Cochrane Database Syst Rev* CD000174, 2002.

Kajino H, Chen YQ, Seidner SR, et al: Factors that increase the contractile tone of the ductus arteriosus also regulate its anatomic remodeling, *Am J Physiol Regul Integr Comp Physiol* 281:R291-R301, 2001.

Keller RL, Tacy TA, Fields S, et al: Combined treatment with a non-selective nitric oxide synthase inhibitor (L-NMMA) and indomethacin increases ductus constriction in extremely premature newborns, *Pediatr Res* 58:1216-1221, 2005.

Schmidt B, Davis P, Moddemann D, et al: Long-term effects of indomethacin prophylaxis in extremely-low-birth- weight infants, *N Engl J Med* 344:1966-1972, 2001.

Seidner SR, Chen Y-Q, Oprysko PR, et al: Combined prostaglandin and nitric oxide inhibition produces anatomic remodeling and closure of the ductus arteriosus in the premature newborn baboon, *Pediatr Res* 50:365-373, 2001.

Thebaud B, Michelakis ED, Wu XC, et al: Oxygen-sensitive K_V channel gene transfer confers oxygen responsiveness to preterm rabbit and remodeled human ductus arteriosus: implications for infants with patent ductus arteriosus, *Circulation* 110:1372-1379, 2004.

Thebaud B, Wu XC, Kajimoto H, et al: Developmental absence of the O_2 sensitivity of L-type calcium channels in preterm ductus arteriosus smooth muscle cells impairs O_2 constriction contributing to patent ductus arteriosus, *Pediatr Res* 63:176-181, 2008.

Vohr BR, Allan WC, Westerveld M, et al: School-age outcomes of very low birth weight infants in the indomethacin intraventricular hemorrhage prevention trial, *Pediatrics* 111:e340-e346, 2003.

Complete references used in this text can be found online at www.expertconsult.com

CONGENITAL HEART DISEASE

Thomas D. Scholz and Benjamin E. Reinking

Congenital heart disease (CHD) is the most common birth defect encountered in the clinical setting. The prevalence of all forms of congenital heart lesions is approximately 1% of live births, although estimates in the newborn are likely to be compromised by underdiagnosis of some lesions such as bicuspid aortic valve and overdiagnosis of normal structures that are in transition, including the foramen ovale and ductus arteriosus. The presentation of the newborn with CHD can range from absence of symptoms to complete cardiovascular collapse. Most commonly, neonates with CHD present with a murmur, cyanosis, and/or congestive heart failure. Lesions that result in each of these clinical findings are considered separately here, although considerable overlap exists among the three groups.

GENERAL CONSIDERATIONS

FETAL-TO-POSTNATAL TRANSITION

The hemodynamic state of the fetus is much different from that of the newborn. In the fetus, a relatively low systemic resistance exists because of the presence of the placenta, and the pulmonary vasculature maintains a high resistance. Central shunts exist that provide alternate routes on the venous side (ductus venosus), within the heart (foramen ovale), and on the arterial side of the circulation (ductus arteriosus).

The ductus venosus predominantly collects oxygen- and nutrient-rich blood from the placenta via the umbilical vein and delivers this blood directly to the right atrium, largely bypassing the hepatic and portal venous systems. As indicated by based on studies in fetal sheep, less than one half of the umbilical venous return enters the left lobe of the liver and reaches the ductus venosus near its insertion into the inferior vena cava (IVC), returning as relatively nutrient-rich blood (Edelstone et al, 1978). The lateral position of the IVC within the right atrium results in streaming of this nutrient-rich blood across the foramen ovale and into the left atrium. The most desaturated blood to return to the right atrium comes from the coronary sinus, which combines with the venous return from the superior vena cava and is directed across the tricuspid valve into the right ventricle.

In the fetus, the presence of the ductus arteriosus, which is nonrestrictive, results in the subjection of both ventricles to a comparable afterload. Compared with that in the postnatal heart, this results in an increase in right ventricular workload and some restriction to filling of the right ventricle. The nutrient-rich blood from the umbilical vein that has crossed the foramen ovale to enter the left side of the heart predominantly supplies the heart and brain. Output from the right ventricle supplies the lungs (less than 8% of the combined cardiac output) and flows right to left through the ductus arteriosus to supply the remainder of the body.

At birth, several important transitions take place that allow the fetus to adapt to extrauterine life. First, the gradual decline in pulmonary vascular resistance that was occurring during the last trimester of pregnancy undergoes an abrupt drop with the first breath taken by the newborn (Figure 55-1). The decline in pulmonary vascular resistance results in a more than 20-fold increase in pulmonary blood flow and reversal of flow (left to right) in the ductus arteriosus before its closure (Teitel, 1988). Second, the central shunts present in the fetus undergo closure such that blood flows in series through the body. The ductus venosus closes largely because of lack of flow after separation of the placenta, although some contractile elements may be present in the vessel wall (Adeagbo et al, 2004). The foramen ovale becomes occluded as the flap of the septum primum abuts the septum secundum following the increased pulmonary blood flow that increases filling of the left atrium. Small residual left-to-right shunts at the foramen ovale may persist, although these will generally decrease with time (see later discussion of atrial septal defects). Closure of the ductus arteriosus is mediated by a variety of pathways, although patency of the ductus can usually be maintained by exogenous prostaglandin administration. The third important transition at birth is an increase in the combined ventricle output as the metabolic demands of the body increase at birth.

The dramatic hemodynamic changes that occur at birth continue to evolve over the first few months of life. There is a continued decline in pulmonary vascular resistance for the first 6–8 weeks of life. In addition, the right ventricle remodels to a thinner and more compliant ventricle. Probe patency of the foramen ovale may persist for years, although in most individuals the septa become adherent.

NOMENCLATURE

The complete description of any heart requires more than a description of the presence or absence of a specific congenital heart defect. Each heart has a specific set of structures and connections that may be normal or abnormal. Although the terminology used for the various lesions that affect the heart is relatively consistent among pediatric cardiologists, various nomenclatures have been developed to completely define the cardiac anatomy. The various systems that have evolved are based on surgical approaches, embryologic origins, or spatial relationships and have hampered communication between individuals and institutions. A common method of describing cardiac anatomy would be a benefit but seems unlikely to be agreed on in the near future. Although the brief summary of nomenclature that is given here is based on the segmental approach of Anderson's group (Anderson et al, 1984), the embryologic approach of Van Praagh is equally valid and used by several institutions (Van Praagh, 1972).

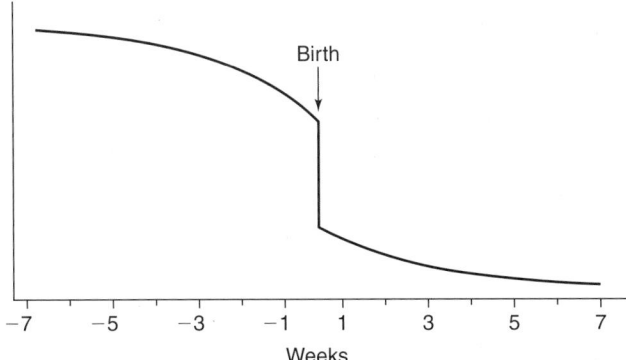

FIGURE 55-1 **Change in pulmonary vascular resistance.** A gradual decline in pulmonary vascular resistance is seen during the latter part of gestation followed by an abrupt decline at birth. A gradual decline occurs postnatally over the next 6 to 8 weeks.

The segmental approach to describing cardiac anatomy includes the following elements:

1. Cardiac position
2. Visceral sidedness
3. Systemic and pulmonary venous connections
4. Atrial sidedness and atrial connections
5. Atrioventricular (AV) valves
6. Ventricle sidedness
7. Ventriculoarterial connections
8. Great vessel number and position

The description of cardiac position in the chest can be separated into where the heart is located and the direction in which the apex of the heart is pointed. Normally, the heart is in the left chest with the apex pointed to the left. Dextro- (right) or meso- (midline) position of the heart can occur with decreased right lung volume, severe scoliosis, or an elevated left diaphragm. Typically, the position of the heart in the chest is determined by chest radiography. The normal leftward-pointing apex of the heart (levocardia) can vary to mesocardia (in various heterotaxy syndromes) or dextrocardia (in situs inversus). The orientation of the apex of the heart is usually defined by echocardiography.

Visceral sidedness is often defined separately for the abdominal organs, the cardiac structures, and the lungs, although they frequently share the same destination. Sidedness is referred to as solitus (normal), inversus (mirror image), or ambiguus (isomerism or indeterminate). In the last situation, effort is made to define whether the organs that appear on both sides are right-sided (liver, right atrium, and trilobed lung) or left-sided (stomach/spleen, left atrium, bilobed lung) structures, because this can have prognostic and therapeutic importance. For instance, patients with bilateral right-sidedness typically lack a spleen, require lifelong prophylactic antibiotics for encapsulated organisms, and have malrotation of the intestine.

Venous connections of the superior and inferior venae cavae must also be delineated. The usual connection of the superior vena cava (SVC) to the right atrium may also be accompanied by a persistent left SVC to the coronary sinus, with or without a bridging brachiocephalic vein. The inferior vena cava is derived from various embryologic vessels and can have its suprahepatic segment interrupted, in which case the normal connection of the IVC to the right atrium does not occur. In this case, lower extremity blood

flow is routed to the SVC through the azygous or hemiazygous systems. Various pulmonary venous connections are described next.

Atrial sidedness can be solitus with the morphologic right atrium on the right (normal), inversus, mirror-image, common, or, rarely, indeterminate. The right atrium is typically identified by its venous connections (in particular, the coronary sinus), the presence of the crista terminalis, the large sail-shaped appendage, and the coarse pectinate muscles of the free wall. The left atrium is characterized by its smooth walls and narrow, finger-shaped appendage. Atrial morphology can typically be discerned by echocardiography, although angiography may also aid in their distinction. When the morphologic right atrium connects to the morphologic right ventricle (and similarly on the left), the connection is concordant. A discordant connection occurs when the morphologic right atrium connects to the morphologic left ventricle, as in corrected transposition of the great arteries. When both atria connect to one ventricle (as in double-inlet left ventricle) or a single ventricle, the type of connection is referred to as univentricular. An ambiguous connection occurs in cases of atrial isomerism.

The AV valves usually travel with their ventricle. Thus, the tricuspid valve, when present, connects to the morphologic right ventricle and the mitral valve connects to the morphologic left ventricle. The tricuspid valve has three leaflets and is distinguished from the mitral valve by the septal attachments of its papillary muscles and the slight, inferior position of the septal leaflet of the tricuspid valve relative to the anterior leaflet of the mitral valve. When the AV valves fail to undergo septation, a common AV valve is found, as in children with a complete AV septal defect. The position of the AV valves and their chordal attachments are used to define whether the valves are malaligned or straddling. A malaligned AV valve is not completely positioned over its respective ventricle, which is sometimes referred to as overriding. If the chordal attachments of an AV valve cross the septum and connect to the other ventricle, an AV valve is referred to as straddling.

The morphology of the ventricles, the associated AV valve, and the outflow portion of the ventricle can generally be used to identify the right and left ventricles. The right ventricle, besides being associated with the tricuspid valve, is more heavily trabeculated at its apex and anterior free wall than the left ventricle. In addition, an infundibular or conus ring exists in the right ventricle that separates the tricuspid and semilunar valves. The left ventricle, besides being more smooth-walled with finer trabeculations at its apex than the right ventricle, demonstrates fibrous continuity between the mitral and semilunar valves. When the ventricular morphology is uncertain, the ventricles are said to be indeterminate. A common ventricle is defined by virtual absence of the interventricular septum.

The great vessels are largely defined by their branching pattern. The pulmonary artery bifurcates shortly after exiting the heart into the right and left pulmonary arteries, which undergo subsequent branching to supply the segments of the lung. The right pulmonary artery is positioned anterior to the right upper bronchus, whereas the left pulmonary artery is posterior to the left upper bronchus. The pulmonary arteries typically follow the situs of the lungs such that mirror-image pulmonary artery branching is seen in situs inversus, bilateral branch pulmonary arteries anterior to the upper bronchus are seen in right isomerism, and branch pulmonary arteries posterior to the upper bronchus are seen in left isomerism. The aorta is normally left-sided, traveling to the left of the main bronchus, and gives rise to the three arch vessels. A right aortic arch passes to the right of the main bronchus before crossing back to the left side of the spine in the thorax and gives rise to mirror-image arch vessels such that the first arch vessel, the brachiocephalic artery, bifurcates to give rise to the right subclavian and right carotid. Although the aorta is typically posterior and rightward to the main pulmonary artery, the relative position of the vessels can vary greatly. Most commonly, in d-transposition of the great arteries, the aorta is anterior and rightward to the main pulmonary artery. In situations where only a single semilunar valve is present, a truncus arteriosus (or common truncal artery) is found that gives rise to both the aorta and pulmonary artery.

The ventriculoarterial connections are said to be concordant when the right ventricle connects to the pulmonary artery and the left ventricle gives rise to the aorta. The ventriculoarterial connection is discordant when the opposite occurs. The ventriculoarterial connection can also be double, single, or common. If both great arteries arise from one ventricle, a double outlet occurs. The definition of a double-outlet connection is somewhat controversial. For example, in the case of double-outlet right ventricle (DORV) with normally related great vessels, some clinicians have proposed basing the definition on whether greater than 50% of the aorta overrides the right ventricle, whereas others define the double outlet on the basis of presence of a subaortic conus exists that results in mitral-aortic discontinuity. From a clinical management perspective, both situations are relevant for either placement of the ventricular septal defect (VSD) patch or the potential for development of subaortic obstruction, respectively. A single outlet results when severe pulmonary hypoplasia occurs such that no main pulmonary artery segment is present. A common outlet occurs in truncus arteriosus.

CLINICAL EVALUATION OF THE NEWBORN

Even with the technologic advances in pre- and postnatal echocardiography and genetic testing, a careful history and physical examination is needed in every newborn with suspected congenital heart disease. Birth history including complications during pregnancy, labor, and delivery is important to document. Often, the child with cyanosis due to structural heart disease has an unremarkable birth history. A difficult labor or delivery may point toward noncardiac causes of cyanosis such as persistent fetal circulation, infection, or pneumothorax. For the child with poor systemic perfusion, a history of premature rupture of membranes or maternal fever may suggest sepsis as a cause for the diminished cardiac function. Hematologic abnormalities that may cause cardiovascular dysfunction in the neonate, such as polycythemia or anemia, may be suggested by a history of placental abruption or twin-twin transfusion.

Family history is critical to review with the biologic parents. There is a genetic basis for a growing number of congenital heart defects (see later discussion). CHD in a sibling more than doubles the risk of CHD in future children (Nora and Nora, 1988). A history of congenital heart disease in either of the parents also increases the chance of developing a congenital heart lesion (Nora and Nora, 1987; Whittemore et al, 1994).

Physical examination of the newborn should initially include a general assessment looking for dysmorphic features and the degree of distress of the infant. The child with cardiac obstructive physiology may have shallow, rapid respirations with intercostal and suprasternal retractions. Cyanosis may or may not be seen, depending on the degree of hemoglobin desaturation (roughly 5 g of hemoglobin must be desaturated to be clinically evident). Vital signs, including four extremity blood pressures, should be determined along with pre- and post-ductal oxygen saturation measurement. Palpation of the precordium may identify an overactive or displaced cardiac impulse or the sensation of a thrill due to turbulent flow. Palpation of the abdomen for a liver edge or spleen tip can often provide an indication of volume overload or neonatal infection. Assessment of femoral and upper extremity pulses is essential. Simultaneous palpation of the right brachial and right femoral pulses allows assessment of comparable timing and intensity of the pulsations. Perfusion and capillary refill of the extremities is also important to determine.

Auscultation is often challenging in the sick neonate. However, characterizing the presence, timing, intensity, position, and radiation of murmurs that are present may provide a clue to the underlying diagnosis. In the tachypneic and tachycardic child, it is critical to listen over the head and liver for a continuous murmur that may indicate an arteriovenous malformation. The presence of a click or gallop over the precordium may indicate valvular disease or cardiac failure. Assessment of the second heart sound is particularly important. It has been suggested that the presence of physiologic splitting of the second heart sound nearly always suggests a structurally normal heart (El-Segaier et al, 2007).

Signs of congestive heart failure in the newborn may be subtle and include resting tachypnea with no periodic variation, sinus tachycardia, and enlarged liver. Tachypnea may be accompanied by nasal flaring and inter- and subcostal retractions, particularly if elevated pulmonary venous pressures are present. Grunting respirations are a particularly concerning sign in a newborn that often accompanies severe heart failure and decreased systemic perfusion.

LABORATORY ASSESSMENT OF THE NEONATE

As mentioned earlier, initial laboratory assessment should include measurement of preductal (right hand) and postductal (foot) oxygen saturations. Values less than 93% are considered abnormal. The oxygen challenge test is performed by increasing the inspired oxygen concentration to 100% for at least 5 minutes. Oxygen saturation values that increase into the normal range may be useful to distinguish an admixture, cyanotic heart lesion from lung disease, although this test does not discriminate perfectly.

TABLE 55-1 Electrocardiogram Standards

Age Group	QRS Axis	PR1	QRSD	QV6 (mm)	RV1 (mm)	SV1 (mm)	RV6 (mm)	SV6 (mm)	SV1+RV6
<1 day	59–163	0.08–0.16	.031–.075	2	5–26	0–23	0–11	0–9.5	28
1–2 days	64–161	0.08–0.14	.032–.066	2.5	5–27	0–21	0–12	0–9.5	29
3–6 days	77–163	0.07–0.14	.031–.068	3	3–24	0–17	0.5–12	0–10	24.5
1–3 weeks	65–161	0.07–0.14	.036–.08	3	3–21	0–11	2.5–16.5	0–10	21
1–2 months	31–113	0.07–0.13	.033–.076	3	3–18	0–12	5–21.5	0–6.5	29
3–5 months	7–104	0.07–0.15	.032–.08	3	3–20	0–17	6.5–22.5	0–10	32
6–11 months	6–99	0.07–0.16	.034–.076	3	1.5–20	0.5–18	6–22.5	0–7	32
1–2 years	7–101	0.08–0.15	.038–.076	3	2.5–17	0.5–21	6–22.5	0–6.5	39
3–4 years	6–104	0.09–0.16	.041–.072	3.5	1–18	0.2–21	8–24.5	0–5	42
5–7 years	11–143	0.09–0.16	.042–.079	4.5	0.5–14	0.3–24	8.5–26.5	0–4	47
8–11 years	9–114	0.09–0.17	.041–.085	3	0–12	0.3–25	9–25.5	0–4	45.5
12–15 years	11–130	0.09–0.18	.044–.087	3	0–10	0.3–21	6.5–23	0–4	41
Adult	–30–90	0.12–0.2	0.05–0.1		0–10	0.5–23	4–23	0–4	35

Normal ranges of electrocardiogram measurements (made at full standard) are given. The values vary throughout childhood, because the in utero right ventricular dominance decreases postnatally.

History and physical examination should be included and guide the need for further evaluation. A decrease in postductal oxygen saturations compared to preductal values suggests right-to-left shunting due to an increase in pulmonary vascular resistance. The unusual situation where the preductal saturation is less than the postductal reading occurs with transposition of the great arteries and pulmonary hypertension with a patent ductus arteriosus (PDA).

An electrocardiogram (ECG) should be obtained in the initial evaluation of the newborn with suspected CHD although, in the absence of an arrhythmia, it rarely provides a specific diagnosis. The neonatal ECG demonstrates prominent rightward forces and may have an upright T wave in the right precordial leads in the first few days of life and still not be diagnostic of right ventricular hypertrophy. Age-dependent standards are available and should be referred to when evaluating the ECG (Table 55-1). Certain lesions may be associated with distinctive findings on ECG such as extreme right axis deviation and q waves in leads I and aVL (complete AV canal), preexcitation and right atrial enlargement (Ebstein's anomaly), and q waves in leads V1 to V3 (corrected transposition of the great arteries).

A chest radiograph should also be obtained in every newborn who is evaluated for CHD. The chest radiograph may help to determine if lung disease is contributing to cyanosis. The heart size, shape, and border contours should be evaluated on the chest radiograph along with pulmonary vascular markings. A prominent thymic shadow in the newborn may make identification of classic chest radiography findings difficult (such as the "boot-shaped" heart in tetralogy of Fallot (TOF), the "egg on a string" in transposition, and the "snowman" appearance in supracardiac total anomalous pulmonary venous return), although the massively increased heart size typically found with Ebstein's anomaly (see later discussion) will not be missed. An absent thymic shadow may suggest DiGeorge syndrome (22q11 deletion), although genetic testing is still required. Increases in pulmonary vascular markings typically found in left-to-right shunt lesions may

not be immediately apparent in the newborn because of the relatively high pulmonary vascular resistance and may take days or weeks to evolve. Often, decreased pulmonary vascular markings in lesions with diminished pulmonary blood flow, such as tricuspid or pulmonary atresia, will be apparent in the newborn period. Presence of a PDA, however, will improve pulmonary blood flow in these lesions.

Echocardiography is truly the mainstay in the diagnosis of congenital heart disease in the neonate (described in detail in Chapter 53). Although we encourage complete cardiovascular evaluation and consultation with a pediatric cardiologist in all children with suspected CHD, more programs are performing echocardiograms in neonates without direct evaluation of the newborn by a pediatric cardiologist. In such instances, it is critical to have the echocardiographic examination reviewed by a pediatric cardiologist with some knowledge of the clinical condition of the child. Furthermore, the pediatric cardiologist reading the echocardiogram should discuss the findings directly with the caregivers in order for the team to define relevant therapy and follow-up.

GENETICS AND CONGENITAL HEART DISEASE

Our understanding of the genetic basis of CHD is progressing at a rapid pace. The early identification of the association of specific syndromes with CHD suggested that it would be possible to identify genes relevant to abnormal cardiac morphogenesis. With the completion of the Human Genome Project and the availability of large-scale sequencing techniques, it is expected that genetic causes for CHD will continue to become more highly refined, as will the identification of novel gene-environment interactions that alter cardiac development. A child with suspected CHD should be carefully evaluated for dysmorphic features that may indicate an associated syndrome. The converse is also true in that if a newborn is suspected to have a syndrome, careful cardiac evaluation, including an echocardiogram, should be considered.

Screening for chromosomes is an important initial step in the genetic evaluation of the newborn with a presumed syndrome. Well-described associations of congenital cardiac lesions with chromosome abnormalities include trisomy 21 with complete AV septal defect, Turner's syndrome (45 XO) with coarctation of the aorta, Williams syndrome (7q11 deletion) with valvar and supravalvar pulmonic stenosis, and DiGeorge or velocraniofacial syndrome (22q11 deletion) with conotruncal anomalies. These syndromes, and others, make karyotype analysis with fluorescence in situ hybridization (FISH) analysis an important initial step in the workup of infants with these lesions.

A number of single-gene disorders that are associated with CHD have now been defined using direct sequencing of chromosome regions associated with specific syndromes, linkage analysis based on data for large kindreds with a congenital heart lesion, and genome-wide association studies using microarrays or single-nucleotide polymorphisms (SNPs). Included in this list of syndromes and cardiac lesions due to single-gene defects are Noonan's syndrome (pulmonic stenosis), Holt-Oram syndrome (atrial septal defect), Alagille syndrome (peripheral pulmonic stenosis), Ellis-van Creveld syndrome (common atrium), and CHARGE syndrome (embodying variety of lesions). Syndromes and single-gene disorders and their associated CHD have been well tabulated, and the reader is referred to these references for complete listings (Allen et al, 2008).

Genetic testing should be done in all newborns with suspected syndromes whether or not CHD is present. FISH studies for 22q11 deletions should be performed in all infants with conotruncal anomalies such as tetralogy of Fallot, truncus arteriosus, and interrupted aortic arch. Other FISH studies can be specifically ordered at most institutions, although the maximum number of fluorescent probes is typically four or five because of detection limitations of the range of wavelengths available. Genome-wide chromosome microarray screening is now also available that can detect deletions and duplications across the genome, although results take approximately 1 week to generate, and the amount of blood needed for the study may be a limitation in some infants.

The usefulness of genetic testing is not only to help to provide prognostic information for a specific patient, but to provide counseling for the family. Consulting genetics faculty should be considered whenever a karyotype, FISH study, or genome-wide chromosome microarray is found to be abnormal. Consideration of services available to the infant, screening of additional family members, and risk to future pregnancies should be reviewed during the genetics consultation that will affect the overall care of the patient.

MURMURS IN THE NEWBORN: CONGENITAL CARDIAC LESIONS

PATENT DUCTUS ARTERIOSUS AND AORTOPULMONARY WINDOW

As discussed earlier, every child is born with a PDA that typically closes within the 1st week of life. Prematurity is a risk factor for a persistent PDA and is covered in Chapter 54. Persistent PDA in term infants occurs more commonly in females and, in some patients, may have a genetic component,

as suggested by an animal model of inbred poodles (Knight et al, 1973) and linkage to chromosome 12 (Mani et al, 2002).

The pathophysiology of a PDA largely depends on the degree of shunting from the aorta to the pulmonary artery, which is determined by the inner diameter and length of the PDA and the relative pulmonary and systemic resistances. If the PDA diameter is small, the ductus itself will provide the primary site of resistance to flow and the shunt will be small. In the case of a larger PDA, low pulmonary vascular resistance may allow for a significant shunt that places the patient at risk for developing heart failure and, eventually, pulmonary vascular occlusive disease. The low-resistance pathway through the lungs provides a route for diastolic runoff from the aorta that can result in decreased coronary perfusion pressure. The diastolic steal by the pulmonary artery can lead to myocardial ischemia.

Clinically, patients with a small shunt will be asymptomatic. With a larger PDA shunt, the progressive decline in pulmonary vascular resistance postnatally will cause an increase in left-to-right shunt flow with signs of increasing heart failure. The murmur in a child with a PDA is generally continuous and has been described as a "machinery" murmur in the left infraclavicular region. The character of the murmur, however, varies greatly, although the continuous nature is generally present once the pulmonary vascular resistance has declined. Examination of the patient with a PDA will also include a wide pulse pressure due to decreased diastolic pressure and bounding pulses.

The diagnosis of PDA, when suspected on examination, can nearly always be confirmed by echocardiography. Even in the face of high pulmonary vascular resistance with limited left-to-right shunting, differences in the pulse waveforms between the aorta and pulmonary artery will allow left-to-right and/or right-to-left shunting to be observed by color Doppler imaging. Echocardiography can also provide information regarding the degree of left-to-right shunting as the dimensions of the left atrium and left ventricle are increased, and the left atrium–to–aorta ratio is increased. In addition, retrograde flow will be seen in the proximal descending aorta when a large shunt is present. Cardiac catheterization is rarely needed unless coil closure of the PDA is considered.

The prognosis for small PDAs is quite good, and debate exists as to whether closure of "silent" PDAs incidentally identified by echocardiography should be undertaken (Giroud and Jacobs, 2007). With the most recent recommendations from the American Heart Association suggesting that PDAs do not require subacute bacterial endocarditis prophylaxis (Wilson et al, 2007), the need to close these small vessels is low.

Because of long-term concerns with pulmonary over-circulation and the development of pulmonary vascular occlusive disease, closure of PDAs by 1 year of age is recommended when a significant left-to-right shunt is present. Surgical ligation and division can readily be performed through a lateral thoracotomy. However, coil or device closure in the catheterization labratory has a lower morbidity and success rates equal to those with surgery (Arora, 2005). As a result, catheter closure of PDAs has become the preferred method in nonpremature infants.

Aortopulmonary (AP) window occurs when there is direct communication between the aorta and main pulmonary artery and is a rare lesion that can readily be confused with

PDA on both physical and laboratory evaluation. Nearly half of patients with an AP window have an associated cardiac anomaly. These lesions nearly always result in a large degree of left-to-right shunting. Patients will show signs of congestive heart failure on examination, and physical and laboratory findings will be similar to those with a large PDA. Generally, all AP windows should be closed when they are identified. Closure of an AP window must be done surgically, with patch closure from the pulmonary artery side generally being the preferred technique.

VENTRICULAR SEPTAL DEFECT

VSDs are the most common type of congenital heart disease (excluding bicuspid aortic valve). Generally, VSDs are classified into four types (Figure 55-2):
- Perimembranous
- Muscular
- Inlet
- Outlet

The perimembranous VSD is the most common of the four types and has variably been referred to as membranous, paramembranous, and infracristal. From the right ventricular side of the heart, these defects lie under the septal leaflet of the tricuspid valve below the crista supraventricularis and posterior to the papillary muscle of the conus. Muscular VSDs can occur in isolation or as multiples ("Swiss cheese septum") and, as the name implies, can occur anywhere in the muscular septum. Apical muscular VSDs are the most common and are sometimes difficult to accurately size by echocardiography because of the heavy trabeculations at the apex of the right ventricle. Inlet VSDs are located posterior and inferior to perimembranous defects; although the nomenclature is controversial, this is the location of the defect in patients with complete AV septal defects (see later discussion). The location of the VSD in patients with outlet defects is above the crista supraventricularis and typically undermines the right aortic valve leaflet. A variety of synonyms have been used for outlet VSDs, including subarterial, subaortic, supracristal, and conal VSD.

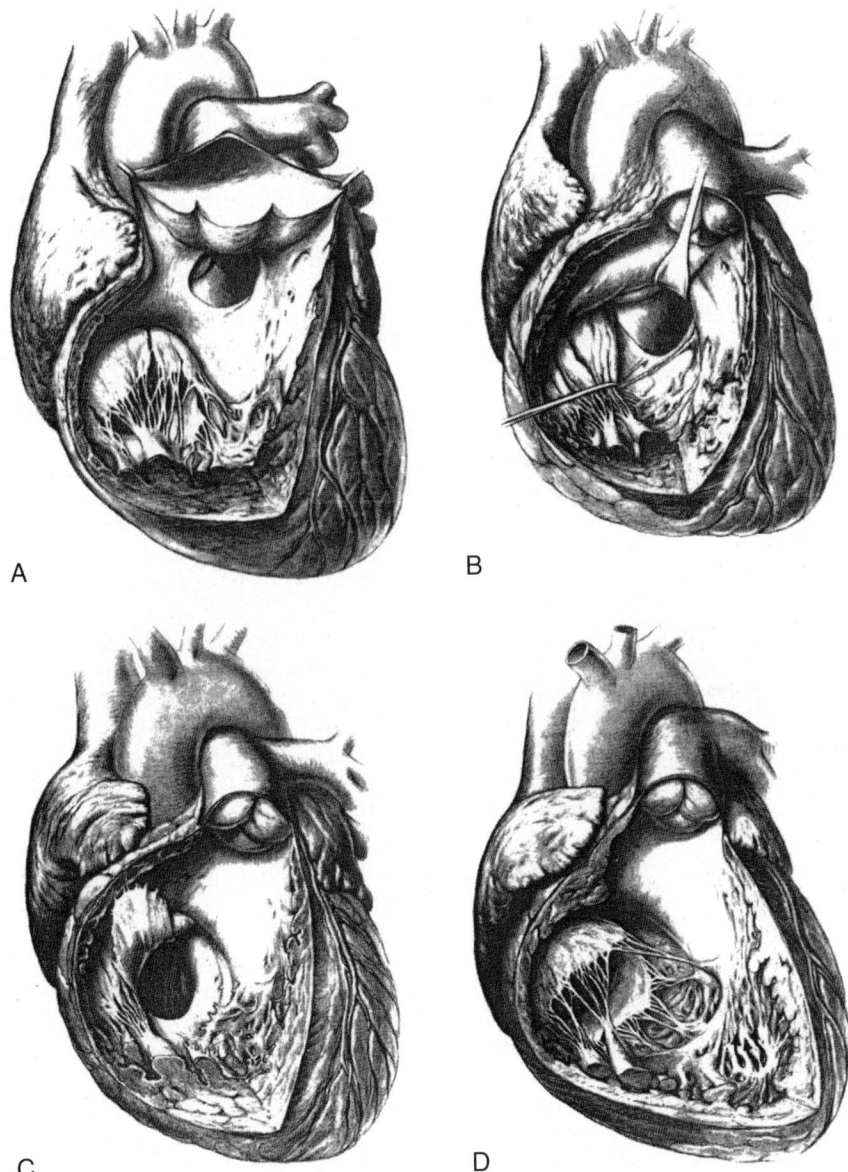

A

B

C

D

FIGURE 55-2 Anatomic varieties of ventricular septal defect. A, Subpulmonary defect; **B,** membranous defect; **C,** inlet (atrioventricular septal defect type) defect; **D,** apical muscular defects. *(From Mavroudis C, Backer CL:* Pediatric cardiac surgery, *St. Louis, 1994, Mosby-Year Book.)*

The clinical importance of any VSD is dependent on the size of the defect and the relative pulmonary-to-systemic vascular resistance, which together determine the degree of left-to-right shunting. An additional consideration with outlet VSDs is the degree to which the right coronary cusp of the aortic valve prolapses into the defect and results in aortic insufficiency. Defects whose cross-sectional area is equal to or greater than the cross-sectional area of the aortic valve will not restrict flow leaving the left ventricle and entering the right ventricle. In this case, the degree of shunting will be determined by the relative resistance to flow in the pulmonary and systemic vascular beds. The normal postnatal decline in pulmonary vascular resistance will result in a progressive increase in left-to-right shunting and signs of congestive heart failure. A small percentage of children do not experience the usual postnatal decline in pulmonary vascular resistance and may never develop signs of pulmonary overcirculation and heart failure despite the presence of a large VSD. As discussed later, this is an indication for early surgical closure of the defect.

When the VSD is small relative to the aortic valve, the defect itself will be the primary point of resistance to shunt flow. In this case, changes in pulmonary vascular resistance will have little impact on the degree of left-to-right shunting.

An important associated lesion that is critical to rule out is coarctation of the aorta. The coarctation results in a fixed, elevated systemic vascular resistance that can lead to important left-to-right shunting even in the presence of a small VSD. In this case, medical therapy is often unable to control congestive heart failure symptoms, and surgery is needed.

The volume of shunted blood is most accurately quantitated at cardiac catheterization based on step-up in oxygen saturation from the right atrium (mixed venous) to the pulmonary artery and is represented as the ratio of pulmonary-to-systemic blood flow (Qp:Qs). Generally, a Qp:Qs <1.5 is considered below the threshold for surgery, whereas a Qp:Qs >2.0 is an indication for surgery. The Qp:Qs can also be estimated by echocardiography and by magnetic resonance imaging.

The examination of the patient with a VSD depends on the magnitude of the shunt. Small defects that provide considerable restriction to flow often have the loudest murmur. The rapid drop in pulmonary vascular resistance immediately after birth allows VSD murmurs to often be heard in the newborn nursery, although the full extent of the murmur, and perhaps a thrill at the lower left sternal border, may not be appreciated for several weeks. The murmur may have a more ejection quality in the newborn nursery in the face of high pulmonary vascular resistance and somewhat elevated right ventricular pressure. The more typical holosystolic murmur will be more apparent as the pulmonary vascular resistance falls.

With large VSDs, little or no murmur may be heard, depending on the pulmonary vascular resistance. With low pulmonary vascular resistance, signs of heart failure will likely be present, including tachypnea with nasal flaring and retractions, tachycardia, diaphoresis, poor feeding, and diminished weight gain. A systolic murmur at the lower left sternal border (due to flow across the VSD) or upper left sternal border (due to increased flow across

the right ventricular outflow tract [RVOT]) may be heard along with a diastolic inflow rumble (an absence of silence) at the apex. If pulmonary vascular resistance is high, the pulmonic component of the second heart sound may be increased, although difficult to appreciate. Occasionally, large defects may allow transient right-to-left shunting to occur, particularly when the infant is crying.

In patients with an outlet VSD, the holosystolic murmur is often present, but the murmur is located higher on the left sternal border. Care should be taken to listen for the diastolic decrescendo of aortic insufficiency at the mid-left sternal border or at the apex.

The laboratory evaluation of the infant with a suspected VSD should include an ECG, chest radiograph, and echocardiogram. In infants, the ECG may not be distinctive unless an inlet VSD is present (see later discussion). The chest radiograph, even in the neonate, is important to obtain to assess heart size and pulmonary vascular markings. The chest radiograph can be an important tool in the followup of newborns with VSDs to assess progression in left-to-right shunting as the pulmonary vascular resistance declines. Echocardiography is the definitive diagnostic modality for characterizing the location and size of the VSDs. Associated lesions, such as coarctation of the aorta, can also be readily assessed by echocardiography. Doppler studies can estimate the degree of restriction by calculating the pressure drop at the defect (see Chapter 53). M-mode measurements can be used to determine left ventricular dimensions, which will be increased when a significant left-to-right shunt is present. As mentioned earlier, cardiac catheterization can accurately quantitate the degree of shunting but is rarely needed in the initial assessment of the newborn with VSD.

Up to 80% of small, muscular VSDs and 30% to 50% of perimembranous defects will close spontaneously. It is uncommon for these defects to increase in size, although the degree of left-to-right shunting can increase as pulmonary vascular resistance drops. Occasionally, inlet VSDs will undergo closure secondary to chordal attachments of the AV valves, but closure is generally present at birth if it is going to occur. Outlet VSDs virtually never close and have the associated risk of progressive aortic insufficiency due to prolapsing of the right coronary cusp into the defect.

The short-term consideration in following patients with VSDs is the management of congestive heart failure if the left-to-right shunt is excessive. Medications that are used include furosemide (typically 1 mg/kg/dose bid), digoxin (5 µg/kg/dose bid), and afterload reduction with enalapril (initial dose of 0.05 mg/kg/dose bid up to 0.25 mg/kg/dose bid—monitoring blood pressure). The primary goal in controlling congestive heart failure is to allow the newborn to grow adequately and, it is hoped, allow progressive closure of the VSDs. Weight gain is a useful and objective measure to follow.

The long-term goal of therapy or intervention is to prevent the development of irreversible pulmonary vascular occlusive disease. Shunts with a Qp:Qs >2 are at long-term risk for development of Eisenmenger's syndrome, and closure of the defect is warranted beyond 2 to 4 years of age when further decline in defect size is unlikely.

If medical therapy fails to control heart failure and the infant has failure to thrive, surgical closure of the defect in the first 6 months of life is needed. Surgical closure is also indicated in the 6- to 12-month-old child with a large VSD who has not demonstrated signs and symptoms of congestive heart failure due to lack of decline in pulmonary vascular resistance. In these infants, irreversible changes in the pulmonary vasculature may occur if the pressure load is not taken off the lungs. As mentioned earlier, defects with a Qp:Qs >2 and outlet defects also require closure. The use of pulmonary artery banding is falling out of favor for palliation of patients with VSDs unless the patient's clinical condition makes complete repair untenable. There is growing use of hybrid procedures where the surgeon and interventional cardiologist work together to close defects in small children (Contrafouris et al, 2009). This combined approach has successfully been applied to the closure of muscular VSDs in infants that are positioned in a location that is difficult for the surgeon to visualize from a right atrial approach. Additional indications for the hybrid approach to VSD closure will likely be determined in the coming years.

ATRIAL SEPTAL DEFECTS

Although atrial septal defects (ASDs) rarely produce a murmur in the neonatal period, the systolic murmur they generate later in life makes them appropriate for this section. As discussed previously, atrial-level shunting through the foramen ovale in utero allows the nutrient-rich placental blood to gain access to the left ventricle and ascending aorta. In the immediate postnatal period, careful echo examination of the interatrial septum will usually identify residual left-to-right or bidirectional shunting through the foramen ovale. Measurement of the size of the shunt provides an indication of whether there will be a persistent septal defect. An opening less than 6 mm in a term infant will most likely close and is referred to as a patent foramen ovale in order to distinguish it from a true atrial septal defect. Atrial septal defects that represent congenital lesions are classified as follows:

- Secundum
- Primum
- Sinus venosus
- Coronary sinus

Secundum defects are the most common and, when present in the neonate, allow for left-to-right or bidirectional shunting. The direction of the shunt, and the reason an ASD murmur is typically not heard in the neonate, is that right ventricular compliance remains low until the right ventricle remodels postnatally. The reduced right ventricular compliance increases right atrial pressure and limits the amount of left-to-right atrial-level shunting. Secundum ASDs are associated with Holt-Oram syndrome (abnormal radii, first-degree AV block, and ASD). Primum ASDs are in the spectrum of AV septal defects and are considered in the next section. Sinus venosus defects occur when the wall separating the upper or lower right pulmonary vein is deficient so that pulmonary venous return from either or both veins spills into the right atrium. This results in a left-to-right shunt. This variant of anomalous pulmonary venous return is considered in greater detail later. Coronary sinus defects result from an "unroofing" of the coronary sinus so that the coronary sinus enters at the left-right

atrial junction where the septum is deficient. Often, this lesion is associated with a persistent left superior vena cava that enters into the coronary sinus.

In later childhood when the compliance of the right ventricle increases and left-to-right shunting through an ASD increases, the classic physical findings of fixed splitting of S2, a systolic ejection murmur at the left upper sternal border, and a diastolic right ventricular inflow murmur at the lower left sternal border become apparent in lesions with a Qp:Qs >2. Electrocardiography will often demonstrate an rsR' pattern in the right precordial leads with evidence of right ventricular hypertrophy. Cardiomegaly with a prominent pulmonary artery segment and increased vascular markings will be seen on chest radiograph. Echocardiogram remains the gold standard for identifying and sizing the defects.

It is uncommon for infants and children with an isolated ASD to develop heart failure. Typically, intervention for a significant ASD is performed to prevent the long-term sequelae of pulmonary vascular occlusive disease. Thus, closure is rarely performed before the age of 3 or 4 years. Device closure of secundum ASDs is now routinely performed in the catheterization laboratory in children weighing more than 15 kg, although surgical closure is still performed when lesions are large or the rim of tissue between the ASD and aorta is deficient.

ATRIOVENTRICULAR SEPTAL DEFECTS

A variety of terms have been used to describe AV septal defects including AV canal defect, endocardial cushion defect, and common AV orifice. In addition, there is a spectrum of AV septal defects:

- Complete: a common AV valve is present along with a significant primum ASD and inlet VSD
- *Intermediate*: a common AV valve annulus although separate AV valves along with a primum ASD and inlet VSD
- Transitional: completely separate AV valves along with a primum ASD and inlet VSD
- Partial: separate AV valves with a primum ASD and no VSD

These four groups have some therapeutic relevance with regard to the degree of AV valve abnormality that must be considered at surgery, although each has a cleft between the anterior bridging leaflet and the lateral leaflet of the left-sided (mitral) valve that must be addressed. In infants with a complete AV septal defect, it is important to assess whether the right and left ventricles are *balanced*, that is, equally developed so that a two-ventricle repair is possible, and also to determine the degree of AV insufficiency, which has prognostic importance in the surgical outcome. The association of AV septal defects with Down syndrome has been addressed previously.

In the immediate postnatal period, variations in pulmonary vascular resistance that occur, particularly in infants with Down syndrome, can result in a right-to-left shunt through a nonrestrictive primum ASD and/or inlet VSD and result in systemic desaturation. Many infants with complete AV septal defects will develop heart failure in the first 2 months of life as pulmonary vascular resistance falls. A small percentage of infants will not have a decline in pulmonary vascular resistance, making the lack of heart

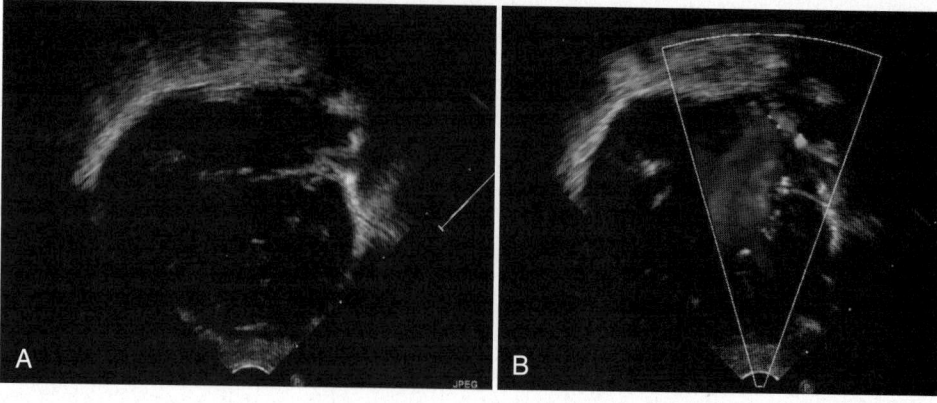

FIGURE 55-3 *(Supplemental color version of this figure is available online at www.expertconsult.com.)* **Echocardiographic view of complete atrioventricular septal defect. A,** Four-chamber view showing the common AV valve that separates the atria and ventricles (RV, right ventricle; LV, left ventricle) which in this patient are well balanced. The large primum ASD and inlet VSD are seen. **B,** With color Doppler, inflow across the AV valve is seen.

failure a troubling sign and an indication for early surgical repair.

Although diagnosis largely rests on the echocardiogram, AV septal defects can be suspected on ECG with the presence of a superior frontal QRS axis (ranging from –30 to –120 degrees), evidence of right ventricular hypertrophy, and Q waves in leads I and aVL. Echocardiography is used to define the type of AV septal defect and identify associated anomalies (Figure 55-3). As mentioned earlier, critical assessment of relative ventricular sizes and the degree of AV valve insufficiency is necessary. Interrogation of the right ventricular outflow tract (RVOT) is also needed due to the associated pulmonic stenosis or tetralogy of Fallot that can occur with complete AV septal defects.

Correction of complete AV septal defects is done surgically at 4 to 6 months of age. While awaiting surgery, care must be taken not to treat minor desaturation episodes with excessive oxygen because oxygen-induced lowering of pulmonary vascular resistance can rapidly worsen heart failure and lead to further desaturation, a spiral that can be difficult to reverse. Furosemide, digoxin, and afterload reduction are often needed to control heart failure, and some cardiologists will start these medications in the immediate postnatal period because of the high likelihood of infants developing congestive heart failure. Complete repair (septation of atrial, AV valves, and ventricles) is preferred. It is very rare that palliative banding of the pulmonary artery is needed to control heart failure symptoms. As mentioned previously, early repair should be considered in the infant who does not have a decline in pulmonary vascular resistance and the development of heart failure because of the concern of early development of irreversible increases in pulmonary vascular resistance, particularly in non–Down syndrome complete AV septal defect patients.

PERIPHERAL PULMONIC STENOSIS

Peripheral pulmonic stenosis (PPS) can range widely in its severity. In many instances, mild narrowing of the branch pulmonary arteries occurs in the neonate and produces a murmur that is heard widely throughout the chest. The murmur due to this mild PPS is considered by some to be an "innocent murmur" of infancy and usually resolves by 2 to 4 months of age. This lesion likely reflects mild hypoplasia of the branch pulmonary arteries due to decreased in utero pulmonary blood flow and the postnatal transition where these vessels must accommodate the entire cardiac output.

More severe PPS is seen in cases of congenital rubella syndrome or in association with Williams or Noonan's syndrome. Branch pulmonary artery stenoses can also occur with tetralogy of Fallot. In these cases, multiple levels of obstruction may exist that require catheterization or surgical intervention.

In isolated or mild PPS, minimal right ventricular pressure overload occurs. With increasing stenosis, right ventricular pressure overload will result in right ventricular hypertrophy and, in later stages, right atrial enlargement on ECG. Echocardiography can interrogate the proximal pulmonary arteries, but more distal lesions require other imaging modalities such as magnetic resonance imaging or cardiac catheterization.

Intervention to treat severe branch stenoses should be considered when right ventricular pressure is greater than 75% of systemic pressure or any clinical or laboratory evidence of right ventricular dysfunction is present. Surgical management is possible for proximal areas of stenosis, although the treatment preferred by most clinicians is balloon dilation or expandable stent placement in the cardiac catheterization laboratory. Repeated interventions may be needed to enlarge vessels as the patient grows or to dilate other areas of stenosis that develop.

PULMONIC STENOSIS

Isolated pulmonary valve stenosis is a common cause of a systolic ejection murmur in the neonatal period. Although cases typically occur sporadically, more than 50% of infants with Noonan's syndrome will have pulmonic stenosis, and thus the pulmonary valve should be evaluated in all these children.

The degree of pulmonic stenosis determines the pathophysiology of the disease process. As the stenosis of the valve worsens, right ventricular pressure increases along with the degree of right ventricular wall stress. Right ventricular hypertrophy will develop if the stenosis is left untreated. In severe, or critical, pulmonic stenosis (discussed later), heart failure can develop in the neonate accompanied by cyanosis due to right-to-left shunting at the atrial level.

The degree of stenosis is generally classified based on the pressure drop across the pulmonic valve, with mild stenosis defined as a gradient <30 mm Hg, moderate stenosis as a gradient of 30 to 60 mm Hg, and severe stenosis as >60 mm Hg. Although these definitions were initially based

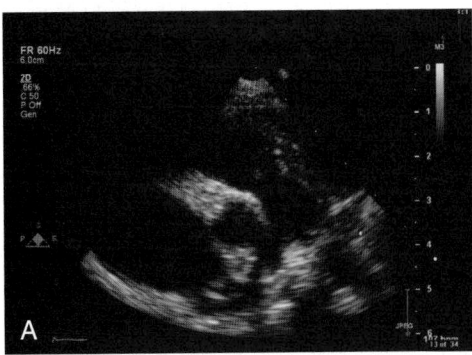 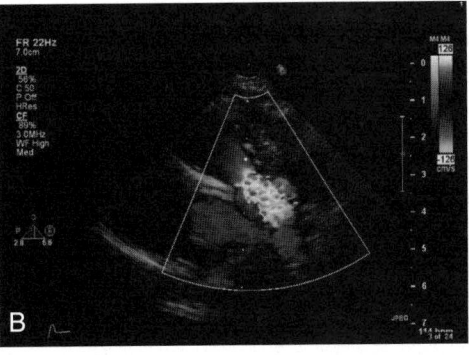

FIGURE 55-4 *(See also Color Plate 22.)* **Pulmonic stenosis. A,** Short-axis view of pulmonic stenosis with a thickened appearing pulmonic valve (PV). **B,** Using color Doppler imaging, turbulence in the main pulmonary artery is seen above the pulmonic valve.

on cardiac catheterization, current follow-up of patients with pulmonic stenosis utilizes echocardiogram, which overestimates the gradient compared to direct hemodynamic measurement at catheterization. Thus, some use an *echo gradient* of <40 mm Hg as mild pulmonic stenosis.

Consideration of the valve gradient is critical because of the prognostic significance of the value. In older children, mild stenosis rarely progresses (Nugent et al, 1977). In infants, however, follow-up of patients with echo gradients <40 mm Hg found that 29% developed progressive valve stenosis, with half of those showing an increase in the first 6 months of life (Rowland, 1997). Neonates with moderate valve stenosis may face an even greater likelihood of developing progressive stenosis, although limited data exist.

A systolic ejection murmur of pulmonic stenosis can be heard in the neonatal period at the upper left sternal border. Typically, although the fast heart rate in the neonate may make it difficult to appreciate, a systolic ejection click just after the first heart sound (S1) can be heard in most of these infants and is an important feature to distinguish pulmonic stenosis from other lesions. Much as in PPS (see earlier discussion), the murmur of pulmonic stenosis radiates throughout the lung fields. As the gradient across the valve worsens, a thrill may be palpable at the upper left sternal border. As the degree of stenosis progresses further and becomes severe, the murmur and click will diminish and may even be absent as right ventricular dysfunction worsens. Of note is that while progressive pulmonic stenosis may be able to be estimated on the basis of the murmur, the clinical condition of the infant may not change appreciably until the degree of stenosis becomes severe.

The findings on laboratory studies in infants with pulmonic stenosis will vary depending on the degree of stenosis. Electrocardiogram will demonstrate right ventricular hypertrophy in most patients with moderate stenosis, although the study may be normal when mild stenosis is present. Chest radiography is often normal unless poststenotic dilation of the main pulmonary artery has developed. Echocardiography will be diagnostic. The valve will have varying degrees of dysplasia that is characterized by thickened, poorly mobile leaflets that dome during systole. Turbulence distal to the valve will be seen by color Doppler imaging (Figure 55-4), while pulsed-wave Doppler is used to determine the degree of stenosis. As discussed earlier, Doppler echo generally gives a value of stenosis that is 20% to 30% higher than the peak-to-peak pressure gradient measured as cardiac catheterization.

Treatment of isolated pulmonic stenosis, even in the neonate, can readily be performed by balloon valvotomy in the cardiac catheterization laboratory. The exception may be in infants with Noonan's syndrome where the degree of valvar dysplasia may prevent an adequate result, although most will initially attempt a balloon valvotomy before progressing to surgery. Valvotomy should be considered in infants with more than mild stenosis. Mild or moderate pulmonary insufficiency, should it develop after balloon valvotomy, is usually well tolerated. Recurrent stenosis and more significant pulmonic insufficiency are found more often when valvotomy is needed in the neonatal period (Garty et al, 2005).

AORTIC STENOSIS

Like stenosis of the pulmonic valve, aortic valve stenosis can produce a murmur in the neonatal period. However, aortic stenosis is more likely to be progressive than pulmonic stenosis. Levels of obstruction of the left ventricular outflow tract can also occur at the subvalvar and supravalvar levels. Subvalvar stenosis is rarely diagnosed in the neonatal period, but often progresses later in life as a fibromuscular ridge beneath the aortic valve. Supravalvular stenosis can present in the newborn period and is often associated with Williams syndrome.

As with pulmonic stenosis, the pathophysiology and physical findings associated with aortic valve stenosis depend on the degree of obstruction. Certainly the most common aortic valve abnormality addressed in the neonatal period is critical aortic stenosis associated with decreased left ventricular function. This medical emergent situation is addressed in detail later. Mild (aortic valve gradient <30 mm Hg) and moderate (valve gradient of 30 to 60 mm Hg) aortic valve stenosis is not commonly encountered in the neonatal period. When it is, these milder forms of stenosis are generally associated with a bicuspid aortic valve and tend to progress with age. The rate of change of progression throughout infancy and childhood is quite variable and necessitates frequent follow-up of these patients.

The murmur in the newborn with aortic stenosis may be difficult to localize to the upper right sternal border as in older children. A thrill is usually palpable at the suprasternal notch with even mild aortic valve stenosis with a precordial thrill felt as the degree of stenosis increases. Usually a click from the stenotic aortic valve is heard at the apex or lower left sternal border.

Electrocardiography may be of limited benefit in the newborn with mild or even moderate aortic valve stenosis, although some degree of left ventricular hypertrophy may be seen. Chest radiograph is of limited benefit in following these patients, with the focus of the diagnostic assessment being the echocardiogram. On echocardiogram, the aortic valve can be characterized. Fused leaflets that are thickened and domed are seen. Pulsed Doppler is used to determine the gradient across the valve; color Doppler imaging can define the presence of aortic insufficiency.

Initial management of moderate aortic valve stenosis is balloon valvotomy in the cardiac catheterization laboratory. The balloon is sized in an effort to limit aortic insufficiency, which is much less well tolerated than insufficiency of the pulmonic valve. If significant aortic valve insufficiency is present or develops, surgical repair or valve replacement is needed. In neonates and infants, the Ross procedure is usually the procedure of choice (Elkins et al, 1994). In this procedure, the pulmonary valve is removed intact from the patient and sewn into the aortic position, and a homograft is placed in the pulmonic position. Interestingly, the pulmonary autograft generally demonstrates good growth and excellent function in the aortic position. Although the child will outgrow the pulmonary homograft, replacing it and managing progressive pulmonic stenosis is much easier than addressing the aortic valve.

CYANOSIS IN THE NEWBORN

Congenital heart defects that present with cyanosis do so because of a right-to-left shunt. The shunt results in mixing of the systemic and pulmonary venous returns that can occur between the atria and ventricles or great vessels. Defects manifesting predominantly with cyanosis can be further subclassified by the amount of associated pulmonary blood. If there is no restriction to pulmonary blood flow, cardiac output to the lungs will increase as the normal postnatal drop in pulmonary vascular resistance occurs. Clinically, this results in tachypnea, poor feeding, hepatomegaly, and pulmonary edema. Much of the neonatal management is aimed at balancing the ratio of systemic to pulmonary blood flow. Defects with restriction to pulmonary blood flow typically present with cyanosis without associated symptoms of congestive heart failure. If the restriction is severe, pulmonary blood flow may be dependent on a left-to-right shunt through the ductus arteriosus. These patients typically have some degree of right ventricular hypertension. If the ductus closes, profound cyanosis results. Lesions presenting primarily with cyanosis in the newborn period are discussed below.

TRANSPOSITION OF THE GREAT ARTERIES

Transposition of the great arteries (TGA) accounts for 5% of all cases of cyanotic congenital heart disease and is the most common cyanotic cardiac defect in the newborn. There is a strong male predominance (60% to 70%), but no other clear association between TGA and maternal conditions, teratogen exposure, or genetic abnormalities. TGA is typically an isolated defect, with <10% of cases associated with extracardiac malformations.

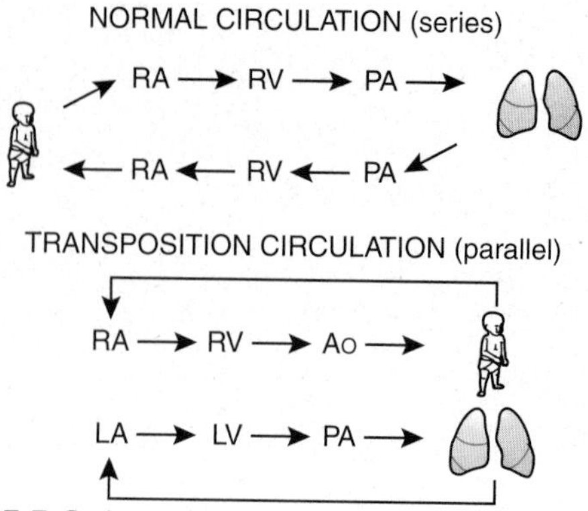

FIGURE 55-5 **Series and parallel circulations.** The series circulation in the normal newborn is compared with the parallel circulation in transposition of the great arteries (TGA). In TGA, survival after birth is dependent on mixing at either the atrial, ventricular, or great vessel level. *(From Wernovsky G: Transposition of the great arteries. In Allen HD, Gutgesell HP, Clark EB, et al, editors: Moss and Adams' heart disease in infants, children, and adolescents: including the fetus and young adult, ed 6, Philadelphia, 2001, Lippincott Williams & Wilkins, pp 1027-1084.)*

In the most common form of TGA (d-TGA, complete transposition, or simple transposition), the aorta arises from the right ventricle anteriorly and slightly rightward of the pulmonary artery, which arises from the left ventricle. Desaturated blood returns to the right ventricle and is recirculated to the body via the aorta, while oxygenated blood returns to the left ventricle and is recirculated to the lungs. The end result is separate, parallel circulations (Figure 55-5). Survival is dependent on communication between the two circulations, typically in the form of bidirectional shunting at the patent foramen ovale (PFO) and PDA. With absent or small communications between the circulations, severe systemic acidosis and hypoxia develop after birth, resulting in death.

Cyanosis is apparent within the first few hours of life and is not responsive to oxygen. Cardiac examination is typically normal with the exception of a loud single S2. Because of the arrangement of the great vessels, the louder closure of the anterior aortic valve obscures closure of the more posterior pulmonary valve. Chest radiograph may be normal or reveal a narrow mediastinum with slight predominance of the right ventricle resulting in an "egg on a string" appearance. Pulmonary vascular markings are normal to slightly increased. ECG is typically normal but may reveal right ventricular hypertrophy. Echocardiogram reveals the transposed great vessels and is used to determine the size of the PFO and PDA and to define any associated cardiac defects.

Initial management of infants with TGA is aimed at maintaining communication between the systemic and pulmonary circulations. Prostaglandin E_1 is started to maintain patency of the ductus arteriosus (dose of 0.05 to 0.1 µg/kg/min). In patients with a restrictive patent foramen ovale, or with persistent hypoxia and acidosis despite a PDA, a balloon atrial septostomy is performed within the first 24 to 48 hours of life to encourage mixing at the atrial level. In the setting of adequate mixing, pulmonary overcirculation may develop as pulmonary vascular resistance drops. Surgical treatment is the arterial switch procedure (Figure 55-6), typically performed within the 1st week of life (Castaneda et al, 1989; Prifti et al, 2002).

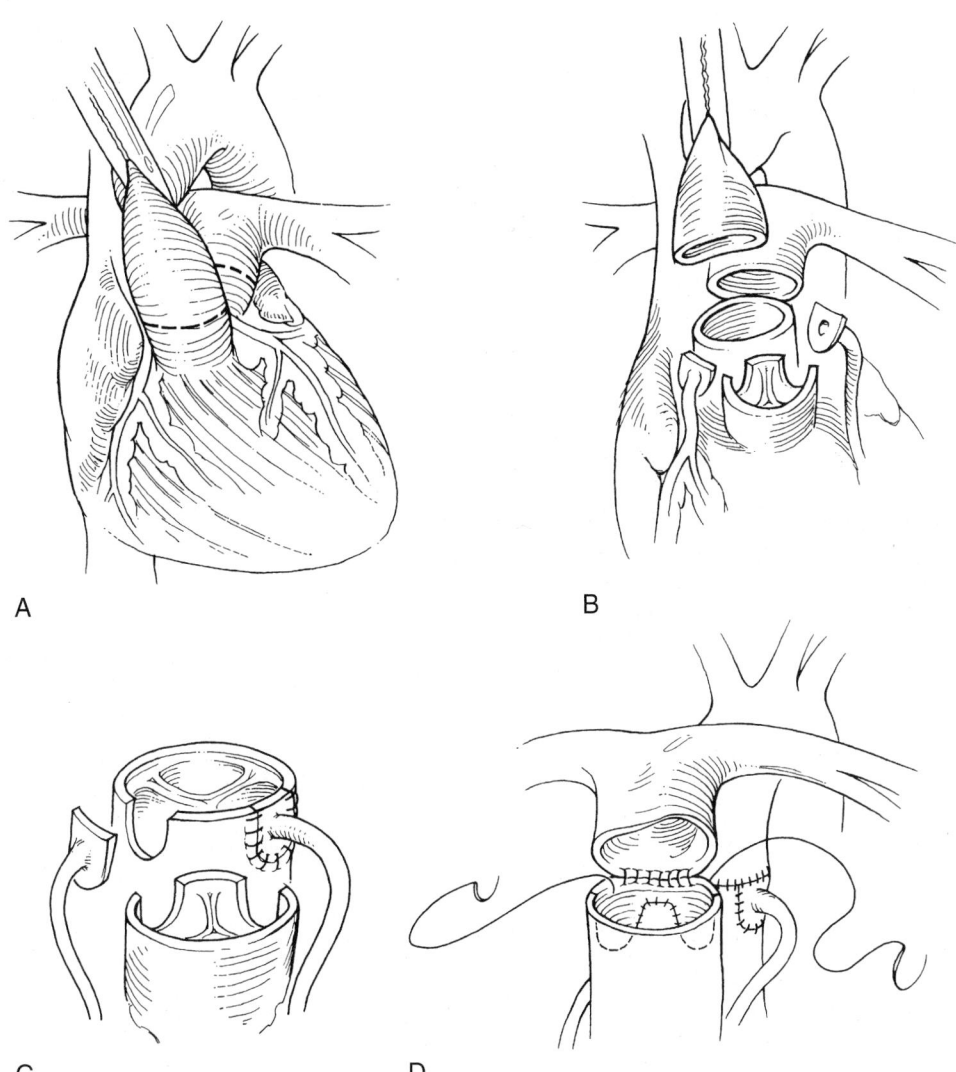

A

B

C

D

FIGURE 55-6 **Arterial switch operation for d-transposition of the great arteries. A,** The *dashed lines* depict the planned location of transection of the great vessels. **B,** The coronary arteries are removed with surrounding aortic wall as "buttons." **C,** The coronary buttons are translocated to the posterior neoaortic root. **D,** The Lecompte maneuver brings both pulmonary arteries anterior to the neoaorta. The aortic suture line is completed, incorporating the coronary buttons. The coronary donor sites are filled in with patches of autologous pericardium, and the pulmonary anastomosis is completed. *(From Wernovsky G, Jonas RA: Transposition of the great arteries. In Chang AC, Hanley FL, Wernovsky G, et al, editors:* Pediatric cardiac intensive care, *Baltimore, 1998, Williams & Wilkins, pp 289-301.)*

Although TGA is usually an isolated lesion, 40–45% of patients have an associated ventricular septal defect, 10% have a ventricular septal defect with left ventricular outflow tract obstruction, and 5% have left ventricular outflow tract obstruction alone. In addition, there is a wide variety in coronary artery anatomy in patients with TGA. The clinical presentation of patients with TGA and VSD depends on the size of the VSD. Those with a restrictive VSD present like patients with TGA and intact ventricular septum. Those with a large VSD may not experience any symptoms initially. As pulmonary vascular resistance drops, symptoms of pulmonary overcirculation develop. Patients with restricted pulmonary blood flow (TGA with VSD and pulmonic stenosis) appear clinically similar to patients with tetralogy of Fallot. The timing and type of surgical repair in patients with complex TGA is variable and beyond the scope of this chapter.

DOUBLE-OUTLET RIGHT VENTRICLE

Double-outlet right ventricle (DORV) is relatively rare and consists of a diverse group of lesions characterized by the origination of both great vessels from the right ventricle and by the persistence of the subaortic and subpulmonary conus. There are multiple anatomic variations of this lesion, which are commonly classified by the relationship of the great vessels to one another and/or by the location of the ventricular septal defect to the great vessels (Figure 55-7) (Anderson et al, 1983; Mahle et al, 2008; Stellin et al, 1991). Accordingly, there are four types of DORV, each with a slightly different neonatal presentation and surgical management.

DORV of the tetralogy type typically has normally related great vessels with a subaortic VSD. Because the subaortic conus is pulled anteriorly, the subpulmonary conus is typically smaller, resulting in variable obstruction

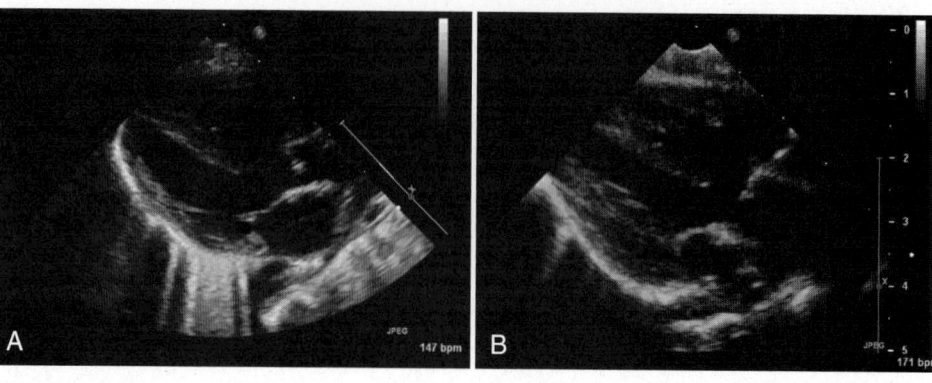

FIGURE 55-7 Echocardiographic views of double outlet right ventricle. **A,** The aorta is committed to the right ventricle and the ventricular septal defect is below the aortic valve. **B,** The great vessels are transposed in this patient with the pulmonary artery overriding the ventricular septal defect.

to pulmonary blood flow. The clinical presentation and surgical management are similar to those of tetralogy of Fallot.

DORV of the transposition type typically has malposed great vessels with the aorta located either anterior to or rightward of the pulmonary artery. The ventricular septal defect is subpulmonary and directs flow into the pulmonary artery, resulting in transposition-like physiology. This lesion is frequently associated with variable obstruction to aortic blood flow and coarctation of the aorta. Surgical repair consists of baffling the VSD to the pulmonary valve and performing an arterial switch. In the setting of coronary artery anomalies that prevent an arterial switch, the left ventricle is baffled to both the aortic and pulmonary valves and a right ventricle to pulmonary artery conduit is placed. Arch obstruction is corrected if needed.

In DORV with a "doubly committed" VSD, the VSD is below both great vessels. The physiology and clinical presentation are variable, depending on the size and orientation of the VSD and the degree of outflow tract obstruction. Surgical repair is directed at closing the interventricular communication without obstructing either ventricular outflow.

The least common variety of DORV is that in which the VSD is remote from both great vessels. Because of the distance between the VSD and the great vessels, a two-ventricle repair is difficult and often impossible. Pulmonary banding is frequently performed in the newborn period to limit pulmonary blood flow, delaying attempts at a biventricular repair or single ventricle palliation until several months of age. Recently, there has been increasing interest in biventricular repair for this lesion through creation of intracardiac baffles (Lacour-Gayet, 2002).

TRUNCUS ARTERIOSUS

In truncus arteriosus, a single arterial trunk gives rise to the pulmonary, systemic, and coronary circulation. The arterial trunk typically overrides a ventricular septal defect. Truncus is classified by the origin of the pulmonary arteries (Figure 55-8). In type I, a small pulmonary artery arises from the arterial trunk and bifurcates in the right and left branch pulmonary arteries. The right and left pulmonary arteries can also arise from separate ostia that are either close to one another (type II) or some distance apart (type III) (Collett, 1949). Type IV is similar to tetralogy of Fallot with pulmonary atresia (see later discussion). The truncal valve has between one and six cusps. It is occasionally

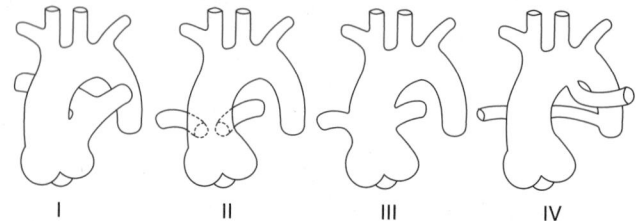

I   II   III   IV

FIGURE 55-8 Types of truncus arteriosus. The classification of truncus arteriosus is determined by the origin of the pulmonary arteries (see text for details).

insufficient, but rarely stenotic. Truncus usually occurs as an isolated cardiovascular defect, although it has been associated with microdeletion of chromosomal region 22q11 (McElhinney et al, 2003).

As the pulmonary vascular resistance drops over the first several weeks of life, increased shunting from the arterial trunk to the pulmonary arteries occurs, and pulmonary overcirculation develops. If left untreated, symptoms of heart failure develop. Long-term pulmonary vascular obstructive disease occurs.

The clinical presentation of truncus changes with the pulmonary vascular resistance. Initially, infants are minimally cyanotic and do not appear to be in distress. As pulmonary overcirculation occurs, symptoms of heart failure develop. Cardiac examination reveals a hyperdynamic precordium and a loud single S2. As pulmonary vascular resistance drops, the pulses become bounding and the pulse pressure widens because of runoff into the pulmonary arteries. A low-pitched diastolic inflow rumble may be heard at the apex. In addition, a systolic ejection murmur may be present, and a medium- to high-pitched diastolic murmur may be heard from truncal valve insufficiency. Chest radiograph typically reveals cardiomegaly with pulmonary vascular markings that increase over the first few weeks of life. ECG demonstrates right, left, or biventricular hypertrophy. Echocardiography is used to demonstrate the anatomy and evaluate for associated cardiac defects such as right aortic arch, coronary artery anomalies, interrupted aortic arch, and secundum atrial septal defects.

Initially, heart failure symptoms are managed with anticongestive medications. Surgical repair is typically performed within the first 2 months of life because of difficulty in controlling heart failure. The usual repair involves closure of the ventricular septal defect so that the arterial trunk arises from the left ventricle. A right ventricle–to–pulmonary artery conduit is then placed

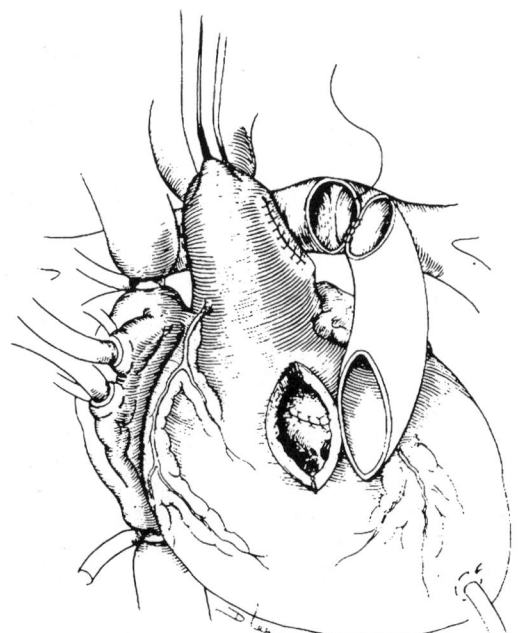

FIGURE 55-9 Anatomy and repair of truncus arteriosus. After the branch pulmonary arteries are removed from the common trunk (and the resulting aortic defect is closed), a ventriculotomy is performed. The ventricular septal defect is closed through this incision, and a conduit is placed from the right ventricle to the pulmonary arteries. *(From Behrendt DM, Dick M: Truncus repair with a valveless conduit in neonates, J Thorac Cardiovasc Surg 110:1148-1150, 1995.)*

(Figure 55-9). This conduit needs to be replaced several times over the course of the patient's life.

TOTAL ANOMALOUS PULMONARY VENOUS RETURN

In total anomalous pulmonary venous return (TAPVR) the pulmonary veins return to a systemic vein or directly to the right atrium, rather than the left atrium. Both systemic and pulmonary venous return pass through the right atrium, right ventricle, and pulmonary artery, creating pulmonary overcirculation and right heart volume overload. An atrial septal defect is present in all cases. The right atrium–to–left-atrium shunt supplies the systemic cardiac output. If the atrial septal defect is restrictive, then systemic output will be limited.

Several common patterns of anomalous pulmonary venous return are seen (Figure 55-10) (Edwards and Helmholz, 1956). Most commonly, the anomalous veins drain in a supracardiac fashion, entering the left innominate vein or superior vena cava via a vertical vein, and draining into the right atrium via the superior vena cava. Cardiac drainage occurs when the anomalous veins drain into the right atrium via the coronary sinus. Alternatively, a descending vein may pass through the diaphragmatic hiatus and enter the hepatic or portal venous system, resulting in infracardiac drainage. Rarely, a mixed pattern of drainage may exist, or the anomalous veins may drain directly to the right atrium. Drainage directly into the right atrium occurs almost exclusively in patients with heterotaxy.

The clinical presentation of TAPVR varies, depending on the degree of obstruction to pulmonary venous flow.

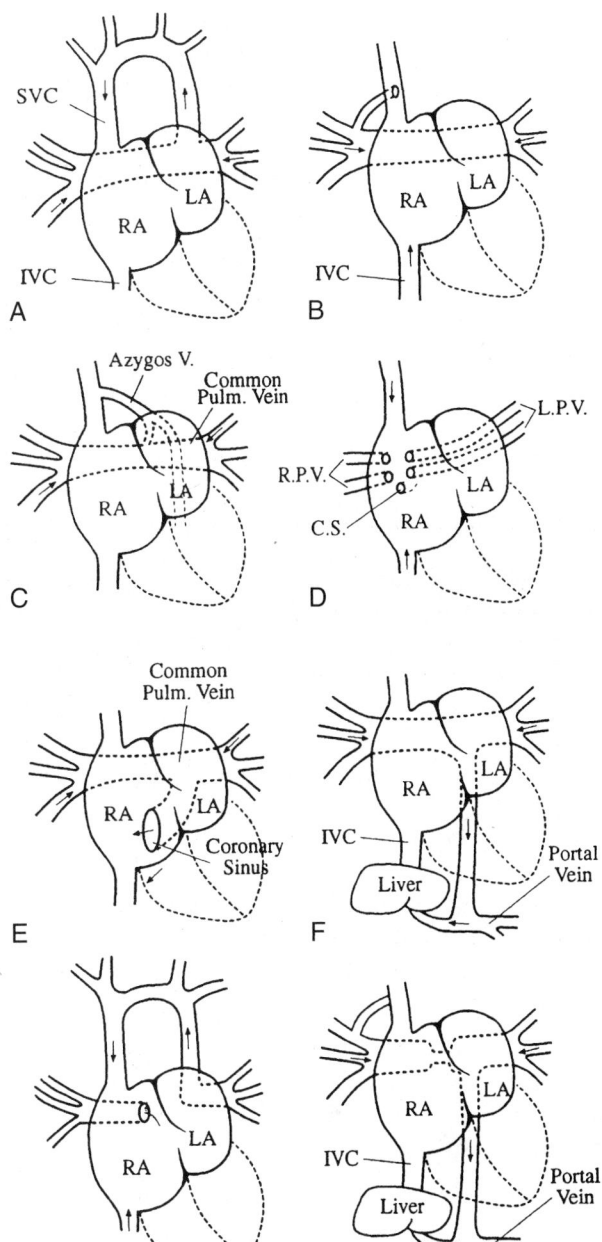

FIGURE 55-10 Anatomic varieties of total anomalous pulmonary venous return: **A** to **C,** Supracardiac; **D** and **E,** cardiac; **F,** infracardiac; **G** and **H,** mixed. See text for details. *CS,* Coronary sinus; *IVC,* inferior vena cava; *LA,* left atrium; *LPV,* left pulmonary vein; *RA,* right atrium; *RPV,* right pulmonary vein; *SVC,* superior vena cava. *(From Eimbcke F, Enriquez G, Gomez O, et al: Total anomalous pulmonary venous connection. In Moller JH, Hoffman JIE, editors: Pediatric cardiovascular medicine, Philadelphia, 2000, Churchill Livingstone, pp 409-420.)*

Patients with unobstructed pulmonary venous flow will have minimal symptoms in the newborn period, and cyanosis is usually not apparent. Symptoms of right heart failure develop over time owing to the progressive right heart volume overload. Physical examination may reveal a right ventricular heave, fixed split S2, and a soft systolic ejection murmur in the pulmonic area. Chest radiograph may demonstrate cardiomegaly due to an enlarged right atrium, right ventricle, and main pulmonary artery. Pulmonary vascular markings increase over time. ECG reveals

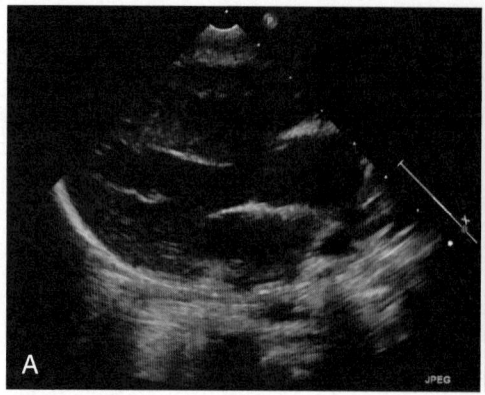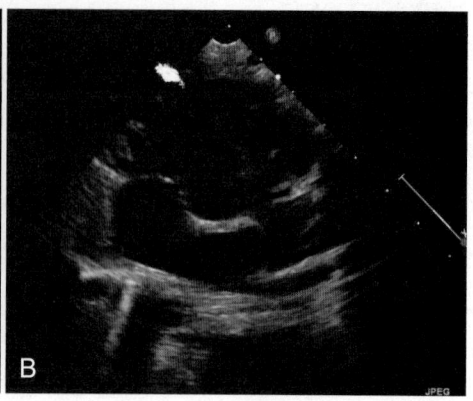

FIGURE 55-11 Echocardiographic view of tetralogy of Fallot. **A,** Some of the anatomic features of tetralogy of Fallot are readily demonstrated on the long-axis echocardiographic view including the hypertrophy of the right ventricle, the ventricular septal defect (VSD), and the aorta overriding the VSD. **B,** The short-axis view on echo shows the infundibular or right ventricular outflow tract stenosis.

peaked p waves and right ventricular hypertrophy. Patients with moderate restriction to pulmonary blood flow are typically cyanotic in the newborn period. There is usually adequate mixing of venous return to allow for oxygen delivery to tissues. These patients may, however, benefit from supplemental oxygen, mechanical ventilation, and sedation to decrease oxygen consumption. The presentation of patients with obstructed pulmonary blood flow is discussed later in this chapter under obstructive lesions.

Treatment of TAPVR is surgical. In most cases, a pulmonary venous confluence is seen near the left atrium. Cardiac catheterization is used to define pulmonary venous anatomy if the pulmonary veins are not well seen by echocardiography. During surgery, the pulmonary venous confluence is anastomosed to the left atrium, the atrial septal defect is closed, and the connections to systemic veins are ligated. In the absence of pulmonary venous obstruction and in the setting of uncomplicated anatomy, surgical mortality is low and long-term results are good. Late pulmonary venous obstruction occurs in approximately 20% of cases, with relatively poor surgical and interventional cardiac catheterization results.

TETRALOGY OF FALLOT

Tetralogy of Fallot (TOF) consists of a ventricular septal defect, overriding aorta, RVOT obstruction, and right ventricular hypertrophy (Figure 55-11). The severity and location of the RVOT obstruction are variable. Infundibular hypertrophy, a small, frequently bicuspid pulmonary valve, and small main pulmonary artery can jointly or independently create obstruction at the subvalve, valve, or supravalve level, respectively. Complete obstruction of the right ventricular outflow tract (pulmonary atresia) with a ventricular septal defect is an extreme form of TOF. TOF is associated with a right aortic arch in 20% of cases and aberrant coronary arteries in 5–10% of cases, both of which can affect surgical planning. The etiology of TOF is heterogeneous. Maternal diabetes, phenylketonuria, and retinoic acid exposure have been associated with TOF. In addition, genetic syndromes including 22q11 deletion, Alagille syndrome, and VACTERL/VATER sequence have been associated with TOF.

The pathophysiology and clinical presentation of TOF are directly tied to the severity of the RVOT obstruction. With mild RVOT obstruction, the predominant shunt through the VSD is left to right. Cyanosis is minimal, and

symptoms of heart failure are the typical presenting manifestations. The main and branch pulmonary arteries are usually of normal size. With moderate RVOT obstruction, the shunt through the VSD is right to left but the prograde flow through the RVOT is adequate, resulting in mild cyanosis. The main and branch pulmonary arteries may have areas of focal stenosis or be diffusely small. With severe RVOT obstruction, there is minimal or no prograde flow across the RVOT. Pulmonary blood flow is thus dependent on left-to-right shunt through the PDA. Patients are severely cyanotic. PDA closure leads to cardiovascular collapse. The main and branch pulmonary arteries may be confluent and small. With pulmonary atresia (pulmonary atresia VSD or tetralogy pulmonary atresia), the pulmonary vascular bed is variable. The pulmonary arteries can be confluent, normal-sized, and fed entirely by the ductus arteriosus; confluent, small, with a small ductus; or virtually absent with pulmonary blood flow supplied by multiple aortopulmonary collateral vessels (MAPCAs).

Initial management depends on the amount of pulmonary blood flow. Patients without significant symptoms or hypoxemia undergo a complete repair in the first 6 months of life. Complete repair consists of VSD closure and relief of RVOT obstruction through a combination of infundibular muscle resection, pulmonary valvotomy, or RVOT patch that can extend out to the branch pulmonary arteries as needed (Figure 55-12). In patients with significant cyanosis or ductal dependent circulation, management options include palliation with a systemic–to–pulmonary artery shunt in the newborn period (modified Blalock-Taussig shunt) and complete repair at a later date or a complete anatomic correction in the newborn period. The recent trend has been toward earlier complete correction in symptomatic infants (Ooi et al, 2006; Reddy et al, 1995; Tamesberger et al, 2008).

TETRALOGY OF FALLOT WITH ABSENT PULMONARY VALVE

ToF with absent pulmonary valve (APV), or APV syndrome, is a spectrum of disorders with a rudimentary pulmonary valve. The resultant pulmonary valve stenosis and insufficiency cause dilation of the right ventricle and main and branch pulmonary arteries that is apparent in utero (Figure 55-13). The vast majority of cases also have a malalignment ventricular septal defect. Presumably secondary to airway compression by the dilated pulmonary

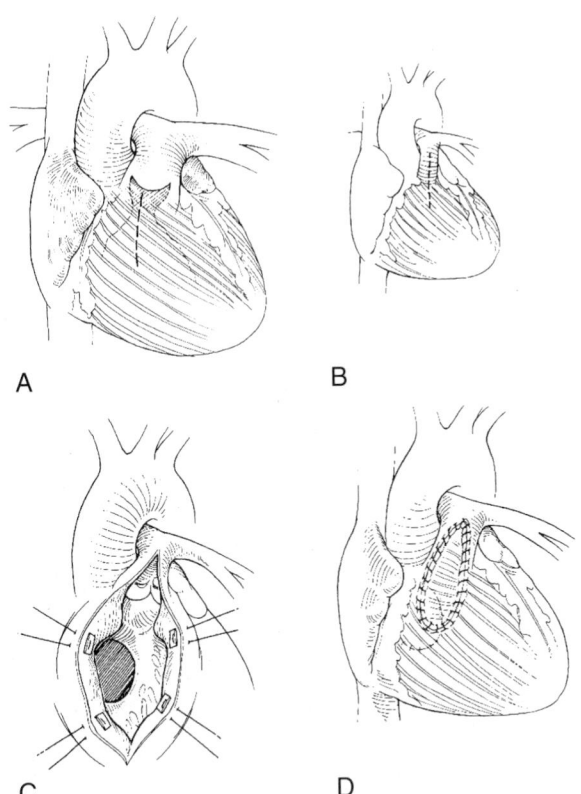

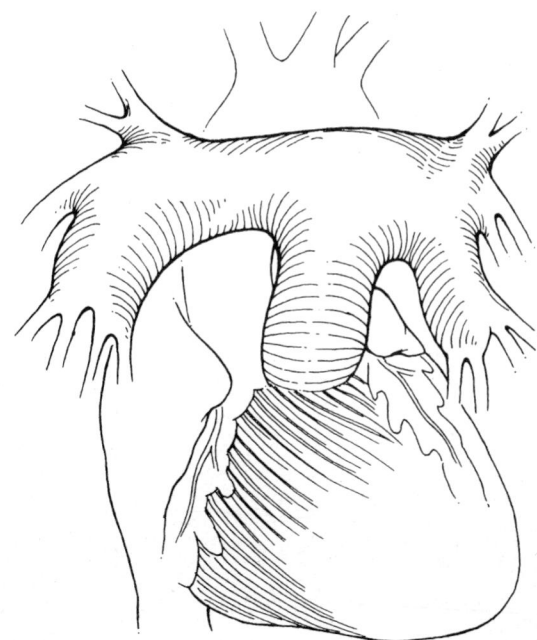

FIGURE 55-13 Tetralogy of Fallot with absent pulmonary valve. Severe dilatation of the main and branch pulmonary arteries is seen and is frequently with associated bronchial compression and large and small airway disease. The intracardiac anatomy is usually similar to that in standard tetralogy of Fallot. *(From Spray TL, Wernovsky G: Right ventricular outflow tract obstruction. In Chang AC, Hanley FL, Wernovsky G, et al, editors:* Pediatric cardiac intensive care, *Baltimore, 1998, Williams & Wilkins, pp 257-270.)*

FIGURE 55-12 Repair of tetralogy of Fallot. **A,** *Dashed line* depicts nontransannular incision, used when the pulmonary valve and annulus are of adequate size. **B,** A transannular incision *(dashed line)* is used when there is annular hypoplasia. **C,** An example of transventricular exposure of the ventricular septal defect (VSD). Alternatively, the VSD may be closed via a right atriotomy through the tricuspid valve. **D,** External view of patch closure of the transannular incision. *(From Spray TL, Wernovsky G: Right ventricular outflow tract obstruction. In Chang AC, Hanley FL, Wernovsky G, et al, editors:* Pediatric cardiac intensive care, *Baltimore, 1998, Williams & Wilkins, pp 257-270.)*

vasculature, this syndrome is commonly associated with airway anomalies. There is a high prevalence of 22q11 deletion among patients with APV.

Physical examination reveals a characteristic to-and-fro murmur of pulmonary stenosis and insufficiency. A prominent right ventricular heave and hepatomegaly are present secondary to the right ventricular volume overload. There is a wide range of symptoms, depending on the degree of right ventricular volume overload and degree of airway disease. At one end of the spectrum is an asymptomatic neonate with mild cyanosis and the gradual development of heart failure symptoms during the normal postnatal decline in pulmonary vascular resistance. At the other end of the spectrum is a critically ill infant with severe cyanosis and respiratory failure due to the combination of right-to-left shunt through the VSD and underlying airway disease. Mechanical ventilation is necessary and occasionally unsuccessful because of airway compression by the dilated pulmonary vasculature. Urgent surgery is required in these infants.

Surgery consists of VSD closure, pulmonary artery plication, relief of RVOT obstruction, and insertion of a valve or homograft in the RVOT position. There is significant variation in surgical technique between centers (Alsoufi et al, 2007; Tissot et al, 2007). The surgical mortality and

short- and long-term outcomes are related primarily to the severity of pulmonary artery dilation and airway compression. More severely affected infants have a higher surgical mortality and need for prolonged postoperative ventilation. Those with less significant pulmonary artery dilation have low postoperative mortality and long-term outcomes similar to those with TOF.

PULMONARY ATRESIA WITH INTACT VENTRICULAR SEPTUM

In pulmonary atresia with intact ventricular septum, the pulmonary valve leaflets are fused or fail to form. Without egress from the right ventricle, systemic venous return passes through the patent foramen ovale and mixes with pulmonary venous return. Pulmonary blood flow is dependent on the PDA, with the left ventricle providing cardiac output to both the systemic and pulmonary circulations. Tricuspid valve and right ventricular size vary, ranging from nearly normal-sized structures to a nearly atretic tricuspid valve and diminutive right ventricular chamber. The latter patients may have sinusoidal channels in the right ventricular myocardium that communicate with the coronary circulation. The high right ventricular pressure results in retrograde perfusion of the coronary arteries, resulting in right ventricle-dependent coronary circulation (Figure 55-14).

Pulmonary atresia with intact ventricular septum presents with cyanosis. Cardiac examination reveals a single loud second heart sound. A murmur is typically not present, other than from the PDA. ECG typically reveals a relative lack of right-sided forces with a QRS axis between 0 and 90 degrees. The p wave is peaked from right atrial

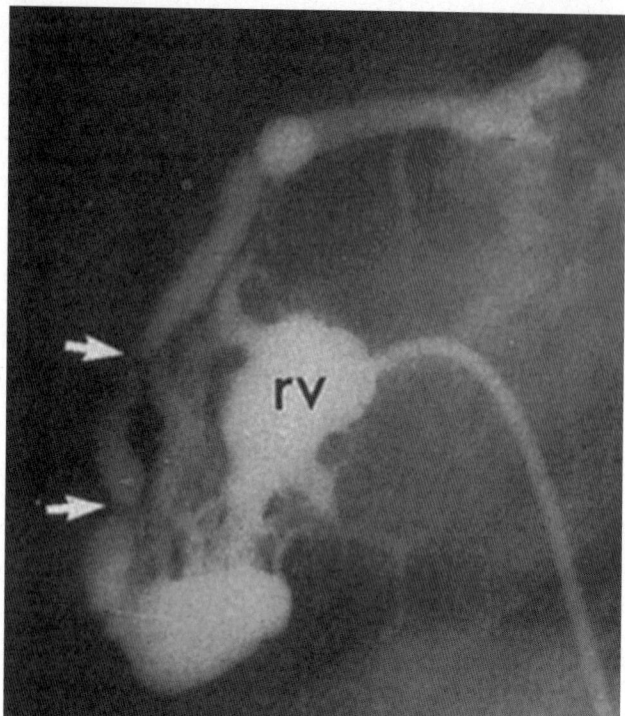

FIGURE 55-14 Lateral angiogram from a newborn with pulmonary atresia and intact ventricular septum. After injection of contrast through the hypertrophied and diminutive right ventricle *(rv)*, there is retrograde filling of tortuous coronary arteries through sinusoidal connections to the right ventricle *(arrows)*.

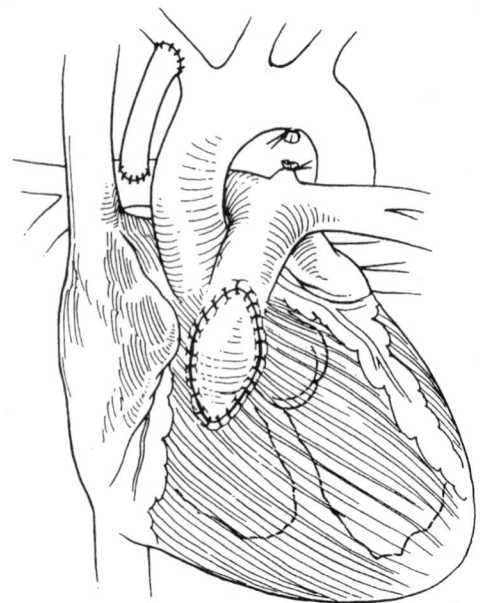

FIGURE 55-15 Newborn surgical palliation for pulmonary atresia with intact ventricular septum and normal coronary arteries. A right ventricular outflow tract patch is placed, the ductus is ligated and divided, and a modified Blalock-Taussig shunt is placed. *(From Wernovsky G, Hanley FL: Pulmonary atresia with intact ventricular septum. In Chang AC, Hanley FL, Wernovsky G, et al, editors:* Pediatric cardiac intensive care, *Baltimore, 1998, Williams & Wilkins, pp 265-270.)*

enlargement. Pulmonary vascular markings on chest radiograph are typically decreased. Echocardiography confirms the diagnosis and can be used to look for coronary sinusoids. Cardiac catheterization is performed in patients where coronary sinusoids are known or suspected to completely define the extent and connections of the sinusoids.

Initially, prostaglandin E_1 (PGE$_1$) is used to maintain ductal patency until a more permanent source of pulmonary blood flow is provided. In patients with right ventricle-dependent coronary circulation, the outcome of surgical repair is often poor. A systemic-to-pulmonary shunt followed by staged single-ventricle palliation may be tried, but proceeding directly to heart transplantation may be appropriate. In patients without right ventricular coronary-dependent circulation, an egress from the right ventricle to pulmonary arteries is created by surgical valvotomy or RVOT augmentation, or valve perforation and valvuloplasty are performed in the catheterization lab (Figure 55-15) (Justo et al, 1997). At times, additional pulmonary blood flow is provided by a modified Blalock-Taussig or other systemic-to-pulmonary shunt. The postoperative course can be complicated by low cardiac output or a circular shunt.

TRICUSPID ATRESIA

In tricuspid atresia, there is no outlet from the right atrium to the right ventricle. Systemic venous return passes from the right atrium, through a PFO or ASD, to the left ventricle. More than 90% of patients with tricuspid atresia have an associated VSD, allowing blood to pass from the left

ventricle to the pulmonary arteries (Figure 55-16). The size of the ventricular septal defect determines the amount of pulmonary blood flow. Patients with a small or absent VSD have a very hypoplastic right ventricle and pulmonary artery. The major portion of pulmonary blood flow passes through the PDA. If a large VSD is present, pulmonary blood flow is prograde through the pulmonary valve, and the ductus is not necessary. A variant of tricuspid atresia is associated with transposition of the great vessels. Pulmonary blood flow is derived from the left ventricle, and systemic blood flow must pass through the VSD. There may be an associated coarctation or hypoplastic aortic arch in these patients.

Clinically, cyanosis is present at birth, the degree of which is dependent on the degree of restriction to pulmonary blood flow. A holosystolic murmur consistent with a VSD and a prominent left ventricular impulse are present on examination. Electrocardiography is nearly diagnostic and reveals left axis deviation and left ventricular hypertrophy. Chest radiography reveals variable pulmonary vascular markings, depending on the size of the VSD and relationship of the great vessels. Echocardiography demonstrates a fibromuscular plate in place of the tricuspid valve and a variably small right ventricle and pulmonary valve. The relationship of the great vessels can also be determined by echo. The degree of obstruction at the VSD or across the RVOT can be evaluated.

PGE$_1$ is used initially to maintain a PDA. If there is restriction to flow at the atrial level, a balloon septostomy is performed. Further management depends on the amount of pulmonary blood flow and the relationship of the great vessels. Patients with ductal dependent pulmonary blood flow have a systemic-to-pulmonary-artery shunt placed (modified Blalock-Taussig shunt).

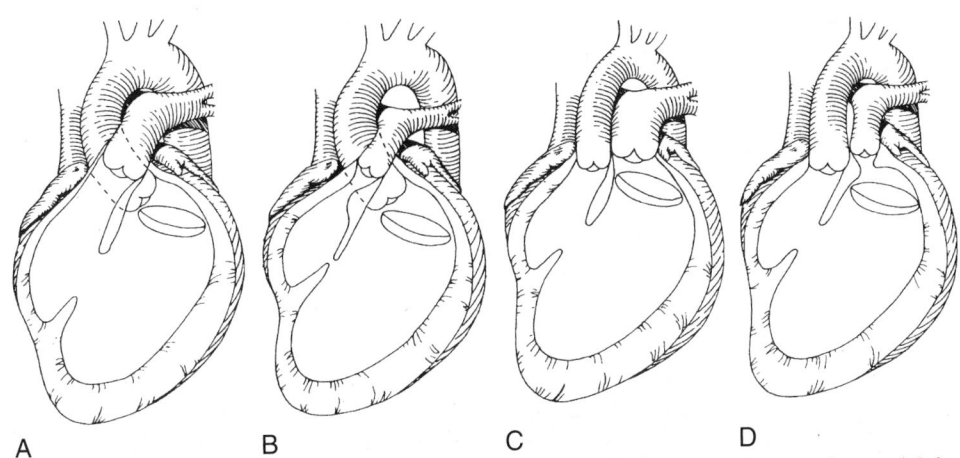

FIGURE 55-16 Anatomic variants in tricuspid atresia. **A,** Normally related great vessels with a large ventricular septal defect (VSD) and normal-sized pulmonary arteries (PAs). **B,** Normally related great vessels with a small VSD and PAs. **C,** Transposed great arteries (left ventricle aligned with the PA, right ventricle with the aorta) with a relatively small VSD and aorta. Many patients with this variant have coarctation as well (see text). **D,** Transposed great vessels with a VSD, subpulmonary obstruction, and small PAs. *(From Fyler DC: Tricuspid atresia. In Fyler DC, editor: Nadas' pediatric cardiology, Philadelphia, 1992b, Hanley & Belfus, pp 659-667.)*

Those with adequate pulmonary blood flow undergo a superior vena cava–to–pulmonary artery anastomosis (bidirectional Glenn) at approximately 6 months of age, with completion of the Fontan procedure around 3 years of age. Patients with transposition, or more complex anatomy, undergo more extensive palliative procedures initially, but continue down the pathway to Fontan palliation.

EBSTEIN'S ANOMALY OF THE TRICUSPID VALVE

Ebstein's anomaly is a rare form of congenital heart disease with variable presentation. Dysplasia of the tricuspid valve, with downward displacement of the septal and posterior leaflets, is the defining feature (Figure 55-17). The anterior leaflet, although normally positioned in the valve annulus, frequently has abnormal chordal attachments and is large and redundant. The tricuspid valve abnormality can be accompanied by tricuspid regurgitation, right atrial dilation, abnormal right ventricular myocardium, and an increased risk for Wolf-Parkinson-White syndrome. In addition, functional and true pulmonary atresia can occur with severe Ebstein's malformation. With displacement of the tricuspid valve, a significant portion of the right ventricle becomes atrialized, making it an ineffective pumping chamber. In this setting, it can be difficult to differentiate functional pulmonary atresia from true pulmonary atresia. Severe Ebstein's anomaly of the tricuspid valve is associated with heart failure in utero (Tongsong et al, 2005).

The clinical presentation is variable and depends on the degree of displacement of the tricuspid valve and severity of RVOT obstruction. In many patients, symptoms are mild and do not manifest until later in life. In more severe disease, cyanosis results when a right-to-left shunt occurs at the atrial level, secondary to the tricuspid regurgitation and elevated right atrial pressures. Cardiac examination reveals a holosystolic murmur at the lower left sternal border with associated gallop and clicks. Neonates with severe Ebstein's anomaly present with marked cyanosis, cardiomegaly, and ductus dependent pulmonary blood flow. Chest radiograph appearance is characteristic in severe cases, with massive

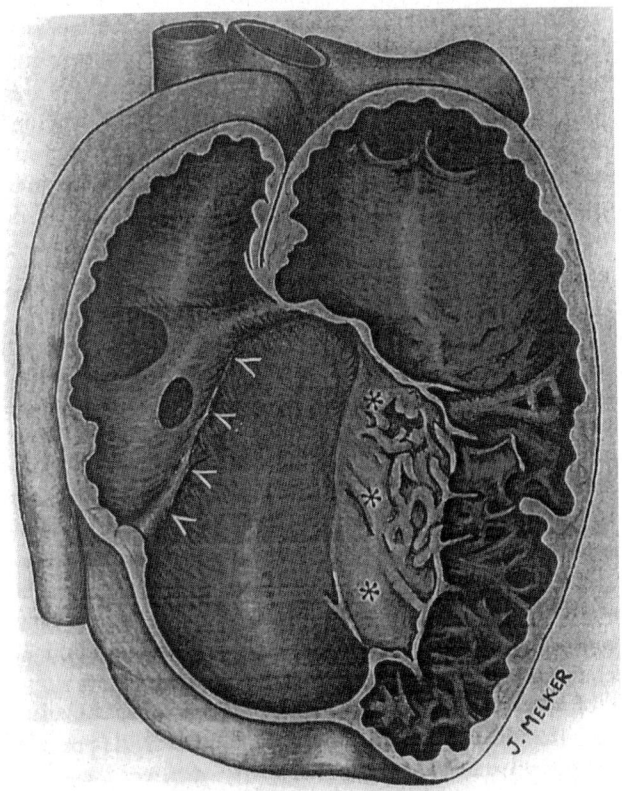

FIGURE 55-17 Inferior displacement of tricuspid valve leaflet (*) into the right ventricular cavity. The *white arrowheads* indicate the normally positioned tricuspid valve annulus. The area between the true annulus and the displaced valve leaflet is considered "atrialized." *(From Epstein ML: Congenital stenosis and insufficiency of the tricuspid valve. In Allen HD, Gutgesell HP, Clark EB, Driscoll DJ, editors: Moss and Adams' heart disease in infants, children, and adolescents: including the fetus and young adult, ed 6, Philadelphia, 2001, Lippincott Williams & Wilkins, pp 810-819.)*

cardiomegaly evident at birth (Figure 55-18). Death can occur from the significant heart failure and hypoxemia. Clinical improvement may occur as the pulmonary vascular resistance drops, improving the right ventricle's ability to contribute to pulmonary blood flow.

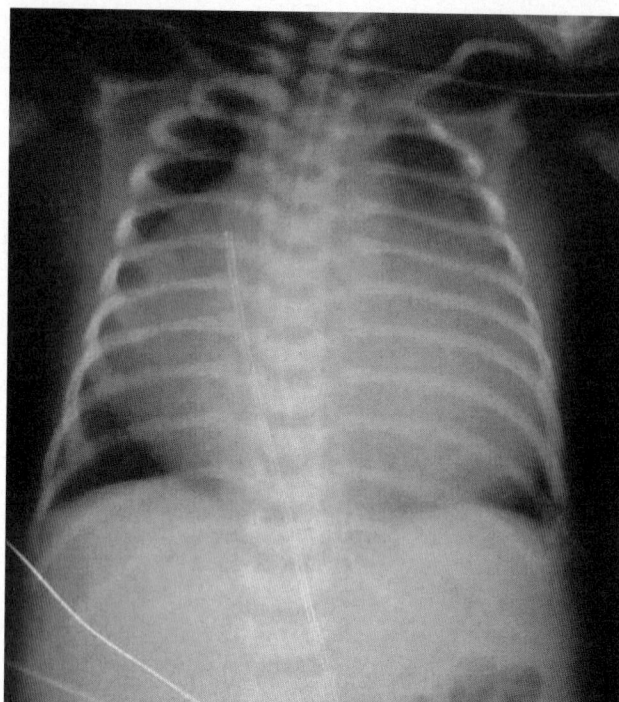

FIGURE 55-18 Chest radiograph in a 1-day-old newborn with Ebstein's anomaly of the tricuspid valve. Note the massive cardiomegaly and relative pulmonary oligemia and hypoplasia.

Initially, management of the severely cyanotic infant is aimed at promoting pulmonary blood flow. PGE$_1$ is used to maintain ductal patency. Supplemental oxygen, inhaled nitric oxide, and mild respiratory alkalosis can have marginal success in improving pulmonary blood flow by lowering pulmonary vascular resistance. After several days, attempts are made at weaning from the PGE$_1$. If this is unsuccessful, surgical options are considered. Options include tricuspid valve repair or replacement, 1½ ventricle repair, or other palliative procedures such as right ventricular exclusion with a fenestrated patch and placement of a modified Blalock-Taussig shunt (Reemtsen et al, 2007). Although surgical outcomes have improved, a neonatal repair for symptomatic disease remains a risk factor for death (McElhinney et al, 2005; Sarris et al, 2006).

LESIONS THAT MANIFEST PRIMARILY WITH HEART FAILURE

HYPOPLASTIC LEFT HEART SYNDROME

Hypoplastic left heart syndrome (HLHS) is an anatomically heterogeneous lesion characterized by a variable degree of underdevelopment of the left ventricle, hypoplasia or atresia of the aortic and mitral valves, and hypoplasia of the aortic arch. Although HLHS accounts for only 1.4% to 3.8% of all congenital heart defects, it accounts for 23% of cardiac deaths in the 1st week of life and 15% of cardiac deaths in the 1st month of life (Samanek, 2000). HLHS likely is multifactorial in etiology. There is a slight male predominance. Although there is no clear genetic etiology, familial clustering of various left heart obstructive lesions has been noted.

It is theorized that the growth of developing vascular structures is dependent on flow. HLHS probably results from in utero obstruction of left ventricular inflow or outflow. The fetal left ventricle is predominantly filled with blood that passes through the foramen ovale. Restriction to flow or reversal of flow through the foramen ovale could then result in decreased flow to the left heart and its underdevelopment. Similarly, several studies have documented the progression of severe aortic stenosis to hypoplastic left heart syndrome in utero (Danford and Cronican, 1992; Hornberger et al, 1995). The progressive left ventricular hypertrophy, dilation, and fibrosis associated with severe aortic stenosis can lead to decreased ventricular compliance, elevated left atrial pressures, and reversal of flow through the foramen ovale in utero. Prenatal cardiac intervention is still in its infancy, but recent successes with in utero balloon dilation of the aortic valve suggest that the progression to HLHS can be altered (Makikallio et al, 2006).

Because of the underdevelopment of the left heart structures, pulmonary venous return must exit the left atrium through the foramen ovale. Pulmonary venous blood then mixes with systemic venous return in the right atrium and enters the right ventricle. Right ventricular output then passes either to the pulmonary circulation or through the ductus arteriosus to the systemic circulation. That is, the pulmonary and systemic circulations are in parallel. The ratio of systemic to pulmonary blood flow is determined by the relative resistances of the vascular beds. As the normal postnatal drop in pulmonary vascular resistance occurs, pulmonary flow increases at the expense of systemic flow. Thus, the management of HLHS is dependent on an adequate egress from the left atrium and balancing the resistances of the pulmonary and systemic vascular beds.

Most cases of HLHS are now diagnosed prenatally when an abnormal four-chamber view is noted on a screening obstetric ultrasound examination. Ideally, delivery is planned and occurs at a tertiary care center. Postnatally, prostaglandins are immediately started to maintain ductal patency and an echocardiogram is obtained to confirm the diagnosis. The cardiothoracic surgeon and the interventional cardiologist should be made aware and available at the time of delivery.

In the absence of prenatal diagnosis, postnatal presentation is somewhat variable and dependent on ductal patency and the degree of restriction to flow at the atrial septum. The infant with an unrestrictive atrial septum and PDA is largely asymptomatic at birth and may be missed in the newborn period. Cyanosis is minimal and pulmonary overcirculation is mild whereas pulmonary vascular resistance is high. Cardiac exam is relatively unremarkable. The second heart sound is single and loud. A third heart sound becomes apparent as heart failure develops. As pulmonary vascular resistance drops and ductal closure occurs, feeding difficulties and respiratory distress become apparent with rapid progression to cardiovascular collapse. Physical exam after ductal restriction is significant for lethargy, pallor, and diminished or absent pulses. Chest radiograph typically reveals relatively normal-sized heart and pulmonary edema. ECG is nonspecific but may reveal relative lack of left-sided forces.

The patient with a restrictive atrial septum presents with tachypnea and profound cyanosis shortly after birth. The elevated left atrial and pulmonary venous pressures result in pulmonary venous congestion that is apparent on chest radiograph.

The preoperative management of patients with HLHS is directed at balancing the ratio of pulmonary-to-systemic blood flow (Qp:Qs) to allow for sufficient oxygenation of blood while maintaining adequate systemic cardiac output. Prostaglandins should be started immediately postnatally to ensure ductal patency. Echocardiography is utilized to confirm cardiac anatomy and determine the degree of restriction to flow through the foramen ovale. If the atrial-level shunt is restrictive with profound cyanosis and metabolic acidosis, a balloon atrial septostomy, surgical septectomy, or emergent stage I palliation should be performed (see later discussion). If the restriction was present in utero, pathologic fibrosis and arterialization of the pulmonary veins and medial hypertrophy of the pulmonary arterioles occurs. Even after atrial septostomy, lung disease can persist and pulmonary vascular resistance can remain high. Oxygen may be needed to maintain saturations in an appropriate range. This subset of patients has a high mortality rate.

A small group of patients will have adequately balanced pulmonary and systemic blood flow at the time of presentation. A small degree of restriction to flow through the foramen ovale may be associated with slight cyanosis but has the beneficial effect of restricting pulmonary blood flow. In the absence of acidosis or end organ dysfunction, this state is generally tolerated until stage I palliation is performed.

An unrestrictive atrial septal defect allows increased pulmonary blood flow as the pulmonary vascular resistance falls. Because of the parallel arrangement of the circulations, increasing pulmonary flow decreases systemic flow. In this setting, there is increasing oxygen saturation associated with inadequate oxygen delivery to the tissues. Worsening metabolic acidosis and end-organ dysfunction ensue. The ratio of pulmonary to systemic blood flow is balanced by manipulating the resistances of the pulmonary and systemic vascular beds. The success of these therapies is monitored using oxygen saturation, mixed venous saturation, lactate, and arterial blood gases.

Pulmonary vascular resistance can be manipulated through mechanical ventilation and alteration in the amount of oxygen delivered. Mechanical ventilation with high positive end-expiratory pressure (PEEP) can limit pulmonary blood flow. Pulmonary vascular resistance can also be increased by adding CO_2 (FiCO$_2$ 0.03) or nitrogen (FiO$_2$ 0.17) to the ventilator circuit (Riordan et al, 1996; Shime et al, 2000). Both CO_2 and nitrogen have been shown to decrease the Qp:Qs and decrease oxygen saturations. Only hypercarbia has been shown to improve systemic oxygen delivery (Tabbutt et al, 2001). The goal of this therapy is to maintain normal lactate, systemic oxygen saturation at 75–85%, and mixed venous oxygen saturation approximately 25 percentage points lower than systemic saturations.

Vasoactive medications can be used to alter systemic vascular resistance and improve ventricular function. Use of these medications is determined by clinical presentation and echocardiographic findings. Milrinone can be used to provide some afterload reduction, if tolerated by blood pressure. The inotropic effects of milrinone are also an advantage if ventricular function is poor. In addition to decreasing pulmonary blood flow, afterload reduction has the added benefit of decreasing tricuspid valve regurgitation if it is present. Milrinone also dilates the pulmonary vascular bed, so care should be taken when it is used. Although counterintuitive, when faced with an unoperated patient with high oxygen saturations and low peripheral blood pressure, the gentle addition of milrinone may improve blood pressure simply by increasing systemic blood flow.

The immediate goal of surgical palliation is to provide stable unrestricted systemic and coronary blood flow and reliably restricted pulmonary blood flow. There are several strategies for stage I palliation. Traditionally, aortic arch reconstruction was performed using pulmonary artery tissue and pulmonary blood flow was supplied using a modified BT shunt (Norwood procedure) (Figure 55-19). A recent modification of a right ventricle-to-pulmonary artery conduit has been used to supply pulmonary blood flow — the Sano modification; Figure 55-20). The Sano modification has the presumed benefit of providing pulsatile flow to the pulmonary arteries without aortopulmonary diastolic run off and coronary steal. The downside of this procedure is the need for a ventriculotomy. A hybrid procedure that combines stent placement in the ductus arteriosus by the cardiologist and pulmonary artery banding by the surgeon is an approach being taken by a number of institutions that provides a relatively noninvasive stage I palliation for hypoplastic left heart syndrome (Caldarone et al, 2007). Each of these procedures has its pros and cons and its advocates and detractors (Caldarone et al, 2007; Ghanayem et al, 2006; Malec et al, 2003). Longer-term prospective studies are needed to determine the optimal approach to stage I palliation. In the low-risk patient, survival after the first stage nears 80–90%.

The remaining palliative surgeries occur outside the newborn period. Stage II palliation unloads the right ventricle and begins to separate the pulmonary and systemic circulations. The superior cavopulmonary anastomosis (bidirectional Glenn) is usually performed between 4 and 6 months of age. During this procedure, the conduit providing pulmonary flow is removed and the superior vena cava is anastomosed to the pulmonary artery.

Stage III palliation completely separates the pulmonary and systemic circulations. An inferior cavopulmonary anastomosis (Fontan completion) is performed by one of several techniques.

OBSTRUCTED TOTAL ANOMALOUS PULMONARY VENOUS RETURN

Obstructed total anomalous pulmonary venous return (TAPVR) represents one of the few remaining neonatal surgical emergencies in pediatric cardiology. Although obstruction can occur with any type of TAPVR, it is most common in infradiaphragmatic TAPVR. Physiologically, obstruction to pulmonary venous flow results in pulmonary venous hypertension that is transmitted to the pulmonary capillary bed, resulting in pulmonary edema.

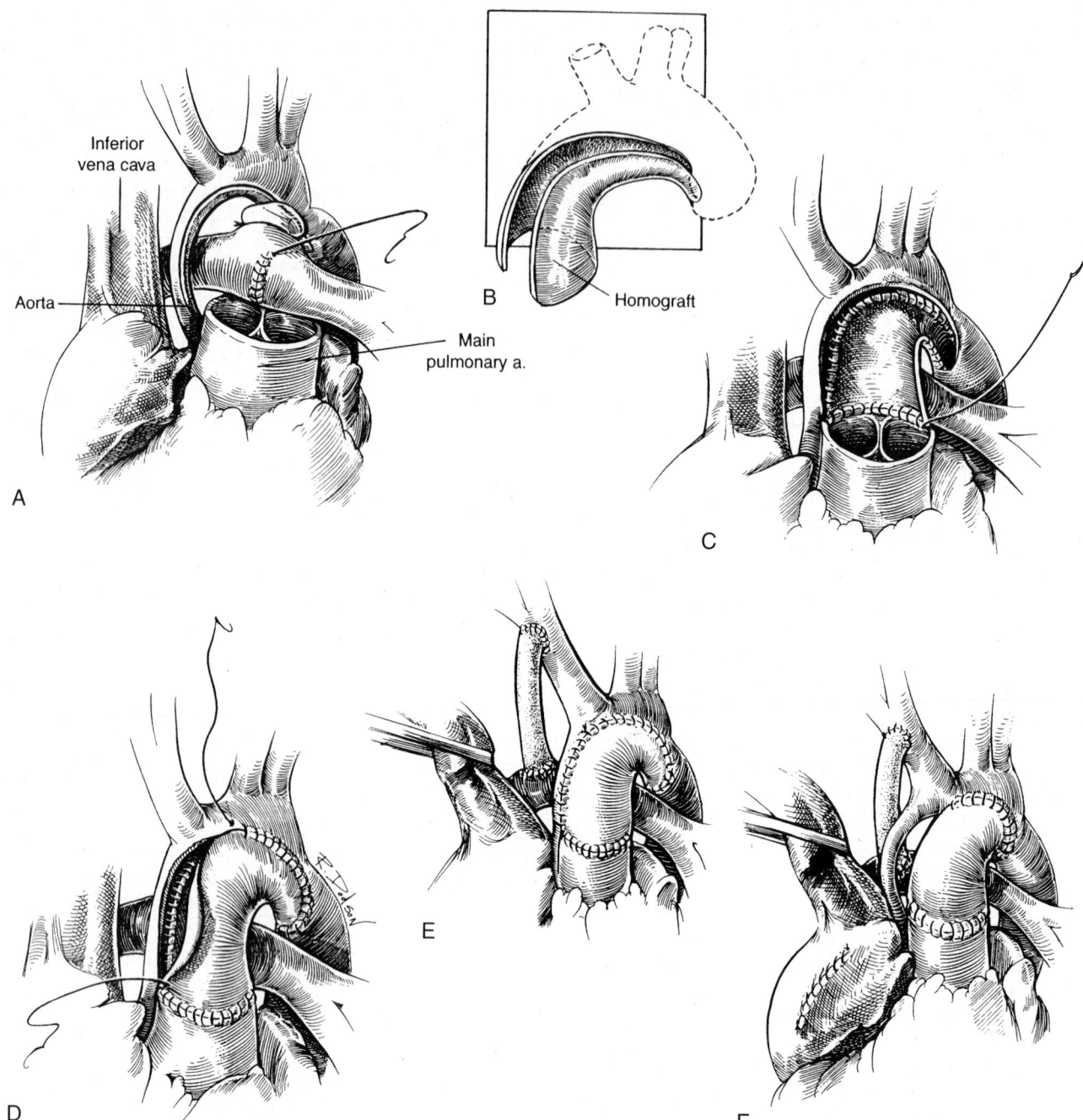

FIGURE 55-19 **Stage I palliation for hypoplastic left heart syndrome: classic Norwood procedure. A,** The main pulmonary artery is transected, and the distal end oversewn. The ductus arteriosus is ligated, and an incision is made from the proximal ascending aorta around the aortic arch to the level of the ductus. **B,** A pulmonary homograft is utilized to create a patch to reconstruct the neoaorta. **C** and **D,** This homograft patch is used to connect the proximal main pulmonary artery and pulmonary (neoaortic) valve to the ascending aorta and transverse arch. **E,** A modified Blalock-Taussig shunt is placed from the base of the innominate artery to the right pulmonary artery. **F,** An alternative technique utilizing a circumferential tube graft from the proximal main pulmonary artery to the distal transverse aortic arch. *Not shown*: Atrial septectomy is performed to provide unobstructed egress from the pulmonary veins to the right ventricle. *(From Castañeda AR, Jonas RA, Mayer JE Jr, et al:* Cardiac surgery of the neonate and infant, *Philadelphia, 1994, WB Saunders.)*

Pulmonary blood flow is severely limited. Newborns thus present with profound cyanosis and respiratory distress that is not responsive to medical management. Prostaglandins may help minimize the obstruction by maintaining patency of the ductus venosus, but patency of the ductus arteriosus does not improve the clinical picture, because the limitation to pulmonary blood flow is not due to insufficient antegrade flow, but rather obstructed outflow.

Chest radiograph reveals a normal cardiac silhouette with pulmonary venous congestion that may be interpreted as interstitial pneumonia (Figure 55-21). Echocardiography can be challenging in these patients. The pulmonary veins can be small because of limited flow, making them difficult to detect by two-dimensional and color Doppler imaging. Surgical treatment is the same as for unobstructed TAPVR. The postoperative course is frequently marked

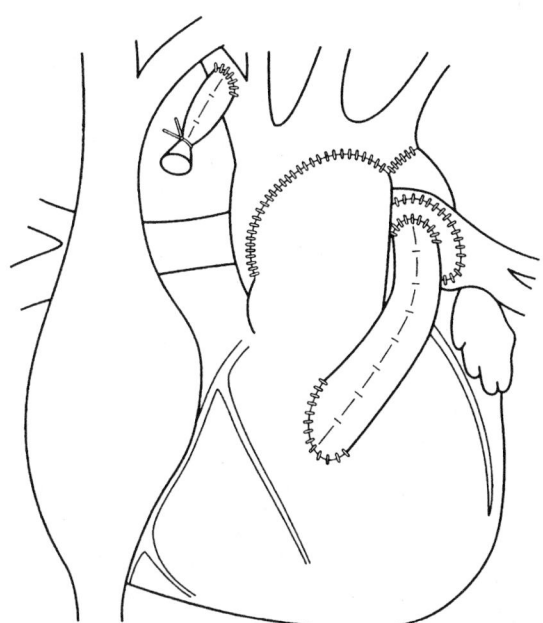

FIGURE 55-20 Right ventricle-pulmonary artery, or Sano, modification of stage I reconstruction. The arch reconstruction is similar to that shown in Figure 57-20. The Blalock-Taussig shunt is replaced with a Gore-Tex tube inserted from the right ventricle to the main pulmonary artery. *(From Sano S, Ishino K, Kawada K, et al: Right ventricle-pulmonary artery shunt in first-stage palliation of hypoplastic left heart syndrome, J Thorac Cardiovasc Surg 126:504-510, 2003.)*

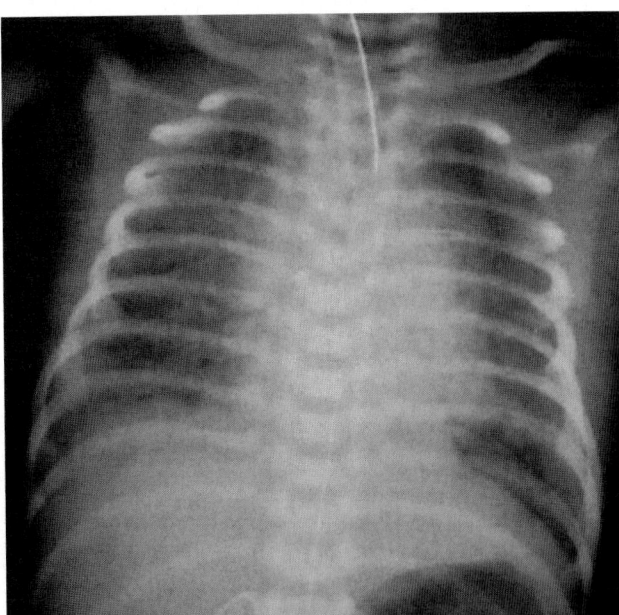

FIGURE 55-21 Chest radiograph in a 1-day-old infant with obstructed total anomalous pulmonary venous return.

by pulmonary vascular resistance lability, right ventricular hypertension, and low cardiac output syndrome.

COR TRIATRIATUM

Embryologically, the pulmonary veins enter a common pulmonary vein that initially has no connection to the left atrium (Neill, 1956). During normal development, the common pulmonary vein becomes incorporated into the left atrium, resulting in the usual pattern of two right and two left pulmonary veins entering the left atrium. Abnormal incorporation of the common pulmonary vein can result in cor triatriatum, a condition in which the common pulmonary vein joins the left atrium through a single opening. If the opening is small and restrictive, the clinical presentation is similar to that in obstructed TAPVR. If the opening is nonrestrictive, no symptoms are present. Surgical resection of the membrane that separates the left atrium and common pulmonary vein is an effective treatment. Significant preoperative pulmonary venous obstruction increases surgical mortality.

MITRAL STENOSIS

Congenital mitral stenosis is a rare form of congenital heart disease with several subtypes. The stenosis can occur in the supravalvular region, at the valve annulus, or within the mitral valve support apparatus. Typical congenital mitral stenosis is characterized by thickened leaflets, short or absent chordae tendineae, obliteration of interchordal spaces, and two separate papillary muscles. Supravalvar mitral ring occurs when there is connective tissue outgrowth on the atrial surface of the mitral valve leaflets,

leading to a decreased mitral valve orifice. The mitral valve orifice can also be stenotic secondary to a parachute mitral valve, when most or all chordae tendineae insert onto only one papillary muscle. Another form of obstruction occurs with a double orifice mitral valve, where a tongue of tissue connects the anterior and posterior mitral valve leaflets. A mitral arcade or hammock occurs when the leaflets are connected directly or by short chordae to the papillary muscles. Congenital mitral stenosis frequently occurs in conjunction with other left-sided obstructive lesions.

Symptoms from mitral stenosis usually occur in the first 2 years of life and may consist of shortness of breath, respiratory distress or wheezing, cyanosis, and pallor. Cardiac exam reveals a rumbling apical diastolic murmur, loud first heart sound, and loud split second heart sound. Opening snap of the mitral valve may be heard. Chest radiograph reveals left atrial enlargement and pulmonary venous congestion. ECG reveals right ventricular hypertrophy with normal, bifid, or spiked P waves suggesting left atrial enlargement. Echocardiogram is used to define mitral valve anatomy and localize the area of obstruction. Doppler can be used to determine valve gradient and estimate right ventricular pressure.

Treatment options for congenital mitral valve stenosis include balloon mitral valvuloplasty, surgical mitral valvuloplasty, and mitral valve replacement. Despite recent improvements in outcomes, intervention and mitral valve replacement have relatively poor short-term outcomes (McElhinney et al, 2005). Patients with additional left-sided obstructive lesions or associated defects frequently require single-ventricle palliation.

CRITICAL AORTIC STENOSIS

Patients with critical aortic stenosis have severe left ventricular outflow tract obstruction that limits systemic cardiac output (Figure 55-22). The result is ductus dependent systemic perfusion. Although the obstruction can occur

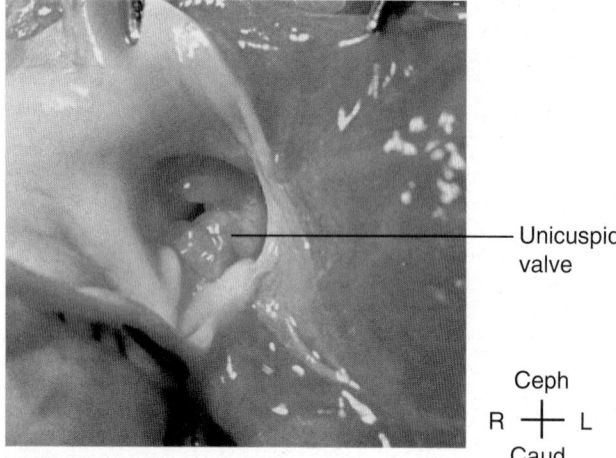

— Unicuspid valve

Ceph

R ┼ L

Caud

FIGURE 55-22 **Congenital aortic stenosis.** Frontal view through opened aorta demonstrates stenotic and dysmorphic aortic valve with commissural fusion. *(From Litwin SB:* Color atlas of congenital heart surgery, *St. Louis, 1996, Mosby.)*

below the valve, at the valve, above the valve, or a combination of these, this section focuses on outflow tract obstruction resulting from morphologic problems of the aortic valve. Severe aortic valve stenosis is defined as a Doppler-derived pressure gradient greater than 60 mm Hg. Moderate stenosis is defined as gradient of 30 to 60 mm Hg, whereas mild stenosis is a peak gradient less than 30 mm Hg. In the setting of depressed left ventricular function, the Doppler echo-derived gradient may be significantly lower and underestimate the severity of the stenosis.

Aortic valve stenosis is detectable in utero. The long-standing pressure overload on the left ventricle causes left hypertrophy and left ventricular scarring (endocardial fibroelastosis). In some cases, as discussed earlier, the disease progresses to hypoplastic left heart syndrome. Attempts have been made to identify fetuses at high risk for progressing to hypoplastic left heart syndrome and then perform an in utero valvuloplasty with the hope of alleviating the obstruction and altering the course of the disease (Makikallio et al, 2006). Although initial results with this procedure are promising, more work is needed in this area.

Clinically, critical aortic stenosis manifests in the newborn period with signs of decreased systemic perfusion: pallor, decreased pulses, and prolonged capillary refill. A harsh ejection-quality murmur is heard on exam in the aortic area. The volume and quality of the murmur correlate with the severity of stenosis in the setting of normal left ventricular function. If left ventricular function is depressed, the murmur may be soft despite severe stenosis. Electrocardiogram reveals left ventricular hypertrophy with possible T-wave abnormalities. Heart size is typically normal on chest film, although the aortic knob may be prominent and pulmonary congestion may be present. Echocardiogram is used to define the location and severity of the left ventricular outflow tract obstruction. Aortic stenosis is commonly found with other left-sided obstructive lesions, with possible underdevelopment of left heart structures. These findings may alter the treatment plan and lead to single-ventricle palliation. Published models have attempted to identify echocardiographic findings that predict the suitability of a two-ventricle repair in neonates with critical aortic stenosis (Colan et al, 2006; Lofland et al, 2001; Rhodes et al, 1991).

Initial management of infants with critical aortic stenosis is directed at the treatment of cardiogenic shock. Intubation, mechanical ventilation, stable vascular access, inotropic support, sedation, and paralysis are all frequently necessary. PGE_1 maintains ductal patency and provides systemic output. A small patent foramen ovale must be present for pulmonary venous return to cross the atrial septum and enter the systemic vasculature via the right ventricle and ductus arteriosus. A balloon septostomy may be necessary to decompress the left atrium.

Further management depends on left ventricular size and the presence of other left heart obstructive lesions. Patients with multiple levels of left heart obstruction, a small mitral valve, hypoplastic aortic arch, or small left ventricle may be best suited for single-ventricle palliation. Options for two-ventricle palliation include balloon valvuloplasty in the cardiac catheterization lab, surgical valvotomy, or neonatal Ross procedure (Figure 55-23) (Alsoufi et al, 2007). Outcomes of all procedures depend, in part, on relief of obstruction, presence of aortic valve regurgitation, associated cardiac lesions, and severity of end-organ dysfunction at the time of initial presentation. The mortality of each of the interventions is relatively high. Regardless of the treatment chosen, critical aortic stenosis is a lifelong illness. Patients require close follow-up and multiple procedures throughout their lifetimes.

COARCTATION OF THE AORTA

Coarctation may occur anywhere from the transverse aortic arch to the bifurcation of the iliac arteries. Most commonly, there is a discrete narrowing distal to the left subclavian artery, across from the aortic insertion of the ductus arteriosus in a *juxtaductal* position. Conversely, there can be long-segment narrowing of the transverse aortic arch, otherwise referred to as a hypoplastic aortic arch. A bicuspid aortic valve occurs in 70% of cases. Other left-sided obstructive lesions tend to occur with coarctation of the aorta. There is a 2:1 male-to-female preponderance and an association with Turner's syndrome.

In neonates with a discrete juxtaductal narrowing, the PDA widens the narrowed area and provides relief from the obstruction. The net shunt through the PDA is left to right. These patients have equal oxygen saturations in the upper and lower extremities. In patients with a severe coarctation or a diffusely hypoplastic arch, descending aortic flow originates from a right-to-left shunt through the ductus arteriosus. Differential upper and lower extremity oxygen saturations occur in these patients, with the upper extremities having greater saturation than the lower extremities.

The clinical presentation of coarctation of the aorta depends on the severity of the narrowing. Mild coarctation often does not manifest in infancy. Detection typically occurs when upper extremity hypertension and diminished or absent femoral pulses are noted on exam. Infants with more severe coarctation or aortic arch hypoplasia present with diminished lower extremity perfusion after ductal closure. Physical exam reveals an infant in extremis with

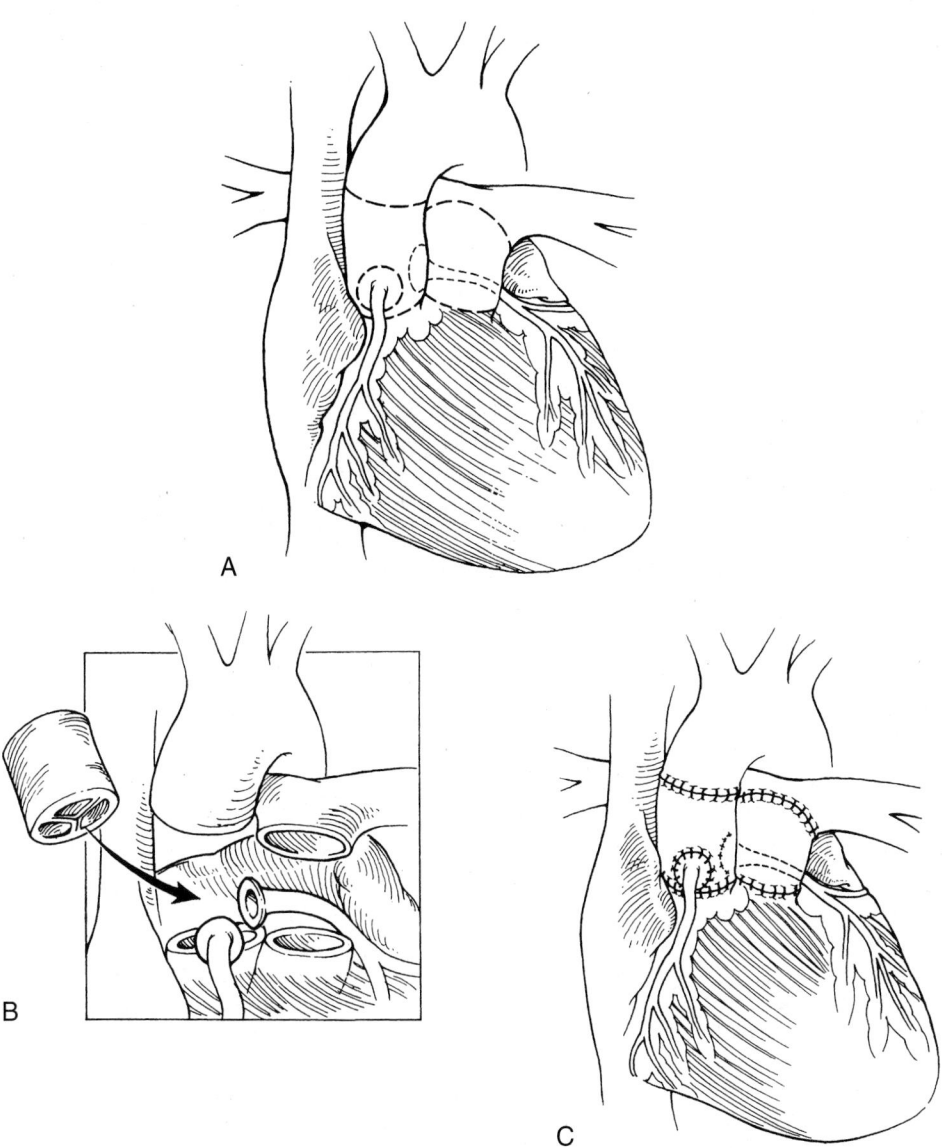

A

B

C

FIGURE 55-23 Ross procedure: "Autograft" aortic valve replacement. **A,** *Dotted lines* depict surgical incisions around coronary arteries, aorta, and pulmonary artery. **B,** After removal of the coronary arteries and adjacent "buttons" and the diseased aortic valve, the patient's native pulmonary valve ("autograft") is positioned in the aortic root. **C,** Completed repair with reimplanted coronary arteries and a cadaveric homograft valve inserted in the pulmonary position. *(From Chang AC, Burke RP: Left ventricular outflow tract obstruction. In Chang AC, Hanley FL, Wernovsky G, et al, editors:* Pediatric cardiac intensive care, *Baltimore, 1998, Williams & Wilkins, pp 233-256.)*

poor perfusion and absent femoral pulses. Cardiac exam may reveal a systolic ejection click if a bicuspid aortic valve is present. A systolic ejection-quality murmur is heard that radiates to the back and left infraclavicular area. Chest radiograph demonstrates a large heart with increased pulmonary vascular markings. ECG reveals right ventricular hypertrophy. Echocardiography is used to define the location and extent of aortic narrowing. Additional left-sided obstructive lesions are ruled out. Right ventricular hypertrophy and right ventricular hypertension are also frequently noted.

Treatment of the infant presenting with coarctation of the aorta is similar to that of infants with aortic stenosis. Intubation and mechanical ventilation are necessary. Vascular access is obtained for inotropes. PGE_1 is started to open the ductus arteriosus. Metabolic derangements are corrected. Ideally, the infant is stabilized before surgery. Surgery is typically indicated at the time of diagnosis, even in relatively asymptomatic patients. In most cases, a lateral thoracotomy is performed, the area of coarctation is excised, and an end-to-end anastomosis is performed. If long-segment narrowing is present, patch material may be used to augment the arch and a more extended end-to-end

anastomosis is performed. Balloon angioplasty of native coarctation is not typically performed in infancy because of the risk of aneurysm, recoarctation, and vascular injury at the site of access.

Surgical mortality is slightly greater than 5% (Gutgesell et al, 2001). Recoarctation occurs in 10% to 15% of children and is successfully managed with balloon angioplasty. If a ventricular septal defect is present, this is typically closed at the time of surgery.

INTERRUPTED AORTIC ARCH

Interrupted aortic arch is a relatively rare anomaly that is defined simply as complete separation of the ascending and descending aorta. Interrupted aortic arch can be classified by the location of the interruption relative to the head and neck vessels (Figure 55-24): type A, distal to the left subclavian artery; type B, between the left subclavian and left carotid arteries; and type C, between the left carotid and innominate arteries. All types of interruption occur in conjunction with posterior malalignment of the infundibular septum; this results in a ventricular septal defect and

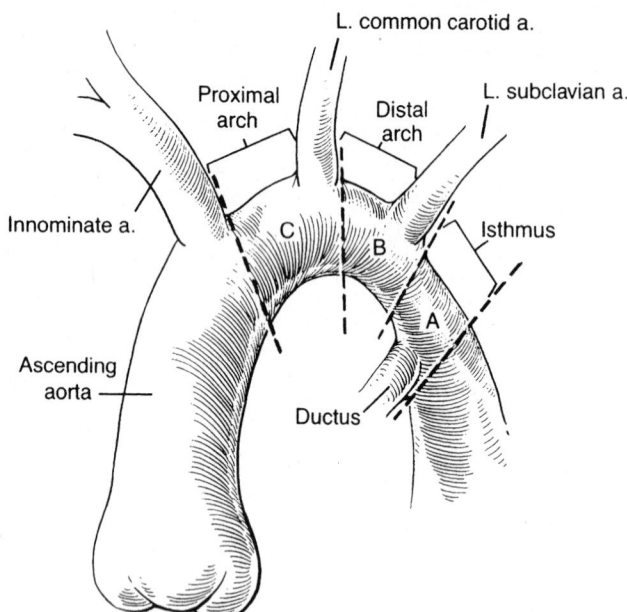

FIGURE 55-24 **Anatomic classification of interrupted aortic arch.** *Dashed lines* indicate the potential areas of discontinuity (interruption) in the aortic arch. See text for details. *(From Castañeda AR, Jonas RA, Mayer JE Jr, et al: Cardiac surgery of the neonate and infant, Philadelphia, 1994, WB Saunders.)*

various degrees of left ventricular outflow tract obstruction. Aberrant arrangements of the head and neck vessels are common, with 50% of patients with type B interruption having an aberrant right subclavian artery that arises from the descending aorta. Interrupted aortic arch is associated with 22q11 deletion.

The clinical presentation of interrupted aortic arch is similar to that of other left-sided obstructive lesions. Descending aortic flow is entirely dependent on right-to-left shunting through the PDA. Ductal closure causes cardiovascular collapse. Initial management is as described for coarctation of the aorta. PGE$_1$ should be started as soon as possible, because all other resuscitative efforts will have no benefit until postductal circulation is established.

Surgical repair is performed after metabolic acidosis resolves and end-organ function is improved. Continuity is established between the ascending and descending aorta via end-to-end anastomosis, homograft insertion/patch augmentation to connect the two segments, or jump grafts (Figure 55-25). The ventricular septal defect is typically closed. In patients with severe left ventricular hypoplasia, a two-ventricle repair may not be possible and a staged repair or single-ventricle palliation is performed (Tchervenkov et al, 2005). Surgical mortality is less than 10%, but higher in patients with additional anomalies (Brown et al, 2006). Repeat operation due to left ventricular outflow tract obstruction and balloon angioplasty for recurrent arch obstruction are both common.

ANOMALOUS ORIGIN OF THE LEFT CORONARY ARTERY FROM THE PULMONARY ARTERY

When the left coronary artery arises from the pulmonary artery, inadequate oxygen delivery to the left ventricle results. Coronary artery perfusion occurs primarily during diastole. As pulmonary artery pressures drops postnatally, perfusion pressure of the left coronary artery falls, resulting in ischemia and infarction of the left ventricle. If collateral vessels connect the right and left coronary circulations, flow in the left coronary artery reverses. A left-to-right shunt occurs, resulting in coronary artery steal. Mitral valve regurgitation secondary to papillary muscle ischemia and left ventricular dilation develops.

Clinically, symptoms typically develop in the 1st month of life. If adequate collateral vessels and myocardial oxygen delivery exist, the patient may present later in life with angina-like symptoms. In the infant, attacks of irritability, pallor, and diaphoresis with feeds are a common presentation. Cardiac examination reveals a displaced point of maximum impulse, gallop rhythm, and nonspecific murmur. If mitral regurgitation is present, a holosystolic, regurgitant-quality murmur is heard. Chest radiograph reveals massive cardiomegaly. The ECG demonstrates a QR pattern and inverted T waves in leads I and aVL. Leads V$_5$ and V$_6$ may also show deep Q waves, inverted T waves, and ST segment depression. Echocardiography may suggest the diagnosis but is not always reliable, because the left coronary occasionally appears to arise from the aorta. Color Doppler may demonstrate retrograde flow in the left coronary with flow into the pulmonary artery. Cardiac catheterization is diagnostic.

Symptoms of congestive heart failure are managed medically. Surgical reimplantation of the left coronary artery to the aorta restores normal coronary perfusion pressure. If the usual two-vessel coronary blood supply is reestablished, there is gradual normalization of left ventricular size and function by echocardiography (Kuroczynski et al, 2008; Lange et al, 2007). If myocardial damage is severe or the left coronary artery is unable to be reimplanted surgically, cardiac transplantation is performed.

SYSTEMIC ARTERIAL MALFORMATIONS

Vascular anomalies are placed in two major groups: hemangiomas and malformations. Hemangiomas are tumors that demonstrate endothelial hyperplasia and undergo a period of proliferation and involution. Malformations result from abnormal vascular morphogenesis. They have normal endothelial cell turnover and grow accordingly with surrounding structures. Vascular malformations are further subcategorized by the type of vascular tissue involved (arterial, venous, and lymphatic). Because of their association with high output failure in the newborn period, two types of systemic vascular malformations are discussed further: arteriovenous malformations (AVMs) and arteriovenous fistulas (AVFs). An AVM results from multiple microfistulas between small arteries and veins. An AVF results from a connection between a large artery and vein.

Hemodynamically significant AVFs and AVMs manifest with high-output heart failure and cyanosis in the newborn period. An effective large left-to-right shunt occurs through the direct arterial-venous connections. Heart rate, stroke volume, plasma volume, and cardiac output are increased. The fistulous connection lowers systemic vascular resistance, promoting a right-to-left shunt through the ductus arteriosus, particularly if the normal postnatal

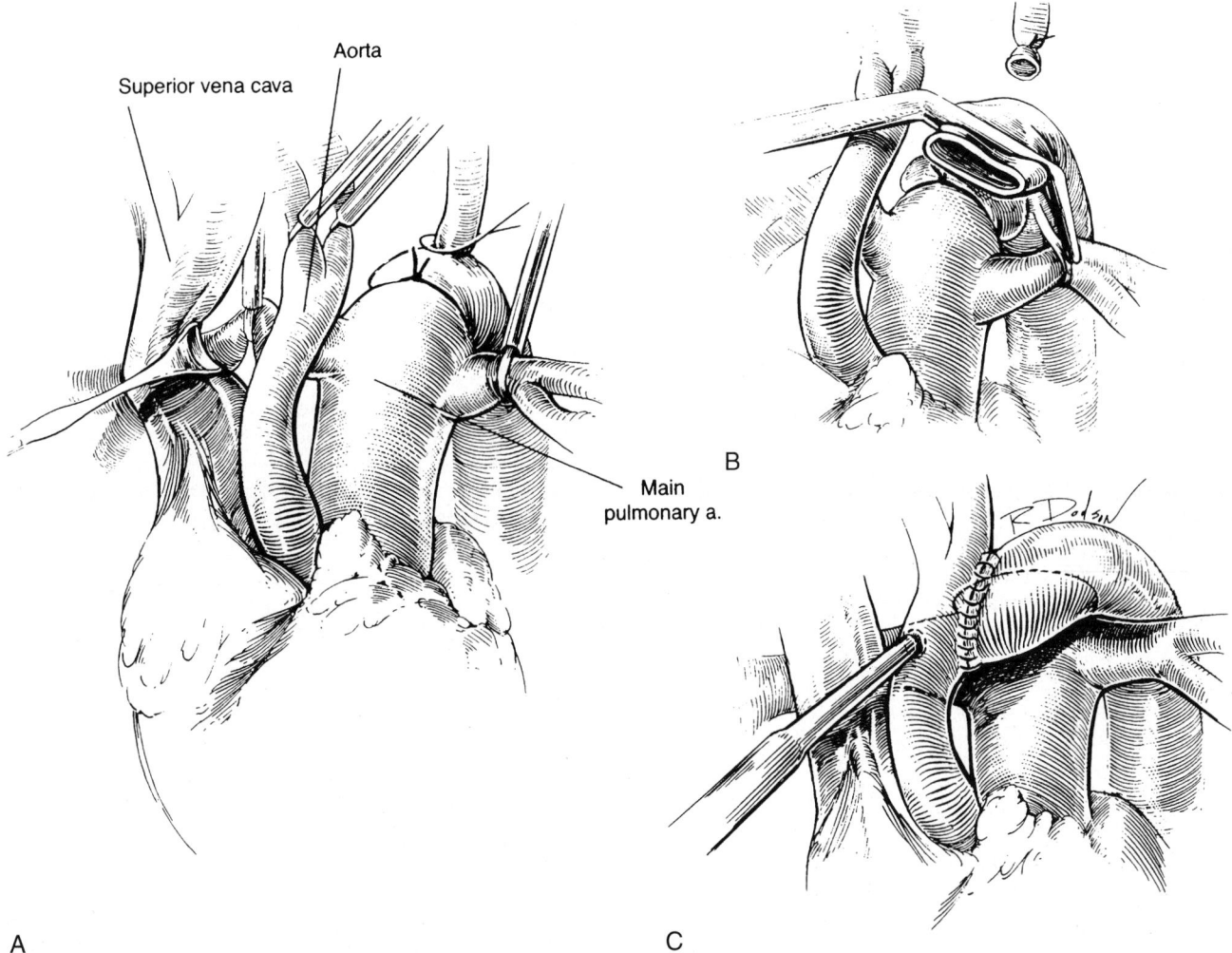

FIGURE 55-25 Surgical repair of interrupted aortic arch, type B. A, The branch pulmonary arteries and arch vessels are snared, and a ligature is placed around the ductus arteriosus. **B,** The proximal descending aorta is controlled with a clamp. To adequately mobilize the descending aorta, the left subclavian artery may need to be divided (as shown). After resection of the ductus arteriosus, the proximal (pulmonary artery) end is oversewn. **C,** The descending aorta is anastomosed directly to the ascending aorta. An alternative strategy is anastomosis of the left subclavian and left common carotid arteries combined with homograft patch augmentation of the inferior surface of the arch. Ventricular septal defect closure, when present, is also performed (not shown). *(From Castañeda AR, Jonas RA, Mayer JE Jr, et al: Cardiac surgery of the neonate and infant, Philadelphia, 1994, WB Saunders.)*

drop in pulmonary vascular resistance has not occurred. The increased systemic venous return increases right atrial pressures and promotes right-to-left shunting through the foramen ovale.

Cardiac examination reveals a hyperdynamic precordium. A prominent second heart sound, S3, and S4 may be heard. Systolic murmurs may be present secondary to tricuspid valve regurgitation or increased flow across the pulmonary valve. Increased tricuspid valve flow may create a diastolic sound. Bruits may be heard over the vascular malformation. When a malformation is suspected, care must be taken to auscultate areas where malformations are likely, such as the head, liver, and chest. Arteries proximal to the malformation are typically dilated with bounding pulses, whereas those distal are small with diminished pulses. ECG is nonspecific and may demonstrate right atrial and right ventricular enlargement. Chest radiograph reveals cardiomegaly with increased pulmonary vascular markings. Echocardiography demonstrates generalized cardiomegaly. Treatment, if necessary, requires

interventional closure or surgical ligation of the anomalous vascular connections.

CARDIOMYOPATHY

A large body of literature exists describing the diagnosis and management of structural congenital heart disease in the fetus and newborn. There is a paucity of information, however, regarding the diagnosis and management of fetal and newborn cardiomyopathy. In evaluating a newborn infant with signs of congestive heart failure, structural heart disease should be ruled out. In the absence of structural problems, the diagnosis of cardiomyopathy should be considered. The etiology of neonatal cardiomyopathy includes prenatal infections (with cytomegalovirus, human immunodeficiency virus, enterovirus, or parvovirus); familial or genetic causes; maternal autoimmune disease with anti-Ro or anti-La antibodies; prenatal drug exposure; arrhythmia-induced cardiomyopathy; and twin-twin transfusion. Postnatal evaluation should include a search for the underlying cause.

TABLE 55-2 Availability of Infant Heart Donors

Year	1999	2000	2001	2002	2003	2004	2005	2006	2007	2008
Donors	53	62	59	62	62	66	71	88	80	88

Data from the Organ Procurement and Transplant Network Database (http://optn.transplant.hrsa.gov/).

Initial management is similar to that for other types of heart disease. Initial stabilization may require mechanical ventilation, the use of ionotropes, afterload reduction, and diuresis. Long-term treatment is dependent somewhat on the specific cause of the cardiomyopathy, because some forms may be reversible. Cardiac transplantation should be considered if cardiac function is poor or improvement is not noted.

HEART TRANSPLANTATION

The first heart transplant procedure in an infant was reported in 1968 (Kantrowitz et al, 1968). Since then, improved understanding of transplant immunology and medical management has made heart transplantation in infants and children an important option in inoperable patients or those with end-stage cardiac disease. In a recent scientific statement from the American Heart Association, the indications for pediatric heart transplantation were defined (adapted from Canter et al, 2007):

1. Need for ongoing intravenous inotropic or mechanical circulatory support
2. Complex CHD not amenable to conventional surgical repair or palliation or for which the surgical procedure carries a higher risk of mortality than transplantation
3. Progressive deterioration of ventricular function or functional status despite optimal medical care
4. Malignant arrhythmia or survival after cardiac arrest unresponsive to medical therapy, catheter ablation, or an automatic implantable defibrillator
5. Progressive pulmonary hypertension that could preclude future transplantation
6. Growth failure secondary to severe congestive heart failure unresponsive to conventional medical therapy
7. Unacceptably poor quality of life

There are a variety of lesions in the neonate for which cardiac transplantation has been used as primary palliation. These have included hypoplastic left heart, pulmonary atresia with intact ventricular septum and presence of coronary sinusoids, complex heterotaxy or unbalanced complete AV canal with poor common AV valve function, and single-ventricle hearts in which the dominant semilunar valve is severely insufficient. In considering transplantation in these patients, there is a balance between the success of palliative surgery and the availability of organs for transplantation. For example, over the past decade, survival of patients undergoing surgical palliation of hypoplastic left heart syndrome has continued to improve (Alsoufi et al, 2007; Gordon et al, 2008). With the availability of infant donors increasing only slightly over this period of time (Table 55-2), the balance for treatment of these newborns has shifted toward surgical palliation with the Norwood or hybrid Norwood procedures.

Patients with the other lesions just noted continue to have relatively poor surgical outcomes, suggesting that palliation with heart transplantation may be the best approach. Given the limited availability of organs, however, it should be recognized that some of these infants will not survive to transplantation (Kirklin et al, 2006). The long-term survival of infants who undergo heart transplantation is quite good. The calculated "half-life" of transplant recipients younger than 1 year of age was 15.8 years, 14.2 years for children between 1 and 10 years, and 11.4 years for children over the age of 10 years (Boucek et al, 2007).

It is interesting that there appears to be a survival advantage in newborns who receive their transplant before 1 month of age versus those between 1 and 12 months (del Rio, 2000). Although the mechanism of the improved survival in the younger neonates is not known, it may reflect an immunologic window where in graft rejection and transplant coronary artery disease are limited.

Complete references and supplemental color images used in this text can be found online at www.expertconsult.com

ARRHYTHMIAS IN THE NEWBORN AND FETUS

Jeremy P. Moore, Gary M. Satou, and Thomas S. Klitzner

Advances in both electrophysiology and fetal echocardiography over the past two decades have substantially enhanced our ability to diagnose and treat arrhythmias in the fetus and newborn. This chapter outlines many of the advances and can serve as a guide to the most modern approaches to the issue of rhythm disturbances in the perinatal period. After a brief introduction to the pathophysiology of arrhythmias, the chapter is divided into sections on the neonate and fetus. Each section is organized to describe the various types of arrhythmias occurring in that period, along with the corresponding management strategies. Of necessity, there is some overlap between the neonatal and fetal sections, which is highlighted when appropriate. Although advances in the field occur frequently, the basic understanding of arrhythmia pathogenesis and the overall principles of treatment outlined here have remained relatively constant for the last 5 to 10 years.

In this chapter, fetal tachycardia is considered a persistent elevation in the heart rate above 180 beats/min and fetal bradycardia is defined as a persistent heart rate below 100 beats/min. After birth, these same definitions apply to the neonate (Davignon et al, 1980).

PATHOPHYSIOLOGY OF ARRHYTHMIAS IN THE NEONATE AND FETUS

Three general mechanisms of arrhythmogenesis have been described and are presumed to be responsible for the majority of tachycardias seen in the fetus and neonate with tachycardia:

- Reentry
- Abnormal automaticity
- Triggered activity

Reentry classically requires several conditions for initiation and maintenance, including multiple pathways for impulse conduction, an area of slow conduction in at least one of these pathways, block in one pathway, and recovery of tissue excitability at the site of origin. These rhythms involve anatomically defined circuits of electrical activity and therefore tend to behave predictably with a stable cycle length and paroxysmal initiation and termination. Reentrant rhythms may be altered or interrupted by premature beats that enter the reentry circuit.

Abnormal automaticity is the result of spontaneous depolarization of a group of myocardial cells known as the automatic focus. Automatic rhythms tend to accelerate on initiation and show variation in rate with changes in external influences, most significantly autonomic tone. However, premature beats do not alter automatic rhythms unless they depolarize the automatic focus, which is unusual.

Triggered activity is due to small, spontaneous depolarizations of the myocardial cell membrane that result in repetitive electrical activity when they reach threshold. Conditions that predispose to triggered arrhythmias are intrinsic myocardial disease, ischemia, digitalis toxicity, and metabolic disturbances.

NEONATAL RHYTHMS

TACHYCARDIAS

Although a host of neonatal tachycardias may be seen in clinical practice, only a few are seen commonly. These more common tachycardias include orthodromic reciprocating tachycardia (ORT) and atrial flutter.

The substrate of ORT is a reentrant circuit that includes the atrium, the atrioventricular (AV) node, and His-Purkinje system in the antegrade direction, and the ventricular myocardium and an accessory pathway in the retrograde direction back to the atrium (Figure 56-1). This is the most common arrhythmia in the newborn period. ORT manifests as a narrow-complex tachycardia with a P wave that occurs more than 70 ms (just under 2 "little" boxes on a standard electrocardiogram [ECG]) after the QRS complex. The heart rate tends to be in the range of 240 to 260 beats/min in the newborn. A large percentage of the accessory pathways responsible for ORT will spontaneously become nonfunctional during the course of infancy as the heart matures.

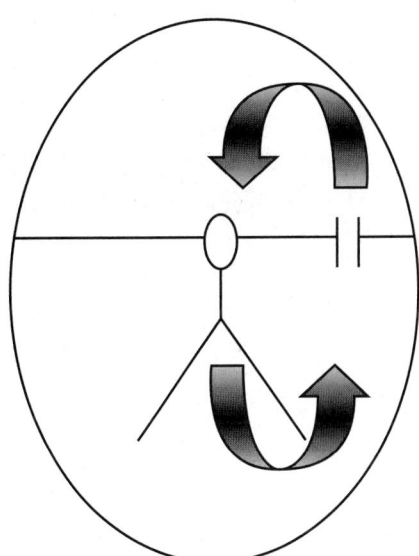

FIGURE 56-1 Mechanism of orthodromic reciprocating tachycardia. The electrical impulse travels down the normal conduction system by way of the AV node and His-Purkinje system to the ventricle, where it returns to the atrium by the accessory pathway (in this case, a left-sided pathway).

Atrial flutter is a reentrant rhythm that requires only the atrium to complete the circuit, with conduction to the ventricles occurring passively over the AV node. Typical circuits travel in a counterclockwise direction around the tricuspid valve annulus, which is responsible for the characteristic appearance on the 12-lead ECG. Features include sawtooth P waves in the inferior leads and positive, generally more discrete, P waves in lead V1. Atrial rates tend to be greater than 300 beats/min, resulting in various degrees of aberrancy (bundle-branch block) and physiologic AV block. In the neonate, classic flutter waves may be absent. Consequently, the atrial rate tends to be the most important clue to the diagnosis (Figure 56-2). After conversion to sinus rhythm, recurrence of atrial flutter is rare in the neonate without structural heart disease (Wren, 2006).

Other tachycardias in the newborn are much less common, but are important to recognize in order for therapy to be administered in a timely manner. They are considered next in their relative order of frequency.

Atrial ectopic tachycardia (AET) is often an incessant rhythm that displays warm-up periods and variable functional AV block at higher rates. The most characteristic feature on the surface ECG is the p-wave axis, which is almost always abnormal. Most foci originate from remnants of embryonic myocardium that insert on extracardiac structures, such as the superior vena cava (SVC), pulmonary veins, coronary sinus, and atrial appendages. The location of these foci tends to dictate the resultant p-wave axis. Incessant tachycardia due to AET carries the associated risk of tachycardia-mediated cardiomyopathy if the rhythm goes undiagnosed for extended periods of time. In patients with AET tachycardia, AV node–blocking medications may result in high-grade AV block with little effect on the underlying atrial rhythm but may be diagnostic (Figure 56-3). This distinction may be especially useful for ectopic tachycardias that originate near the SVC, which otherwise can appear very similar to sinus tachycardia on the surface ECG.

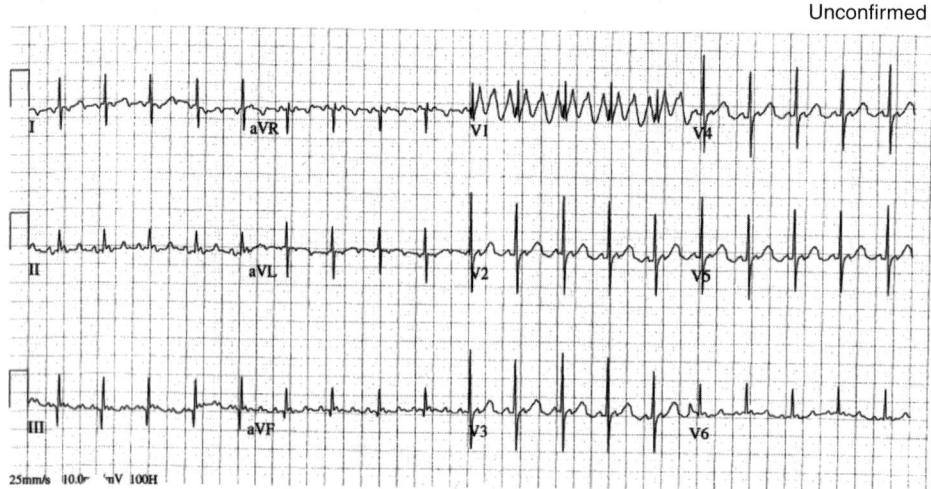

FIGURE 56-2 **12-lead electrocardiogram demonstrating atrial flutter.** The atrial rate is approximately 360 beats/min. Note that the atrioventricular conduction demonstrates 3:1 AV block, resulting in the slower ventricular rate of only 120 bpm. P waves appear discrete and are positive in the inferior leads, as opposed to the classic "sawtooth" pattern seen in older children and adults. *AV,* Atrioventricular; *ECG,* elecrocardiogram.

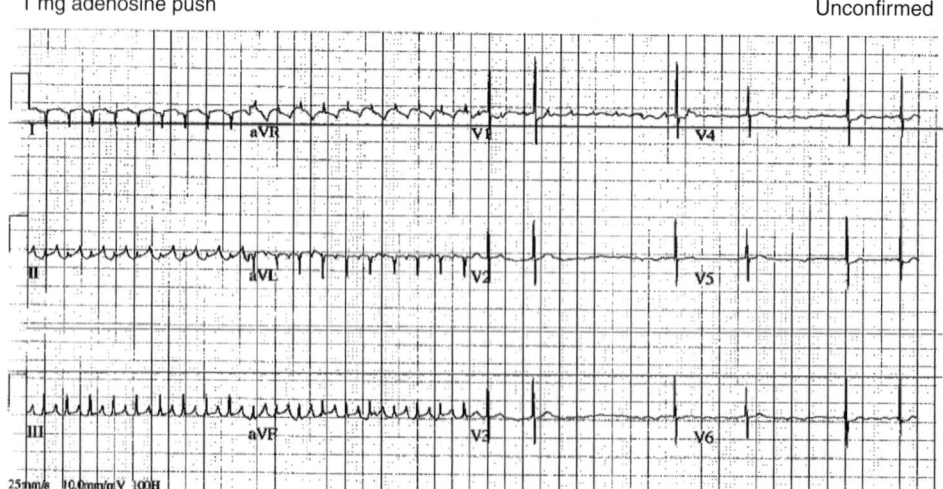

FIGURE 56-3 **12-lead ECG in a patient with atrial ectopic tachycardia.** The P-wave axis suggests a posterior and slightly leftward focus. Note that the ectopic rhythm (best seen in lead V1) is not perturbed by the administration of a bolus of adenosine. *AET,* Atrial ectopic tachycardia; *EGG,* electrocardiogram.

The permanent form of junctional reciprocating tachycardia (PJRT) is a rare reentrant rhythm that uses the AV node and His-Purkinje system as the antegrade pathway and a slowly conducting accessory pathway in the region of the posterior septum of the heart as the retrograde limb. This rhythm often manifests with heart rates in the upper range of normal for the neonate but is typically incessant with frequent interruptions and spontaneous reinitiations. Consequently, PJRT also can result in a progressive cardiomyopathy if it goes unnoticed over extended periods of time. The hallmarks of this rhythm are its sudden onset and termination, as well as the characteristically inverted P-wave axis (sometimes quite large) on the 12-lead ECG (Figure 56-4).

Congenital junctional ectopic tachycardia (JET) is extremely rare, and there are only a few case series describing experience with this rhythm (Coumel et al, 1976; Villain et al, 1990). The arrhythmia is due to abnormal automaticity in the region of the AV junction. The nature of the rhythm results in simultaneous depolarization of atria and ventricles, with subsequent loss of AV synchrony. The rhythm tends to be very resistant to medical management, with the net effect being a predisposition to tachycardia-mediated cardiomyopathy over time.

Ventricular tachycardia (VT) is defined as a ventricular rhythm greater than 20% faster than the underlying sinus rhythm. It is characterized by a wide QRS complex (more than 80 ms, or 2 "little" boxes on the neonatal ECG). It is considered sustained if lasting longer than 30 seconds and incessant if present more than 10% of the time on continuous monitoring. Clues to the diagnosis of VT in the neonate are as follows (Batra and Silka, 2000):

1. The QRS complex has abnormal axis and morphology as compared with sinus rhythm.
2. The first QRS complex occurs earlier than expected and is not preceded by an atrial depolarization.
3. Ventriculoatrial (VA) dissociation or fusion complexes occur.

Not all wide complex tachycardia is VT, however. The differential diagnosis also includes supraventricular tachycardia (SVT) with aberrancy as well as some forms of SVT utilizing an accessory pathway in the antegrade direction. The preceding criteria are often helpful in making the correct diagnosis.

VT has several diverse causes in the neonate. The most common inherited cause of neonatal VT is the long QT syndrome (LQTS). The reported prevalence of this

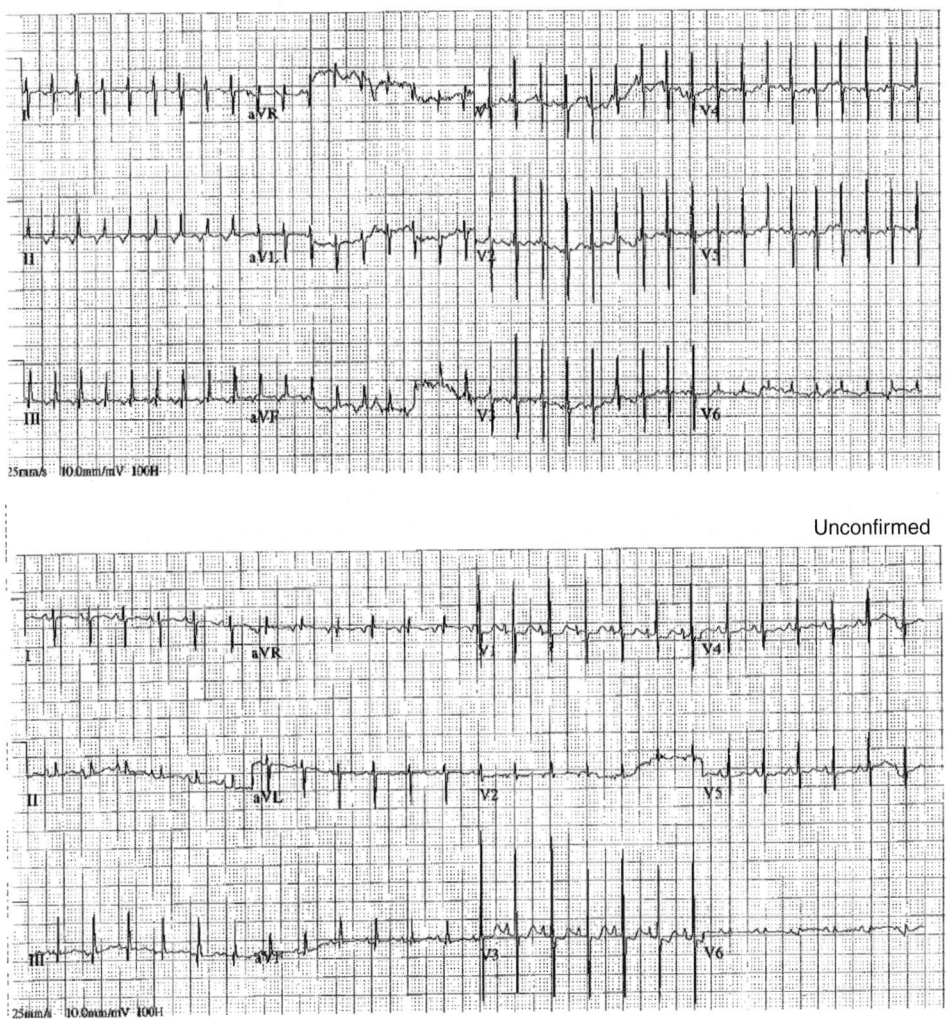

FIGURE 56-4 12-lead electrocardiogram in a neonate with permanent form of junctional reciprocating tachycardia before and after adenosine administration. During tachycardia, the p wave axis is directed superiorly and rightward, consistent with an origin near the "crux" of the heart.

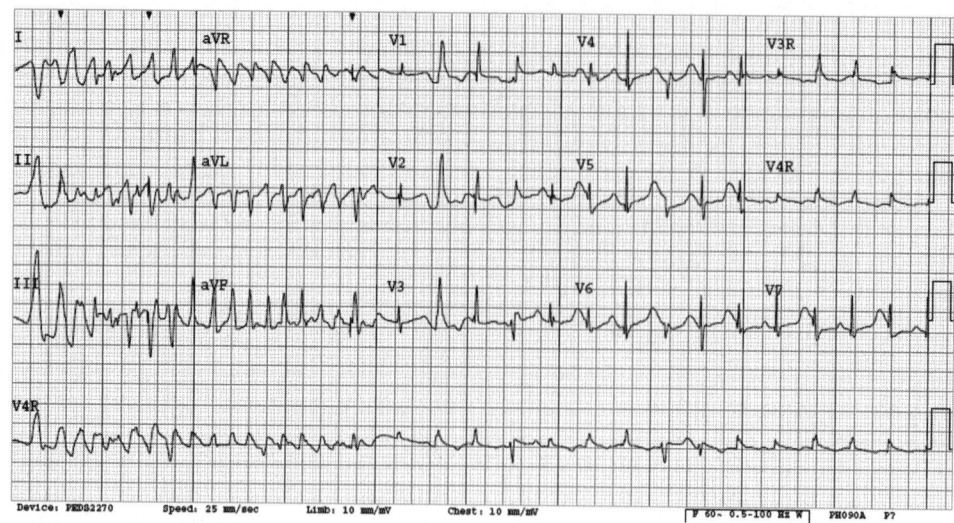

FIGURE 56-5 15-lead electrocardiogram (ECG) and rhythm strip recording of torsades de pointes type ventricular tachycardia in a neonate with congenital long QT syndrome. Note the "twisting" pattern of the QRS complex during tachycardia. The rhythm spontaneously terminates with resumption of sinus rhythm at the beginning of the ECG.

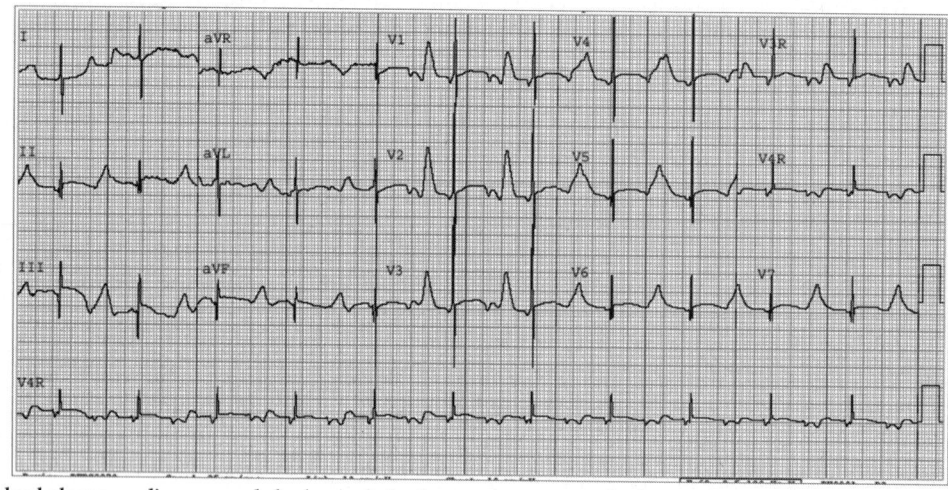

FIGURE 56-6 15-lead electrocardiogram and rhythm strip in the same neonate as in the previous figure. Note the very long QT interval and 2:1 atrioventricular block, owing to the functional refractoriness of the ventricle during the prolonged QT interval.

condition in the general population is approximately 1 in 2500, but prevalence may be higher in the neonate (Collins and Van Hare, 2006). The arrhythmias associated with this condition are related to prolongation of repolarization in the epicardial layer of the heart leading to early afterdepolarizations (a form of triggered activity) and subsequent polymorphic VT (Yan et al, 1998). In patients with LQTS, the VT is described as torsades de pointes (TdP) which literally means "twisting of the points" and displays a classic ECG appearance (Figure 56-5). In any patient presenting with this type of ventricular tachycardia, the diagnosis should be strongly suspected and the baseline 12-lead ECG should be examined for prolongation of the QT interval. In the neonate, the corrected QT interval should be less than 440 ms, regardless of gender (Schwartz et al, 1998). Unfortunately, during the first days to week of life the QTc tends to be highly variable, making this measurement unreliable (Walsh, 1963). Rarely, severely affected neonates may present with 2:1 AV block and bradycardia related to functional refractoriness of ventricular tissue due to the long QT interval (Figure 56-6).

Prolongation of the QT interval can also be acquired, in which case it can be secondary to factors such as medication administration, electrolyte abnormalities, or neurologic injury. Just as with the congenital LQTS, acquired QT prolongation can predispose the neonate to TdP.

Another source of VT in the neonate is the presence of intramyocardial tumors. The most common tumors seen in the newborn period are rhabdomyomas, which typically are multiple and involve the ventricular muscle directly, but occasionally can involve the conduction system as well. VT related to rhabdomyomas may be difficult to control, but typically improves with time because these tumors tend to spontaneously regress. More rarely, neonates may be affected by a disease entity known as histiocytoid cardiomyopathy. This is a genetic disorder characterized by macroscopic yellow-tan nodules, which are Purkinje fibers and scattered clusters of histiocytoid myocytes (Finsterer, 2008). These abnormal cell collections can be the focus of VT in affected neonates and infants.

Neonatal VT may also be a nonspecific response to a variety of systemic insults that include electrolyte

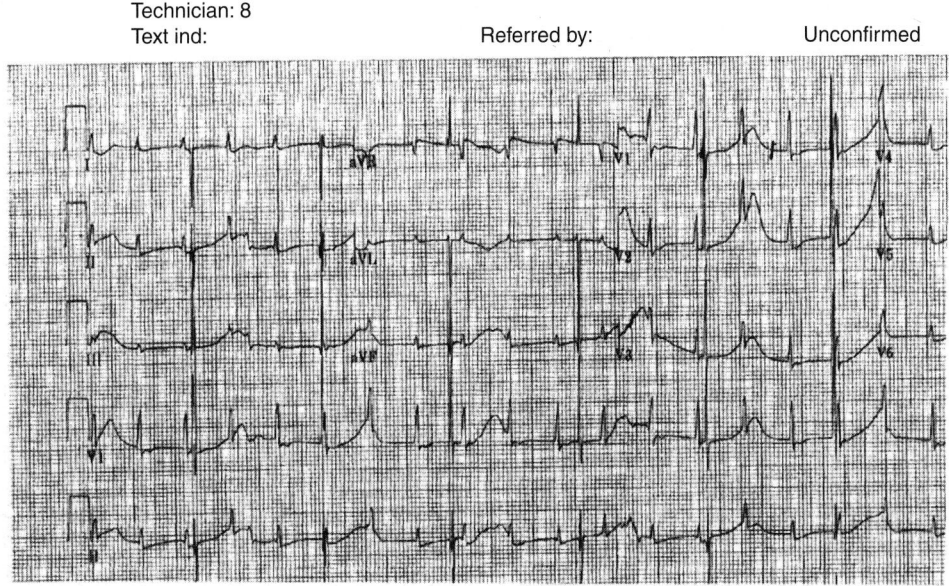

Technician: 8
Text ind: Referred by: Unconfirmed

FIGURE 56-7 Congenital AV block. The atrial rate is 130 beats/min and the ventricular rate is just under 50 beats/min. There is complete dissociation between the atrial and ventricular rhythms. The very tall P waves represent right atrial enlargement.

TABLE 56-1   Echocardiographic Diagnosis of Fetal Tachycardia Subtype Based on the Ventriculoatrial Interval/Duration

VA Relationship	Tachycardia Diagnosis
Short VA (VA<AV)	ORT
Long VA (VA > AV)	AET
	PJRT
	Sinus tachycardia
Simultaneous VA	JET
2:1 AV relationship	AFL
	AET (less likely)
VA dissociation	JET
	VT

AET, Atrial ectopic tachycardia; *AV,* atrioventricular; *JET,* junctional ectopic tachycardia; *ORT,* orthodromic reciprocating tachycardia; *PJRT,* permanent junctional ectopic tachycardia; *VA,* ventriculoatrial.

BOX 56-1   Pathologic Causes of Neonatal Bradycardia

Left atrial isomerism
LQTS with 2:1 block
Sick sinus syndrome
Blocked atrial bigeminy

derangements, acidosis, hypoxia, sepsis, and myocardial ischemia. Correction of the underlying problem usually ameliorates the tachycardia.

Myocarditis is an important cause of neonatal VT, but usually manifests with hemodynamic instability and shock rather than isolated tachycardia. Other electrocardiographic clues to the diagnosis include decreased precordial voltages, various conduction abnormalities, and frequent atrial and/or ventricular ectopy.

Noninfectious cardiomyopathies may manifest with VT, but as with myocarditis, other signs and symptoms are often present to assist in the diagnosis. These may include respiratory distress with inspiratory crackles, cardiomegaly, thready pulse with narrowed pulse pressure, and hemodynamic instability.

Benign forms of "idiopathic VT" can affect healthy neonates with structurally normal hearts. These include idiopathic right ventricular outflow tract (RVOT) tachycardia and left ventricular posterior fascicular VT. Last,

accelerated idioventricular rhythm (AIVR) refers to a ventricular rhythm that is not more than 10–20 beats/min faster than the underlying sinus rate. The QRS axis is most commonly a left bundlebranch block with an inferior axis. This rhythm is generally benign and most often self-limiting.

BRADYCARDIAS

Neonatal bradycardia is defined as a persistent heart rate <100 beats/min. Noncardiac causes are most common and are typically transient. These usually involve situations associated with high vagal tone. Bradycardia in the neonate may also represent a nonspecific response to hypoxia and acidosis, in which case it may be more sustained.

Cardiac causes of fetal and neonatal bradycardia are diverse. The most common is congenital AV block, which occurs in approximately 1:20,000 live births (Michaelsson and Engle, 1972) (Figure 56-7). Other, less frequent cardiac etiologies are listed in Box 56-1. Congenital AV block is generally divided into two broad categories based on the underlying pathophysiology.

Congenital Atrioventricular Block Associated with Structural Heart Disease

The congenital heart defects that are most frequently accompanied by congenital heart block include heterotaxy syndrome (with left atrial isomerism), congenitally corrected transposition of the great arteries, and AV canal defects. Congenital AV block associated with structural heart disease has the highest mortality of the two subtypes, with fetal loss rates as high as 75%. Large clinical studies evaluating the incidence of fetal and neonatal congenital AV block have shown that in utero, the causes of heart block are initially evenly distributed, with 50% of cases due to structural heart disease and 50% due to immune-mediated mechanisms (Machado et al, 1988; Schmidt et al, 1991). Postnatally, however, the incidence of congenital AV block associated with structural heart disease decreases to 30% of cases with the remaining cases related to immune-mediated mechanisms, reflecting the high in utero mortality of the former. Outcomes for a fetus with the combination of congenital AV block, complex congenital heart disease, and hydrops fetalis is particularly dismal, with extremely high rates of fetal loss (Anandakumar et al, 1996).

Immune-Mediated Congenital Atrioventricular Block

The presence of maternal anti-Ro (SSA) or anti-La (SSB) antibodies have been demonstrated in most cases of *isolated* congenital AV block, with the presumed mechanism being that of immunecomplex deposition with specific damage to the fetal cardiac conduction system. Ro-52 specific antibodies have shown a very close association to immune-mediated congenital AV block in recent studies (Salomonsson et al, 2004). The risk of heart block in mothers with anti-SSA and anti-SSB antibodies is approximately 2% to 3%, with recurrence rates after one affected child as high as 14% to 17%. Autopsy specimens typically reveal progressive fibrosis of the AV nodal structures in affected fetuses. The process typically spares the His-Purkinje system, however, so that the slower "escape rhythm" tends to be fairly reliable. In addition, damage to the conduction system is variably accompanied by damage to contractile elements of the heart (Assad et al, 1994; Horsfall et al, 1996; Schmidt et al, 1991; Walkinshaw et al, 1994). Less frequently, a progressive cardiomyopathy develops, unrelated to the heart block, and is marked by sustained high levels of maternal autoantibodies in the affected fetus and neonate (Moak et al, 2001; Taylor-Alber et al, 1997). The risk of transfer of maternal autoantibodies to the fetus seems to be highest between 16 and 26 weeks' gestation (Buyon et al, 1998; Waltuck and Buyon, 1994), and it usually is at this point that affected fetuses will demonstrate manifestations of conduction system disease.

An uncommon cause of neonatal bradycardia is blocked atrial bigeminy, which is a pattern of atrial ectopic beats closely coupled to the preceding QRS complex, in which the AV node is refractory. This results in failure of conduction to the ventricle (Figure 56-8). In most cases, this phenomenon results in bradycardia, but it also predicts a higher risk for progression to sustained tachycardia (Simpson et al, 1996). The underlying pathophysiology is often times reentry from the ventricle to the atrium over an accessory pathway (Kleinman and Nehgme, 2004). In other cases, atrial bigeminy may be caused by a redundant flap of the foramen ovale, which comes in contact with the free wall of the atrium during ventricular systole when the membrane moves away from the septum (Pernot et al, 1984; Phillipos et al, 1994).

NEONATAL MANAGEMENT
NEONATAL TACHYCARDIA MANAGEMENT

The management of neonatal supraventricular tachycardia (SVT) is based on the presumed mechanism of the tachyarrhythmia, with ORT and atrial flutter being most common (Figure 56-9 shows a proposed treatment algorithm and drug dosing). Cases of ORT can often be terminated with vagal maneuvers or adenosine. Digoxin remains first-line therapy for treatment and prevention of both ORT and atrial flutter in many institutions after preexcitation has been excluded on the 12-lead ECG. Digoxin can be administered orally or by the intravenous (IV) route (with IV administration of digoxin being 80% of the enteral dose). The surface electrocardiogram is followed for evidence of PR prolongation, and serum potassium levels are kept in the normal range. Whereas some institutions use propranolol as a first-line agent for neonatal tachycardia, many others reserve propranolol and flecainide for refractory cases of ORT. Atrial flutter responds well to electrical cardioversion if initial therapy with digoxin fails. This is more likely to occur if the rhythm is less organized and resembles atrial fibrillation. In cases of successful electrical cardioversion, flecainide may be used to prevent recurrence. Regardless of the drug chosen, therapy is generally continued for 6 months, after which time recurrence rates decrease significantly (Wren, 2006). Some centers follow a "wait and see" policy after conversion of neonatal atrial flutter to sinus rhythm, given that recurrence rates are low (Jaeggi et al, 1998).

In contrast with neonatal ORT and atrial flutter, atrial ectopic tachycardia is less effectively treated with digoxin and often requires the administration of flecainide or sotalol. In more refractory cases, combination therapy with both agents is required. Alternatively, amiodarone can be used. IV administration of amiodarone is avoided whenever possible, given rare reports of neonatal "gasping

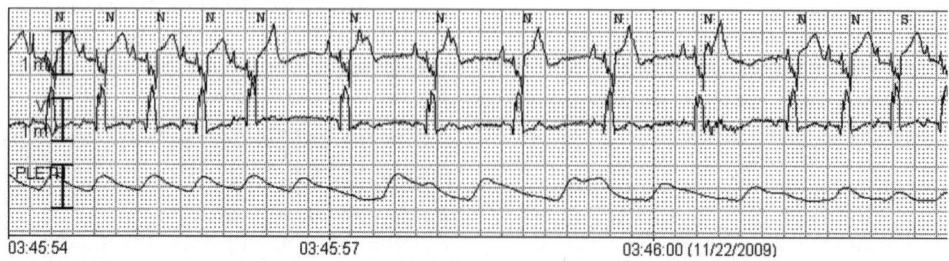

FIGURE 56-8 Two-lead rhythm strip and arterial line trace demonstrating blocked atrial bigeminy in a newborn with intermittent episodes of bradycardia. The blocked atrial extrasystoles can be seen superimposed on the T waves preceding the pauses.

syndrome" and leaching of plasticizers from IV tubing (Centers for Disease Control, 1982; Gershanik et al, 1982; Sabex, 2001). However, it has been used safely in this form when required for more refractory arrhythmias (Perry et al, 1996). Amiodarone is administered with loading doses and is continued at this dose until the atrial rate is in the normal range, or for 10 days, whichever comes first. At this point, the dose of amiodarone is decreased to the maintenance range. If monotherapy is successful, a trial of discontinuation of the drug is attempted at 6 months of age. With combination therapy, a staggered wean is best. For example, one drug can be discontinued at 6 months, and then a trial period discontinuing the remaining medication can be performed several months later.

Congenital JET tends to be a refractory arrhythmia and often does not respond to the usual drug therapies. Amiodarone is the drug most likely to be successful for the treatment of JET. However, in exceptional cases, biventricular pacing and high-dose antiarrhythmic therapy with two separate agents may be required to achieve arrhythmia suppression.

The two ventricular rhythms relevant to the neonatal period are AIVR and VT. In general, AIVR does not require therapy and resolves during infancy. The treatment of VT should be based on the underlying mechanism, but patients with hemodynamically unstable VT/ventricular fibrillation should undergo immediate cardiac defibrillation according to American Heart Association (AHA) guidelines.

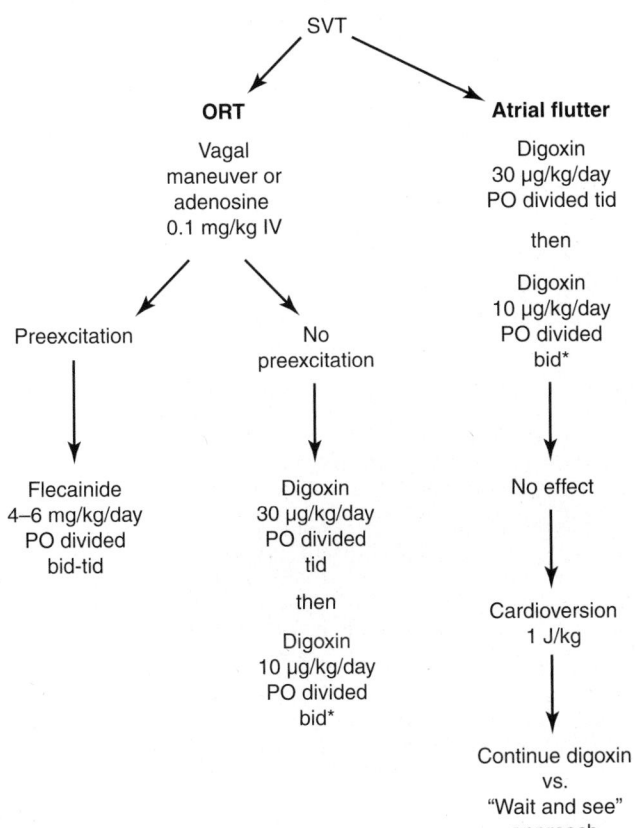

FIGURE 56-9 Suggested neonatal management scheme for the two most common types of Supraventricular tachycardia. Orthodromic reciprocating tachycardia is usually treated medically, whereas atrial flutter may require electrical cardioversion. See text for further details. *Digoxin dose reduction is required in preterm neonates.

In cases in which cardiac defibrillation has been performed, further therapy of TdP consists of IV magnesium. Once rhythm control has been achieved, a continued search should be made for exacerbating factors. Drug-induced TdP usually responds well to removal of the offending medication in addition to aggressive correction of electrolyte disturbances. If the etiologic disorder is determined to be congenital LQTS, therapy relies heavily on the use of beta-blockers, the most common of which is propranolol. Neonates with suspected or proven LQTS should have all QT-prolonging medications stopped. Electrolytes should always be kept in the normal range with special attention to serum potassium levels. Other LQTS-specific treatment modalities for severely affected neonates who experience breakthrough episodes despite beta-blocker therapy include left stellate ganglionectomy as well as implantable cardioverter-defibrillator (ICD) placement (Berul, 2000, Progress Pediatr Cardiol). ICD implantation is typically used only as secondary preventive measure after aborted sudden cardiac death, particularly because ICD shocks have been implicated in creating incessant tachycardia.

Management of VT related to intracardiac tumors often begins acutely with a lidocaine drip. Long term suppression often involves beta-blocker therapy with class Ic agents or amiodarone for more refractory cases. The acute treatment for VT in the setting of myocarditis and dilated cardiomyopathies similarly relies on lidocaine for rapid arrhythmia suppression, whereas amiodarone is often the drug of choice for more long-term suppression.

The management of idiopathic VT in the neonate usually does not require therapy, because these tend to be benign rhythms. Right ventricular outflow tract (RVOT) tachycardia is usually well controlled with beta-blocker therapy if needed.

NEONATAL BRADYCARDIA MANAGEMENT

Congenital AV block in the otherwise healthy neonate with good ventricular function and average heart rates greater than 55 beats/min is generally well tolerated, and follow-up can be performed as an outpatient. Close observation should include serial history and physical examinations, echocardiography, and Holter monitoring. Evidence of an unreliable escape rhythm and progressive cardiac dysfunction suggest the need for pacemaker placement. Consensus guidelines have been published recently regarding indications for pacing (Hui et al, 2008). In infancy, class I indications include the following (Epstein et al, 2008):

1. A wide QRS escape rhythm, complex ventricular ectopy, or ventricular dysfunction
2. An average ventricular rate less than 55 beats/min with isolated heart block
3. An average ventricular rate less than 70 beats/min with associated congenital heart disease

At the time of delivery, any significant pleural effusions related to hydrops fetalis should be drained and medical therapy with isoproterenol can be started if there is evidence of hemodynamic compromise. Epicardial pacing is generally feasible in infants who weigh more than 2 kg, and temporary transvenous pacing can be instituted via an umbilical or femoral venous approach on an emergent basis.

Blocked atrial bigeminy as a cause of bradycardia is generally a benign neonatal rhythm. Treatment is indicated in the occasional neonate in whom the extrasystoles serve as a trigger for recurrent episodes of supraventricular tachycardia. In these cases, conservative management with digoxin is recommended (Fish and Benson, 2001). Because several studies have described an association with these rhythms and the future occurrence of SVT, outpatient follow-up is also warranted.

FETAL RHYTHMS

IRREGULAR RHYTHMS

One of the most common reasons for referral to the fetal cardiologist is irregular fetal heart rhythms, noted in 1–3% of pregnancies (Strasburger, 2005). The causes of these irregular rhythms are often isolated premature atrial beats (Srinivasan and Strasburger, 2008). Rarely, they may be ventricular in origin. Occasionally, they may be related to intermittent disturbances in AV conduction due to primary AV nodal disease or secondarily related to abnormalities in ventricular repolarization. The vast majority of these ectopic beats are benign. Only a very small subset of cases represent underlying cardiac pathology or progress to persistent, sustained tachyarrhythmias.

Investigation of the fetus referred for an abnormal rhythm should focus on causes of impaired AV conduction and causes of abnormal atrial or ventricular ectopy. Etiopathologic disorders include various degrees of AV block, congenital LQTS, myocarditis, and intracardiac tumors, among others. LQTS is suggested by a combination of bradycardia alternating with tachycardia at different times in the same fetus (Strasburger, 2005). The association of an irregular rhythm with one of the foregoing

pathologic entities has been described in 2.6% of fetuses referred for cardiac evaluation (Cuneo et al, 2006). In addition to indicating a specific pathologic diagnosis, the occurrence of frequent benign ectopy such as premature atrial contractions in the fetus has been associated with the subsequent development of sustained tachycardia in 2–3% of affected fetuses (Simpson et al, 1996; Wakai et al, 2003). The presence of cardiomegaly, systolic ventricular dysfunction, AV valve regurgitation, or hydrops suggests the diagnosis of either frequent episodes of SVT or fetal myocarditis. In this circumstance, frequent ultrasound evaluation is required until the ectopy has resolved (Hornberger and Sahn, 2007). Because frequent ectopy may trigger the future occurrence of SVT given the incidence of accessory pathways in the immature heart (Ko et al, 1992; Perry and Garson, 1990; Silver et al, 1973), many institutions recommend providing continued monitoring of the fetal heart on a weekly or biweekly basis (Fouron et al, 2004).

FETAL TACHYCARDIAS

The two most common mechanisms of SVT in utero are ORT in approximately 70% of cases, followed by atrial flutter (AFL) in 20% (Strasburger, 2005) (see Figures 56-10 and 56-11). Less frequent mechanisms make up the remainder. A convenient classification scheme to determine the type of SVT in utero (see Box 56-1) uses the echocardiographic measurement of the interval between the ventricular contraction (V) and the subsequent atrial contraction (A). With this approach, tailored management and prognosis can be assessed for a given fetus based on the suspected type of SVT (Table 56-1). As well, the

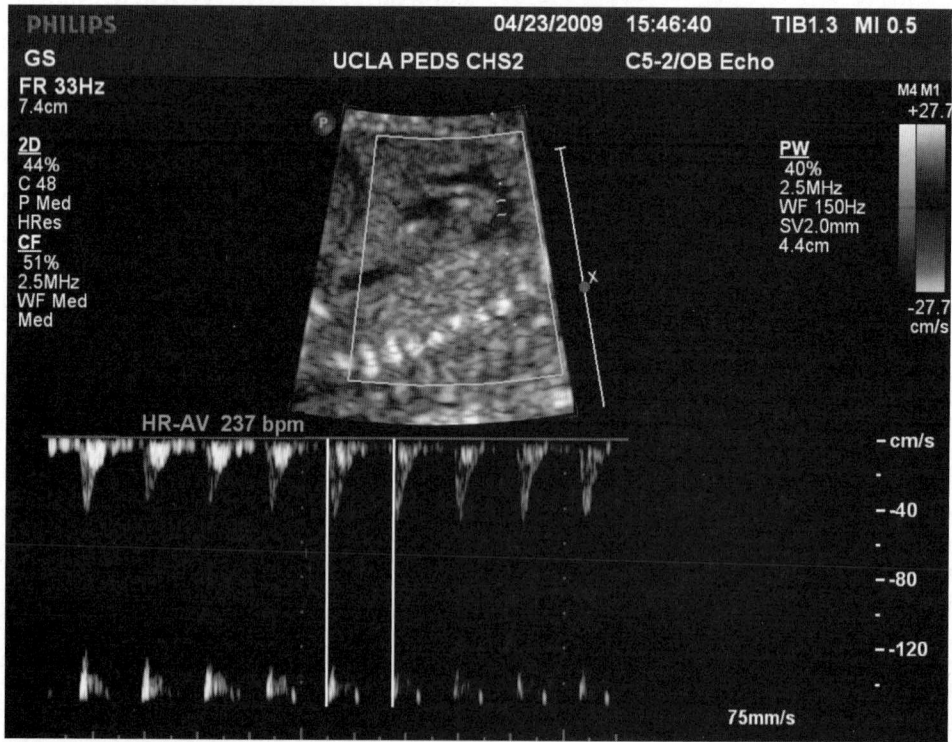

FIGURE 56-10 **Doppler echocardiography recording performed in a fetus with Supraventricular tachycardia.** The pulse Doppler pattern, measured in the aortic arch, demonstrates an elevated ventricular contraction rate at 237 beats/min. Note that the atrial rate is not apparent in this interrogation.

echocardiographic examination can be used serially to monitor treatment outcomes and to detect impaired myocardial function that may develop with sustained tachyarrhythmias.

Because the immature fetal myocardium is intrinsically less compliant than the mature myocardium (Friedman, 1972), persistent tachycardias are not well tolerated and, in protracted cases, can lead to the development of nonimmune hydrops fetalis. Risk factors for the development of hydrops fetalis include early gestational age (<32 weeks) (Hornberger and Sahn, 2007; Naheed et al, 1996) and prolonged duration of tachycardia (Naheed et al, 1996). As the fetal myocardium is challenged by a further reduction in diastolic filling in the setting of tachycardia, atrial pressures increase, with the pulsations of atrial contraction being ultimately transmitted to the umbilical veins (Gudmundsson et al, 1991). Hepatic venous congestion may then result in decreased synthesis of albumin and decreased serum oncotic pressure. When the elevated hydrostatic pressure of myocardial dysfunction exceeds oncotic pressure, extravasation of fluid into the extravascular space ensues, leading to the clinical manifestation of hydrops fetalis (Grossman et al, 1990). This syndrome is defined by the accumulation of fluid in more than two of the following locations: abdomen, skin, pericardium, or pleural space. At the same time, increased placental venous pressure can lead to polyhydramnios and increased risk of premature delivery with its attendant risks of complications (Maxwell et al, 1988). Poor placental transfer of oxygen to the fetus through a congested placental circuit can be a terminal event in this scenario.

In the fetus, ORT usually presents with intermittent or sustained heart rates in the range of 240 to 260 beats/min and a 1:1 AV relationship. Similar to the situation in the newborn and infant, this rhythm results from conduction down the AV node to the ventricles and back up an accessory pathway to the atrium to complete the circuit. In general, ORT presents at an earlier age than AFL, usually at weeks 28 to 33 of gestation (Hornberger and Sahn, 2007). Progression to hydrops is not uncommon, with risk factors being tachycardia duration, fetal immaturity, and concurrent structural heart disease (Hornberger and Sahn, 2007; Naheed et al, 1996). It has also been suggested that pathway location on the left side is a risk factor for progression to hydrops fetalis due to changes in intracardiac hemodynamics (left atrial pressure is transiently elevated above right atrial pressures, thereby restricting flow across the foramen ovale) (Kannankeril et al, 2003).

The second most common mechanism of fetal tachycardia is AFL, which is characterized by atrial rates of 300–500 per minute and slower ventricular rates due to physiologic block in the AV node. This rhythm is more likely to manifest later in pregnancy than ORT, predominantly at 31 to 34 weeks' gestation. (Jaeggi et al, 1998; Strasburger, 2005). A unique feature of the fetal atrium in the latter part of gestation is its ability to sustain high atrial rates and thereby permit this type of tachycardia (Til et al, 1992). The most common presentation of AFL in the fetus demonstrates ventricular rates of 150 to170 per minute. Because the rhythm usually occurs in the more mature fetus and with lower ventricular rates, it is generally a well-tolerated rhythm (Jaeggi et al, 1998). However, the rhythm can go undiagnosed because of the relatively normal ventricular rates (Fouron et al, 2004). In this situation, the lack of variability in heart rate is the primary clue to the diagnosis. An association with accessory pathways has been reported in many fetuses with AFL (Naheed et al, 1996) and ORT has been reported to

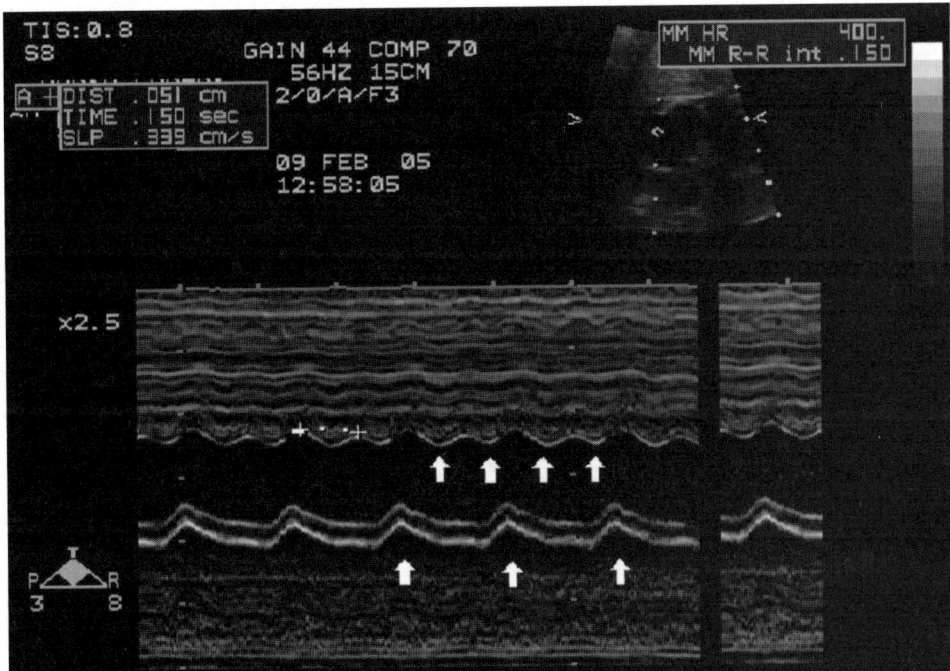

FIGURE 56-11 *(See also Color Plate 23.)* **Fetal M-mode echocardiogram recording of a late second-trimester fetus with atrial flutter.** The ultrasound cursor is positioned through the right atrium, the tricuspid valve, and the right ventricle *(upper right corner)*. The top row of *four arrows* delineates the mechanical right atrial contraction rate, which is faster than the tricuspid valve/right ventricle contraction rate *(bottom three arrows)*.

co-occur spontaneously in 12% to 33% of affected fetuses (Casey et al, 1997; Till and Wren, 1992).

The fetal echocardiogram may suggest less common tachycardias on the basis of an increased fetal heart rate with long ventriculoatrial (VA) times. The differential diagnosis for this group of tachycardias includes AET and PJRT. The latter may be distinguished on the basis of sudden onset, usually triggered by an atrial extrasystole and a consistent heart rate during tachycardia. On the other hand, AET typically demonstrates a gradual warm-up phase with variable physiologic block in the AV node at faster rates. Tachycardia rates with AET are generally on the order of 180 to 250/min (Strasburger, 2005). In general, this class of fetal arrhythmias is the most refractory to treatment both before and after birth.

Occasionally, sinus tachycardia may be confused with AET as noted previously for the newborn. Characteristics specific to sinus tachycardia include a gradual warm-up period, preservation of heart rate variability, and consistently normal conduction through the AV node to the ventricles (Srinivasan and Strasburger, 2008). Causes of fetal sinus tachycardia in excess of 180/min include maternal pyrexia, stimulant medications, and thyrotoxicosis, as well as fetal anemia, distress, and infection (Fisher et al, 1983).

Congenital JET is rare automatic rhythm with a consistent warm-up phase and is generally very resistant to therapy. It has been reported only rarely in utero (Coumel et al, 1976; Villain et al, 1990). As noted previously, JET can be an incessant rhythm that ultimately leads to a secondary cardiomyopathy.

FETAL MANAGEMENT

MANAGEMENT OF IRREGULAR FETAL RHYTHMS

In general, if ectopy is infrequent (i.e., <1 beat per 10 sinus beats), no further investigation is indicated after associated pathologic entities have been ruled out, and follow-up can be handled adequately in the obstetric office (Srinivasan and Strasburger, 2008). With frequent ectopy, however, follow-up auscultation of the fetal heart rate should be performed approximately every 2 weeks, with a repeat echocardiographic examination approximately 4 to 6 weeks to ensure there has been no progression to SVT. Postnatally, an ECG should be obtained to exclude preexcitation (Simpson et al, 1996; Srinivasan and Strasburger, 2008).

FETAL TACHYARRHYTHMIA MANAGEMENT

Management of fetal tachyarrhythmias is generally divided into three categories (Srinivasan and Strasburger, 2008).
1. Observation
2. Transplacental drug therapy
3. Delivery of the fetus

In the situation of intermittent tachycardia (usually defined as lasting less than 12 hours at a time or present during <50% of the echocardiographic examination) (Cuneo et al, 2000; Jaeggi et al, 1998) in a fetus of late gestational age, the rhythm is generally well tolerated and rarely results in myocardial dysfunction. In the absence of hydrops fetalis, many would advocate observation alone

(Cuneo et al, 2000; Srinivasan and Strasburger, 2008; Strasburger, 2005). This consists of a brief observation period in the hospital to document arrhythmia duration and frequency and fetal well-being, followed by repeat obstetrical ultrasounds on an initial daily and then biweekly basis to ensure that clinical deterioration does not occur.

At the other extreme, emergent delivery should be reserved for the hydropic fetus who exhibits persistent, difficult-to-treat arrhythmias, in whom both transplacental and direct therapy have failed. If delivery is to be a viable option, however, the fetus should be of a reasonable gestational age (Srinivasan and Strasburger, 2008).

The remaining subgroup of patients are treated with what is referred to as transplacental drug therapy. Multiple treatment algorithms have been proposed, but there is no universal or standard approach. A suggested management algorithm for fetal tachyarrhythmias is presented in Figures 56-12 and 56-13.

The most commonly used and safest antiarrhythmic agent for the treatment of fetal tachycardia remains digoxin, which is associated with a very low mortality per patient treated (Srinivarsan and Strasburger, 2008). Digoxin monotherapy is very effective for the treatment

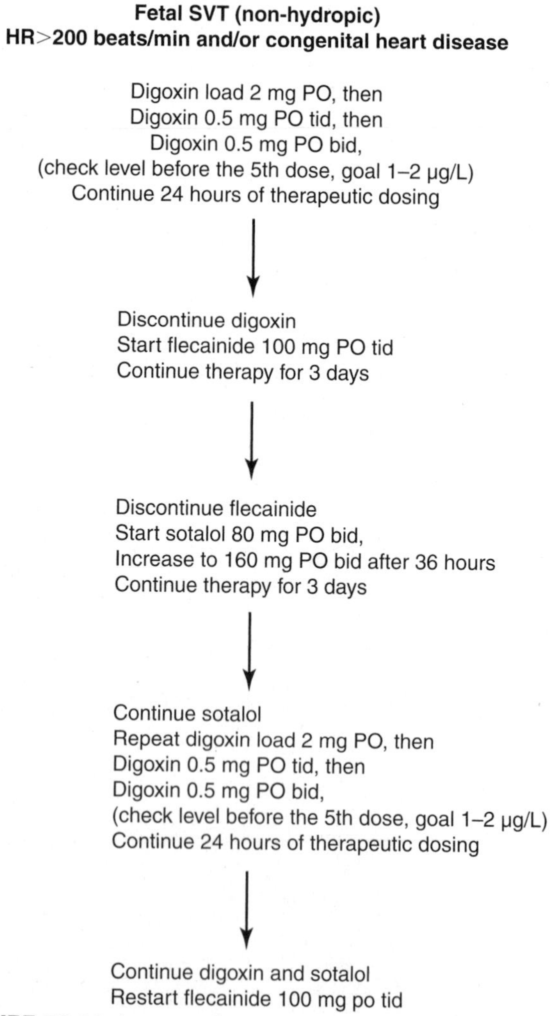

Fetal SVT (non-hydropic)
HR>200 beats/min and/or congenital heart disease

Digoxin load 2 mg PO, then
Digoxin 0.5 mg PO tid, then
Digoxin 0.5 mg PO bid,
(check level before the 5th dose, goal 1–2 µg/L)
Continue 24 hours of therapeutic dosing

↓

Discontinue digoxin
Start flecainide 100 mg PO tid
Continue therapy for 3 days

↓

Discontinue flecainide
Start sotalol 80 mg PO bid,
Increase to 160 mg PO bid after 36 hours
Continue therapy for 3 days

↓

Continue sotalol
Repeat digoxin load 2 mg PO, then
Digoxin 0.5 mg PO tid, then
Digoxin 0.5 mg PO bid,
(check level before the 5th dose, goal 1–2 µg/L)
Continue 24 hours of therapeutic dosing

↓

Continue digoxin and sotalol
Restart flecainide 100 mg po tid

FIGURE 56-12 A suggested management strategy for fetal tachycardia (nonhydropic) with escalation of management for non-responders. *SVT*, Supraventricular tachycardia.

of ORT and, to a lesser degree, AFL. Published series describe an efficacy of 62–100% in the absence of hydrops (Casey et al, 1997; Fouron et al, 2004; Krapp et al, 2003; Simpson and Sharland, 1998). Digoxin is administered to the mother orally or intravenously, depending on institutional preference. Before maternal administration, a maternal 12-lead ECG and cardiology consultation should be obtained to rule out high-risk factors such as preexcitation, or other cardiovascular disease. (This prescreening approach is important when considering any drug for transplacental therapy.) Maternal hypokalemia should also be excluded. Unfortunately, transplacental transfer of digoxin is significantly impaired in the setting of hydrops (Srinivasan and Strasburger, 2008) and efficacy decreases to approximately 25% for hydropic fetuses (Krapp et al, 2003). In this setting, combination therapy is usually required. Of note, some investigators prefer not to use digoxin for the control of fetal arrhythmias unless there is evidence of congestive heart failure because of the very small risk of atrial fibrillation with rapid antegrade conduction across an accessory pathway (Kleinman and Nehgme, 2004).

The most common second-line agent in the treatment of fetal tachycardia is flecainide, a class Ic antiarrhythmic with powerful sodium channel–blocking properties. Flecainide reaches higher concentrations in the placenta in the setting of hydrops fetalis than levels achieved with digoxin and results in cardioversion rate of around 60% of hydropic fetuses with SVT or flutter (Simpson and Sharland, 1998).

Fetal SVT with hydrops

Digoxin load 2 mg PO, then
Digoxin 0.5 mg PO tid, then
Digoxin 0.5 mg po bid,
(check level before the 5th dose, goal 1–2 μg/L)
Continue 24 hours of therapeutic dosing

+

Flecainide 100 mg PO tid
Continue therapy for 3 days

Discontinue digoxin and flecainide
Start sotalol 80 mg PO bid,
Increase to 160 mg PO bid after 36 hours
Continue therapy for 3 days

Continue sotalol
Restart flecainide
Continue therapy for 3 days

Hold flecainide and sotalol for 36 hours
Start amiodarone 150 mg PO bid

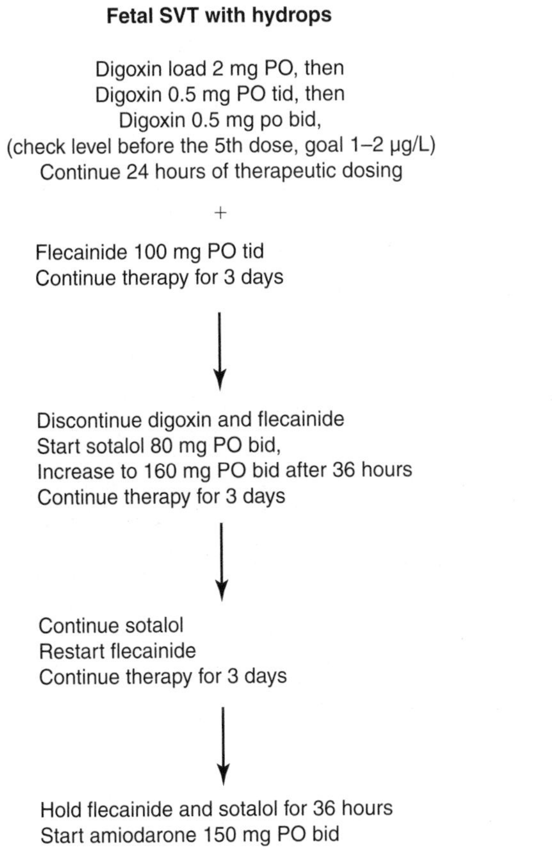

FIGURE 56-13 Suggested management scheme for the fetus with SVT and hydrops fetalis. Combination therapy is recommended up front, because digoxin monotherapy is often ineffective in this setting.

Before initiation of flecainide, the mother should be screened for evidence of structural or ischemic heart disease and a baseline ECG recorded. Renal and hepatic disease should be excluded. The QRS duration should be followed with a decrease in the dosage for >50% increase in duration, or more than 25% if the baseline QRS is >120 ms. Some institutions prefer not to use flecainide because of reports of potential proarrhythmic effects in the neonate (Allan et al, 1991; Fish et al, 1991).

Another second-line agent, sotalol, is the preferred drug at some institutions (Hornberger and Sahn, 2007). Sotalol is a class III antiarrhythmic with beta-blocking properties that has been shown to effectively alter conduction properties in fetal animal models (Houyel et al, 1992). In addition, placental transfer results in a maternal to fetal ratio of nearly 2:1. Maternal renal disease should be excluded before initiating therapy, because this is the major route of elimination, and the maternal ECG should be screened for evidence of QTc prolongation, which can be exacerbated by therapy. If follow-up ECGs demonstrate QTc prolongation >25% above baseline or >500 ms, the drug should be withheld.

One other drug used occasionally in the treatment of fetal tachycardias is amiodarone. Amiodarone has demonstrated safety and efficacy in the control of fetal arrhythmias, but has diminished transplacental transfer and is generally less efficacious. Some centers do not use it at all, whereas others may reserve use for cases in which other pharmacologic approaches have failed.

FETAL BRADYCARDIAS

The pathophysiology and natural history of fetal bradycardia have been discussed earlier. However, the echocardiographic evaluation of the fetus with AV block deserves special mention.

The echocardiographic evaluation of the fetus referred for congenital AV block is based on the search for dissociation of atrial and ventricular contractions with a slow ventricular "escape rhythm." Although scattered case reports and small series have suggested a progressive evolution from first- through third-degree heart block over time, a recent large multiinstitutional retrospective review was unable to demonstrate this pattern in affected fetuses, presumably because of the transient influence of vagal tone as a compounding factor, as well as rapid progression of findings in some cases (Friedman et al, 2008). When congenital AV block is present in a well-compensated fetus, the ejection fraction remains normal with an elevated end-diastolic volume and increased flow across the pulmonary and aortic valves. The cardiothoracic ratio can be determined echocardiographically and followed serially to detect cardiac enlargement and secondary evidence of cardiac decompensation (Paladini et al, 1990). More diffuse sequelae, such as moderate (or greater) tricuspid regurgitation, depressed ventricular systolic function, and atrial endocardial fibroelastosis, as identified in recent studies, are often thought to be secondary to an immune-mediated myocarditis (Friedman et al, 2008). Low fetal heart rate is a well-described risk factor, with values below 55 beats/min associated with increased rates of in utero demise (Schmidt et al, 1991).

FETAL BRADYCARDIA MANAGEMENT

Treatment of immune-mediated congenital AV block is largely empirical and based on fetal hemodynamic status. Although maternal steroid administration has been shown to improve fetal survival (Jaeggi et al, 2004) and even temporarily reverse complete AV block (Jaeggi et al, 2004), multiple adverse effects have been reported, including impairment of postnatal mental development, especially with fluorinated formulations such as dexamethasone (Baud et al, 1999, 2001) and oligohydramnios. Other potential therapies include beta-sympathomimetics (Groves et al, 1995), intravenous immunoglobulin, and plasmapheresis. However, plasmapheresis has generally been found to be ineffective (Buyon et al, 1987). A specific contraindication to beta-sympathomimetics includes congenital LQTS which notably can manifest with 2:1 block. Drug therapy of this type and in this setting can be catastrophic.

Management strategies include surveillance with serial echocardiograms to evaluate the progression of ventricular dysfunction. If decompensation is noted, maternal therapy with betamethasone can be initiated. Fetuses with low or dropping heart rates can be treated with maternal beta-sympathomimetics. Unfortunately, once hydrops fetalis has developed, this latter therapy has not been shown to improve outcomes (Schmidt et al, 1991). Delivery is reserved for cases in which concern for fetal loss is high or if a gestational age of 34–35 weeks has been achieved.

SUGGESTED READINGS

Batra A, Silka MJ: Ventricular arrhythmias, *Prog Pediatr Cardiol* 11:39-45, 2000.

Collins K, Van Hare GF: Advances in congenital long QT syndrome, *Curr Opin Pediatr* 18:497-502, 2006.

Cuneo BF, Strasburger JF: Management strategy for fetal tachycardia, *Obstet Gynecol* 96:575-581, 2000.

Epstein AE, DiMarco JP, Ellenbogen KA, et al: ACC/AHA/HRS 2008 guidelines for device-based therapy of cardiac rhythm abnormalities: A report of the American College of Cardiology/American Heart Association Task Force on Practice Guidelines (Writing committee to revise the ACC/AHA/NASPE 2002 Guideline update for implantation of cardiac pacemakers and antiarrhythmia devices): development in collaboration with the American Association for Thoracic Surgery and Society of Thoracic Surgeons, *Circulation* 117:e350-e408, 2008.

Friedman DM, Kim MY, Copel JA, et al: Utility of cardiac monitoring in fetuses at risk for congenital heart block: the PR interval and dexamethasone evaluation (PRIDE) prospective study, *Circulation* 117:485-493, 2008.

Goves AM, Allan LD, Rosenthal E: Therapeutic trial of sympathomimetics in three cases of complete heart block in the fetus, *Circulation* 1592:3394-3396, 1995.

Hornberger LK, Sahn DJ: Rhythm abnormalities of the fetus, *Heart* 93:1294-1300, 2007.

Jaeggi ET, Fouron JC, Silverman ED, et al: Transplacental fetal treatment improves the outcome of prenatally diagnosed complete atrioventricular block without structural heart disease, *Circulation* 110:1542-1548, 2004.

Kleinman CS, Nehgme RA: Cardiac arrhythmias in the human fetus, *Pediatr Cardiol* 25:234-251, 2004.

Ko JK, Deal BJ, Strasburger JF, Benson DW: Supraventricular tachycardia mechanisms and their age distribution in pediatric patients, *Am J Cardiol* 69:1028-1032, 1992.

Krapp M, Gembruch U, Baumann P: Venous blood flow pattern suggesting tachycardia-induced cardiomyopathy in the fetus, *Ultrasound Obstet Gynecol* 10:32-40, 1997.

Nii M, Hamilton RM, Fenwick L, et al: Assessment of fetal atrioventricular time intervals by tissue Doppler and pulse Doppler echocardiography: normal values and correlation with fetal electrocardiography, *Heart* 92:1831-1837, 2006.

Perry JC, Garson A Jr: Supraventricular tachycardia due to Wolff-Parkinson-White syndrome in children: early disappearance and late recurrence, *J Am Coll Cardiol* 16:1215-1520, 1990.

Schwartz PM, Stramba-Dadiale M, Segantini A, et al: Prolongation of the QT interval and the sudden death syndrome, *New Engl J Med* 338:1709-1714, 1998.

Complete references and supplemental color images used in this text can be found online at www.expertconsult.com

Neurodevelopmental Outcomes in Children with Congenital Heart Disease

Gil Wernovsky

Before the early 1980s, it was uncommon for children with complex congenital heart disease (CHD) to survive into later childhood. The nearly simultaneous advances in congenital cardiac surgery, echocardiography, and intensive care medicine were coupled with the availability of prostaglandins and the developing discipline of interventional cardiology. Together, these factors resulted in a dramatic fall in surgical mortality, with complex repairs taking place at increasingly younger ages. At many large centers, palliative surgery followed by later repair was replaced by primary repair in infancy, while staged reconstructive surgery for various forms of functionally univentricular heart, including those with hypoplastic left heart syndrome (HLHS) was improving with steadily falling rates of surgical mortality. As a result, the early part of the 21st century has seen an increasing number of children with complex CHD entering primary and secondary schooling. Research into their academic and behavioral outcomes has led to some sobering realizations about the outcomes in these children. For the purposes of this chapter, *complex CHD* refers to morphologic abnormalities significant enough to require surgical or catheter intervention as neonates or young infants.

SCOPE OF THE PROBLEM

An estimated 30,000 to 40,000 children are born in North America each year with CHD, and approximately one third require surgical intervention during the 1st year of life. CHD represents a spectrum of anomalies from relatively minor structural defects such as a bicuspid aortic valve or tiny ventricular septal defect through more complex conditions requiring surgical repair in early infancy, such as tetralogy of Fallot (TOF) or HLHS. For this group of children with complex CHD, approximately one half will develop some signs of neurodevelopmental disability as they mature. These typically are mild, but also typically occur in combination, and occasionally they are quite debilitating. Formal evaluations of preschool and school-aged children who were born with complex CHD demonstrate a pattern of neurodevelopmental sequelae that may appear alone or in combination. These include mild cognitive impairment; expressive speech and language abnormalities; impaired visual-spatial and visual-motor skills; attention-deficit/hyperactivity disorder (ADHD); motor delays; and learning disabilities.

The need for early intervention, rehabilitative services, and special education reduces the quality of life for these children and their families, as well as resulting in significant costs to society. As children progress through school, low scores in terms of academic achievement, learning disabilities, behavioral problems, difficulties with social

cognition, and ADHD may result in academic failure, development of poor skills both in the classroom and socially, low self-esteem, behavioral disinhibition, and ultimate delinquency. In view of these findings, there is active interest in better understanding the mechanisms of brain injury in these children, in order to design treatment trials and improve long-term outcomes for future patients. In addition, there is active interest in adapting techniques used to treat these disabilities in children without CHD to this growing population (Table 57-1).

MECHANISMS OF INJURY

Central nervous system (CNS) injury in children with CHD is a result of a complex interaction of patient-specific factors and environmental influences including, but not limited to, the effects of various interventions such as cardiac surgery. The risk of a poor developmental outcome varies according to the specific cardiac defect. In addition, there is significant interindividual variation in developmental outcome, even among children with the same cardiac defect. Cerebral ischemia before, during, and after the surgical repair of CHD has been proposed to be a primary mechanism of CNS injury. However, many factors may contribute to neurologic dysfunction. There is growing recognition that the brain is abnormal at birth in many neonates with complex CHD. These recent studies have identified a surprisingly high incidence of white matter injury, stroke, and hemorrhage, as well as brain immaturity such as an underdeveloped operculum (Licht et al, 2009; Mahle et al, 2002; Miller et al, 2007). These findings are due in part to abnormalities of fetal blood flow and substrate delivery leading to immaturity of the developing CNS (Donofrio et al, 2003; Kaltman et al, 2005; Limperopoulos et al, 2010) and in part due to congenital structural CNS abnormalities (Glauser et al, 1990; Mahle et al, 2002).

FETAL CEREBROVASCULAR PHYSIOLOGY AND OXYGEN DELIVERY

Ultrasound studies in the fetus have revealed that cerebral vascular resistance is altered in the presence of congenital cardiac disease. Fetuses with left-sided disease, for example, hypoplastic left heart syndrome, were shown to have decreased cerebral vascular resistance compared with normal fetuses (Donofrio et al, 2003; Kaltman et al, 2005). In patients with aortic atresia, the fetal cardiac output from the arterial duct must deliver flow cephalic to the brain as well as caudal to the low-resistance placenta. It is speculated that cerebral vascular resistance must therefore

TABLE 57-1   The Neurodevelopmental Challenges Seen in Children With Complex CHD

Age Group	Relevant Domains	Findings and Clinical Impact
Infants and toddlers (approximately 0–3 years)	Behavior and temperament	Negative in mood and difficult to soothe, particularly in infants with forms of single ventricle. High incidence of parental anxiety and clinical depression.
	Gross motor	Hypotonia and hypertonia both described. May have delayed rolling, sitting, crawling, walking, running, and stair skills. Likely less active than peers. Decreased prone skills.
	Fine motor	Delays affect abilities to reach toward objects. These include difficulty with grasp and exploration of toys with both hands, limited ability to operate levers or push buttons on toys, and decreased play skills, including stacking and container play. Decreased self-feeding skills and dressing skills.
	Oral motor	Poorly coordinated suck and swallow as infants.
	Language	Delays in expressive language more prevalent than receptive language. Reduced ability to imitate oral movements and speech sounds.
	Cognition	Difficult to assess in infants; standardized testing has limited predictive validity for later intelligence. Individual scores on the Mental Developmental Index of the Bayley Scales of Infant Development are typically in the normal range, although group mean values are frequently below average. Difficulties have been identified with object permanence, cause-effect, and attention to task.
	Visual-perceptual	Delays lead to decreased ability to target, reach toward toys and other objects. Decreased ability to stack and copy block designs and in prewriting skills such as tracing and copying simple shapes.
	Sensory processing	May have sensitivity to touch, position changes, different textures of toys/clothes, sounds, and bathing.
Preschool children (approximately 3–5 years)	Behavior and temperament	Increased incidence of internalizing (anxiety, depression) and externalizing (hyperactivity, impulsivity, disruptive) behaviors.
	Gross motor	Decreased coordination and balance may lead to "clumsiness" with ball skills, stairs, running, etc. May have difficulty keeping up with peers. Postural challenges and fatigue with tabletop activities.
	Fine motor	Decreased coordination with hands and quality of grasp, leading to challenges with school tasks, including the use of writing utensils, prewriting skills, scissor skills. Difficulties with activities of daily living skills including self-feeding, dressing and fasteners (Velcro, zippers, etc.) may be present.
	Language	Apraxia of speech, or difficulty with the motor planning of speech. Reduced intelligibility of connected speech.
	Cognition	Standardized testing typically at or slightly below average; cognitive delays are rarely significant.
	Visual-perceptual	Difficulties in identifying speed of moving objects, ball catching, tracking moving objects, and color differences, noting things as "similar" or "different." May have difficulties with coloring in lines, puzzles, and connect the dots.
	Sensory processing	May have sensitivity to certain materials used in activities of daily living, school and play tasks. May have decreased awareness of body in space. May seek out and/or avoid sensory input.
Children (approximately 5–12 years)	Behavior	Difficulty sustaining attention to tasks, regulating activity level and emotions. Increased incidence of internalizing (anxiety, depression) and externalizing (hyperactivity, impulsivity, disruptive) behaviors.
	Motor	Decreased balance and strength, as well as higher-level coordination skills. Also may have decreased ability to keep up with peers; may be the "last one chosen for sports activities." Decreased fine motor abilities affecting important school tasks such as handwriting skills, scissors ability, and activities of daily living such as shoe-tying, grooming, and self-care.
	Speech and language	Reduced intelligibility of connected speech. Delays in expressive language that may affect higher-level cognitive, memory and executive functioning. Apraxia of speech, or difficulty with the motor planning of speech. Simplistic story-telling. Echolalia and repetition of questions.
	Cognition	Individual scores on standardized IQ and achievement testing are frequently within normal limits, although group mean values lower than expected.
	Visual-perceptual and problem solving	Decreased handwriting skills, speed of note-taking, and ability to copy notes from board/book. Difficulties in checking work. Difficulty with word searches, hidden picture activities, and mazes.
	Executive function and working memory	Difficulty following multistep instructions, organizing materials, and sequencing tasks. Slower processing of incoming information and written output.
	Personal/social	Deficits in adaptive functioning (activities, social relationships, school performance).

TABLE 57-1 The Neurodevelopmental Challenges Seen in Children With Complex CHD—cont'd

Age Group	Relevant Domains	Findings and Clinical Impact
Adolescents and young adults (>12 years)	Sensory processing	May have sensitivity to certain materials used in activities of daily living, school, and play tasks. May have decreased awareness of body in space. May seek out and/or avoid sensory input.
	Behavior	Increased incidence of internalizing (anxiety, depression) and externalizing (hyperactivity, impulsivity, disruptive) behaviors.
	Motor	If easily fatigued and/or decreased strength, may self-limit and choose activities that do not require physical activity. Decreased handwriting skills. Decreased speed of note taking.
	Speech and language	An early history of speech and language delay or disorders will likely affect higher-level cognitive and executive functioning skills.
	Cognition	Individual scores on standardized IQ and achievement testing are frequently within normal limits, although group mean values lower than expected. Increased prevalence of aptitude-achievement discrepancies.
	Visual-perceptual and problem solving	Decreased speed of note-taking from board/book. Decreased ability to read complex graphs/diagrams. Implicated in difficulties in mathematics.
	Executive function and working memory	Difficulty following multistep instructions, organizing materials, and sequencing tasks. Slower processing of incoming information and written output. Limitations to logical hypothesis generation and testing and to applying principles to solve problems.
	Higher-order theory of mind	Weaknesses in higher order "theory of mind," such as social cognition (understanding what another may be thinking or feeling), empathy, cognitive flexibility, and planning.
	Personal/social	Alexithymia (inability to express feelings with words). Difficulty identifying and describing internal state. Strained interpersonal relationships.

Approximately 50% of children with complex CHD have one or more of these domains affected. This has been termed *high prevalence–low severity* disability. However, although many of these findings are mild individually, in combination they may significantly impair school performance and employment opportunities in adulthood.

be lower than normal to allow adequate blood flow to the developing brain. Fetuses with right-sided obstructive lesions, for example, TOF, were also shown to have increased fetal cerebral vascular resistance (Kaltman et al, 2005). In these children, it is speculated that the obstruction to flow into the pulmonary arteries changes the usual delivery from the patent arterial duct caudal to the placenta. In these cases, the left ventricle must contribute to placental blood flow antegrade from the ascending aorta, with a resultant increase in cerebral vascular resistance. The impact of these alterations in fetal cerebral vascular resistance is unclear, but they almost certainly play a role in subsequent neurologic development.

In the normal fetus, the intracirculatory patterns created by the normal fetal connections result in preferential streaming of the most highly oxygenated fetal blood to the developing brain, and the most desaturated blood to the placenta. When significant structural disease exists within the heart, these beneficial patterns are likely to be altered. Although not yet confirmed by fetal magnetic resonance spectroscopy, fetuses with transposition are likely to have the blood with the lowest saturation of oxygen returning to the ascending aorta and brain, while blood with the highest saturation returns to the abdominal organs and placenta. Speculation on the consequences of the transposed fetal circulation as an explanation for the high incidence of macrosomia in these infants dates back almost 50 years (Naeye, 1966), and this pathomechanism has also been offered as an explanation for the increased incidence of relative microcephaly seen in transposition. Complete mixing, as

seen in fetuses with functionally univentricular hearts, fetal will produce intermediate values of cerebral saturation of oxygen, but lower than those seen in the normal fetus.

It has long been recognized that the neurologic status of newborns with CHD is frequently abnormal before open heart surgery. Gillon (1973) reported neurologic abnormalities including tone abnormalities, abnormal posturing, weak cry, and poor coordination of suck, swallow, and breathing in many infants before open heart surgery. After birth, cerebral blood flow has been shown to be significantly lower than normal in some patients, because of low cardiac output or a low diastolic blood pressure ("steal") secondary to an open ductus arteriosus (Licht et al, 2004). In some lesions, such as total anomalous pulmonary venous return with obstruction and transposition of the great arteries (TGA) for later profound hypoxemia and acidosis may result immediately after birth secondary to the uncorrected CHD. Certain procedures, such as balloon atrial septostomy, have been linked to an increased risk of stroke by some authors (McQuillen et al, 2006; Mukherjee, 2010) but not others (Applegate and Lim, 2010; Petit et al, 2009). Genetic syndromes, present in a significant proportion of children with complex CHD, play a role in abnormalities of brain structure as well as developmental delays (Andelfinger, 2008). A study from Montreal Children's Hospital evaluated 56 consecutive neonates referred for open-heart surgery (Limperopoulos et al, 1999). Neurobehavioral and neurologic abnormalities, including hypotonia, hypertonia, jitteriness, motor asymmetries, and absence of suck reflex, were noted in more than 50% of patients before surgery. Preoperative seizures were present in three patients; 35% were microcephalic, and 12.5% were macrocephalic. Finally, all patients with a right-to-left shunt have the potential for air or particulate emboli to reach the brain from intravenous catheters, whether before or after surgery.

Hypoxemia, low cardiac output, and cardiac arrest in patients with uncorrected CHD may result in CNS ischemia and injury. Aisenberg et al (1982) evaluated mental and motor development in 173 infants with uncorrected CHD. Developmental delay was present in 25% and was apparent as early as 2 months of age. Congestive heart failure and hypoxemia were risk factors for developmental delay. Kurth et al (2001), from The Children's Hospital of Philadelphia, used near infrared spectroscopy (NIRS) to evaluate cerebral oxygenation in 93 infants with heart defects before surgery. Decreased cerebral oxygenation was present in many patients, particularly infants with TOF and those with HLHS or other single-ventricle physiology. Very low cerebral oxygen saturations (<38%) were found in 13 patients, suggesting that patients with CHD are at risk for cerebral ischemia and CNS injury in the preoperative period (Box 57-1).

MICROCEPHALY

Head circumference at birth is a surrogate for growth of the brain, and in neonates without congenital cardiac disease, microcephaly is independently associated with later developmental delays and academic difficulties. The incidence of microcephaly at birth is increased in children with complex CHD, approaching a rate of 25% in some reports (Hinton et al, 2008; Mahle et al, 2002; Miller et al, 2007; Shillingford et al, 2007), and persists into later infancy. Although the causes are speculative, and most certainly multifactorial, a recent report in children with HLHS, in whom the median head circumference was at only the 18th percentile, revealed that patients with microcephaly had significantly smaller ascending aortas than those without, suggesting that reduced flow to the brain from the left ventricle secondary to anatomic hypoplasia of the ascending aorta may result in diminished brain growth (Shillingford et al, 2007).

THE OPEN OPERCULUM

The opercular region is that covering the so-called insula and is made up of frontal, temporal, and parietal cortical convolutions. In magnetic resonance and computed tomography imaging studies of neonates with complex CHD, underdevelopment of the operculum may be seen in nearly one quarter of the patients and is a marker for functional immaturity of the brain. This may be a unilateral or bilateral finding and has been termed underoperculinization, or an open operculum. The operculum is thought to be related to oral motor coordination, taste, and speech, particularly to expressive language. In adults who experience a stroke in this area of the brain, the so-called Foix-Chavany-Marie syndrome, deficits include impairment of voluntary movements such as chewing and deglutition, dysarthria, and problems with taste. In macaque monkeys, receptive fields on the tongue, lips, and palate have been mapped to the operculum. Given the high prevalence of problems with feeding, delay with expressive language, and oral-motor apraxia in children with complex cardiac malformations, as well as the increasing recognition of a high prevalence of an open operculum, one can speculate that some patients with these oral-motor developmental disabilities may have a structural underdevelopment of the operculum. Studies are currently under way to test this hypothesis.

PERIVENTRICULAR LEUKOMALACIA

Injury to the white matter, a common finding in premature infants, has been increasingly recognized in full-term neonates with complex CHD. It has been suggested that decreased blood flow to the brain preoperatively is significantly associated with lesions in the white matter, affecting slightly more than one quarter of neonates before surgery (Mahle et al, 2002). Periventricular leukomalacia was also found in slightly more than half of a cohort of patients who underwent surgery for complex CHD, but was rarely detected in those who underwent surgery between 1 and 6 months of age (Galli et al, 2004). Magnetic resonance imaging has shown not only a high incidence of injury to the white matter but also evidence of immature brain metabolism and microstructure, which are strikingly similar to findings seen in the premature population.

Periventricular leukomalacia is believed to arise from several factors, including the high susceptibility of the immature oligodendrocyte to hypoxic ischemic injury, as well as the watershed distribution of flow of blood to this area between the small arteries that penetrate from the cortex and those that arise centrally and run radially outward. This watershed area is particularly prone to ischemia during decreases in cerebral perfusion pressure. In premature infants, severe degrees of periventricular leukomalacia have been associated with cerebral palsy, whereas mild degrees of injury have been associated with developmental delay, motor difficulties, and behavioral disorders—a developmental "phenotype" remarkably similar to that of school-age children with complex CHD.

THE EFFECT ON THE BRAIN OF CARDIAC SURGERY

Even though there is increasing evidence for congenital and acquired CNS injury in children with CHD before surgery, many investigators still focus on intraoperative management as the primary mechanism of CNS injury. As

---

BOX 57-1   Patient-Specific Risk Factors for Neurodevelopmental Delays in CHD

- Congenital central nervous system abnormalities
- Genetic syndromes
- Genetic susceptibility to cerebral ischemia-reperfusion injury
- Underlying cardiac diagnosis
- Additional congenital anomalies
- Lower birthweight (prematurity and/or intrauterine growth restriction)

opposed to all of the risk factors for abnormal neurologic development discussed thus far, variation in intraoperative support, such as the conduct of cardiopulmonary bypass, is one of the few modifiable risk factors that can be altered to improve long-term neurologic outcomes. Multiple factors may contribute to CNS injury during surgical repair, including hypoxemia, cerebral hypoperfusion, and cerebral embolism (particulate and/or air). Factors that possibly contribute to intraoperative neurologic injury include the type of support during surgery (deep hypothermic circulatory arrest [DHCA] or continuous cardiopulmonary bypass [CPB]), use of hemodilution, the degree of cooling, use of steroids, and type of blood gas management.

Use of CPB exposes the blood to foreign surfaces of the bypass circuit, initiating a systemic inflammatory response characterized by neutrophil activation, complement activation, and increased circulating levels of inflammatory cytokines (du Plessis, 1999). This inflammatory response may result in increased capillary permeability, tissue edema, and organ dysfunction. When continuous CPB is used, perfusion to the body and brain is maintained. When DHCA is used, there is a period of obligate global cerebral ischemia followed by reperfusion. Use of DHCA provides a bloodless surgical field, facilitating meticulous completion of the repair, and decreases the duration of blood exposure to the bypass circuit, but at the cost of a period of global cerebral ischemia. Continuous CPB maintains perfusion to the brain and body but increases the duration of blood exposure to the bypass circuit, which may increase the severity of inflammatory response. Use of continuous CPB avoids the period of cerebral ischemia but results in a greater increase in total body water and more severe dysfunction of other organs, such as the lungs (Skaryak et al, 1996; Wernovsky et al, 1995). These multiple facets of CPB have received considerable attention and have

been the subject of active research. Of the many potential modifiable technical features of cardiopulmonary bypass (Box 57-2), there are three that have been most extensively studied, particularly with randomized clinical trials.

pH MANAGEMENT

In one very important trial at Children's Hospital, Boston (du Plessis et al, 1997), developmental and neurologic outcomes were evaluated in infants undergoing biventricular repair of a variety of cardiac defects at less than 9 months of age who were randomized to either alpha-stat or pH-stat management during deep hypothermic cardiopulmonary bypass. Although there were some benefits reported with the use of pH-stat management for outcomes in the immediate perioperative period, the use of either strategy was not consistently related to either improved or impaired neurodevelopmental outcomes at 1 to 4 years of age (Bellinger et al, 2001). On the Bayley Scales of Infant Development, there was no effect of treatment on the Psychomotor Development Index (PDI). The Mental Development Index (MDI), in contrast, varied significantly depending on the underlying anatomic diagnosis. For patients with transposition and TOF, use of pH-stat resulted in a slightly higher mental developmental index, although the difference was not statistically significant. In patients with a ventricular septal defect, the effect was opposite, with use of alpha-stat management resulting in significantly improved scores. There was a significant effect of cardiac diagnosis on outcomes. Both scores of the Bayley examinations were significantly higher in those with transposition than in those with the other cardiac defects. Despite the equivocal data in this early report, with no longer-term follow-up yet available, many centers are currently using pH-stat management exclusively in all operations on neonates and infants. Further research in this area, based on additional potential modifiers, for example, cardiac diagnosis, age, and severity of preoperative hypoxemia, should continue.

HEMATOCRIT DURING BYPASS

During cardiopulmonary bypass, hemodilution has been widely applied based on the notion that increased viscosity would be detrimental during periods of profound or even moderate hypothermia. Results in animals suggesting that higher hematocrit levels resulted in better cerebral protection were recently investigated in two randomized clinical trials (Jonas et al, 2003; Newburger et al, 2008). The results of these trials indicated that hematocrit levels during bypass below 24% were associated with lower scores in the PDI of the Bayley Scales of Infant Development, although the improvement was not seen at hematocrit levels of 35% versus 25%. In addition, lower hematocrit levels were associated with a more positive fluid balance after surgery and higher serum lactate levels.

DEEP HYPOTHERMIC CIRCULATORY ARREST

Much has been written on the potentially deleterious effects of prolonged circulatory arrest with profound hypothermia in cardiac surgery for neonates and infants. It

---

BOX 57-2   Procedural and Environmental Risk Factors for Neurodevelopmental Delays in CHD

PREOPERATIVE
  Cardiac arrest
  Low cardiac output
  Profound hypoxemia

OPERATIVE
  Longer duration of cardiopulmonary bypass
  Longer duration of deep hypothermic circulatory arrest
  Air or particulate embolization

POSTOPERATIVE
  Hypoxemia
  Hypotension
  Low cardiac output
  Cardiac arrest
  Postoperative seizures
  Air or particulate embolization
  Longer length of hospital stay

OTHER
  Chronic (preoperative/postoperative) hypoxemia
  Lower socioeconomic status
  Higher parental stress

is generally agreed that very prolonged periods of uninterrupted circulatory arrest may have adverse neurologic outcomes. Close inspection of the data shows that the effects of short durations of circulatory arrest are inconsistently related to adverse outcomes, and that the effect of circulatory arrest is not a linear phenomenon. The effects are most likely modified by other preoperative and postoperative factors related to the patient. Some reports, most in an earlier era of cardiac surgery, demonstrate a detrimental effect of circulatory arrest on a variety of outcomes relating to the CNS whereas some demonstrate either an inconsistent effect or no effect. Some have taken the stance that, because a majority of studies suggest a negative effect of circulatory arrest, it should be avoided at all costs. Innovative and challenging strategies have been designed to provide continuous cerebral perfusion during reconstruction of the aortic arch or intracardiac repair. The avoidance of circulatory arrest, however, by necessity requires an increased duration of CPB. This has consistently been shown to have an adverse effect on outcomes in both the short and longer term. A randomized trial comparing circulatory arrest to continuous cerebral perfusion has recently been completed at the University of Michigan (Goldberg et al, 2007). This demonstrated no improvement in developmental scores at 1 year of age. Similar findings were reported in a contemporaneous but nonrandomized study at Children's Hospital of Boston (Visconti et al, 2006). It seems imprudent to change practice based on studies with only short-term developmental assessment. Developmental studies in infants have very limited predictive validity for long-term outcomes, for patients with or without CHD.

Perhaps the best conducted study in this regard, which emphasizes this point, is the Boston Circulatory Arrest Study (Bellinger, 2008; Bellinger et al, 1997, 1999, 2003, 2009; Helmers et al, 1997; Newburger et al, 1993; Rappaport et al, 1998; Wernovsky et al, 1995; Wypij et al, 2003). In this study, a cohort of children with transposition undergoing an arterial switch were randomly assigned to intraoperative support predominantly by DHCA or predominantly by CBP at low flow. Earlier reports suggested that the group as a whole was performing below expectations in many aspects of evaluation, with worse outcomes for those undergoing circulatory arrest in the areas of postoperative seizures and motor skills at 1 year of age, as well as behavior, speech, and language at the age of 4 years. Mean intelligence quotient at the age of 4 was lower than expected, at 93, with no difference according to assignment. Many centers began avoiding even short periods of circulatory arrest based on these and other reports. In 2003, assessments of quality of life and detailed standardized testing were reported. Neurodevelopmental analyses when the patients were aged 8 years revealed that the intelligence quotients for the cohort as a whole were then closer to normal, at 98 versus the population mean of 100. The patients did demonstrate significant deficits in visual-spatial and visual-memory skills, as well as in components of executive functioning such as working memory, hypothesis generation, sustained attention, and higher-order language skills. In other words, the children had difficulty coordinating skills to perform complex operations. Those repaired using circulatory arrest scored worse on motor and speech functioning, whereas those undergoing bypass at low flow demonstrated worse scores for impulsivity and behavior. When compared with a normative sample, parents of the entire cohort reported significantly higher frequencies of attention problems, developmental delay, and problems with learning and speech. More than one third of the population required remedial services at school, and 1 in 10 had repeated a grade. Thus, in this population of patients who underwent the arterial switch operation between 1988 and 1992, there appears to be a correlation between congenital CHD and its surgical repair, with difficulties occurring later with speech and language, behavioral difficulties, and execution planning in childhood. Whether current modifications of techniques will improve the outcomes in the long term remains the subject of ongoing study. This well-designed trial, with superb follow-up, enrolled neonates for whom the management plan included an arterial switch operation between 1988 and 1992. Hence, the results reflect the perioperative and surgical care delivered in that era, and thus may not be generalizable to the current era, or to other congenital cardiac lesions. For example, some features of routine postoperative care in that era, including extension of the anesthetic period for at least 48 hours, active rewarming in the intensive care unit after surgery, and hyperventilation to reduce the risk of pulmonary hypertension, may each independently and adversely affect neurodevelopmental outcomes. In addition, those patients randomized to receive predominantly continuous bypass also underwent a relatively brief period of circulatory arrest. Thus, the study does not compare use of circulatory arrest to no circulatory arrest. The results nonetheless serve to show the multiple factors that influence developmental outcome at school age and show that factors related to poorer outcome, such as use of DHCA, which seem apparent and significant on early testing, may be attenuated or even abolished during longer-term follow-up, as other factors assume a more important role.

POSTOPERATIVE FACTORS

CNS injury may occur or be exacerbated in the postoperative period. Most studies have focused on the operating room as the site of CNS injury; however, events in the cardiac intensive care unit may be equally important. Cerebral ischemia can result from low cardiac output or severe hypoxemia. Postoperative hyperthermia may increase the metabolic needs of the brain, resulting in worsening CNS injury (Shum-Tim et al, 1998). In addition, postoperative cardiac arrest may result in significant CNS injury. After cardiac surgery with CPB with or without DHCA, cerebral autoregulation may be impaired (Bassan et al, 2005). After surgery, especially in neonates and infants, there is a predictable and reproducible fall in cardiac output (Wernovsky et al, 1995). This period of decreased oxygen delivery, usually within the first 24 hours after surgery, represents a particularly vulnerable time for the CNS, especially if associated with increased oxygen consumption (as with fever, pain, seizures, or agitation). At present, studies linking postoperative hemodynamic lability to long-term CNS outcomes are lacking. However, postoperative hypotension has been shown to be related to new or worsened white matter injury (Galli et al, 2004), especially if combined with hyperventilation (Samanta et al, 2009), which may further reduce cerebral blood flow. Finally, there are a growing number of reports that an increased length of stay in the hospital, and in the intensive care unit in particular, is associated with worse long-term outcomes, and this association is *independent* of the reasons for the prolonged length of stay, such as sepsis or low cardiac output (Fuller et al, 2009; Mahle et al, 2006; Matsuzaki et al, 2010; Newburger et al, 2003).

Thus, it may be very difficult to completely define the etiologic factors leading to CNS injury in individual patients with CHD. The neurologic sequelae of cardiac surgery can be subtle in very young infants. The full extent of an injury is often not fully recognized until long after the event, when certain cognitive and higher executive skills are required. Neurologic examination of neonates and infants is limited, and developmental testing, even at 1 year of age, has imprecise predictive value for long-term neurodevelopmental outcomes. Investigators have evaluated potential surrogate measures such as electroencephalographic monitoring and magnetic resonance imaging of the brain. However, the predictive value of these tests in isolation for long-term neurodevelopmental outcome is uncertain. Examination of preschool- and school-aged children provides greater sensitivity and specificity in determination of neurologic defects and remains the standard for evaluation of the neurologic sequelae of infant cardiac surgery.

GENETIC SUSCEPTIBILITY TO NEUROLOGIC INJURY AND DEVELOPMENTAL DYSFUNCTION

All of the foregoing risk factors do not fully explain either the high frequency or the pattern of neurodevelopmental dysfunction described in children with complex CHD, suggesting that other patient-specific factors may be important determinants of neurologic injury. Intellectual development and cognitive function are highly heritable and probably are dependent on multiple genes, as well as on environmental factors. Numerous inherited defects or syndromes that are associated with compromised mental development and intellectual capacity (e.g., Down syndrome, Williams syndrome, DiGeorge syndrome) may have CHD as one of the phenotypic outcomes. Although the genetic basis for most cardiac defects has not been delineated, specific genetic anomalies have been implicated in the pathogenesis of some defects. For example, microdeletions of chromosome 22 are associated with DiGeorge syndrome and a variety of heart defects, including TOF, truncus arteriosus, and interruption of the aortic arch. Developmental abnormalities are present in children with 22q11 microdeletions, even those with no cardiac abnormalities (Gerdes et al, 1999). Thus, children with cardiac defects and 22q11 microdeletions may be developmentally impaired independent of the cardiac defect and cardiac surgery. It may be difficult to separate the adverse developmental sequelae of an underlying genetic anomaly from those related to CHD and cardiac surgery.

Risk of disease or injury in response to an environmental stimulus is a complex interaction between genetic susceptibility and environmental exposures. Interindividual variation in disease risk and in the response to environmental factors is significant. The risk may be modified by age, gender, ethnicity, and the extent of exposure to environmental factors. Multiple genes are involved in determining an individual's response to a specific environmental factor. Interindividual variation in response to environmental exposures, such as cardiac surgery, probably is due in part to genetic polymorphisms. Common genetic variants, often due to single-nucleotide substitutions, occur with a frequency of greater than 1%. For a child with CHD, environmental factors include cardiac surgery, use of DHCA, need for repeated operations, and socioeconomic status. The role of genetic polymorphisms in determining susceptibility to CNS injury in children with CHD is not known.

Recent studies suggest that polymorphisms of apolipoprotein E may be predictors of adverse neurodevelopmental sequelae after infant cardiac surgery (Burnham et al, 2010; Fuller et al, 2009; Gaynor et al, 2003, 2009), as has been similarly reported in adults (Newman, 1995; Steed et al, 2001; Robson et al, 2002). It is likely that multiple genes modulate the CNS response to CPB, DHCA, and other environmental factors modifying the risk and pattern of injury (Ozbek et al, 2005).

The underlying cardiac diagnosis may have a significant and independent impact on neurodevelopmental outcome and may modulate the effects of neuroprotective strategies. Presence of a ventricular septal defect (VSD) in patients with transposition of the great arteries is a significant risk factor for poor developmental outcome (Bellinger et al, 1995, 1999; Newburger et al, 1993). In the pH study mentioned previously, developmental and neurologic outcomes were evaluated in infants undergoing repair of a variety of cardiac defects before the age of 9 months who were randomized to either alpha-stat or pH-stat blood gas management strategy during deep hypothermic CPB (Bellinger et al, 2001). Children with transposition (TGA) with or without VSD, TOF, isolated VSD, atrioventricular canal defect, truncus arteriosus, and total anomalous pulmonary venous return were enrolled. There was no effect of treatment group on the PDI score of the Bayley Scales of Infant Development. The MDI score, however, varied significantly depending on treatment group and diagnosis. For patients with TGA and TOF, use of pH-stat resulted in a slightly higher MDI, although the difference was not statistically significant. Of interest, in the VSD subgroup, the treatment effect was opposite with use of alpha-stat management, resulting in significantly improved scores. Cardiac diagnosis had a significant effect on outcomes: PDI and MDI scores were significantly higher in the TGA group compared with those noted for the other cardiac defects. A study at The Children's Hospital of Philadelphia evaluated the neuroprotective effect of allopurinol, a scavenger and inhibitor of oxygen free radical production, during infant cardiac surgery using DHCA (Clancy et al, 2001). A total of 318 infants (131 with HLHS) underwent surgery. Allopurinol provided significant neuroprotection only in patients with HLHS; no benefit was found in the non-HLHS patients.

HYPOPLASTIC LEFT HEART SYNDROME

Previous studies have suggested that developmental outcome is worst for patients with complex cardiac defects, such as HLHS, who require multiple operations during infancy and early childhood (Wernovsky et al, 2000). Rogers et al (1995) at the Children's Hospital of Buffalo evaluated 11 survivors of staged repair for HLHS at a mean age of 38 months. Seven children (64%) had major developmental disabilities and were considered to be mentally retarded. Two had severe cerebral palsy. Gross motor delays were present in 5 children (45%). At follow-up, microcephaly was present in 8 children (73%) and correlated with cognitive delay. More recent studies, however, suggest that developmental outcomes for these children have improved. Kern et al (1998) at Columbia-Presbyterian Medical Center evaluated early neurodevelopmental outcome after stage I reconstruction for HLHS. Twelve patients who had undergone the Norwood procedure and subsequent surgery were evaluated along with a control group of children including siblings and first cousins. DHCA was used for the stage I reconstruction, with a mean duration of 56 minutes. The median scores for Full-Scale IQ were in the lower range of normal. Although scores for control subjects were generally higher than for patients, the differences between the two groups in intelligence testing did not reach statistical significance. The only statistically significant difference was in adaptive behavior, with the controls scoring higher. There was no correlation between neurologic outcome and bypass time, age at surgery, number of operations, or age at testing. Longer duration of DHCA was a risk factor for lower Full-Scale IQ.

Eke et al (1996) from Loma Linda evaluated the neurologic sequelae of DHCA in patients undergoing neonatal cardiac transplantation. The majority of these patients had HLHS. Developmental outcomes were evaluated using the Bayley Scales of Infant Development. There was no correlation between the duration of DHCA and neurodevelopmental outcome. Mahle et al (2000) at The Children's Hospital of Philadelphia evaluated neurodevelopmental outcomes in school-aged survivors of reconstructive surgery for HLHS. A majority of patients had IQ scores within the normal range; however, mean performance for the study group was lower than population norms. In a multivariable analysis, only the occurrence of a preoperative seizure predicted lower Full-Scale IQ. Duration of DHCA was not a predictor of lower IQ, although this lack of correlation may be due to the narrow spread of DHCA time in the study cohort. Scores on achievement tests (mathematics and reading) were lower than expected for the normal population. Nearly two thirds of the cohort had a clinical diagnosis of ADHD.

In another, more recent cohort, cognitive outcomes in school-age children with HLHS were assessed with the Wechsler Preschool and Primary Scale of Intelligence-Revised (Goldberg et al, 2000). Mean scores for the entire cohort were within the normal range for Full-Scale IQ, Verbal IQ, and Performance IQ. Scores for patients with HLHS were lower than for patients with other defects but were not significantly different from scores for the standard population. Use of DHCA was associated with lower scores. Because of the significant mortality previously associated with staged reconstructive surgery for HLHS, most of these studies evaluated relatively small numbers of young patients. In addition, these studies provide conflicting evidence concerning the significance of DHCA as a risk factor for adverse neurodevelopmental outcomes.

It is of interest to examine the developmental abnormalities seen in children with HLHS who underwent staged surgical reconstruction (Norwood, Glenn, and Fontan procedures) and compare them to the findings after transplantation for the same disease (Mahle et al, 2006). The patterns of dysfunction are remarkably similar, despite the markedly different therapeutic strategies. This similarity suggests that factors other than the surgical approach and intraoperative support, such as congenital CNS disease and the abnormal fetal physiology, may play a more significant role in long-term outcome for these children. Of importance, outcomes for these complex patients have improved in recent years in terms of both mortality and neurodevelopmental outcome. A recently completed randomized trial of surgical strategies for HLHS has reported data on early mortality (Ohye et al, 2010); long-term neurodevelopmental outcomes are being measured during longitudinal follow-up and are likely to represent the largest and most comprehensive study performed in children with HLHS.

FUNCTIONAL STATUS AFTER REPAIR OF COMPLEX CONGENITAL HEART DISEASE

Most studies have focused on delineating cognitive impairments in children who have undergone repair of CHD; however, the impact on the child's functional status and on the child's caregivers has not been as carefully investigated. Recently, parental stress was assessed early after surgery for complex CHD (Torowicz et al, 2010). The demands of care for infants with CHD were a significant source of parental stress compared with those in control parents, especially related to feeding and medication burden. In addition, infants with single-ventricle palliation were more negative in mood and less distractible than those children who underwent biventricular repair. In childhood, developmental delay after cardiac surgery can impair a child's functional status, resulting in a considerable burden for family and caregiver. Limperopoulos et al (2001) from Montreal Children's Hospital evaluated functional limitations and burden of care in 131 infants after surgical repair of CHD, using the WeeFIM (Functional Independence Measure), a pediatric functional assessment designed to assess and track levels of functional independence, and the Vineland Adaptive Behavior Scale. Only 21% of the patients were functioning within their appropriate age range. Moderate disability was noted in 37% and severe disability in 6%. Functional difficulties in daily living skills were documented in 40% of the patients, and greater than 50% had poor socialization skills. Factors that increased the risk of functional disabilities included microcephaly, longer duration of DHCA, longer length of stay in the intensive care unit, and lower level of maternal education. Finally, essentially all studies conducted in school-aged children suggest that between 25% and 40% of school-aged children will require remedial help in school.

SUMMARY

Although children with mild types of CHD appear to have normal CNS and neurodevelopmental outcomes (Quartermain et al, 2010; van der Rijken et al, 2008), children with complex CHD constitute an at-risk population with a significant incidence of adverse developmental outcomes. Current techniques for developmental evaluation in neonates and infants are imprecise predictors of late outcomes. Evaluation of preschool- and school-aged children reveals a pattern of neurodevelopmental dysfunction characterized by mild cognitive impairment, motor dysfunction, impaired visual-spatial and visual-motor skills, and attention and academic difficulties in about one-half of the children. There are significant problems with expressive speech and language and a high incidence of learning disabilities.

The factors resulting in CNS injury and developmental dysfunction in these children are not completely understood. Developmental dysfunction results from a complex interaction between patient-specific factors (genetic susceptibility, cardiac diagnosis) and environmental factors (preoperative events; techniques of support during surgical repair, including the use of DHCA; postoperative events; socioeconomic status). Currently, reported risk factors do not adequately explain the pattern or incidence of CNS injury after cardiac surgery in infants, suggesting that other patient-specific factors may modulate the response to CHD and cardiac surgery, increasing the risk of adverse neurodevelopmental sequelae. Children with CHD are at risk for cerebral ischemia before, during, and after cardiac surgery; therefore, factors, that impair CNS recovery after ischemia may be important determinants of long-term neurologic outcome.

SUGGESTED READINGS

Bellinger DC: Are children with congenital cardiac malformations at increased risk of deficits in social cognition? *Cardiol Young* 18:3-9, 2008.

Bellinger DC, Wypij D, du Plessis AJ, et al: Developmental and neurologic effects of alpha-stat versus pH-stat strategies for deep hypothermic cardiopulmonary bypass in infants, *J Thorac Cardiovasc Surg* 121:374-383, 2001.

Fuller S, Nord AS, Gerdes M, et al: Predictors of impaired neurodevelopmental outcomes at one year of age after infant cardiac surgery, *Eur J Cardiothorac Surg* 36:40-47, 2009.

Gaynor JW, Gerdes M, Zackai EH, et al: Apolipoprotein E genotype and neurodevelopmental sequelae of infant cardiac surgery, *J Thorac Cardiovasc Surg* 126:1736-1745, 2003.

Goldberg CS, Bove EL, Devaney EJ, et al: A randomized clinical trial of regional cerebral perfusion versus deep hypothermic circulatory arrest: outcomes for infants with functional single ventricle, *J Thorac Cardiovasc Surg* 133:880-887, 2007.

Licht DJ, Clancy RR, Shera DM, et al: Brain maturation is delayed in infants with complex congenital heart defects, *J Thorac Cardiovasc Surg* 137:529-536, 2009: discussion 536-527.

Licht DJ, Wang J, Silvestre DW, et al: Preoperative cerebral blood flow is diminished in neonates with severe congenital heart defects, *J Thorac Cardiovasc Surg* 128:841-849, 2004.

McQuillen PS, Hamrick SE, Perez MJ, et al: Balloon atrial septostomy is associated with preoperative stroke in neonates with transposition of the great arteries, *Circulation* 113:280-285, 2006.

Newburger JW, Jonas RA, Wernovsky G, et al: A comparison of the perioperative neurologic effects of hypothermic circulatory arrest versus low-flow cardiopulmonary bypass in infant heart surgery, *N Engl J Med* 329:1057-1064, 1993.

Newburger JW, Wypij D, Bellinger DC, et al: Length of stay after infant heart surgery is related to cognitive outcome at age 8 years, *J Pediatr* 143:67-73, 2003.

Wernovsky G, Stiles KM, Gauvreau K, et al: Cognitive development after the Fontan operation, *Circulation* 102:883-889, 2000.

Complete references used in this text can be found online at www.expertconsult.com

PART XII

NEUROLOGIC SYSTEM

DEVELOPMENTAL PHYSIOLOGY OF THE CENTRAL NERVOUS SYSTEM

Christine A. Gleason, A. Roger Hohimer, and Stephen A. Back

Over the past several decades, numerous important advances have been made in neonatal cardiovascular and pulmonary medicine, that have dramatically improved survival of critically ill term and preterm infants. Attention has now turned increasingly toward improving the neurologic outcome in not only these critically ill high-risk infants but also those born with prenatal brain injuries, brain malformations, or neurodevelopmental disorders. In the first edition of this textbook, limited attention was devoted to neonatal neurology. Beginning with the eighth edition, the book now features a comprehensive neurology section that, in addition to this introductory chapter, includes chapters devoted to neonatal neuroimaging; malformations and deformations of the developing brain; brain injury and neuroprotection; neuromuscular disorders; neonatal seizures; and finally, risk assessment and neurodevelopmental outcomes. This introductory chapter provides an overview of central nervous system (CNS) vascular anatomy and physiology and a discussion of normal principles of regulation of cerebral blood flow (CBF) and energy metabolism. Chapter 60 discusses normal CNS developmental anatomy in the context of the associated major human brain malformations.

CENTRAL NERVOUS SYSTEM VASCULAR DEVELOPMENT

Development of the cerebral vasculature is closely linked with that of neural tissue. Early in development, the CNS is essentially avascular. Blood vessels form as a meshwork in the meninges before growing into the CNS from the pial surface in a caudal-to-rostral progression. The blood-brain barrier is essentially a collection of capillary–endothelial cell tight junctions and develops under the influence of astrocytes. Brain blood vessel formation and blood-brain barrier capacities are present early in the CNS, but maximal capillary sprouting occurs during the period of dendritic growth and glial cell proliferation.

Cerebral vascular development, particularly in the periventricular region, is clinically relevant because the immature infant is susceptible to ischemic injury in the white matter around the ventricles and to hemorrhage in the germinal matrix region (part of the ventricular zone) and into the ventricles (Takashima and Tanaka, 1978a, 1978b). The periventricular white matter has two major blood supplies. Perforating arteries branch from leptomeningeal arteries, penetrate the cerebral cortex, and terminate as capillary beds adjacent to the ventricles. Branches of choroidal and striate arteries project toward the lateral ventricles and then deviate away from the ventricle toward their final termination in vascular capillary beds in the periventricular white matter. It has been proposed that these vascular beds collectively form vascular end zones and border zones that render the periventricular white matter particularly susceptible to ischemia. However, the existence of these border zones remains controversial (Mayer and Kier, 1991; Nelson et al, 1991; Takashima et al, 2009; Volpe, 2008). Recent studies in the preterm fetal sheep measured blood flow in histopathologically defined regions of injury in cerebral cortex and white matter (McClure et al, 2008). Although white matter blood flow is lower than cerebral gray matter, there was no evidence for pathologically significant gradients of fetal blood flow within the periventricular white matter under conditions of ischemia or reperfusion. White matter lesions did not localize to regions susceptible to greater ischemia, nor did less vulnerable regions of cerebral white matter have greater flow during ischemia. An alternative explanation for the topography of cerebral white matter lesions is the distribution of susceptible cell types, particularly late oligodendrocyte progenitors, that are particularly susceptible to hypoxia-ischemia (Back et al, 2005; Riddle et al, 2006).

A current limitation to our understanding of human cerebral vascular development is the lack of approaches that precisely measure regional blood flow in real time in the preterm or term neonate. Magnetic resonance angiography (MRA) has provided structural data on the impact of preterm birth on subsequent vascular development. Preterm survivors studied longitudinally up to 18 months of age demonstrated a persistent reduced tortuosity of proximal segments of all major cerebral arteries (Malamentiniou et al, 2006). Recently, van Kooij et al (2010) assessed the circle of Willis in 72 preterm neonates at term-equivalent age using magnetic MRA. They observed "a high prevalence of variant types of the circle of Willis" with corresponding variations in flow in the internal carotid and basilar artery. The significance of this finding with regard to regional blood flow, brain injury, brain development, or vulnerability to injury later in life is not known.

Venous drainage from the cerebral hemispheres is bidirectional. Cortical and subcortical veins drain in the meningeal direction from cortex and superficial white matter, whereas medullary veins drain in the ventricular direction from the deep white matter. Studies of collagen type 6

811

immunoreactivity suggested that arterial vessels may be more late-maturing relative to venous development in the deep white matter (Takashima et al, 2009). Characteristics of the developing vasculature, such as the fact that the medullary veins in the deeper cerebral white matter are more developed than the veins in the subcortical white matter, may predispose the developing deep white matter to certain types of injury, particularly periventricular venous infarction that occurs in association with intraventricular hemorrhage (Volpe, 2008).

GERMINAL MATRIX

The germinal matrix is supplied by striatal arteries through a dense capillary network that is particularly susceptible to hemorrhage in the preterm infant. Although the germinal matrix is considerably more vascular than the cerebral cortex or white matter, the increased risk for hemorrhage is related to developmental immaturity of the vasculature and the cellular and extracellular matrix elements that make up the blood-brain barrier. The propensity of the matrix to hemorrhage in premature infants less than 34 weeks' gestational age is thus related to a complex interplay between vascular fragility and disturbances in cerebral blood flow that are particularly prominent in the first 3 to 4 postnatal days (Ballabh, 2010; Ment et al, 1995).

In recent years, the relative contributions of several of the key molecular components of the blood-brain barrier to germinal matrix hemorrhage have been studied. The barrier is composed of astrocytic endfeet, pericytes, basement membrane, and endothelial tight junctions. Pericytes are involved in both the initiation of angiogenesis and the later stabilization of blood vessels via the synthesis of components of the extracellular matrix and regulation of endothelial differentiation. Perivascular coverage by astrocytic endfeet and pericytes is reduced in human preterm germinal matrix relative to other brain regions (Braun et al, 2007; El-Khoury et al, 2006).

Studies of the ultrastructural features of the blood-brain barrier in an animal model initially suggested that postnatal endothelial basal lamina deposition occurs before tight junction formation and glial investiture and that basal lamina induction influences the latter two processes (Ment et al, 1995). Various candidate molecules have been proposed to contribute to the stabilization of the matrix vasculature in the first days of life, including laminin, collagen V (Ment et al, 1991), and fibronectin (Xu et al, 2008), all of which increase significantly with advancing age after birth. Enhanced expression of these molecules in the germinal eminence was promoted by indomethacin (Ment et al, 1991) or low-dose prenatal betamethasone (Xu et al, 2008), suggesting that these agents might stabilize the germinal matrix vasculature.

The biology of vascular maturation is an active research area that raises an alternative strategy for prevention of intraventricular hemorrhage. Endothelial proliferation declines in the 1st week of life in human germinal matrix, which supports the notion that angiogenesis is in an active phase around the time of birth (Ballabh et al, 2007). The pronounced angiogenesis in the preterm matrix coincides with the increased expression of the proangiogenic factors vascular endothelial growth factor (VEGF) and angiopoietin-2 in the matrix relative to cerebral cortex and white matter. Moreover, inhibitors of VEGF activity significantly reduced the incidence of intraventricular hemorrhage in a premature rabbit model. Despite the potential benefits of short-term treatment with antiangiogenesis factors, the potential of these agents to cause hypoxia to the germinal matrix or other tissues remains unclear.

REGULATION OF CEREBRAL BLOOD FLOW AND ENERGY METABOLISM

CBF is regulated by many systemic and local factors, including arterial blood pressure, intracranial pressure, arterial O_2 content, hematocrit, and arterial CO_2 tension. Cerebral O_2 consumption (i.e., cerebral metabolic rate, or $CMRO_2$) is an important determinant of CBF. Responsivity of the cerebral circulation to the aforementioned stimuli also is determined in part by $CMRO_2$.

CBF normally is regulated to maintain adequate oxygen and substrate delivery to the brain. When blood flow regulatory limits and oxygen extraction capabilities of the brain are exceeded, the brain sustains tissue hypoxia. When abnormally low CBF is the primary abnormality, then the brain sustains ischemia. In most clinical situations, both hypoxia and ischemia occur, although one may predominate. It should be emphasized that even under conditions of significant hypoxia-ischemia, cerebral injury is often selective rather than diffuse. The timing of an insult during development is a critical factor that contributes to CNS susceptibility to hypoxia-ischemia. For example, under conditions of prolonged global cerebral ischemia, the cerebral cortex is relatively spared in the preterm fetal sheep, whereas panlaminar cortical necrosis occurs in the term animal (Reddy et al, 1998; Riddle et al, 2006). In a fetal rabbit model of placental insufficiency, significant global fetal hypoxia-ischemia caused minimal preterm cerebral white matter injury, but a similar insult three days later in gestation causes pronounced white matter injury (Buser et al, 2010). The timing of appearance of susceptible oligodendroglial progenitors defined the relative susceptibility of the white matter at these two developmental ages. Hence, the extent of the susceptibility to hypoxia-ischemia is related to both the timing and the regional expression of cellular-molecular factors.

AUTOREGULATION

Cerebral autoregulation refers to the maintenance of constant CBF over a range of changes in arterial blood pressure or cerebral perfusion pressure (Lassen and Christensen, 1976; Paulson et al, 1990). This autoregulatory range has both upper and lower limits; above or below these limits, CBF does not remain constant but instead increases or decreases passively, along with changes in arterial blood pressures. Cerebral autoregulation has been demonstrated in several species and across developmental stages, but the mechanism of this important phenomenon remains elusive. It is believed to be an intrinsic property of arterial smooth muscle cells, in which transmural pressure modifies muscle tone, by affecting the activation state of K^+ and Ca^{2+} channels in muscle cells, thereby affecting the cells' membrane potential (Greisen, 2005). Current thinking also supports the notion that autoregulation is mediated by a fine balance between endothelial cell–derived constricting and relaxing factors (Iadecola and Nedergaard, 2007). In adults, CBF remains constant over an autoregulatory range of mean blood pressures from 50 to 150 mm Hg (Paulson et al, 1990). In late fetal lambs, the range is lower and narrower (40 to 80 mm Hg), but more importantly, normal blood pressure is at most 5 to 10 mm Hg above the lower limit of the autoregulatory curve (Papile et al, 1985). Preterm fetal lambs show even less autoregulatory capability (Helou et al, 1994).

Autoregulation of CBF is of considerable interest to neonatologists because of the many clinical circumstances under which it may be impaired with risk for tissue hypoxia-ischemia. Impaired cerebral autoregulation in sick and clinically unstable premature infants was initially studied by means of xenon clearance and Doppler studies and more recently by near infrared spectroscopy and spatially resolved spectroscopy (du Plessis, 2008; Greisen, 2009). Severe perinatal asphyxia, hypoxia, head trauma, and hypercapnic acidosis, even when relatively mild, have been shown to attenuate or even abolish autoregulation (Busija and Heistad, 1984; Jones et al, 1988; Tweed et al, 1986). Nevertheless, considerable controversy remains regarding the role of pressure passivity in the pathogenesis of various forms of brain injury in the sick preterm neonate. This is illustrated, for example, by recent studies that failed to support a role for impaired autoregulation in the pathogenesis of intraventricular hemorrhage (Soul et al, 2007; Wong et al, 2008). Hence, basic questions regarding cerebral autoregulation remain unanswered, including determining the optimal clinical practices for blood pressure regulation (Greisen, 2009).

The Cushing phenomenon is characterized by increasing systemic arterial pressure, enough to maintain cerebral perfusion pressure when intracranial pressure rises. Harris et al (1989) have shown that this response is highly developed in fetal sheep, possibly as an adaptation to the rigors of head compression during labor. If the newborn human Cushing response is similarly well developed, then the newborn brain may be better able to preserve cerebral blood pressure when intracranial pressure rises (as with postasphyxial cerebral edema).

RESPONSE TO HYPOXIA

When arterial oxygen content (CaO_2) decreases, the cerebral circulation responds by increasing CBF to maintain oxygen delivery to the brain. This cerebral vasodilatory hypoxic response is directly related to CaO_2 and not to arterial oxygen tension (PaO_2). Increased CBF preserves cerebral oxygen delivery ($CaO_2 \times CBF$) and cerebral O_2 consumption [($CaO_2 - CvO_2) \times CBF$]. There is a limit beyond which CBF cannot increase, and then O_2 delivery falls. The brain must then increase O_2 extraction to maintain CMRO$_2$. There is a limit to this as well (cerebral venous PO$_2$), and when this is reached, CMRO$_2$ falls and brain tissue hypoxia results.

Jones and colleagues (1981) studied hypoxic hypoxia in neonatal sheep and found that CBF correlates best with CaO_2; as CaO_2 decreases, CBF increases. Studies have shown similar cerebral hypoxic cerebral vasodilatory responses in fetal (Ashwal et al, 1981) and adult sheep (Koehler et al, 1984). Developmental differences have been noted, however, in the regional brain blood flow responses to hypoxia. Ashwal and associates (1981) demonstrated a hierarchy of responsivity in fetal sheep in which the brainstem is more responsive than the subcortex or cortex. Such a hierarchy has not been noted in more mature sheep. Studies in immature fetal sheep (Gleason et al, 1990) have shown that cerebral O_2 delivery is not maintained during hypoxic hypoxia; therefore, fractional O_2 extraction must increase to maintain CMRO$_2$. This finding suggests that important regulatory mechanisms are not fully developed in the immature brain, thus rendering it more vulnerable to hypoxic injury.

Anemic hypoxia produces a rise in CBF similar to that with hypoxic hypoxia so that oxygen delivery is maintained despite reduced CaO_2 (Jones et al, 1981). Arterial PaO_2 changes little, if at all, in anemic hypoxia, and changes in blood viscosity alone are not sufficient to account for the increase. Patchy areas of tissue hypoxia, with some areas receiving only plasma, could produce cerebral vasodilation (Jones et al, 1988).

HYPEROXIA

Several studies have demonstrated a decrease in cerebral blood flow when PaO_2 is raised to relatively hyperoxic levels. Gleason et al (1988) raised fetal PaO_2 from 20 to 73 mm Hg in fetal sheep and noted a 46% drop in CBF. Kennedy et al (1971) showed a 20% to 30% decrease in CBF during extreme hyperoxia (PaO_2 of 349 mm Hg) in neonatal puppies; this CBF response disappeared by 3 weeks of age. Rahilly (1980) demonstrated a 33% drop in cranial blood flow in term infants breathing 100% O_2, and Leahy et al (1980) showed a 15% drop in CBF in preterm infants who received similar treatment. These results are not surprising when the curve for the CBF response to hyperoxia is placed along the inverse hyperbolic hypoxic response curve previously described by Jones et al (1977) for fetal sheep. This potential decrease in CBF with increased O_2 is certainly an important consideration in the decision to use extracorporeal membrane oxygenation in a hypoxemic neonate, during which the carotid PaO_2 may transiently be as high as 500 mm Hg, or in resuscitation of a newborn using 100% oxygen (Gleason, 1993).

POLYCYTHEMIA/HYPERVISCOSITY

Arterial O_2 content increases when the hemoglobin concentration rises, as does whole blood viscosity. An increase in CaO_2 alone results in decreased CBF. The independent effect of hyperviscosity on decreasing CBF in polycythemic animals was studied by Massik et al (1987). In their study in lambs, methemoglobin was used to dissociate the effects of hematocrit and CaO_2 as the hematocrit was raised. Approximately 50% of the decrease in CBF associated with polycythemia was attributed to hyperviscosity and the remainder to increases in CaO_2. In the perinatal period, a number of factors can result in neonatal polycythemia, both chronically (fetal hypoxia) and acutely (umbilical cord clamping). Although neurologic signs may be present, a partial exchange transfusion to reduce the hematocrit has not been shown to be of benefit with short-term or long-term neurologic abnormalities (Rosenkrantz, 2003).

ALTERATIONS IN CEREBRAL OXYGEN CONSUMPTION

CBF normally is coupled with $CMRO_2$, such that when clinical conditions alter $CMRO_2$, CBF is adjusted appropriately (Siesjo, 1984). For example, in the preterm sheep, barbiturate coma lowers $CMRO_2$; therefore, CBF is comparably reduced (Hohimer and Bissonnette, 1989). Donegan et al (1985) studied CBF autoregulation and hypoxic responses during pentobarbital-induced coma in newborn lambs. The CBF response to hypoxia was attenuated during coma, but only in proportion to the decrease in $CMRO_2$. Chronic narcotic infusions in ventilated sick preterm infants may induce a similar response.

Cerebral O_2 consumption increases during neuronal excitation such as seizures (Metzger, 1979; Plum and Duffy, 1975). Increased CBF mirrors the increased $CMRO_2$, but there may not be adequate tissue PO_2. If seizure activity is sustained, the high metabolic rate and potentially maximal CBF may increase the brain's susceptibility to additional hypoxic-ischemic injury (Meldrum and Nilsson, 1976).

CARBON DIOXIDE REACTIVITY

Changes in arterial PCO_2 induce significant cerebral vascular responses in developing animals (Rosenberg, 1982). Hypercapnia is a potent cerebral vasodilator, and hypocapnia is a potent vasoconstrictor (Reivich et al, 1971; Volpe, 2008). Hypocapnia may occur clinically secondary to overventilation or may be induced intentionally, in an attempt to decrease pulmonary vascular resistance. Numerous studies have demonstrated a 30% to 40% reduction in CBF after 15 to 30 minutes of moderately severe hypocapnia ($PaCO_2$ of 15 to 25 mm Hg). A gradual increase in CBF during prolonged hypocarbia has been shown by Gleason et al (1989) in newborn lambs, with CBF gradually returning to baseline during 6 hours of hyperventilation. In these hyperventilated lambs, significant cerebral hyperemia was noted after abrupt discontinuation of hyperventilation. Additional animal studies by Deliveria-Papadopoulos and associates (1988) have suggested that severe hypocapnia ($PaCO_2$ <10 mm Hg) results in tissue ischemia. In newborn piglets, hyperventilation increases the expression of Bax, a pro-apoptotic protein, without simultaneous induction of the anti-apoptotic protein bcl-2 (Greisen, 2009; Lasso Pirot et al, 2007). Clinical studies have shown abnormal electroencephalograms, auditory evoked responses, and abnormal neurodevelopmental outcomes associated with significant hypocarbia.

The effect of hypercapnia on the cerebral circulation has been of interest to neonatologists since the "permissive hypercapnia" ventilatory strategy was introduced in an attempt to minimize lung damage in preterm infants. In newborn sheep, increasing PCO_2 from 37 to 78 mm Hg resulted in a 355% increase in CBF, which remained 195% above baseline after 6 hours. An abrupt return to normocapnia resulted in a return to baseline with no adverse effects on cerebral oxygenation throughout the study (Hino et al, 2000). Clinically, Kaiser et al (2005) used Doppler ultrasound to measure cerebral blood flow velocity during and after tracheal suctioning in preterm neonates and noted that the cerebral circulation became progressively pressure passive with hypercapnia. They recommended careful control of $PaCO_2$ (avoiding both hypercapnia and hypocapnia) during the first week of life to limit brain injury.

BRAIN ENERGY METABOLISM

Oxygen and glucose are the brain's primary energy fuels. Although the requirement for oxygen is absolute, other substrates can replace or augment glucose during special circumstances such as hypoglycemia or anoxia (Jones, 1979). When oxygen delivery to the brain is impaired and oxygen extraction capability is exceeded, tissue hypoxia occurs, and brain damage may be the result. The issue of whether or not newborns have decreased vulnerability or "resistance" to anoxic insult continues to be debated. Increased survivability after prolonged anoxia has been demonstrated in immature animals such as newborn rats, and there have been occasional anecdotal reports of this phenomenon in newborn infants, but whether or not such increased survivability reflects resistance of the *brain* to anoxia is debatable. Nevertheless, immature animals do have better survival, and this has been variously attributed to (1) lower cerebral O_2 consumption, (2) predominance of anaerobic metabolism as an energy source, or (3) circulatory adaptations in immature animals, such as greater stores of cardiac glycogen that enable the heart to sustain the cerebral circulation. None of these possible mechanisms accounts for increased survival in all species, and none has been definitively proved to be important exclusively in immature animals (Gleason, 1993; Jones, 1979).

Hypoglycemia occurs quite commonly in sick newborn infants, although the associated physiologic conditions vary considerably. Poor glycogen stores, increased glucose demands, hyperinsulinism, and poor glucose intake are among the more common of these conditions. Cerebral effects of hypoglycemia may depend in part on the cerebral effects of the associated physiologic conditions. Alternative oxidative substrates are available to the brain, including ketone bodies, lactate, amino acids, and lipids. Owen et al (1967) showed that cerebral ketone body consumption accounts for 50% of cerebral O_2 consumption in obese adults who were starved for 5 to 6 weeks. Hypoglycemia is associated with decreased cerebral glucose consumption but no change in cerebral O_2 consumption (Jones, 1979). Whether this response is adaptive or pathologic is not known.

METABOLIC ALKALOSIS/ACIDOSIS

Cerebrovascular resistance is believed to be directly related to brain interstitial pH (Kontos et al, 1977). Biologic membranes are highly permeable to CO_2, so a change in $PaCO_2$ has an almost immediate effect on interstitial pH and, consequently, on CBF. In contrast, hydrogen and bicarbonate ions do not diffuse as easily through membranes. Therefore, induction of acute metabolic acidosis or alkalosis has not been shown to change CBF or autoregulation

(Harper and Bell, 1963; Hermansen et al, 1984). During hypocapnia, addition of metabolic alkalosis does not alter CBF. However, during hypercapnia, bicarbonate infusion causes a significant decrease in CBF (Arvidsson et al, 1981), suggesting that hypercapnia alters the blood-brain permeability to ions. Such alterations in blood-brain barrier may also be associated with neonatal hypoxic/ischemic brain injury.

Sodium bicarbonate is used clinically to correct metabolic acidosis in neonates, but it has been used with caution since a 1974 report that linked its use with hypernatremia, intracranial hemorrhage, and acute secondary changes in arterial PCO_2 (Simmons et al, 1974). Laptook (1985) evaluated the cerebral effects of sodium bicarbonate (2 mEq/kg given over 3 minutes) administered to paralyzed newborn piglets to correct metabolic acidosis associated with hypoxemia. This investigator noted no alterations in brain blood flow or O_2 delivery. Constant $PaCO_2$ was maintained by increasing the ventilator rate during the bicarbonate infusion. In a study of preterm infants with metabolic acidosis, slow infusion (over 30 minutes) of 4% $NaHCO_3$ was associated with less fluctuation in cerebral hemodynamics (primarily, an increase in cerebral blood volume), compared with a rapid bolus (van Alfen-van der Velden et al, 2006). A 2005 Cochrane Review concluded that there was insufficient evidence to determine whether infusion of sodium bicarbonate reduces morbidity and mortality rates in preterm infants with metabolic acidosis (Lawn et al, 2005). Similarly, there is lack of evidence for efficacy and potential for harm when sodium bicarbonate is given during cardiac arrest. This overall lack of evidence for benefit led Aschner and Poland (2008) to conclude, in a review article on sodium bicarbonate, that "clinicians should resist the common impulse to administer bicarbonate to infants with metabolic acidosis, recognizing the risks of immediate worsening of the intracellular milieu."

SUGGESTED GUIDELINES FOR CEREBROVASCULAR AND METABOLIC CARE IN HIGH-RISK NEWBORNS

Guiding principles for the cerebrovascular and metabolic care of critically ill preterm and term infants may include the following:
1. Maintain stable blood pressure. Severe hypotension is clearly detrimental, but so are rapid increases in blood pressure in a pressure-passive circulation.
2. Maintain stable acid-base balance without rapid corrections.
3. Avoid severe hypoxemia.
4. Avoid marked hyperoxemia (i.e., consider effects of resuscitating with 100% oxygen).
5. Avoid major changes in $PaCO_2$, both hypocapnia and hypercapnia.
6. Correct significant anemia or polycythemia; if the condition is chronic, correct slowly.
7. Consider cerebrovascular and metabolic effects of any new (and existing) drug therapies. Use the lowest effective dose for the shortest period of time.
8. Maintain euglycemia, particularly in asphyxiated newborns.

SUGGESTED READINGS

Back SA, Miller SP: Cerebral white matter injury. The changing spectrum in survivors of preterm birth, *NeoReviews* 8:e418-e424, 2007.

Back SA: Mechanisms of acute and chronic brain injury in the preterm infant. In Miller SP, Shevel M, editors: *International reviews in child neurology*, London, 2011(in press), McKeith Press.

Braun A, Xu H, Hu F, et al: Paucity of pericytes in germinal matrix vasculature of premature infants, *J Neurosci* 27:12012-12024, 2007.

du Plessis AJ: Cerebrovascular injury in premature infants: current understanding and challenges for future prevention, *Clin Perinatol* 35:609-641, 2008.

Greisen G: To autoregulate or not to autoregulate—that is no longer the question, *Semin Pediatr Neurol* 16:207-215, 2009.

Iadecola C, Nedergaard M: Glial regulation of the cerebral microvasculature, *Nat Neurosci* 10:1369-1376, 2007.

Jones MD Jr, Koehler RC, Traystman RJ: Regulation of cerebral blood flow in the fetus, newborn, and adult. In Guthrie RD, editor: *Neonatal intensive care*, New York, 1988, Churchill Livingstone, pp 123-152.

Malamateniou C, Counsell SJ, Allsop JM, et al: The effect of preterm birth on neonatal cerebral vasculature studied with magnetic resonance angiography at 3 tesla, *Neuroimage* 32:1050-1059, 2006.

McClure M, Riddle A, Manese M, et al: Cerebral blood flow heterogeneity in preterm sheep: lack of physiological support for vascular boundary zones in fetal cerebral white matter, *J Cereb Blood Flow Metab* 28:995-1008, 2008.

Ment LR, Stewart WB, Ardito TA, et al: Germinal matrix microvascular maturation correlates inversely with the risk period for neonatal intraventricular hemorrhage, *Dev Brain Res* 84:142-149, 1995.

Takashima S, Itoh M, Oka A: A history of our understanding of cerebral vascular development and pathogenesis of perinatal brain damage over the past 30 years, *Semin Pediatr Neurol* 16:226-236, 2009.

van Alfen-van der Velden AAEM, Hopman JCW, Klaessens JHGM, et al: Effects of rapid versus slow infusion of sodium bicarbonate on cerebral hemodynamics and oxygenation in preterm infants, *Biol Neonate* 90:122, 2006.

Volpe JP: *Neurology of the newborn*, Philadelphia, 2008, WB Saunders.

Complete references used in this text can be found online at www.expertconsult.com

NEONATAL NEUROIMAGING

Sanjay P. Prabhu, P. Ellen Grant, Richard L. Robertson, and George A. Taylor

ULTRASONOGRAPHY

ANATOMIC (GRAY SCALE) SONOGRAPHY

Ultrasonography (US) became a viable tool for imaging the neonatal brain in the late 1970s with the development of real-time capabilities (Pape et al, 1979). Subsequent advances in ultrasound technology have dramatically improved our ability to visualize normal structures and abnormalities in the neonatal brain. As a result, US continues to be an integral part of caring for the critically ill neonate.

Diagnostic US relies on the transmission and reflection of high-frequency sound waves into tissues. The speed and reflectivity of sound differ among various tissues, resulting in acoustic interfaces that can be used to create images of anatomic structures. By convention, tissues with high reflectance, such as clotted blood, are bright, and those with low reflectance, such as cerebrospinal fluid (CSF) or moving blood, are dark. Thick bone and air significantly interfere with the transmission of sound into deeper tissues. Consequently, cranial US requires a coupling agent (gel) between the transducer and the skin to eliminate as much intervening air as possible and most often is performed through an open fontanel.

DOPPLER SONOGRAPHY

Continuous-wave and pulsed-wave Doppler techniques have been used for decades to sample hemodynamics in specific intracranial vessels. The resistive index (RI) and mean blood flow velocity over time (time-averaged velocity) are the most commonly used spectral Doppler measures for monitoring intracranial hemodynamics. The easiest and most reproducible are measures of pulsatility, which are relatively insensitive to differences in angle of insonation and correlate well with acute changes in intracerebral perfusion pressure. As the intracranial pressure rises, arterial flow tends to be more affected during diastole than during systole, resulting in an elevated pulsatility of flow. This phenomenon has been reported in Doppler studies in infants with elevated intracranial pressure (ICP) from a variety of causes including hydrocephalus, cerebral edema, and intracranial hemorrhage. However, elevated ICP may not always be present in infants with abnormal intracranial pressure-volume relationships (decreased cranial compliance). Thus, the RI may be within the normal range in these infants. Doppler examination of the anterior cerebral artery during fontanel compression may be useful in the early identification of infants with abnormal intracranial compliance before the development of increased ICP as shown by elevated baseline RI.

Many factors other than cerebrovascular resistance may affect the RI in an intracranial vessel, including the presence of a patent ductus arteriosus, alterations in heart rate and cardiac output, and the amount of pressure applied on the fontanel during scanning (Perlman et al, 1981; Taylor, 1992a; Taylor et al, 1989, 1996).

Although reproducible and easy to obtain, the RI is only a weak predictor of cerebrovascular resistance under most physiologic conditions. Mean blood flow velocity measures are the most informative indices of cerebral blood flow (CBF). A strong correlation has been demonstrated between mean blood flow velocity and changes in global CBF under a variety of clinical and experimental conditions (Taylor et al, 1990).

The introduction of color Doppler technology in 1989 has made imaging and reliable hemodynamic sampling of the intracranial vasculature routinely possible in the normal newborn (Dean and Taylor, 1995; Mitchell et al, 1988, 1989; Taylor, 1992b). Standard color Doppler sonography is based on an estimate of the mean frequency shift created by the movement of red blood cells at different velocities within the tissue or blood vessel being examined. Flow is generally depicted as variations of red or blue color, depending on the degree of shift from the baseline frequency, and on the direction of the moving red cells.

EQUIPMENT AND SCANNING TECHNIQUE

Transducers

In the premature infant, transducers operating at a higher frequency range (7 to 10 MHz) are recommended because of their higher spatial resolution. Lower-frequency transducers (3.5 to 5 MHz) are often used in larger infants to obtain adequate sound penetration. Sector transducers with a 120-degree imaging field are most useful for imaging through the anterior and posterior fontanels.

Scanning Technique

For sonographic examination of the neonatal brain, standardized coronal and sagittal images are obtained through the anterior fontanel. Coronal images are obtained by placing the transducer transversely across the fontanel and sweeping it in an anteroposterior direction to cover the entire brain (Figure 59-1). The transducer should be carefully held to produce symmetric imaging of both hemispheres.

At least six angled images are obtained. The most anterior image is anterior to the frontal horns of the lateral ventricles at the level of the orbits. The frontal lobes and anterior portion of the interhemispheric fissure can be visualized. The second image is obtained through the anterior horns of the lateral ventricles at the level of the suprasellar cistern. This structure has the appearance of

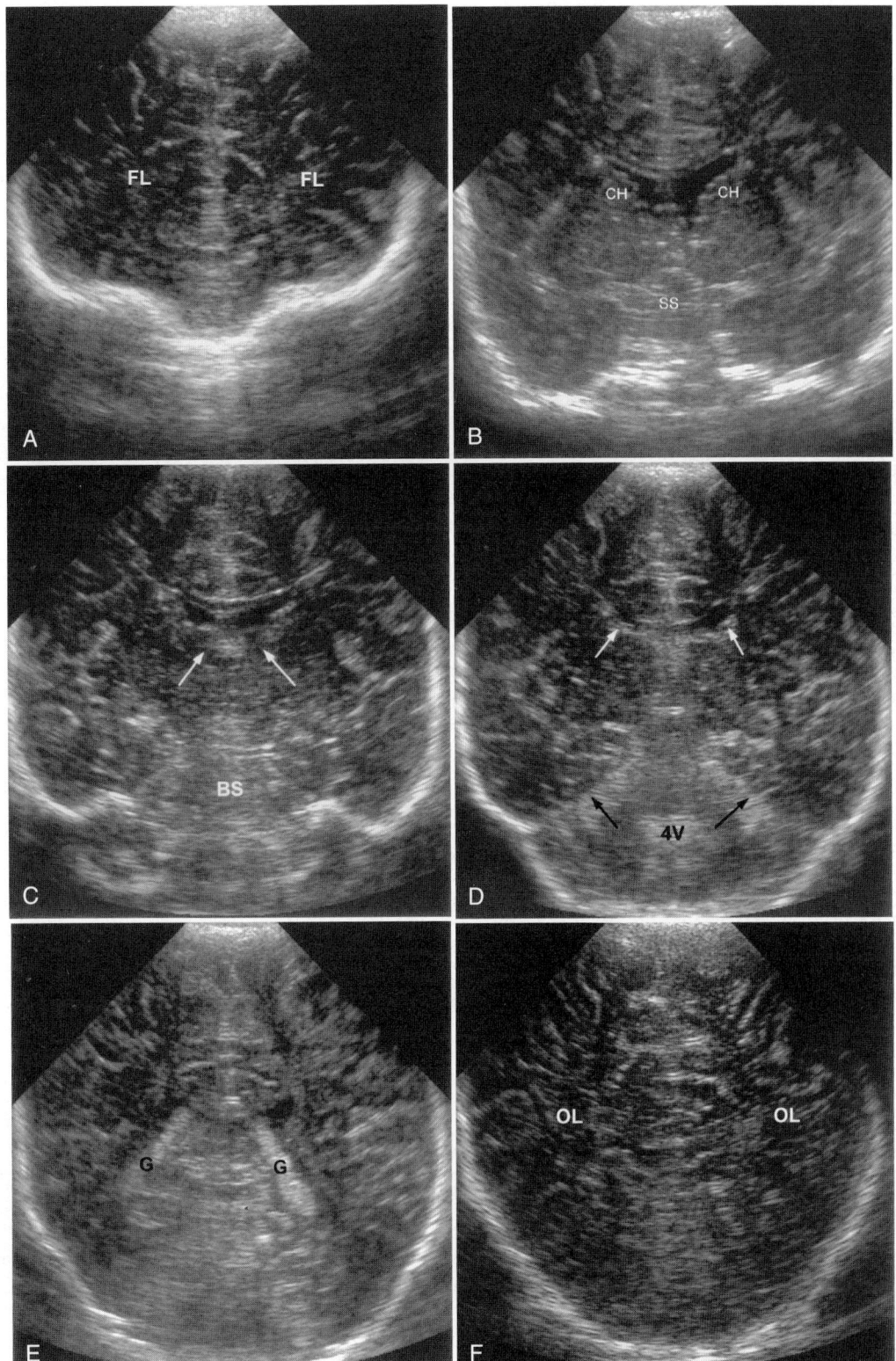

FIGURE 59-1 Standard coronal planes of cranial sonography performed through the anterior fontanel. A, Plane 1 is angled anteriorly to include the frontal lobes (*FL*) and orbits. **B,** Plane 2 demonstrates the caudate heads (*CH*) and the suprasellar cistern (*SS*). **C,** Plane 3 passes through the foramina of Monro (*arrows*) and the brainstem (*BS*). **D,** Coronal plane 4 shows the rounded echogenic choroid plexus within the body of the lateral ventricles (*white arrows*), the fourth ventricle (*4V*), and the tentorium (*black arrows*). **E,** Plane 5 includes the glomus (*G*) of the choroid plexus in the trigones of the lateral ventricles. **F,** Plane 6 is angled posteriorly to include the occipital lobes (*OL*).

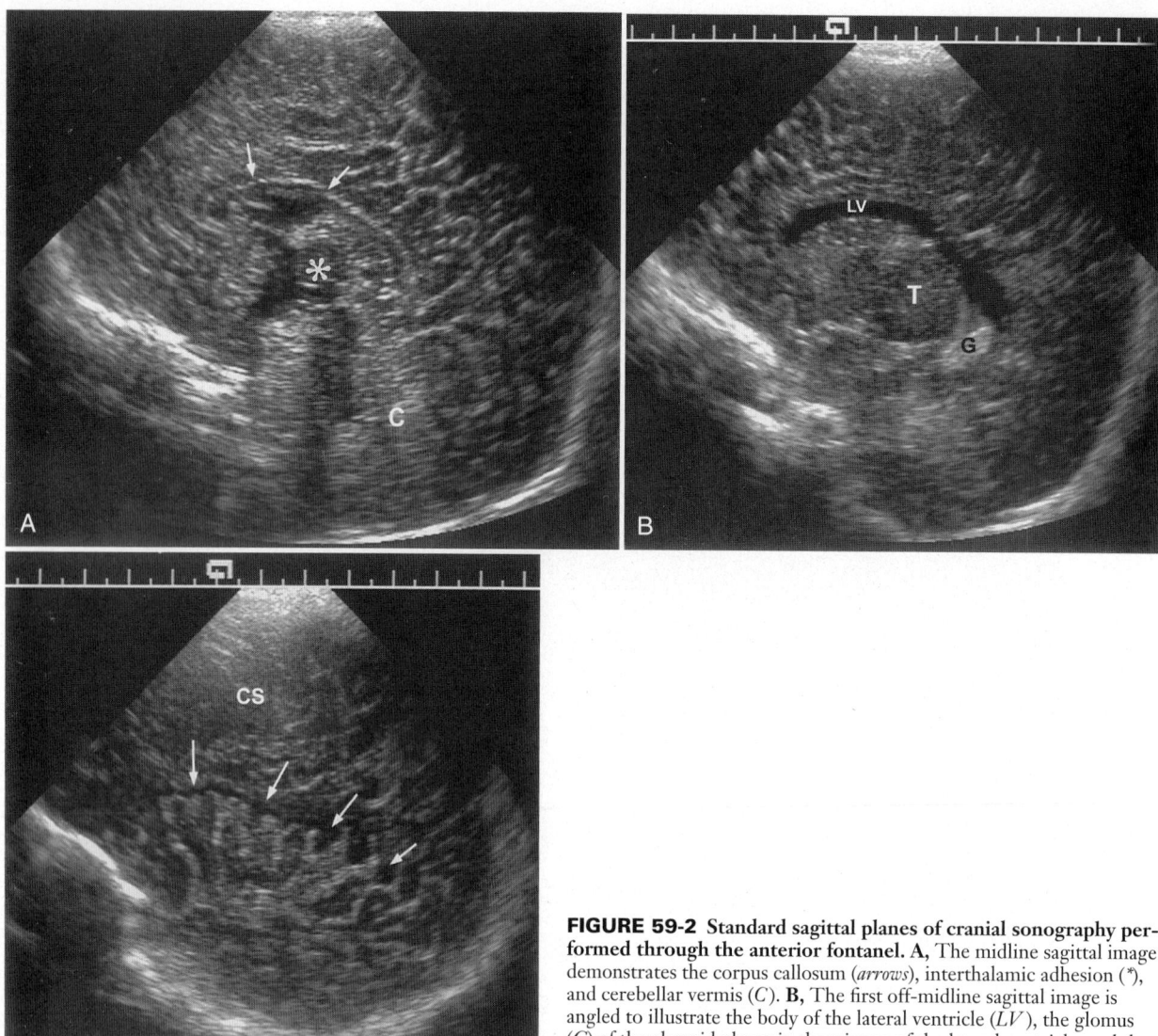

FIGURE 59-2 Standard sagittal planes of cranial sonography performed through the anterior fontanel. **A,** The midline sagittal image demonstrates the corpus callosum (*arrows*), interthalamic adhesion (*), and cerebellar vermis (*C*). **B,** The first off-midline sagittal image is angled to illustrate the body of the lateral ventricle (*LV*), the glomus (*G*) of the choroid plexus in the trigone of the lateral ventricle, and the thalamus (*T*). **C,** The far-lateral sagittal image includes the sylvian fissure (*arrows*).

an echogenic five-pointed star. The hypoechoic caudate nucleus can be seen inferior and lateral to the comma-shaped lateral ventricles. The ventricles are separated from each other by the centrally positioned cavum of the septum pellucidum. Basal ganglia, frontal and temporal lobes, insula, and T-shaped sylvian fissure can be identified in this plane. The next image is obtained more posteriorly through the body of the lateral ventricles at the level of the paired foramina of Monro and brainstem. The anterior portion of the choroid plexus can identified as three small echogenic structures along the inferomedial aspect of the lateral ventricles, and paired thalami can be seen lateral to the third ventricle. Lateral and superior to the lentiform nuclei is a region of the deep white matter called the centrum semiovale. The fourth image is obtained with the transducer angled slightly more posteriorly. At this level, the lateral ventricles have a more rounded appearance, and the choroid plexus is seen as a more prominent echogenic structure along the floor of the ventricles. The

confluence of frontal, parietal, and temporal lobes can be seen as well as the echogenic tentorium cerebelli and the anterior portion of the cerebellum and fourth ventricle. The transducer sweep is continued posteriorly until the prominent paired echogenic structures of the glomus of the choroid plexus are seen in the atrium of the lateral ventricles. The parietal and posterior aspects of the temporal lobe and sylvian fissure can be visualized, along with the echogenic cerebellum inferiorly. The last coronal image is obtained posterior to the lateral ventricles. The posterior aspect of the interhemispheric fissure and the occipital lobes are seen on this view.

Sagittal images are obtained by placing the transducer longitudinally along the anterior fontanel (Figure 59-2). A total of five images are usually obtained, one along the midline and two on each side by angling the transducer laterally. True midline can be established by identifying the curved corpus callosum and echogenic cerebellar vermis on the same imaging plane. The cingulate gyrus can be seen as an undulating echogenic line superior to the corpus callosum. The medial aspect of the paired thalamic nuclei, the tectum of the midbrain, and fourth ventricle can be identified on this image. The transducer is swept laterally approximately 10 degrees to show the body of the lateral ventricle. Because the lateral ventricles are not located in a straight anteroposterior line, the transducer must be slightly angled so that the posterior aspect of the probe is positioned more laterally than its anterior aspect. The echogenic choroid plexus is C-shaped and cups the thalamus like a baseball in a catcher's mitt. Its superior limb extends anteriorly to the caudothalamic notch immediately posterior to the head of the caudate nucleus. Its inferior limb extends well into the temporal horn. The second angled sagittal image is obtained with the transducer angled lateral to the body of the lateral ventricle. The centrum semiovale is well shown, and the sylvian fissure can be seen separating the parietal and temporal lobes (Naidich and Yousefzadeh, 1986; Siegel, 2001).

Although scans through the anterior fontanel provide adequate views of the cerebral hemispheres, images of the convexities, midbrain and posterior fossa are often limited. Four additional scanning approaches through the midline posterior fontanel, the squamosal suture, the posterolateral or mastoid fontanel, and the foramen magnum can be very useful as additional problem-solving tools in selected patients with suspected or poorly delineated posterior fossa and midbrain lesions (Buckley et al, 1997; Luna and Goldstein, 2000) (Figure 59-3).

COMPRESSION DOPPLER

Color Doppler is used to identify the pericallosal portion of the anterior cerebral artery (ACA) in midline sagittal projection using a 7- to 8-MHz vector transducer. A baseline Doppler spectrum is obtained while no pressure is exerted over the fontanel. The fontanel is then completely depressed with the transducer such that any additional pressure results in no further depression of the fontanel. During compression, the Doppler range gate is repositioned over the same portion of the ACA, and a second Doppler spectrum is obtained. The duration of each pressure episode should not exceed 3 to 5 seconds.

CLINICAL INDICATIONS

The most common indication for cranial US in the newborn is screening for suspected intracranial hemorrhage and periventricular leukomalacia (PVL) in the premature infant. Once either is detected, US is an excellent method for monitoring the progression or resolution of the pathologic process as well as for detecting the attendant complications of ventricular dilatation and progressive hydrocephalus. Sonography also is a very useful tool in the identification of focal infarction and hemorrhagic lesions in the term or near-term infant, as well as congenital midline anomalies, cystic lesions, vascular malformations, and intracranial calcifications, and in the definition of extraaxial fluid collections. The portable, noninvasive nature of cranial US allows for the cribside identification of many important lesions on an urgent basis without need for transport of the unstable or critically ill newborn.

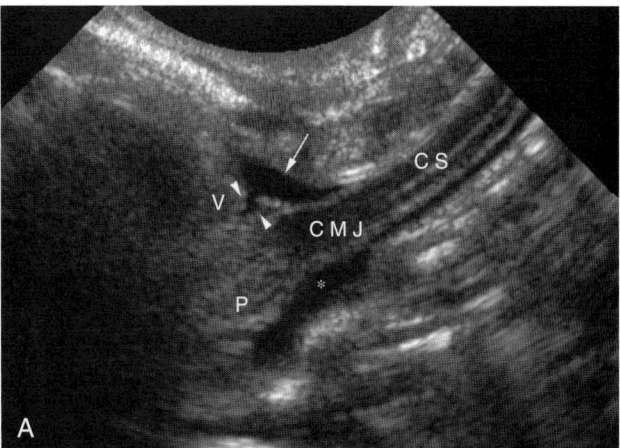

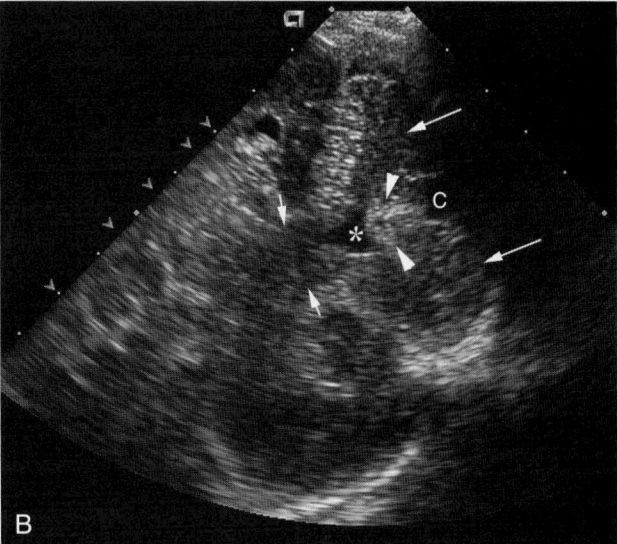

FIGURE 59-3 **Cranial sonography performed using alternate imaging approaches. A,** Midline sagittal image obtained through the foramen magnum shows the cervical spine (*CS*), cervico-medullary junction (*CMJ*), pons (*P*), cerebellar vermis (*V*), vallecula (*arrowheads*), cisterna magna (*arrow*), and pre-pontine cistern (***). **B,** Oblique axial image obtained through the mastoid fontanel demonstrates the cerebellar lobes (*long arrows*), cerebellar vermis (*arrowheads*), midbrain (*short arrows*), fourth ventricle (***), and cisterna magna (*C*).

A more definitive characterization of a sonographic finding or suspected lesion can be performed subsequently with magnetic resonance imaging (MRI) or computed tomography (CT) once the infant is more stable.

COMPUTED TOMOGRAPHY

CT uses a narrowly collimated x-ray beam in conjunction with a digital detector array to produce a cross-sectional anatomic image (Boyd, 1995) (Figure 59-4). Although employing ionizing radiation, current-generation CT scanners effectively limit exposure to the immediate volume of interest (Raj et al, 2000). Tissue contrast in CT is dependent on differential attenuation of the x-ray beam. Tissues with high electron density, such as bone, markedly attenuate the beam, whereas brain and other soft tissues absorb fewer photons. Relative tissue densities on CT images are, by convention, measured in Hounsfield units (HU). After acquisition of the digital data, the images can

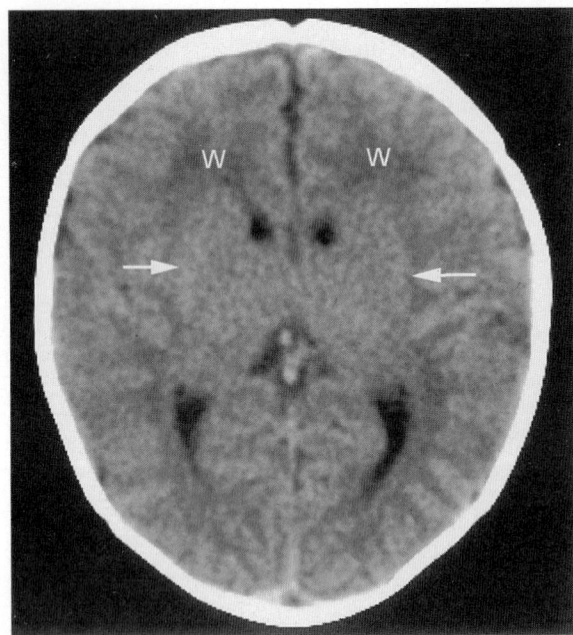

FIGURE 59-4 Axial computed tomographic image in a normal term newborn. Unmyelinated white matter is characterized by low density (*W*), whereas cortex and deep gray matter (*arrows*) are slightly denser.

be adjusted to emphasize different tissues such as bone or soft tissue.

TECHNIQUES

CT images are typically acquired in the axial plane. In most systems, the patient lies supine on a specialized scan table while the x-ray tube and detector array are rotated through a 360-degree arc. The scan table is then advanced several millimeters, and the next image slice is obtained. With current-generation scanners, the images are often acquired in a spiral (helical) or volumetric fashion with continuous rotation of the x-ray tube-detector array and uninterrupted scan table advancement.

Brain CT in the newborn is usually performed without the administration of intravenous contrast. Intravenous contrast may be used in CT for the evaluation of blood-brain barrier breakdown and as a blood pool agent for vascular imaging. Most often, however, the relevant clinical questions regarding the presence of hemorrhage, masses, or infarctions or ventricular dilatation can be answered without the use of contrast or are more fully evaluated with MRI (Cowan and MacDonald, 1999; Haring et al, 1999).

RISKS OF RADIATION

Children are at greater risk than adults from a given dose of radiation. This is explained by the inherent radiosensitivity of their young, developing tissues and because they have more remaining years of life during which a radiation-induced cancer could develop (Brenner and Hall, 2007). Further, although absolute energy imparted from a CT is smaller in children because of the smaller volume of tissues exposed, the effective dose is significantly higher than in an adult, for a similar amount of radiation used (Vock, 2005). Therefore, weight-based protocols to scan neonates to minimize the risks of radiation to the neonate have been suggested. It is important to justify a CT exam, and when one is performed, every attempt must be made to minimize the area scanned and to reduce the radiation dose as much as reasonably acceptable by selecting optimal parameters for age and size of the child and avoiding multiple scanning of the same area.

CLINICAL INDICATIONS

In addition to the dangers of radiation exposure and attendant risks associated with the use of CT and the relatively limited tissue information obtained, there are now few indications for CT of the neonatal brain. Both US and MRI provide imaging of the brain without the use of ionizing radiation. The multiple tissue parameters interrogated with MRI and the ability to generate multiplanar images make it the preferred modality for evaluation of the neonatal central nervous system (CNS). US is sufficient for addressing many causes of an acute change in neurologic status and is a useful tool for evaluating the neonate who is too unstable to undergo MRI. The primary indication for brain CT in a neonate is to evaluate potential causes of neurologic findings, when information from US is insufficient to fully answer the clinical questions and when the child's condition is not stable enough to safely undergo an MRI exam or when MRI is not readily available. CT is particularly useful for the detection of hemorrhage, calcification, or mineralization and delineation of craniofacial osseous anomalies. Although CT can be used for detection of infarction, its sensitivity in the early stages of stroke is significantly limited, and MRI is the investigation of choice in cases of suspected ischemic injury.

CT venography may be used to assess patency of the dural venous sinuses in the neonate; however, MR venography or Doppler sonography provides similar information without the use of ionizing radiation.

MAGNETIC RESONANCE IMAGING

MRI is an established technique based on the principles of nuclear MR. Clinical MRI uses a radiofrequency (RF) pulse to interrogate the properties of water protons in an applied external magnetic field (Balter, 1987; Mulkern and Chung, 2000). The behavior of the protons is determined by both the applied external magnetic field and the local magnetic field produced by neighboring protons. Image signal intensity (brightness) is related to the overall water content of the tissue as well as the inherent tissue properties: T1, T2, proton flow, proton diffusion, paramagnetism, magnetic susceptibility, and chemical shift (Barnes and Taylor, 1998). MR contrast is determined by the relative emphasis (i.e., weighting) placed on these various factors during image acquisition (Figs. 59-5 to 59-8). The manipulation of multiple tissue properties in MRI provides greater flexibility in imaging than is available with the single tissue property used in US (acoustic impedance) or CT (x-ray attenuation). MR images may be obtained in any desired anatomic plane without repositioning the patient. With few exceptions (e.g., Sturge-Weber syndrome, tumor, infection, intra- and extraaxial collections), neonatal brain MRI does not require the use of intravenous contrast.

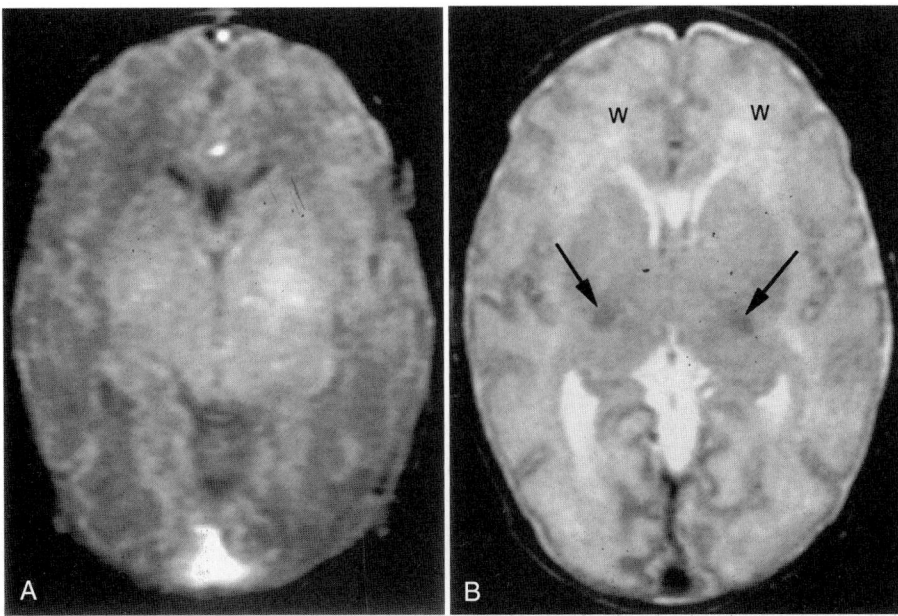

FIGURE 59-5 Axial images in a normal 34-week-gestation preterm neonate. **A,** Unmyelinated subcortical white matter appears hypointense (dark) on T1-weighted imaging, while the cortical and deep gray matter exhibit higher signal intensity. **B,** Unmyelinated subcortical white matter (*W*) appears markedly hyperintense (bright) on the T2-weighted fast spin echo image, while areas of early myelination, such as in the lateral thalamus (*arrows*), are of lower signal intensity. Loss of this focus of hypointensity is one of the earliest indicators of hypoxic-ischemic injury on T2-weighted images.

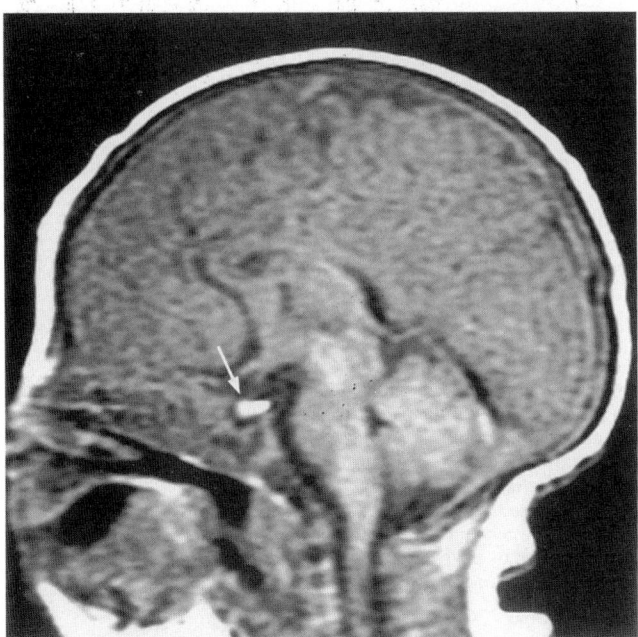

FIGURE 59-6 Midline sagittal T1-weighted image from a normal term neonate. Midline structures such as the corpus callosum, brainstem, and cerebellar vermis are well seen in the newborn. Of note, the anterior pituitary (*arrow*) is diffusely hyperintense because of hormonal activity. Note that the posterior pituitary gland (*arrow*) is intensely bright.

TECHNIQUES

Anatomic Magnetic Resonance Imaging

In general, conventional MR spin echo imaging is not as rapid as US or CT. In recent years, however, a number of fast imaging pulse sequences such as fast spin echo, fast spoiled gradient-recalled imaging have been developed (see Figs. 59-6 and 59-7, *A-C*). The use of these techniques in conjunction with higher-field-strength MR units,

parallel imaging, and multichannel coils has helped reduce scan acquisition times significantly. As a result of these developments, imaging can be performed without sedation or anesthesia in the vast majority of neonates. Appropriate patient positioning and immobilization is typically adequate to permit diagnostic imaging, although sedation or anesthesia may still be required in some cases to provide motion-free imaging. More recently, MR-compatible incubators and monitoring systems have been developed to enable imaging studies of critically ill preterm and term neonates, with continued full clinical support while undergoing MR imaging studies. MR-compatible incubators can enable control of airflow, humidity and temperature regulation, monitoring and respiratory devices and can provide a safe and controlled environment for critically ill preterm and term newborns (Panigrahy et al, 2010). Such MRI-compatible neonatal incubators are currently in use in a number of centers in the United States. The use of the integrated RF head and body coils optimized for newborns has also been shown to improve the quality of MR imaging.

MRI has superseded CT in demonstrating features of acute focal cerebral ischemia, hypoxic ischemic brain injury, congenital malformations, vascular anomalies, hemorrhages, infections, and neoplasia.

MR angiography (MRA) and MR venography (MRV) may be used to demonstrate the intracranial arteries and veins of the neonatal brain without the use of intravenous contrast. Vascular imaging is usually performed by exploiting the time-of-flight (TOF) effect that occurs when stationary tissues are repeatedly excited with RF pulses causing their signal to be suppressed. Signal suppression in stationary tissues occurs due to the relatively long T1 of the brain and a consequent inability of protons to regain magnetization between RF pulses. The use of short interval RF pulses leaves only previously unexcited protons in blood moving into the imaging volume free to generate signal. This signal can be used to create a representation of either arterial or venous structures.

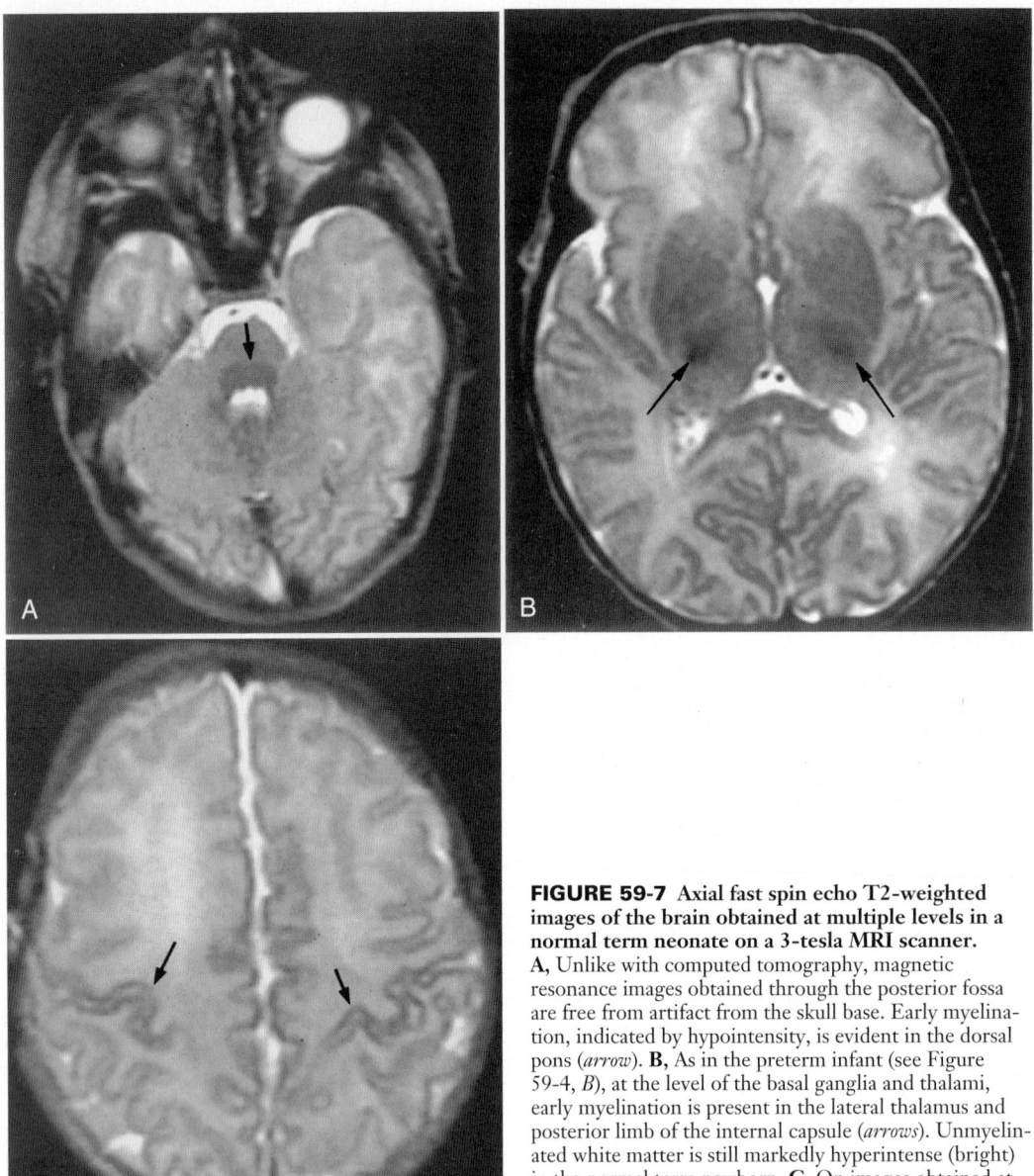

FIGURE 59-7 **Axial fast spin echo T2-weighted images of the brain obtained at multiple levels in a normal term neonate on a 3-tesla MRI scanner.** **A,** Unlike with computed tomography, magnetic resonance images obtained through the posterior fossa are free from artifact from the skull base. Early myelination, indicated by hypointensity, is evident in the dorsal pons (*arrow*). **B,** As in the preterm infant (see Figure 59-4, *B*), at the level of the basal ganglia and thalami, early myelination is present in the lateral thalamus and posterior limb of the internal capsule (*arrows*). Unmyelinated white matter is still markedly hyperintense (bright) in the normal term newborn. **C,** On images obtained at the level of the centrum semiovale, the rolandic cortex is easily identified by its low signal intensity (*arrows*) caused by early myelination.

Advanced MRI Techniques

Advanced MRI techniques that are useful in evaluating the normally developing or injured neonatal brain include diffusion-weighted and diffusion-tensor imaging (DWI and DTI), arterial spin labeling (ASL), perfusion-weighted imaging and susceptibility-weighted imaging (SWI), and volumetric imaging. Postprocessing of these imaging data often yield additional information about the structure or function of the brain beyond that provided by the image acquisitions themselves. For example, insights into increases in the overall cortical surface area and cortical thickness in the premature period have emerged from the use segmentation algorithms applied to volumetrically acquired imaging data.

These newer sequences have been made possible in large part by the development of ultrafast imaging such as echo

planar MRI and the improved uniformity of the magnetic field available with newer MR scanners. Used in adults and older children for several years, functional techniques are also now being applied in the newborn.

DIFFUSION IMAGING

Initially popularized for its usefulness in the evaluation of acute stroke in adults, diffusion imaging (DI) is now widely utilized to provide information about both normal and abnormal processes, in the neonatal brain (Robertson et al, 1999; Rutherford et al, 1995). In DI, supplemental MR gradients are applied during the image acquisition. The motion of protons during the application of these gradients affects the signal in the image, thereby, providing information on molecular diffusion. DI may be performed

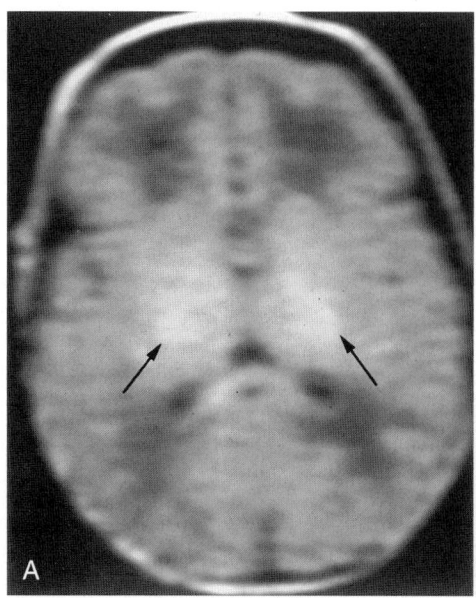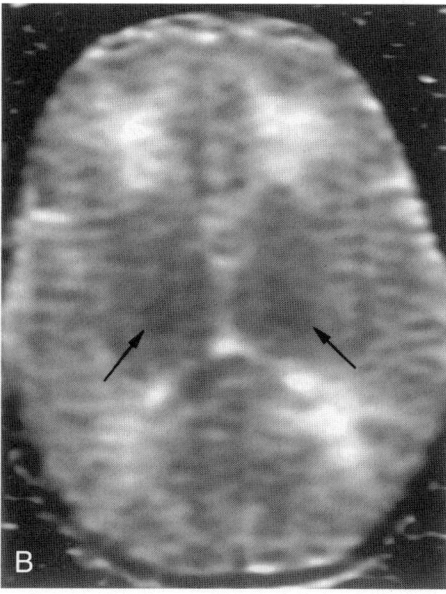

FIGURE 59-8 Axial diffusion-weighted imaging in a normal term newborn. **A,** Isotropic diffusion-weighted image at the level of the basal ganglia. Unmyelinated white matter has very low signal intensity because of the rapid diffusion of water in these regions, whereas areas that have already begun to myelinate, such as the lateral thalamus and posterior limb of the internal capsule (*arrows*), have more restricted diffusion and increased signal. **B,** Corresponding processed apparent diffusion coefficient (ADC) map. These maps are produced to limit T2 effects in the images. Areas with relatively restricted molecular diffusion are, by convention, depicted as lower pixel values (*arrows*).

using one of several techniques. In diffusion-weighted imaging, the supplemental gradients are employed in one to three directions. DWI is often used to evaluate pathologic processes such as brain infarction but provides limited information on brain structure. In diffusion-tensor imaging, the supplemental gradients are employed in many more directions, typically from 6 to 35 or more. Using DTI, differences in regional diffusion due to inherent brain structure can begin to be resolved and mapped. This information, can, for example, be used to generate images of white matter fiber tracts. A new diffusion imaging technique, diffusion-spectrum imaging (DSI), provides even more information by directly measuring three dimensional-spin diffusion probability. By exploring the orientation contrast information in DSI, it is possible to resolve intravoxel fiber crossing more accurately than with DTI, allowing improved delineation of white matter tracts.

In newborns, DI has been used to study normal brain myelination as well as ischemic and nonischemic CNS disorders. The immature brain is characterized by a high water content and relatively rapid molecular diffusion (Robertson and Robson, 2001; Robertson et al, 1999; Sakuma et al, 1991) (see Figure 59-7). The bulk of the water in the neonatal brain is within the extracellular space (Barlow et al, 1961). As the brain matures, a gradual decline in the extracellular volume fraction occurs because of the hydrophobic nature of myelin. Myelin also impairs the exchange of water molecules across the cell membrane. Because the movement of water within the cell is limited by its interaction with intracellular structures and the cell membrane, the apparent diffusion coefficient (ADC) of intracellular water is lower than that of extracellular water. Consequently, the ADC of myelinated white matter is lower than that of unmyelinated white matter. In addition, because of cellular structure, the direction of movement of intracellular water is preferentially along the length of the axon rather than perpendicular to it. Therefore, the relative anisotropy (RA), a measure of the inequality of diffusibility in different directions, increases as the proportion of intracellular water increases (Takeda et al, 1997; Toft et al, 1996).

Interestingly, there is a striking decrease in the overall diffusion (decreased ADC) in the central white matter between 28 and 40 weeks of postconceptional age. This occurs even though there is very little myelin deposition during this stage of brain development. This reduction in water diffusivity is accompanied by increased directionality of diffusion (increased RA). Factors that are believed to increase RA during this stage of development include neurofilament development, axon alignment, a growing number of membrane barriers, greater cohesiveness and compactness of the fiber tracts, reduced extraaxonal space (i.e., greater packing), and changes in extracellular and intracellular matrix (Huppi et al, 1998).

PERFUSION IMAGING

Cerebral perfusion may be assessed on MR either by imaging during the administration of an exogenous contrast agent in dynamic susceptibility contrast-enhanced perfusion imaging (DSCE) or RF "tagging" of in-flowing protons in ASL. In DSCE, rapid imaging is performed during the bolus administration of a susceptibility contrast agent, such as gadolinium-DPTA. The passage of contrast through the microvasculature leads to decreases in signal intensity proportional to regional tissue perfusion. Analysis of the change in signal intensity over time can provide information on the time to peak contrast concentration, cerebral blood flow, cerebral blood volume, and mean transit time of the contrast (Laswad et al, 2009). Although DSCE can be performed in neonates, successful imaging requires a rapid injection of a relatively large volume of contrast material. The limited, small-gauge intravenous access frequently available in the neonate is not optimal for DSCE perfusion-weighted imaging.

ARTERIAL SPIN LABELING

ASL is a technique assessing cerebral perfusion without the use of intravenous contrast. It is carried out by labeling protons of the intravascular arterial blood using one or two radiofrequency pulses that invert the longitudinal magnetization of protons in arterial blood just upstream of the region of interest. The measurable magnetization and T1 relaxation time of the labeled blood will thus be modified. During acquisition (ultrafast echo planar type sequences), the signal obtained is the sum of the measurable magnetization of the region of interest and the magnetization from the labeled blood pool present in the explored volume. A second unlabeled acquisition serves as a reference to then calculate the perfusion images. The ability to assess perfusion without use of intravenous contrast medium and the relatively rapid acquisition times make ASL an attractive technique for use in the ill neonate. However, the signal intensity changes associated with perfusion in ASL are relatively modest, making the technique challenging to perform successfully.

SUSCEPTIBILITY-WEIGHTED IMAGING

All MRI techniques are susceptible to signal losses due to static inhomogeneities in the magnetic field. Mineralization and blood products cause local distortions in the magnetic field that can affect the MR image. The relative sensitivity of the MR image to perturbations in the magnetic field varies by sequence type. Gradient echo (GRE) imaging is particularly sensitive to static local magnetic field inhomogeneities and has long been used to detect regions of mineralization or prior hemorrhage. More recently, a newer technique, SWI, has been developed that provides both a greater sensitivity to magnetic field inhomogeneities and an ability to distinguish between blood products and mineralization by capturing information on proton spin phase. Although both paramagnetic substances (e.g., blood products) and diamagnetic substances (e.g., mineralization) alter proton spins, they do so in an opposite manner. Calcification and blood products, both of which cause a loss of signal on the MR image, can be distinguished from one another by evaluating the effect of their presence on proton spin phase images.

FUNCTIONAL MRI TECHNIQUES

Use of functional techniques such as magnetic resonance spectroscopy (MRS) and brain activation functional MRI (fMRI) using the blood oxygen level–dependent (BOLD) technique have increased the understanding of the biochemical and physiologic changes occurring in the neonatal brain in the first weeks to month of life. The following paragraphs discuss the value of some of these techniques.

Magnetic Resonance Spectroscopy

Proton MRS exploits the minute differences in magnetic moments of hydrogen atoms reflecting differences in their local chemical environment to produce spectra characteristic of a variety of metabolites (Keevil et al, 1998) (Figure 59-9). Because of its ability to detect both normal and abnormal metabolites in the brain, MRS is popular in the MR assessment of a number of processes affecting the newborn (Vigneron et al, 2001).

With most proton MRS techniques, the signal from water protons must be suppressed to demonstrate

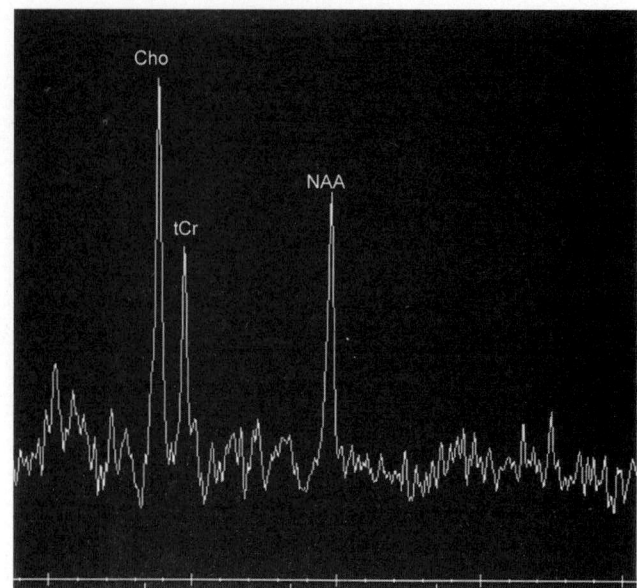

FIGURE 59-9 Single-voxel proton spectroscopy of the brain from a normal term neonate. The spectra were obtained with an echo time of 144 ms. Three prominent peaks are identified: At 3.2 ppm is choline *(Cho)*. Choline compounds are involved in the metabolism of membrane lipids. At 3.0 ppm is total creatine *(tCr)*. Creatine and phosphocreatine are involved in ATP metabolism. At 2.0 ppm is *N*-acetyl aspartate *(NAA)*. NAA is an intracellular compound found primarily in neurons. Note that lactate, which would appear, if present, as an inverted doublet at 1.3 ppm, is not seen in the normal newborn.

biologically interesting metabolites that are present in very small quantities. This requires a very homogeneous magnetic field that is generally found only in newer and higher-field-strength MR systems. Because of the tiny amount of signal emanating from the metabolites of interest, relatively large voxels (1 to 2 cm^3) must be acquired to obtain adequate signal intensity. MRS may be performed using single voxels, which sample a small region of the brain, or multiple voxels, by which many areas may be interrogated during a single acquisition (Vigneron et al, 2001). Typically, single-voxel MRS provides higher quality spectra than those available with multiple-voxel techniques.

Three metabolites are most apparent in the normal neonatal brain proton spectra: choline (3.2 ppm), total creatine (3.0 ppm), and *N*-acetyl aspartate (NAA) (2.0 ppm) (Heerschap and van den Berg, 1994). Choline compounds are central in the metabolism of membrane lipids and tend to be elevated in processes that result in rapid cell turnover. As a consequence of membrane development during myelination, the amount of choline present in the neonatal brain tends to be relatively large. The total creatine peak is composed of creatine and phosphocreatine, which serve as a reserve for high-energy phosphates in neurons and also as an ATP/ADP buffer. Total creatine tends to remain relatively constant in most intracranial processes (Govindaraju et al, 2000). NAA is an intracellular compound found primarily in neurons, although its biologic function is largely unknown (Miller, 1991). NAA is present in smaller quantities in the neonate than in the older child or adult.

Lactate is a terminal product of glycolysis. The tissue concentration of lactate can vary from minute to minute, depending on the status of a number of major metabolic pathways.

Lactate is not demonstrated on proton MRS in the normal newborn brain but may be seen as a prominent doublet at 1.3 ppm in certain pathologic conditions such as energy exhaustion due to ischemia/infarction or certain metabolic disorders. Depending on the parameters chosen for imaging, the lactate peaks may project above or below the baseline.

Brain Activation Function Magnetic Resonance Imaging

MR brain activation studies have been performed successfully in the neonate, albeit in limited scope (Anderson et al, 2001; Benaron et al, 2000; Born et al, 1998). The use of MRI to indirectly demonstrate cortical activation is based on the observation that regional blood flow varies with neuronal activity. That is, in areas of the brain that are activated, there is an increase in blood flow. During brain activation, the oxygen extraction fraction remains constant. Consequently, there is an increase in the local concentration of oxyhemoglobin and a decrease in the local concentration of deoxyhemoglobin in regions of activation (Buchbinder and Cosgrove, 1998). Deoxyhemoglobin has susceptibility effects that cause minor perturbations in the magnetic field, leading to signal loss. The increase in oxyhemoglobin that accompanies brain activation causes a local increase in signal intensity. These changes form the basis of the BOLD MRI technique. Because the signal changes associated with brain activation are quite small, a number of images must be averaged together to demonstrate cortical activation. Typically, therefore, BOLD imaging requires that the subject cooperate with repetitive tasks to demonstrate brain activation. Because the neonate is unable to perform such tasks, only those stimuli that produce an involuntary response, such as visual cortical activation with strobe light flashes, may be tested. Despite these limitations, the use of BOLD MRI to evaluate neonatal brain activation is an active area of research (Anderson et al, 2001; Benaron et al, 2000; Born et al, 1998).

NEAR INFRARED SPECTROSCOPY AND QUANTITATIVE DETERMINATIONS OF OXYGENATED HEMOGLOBIN

NIRS is a noninvasive optical imaging technique used to measure hemoglobin oxygenation in the blood in vivo. It can provide useful information about cerebral hemoglobin oxygen saturation, cerebral blood volume, cerebral blood flow, cerebral venous oxygen saturation, and cerebral oxygen availability and utilization (Franceschini et al, 2007).

The NIRS technique is based on the fact that light in the near-infrared range can pass relatively easily through the skin, bone, and other tissues in a newborn infant, and on the property of hemoglobin to absorb light in the near-infrared range. Appropriate selection of near-infrared wavelengths allows detection of the characteristic changes in light absorption of oxygenated and deoxygenated hemoglobin and oxygenated cytochrome aa_3. This in turn allows quantification of oxygenated and deoxygenated hemoglobin and determines the oxidation-reduction state of cytochrome oxidase. NIRS data is expressed as a percentage of HbO_2 saturation, or absolute changes in HbO_2, deoxyhemoglobin, and total hemoglobin in micromolar concentrations, referenced to an arbitrary baseline.

Significant advances in NIRS technique include development of frequency-domain and time-domain (FD-NIRS and TD-NIRS) devices that allow quantification of brain tissue oxygen (StO_2) and total hemoglobin concentration (HbT). Recently, FD-NIRS has been looked at in assessing neonatal brain injury (Grant et al, 2009). The results from early studies indicate that there is no significant difference in measured StO_2 between brain-injured and normal neonates, suggesting that StO_2 alone may be insensitive to evolving brain injury. Combining cerebral blood volume (CBV) and regional cerebral oxygen consumption ($CMRO_2$) has been shown in encouraging sensitivity and specificity values for FD-NIRS for detecting brain injury within the first 2 weeks of life (Grant et al, 2009).

CHOOSING THE APPROPRIATE TEST

Ultrasound is the modality of choice for monitoring and screening for suspected intracranial hemorrhage and PVL in the premature infant, and for detecting the subsequent complications of ventricular dilatation and progressive hydrocephalus. In the hands of skilled operators, it can be a very useful tool in the identification of congenital midline anomalies, cystic lesions, vascular malformations, and intracranial calcifications and in the definition of extraaxial fluid collections.

CT is superior to MRI, and remains the study of choice, for the detection of parenchymal calcification and demonstration of bone abnormalities. However, it is important to note that potential late untoward effects of radiation used for diagnostic CT scanning have been highlighted by a number of studies (Donnelly and Frush, 2001; Hall, 2007). The theoretical risk of malignancy related to exposure to ionizing radiation is highest in the neonate. Given that significant intracranial hemorrhage is detected by MRI as well as by CT, an argument can be made for eliminating CT for the evaluation of the encephalopathic term neonate, thereby avoiding the potential risks of ionizing radiation altogether (Robertson et al, 2003).

In addition to its ability to detect focal cerebral infarcts earlier than CT, MRI is superior to CT in detecting disorders of neuronal migration, abnormal myelination, arteriovenous malformations, venous thrombosis, differentiating hemorrhagic infarction from primary parenchymal hemorrhage, posterior fossa lesions (Figure 59-10), and almost all spinal cord abnormalities (Volpe, 2008).

IMAGING APPLICATIONS

NORMAL PRETERM VERSUS TERM INFANTS

The most obvious difference between the preterm and the term neonatal brain is relative maturation of the sulcal/gyral architecture. As with fetal imaging, the cerebral cortex of the preterm infants studied at 25 weeks of gestational age equivalent has a very smooth cortical mantle with a largely uncovered sylvian fissure and very few developed gyri. At this age, demonstration of lissencephaly and of some localized anomalies of cortical development is not possible with US and may be difficult with more advanced imaging techniques as well. Cortical maturation proceeds in a predictable fashion and should attain a fully developed

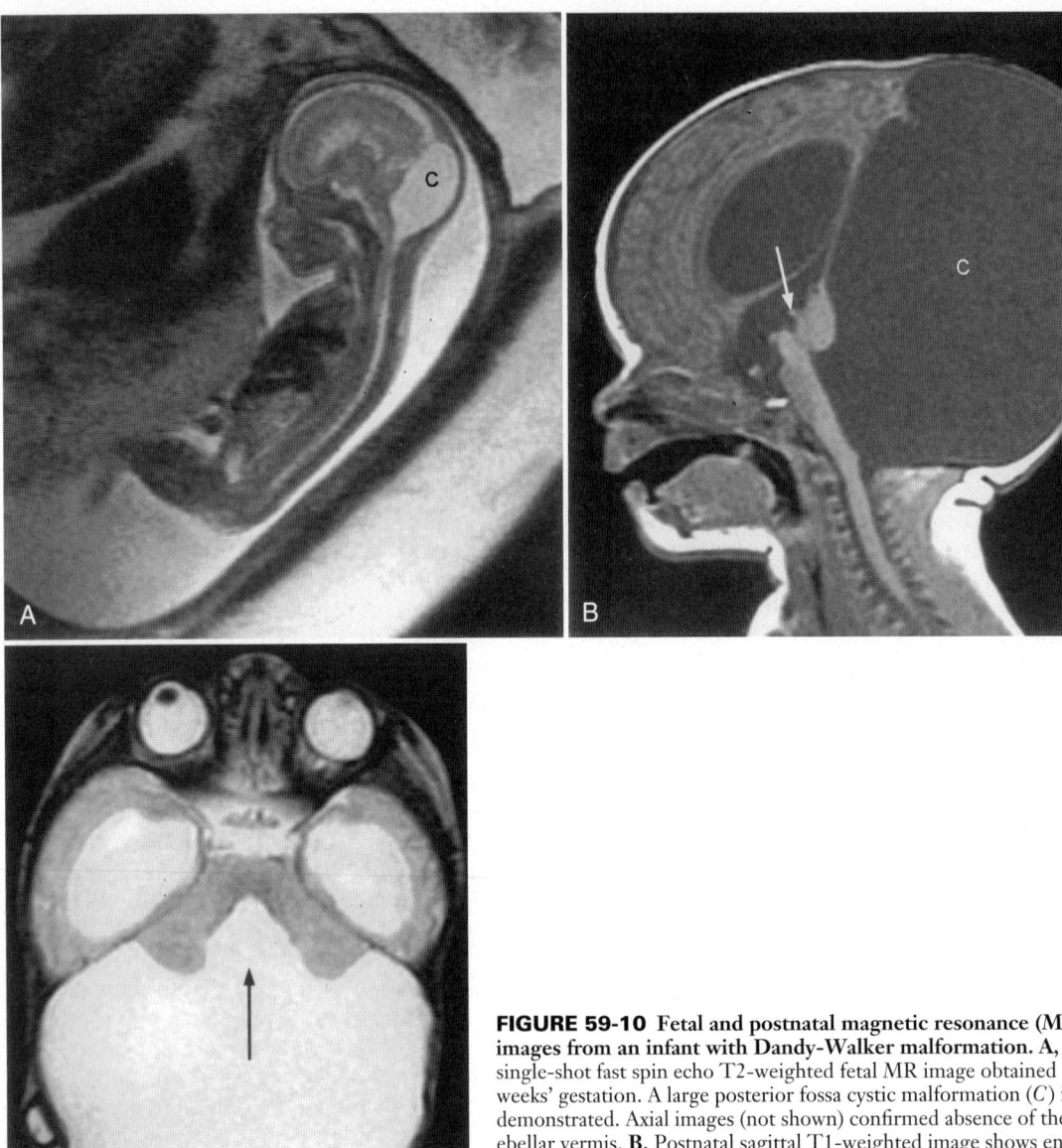

FIGURE 59-10 Fetal and postnatal magnetic resonance (MR) images from an infant with Dandy-Walker malformation. **A,** Sagittal single-shot fast spin echo T2-weighted fetal MR image obtained at 19.5 weeks' gestation. A large posterior fossa cystic malformation (*C*) is clearly demonstrated. Axial images (not shown) confirmed absence of the cerebellar vermis. **B,** Postnatal sagittal T1-weighted image shows enlargement of the posterior fossa cyst (*C*). There is dilatation of the lateral and third ventricles due to aqueductal stenosis indicated by elevation of the tectum (*arrow*). **C,** Absence of the cerebellar vermis is apparent on the axial T2-weighted image (*arrow*).

secondary sulcal/gyral pattern by 40 to 44 weeks of gestational age (Chi et al, 1977). On US, gyri are depicted as linear echoes that increase in length, undulation, and branching as the infant matures.

A prominent feature of both the preterm and the term neonatal brain is the very high water content of the unmyelinated subcortical white matter. In the premature infant, there is little difference in echogenicity between gray and white matter until 32 to 34 weeks' gestation. In the near-term infant, the cortical ribbon is hypoechoic in relation to the underlying white matter. Beyond 40 weeks' gestation, the overall echogenicity of white matter structures increases markedly, and visualization of deeper structures may become more difficult. On CT, unmyelinated white matter is hypodense relative to cortex and deep central gray matter. On MRI, the high water content of unmyelinated white matter produces marked prolongation of T1 and T2, causing the white matter to be hypointense to gray matter on T1-weighted imaging and hyperintense to gray matter on T2-weighted imaging. This pattern is the inverse of signal intensities of gray and white matter present in the fully myelinated brains of older children and adults (Barkovich, 2000; Barkovich et al, 1988). Because many pathologic processes result in edema, seen as low density on CT studies and resulting in T1 and T2 prolongation on MR images, these lesions are especially difficult to see in the neonatal white matter.

INTRACRANIAL HEMORRHAGE

Acute intracranial hemorrhage in the neonate may be epidural, subdural, subarachnoid, or parenchymal in location. Hemorrhages may be small and noted incidentally on

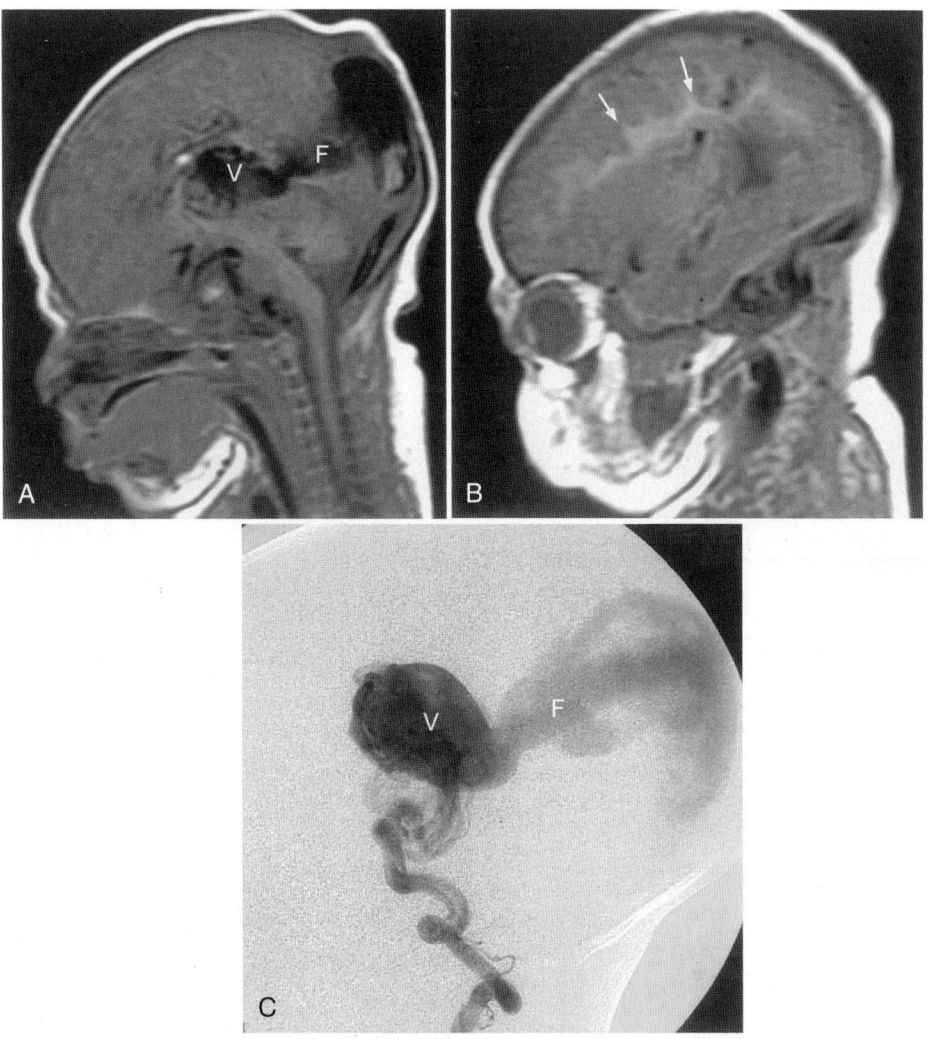

FIGURE 59-11 The patient was a neonate with congestive heart failure due to a Galenic arteriovenous malformation (also called vein of Galen aneurysm). **A,** Midline sagittal T1-weighted magnetic resonance (MR) image shows a signal void within the median prosencephalic vein (*V*), the embryologic precursor to the vein of Galen, and the persistent falcine sinus (*F*). **B,** Parasagittal T1-weighted MR image shows hyperintensity of the subcortical white matter (*arrows*) due to chronic ischemic injury. **C,** Selective vertebral artery conventional angiogram performed as part of a transcatheter therapeutic procedure shows flow within the varix (*V*) and draining sinus (*F*). Note that although the feeding arteries are markedly dilated because of the massive intracranial flow that is present, all of the blood flow is diverted through the fistulas, and there are no brain parenchymal branches filling. This "steal" phenomenon produces the ischemic changes that can be demonstrated with computed tomography and MR imaging.

imaging performed for other reasons or may be large and produce acute neurologic symptoms.

Small parturitional subdural hemorrhages are common even in the absence of a traumatic birth history and are often asymptomatic (Holden et al, 1999). Significant subdural hemorrhages are most frequently encountered in the setting of traumatic delivery, accidental trauma or, occasionally, nonaccidental trauma. Laceration of the falx cerebri or the tentorium cerebelli may produce large or rapidly expanding subdural hematomas. Larger subdural hematomas may be associated with acute or progressive symptoms due to intracranial mass effect.

A small amount of parturitional subarachnoid bleeding is not uncommon. Subarachnoid hemorrhage with larger amounts of bleeding may occasionally occur in conjunction with vascular malformations. The most common symptomatic intracranial vascular malformation in the newborn is the vein of Galen malformation (Figure 59-11). Although most newborns with vein of Galen

malformations present with cardiopulmonary distress due to high-output cardiac failure resulting from arteriovenous shunts, massive subarachnoid bleeding may occasionally occur from either spontaneous or iatrogenic perforation of the varix or feeding arteries.

Parenchymal hemorrhage in the preterm infant occurs most often in or around the highly cellular, gelatinous, and highly vascularized subependymal germinal matrix. Although its pathogenesis is multifactorial (Volpe, 2008), a common final pathway seems to be microscopic perivenular hemorrhage in the highly vascular germinal matrix (Ghazi-Birry et al, 1997).

The classification originally proposed by Papile and colleagues remains the most widely accepted method of grading the severity of germinal matrix hemorrhage in the preterm infant (Papile et al, 1983). Grade I consists of subependymal hemorrhage only (Figures 59-12 and 59-13). On US, grade I hemorrhages appear as bright echogenic foci in the subependymal area typically located in or

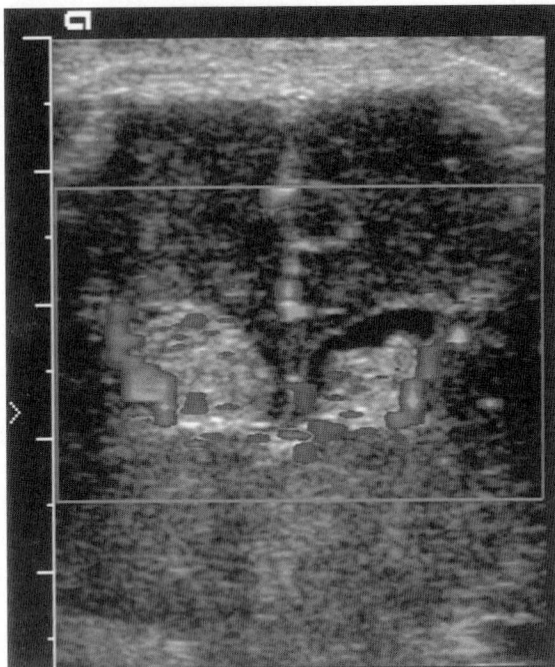

FIGURE 59-12 *(See also Color Plate 24.)* **Coronal color Doppler image of bilateral grade I germinal matrix hemorrhages.** The hemorrhages are echogenic. Although flow is confirmed within the terminal veins (*blue*), the veins are laterally displaced by the subependymal hemorrhages.

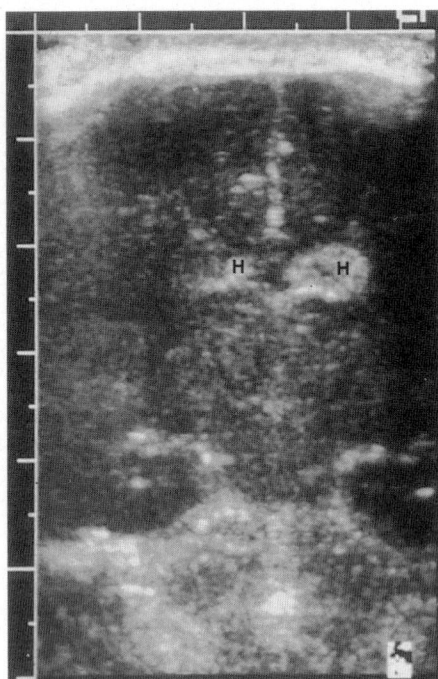

FIGURE 59-14 **Coronal ultrasound study of bilateral grade II intracranial hemorrhage in the preterm neonate.** Echogenic subependymal hemorrhages (*H*) are seen extending into the lateral ventricles. There is no hydrocephalus.

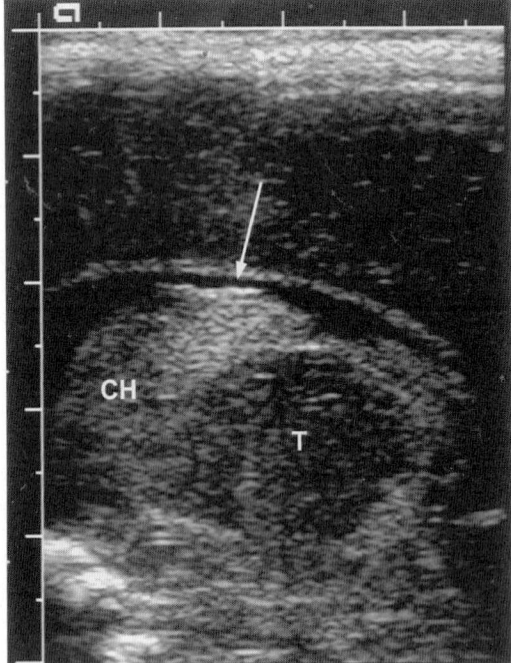

FIGURE 59-13 **Sagittal ultrasound study of grade I germinal matrix hemorrhage.** Echogenic hemorrhage (*arrow*) is seen at the caudothalamic notch situated between the caudate head (*CH*) anteriorly and the thalamus (*T*) posteriorly.

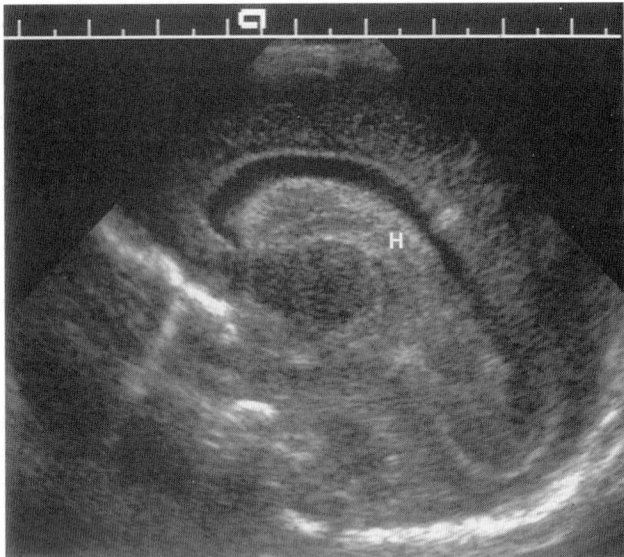

FIGURE 59-15 **Sagittal ultrasound study of grade III intracranial hemorrhage.** The lateral ventricle is moderately dilated and filled with echogenic blood (*H*).

anterior to the caudothalamic notch. Grade II is defined as subependymal and intraventricular hemorrhage without ventricular dilatation (Figure 59-14). Grade III is the combination of subependymal and intraventricular hemorrhage with ventricular dilatation by clot (Figure 59-15).

Small choroid plexus hemorrhages may be difficult to distinguish from a normal "lumpy bumpy" choroid plexus, because both are brightly echogenic. Larger, acute intraventricular clots can be identified as echogenic irregular and asymmetrical masses. Poorly clotted blood will often result in a fluid-debris level within the ventricle that disappears or is redistributed when the baby is repositioned and blood is remixed with CSF. In critically ill premature infants it is important to distinguish progression of a grade II hemorrhage to grade III from the development of

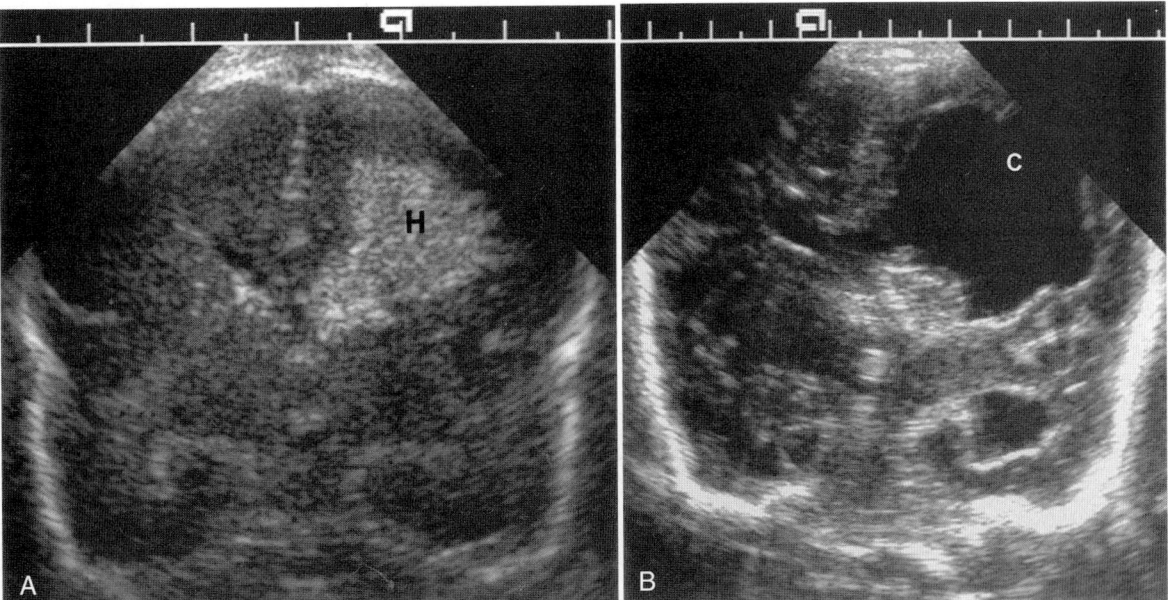

FIGURE 59-16 Coronal ultrasound study of intraparenchymal hemorrhage. **A,** Initially the parenchymal hemorrhage (*H*) is echogenic. **B,** As the hematoma ages, liquefaction occurs and the hematoma becomes echolucent with the development of a porencephalic cyst (*C*).

posthemorrhagic hydrocephalus. Both entities are associated with intraventricular clot and dilatation of the ventricular system. However, in grade III hemorrhage, the ventricle is almost completely distended by clot, whereas the ventricle in posthemorrhagic hydrocephalus is often primarily distended with CSF. The size of the obstructing intraventricular clot may be relatively small. The distinction is important because ventricular dilatation caused by increasing hemorrhage may have therapeutic implications different from those associated with posthemorrhagic hydrocephalus.

Destruction of the germinal matrix and the precursor glial cells within it is the most consistent consequence of the periventricular hemorrhage. This destruction of glial cells has an adverse effect on subsequent brain development (Volpe, 2008).

Up to 15% of very low birthweight infants with intraventricular hemorrhage develop hemorrhagic necrosis in the periventricular white matter. A number of neuropathologic studies have shown that simple extension of blood into the periventricular white matter does not account for this periventricular hemorrhagic necrosis. Instead, this finding is now believed to be a hemorrhagic infarction, resulting from venous congestion of the terminal medullary veins in the region of residual germinal matrix at the caudothalamic groove (see Figure 59-11). This hemorrhagic venous infarction can be depicted with color Doppler techniques (Taylor, 1995, 1997). The most common result of the periventricular hemorrhagic infarction is a large porencephalic cyst, either alone or in combination with other smaller cysts.

Periventricular hemorrhagic infarction (PVHI), formerly described as a grade 4 germinal matrix hemorrhage (GMH) in the original classification, is now thought to be caused by pressure of the GMH on the periventricular terminal medullary veins that drain the cerebral hemispheres (Volpe, 1998). This leads to venous congestion in the periventricular white matter and subsequently to

ischemia and hemorrhage (see Figure 59-15). PVHI, or venous infarction, is now considered a complication of the GMH instead of an extension of the GMH. PVHI is seen in 10% to 15% of preterm infants with germinal matrix hemorrhage and is, on occasion, documented in the fetus on obstetrical sonography or fetal MRI.

In the term infant, lobar parenchymal and subpial hemorrhages are occasionally encountered (Koenigsberger, 1999) (Figure 59-16). These hemorrhages appear to occur spontaneously in the first few days of life in otherwise healthy babies.

Spontaneous superficial parenchymal and leptomeningeal hemorrhage occurs in otherwise healthy term neonates (Figure 59-17). The hemorrhage is most often in the temporal lobe and in proximity to sutures, often accompanied by minor overlying soft tissue swelling and subjacent decreased diffusion in the brain parenchyma. This pattern suggests the possibility of local trauma with contusion or venous compression or occlusion as contributing to the development of these hemorrhages (Huang and Robertson, 2004).

Color Doppler US may be used to characterize extracerebral fluid collections as subarachnoid, subdural, or combined. Because superficial cortical blood vessels lie within the pia-arachnoid, fluid in the subarachnoid space lifts the cortical vessels away from the brain surface, whereas fluid in the subdural space approximates cortical vessels to the brain surface and is separated from these vessels by a thin membrane (Figure 59-18). Correlation with MRI and CT suggests that color Doppler is reliable in making this differentiation (Chen et al, 1996).

Suspected intracranial hemorrhage remains one of the most common indications for brain CT in the neonate. On CT, acute hemorrhage appears hyperdense relative to the brain parenchyma (see Figure 59-18). Of note, the dural venous sinuses and cortical veins appear relatively dense during the first few days of life as a result of high hematocrit levels. This normal density of the venous structures

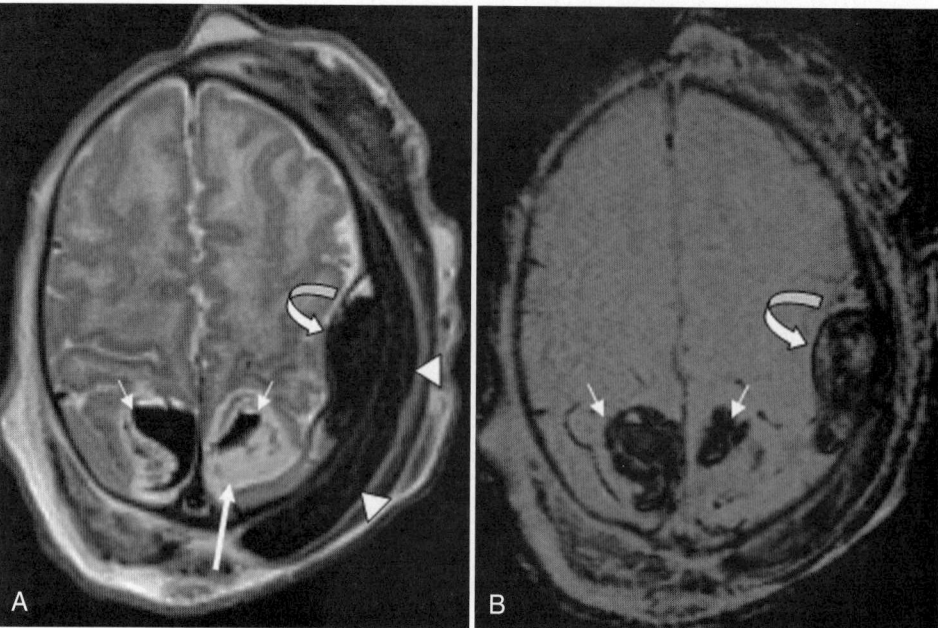

FIGURE 59-17 The patient is a term neonate scanned on day 2 after a failed forceps delivery and low Apgar scores and acidosis at birth. **A,** Axial T2-weighted image shows bilateral parasagittal right and left subpial hemorrhages (*arrows*) with surrounding edema (*long arrow*). There is a left frontoparietal epidural hematoma (*curved arrow*) and a large subgaleal hematoma (*arrowheads*) as well. **B,** Corresponding susceptibility-weighted image shows large areas of susceptibility corresponding to the areas of subpial (*arrows*), epidural (*curved arrow*), and subgaleal hemorrhage (*arrowheads*).

should not be mistaken for subdural bleeding or dural venous sinus thrombosis on CT. As blood ages, the density of the clot will decrease. In the chronic phase, sites of extraaxial or parenchymal hemorrhage have decreased density relative to the brain parenchyma. Parturitional subdural hemorrhages are typically completely resolved by 6 to 8 weeks of life.

Until recently, MRI was considered to be less sensitive for the detection of acute intracranial hemorrhage than CT. However, if either gradient echo sequences or the more recently described SWI technique is used, all significant intracranial hemorrhages in the newborn are reliably demonstrated by MRI (Blankenberg et al, 2000; Robertson et al, 2003). On MRI, the signal intensity of blood varies with age.

Although the timing for the development of the various stages of hemorrhage in the neonate may differ from that in the adult, the signal intensity changes are similar. With hyperacute hemorrhage, unclotted blood appears similar to free fluid (i.e., low signal intensity on T1-weighted images and high signal intensity on T2-weighted images). Within hours, oxyhemoglobin is converted to deoxyhemoglobin. Deoxyhemoglobin within the red blood cells causes susceptibility artifact that produces low signal intensity on T2-weighted images (Figure 59-19). Over the first several days, deoxyhemoglobin is converted to methemoglobin, which results in high signal intensity on T1-weighted images and low signal intensity on T2-weighted images. Subsequently, the red blood cells lyse, and an increase in signal intensity is observed on the T2-weighted images. Chronically, hemosiderin staining occurs, which appears dark on both T1-weighted and T2-weighted images.

The administration of contrast agent is not usually required in the MRI investigation of hemorrhage, except in the rare case of suspected underlying tumor. When tumor is present, it is imperative that spinal imaging also be performed because most brain tumors discovered in the newborn period have a propensity to seed the CSF.

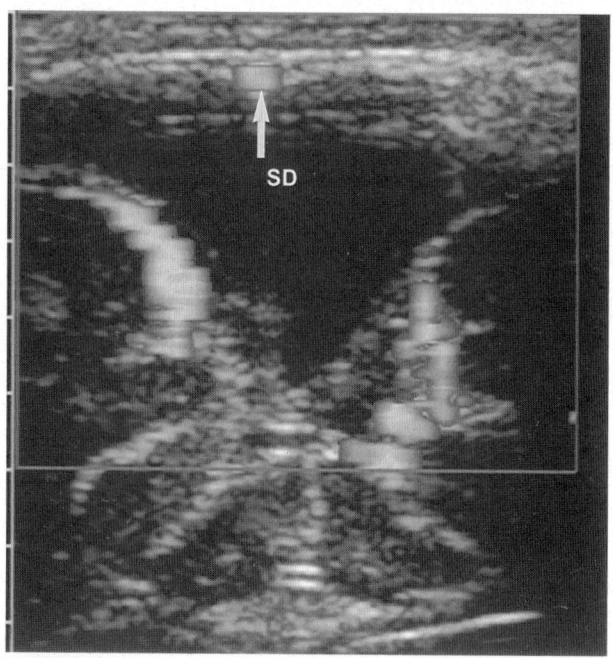

FIGURE 59-18 *(See also Color Plate 25.)* Coronal color Doppler ultrasound study shows that the vessels (color) are displaced toward the brain parenchyma by the subdural fluid (*SD*). Note flow in the superior sagittal sinus (*arrow*).

NEONATAL CEREBRAL INFARCTION

Neonatal cerebral infarction is a common cause of infant morbidity and mortality (Rivkin, 1997; Volpe, 2008). Infarctions in the newborn may be due to global transient decreases in blood flow or in oxygen delivery to the brain (hypoxic-ischemic injury) (Figure 59-20) or to focal arterial or venous occlusions (Figures 59-21 to 59-23). Hypoxia-ischemia tends to produce bilaterally symmetric lesions, whereas arterial or venous occlusions are associated with focal or asymmetric multifocal areas of

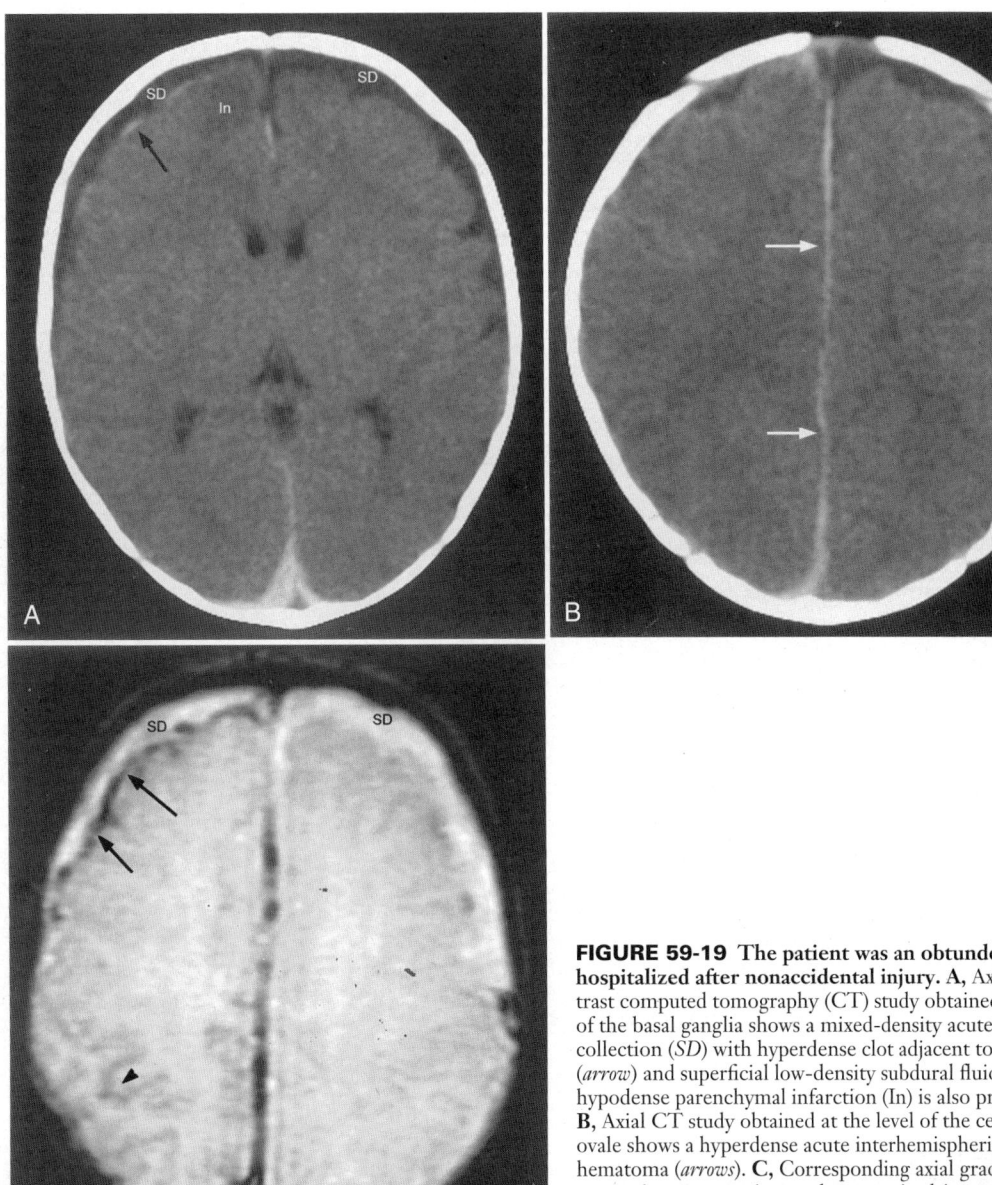

FIGURE 59-19 **The patient was an obtunded neonate hospitalized after nonaccidental injury. A,** Axial noncontrast computed tomography (CT) study obtained at the level of the basal ganglia shows a mixed-density acute subdural collection (*SD*) with hyperdense clot adjacent to the brain (*arrow*) and superficial low-density subdural fluid. A small hypodense parenchymal infarction (In) is also present. **B,** Axial CT study obtained at the level of the centrum semiovale shows a hyperdense acute interhemispheric-subdural hematoma (*arrows*). **C,** Corresponding axial gradient-echo magnetic resonance image shows a mixed-intensity subdural collection with hypointense clot (*arrows*) adjacent to the brain and hyperintense supernatant (*SD*). A small amount of subarachnoid blood is also present (*arrowhead*).

infarction. A variety of imaging appearances of infarction may be observed at a given postnatal age, and lack of specificity in the clinical presentation may further complicate the interpretation of the imaging (Robertson and Robson, 2001).

In the term infant, the vascular border-zone territories are in a parasagittal location, anteriorly between the major branches of the anterior and middle cerebral arteries and posteriorly between the branches of the anterior, middle, and posterior cerebral arteries. In our experience, border-zone ischemic injury in the term neonate most often occurs in conjunction with deep central gray and white matter injury in cases of profound hypoxia-ischemia.

Profound hypoxia-ischemia in the preterm or term infant tends to affect those regions of the brain with the greatest metabolic requirements. These include areas with high concentrations of excitatory neurotransmitters or regions that are actively myelinating (Rivkin, 1997; Volpe, 1997). The dorsal brainstem, thalami, posterior portions of basal ganglia, posterior limb of internal capsule, corona radiate, and mesial temporal lobes are especially susceptible to injury (see Figure 59-19). The medial portions of the cerebellar hemispheres and cerebellar vermis are also commonly affected. Areas of the brain with lower energy requirements, such as unmyelinated white matter and cortex, tend to be relatively spared unless the ischemia is particularly severe. After severe hypoxia-ischemia, the pattern of tissue injury is variable. In some infants, a deep central gray matter distribution of injury with relative preservation of the cortex and subcortical white matter is present (Roland et al, 1998). In other infants, there is widespread necrosis, ultimately producing a pattern of cystic encephalomalacia.

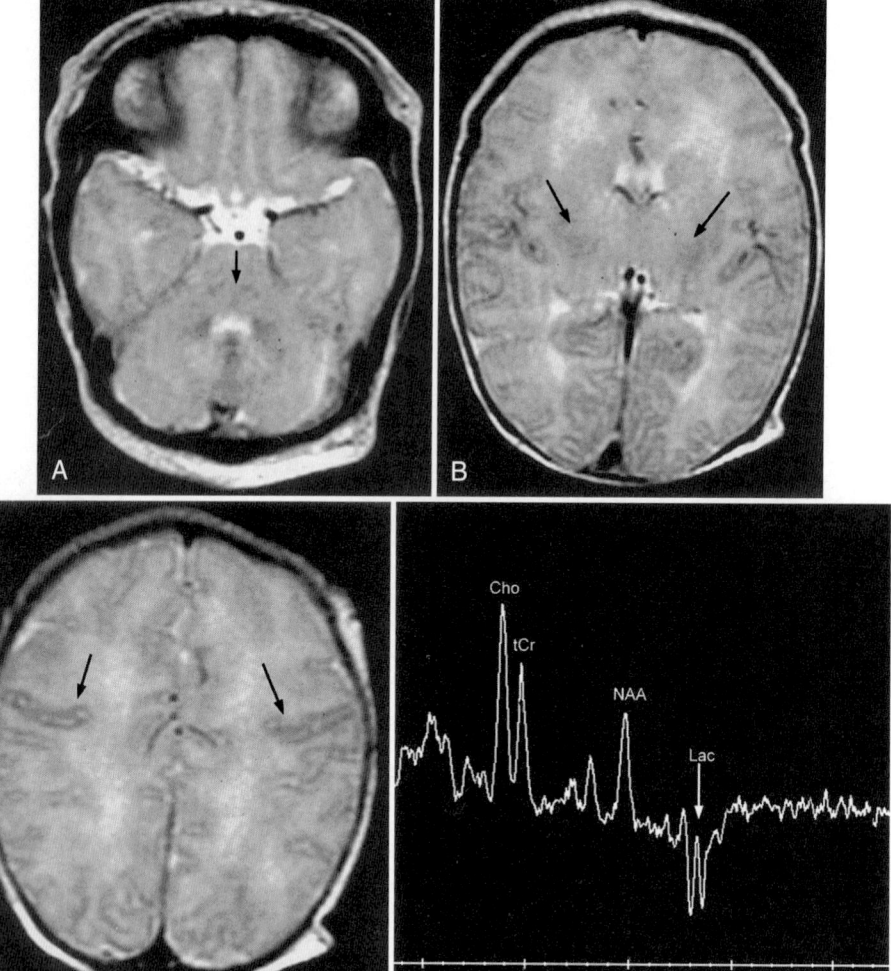

FIGURE 59-20 Magnetic resonance images obtained at 24 hours of life in a neonate with profound hypoxic-ischemic brain injury. Compare with normal T2-weighted and diffusion images (see Figures 59-6 and 59-7). **A** to **C**, T2-weighted images demonstrate edema with loss of normal hypointensity in the dorsal pons (*arrow*) **(A)** and the lateral thalami and internal capsule (*arrows*) **(B)**. Markedly decreased diffusion is seen in the lateral thalami and internal capsule on the apparent diffusion coefficient maps (*arrows*) **(C)**. **D**, Single-voxel spectroscopy obtained from the left basal ganglia demonstrates a prominent lactate doublet (*Lac*). The peaks project above the baseline because of the echo time used (TE = 270 ms). *Cho,* Choline; *NAA, N*-acetyl aspartate; *Cr1* and *Cr2,* two peaks of creatine.

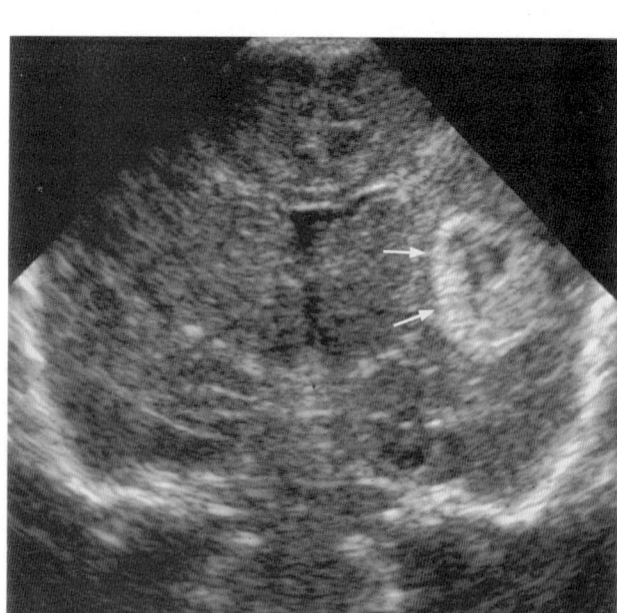

FIGURE 59-21 Coronal ultrasound image shows an echogenic left middle cerebral artery distribution infarction (*arrows*).

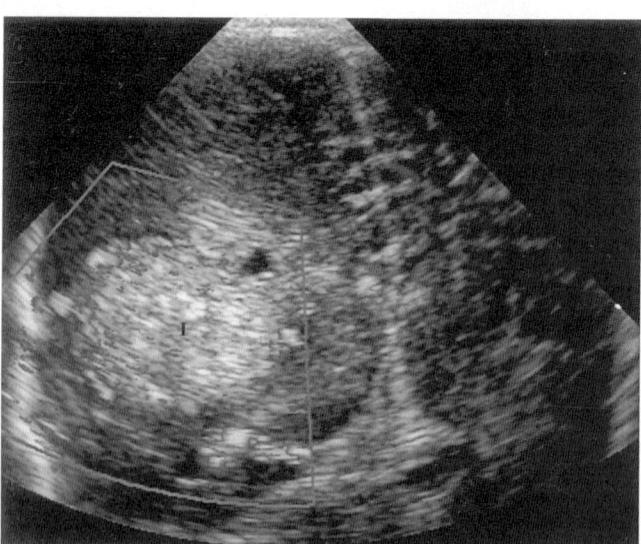

FIGURE 59-22 *(See also Color Plate 26.)* **The patient was a neonate with a focal right occipital infarction with surrounding "luxury perfusion."** A coronal ultrasound image obtained through the anterior fontanel shows a hyperechoic right occipital infarction (*I*) surrounded by increased flow on color Doppler examination.

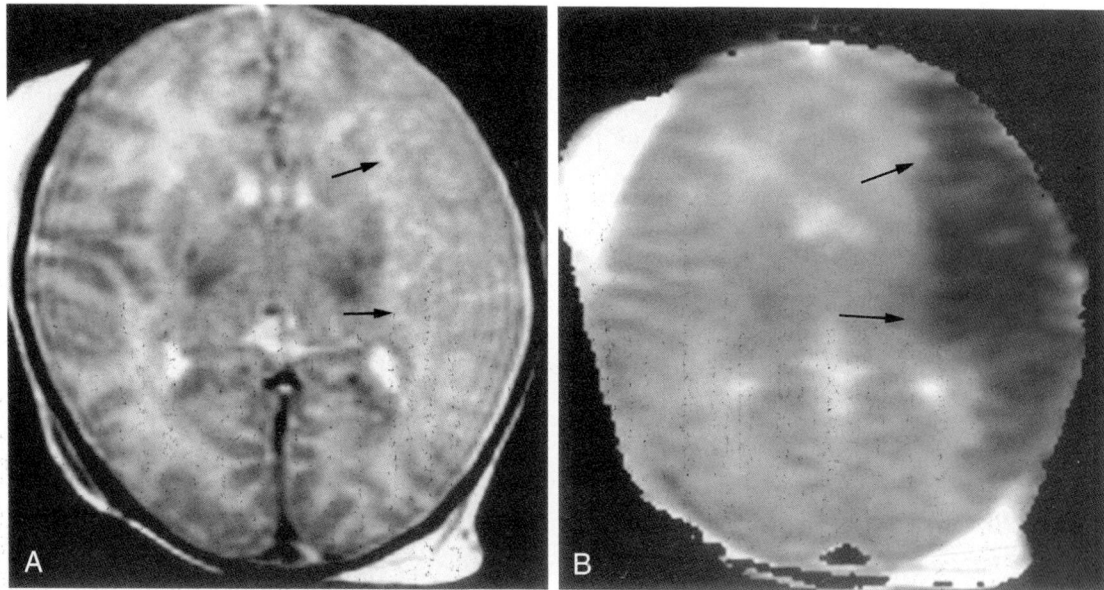

FIGURE 59-23 Magnetic resonance imaging of a focal left middle cerebral artery infarction in a 6-day-old neonate. **A,** Axial T2-weighted image shows edema and loss of the cortical ribbon in the left middle cerebral artery territory (*arrows*). **B,** Apparent diffusion coefficient (ADC) map shows markedly restricted diffusion (hypointensity) in the area of infarction (*arrows*).

The deep central pattern of injury is associated with a variable outcome, whereas widespread encephalomalacia more consistently portends a poor prognosis.

On cranial US, ischemic areas of thalamus and basal ganglia may appear focally or diffusely echogenic. US findings may be quite variable in time of onset and are insensitive to the extent of injury compared to CT or MRI.

In the first few hours after hypoxia-ischemia, brain CT findings are usually normal. Depending on the severity of the insult, changes may begin to be apparent in 24 to 48 hours. In severe hypoxia-ischemia, the thalami and basal ganglia develop low density. The cortical ribbon may become indistinct or even indistinguishable from the subcortical white matter. A subset of babies with hypoxia-ischemia will develop mineralization and hypermyelination in the deep gray matter structures, producing hyperdensity in these structures, an appearance termed status marmoratus.

Although there is considerable variability in the MR appearance of hypoxia-ischemia, some general trends may be observed (Johnson et al, 1999; Robertson et al, 1999; Rutherford et al, 1995; Wolf et al, 2001). Up to 15 to 18 hours after the ischemic event, the diffusion-weighted imaging is often normal. At this time, T1- and T2-weighted sequences typically also fail to show any abnormality. Some studies indicate that measuring the ADC values in visibly normal appearing brain, particularly in the basal ganglia and brainstem, may correlate with outcome (Liauw et al, 2009). Progressively over the next 24 to 48 hours, restricted diffusion develops within the regions of the brain with the highest metabolic requirements (Robertson and Robson, 2001). During this time, the T1- and T2-weighted images also become abnormal (Barkovich et al, 1995). Toward the end of the 1st week, it is not uncommon to demonstrate decreased diffusion in the subcortical white matter in areas that on early examinations showed normal or even increased diffusion (Robertson

et al, 1999). These white matter regions typically show hyperintensity on T2-weighted sequences in advance of the development of decreased diffusion. By 10 to 14 days, the diffusion abnormalities typically normalize, and ultimately, increased diffusion may be present. Chronically, T1-weighted and T2-weighted sequences show areas of signal abnormalities related to gliosis, mineralization, or hypermyelination associated with variable tissue loss.

MRS also has been used to evaluate neonates with hypoxia-ischemia (Barkovich et al, 1999; Cady, 2001). The observed changes on MRS in newborns with hypoxia-ischemia include the presence of lactate, indicating energy failure, and a decrease in NAA, suggesting decreased neuronal density or activity (see Figure 59-19). The demonstration of lactate requires the use of a long echo sequence (e.g., echo time [TE] of 135 ms or 270 ms). On the 135-ms TE acquisition, lactate is seen as a doublet peak projecting below the baseline at 1.3 ppm (lactate peaks project above the baseline at the 270-ms TE). Lactate is evident within the first few hours after onset of hypoxia-ischemia. The amount of lactate slowly diminishes over the ensuing several days. Occasionally, elevation of lactate levels will recur several weeks after the insult (Hanrahan et al, 1998). The etiology of this delayed appearance of lactate is uncertain, but it may be due to the production of lactate by macrophages moving into the area of infarction as part of the reparative process. Studies have shown that the presence of lactate within the basal ganglia or as a delayed finding is associated with an abnormal neurologic outcome at 1 year of age (Barkovich et al, 1999; Hanrahan et al, 1998).

Focal infarctions most often occur in a middle cerebral artery distribution (de Vries et al, 1997, 1999; Sreenan et al, 2000) (see Figures 59-20 and 59-21). Focal infarcts may be small and involve the cortex only, or they may involve the subcortical white matter, internal capsule, and basal ganglia. Infarcts that are confined to the cortex tend to carry a relatively good prognosis. Lesions also involving the internal capsule and basal ganglia are usually associated with a persistent hemiparesis (de Vries et al, 1999; Mercuri et al, 1999).

Sonographically, focal infarcts initially manifest as geographic areas of increased echogenicity, followed by progressively increased echogenicity and loss of gyral and sulcal definition (see Figure 59-21). Mass effect and effacement of the ventricular system are often present. Initially there is diminished flow demonstrated on duplex and color Doppler US. Over time, increased flow in the surrounding tissues consistent with "luxury perfusion" can be seen on color Doppler US (see Figure 59-22) (Hernanz-Schulman et al, 1988; Taylor, 1994).

On CT, focal infarcts appear as localized regions of hypodensity with loss of the cortical ribbon. Hemorrhagic conversion of an arterial infarction in the newborn is uncommon.

On MRI, focal infarcts are seen as regions of low signal intensity on T1-weighted sequences and high signal intensity on T2-weighted sequences (see Figure 59-23). Signal alterations occur earlier and more consistently on both diffusion and conventional MRI in focal infarctions than in hypoxia-ischemia (Robertson et al, 1999).

Unlike imaging in hypoxia-ischemia, even on the first day of life, the diffusion and the conventional imaging will typically demonstrate focal infarctions (Robertson et al, 1999). Also unlike hypoxia-ischemia, focal infarctions in the neonate do not usually show an increase in extent on follow-up imaging. The diffusion abnormality tends to normalize by 10 to 14 days. Atrophic changes are generally apparent on follow-up T1- and T2-weighted images; however, the degree of accompanying gliosis is variable. At times, chronic infarcts may appear simply as focally prominent sulci.

Venous infarction resulting from thrombosis of the internal cerebral veins and perimedullary veins must be considered in neonates presenting with hemorrhagic infarcts, particularly around the thalamus (Figure 59-24).

PERIVENTRICULAR LEUKOMALACIA

Periventricular leukomalacia is the most common form of white matter injury of prematurity (Inder et al, 1999; Volpe, 1997). PVL is characterized by focal necrotic lesions in the periventricular white matter, optic radiations, and acoustic radiations and less prominent, more diffuse cerebral white matter injury. In the premature infant, these sites have in common their location in vascular border zones, lying between the long penetrating branches of the middle, anterior, and posterior cerebral arteries that pierce the cortex from the pial surface and the basal penetrating vasculature suggesting an ischemic origin of the lesions (e.g., lenticulostriate and choroidal vessels) (Shuman and Selednik, 1980; Volpe, 2008). As the fetus or infant approaches term, there is a gradual shift in these border zone territories toward a parasagittal location. Neuropathologically, PVL is characterized in the acute phase by coagulation necrosis and neuroaxonal swelling (Volpe, 2008). A variable amount of hemorrhage may be present. In the subacute stage, cysts may form in the larger lesions. Ultimately, astrogliosis develops and the cysts become less apparent.

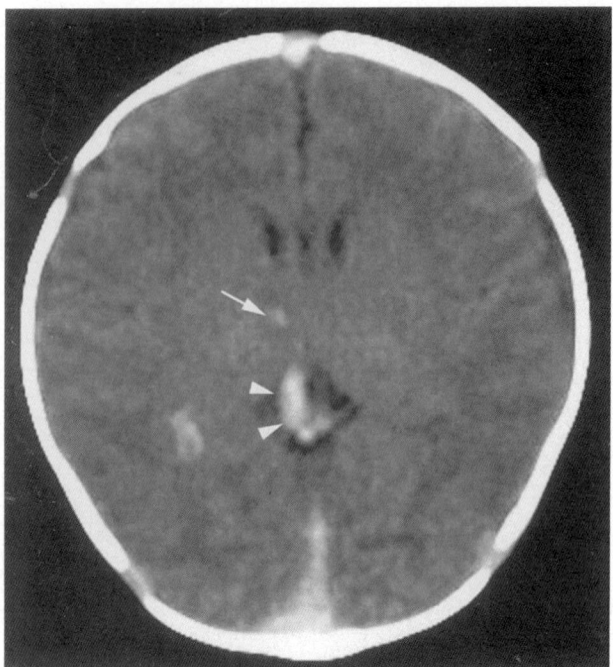

FIGURE 59-24 The patient was a newborn with sagittal sinus, straight sinus, and right internal cerebral vein thrombosis and right thalamic hemorrhagic venous infarction. An axial, non–contrast-enhanced CT scan shows high-density clot (*arrowheads*) in the right internal cerebral vein and a small hemorrhagic infarction (*arrow*) in the right thalamus.

The US appearance of the brain may be normal within the first 2 weeks after the inciting event. After 10 to 14 days, the echogenicity of affected areas of deep white matter increases. These areas of abnormality may be focal or diffuse, symmetrical or asymmetrical. They are typically located along the trigones of the lateral ventricles but can involve extensive areas of white matter. PVL is seldom associated with mass effect and displacement of surrounding structures. Cystic encephalomalacia appears in the areas of increased echogenicity within 2 to 3 weeks after the initial insult (Figure 59-25). These are characterized by cysts ranging between 1 mm and 2-3 cm in size. They may be single or multiple and may occasionally communicate with the ventricular system. Focal or hemispheric atrophy is the final stage of PVL and is characterized by dilatation of the ipsilateral ventricle and prominence of the sulci and interhemispheric fissure (Schellinger et al, 1984).

White matter lesions, including those due to PVL, are difficult to detect in the neonate using either CT or MRI because of the inherent high water content of unmyelinated white matter. On CT, even relatively large cysts may be inapparent. Occasionally, the cystic areas may appear slightly more lucent (hypodense) than the surrounding parenchyma. Acute hemorrhagic lesions are hyperdense. The cystic phase of PVL is also difficult to identify on MRI, because the cysts are characterized by long T1 (hypointensity) and long T2 (hyperintensity), similar to normal unmyelinated white matter. Hemorrhagic lesions appear as foci of hyperintensity on T1-weighted sequences and hypointensity on T2-weighted sequences (Figure 59-26). PVL has been reported to show decreased diffusion in the acute phase (Inder et al, 1999).

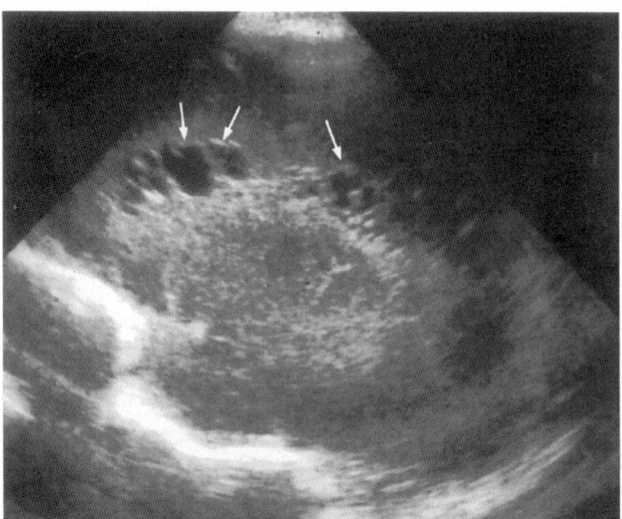

FIGURE 59-25 Sagittal ultrasound image of cystic periventricular leukomalacia demonstrates multiple echolucent periventricular cysts (*arrows*) involving the frontal, parietal, and occipital white matter.

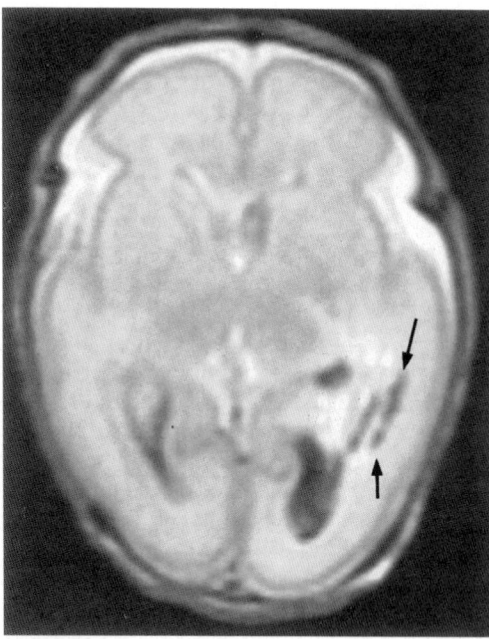

FIGURE 59-26 Axial T2-weighted magnetic resonance image from a 26-week-gestation premature infant. Hemorrhagic PVL is indicated by periventricular hypointensity (*arrows*). Intraventricular hypointense hemorrhage is also present in this neonate.

CONGENITAL MALFORMATIONS

Although use of cranial sonography is limited by the available acoustic windows, many structural anomalies of the brain can be well characterized by this portable technique. However, for most congenital anomalies, MRI has become the most definitive imaging examination (Barkovich, 1988). The multiplanar capability and inherent high tissue contrast of MRI make it superior to CT for the delineation of most congenital malformations. Additionally, unlike CT, MR images are not degraded by artifact from bone. Therefore, MRI is able to provide a detailed evaluation of the regions of the supratentorial brain near the skull base and the posterior fossa.

For most congenital brain malformations, standard T1-weighted and T2-weighted images are sufficient to characterize the anomaly with MRI. Multiplanar conventional imaging is usually all that is required to characterize disorders of structural development including the holoprosencephaly spectrum, malformations of the corpus callosum, leptomeningeal malformations, and posterior fossa malformations (Dodge and Dobyns, 1995; Lena et al, 1995; Rubinstein et al, 1996; Smith et al, 1996) (see Figure 59-9). Thin-section, high-resolution volumetric images may be reformatted in multiple planes to show structural relationships. Intravenous contrast is not usually required for the MR evaluation of congenital brain anomalies.

Although CT is not considered the imaging modality of choice for most congenital brain malformations, it may be used to assess bone integrity and to search for parenchymal calcifications. CT is useful in the assessment of scalp lesions and for calvarial or skull-base defects in the setting of certain intracranial lesions such as cephaloceles and dermoids (Ruge et al, 1988). Sutural synostosis, although only occasionally presenting in the newborn, is best assessed with three-dimensional CT. Cutis aplasia may require CT evaluation to determine the extent of underlying bone deficiency (Madsen et al, 1998).

High-resolution CT is useful for anatomic delineation of facial and temporal bone lesions (Vanzieleghem et al,

2001). Choanal atresia, especially if bilateral, may require urgent CT assessment. Nasal pits or dermoids are typically evaluated using a combination of high-resolution CT for bone detail and MRI for soft-tissue extent of the lesion (Lusk and Lee, 1986). Most temporal bone anomalies do not require intervention during the neonatal period; therefore, CT studies are usually deferred until later in infancy.

VASCULAR MALFORMATIONS

Vascular malformations are classified on the basis of hemodynamics as high-flow or low-flow anomalies (Meyer et al, 1991). High-flow lesions include arteriovenous fistula, with direct, macroscopic connections between arteries and veins, and arteriovenous malformation, with a meshwork of dysplastic vessels termed a *nidus* interposed between the supplying artery and the draining vein. Low-flow vascular malformations include cavernous malformation, developmental venous anomaly, and capillary telangiectasia. Both high- and low-flow intracranial vascular malformations may be present in the newborn; however, it is typically the high-flow lesions that are likely to be symptomatic during the neonatal period.

Many high-flow vascular malformations are now diagnosed in utero using fetal US or MRI. A majority of high-flow vascular malformations manifest in the neonate with symptoms related to high-output cardiac failure (Lasjaunias et al, 1986). CT and postnatal MRI are not typically required to diagnose the presence of the malformation but may provide useful information with respect to prognosis. In high-flow lesions, blood flow is diverted away from the brain parenchyma and through the shunt(s), so that ischemic brain injury may result (see Figure 59-11).

The presence of encephalomalacia and parenchymal calcification on CT indicates chronic ischemic injury and is associated with a poor neurologic outcome (Brunelle, 1997). CT angiography (CTA) and CT venography (CTV) may occasionally be performed to characterize the arterial supply and size of shunts before intervention.

MRI will show changes similar to those seen with CT including parenchymal ischemic changes (see Figure 59-11, *B*). MRA/MRV can be used in a similar fashion to that for CTA/CTV to characterize the vascular anomaly. However, MRA/MRV is prone to signal loss related to turbulent flow and may therefore be less reliable than CTA/CTV in high-flow lesions.

Conventional catheter angiography is usually performed as a part of a planned endovascular approach to therapy. Subselective vascular injections are used to carefully define the anatomy of the arteriovenous shunts. The choice of embolic material employed depends on the nature and location of the shunts. Sonography with color and duplex Doppler techniques may be used as an adjunct to monitor changing cerebral hemodynamics and complications during endovascular procedures.

Low-flow intracranial vascular anomalies are occasionally encountered as incidental findings on brain CT and MRI in the newborn. Hemorrhage due to low-flow vascular anomalies is exceedingly rare in the neonate.

HYDROCEPHALUS

Hydrocephalus is one of the most common reasons to perform brain imaging in the newborn. Hydrocephalus is nearly always due to an obstruction of CSF resorption. The blockage may occur within the ventricles or in the extracerebral CSF spaces. Hydrocephalus due to the overproduction of CSF is exceedingly rare but may occasionally occur with choroid plexus papilloma or choroid plexus hyperplasia (Figure 59-27).

Hydrocephalus may be either congenital or acquired. Congenital causes of hydrocephalus include Chiari II malformation, aqueductal stenosis, encephalocele, universal craniosynostosis, and skull base dysplasia with jugular venous stenosis as in Crouzon syndrome (McLone and Naidich, 1992; Naidich et al, 1992; Robson et al, 2000). Acquired hydrocephalus may be due to hemorrhage, infection, mass effect from tumor, or venous hypertension (Brann et al, 1990; Hedlund and Boyer, 1999).

Sonography plays an important role in the evaluation of posthemorrhagic hydrocephalus (Figure 59-28). The goals of the US examination are to determine the presence and severity of ventricular dilatation, to identify the location and cause of obstruction (ependymitis vs. clot), to monitor the adequacy of treatment, and to identify potential complications of therapy. The evaluation of the ventricular system in the neonate should include standardized measurements of the lateral ventricles. Although the atria dilate early in the course of ventriculomegaly, measurements of the lateral ventricles on parasagittal images are the most variable in clinical practice (Shackleford, 1986). We use the maximal width of the frontal horns measured at the level of the foramen of Monro to follow ventricular size. This measurement was chosen because it uses reproducible landmarks that are not affected by angulation of the transducer and provide independent measures of each lateral ventricle. In our experience, it provides the most useful measurement for monitoring change in ventricular size.

In general, dilatation tends to be greatest in the ventricle just proximal to the point of obstruction to flow. For example, the normal aqueduct of Sylvius is a narrow passage and often not clearly visible on US. It typically does not become distended by clot. However, when an obstruction to CSF flow exists at the level of the fourth ventricle or beyond, the aqueduct may become markedly distended and is then easily depicted (Taylor, 2001) (Figure 59-29). Early detection of a dilated fourth ventricle may have important therapeutic implications, especially when accompanied by clot or absence of CSF in the cisterna magna. This combination of findings strongly suggests the presence of a blockage to CSF flow into the spinal subarachnoid space (Hall et al, 1992) and the probable failure of serial lumbar punctures as a therapeutic option.

As the ICP rises, arterial flow tends to be more affected during diastole than during systole, resulting in an elevated pulsatility of flow. Seibert and colleagues (1989) have shown that increasing RI on pulsed Doppler interrogation correlates well with elevation in ICP in an animal model of acute hydrocephalus. They and others also have shown a significant drop in pulsatility following ventricular tapping and shunting in infants with hydrocephalus (Bada et al, 1982). However, elevated ICP may not always be present in infants with ventricular dilatation, and the RI may be well within the normal range. Doppler examination of the anterior or middle cerebral artery during fontanel compression may be useful in the early identification of infants with abnormal intracranial compliance before the development of increased ICP as shown by elevated baseline RI (Taylor et al, 1994). According to the Monro-Kellie hypothesis, the volume of brain, CSF, blood, and other intracranial components is constant (Bruce et al, 1977). During graded fontanel compression in normal infants, CSF or blood can be readily displaced to compensate for the small increase in volume delivered by compression of the anterior fontanel, resulting in no increase in ICP. In infants with hydrocephalus, however, the increase in intracranial volume with fontanel compression is translated into a transient increase in ICP and an acute increase in arterial pulsatility (Figure 59-30). Serial examinations using this technique can also be used to follow an individual infant's ability to compensate for minor changes in intracranial volume and thus serve as a noninvasive indirect measure of intracranial compliance (Taylor and Madsen, 1996).

In our experience, transient (3 to 5 seconds) fontanel compression is a safe and well-tolerated procedure, even in critically ill premature infants. However, prolonged compression of the fontanel should be avoided. Pressure should be immediately released if heart rate significantly decreases during Doppler examination. In addition, the presence of reversed flow during diastole in a Doppler study obtained without fontanel compression is strongly suggestive of elevated ICP, and fontanel compression is not necessary or recommended in these patients.

Imaging of hydrocephalus is carried out before shunting to determine the cause of ventricular dilatation, to identify the site of obstruction, and to differentiate hydrocephalus from other intracranial abnormalities, such as holoprosencephaly and hydranencephaly, that may mimic severe

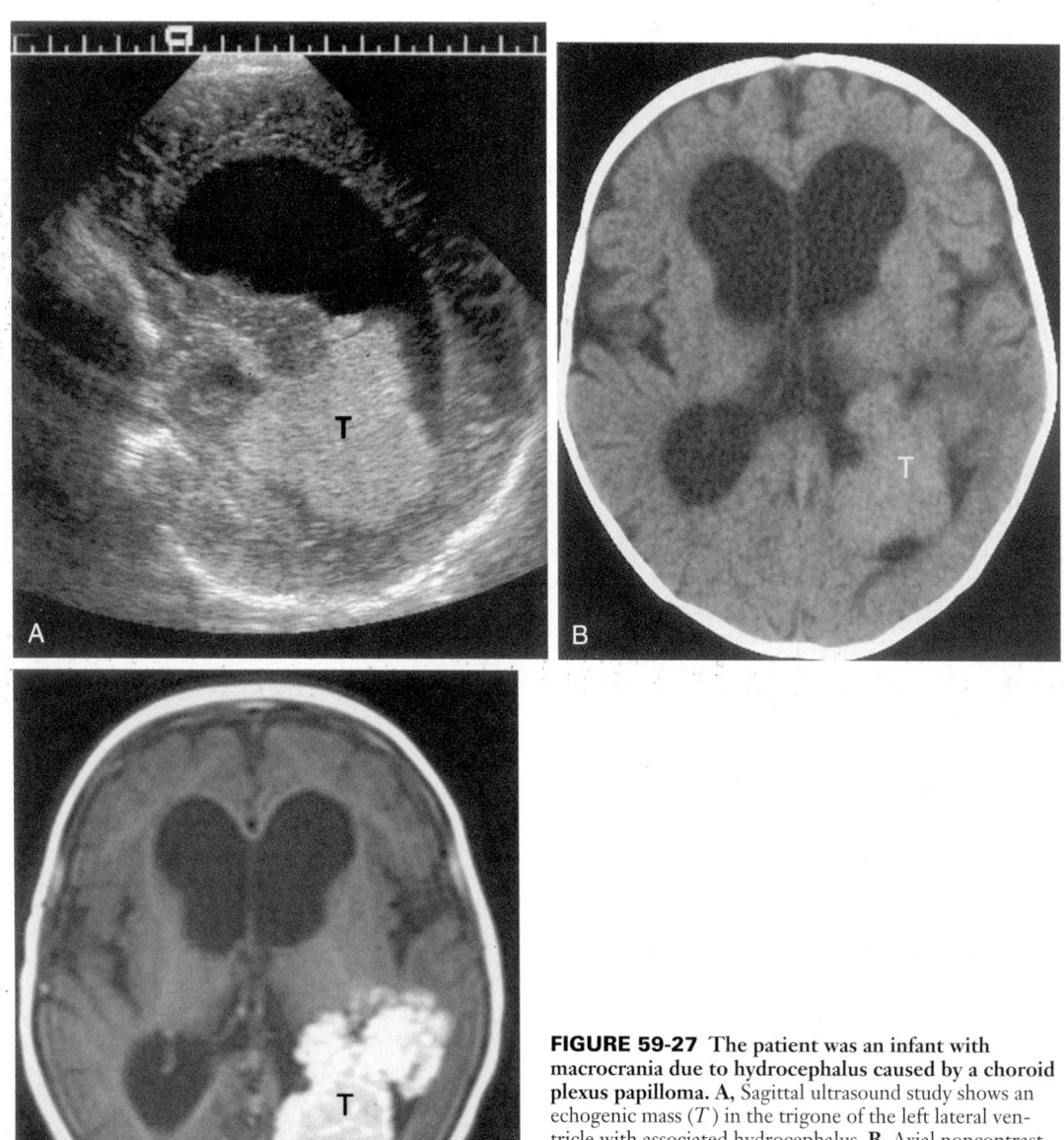

FIGURE 59-27 **The patient was an infant with macrocrania due to hydrocephalus caused by a choroid plexus papilloma. A,** Sagittal ultrasound study shows an echogenic mass (*T*) in the trigone of the left lateral ventricle with associated hydrocephalus. **B,** Axial noncontrast computed tomographic study shows an isodense mass (*T*) filling the trigone of the left lateral ventricle. The lateral ventricles are dilated bilaterally without an obvious cause of obstruction. **C,** Contrast-enhanced T1-weighted magnetic resonance image shows intense enhancement of the tumor (*T*) typical of choroid plexus papilloma.

hydrocephalus. After shunt placement, imaging is carried out to evaluate ventricular decompression and shunt position, and to assess for the presence of surgical complications and for the development of extraaxial collections.

MRI is the preferred examination for preoperative assessment of hydrocephalus. Thin-section T1- or T2-weighted images, three-dimensional constructive interference in steady-state (3D-CISS) or three-dimensional fast imaging employing steady-state acquisition (3D FIESTA) sequences provide excellent CSF-to-aqueduct contrast. We have found these sequences especially useful in assessing the aqueduct and obstructive membranes in CSF pathways, especially in the fourth ventricular exit foramina and the basal cisterns. By revealing these obstructive membranes, use of these sequences can alter patient treatment and prognosis (Dincer et al 2009).

On MRI, the findings in aqueductal stenosis include loss of the normal signal void within the aqueduct and elevation of the superior tectal plate (see Figure 59-9). Occasionally, high signal intensity suggesting gliosis is seen in the periaqueductal gray matter. Tectal tumors are rarely encountered in neonates. CSF flow studies may be performed to corroborate lack of flow within the aqueduct in equivocal cases. Use of contrast media may be required to evaluate congenital tumors causing hydrocephalus and to search for leptomeningeal metastases.

NEONATAL INFECTION

Congenital cytomegalovirus (CMV) infection is associated with anomalies of cortical development, diminished white matter volume, delayed myelination, variably small

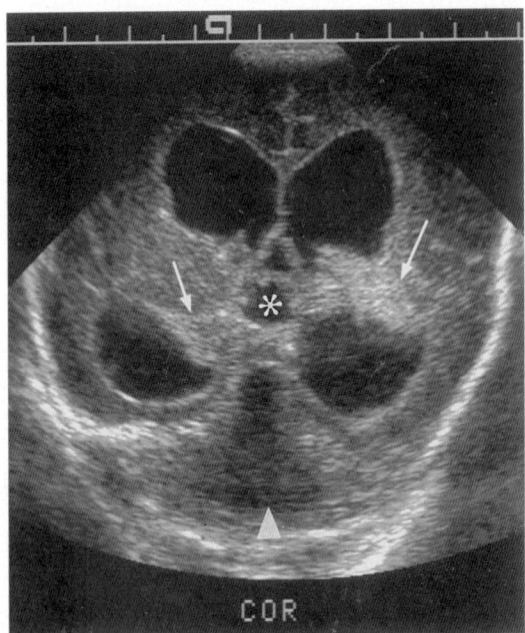

FIGURE 59-28 **Coronal ultrasound study of posthemorrhagic hydrocephalus obtained through the anterior fontanel.** Adherent, nondependent echogenic clot (*arrows*) is present within the dilated lateral ventricles. The absence of positional change in location of the echogenic material helps to differentiate blood clot from debris in ventriculitis. Note the dilated third ventricle (***) and fourth ventricle (*arrowhead*).

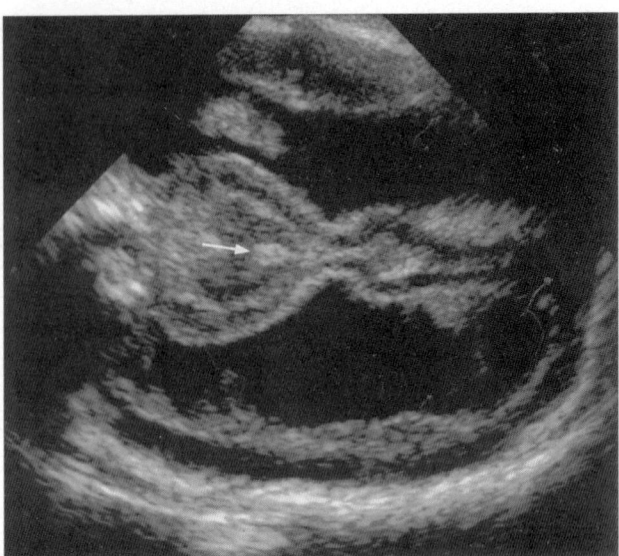

FIGURE 59-29 Axial ultrasound image from an infant with posthemorrhagic hydrocephalus. Due to obstructing clot at the level of the aqueduct of Sylvius (*arrow*), the lateral ventricles and upper aqueduct are distended.

cerebella, parenchymal calcification, and mild ventriculomegaly (Barkovich and Lindan, 1994).

Whereas both CT and US may demonstrate parenchymal calcifications, multiplanar MRI provides superior delineation of the anomalies associated with congenital CMV infection of the CNS. Conventional imaging including coronal T2-weighted images is useful in defining the anatomic abnormalities. We have noted increased diffusion in the regions of delayed myelination. DI findings have otherwise been unremarkable. Findings on high-resolution temporal bone MRI performed in infants with associated hearing loss are typically normal. One recent study in patients with CMV infection demonstrated increased diffusion in the white matter, decreased fractional anisotropy and reduced concentrations of total *N*-acetyl aspartate and choline-containing compounds and slightly increased myoinositol concentration on MRS (Van der Voorn et al, 2009). It has been suggested that the pathology of the white matter lesions in congenital CMV infections is characterized by axonal losses, lack of myelin deposition due to oligodendrocytic losses, and astrogliosis and is similar to the changes seen in PVL: Both congenital CMV infection and PVL affect the cerebral white matter in the same developmental period when immature oligodendrocytes are particularly vulnerable.

Neonatal herpes simplex virus (HSV) infection may involve any region of the brain and is typically multifocal (unlike HSV infection in adults, which has a predilection for the temporal lobes) (Baskin and Hedlund 2007).

Brain CT in HSV infection usually shows multifocal low density in the cortex and subcortical white matter. Occasionally, petechial hemorrhage may occur. Conventional MRI demonstrates multiple areas of cortical and

deep gray matter of low signal intensity on T1-weighted images and high signal intensity on T2-weighted images (Figure 59-31). Hemorrhage produces shortening of T1 (hyperintensity) and T2 (hypointensity). On DI, sites of involvement typically have decreased diffusion during the acute phase of the illness. The decreased diffusion is presumably due to necrosis.

Congenital human immunodeficiency virus (HIV) infection remains prevalent in regions including many Asian countries, sub-Saharan Africa, and parts of Latin America. The number of children diagnosed with HIV has decreased significantly. However, despite the fact that more than 90% of all childhood HIV infections are due to in utero transmission, neurologic and imaging manifestations of HIV infection in the immediate neonatal period are rare (Volpe, 1995). Neuroimaging abnormalities develop mainly after the neonatal period, with atrophy and white matter changes seen on MRI and cerebral and basal ganglia calcifications seen on CT (Volpe, 2008).

Neonatal bacterial CNS infections are rarely associated with imaging abnormalities. However, some bacteria such as *Citrobacter* species, *Serratia marcescens*, *Proteus*, *Pseudomonas aeruginosa*, and members of family Enterobacteriaceae may produce parenchymal necrosis and abscess formation (Figure 59-32). Thrombosis of cortical and subependymal veins may also occur. By both CT and MRI, leptomeningeal enhancement may be seen after the administration of intravenous contrast. If cerebritis develops, the cortex and subcortical white matter are seen as areas of low density on CT and of increased signal intensity on T2-weighted MRI. Abscesses are demonstrated as rim-enhancing lesions on both CT and MRI. These lesions, along with the surrounding hyperemia, can also be well demonstrated by cranial US. Widespread malacic changes may be seen on late follow-up imaging after necrotizing CNS infections.

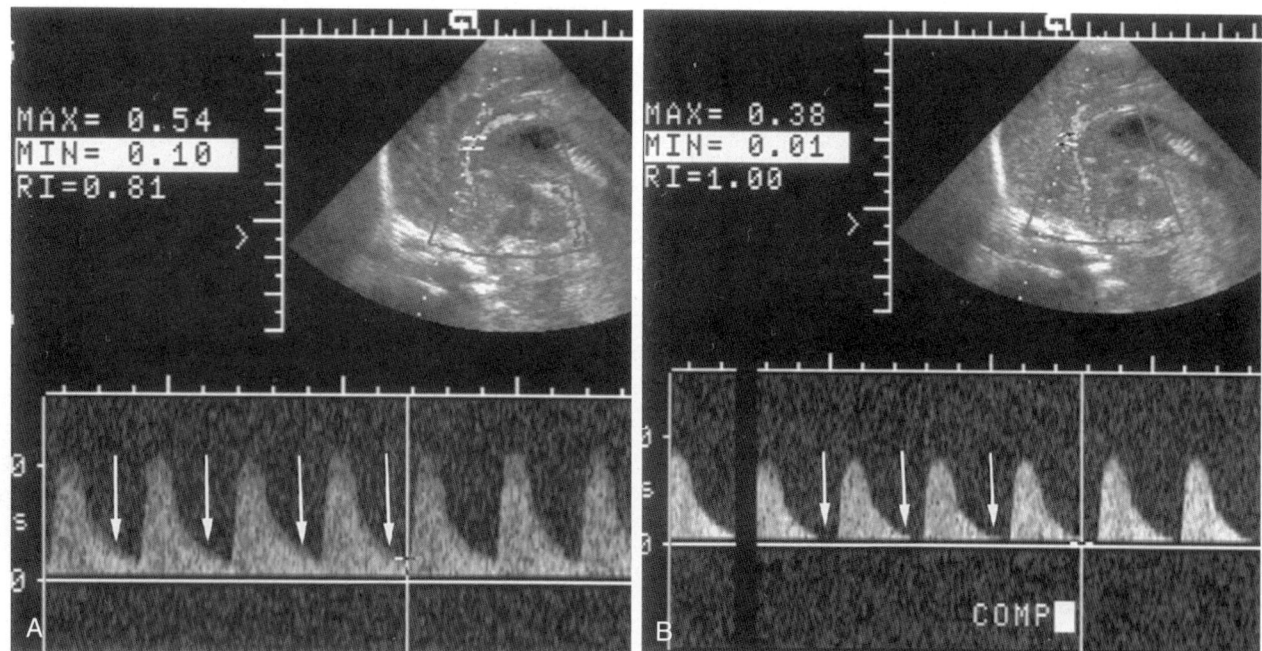

FIGURE 59-30 Positive Doppler ultrasound compression study in hydrocephalus. **A,** Baseline examination of blood flow within the anterior cerebral artery without fontanel compression shows a low resistance pattern with flow during both systole and diastole (resistive index = 0.81). **B,** Examination during transient compression of the anterior fontanel using the ultrasound transducer results in a loss of diastolic flow resulting from increased intracranial pressure (resistive index = 1.0).

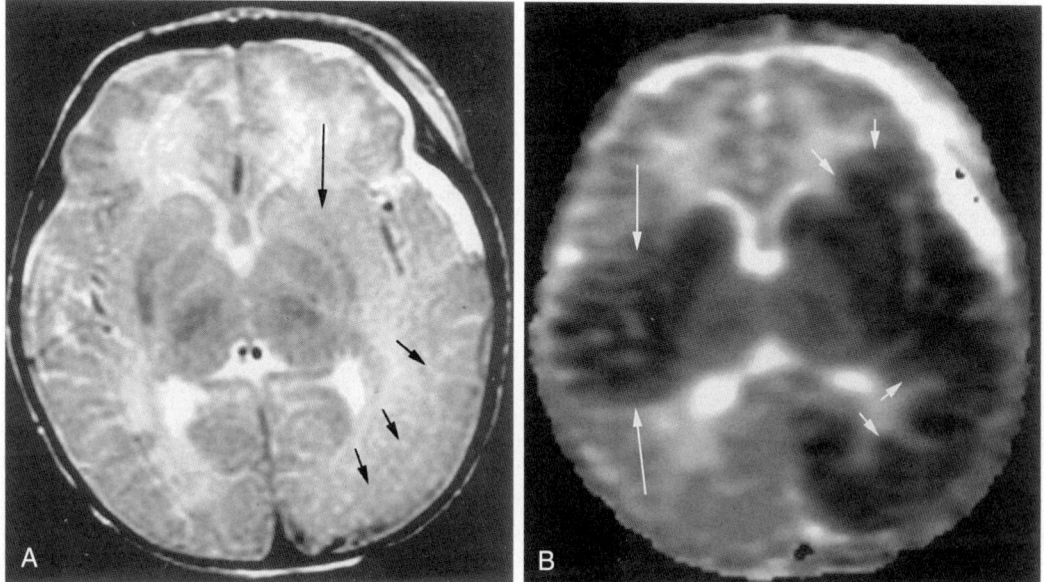

FIGURE 59-31 Magnetic resonance images from a term neonate with herpes simplex virus (HSV) encephalitis. **A,** Axial T2-weighted image shows high signal intensity in the left basal ganglia (*long arrow*) and loss of the cortical ribbon in the left cerebral hemisphere (*short arrows*). Unlike HSV infection in adults, neonatal herpes is not confined to the temporal and subfrontal lobes, and basal ganglia involvement is common. **B,** Apparent diffusion coefficient (ADC) map from the same examination shows extensive restricted diffusion (hypointensity) involving the areas on the left seen on the T2-weighted images (*short arrows*) and additional right hemispheric cortical (*long arrows*) and deep gray matter involvement.

NEONATAL BRAIN TUMORS

Brain tumors are rare in the newborn. When they occur, they are most often supratentorial, large, high-grade lesions such as primitive neuroepithelial tumors and choroid plexus carcinoma (Figure 59-33).

The imaging appearance of brain tumors is variable depending on the cellularity of the lesion and the presence or absence of necrosis (Klisch et al, 2000) (see Figure 59-32). Low-grade, less cellular tumors tend to have low density on CT, high signal intensity on T2-weighted MRI, and increased diffusion relative to normal brain. High-grade, densely cellular tumors generally are hyperdense on CT and of low signal intensity on T2-weighted MRI and have decreased diffusion relative to normal

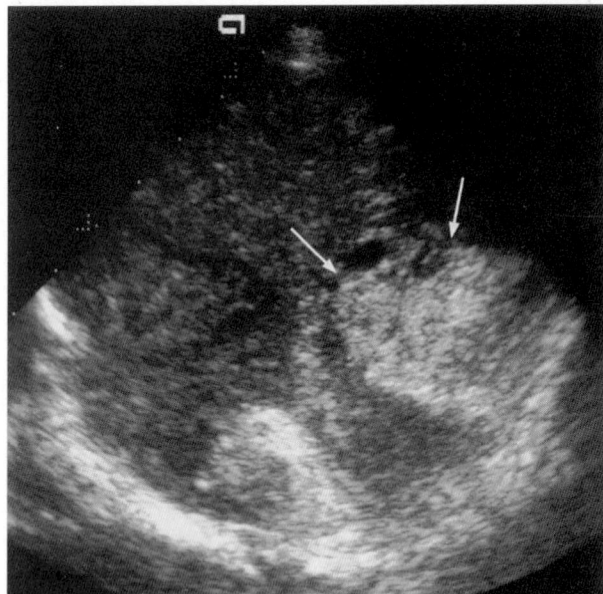

FIGURE 59-32 **Ultrasound study of abscess due to *Citrobacter* infection.** A large echogenic mass/abscess (*arrows*) is clearly demonstrated. Abscess formation is most often associated with bacterial infections, such as that due to *Citrobacter* species, that cause parenchymal necrosis.

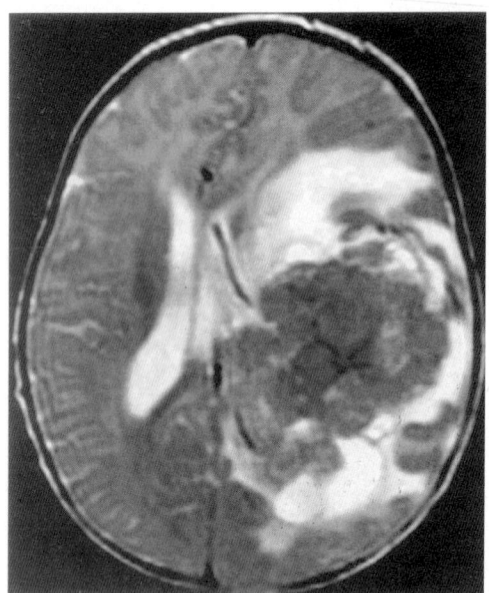

FIGURE 59-33 **The patient was a 1-month-old infant with choroid plexus carcinoma.** A large left hemispheric mass with regions hypointensity densely cellular tumor is evident on T2-weighted magnetic resonance image.

brain. Enhancement of the tumors is variable but tends to increase with increasing malignancy of the tumor. Important exceptions to this general rule are pilocytic astrocytoma and choroid plexus papilloma (see Figure 59-33), which, despite their low grade, tend to avidly enhance after contrast administration.

Malformative masses such as dermoid, epidermoid, and teratoma are occasionally detected in the neonate (Figure 59-34) (Haddad et al, 1991). These lesions may be associated with other markers of cerebral dysgenesis such as anomalies of the corpus callosum or pericallosal lipoma.

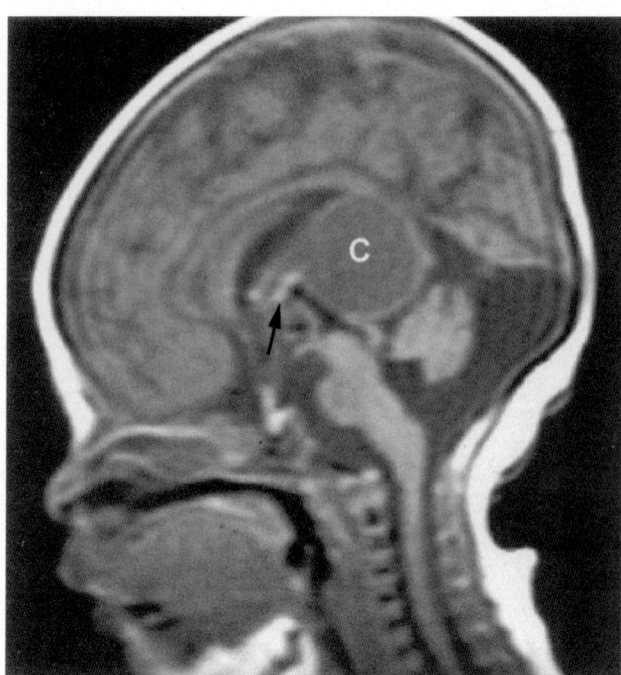

FIGURE 59-34 **The patient was a neonate with a pineal region teratoma.** Sagittal T1-weighted image shows a large cystic lesion (*C*). The mass contains a small amount of high signal intensity (*arrow*) due to the presence of fat, which strongly suggests the diagnosis of teratoma.

A dermal sinus tract is often present in association with midline cysts.

Malformative masses often have a characteristic appearance on imaging as a result of the presence of fat and/or calcification within the lesion (Smirniotopoulos and Chiechi, 1995). Both dermoid and epidermoid tend to be of low density on CT. Calcification is sometimes seen within the cyst wall. Teeth formed within a teratoma will produce dense calcification on CT, whereas foci of fat have very low density, comparable to that of subcutaneous fat. CT is also used to document associated bone defects that accompany dermal sinus tracts.

On MRI, epidermoids tend to be similar to CSF in signal intensity on T1- and T2-weighted sequences and usually show increased signal (decreased diffusion) relative to CSF on DI. Occasionally, the cyst wall may enhance after intravenous contrast administration. Dermoid cysts containing fat have high signal intensity on T1-weighted sequences. High-resolution MRI may occasionally be required to demonstrate an associated dermal sinus tract. Teratomas may have foci of fat that produce high signal intensity on T1-weighted sequences. Calcifications appear as rounded signal voids on both T1-weighted and T2-weighted sequences.

HYPOGLYCEMIA

Severe perinatal hypoglycemia may result in energy exhaustion and parenchymal infarction in the neonate. In severe hypoglycemia, diffuse cortical and subcortical white matter damage may be evident, with the parietal and occipital lobes most severely affected (Barkovich et al, 1998). Globus pallidus injury has been observed in patients with the most severe cortical injury (Barkovich et al, 1998). Initially,

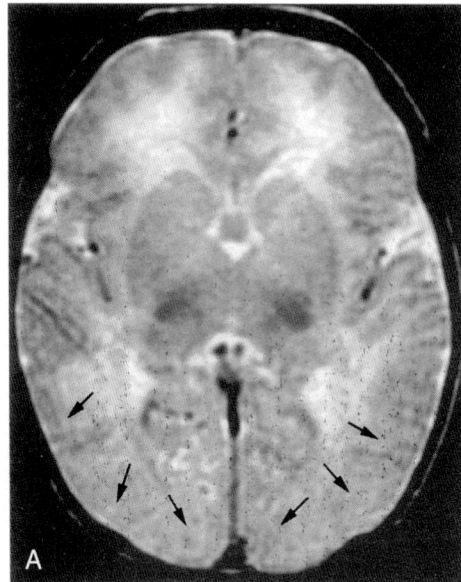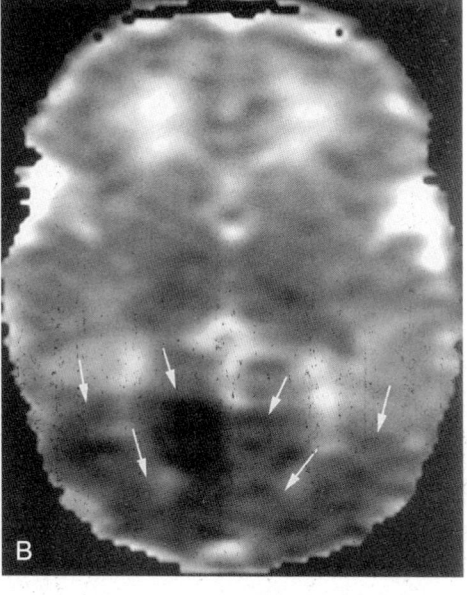

FIGURE 59-35 Term newborn with marked hypoglycemia and seizures. **A,** Bilaterally symmetric loss of the cortical ribbon is apparent in the parietal and occipital lobes on T2-weighted imaging (*arrows*). **B,** Decreased ADC values are present in corresponding regions of the parietal and occipital cortex (*arrows*).

on CT and MRI, cortical edema is present within the parietal and occipital regions of the cortex (Figure 59-35). As with other causes of infarction, decreased diffusion is usually observed acutely (Barkovich et al, 1998). Chronically, tissue loss is present in the areas that earlier showed edema and abnormal diffusion (Sugama et al, 2001).

HYPERBILIRUBINEMIA

In newborns, severe hyperbilirubinemia and consequent kernicterus may develop. The findings on brain MRI in patients with kernicterus are characteristic. Unlike hypoxia-ischemia, which tends to primarily affect the putamen and thalamus, hyperbilirubinemia selectively affects the globus pallidus. Recently, it has been suggested that the high resting neuronal activity in the globus pallidus might make it more vulnerable to less intense, subacute oxidative stresses from mitochondrial toxins such as bilirubin (Johnston and Hoon, 2000). The imaging findings in kernicterus are most apparent on MRI, with hyperintensity at the posterior margin or throughout the globi pallidi on T2-weighted sequences (Sugama et al, 2001).

NEUROCUTANEOUS DISORDERS

Of the phakomatoses, the two for which imaging is most commonly required in the neonate are tuberous sclerosis and Sturge-Weber syndrome. Because the outwardly apparent clinical features of tuberous sclerosis, such as adenoma sebaceum, are not usually apparent until late childhood or adulthood, early brain imaging is most often requested when cardiac tumors are identified on prenatal US or when there is a positive family history. The intracranial manifestations of tuberous sclerosis include cortical tubers, subependymal hamartomas, subependymal giant cell tumors, and abnormal neuronal and glial cells in the white matter.

On brain CT in the neonate, there is variable calcification of subependymal nodules that appear as small nodular densities projecting into the lateral ventricles (Griffiths

and Martland, 1997) (Figure 59-36). The appearance may be similar to that of periventricular calcifications seen with congenital infections such as with CMV but can be differentiated from the latter on the basis of the projection of the lesions into the lateral ventricles and demonstration of cortical tubers. White matter abnormalities are extremely difficult to demonstrate because of the normal low density of unmyelinated neonatal white matter. Likewise, cortical tubers, which are not usually calcified in the newborn, may be difficult to demonstrate with CT, because the affected gyri may simply appear mildly broadened.

On brain MRI in the newborn, subependymal hamartomas may be quite subtle in appearance and must be carefully searched for. The cortical lesions of tuberous sclerosis have variable signal intensity. Cortical tubers appear may appear hyperintense or hypointense to unmyelinated white matter on T1-weighted images. The cortical tubers may be difficult to identify on T2-weighted images in the neonate, because their signal intensity is often similar to that of the unmyelinated subcortical white matter (see Figure 59-36).

Sturge-Weber syndrome (SWS) (i.e., encephalotrigeminal angiomatosis) is a neurocutaneous disorder comprising a facial capillary malformation in the distribution of branches of the trigeminal nerve and an intracranial leptomeningeal capillary-venous malformation. Clinically, patients present with a "port-wine facial nevus" and seizures (Pascual-Castroviejo et al, 1993). Intracranial manifestations of SWS are found in only a small minority of patients with facial capillary malformations.

On brain CT, SWS in the newborn may be difficult to detect. Gyral calcification, a radiographic hallmark of this disorder, may or may not be present. Even when present, the extent of the calcification may not reflect the entire distribution of the vascular malformation. Because of the abnormal development of the cortical venous drainage system, the medullary veins that serve as collateral venous pathways are enlarged and the ipsilateral choroid plexus is engorged and appears enlarged. Hemiatrophy of the brain and overgrowth of the skull are manifestations of long-term ischemic brain injury due to impaired tissue

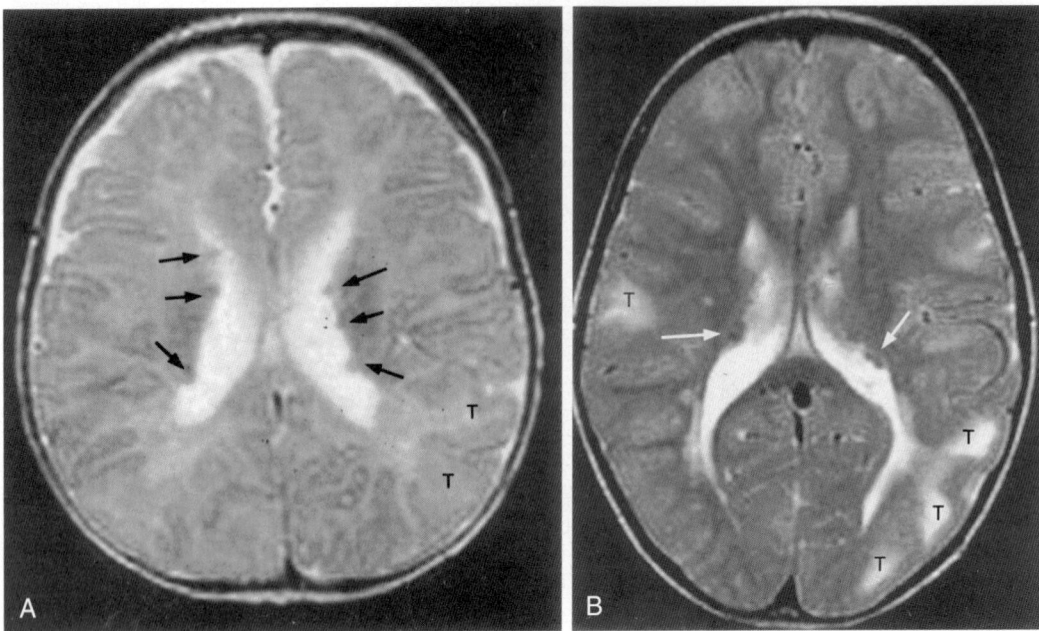

FIGURE 59-36 **The patient was a term neonate with cardiac rhabdomyomas. A,** Axial T2-weighted magnetic resonance (MR) image obtained at 2 weeks of age shows subependymal nodules (*arrows*) indicative of tuberous sclerosis. Note that the cortical tubers (*T*) may be difficult to see in the newborn. **B,** Follow-up T2-weighted MR image in the same child at 5 years of age shows hypointense subependymal nodules (*arrows*). The cortical tubers (*T*) are now much more obvious.

perfusion and are a hallmark of SWS in older infants or children but are usually not apparent in the newborn.

Contrast-enhanced brain MRI is considered the imaging modality of choice for evaluation of SWS (Elster and Chen, 1990; Pascual-Castroviejo et al, 1993). T1-weighted imaging after the administration of intravenous gadolinium provides the best depiction of the extent of the leptomeningeal vascular anomaly (Figure 59-37). Although gradient echo MRI may be less sensitive than CT for the demonstration of gyral calcification, it is often useful in demonstrating the presence of cortical mineralization. More recently, we have found that SWI can provide useful and unique information complementary to conventional contrast-enhanced T1-weighted MRI for characterizing SWS. We advocate the incorporation of the SWI sequence into routine clinical MRI protocols for suspected SWS. Recent studies have suggested that SWI is superior to gadolinium-enhanced T1 images in identifying the enlarged transmedullary veins, abnormal periventricular veins, cortical gyriform abnormalities, and gray matter–white matter junction abnormalities. Conversely, the gadolinium-enhanced T1 images were found to be better than SWI in identifying enlarged choroid plexus and leptomeningeal abnormalities (Hu et al, 2008).

ADVANTAGES AND DISADVANTAGES OF NEUROIMAGING TECHNIQUES

ULTRASONOGRAPHY

The most significant advantages of US are its portability, lack of ionizing radiation, relative availability and affordability, and ability to depict hemodynamics of blood flow in real time. The most serious disadvantages are its relative lack of spatial resolution compared with CT and MRI, the need for an acoustic window, its operator dependence, and the nonspecificity of many US findings. In addition, the differentiation between bland and hemorrhagic lesions is often difficult, and it is an insensitive tool for the diagnosis of neuronal migration disorders and diffuse neuronal injury.

COMPUTED TOMOGRAPHY

Advantages of CT include availability, compatibility with life support systems, rapid image acquisition, and relative lack of operator dependency.

Unfortunately, CT offers more limited soft tissue contrast than that provided by MRI and is prone to beam-hardening artifact from the skull base such that there is limited detail of the posterior fossa and temporal lobes. In addition, imaging can be acquired only in the axial or coronal plane. The risks associated with exposure to ionizing radiation from CT have come under increased scrutiny as described in an earlier section (Brenner et al, 2001; Huda et al, 2001). It appears that the long-term risk of malignancy due to x-ray exposure may be greatest in the newborn and gradually diminishes with age (Brenner et al, 2001; Brenner and Hall, 2007). The decision to perform CT for neonatal brain imaging should be made on a case-by-case basis, with recognition of the potentially significant medical benefit of performing the study compared with a small theoretical risk of the development of malignancy over the patient's lifetime. When appropriate, it may be prudent to consider using MRI or US, because neither employs ionizing radiation.

Although most brain CT studies in the neonate do not require the administration of intravenous contrast, occasionally, as with suspected dural venous sinus thrombosis, contrast may be of benefit. Because the primary route of

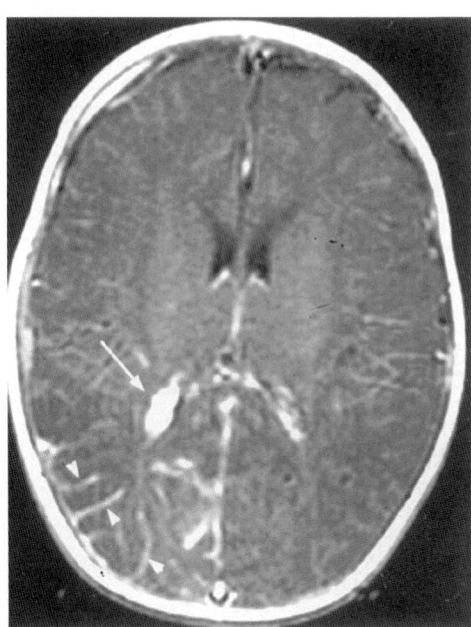

FIGURE 59-37 The patient was a term neonate with seizures and facial capillary nevus. Axial T1-weighted post-gadolinium magnetic resonance image demonstrates asymmetric leptomeningeal enhancement (*arrowheads*) in the right parietal and occipital lobes due to the presence of the leptomeningeal capillary-venous malformation that defines Sturge-Weber syndrome. The choroid plexus ipsilateral (*arrow*) to the leptomeningeal anomaly is typically enlarged. Note that the brain is not yet atrophic in the area of the malformation.

contrast excretion is via the kidney, the renal status must be considered in the newborn, just as in the older child or adult. Typically, nonionic contrast is used, to decrease the risk of side effects related to the high osmolality of the ionic agents.

MAGNETIC RESONANCE IMAGING

Advantages of MRI include superior image detail compared with CT and US and the possibility of evaluating multiple tissue parameters. As with US, MRI does not carry the theoretical risks associated with the use of ionizing radiation. In addition, both anatomic and functional information may be obtained from MRI during the same examination. Moreover, MRI offers improved delineation of the posterior fossa structures without significant artifact from the skull base as occurs with CT, and without the need for an appropriate acoustic window as is essential with US.

The single biggest disadvantage of MRI is the requirement for a strong magnetic field. As a result, the MRI examination room must be magnetically shielded, and all equipment entering the room must be nonferromagnetic. For these reasons, the imaging of the ill neonate can be difficult. Additionally, because of the relatively long time for image acquisition, sedation or anesthesia is often required. However, generally, the additional information obtained

with MRI over CT warrants the added inconvenience of the examination, provided that the imaging suite and personnel are equipped to handle the unique requirements of neonatal brain MRI.

SUMMARY OF NEUROIMAGING PRACTICE GUIDELINES

A multidisciplinary group reviewed the literature and established guidelines for neuroimaging in the neonate (Ment et al, 2002). This practice parameter is endorsed by the American Academy of Pediatrics, the American Society of Pediatric Neuroradiology, and the Society for Pediatric Radiology and was subsequently reaffirmed in 2005. The practice parameter recommendations for imaging of the preterm neonate are that routine cranial US screening be performed in all infants born at less than 30 weeks of gestational age once between days 7 and 14 of life and repeated between 36 and 40 weeks of postmenstrual age. For term infants, the recommendations are that noncontrast CT be performed to detect hemorrhagic lesions in the encephalopathic newborn with a history of birth trauma, low hematocrit, or coagulopathy. If CT is inconclusive, then MRI should be performed between days 2 and 8 of life to assess the location and extent of injury.

We emphasize that these practice parameters reflect a review of available literature that was examined by the panel in 2005. With the increased availability of 3-tesla MRI scanners and the newer techniques described earlier, the algorithm for imaging the sick neonate may need revision in the near future.

SUGGESTED READINGS

Franceschini Ma, Thaker S, Themelis G, et al: Assessment of infant brain development with frequency-domain near-infrared spectroscopy, *Pediatr Res* 61:546-551, 2007.
Grant PE, Roche-Labarbe N, Surova A, et al: Increased cerebral blood volume and oxygen consumption in neonatal brain injury, *J Cereb Blood Flow Metab* 29:1704-1713, 2009.
Liauw L, van Wezel-Meijler G, Veen S, et al: Do apparent diffusion coefficient measurements predict outcome in children with neonatal hypoxic-ischemic encephalopathy? *AJNR Am J Neuroradiol* 30:264-270, 2009.
Luna JA, Goldstein RB: Sonographic visualization of neonatal posterior fossa abnormalities through the posterolateral fontanelle, *AJR Am J Roentgenol* 174:561-567, 2000.
Panigrahy A, Borzage M, Blüml S: Basic principles and concepts underlying recent advances in magnetic resonance imaging of the developing brain, *Semin Perinatol* 34(1):3-19, 2010.
Robertson RL, Robson CD: Diffusion imaging in neonates, *Neuroimag Clin North Am* 12:55-70, 2002.
Robertson RL, Robson CD, Antiles S, et al: CT versus MR in neonatal brain imaging at term, *Pediatr Radiol* 33:442-449, 2003.
Taylor GA: Doppler of the neonatal and infant brain. In Rumack CM, Wilson SR, Charboneau JW, editors: *Diagnostic ultrasound*, St. Louis, 1998, Mosby, pp 1503-1525.
Taylor GA: Sonographic assessment of posthemorrhagic ventricular dilatation, *Radiol Clin North Am* 39:541-551, 2001.
Vigneron DB, Zimmerman RA, Noworolski SM, et al: Three-dimensional proton MR spectroscopic imaging of premature and term neonates, *AJNR Am J Neuroradiol* 22:1424-1433, 2001.
Vock P: CT dose reduction in children, *Eur Radiol* 15:2330-2340, 2005.
Wolf RL, Zimmerman RA, Clancy R, et al: Quantitative apparent diffusion coefficient measurements in term neonates for early detection of hypoxic-ischemic brain injury: initial experience, *Radiology* 218:825-833, 2001.

Complete references used in this text can be found online at www.expertconsult.com

CONGENITAL MALFORMATIONS OF THE CENTRAL NERVOUS SYSTEM

Stephen A. Back and Lauren L. Plawner

Throughout fetal gestation, the sequence of events that direct the formation of the central nervous system CNS may be interrupted by deleterious intrinsic events or extrinsic insults that result in malformations. This chapter examines those disorders that are more commonly encountered in neonatology. An understanding of the origins and consequences of these disorders are considered within the context of normal CNS development. The peak timing of these events during fetal gestation is summarized in Table 60-1 together with some of the more commonly associated CNS malformations. Remarkable progress in basic developmental neurobiology in the past decade has translated into rapid advances in our understanding of the molecular and genetic basis of many of these previously perplexing disorders. Although a majority of these disorders arise from adverse events that occur during the early phases of pregnancy, these new insights begin to provide a more rational basis for the assessment of prognosis, as well as for the management of future pregnancies.

A true CNS malformation may be multifactorial in origin and results when a disruption occurs in an intrinsic developmental process. Acquired defects occur when an already normally formed brain is injured by a secondary process, such as vascular compromise, hypoxia ischemia, infection, toxic exposure, physical compression or trauma. The nature of acquired malformations is closely related to the stage of development at which the injury occurs, as well as the duration of the insult. Although acquired lesions are usually *encephaloclastic* in nature, which means that destruction of normal brain tissue has occurred, they can resemble primary developmental lesions in some cases (Roessmann, 1995).

PRIMARY AND SECONDARY NEURAL TUBE FORMATION (NEURULATION)

The earliest developmental stages include the one celled embryo, the cleaving embryo, the blastocyst, the process of implantation and development of the amniotic cavity, the formation of chorionic villi, and the formation of axial features (right and left sides, rostral and caudal ends). All of these events occur during the first 14 postconceptual days. At 16 days, the site of the future neural plate can be defined by autoradiographic means, and at about 18 days, the neural groove can be seen (England, 1988; O'Rahilly and Muller, 1994).

Neural tube formation (neurulation) occurs through an inductive process that stimulates the dorsal aspect of the embryo to form the brain and spinal cord. Initial events involve formation of the brain and much of the spinal cord, with the exception of the sacral-coccygeal segments (primary neurulation). Later in embryogenesis, the lower sacral segments of the spinal cord are formed (secondary

neurulation). Disruption of primary and secondary neurulation results in distinctly different malformations that are considered separately.

PRIMARY NEURAL TUBE FORMATION

This process forms the brain and spinal cord, with the exception of the most caudal (sacral-coccygeal) segments of the spinal cord. Primary neurulation spans from approximately 18 days' gestation to the end of the 4th gestational week. It involves a complex series of morphogenetic events directed by cell proliferation and apoptosis as well as changes in cell shape and adhesion that regulate cell migration. As discussed later, mutations in the genes that regulate these processes underlie a variety of neural tube defects. During gastrulation, an area of thickened neuroectoderm, the neural plate, is initially formed via induction by the underlying axial mesoderm (notochord and prechordal plate (Figure 60-1, *A*). The nascent neural plate is induced by fibroblast growth factor-8 (FGF-8) activity derived from the primary endoderm (Stern, 2005). It now appears that the ectodermal cells of the neural plate are intrinsically programmed to differentiate along neural lineages. In fact, suppression of this differentiation by various members of the bone morphogenetic proteins (BMPs) is required to generate epidermis from the lateral ectoderm. Hence, endoderm-derived FGFs and lateral ectoderm-derived BMPs, as well as BMP-inhibitory factors from Hensen's node, interact to establish the initial dorsoventral polarity and anterior-posterior regionalization of the neural plate (reviewed in Vieira et al, 2010). At 20 to 21 days, the neural groove forms in the midline with a neural fold on either side (see Figure 60-1, *B*). Elevation of the neural folds coincides with formation of a midline medial hinge point and paired dorsolateral hinge points. Areas destined to become the forebrain, midbrain, and hindbrain can be identified at this early stage. By day 22, the neural folds are beginning to fuse to form the neural tube and central canal (England, 1988; O'Rahilly and Muller, 1994).

The fusion of the neural tube coincides with further planar segregation of the tube into dorsal and ventral domains (Vieira et al, 2010). Central to this process are two key signaling molecules that establish the dorsoventral plane of the neural tube: BMPs derived from the roof plate in the dorsal midline and Sonic hedgehog (Shh) derived from the floor plate in the ventral midline (see Figure 60-1, *B*). Thus, gradients of BMP and Shh induce the formation of the alar and basal plates, respectively, which comprise the future brainstem and spinal cord. In broadest terms, the alar plate gives rise to neurons that are mainly related to sensory functions whereas the basal plate gives rise to motor neurons and interneurons.

TABLE 60-1 Timing of the Major Gestational Events in Human Brain Development and Representative Examples of Significant Related Disorders

Major Developmental Event	Window in Development
Primary Neurulation	**3–4 weeks**
Craniorachischisis totalis Anencephaly Encephalocele Myeloschisis Myelomeningocele/Arnold-Chiari malformation	
Prosencephalic Development	**4–8 weeks**
Holoprosencephaly Agenesis of the corpus callosum Agenesis of septum pellucidum/septo-optic dysplasia	
Hindbrain Development	**3–12+ weeks**
Dandy-Walker malformation Malformations associated with cerebellar vermis hypoplasia Malformations associated with the molar tooth sign (Joubert's syndrome)	
Neuronal Proliferation	**8–12 weeks**
Micrencephaly (micrencephaly vera, radial microbrain) Human autosomal recessive primary micrencephaly types 1–5 Macrencephaly Hemimegalencephaly	
Neuronal Migration	**8–16 weeks**
Schizencephaly Polymicrogyria Lissencephaly/pachygyria Lissencephaly with cerebellar hypoplasia Cobblestone complex syndromes Neuronal heterotopias Cortical dysplasia	

NEURAL TUBE CLOSURE AND NEURAL CREST MIGRATION

Primary neurulation concludes with a series of critical events that result in closure of the neural tube. The neural folds fuse first in the nascent occipitocervical region. Current studies no longer support the "zipper" concept of closure of the neural tube. Rather, fusion occurs at three major sites, with the closure of the cranium being the most complex. Closure site 1 is located at the junction of the hindbrain and spinal cord. Closure site 2 resides at the junction of the midbrain and forebrain and site 3 is at the most rostral extent of the forebrain. At each site, closure proceeds simultaneously both rostrally and caudally. Inbred strains of mice show differences in the timing of the various closure sites and in the exact locations and sequences of closure, all of which are dependent on specific genes (Harris and Juriloff, 2007; Van Allen et al, 1993; Vieira et al, 2010; Zohn and Sarkar, 2008). Analysis of the locations where human anterior neural tube defects occur further supports the notion that anterior neural tube closure proceeds simultaneously at multiple sites (Golden and Chernoff, 1995). Disturbances in human neural tube closure appear to occur by failure of closure at one or more sites or by defective fusion adjacent to sites of closure.

By days 24 to 25, fusion progresses rostrally to the level of the colliculi, and fusion continues rostrally and caudally until only the anterior neuropore and the posterior neuropore are open (Figure 60-2). By day 24, the anterior neuropore has closed; by day 26, the posterior neuropore has closed at the site corresponding to around S2 (O'Rahilly and Muller, 1994). The skull, vertebrae, and dura form through interactions between the neural tube and the adjacent mesoderm. As the rostral parts of the neural folds fuse, the neural crest is formed from ectodermal cells on both sides of the neural tube. The neural crest cells migrate shortly after neural tube closure. They give rise to sensory, sympathetic, and parasympathetic ganglia; chromaffin cells of the adrenal medulla; skin melanocytes; enteric neurons in the gastrointestinal tract; and facial connective tissue (Hall, 2008; O'Rahilly and Muller, 1994).

SECONDARY NEURAL TUBE FORMATION AND CAUDAL REGRESSION

The process of secondary neural tube formation occurs approximately between gestational days 30 to 50, during which vacuoles form in a caudal cell mass that surrounds the lower neural tube. The vacuoles coalesce and connect with the central canal of the already present neural tube. At postconceptual days 41 to 51, the caudalmost part of the neural tube and central canal begins to regress as the tail of the embryo disappears. Atrophy of the caudal neural tube results in formation of a fibrous strand called the filum terminale, which is present throughout life. As the vertebral bodies grow, the end of the central canal (the conus medullaris) becomes placed higher in the vertebral column, eventually reaching the L1-2 level (usually by 2 weeks postnatally). This may be caused by proportionately greater lengthening of the spinal vertebrae compared with the spinal cord (England, 1988; O'Rahilly and Muller, 1994). Disorders of secondary neurulation give rise to several clinically significant occult dysraphic states, discussed later.

NEURAL TUBE DEFECTS

Neural tube defects result from a failure of primary neural tube closure during the 4th week of human gestation (Roessmann, 1995). Most of these defects are related to some degree of failure of anterior or posterior neuropore closure. The clinical spectrum of brain malformations associated with disrupted anterior neuropore closure are, in order of decreasing severity: anencephaly and the encephaloceles. Myeloschisis and myelomeningoceles with the associated Arnold-Chiari malformations encompass the spectrum of spinal cord defects associated with failure of posterior neuropore closure. In addition, craniorachischis totalis is a severe malformation of the brain and spinal cord, which essentially involves complete failure of neural tube closure, and usually results in spontaneous abortion during embryogenesis or early fetal development. Similarly, myeloschisis commonly results in stillbirth, as a result of extensive malformation of large portions of the spinal cord. The remainder of the neural tube defects to be discussed result in malformations of the CNS and the overlying axial skeleton, meninges, and skin that are associated with varying degrees of viability in the newborn period.

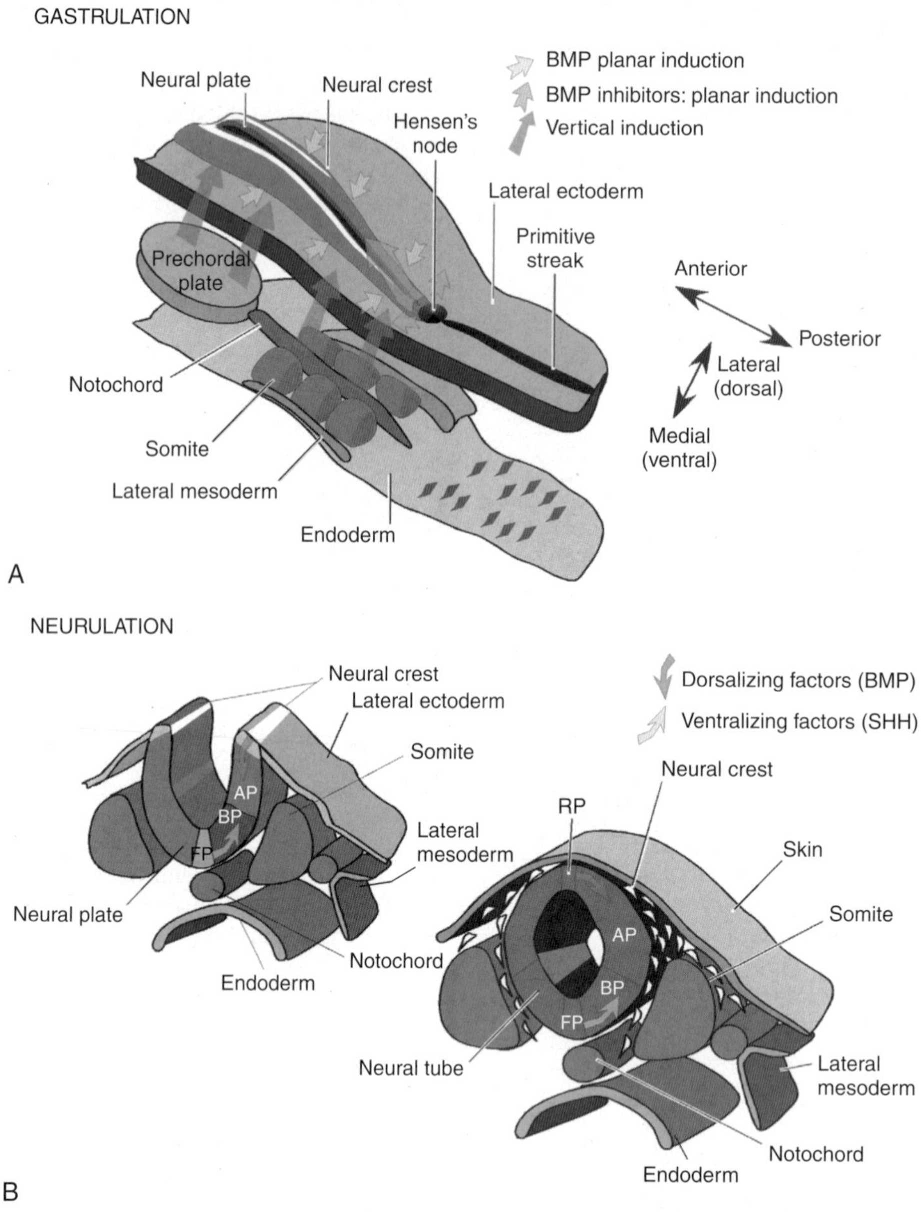

GASTRULATION

A

NEURULATION

B

FIGURE 60-1 *(See also color plate 27.)* **Formation of the neural tube. A,** During gastrulation, at the neural plate stage, dorsoventral polarity and early anteroposterior regionalization is defined by a process of vertical induction by fibroblast growth factor-8 (FGF-8) and other factors (*long gray arrows*) derived from mesendoderm (notochord and prechordal plate). Planar induction occurs via BMPs and BMP inhibitors that are derived from lateral ectoderm (*short light gray arrows*) and Hensen's node (*short dark gray arrows*), respectively. **B,** The process of neurulation proceeds with the approximation of the neural folds toward the dorsal midline. Before closure of the neural tube, neural crest cells delaminate and migrate from the neural folds. Dorsalizing factors (BMPs; *dark gray arrow*) derived from the dorsal midline roofplate (RP) and ventralizing factors (SHH; *light gray arrow*) from the floor plate (FP) establish dorsal-ventral gradients of these key signaling molecules that induce formation of the alar plate (AP) and the basal plate (BP) from the lateral wall of the neural tube. *(From: Vieira C, Pombero A, Garcia-Lopez R, et al: Molecular mechanisms controlling brain development: an overview of neuroepithelial secondary organizers, Int J Dev Biol 54:7-20, 2010; courtesy Dr. Salvador Martinez, Institute of Neuroscience, Universidad Miguel Hernandez, San Juan de Alicante, Spain.)*

EPIDEMIOLOGY

Neural tube defects remain one of the most common congenital malformations encountered in newborns. Despite a recent decline in prevalence, 0.5 to 2 per 1000 pregnancies are affected worldwide (Au et al, 2010; Mitchell, 2005). Because many congenital malformations occur during embryonic development, incidence data are essentially impossible to ascertain. Nevertheless, the prevalence of neural tube defects varies widely and is particularly influenced by race, ethnicity, geographical area, and

socioeconomic status (Frey and Hauser, 2003). In the United States, for example, the risk for neural tube defects is higher for Hispanics but lower for African Americans. Geographically, one of the higher prevalence rates occurs in the United Kingdom; distinct geographic gradients also exist within this region. For unclear reasons, after the first affected pregnancy, the risk of recurrence increases at a disproportionately higher rate with each subsequent pregnancy and remains markedly higher than the baseline risk for the relevant general population. In fact, the risk may

A

B

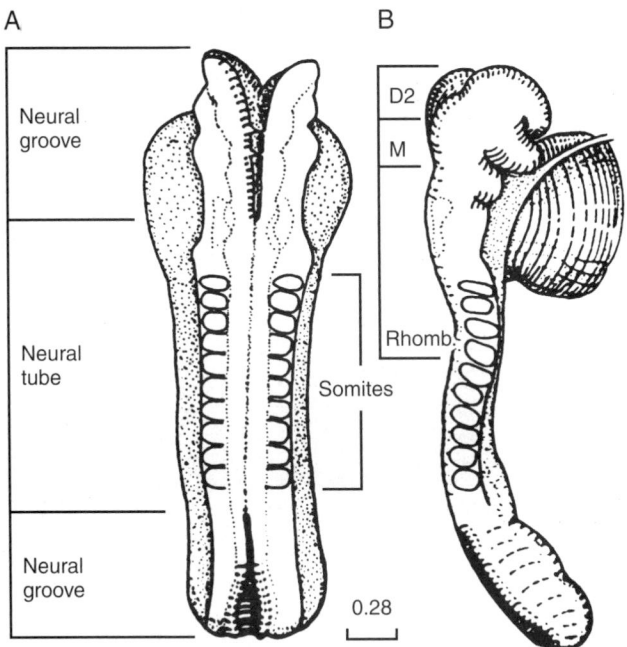

FIGURE 60-2 Positions of anterior and posterior neuropores. *(From O'Rahilly R, Muller F:* The embryonic human brain, *New York, 1994, Wiley-Liss, p 45.)*

nearly triple after each subsequent pregnancy (Elwood et al, 1992).

There has been a marked decline in prevalence at birth of both anencephaly and spina bifida. In 1960, the prevalence for England and Wales was about 6 in 1000 births; in 1990, this rate dropped to about 1 in 1000. The lower rates reflect two major interventions: in utero diagnosis with termination of affected pregnancies and maternal periconceptional folate therapy. The latter is estimated to prevent ~60–70% of neural tube defects (Castilla et al, 2003; Czeizel and Dudas, 1992; Frey and Hauser, 2003; Mills and Signore, 2004; MRC Vitamin Study Research Group, 1992; Oakley et al, 1994; Smithells et al, 1981; Wolff et al, 2009). The mechanisms by which folate prevents defects in neural tube closure remain unclear. There are approximately 200 known genes required for neurulation, many of which are involved in folic acid metabolism or transport (Juriloff and Harris, 2007). Folate deficiency does not cause neural tube defects in mice that lack genetic predisposition (Burren et al, 2008). Although the basis for folate-resistant neural tube defects is unclear, inositol deficiency can trigger neural tube defects in rodents, and inositol supplementation prevents a significant proportion of spinal defects in a mutant mouse model (Copp and Greene, 2009). However, only folate supplementation (0.4 to 0.8 mg daily) is currently recommended for women of childbearing age in the United States (U.S. Preventive Task Force, 2009).

ETIOLOGY

The etiology of neural tube defects is complex and clearly multifactorial. Genetic and environmental factors operate independently to determine individual and population risk. The majority of defects occur sporadically. Although numerous genetic syndromes are associated with familial

forms of neural tube defects, they uncommonly come to term and appear to comprise a very small percentage of all cases (Au et al, 2010; Blom, 2009; Hall and Solehdin, 1998). Such defects have been informative, however, in the identification of many human gene defects that have been confirmed to disrupt key neurulation events in mouse models (Harris and Juriloff, 2007). For example, multiple human gene defects have recently been identified in a noncanonical Wnt signaling pathway shown to regulate cell polarity (Zohn and Sarkar, 2008). Mutations in this pathway disrupt neural tube closure in lower vertebres via a failure of axial elongation or inability of the neural folds to merge in the dorsal midline. Defects range from severe craniorachischisis to spina bifida and exencephaly. One widely studied mouse model is the curly tail (*ct*) variant. The responsible *ct* gene localizes to the distal arm of chromosome 4 and has at least three modifier loci that influence the incidence of neural tube defects (Neumann et al, 1994). An important concept to emerge is that individual gene defects may cause mild or insignificant neurulation defects, whereas compound mutations result in highly penetrant severe defects (Zohn and Sarkar, 2008).

Among the numerous environmental risk factors that have been linked to neural tube defects, the most prominent include maternal febrile illness, maternal heat exposure in the first trimester (e.g., sauna or hot tub use), hyperglycemia from maternal diabetes mellitus or obesity, lower socioeconomic status, dietary factors (prenatal tea but not caffeine consumption), and prenatal exposure to a number of drugs including antiepileptic medications (Au et al, 2010; Blom, 2009; Frey and Hauser, 2003). Valproate and carbamazepine are both associated with an increased risk of neural tube defects (Jones et al, 1989; Yerby, 2003).

DISORDERS OF PRIMARY NEURULATION

Anencephaly

Anencephaly accounts for roughly more than half of all human neural tube defects, which have a worldwide incidence that ranges from 1.0 to 10.0 per 1,000 live births (Au et al, 2010). As an early neurulation defect, it occurs no later than 24 days of gestation. Anencephaly is the most severe and common of the disorders of anterior neural tube closure (Figure 60-3). Both anencephaly and occipital encephaloceles (discussed later) affect girls more than boys. A majority of infants are stillborn. Moreover, it is uniformly lethal within the first 2 months of life in the roughly 25% of cases that survive into the neonatal period (Baird and Sadovnick, 1984; Peabody et al, 1989). The duration of survival is critically related to intensive care support. Without intensive care, survival has not been reported beyond 14 days of life. Survival is related in part to persistence of rudimentary brainstem function. This finding is inconsistent with the diagnosis of brain death in the United States, which is a requirement for organ donation (AAP Committee on Bioethics, 1992; McAbee et al, 2000).

Anencephaly most commonly involves the forebrain and upper brainstem, which accounts for the devastating outcome. It is characterized by absence of the calvaria,

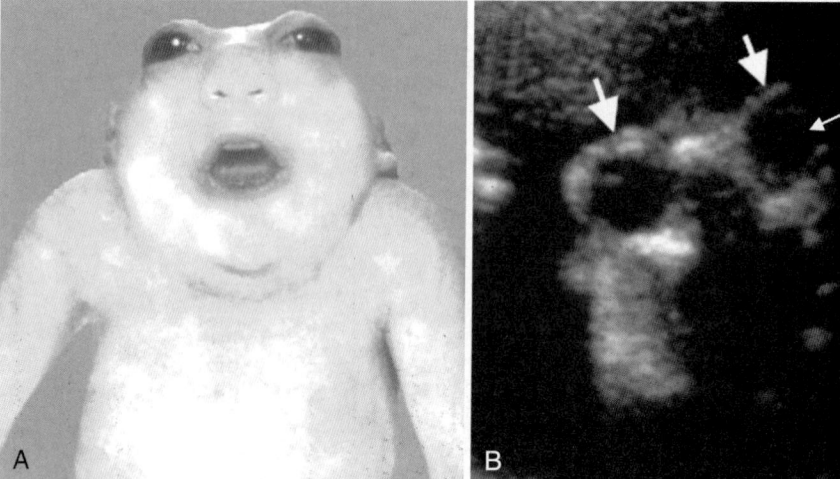

FIGURE 60-3 A, An anencephalic infant. **B,** Ultrasonogram of anencephaly. Note the absence of the normal cranial structures (*large arrows*) superior to the orbits (*O*). (*Courtesy Dr. Marjorie Grafe, Department of Pathology, Oregon Health and Science University.*)

and the intracranial contents are replaced by vascularized, disorganized glial tissue (area cerebrovasculosa) (Menkes, 1991; Roessmann, 1995). The hypothalamus and cerebellum are usually malformed, the anterior lobe of the pituitary is present, and the internal carotid arteries are hypoplastic, which may be secondary to abnormal brain formation. Because the anencephalic infant has a period of exencephaly, in which the brain tissue extrudes through the unformed calvaria and then is degraded by exposure to the amniotic fluid, some investigators have hypothesized that the primary defect is the abnormal skull formation. There are some cases in which remnants of calvarial bones are present, with normal brain under the protective bones (Roessmann, 1995).

Anencephaly can be diagnosed by fetal ultrasound examination (see Figure 60-3, *B*) in the second trimester of gestation (Crane, 1992; Goldstein and Filly, 1988). Polyhydramnios is frequently associated. Anencephaly is also suspected by measurement of alpha-fetoprotein (AFP) in maternal serum. AFP is the major serum protein in the early embryo and is fetus specific. It normally passes from the fetal serum into fetal urine and then into amniotic fluid; in the amniotic fluid, it is swallowed by the fetus and metabolized in the fetal gastrointestinal tract (Brock, 1976). In anencephaly, open spina bifida, and open encephalocele, there is leakage of fetal serum directly into the amniotic fluid, and the level of AFP is elevated in the amniotic fluid, as are maternal serum protein levels. By contrast, when a neural tube defect is closed (i.e., covered by intact skin), the AFP level is not elevated. This occurs in about 5% of neural tube defects (Milunsky et al, 1980).

Encephalocele

In contrast to anencephaly, encephalocele appears to arise from a restricted rather than diffuse failure of anterior neuropore closure around 26 days' gestation. Encephaloceles typically present as a cranial defect through which brain tissue protrudes. Less severe defects may occur with later onset. These include cranium bifidum, where there is a failure of midline fusion of the skull, and cranial

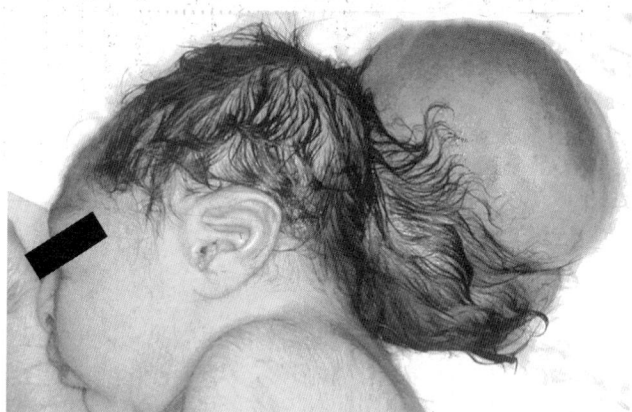

FIGURE 60-4 Newborn infant with a large occipital encephalocele. (*Courtesy Dr. Marjorie Grafe, Department of Pathology, Oregon Health and Science University.*)

meningoceles that contain meningeal but not neural tissue. In up to 80% of cases, encephaloceles occur in the occipital region (Figure 60-4), with the remainder in the parietal, frontonasal, intranasal, or nasopharyngeal regions. Although the precise pathogenetic mechanism remains unclear, geographical or ethnic-genetic factors appear to influence the location of the lesion. Frontal encephaloceles are more prevalent in Southeast Asia, for example, whereas lesions that involve the occipital lobe are more common in Western populations (Mahapatra and Agrawal, 2006). A role for genetic factors is supported by a number of autosomal recessive syndromes where encephalocele is present (e.g., Meckel's syndrome and Walker-Warburg syndrome). Overall, about one half of infants with encephaloceles have other major congenital anomalies that include microcephaly, arhinencephaly, anophthalmia, cleft lip or palate, craniosynostosis, complex congenital heart disease, and other systemic abnormalities (Brown and Sheridan-Pereira, 1992).

Encephaloceles are also associated with various other CNS defects that influence the severity of the outcome as well as the surgical management. These include anomalous draining veins, as well as hydrocephalus, which is observed in up to 50% of cases (Diebler and Dulac, 1987; Menkes, 1991). The occurrence of lower occipital lobe encephalocele with skull base defects and malformations of the cerebellum and lower brainstem characterizes Chiari type III malformations (see later discussion of Chiari type II malformations that occur in association with myelomeningocele). Partial or complete agenesis of the corpus callosum and subependymal nodular heterotopias are other frequently associated CNS malformations, as discussed later.

Evaluation of the infant with an encephalocele can be aided by transillumination, skull radiographs, cranial ultrasound, computed tomography (CT) scan, and magnetic resonance imaging (MRI). Decisions about the appropriate modality depend on the individual cases and whether other cerebral anomalies or hydrocephalus is suspected. Fronto-nasal encephaloceles pulse or bulge with brief bilateral jugular vein compression, indicating communication with the subarachnoid space. Nasal *gliomas*, dermoids, and teratomas can all occur in the same region. Intranasal encephalocele should be suspected when an intranasal mass is found in a child with a broad nasal bridge and widely spaced eyes. Some of these children may also present with recurrent meningitis (Menkes, 1991). Basal encephaloceles are not usually diagnosed until childhood and can be located in the nasopharynx, sphenoid sinus, or posterior orbit.

In the majority of patients, neurosurgical management is indicated early in life. However, large lesions or other severe CNS anomalies may preclude intervention. Early intervention is imperative for those infants at high risk for meningitis caused by lesions that externally communicate and leak CSF. Encephaloceles can trigger medically intractable seizures, which may be responsive to surgical resection (Faulkner et al, 2010). Survival and outcome remain difficult to predict because of the variability of presentation and surgical selection bias. One study of a series of children with encephaloceles reported overall mortality at 29% (45% in infants with posterior defects; 0% in infants with anterior defects) (Brown and Sheridan-Pereira, 1992). Neurologic deficits were severe in 33% of survivors with anterior defects and in 33% of survivors with posterior defects. Mild neurologic deficits were found in 17% of survivors of anterior defects and in 50% of survivors of posterior defects.

Myeloschisis

Myeloschisis may be regarded as being at the more severe end of the spectrum of malformations of the spinal cord that arise from failure of posterior neuropore closure no later than 24 days' gestation. Hence, myeloschisis arises from an extensive failure of posterior neuropore closure, whereas myelomeningocele (see next section) arises from more restricted disturbances in posterior neuropore closure. Myeloschisis manifests as a severely malformed spinal cord with an exposed primitive neural plate–like structure that lacks overlying vertebrae and skin. At the level of the malformed upper cervical cord, there may often be associated malformations of the base of the skull that result in retroflexion of the head on the cervical spine (iniencephaly). Not unexpectedly, a majority of infants with myeloschisis are stillborn.

Myelomeningocele

Myelomeningocele and other associated malformations of the spinal cord arise from restricted failure of posterior neuropore closure probably no later than day 26 of gestation. The incidence of myelomeningocele has fallen substantially since the recognition that maternal folate plays a critical role in neural tube closure. Consequently, in the United States, the prevalence of spina bifida was reported in 2005 to be 2 in 10,000 live births and fell approximately 23% between 1995 and 2003 (Au et al, 2010). The spectrum of these spinal cord malformations includes myelomeningocele and meningocele. Myelomeningocele is characterized by herniation of the meninges and spinal cord at the site of the defect. Myelomeningoceles are usually exposed lesions on the back without vertebral or dermal covering (Figure 60-5), unless a lipoma overlies the defect (i.e., a lipomyelomeningocele) (Menkes, 1991). A meningocele is a restricted herniation of the meninges at the defect site. It is usually covered by skin, and neurologic function is often normal. Myelomeningoceles are about 4 times more common than meningoceles (Friede, 1989; Menkes, 1991). These lesions most often occur in the lumbar or lumbosacral regions (69% of cases), which supports the concept that the site of final closure of the posterior neuropore is in the lumbar region.

Myelomeningocele is rarely an isolated malformation, but is usually accompanied by other clinically significant CNS abnormalities. Of major importance is hydrocephalus, which is frequently associated with the Arnold-Chiari II malformation, discussed later (Del Bigio, 2010). Hydrocephalus is not universal, and its development in myelomeningocele correlates with the site of the lesion. Sixty percent of patients with occipital, cervical, thoracic, or sacral lesions develop hydrocephalus, whereas 90% of those with thoracolumbar, lumbar, or lumbosacral lesions do so (Lorber, 1961). Increased intracranial pressure is present in about 15% of newborns with myelomeningocele. In some infants, there are no signs of increased pressure because of decompression due to leakage of cerebrospinal fluid (CSF) from the myelomeningocele (Stein and Schut, 1979). In these infants, hydrocephalus and increased pressure may become evident later after surgical closure of the myelomeningocele. Most infants with hydrocephalus develop an abnormal increase in head circumference within a month after birth (Stein and Schut, 1979).

As in anencephaly, fetal diagnosis of an open myelomeningocele is suspected by detection of an elevation in AFP in maternal serum and can be confirmed by fetal ultrasound or MRI (see Figure 60-5, *A*) (Cameron and Moran, 2009). Screen for AFP is usually performed in the second trimester together with three additional markers (human chorionic gonadotropin [hCG], unconjugated estriol [ue(3)], and inhibin A) that collectively comprise the "quadruple screen." This screen is designed to detect open neural tube defects and Down syndrome (Anderson and Brown, 2009). A false-positive AFP result occurs with misdating of the fetus (older than predicted) and multiple gestation pregnancy (Brock, 1976). Other causes of a high maternal serum AFP include contamination of the amniotic fluid by fetal blood, which may occur in cases of esophageal and duodenal atresia, annular pancreas, omphalocele, gastroschisis, congenital nephrosis, polycystic kidneys, renal

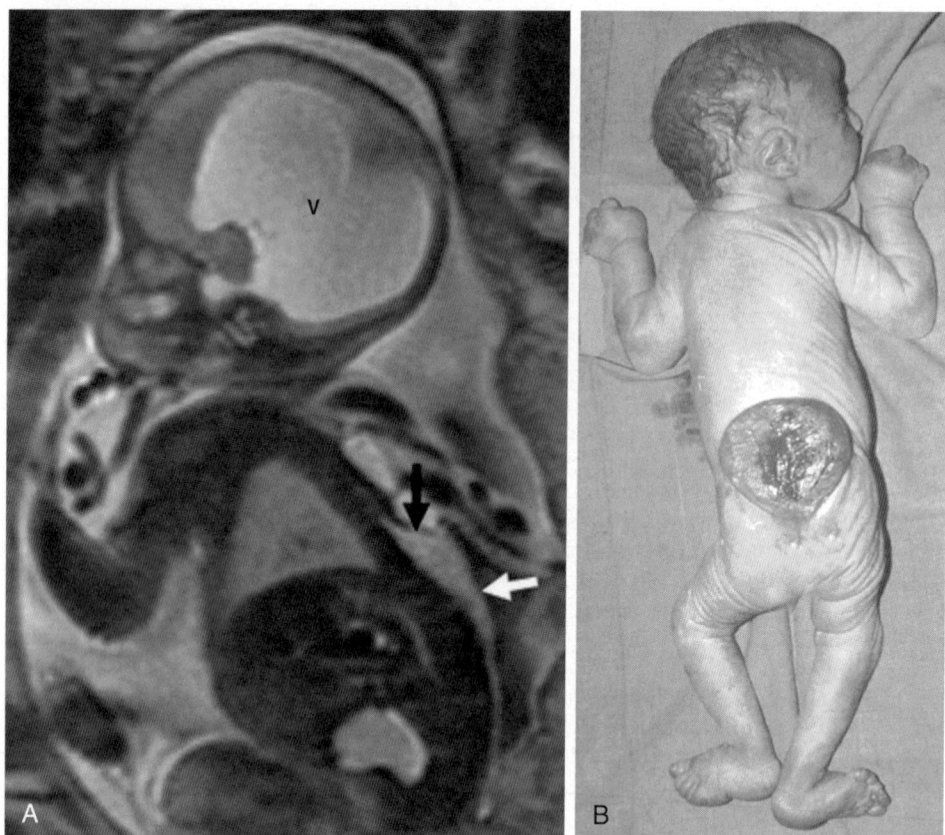

FIGURE 60-5 **A,** Fetal magnetic resonance image of a thoracolumbar dysraphism. The *black arrow* marks the upper limit of the dysraphism and the *white arrow* indicates the meningocele. Note the severe ventriculomegaly *(V).* **B,** Newborn infant with a large thoracolumbar myelomeningocele. There is weakness of the distal musculature in the lower extremities. (*A, Courtesy Dr. Dianna M. E. Bardo, Department of Radiology, Oregon Health and Science University. **B,** Courtesy Dr. Marjorie Grafe, Department of Pathology, Oregon Health and Science University.*)

agenesis, or fetal demise. The optimal time for determination in maternal serum is 16 to 18 weeks' gestation and in amniotic fluid at 14 to 16 weeks' gestation.

Clinical management of the newborn with a neural tube defect must be individualized. In the past, selective aggressive treatment was instituted for infants anticipated to have a better outcome. At present, aggressive surgical therapy is advocated for most infants; to date, this has resulted in patients with increased cognitive abilities, increased ambulation, a lower incidence of incontinence, and lower mortality (Hunt and Holmes, 1975; McLone 1992; Stein et al, 1975).

Prenatal fetoscopic surgical repair of myelomeningocele is under active investigation as a means to reduce direct injury that is suspected to occur as a result of chronic exposure of neural tissue to amniotic fluid (Hirose and Farmer, 2009). Preliminary studies found no consistent evidence for improved urologic or neurologic function and identified concerns for maternal safety. An ongoing multicenter trial seeks to identify a subset of patients for whom there is potential benefit (Hirose and Farmer, 2009).

Arnold-Chiari Malformation

The Arnold-Chiari malformation occurs in at least 95% of children with a myelomeningocele that includes a lumbar lesion (Figure 60-6). This malformation results in two types of serious complications (hydrocephalus and

brainstem dysfunction) that are a significant cause of morbidity and mortality in infants with a myelomeningocele. The clinical sequelae of this class of malformations are best understood in the context of the principal types of associated anatomical abnormalities (Juranek and Salman, 2010). Hindbrain malformations involve both the brainstem and the cerebellum. Brainstem abnormalities include downward displacement of the medulla and the fourth ventricle through the foramen magnum into the upper cervical canal, which results in obstruction of the fourth ventricle and compression of the upper cervical cord. The resultant downward stretch of the cervical roots causes them to project cranially to their foramina rather than to follow their normal lateral or descending course. The caudal displacement of the brainstem thins and elongates the lower pons and upper medulla, which may compress brainstem nuclei as well as compromise the roots of the cranial nerves (Blaauw, 1971; Friede, 1989; Naidich et al, 1980). The herniation of the cerebellar tonsils through the foramen magnum and flattening of the lower cerebellar hemispheres are frequently associated with the caudal displacement of the brainstem. A variety of bony malformations are observed that include enlargement of the foramen magnum, defects of the occiput, and anomalies of the cervical vertebrae. Finally, cortical neuronal migration abnormalities (cerebral cortical dysplasia or polymicrogyria) are frequently associated with Chiari malformations and may account for cognitive deficits and epilepsy seen in some patients.

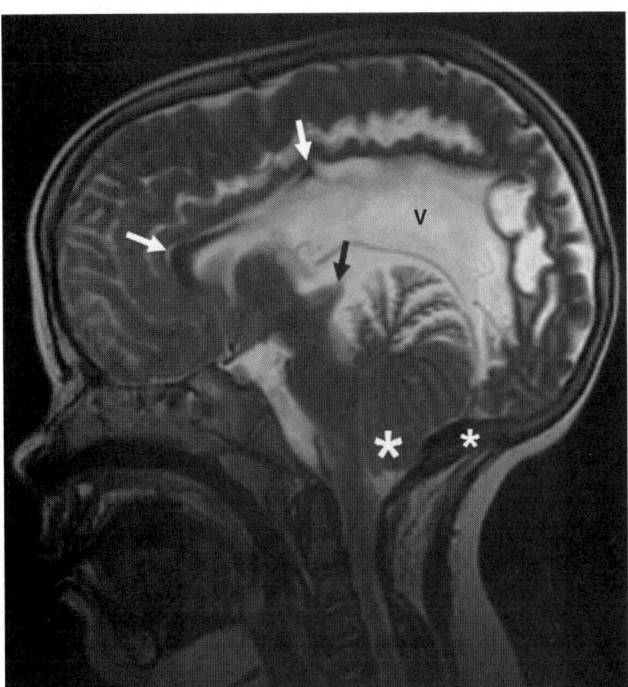

FIGURE 60-6 Sagittal magnetic resonance image (T2) of a child with myelomeningocele and a Chiari II malformation with downward displacement of the cerebellar tonsils (*large asterisk*) and a low position of the torcula (*small asterisk*). Note the pronounced hydrocephalus and ventriculomegaly *(V)*, dysplastic corpus callosum (*white arrows*), and the beaked tectum (*black arrow*). *(Courtesy Dr. Dianna M. E. Bardo, Department of Radiology, Oregon Health and Science University.)*

It follows from this constellation of hindbrain abnormalities that hydrocephalus is commonly associated with Chiari malformations (Del Bigio, 2010). The hydrocephalus may arise from compression of the fourth ventricle or obstruction of CSF outflow through the foramen magnum. In addition, many patients also have aqueductal stenosis or uncommonly, aqueductal atresia (Gilbert et al, 1986; Peach, 1965; Stein and Schut, 1979). A less well recognized but potentially fatal complication of hindbrain abnormalities is primary dysfunction of the brainstem. This can manifest as apneic episodes with cyanosis, vocal cord paralysis with laryngeal stridor, or feeding disturbances that result in aspiration related to reflux. Ventilatory disturbances may be either obstructive or central and, thus, prominent during sleep. These disturbances may be identified by polysomnography and pulmonary function studies (Kirk et al, 1999).

Occult Spinal Dysraphisms

Occult spinal dysraphic states are the result of defects in caudal neural tube formation (i.e., secondary neurulation). As discussed previously, development of the sacral and coccygeal segments of the spinal cord involves a process of canalization and caudal regression of the distal neural tube. In contrast to defects in primary neural tube formation, these defects thus uniformly localize to the distal cord and are closed defects with an intact dermal covering. In some instances, these defects are truly occult without any overlying abnormalities of the skin and may go undetected until symptomatic. However, in the majority of newborn

infants a lumbosacral midline cutaneous lesion may indicate an occult spinal dysraphism (Figure 60-7). These lesions include abnormal hair tufts, hemangiomas, pigmented spots, skin tags, aplasia cutis congenita, cutaneous dimples or tracts, or a subcutaneous mass (Albright et al, 1989; Hall et al, 1981; Scatliff et al, 1989).

The spinal cord lesions associated with occult dysraphisms include myelocystocele; diastematomyelia-diplomyelia; meningocele-lipomeningocele; lipoma, teratoma, and other tumors; dermal sinus with or without dermoid or epidermoid cyst formation; and tethered cord (Anderson, 1975; Menkes, 1991) (Figure 60-8). More severe lesions include neurenteric cyst, anterior meningocele, and the findings of the caudal regression syndrome (dysraphia of sacrum and coccyx, atrophy of muscles and bones of the legs, fusion of spinal nerves and sensory ganglia, or agenesis of the distal spinal cord) (Towfighi and Housman, 1991). Infants of diabetic mothers are at increased risk for these lesions as well as for more severe neural tube defects (Becerra et al, 1990).

Regardless of the caudal neural tube malformation, an almost invariate feature is an abnormal conus and a thickened filum. A symptomatic tethered cord is a common presentation after surgical repair of myelomeningocele (Bowman et al, 2009). The movement of the filum is commonly restricted or "tethered" by fibrous bands or masses (e.g., a lipoma or teratoma) that can be diagnosed prenatally (Sohaey et al, 2009). Consequently, during growth of the lower spinal cord, progressive functional impairment can occur as the cord is stretched against the fixed filum (Lew and Kothbauer, 2007). Neurologic impairment rarely presents in the newborn period (Hertlzer et al, 2010). Deficits related to these lesions, which occur in infancy and childhood, include delay in walking, disturbed sphincter control, anatomic abnormalities of the feet or legs, and pain in the back or legs. Gait and sphincter abnormalities, foot deformities, and scoliosis are more common in older patients. Recurrent meningitis and rapid loss of function are rare but serious presentations. In the newborn period, a diagnostic evaluation of occult dysraphisms is indicated because early surgical intervention now carries a low risk of morbidity and can preclude sudden neurologic deterioration and the development of permanent deficits (Gower et al, 1988; Hertzler et al, 2010; Scatliff et al, 1989). In neonates, this evaluation may be facilitated by spinal radiographs or CT, which may detect vertebral anomalies; spinal ultrasonography, which permits a dynamic evaluation of lower spinal cord mobility; and MR imaging to define structural anomalies of the cord. After the age of 3 to 4 months, the ossification centers of the spine interfere with visualization of the conus medullaris and its normal motion by ultrasonography. Hence, high-resolution MRI with thin slices (2.5 to 3.0 mm) is the preferred study to evaluate tethered cord and lipomas of the filum. MRI is currently under investigation to evaluate movement-dependent changes in position of the conus medullaris in relation to the dorsal dural surface of the thecal sac.

DISORDERS OF NEURAL CREST MIGRATION

As the neural tube begins to fuse, the neural crest forms as a distinct region of neuroectoderm at the junction between the neural plate and the lateral ectoderm (see

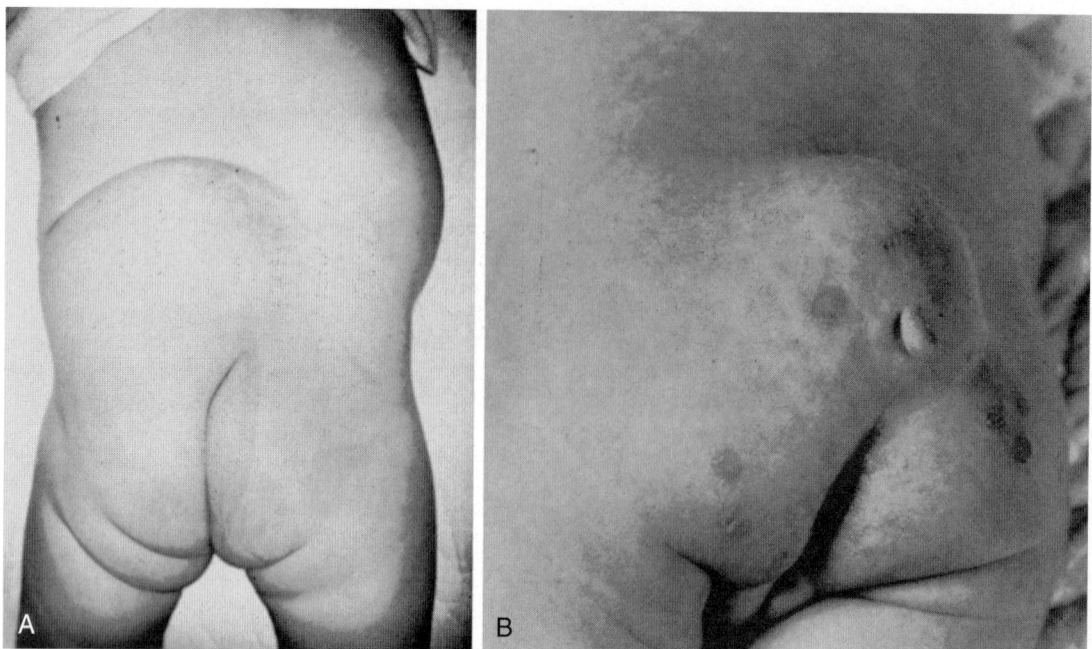

FIGURE 60-7 **A** and **B, Two examples of lipomeningocele.** Each presented in the left buttock as a firm, well-circumscribed, lobulated tumor that became tense when the infant cried. **B** shows macular erosions and a congenital skin tag and dimple over the surface. This last feature may be a pilonidal dimple displaced by the tumor.

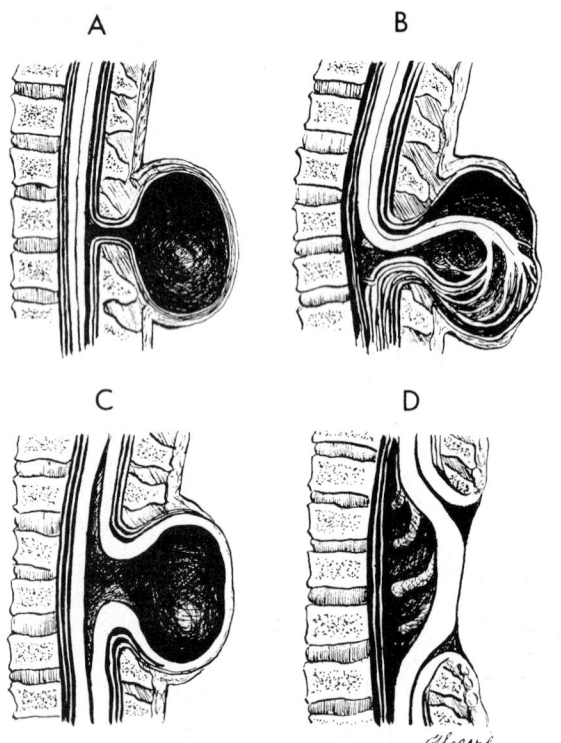

FIGURE 60-8 **Diagram of meningoceles. A,** Meningocele: Through the bony defect (spina bifida), the meninges herniate and form a cystic sac filled with spinal fluid. The spinal cord does not participate in the herniation and may or may not be abnormal. **B,** Myelomeningocele: Spina bifida with myelomeningocele; the spinal cord is herniated into the sac and ends there or may continue in an abnormal way further downward. **C,** Myelocystocele or syringomyelocele: The spinal cord shows hydromyelia; the posterior wall of the spinal cord is attached to the ectoderm and undifferentiated. **D,** Myelocele: The spinal cord is araphic; a cystic cavity is in front of the anterior wall of the spinal cord. *(From Benda CE:* Developmental disorders of mentation and cerebral palsies, *New York, 1952, Grune and Stratton.)*

Figure 60-1, *B*). This special population of cells gives rise to a remarkably large and diverse number of structures within and outside of the nervous system. There are four major derivatives of the neural crest: the cranial, the vagal and sacral, the truncal, and the cardiac (Hall, 2008). Neural crest derivatives that contribute to the nervous system include the sensory ganglia of cranial nerves V, VI, IX, and X (cranial neural crest); parasympathetic ganglia (vagal neural crest); dorsal root ganglia; sympathetic ganglia (truncal neural crest); and celiac, mesenteric, and aorticorenal ganglia (cardiac neural crest). The truncal neural crest becomes fragmented along with the truncal somites. After the neural crest anlage are formed, neural crest cells migrate throughout the entire embryo. Migration is rostrocaudal, along the medial axis of the embryo (LeDouarin, 1982). After migration is complete, the neural crest cells contributes to five major systems: (1) nervous system: meningioblasts, Schwann cells, ganglia (including enteric ganglion cells of the digestive tract); (2) endocrine system: chromaffin cells of the adrenal medulla and several types of endocrine and paraendocrine cells; (3) melanoblasts in all tissues except the retina; (4) the skeletal system of the head, face, and neck; and (5) cardiac system: connective tissue of the great vessels, aorticopulmonary septum, and smooth muscle of the great arteries.

Abnormalities thus can arise in the migration or differentiation of the neural crest cells, or neural crest derivatives may develop tumors (Jacobson, 1991; Reznik and Pierard, 1995). Disorders related to abnormalities of neural crest formation, migration, proliferation, or differentiation include the LEOPARD syndrome, multiple lentigines syndrome, NAME syndrome, LAMB syndrome, Peutz-Jeghers-Touraine syndrome, and Treacher–Collins syndrome (Reznik and Pierard, 1995). Tumors derived from neural crest cells include those arising from Schwann cells, perineural cells, or fibrocytes; from neural sense organs; from ganglionic or neuroendocrine cells; or from melanogenic cells (Louis and von Deimling, 1995; Reznik and Pierard, 1995). Neuroblastoma is a neuroectodermal tumor that occurs mostly in children. It usually arises from the adrenal gland but can arise from sympathetic ganglia, the neuroendocrine system, or the ovary (Maris, 2010). It is sometimes seen in association with neurofibromatosis. Cutaneous metastases from neuroblastoma can occur as multiple skin nodules and have been seen in the newborn.

Hirschsprung's disease is a disorder of neural crest stem cells that occurs in 1 in 5000 births (Mundt and Bates, 2010). It is characterized by absence of hindgut intramural ganglion cells, which causes intestinal obstruction in the neonatal period. A gene associated with some cases of Hirschsprung's disease has been mapped to chromosome 10 and localized to the *RET* proto-oncogene (Edery et al, 1994; Moore and Zaahl, 2008; Romeo et al, 1994; Yin et al, 1994). Mutations that affect the RET protein also occur in patients with multiple endocrine neoplasia type 2A (Donis-Keller et al, 1993; Moore and Zaahl, 2008; Mulligan et al, 1993).

PROSENCEPHALIC CLEAVAGE AND RELATED EVENTS

NORMAL PROSENCEPHALIC DEVELOPMENT

The prosencephalon refers embryologically to the telencephalon and the diencephalon, the future forebrain. The telencephalon gives rise to the cerebral hemispheres; the diencephalon gives rise to the thalamus and hypothalamus. Prosencephalic development begins shortly after the closure of the anterior neuropore. The prosencephalon arises through developmental processes that induce the bifurcation of the rostral extent of the fluid-filled neural tube to form the right and left forebrain structures (Rubenstein and Beachy, 1998). This process thus involves the duplication of structures along the midline. The inductive processes that direct forebrain development also control craniofacial development. Hence, disruption of prosencephalic development is frequently associated with midline anomalies of both the forebrain and the face.

During the 5th to 6th weeks of development, the ultimate structure of the forebrain is defined by the sequential cleavage of the forebrain along three major planes. As the anterior neuropore is closing, the first major event is formation of the optic vesicles and nasal placodes, separated along the *horizontal* plane, which will give rise to the neural and craniofacial structures of the visual and olfactory systems, respectively. Shortly thereafter, when the embryo has reached a length of about 5 mm, both neuropores have closed, thus isolating the developing ventricular system from the amniotic fluid. At this time, the retinal and lens placodes are developing. Concurrently, in the brainstem, the cerebellum begins to form, as well as some somatic and visceral efferent nuclei, the common afferent tract, and the ganglia for most of the cranial nerves.

At about day 32 of gestation, when the embryo is 5 to 7 mm long, the second major event in forebrain development occurs when the forebrain is cleaved in the *sagittal* plane to give rise to the paired cerebral hemispheres, lateral ventricles, and basal ganglia. Specific areas, such as the

hypothalamic, amygdaloid, hippocampal, and olfactory regions, can be defined. Shortly thereafter, the third major event in forebrain development occurs when the forebrain is cleaved in the *coronal* or *transverse* plane to separate the telencephalon from the diencephalon, thus defining the epithalamus, subthalamus, and hypothalamus.

During the remainder of the 2nd and 3rd months of gestation, the subsequent events in forebrain development occur along the midline to generate three major structures: the corpus callosum, the optic nerve/chiasm, and the hypothalamus. Disturbances in the formation of these midline structures, in particular the corpus callosum and the optic chiasm, are reflected in abnormal axon "pathfinding" to the midline and the failure of hemispheric and optic fibers to cross to the opposite hemisphere.

DISORDERS OF STRUCTURES DERIVED FROM THE PROSENCEPHALON

Holoprosencephaly

Holoprosencephaly (HPE) is the most common brain malformation (Barr and Cohen, 1999; Norman et al, 1995a) in that it has a prevalence of 1 in 250 in the developing embryo. However, many of these conceptuses do not survive to term, resulting in a live birth prevalence of 1 in 10,000 to 1 in 20,000 (Croen et al, 1996; Croen et al, 2000; Orioli and Castilla, 2010; Rasmussen et al, 1996). The abnormality in HPE is a variable degree of incomplete separation of the prosencephalon along one or more of its three major planes. HPE represents a continuum of prosencephalic nonseparation that is traditionally divided into alobar, semilobar, and lobar types (Figure 60-9). In *alobar* HPE (Figure 60-10), the most severe type, a single anterior ventricle is contained within a holosphere (i.e., there is a complete lack of separation of the prosencephalon into two distinct hemispheres, which manifests as the absence of the interhemispheric fissure). There is complete agenesis of the corpus callosum, the thalami usually are fused, and the basal ganglia are a single mass. Milder presentations involve partially formed hemispheres—*semilobar* HPE—and *lobar* forms, in which the distinct hemispheres can be distinguished and a portion of the posterior corpus callosum is present. In addition to these traditional HPE categories, a "middle hemispheric variant" has been described in which the posterior frontal and parietal lobes (i.e., the "midsections" of the brain) fail to separate, with absence of the body of the corpus callosum but presence of the genu and splenium (Barkovich and Quint, 1993; Lewis et al, 2002).

Associated with this midline brain malformation in HPE are often midline craniofacial anomalies. This may range from cyclopia (a single central eye) with a noselike structure (proboscis) above the eye, to cebocephaly (a flattened single nostril situated centrally between the eyes), to median cleft lip. Mildly affected infants may display a single central incisor or hypotelorism. It is often stated that "the face predicts the brain," referring to the fact that more severe facial malformations are often associated with more severe brain malformations. There are exceptions to this rule, however, with patients with lobar HPE having normal facies, and those with alobar HPE having

FIGURE 60-9 The spectrum of holoprosencephaly as demonstrated by magnetic resonance imaging. **A** and **B,** Magnetic resonance images of the brain in a patient with alobar HPE. T1-weighted axial image **(A)** reveals lack of separation of the two hemispheres and deep gray nuclei. Large dorsal cyst (dc) is observed posteriorly. T1-weighted sagittal image **(B)** reveals a midline ventricle, a monoventricle (mv), that communicates posteriorly with the dorsal cyst *(dc)*. **C** and **D,** Magnetic resonance imaging of a patient with semilobar HPE. T2-weighted axial image **(C)** indicates separation of the hemispheres posteriorly but not anteriorly. Anterior horns of the lateral ventricles are absent, whereas the posterior horns are well formed and separated. There is also an incomplete separation of the basal ganglia. T2-weighted coronal image **(D)** reveals a lack of interhemispheric fissure and a monoventricle *(mv)*. **E** and **F,** Magnetic resonance imaging of the brain in a patient with lobar HPE. T1-weighted axial image **(E)** reveals that two hemispheres are fairly well separated as manifested by the presence of an interhemispheric fissure both anteriorly and posteriorly. Note that the frontal horns of the lateral ventricles are only rudimentary *(arrowheads)*. T1-weighted coronal image **(F)** documents incomplete separation of the inferior frontal lobes near the midline. **G** and **H,** Magnetic resonance imaging of the brain in a patient with the middle interhemispheric variant of HPE. T1-weighted axial **(G)** and coronal **(H)** images demonstrate the continuity of gray matter in the posterior frontal lobes across the midline *(arrows)*. For T1-weighted images, TR of 600–630 ms and TE of 10–16 ms were used. For T2-weighted images, TR of 3000 ms and TE of 120 ms were used. *(From Hahn JS, Plawner LL: Evaluation and management of children with holoprosencephaly,* Pediatr Neurol *31:79-88, 2004.)*

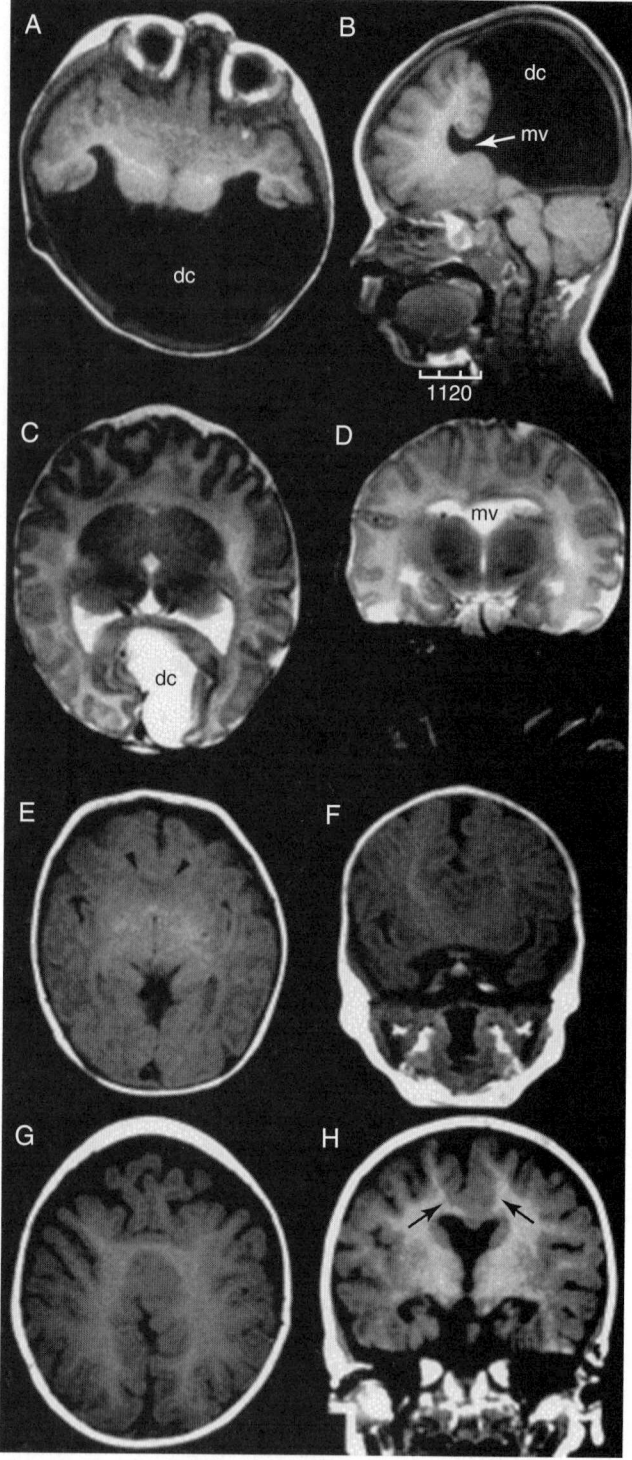

more severely abnormal facies (Cohen, 1989; DeMyer et al, 1964; Plawner et al, 2002).

Clinical Features

Early literature indicated that children with HPE uniformly died during infancy. This statement may have been due to identification of only the most severe cases. Early death is typical for most cytogenetically abnormal children (Croen et al, 1996). However, of cytogenetically normal patients with all types of HPE, more than 50% are alive at 12 months (Barr and Cohen, 1999; Olsen et al, 1997). Survival into late adolescence and adulthood has been reported (Levey et al, 2010; Plawner et al, 2002).

Children with HPE face many medical and neurologic problems. The severity of their symptoms is often correlated with the degree of brain malformation. Microcephaly is the rule, except when hydrocephalus results (Hahn and Plawner, 2004). It has been hypothesized that hydrocephalus results from the blockage of CSF flow through the fused thalami, and the development of a large dorsal cyst (Simon et al, 2001). If there is clinical evidence that these fluid collections are under pressure, placement of ventriculoperitoneal shunts can improve symptoms (Levey et al, 2010).

As with other midline brain defects, endocrinologic abnormalities are very common. Diabetes insipidus occurs in up to 70%, with hypothyroidism, hypoadrenocorticism, and growth hormone deficiency being much less common (Hahn et al, 2005). Diabetes insipidus should be screened for intermittently because it may develop over time. Hypothalamic dysfunction also may cause irregularities of sleep, temperature regulation, appetite, and thirst.

Despite the significant brain malformations in HPE, only about 40% of children will have epilepsy; about one third of these will have intractable epilepsy (Plawner et al, 2002; Levey et al, 2010). Seizures may also be provoked

by endocrinologic abnormalities such as hypernatremia or hypoglycemia. Abnormal muscle tone and motoric dysfunction are very common in children with HPE. Hypotonia is most common during infancy, with the development of spasticity and dystonia as the child develops. The motor dysfunction also causes poor oromotor function, and about two thirds of children with HPE will require gastrostomy tube placement.

Delayed development and cognitive disability are very frequent in HPE and are related to the degree of brain

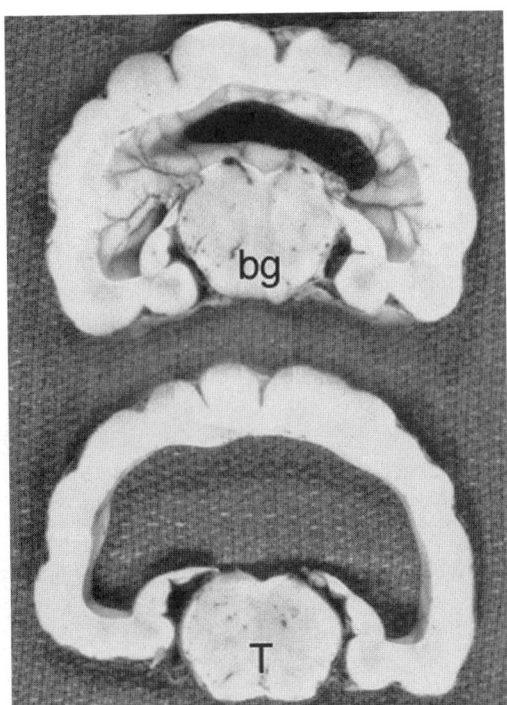

FIGURE 60-10 Alobar holoprosencephaly. Coronal views demonstrate a single anterior ventricle. Note the complete lack of separation of the forebrain into two distinct hemispheres. There is agenesis of the corpus callosum, the basal ganglia are a single mass (*bg*), and the thalami (*T*) are usually fused. (*Courtesy Dr. Marjorie Grafe, Department of Pathology, Oregon Health and Science University.*)

malformation. Alobar HPE patients are nonambulatory. Patients with lobar HPE may ambulate, have functional hand use, and some degree of verbal communication. In all types of HPE there are relative strengths in receptive language and socialization (Kovar et al, 2001).

Etiology and Epidemiology

The etiology of HPE clearly is multifactorial, and both genetic and environmental factors appear to contribute to the extremely variable spectrum of forebrain and craniofacial malformations (Golden, 1998; Muenke and Beachy, 2000; Norman et al, 1995a). It has been appreciated for over a century that a wide variety of environmental insults (e.g., ethanol, vitamin A toxicity related to elevated retinoic acid levels) applied experimentally can produce cyclopia during the early phase of gastrulation in vertebrate embryos. Maternal diabetes mellitus increases the risk for HPE about 200-fold, to approximately 1% to 2% of all pregnancies. Cholesterol-lowering agents have recently been associated with HPE, by a mechanism described later (Edison and Muenke, 2003).

The genetic basis of HPE has been an area of very active and fruitful research. HPE may be caused by an abnormality in chromosome number, or a single-gene mutation. Abnormalities in single genes may causes either "syndromic" (i.e., associated with multiple other congenital anomalies), or "nonsyndromic" HPE. The most common disorders of chromosomal number that manifest with HPE are triploidy and trisomies 13 and 18. These abnormalities often result in pregnancies that do not survive to term, so the incidence is higher in studies looking at conceptuses

rather than live births. Approximately 18% to 25% of HPE result from a mutation in a single gene, which causes syndromic HPE such as the Smith-Lemli-Opitz, Rubenstein-Taybi, Kallman, and Pallister-Hall syndromes (Muenke and Beachy, 2000). Six genes have been well established to cause nonsyndromic HPE: *Shh*, *ZIC2*, *SIX3*, *TGIF*, *GLI2*, and *PTCH1*). Shh was the first identified, best studied, and accounts for up to 40% of familial cases of HPE (Nanni et al, 1999; Roessler et al, 1996). Several of the other genes just listed are involved in the Shh pathway (see later discussion). Five other genes have been associated with HPE, but they are rare, and putative pathophysiologic pathways have not been well established.

HPE is characterized by extreme intrafamilial variability. Asymptomatic or mildly affected family members may carry a deletion for a gene associated with HPE, whereas in a subsequent generation, offspring with the same gene may be severely affected. One explanation for these paradoxical observations comes from studies supporting that the mode of inheritance for HPE may be multigenic transmission (Ming and Muenke, 2002). Mouse models of HPE exist in which mutations in two distinct genes are required to cause HPE. Several affected patients have been identified in whom abnormal alleles for two separate genes were identified. In these cases, a phenotypically normal parent carried a mutation for one gene but not the other (Nanni et al, 1999; Roessler et al, 1996). Hence, the severity of expression of the HPE phenotype throughout a given family may be influenced by the additive contributions from multiple environmental/teratogenic and genetic factors, which may be weighted differently in each affected family member.

Despite the wide intrafamilial variability, some genotype-phenotype correlations have emerged. For example, patients with ZIC2 mutations can have a characteristic facial appearance consisting of bitemporal narrowing, upslanting palpebral fissures, large ears, and a short nose with anteverted nares. ZIC2 mutations also appear to be the most common de novo mutation and have a high penetrance (Solomon et al, 2009, 2010).

Related Molecular Genetic Events

It was recognized decades ago that experimental ablation of the prechordal mesoderm, a mesodermal cell group under the ventral forebrain, disrupted the formation of the chiasmatic plate and optic vesicles and produced cyclopia. It was proposed that the prechordal plate induced the formation of ventral forebrain structures and directed the segmentation of the developing optic fields. Only recently has this complex picture begun to be clarified by the identification of multiple genes expressed in the prechordal plate that directly or indirectly regulate the development of the ventral forebrain. Many of these genes were identified in chromosomal regions with known deletions associated with HPE.

Shh is a signaling molecule secreted in the prechordal mesoderm that directs early embryonic patterning of the ventral forebrain. Mutations of the gene for Shh were the first identified to cause human HPE (Nanni et al, 1999; Roessler et al, 1996). Subsequently, mutations in other genes in the Shh signaling pathway also were identified, underscoring the importance of defects in Shh signaling in the pathogenesis of HPE (Muenke and Beachy, 2000). These include mutations in the receptor for Shh, PTCH1 (Patched), in GLI2, which is a zinc finger transcription factor that mediates Shh signaling, and in ZIC2, which may mediate the response to Shh protein signaling (Warr et al, 2008).

Cholesterol is necessary for Shh functioning, which has implications for both genetic and environmental causation of HPE. Smith-Lemli-Opitz syndrome arises from a defect in the terminal step in cholesterol biosynthesis (7-dehydrocholesterol reductase); approximately 5% of cases of this syndrome manifest with HPE. Additionally, two plant alkaloids—cyclopamine and jervine—have been identified that caused epidemics of cyclopia in sheep that ingested plants rich in these compounds. Both compounds disrupt the Shh signaling pathway via inhibition of cholesterol biosynthesis. A recent study of cholesterol synthesis in patients with HPE showed that 10% had abnormalities in cholesterol production. About a quarter of these also had a mutation in one of the known HPE genes (Hass et al, 2007). Such findings support that the interactions of multiple environmental/teratogenic and genetic variables are likely to account for the considerable heterogeneity in the phenotypic expression of HPE within families and populations.

Agenesis of the Corpus Callosum

The corpus callosum is the largest of the cerebral commissures and consists of 190 million axons. The formation of the corpus callosum is a complex, multistep process that involves cellular proliferation, cellular migration, axonal growth, and midline patterning. This process is mediated by many genes and takes at least 11 weeks to complete. Thus, there are many genetic as well as environmental factors that can affect callosal formation and result in complete callosal agenesis (ACC) or callosal hypoplasia (Figure 60-11). At least 12 genomic loci are consistently associated with ACC, many of which appear to confer susceptibility to other brain malformations such as cerebellar hypoplasia, microcephaly, and polymicrogyria (O'Driscoll et al, 2010).

Agenesis of the corpus callosum may be difficult to distinguish from conditions in which dysgenesis, hypoplasia, or destructive lesions have occurred. The anatomic features of true agenesis of the corpus callosum include abnormal gyration of the medial portion of each hemisphere, eversion of the cingulate gyri, and sulcation that is perpendicular to the long axis of the hemisphere (Barkovich and Norman, 1988). The external angles of the lateral ventricle are oriented parallel and upward, toward the vertex, and the fornices are widely separated (Figure 60-12). When present, a useful distinguishing feature is Probst's bundles, which are fiber bundles that run parallel to the ventricle and carry callosal fibers in an anterior-to-posterior direction. Agenesis of the corpus callosum can be total or partial; when it is partial, the splenium is involved, and the genu remains intact (Roessmann, 1995; Schaefer, 1991).

Agenesis of the corpus callosum is a feature of dozens of different disorders. It is a primary feature of several important genetic syndromes such as Mowat-Wilson, Aicardi's syndrome, and X-linked lissencephaly with ACC

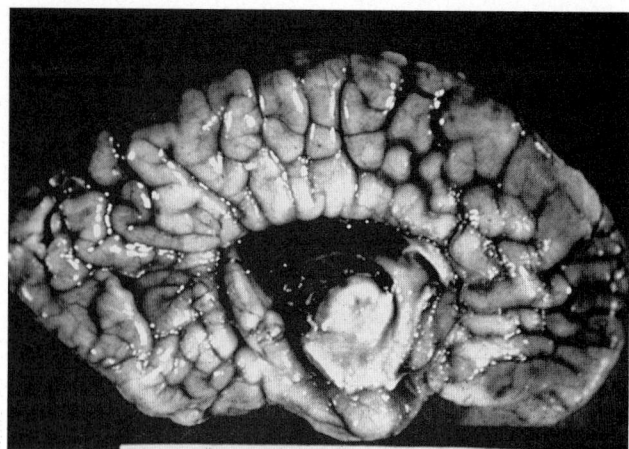

FIGURE 60-11 Agenesis of the corpus callosum. *(Courtesy Dr. Dawna L. Armstrong, Department of Pathology, Texas Children's Hospital.)*

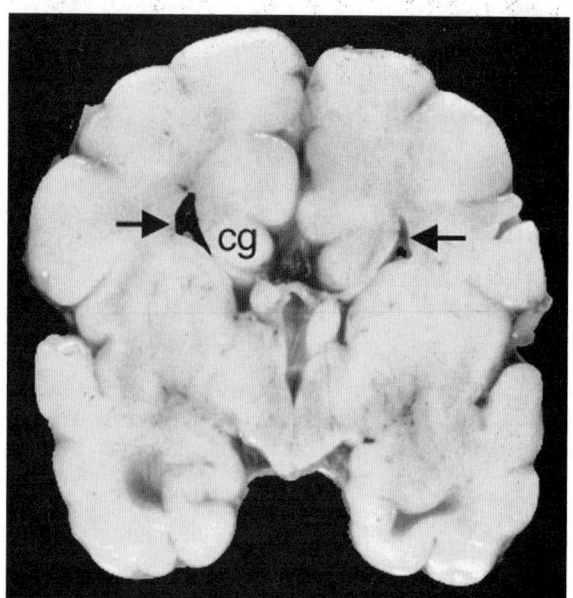

FIGURE 60-12 Agenesis of the corpus callosum. Note the eversion of both of the cingulate gyri *(cg)*. The lateral ventricles are oriented parallel and pointed upward toward the vertex *(arrows)*. Probst's bundles are not apparent in this immature brain. *(Courtesy Dr. Marjorie Grafe, Department of Pathology, Oregon Health and Science University.)*

and ambiguous genitalia (XLAG). It can also be seen as a nonspecific finding, such as in Sotos' or Wolf-Hirschhorn syndromes (Table 60-2). A recent population-based study (Glass et al, 2008) found that callosal anomalies were associated with a chromosomal abnormality 17% of the time, commonly aneuploidy (chromosomes 13, 18, 21). Environmental influences (e.g., teratogens or in utero infections) have also been implicated in the causation of ACC. Ethanol exposure has the strongest association with ACC and is seen in 7% of children with fetal alcohol syndrome (Roebuck et al, 1998).

ACC is associated with other CNS malformations 29 to 80% of the time and with musculoskeletal and cardiac abnormalities 34% and 28% of the time, respectively (Glass et al, 2008; Jeret et al, 1987; Parish et al, 1979). The concurrent CNS malformations seen with ACC are diverse and include heterotopia, abnormal sulcation, commissural

TABLE 60-2   Partial List of Syndromes Associated With Agenesis of the Corpus Callosum (ACC)

Syndrome	Gene	Features
Mowat-Wilson syndrome	ZEB2	ACC, mental retardation, Hirschsprung's disease, heart defects, genitourinary defects
X-linked lissencephaly with ambiguous genitalia (XLAG)	ARX	ACC, lissencephaly, epilepsy, abnormal genitalia
L1 syndrome	L1CAM	ACC, spastic paraparesis, mental retardation
Andermann syndrome	SLC12A6	ACC, progressive neuropathy
FG syndrome	MED12	ACC, hypotonia, mental retardation, dysmorphisms, constipation
Acrocallosal syndrome	Unknown	ACC, polydactyly, mental retardation
Aicardi's syndrome	Unknown	ACC, chorioretinal lacunae, infantile spasms, mental retardation
Fryns syndrome	Unknown	Dysmorphisms, congenital diaphragmatic hernia, pulmonary hypoplasia
Sotos' syndrome	NSD1	Somatic overgrowth, learning disabilities, dysmorphisms, ACC
Pyruvate decarboxylase deficiency	Specific gene unknown	Lactic acidosis, mental retardation, ACC
Wolf-Hirschhorn syndrome	On chromosome 4p16	Growth deficiency, dysmorphisms, mental retardation, seizures, ACC
Opitz G	Unknown	Dysmorphisms, laryngotracheoesophageal defects, genitourinary defects, ACC

and white matter abnormalities, and malformations of the posterior fossa (Hetts et al, 2006).

Consistent with the broad range of genetic factors and other concurrent malformations, the neurologic and developmental consequences of ACC are varied. Shevell (2002) found in his practice-based retrospective study that almost one third of patients with ACC were either developmentally normal or had mild developmental delay. Factors predictive of adverse developmental outcome were microcephaly, epilepsy, cerebral palsy, and cerebral dysgenesis. The outcome of isolated ACC is less clear. Prognosis is generally good, but neuropsychologic testing shows cognitive and behavioral deficits in many. IQ is typically normal, but lower than expected based on family history (Chiarello, 1980). Moutard et al (2003) prospectively studied 17 children with prenatally diagnosed isolated ACC through 6 years of age. All had IQs in the normal range, but there was a tendency for the IQ to decrease with age, and behavioral difficulties were common. For example, at 2 years of age attention difficulty was seen in 25%; by 4 years this was a problem in 44%. Neuropsychologic studies have shown specific impairment in abstract reasoning, problem solving, and category fluency (David et al, 1993; Fischer et al, 1992). Word generation is generally normal in patients with ACC, but there is difficulty with higher-level language such as comprehension of syntax and linguistic pragmatics (i.e., understanding idioms and humor) (Banich et al, 2000).

Agenesis of the Septum Pellucidum and Septo-optic Dysplasia

Septo-optic dysplasia (SOD) is the triad of absence of the septum pellucidum, optic nerve hypoplasia, and pituitary dysfunction. The diagnosis is made clinically when two or more features of the triad are present. Only 30% of patients have all three features (Morishima et al, 1986). Frequently, other cerebral abnormalities are present, including schizencephaly and absence of the pituitary infundibulum. The severity of the clinical features is quite variable. Children with SOD may be blind or have reduced vision and nystagmus. Neurodevelopmental prognosis is controversial. In early studies, cerebral palsy was found in 57%, mental retardation in 71%, epilepsy in 37%, and behavior problems in 20% of children with SOD (Acers, 1981; Margalith et al, 1984). A later neurodevelopmental study of seven children with unilateral or bilateral optic nerve hypoplasia, whose only other documented CNS abnormality was absence of the septum pellucidum, found normal cognitive development, intact neurologic status, normal language development, and age-appropriate behavior in six of the seven (Williams et al, 1993). Conversely, a descriptive series of three children with SOD plus cortical dysplasias, showed that all three had abnormal development and neurologic exams (Miller et al, 2000). Thus, the abnormalities found in many patients with SOD are likely caused by other associated brain lesions.

HESX1 is the only gene identified thus far as a likely cause of SOD. HESX1 is a transcriptional repressor and is a homeobox gene whose mouse homologue has important roles in forebrain, midline, and pituitary development. Mutations in this gene have led to both homozygous and heterozygous forms of SOD. The homozygous mutations are fully penetrant and are associated with more severe disease (Dattani et al, 1998; Thomas et al, 2001). The contribution of mutations in HESX1 to the cause of SOD appears to be less than 1% (McNay et al, 2007). Mutations in HESX1 may also cause isolated pituitary dysfunction. In addition to genetic causes, some cases of SOD have been implicated to have antenatal drug and alcohol abuse or a vascular pathogenesis (Lippe et al, 1979; Lubinsky, 1997; Stevens et al, 2004).

The cavum septi pellucidi is an opening formed by the separation of the lamellae of the septum pellucidum; the lamellae fuse as the fetal brain matures. The cavum septi pellucidi may persist into extrauterine life, especially in preterm infants. Mott et al (1992) have documented the presence of a cavum septi pellucidi in all infants born at less than 36 weeks' gestation routinely studied by cranial sonographic examination. A cavum septi pellucidi was

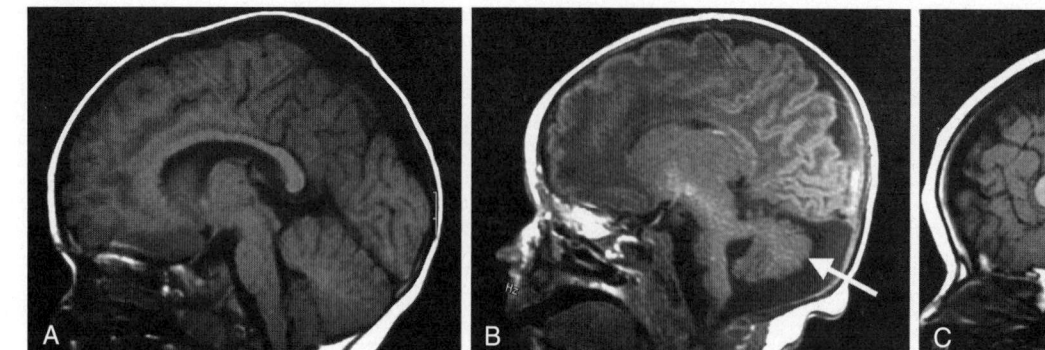

FIGURE 60-13 Dandy-Walker malformation (DWM). Sagittal images of a normal brain **(A)**, the brain of a child with Joubert's syndrome **(B)**, and the brain of a child with DWM **(C)** illustrate that features of the hindbrain malformations seen in the DWM overlap with that of other disorders. Note the presence of cerebellar vermis hypoplasia (*arrow*) in both **B** and **C**. By contrast, the patient with Joubert's syndrome **(B)** has only a slightly enlarged fourth ventricle, whereas in the DWM **(C)** the fourth ventricle is massively dilated. *(Courtesy Dr. Joseph G. Gleeson, Department of Neurology, University of California, San Diego, School of Medicine, and Dr. William B. Dobyns, The University of Chicago School of Medicine.)*

present in 36% of term newborns in the series reported by these investigators.

MALFORMATIONS OF STRUCTURES IN THE POSTERIOR FOSSA

NORMAL HINDBRAIN DEVELOPMENT

Malformations of the posterior fossa comprise an embryologically diverse group of disorders. Because these disorders are frequently associated with compromise to vital functions of the brainstem, management may focus on concerns for apnea and hydrocephalus, for example. Controversies will undoubtedly persist regarding the appropriate classification of these disorders until such time as the molecular genetic basis is further resolved.

The development of posterior fossa structures begins shortly after closure of the neural tube and coincides with the onset of prosencephalic development (ten Donkelaar and Lammens, 2009). At this time, the primary brain vesicles of the primitive hindbrain (rhombencephalon) emerge distal to the prosencephalon along an anterior-posterior axis. The midbrain derives from the mesencephalon and is embryologically distinct from the rhombencephalon from which the major hindbrain structures derive (cerebellum, pons [metencephalon], and medulla [myelencephalon]). Between 3 and 5 weeks' gestation, the rhombencephalon can be identified between the cranial and cervical flexures of the neural tube. Eight distinct rhombomeres have been defined in the rhombencephalon. The alar plate of rhombomere 1 gives rise to the cerebellum and rhombomeres 2 to 8 to the pons, medulla, and cranial nerves 5 to 10.

MALFORMATIONS WITH MAJOR CEREBELLAR INVOLVEMENT

Acquired malformations typically are unilateral or asymmetric, whereas inherited abnormalities symmetrically involve both cerebellar hemispheres, the vermis, or midline. The involvement of the cerebellum plus pontine hypoplasia comprises a distinct group of malformations (i.e., the pontocerebellar hypoplasias). Global cerebellar hypoplasia may also occur as a consequence of intrauterine

insults such as toxins or irradiation and in association with chromosomal syndromes such as trisomy 13, 18, or 21.

Of the cerebellar malformations associated with significant posterior fossa cerebrospinal fluid collections, the prototype is the Dandy-Walker malformation (DWM), discussed later. A number of other posterior fossa malformations share similar embryologic derivatives or similar anatomical features with the DWM (Figure 60-13). These variants of the DWM include several syndromes of cerebellar vermis hypoplasia and dysplasia, syndromes that involve diffuse cerebellar hypoplasia and syndromes with normal cerebellar size and architecture, but with a large posterior fossa fluid collection that does not communicate with the fourth ventricle (e.g., mega cisterna magna or arachnoid cyst) (Altman et al, 1992; Barkovich et al, 2009; Niesen, 2002; Parisi and Dobyns, 2003; Patel and Barkovich, 2002; ten Donkellaar and Lammens, 2009). Moreover, numerous chromosomal anomalies, such as trisomy 9, 13, and 18, present with the DWM.

The DWM has also been described in association with a variety of genetic syndromes. One of these is the Walker-Warburg syndrome, which is characterized not only by extensive brainstem and cerebellar hypoplasia, but also by ocular anomalies, congenital muscular dystrophy, cortical migration abnormalities, and encephalocele. These have led to a variety of attempts to develop unifying classification schemes under the rubric of "DWM and its variants." Because the molecular mechanisms that underlie these malformations are mostly unknown, there is currently no basis for linking them as a spectrum. It should be emphasized that a more unfavorable outcome is related to the extent of other posterior fossa and CNS malformations. Hence, when "DWM" is diagnosed, prenatal and postnatal management and prognosis depend on precise definition of the particular anatomical abnormalities present. Prenatal ultrasound and MRI are increasingly employed, but both have continued challenges for the precise anatomical definition of these malformations (Malinger et al, 2009). Moreover, a number of clinically significant malformations accompany these hindbrain variants, notably agenesis of the corpus callosum and cerebral neuronal migration disturbances (polymicrogyria and heterotopias). Hence, establishing prognosis for DWM and other cerebellar malformations during pregnancy can be difficult.

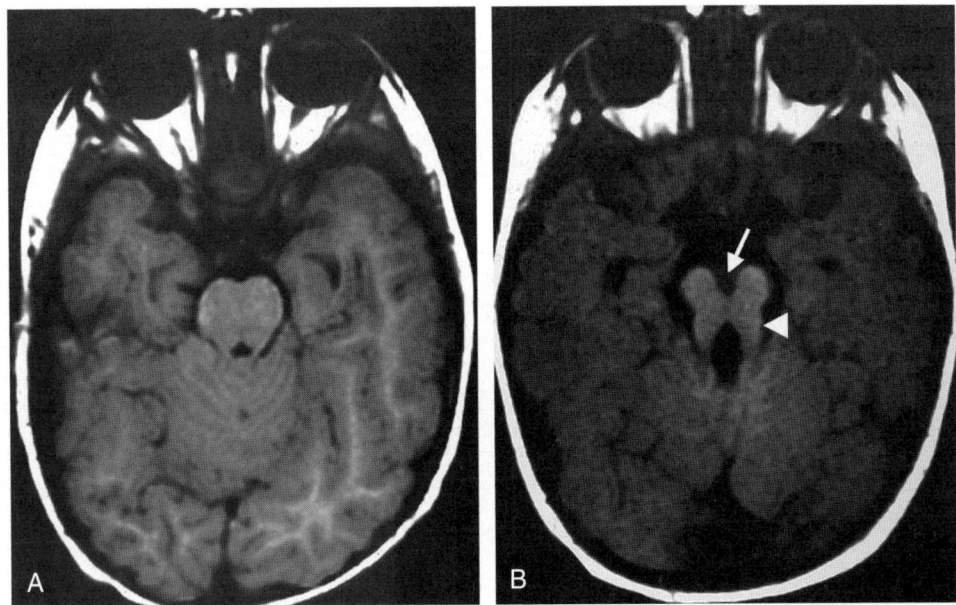

FIGURE 60-14 Molar tooth sign (MTS). Comparison of axial images from a normal brain (A) with that of a child with Joubert's syndrome (B). Note two key features of the MTS: a deepened interpeduncular fossa (*arrow*) and the elongated superior cerebellar peduncles (*arrowhead*). The third feature, cerebellar vermis hypoplasia, is seen in Figure 60-13, *B*. (*Courtesy Dr. Joseph G. Gleeson, Department of Neurology, University of California, San Diego, School of Medicine.*)

Children with isolated inferior vermis hypoplasia or mega cisterna magna have better neurodevelopmental outcomes compared with those with DWM or other hindbrain malformations (Bolduc and Limperopoulos, 2009).

Pontocerebellar hypoplasia is a diverse group of largely autosomal recessive disorders characterized by a reduction in pontine volume and a variable degree of cerebellar hypoplasia (for review, see ten Donkellaar and Lammens, 2009). A majority lack a clear etiology. At least five types have been described with associated features such as spinal muscular atrophy or extrapyramidal motor features. Some cases occur in association with congenital disorders of glycosylation, mitochondrial diseases, and congenital muscular dystrophies.

Dandy-Walker Malformation

Precise estimates of the incidence of Dandy-Walker malformation (DWM) are clearly affected by the lack of agreement regarding the definition of DWM. Nevertheless, DWM appears to occur in at least 1 in 5000 liveborn infants (Parisi and Dobyns, 2003). Inheritance is usually sporadic with a low risk of recurrence. The etiology is unknown. Two genetic loci have been identified for DWM. Recently, mutations in the human gene FOXC1 have been associated with DWM as well as cerebellar vermis hypoplasia and mega–cisterna magna (Aldinger et al, 2009). The invariant features of the DWM are aplasia or hypoplasia of the vermis of the cerebellum, cystic dilation of the fourth ventricle, and enlargement of the posterior fossa with upward displacement of the lateral sinuses, tentorium, and torcular (Benda, 1954; D'Agostino, 1963; Friede, 1989; Hart et al, 1972). The enlargement of the posterior fossa and displacement of its contents is related to communication of the fourth ventricle with a retrocerebellar cyst, which may be of considerable size. Communicating hydrocephalus

with dilated lateral ventricles is also a common feature that may present in the neonatal period with macrocephaly. In fact, a majority of cases of DWM present with symptoms related to hydrocephalus (Costa and Hauw, 1995; Hart et al, 1972). There is no general agreement regarding the optimal management of hydrocephalus in DWM, which usually involves some combination of ventricular or posterior fossa shunt placement. Other prominent neurologic features include ataxia, nystagmus, apnea, cranial neuropathies, and developmental delay.

Syndromes Associated With the Molar Tooth Sign

The molar tooth sign (MTS) is defined as the triad of cerebellar vermis hypoplasia, and two mid-hindbrain malformations (an abnormally deep interpeduncular fossa and elongated cerebellar peduncles). When viewed on axial MRI images (Figure 60-14), the brainstem malformations have the distinctive appearance of a molar tooth. Abnormalities of the cerebellum are also found in Joubert's syndrome, which is the most extensively studied of several uncommon autosomal recessive cerebello-oculo-renal syndromes associated with the molar tooth sign (MTS) (Parisi and Dobyns, 2002). The cerebellar lesion usually involves complete or partial agenesis of the vermis (see Figure 60-13, *B*), but there may also be dysplasia of the dentate nucleus, cerebellar heterotopias, anomalies of brain stem nuclei, and absence of decussation of the pyramidal tracts (Curatolo et al, 1980).

Joubert's syndrome (JS) is a rare autosomal recessive disorder. It is the prototype for a recently identified group of disorders known as "ciliopathies," in which defects occur in the structure or function of the cellular primary cilium (Lee and Gleeson, 2010; Nigg and Raff, 2009). At least seven genes have been identified for various subtypes of JS, which subserve signal transduction pathways at the primary cilium. Primary cilia are found in both Purkinje cells and granule cell progenitors. Defective ciliary function is also a feature of retinal dystrophy and fibrocystic renal disease, thus providing a unifying mechanism for many of the multisystem abnormalities seen in patients with JS.

The most prominent clinical features of JS are hypotonia, abnormal eye movements (horizontal nystagmus and oculomotor apraxia), ataxia, abnormal breathing patterns (periods of hyperpnea alternating with apnea) and cognitive delays/mental retardation (Joubert et al, 1969). Variable features of Joubert's syndrome include occipital encephalocele, microcephaly, low-set ears, polydactyly, and pigmentary retinopathy (Egger et al, 1982; Friede and Boltshauser, 1978). Renal disease in Joubert's syndrome includes cystic dysplasia of the kidneys and juvenile nephronophthisis. The latter is a form of medullary cystic renal disease that progresses to chronic renal failure (Satran et al, 1999).

CENTRAL NERVOUS SYSTEM DEVELOPMENT IN THE POSTEMBRYONIC PERIOD
NORMAL DEVELOPMENT OF THE CORTICAL PLATE

Proliferative Events

Four transient tangential layers form during the process of cerebral cortical development. These (from the ventricle to the brain surface) are the ventricular, subventricular, intermediate, and marginal zones. Initially, the nascent cortical plate derives from the ventricular zone (VZ). The VZ is the site of earliest proliferation of neuronal and radial glial progenitor cells in the wall of the neural tube. As the cerebral wall expands, the subventricular zone becomes a secondary site of later neuronal and glial proliferation. These proliferative events occur roughly between 4 and 16 weeks' gestation. Peak cell proliferation occurs around 8 to 16 weeks. This coincides with the expansion of the cortical plate, which appears when the embryo is about 22 to 24 mm long, at about 52 days' gestation.

The initial cycles of neural progenitor proliferation in the VZ result in the symmetrical expansion of the stem cell pool such that each mitotic event results in the generation of two additional stem cells (Caviness, 1995; Rakic, 1995). This process determines the total pool of stem cells, or so-called proliferative units from which the cortical plate will form. Once the generation of this stem cell pool stabilizes, a second phase of proliferation begins during which individual stem cell clones begin to divide asymmetrically. During this phase of clonal expansion, each mitosis generates an additional stem cell and another neuronal cell that withdraws from the cell cycle. The latter postmitotic neuron then begins migration from the VZ to the outer wall of the neural tube. Hence, this second phase of asymmetric cell division results in the expansion of each individual stem cell clone or proliferative unit. Eventually, this phase results in a proportionately larger number of postmitotic cells that all derive from the same proliferative unit.

Migrational Events

Rakic first proposed that the postmitotic neurons that derive from an individual clonal population in the VZ migrate together along the same radial glia fiber to generate individual columns of cells within the cortical plate (Rakic, 1998). The radial glia processes extend from the VZ to the outer wall of the neural tube and serve as a scaffold to guide the migration of individual clones of postmitotic neurons to form the preplate. Migration of neurons from the VZ occurs in an "outside-in" fashion, such that the neurons furthest from the ventricle migrate first and those closest to the ventricle migrate last.

As neuronal migration proceeds, the preplate is split by the arrival of subsequent populations of neuronal progenitors that will form the cortical plate. The cortical plate ultimately gives rise to cortical layers II–VI. The splitting of the preplate results in the formation of the marginal zone (future cortical layer I) and the subplate, which resides between the intermediate zone (the future cerebral white matter) and the bottom of the cortical plate (Marin-Padilla, 1988, 1998). The Cajal-Retzius neurons of the marginal zone and the subplate neurons play critical roles in neuronal migrations, as discussed later.

As neuronal migration progresses, each subsequent group of neurons migrates past the neurons that migrated earlier. Hence, the earliest neurons to migrate eventually reside in the deepest cortical layer. Because the last neurons to migrate reside the closest to layer 1, the cortical layers are thereby formed in an "inside-out" sequence. The major events involved in formation of the cortical layers are occurring between approximately 7 and 11 weeks.

Subplate Neurons and Establishment of Thalamocortical Connections

As emphasized earlier, the cortical plate develops from within the preplate. The preplate consists of the earliest generated neurons and a plexus of nerve fibers. With subsequent waves of neuronal migration, the preplate is split into the marginal zone (i.e., a superplate) and a subplate. Hence, the cells in these layers are among the earliest generated neurons. In the second trimester, two subcortical afferent systems are present in the subplate (Allendoerfer and Shatz, 1994). These are thalamocortical fibers and basal forebrain fibers, which remain in the subcortical region for a period of time before their fibers penetrate the cortical plate. The neurons of layer IV in the cortex receive their predominant ascending inputs from the thalamus. Interestingly, however, the thalamic axons are present in the cortex long before the layer IV neurons have reached the cortical plate. These axons reside in the subplate for a period of weeks in proximity to postmitotic neurons in the subplate. Most of these early maturing subplate neurons undergo programmed cell death after the thalamic axons have grown into the cortical plate (Chun et al, 1987).

Hence, subplate neurons transiently appear during a critical window in development, and few are present in the adult neocortex. In human, the subplate achieves its peak size by 24 weeks' gestation and declines thereafter (Kostovic and Rakic, 1990; Kostovic and Vasung, 2009). The hypothesis that these subplate neurons play a critical role in thalamocortical development by guiding thalamic axons into the cortical plate has been substantiated by studies that have shown that deletion of the early subplate neurons prevents the thalamic axons from innervating the cortex. Thus, the transient subplate neurons play an important role in establishing both thalamocortical and cortico-cortical connections (Ghosh et al, 1990; Kanold et al, 2003).

DISORDERS OF NEURONAL PROLIFERATION

Micrencephaly

Micrencephaly is a disorder in which the primary defect is a marked reduction in the size of the brain or of the cerebral hemispheres. Microcephaly denotes a small cranial vault (<-2 standard deviations [SD] below normative curves for age) that is related either to micrencephaly or acquired brain atrophy (e.g., multicystic encephalopathy, hydranencephaly, diffuse cortical atrophy). Until recently, micrencephaly was considered to be an isolated defect of either decreased neuronal proliferation or increased apoptosis (programmed cell death). Representative examples are radial microbrain and micrencephaly vera (Evrard et al, 1989; Rakic, 1988). However, MRI studies have begun to define greater heterogeneity in the types of malformations that are associated with micrencephaly (Barkovich et al, 2001; Tarrant et al, 2009). Associated malformations include simplified gyral patterns, microlissencephaly with thickened cortical gray matter, and polymicrogyria (Barkovich et al, 1998; Peiffer et al, 1999; Sztriha et al, 1998). The association of micrencephaly with features of cortical neuronal migration abnormalities suggests overlap in the mechanisms that direct neuronal proliferation and migration in humans.

Two subgroups of isolated micrencephaly, radial microbrain and micrencephaly vera, provide insight into mechanisms of isolated disturbances of neuronal proliferation. Radial microbrain appears to be related to a reduced *number* of proliferative units. By contrast, micrencephaly vera appears to be related to a reduced *size* of proliferative units (Evrard et al, 1989; Rakic, 1988). Radial microbrain is a rare familial condition characterized by a normal gyral and cortical lamination pattern, but an abnormal number of cortical neuronal columns. The number of cells per column is normal, implying that the defect resides in early neural stem cell division with an impact on the ultimate number of "proliferative units" available to generate the cortical columns.

Micrencephaly vera describes a variety of conditions with small brain size where the underlying etiology may be related to a disturbance in neuronal proliferation. Cases of autosomal recessive micrencephaly vera have a simplified gyral pattern. The number of cortical neuronal columns is normal, but the cell number in each column is reduced (Evrard et al, 1989). This constellation of findings most likely occurs between 6 and 18 weeks' gestation, when later proliferative events occur.

The potential etiologies for microcephaly are diverse. It is associated with hundreds of genetic syndromes. Autosomal dominant, autosomal recessive, and X-linked recessive inheritance patterns have been described (Robain and Lyon, 1972; Warkany et al, 1981). Irradiation before 18 weeks' gestation is a well-known teratogenic agent that can produce micrencephaly. Exposure to alcohol and cocaine during this time can also result in micrencephaly

(Gieron-Korthals et al, 1994; Peiffer et al, 1979). Maternal hyperphenylalaninemia has also been associated with these defects in nonphenylketonuric offspring (Lenke and Levy, 1980; Waisbren and Levy, 1990).

A recent large retrospective review found that the prognosis for microcephaly is closely related to the severity of the reduction in head circumference (Ashwal et al, 2009). Developmental disabilities and imaging abnormalities are seen in approximately 80% of children with severe microcephaly defined as a head circumference <-3 SD. The major comorbid conditions are mental retardation (approximately 50%), epilepsy (approximately 40%), cerebral palsy, and ophthalmologic disorders (each approximately 20%).

Eight genetic loci and five genes for human autosomal recessive primary microcephaly have been mapped (Thornton and Woods, 2009). All result in a small but structurally normal-appearing brain and a similar range of mental retardation without other neurologically distinguishing features. Although all the proteins identified to date are ubiquitously expressed and operate in diverse pathways, all are associated with the centrosome, suggesting a common mechanism to regulate neurogenesis.

Macrencephaly

Macrencephaly refers to a diverse group of conditions characterized by a large brain. Although it has been hypothesized that macrencephaly is related to an aberrant increase in neuronal proliferation, quantitative neuropathologic studies are lacking. Macrencephaly manifests most commonly as an isolated finding in familial (autosomal dominant or autosomal recessive) and sporadic cases. Among the other diverse conditions that are associated with macrencephaly are chromosomal disorders (fragile X syndrome and Klinefelter's syndrome) and neuroendocrine disorders related to a generalized disturbance in growth (Beckwith-Wiedemann syndrome, cerebral gigantism, and achondroplasia) (DeMyer, 1972; Dodge et al, 1983).

At birth, the head circumference in about half of cases is greater than the 90th percentile. The diagnosis of autosomal dominant macrencephaly is greatly favored by the finding of a large head circumference (macrocephaly) in either parent. Autosomal dominant inheritance is generally associated with a more favorable outcome, whereas the rare cases of autosomal recessive inheritance are commonly associated with mental retardation and epilepsy. One generally benign form of autosomal dominant macrencephaly is accompanied by extracerebral fluid collections that enlarge the subarachnoid spaces (Alvarez et al, 1986). Erroneously referred to as "external hydrocephalus," there is rarely an indication for placement of a shunt to drain this fluid. Rather, the initial acceleration in head circumference generally arrests spontaneously by around the 1st year of life, and thereafter the fluid collections become smaller. These fluid collections appear to be related to an imbalance in cerebrospinal fluid generation at birth related to developmental immaturity of the subarachnoid granulations that resorb this fluid (Neveling and Truex, 1983; Barlow, 1984).

Hemimegalencephaly (Figure 60-15) refers to a rare malformation of unilateral macrencephaly related to enlargement of some portion of one cerebral hemisphere and accompanied by increased cortical thickness and abnormal

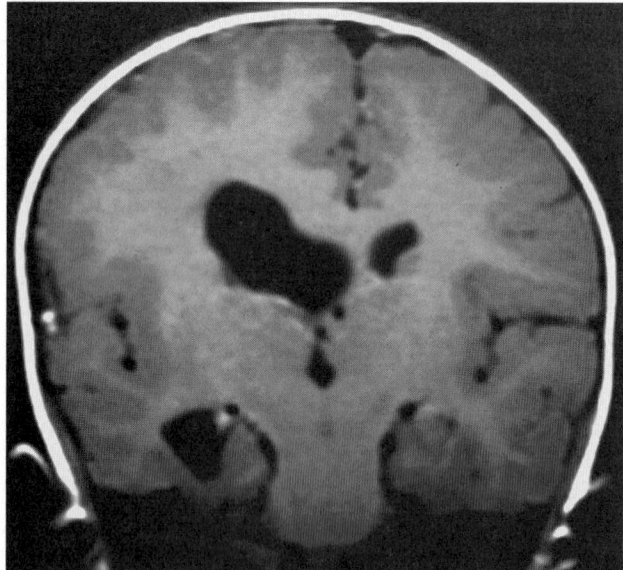

FIGURE 60-15 Magnetic resonance image scan, hemimegalen-cephaly. Note the marked asymmetry of the two cerebral hemispheres with the pronounced enlargement *on the left.* *(Courtesy Dr. Martin Salinsky, Department of Neurology, Oregon Health and Science University.)*

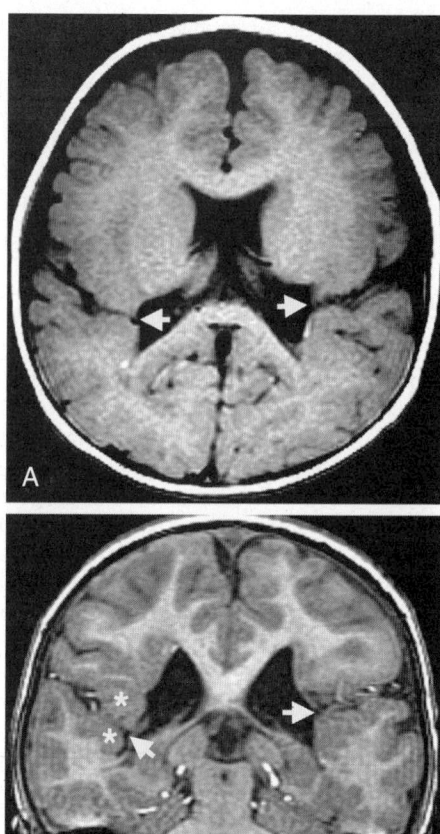

FIGURE 60-16 Magnetic resonance image scan, bilateral open-lip schizencephaly. A, Axial T1 weighted image. Note that the bilateral clefts (*arrows*) extend to the lateral ventricles. **B,** Coronal T1-weighted image. Note that the clefts (*arrows*) are lined with gray matter (*). *(Courtesy Dr. A. James Barkovich, Department of Radiology, University of California, San Francisco, School of Medicine.)*

cortical gyration (Robain et al, 1972). The pathologic features include apparent disturbances in astroglia proliferation and morphology as well as neuronal heterotopias in subcortical white matter (De Rosa et al, 1992). The usual onset for intractable epilepsy is in the neonatal period (Ohtsuka et al, 1999). A markedly improved outcome may be achieved in selected patients after hemispherectomy as early as the neonatal period (Battaglia et al, 1999). The primary genetic defect is unknown. It has been noted in association with neurocutaneous disorders including the sebaceous nevus syndrome (Dodge and Dobyns, 1995) and hypomelanosis of Ito (Montagna et al, 1991).

DISORDERS OF NEURONAL MIGRATION

Neuronal migration disorders are characterized anatomically by defects in the lamination of the cerebral cortex. Most of these defects are related to some degree of failure of neurons to migrate to their appropriate target positions within the normal six layers of the developing cerebral cortex. The clinical spectrum of brain malformations associated with disrupted neuronal migration ranges from complete focal agenesis of an entire region of the cerebral cortex in schizencephaly to more subtle abnormalities where heterotopic clusters of neurons are retained in abnormal locations within the subcortical white matter (see Table 60-1). In many disorders, there are prominent disturbances in the formation of the cortical surface that manifest as gyral abnormalities. In the extreme, there is a complete absence of gyri and a smooth cortical surface (lissencephaly). At the other extreme is an excess of small gyral convolutions (polymicrogyria). The fact that these gyral abnormalities are often accompanied by other malformations, such as hypoplasia or agenesis of the corpus callosum, points to a complex interplay between the mechanisms that determine neuronal migration and axon pathfinding. This is consistent with the fact that the timing of

neuronal migration and midline prosencephalic development overlap. Hence, disturbances in neuronal migration would be anticipated to have a deleterious impact on the axonotropic signaling required for establishment of inter- and intrahemispheric cortical connections.

Schizencephaly

Schizencephaly (i.e., split brain) is characterized by severe focal malformations of the cerebral cortex that result in complete agenesis of all layers of the cortical wall. The resultant defect is a cleft in the cerebral cortex in one or both hemispheres, which thus connects the lateral ventricle with the extracerebral space (Figure 60-16). When the defect is wide (separated-lip or open-lip schizencephaly), the malformation may be confused with a lesion caused by a severe destructive process. However, a feature of schizencephaly that differentiates it from an encephaloclastic lesion (e.g., hydrancephaly, porencephaly) is that on histologic examination, the cleft has features of a migrational disturbance, such as large neuronal heterotopias bordered by adjacent polymicrogyria. When the defect is narrow (closed-lip schizencephaly), it has the appearance of a narrow groove in the cortical mantle. The morphologic features of schizencephalic clefts by neuroimaging are best delineated by MRI, which has demonstrated the common occurrence of subependymal heterotopias and polymicrogyria and the universal finding of diminished volume of the cerebral white matter (Hayashi et al, 2002a). In addition, a wide range of anomalies related to disturbances of prosencephalic development may occur in association with schizencephaly. These include holoprosencephaly, agenesis of the corpus callosum, and agenesis of the septum pellucidum.

Schizencephaly occurs with a wide range of clinical severity that is related to the size and distribution of the cerebral clefts and the extent of associated malformations (Barkovich and Kjos, 1992; Packard et al, 1997). Significant cognitive impairment is almost universal with bilateral anomalies but occurs in a minority of cases with unilateral lesions. Motor disturbances (spasticity, hemiparesis) are common with both unilateral and bilateral lesions; this finding is likely related to the predilection for frontal lesions. Epilepsy is common in schizencephaly, present in 37% to 65% of patients in case series (as reviewed by Granata et al, 2005). A wide variety of seizure types may manifest, including focal seizures, generalized seizures and infantile spasms. Of interest, some groups have found that the severity of the epilepsy is not correlated with the severity of the brain malformation; patients with unilateral schizencephaly had earlier age of seizure onset and more refractory epilepsy than those with bilateral schizencephaly (Denis et al, 2000; Granata et al, 1996). Hydrocephalus is seen almost exclusively with separated-lip lesions.

The etiology of schizencephaly remains controversial. Many feel that schizencephaly can result from various types of injury to the developing cortex, but the degree to which genetic mutations may cause this defect in neuronal migration is unclear. In utero exposure to toxins and infection is associated with schizencephaly (Iannetti et al, 1998; Takano et al, 1999). It has been suggested that ischemic injury (from toxin, infection, or hypoxia) early in gestation could damage the radial glial fibers resulting in the full-thickness cortical cleft (Barkovich and Kjos, 1992). The possible role of the human homeobox gene *EMX2* in schizencephaly is unclear. Initial reports found some familial cases with *EMX2* mutations (Brunelli et al, 1996; Faiella et al, 1997; Granata et al, 1997). However, further studies have suggested that these mutations were unlikely to be pathogenic, because they did not result in truncation of the protein or a change in protein function, and no mutations in the *EMX2* gene were found in 39 patients with schizencephaly (Merello et al, 2008). Additionally, *EMX2* mutations have not been reported in additional families with schizencephaly. Moreover, the same initially described mutations were seen in unaffected family members, which suggests that the mutation may instead represent a polymorphic variant. Mouse models of *EMX2* deletions also do not result in schizencephaly (Pellegrini et al, 1996; Yoshida et al, 1997).

Polymicrogyria

Polymicrogyria constitutes a heterogeneous group of malformations where an excessive number of small and partially fused gyri are separated by shallow sulci (Figure

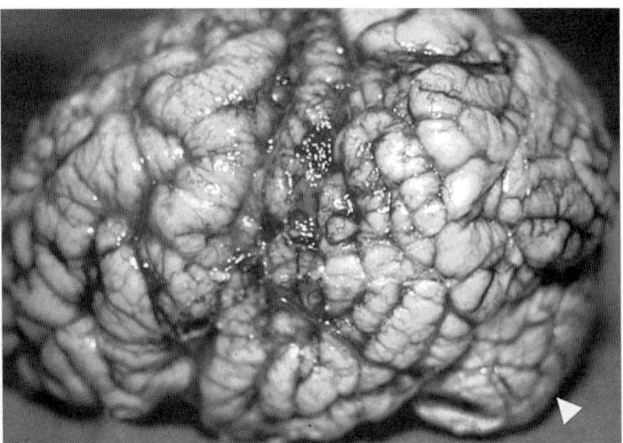

FIGURE 60-17   Polymicrogyria. Much of the cerebral cortex in this photograph shows the irregular, "cobblestone" appearance of polymicrogyria. More normal gyri are present at the frontal pole (*lower left*). The cerebellum is indicated at lower right (*arrowhead*). (*Courtesy Dr. Marjorie Grafe, Department of Pathology, Oregon Health and Science University.*)

60-17). It is thought to result from an injury or genetic disorder that occurs towards the end of neuronal migration or the beginning of cortical organization. Consequently, the normal six-layered cortical lamination pattern is disrupted.

Polymicrogyria is diverse both in terms of etiology and histologic features. Causes may be environmental such as intrauterine infection or ischemia (Barkovich and Lindan, 1994; Barkovich et al, 2010), or genetic. Histopathologically, there are two major types of polymicrogyria, layered and unlayered. In *layered polymicrogyria*, four distinct cortical layers form instead of the normal six layers. This "classic" form is not associated with other migrational abnormalities but often is more diffusely localized adjacent to regions of encephalomalacia related to infection (e.g., toxoplasmosis, cytomegalovirus infection) or ischemia with cortical laminar necrosis.

Unlayered polymicrogyria is characterized by a markedly disorganized cortex that lacks distinct cortical layers. The timing of appearance of this form appears to be no later than 4 to 5 months' gestation. Unlayered polymicrogyria is associated with other migrational disturbances, particularly subcortical nodular heterotopias, lissencephaly, and schizencephaly. A genetic basis is suggested by syndromic associations (e.g., Zellweger's syndrome, Miller-Dieker syndrome, DiGeorge syndrome); familial transmission; and sporadic cases with X-linked, autosomal recessive, and autosomal dominant inheritance patterns (Barkovich et al, 1999; Ross and Walsh, 2001).

Delineation of the spectrum of CNS malformations associated with polymicrogyria has been greatly advanced by MRI. Importantly, if thick sections (>4 mm) are acquired, these anomalies may resemble focal pachygyria, abnormally thick large gyri, because of signal averaging from the microgyri. Barkovich (2010) recommends image acquisition in three planes with thinner slice thickness and sequences that provide optimal gray matter–white matter contrast (such as volume 3DFT spoiled gradient acquisition and volume 3DFT fast spin echo images with 1.5-mm slices). Polymicrogyria shows a strong predilection for the

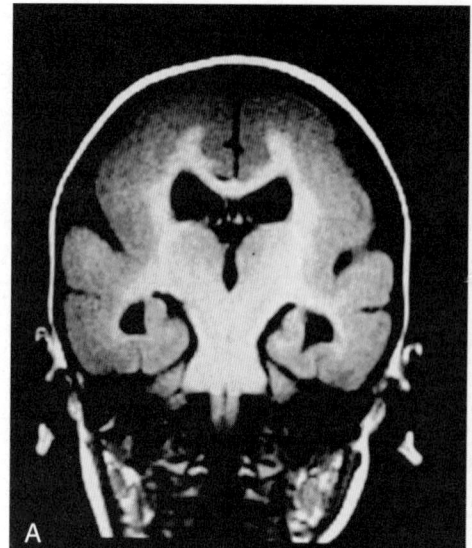
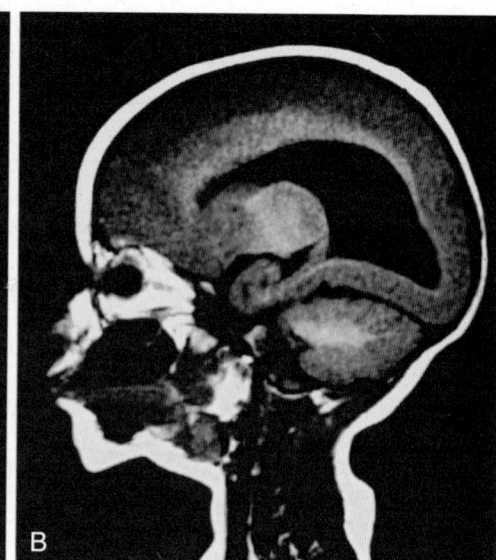

FIGURE 60-18 T1-weighted MR images of the brain of a child with classical lissencephaly. **A,** Coronal view. **B,** Sagittal view. Note the pronounced thickening of the cerebral cortex and the striking reduction in cortical gyration. *(Courtesy Dr. C. McCluggage, Department of Radiology, Texas Children's Hospital.)*

sylvian fissure and adjacent regions of frontal and parietal cortex (80% of cases), whereas the cingulate cortex, striate cortex, gyrus rectus, and hippocampus are spared. Polymicrogyria is bilateral in 60% of cases (Hayashi et al, 2002b). Often, an additional associated feature is a decrease in cerebral white matter volume adjacent to the dysplastic cortex.

The clinical features of patients with polymicrogyria are variable and relate in part to the extent and distribution of cortical dysplasia. Bilateral polymicrogyria and polymicrogyria that involves more than half of a single hemisphere carry a poor prognosis related to moderate to severe developmental delay and significant motor dysfunction (Barkovich, 2005). Because frontal cortical lesions are common, hemiparesis or quadriparesis is often seen. Epilepsy, notably partial complex seizures, multiple generalized seizure types, or refractory epilepsy, is common but may be delayed in onset beyond the neonatal period.

There are several common syndromes of bilateral symmetrical polymicrogyria. Bilateral perisylvian symmetrical polymicrogyria results in oropharyngeal dysfunction in all patients, because the perisylvian cortex subserves oromotor control and the motor programs of language. Discoordination of suck and swallow is common in the neonate. Epilepsy is seen in 80% of patients and mental retardation in 50–80% (Guerreiro et al, 2000; Guerrini et al, 1992; Kuzniecky et al, 1993). Gene loci linked to this syndrome are Xq21.33, 22q11.2 and Xq28 (Robin et al, 2006; Roll et al, 2006; Villard et al, 2002). In bilateral frontoparietal polymicrogyria, consistent findings include global developmental delay, dysconjugate gaze/esotropia, and bilateral pyramidal and cerebellar motor signs (Chang et al, 2003). Abnormalities in the G protein–coupled receptor GPR56 (16q12.2) have been implicated in this form of polymicrogyria (Chang et al, 2003; Piao et al, 2002). In addition to the polymicrogyria, neuroimaging shows bilateral white matter signal changes, a small brainstem, and a small dysmorphic cerebellum, which is unique for the polymicrogyria syndromes (Barkovich, 2010).

Lissencephaly and Pachygyria

The lissencephalies are a class of neuronal migrational disorders characterized by a paucity or absence of gyri (*agyria*), which gives the cortical surface a smooth or nearly smooth appearance (Kato and Dobyns, 2003). In most patients, lissencephaly is characterized by an abnormally thick cortex and disturbances in the organization of the cortical layers that may be accompanied by diffuse neuronal heterotopias (Figure 60-18). The spectrum of gyral malformations includes *pachygyria*, characterized by regions of cortex with a reduced number of coarse, broadened gyri, and *subcortical band heterotopia* ("double cortex"), where a circumferential band of heterotopic neurons resides within the subcortical white matter directly beneath a relatively normal cortex.

The classification of the lissencephalies has undergone major revision to reflect the rapidly evolving molecular basis of these disorders (Barkovich et al, 2001; Jissendi-Tchofo et al, 2009). A majority of cases are subsumed under the classical lissencephaly/subcortical band heterotopia spectrum (previously type 1). There are currently five genes that cause or contribute to lissencephaly in humans (Kato and Dobyns, 2003). Three genes, *LIS1*, *DCX*, and *TUBA1A*, account for a majority of cases of classical lissencephaly (Kerjan and Gleeson, 2007a). Mutations of the LIS1 gene were first detected in the Miller-Dieker syndrome (severe lissencephaly and distinct craniofacial abnormalities) after identification of chromosome 17p13.3 deletions in over 90% of these patients (Ledbetter et al, 1992). This syndrome is always associated with a more severe lissencephaly phenotype, which appears to reflect the fact that the 17p deletion also contains the 14-3-3ε gene, which is also implicated in neuronal migration. Subsequent studies determined that sporadic cases of isolated lissencephaly were caused by LIS1 mutations, as well. LIS1 encodes a noncatalytic subunit of a ubiquitously expressed enzyme, platelet-activating factor acetylhydrolase. The mechanisms by which LIS1 mutations disrupt neuronal migration relate in part to its roles in cell motility as well

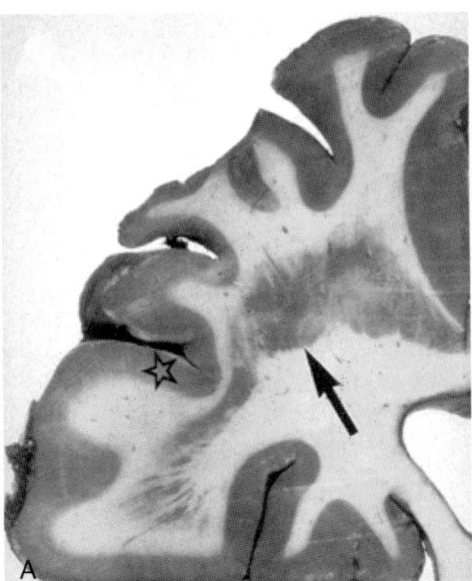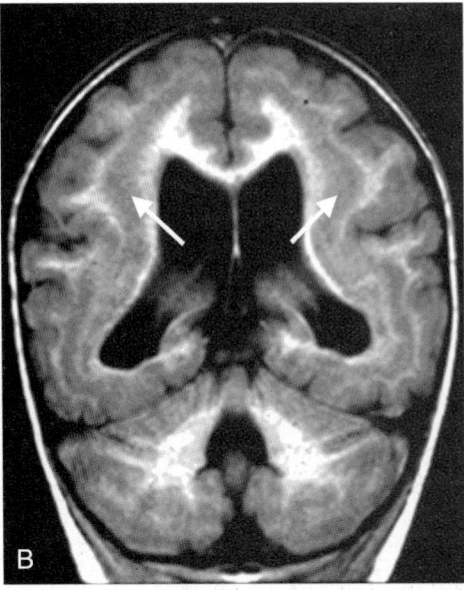

FIGURE 60-19 Subcortical band heterotopia in two female patients diagnosed with a DCX mutation. **A,** This histologic specimen demonstrates the presence of a broad band of heterotopic gray matter (*arrow*) that is situated within the cerebral white matter and distinct from the cerebral cortex (*star*). **B,** T1-weighted axial magnetic resonance image demonstrates the circumferential nature of the subcortical band heterotopia (*arrows*). *(Courtesy Dr. Joseph G. Gleeson, Department of Neurology, University of California, San Diego, School of Medicine; M. Elizabeth Ross, Department of Neurology, University of Minnesota; Christopher A. Walsh, Department of Neurology, University of Minnesota; and Christopher A. Walsh, Department of Neurology, Harvard Medical School.)*

as mitosis (neurogenesis). The DCX gene was first demonstrated to cause X-linked lissencephaly and subcortical band heterotopia. DCX encodes the doublecortin protein, which is a neuron-specific protein that functions in part in microtubule polymerization and may interact with LIS1 (des Portes et al, 1998; Gleeson et al, 1998). Mutations in the ARX gene result in another form of X-linked lissencephaly with abnormal genitalia and is further characterized by abnormal basal ganglia, often with small cysts, immature white matter, and agenesis of the corpus callosum (Kitamura et al, 2002). ARX is a homeobox gene specifically expressed in forebrain interneurons and the male gonads, where it directs differentiation of the testes. ARX functions in proliferation of neuronal progenitors and in differentiation and migration of interneurons. TUBA 1 encodes alpha-1a tubulin and appears to be the least common of the mutations associated with classical lissencephaly (Morris-Rosendahl et al, 2008). The spectrum of malformations associated with TUBA 1 mutations is broad and commonly includes congenital microcephaly, callosal dysgenesis, and cerebellar hypoplasia.

LIS1, DCX, and other proteins implicated in neuronal migration appear to interact via functionally complex signaling mechanisms to modulate alterations in cell shape at the level of the actin and microtubule-based cytoskeleton (Ross and Walsh, 2001). It is thus not surprising that LIS1 and DCX mutations are associated with considerable variation in the phenotypic expression of classical lissencephaly. Six distinct grades of morphologic severity have been defined that overlap among agyria, pachygyria, and subcortical band heterotopia (Kato and Dobyns, 2003). The most severe form (grade 1) is usually associated with either the Miller-Dieker syndrome or a severe mutation of DCX. Moreover, the gyral malformations associated with LIS1 mutations are more pronounced posteriorly

than anteriorly, whereas the gradient of injury is reversed with DCX mutations. The picture is further complicated in X-linked dominant lissencephaly insofar as males and females typically display different phenotypes related to DCX mutations. Because of hemizygosity for DXC on the X chromosome, males often display severe lissencephaly that resembles that seen in LIS1 mutations. Because of lyonization (random X-inactivation), females, however, typically display the subcortical band heterotopia phenotype (Figure 60-19). However, when mosaicism for the aberrant DCX allele predominates, some DCX females can display severe lissencephaly.

Although predictions of genotype are not readily feasible based on the pattern of malformations present, *clinical features* more consistently correlate with the lesions present. Superior definition of malformations is achieved by MRI. In the newborn, the typical presentation of isolated lissencephaly is pronounced hypotonia accompanied by a lack of motor activity. Only later in the first year may spasticity develop. Depending on the nature of the LIS1 mutation on chromosome 17, craniofacial anomalies can be subtle (bitemporal hollowing and a small jaw) or the full expression of the Miller-Dieker syndrome (Dobyns et al, 1984). Head circumference is typically normal at birth, but progressive microcephaly occurs during the first year of life. Although neonatal seizures may occur, severe myoclonic epilepsy typically develops in the latter half of the first year (e.g., infantile spasms or Lennox-Gastaut syndrome) (Guerrini and Carrozzo, 2001). Isolated lissencephaly carries a poor long-term prognosis dominated by mental retardation, spastic quadriparesis, and epilepsy. The severity of clinical deficits is typically less for infants with focal pachygyria. Patients with subcortical band heterotopia are much less affected than those with isolated lissencephaly. Although they may develop seizures and cognitive impairment, roughly 25% of patients have normal or near-normal intelligence. Neurologic deficits roughly correlate with the thickness and extent of the subcortical band (Dobyns et al, 1996).

Lissencephaly With Cerebellar Hypoplasia

This group encompasses six broad classes (a–f) of malformations that share a lissencephaly spectrum of agyria-pachygyria plus some degree of cerebellar hypoplasia (Barkovich et al, 2001; Jissendi-Tchofo et al, 2009; Kato and Dobyns, 2003; Ross et al, 2001). Individual classes are defined on the basis of additional defining malformations (e.g., brainstem hypoplasia, agenesis of the corpus callosum). The prototype for these disorders is LCHb, in which lissencephaly is accompanied by severe global cerebellar hypoplasia and a very malformed hippocampus. The lissencephaly is characterized by a moderately thick cortex that has an anterior greater than posterior gradient of severity. Several patients with LCHb have proven mutations in the *RELN* gene, which encodes reelin, a large extracellular matrix protein (Hong et al, 2000; Ross and Walsh, 2001). This is notable, because the mouse homologue of the *RELN* gene was shown to account for the phenotype of the reeler mouse, a severely ataxic mutant mouse strain in which the cerebral and cerebellar cortex display an inversion of the normal mammalian "inside-out" laminar organization pattern (Rakic and Caviness, 1995). A role for reelin in neuronal migration is supported by the observation that it is secreted by the Cajal-Retzius cells of the embryonic preplate as well as cerebellar external granule cell layer neurons and pioneering cells of the hippocampus. The distribution pattern of reelin is, thus, consistent with the pattern of malformations seen in LCHb. Functionally, reelin activates a signal transduction pathway via two distinct membrane-associated lipoproteins, the apolipoprotein E2 and the very low-density lipoprotein receptors. These receptors direct the phosphorylation of mDab1, which, on activation, participates in actin polymerization, an integral event in cell migration (Kerjan and Gleeson, 2007b). Of interest, abnormalities very similar to the reeler mouse are observed in mutant mouse strains with disruptions of mDab1 or both lipoprotein receptors.

Cobblestone Complex Syndromes

The cobblestone complex syndromes are included here because they all involve abnormal neuronal migration and were previously classified with type II lissencephaly (Barkovich et al, 2001). Three congenital muscular dystrophy syndromes are represented: Walker-Warburg syndrome, muscle-eye-brain disease, and Fukuyama congenital muscular dystrophy (FCMD). The isolated cobblestone complex malformation without retinal or muscle involvement is rare. The neuronal migration anomaly in the cobblestone complex arises because of failure of early migrating neurons to arrest at the marginal zone (the future layer 1 of the cerebral cortex). Rather, these heterotopic neurons migrate farther through a defective glial limiting membrane into the leptomeninges, which thicken and adhere to the cortical surface—hence the term

cobblestone lissencephaly. These collections of leptomeningeal neurons can be sufficiently large to obliterate the subarachnoid spaces, with resultant communicating hydrocephalus related to disruption of CSF resorption. The organization of the cerebral cortex is markedly more abnormal than in classical lissencephaly and is characterized by large ectopic clusters of neurons with no discernible lamination pattern.

Walker-Warburg syndrome is the most severe of the three cobblestone complex congenital muscular dystrophy syndromes (Warburg, 1987). Several clinical features distinguish it from those seen with classical lissencephaly. Macrocephaly is commonly present at birth or develops in the 1st year of life. The macrocephaly is typically related to communicating hydrocephalus as well as dilation of the third and fourth ventricles when a retrocerebellar cyst is present (see later discussion). In addition to lissencephaly, cerebellar/hindbrain and oculoretinal malformations and congenital muscular dystrophy are also universal and required for the diagnosis. Cerebellar malformations were discussed earlier, in the context of the DWM, and include midline cerebellar hypoplasia and retrocerebellar cyst. Protrusions of the latter through a skull defect can result in a posterior encephalocele. Ocular anomalies include retinal detachment, optic nerve hypoplasia, microphthalmia, and colobomas. The muscular weakness is typically severe and is associated with elevated serum creatine kinase. The prognosis for survival beyond the 1st year is poor. This complex constellation of features may be recalled by the eponym CHARM ± E (*c*erebellar, *h*ydrocephalus, *a*gyria, *r*etinal, *m*uscle, *e*ncephalocele) (Volpe, 2000).

The spectrum of brain malformations in muscle-eye-brain disease is generally less severe than in Walker-Warburg syndrome. These include milder lissencephaly with frontal pachygyria and less severe occipital gyral dysplasia. Midline cerebellar hypoplasia is more variable, and the retrocerebellar cyst and encephalocele are not seen. Ocular abnormalities include retinal and optic nerve hypoplasia, cataracts and glaucoma. The cobblestone complex malformations are generally least severe in FCMD, and the eye abnormalities are minor or do not occur (Fukuyama et al, 1984). However, the cortical dysplasia in FCMD is sufficiently severe to produce severe mental retardation in at least half of patients. Hence, it can be difficult clinically to distinguish between patients with severe FCMD and those with mild Walker-Warburg syndrome.

Despite overlap in their clinical features, current data support that the cobblestone complex muscular dystrophy syndromes are genetically distinct autosomal recessive disorders (Cormand et al, 2001). These disorders belong to a new class of glycosylation-deficient muscular dystrophies, the dystroglycanopathies that are related to mutations in enzymes that catalyze the post-translational *O*-glycosylation of a small number of mammalian glycoproteins (Grewal and Hewitt, 2003; Toda et al, 2005). Mutations have been described in at least six different genes (Clement et al, 2008). Point mutations in *POMT1*, encoding a putative *O*-mannosyltransferase, account for approximately 20% cases of Walker-Warburg syndrome, which displays reduced glycosylation of alpha-dystroglycan (Beltran-Valero de Barnabe et al, 2002). The defect in muscle-eye-brain disease is *POMGnT1*, the

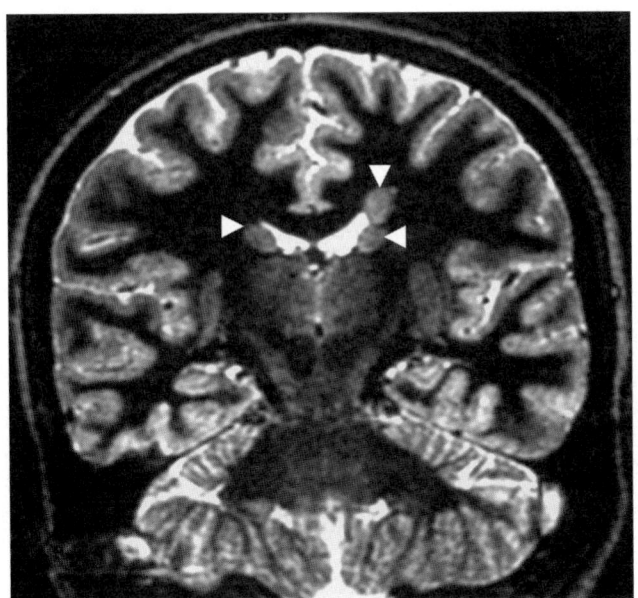

FIGURE 60-20 **Magnetic resonance image scan, periventricular nodular heterotopia.** Three discrete periventricular nodular masses (*arrowheads*) are visualized adjacent to the lateral ventricles in this T2-weighted coronal image. Note the otherwise normal convolutional pattern of the cerebral cortex. *(Courtesy Dr. Martin Salinsky, Department of Neurology, Oregon Health and Science University.)*

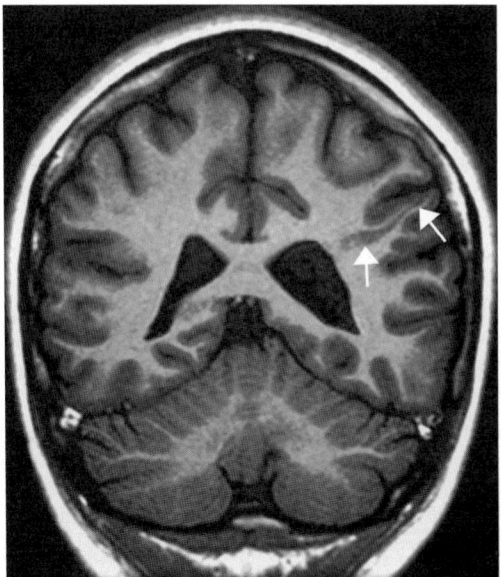

FIGURE 60-21 **Magnetic resonance image scan, subcortical white matter heterotopia.** This T1-weighted coronal image shows a diffuse stream of heterotopic gray matter (*arrows*) that spans from near the ventricular surface to the cerebral cortex. The appearance of this focal disturbance of neuronal migration suggests that the neurons were "hung up" in their migration from the ventricular surface to the cerebral cortex. *(Courtesy Dr. Martin Salinsky, Department of Neurology, Oregon Health and Science University.)*

gene for a definitive mannosyltransferase, *O*-linked mannose β1,2-*N*-acetylglucosaminyltransferase 1 (Taniguchi et al, 2003). The defect in FCMD resides in the protein fukutin (Kobayashi et al, 2000), a putative phospholigand transferase that shares homology with microbial proteins involved in mannosyl phosphorylation. Hence, the overlapping clinical phenotypes for the three cobblestone complex muscular dystrophies appear to be related in part to defects in a common glycosylation pathway that involves *O*-mannosylation of proteins.

Neuronal Heterotopia

Heterotopias are displaced collections of neurons that have failed to complete their normal migration from the ventricular zone. They are most commonly observed in periventricular white matter, where they comprise nodular collections of cells ("periventricular nodular heterotopia") (Figure 60-20), or in the subcortical white matter, where they may be nodular or diffuse (Figure 60-21). Heterotopias are, in fact, a feature of virtually all of the migrational disorders. In addition, they are often the primary migrational disturbance associated with a wide range of disorders. These include metabolic disorders; fetal toxic exposures; and neurocutaneous, multiple congenital, and chromosomal syndromes (Volpe, 2000). Hence, the clinical significance of heterotopic neurons in these conditions may be as an overt sign of a more serious underlying neurologic condition.

As isolated disorders, the heterotopias are clinically and pathologically less severe than the subcortical band heterotopias, separate disorders that are variously expressed in the spectrum of classic lissencephaly, discussed earlier. The isolated heterotopias are classified with regard to a primary periventricular (subependymal), subcortical white matter, or

marginal (superficial cortical/leptomeningeal) site of pathology (Barkovich et al, 2001). Typically, superficial cortical neuronal heterotopias are an incidental finding at autopsy. However, glial-neuronal heterotopias that infiltrate the leptomeninges occur in association with fetal exposure to teratogens such as methylmercury (Choi et al, 1978) or as seen in the fetal alcohol syndrome (Norman et al, 1995b).

The nodules are composed of highly differentiated neurons that can form complex networks and elaborate dense synaptic terminals (Eksioglu et al, 1996). Epileptic discharges have been recorded from the nodules, and it is felt that the seizures that occur in patients with heterotopias originate from the nodules themselves (Li et al, 1997).

Two genes have been identified that cause periventricular heterotopia. The most well-characterized isolated heterotopia syndrome is the bilateral periventricular nodular heterotopia syndrome (Ross and Walsh, 2001), which is caused by mutations in filamin A (FLNA). This is inherited as an X-linked dominant disorder that therefore occurs in females and usually is embryonic lethal in males. FLNA is an actin cross-linking phosphoprotein that appears to function in the actin remodeling required for cell migration out of the ventricular zone (Fox et al, 1998). The usual phenotype of FLNA mutations is a female with seizures and/or psychiatric difficulty with normal or near-normal intelligence. Patients may also have specific difficulty with dyslexia (Chang et al, 2005). There is a suggestion that FLN A mutations may also result in cardiovascular abnormalities, because there have been case reports of individuals with strokes at early ages, aneurysms, and early death (Fox et al, 1998).

Periventricular heterotopia has also been linked to mutations in ARFGEF2 (adenosine diphosphate–ribosylation factor guanine exchange factor 2) (Sheen et al, 2004).

This gene is located on chromosome 20 and inherited in an autosomal recessive fashion. Heterozygous parents are asymptomatic; homozygous offspring have heterotopias, microcephaly, and severe developmental delay. Abnormalities in this gene have thus far been identified only in two consanguineous families. The ARFGEF2 protein (BIG2) regulates vesicular transport. It is hypothesized that BIG2 may affect the vesicle trafficking of adhesion molecules that are required for the movement of neurons from the ventricular zone (Pacheco-Rodriguez et al, 2002; Sheen et al, 2004).

Periventricular heterotopia has also been associated with duplications of 5p, although no specific gene has so far been identified (Sheen et al, 2003). Of all cases of familial periventricular heterotopia, 80% have *FLNA* mutations. Only 20% of sporadic cases have *FLNA* mutations, indicating the importance of environmental influences, or genetic causes not yet identified (Lu and Sheen, 2005).

SUMMARY

Advances in human genetics have led to continued rapid progress toward improved understanding of the cellular and molecular pathogenesis of human brain malformations. These advances are providing a more rational means to approach both prenatal and postnatal diagnosis, which is increasingly allowing for a more realistic assessment of prognosis. Although therapy for brain malformations is still largely focused on treatment of adverse symptoms and sequelae, recent experimental studies suggest that the migration of some populations of neurons may not be permanently arrested. For example, in a rat model of subcortical band heterotopia, some neuronal migration abnormalities were reduced when the doublecortin gene was reexpressed in neurons during a postnatal window during which they were still receptive to reinitiation of migration. This led to diminution of seizures (Manent et al, 2009). Such studies underscore the critical need for ongoing basic research in developmental neurobiology to accelerate progress toward both better diagnosis and treatment of these devastating disorders.

Complete references used in this text can be found online at www.expertconsult.com

CENTRAL NERVOUS SYSTEM INJURY AND NEUROPROTECTION

Sonia L. Bonifacio, Fernando Gonzalez, and Donna M. Ferriero

INJURY AND PROTECTION IN THE DEVELOPING NERVOUS SYSTEM

Injury to the developing brain from a variety of factors (hypoxia-ischemia, infections, inflammation) results in predictable pathologic patterns based on age at the time of insult, and the severity of the insult. This is due to the selective vulnerability of populations of cells undergoing active metabolic change during these time periods. The most common type of injury in the preterm brain is intraventricular hemorrhage (IVH) from germinal matrix bleeding, and white matter injury due to hypoxia-ischemia and infections. In the term brain, the deep gray matter is more likely to be affected by a severe insult. A variety of patterns of cortical and subcortical parenchymal injuries can be seen, depending on how blood flow or metabolism is disrupted. Perinatal arterial ischemic stroke, sinovenous thrombosis and perinatal hemorrhagic stroke occur in both preterm and term newborns. A number of traumatic injuries also can occur in the neonatal period, including damage to the calvaria, cranial nerves, spinal cord, and peripheral nerves. The ability to protect against the adverse sequelae of these varied types of injuries will depend on the timing of injury accurate diagnosis, careful early management, and the development of age-appropriate therapies. New therapies for brain injury in newborns, such as hypothermia for term neonatal encephalopathy, are being implemented, and adjunctive therapies continue to be studied in animal models.

INTRAVENTRICULAR AND PERIVENTRICULAR HEMORRHAGE IN THE PRETERM INFANT

Pathogenesis

IVH is a common injury in the preterm brain, originating in the subependymal germinal matrix. Cortical neuronal and glial cell precursors develop from the germinal matrix and adjacent ventricular germinal zone during the late second and early third trimesters. The subependymal germinal matrix is a highly vascularized region whose arterial supply is derived from the anterior and middle cerebral arteries as well as the anterior choroidal artery. These arteries feed an elaborate capillary network of thin-walled vessels that is continuous with a deep venous system that terminates in the vein of Galen. The terminal, choroidal, and thalamostriate veins course anteriorly to form the internal cerebral vein, which courses posteriorly to join the vein of Galen, thus leading to a U-shaped turn in the direction of blood flow. Involution of the germinal matrix occurs with advancing gestation.

The predisposition of the premature infant to IVH is due to several factors. A pressure-passive state exists due to the lack of autoregulation of cerebral blood flow in the cerebral arterioles in the premature brain. In the presence of a highly vascularized subependymal germinal matrix, the lack of a supporting basement membrane in the blood vessels of the germinal matrix and an increased amount of fibrinolytic activity in the germinal matrix region also predispose to the development of IVH. Extravascular tissue pressure decreases in the first few days of extrauterine life, and in the setting of elevation of venous pressure or an increase in fluctuations in cerebral blood flow velocity from a variety of factors (respiratory distress, pneumothorax, asphyxia, myocardial failure, patent ductus arteriosus, hypotension, hypothermia, hyperosmolarity), IVH may occur (Ment and Schneider, 1993). Fluctuating pressure passivity is common in premature infants and may be associated with IVH (O'Leary et al, 2009; Soul et al, 2007).

IVH has been produced experimentally after hypotension followed by reperfusion (Goddard-Finegold et al, 1982; Ment et al, 1982). These studies support the observation that infants with IVH are more likely to have had an early period of prolonged hypotension followed by an increase in blood pressure (Miall-Allen and Whitelaw, 1987; Miall-Allen et al, 1987). Isolated hypertension associated with seizures, intubation, and suctioning also predispose the brain to IVH. Even gavage feeding and surfactant administration can lead to changes in cerebral hemodynamics as measured by near-infrared spectroscopy (NIRS) that may result in IVH (Baserga et al, 2003; Kaiser et al, 2004; Roll et al, 2000).

Box 61-1 lists the different factors that may interact in an individual case to produce IVH.

Cellular injury in infants with grade III or IV (PVHI) IVH may occur from ischemic injury that may precede the bleed, from a decrease in cerebral blood flow, or from increased intracranial pressure, as well as vasospasm. Posthemorrhagic hydrocephalus is a common sequela of periventricular venous infarction (grade IV). These severe IVH grades are associated with periventricular white matter injury and sometimes pontine neuronal necrosis (Volpe, 2008). In this setting, venous infarction leads to neuronal as well as oligodendroglial cell death (Craig et al, 2003).

Site, Incidence, and Timing of Hemorrhage

In preterm infants, germinal matrix hemorrhage is most commonly seen at the junction of the terminal, choroidal, and thalamostriate veins in the germinal matrix over the body of the caudate nucleus at the level of the foramen of Monro. Parenchymal hemorrhage occurs most commonly

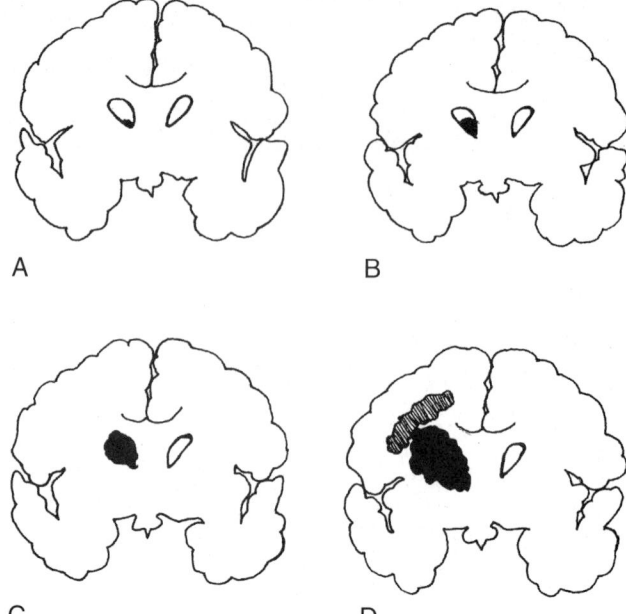

FIGURE 61-1 **Illustration of intraventricular hemorrhage (IVH) grades as determined by degree of hemorrhage** (see Table 61-1). **A,** Grade I hemorrhage involves less than 10% of the ventricular volume in the lateral ventricles; **B,** grade II hemorrhage involves 10% to 50%; **C,** grade III involves greater than 50% of the ventricular volume and is often associated with some ventricular dilatation; and **D,** grade IV (Papile et al, 1978) or unclassified (Volpe, 2009) is associated with parenchymal echodensities on head ultrasound study, indicating parenchymal infarction.

in the frontoparietal region, in approximately 15% of cases, and is thought not to be an extension of the IVH but rather, a separate process—a hemorrhagic infarction. The hemorrhage is more often unilateral or, in less than 30% of cases, asymmetrically bilateral.

The incidence and severity of IVH increase with decreasing gestation. It occurs in approximately 4.6% of term newborns and was previously reported to occur in 40% to 60% of very low-birthweight (VLBW) infants (less than 1500 g birthweight). An overall reduction of IVH in this population to 15% to 25% has been observed in the past two decades (McCrea and Ment, 2008; Paneth et al, 1993; Vohr et al, 2000). Although there has been a gradual decline in the incidence of all grades of IVH, the increased survival of VLBW infants has resulted in an increase in the absolute number of infants with IVH. The risk period for the occurrence of IVH is highest in the first 3 or 4 days of life. Hemorrhage is rarely seen at birth, although it has been reported as early as within the 1st hour of age (Ment et al, 1984). Antenatal hemorrhages can occur, especially in the setting of neonatal alloimmune thrombocytopenia. Twenty-five percent of hemorrhages occur by the 6th hour and 50% of hemorrhages occur during the first 24 hours of life. Less than 5% of infants develop IVH after the 4th or 5th day of life (Ment and Schneider, 1993). Extension of the hemorrhage may occur over the first few days secondary to events leading to alterations in cerebral blood flow.

Clinical Presentation

The clinical presentation of IVH in the newborn depends on the extent of the hemorrhage and may vary from asymptomatic to a sudden and catastrophic deterioration that manifests with neurologic signs such as stupor or coma, seizures, decerebrate posturing, or apnea. A full fontanel along with a sudden drop in hematocrit, hyperglycemia, hyperkalemia, hypotension, and bradycardia all can herald an IVH. Inappropriate secretion of antidiuretic hormone may be present. The more common presentation, however, is that of a gradual clinical deterioration with an altered level of consciousness, hypotonia, abnormal extremity, or eye movements. In 25% to 50% of cases, clinical correlation is lacking (Dubowitz et al, 1998).

Grading of Intraventricular Hemorrhage

Ultrasound examination is a reliable and sensitive technique for evaluating the severity of IVH in the newborn nursery (Pape et al, 1983, 1979). Papile and associates

adapted the standard grading system originally applied to computed tomographic images of IVH to ultrasound images and classified IVH into four different grades of severity depending on the location and extent of the bleed (Papile et al, 1978) (Figure 61-1; Table 61-1). Outcome studies performed over the past two decades use this system for classification. In the preferred grading system used by Volpe (2008), the presence of intracerebral hemorrhage or parenchymal lesions is mentioned separately and not designated as grade IV. This system relies on the head ultrasound examination as the diagnostic measure and more accurately defines IVH based on the extent of the ventricular hemorrhage. Because parenchymal involvement is a distinct process, it is not included in the continuous grading (see Table 61-1). In VLBW infants, 10% to 15% suffer from the more severe hemorrhages (McCrea and Ment, 2008).

Outcome and Prognosis

Grade I hemorrhage and grade II hemorrhage generally are followed by resolution. Grade III hemorrhage evolves over a period of 1 to 3 weeks and in some cases produces a fibrotic reaction that obliterates the subarachnoid space and leads to ventricular dilatation and hydrocephalus. Traditional clinical criteria of increasing ventricular dilatation such as rapid head growth, full anterior fontanel, and separated cranial sutures often appear days or even weeks after the dilatation begins. This delayed appearance is due to the presence of a large subarachnoid space as well as the paucity of myelin in premature infants. In 15% of cases

TABLE 61-1   Grading of Intraventricular Hemorrhage (IVH) by Cranial Ultrasound Findings

Papile Grading System		Volpe Grading System*	
I	Subependymal hemorrhage with minimal or no IVH	I	Germinal matrix hemorrhage <10% IVH
II	Definite IVH without distention of the ventricles	II	IVH 10% to 50%
III	Enlargement of the ventricles secondary to distention with blood	III	IVH >50%, usually with distention of lateral ventricle
IV	Extension of the hemorrhage into the parenchyma along with IVH and enlargement	Separate notation	Periventricular echodensity signifying parenchymal lesion

IVH, Intraventricular hemorrhage.
*By cranial ultrasound.

of IVH, areas of periventricular hemorrhagic involvement are noted (Volpe, 2008). This finding is believed to be due to an independent venous infarct of the periventricular white matter and not a direct extension of the IVH into the parenchyma (Volpe, 2008). Intraparenchymal hemorrhage is followed in 1 to 8 weeks by tissue destruction and formation of a porencephalic cyst. Outcomes vary between studies, but in general, mortality rates are not significantly increased in infants with a grade I or II hemorrhage. Grades III and IV are associated with increased mortality, with mortality rates in neonates suffering hemorrhagic infarction approaching 50% (Brouwer et al, 2008; Sarkar et al, 2009).

Several studies have focused on the relationship between IVH and subsequent neurologic dysfunction. Although grade I and grade II IVH are not associated with significant morbidity, grade III is associated with neurologic sequelae in up to 35% of infants, and grade IV is associated with sequelae in as many as 55% of affected infants (Brouwer et al, 2008). The severity of neurologic sequelae such as seizures, severe motor handicap, and severe hearing and vision impairment increases in infants with grade III or IV hemorrhage in whom persistent ventriculomegaly develops. The presence of hydrocephalus with or without shunting at term increases the odds of a poor neurodevelopmental outcome. Vohr et al (2000), in a longitudinal study of 90 preterm infants with birthweights of less than 1750 g, reported that by 2 years of age, only infants with grade III and grade IV differed in neurologic examination findings from the term control infants. Unlike motor function, cognitive function as assessed by the Bayley scores deteriorates in the first 18 months of life. Infants with grade I and grade II IVH have lower scores than those infants with no IVH or normal term infants. In another study of extremely low-birth weight (ELBW) infants (weight <1000 g at birth), those with grade I or II hemorrhage had an increased risk for major neurodevelopmental impairment (odds ratio [OR] 1.83, 95% confidence interval [CI] 1.11 to 30.03, p <0.05) when

compared with those with normal cranial ultrasounds findings (Patra et al, 2006). This increased risk of abnormal outcome may be related to underrecognized white and gray matter injury (Inder et al, 1999b). Follow-up studies have shown that the degree of IVH at birth and the presence of ventriculomegaly are predictors of neurologic status at 24 months' corrected age (Brouwer et al, 2008).

Prevention

Prevention of preterm birth is the most effective method of reducing the incidence of IVH. In the event of preterm labor it is advisable that the infant be born at a center specializing in high-risk deliveries. The risk of IVH is higher in infants who are transported after birth. Adequate management of labor and delivery is essential. Studies of antenatal steroids have demonstrated decreased risk of IVH and cerebral palsy (Leviton et al, 1999). A recent trial of antenatal magnesium sulfate showed a reduction in cerebral palsy but no difference in the rates of IVH (Rouse et al, 2008). Appropriate resuscitation of the preterm infant and vigilance in avoiding hyperventilation and low Pco_2 or hypoxia, maintaining adequate mean arterial pressure, and avoiding elevations in cerebral blood flow by excessive handling or tracheal suctioning are vital. Prevention of pneumothorax and acidosis and avoidance of rapid infusions of sodium bicarbonate or volume expanders also are critical. Because of the increased risk of neurodevelopmental sequelae in infants with IVH, several clinical trials have studied the effects of various pharmacologic interventions to reduce the incidence of IVH. Several clinical trials have been done to evaluate the role of prolonged neuromuscular paralysis in preterm infants. A metaanalysis of five trials concluded that although neuromuscular paralysis with pancuronium may help decrease IVH and pneumothorax in asynchronously breathing infants, its routine use cannot be recommended because of concerns about safety and long-term pulmonary and neurologic effects (Cools and Offringa, 2000).

A low mean arterial blood pressure (MAP) and an increase in fluctuation of blood pressure have been associated with an increased risk of IVH. Close monitoring of the MAP is recommended; however, there is no evidence suggesting that pharmacologic manipulation of the MAP (e.g., with pressors, steroids, or volume expanders) to achieve a set goal (e.g., MAP >30 mm Hg) alters the incidence of IVH or improves neonatal outcome. Phenobarbital administration was shown in early studies to be beneficial by preventing fluctuations in blood pressure (Donn et al, 1981). Subsequently, the results of multicenter trial testing the effect of antenatal administration of phenobarbital (10 mg/kg) to 110 women on the frequency of IVH in infants between 24 and 33 weeks of age showed no decrease in IVH in infants born to mothers treated with phenobarbital (Kaempf et al, 1990). A larger trial confirmed these findings, and long-term follow-up at 18 to 22 months of these infants found no difference in neurodevelopment (Shankaran et al, 1997, 2002). A metaanalysis of 10 trials of postnatal phenobarbital showed no difference in the rates of severe IVH or ventriculomegaly. Therefore, postnatal administration of phenobarbital for reduction of IVH is not recommended (Whitelaw and Odd, 2007).

Pharmacologic doses of vitamin E, an antioxidant, have been associated with a reduction in the incidence of IVH in LBW infants when given intramuscularly (Speer et al, 1984). However, after reports of the association of such large doses of vitamin E with sepsis and necrotizing enterocolitis, its use for prevention of IVH was curtailed (Finer et al, 1984; Johnson et al, 1985). There has been little reported in the literature since these studies.

Indomethacin, a prostaglandin synthetase inhibitor, had originally been shown to decrease the incidence of IVH in infants weighing less than 1250 g (Ment et al, 1985). A recent study on the long-term effects of indomethacin prophylaxis in ELBW infants showed no improvement in the rate of survival without neurosensory impairment at 18 months, despite the reduction in severe IVH (Schmidt et al, 2001). A metaanalysis of 19 trials and 2872 infants found an increased risk of oliguria that was, however, not associated with major renal impairment; no difference in the incidence of necrotizing enterocolitis; a modest reduction in the number of infants with severe IVH; but no difference in long-term neurosensory impairments (Fowlie and Davis, 2002).

Use of antenatal steroids (Canterino et al, 2001; Elimian et al, 2000; Smith et al, 2000) and surfactant replacement therapy have been shown to decrease the incidence of IVH as well as neonatal mortality in LBW infants (Soll and Dargaville, 2000). The increase in IVH reported with surfactant administration may occur as a result of the mode of instillation (Cowan et al, 1991; Hellstrom-Westas et al, 1991, 1992) and the drop in $Paco_2$ with improved ventilation. A significant drop in MAP and cerebral blood flow volume can occur during surfactant administration; attention should be paid to the speed and volume of instillation.

Several studies have been done to evaluate the early use of high-frequency ventilation versus conventional ventilation for infants with respiratory distress syndrome. One of these studies have shown an increased incidence of IVH with high-frequency oscillatory ventilation (HFOV) (HIFI Study Group, 1989, Moriette et al, 2001), whereas another study of jet ventilation did not find an increase in IVH (Keszler et al, 1997). Overall there is no evidence of decreased or increased risk of severe IVH in those treated with high-frequency versus conventional ventilation.

It is important to avoid both hypocarbia (Pco_2 <30 mm Hg) or hypercarbia (Pco_2 >55 mm Hg) because of their significant effects on cerebral blood flow. Hypocarbia is associated with hypotension as well as an acute decrease in cerebral blood flow. Avoiding low Pco_2 has been shown to be neuroprotective in animal studies (Sola et al, 1983; Vannucci et al, 1995). Although the effect of low Pco_2 levels has not been systematically studied in preterm infants, low levels have been shown to be deleterious in term infants with pulmonary hypertension (Ferrara et al, 1984). Hypercarbia leads to increases in cerebral blood flow, which in the presence of other therapies aimed at increasing blood pressure, may be damaging to the central nervous system (CNS).

Free radicals and iron have been shown to be damaging to oligodendrocytes in both cell culture and animal studies (Back et al, 1998; Dommergues et al, 1998). Also, iron-chelating agents such as deferoxamine have been shown to be neuroprotective in animal models (Sarco et al, 2000). It may be wise to prevent iron overload during the period of critical cortical development (Gressens et al, 2002). Similarly, avoiding hyperoxia is important to prevent free radical injury.

Several of the medications that are used frequently in LBW infants may have effects on neurodevelopment. Caffeine therapy for apnea in VLBW infants has been shown in a randomized controlled trial to reduce the incidence of cerebral palsy and neurodevelopmental delay at 18 to 21 months of age (Schmidt et al, 2007). Postnatal steroid use in preterm infants has been found to be associated with an increased risk of periventricular leukomalocia (PVL) and poor neurodevelopment (Merz et al, 1999; Murphy et al, 2001). Pain medications such as morphine, fentanyl, and midazolam are often used for analgesia in ventilated preterm infants. However, there is increasing concern regarding the potential detrimental effects of this practice on the developing brain. Recently, Simons et al (2003) found that routine morphine infusion in ventilated preterm newborns had no measurable analgesic effect and no beneficial effect on neurodevelopment. More controlled studies are needed comparing the efficacy and safety of different analgesic practices in the preterm population.

Management

Infants with birthweights of less than 1500 g or gestational age of less than 32 weeks should have a screening ultrasound performed to detect IVH. A scan on the 4th postnatal day detects 90% of lesions. Because extension of the bleed sometimes occurs over the next few days, a repeat ultrasound examination after 5 days is necessary to establish the extent of the bleed.

The decision to continue intensive care support depends on the severity of the bleed as assessed by head ultrasound examination as well as the infant's gestational age and clinical condition. Parents should be informed regarding the presence of IVH and the prognosis of the infant.

Acute management is mainly supportive and requires control of ventilation, maintenance of a normal metabolic status and optimal nutritional state, and detection and treatment of seizures. Systemic blood pressure should be maintained with cautious attention to the rate of administration of fluid. Consideration of the aforementioned risk factors is important to prevent ischemia.

Of the infants in whom enlargement of the ventricles occurs, approximately 50% develop rapidly progressive ventricular dilatation over the next 4 to 8 weeks. Regular measurement of head circumference and examination of the fontanel and clinical status are recommended in the first 4 weeks in cases of slowly progressive hydrocephalus. Serial lumbar puncture or use of carbonic anhydrase inhibitors has been recommended by some clinicians. A randomized controlled trial of the combined use of furosemide and acetazolamide in 177 infants with posthemorrhagic hydrocephalus concluded that this treatment is ineffective in decreasing the need for shunt placement and is associated with increased risk of a poor neurologic outcome (Kennedy et al, 2001). Use of streptokinase immediately after an IVH with development of posthemorrhagic hydrocephalus has been advocated by some to be beneficial. The studies to date have been too small to allow reasonable conclusions (Haines and Lapointe, 1999; Luciano et al, 1998, Whitelaw, 2001). One randomized multi-center trial of drainage, irrigation, and fibrinolytic therapy compared with tapping of excess cerebral spinal fluid to prevent shunt dependence showed no benefit (Whitelaw et al, 2007).

In infants with rapidly progressive hydrocephalus that does not respond to serial lumbar punctures, placement of an external ventriculostomy is necessary as a temporizing measure. Placement of a ventriculoperitoneal shunt that diverts cerebrospinal fluid (CSF) from the lateral ventricles to the peritoneal cavity in a premature infant is problematic because of the risk of skin breakdown, shunt obstruction, and/or infection. However, some centers are placing subgaleal shunts as a temporizing measure in these infants; these shunts may be associated with significantly fewer complications (Fulmer et al, 2000).

WHITE MATTER INJURY

In the premature newborn, white matter injury (WMI) consists of discrete (focal) areas of magnetic resonance (MR) signal abnormality. With the increasing use of MR imaging (MRI) in the clinical assessment of brain injury in the premature newborn, "focal non-cystic white matter injury" is recognized as the most common pattern of brain injury in this population (Cornette et al, 2002; Miller et al, 2005a). On conventional MRI, focal noncystic WMI appears as areas of hyperintensity on T1-weighted MR images (Figure 61-2). This type of WMI is distinct from cystic PVL, a more severe abnormality that refers specifically to cystic regions of necrosis in the periventricular white matter that are well detected by brain ultrasound (Volpe, 2009). However, most children who exhibit deficits in motor and cognitive outcomes do not have sonographically-identified PVL (Aziz et al, 1995; Hamrick et al, 2004). As focal non-cystic WMI is observed in half of premature newborns on MRI, this type of white matter injury has been under-recognized (Miller et al, 2003, 2005a).

Premature newborns may have diffuse impairments in the progression and rate of brain development. These acquired developmental brain abnormalities may be even more common than the focal "injuries" identified on MRI and are not limited to the white matter. When severe, these diffuse abnormalities are apparent on MRI by a paucity of white matter, ventriculomegaly, impaired gyral development, or enlarged subarachnoid spaces (Inder et al, 2003). However, most premature newborns do not have these dramatic abnormalities, and up to 20% with adverse outcomes do not have significant qualitative abnormalities on MRI (Boardman et al, 2007; Miller et al, 2005a). One possibility is that the brain is imaged at a time when signal abnormalities have been replaced by tissue loss that is not as easily detected on qualitative MRI.

Clinical Factors Important for White Matter Injury

There is now evidence that the risk of brain injury and abnormal brain development is altered by systemic illness and by critical care therapies. For example, the severity of

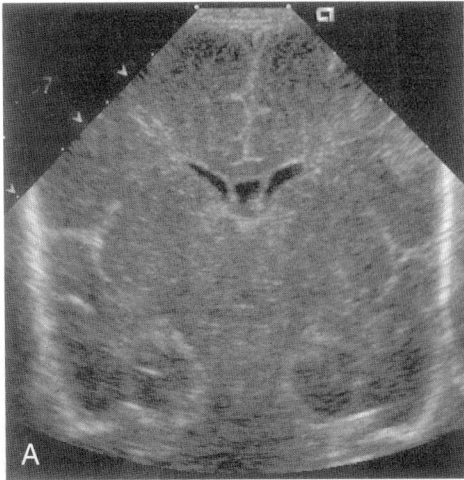

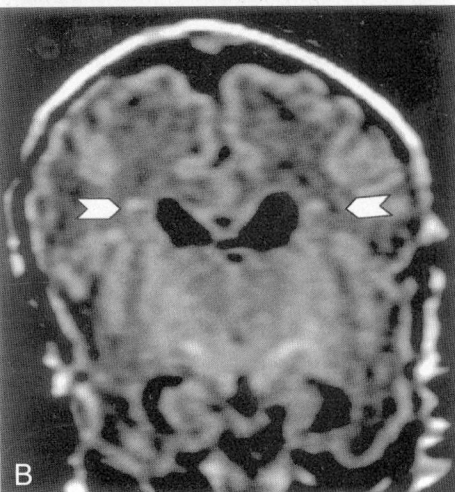

FIGURE 61-2 A, Head ultrasound image with no evidence of periventricular leukomalacia. **B,** Abnormalities are well seen on T1-weighted magnetic resonance image (*arrows*) in the same patient.

chronic lung disease predicts cognitive outcome at 8 years of age, even after controlling for birthweight and neurological complications (Short et al, 2003). Postnatal infection in preterm newborns is also associated with impaired neurodevelopmental outcomes (Stoll et al, 2004). Recurrent postnatal infection is an important risk for progressive WMI (Glass et al, 2008). Recent observations suggest that motor impairments seen more commonly in preterm infants with sepsis are mediated by white matter abnormalities (Shah et al, 2008). However, other studies suggest that both postnatal infection and WMI are *independently* associated with adverse neurodevelopmental outcomes (Miller et al, 2005a). In regard to critical care therapies, postnatal exposure to corticosteroids for the prevention and treatment of chronic lung disease may impair brain growth, though this effect may be limited to treatment with dexamethasone (Lodygensky et al, 2005; Murphy et al, 2001). A dramatic decline in the incidence of cystic PVL may be related to a decrease in days of mechanical ventilation (Hamrick et al, 2004), possibly by avoiding hypocarbic alkalosis (Fujimoto et al, 1994). In an observational study, less WMI was seen in premature newborns exposed to prolonged indomethacin therapy for patent ductus arteriosus (Miller et al, 2006). Clinical features of

WMI in the premature infant may involve impairment of gaze and hearing, weakness, or altered muscle tone. Long-term problems may include spastic diplegia and visual and auditory impairment.

Pathogenesis of White Matter Injury

Important work regarding the pathogenesis of WMI has been performed in the last decade. It appears that the late oligodendrocyte progenitors that populate human cerebral white matter during the high-risk period for white matter injury are the major target of ischemic, free radical, or cytokine injury (Back et al, 2001, 2002, 2007). However, recent studies show that injury may be due to lack of oligodendrocyte maturation, resulting in decreased myelination and subsequent axonal injury (Segovia et al, 2008). Some data suggest vulnerability of the subplate neurons as well (McQuillen et al, 2003). Tissue damage is associated with proliferation of astrocytes and microglial cells in areas of subcortical degeneration. Increasingly, injury to the developing gray matter is also being identified in the setting of white matter injury and is recognized both in neuropathologic studies and with advanced imaging techniques (Inder et al, 2005; Pierson et al, 2007). The mechanisms of neuronal injury are likely to be similar to those causing injury of the white matter and the preoligodendrocytes.

IMAGING FOR DIAGNOSIS OF INTRAVENTRICULAR HEMORRHAGE AND WHITE MATTER INJURY

A practice parameter published jointly by the American Academy of Pediatrics, the American Society of Pediatric Neuroradiology, and the Society for Pediatric Radiology recommends routine screening with cranial ultrasonography for all infants of less than 30 weeks' gestation between 7 and 14 days of age. A repeat ultrasound examination is recommended between 36 and 40 weeks of postmenstrual age (Ment et al, 2002c). However, considerable advances in the field of MRI in premature infants have been made recently (Miller et al, 2002). Several studies have focused on determining the spectrum of white matter injury detected by MRI and its effect on neurodevelopment (Groenendaal et al, 1997; Hüppi et al, 1998; Inder et al, 1999a; Maalouf et al, 2001, 1999; Ment et al, 2002; van Wezel-Meijler et al, 1998). Newer techniques such as diffusion tensor imaging (DTI) have been shown to be helpful in defining areas of the brain at risk for damage (Barkovich et al, 2001; Huppi and Inder, 2001). DTI can also be used to monitor normal development of pathways using the apparent diffusion coefficient and anisotropy in certain regions (Miller et al, 2002c). In a comparison of head ultrasound examination with MRI, MRI was more sensitive in identifying PVL (Rijn et al, 2001). Lesions on MRI also show a stronger correlation with school age outcome than lesions on ultrasound (Rademaker et al, 2005). It is now becoming clear that lesions that affect developmental outcome and that are not present on cranial ultrasound images can be detected by MRI (Miller et al, 2005a; Woodward et al, 2006). Given the foregoing studies, MRI should be considered in all ELBW infants at 36 to 40 weeks' postmenstrual age if clinical suspicion

for parenchymal brain injury exists. As MRI technology continues to evolve and methods of obtaining scans in this patient population are also improving, including the development of MRI-compatible incubators and specialized neonatal head coils, we will continue to gain insight into injury patterns in the developing brain.

HYPOXIC-ISCHEMIC REPERFUSION INJURY IN THE NEWBORN

Perinatal hypoxic-ischemic reperfusion (HI-R) injury may result in neonatal hypoxic-ischemic encephalopathy (HIE), which is a significant cause of neonatal morbidity and mortality and can lead to severe long-term neurologic deficits. The incidence of HIE is approximately 6 in 1000 term infants, with the incidence of death or severe neurologic deficit being 1 in 1000 (Levene and Evans, 1985).

Etiology

Hypoxic-ischemic brain injury results when the decrease in cerebral perfusion is severe enough to overwhelm the ability of tissue to extract oxygen from the blood, thereby leading to a mismatch between cerebral blood flow and oxidative metabolism. Although the final pathways leading to cerebral brain death are remarkably similar regardless of the instigating event, the extent, location, and evolution of cell death probably are determined by the nature of the insult. The etiology of HIE is multifactorial. In a study of risk factors for neonatal encephalopathy, antepartum risk factors such as maternal hypotension, infertility treatment, and thyroid disease were present in 69% of cases; both antepartum and intrapartum risk factors were present in 24%; and a history of an intrapartum event such as maternal fever, difficult forceps delivery, breech extraction, cord prolapse, or abruptio placentae was present in 5% of cases (Badawi et al, 1998). Postnatal events such as severe respiratory distress or congenital heart disease, sepsis, and shock are responsible for fewer than 10% of cases of HIE.

Clinical Signs and Symptoms

The clinical signs and symptoms depend on the severity, timing, and duration of the insult. The infant's gestational age needs to be taken into consideration in the evaluation. Symptoms usually evolve over a period of 72 hours (Sarnat and Sarnat, 1976) (Table 61-2).

During the first 12 hours after birth, the signs and symptoms are secondary to cerebral hemisphere depression, although signs of brainstem involvement may be present. During this period, the infant is not easily arousable. This alteration in consciousness is attributed to the involvement of the cerebral hemispheres, the reticular activating system, or the thalamus. Periodic breathing with apnea or bradycardia is usually present. The infant has intact pupillary responses and may have spontaneous eye movements, depending on involvement of cranial nuclei 3, 4, and 6. Cerebral cortical or cerebellar cortical involvement may manifest as hypotonia with decreased movement or as jitteriness or seizure activity, which is seen in 50% of severely affected infants by 6 to 12 hours after birth. The Moro, grasp, and suck and swallow reflexes may be absent

TABLE 61-2   Clinical Staging of Hypoxic-Ischemic Encephalopathy

Factor	Stage 1	Stage 2	Stage 3
Level of consciousness	Alert	Lethargy	Coma
Muscle tone	Normal	Hypotonia	Flaccidity
Tendon reflexes	Normal/increased	Increased	Depressed/absent
Myoclonus	Present	Present	Absent
Complex reflexes			
Sucking	Active	Weak	Absent
Moro	Exaggerated	Incomplete	Absent
Grasping	Normal/exaggerated	Exaggerated	Absent
Oculocephalic (doll's eyes)	Normal	Overreactive	Reduced/absent

Data from Sarnat NB, Sarnat MS: Neonatal encephalopathy following distress, *Arch Neurol* 33:696-705, 1976.

or depressed. In cases of severe asphyxia, seizures may be seen within 2 to 3 hours following the insult. Seizure onset usually occurs within the first 24 hours of life. Seizure activity in a term infant can be multifocal or focal in nature. Subtle seizures may also manifest as ocular movements such as tonic horizontal deviation of the eyes or sustained eye opening or blinking; orolingual movements such as tongue or lip smacking or sucking, or rowing or bicycling movements of the extremities, or as recurrent apnea (Mizrahi and Kellaway, 1987). Electrographic seizures without clinical correlate may also be present, and therefore the newborn with moderate encephalopathy should be monitored for seizures in the form of a complete electroencephalogram (EEG) or amplitude-integrated electroencephalography (EEG) (aEEG). Brainstem release phenomena are common in severely asphyxiated newborns and may be misinterpreted as seizures.

During the 12- to 24-hour period after the injury, there is an apparent increase in the level of alertness, but this is not associated with other signs of improvement in neurologic function. This period is accompanied by seizures in 15% to 20% of infants, apneic episodes in 50%, and jitteriness as well as weakness in the proximal limbs in 35% to 50%. The Moro reflex is exaggerated, the infant's cry is shrill and monotonous, and the deep tendon reflexes are exaggerated.

After 24 to 72 hours, the infant's level of consciousness deteriorates. This is followed by respiratory arrest and signs of brainstem dysfunction such as loss of responsiveness to the doll's eyes maneuver, fixed and dilated pupils, and sometimes death. Infants who survive until 72 hours continue in stupor with disturbed suck, swallow, and gag reflexes; hypotonia; and weakness of the proximal limbs and especially facial and bulbar musculature.

Diagnosis

The diagnosis of HIE is made through a careful history, laboratory studies, and neurologic examination. Metabolic abnormalities, cerebral dysgenesis, and infection can

mimic HIE. There is sometimes a history of intrauterine distress, as evidenced by abnormalities on the fetal heart tracing, passage of meconium, or a history of difficult labor or delivery with a decrease in placental or fetal blood flow. A history of a difficult resuscitation that includes the use of cardiopulmonary resuscitation, medications in the delivery room, and intubation and assisted ventilation at birth and low extended Apgar scores after 5 minutes of age are associated with HIE. Excessive jitteriness, seizures, apneic episodes, or abnormal cry are signs of injury.

The neurologic examination provides important information for prognosis. Laboratory tests can be helpful in diagnosing HIE. Metabolic complications such as hypoglycemia, hypocalcemia, hyponatremia, hypoxemia, and acidosis are frequently seen. Several other metabolic parameters such as serum brain-specific creatine kinase (BB fraction), serum hypoxanthine, and serum lactate also are elevated. Lumbar puncture should be performed if the history is not consistent with perinatal distress, to rule out conditions that may mimic HIE. Lumbar puncture should be used to measure cell count, protein and glucose levels, and ratio of lactate to pyruvate, as well as brain-specific creatine kinase. A CSF protein level above 150 mg/dL is considered abnormal. Urinary lactate-to-creatine ratios have been shown to be elevated in asphyxiated infants (Huang et al, 1999). Elevated urinary S100B protein may also serve as a marker of severe perinatal asphyxia (Gazzolo et al, 2004).

Changes on the EEG can be helpful in determining the severity of the insult. The initial change is a suppression of amplitude and frequency. This is followed after 24 hours by a periodic pattern that consists of periods of greater voltage suppression interspersed with bursts of sharp and slow waves. Subsequently, a "burst suppression" pattern with fewer bursts and more severe voltage depression is seen, followed by an isoelectric tracing. The EEG is helpful in supporting the diagnosis of HIE, and amplitude-integrated electroencephalography has been used in both animal and human studies as an aid to identify newborns moderately to severely compromised by hypoxic-ischemic injury (al Naqeeb et al, 1999; Toet et al, 1999). Both aEEG and conventional EEG are useful in monitoring the evolution of encephalopathy, in monitoring for seizures as there can be a high rate of electrographic seizures without clinical correlate, and in predicting outcome. EEG monitoring is critically important after administration of an antiseizure medication, such as phenobarbital, as there is a high likelihood of electroclinical dissociation (Biagioni et al, 1998).

Neuroimaging has become increasingly useful for the accurate diagnosis of HIE. Computed tomography (CT) often is not helpful in making a diagnosis because it is insensitive to changes in water content. Also, especially in the posterior fossa, injury can be obscured by bone artifact. CT is best used to determine the extent of bleeding in an emergency situation when MRI is not available.

MRI has proved to be a sensitive technique to determine injury in the term infant brain. Absence of signal in the posterior limb of the internal capsule is strongly associated with poor neurologic outcome (Rutherford et al, 1995). MRI performed as early as 4 days to as late as 2 to 3 weeks of life, dependent on the techniques used, can be highly predictive of outcome at 18 months of age, even following hypothermia therapy (Barkovich et al, 2006; Miller et al, 2005b; Rutherford et al, 2010).

Ultrasonography is extremely useful for imaging the unstable patient if performed with high-resolution transducers (de Vries et al, 1997). Injury to the basal ganglia, periventricular echodensities, and presence of focal or multifocal ischemic parenchymal lesions suggest neurologic deficits. Ultrasound is insensitive to cortical damage; therefore, in term infants, ultrasound findings may underrepresent the extent of the lesion.

Proton magnetic resonance spectroscopy (MRS) also has been useful for depicting age-dependent changes in preterm infants and can be a powerful tool for diagnosing early damage in both preterm and term infants (Vigneron et al, 2001). MRS provides a quantitative in vivo measure of brain biochemistry. At long echo times, it can measure resonance intensities for N-acetyl aspartate (NAA), creatinine (Cr), phosphocreatine, choline (Cho), and lactate. The measure of NAA in reference to baseline Cr or Cho has provided a sensitive indicator of neuronal integrity, whereas lactate has indicated the presence of oxidative stress or ongoing injury. MRS is now being used more extensively to identify areas at risk in perinatal HIE (Holshouser et al, 2000).

NIRS is a noninvasive technique that holds promise in the future. It can be used at the bedside to provide information regarding cerebral oxygen delivery. However, this modality is not quantitative and is not available at many centers.

Patterns of Injury and Pathology

The mechanism of injury can be one of several types. Different patterns of injury may result, depending on the duration and severity of the insult.

Global hypoxia-ischemia develops when the oxygen requirements for cerebral metabolism are unable to be met by cerebral perfusion pressure, as is seen with a decrease in cerebral arterial pressure or an increase in cerebral venous pressure. Although the injury may be transient, it sets into motion a cascade of events that ultimately lead to neuronal death. The duration of the insult necessary to produce brain injury is inversely proportional to the gestational age of the fetus. The extent and location of the injury can be patchy bilaterally, or diffuse and involve the entire cortex. The latent period to neuronal cell death produced by a global insult can range from hours to days and is determined by a complex interaction among various vascular, cellular, and metabolic factors (see later). In some circumstances, lesions may involve the brainstem (*pontosubicular necrosis*) or the cerebellum. Infants with pontosubicular necrosis have impairment of the cranial nerve nuclei and will exhibit ptosis and facial diparesis.

Focal ischemia occurs when the arterial or venous blood supply to a region is compromised. The degree of injury is dependent on the collateral blood supply to this region. The injured region typically consists of a central dense region of ischemia that undergoes rapid cell death—the core—surrounded by a region of evolving cell injury—the *penumbra*. The cells in the penumbral region initially are sustained by anaerobic glycolysis. However, within

hours the injury becomes irreversible, thus bringing the penumbra into the gradually enlarging area of infarction. This period of delay in cell death provides an opportunity for therapeutic intervention and prevention of further cell damage. Partial asphyxia without acidosis, as occurs in response to impairment of placental gas exchange by uterine contractions, maternal hypotension, or impairment in maternal placental circulation, can produce either widespread cerebral cortical necrosis or a more focal injury to the posterior parietal parasagittal regions. Partial asphyxia with acidosis has been shown to cause white matter injury.

Focal and multifocal cerebral necroses occur secondary to an embolus or thrombus (see Perinatal Stroke, later). There are often underlying problems such as thrombophilias, maternal idiopathic thrombocytopenic purpura, vascular maldevelopment, or history of maternal cocaine use. Infants may present with unilateral, focal seizures or display asymmetric motor function, or they may be asymptomatic.

Selective neuronal necrosis can involve specific regions of the cortex, thalamus, brainstem, cerebellum, or hippocampus. An acute global injury such as is seen with uterine rupture or cord prolapse causes injury to the basal ganglia, thalamus, and brainstem, whereas a prolonged partial injury affects mainly the cortex and subcortical white matter. Damage is more extensive in the posterior parietal-occipital region than in the anterior cortical areas. Clinical signs in the infant relate to the site of injury. Seizures are a feature of cortical injury, whereas irritability, posturing, and brainstem dysfunction are seen with infarcts affecting the basal ganglia and thalamus. Long-term sequelae of such an injury include cerebral atrophy and multicystic encephalomalacia. *Status marmoratus* refers to the marbled appearance of the basal ganglia, thalamus, and cerebral cortex in response to the injury. This appearance results from gross shrinkage of the striatum and defects in myelination. It may relate to the type of insult or the density of glutaminergic receptors in the basal ganglia (Johnston, 1995). Although the clinical correlate of this condition in the newborn is not well defined, it is seen in children with choreoathetoid cerebral palsy.

Cerebral blood flow is closely autoregulated over a wide range of systemic blood pressure by either vasoconstriction or dilatation of cerebral arterioles. However, this mechanism is imperfect in the newborn. Therefore, rapid changes in cerebral perfusion pressure can occur in response to changes in systemic blood pressure, as well as changes in cerebral PaO_2 and $PaCO_2$. Injury typically tends to occur in the watershed regions, which in the term newborn are located in the parasagittal regions of the cerebral cortex. The periventricular white matter is the most vulnerable region in preterm newborns.

Clinical features of *parasagittal injury* include hypotonia and weakness, especially in the upper trunk. Cortical infarcts usually occur in the watershed region supplied by the most peripheral branches of the anterior, middle, and posterior cerebral arteries.

Spinal cord ischemia is not uncommon after HI-R injury. In patients with hyporeflexia or areflexia, spinal cord pathology should be considered. Ischemic necrosis occurs in spinal cord gray matter (Clancy et al, 1989).

Cellular Mechanisms

The immature brain is more susceptible to hypoxic-ischemic injury for several reasons, including immaturity of vascular regulation, along with maturational differences in metabolic oxidative function between the newborn and adult brain (Ferriero, 2001).

Although overall cerebral O_2 demands are lower in the infant than in the adult, cerebral oxidative metabolism is considerably increased in areas of active neural development that are associated with either synapse formation or activation of enzymes required for ion homeostasis. Glucose is the primary source of energy in cerebral metabolism, and although the newborn brain is capable of utilizing alternative energy substrates such as ketones, lactate, and free fatty acids, glucose uptake mechanisms are relatively underdeveloped (Cremer et al, 1979; Gregoire et al, 1978). Absence of energy stores makes the brain dependent on sustained perfusion. Animal studies have shown that this impaired uptake of glucose can impair cerebral metabolism even before oxygen depletion (Yager et al, 1996).

Vasoautoregulation in response to increased cerebral blood pressure or flow is relatively underdeveloped in the newborn, thus rendering the infant more vulnerable to ischemic events. The gradual increase in vascularity of the developing brain leads to the creation of watershed areas (i.e., areas not well vascularized). These regions are more vulnerable to global ischemic events. These global events lead to patterns of focal injury that are dependent on maturational processes. The similarities between processes essential for brain development and those mediating cellular injury make the immature brain particularly vulnerable to ischemic insult. These similarities include an increased density of glutamate receptors, an increase in glutaminergic synapses in particular regions of the immature brain, and enhanced accumulation of cytosolic calcium after activation of the glutamate receptor. It has been shown that there are proportionally more glutamate receptors in the immature rat brain than in the mature rat brain and that the developing rat brain is much more sensitive to injury than the newborn or adult brain (Yager et al, 1996). HI-R injury triggers a complex series of cellular events that evolve rapidly through amplifying cascades, eventually leading to severe cerebral damage. A gradual or sudden decrease in cerebral oxygen and energy substrates initially leads to synaptic inactivation, which is a reversible and adaptive response to HI-R injury. Decreased cerebral energy stores lead to membrane pump failure and the subsequent inability to maintain normal ion gradients (Figure 61-3). This is followed by neuronal membrane depolarization and release of neurotransmitters such as glutamate, which increase cytosolic calcium and induce destructive enzymes and free radicals. Reoxygenation after the ischemic episode plays a significant role in cellular injury. The pathogenesis of HI-R injury can be divided arbitrarily into four phases (Box 61-2; see also Figure 61-3):

1. A decrease in cerebral energy and membrane depolarization
2. A phase of increased release of neurotransmitters and neuronal damage
3. A period of reperfusion
4. A final phase of irreversible cell death

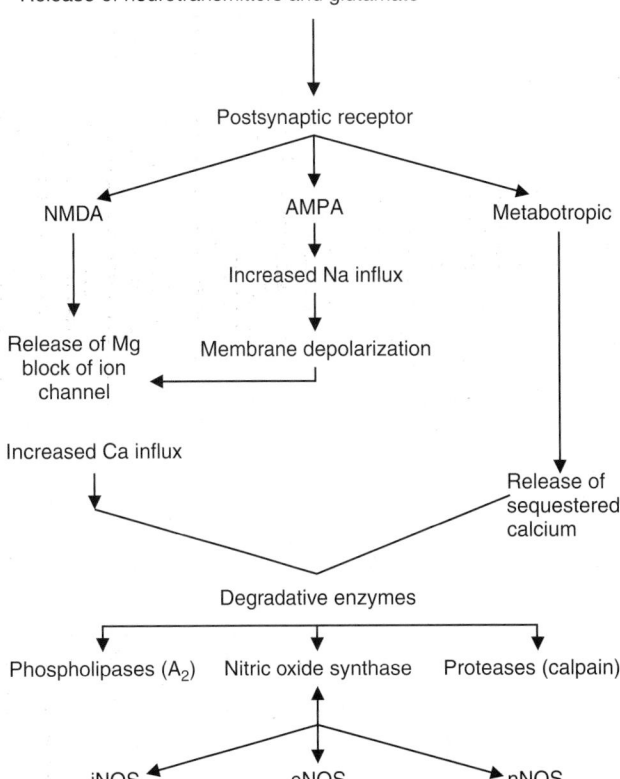

FIGURE 61-3 Flow diagram of events occurring after hypoxic-ischemic/reperfusion injury leading to energy depletion, membrane polarization, neurotransmitter release, calcium influx, and intracellular enzymatic activation leading to cell death.

Decrease in Cerebral Energy and Membrane Depolarization

HI-R injury is followed by a depression of brain function that probably is a protective mechanism to preserve energy. In the normal state, glucose and oxygen are the main requirements for brain energy production, which occurs by oxidative phosphorylation. Glucose is taken up by a carrier-mediated diffusion process and phosphorylated to glucose 6-phosphate, the major portion of which enters the glycolytic pathway to form pyruvate. Pyruvate enters the mitochondria and is converted to acetyl coenzyme A (acetyl CoA); acetyl CoA enters the citric acid cycle and undergoes oxidation to CO_2. The electrons generated get transported through several carrier proteins such as (reduced) nicotinamide adenine dinucleotide (NADH) within the mitochondria. NADH couples to molecular oxygen and forms ATP through phosphorylation of ADP by adenine kinase. Phosphocreatine also can serve as a store of energy that can transfer phosphorus to generate ATP. HI-R injury is followed by a decrease in brain glucose and ATP. Anaerobic glycolysis is much less efficient at ATP production. Aerobic glycolysis generates 38 moles of ATP per mole of glucose, compared with 2 moles of ATP produced by anaerobic glycolysis.

A decrease in ATP affects the Na/K ATPase pump that helps to maintain the state of polarization of the neuronal membrane. A failure of the pump leads to an influx of sodium into the cell and potassium outside the cell. Associated glial uptake of sodium and water leads to astrocytic swelling that in turn decreases diffusion of oxygen and glucose to the neurons.

Accumulation of lactate secondary to anaerobic glycolysis leads to tissue acidosis, which inhibits both vascular autoregulation and phosphofructokinase, the rate-limiting enzyme in glycolysis. In immature animals, hypoglycemia has been shown to be damaging; pretreating animals with glucose decreases the impact of the injury when given before, but not during, the injury (Sheldon et al, 1992; Vannucci and Vannucci, 2000). This is in contrast with the effect of glucose administration in mature animals.

Excitotoxicity

There is sufficient evidence that excitatory neurotransmitters play a major role in HI-R injury. Excitotoxicity refers to excessive glutamatergic activation that leads to cell injury and death (Olney, 2003). Neuronal injury is initiated by release of glutamate and other excitatory neurotransmitters from the presynaptic neurons. Initially the decrease in energy supply decreases ATP-dependent exocytosis of glutamate and decreases activity of glutamate synthetase, the enzyme responsible for converting glutamate to nontoxic glutamine. Subsequently, glutamate release occurs by both a reversal of normal glutamate uptake mechanisms by the nerve terminals and glia, and membrane leakage. A secondary increase in glutamate occurs during the phase of reoxygenation.

Glutamate receptors are of three subtypes: N-methyl-D-aspartate (NMDA), amino-3-hydroxy-5-methyl-4-isoxazole propionic acid (AMPA), and the G protein–associated metabotropic receptor. The NMDA receptor is a postsynaptic receptor that is activated by glutamate and has been shown to play an important role in normal brain development including neuronal survival, differentiation,

arborization of dendrites, growth of axons, and development of synapses. The expression of NMDA receptor subtypes as well as the subunit composition of the glutamate receptors changes with maturation (Johnston, 1995; MacDonald and Nowak, 1990). The density of receptors is higher in regions of active development, and the different subtypes vary in different regions of the brain at different gestational ages. Several features in the subunit composition of the immature NMDA receptor result in enhanced opening and influx of calcium into the ion channels (Andersen et al, 1995; Ben-Ari et al, 1988; Morrisett et al, 1990). Activation of any of the three subtypes of glutamate-activated postsynaptic neuron receptors leads to an influx of calcium into the postsynaptic neurons. Activation of the NMDA receptor releases the magnesium block within the ion channel and leads to the entry of calcium into the ion channel. Activation of the AMPA receptor mediates fast excitatory neurotransmission by triggering an influx of sodium. The resulting membrane depolarization opens calcium channels and releases the magnesium block of the NMDA channel, thereby leading to cytosolic accumulation of calcium. Activation of the metabotropic receptor results in the generation of inositol triphosphate, which triggers release of sequestered calcium.

The increase in intracellular calcium sets into motion an irreversible cascade of events that leads to cell injury. Calcium activates several degradative enzymes such as phospholipases, proteases, and endonucleases. Activated phospholipases such as phospholipase A_2 hydrolyze membrane phospholipid, thereby releasing free fatty acids such as arachidonic acid. Arachidonic acid can mediate injury by several mechanisms, including increased release of glutamate, uncoupling of oxidative phosphorylation, and inactivation of membrane Na/K ATPase. Proteases degrade cytoskeletal and other proteins. Cyclooxygenase stimulates production of arachidonic acid and prostaglandins. Enzyme activation as well as activation of xanthine and prostaglandins generates free radicals that perpetuate the injury by lipid membrane peroxidation. Hypoxic-ischemic injury also leads to a change in iron homeostasis. Iron is usually maintained in a nontoxic "ferric" state but is reduced into the injurious "ferrous" form, which can react with oxygen-reactive species to propagate further injury.

Oxidative Stress

Nitric oxide synthase (NOS), one of the enzymes that is released during HI-R injury, has been identified as a mediator of cellular injury. NO causes cellular injury by various mechanisms: combining with superoxide to form a peroxynitrite radical that causes lipid peroxidation, generating free radicals by stimulation of cyclooxygenase activity, direct DNA damage, and participating in the neurotransmitter response by reentering the presynaptic neuron and further increasing release of glutamate.

NO may mediate both the initial reperfusion by vasodilatation and the later mitochondrial enzyme inhibition. During the initial period of reperfusion there is a clearance of glutamate (Takahashi et al, 1997). Several mechanisms that have been proposed to explain the ultimate increase in calcium influx and perpetuation of injury have been the subject of excellent reviews (Inder and Volpe, 2000, White et al, 2000). Some of the mechanisms proposed include a long-term potentiation of NMDA receptors to low levels of extracellular glutamate, which can then lead to an exaggerated calcium influx, an impairment of the Na/K ATPase pump from delayed energy failure (Obrenovitch and Urenjak, 1997), and enhanced release of glutamate by NO. Generation of free radicals during this phase occurs by two methods: free fatty acids enter the cyclooxygenase pathway and generate arachidonic acid and prostaglandins, and xanthine oxidase converts hypoxanthine to uric acid. Free radicals activate adhesion molecules in platelets and leukocytes, which increases occlusion of the microvasculature, thereby perpetuating injury.

Cell Death

Cell death can occur as necrosis or apoptosis after ischemia. *Apoptosis* refers to programmed cell death, a mechanism that is ongoing during the process of brain maturation. Apoptotic cells are characterized by nuclear shrinkage, chromatin condensation, and DNA fragmentation. Necrotic cells are characterized by cellular swelling, fracture of cell membranes, and an inflammatory cellular reaction. It is hypothesized that a severe insult leads to necrosis, as is seen in the central area of injury, whereas a longer duration of a less severe injury may lead to apoptosis, as seen in the penumbra. In the immature brain, a third pathologic form of injury has been described: the apoptotic-necrotic continuum (Portera-Cailliau et al, 1997). This particular pattern may represent the predominant form of injury (Northington et al, 2001a, 2001b). It has recently been shown in animal models that there is a prolonged period of delayed cell death due to apoptosis (Nakajima et al, 2000; Northington et al, 2001a). This exciting finding suggests that there is a prolonged window of opportunity for interventional strategies.

Management of Hypoxic-Ischemic Encephaolpathy

The immediate management of HIE requires securing an appropriate airway and maintaining adequate circulation. Cerebral edema resulting from hypoxia-ischemia is maximal between 36 and 96 hours and can impair cerebral blood flow secondary to increased intracranial pressure. There is no consensus regarding the need to treat cerebral edema aggressively, because its role in producing neurologic sequelae is debatable. Although steroids have been shown to be beneficial in vasogenic cerebral edema, most investigators agree that corticosteroids are not beneficial for cerebral edema arising from hypoxic-ischemic injury. Attempts to decrease intracranial pressure by controlled hyperventilation ($Paco_2$ of 20 to 25 mm Hg) as well as by the use of furosemide or mannitol may actually be harmful (Collins et al, 2001). Because there is accumulating animal and human evidence of the detrimental effect of seizures, seizure activity should be controlled to limit further compromise of neurologic status, and electroencephalography in the form of aEEG or EEG should be used to monitor for subclinical seizures (Bjorkman et al, 2010; Glass et al, 2009; Miller et al, 2002d; van Rooij et al, 2010). Multiorgan function must be monitored

carefully. Maintenance of adequate cerebral perfusion is necessary, and inotropic agents need to be used in patients with evidence of myocardial dysfunction. It is important to avoid both systemic hypotension and hypertension. Infants with hypoxic-ischemic injury can develop hyponatremia from syndrome of inappropriate secretion of antidiuretic hormone (SIADH). Hypoglycemia in an immature animal model during the evolution of HIE has been found to aggravate the insult (Sheldon et al, 1996). Therefore, fluid overload should be avoided, and serum glucose and electrolytes should be monitored closely. Body temperature should be closely monitored and hyperthermia avoided. Moderate hypothermia therapy in the form of whole-body or selective head cooling is being rapidly implemented as part of routine care in many nurseries for infants with moderate to severe encephalopathy and evidence of perinatal asphyxia. Those with moderate to severe encephalopathy should be referred and transferred to an institution with a hypothermia program within the first 6 hours of life. There are currently ongoing studies evaluating whether or not institution of hypothermia, delayed prolonged, or deeper, or hypothermia plus other agents (e.g., xenon, erythropoietin), is neuroprotective for newborns with HIE.

Prognosis

Outcome of HIE depends on the severity of the initial insult and the degree of brain damage. Several factors such as maturity of the infant, placental-fetal blood flow, energy reserves, or presence of cerebral anomalies can affect the final outcome. It is often difficult to determine the duration of the insult because the vast majority of insults occur in utero and because accurate fetal surveillance is difficult. Certain clinical factors as well as the results of brain imaging studies can help identify infants with a poor prognosis (Barkovich et al, 1995; Biagioni et al, 2001). Seizures should be treated, because they have been associated with increased lactate and poor neurodevelopmental outcome. The presence of seizures is perhaps the best clinical indicator of adverse outcome, especially if seizure activity occurs in the first 12 hours of life or if seizures are difficult to control (Miller et al, 2002d).

The Apgar score is not a good predictor of outcome. This measure is affected by the use of maternal drugs or anesthesia, and by the vagal-induced respiratory depression that occurs from the use of suction catheters or from oropharyngeal secretions. There is also considerable variation among personnel in assigning the Apgar score, and all of the five different parameters that make up the Apgar score are not equally weighted for neurologic outcome. Although the Apgar score at 1 minute is not predictive of a poor outcome, the predictive ability does increase with a continued depressed score with increasing age of the infant. It has been shown that infants with Apgar scores of less than 6 at 5 minutes are three times more likely to have abnormalities on neurologic examination than are infants with scores greater than 6 (Levene et al, 1986). However, if the infant shows no neurologic symptoms in the perinatal period, the outcome is often normal. Ekert et al (1997) built a model to predict severe adverse outcome within 4 hours of birth in neonates with HIE and found that delayed onset of breathing, need for chest compressions, and seizures had a sensitivity of 85% and specificity of 68%. In another predictive model, the following factors were included: the need for chest compressions for >1 minute, delayed onset of respirations >30 minutes, and base deficit >16 within the 1st hour of life, were predictive of poor outcome. When none of the factors were present, the rate of adverse outcome was 46% (95% CI, 33% to 58%) with none of the 3 factors, 64% (95% CI, 54% to 73%) with any 1 factors, 76% (95% CI, 66% to 85%) with any 2 factors, and 93% (95% CI, 81% to 99%) with all of the 3 factors present (Shah et al, 2006).

The duration of the neurologic abnormalities is usually helpful in predicting long-term neurologic disability. In two separate studies, normal examination findings at 1 week and at 2 weeks of age correlated with a good outcome (Robertson and Finer, 1985; Sarnat and Sarnat, 1976). Hypothermia treatment may confound the predictability of level of encephalopathy at the completion of therapy. In a secondary analysis of the Cool-Cap hypothermia trial, the outcomes for newborns after therapy was not necessarily reflected in improvement in the grade of encephalopathy, which may be due to other factors such as the use of morphine or other sedating drugs during cooling (Gunn et al, 2008). Other clinical tools used include the presence of impairment of other organ systems and the Score for Neonatal Acute Physiology–Perinatal Extension (SNAP-PE), a physiologic assessment score done within the first 24 hours of life (Newton et al, 2001). As with other clinical measures, neither of these tools is able to prognosticate outcome in the moderately asphyxiated newborn.

Predicting Outcome With Diagnostic Tests
Electroencephalography
The rate of recovery of the EEG to normal baseline activity and the severity of neonatal encephalopathy can be helpful in establishing the neurologic prognosis (Biagioni et al, 2001).

Amplitude Integrated Electroencephalogram
Amplitude-integrated EEG is a bedside monitor that is useful in assessing the background activity of the brain and in identifying seizures. It is easily interpreted by those with limited training. It is complementary to conventional EEG, may be used as a screening test for those with possible seizures or in monitoring for seizures in an acutely ill or paralyzed neonate, and can help monitor response to antiepileptic medications; also, the rate of recovery of the background in HIE is associated with outcome (Hellstrom-Westas et al, 1995; Toet et al, 1999; van Rooij et al, 2005; van Rooij et al, 2010).

Magnetic Resonance Imaging
MRI has been shown in a variety of studies to be useful in predicting outcome in neonates with HIE (Barkovich et al, 1998; Biagioni et al, 2001; Ment et al, 2002; Rutherford et al, 2006). In particular, absence of the signal in the posterior limb of the internal capsule has been associated with poor neurodevelopmental outcome. A joint statement from the American Academy of Pediatrics, the American Society of Pediatric Neuroradiology, and the Society for Pediatric Radiology recommends that a noncontrast CT

study be performed to detect hemorrhagic lesions in term infants with encephalopathy and a birth history of trauma, coagulopathy, or low hematocrit. If the CT findings are inconclusive, MRI is recommended between days 2 and 8 to assess location and extent of injury (Ment et al, 2002). Because the CT scan does not compare favorably with MRI for confirming the diagnosis of hypoxic-ischemic injury or for providing prognostic information, Miller et al (Miller et al, 2002a) recommend that an MRI study be performed in the first week of life for establishing the diagnosis in an encephalopathic newborn (Figure 61-4, *A*).

Magnetic Resonance Spectroscopy
MRS has been shown to correlate with neurologic outcome and may be more sensitive in identifying injury and metabolic disturbances from seizures than standard imaging (Miller et al, 2002d) (see Figure 61-4, *B*). Abnormalities seen on MRS have been significantly associated with both neurologic and cognitive outcomes. Both high lactate and low NAA levels have been associated with persistent injury (Barkovich et al, 2001; Miller et al, 2002b). Study results have varied in accordance with the timing of the scan in relation to the injury. It has been reported that the lactate level of the injured brain increases within the first 24 hours and remains elevated thereafter, presumably because of energy failure and the necessity to metabolize glucose anaerobically (Hanrahan et al, 1996; Penrice et al, 1996). However, the NAA level does not diminish significantly until sometime beyond 48 hours (Penrice et al, 1997). The precise time at which NAA begins to diminish in asphyxiated neonates is not precisely known.

Outcome
The outcome for hypoxic-ischemic brain injury differs substantially for the preterm infant and the term infant. Although more preterm infants survive such an insult than term infants, preterm survivors are more likely to have neurodevelopmental disabilities. In a recent study of extremely preterm children, 49% had disabilities, with 23% meeting criteria for severe disabilities (Wood et al, 2000). In term infants with neonatal encephalopathy, the presence of seizures and the severity and duration of encephalopathic state are predictors of poor outcome (Glass et al, 2009; Robertson et al, 1989; Thornberg et al, 1995). Infants with mild neonatal encephalopathy syndromes usually have no deficits, whereas those with severe encephalopathy die or are severely impaired with spastic quadriparesis, cortical visual impairment, and seizure disorders. Those with moderate degrees of encephalopathy can be normal to severely abnormal, depending on the pattern of injury seen on MRI and MRS and the persistence of EEG abnormalities (Barkovich et al, 2001; Biagioni et al, 2001). The neurologic examination at 3 months may be a good prognostic indicator (Hajnal et al, 1999). In one cohort study, those with predominant injury to the deep grey nuclei experienced more severe outcomes at 30 months compared to those with predominant watershed region injury (Miller et al, 2005b). Using a separate MRI scoring system, in a cohort of 73 neonates with HIE, abnormalities of the posterior limb of the internal capsule were predictive of poor outcome at 1 year of age (Rutherford et al, 1998). Hypothermia is associated with an

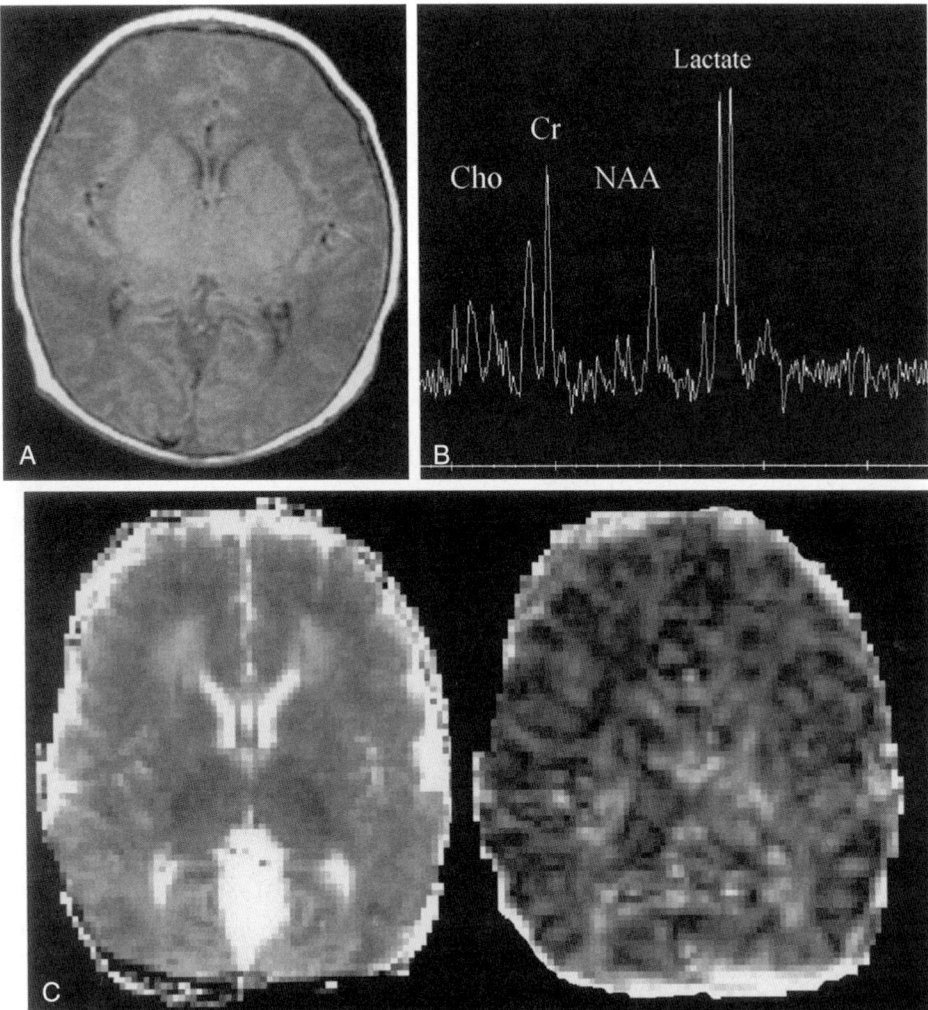

FIGURE 61-4 Magnetic resonance (MR) spectra and diffusion-weighted images obtained on day 2 of life in a term infant with moderate hypoxic-ischemic encephalopathy. **A,** MR image shows loss of signal intensity in the posterior limb of the internal capsule. **B,** The MR spectra show elevated lactate and decreased *N*-acetyl aspartate *(NAA)* peaks in the basal ganglia in that area; **C,** diffusion-weighted images show restricted diffusion on the apparent diffusion coefficient (ADC) image *(left)* and loss of anisotropy *(right)*.

increase in number of infants with a normal scan, a reduction in severity or basal ganglia/thalamic and cortical injury, and these findings are still predictive of outcome (Bonifacio et al, 2011; Inder et al, 2004; Rutherford et al, 2005, 2010).

PERINATAL STROKE

Perinatal strokes can be arterial or venous in nature (Figure 61-5). Perinatal stroke is defined as an ischemic event that occurs between 28 weeks' gestation and 7 days of age and includes in utero strokes. The term *neonatal stroke* is reserved for events occurring between birth and the end of the 1st month of life (Raju et al, 2007). It is difficult to establish the exact prevalence of perinatal stroke. Using studies of children with neonatal seizures, prevalence has been estimated to be roughly 12% of neonates greater than 31 weeks' gestation who present with seizures (Lynch et al, 2002). Perinatal stroke is increasingly recognized in full-term infants with an incidence of 1 per 2300 to 4000 liveborn infants (Kirton and deVeber, 2009; Nelson and Lynch, 2004; Schneider et al, 2004; Schulzke et al, 2005).

In the newborn period, seizures are the most common presenting symptom. Other symptoms include encephalopathy, abnormalities of tone, feeding problems, or apnea. However, there is a subgroup of neonates who do not present with evidence of injury until late infancy because the neurologic examination findings are normal in the newborn period. This is referred to as presumed perinatal stroke. These infants present later with pathologic early hand preference and/or seizures (Golomb et al, 2001). Stroke in the newborn has a slight male predominance, and there is a tendency toward left-sided lesions (Golomb, 2009; Golomb et al, 2001; Trauner et al, 1993).

The U.S. infant mortality rate for years 1995 to 1998 due to stroke (ICD-9 CM 430-437) is 5.33/100,000 per year, perinatal mortality is 2.21/100,000, and neonatal mortality is 3.49/100,000 live births per year (Lynch and Nelson, 2001). The National Hospital Discharge Survey, from 1980 through 1998, determined that for infants younger than 30 days of age, the in-hospital mortality rate for neonatal stroke was 10.1%, or 2.67/100,000 live births (Lynch and Nelson, 2001; Lynch et al, 2002).

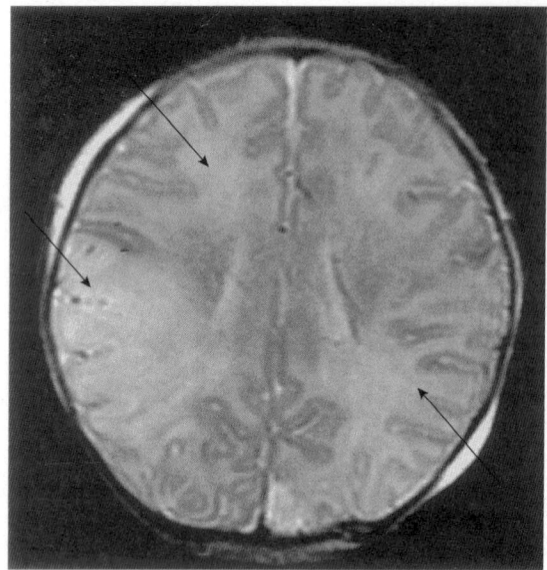

FIGURE 61-5 Brain magnetic resonance T2-weighted image in term neonate who suffered ischemic arterial stroke. Increased signal intensity is seen in the right parietal and frontal areas and the left posterior parietal region.

Cerebral Venous Thrombosis

Sinovenous thrombosis (SVT) is an important cause of stroke in the neonate. It is being increasingly diagnosed in recent years, probably reflecting the use of more sensitive neuroimaging techniques. In a retrospective series of children with abnormal imaging studies suggestive of SVT, 61% were neonates (Carvalho et al, 2001). The Canadian Pediatric Ischemic Stroke Registry (CPISR) identified 0.67 case per 100,000 per year, with neonates the most commonly affected (43%) (deVeber and Andrew, 2001). Most recently in a non–population-based study of 84 neonates with symptomatic SVT, 61% presented within the 1st week of life (Jordan et al, 2010). Risk factors are similar to those for ischemic stroke, with thrombophilias, asphyxial stress, dehydration, and infection being more common in the neonate (Fitzgerald et al, 2006; Kenet et al, 2007). Often, more than one risk factor is present (Wu et al, 2002).

Neonates present with seizures as the most common sign. The head ultrasound examination often reveals an IVH. Further neuroimaging with MRI and MR venography will reveal the site of the venous thrombosis and may also show other parenchymal abnormalities, such as thalamic hemorrhage (Wu et al, 2003b) (Figure 61-6).

Risk Factors

A number of different types of studies of infants with perinatal stroke has found an association with cardiac disorders, blood disorders, infection, trauma, drugs, maternal and placental disorders, catheterization, extracorporeal membrane oxygenation, and perinatal asphyxia. In some studies, the occurrence of multiple risk factors has been noted, especially blood disorders and asphyxial stress (Golomb et al, 2001; Lee et al, 2005).

Outcome

A review of the literature for case reports, series, and case-control studies of perinatal or neonatal stroke, which included 572 infants with perinatal stroke, revealed that 40% of infants with perinatal stroke were neurologically normal, 56% were abnormal (having neurologic or cognitive abnormalities), and 3.0% had died by the outcome evaluation period (Lynch et al, 2002). A similar review concluded that more than 50% of children with neonatal stroke appear normal by 12 to 18 months of age (de Vries et al, 1997). The majority of children did not have recurrent seizures. In the CPISR, the recurrence rate among children with neonatal stroke was 3% to 5%, and among survivors, outcome was normal in 33% (deVeber and Andrew, 2001). In one case series of 24 infants with MRI-confirmed cerebral infarction, 64% of the neonates had neurodevelopmental sequelae. Despite these impairments, most children walk independently by 2 years of age (Golomb, 2009). The presence of prothrombotic disorders, especially presence of factor V Leiden deficiency, was associated with poor outcome in term infants (Mercuri, 2001).

The neurodevelopmental outcome of neonates with SVT is reported to be normal in 77% to 82%. Presence of venous infarction and refractory seizures has been associated with neurologic sequelae (Carvalho et al, 2001; deVeber and Andrew, 2001; Shevell et al, 1989).

Management

There are no randomized trials for acute or chronic therapy following perinatal stroke. The use of anticoagulation therapy for the newborn is based on case series and expert opinion but is still not determined. Recently, guidelines regarding management, diagnostic evaluation, and therapy were published by the American Heart Association Stroke Council (Roach et al, 2008). It is difficult to extrapolate from adult or even nonneonatal pediatric studies. In the acute phase, treatment is mostly supportive. Hydration status, monitoring and treatment of seizures, and antibiotics may be important. Serial imaging may be used to identify extension of thrombi. In neonates with arterial ischemic stroke, anticoagulation may be considered in those with an ongoing cardioembolic source or recurrent stroke. In those with SVT without significant intracranial hemorrhage, the American College of Chest Physicians (ACCP) recommends treatment with unfractionated heparin or low-molecular-weight heparin (LMWH) followed by LMWH or vitamin K antagonists for 6 to 12 weeks (Monagle et al, 2008). Currently a study is being planned for the use of anticoagulation in VST.

PERINATAL TRAUMA

Injuries of the cranial structures and the brain can occur secondary to trauma during the process of birth. Perinatal trauma can result from various causes in utero, during labor, and postnatally. The nature of the trauma can be either mechanical or vascular. Embolism and thrombosis can result from placental infarcts or absorption of material from a macerated twin fetus, or with disorders of

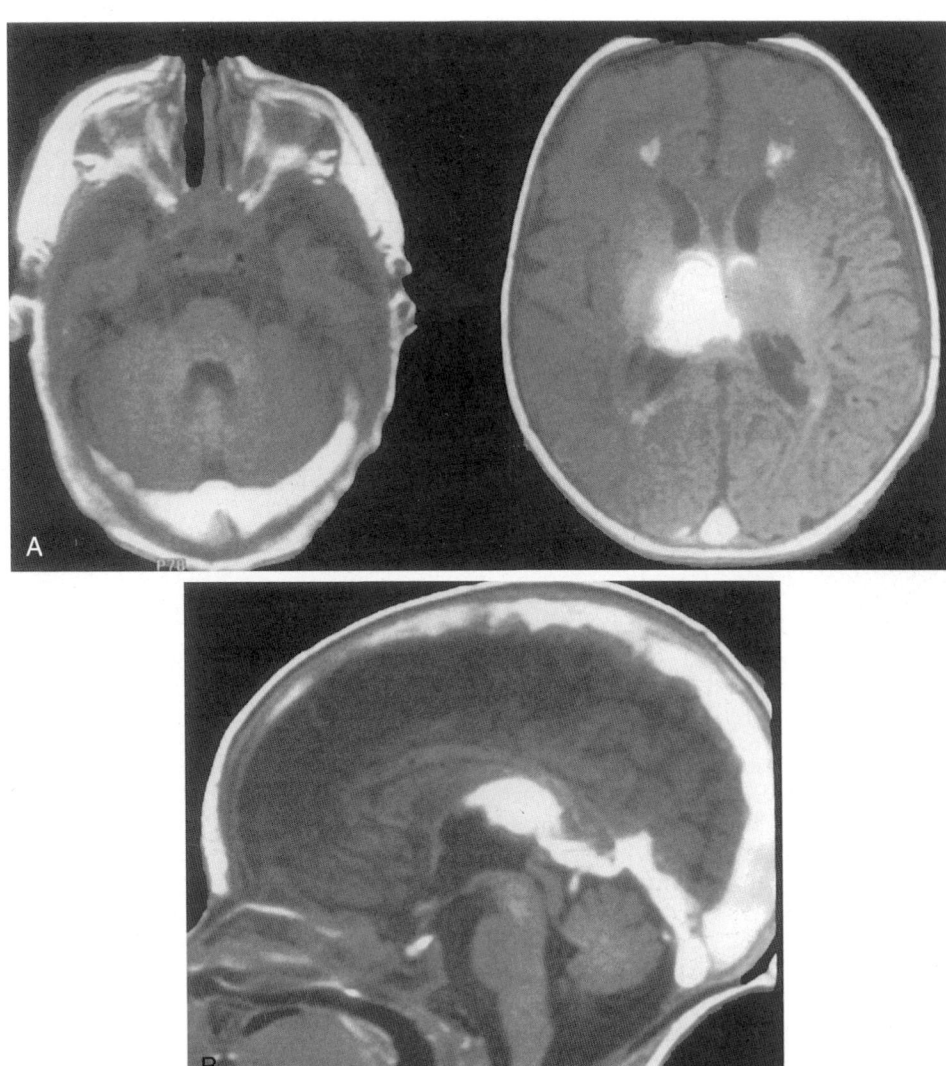

FIGURE 61-6 **Brain magnetic resonance (MR) images of sinovenous thrombosis with thalamic infarction in a term neonate. A,** Right thalamic infarction and hemorrhage seen on axial T1-weighted MR image; **B,** thrombosis of entire venous system seen on sagittal T1-weighted MR image.

coagulation or sepsis. Mechanical trauma can cause injury to both cranial and extracranial structures as well as the spinal cord and peripheral nerve structures.

Mechanical Trauma

Mechanical trauma can result in damage to extracranial structures, cranial structures, intracranial structures, spinal cord, or peripheral nerves.

Molding of the Head and Caput Succedaneum

Molding of the head is frequently seen in the newborn delivered either vaginally or by cesarean section. It refers to the asymmetrical shape of the head that results from mechanical pressure exerted during passage through the birth canal or during extraction by cesarean section. Caput succedaneum refers to the edematous soft tissue swelling that is often associated with bruising over the molded region. Although this condition is generally benign and resolves with time, abrasions over the area can become infected, and hyperbilirubinemia may develop with resolution of bruising (Figure 61-7).

Subgaleal Hemorrhage

In certain cases the trauma may be severe enough to cause a subgaleal hemorrhage, which consists of extension of the bleeding beneath the scalp aponeurosis to the nape of the neck. This condition needs to be recognized immediately because it can lead to severe blood loss and shock. The coagulation status should be evaluated, because subgaleal hemorrhage may be a presenting sign of hemophilia, hemorrhagic disease of the newborn, or other coagulation disorders. A CT scan or MRI is indicated, especially in conditions associated with an enlarging scalp swelling, altered mental status, and/or decreasing hematocrit with signs of hemorrhagic shock. Maintenance of the circulatory status of the infant is critical and may require use of packed cells or plasma to correct hypovolemia and any coagulopathy. Because of the nature of the subgaleal space, a neonate's entire blood volume can enter this space and lead to significant shock with resulting hypoxic-ischemic brain injury. Occasionally, severe trauma can lead to tearing of either the tentorium or the falx cerebri. A subdural hematoma may occur in cases with venous lacerations.

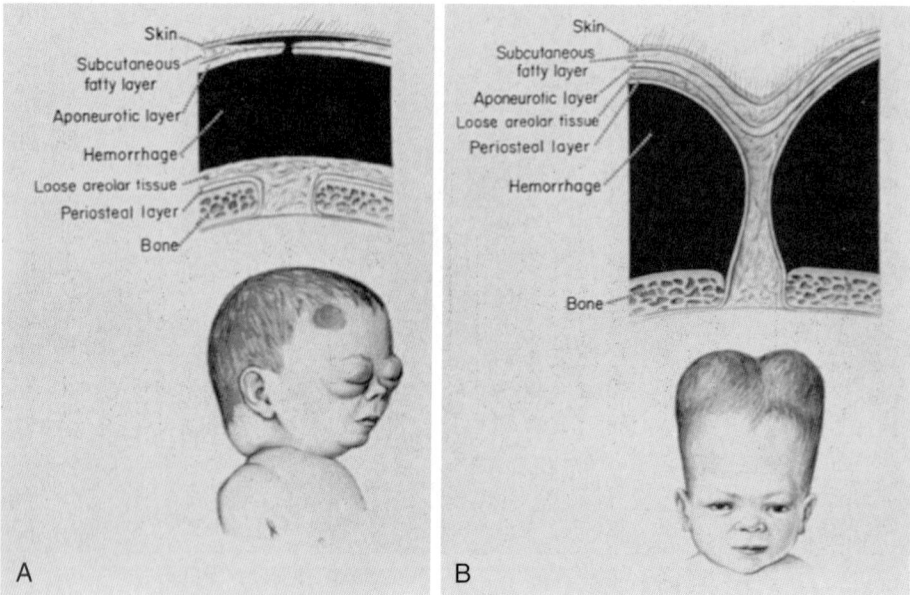

FIGURE 61-7 **A,** Location of edema and hemorrhage seen with a caput succedaneum. **B,** Location of hemorrhage seen with a cephalohematoma.

Cephalohematoma

Hemorrhage beneath the subperiosteum of the scalp leading to an elevation in usually the parietal region of the skull is called a cephalohematoma. It is distinguished from a caput as follows: it does not cross suture lines, it manifests as a firmer swelling that does not transilluminate, and it has a well-defined edge (Figure 61-7). Rarely, it is seen in the occipital region as a soft swelling that needs to be distinguished from an encephalocele. The incidence of cephalohematoma is estimated to be 1.5% to 2.5% of all deliveries. It is seen twice as frequently in male infants and presents bilaterally in 15% of patients. Linear fractures are seen in 5% of unilateral lesions and in 18% of bilateral lesions.

A cephalohematoma generally resolves over a period of 2 to 8 weeks. It often leaves behind a sharp palpable ridge due to calcium deposition. Resorption of the extravasated blood can lead to hyperbilirubinemia, and infants should be observed for jaundice. A severe bleed can lead to anemia. Infection of the mass with formation of an abscess and associated osteomyelitis can occur in rare cases. It should be suspected in the event of an enlarging mass manifesting with fever and laboratory results suggestive of an infection. A skull radiograph or a CT scan is indicated in cases in which a fracture is suspected. Hyperostosis and thickening of the parietal region, calcium deposition, or cystic defects within the hematoma may be seen on neuroimaging studies.

Skull Fractures

Several features of the skull of the newborn make it less likely to sustain fractures, even in the presence of considerable pressure during the process of birth. The presence of unossified sutures and decreased mineralization makes the neonatal skull less rigid and more amenable to temporary distortion. However, fractures do occur in deliveries, especially those associated with forceps or blunt abdominal trauma to the mother. Fractures can also occur simply

from pressure of the head against the sacral promontory during delivery from forceful uterine contractions.

Fractures may be linear or depressed and usually occur in the frontal or parietal region. Linear fractures are more common and, if nondisplaced, usually do not pose a problem and do not need treatment. They are seen as a linear region of decreased density on a skull radiograph. Some fractures can be associated with a leptomeningeal cyst when it occurs near suture lines ("growing fracture of the skull").

Depressed skull fractures associated with application of pressure over the parietal region are seen on the anteroposterior skull radiograph as a linear region of increased density. These may not be visualized on the lateral film. A depressed fracture can serve as a focus for seizure activity, and it is therefore recommended that the region be elevated by a surgical procedure.

Subdural Hemorrhage

The dura mater, the outer meningeal layer, lies immediately below the bony layer of the skull and contains several blood vessels. It also encloses the major sinuses between its two layers. Severe compression and stretching can lead to tears of the falx cerebri or the tentorium cerebelli, especially at the site at which the falx meets the tentorium. Risk factors include macrosomia, cephalopelvic disproportion, shoulder dystocia, forceps delivery, and premature delivery. Hemorrhage can occur by injury to the dural sinuses, the major cerebral veins, or the vein of Galen. Injury of the superficial cerebral veins leads to hemorrhage over the cerebrum. Injury to the straight sinus or the vein of Galen can cause extension of a subdural hemorrhage from the base of the brain into the posterior fossa. Damage to the sagittal sinus from overriding parietal bones, and damage to the occipital sinus in conditions leading to separation of the squamous from the lateral parts of the occipital bone, can be seen with breech presentation.

A subdural hemorrhage should be suspected in cases in which there is a history of trauma or a difficult delivery with development of focal cerebral signs such as unequal pupils, deviation of the eyes, or hemiparesis. Symptoms may present over a period of a few hours to days. Often the infant presents with nonspecific signs such as pallor, lethargy, irritability, and a decreased Moro response. A bulging anterior fontanel may be the sign of an acute bleed. Posterior fossa hemorrhages, which can be accompanied by cerebellar hemorrhages or IVH, may manifest later with opisthotonos, apnea and bradycardia, altered mental status, and seizures. Pressure on the fourth ventricle can lead to signs of increased intracranial pressure and apnea.

Ultrasonography is inadequate for demonstrating the presence of a subdural bleed. MRI is a more appropriate imaging study for this purpose and should be undertaken if the diagnosis is suspected.

No surgical treatment is recommended in asymptomatic cases. Evacuation of a posterior fossa bleed can sometimes be lifesaving, although surgical evacuation is not effective in the case of a large subdural hemorrhage. Close monitoring is necessary to detect signs of deterioration in neurologic status. Presence of increased intracranial pressure may require a subdural tap or placement of a subdural shunt.

Subarachnoid Hemorrhage

Subarachnoid hemorrhage occurs as a result of damage to veins traversing the subarachnoid space. This type of injury is fairly common and may manifest as seizures. Diagnosis is suspected when frank blood or blood-tinged fluid is obtained on lumbar puncture. No treatment is needed, because the condition usually resolves spontaneously.

Spinal Cord Injury

Spinal cord injury was first described in the 1800s and is a relatively rare event now because of improved obstetric practices. In a review of studies of cerebral palsy, spinal cord injury was noted to account for just 0.6% of injuries. It is most commonly associated with breech delivery and occurs secondary to either a lateral or longitudinal stretching force or torsion of the neck during delivery. It can also be seen in premature infants as a result of extension of an intracranial hemorrhage. Damage occurs to the cord, the covering meninges, nerve roots, and blood vessels.

The pathologic findings may include laceration of the cord, epidural hemorrhage, laceration of the dura with a subdural hemorrhage, and tears of the nerve roots, as well as focal hemorrhages within the cord.

Most patients with a severe spinal cord injury do not survive. The cervical and upper thoracic segments of the spine are most commonly affected. The condition should be suspected in any infant with a breech presentation who has poor muscle tone and flaccid weakness of the extremities. The presentation in many cases is that of spastic paraparesis with respiratory depression and hypotonia. There is often involvement of both the motor and the sensory systems. Urinary retention and abdominal distention with paradoxical respirations may be present. The neurologic examination is significant for an absence of sensation below the level of the injury. This can manifest as reduced skin temperature and decreased tendon reflexes in the acute phase, followed by the appearance of triple-flexion withdrawal movements.

The differential diagnosis includes neuromuscular disorders such as spinal muscular atrophy, congenital myasthenia gravis, and a tumor of the cervical or lumbar region of the cord. Spinal muscular atrophy is usually not associated with loss of sensation or bladder control. A tumor of the spinal cord is usually associated with midline skin abnormalities such as dimpling, hemangioma, or tufts of hair.

Treatment is usually supportive and may require intubation for respiratory support. No specific treatment is available. Most cases are severe and irreversible, although milder degrees of injury are potentially reversible.

Cranial Nerve Injury
Facial Nerve Injury

Facial nerve injury is the most common cranial nerve injury seen secondary to birth trauma. Contrary to common belief, forceps application is not associated with an increased incidence of facial nerve palsy. The site of injury and the precise timing of injury are controversial. The nerve is most commonly injured at the point where it emerges from the stylomastoid foramen, and the lesion is therefore similar to a lower motor neuron lesion. The signs and symptoms include difficulty in closing the eyelid on the affected side, loss of the normal nasolabial fold, and an asymmetrical crying facies. The forehead is spared, because it is innervated by the opposite facial nerve. The injury occurs as a result of compression of the nerve against the sacral promontory, especially in cases in which presentation of the fetal head leads to compression of the mandible and the neck against the shoulder. Usually, compression of the nerve occurs after it has exited the mastoid canal, although occasionally the portion within the mastoid can also be affected.

Nerve excitability or conduction tests are not usually recommended unless there is no improvement over 3 to 4 days. Most lesions begin to resolve after 1 week. Nerve excitability tests are usually helpful in distinguishing partial from complete denervation. In the case of partial injury, nerve stimulation can lead to some muscular contraction. However, the lack of response to nerve stimulation does not necessarily predict a poor outcome. A neurology consultation should be obtained in cases that do not show resolution within a few weeks. Methyl cellulose eye drops should be used on the affected side to prevent irritation from dryness of the conjunctiva. In severe cases, surgery may be necessary to repair a severed nerve.

Congenital Hypoplasia of the Depressor Anguli Oris Muscle

Congenital hypoplasia of the depressor anguli oris muscle is not due to perinatal trauma but is included here for differential diagnosis purposes. In affected infants, unilateral congenital absence of the depressor anguli oris muscle leads to an inability of contraction and eversion of the lower lip on the same side during crying episodes. The infant thus appears to have an asymmetrical face while crying. The condition becomes less prominent with age, as episodes of crying are reduced in the older child. This condition can occur as an isolated anomaly or be associated with other anomalies. In a review of data for 41 infants with the condition, 27 had associated genitourinary, respiratory, or cardiovascular abnormalities (Pape and Pickering, 1972). Congenital heart disease, especially a ventricular septal defect, is the most common associated anomaly.

Injury to Other Cranial Nerves

Injury of other cranial nerves secondary to birth trauma is rare. Transient ptosis may be seen as a result of damage to the oculomotor nerve. Unilateral as well as bilateral optic nerve atrophy has been reported to occur from orbital fracture.

Peripheral Nerve Injury
Brachial Plexus Injury

Injury to the brachial plexus usually results from the prolonged vaginal extraction of a macrosomic infant. Traction of the shoulder in a breech presentation as well as turning away of the head in a difficult vertex presentation leads to stretching of the plexus. In most cases, the condition is unilateral; it is located on the right twice as often as on the left. In the mildest cases, nerves C5 and C6 are affected, followed by additional nerves in more severe cases. The nerve is compressed within the nerve sheath from hemorrhage and edema. In severe cases, there may be avulsion of the nerve from the spinal cord. Improvement in obstetric care has resulted in a decrease in incidence of this condition.

Erb-Duchenne paralysis refers to the paralysis of the upper brachial plexus involving nerves C5 and C6. Weakness of the deltoid, biceps, brachioradialis, and supinator muscles leads to the classic clinical picture in which the infant holds the affected arm in a position of tight adduction and internal rotation of the shoulder along with extension and pronation of the elbow. Involvement of C7 can lead to a weakness of the extensors and exaggerated flexion of the wrist. The Moro reflex is asymmetrical and absent on the affected side, and the biceps reflex is weak or absent. The grasp reflex is usually present. The injury may be associated with a fracture of the clavicle or humerus, displacement of the radial head, or shoulder dislocation. Injury of C4 can lead to phrenic nerve paralysis, which manifests as rapid, shallow breathing and decreased movement of the diaphragm on the affected side.

Klumpke paralysis results from injury to the lower brachial plexus and accounts for 2.5% of cases of brachial plexus injury. It is associated with weakness of the flexor muscles of the wrist as well as the intrinsic muscles of the hand. The grasp reflex is absent, and there may be loss of sensation over the hand. Involvement of the cervical sympathetic nerves can lead to unilateral miosis (Horner syndrome). Complete paralysis of the arm is seen in cases in which the entire brachial plexus is damaged.

The diagnosis can be made on the basis of the history of difficult delivery, posture of the affected arm, and the loss of voluntary and reflex movements. Radiographic examination performed with fluoroscopy or ultrasonography can help make the diagnosis of phrenic nerve injury.

Radiographic studies can also detect any associated fractures or dislocations. Use of somatosensory evoked potentials may help to distinguish completed avulsion at the spinal cord from a more distal lesion. MRI also can be used to demonstrate root avulsion. The extent of denervation can be demonstrated by performing an EEG 2 to 3 weeks after the injury.

The treatment is mainly supportive and consists of physical therapy to avoid the development of contractures. The arm should be kept in a natural position and not be over-immobilized. Passive exercises should be started 1 week after birth. The timing of recovery is dependent on the extent of the lesion. In mild partial plexus injury and Erb-Duchenne injury, improvement is seen by 1 or 2 weeks after birth, and recovery is complete by 1 to 18 months. Prognosis is poorer in Klumpke paralysis and in cases of complete plexus damage. Recovery is rarely complete in these infants, and sequelae may include muscle atrophy and contractures. Return of neuromuscular function is not always associated with return of normal movements of the extremities due to early deprivation of sensorimotor function.

STRATEGIES FOR NEUROPROTECTION

Considerable advances have been made in recent years in elucidating the cellular and vascular mechanisms of hypoxic-ischemic brain injury. Anticipation and prevention of conditions that cause HIE constitute the best neuroprotective strategy. Many potential strategies have been studied in animal or adult models of disease. Extrapolating the effects of these studies to the human newborn is difficult because the mechanism of injury in experimental animal models is not necessarily similar to that in infants, and several features of the newborn developing brain make it uniquely more susceptible to injury than the adult brain. Therefore, these therapies must be tested in the neonatal population (Box 61-3).

Early identification of infants with a moderately severe insult is necessary in order to initiate appropriate therapy within the narrow therapeutic window, although it is difficult to assess the degree of encephalopathy initially. In addition to our lack of ability to select neonates for neuroprotective therapies, interruption of the injurious events by neuroprotective agents may also simultaneously affect normal developmental processes. Another important issue relates to the route and timing of intervention. Asphyxia in neonates is often associated with multiorgan dysfunction, which can affect the pharmacokinetics of drug therapies. Side effects of these agents can include hypotension and cardiac depression, exacerbating the initial injury by reducing cerebral perfusion pressure.

Several strategies for neuroprotection exert their effects at different stages of the cascade of events that is initiated after injury. These strategies include methods to reduce depletion of ATP stores, both in cases in which hypoxic-ischemic insult is predictable and in the early postinsult phase, to reduce membrane depolarization, to inhibit glutamate release, to inhibit accumulation of intracellular calcium, to block glutamate-responsive NMDA and AMPA receptors, to prevent release of degradative enzymes, to sequester free radicals, to use thrombolytic agents, and to

BOX 61-3   Possible Neuroprotective Strategies

Hypothermia
Glutamate receptor antagonists
    NMDA receptor antagonists
        Glutamate-binding site
        Glycine, phencyclidine, magnesium-binding sites
    AMPA receptor antagonists
Erythropoietin
GABA antagonists
Calcium channel blockers
Nitric oxide synthase inhibitors
Other free radical inhibitors
    Allopurinol
    Vitamin E
Metalloporphyrins
Deferoxamine
Growth factors
Caspase inhibitors

AMPA, Amino-3-hydroxy-5-methyl-4-isoxazole propionic acid; *GABA*, gamma-aminobutyric acid; *NMDA*, N-methyl-D-aspartate.

prevent the reperfusion injury by inhibition of xanthine oxidase. The following discussion examines some of these methods in more detail.

MAINTAINING ENERGY STORES

Prevention of depletion of cerebral energy stores is a strategy that can be utilized in cases in which injury is anticipated (e.g., cardiac surgery requiring placement of the infant on cardiopulmonary bypass). It is recommended that seizures and conditions that exacerbate energy depletion, such as hyperthermia, be avoided in cases of HI-R injury.

HYPOTHERMIA

Mild sustained hypothermia is one of the most exciting and viable neuroprotective strategies for limiting neonatal HI-R injury to emerge from the laboratory in recent years. Cerebral metabolism after the initial phase of energy failure during asphyxia may recover in a latent phase but then deteriorate in a secondary phase of brain injury 6 to 15 hours later. In studies in cell culture and in vivo models of focal and global cerebral ischemias in both adults and immature animals, hypothermia has been shown to have a neuroprotective effect (Coimbra and Wieloch, 1994; Colbourne and Corbett, 1994; Sirimanne et al, 1996). Experimental studies in animal models have shown that moderate hypothermia established within 30 minutes after the HI-R injury is neuroprotective (Edwards et al, 1995; Haaland et al, 1997; Thoresen et al, 1995, 1996; Tooley et al, 2003). These and other studies have shown that hypothermia inhibits early adverse events as well as later events such as secondary energy failure and apoptosis. Studies in fetal sheep have shown that prolonged cerebral cooling starting 5.5 hours but not 8.5 hours after cerebral ischemia may still be associated with neuronal rescue (Gunn et al, 1997).

The possible mechanisms by which hypothermia helps in neuroprotection are inhibition of glutamate release, decreased metabolism and energy conservation, decreased metabolic acidosis, decreased free radical generation, prevention of energy failure and apoptosis, and inhibition of effects of adhesion molecules at the microvascular level, thereby inhibiting the breakdown of the blood-brain barrier and reducing brain edema. Some studies indicate that hypothermia delays but does not prevent the cellular or vascular outcome of HIE. However, even delaying onset of damage can be helpful in prolonging the therapeutic window for other therapies to take effect.

Hypothermia was first reported in the therapy of infants after perinatal asphyxia in 1959, but these experiments did not have a group of control infants (Westin et al, 1959). The adverse consequences of hypothermia and the importance of maintaining infants in a normothermic environment are well known. Metabolic, cardiovascular, pulmonary, coagulation, and immunologic disturbances all have been reported with hypothermia, although the results of the trials demonstrate few complications. A prospective randomized trial conducted to identify the adverse effects of hypothermia showed that selective head cooling was safe, with minimal systemic toxicity (Gunn et al, 1998). Mild hypothermia in this study was induced by application of a water-cooled coil to the infant's head, thereby lowering the cranial temperature to 34.5° C for 72 hours within 2 to 5 hours after the injury. Rectal temperature was maintained up to 35.7° C. The results of this and other studies led to the initiation of several multicenter clinical trials for neuroprotective efficacy.

There have now been four large randomized trials of moderate hypothermia for HIE (Azzopardi et al, 2009; Eicher et al, 2005; Gluckman et al, 2005; Shankaran et al, 2005). Trials of both selective head cooling and whole-body cooling have demonstrated benefit in those with moderate encephalopathy. The therapeutic benefit on those with severe encephalopathy differs between the studies. In a metaanalysis of 8 trials, including 638 infants, hypothermia for moderate/severe neonatal encephalopathy in neonates with evidence of perinatal asphyxia resulted in a significant reduction in mortality or major neurodevelopmental disability to 18 months of age (relative risk [RR] 0.76, 95% CI 0.65, 0.89, number needed to treat [NNT] 7, 95% CI 4, 14) (Jacobs et al, 2007). Cooling also resulted in statistically significant reductions in mortality (typical RR 0.74, 95% CI 0.58, 0.94, NNT 11, 95% CI 6, 50) and in neurodevelopmental disability in survivors (typical RR 0.68; 95% CI 0.51, 0.92), typical RD –0.13, 95% CI –0.23, –0.03, NNT 8, 95% CI 4, 33). Given these findings and because there are currently no other effective therapeutic options, hypothermia is being implemented in many NICUs as a neuroprotective strategy for HIE (Jacobs et al, 2007).

PRECONDITIONING AND GROWTH FACTORS

The response of the neonatal brain to milder forms of injury can help us learn about mechanisms that the brain uses to protect itself from insults. Genes upregulated by stress, such as those that induce growth and differentiation, have been shown to be neuroprotective in animal models (Han and Holtzman, 2000). Animals treated with sublethal stress are protected from subsequent insults that would otherwise be deadly (Bergeron et al, 2000; Sheldon et al, 2007). Immature rats that are exposed to hypoxia have reduced brain injury following HI that occurs 24 hours after this preconditioning stimulus, with protection that persists 1 to 3 weeks later (Gidday et al, 1994; Vannucci et al, 1998). It is possible that injury may only be delayed, and protection may not be permanent; however, hypoxic preconditioning does provide long-lasting histological and functional protection for up to 8 weeks after neonatal rodent HI (Gustavsson et al, 2005).

Hypoxia-inducible factor 1α [HIF-1α] activation is a key modulator of the protection against subsequent HI injury that is induced by hypoxic preconditioning (Bergeron et al, 2000; Ran et al, 2005). HIF-1α is a neuronal transcription factor that stabilizes during hypoxia by binding to HIF-1β. Following stabilization, it produces a variety of downstream targets that are neuroprotective, including insulin-like growth factor-1 (IGF-1), vascular endothelial growth factor (VEGF), and erythropoietin (EPO).

EPO is a glycoprotein that was originally identified for its role in erythropoiesis. Functions include modulation of the inflammatory and immune responses (Villa et al, 2003), vasogenic and proangiogenic effects through its interaction with VEGF (Chong et al, 2002; Wang et al, 2004b), as well as effects on CNS development and repair. EPO and EPO receptor are expressed by a variety of different cell types in the CNS with changing patterns during development (Juul et al, 1999). EPO plays a key role in neural differentiation and neurogenesis early in development, promoting neurogenesis in vitro and in vivo (Shingo et al, 2001).

Postinjury treatment protocols with exogenously administered EPO has a protective effect in a variety of different models of brain injury in newborn rodents with both short- and long-term histological and behavioral improvement (Sola et al, 2005b). A single dose of EPO given immediately after neonatal hypoxic-ischemic injury in rats significantly reduces infarct volume and improves long-term spatial memory (Kumral et al, 2004). Single- and multiple-dose treatment regimens of EPO following neonatal focal ischemic stroke in rats reduce infarct volume (Sola et al, 2005a) and improve both short-term sensorimotor (Chang et al, 2005) and long-term cognitive (Gonzalez et al, 2009) outcomes, but there may be more long-lasting behavioral benefit in female rats (Wen et al, 2006). EPO treatment initiated 24 hours after neonatal HI also decreases brain injury (Sun et al, 2005). In addition, EPO enhances neurogenesis and directs multipotential neural stem cells toward a neuronal cell fate (Gonzalez et al, 2007; Shingo et al, 2001; Wang et al, 2004b). Following transient ischemic stroke, there is a temporary precursor cell proliferation in the rodent subventricular zone (SVZ), a source of endogenous precursor cells throughout the life of the rodent, with this precursor cell proliferation and differentiation favoring gliogenesis (Plane et al, 2004). EPO has been shown to enhance neurogenesis in vivo in the SVZ after stroke in the adult rat (Wang et al, 2004b). Neurogenesis has also been demonstrated following EPO treatment with an increase in newly generated cells from precursors, and possibly also an effect on cell fate commitment in vitro (Lu et al, 2005; Osredkar et al, 2010; Shingo et al, 2001; Wang et al, 2004b).

In humans, EPO is safely used for treatment of anemia in premature infants (Aher and Ohlsson, 2006).

EPO for neuroprotection is given in much higher doses (1000–5000 U/kg/dose) than for anemia to enable crossing of the blood-brain barrier with unknown pharmacokinetics in humans (Chang et al, 2005; Demers et al, 2005; McPherson and Juul, 2007). Recently, ELBW infants tolerated doses between 500 and 2500 U/kg/dose (Juul et al, 2008), and studies are ongoing. There has been one trial of EPO following neonatal HI, showing promising results. Repeated low-dose EPO over the first 2 weeks of life resulted in a reduction in death or moderate/severe disability at 18 months of age (Zhu et al, 2009). Further studies evaluating the safety, optimal dosage, and use in conjunction with hypothermia therapy are needed before implementation. A multicenter safety and pharmacokinetics trial is currently underway.

VEGF is a regulator of angiogenesis and is also involved in neuronal cell proliferation and migration (Zachary, 2005). The endothelial microenvironment establishes a vascular niche that promotes survival and proliferation of progenitor cells, which is tightly coordinated with angiogenesis (Palmer et al, 2000). VEGF-A is the most important member of a family of growth factors and is expressed in cortical neurons during early development, switching to mature glial cells near vessels during maturation. After exposure to hypoxia, there is increased neuronal and glial expression of VEGF-A, directing vascularization and stimulating proliferation of neuronal and nonneuronal cell types (Forstreuter et al, 2002; Jin et al, 2002; Krum and Rosenstein, 1998; Mu et al, 2003). VEGF also has chemotactic effects on neurogenic zones in the brain, increasing migration of stem cells during anoxia (Bagnard et al, 2001; Maurer et al, 2003; Yang and Cepko, 1996). VEGF-knockout mice have severe impairments in vascularization, neuronal migration, and survival (Raab et al, 2004).

Timing of VEGF administrations is important. In adult ischemia models, intravenous VEGF administered 1 hour after insult increases blood-brain barrier leakage and lesion size, but late administration 48 hours after ischemia enhances angiogenesis and functional performance (Zhang et al, 2000). Both topical and intracerebroventricular injection reduced infarct volume, and benefit has been shown in neurodegenerative and traumatic models of injury as well (Harrigan et al, 2003; Hayashi et al, 1998). VEGF overexpression confers direct neuroprotection resulting from inhibition of apoptotic pathways (Zachary, 2005).

Other factors have also shown promise, but given their role in normal neurodevelopment, the effects of treatment are not known. IGF-1 is important for growth and maturation of the fetal brain, as well as differentiation of oligodendrocyte precursors (D'Ercole et al, 1996). IGF-1 has prosurvival properties that can prevent perinatal hypoxic and excitotoxic injury, and it is also effective after intranasal administration (Johnston et al, 1996; Pang et al, 2007; Lin et al, 2009). Brain-derived neurotrophic factor is a neurotrophin that also provides neuroprotection in neonatal HI (Cheng et al, 1997; Cheng et al, 1998; Holtzman et al, 1996; Husson et al, 2005). It prevents spatial learning and memory impairments after injury, but its effectiveness is limited by the stage of development (Husson et al, 2005; Cheng et al, 1998). Although protective in mice when given on postnatal day 5 (P5), it has no effect at later time points and actually exacerbates excitotoxicity if given on the day of birth (Husson et al, 2005).

ANTIOXIDANTS

Antioxidant defenses such as superoxide dismutase, glutathione peroxidase, catalase, and compounds such as vitamins A, C, and E, as well as beta-carotene, glutathione, and ubiquinones scavenge free radicals (FRs) under normal conditions. Damage occurs when there is an imbalance between their generation and uptake (Fridovich, 1997). Following HI, there is an increase in superoxide and hydroxyl radical production and rapid depletion of antioxidant stores, which leads to cell membrane damage, excitotoxic energy depletion, cytosolic calcium accumulation, and activation of proapoptotic genes that cause damage to cellular components and result in cell death (Taylor et al, 1999).

In an effort to reduce oxidative damage to the neonate, a number of strategies have been employed including reactive oxygen species (ROS) scavengers, lipid peroxidation inhibitors, FR reducers, and nitric oxide synthase (NOS) inhibitors. NOS catalyzes the synthesis of NO from the conversion of arginine to citrulline (Boucher et al, 1999). NO plays an important role in pulmonary, systemic, and cerebral vasodilation and is constitutively produced in response to increased intracellular calcium by endothelial nitric oxide synthase (eNOS) in endothelial cells and by neuronal nitric oxide synthase (nNOS) in astrocytes and neurons. An inducible isoform of nitric oxide synthase (iNOS) also produces NO in response to cellular stress, which initiates neuronal damage when converted to secondary reactive nitrogen species that facilitate nitration and nitrosylation reactions (Beckman and Koppenol, 1996). Early endothelial NO is protective by maintaining blood flow, but early neuronal NO and late inducible NO promote cell death (Iadecola et al, 1997). Selective inhibition of nNOS or iNOS has shown potential as a neuroprotective strategy (van den Tweel et al, 2005). Regions expressing nNOS correspond to those that are susceptible to excitotoxicity, expressing NMDA receptors in vivo and in vitro (Black et al, 1995; Dawson et al, 1993; Ferriero et al, 1996). Destruction of neurons containing nNOS or targeted disruption of the nNOS gene protects animals from HI injury (Ferriero et al, 1995, 1996), but nonspecific blockade of nNOS and eNOS is not protective (Marks et al, 1996). There have been few studies in human newborns examining cerebral NO production. CSF NO levels increase with severity of HIE at 24 to 72 hours after asphyxia (Ergenekon et al, 1999), with increased NO and nitrotyrosine levels in the spinal cord as well (Groenendaal et al, 2008). Initial results in premature infants treated with inhaled NO for prevention of bronchopulmonary dysplasia show reductions in ultrasound diagnosed brain injury and improvements in neurodevelopmental outcomes at 2 years of age, but long-term results are still pending (Ballard et al, 2006; Schreiber et al, 2003).

Other antioxidant strategies that either block FR production or increase antioxidant defenses include melatonin, allopurinol, and deferoxamine. Melatonin is an indoleamine that is formed in higher quantities in adults and functions as a direct scavenger of ROS and NO. It has been found to provide long-lasting neuroprotection in experimental HI and focal cerebral ischemic injury, and human neonates treated with melatonin were also found to have decreased proinflammatory cytokines (Carloni et al, 2008; Gitto et al, 2004, 2005; Koh, 2008). Allopurinol has mixed effects that have shown promise in animal and human studies. Xanthine oxidase–derived superoxide and H_2O_2 react with NO to form damaging reactive nitrogen species. Allopurinol reduces FR production by inhibiting xanthine oxidase while also scavenging hydroxyl radicals. High-dose allopurinol given 15 minutes after HI in P7 rats decreases acute edema and long-term infarct volume (Palmer et al, 1993). Short-term benefits have also been seen in neonates undergoing cardiac surgery for hypoplastic left heart syndrome (Clancy et al, 2001). Early allopurinol in asphyxiated infants improved short-term neurodevelopmental outcomes and decreased serum NO levels after administration; however, there may only be a brief window for benefit, because no improvement in long-term outcomes was seen with later treatment after birth asphyxia (Benders et al, 2006). Deferoxamine (DFO) is an iron chelator that decreases FR production by binding with iron and decreasing the production of OH^- that occurs via the Fenton reaction, while also stabilizing HIF-1α to produce its downstream products VEGF and EPO (Hamrick et al, 2005; Mu et al, 2005). DFO is protective during exposure to H_2O_2 or excitotoxicity in vitro, and in animal models of HI and transient ischemic stroke in vivo (Almli et al, 2001; Mu et al, 2005; Palmer et al, 1994; Sarco et al, 2000). N-Acetylcysteine (NAC) is a glutathione precursor and FR scavenger that attenuates lipopolysaccharide-induced white matter injury in newborn rats (Aruoma et al, 1989; Paintlia et al, 2004), but results for other antioxidant compounds, such as vitamin E, have been inconclusive (Brion et al, 2003).

ANTIEXCITOTOXICITY

There has long been a search for agents that decrease brain injury by decreasing excitotoxicity. Dizocilpine (MK801) is a noncompetitive NMDA receptor antagonist that has been studied in humans, but is poorly tolerated and has also been shown to increase apoptosis and decrease neuronal migration in animal models (Ikonomidou and Turski, 2002). Memantine is a low-affinity noncompetitive NMDA receptor antagonist that is well tolerated in adults for Alzheimer's-type dementia (Chen and Lipton, 2006). Post-HI treatment with memantine attenuates acute white matter injury in P6 rats, resulting in long-term histological improvement in vivo and restoring neuronal migration in vitro (Chen et al, 1998; Manning et al, 2008; Volbracht et al, 2006). Another method to decrease excitotoxicity is the use of topiramate, an AMPA-kainate receptor antagonist that is an FDA-approved antiepileptic for patients more than 2 years of age. It has been shown to protect newborn rodents from excitotoxic brain lesions, reducing brain damage and cognitive impairment when administered within 2 hours of the insult (Noh et al, 2006; Sfaello et al, 2005). An intravenous preparation of topiramate does not yet exist for human use, but this treatment shows potential as a therapy for early newborn seizure and injury.

Magnesium sulfate has shown some benefit in preventing white matter damage in animal models, and one possible mechanism of its neuroprotection is the blockade of NMDA receptors (Khashaba et al, 2006; Marret et al, 1995; Spandou et al, 2007; Turkyilmaz et al, 2002). In a multicenter clinical trial of mothers treated with magnesium who were at risk for preterm delivery, no perinatal side effects were seen, and there was some benefit for the neurodevelopment of survivors (Crowther et al, 2003). However, magnesium administered to asphyxiated term neonates did not result in improvements in aEEG patterns and when given in larger doses was associated with profound hypotension (Groenendaal et al, 2002; Levene et al, 1995).

ANTI-INFLAMMATORY THERAPY

Maternal infection is a known risk factor for white matter damage and poor outcomes, such as cerebral palsy (Dammann et al, 2002; Wu et al, 2003a; Wu and Colford, 2000). The inflammatory response and cytokine production that accompanies infection may play a large role in cell damage and loss (Stirling et al, 2005). Local microglia is activated early and produces proinflammatory cytokines such as TNF-α, IL-1β, and IL-6, as well as glutamate, FRs, and NO. Systemic administration of these cytokines increases excitotoxic lesions (Dommergues et al, 2000), whereas therapies that block microglial activation and cytokine release protect the brain from excitotoxic damage (Dommergues et al, 2003).

Minocycline crosses the blood-brain barrier and has anti-inflammatory effects, including decreasing microglial activation and caspase-3 expression (Chen et al, 2000; Zhu et al, 2002), lipid peroxidation (Pruzanski et al, 1992), and other proinflammatory activity (Machado et al, 2006) while increasing antiapoptotic gene expression (Scarabelli et al, 2004; Wang et al, 2004a). It has shown promise in a number of animal models of neurodegenerative or ischemic disease (Chen et al, 2000; Choi et al, 2007; Du et al, 2001; Popovic et al, 2002; Yrjanheikki et al, 1999). In the neonatal brain, it appears to decrease tissue damage and caspase-3 activation in rodents when given immediately before or after injury, but results are inconsistent (Arvin et al, 2002; Cai et al, 2006; Fox et al, 2005). Low- and high-dose regimens are effective in reducing short-term HI-induced inflammation, protecting developing oligodendrocytes (Cai et al, 2006) and myelin content in neonatal rats (Carty et al, 2008), but this effect was only transient in another study of neonatal rodent stroke (Fox et al, 2005). Delayed therapy has been found to decrease TNF-α and matrix metalloproteinase MMP-12, but efficacy was lost when treatment was extended for a week after stroke (Wasserman et al, 2007). These effects also appear to be species dependent, with an increase in injury in developing C57B1/6 mice (Tsuji et al, 2004).

CELL DEATH INHIBITORS

Although necrosis plays a major role in early neuronal death following injury (Northington et al, 2001b), there is a spectrum of cell death that includes apoptosis (Portera-Cailliau et al, 1997) that may result in heterogeneous responses to antiapoptotic therapies (Northington et al, 2005). It is also probable that apoptosis and cleavage and activation of caspase-3 are responsible for more of the cell death that occurs in delayed phases of injury and neurodegeneration (Hu et al, 2000).

Specific and nonspecific inhibition of caspases or cysteine proteases has been attempted with some success (Blomgren et al, 2001; Feng et al, 2003; Han et al, 2002; Ostwald et al, 1993). For example, calpain or caspase-3 inhibitors such as MDL 28710 and M826 protect neonatal rats after HI (Han et al, 2002; Kawamura et al, 2005). Pretreatment with the hormone 17β-estradiol is neuroprotective in immature rats and appears to work through both antiapoptotic and FR-scavenging pathways (Nunez et al, 2007). In addition, the nuclear enzyme poly(ADP-ribose) polymerase (PARP) is activated during stress and enables DNA repair; however, the PARP-1 isoform also contributes to ischemic neuronal injury by depleting energy stores and activating microglia, leading to cell death. PARP-1 is more abundant in the immature brain, and its blockade protects against excitotoxicity and ischemic injury (Hagberg et al, 2004). The PARP-1 inhibitor 3-aminobenzamide reduces injury after focal ischemia in P7 rats (Ducrocq et al, 2000), but PARP-1 blockade appears to preferentially protect males (Hagberg et al, 2004).

STEM CELL THERAPY

Neural stem cells (NSCs) are multipotent precursors that self-renew and retain the ability to differentiate into a variety of neuronal and nonneuronal cell types in the CNS. They reside in neurogenic zones throughout life, such as the SVZ and the dentate gyrus of the hippocampus. In rodents, NSC transplantation has shown potential as a therapeutic strategy in adult animal models of brain injury. Implanted cells integrate into injured tissue (Park et al, 2002), decreasing volume loss and improving behavioral outcomes (Capone et al, 2007; Hicks et al, 2007; Hoehn et al, 2002; Park et al, 2006a, 2006b). In neonatal models, intraventricular implantation of NSCs after HI results in their migration to injured areas (Park et al, 2006a,b) and differentiation into neurons, astrocytes, oligodendrocytes, and undifferentiated progenitors. These cells promote regeneration, angiogenesis, and neuronal cell survival in both rodent and primate models, and nonneuronal progeny inhibit inflammation and scar formation (Imitola et al, 2004; Mueller et al, 2006). Although complications of implantation have not been noted in these models, efficacy does depend on time of implantation, and the therapeutic window is not known. More recent technology enables labeling of stem cells, which can then be tracked from the site of implantation through their migratory path into the ischemic tissue, making their identification and eventual outcome in humans feasible (Guzman et al, 2007; Modo et al, 2004; Rice et al, 2007).

COMBINATION THERAPY

Therapeutic hypothermia has become common practice in many institutions since showing benefit in moderately to severely encephalopathic newborns; however, it does not completely protect or repair an injured brain, so the search for adjuvant therapies continues. Combinatorial therapy may provide more long-lasting neuroprotection, salvaging the brain from severe injury and deficits while also enhancing repair and regeneration, possibly providing additive, if not synergistic, protection.

Xenon is approved for use as a general anesthetic in Europe and has shown promise as a protective agent. It is an NMDA antagonist, preventing progression of excitotoxic damage. It appears to be superior to other NMDA antagonists, possibly through inhibition of AMPA and kainate receptors, reduction of neurotransmitter release, or effects on other ion channels (Dinse et al, 2005; Gruss et al, 2004; Ma and Zhang, 2003). In rats, combination xenon and hypothermia initiated 4 hours after neonatal HI provided synergistic histologic and functional protection when evaluated at 30 days after injury (Ma et al, 2005). Hypothermia does reduce glutamate and glycine release (Busto et al, 1989), and NMDA receptor antagonism may explain these effects. More recently, an additive effect was shown after HI in P7 rats that were cooled to 32°C and received 50% xenon, with improvement in long-term histology and functional performance that exceeded the individual benefit of either (Hobbs et al, 2008). More extensive studies on xenon use in human neonates are necessary.

As mentioned earlier, NAC is a medication approved for neonates that is a scavenger of oxygen radicals and restores intracellular glutathione levels, attenuating reperfusion injury and decreasing inflammation and NO production in adult models of stroke (Khan et al, 2004; Sekhon et al, 2003). Adding NAC therapy to systemic hypothermia reduced brain volume loss at both 2 and 4 weeks after neonatal rodent HI, with increased myelin expression and improved reflexes (Jatana et al, 2006). Inhibition of inflammation with MK-801 has also been effective when combined with hypothermia in neonatal rats post HI injury (Alkan et al, 2001). In P7 rats that underwent HI followed by early topiramate and delayed hypothermia, improved short-term histology and function was seen (Liu et al, 2004). This may provide a window for protection if hypothermia is delayed, which is possible given difficulty in initiation of cooling if infants are born at an outside hospital or transport is delayed.

SUMMARY

There continues to be an explosion of information regarding the pathophysiology and possible therapy of ischemic and traumatic injuries to the developing nervous system. The realization that the immature brain exhibits different pathogenetic mechanisms in response to these insults has led investigators to think differently about designing therapies for the immature brain. With continued investigations regarding the mechanisms of cell death in the immature brain, the development of age-appropriate neuroprotective strategies is not far behind.

SUGGESTED READINGS

Back SA, Riddle A, McClure MM: Maturation-dependent vulnerability of perinatal white matter in premature birth, *Stroke* 38(2 Suppl):724-730, 2007.
Barkovich AJ, Miller SP, Bartha A, et al: MR imaging, MR spectroscopy, and diffusion tensor imaging of sequential studies in neonates with encephalopathy, *AJNR Am J Neuroradiol* 27:533-547, 2006.
Hellstrom-Westas L, Rosen I, Svenningsen NW: Predictive value of early continuous amplitude integrated EEG recordings on outcome after severe birth asphyxia in full term infants,, *Arch Dis Child Fetal Neonatal Ed* 72:F34-38, 1995.
Jacobs S, Hunt R, Tarnow-Mordi W, et al: Cooling for newborns with hypoxic ischaemic encephalopathy. *Cochrane Database Syst Rev* (4)CD003311, 2007.
Miller SP, Ferriero DM, Leonard C, et al: Early brain injury in premature newborns detected with MRI: relationship with early neurodevelopmental outcome, *J Pediatr* 147:609-616, 2005.
Papile LA, Burstein J, Burstein R, Koffler H: Incidence and evolution of subependymal and intraventricular hemorrhage: a study of infants with birth weights less than 1,500 gm, *J Pediatr* 92:529-534, 1978.
Rutherford M, Ramenghi LA, Edwards AD, et al: Assessment of brain tissue injury after moderate hypothermia in neonates with hypoxic-ischaemic encephalopathy: a nested substudy of a randomised controlled trial, *Lancet Neurol* 9:39-45, 2010.
Sarnat HB, Sarnat MS: Neonatal encephalopathy following fetal distress. A clinical and electroencephalographic study, *Arch Neurol* 33:696-705, 1976.
Tooley JR, Satas S, Porter H: Head cooling with mild systemic hypothermia in anesthetized piglets is neuroprotective, *Ann Neurol* 53:65-72, 2003.
van Rooij LG, Toet MC, van Huffelen AC, et al: Effect of treatment of subclinical neonatal seizures detected with aEEG: randomized, controlled trial, *Pediatrics* 125:e358-e366, 2010.
Volpe JJ: Brain injury in premature infants: a complex amalgam of destructive and developmental disturbances, *Lancet Neurol* 8:110-124, 2009.
Woodward LJ, Anderson PJ, Austin NC, et al: Neonatal MRI to predict neurodevelopmental outcomes in preterm infants, *N Engl J Med* 355:685-694, 2006.

Complete references used in this text can be found online at www.expertconsult.com

NEONATAL NEUROMUSCULAR DISORDERS

Eugenio Mercuri and Marika Pane

In the past two decades, more than 200 loci responsible for neuromuscular disorders have been identified. This has resulted in new approaches to their classification and in a better definition of phenotype-genotype correlations and of the clinical and histopathologic features for each form. Although by definition all of the genetically inherited disorders should be considered congenital, in clinical practice the term *congenital* is generally applied to the forms with overt clinical signs in the neonatal period or in the first months after birth. These include disorders with primary muscle involvement, such as congenital myopathies and muscular dystrophies, motoneuron disorders, and disorders of the neuromuscular junction, such as neonatal myasthenia.

This chapter reviews the current state of knowledge of the neuromuscular disorders with neonatal onset, providing clinical, pathologic, and, when appropriate, radiologic details for each form. The final part of the chapter summarizes the steps in the diagnostic evaluation of hypotonic neonates in whom a neuromuscular disorder is suspected.

PRIMARY MUSCLE DISORDERS

There are a number of primary muscle disorders with early neonatal onset. These can be broadly subdivided into two groups: muscular dystrophies and congenital myopathies. Congenital muscular dystrophies (CMDs) and congenital myotonic dystrophy are the most common forms of dystrophies with neonatal onset, whereas other dystrophies that are overall more frequent in the pediatric population are, with a few exceptions, generally not clinically symptomatic in the first year. Whereas muscular dystrophies share severe disruption, with a typical "dystrophic pattern" on muscle biopsy, congenital myopathies generally have better preservation of the architecture of muscle fibers and less severe changes such as fiber type dysproportion.

In the past several years there has been increasing evidence that each of these two groups has a quite wide genetic heterogeneity. Although until recently their classification has been based mainly on histopathologic findings, after the recent discoveries of the underlying gene defects, the most recent classifications take into account and combine both histopathologic and genetic findings.

MUSCULAR DYSTROPHIES

Congenital Muscular Dystrophies

Congenital muscular dystrophies represent a heterogeneous group of disorders sharing some features, namely dystrophic changes on muscle biopsy and neonatal or early onset of weakness and often contractures (Dubowitz, 1994). Until recently, classification of CMD was based primarily on the presence or absence of merosin, an extracellular matrix protein found to be missing in approximately

35% to 45% of cases of CMD (Dubowitz, 1994; Tome et al, 1995) or on the presence of associated structural brain abnormalities (Dubowitz, 1994; Mercuri et al, 2001; Muntoni et al, 2002, 2004). In the past few years, the identification of several genes responsible for distinct clinical entities has helped to better classify these forms and to better understand the mechanisms underlying the different disorders.

We now recognize nine forms of CMD for which the genetic defect is known. Several additional forms will likely be discovered, based on their unique clinical and immunohistopathologic features. Table 62-1 shows the classification of the currently identified CMD forms. A comprehensive review of all the CMD forms is beyond the scope of this chapter and we will therefore describe the forms associated with alpha-dystroglycan (α-DG) deficiency and those with merosin deficiency that are the most commonly observed.

Alpha-Dystroglycanopathies

The major contribution to the new classification comes from the identification of a family of genes directly involved in the glycosylation of α-DG. Six of the nine genes identified so far are involved in this process and the forms of muscular dystrophies associated with them are collectively designated as alpha-dystroglycanopathies. These are a clinically and genetically heterogeneous group of autosomal recessive muscular dystrophies with variable neurologic and ophthalmic involvement sharing the common feature of hypoglycosylation of α-DG on skeletal muscle biopsy (Muntoni et al, 2002). To date, mutations in six known or putative glycosyltranferase genes have been identified in these disorders (Beltran-Valero de Bernabe et al, 2002; Brockington et al, 2001a; Kobayashi et al, 1998; Longman et al, 2003; van Reeuwijk et al, 2005a, 2005b; Yoshida et al, 2001).

1. Protein-O-mannosyl transferase 1 (*POMT1*; OMIM 607423)
2. Protein-O-mannosyl transferase 2 (*POMT2*; OMIM 607439)
3. Protein-O-mannose 1,2-N-acetylglucosaminyltransferase 1 (*POMGnT1*; OMIM 606822)
4. Fukutin (OMIM 607440)
5. Fukutin-related protein (*FKRP*; OMIM 606596)
6. LARGE (OMIM 603590)

The phenotypic severity of these forms is extremely variable. At the most severe end of the clinical spectrum are disorders characterized by CMD with severe structural brain and eye abnormalities including Walker-Warburg syndrome (WWS), muscle-eye-brain (MEB) disease, and Fukuyama congenital muscular dystrophy (FCMD). Individuals at the mildest end of the clinical spectrum may present in adult life with limb-girdle muscular dystrophies, with no associated brain or eye involvement (Brockington et al, 2001b).

Recent studies on large populations of patients have reported that known mutations can be detected in only about half the patients with clinical signs suggestive of an alpha-dystroglycanopathy, suggesting that other still-unknown genes are involved (Geodfrey et al, 2007; Mercuri et al, 2009).

As a group, patients with these forms of CMD often have relative hypertrophy of the lower limbs and wasting of the upper limbs and often have structural brain involvement. After the genes were identified, it was initially thought that each gene could be associated with distinct clinical entities, but it is now increasingly obvious that each of the six genes associated with α-DG deficiency may give rise to different phenotypes and, conversely, that each phenotype can be associated with mutations in any of the six genes (Clements et al, 2008; Mercuri et al, 2006, 2009).

We now describe the three forms that have been classically associated with specific structural brain and eye abnormalities (WWS, MEB, FCMD), but other patterns of brain involvement have also been identified (Clements et al, 2008).

Walker-Warburg Syndrome

Walker-Warburg Syndrome (WWS) is the most severe of the congenital muscular dystrophies with central nervous system (CNS) involvement. Severe weakness and neonatal hypotonia, associated with clinical signs of CNS involvement such as poor visual attention and decreased alertness, are invariably present (Dobyns et al, 1989). Ocular abnormalities, such as retinal dysgenesis, microphthalmia, and anterior chamber malformations, are also consistent findings.

Brain magnetic resonance imaging (MRI) (Figure 62-1) shows a type II lissencephaly with the typical micropolygyric cobblestone cortex; the white matter is also severely abnormal, showing dysmyelination or cystic changes (Dobyns et al, 1989). Cerebellar and brainstem hypoplasia is also always present.

Affected infants are often thought have an isolated CNS malformation until a markedly elevated serum creatine kinase (CK) suggests the presence of skeletal muscle involvement as well. The congenital muscular dystrophy diagnosis is then confirmed by pathologic studies.

Initially associated with mutations in the *POMT1* gene (Beltran Valero et al, 2002), the Walker-Warburg phenotype has now been associated with mutations in five of the α-DG genes (Clements et al, 2008; Geodfrey et al, 2007; Mercuri et al, 2006).

Muscle-Eye-Brain Disease

Clinical signs are usually present at birth or in the first months of life with hypotonia and weakness often associated with ocular abnormalities that may be milder than in WWS and may become evident only after the first years of life (Santavuori et al, 1989). Brain MRI shows extensive abnormalities of neuronal migration, such as pachygyria and polymicrogyria and often brainstem and cerebellar hypoplasia and periventricular white matter changes. Initially associated with mutations in the POMGnT1 gene (Yoshida et al, 2001), the muscle-eye-brain (MEB) phenotype has also been associated

TABLE 62-1 Congenital Muscular Dystrophy (CMD) Forms With Known Genetic Defects

Chromosome Locus	Gene	Protein Defect	Disease Phenotype(s)
6q22-23	*LAMA2*	Laminin α2	Primary merosin deficiency (MDC1A)
21q22.3 2q37	*COL6A1, A2 COL6A3*	Collagen VI	Ullrich CMD
12q13	*ITGA7*	Integrin α7	Integrin α7-related CMD
9q31	*FCMD*	Fukutin	Fukuyama CMD Walker-Warburg syndrome
1q32-34	*POMGnT1*	Protein-*O*-mannose β1,2 *N*-acetylglucosaminyltransferase1	Muscle-eye-brain disease Walker-Warburg syndrome
9q34.1	*POMT1*	Protein-*O*-mannosyltransferase 1	CMD with distinct CNS abnormalities Other phenotypes
14q24.3	*POMT2*	Protein-*O*-mannosyltransferase 2	
1q42	—	Presumed glycosyltransferase	
19q13.3	*FKRP*	Fukutin-related protein FKRP	
22q12.3-13.1	*LARGE*	LARGE	
1p35-36	*SEPN1*	Selenoprotein N	CMD with spinal rigidity (RSMD1)
4p16.3	Unknown	Unknown	Merosin-positive CMD

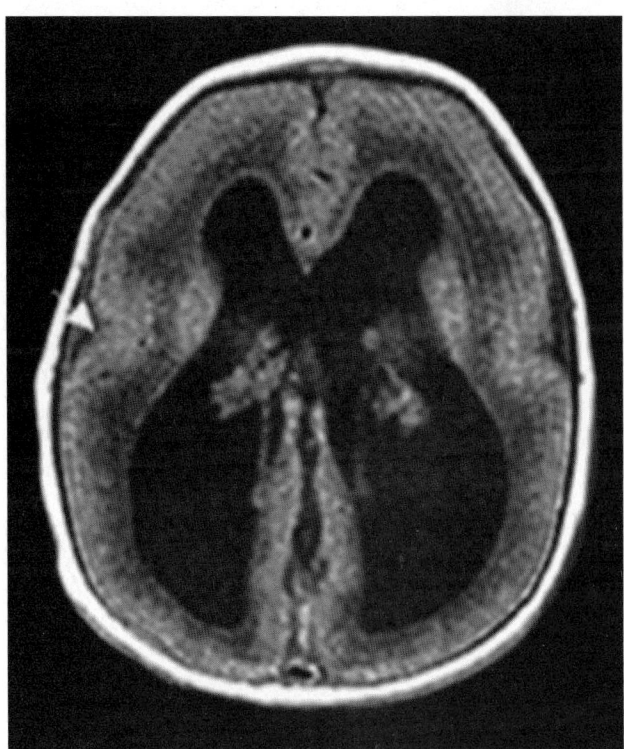

FIGURE 62-1 Brain magnetic resonance imaging showing lissencephaly in Walker-Warburg syndrome.

with mutations in all five of the other α-DG genes (Clements et al, 2008; Geodfrey et al, 2007; Mercuri et al, 2006).

Fukuyama Congenital Muscular Dystrophy

Fukuyama congenital muscular dystrophy (FCMO) is very rare outside of Japan. Clinical features include mild to moderate hypotonia at birth and progressive deterioration with increasing weakness, joint contractures, high CK levels, moderate to severe mental retardation, and frequent association with epilepsy. Ocular abnormalities occur in approximately 70% of these children but are rarely severe. Brain MRI shows structural changes consisting of pachygyria and polymicrogyria and low-density white matter areas. The gene responsible for FCMD is another glycosyltransferase named fukutin (Osawa et al, 1997).

Other Forms of Alpha-Dystroglycanopathies

Some patients with alpha-dystroglycanopathies may have cerebellar hypoplasia or dysplasia that can be present in isolation (Topaloglu et al, 2003) or associated with more diffuse structural brain changes (Clements et al, 2008; Mercuri et al, 2006).

As a rule of thumb, whenever an infant has structural brain abnormalities, especially if associated with eye abnormalities and clinical signs of weakness, it is useful to obtain serum CK levels. With very few exceptions, all reported cases have increased serum CK levels (>5 times the normal levels).

Merosin-Deficient Congenital Muscular Dystrophy

Merosin-deficient congenital muscular dystrophy, classified as MDC1A, is an autosomal recessive form due to mutations in the *LAMA2* gene on chromosome 6, encoding merosin (laminin a2), an extracellular matrix protein (Tome et al, 1994).

Children with merosin deficiency are usually symptomatic at birth or in the first few weeks of life with hypotonia and muscle weakness, weak cry and, in 10–30% of cases, contractures. Weakness often affects upper limbs more than lower limbs. These infants may present with feeding and respiratory problems, although these tend to resolve in the first months. Serum CK levels in these children are always grossly elevated (10 times the normal values). There is severe motor delay, and children never acquire independent ambulation (Philpot et al, 1995).

Brain MRI (Figure 62-2) shows diffuse white matter changes that are a typical feature of merosin-deficient CMD (Philpot et al, 1995). However, these changes become evident only at about 6 months of age. These findings are not obvious on conventional MRI scans performed in the first months of life (Mercuri et al, 1996), though they can be suspected with use of more sensitive T2-weighted images (Mercuri et al, 2000).

Some studies have demonstrated that other patterns of brain lesions, such as cerebellar hypoplasia and/or cortical dysplasia (Sunada et al, 1995), can be observed in approximately 10% of children with merosin-deficient congenital muscular dystrophy.

Congenital Myotonic Dystrophy

The neonatal form of myotonic muscular dystrophy differs from the adult form both clinically and pathologically. Infants with congenital myotonic dystrophy are often born after a pregnancy complicated by polyhydramnios and reduced fetal movements. At birth, clinical signs include weakness, hypotonia, and often severe contractures affecting feet (bilateral equinovarus talipes deformity), knees, and hips, at times dislocated. Marked difficulty in sucking and swallowing is often present in association with striking facial weakness, with a triangular open mouth.

There is also often respiratory muscle weakness, and mechanical ventilation is often required at least in the first weeks of life. Severe neonatal feeding difficulties are also present and require nasogastric tube feeding for several months even in infants who breathe spontaneously.

Both respiratory and feeding difficulties tend to lessen over the first months of life, and gastrostomy tube placement is very rarely needed. The duration and severity of respiratory involvement are important determinants of the long-term survival of these infants. Previous studies have indicated that need for mechanical ventilation for more than 4 weeks in a term infant is a negative prognostic factor for long-term survival (Rutherford et al, 1989).

It is important to recognize that many of the signs invariably present or frequently found in the adult form (such as clinically evident myotonia or cardiac and ocular abnormalities) are often not present in the neonatal period.

The muscle biopsy is not needed in children with congenital myotonic dystrophy. A detailed pedigree and the examination of the mother are generally strongly indicative of the diagnosis because, although myotonic dystrophy is an autosomal dominant trait, the mother is the transmitting parent in 94% of cases (Harper et al, 1992). On detailed examination, the mother generally has features such as facial weakness, mild ptosis, a stiff smile, an inability to bury the eyelashes, and/or or grip myotonia. In most cases, maternal signs are very mild, and the mother is often unaware of being affected.

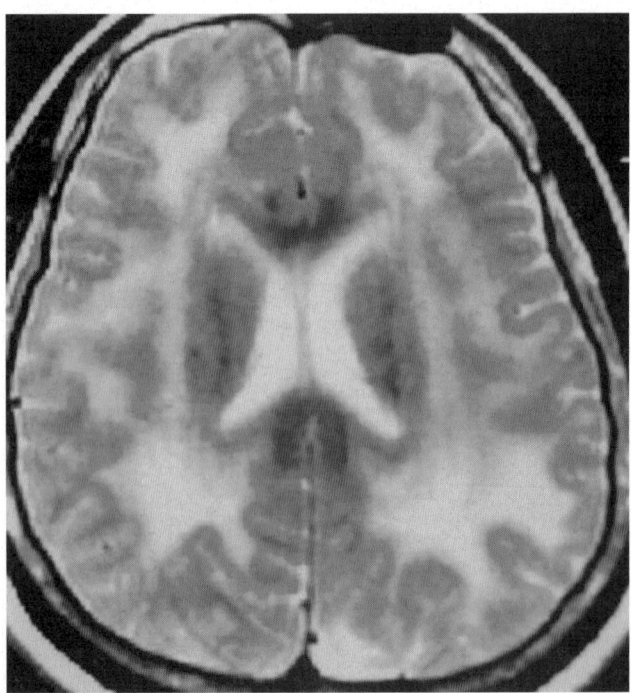

FIGURE 62-2 Brain MRI showing diffuse white matter changes in merosin-deficient congenital muscular dystrophy.

Percussion myotonia on clinical examination and myotonic discharge on electromyography (EMG) will help to further support the diagnosis, which can then be confirmed by molecular genetic testing. This latter is performed by looking at the expansion (increase in the number of CTG trinucleotide repeats) in the *DMPK* gene on chromosome 19. The female locus is more unstable than the male locus—hence the predominance of maternal transmission (Mulley et al, 1993).

Other Forms of Muscular Dystrophies

In the most common forms of muscular dystrophies occurring in pediatric population, such as Duchenne or limb girdle muscular dystrophies, the onset of clinical signs is generally well beyond the 1st year of age. However, it should be mentioned that neonatal or early onset has occasionally been reported in individual cases of specific late-onset forms such as facioscapuloperoneal muscular dystrophy. We and others have found that the dominantly inherited form of Emery-Dreifuss muscular dystrophy, caused by mutations in the LMNA gene, can have a very early presentation with reduced fetal movements and severe hypotonia and weakness at birth with marked involvement of the neck muscles (D'Amico et al, 2005; Mercuri et al, 2004; Quijano-Roy et al, 2008).

An important clinical issue is whether to perform diagnostic screening in an asymptomatic neonate with a positive family history, and if so, when. Performing genetic testing without muscle biopsies makes it easier to have an early diagnosis if the parents are concerned or if this is desired for prognosis, management, or genetic counseling.

CONGENITAL MYOPATHIES

The term *congenital myopathies* refers to a group of genetically inherited primary myopathies characterized by "nondystrophic" changes on muscle biopsies (for a recent review, see Sewry et al, 2008). Unlike muscular dystrophies, these myopathies tend to be relatively nonprogressive even though respiratory muscle weakness may affect prognosis.

This group of disorders is clinically, biochemically, and genetically very heterogeneous. Until recently, the classification of congenital myopathies was based mainly on clinical criteria and histopathologic findings, and the names of these conditions derive from the typical muscle histopathologic findings, which separated those forms with rods from those with cores. However, identification of mutations in different genes has dramatically advanced our understanding of their molecular basis. As with CMDs, there is increasing evidence that the boundaries between defined conditions are often indistinct. Mutations in the same gene can give rise to diverse clinical and histopathologic phenotypes, and conversely, the same phenotype can arise from mutations in a variety of genes (Sewry et al, 2008).

The generic term *congenital myopathy* for the group as a whole is probably a reasonable one, although not all cases are strictly "congenital" with symptoms presenting at birth. Indeed, many cases clinical manifestations may appear much later (Dubowitz, 1995). In order of frequency, the conditions that are more frequent in the neonatal period are nemaline myopathy, central core disease, myotubular myopathy, and minicore disease. Both minicore and central core disease manifest more frequently in early infancy than in the neonatal period, although earlier presentation is possible (Jungbluth, 2004).

Clinically, there are some common presenting features that point to a diagnosis of congenital myopathy, although it is difficult to distinguish among the individual diseases. In neonatal-onset forms, the primary clinical signs are floppiness, often associated with contractures, and weakness that often affects the facial muscles. In nemaline myopathy, minicore disease, and myotubular myopathy, there is a significant tendency to develop progressive respiratory failure, probably related to diaphragmatic involvement. Unlike the muscular dystrophies, the serum CK levels are frequently normal or only mildly elevated. The electromyography (EMG) traces may also be normal or may show mild, nonspecific changes. In all cases, these clinical findings alone will not be enough, and muscle biopsy is the only way to make a definitive diagnosis. It also helps in selecting the most appropriate genetic tests.

Table 62-2 shows a summary of the conditions that have been recognized to date. Generally, the names reflect the underlying structural change.

Nemaline Myopathy

Nemaline myopathy takes the name from the rods observed on muscle biopsy resembling threadlike structures (Greek: *nema*, "thread"). The clinical spectrum of nemaline myopathies is wide, ranging from early-onset neonatal forms to others in which affected individuals develop mild weakness only much later in life. In the neonatal period, there are two main modalities of presentation. In the "classical" congenital form, infants show hypotonia, general weakness predominantly affecting facial and axial muscles, and bulbar and feeding difficulties, requiring frequent suctioning, tube feeding, and gastrostomy. The other form is even more severe: Affected infants have a history of polyhydramnios and, at birth, present with arthrogryposis, severe weakness with complete immobility and respiratory failure, and severe feeding difficulties. Mild dysmorphic features compatible with a fetal akinesia sequence are common. There are cases in between the "classical" variant and this severe form.

The prognosis is always poor for children with the severe congenital form, and fetal akinesia without any improvement of tone, weakness, or bulbar and respiratory function even after several months. The prognosis for the classical form is in contrast much better, with steady improvement most children acquire independent ambulation, even though other signs of the disease such as failure to thrive, scoliosis, and nocturnal hypoventilation are frequent, even in ambulant children.

The serum CK levels are usually normal or only mildly elevated. The muscle biopsy typically shows a well-formed muscle with mild or moderate variability of fiber size, no necrosis or degenerative change, and an abundance of rod-like structures in muscle.

TABLE 62-2 The Most Common Congenital Myopathies With Known Gene Defects

	Gene	Chromosomal Locus	Inheritance*	Protein
Nemaline Myopathy	ACTA1	1q42	AD or AR	Skeletal α-actin
	NEB	2q2	AR	Nebulin
	TPM3	1q2	AD	α-Tropomyosin
	TPM2	9p13	AD	β-Tropomyosin
	TNNT1	19q13	AR	Troponin T
	CFL2	14q12	AD	Cofilin-2
Congenital Myopathies With Cores				
Central core disease	RYR1	19q13	AD or AR	Ryanodine receptor
Multiminicore disease	SEPN1	1P36	AR	Selenoprotein N1
Central Nuclei and Centronuclear Myopathies				
Myotubular myopathies	MTM1	Xq28	XLR	Myotubularin
Centronuclear myopathies	DNM2	19q13	AD	Dynamin 2
	BIN1	2q14	AR	Amphiphysin
	RYR1	19q13	AR	Ryanodine receptor

*AD, Autosomal dominant; AR, autosomal recessive; XLR, X-linked recessive.

Nemaline myopathy is genetically heterogeneous, with at least five genes now implicated in its pathogenesis:

1. Slow α-tropomyosin (TPM3) (Laing et al, 1995)
2. Nebulin (NEB) (Pelin et al, 1999)
3. Skeletal muscle α-actin (ACTA1) (Nowak et al, 1999)
4. β-tropomyosin (TPM2) (Donner et al, 2002)
5. Muscle troponin T (TNNT1) (Johnston et al, 2000)

Prenatal diagnosis is therefore now available for the genetically defined variants. For example, most of the classical milder congenital forms are due to recessive mutations in the NEB gene (Pelin et al, 1999), whereas the great majority of the severe forms have de novo dominant mutations in the ACTA1 gene (Nowak et al, 1999). Recessive mutations in the slow α-tropomyosin (TPM3) gene have been implicated in one homozygous case with early severe presentation (Tan et al, 1999). With few exceptions, the rest do not have mutations in the five known genes and are probably due to mutations in an as yet unidentified gene.

Central Core Disease

Central core disease (CCD) is the most common congenital myopathy. Several hundred cases have now been documented, but this most common form does not always have a neonatal onset. Delayed motor milestones and weakness usually occur in infancy or early childhood, although contractures at birth (equinovarus foot deformity, hip dislocation) are frequently found. However, a number of patients at the severe end of the spectrum have early neonatal presentation with severe arthrogryposis and scoliosis. Severe facial and respiratory muscle weakness and bulbar dysfunction are also present (Sewry et al, 2002).

A novel severe dominant and recessive variant of early-onset central core disease with antenatal onset, fetal akinesia, and, in addition to weakness and severe contractures, severe facial weakness and ptosis has also been reported (Romero et al, 2003).

The prognosis of these forms is variable and often reflects the severity of presentation. In milder forms, the natural course is static or only slowly progressive, with most affected individuals achieving the ability to walk. In the severe form, most affected children die in infancy, although in some patients the long-term outcome can be less severe (Romero et al, 2003).

Serum CK activity is usually normal or only moderately elevated. The biopsy typically shows massive type I myofiber predominance, and predominantly central, corelike areas on oxidative stains; however, these striking abnormalities may develop only after several years despite the congenital onset of muscle weakness. Marked type I predominance or uniformity may be the only abnormal feature in these cases at an early age. CCD is commonly transmitted as an autosomal-dominant trait with variable penetrance, and examination of the parents and a detailed family history may help to clarify the diagnosis.

Malignant hyperthermia susceptibility is a common complication, and all patients should thus be considered at risk. In most affected cases, genetic analysis shows dominant missense mutations in the ryanodine receptor (RYR1) gene at 19q13.1, the same genetic mutation as in malignant hyperthermia. The gene encodes a tetramer "ryanodine" receptor to a calcium channel of the sarcoplasmic reticulum within the myofiber (Ferreiro et al, 2002; Jungbluth et al, 2002).

De novo dominant mutations are common and account for a majority of sporadic cases, even though recessive pedigrees have also been reported (Jungbluth et al, 2007).

Minicore Myopathy (Multicore Disease)

Minicore myopathy is a rare condition, that usually does not manifest clinically in the neonatal period. The most common phenotype features marked axial weakness with spinal rigidity, scoliosis, and respiratory failure in late childhood. At least two genes are responsible for minicore disease: (1) the *SEPN1* gene (the same gene that, when disrupted, can give rise to rigid spine syndrome, suggesting that the two conditions are allelic) and (2) recessive *RYR1* gene mutations (Ferreiro et al, 2002; Jungbluth et al, 2007).

Myotubular (Centronuclear) Myopathy

Myotubular myopathy derives from its muscle biopsy description: numerous centrally placed (centronuclear) nuclei with a surrounding central zone devoid of oxidative enzyme activity. The clinical phenotype of myotubular (centronuclear) myopathy is highly variable, ranging from severe neonatal forms to milder forms with later onset, depending in part on the mode of inheritance. The severe neonatal phenotype is due to the more common X-linked form and is characteristically that of a male infant presenting with polyhydramnios, reduced fetal movement, and, after birth, with marked hypotonia, a variable degree of external ophthalmoplegia, respiratory failure, dysphagia, and often undescended testes (Barth et al, 1975; Sarnat et al, 1990, 1994). The disease is often fatal, but severely affected infants who are ventilator-dependent in the neonatal period may survive if they are maintained on a ventilator, although they will have almost complete lack of motor developmental progress. The autosomal recessive forms are more variable, ranging from early presentation with marked weakness and inability to walk to milder variants. The gene for the X-linked variant is the myotubularin gene (*MTM1*) on chromosome X a q28 (Laporte et al, 1997).

MOTOR NEURON DISORDERS

SPINAL MUSCULAR ATROPHY

The term *spinal muscular atrophy* (SMA) includes a group of disorders characterized by a progressive degenerative disease of spinal and brainstem motoneurons. The most frequent forms of motoneuron involvement in infancy are related to mutations in the survival motor neuron (SMN) gene on chromosome 5. This includes a wide range of clinical forms ranging from severe neonatal-onset forms to those occurring only in adulthood with very mild signs. From a practical standpoint, the classification of SMA takes into account the age at onset and the child's ability to sit unaided and to stand and walk unaided:

1. Severe: Unable to sit unsupported, with onset at birth or in the first months.
2. Intermediate: Able to sit unsupported. Unable to stand or walk unaided.
3. Mild: Able to stand and walk.

This classification is useful in clinical practice (Dubowitz, 1995), but it should be recognized that within each subdivision, there is a wide variability with an overall continuum of severity.

In severe SMA, also called Werdnig-Hoffmann disease or type I SMA, the onset is early, either in utero or within the first 2–3 months of life. In infants who do not show overt clinical signs at birth, the onset may be sudden, and a previously active infant may suddenly lose the ability to move the limbs.

The clinical features in type I SMA are very typical. The posture is characterized by involvement of the internal rotators of the shoulders that gives the arms an internally rotated, "jug-handle" position by the side of the body, with the hands facing outward. This posture is secondary to weakness and not to contractures, because these are not features of severe SMA, even though mild contractures may occur in patients who are not adequately mobilized.

Strikingly, there is no facial weakness, and the child's expression appears normal, this being in contrast with the severe weakness affecting the axial and limb muscles. There is generalized marked hypotonia with almost complete absence of movements and marked weakness that involves both axial and limb muscles (Figure 62-3, *A* and *B*). In the neonatal-onset forms, infants with type I SMA generally do not achieve good head control, although this milestone can be achieved and maintained in a proportion of those who have onset after the neonatal period.

The lower limbs are more affected than the upper, and the proximal muscles more than distal. Very often the movements are restricted to the feet and to the distal part of both upper and lower limbs, with some antigravity movements of fingers and toes. Some infants may also be able to flex and extend the elbows, but without any antigravity movements at the shoulders or upper arm level or in the legs. These infants never achieve the ability to roll over spontaneously. Tendon reflexes are always absent. The intercostal muscles are also severely affected, and

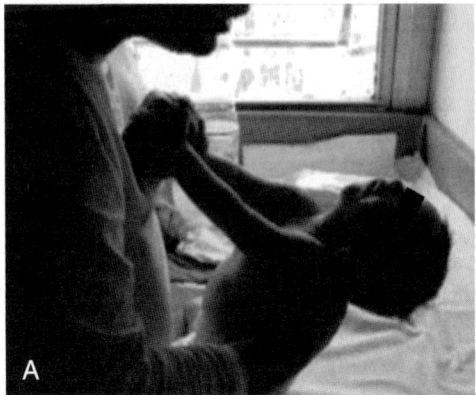
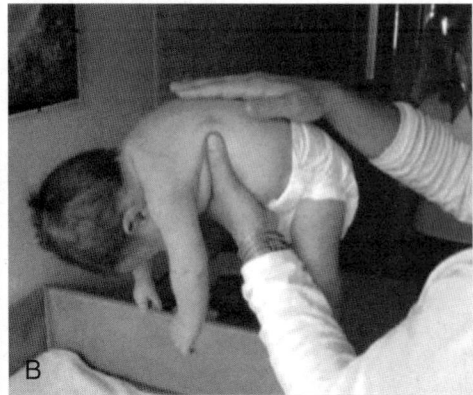

FIGURE 62-3 Severe hypotonia and weakness affecting axial muscles **(A)** and limbs **(B)** in an infant affected by spinal muscular atrophy.

breathing is almost entirely diaphragmatic. This gives the chest a bell-shaped appearance with costal recession and with associated distention of the abdomen with inspiration.

A classic feature of infantile SMA is bulbar weakness with difficulty in sucking and swallowing and an associated accumulation of mucus in the pharynx. These signs may occur at presentation or later during the 1st year and help to distinguish the disease from other neuromuscular disorders presenting in early infancy, which do not have this selective respiratory muscle involvement and frequently have evidence of diaphragmatic weakness. In SMA patients, the cry is often weak and ineffectual, as is any effort at coughing.

The combination of severe weakness and hypotonia, typical posture, absence of tendon reflexes, sparing of the facial muscles, and bell-shaped chest with predominant diaphragmatic breathing pattern are fairly consistent features of SMA and are strongly suggestive of the diagnosis on initial neonatal assessment. EMG shows fibrillation potentials and other signs of denervation of muscle, but findings are often nonspecific in neonates. In the past, when genetic testing was not available, a muscle biopsy was routinely performed, showing a characteristic pattern of peripheral denervation. With genetic testing now readily available and providing reliable results in approximately 95% of cases, muscle biopsy is no longer performed and the diagnosis is made by finding deletions in the SMN gene (Wang et al, 2007).

Until recently, studies of the natural history of type I SMA reported a very poor prognosis with a mean age at death of approximately 8 months. Affected infants are prone to recurrent respiratory infections and rarely survived beyond the first 2 years of life unless tracheotomy was performed. For many years, management of tracheotomy and chronic mechanical ventilation was the only option available to prolong survival. This approach was strongly discouraged by most clinicians because of quality-of-life concerns. However, the natural history of type I SMA has recently changed considerably (Oskoui et al, 2007). In the past few years there has been increasing evidence that infants with type I SMA should be treated with noninvasive ventilator support as early as possible, because this prevents intermittent hypoxia and hypercapnia (especially at night) and also helps to expand the chest muscles. Other measures, such as performing gastrostomy at the onset of swallowing problems or even before their onset, have further decreased the chances of reduced survival related to poor growth and aspiration. Although there are no systematic double-blind studies to establish the long-term effect of these management strategies on survival, they have become routine in many centers. Recent reports have shown clearly increased overall survival rates for these children and improved recovery from acute respiratory infections (Bertini et al, 2005; Wang et al, 2007).

NONSPINAL MUSCULAR ATROPHY MOTOR NEURON DISEASES

Motor neuron diseases that are not linked to mutations in chromosome 5 are rare in neonates. Among these, two often have onset at birth and should be taken into account when dealing with infants with clinical and neurophysiologic signs of motoneuron involvement. In both, there are signs that are different from those found in type I SMA that help in the differential diagnosis. The two forms include *diaphragmatic SMA* (Grohmann et al, 2001; Mercuri et al, 2000) and the form with *pontocerebellar hypoplasia* (Barth et al, 1993).

Diaphragmatic Spinal Muscular Atrophy

Diaphragmatic SMA, also known as spinal muscular atrophy with respiratory distress (SMARD), is also characterized by motoneuron involvement, but unlike the "classical SMA" linked to chromosome 5, in this form there is diaphragmatic weakness, with early onset of life-threatening respiratory failure (Rudnik-Schöneborn et al, 2004). This is due to severe diaphragmatic paralysis with elevation of both hemidiaphragms on chest radiograph. In typical SMA, the diaphragm is spared and the intercostal muscles are more severely affected. The distribution of weakness is another marked difference between the classical SMA, because in SMARD the distal and not the proximal muscles are predominantly involved. SMARD is a clinically and genetically heterogeneous condition. SMARD1 results from mutations in the gene encoding the immunoglobulin-binding protein 2 (*IGHMBP2*) on 11q13 (Groham et al, 2001; Guenther et al, 2007).

Pontocerebellar Hypoplasia

Pontocerebellar hypoplasia is a progressive degenerative disease involving both motoneurons and the CNS, the latter including hypoplasia of the cerebellar vermis and often of the cerebellar hemispheres, associated with a thin brainstem and pons (Barth et al, 1993). In affected infants, clinical signs relate to both motoneuron and CNS involvement. The clinical course is progressive, and respiratory and feeding difficulties, already present at birth or in early infancy, become increasingly severe. This form is not allelic to SMA, and the genetics of these forms have only recently been identified (Budde et al, 2008; Renbaum et al, 2009).

Finally, it should be mentioned that involvement of motor neurons can also be found in the Pena-Shokeir sequences with motoneuron signs associated with arthrogryposis and with normal *SMN* gene expression (Hageman et al, 1987) and in several metabolic diseases of the nervous system, even though the signs of denervation are often obscured by the more prominent CNS or muscle involvement.

MYASTHENIA GRAVIS

TRANSIENT NEONATAL MYASTHENIA

Approximately 20% of infants born to mothers with acquired myasthenia gravis may have transient signs of myasthenia for several days to weeks, as a result of transplacental transfer of maternal antibodies directed against the acetylcholine receptor (AChR). There is no direct correlation between the severity of maternal myasthenia and neonatal clinical signs. In fact, neonatal myasthenia may occur not only in mothers with a known diagnosis but in infants born to undiagnosed mothers who have subclinical disease but are positive for AchR antibody (Papazian et al, 1992). Onset of clinical signs generally occurs within several hours after birth and always within the first 3 days and include respiratory insufficiency, inability to suck or swallow, and generalized hypotonia and weakness with facial involvement. Ptosis is not always present, but signs of fatigability can be observed, especially during feedings. Ventilatory support and feeding by gavage may be needed during this period. Recovery is anticipated by 2 months in 90% and by 4 months in most infants.

Once the first signs appear, diagnosis can be confirmed by anticholinesterase administration. Positive AchR antibodies in the infant or the mother provide further evidence, but their absence does not rule out the diagnosis. Overall management aims at supporting feeding and ventilation until spontaneous recovery occurs. In symptomatic infants, neostigmine (or pyridostigmine) should be given orally or by nasogastric tube until the infant is no longer symptomatic.

CONGENITAL MYASTHENIC SYNDROMES

Congenital myasthenic syndromes are inherited disorders resulting in neuromuscular transmission dysfunction. These are not related to maternal myasthenia and are nearly always permanent disorders (Engel et al, 2001, 2003). Inheritance is autosomal recessive, except with slow channel syndrome, which is autosomal dominant. Depending on the site and mechanism of the neuromuscular transmission defect, they are classified into presynaptic, synaptic, and postsynaptic categories. Presentation in the early neonatal period is less common and is mainly limited to the forms with episodic apnea (familial infantile myasthenia) and endplate acetylcholinesterase deficiency. Neonates with congenital myasthenia gravis do not experience myasthenic crises or exhibit elevations of AChR antibodies in plasma.

Most of the syndromes will respond to acetylcholinesterase inhibitors. An exception is the slow channel syndrome. Patients with this form do not respond to acetylcholinesterase inhibitors, and in some cases a worsening has been reported after their administration.

INVESTIGATION OF NEUROMUSCULAR DISEASES IN THE NEONATE

The field of inherited muscle disorders has become increasingly complex. The level of genetic heterogeneity is far greater than initially appreciated, and genetically different conditions often share similar clinical and histopathologic phenotypes. For disorders in which the genetic defect is known, a definitive diagnosis can be made by screening for the known genes. However, as the number of proteins and genes that can be potentially screened for enlarges, additional tools for selecting the appropriate genetic and biochemical markers are required. Muscle biopsy generally provides important clues for determining the most appropriate investigations, but clinical examination still plays an important role both in detecting a neuromuscular disorder and in the differential diagnosis with other causes of hypotonia in the newborn infant. Hypotonia is the most

typical and common sign of neuromuscular involvement in the newborn infant but can also present in many nonneuromuscular disorders, and, in some cases, the differential diagnosis can be quite difficult.

CLINICAL EXAMINATION

A detailed clinical examination and a good clinical and obstetric history provide in many cases the foundation to distinguish infants with peripheral involvement from those with CNS involvement, and, in some cases, provide important clues for a more specific diagnosis.

In a large cohort of 83 infants referred for evaluation of hypotonia, neuromuscular disorders were identified in 47% of infants. The investigators found that the presence of weakness and contractures had a very high sensitivity and high specificity to detect neuromuscular disorders (Vasta et al, 2005). Other presenting signs of neuromuscular disorders included arthrogryposis, feeding difficulties, sudden episodes of collapse, and unexplained respiratory failure. Reduced fetal movements and polyhydramnios are also frequent in infants with neuromuscular disorders and suggest weakness with onset in utero (Vasta et al, 2005).

CREATINE KINASE

The chances of detecting a neuromuscular disorder further increase if the infant's serum CK levels are increased. However, a normal CK level does not exclude the possibility of a neuromuscular disorder, because the enzymatic levels are normal or only mildly elevated in congenital myopathies such as SMA.

ELECTROMYOGRAPHY

EMG may help at this stage in patients with motor neuron disorders and in other primary myopathies, but it is considered less reliable than at older ages both for technical reasons and because some features may not develop until the pathologic process has progressed further.

MUSCLE BIOPSY AND GENETIC STUDIES: WHICH ONE COMES FIRST?

Muscle biopsy is generally the next step. However, before performing the biopsy, one should exclude disorders that can be suspected from clinical examination and confirmed by genetic analysis, in which case muscle biopsy can be avoided. The two disorders that can be more easily diagnosed on clinical examination are type I SMA and congenital myotonic dystrophy. In SMA, the combination of these clinical signs previously described with evidence of denervation on EMG is a very strong indicator of the disease, which can then be confirmed by genetic analysis (see earlier discussion). Similarly, weakness and hypotonia in an infant with contractures (sometimes associated with facial weakness and respiratory and bulbar involvement) should prompt an investigation of the mother, who may show clinical or EMG signs of myotonia. These cumulative findings may then point to a diagnosis of congenital myotonic dystrophy which can be confirmed by genetic analysis.

In contrast, when the clinical examination, serum CK levels, and possibly the EMG are suggestive of a congenital myopathy or a congenital muscular dystrophy, a muscle biopsy should be done. The biopsy is needed not only to confirm possible muscle involvement but also to detect possible structural changes that may help to define the type of myopathy (e.g., rods, cores, fiber predominance); to study the expression of proteins such as merosin or α-DG; and to ultimately determine the definitive diagnosis and select the most appropriate genetic investigations.

IMAGING STUDIES

In view of all the recent findings on the forms of CMDs associated with CNS involvement, it has become mandatory to perform imaging studies in hypotonic infants in order to detect possible major or minor brain abnormalities that will help determine a diagnosis. Conversely, in infants in whom brain imaging has shown cerebellar hypoplasia or other structural brain abnormalities, it is important to perform appropriate clinical investigations to detect possible signs of weakness and or contractures that may suggest possible muscle involvement. In these patients, the evaluation of serum CK may provide additional information, because with few exceptions, all forms of congenital muscular dystrophies with structural brain involvement reported thus far have very high serum enzymatic levels (Geodfrey et al, 2007; Mercuri et al, 2009).

SUGGESTED READINGS

Clements E, Mercuri E, Godfrey C, et al: Brain involvement in muscular dystrophies with defective dystroglycan glycosylation, *Ann Neurol* 64:573-582, 2008.

Ferreiro A, Quijano-Roy S, Pichereau C, et al: Mutations of the selenoprotein N gene, which is implicated in rigid spine muscular dystrophy, cause the classical phenotype of multiminicore disease: reassessing the nosology of early-onset myopathies, *Am J Hum Genet* 71:739-749, 2002.

Godfrey C, Clement E, Mein R, et al: Refining genotype phenotype correlations in muscular dystrophies with defective glycosylation of dystroglycan, *Brain* 130:2725-2735, 2007.

Grohmann K, Schuelke M, Diers A, et al: Mutations in the gene encoding immunoglobulin mu-binding protein 2 cause spinal muscular atrophy with respiratory distress type 1, *Nat Genet* 29:75-77, 2001.

Jungbluth H: Multi-minicore disease. Review, *Orphanet J Rare Dis* 2:31, 2007.

Mercuri E, Messina S, Bruno C, et al: Congenital muscular dystrophies with defective glycosylation of dystroglycan: a population study, *Neurology* 72:1802-1809, 2009.

Muntoni F, Voit T: The congenital muscular dystrophies in 2004: a century of exciting progress, *Neuromuscul Disord* 14:635-649, 2004.

Romero NB, Monnier N, Viollet L, et al: Dominant and recessive central core disease associated with RYR1 mutations and fetal akinesia, *Brain* 126:2341-2349, 2003.

Rudnik-Schöneborn S, Stolz P, Varon R, et al: Long-term observations of patients with infantile spinal muscular atrophy with respiratory distress type 1 (SMARD1), *Neuropediatrics* 35:174-182, 2004.

Tome FM, Evangelista T, Leclerc A, et al: Congenital muscular dystrophy with merosin deficiency, *C R Acad Sci III* 317:351-357, 1994.

Vasta I, Kinali M, Messina S, et al: Can clinical signs identify newborns with neuromuscular disorders? *J Pediatr* 146:73-79, 2005.

Wang CH, Finkel RS, Bertini ES, et al: Participants of the International Conference on SMA Standard of Care. Consensus statement for standard of care in spinal muscular atrophy, *J Child Neurol* 22:1027-1049, 2007.

Complete references and supplemental color images used in this text can be found online at www.expertconsult.com

NEONATAL SEIZURES

Mark S. Scher

Neonatal seizures are one of the few neonatal neurologic conditions that require immediate medical attention. Although prompt diagnostic and therapeutic interventions are needed, multiple challenges impede the physician's evaluation and management of the newborn with suspected seizures (Table 63-1) (Scher, 1997a, 2001b, 2002; Scher and Beggarly, 1989). Clinical and electroencephalographic manifestations of neonatal seizures vary dramatically from those in older children, and seizure recognition remains the foremost challenge to overcome. This dilemma is underscored by the brevity and subtlety of the clinical repertoire of the neonatal neurologic examination. Environmental restrictions in an intensive care setting—the sick infant may be confined to an incubator, intubated, and attached to multiple catheters—limit accessibility by caregivers. Medications alter arousal and muscle tone and limit the clinician's ability to detect clinical neurologic signs reflective of the underlying disease state. Brain injury from antepartum factors may precipitate neonatal seizures as part of an encephalopathic clinical picture during the intrapartum and neonatal periods (Scher, 1994, 2006), well beyond when brain injury occurred. Overlapping medical conditions from fetal through neonatal periods must be factored into the most appropriate etiologic algorithm that explains seizure expression before application of the most accurate prognosis. Medication options that effectively treat seizures remain elusive and may need to be designed and utilized on the basis of the underlying diagnosis (Scher, 2001a, 2006; Silverstein et al, 2008). This chapter presents issues regarding recognition, differential diagnosis, prognosis, and treatment of neonatal seizures, in the context of current neurobiologic and pathophysiologic explanations or causes for neonatal seizures and consequential brain injury.

DIAGNOSTIC DILEMMAS: CLINICAL VERSUS ELECTROENCEPHALOGRAPHIC CRITERIA

Because neonatal seizures are generally brief and subtle in clinical appearance, unusual behaviors may be difficult to recognize and classify. The most common practice in many neonatal intensive care units (NICUs) is to rely on clinical behaviors to identify seizures, without confirmation by electroencephalography (EEG). Motor or autonomic behaviors, however, may represent normal gestational age- and state-specific behaviors in healthy infants or, alternatively, nonepileptic paroxysmal conditions in encephalopathic infants. Medical personnel also vary significantly in their ability to recognize suspicious behaviors; this variability will contribute to overdiagnosis or underdiagnosis. Therefore, confirmation of suspicious clinical events as seizures using coincident EEG recordings is now

strongly recommended. Using either routine EEG studies (Glauser and Clancy, 1992) or continuous synchronized video-EEG-polygraphic recordings (Mizrahi and Kellaway, 1998), more reliable start and end points of electrographically confirmed seizures can be established before decisions are made regarding treatment intervention. Rigorous physiologic monitoring of non–central nervous system (CNS) measures also assists in the recognition and management of seizures.

CLINICAL SEIZURE CRITERIA

The International League Against Epilepsy's classification adopted by the World Health Organization still considers neonatal seizures within an unclassified category (Commission, 1981). A more recent classification scheme suggests a stricter distinction of clinical seizure (nonepileptic) events from electrographically confirmed (epileptic) seizures with respect to possible treatment interventions (Mizrahi and Kellaway, 1998). Continued refinement using novel seizure classifications is needed to reconcile disagreements between clinical and EEG criteria, which impede a correct seizure diagnosis.

Several caveats useful in the evaluation for suspected neonatal seizures are listed in Box 63-1.

Clinical criteria for neonatal seizure diagnosis were historically subdivided into five categories: focal clonic, multifocal or migratory clonic, tonic, myoclonic, and subtle seizures (Volpe, 2001). A more recent classification expands these clinical subtypes, adopting a strict temporal occurrence of specific clinical events with coincident electrographic seizures, to distinguish neonatal clinical "nonepileptic" seizures from "epileptic" seizures (Mizrahi and Kellaway, 1998) (Table 63-2).

Subtle Seizure Activity

Subtle seizure activity—now termed *motor automatisms and buccolingual movements*—is the most frequently observed category of neonatal seizures. Before a seizure evaluation is initiated, the normal occurrence of alterations in cardiorespiratory regularity, body movements, and other behaviors during active sleep (rapid eye movement [REM] sleep), quiet sleep (non-REM [NREM] sleep), or waking states should be appreciated (Da Silva et al, 1998; Scher, 1996). In any event, paroxysmal activity that interrupts the expected behavioral repertoire of the newborn infant and appears stereotypic or repetitive should heighten the clinician's level of suspicion for seizures. Repetitive buccolingual movements, orbital-ocular movements, unusual "bicycling" or "pedaling," and autonomic signs are examples of this seizure category (Figure 63-1). Periodic alterations in heart rate, blood pressure, or oxygenation or other autonomic signs are particularly helpful clues to seizure

TABLE 63-1 Dilemmas Regarding Neonatal Seizures

Diagnostic choices	Reliance on clinical vs. electroencephalographic criteria
Etiologic explanations	Multiple prenatal/neonatal conditions with variable times of onset and duration
Treatment decisions	Who, when, how, and for how long?
Prognostic questions	Consider mechanisms of injury based on underlying disorder vs. intrinsic vulnerability of the immature brain to prolonged seizures

---

BOX 63-1　Caveats Concerning Recognition of Neonatal Seizures

- Stereotypic behaviors occur in association with normal neonatal sleep or waking states, medication effects, and gestational maturity.
- Any abnormal repetitive activity may be a clinical seizure if out of context for expected neonatal behavior.
- Document coincident electrographic seizures with the suspected clinical event.
- Abnormal behavioral phenomena with inconsistent relationships with coincident electroencephalographic seizures suggest a subcortical seizure focus.
- Nonepileptic pathologic movement disorders are independent of the seizure state.

---

activity during pharmacologic paralysis for ventilatory care. Autonomic expressions, however, also are intermixed with somatic findings. Isolated autonomic signs such as apnea are rarely associated with coincident electrographic seizures (Fenichel et al, 1980). Synchronized video-EEG-polygraphic recordings are now preferred to document temporal relationships between clinical and electrographic events (Mizrahi and Kellaway, 1998; Scher, 1997a, 2001b). Despite the "subtle" expression of this seizure category, affected children may suffer significant brain injuries.

Clonic Seizures

Rhythmic movements of body parts that consist of a rapid flexion phase followed by a slower extensor movement may be *clonic seizures*, to be distinguished from the symmetric "to-and-fro" movements of nonepileptic tremulousness or jitteriness (Scher, 2001b). Gentle flexion of the affected body part easily suppresses the tremor, whereas clonic seizures persist. Clonic movements can involve face, arm, leg, or respiratory or pharyngeal muscles (Figure 63-2, *A* and *B*). Generalized clonic activities also can occur but rarely consist of the classic tonic followed by clonic phases, characteristic of the generalized motor seizure noted in older children and adults. Focal clonic and hemiclonic seizures have been described with localized brain injury, usually from cerebrovascular lesions (Clancy et al, 1985; Levy et al, 1985; Scher et al, 1986), but also can be seen with generalized or multifocal brain abnormalities. As with older patients, focal seizures in the neonate can be followed by transient motor weakness, historically referred to as a transient Todd's paresis or paralysis, characterized by a more persistent hemiparesis over days to

TABLE 63-2 Classification and Clinical Characteristics of Neonatal Seizures

Seizure Class	Characterization
Focal clonic	Repetitive, rhythmic contractions of muscle groups of the limbs, face, or trunk May be unifocal or multifocal May occur synchronously or asynchronously in muscle groups on one side of the body May occur simultaneously but asynchronously on both sides Cannot be suppressed by restraint *Pathophysiology:* epileptic
Focal tonic	Sustained posturing of single limbs Sustained asymmetric posturing of the trunk Sustained eye deviation Cannot be provoked by stimulation or suppressed by restraint *Pathophysiology:* epileptic
Generalized tonic	Sustained symmetric posturing of limbs, trunk, and neck May be flexor, extensor, or mixed extensor/flexor May be provoked or intensified by stimulation May be suppressed by restraint or repositioning *Presumed pathophysiology:* nonepileptic
Myoclonic	Random, single, rapid contractions of muscle groups of the limbs, face, or trunk Typically not repetitive or may recur at a slow rate May be generalized, focal, or fragmentary May be provoked by stimulation *Presumed pathophysiology:* may be epileptic or nonepileptic
Spasms	May be flexor, extensor, or mixed extensor/flexor May occur in clusters Cannot be provoked by stimulation or suppressed by restraint *Pathophysiology:* epileptic
Motor automatisms	
Ocular signs	Random and roving eye movements or nystagmus (distinct from tonic eye deviation) May be provoked or intensified by tactile stimulation *Presumed pathophysiology:* nonepileptic
Oral-buccal-lingual movements	Sucking, chewing, tongue protrusions May be provoked or intensified by stimulation *Presumed pathophysiology:* nonepileptic
Progression movements	Rowing or swimming movements Pedaling or bicycling movements of the legs May be provoked or intensified by stimulation May be suppressed by restraint or repositioning *Presumed pathophysiology:* nonepileptic
Complex purposeless movements	Sudden arousal with transient increased random activity of the limbs May be provoked or intensified by stimulation *Presumed pathophysiology:* nonepileptic

From Mizrahi EM, Kellaway P: *Diagnosis and management of neonatal seizures,* Philadelphia, 1998, Lippincott-Raven, pp 1-155.

weeks. Clonic movements without EEG-confirmed seizures have been described in neonates with normal EEG background rhythms, in whom neurodevelopmental outcome can be normal (Rose and Lombroso, 1970). The less experienced clinician may misclassify myoclonic as clonic movements.

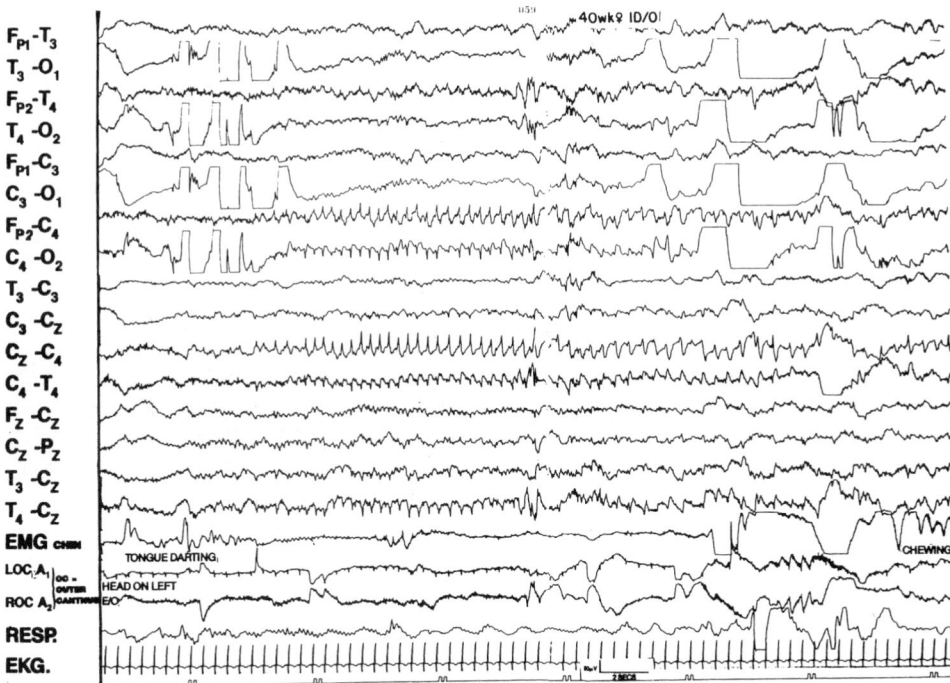

FIGURE 63-1 Segment of electroencephalogram (EEG) from a 40-week-gestation, 1-day-old female infant after severe asphyxia resulting from rupture of velamentous insertion of the umbilical cord during delivery. An electrical seizure in the right central/midline region is recorded coincident with buccolingual and eye movements (see comments and eye channels on record). *(From Scher MS, Painter MJ: Electrographic diagnosis of neonatal seizures: issues of diagnostic accuracy, clinical correlation and survival. In Wasterlain CG, Vert P, editors:* Neonatal seizures, *New York, 1990, Raven Press, p 17.)*

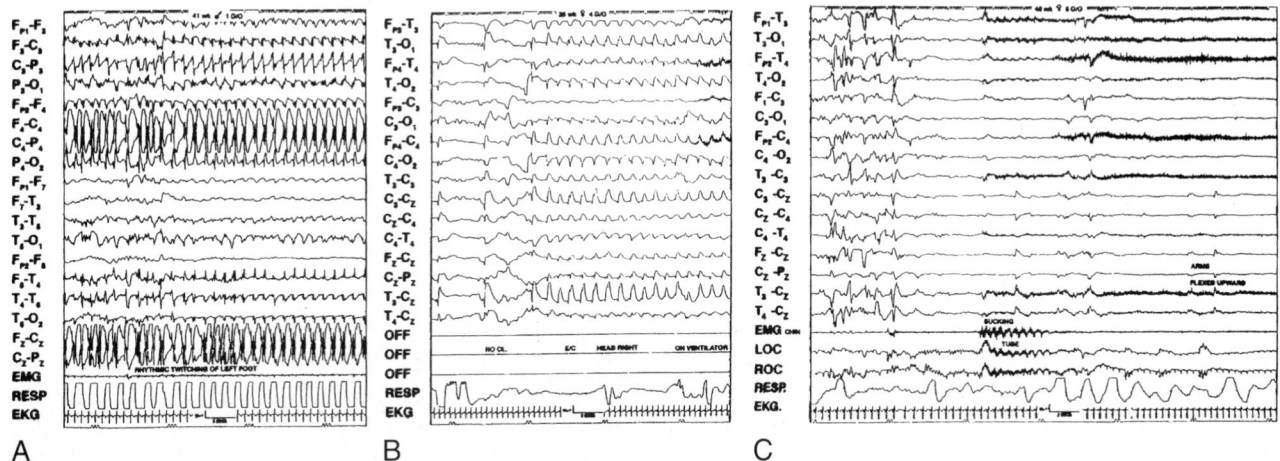

FIGURE 63-2 A, Segment of electroencephalogram (EEG) from a 41-week-gestation, 1-day-old male infant with an electroclinical seizure characterized by rhythmic clonic movements of the left foot coincident with bihemispheric electrographic discharges of higher amplitude in the right hemisphere. This seizure was documented before administration of antiepileptic medication. **B,** Segment of EEG from a 25-week-gestation, 4-day-old female infant with an electrographic seizure without clinical accompaniments. **C,** Segment of EEG from a 40-week-gestation, 6-day-old infant with stereotypic flexion posturing in the absence of electrographic seizures (note muscle artifact). *(From Scher MS: Pediatric electroencephalography and evoked potentials. In Swaiman KS, editor:* Pediatric neurology: principles and practice, *St. Louis, Mo, 1999, CV Mosby, p 164.)*

Multifocal (Fragmentary) Clonic Seizures

The word *fragmentary* was historically applied to distinguish multifocal clonic seizures from the more classic generalized tonic-clonic seizure seen in the older child. Multifocal or migratory clonic activities spread over body parts in either a random or an anatomically appropriate fashion. Seizure movements may alternate from side to side and appear asynchronously between the two halves of the child's body. Multifocal clonic seizures may be misclassified as myoclonic seizures, and

video-EEG documentation helps with proper identification. Neonates with this seizure description often suffer death or significant neurologic morbidity (Rose and Lombroso, 1970).

Tonic Seizures

Tonic seizure refers to a sustained flexion or extension of axial or appendicular muscle groups (Figure 63-3, *A* and *B*). Tonic movements of a limb or sustained head or eye

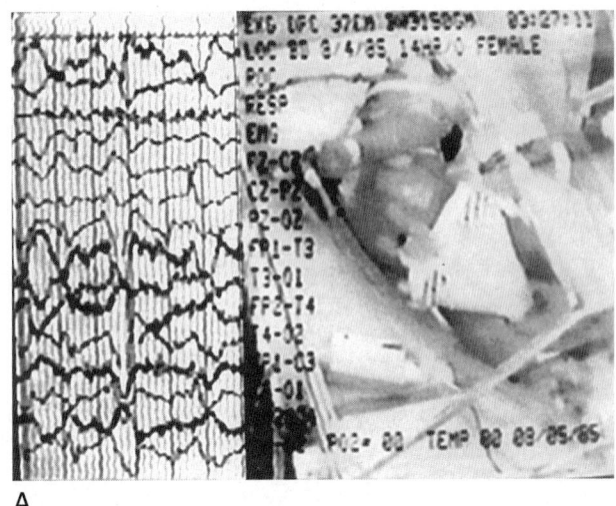 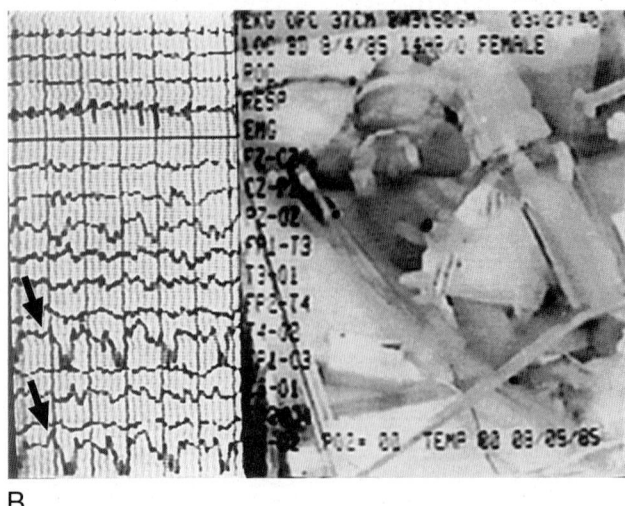

FIGURE 63-3 **A,** Segment of a synchronized video-electroencephalographic recording from a 37-week-gestation, 1-day-old female infant who suffered asphyxia demonstrates prominent opisthotonos with left arm extension in the absence of coincident electrographic seizure activity. **B,** Synchronized video-electroencephalographic recording from the same patient as in **A,** documenting electrographic seizure in the right posterior quadrant (*arrows*), after cessation of left arm tonic movements and persistent opisthotonos. *(From Scher MS, Painter MJ: Controversies concerning neonatal seizures. In Pellock JM, editor: Seizure disorders, Pediatr Clin North Am 36:292, 1989.)*

turning may also be noted. Documentation of tonic activity during coincident EEG recording is needed, because 30% of such movements lack a temporal correlation with electrographic seizures (Kellaway and Hrachovy, 1983). Such nonepileptic activity is referred to as "brainstem release" resulting from functional decortication after severe neocortical dysfunction or damage. Extensive neocortical damage or dysfunction permits the emergence of uninhibited subcortical expressions of extensor movements (Sarnat, 1984). Tonic seizures may also be misidentified when nonepileptic movement disorders consisting of dystonia are more appropriate behavioral descriptions. Both tonic movements and dystonic posturing may simultaneously occur in the same neonate.

Myoclonic Seizures

Myoclonic movements are rapid, isolated jerks that can be generalized, multifocal, or focal in an axial or appendicular distribution. Myoclonus lacks the slow return phase of the clonic movement complex. Healthy preterm infants commonly exhibit myoclonic movements without seizures or a brain disorder. An EEG, therefore, is recommended to confirm the coincident appearance of electrographic discharges with these movements (Figure 63-4, *A*). Pathologic myoclonus in the absence of electrographically confirmed seizures also can occur in severely ill preterm or full-term infants after severe brain dysfunction or damage (Scher, 1985). As with older children and adults, myoclonus may reflect injuries at multiple levels of the neuraxis, from spinal cord to brainstem to cortical regions. Stimulus-evoked myoclonus with either single coincident spike discharges or sustained electrographic seizures has been reported (Scher, 1997b). An extensive evaluation must be initiated to exclude metabolic, structural, and genetic causes. Rarely, healthy sleeping neonates exhibit abundant myoclonus

that subsides on arousal to the waking state (Resnick et al, 1986); this entity is termed benign *sleep myoclonus of the newborn.*

NONEPILEPTIC BEHAVIORS OF NEONATES

Nonepileptic neonatal movement repertoires continue to challenge the physician's attempt to accurately diagnose seizures. Coincident synchronized video-EEG-polygraphic recordings are now suggested to confirm the temporal relationships between the suspicious clinical phenomena and electrographic expression of seizures (Mizrahi and Kellaway, 1998; Scher 1997a, 2001b).

Tremulousness or Jitteriness Without Coincident Electrographic Seizures

Tremors are frequently misidentified as clonic activity by inexperienced medical personnel. The flexion and extension phases of tremor are equal in amplitude, unlike the unequal phases of clonic movements. Children are generally alert or hyperalert but may also appear somnolent or lethargic as part of an encephalopathy. Passive flexion and repositioning of the affected tremulous body part will diminish or eliminate the movement. Such movements usually are spontaneous but can be provoked by tactile stimulation. This movement may also appear asymmetric, with decreased expression in a weak limb after a brain injury or peripheral neuropathy. Metabolic or toxin-induced encephalopathies, including those due to mild asphyxia, drug withdrawal, hypoglycemia or hypocalcemia, intracranial hemorrhage, hypothermia, and growth restriction, are common clinical scenarios in which tremulous movements occur. Neonatal tremors generally diminish with increasing postconceptional age, spontaneously resolving over days to weeks, with normal neurologic outcome (Parker et al, 1990).

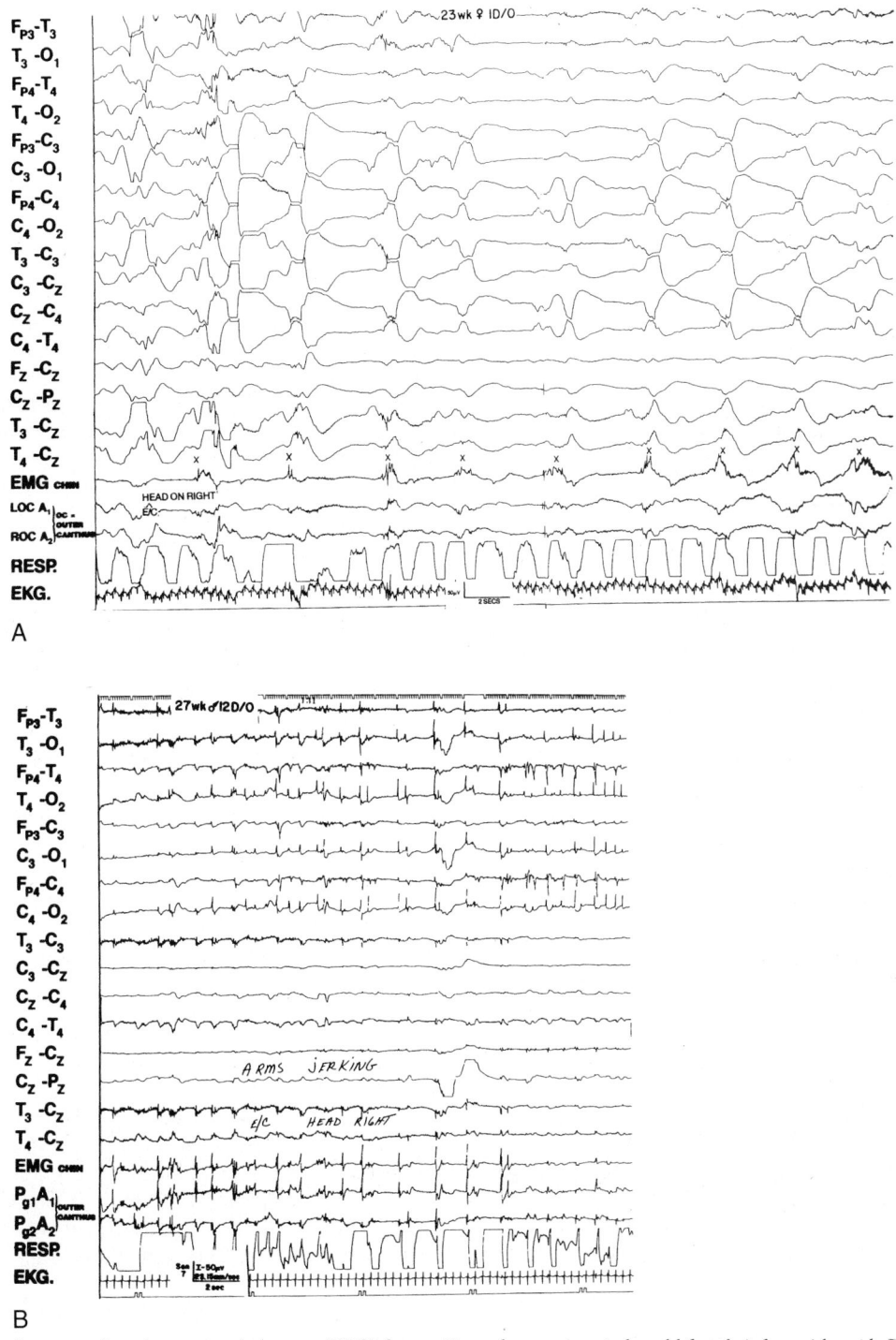

FIGURE 63-4 A, Segment of an electroencephalogram (EEG) from a 23-week-gestation, 1-day-old female infant with grade III intraventricular hemorrhage and progressive ventriculomegaly. An electroclinical seizure is noted coincident with myoclonic movements of the diaphragm (*x marks*). **B,** Segment of an EEG from an encephalopathic 27-week-gestation, 12-day-old male infant with herpes encephalitis who exhibits nonepileptic multifocal myoclonus (myogenic potentials as electroencephalographic artifacts). (*A, From Scher MS: Pathological myoclonus of the newborn: electrographic and clinical correlations,* Pediatr Neurol *1:342-348, 1985, with permission.*)

Neonatal Myoclonus Without Coincident Electrographic Seizures

Myoclonic movements can be bilateral and synchronous or asymmetric and asynchronous in appearance. Benign myoclonic activity occurs more frequently during active (REM) sleep and is more predominant in the preterm infant (Hakamada et al, 1981; Scher, 1996), as well as rarely in healthy full-term infants; movements are not stimulus sensitive, have no coincident electrographic seizure correlates, are not associated with EEG background abnormalities, and are suppressed during wakefulness. Benign neonatal sleep myoclonus must be a diagnosis of exclusion.

Infants with severe CNS dysfunction may present with nonepileptic spontaneous or stimulus-evoked pathologic myoclonus (see Figure 63-4, *B*). Neonates with different forms of metabolic encephalopathies such as glycine encephalopathy, cerebrovascular lesions, brain infections, or congenital malformations can present with nonepileptic pathologic myoclonus (Scher, 1985, 1997b). Encephalopathic neonates may respond to tactile or painful stimulation by isolated focal, segmental, or generalized myoclonic movements. Rarely, cortically generated spike or sharp wave discharges, as well as seizures, also may be noted on the EEG recordings that are coincident with these myoclonic movements. Medication-induced myoclonus and other stereotypic movements also have been described (Sexson et al, 1995); these abnormalities resolve when the drug is withdrawn.

Neonatal Dyskinesias: Dystonia or Choreoathetosis Without Coincident Electrographic Seizures

Dystonia and choreoathetosis are commonly occurring movement disorders that are often misdiagnosed as seizures. These nonepileptic movement disorders are associated with either acute or chronic disease states involving basal ganglia structures or the extrapyramidal pathways that innervate these regions. Dystonia is one of three clinical expressions of neonatal hypertonic states that often reflect antepartum timing to brain injury (Scher, 2008a,b). However, either antepartum or intrapartum adverse events such as severe asphyxia can damage the basal ganglia (i.e., status marmoratus) (Volpe, 2001), as expressed as dyskinesias. Rarely, specific inherited metabolic diseases (Barth, 1992) (e.g., glutaric aciduria) also can injure these structures. Sustained posturing or dystonia often reflects functional disinhibition of subcortical motor pathways due to disease or malformation of the neocortex (Sarnat, 1984) (see Figure 63-2, *C*). Documentation of electrographic seizures by coincident video-EEG-polygraphic recordings will help avoid misdiagnosis and inappropriate treatment of nonepileptic dyskinesias (see Figure 63-3, *A* and *B*).

ELECTROGRAPHIC SEIZURE CRITERIA

Over the past several decades, electrographic/polysomnographic studies have become invaluable tools for the assessment of suspected seizures (Mizrahi and Kellaway, 1998; Pope et al, 1992; Scher, 1999, 2001b). Technical and interpretive skills for assessment of normal and abnormal neonatal EEG sleep patterns must be mastered to develop a confident visual analysis style for seizure recognition. Corroboration with the EEG technologist is always an essential part of the diagnostic process, because physiologic and nonphysiologic artifacts can masquerade as electrographic seizures. The physician also must anticipate expected behaviors for the child for gestational maturity, medication use, and state of arousal, in the context of potential artifacts.

As with the epileptic older child and adult, it is generally accepted that the neonatal epileptic seizure is a clinical paroxysm of altered brain function with the simultaneous presence of an electrographic event on an EEG recording. For assessment of the suspected clinical event in the neonate, synchronized video-EEG-polygraphic monitoring is

a useful tool to distinguish an epileptic from a nonepileptic event. Single-channel computerized devices for continuous prolonged monitoring (Hellstrom-Westas, 1992) are useful as screening tools but may fail to detect focal or regional seizures if the single-channel recording is distant from the brain region involved with seizure expression. Neonatal electrographic seizures commonly arise focally from a single brain region. One brain study described 56% of neonatal seizures presenting in a single location, with the remainder occurring in multiple locations (Bye and Flanagan, 1995). In another study, only one third of neonatal EEG seizures displayed clinical signs on simultaneous video recordings, and two thirds went unrecognized or were misinterpreted by experienced neonatal staff (Murray et al, 2008). In the recognition and management of neonatal seizures, clinical diagnosis alone is not enough. Although amplitude-integrated EEG (aEEG) provides simplified bedside monitoring of cerebral functioning, proposed schemes are needed to combine screening with aEEG followed by conventional EEG monitoring (El-Dib et al, 2009).

Ictal Electroencephalographic Patterns: A More Reliable Marker for Seizure Onset, Duration, and Severity

Neonatal electroencephalographic seizure patterns commonly consist of a repetitive sequence of waveforms that evolve in frequency, amplitude, electrical field, and/or morphology. Four types of ictal patterns have been described: focal ictal patterns with normal backgrounds, focal patterns with abnormal backgrounds, multifocal ictal patterns, and focal monorhythmic periodic patterns of various frequencies (Scher, 2001b). It is generally suggested that a minimal duration of 10 seconds for the evolution of discharges is required to distinguish electrographic seizures from repetitive but nonictal epileptiform discharges (Bye and Flannagan, 1995; Clancy and Legido, 1987; Scher et al, 1993) (see Figure 63-1). Clinical neurophysiologists alternatively classify brief or prolonged repetitive discharges that lack this electrographic evolution as nonictal abnormal epileptiform patterns, which does not conform to the seizure definition.

For the older patient, status epilepticus is defined as at least 30 minutes of continuous seizures or two consecutive seizures with an interictal period during which the patient fails to return to full consciousness. This definition, however, does not easily apply to the neonate because levels of arousal are difficult to assess, particularly if sedative medications are given. Neonatal status epilepticus was reported in one third of full-term infant EEG recordings and in 20% of the total cohort of preterm and full-term infant EEG recordings (Scher et al, 1993) using a definition of status epilepticus as continuous seizure activity for 30 minutes or 50% of the recording time. If clinicians relied only on clinical criteria, status epilepticus would be underdiagnosed. Without EEG confirmation, the underdiagnosis of status epilepticus would contribute to brain injury, as discussed later in the section "Effects of Neonatal Seizures on Brain Development: Consequences of Underdiagnosis."

Uncoupling of the clinical and electrographic expressions of neonatal seizures after antiepileptic medication

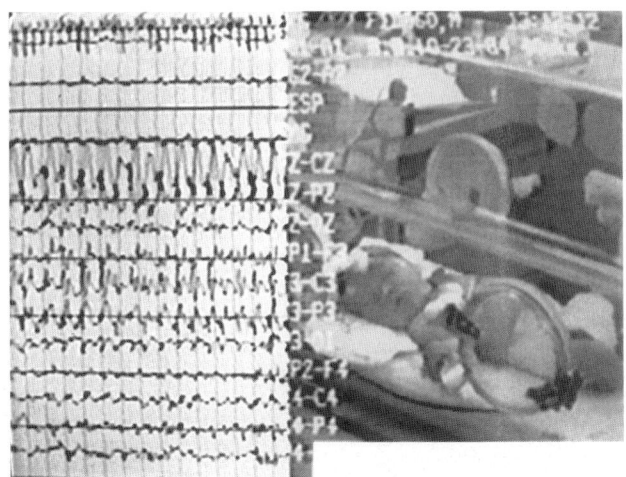

FIGURE 63-5 Segment of a synchronized video-electroencephalographic recording from a 40-week-gestation, 1-day-old male infant with electrographic status epilepticus noted in the left central/midline regions, after antiepileptic medication administration. Focal right shoulder clonic activity was only intermittently noted, while continuous electrographic seizures were documented mostly without clinical expression. This phenomenon of uncoupling of electrical and clinical seizure activities is associated with antiepileptic drug administration (see text). *(From Scher MS, Painter MJ: Controversies concerning neonatal seizures. In Pellock JM, editor: Seizure disorders, Pediatr Clin North Am 36:290, 1989.)*

administration also contributes to the underestimation of the true seizure duration and frequency of status epilepticus (Figure 63-5). One study estimated that 25% of neonates expressed persistent electrographic seizures despite resolution of their clinical seizure behaviors after receiving one or more antiepileptic medications (Scher, 1994); this phenomenon is termed *electroclinical uncoupling.*

The neonate may alternately express or sustain repetitive or periodic discharges greater than 10 seconds in duration that do not satisfy the electrographic criteria for seizures. The same neonate may express both periodic discharges and electrographic seizures at other times during the same EEG recording (Scher and Beggarly, 1989).

At the opposite end of the spectrum from periodic discharges, brief rhythmic discharges that are less than 10 seconds in duration also do not satisfy electroencephalographic criteria for seizures. Some neonates with electrographic seizures also may exhibit these brief discharges. Both periodic and brief discharges are associated with compromised neurodevelopmental outcome (Oliveira et al, 2000; Scher and Painter, 1989).

Subcortical Seizures versus Nonictal Functional Decortication

Experimental animal models offer conflicting evidence regarding suspicious clinical events for which coincident electrographic confirmation of seizures is absent (Scher, 2001b). Most neurologists prefer documentation of an ictal pattern by surface EEG electrodes before diagnosing a seizure. However, subcortical seizures with or without intermittent propagation to the surface may also occur. Electroclinical disassociation (ECD) is one proposed mechanism by which subcortical neonatal seizures intermittently appear on surface-recorded EEG studies

(Biagioni et al, 1998; Weiner et al, 1991). ECD is defined as a reproducible clinical event that occurs both with and without coincidental electrographic seizures, documented in one study as 34% of 51 neonates (Weiner et al, 1991). A clinical seizure precedes the electrographic expression, suggesting a subcortical onset before propagation to the cortical surface.

Some investigators have proposed a nonictal "brainstem release" phenomenon that explains suspicious clinical events that never have coincident EEG seizures expressed on surface recording (Mizrahi and Kellaway, 1998). These authors argue, for example, that motor automatisms have an inconsistent relationship with coincident EEG seizure activity. They alternatively speculate that functional nonictal decortication resulting from neocortical damage best explains these movements, without diagnosing epileptic seizures (Kellaway and Hrachovy, 1983).

This dilemma should encourage the clinician to use the EEG as a neurophysiologic yardstick by which more exact seizure start and end points can be assigned, before offering pharmacologic treatment with antiepileptic drugs (AEDs). Neonates can exhibit electrographic seizures that will go undetected unless EEG studies are utilized (O'Meara et al, 1995; Scher et al, 1993) (Figure 63-6; see also Figure 63-5). For example, in neonates who have been pharmacologically paralyzed for ventilatory assistance or in those who have received AEDs, clinical expression of seizures will be suppressed. In one cohort of 92 infants, 60% were pretreated with antiepileptic medications, and 50% of the cohort had electrographic seizures with no clinical accompaniment. Both clinical and electrographic seizure criteria were noted for 45% of 62 preterm infants and 53% of 30 full-term infants. Seventeen infants were pharmacologically paralyzed when the electrographic seizure was first documented. In a another cohort of 60 infants who were not pretreated with antiepileptic medications, 7% of infants had only electrographic seizures before AED administration, and 25% expressed electroclinical uncoupling after AED use (Scher, 1994).

Both overestimation and underestimation of neonatal seizure incidences are reported, depending on whether clinical or electrical criteria are used. Based on clinical criteria, seizure incidences ranged from 0.5% in term infants to 22.2% in preterm neonates (Lanska et al, 1995; Ronen et al, 1999; Seay and Bray, 1977). Discrepancies in incidence estimates reflect varying postconceptional ages of the study populations chosen, interobserver variability, and the hospital setting in which the diagnosis was made. Hospital-based studies, which will include a greater incidence of high-risk deliveries, generally report a higher seizure incidence. Population studies that include less medically fragile infants from general nurseries report lower percentages. Incidence figures based only on clinical criteria without EEG confirmation include "false positives," consisting of cases in which the neonates had either normal or nonepileptic pathologic neonatal behaviors. Conversely, the lack of electrographic seizures may include a subset of "false negatives," in which the infants express seizures only from subcortical brain regions, without propagation to the cortical surface. Consensus between clinical and EEG criteria, therefore, is still needed to reach the best incidence estimate.

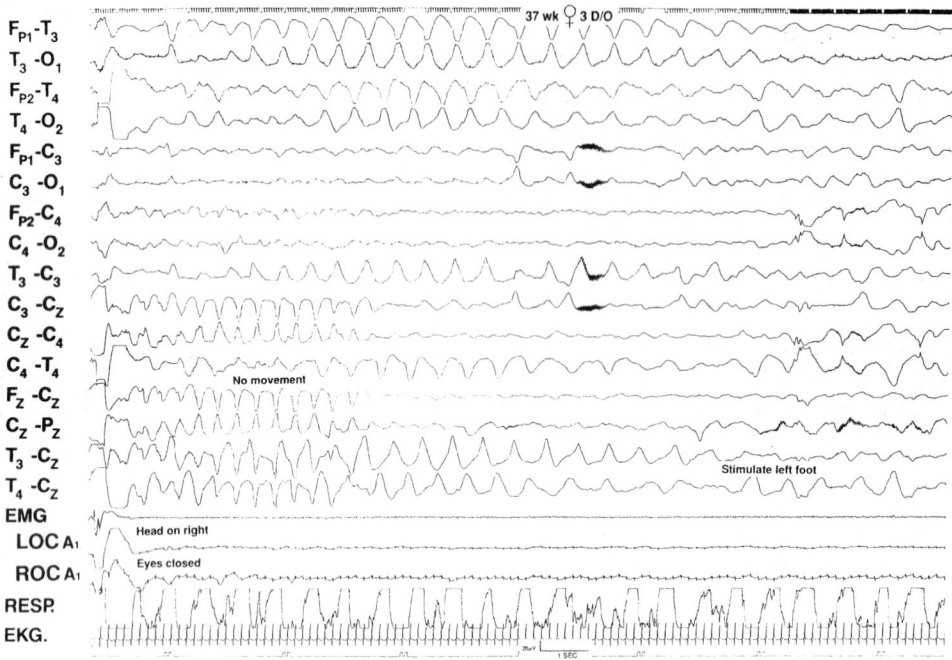

FIGURE 63-6 Segment of a synchronized video-electroencephalographic recording from a 37-week-gestation, 3-day-old female infant who was pharmacologically paralyzed for ventilatory care. A seizure is noted in the right posterior quadrant and midline. *(From Scher MS, Painter MJ: Controversies concerning neonatal seizures. In Pellock JM, editor: Seizure disorders,* Pediatr Clin North Am *36:290, 1989.)*

Interictal Electroencephalographic Abnormalities

Besides use of the EEG to diagnose seizures, documentation of interictal EEG abnormalities is extremely useful for patient management and prognosis. Interictal EEG findings are not pathognomonic for particular etiologic disorders, mechanisms, or timing (Scher, 1994). The clinician must integrate historical, physical examination, and laboratory findings with the electrographic interpretation of both seizure and nonseizure pattern findings for the particular child. The depth and the severity of neonatal brain disorders, as measured by the markedly abnormal interictal findings, help to predict subsequent development of seizures (Laroia et al, 1998). Serial EEG studies help the clinician to predict long-term outcome (see later section on prognosis).

DIAGNOSTIC DILEMMAS: IDENTIFYING CAUSES FOR SEIZURES

Diverse medical conditions in the newborn can be associated with seizure activity (Adamson et al, 1995; Kellaway and Hrachovy, 1983) (Table 63-3). Asphyxia is traditionally introduced as the representative etiologic disorder that exemplifies when seizures may occur. The asphyxial condition, however, encompasses heterogeneous conditions associated with hypoxia-ischemia, which may lead to seizures over a variable timeline encompassing antepartum, intrapartum, and neonatal periods.

Neonatal seizures are not disease-specific and can be associated with a variety of medical conditions occurring before, during, or after parturition. Seizures may occur as part of an asphyxial brain disorder that is expressed after birth (i.e., hypoxic-ischemic encephalopathy). Alternatively,

neonatal encephalopathies may represent other etiologic disorders with incidental asphyxia. Finally, seizures can present as an isolated clinical sign secondary to a remote antepartum asphyxial stress without other signs of a postnatal encephalopathy. A logistic model developed to predict seizures emphasizes the accumulation of both antepartum and intrapartum factors that increase the likelihood of neonatal seizure occurrence in the context of asphyxia (Patterson et al, 1989). Although separately these same factors have low positive predictive values, a significant cumulative risk profile results when maternal anemia, vaginal bleeding, asthma, meconium-stained amniotic fluid, abnormal fetal presentation, fetal distress, and shoulder dystocia all are considered. Another study of 40 neonates with clinical seizures indicated that only 37.5% of the seizures were associated with asphyxia, whereas a majority of term infants had early-onset seizures due to malformation, stroke, infection, or hemorrhage (Lien et al, 1995). In a population-based study, several antepartum and intrapartum factors increased the risk of neonatal seizures during the birth admission (Glass et al, 2009b). Infants of women whose age was 40 years and older who were nulliparous, had diabetes mellitus, intrapartum fever, or infection or delivered at greater than 42 weeks had an increased risk of seizures.

HYPOXIA-ISCHEMIA

Hypoxia-ischemia or asphyxia is nonetheless traditionally considered the most common cause of neonatal seizures (Brown et al, 1972, 1974; Sarnat and Sarnat, 1976; Volpe, 2001). However, infants can suffer asphyxia before as well as during parturition, and 10% of neonatal asphyxia cases also result from postnatal causes (Volpe, 2001). When asphyxia is suspected during the labor and delivery

TABLE 63-3 Differential Diagnosis of Neonatal Seizures*

Metabolic	Congenital infections
Hypoxia-ischemia (i.e., asphyxia)	Herpes simplex
Hypoglycemia	Syphilis
Hypocalcemia	Cytomegalovirus infection
Hypomagnesemia	Coxsackievirus
Hypoglycemia	Meningoencephalitis
Glycogen storage disease	Toxoplasmosis
Galactosemia	Acquired immunodeficiency syndrome (AIDS)
Idiopathic	Brain abscess
Hypomagnesemia	Brain anomalies (i.e., cerebral dysgenesis from either congenital or acquired causes)
Infant of a diabetic mother	
Neonatal hypoparathyroidism	
Maternal hyperparathyroidism	Drug withdrawal or toxins
	Prenatal exposure to substances of abuse—methadone, heroin, barbiturate, cocaine
High phosphate load	
Other electrolyte imbalances	Prescribed medications— propoxyphene, isoniazid
Hypernatremia	
Hyponatremia	Local anesthetics
Intrauterine growth restriction	Hypertensive encephalopathy
Infant of a diabetic mother	Amino acid metabolism
Intracranial hemorrhage	Branched-chain amino acidopathies
Subarachnoid hemorrhage	
Subdural/epidural hematoma	Urea cycle abnormalities
Intraventricular hemorrhage	Nonketotic hyperglycinemia
Cerebrovascular lesions (other than trauma)	Ketotic hyperglycinemia
	Familial seizures
Cerebral infarction (thrombotic vs. embolic causes)	Neurocutaneous syndromes
	Tuberous sclerosis
Ischemic vs. hemorrhagic lesions	Incontinentia pigmenti
	Autosomal dominant neonatal seizures
Cortical vein thrombosis	
Circulatory disturbances from hypoperfusion	Selected genetic syndromes
	Zellweger's syndrome
Trauma	Neonatal adrenoleukodystrophy
Infections	
Bacterial meningitis	Smith-Lemli-Opitz syndrome
Viral encephalitis	

*Etiology independent of timing from fetal to neonatal periods.
Adapted from Scher MS: Neonatal seizures: an expression of fetal or neonatal brain disorders. In Stevenson DK, Benitz WE, Sunshine P, editors: *Fetal and neonatal brain injury: mechanisms, management and the risks of practice,* ed 3, Cambridge, UK, 2002, Cambridge University Press, pp 735-784.

process, biochemical confirmation is required. This metabolic definition of asphyxia represents the cardinal feature of hypoxic-ischemic encephalopathy (HIE).

The American College of Obstetricians and Gynecologists (ACOG) initially published guidelines that suggest four cardinal criteria to define postasphyxial neonatal encephalopathy—that is, HIE—after significant clinical depression noted at birth (ACOG, 2003). These four criteria include:

1. Profound metabolic or mixed acidemia with a pH of less than 7.00 in umbilical cord blood
2. Persistence of an Apgar score of 0 to 3 for longer than 5 minutes
3. Neonatal neurologic sequelae (i.e., seizures, coma, and hypotonia)
4. Multiorgan system dysfunction (i.e., significant cardiovascular, gastrointestinal, hematologic, pulmonary, and renal involvement)

More recent guidelines have been published that suggest stricter criteria, including the four cardinal criteria as well

as four collective criteria. Clinicians now recognize that antepartum etiologies from maternal, placental, and/or fetal conditions explain 85% to 90% of HIE, whereas intrapartum etiologies account for a minority of HIE cases, between 10% and 15% (Graham et al, 2008).

OTHER CAUSES OF NEONATAL ENCEPHALOPATHY

Diverse etiologic disorders and conditions occurring in the antepartum, intrapartum, and neonatal periods may cause neonatal encephalopathies, with or without accompanying seizures. Children certainly may exhibit altered arousal and muscle tone, as well as seizures, without meeting the suggested criteria for HIE from intrapartum causes (ACOG, 2003). These children can appear neurologically abnormal based on antepartum conditions involving maternal, placental, or fetal diseases (Adamson et al, 1995).

A case-control study of term infants with clinical seizures reported a fourfold increase in the risk of unexplained early-onset seizures after intrapartum fever (Lieberman et al, 2000). All known causes of seizures were eliminated including meningitis and sepsis. Compared with 152 controls, the 38 newborns experienced intrapartum fever as an independent risk factor on logistic regression analysis that predicted seizures. The authors speculated on the role of circulating maternal cytokines that triggered "physiologic events" contributing to neonatal encephalopathy seizures, which did not occur from asphyxia.

Postnatal medical illnesses also cause or contribute to asphyxia-induced brain injury and seizures without intrapartum HIE. Persistent pulmonary hypertension of the newborn (PPHN), cyanotic congenital heart disease, sepsis, and meningitis are several examples. In one hospital-based study conducted over a 14-year period, 62 of 247 infants presented with EEG-confirmed seizures after an uneventful delivery without fetal distress during labor or neonatal depression at birth. Twenty of these 62 infants (32%) later presented with postnatal onset of pulmonary disease, sepsis, or meningitis (Scher, 1994).

Placental findings may reflect chronic disease states at antepartum time points with or without metabolic acidosis and evolving HIE after birth (Scher, 2002). Although meconium passage more commonly occurs in otherwise healthy newborns, meconium-stained skin also may be associated with meconium-laden macrophages within placental membranes in the depressed newborn. Meconium staining through the chorionic to amnion layers suggests a longer-standing asphyxial stress over a 4- to 6-hour period, which may precede the labor period.

Placental weights below the 10th or above the 90th percentile suggest chronic perfusion abnormalities to the fetus over weeks. Microscopic evidence of lymphocytic infiltration, altered villous maturation, chorangiosis, and erythroblastic proliferation of villi of the placenta support chronic asphyxial stresses to the fetus. In a study of preterm and full-term neonates (23 to 42 weeks of chronologic age) with electrographically confirmed seizures, a significant association between seizures and chronic (with or without acute) placental lesions was noted by calculated odds-risk ratios, increasing to a factor of 12.1 (P <.003) by term age. In contrast, odds ratios were not significant for infants with seizures and exclusively acute placental lesions, presumably from events closer to labor and delivery (Scher et al, 1998).

Clinical examination findings in the depressed neonate with suspected HIE may reflect antepartum disease states rather than evolving HIE (Ajayi et al, 1998). Intrauterine growth restriction, hydrops fetalis, and joint contractures (including arthrogryposis) are findings that suggest intrauterine disease conditions associated with antepartum disease states. Later intrapartum fetal distress with or without asphyxia and neonatal depression also may occur with subsequent neonatal seizures (Scher, 2001a, 2001c). Hypertonicity, often with cortical thumbs (i.e., severely adducted across closed palms), in a depressed child who then rapidly recovers over hours after a successful resuscitative effort also suggests a longer-standing fetal brain disorder. Sustained hypotonia and unresponsiveness for 3 to 7 days constitute the expected clinical repertoire of HIE after an intrapartum asphyxial stress, either with or without coincident brain injury. In encephalopathic newborns, depressed arousal and hypotonia nonetheless also may reflect an antepartum disease process with neonatal dysfunction or superimposed injury after a stressful intrapartum period. For example, this was described in 10 of 20 neurologically depressed infants with electrographic seizures and isoelectric interictal EEG pattern abnormalities, who were comatose and flaccid for days, requiring ventilator assistance after difficult deliveries (Barabas et al, 1993). All children appeared neurologically depressed after asphyxial stress during the intrapartum period (i.e., depressed Apgar scores and metabolic acidosis). Fetal brain injury from preexisting maternal-placental diseases was documented by evidence of chronic brain lesions on neuroimaging studies and/or neuropathologic postmortem findings. Although intrapartum asphyxial stress may worsen brain injury in some children, it was impossible to differentiate the neonatal encephalopathy from preexisting antepartum brain injury for these 10 children.

HYPOGLYCEMIA

Hypoglycemia is generally defined as glucose levels of less than 20 mg/dL in preterm infants and less than 30 mg/dL in term infants (Cornblath and Schwartz, 1967; Milner, 1972). No clear consensus exists concerning a direct cause and effect for hypoglycemia with seizure occurrence (Sencor, 1973). Methods of glucose determination (i.e., point-of-care blood sampling versus laboratory serum sampling) will affect the accuracy of the value. Also, associated disturbances may coexist, such as hypocalcemia, craniocerebral trauma, cerebrovascular lesions, and asphyxia, which may contribute to lowering the threshold for seizures. Infants born to diabetic or preeclamptic mothers, particularly those who were small for gestational age, also are at risk for hypoglycemia. Jitteriness, apnea, and altered tone are clinical signs that may appear in children with hypoglycemia, but they are not representative of a seizure state. Cerebrovascular lesions in posterior brain regions have been reported in children who suffer hypoglycemia (Griffiths and Laurence, 1974). Vulnerability of brain to ischemic insults is enhanced by concomitant hypoglycemia, as reported in mature animals (Siemkowicz and Hansen, 1978) and neonatal infants (Griffiths and Laurence, 1974).

HYPOCALCEMIA

Total serum calcium levels of less than 7.5 mg/dL in preterm and less than 8 mg/dL in the term infant generally define hypocalcemia. The ionized fraction is a more sensitive indicator of seizure vulnerability. As with hypoglycemia, the exact level of hypocalcemia at which seizures occur is debatable. An ionized fraction of 0.6 or less may have a more predictable association with the occurrence of seizures. Late-onset hypocalcemia due to use of high-phosphate infant formula has been previously cited as a common cause of seizures (Keen and Lee, 1973; McInerny and Schubert, 1969; Rose and Lombroso, 1970). However, hypocalcemia now more commonly occurs in infants with trauma, hemolytic disease, or asphyxia and may coexist with hypoglycemia or hypomagnesemia. Rarely, congenital hypoparathyroidism occurring in association with other genetic abnormalities such as DiGeorge syndrome (i.e., velocardiofacial syndrome, with a 22q11 deletion associated with cardiac and brain anomalies) must be considered. Affected infants may have severe congenital heart disease, as well as hypoparathyroid state with hypocalcemia and hypomagnesemia, which precipitates seizures (Lynch and Rust, 1994). Hypocalcemia of unknown etiology in infants also may be the result of maternal hypercalcemia. Ascertainment of the mother's calcium status should be considered, because maternal hypercalcemia can suppress fetal parathyroid development.

HYPONATREMIA AND HYPERNATREMIA

Hyponatremia is a metabolic disturbance that may result from inappropriate secretion of antidiuretic hormone after severe brain trauma, infection, or asphyxia (Volpe, 2001) but is an uncommon isolated cause of neonatal seizures. Hypernatremia also is a rare cause of seizures, usually associated with congenital adrenal abnormalities or iatrogenic disturbance of serum sodium balance, from the use of intravenous fluids with high concentrations of sodium.

CEREBROVASCULAR LESIONS

Hemorrhagic or ischemic cerebrovascular lesions are associated with neonatal seizures, on either an arterial or a venous basis (Clancy et al, 1985; Levy et al, 1985; Ment et al, 1984; Rivkin et al, 1992; Scher and Beggarly, 1989; Scher et al, 1986). Intraventricular or periventricular hemorrhage (IVH or PVH) is the most common intracranial hemorrhagic lesion in the preterm infant and has been associated with seizures in as much as 45% of a preterm population with EEG-confirmed seizures (Scher et al, 1993). In a cohort of newborns with clinical seizures, IVH was the predominant cause of seizures in preterm infants of less than 30 weeks' gestational age (Sheth et al, 1999). Intracranial hemorrhage is usually expected within the first 72 hours of life of the preterm infant. Although IVH-PVH may occur in otherwise asymptomatic infants, the neonate with a catastrophic deterioration of clinical status will exhibit signs of apnea, bulging fontanel, hypertonia, and seizures (Volpe, 2001). Seventeen percent of preterm infants with IVH may have acute seizures during the 1st month of life; 10% of one cohort suffered remote seizures

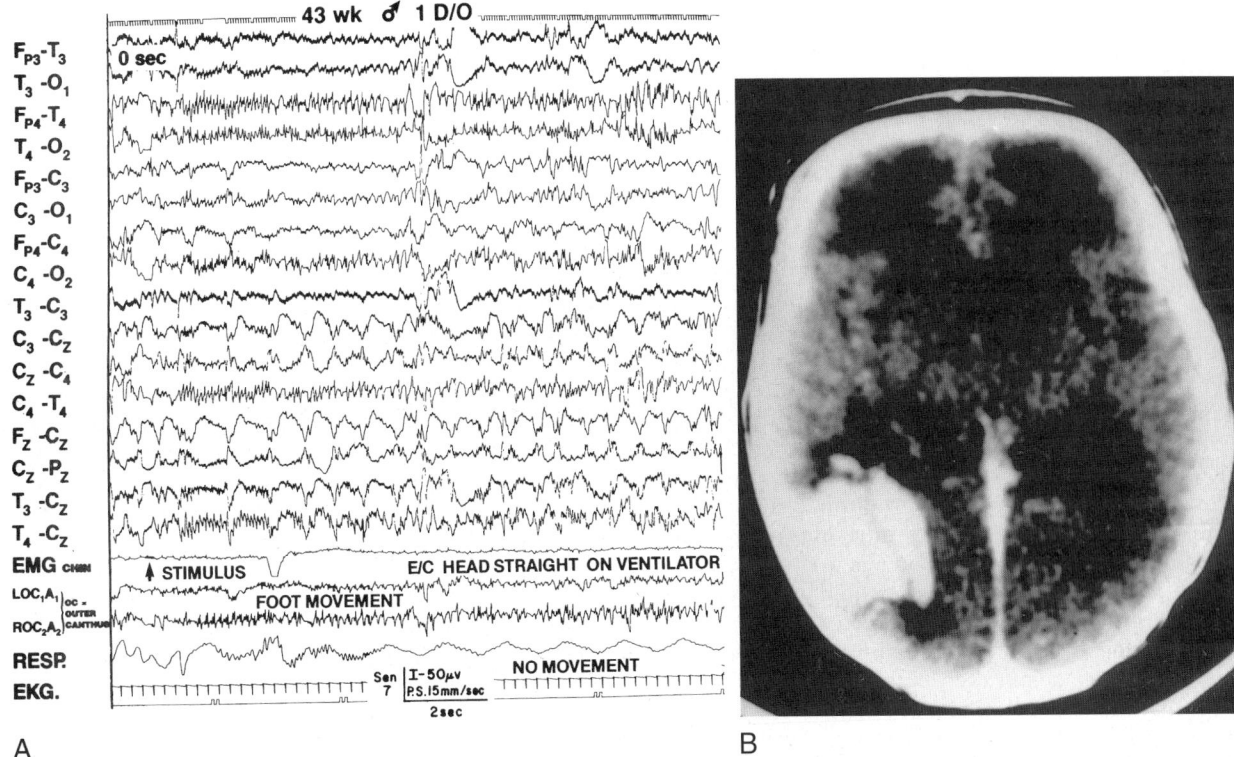

A   B

FIGURE 63-7 **A,** Segment of an electroencephalographic recording from a 43-week-gestation, 1-day-old male infant with a stimulus-evoked electrographic seizure (*arrow*) in the right temporal region, without clinical accompaniments. The child required ventilatory care for persistent pulmonary hypertension of the neonate (see text). **B,** Computed tomography scan on day 6 from the patient in **A,** documenting a hemorrhagic infarction in the right posterior quadrant with surrounding edema. *(From Scher MS, Klesh KW, Murphy TF, Guthrie RD: Seizures and infarction in neonates with persistent pulmonary hypertension,* Pediatr Neurol *2:332-339, 1986, with permission.)*

(after hospital discharge) (Strober et al, 1997). Full-term infants present less commonly with IVH, which usually originates from the choroid plexus or thalamus.

Another site of intracranial hemorrhage is the subarachnoid space; hemorrhage in this location may result in seizures but generally is associated with a more favorable outcome. Subdural hematoma, whether spontaneous or with craniocerebral trauma, should always be considered, particularly when focal trauma to the face, scalp, or head has occurred; simultaneous occurrences of cerebral contusion and infarction also should be considered.

Cerebral infarction has been described in neonates with seizures and can result from events during the antepartum, intrapartum, or neonatal period. Either preterm or term neonates with infarction also may present without seizure expression (De Vries et al, 1997). Seizures also can occur in otherwise healthy infants, suggesting an antepartum occurrence of cerebral infarction (Mercuri et al, 1995; Scher et al, 1991). Aggressive use of neuroimaging during the antepartum period by fetal sonography or magnetic resonance (MR) techniques, or within the first days after birth, may document remote brain lesions (Scher, 2001a,c). In a group of 62 healthy infants with electrographic seizures after an uneventful delivery, 23 (37%) had cerebrovascular lesions, and 18 of the 23 had ischemic brain lesions (Scher et al, 1993). Destructive lesions such as evolving porencephaly require approximately 5 to 7 days before becoming radiographically evident. The occurrence of injury during more recent intrapartum or neonatal periods can be supported by the presence of

early cerebral edema using diffusion-weighted MR images (Forbes et al, 2000). Cerebral infarction also may occur during the postnatal period from asphyxia, polycythemia, dehydration, or coagulopathy.

PPHN with severe and recurrent hypoxia also can be associated with cerebrovascular lesions and seizures (Scher et al, 1986) (Figure 63-7, *A* and *B*). Certain infants with PPHN will require extracorporeal membrane oxygenation (ECMO) to treat severe forms of this pulmonary disease, which does not respond to traditional ventilatory therapy. Radiographic documentation of brain lesions is needed before initiation of ECMO, because the anticoagulation required for ECMO may convert "bland" or ischemic infarctions to hemorrhagic forms, with greater risk for cerebral edema and herniation. Although meconium aspiration syndrome has historically been identified with an intrapartum/neonatal presentation of PPHN, in most affected children this lung disease generally is secondary to antepartum maternal/fetal or placental conditions that predispose the fetus to thickening of the muscular layers of the pulmonary arteries in utero, with resultant sustained increased pulmonary vascular resistance after birth (Benitz et al, 1997).

Cerebral infarction in the venous distribution of the brain may also lead to neonatal seizures (Rivkin et al, 1992; Shevell et al, 1989). Lateral or sagittal sinus thrombosis after coagulopathy can occur secondary to systemic infection, polycythemia, or dehydration. Venous infarction within the deep white matter of the preterm infant's brain also occurs in association with IVH.

INFECTION

Central nervous system infections during the antepartum or postnatal period can be associated with neonatal seizures (Kairam and De Vivo, 1981). A specific group of congenital infections—toxoplasmosis, rubella, cytomegalic inclusion disease, and herpes (the TORCH infections)—can produce severe encephalopathic damage that results in seizures, as well as more diffuse brain disorders. Other congenital infections include those due to enteroviruses and parvoviruses. Specific infections—for instance, neonatal herpes encephalitis—may be associated with severe EEG pattern abnormalities (Mizrahi and Tharp, 1982). Rubella, toxoplasmosis, and cytomegalic inclusion disease each also can lead to devastating encephalitis, usually manifesting with microcephaly, jaundice, body rash, hepatosplenomegaly, and/or chorioretinitis. Increasing lethargy and obtundation with or without seizures may suggest the subacute presentation of encephalitis during the postnatal period. Serial cerebrospinal fluid (CSF) analyses document progressively increasing protein levels and/or pleocytosis.

Bacterial infections from either gram-negative or gram-positive organisms, acquired in utero or postnatally, also are associated with neonatal seizures. Infection with some organisms, such as *Escherichia coli*, group B streptococci, *Listeria monocytogenes*, and *Mycoplasma*, may produce severe leptomeningeal infiltration, with possible abscess formation and cerebrovascular occlusions. A high percentage of survivors suffers significant neurologic sequelae.

CENTRAL NERVOUS SYSTEM MALFORMATIONS

Disorders occurring during the stages of induction, segmentation, proliferation, migration, myelination, and synaptogenesis can contribute to brain malformations. The neonate with such malformations is at increased risk for seizures in association with the stress experienced around the time of birth (Palmini et al, 1994), which presumably lowers seizure thresholds. Brain anomalies may occur as a result of either genetic causes from conception and/or acquired defects early during gestation. Specific dysgenesis syndromes, such as holoprosencephaly and lissencephaly, can be associated with characteristic facial or body anomalies. Cytogenetic studies may document trisomies or deletion defects. Unfortunately, infants may lack physical clues to the presence of a brain malformation. Therefore, a high index of clinical suspicion for this entity is warranted in evaluating neonates with persistent seizures. In one study, 9% of 356 infants who presented with neonatal seizures were found to have brain malformations (Sheth et al, 1999). Neuroimaging, preferably with MR techniques, documents brain dysgenesis in children who may also express severe electrographic disturbances including seizures. Local or regional brain malformations are rare causes of early-onset epilepsy in neonates and young infants (Aicardi, 1985; Ohtahara, 1978). Functional imaging studies such as positron emission tomography scans (Chugani et al, 1994) may identify localized areas of altered brain metabolism, which can assist in a neurosurgical approach to seizure management, even in young

children who fail to respond to AED maintenance (Pedespan et al, 1995).

INBORN ERRORS OF METABOLISM

Inherited biochemical abnormalities are rare causes of neonatal seizures (Scher, 2001b). Intractable seizures associated with elevated lactate and pyruvate levels in blood and CSF may reflect specific inborn errors of metabolism. Dysplastic or destructive brain lesions, as documented on neuroimaging, may be associated with specific biochemical defects, such as glycine encephalopathy or branched-chain aminoacidopathies. Pregnancy, labor, and delivery histories for affected infants are commonly uneventful. The emergence of poor feeding and also increasing lethargy, stupor, coma, and seizures are early indications of an inborn metabolic disturbance during the first few days of life. The newborn with an inherited metabolic disorder may initially present as a neurologically depressed and hypotonic child with asphyxia and seizures (Barth, 1992). Some children respond to specific dietary therapies, including vitamin supplementation (Painter et al, 1984), depending on the enzymatic defect. Specific urea cycle defects such as carbamoylphosphate synthetase deficiency may manifest as coma and seizures during the first 2 days of life, with marked elevations in plasma ammonia levels. Affected infants may respond to aggressive treatment with exchange transfusion, dialysis, and appropriate dietary adjustments.

Pyridoxine (vitamin B_6) dependency is an uncommon cause of neonatal seizures. Pyridoxal-5′-phosphate is the cofactor for more than 100 enzymatic reactions, of which several are important for the central nervous system metabolism of various amino acids and neurotransmitters. Infants with pyridoxine-dependent epilepsy (PDE) generally present with anticonvulsant resistant seizures within the first several days of life, frequently associated with signs of encephalopathy including irritability, sleeplessness, and hypotonia (Gospe, 2010). In retrospect, some mothers will occasionally report paroxysmal fetal movements. In this clinical setting, the infant who is unresponsive to conventional antiepileptic medications should promptly receive an intravenous injection of 100 mg of pyridoxine; up to 500 mg administered over 30 minutes may be needed to obtain a clinical response. Although a pathognomonic EEG pattern is not seen in this disorder, concomitant EEG monitoring may be helpful to evaluate the extent of electrographic seizure activity and to aid in following the clinical response to pyridoxine administration (Schmitt et al, 2010). Termination of clinical seizures within minutes to hours as well as improvement in the EEG supports a clinical diagnosis of PDE. For these patients, pyridoxine administered in pharmacologic doses of 15 mg/kg/day is needed to maintain seizure control. PDE is an autosomal recessive disorder due to mutations in the *ALDH7A1* gene, and affected patients have elevated levels of α-aminoadipic semialdehyde in blood and urine. Patients with clinically suspected PDE should have molecular and/or biochemical confirmation of the disorder (Gospe, 2001).

Other rare causes of seizures include disorders of carbohydrate metabolism with coincident hypoglycemia (Scher, 2002) as well as peroxisomal disorders such as neonatal adrenoleukodystrophy or Zellweger's syndrome. A defect in a glucose transporter protein necessary to move glucose across the blood-brain barrier also has been reported, which results in hypoglycorrhachia and seizures (De Vivo et al, 1991). Affected children may achieve seizure control with a ketogenic diet but nonetheless suffer delayed development.

Molybdenum cofactor deficiency and isolated sulfite oxidase deficiencies are other rare metabolic defects that cause neonatal seizures and associated destructive changes on neuroimaging, which may resemble findings in cerebrovascular disease or asphyxia (Slot et al, 1993).

DRUG WITHDRAWAL AND INTOXICATION

Newborns born to mothers with a history of prenatal substance abuse may be at increased risk for neonatal seizures (Herzlinger et al, 1977; Zelson et al, 1971). Exposure to barbiturates, alcohol, heroin, cocaine, or methadone commonly results in neurologic abnormalities that include tremors and irritability. More recently, withdrawal movements such as tremors have been identified with selective serotonin reuptake inhibitors (SSRIs) (Kuschel, 2007). Although noted during the immediate postnatal period, withdrawal symptoms may also occur as long as 4 to 6 weeks after birth (Kandall and Gartner, 1974; Zelson et al, 1971); EEG studies are useful to corroborate such movements with coincident electrographic seizures. Certain drugs such as short-acting barbiturates may be associated with seizures within the first several days of life (Bleyer and Marshall, 1972). Seizures may occur directly after substance withdrawal or may be associated with longer-standing uteroplacental insufficiency, promoted by chronic substance use and poor prenatal health maintenance by the mother. Careful review of placental/cord specimens may reveal chronic or acute pathologic lesions that contribute to antepartum or intrauterine asphyxia.

Inadvertent fetal injection with a local anesthetic agent during delivery may induce intoxication, which is a rare cause of seizures (Dodson, 1976; Hillman et al, 1979). Patients present during the first 6 to 8 hours of life with apnea, bradycardia, and hypotonia and are comatose, without brainstem reflexes. If the obstetric history indicates pudendal administration of an anesthetic to the mother, a careful examination of the child's scalp or body for puncture marks is indicated. Determination of plasma levels of the suspected anesthetic agent will establish the diagnosis. Treatment consists of ventilatory support and removal of the drug by therapeutic diuresis, acidification of the urine, or exchange transfusion. Antiepileptic medications are rarely indicated.

PROGRESSIVE NEONATAL EPILEPTIC SYNDROMES

Progressive epileptic syndromes rarely manifest during the 1st month of life (Mizrahi and Clancy, 2000). These children usually exhibit myoclonic or migratory seizures that are poorly controlled by antiepileptic medications, with brain malformations often demonstrable on brain imaging (Ekert et al, 1997; Ohtahara, 1978). These neonatal epileptic syndromes are termed *early myoclonic encephalopathy* or *early infantile epileptic encephalopathy* (Ohtahara syndrome), and the EEG commonly documents burst suppression or markedly disorganized background rhythms. Rarely, a neonate with idiopathic localization-related or partial seizures without neuroimaging abnormalities presents with intractable epilepsy (Natsume et al, 1996).

With neurocutaneous syndromes such as incontinentia pigmenti and tuberous sclerosis, symptomatic epilepsy during the neonatal period may be the presenting clinical manifestation of either of these genetic disorders. Incontinentia pigmenti is accompanied by a vesicular crusting rash, which initially mimics a herpetic infection. Seizures may or may not be present. The skin lesions evolve into lightly pigmented, raised sebaceous lesions in older infants and children. Tuberous sclerosis also rarely manifests with skin lesions in the newborn period. Hypopigmented lesions, initially noted under ultraviolet light, usually appear later during infancy. Two fetal presentations of tuberous sclerosis are that of the more common cardiac tumor, usually a rhabdomyoma, and rarely that of a congenital brain tumor, both noted on fetal sonography. Neonatal seizures also may be the presenting feature (Miller et al, 1998), with documentation of intracranial lesions on postnatal neuroimaging.

BENIGN FAMILIAL NEONATAL SEIZURES

The autosomal dominant form of neonatal seizures is a rare genetic epilepsy that should be considered in the context of a positive family history (Bjerre and Corelius, 1968; Pettit and Fenichel, 1980; Ryan et al, 1991). Exclusion of infectious, metabolic, toxic, or structural causes needs to be completed before this entity is considered in the diagnosis. The genetic defect was first described on chromosome 20q, specifically at the D20S19 and D20S20 loci, as well as a locus EBN2 on chromosome 8q24. By positional cloning, a potassium channel gene (*KCNQ2*) located on 20q13.3 was first isolated and found to be expressed in the brain (Bjerre and Corelius, 1968). A second potassium channel gene (*KCNQ3*) also has been described and may explain the variability in phenotypic expression of seizures and outcome (Leppert and Singh, 1999). Recently, mutations in ion channels also have been implicated in Jervell and Lange-Nielsen syndrome, whose symptoms include congenital deafness and cardiac arrhythmias (Jentsch et al, 2000). Infant outcomes range from excellent to guarded, depending on the persistence of seizures beyond the neonatal period. Response to antiepileptic medication is generally good, although some clinicians describe variable success. Further studies are needed to clarify the relationship between phenotypic and genotypic expressions of this disorder.

SEIZURES REFLECTING FETAL OR NEONATAL BRAIN DISORDERS: GUIDE TO DIFFERENTIAL DIAGNOSIS

The neurologist must place EEG-confirmed seizures in the context of historical, clinical, and laboratory evidence to determine both the pathogenesis and timing of a brain disorder. Seizures occurring in neonates who have experienced asphyxia support either acute intrapartum events or antepartum disease processes, or both. Does the child with seizures also have clinical and laboratory signs of evolving cerebral edema? The presence of a bulging fontanel with neuroimaging evidence of increased intracranial pressure and cerebral edema (i.e., obliterated ventricular outline and abnormal diffusion-weighted MR images), hyponatremia, and increased urine osmolality (i.e., the syndrome of inappropriate secretion of antidiuretic hormone) more strongly suggest a more recent asphyxial disease process, in or around the intrapartum period, causing acute or subacute cerebral edema.

Alternatively, failure to document evolving cerebral edema during the first 3 days after asphyxia or documentation of encephalomalacia or cystic brain lesions on neuroimaging shortly after birth (even in the encephalopathic newborn) suggests a more chronic disease process with remote antepartum brain injury. Liquefaction necrosis requires 2 weeks or longer after a presumed asphyxial event to produce a cystic cavity (Friede, 1975) before becoming visible on neuroimaging.

Isolated seizures in an otherwise asymptomatic neonate also suggest a disease process that occurred during either the postnatal or the antepartum period. Neonates present with seizures as a result of postnatal illnesses from intracranial infection, cardiovascular lesions, drug toxicity, or inherited metabolic diseases. Children with antepartum injuries may express isolated seizures after in utero cerebrovascular injury secondary to thrombolytic and/or embolic disease of the mother, placenta, or fetus. Fetal injury alternatively may occur after ischemia-hypoperfusion events from circulatory disturbances such as maternal shock, chorioamnionitis, or placental fetal vasculopathy (Miller, 2000).

Only a fraction of neonates with cerebrovascular disease present with neonatal seizures (De Vries et al, 1997). Why some children remain asymptomatic until later during childhood is unknown. Neonatal expression of seizures may reflect superimposed stress during parturition, which lowers seizure threshold in susceptible brain regions that have been previously damaged.

After a careful review of the medical histories of the mother, fetus, and newborn, determination of serum glucose, electrolytes, ammonia, lactate, pyruvate, magnesium, calcium, and phosphorus levels may diagnose correctable metabolic conditions in newborns with seizures who will not require antiepileptic medications. CSF analyses including cell count, protein, glucose, lactate, pyruvate, amino acids, and culture studies are performed to assess for CNS infection, intracranial hemorrhage, and metabolic disease. Alternatively, metabolic acidosis on serial arterial blood gas determinations may suggest an inherited metabolic disease, particularly if intrapartum asphyxia was not judged to be severe. Absence of multiorgan dysfunction may alert the clinician to other potential causes of seizures besides intrapartum asphyxia. Signs of chronic in utero stress such as growth restriction, early hypertonicity after neonatal depression, joint contractures, or elevated nucleated red blood cell values all suggest longer-standing antepartum stress to the fetus. Genetic or syndromic conditions may contribute to the expression of neonatal encephalopathies independent of asphyxial injury (Felix et al, 2000). Careful review of placental and cord specimens also can be

extremely useful to help time a brain insult. Neuroimaging, preferably using MR techniques, can locate, grade the severity of, and possibly time an insult (Leth et al, 1997) (i.e., using diffusion-weighted images). Ancillary studies may also include measurement of long-chain fatty acid and chromosomal/DNA analyses, as deemed necessary by family and clinical history. Finally, serum and urine organic acid and amino acid determinations may be needed to delineate a specific biochemical disorder for the child with a persistent metabolic acidosis. Lysosomal enzyme studies also are occasionally considered to diagnose specific enzymatic deficiencies in children with neonatal seizures.

CHALLENGES REGARDING PROGNOSTIC ASSESSMENTS

The mortality rate among infants who present with clinical neonatal seizures has declined from 40% to 15% (Volpe, 2001). Studies of EEG-confirmed seizures documented mortality rates of 50% in preterm and 40% in full-term infants during the 1980s (Scher and Painter, 1989; Scher et al, 1993), with the mortality rate dropping below 20% in the 1990s in the same obstetric center (Scher, 1997a). The incidence of adverse neurologic sequelae, however, remains high; approximately two thirds of survivors are so affected. Even if major neurodevelopmental sequelae such as motor deficits and mental retardation were avoided in survivors after neonatal seizures, subtle neurodevelopmental vulnerability may manifest in late teenage years as specific learning difficulties or poor social adjustment (Temple et al, 1995), underscoring more recent experimental findings of long-term deficits in animal populations (Holmes and Ben-Ari, 2001). The poor prognosis for premature infants with seizures is reflected in high rates of subsequent disability and mortality, suggesting that severity and timing of the pathologic process continue to be major determinants for outcome (Ronen et al, 2007).

Prediction of outcome should also consider the etiologic disorder for the seizures, such as severe asphyxia, significant craniocerebral trauma, and brain infections. More accurate imaging procedures (magnetic resonance imaging [MRI] in particular) have increased our awareness of destructive and congenital brain lesions with a higher risk for compromised outcome.

Interictal EEG pattern abnormalities are also extremely helpful in predicting neurologic outcome in the neonate with seizures (Bye et al, 1997; Monod et al, 1972; Sinclair et al, 1999; Tharp et al, 1981). Major background disturbances such as burst suppression are highly predictive of poor outcome, particularly when persistent abnormalities are still present on serial EEG studies into the 2nd week of life. Seizure patterns alone, however, are not accurate to predict outcome, unless quantified to high numbers, long durations, and multifocal distribution (McBride et al, 2000). In one study, normal findings on interictal EEGs were associated with an 86% chance of normal development at 4 years of age in 139 neonates with seizures (Rose and Lombroso, 1970); by contrast, neonates with markedly abnormal EEG background disturbances had only a 7% chance for normal outcome. Another study (Rowe et al, 1985) reported outcome in term and preterm infants with seizures, concluding that the EEG background was more predictive of outcome than the presence of isolated sharp wave discharges. Even severe electroencephalographic abnormalities on single-channel spectral EEG recordings after asphyxia carry a higher risk for sequelae (Hellstrom-Westas, 1992).

Neonates with seizures have an increased risk for epilepsy during childhood (Watanabe et al, 1982). On the basis of clinical seizure criteria, 20% to 25% of neonates with seizures later develop epilepsy (Holden et al, 1982). Excluding febrile seizures, the prevalence of epilepsy by 6 to 7 years of age is estimated to be between 15% and 30%, based on EEG-confirmed seizures for an inborn hospital population; two thirds of this cohort were preterm neonates (Scher et al, 1993). These findings are in contrast with an incidence of 56% with epilepsy for an exclusively outborn neonatal population of primarily full-term newborns with seizures (Clancy and Legido, 1991). Epilepsy risk therefore reflects selection bias of specific study groups, as well as referral patterns in different hospital settings. For example, low birthweight, short gestational age, and intrauterine growth restriction are associated with an increased risk of epilepsy (Sun et al, 2008).

DIAGNOSTIC DILEMMAS REGARDING TREATMENT CHOICES

CORRECTIVE THERAPIES

Rapid infusion of glucose or other supplemental electrolytes should be initiated before antiepileptic medications are considered. Hypoglycemia can be readily corrected by intravenous administration of 5 to 10 mg/kg of a 10% to 15% dextrose solution, followed by an infusion of 8 to 10 mg/kg/minute. Persistent hypoglycemia may require more hypertonic glucose solutions. Rarely, prednisone, 2 mg/kg/day, may be needed to establish a glucose level within the normal range (Scher, 2001b).

Hypocalcemia-induced seizures should be treated with an intravenous infusion of 200 mg/kg of calcium gluconate. This dosage should be repeated every 5 to 6 hours over the first 24 hours. Serum magnesium concentrations also should be measured, because hypomagnesemia may accompany hypocalcemia; 0.2 mg/kg of magnesium sulfate should be given by intramuscular injection (Scher, 2001b).

Disorders of serum sodium are rare causes of neonatal seizures. Either fluid restriction or replacement with hypotonic solutions is generally the mode of therapy for correcting sodium dysmetabolism.

Pyridoxine dependency requires the injection of 50 to 500 mg of pyridoxine during a seizure with coincident EEG monitoring. A beneficial pyridoxine effect occurs either immediately or over the first several hours. A daily dose of 50 to 100 mg of pyridoxine should then be administered (Scher, 2001b).

ANTIEPILEPTIC MEDICATIONS

If the decision to treat neonates with AEDs is reached, important questions must be addressed with respect to who should be treated, when to begin treatment, which drug to use, and for how long. Some clinicians suggest that only neonates with clinical seizures should receive medications; brief electrographic seizures need not be treated. Others suggest more aggressive treatment of electrographic seizures, because uncontrolled seizures potentially have an adverse effect on immature brain development (Dwyer and Wasterlain, 1982; Wasterlain, 1997). Others warn that early administration of an AED, such as phenobarbital, even before signs of HIE appear, may have adverse effects on outcome in term infants (Ajayi et al, 1998).

Phenobarbital and phenytoin, nonetheless, remain the most widely used AEDs; use of benzodiazepines, primidone, and valproic acid has been anecdotally reported (Scher, 2001b). The half-life of phenobarbital ranges from 45 to 173 hours in the neonate (Lockman et al, 1979; Painter et al, 1978, 1981); the initial loading dose is recommended at 20 mg/kg, with a maintenance dose of 3 to 4 mg/kg/day. Therapeutic levels are generally suggested to be between 16 and 40 µg/mL; however, there is no consensus with respect to drug maintenance.

The preferred loading dose of phenytoin is 15 to 20 mg/kg (Painter et al, 1978, 1981). Serum levels of phenytoin are difficult to maintain because this drug is rapidly redistributed to body tissues. Blood levels cannot be well maintained using an oral preparation. A water-soluble form, fosphenytoin, may be administered at the same loading dose. This specific agent has less harmful effects on the vein where it is injected.

Benzodiazepines also may be used to control neonatal seizures. The drug most widely used is diazepam. One early study suggests a half-life of 54 hours in preterm infants to 18 hours in full-term infants (Smith and Masotti, 1971). Intravenous administration is recommended because the drug is absorbed slowly after an intramuscular injection. Diazepam is highly protein-bound; alteration of bilirubin binding is low. Recommended intravenous doses for acute management should begin at 0.5 mg/kg. Deposition into muscle precludes its use as a maintenance antiepileptic medication, because profound hypotonia and respiratory depression may result, particularly if barbiturates also have been administered.

Efficacy of Treatment

Conflicting studies report varying efficacy with phenobarbital or phenytoin. Most studies only apply a clinical end point to seizure cessation. One study (Painter et al, 1978) found that only 36% of neonates with clinical seizures responded to phenobarbital; another study noted cessation of clinical seizures with phenobarbital in only 32% of neonates (Lockman et al, 1979). With doses as high as 40 mg/kg (Gal et al, 1982), the rate of clinical seizure control was reported to be 85%. A more recent study reported that the earlier administration of high-dose phenobarbital in a group of asphyxiated infants was associated with a 27% reduction in clinical seizures and better outcomes than in a group of infants who did not receive high dosages (Hall et al, 1998). However, coincident EEG studies are now suggested to verify the resolution of electrographic seizures. A recent report suggests that 25% of neonates have persistent electrographic seizures after suppression of clinical seizure behaviors following drug administration (Scher, 1994). With use of the EEG to judge cessation of seizures, neither phenobarbital nor phenytoin was effective in controlling seizure activity (Painter et al, 1999).

The use of free or drug-bound fractions of AEDs has been suggested to better assess both efficacy and potential toxicity of these drugs in pediatric populations (Painter et al, 1987). Drug binding in neonates with seizures has only recently been reported and can be altered in a sick neonate with organ dysfunction. Toxic side effects may result from elevated free fractions of a drug, which may adversely affect cardiovascular and respiratory functions. To guard against untoward effects, evaluation of treatment and efficacy must take into account both total and free AED fractions, in the context of the newborn's progression or resolution of systemic illness.

Novel Antiepileptic Drug Approaches

Mechanisms of seizure generation, propagation, and termination are different during early brain development as compared with more mature ages. These age-related mechanisms have partially been elucidated (Jensen, 1999; Sanchez and Jensen, 2001). Given that traditional antiepileptic medications have unacceptable efficacy to stop neonatal seizures for specific subsets of newborns, alternative medication options must be developed.

New antiepileptic alternatives to treat neonatal seizures are now being studied. One class of medications are the N-methyl-D-aspartate (NMDA) antagonists such as topiramate (Koh and Jensen, 2001). Experimental animal models of asphyxia-induced seizure activity in immature brains have indicated a certain degree of efficacy. Such models provide data regarding pharmacologi and physiological characteristics of neuronal responses after an asphyxial stress that cause excessive release of excitotoxic neurotransmitter (Jensen and Wang, 1996) such as glutamate. Specific cell membrane receptors termed metabotropic glutamate receptors (MGluRs) are sensitive to extracellular glutamate release and may play a role in epileptogenesis and seizure-induced brain damage (Aronica et al, 1997). One class of membrane receptor, for example, has been studied in rat pups after hypoxia-induced seizures, suggesting that MGluR downregulation can be associated with epileptogenesis in the absence of cell loss (Sanchez and Jensen, 2001). Subclasses of MGluRs will lead to investigations of novel drugs that block these membrane receptors as the mode of treatment for neonatal seizures (Lie et al, 2000).

Another therapeutic approach is suggested by experimental studies that demonstrate enhanced seizure susceptibility in the developing brain because γ-aminobutyric acid (GABA) exerts a depolarizing excitatory rather than repolarizing inhibitory action in immature subjects (Brooks-Kayal, 2005). This paradoxical action of GABA early in development may be due in part to age-related differences in chloride homeostasis (Lie et al, 2000). Chloride transport is a function of two membrane pumps with different time courses of expression. Early in development (i.e., in the rat, P3-P15 after birth), the Na^+-K^+-$2Cl^-$ cotransporter (NKCC1) imports large amounts of chloride into the neuron (along with sodium and potassium to maintain electroneutrality). This pump sets the chloride equilibrium potential positive to the resting potential so

that when the $GABA_A$ receptor is activated, chloride flows out of the neuron, depolarizing it. Differences in cortical versus subcortical GABAergic signaling from this chloride transporter have been demonstrated, suggesting that electroclinical uncoupling of neonatal seizures occurs more likely in cortical regions where NKCC1 cotransporter is more active (Glykys et al, 2009). Over time, NKCC1 expression diminishes, and another chloride transporter, KCC2, is expressed. KCC2 has the opposite effect; it extrudes chloride out of the neuron, placing the equilibrium potential more negative than the resting potential so that $GABA_A$ receptor activation allows extracellular chloride to flow into the neuron, hyperpolarizing it and endowing GABA with inhibitory action.

Researchers have termed this the developmental "switch" in chloride homeostasis. This maturational aspect to the chloride ion may influence seizure susceptibility in the neonatal brain. The additional depolarization that is due to $GABA_A$ receptor activation augments excitation that may be initiated by the glutamate neurotransmission. As a result, there is a shift in the excitation-inhibition balance toward excessive excitation, and thus toward seizure activity. These conclusions have been suggested by Dzhala et al (2005), who described the developmental profile of NKCC1 in the human neonate. In the early postnatal period, NKCC1 rises to a peak and then declines to adult levels. This rearrangement of membrane receptors occurs over the first several months of life. In the same time period, KCC2 expression gradually rises to adult levels. Blocking NKCC1 function with a commonly used diuretic known as bumetanide prevents the accumulation of intercellular chloride and therefore counteracts the depolarizing action of $GABA_A$ receptor activation. Bumetanide reduces kainate-induced seizures in neonatal but not adult rats and bursts firing in hippocampus slices. As further evidence, in genetically engineered mice that lack NKCC1, bumetanide is not effective in ameliorating seizures, supporting its role as a specific inhibitor of NKCC1. Therefore, bumetanide is now considered a promising antiepileptic drug with a developmental target, namely the immature chloride cotransporter NKCC1. Some claim that this particular diuretic can be safely used in the neonate, although its long-term safety profile needs to be better studied. It has also been recently suggested that pharmacologic agents that can diminish bursting behavior in neonatal neurons can add an additional level to the control of seizures. Dzhala et al (2005) demonstrated that bumetanide rapidly suppresses synchronous bursts of network activity in P4-P8 hippocampus slices in the rat model. This supports the use of this agent as a potential antiepileptic medication in this age group. Clinical trials need to demonstrate that bumetanide or other similar diuretics can inhibit seizure activity, with or without conventional medications such as phenobarbital (Haglund and Hochman, 2005). It will be necessary to establish that these agents can reach the brain in appropriate concentrations and lack short- as well as long-term side effects.

There are still crucial issues regarding the theory that GABA-mediated excitation may play an important role in human neonatal seizures which may be amenable to treatment as discussed earlier. It is yet unknown why some GABA-ergic agents such as phenobarbital and benzodiazepine fail to have adequate efficacy for human neonatal seizure control for a substantial subset of patients. Though seizures can be halted in a percentage of newborns, additional understanding of epileptogenesis in the immature brain must consider the timing and etiology-specific aspects of GABA-mediated mechanisms of seizures as they relate to asphyxia, infection, or trauma. A specific etiology may alter seizure threshold by epigenetic modification, changing the specific genetic variability within individuals in a time-sensitive manner. Based on up- or downregulation of genetic expression, individuals who suffer asphyxia, infection, or trauma may have variable vulnerability or resistance to GABA-mediated mechanisms for seizures. This generalization is further complicated by not only the timing of injury but also the specific brain region of damage, which may have occurred remotely either during the antepartum or during the intrapartum or neonatal period. Seizures from selectively damaged deep gray matter, neocortical layers, or white matter regions may respond differently to similar antiepileptic drug regimens. Therefore, one must consider whether neonatal seizures represent novel brain injury or are surrogates of injury resulting from etiologies either varied in brain location or during time periods beginning during fetal life (Scher, 2003). The neurologist must place events leading to seizures in the context of clinical, historical, and laboratory findings to determine both the pathogenesis and timing of an encephalopathic process in a neonate who is symptomatic with seizures. A new classification of neonatal seizures that integrates electrographic expression, brain region, etiology, and timing may then have more relevance to the choice of antiepileptic medication (Scher, 2006).

Discontinuation of Drug Use

The clinician's decision to maintain or discontinue AED use is also uncertain. Discontinuation of drugs before discharge from the NICU is generally recommended, because then clinical assessments of arousal, tone, and behavior will not be hampered by medication effect. However, newborns with congenital or destructive brain lesions on neuroimaging or those with persistently abnormal findings on neurologic examination at the time of discharge may require a slower taper off medication over several weeks or months. In most children with neonatal seizures, the seizures rarely reoccur during the first 2 years of life, and prophylactic AED administration need not be maintained past 3 months of age, even in the child at risk. This recommendation is supported by a recent study suggesting a low risk of seizure recurrence after early withdrawal of AED therapy in the neonatal period (Hellstrom-Westas et al, 1995). Also, older infants who present with specific epileptic syndromes, such as infantile spasms, will not respond to the conventional AEDs that were initially begun during the neonatal period. This honeymoon period without seizures commonly persists for many years in most children, before isolated or recurrent seizures appear.

The potential for damage to the developing CNS from AEDs also emphasizes the need to consider early discontinuation of these agents in the newborn period. Adverse effects on the morphology and metabolism of neuronal cells have been extensively reported from collective research performed over the past several decades (Mizrahi, 1999).

EFFECTS OF NEONATAL SEIZURES ON BRAIN DEVELOPMENT: CONSEQUENCES OF UNDERDIAGNOSIS

Embedded within the controversy regarding how to diagnose neonatal seizures (i.e., clinical vs. electroencephalographic) is the association of repetitive or prolonged seizures with brain damage both acutely and as a result of altered brain development. Linked to the clinician's concern for seizure duration is an appreciation of the diverse neuropathologic processes and etiologic disorders that cause neonatal seizures with resultant neurologic sequelae (Lien et al, 1995). CNS infections and severe asphyxia are two etiologic disorders that exemplify underlying pathophysiologic mechanisms responsible for brain damage in neonates independent of or with seizure expression.

During the acute phase of a neonatal brain disorder, seizures can cause or contribute to brain damage by drastically impairing the neurovascular unit. Such a unit is composed of pial and intraparenchymal cerebral arteries and arterioles, the extrinsic and intrinsic innervation of these vessels, and the perivascular astrocytes and neurons. Seizures can dramatically increase brain metabolism and cerebral blood flow during the ictal period, disrupt the blood-brain barrier, and cause an acute loss of cerebral pressure autoregulation, as well as a delayed impairment of cerebrovascular reactivity to various stimuli (Zimmerman et al, 2008). In addition to blood flow–related brain injury from seizure activity, seizures are associated with brain injury severity in a neonatal model of asphyxia. On postmortem examination, animals with seizures after asphyxia showed the greatest degree of neuropathologic injury compared to animals without seizures. Furthermore, animals with electrographic seizures with clinical signs had significantly greater histological damage compared to those with electrographic seizures alone, not apparent on MRI or spectroscopy. These results need to be duplicated in other animal studies as well as verified in human protocols involving seizures caused by multiple etiologies.

Adverse long-term effects of the seizure state on the developing brain have been reviewed (Holmes and Ben-Ari, 2001). Seizures can disrupt a cascade of biochemical and molecular pathways that normally are responsible for the plasticity or activity-dependent development of the maturing nervous system. Depending on the degree of brain immaturity, seizures may disrupt the processes of cell division, migration, and myelination; sequential expression of receptor formation; and stabilization of synapses—each of which contributes to the risk of neurologic sequelae, to varying degrees (Holmes, 2009; Holmes et al, 1998).

Experimental models of seizures in immature animals suggest comparatively less vulnerability to seizure-induced brain injury than in mature animals (Huang et al, 1999). In adult animals, seizures alter growth of hippocampal granule cells and of axonal and mossy fibers, resulting in long-term deficits in learning, memory, and behavior. A single prolonged seizure in an immature animal, on the other hand, results in less cell loss or fiber sprouting and consequentially fewer deficits in learning memory and behavior. Resistance to brain damage from prolonged seizure activity, however, is age-specific, as evidenced by increased cell damage after only 2 weeks of age (Sankar et al, 2000). A 2001 study examined developmental changes in epileptiform activity in neocortical preparations in four different age groups and using four different pharmacologic models. The study confirmed that there are definite age-dependent differences in susceptibility to epileptiform activity in the neocortex. These developmental changes seem to relate to intrinsic network properties of the neocortex that are independent of ontogenetic differences in any specific neurotransmitter system (Wong and Yamada, 2001). Nonetheless, experimental neonatal status epilepticus in a rodent model resulted in classic hippocampal sclerosis and temporal lobe epilepsy (Dunleavy et al, 2009), suggesting there may be a threshold for recurrent seizures in an immature brain above which altered neuronal network connectivity leads to epilepsy at older ages.

Repetitive or prolonged neonatal seizures alternatively can increase the susceptibility of the developing brain to suffer subsequent seizure-induced injury during adolescence or early adulthood, by altering neuronal connectivity rather than increasing cell death (Holmes and Ben-Ari, 2001; Holmes et al, 1998; Koh et al, 1999). Neonatal animals subjected to status epilepticus have reduced seizure thresholds at later ages and demonstrate impairments of learning, memory, and activity levels after suffering seizures as adults. Proposed mechanisms of injury also include reduced neurogenesis in the hippocampus, for example, possibly because of ischemia-induced apoptosis, as well as necrotic pathways (McCabe et al, 2001). Other suggested mechanisms of injury include effects of nitric oxide synthase inhibition on cerebral circulation, which then contributes to ischemic injury (Takei et al, 1999). Neonatal seizures, therefore, may initiate a cascade of diverse changes in brain development that become maladaptive at older ages and increase the risk of subsequent damage after subsequent insults. Destructive mechanisms such as mossy fiber sprouting in the hippocampus or increased neuronal apoptosis may explain mutually exclusive pathways by which the immature brain suffers altered connectivity and reduced cell number, which is then "primed" for later seizure-induced cell loss at older ages.

The critical duration of seizures, whether cumulative or continuous, remains elusive with respect to resultant brain injury. Given that as many as one third of full-term infants experience electrographic seizures that satisfy a definition of status epilepticus (Scher et al, 1993), EEG documentation appears crucial to assign seizure duration. A study of 10-day-old rat pups indicated that prolonged seizures for 30 minutes after asphyxia resulted in exacerbation of brain injury specific to the hippocampus, while sparing the neocortex. Prolonged neonatal seizures do worsen damage incurred by an already compromised brain (Wirrell et al, 2001) in a region-specific manner. In a neonatal rodent model of brief recurrent seizures, Landrot et al (2001) demonstrated increased mossy fiber sprouting in the granule cells of the hippocampus, which

correlated with impaired cognition and reduced EEG power spectra during adolescence. A companion study from the same laboratory demonstrated alterations in cognition and seizure susceptibility within 2 weeks of the last seizure before the adult pattern of mossy fiber distribution is achieved. Therefore, therapeutic strategies to alter the adverse outcomes of neonatal seizures must be initiated during or shortly after the seizures.

The overlapping effects of brain dysgenesis or injury from specific etiologic disorders versus seizure-induced brain damage make it difficult to differentiate preexisting brain lesions from the direct injurious effects of seizures themselves. The use of microdialysis probes in white and gray matter of piglet brains subjected to hypoxia indicates elevated lactate-pyruvate ratios after hypoxia but no direct association with seizure activity (Thoresen et al, 1998). These findings support the conclusion that seizures themselves may not always be injurious to brain.

The dearth of well-designed clinical investigations of outcome after neonatal seizures in humans unfortunately does not permit broad confirmation of these experimental findings. Better definitions of neonatal seizure severity, including electrographic expression and seizure duration, are required to help resolve this controversy. An investigation in human newborns with perinatal asphyxia suggests that seizure severity is independently associated with brain injury as measured by MR spectroscopy (Miller et al, 2002) and worse neurodevelopmental outcome (Glass et al, 2009a,b), but not all subjects had electrographic confirmation of seizures. Another study, however, used EEG confirmation of electrical status epilepticus and reported more severe neurodevelopmental disability and postnatal epilepsy (Pisani et al, 2007).

Aggressive use of antiepileptic medications without electroencephalographic confirmation contributes to the inaccurate estimate of seizure severity in neonates and possible medication-induced brain injury. Intractable seizures generally require the use of multiple antiepileptic medications, which may still not effectively control seizures (Painter et al, 1999). Drugs also may impede the clinician's ability to recognize persistent seizures, because of the uncoupling phenomenon in which the clinical expression is suppressed while the electrical expression of seizures continues. Clinical definitions of seizure occurrence and duration consequently underestimate seizure severity, which may be associated with increased risk for brain damage (Ekert et al, 1997). AED use also has secondary harmful effects on cardiac and respiratory functions, with resultant circulatory disturbances that will contribute to brain injury because of hypoperfusion (Lien et al, 1995). Finally, AED use may have teratogenic effects on brain development with exposure over long periods of time.

SUGGESTED READINGS

Da Silva O, Collado Guzman GM, Young GB: The value of standard electroencephalograms in the evaluation of the newborn with recurrent apneas, *J Perinatol* 18:377-380, 1998.
Dunleavy M, Shinoda S, Schindler C, et al: Experimental neonatal status epilepticus and the development of temporal lobe epilepsy with unilateral hippocampal sclerosis, *Am J Pathol* 176:330-342, 2009.
El-Dib M, Chang T, Tsuchida TN, et al: Amplitude-integrated electroencephalography in neonates, *Pediatr Neurol* 41:315-326, 2009.

Glass HC, Glidden D, Jeremy RJ, et al: Clinical neonatal seizures are independently associated with outcome in infants at risk for hypoxic-ischemic brain injury, *J Pediatr* 155:318-323, 2009a.

Glass HC, Pham TN, Danielsen B, et al: Antenatal and intrapartum risk factors for seizures in term newborns: a population-based study, California 1998-2002, *J Pediatr* 154:24-28, 2009b.

Holmes GL: The long-term effects of neonatal seizures, *Clin Perinatol* 36:901-914, 2009: vii.

Lynch BJ, Rust RS: Natural history and outcome of neonatal hypocalcemic and hypomagnesemic seizures, *Pediatr Neurol* 11:23-27, 1994.

Murray DM, Boylan GB, Ali I, et al: Defining the gap between electrographic seizure burden, clinical expression and staff recognition of neonatal seizures, *Arch Dis Child Fetal Neonatal Ed* 93:F187-F191, 2008.

Painter MJ, Scher MS, Stein AD, et al: Phenobarbital compared with phenytoin for the treatment of neonatal seizures, *N Engl J Med* 341:485-489, 1999.

Scher M: Neonatal seizures: an expression of fetal or neonatal brain disorders. In Stevenson DE, Benitz WE, Sunshine P, editors: *Fetal and neonatal brain injury mechanisms, management and the risks of practice*, Cambridge, UK, 2002, Cambridge University Press, pp 735-784.

Schmitt B, Baumgartner M, Mills PB, et al: Seizures and paroxysmal events: symptoms pointing to the diagnosis of pyridoxine-dependent epilepsy and pyridoxine phosphate oxidase deficiency, *Dev Med Child Neurol* 52:e133-e142, 2010.

Silverstein FS, Jensen FE, Inder T, et al: Improving the treatment of neonatal seizures: National Institute of Neurological Disorders and Stroke workshop report, *J Pediatr* 153:12-15, 2008.

Complete references used in this text can be found online at www.expertconsult.com

RISK ASSESSMENT AND NEURODEVELOPMENTAL OUTCOMES

Mary Leppert and Marilee C. Allen

RISK OF NEURODEVELOPMENTAL DISABILITY

"Will my child survive?" "How will this illness influence my child's life?" These are the two questions most frequently asked by parents of infants in a neonatal intensive care unit (NICU). As difficult as it is to predict survival of a sick or very preterm infant, it is far more difficult to answer questions regarding quality of life for the infant who survives. How much recovery will there be? Will the child develop further complications? Most important, how will this early illness influence the child's neurologic, sensory, and cognitive development? For most conditions requiring neonatal intensive care, it is difficult to define the full extent (if any) of damage to or malformation of an infant's organ systems. Newborns have a remarkable potential for recovery, but how organs recover is poorly understood. Predicting the outcome for an individual NICU infant is therefore difficult.

Most commonly, *high risk* refers to the likelihood of neurodevelopmental disability, which is a group of interrelated, chronic, nonprogressive disorders of the central nervous system (CNS) caused by injury to or malformation of the developing brain. They form a spectrum ranging from cerebral palsy (motor impairment) and intellectual disability (cognitive impairment), to sensory impairment, to the more subtle disorders of CNS function (Table 64-1) (Accardo, 2008). These more subtle disorders of higher cortical function include language disorders, visual-perceptual problems, learning disability, minor neuromotor dysfunction, attention deficits, executive dysfunction, and behavioral problems. They have a lesser severity but a higher prevalence in the general population than is the case for the major disabilities (i.e., cerebral palsy and intellectual disability). *Intellectual disability* has supplanted the more stigmatic term *mental retardation*. Neurodevelopmental impairment (NDI) generally refers to cerebral palsy (CP), intellectual disability, severe hearing impairment, and severe visual impairment, and at times it may include severe learning disability, seizure disorder, or hydrocephalus.

Although preterm infants and sick full-term infants who required neonatal intensive care have an increased risk of neurodevelopmental disabilities compared with the general population, most do not develop major disability or NDI (Darlow et al, 2009). Although most children with disability manifest initial developmental delay, some have functional limitations without delay in milestone attainment. A preterm infant who was born at 27 weeks' gestation and had a right intraparenchymal hemorrhage had no delays when seen on follow-up at 14 months corrected for degree of prematurity. He walked independently, had a right pincer grasp, and said three meaningful words.

On careful inspection, however, circumduction of his left foot was evident when he walked, and he had only a raking grasp with his left hand. Findings on examination—a tight left heel cord and some increased tone at his hips and on pronation and supination of his left arm—were consistent with a left spastic hemiplegia. Children with complex medical conditions may initially demonstrate developmental delay but not have long-term disability. An infant with chronic lung disease and mild hypotonia who is not rolling over by 6 months corrected for degree of prematurity has delayed development and is at risk for motor and language impairment. However, treatment of his lung disease may be associated with improved rate of attainment of developmental milestones, and he may have no or very mild impairment.

A large number of perinatal and demographic risk factors with differing capacities to predict neurodevelopmental disabilities have been identified and are summarized in Box 64-1. Multiple risk factors further increase risk of developmental disability (Behrman et al, 2007; Schmidt et al, 2003). Poverty increases the risks of prematurity and intrauterine growth restriction; low socioeconomic status, poor parental education, and maternal depression all have adverse effects on infant cognitive development and behavior (Behrman et al, 2007; Gray et al, 2004; Weisglas-Kuperus et al, 2009; Wood et al, 2005). A number of obstetric conditions (e.g., abruptio placentae, maternal antepartum hemorrhage) may be catastrophic, but prompt intervention can circumvent death and disability. Abnormalities on neonatal neurologic examination and neuroimaging studies are better predictors of outcome than preceding obstetric conditions, electronic fetal heart rate abnormalities, metabolic acidosis, or Apgar scores at birth (Graham et al, 2006, 2008; Handley-Derry et al, 1997; Lindstrom et al, 2008; Logitharajah et al, 2009; Nelson, 2002). As birthweight and gestational age decrease, rates of complications of prematurity and neurodevelopmental disability increase (Behrman et al, 2007). Rates of CP, cognitive impairment, and other neurodevelopmental disabilities increase with number and severity of neonatal complications, severity of neonatal encephalopathy, abnormalities on neonatal neurodevelopmental assessments, and neuroimaging abnormalities (Aarnoudse-Moens et al, 2009b; Allen and Capute, 1989; Amess et al, 1999; Behrman et al, 2007; Dixon et al, 2002; Handley-Derry et al, 1997; Krageloh-Mann and Cans, 2009; Marlow and Budge, 2005; Marret et al, 2007; Miller et al, 2005; Schmidt et al, 2003; Vohr et al, 2005b; Wyatt et al, 2007).

Neither risk nor statistical association implies causation, but studies of risk factors can provide important insights into etiology of neurodevelopmental disability (Allen, 2002; Behrman et al, 2007; Nelson, 2002; O'Shea, 2002).

TABLE 64-1 Prevalence of Neurodevelopmental Disabilities in the General Population

Disability	Prevalence per 1000 Children*
Cerebral palsy	1–4
Intellectual disability	7–40
Severe intellectual disability	4–5
Hearing impairment	1–3.1
Visual impairment	0.4–1.0
Specific learning disability	40–175
Speech and language disorders	20–74
Attention deficit hyperactivity disorders	14–74
Behavior disorders	3–15
Minor neuromotor dysfunction/ coordination disorder	50–150
Autism	2–7
Special education for disability	88
Cerebral palsy, intellectual disability, autism, *or* hearing *or* visual impairment	19

*Accardo PJ: *Capute and Accardo's neurodevelopmental disabilities in infancy and childhood,* ed 3, Baltimore, 2008, Paul H. Brookes.

BOX 64-1   Categories of Perinatal Risk Factors

BACKGROUND CHARACTERISTICS

Socioeconomic status, social class, parental education, race, ethnic group

PRENATAL AND OBSTETRIC COMPLICATIONS

Maternal acute or chronic illness, maternal ingestion of drugs
Congenital infection, maternal urinary tract infections, chorioamnionitis
Multiple gestation, intrauterine death of a co-twin
Placental and cord problems (e.g., placental abruption, prolapsed cord)
Labor and delivery complications

PHYSICAL CHARACTERISTICS

Gender
Congenital anomalies, dysmorphic features, genetic syndromes
Prematurity, postmaturity
Intrauterine growth restriction/small for gestational age, microcephaly

CONDITION AT BIRTH

Apgar scores, cord pH, meconium staining, need for and response to resuscitation

NEONATAL COMPLICATIONS

Hypoxia, acidosis, hypotension/shock
Chronic lung disease/bronchopulmonary dysplasia, hypoxic respiratory failure, apnea
Sepsis, meningitis, necrotizing enterocolitis
Retinopathy of prematurity

MEASURES OF CENTRAL NERVOUS SYSTEM STRUCTURE AND FUNCTION

Clinical: stage of neonatal encephalopathy, neurodevelopmental examination, seizures
Neuroimaging: intraventricular hemorrhage, intraparenchymal hemorrhage, periventricular leukomalacia or evidence of white matter injury, encephalomalacia, ventricular dilation, cortical atrophy, hydrocephalus, injury to the deep gray nuclei and posterior limb of the internal capsule
EEG: burst-suppression pattern, low amplitude

An abnormal fetus with an unrecognized genetic disorder, prenatal insult, or malformation may grow poorly in utero, precipitate preterm delivery, fail to turn or descend properly, need stimulation to breathe at birth, and/or nipple-feed poorly. As many as 50% to 65% of children with CP were born at term, and many have evidence of intrauterine infection, coagulopathy, placental pathology, or death of a co-twin (Himmelmann et al, 2010; Nelson, 2002; Sellier et al, 2010). In a European collaborative study of 4002 children with CP who had birthweight (BW) at or above 2500 g, only 24% had received neonatal intensive care (Sellier et al, 2010). Strong evidence links cerebral palsy in preterm infants to ischemic and/or cytokine-mediated brain injury, with perhaps also a role for insufficient levels of developmentally regulated neuroprotective substances (e.g., thyroxine, hydrocortisone) (Mann et al, 2009; O'Shea, 2002; O'Shea et al, 2009).

The presence or absence of perinatal and neonatal risk factors can neither diagnose neurodevelopmental disability nor ensure normal development. Uncertainty regarding a child's outcome is difficult for both parents and professionals. Helping parents to recognize and cope with their fears allows development of a realistic plan for the future, including identifying family support systems, early intervention strategies, and community resources. The clinician should begin by describing the range of possible outcomes to parents. Mildly increased risk for disability should be acknowledged but put into perspective. Parents of infants with significant or multiple risk factors should be offered focused neurodevelopmental follow-up evaluation and support, especially during critical early years. A comprehensive, developmentally based, family-oriented follow-up clinic helps to ensure early diagnosis of neurodevelopmental disability, shape early intervention strategies to meet the infant's and family's evolving needs, and provide parents with continuity and ongoing support during a difficult period of uncertainty and adjustment.

NEURODEVELOPMENTAL OUTCOME

This section describes the outcome for several groups of high-risk infants cared for in the NICU. The reported incidences of disability differ from study to study because of variations in a number of factors: study criteria, ethnic and demographic composition of the study population, obstetric and neonatal care practices, follow-up rate, length of follow-up, and assessment methodologies. High follow-up rates are preferable but difficult to attain. Low follow-up rates raise concerns about bias—for example, one study found difficulty with follow-up to be associated with lower intelligence quotient (IQ), greater degree of disability, and single parents with less education (Callanan et al, 2001).

How the children are followed, and for how long, influences what neurodevelopmental disabilities are detected. Studies that evaluate infants up to 1 year focus on the major disabilities, particularly motor and sensory disabilities, but are inadequate for assessing mild CP, mild intellectual disability, or borderline intelligence. Mild to moderate sensory impairments may be missed if specific evaluations of hearing and vision are not performed after initial screening in the NICU. Evaluating older children improves diagnostic accuracy and recognition of mild disabilities, but can lower follow-up rates. Follow-up assessments from 2 to 6 years can detect mild intellectual disabilities, minor neuromotor dysfunction, behavioral problems, attention deficits, and language delay. Questions about learning disability and other school-related problems require follow-up to school age. Longitudinal studies have found an increased incidence of school problems with longer periods of follow-up evaluation (Aylward, 2002; Msall and Tremont, 2002). The younger child with more subtle impairments often has some ability to compensate for learning difficulties or inefficiencies initially, but experiences difficulties when work becomes more complex, abstract thought and expression are required, and efficiency becomes important in completing homework and test-taking. Follow-up to adolescence and adulthood addresses questions about functional abilities, independence, and quality of life.

PRETERM INFANTS

Prematurity is a common, complex condition due to multiple gene-environmental interactions, including both maternal and fetal genomes, the intrauterine environment, and the mother's environment (Behrman et al, 2007). Prematurity is a major public health problem in the United States: it accounts for 64% to 75% of infant deaths, 42% to 47% of children with CP, 27% of children with significant cognitive impairments, and 23% to 37% of children with significant sensory impairments. A conservative estimate by the Institute of Medicine found the annual economic burden for preterm births in 2005 to be $26.2 billion ($51,600 per preterm infant born) over that of a full-term infant. The population of preterm infants is remarkably heterogeneous with respect to etiology, complications, and outcomes. Although it was initially defined by birthweight (BW <2500 g), and now by gestational age (GA <37 weeks), prematurity's defining characteristic is immature organ development for extrauterine life. Just as BW varies with GA, there is individual variation in degree of maturity for both BW and GA (Allen, 2005). Final common pathways to preterm delivery include spontaneous preterm labor, preterm rupture of membranes, and indicated preterm delivery for maternal or fetal health (Behrman et al, 2007). The multiple risk factors identified for each pathway overlap, yet the strongest predictor is a prior preterm birth. Inflammation and infection have been implicated as etiologies for preterm birth, complications of prematurity (e.g., chronic lung disease), and neurodevelopmental disability.

MOTOR IMPAIRMENT

Preterm infants exhibit a range of neuromotor abnormalities on exam, which often persist and may be accompanied by motor delay and/or motor impairment, as well as fine motor impairment, visual-spatial deficits, executive dysfunction, visual-perceptual impairment, and problems with motor planning and visual navigation (Bracewell and Marlow, 2002; Davis et al, 2007; Hadders-Algra, 2002; Johnson et al, 2009; Marlow et al, 2007; Mikkola et al, 2005; Pavlova et al, 2007; Samsom et al, 2002; Schmidhauser et al,

2006; Sigurdardottir et al, 2009; Venkateswaran and Shevell, 2008; Vohr et al, 2005a; Williams et al, 2010). Motor impairments in children born preterm range from severe to mild CP, to mild functional motor impairment, termed minor neuromotor dysfunction (MND) or developmental coordination disorder (DCD). For many preterm children with CP or MND/DCD, their motor impairment is far less disabling than their associated impairments (e.g., executive dysfunction, cognitive impairments, fine motor difficulties) and that lead to difficulties in the classroom and with their peers.

Most preterm infants do not develop CP (Tables 64-2 and 64-3). The risk for CP increases with decreasing GA and BW (see Tables 64-2 and 64-3). In large regional population studies, the prevalence of CP increased from 0.9 to 1.5 per 1000 live births of children born full term with normal BW, to 6.1 to 6.7 per 1000 live births at 32 to 36 weeks' gestation, 18.1 to 21.6 at 28 to 36 weeks' gestation, and 40.4 to 43.7 at 28 to 31 weeks' gestation; and from 6.7 to 10.5 per 1000 live births with BW 1500 to 2499 g, 39.5 to 50.6 for BW <1500 g, and 58.3 to 80 for BW <1000 g (see Table 64-2) (Dolk et al, 2006; Himmelmann et al, 2005, 2010; Platt et al, 2007; Sellier et al, 2010; Sigurdardottir et al, 2009; Surman et al, 2009). The preterm outcome studies in Table 64-3 reported the rate of CP in survivors (not per live births); this is an important distinction, because many infants born at 22 to 25 weeks' gestation die in the delivery room, in the NICU, and before follow-up studies assess their development (Bodeau-Livinec et al, 2008; Doyle, 2001; Groenendaal et al, 2010; Kutz et al, 2009; Marlow et al, 2005b; Wood et al, 2000). Two studies reporting rate of CP in survivors by each week of gestation found a progressive increase as GA decreased, from 0.7% at 34 weeks GA, to 4% at 32 weeks GA, to 19% at 26 weeks GA (Ancel et al, 2006; Marret et al, 2007). At the limit of viability, 12% to 23% of survivors born before 26 weeks' gestation had CP, and up to half had severe functional motor impairment (i.e., spastic quadriplegia or nonambulatory spastic diplegia) (Bodeau-Livinec et al, 2008; Hintz et al, 2005; Johnson et al, 2009; Marlow et al, 2005b; Stahlmann et al, 2009; Steinmacher et al, 2008; Voss et al, 2007; Wilson-Costello et al, 2005, 2007).

Spastic diplegia, with greater spasticity in the legs and no to minimal involvement of the arms, occurs in 44% to 68% of preterm children (Ancel et al, 2006; Behrman et al, 2007; Mikkola et al, 2005; Sigurdardottir et al, 2009; Wood et al, 2000). Some preterm outcome studies distinguish between disabling, moderate to severe motor impairment or nonambulatory CP and mild CP (Marlow et al, 2005b; Stahlmann et al, 2009). There is some disagreement as to the distinction between mild CP and MND. A child with tight heel cords and hyperreflexia who toe-walks initially but walks independently with heels down by age 2 may be classified as having either mild CP or MND. Some of these children require physical therapy and/or bracing with ankle-foot orthoses, but with age they improve and their gross motor dysfunction is much less obvious (their mild CP disappears).

Many preterm outcome studies have reported more mild gross and fine motor impairments and visual-perceptual and visual-spatial deficits in preterm infants, even those without CP or intellectual disability, than in full-term

TABLE 64-2   Prevalence of Cerebral Palsy (CP) by Gestational Age (GA) and Birthweight (BW) Categories

Study	Region	Ages (years)	Years of Birth	GA (weeks)	BW (g)	CP per 1000 Live Births	CP, % Live Births
Himmelmann et al, 2010	Sweden	4–8	1999–2002	≥37		1.43	0.1%
				32–36		6.1	0.6%
				28–31		43.7	4.4%
				<28		55.6	5.6%
					≥2500	1.44	0.1%
					1500–2499	9.9	1.0%
					1000–1499	44	4.4%
					<1000	58.3	5.8%
Himmelmann et al, 2005	Sweden	4–8	1995–1998	≥37		1.11	0.1%
				32–36		6.7	0.7%
				28–31		40.4	4.4%
				<28		76.6	7.7%
					≥2500	1.2	0.1%
					1500–2499	6.7	0.7%
					1000–1499	54.4	5.4%
					<1000	82	8.2%
Sigurdardottir et al, 2009	Iceland	4–8	1997–2003	≥37		0.9	0.1%
				28–36		21.6	2.2%
					≥2500	1.1	0.1%
					1500–2499	15	1.5%
					<1500	104.2	10.4%
	Iceland	4–8	1990–1996	≥37		1.5	0.2%
				28–36		18.1	1.8%
					≥2500	1.5	0.2%
					1500–2499	17.3	1.7%
					<1500	46.3	4.6%
Dolk et al, 2006	Northern Ireland	≥5	1994–1997		≥2500	1.2	0.1%
					1500–2499	10.5	1.0%
					<1500	44.5	4.5%
Sellier et al, 2010	Europe	≥4	1998		≥2500	0.99	0.1%
			1980–1998		≥2500	1.14	0.1%
Platt et al, 2007	Europe	≥4	1996		≤1500	39.5	4.0%
			1980–1996	<28		48.6	4.9%
					≤1500	50.6	5.1%
Surman et al, 2009	United Kingdom		1976–1999		≥2500	1.2	0.1%
					<2500	16	1.6%

comparison children (Behrman et al, 2007; Bracewell and Marlow, 2002; Breslau et al, 2000; Davis et al, 2007; Goyen et al, 1998; Marlow et al, 2007; Mikkola et al, 2005; Pavlova et al, 2007; Schmidhauser et al, 2006; Williams et al, 2010). Asymmetric leg or hand function, balance problems, incoordination, poor postural stability, difficulty with motor planning (figuring out how to perform complex motor tasks), sensory-motor integration problems (e.g., difficulty tolerating certain textures of foods, touch or sounds) and fine motor dysfunction can interfere with development of self-help skills, ability to play on the playground, peer relationships, and self-esteem. These subtle impairments can lead to problems with dressing, cutting with scissors, handwriting, academic learning, and behavior. Prevalence varies with how the population is

defined, age at evaluation, and assessment methods: 70% of 11- to 13-year-olds with BW below 1000 g had definite motor problems compared with 22% of controls, OR 9.5 (95% confidence intervals [CI] 3.7 to 24.3) (Burns et al, 2009); 9.5% of 8- to 9-year-olds with GA below 28 weeks had DCD compared with 2% of controls ($p=0.001$) (Davis et al, 2007); 20% to 30% of children born at 32 to 36 weeks' gestation had difficulty with fine motor coordination and visual-motor tasks (Huddy et al, 2001). In the EPICure longitudinal study, children born before 26 weeks GA in 1995 had much poorer performance on a variety of motor tasks than full-term controls, including sensorimotor difficulties, visuospatial problems, and overflow movements during motor tasks, as well as a higher prevalence of left-handedness (28% vs. 10%) (Marlow et al, 2007).

TABLE 64-3   Rates of Neurodevelopmental Disability in Preterm Infants

Study	Ages (years)	Birth Years	F/U Rate	n	GA (weeks)	BW (g)	CP	IQ <70	IQ <85	Mean IQ ±SD	VI	HI	NDI	Normal
Netherlands														
Groenendaal et al, 2010	>2	2002–2006		422	25–29.9		3.4%							
	>2	1997–2001		356	25–29.9		6.8%							
	>2	1991–1996		434	25–29.9		5.8%							
Claas et al, 2010	2	2001–2005	91%	56	≥24	≤750		8.9%	33.9%	92.8 ± 17.7				
	2	1996–2000	91%	45	≥24	≤750		0	15.6%	97.6 ± 9.8				
Finland														
Munck et al, 2010 (PIPARI)	2	2001–2003	96%	192	≥37					109.8 ± 11.7				
	2	2001–2006	94%	182		<1500	7.1%	3.3%		101.7 ± 15.4	0	2.2%	10%	
	2			106		1001–1500		1.9%		105.4 ± 12.6			7%	
	2			76		≤1000		5.3%		96.7 ± 17.3			15%	
Mikkola et al, 2005	5	1996–1997		351		≤1000	14.0%	9.0%		96 ± 19	0.6%	4.0%	20%	
	5			103	≤27		19.0%	12.0%		96 ± 19		6.7%		26%
United States														
Bode et al, 2009	2	2005–2006	97%	172	≤30	<1000	5.0%	10.0%			1.0%	1.0%	9%	
Wilson-Costello et al, 2007	1.8	2000–2002	92%	161		<1000	5%	21%	43%	85.9 ± 20	1%	1%	23%	
Hintz et al, 2005[†]	1.8	1996–1999	89%	473	<25		21.0%	47.0%	71.0%	72* (57–87)	1.1%	2.6%	58%	21%
	1.8	1993–1996	80%	366	<25		23.0%	40.0%	70.0%	75* (63–86)	2.3%	4.3%	55%	21%
Vohr et al, 2005[†]	1.8	1997–1999	84%	910	≤27	≤1000	18.1%	37.2%			1.0%	1.8%	45%	
	1.8	1995–1996	84%	716	≤27	≤1000	18.7%	38.5%			1.5%	2.3%	47%	
	1.8	1993–1994	74%	665	≤27	≤1000	20.1%	41.8%			2.3%	3.4%	50%	
Wilson-Costello et al, 2005[†]	1.8	1990–1998	90%	417		<1000	14.0%	26.0%	44.0%	83.6 ± 19	1.0%	7.0%	36%	
	1.8			272		750–999	15.0%	22.0%	40.0%	85.3 ± 19	1.0%	6.0%	32%	
	1.8			145		500–799	12.0%	34.0%	51.0%	80.3 ± 20	1.0%	10.0%	43%	
Hack et al, 2005	8	1992–1995		176		>2500				99.8 ± 15				
	8	1992–1995	92%	200		<1000	16.0%	16.0%	37.0%	87.8 ± 19	0	1.5%		
	1.8	1992–1995	92%	200		<1000	15.0%	39.0%	67.0%	75.6 ± 16	0.5%	5.0%		
Australia														
Doyle et al, 2010	2	2005	91%	202	≥37		0	2.0%	20.3%	108.9 ± 14.3	0	0.5%	3%	79%
	2		95%	163	22–27		9.8%	16.0%	47.9%	97.5 ± 12.6	0	2.5%	20%	51%
Roberts et al, 2010	8	1997	87%	173	≥37		0	3.0%	12.9%	105.6 ± 12.4	0	0	3%	87%
	8	1997	94%	189	22–27	500–999	11.9%	14.8%	53.5%	93.1 ± 16.1	1.6%	2.1%	19%	41%

Study													
Roberts et al, 2009	8	1997	94%	160	500–999	9.7%	11.4%	50.3%	94.1 ± 14.3	1.8%	2.4%	18%	45%
	8	1991–1992	93%	224	500–999	10.7%	16.5%	41.5%	94.9 ± 15.8	1.1%	1.5%	19%	56%
Doyle et al, 2001	5	1991–1992	98%	221	<28	11.3%	15.4%			1.8%	0.9%	20%	
Poland													
Stoinska et al, 2010	2	1999–2003		450	<1500	16.7%			78.0 ± 14.9	4.8%	1.6%		
Austria													
Sommer et al, 2007	2	1996–2001	91%	48	≤26	6.0%	54.0%			6.0%	6.0%		
New Zealand													
Woodward et al, 2009	4	1998–2000	96%	107	≥37	0.9%		13.1%	104.7 ± 13.5				74%
	4		98%	105	≤33	16.2%		34.3%	94.9 ± 15.5				40%
	4			62	28-33	14.5%		35.5%	95.7 ± 13.9				45%
	4			43	23-27	18.6%		32.6%	93.9 ± 17.6				33%
Germany													
Stahlmann et al, 2009	7–9	1997–1999	82%	75	<27	15.0%	26.0%	48.7%		2.0%	0	20%	36%
Steinmacher et al, 2008	5.6	1996–1999	96%	67	≤25	12.0%	27.0%	43.0%	82 ± 23	4.0%	1.0%	18%	43%
Voss et al, 2007	6–10	1993–1998	75%	129	<1000	9.3%	13.2%			0	0	17%	45%
France (Epipage)													
Bodeau-Livinec et al, 2008	5	1997–1998	57%	74	≤25	15.9%	13.5%	45.9%	86.9 ± 16.1				
Larroque et al, 2008	5	1997	60%	396	39-40		3.0%	12.0%					
	5		77%	1817	<33	9.0%	12.0%	32.0%				14%	
	5				29-32							36%	
	5				<29							49%	
Marret et al, 2007	2	1997	61%	140	34	0.7%	5.3%	23.9%	98 ± 17	0.8%	1.5%		
	2		69%	135	33	3.7%	8.2%	22.8%	97 ± 18	2.3%	0		
	2		76%	513	32	4.1%	8.1%	25.8%	97 ± 18	1.9%	0.2%		
	2		72%	379	31	8.7%	10.7%	33.2%	93 ± 18	2.2%	0.3%		
	2		76%	288	30	6.3%	9.9%	35.3%	94 ± 19	0.7%	0.3%		
Ancel et al, 2006	2	1997		1954	≤32	8.2%							
	2			424	31	6.8%							
	2			315	30	8.3%							
	2			196	29	8.2%							
	2			191	28	11.0%							
	2			146	27	12.3%							

Continued

TABLE 64-3 Rates of Neurodevelopmental Disability in Preterm Infants—cont'd

Study	Ages (years)	Birth Years	F/U Rate	n	GA (weeks)	BW (g)	CP	IQ <70	IQ <85	Mean IQ ±SD	VI	HI	NDI	Normal
	2			82	26		22.0%							
	2			62	≤25		19.4%							
British Isles (EPICure)														
Johnson et al, 2009	11	1995		153	≥37		0	1.3%		104 ± 11	0	0	1%	71%
	11		71%	219	≤25		17.4%	40.0%		84 ± 18	9.0%	2.0%	45%	16%
Marlow et al, 2005†	6	1995		160	≥37		0	1.3%		105.7 ± 11.8	0	1%	1.3%	94%
	6		78%	241	≤25		20.0%	20.7%	46%	82.1 ± 19.2	7%	6%	24.5%	46%
Wood et al, 2000	2.5	1995	92%	283	≤25		18.0%	30.0%		84 ± 12	2.0%	3.0%		49%

CP, Cerebral palsy (children with mild to severe CP/survivors assessed); F/U Rate, follow-up rate (number of children seen for assessment/number of survivors); HI, hearing impairment, generally severe (severe hearing loss, required hearing aids); IQ, intelligence quotient or equivalent (intellectual disability is IQ <70; borderline intelligence is IQ 70-84); n, number of children assessed per group; NDI, neurodevelopmental Impairment (generally CP, IQ <70, severe visual impairment and/or hearing impairment); Normal, as defined in each study (no mild, moderate, or severe neurodevelopmental disability); VI, visual impairment, generally severe (very poor visual acuity, blind or no light perception).

*Median (interquartile range).

†Data from the National Institute of Child Health and Development Neonatal Research Network.

The prevalence of mild to moderate motor impairment in children born preterm who did not have CP was estimated at 40.5/100 (95% CI 32.1, 48.9) from pooled data in a random effects metaanalysis of 15 published studies (Williams et al, 2010). Their estimate of the prevalence of moderate motor impairment from pooled data was 19.0/100 (95% CI 14.2, 23.8).

COGNITIVE IMPAIRMENT

Populations of preterm children demonstrate a normal range of intelligence, but with lower means than those of full-term controls, even after adjustment for socioeconomic status and neurologic injury or impairment (Aylward, 2002; Behrman et al, 2007; Bhutta et al, 2002; Charkaluk et al, 2010; Johnson, 2007; Johnson et al, 2009). The significance of a lower mean IQ is in the greater proportion of children with intellectual disability, borderline intelligence, and low average intelligence who have difficulties functioning at school and in society. A Norwegian study found that prevalence of intellectual disability was 1.4 times higher for children born at 32 to 36 weeks GA and increased to 6.9 times higher for children born before 32 weeks GA (Stromme and Hagberg, 2000). Two studies found that preterm children did much better on cognitive tests at school age compared with their performance on the Bayley Scale of Infant Development at age 2, especially in the children who had no neurologic impairment and mothers with a high educational level (Hack et al, 2005; Roberts et al, 2010).

Cognitive impairments are the most common disabilities in preterm children, and their prevalence increases with decreasing GA and BW categories (see Table 64-3) (Behrman et al, 2007; Bhutta et al, 2002; Johnson, 2007; Johnson et al, 2009; Kirkegaard et al, 2006; Stoinska and Gadzinowski, 2010; Weisglas-Kuperus et al, 2009). Most preterm outcome studies report that 8% to 11% of children born before 28 to 32 weeks' gestation and 14% to as high as 54% of children born before 26 to 28 weeks' gestation had cognitive scores more than 2 standard deviations (SD) below the test mean (i.e., IQ <70), in comparison with only 1% to 2% of full-term controls (Bode et al, 2009; Doyle and Anderson, 2005; Doyle et al, 2010; Hintz et al, 2005; Johnson et al, 2009; Larroque et al, 2008; Marlow et al, 2005b; Marret et al, 2007; Roberts et al, 2010; Sommer et al, 2007; Vohr et al, 2005b). In the EPICure study, 21% of 6-year-olds born before 26 weeks GA had IQ scores more than 2 SD below the test mean, 25% had IQ scores 1 to 2 SD below the mean, and only 54% had IQ scores in the normal range (i.e., above 1 SD below the mean), as compared with 0, 2%, and 98%, respectively, of full-term controls (Marlow et al, 2005b). The mean IQ of the full-term controls was 106 (SD 12): 41% of preterm children had IQ scores more than 2 SD below the mean of the full-term controls, and 71% had IQ scores more than 1 SD below their mean. In a Finnish preterm outcome study, full-term controls had a mean IQ of 110 (SD 12): Only 3.3% of children with BW below 1500 g had IQ scores more than 2 SD below test norms, but using data from their full-term control sample, this increased to 15.4% (Munck et al, 2010). The lower mean IQ in the preterm population is not due solely to neurologic

impairment: a metaanalysis of 16 case-control studies of children 5 years or older found a persistently lower mean IQ score for preterm infants, and when children with neurologic impairment were excluded, the weighted mean difference decreased only from 10.9 (95% CI 9.2, 12.5) to 10.2 (95% CI 9.0, 11.5) (Bhutta et al, 2002).

Intelligence scores are a composite of scores on multiple cognitive processing subtests; many preterm children with normal IQ scores have problems with attention, memory, complex language processing, nonverbal reasoning, visual-perceptual abilities, and/or executive function that interfere with learning, behavior, and school performance (Aarnoudse-Moens et al, 2009a; Behrman et al, 2007; Bhutta et al, 2002; Caravale et al, 2005; Charkaluk et al, 2010; Grunau et al, 2002; Johnson, 2007; Litt et al, 2005; Marlow et al, 2007; Mulder et al, 2010). Difficulty in processing complex language makes it more difficult for a child to comprehend and follow school lessons or even directions. Early language disorders place children at higher risk for later language-based learning disability (reading and written language). Problems with visual perceptual abilities, visuospatial skills, and fine motor function contribute to difficulties with reading and writing. Processing speed, attention, working memory, flexibility generating ideas, organizing information, adaptability, and planning a sequence of actions in advance were much more difficult for 8-year-olds born before 28 weeks GA than for normal BW controls (Anderson and Doyle, 2003). A metaanalysis of 12 studies of executive function in preterm children born before 34 weeks' gestation and/or with BW <1500 g found that combined effect sizes were lower than those for full-term controls in measures of executive function: they had a decrement of 0.57 SD for verbal fluency, 0.36 SD for working memory, and 0.49 SD for cognitive flexibility (Aarnoudse-Moens et al, 2009b).

As many as 25% to 40% of children with BW below 1000 g have learning disabilities, especially in math or reading, and 50% to 70% require special education in school (Anderson and Doyle, 2003; Bhutta et al, 2002; Grunau et al, 2002; Litt et al, 2005; Saigal et al, 2000). A metaanalysis of 14 published papers on academic achievement of children born very preterm (before 34 weeks' gestation) and/or with BW at or below 1500 g found combined effect sizes that show that preterm children score 0.6 SD below full-term peers on mathematics tests, 0.48 SD below on reading tests, and 0.76 SD below on spelling tests (Aarnoudse-Moens et al, 2009b). Rates of learning disabilities, executive dysfunction, and school and behavior problems increase with decreasing GA and BW categories (Aarnoudse-Moens et al, 2009b; Anderson and Doyle, 2004; Behrman et al, 2007; Grunau et al, 2002; Johnson, 2007; Kirkegaard et al, 2006; Pinto-Martin et al, 2004; Saigal et al, 2000).

Behavioral problems are also more common in children born preterm than in full-term controls (Grunau et al, 2004; Johnson, 2007; Marlow et al, 2007; Stahlmann et al, 2009; Woodward et al, 2009). A metaanalysis of 16 case-control school-age outcome studies found higher prevalence of attention deficit hyperactivity disorder, externalizing symptoms (e.g., delinquency), and internalizing symptoms (e.g., anxiety, depression) in 67%, 69%, and 75% of studies, respectively (Bhutta et al, 2002). A more recent metaanalysis of nine studies on behavioral problems of children born preterm found that attention problems were most pronounced in very preterm children and/or children with BW <1500 g (Aarnoudse-Moens et al, 2009b). Ratings by teachers and parents were 0.43 and 0.59 SD higher, respectively, than for controls. In contrast, the combined effect sizes for internalizing or externalizing behaviors were relatively small, <28.0 and <0.09, respectively. Children born preterm often have attention problems without hyperactivity and without disruptive behavior or conduct disorders (Johnson, 2007).

SENSORY IMPAIRMENTS

Retinopathy of prematurity continues to be a cause of severe visual impairment, especially in the most immature and smallest preterm infants (see Table 64-3). Myopia and strabismus are common in preterm infants and generally necessitate intervention. The incidence of hearing impairment in very preterm infants ranges from 1% to 11%, depending on the population and definitions used. Sensory input is crucial for learning, therefore sensory impairments are important to diagnose as early as possible. Yoshinaga-Itano et al (1998) found better cognitive and language scores in children who had their hearing impairment diagnosed and treated by 6 months than in children whose hearing impairment was identified later. Now, with universal hearing screening, all infants have their hearing screened in the neonatal period, but hearing should also be reevaluated whenever language delay is detected.

FUNCTION IN ADOLESCENCE AND ADULTHOOD

Most adolescents and adults born preterm demonstrate a normal range of intelligence, and most (56% to 82%) graduate from high school (Hack et al, 2002; Lefebvre et al, 2005; Saigal et al, 2006a). They require more special education support, however, and their competitive disadvantage persists. They continue to have lower mean cognitive scores than full-term controls: 87 versus 92 for 18-year-olds with BW below 1500 g (Hack et al, 2002); 94 versus 108, p <0.0001, for those with BW below 1000 g (Lefebvre et al, 2005), and 99 vs. 104, p <0.001. for adolescents with BW below 1000 g and who had no neurosensory impairment (Saigal et al, 2006b). In young adulthood, 11% with BW below 1500 g and 27% with BW below 1000 g continued to demonstrate neurosensory impairment; half of the young adults with BW below 1000 g who did not graduate from high school had neurosensory impairments (Hack et al, 2002; Saigal et al, 2006b). Young adult men born very preterm were significantly less likely to achieve high school or a postgraduate education than women. Compared with full-term control subjects, 20-year-olds with BW below 1500 g had lower math and reading academic achievement scores, fewer who graduated from high school (74% vs. 83%), and higher mean age at graduation (18.2 vs. 17.9 years) (Hack et al, 2002). A British educational study found lower test scores for the General Certificate of Secondary Education in graduates with BW below 1500 g than in control subjects born full-term (Pharoah et al, 2003).

Social-emotional and behavioral issues are more common in school-aged children born preterm: in a metaanalysis,

81% of studies reviewed found more behavior problems than controls, 67% found a higher prevalence of attention deficit disorder, 69% found a higher prevalence of externalizing symptoms (e.g., delinquency), and 75% found a higher prevalence of internalizing symptoms (e.g., anxiety, depression) (Bhutta et al, 2002). A study of children born before 29 weeks GA noted that they were more often the target of bullying (Nadeau et al, 2004). Teens and young adults born preterm (i.e., BW below 800 g, 1000 g and 1500 g, or GA below 35 weeks) report less confidence with their attractiveness, athletics, academic achievement, and romance than full-term controls, but similar self-esteem, social activities, and sense of their own quality of life (Cooke, 2004; Grunau et al, 2004; Saigal et al, 2006a). A study of young adults with BW below 1500 g found higher prevalence of anxiety/depression and withdrawal and fewer friends in women (but not in men) compared with full-term controls (Hack et al, 2004). However, compared with full-term controls, young adults with BW below 1500 g have the same or lower prevalence rates of delinquency, teen pregnancies, cigarette smoking, alcohol abuse, and illicit drug use, even when those with neurosensory impairments were excluded from analysis (Bjerager et al, 1995; Cooke, 2004; Gaddlin et al, 2009; Hack et al, 2002).

Although some outcome studies have found lower rates of educational attainment and employment in young adults with BW below 1500 g, a study of young adults born in the McMaster Health Region in Canada with BW below 1000 g found no significant differences in rates of high school graduation, enrollment in higher education, paid employment, living independently, marriage or cohabitation, or parenthood compared with full-term controls (Cooke, 2004; Hack et al, 2002; Saigal et al, 2006b). A 31-year follow-up study of offspring of mothers enrolled in an antenatal steroid trial found no differences between 126 adults born preterm and 66 full-term controls with respect to educational attainment, socioeconomic status, cognitive functioning, working memory, attention, psychiatric symptoms, or marital status (Dalziel et al, 2007). However, a very large population-based Norwegian study of adults born 1967–1976 and followed through 2004 found that rates of high school graduation, graduate education, and having children increased with increasing GA: the lowest rates were in those born at 22 to 27 weeks GA (Swamy et al, 2008). Reproductive rates were only 25% for women and 14% for men born at 22 to 27 weeks GA, compared with 68% for women and 50% for men born at term. Women born preterm were more likely to have preterm infants, and women born at 28 to 32 weeks GA were more likely to have a fetus or infant die.

SMALL-FOR-GESTATIONAL-AGE INFANTS

The term *small for gestational age* is an arbitrary classification that refers to an infant whose intrauterine growth is less than expected for gestational age at birth. It is, in fact, a heterogeneous category, with a wide range of causes, risk of perinatal complications, and outcomes. Small size at birth may be due to parental (especially maternal) small size; insult or injury to the fetus; fetal maldevelopment; congenital infection; maternal ingestion (e.g., cigarettes, alcohol, narcotics); or deprivation of supply of oxygen or nutrients due to placental insufficiency or maternal illness. Magnitude of risk for death, perinatal complications, and neurodevelopmental disability varies with the cause of the intrauterine growth restriction (IUGR), the timing of the insult (if any), and the perinatal complications that the child encounters.

The small-for-gestational-age (SGA) infant whose mother is small is likely to be only mildly growth-restricted and have no increased risk of neurodevelopmental disability. With trisomy 18, poor fetal growth early in pregnancy is likely, with death within the first several months, or the affected child will develop multiple severe neurodevelopmental disabilities. The SGA infant with fetal alcohol syndrome has prenatal and postnatal growth deficiencies and an increased risk of congenital anomalies (e.g., characteristic facies, joint anomalies, ventricular septal defect) and CNS dysfunction (e.g., mild to moderate intellectual disability, tremors, fine motor incoordination, hyperactivity). Uteroplacental insufficiency often manifests later in pregnancy (after 27 or 28 weeks of gestation) and often causes asymmetric growth restriction with sparing of head growth. IUGR from uteroplacental insufficiency can be viewed as an adaptation to restricted supply of nutrients. Although it may be an effective human adaptation to adverse intrauterine circumstances, most IUGR infants survive, but they can have significant morbidity: perinatal complications (e.g., perinatal asphyxia, hypoglycemia), hypertension later in life (related to rapid postnatal weight gain), short stature, and school problems (Farfel et al, 2009; Hollo et al, 2002; Larroque et al, 2001; Low et al, 1992; Paz et al, 2001; Pryor et al, 1995; Rosenberg, 2008; Singhal et al, 2007; Strauss, 2000).

Studies that report developmental outcome of SGA infants generally exclude infants with congenital anomalies, genetic syndromes, or congenital infections. They follow primarily infants with placental insufficiency or unknown cause of IUGR, and they distinguish between the full-term and the preterm SGA infant. A population-based case-control study found a five- to sevenfold increased risk of developing CP in full-term singleton children born with severe IUGR compared with matched appropriate birthweight for gestational age (AGA) controls (Jacobsson et al, 2008). Prospective studies of children and adolescents born full term with IUGR find a slightly lower mean IQ score and higher incidences of academic failure (as high as 25% to 35%) and behavior problems in full-term SGA children than in full-term AGA children (Hollo et al, 2002; Larroque et al, 2001; Low et al, 1992; Paz et al, 2001; Pryor et al, 1995; Strauss, 2000). Despite having shorter stature, more academic problems, and lesser academic and professional achievements, adults born IUGR at term report being employed, married, and satisfaction with life at rates similar to those for AGA control subjects (Larroque et al, 2001; Strauss, 2000).

The preterm SGA infant has the disadvantages of both prematurity and IUGR; many are born preterm because of hostile intrauterine conditions causing signs of fetal distress. Their IUGR occurs earlier in the pregnancy and is more severe than the IUGR of full-term infants. Their IUGR status does not appear to increase their risk of CP over the risk of AGA preterm infants, but there is some evidence that they have a lower rate of normal neurodevelopmental outcome (Claas et al, 2010; Gray et al, 1998; Jacobsson et al, 2008). In a longitudinal study, young adults born with symmetric IUGR (i.e., head proportional with size at birth) had lower mean IQ scores than those in affected persons who had evidence of brain sparing, with asymmetric IUGR (Weisglas-Kuperus et al, 2009). Worsening uteroplacental insufficiency can accelerate fetal brain and lung maturation during the third trimester (Amiel-Tison et al, 2004a, 2004b; Scherjon et al, 2000). This adaptive response to increase survival if delivery is preterm has a cost in brain development, in terms of intelligence and behavior. Worsening intrauterine circumstances can overcome compensatory mechanisms. Infants born after detection by Doppler of abnormal blood flow patterns in the umbilical and fetal arteries tend to have reduced brain volumes and worse neurodevelopmental outcomes (Fouron et al, 2001, 2005; Maunu et al, 2007; Shand et al, 2009).

SICK FULL-TERM INFANTS

The full-term infant may require neonatal intensive care for a variety of reasons, including complications of IUGR, perinatal asphyxia, maternal substance abuse, congenital anomalies, or infection. It is most difficult to predict outcome in infants with poorly understood illness such as the newborn with sluggish but eventually good response in the delivery room, the newborn who appears septic but has negative culture results, the newborn who does not feed well initially, and others with undefined illness. Under most circumstances, these children will do well, but for some, initial illness may be a sign of a CNS disorder or systemic illness that contributes to abnormal outcome. Maternal drug use, infection, or congenital anomalies may underlie conditions that require neonatal intensive care, thereby adding to risk for disability.

HYPOXIC RESPIRATORY FAILURE

The most frequent cause of hypoxic respiratory failure requiring neonatal intensive care in full-term and late preterm infants (born after 33 weeks GA) is persistent pulmonary hypertension of the newborn, either as a primary disorder of neonatal adaptation or associated with meconium aspiration, pneumonia, sepsis, pulmonary hypoplasia, or respiratory distress syndrome. Follow-up of neonates who participated in trials of treatment with inhaled nitric oxide (iNO) or extracorporeal membrane oxygenation (ECMO) provides current data on neurodevelopmental outcomes in this population. Metaanalyses of randomized controlled trials (RCTs) found ECMO to be effective in reducing mortality and iNO to be effective in reducing need for ECMO, without adverse effects on neurodevelopmental outcomes (Finer and Barrington, 2006; Mugford, 2008). A large British RCT of ECMO versus conventional management found no differences in neurodevelopmental outcomes at 1, 4, and 7 years, but only half of assessed survivors (55% vs. 50%) had no disability (McNally et al, 2006). Neuromotor abnormalities were common (60%), but motor disability was moderate to severe in only 6% and mild in 10%. Most (76%) had normal cognitive scores, and 13% had cognitive scores below

2 SD below the mean. Many had difficulty with reading comprehension, visuospatial tasks, and verbal memory (39%, 26%, and 39% scored below the 10th percentile, respectively). A few had sensory impairments: 2% had significant visual impairment, 13% wore glasses, and 6% required hearing aids. The finding of a progressive hearing loss in children between 4 and 7 years highlights the need for serial audiologic evaluations in addition to neurodevelopmental follow-up evaluation in children who had hypoxic respiratory failure or persistent pulmonary hypertension as neonates.

RCT follow-up studies of iNO report that 7% to 13% developed CP, 22% to 30% had cognitive impairment, 2% had severe visual impairment, 7% to 19% had hearing impairment, 22% to 30% had intellectual disability, and 26% to 54% had some neurodevelopmental impairment (Konduri et al, 2007; Lipkin et al, 2002). A small study of 29 full-term infants with meconium aspiration syndrome (only 1 treated with iNO, 2 with ECMO) found that 7% developed CP by 3 years, 14% had intellectual disability, and 41% had mild deficits (i.e., hypotonia and/or mild speech delay) (Beligere and Rao, 2008).

NEONATAL ENCEPHALOPATHY

One recurring scenario in the NICU is that of the full-term infant who has either subtle or florid signs of neonatal encephalopathy (see Chapter 61). Neonatal encephalopathy is characterized by clinical findings (e.g., hyperexcitability, coma, seizures) that are used to categorize infants as to severity of encephalopathy (Sarnat and Sarnat, 1976). Not every neonate with encephalopathy has hypoxic-ischemic encephalopathy (HIE), and not every infant with obstetric or perinatal histories suggestive of hypoxia-ischemia has encephalopathy (Graham et al, 2006, 2008; Rafay et al, 2009). Although infants with low Apgar scores have increased risk of mortality and morbidity, these scores are very poor predictors of neurodevelopmental outcome unless they are persistently very low (Moster et al, 2001; Patel and Beeby, 2004). Increasing attention to the difficulties of defining encephalopathy has led to an appreciation of the complexities of determining causes, effects, and outcomes (Dixon et al, 2002; Nelson, 2002; Nelson and Lynch, 2004; Rafay et al, 2009; Shalak et al, 2003). In one study of neonates with cerebral infarctions, 52% had signs of fetal distress (e.g., abnormalities of fetal heart rate patterns), 56% required resuscitation at delivery, 56% developed encephalopathy, and 91% had seizures; on follow-up to 18 months, 48% developed CP, 41% had intellectual disability, 15% had visual impairments, and 50% had multiple impairments (Sreenan et al, 2000). Identifying the etiology of neonatal encephalopathy (e.g., HIE, stroke, meningitis) has important implications for immediate and long-term management. A number of recent randomized controlled trials of hypothermia to treat late preterm and full-term infants with perinatal HIE have demonstrated statistically significant decreases in mortality, neurodevelopmental disability, and combined outcome of death or neurodevelopmental disability (Azzopardi et al, 2009; Gluckman et al, 2005; Jacobs, 2007; Shankaran et al, 2008).

Severity of neonatal encephalopathy remains the best predictor of neurodevelopmental outcome, with or without therapeutic hypothermia (Dixon et al, 2002; Marlow et al, 2005a; Robertson et al, 1989; Ronen et al, 2007; van Kooij et al, 2010; Wyatt et al, 2007). The majority of infants with severe encephalopathy who survive develop major disabilities: 41% to 56% disabling CP (often spastic quadriplegia or mixed CP), 41% to 67% intellectual disability, 6% to 18% hearing impairment, 13% to 25% blindness (often cortical blindness), and 24% to 29% seizure disorder; 35% to 56% had multiple impairments, and at school age, only 21% had no academic special needs (Marlow et al, 2005a; Shankaran et al, 2008). Children with moderate encephalopathy fare somewhat better, but 6% to 21% have disabling CP, 21% to 30% have intellectual disability, 10% to 12% have sensory impairments, 15% to 21% have seizure disorder, and many of those without major disabilities have lower scores on tests of intelligence, visual-motor integration, vocabulary, reading, spelling, and arithmetic than such scores achieved by either healthy peers or children with mild encephalopathy (Handley-Derry et al, 1997; Marlow et al, 2005a; Shankaran et al, 2008). Of survivors treated with therapeutic hypothermia for HIE, 19% to 28% had disabling CP, 24% to 30% had intellectual disability, 7% to 10% had severe visual impairment, 4% to 8% had hearing impairment, 10% to 15% had a seizure disorder, and 19% to 21% had multiple impairments (Azzopardi et al, 2009; Gluckman et al, 2005; Shankaran et al, 2008).

The presence of seizures, abnormalities on neonatal neurodevelopmental examination, neuroimaging studies (especially magnetic resonance imaging [MRI]), and electroencephalography (EEG) can be helpful in predicting neurodevelopmental outcome for infants with neonatal encephalopathy. Of 62 full-term survivors who had had neonatal seizures, 17% developed CP, 14% had intellectual disability, 18% had seizure disorder, and 27% had learning disability (Ronen et al, 2007). Absence of seizures, higher amplitude on amplitude-integrated EEGs, and sleep-wake cycling on EEG by 36 hours are associated with better neurodevelopmental outcomes (Gluckman et al, 2005; Osredkar et al, 2005; Ronen et al, 2007; Wyatt et al, 2007). Severe motor and cognitive impairments are associated with injury to the deep gray nuclei, perirolandic cortex, and posterior limb of the internal capsule (Miller et al, 2005; Rutherford et al, 1998). Infants with a watershed pattern of injury to predominantly the white matter have more cognitive dysfunction than infants with encephalopathy who had normal neonatal MRIs (Miller et al, 2005). Clinical assessments of full-term infants with encephalopathy are also predictive of neurodevelopmental outcome: In addition to the Sarnat scoring system, the Amiel-Tison Neurological Assessment at Term and Prechtl's Assessment of General Movements are independent assessment tools that can improve prediction when used serially, or when combined with neuroimaging studies and/or EEGs (Amess et al, 1999; Cioni et al, 1997; Einspieler and Prechtl, 2005; Gosselin et al, 2005; Murray et al, 2010; Paro-Panjan et al, 2005). Assessments of neonatal brain structure and function using neuroimaging, EEG, and clinical assessments can be useful in determining timing, nature, and recovery from brain injury (Amiel-Tison, 2002; Chau et al, 2009; Liauw et al, 2009; Murray et al, 2010; Parikh et al, 2009).

CONGENITAL ANOMALIES

Congenital anomalies increase an infant's risk of CP and intellectual disability (Croen et al, 2001; Jelliffe-Pawlowski et al, 2003; Walden et al, 2007). Some studies of specific anomalies report neurodevelopmental outcomes, but more research is needed to define the scope of neurodevelopmental disabilities in these and other congenital anomalies requiring neonatal intensive care. A study of 17 infants with gastroschisis (11 preterm, 6 SGA) followed to a mean age of 20 months found their mean cognitive score was normal (101); 1 had a cognitive score below 70, and 2 had cognitive scores between 70 and 85 (South et al, 2008). Most (82%) continued to have bowel dysfunction.

A Dutch study of 33 children with congenital diaphragmatic hernia (not treated with ECMO) followed for 6 to 16 years found a normal mean IQ score for the group (100 ± 13.2), and 4 children had IQ scores more than 1 standard deviation below the mean (Peetsold et al, 2009). They had normal visual-motor integration abilities, but many had problems with sustained attention (39%), behavior (21%), and learning (30%).

Children with congenital heart disease have a higher prevalence of brain abnormalities on neuroimaging than controls, including evidence of white matter injury (32% vs. none in the controls) (Miller et al, 2007). Children with congenital heart disease may have cognitive, adaptive, and behavioral abnormalities related to brain malformations, brain maldevelopment due to differences in cardiovascular flow in utero, hypoxia/ischemia, and/or a prolonged circulatory arrest time or other problems during cardiac surgery (Goldberg, 2007; Ikle et al, 2003; Limperopoulos et al, 2000, 2002; Rudolph, 2010). In a study of infants with hypoplastic left hearts, neonatal assessment (before surgery) noted neurologic abnormalities in 56%, microcephaly in 36%, feeding abnormalities in 34%, and seizures in 7% (Limperopoulos et al, 2000). An evaluation several days before surgery (at a mean age of 7 months) revealed neuromotor abnormalities in 38%, microcephaly in 25%, gross motor delays in 26%, and fine motor delays in 23%. Postoperative findings were very similar to preoperative assessments: Only 12% developed neurologic abnormalities after surgery. The strongest predictors were preoperative abnormalities, cardiorespiratory status (neurologic abnormalities were present in 64% with preoperative O$_2$ saturations *below* 85% vs. 31% with preoperative O$_2$ saturations *above* 85%), and longer time on perioperative cardiopulmonary bypass.

Malformations of the nervous system are generally associated with increased risk of neurodevelopmental disability. In a study of 20 children with prenatally diagnosed isolated agenesis or hypoplastic corpus callosum who were followed for 3 to 16 years, 20% had severe disability, 25% had moderate disability, and 55% had normal neurodevelopmental outcome (including 73% with complete agenesis of the corpus callosum) (Chadie et al, 2008). A postnatal MRI showed additional major cerebral abnormalities in 3 of the 4 children with severe disability. Neuromotor dysfunction in children with meningomyelocele is determined by the level of the spinal cord lesion; 30% have intellectual disability due to malformations or effects of hydrocephalus, and many of those with normal intelligence have specific learning disabilities (Barf et al, 2003; Oakeshott and Hunt, 2003). Neurodevelopmental outcome for children with encephalocele is determined by degree and area of herniation of brain tissue and whether there are other associated brain malformations. Children with congenital hydrocephalus have a high incidence of mild neurocognitive impairment, but their prognosis is worse if they had significant prolonged increased intracranial pressure, infections, asphyxia, intracranial hemorrhage, or other brain anomalies (Mataro et al, 2001).

HEALTH AND GROWTH

Although NICU infants are much improved at the time of discharge, many have lingering medical problems that require close follow-up evaluation by their primary care providers (Behrman et al, 2007; Doyle et al, 2003; Huddy et al, 2008; Lipkin et al, 2002; McNally et al, 2006; Walden et al, 2007). They remain vulnerable to infections, further complications, difficulty feeding, and poor growth. Rehospitalization for illness (especially respiratory illness) or surgery (e.g., umbilical hernia repair, gastrostomy, Nissen fundoplication) is common. Adequate nutrition is essential for growth of the developing infant, especially for lung and brain growth. Good weight gain, linear growth, and head growth are reassuring that the child is doing well. Although most infants catch up in their growth within several years, some infants with extreme prematurity, IUGR, severe neonatal illness, or syndromes such as fetal alcohol syndrome always remain small for their age (Farfel et al, 2009; Hack et al, 2002; Pryor et al, 1995; Saigal et al, 2001; Strauss, 2000).

Infants who exhibit significant deviation below normal on growth curves should be evaluated for undetected or inadequately treated gastrointestinal, pulmonary, urologic, or cardiac conditions. Gastroesophageal reflux can lead to discomfort from esophagitis, irritability, extensor posturing, and poor growth. Some children with genetic syndromes or who were critically ill as newborns demonstrate decreased appetite, food refusal, and poor growth. Oromotor dysfunction, with poorly coordinated suck and swallow, must be considered in NICU newborns with poor growth, food refusal behaviors, or neurologic abnormalities. Infants with chronic lung disease or congestive heart failure may tire with feedings and require frequent interruptions because of exercise intolerance.

An oromotor evaluation by an occupational therapist or speech pathologist may include a radiographic swallow study to pinpoint the problem, to determine whether oral feeding is safe, and to assess how the infant handles liquids versus solid foods. The cause of the feeding problem determines treatment: positioning, thickening liquids, medications, and possibly surgery for infants with gastroesophageal reflux; calorically dense food for poor appetite and growth; behavior management program for food refusal behavior not due to organic causes; supplemental oxygen for children with intermittent hypoxia; and gastrostomy for children who chronically aspirate, have severe oromotor dysfunction, or demonstrate food refusal unresponsive to behavioral interventions. Children fed totally or primarily by gastrostomy require an oromotor stimulation program to maintain feeding skills and prevent oromotor hypersensitivity. When NICU infants are discharged with gastrostomy, continuous feedings, special formulas, or dietary supplements, they require specific nutritional or gastrointestinal follow-up evaluation to address changing needs and parental concerns.

Chronic lung disease (i.e., bronchopulmonary dysplasia) is a complication of prematurity and respiratory failure in full-term newborns (Behrman et al, 2007; Doyle et al, 2003; McNally et al, 2006; Peetsold et al, 2009). These children are vulnerable to respiratory infections, and they frequently require bronchodilators, oxygen supplements, or diuretics. The experienced clinician uses clinical history, physical examination, evidence of growth, signs of exercise intolerance, and pulse oximetry (especially during feeding and sleep) in making decisions regarding tapering oxygen supplements and diuretics. Infants who are well oxygenated at rest may be relying on their reserves and have difficulties when nipple feeding or sleeping. Some infants with chronic lung disease have transient increases in oxygen requirements during periods of accelerated growth.

Developmental interventions for medically fragile infants should be home based whenever possible to reduce the risks of infection. Infants should be shielded from friends and family with infectious illnesses. Therapists who provide early intervention should be skilled in working with these infants, should recognize the signs of exercise intolerance or increasing distress, and should be trained in how to respond promptly in an emergency (e.g., cardiopulmonary resuscitation training). Infants on supplemental oxygen may need an increase in oxygen when handled.

Preterm infants and other high-risk infants need the protection from childhood illnesses that is conferred by immunization. Immunizations should be given according to the recommended schedule (Saari and the Committee on Infectious Diseases, 2003). Even in extremely preterm infants, full doses appropriate for chronologic age should be used. Infants who are still in the NICU or who are immunocompromised (or whose family includes an immunocompromised person) should not be given live viral vaccines. Pertussis protection should be deferred only for infants with signs of neurologic deterioration or uncontrolled seizure disorder, although it may be postponed pending diagnostic evaluation in a child with recent onset of seizures.

FOLLOW-UP EVALUATION OF THE HIGH-RISK INFANT

The American Academy of Pediatrics has established a policy for the screening and surveillance of developmental concerns in all children in the primary care setting (Council on Children with Disabilities et al, 2006). This policy is most germane to the high-risk NICU infant whose medical problems, increased risk of neurodevelopmental disability, and uncertainty regarding outcome necessitate long-term follow-up in a specialized, multidisciplinary setting.

IMPORTANCE OF DISCHARGE PLANNING

Good discharge planning aims to smooth the infant's transition from hospital to home and to provide the health care, developmental, and parental supports needed by the infant and family. A parent conference that reviews the infant's hospital course and plans for discharge provides an opportunity to discuss the infant's risk status, to assess the parents' understanding, to appreciate the infant's progress, and to begin to make plans for discharge home. In the review of the infant's various risk factors, an honest but sensitive discussion puts the infant's risk for neurodevelopmental disabilities into perspective, giving the range of possible outcomes. Parents should be reassured whenever possible, given the opportunity to hope, and provided with perspective on their infant's risks.

Discharge teaching includes well-baby care (for first-time parents); techniques of cardiopulmonary resuscitation (useful for all parents); use of any special equipment or medication; and recommendations regarding infant car seats, bedding, feeding, positioning, and handling. Plans for follow-up care after hospital discharge should address both the infant's and the family's special needs. All infants discharged from a NICU should have a designated primary care provider who can follow the infant closely and address the infant's special needs as they emerge. Preterm infants with retinopathy of prematurity, incompletely vascularized retinas, congenital infection, or cortical abnormalities require ophthalmologic follow-up evaluation. Infants who failed or did not receive audiologic screening require audiologic follow-up evaluation. Infants with specific medical conditions may require pediatric surgical, pulmonary, gastrointestinal, nutritional, cardiac, neurologic, orthopedic, or other subspecialty follow-up evaluations.

COMPREHENSIVE DEVELOPMENTAL FOLLOW-UP EVALUATION

Criteria for referral of high-risk NICU infants for comprehensive developmental follow-up vary widely, based on available resources, funding, geography, and family needs. Ideally, all NICU infants should be viewed as high risk and offered comprehensive developmental follow-up evaluations through school age. Incentives for families to return for follow-up evaluations encourage high follow-up rates, thereby providing NICUs with accurate outcome data for specific conditions. Close relationships between a NICU follow-up clinic and community health, educational, and social services promote coordination of intervention services based on the child's and family's needs. Limited resources and funding, organizational difficulties, and time constraints all interfere with ideal comprehensive, coordinated, family-focused follow-up and intervention efforts. Although often considered dispensable, developmental follow-up evaluations and early intervention should be viewed as an essential part of the continuum of care provided to high-risk infants and their families.

The goals of comprehensive, coordinated developmental follow-up are to help the family optimize the child's growth and development; to help integrate the child into the family, school, and community; and to intervene when possible to reduce future medical, social, and emotional costs. These goals are promoted by the recognition that each child is an individual with unique qualities, strengths, impairments, and abilities, and that each family differs in background, social supports, finances, and personal coping mechanisms.

Follow-up is a dynamic process that evolves as the child grows, develops, and increasingly interacts with his or her environment. Recognition of impairments, disabilities, and handicaps relies on parental reports, an appreciation of individual variability in the normal pattern of development over time, and the examiner's assessment skills and ability to determine the significance of abnormalities or deviations from the normal pattern. Once recognized, problems should be discussed with parents, including a nonmedical definition of specific diagnoses (e.g., CP, learning disability) and identification of specific intervention strategies.

Assessing the development of the high-risk infant relies on the basic tools of medicine: the history and the physical examination. The focus of the developmental history is to obtain information about the infant's behavior (e.g., sleep, feeding, temperament, behavior problems) and developmental milestone acquisition. A history of milestone attainment is most effective when obtained at each follow-up visit (Accardo, 2008; Accardo and Capute, 2005; Allen and Alexander, 1997). The physical examination is expanded to a neurodevelopmental examination that includes an assessment of posture, muscle tone, reflexes, and functional abilities (Accardo, 2008; Amiel-Tison and Gosselin, 2001). Many follow-up clinics rely on neuropsychologists to evaluate the cognition of high-risk infants, either with sequential assessments or with one or two carefully timed assessments (e.g., at 12 or 24 months).

The developmental milestones should be viewed in terms of the major streams of development: gross motor, fine motor, adaptive, and language abilities (Accardo, 2008; Accardo and Capute, 2005). Gross and fine motor abilities are used to assess motor development and to screen for CP and minor neuromotor dysfunction. Children with CP generally have significant motor delay and persistent neuromotor abnormalities. Children with minor neuromotor dysfunction have milder or no delay and mild neuromotor abnormalities on examination. Delay in adaptive, or self-help, skills may be seen with intellectual disability, CP, minor neuromotor dysfunction, or environmental or behavioral causes. For example, not using a fork for eating may be because the child's mother did not introduce a fork (environmental) or because the child refuses to use a fork (behavioral). Delay in language abilities can signal intellectual disability, hearing impairment, language disorder, or autism spectrum and requires an audiologic evaluation as an initial assessment.

Assessing milestone acquisition in preterm infants raises the controversial question of whether to correct for the degree of prematurity. This issue is most important early in life and in extremely preterm infants. Consider the following example: An infant born at 27 weeks' gestation is now 6 months old and not yet rolling over, but she plays with her hands in midline and can support herself on her forearms in prone position. Her motor quotient (i.e., developmental age divided by chronologic age) is 50 (i.e., 50% of normal—therefore, delayed). If one corrects for degree of prematurity (using her term age equivalent/adjusted age/corrected age), her motor quotient is 100 (i.e., normal). Her developmental status at this age is determined by whether one corrects for degree of prematurity. As children age, the numeric difference in the adjusted and chronologic age developmental quotient becomes less significant, so correction for prematurity is no longer important by age 5 years.

When considering correction for degree of prematurity, the clinician should evaluate each stream of development separately because these may differ in responsiveness to environmental stimulation. Earlier exposure to the extrauterine environment may have greater effect on the development of language than on motor development. There is strong evidence that for motor abilities, one should fully correct for degree of prematurity (Allen and Alexander, 1990, 1992; Palisano, 1986). Language, a component of cognition, may be accelerated by early extrauterine experience. Traditionally, psychologists do correct for degree of prematurity in preterm infants when assessing cognition. They do not agree on full versus partial correction or on how long to correct: for 1 year, 2 years, or indefinitely (Allen, 2002; Aylward, 2002). There is some concern that correcting for degree of prematurity overestimates a child's cognitive abilities and may fail to identify those infants who would benefit from early intervention (Den Ouden et al, 1991; Thompson et al, 1993). Nevertheless, most agree to correct for degree of prematurity for at least 2 years. This issue is important early in infancy and with the most immature infants, but it influences outcomes until 8.5 years (Rickards et al, 1989). Preterm children with language or cognitive abilities consistently below those for their age corrected for degree of prematurity should be referred for multidisciplinary evaluation and early intervention.

Eligibility for surveillance or services for preterm infants differs in different geographic areas. Part C services (birth to 3 years) are required in every state of the United States, under federal law, but the terms of services differ. Some states offer periodic developmental surveillance for children born with any risk (established, biologic/medical, or environmental) of developmental delays, whereas other states do not. Furthermore, the criteria for service eligibility vary widely. Some states provide intervention services to children with delay based on chronologic age, other states wait until a child is delayed with respect to adjusted age, and still other states use a sliding scale correction of prematurity. The very definition of delay also varies by state: for some states a 25% delay in any expected stream of development qualifies a child for services, whereas in other areas children must demonstrate as much as 50% delay in one or more streams of development to qualify for intervention services (Shackelford, 2006).

REFERRAL FOR MULTIDISCIPLINARY EVALUATION AND EARLY INTERVENTION SERVICES

Infants with identified developmental delays should be referred for a multidisciplinary evaluation that assesses all aspects of development. Brain injury is more likely to be diffuse than focal, and more than one stream of development may be affected to varied degrees. Although the most obvious abnormality is identified first, this may not be the most disabling of the child's problems. A preterm infant who presents with delayed walking and tight heel cords may be diagnosed with mild spastic diplegia. This child has an excellent prognosis for walking, running, and good motor function. Problems associated with CP (e.g., learning disability, myopia, attention deficit) may have far more impact on the child's quality of life and adult functioning than will the presenting motor impairment.

Part H of Public Law (PL) 99-157 passed by the U.S. Congress in 1986, followed by the Individuals with Disabilities Education Act (IDEA, PL 101-476 and PL 102-119) in 1990, encouraged and then required states to provide a comprehensive, coordinated interagency system of early intervention services for infants and toddlers with developmental delays and with conditions that lead to developmental delays (e.g., Down syndrome, fetal alcohol syndrome). Some states also provide services for high-risk infants and their families. Infants may be referred by NICUs, NICU follow-up clinics, pediatricians, or families. Each child who is referred is entitled to a multidisciplinary assessment and a service coordinator to help coordinate the assessment and services. If the child is eligible for the program, the parents, service coordinator, and multidisciplinary team devise an individualized family service plan that identifies the child's and family's needs and what services will be used to address these needs. This program recognizes the importance of (1) viewing each child as a unique individual, (2) evaluating not only needs but also strengths, (3) including the family in the planning process, and (4) coordinating all intervention services. Early intervention strategies minimize secondary complications and provide much-needed parental support in coping with disability or uncertainty. The choice of interventions is determined by the individual child's developmental profile and health, the needs of the family, and available resources. Programs or services that enable the family to meet the child's needs better (e.g., drug counseling, transportation, parent support groups) also are identified.

Pediatricians and clinicians privileged with the care of children are encouraged to become familiar with the availability of early intervention services and how to access and collaborate with these services and their providers. The AAP stated that an environment should be created in which the physician, family, and other service providers work together in a caring, collegial and compassionate atmosphere that ensures that early intervention services are of high quality, accessible, continuous, comprehensive, and culturally competent (Duby, 2007).

Although a number of studies have demonstrated beneficial effects of early intervention programs, there is no proof that early intervention prevents neurodevelopmental disability (Achenbach et al, 1993; Bennett, 1991; Brooks-Gunn et al, 1994; Infant Health and Development Program, 1990; Palmer, 1988; Piper et al, 1986; Ramey et al, 1992; Rothberg et al, 1991). One difficulty lies with the use of the global term *early intervention*, which covers many different intervention strategies. Early intervention can be as nonspecific as providing social work support and parent classes on infant development or as specific as a physical therapy intervention aimed at facilitating coming to a sitting position from supine in a child with the prerequisite skills and postural reactions. Early intervention for a child with severe spastic quadriplegia would include recommendations for positioning and handling the child and providing adaptive equipment for sitting, traveling, eating, and communication. Designing good intervention trials that evaluate the efficacy of specific intervention strategies is complicated by the fact that each person is unique. This makes it difficult to define study sample criteria and outcomes and to match disabled children for randomization.

Nevertheless, each intervention strategy must be evaluated for efficacy in a well-defined population. Both hearing and visual impairments are responsive to early intervention services that can dramatically improve the child's functioning and quality of life, especially if begun early. Infants with severe hearing impairments may benefit from wearing hearing aids, learning to respond to and to use sign language, specific educational interventions using multiple sensory modalities and parental support. Studies have shown that a focused educational intervention for preterm infants has beneficial initial effects on cognition and behavior, although long-term benefits have not been proved (Achenbach et al, 1993; Brooks-Gunn et al, 1994; Infant Health and Development Program, 1990; Ramey et al, 1992). Few early intervention studies have evaluated whether there is an effect on function at school or at home. These functional abilities may be not only the most responsive to early intervention but also the most important outcome variables. Studies have been limited to short-term interventions. It stands to reason that the most benefit can be derived from long-term, continuous interventions.

SUMMARY

Although children who require neonatal intensive care have a higher incidence of neurodevelopmental disabilities and health sequelae, most survivors are healthy and function well. The likelihood, type, and severity of disability vary with the condition requiring neonatal intensive care, with various perinatal and demographic risk factors, and perhaps with availability of developmental supports for the child and social supports for the family. It is impossible to diagnose neurodevelopmental disabilities with certainty in the neonatal period. Absence of risk factors and neurologic abnormalities is reassuring. Multiple or severe risk factors can identify infants at high risk for disability.

The uncertainty regarding an infant's outcome and the dynamic nature of early infant and child development necessitate careful medical and developmental follow-up evaluation of high-risk NICU infants during infancy and childhood. Survival is not the only goal of neonatal intensive care. Because the NICU is but the first step in an infant's life, follow-up (or perhaps follow-through) is an important component of the continuum of care that should be offered to high-risk infants. The goals of follow-up are to assist the family to optimize the child's growth and development so that the child is as functional as possible and to help integrate the child into the family, school, and community.

Subtle cognitive, sensorimotor, and neurologic abnormalities can have a devastating impact on self-esteem, peer relationships, and school performance. Alerting parents, teachers, and friends about a child's difficulties and frustrations, and the impact of these on the child's self-esteem, allows them to provide a more supportive environment. By helping to maintain a child's self-esteem and to improve the child's ability to cope with the demands of school and playground, many secondary social and emotional problems can be prevented or ameliorated. Work to improve NICU outcomes includes developing both better neuroprotection strategies for the fetus and sick neonate and better methods of supporting developing infants and their families.

SUGGESTED READINGS

Allen MC, Capute AJ: Neonatal neurodevelopmental examination as a predictor of neuromotor outcome in premature infants, *Pediatrics* 83:498-506, 1989.

Amiel-Tison C, Gosselin J: *Neurologic development from birth to six years*, Baltimore, 2001, Johns Hopkins University Press.

Aylward GP: Cognitive and neuropsychological outcomes: more than IQ scores, *Ment Retard Dev Disabil Res Rev* 8:234-240, 2002.

Behrman RE, Butler AS, editors: *Preterm birth: causes, consequences, and prevention*, Washington, DC, 2007, National Academies Press.

Doyle LW, Roberts G, Anderson PJ for the Victorian Infant Colaborative Study Group: Outcomes at age 2 years of infants <28 weeks' gestational age born in Victoria in 2005, *J Pediatr* 156:49-53, 2010.

Hack M, Youngstrom EA, Cartar L, et al: Behavioral outcomes and evidence of psychopathology among very low birth weight infants at age 20 years, *Pediatrics* 114:932-940, 2004.

Marlow N, Hennessy EM, Bracewell MA, Wolke D: EPICure Study Group: Motor and executive function at 6 years of age after extremely preterm birth, *Pediatrics* 120:793-804, 2007.

Nelson KB: The epidemiology of cerebral palsy in term infants, *Ment Retard Dev Disabil Res Rev* 8:146-150, 2002.

Saigal S, Stoskopf B, Streiner D, et al: Transition of extremely low-birth-weight infants from adolescence to young adulthood: comparison with normal birth-weight controls, *JAMA* 295:667-675, 2006b.

Shackelford J: *State and jurisdictional eligibility definitions for infants and toddlers with disability under IDEA.* NECTAC notes (No. 21), 2006, The University of North Carolina FGP Child Development Institute, National Early Childhood Technical Assistance Center.

Sigurdardottir S, Thorkelsson T, Halldorsdottir M, et al: Trends in prevalence and characteristics of cerebral palsy among Icelandic children born 1990 to 2003, *Dev Med Child Neurol* 51:356-363, 2009.

Vohr BR, Wright LL, Poole WK, McDonald SA: NICHD Neonatal Research Network Follow-up Study: Neurodevelopmental outcomes of extremely low birth weight infants <32 weeks' gestation between 1993 and 1998, *Pediatrics* 116:635-643, 2005b.

Complete references used in this text can be found online at www.expertconsult.com

BREASTFEEDING

Lydia Furman and Richard J. Schanler

Exclusive breastfeeding through 6 months, with continued breastfeeding to 12 months and beyond, is recommended for all infants by the World Health Organization (WHO, www.who.int/topics/breastfeeding/en), the American Academy of Pediatrics (AAP, www.aap.org/breastfeeding), and other professional organizations. The success of adequate lactation depends on supportive attitudes of professional personnel in pediatrics and obstetrics, and on hospital routines and practices that are conducive to initiation and maintenance of breastfeeding, as well as awareness that many mothers will need instruction and assistance to establish breastfeeding. Much information must be shared with new parents in the short postpartum hospital stay, so both prenatal and postdischarge breastfeeding education and support are necessary. Caregivers should be trained to observe and document breastfeeding, and infants should have early follow-up at 3 to 5 days of age with a knowledgeable health care provider (AAP, 2005).

RATES OF BREASTFEEDING IN THE UNITED STATES

Although breastfeeding was the norm in the early part of this century, rates declined after World War II, likely because of the availability of commercial formulas. However, recognition of breastfeeding benefits grew during the 1970s, and rates more than doubled in the United States from 24.7% in 1971 to 59.7% in 1984 (Wright, 2001). The U.S. Centers for Disease Control and Prevention began monitoring annual breastfeeding rates through the National Immunization Survey (NIS), and these figures can be compared with the Department of Health and Human Services' Healthy People 2010 breastfeeding goals, which aimed for a 75% breastfeeding initiation rate in the postpartum period, and 50% and 25% of mothers to continue any breastfeeding at 6 and 12 months, respectively (Table 65-1) (U.S. DHHS and Office on Women's Health, 2000). New Healthy people 2020 goals seek to increase further the proportion of infants who are breastfeed, and aim for 82% initiation and 46% and 26% exclusive breastfeeding at 3 and 6 months, respectively (U.S DHHS, 2011). National rates of breastfeeding have increased since 1990 but do not yet meet Healthy People goals for initiation, duration, and exclusivity. One in four infants receives formula supplementation within 2 days of birth, and almost half (45.9%) receive formula before 6 months of age (Breastfeeding Data and Statistics, 2009). Although some states and population subgroups have met initiation and continuation goals, disparities related to race, ethnicity, age, and socioeconomic status have not been eliminated. Non-Hispanic African Americans and economically disadvantaged populations have the lowest breastfeeding rates for all measures at all infant ages, and women who are younger, unmarried, receive or are eligible for WIC, and who have a lower educational level are less likely to initiate or continue breastfeeding (Table 65-2) (Ryan and Zhou, 2006). Culturally specific feeding beliefs may also influence breastfeeding choice (Scrimshaw, 1984). Such an example from the Navajo culture is the belief that either negative emotions or, by contrast, positive maternal attributes, can be transmitted through breast milk (Wright et al, 2003). Racial and ethnic disparities in breastfeeding rates are an important arena for public health initiatives, and their elimination is a part of the Healthy People goals.

INTERVENTIONS TO SUPPORT BREASTFEEDING INITIATION AND CONTINUATION

In response to extensive formula marketing in the developing world with resulting high rates of infant morbidity and mortality, the World Health Assembly created The International Code of Marketing of Breastmilk Substitutes (1981) to promote ethical marketing of formula products (White, 2001). In 1992 UNICEF and WHO developed the Baby Friendly Hospital Initiative, an international program to promote breastfeeding supportive policies for birthing hospitals (Box 65-1). The BFHI ten steps in combination with an eleventh step, International Code adherence fulfilled by purchasing hospital formula rather than receiving it free, effectively increased breastfeeding rates worldwide (Merten et al, 2005). U.S. hospitals that adhere to evidence-based maternity practices significantly increase the likelihood of mothers initiating breastfeeding, exclusively breastfeeding, and breastfeeding beyond 6 weeks (DiGirolamo et al, 2008). Effective practices include BFHI recommendations such as initiating breastfeeding within 1 hour of birth, 24-hour rooming in, breastfeeding on demand, and avoidance of supplementation that is not medically necessary, as well as skin-to-skin (i.e., kangaroo) care and discontinuation of commercial gift bags with free formula samples (U.S. DHHS, CDC, 2008).

The combination of prenatal and postnatal assistance, breastfeeding support groups, educational interventions for fathers, and breastfeeding peer counselors (trained lay persons of a racial, economic, and ethnic background similar to the mother) are associated with increased breastfeeding duration and exclusivity (Britton et al, 2007; Chung et al,

TABLE 65-1   Healthy People Breastfeeding Goals and Rates of Breastfeeding in the United States[*]

Healthy People 2020 Objectives	2000	2001	2002	2003	2004	2005	2006
Breastfeeding Initiation and Duration							
82% initiation postpartum	70.9 ± 1.9	71.6 ± 1.0	71.4 ± 0.9	72.6 ± 0.9	73.1 ± 0.8	74.2 ± 1.2	74.0 ± 0.9
66% any breastfeeding at 6 months	34.2 ± 2.0	36.9 ± 1.2	37.6 ± 1.0	39.1 ± 0.9	42.1 ± 0.9	43.1 ± 1.3	43.5 ± 1.1
34% any breastfeeding at 12 months	15.7 ± 1.5	18.2 ± 0.9	19.0 ± 0.8	19.6 ± 0.8	21.4 ± 0.8	21.4 ± 1.1	22.7 ± 0.9
Exclusive Breastfeeding							
46% exclusive breastfeeding at 3 months	NA	NA	NA	29.6 ± 1.5	31.5 ± 0.9	31.5 ± 1.3	33.6 ± 1.0
26% exclusive breastfeeding at 6 months	NA	NA	NA	10.3 ± 1.0	12.1 ± 0.7	11.9 ± 0.9	14.1 ± 0.8

NA, Data were not collected and are not available.
Numbers represent percent of U.S. children who were breastfed, by birth year, National Immunization Survey, United States (percent ± half 95% confidence interval)
[*]Centers for Disease Control and Prevention: *Breastfeeding among U.S. children born 1999-2007*, CDC National Immunization Survey. Available at www.cdc.gov/breastfeeding/data/NIS_data/ and www.healthypeople.gov/2020/topicsobjectives2020/objectives list.aspx?topicid=26. Accessed May 17, 2011.

2008). Maternal employment is associated with decreased breastfeeding: initiation rates are significantly lower if the mother intends to return to work before 6 weeks postbirth, and breastfeeding continuation is lower among mothers working >20 hours per week (Meek, 2001; Wright, 2001). Workday strategies that include feeding the infant directly from the breast appear more effective than pumping only (Fein et al, 2008). Public policy changes may improve breastfeeding rates, because maternity leaves of <12 weeks are associated with increased risk of breastfeeding failure, whereas an increase in maternity leave time is associated with attainment of national goals for breastfeeding duration (Baker and Milligan, 2008; Guendelman et al, 2009).

THE EVIDENCE TO SUPPORT BREASTFEEDING

Each year approximately 10 million childhood deaths occur, largely due to diarrhea, malnutrition, malaria, acquired immunodeficiency syndrome, pneumonia, and measles, 90% in the 42 poorest countries in the world. Exclusive breastfeeding through 6 months of age has the potential to prevent 13% of these deaths and is the most effective international preventive health intervention for children under age 5 years (Jones et al, 2003). Human milk has widely acknowledged benefits across economic strata with respect to infant nutrition, gastrointestinal function, host defense, neurodevelopment, and psychological well-being for full-term and premature infants. The benefits of any breastfeeding as compared to no breastfeeding, as well as a "dose-dependent" effect of breastfeeding duration and exclusivity, are well documented. Maternal health benefits appear to increase with months of lactation and are also well described (Ip et al, 2007; Kramer et al, 2001). The resulting societal and economic benefits of full breastfeeding are significant.

NUTRITIONAL ASPECTS

The human milk model is used to design the composition of breast milk substitutes, because the goal for infant nutrition through the first year is to mimic the body composition of the breastfed infant. Human milk has a dynamic nutrient composition that changes through lactation, over the course of a day, and within a feeding, and differs between women. Components of human milk exert dual roles, active in both nutrition and immune function. A reference tabulation of the composition of human milk comparing early and more mature milk is given in Table 65-3 (Picciano, 2001). In the first few weeks after birth, the total nitrogen content of milk from mothers who deliver prematurely (preterm milk) is greater than milk obtained from women delivering at term (term milk) (Schanler, 1995). The total nitrogen content in both milks, however, declines similarly to approach what is called mature milk (Blanc, 1981).

The protein quality of human milk (whey 70% and casein 30%) differs from that of bovine milk (82% casein, 18% whey). Caseins are proteins with low solubility in gastric acid, whereas whey proteins remain in solution after acid precipitation. The whey protein fraction is more easily digested and promotes rapid gastric emptying. It also provides lower concentrations of phenylalanine, tyrosine, and methionine and higher concentrations of taurine than the casein fraction and serves as a model for enteral and parenteral amino acid mixtures. The major whey protein in human milk is α-lactalbumin, whereas that of bovine milk is β-lactoglobulin, the protein associated with cow's milk allergy. Lactoferrin, lysozyme, and secretory immunoglobulin A (sIgA) are specific immunoactive human whey proteins that resist proteolytic digestion and thus serve as a first line of defense by lining the gastrointestinal tract (Goldman et al, 1994). The lipid system in human milk, responsible for providing approximately 50% of the calories in the milk, is structured to facilitate fat digestion and absorption. The lipid system is composed of an organized milk fat globule, heat-labile bile salt-stimulated lipase, and a pattern of fatty acids (high in palmitic [C16:0], oleic [C16:1ω9], linoleic [C18:2ω6], and linolenic [C18:3ω3] acids) characteristically distributed on the triglyceride molecule (C16:0 at the 2-position of the molecule). The fat blends in formula are modified to contain greater medium and intermediate chain-length fatty acids, which are absorbed passively, in an attempt to mimic the superior fat absorption from human milk. The pattern of fatty acids in human milk also is unique in its composition of very long-chain polyunsaturated fatty acids. Arachidonic acid (C20:4ω6) and docosahexaenoic acid (C22:6ω3),

TABLE 65-2   Final Breastfeeding Rates by Socio-Demographic Factors, among Children Born in 2005 (Percent ± Half 95% Confidence Interval)

Socio-Demographic Factors	Number	Ever Breastfeeding	Breastfeeding* at 6 Months	Breastfeeding* at 12 Months
U.S. national	23,714	74.1 ± 1.0	42.9 ± 1.1	21.5 ± 0.9
Race/ethnicity				
American Indian or Alaskan	830	64.9 ± 6.6	34.9 ± 6.3	15.0 ± 3.9
Asian or Pacific Islander	1,571	81.9 ± 3.9	56.4 ± 4.6	32.1 ± 4.2
Black or African American	3,423	59.8 ± 2.6	31.1 ± 2.5	15.8 ± 2.0
White	19,216	76.9 ± 1.0	44.7 ± 1.2	22.2 ± 1.0
Hispanic or Latino	4,839	80.7 ± 1.9	45.9 ± 2.5	23.7 ± 2.1
Not Hispanic or Latino (NH)	18,875	71.5 ± 1.1	41.7 ± 1.1	20.6 ± 0.9
NH Black or African American	2,977	57.2 ± 2.8	29.5 ± 2.5	14.8 ± 2.1
NH White	15,011	74.6 ± 1.2	43.8 ± 1.3	21.2 ± 1.0
Receiving WIC†				
Yes	9,933	67.4 ± 1.5	33.9 ± 1.6	16.9 ± 1.3
No, but eligible	1,124	75.1 ± 4.2	53.0 ± 5.1	32.4 ± 5.0
Ineligible	11,531	82.6 ± 1.2	52.9 ± 1.5	25.7 ± 1.3
Maternal Age, Years				
<20	518	51.8 ± 7.3	18.6 ± 5.6	8.9 ± 4.0
20–29	8,187	69.7 ± 1.7	35.1 ± 1.8	15.4 ± 1.3
>=30	15,009	78.4 ± 1.1	49.8 ± 1.4	26.4 ± 1.2
Maternal Education				
Not a high school graduate	2,813	66.3 ± 2.8	36.4 ± 3.0	19.7 ± 2.4
High school graduate	4,347	67.5 ± 2.0	33.9 ± 2.2	16.4 ± 1.7
Some college	6,504	74.1 ± 1.7	38.9 ± 2.0	18.6 ± 1.7
College graduate	10,050	86.1 ± 1.1	59.1 ± 1.5	29.7 ± 1.4
Maternal Marital Status				
Married	18,003	79.4 ± 1.0	49.5 ± 1.2	25.1 ± 1.1
Unmarried‡	5,711	61.9 ± 2.0	27.8 ± 2.0	13.1 ± 1.6
Poverty Income Ratio,§ %				
<100%	4,288	66.6 ± 2.3	35.7 ± 2.5	18.8 ± 2.1
100%–184%	3,573	70.2 ± 2.5	37.6 ± 2.8	20.0 ± 2.3
185%–349%	5,601	75.5 ± 1.9	44.7 ± 2.1	22.8 ± 1.7
≥350%	8,136	82.6 ± 1.4	51.6 ± 1.8	23.7 ± 1.5

Source: National Immunization Survey, Centers for Disease Control and Prevention, Department of Health and Human Services. Sample sizes appearing in the NIS breastfeeding tables are slightly smaller than the numbers published in other NIS publications because in the DNPAO breastfeeding analyses, the sample was limited to records with valid responses to the breastfeeding questions.

Abstracted from Centers for Disease Control and Prevention National Immunization Survey data. Available at www.cdc.gov/breastfeeding/data/NIS_data/2005/socio-demographic.htm. Accessed May 12, 2011.

*Breastfeeding with or without the addition of complementary liquids or solids.

†WIC, Special Supplemental Nutrition Program for Women, Infants, and Children.

‡Unmarried includes never married, widowed, separated, divorced.

§Poverty Income Ratio, Ratio of self-reported family income to the federal poverty threshold value depending on the number of people in the household.

derivatives of linoleic and linolenic acids, respectively, are found in human but not bovine milk and have recently been added to formula. Arachidonic and docosahexaenoic acids are constituents of retinal and brain phospholipid membranes and have been associated with improved visual function and, potentially, neurodevelopmental outcome.

The carbohydrate composition of human milk is important as a nutritional source of lactose and for the presence of oligosaccharides. A softer stool consistency, more non-pathogenic fecal flora, and improved mineral absorption have each been attributed to small quantities of unabsorbed lactose. Oligosaccharides are carbohydrate polymers (also including glycoproteins) that, in addition to their role in nutrition, help protect the infant because their structure mimics specific bacterial antigen receptors and prevents bacterial attachment to the host mucosa. Fucosylated glycans specifically inhibit binding by Haemophilus influenzae, Campylobacter jejuni, and viral agents (Morrow et al, 2005). Oligosaccharides also are the prebiotics that stimulate the growth of nonpathogenic bifidus bacteria. The concentrations of calcium and phosphorus in human milk are significantly lower than in other milks because they are present in more bioavailable forms: bound to digestible proteins and in complexed and ionized states (Neville and Waters, 1983). Thus, despite differences in mineral intake, bone mineral content of breastfed infants is similar to that of infants fed formula (Venkataraman et al, 1992). The concentrations of copper and zinc, despite their decline through lactation, appear adequate to meet the infant's nutritional needs, but the concentration of iron does not meet the growing infant's needs beyond 6 months, so a supplement in the form of iron-containing complementary feedings is indicated to prevent subsequent iron deficiency anemia (Casey et al, 1985; Dallman et al, 1980; Lönnerdal and Hernell, 1994).

Vitamin K deficiency may be a concern in the infant because bacterial flora are responsible for ensuring vitamin K adequacy. The intestinal flora of the breastfed infant make less vitamin K and its content in human milk is low; thus, a single dose of vitamin K should be given at birth (Greer and Suttie, 1988). The content of vitamin D in human milk is dependent on maternal vitamin D status. However, many women have insufficient vitamin D stores and their infants do not receive adequate sun exposure to permit skin production of vitamin D precursors. Vitamin D deficiency leading to rickets has been reported in breastfed infants, especially those with dark skin pigmentation, little exposure to sunlight, or associated with the appropriate use of sunscreen ointments (Kreiter et al, 2000). Infant supplementation with 400 IU of vitamin D daily is indicated (Wagner and Greer, 2008).

NUTRITIONAL IMPLICATIONS FOR THE PREMATURE INFANT

The nutritional adequacy of human milk for premature infants may be limited for several reasons. The energy and protein contents of breast milk aliquots brought to the neonatal nursery by the mother are highly variable (Polberger and Raiha, 1995). The most variable nutrient in human milk is fat, the content of which differs during lactation, throughout the day, from mother to mother, and within a single milk expression (Neville et al, 1984). Because human milk is not homogenized, the fat content separates from the body of milk during standing and may be lost if continuous tube feeding is used. In fact, much of the variation in energy content of milk as used in the nursery is a result of differences in and/or losses of fat in the unfortified milk (Greer et al, 1984; Schanler, 1988). Although concentrations of protein, sodium, and zinc decline through lactation, the nutrient needs of the premature infant remain higher than those of term infants until sometime after term postmenstrual age. Therefore, the physiologic decline in milk concentration of protein and micronutrients precedes any reduction in the infant's needs and results in an inadequate nutrient supply from human milk for the premature infant. With feeding of unfortified human milk, protein insufficiency is manifest by declines in growth rates and by lowered biochemical indicators of protein status (blood urea nitrogen and serum prealbumin) (Cooper et al, 1984; Kashyap et al, 1986; Tyson et al, 1983). The absolute inadequate intake of calcium and phosphorus results in a progressive decrease in serum phosphorus and increases in serum calcium and alkaline phosphatase activity compared with infants fed preterm formula (Pettifor et al, 1986; Rowe et al, 1979). Follow-up of premature infants fed unfortified human milk finds reduced linear growth at 18 months and relationships to adolescent height (Lucas et al, 1989).

Thus, premature infants weighing less than 1500 g at birth should receive human milk fortifier, a multinutrient supplement designed to meet their nutritional needs and prevent clinical deficiency diseases and growth failure. The fortifier adds not only protein, calcium, phosphorus, and calories but other micronutrients (Table 65-4). Results from individual studies were confirmed by a systematic review that addressed multinutrient fortification of human milk and included a metaanalysis of controlled trials of human milk fortification compared with the feeding of unfortified human milk (Kuschel and Harding, 2005). The addition of multinutrient fortifiers to human milk resulted in short-term improvements in weight gain, increments in length and head circumference, and bone mineral content during hospital stay (Kashyap et al, 1990; Kuschel and Harding, 2005; Schanler et al, 1985).

Human milk fortifier usually is added once the premature infant is tolerating tube feeding of approximately 100 mL/kg/day and continued until the infant has achieved all oral feedings, a body weight of 1800 g, or is near discharge from the hospital. Subsequently, the infant may be fed unfortified breast milk, although monitoring of infant weight gain to achieve >20 g/day, linear growth of 0.5 cm/week, and of alkaline phosphatase levels, aiming for <450 IU/L, is suggested (Hall, 2001).

GASTROINTESTINAL FUNCTION

Many factors in human milk may stimulate gastrointestinal growth and motility and enhance maturity of the gastrointestinal tract. Bioactive factors such as lactoferrin may affect intestinal growth, glutamine affects intestinal

TABLE 65-3 Representative Values for Constituents of Human Milk*

Constituent (per liter)[†]	Early Milk	Mature Milk	Constituent (per liter)[†]	Early Milk	Mature Milk
Energy (kcal)		650–700	Total ω6 fatty acids (%)	11.6	13.06
Carbohydrate			Linoleic acid (C18:2ω6)	8.9	11.3
Lactose (g)	20–30	67	Arachidonic acid (C20:4ω6)	0.7	0.5
Glucose (g)	0.2–1.0	0.2–0.3	Water-soluble vitamins		
Oligosaccharides (g)	22–24	12–14	Ascorbic acid (mg)		100
Total nitrogen (g)	3.0	1.9	Thiamine (µg)	20	200
Nonprotein nitrogen (g)	0.5	0.45	Riboflavin (µg)		400–600
Protein nitrogen (g)	2.5	1.45	Niacin (mg)	0.5	1.8–6.0
Total protein (g)	16	9	Vitamin B_6 (mg)		0.09–0.31
Casein (g)	3.8	5.7	Folate (µg)		80–140
β-Casein (g)	2.6	4.4	Vitamin B_{12} (µg)		0.5–1.0
κ-Casein (g)	1.2	1.3	Pantothenic acid (mg)		2–2.5
α-Lactalbumin (g)	3.62	3.26	Biotin (µg)		5–9
Lactoferrin (g)	3.53	1.94	Fat-soluble vitamins		
Albumin (g)	0.39	0.41	Retinol (mg)	2	0.3–0.6
sIgA (g)	2.0	1.0	Carotenoids (mg)	2	0.2–0.6
IgM (g)	0.12	0.2	Vitamin K (µg)	2–5	2–3
IgG (g)	0.34	0.05	Vitamin D (µg)		0.33
Total lipids (%)	2	3.5	Vitamin E (mg)	8–12	3–8
Triglyceride (% total lipids)	97–98	97–98	Minerals		
Cholesterol[‡] (% total lipids)	0.7–1.3	0.4–0.5	Calcium (mg)	250	200–250
Phospholipids (% total lipids)	1.1	0.6–0.8	Magnesium (mg)	30–35	30–35
Fatty acids (weight %)	88	88	Phosphorus (mg)	120–160	120–140
Total saturated fatty acids (%)	43–44	44–45	Sodium (mg)	300–400	120–250
Palmitic acid (C16:0)		20	Potassium (mg)	600–700	400–550
Monounsaturated fatty acids (%)		40	Chloride (mg)	600–800	400–450
Oleic acid (C18:1ω9)	32	31	Iron (mg)	0.5–1.0	0.3–0.9
Polyunsaturated (PUFA) fatty acids (%)	13	14–15	Zinc (mg)	8–12	1–3
Total ω3 fatty acids (%)	1.5	1.5	Copper (mg)	0.5–0.8	0.2–0.4
Linolenic acid (C18:3ω3)	0.7	0.9	Manganese (µg)	5–6	3
Eicosapentaenoic acid (C22:5ω3)	0.2	0.1	Selenium (µg)	40	7–33
Docosahexaenoic acid (C22:6ω3)	0.5	0.2	Iodine (µg)		150
			Fluoride (µg)		4–15

Adapted from American Academy of Pediatrics, American College of Obstetricians and Gynecologists: *Breastfeeding handbook for physicians*, Elk Grove Village, Ill., 2006, American Academy of Pediatrics.
*Adapted from Picciano MF: Appendix: Representative values for constituents of human milk, *Pediatr Clin North Am* 48:263-272, 2001.
[†]All values are expressed per liter of milk with the exception of lipids, which are expressed as a percentage on the basis of milk volume or weight of total lipids.
[‡]The cholesterol content of human milk ranges from 100 to 200 mg/L in most samples of human milk after day 21 of lactation.

cellular metabolism, and nucleotides affect fecal flora. Gastric emptying is faster after infants are fed human milk than when they are fed commercial formula, and large gastric residual volumes are less frequent in preterm infants fed human milk (Schanler et al, 1999).

HOST DEFENSE

Specific factors such as sIgA, lactoferrin, lysozyme, oligosaccharides, growth factors, and cellular components augment the infant's active host defenses (Table 65-5) (Hamosh, 2001). The infant also receives specific passive immunity via the enteromammary immune system in which the mother produces sIgA antibody in response to foreign antigens, and specific antibodies are then elaborated at

mucosal surfaces and in her breast milk (Kleinman and Walker, 1979).

In Brazil, infants who were completely weaned had 14.2 times the risk of death from diarrhea and 3.6 times the risk of respiratory infection compared with exclusively breast-fed infants (Victora et al, 1987). Not only in developing countries, but also in the United States and other developed countries, there is a reduction in the incidence of gastrointestinal and respiratory diseases and otitis media that is directly attributed to breastfeeding (Dewey et al, 1995; Pisacane et al, 1992). As compared to infants who received no breast milk, a lower risk of otitis media is found among infants who received any breast milk (odds ratio [OR] = 0.77, 95% confidence interval = 0.64 to 0.91) and among those exclusively breastfed for >3 or >6 months (OR = 0.5,

TABLE 65-4 Nutrient Composition of Human Milk and Selected Fortified Human Milk[147-151]

	Preterm Human Milk (1 week)	Mature Preterm Human Milk (1 month)	Mature Preterm Human Milk + Human Milk Fortifier*
Volume, mL	100	100	100
Energy, kcal	67	69	83
Protein, g	2.4	1.5	2.5—2.6
Whey/casein (%)	70/30	70/30	70/30
Fat, g	3.8	3.6	4.0–4.6
MCT (%)	2	2	11–17
Carbohydrate, g	6.1	6.7	7.1–8.5
Lactose (%)	100	100	80–85
Calcium, mg	25	29	119-146
Phosphorus, mg	14	9.3	59–76
Magnesium, mg	3.1	2.4	3.4–9.4
Sodium, mEq (mmol)	2.2	0.9	1.6
Potassium, mEq (mmol)	1.8	1.3	2–2.9
Chloride, mEq (mmol)	2.6	1.5	1.9–2.6
Zinc, μg	500	215	935–1215
Copper, μg	80	51	95–221
Vitamin A, IU	560	227	847–1177
Vitamin D, IU	4	1.2	122–151
Vitamin E, mg	1.0	0.3	3.5–4.9

MCT, Medium-chain triglycerides.

*Enfamil Human Milk Fortifier (Mead Johnson Nutritionals, Evansville, Ind) or Similac Human Milk Fortifier (Ross Laboratories, Columbus, Ohio); 4 packets + 100 mL mature preterm human milk.

TABLE 65-5 Selected Bioactive Factors in Human Milk

Secretory IgA	Specific antigen-targeted antiinfective action
Lactoferrin	Immunomodulation, iron chelation, antimicrobial action, antiadhesive, trophic for intestinal growth
Lysozyme	Bacterial lysis, immunomodulation
κ-casein	Antiadhesive, bacterial flora
Oligosaccharides	Bacterial attachment
Cytokines	Antiinflammatory, epithelial barrier function
Epidermal growth factor	Luminal surveillance, repair of intestine
Transforming growth factor suppresses lymphocyte function	Promotes epithelial cell growth (TGF-β) (TGF-β), (TGF-α)
Nerve growth factor	
PAF-acetylhydrolase	Blocks action of platelet activating factor
Glutathione peroxidase	Prevents lipid oxidation
Nucleotides	Enhance antibody responses, bacterial flora
Vitamin A, E, C	Antioxidants
Glutamine	Intestinal cell fuel, immune responses
Lipids	Antiinfective properties

Adapted from American Academy of Pediatrics, American College of Obstetricians and Gynecologists: *Breastfeeding handbook for physicians*, Elk Grove Village, Ill., 2006, American Academy of Pediatrics; Hamosh M: Bioactive factors in human milk, *Pediatr Clin North Am* 48:69-86, 2001.

95% CI = 0.36 to 0.70) (Ip et al, 2007). In an international study including developed and developing countries, comparing infants receiving no breast milk with those exclusively breastfed for 6 months, the median relative risk of diarrheal morbidity was 3.5 to 4.9 (Feachem and Koblinsky, 1984). Considering only infants in the developed world, the benefit of breastfeeding is maintained: the risk of non-specific gastrointestinal disease is lower in the 1st year of life among infants who receive exclusive or partial breastfeeding compared with those who received formula only (OR = 0.36, 95% CI = 0.32 to 0.41) for cohort studies) (Ip et al, 2007). Even after adjusting for relevant confounders such as daycare and smoke exposure and socioeconomic status, the risk of hospitalization due to lower respiratory infection (in developed countries) is significantly lower among infants exclusively breastfed for 4 months as compared to those receiving no breast milk (relative risk = 0.28, 95% CI = 0.14 to 0.54) (Ip et al, 2007). Lower respiratory tract illnesses in the first 4 months of life are less common and less severe among infants breastfed for 1 month or longer (Chantry et al, 2006) (Box 65-2).

Breastfeeding also confers a strong protective effect against Haemophilus influenzae type b infection (Arnold et al, 1993; Peterson et al, 1991). Urinary tract infections have been reported to be more frequent among formula-fed infants than among breastfed infants (Marild et al, 1990; Pisacane et al, 1992). Reduced adhesion to uroepithelial cells by pathogens as mediated by oligosaccharides, sIgA, or lactoferrin has been hypothesized as mechanisms for this protective effect (Coppa et al, 1990; Goldblum a threshold for protection (Furman et al, 2003; Schanler et al, 1999).

Finally, breastfeeding appears to be protective against sudden infant death syndrome (SIDS) (Ford et al, 1993; Ip et al, 2007). A metaanalysis of seven case-control studies found that infants with a history of being breastfed had a 36% reduction in risk for SIDS as compared with infants never breastfed (Ip et al, 2007). Without a known mechanism for this effect, it is possible that breastfeeding serves as a marker for other unmeasured maternal behaviors that reduce the risk of SIDS.

CHRONIC DISEASES OF CHILDHOOD

Data from epidemiologic studies suggest that certain chronic disorders have a lower incidence in children who were breastfed as infants (see Box 65-2). Because of the nature of these studies, causal relationships between breastfeeding and the health outcomes of interest are difficult to infer. Among these disorders are Crohn's disease, celiac disease, lymphoma, and leukemia (Akobeng et al, 2006; Koletzko et al, 1989; Kwan et al, 2004; Martin et al, 2005). A small protective effect of exclusive breastfeeding for >3 months against the development of type 1 diabetes has been reported, although this remains controversial (Caicedo et al, 2005; Ip et al, 2007; Norris and Scott, 1996). The cross-reaction of bovine milk β-lactoglobulin antibodies with pancreatic insulin–producing cell antibodies offers a possible mechanism (Karjalainen et al, 1992). There are also conflicting data regarding the protection afforded by breastfeeding against allergic disease (Friedman and Zeiger, 2005; Kramer, 1988). However, metaanalysis of prospective cohort studies supports the conclusion that exclusive breastfeeding for >3 months lowers the risk of atopic dermatitis (OR = 0.68, 95% CI = 0.52 to 0.88) and asthma (OR = 0.70, 95% CI = 0.60 to 0.81); risk is lowered further in the presence of a family history of atopy (atopic dermatitis [OR = 0.58 and asthma OR = 0.52]) (Arenz et al, 2004; Gdalevich et al, 2001a,b; Ip et al, 2007).

Several reports suggest a significant inverse relationship between breastfeeding duration and the development of overweight and obesity in adolescents and young adults (Gillman et al, 2001; von Kries et al, 1999). A significant reduction in the risk of overweight in later life was reported in two metaanalyses using good to moderate-quality studies that compared any breastfeeding to no breastfeeding (pooled adjusted ORs = 0.76 and 0.93) (Arenz et al, 2004; Owen et al, 2005). Most but not all studies also endorse a protective effect of breastfeeding against overweight/obesity in preschool and school-aged children. Although it is difficult to eliminate the possibility of residual confounding by unmeasured lifestyle factors, metaanalysis results in favor of this effect have been adjusted for the critical confounder of maternal body mass index, as well as many other confounders including birthweight for gestational age, race and ethnicity, and socioeconomic factors (Ip et al, 2007). It is speculated that breastfeeding promotes internal self-regulation of energy intake and less rapid early weight gain, is associated with lower rates of diabetes, and affects long-term programming of leptin metabolism (Dewey and Lönnerdal, 1986; Heinig et al, 1993; Singhal et al, 2002; Stettler et al, 2002).

et al, 1989). Clinical studies throughout the world have also suggested a decrease in the rate of infection-related events in human milk–fed premature infants as compared with those fed formula (El-Mohandes et al, 1998; Hylander et al, 1998; Narayanan et al, 1980; Ronnestad et al, 2005; Schanler et al, 1999). Methodologic issues, including inability to truly randomize receipt of own mother's milk, varying definitions of human milk (mother's own vs. donor, frozen vs. fresh, mixed with formula), of volume of human milk intake (mL/kg/day vs. daily percent of enteral or all intake), and outcome (blood culture positive or infection at other sites) create difficulty interpreting results (de Silva et al, 2004; Schanler et al, 1999). However, lack of an exclusively human milk–fed cohort, for example, tends to strengthen not weaken positive studies, and the preponderance of available data appears to support a role for human milk in reducing episodes of late-onset sepsis. Fewer and less severe episodes of necrotizing enterocolitis are reported in premature infants who receive human milk, and this conclusion has stood up to metaanalysis (Furman et al, 2003; Ip et al, 2007; Lucas and Cole, 1990; Schanler et al, 1999; Schanler et al, 2002). Data from studies that quantified human milk intakes suggest that its protective effect (1) is optimized by exclusive human milk feeding, as in term infants, and (2) is likely dose-dependent with

NEUROBEHAVIORAL ASPECTS

Whether or not an improvement in cognitive ability is attributable to breastfeeding and human milk is difficult to determine. A small but significant increase in intelligence quotient has been associated with duration of breastfeeding among full-term and low-birthweight infants in some but not all studies and metaanalyses (Anderson et al, 1999; Horwood and Fergusson, 1998; Ip et al, 2007; Jain et al, 2002; Rogan and Gladen, 1993). Disagreement remains even (1) when results are adjusted for the key confounders of maternal intelligence, maternal education, and socioeconomic class, and (2) when only studies meeting strict clinical epidemiologic standards are included (Ip et al, 2007). Residual confounding due to unmeasured factors is difficult to exclude. Among premature infants, factors related to neonatal morbidity such as chronic lung disease and intraventricular hemorrhage must also be considered. Early work with premature infants suggested a benefit of human milk as compared to term formula on intelligence at age 8 years, but these results are difficult to extrapolate to the present because both formula and breast milk are now fortified (Lucas et al, 1992). More recently, significantly improved neurodevelopment among extremely low-birthweight infants as measured by the Bayley Scales of Infant Development II at 18 to 22 and 30 months of age has been correlated with the receipt of fortified human milk during hospitalization. The magnitude of the effect at 18 to 22 months was greatest in the highest quintile (>80%), which averaged 110 mL/kg/day of human milk, and at 30 months the effect persisted such that for every 10 mL/kg/day increase in human milk, the Mental Developmental Index increased by 0.59 points, the Psychomotor Developmental Index by 0.56 points, and the total behavior percentile score by 0.99 points (Vohr et al, 2006, 2007). Finally, maternal-infant bonding is enhanced during breastfeeding. The likely biologic basis for this universal observation is oxytocin, which causes the milk ejection reflex during nursing and serves as a central neurotransmitter that directly affects maternal nurturing behaviors, maternal-infant social interaction, gaze, vocalizations, and affectionate touch (Feldman et al, 2007).

MATERNAL BENEFITS

There are multiple positive effects of breastfeeding for the mother (see Box 65-2). Many clinicians believe that postpartum weight loss and uterine involution are more rapid while breastfeeding (Heinig and Dewey, 1997; Ip et al, 2007). Lactation has a beneficial effect on lipid and glucose metabolism and is associated with a reduction in type 2 diabetes and a lower risk of cardiovascular morbidities (Schwarz et al, 2009; Stuebe et al, 2005). Exclusive breastfeeding delays the resumption of normal ovarian cycles and the return of fertility in most mothers, likely because of an elevated prolactin level (McNeilly, 1993). The lactational amenorrhea method (LAM) is a highly effective global contraceptive program with efficacy rates of 98.5% to 100% (Labbok, 2001). The three criteria that ensure the lowest pregnancy rate are full breastfeeding (round-the-clock), no resumption of menses, and infant age <6 months (Labbok, 2001). Breastfeeding can therefore contribute to global child spacing, which additionally improves

maternal health. Epidemiologic studies have documented a decreased incidence of premenopausal breast cancer and ovarian cancer in women who have breastfed (Collaborative Group on Hormonal Factors in Breast Cancer, 2002; Ip et al, 2007; Rosenblatt et al, 1993). Lactation also appears to protect against osteoporosis, because during lactation maternal bone density declines, yet it is normal in the postweaning period, suggesting mechanisms for catch-up mineralization (Kalkwarf et al, 1997; Specker et al, 1991).

SOCIETAL IMPACT OF BREASTFEEDING

The economic advantages of breastfeeding can be tangibly calculated. From a national economic perspective, it has been estimated that if 50% of infants enrolled in the WIC program were breastfed exclusively for just the first 3 months of life, a savings of approximately $4 million per month would be realized (Montgomery and Splett, 1997). These savings would accrue from a combined reduction in household expenditure on formula, as well as reductions in health care expenditures and reduced parental work absence due to the decreased rates of illness experienced by breastfed infants. It is estimated that health care costs significantly decrease with every additional month of breastfeeding and with each month delay in return to work after 3 months (Cattaneo et al, 2006). The U.S. Department of Agriculture Economic Research Service estimated that if levels of breastfeeding in the United States were elevated to the Healthy People 2010 (unrevised) goals, $3.6 billion would be saved (Weimer, 2001). Thus, extraordinary societal and economic incentives support attainment of full breastfeeding for each infant.

CONTRAINDICATIONS TO BREASTFEEDING

Few true contraindications to breastfeeding exist (Box 65-3). Mothers with fever or other minor illness should be permitted to breastfeed, because the infant has already been exposed to the infectious agent and will be able to benefit from the mother's developing immunity if breastfeeding can continue. Few maternal medications contraindicate breastfeeding, and alternative drug choices are available in most cases (U.S. National Library of Medicine, 2009). Mothers who have undergone breast reduction or breast implant surgery can breastfeed, but should work closely with a lactation consultant because milk supply may be negatively affected if ducts or nerves were severed during surgery.

ANATOMY AND PHYSIOLOGY OF LACTATION

Breast milk is produced by the mammary alveolar cells of the breast after childbirth. The mammary gland is a highly evolved skin gland, and its rudiments are first seen during the 6th week in utero. Mammogenesis, or breast development, begins during puberty with increased breast size due mainly to estrogen and lobuloalveolar development facilitated predominantly by progesterone. During pregnancy, with the support of these hormones and others including prolactin and placental lactogen, breast glandular tissue further differentiates, and the alveolar epithelium proliferates and then becomes secretory. Research using ultrasound technology has changed understanding of breast anatomy (Figure 65-1) (Ramsay

et al, 2005). It now appears that the milk ducts branch close to the nipple, that their number is lower and more variable than previously believed, that most glandular tissue is close to the nipple, and that the lactiferous sinuses, which were thought to store milk, do not exist. These findings have implications for hand expression of breast milk as well as for breast augmentation or reduction surgery.

The capability to secrete milk, or lactogenesis, begins by midpregnancy, although actual milk secretion does not occur at this time because of high circulating levels of progesterone (and probably estrogen). During pregnancy, secretory differentiation of the mammary epithelial cells into lactocytes that have the ability to produce milk components occurs: this is known as lactogenesis I. At the end of gestation, the alveoli are filled with proteins, including secretory IgA and leukocytes and desquamated cells. This initial glandular fluid is colostrum. Lactogenesis II or secretory activation of the lactocytes, also known as the milk coming in, occurs shortly after delivery, usually between days 2 and 8. This phase, defined by the copious onset of milk secretion, is triggered by birth and the drop in progesterone associated with removal of the placenta. The hormonal support of adequate circulating prolactin and cortisol are both required, and other hormones, including insulin and thyroid hormone, likely play a supporting role. During this time milk volume increases from about 50 to 100 mL per day to 500 mL per day, and transitional milk is produced, a descriptor for milk that is literally transitioning from colostrum to mature milk in composition (Neville et al, 2001).

The control of lactogenesis is completely hormonal. Evidence suggests that milk removal or infant suckling are not needed for the programmed changes of lactogenesis, although it is possible that milk removal improves the efficiency of early milk secretion (Pang and Hartman, 2007). Delayed lactogenesis II has been associated with placental retention (failure of progesterone to decline postpartum),

BOX 65-3 Contraindications to Breastfeeding

MATERNAL

Untreated active maternal miliary tuberculosis: Refrain from breastfeeding or infant contact until treated and no longer contagious—approximately 2 weeks

Active herpetic lesions on the breast: Refrain from breastfeeding until active lesions on breast and nipple have resolved. Vaginal herpes is not a contraindication

Active varicella (chickenpox) lesions on the breast: Express milk until lesions are crusted over, administer varicella immunoglobulin to infant

Active human immunodeficiency virus (HIV) infection: Active HIV is not an absolute contraindication in developing countries*

Active human T-lymphotrophic virus (HTLV, types 1 and 2) infection

Use of illicit drugs is an absolute contraindication: Drug-free methadone-maintained women can breastfeed

Chemotherapy: For duration of treatment; seek consultation for diagnostic studies utilizing radiation so as to determine duration of express and discard required

INFANT

Galactosemia: Lactose cannot be ingested and is the carbohydrate of breast milk

Other inborn errors of metabolism require consultation based on the specific metabolic defect

Adapted from Pickering LJ, Baker CJ, Long SS, McMillan JA: *Red book: 2006 report of the Committee on Infectious Diseases,* Elk Grove, Ill., 2006, American Academy of Pediatrics; Jansson LM, Choo R, Velez ML, et al: Methadone maintenance and breastfeeding in the neonatal period, *Pediatrics* 121:106-114, 2008.
*"Exclusive breastfeeding is recommended for HIV-infected women for the first six months of life unless replacement feeding is acceptable, feasible, affordable, sustainable and safe for them and their infants before that time." World Health Organization recommendation. www.who.int/child_adolescent_health/topics/prevention_care/child/nutrition/hivif/en/index.html. Accessed April 1, 2011.

OLD 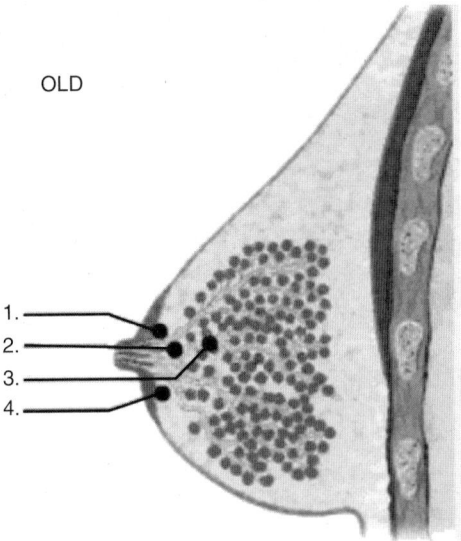 NEW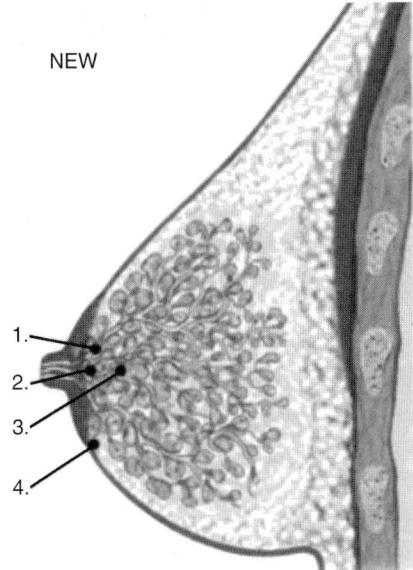

FIGURE 65-1 Anatomy of the breast (Ramsay et al, 2005). *From Medela AG:* Old vs New Anatomy, *Switzerland, 2006. PDF available at www.medela breastfeedingus.com/for-professionals/cbe-information/106/breast-anatomy-research. Accessed April 1, 2011.*

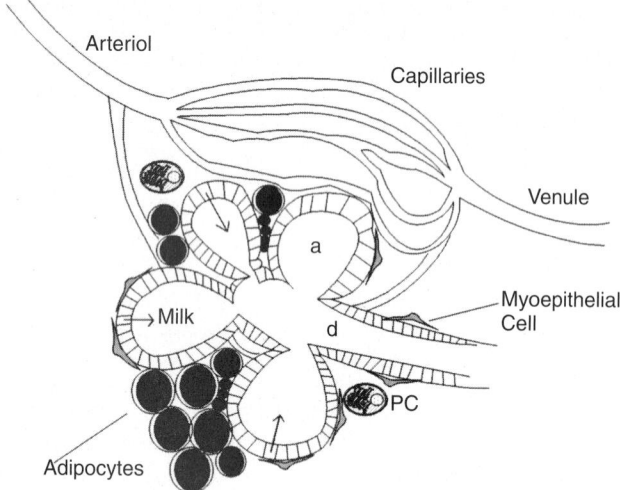

FIGURE 65-2 The milk secreting unit: the terminal duct lobular unit. *a*, Alveoli; *d*, ductule. (*From Neville MC: Milk secretion: an overview. Available at http://mammary.nih.gov/reviews/lactation/Neville001/ images/Modmgalv.jpg. Accessed April 1, 2011*).

hypothyroidism, and theca lutein ovarian cysts, and for unknown reasons there are associations with cesarean delivery, premature delivery, and maternal insulin-dependent diabetes.

If the mother begins to feed her infant at the breast (or to express milk from the breast), then the next phase of lactation, called galactopoiesis or maintenance of milk secretion, starts at approximately day 9 postpartum and continues until weaning and involution of the breast. The control of galactopoiesis is both endocrine and autocrine. Prolactin and cortisol are necessary for milk production: prolactin binds to epithelial cell receptors and is responsible for activating the milk protein genes for alpha-lactalbumin and casein. Milk synthesis remains near 700 to 800 mL/day throughout lactation, but the actual volume of milk produced is dependent on milk removal. With decreased removal or incomplete emptying of the breast due to infrequent or inefficient infant sucking, milk synthesis is adjusted downward because of a locally produced whey protein called feedback inhibitor of lactation (FIL). FIL appears to act on alveolar cell receptors to decrease their sensitivity to prolactin and therefore to decrease milk production. The cellular mechanisms for milk synthesis and secretion are described elsewhere (Neville, 2001; Neville et al, 2001).

Milk that was accumulated in the alveoli cannot flow passively into the ducts. Actual milk ejection or galactokinesis is dependent on the hormone oxytocin, which is produced in the posterior pituitary. Oxytocin secretion is stimulated by infant suckling and other sensory inputs that mimic the infant, such as cry, sight, smell, and touch. Stretch receptors in the cannulicular ductal system are activated, and afferent nerve endings send a signal to the central nervous system. The alveolar lactocytes are wrapped with myoepithelial cells that lack innervation but have oxytocin receptors (Figure 65-2). In the presence of oxytocin, they squeeze milk into the ducts, leading to milk ejection. Prolactin originates in the anterior pituitary, and although secretion is also stimulated by sucking, its production is not inhibited by pain and stress like that of oxytocin, and the milk ejection reflex, or let down does not directly depend on it.

During weaning or extended periods of infrequent sucking at the breast, levels of prolactin drift downward. The tight junctions between alveolar lactocytes appear to open and allow for passage of electrolytes including sodium and chloride. Elevated breast milk sodium is associated with several clinical situations, including involution and remodeling of the mammary gland, which occurs with cessation of milk secretion.

THE MANAGEMENT OF BREASTFEEDING

The successful management of lactation begins before and during pregnancy (Freed et al, 1991; Lawrence, 1994). Formal prenatal breastfeeding education, in addition to the personalized information offered during prenatal visits, positively affects exclusive breastfeeding and breastfeeding at 6 months (Noel-Weiss et al, 2006). Ideally, breastfeeding education should precede pregnancy and be taught in secondary school and throughout the reproductive life cycle. Pediatricians have many opportunities to promote and normalize breastfeeding at the prenatal visit, if one is conducted, and during health maintenance visits at all ages. Prenatal obstetric visits provide significant opportunities for the obstetrician or nurse-midwife to promote and encourage breastfeeding. In support of this approach, maternal prenatal intention to breastfeed appears to be the best predictor of breastfeeding initiation and duration. A study of 10,548 women examined only intended duration of breastfeeding as an explanatory variable and correctly predicted 91.4% of breastfeeding initiation and 72.2% of infant feeding at 6 months (Donath and Amir, 2003).

HOSPITAL CARE

Hospital management of delivery room and postpartum routines has been shown to affect rates of breastfeeding (DiGirolamo et al, 2008). Optimal written hospital guidelines should seek to promote and support breastfeeding for each mother-infant dyad per recommendations of the American Academy of Pediatrics and the World Health Organization; maximize each mother's ability to meet her own breastfeeding goals; and maximize each infant's opportunity to receive full feeds of breast milk. Collaboration between all health professionals and staff interacting with the mother and infant is essential. The "ten steps" of the Baby Friendly Hospital Initiative serve as a useful and evidence-based guide to hospital policy (see Box 65-1). Each step may require changes in hospital routines that have endured over many years but are not conducive to breastfeeding. For example, mothers should be encouraged to put the infant to breastfeed within the 1st hour after birth. Newborns who are placed skin-to-skin on the mother's abdomen minutes after birth are able to initiate a crawl toward the breast and nipple, latch on, and begin sucking. The necessary medical routines of infant identification, drying, warmth, assessment, and administration of prophylactic eye drops and vitamin K can be performed without losing the opportunity for breastcrawl. Other Baby Friendly "steps" that promote breastfeeding include avoidance of supplements (formula or water) unless medically necessary, 24-hour infant rooming in, and avoidance of pacifiers until breastfeeding is well established. If well-meaning health providers offer bottles or pacifiers, or hustle infants back to the nursery to facilitate morning report or other routines, mothers have fewer opportunities to read early infant hunger cues, to put the baby to breast, and to get the assistance that builds their confidence, and supplementation is likely to interfere with milk supply. Birthing hospitals that have been certified as Baby Friendly and thus adhere to the ten steps have sustained improvements in rates of breastfeeding initiation, even among high-risk maternal populations (Merewood et al, 2005). These benefits may extend to mother-infant dyads in adjoining neonatal intensive care units, although necessary modifications to the ten steps that accommodate the needs of premature infants have been proposed (Nyqvist, 2008).

INITIAL MANAGEMENT

Normal healthy infants are able to latch on to the breast in the first hour after birth (AAP, 2005). The goals for the infant during the postpartum stay include: (1) achievement of latch on to the breast within the first 6 hours of life, (2) feeding every 2 to 3 hours at the breast (8 to 10 times per 24 hours), (3) nursing at both breasts each feeding for up to 15 to 20 minutes per side, (4) ability to transfer milk (or colostrum) adequately at each feeding, and (5) that the mother will feel comfortable with the infant feeding at the breast. Maternal and infant risk factors for lactation difficulty (Box 65-4) should be identified within the first hours after birth so that interventions to promote maternal and infant health and the breastfeeding process can be promptly initiated, and this assessment process should be ongoing through the hospital stay.

LATCH-ON

Good latch is the cornerstone of successful breastfeeding because it permits adequate milk transfer to the infant and prevents excessive nipple pain for the mother. Brief videos are available that demonstrate how to assist a mother achieve latch. Nursing at the breast is fundamentally different from bottle-feeding in that the infant pumps the milk from behind the nipple while nursing rather than sucking on the nipple to elicit flow. There are several ways to hold an infant to breastfeed, but to achieve good latch, the mother and infant should be tummy-to-tummy, regardless of the holding position, with the infant facing the mother's body. The mother can hold her breast well behind the areola using a C hold with four fingers under the nipple and the thumb above. She then strokes the infant's mid upper lip with her nipple, and once rooting is elicited and the infant opens his mouth, she can promptly bring the infant in so he takes in the breast including the areola, not just the nipple. The mother's nipple is protected because it is well back in the infant's mouth, and the infant's jaw massages milk from behind the areola. The infant's nose and chin will contact the mother's skin and the mother should not have pain with infant sucking. Many women do acknowledge that breastfeeding is initially painful to just uncomfortable, including the uterine contractions elicited by oxytocin during let-down, but if breast or nipple pain persists, prompt breastfeeding assistance is needed.

BOX 65-4 Risk Factors for Lactation Failure or Difficulty

MATERNAL FACTORS
Maternal chronic illness (e.g., cystic fibrosis, diabetes type 1 or 2)
Anatomic
  Prior breast surgery
  Inverted nipples, nipple size mismatch with infant mouth
  Tubular or variant breast shape (size per se is not a factor)
Obesity
History of prior breastfeeding difficulty
Perinatal complications (e.g., hemorrhage, hypertension/preeclampsia, shock, infection)
Cesarean delivery
Multiples (twins, triplets, etc.)
Maternal-infant separation
Secondary—nipple trauma, nipple pain, engorgement

INFANT FACTORS
Premature delivery <34 weeks
Late preterm delivery (34 to 36 weeks' gestation)
Term delivery at 37 weeks (some infants)
Birthweight large or small for gestational age (LGA or SGA)
No effective latch in the first 24 hours
Anatomic or congenital anomaly
  Trisomy
  Major congenital malformation
  Micrognathia, Pierre-Robin sequence
  Cleft palate or lip
  Macroglossia or ankyloglossia
Neurologic abnormality with hypotonia or hypertonia
Neonatal intensive care unit admission/perinatal complications (e.g., hypoxic-ischemic encephalopathy; pneumonia)
Sleepy infant of any cause
Maternal-infant separation
Secondary—supplemented more than once in 24 hours, weight >7% below birthweight, excessive pacifier use

THE FIRST 2 WEEKS TO 2 MONTHS

Each hospital should establish breastfeeding support groups or work with organized community support groups so that families have a resource on leaving the hospital. All breastfed infants should be seen by a knowledgeable health care professional at 3 to 5 days of age to avoid potential problems of dehydration and severe jaundice (AAP, 2005).

The nursing history varies from infant to infant and over any 24-hour period, so although nursing every 1.5 to 3 hours is the average, some infants will "cluster feed," nursing more frequently for short periods. Without anticipatory guidance, new mothers may compare their infants to bottle-fed infants and misinterpret the normal frequency of breastfeeding to mean that they have insufficient milk. As infants get older, they nurse more efficiently, and the frequency and duration of feedings decrease. New parents may expect their baby to cry when he is hungry and need guidance that crying is a late sign of hunger and can result in an infant who is difficult to calm and latch. Earlier hunger signs include rooting, finger and fist sucking and lip smacking. Pacifiers may be a marker for breastfeeding difficulty, but because their use is associated with a possible reduction in SIDS risk, a pacifier can be introduced if desired once breastfeeding is well established after 2 to 3 weeks of age.

Once lactogenesis stage II is completed, an infant who did not lose excessive weight and who is nursing effectively should obtain enough milk to begin gaining weight, 15 to 30 grams per day, by day 4 or 5. At this rate, most breast-fed infants will exceed their birthweight by 10 to 14 days, and gain 150 to 210 grams per week for the first 2 months. A breastfed infant who weighs less than birthweight at 2 weeks requires evaluation and intervention. Infants must receive vitamin K at birth and 400 IU of vitamin D daily (Wagner and Greer, 2008). Anticipatory guidance should include information about growth spurts, in which infants are restless and breastfeed more often than usual for 2 to 3 days. These typically occur at approximately ages 3 weeks, 6 weeks, 3 months, and every few months, and they may be exhausting for the mother. Because milk supply depends on infant demand, permitting the infant to breastfeed as needed is optimal. In addition, screening for maternal depression, which is associated with a decreased duration of breastfeeding, and for maternal concerns that can become barriers to continued breastfeeding, such as sore nipples, is critical (Dennis and McQueen, 2009).

Mothers who seek to combine breast and bottle or who face return to work can offer one bottle of expressed milk daily from the time breastfeeding is established at 2 to 3 weeks of age: many clinicians and mothers report that infants who are unaccustomed to a bottle will refuse one if not introduced before 1 month of age. Although exclusive breastfeeding through 6 months with addition of complementary feeds and continued breastfeeding until 1 to 2 years of age is clearly an evidence-based medical recommendation, mothers face many family and work constraints. Good information should be provided in a supportive nonjudgmental context about flexible ways to combine working outside the home with breastfeeding, especially because out-of-home employment is a risk factor for premature weaning. In addition to expressing and storing milk for bottle-feeding, mothers may want to identify reduced or flexible hours, take the infant to work, or breastfeed during breaks at a nearby childcare facility (Fein et al, 2008; Li et al, 2008).

BREASTFEEDING THE LATE PRETERM INFANT

Late preterm infants (34⁷⁄ to 36⁷⁄ weeks' gestation) are at high risk for complications of insufficient breast milk intake, including dehydration, hypernatremia, severe jaundice, and poor weight gain, and their mothers are at high risk for lactation failure due to immature and ineffective infant sucking (Raju, 2006; Watchko, 2006). Interventions to support breastfeeding in the late preterm infant include providing (1) positive personal support to the mother, (2) hands-on assistance with latch and infant positioning each feed, (3) encouragement of milk expression using a breast pump after each feed and every 2 to 3 hours (8 to 10 times per day) for 10 to 15 minutes, and (4) continuing rooming-in and skin-to-skin care as often as possible. Within hours of birth, the mother can be taught to hand-express colostrum to feed the baby, and within 24 hours of birth she can begin breast milk expression every 2 to 3 hours after breastfeeding using a hospital grade electric pump. Infant interventions include waking the infant to feed and providing supplementation with or after each feeding at least every 2 to 3 hours with expressed colostrum or breast milk (mixed with formula if there is not yet enough breast milk). The infant may appear sleepy and not awake spontaneously for feeds, so he or she should be waked on this schedule and supplemented after each breastfeed using a supplemental nursing system, bottle, cup, or syringe, to give a standardized quantity of milk. Some clinicians recommend 3 to 5 mL per kg per feed every 2 to 3 hours after day 1, whereas others recommend a schedule of 5 to 10 mL per feed on day 1, 10 to 20 mL per feed on day 2, 20 to 30 mL on day 3, and so forth, based on breastfeeding ability. This trio of nursing at the breast followed by supplementation (or simultaneous with nursing if a supplemental nursing system is used) and then maternal milk expression, comprises "triple feeds," a bridge to successful lactation for the at-risk maternal-infant dyad. In this manner the mother's milk supply is not at risk or diminished because of ineffective or infrequent sucking, and the physiologically immature infant is guaranteed sufficient intake. Whether intervention is required or breastfeeding appears to proceed smoothly, a breastfeeding management plan for discharge should be established before discharge.

MATERNAL BREASTFEEDING ISSUES

NIPPLE PAIN

Sore nipples and pain are the most common complaint of breastfeeding mothers in the immediate postpartum period. Early, mild discomfort is common, but severe nipple pain, the presence of cracks or bruises and skin lesions, or discomfort that continues throughout a feeding or that is not improving at the end of the 1st week should not be considered normal. The most common cause of nipple pain is difficulty with breastfeeding technique, specifically, poor position and/or improper latch, and prompt skilled help is the primary intervention. Limited milk transfer occurs when the infant is attached incorrectly, resulting in poor infant weight gain and impaired milk production. Potential causes of nipple pain include not releasing suction before taking the infant off the breast, overzealous breast cleansing, skin irritant preparations, unique skin sensitivity, skin trauma leading to impetigo, and Candida infection. Treatment for nipple pain depends on the underlying etiology. If severe trauma exists, it may be necessary either to express milk or use a nipple shield with guidance from a lactation consultant until healed.

ENGORGEMENT AND BLOCKED DUCTS

Physiologic breast fullness occurs due to vascular congestion during lactogenesis II. Pathologic engorgement, in which the infant cannot initially remove milk, is the firm, diffuse, and painful overfilling and edema of breasts usually due to rapid increase in milk volume, or to a skipped feeding. The best treatments for engorgement are a warm shower and gentle hand massage to soften the areola and permit the infant to attach, frequent effective breastfeedings (or milk expression with a pump if the infant is not able), and cold packs for 5 minutes after each feeding. Engorgement should not be confused with a plugged milk duct, which can result in a localized lump in one area of the breast, usually due to infrequent or ineffective feedings or local pressure due to constrictive clothing. Treatment includes warm packs, gentle massage from the painful area toward the nipple, frequent effective feedings using different infant positions to facilitate emptying, and discontinuation of tight or underwire bras.

MASTITIS

As a single area of localized warmth, tenderness, edema, and erythema in one breast more than 10 days after delivery, mastitis may present with a sudden onset of breast pain, myalgia, and fever, or with flulike symptoms such as fatigue, nausea, vomiting, and headache. The infection commonly enters through a break in the skin, usually a cracked nipple. However, milk stasis and congestion from engorgement, or obstruction from plugged ducts, also can lead to mastitis. The treatment of mastitis includes antibiotics, and continuation of breastfeeding with frequent feeding (or pumping) to allow the drainage of the affected breast. Additional therapy includes the encouragement of fluid intake, bed rest, and pain control.

LOW MILK SUPPLY

Actual low milk supply most often results from infrequent and/or ineffective feedings at the breast, introduction of formula supplementation that decreases breastfeeding frequency, or early (before 3 weeks) introduction of bottles, each of which decrease milk supply because of inadequate milk removal. Primary treatment includes increased effectiveness and frequency of milk removal; galactagogues, such as metoclopramide, occasionally may be helpful if use is temporary and supervised. Maternal factors reducing milk supply during or after the postpartum period include primary or secondary hypoprolactinemia, absence of an intact adenohypophyseal axis, severe maternal illness including sepsis or hemorrhage, prior breast surgery, obesity (due to a decreased prolactin response to suckling), estrogen-containing contraceptives, and severe fatigue, stress, or pain (Rasmussen and Kjolhede, 2004). It is not clear whether maternal smoking actually reduces milk supply or is a behavioral risk factor for decreased duration of breastfeeding. Perceived low milk supply, in which the infant has a normal growth pattern but the mother believes she does not have sufficient milk, can result from growth spurts leading to increased infant demand, changes in the efficiency of the breast around 4 weeks leading to decreased apparent fullness before nursing, or increased efficiency of infant nursing beginning at 2 to 3 months leading to less frequent or shorter breastfeeding sessions. Infant weight check is diagnostic.

CONTRACEPTION

Data regarding the effect of hormonal contraception on milk supply is limited and contemporary studies are needed. There is clinical agreement that LAM (lactational amenorrhea method; see earlier discussion) and nonhormonal methods of contraception are preferable during breastfeeding. Data from WHO that are now more than 25 years old showed that estrogen-containing contraceptives significantly decrease milk supply, although they do not appear to affect infant growth (Tankeyoon et al, 1984). Limited evidence suggests no effect of progestin-only oral or injectable contraceptives on milk supply if initiated after milk supply is established; however, large prospective trials are needed (Perheentupa et al, 2003).

JAUNDICE AND BREASTFEEDING

The association between breastfeeding and jaundice is observed in two distinct entities: breastfeeding jaundice and breast-milk jaundice.

BREASTFEEDING JAUNDICE

Severe jaundice is the most frequent reason for readmission of late preterm and term infants, most of whom are breastfeeding. If there is any delay in lactogenesis II or if the infant has ineffective milk removal or infrequent sucking, less milk will be ingested and consequently less milk will be produced, leading to a cycle of decreased demand and decreased supply, with consequent starvation jaundice or breast-nonfeeding jaundice. The most common risk factor for inadequate milk removal is late preterm birth. Lack of milk leads to intestinal milk stasis. The neonatal intestine has highly active glucuronidases that cleave conjugated bilirubin to unconjugated bilirubin. The unconjugated bilirubin is readily reabsorbed and recirculated to the liver for conjugation. Milk, by providing calories and gastrocolic stimulation, alleviates the recirculation of bilirubin. Thus, the treatment focuses on improving maternal lactation and providing milk (expressed human milk, donor milk, or formula) to the infant.

Notably almost every reported case of kernicterus over the past two decades has been in breastfed infants, with late preterm infants overrepresented in the U.S. Pilot Kernicterus Registry (Bhutani and Johnson, 2006; Newman et al, 2003). Thus, primary prevention of "breast-nonfeeding jaundice" includes the measurement of total serum bilirubin at discharge to predict future therapy and establishment of optimal lactation. These factors need to be reassessed at the 3- to 5-day follow-up visit (AAP, 2005).

BREAST MILK JAUNDICE

In breastfed infants, total serum bilirubin concentrations remain elevated, and in a few infants this may last for as long as 12 weeks. In formula-fed infants, serum bilirubin declines, reaching values of less than 1.5 mg/dL by the 11th or 12th day after birth. It has been suggested that the elevation in serum bilirubin may be protective against oxidative injury because it has been shown to be an effective antioxidant in vitro. Because this is a normal response to breastfeeding, other than the jaundice the infants appear healthy. The infants have a normal physical exam and are growing normally. Mature human milk contains an unidentified factor that enhances the intestinal absorption of bilirubin in a susceptible host infant to produce jaundice. As the production of the factor diminishes over time and the liver matures, the serum bilirubin concentration eventually returns to normal. Prolonged unconjugated hyperbilirubinemia in an outpatient infant may also be a result of galactosemia, hypothyroidism, urinary tract infection, pyloric stenosis, or low-grade hemolysis.

Breastfeeding should be continued and parents should be reassured. Persistent rise in serum bilirubin may necessitate a diagnostic challenge by interrupting breastfeeding for 24 to 48 hours. Following interruption of breastfeeding, the total serum bilirubin will decline markedly and not rise to prior levels with resumption of breastfeeding. If breastfeeding is interrupted, the mother should be encouraged and helped to maintain her milk supply. The mother may be reluctant to resume breastfeeding because of the association between breastfeeding and jaundice. A positive attitude on the part of the health care practitioners and assurance that this will not occur later may avoid termination of breastfeeding.

GROWTH OF THE BREASTFED INFANT

The rate and pattern of weight gain of breastfed infants differs from that of infants fed formula, and several studies have concluded that the breastfed infants should be considered the norm (Butte et al, 1984, 1990; Dewey et al, 1991, 1992). The World Health Organization recently published a new international growth reference based on the growth of healthy infants who were breastfed throughout the 1st year of life (de Onis et al, 2006). The new WHO Child Growth Standards (www.who.int/childgrowth) set the benchmark for growth and development of all children from birth to age 5, replacing old references, such as the U.S.-based National Center for Health Statistics (NCHS) growth charts, which were based on cross-sectional samples of children receiving both formula and breast milk and were specific to both time and place. The WHO Multicentre Growth Reference Study (MGRS) was undertaken between 1997 and 2003 and gathered primary longitudinal growth data from about 8500 children of differing ethnic, racial, and cultural backgrounds (Brazil, Ghana, India, Norway, Oman, and the United States). The participating children were selected based on the criteria for optimum environments for healthy development, including healthy feeding practices (specifically breastfeeding and good complementary feeding), good health care (including vaccinations and immunization), and mothers who did not smoke. The MGRS growth charts are based on the breastfed infant as the normative growth model and represent the current evidence-based standard for growth of the healthy child.

Clinicians occasionally are in doubt as to when to intervene if a breastfed infant is not gaining adequate weight (Powers, 2001). A newborn infant less than 2 weeks of age whose weight is more than 10% below birthweight must be evaluated, and an older infant who fails to regain birthweight by 2 weeks or is not gaining a minimum of 20 grams per day should be evaluated. The infant with growth faltering, when the weight-for-age (or weight-for-length) is more than 2 standard deviations below the mean or weight-for-age that crosses more than 2 percentile channels downward on the growth chart, should also be evaluated. Assessments of milk supply and intake, appropriateness of complementary foods, and the feeding environment all are

part of evaluation of slow weight gain or faltering growth. Causes of growth problems not related to breastfeeding must be considered—for example, cystic fibrosis—as well as issues specific to breastfeeding, such as ankyloglossia.

COLLECTION AND STORAGE OF HUMAN MILK

Electric breast pumps enable optimal milk production for mothers separated, by either employment or hospitalization, from their infants. Mothers should maintain a milk pumping frequency of 6 to 8 times per day to achieve and maintain their milk production. Milk volume on day 4 may be predictive of supply at 6 weeks. Low milk production may be a problem in mothers of hospitalized newborns. Factors implicated in low supply include biologic immaturity of the mammary gland, maternal stress and/or illness, and difficulty maintaining a supply without a suckling infant. Hospital-based lactation programs and skin-to-skin care have been shown to increase duration of lactation (Bier et al, 1996; Meier and Engstrom, 2007).

There are many instances when mothers will be separated from their infants, and prior knowledge allows them to select methods to express and store their milk for future use. Return to work or school, illness, and hospitalization are some of the common reasons encountered by mothers who wish to learn about the methods for milk collection and storage. General techniques for ensuring cleanliness during milk expression begin with good hand washing with soap and water. Electric breast pumps generally are more effective than mechanical pumps or manual expression. Bicycle horn-type hand pumps may cause breast trauma and contamination of milk and should not be used. Many mothers find the double-collecting kits that enable simultaneous breast pumping from both breasts more efficient for milk expression. Collection kits should be rinsed, cleaned with hot soapy water, and dried in the air. Dishwasher cleaning is also adequate. Glass or hard plastic containers should be used for milk storage. Bacteriologic testing is not necessary for milk collected for feeding to a mother's own infant unless caregivers suspect that the technique for milk collection is not optimal. Milk to be fed within 5 days of collection can be refrigerated without significant bacterial proliferation.

Freezing is the preferred method of storing milk that will not be fed. Single milk expressions should be packaged separately for freezing and labeled with the date (and name of the infant if the infant is cared for in a child care center or hospital). Unlike heat treatment, freezing preserves many of the nutritional and immunologic benefits of human milk. When frozen appropriately, milk can be stored for as long as 3 to 6 months. Milk should be thawed rapidly, usually by holding the container under running tepid (not hot) water. Milk should never be thawed in a microwave oven. After milk is thawed, it should not be refrozen. Thawed milk should be used completely within 24 hours.

DONOR HUMAN MILK

Donor human milk has been increasingly offered and utilized in settings in which breast milk would benefit the infant, but the mother is unable to provide her milk, most frequently in the NICU (Schanler et al, 2005). A Cochrane review concluded that feeding of preterm and low-birth-weight infants with donor milk as compared to preterm formula resulted in a lower risk of developing necrotizing enterocolitis but also led to lower rates of short-term growth (Quigley et al, 2007). A recent development in processing technology has enabled the use of an exclusively human milk diet composed of pasteurized donor human milk and human milk-based fortifier. When studied in extremely premature infants, the exclusively human milk–based diet was associated with lower rates of necrotizing enterocolitis than a diet containing any bovine milk–based products (Sullivan et al, 2009). This promising technology now allows the premature infant to receive a diet of exclusively human milk.

CONCLUSION

In summary, worldwide infant mortality rates are lower in breastfed infants compared with those fed formula, and evidence is compelling that breastfeeding significantly reduces the number and severity of infections in both term and preterm infants in developed and developing countries (Bahl et al, 2005; Chen and Rogan, 2004; Ip et al, 2007; Jones et al, 2003). Strong evidence demonstrates that breastfeeding also promotes maternal health. Breastfeeding also may be associated with long-term beneficial effects on infant health, growth, and development. Substantial improvements are needed in rates of breastfeeding, particularly among racial, ethnic, and socioeconomic subpopulations that suffer the highest infant morbidity and mortality rates. Health care practitioners are uniquely positioned to influence women in their decision to breastfeed. Practitioners should also be prepared to assist in the management of breastfeeding problems and in the logistics of breastfeeding. Discussion regarding the benefits of breastfeeding permits the mother to make an informed infant feeding choice, and for many women, physician support of breastfeeding is critical to their success in providing the best possible means of nourishing their infant.

SUGGESTED READINGS

American Academy of Pediatrics: Section on Breastfeeding: Breastfeeding and the use of human milk, *Pediatrics* 115:496-506, 2005.
Britton C, McCormick FM, Renfrew MJ, et al: Support for breastfeeding mothers. *Cochrane Database Syst Rev* 1:CD001141, 2007.
Chung M, Raman G, Trikalinos T, et al: Interventions in primary care to promote breastfeeding: an evidence review for the U.S. Preventive Services Task Force, *Ann Intern Med* 149:565-582, 2008.

DiGirolamo AM, Grummer-Strawn LM, Fein SB: Effect of maternity-care practices on breastfeeding, *Pediatrics* 122:S43-S49, 2008.
Ip S, Chung M, Raman G, et al: *Breastfeeding and maternal and infant health outcomes in developed countries*, Tufts-New England Medical Center Evidence-Based Practice Center. Rockville, MD, 2007, Agency for Healthcare Research and Quality Publication 153. Agency for Healthcare Research and Quality, pp 1-186.
Jones G, Steketee RW, Black RE, et al: How many child deaths can we prevent this year? *Lancet* 362:65-71, 2003.
Kramer MS, Chalmers B, Hodnett ED, et al: Promotion of Breastfeeding Intervention Trial (PROBIT): A randomized trial in the Republic of Belarus, *JAMA* 285:413-420, 2001.
Schanler RJ, Atkinson SA: Human milk. In Tsang RC, Uauy R, Koletzko B, Zlotkin S, editors: *Nutrition of the preterm infant. Scientific basis and practical guidelines*, Cincinnati, Ohio, 2005, Digital Educational Publishing, pp 333-356.
Schwartz EB, Ray RM, Stuebe AM, et al: Duration of lactation and risk factors for maternal cardiovascular disease, *Obstet Gynecol* 113:974-982, 2009.
U.S. Department of Health and Human Services: Centers for Disease Control and Prevention: Breastfeeding-related maternity practices at hospitals and birth centers—United States 2007, *MMWR* 57:621-625, 2008.
Wagner CL, Greer FR: Prevention of rickets and vitamin D deficiency in infants, children and adolescents, *Pediatrics* 122:1142-1152, 2008.

SUGGESTED INTERNET RESOURCES

This list is neither exhaustive nor presented in a specific order, but is intended as an introduction to web-based educational materials that promote or inform about breastfeeding.

"*Breastfeeding Basics* is an academic, non-commercial, short course on the fundamentals of breastfeeding. It is geared primarily for the medical practitioner, although anyone is welcome to browse or take the course." Authored by Mary O'Connor, M.D., Available at: *http://www.breastfeedingbasics.org/*

The Stanford School of Medicine, Newborn Nursery at Lucile Packard Children's Hospital website "is designed to support the educational goals of our pediatric trainees and provide a useful resource for health care professionals worldwide who are caring for newborns" and is Available at: *http://newborns.stanford.edu/Breastfeeding/*

The New 3rd Edition of Wellstart's Lactation Management Self-Study Modules, Level 1, is an educational tool with clinical cases in a question-answer format and is intended for health professionals interested in breastfeeding. This link provides access to a free download for the first three modules: *http://www.wellstart.org/*

Wellstart provides a webpage of links to sites that support breastfeeding and promote breastfeeding education, available at: *http://www.wellstart.org/links.html*

The Academy of Breastfeeding Medicine has clinical protocols related to breastfeeding, which are not intended as standards of care but offer informative guidelines. These are available at: *www.guideline.gov and at http://www.bfmed.org/Resources/Protocols.aspx*

The American Academy of Pediatrics has created The Breastfeeding Residency Curriculum Online Resource for program directors and other faculty. This resource offers "tools and resources about breastfeeding including clinical and cultural cases, prepared presentations about breastfeeding management, and evaluation and tracking tools" and is available at: *http://www.aap.org/breastfeeding/curriculum/*

LaLeche League is an international organization dedicated to providing information and support to breastfeeding mothers, at: *http://www.llli.org/*

The International Lactation Consultant Association (ILCA) is "the professional association for International Board Certified Lactation Consultants (IBCLCs) and other health care professionals who care for breastfeeding families" and is available at: *http://www.ilca.org/*

LactMed is a data base with information on safe use of medications during lactation and is located on the National Library of Medicine's ToxNet at *http://toxnet.nlm.nih.gov/cgi-bin/sis/htmlgen?LACT*

Complete references and supplemental color images used in this text can be found online at www.expertconsult.com

ENTERAL NUTRITION FOR THE HIGH-RISK NEONATE

Brenda B. Poindexter and Richard J. Schanler

Providing optimal enteral nutrition to high-risk premature neonates is a difficult clinical challenge. In order to achieve optimal growth, nutritional needs in the early neonatal period are greater than at any other time in life. The circumstance of premature delivery results in decreased nutrient deposition in the infant. Critical illness and immature gut motility and function often preclude intended delivery of nutrition. Despite the lack of evidence, fear of necrotizing enterocolitis if feedings are advanced too quickly may also limit provision of optimal enteral nutrition. Consequently, the premature infant requires specialized nutritional support to meet these great demands for growth.

Current recommendations for provision of enteral nutrition to premature infants are based on the goal of duplicating rates of intrauterine accretion of the fetus at the same postmenstrual age. However, this goal is rarely accomplished and the incidence of postnatal growth failure in very low-birthweight (VLBW) infants remains unacceptably high. Recent data from the NICHD Neonatal Research Network report that 91% of VLBW infants weigh less than the 10th percentile at 36 weeks' postmenstrual age (Fanaroff et al, 2007). Infants who experience one or more major morbidities such as bronchopulmonary dysplasia, severe intraventricular hemorrhage, necrotizing enterocolitis, or late-onset sepsis are at increased risk for growth failure. The association between suboptimal postnatal growth and poor neurodevelopmental outcomes at 18 to 22 months' corrected age is especially worrisome and emphasizes the importance of optimizing nutritional support for infants born prematurely.

Special considerations regarding nutrient needs of premature infants arise at birth. Because of limited body stores, increased energy expenditure, severity of illness, and/or immaturity and inability to tolerate enteral feedings, premature infants are given parenteral nutrition immediately from birth. Enteral feedings are often precluded because of the multiplicity of medical problems, but gastrointestinal priming with minimal quantities of milk is used to stimulate intestinal function. As the infant matures physiologically and the medical condition stabilizes, parenteral nutrition is slowly replaced with enteral nutrition. This chapter describes the basis of recommendations for enteral nutrient support for high-risk neonates. In addition, evidence regarding the initiation and advancement of enteral feedings in premature infants is discussed. Finally, special considerations for enteral nutrition after discharge from the neonatal intensive care unit are reviewed.

MACRONUTRIENT REQUIREMENTS IN THE ENTERALLY FED PREMATURE NEONATE

PROTEIN

When fetal life is interrupted by premature birth, significant protein deficits can occur and can be difficult if not impossible to recoup (Embleton et al, 2001). In several observational studies, early protein intake has been associated with postnatal growth in extremely premature infants. In fact, protein intake in the first 2 weeks of life in extremely low-birthweight infants is an independent prognostic determinant of growth (Berry et al, 1997). In addition, differences in weight gain velocity in these infants can be predicted by early protein intake (Berry et al, 1997; Olsen et al, 2002). Finally, there is increasing evidence that the amount of protein intake early in life correlates with improved neurodevelopmental outcomes. In order to optimize growth outcomes, particular focus must therefore be given to enteral protein intake.

The most commonly accepted goal of provision of enteral nutrition to premature infants is to achieve growth comparable to the fetus. At 26 weeks' gestation, the fetus accretes approximately 2.2 g/kg per day of protein; by term, this amount declines to approximately 0.9 g/kg per day. Protein losses are inversely related to gestational age, providing an explanation of higher protein requirements in extremely premature neonates. Accretion of protein is dependent on protein quantity and quality, energy intake, and underlying disease states (such as sepsis or surgical stress), as well as concomitant medications (such as systemic steroids, fentanyl, and insulin).

Using the factorial approach, Ziegler has estimated protein (and energy) requirements of VLBW infants to approximate the rate of fetal growth (Ziegler, 2007; Ziegler et al, 2002). In this model, protein requirements are estimated as the sum of needs for growth in addition to needs for replacement of protein losses. Based on this model, protein requirements for premature infants weighing 500 to 1200 grams are 4.0 g/kg per day; with increasing body weight, protein requirements determined by the factorial approach decrease. Enteral protein (and energy) requirements using the factorial approach are shown in Table 66-1. Protein and energy needs should be considered hand in hand, because protein synthesis requires energy. Extremely premature infants require a higher protein to energy ratio for optimal growth (also discussed in section on enteral energy requirements).

TABLE 66-1 Estimated Protein and Energy Requirements to Achieve Fetal Growth*

Weight (g)	Protein (g/kg/d)	Energy (kcal/kg/d)	Protein:Energy (g/100 kcal)
500–700	4.0	105	3.8
700–900	4.0	108	3.7
900–1200	4.0	119	3.4
1200–1500	3.9	125	3.1
1500–1800	3.6	128	2.8
1800–2200	3.4	131	2.6

*Based on factorial method (Ziegler EE, Thureen PJ, Carlson SJ: Aggressive nutrition of the very low birthweight infant, *Clin Perinatol* 29:225-244, 2002).

Protein retention, or balance, generally is a function of protein intake if energy intake is adequate (Zlotkin et al, 1981). Enteral protein requirements are calculated to be higher than parenteral, because only approximately 85% of enteral protein is absorbed. In contrast to empiric methods, this approach does not take into consideration nutrient requirements for catch-up growth.

The Canadian Paediatric Society, the Life Sciences Research Office of the American Society for Nutritional Sciences, the American Academy of Pediatrics Committee on Nutrition, and the European Society for Paediatric Gastroenterology, Hepatology, and Nutrition (ESPGHAN) Committee on Nutrition have all made recommendations regarding enteral protein intakes for VLBW infants; these recommendations are shown in Table 66-2. The recently updated commentary from the ESPGHAN Committee (Agostoni et al, 2010) has recommended the highest protein intake for infants up to 1000 g at 4.0 to 4.5 g/kg per day.

Further studies are required to more clearly define the upper limit of enteral protein intake in premature neonates to optimize growth and neurodevelopmental outcomes.

ENERGY

In utero, the fetus utilizes both glucose and amino acids as a source of energy. If energy intake is not adequate, protein utilization is not efficient, resulting in lower retention of nitrogen. As shown in Table 66-1, Ziegler and colleagues have estimated that energy requirements are lower in infants with lower body weight. Coupled with the inverse relationship between protein requirements and weight, the protein-to-energy ratio required to achieve fetal growth is highest in the most premature. The recommended energy intake for enterally fed premature infants ranges between 110 and 135 kcal/kg per day (Agostoni et al, 2010).

The optimal ratio of enteral protein to energy intake must be defined not only in terms of optimizing weight gain, but also by that which achieves optimal body composition. Consequently, attempting to duplicate the intrauterine environment may not be appropriate for extrauterine life, given differences in nutrient supply and metabolism. Changes in body composition in response to energy intake are an important consideration, because excessive energy intake can contribute to excessive fat

TABLE 66-2 Recommended Enteral Protein Intakes for Very Low-Birthweight Infants

	g/kg/d
Canadian Paediatric Society, 1995*	
Birthweight <1000 g	3.5–4.0
Birthweight ≥1000 g	3.0–3.6
Life Sciences Research Office, 2002†	3.4–4.3
AAP Committee on Nutrition, 2004‡	3.5–4.0
ESPGHAN, 2010§	
Weight up to 1000 g	4.0–4.5
Weight 1000-1800 g	3.5–4.0

*From Canadian Paediatric Society, NC: Nutrient needs and feeding of premature infants, Nutrition Committee, Canadian Paediatric Society, *CMAJ* 152:1765-1785, 1995.
†From Klein CJ: Nutrient requirements for preterm infant formulas, *J Nutr* 132 (Suppl 1):1395S-1577S, 2002.
‡From American Academy of Pediatrics: *Pediatric nutrition handbook*, Elk Grove Village, Ill, 2004, American Academy of Pediatrics.
§From Agostoni C, Buonocore G, Carnielli VP, et al: Enteral nutrient supply for preterm infants: commentary from the European Society for Paediatric Gastroenterology, Hepatology, and Nutrition Committee on Nutrition, *J Pediatr Gastroenterol Nutr* 50:85-91, 2010.

TABLE 66-3 Estimated Energy Requirements for Premature Infants

Factor	kcal/kg/d
Energy expenditure	
Resting metabolic rate	40–60
Activity	0–5
Thermoregulation	0–5
Synthesis/energy cost of growth	15
Energy stored	20–30
Energy excreted	15
Total energy requirement	90–120

deposition, and recent studies have suggested that rapid weight gain may be associated with adverse outcomes.

The energy needs of the neonate are derived from a computation of the energy expenditure, energy storage, and energy losses. Energy expenditure consists of the energy needed to cover the resting metabolic rate, activity, thermoregulation, and the energy cost of growth. Energy storage consists of the energy (fat and lean mass) deposited for growth. Energy losses usually are due to incomplete absorption of nutrients and are greater in premature infants than in term infants or adults. The daily energy needs for the growing premature infant are summarized in Table 66-3. The largest component of the total estimated energy requirement is that needed for the resting metabolic rate. When nourished parenterally, the premature infant has less fecal energy loss, generally fewer episodes of cold stress, and somewhat lesser activity so that the actual energy needs for growth are lowered to approximately 80 to 100 kcal/kg/day. In circumstances of chronic disease, such as bronchopulmonary dysplasia, the resting energy expenditure rises significantly. Total energy needs in premature infants with bronchopulmonary dysplasia are increased because of greater energy expenditure, activity, and fecal energy losses. It is not surprising to find that these infants may require 150 kcal/kg/day to achieve weight gain.

CARBOHYDRATES

The main carbohydrate in human milk is lactose, supplying nearly half of the total calories. Lactase (β-galactosidase) is an intestinal enzyme that hydrolyzes lactose to glucose and galactose in the small intestine. Despite lower levels of intestinal lactase activities in premature infants, premature infants are able to efficiently digest lactose. Nonetheless, many infant formulas designed for premature infants supply glucose polymers. Glucose polymers are digested by α-glucosidases; the activity level of these enzymes approximates adult levels much sooner than β-galactosidase, which theoretically makes glucose polymers easier for the premature infant to digest than lactose. Glucose polymers also have an advantage in that they increase caloric density without a rise in osmolality. Recommended carbohydrate intake for premature infants is 11.6 to 13.2 g/kg per day (Agostoni et al, 2010). This amount of intake will provide sufficient glucose to meet needs for total energy expenditure.

FAT

Fat provides a substantial source of energy for growing premature infants. Premature infants have low levels of pancreatic lipase, bile acids, and lingual lipase. Human milk, however, supplies a variety of lipases, including lipoprotein lipase, bile salt esterase, and nonactivated lipase. The composition of dietary fat affects absorption and digestion. The absorption of fatty acids increases with decreasing chain length and with the degree of unsaturation. Consequently, medium-chain triglycerides (6- to 12-carbon chain length) are hydrolyzed more readily than long-chain triglycerides. In contrast to formulas designed for term infants, premature infant formulas supply medium-chain triglycerides. Human milk supplies 8% to 12% of fat as medium-chain triglycerides. Recommended intake for lipid in enterally fed premature infants ranges between 4.8 and 6.6 g/kg per day. Of this amount, medium-chain triglycerides should be less than 40% of total intake (Agostoni et al, 2010).

COMPOSITION OF HUMAN MILK AND PREMATURE FORMULAS

Human milk is the preferred source of enteral nutrition for premature infants. However, as discussed later, in order to meet nutrient requirements and support optimal rates of growth and bone mineralization, fortification of human milk is recommended. The compositions of human milk/human milk fortifiers are shown in Table 66-4; the compositions of commercially available premature formulas are shown in Table 66-5.

PROTEIN

In the first few weeks after birth, the protein content of milk from mothers who deliver premature infants (preterm milk) is greater than that of milk obtained from women delivering term infants (term milk). The protein content of both preterm and term milk declines over time, such that beyond 2 weeks it levels off to that of what we call mature milk. The quality of protein—the proportion of whey and casein—in human milk is particularly suitable for the premature infant. Human milk contains 70% whey and 30% casein, whereas bovine milk contains 18% whey and 82% casein. A whey-or casein-dominant commercial formula, therefore, refers to these proportions of bovine milk. The whey fraction of milk consists of soluble proteins that are digested more easily. Human milk and then whey-dominated bovine milk, in that order, promote more rapid gastric emptying than occurs with casein-dominated milk.

The compositions of the whey fractions of human and bovine milks differ significantly. The major human whey protein is α-lactalbumin, a nutritional protein for the infant and a component of mammary gland lactose synthesis. Lactoferrin, lysozyme, and secretory immunoglobulin A are specific human whey proteins that are particularly resistant to hydrolysis, and, as such, line the gastrointestinal tract to play a primary role in host defense. These proteins, therefore, may be suitable for the premature infant who is exposed to multiple pathogens in the nursery environment. The three host defense proteins are present in only trace quantities in bovine milk.

The major amino acid for the fetus and in human milk is glutamine, which is not found in commercial formula because of problems with stability of the free amino acid. Glutamine, however, is an important amino acid for cell growth, specifically intestinal epithelial growth; has a role in immune function; and is a precursor in glutathione synthesis. When commercial formula was supplemented with glutamine under experimental conditions, although there was no difference in rates of sepsis, premature infants who received enteral glutamine supplementation had less feeding dysfunction than those who received unsupplemented formula (Vaughn et al, 2003). Further research efforts are under way to define how to supply this amino acid if human milk is not fed to premature infants.

The protein content of currently available premature formulas and human milk fortifiers when fed at 120 kcal/kg per day is shown in Table 66-6. Given the protein content of these current options, delivery of recommended amounts of enteral protein is a significant clinical challenge. Embleton and colleagues have reported that intake of both protein and energy in infants less than 30 weeks' gestation is consistently less than what is recommended (Embleton et al, 2001).

Although the protein content of human milk from mothers who deliver prematurely is higher than the protein content of human milk from mothers who deliver at term, the protein content of preterm human milk declines over time (from approximately 1.9 g/dL at 7 days of age to approximately 1.2 g/dL by 30 days). Consequently, human milk fortifiers are necessary to provide additional protein in an effort to meet the growth needs of the premature infant receiving human milk. Using standard human milk fortifier (4 packets per 100 mL of human milk), the protein content of preterm human milk at 1 month postnatal age can be increased to 2.14 g/dL (providing 3.3 g protein/kg per day if fed at 120 kcal/kg per day). However, to achieve

TABLE 66-4　Composition of Human Milk and Human Milk Fortifiers

	Preterm Human Milk	Similac HMF 4 pkt*	Similac HMF 4 pkt + 100 mL PTHM*	Enfamil HMF 4 pkt†	Enfamil HMF 4 pkt + 100 mL PTHM†	ProLact+4‡	ProLact+4 4:1 Ratio PTHM‡
Energy, (cal)	67	100	14	81	14	81	28.3	83
Volume, (mL)	100	149		100		100	20	80 + 20
Protein, g	1.4	2.1	1	2.4	1.1	2.5	1.2	2.3
Fat, g	3.9	5.8	0.36	4.3	1	4.89	1.8	4.9
Carbohydrate, g	6.6	9.9	1.8	8.4	<0.4	7.04	1.8	7.3
Vitamin A, IU	390	581	620	1010	950	1340	59.6	
Vitamin D, IU	2	3	120	122	150	152	26	
Vitamin E, IU	1	1.6	3.2	4.2	4.6	5.7	0.4	
Vitamin K, µg	0.2	0.3	8.3	8.5	4.4	4.6	<0.2	
Thiamin (vitamin B$_1$), µg	21	31	233	254	150	171	4	
Riboflavin (vitamin B$_2$), µg	48	72	417	465	220	268	15	
Vitamin B$_6$, µg	15	22	211	226	115	130		
Vitamin B$_{12}$, µg	0.05	0.07	0.64	0.69	0.18	0.23		
Niacin, µg	150	224	3570	3720	3000	3150	52	
Folic acid, µg	3.4	5	23	26.4	25	28.4		
Pantothenic acid, µg	181	269	150	331	730	910	75	
Biotin, µg	0.4	0.6	2.6	2.64	2.7	3.1	0.2	
Vitamin C, µg	11	16	25	36	12	23	<0.2	
Choline, mg	9.4	14						
Inositol, mg	14.7	22.0						
Calcium, mg	25	37	117	142	90	115	117	128
Phosphorus, mg	13	19	67	80	50	63	70	70
Magnesium, mg	3.1	4.6	7	10	1	4.1	5.1	8
Iron, mg	0.12	0.18	0.35	0.47	1.44	1.56	0.1	0.2
Zinc, mg	0.34	0.51	1	1.3	0.72	1.06	0.5	0.74
Manganese, µg	0.67	1	7.2	7.9	10	10.7	<12	2.4
Copper, µg	64.4	96	170	234	44	108	60.8	67
Iodine, µg	11	16						
Selenium, µg	1.5	2.2						
Sodium, mg	25	37	15	40	16	40.8	37	54
Potassium, mg	57	85	63	120	29	86	34.4	71
Chloride, mg	55	82	38	93	13	68	38.6	83
Osmolality, mOsm/kg H$_2$O	290	290		385		350		<335

HMF, Human milk fortifier; *PTHM*, preterm human milk.

* www.abbott.com, Pediatric Nutritionals Product Guide July 2007. Ross Products Division. Abbott Laboratories 70092-001/50936/July 2007; Product Label 4/09.

†www.meadjohnson.com, Pediatric Products Handbook LB5 Rev 8/07; Product Label 4/09.

‡www.prolacta.com

4.0 g/kg per day of protein with human milk, many units use additional powder fortifier, fortified donor milk, 30 kcal/oz preterm formula, or the addition of a protein supplement. Recently, a pasteurized donor human milk–based human milk fortifier (Prolact-Plus, Prolacta Bioscience) was evaluated in extremely premature infants. Compared to infants receiving a mother's milk–based diet that also included bovine milk–based products, an exclusively human milk–based diet was associated with lower rates of necrotizing enterocolitis (Sullivan et al, 2010).

The Life Sciences Research Office of the American Society for Nutritional Sciences published guidelines for nutrient requirements of preterm infant formulas in 2002 (Klein, 2002). In order to meet the recommended intake of enteral protein, premature formula or human milk would need to supply 3.2 to 4.1 g protein per 100 kcal. When 24 calorie/oz preterm formula is fed at 120 kcal/kg per day, only one currently available formula supplies 4 g/kg per day of protein (Similac Special Care High Protein; Abbott Nutrition). The use of a higher-protein premature formula (3.6 g protein/100 kcal) was studied by Cooke and Embleton (Cooke et al, 2006). Compared with use of standard preterm formula (3.0 g/100 kcal), use of the higher-protein formula resulted in increased protein accretion

TABLE 66-5 Composition of Premature Formulas (per 100 kcal)

	Similac Special Care (Abbott/Ross)		Enfamil Premature (Mead Johnson)		Good Start Premature 24 (Nestle)
	24 kcal/oz High Pro	24 kcal/oz	30 kcal/oz	24 kcal/oz	24 kcal/oz
Volume (mL)	123	123	99	124	125
Protein					
Content (g)	3.3	3	3	3	3
% Energy (cal)	13.2	12	12	12	12
Whey-casein ratio	60:40	60:40	60:40	60:40	100:0
Lipid					
Content (g)	5.43	5.43	6.61	5.1	5.2
% Energy	49	47	57	44	46
Source					
Medium-chain triglycerides (MCT) (%)	50	50	50	40	40
Coconut (%)	20	20	18	0	
Soybean (%)	30	30	30	30	29
Oleic (%)	27				
Safflower (%)	29				
Docosahexaenoic acid (DHA) (%) FA	0.25	0.25	0.25	0.33	0.32
Arachidonic acid (AA) (%) FA	0.4	0.4	0.4	0.67	0.64
Carbohydrate					
Content (g)	10	10.3	7.73	11	10.5
% Energy (cal)	40	41	31	44	42
Minerals and Trace Elements					
Calcium (mg)	180	180	180	165	164
Chloride (mg)	81	81	81	90	85
Copper (μg)	250	250	250	120	150
Iodine (μg)	6	6	6	25	35
Iron (mg)	1.8	1.8	1.8	1.8	1.8
Phosphorus (mg)	100	100	100	83	85
Potassium (mg)	129	129	129	98	120
Magnesium (μg)	12	12	12	9	10
Manganese (μg)	12	12	12	6.3	7
Selenium (μg)	1.8	1.8	1.8	2.8	2
Sodium (mg)	43	43	43	58	55
Zinc (mg	1.5	1.5	1.5	1.5	1.3
Vitamins					
Fat-Soluble					
Vitamin A (IU)	1250	1250	1250	1250	1000
Vitamin D (IU)	150	150	150	240	180
Vitamin E (IU)	4	4	4	6.3	6
Vitamin K (μg)	12	12	12	8	8
Water-Soluble					
Vitamin B_6 (μg)	250	250	250	150	200
Vitamin B_{12} (μg)	0.55	0.55	0.55	0.25	0.25
Vitamin C (mg)	37	37	37	20	30
Biotin (μg)	37	37	37	4	5
Folic acid (μg)	37	37	37	40	45

TABLE 66-5   Composition of Premature Formulas (per 100 kcal)—cont'd

	Similac Special Care (Abbott/Ross)		Enfamil Premature (Mead Johnson)		Good Start Premature 24 (Nestle)
	24 kcal/oz High Pro	24 kcal/oz	30 kcal/oz	24 kcal/oz	24 kcal/oz
Niacin (mg)	5	5	5	4	4
Pantothenic acid (mg)	1.9	1.9	1.9	1.2	14
Riboflavin (µg)	620	620	620	300	300
Thiamine (µg)	250	250	250	200	200
Other					
Carnitine (mg)	5.9	5.9	5.9	2.4	
Choline (mg)	10	10	10	20	15
Inositol (mg)	40	40	40	44	35
Taurine	(mg)	6.7	6.7	6.7	6
Osmolality(mOsmol/kg H₂O) 280	280	325	300	275	

TABLE 66-6   Protein Content of Enteral Nutrition Options for Premature Infants (When Providing 120 kcal/kg/d)

	g/kg/d
Preterm Human Milk (1 month)	
Unfortified	2.4
Fortified	3.6
24 cal/oz Premature Formula	
Enfamil Premature	3.6
Similac Special Care	3.6
Similac Special Care "high protein"	4.0
27 cal/oz Premature Formula	
24 cal standard + 30 cal	3.6
24 cal SSC high protein + 30 cal	3.8
30 cal/oz Premature Formula	
Ready-to-feed	3.6
24 cal formula + polycose + MCT oil	2.8

MCT, Medium-chain triglyceride; *SSC*, Similac Special Care.

and improved weight gain without evidence of toxicity. Many strategies are employed at various neonatal intensive care units to increase protein intake, most requiring the addition of a protein supplement to enteral nutrition. It is important to point out that increasing caloric density with only carbohydrate and fat (such as adding polycose and/or medium chain triglyceride oil) results in a protein content that is significantly less than the amount required by extremely premature infants. Calorically dense feedings (greater than 24 kcal/oz) should be considered for infants who cannot meet their needs for growth using standard preterm formula (or standard fortified breast milk). In these situations, proportional growth should be considered more than absolute weight gain.

FAT

The lipid system in human milk is structured in a way that facilitates fat digestion and absorption. In human milk, fat exists as organized fat globules containing an outer protein coat and an inner lipid core. The type of fatty acids (high palmitic 16:0, oleic 18:1, linoleic 18:2ω-6, and linoleic 18:3ω-3), their distribution on the triglyceride molecule (16:0 at the 2 position of the molecule), and the presence of bile salt–stimulated lipase are important components of the lipid system in human milk. Because the lipase is heat-labile, the superior fat absorption from human milk is reported only when unprocessed milk is fed.

The most variable nutrient component in human milk is fat, the major energy source, making up nearly 50% of the calories. The fat content of human milk varies among women, changes during the day, rises slightly during lactation, and increases dramatically within a single milk expression. The variability in total fat content is unrelated to maternal dietary fat intake. Because it is not homogenized, the fat separates out of human milk on standing. The separated fat may adhere to collection containers, feeding tubes, and syringes. If significant fat is lost, energy intake may be compromised in the premature infant.

Manufacturers of infant formulas modify their fat blends to mimic the fat absorption from human milk. This accounts for differences in the constituent fatty acids between human milk and cow's milk–based formulas. Generally, commercial formulations have a greater quantity of medium-chain fatty acids (MCFAs) to compensate for the absence of lipase and the unique structure of triglycerides in human milk. In human milk, saturated fatty acids, particularly palmitic acid, are esterified in the 2 position of the triglyceride molecule. The end product of digestion of the triglyceride is a 2-monoglyceride and minimal free fatty acid. The 2-monoglyceride is absorbed better than the free fatty acid. This enhanced absorption is important because free palmitic acid has a great tendency to bind with minerals to form soaps. In that event, both fat and mineral absorption would be limited. Thus, the overall structure of human milk is designed to provide optimal fat and mineral absorption.

Essential Fatty Acids

The essential fatty acids, linoleic and linolenic acids, are present in ample quantities in human milk and commercial formula. Without an adequate intake of these fatty acids, essential fatty acid deficiency (thrombocytopenia, dermatitis, increased infections, and delayed growth) can develop in as little as 1 week. Only 0.5 g/kg/day (~4% of total energy intake) of essential fatty acids will prevent the deficiency. α-Linolenic acid is an important precursor for synthesis of both eicosapentaenoic acid and docosahexaenoic acid (DHA). The very long-chain polyunsaturated fatty acids arachidonic acid (20:4ω-6) and DHA (22:6ω-3) are found in human but not bovine milk and are components of phospholipids found in brain, retina, and red blood cell membranes (Uauy and Hoffman, 1991). Arachidonic and docosahexaenoic acids functionally have been associated with body growth, vision, and cognition (Carlson et al, 1996a, 1996b). In addition, the fatty acids are integral parts of prostaglandin metabolism. When their diet was supplemented with polyunsaturated fatty acids, formula-fed premature infants had red blood cell concentrations of DHA paralleling those of similar infants fed human milk. Follow-up studies of such supplemented infants suggest improvements in visual acuity compared with unsupplemented infants, but of similar magnitude to that in infants fed human milk (Heird and Lapillonne, 2005). Improvement in cognitive measures during the 1st year of life have also been shown. Both arachidonic acid (AA) and DHA are now added to premature formula. Recommended intakes for DHA and AA are 11 to 27 mg/100 kcal and 16 to 39 mg/100 kcal, respectively (Agostoni et al, 2010).

Medium-Chain Fatty Acids

The proportion of MCFAS, here defined as carbon length 6:0 to 12:0, is less than 12% of total fatty acids in human milk but approaches 50% in preterm formulas. MCFAs are not essential fatty acids. Previous reports suggested that MCFAs were absorbed passively and to a greater extent than long-chain fatty acids (LCFA) and affected growth and mineral absorption positively. However, when added exogenously to milk, MCFAs have been reported to adhere to feeding tubes, thereby diminishing fat delivery to the infant. No compelling data exist to suggest that a high proportion of MCFAs is needed for preterm formulas. Indeed, formulas containing a very high proportion of MCFAs (>80%) may produce essential fatty acid deficiency if fed for a prolonged period of time.

The variability in the fat content of human milk may be used to advantage in the premature infant. Most milk transfer during a feeding occurs in 10 to 15 minutes, but continued milk expression yields a milk with a progressively higher fat content—the hindmilk—than the earlier foremilk. The fat content of hindmilk may be 1.5- to 3-fold greater than that of foremilk. The use of hindmilk

in selected cases may provide the premature infant with additional energy. Fractionation of each milk expression into two portions, foremilk and hindmilk, is practical if the mother's milk production is greater than that needed by the infant. No differences between fractions were observed for the concentration of nitrogen, calcium, phosphorus, sodium, or potassium. Copper and zinc concentrations declined by approximately 5% from foremilk to hindmilk.

The differences between foremilk and hindmilk also should be considered in terms of the distribution of calories. Fat and protein compose 42% and 12%, respectively, of calories in foremilk and 55% and 9% of calories in hindmilk. Theoretically, the long-term feeding of hindmilk could exert a negative effect on protein status. A greater proportion of protein calories (10% to 12%) is recommended for premature infants.

CARNITINE

Carnitine is synthesized from lysine and methionine and serves as an important effector of fatty acid oxidation in the mitochondria. The provision of carnitine in the diet results in improved fatty acid oxidation. Human milk contains abundant carnitine, and all infant formulas are supplemented with carnitine.

INITIATION AND ADVANCEMENT OF ENTERAL FEEDS

In early postnatal life, extremely premature infants are dependent on the parenteral route if nutrient requirements are to be met. The strategy employed to transition to full enteral feeds is the source of much debate, and there is considerable variation in practice among different neonatal intensive care units. The primary questions that clinicians must consider include when to initiate enteral feeds, how to advance feedings (continuously or more slowly at first), and how rapidly to advance the enteral feeding volume. These questions have been difficult to study in a rigorous manner but have been addressed in a series of Cochrane systematic reviews by Kennedy and Tyson (Kennedy et al, 2000; Tyson and Kennedy, 2000). The primary question is to determine the optimal feeding regimen that does not increase the incidence of necrotizing enterocolitis.

GASTROINTESTINAL PRIMING

The lack of enteral nutrients poses several problems for the development of the intestinal tract. In several animal species, the absence of enteral nutrients is associated with diminished intestinal growth, atrophy of intestinal mucosa, delayed maturation of intestinal enzymes, and increases in permeability and bacterial translocation. A lack of enteral nutrients also affects intestinal motility, perfusion, and hormonal responses. The hormonal response to feeding premature infants has been evaluated by measuring the plasma concentrations of a variety of gastrointestinal hormones in response to milk feeding during the 1st week after birth (Lucas et al, 1986). Significant hormonal surges were noted after milk feeding, but no response was observed in the absence of feeding. In further investigations, it was observed that hormonal surges of gastrin, gastric inhibitory polypeptide, and enteroglucagon occurred after the feeding of small quantities of milk (24 mL), but motilin surges were not observed until the cumulative milk intake was 700 mL.

The foregoing observations prompted prospective randomized clinical studies of the effects of small volumes of milk given as early minimal enteral feeding, or trophic feeding, in premature infants. When studied in the 1st or 2nd week after birth, infants who received "early" milk feedings had a better feeding tolerance when feedings were advanced, required a shorter duration of parenteral nutrition, and had a lower incidence of conjugated hyperbilirubinemia compared with similar infants given only parenteral nutrition during the same interval (Slagle and Gross, 1988). The lower alkaline phosphatase activity, primarily of bone origin, was observed for 14 weeks, well beyond the initial intervention in the 1st week. Significant stimulation of gastrointestinal hormones, such as gastrin and gastric inhibitory polypeptide, also was reported after the early feeding of small quantities of milk (Meetze et al, 1992). Intestinal motility patterns matured more rapidly in premature infants receiving early enteral feeding (Berseth, 1992). Subsequent investigations demonstrated that trophic feeding was associated with greater absorption of calcium and phosphorus, greater lactase activity, and reduced intestinal permeability. The metaanalysis of several studies of gastrointestinal priming indicated that its use was associated with a shorter time to regain birthweight, fewer days when feeding was withheld, and a shorter duration of hospitalization, but no increase in the incidence of necrotizing enterocolitis. The infants also had the usual pathologic conditions of patent ductus arteriosus, intraventricular hemorrhage, or systemic hypotension.

MINERAL, VITAMIN, AND TRACE ELEMENT SUPPLEMENTATION

The recommended oral intake for vitamins is shown in Table 66-7; recommended intake for minerals and trace elements is shown in Table 66-8.

CALCIUM AND PHOSPHORUS

Calcium and phosphorus are primary components of the skeleton, accounting for 99% and 85%, respectively, of bone mass. The goal for premature infant nutrition is to achieve a bone mineralization pattern similar to that in the fetus, to avoid osteopenia and fractures. Preterm human milk contains approximately 250 mg/L and 140 mg/L, respectively, of calcium and phosphorus. In contrast, the calcium and phosphorus contents of enteral products designed for premature infants in the United States are significantly greater. In human milk, calcium and phosphorus exist in ionized and complexed forms that are easily absorbed. Thus, in the design of commercial formulas, greater quantities of these minerals are added to compensate for their poorer bioavailability. However, distinct from the term infant, the premature infant requires significantly greater quantities of calcium and phosphorus than can be provided in human milk.

TABLE 66-7   Recommended Oral Intake of Vitamins for Preterm Infants

Vitamin (per 100 kcal)	AAP*	ESPGHAN†
Fat Soluble		
Vitamin A (IU)	467–1364	1210–2466
Vitamin D (IU)	100–364	100–350 (800–1000/d)
Vitamin E (IU)	4–10.9	2–10 mg alpha TE
Vitamin K (μg)	5.3–9.1	4–25
Water Soluble		
Vitamin B$_6$ (μg)	100–191	41–330
Vitamin B$_{12}$ (μg)	0.2–0.27	0.08–0.7
Vitamin C (mg)	12–21.8	10–42
Biotin (μg)	2.4–5.5	1.5–15
Folic acid (μg)	17–45	32–90
Niacin (mg)	2.4–4.4	0.345–5
Pantothenate (mg)	0.8–1.5	0.3–1.9
Riboflavin (μg)	167–327	180–365
Thiamin (μg)	120–218	125–275

*From American Academy of Pediatrics: *Pediatric nutrition handbook*, Elk Grove Village, Ill, 2009, American Academy of Pediatrics.
†From Agostoni C, Buonocore G, Carnielli VP, et al: Enteral nutrient supply for preterm infants: commentary from the European Society for Paediatric Gastroenterology, Hepatology, and Nutrition Committee on Nutrition, *J Pediatr Gastroenterol Nutr* 50:85-91, 2010.

TABLE 66-8   Recommended Oral Intake of Minerals and Trace Elements for Preterm Infants

Mineral/Trace Element (per 100 kcal)	AAP*	ESPGHAN†
Calcium (mg)	67–200	110–130
Chloride (mEq)	2–6.5	1.7–4.6
Magnesium (mg)	5.3–13.6	7.5–13.6
Phosphorus (mg)	40–127	55–80
Potassium (mEq)	1.3–2.7	1.5–4.1
Sodium (mEq)	2–4.6	1.7–2.7
Iron (mg)	1.33–3.64	1.8–2.7
Chromium (μg)	0.07–2.05	0.027–1.12
Copper (μg)	80–136	90–120
Fluoride (μg)		1.4–55
Iodine (μg)	6.7–54.5	10–50
Manganese (μg)	0.5–6.8	6.3–25
Molybdenum (μg)	0.2–0.27	0.27–4.5
Selenium (μg)	0.9–4.1	4.5–9
Zinc (mg)	0.34–2.7	1–1.8

*From American Academy of Pediatrics: *Pediatric nutrition handbook*, Elk Grove Village, Ill, 2009, American Academy of Pediatrics.
†From Agostoni C, Buonocore G, Carnielli VP, et al: Enteral nutrient supply for preterm infants: commentary from the European Society for Paediatric Gastroenterology, Hepatology, and Nutrition Committee on Nutrition, *J Pediatr Gastroenterol Nutr* 50:85-91, 2010.

For the human milk–fed premature infant, calcium and phosphorus are deficient throughout lactation, and levels are far below those necessary to achieve respective intrauterine accretion rates. Deficient intakes of calcium and phosphorus are associated with biochemical markers such as low serum and urine phosphorus concentrations, elevated serum alkaline phosphatase activity, and elevated serum and urine calcium concentrations. Usually, serum phosphorus concentrations are the best indicators of calcium and phosphorus status in human milk–fed premature infants. Prolonged deficiency of these minerals tends to stimulate bone resorption to normalize serum calcium concentrations. This bone activity often is correlated with elevated serum alkaline phosphatase activity. It has been reported that a majority of premature infants who had an elevated serum alkaline phosphatase activity were those fed human milk. Moreover, follow-up evaluations of the same infants at 9 and 18 months noted that linear growth was significantly lower in the group that had the higher serum activity of alkaline phosphatase in the neonatal period. A high alkaline phosphatase value in the neonatal period is a negative predictor of height in 9- to 12-year-old adolescents (Fewtrell et al, 2000).

The supplementation of human milk with both calcium and phosphorus not only improves the net retention of both minerals but also improves bone mineral content. Current management of human milk–fed premature infants emphasizes the need for supplements of both calcium and phosphorus. A linear relationship exists between calcium (or phosphorus) intake and net retention in enterally fed premature infants. Premature infants receiving unfortified human milk never achieve intrauterine accretion rates for calcium and phosphorus. Intakes of approximately 200 and 100 mg/kg/day, respectively, of calcium and phosphorus can be achieved with the use of specialized human milk fortifiers and preterm formulas, thus making it possible to meet intrauterine estimates. However, term infant formulas and specialized (not "preterm") formulas provide inadequate quantities of calcium and phosphorus to meet the needs of growing premature infants. Several factors affect the absorption of calcium and phosphorus, including postnatal age and intake of calcium, phosphorus, lactose, fat, and vitamin D. Vitamin D, however, is responsible for only a small component of calcium absorption in premature infants.

The time to supply sufficient calcium and phosphorus stores for premature infants is during the initial hospitalization, before their discharge and the beginning of exclusive breastfeeding. However, because of the need for prolonged parenteral nutrition and the inability to provide "catch-up" quantities of calcium and phosphorus in milk, some infants may benefit from additional calcium and phosphorus after hospital discharge.

MAGNESIUM

Approximately 60% of body magnesium is in bone. Preterm human milk contains approximately 30 mg/L of magnesium. The absorption of magnesium is significantly greater from unfortified human milk than from formula. Net magnesium retention in human milk–fed premature infants meets intrauterine estimates.

TRACE ELEMENTS

Zinc

Several factors affect the zinc needs of the enterally fed premature infant. Fetal accretion of zinc is approximately 0.85 mg/kg/day. Growth is a major determinant of zinc needs. The major excretory route is via the gastrointestinal tract. Infants with large gastrointestinal fluid losses may become zinc deficient. Premature infants receiving pooled pasteurized human milk (zinc intake of approximately 0.7 mg/kg/day) are in negative zinc balance for 60 days postnatally and never meet the intrauterine accretion rate. In contrast, intakes of 1.8 to 2 mg/kg/day are associated with a net retention of zinc that surpasses intrauterine accretion rates. The classic signs of zinc deficiency include an erythematous skin rash involving perioral, perineal, and facial areas, as well as the extremities. Although there are limitations to the assay, plasma zinc values lower than 50 μg/dL are highly suggestive of deficiency. A very low activity of serum alkaline phosphatase, a zinc-dependent enzyme, also is suggestive of deficiency. Reports of symptomatic zinc deficiency in unsupplemented human milk–fed premature infants serve as a reminder of the decline in milk zinc concentration as lactation advances.

Copper

No universally accepted methods exist to assess copper status clinically. Balance study data provide only an estimate of copper retention at one point in time. Premature infants receiving pooled pasteurized human milk (copper intakes of approximately 85 μg/kg/day) are in negative copper balance for 30 days postnatally and never meet the intrauterine accretion rate. Human milk fortifier supplies additional copper. Symptoms of copper deficiency include osteopenia, neutropenia, and hypochromic anemia. Because copper is excreted in bile, cases of severe cholestasis warrant limiting copper intakes.

Iron

The iron needs of the premature infant are determined by birthweight, initial hemoglobin, rate of growth, and magnitude of iron loss and/or volume of transfused blood. Postnatal iron metabolism occurs in three phases. In the first phase, there is decreased erythropoiesis. The hemoglobin concentration declines to a nadir, physiologic anemia of prematurity, which is at approximately 2 to 3 months of postnatal age. In the second phase, the hemoglobin rises as active red cell production is occurring. In this phase, iron is needed. The third phase is an exhaustion of iron stores, or late anemia of prematurity, observed if iron supplementation is inadequate.

The concentration of iron in human milk declines through lactation. Premature infants fed human milk are in negative iron balance, which, in the absence of transfusion, can be corrected with iron supplements. Iron absorption also appears to be facilitated by a modest degree of anemia. Thus, the usual recommendations for premature infants suggest delaying iron supplementation until 2 to 3 months of postnatal age, when hemoglobin concentrations are at a nadir.

Generally, ferrous sulfate (elemental iron, 2 mg/kg/day) drops are used in human milk–fed premature infants beginning soon after the achievement of complete enteral feedings. Formula-fed premature infants should receive iron-fortified formula from the onset of milk feeding.

Sodium and Potassium

Premature infants generally need more sodium per unit of body weight than is needed by term infants. This increased need is due to immature renal sodium conservation mechanisms. Sodium wasting is inversely related to gestational age. A comparison of sodium intakes of 2.9 and 1.6 mEq (mmol)/kg/day in premature infants suggested that the former intake provided more appropriate serum sodium concentrations. Hyponatremia also may occur in premature infants primarily fed human milk because the sodium content of preterm milk continues to decline through lactation. The need for these electrolytes may increase during or after diuretic usage.

Vitamins

The fat-soluble vitamins A, D, E, and K are stored in the body, and large doses may result in toxicity. Water-soluble vitamins—thiamine, riboflavin, niacin, vitamin B_6, folate, vitamin B_{12}, pantothenic acid, biotin, and vitamin C—are not stored in the body, and excess intakes are excreted in the urine or bile (vitamin B_{12}). The intake of water-soluble vitamins, therefore, should be at frequent intervals to avoid deficiency states. Vitamin A and riboflavin concentrations decline in human milk under conditions of light exposure and after passage through feeding tubes. As a consequence of exposure to air, ascorbic acid concentrations are lower in pooled human milk. Supplementary vitamins are provided in human milk fortifiers and in preterm formulas. Once feedings in the premature infant change to unfortified human milk or standard formula, a multivitamin supplement should be added.

The American Academy of Pediatrics Committee on Nutrition recently issued new guidelines doubling the amount of recommended vitamin D to 400 IU per day for infants (American Academy of Pediatrics, 2009). The recommendation applies to infants receiving human milk and those who are consuming less than 1 quart of infant formula per day. The change in the recommendation is based in part on the risk of rickets in exclusively breastfed infants who are not supplemented with 400 IU of vitamin D per day.

POSTDISCHARGE NUTRITION FOR THE PREMATURE INFANT

Growing evidence suggests that the quality of early nutrition support has long-term implications for infant health and development. The goal of in-hospital nutritional support is to meet intrauterine rates of nutrient accretion. Accordingly, the premature infant should receive fortified human milk or preterm formula during the hospitalization period. Hospital discharge, however, frequently occurs before the completion of the intrauterine growth phase (up to approximately 36 weeks). Moreover, during hospitalization, despite what we may consider to be optimal nutrient support, growth deficits emerge, such that at discharge the infant is well below the 10th percentile on corresponding growth charts. Thus, concerns about nutrition support extend into the postdischarge period. Unfortunately, unlike in the term infant, whose needs are modeled after the healthy breastfed infant, and the premature infant, whose needs are determined by the intrauterine growth model, there are no references to determine the nutritional needs of the premature infant at discharge.

The 1st year of life represents a crucial time of brain growth. Observational studies have found that failure to catch up in weight by 8 months of age was associated with lower scores on the Bayley Scales of Infant Development, poor head circumference growth, and higher rates of neurosensory impairment (Hack et al, 1982).

The composition of postdischarge formulas designed for the premature infant are shown in Table 66-9. These formulas supply more energy (22 calories/oz), protein (2.8 g/100 kcal), calcium, phosphorus, and zinc. Compared to term formula, these formulas provide 49% more protein, 10% more calories, 48% more calcium, 62% more phosphorus, and 75% more zinc. Ongoing fortification of human milk should also be considered for premature infant and can be accomplished in a variety of ways, including the addition of a postdischarge formula to human milk in order to increase energy, protein, calcium, and phosphorus intake.

Carver and colleagues performed a clinical trial in which infants with birthweight less than 1800 grams were randomized to receive term formula or a nutrient-enriched formula until 12 months corrected age. These workers found that infants who received the nutrient-enriched formula had improved proportional growth, because they weighed more at 6 and 12 months corrected age, had greater body length at 6 months corrected age, and were found to have better head circumference growth at term and at 1, 2, 6, and 12 months corrected age. The nutrient-enriched formula was of particular benefit to infants with birthweight less than 1250 grams (Carver et al, 2001). Bishop and colleagues found increased bone mineral content up to 9 months corrected age in infants who received nutrient-enriched formula compared to term formula (Bishop et al, 1993).

Nutrition should be discussed during the discharge planning process with the families of former premature infants. In addition, these plans should be discussed with the primary medical caregiver to ensure a smooth transition to the outpatient setting. Premature infants who are formula-fed should be fed nutrient-enriched postdischarge formula for the 1st year of life. The duration of use will vary depending on the severity of postnatal growth failure, bone health, and proportional growth after NICU discharge. Likewise, growth of premature infants who are discharged on human milk should be closely monitored to ensure optimal proportional growth.

TABLE 66-9   Composition of Premature Postdischarge Formulas (per 100 kcal)

	Similac Neosure Advance (Abbott) 22 kcal/oz	Enfacare Lipil (Mead Johnson) 22 kcal/oz		Similac Neosure Advance (Abbott) 22 kcal/oz	Enfacare Lipil (Mead Johnson) 22 kcal/oz
Volume (mL)	134	136	Magnesium (µg)	9	8
Protein			Manganese (µg)	10	15
Content (g)	2.8	2.8	Selenium (µg)	2.3	2.8
% Energy	11	11	Sodium (mg)	33	35
Whey:casein	50:50	60:40	Zinc (mg)	1.2	1.25
Lipid			**Vitamins**		
Content (g)	5.5	5.3	**Fat-Soluble**		
% Energy	49	47	Vitamin A (IU)	460	450
Source			Vitamin D (IU)	70	70–80
Medium-chain triglycerides (MCTs) (%)	25	20	Vitamin E (IU)	3.6	4
Coconut (%)	29	15	Vitamin K (µg)	11	8
Soybean (%)	45	29	**Water-Soluble**		
Oleic (%)	34		Vitamin B$_6$ (µg)	100	100
Docosahexaenoic acid (DHA) (mg)	8	17	Vitamin B$_{12}$ (µg)	0.4	0.3
Arachidonic acid (AA) (mg)	22	34	Vitamin C (mg)	15	16
Carbohydrate			Biotin (µg)	9	6
Content (g)	10.1	10.4	Folic acid (µg)	25	26
% Energy	40	42	Niacin (mg)	1.95	2
Minerals and Trace Elements			Pantothenic acid (mg)	0.8	0.85
Calcium (mg)	105	120	Riboflavin (µg)	150	200
Chloride (mg)	75	78	Thiamine (µg)	220	200
Copper (µg)	120	120	**Other**		
Iodine (µg)	15	21	Carnitine (mg)	7.7	2
Iron (mg)	1.8	1.8	Choline (mg)	16	24
Phosphorus (mg)	62	66	Inositol (mg)	35	30
Potassium (mg)	142	105	Taurine (mg)	10.7	6
			Osmolality (mOsmol/kg)	250	250–300

SUGGESTED READINGS

Agostoni C, Buonocore G, Carnielli VP, et al: Enteral nutrient supply for preterm infants: commentary from the European Society for Paediatric Gastroenterology, Hepatology, and Nutrition Committee on Nutrition, *J Pediatr Gastroenterol Nutr* 50:85-91, 2010.

Carver JD, Wu PY, Hall RT, et al: Growth of preterm infants fed nutrient-enriched or term formula after hospital discharge, *Pediatrics* 107:683-689, 2001.

Cooke R, Embleton N, Rigo J, et al: High protein pre-term infant formula: effect on nutrient balance, metabolic status and growth, *Pediatr Res* 59:265-270, 2006.

Embleton NE, Pang N, Cooke RJ: Postnatal malnutrition and growth retardation: an inevitable consequence of current recommendations in preterm infants? *Pediatrics* 107:270-273, 2001.

Kennedy KA, Tyson JE, Chamnanvanakij S: Rapid versus slow rate of advancement of feedings for promoting growth and preventing necrotizing enterocolitis in parenterally fed low-birth-weight infants, *Cochrane Database Syst Rev* (2): CD001241, 2000.

Olsen IE, Richardson DK, Schmid CH, et al: Intersite differences in weight growth velocity of extremely premature infants, *Pediatrics* 110:1125-1132, 2002.

Tyson JE, Kennedy KA: Minimal enteral nutrition for promoting feeding tolerance and preventing morbidity in parenterally fed infants. *Cochrane Database Syst Rev* (2):CD000504, 2000.

Ziegler EE: Protein requirements of very low birth weight infants, *J Pediatr Gastroenterol Nutr* 45(Suppl 3):S170-S174, 2007.

Ziegler EE, Thureen PJ, Carlson SJ: Aggressive nutrition of the very low birth-weight infant, *Clin Perinatol* 29:225-244, 2002.

Complete references used in this text can be found online at www.expertconsult.com

PARENTERAL NUTRITION

Brenda B. Poindexter and Scott C. Denne

Effective nutritional support of premature and critically ill infants is largely dependent on parenteral nutrition, especially in early postnatal life. In practice, the supply of nutrients to preterm neonates—especially extremely low-birthweight (ELBW) infants—is rarely adequate, and these infants accumulate major deficits in early postnatal life (Berry et al, 1997; Embleton et al, 2001; Olsen et al, 2002). A high proportion of ELBW infants exhibit poor growth in the neonatal intensive care unit (NICU), with those at the lowest gestational age and birthweight at greatest risk (Clark et al, 2003; Fanaroff et al, 2007). However, growing evidence indicates that early use of parenteral nutrition may minimize protein losses and improve growth outcomes (Poindexter, 2005; Stephens et al, 2009; Thureen et al, 2003; Wilson et al, 1997). For example, Wilson et al (1997), in a randomized clinical trial in 125 sick very low-birthweight (VLBW) infants, demonstrated that early aggressive parenteral nutrition combined with early enteral feeding reduced growth failure without an increased incidence of adverse clinical consequences or metabolic derangements. More recent observational studies have produced similar results (Poindexter, 2005; Valentine et al, 2009). In addition to improved growth outcomes, Stephens et al (2009) found an association between increased protein and energy intake in the 1st week of life and higher Bayley Mental Development Index scores at 18 months corrected age. Parenteral nutrition solutions, although still imperfect, have improved markedly from the early days of use, and complications are less common. At present, improved growth outcomes in preterm infants appear to require a more sustained effort at providing parenteral nutritional support, especially in early postnatal life. This means initiating parenteral nutrition within the first 24 hours, continuing until enteral nutrition supplies at least 75% of the total protein and energy requirements, and reinstituting parenteral nutrition quickly whenever enteral feeding is suspended.

COMPONENTS OF PARENTERAL NUTRITION

PROTEIN

The initial goal of parenteral nutrition is to minimize losses and preserve existing body stores; this is particularly important for protein. Protein losses are significant in all neonates in the absence of amino acid intake, and these losses are the highest in the most immature neonates. For example, 26-week-gestation infants lose 1.5 g/kg/day of body protein; protein losses in term infants are approximately half that rate (0.7 g/kg/day) (Denne et al, 1996). These high rates of loss in extremely premature infants result in substantial protein deficits. If extremely premature infants are provided with no amino acid supply, they lose over 1.5% of their body protein per day when they should be accumulating protein at a rate of 2% per day. After only 3 days of no protein intake, a 10% protein deficit results.

Fortunately, there is good evidence that early amino acid intake can compensate for high rates of protein loss and thus preserve body protein, even at low caloric intakes (Kashyap and Heird, 1994; Rivera et al, 1993; Saini et al, 1989; Van Lingen et al, 1992). Amino acid intakes of 1.1 to 2.3 g/kg/day at caloric intakes of 30 to 50 kcal/kg/day change the protein balance from significantly negative to neutral or positive in sick VLBW infants (Rivera et al, 1993; Saini et al, 1989; Van Lingen et al, 1992). More recently, Thureen et al (1998) conducted a randomized trial of 1 g/kg/day versus 3 g/kg/day amino acid intake immediately after birth in extremely premature infants. Despite a modest caloric intake in both groups (approximately 50 kcal/kg/day), protein accretion was significantly greater in the higher amino acid intake group. In all these studies evaluating the effect of early amino acid intake in premature infants, no differences in ammonia concentrations or acid-base status were observed between infants who received amino acids and those who did not (Paisley et al, 2000; Rivera et al, 1993; Saini et al, 1989; Van Lingen et al, 1992). In addition, these studies demonstrated no relationship between amino acid intake and blood urea nitrogen (BUN), although two recent studies reported modestly elevated BUN levels in infants receiving higher amino acid intakes at 7 days of age (Blanco et al, 2008; Clark et al, 2007). The fact that BUN concentrations do not usually correlate with amino acid intake in early postnatal life suggests these levels are related primarily to fluid status and that increased BUN levels should not be used as an indication of protein excess. These data indicate that providing parenteral amino acids at a rate of 2 to 3 g/kg/day as soon as possible after birth (within hours) can preserve limited body protein stores in sick premature and ELBW infants, even at low caloric intakes.

It is important to point out that even though parenteral amino acid administration is beneficial at low caloric intakes, increasing caloric intake is likely to improve protein accretion. Older studies in premature infants have suggested that increasing caloric intake from 50 to 80 kcal/kg/day can significantly improve protein balance (Pineault et al, 1988; Zlotkin et al, 1981). Based on currently available data, 70 to 80 kcal/kg/day may be sufficient to maximize protein accretion. However, additional energy beyond this amount probably is necessary to produce appropriate fat accretion (see "Energy" section).

The ultimate goal of parenteral amino acid administration is to achieve the rate of fetal protein accretion. Based on a variety of studies measuring protein losses and balance, 3.5 to 4.0 g/kg/day of amino acids is a reasonable estimate of parenteral protein requirements in ELBW infants (Ziegler, 2007) (Table 67-1). Recent evidence suggests that up to 4.0 g/kg/day of amino acids is well tolerated by ELBW infants (Porcelli and Sisk, 2002). For premature infants with birthweights of over 1000 g, estimated parenteral protein requirements are 3.0 to 3.5 g/kg/day. Estimates for term infants are 2.5 to 3 g/kg/day. Parenteral protein intake recommendations for premature infants are shown in Table 67-1.

The composition of currently available amino acid solutions is shown in Table 67-2. These amino acid solutions were designed to mimic plasma amino acid concentrations in healthy 30-day-old breastfed term infants (TrophAmine) or fetal or neonatal cord blood amino acid concentrations (Primene). No convincing information exists to support the superiority of one neonatal amino acid solution over another.

Although the current neonatal amino acid solutions represent a substantial advance over previous casein

TABLE 67-1 Suggested Daily Parenteral Intakes for ELBW and VLBW Infants

Component (units/kg/day)	ELBW			VLBW		
	Day 0*	Transition†	Growing	Day 0*	Transition†	Growing
Energy (kcal)	40–50	70–80	100–110	40–50	60–70	90–100
Protein (g)	2–3	3.5	3.5–4	2–3	3.0–3.5	3.0–3.5
Glucose (g)	7–10	8–15	13–17	7–10	8–15	13–17
Fat (g)	1	1–3	3–4	1	1–3	3
Na (mEq)	0–1	2–4	3–7	0–1	2–4	3–5
Potassium (K) (mEq)	0	0–2	2–3	0	0–2	2–3
Chloride (mEq)	0–1	2–4	3–7	0–1	2–4	3–7
Calcium (mg)	20–60	60	60–80	20–60	60	60–80
Phosphorus (mg)	0	45–60	45–60	0	45–60	45–60
Magnesium (mg)	0	3–7.2	3–7.2	0	3–7.2	3–7.2

ELBW, Extremely low-birthweight: <1000 g; *VLBW*, very low-birthweight, <1500 g.
*Recommended parenteral intakes on the first day of life.
†Period of transition to physiologic and metabolic stability. For most premature neonates, this occurs between 2 and 7 days.

TABLE 67-2 Composition of Commercial Parenteral Amino Acid Solutions

Amino Acid*	Concentration: mg/dL			
	Aminosyn-PF (Abbott)	TrophAmine (B. Braun)	Primene (Baxter)†	Premasol (Baxter)†
Histidine	312	480	380	480
Isoleucine	760	820	670	820
Leucine	1200	1400	1000	1400
Lysine	677	820	1100	820
Methionine	180	340	240	340
Phenylalanine	427	480	420	480
Threonine	512	420	370	420
Tryptophan	180	200	200	200
Valine	673	780	760	780
Alanine	698	540	800	540
Arginine	1227	1200	840	1200
Proline	812	680	300	680
Serine	495	380	400	380
Taurine	70	25	60	25
Tyrosine	44	240‡	45	240‡
Glycine	385	360	400	360
Cysteine	—	<16	189	<16
Glutamic acid	820	500	1000	500
Aspartic acid	527	320	600	320

Data from the American Hospital Formulary Service: Drug information. Bethesda, Md, 2000; Drug Product Database; and Premasol package insert (Deerfield, Ill, 2003, Baxter Healthcare Corporation).
*All amino acid mixtures shown are 10% solutions.
†Primene available in Canada; Premasol available in the United States.
‡Mixture of L-tyrosine and N-acetyltyrosine.

hydrolysates and early crystalline amino acid mixtures, specific deficiencies remain. Glutamine, an amino acid abundantly supplied by breast milk and potentially conditionally essential in premature infants, is not included in any available amino acid solution because of issues of stability. However, the NICHD Neonatal Research Network conducted a multicenter, randomized clinical trial of parenteral glutamine supplementation and found that parenteral glutamine supplementation did not decrease mortality or the incidence of late-onset sepsis in ELBW infants (Poindexter et al, 2004). In addition, glutamine had no effect on tolerance of enteral feeds, necrotizing enterocolitis, or growth. Tyrosine has very limited solubility, so little is included in current amino acid solutions. TrophAmine contains a soluble derivative of tyrosine (N-acetyltyrosine), but this derivative appears to have poor bioavailability. A variety of studies in premature infants suggest that the tyrosine supply may not be optimal in current amino acid solutions (Brunton et al, 2000). Cysteine is not included in most amino acid solutions because it is not stable for long periods. However, a cysteine hydrochloride supplement that can be added to the parenteral nutrition solution just before delivery is commercially available. There is evidence to support that when cysteine hydrochloride supplements are added to parenteral nutrition, nitrogen retention is improved in premature infants (Soghier and Brion, 2006). The addition of cysteine hydrochloride also improves the solubility of calcium and phosphorus in parenteral nutrition solutions and also may improve the status of the important antioxidant glutathione. For these reasons, the addition of cysteine hydrochloride (40 mg/g of amino acid, up to a maximum of 120 mg/kg) is recommended. Cysteine hydrochloride can result in metabolic acidosis, but this possibility can be appropriately countered by the use of acetate in the parenteral nutrition solution as a buffer (Peters et al, 1997).

ENERGY

The initial goal of parenteral nutrition in early postnatal life is to provide sufficient energy intake to at least match rates of energy expenditure in order to preserve body energy stores. Measures of energy expenditure in premature infants have ranged between 30 and 70 kcal/kg/day; energy expenditure increases with energy intake and with advancing postnatal age (Bauer et al, 2003a, 2003b; Torine et al, 2007; Weintraub et al, 2009). Energy expenditure also appears to be greater at lower birthweights (Weintraub et al, 2009). An intake of approximately 70 kcal/kg/day is a reasonable clinical goal to achieve neutral or slightly positive energy balance, although because of glucose and lipid intolerance, this intake may not be able to be achieved for a number of days after birth. Nevertheless, maximizing energy intake within the limits of glucose and lipid tolerance can minimize accumulating energy deficits. It is also important to note that common clinical conditions such as sepsis and chronic lung disease can significantly increase energy expenditure, which can further exaggerate energy deficits (Bauer et al, 2003c; Torine et al, 2007).

To support normal rates of growth, a positive energy balance of 20 to 25 kcal/kg/day must be achieved (Denne, 2001). This requires 90 to 100 kcal/kg/day for preterm infants with birthweights of less than 1000 g and 100 to 110 kcal/kg/day for ELBW infants (see Table 67-1). A parenteral intake of 80 to 90 kcal/kg/day is most often sufficient for term infants. Most of the parenteral calories are best supplied by a balanced caloric intake of lipid and glucose. Parenteral energy requirements are less than those required for enteral nutrition because no energy is lost in the stools. Recommendations for parenteral energy intake are shown in Table 67-1.

GLUCOSE

Glucose is typically the first parenteral nutrient provided to the preterm infant, and glucose administration is begun minutes after birth in order to maintain glucose homeostasis and preserve endogenous carbohydrate stores. Although the precise definitions of hypoglycemia and hyperglycemia remain a topic of debate, maintaining glucose concentrations of above 40 mg/dL and below 150 to 200 mg/dL is a reasonable clinical goal (Cornblath et al, 2000). Hypoglycemia is easily avoided in preterm infants by maintaining a constant intravenous glucose delivery, but hyperglycemia is more often problematic, especially in ELBW infants shortly after birth. Hyperglycemia is very common in this population in early postnatal life, with more than three fourths of ELBW infants having glucose concentrations exceeding 150 mg/dL, and a third of infants with frequent glucose concentrations over 180 mg/dL (Beardsall et al, 2008; Blanco et al, 2006).

Glucose infusion rate of 4 to 7 mg/kg/minute (70 to 110 mL/kg/day of 10% dextrose in water [$D_{10}W$]) is an appropriate starting point for most infants. This rate of glucose infusion approximates or slightly exceeds the rate of endogenous glucose release from the liver in term and premature infants with birthweights above 1000 g; therefore, this rate of glucose infusion serves to preserve the limited carbohydrate stores in these infants. For ELBW infants, a rate of 8 to 10 mg/kg/minute is required to match endogenous glucose production (Hertz et al, 1993). Unfortunately, many infants will not tolerate this rate of glucose infusion for several days without hyperglycemia. Because ELBW infants can have fluid requirements in excess of 100 mL/kg/day, beginning with 5% dextrose may be necessary to maintain glucose infusion rates in the range of 4 to 7 mg/kg in order to achieve glucose homeostasis.

A gradual increase in glucose intake over 2 to 7 days, up to 13 to 17 g/kg/day, is usually tolerated when the glucose is combined with amino acid intake. An infusion rate of 18 g/kg/day is a reasonable maximum for intravenous glucose delivery, because higher rates probably exceed the glucose oxidative capacity (Chessex et al, 1995; Jones et al, 1993). Exceeding glucose oxidative capacity will drive extensive lipogenesis, an energy-expensive process. Supplying appropriate amounts of glucose rarely requires glucose solution concentrations in excess of 12.5%, unless infants are fluid-restricted. Recommendations for glucose intake during parenteral nutrition are provided in Table 67-1.

Some ELBW infants have difficulty tolerating even moderate rates of glucose delivery. This problem usually can be overcome by a temporary reduction in the glucose infusion rate. The use of insulin in this situation remains a controversial practice. Collins et al (1991), in a small randomized controlled trial, demonstrated increased weight gain in infants who received insulin infusions. No differences in head circumference or length were observed between these infants and controls, suggesting that insulin may have produced increases in fat mass but not in lean tissue. Poindexter et al (1998) evaluated the effect of insulin on protein metabolism using a euglycemic hyperinsulinemic clamp. Insulin infusion resulted in no improvement in protein balance and unexpectedly produced significant lactic acidosis. An international, randomized clinical trial was recently conducted to determine whether early insulin therapy would reduce hyperglycemia and improve outcomes in VLBW infants (Beardsall et al, 2008). The study demonstrated no improvements in mortality, sepsis, growth, intracranial disease, necrotizing enterocolitis, or chronic lung disease and was terminated early because of futility concerns. The authors concluded that there is little clinical benefit of routine early insulin administration; although insulin may decrease the incidence of hyperglycemia, early insulin may also increase the number of episodes of hypoglycemia. Nevertheless, there are rare ELBW infants who remain hyperglycemic despite very low glucose infusion rates; these infants may require exogenous insulin beginning at 0.05 unit/kg/hour for a short period of time to produce normoglycemia.

Meeting the goal of 13 to 17 g/kg/day of intravenous glucose will result in a caloric intake of 45 to 60 kcal/kg/day, which is insufficient by itself to meet total energy needs. Intravenous lipids are necessary to supply the rest of the nonprotein calories. A balanced glucose and lipid approach to supplying nonprotein calories has a number of advantages: it better approximates the carbohydrate-to-fat ratio in enteral feedings, it may improve overall protein accretion, and it minimizes overall energy expenditure (Nose et al, 1987; Van Aerde et al, 1989).

LIPIDS

Intravenous lipids are made up of triglycerides, phospholipids from egg yolk to emulsify, and glycerol, which is added to achieve isotonicity. Intravenous lipid solutions commercially available in the United States are derived from soybean oil (Intralipid) or a combination of soybean oil and safflower oil (Liposyn II); these solutions contain long-chain triglycerides. Differences in lipid source result in a slightly different fatty acid profile; the compositions of intravenous lipid solutions are shown in Table 67-3. All available intravenous lipid products have a fatty acid profile substantially different from that of human milk. At present, there is not convincing information that any of the solutions produce clinically different outcomes.

Intravenous lipid solutions contain lipid particles similar in size to endogenously produced chylomicrons. These particles are hydrolyzed by lipoprotein lipase into free fatty acids. Lipoprotein lipase activity and triglyceride clearance are reduced in preterm infants of less than 28 weeks' gestation (Brans et al, 1986). Although heparin can release lipoprotein lipase from the endothelium into the circulation, at present no evidence exists that this increases lipid utilization in preterm infants (Spear et al, 1988). In the absence of any information demonstrating clinical benefit

TABLE 67-3 Composition of Parenteral Lipid Emulsions

	Intralipid 20%	Liposyn-II 20%	Omegaven*
Oil			
Soybean	20	10	—
Safflower	—	10	—
Fish	—	—	10
Fats (%)			
Linoleic	50	65	0.1–0.7
α-Linolenic	9	4	<0.2
EPA	—	—	1.3–2.8
DHA	—	—	1.4–3.1
Arachidonic acid	—	—	0.1–0.4
Glycerol	2.3	2.5	2.5
Egg phospholipid	1.2	1.2	1.2
Phytosterols, mg/L	348 + 33	383	0

DHA, Docosahexaenoic acid; *EPA*, eicosapentaenoic acid.
*Omegaven is not approved for use in the United States and is only available under experimental or compassionate use protocol. Omegaven is only available as a 10% solution (10 g lipid per 100 mL).

of heparin administration, the routine addition of heparin in lipid infusions is not recommended.

Linoleic and linolenic acids cannot be endogenously synthesized and therefore are essential fatty acids for humans. Biochemical evidence of essential fatty acid deficiency may be noted in preterm infants within 72 hours of birth (Foote et al, 1991). Essential fatty acid deficiency can be avoided if 0.5 to 1.0 g/kg/day of intravenous lipid is provided. Additional intravenous lipid beyond these amounts is necessary if the energy requirements of preterm infants are to be met in early postnatal life.

The early administration of intravenous lipids to preterm infants has been the subject of discussion and debate; this debate has centered primarily on the acute metabolic effects of early intravenous lipids and the potential long-term consequences. Gilbertson et al (1991) evaluated the short-term metabolic effects of early intravenous lipids in a randomized controlled trial. This study examined 29 infants requiring mechanical ventilation with an average gestational age of 28 weeks and an average birthweight of 1.1 kg. One group received intravenous lipid at 1.0 g/kg/day beginning on day 1; this was gradually increased to 3.0 g/kg/day by day 4. The control group received intravenous lipid only after day 8. There were no differences in PO_2, PCO_2, hyperglycemia, bilirubin concentrations, thrombocytopenia, or free fatty acid concentrations between the two groups. In addition, triglyceride concentrations were similar in both groups. Another trial using a slightly different study design produced similar results (Murdock et al, 1995). Current evidence strongly suggests that intravenous lipids can be administered to sick preterm infants in early postnatal life without causing acute metabolic derangements.

Concern about the long-term safety of early intravenous administration of lipids, particularly the possibility of an increase in mortality and bronchopulmonary dysplasia, was raised by some early observational studies. A recent metaanalysis of randomized controlled studies found no increase in chronic lung disease resulting from early lipid administration to premature infants (Simmer and Rao, 2005). In view of these data and of the essential fatty acid and caloric needs of sick premature infants, early intravenous lipid administration (on day 1 of life) is a recommended clinical practice.

The rate of intravenous lipid infusion is important, and plasma lipid clearance is improved when intravenous lipid is given as a continuous infusion over 24 hours (Putet, 2000). Lipid infusion rates in excess of 0.25 g/kg/hour are associated with decreases in PO_2 (Brans et al, 1986). Lipid infusion rates well under this value can easily be achieved in clinical practice if lipids are provided over 24 hours in an amount not exceeding 3 to 4 g/kg/day. This level of lipid intake is usually sufficient to supply the caloric needs of preterm infants (in combination with glucose) and is usually tolerated by premature infants. Triglyceride concentrations are most often used as an indication of lipid tolerance, and maintaining triglyceride concentrations below 150 to 200 mg/dL seems desirable. Recommendations for parenteral lipid intake are provided in Table 67-1.

Numerous studies have documented superiority of 20% over 10% lipid emulsions (Putet, 2000). Lipid clearance is improved with the 20% solutions because these solutions have half the amount of phospholipid emulsifier relative to the same amount of triglycerides. Phospholipids can combine with cholesterol to form lipoprotein X, which ultimately interferes with the clearance of infused triglycerides. Consequently, the use of 10% lipid emulsions should be avoided. A 30% lipid solution has recently become available and may confer even more advantages, although there currently are no comparative data.

Concern has been expressed about the use of intravenous lipids in infants with hyperbilirubinemia, because free fatty acids may displace bilirubin from albumin-binding sites, potentially increasing the risk of kernicterus. A recent study that measured free bilirubin in relation to intravenous lipid intake in premature infants less that 33 weeks' gestation demonstrated an increase in free bilirubin with higher intravenous lipid intakes in infants less than 29 weeks' gestation, but not for those at higher gestational ages (Amin et al, 2009). Although the clinical significance of this finding is uncertain, it may be reasonable to consider reducing intravenous lipids in extremely premature infants with significant hyperbilirubinemia.

Intravenous lipid emulsions may undergo lipid peroxidation, with the formation of organic free radicals, potentially initiating tissue injury. Light, especially phototherapy, may play some role in increasing lipid peroxidation in intravenous lipid emulsions (Neuzil et al, 1995). However, multivitamin preparations included in the intravenous solutions are major contributors to generation of peroxides, and lipid emulsions may have only a minor additive effect (Lavoie et al, 1997). Some small studies have suggested that light protection may reduce chronic lung disease, but these results have not been consistent (Bassiouny et al, 2009; Chessex et al, 2007; Sherlock and Chessex, 2009). On the basis of these findings, some clinicians protect intravenous lipid solutions from light, although the importance or clinical efficacy of this practice remains in doubt. Only a large randomized clinical trial is likely to resolve this issue (Sherlock and Chessex, 2009).

Carnitine facilitates transport of long-chain fatty acids through the myocardial membrane and thereby plays an important role in their oxidation. Premature infants receiving parenteral nutrition have low carnitine levels, but the clinical significance of this finding remains uncertain. Metaanalysis of the studies evaluating carnitine supplementation in parenteral nutrition showed no evidence of effect on ketogenesis, lipid utilization, or weight gain (Cairns and Stalker, 2000). At present, insufficient information is available to support a recommendation for the routine supplementation of parenterally fed neonates with carnitine.

ELECTROLYTES, MINERALS, TRACE ELEMENTS, AND VITAMINS

Sodium needs are low in the first few days of life because of the expected free water diuresis. For ELBW infants, addition of sodium to the parenteral nutrition solution may not be necessary until about day 3 of life. It is, however, necessary to frequently measure sodium concentrations and water balance. After the initial diuresis, 2 to 4 mEq/kg/day is usually sufficient to maintain serum sodium in the normal range, but ELBW infants sometimes require higher sodium intakes to compensate for larger renal sodium losses. Chloride requirements follow the same time course as for sodium requirements and also are 2 to 4 mEq/kg/day. Once electrolytes are added to the parenteral nutrition solution, chloride intake should not be less than 1 mEq/kg/day, and all chloride should not be omitted when sodium bicarbonate or acetate is given to correct metabolic acidosis. Potassium requirements again are low in the first few days of life, and potassium should probably be omitted from parenteral solutions in ELBW infants until renal function is clearly established. Potassium intakes of 2 to 3 mEq/kg/day are usually adequate to maintain normal serum potassium concentrations.

Parenteral nutrition solutions usually require the addition of anions, as either acetate or chloride. In general, excess anions should be provided as acetate in order to prevent hyperchloremic metabolic acidosis. A randomized controlled trial demonstrated that acetate in parenteral nutrition solutions effectively ameliorates acidosis (Phelps and Cochran, 1989).

Supplying calcium and phosphorus in parenteral nutrition remains a significant clinical challenge because of limited solubility. It is currently not possible to supply enough calcium and phosphorus to support adequate bone mineralization in preterm infants using the solutions available in the United States. In other countries, organophosphate preparations are available (e.g., glycerophosphate), and calcium and phosphorus can be supplied in parenteral nutrition solutions in amounts that approximate enteral intakes. Precipitation of calcium and phosphorus remains an issue in the United States, however, and the solubility of calcium and phosphorus in parenteral nutrition solutions depends on temperature, type and concentration of amino acid, glucose concentration, pH, type of calcium salt, sequence of addition of calcium and phosphorus to the solution, the calcium-to-phosphorus ratio, and the presence of lipid. Adding cysteine to parenteral nutrition solutions lowers the pH, which improves calcium and phosphorus solubility. Intakes of 60 to 80 mg/kg/day of elemental calcium (1.5 to 2.0 mmol/kg/day) and 48 to 60 mg/kg/day of phosphorus (1.5 to 2.0 mmol/kg/day) have been recommended for premature infants receiving parenteral nutrition (Atkinson and Tsang, 2005). A calcium-to-phosphorus ratio of 1.7:1 by weight (1.3:1 by molar ratio) may be optimal for bone mineralization, but it appears that neonates can tolerate and adjust to molar ratios over the range of 0.8 to 1.5 (Atkinson and Tsang, 2005). In general, calcium and phosphorus should be added to parenteral nutrition solutions in early postnatal life. Magnesium also is a necessary nutrient and should be supplied at 3 to 7.2 mg/kg/day. Calcium, phosphorus, and magnesium serum concentrations should be frequently monitored.

Recommendations for trace elements in term and preterm infants are primarily derived from the American Society for Clinical Nutrition (ASCN) guidelines from 1988 (Greene et al, 1988). There is reasonable consensus that zinc should be included early in parenteral nutrition solutions (250 μg/kg/day for term infants, 400 μg/kg/day for preterm infants). Other trace elements probably are not needed until after the first 2 weeks of life.

The recommended intakes of trace elements for term and preterm infants are shown in Table 67-4. Zinc and copper are available in the sulfate form and can be added separately to parenteral solutions. Several pediatric trace metal solutions are available that contain zinc, copper, magnesium, and chromium in various proportions; these solutions are usually provided at 0.2 mL/kg/day. When trace metal solutions are used, additional zinc usually is needed to provide the recommended intake for preterm infants. Supplementation with selenium is suggested after 2 weeks of age, because preterm infants can become selenium deficient after 2 weeks of exclusive parenteral nutrition. In infants with cholestasis, copper and manganese should be discontinued, and chromium and selenium should be used with caution and in smaller amounts in infants with renal dysfunction. At present, parenteral iron is recommended only when preterm infants are nourished exclusively by parenteral solutions for the first 2 months of life.

The recommended intakes of vitamins for term and preterm infants on parenteral nutrition are shown in Table 67-5. Currently only one pediatric multivitamin preparation is available, and it is delivered with a standard dosage of 2 mL/kg/day (maximum 5 mL/day) in preterm infants and 5 mL/day in term infants. These dosages provide higher amounts of most of the B vitamins and lower amounts of vitamin A relative to the recommendations.

COMPLICATIONS OF PARENTERAL NUTRITION

Although a wide variety of complications associated with parenteral nutrition were reported in the early days of use, most of these are now rare with current parenteral solutions. Many of the complications (electrolyte and glucose imbalance) can be prevented or corrected by manipulating the constituents of the infusate. The primary complications of parenteral nutrition as currently used are cholestasis and those related to the infusion catheter.

Cholestatic jaundice as a result of hepatic dysfunction is a well-recognized complication of parenteral nutrition.

TABLE 67-4 Recommended Parenteral Intake of Trace Elements for Term and Preterm Infants

Trace Element	Term (μg/kg/day)	Preterm (μg/kg/day)
Chromium*	0.20	0.2
Copper†	20	20
Iron‡	—	—
Fluoride§	—	—
Iodide	1	1
Manganese†	1	1
Molybdenum	0.25	0.25
Selenium*	2	2
Zinc ‖	250	400

Data from the American Society for Clinical Nutrition, Subcommittee on Pediatric Parenteral Nutrient Requirements, from the Committee on Clinical Practice Issues: *Am J Clin Nutr* 48:1324-1343, 1988.
ASCN, American Society for Clinical Nutrition; *TPN,* total parenteral nutrition.
*Renal dysfunction can cause toxicity.
†Impaired biliary excretion can cause toxicity.
‡Recommendation is made with caution because of very limited experience with intravenous iron in infants and lack of a safe, acceptable intravenous preparation (estimated daily intravenous requirement is 100 μg/kg for term infants and 200 μg/kg for preterm infants).
§Because of a lack of information on the compatibility of fluoride with TPN and on the contamination level of fluoride in TPN solutions, firm recommendations cannot be made; with long-term TPN (longer than 3 months), a dosage of 500 μg/day may be important in preterm infants, who already have a higher incidence of subsequent dental caries.
‖ The only trace element recommended on day 1 of parenteral nutrition. If the infant requires TPN for longer than 3 months, the dosage must be reduced to 100 μg/kg/day.

The initial histologic lesion is cholestasis, both intracellular and intracanalicular, followed by portal inflammation and progression to bile duct proliferation after several weeks of parenteral nutrition. Cholestasis most often resolves after discontinuation of parenteral nutrition and initiation of enteral feedings. Some rare instances of irreversible liver failure have been documented, but this seems to occur only after several months of use.

The etiology of parenteral nutrition–associated liver disease (PNALD) cholestasis is unknown and most likely multifactorial. The patients at greatest risk are critically ill premature infants who are susceptible to multiple insults, such as hypoxia, hemodynamic instability, and sepsis. The most frequently identified risk factors in parenteral nutrition–associated cholestasis are duration of parenteral nutrition, degree of immaturity, and delayed enteral feeding (Steinbach et al, 2008). There is also evidence that being small for gestational age is also an independent risk factor for PNALD (Robinson and Ehrenkranz, 2008). The incidence of cholestasis in premature infants less than 30 weeks' gestation has recently been estimated at 11% (Steinbach et al, 2008).

There is expanding evidence that even small-volume enteral feedings can reduce the incidence of cholestasis. Early studies of parenteral nutrition suggested a possible relationship between the quantity of amino acids and hepatic dysfunction. More recent studies, using historical controls, suggest that the newer amino acid solutions may result in less cholestasis (Heird et al, 1987). The specific role of the quantity and composition of parenteral amino acids in the cause of cholestatic jaundice in premature infants remains unclear. Some investigators have

TABLE 67-5   Recommended Parenteral Intake of Vitamins for Term and Preterm Infants

Vitamin	Term (daily dose)		Preterm (dose/kg/day)*	
	Recommended	**MVI-Pediatric (1 vial: 5 mL)**	**Recommended**	**MVI-Pediatric (40% of vial: 2 mL/kg/day)**
Fat-Soluble				
Vitamin A (IU)	2300	2300	1640	920
Vitamin D (IU)	400	400	160	160
Vitamin E (IU)	7	7	2.8	—
Vitamin K (µg)	200	200	80†	80
Water-Soluble				
Vitamin B_6 (µg)	1000	1000	180	400
Vitamin B_{12} (µg)	1	1	0.3	0.4
Vitamin C (mg)	80	80	25	32
Biotin (µg)	20	20	6	8
Folic acid (µg)	140	140	56	56
Niacin (mg)	17	17	6.8	6.8
Pantothenate (mg)	5	5	2	2
Riboflavin (µg)	1400	1400	150	560
Thiamin (µg)	1200	1200	350	480

Data from the American Society for Clinical Nutrition, Subcommittee on Pediatric Parenteral Nutrient Requirements, from the Committee on Clinical Practice Issues: *Am J Clin Nutr* 48:1324-1343, 1988.

*Maximum not to exceed dosage for term infant. *Note*: American Society for Clinical Nutrition (ASCN) recommendations (1988) currently are not achievable because no ideal intravenous vitamin preparation is available for preterm infants; 40% of a vial (2 mL/kg/day) of MVI-Pediatric (Armor, USA; Rorer, Canada) is the closest intake that can be achieved.

†This does not include the 0.5 to 1 mg of vitamin K to be given at birth, as recommended by the American Academy of Pediatrics.

hypothesized that fish-oil lipid emulsions prevent steatosis, potentially through improved triglyceride clearance and antiinflammatory properties (Alwayn et al, 2005).

There have been several reports in infants of improvement in PNALD with the fish oil–based product Omegaven (Diamond et al, 2009; Gura et al, 2008; Puder et al, 2009). Puder et al (2009) performed an open label trial of Omegaven in 42 infants with short bowel syndrome with PNALD, and compared them with a similar cohort of short bowel syndrome infants who received only soy-based intravenous lipids. The group receiving Omegaven had lower rates of mortality and liver transplantation, and a higher rate of cholestasis reversal. However, this therapy is currently only available in the United States through research or compassionate use protocols. Data from randomized clinical trials are needed before recommending change in clinical practice to include Omegaven for the treatment of PNALD.

Some infants with cholestasis will require continued parenteral nutrition. In these infants, the use of small-volume enteral feeding in combination with parenteral nutrition may stabilize or improve hepatic function. The use of phenobarbital and ursodeoxycholic acid has been shown to be beneficial in some studies of older children and adults. However, a recent study in preterm infants demonstrated that tauroursodeoxycholic acid did not prevent the development of parenteral nutrition-associated cholestasis and was ineffective in reducing cholestasis once it occurred (Heubi et al, 2002). At present, the routine use of ursodeoxycholic acid or phenobarbital in parenteral nutrition-associated cholestasis cannot be recommended.

Catheter-related complications remain an important problem with parenteral nutrition; the major complication

is infection. Two of the most common bacterial pathogens are *Staphylococcus epidermidis* and *Staphylococcus aureus*. Fungal infections also occur, *Candida albicans* and *Malassezia furfur* being the most common agents. The incidence of sepsis during parenteral nutrition is higher at the lower gestational ages and also increases with the duration of parenteral nutrition. Parenteral nutrition–associated sepsis is likely to be a product of many factors, not the least of which is that the most immature and critically ill patients are most likely to receive parenteral nutrition for prolonged periods. In infants who have developed cholestasis while receiving parenteral nutrition, the rate of sepsis may be increased. The infusate itself also may play a role in the development of sepsis; an association has been reported between the use of intravenous lipid and coagulase-negative staphylococcal bacteremia and *M. furfur* fungemia (Freeman et al, 1990; Redline et al, 1985). At present, avoiding parenteral nutrition–associated infections is best accomplished by meticulous attention to sterile technique in catheter care and early initiation and advancement of enteral nutrition. Prophylactic low-dose vancomycin may diminish the incidence of parenteral nutrition-associated sepsis, but in view of concerns about toxicities and the potential for antibiotic resistance, this approach cannot be recommended (Craft et al, 2002).

Complications specifically related to the catheter also have been reported. Broviac catheters are difficult to place and are associated with thrombosis in neonates (Sadiq et al, 1987). In most NICUs, Broviac catheters have largely been replaced by small-bore Silastic catheters placed percutaneously. However, all central catheters, including the small-bore variety, have produced life-threatening complications. Pericardial tamponade and significant pleural effusions are known complications of the use of central catheters in neonates (Aiken et al, 1992; Giacoia 1991). Although these are uncommon events, clinical awareness and early recognition of these complications can prevent mortality.

USE OF PARENTERAL NUTRITION IN THE NEONATAL INTENSIVE CARE UNIT: A PRACTICAL APPROACH

The preceding portion of this chapter has presented the scientific basis for recommendations regarding provision of parenteral nutrition to neonates. The following paragraphs present a practical approach to the administration of parenteral nutrition, with a particular emphasis on ELBW infants.

Every clinician caring for ELBW infants must recognize the urgent need to initiate intravenous amino acids shortly after birth. As mentioned previously, the ELBW infant loses 1.5% of total body protein each day that amino acids are withheld. Consequently, the goal of early parenteral nutrition should be to limit catabolism and preserve endogenous protein stores. Numerous studies have clearly demonstrated both the safety and efficacy of early amino acids in accomplishing this goal, even at low caloric intakes.

We recommend starting 3.0 g/kg/day of amino acids on the 1st day of life. This can be accomplished simply by adding one of the crystalline amino acid solutions designed for use in neonates (Aminosyn-PF, Primene, Premasol, or TrophAmine) to glucose to use as the initial maintenance fluid in ELBW infants. We recommend developing a neonatal amino acid stock solution, made in advance in the pharmacy. The solution contains amino acids in a 7.5% dextrose that, when delivered at 60 mL/kg/day, provides 3 g/kg/day of amino acids. Additional fluids with or without electrolytes and/or a higher concentration of dextrose are "Y'd in," with adjustments as needed for the individual infant's fluid, dextrose, and electrolyte requirements, eliminating the need to discard the bag of parenteral nutrition fluid for such changes in status. It is important to note that this stock solution should not be increased beyond 60 mL/kg/day; any alterations to total fluids must be made with ancillary fluids This mixture of glucose and amino acids can be given via a peripheral intravenous line, umbilical venous line, or percutaneous central venous catheter. Increased use of percutaneously placed central venous catheters has certainly facilitated early and widespread use of parenteral nutrition in premature infants. In our nursery, strong consideration is given to percutaneous central venous line placement in ELBW infants early in their postnatal course.

To meet growth requirements, 3.5 to 4.0 g/kg/day of amino acids is required. It is important to point out that such amounts are merely estimates, and protein requirements to sustain optimal growth in ELBW infants might be even higher. Once administration of amino acids is initiated, intake can be advanced to meet requirements for growth over a relatively short period. We typically advance amino acid intake 3.5 g/kg/day by the 2nd day of life. Given the available data, we also recommend the addition of cysteine to the amino acid solution (40 mg/g of

amino acids, to a maximum of 120 mg). However, we delay adding cysteine until other electrolytes are included in the parenteral nutrition solution so that acetate can be added to buffer the cysteine acid load.

Glucose should be supplied in a quantity sufficient to maintain normal plasma glucose concentrations. As discussed previously, glucose production and utilization rates are highest in the most premature infants; their glucose needs are in the range of 6 to 8 mg/kg/minute, whereas the term infant's needs are approximately 3 to 4 mg/kg/minute. Giving 10% dextrose at 100 mL/kg/day provides a glucose infusion rate of 7 mg/kg/minute. Starting infants with birthweights less than 1000 g on 5% dextrose is likely to be prudent if their total fluid requirements are greater than 120 to 150 mL/kg/day.

Lipids should be started within the first 24 hours of life, usually at 1.0 g/kg/day. We typically start lipids at 1.0 g/kg/day and advance by 0.5 to 1.0 g/kg/day to a usual maximum of 3 g/kg/day while monitoring and maintaining serum triglycerides at less than 200 mg/dL. Given the numerous advantages over 10% solutions, 20% lipid emulsions should always be used. To facilitate clearance and to avoid impairment of oxygenation, lipids should be infused over a 24-hour period. There is currently no evidence to support the use of cyclic infusion in the acute setting of the NICU.

Caloric goals during parenteral nutrition are lower than with enteral feeds. To achieve optimal protein retention, approximately 70 to 80 kcal/kg/day is a reasonable goal. To optimize growth, somewhat higher caloric intakes may be necessary. The nonprotein balance between carbohydrate and lipid should be approximately 60:40. These goals can usually be achieved using glucose solutions with concentrations no greater than 12.5% (Table 67-6).

There is a paucity of data related to monitoring laboratory tests during provision of parenteral nutrition. Suggested monitoring for infants receiving parenteral

TABLE 67-6 Caloric Value of Parenteral Nutrition Solutions

Composition*	kcal/kg/day	% of Nonprotein Calories
Example 1: Total Fluids at 110 mL/kg/day		
10% dextrose	37	55
3 g/kg/day lipid	30	45
3.5 g/kg/day amino acids	14	—
Total	81	—
Example 2: Total Fluids at 80 mL/kg/day		
12.5% dextrose	34	53
3 g/kg/day lipid	30	47
3.5 g/kg/day amino acids	14	—
Total	78	—
Example 3: Total Fluids at 140 mL/kg/day		
12.5% dextrose	60	67
3 g/kg/day lipid	30	33
3.5 g/kg/day amino acids	14	—
Total	104	—

*Dextrose: 3.4 kcal/g; protein: 4 kcal/g; lipid (20% emulsion): 10 kcal/g.

TABLE 67-7 Suggested Monitoring During Parenteral Nutrition

Parameter	Frequency
Weight	Daily
Length and OFC	Weekly
Serum glucose	1×/shift during week 1, then daily
Serum Na, K, Cl, BUN, Ca, P, Mg, hematocrit	2–3×/week during week 1, then weekly
Alkaline phosphatase, ALT (SGPT), GGT, fractionated bilirubin	Weekly

ALT, Alanine aminotransferase; *BUN*, blood urea nitrogen; *GGT*, gamma-glutamyl transferase; *OFC*, occipitofrontal circumference; *SGPT*, serum glutamate-pyruvate aminotransferase.

nutrition is shown in Table 67-7. All of these laboratory tests may not be appropriate in ELBW infants because of constraints related to blood sampling.

The use of parenteral nutrition should be accompanied by the early initiation of enteral feeds (within the first 1 to 3 days of life). Parenteral nutrition should be continued until enteral feedings are well established and providing approximately 100 to 110 kcal/kg/day, although availability of intravenous access may necessitate earlier termination of parenteral nutrition in some circumstances. As enteral feeds are advanced, the protein and lipid contents of the parenteral nutrition can be gradually decreased. In addition, careful and prompt attention to reinstitution of parenteral nutrition during episodes of intolerance of enteral feeds cannot be overemphasized. Infants with intolerance of enteral feeds in whom nothing-by-mouth (NPO) status is frequently necessary present an additional challenge. In such infants, it may be prudent to determine full-volume parenteral nutrition needs as for NPO status and to then run the parenteral nutrition solution at a lower rate if enteral feeds are administered. With this approach, if a change to NPO status becomes necessary after administration of the parenteral nutrition fluid has begun, the volume can be safely increased without compromising caloric and protein intake.

SUGGESTED READINGS

Bauer J, Maier K, Hellstern G, et al: Longitudinal evaluation of energy expenditure in preterm infants with birth weight less than 1000 g, *Br J Nutr* 89:533-537, 2003.

Beardsall K, Vanhaesebrouck S, Ogilvy-Stuart AL, et al: Early insulin therapy in very-low-birth-weight infants, *N Engl J Med* 359:1873-1884, 2008.

Clark RH, Thomas P, Peabody J: Extrauterine growth restriction remains a serious problem in prematurely born neonates, *Pediatrics* 111:986-990, 2003.

Denne S: Protein and energy requirements in preterm infants, *Semin Neonatol* 6:377-382, 2001.

Fanaroff AA, Stoll BJ, Wright LL, et al: Trends in neonatal morbidity and mortality for very low birthweight infants, *Am J Obstet Gynecol* 196:147, 2007.

Poindexter BB: Early amino acid administration for premature neonates, *J Pediatr* 147:420-421, 2005.

Putet G: Lipid metabolism of the micropremie, *Clin Perinatol* 27:57, 2000.

Simmer K, Rao SC: Early introduction of lipids to parenterally-fed preterm infants, *Cochrane Database Syst Rev* 2:CD005256, 2005.

Steinbach M, Clark RH, Kelleher AS, et al: Demographic and nutritional factors associated with prolonged cholestatic jaundice in the premature infant, *J Perinatol* 28:129-135, 2008.

Stephens BE, Walden RV, Gargus RA, et al: First-week protein and energy intakes are associated with 18-month developmental outcomes in extremely low birth weight infants, *Pediatrics* 123:1337-1343, 2009.

Thureen PJ, Melara D, Fennessey PV, et al: Effect of low versus high intravenous amino acid intake on very low birth weight infants in the early neonatal period, *Pediatr Res* 53:24-32, 2003.

Torine IJ, Denne SC, Wright-Coltart S, et al: Effect of late-onset sepsis on energy expenditure in extremely premature infants, *Pediatr Res* 61:600-603, 2007.

Complete references used in this text can be found online at www.expertconsult.com

CHAPTER
68

DEVELOPMENTAL ANATOMY AND PHYSIOLOGY OF THE GASTROINTESTINAL TRACT

Reed A. Dimmitt and Eric Sibley

STRUCTURAL AND FUNCTIONAL DEVELOPMENT

Understanding the development of the human gastrointestinal tract, from both an anatomic and cellular basis, has a long history, dating back more than a century. This knowledge encompasses prenatal in utero and postnatal processes. Changes in both morphogenesis and cellular differentiation drive structural formation of the gastrointestinal tract in the developing embryo. Digestive function continues to develop following birth. Advances in molecular biology have revealed that specific aspects of gastrointestinal tract development involve genetically controlled interaction between trophic compounds and cellular receptors, as described later for the different organs of the gastrointestinal tract.

From a global perspective, the gastrointestinal tract results from embryonic invagination and folding during week 4 of gestation. Eventually, the buccopharyngeal and cloacal membranes rupture, permitting a direct communication between the fetal gastrointestinal tract and the in utero environment. A series of folding, lengthening, and luminal dilation events result in the formation of the foregut (esophagus, stomach, duodenum, liver, and pancreas); the midgut (jejunum, ileum, ascending colon, and transverse colon); and hindgut (descending colon, sigmoid colon, and rectum). With additional elongation and growth during the first trimester, the developing gut migrates into the umbilical cord. It returns to the fetal abdominal cavity and rotates counterclockwise around the axis of the superior mesenteric artery around 20 weeks' gestation (Figure 68-1). Thus, by the second trimester, basic morphogenesis of the fetal gastrointestinal tract is complete. Additional in utero and postnatal functional maturation is still necessary. For example, gastrointestinal motility is markedly disorganized at 24 weeks' gestation. Although dysmotility is a normal developmental "milestone" in the fetal environment, uncoordinated peristalsis in the extremely low-birthweight infant is associated with significant postnatal problems.

Knowledge of the cellular and molecular processes of early morphogenesis is rapidly expanding and involves crosstalk between maternal and fetal factors during development. We first discuss the embryology of the gastrointestinal tract in advance of discussing functional development including digestion.

FOREGUT

ESOPHAGUS

The normal morphogenesis of foregut can be subdivided into five successive developmental stages (Kluth et al, 2003). In the first stage, occurring at days 22–23, the primitive foregut differentiates into ventral and dorsal structures, termed the lung field and esophageal area, respectively. The esophageal area has one cell layer consisting of 10 somites. In the second stage, the lung bud develops from the caudal lung field proximal to the liver. Next, in the third stage, longitudinal ridges appear inside the lumen of the developing foregut, which results in a distinct and separate dorsal esophageal area. The fourth stage involves proliferation of the longitudinal ridges, resulting in a tracheoesophageal septum. Subsequently, apoptosis in the central section of the septum begins the initial separation of the dorsal and ventral compartments. In the fifth stage, there is the formation of definitive respiratory and esophageal structures between weeks 6 and 7 of gestation.

Researchers utilizing *Drosophila* and murine models have identified a myriad of key signaling pathways in foregut development. For example, the hedgehog signaling pathway appears to be essential for maintaining stem cell niches as well as directing developmental axes (Figure 68-2) (Lees et al, 2005). Hedgehog binds to a cell membrane receptor Patched (Ptc) resulting in downstream signaling and transcription factor mediated cell differentiation. Defects in this pathway are associated with congenital anomalies of the foregut.

STOMACH

By week 6 of gestation, the fetal stomach is well defined. The muscular layers (the inner circular and outer longitudinal) become visible by 9 weeks. By week 12 of gestation, the gastric mucosa has differentiated into the various types of epithelium: the zymogen, endocrine, mucous, and parietal cells. By 16 weeks, all of these cells are secreting their respective cellular products.

Several trophic factors have been shown to be involved in gastric epithelial differentiation. Crosstalk between transforming growth factor-β1 and basement membrane

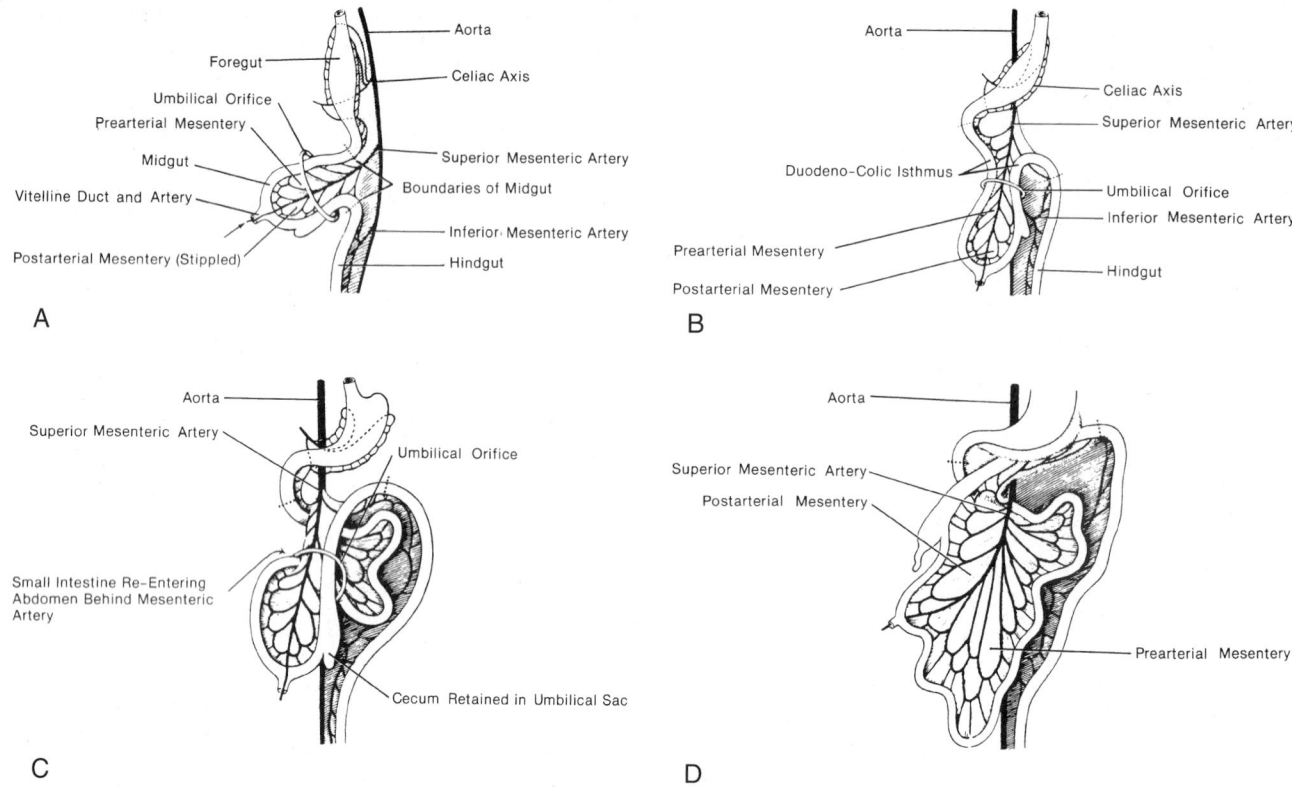

FIGURE 68-1 **Diagrams showing normal rotation of alimentary tract. A,** Fifth week of intrauterine life *(lateral view)*. The foregut, midgut, and hindgut are shown with their individual blood supply supported by the common dorsal mesentery in the sagittal plane. The midgut loop has been extruded into the umbilical cord. **B,** Eighth week of intrauterine life *(anteroposterior view)*. The first stage of rotation is being completed. Note the narrow duodenocolic isthmus from which the midgut loop depends and the right-sided position of the small intestine and left-sided position of the colon. Maintenance of this position within the abdomen after birth is termed *nonrotation*. **C,** About the 10th week of intrauterine life, during the second stage of rotation *(anteroposterior view)*. The bowel in the temporary umbilical hernia is in the process of reduction; the most proximal part of the prearterial segment entering the abdomen to the right of the superior mesenteric artery is held forward close to the cecum and ascending colon, permitting the bowel to pass under it. As the coils of small intestine collect within the abdomen, the hindgut is displaced to the left and upward. **D,** Eleventh week of intrauterine life at the end of the second stage of rotation. From its original sagittal position, the midgut has rotated 270 degrees in a counterclockwise direction about the origin of the superior mesenteric artery. The essentials of the permanent disposition of the viscera have been attained. *(A to D, From Gardner CE Jr, Hart D: Anomalies of intestinal rotation as a cause of intestinal obstruction,* Arch Surg *29:942-946, 1934. Copyright 1934, American Medical Association.)*

proteins called laminins are important mediators of gastric epithelial polarity (Basque et al, 2002). Fibroblast growth factors 10 and 2, proteins in the hedgehog pathway, are strong determinants of gastric epithelial differentiation, in particular with parietal cell differentiation (Spencer-Dene et al, 2006).

LIVER AND PANCREAS

The liver and pancreas develop from two different anatomical domains of the definitive endodermal epithelium of the embryonic foregut. Fate-mapping experiments demonstrate that the liver arises from precursor cells in the developing ventral foregut as well as from a small group of endodermal cells tracking down the ventral midline. During foregut closure, the medial and lateral domains come together. The pancreas is also induced in lateral endoderm domains, adjacent and caudal to the lateral liver domains, and in cells near the dorsal midline of the foregut (Zaret and Grompe, 2008).

After the initial differentiation, several transcription factors shape the developing liver precursor cells into hepatocytes and bile duct cells. In an even more complex process,

the pancreatic cells are induced to become specific endocrine, acinar, or ductal cells (Figure 68-3).

From an organogenesis aspect, rotation and fusion of the dorsal and ventral pancreatic buds occur by 7 weeks' gestation. By 14 weeks, immunoreactive insulin can be detected and pancreatic zymogen granules are present in the acinar cells. By 16 weeks, amylase is present. Trypsin, lipase, and amylase are secreted into the duodenum by 31 weeks (Zoppi et al, 1972). As mentioned earlier, the liver is derived as an outbudding from the foregut. The cranial portion of the bud differentiates into hepatic parenchyma, and the caudal portion into the gallbladder. Specific hepatic lobules and bile canaliculi can be detected by 6 weeks. Bile acids are present in the liver by 12 weeks and are actively secreted into the small intestine by 22 weeks' gestation.

MIDGUT AND HINDGUT

Although portions of the small intestine are derived from the foregut and midgut and portions of the colon are derived from the midgut and hindgut, we discuss these portions of the gastrointestinal tract from an end-organ perspective.

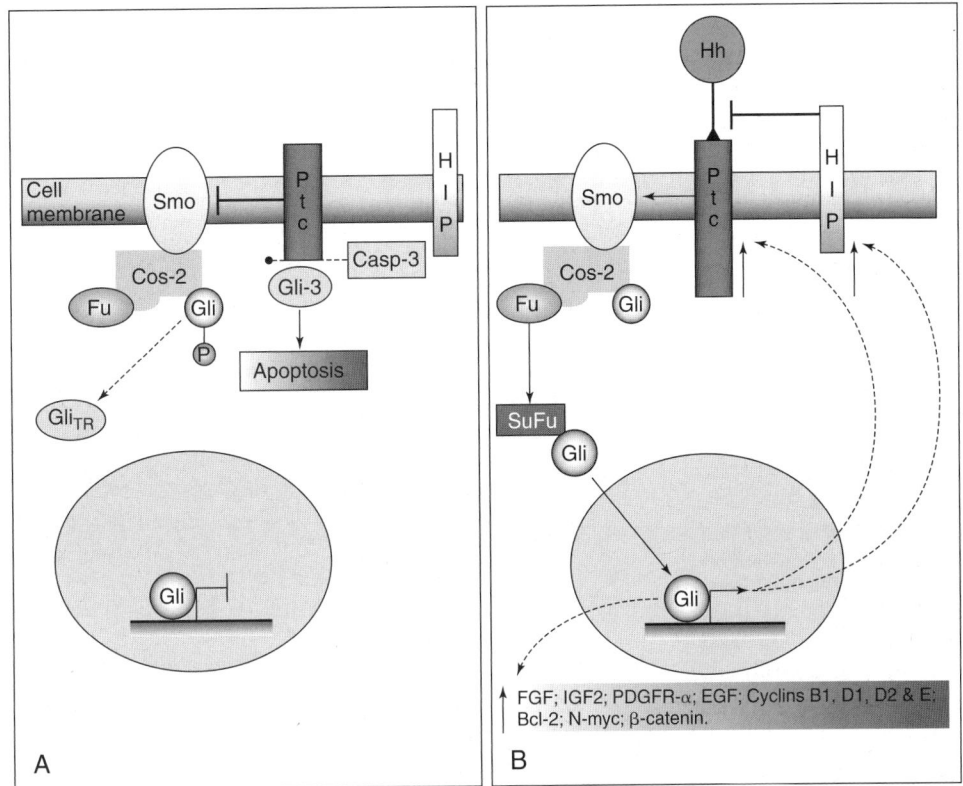

FIGURE 68-2 Hedgehog (Hh) signaling in mammalian cells. In the absence of Hh **(A)**, the receptor Patched *(Ptc)* exerts an inhibitory effect on Smoothened *(Smo)*, a transmembrane protein with homology to G-protein-coupled receptors. In the presence of Hh ligand-binding **(B)**, the inhibitory action of Ptc on Smo is released. The full Gli product is now stabilized and transferred to the nucleus. Once in the nucleus, the full Gli product binds to and upregulates transcriptional targets, including Ptc and another Hh-binding protein, *HIP*. In this manner, excess Hh is sequestered and the pathway regulated.

SMALL INTESTINE

The ultimate digestive function of the small intestine requires intestinal epithelium to secrete digestive enzymes and to provide sufficient surface area to absorb nutrients. Therefore, it is important to understand the development of the cellular differentiation as well as overall intestinal length.

As previously mentioned, the hedgehog signaling pathway is also important in endodermal and mesodermal differentiation in small intestinal development. In addition, the genes encoding for the transcription factors *Sox9*, *Sox17*, and *SRY* have been shown to be essential in endoderm differentiation, whereas the *Hox* family of transcription factors are involved in mesodermal differentiation (de Santa Barbara et al, 2003).

After differentiation, the intestinal villous and crypt development is under the control of several growth factors that are secreted in autocrine, paracrine, endocrine, and exocrine pathways (Ménard, 2004). Glucagon-like peptide 1 and 2 are secreted by intestinal neurons and L cells, respectively, and are associated with increased intestinal length (Sigalet et al, 2004). Clinical trials in adults are underway administering glucagon-like peptide 2 in patients with short bowel syndrome and may eventually show promise in pediatric patients with intestinal failure.

The small intestine is well developed after its extracorporeal migration into the umbilical cord. Rapid epithelial proliferation occludes the small-intestinal lumen early in development, but the lumen becomes patent at 12 weeks' gestation. There is a gradual development of digestive function that is not fully complete until 34 weeks' gestation, thus posing additional problems regarding administering enteral nutrition to premature infants.

COLON

The hindgut is formed by an early dilatation of the fetal cecum at 4 weeks' gestation. By 12 weeks, this primitive structure takes on the gross anatomic features of the colon. At this same time, the midgut rotation is completed, resulting in the cecum being located in the right lower abdominal space. The hallmark of colonic function is coordinated motility, especially in the development of the rectum. The rectum forms by 8 weeks, and formation of complete muscle layers and neural migration of neural crest cells are accomplished by 24 weeks. By 22 weeks, the premature colon maintains some aspects of the small intestine, including villi and disaccharidase function. With developmental maturation, the colonic crypt structures dominate the mucosal surface, and the intestinal characteristics diminish (Raul et al, 1986).

From a cellular developmental aspect, several trophic factors have been linked to colonic differentiation. Elf-3, a member of the Ets transcription factor family, controls intestinal epithelial differentiation during development by regulating the expression of growth factor receptors in

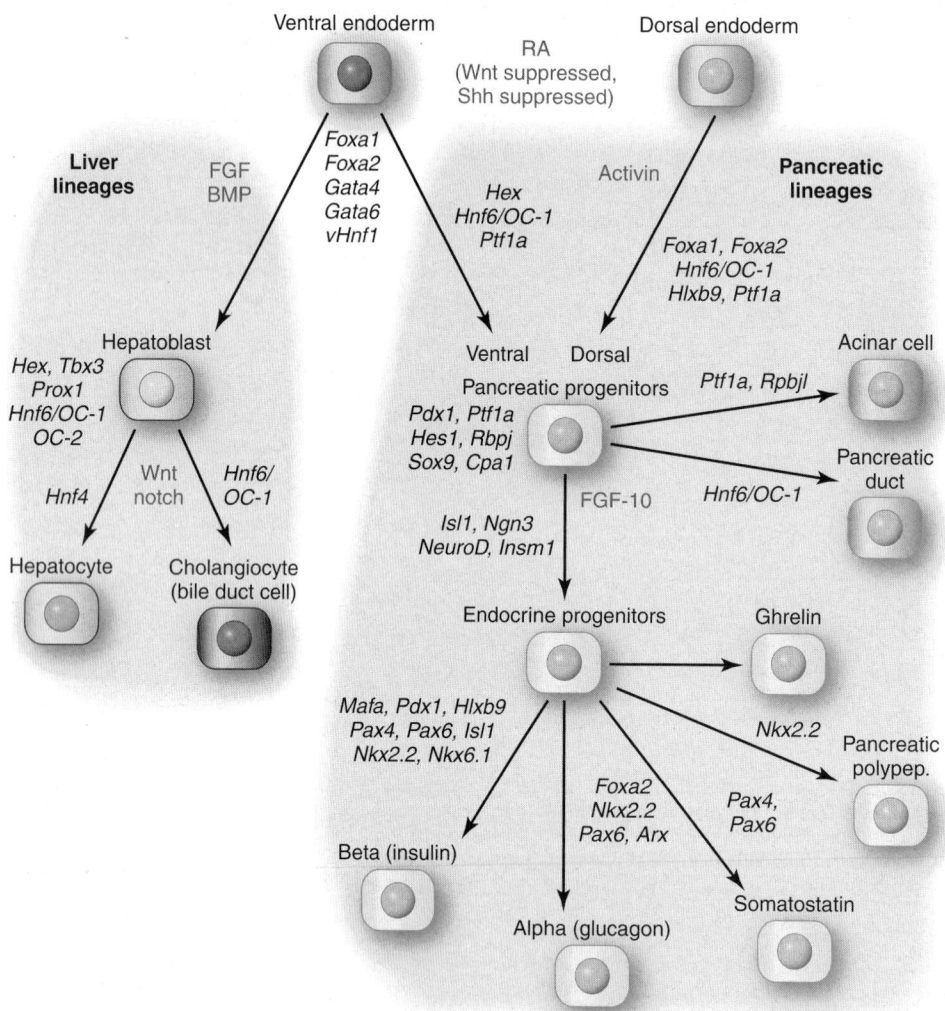

FIGURE 68-3 Regulatory factors controlling cell type lineages within the liver and pancreas. Transcription factor genes involved in differentiation are noted in italics. *(From Zaret KS, Grompe M: Generation and regeneration of cells of the liver and pancreas,* Science *322:1490-1494, 2008.)*

epithelial cells (Jedlicka and Gutierrez-Hartmann, 2008). Recently identified molecules termed micro-RNAs have been shown to regulate cell differentiation and maintenance of the pluripotent stem cells (Monzo et al, 2008).

The developing enteric nervous system is derived in a large part from the vagal neural crest cells with additional contribution from migration of the precursor cells from the sacral region. Molecules that have been shown to control the migration of ganglion cells include the RET/ GFRa1/GDNF and endothelin receptor-B/endothelin-3 signaling pathways, transcription factors such as Phox2b, Sox10, Pax3, Mash1, Hox11L1 and Sip1, the hedgehog signaling system, neurotrophins, and bone morphogenetic proteins (Burns and Thapar, 2006). Defects in these molecules may be related to congenital colonic disease, including Hirschsprung's disease.

MUCOSAL IMMUNE SYSTEM DEVELOPMENT

The gastrointestinal tract is the largest immune organ in the body and thus warrants review of its development. As with other aspects of gastrointestinal tract development, the mucosal immune system undergoes both fetal and

postnatal changes. The dramatic changes following exposure to food and bacterially derived molecules after birth have been shown to be a major determinant in ongoing mucosal immune modification.

Mucosal immunity is composed of innate and adaptive arms. The innate immune system includes a chemical/noncellular component (e.g., gastric acid, intestinal mucous layer, epithelial barrier function, and defensins), as well as a cellular compartment (e.g., neutrophils, macrophages, and antigen-presenting cells). The adaptive immune system is made up of T cell lymphocytes and B cell–mediated humoral immunity.

Although primarily considered to be involved in digestion, gastric acid, bile salts, and pancreatic secretions function to inhibit potential pathogenic bacterial growth. Clinical investigators have demonstrated that delaying feedings in premature infants results in decreased gastric acid secretion, possibly the mechanism whereby trophic feedings prevent necrotizing enterocolitis (NEC) (Berseth et al, 2005; Hyman et al, 1983). In addition, administering histamine H_2 blockers to premature infants is associated with increased sepsis (Beck-Sague et al, 1994) and NEC (Guillet et al, 2006).

Mucins, glycoproteins, immunoglobulins, glycolipids, trefoil factors, and albumin are all constituents of the luminal mucus layer. Previously, it was believed that mucus functions in a nonspecific manner to prevent bacterial adhesion and expel potential pathogens. It is now clear that certain components of the mucus layer are involved in mucosal healing. Specifically, the trefoil factor family has proangiogenic and antiapoptotic qualities, as well as modulating cell-to-cell contacts and potentiating epidermal growth factor (Hoffmann, 2005).

The epithelial barrier function is accomplished by intracellular proteins that anchor the cells to each other, preventing large molecules from penetrating. Recently, it has been shown that these proteins are not just "spot welds" but are dynamic in nature and respond to physiologic and pathologic stimuli (Graham et al, 2009). In addition, dendritic cells, a type of antigen-presenting cells, can sample the microbiota of the intestinal lumen by sending "periscopes" through the tight junctions, suggesting an epithelial-immune cell interaction.

Defensins are antimicrobial proteins secreted by specialized intestinal epithelium called Paneth cells. It appears that defensins are uniformly expressed in the gastrointestinal tract at 14 weeks' gestation but are restricted to the small intestine by 17 weeks. The number of Paneth cells and expression of defensins in 24-week infants is significantly lower than in term infants and may be associated with increased sepsis and NEC in premature infants (Mallow et al, 1996).

The cellular components of innate immunity include macrophages and granulocytes. Macrophages are present in the fetal intestine as early as week 11 of gestation. A recent study has demonstrated that chemerin is a potent recruiter of intestinal macrophages with peak level production at 20–24 weeks (Maheshwari et al, 2009).

Previously, the cells of the innate immune system were believed to act in a nonspecific manner in response to pathogenic stimuli. It is now clear that specific bacterial components signal through membrane-associated receptors termed toll-like receptors (TLRs). For example, lipopolysaccharide from gram-negative bacteria is the ligand for TLR-4, which results in a downstream inflammatory response. TLRs are expressed by both immune cells and gastrointestinal epithelial cells. TLR4 is expressed on fetal enterocytes as early as 18 weeks' gestation (Fusunyan et al, 2001) and may be induced following birth with the acquisition of the intestinal microbiota.

The adaptive immune system of host defense is composed of T cells and humoral immunity. Lymphocytes have been shown to proliferate in response to mitogenic stimuli at 12 weeks' gestation. Peyer's patches are lymphoid tissue that process lumen antigens. M cells are differentiated intestinal epithelia that function to process antigens to lymphocytes and other cells in Peyer's patches and can be observed at 17 weeks' gestation. Peyer's patches are essential for the production of plasma cells that secrete mucosal associated immunoglobulins.

Once naive T cells interact with antigen, they develop into specific phenotypes based on their cytokine production. Currently, T cell subsets include T-helper cell 1 (Th1), Th2, Th17 (producing IL-17), and regulator T cells (Weaver et al, 2006). In the sterile in utero environment,

T cells are predominantly Th2, promoting a symbiosis between fetus and mother. On presentation with antigen, there is a switch to the more mature cells. The gestational age at which this T cell commitment can occur is unknown and is a fertile area for future research.

GASTROINTESTINAL MICROBIOTA

The newborn infant is born with a sterile gut that acquires its microbiota in the postnatal period. On the basis of some classic culture-based studies performed in the 1970s and 1980s, the term infant microbiota was determined. The composition of the infant microbiota is less complex and features a higher proportion of facultative bacteria than in the adult. The facultative bacteria are the first to colonize secondary to the oxygen content of the intestine, which prevents the growth of obligate anaerobic bacteria. Thus, after the acquisition and expansion of facultative *Escherichia coli* and *Enterococcus* spp., the intestinal oxygen is consumed, thereby allowing for subsequent colonization by anaerobic *Bifidobacterium*, *Bacteroides*, and *Clostridium* spp. (Adlerberth, 2008).

DIGESTIVE PHYSIOLOGY

The human gastrointestinal tract functions to digest and absorb nutrients consumed in food. Nutrient digestion consists of breaking down carbohydrates, proteins, and fats to smaller component molecules (monosaccharides, oligopeptides and amino acids, and free fatty acids and monoglycerides) that can be transported into absorptive intestinal epithelial cells and then into the portal circulation. Human digestive function matures throughout embryogenesis as the gastrointestinal organs develop and acquire different digestive capacities.

CARBOHYDRATE DIGESTION

Carbohydrates supply approximately 40% of ingested calories in term infants. Dietary carbohydrates consist of sugars and starches. Lactose is the predominant sugar in human breast milk and most milk-based infant formulas. Before absorption of its constituent glucose and galactose monosaccharides, the lactose disaccharide must be hydrolyzed by the enzymatic action of the intestinal lactase enzyme. Lactase is a membrane-bound protein present on the apical surface of enterocytes, the intestinal absorptive cells. During early fetal life, lactase gene is expressed in the colon and small intestine. By term, however, a spatial gradient of lactase gene expression is established, with peak expression in the proximal intestine (Raul et al, 1986). Lactase activity increases during fetal maturation, with the greatest increase, about fourfold, occurring during the third trimester (Weaver et al, 1986). In the absence of sufficient lactase hydrolysis, undigested lactose can result in an osmotic diarrhea. Although preterm infants have relatively low levels of lactase activity, they are often able to sustain normal growth with little diarrhea when fed breast milk or lactose-containing formula (MacLean and Fink, 1980). Some formulas also contain complex carbohydrates in the form of glucose polymers. Glucose polymers require amylase for hydrolysis. The process of complex carbohydrate digestion is initiated in the lumen of the gastrointestinal tract by the action of alpha-amylases secreted by the salivary gland and the pancreas. Because pancreatic amylase levels are low in neonates, salivary amylase supports a significant amount of glucose polymer digestion along with the mucosal glucoamylase enzyme (Hodge et al, 1983). Glucoamylase is a membrane-bound hydrolase synthesized by the enterocyte that removes single glucose residues from alpha (1–4) chains of glucose polymers. Glucoamylase activity is detectable as early as 13 weeks' gestation and increases two- to threefold in the near-term newborn (Ménard, 1994).

The monosaccharide products of luminal and membrane-bound hydrolysis of carbohydrates are transported across both the apical and basolateral enterocyte membranes and into the portal circulation. Active glucose and galactose transport into enterocytes is carried out predominantly by the apical sodium-glucose cotransport protein, SGLT1. Glucose and galactose are transported out of the enterocyte by the basolateral GLUT2 transport protein. Congenital defects of the SGLT1 protein result in rare cases of glucose-galactose malabsorption characterized by severe, watery, acidic diarrhea in the newborn period (Martín et al, 1996). Treatment consists of a glucose- and galactose-free diet, initially given as a fructose-based formula.

PROTEIN DIGESTION

Proteins contribute less than 10% of ingested calories in infants. Many of the amino acids used for protein synthesis are produced within the body. Essential amino acids, however, must be provided through dietary protein. Similar to digestion of complex carbohydrates, protein digestion involves both luminal and mucosal enzymatic hydrolysis. Proteins are initially digested within the intestinal lumen by proteases secreted by the stomach (pepsin) and pancreas (trypsin, chymotrypsin, carboxypeptidase, elastase). The final products of luminal digestion are amino acids and oligopeptides composed of 2- to 6-amino-acid residues. Digestion of oligopeptides greater than two residues is performed by mucosal membrane-bound brush-border peptidases. Bi- and tripeptides can be transported through the enterocyte membrane via the proton-coupled PEPT1 transporter and may be further hydrolyzed by cytosolic peptidases that exist within the cell or transported out of the cell and into the portal system as peptides (Liang et al, 1995). Amino acids are transported into enterocytes by a great variety of amino acid transporters. The activities of most of the brush-border and cytosolic peptidases are well developed in the preterm infant. There is evidence, however, that some milk proteins may be absorbed intact into the circulation (Kuitunen et al, 1994).

FAT DIGESTION

Fat provides 40 to 50% of the caloric intake of the newborn. Similar to carbohydrate and protein digestion, fat processing is initiated in the lumen before mucosal absorption. By means of enzymatic action, lingual, gastric, and pancreatic lipases function to hydrolyze fat to its constituent free fatty acids and monoglycerides. Pancreatic lipases are in relatively low concentration at birth. Lingual lipases and gastric lipases, however, are present by 26 weeks' gestation and thus contribute significantly to neonatal fat digestion (Hamosh et al, 1981). In addition, a bile salt–dependent lipase present in human milk is capable of hydrolyzing fats (Freed et al, 1987). Bile salts secreted by the liver and gallbladder are necessary for efficient absorption of fats and function to emulsify fat in the intestinal lumen. Bile flow to the intestine increases rapidly after birth and initiation of feeding. After luminal hydrolysis of fat, mixed micelles of fatty acids and monoglycerides diffuse directly across the cell membrane of mucosal intestinal cells.

SUGGESTED READINGS

Briana DD, Malamitsi-Puchner A: The role of adipocytokines in fetal growth, *Ann N Y Acad Sci* 1205:82-87, 2010.

Burns AJ, Roberts RR, Bornstein JC, et al: Development of the enteric nervous system and its role in intestinal motility during fetal and early postnatal stages, *Semin Pediatr Surg* 18:196-205, 2009.

Gerritsen J, Smidt H, Rijkers GT, et al: Intestinal microbiota in human health and disease: the impact of probiotics, *Genes Nutr*, 2001.

Green AS, Rozance PJ, Limesand SW: Cionsequences of a compromised intrauterine environment on islet function, *J Endocrinol* 205:211-224, 2010.

Kinroos JM, Darzi AW, Nicholson JK: Gut microbiome-host interactions in health and disease, *Genome Med* 3:14m, 2011.

Kung JW, Currie IS, Forbes SJ, et al: Liver development, regeneration and carcinogenesis, *Biomed Biotechnol* 20010:984248, 2010.

Lebenthal A, Lebenthal E: The ontogeny of the small intestinal epithelium, *J Parenter Enteral Nutr* 23:S3-S6, 1999.

Lebenthal E, Lee PC: Gastrointestinal physiologic considerations in the feeding of the developing infant, *Curr Concepts Nutr* 14:125-145, 1985.

Murtaugh LC: The what, where, when and how of Wnt/beta-catenin signaling in pancreas development, *Organogenesis* 4:81-86, 2008.

Ratcliffe EM: Molecular development of the extrinsic sensory innervation of the gastrointestinal tract, *Auton Neurosci* 161:1-5, 2011.

Complete references and supplemental color images used in this text can be found online at www.expertconsult.com

CHAPTER 69

STRUCTURAL ANOMALIES OF THE GASTROINTESTINAL TRACT

Clara Song, Jeffrey S. Upperman, and Victoria Niklas

DISORDERS OF THE MOUTH AND NECK

MOUTH

Small nodules are present on the hard palate and mandibular and maxillary ridges in 80% of newborns. Nodules on the hard palate are called *Epstein's pearls*, whereas those on the mandibular and maxillary alveolar ridges are called *Bohn's nodules*. Both types of nodules are generally 1–3 mm in size and are thought to be remnants of salivary gland tissue. Most nodules usually disappear spontaneously within the first 3 months of life.

Cysts filled with mucus within the floor of the mouth are called *ranulas*. Clinically, ranulas are classified into two types, simple ranulas or superficial ranulas or plunging or cervical ranulas. Simple ranulas are usually pea-sized, disappear spontaneously, and are generally of no consequence. Plunging ranulas generally involve the submandibular and submental space of the neck, and although some of these cysts resolve, a large or persistent ranula may lead to feeding difficulties, thereby requiring surgical excision or marsupialization (Patel et al, 2009; Zhi et al, 2008).

Malignant tumors of the mouth are rare in the newborn. An *epignathus* is any tumor that arises from the upper jaw or palate and projects from the mouth. These tumors may be polyps, dermoids, adenomas, or teratomas, or rarely a granulosa cell tumor called *epulis* (Kumar and Sharma, 2008). In addition to a careful physical examination, these tumors should be evaluated with computed tomography (CT) or magnetic resonance imaging (MRI) so as to fully define the extent of the tumor and to determine whether it impinges on the nasopharynx, airway, or esophagus. Tumors that impinge on the nasopharynx, airway, or esophagus or those with in infants with clinical signs and symptoms such as respiratory distress or feeding difficulties will need definitive treatment by surgical removal.

Tumors of the salivary gland (with the parotid gland being most commonly affected) may arise anywhere in the gland. Although they are typically confined to the intracapsular portion of the gland, sentinel lesions on the surface of the gland may be present (Bradley et al, 2007; Mehta and Willging, 2006; Myer and Cotton, 1986). These tumors should be evaluated by Doppler ultrasound and then further evaluated with CT or MRI (Lowe et al, 2001). Histologic diagnosis may be confirmed by open biopsy or excision. Hemangioma-endothelioma and mixed tumors are the most common noninflammatory tumors. Hemangiomas often give a bluish hue to overlying skin and may transiently increase in size with crying because of blood-filling by the cavernous tissue component of the tumor. Juxtaparotid lymphangiomas are rare, but they tend to be multiloculated and composed of cystic spaces of varying sizes that may increase in size because of an upper respiratory tract infection. Local resection is generally the treatment of choice (Har-El et al, 1985; Thompson, 2002).

Infection of the parotid gland (suppurative parotitis) or salivary gland (sialadenitis) should be considered in cases in which these glands rapidly enlarge and display signs of inflammation during the 1st month of life. Primary sialadenitis, however, is extremely rare, and most cases of sialadenitis in the submaxillary gland result as extensions from the parotid gland. The diagnosis may be confirmed by applying gentle pressure on the gland and expressing pus from the Stensen duct. *Staphylococcus aureus* or *Escherichia coli* is commonly isolated, but broad-spectrum antimicrobial coverage should be started until the organism has been identified and sensitivities have been established, because sepsis and extension to include the salivary glands are not uncommon.

TONGUE

Congenital disorders of the tongue include agenesis, true hypertrophy, enlargement due to lymphangiomas, aberrant thyroid tissue and abnormalities of fixation. Abnormalities of the tongue may also be associated with breathing or feeding difficulties. Aglossia congenita, or congenital absence of the tongue, is extremely rare, but affected infants retain taste sensation and can learn to speak. Ankyloglossia inferior ("tongue-tie") is also common in newborns (Hall and Renfrew, 2005). The short frenulum, however, does not usually interfere with sucking and swallowing, and the frenulum usually lengthens with age.

Ankyloglossia superior, attachment of the tongue to the roof of the mouth, is a rare anomaly that must be recognized at birth because respiratory obstruction may occur (Bolling et al, 2007). Other lesions, such as micrognathia, macroglossia, and cleft palate, are frequently associated with this anomaly.

Neonates with true macroglossia, or enlargement of the tongue, often have continuous protrusion of the tongue and associated difficulties with feeding as well as noisy respirations and possible respiratory failure. These infants often have Down or Beckwith-Wiedemann syndrome. Lymphangioma and idiopathic muscular hypertrophy are additional common causes of macroglossia. A tongue with lymphangioma appears as a raised, firm mass with a warty-looking surface. The treatment for lymphangioma is surgical removal, if possible, or reduction of the tumor bulk with reshaping of the tongue. Infants with idiopathic muscular hypertrophy should be treated conservatively, because the relative size of the tongue often decreases as the mandible grows during infancy.

Thyroid tissue may be present as a solid or cystic mass in the posterior midline of the tongue or under it. If

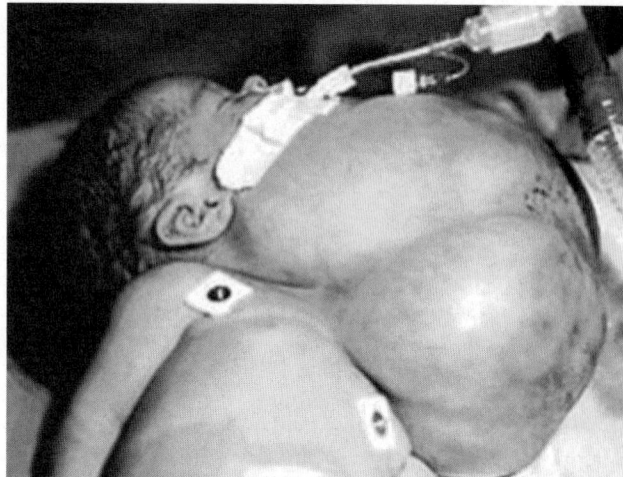

FIGURE 69-1 *(See also Color Plate 28.)* **Cystic hygroma of the face and neck.** Prenatal diagnosis of this large lesion led to the delivery of this infant using ex utero intrapartum treatment. *(From* Archives of Pediatrics & Adolescent Medicine, *155:1271-1272, 2001, Copyright 2001, American Medical Association. All rights reserved.)*

enlargement of the tongue is due to ectopic thyroid tissue, no other thyroid tissue may exist. Normal migration of the thyroid gland did not occur during development. Therefore, before resection of any midline lingual tumor, a thyroid scan should be performed to rule out a lingual thyroid gland.

NASOPHARYNX

Nasopharyngeal tumors are rare and may include polyps, dermoids, or teratomas. Often these tumors are on a stalk and project into the mouth. Those not projecting externally may be palpated as movable, sausage-shaped masses in the pharynx. These tumors should be excised urgently because they often cause respiratory distress from upper airway obstruction. Intubation under direct laryngoscopy may be warranted.

NECK

Cystic hygroma is the most common lateral neck mass in the newborn (Figure 69-1). Cystic hygromas are derived from lymphatic tissue and are present as multilobular, multicystic masses that may rapidly enlarge and cause severe respiratory compromise. Dynamic MRI or CT imaging is useful in identifying the extent and intrathoracic course of these masses. Excision is the treatment of choice, although sclerotherapy has been used for very large or recurrent tumors (Samuel et al, 2000). Infants diagnosed prenatally with giant lymphangiomas (or other giant tumors of the neck) benefit from controlled cesarean section delivery using an ex-utero intrapartum treatment (EXIT) procedure. In these cases, intubation through a tracheotomy after partial dissection of the mass away from the trachea is life-saving (Mychaliska et al, 1997).

Branchial cleft anomalies may manifest as skin tags, pits, sinuses, fistulas, or cysts in the preauricular and lateral cervical regions. Most lesions are remnants of the second branchial cleft and pouch, and 10% to 15% occur bilaterally (Bill and Vadheim, 1955). Sinuses and fistulas may

be discovered during the newborn period, but cysts often require time to fill and usually are not recognized until later in childhood. Ultrasound or CT scan of the neck may be useful to define anatomic relationships, and surgical removal is the treatment of choice.

The so-called sternomastoid tumor, also called the "pseudotumor" of infancy, can be seen and palpated as a smooth oval mass within the body of the sternocleidomastoid muscle. The cause is unknown, but the incidence is seven times higher after breech delivery (Ling and Low, 1972) and among infants who have had specific fetal positioning in utero (Rosegger and Steinwendner, 1992). Histopathology suggests that it results from endomysial fibrosis characterized by deposition of collagen and fibroblasts around individual muscle fibers that subsequently undergo atrophy. Torticollis may develop in up to 20% of cases, and in those cases, hip dysplasia may be present (Porter et al, 1995). Even if torticollis is not present, the head may still be rotated to the side opposite to that of the tumor. If cranial and facial asymmetry result in severe hemihypoplasia, cosmetic surgical correction may be indicated if the hemihypoplasia does not resolve within 6 to 12 months (Wirth et al, 1992).

Midline neck masses in newborns include cystic hygromas, hemangiomas, dermoid cysts, teratomas, enlarged thyroid tumors or goiters, and ectopic thyroid or thymic tissue. Goiters visible at birth may be associated with maternal hypothyroidism, hyperthyroidism, or euthyroidism. The second most common location for ectopic thyroid tissue, after the base of the tongue, is the anterior midline of the neck, just at or below the hyoid bone (Meyerowitz and Buchholz, 1969). Although this tissue may be easily mistaken for a thyroglossal duct cyst, such cysts rarely are present in the newborn. Therefore, before removal of ectopic thyroid tissue, a thyroid scan should be performed to determine if the ectopic thyroid is the infant's only functioning thyroid tissue. Thymic tissue arises high in the cervical region of the embryo as two lateral buds. The buds migrate caudad and join in the anterior mediastinum. Abnormal migration results in ectopic location or cyst formation (or both); the aberrant tissue or cyst may manifest as a lateral or midline neck mass and require surgical removal (Thompson and Love, 1972).

DISORDERS OF THE ESOPHAGUS
ESOPHAGEAL ATRESIA WITH TRACHEOESOPHAGEAL FISTULA

Definition

Esophageal atresia (EA) and tracheoesophageal fistula (TEF) may occur as separate congenital defects, but more frequently they are seen together as a compound defect. Esophageal atresia with a distal tracheoesophageal fistula is by far the most common form, accounting for 85% of cases (Figure 69-2) (Raffensperger, 1990).

Epidemiology

The incidence of EA with TEF ranges from 1 in 3000 to 1 in 4000 live births (Raffensperger, 1990). Most series show a slight male predominance and an increased incidence

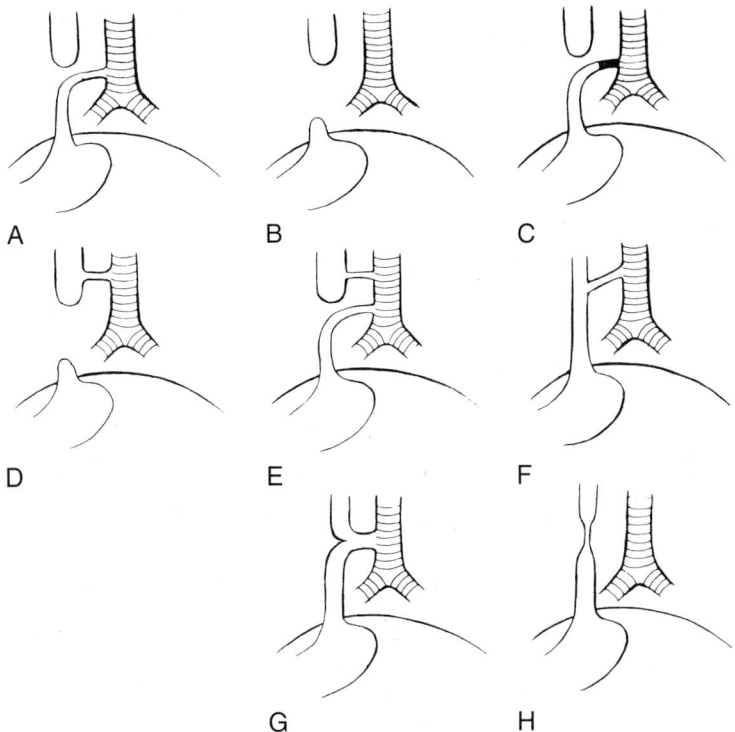

FIGURE 69-2 **Types of tracheoesophageal fistulas. A** is overwhelmingly the most common, accounting for 85% of esophageal malformations. **B** is next most common and can be distinguished from **A** by the absence of air in the intestinal tract on radiographs. All of the other types have been noted sporadically. *(From Avery ME, et al:* The lung and its disorders in the newborn infant, *ed 4, Philadelphia, 1981, WB Saunders.)*

in premature infants (Reckham, 1981). The role of genetic factors is unclear, although this anomaly has been described in siblings as well as in identical twins (Hausmann et al, 1957; Woolley et al, 1961). In addition, two kindreds with autosomal dominant transmission have been reported (Pletcher et al, 1991).

Etiology

The anomaly occurs before the 8th week of gestation, although the exact mechanism is unknown. It is thought to result from abnormal division or compression at the time the foregut divides into a ventral and a dorsal tube, giving rise to the trachea and esophagus. When this process of division is abnormal or when there is compression of these primitive tubes by an extrinsic structure such as an anomalous blood vessel, EA or TEF, or both, may result.

Diagnosis

Polyhydramnios is present in approximately one third of pregnancies with EA because the fetus is unable to swallow amniotic fluid. Within hours after birth, infants with EA accumulate large amounts of oral secretions, which may precipitate coughing or choking, with consequent respiratory distress. Infants vomit when they are fed, and in cases with a distal tracheoesophageal connection, abdominal distention may ensue as the intestine fills with air. The presence of a flat or gasless abdomen should suggest an isolated EA without a distal TEF (see Figure 69-2). Some patients with a gasless abdomen, however, may have a TEF that is partially obliterated but that will still require

surgical ligation (Goh et al, 1991). The most dramatic presentation of TEF occurs when the fistula is proximal to the EA. Affected infants develop life-threatening respiratory failure from aspiration almost immediately after birth. Infants with the so-called H-type TEF (see Figure 69-2) usually do not develop symptoms in the newborn period. Instead, these infants frequently present with a history (over months to years) of mild respiratory distress related to feeding or recurrent pneumonia.

If a diagnosis of EA is suspected, a soft 5 or 8 French feeding tube can be passed into the esophagus until it meets resistance. On occasion, the tube will coil in a blind pouch, creating the false impression that the esophagus is patent. In such cases a plain x-ray film confirms coiling of the feeding tube, frequently in an air-filled upper esophageal pouch (Figure 69-3). The presence of gas in the abdomen suggests that a distal TEF is present.

Treatment

Preoperative care of the infant with EA includes the insertion of a sump suction catheter into the proximal esophageal pouch for the continuous evacuation of secretions. The preoperative pulmonary complications associated with EA/TEF occur because of aspiration of oral contents or reflux of gastric contents into the airway. Placing a tube with continuous suction into the proximal esophageal pouch can minimize the aspiration of saliva. The infant also should be maintained in an upright position to decrease reflux of gastric secretions through the fistula and into lungs. In addition, minimizing positive-pressure ventilation can minimize gastric distention and reflux of

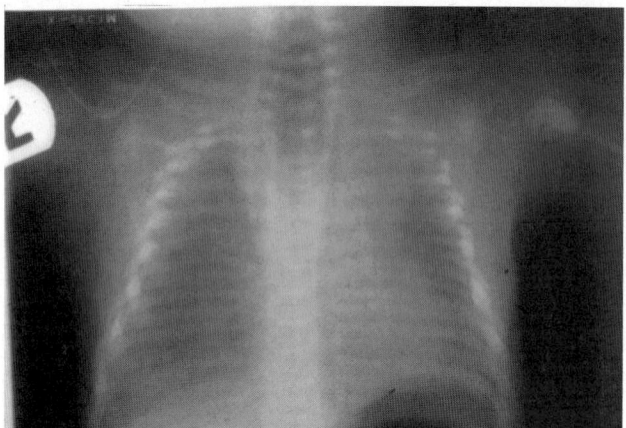

FIGURE 69-3 **Anteroposterior view of the chest of a female infant with esophageal atresia and tracheoesophageal fistula.** A large upper pouch is outlined by air and by a curled nasogastric tube. Air is seen within the abdomen, indicating a tracheoesophageal fistula.

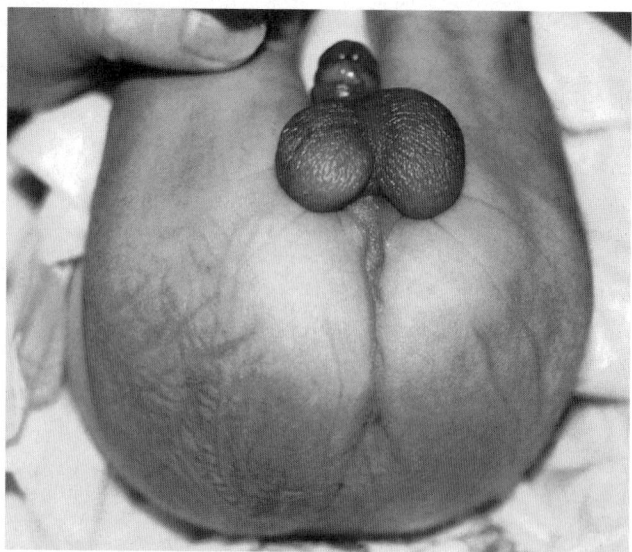

FIGURE 69-4 Perineum of male newborn with an imperforate anus.

gastric contents. Treatment with systemic antacids can also reduce reflux of acidic gastric contents into lung or distal esophageal pouch. Hydration is maintained by intravenous fluids, and surgical repair is undertaken as soon as the infant's general condition permits.

If progressive gastric distention occurs, a decompressive gastrostomy can be performed. An associated duodenal atresia should also be considered in severe cases of gastric distention necessitating emergent placement of a gastrostomy tube (Holder, 1993). If the fistula is large, there may be significant loss of tidal volume if the infant requires positive pressure ventilation. This volume loss can usually be controlled by connecting the gastrostomy to a chest tube system under water seal (Fann et al, 1988). In extreme cases in which the infant may not tolerate a thoracotomy and definitive procedure, a Fogarty catheter can be passed with a bronchoscope to occlude the fistula (Filston et al, 1982).

Preoperative evaluation in infants with EA/TEF should include an evaluation for other major anomalies, as they occur in 50% to 70% of these patients (Harmon and Coran, 1999; Holder, 1993; Rejjal, 1999). The VACTERL association consists of *vertebral anomalies, anal agenesis* (imperforate anus) (Figure 69-4), *cardiac defects* (most commonly patent ductus arteriosus, atrial septal defect, and ventricular septal defect), *tracheo esophageal fistula, renal anomalies,* and *limb anomalies* (most often radial anomalies) and is present in 25% to 30% of children with EA/TEF (Corsello et al, 1993; Harmon and Coran, 1999; Manning et al, 1986; Quan and Smith, 1973). Infants with EA/TEF within the VACTERL association tend to have higher proximal pouches, more complications, and a higher mortality than those in infants with isolated EA/TEF (Greenwood and Rosenthal, 1976; Holder, 1993; Touloukian and Keller, 1988; Weber et al, 1980). In particular, the presence of cardiac defects has a significant impact on mortality rates in EA/TEF (Spitz, 1993). Gastrointestinal anomalies occur in 15% of patients, with anal atresia being the most common, although duodenal atresia may also occur (Harmon and Coran, 1999; Holder, 1993).

Operative strategy in EA/TEF is based on the anatomy and whether other anomalies are present. In general, the

infant who lacks other anomalies and has a reasonably stable pulmonary status should undergo primary repair of the atresia and ligation of the fistula soon after birth. To accomplish this, an extrapleural or transpleural approach is used, the fistula is divided, and an anastomosis between the proximal and distal esophageal segments is achieved using an end-to-end anastomosis. In infants with extreme pulmonary compromise or significant associated anomalies, an initial gastrostomy for decompression with later repair of the EA/TEF may be indicated. Infants with the lowest probability of survival are likely to benefit from a staged approach (Alexander et al, 1993; Spitz et al, 1987).

Postoperative care consists of respiratory support, antibiotics, and intravenous nutritional support. Enteral feedings via a gastrostomy or a transpyloric tube may be started on the 3rd or 4th postoperative day. These feedings initially are given by continuous infusion because the stomach is often small. Bolus feedings are usually introduced once full enteral feeds are established, with oral feedings 7 to 10 days postoperatively after confirmation by a radiographic contrast study that there are no esophageal anastomotic leaks. Some investigators have questioned whether contrast studies are necessary for infants who remain free of clinical symptoms related to postoperative complications (Yancher et al, 2001).

Complications after repair of EA/TEF include esophageal anastomotic leak, esophageal stricture, gastroesophageal reflux, recurrent fistula, and tracheal obstruction. The incidence of anastomotic leak is 10% to 15% (Harmon and Coran, 1999). The diagnosis may be made by noting the presence of saliva in the chest tube, but it is confirmed by a contrast swallow study. Management is expectant because most of these leaks close spontaneously. A minor esophageal stricture is almost universal after repair of an EA/TEF. Significant strictures occur in 5% to 10% of infants (Harmon and Coran, 1999). The diagnosis is confirmed by barium swallow examination. Treatment of esophageal strictures is with serial esophageal dilatation, either with Jackson dilators or by balloon dilatation (Benjamin et al, 1993; Shah and Berman, 1993). Esophageal strictures are also one of the most common late complications of EA repair and manifest with abnormal esophageal motility and dysphagia. Esophageal strictures at the anastomotic site should be suspected if feeding difficulty develops, particularly after the 3rd week. Repeated balloon dilation may be necessary to relieve the stricture, although residual esophageal dysmotility may persist for a lifetime. Gastroesophageal reflux occurs in 40% to 70% of these children because of an abnormal angle and incompetence of the lower esophageal sphincter in addition to abnormal motility in the body of the esophagus across the anastomosis (Holder, 1993; Jolley et al, 1980; Pieretii et al, 1974; Whitington et al, 1977). Medical therapy with antacids and intestinal motility agents may be successful initially, but many patients require antireflux surgery. Clinically significant tracheal obstruction may occur in as many as 25% of children with EA/TEF as a consequence of tracheomalacia (Corbally et al, 1993; Harmon and Coran, 1999). The onset of respiratory symptoms with or immediately after feeding usually occurs in the months after repair of EA/TEF but may be in the immediate postoperative period (Holder, 1993). The diagnosis of tracheal obstruction due to tracheomalacia is made by bronchoscopy (Holder, 1993). In the child without significant distress, most symptoms subside over the first year or two of life (Holder, 1993). The surgical treatment of severe tracheomalacia is aortopexy, or suspension of the aorta (and therefore the anterior trachea) to the posterior surface of the sternum (Corbally et al, 1993; Holder, 1993). The incidence of recurrent fistula is probably less than 10% (Harmon and Coran, 1999). Recurrence of TEF usually occurs in the immediate postoperative period, but the diagnosis may not be made for months or years. The manifestations of a recurrent fistula are similar to aspiration with gastroesophageal reflux: coughing with feeds and recurrent pulmonary infections. Small fistulas may close spontaneously, but if a fistula persists for longer than 4 weeks, surgical closure is indicated (Harmon and Coran, 1999). Most surgeons prefer to wait 3 to 6 months after the initial EA/TEF repair, if possible, allowing inflammation and edema to decrease (Holder, 1993).

Prognosis

The overall survival rate in term infants without respiratory complications preoperatively approaches 95% (Holder and Ashcraft, 1970). Among premature infants or those with moderate to severe respiratory disease, survival is 85%. Infants with multiple anomalies or those with severe respiratory disease have a 75% survival rate. Infants with a birthweight less than 1500 g and a major cardiac anomaly have a significantly lower survival rate of 50% (Spitz et al, 1987).

TRACHEOESOPHAGEAL FISTULA WITHOUT ESOPHAGEAL ATRESIA

Only 5% of TEFs occur in the absence of EA. Symptoms include coughing and cyanosis with feeding and recurrent episodes of pneumonia. If the diagnosis of TEF is suspected, oral feedings should be withheld, and a specialized contrast esophagram using a catheter gradually withdrawn

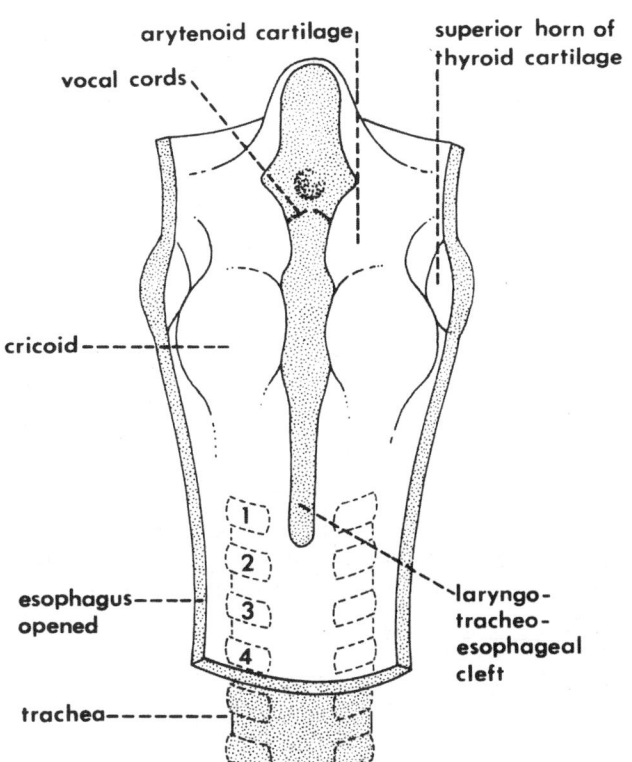

FIGURE 69-5 Illustration of the anatomy of a laryngotracheoesophageal cleft. (*From Burroughs N, Leape LL: Laryngotracheoesophageal cleft: report of a case successfully treated and review of the literature,* Pediatrics *53:517, 1974. Reproduced by permission of* Pediatrics.)

through the esophagus should be performed in an attempt to demonstrate the fistula. If this is unsuccessful, simultaneous endoscopic examinations of the trachea and esophagus may be done with instillation of small amounts of methylene blue into the trachea while simultaneously evaluating for its appearance in the esophagus. Most of these fistulas are located superior to the second thoracic vertebra and can be repaired through a right cervical neck incision.

LARYNGOTRACHEOESOPHAGEAL CLEFT

Laryngotracheoesophageal cleft is a communication of the larynx and trachea with the esophagus. The defect varies in length, with the shortest being the length of the arytenoid cartilages and the longest extending the entire length of the trachea (Figure 69-5). These clefts form between the 5th and 7th weeks of gestation when there is a failure of the rostral advance and fusion of lateral ridges of the laryngotracheal groove. One fifth of the clefts are associated with EA and TEF. Clinical presentation occurs early in the newborn period and is similar to that for EA/TEF, except that stridor also may be present. A carefully done esophageal dye study should establish the diagnosis. Tracheal spillover, however, may be misinterpreted to be due to the presence of a high H-type fistula or the presence of incoordination of the swallowing mechanism. Patients with clefts should undergo bronchoscopic evaluation with immediate surgical repair. A temporary tracheostomy is often placed because breakdown of the closure is common.

CONGENITAL ESOPHAGEAL STENOSIS

Congenital esophageal stenosis is a very rare anomaly caused by inborn malformation of the esophageal wall musculature (Nihoul-Fekete et al, 1987). It may take the form of a membranous web or diaphragm or a fibromuscular thickening or may be secondary to tracheobronchial remnants in the wall of the esophagus. The last-named is the most common form and typically occurs in the distal esophagus. This condition may also be associated with EA (Ibrahim et al, 2007). Many infants are asymptomatic until solid foods are introduced into the diet. In the neonatal period, the condition may manifest with severe regurgitation and respiratory distress. The diagnosis may be difficult to establish, although a contrast esophagram will usually reveal the narrowing. Fibromuscular hypertrophy and occasionally webs can be treated with repeated dilatations; surgical resection is the treatment of choice for all other lesions. An antireflux procedure is added for distal lesions but should be avoided before definitive surgery in the presence of stricture, gastroesophageal reflux or dysmotility (Ibrahim et al, 2007).

ESOPHAGEAL DUPLICATION CYSTS

Esophageal duplications are very rare and represent 10% to 15% of all gastrointestinal duplications. The overall incidence of esophageal duplications is approximately 1 in 8200, with a majority occurring in males (Arbona et al, 1984). The incidence of cystic duplications is even less common. The duplications occur when ventral budding of the lung primordium from the embryonic foregut at 3 to 4 weeks' gestation does not occur normally (Phillapart and Farmer, 1998). This results in the formation of vacuoles and in the obliteration of the esophageal lumen during early development. If vacuoles coalesce during recanalization, duplications are formed. The cysts are usually small and may be located anywhere in the posterior mediastinum or neck. Other associated congenital anomalies include EA, TEF, intestinal duplications, and spinal/vertebral anomalies (Eichmann et al, 2001). Cysts often manifest asymptomatically during childhood, or with digestive or respiratory signs and symptoms even in the neonatal period (Stewart et al, 1993). These signs and symptoms can include stridor, respiratory distress, difficulty swallowing, failure to thrive, or cough due to displacement of mediastinal structures (Eichmann et al, 2001). Associated vertebral anomalies suggest the presence of a neurenteric cyst, which may have a connection to the spinal canal. Diagnosis is confirmed by CT, and treatment involves surgical excision.

RUPTURE OF THE ESOPHAGUS

Esophageal perforation most commonly occurs in premature infants after placement of a nasogastric tube or occur secondary to esophageal intubation with an endotracheal tube (Krasna et al, 1987), although spontaneous rupture of the esophagus has been described. The inability to advance a nasogastric tube, hematemesis, and hydropneumothorax may be presenting manifestations. An esophagram can confirm the diagnosis, and urgent cessation of feeding and surgical repair are indicated; often a later contrast swallow study is indicated.

DISORDERS OF THE STOMACH

GASTRIC DUPLICATION

Gastric duplications are spherical or hollow tubular structures that are contiguous with the stomach wall and are lined by a mucosal layer from gastric, small bowel, or colonic epithelium but contain a smooth muscle coat contiguous with the muscle of the stomach. Most duplications do not communicate with the gastric lumen and are located along the greater curvature of the stomach. Embryologically they arise during the 4th week of gestation, when the embryonic notochordal plates and endoderm normally separate. A band between them may cause a traction diverticulum, leading to cyst formation. In addition, communication between the duplication and the pancreatic duct may lead to pancreatitis (Kaneko et al, 1999). Associated anomalies occur in 50% of these patients, the most common being esophageal duplication and vertebral abnormalities. Patients usually present at less than a year of age with vomiting, poor feeding, and failure to gain weight. Infants may also present with an abdominal mass or gastric outlet obstruction that may be confused with pyloric hypertrophy. The mucosal lining of cysts is often gastric, which can lead to melena or hematemesis from chronic "gastritis" (Holcomb et al, 1989). Treatment is complete surgical excision of the duplication and any accompanying cysts.

CONGENITAL GASTRIC OUTLET OBSTRUCTION

This rare condition may be caused by either a membrane or atresia, located in either the antrum or pylorus. An incomplete web or diaphragm may also be present, causing partial obstruction. Maternal polyhydramnios occurs in half of the cases. The defect may be due to vascular compromise early in gestation, similar to that causing intestinal and colonic atresias. Associated anomalies are frequent, including epidermolysis bullosa (Okoye et al, 2000). The presence of a gasless abdomen on plain film and the failure of contrast material to leave the stomach on an upper gastrointestinal series are suggestive of the diagnosis and warrant urgent operative intervention. Treatment involves excision of the defect with pyloroplasty, but some patients may require a gastroduodenostomy.

PYLORIC STENOSIS

Definition and Epidemiology

Idiopathic hypertrophy of the pyloric muscle in early infancy results in partial gastric outlet obstruction. The incidence is 1 in 1000 to 3 in 1000 live births, and males are affected four times more often than females. First-born infants account for half of the cases. Whites are at greater risk than African American infants. Premature infants are affected with the same frequency as for term infants (Laron and Horne, 1957).

Etiology

The exact cause of pyloric stenosis is unknown. Hereditary factors may play a role because there is a 7% incidence of pyloric stenosis among the siblings of affected patients. Pyloric stenosis has been documented in the literature to have an association with prostaglandin infusion, erythromycin administration, esophageal atresia, cystic fibrosis, Gilbert syndrome, epidermolysis bullosa, and Jacobsen syndrome (Callahan et al, 1999; Czernik and Raine, 1982; Dereure et al, 2001; Honein et al, 1999; Kakishi, 2002; Murthi and Nour, 2004; Schinzel et al, 1977; Trioche et al, 1999).

Diagnosis

Nonbilious emesis is the primary presenting symptom. It may occur from birth to 12 weeks, but most often the onset is between the 3rd and 5th week of postnatal life. In premature infants, the onset follows the same pattern postnatally, regardless of the postconceptional age. At first, vomiting may occur infrequently. With time, the frequency, volume, and projectile nature of emesis become characteristic. Weight loss, dehydration, and a hypokalemic, hypochloremic metabolic alkalosis may occur as a consequence of the vomiting. Gastric peristaltic waves may be seen passing obliquely from the left upper quadrant across the midline when the infant is fed. In most instances of pyloric stenosis, a definite tumor, or "olive," can be palpated in the epigastric area or just to the right of the midline in the right upper quadrant. Jaundice may occasionally occur, but indirect hyperbilirubinemia recedes 5 to 10 days after pyloromyotomy. Ultrasound examination is confirmatory, having replaced the upper gastrointestinal series as the diagnostic modality of choice (Figure 69-6) (Hallam et al, 1995). Infants with other primary surgical conditions may not present with signs and symptoms typical of pyloric stenosis. Emesis or increased residuals in these patients are often falsely attributed to postsurgical ileus, and electrolyte abnormalities are often precluded by postoperative fluid and electrolyte management (Murthi et al, 2004).

Differential diagnosis of pyloric stenosis includes infantile pylorospasm, which is distinguished from pyloric stenosis by ultrasonographic evaluation (Cohen et al, 1998). The cause of pylorospasm is unknown. In infants with both pylorospasm and infantile pyloric stenosis, some data suggest that a lack of nitric oxide synthase in pyloric tissue may be involved (Vanderwinden et al, 1992). Conservative medical management consisting of treatment with antacids, histamine H_2 receptor blockers, and metoclopramide may relieve the spasm. Pylorospasm usually is transient and resolves within 1 to 2 weeks.

Treatment

The stomach should be decompressed with a tube placed and connected to low intermittent suction; dehydration and accompanying metabolic alkalosis should be corrected with intravenous fluids before surgery. Pyloromyotomy involves splitting the hypertrophied pyloric muscle, and may be performed through a periumbilical incision or laparoscopically (Shankar et al, 2000). Feedings may be resumed 6 to 12 hours after surgery and advanced toward a regular schedule.

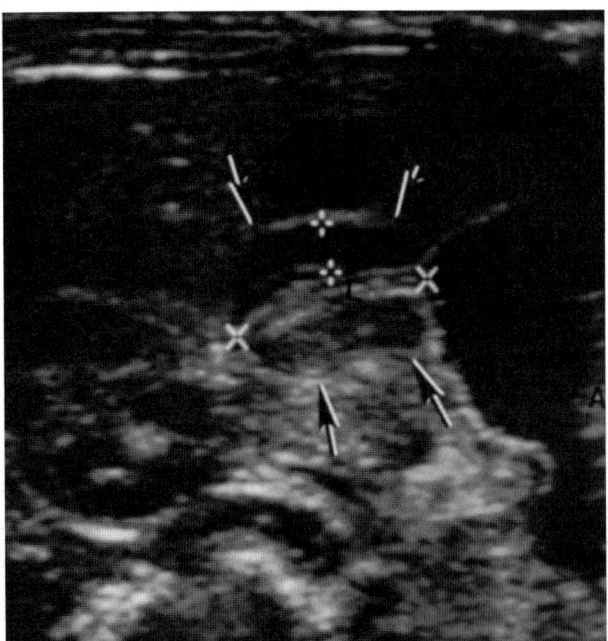

FIGURE 69-6 Ultrasonographic study of the right upper quadrant in a 1-month-old infant with a 1-week history of vomiting. The length (from + to +) of the pylorus is 18.4 mm (normal up to 16 mm), and wall thickness (H) is 4.5 mm (normal is up to 4.0 mm). The *arrows* outline the muscular wall and point to the lumen (*L*). *A* is the antral lumen. (*Courtesy of Dr. Ronald M. Cohen, Children's Hospital, Oakland, Calif.*)

Prognosis

Surgery is curative. Complications may include incomplete pyloromyotomy and perforation.

GASTRIC PERFORATION

Spontaneous perforation of the stomach in the newborn occurs most often during the first few days of life (Figure 69-7) (St. Vil et al, 1992). Perinatal stress leading to localized ischemia appears to be the causative mechanism in most cases, although in some, no cause can be identified. Potential causes include rapid overdistention of the stomach, trauma from passage of a nasogastric tube, and spontaneous rupture of weak points in the gastric wall along the greater curvature where muscle is deficient. Rates of mortality are notably higher in preterm infants and infants born with lower birthweight (Lin et al, 2008).

Signs and symptoms typically occur by the 2nd to 5th day and include refusal to feed, vomiting, respiratory distress, decreased activity and abdominal distention. Plain x-ray films of the abdomen show the presence of free air. Immediate decompression, fluid resuscitation, and broad-spectrum antibiotic administration should be followed by immediate surgical exploration and repair . Early recognition and treatment result in a higher survival rate.

DISORDERS OF THE INTESTINE

MECHANICAL OBSTRUCTION

Complete or partial obstruction of the small bowel or colon is not unusual in the newborn. A variety of lesions, intrinsic or extrinsic, may be responsible (Table 69-1).

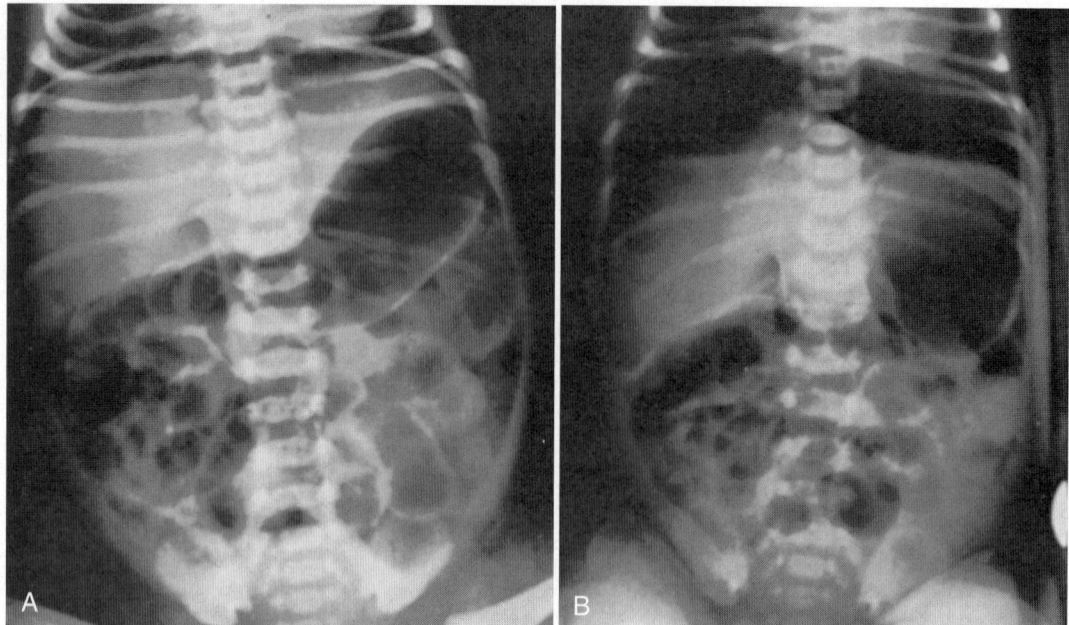

FIGURE 69-7 A, Anteroposterior view of abdomen of an infant in erect position at 72 hours of life shows air underneath the diaphragms as well as air within the stomach and small intestine. **B,** Ten hours later, the radiograph reveals progressive accumulation of free peritoneal air under the diaphragm.

TABLE 69-1   Causes of Intestinal Obstruction in the Newborn

Congenital	Acquired	Functional
Atresia	Necrotizing	Hirschsprung's
Stenosis	enterocolitis	disease
Meconium ileus	Intussusception	Meconium plug
Anorectal	Peritoneal	syndrome
malformations	adhesions	Ileus
Enteric duplications		Peritonitis
Volvulus		
Peritoneal bands		
Annular pancreas		
Cysts and tumors		
Incarcerated hernias		

Success or failure in terms of morbidity and mortality depends not so much on pinpointing the exact location of the lesion as on correctly diagnosing obstruction as the cause of clinical symptoms and then instituting prompt operative intervention.

Bilious emesis with abdominal distention and the failure to pass meconium are highly suggestive of the presence of intestinal obstruction. If the obstruction is high or complete, symptoms start soon after birth. Bilious emesis suggests that the lesion is located distal to the ampulla of Vater, whereas sporadic vomiting may be seen in patients with partial obstruction caused by malrotation, intestinal duplication, or annular pancreas. Abdominal distention may be present soon after birth, reaching a peak at 24 to 48 hours with visible peristaltic waves. Failure to pass meconium within 24 hours after birth suggests the presence of a lower intestinal or colonic obstruction. Infants with high obstruction, or even those with obstruction as low as the ileum, may still pass meconium, so this finding by itself does not exclude obstruction. Prenatal diagnosis of gastrointestinal obstruction by fetal ultrasound imaging

has been successful (Langer et al, 1989) and has become more common.

The initial radiographic studies should be plain x-ray films obtained with the infant in supine and left lateral positions. Normally, air fills the stomach immediately after birth, the small bowel within 12 hours, and the colon within 24 hours. When obstruction exists, the air pattern stops abruptly at that point, leaving the remainder of the bowel airless. Obstruction at the pylorus produces one large bubble outlining the dilated stomach, whereas duodenal obstructions produce a "double-bubble" appearance (Figure 69-8). Distal obstructions show a series of dilated, air- and fluid-filled loops of intestine. Obstruction resulting from meconium ileus is an exception in that air-fluid levels are not usually seen. In an incomplete obstruction, gas may be seen distal to dilated loops of bowel.

If the diagnosis is in doubt or a meconium plug is suspected, a contrast enema can be done. The finding of a microcolon is consistent with smalle-intestinal atresia or meconium plug with ileus. An upper gastrointestinal series is done only if the plain film and enema are nondiagnostic.

ATRESIAS

Definition and Etiology

Atresia, complete obstruction of the lumen of bowel, should be distinguished from *stenosis*, which is a narrowing of the lumen. Atresias account for one third of all intestinal obstructions in the newborn, occurring in 1 of every 1500 live births. Sites of occurrence, in order of frequency, are jejunoileal, duodenal, and colonic. Failure of the gut to recanalize during the 8th to 10th weeks of gestation seems to be the most likely cause for duodenal atresia. In the jejunum, ileum, and colon, intrauterine vascular compromise may be responsible for bowel atresias (Louw,

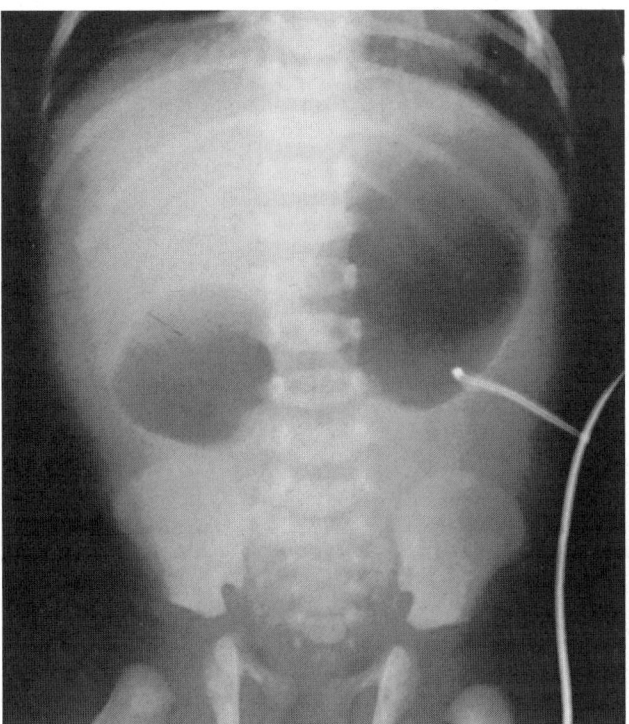

FIGURE 69-8 Abdominal film from a 12-hour-old infant with vomiting. A "double-bubble" sign is present. At laparotomy, duodenal atresia was found. *(Courtesy of Dr. Ronald M. Cohen, Children's Hospital, Oakland, Calif.)*

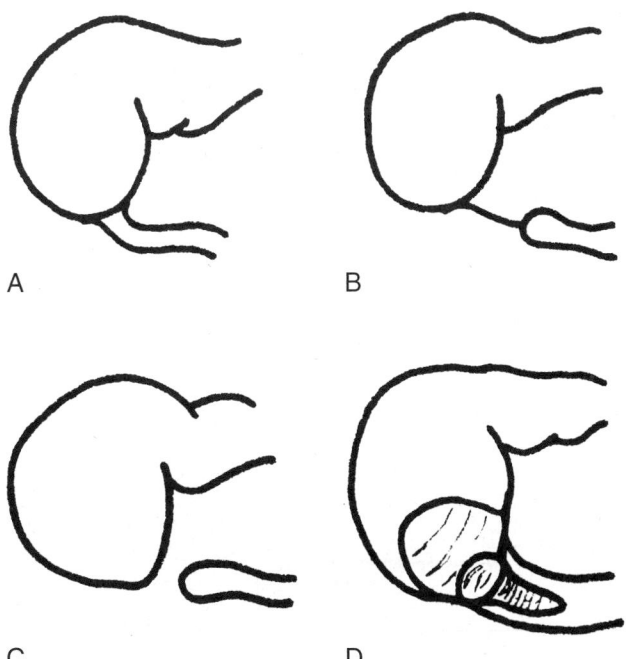

FIGURE 69-9 Forms of intrinsic duodenal obstruction. **A,** Duodenal atresia with continuity of the bowel wall. **B,** Duodenal atresia with a fibrous cord joining segments. **C,** Complete atresia with two separate segments. **D,** Windsock deformity.

1966). Other potential causes in utero include incarceration of the physiologic umbilical hernia, localized volvulus, intussusception, focal peritonitis, and peritoneal band formation. Mortality is low, regardless of location of atresia, but increases if there are associated congenital anomalies and in low-birthweight infants (less than 2 kg) (Piper et al, 2008).

Duodenal Atresia

Thirty percent of all atresias occur in the duodenum, and most are distal to the ampulla of Vater. Incidence of duodenal atresia ranges from 1 in 5000 to 1 in 10,000 live births, with males slightly more affected than females (Choudhry et al, 2009; Kimura and Loening-Baucke, 2000). Many infants with duodenal atresia have a history of polyhydramnios and are born before term (Dalla Vecchia et al, 1998). Other associated anomalies include Down syndrome, cardiovascular malformations, malrotation, EA, TEF, small-bowel lesions, anorectal lesions, renal anomalies, and VACTERL association (Choudhry et al, 2009; Dalla Vecchia et al, 1998). Congenital duodenal obstruction can be due to an atretic lesion or duodenal web, duodenal stenosis, and annular pancreas, which can also be found incidentally and may not be the actual cause of obstruction. Anatomically, duodenal atresia may occur in several forms (Figure 69-9). Prenatal diagnosis by fetal ultrasound is becoming increasingly frequent (Stoll et al, 1996).

Bilious emesis on the first day of life and a history of polyhydramnios are common presenting features. Abdominal distention is usually absent. Dehydration with metabolic alkalosis rapidly ensues. The diagnosis may be made on plain abdominal radiographs with the appearance of the "double-bubble" sign (see Figure 69-8). Overall survival rate is high, with reported mortality rates of 5% or less. Mortality rate increases if congenital anomalies, especially cardiac lesions, are present (Choudhry et al, 2009; Escobar et al, 2004). Long-term follow-up is important because late complications, such as gastroesophageal reflux disease, delayed gastric emptying, peptic ulcer disorders, megaduodenum, and intestinal obstructions due to adhesions, may occur into adulthood (Escobar et al, 2004).

Medical therapy consists of the passage of a nasogastric tube and correction of dehydration and electrolyte abnormalities. Prompt surgical intervention is necessary, although with a clear diagnosis, surgery may be delayed in very low-birthweight infants. Because of the high incidence of multiple atresias (15%), inspection of the entire bowel is carried out before bypassing the obstruction with a duodenoduodenostomy (Weber et al, 1986). An excessively distended proximal duodenum may need to be tapered as well, in an effort to reduce the duodenal dysmotility that often delays the start of normal feeds. The outcome for these infants generally is good but depends on their associated anomalies.

Jejunoileal Atresia

Fifty percent of intestinal atresias occur in the jejunum or ileum. Incidence of jejunoileal atresia is reported between 1 in 330 and 1 in 1500 live births (Sai Prasad and Bajpai, 2000). Premature birth is not uncommon (Stollman et al, 2009). Associated extraintestinal anomalies are infrequent but can include cardiac, renal, skeletal, and central nervous

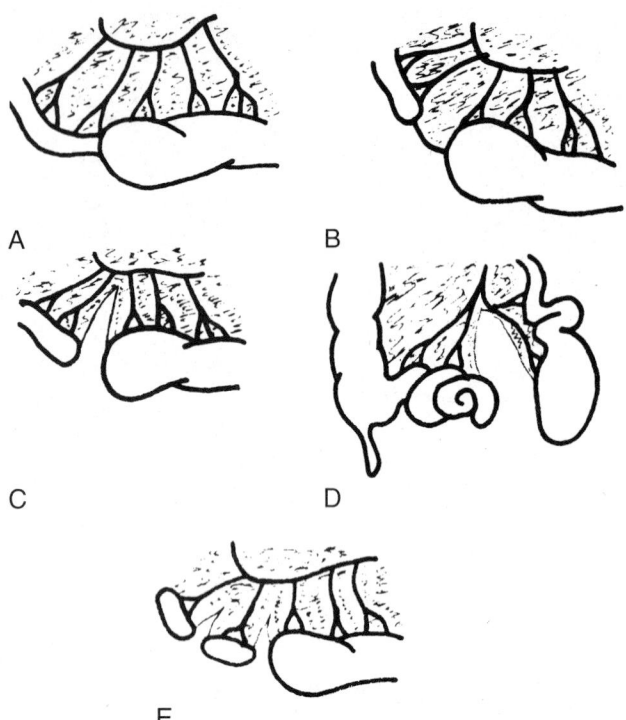

FIGURE 69-10 Classification of intestinal atresias. **A,** Mucosal atresia with intact bowel wall and mesentery. **B,** Blind ends joined by a fibrous cord. **C,** Blind ends separated by a mesenteric defect. **D,** Blind ends with the "apple peel" atresia. **E,** Multiple atresias.

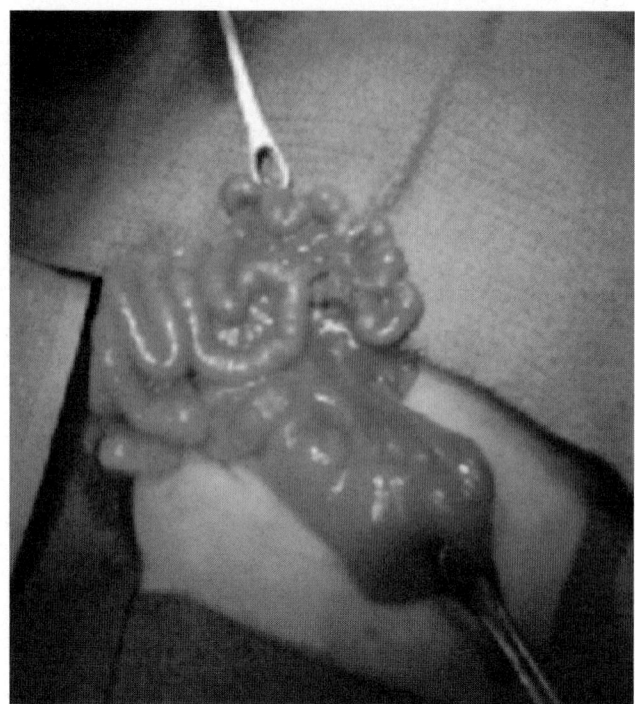

FIGURE 69-11 **Multiple intestinal atresias are visualized at laparotomy.** Dilated loops of the bowel are seen proximal to the obstruction.

system abnormalities (occurring in 7% of cases) (Dalla Vecchia et al, 1998). Anomalies of the gastrointestinal tract can occur in up to 24% of infants and can include gastroschisis, omphalocele, malrotation, Meckel's diverticulum, biliary atresia, situs inversus abdominalis, ectopic pancreas, and abnormal gallbladder. Numerous studies have also reported an association with cystic fibrosis (CF) (Stollman et al, 2009). Jejunoileal atresias are thought to result from a late intrauterine mesenteric vascular accident. Jejunoileal atresias are equally distributed between the jejunum and ileum and are multiple in 10% to 20% of cases (Grosfeld et al, 1979). A useful classification is shown in Figure 69-10 (Grosfeld et al, 1979). Intestinal length may be significantly decreased in type IIIb atresias ("apple peel" or "Christmas tree" deformity) and in type IV multiple atresias ("string of sausages" appearance). Prenatal ultrasound diagnosis is possible but is less accurate than in duodenal atresia (Figure 69-11).

Signs and symptoms of small bowel atresia include maternal polyhydramnios, bilious vomiting, abdominal distention (which may not become obvious until the 2nd or 3rd day of life), failure to pass meconium, and jaundice. Passage of meconium does not exclude atresia, because 20% to 40% of newborns with the condition will pass some meconium. Plain abdominal radiographs show varying amounts of dilated, thumb-sized loops of bowel ("rule of thumb"), air-fluid levels, and absence of rectal gas (Figure 69-12). Peritoneal calcification signifies the presence of meconium peritonitis, the result of a prenatal intestinal perforation. Contrast enema (usually using water-soluble contrast material) is the diagnostic test of choice. Contrast material may not reach the obstruction,

but the appearance of a microcolon in the normal anatomic position is strong evidence that other lesions, such as malrotation, colonic atresia, and aganglionosis, are unlikely. Meconium ileus, or a functional obstruction by inspissated meconium, should be excluded by careful evaluation of clinical and diagnostic tests, because in most such cases, this condition can be managed nonoperatively.

The type of surgical procedure used to repair intestinal atresias will depend on the lesion, but most often it involves resection of the atretic segment(s) with primary end-to-end anastomosis or an intercurrent enterostomy with a take-down at a later date. Significant luminal discrepancies between the proximal and distal ends are addressed by amputation of large blind pouches, tapering enteroplasty, and/or end-to-oblique anastomosis at the time of the primary surgery or more commonly on take-down of the enterostomy. A certain degree of functional obstruction may still be encountered postoperatively, especially in proximal atresias. Prognosis is excellent, except with types IIIb and IV atresias, in which significant mesenteric defects may result in short bowel syndrome. Postoperative complications include sepsis, anastomotic leak, wound infection, necrotizing enterocolitis, bowel obstruction, and vitamin B_{12} deficiency. Mortality is low, but is higher in cases that result in short bowel syndrome (Stollman et al, 2009).

Colonic Atresia

Fewer than 10% of cases of intestinal atresia occur in the colon, and stenosis is even less common. Associated anomalies may occur in one third of the infants, and up to 20% of cases may be accompanied by other intestinal atresias. Clinical signs and symptoms of colonic atresia

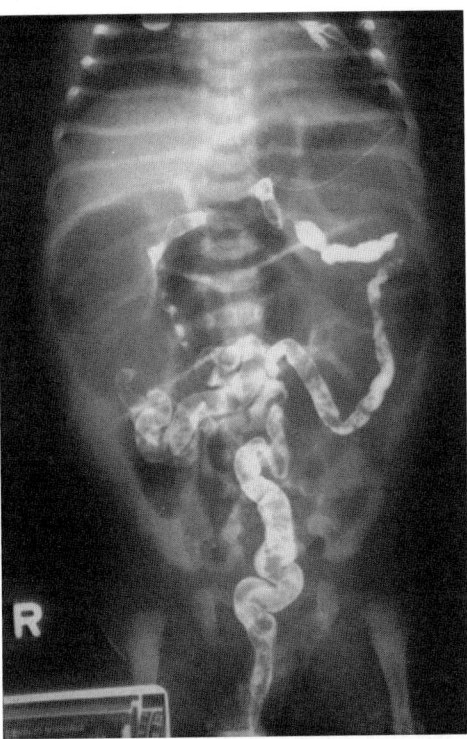

FIGURE 69-12 **Anteroposterior view of abdomen of male newborn with intestinal atresia.** Multiple dilated bowel loops are present. Microcolon is evident from the contrast enema.

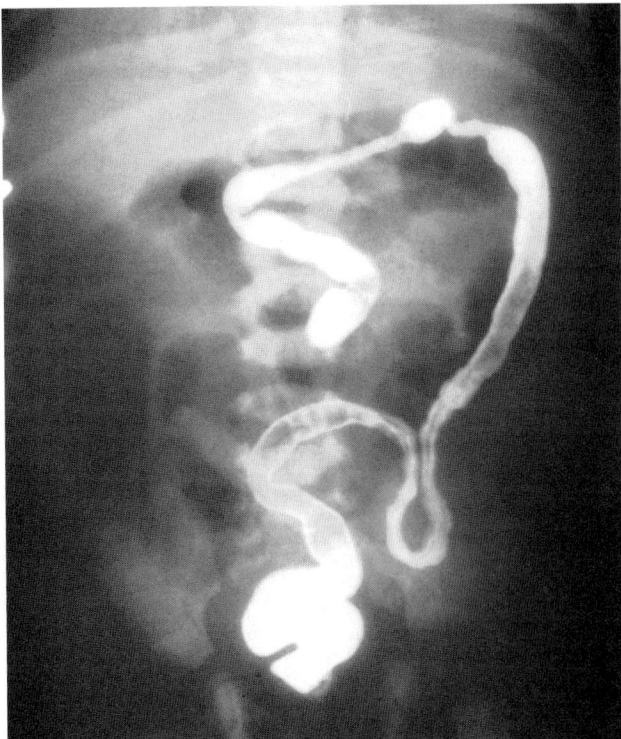

FIGURE 69-13 **Anteroposterior view of abdomen of newborn with colonic atresia.** Distal microcolon is evident by contrast enema.

include abdominal distention and vomiting beginning on the 2nd or 3rd day of life and failure to pass meconium. On plain radiographs, dilated loops of bowel are present, often with a distal cutoff (Figure 69-13). Pneumoperitoneum from intestinal perforation is found in 10% of cases. A contrast enema is essential for diagnosis, showing a distal microcolon, although the atretic segment may be visualized directly (Figure 69-14). The preferred surgical approach involves resection of the atretic segment and primary anastomosis (Davenport et al, 1990). This approach has replaced various staging procedures in stable patients without peritonitis. Outcome generally is very good.

MECONIUM ILEUS

Definition and Etiology

Meconium ileus refers to an intraluminal intestinal obstruction produced by thick inspissated meconium. Ninety percent of patients with meconium ileus have CF, and 10% to 15% of these infants have a history of meconium ileus. More than 70% of cases of CF are associated with a deletion of three nucleotides in the cystic fibrosis transmembrane conductance regulator gene *(CFTR)* on the long (q) arm of human chromosome 7, although other mutations have been described; not all variants are associated with meconium ileus (Mornet et al, 1988; Rommens et al, 1989). In utero, some CF fetuses produce exceptionally viscid secretions from the mucous glands of the small intestine. The meconium formed is dry and contains higher-than-usual concentrations of protein, including albumin (Schwachmann and Antonowicz, 1981). The abnormal meconium adheres firmly to the mucosal surface of the distal small

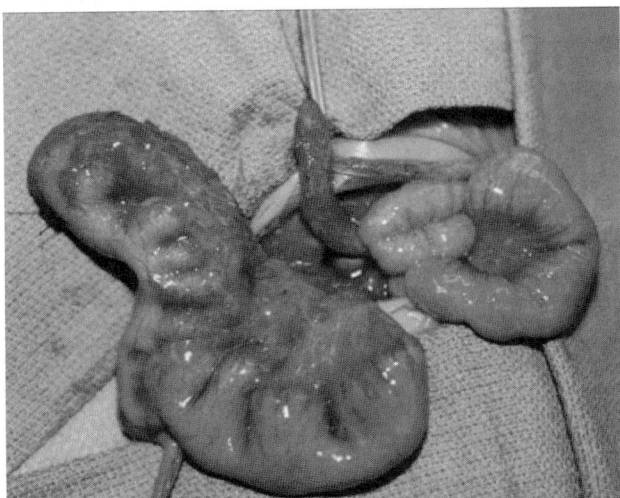

FIGURE 69-14 **Colonic atresia is visualized at laparotomy.** Proximal dilated bowel is evident.

bowel, creating an intraluminal obstruction. Histologically, the goblet cells and mucous glands are prominent and distended with an eosinophilic material that merges with intraluminal meconium for a cast of the crypts and villi. Proximal to the obstruction, there may be intestinal muscular hypertrophy.

Diagnosis

Meconium ileus often manifests with signs of obstruction, but without perforation within the first 48 hours in an otherwise healthy-appearing infant. Obstruction

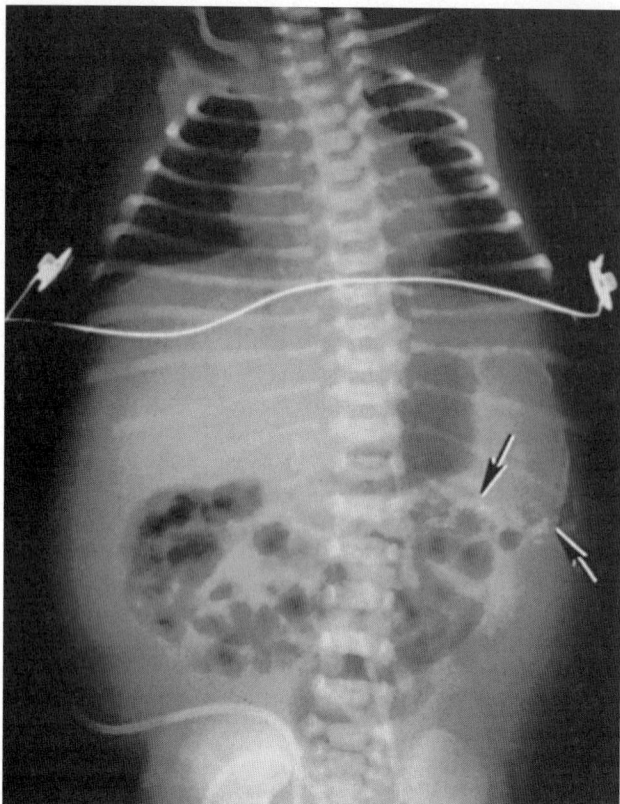

FIGURE 69-15 Radiographic appearance of ascites and abdominal calcifications (*arrows*) secondary to meconium peritonitis in a newborn infant. No gas is present in the rectum. The infant had ileal atresia, and a subsequent sweat chloride test was positive for cystic fibrosis. (*Courtesy of Dr. Ronald M. Cohen, Children's Hospital, Oakland, Calif.*)

usually occurs in the middle and distal ileum. Abdominal distention generally develops between 12 and 24 hours of life with no passage of meconium, although vomiting is uncommon. Physical examinations may reveal firm palpable masses throughout the abdomen that are freely movable in any direction (i.e., doughy abdomen). Meconium ileus complicated by volvulus, atresias, perforation and meconium peritonitis, or pseudocyst formation is found in 30% to 50% of the cases (Rescorla and Grosfeld, 1993). Newborns with the latter complications present earlier and appear more ill—often with severe vomiting, signs of neonatal sepsis, and more marked abdominal distention causing respiratory distress—than those with simple meconium ileus.

Radiographic examination shows dilated loops of bowel. Fluid levels are inconspicuous because of the viscous nature of meconium, which produces a coarse granular appearance ("ground-glass" appearance or "soap bubble" sign), typically in the right lower quadrant. The abdominal film may show, in addition to distended gas-filled loops, intraabdominal calcification indicative of intrauterine perforation and meconium peritonitis (Figure 69-15). The presence of air-fluid levels suggests the presence of jejunal or ileal atresia. The presence of a single grossly distended loop of bowel suggests the presence of postnatal volvulus. Perforations after birth result in free intraperitoneal air. Newborns suspected of having meconium ileus or any other distal bowel obstruction should undergo a contrast enema study. In meconium ileus, this study typically shows a microcolon and obstruction by multiple filling defects in the terminal ileum.

All newborns with meconium ileus should be evaluated for CF. Boat and co-workers (1989) have reviewed the clinical, physiologic, and genetic aspects of CF. The identification and cloning of the primary CF gene and the ability to identify mutations causing CF have advanced the clinician's ability to provide accurate diagnosis as well as counseling (Kerem et al, 1989b; Lemna et al, 1990; Rommens et al, 1989).

Treatment

In simple meconium ileus, approximately 60% of infants have their obstruction successfully relieved by the diagnostic contrast enema, ideally using a water-soluble contrast agent (Kao and Franken, 1995). Before the hyperosmolar enema is given, other complications such as perforation, volvulus, or atresia must be excluded. The hypertonic enema draws water into the intestinal tract, dislodging and breaking up meconium. Because of rapid fluid shifts, great care must be taken to maintain fluid and electrolyte balance. Failure of the contrast to dislodge the inspissated meconium after two attempts is an indication for surgical intervention. If the enema is successful, acetylcysteine, 5 mL every 6 hours, may be given via a nasogastric tube to help complete the clean-out.

Surgical intervention in simple meconium ileus usually consists of enterotomy with acetylcysteine irrigation and immediate closure. Other procedures such as resection of the ileum, with or without construction of various defunctioning ileostomies, are rarely indicated (Rescorla and Grosfeld, 1993). Complicated meconium ileus always requires surgical intervention, and the choice of operative procedure depends on the pathologic findings.

Prognosis

Operative mortality is minimal for simple meconium ileus. Perforation and electrolyte imbalance are the main complications of hyperosmolar enemas (Kao and Franken, 1995). Long-term outcome is influenced by the severity of pulmonary involvement.

Meconium plug syndrome is a similar entity not related to CF. Affected infants present similarly clinically, yet on contrast enema the obstruction is colonic and uniformly relieved during the study. Because of the diagnostic similarity and the fact that some children with CF may present with this pattern, testing for CF is indicated in all newborns with meconium obstruction (Rosenstein, 1978).

ANORECTAL MALFORMATIONS

Definition and Epidemiology

Anorectal anomalies occur in 1 of every 5000 births and are slightly more common in males (deVries and Cox, 1985). Associated anomalies occur in more than half of affected infants and are more frequent in "high" forms (see Etiology). Most frequent are vertebral, genitourinary, and gastrointestinal malformations (Kiely and Pena, 1998).

In infants with trisomy 21, 95% of those with anorectal malformations have imperforate anus without fistulas, as opposed to only 5% of all patients with anorectal anomalies (Levitt and Pena, 2007).

Etiology

The proctoderm comprises the anus and a canal that extends cephalad a short distance to meet the blind end of the hindgut, which has simultaneously moved caudad. Around weeks 7 to 8 of gestation, these should make contact, separated only by an anal membrane. At the same time, the lower urinary tract develops alongside the lower intestinal tract, separated by the urorectal membrane. Anal malformations arise locally from maldevelopment within the proctoderm. Atresias, stenoses, and fistulas arise from imperfect resolution of the anorectal membrane with or without concomitant failure of the urorectal membrane to separate completely the rectal and genitourinary components.

Anorectal malformations have traditionally been classified on the basis of the level of the rectal pouch (above the levator sling, or "high"; below it, or "low"; or at the level, "intermediate") and the presence or absence of an associated fistula (Levitt and Pena, 2007; Pena, 1997). A fistula is present in 95% of the cases, either externally as an anocutaneous fistula or internally as a rectourethral or rectovesical fistula.

Diagnosis and Treatment

Diagnosis is based on careful perineal examination, with imaging studies reserved for cases of diagnostic uncertainty and for evaluation of associated anomalies. The two key considerations in the assessment are the need for a colostomy and the presence of significant associated anomalies. The level of the defect may be clinically identifiable. Infants with low defects may have cutaneous fistulas, meconium present at the perineum, a bulging anal membrane, and well-formed buttocks. Females will often pass meconium through a perineal, vestibular, or vaginal fistula, or the anomaly may manifest as a cloaca (i.e., one-hole perineum). Male infants with low defects may have a bucket-handle malformation (a midline bridge of skin) or cutaneous fistulas that may track along the midline raphe toward the penis, discharging a tiny epithelial pearl or a meconium drop (see Figure 69-4) (Levitt and Pena, 2007). Finding meconium in the urine or air in the bladder may identify the presence of an internal fistula.

Plain abdominal radiographs may show progressive distal bowel obstruction. The traditional "invertogram" used to identify the distance between the rectal pouch and the skin has been replaced by a cross-table prone film obtained with the pelvis elevated, although this study should not be done in the first 24 hours of life, because the radiographic appearance may suggest a falsely increased gap (Kiely and Pena, 1998). Perineal ultrasound examination may prove to be more accurate than plain films. Abdominal ultrasonography, cardiac echography, and skeletal films may be required to rule out associated anomalies. The management of low defects includes several procedures aimed at restoring the anorectal canal, by cut-back of a cutaneous

fistula, anal transposition, or limited posterior sagittal anorectoplasty (Kiely and Pena, 1998). High and so-called intermediate defects require an immediate colostomy, followed by elective repair. Before the final repair, a distal colostogram allows precise localization of the fistula. Although there are multiple approaches to the definitive correction of anorectal malformations, the aim of all is to close any fistula and then tunnel the rectal pouch through the anatomic sphincter muscle to the anoderm. The posterior sagittal anorectoplasty popularized by Pena has become the most frequently performed procedure worldwide (Kiely and Pena, 1998).

Prognosis

Although the surgical mortality rate is low and primarily dependent on associated anomalies, functional long-term results are variable. Children born with low defects often will be chronically constipated; incontinence may occur in 30% to 35% of patients with high defects (Ditesheim and Templeton, 1987). Furthermore, quality of life correlates closely with whether continence can be established (Ditesheim and Templeton, 1987). Nevertheless, a majority of these children can be rendered functionally continent through a bowel management program, anorectal biofeedback, and antegrade enemas via a cecostomy in selected patients (Paidas, 1997).

ENTERIC DUPLICATIONS

Duplications of the gastrointestinal tract are relatively rare. Developmentally, the most favored hypothesis is the split notochord, resulting from adherence between ectoderm and endoderm in the neural plate (Pang et al, 1992).

Duplications may occur anywhere from the mouth to the rectum, although a majority are found in the small bowel. Associated anomalies, especially of the intestinal tract, are common. Duplications are generally located on the mesenteric side of the lumen, are lined by intestinal mucosa, and share a common wall and mesenteric blood supply with the adjacent intestine. Most duplications are spherical, presenting as cysts occasionally communicating with the main enteric lumen. Tubular duplications may involve long segments of bowel but are rare.

Many duplications manifest in the neonatal period, usually with obstructive signs in the presence of a palpable mass (Stringer and Spitz, 1995). Esophageal duplications may cause respiratory distress, whereas ectopic gastric tissue may cause rectal bleeding from peptic ulceration. Plain films of the abdomen may show displacement of adjacent viscera by a mass. Upper and/or lower gastrointestinal contrast studies may demonstrate a filling defect or, rarely, a communication between the cyst and normal bowel. Ultrasound diagnosis is possible both prenatally and postnatally, based on a characteristic appearance of the wall of the mass. CT or MRI is the modality of choice for imaging thoracic duplications.

The treatment of choice is surgical excision with primary anastomosis, although partial excision with destruction of residual enteric lining may be necessary for long tubular duplications (Stringer and Spitz, 1995).

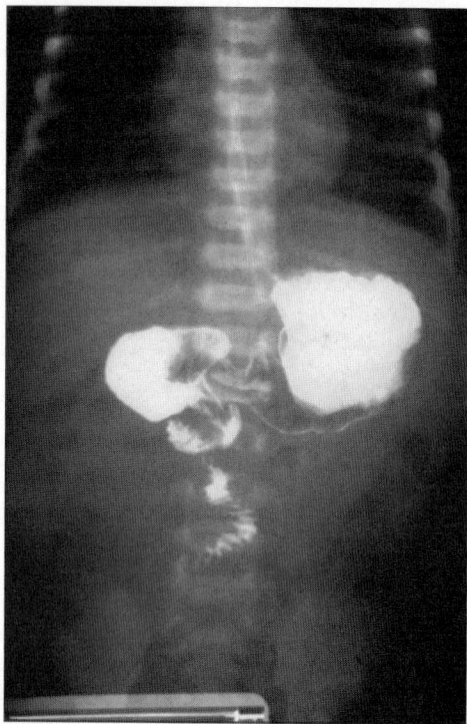

FIGURE 69-16 Anteroposterior view of abdomen of male infant with midgut volvulus. The contrast shows the duodenojejunal junction to be to the right of the spine, indicative of underlying malrotation. The proximal jejunum is obstructed in the "coil spring" appearance of acute midgut volvulus.

MALROTATION AND MIDGUT VOLVULUS

Presentation

Anomalies of intestinal rotation occur in 1 in 6000 live births. Malrotation of the gut occurs between 8 and 10 weeks of gestation, when the elongating intestine returns to the abdominal cavity. If the mesenteric attachments do not develop properly, the midgut lies free, attached to the posterior abdominal wall at only two points: the duodenum and the proximal colon. It may therefore twist in either direction, but when volvulus occurs, it is usually in the clockwise direction. Midgut volvulus may occur any time postnatally, but 80% of cases are found in the neonatal period (Seashore and Touloukian, 1994). Although rare, cases of fetal volvulus with and without malrotation have been reported. Signs develop with or immediately after delivery and include a tense and distended abdomen, bloody stools, and dark discoloration of the abdominal wall (Cullen's sign). Other signs may include maternal polyhydramnios, presence of an abdominal mass, ascites, bilious emesis and/or gastric aspirate, peritoneal calcifications signifying meconium peritonitis after intrauterine intestinal perforation, or even systemic shock. Fetal volvulus has been associated with hydrops fetalis, preterm delivery, fetal demise, and spontaneous abortion (Morikawa, 1999). Morbidity and mortality with fetal volvulus are high, largely because of late diagnosis. Infants with malrotation and midgut volvulus may have other associated congenital anomalies, such as intestinal atresias, gastroschisis, omphalocele, congenital diaphragmatic hernia, and annular pancreas, as well as

chromosomal abnormalities, namely trisomies (Molvarec et al, 2007).

The newborn with midgut volvulus presents with high intestinal obstructive symptoms, often in the 1st week of life. Sudden bilious vomiting with abdominal distention in a previously well newborn is particularly suggestive. Mesenteric vascular compromise of the midgut leads to rapidly progressive intestinal ischemia and necrosis, peritonitis, sepsis, and shock. Laboratory investigations usually reveal biochemical signs of visceral ischemia, coagulopathy, and sepsis.

Plain abdominal films may show a high intestinal obstruction, although the closed-loop obstruction produced may fail to show air-fluid levels, because the compromised bowel often is filled with fluid alone (Figure 69-16). Findings on plain radiographs may therefore be variable and cannot be used to rule out a midgut volvulus. A "gasless abdomen" finding is particularly worrisome. A "double-bubble sign" on radiograph suggesting duodenal atresia has been described in the literature to be malrotation with volvulus (Gilberson-Dahdal et al, 2009). If surgical treatment is delayed in these cases, an ultrasound examination should be performed to evaluate for volvulus. The stable infant with suspected volvulus should undergo an urgent upper gastrointestinal contrast study to document the position of the duodenojejunal flexure and to identify any proximal obstruction. Ultrasound examination may reveal the "whirlpool sign" in an acute volvulus or may document the correct or reversed position of the superior mesentery artery and vein (Pracros et al, 1992). The infant with peritonitis and suspected midgut volvulus should be promptly resuscitated and taken for immediate laparotomy.

Treatment

At laparotomy, the volvulus is reduced by counterclockwise rotation, and intestinal viability is carefully assessed. Frank necrotic bowel is removed, followed by either primary anastomosis or stoma creation. A Ladd's procedure is also carried out, including lysis of peritoneal bands, appendectomy, and replacement of the bowel in a malrotated position with the cecum on the left lower quadrant. An appendectomy is carried out because a subsequent diagnosis of appendicitis may be difficult (the appendix will not be located in the lower right quadrant). Recurrent volvulus after this procedure is very unusual (Yu et al, 2009).

The infant with necrosis of the entire midgut presents a particularly challenging problem. A second-look laparotomy in 12 to 36 hours is often undertaken to assess intestinal viability. Options in the case of minimal intestinal recovery include intestinal failure protocols and bowel-lengthening procedures, intestinal transplantation, and compassionate care alone.

INTUSSUSCEPTION

Intussusception is the telescoping of one loop of bowel into another loop of bowel. Although intussusception is a relatively common cause of intestinal obstruction in infants 6 to 18 months of age, it is very rare in neonates. Prenatal intussusception is responsible for some cases of intestinal atresia (Wang et al, 1998). In premature infants, intussusception may manifest without a specific leading point and with a picture mimicking that of necrotizing enterocolitis (Mooney et al, 1996). In the full-term newborn, a colonic leading point is often encountered (Wang et al, 1998). Should a diagnosis of intussusception be entertained, ultrasound examination and/or contrast enema are indicated. Hydrostatic reduction is not usually successful in neonates, and therefore a laparotomy with operative reduction or resection is necessary.

SUGGESTED READINGS

Agostino P, Halla NJ, Chowdhury MM: Gastrointestinal surgery in the neonate, *Curr Paediatr* 16:153-164, 2006.

Bill AH, Vadheim JL: Cysts, sinuses and fistulas of the neck arising from the first and second branchial clefts, *Am Surg* 42:904-908, 1955.

Chappuis JP: Current aspects of cystic lymphangioma in the neck, *Arch Pediatr* 1:186-192, 1994.

Choudhry MS, Rahman N, Boyd P, et al: Duodenal atresia: associated anomalies, prenatal diagnosis and outcome, *Pediatr Surg Int* 25:727-730, 2009.

Hallam D, Hansen B, Bodner B, et al: Pyloric size in normal infants and infants suspected of having hypertropic pyloric stenosis, *Acta Radiol* 36:261-264, 1995.

Harmon CM, Coran AG: Congenital anomalies of the esophagus. In O'Neill JA, Rowe MI, Grosfeld JL, et al: *Pediatric surgery*, St. Louis, Mo, 1999, Mosby–Year Book, pp 941-967.

Koch BL, Myer C III, Egelhoff JC: Congenital epulis, *AJNR Am J Neuroradiol* 18:739-741, 1997.

Kumar B, Sharma SB: Neonatal oral tumors. Congenital epulis and epignathus, *J Pediatr Surg* 43:9-11, 2008.

Martin LW, Zerella JT: Jejunoileal atresia: a proposed classification, *J Pediatr Surg* 11:399-403, 1976.

Mehta D, Willging LP: Pediatric salivary gland lesions, *Semin Pediatr Surg* 15:76-84, 2006.

Pena A: Advances in anorectal malformations, *Semin Pediatr Surg* 6:165-169, 1997.

Piper H, Alesbury J, Waterford S, et al: Intestinal atresias: factors affecting clinical outcomes, *J Pediatr Surg* 43:1244-1248, 2008.

Raffensperger JG: Esophageal atresia and tracheoesophageal stenosis. In Raffensperger JG, editor: *Swenson's pediatric surgery*, ed 5, Norwalk, Conn, 1990, Appleton & Lange, pp 697-717.

Complete references and supplemental color images used in this text can be found online at www.expertconsult.com

INNATE AND MUCOSAL IMMUNITY IN THE DEVELOPING GASTROINTESTINAL TRACT: RELATIONSHIP TO EARLY AND LATER DISEASE

Camilia R. Martin and W. Allan Walker

The fully developed gastrointestinal (GI) tract reaches a total length of approximately 22 to 30 feet (Hounnou et al, 2002) and has a mucosal surface area of 300 to 400 m² (DeWitt and Kudsk, 1999), which is equivalent to the size of a singles tennis court. Coexistent within the intestinal tract is a diverse microbial community with an abundance of organisms that exceeds the number of cells in the entire human body by 10-fold (Bjorksten, 2004). During development of the GI tract, the interaction between this microbiome and the intestinal mucosal epithelium is an essential component in the education of the host's immune and inflammatory responses against foreign antigens.

The anatomic and functional development of the GI tract begins during early embryogenesis and continues well into childhood. In addition to the essential digestive and absorptive capacities provided by the gastrointestinal system, the intestinal tract will also become the largest defense barrier and immune organ in the body. Its complex anatomic structures and dynamic functions protect the host from an onslaught of dietary and environmental antigens, which begins immediately after birth. These multiple layers of intestinal defenses are elegantly coordinated and tightly regulated. The immune and inflammatory responses initiated by the intestinal mucosa must constantly balance between eliciting a tolerant response to environmental antigens that facilitate further intestinal development with a more aggressive inflammatory attack against potential pathogens that risk the health of the host.

Abnormal development and regulation in the balance between immune tolerance and inflammatory responsiveness result in an inappropriate host response to antigenic challenges. This increases the vulnerability of the host to diseases of chronic, unregulated inflammation and dysregulated immunity.

DEVELOPMENT OF THE INTESTINAL TRACT

The development of the intestinal tract spans the periods of early embryogenesis (i.e., fetal development) to the introduction of solid foods (i.e., late infancy to early childhood). This period of ontogeny can be separated into five developmental phases (Table 70-1) (Wagner et al, 2008). Embryonic organogenesis and primitive gut formation is established in phase I. In phase II, the GI tract becomes a tubular structure, anatomic development (elongation and formation of villus structures) continues, and the functional role of the intestinal epithelium is initiated. Phase III is characterized by rapid linear growth, continued anatomic development of the villus architecture, and ongoing cellular differentiation with maturation of specific cellular physiologic functions. Phase IV begins immediately after birth when postnatal structural and immune development are mediated by the interaction between the host and exogenous, environmental exposures. This developmental phase is mostly directed by the establishment of the intestinal microbiome and the response to dietary factors present in human milk and/or formula. Weaning from human milk or formula and the introduction of solid foods signal is the beginning of phase V. During this period, structural development of the intestines and maturation of mucosal immunity are refined.

FETAL DEVELOPMENT

The first three phases of intestinal development occur in utero. By the end of the first trimester many of the epithelial cellular elements, including specialized cells, have made their appearance (Table 70-2). During this same period of embryogenesis, development of the anatomic structures necessary for optimal function of the GI tract is established, including formation of tight junctions and crypt villi. Also in the first trimester and into the early part of the second trimester, additional specialized cells establish their presence; the products of these specialized cells begin to be metabolized and secreted (e.g., mucin, defensins, lysozymes), and cell surface receptors can be identified (e.g., Toll-like receptor [TLR]-2, TLR-4) (Buisine et al, 1998; Fusunyan et al, 2001; Louis and Lin, 2009; Mallow et al, 1996; Neu and Li, 2003; Rumbo and Schiffrin, 2005).

ROLE OF AMNIOTIC FLUID IN EARLY GASTROINTESTINAL DEVELOPMENT

The development, maturation, and maintenance of the intestinal tract's complex functions require interaction with environmental exposures. This process will repeat itself with each changing environment and antigenic exposure; these periods include intrauterine life (fetus), postnatal introduction to the environment and to human milk or formula as the sole dietary source (early infancy), transition to solid foods (late infancy), and expansion of the dietary repertoire and thus the diversity of antigenic exposure (early childhood).

Therefore, one of the first influential factors in the development of intestinal structure and function is exposure to amniotic fluid. The amniotic fluid cavity is identified early

TABLE 70-1 Phases of Gut Development

Phase	Time Period	Development
Phase I	0–5 weeks' gestation	Embryonic phase of organogenesis
		Primitive gut forms
Phase II	Early to mid-gestation	Entrance and exit sites of gastrointestinal tract form
		Selective growth and apoptosis with formation of rudimentary primitive gut tube
		Formation of mouth and anus
		Swallowing begins
Phase III	Late gestation	Characterized by active differentiation
		Crypts increase in cell number causing cells to migrate up villi
		Starts several weeks before birth
		Characterized by more rapid growth than fetal body as a whole
		Rate of growth continues through the first feedings
		Growth accompanied by selective apoptosis; occurs not only at the tips of villi but in crypts as well
Phase IV	Birth–6 months	Begins after birth with exposure to enteral nutrition
		Human milk feedings bring about more rapid mucosal differentiation and development than artificial feedings
		Mucosal growth continues during infancy: fission and deepening of crypts, increasing villus width and number, and the appearance of submucosal folds
		GI tract is confronted with largest antigenic load to body in form of dietary proteins, commensal organisms, and pathogens: greater antigenic load with artificial feedings
		Mucosal immune system of gut develops extraordinary ability to distinguish between foreign pathogens and safe nutrient proteins and commensal organisms: process facilitated by human milk, leads to effective oral tolerance; success of such local interactions between local innate and specific immunity becomes the prerequisite for lifelong health
Phase V	>6 months	Occurs during weaning phase in late infancy/early childhood during transition from milk feedings to complementary, solid foods
		Second phase of mucosal expansion associated with epithelial hyperplasia that renders the gut similar in function to that of older children and adults

Modified from Wagner CL, Taylor SN, Johnson D: Host factors in amniotic fluid and breast milk that contribute to gut maturation, *Clin Rev Allerg Immunol* 34:191-204, 2008.

in embryogenesis, and amniotic fluid rapidly accumulates during early gestation (Underwood and Sherman, 2006). Initially, amniotic fluid is predominantly composed of water and solute from maternal plasma that is delivered to the fetus via the placenta and diffuses from the nonkeratinized fetal tissues into the amniotic space. As gestation lengthens, there are other contributors to the contents of amniotic fluid, including the placenta, amniotic membranes, and the fetus. It is not until the second half of pregnancy that the fetus actively and significantly contributes to the volume and composition of the amniotic fluid, mainly through swallowing and urination (Underwood et al, 2005).

Amniotic fluid is a complex, dynamic fluid whose composition varies over the gestational period. Proteomic analysis of amniotic fluid at 16 to 18 weeks' gestation identified more than 500 proteins, although many more are likely to exist (Cho et al, 2007). Amniotic fluid is enriched with hormones, trophic or growth factors, nutrients and other plasma proteins, modulators of coagulation, modulators of immunity and inflammation, and mediators of cell growth and differentiation, which together facilitate the development of many organ systems, especially the gastrointestinal system (Box 70-1) (Cho et al, 2007; Underwood et al, 2005; Underwood and Sherman, 2006; Wagner et al, 2008). However, additional studies are needed to further characterize the changes in the relative concentrations of trophic factors and cytokines in amniotic fluid

across gestational ages and its specific effects on intestinal development.

In week 16, the fetus begins to swallow amniotic fluid, ingesting approximately 450 to 1000 mL per day during the third trimester and in late gestation (Louis and Lin, 2009; Montgomery et al, 1999; Neu and Li, 2003; Rumbo and Schiffrin, 2005). Thus, early in the second trimester until parturition, the intestinal tract of the fetus is continuously bathed in amniotic fluid, and the presence of this flow as well as the exposure to its complex components is essential for its proper growth and differentiation. When the flow of amniotic fluid to the GI tract is disrupted, intestinal development is hampered, with reduced intestinal growth and decreased digestive and absorptive capabilities (Mulvihill et al, 1985, 1986; Sangild et al, 2002; Trahair and Sangild, 2000; Wagner et al, 2008). Many of the proteins found in amniotic fluid also have a direct role in facilitating intestinal development and likely work optimally in concert with each other rather than alone (Wagner et al, 2008). More specifically, the trophic factors epidermal growth factor (EGF), transforming growth factor (TGF)-β, TGF-β_1, insulin-like growth factor (IGF)-1, granulocyte colony-stimulating factor (G-CSF), and erythropoietin (EPO) have been shown to be important for stimulating intestinal growth, cellular differentiation, and maturation of cellular absorptive and secretive functions (Underwood and Sherman, 2006).

TABLE 70-2 Fetal Development of the Intestinal Tract

Developmental Feature	Gestational Age, Weeks
Specialized Cells	
Intraepithelial lymphocytes	8
Intestinal absorptive epithelium	9
Goblet cells	8–10
Enteroendocrine cells	9–11
Paneth cells	11–12
Microfold cells (M cells)	17
Dendritic cells	19
Advanced Structural Components	
Tight junctions	10
Crypt-villus architecture	12
Peyer's patches	19
Elements of Innate Mucosal Immunity	
Mucin	8–10*
Defensins	13
Lysozyme	20
Toll-like receptors: TLR2, TLR4	20

Data from Buisine MP, Devisme L, Savidge TC, et al: Mucin gene expression in human embryonic and fetal intestine, *Gut* 43:519-524, 1998; Fusunyan RD, Nanthakumar NN, Baldeon ME, Walker WA: Evidence for an innate immune response in the immature human intestine: toll-like receptors on fetal enterocytes, *Pediatr Res* 49:589-593, 2001; Louis NA, Lin PW: The intestinal immune barrier, *NeoReviews* 10:e180-190, 2009; Mallow EB, Harris A, Salzman N, et al: Human enteric defensins. Gene structure and developmental expression, *J Biol Chem* 271:4038-4045, 1996; Neu J, Li N: The neonatal gastrointestinal tract: developmental anatomy, physiology, and clinical implications, *NeoReviews* 4:e7-13, 2003; Rumbo M, Schiffrin EJ: Ontogeny of intestinal epithelium immune functions: developmental and environmental regulation, *Cell Mol Life Sci* 62:1288-1296, 2005.
*Some investigators note the presence of mucin as early as 6–7 weeks' gestation (Buisine MP, Devisme L, Savidge TC, et al: Mucin gene expression in human embryonic and fetal intestine, *Gut* 43:519-524, 1998).

INNATE AND MUCOSAL IMMUNITY OF THE INTESTINAL TRACT

Soon after delivery, phase 4 of gastrointestinal development begins. During this phase, the infant is rapidly presented with environmental and dietary stimuli (e.g., microorganisms, food antigens, and xenobiotics) that directly influence ongoing intestinal development and maturation of physiologic functions and mucosal immunity. The successful interaction between these antigenic exposures and the host's cellular responses is essential for the development of the innate and adaptive mucosal immunity of the GI tract and ultimately long-term protection of the host. An inappropriate intestinal response to environmental challenges may lead to altered immune and inflammatory regulation with local (GI) and systemic consequences.

However, before understanding the potential influences of environmental exposures on intestinal development and mucosal immunity, the specific structures that exist to coordinate this interaction must be reviewed. The intestinal components that make up the layers of defense and mediate appropriate oral tolerance or aggressive responsiveness can be found within the single-layer epithelial cell wall and within the structures that comprise the gut-associated lymphoid tissue (GALT).

INTESTINAL BARRIER FUNCTION: THE EPITHELIAL CELL LAYER AND TIGHT JUNCTIONS

The intestinal epithelium is a single layer of cells composed of multiple cell types, including enterocytes; enteroendocrine cells; intraepithelial lymphocytes; goblet cells; Paneth cells; and microfold or M cells (Figure 70-1)

BOX 70-1*   Amniotic Fluid Composition

HORMONES
GH
GRP
Prolactin

TROPHIC OR GROWTH FACTORS
EGF
TGF-α
TGF-β₁
IGF-1
Erythropoietin
G-CSF
HGF
Vasoactive endothelial growth factor

NUTRIENTS AND OTHER PROTEINS
Water
Electrolytes
Carbohydrates
Amino acids
Lipids
Albumin
Serotransferrin
Ceruloplasmin
α-Fetoprotein
Vitamin D–binding protein
Apolipoprotein A-1

MODULATORS OF IMMUNITY AND INFLAMMATION
Immunoglobulins
Interleukins
Complement
α-Defensins
Lactoferrin
Lysozyme
Calprotectin
Cathelicidin
α1-Antitrypsin
α1-Microglobulin

CELL GROWTH AND DIFFERENTIATION
Fibronectin
Periostin
TGFβ-induced protein Ig-h3 precursor
Polyamines

MODULATORS OF COAGULATION
Antithrombin III
Plasminogen

EGF, Epidermal growth factor; *G-CSF*, granulocyte colony-stimulating factor; *GH*, growth hormone; *GRP*, gastrin-releasing peptide; *HGF*, hepatocyte growth factor; *IGF-1*, insulin-like growth factor 1; *TGF-α*, transforming growth factor-α; *TGF-β₁*, transforming growth factor-β1.
*Bold proteins are in the top 15 in abundance at 16–18 weeks' gestation.
Data from Cho CK, Shan SJ, Winsor EJ, et al: Proteomics analysis of human amniotic fluid, *Mol Cell Proteomics* 6:1406-1415, 2007; Underwood MA, Gilbert WM, Sherman MP: Amniotic fluid: not just fetal urine anymore, *J Perinatol* 25:341-348, 2005; Underwood MA, Sherman MP: Nutritional characteristics of amniotic fluid, *NeoReviews* 7:e310-316, 2006; Wagner CL, Taylor SN, Johnson D: Host factors in amniotic fluid and breast milk that contribute to gut maturation, *Clin Rev Allergy Immunol* 34:191-204, 2008.

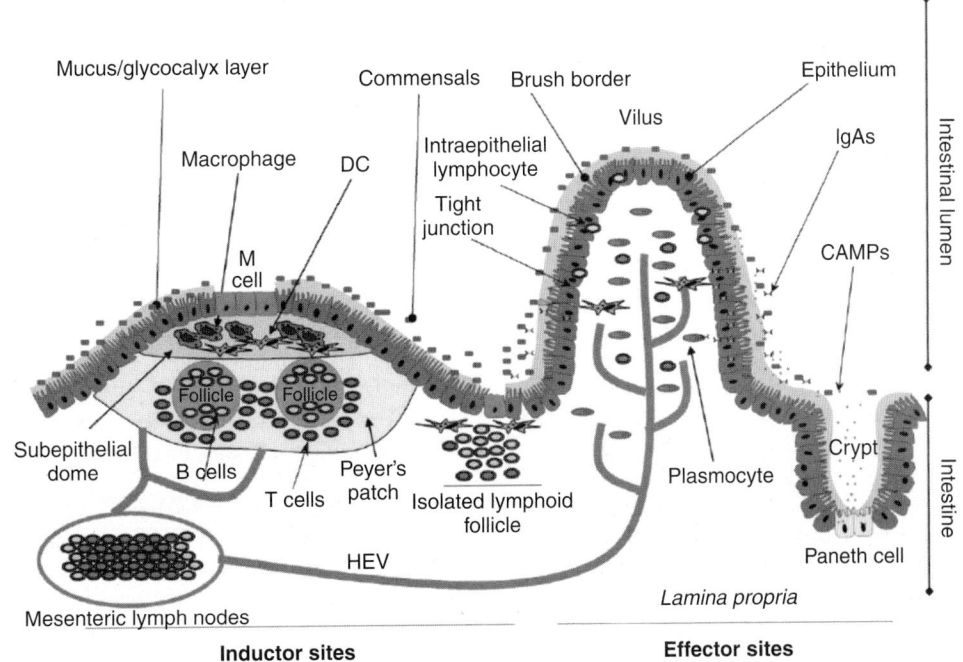

FIGURE 70-1 **Structural components of the intestinal epithelial barrier and immune system.** Epithelial cell layer: enterocytes, enteroendocrine cells, intraepithelial lymphocytes, goblet cells, Paneth cells, and microfold or M cells. Gut-associated lymphoid tissue (GALT): *inductor sites*: mesenteric lymph nodes, Peyer's patches, isolated lymphoid follicles; *effector sites*: epithelium (intraepithelial lymphocyte) and lamina propria IgA-producing plasma cells, primed T cells, monocytes, and mast cells. *(From Magalhaes JG, Tattoli I, Girardin SE: The intestinal epithelial barrier: how to distinguish between the microbial flora and pathogens, Semin Immunol 19:106-115, 2007.)*

(Lievin-Le Moal and Servin, 2006; Magalhaes et al, 2007; Yu and Yang, 2009). Each of these cells has individualized specialized functions (discussed in further detail below); together their cell-to-cell interactions and adherence form the basis of the intestinal cell barrier and the first-line defense against the potential penetration of pathogenic bacteria and antigens into the underlying mucosa.

The intestinal barrier is maintained by regulation and maintenance of two pathways: the transcellular pathway and the paracellular pathway (Groschwitz and Hogan, 2009). Three junctional complexes regulate the paracellular pathway: tight junctions (TJs), adherens junctions (AJs), and desmosomes. These junctional complexes serve as trafficking police by not allowing passage of macromolecules but allowing for essential transfer of fluids, electrolytes, and small peptides. Forty different proteins have been found to be important components of TJs, including ZO-1, -2, and -3 linker proteins, occludins, and claudins. AJs consist of cadherin-catenin complexes (Lievin-Le Moal and Servin, 2006). This dynamic and complex network of proteins interacts with each other but is also influenced by external factors. For example, permeability may be altered by pathologic insults or by other factors such as zonulin, a protein that appears to increase permeability across tight junctions and has been implicated in the pathogenesis of celiac disease and type-1 diabetes (Fasano and Shea-Donohue, 2005; Vaarala et al, 2008). In addition, tumor necrosis factor (TNF)-α, interferon (IFN)-γ, and nitric oxide have all been shown to cause barrier dysfunction, whereas TLR2-activated protein kinase C isoforms influence arrangement of ZO-1 junction proteins, increasing barrier integrity. Optimization of tight junctions is also

mediated by the short-chain fatty acid butyrate and the amino acid glutamine (Fasano and Shea-Donohue, 2005; Neu and Mackey, 2003)

SPECIALIZED EPITHELIAL IMMUNE CELLS

Goblet cells originate from crypt stem cells and migrate along the crypt-villus axis as they mature (Lievin-Le Moal and Servin, 2006). Goblet cells secrete mucins, which are high-molecular-weight glycoproteins that form a protective layer against offending antigens. Mucin is a complex matrix of water, electrolytes, mucins, glycoproteins, immunoglobulins (sIgA), glycolipids, and albumin (Neu and Mackey, 2003). Mucin binds to bacteria and prevents direct epithelial binding by microorganisms; facilitates bacterial removal by the luminal stream; and binds to trophic and other factors (e.g., epidermal growth factor, intestinal trefoil factor) that are critical for intestinal development, maintenance of intestinal health, and intestinal repair (Louis and Lin, 2009). More than 20 mucin genes have been identified, with MUC2 being the predominant mucin produced by intestinal goblet cells. There is a continuous production of mucins to maintain a constant mucin layer; however, mucin production can also be upregulated with exposure to specific bioactive factors such as hormones, inflammatory mediators, and factors derived from microbial residents of the GI tract (e.g., lipopolysaccharides, flagellin A, lipoteichoic acids) (Dharmani et al, 2009). In addition to mucins, intestinal goblet cells also produce intestinal trefoil factor (TFF), specifically TFF3, and resistin-like molecule-β (RELM-β) (Dharmani et al, 2009). Potential roles of TFF include stabilization of the mucin layer and reparation of mucosal injury. In addition to regulation of barrier function, RELM-β also appears to be involved in positive feedback to the goblet cell to increase mucin production.

Paneth cells are located in the crypt bases and, unlike goblet cells, do not migrate up the crypt-villus axis (i.e., they remain in the crypt base). Paneth cells produce antimicrobial peptides (AMPs) in response to lipopolysaccharide (LPS) and other enteric pathogen exposures. Their position in the crypt bases near stem cells allows them to protect these nondifferentiated cells from microbes and preserves the regenerative ability of the intestinal epithelium (Keshav, 2006). Of note, additional observations suggest that other intestinal epithelial cells besides Paneth cells can produce AMPs (Lievin-Le Moal and Servin, 2006). AMPs are currently categorized into two main families: defensins (α and β) and cathelicidins. They appear to exert their antimicrobial effects by incorporating into the cell membrane and creating pores allowing for the influx of anions and killing of the offending organism (Louis and Lin, 2009). α-Defensins, also known as cryptidins, are activated by matrix metalloprotease-7 (MMP-7) to microbicidal peptides (Schenk and Mueller, 2008). Other bactericidal compounds found in Paneth cells include lysozyme and phospholipase A2 type IIA (Keshav, 2006).

Microfold or M cells reside within the epithelial cell layer overlying organized foci of lymphoid tissue. Similar to goblet cells, M cells originate from the crypt, differentiate, and migrate along the crypt-villus axis. However, unlike their neighboring cells, M cells lack microvilli on their luminal surfaces. Rather, the luminal surface has microfolds, giving rise to its name. Additionally, on the basolateral surface, there are multiple invaginations that house immune cells such as lymphocytes and macrophages. Via phagocytosis, M cells sample and engulf luminal antigens and microorganisms and present them to the underlying effector immune cells (Hathaway and Kraehenbuhl, 2000; Miller et al, 2007).

GUT-ASSOCIATED LYMPHOID TISSUE

GALT has two main components: the inductor sites and the effector sites (see Figure 70-1) (Magalhaes et al, 2007). The inductor sites represent the structures where immune responses are initiated, namely antigen uptake and processing (Magalhaes et al, 2007; Neurath et al, 2002). It is within these structures that antigen-presenting cells (APCs) activate CD4 T cells, CD8 T cells, and B cells. The inductor sites consist of mesenteric lymph nodes, Peyer's patches, isolated lymphoid follicles (ILFs), and cryptopatches, which are clusters of immature lymphocytes that give rise to ILFs.

Effector cells are the immune cells, which, once activated, modulate downstream immune and inflammatory signaling. Effector sites are the locations where these effector cells reside; these include the epithelium and the lamina propria. The primary effector cell within the epithelium is the intraepithelial lymphocyte. These are scattered T lymphocytes that are situated along the basolateral side of the single epithelial cell layer and are capable of producing cytokines. The lamina propria is home to numerous effector cells, including IgA-producing plasma cells, primed T cells, monocytes, and mast cells (Magalhaes et al, 2007).

Monocytes give rise to macrophages and dendritic cells. *Macrophages* are preferentially positioned in the subepithelial region but may also reside in the intraepithelial region. Macrophages rapidly phagocytose invading bacteria and subsequently eradicate the organism by generation of superoxide and inducible nitric oxide (Schenk and Mueller, 2008). In addition, macrophages serve to scavenge dying cells and foreign debris and remodel tissue after inflammatory damage (Schenk and Mueller, 2008). Intestinal macrophages are able to perform these duties without cell activation or cytokine production because they lack pathogen recognition receptors, Fc receptors for IgA and IgG, and complement receptors (Schenk and Mueller, 2008). *Dendritic cells* are APCs that reside in Peyer's patches as well as scattered throughout the GI tract. The scattered dendritic cells insert their dendritic extensions between the epithelial cells across the tight junctions to sample luminal antigens (Schenk and Mueller, 2008).

Mast cells bind IgE via Fc epsilon receptors and release histamine and serotonin. These mediators upregulate mucin production, increase intestinal permeability, contract smooth muscle cells, and are a chemoattractant for granulocytes (Neu and Mackey, 2003).

COORDINATED LAYERS OF DEFENSE: PUTTING IT ALL TOGETHER

NONSPECIFIC PHYSICAL AND CHEMICAL BARRIERS

On entering the intestinal lumen, a foreign antigen (e.g., bacterial pathogen, food antigen, or xenobiotic) encounters many tightly coordinated layers of mucosal defenses. The first layer of defense is a series of physical and chemical barriers designed to provide constant surveillance and prevent epithelial adherence and translocation of the potential pathogens or passage of these antigens between the paracellular spaces. Within this first line of defense are the acidic environment of the stomach, the numerous digestive enzymes that exist along the entire GI route, and bile salts (Martin and Walker, 2006). These factors serve to digest dietary nutrients, but a side benefit of this digestive process is the destruction of ingested pathogens and other potentially immunogenic proteins into small, nonimmunogenic molecules of less than approximately 10 amino acids in length (Mayer, 2003). Additional mechanisms of the initial mucosal defense include production of mucus by goblet cells to inhibit microbial adherence, presence of polymeric secretory IgA within this mucus layer to bind luminal antigens, peristalsis to facilitate removal of antigen-antibody complexes (Walker, 2002; Winkler et al, 2007), secretion of antimicrobial peptides by Paneth cells (Keshav, 2006), and maintenance of tight junctions to prevent paracellular passage (Groschwitz and Hogan, 2009).

ANTIGEN SAMPLING AND PRESENTATION

Bacterial, dietary, and/or xenobiotic antigens that are present in the intestinal lumen are internalized and processed by several pathways: the M cell pathway; the intraepithelial dendritic cell pathway; and the enterocyte pathway

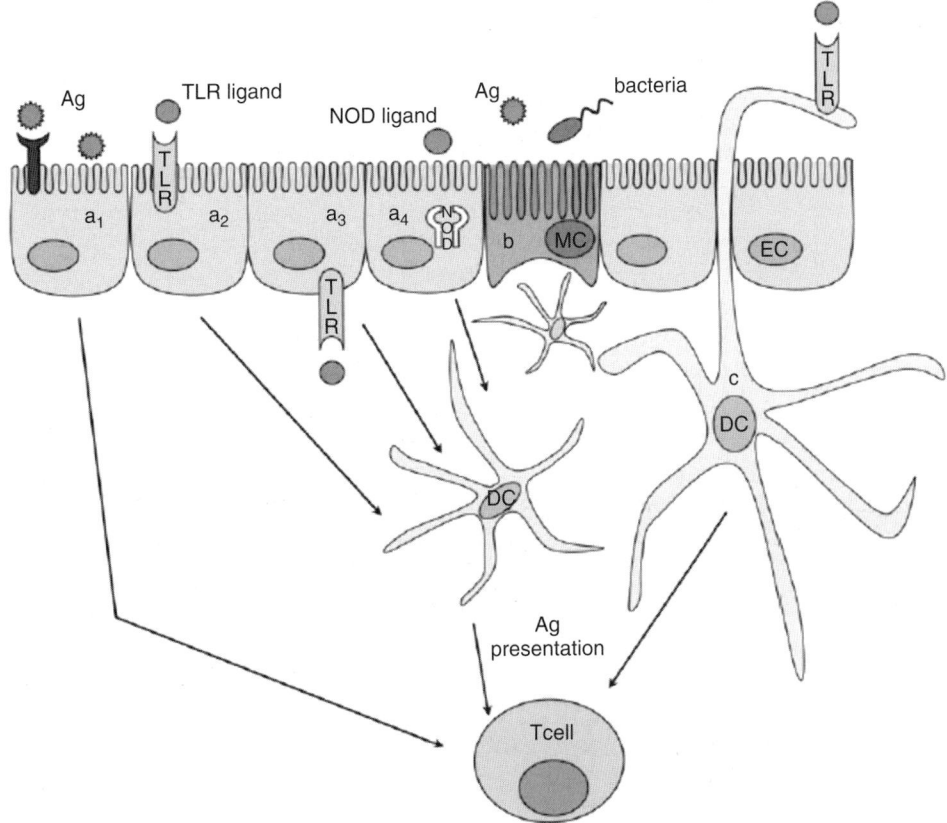

FIGURE 70-2 Antigen (Ag) sampling. *a*, enterocyte pathway; *a₁*, pinocytosis, receptor-mediated endocytosis; *a₂*, apical Toll-like receptor (TLR) recognition; *a₃*, basolateral TLR recognition; *a₄*, nucleotide-binding oligomerization domain (NOD) receptor recognition; *b*, M cell pathway; *c*, intraepithelial dendritic cell pathway. *(From Winkler P, Ghadimi D, Schrezenmeir J, Kraehenbuhl JP: Molecular and cellular basis of microflora-host interactions,* J Nutr *137:756S-772S, 2007.)*

by nonspecific pinocytosis, receptor-mediated endocytosis, toll-like receptor (TLR) recognition, or nucleotide-binding oligomerization domain (NOD) receptor recognition (Figure 70-2) (Winkler et al, 2007).

M Cell and Dendritic Cell Pathway

As previously described, M cells reside within the single-cell epithelial layer and are uniquely positioned over organized sections of lymphoid tissue and Peyer's patches. M cells sample antigens, actively transport them into the submucosa, and present them to effector cells, such as dendritic cells and lymphocytes. This process leads to T cell differentiation and B cell activation. Similarly, dendritic cells that have interdigitated their dendritic extensions across the paracellular junctions sample luminal antigens and migrate to lymphoid structures to participate in T and B cell activation.

Receptor-Mediated Endocytosis and Processing: Toll-like and NOD Receptors

Pattern recognition receptors (PRRs), such as TLRs, formylated peptide receptors, and NOD receptors, recognize and bind to highly conserved specific pathogen regions or molecular motifs, commonly referred to as pathogen-associated molecular patterns (PAMPs) or microb associated

molecular patterns (MAMPs). The conservation of these molecular motifs among microorganisms of the same class allows the mucosal cell to recognize most microorganisms by using a select group of PRRs. General classes of PAMPs include nucleic acids (e.g., dsRNA in viral organisms), polypeptides (e.g., flagellin), and macromolecules (e.g., lipopolysaccharide in the bacterial cell wall of gram-negative organisms and peptidoglycan in the bacterial cell wall of gram-positive organisms) (Louis and Lin, 2009).

TLRs are transmembrane proteins that are expressed on the luminal or basolateral surfaces of host defense cells. The extracellular component of leucine-rich repeat recognition domain binds to the specific PAMP, while the intracellular interleukin-1 receptor-like domain activates cytoplasmic proteins responsible for downstream signaling (Louis and Lin, 2009; Macdonald and Monteleone, 2005). To date, 11 TLRs have been identified. Each TLR recognizes and binds with specific PAMPs, some unique to that particular TLR and some overlapping with other TLRs. TLR4 is preferentially expressed by enterocytes within crypts, whereas TLR2, TLR3, and TLR5 are preferentially expressed on the villus enterocytes (Fusunyan et al, 2001; Winkler et al, 2007). Of note, TLR5 is unique in that it is situated at the basolateral surface below the tight junctions. NODs are distinct from TLRs in that they reside within the cell's cytoplasm. Of special interest to the intestinal tract, NOD1 and NOD2 (also known as caspase recruitment domain 4 [CARD4] and CARD15) are

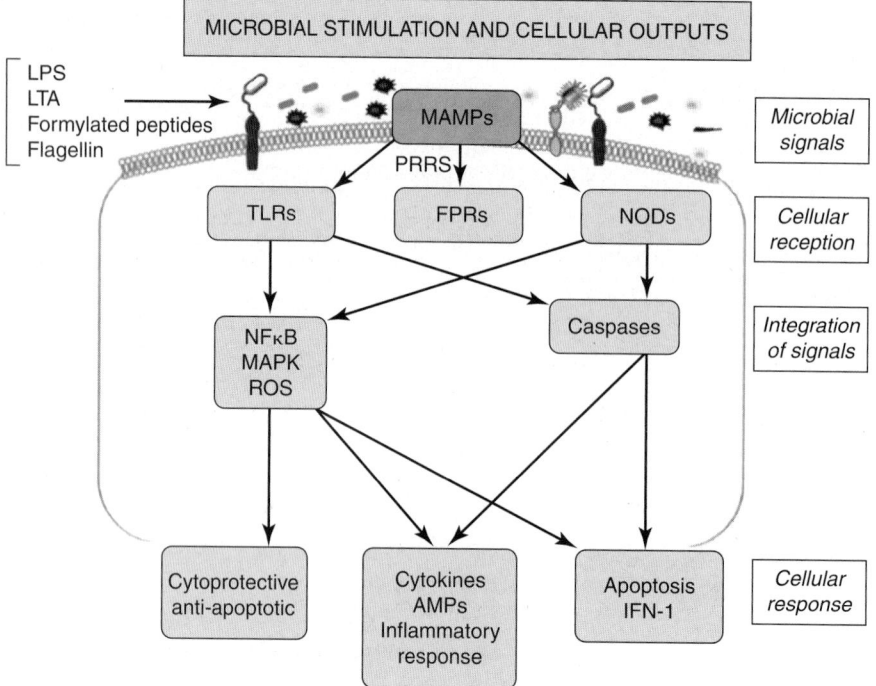

FIGURE 70-3 PRR-PAMP (MAMP) complex activation and downstream signaling. Microbial components such as lipopolysaccharide *(LPS)*, lipoteichoic acid *(LTA)*, formylated peptides, and flagellin serve as microbial-associated molecular patterns *(MAMPs)* and signal pattern-recognition receptors *(PRRs)* including toll-like receptors *(TLRs)*, formylated peptide receptors *(FPRs)*, or nucleotide-binding oligomerization domain-like receptors *(NODs)*. Integration of these signals evokes cellular outputs based on the initial perception of the triggering organism. Output can be a protective response to commensal microbiota or an inflammatory response to pathogenic organism(s), or it can trigger apoptosis. *(From Sharma R, Tepas JJ 3rd: Microecology, intestinal epithelial barrier and necrotizing enterocolitis,* Pediatr Surg Int *26:11-21, 2010.)*

expressed within intestinal antigen-presenting cells and epithelial cells (Winkler et al, 2007).

The PAMP–PRR complex results in the activation of several, well-described cytoplasmic signaling pathways. These pathways include activation of nuclear factor kappa B (NF-κB), mitogen-activated protein kinase (MAPK), and interferon regulatory factor (IRF) (Louis and Lin, 2009; Neish, 2009). Modulation of these pathways involves a regulated series of phosphorylation and ubiquitination. With ubiquitination, NF-κB, MAPK, and IRF are free to translocate into the cell's nucleus and upregulate the production of downstream molecules that combine to initiate an inflammatory response to effectively rid the body of the invading pathogen. This diverse group of molecules includes cytokines, antimicrobial peptides, chemotactic messengers, adhesion molecules, and other acute-phase reactants (Louis and Lin, 2009; Sharma and Tepas, 2010). Concomitant with activation of these proinflammatory pathways is the stimulation of apoptotic pathways (via caspases) to assist in the removal of infected or injured cells (Figure 70-3) (Louis and Lin, 2009; Sharma and Tepas, 2010).

Th1/Th2 Polarization

Downstream signaling mediated by PRR-PAMP complexes activates APC differentiation, which in turn modulates the differentiation of T-helper (Th) cells. The specific class of APC mediates the type of differentiation that the T-helper cells will undergo. For example, the CD8+ dendritic cell regulates the maturation of the Th cell to a Th1

cell, whereas the CD8− dendritic cell activates Th2 cells. Th1 cells increase cytokine production of IFN-γ and lymphotoxin, activate macrophages, and are associated with delayed-type hypersensitivity. Th2 cells increase the production of interleukin (IL)-4, IL-5, IL-9, and IL-13. Th-2 cells mediate allergic responses and facilitate antibody production, mast-cell degranulation, and eosinophil activation (Neurath et al, 2002) (Figure 70-4).

EXOGENOUS EXPOSURES AND THEIR IMPACT ON INNATE INTESTINAL IMMUNE DEFENSES

BACTERIAL COLONIZATION

Ultimately the intestinal microbiota will consist of 10^{13} to 10^{14} microorganisms representing 800–1000 species of bacteria that encode millions of genes. The abundance of microorganisms increases distally along the intestinal tract (Martin and Walker, 2008). Interestingly, colonization profiles are unique to the location within the intestinal tract, and this is true not just across the major divisions (e.g., ileum vs. colon), but also across the microstructures within the gut (e.g., microbiota within the lumen, vs. within the mucus layer, vs. within the crypts, vs. colonization and adherence on the intestinal epithelial cells) (Lievin-Le Moal and Servin, 2006).

Establishment of the microbial ecosystem begins soon after delivery, when the newborn gut leaves a predominantly sterile environment and is rapidly exposed to environmental bacteria. If the infant was born by vaginal

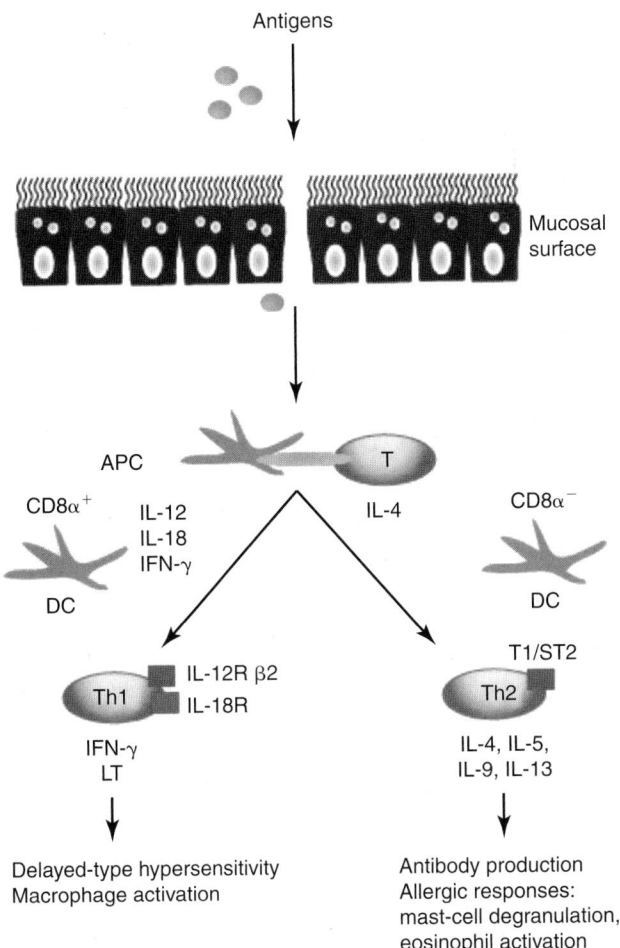

Antigens

Mucosal surface

APC

T

CD8α+   IL-12   IL-4   CD8α−
            IL-18
            IFN-γ

DC   DC

                                    T1/ST2

Th1   IL-12R β2   Th2
         IL-18R

IFN-γ   IL-4, IL-5,
LT   IL-9, IL-13

Delayed-type hypersensitivity   Antibody production
Macrophage activation   Allergic responses:
                                     mast-cell degranulation,
                                     eosinophil activation

FIGURE 70-4 Th1/Th2 polarization. *(From Neurath MF, Finotto S, Glimcher LH: The role of Th1/Th2 polarization in mucosal immunity, Nat Med 8:567-573, 2002.)*

delivery, this first exposure is dominated by the microorganisms that make up the mother's vaginal and fecal microflora. Subsequent to this exposure, microorganisms are introduced into the intestinal tract with the commencement of enteral feedings.

To effectively colonize the intestinal epithelium, bacteria adhere in a lectin-like manner to carbohydrate receptors or glycoconjugates. Glycoconjugate expression is controlled by glycosyltransferase enzymes, which are developmentally regulated, and ongoing maturation of this process is stimulated by colonizing bacteria (Forchielli and Walker, 2005; Walker, 2002).

During the 1st week of life, the bacterial colonization profile of a healthy, full-term infant is unstable and constitutes a simple array of organisms. This is quickly followed by a persistent, more stable colonization density in the range of 10^9–10^{10} per gram of stool (Favier et al, 2002; Palmer et al, 2007). Once the intestinal flora pattern is established, there is relative stability in this microbial population, with very few shifts in colonization profiles over time. However, shifts do occur, mainly in response to major changes in dietary intake such as introduction of solid foods (Palmer et al, 2007; Stark and Lee, 1982b) or with medication use (antibiotics). Within a short period of time after the initiation of a microbial

shift, stability is reestablished (Palmer et al, 2007). By the end of the 1st year of life, colonization patterns begin to mirror those seen in adults (Palmer et al, 2007; Stark and Lee, 1982b).

The timing of microbial colonization and the specific composition of the established microbiome vary with mode of delivery, diet, and other environmental exposures (hospital environment, antibiotic use).

Mode of Delivery

Infants born by vaginal delivery possess a microbiome pattern that is similar to the mother's vaginal and fecal microflora (Mandar and Mikelsaar, 1996; Palmer et al, 2007). In contrast, infants delivered by cesarean section demonstrate delayed colonization and lack of microbial diversity (Fanaro et al, 2003; Palmer et al, 2007). Once colonization does occur, patterns tend to reflect the indigenous microbial population that resides in the infant's environment, with low levels of strict anaerobes (Bennet and Nord, 1987; Neut et al, 1987; Penders et al, 2006) such as *Bifidobacterium* and *Bacteroides*, and a higher proportion of *Clostridium difficile* (Penders et al, 2006).

Diet

Infants fed human milk tend to demonstrate *Bifidobacterium*, a commensal organism with multiple immune benefits, as the predominant organism within their intestinal microbiota. Other organisms that may be present in lesser quantities include staphylococci, streptococci, and lactobacilli (Balmer and Wharton, 1989; Harmsen et al, 2000). Other obligate anaerobes are rare (Balmer and Wharton, 1989; Fanaro et al, 2003; Hopkins et al, 2005; Penders et al, 2006). In contrast, the intestinal flora of formula-fed infants is more likely to have a greater number of pathogenic species such as enterococci, coliforms, and clostridia (Balmer and Wharton, 1989; Benno et al, 1984; Fanaro et al, 2003; Harmsen et al, 2000; Hopkins et al, 2005; Penders et al, 2005, 2006; Yoshioka et al, 1983). The unique contributions of breast milk, such as the presence of oligosaccharides and immunomodulators, likely explain, in part, the disparate colonization patterns observed between breastfed and formula-fed infants (Agostoni et al, 2004).

Environment

The environment in which the infant resides exerts a strong influence over the final composition of the intestinal microbiota. Important for the preterm or ill term newborn, hospitalized infants tend to have a predominance of pathogenic organisms, such as coliforms, *Bacteroides*, and *Clostridium* organisms (Fanaro et al, 2003; Penders et al, 2006), a pattern reflective of their high-risk residence. In addition, infants who reside in the same environment share similar microbiotas. This is best demonstrated in sibling studies and in studies of infants hospitalized in the same institution or ward. These observations all support the profound impact the physical environment exerts on establishment of the intestinal microbiota (Fanaro et al, 2003; Lundequist et al, 1985; Palmer et al, 2007).

Antibiotic Use

Antibiotics influence both the density and composition of microorganisms within the intestinal tract (Palmer et al, 2007). As would be expected, antibiotics tend to ameliorate commensal, low-resistance organisms while leaving behind more pathogenic organisms. As an effect potentially detrimental to the host, organisms such as *Bifidobacterium* and *Bacteroides* are significantly reduced (Bennet and Nord, 1987; Penders et al, 2006). And, perhaps even more concerning, after the course of antibiotics has been completed, there is slow restoration of the *Bifidobacterium* population, and the *Bacteroides* population is unlikely to be reestablished (Bennet and Nord, 1987). Additionally, delayed colonization with *Lactobacillus* spp., increased *Klebsiella* spp., and rapid colonization with staphylococci have been observed with antibiotic use (Magne et al, 2005).

The Intestinal Microbiota and Gut Immunity and Inflammation

Although the gut serves as the largest defense barrier and actively protects itself from invasion by pathogenic organisms, establishment of a stable and diverse intestinal microflora and the ensuing "microbial-epithelial crosstalk" between colonizing, commensal bacteria and the intestinal epithelium is essential for optimal development of mucosal immunity and regulation of intestinal inflammation. This interaction is essential for proper development of host immunity (Artis, 2008; Macpherson and Harris, 2004; Vanderhoof and Young, 2002). A diverse array of organisms within the intestinal microbiota allowing for a healthy microbial-epithelial interaction enables many downstream benefits to intestinal development and mucosal immunity. These benefits include: maintaining mucosal barrier integrity by reducing mucosal permeability, increasing mucus production, strengthening intestinal tight junctions, increasing the production of small proline-rich protein-2a (sprp2a), and inhibiting bacterial translocation (Deplancke and Gaskins, 2001; Kennedy et al,

2002; Lievin-Le Moal and Servin, 2006; Mack et al, 1999; Madsen et al, 2001; Orrhage and Nord, 1999; Panigrahi et al, 1994; Schenk and Mueller, 2008; Stratiki et al, 2007); regulating bacterial adherence and colonization of pathogenic organisms by producing antimicrobial peptides such as defensins, reducing intraluminal pH, and competing for cell surface binding sites; collectively, this protective role is also known as "colonization resistance" (Bernet et al, 1994; Collins and Gibson, 1999; Ouellette, 2004; Vollaard and Clasener, 1994); enhancing intestinal immune defenses by increasing production of IgA, short-chain fatty acids, and blood leukocyte phagocytosis (Fukushima et al, 1998; Schiffrin et al, 1995; Sudo et al, 1997; Viljanen et al, 2005; Weng et al, 2007); and regulating intestinal inflammation by mediating Th-cell differentiation, increasing antiinflammatory cytokine production, and decreasing the production of proinflammatory cytokines (Caplan and Jilling, 2000; Fujii et al, 2006; Klinman et al, 1996; Marin et al, 1998; Millar et al, 2003; Murch, 2001; Takeda et al, 2006). In the last scenario, one mechanism by which commensal bacteria reduce the production of proinflammatory mediators is by inhibiting the activation of NF-κB. This is in contrast to the proinflammatory upregulation of NF-κB by pathogenic organisms and associated antigens (LPS) (Claud and Walker, 2001; Magalhaes et al, 2007; Walker, 2002).

DIET: HUMAN MILK AND INFANT FORMULA

Similar to amniotic fluid, breast milk is rich with bioactive components that are essential in providing the immature newborn a complement of innate immune functions during the early postnatal transitional period while the immature newborn develops its own innate immune defenses (Newburg and Walker, 2007). The factors in breast milk have been shown to promote postnatal structural development of the intestinal tract; yield a favorable, beneficial bacterial colonization pattern; deliver bactericidal proteins; and provide other immune defenses (Box 70-2)

(Donovan, 2006). In addition, human milk adapts to meet the needs of the infant and to appropriately provide the essential nutrients to optimize the infant's developmental stage. For example, growth and immune factors tend to be higher in preterm milk than in term milk (Donovan, 2006; Walker, 2010).

Factors present in breast milk have been shown in piglet and rodent models to contribute to the ongoing structural development of the intestinal tract. When provided breast milk (especially colostrum) versus formula or in the absence of any enteral substrate, animals receiving breast milk demonstrate an increase in mucosal mass and villus height (Sangild, 2006). Morphologic studies of human infants to examine the potential benefits of breast milk are more difficult to perform for obvious reasons. However, studies evaluating diet and intestinal barrier function have been performed in human infants and can be used as an indirect measure for morphologic development and integrity. Indeed, infants fed predominantly formula versus breast milk demonstrated increased intestinal permeability, suggesting compromise in intestinal barrier function (Taylor et al, 2009).

As described, infants fed breast milk exhibit a greater representation of commensal organisms, such as *Bifidobacterium* and *Lactobacillus*, conferring multiple benefits to the developing intestinal tract and accompanying mucosal immunity. Many bioactive compounds in breast milk contribute to the beneficial microbial-epithelial interaction, such as the presence of oligosaccharides and other natural prebiotics. Interestingly, the microbiome that exists within breast milk itself may also be important in providing immunologic immunity to the infant. Commensal bacterial isolates, such as certain *Staphylococcal* species, streptococci, and *Lactobacillus*, have been found in breast milk, and these organisms have been shown to be bactericidal against *Staphylococcus aureus*, an important pathogen in neonates. Also observed in this study was the *production* of nicin, a known bactericidal agent, by the breast milk isolate *L. lactis* (Heikkila and Saris, 2003). Other bactericidal agents that have been found in breast milk include defensins and cathelicidin, which also demonstrate antimicrobial activity against neonatal pathogens such as *Staphylococcus aureus*, group A *Streptococcus*, and *Escherichia coli* (Murakami et al, 2005). In addition to antimicrobial peptides, breast milk contains a host of other immunomodulators (including nutritional) that ultimately benefit the infant.

Over time, the composition of formula has been iteratively modified; however, formula continues to fall short of being able to provide the multitude of factors that are present in breast milk, and thus, infants fed formula fail to share the same health benefits seen in breastfed infants. Infants fed predominantly breast milk have a reduced incidence of infections (e.g., diarrhea, upper respiratory illness, otitis media, urinary tract infections, bacteremia) (Hengstermann et al, 2010; Quigley et al, 2009), atopic illnesses (e.g., eczema, asthma) (Bener et al, 2007), and autoimmune diseases (e.g., celiac disease, type 1 diabetes mellitus) (Auricchio et al, 1983; Sadauskaite-Kuehne et al, 2004). Specifically for the preterm infant, infants fed breast milk are less likely to develop necrotizing enterocolitis (NEC) compared to infants fed formula (Schanler et al, 1999).

TABLE 70-3   NICU Exposures and Potential Consequences on Intestinal Barrier Defense and Bacterial Colonization in Premature Infants

	Exposure	Potential Consequences
Nonspecific barrier defense	Prematurity	↓ immunoglobulin levels
		↓ production of digestive enzymes
		↓ production of mucus
		Dysfunctional peristalsis
	Delayed feeding	Villous atrophy
		↓ production of digestive enzymes
		↓ production of mucus
		↓ peristalsis
	Medications	
	Histamine H₂ receptor blockers	↓ gastric acidity
	Vasopressors and Indocin	↑ risk for intestinal ischemia and enterocyte injury
	Sedatives and paralytic agents	↓ peristalsis
Bacterial colonization	Prematurity	Accentuated inflammatory response
		Abnormal glycosylation pattern
	Delayed feedings	Delay in bacterial colonization
	Broad-spectrum antibiotics	Prolonged sterilization of gut
		Delayed colonization of beneficial, commensal bacteria
		Preferred bacterial colonization of pathogenic bacteria
	Formula feeding and hospitalization	Preferred bacterial colonization of pathogenic bacteria

From Martin CR, Walker WA: Intestinal immune defences and the inflammatory response in necrotising enterocolitis, *Semin Fetal Neonatal Med* 11:369-377, 2006.

IMPACT OF ALTERED MUCOSAL IMMUNITY ON EARLY AND LATER DISEASE
PREMATURITY AND NECROTIZING ENTEROCOLITIS

Inadequate Physical and Chemical Barriers

Developmental immaturity of the immune system, hospital environmental exposures, and medical interventions combine to hamper postnatal development of innate and mucosal immunity in the preterm infant (Table 70-3) (Martin and Walker, 2006). These factors pose potential threats to the preterm infant, particularly to conditions mediated by altered mucosal immunity and intestinal bacterial colonization.

The first line of defense of nonspecific physical and chemical barriers is disrupted because of inadequate production of gastric acidity, digestive enzymes, mucus, immunoglobulins, and decreased peristalsis. In addition, common medication exposures (antibiotics, histamine H₂ receptor blockers, vasoconstrictors, sedatives, and paralytics) decrease these inherent defenses by decreasing expression of antibacterial peptides (Louis and Lin, 2009; Schumann et al, 2005), altering natural acidity, and decreasing peristalsis. As a result, there is a reduced ability to eliminate pathogenic organisms, allowing for increased epithelial adherence and bacterial translocation. Inadequate development of mucosal immunity is further exacerbated by induced mucosal and villus atrophy that likely develops as a consequence of prolonged absence of enteral feedings (Niinikoski et al, 2004).

Abnormal Colonization of the Preterm Gut

Although it was once thought that the in utero environment was sterile, bacteria have been identified in early meconium samples in preterm infants, suggesting a potential prenatal influence on early intestinal bacterial colonization (Mshvildadze et al, 2008). Once a more broad microbial community has been established, the fecal organisms commonly observed in preterm infants include enterococci, members of Enterobacteriaceae, *E. coli*, staphylococci, streptococci, *Clostridium*, and *Bacteroides* (Millar et al, 2003; Penders et al, 2006; Schwiertz et al, 2003; Stark and Lee, 1982a). This bacterial profile is distinctly different from those seen in breastfed term infants, yet, similar to patterns exhibited by formula-fed full-term infants. However, in contrast to formula-fed term infants, the colonization by these pathogenic bacteria persists longer (Sakata et al, 1985) and there was slow development of colonization by the commensal bacterium *Bifidobacterium* (Stark and Lee, 1982b).

The differences in bacterial colonization patterns between healthy, full-term infants and preterm infants can be partially explained by the inadequate physical and chemical barriers described earlier, which allow for greater penetration and adherence by pathogenic organisms; immaturity of epithelial glycoconjugate expression (an important modulator of bacterial adherence) (Claud et al, 2004; Walker, 2002); and the unique environmental exposures experienced by the preterm infant. Almost universally, preterm, low-birthweight infants experience delayed enteral feedings, are exposed to early and prolonged broad-spectrum antibiotics, and are introduced to residential hospital flora. Each of these factors contributes to delayed intestinal colonization by commensal, nonpathogenic bacteria, a predominance of pathogenic bacteria, and a lack of microbial diversity (Agarwal et al, 2003; Butel et al, 2007; Fanaro et al, 2003; Magne et al, 2005).

As reviewed, in the mature enterocyte, commensal bacteria inhibit the activation of NF-κB, which is in contrast to pathogenic bacteria that activate NF-κB (Claud and Walker, 2001; Walker, 2002). Of particular importance to the premature neonate is the developmentally reduced expression of inhibitor kappa B (IκB), an inhibitory protein to NF-κB, which, when bound, inhibits NF-κB translocation into the cell nucleus and transcription of proinflammatory mediators. As a result, the immature enterocyte is in an activated, proinflammatory state, and this excessive inflammatory response is seen with both commensal and pathogenic bacteria (Claud et al, 2004).

Necrotizing Enterocolitis

NEC is a devastating gastrointestinal disease predominantly observed in preterm infants. The pathogenesis is incompletely understood and is likely multifactorial. As discussed, the preterm infant possesses and experiences multiple perturbations to postnatal intestinal and immune development, all of which likely work in concert with one another to increase the vulnerability of the preterm infant to NEC. Just a few examples that illustrate this are: the increased prevalence in formula-fed infants (lack of exposure to the bioactive compounds found in breast milk); the disparate intestinal bacterial colonization profiles observed in infants who developed NEC versus control infants (Wang et al, 2009) (lack of benefits offered by commensal bacteria and increased risk of increased inflammation and bacterial translocation by pathogenic bacteria); the reduction of NEC with the use of probiotics; and the increased incidence of NEC after exposure to prolonged antibiotics (delayed bacterial colonization with preference for pathogenic microorganisms) and to H_2 blockers (decrease gastric acidity, thus dampening one component of the first line of defense against pathogenic antigens provided by the intestinal tract) (Cotten et al, 2009; Guillet et al, 2006).

In the absence of TLR4, as demonstrated by the TLR4 knockout mouse, the development of NEC is prevented (Leaphart et al, 2007). This supports the general hypothesis that the expression and modulation (i.e., suppression or activation) of TLR4 are important in the pathogenesis of NEC. Downregulation of TLR4 suppresses downstream proinflammatory signaling as observed with postnatal intestinal bacterial colonization by commensal organisms, whereas TLR4 activation results in increased proinflammatory signaling. In addition, TLR4 activation may mediate other downstream pathways, reducing the epithelial cells' capacity for regeneration and proliferation (Sodhi et al, 2010). Activation of TLR4 is mediated by LPS and possibly other stressors such as hypoxia, conditions often utilized to induce NEC in animal models, and shared risk factors in preterm infants at risk for NEC. Thus, the balance between TLR4 suppression and activation is likely to be critical in determining the postnatal susceptibility to NEC in the preterm infant (Abreu, 2010).

ATOPIC DISEASES

The incidence of allergic diseases has dramatically increased over the past several decades in developed countries. The potential mechanism for this phenomenon has been termed the *hygiene hypothesis* (Bach, 2002; von Mutius, 2007). The interaction with microbes and subsequent colonization by these organisms are essential in the development of mucosal immunity. With colonization of a diverse microbial population, the newborn shifts from a predominant Th2 cellular response (conditioned during fetal development to prevent maternal rejection of the fetus) (Morein et al, 2007), to a Th1 cellular response. However, in developed countries with improved hygiene and sanitation, the diversity of microbes in the intestinal ecosystem is lacking, and Th2 cellular responses continue to dominate (Tlaskalova-Hogenova et al, 2002). Supporting the vital contribution that the intestinal ecosystem plays in development of allergic responses are the observations of different colonization patterns observed in atopic subjects versus healthy controls (Bjorksten, 2004; Vaarala et al, 2008) and the reduction of atopic diseases with probiotic supplementation (Bjorksten, 2005). Other defects in mucosal immunity observed that allergic individuals have increased intestinal permeability and a deficiency of IgA.

DISEASES OF AUTOIMMUNITY: INFLAMMATORY BOWEL DISEASE, CELIAC DISEASE, AND TYPE 1 DIABETES

Alterations in several areas of innate mucosal immunity play a significant role in the pathogenesis of Crohn's disease, celiac disease, and type 1 diabetes mellitus. Individuals with Crohn's disease have impaired intestinal barrier function; differential expression in toll-like receptors (TL3, TL4); and Th1-dominated cellular responses. Differential expression in TLRs and Th1-dominated cellular responses likely contribute to the inappropriate, excessive inflammatory response to antigenic stimuli (toward *both* commensal and pathogenic bacteria), which is one of the hallmarks of this disease (Cario and Podolsky, 2000; Sartor, 2008). IL-12 and STAT4 activation are important for Th1 T-cell differentiation. Increased IL-12 production noted in Crohn's patients and in animal models, in addition to the observation of successful suppression of intestinal inflammation with IL-12 agonists, provides supporting evidence for the importance of Th1-mediated chronic intestinal inflammation (Macdonald and Monteleone, 2005; Neurath et al, 2002). An imbalance in Th1/Th2 cellular responses in Crohn's patients is further suggestive with the finding that a genetic mutation in the nucleotide-binding oligomerization domain 2 (NOD2) gene, a protein that in its native form inhibits TLR2 activation, is more common in patients with Crohn's disease compared to controls (O'Neill, 2004).

The role of impaired intestinal barrier function has been well established in Crohn's disease (Schulzke et al, 2009). The presence of a "leaky gut" also has been established to be important in the pathogenesis of other autoimmune diseases such as celiac disease and type 1 diabetes mellitus. Furthermore, barrier dysfunction and increased intestinal permeability likely precede the clinical presentation of these autoimmune diseases.

The process by which a breach in intestinal barrier function leads to celiac disease has become the model of intestinally mediated autoimmune diseases. Gliadin (the protein in wheat, barley, and rye) activates myeloid differentiation primary-response gene 88 (MyD88), which, in turn, upregulates the release of zonulin. Zonulin upregulation opens the tight junctions, allowing for intraepithelial passage of gliadin into the intestinal submucosa to interact with effector immune cells and increase the production of proinflammatory cytokines, ultimately leading to intestinal inflammation and cell damage (Fasano and Shea-Donohue, 2005). Removal of gluten from the diet halts this process, allowing for restoration of intestinal barrier function and intestinal recovery.

The interplay among altered intestinal bacterial colonization, impaired barrier function, and a dysregulated proinflammatory response has been implicated in the pathogenesis of type 1 diabetes mellitus (Vaarala et al,

2008). However, currently much of the evidence for aberrant intestinal microbiota comes from animal models where the microbial composition and the microbial-epithelial interaction are manipulated by antibiotic administration in non-obese diabetic mice. Similar to subjects with Crohn's disease, compared with controls, individuals with type 1 diabetes mellitus have impaired intestinal barrier function as demonstrated by permeability studies using mannitol and lactulose. Altered barrier function has also been shown in animal models in those that eventually develop diabetes. Diabetic animals have decreased expression of claudin, an important protein in tight junction complexes, before the onset of disease. Finally, examination of intestinal biopsies from children with type 1 diabetes mellitus demonstrated an increased presence and expression of inflammatory cells and biomarkers (e.g., HLA class II molecules, intercellular adhesion molecule [ICAM]-1, IL-4, IL-1α) within the villus architecture.

OBESITY

Altered bacterial colonization patterns are evident in obesity. In animal models of genetic obesity, obese mice have distinctly different microbial colonization patterns compared to their lean littermates with bacteria counts higher in Firmicutes and lower in Bacteroidetes. These microbial shifts are also seen in diet-induced animal models of obesity by placing the mice on a prolonged Western diet (Reinhardt et al, 2009). In humans, childhood obesity is increased in formula versus breastfed infants. And, as discussed earlier, different microbial colonization patterns exist between these two groups, suggesting that their ecosystem may play a role in the propensity for obesity. In a longitudinal study of childhood obesity, infants who later developed obesity, compared to infants who maintained a normal weight in childhood, had a fecal microbial pattern that contained lower concentrations of *Bifidobacterium* and higher concentrations of *S. aureus*. Obesity has been associated with low-grade chronic inflammation; thus, the reduction of the commensal organism *Bifidobacterium* and the increased presence of the pathogenic organism *S. aureus* may, in part, contribute to the pathogenesis of chronic inflammation (Kalliomaki et al, 2008).

In addition, the intestinal ecosystem is an important modulator of the host's metabolic activities, some of which are important to the pathogenesis of obesity. Metagenomic studies of the microbiota in obese patients demonstrate an increased presence of genes that are involved in energy harvest. Other metabolic pathways mediated by the microbiota include increased hepatic lipogenesis; decreased fatty acid oxidation in skeletal muscle; and LPS-mediated chronic inflammation in adipose tissue (Reinhardt et al, 2009).

CONCLUSION

The GI tract serves many complex nutritional and immune functions critical for survival. The morphologic development of the intestinal tract to serve these specialized functions begins in early embryogenesis and continues throughout childhood. Exposure to amniotic fluid followed by postnatal exposures to human milk, formula, and environmental microorganisms is essential for the continued anatomic differentiation of the intestinal tract and development of mucosal immunity. Ultimately, multiple layers of immunologic defenses and a balance between oral tolerance and inflammatory responsiveness are established and maintained throughout the life of the host. Perturbations to this balance or to any component of the multiple layers of mucosal defenses increase the vulnerability of the host to atopic diseases, autoimmune disorders, or conditions mediated by chronic, unregulated inflammation.

SUGGESTED READINGS

Artis D: Epithelial-cell recognition of commensal bacteria and maintenance of immune homeostasis in the gut, *Nat Rev Immunol* 8:411-420, 2008.

Bach JF: The effect of infections on susceptibility to autoimmune and allergic diseases, *N Engl J Med* 347:911-920, 2002.

Donovan SM: Role of human milk components in gastrointestinal development: current knowledge and future NEEDS, *J Pediatr* 149:S49-S61, 2006.

Magalhaes JG, Tattoli I, Girardin SE: The intestinal epithelial barrier: how to distinguish between the microbial flora and pathogens, *Semin Immunol* 19:106-115, 2007.

Neurath MF, Finotto S, Glimcher LH: The role of Th1/Th2 polarization in mucosal immunity, *Nat Med* 8:567-573, 2002.

Sharma R, Tepas JJ 3rd: Microecology, intestinal epithelial barrier and necrotizing enterocolitis, *Pediatr Surg Int* 26:11-21, 2010.

Wagner CL, Taylor SN, Johnson D: Host factors in amniotic fluid and breast milk that contribute to gut maturation, *Clin Rev Allergy Immunol* 34:191-204, 2008.

Winkler P, Ghadimi D, Schrezenmeir J, Kraehenbuhl JP: Molecular and cellular basis of microflora-host interactions, *J Nutr* 137(Suppl 2):756S-772S, 2007.

Complete references and supplemental color images used in this text can be found online at www.expertconsult.com

ABDOMINAL WALL PROBLEMS

DISORDERS OF THE UMBILICAL REGION

The umbilical region is the site of intricate, complex activity during embryonic life. Early in gestation, a widely open communication exists between the yolk sac and primitive gut. Later, the entire midgut passes through this communication to form a large physiologic umbilical hernia that persists in utero for several weeks. Thereafter, the gut returns to its position in the abdominal cavity. By the third trimester, the aperture around the vessels, omphalomesenteric (vitelline) duct, and urachus begins to narrow. After birth, the umbilical arteries contract, blood flow ceases, their intimal and medial layers undergo aseptic necrosis, and the stump separates. Alterations in this orderly but complex sequence of events result in serious congenital anomalies.

UMBILICAL CORD LESIONS

NONCOILED UMBILICAL BLOOD VESSELS

The three vessels within the cord are coiled to form a helical structure. The number of twists can vary greatly (ranging from 0 to 40) and, rarely, reaches 380 per cord (Donlon and Furdon, 2002). Left-twisted vessels outnumber right-twisted vessels 7 to 1. Absence of any twists occurs in about 4% of pregnancies (Strong et al, 1993). The helical structure is identifiable by ultrasound examination by the end of the first trimester. Although how the vessels come to have this geometric arrangement has not been established, such a configuration—like that of a telephone cord—is more able to resist external compression, stretch, or torsion, and the cord remains flexible (Strong et al, 1993). The absence of coils is associated with increased abnormalities that include single umbilical artery, trisomy 21, and coarctation of the aorta. Approximately 10% of infants without coils are stillborn, and the incidence of preterm birth is greater than expected.

SINGLE UMBILICAL ARTERY

Normally the umbilical cord is composed of two arteries and a vein. A single umbilical artery occurs in 1% of single births and in 7% of twin births. The presence of a single umbilical artery is higher among aborted fetuses and thus is thought to be a marker for increased fetal risk (Deshpande et al, 2009; Mu et al, 2008). Among newborns with single umbilical artery, there is a higher incidence of poor fetal growth and a slightly increased risk for renal anomalies. Therefore, the presence of a single umbilical artery warrants careful intrauterine monitoring, although postpartum imaging may not be warranted (Deshpande et al, 2009).

UMBILICAL GRANULOMA AND POLYP

If the separation of the umbilical stump is delayed beyond 5 to 8 days after birth, granulation tissue may be produced, delaying epithelialization (Figure 71-1). Judicious desiccation with silver nitrate is the treatment of choice if the granuloma does not resolve.

Granulomas must be differentiated from umbilical polyps, which typically contain gastric or intestinal mucosa (Figure 71-2). Treatment is surgical excision, without need of exploring the peritoneal cavity (Pacilli et al, 2007).

DELAY IN SEPARATION OF THE CORD

If the umbilical cord fails to separate after more than 14 days, investigation for a possible defect in neutrophil function and chemotaxis should be undertaken.

ABDOMINAL WALL DEFECTS

UMBILICAL HERNIA

The umbilical ring is formed when the mesoderm of the muscle and fascia around the umbilical vessels and urachus contracts. Umbilical hernias are caused by failure of closure of the umbilical ring; unlike the case of omphaloceles, skin and subcutaneous tissue cover the defect. These lesions are found in 30% of African American infants and in 4% of white infants; there is a high familial incidence. The condition is more common in low-birthweight babies and in infants with trisomy 21.

The actual fascial defect varies in size, ranging from 1 to 4 cm in diameter. The sac may contain a loop of bowel that is easily pushed back into the abdomen, or preperitoneal fat. Approximately 80% of these hernias close spontaneously by 3 to 4 years, and the risk of incarceration is exceedingly low. Spontaneous closure is less likely in hernias with fascial defects greater than 1.5 cm. Surgical correction is therefore only indicated in large-defect hernias, in children over 4 to 6 years of age, or if symptoms occur (Poenaru, 2001).

OMPHALOCELE

Definition and Epidemiology

Omphalocele refers to a congenital defect in the formation of the umbilical portion of the abdominal wall that is larger than 4 cm in diameter (Table 71-1; Figure 71-3). The defect occurs in 1 in 6000 to 1 in 10,000 live births. Although many omphaloceles are isolated defects, some are part of a constellation of malformations (such as the Beckwith-Wiedemann syndrome or trisomy 18), and a few cases are associated with maternal ingestion of valproic acid

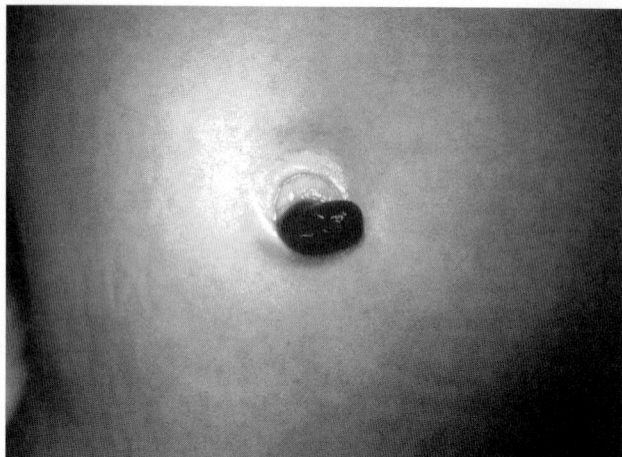

FIGURE 71-1 Umbilical granuloma, characterized by fleshy appearance but without any central depression or lumen.

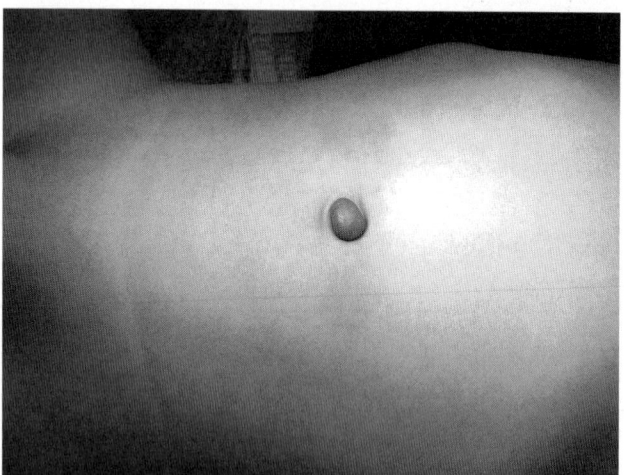

FIGURE 71-2 Umbilical polyp. The lesion is skin-covered.

TABLE 71-1   Characteristics of Gastroschisis and Omphalocele

Defect	Gastroschisis	Omphalocele
Covering sac	Absent	Present, but may be torn
Fascial defect	Small	Small or large
Cord attachment	Onto the abdominal wall	Onto the sac
Herniated bowel	Edematous	Normal
Prematurity (%)	50–60	10–20
Associated anomalies (%)	10–15	45–55
Gastrointestinal	18	37
Cardiac	2	20
Trisomy syndromes	—	30
Necrotizing enterocolitis (%)	18	Only if sac is ruptured
Malabsorption	Common	Only if sac is ruptured

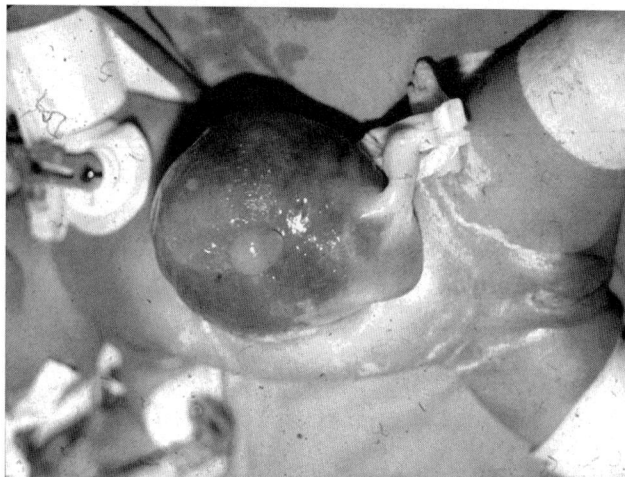

FIGURE 71-3 *(See also Color Plate 29.)* **Female newborn with omphalocele.** The fascial defect is large, situated at the base of the umbilical cord, covered by a glistening membrane and containing both liver and bowel.

for seizure control (Boussemart et al, 1995). Omphalocele is also present in infants who have the OEIS complex, a constellation of anomalies that includes omphalocele, bladder exstrophy, imperforate anus, and spinal defects (Tiblad et al, 2008). Associated malformations are present in 75% of the patients, compared to only 15% in the case of gastroschisis (Stoll et al, 2008). By the very nature of the developmental defect (see later discussion), all infants with omphalocele have malrotation.

Etiology

Early in fetal life, the small intestine lies outside of the abdominal cavity. By the 10th week, the midgut returns to the abdomen, and the somatic layers of the cephalic, caudal, and lateral folds join to close the defect in the abdominal wall. For unknown reasons, this closure may not occur. Several types of omphalocele are recognized, based on the specific fold that fails to close. *Epigastric omphalocele* occurs when there is abnormal closure of the cephalic fold. Because these somites also form the lower thoracic wall, failure of closure results in the Cantrell pentalogy, which includes cleft sternum, diaphragmatic defects, pericardial defects, cardiac anomalies, and omphalocele. *Classic*

omphalocele occurs when there is an interruption in lateral fold development, resulting in an abdominal wall defect that lies between the epigastric and hypogastric regions. In addition to loops of bowel, liver also may herniate through the abdominal wall defect. The umbilicus arises from an anterior position on the omphalocele, and the muscular abdominal wall is normal. Failure in closure of the caudal fold results in a *hypogastric omphalocele*. Associated defects include bladder exstrophy and imperforate anus.

Diagnosis

Alpha-fetoprotein (AFP) is synthesized in the fetal liver and is excreted by the fetal kidneys. It also crosses the placenta and appears in the maternal circulation by 12 weeks' gestation. Maternal plasma levels of AFP are elevated when fetuses have neural tube defects, abdominal wall defects, or atresia of the duodenum or esophagus. Maternal serum AFP is used as a screening test, although there is a 40% rate of false-positive results. Analysis of amniotic AFP and acetyl-cholinesterase-pseudocholinesterase levels can be sensitive in detecting abdominal wall defects, especially gastroschisis (Saleh et al, 1993; Saller et al, 1994). Human chorionic gonadotropin levels have shown promise in small series in detecting abdominal wall defects (Schmidt et al, 1993).

Ultrasound evaluation is not useful during the first trimester, when the midgut is normally herniated. Beyond 14 weeks, however, this modality has a 96% sensitivity (Patel et al, 2009). The combined use of maternal serum AFP and ultrasound examination at 19 weeks has been shown in a series of 8000 patients to have excellent sensitivity in identifying abdominal wall defects (Luck, 1992). Once an abdominal wall defect has been identified, ultrasound examination often can distinguish omphalocele from gastroschisis. Because the association of cardiac anomalies and chromosomal disorders is high, fetal echocardiography and amniocentesis should also be performed. Vaginal delivery does not adversely affect outcome; therefore, the need for cesarean section should be based on obstetric indications alone (Segel et al, 2001). If not discovered prenatally, the diagnosis is obvious at birth. If the sac ruptures, the bowel loops may become edematous and matted together, mimicking gastroschisis.

Treatment

The presence of exteriorized bowel results in heat loss and extravasation of fluid and provides a major portal of entry for bacteria. When the omphalocele is first seen, the sac should be kept moist by wrapping it with gauze sponges that have been soaked in warmed normal saline. A plastic covering is then wrapped around the defect to limit water and heat loss (Figure 71-4). Care should be taken to prevent angulation of the sac when the child is prone, to prevent kinking of mesenteric vessels. Alternatively, the infant can be positioned on the side, with the exteriorized bowel in an anterior position. A nasogastric tube is passed to decrease the accumulation of air in the bowel. The infant should be given 1.5 times the maintenance intravenous fluid volume and broad-spectrum antibiotics. Thereafter, any inspection and manipulation of the abdominal contents should be done with sterile gloves.

Operative repair should be undertaken as soon as possible, ideally within 2 to 4 hours of birth. Small defects can be closed with a single-stage repair. For larger defects, primary repair may cause respiratory failure and abdominal compartment syndrome because the abdominal cavity is too small to accommodate the bowel. Complications of compartment syndrome include renal failure, hypotension from compression of the vena cava, hepatic ischemia, and intestinal ischemia. In affected infants, a staged repair is performed using a prosthetic device called a *silo* to cover the defect (Figure 71-5). Final closure can then be achieved after gradual reduction of the bowel into the abdominal cavity over 7 to 10 days (Dunn and Fonkalsrud, 1997). Selected "giant omphaloceles" can also be initially managed non-operatively with silver sulfadiazine, followed by abdominal wall closure later in infancy (Lee et al, 2006)

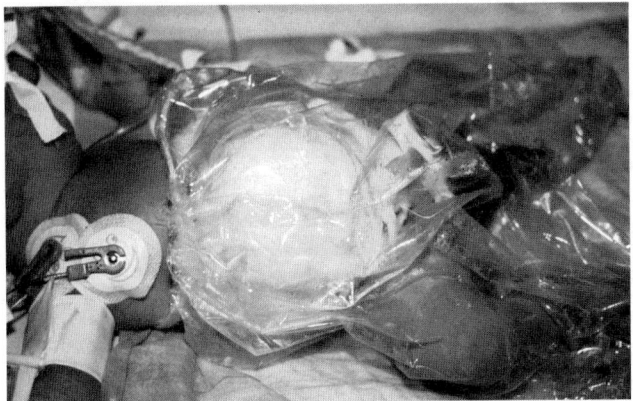

FIGURE 71-4 **Newborn with gastroschisis managed in a sterile bag (bowel bag) up to the nipple line.** The bag protects the baby from heat and water loss while allowing good visualization of the herniated bowel.

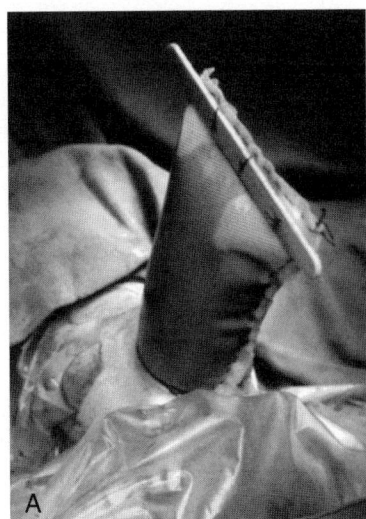
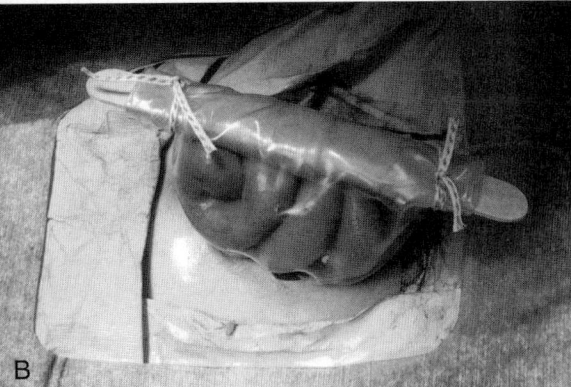

FIGURE 71-5 **Use of a Silastic silo in the management of gastroschisis. A,** Sutured silo immediately after construction. **B,** Ready-made silo after several reduction turns.

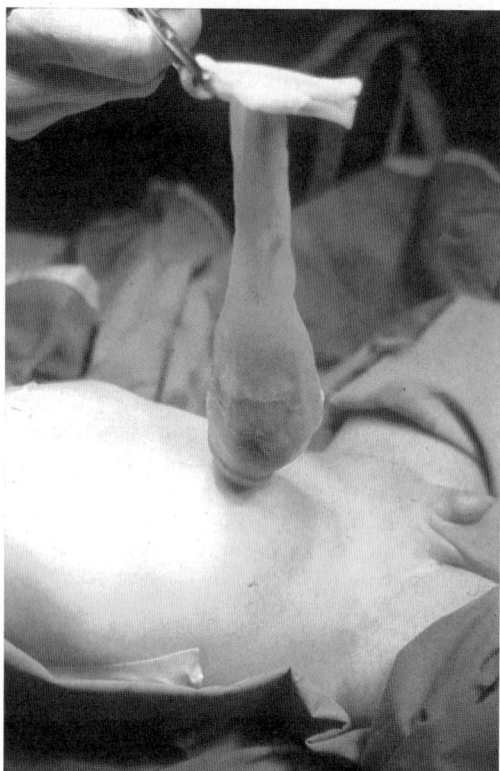

FIGURE 71-6 Hernia of the umbilical cord. This is in fact a small omphalocele, containing only bowel loops in a small sac within the umbilical cord.

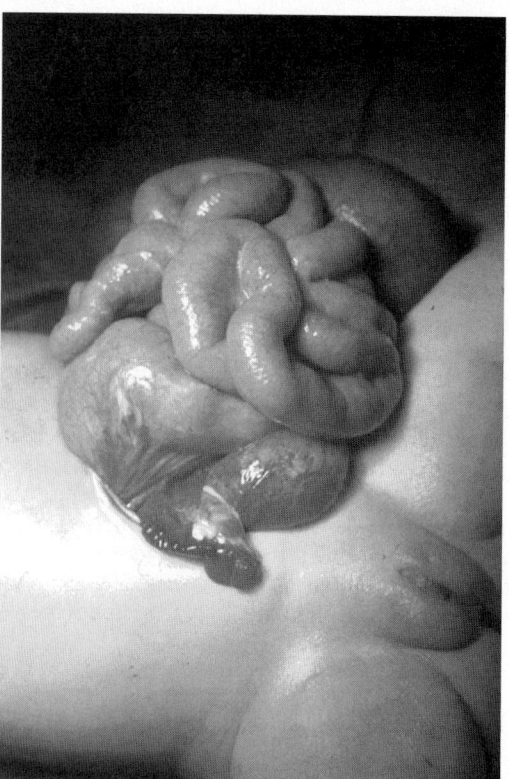

FIGURE 71-7 *(See also Color Plate 30.)* **Female newborn with gastroschisis.** The fascial defect is relatively small and situated to the right of the umbilical cord and contains exposed bowel (as well as an ovary in this instance).

Postoperatively, protracted ileus may occur, necessitating prolonged parenteral nutrition. Attention must also be directed to the diagnosis and management of associated anomalies.

Prognosis

The mortality rate with associated heart disease is 80%. In the absence of heart disease, 70% to 90% of infants with omphalocele survive (Forrester and Merz, 1999; Kitchanan et al, 2000).

CORD HERNIA

A small omphalocele is called a *cord hernia*. By definition, the defect in the abdominal wall is less than 4 cm in diameter, and the exteriorized sac contains only loops of bowel (Figures 71-6). This defect arises between the 8th and 10th weeks as a result of failure of closure of the umbilical ring. Cord hernias can be missed at birth, and the intestine can be injured by careless proximal application of the cord clamp. Otherwise, these defects are easily managed by primary closure at birth and have an excellent outcome.

GASTROSCHISIS

Definition and Epidemiology

Gastroschisis is the herniation of abdominal contents through an abdominal wall defect, usually occurring on the right side of a normally positioned umbilical cord

(Figure 71-7). This lesion was traditionally less frequent than omphalocele, but its incidence is increasing worldwide (Srivastava et al, 2009; Vu et al, 2008). The defect appears most common among young mothers and those of low gravidity (Fillingham and Rankin, 2008). Associated anomalies are found in only 15% of patients, the vast majority being intestinal atresias (Stoll et al, 2008). Infants with gastroschisis tend to have intrauterine growth restriction (Santiago-Munoz et al, 2007) .

Etiology

Although the cause of these lesions is not known, many investigators speculate that they may be of vascular origin. Intrauterine interruption of the omphalomesenteric artery has been proposed, an explanation that accounts for many of the clinically observed differences between this lesion and omphalocele (Hoyme et al, 1981).

Diagnosis and Treatment

As described for omphalocele, gastroschisis can be correctly diagnosed prenatally (Figure 71-8). Because the peritoneal sac is absent, the fetal bowel is continuously bathed in amniotic fluid, which results in a significant intestinal "peel," causing poor intestinal motility. As with omphalocele, the need for cesarean section should be restricted to obstetric indications only, despite some evidence that prelabor cesarean section results in better outcome because of the ensuing absence of the fibrous peel (Serra et al, 2008).

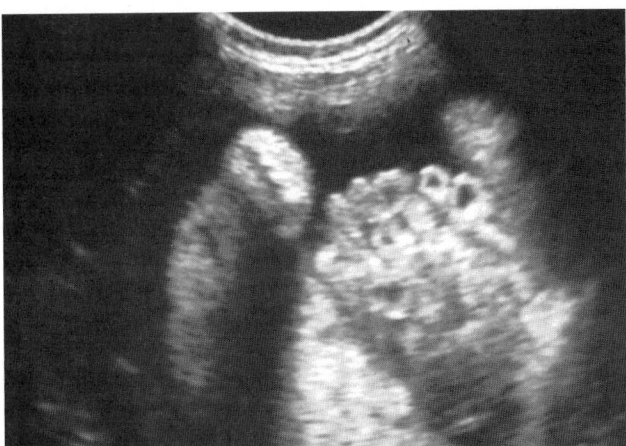

FIGURE 71-8 **Ultrasound image of fetus with gastroschisis.** The intestinal loops are seen free in the amniotic sac.

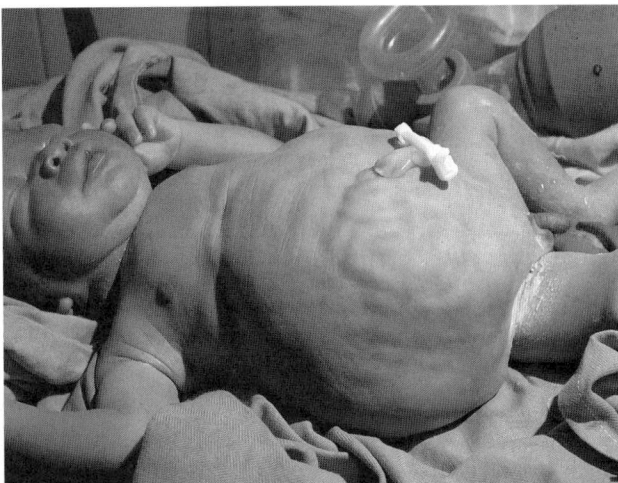

FIGURE 71-9 *(See also Color Plate 31.)* **Newborn with prune-belly syndrome.** The laxity of the abdominal wall musculature is obvious.

The diagnosis is readily made at birth. The entire gastrointestinal tract usually is eviscerated, but unlike with omphalocele, the liver is not exteriorized. The intestinal loops usually are covered by a thick fibrous "peel," which makes them firm, often with a cauliflower-like appearance. Intestinal atresias may be apparent as well. Rare complications include intrapartum mesenteric disruption, prenatal volvulus, and closure of the abdominal wall defect around the exteriorized gut (i.e., closing gastroschisis) (Houben et al, 2009). All of these events can cause catastrophic intestinal loss.

As described for omphalocele, the bowel contents should be kept moist and relatively sterile at birth. A nasogastric tube is passed for decompression, and 1.5 times the maintenance intravenous fluid volume is given. Broad-spectrum antibiotics also should be started. Because the abdominal wall defect often is small, vascular compromise occurs more readily, and great care should be taken to position the infant and the exteriorized bowel to prevent kinking of mesenteric vessels. Unlike with omphalocele, primary closure is possible in 90% of patients, but larger defects may require staged repair. A spring-loaded Silastic silo device that can be placed at the bedside allows early closure of the defect and avoids the need for emergency surgery (Jensen et al, 2009; Pastor et al, 2008). Alternatively, simple cases of gastroschisis can be managed with a sutureless bedside technique not requiring general anesthesia (Sandler et al, 2004). All techniques of intestinal protection and abdominal wall closure appear, however, to be equally effective, and only failure to obtain primary closure is associated with significant delays in resuming intestinal function (Weinsheimer et al, 2008). Postoperatively, prolonged ileus often occurs because of intestinal dysmorphology, which often includes the myenteric plexus. Despite this ileus, minimal enteral feeding in the early postoperative period can decrease time to discharge and overall mortality (Walter-Nicolet et al, 2009). Affected infants are at increased risk for necrotizing enterocolitis (Oldham et al, 1988). Intestinal atresias usually are not repaired at the initial procedure because of the fibrous peel and therefore require repair at 3 to 4 weeks of age (Snyder et al, 2001). One third of babies with gastroschisis will experience growth delay in infancy, and prolonged intestinal dysmotility is common (Phillips et al, 2008; South et al, 2008).

Prognosis

Mortality rates have decreased to 5% to 10% (Fillingham and Rankin, 2008; Kitchanan et al, 2000). Postoperative recovery may be longer in infants undergoing repair of gastroschisis than in those with omphalocele. Enteral feedings may not be established until 2 months after operation, and some infants will require home parenteral nutrition (Molik et al, 2001). In spite of these initial feeding difficulties, most gastroschisis survivors maintain normal growth during infancy and childhood (Davies and Stringer, 1997).

PRUNE-BELLY SYNDROME

Prune-belly syndrome refers to a triad of anomalies consisting of a deficiency of abdominal musculature, cryptorchidism, and urinary tract abnormalities—in fact, it has also been called the "triad syndrome." The most common urinary tract anomalies seen are megaloureter, cystic renal dysplasia, urethral obstruction, and megacystis (Woods and Brandon, 2007). Malrotation occurs in 30% of cases, and cardiac anomalies in 20%. The syndrome rarely occurs in females, and its exact cause is unknown. Theories include failure in the development of the abdominal wall between the 6th and 8th weeks of gestation and primary urethral obstruction with early bladder distention (Woods and Brandon, 2007). At birth, the defect is obvious on inspection. The abdomen is shapeless, and the skin hangs in wrinkled folds (Figure 71-9). There may be an open patent urachus, which by itself signals a poor prognosis. Of immediate concern is evaluation for and relief of urinary tract obstruction. Approximately 20% of patients with prune-belly syndrome die in the neonatal period from renal dysplasia or pulmonary hypoplasia, but of those who survive, 30% develop renal failure during childhood (Burbige et al, 1987). Surgical management of the genitourinary tract remains controversial, with advocates of both watchful waiting and major reconstruction. The latter should be performed only where specialized surgical and anesthesia expertise are available, because the surgery is challenging and postoperative complications are frequent.

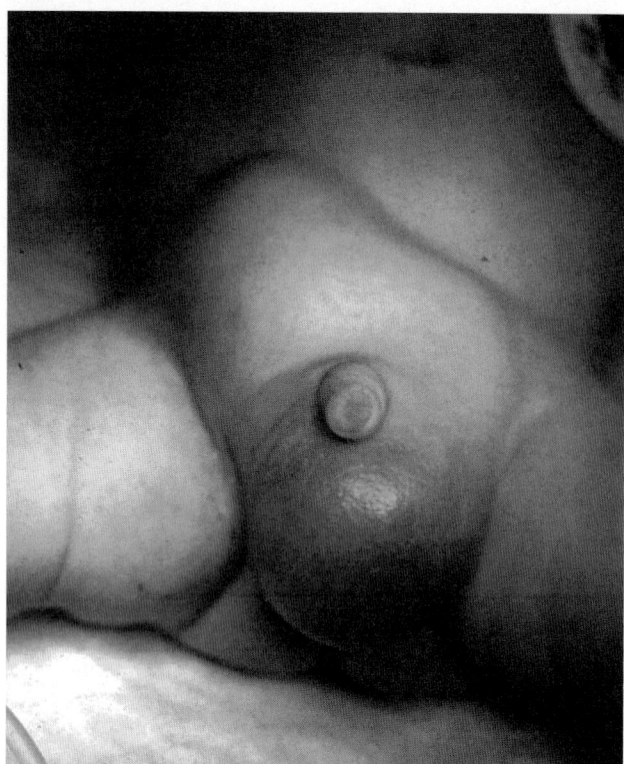

FIGURE 71-10 Infant with large right-sided inguinal hernia. The right inguinal canal is visibly distended by the herniated bowel.

The undescended testes are corrected in childhood for monitoring and psychological reasons.

INGUINAL HERNIA

The gonads are formed during weeks 5 to 12 of gestation. The testes descend through the internal ring at 28 weeks. In the general population, inguinal hernias occur in 1% of all live births. The incidence of inguinal hernia in low-birthweight infants varies between 3% for birthweights of 1500 to 2000 g to 42% for birthweights of 500 to 1000 g (Peevy et al, 1986). With preterm delivery and the accompanying increase in intraabdominal pressure, testicular descent and inguinal canal closure are impaired, thus explaining the increased incidence of inguinal hernia (Figure 71-10).

Additional risk factors for inguinal hernias are cystic fibrosis, congenital dislocation of the hip, presence of a ventriculoperitoneal shunt, and abdominal wall defects. Incarceration and strangulation are common in infant hernias. The combined incidence of these complications is as high as 30% (Rowe and Clatworthy, 1970), although it appears to be lower in preterm infants. Therefore, repeated examinations may be necessary, particularly if the infant's clinical status becomes unstable or if a tense, fluctuant scrotal mass or vomiting develops. Most of these incarcerated hernias may be reduced nonoperatively by placing the infant in the Trendelenburg position with sedation and application of an ice pack to the inguinal-scrotal area. Successful reduction should be followed by surgical repair in 24 to 48 hours (allowing for resolution of local edema). Failure of reduction necessitates immediate surgical repair.

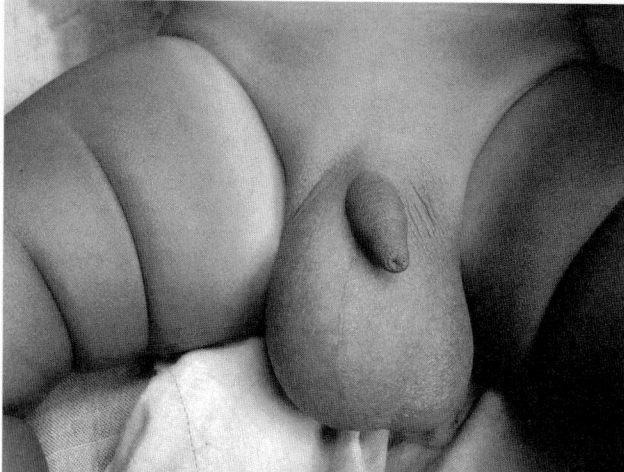

FIGURE 71-11 *(See also Color Plate 32.)* **Bilateral infantile hydroceles.** The scrotum is distended by fluid, whereas the inguinal canals are normal.

Nonincarcerated hernias in infants require repair as soon as convenient, preferably within 1 to 2 weeks of diagnosis (Zamakhshary et al, 2008). Premature babies are traditionally operated on just before their discharge from the neonatal intensive care unit, or very soon afterward—although earlier repair may be technically easier for large hernias (Ein et al, 2006). Postoperative apnea occurs in about 5% of preterm infants, particularly those with a history of apneas (Murphy et al, 2008). Postoperative overnight admission for apnea monitoring is therefore indicated for higher-risk outpatients until 48 weeks of postconceptional age. The lowest incidence of apneas occurs with surgery performed using spinal block without sedation (Somri et al, 1998). Other specific postoperative complications include persistent scrotal swelling, recurrence, testicular atrophy, and injury to the vas deferens. Recurrence is highest in premature babies (Vogels et al, 2009). Contralateral exploration is probably not indicated in most cases, because the actual risk of a metachronous hernia has been generally estimated at below 10% (Ein et al, 2006; Zamakhshary et al, 2009).

HYDROCELE

A *hydrocele* is a collection of fluid in the scrotum without an obvious inguinal hernia. The typical hydrocele is noted at or shortly after birth as a unilateral or bilateral swelling in the scrotum, which may fluctuate in size.

The scrotum is enlarged, may be very tense with fluid, and usually is nontender, often with a bluish appearance; the inguinal canal is normal (Figure 71-11). Differentiation between hydrocele and hernia is critical and may be difficult in the infant. Transillumination is useful, but findings must be interpreted cautiously, because fluid or gas-filled bowel may transilluminate in small infants. An irreducible yet nontender groin or scrotal mass probably is a hydrocele.

The recommended management of a hydrocele is observation during the first 1 or 2 years of life, unless a hernia cannot be excluded. Hydroceles that persist or appear beyond that age are unlikely to resolve spontaneously, and affected infants should therefore undergo elective surgical repair.

URACHAL LESIONS

The urachus is the remnant of the allantois that extends from the bladder portion of the cloaca to the umbilicus. The urachus may remain completely patent throughout its length or fail to obliterate (Figures 71-12 and 71-13). All varieties of this defect are rare, and treatment is customized to each patient (Galati et al, 2008).

COMPLETELY PATENT URACHUS

A completely patent urachus manifests with the passage of urine from the umbilicus. Radiopaque contrast material injected into the orifice outlines the urachal tract and fills the bladder. Treatment consists of surgical excision of the umbilicus along with the entire urachus down to the bladder. Results are typically good.

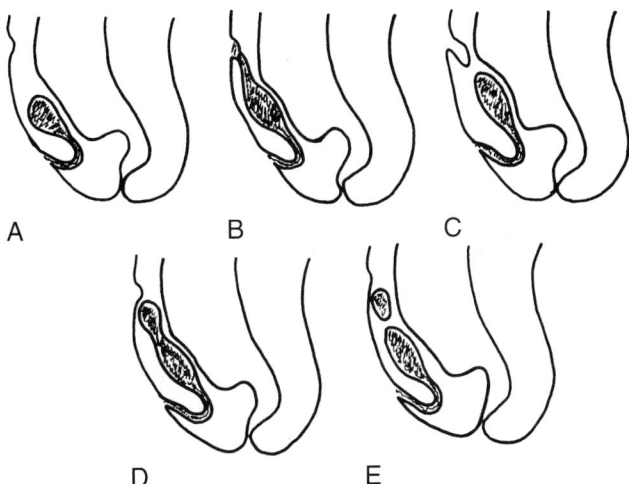

FIGURE 71-12 **Urachal anomalies. A,** Normal anatomy. **B,** Completely patent urachus. **C,** Blind external tract: urachal sinus. **D,** Blind internal tract: bladder diverticulum. **E,** Urachal cyst.

BLIND EXTERNAL URACHUS

When only the distal end of the urachus fails to obliterate, a draining sinus results. Drainage of urine begins sometime after the cord separates. Surgical excision of the sinus tract is required if it persists beyond 6 months of life (Galati et al, 2008).

BLIND INTERNAL URACHUS

Failure of obliteration of the proximal end of the urachus results in a bladder diverticulum. It produces no symptoms and may be coincidentally discovered on cystogram. Nothing needs to be done surgically.

URACHAL CYST

Incomplete obliteration of the midportion of the urachus leads to the development of a urachal cyst. Cysts may present at birth or may grow slowly and become obvious at any time during infancy or childhood, often through infection. Ultrasound examination is diagnostic. Treatment involves surgical resection, which may be preceded by incision and drainage of the superimposed abscess.

MALFORMATIONS OF THE OMPHALOMESENTERIC DUCT

In the developing embryo, the omphalomesenteric (vitelline) duct connects the yolk sac to the primitive midgut through the umbilical cord. In the normal course of ontogeny, the duct becomes obliterated and disappears. Under certain circumstances however, all or portions of the duct may persist (Figures 71-14 and 71-15). This may cause symptoms through drainage, infection, and intestinal obstruction. As with urachal remnants, presentation and management vary with each type (Snyder, 2007).

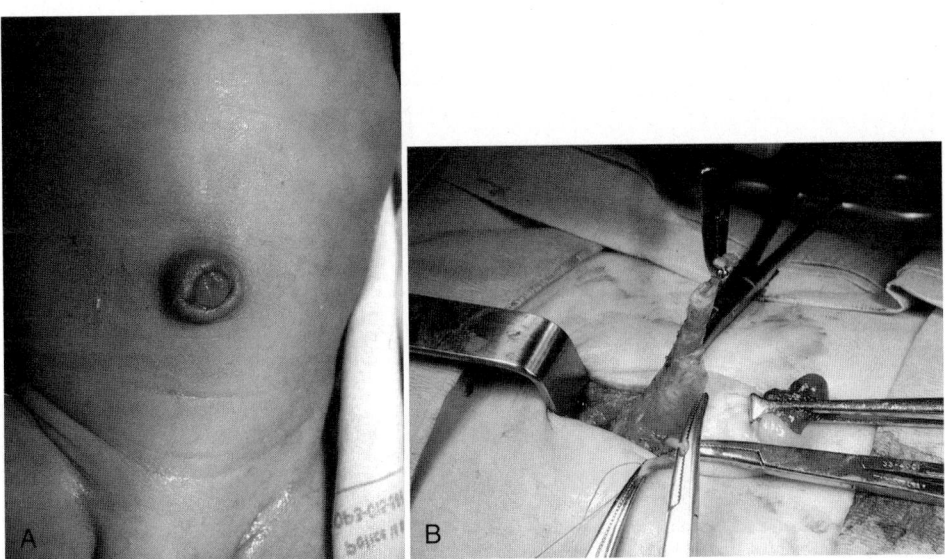

FIGURE 71-13 **Patent urachus. A,** Appearance of defect. **B,** Operative photograph of the urachal remnant with wide attachment to the bladder.

PATENT OMPHALOMESENTERIC DUCT

Patent omphalomesenteric duct is an enteroumbilical fistula, manifesting with the passage of meconium or fecal matter through the umbilicus. The condition may begin at birth or occur within 1 to 2 weeks. The most significant danger with this lesion is evagination (prolapse) of the small bowel through the umbilical orifice, with a significant increase in mortality. Once this lesion is diagnosed, it should be corrected by surgical excision of the umbilicus and the duct.

OMPHALOMESENTERIC SINUS

Failure of distal closure of the omphalomesenteric duct leads to the formation of a sinus. Persistent watery discharge from the umbilical cord is the initial presentation. Examination of the umbilicus reveals a red nodule projecting from the base. Gentle massage results in the extrusion of mucus, which differentiates this lesion from an umbilical granuloma. Injection of radiopaque contrast material outlines the sinus tract. Treatment consists of surgical excision.

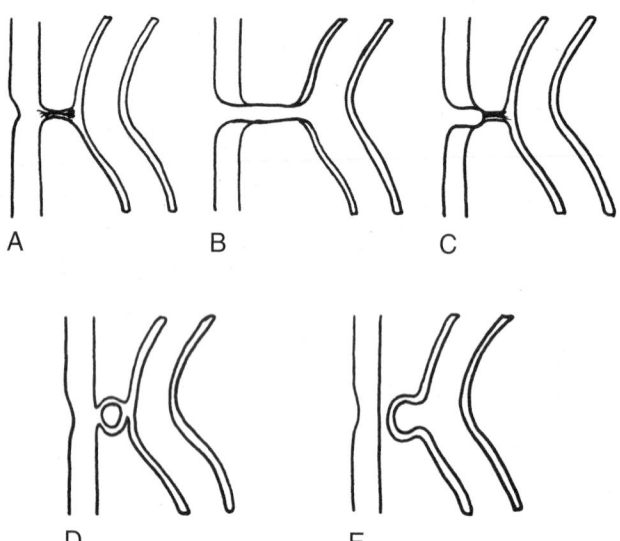

FIGURE 71-14 Omphalomesenteric (vitelline) duct anomalies. A, Normal anatomy. **B,** Patent omphalomesenteric duct. **C,** Blind external tract: umbilical sinus. **D,** Omphalomesenteric duct cyst. **E,** Blind internal tract: Meckel's diverticulum.

OMPHALOMESENTERIC DUCT CYST

When the middle portion of the omphalomesenteric duct persists and eventually fills with secretions, a cyst forms. This lesion may be detected as an enlarging umbilical mass. Treatment consists of surgical excision.

MECKEL'S DIVERTICULUM

When the proximal, or intestinal, end of the omphalomesenteric duct fails to become obliterated completely, an outpouching of the ileum persists. The diverticulum may vary in size, shape, and point of attachment, although the junction usually lies at some point in the distal ileum (Figure 71-16). It must arise from the antimesenteric side of the bowel, a feature that distinguishes Meckel's diverticulum from enteric duplications. Its distal end usually lies free in the peritoneal cavity, but in some cases it is attached to the umbilicus by a fibrous cord and in a small minority remains patent to the umbilicus (omphalomesenteric fistula). Twenty percent of these diverticula contain ectopic pancreatic or gastric tissue.

Incidence

Meckel's diverticula can be discovered in 1.5% to 2% of all persons. Only a small proportion of these diverticula ever become symptomatic, and when they do, this usually happens beyond the age of 4 months. Only exceptionally do they cause illness in the neonatal period. Affected males outnumber females in a ratio of 3:1 to 5:1.

Meckel's diverticulum manifests clinically with bowel obstruction, intestinal bleeding, inflammation, or perforation (Menezes et al, 2008). A pancreatic or gastric mass may act as a leading point to produce intussusception. Gastric mucosa may cause peptic ulceration and bleeding; the latter is almost always the presenting sign if Meckel's diverticulum becomes symptomatic. The fibrous cord, if present, may produce intestinal obstruction. Rarely, inflammation of the diverticulum may lead to peritonitis.

Diagnosis

Hemorrhage from the bowel is the definitive sign of a Meckel's diverticulum. Older children and adults may present with signs and symptoms of diverticulitis, but this

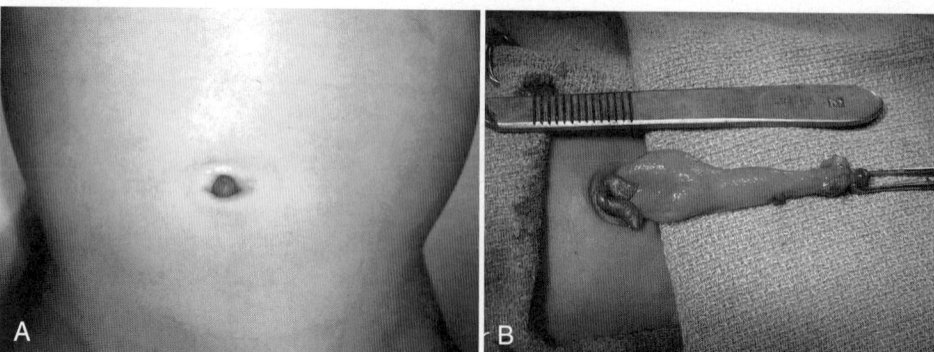

FIGURE 71-15 Omphalomesenteric duct remnant. A, Appearance of the umbilicus. **B,** Operative picture of wide patent remnant attached to anti-mesenteric side of the ileum.

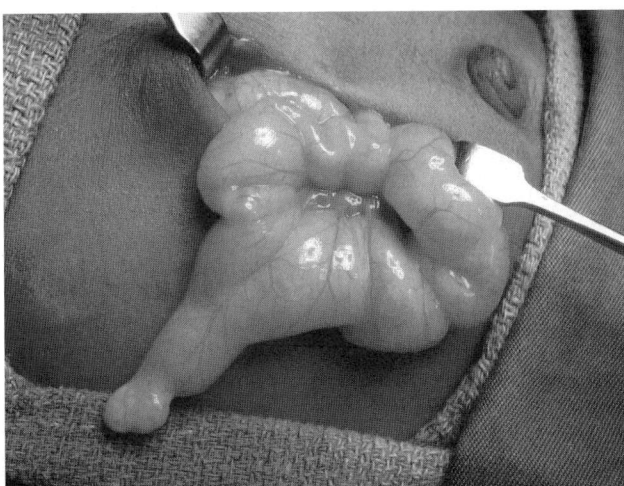

FIGURE 71-16 **Meckel's diverticulum.** Note the solid tip of the diverticulum, which probably is filled by ectopic gastric or pancreatic tissue.

condition has never been described in young infants. Hemorrhage is often sudden and catastrophic, causing a precipitous fall in the hematocrit and a shock-like state within a few hours. The first few stools passed may be composed almost entirely of unchanged blood; later, they become burgundy-colored and then tarry. In other instances, bleeding is constant and occult. About 25% of persons with Meckel's diverticulum present with intussusception.

Meckel's diverticulum must be differentiated from other disorders that produce gross bleeding from the bowel: peptic ulcer, enteric duplication, intestinal polyp, intussusception, and intestinal hemangioma. Anal fissure, proctitis, and ulcerative colitis ordinarily do not lead to gross hemorrhage, blood loss being confined to the passage of bloody mucus or of stools containing a surface accumulation of blood. The most useful point in the differential diagnosis is that hematemesis usually coexists with rectal bleeding when peptic ulcer is present, whereas hematemesis rarely occurs with Meckel's diverticulum. Enteric duplications are often palpable.

The diagnostic test of choice for Meckel's diverticulum is a technetium-99m pertechnetate scan ("Meckel scan"), which detects the ectopic gastric mucosa. This test is most useful in patients presenting with rectal bleeding—the false-negative rate is high in patients with other symptoms (Menezes et al, 2008). Pentagastrin or cimetidine is useful in enhancing the image of gastric mucosa on subsequent technetium scans.

Treatment

Resuscitation and blood replacement therapy is the initial treatment regardless of the cause of bleeding. If bleeding ceases, careful observation for recurrence of bleeding is often all that is indicated, because peptic ulcer rarely recurs. A second episode of bleeding, however, strongly suggests that other diagnostic procedures may be needed, including endoscopy, laparoscopy, and laparotomy. Surgical treatment is generally reserved for symptomatic diverticula and those thought to contain ectopic tissue (Snyder, 2007). Diverticulectomy is increasingly performed by laparoscopy.

SUGGESTED READINGS

Burbige KA, Amodio J, Berdon WE, et al: Prune-belly syndrome: thirty-five years of experience, *J Urol* 137:86-90, 1987.

Ein SH, Njere I, Ein A: Six thousand three hundred sixty-one pediatric inguinal hernias: a 35-year review, *J Pediatr Surg* 41:980-986, 2006.

Galati V, Donovan B, Ramji F, et al: Management of urachal remnants in early childhood, *J Urol* 180:S1824-S1826, 2008.

Islam S: Clinical care outcomes in abdominal wall defects, *Curr Opin Pediatr* 20:305-310, 2008.

Kitchanan S, Patole SK, Muller R, et al: Neonatal outcome of gastroschisis and exomphalos: a 10-year review, *J Paediatr Child Health* 36:428-430, 2000.

Lau ST, Lee YH, Caty MG: Current management of hernias and hydroceles, *Semin Pediatr Surg* 16:50-57, 2007.

Mann S, Blinman TA, Douglas Wilson R: Prenatal and postnatal management of omphalocele, *Prenat Diagn* 28:626-632, 2008.

Menezes M, Tareen F, Saeed A, et al: Symptomatic Meckel's diverticulum in children: a 16-year review, *Pediatr Surg Int* 24:575-577, 2008.

Snyder CL: Current management of umbilical abnormalities and related anomalies, *Semin Pediatr Surg* 16:41-49, 2007.

Suita S, Nagasaki A: Urachal remnants, *Semin Pediatr Surg* 5:107-115, 1996.

Complete references and supplemental color images used in this text can be found online at www.expertconsult.com

THE DEVELOPING INTESTINAL MICROBIOME:
IMPLICATIONS FOR THE NEONATE

Josef Neu, Christopher M. Young, and Volker Mai

The recent development of non–culture-based-techniques to evaluate the microbial genome is providing new insights into the relationship that exists between microbes and their mammalian hosts, especially the microbes that reside in the gastrointestinal (GI) tract (Gill et al, 2006). Using this technology has shown that the gene pool contributed by the gut microbiota vastly exceeds that of the human genome. It has been suggested that of the cells in the average human, only 10% are mammalian and the rest are microbial (Gill et al, 2006; Xu and Gordon, 2003). These organisms mostly reside within their host in a symbiotic and/or commensal manner. During the course of evolution, the host has developed defensive responses against microbes that are considered foreign, but at the same time has developed a mechanism that provides not only tolerance but a welcoming environment that benefits both microbes and the host (Bäckhed et al, 2005; Hooper, 2004; Hooper and Gordon, 2001; Hooper et al, 2002). This chapter provides an overview of the current knowledge of the intestinal microbiome and how it relates to neonatal and subsequent health via its interaction with the developing GI tract. Included is a brief description of new and developing technologies that are rapidly advancing this field. This chapter also provides brief overviews of several clinical aspects of microbe/host interaction, including basic interactions between the microbiome and the intestinal immune system; intrauterine and fetal life as it relates to premature labor; maternal and perinatal influences on postnatal health in the premature and term infant; and disease entities such as necrotizing enterocolitis (NEC) and sepsis.

THE MICROBIOME

BEYOND CULTURE

In 1683, Antonie van Leeuwenhoek wrote about his observations of the microorganisms associated with his own teeth. These were the first recorded observations of bacteria living in a human host (Gest, 2004). In the field of digestive physiology, it has long been known that microbes are abundant in the intestine, but they were initially considered to have no beneficial effect for the host. This concept is changing. New technologies are rapidly deepening our knowledge and appreciation of our microbial companions. These non–culture-based methods have shown that the majority of microbes in the intestine cannot be cultivated and isolated in culture with current methods. New information is emerging about the extensive role microbes play in human physiology, health, and disease. It is estimated that there are thousands of bacterial species within our bodies, most of them in our intestines. Recent studies have shown that the communities of microbes in the intestine have a profound effect on digestive physiology,

development, and health of the host (Dethlefsen et al, 2007; Gill et al, 2006; Hooper, 2004; Stappenbeck et al, 2002). This finding has led to the concept of a microbiome, which includes the microbiota and their complete genetic elements. The microbial metagenome is defined as the totality of microbes, their genetic elements (genomes), and their environmental interactions in a defined environment. A defined environment could, for example, be the gut of a human being or a soil sample.

Efforts to sequence the human intestinal microbiome are revealing a high degree of complexity, and additional technologies are emerging that will help to describe not only the composition of the human intestinal microbiota, but also the molecular, immunologic, and metabolic interactions that these organisms have with their host, along with their functional implications. The success of newly developed technologies has laid the groundwork for studies related to the Human Microbiome Project (Turnbaugh et al, 2007) that intend to further characterize the human microbiome as well as develop a better understanding of its role in health and disease.

NEW TECHNOLOGIES FOR ANALYSIS OF THE HUMAN MICROBIOME

Until the beginning of the last decade, culture-based techniques were the mainstay of evaluating intestinal microbes and still form the basis for diagnostic clinical microbiology. However, a majority of bacterial cells seen microscopically in feces cannot currently be cultured in the laboratory (Ben-Amor et al, 2005). The recently developed high-throughput molecular techniques analyze microbial DNA and RNA and can be divided into 16S rRNA–based and metagenomic approaches. The 16S rRNA gene is used as a stable phylogenetic marker to define which microbes are present in a sample and in what proportion (Pace, 1997). More complex metagenomic studies, in which community DNA is subjected to shotgun sequencing, can give additional insight into the metabolic potential of the microbiome (Rondon et al, 2000). A comprehensive review of these techniques is beyond the scope of this chapter, but we offer a brief summary of some of the more commonly used techniques in Table 72-1.

Both methods include the extraction of community DNA or RNA from feces or other samples of interest. The 16S rRNA is a part of the ribosomal RNA. It is commonly used for phylogenetic studies, because some regions of the gene encoding it are highly conserved and can act as primer binding sites, whereas other regions containing phylogenetic information are highly variable. As a result, various 16S rRNA–based methods have been incorporated into diagnostic clinical microbiology as a rapid, accurate alternative to phenotypic culture-based methods of bacterial identification.

TABLE 72-1   Summary of Selected 16S rRNA–Based Techniques Used for Identifying Intestinal Microbiota

Technique	Primary Function	Advantage(s)	Disadvantage(s)
DGGE/TGGE/ ARISA	Qualitative determination of dominant microbes and of overall microbiota diversity	Diversity analyses	Does not provide direct identification of microbes
Fluorescence in situ hybridization (FISH)	Quantitative analysis of total fecal bacteria and of targeted groups of bacteria	Analysis of targeted bacteria using specific probes Not based on PCR, thus free of PCR bias	Requires a priori knowledge of target bacterial 16S rRNA sequences for design of probes Only a few probes can be used for one analysis
16S rRNA pyroseqencing	Comprehensive analysis of 16S rRNA content in community DNA for detection of known as well as unknown bacteria	Provides a comprehensive overall analysis of microbes Currently one of the best techniques for identification of microbes that cannot be analyzed by culture-based methods	Currently very costly, but high-throughput, automated technology is increasing the efficiency and utility

Following DNA extraction from fecal samples, amplification of the targeted 16S rRNA genes can be achieved with universal polymerase chain reaction (PCR) primers capable of amplifying rRNA genes from most bacteria with similar efficiency. Alternatively, specific primers designed to amplify rRNA genes from a particular bacterial group of interest can be used to test for their presence by conventional PCR assay or to enumerate them using a quantitative PCR approach. PCR amplicons can also be sequenced using novel high-throughput pyrosequencing technology. Based on the degree of nucleotide similarity (usually between 95% and 99%), sequences can be separated into operational taxonomic units that form the basis for comparisons of microbiota composition and diversity between samples.

Profiling approaches include denaturing gradient gel electrophoresis (DGGE), temperature gradient gel electrophoresis (TGGE), and automated ribosomal interspacer analysis (ARISA) (Fisher and Triplett, 1999; Muyzer, 1999). These techniques allow for an efficient qualitative initial profiling of microbiota composition that can be applied to large studies. In DGGE, DNA isolated from fecal samples and variable region(s) of the 16S rRNA are amplified with universal or group specific primers, one of which contains a GC clamp to facilitate stronger adherence of the two DNA strands (PCR) (Muyzer, 1999). The products are then separated on a denaturing gradient gel that achieves separation of same-sized DNA fragments present in the mixed pool of DNA fragments based on the differences in melting characteristics that are due mainly to varying GC content. The resulting separated bands can be cut and eluted from the gel, followed by sequencing to identify the bacterial group or species that contributed to the template DNA. These fingerprinting methods, although efficient for initial screening, are limited in that only the most abundant members of the community can be observed.

Currently any in-depth analysis of microbial community composition, such as that present in the intestine, takes advantage of high-throughput sequencing for both 16S rRNA and metagenomic approaches, mainly through 454 illumina sequencing (Tringe and Hugenholtz, 2008). This technique allows for the simultaneous identification of the bacterial lineages that are present in a complex community DNA sample at a depth that exceeds conventional Sanger sequencing by many fold. An in-depth description goes beyond the scope of this chapter but can be obtained at http://www.454.com. Briefly, a PCR amplification step occurs in microreactors (emulsions) surrounding microbeads. The amplified DNA can then be sequenced based on the light-emitting pyrosequencing technique. Sequences from multiple samples can be barcoded and pooled, reducing the sequencing cost per sample. Sequences can then be classified according to taxonomy (16S) and function (metagenomics). Sequencing is especially useful when determining which specific species, genes, or pathways differ between communities.

Another molecular technique that does not require PCR or sequencing, fluorescence in situ hybridization (FISH), uses group- or species-specific labeled probes designed with data previously derived from sequencing (Zoetendal et al, 2004) to quantify microbiota composition. The probes are tagged with a 5′ fluorescent dye that permits both detection and quantification of the specific bacterial populations. Other microbiota analysis approaches include short sequence tags (Fisher and Triplett, 1999) and microarrays (He et al, 2007). The latter approach was recently used by Palmer et al (2007) to track development of the human intestinal microbiota in infancy.

All of these techniques have advantages and disadvantages including various biases. Cutting costs of the more in-depth sequencing techniques and data analysis using advanced bioinformatics tools remains a huge challenge.

THE "OMES"

The foregoing discussion underlines the fact that the human organism is composed of and controlled by not only its mammalian genetic complement (human genome) but also the microbial genetic component (microbiome). These synergize with the environmental factors, such as nutrition, to make up the epigenome, proteome, transcriptome, and metabolome. Alterations in the intestinal microbiome have been linked to numerous pathologic processes and conditions such as obesity, autoimmune diseases, allergy, asthma, eczema, and even the induction of premature labor, some of which are described in this chapter. The role of intestinal microbes, especially during early development in these highly interrelated components, is in its early phases of understanding but is clearly related to human health and disease and is fertile for future investigation (Turnbaugh and Gordon, 2008).

ACTIVITIES OF THE INTESTINAL MICROBIOME

Using the aforementioned techniques, the investigation of the biomes and how they interact within the intestine is becoming progressively more feasible. The human meta-organism contains a prokaryotic component in the intestine that comprises nearly 10^{14} (Muyzer, 1999) cells that weigh over 1 kg in the adult. There is a marked aboral gradient in the number and types of microbes in different regions of the intestine, with 10^{11} (Ben-Amor et al, 2005) in the ascending colon, 10^{7-8} (Dethlefsen et al, 2007; Gest, 2004) in the distal ileum, and 10^3 (Bäckhed et al, 2005; Xu and Gordon, 2003) in the jejunum. A better understanding of many of the activities of the microbiota in the GI tract (Box 72-1) is emerging. Here we describe functional aspects of the microbiome and interactions with the intestinal epithelium by anatomic site: the small intestine primarily as the site of immunoreactivity and the large intestine functioning as a bioreactor (Neish, 2009).

INFLAMMATION AND IMMUNITY

The intestinal microbes represent a key regulatory element for the appropriate development of the adaptive immune system and also for the innate inflammatory response. For the innate component, the intestinal epithelium partially relies on various receptors, such as the Toll-like receptors (TLRs), to act as an interface between the luminal microbiota and signal transduction pathways. As various studies have shown, TLRs are cell-surface receptors that recognize specific microbial ligands from both pathogens and commensals, enabling the innate immune system to recognize nonself and activating both innate and adaptive immune responses (Takeda et al, 2003). Nucleotide-binding oligomerization domains (NODs) have a similar function with recognition of foreign molecules within the cellular compartment. These studies suggest that the epithelium and resident immune cells do not simply tolerate commensal microorganisms but are dependent on them for the appropriate induction of immune responses. Commensal bacteria contain a variety of molecules such as lipopolysaccharide (LPS), lipoteichoic acid, and short nucleotide multimers that, on lysis of bacteria, can interact in the normal intestine with a population of surface TLRs.

The resultant ongoing signaling enhances the ability of the epithelial surface to withstand injury while also priming the surface for enhanced repair responses (Madara, 2004; Strober, 2004). Therefore, either the disruption of TLR signaling or the removal of TLR ligands compromises the ability of the intestinal surface to protect and repair itself in the face of inflammatory or infectious insult (Rakoff-Nahoum et al, 2004).

THE BIOREACTOR FUNCTION

Complex carbohydrates are poorly digested by the human digestive system and require the intestinal microbiota for breakdown via fermentation. In the distal intestine, primarily the proximal colon, the intestinal microbiome is highly metabolically active; these activities might best be studied using metabolomic methodologies. The fermentation end products include short-chain fatty acids (SCFAs) such as acetate, propionate, and butyrate. The SCFAs influence various aspects of intestinal physiology beyond being a main caloric source, especially for the epithelial colonocytes (they supply an estimated 5–15% of human energy requirements). The various SCFAs possess differentiating and growth-promoting activities that are thought to be related to their effects on histone deacetylase activity; they may also have epigenetic effects. SCFAs have immunomodulatory effects and major effects on the interepithelial tight junctions. Examples of processes that can be mediated via the gut microbiota's metabolic functions include how differences in the microbial population affect obesity, non–insulin-dependent diabetes, and atherosclerosis (Ley et al, 2006). In the distal intestine, primarily the colon, undigested complex carbohydrates in the weaned individual are primarily vegetable fibers, whereas in the infant, it is primarily undigested human milk oligosaccharide and in some cases, primarily very preterm infants, nonabsorbed lactose. Thus, even if there is a deficiency of lactase activity in the small intestine of very premature neonates, a healthy distal intestinal flora is able to "salvage" some of the undigested lactose into absorbable and usable two- to four-carbon energy sources (Figure 72-1) (Kien, 1996).

DEVELOPMENT OF THE INTESTINAL MICROBIOME

THE FETAL MICROBIOME AND PRETERM BIRTH

Preterm birth is a leading cause of infant death and also major lifelong health problems, which include cerebral palsy and neurodevelopmental delays, vision loss, and GI problems related to short-gut syndrome. There appear to be several predisposing factors for preterm birth, but one component that clearly plays a role is the so-called fetal inflammatory response syndrome (FIRS).

Emerging evidence suggests that microbes may play a role in premature labor through interactions with fetal intestine that result in an inflammatory immune response (Figure 72-2). This hypothesis is supported by (1) the association between microbial colonization of the amniotic fluid, FIRS, and premature labor (Andrews et al, 1995; Bobitt and Ledger, 1997; Goldenberg et al,

2008; Romero et al, 1988, 1998, 2007), (2) the observation that the fetus swallows large quantities of amniotic fluid during the late second and third trimesters of pregnancy (Brace and Wolf, 1989; Gilbert and Brace, 1993), and (3) the induction of systemic inflammation to be derived from the GI tract (Carrico et al, 1986), especially that of the fetus in utero (Nanthakumar et al, 2000). Recent studies using non–culture-based techniques reveal a significant prevalence of microbes in amniotic fluid that cannot be readily cultured using standard laboratory techniques (DiGiulio et al, 2008; Han et al, 2009). These observations are in contrast to results from earlier culture-based studies that did not detect microbial presence in amniotic fluid and can be rationalized by the conclusion that in the amniotic fluid of many women who deliver prematurely, there are bacteria present that have not previously been cultured by standard techniques. Furthermore, it has been suggested that a greater degree of prematurity is associated with the 16S rRNA bacterial load in the amniotic fluid, even in the absence of ruptured membranes (DiGiulio et al, 2008).

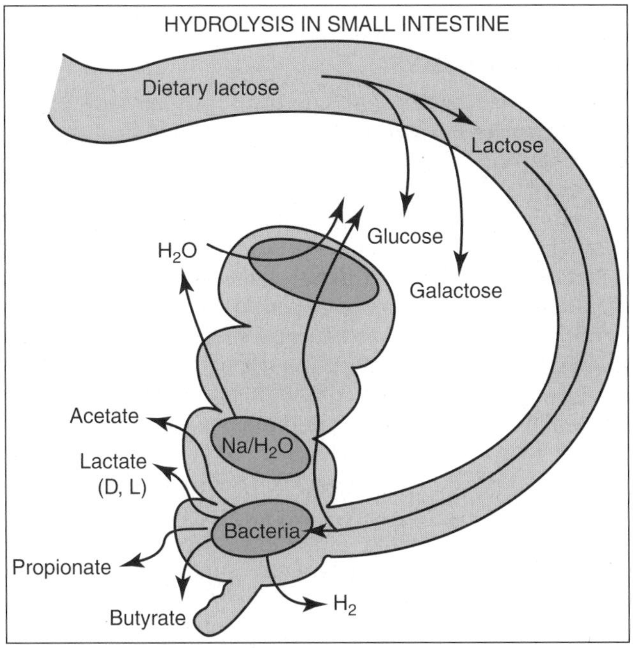

Although the inflammatory mediators that are related to premature delivery could originate from the placenta, the fetal GI tract is a more likely origin of the inflammatory response and to our knowledge has not been previously implicated in FIRS. Evidence for a fetal origin stems from several studies, including the original findings of elevated proinflammatory cytokines obtained by cordocentesis (Gomez et al, 1998; Pacora et al, 2002; Romero et al, 2007), suggesting a fetal origin. The fact that the white blood cells found in amniotic fluid are predominantly of fetal origin is also germane (Sampson et al, 1997). More recent studies underscore the important role of the fetus in initiation of the cascade of responses causing premature labor.

This concept of the fetal intestinal origin of FIRS stems from the observation that the fetus is known to swallow large quantities of amniotic fluid (Brace and Wolf, 1989; Gilbert and Brace, 1993). This amniotic fluid subsequently reaches the fetal distal small intestine, an organ that was initially found in rodents to be significantly more sensitive to inflammatory stimuli than more mature intestines (Chan et al, 2002). In humans, the fetal intestine has also been found to respond to stimuli such as LPS even more robustly than more mature intestine (Nanthakumar et al, 2000). The fact that the intestine has been called the "motor that drives systemic inflammation and multiple organ failure" (Carrico et al, 1986) is highly relevant to our hypothesis because this "motor" could be driving the fetal inflammatory response that leads to premature labor. This fetal inflammatory response not only is critical in terms of premature labor, but has also been linked to other morbidities affecting multiple organ systems in the neonate (Dammann et al, 2001, 2002; Gotsch et al, 2007; Nelson et al, 1998; Yoon et al, 2003, 2000).

FIGURE 72-1   Fate of unhydrolyzed lactose in the intestine. Dietary lactose that is not hydrolyzed and absorbed in the small intestine passes to the distal intestine, where it is broken down into the short-chain fatty acids acetate, propionate, and butyrate, which can act as substrates for energy production and play other important roles such as controlling proliferation and differentiation and maintaining integrity of intercellular junctions.

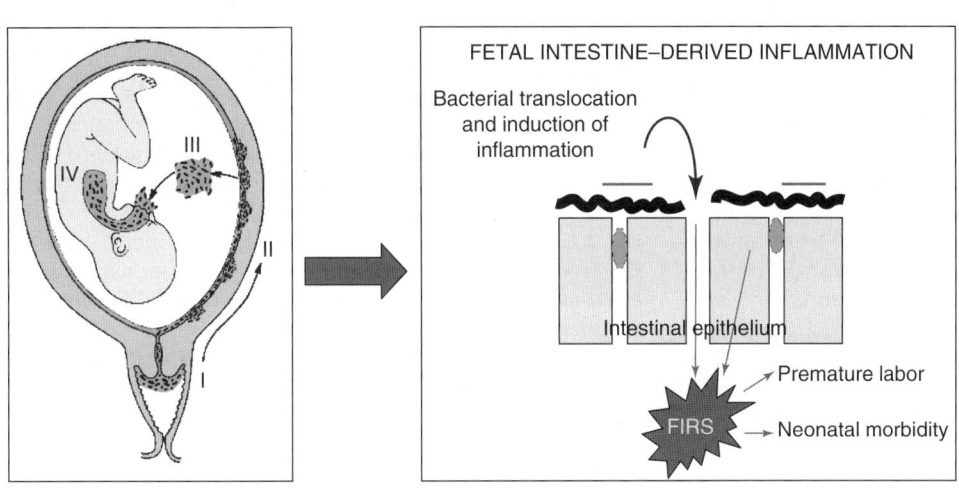

FIGURE 72-2   Proposed fate of microbes in amniotic fluid. Microbes in amniotic fluid are swallowed by the fetus, and these in turn can be translocated through the intestinal epithelium and incite inflammation that may affect distal organs as well as potentially incite uterine contraction and premature delivery.

THE PREMATURE INFANT MICROBIOME

The microbial population of the developing GI tract of the premature infant affects maturation and optimal function of the intestinal innate and adaptive immune system. Because a major role has been ascribed to systemic (usually intestine derived) inflammation on several neonatal diseases including NEC, chronic lung disease, intraventricular hemorrhage, periventricular leukomalacia, and hematopoietic abnormalities, factors that may modulate these responses originating in the intestine are of interest.

Over the past few years, a body of literature has emerged supporting that overproduction of interleukin-8 (IL-8) is a critical, and arguably the most important, component of the systemic inflammatory response in neonates. The role of IL-8 in chorioamnionitis, intracerebral hemorrhage, and lung disease is compelling (De Dooy et al, 2001; Kohse et al, 2002; Shalak et al, 2002; Tauscher et al, 2003; Yoon et al, 2003). High concentrations of IL-8 are frequently noted in the plasma and affected tissues of patients who exhibit these problems. This leukocyte chemoattractant chemokine, which can be produced in large quantities by the intestine, has thus been causally linked to some of these problems, implying that modulation of intestinal production of IL-8 may be a key to prevention. It is notable that infant intestine appears to be much more sensitive to stimuli, such as LPS and flagellin that induce IL-8, than is adult intestine (Claud et al, 2004; Nanthakumar et al, 2000). The relationship of this and other inflammatory mediators and the intestinal microbiota as they relate to neonatal inflammatory conditions remains to be elucidated.

NUTRITION AND THE DEVELOPING INTESTINAL MICROBIOME

A more specific understanding of the neonatal intestinal microecology as it relates to inflammatory mechanisms may lead to measures that can prevent diseases. In the premature infant, the reliance on parenteral nutrition while providing few or no enteral nutrients may be highly significant in the promotion of intestinal inflammation, because the presence of enteral nutrients can prevent gut-derived inflammation (Kudsk, 2002). Whether this is partially due to stimulation of commensal bacterial growth is speculative. Several in vitro studies have shown that probiotics (live, heat-killed, and DNA from probiotic bacteria) can downregulate intestinal IL-8 production (Bai et al, 2004; Jijon et al, 2004; Li et al, 2009; Lopez et al, 2008; Ma et al, 2004; Rachmilewicz et al, 2004; Zhang et al, 2005) induced by proinflammatory stimuli such as LPS.

Human milk contains a wide array of biologically active components. The growth of pathogenic bacteria and viruses is known to be inhibited by proteins such as lactoferrin, secretory IgA, and peptides formed from human milk during digestion (Lonnerdal, 2004). Human milk is an important factor in the initiation, development, and composition of the neonatal gut microbiota. It has been found to be a significant source of lactic acid bacteria that appear to be of endogenous origin and not contaminants from the breast skin (Martin and Walker, 2006; Perez et al, 2007). The lactobacillus isolated from milk of healthy mothers is phylogenetically related to strains commonly used in commercial probiotic products and shares characteristics such as survival in GI tract conditions, production of antimicrobial compounds, adherence to intestinal cells, production of biogenic amines, and patterns of antibiotic resistance. Among the numerous substances present in human milk, some of the oligosaccharides have a prebiotic effect, stimulating the development of bifidobacteria in the colon (Coppa et al, 2004). Breastfed infants, unlike those who are formula fed, have an intestinal ecosystem characterized by a strong prevalence of bifidobacteria and lactobacilli (Bourlioux et al, 2003; Saavedra, 2001). Human milk can be considered a synbiotic (Coppa et al, 2004), because it contains live beneficial bacteria (probiotics) as well as nutrients that can enhance their growth (prebiotics).

PROBIOTICS

Probiotics are dietary supplements of live microorganisms thought to be healthy for the host organism. According to the currently adopted definition by FAO/WHO, probiotics are "live microorganisms which, when administered in adequate amounts, confer a health benefit on the host" (FAO/WHO, 2001). There is an increasing body of evidence supporting the health benefits of probiotics for premature infants. The decrease in NEC incidence and overall mortality reported from a small number of these studies has catalyzed the routine use of these agents. However, sufficient evidence of both short- and long-term safety and health effects beyond infancy is lacking.

CONCERNS ABOUT ADMINISTRATION OF LIVE MICROBES (PROBIOTICS)

Despite the large body of evidence supporting the health benefits of probiotics, several concerns have been raised about the possibility of unwanted side effects. This concern is especially valid in sick patients or very young individuals where microbiota manipulation may result in adverse effects (Besselink et al, 2008; Boyle et al, 2006; Honeycutt et al, 2007; Neu, 2007; Singhi, 2007; Taylor et al, 2007). Another key issue concerns the safety aspects of bacteria added to particular products marketed for improvement of general health or treatment of (post) infectious symptoms. In some cases, virulence potential has been detected in probiotic bacterial strains. There is also concern that horizontal gene transfer can result in acquisition of virulence genes or antimicrobial resistance in probiotic bacteria (Wassenaar et al, 2008). Antimicrobial resistance in these probiotic bacteria can potentially aid the spread of undesired resistance in intestinal bacterial populations.

One of the known mechanisms of probiotics is the capability of modulating an overaggressive inflammatory response (Claud et al, 2004; Neish, 2002; Zhang et al, 2005), but under certain circumstances probiotics may actually incite an inflammatory response of their own, especially in highly susceptible individuals (Boyle et al, 2006; Liong, 2008). There is some concern that probiotic bacteria may translocate to the locally draining tissues and circulatory system, causing bacteremia, especially in immunocompromised individuals. Contrary to some of the initial studies that demonstrated positive benefits of probiotics in patients with atopic dermatitis, considerable controversy is rising, as studies are beginning to show that there may be detrimental effects at later stages of life (Boyle et al, 2008). For example, in one study supplementation with *Lactobacillus rhamnosus* GG during pregnancy and early infancy neither reduced the incidence of atopic dermatitis nor altered its severity in affected children, but was associated with an increased rate of recurrent episodes of wheezing bronchitis (Kopp and Ghosh, 1995).

Despite justified enthusiasm for the beneficial use of probiotics in premature infants for the prevention of NEC based on randomized controlled trials (Bin-Nun et al, 2005; Lin et al, 2005), data from one of the most recent multicenter trials suggests that the group with the smallest infants with birthweights (<750 g) may actually be at *increased* risk for sepsis (12 infants in the probiotic group and 1 infant in the control group developed sepsis) when given prophylactic probiotics (Lin et al, 2008).

There is concern that probiotics may establish inappropriate residence in the gut that prevents normal colonization of other microflora in the GI tract, resulting in subsequent alteration of normal immune system development (Neu, 2007). There is also concern that manipulation before establishment of a normal core microbiome in newborns may incur risks such as consequences of imbalanced fermentation profiles (Neu, 2007).

These concerns prompt consideration of alternative agents such as prebiotics, which are usually indigestible oligosaccharides that prompt growth of resident (and, it is hoped, beneficial) microorganisms. "Postbiotics," products of microbial fermentation, such as the SCFAs acetate, propionate, and butyrate, may also provide beneficial effects (Roy et al, 2006). Accumulating evidence suggests that other small molecules derived from lysed microorganisms (usually molecules acting on Toll-like and other signal transduction receptors in the intestinal epithelium, dendritic cells, and other immunoreactive intestinal cells) may confer the same benefits as probiotics without incurring the risks associated with a live organism.

CONCLUSION

The ongoing revolution in microbial genomics and metabolomics as applied to the developing intestinal microbiota provides exciting avenues for studying basic scientific processes and applications to the prevention and treatment of diseases. We are just beginning to scrape the surface of the potential application of this emerging science as it pertains to the newborn infant. The relationship of the developing microbiome to intestinal development, nutrition, inflammation, the immune system, and how it relates to numerous diseases in the infant as well as subsequent health in the adolescent and adult is rapidly emerging. It is likely that our understanding of the developing microbiome will offer revolutionary means to prevent disease and promote future health.

SUGGESTED READINGS

Bäckhed F, Ley RE, Sonnenburg JL, et al: Host-bacterial mutualism in the human intestine, *Science* 307:1915-1920, 2005.

Carrico CJ, Meakins JL, Marshall JC, et al: Multiple-organ-failure syndrome. The gastrointestinal tract: the "motor" of MOF, *Arch Surg* 121:196-208, 1986.

Claud EC LL, Anton PM, Savidge T, et al: Developmentally regulated IκB expression in intestinal epithelium and susceptibility to flagellin-induced inflammation, *Proc Natl Acad Sci U S A* 101:7404-7408, 2004.

Dethlefsen L, McFall-Ngai M, Relman DA: An ecological and evolutionary perspective on human-microbe mutualism and disease, *Nature* 449:811-818, 2007.

DiGiulio DB, Romero R, Amogan HP, et al: Microbial prevalence, diversity and abundance in amniotic fluid during preterm labor: a molecular and culture-based investigation, *PLoS ONE* 3:33056, 2008.

Hooper LV: Bacterial contributions to mammalian gut development, *Trends Microbiol* 12:129-134, 2004.

Lopez M, Li N, Kataria J, et al: Live and ultraviolet-inactivated *Lactobacillus rhamnosus* GG decrease flagellin-induced interleukin-8 production in Caco-2 cells. *J Nutr* 138:2264-2268, 2008.

Madara J: Building an intestine: architectural contributions of commensal bacteria, *N Engl J Med* 351:1685-1686, 2004.

Neish AS: The gut microflora and intestinal epithelial cells: a continuing dialogue, *Microbes Infect* 4:309-317, 2002.

Rakoff-Nahoum S, Paglino J, Eslami-Varzaneh F, et al: Recognition of commensal microflora by toll-like receptors is required for intestinal homeostasis, *Cell* 118:229-241, 2004.

Strober W: Epithelial cells pay a Toll for protection, *Nat Med* 10:898-900, 2004.

Turnbaugh PJ, Gordon JI: An invitation to the marriage of metagenomics and metabolomics, *Cell* 134:708-713, 2008.

Complete references and supplemental color images used in this text can be found online at www.expertconsult.com

NECROTIZING ENTEROCOLITIS AND SHORT BOWEL SYNDROME

Michael Caplan

NECROTIZING ENTEROCOLITIS

Necrotizing enterocolitis (NEC) is an acute inflammatory necrosis of the bowel that primarily afflicts preterm infants. Although there is significant geographic variation, the incidence ranges between 7% and 10% for infants born weighing less than 1500 g. Of the infants in whom NEC develops, the mortality rate ranges from 25% to 30%, and up to 50% receive a surgical procedure. NEC survivors have a significant risk for gastrointestinal complications such as intestinal stricture or short bowel syndrome (SBS), and the risk for abnormal neurodevelopmental outcome is significantly increased, particularly in patients with NEC requiring surgery. Although still under investigation, it appears that probiotic supplementation in high-risk premature infants may significantly reduce the risk of disease in this fragile population.

EPIDEMIOLOGY AND PATHOGENESIS

The incidence of NEC varies geographically and temporally; it ranged between 2% and 22% in an NICHD observational study of very low-birthweight (VLBW) infants (Uauy et al, 1991) and was reported to be 28% in Hong Kong (Siu et al, 1998), 14% in Argentina (Halac et al, 1990), and 7% in a cohort of <2000-g preterm infants from Austria (Eibl et al, 1988). Although NEC is infrequent in full-term infants (5% to 10% of reported cases), in this population it is often associated with other conditions such as congenital heart disease, birth asphyxia, polycythemia, exchange transfusion, or intrauterine growth restriction (Bolisetty and Lui, 2001). In preterm infants, the incidence of NEC varies inversely with gestational age and birthweight, and studies suggest a higher incidence in boys and African-American infants (Ryder et al, 1980).

The age at onset of NEC is inversely related to gestational age, with a mean age of 3 to 4 days for term infants and 3 to 4 weeks for infants born at less than 28 weeks' gestation. Most patients with NEC have been previously fed via the enteral route. Although NEC does occur in unfed premature infants, spontaneous intestinal perforation (SIP), a distinct pathologic entity, commonly presents in extremely low-birthweight (ELBW) infants during the first couple of weeks after birth and before the initiation of feeding (Gordon, 2009; Swanson et al, 2009). Patients with SIP present earlier and seem to have a better prognosis than those who develop the clinical and pathologic hallmarks of NEC (Table 73-1).

NEC cases typically present sporadically and without warning in neonatal intensive care units, but occasionally are associated with epidemics related to a specific pathogen. A wide variety of organisms have been associated with these outbreaks, including *Klebsiella pneumoniae*, *Escherichia coli*, clostridia, coagulase-negative staphylococci, and rotavirus. It is currently hypothesized that NEC is not directly caused by infectious agents, but the presence of abnormal microbial flora with additional risk factors of bowel ischemia, immaturity of host mucosal defense, and enteral feedings is thought to contribute to the initiation and pathogenesis of disease, presumably due to the activation of the inflammatory response (Frost et al, 2008).

Bowel Ischemia

Early observations suggested that profound intestinal ischemia led to intestinal necrosis similar to NEC in situations associated with birth asphyxia and shock associated with other conditions. Similar to the "diving reflex" observed in aquatic mammals, it was hypothesized that in periods of stress, blood flow was diverted away from the splanchnic circulation, resulting in bowel injury (Touloukian et al, 1972). Neonatal animals have been shown to have abnormal regulation of the intestinal circulation that may predispose them to NEC. The basal intestinal vascular resistance is elevated in the fetus and soon after birth decreases significantly, allowing for the rapid increase in intestinal blood flow that is necessary for robust intestinal and somatic growth (Nowicki and Miller, 1988). It has been shown that this change in the resting vascular resistance is dependent on the balance between dilator (nitric oxide) and constrictor (endothelin) mediators and the myogenic response, and altered levels of these vasoactive mediators are observed in human patients with NEC (Nowicki et al, 2005, 2007). In response to circulatory stress, neonates respond with compromised intestinal flow and/or vascular resistance. In response to hypotension, newborn animals (3-day-old but not 30-day-old swine) appear to have defective pressure-flow autoregulation, resulting in compromised intestinal oxygen delivery and tissue oxygenation (Nowicki and Minnich, 1999). There are multiple chemical mediators (nitric oxide, endothelin, substance P, norepinephrine, and angiotensin) that affect intestinal vasomotor tone, and in the stressed newborn, abnormal regulation of these may result in compromised circulatory autoregulation, leading to perpetuation of intestinal ischemia and tissue necrosis.

Clinical factors associated with altered intestinal blood flow might influence the risk for NEC. Umbilical arterial catheters might pose a threat to the intestinal vasculature, although there is no clear data that demonstrate a higher risk for NEC in patients with these devices (Davey et al, 1994). The presence of the patent ductus arteriosus (PDA) and a left-to-right shunt results in compromised blood flow to the intestine during diastole. In a randomized, controlled trial in infants whose birthweights were less than 1000 g, prophylactic closure of the ductus arteriosus by surgical ligation reduced the rate of NEC from 30% in the control group, compared with 8% in the early-closure group

TABLE 73-1 Clinical Differences between Necrotizing Enterocolitis (NEC) and Spontaneous Intestinal Perforation (SIP)

	NEC	SIP
Incidence <1500 g	7–10%	2–3%
Age at onset	2–6 weeks	0–14 days
Pneumatosis	Yes	No
Enteral feedings	Yes	No
Histologic evidence of villus necrosis	Yes	No
Mortality	10–30% above baseline	5–10% above baseline

(Cassady et al, 1989). Other studies suggest that treatment of the PDA with indocin, rather than the PDA itself, increases the risk for disease due to the effects of indocin on the intestinal circulation (Fowlie, 2000). Maternal cocaine use can cause fetal intestinal vasoconstriction and, in some animal studies and preterm human observational trials, is associated with an increased risk for NEC (Kilic et al, 2000). Finally, recent studies have suggested an association between packed red blood cell transfusions and an increased risk for NEC, and in these patients it is surmised that the rapid correction of significant anemia may influence intestinal vascular autoregulation (Mally et al, 2006).

Host Defense Factors

As reviewed in Chapter 70, host defense in the preterm gastrointestinal tract is markedly impaired. In order to prevent pathogens from invading the mucosal lining and causing invasive infection, intestinal host defense is exceedingly complex and includes (1) physical barriers such as skin, mucous membranes, intestinal epithelia and microvilli, epithelial cell tight junctions, and mucin; (2) immune cells such as polymorphonuclear leukocytes, macrophages, eosinophils, and lymphocytes; and (3) multiple biochemical factors. Intestinal permeability is impaired in the neonate, and especially the preterm neonate, and allows immunoglobulins, proteins, and carbohydrates to traverse into the systemic circulation (Piena-Spoel et al, 2001). Intestinal mucus, a complex gel consisting of water, electrolytes, mucins, glycoprotein, immunoglobulins, and glycolipids, protects against bacterial and toxin invasion and is abnormal in developing animals and perhaps premature infants (Clark et al, 2006). Additionally, key bacteriostatic proteins are secreted from epithelium that bind to or inactivate the function of invading organisms. Human defensins and intestinal trefoil factor are proteins that are developmentally regulated and might play a role in the development of NEC (Salzman et al, 2007; Shi et al, 2007).

Immunologic factors that contribute to host defense are compromised in developing animals. For example, intestinal intraepithelial lymphocytes (IELs) are decreased in neonates (B and T cells) and do not approach adult levels until 3 to 4 weeks of life (Kuo et al, 2001). Newborns have markedly reduced secretory immunoglobulin A (IgA) in salivary samples, reflecting the decreased activity presumed in intestine (Eibl et al, 1988). Breast milk feeding provides significant

supplementation; formula-fed neonates have impaired intestinal humoral immunity, and this deficiency may predispose to the increased incidence of infectious diseases and NEC noted in this population. Of interest, oligosaccharides have recently been added to neonatal formula to approximate human milk, and this supplementation appears to increase secretory IgA as well as alter the microbial flora to resemble that observed in a breastfed infant; it could also influence the development of intestinal infection and inflammation (Scholtens et al, 2008).

Multiple biochemical factors contribute to the maintenance of gut health and integrity, and many are suppressed in the preterm newborn patient or animal. Critical factors that appear to influence mucosal homeostasis include lactoferrin (Yen et al, 2009), glutamine (Neu, 2001), growth factors such as epidermal growth factor (EGF) (Halpern et al, 2006a), heparin-binding (HB)-EGF (Feng et al, 2006), transforming growth factor (TGF) (Claud et al, 2003), insulin-like growth factor (IGF) (Ozen et al, 2005), erythropoietin (EPO) (Ledbetter and Juul, 2000), gastric acid, polyunsaturated fatty acids (Carlson et al, 1998; Lu et al, 2007), nucleotides, and many others. These factors contribute to gut maturation and regulation of the inflammatory cascade, a complex system that is altered in the neonate and are discussed in detail in a subsequent section.

Because NEC occurs less frequently among infants fed breast milk, and because breastfeeding appears to protect infants from a number of diseases, numerous investigators have attempted to delineate the factors in breast milk that contribute to neonatal host defense. As detailed in Chapter 65, breast milk contains immunoglobulins, leukocytes, and numerous antibacterial agents that are not present in artificial cow's milk–based formula. In a variety of animal studies and human trials, supplementation with substances present in human milk has reduced the risk for NEC, including IgA/IgG, leukocytes, lactoferrin, polyunsaturated fatty acids, platelet-activating factor (PAF)-acetylhydrolase, EGF, HB-EGF, and EPO (see references just given).

Enteral Feeding

Most infants who develop NEC have begun enteral feeding. The mechanism whereby feeding promotes the initiation of disease is not clear, although reports have suggested potential mechanisms such as osmolar stress (Willis et al, 1977), by-product synthesis of toxic short-chain fatty acids (Nafday et al, 2005), intestinal distention following rapidly advancing feeding volumes leading to abnormal vascular regulation, activation of gut hormones and mediators, and altered bile acid metabolism (Halpern et al, 2006b). Early studies suggested that delaying the initiation of feeding reduced the incidence of NEC; however, more recent reports have not confirmed these observations, and multiple trials to evaluate the safety and benefit of early hypocaloric feedings suggest that these are well tolerated and provide beneficial effects (Tyson and Kennedy, 2000). Nonetheless, these studies have not been appropriately powered to identify an increased rate of NEC, and in one trial the prolonged use of small enteral feeding volumes for the first 10 feeding days reduced the incidence of NEC compared to infants whose feeding volumes were increased daily by 20 mL/kg/day increments (Berseth et al, 2003). Precise recommendations regarding feeding volumes, time of feeding initiation and advancement, fortification strategies, and feeding strategies during times of additional risk factors such as PDA, indocin treatment, and the presence of an umbilical arterial catheter will require additional information.

BACTERIAL COLONIZATION AND THE PRO-INFLAMMATORY RESPONSE

As compared to full-term, nursing infants, who have a rich diversity and large quantities of bacteria colonizing their distal intestinal tracts, preterm infants have significantly fewer bacterial species and numbers, and less diversity (Gewolb et al, 1999; Palmer et al, 2007). Of interest, a recent study demonstrated that patients with NEC had even less microbial diversity than gestational age–matched controls, suggesting that the total bacterial milieu might influence the development of intestinal injury in this population (Wang et al, 2009). Although commensal organisms that promote intestinal health and protect against inflammatory responses are prominent in full-term neonatal flora, as in older children and adults, in preterm infants these organisms, including *Bifidobacteria* spp. and *Lactobacillus* spp., are distinctly uncommon (Gewolb et al, 1999). These features of the bacterial flora unique to the VLBW infant are thought to initiate pro-inflammatory signaling in the context of formula feeding, intestinal ischemic stress, and deficient host mucosal immune responses.

It is now well recognized that bacteria and other pathogens initiate a complex signaling cascade via the binding to and activation of specific pattern recognition receptors, called human Toll-like receptors (TLRs), that are present on most cells and tissues (Akira and Hemmi, 2003; Gribar et al, 2008). In the case of gram-negative enteric bacteria such as *Escherichia coli*, cell wall lipopolysaccharide (LPS) activates the specific TLR4 on inflammatory and immune cells, and a series of signal transduction events ultimately result in the nuclear translocation of nuclear factor kappa B (NF-κB) and transcription of proinflammatory genes such as interleukin (IL)-1, IL-8, tumor necrosis factor, inducible nitric oxide synthase (iNOS), and phospholipase A_2. These mediators have been shown to be elevated in preterm infants with NEC, and they ultimately result in a robust inflammatory response (Caplan et al, 1990b; Edelson et al, 1999; Harris et al, 1994). Although proinflammatory activation appropriately protects against bacterial invasion at the mucosal environment in normal circumstances, in the setting where antiinflammatory signaling is inadequate, overzealous responses can lead to intestinal inflammation and necrosis.

It is theorized that the premature infant is more prone to proinflammatory signaling without balanced antiinflammatory responses following bacterial-TLR activation, and that these differences contribute to the pathogenesis of NEC. When counterregulatory responses are insufficient, pathologic changes to gut mucosa occur and may include accentuated apoptosis of epithelial cells (Jilling et al, 2004), perturbation of tight junctional proteins and complexes (Clark et al, 2006), increased mucosal permeability (Langer et al, 1993), bacterial translocation (Deitch et al, 1991), alterations of vascular tone and microcirculation (Reber et al, 2002), and additional neutrophil infiltration

and accumulation leading to intestinal necrosis. Specific alterations in neonatal anti-inflammatory responses have been identified, and include (1) propensity to synthesize IL-8 in response to bacterial stress (Claud et al, 2004); (2) deficiency in PAF-acetylhydrolase activity, the degrading enzyme for PAF, a potent phospholipid mediator shown to initiate mucosal injury (Caplan et al, 1990a); and (3) increased activity of intestinal NF-κB due to inhibition of inhibitory protein IκB (De Plaen et al, 2007). Recent studies have shown that although epithelial cells normally do not express TLR4 on the mucosal surface, in stressed neonatal animals and in preterm infants with NEC, TLR4 expression is upregulated on the apical surface of epithelial cells (Jilling et al, 2006; Leaphart et al, 2007). This finding may further explain the robust and unusual proinflammatory response observed in neonates with necrotizing enterocolitis. Finally, because epidemiologic studies suggest an increased risk of disease depending on gender, race, and twin siblings of affected patients (Holman et al, 1997), single-nucleotide polymorphisms have been evaluated in this context, and polymorphisms of several inflammatory genes have been identified that might lead toward a predilection of NEC (Young et al, 2009).

CLINICAL PRESENTATION

The clinical signs and symptoms of NEC are variable and can include abdominal distention, vomiting or increased gastric residuals, bilious drainage from enteral feeding tubes, or hematochezia, and in some cases tenderness and discoloration (Figure 73-1). Frequently present are nonspecific systemic signs that may include temperature instability, apnea, lethargy, poor perfusion, or hypotension. Similar to patients with septic shock who demonstrate a robust inflammatory response, NEC patients can have abnormal white blood cell counts, thrombocytopenia, capillary leak, intravascular volume depletion, metabolic acidosis, acute tubular necrosis, respiratory failure, hypotensive shock, and death.

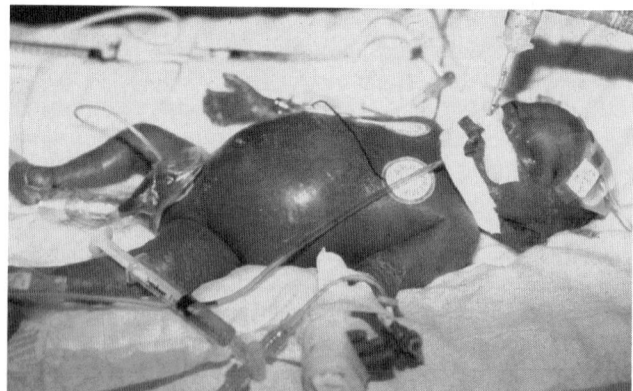

FIGURE 73-1 Clinical presentation of a preterm infant with necrotizing enterocolitis. This infant was born at 28 weeks' gestation and had been receiving enteral feedings for 1 week when he developed acute abdominal distention, hematochezia, and vomiting. Note the discoloration of the skin overlying the abdomen. Also, this infant required endotracheal intubation because of respiratory compromise that occurred as a result of the upward pressure of the abdominal contents on the diaphragm. *(Courtesy Dr. Lalo Cabrera-Meza, Baylor College of Medicine, Houston, Texas.)*

TABLE 73-2   Modified Bell's Staging Criteria for Necrotizing Enterocolitis

Stage	Systemic Signs	Intestinal Signs	Radiologic Signs	Treatment
I: Suspected				
A	Temperature instability, apnea, bradycardia	Elevated pregavage residuals, mild abdominal distention, occult blood in stool	Normal or mild ileus	NPO, antibiotics × 3 days
B	Same as for IA	Same as for IA, plus gross blood in stool	Same as for IA	Same as for IA
II: Definite				
A: Mildly ill	Same as for IA	Same as for I, plus absent bowel sounds, abdominal tenderness	Ileus, intestinal pneumatosis	NPO, antibiotics × 7–10 days
B: Moderately ill	Same as for I, plus mild metabolic acidosis, mild thrombocytopenia	Same as for I, plus absent bowel sounds, definite abdominal tenderness, abdominal cellulitis, right lower quadrant mass	Same as for IIA, plus portal vein gas, with or without ascites	NPO, antibiotics × 14 days
III: Advanced				
A: Severely ill bowel intact	Same as for IIB, plus hypotension, bradycardia, respiratory acidosis, metabolic acidosis, disseminated intravascular coagulation, neutropenia	Same as for I and II, plus signs of generalized peritonitis, marked tenderness, and distention of abdomen	Same as for IIB, plus definite ascites	NPO, antibiotics × 14 days, fluid resuscitation, inotropic support, ventilator therapy, paracentesis
B: Severely ill, bowel perforated	Same as for IIIA	Same as for IIIA	Same as for IIB, plus pneumoperitoneum	Same as for IIIA, plus surgery

From Walsh MC, Kliegman RM, Fanaroff AA: Necrotizing enterocolitis: a practitioner's perspective, *Pediatr Rev* 9:225, 1988. Reproduced with permission from *Pediatrics*.
NPO, Nulla per os (nothing by mouth).

The diagnostic radiographic hallmark of NEC is the presence of pneumatosis intestinalis, and this finding has been clearly established as a critical diagnostic criterion in the staging system suggested by Bell et al and modified by Walsh and Kliegman (Bell et al, 1978; Walsh and Kliegman, 1986) (Table 73-2). Pneumatosis represents gas accumulation in the bowel wall that includes hydrogen gas that is produced from bacterial metabolism of carbohydrate substrate (Figure 73-2). Portal venous gas is also diagnostic of NEC even in the absence of pneumatosis intestinalis, and early studies suggested that this presentation carried a worse prognosis (Figure 73-3) (Molik et al, 2001). If NEC progresses to bowel perforation, pneumoperitoneum may be identified. Most typically, free air is visualized on a cross-table lateral or right lateral decubitus film (Figure 73-4). Occasionally, free air can be visualized as a central periumbilical collection on an anteroposterior film—the "football sign" (see Figure 73-4, *B*). Recent studies have demonstrated that ultrasonographic findings of pneumatosis and portal venous air are easily appreciated by the trained observer, and that abdominal ultrasound imaging may allow for earlier and more precise diagnosis, and in cases of medical NEC that improve, quicker advancement toward enteral feeding (Bohnhorst et al, 2003; Dordelmann et al, 2008).

TREATMENT

Medical Management

The medical management of NEC is focused on providing aggressive supportive care, because no specific interventions have been shown to limit the progression of disease. Initial treatments include the discontinuation of enteral feedings, decompression of intestinal contents with nasogastric drainage, and broad-spectrum antibiotic therapy. Antibiotic regimens should cover typical nursery enteric flora and may include ampicillin/aminoglycoside, ampicillin-cephalosporin, or, in settings with frequent staphylococcal colonization, vancomycin-aminoglycoside. Although only 20% to 30% of NEC cases identify positive blood cultures (Kliegman and Fanaroff, 1984), treatment usually continues for 7 to 10 days even with sterile blood cultures; however, the utility of this approach has not been carefully studied. Because NEC is an inflammatory process that results in substantial third-space fluid loss, liberal use of volume support may be needed during the first 48 to 72 hours of treatment, even without overt intravascular volume depletion. In addition to the aggressive use of fluids and volume expanders such as albumin, pressor agents such as dopamine may be required to maintain the infant's blood pressure and peripheral perfusion. Because many infants with NEC develop apnea or respiratory compromise owing to abdominal distention and upward compression on the diaphragm, intubation and ventilatory support may be required. Frequent monitoring of blood gases, complete blood counts, electrolytes, and serum glucose is essential in these critically ill patients, who develop metabolic acidosis, hyperkalemia, thrombocytopenia, neutropenia, hyper- or hypoglycemia, and anemia with disseminated intravascular coagulation.

Surgical Management

Despite optimal neonatal intensive care, between 10% and 30% of patients with NEC will succumb to this disease (Badowicz and Latawiec-Mazurkiewicz, 2000; Lin and

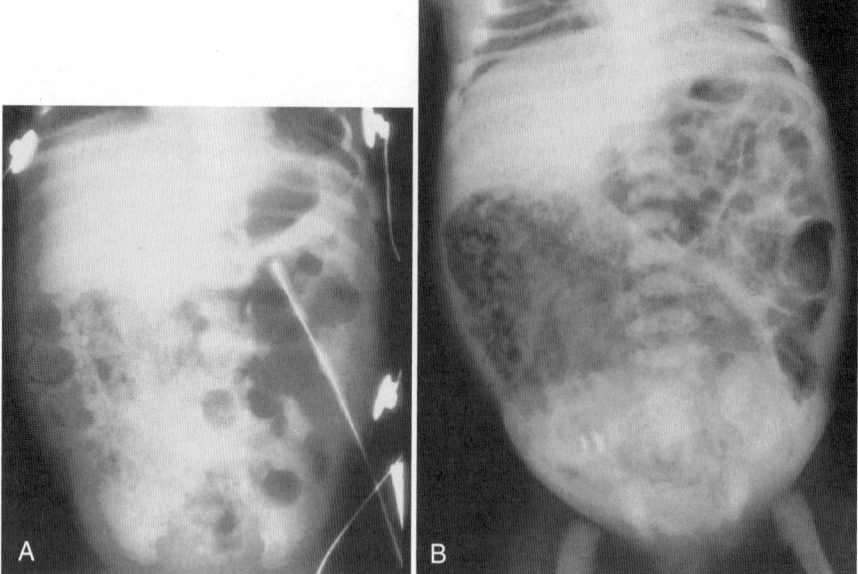

FIGURE 73-2 **A,** Typical abdominal radiographic appearance of intestinal pneumatosis seen in necrotizing enterocolitis: dark concentric rings around the bowel loops in the right upper quadrant. **B,** This radiograph displays the *bubbly gas* pattern occasionally seen in necrotizing enterocolitis. *(Courtesy Dr. Lalo Cabrera-Meza, Baylor College of Medicine, Houston, Texas.)*

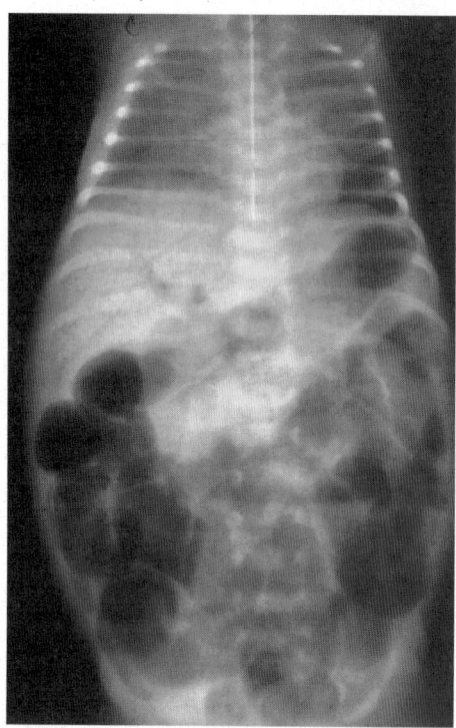

FIGURE 73-3 This radiograph displays the presence of portal gas, which is seen as linear dark streaks within the hepatic density. *(Courtesy Dr. Lalo Cabrera-Meza, Baylor College of Medicine, Houston, Texas.)*

obtained by paracentesis, but none of these are absolute. The goals of surgery are to resect necrotic bowel, to decompress the intestine and free intraperitoneal air, and to preserve as much bowel length as possible.

Because surgical intervention does not appear to alter the progression of ongoing inflammation and disease, the timing, benefit, and approach for surgery in NEC cases remains controversial. Although most physicians agree that a procedure is indicated in a case of NEC with perforation, the utility and effectiveness of these interventions have not been well studied. Yet, it is thought that decompression with a percutaneous drain might be as effective as an exploratory laparotomy. A peritoneal drain allows for decompression of intraabdominal gas that might impede respiratory function and, in these situations, appears to provide time for natural healing to occur. In several studies, including an observational prospective trial (Blakely et al, 2006), a randomized trial (Moss et al, 2006), and an international randomized trial (Rees et al, 2008), there were no differences in effect between peritoneal drain and laparotomy on mortality or short-term gastrointestinal function in cases of NEC with perforation, or NEC with worsening clinical signs and symptoms. Of note, in these studies, many patients with a percutaneous drain never required additional surgical exploration, suggesting that definitive intervention was not required and in fact might not alter the outcome of the disease.

LONG-TERM COMPLICATIONS

Although more than 70% of patients with NEC survive, long-term gastrointestinal complications include intestinal strictures and SBS. Strictures result from fibrotic healing of inflamed intestine and occur in 10% to 35% of patients with medical and surgical disease (Horwitz et al, 1995). Patients with strictures typically develop recurrent abdominal distention 2 to 3 weeks after recovery from NEC, but

Stoll, 2006). One third of the patients present with a milder form of disease that resolves with medical therapy alone, and approximately 50% of cases require surgical intervention. The most common indication for surgery is the presence of pneumoperitoneum. Other indications may be the presence of clinical deterioration despite aggressive medical therapy, the presence of a fixed dilated loop of bowel on serial radiographs, and evidence of peritonitis and gangrenous bowel

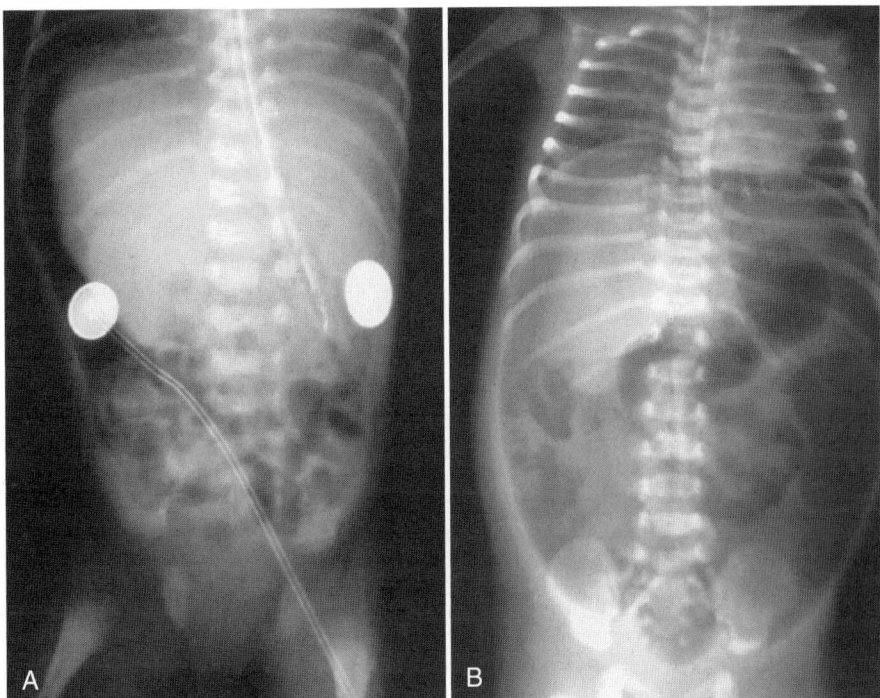

FIGURE 73-4 A, This radiograph demonstrates intestinal perforation as displayed by the presence of a gas lucency that lies between the hepatic density and the outer abdominal wall. **B,** This radiograph is from another infant whose bowel is perforated. In **B,** air lies anterior to the loops of intestine as well as along the right abdominal wall, where it is displacing loops of bowel medially. *(Courtesy Dr. Lalo Cabrera-Meza, Baylor College of Medicine, Houston, Texas.)*

these can be diagnosed months or years after the initial presentation (Figure 73-5). Many cases can be managed medically, but if the narrowing is severe, surgical resection is often required.

SBS occurs when inadequate bowel remains following NEC with or without surgery to allow normal growth on enteral nutrition. Although there is controversy regarding the amount of bowel length needed to support adequate growth, it is estimated that infants require a minimum of 25 to 40 cm of viable small intestine (Galea et al, 1992). As outlined in a subsequent section, medical and surgical management must address issues related to malabsorption, bacterial overgrowth, and alterations in intestinal transit.

Neurodevelopmental impairment (NDI) is observed with increased frequency following the diagnosis of NEC in premature infants. In a series of observational trials, the risk of cerebral palsy and/or mental retardation in afflicted patients is as high as 57% compared with gestational age– and birthweight-matched controls with much lower rates, and patients with surgical NEC have a 1.8 relative risk of NDI compared with age-matched controls (Hintz et al, 2005). The etiology of this serious long-term complication is thought to be related to white matter injury following systemic inflammatory activation and/or nutritional deficiencies associated with prolonged lack of enteral nutrition. Further studies are needed to define the pathogenesis and to establish preventive approaches, but caution should be used in counseling parents of these high-risk patients.

PREVENTIVE STRATEGIES

Because the onset of NEC is typically acute and disease progresses rapidly, no therapeutic intervention introduced after confirmation of the diagnosis has been efficacious.

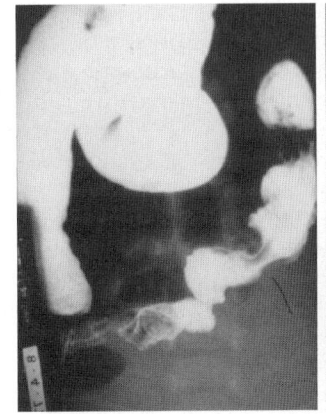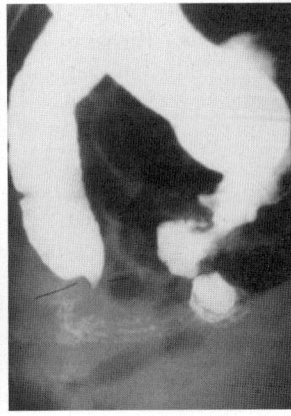

FIGURE 73-5 This barium study was obtained in an infant who had recovered from necrotizing enterocolitis and was experiencing intermittent episodes of abdominal distention when enteral feedings were given. Note that multiple areas of stricture are present. *(Courtesy Dr. Lalo Cabrera-Meza, Baylor College of Medicine, Houston, Texas.)*

Nonetheless, many approaches have been attempted to prevent NEC in animal and human studies, but there are no currently accepted strategies that are deemed standard-of-care, besides judicious human milk feeding. Nonetheless, although human milk feeding for preterm infants in neonatal intensive care units throughout the United States has increased dramatically over the past decade, there has not been a reduction in the overall incidence of NEC, and therefore new preventive strategies are desperately needed. Lower rates of NEC have been shown in animal models following breast milk feeding (Dvorak et al, 2004), IgA supplementation (Barlow et al, 1974), antibiotic prophylaxis, steroids (Israel et al, 1990), probiotics (Caplan et al, 1999; Siggers et al, 2008), polyunsaturated fatty acids (Lu et al, 2007), PAF antagonists (Caplan et al, 1997a), PAF-acetylhydrolase (Caplan et al, 1997b), EGF (Dvorak et al, 2008), trefoil factor (Shi et al, 2007), leukocyte depletion (Sun et al, 1996), bile acid transport inhibitors (Halpern et al, 2006b), and oxygen radical scavengers (Cueva and Hsueh, 1988). In human studies, prevention trials with IgA/IgG (Eibl et al, 1988), steroids (Halac et al, 1990), polyunsaturated fatty acids (Carlson et al, 1998), arginine (Amin et al, 2002), donor human milk (Lucas and Cole, 1990), and antibiotics (Siu et al, 1998) have been conducted with limited success, but because of various problems, including poor study design, risks of intervention, lack of reproducibility, and weak statistical power, these approaches have yet to become routine strategies in the neonatal intensive care unit for preterm infants. A recent study suggests that lactoferrin, an iron transport protein that has additional antiinflammatory and antimicrobial activity, not only reduces the risk of late-onset sepsis in preterm infants, but also might lower the incidence of NEC.

Probiotic supplementation is a promising approach for the prevention of NEC in VLBW infants (Caplan, 2009). Studies suggest that probiotic colonization in VLBW infants is abnormal, and multiple biologic mechanisms have been identified that could explain their effects on proinflammatory signaling and disease (Walker, 2008). There have now been several international trials that demonstrate the efficacy of probiotic prophylaxis for the prevention of NEC (Bin-Nun et al, 2005; Dani et al, 2002; Hoyos, 1999; Lin et al, 2005, 2008; Samanta et al, 2009; Walker, 2008), and although the specific probiotic species and dosing varies between studies, the cumulative results identified a reduction in NEC from 142 of 2143 controls (6.6%) to 53 of 2093 treated patients (2.5%, p <0.01). Despite these exciting results, additional studies are warranted before clear standard-of-care can be recommended, because of some potential concerns. First, probiotic preparations have not been carefully regulated, and because some studies have shown inaccuracies in the reported organism species and content, appropriate quality control measures are warranted. Second, various probiotic species have differing effects, and the optimal probiotic combination and optimal dosing strategy are not clearly elucidated. Third, recent studies have shown potential harm with probiotic prophylaxis, with increased mortality in critically ill adult patients with pancreatitis (Besselink et al, 2008), and increased asthma in childhood (Kalliomaki et al, 2007). Finally, although probiotic sepsis has not been observed in the NEC prevention trials, careful culturing strategies are not routinely used, and studies have now identified probiotic sepsis in neonatal patients in other clinical situations, so appropriate vigilance is essential.

SHORT BOWEL SYNDROME

The normal small intestine length in the term infant is 200 to 300 cm. The most common causes of short gut in the newborn is bowel resection after NEC, midgut volvulus, or congenital anomalies such as jejunal or ileal atresia and gastroschisis. Thus, newborns most typically have a short gut characterized by losses of ileum and the ileocecal valve (ICV). Estimates suggest that 25 cm of bowel with

an intact ICV and 42 cm without an ICV is the minimum for successful survival and adaptation in full-term neonates (Galea et al, 1992). Nonetheless, the diagnosis of SBS is made using functional criteria rather than on actual gut length, and typically is based on the prolonged need for parenteral nutrition for more than 6 weeks (Ching et al, 2007).

SBS is more common in VLBW infants observed in the neonatal intensive care unit setting, and most of these are due to NEC (96%). Information from a recent cohort identified that 0.7% of these patients had SBS, and it was more common in ELBW infants, boys, and patients that were small for gestational age (Cole et al, 2008). Follow-up of these patients demonstrated, not surprisingly, an increased risk for death and at, 18 to 22 months of life, an increased need for tube feedings, rehospitalization, and growth delay.

TREATMENT

Multidisciplinary care is essential for patients with SBS and requires parenteral and enteral nutritional support, management of ongoing medical issues including cholestasis, in some cases surgical intervention with intestinal lengthening procedures, and occasionally intestinal or intestinal/hepatic transplantation (Goulet et al, 2009; Gupte et al, 2006).

Because bile salts, fat-soluble vitamins, and trace minerals are absorbed in the distal ileum, infants with SBS are prone to steatorrhea and specific vitamin and mineral deficiencies. Cholestyramine, an ion-exchange resin that binds bile salts, often is used to reduce steatorrhea. Fat malabsorption is common, and replacements should be provided with careful monitoring. Recent reports suggest that patients with SBS and severe cholestasis on complete intravenous nutrition are deficient in omega-3 fatty acids, and that intravenous fish oil supplementation can markedly improve the clinical status of these patients, particularly in regard to liver failure (Gura et al, 2008). Deficiencies of vitamins A, D, E, K, and B_{12} as well as zinc and magnesium all have been described in infants with short gut. Therefore, levels of all of these substrates should be monitored and supplemented appropriately.

Bacterial overgrowth can occur as a result of reflux of colonic contents into the distal ileum in the absence of an ileocecal valve, in abnormal peristalsis, or in the presence of fistulas (Cole and Ziegler, 2007). Bacterial overgrowth can impair fat and vitamin B_{12} absorption and depress mucosal function, resulting in malabsorption and profound diarrhea. Symptomatic improvement with antibiotic regimens such as metronidazole or vancomycin may occur, and recently clinicians have utilized probiotics for this clinical situation (De Groote et al, 2005).

Tolerance of enteral feedings with adequate growth is not easily achieved in many cases. In a recent report, remaining bowel length and plasma bilirubin level correlated with ultimate success in transitioning from intravenous to enteral feeding (Nucci et al, 2008). To enhance mucosal growth and improve bowel function, the use of additives such as glutamine and IGF-1 has been attempted, with equivocal results (Chu et al, 2004). One recent report showed benefit with EGF in five patients with SBS, particularly on nutrient absorption, but without beneficial effects on weight gain or liver function tests (Sigalet et al, 2005).

Although most infants can be managed medically until intestinal adaptation occurs, approximately 10–15% are dependent on total parenteral nutrition. Several surgical options are available for this group of patients (Hosie et al, 2006; Javid et al, 2005; Misiakos et al, 2007). Techniques include reversal of a small segment of bowel to slow transit, tapering or plicating dilated loops of intestine to improve motility, and intestinal lengthening procedures such as Bianchi's isoperistaltic doubling and Kimura's isolated segments technique. Experience with these procedures remains limited, and their associated complication and failure rates are high; still, they constitute a less invasive option than intestinal transplantation, which can be considered for selected patients. A review by one center reported a 3-year survival rate of 60% for intestinal transplantation used in SBS patients following the diagnosis of NEC (Vennarecci et al, 2001). Because of the lack of adequate donors and the guarded long-term prognosis for these complex patients, individual decision making is difficult and requires the coordinated efforts of multiple health care professionals in selected centers.

SUGGESTED READINGS

Caplan MS: Probiotic and prebiotic supplementation for the prevention of neonatal necrotizing enterocolitis, *J Perinatol* 29:S2-S6, 2009.

Gordon PV: Understanding intestinal vulnerability to perforation in the extremely low birth weight infant, *Pediatr Res* 65:138-144, 2009.

Gribar SC, Anand RJ, Sodhi CP, Hackam DJ: The role of epithelial Toll-like receptor signaling in the pathogenesis of intestinal inflammation, *J Leukoc Biol* 83:493-498, 2008.

Lin PW, Stoll BJ: Necrotising enterocolitis, *Lancet* 368:1271-1283, 368.

Misiakos EP, Macheras A, Kapetanakis T, Liakakos T: Short bowel syndrome: current medical and surgical trends, *J Clin Gastroenterol* 41:5-18, 2007.

Young C, Sharma R, Handfield M, et al: Biomarkers for infants at risk for necrotizing enterocolitis: clues to prevention? *Pediatr Res* 65:91R-97R, 2009.

Complete references used in this text can be found online at www.expertconsult.com

DISORDERS OF THE LIVER

Frederick J. Suchy and Nanda Kerkar

Liver disease in the newborn has long been a challenge, and can present with a clinical spectrum ranging from asymptomatic abnormalities on liver biochemical tests to fulminant hepatic failure. Cholestasis is usually present, because of the immaturity of hepatic excretory function (Balistreri, 2002). Indeed, there are more distinct and unique causes of cholestatic jaundice in the neonate than at any other time of life (Suchy, 2004). The ability to make a specific diagnosis is complicated by similar clinical and biochemical features of neonatal liver disease caused by congenital malformations, inborn errors of metabolism, genetic cholestatic syndromes, and perinatal infections. Early diagnosis may allow treatment of some metabolic or infectious disorders and surgical management of biliary anomalies.

APPROACH TO THE NEWBORN WITH LIVER DISEASE

Jaundice persisting beyond 2 weeks is considered to be prolonged jaundice. Cholestasis is present if more than 20% of an elevated total bilirubin is conjugated. The common causes of neonatal cholestasis are listed in Boxes 74-1 and 74-2 and in Table 74-1. The amount of blood that can be drawn from a small infant is limited, and hence it is important to prioritize laboratory tests based on the clinical scenario, including whether the infant is sick with/without liver failure, is premature in the neonatal intensive care unit, or is a relatively well term infant.

In an infant with liver failure, effort should be focused on excluding life-threatening, treatable causes of liver dysfunction such as sepsis, neonatal hemochromatosis, metabolic/endocrine problems, and bleeding from vitamin K deficiency. History of consanguineous marriages and neonatal deaths should be solicited. Bacterial infections with both gram-positive and gram-negative organisms and viral infection with herpes simplex or an enterovirus should be excluded, especially if there is concern about sepsis. Neonatal hemochromatosis is a rare but important cause of liver failure in infancy that is diagnosed by demonstrating iron deposition in extrahepatic areas, particularly salivary gland (buccal biopsy) and heart/pancreas (magnetic resonance imaging [MRI]). If the cholestatic infant is also hypoglycemic and/or hypotensive, endocrine problems such as hypopituitarism or metabolic problems such as galactosemia should be considered, and excluded by pituitary function tests and galactose-1-phosphate uridyl transferase enzyme analysis. Nonketotic hypoglycemia is usually indicative of fatty acid oxidation defects, and acyl carnitine profile is a good screening test. Tyrosinemia and inborn errors of bile acid metabolism can lead to liver failure, and testing urine for organic acids and abnormal bile acid metabolites can be diagnostic. Sometimes liver failure can be part of a systemic disease, that is, mitochondrial disease—lactic acidosis is characteristic, and the pH and lactate/pyruvate ratio should be tested in such infants.

BOX 74-1   Infections Associated With Neonatal Liver Disease

BACTERIAL AND PARASITIC

Bacterial sepsis
Syphilis
Listeriosis
Tuberculosis
Urinary tract infection
Toxoplasmosis
Malaria

VIRAL

Cytomegalovirus
Herpes (simplex, zoster, human herpes virus 6)
Rubella
Reovirus
Adenovirus
Enteroviruses
Parvovirus B6
Syncytial giant cell hepatitis with paramyxoviral-like inclusions
Hepatitis B
Hepatitis E

BOX 74-2   Biliary Tract Disorders of the Newborn

Biliary atresia
Choledochal cysts
Spontaneous perforation of the common bile duct
Mucous plug syndrome
Neonatal sclerosing cholangitis
Paucity of intrahepatic bile ducts (nonsyndromic)
Alagille syndrome
Caroli's disease/syndrome
Cystic fibrosis
Idiopathic bile duct stricture (possibly congenital)
Cholelithiasis
Acute cholecystitis
Chronic cholecystitis
Acalculous cholecystitis
Acute hydrops of the gallbladder

Infants with liver failure often are listed for liver transplantation, but it is important to rapidly establish that there are no contraindications for transplantation, such as sepsis, systemic disease, or hemophagocytic lymphohistiocytosis. The last should be suspected if there is fever in association with liver failure, characteristically with pancytopenia, hypofibrinogenemia, and hypertriglyceridemia. The bone marrow histology is useful in ruling out storage disorders such as Niemann-Pick disease and Gaucher's disease.

If the infant is a stable premature infant, the duration of total parenteral nutrition, the lack or amount of enteral feeding, episodes of sepsis, medications causing cholestasis

TABLE 74-1   Inborn Errors of Metabolism With a Neonatal Hepatic Phenotype

Disorder	Defect	Clinical Features
Galactosemia*	Galactose-1-phosphate uridyl transferase	Jaundice, hepatomegaly, vomiting, hypoglycemia, *Escherichia coli* sepsis
Tyrosinemia*	Fumarylacetoacetate hydrolase	Jaundice, hepatosplenomegaly, failure to thrive, ascites, coagulopathy, and rickets
Fructosemia	Fructose-1,6-biphosphate aldolase	Vomiting, hypoglycemia, and hypophosphatemia, hepatomegaly jaundice on exposure to fructose
Niemann-Pick disease type C	Defective lipid trafficking/storage	Cholestasis, hepatomegaly, fetal ascites, neurodegeneration
Gaucher disease type 2	Acid β-glucosidase	Cholestasis, hepatomegaly, neurodegeneration
α₁-Antitrypsin deficiency	α₁-Antitrypsin	Cholestasis
Bile acid synthetic defects	Multiple enzymatic defects	Cholestasis, liver failure, fat-soluble vitamin deficiencies
Mitochondrial respiratory chain defects	Complexes I, III or IV, or mtDNA depletion/mutation	Liver failure, lactic acidosis, multisystem disease
Citrin deficiency	Mitochondrial aspartate-glutamate transporter	Cholestasis, coagulopathy, failure to thrive, hypoglycemia, fatty liver, hyperaminoacidemia
Disorders of fatty acid oxidation*	Multiple enzymatic and transport defects	Nonketotic hypoglycemia, cholestasis, coagulopathy, multisystem disease
Glycogen storage diseases	Multiple enzymatic defects	Hepatomegaly, hypoglycemia, hyperuricemia in type 1, hyperlipidemia, lactic acidosis
Wolman disease	Lysosomal acid lipase	Cholestasis, hepatomegaly, vomiting, diarrhea, adrenal calcifications
Zellweger's syndrome	Peroxisomal biogenesis	Cholestasis, hepatomegaly, severe neurologic dysfunction, hypotonia, craniofacial abnormalities

*Detected by newborn screening in some states.

including trimethoprim-sulfamethoxazole, cephalosporin, anticonvulsants, and episodes of significant hypoxia or hypotension should be carefully assessed. Inspissated bile syndrome is the transient conjugated hyperbilirubinemia that occurs during the recovery phase of hemolysis, when it appears that the bilirubin is conjugated more rapidly that it can be excreted (Hickey and Power, 1956). In the term infant, presence of dark urine and acholic stools should raise the index of suspicion for an obstructive cause of jaundice—biliary atresia, choledochal cyst, or biliary stricture. Older infants may have pruritus; failure to thrive; bleeding from vitamin K deficiency; problems related to fat malabsorption such as steatorrhea and vitamin A, D, E, and K deficiency; and complications related to portal hypertension such as ascites, gastrointestinal bleeding, and hypersplenism. During the physical examination, syndromic features should be looked for—Alagille syndrome and Down syndrome are associated with cholestasis. Laboratory investigations include complete blood count, international normalized ratio, liver function tests with fractionated bilirubin, α₁-antitrypsin phenotype, thyroxine, thyroid-stimulating hormone, cortisol, iron, ferritin, immunoreactive trypsin, galactose-1-phosphate uridyl transferase, cholesterol, triglycerides, TORCH, hepatitis B virus, parvovirus, human immunodeficiency virus, serum and urinary organic acids, amino acids, and bile acid metabolites (Suchy, 2004). In the sick infant, blood glucose, lactate, ammonia, pH, paracentesis, and blood and urine culture are also necessary. A chest x-ray and abdominal ultrasonography should be requested. If there is history of meconium ileus, screening tests for cystic fibrosis should be performed. If cholestasis is associated with a low serum γ-glutamyl transpeptidase, then progressive familial

intrahepatic cholestasis or a bile acid synthetic defect are high in the differential diagnosis. Liver biopsy is essential in persistent cholestatic jaundice, unless the infant's condition precludes the procedure. Bone marrow biopsy and skin fibroblast culture may be necessary in storage disorders. Hepatobiliary scintigraphy, endoscopic retrograde cholangiopancreatography, and MRI may also be helpful in select cases. Exploratory laparotomy and intraoperative cholangiogram is the gold standard for diagnosis of biliary atresia.

INFECTIONS OF THE LIVER IN THE NEWBORN

Idiopathic neonatal hepatitis should be considered an obsolete and misleading term that was once used to denote the process of intrahepatic cholestasis and giant cell transformation of hepatocytes (Balistreri, 2002; Balistreri and Bezerra, 2006). It is now recognized that multinucleated giant cells are a prototypical response of the immature liver to a wide range of injuries, including biliary obstruction, infection, and metabolic diseases. A disorder should now be designated as neonatal hepatitis only if an infectious disorder has been documented or considered likely on the basis of other clinical features associated with congenital infection (Balistreri, 2002; Balistreri and Bezerra, 2006). Box 74-1 lists the infectious disorders that can be associated with neonatal hepatitis and includes the complex of toxoplasmosis, rubella, cytomegalovirus, herpes, and others designated by the acronym *TORCH*. Specific culture, serologic studies and approaches in molecular microbiology such as the polymerase chain reaction are used to establish a specific diagnosis.

BACTERIAL INFECTIONS

Cholestatic jaundice has long been associated with severe bacterial infections in the neonate (Balistreri, 2002). Both gram-positive and gram-negative organisms have been implicated. Cholestasis results from the effects of circulating endotoxin from bacteria that significantly alters the expression of transporters that contribute to bile formation. The release of cytokines in response to the infection also impairs hepatobiliary function. Septicemia is often present, but cholestasis can also be observed with urinary tract infections in the absence of a positive blood culture (Garcia and Nager, 2002). Liver dysfunction rapidly improves with appropriate antibiotic therapy.

CONGENITAL SYPHILIS

Despite routine maternal screening, congenital syphilis remains a significant perinatal infection that should be considered in the differential diagnosis of any neonate with hepatitis (Walker and Walker, 2007). Florid cases with typical findings in bone, skin, central nervous system, and liver may be obvious to the clinician, but milder cases may present with hepatitis, skin rash, and failure to thrive with or without a purulent nasal discharge. Hepatosplenomegaly is usually present (Chakraborty and Luck, 2008). Laboratory studies reveal modest elevation of serum aminotransferases and conjugated hyperbilirubinemia. Liver biopsy usually shows a diffuse mononuclear cell infiltration and a dissecting lobular fibrosis. Spirochetes may be identified using silver stains. A definitive diagnosis can be made by finding spirochetes in exudates from skin or mucosal lesions on dark field microscopy or a direct fluorescent antibody test. The well-known nontreponemal antibody tests (VDRL, rapid plasma reagin [RPR], and automated RPR test [ART]) should be positive. The fluorescent treponemal antibody absorption and *Treponema pallidum* particle agglutination tests should provide a presumptive diagnosis. Treatment with penicillin is highly effective. Liver dysfunction may take several months to resolve (Long et al, 1984).

CYTOMEGALOVIRUS

Congenital cytomegalovirus (CMV) infection affects 1% to 2% of newborns, but only about 10% of infected infants are symptomatic at birth with intrauterine growth retardation, microcephaly, intracerebral calcifications, jaundice, retinitis, and hepatosplenomegaly. Fetal ascites and hydrops may occur (Kenneson and Cannon, 2007). Conjugated hyperbilirubinemia and elevated aminotransferase values are typical (Fischler et al, 1999). Liver biopsy may show giant cell transformation, portal inflammatory infiltrates, extramedullary hematopoiesis, bile ductular proliferation, and portal or interstitial fibrosis. Large intranuclear inclusions are typically found in bile duct epithelium and to a lesser extent in hepatocytes.

Perinatal infection with CMV may also occur in infants as early as 3 weeks of age from exposure to maternal secretions, from ingestion of breast milk, or from blood products (Capretti et al, 2009; Kenneson and Cannon, 2007). Although most babies are asymptomatic, a sepsis-like condition can occur with hepatosplenomegaly, elevated serum aminotransferases, pneumonitis, leukopenia, and thrombocytopenia. Very low-birthweight infants are particularly prone to develop symptomatic illness (Capretti et al, 2009).

CMV may be isolated from multiple sites including the nasopharynx, urine, peripheral blood leukocytes, and liver tissue (Maine et al, 2001; Mendelson et al, 2006). Detection of the viral genome in urine or serum by PCR may be used to diagnose congenital and perinatal CMV infection (Soetens et al, 2008).

Ganciclovir has been used to treat some congenitally and perinatally infected infants, but its efficacy and safety in this age group remain unsettled. Infants with severe systemic disease including hepatitis may benefit (Ozkan et al, 2007). Although some treated infants have had improvement or maintenance of normal hearing when tested later, the effect on liver disease remains to be demonstrated (Fischler et al, 2002). Cirrhosis and noncirrhotic portal hypertension occur rarely (Ghishan et al, 1984).

HERPES SIMPLEX

Herpes simplex may cause hepatitis as part of a disseminated infection in the newborn. Although in utero infection can occur, most herpes infections are transmitted at birth and are associated with primary infection in the mother rather than reactivation of a previous infection (30% to 50% vs. approximately 5% or less). Neonates with disseminated disease may not manifest skin lesions initially, so herpes simplex infection should be considered in any newborn who appears septic, particularly with severe hepatic dysfunction (Caviness et al, 2008). Involvement of the central nervous system often occurs and may present with seizures. Although liver tests may be mildly abnormal, infants often present with jaundice, hepatosplenomegaly, markedly elevated aminotransferases, and coagulopathy (Verma et al, 2006).

Diagnosis relies on positive cultures from secretions, blood, urine, cerebrospinal fluid, and scrapings from vesicles. Direct fluorescent antibody staining of vesicle contents may facilitate a more rapid diagnosis. Polymerase chain reaction analysis may be used to detect herpes simplex virus DNA in CSF and blood. Liver histopathology shows extensive bland necrosis, often with hemorrhage and minimal inflammation. Intranuclear acidophilic inclusions are found in hepatocytes.

Parenteral treatment with acyclovir may be life-saving, but many infants with disseminated disease and encephalitis have significant neurologic sequelae (Kimberlin et al, 2001a). Approximately one fourth of infants will still die despite antiviral therapy (Kimberlin, 2001; Kimberlin et al, 2001b). Liver transplantation has been successful in a few neonates with fulminant hepatic failure without severe encephalitis (Lee et al, 2002; Twagira et al, 2004).

HEPATITIS VIRUSES (A, B, C, D, AND E)

The classic hepatitis viruses (A, B C, D and E) are rarely a cause of significant liver disease in the neonate, but there are several issues of importance to be considered in the newborn.

Acute hepatitis A during pregnancy is associated with a high risk of maternal complications and preterm labor (Elinav et al, 2006). Hepatitis A infection may be acquired in the neonate via the fecal-oral route or by blood transfusion from a blood donor incubating the infection. These infants are virtually always asymptomatic, but present a hazard for transmission to adults, particularly to caretakers in the nursery (Chodick et al, 2006).

Materno-fetal transmission of hepatitis E virus (HEV) occurs, but the virus is particularly dangerous for the mother, resulting in a mortality rate of 25% to 45% if the acute infection occurs during the third trimester of pregnancy (Khuroo and Kamili, 2009). Vertically transmitted HEV infection can cause clinical hepatitis or even fulminant hepatic failure in neonates. The hepatitis and viremia resolve in surviving infants.

Newborns have a 95% chance of acquiring hepatitis B if the mother is chronically infected with hepatitis B or suffers acute hepatitis B in the third trimester or early in the postpartum period (Shah et al, 2009). In utero transmission is rare and is not preventable with postnatal immunoprophylaxis. Most cases of vertical transmission occur during delivery and can be prevented by prompt postnatal administration of hepatitis B immunoglobulin and hepatitis B vaccine. Infants acquiring hepatitis B are usually asymptomatic and immunotolerant in that they have normal or near-normal liver tests and very high levels of hepatitis B DNA in blood (Chang, 2007). Fulminant hepatitis B has been reported rarely in infants born to mothers with precore mutations in hepatitis B DNA.

Transmission of hepatitis C occurs only in about 5% of infants born to infected mothers (Indolfi and Resti, 2009). The risk of transmission correlates with the degree of maternal viremia. Mothers infected with the human immunodeficiency virus often manifest high levels of hepatitis C RNA, and are more likely to transmit infection to their newborns (Marine-Barjoan et al, 2007). Infants infected with hepatitis C are generally asymptomatic and have normal liver tests. In infants born to infected mothers, passively acquired maternal serum antibody to hepatitis C virus may persist for up to 18 months. If there is reason to exclude infection with hepatitis C at an earlier time, measurement of hepatitis C RNA in serum is feasible. Hepatitis C infection is not a contraindication to breastfeeding if the mother's nipples are not damaged.

ENTEROVIRAL INFECTIONS

Disseminated enteroviral infections with fulminant hepatic failure occurs predominantly in newborns (Abzug, 2004). Risk factors for severe enteroviral disease include prematurity, absence of neutralizing antibody from the mother to the infecting serotype, and maternal illness before and around the time of delivery. Infants appear septic with fever, irritability, lethargy, anorexia, and rash. The polymerase chain reaction is more sensitive and rapid than viral culture for detecting enteroviruses in cerebrospinal fluid, blood, urine, and throat specimens. Intravenous immunoglobulin has been used as a therapeutic agent for neonates with life-threatening infections, but clinical efficacy has not been established. Pleconaril, an investigational agent that inhibits viral attachment to host cell receptors and uncoating of viral nucleic acid, has shown some success in treating neonates with severe hepatitis and/or myocarditis in uncontrolled reports (Bauer et al, 2002). It was not effective in a double-blind placebo-controlled trial in infants with enterovirus meningitis (Abzug et al, 2003).

DISORDERS OF THE BILE DUCTS

There are many disorders that primarily and secondarily involve bile ducts in the newborn (see Box 74-2) (Birnbaum and Suchy, 1998). The intra- and extrahepatic bile ducts may be affected by abnormal morphogenesis and are particularly susceptible to injury from infection, inborn errors of metabolism, or even the immune system.

BILIARY ATRESIA

Biliary atresia (BA) is the most common cause of end-stage liver disease in infants and is the leading indication for liver transplantation in pediatrics. The incidence is estimated to be between 1 in 8000 and 1 in 12,000 live births and has a female predominance. BA appears to be secondary to an inflammatory process of unknown etiology resulting in fibrous obliteration of the biliary tract. There is no excretion of bile from the liver into duodenum leading to cholestasis, fibrosis and ultimately cirrhosis. Anatomically, BA has been classified into three types based on the extent and site of fibrosis in the biliary tree, based on data produced by the Japanese Society of Pediatric surgeons (Kasai et al, 1976):

Type 1: Atresia of the common bile duct with patent proximal ducts
Type 2: Atresia involving the hepatic duct but with patent proximal ducts
Type 3: Atresia involving the right and left hepatic ducts at the porta hepatis

Type 3 is the most common (88%) and has the worst prognosis. The term *extrahepatic biliary hypoplasia* refers to the cholangiographic demonstration of a patent but narrow biliary tree. The term *intrahepatic biliary atresia* is a misnomer and should be replaced by *paucity of intrahepatic bile ducts* or *intrahepatic bile duct hypoplasia* (Mowat, 1994).

Two forms of biliary atresia have been described based on clinical features: the more common perinatal or acquired form (80%) and the rarer fetal or embryonic form (20%) (Suchy et al, 2007), which is associated with congenital abnormalities. In 51 of 251 (20%) patients with BA, (a) single or dual anomalies involving cardiac, gastrointestinal, or urinary systems were found in 30 (59%); (b) combinations of anomalies within the laterality sequence (polysplenia, cardiovascular defects, asplenia, abdominal situs inversus, intestinal malformation, and anomalies of the portal vein and hepatic artery) were present in 15 (29%); and (c) intestinal malrotation occurred in 6 (12%), some with preduodenal portal vein. The term *BASM* (biliary atresia splenic malformation syndrome) has been proposed to describe a subgroup of infants with BA who also had a macroscopic splenic anomaly (Davenport et al, 2006). Of 548 infants with BA studied in a single institution, 56 (10.2%) had BASM and 37 were females. Splenic abnormalities included polysplenia (n = 43, 77%), double spleen (n = 7, 12%), and asplenia (n = 6, 11%). Situs inversus abdominis was noted in 21 cases (37%). The portal vein was abnormal in 35 (61%) of the infants, and the inferior vena cava was absent in 22 (39%). Structural cardiac anomalies were noted in 25 (45%) infants. Maternal diabetes mellitus was noted in 12.5% of pregnancies, and this may be of significance because a relationship between maternal diabetes and experimental situs inversus (Maeyama et al, 2001) as well as human L/R asymmetry malformations has been reported (Martinez-Frias, 2001). The prognosis of infants with BASM was appreciably worse (Davenport et al, 2006).

Pathogenesis

The cause of biliary atresia is unknown. The disease is not inherited, and there have been several reports of dizygotic and monozygotic twins discordant for biliary atresia (Bezerra, 2005). There is no evidence that biliary atresia results from a failure in morphogenesis or recanalization of the bile duct during embryonic development. An ischemic or toxic origin of extrahepatic bile duct injury is unlikely. Congenital infections with cytomegalovirus, rubella virus, reovirus 3, human herpesvirus 6, and papillomavirus occasionally have been implicated in some infants (Sokol and Mack, 2001). Initial reports of the involvement of group C rotavirus in biliary atresia have not been confirmed (Bobo et al, 1997). Clinical features support the view that in most cases, injury to the biliary tract occurs after birth (Sokol and Mack, 2001).

Human leukocyte antigen B12 (HLA-B12) has been found more frequently among biliary atresia patients without associated anomalies. The HLA haplotypes -A9, -B5, -A28, and -B35 occur more frequently (Silveira et al, 1993). Microarray gene chip analysis of cRNA from livers of infants with biliary atresia has revealed a coordinated activation of genes involved in lymphocyte differentiation and inflammation (Bezerra et al, 2002). The overexpression of osteopontin and interferon (IFN)-γ suggests a potential role of Th1-like cytokines in disease pathogenesis. Oligoclonal expansions of CD4 and CD8 T cells in liver and extrahepatic bile duct remnant tissues also have been found, indicating the presence of activated T cells reacting to specific antigenic stimulation in biliary atresia (Mack et al, 2007). Even after restoration of bile flow by portoenterostomy, circulating markers of inflammation persist, with clear progressive elevation in both Th1 effectors (interleukin [IL]-2 and IFN) and some Th2 effectors (IL-4), as well as the macrophage marker (TNFα). Increased expression of soluble cell adhesion molecules, sICAM-1 and sVCAM-1, likely reflects ongoing recruitment of circulating inflammatory/immunocompetent cells into target tissues (Nararyanaswamy et al, 2007). It remains unknown whether this immune response is induced by a viral infection or reflects a genetically programmed response to an infectious or environmental exposure. Maternal microchimerism has been demonstrated in BA, and it has been suggested that maternal cells could elicit an immune response similar to graft-versus-host disease (Kobayashi et al, 2007; Mieli-Vergani and Vergani, 2009).

Extrahepatic anomalies occur in 10% to 25% of patients and include cardiovascular defects, polysplenia, malrotation, situs inversus, and bowel atresias (Tanano, 1999). Loss of function mutations in the *CFC1* gene have been found in some patients who have heterotaxia, including an infant with biliary atresia and polysplenia (Bamford et al, 2000). This gene encodes for CRYPTIC, a protein that is involved in establishing the left-right axis during morphogenesis. However, mutations in the *INV* gene, which is also involved in determining laterality, were not found in limited studies of infants with biliary atresia and heterotaxia (Schon et al, 2002). In a microarray analysis of liver tissue from infants with the embryonic form of biliary atresia, often associated with extrahepatic malformations, a unique pattern of overexpression of genes involved in chromatin structure/histone deacetylation and of imprinted genes was found, implying a failure to downregulate embryonic gene programs that influence development of the liver and other organs (Zhang et al, 2004). There have been reports of identifying Jagged1 missense mutation in 10% of patients with BA (Kohsaka et al, 2002) and higher frequency of α₁-antitrypsin heterozygosity in children with BA (Campbell et al, 2007), both of which were associated with worse prognosis, but larger studies are needed to confirm these findings (Mieli-Vergani and Vergani, 2009).

Clinical Features

Infants with BA are typically born at term, with normal birthweight, and present in the first few weeks of life with history of jaundice lasting for more than 2 weeks, pale stools, and dark urine (Sokol et al, 2003). Occasionally, infants may present with bleeding secondary to vitamin K deficiency. In the fetal/embryonal type, infants are usually jaundiced with acholic stools from birth, whereas in the more common perinatal type, stools are pigmented at birth and then become acholic with progressive jaundice in the first few weeks of life (Suchy, 2004). On physical examination, there may be hepatomegaly or hepatosplenomegaly and ascites.

Laboratory studies initially reveal evidence of cholestasis, with a serum bilirubin level of 6 to 12 mg/dL, at least 50% of which is conjugated (Sokol et al, 2003). Serum aminotransferase and alkaline phosphatase levels are moderately elevated. Serum γ-glutamyl transpeptidase and 5′ nucleotidase levels may be markedly elevated.

Diagnosis

The gold standard for making a diagnosis of BA is exploratory laparotomy with intraoperative cholangiogram, because sometimes even the histology on liver biopsy can be ambiguous. BA is the most common surgically correctable liver disorder in infancy (Sokol et al, 2003). Outcome after Kasai portoenterostomy is dependent on the timing of the procedure, with best results achieved earlier in the course of the disease. However, establishing a diagnosis early remains a challenge, because there are no convenient means of screening newborns. The American Academy of Pediatrics currently recommends that infants who are jaundiced at 3 weeks of age should have a measurement of total and conjugated bilirubin (Sokol et al, 2007). A conjugated bilirubin that is more than 20% of an elevated serum bilirubin is diagnostic of cholestasis and potentially serious liver disease. Asking about the color of stools and examining the color of a fresh specimen of stool is helpful in distinguishing between cholestasis (acholic, pale) and unconjugated hyperbilirubinemia (pigmented, green/yellow). In some countries, especially in Asia, a stool card is used to allow identification of acholic stools by parents to facilitate early diagnosis of BA (Hsiao et al, 2008).

Ultrasonography plays an important role in distinguishing BA from other causes of neonatal cholestasis. Using the gallbladder shape and wall structure sonography could identify BA with a sensitivity of 90% and specificity of 92.4% in 346 infants with conjugated hyperbilirubinemia (Farrant et al, 2000). Some find the triangular cord sign, which represents a cone-shaped fibrotic mass cranial to the bifurcation of the portal vein, very useful in the diagnosis of BA (Choi et al, 1996), but others are unable to detect it sonographically (Shneider et al, 2006a). Absence of the common bile duct can sometimes be defined on imaging, as can situs inversus and some of the other malformations associated with the fetal type and the BASM subgroup in BA. On T2-weighted MRI, moderately high signal intensity along the portal tract that extends from the porta hepatis correlated with periductal edema and inflammatory cell infiltration (Schneider et al, 2006). Although BA can be diagnosed on the basis of lack of visualization of either common bile duct or the common hepatic duct, findings on MRI should always be interpreted in conjunction with the clinical information.

Hepatobiliary scintigraphy is a noninvasive way for ruling out extrahepatic biliary atresia. Technetium-99m iminodiacetic acid derivatives are excreted from the blood by hepatocytes and excreted into the bowel through the biliary system. Infants characteristically need to be primed with phenobarbitone for 3 to 5 days before the test, because it increases bilirubin conjugation and has a choleretic effect. If there is excretion of labeled tracer in the intestine, then BA is ruled out. Conversely, if there is no excretion of tracer, then the diagnosis is not necessarily BA, but is also seen in severe neonatal hepatitis and interlobular bile duct paucity (Gilmour et al, 1997). The scintigraphy test is of value in infants in the intensive care unit who are of low birthweight or on oxygen where excretion of tracer in the gut rules out BA and allows the liver biopsy to be postponed/avoided. In the older infant above 6 to 7 weeks, the test may not be as useful, because it causes delay by a week, given the need for phenobarbitone priming and the fact that a definitive diagnosis is not possible without a liver biopsy with or without an intraoperative cholangiogram. Some have used scintigraphy in combination with serum γ-glutamyl transpeptidase levels (Arora et al, 2001; Stipsanelli et al, 2007), and others have primed with ursodeoxycholic acid in an effort to improve sensitivity of the test (Poddar et al, 2004). Duodenal fluid may be obtained to assess the bilirubin content, and if fluid is bile stained, then BA is ruled out. Endoscopic retrograde cholangiopancreatography permits visualization of the biliary tree in young infants, but is technically challenging in the newborn (Guelrud et al, 1991).

Liver biopsy is an essential tool in the evaluation of an infant with conjugated hyperbilirubinemia and should be performed preferably before 8 weeks of age. The histologic features of BA (Figure 74-1) include cholestasis, periportal ductular proliferation, and the presence of bile plugs in cholangioles and interlobular bile ducts (Ishak

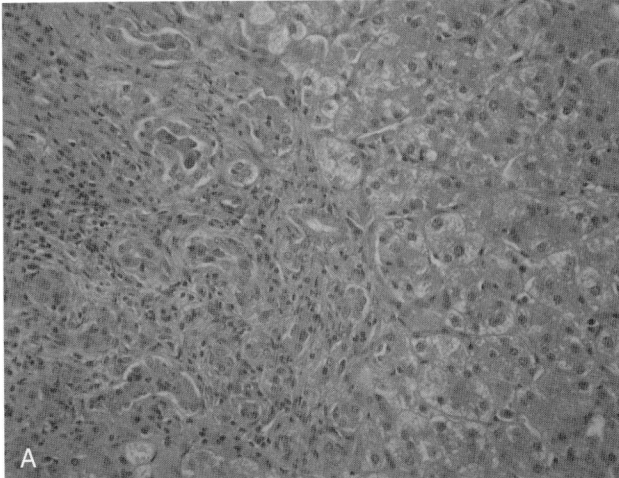
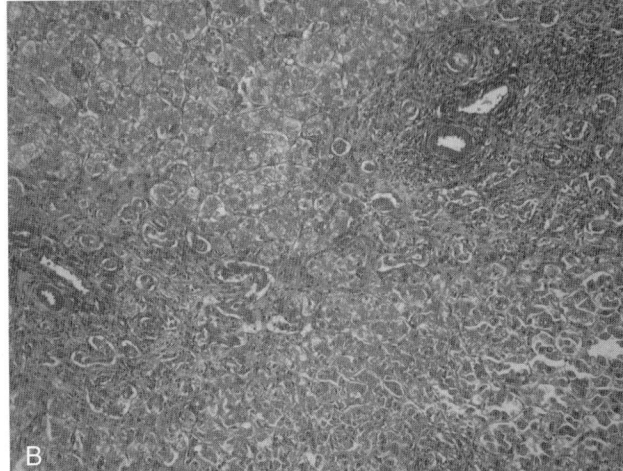

FIGURE 74-1 Liver biopsy from an infant with biliary atresia.
A, Portal tracts are expanded by bile ductular proliferation and fibrosis. Bile ductules contain bile plugs. **B,** *(See also Color Plate 33.)* Trichrome stain demonstrates portal tract fibrosis.

and Sharp, 2002). These findings are highly suggestive of biliary obstruction, but bile ductular proliferation can also be seen in α₁-antitrypsin deficiency. Giant-cell transformation is seen in 15% of cases. Fibrosis is progressive with eventual development of biliary cirrhosis (Lefkowitch et al, 1998).

Management

Based on results of laboratory tests, imaging, and liver histology, when clinical suspicion for BA is high, exploratory laparotomy is planned. If the diagnosis of BA is confirmed on intraoperative cholangiography, the Kasai hepatoportoenterostomy (HPE) procedure is performed. In the Kasai portoenterostomy, an anastomosis between the porta hepatis and a retrocolic Roux-en-Y loop of jejunum is fashioned (Ishak and Sharp, 2002). If successful, bile flow is restored from the intrahepatic ducts to the bowel. The outcome after surgery correlates to timing of surgery. Some series have reported that bile flow can be reestablished in 80% of the infants if surgery is performed early, that is, before 60 days, but the biliary drainage can decrease considerably when surgery is performed later, between 90 and 120 days of life (Balistreri et al, 1996; Mieli-Vergani et al, 1989). A simple rule of thumb for estimating outcome after Kasai portoenterostomy is that two thirds of infants will have successful drainage, but despite this, two thirds of those with bile drainage will require liver transplantation at some stage in their lives. When there is no biliary drainage established for up to 8 weeks after the procedure, infants require liver transplantation. Results are best if the surgeon is experienced and the operation performed in a specialist center. Some have used the size of the bile duct remnant at the hilum to predict outcome, those with diameter above 150 μm having increased chance of good bile flow (Chandra and Altman, 1978). Parameters associated with poor outcome include white race, the severity of the intrahepatic biliary cholangiopathy, the presence of cirrhosis on initial liver biopsy, and absence of ducts at the hilum (Balistreri et al, 1996). Growth failure after HPE was associated with transplantation or death by 24 months of age (DeRusso et al, 2007). There was markedly improved survival in children with total bilirubin level <2 mg/dL at 3 months after HPE (Shneider et al, 2006b).

Attempts have been made over the years to use corticosteroids after HPE to reduce the inflammatory cascade in an attempt to reduce future fibrosis, with varying results (Davenport et al, 2007; Dillon et al, 2001; Kobayashi et al, 2005). Postoperatively, infants are typically maintained on a formula containing high levels of medium-chain triglycerides, supplemented with fat-soluble vitamins, and ursodeoxycholic acid to stimulate bile flow (Sokol, 1994).

The life expectancy without surgery in BA is at most 2 years. In the United States, BA remains the most frequent indication for liver transplantation in pediatrics. Indications for liver transplantation in BA include failed Kasai hepatoportoenterostomy; increasing cholestasis, pruritis, and/or failure to thrive; recurrent cholangitis with bile lakes in the liver on imaging studies; complications related to portal hypertension, including gastrointestinal bleeding not controlled with medical management and decompensated liver disease with ascites; worsening synthetic function (prolonged international normalized ratio and low albumin); and encephalopathy (Shneider and Mazariegos, 2007).

CHOLEDOCHAL CYSTS

Choledochal cysts are congenital anomalies of the biliary tract with dilatations of the extrahepatic and sometimes intrahepatic biliary system (Miyano and Yamataka, 1997). After BA, choledochal cyst is the most common surgical cause of obstructive jaundice in the newborn period. The frequency of choledochal cysts is about 1 in 15,000 live births in Western countries, and as high as 1 in 1000 live births in Japan (Suchy et al, 2001). There is a marked female predominance (4:1), regardless of racial origin. The etiology of choledochal cyst is not known. An anomalous pancreaticobiliary ductal anatomy (with a long common channel before it enters the duodenum) is reported in 70% to 90% of patients with choledochal cyst (Mackenzie et al, 2001; McWhorter, 1924). This may allow reflux of pancreatic enzymes into the common bile duct, resulting in inflammation, weakness, and dilatation. Other etiologic mechanisms include congenital weakness of the common bile duct and obstruction of the distal common bile duct

leading to dilatation (Balistreri et al, 1996). Predominant extrahepatic biliary dilatation has been found in several patients with autosomal recessive polycystic kidney disease (Goilav et al, 2006).

Depending on the extent and shape of the biliary dilatation, choledochal cysts have been classified into several types (Todani et al, 1977). Type Ia is a cystic dilatation of the common bile duct, Ib a focal segmental dilatation of the distal common bile duct, and Ic a fusiform dilatation of both the common hepatic duct and common bile duct. In type II, the cyst forms a diverticulum from the extrahepatic bile duct. Type III, also known as choledochocele, is a dilatation of the distal common bile duct lying mainly within the duodenal wall. Type IV is essentially type I anatomy with either intrahepatic bile duct cyst (IVa) or choledochocele (IVb). Some authors refer to Caroli's disease with multiple cystic dilatations of the intrahepatic biliary tree as type V choledochal cyst. Type Ia is seen most frequently.

Cholestasis is a common presenting feature, and one fifth of those diagnosed with choledochal cyst are jaundiced in the 1st year of life (Altman, 1992). The classic triad of symptoms—intermittent obstructive jaundice, abdominal pain, and a cystic abdominal mass—rarely present in infancy. Care must be taken during examination that the choledochal cyst is not ruptured during palpation.

Ultrasonography is most frequently done to diagnose a choledochal cyst and has even been used to detect a choledochal cyst in the fetus (Bancroft et al, 1994; Kim et al, 1995). Magnetic resonance cholangiography is being used increasingly to evaluate the extent of the cyst and defects within the biliary tree and to detect an anomalous junction of the pancreaticobiliary duct (Kim et al, 2000).

Complications include recurrent cholangitis, biliary cirrhosis, rupture with bile peritonitis, pancreatitis, portal vein thrombosis, hepatic abscess, gallstones, and later cholangiocarcinoma of the cyst wall.

An operative cholangiogram is done to define the extent of intrahepatic and extrahepatic disease. Complete excision of the cyst mucosa is considered essential for successful management of choledochal cysts, as cholangiocarcinoma has been reported in up to one fourth of patients with residual cystic tissue (Todani et al, 1977). Biliary tract continuity is maintained through a choledochojejunostomy with Roux-en-Y anastomosis (McWhorter, 1924). For symptomatic patients, especially when BA is high in the differential, it is advisable to perform surgery before 2 months of age to prevent progressive liver damage and fibrosis (Davenport et al, 2003).

NEONATAL SCLEROSING CHOLANGITIS

Primary sclerosing cholangitis may present in the neonatal period and, in contrast to older children, is not associated with inflammatory bowel disease or autoimmune markers (Amedee-Manesme et al, 1987). Cholestatic jaundice and acholic stools occur within the first weeks of life (Batres et al, 2005). Cholangiography demonstrates a patent biliary system, but with rarefaction of segmental branches, stenosis, and focal dilatation of the intrahepatic bile ducts (Debray et al, 1994). The extrahepatic bile ducts may be involved in most patients. Jaundice may subside spontaneously, but progression to biliary cirrhosis may still occur later in childhood.

The neonatal ichthyosis–sclerosing cholangitis syndrome is a rare autosomal recessive syndrome characterized by scalp hypotrichosis, scarring alopecia, ichthyosis, and sclerosing cholangitis. Mutations in the gene coding for the tight junction protein claudin-1 have been found in these patients (Hadj-Rabia et al, 2004).

SPONTANEOUS PERFORATION OF COMMON BILE DUCT

Spontaneous perforation of common bile duct is a rare cholestatic disorder of infancy (Chardot et al, 1996). The perforation usually occurs at the junction of the cystic and common ducts. The cause is unknown, but congenital or acquired weakness at the site, obstruction at the distal end of the common bile duct from stenosis, or inspissated bile have been proposed (Sahnoun et al, 2007).

Infants present with poor weight gain, jaundice, acholic stools, dark urine, and ascites. Progressive abdominal distention usually occurs due to ascites with bile staining of umbilical and inguinal hernias.

Mild to moderate conjugated hyperbilirubinemia with minimal elevation of serum aminotransferase levels is typical. Abdominal paracentesis reveals clear bile-stained ascitic fluid, which usually is sterile. Ultrasonography confirms ascites, which is sometimes loculated in the right upper quadrant. There is no biliary dilatation. Hepatobiliary scintigraphy is diagnostic, showing free accumulation of isotope within the peritoneal cavity (Ford et al, 1988).

Operative cholangiography is required to demonstrate the site of the perforation. At laparotomy, drainage of bilious ascites and repair of the perforation usually provide effective treatment (Davenport et al, 1991). Cholecystojejunostomy may be required in some infants with stenosis of the common bile duct.

PAUCITY OF INTERLOBULAR BILE DUCTS

Paucity of interlobular bile ducts on a liver biopsy has been defined as the ratio of the number of interlobular bile ducts to the number of portal tracts of less than 0.4 (Kahn, 1991). It may be an isolated and unexplained finding in idiopathic neonatal cholestasis or a feature of a heterogeneous group of disorders that include congenital infections with rubella and cytomegalovirus and genetic disorders such as α_1-antitrypsin deficiency and inborn errors of bile acid metabolism (Kahn et al, 1986).

ALLAGILLE SYNDROME

Alagille syndrome, or syndromic paucity of interlobular bile ducts, is the most common form of familial intrahepatic cholestasis (Alagille et al, 1987). This disorder is characterized by chronic cholestasis, a decreased number of interlobular bile ducts, and a variety of other congenital malformations.

An autosomal dominant mode of transmission with incomplete penetrance and variable expressivity has been established. Mutations in the *jagged1* (*JAG1*) gene on the short arm of chromosome 20 have been identified in approximately 94% of affected patients (Colliton et al, 2001). *JAG1* encodes a ligand in the Notch signaling pathway that is involved in cell fate determination during development. Mutations in the gene encoding for the NOTCH2 receptor have recently been found in patients with Alagille syndrome who were negative for JAG1 mutations (McDaniell et al, 2006).

Chronic cholestasis of varying severity affects 95% of patients (Emerick et al, 1999). Onset in the neonate is common with jaundice and clay-colored stools. Intense pruritus and xanthomata develop later. The liver and spleen are often enlarged. Dysmorphic facies may be difficult to recognize in the newborn, but become more characteristic with age (Emerick et al, 1999, Kamath et al, 2002). The forehead is typically broad; the eyes are deeply set and widely spaced. The mandible is somewhat small and pointed, imparting a triangular appearance to the face. Other extrahepatic anomalies occur variably and commonly include congenital heart disease, particularly peripheral pulmonic stenosis; butterfly vertebrae; posterior embryotoxon of the eye; and impaired growth. Abnormalities of the kidney, the systemic vasculature, and pancreas are other manifestations (Emerick et al, 1999).

There is variable elevation of the serum conjugated bilirubin concentration. Serum alkaline phosphatase, bile acids, γ-glutamyl transpeptidase, and 5′-nucleotidase levels may be extremely high. Serum aminotransferase levels are mildly to moderately increased. Serum cholesterol levels may be 200 mg/dL or higher. Serum triglyceride concentrations of 500 to 1000 mg/dL are commonly found.

The nonspecific histologic features during the first months of life may include ballooning of hepatocytes, cholestasis, portal inflammation, and giant-cell transformation (Kahn, 1991). The number of interlobular bile ducts may not be decreased on initial liver biopsy, but bile duct injury may be present, consisting of lymphocytic infiltration, pyknosis of biliary epithelium, and periductal fibrosis. Serial liver biopsies may show progressive loss and paucity of bile ducts by the age of 6 months. The extrahepatic bile ducts are patent but usually narrowed or hypoplastic.

The mechanisms involved in the pathogenesis of bile duct paucity and cholestasis have not been defined. It is also unknown how the hepatobiliary disease relates to the multiplicity of congenital anomalies found in other organ systems. Notch signaling has an important role in the differentiation of biliary epithelial cells and is essential for their tubular formation during development. A lack of branching and elongation of bile ducts during postnatal liver growth likely contributes to peripheral bile duct paucity and cholestasis (Libbrecht et al, 2005).

Varying degrees of cholestasis, sometimes worsened by intercurrent viral infections, typically occur. Pruritus, cutaneous xanthomata, and neuromuscular symptoms related to vitamin E deficiency may cause significant morbidity. Provision of an adequate caloric intake, prevention or correction of fat-soluble vitamin deficiencies, and symptomatic measures to relieve pruritus are important. The long-term prognosis depends on the severity of the liver disease and associated malformations (Lykavieris et al, 2001). Neonatal cholestatic jaundice has been associated with poorer survival with native liver (Lykavieris et al,

2001). Survival and candidacy for liver transplantation may be limited by the severity of associated cardiovascular anomalies.

CYSTIC DILATATION OF THE INTRAHEPATIC BILE DUCTS

Cystic dilatation of the intrahepatic bile ducts is an inherited disorder characterized by saccular dilatation of several segments of the intrahepatic bile ducts (Desmet, 1998). There are two variants: Caroli's disease, characterized by ectasias of the intrahepatic bile ducts without other abnormalities and Caroli's syndrome, in which congenital ductal dilatation is associated with features of congenital hepatic fibrosis and the renal lesion of autosomal recessive polycystic renal disease (ARPKD) (Bergmann et al, 2004). Caroli's syndrome is more common, but both varieties are inherited in an autosomal recessive fashion.

Patients may present in the newborn period with cholestasis from ascending cholangitis and calculus formation within the abnormal bile ducts (Guay-Woodford and Desmond, 2003; Keane et al, 1997). Caroli's disease has been detected in utero with fetal ultrasound findings of a cystic liver mass and echogenic kidneys (Sgro et al, 2004). Fever, abdominal distention, jaundice, and an enlarged, tender liver are typical. Markedly enlarged kidneys from ARPKD can be palpated.

Elevated serum alkaline phosphatase activity, direct-reacting bilirubin levels, and leukocytosis may be observed during episodes of acute infection. Ultrasonography shows the dilated intrahepatic ducts with intraductal lithiasis and sludge and cystic renal disease, but definitive diagnosis and extent of disease must be determined by percutaneous transhepatic or magnetic resonance cholangiography (Brancatelli et al, 2005). Most patients with Caroli's syndrome have mutations in the *PKHD1* (polycystic kidney and hepatic disease 1) gene (Bergmann et al, 2005).

Cholangitis and sepsis are treated with broad-spectrum antibiotics. Ursodeoxycholic acid therapy may help to inhibit formation of biliary sludge and promote bile flow. Intraductal calculi may require surgery (Arnold and Harrison, 2005).

PARENTERAL NUTRITION ASSOCIATED CHOLESTASIS

Parenteral nutrition–associated cholestasis (PNAC) is frequently seen in newborn infants. Premature infants and those with short bowel syndrome are particularly susceptible (Robinson and Ehrenkranz, 2008). Additional risk factors include an immaturity of liver function, repeated bouts of infection, exposure to endotoxin from bacterial overgrowth of the intestine, lack of enteral feeding, and possibly toxicity from some of the components of the parenteral nutrition solution (Forchielli and Walker, 2003).

The pathophysiology of PNAC has not been completely defined and is likely to be multifactorial. Enteral feedings are trophic for biliary secretion through the release of gastrointestinal hormones such as cholecystokinin, glucagon, gastrin, and enteroglucagon. Biliary stasis leading to gallbladder sludge and stones reflects decreased gallbladder contraction from the lack of enterally stimulated cholecystokinin release. Endotoxin resulting from bacterial overgrowth of the small intestine and from sepsis is a potent inhibitor of transporters for bile acids and other organic anions that are essential for bile formation. Lipid emulsions used in parenteral nutrition have recently been implicated in contributing to cholestasis (Shin et al, 2008). Stigmasterol, a soy lipid-derived phytosterol, has been found to potently antagonize the expression of several critical bile acid transport proteins, including the bile salt export pump and the organic solute transporter (Carter et al, 2007).

Cholestasis typically develops with prolonged use of parenteral nutrition. The clinical features are similar to other cholestatic disorders of the newborn and include elevated serum concentrations of bilirubin, bile acids, and aminotransferases. Alternative causes of cholestasis must be excluded, including biliary tract disorders, perinatal infections, and inborn errors of metabolism.

Hepatocellular and canalicular cholestasis, steatosis, and periportal fibrosis are seen on liver biopsy. Bile ductular proliferation and giant-cell transformation of hepatocytes can also be observed. Evolution to biliary cirrhosis can occur with continued use of parenteral nutrition.

Without a precise knowledge of the factors that cause PNAC, the prevention and treatment of the condition remain problematic. Enteral feedings are extremely important not only for stimulating bile flow, but also for promoting intestinal adaptation in infants with short gut syndrome. Even nutritionally insignificant amounts of enteral feedings may be beneficial. Ursodeoxycholic acid given in doses of 10 to 20 mg/kg of body weight may be helpful in stimulating bile flow and diminishing cytotoxicity from more hydrophobic bile salts (Arslanoglu et al, 2008; Chen et al, 2004a). There is increasing interest in replacing soy-based lipid emulsions with fish oil–based lipid emulsions (Cheung et al, 2009; Gura et al, 2008). Prevention or even reversal of PNAC has been observed in a limited number of infants (de Meijer et al, 2009). Liver transplantation or combined liver-intestinal transplantation may be the only option in patients with end-stage liver disease and extreme short bowel syndrome.

CYSTIC FIBROSIS

Infants with cystic fibrosis may present with cholestasis during the first weeks of life (Colombo, 2007; Lamireau et al, 2004). Meconium ileus may be associated and provide a clue to the underlying diagnosis (Lamireau et al, 2004). Variants in mannose binding lectin and ABCB4 genes may be genetic modifiers influencing the risk for liver disease in CF (Tomaiuolo et al, 2009). Conjugated hyperbilirubinemia and modest elevation of aminotransferases may be observed in the newborn. Serum cholesterol may be low. Liver biopsy shows cholestasis and bile ductular proliferation consistent with an obstructive process (Brigman and Feranchak, 2006). The findings may mimic biliary atresia, and the typical mucus plugs observed later in bile ducts may not be present in the newborn with cystic fibrosis. Meconium ileus may be another diagnostic clue. Operative cholangiography may sometimes be required to exclude biliary atresia. However, neonatal screening tests and eventual sweat chloride analysis should be diagnostic.

Treatment with ursodeoxycholic acid (20 to 40 mg/kg/day) usually leads to improvement in liver biochemical tests, but it is uncertain whether the course of the liver disease is altered (Cheng et al, 2000). The jaundice often resolves even without treatment and does not predict severe liver disease later in life (Shapira et al, 1999).

PROGRESSIVE FAMILIAL INTRAHEPATIC CHOLESTASIS (PFIC)

It has long been recognized that progressive, intrahepatic cholestasis may have a genetic basis, and have its onset in the newborn period. Mutations in several genes encoding transport proteins that contribute to bile formation have been defined in recent years (Alissa et al, 2008).

PFIC1

Patients with PFIC1 (also called Byler disease) present in the newborn or by the age of 1 year with severe cholestasis that progresses to cirrhosis at a variable rate (van Mil et al, 2001). Hepatosplenomegaly, diarrhea, malabsorption, and failure to thrive are common in the first months of life. Fat-soluble vitamin deficiencies occur, resulting in rickets and coagulopathy. Intractable pruritus, a dominant feature of the disease, is generally not observed until approximately 3 months of age,

Serum γ-glutamyl transpeptidase activity and cholesterol concentration are paradoxically normal. The serum bile acid concentration is elevated. Serum aminotransferases are moderately elevated.

A bland hepatocellular, canalicular cholestasis is typical on liver biopsy early in the course of the disease. Cirrhosis eventually occurs. Electron microscopy shows distended bile canaliculi containing unusually coarse and granular bile.

Patients with PFIC1 have mutations in the gene encoding ATP8B1, a P-type ATPase, that is an aminophospholipid flippase localized to the liver canalicular, cholangiocyte, and intestinal apical membranes (Bull et al, 1998). It remains unsettled as to how mutations in the ATP8B1 gene lead to progressive cholestasis. The ordering of aminophospholipids in lipid bilayers in part mediated by ATP8B1 may play a role in regulating important lipid-dependent signaling pathways and the activity of membrane receptors and transport proteins, including those involved in regulating bile acid homeostasis (Chen et al, 2004b). Moreover, the loss of canalicular phospholipid membrane asymmetry may also render the canalicular membrane susceptible to the damaging effects of hydrophobic bile salts. The FIC1 gene is also highly expressed in other organs, including the lungs, small intestine, pancreas, and kidneys, which may account for the extrahepatic manifestations of the disease such as lung disease and diarrhea.

Biliary diversion or ileal bypass may be successful in decreasing pruritus and slowing the progression of liver injury by depleting the liver and intestines of hydrophobic bile acids (Arnell et al, 2008). Liver transplantation may be required in patients with cirrhosis or pruritus refractory to other therapies. Patients may still manifest growth failure, malabsorption, and pancreatitis after an otherwise successful liver transplant because of the extrahepatic expression of ATP8B1.

PFIC2

PFIC2 is caused by mutations in *ABCB11*, which codes for the bile salt export pump (BSEP), the predominant transporter for bile acids on the liver canalicular membrane (Jansen et al, 1999, Suchy and Ananthanarayanan, 2006). Bile secretory failure occurs leading to retention of bile salts and other biliary constituents in the hepatocyte and progressive liver damage (Strautnieks et al, 1998, 2008).

Severe cholestasis begins in the newborn. Jaundice, failure to thrive related to fat malabsorption, and poor intake occur. Fat-soluble vitamin deficiencies are common. Hepatosplenomegaly is usually present. Severe pruritus develops in the first months of life. Progression to cirrhosis is rapid without therapy. Hepatocellular carcinoma and cholangiocarcinoma may occur, even in the 1st year of life (Knisely and Portmann, 2006).

Similar to patients with PFIC-1, serum γ-glutamyl transpeptidase is low, and serum cholesterol levels are normal or near normal. In contrast to patients with PFIC-1, serum aminotransferase levels are usually elevated to over five times normal values.

The histopathology of PFIC2 shows a marked, nonspecific giant-cell hepatitis and lobular cholestasis, similar to many liver diseases of the neonate. Electron microscopy demonstrates dilated bile canaliculi that contain finely granular or filamentous bile. The lack of BSEP immunohistochemical staining on the canalicular membrane is useful diagnostically (Jansen et al, 1999).

Intractable pruritus and progressive liver disease have also been treated with biliary diversion or ileal exclusion. A risk for liver cancer may still exist despite clinical improvement. Liver transplantation is required in many patients.

PFIC3

This disorder is due to mutations in the *MDR3* gene, which encodes a transporter required for biliary phosphatidylcholine secretion (Jacquemin et al, 1999). The age of onset of PFIC3 with jaundice, hepatomegaly, growth failure and acholic stools is extremely broad, but onset has been observed in the 1st month of life (mean age approximately 3.5 years). Pruritus is usually mild. Liver disease tends to evolve slowly to biliary cirrhosis.

In contrast to the other forms of PFIC, the serum concentration of γ-glutamyl transpeptidase is elevated in PFIC3, often over 10 times the normal value (Jacquemin et al, 2001). Other liver tests are variable. Serum cholesterol concentration is usually normal. The cardinal feature of PFIC3 is markedly reduced concentrations of biliary phospholipids (Oude Elferink and Paulusma, 2007).

The histopathology of PFIC3 shows bile ductular proliferation and mixed inflammatory infiltrates. Periductal sclerosis affecting the interlobular bile ducts eventually occurs. Extensive portal fibrosis evolves into biliary cirrhosis in older children.

Oral administration of ursodeoxycholic acid appears to be of value in some patients, particularly those with mild MDR3 mutations and residual biliary phospholipid secretion (Jacquemin et al, 1997). The rationale underlying this therapy is that enrichment of bile with this hydrophilic bile acid reduces cytotoxic injury to hepatocytes and bile ducts and stimulates bile flow. Other patients progress to biliary cirrhosis and ultimately require liver transplantation.

METABOLIC LIVER DISEASE

The liver is involved primarily or secondarily in many inborn errors of metabolism that often present in the first weeks of life, as the infant adjusts to the extrauterine environment. Establishing a specific diagnosis is critically important for genetic counseling and to allow specific therapy in some cases or liver transplantation if the disease is restricted to the liver. Presymptomatic diagnosis and early treatment made possible by newborn screening has changed the natural history of several disorders such as galactosemia and tyrosinemia.

In inborn errors of metabolism such as hereditary tyrosinemia, the absence of a critical enzyme may cause an accumulation of toxic metabolites that damage the liver and other organs. In other disorders, progressive liver injury may occur because of failure to produce essential compounds necessary for normal hepatic function. For example, an inborn error of bile acid metabolism leads to progressive cholestasis because of a lack of bile acid synthesis and impairment of bile flow. Severe liver injury may also result from sequestration of an abnormally synthesized product within the liver, as observed in α_1-antitrypsin deficiency or lysosomal storage disorder.

Clinical features of metabolic liver disease may be nonspecific and can overlap with other hepatic disorders, including viral hepatitis or drug-induced liver injury, or mimic septicemia. Jaundice, vomiting, hepatosplenomegaly, failure to thrive, developmental delay, hypotonia, seizures, and progressive neuromuscular dysfunction may occur (see Table 74-1). Initial laboratory studies are often nonspecific and may include jaundice, hypoglycemia, hyperammonemia, increased aminotransferase levels, acidosis, and hypoprothrombinemia.

HEREDITARY TYROSINEMIA TYPE I

Hereditary tyrosinemia type I is an autosomal-recessive disorder of the tyrosine degradation pathway caused by deficiency of fumarylacetoacetate hydrolase (Mitchell et al, 2007). Highly reactive, electrophilic metabolites of tyrosine, succinyl acetate, succinyl acetone, fumaryl acetoacetate, and maleyl acetoacetate, accumulate and bind to sulfhydryl groups, leading to tissue injury. Many secondary enzymatic and biochemical defects occur in tyrosinemia as a result of the accumulation of these precursor compounds. Succinyl acetoacetate is one example that can inhibit the enzyme porphobilinogen synthase, leading to the accumulation of 5-aminolevulinic acid and symptoms of acute, intermittent porphyria (Grompe, 2001). A transient, benign form of hypertyrosinemia is a self-limiting condition primarily of premature infants, probably caused by an immaturity of tyrosine degradation pathway.

The acute form of the disease presents in the first weeks of life with jaundice, hepatosplenomegaly, failure to thrive, anorexia, ascites, coagulopathy, and rickets. The disorder may begin in utero as evidenced by the presence of cirrhosis and ascites at the time of birth.

Laboratory studies usually show compromise of hepatic synthetic function with hypoalbuminemia and a decrease in vitamin K–dependent coagulation factors (Grompe, 2001). Serum aminotransferase values are mildly to moderately increased. Total and direct bilirubin concentrations are variably increased. Hypoglycemia is common. Hemolytic anemia may occur. Fanconi's syndrome resulting from renal tubular dysfunction may lead to hyperphosphaturia, glucosuria, proteinuria, and aminoaciduria. Serum tyrosine and methionine concentrations are markedly elevated (Russo et al, 2001). Serum α-fetoprotein concentrations are often markedly elevated even in cord blood, supporting the prenatal onset of liver disease.

Phenolic acid by-products of tyrosine metabolism, succinyl acetone and succinyl acetoacetate, are excreted in urine and are diagnostic of this disorder.

Histologic examination of the liver reveals fatty infiltration, iron deposition, varying degrees of hepatocyte necrosis, and pseudoacinar formation. Significant fibrosis may be present early in life with gradual evolution to multinodular cirrhosis. Regenerative nodules mimicking neoplasms may be present in some patients. Hepatocellular carcinoma (HCC) may develop later.

The acute form of type 1 tyrosinemia is usually fatal in the 1st year of life without therapy (Ashorn et al, 2006). Dietary restriction of phenylalanine, methionine, and tyrosine does not prevent progression of the liver disease or development of hepatocellular carcinoma. Medical therapy with 2-(2-nitro-4-trifluoromethylbenzoyl)-1,3-cyclohexanedione (NTBC) is effective in reversing the metabolic abnormalities in hereditary tyrosinemia type 1 (Santra and Baumann, 2008). NTBC treatment reduces flux through the tyrosine degradation pathway, preventing formation of toxic metabolites. With NTBC treatment, serum α-fetoprotein levels decrease and liver synthetic function normalizes. NTBC usually provides protection against HCC if it is started in infancy, but cases of HCC have occurred even when NTBC was started at 5 months of age. AFP is a marker for both the development of liver cancer and the inadequate control of metabolic derangement of tyrosinemia type I itself. Liver transplantation will be required in such cases (Lam et al, 2002).

In asymptomatic newborns identified by newborn screening in Quebec and treated with NTBC within 1 month, none have developed hepatic dysfunction or liver nodules over a follow-up period of up to 9 years (Mitchell et al, 2007). However, the long-term risk for developing hepatocellular carcinoma even in patients who were treated early remains unknown.

α_1-ANTITRYPSIN DEFICIENCY

Antitrypsin is the principal serum protease. α_1-Antitrypsin deficiency can be associated with cholestatic jaundice in the neonate. Patients with homozygous deficiency of this protein (the PiZZ phenotype) have low serum α_1-antitrypsin activity, usually in the range of 10% to 15% of normal values (Kohnlein and Welte, 2008). The incidence of the most common deficiency phenotype, PiZZ, is 1 in 2000 to 1 in 4000 live births.

Measurement of α_1-antitrypsin concentration alone is unreliable for diagnosis because the protein is an acute-phase reactant and may be elevated in the presence of inflammation (Perlmutter et al, 2004). Heterozygotes with the SZ and MZ phenotypes have a less severe reduction in serum α1-antitrypsin concentration and do not develop liver disease. However, α1-antitrypsin heterozygosity may be a modifier for other liver diseases.

Cholestatic jaundice occurs in approximately 10% to 15% of infants with the PiZZ phenotype (Teckman and Lindblad, 2006). Hepatomegaly and acholic stools may occur. Patients rarely may present with signs of advanced liver disease such as ascites or gastrointestinal bleeding. Although asymptomatic, another 40% to 50% of homozygous infants have abnormal liver biochemical tests in the first months of life.

Giant-cell hepatitis is a typical histologic finding in the neonate. Bile ductular proliferation may be observed initially; later, paucity of bile ducts may be found. Periodic-acid-Schiff–positive, diastase-resistant inclusions within hepatocytes, especially in the periportal region, represent the abnormal α1-antitrypsin accumulation but are not prominent before 4 months of age (Teckman, 2007). Fibrosis is variable, but cirrhosis has been reported rarely in the neonatal period.

It is unknown why only 10 to 15% of neonates with the homozygous deficiency manifest liver disease. The PiZZ defect is caused by substitution of a lysine for a glutamate at position 342, leading to misfolding of the protein and its retention in the endoplasmic reticulum (Perlmutter, 2006; Perlmutter et al, 2007). Mutant α1-antitrypsin molecules polymerize in the ER by a loop-sheet insertion mechanism, and are toxic to hepatocytes (Kohnlein and Welte, 2008).

The outcome of neonatal liver disease related to α1-antitrypsin deficiency is variable (Perlmutter, 2002, 2004). Patients may present with or develop cirrhosis within the first months of life. However, in most infants, the jaundice clears by 4 months of age, but variable liver test abnormalities may persist. There is no specific treatment for α1-antitrypsin deficiency. Liver transplantation is curative for patients with end-stage liver disease; the recipient assumes the Pi type of the donor organ.

INBORN ERRORS OF BILE ACID METABOLISM

Bile acids are required to drive bile secretion, and thus any impairment in bile acid biosynthesis or transport can result in cholestasis. At least 14 enzymatic steps are required in the liver to convert cholesterol into the primary bile acids cholic and chenodeoxycholic acid. Inherited defects in nine of these enzymes have now been described that often result in neonatal liver disease (Bove et al, 2000, 2004).

Primary defects in bile acid biosynthesis generally present with intrahepatic cholestasis (Heubi et al, 2007). A severe giant cell hepatitis is often found on liver biopsy. The serum γ-glutamyl transpeptidase concentration is paradoxically normal. The enzymatic block in bile acid synthesis results in a failure to produce normal primary bile acids required for generating bile flow and in accumulation in the liver of bile acid precursors that are intrinsically cholestatic and hepatotoxic. In marked contrast to other cholestatic disorders, inborn errors of bile acid biosynthesis are not associated with pruritus (Setchell and

Heubi, 2006). Measurement of serum bile acids by standard methods can be a useful initial screening test for these disorders in that primary bile acids are very low to absent, even in the face of severe cholestasis. These defects are detected by analysis of urine in reference laboratories by liquid secondary ionization mass spectrometry. Gas chromatography–mass spectrometry of urine, serum, and bile as well as enzymatic and molecular assays for some of the defects are used to establish a specific diagnosis.

Prompt diagnosis of an inborn error of bile acid metabolism is important because several of these disorders can be treated with oral bile acid replacement (Heubi et al, 2007). Treatment with the primary bile acid, cholic acid, has been particularly successful in patients with 3β-hydroxy-C27-steroid oxidoreductase deficiency and Δ4-3-oxosteroid-5-β-reductase deficiency. Cholic acid provides the missing end product required to generate bile flow and downregulates the production of toxic bile acid precursors. Therapy is lifelong. Ursodeoxycholic acid, which is commonly used in other forms of cholestasis even in newborns, is ineffective because it does not inhibit the bile acid synthetic pathway and production of toxic intermediates.

GALACTOSEMIA

Galactosemia is caused by a genetic defect in the metabolism of monosaccharide galactose, which is a constituent of lactose, the main carbohydrate of milk (Bosch et al, 2006). Galactose is normally metabolized to glucose via three separate enzymatic reactions involving galactokinase, galactose-1-phosphate uridyl transferase, and uridine diphosphate galactose-4-epimerase. The most common severe defect involves a deficiency of galactose-1-phosphate uridyl transferase. The enzymatic defect results in the accumulation of toxic metabolites, galactose-1-phosphate and galactitol (Leslie et al, 2003). Inheritance is in an autosomal-recessive fashion.

The clinical presentation of galactosemia occurs in the newborn period after ingestion of galactose. Early manifestations include jaundice, lethargy, vomiting, acidosis, cataracts, failure to thrive, and bleeding. Indirect hyperbilirubinemia is commonly seen and can be accompanied by coagulopathy (Leslie et al, 2003). Gram-negative sepsis is also a common presenting feature. Untreated disease is likely to result in liver failure and severe neurologic injury.

Even though many states now screen for galactosemia, clinicians should not wait for these results to begin therapy in infants with suggestive symptoms. Urine reducing substances are detected in infants fed galactose-containing formulas, although urine glucose dipsticks are negative. Measurement of galactose-1-phosphate uridyl transferase activity should ultimately be performed using red blood cells in all cases. Mutation analysis is also feasible.

Treatment consists of strict elimination of galactose from the diet (Bosch, 2006). This should be initiated as soon as the diagnosis is suspected in order to prevent liver failure. This will normally reverse the hepatic dysfunction associated with galactosemia. Dietary therapy is not entirely successful in the long term, in that patients may still manifest some degree of growth impairment, developmental retardation, motor dysfunction, and hypogonadism (Hughes et al, 2009; Panis et al, 2007).

GLYCOGEN STORAGE DISEASE

The glycogen storage diseases result from inherited, enzymatic defects in glycogen metabolism. Clinical phenotypes result from the inability to utilize glycogen stores, accumulation of glycogen within the liver and/or other tissues, and the toxic effects of certain abnormal types of glycogen.

Type I glycogen storage disease may present in the neonate with hypoglycemia and lactic acidosis (Melis et al, 2005). Hepatomegaly, hyperuricemia, and hyperlipidemia typically occur. Two forms of type I disease exist: deficiencies in glucose-6-phosphatase (type Ia) and glucose-6-phosphate translocase (type Ib). Fasting hypoglycemia can be life threatening in both variants. Significant hypoglycemia may also be seen in glycogen storage disease types III (debranching deficiency), VI (liver phosphorylase deficiency), and IX (hepatic phosphorylase kinase deficiency) (Janecke et al, 2004).

Hepatomegaly can also be seen in types III, IV (branching deficiency), and VI, where normal glycogen breakdown is impaired.

Diagnosis of the specific type of glycogen storage disease is critical for proper treatment and for prediction of prognosis and potential complications. Specific enzymatic assays and DNA diagnostic tests are available in specialty laboratories for each of the disorders, using liver, muscle, leukocytes, and fibroblasts.

Treatment in many of these disorders, particularly glycogen storage disease type I, is directed at maintaining normal blood sugar levels. Frequent feeding of high-carbohydrate-containing foods and nocturnal administration of slow-release glucose polymers, such as uncooked cornstarch, are utilized (Correia et al, 2008; Heller et al, 2008). This prevents the development of hypoglycemia and also limits incorporation of excess dietary glucose into glycogen.

PRIMARY MITOCHONDRIAL DISORDERS

Neonatal liver failure may occur in association with deficiency of complexes I, III or IV (cytochrome c oxidase) of the respiratory chain (Lee and Sokol, 2007). Activities of mitochondrial respiratory chain enzymes can be measured in affected tissues. Point mutations in mitochondrial or nuclear DNA have been detected in some patients with neonatal liver failure. Because of heteroplasmy, mitochondrial DNA (mtDNA) mutations are not uniform in all tissues, so patients may present exclusively with liver disease or with variable involvement of other organ systems.

Lethargy, hypotonia, vomiting, seizures, and poor feeding may be present from birth. Evidence of liver synthetic failure may occur with hypoglycemia, hypoproteinemia, hyperbilirubinemia, hyperammonemia, and coagulopathy (Lee and Sokol, 2007). Prenatal onset with fetal hydrops and congenital ascites has been reported. A key diagnostic feature in these patients is the presence of lactic acidosis and an elevated molar ratio of plasma lactate to pyruvate (normal <20:1) (Lee and Sokol, 2007).

Microvesicular and macrovesicular steatosis with abnormally increased mitochondrial density and swelling is typical on liver biopsy or postmortem specimens. Cholestasis, bile ductular proliferation, and fibrosis or even cirrhosis may be present.

The prognosis for patients with acute liver failure secondary to a mitochondrial disorder is extremely poor. There is no proven medical therapy. Liver transplantation has been successful in patients whose disease is restricted to the liver. MRI and magnetic resonance spectroscopy are critical in patients with acute liver failure as part of the pretransplant evaluation of the central nervous system (Lee and Sokol, 2007). Neurologic deterioration may still occur later even after an initially normal study.

Citrin deficiency is an autosomal recessive disorder that presents in the neonate with cholestasis, coagulopathy, failure to thrive, hypoglycemia, fatty liver, and hyperaminoacidemia (Hutchin et al, 2009; Tamamori et al, 2002). The majority of patients have been of Asian descent. Citrin is a mitochondrial aspartate-glutamate transporter, SLC25A13, which acts as part of the malate-aspartate shuttle in the liver and is thus important for aerobic glycolysis and gluconeogenesis. The varied clinical features may be confusing and mimic many neonatal cholestatic disorders (Sokol and Treem, 1999). Histopathology shows hepatocellular steatosis and cholestasis (Song et al, 2009). Increased serum citrulline and arginine together with galactosuria are nonspecific biochemical markers. The diagnosis can be confirmed by mutation analysis. Liver disease is rarely progressive. Clinical and biochemical abnormalities inexplicably resolve, usually without special treatment, by the age of 1 year in most patients (Tamamori et al, 2002).

CHOLESTASIS AND CONGENITAL HYPOPITUITARISM

Hypopituitarism should be considered in infants presenting with cholestasis and hypoglycemia (Binder et al, 2007). The combined or isolated hormonal deficiencies that may be associated with cholestasis include decreased production of growth hormone, cortisol, and thyroid hormone. Many of these infants have structural abnormalities of the brain on MRI, including hypoplasia of the optic nerves and optic chiasm, agenesis of septum pellucidum, and abnormalities of the corpus callosum and hypothalamopituitary axis (Webb and Dattani, 2010). These are key features of septo-optic dysplasia. There may be a wide spectrum of abnormalities present on imaging that may be limited to hypoplasia or aplasia of the anterior pituitary. Intrahepatic cholestasis may be seen in this disorder. Pituitary hormones may have a trophic effect on bile secretion, but the cholestatic liver disease cannot be solely explained on the basis of hormonal deficiencies. Liver biopsies may show giant-cell transformation of hepatocytes, but paucity of the intralobular bile ducts has also been observed (Binder et al, 2007). Hormone replacement usually leads to resolution of the cholestasis. Septo-optic dysplasia has been associated in some cases with mutations in two genes encoding the transcription factors, *HESX1* and *SOX2*.

HEMOPHAGOCYTIC LYMPHOHISTIOCYTOSIS

Hemophagocytic lymphohistiocytosis (HLH) is a disorder characterized by systemic inflammation caused by the uncontrolled proliferation of activated lymphocytes and histiocytes with massive release of inflammatory cytokines

(Filipovich et al, 2008). In the newborn, the acquired and genetic forms of the disorder are triggered by infections including enterovirus, herpes viruses, and CMV (Suzuki et al, 2009; Tanoshima et al, 2009). The process can begin in utero with nonimmune hydrops fetalis. The liver is invariably involved, even to the point of hepatic failure. Prolonged fever, hepatosplenomegaly, rashes, neurologic dysfunction, lymphadenopathy, and jaundice typically occur. Pancytopenia, elevated serum aminotransferases, bilirubin, elevated triglycerides and ferritin, and low fibrinogen are markers of the disorder. Hemophagocytosis by activated, morphologically normal macrophages is a cardinal feature that may be difficult to demonstrate in the bone marrow or on a liver biopsy early in the course of the disease (Janka, 2007).

Impaired function of natural killer cells and cytotoxic T cells reflect underlying immune dysfunction in genetic and acquired cases (Filipovich, 2008). The genetic disorders associated with HLH discovered so far all disrupt the pathway for granule-mediated cytotoxicity of target cells and eventual activation-induced apoptosis of activated T cells. Defects affect intracellular membrane trafficking mediated by Syntaxin 11, granule exocytosis mediated by MUNC 13-4, or pore-forming cytolysis by perforin (Horne et al, 2008). Mutation analysis may provide a specific diagnosis.

The prognosis for untreated HLH, particularly the familial cases, is extremely poor (Janka, 2007). However, the basis of initial therapy of HLH consists of combinations of proapoptotic chemotherapy and immunosuppressive drugs including corticosteroids targeting the hyperactivated T cells and histiocytes. For patients with a genetic cause, hematopoietic stem cell therapy offers the only possibility for definitive therapy (Cesaro et al, 2008).

NEONATAL HEMOCHROMATOSIS

Neonatal hemochromatosis is a form of neonatal liver failure caused by maternal-fetal alloimmune injury to hepatocytes (Whitington, 2007). Although there is in utero onset of hepatic and extrahepatic hemosiderosis, this entity is not related to hereditary hemochromatosis and is not caused by a primary defect in fetal iron metabolism. As is the case with other alloimmune disorders, the rate of occurrence of severe disease in subsequent newborns after the index case is 60% to 80%. A recent study has shown that occurrence of severe neonatal hemochromatosis in at-risk pregnancies can be significantly reduced by treatment with high-dose intravenous immunoglobulin during gestation (Whitington and Kelly, 2008).

Cholestatic jaundice with coagulopathy and/or ascites at birth is typical. Hypoalbuminemia, hypoglycemia, hyperammonemia, and high iron saturation and serum ferritin levels support the diagnosis. Extrahepatic siderosis can be found on biopsy of a minor salivary gland or MRI of the pancreas and/or heart. Liver histology reveals nonspecific findings of well-established fibrosis or cirrhosis, significant hepatocellular loss, and reactive bile ductular proliferation.

Infants with neonatal hemochromatosis have an expected mortality of more than 90% unless prompt medical treatment and/or liver transplantation is undertaken (Rodrigues et al, 2005). Early recognition of neonatal hemochromatosis is a requisite for survival. Medical

therapy consists of a combination of antioxidants (vitamin E in the form of tocopheryl polyethylene glycol succinate, selenium, and N-acetylcysteine), membrane stabilizers (prostaglandin E₁), and iron chelators (deferoxamine) (Grabhorn et al, 2006). The efficacy of this therapy alone is uncertain, but at least it appears to stabilize infants as a bridge to liver transplantation. In a recent study the addition of intravenous immunoglobulin markedly improved survival without liver transplantation (Rand et al, 2009). Liver transplantation has been successful, but mortality in these acutely ill babies may still exceed 50%. Recurrence of the disease after successful medical therapy or after liver transplantation has not been reported (Heffron et al, 2007).

LYSOSOMAL STORAGE DISEASES

There are more than 50 different lysosomal storage diseases that are caused by enzymatic defects leading to the accumulation of specific substrates that determine their clinical features and outcome (Ballabio and Gieselmann, 2009; Staretz-Chacham et al, 2009). Affected neonates often appear normal at birth, but some babies may demonstrate subtle features and may be mildly symptomatic in the newborn period. Although a detailed discussion of these diseases is beyond the scope of this chapter, it is important to consider that many lysosomal storage diseases may present in the newborn period with involvement of the liver.

Hepatosplenomegaly is a regular presenting feature. A lysosomal storage disease should be considered, particularly if perinatal viral infections, sepsis, and biliary obstruction are excluded. Extrahepatic features such as hypotonia and seizures may be present. Coarse facial features may also be recognized. Several disorders have been associated with nonimmune fetal hydrops and congenital ascites including type 2 Gaucher's disease, sialidosis type II, galactosialidosis, infantile sialic acid storage disease, Salla disease, mucopolysaccharidosis types IV and VII, GM1 gangliosidosis, I-cell disease, Niemann-Pick types A and C, Wolman's disease, and Farber's disease. Neonatal cholestasis has been described in Niemann-Pick type C, I-cell disease, and Gaucher's disease (Garver et al, 2007).

Early diagnosis is critical for genetic counseling, providing a prognosis, and maximizing the potential benefit from emerging enzyme-replacement, cell-based, and pharmacologic therapies (Platt and Lachmann, 2009; Wynn et al, 2009). Owing to the overlap of clinical features in many of these diseases, it is difficult to establish a diagnosis based solely on clinical presentation and findings on a liver biopsy. A specific diagnosis often relies on laboratory assays for detection of the stored product including urinary excretion, enzymatic assays on leukocytes or cultured fibroblasts, and DNA mutational analysis.

CONGENITAL DISORDERS OF GLYCOSYLATION

Congenital disorders of glycosylation (CDG) are inborn errors of metabolism caused by defective N-glycosylation of proteins (Collins and Ferriero, 2005). Because glycoproteins are critically important in metabolism, cell recognition and adhesion, membrane trafficking, host defense, and antigenicity, it is not surprising that CDG can affect multiple organ systems including the liver, with protean clinical manifestations even in the newborn.

At least 12 of the 30 known subtypes involve the liver (Iancu et al, 2007). Hepatomegaly and elevated serum aminotransferases are common. Other common clinical features include dysmorphic facies, mental retardation, failure to thrive, seizures, hypotonia, diarrhea, protein-losing enteropathy, recurrent infection, and coagulopathy. The histopathology is not well defined in most subtypes, but steatosis, fibrosis, and even cirrhosis have been described. A process similar to congenital hepatic fibrosis occurs in CDG-1b.

CDG should be considered in any infant with cryptogenic liver disease. Isoelectric focusing to detect the abnormally glycosylated transferrin is the commonly used diagnostic test, but some forms cannot be detected using this method. Mass spectroscopy and mutation analysis may be of value in some cases (Biffi et al, 2007). There is no specific treatment for most of these disorders.

DISORDERS OF FATTY ACID OXIDATION

Acute liver injury can occur in infants from inherited defects in fatty acid oxidation, resulting from energy deprivation and the accumulation of toxic metabolites of fatty acid oxidation (Rinaldo and Matern, 2000). The liver is central to fatty acid metabolism and requires fatty acid transport into hepatocytes and mitochondria and a series of enzymatic steps that generate energy from oxidation of fatty acids. Hepatopathy has been described in two thirds of the more than 20 defects in fatty acid oxidation. At least six disorders cause relatively severe liver disease, including a long-chain fatty acid transport defect, carnitine palmitoyltransferase deficiency, long-chain hydroxyacyl-CoA-dehydrogenase deficiency, α and β trifunctional protein defects, and short-chain hydroxyacyl-CoA-dehydrogenase deficiency (Rinaldo et al, 2002).

The typical case of severe liver disease often follows the catabolic stress of fasting or intercurrent illness. Nonketotic hypoglycemia is a hallmark feature of these disorders. Serum aminotransferase levels are often markedly elevated with variable degrees of cholestasis and coagulopathy. Myopathy (skeletal and/or cardiac) may be an accompanying feature.

Prompt recognition of defects in fatty acid metabolism is critical for proper treatment. Diagnostic assays that examine intermediate metabolites of fatty acid oxidation need to be performed during illness, because many of the metabolites will rapidly clear with treatment. Nonspecific screening assays and more specific enzymatic and DNA diagnostic tests are used in the evaluation (Gregersen et al, 2001). Initial studies should include assays of plasma carnitine, acylcarnitines, free fatty acids, urine organic acids, and acylglycines. Microvesicular steatosis is a common although not universal feature in fatty acid oxidation defects.

Treatment focuses on stopping ongoing fatty acid oxidation and fat catabolism through the intravenous infusion of 12 to 15 mg/kg/min of glucose. Subsequent avoidance of fasting is crucial, but the benefits of carnitine administration and specific dietary fat restrictions or supplementation

are uncertain (Spiekerkoetter et al, 2009a, 2009b). In cases of liver failure or recurrent bouts of severe hepatic injury, liver transplantation should be considered if there is no evidence of severe systemic or neurologic disease (Alonso, 2005).

GALLSTONES AND CHOLECYSTITIS

Gallstones are rarely detected on a fetal ultrasound (Munjuluri et al, 2005). Most of these infants are asymptomatic postnatally and may have spontaneous disappearance of gallstones over the first few months of life.

Gallstones and calculous cholecystitis occur particularly in premature infants, who have undergone a period of prolonged fasting on parenteral nutrition without frequent gallbladder stimulation (Wilcox et al, 1997). Additional risk factors for development of gallstones in these infants include frequent blood transfusions, episodes of sepsis, abdominal surgery, and use of diuretics and narcotic analgesics. The composition of gallstones in such cases has not been well studied, but limited data suggest they are mixed cholesterol–calcium bilirubinate stones. Asymptomatic gallstones may disappear spontaneously, but may be associated with biliary obstruction and cholecystitis requiring surgical intervention.

Brown pigment gallstones have been associated with biliary obstruction in infants, and are composed of varying proportions of calcium bilirubinate, calcium phosphate, calcium palmitate, cholesterol, and organic material (Treem et al, 1989). In several cases, there was high β-glucuronidase activity in bile, possibly related to bacterial infections of the biliary tract.

LIVER TUMORS

Infantile hemangiomas and hemangioendotheliomas are benign vascular tumors of the liver and account for almost one fifth of liver tumors in childhood (Lopez-Terrada and Finegold, 2007). The presence of visible cutaneous strawberry hemangiomas may suggest the presence of a vascular tumor in the liver. Measuring thyroid function can be very useful as the hemangiomatous tissue produces high levels of type 3 iodothyronine deiodinase, causing hypothyroidism (Huang et al, 2000). A serious complication is high-output cardiac failure and the Kasabach-Merritt syndrome with consumptive coagulopathy, anemia, and thrombocytopenia (Beller and Ruhrmann, 1959). Medical treatment is with steroids. Diuretics, digoxin, hepatic artery ligation, and surgical resection are used if there is heart failure. Liver transplantation is an option when medical treatment fails or there is concern for angiosarcoma.

Malignant liver tumors account for 1.1% of all childhood tumors in the United States (Lopez-Terrada and Finegold, 2007). Hepatoblastoma is the commonest and has a strong association with prematurity; the majority are diagnosed by 1 year of age. Elevated levels of serum α-fetoprotein are associated with 80% to 90% of hepatoblastomas. Treatment is complete resection with or without chemotherapy. Liver transplantation is indicated when tumor resection is not feasible, provided there is no extrahepatic metastasis at the time of transplant.

SUGGESTED READINGS

Alissa FT, Jaffe R, Shneider BL: Update on progressive familial intrahepatic cholestasis, *J Pediatr Gastroenterol Nutr* 46:241-252, 2008.

Colombo C: Liver disease in cystic fibrosis, *Curr Opin Pulm Med* 13:529-536.

Davenport M, Betalli P, D'Antiga L, et al: The spectrum of surgical jaundice in infancy, *J Pediatr Surg* 38:1471-1479, 2003.

Emerick KM, Rand EB, Goldmuntz E, et al: Features of Alagille syndrome in 92 patients: frequency and relation to prognosis, *Hepatology* 29:822-829, 1999.

Lee WS, Sokol RJ: Liver disease in mitochondrial disorders, *Semin Liver Dis* 27:259-273, 2007.

Russo PA, Mitchell GA, Tanguay RM: Tyrosinemia: a review, *Pediatr Dev Pathol* 4:212-221, 2001.

Setchell KD, Heubi JE: Defects in bile acid biosynthesis—diagnosis and treatment, *J Pediatr Gastroenterol Nutr* 43(Suppl 1):S17-S22, 2006.

Sokol RJ, Mack C: Etiopathogenesis of biliary atresia, *Semin Liver Dis* 21:517-524, 2001.

Staretz-Chacham O, Lang TC, LaMarca ME, et al: Lysosomal storage disorders in the newborn, *Pediatrics* 123:1191-1207, 2009.

Suchy FJ: Neonatal cholestasis, *Pediatr Rev* 25:388-396, 2004.

Teckman JH: Alpha1-antitrypsin deficiency in childhood, *Semin Liver Dis* 27:274-281, 2007.

Whitington PF: Neonatal hemochromatosis: a congenital alloimmune hepatitis, *Semin Liver Dis* 27:243-250, 2007.

Complete references and supplemental color images used in this text can be found online at www.expertconsult.com

PART XV

HEMATOLOGIC SYSTEM AND DISORDERS OF BILIRUBIN METABOLISM

CHAPTER 75

DEVELOPMENTAL BIOLOGY OF THE HEMATOLOGIC SYSTEM

Annie Nguyen-Vermillion and Sandra E. Juul

EMBRYONIC HEMATOPOIESIS

Hematopoiesis is the overall process by which self-renewing multipotential stem cells give rise to the multiple lineages of differentiated blood cells (Figure 75-1). This complex process is guided by the coordinated expression of growth factors, some of which act on primitive progenitor cells that can give rise to multiple cell lineages, and others of which support lineage-committed multipotential hematopoietic stem cells (HSCs). Hematopoiesis begins early in embryonic life, with the first hematopoietic cells appearing in the mouse yolk sac at embryonic day 7.5 (Palis and Yoder, 2001; Yoshimoto and Yoder, 2009). By day 10 of mouse gestation, HSCs are present in the aorto-gonado-mesonephron (AGM); activity then shifts to the liver, and finally to the bone marrow (Charbord et al, 1996). Each cell line undergoes developmental changes that are unique and specific. The details of these systems and the resulting clinical impact of these changes are reviewed individually in the following chapters.

STEM CELL BIOLOGY

Pluripotential stem cells sustain marrow function throughout a person's lifetime. A unique characteristic of these cells is that their direct offspring include at least one identical daughter cell, thus perpetuating the population. In contrast, progenitor cells are more differentiated and give rise only to cells more differentiated than themselves. The fate of any particular developing cell is determined by its microenvironment.

The developmental changes in the number, function, and location of HSCs are of great interest to transplantation biologists and gene therapists. The cycling potential and proliferative capacity of HSCs vary with the anatomic source of the cells, and with the age at which the cells are harvested. The sensitivity of these cells to recombinant cytokines also changes with age. Thus, improving the understanding of the ontogeny of these cells will be helpful in optimizing their clinical use.

Embryonic and fetal HSCs are capable of repopulating an adult organism (Fleischmann et al, 1984). In contrast, transplanted adult stem cells have a lower capacity for self-renewal, often resulting in late graft failure. This may be because the adult stem cells continue to express the adult differentiation program despite the fetal environment, indicating an irreversible change in gene expression (Fleischmann et al, 1984). Other explanations for the decrease in proliferative potential may have to do with the accrual of DNA damage over time and loss of telomere repeats with each stem cell division, limiting the replicative potential of stem cells (Notaro et al, 1997; Vaziri et al, 1994; Warren and Rossi, 2009). The increase in cell replication required after engraftment may impose replicative stress on the HSC, decreasing telomere length and resulting in a pronounced aging effect (Wynn et al, 1998).

There is ongoing research focused on optimizing stem cell harvesting techniques. Cell surface markers, which are dependent on cell maturity and gestational age, are often used to identify and separate HSCs using monoclonal antibodies and FACS analysis. For example, CD34, a cell-surface sialomucin, is an antigen commonly used to select hematopoietic stem cells and early erythropoietic progenitor cells. Combining CD34 positivity with the absence of lineage-specific markers (lin–) allows one to select a cell population highly enriched for the cells desired for transplantation. Research is also focused on optimizing stem cell harvest sites. Both bone marrow and cord blood are rich in stem cells and have long been used as progenitor cell pools. The collection of stem cells from peripheral blood by stimulated apheresis, with ex vivo expansion of select populations, is now also a viable option (Brugger et al, 2000; Pettengell et al, 1994a, 1994b).

Umbilical cord blood (UCB) is a source of HSCs that can be harvested and used for transplantation in patients with bone marrow failure, malignancies, and immunodeficiencies (Warwick and Armitage, 2004). UCB can be harvested directly from the umbilical cord after birth. Although small volumes are collected, the cells have a high proliferation index, so fewer cells can be used when compared to bone marrow transplantation (Schoemans et al, 2006). Because of the presumed immaturity of the cord blood cells, human leukocyte antigen (HLA) matching is less stringent for UCB (Rubinstein et al, 1998), allowing for more efficient donor unit identification compared with using a bone marrow registry (Barker et al, 2002; Beatty et al, 2000). This feature of UCB also allows for improved matching ability for patients in minority ethnic populations, because bone marrow registry matches are frequently in short supply. Promising strategies to increase cells available for transplantation include combining multiple units

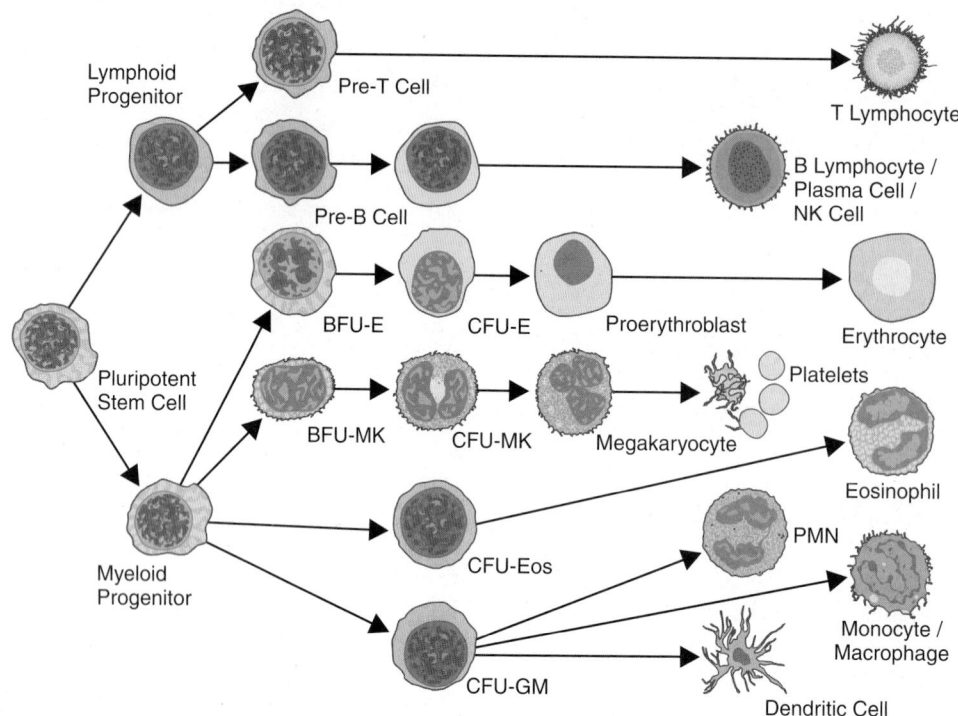

FIGURE 75-1 Overview of hematopoiesis. Hematopoietic lineages are outlined in this simplified overview of hematopoiesis. *BFU*, Burst-forming unit; *CFU*, colony-forming unit; *E*, erythroid; *GM*, granulocyte-macrophage; *MK*, megakaryocyte; *NK*, nonkiller; *PMN*, polymorphonuclear. *(Courtesy Alexander R. Vermillion.)*

of UCB (Barker et al, 2005) and ex vivo expansion of UCB units (Papassavas et al, 2008).

The first successful use of UCB for HSC transplantation purposes was in 1989 between HLA-identical siblings for severe aplastic anemia from Fanconi's anemia (Gluckman et al, 1989). Since then, thousands of UCB transplantations have been done to treat malignancies such as acute lymphoblastic leukemia, acute myeloid leukemia, and chronic myeloid leukemia; bone marrow disorders such as Fanconi's anemia; immunodeficiencies such as severe combined immune deficiency; metabolic disorders; and hemoglobinopathies (Prasad and Kurtzberg, 2009).

UCB can be stored in public or private commercial banks. Donation of harvested cells to public cord blood banks allows for storage in a central repository available to all individuals in need of transplantation. Private banking makes the stored UCB available at a cost for future use by individuals or family. However, there is a low likelihood of any one individual needing an autologous cord blood transplant (Johnson, 1997).

The optimal timing of umbilical cord clamping is controversial. Delaying cord clamping by 30 seconds to 1 minute provides increased blood volume to the neonate, but less is then available for UCB collection, whereas early cord clamping enables significantly more blood to be collected from the placenta after birth but less for the infant. A 2004 Cochrane review suggests that delayed clamping is associated with less intraventricular hemorrhage and fewer transfusions (Rabe et al, 2004). Recent studies have shown only a modest decrease in need for blood transfusions after delayed cord clamping, despite the improvement in red blood cell volume and hematocrit (Strauss et al, 2008).

DEVELOPMENTAL ASPECTS OF ERYTHROPOIESIS

Erythropoiesis is the process of perpetual production of red blood cells (*erythro*, "red"; *poiesis*, "growth"). Serial adaptations occur throughout development so as to meet the changing oxygen demands of the embryo, fetus, and neonate. The type of cells produced, the locations in which they are produced, and even the microenvironments within these locations change as development proceeds (Figure 75-2). The molecular mechanisms involved in instituting, regulating, and maintaining these adaptations are complex.

PRIMITIVE AND DEFINITIVE ERYTHROPOIESIS

During development, two types of red blood cells are formed: primitive and definitive erythrocytes. The liver is the primary organ of hematopoiesis during fetal life, but before the liver is formed, primitive red cells are formed in the yolk sac (Yoshimoto and Yoder, 2009). Hemogenic endothelium, a subset of early endothelium, gives rise to HSCs (Chen et al, 2009; Eilken et al, 2009; Lancrin et al, 2009). Large primitive red cells are produced in blood islands of the yolk sac days after implantation of the embryo. These cells enter the newly formed vasculature of the embryo, where they continue to divide and differentiate for several days. This process is only minimally responsive to the growth factor erythropoietin (EPO) (Lin et al, 1996; Wu et al, 1995b). Primitive erythroblasts are large (>20 μm), CD34-negative, and contain predominantly embryonic hemoglobin. Hemoglobin synthesis continues until cell replication ceases (Boussios and Bertles, 1988).

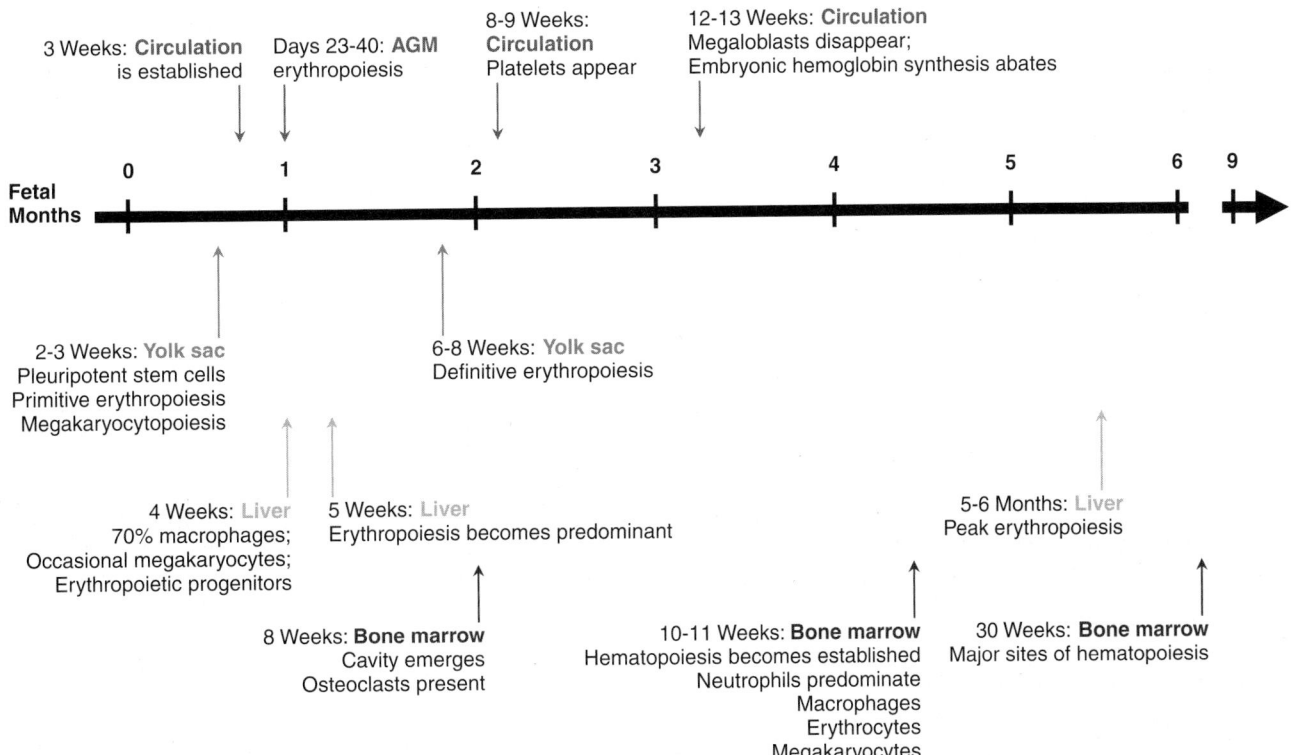

FIGURE 75-2 Changing sites of hematopoiesis during human gestation. Fetal gestation is shown in months along the central horizontal arrow. The timing of significant events during hematopoiesis is shown, beginning with primitive erythropoiesis and megakaryocytopoiesis in the yolk sac and ending with definitive hematopoiesis in the bone marrow during late gestation. *AGM,* Aorto-gonado-mesonephron.

In mice, a transition to definitive erythropoiesis occurs at embryonic day 13.5 (full gestation is 21 days). Definitive erythropoiesis is characterized by smaller (<20 μm) CD34⁺ erythroblasts, which produce fetal and adult hemoglobins, extruding their nuclei when mature. Unlike primitive erythropoiesis, this process is dependent on Janus kinase (JAK) signal transduction and EPO stimulation (Neubauer et al, 1998; Tavassoli, 1991; Wu et al, 1995b). Primitive erythroblasts normally undergo apoptosis, becoming extinct during fetal life, whereas definitive erythroblasts are able to self-renew (Dieterlen-Lievre, 1997).

SWITCH OF THE PRIMARY SITE OF ERYTHROPOIESIS

Humans have four main sites of embryonic and fetal erythropoiesis: yolk sac, aorta (ventral aspect), liver, and bone marrow. In rodents, the spleen is also an important site of hematopoiesis, but there is no evidence for this in healthy humans (Calhoun et al, 1996; Wolf et al, 1983). Studies using an in vitro embryonic stem cell differentiation system have shown that endothelial cells, primitive hematopoietic cells, and definitive blood-cell colonies arise from a common *Flk-1* expressing progenitor (Lancrin et al, 2009). Between embryonic days 8 and 11.5, *Runx 1*, a transcription factor, is required for the formation of HSCs and their progenitors (Chen et al, 2009). Primitive progenitor cells first develop in the yolk sac, followed by the rise of definitive progenitors, also in the yolk sac (Palis, 2008; Palis et al, 2001). Another source of the early definitive progenitors is along the ventral aspect of the embryonic aorta

(Palis, 2008; Tavian et al, 1996; Tavian and Peault, 2005). Once circulation is established, progenitors from all lineages are detected in the blood, then in the fetal liver, and finally in the marrow (Palis et al, 1999; Tavian et al, 2001).

Yolk Sac

The yolk sac is an extraembryonic structure that can be subdivided into the primary and secondary yolk sac. The primary yolk sac is transient and has no known hematopoietic function. In humans, it forms by proliferation and differentiation of primitive endodermal cells 7 to 8 days after conception. These endodermal cells give rise to mesodermal precursors (intermediate cells). The primary yolk sac then collapses into small vesicles, and the secondary yolk sac is formed from its remnants at 12 to 15 days postconception. By 16 to 19 days postconception, primitive erythropoiesis is found in the human yolk sac (Kelemen et al, 1979; Kennedy et al, 1997; Tavassoli, 1991). The secondary yolk sac is an active site of protein synthesis, nutrient transport, and hematopoiesis (Enders and King, 1993). Primitive hematopoietic cells, adherent to surrounding endothelial cells, are first observed at day 16 in the mesodermal layer. These hematopoietic-endothelial cell masses have been described as blood islands (Zon, 1995). As maturation proceeds, these blood islands migrate toward each other, merging to form a network of capillaries. Small clusters of undifferentiated cells, the hemangioblasts, and clusters of primitive erythroblasts are observed in the small vessels present at this developmental stage (Enders and King, 1993). As differentiation proceeds, endothelial and hematopoietic cell lineages emerge. These cell lines share common molecular markers and responsiveness to a cohort of growth factors, and, depending on the microenvironment, they can be derived from a common stem cell in culture (Choi, 1998; Choi et al, 1998; Eichmann et al, 1997; Lancrin et al, 2009; Lux et al, 2008; Palis and Yoder, 2001; Robertson et al, 1999).

After the 6th week postconception, definitive erythroblasts are found in the yolk sac. A decline in yolk sac hematopoiesis is observed after the 8th week of gestation (Enders and King, 1993). There are in vivo differences in the hematopoietic potential of yolk sac cells, compared to those in the liver. Yolk sac–derived hematopoietic cells have more restricted potential in vivo, because only red cells and macrophages are present in the yolk sac (Enzan, 1986), while progenitor cells in the liver develop into the full spectrum of hematopoietic lineages (Palis et al, 1999). However, when yolk sac–derived stem cells are cultured in vitro or are transplanted, they are multipotent, illustrating the importance of the microenvironment in the development of committed cell lineages (Tavassoli, 1991).

Aorto-Gonado-Mesonephron (AGM)

Another site of early erythropoietic activity in the developing human embryo is the ventral aspect of the aorta, in the periumbilical region (Huyhn et al, 1995; Tavian and Peault, 2005). At around the 23rd postconceptional day in humans, the multipotent hematopoietic progenitor cells in this region are more numerous than in the yolk sac or the liver (Huyhn et al, 1995). By day 40 of gestation, hematopoiesis in this site is concluded.

Liver

A short time after the onset of blood circulation (4 to 5 weeks' gestation), erythropoiesis begins in the liver (Kelemen et al, 1979). As in the yolk sac, primitive erythroblasts predominate in early erythropoiesis. However, over the next 4 weeks, definitive erythrocytes become the predominant red cell form. During this time, the liver mass increases 40-fold, with hematopoietic cells comprising 60% of the liver by weeks 11 to 12 (Thomas and Yoffey, 1964). Meanwhile, other hematopoietic cell lineages are also produced in the liver. Early in this process (5 weeks), macrophages predominate, with approximately 1 granulocyte to every 9 macrophages (Slayton et al, 1998). In contrast to the yolk sac, during the period of peak hepatic hematopoiesis (weeks 6 to 18), production of all hematopoietic cell lines (erythrocytes, macrophages, megakaryocytes, granulocytes, and lymphocytes) occurs. Between 18 and 21 weeks' gestation, hematopoiesis in the liver diminishes, but the liver continues as an erythropoietic organ until term.

Bone Marrow

As hepatic hematopoiesis diminishes, the bone marrow becomes the primary site of erythropoiesis and remains so throughout postnatal life. The process of erythropoiesis in marrow begins at about 8 weeks, again, with primitive erythrocytosis (Kelemen et al, 1979). Over the next several gestational weeks, a switch to definitive erythropoiesis occurs, and by 14 weeks, only definitive erythroblasts are present. As with the liver, production of all hematopoietic cells occurs in bone marrow. Erythropoietic cells constitute a maximum of 35% of total bone marrow cells at week 12 of gestation, falling to between 20% and 30% thereafter (Charbord et al, 1996; Thomas and Yoffey, 1962).

FACTORS INFLUENCING THE SITES OF ERYTHROPOIESIS

The microenvironment at each site of hematopoiesis influences the type and timing of hematopoietic development. The microenvironment includes hematopoietic growth factors and cytokines, as well as the extracellular matrix in which the cells proliferate.

Growth factors are thought to act mainly as permissive and/or selective signals, allowing already committed cell types to proliferate and differentiate. Growth factors important for definitive erythropoiesis include EPO, stem cell factor (SCF) (c-kit), interleukin-3 (IL-3), thrombopoietin (TPO), and possibly insulin, and insulin-like growth factor 1 (IGF-1), both of which act as nonessential survival factors for CD34+ cells (Muta and Krantz, 1993; Muta et al, 1994; Ratajczak et al, 1998). These growth factors work in concert to promote definitive erythropoiesis. However, EPO is the primary growth factor: in the absence of EPO signaling, as in the case for both EPO and EPO receptor null mutations, definitive erythropoiesis does not occur. Null mutations of either EPO or its receptor are lethal at 13.5 days' gestation in the mouse, because of severe anemia (Wu et al, 1995a, 1995b).

EXTRAMEDULLARY HEMATOPOIESIS

After the bone marrow has been established as the primary site of erythropoiesis, extramedullary hematopoiesis occasionally occurs as a pathologic process. This can occur with severe bone marrow failure of any etiology, but common causes include congenital rubella, cytomegalovirus, and parvovirus B19 infection. Extramedullary hematopoiesis has been documented in many tissues, including the liver, spleen, adrenal glands, pancreas, thyroid gland, endocardium, testes, uterus, skin, and brain. When the skin is involved, this results in the classic "blueberry muffin" rash seen in newborns with congenital rubella or CMV infection.

ONTOGENY OF ERYTHROCYTES

The earliest precursor cells specific to the erythroid lineage are the burst-forming unit-erythroid (BFU-E). BFU-E have low numbers of EPO receptors (Sawada et al, 1988, 1990) and respond to EPO, as well as GM-CSF and IL-3. As these cells mature into colony-forming unit-erythroid (CFU-E) and proerythroblasts, they become highly dependent on EPO, which is reflected by the high density of EPO receptors on the cell membrane (up to 1000 per cell) (Broudy et al, 1991). Mature erythroblasts have fewer EPO receptors and therefore are less sensitive to EPO stimulation, and reticulocytes and erythrocytes have no EPO receptors and are unresponsive to EPO. These mature cells are unique, in that they do not have a nucleus, DNA, RNA, ribosomes, or mitochondria. The principal functions of mature erythrocyte metabolism are to maintain adequate adenosine triphosphate (ATP) stores, to produce reducing substances to act as antioxidants, and to produce 2,3-diphosphoglycerate (2,3-DPG), which modifies the oxygen affinity of hemoglobin.

Important developmental changes occur in hematocrit, reticulocyte count, red cell morphology, membrane content, deformability, life span, and metabolism. Over the course of gestation, there is a rise in expected hematocrit, from 36% ± 3% at 18 to 20 weeks' gestation (fetal samples) to 55% ± 6% (Jopling et al, 2009) expected at term birth. In order to maintain this increase in hematocrit and blood volume (up to 7 mL/day during the last trimester) associated with fetal growth, the production of approximately 50×10^9 erythrocytes per day is required, based on animal experiments (Bell and Wintour, 1985). During this same period of fetal development, erythrocyte size (the mean cell volume) decreases from 134 ± 9 fL to 119 ± 9 fL (Forestier et al, 1991; Zaizov and Matoth, 1976). A recent study examined erythrocyte indices over a wide range of gestational ages to develop new reference ranges (Christensen et al, 2009). Christensen et al (2009) showed erythrocytes to be very large in neonates at the limits of extrauterine viability, with a steady decrease in size as gestational age increases. At term, the mean cell volume remains larger than that of normal healthy adults. Mean cell volume continues to drop postnatally, reaching a nadir at 4 to 6 months of life. It then increases to reach adult values (88 ± 8 fL) by approximately 1 year of life.

Reticulocytes are near-mature erythrocytes released from the bone marrow into the circulation. Although the nucleus has been extruded, they retain cytoplasmic organelles such as ribosomes, mitochondria, and Golgi bodies for approximately 24 hours. These newly released cells can be differentiated from mature red blood cells by staining with new methylene blue or brilliant cresyl blue, which stain the nucleic acid within the cells. Evaluation of a patient's reticulocyte count can be used to assess the level of erythrocyte production, because high values indicate active erythropoiesis, whereas depressed numbers indicate low levels of erythropoiesis. At birth, reticulocyte counts in preterm infants tend to be higher than in term infants (400,000 to 550,000 vs. 200,000 to 400,000) (Christensen, 2000). Absolute reticulocyte counts, reticulocyte percentage of total red cells, and corrected reticulocyte counts can be obtained. In general, when evaluating neonates, the corrected reticulocyte count is the most helpful, because this reflects the reticulocyte response relative to the hematocrit. This corrected value is calculated as: patient's reticulocyte percentage (%) × patient's hematocrit (%) ÷ desired or optimal hematocrit (45%). Some laboratories also report a reticulocyte production index (RPI), which corrects, in addition, for reticulocyte maturation or shift. This can be helpful in differentiating hypoproliferative anemia (RPI <2) from a hyperproliferative or hemolytic anemia (RPI >3).

Red cell morphology is quite heterogeneous in preterm and term infants as compared with adults. Irregularly shaped cells such as poikilocytes, acanthocytes, schizocytes, and burr cells are common in the blood smears of neonates. This reflects developmental changes in cell membrane deformability and flexibility. The neonatal red blood cell membrane has decreased deformability, which contributes to its decreased life span of approximately 70 days as compared to 120 days for the adult red blood cell. Membrane characteristics become more adultlike by 4 to 6 weeks of age.

DEVELOPMENTAL CHANGES IN THE REGULATION OF ERYTHROPOIESIS

The principal growth factor that regulates erythropoiesis is EPO. This 30.4-kDa glycoprotein contains 165 amino acids and is extensively glycosylated, with 40% carbohydrate content. EPO maintains red cell production during fetal, neonatal, and adult life by inhibiting apoptosis of erythroid progenitors and by stimulating their proliferation and differentiation into normoblasts (Jelkmann, 1992; Moritz et al, 1997; Palis and Segel, 1998). Because very little EPO crosses the placenta, the EPO concentrations measured in the fetus reflect fetal synthesis (Eichhorn et al, 1993; Widness et al, 1991). EPO production begins early in fetal life, and it has been identified in extraembryonic coelomic fluid and amniotic fluid (Campbell et al, 1992). The primary site of EPO production during fetal life is the liver, with transition to the kidney postnatally (Fahnenstich and Dame, 1996; Koury and Koury, 1993; Koury et al, 1993). This transition is mediated in part by expression of GATA-4 (Dame et al, 2004). Production of EPO is stimulated by hypoxia via hypoxia-inducible factor (HIF) 1 and 2 pathways (Dioum et al, 2009; Fisher et al, 2009; Lam et al, 2009; Semenza, 2009; Webb et al, 2009). HIF is a DNA-binding complex composed of two subunits: HIF-1b, which is not oxygen responsive and is constitutively expressed, and either HIF-1a or HIF-2a, both of which are highly oxygen sensitive. The HIF complex is, in turn, regulated by prolyl hydroxylase domain enzymes 1 to 3 (Weidemann and Johnson, 2009). Elevated EPO concentrations (up to 8000 μ/mL) have been reported in pathologic states such as fetal hypoxia, anemia, and placental insufficiency and in infants of diabetic mothers (Buescher et al, 1998; Stangenberg et al, 1993).

During fetal development, circulating EPO concentrations range from 4 μ/mL at 16 weeks' gestation to 40 μ/mL at term (Clapp et al, 1995; Fahnenstich et al, 1996; Forestier et al, 1991). An unhealthy intrauterine environment can result in increased EPO production, reflecting fetal hypoxemia (Halmesmäki et al, 1990; Ruth et al, 1990; Teramo et al, 1987). After birth in healthy term infants, serum EPO concentrations decrease at birth to reach a nadir between the 4th and 6th weeks after birth (Brown et al, 1983; Ruth et al, 1990). By 10 to 12 weeks of age they reach adult concentrations (approximately 15 μ/mL) (Kling et al, 1996). These changes in EPO concentrations are consistent with the changes in hemoglobin and hematocrit seen following term birth (physiologic anemia). In preterm infants, the anemia is more severe and persists longer, leading to the anemia of prematurity described earlier. EPO concentrations in these infants are inappropriately low, forming the rationale for recombinant human EPO therapy.

ONTOGENY OF HEMOGLOBIN CHAINS

Organization and Structure of the Hemoglobins

Hemoglobin is a tetrameric molecule comprised of two pairs of polypeptide subunits. As development proceeds, various hemoglobins are constructed by combining two α-like globins (ζ or α) with two β-like globins (ε, γ, δ, or β) to form a hemoglobin tetramer. These tetramers include the embryonic hemoglobins, Hb Gower 1 ($\zeta_2\varepsilon_2$), Hb Gower 2 ($\alpha_2\varepsilon_2$), and Hb Portland 1 ($\zeta_2\gamma_2$), fetal hemoglobin (Hb F) ($\alpha_2\gamma_2$), and the adult hemoglobins Hb A ($\alpha_2\beta_2$) and Hb A$_2$ ($\alpha_2\delta_2$). Their expression and proportion depend on gestational age but can, in part, be modified by external mechanisms. The basic function of the various hemoglobins is similar, but their oxygen affinity differs. As the hemoglobins switch from embryonic to fetal to adult forms, oxygen affinity decreases. Thus, the switch from embryonic to fetal to adult hemoglobin synthesis is a major mechanism by which the developing fetus adapts from the hypoxic intrauterine to the oxygen-rich extrauterine environment (Bard, 2000).

Changes in Hemoglobin Synthesis With Development

The genes within the α- as well as the β-globin families are expressed according to a strict ontogenetic schedule, and the quantitative expression of the genes from each of these families is strictly balanced and coordinated (Bard, 2000). Hemoglobin synthesis begins around 14 days postconception, with synthesis of ζ- and ε-globin chains. These are replaced by the synthesis of α- and γ-globin chains by the 5th to 7th week of gestation (Hb Gower 2, Hb Portland 1, and Hb F become predominant) (Gale et al, 1979). By 12 weeks' gestation, Hb F ($\alpha_2\gamma_2$) accounts for almost all of the hemoglobin produced (Cividalli et al, 1974). After the 20th week of gestation, no ε-globin chains are produced, but the production of the ζ-globin chains can persist through the last trimester in pathologic conditions such as homozygous α-thalassemia. Expression of the γ-globin gene peaks during mid-gestation and declines rapidly during the last month of fetal gestation. β-Globin synthesis, required for Hb A, starts at the 6th week of gestation, increasing as γ-globin synthesis declines, a transition that continues to the 6th month of life (Bard, 1975; Kazazian and Woodhead, 1973). Thus, Hb A synthesis quantitatively increases first after the 30th week of gestation. At the end of the last trimester, a rapid switch from the synthesis of fetal hemoglobin to adult hemoglobin occurs, falling from 85% at 34 weeks' gestation, to 60% to 80% at birth (Peri et al, 1998). The synthesis of δ-globin chains, required for HbA$_2$ ($\alpha_2\delta_2$), begins at the 34th to the 35th week of gestation. After birth, a rapid increase in HbA and HbA$_2$ occurs.

RED BLOOD CELL TRANSFUSION

Transfusion of red blood cells (RBCs) increases blood volume and red blood cell content, thereby increasing oxygen-carrying capacity. We have had the capacity to store blood for future transfusions since the early 1900s (Rous and Turner, 1916a, 1916b). In the early years, cells were kept viable in a citrate and glucose solution, but current solutions make it possible to store cells for more prolonged periods (up to 42 days): citrate-phosphate-dextrose (CPD), citrate-phosphate-dextrose-adenine (CPDA), and various additive solutions (AS), which may contain additional dextrose, mannitol, and adenine (Hess, 2009). The hematocrit of "packed RBCs" ranges from 50% to 80%. During storage, the RBCs undergo metabolic and structural changes. 2,3-DPG, antioxidant, and ATP content decrease, glycolysis decreases, osmotic fragility increases, and deformability decreases (Högman et al, 1985; Lockwood et al, 2003). ATP-dependent membrane pumps are dysfunctional, so extracellular potassium increases at 1 mEq/day, which can be dangerous when transfusing large volumes (Hall et al, 1993; Hess, 2009). Oxidative damage occurs in lipids and proteins during storage and irradiation (Dumaswala et al, 2000; Sharifi et al, 2000). Proinflammatory compounds accumulate during storage of blood, particularly if it is not leukoreduced. After an RBC transfusion, the mean potential life span of the RBC is 85 days with a mean half-life of 43 ± 11 days (Strauss et al, 2004).

Risks of RBC transfusion may be due to the storage process, the transfusion itself, and the association with oxidative damage. Because of the storage process and increasing age of the stored blood, RBC transfusion exposes the recipient to high levels of potassium, glucose, hydrogen, and lactic acid; the clinical significance depends on the age of the blood and the volume transfused (Sümpelmann et al, 2001). Although rare, transfusion-transmitted bacterial infections can occur as a result of bacterial contamination of stored blood (Niu et al, 2006; Wagner, 2004). Other risks of RBC transfusion include viral infections, transfusion-related acute lung injury (TRALI), and graft-versus-host reaction. Multiple RBC transfusions may also put the patient at risk for iron overload and oxidative injury (Sullivan, 1988). There are 200 mg of iron in a 420-mL unit of whole blood, which is then processed into 250-mL units of packed RBCs (Porter, 2001), so a unit of blood with a hematocrit of 60% contains 0.7 mg/mL of iron, which becomes available as the cells turn over. There is increased unbound iron in stored blood, which may increase reactive oxygen species (Hirano et al, 2001). In retrospective and observational studies, increased numbers of RBC transfusions have been associated with retinopathy of prematurity (Dani et al, 2001; Hesse et al, 1997), bronchopulmonary dysplasia, necrotizing enterocolitis, and diuretic use (Valieva et al, 2009).

Optimal hematocrit values and indications for transfusions in infants in the neonatal intensive care unit (NICU) remain controversial. In the past, infants were transfused for hematocrits less than 40%. Because of the risk of transfusions and lack of evidence for benefit, more restrictive transfusion guidelines have been proposed. Most studies comparing restrictive to liberal transfusion practices in premature infants have not demonstrated any benefit to maintaining higher hemoglobin levels (Bell et al, 2005; Brooks et al, 1999; Kirpalani et al, 2006). However, restrictive guidelines were associated with increased periventricular leukomalacia and severe intracranial hemorrhage in one trial of restrictive versus liberal transfusion guidelines for premature infants (Bell et al, 2005). Unfortunately, because brain injury was not a primary outcome variable for the study, no baseline cranial ultrasounds were done before study entry, so it is not clear whether the increased morbidity was transfusion related (Bell et al, 2005). Currently, there is no ideal marker to identify the need for transfusions in neonates, although the following have been studied: clinical indicators (Bifano et al, 1992; Wardle and Weindling, 2001), lactic acid concentration (Frey and Losa, 2001; Izraeli et al, 1993; Möller et al, 1996; Takahashi et al, 2009; Wardle and Weindling, 2001), and echocardiographic findings (Alkalay et al, 2003; Böhler et al, 1994; Nelle et al, 1997). Delayed cord clamping has also been studied as a means to increase the baseline hematocrit value in newborns with modest clinical benefits (Rabe et al, 2004; Strauss et al, 2008). The collection of UCB for autologous blood transfusions in premature infants and neonates with known surgical diseases has been proposed but is not generally practiced (Ballin et al, 1995; Imura et al, 2001; Jansen et al, 2006; Khodabux and Brand, 2009; Khodabux et al, 2008). Current practices focus on minimizing phlebotomy losses, minimizing exposures to multiple donors with the use of divided aliquots from single donors (Mangel et al, 2001), using EPO to increase endogenous red blood cell production, and tolerating lower hematocrit values in clinically stable patients (Bishara and Ohls, 2009).

BILIRUBIN METABOLISM

The primary source of bilirubin in the fetus and newborn is from the breakdown of heme derived from hemoglobin in circulating erythrocytes. Heme is a porphyrin ring surrounding a ferric (Fe^{3+}) ion. The rate-limiting step in the breakdown of this molecule is the formation of biliverdin, a process controlled by heme oxygenase (Beri and Chandra, 1993; Rodgers and Stevenson, 1990). The iron molecule is recycled, and biliverdin is then reduced to bilirubin IXα by biliverdin reductase. In utero, unconjugated bilirubin is processed by the mother after placental transfer. Thus under normal circumstances, the fetal liver plays only a minor role in bilirubin excretion. Unconjugated bilirubin is lipophilic and is tightly bound to albumin in the circulation. The conjugation of bilirubin results in a relatively polar, water-soluble molecule, bilirubin diglucuronide, which can be excreted. This process occurs in the liver and is dependent on ligandin, a transfer protein, and uridine diphosphoglucuronyl transferase. The conjugating ability of the fetus and newborn is impaired relative to older cohorts because of reduced transferase activity and low levels of uridine diphosphoglucuronic acid (Dennery et al, 2001).

DEVELOPMENTAL ASPECTS OF MEGAKARYOCYTOPOIESIS

Platelets are small (average volume of 7.5 fL) anucleated fragments of megakaryocytes, which circulate as smooth disks when unactivated. The normal circulating life span of a platelet is 10 days. Platelets provide the first line of defense in hemostasis. When a breach of the vascular endothelial lining occurs, platelets are activated and adhere to the exposed subendothelium. These activated platelets generate various mediators, including the potent vasoconstrictor thromboxane A2, and ADP, both of which further contribute to hemostatic plug formation.

SITES OF MEGAKARYOCYTE PRODUCTION

Megakaryocytopoiesis is the process by which megakaryocytes and ultimately platelets develop. As with erythropoiesis, the sites of megakaryocytopoiesis change during embryonic and fetal development. In mouse development, megakaryocytes have been identified in the early yolk sac (McGrath and Palis, 2005). These cells, when cultured in the presence of SCF, IL-3, IL-6, EPO, TPO, and G-CSF, can produce not only erythroid bursts but also megakaryocyte colonies. The megakaryocyte progenitors share a common progenitor with primitive hematopoietic cells (McGrath and Palis, 2005). In humans, electron micrographic studies have shown megakaryocytes present in the liver and circulatory system as early as 8 weeks postconception (Hesseldahl and Falck Larsen, 1971).

MEGAKARYOCYTE PRECURSORS

Megakaryocytopoiesis begins with the pluripotent hematopoietic stem cells, which give rise to myeloid progenitor cells (CFU-S), then burst-forming unit-megakaryocyte (BFU-MK) cells, followed by colony-forming unit-megakaryocyte (CFU-MK) cells (see Figure 75-1). Further maturation brings these small mononuclear cells, which are largely indistinguishable from monocytes, to large polyploid cells that are easily recognized based on their phenotype. The process of megakaryocyte differentiation has been separated into four stages. Stage I cells, or megakaryoblasts, are the smallest and most immature. As cells mature through stages II (promegakaryocytes), III (granular megakaryocytes), and IV (mature megakaryocytes), the nucleus becomes multilobed, the cytoplasm becomes increasingly eosinophilic by Wright-Giemsa staining, and cellular size increases from 6 to 24 μm up to as great as 50 μm. The presence of granules increases steadily until in the mature cells they become organized into "platelet fields." Unlike other cell lines, as the nucleus of a megakaryocyte matures, it undergoes endomitosis or endoreduplication, a process by which cell ploidy is increased in the absence of cell division. Megakaryocytes from adults typically have a modal ploidy of 16N, whereas comparable samples from preterm or term infants have a significantly lower ploidy of <8N (Slayton et al, 2005). Megakaryocytes from newborns are also typically smaller than in adults, although they manifest features of mature megakaryocytes. Adult-sized megakaryocytes appear by 2 years of age. Typically, smaller cells with lower ploidy produce less platelets than do larger cells with higher ploidy. Despite this, the platelet count in fetuses and newborns is near the normal adult range (Wiedmeier et al, 2009).

CONTROL OF MEGAKARYOCYTOPOIESIS

Multiple cytokines participate in the process of megakaryocytopoiesis; however, TPO is the principal one. SCF, IL-3, and IL-6 increase ploidy and size of megakaryocytes.

IL-11 also stimulates the proliferation of megakaryocyte progenitors and induces megakaryocyte maturation, while still other growth factors such as EPO, Kit ligand, GM-CSF, IL-1, basic fibroblast growth factor, platelet-derived growth factor, and interferon-γ have a less clearly defined role. Some cytokines inhibit thrombopoiesis, including TGF-β and platelet factor-4 (Gewirtz et al, 1995). The magnitude of the influence of these growth factors changes with development.

THROMBOPOIETIN

The presence of a growth factor to regulate platelet formation was first hypothesized in the 1950s, but it was not actually realized until 1994, when the protein was isolated by five independent laboratories (Kaushansky, 2006; Kaushansky et al, 1995). TPO is composed of 332 amino acids and contains two domains. The amino-terminal is the active domain (153 amino acids) and bears marked homology to EPO. TPO is produced primarily by the liver and kidney, although other tissues express small amounts. TPO acts as a potent stimulator of all stages of megakaryocyte growth and development by binding to its specific cell surface receptor, c-mpl. In TPO and c-mpl knockout models, platelet production is 10% to 15% of controls, confirming that TPO is the primary regulator of platelet production, but also indicating that alternative pathways exist for megakaryocytopoiesis. Regulation of TPO is unusual: TPO is bound to the surface of platelets by its receptor and destroyed, thereby reducing megakaryocyte exposure to the hormone (Kaushansky, 1998). Serum TPO concentrations tend to be lower in preterm infants than in older infants and children, and the TPO response to thrombocytopenia is less robust as gestational age decreases. This is counterbalanced by an increased sensitivity of megakaryocyte precursors to TPO (Sola et al, 1999, 2000).

DEVELOPMENTAL CHANGES IN PLATELET COUNT

Fetal platelet counts increase with gestation. At 15 weeks' gestation, average platelet counts are 187,000/μL, increasing to 274,000/μL at term. Overall, however, preterm infants have somewhat lower platelet counts than those of adults with a broader range of normal (100,000 to 450,000/μL) (Wiedmeier et al, 2009).

PLATELET TRANSFUSIONS

Clinical practice regarding platelets and platelet transfusion is quite variable because no evidence-based guidelines are available. In a 2005 Web-based survey of neonatologists in the United States and Canada, wide variations in practice were noted in both countries, with platelet transfusions frequently administered to nonbleeding neonates with platelet counts greater than 50,000/μL. This practice was particularly common during indomethacin treatment, before or after procedures or operations, or after diagnosing intraventricular hemorrhages (Josephson et al, 2009). This is of concern because several studies have shown a correlation between the number of platelet transfusions received by hospitalized neonates and mortality rate

(Baer et al, 2007; Garcia et al, 2001). For example, in a study of 1600 thrombocytopenic NICU patients, those who received platelet transfusions had higher mortality rates: 2% with no transfusions, 11% with 1 or 2 transfusions, 35% with >10 transfusions, and 50% with ≥20 platelet transfusions (Baer et al, 2007). Clearly, this was partially due to the underlying illness that required the infant to be transfused. However, because transfusion practices vary so widely, investigators were able to ascribe some of the increased mortality risk to harmful effects of multiple platelet transfusions (Baer et al, 2007). In an attempt to create a reasonable yet safe approach to platelet transfusions, two guidelines were prospectively compared: one based on platelet count and the other on platelet mass (platelet count times mean platelet volume). Although the number of platelet transfusions per patient remained the same, fewer patients were transfused when platelet mass was used as a transfusion trigger (Gerday et al, 2009). In a thorough review by Roberts et al (2008), it was recommended that prophylactic transfusions of platelets be avoided after the 1st week of life unless the platelet count falls below 30,000/μL. During the 1st week of life, for preterm infants, in the absence of better data, these workers recommend a transfusion trigger threshold of 50,000/μL. For patients with platelet counts greater than 50,000/μL, transfusions should be reserved for those with active serious bleeding. Another controversy concerns what kind preparation of platelets to transfuse in volume-sensitive neonates: single-donor, multiple-donor, single-unit, or volume-reduced multiple-unit preparations. In general, 10 to 20 mL/kg of single-donor platelets should raise the platelet count by more than 100,000/μL. In the absence of consumption, platelets should remain in circulation approximately 1 week. Volume-reduced or pooled platelets should be avoided when possible, because such processing results in platelet activation and decreased function, with no evidence of benefit.

DEVELOPMENTAL ASPECTS OF GRANULOCYTOPOIESIS

Early hematopoiesis is characterized almost exclusively by erythropoiesis, although a small number of macrophages are produced in the yolk sac. After circulation begins in the 4th to 5th week of gestation, macrophages appear in the liver, brain, and lungs. During the 5th week, hematopoiesis begins in the liver, and the first hematopoietic cells to appear are macrophages (Kelemen and Janossa, 1980). Whether Kupffer cells originate in the yolk sac and migrate to the liver or rise de novo in the liver is unknown. The marrow space begins to develop around the 8th week after conception, and, as is true in the liver, the first hematopoietic cells to appear in the bones are phagocytes (Kelemen and Janossa, 1980; Slayton et al, 1998b). These phagocytic osteoclasts seem to core out the marrow space. When hematopoiesis is established in the marrow at 10 to 11 weeks postconception, primarily neutrophils are produced, in contrast to the liver, where primarily macrophages are present (Slayton et al, 1998a, 1998b).

The thymus appears around 8 weeks postconception. T-cell progenitors are thought to migrate from the fetal liver to the thymus at 8 to 9 weeks postconception (Haynes et al, 1989), and by the 10th week, lymphoid cells constitute 95% of this organ, with granulocyte precursors and macrophages making up the remainder. B cell precursors first appear in the omentum and the fetal liver at 8 weeks postconception. B cell production in the omentum occurs transiently from 8 to 12 weeks (Solvason and Kearney, 1992), while production continues in the fetal liver. Regulatory T cells are found in the thymus and secondary lymphatic organs in the early second trimester and are proposed to be involved in self-reactivity and immune tolerance (Cupedo et al, 2005; Izcue and Powrie, 2005).

The spleen is an important secondary lymphatic organ in humans. The spleen does not have intrinsic granulocytopoiesis and erythropoiesis activities or produce hematopoietic growth factors (Calhoun et al, 1996), and lymphocytes appear to migrate there through fetal blood. Lymphocytes begin to appear in the spleen around 11 weeks postconception. By the 22nd week, 70% of the cells are lymphocytes (Kelemen et al, 1979).

OVERVIEW OF HEMATOPOIETIC CYTOKINES

Hematopoietic growth factors can be classified into two groups: those responsible for the regulation of myeloid and erythroid growth and differentiation, called colony-stimulating factors (CSFs), and those concerned with immunity, called lymphokines. Once sequenced, lymphokines are assigned interleukin (IL) numbers. There is a great deal of functional overlap between hematopoietic growth factors (redundancy), and each growth factor has a multiplicity of biological actions (pleiotropy). Thus, more than one cytokine controls cells in any cell lineage, and most factors affect cells in more than one lineage (Kaushansky, 2006).

EPO, GM-CSF, and G-CSF belong to a family of hematopoietic cytokines that share a predicted tertiary structure and function by binding to specific cell surface receptors. Specific ligand binding results in allosteric changes in the receptor molecules, which, depending on the type of receptor, results either in protein kinase activation, as with macrophage-colony stimulating factor (M-CSF) (Nicola et al, 1997), or in a cascade of intracellular signaling via the JAK-2 kinase mechanism, as is characterized by EPO (Watowich et al, 1996).

Many of the hematopoietic cytokines were discovered by virtue of their growth-promoting effects on hematopoietic cell lines, or their specific immune functions. It was initially assumed that their effects were specific to the hematopoietic system. This view has been challenged, because functional receptors are expressed by other cell types, with clear nonhematopoietic functions as reviewed by Schneider et al (2005) and Juul (2004). For example, both glia and neurons produce many of the cytokines once thought restricted to the hematopoietic system and, furthermore, they express receptors for these peptides, suggesting the capability of both paracrine and autocrine interaction (Konishi et al, 1993; Masuda et al, 1993). EPO and G-CSF are both available in recombinant form and are FDA-approved for clinical use.

ACKNOWLEDGMENT
Supported in part by NICHD grant R01HD052820.

SUGGESTED READINGS

Bell EF, Strauss RG, Widness JA, et al: Randomized trial of liberal versus restrictive guidelines for red blood cell transfusion in preterm infants, *Pediatrics* 115:1685-1691, 2005.
Brugger W, Scheding S, Ziegler B, et al: Ex vivo manipulation of hematopoietic stem and progenitor cells, *Semin Hematol* 37:42-49, 2000.
Chen MJ, Yokomizo T, Zeigler BM, et al: Runx1 is required for the endothelial to haematopoietic cell transition but not thereafter, *Nature* 457:887-891, 2009.
Eilken HM, Nishikawa S, Schroeder T: Continuous single-cell imaging of blood generation from haemogenic endothelium, *Nature* 457:896-900, 2009.
Fisher TS, Lira PD, Stock JL, et al: Analysis of the role of the HIF hydroxylase family members in erythropoiesis, *Biochem Biophys Res Commun* 388:683-688, 2009.
Kaushansky K: Lineage-specific hematopoietic growth factors, *N Engl J Med* 354:2034-2045, 2006.
Kennedy M, Firpo M, Choi K, et al: A common precursor for primitive erythropoiesis and definitive haematopoiesis, *Nature* 386:488-493, 1997.
Khodabux CM, Brand A: The use of cord blood for transfusion purposes: current status, *Vox Sang* 97:281-293, 2009.
Kirpalani H, Whyte RK, Anderson C, et al: The Premature Infants in Need of Transfusion (PINT) study: a randomized, controlled trial of a restrictive (low) versus liberal (high) transfusion threshold for extremely low birth weight infants, *J Pediatr* 149:301-307, 2006.
Palis J, Yoder MC: Yolk-sac hematopoiesis: the first blood cells of mouse and man, *Exp Hematol* 29:927-936, 2001.
Warren LA, Rossi DJ: Stem cells and aging in the hematopoietic system, *Mech Ageing Dev* 130:46-53, 2009.
Yoshimoto M, Yoder MC: Developmental biology: birth of the blood cell, *Nature* 457:801-803, 2009.

Complete references and supplemental color images used in this text can be found online at www.expertconsult.com

CHAPTER 76

HEMOSTATIC DISORDERS OF THE NEWBORN

Guy Young

OVERVIEW OF HEMOSTASIS

Hemostasis refers to the process in which bleeding is staunched at the site of damaged and disrupted endothelium (Roberts et al, 2006). The process is the result of a dynamic interplay among the subendothelium, the endothelium, and circulating cells and proteins. When blood vessel injury occurs, an immediate response of plasma and cellular components must occur in order to minimize bleeding and begin tissue repair; however, this process must be confined to the area of injury so that pathologic thrombosis does not occur. The hemostatic (coagulation) process is often described in three phases—the vascular phase, the platelet phase, and the plasma phase, all of which occur essentially simultaneously. The vascular phase is mediated by the release of local vasoactive agents and results in vasoconstriction at the site of injury, resulting in a reduction in blood flow. Although an intact endothelial cell lining promotes the fluidity of blood by secreting substances such as prostaglandin I_2 (which inhibits platelet aggregation) once blood vessel injury occurs, the underlying subendothelium is exposed, and procoagulant proteins such as tissue factor, collagen, and von Willebrand factor (VWF) come into contact with blood. Circulating VWF comes into contact with collagen in the subendothelium, leading to unfolding of this large multimeric protein, which exposes the platelet receptor, glycoprotein Ib. Platelets then bind to VWF forming a layer bound to the subendothelium in a process termed *platelet adhesion*. Once platelets are bound to the subendothelium, they are activated, resulting in a shape change and release of vasoactive and hemostatic substances, including thromboxane A_2, serotonin, and adenosine diphosphate (ADP), leading to additional vasoconstriction and platelet aggregation thus forming the platelet plug.

The plasma phase of coagulation occurs initially as a result of the exposure of tissue factor in the subendothelium. Tissue factor (TF) binds to and activates factor VII to form the TF:FVIIa complex (also called the extrinsic tenase), which then binds to and activates factor X (FX) to FXa. The TF:FVIIa:FXa converts a small amount of prothrombin to thrombin. This relatively small amount of thrombin then results in a number of reactions aimed at generating a large amount of thrombin, known as the thrombin burst, which is required for normal clot formation. These reactions include platelet activation, resulting in the expression of platelet factor V on the surface of the platelet, as well as activation of (FV) to FVa. In addition, thrombin leads to the activation of factor VIII (FVIII) by its release from VWF and activates FXI. The TF:FVIIa complex mentioned earlier also activates factor IX (FIX) to FIXa, which then binds to the surface of activated platelets at the site of bleeding. Activated FVIII then binds to FIXa, forming the potent intrinsic tenase complex and resulting in the conversion of large amounts of FX to FXa, which then associates with FVa on the activated platelet surface, resulting in the thrombin burst.

The rapid generation of a large amount of thrombin then results in reactions that lead to the formation of a stable fibrin clot. First, thrombin cleaves fibrinogen to form the insoluble fibrin strands that make up the structural element of the fibrin clot. The thrombin burst also leads to two important steps that are important in rendering the clot more resistant to fibrinolysis. Thrombin activates factor XIII which leads to crosslinking of the fibrin monomers into stable fibrin polymers. Second, thrombin activates thrombin-activatable fibrinolysis inhibitor (TAFI), further changing the structure of fibrin and enhancing its resistance to tissue plasminogen activator (tPA)-mediated fibrinolysis, ultimately resulting in a stable clot. This fibrin clot is what results in the cessation of bleeding and acts as the scaffold for tissue repair, which eventually leads to complete restoration of the endothelial lining.

As part of the repair process, the fibrin clot undergoes fibrinolysis, resulting in a blood vessel segment indistinguishable from that which was in place before the injury. The fibrinolytic process is a simpler process with fewer proteins and is initiated by the release of tPA near the site of injury. This leads to the conversion of plasminogen to plasmin, which via interactions with lysine and arginine residues on fibrin is able to cleave fibrin into fragments that then dissolve into the blood.

Both the hemostatic and fibrinolytic processes are regulated by inhibitors whose function is to contain these processes to the site of injury and to quench the reactions, thus preventing them from becoming systemic and pathologic. The hemostatic system has two major inhibitors: (1) antithrombin and (2) the protein C–protein S complex. Antithrombin is released at the margins of endothelial injury and binds in a 1:1 complex with thrombin, resulting in inactivation of any thrombin that is not bound by the forming clot. Any excess free thrombin at the margins of the forming clot binds to thrombomodulin, a receptor on the surface of intact endothelial cells, resulting in a complex that then activates protein C to activated protein C, which in conjunction with protein S inactivates activated FV and FVIII. This negative feedback then leads to a reduction in further thrombin generation, resulting in the quenching of the formation of fibrin. The fibrinolytic system also has inhibitors—principally—plasminogen activator inhibitor-1 (PAI-1), which as its name implies inhibits tPA, and α_2-antiplasmin, which inhibits plasmin.

This intricate system is designed to allow for hemostasis to take place only at the site of injury and for fibrinolysis to follow the formation of the fibrin clot as part of the tissue repair process. Disorders resulting in excessive bleeding can occur secondary to a malfunction of any of the foregoing processes and may be the result of either congenital or acquired conditions. For example, conditions resulting in either a reduced number or a dysfunction of platelets or a reduced amount of or abnormally formed VWF will result in what are termed *disorders of primary hemostasis*, which

1056

collectively manifest with similar symptoms. In addition, deficiencies of clotting factors can be the result of acquired or congenital defects, and such deficiencies can lead to a wide variety and severity of bleeding symptoms. Note, disorders resulting in excess fibrinolysis can be due to either an overabundance of fibrinolytic proteins such as tPA or a deficiency of inhibitors to fibrinolysis such as PAI-1.

Defects in the inhibitory proteins of the hemostatic system can result in a predisposition to thrombosis. These conditions include deficiencies of antithrombin or proteins C and S, molecular defects in prothrombin and factor V, elevations in homocysteine leading to endothelial damage, and reduced fibrinolytic capacity secondary to elevations in lipoprotein(a). This chapter discusses the pathophysiology, clinical presentation, diagnosis, prognosis, and treatment of defects in the coagulation system resulting in disorders of excessive bleeding or thrombosis.

DEVELOPMENTAL HEMOSTASIS

There are major differences between the neonatal hemostatic system and that of adults (or even older children) (Andrew, 1995, 1997). Although the general structure and function of the subendothelium and endothelium is felt to be the same in neonates as in older children, this is a difficult area to study. The number of platelets throughout late fetal life and the neonatal period is the same. However, there appears to be a deficit in platelet function in platelet aggregation studies, and the platelet function analyzer (PFA-100) and bleeding times in neonates are shorter than in older children and adults, probably because of their higher hematocrit and VWF levels. It is not clear whether neonatal platelets function differently from those of older children and adults (Israels, 2009). With the exception of fibrinogen, circulating levels of most coagulation proteins are different from those of adults (Andrew, 1995). Although levels of FVIII and VWF are normal to elevated in the immediate newborn period, levels of the other procoagulant clotting factors are lower. In addition, levels of the natural inhibitors to coagulation (antithrombin, protein C, and protein S) are also lower, resulting in a hemostatic system that is balanced (similar to the adult system). However, that balance is more precarious, because relatively small changes in one protein or another result in a more significant relative change of this balance. Thus, neonates are at increased risk for bleeding as well as thrombosis. Last, the fibrinolytic capacity of neonates is less than that of adults because there is a relative (physiologic) plasminogen deficiency in neonates. This in part probably accounts for the increased incidence of thrombosis in neonates.

INTRODUCTION TO BLEEDING DISORDERS

Excessive bleeding may occur in the immediate newborn period (uncommonly even in utero) or anytime thereafter. Bleeding symptoms may result from derangements in the hemostatic system or secondary to anatomic defects, surgery, or trauma. Furthermore, bleeding symptoms may be confined to specific anatomic sites or may occur in multiple sites. Finally, bleeding symptoms may be present in multiple family members or may occur in the absence of a family history. All of this information is important for clinicians to arrive at a correct diagnosis rapidly and with minimal yet correctly sequenced laboratory testing. Thus, a detailed patient and family history is a vital part of the approach to each patient with a potential bleeding disorder.

Obtaining a detailed patient and family history is crucial regardless of previous laboratory testing. The history includes a detailed discussion of specific bleeding symptoms or abnormalities. Information regarding bleeding symptoms should include location, frequency and pattern, and duration in terms of both appearance of symptoms and time required for cessation. The location may suggest the part of the hemostatic system affected—patients with disorders of primary hemostasis (platelets and VWF) often experience mucocutaneous bleeding, including easy bruising and mucous membrane bleeding, whereas patients with disorders of secondary hemostasis (coagulation factor deficiencies) may experience deep tissue bleeding including the joints, muscles, and central nervous system. Additional important information to be collected includes the current medications the patient is receiving, because these may affect the hemostatic system; the presence or absence of a family history of bleeding; and a history of hemostatic challenges, including surgery, trauma, and perinatal bleeding. The goal at the end of the history is to establish the likelihood of a bleeding disorder, because this judgment determines the required laboratory investigation.

The laboratory evaluation includes performance of initial screening tests. The most common screening tests used include the complete blood count (CBC), prothrombin time (PT), activated partial thromboplastin time (aPTT), and a screening test of platelet function such as the platelet function analyzer (PFA). Of note, the PFA may not be sufficiently sensitive or specific to be useful, and its inclusion as a screening test is controversial. Assaying for specific factors and more detailed examination of platelet function can be performed if indicated by the results of the screening tests. It is important to note that these screening tests are not sensitive to all abnormalities associated with a bleeding disorder, including von Willebrand's disease (VWD), FXIII, PAI-1, and α_2-antiplasmin deficiencies; therefore, a patient history suggestive of a bleeding disorder always warrants further testing regardless of the results of these screening tests. Abnormalities of screening tests do not necessarily represent the presence of a pathologic process, because these tests are sensitive to handling, may vary in reliability based on laboratory, and may be influenced by medications including herbal therapies, as well as other issues. Specific examples of artifactually abnormal results include an elevated PT and/or PTT secondary to poor specimen handling or an abnormal PFA secondary to the ingestion of medications or supplements known to affect platelet function. Finally, as previously mentioned, the normal ranges for the prothrombin time and activated partial thromboplastin time are different from those of adults, and the normal ranges provided by most laboratories are based on adult normative values. It is important to refer to the normal ranges for the specific neonatal age when determining whether either of these assays or specific factor assays are abnormal. See Figure 76-1 for an algorithmic approach to the bleeding patient.

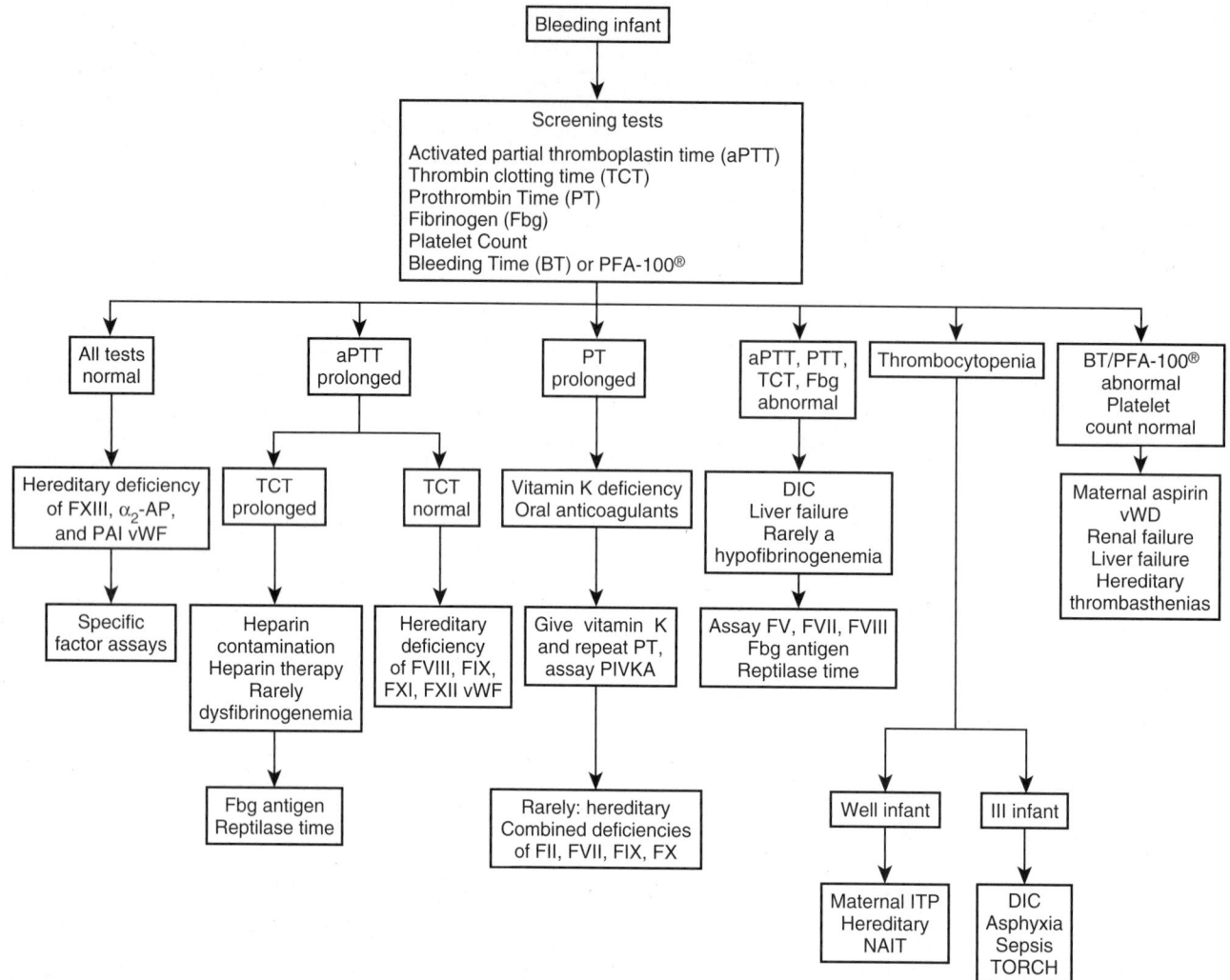

FIGURE 76-1 An algorithmic approach to the patient with excessive bleeding. α_2AP, α_2-antiplasmin; *aPTT*, activated partial thromboplastin time; *BT*, bleeding time; *DIC*, disseminated intravascular coagulation; *F*, factor; *Fbg*, fibrinogen; *FSPs*, fibrin split products; *ITP*, idiopathic thrombocytopenic purpura; *NAIT*, neonatal alloimmune thrombocytopenia; *PAI*, plasminogen activator inhibitor; *PIVKA*, protein induced in the absence of vitamin K; *PT*, prothrombin time; *TCT*, thrombin clotting time; *TORCH*, toxoplasmosis, other infections, rubella, cytomegalovirus infection, herpes simplex; *vWD*, von Willebrand's disease; *vWF*, von Willebrand factor. (*Data from Kisker C: Pathophysiology of bleeding disorders in the newborn. In Polin RA, Fox WW, editors: Fetal and neonatal physiology, Philadelphia, 1998, WB Saunders, pp 1848-1861.*)

HEMORRHAGIC DISORDERS
THROMBOCYTOPENIA

Etiology/Pathophysiology

Thrombocytopenia is a common occurrence in the neonatal intensive care unit, and there are many conditions that can result in neonatal thrombocytopenia (Bussel and Sola-Visner, 2009; Sola-Visner et al, 2009). The conditions that lead to thrombocytopenia can be separated in two ways. One approach is to distinguish these based on whether thrombocytopenia is likely caused by a hematologic disorder, so-called primary thrombocytopenia, or whether the thrombocytopenia is due to nonhematologic conditions, medications, or procedures such as extracorporeal membrane oxygenation (ECMO), which is referred to as secondary thrombocytopenia. Another approach is to separate the disorders according to those that are congenital (Table 76-1) versus those that are acquired (Table 76-2). One can arrive at a reasonable differential diagnosis using either

approach. In general, otherwise-well neonates presenting with thrombocytopenia (either noted incidentally or in association with bleeding symptoms) will be found to have primary thrombocytopenia, whereas ill neonates (often premature) have multiple conditions or medications that are associated with or can lead to thrombocytopenia such that it is difficult to discern one specific underlying cause. It is important to make this distinction in order to pursue a reasonable evaluation that will have a high probability of determining a diagnosis without requiring numerous unnecessary laboratory assays. For the otherwise-well neonate, a detailed approach (see later discussion) will likely lead to a diagnosis from which one can determine the prognosis and treatment, if necessary. If secondary thrombocytopenia is suspected, the prudent approach would be to treat the underlying disorders with the expectation of normalization of the platelet count once the patient improves. Such an approach will also avoid many unnecessary blood tests. If the thrombocytopenia persists after improvement

TABLE 76-1 Congenital Causes of Thrombocytopenia

Small Platelets	Normal-Sized Platelets	Large Platelets
Wiskott-Aldrich syndrome Thrombocytopenia–absent radius (TAR) syndrome	Congenital amegakaryocytic thrombocytopenia (CAMT) Thrombocytopenia associated with trisomies (13, 18)	MYH9-associated thrombocytopenia (May-Heggelin anomaly, Fechtner syndrome, Epstein's syndrome, Sebastian syndrome) Bernard-Soulier syndrome X-linked macrothrombocytopenia

TABLE 76-2 Acquired Causes of Thrombocytopenia

Immune-Mediated	Nonimmune
Passive transfer immune-mediated thrombocytopenia (ITP) Neonatal alloimmune thrombocytopenia Heparin-induced thrombocytopenia Maternal systemic lupus erythematosus	Infections (bacterial, viral, TORCH) Disseminated intravascular coagulation Kasabach-Merritt syndrome Medication Maternal preeclampsia/eclampsia Thrombosis Perinatal hypoxia Respiratory distress syndrome Necrotizing enterocolitis

of the neonate's condition, then a thorough evaluation for primary disorders can be undertaken.

Primary thrombocytopenia can be due to congenital or acquired disorders. Some congenital conditions will be obvious immediately (thrombocytopenia–absent radius [TAR] syndrome), whereas others (congenital amegakaryocytic thrombocytopenia [CAMT]) will require specialized testing (Geddis, 2009). Although congenital thrombocytopenias are rare, several acquired conditions are not uncommon with the most important of these being the immune thrombocytopenias (Bussel and Sola-Visner, 2009). There are two forms of this condition. The first form occurs when the mother has autoimmune thrombocytopenia, either pre existing or developing during pregnancy, resulting in transplacental transfer of her autoantibodies which react with the newborn's platelets resulting in what can be termed passive transfer immune thrombocytopenic purpura (ITP). The second form, termed neonatal alloimmune thrombocytopenia (NAIT), results from the passive transfer of maternal alloantibodies directed against paternally derived platelet antigens that are present on the neonate's platelets. In the first form, the mother most often has thrombocytopenia herself whereas in the second form, the mother's platelet count is normal. Other hematologic disorders resulting in acquired thrombocytopenia include disseminated intravascular coagulation (DIC), which itself has many causes, and certain vascular malformations (kaposiform hemangioendotheliomas and tufted angiomas), which result in platelet consumption (Hall, 2001). In addition, deep vein thrombosis (DVT) in the neonatal period often results in thrombocytopenia. These conditions may be considered secondary causes in some respects; however, because they have a defined hematologic cause, they are grouped with the primary disorders.

There are numerous causes of acquired thrombocytopenia (see Table 76-2) (Sola-Visner et al, 2009). The most common are sepsis (bacterial or viral), congenital viral infections (i.e., TORCH [toxoplasmosis, other infections, rubella, cytomegalovirus, herpes simplex]), necrotizing enterocolitis, chronic lung disease, and certain medications. Often, an ill neonate with thrombocytopenia will have multiple possible causes of thrombocytopenia, and it is difficult to point to one specific problem as the main culprit. In such situations, successful treatment of the underlying condition should result in resolution of the thrombocytopenia, and a detailed evaluation is rarely fruitful and generally unnecessary. One exception to the foregoing is identifying a specific medication that clearly causes thrombocytopenia, in which case elimination or substitution of this medication by another may result in improvement in the platelet count.

Clinical Presentation

Newborns with thrombocytopenia may present with signs of bleeding (most often mucocutaneous), or the discovery of low platelets may be an incidental finding on a CBC performed for other reasons (i.e., presumed sepsis). When newborns have bleeding attributed solely to thrombocytopenia, the platelet count is usually substantially reduced ($<30 \times 10^9$/L). Patients presenting with bleeding may be recognized immediately after birth by bruising on the face or head related to the trauma associated with delivery or may have a cephalhematoma. Bruising and petechiae also may be seen on other parts of the body. Occasionally, internal hemorrhage may have occurred pre- or perinatally, and in such circumstances, clinical signs will relate to the site of bleeding. Intracranial hemorrhage can manifest with a bulging fontanel or with signs of neurologic compromise such as seizures, apnea, or respiratory distress. It should be noted that for patients with NAIT, the incidence of intracranial hemorrhage (ICH) is 25%, although often this occurs in utero. Other deep tissue bleeding occurs only rarely and may present with bloody stools, abdominal distention or gross hematuria. It is incumbent on the physician to request appropriate diagnostic imaging studies if internal hemorrhage is suspected, particularly in a thrombocytopenic neonate. When bleeding occurs outside the immediate newborn period, the symptoms are generally similar to those described earlier, with the exception of the presence of birth trauma. Again, mucocutaneous bleeding is the most common manifestation of bleeding due to thrombocytopenia, although internal hemorrhage should be considered if there are suggestive clinical signs.

Thrombocytopenia may also present as an incidental finding or rarely as a result of a known family history of a thrombocytopenic disorder. When thrombocytopenia presents incidentally, the platelet count tends to be higher (usually $>50 \times 10^9$/L). When this occurs, a thorough evaluation of the patient's history up to this point is warranted to see if a secondary cause can be identified. For example, one should consider why the CBC was performed in the first place. For example, was there a concern for sepsis or other infection? Most often, a secondary cause can be identified, and thus further evaluation is not necessary. In such cases, the thrombocytopenia will presumably resolve once the secondary cause is resolved.

Rarely, when a newborn is found to have thrombocytopenia, incidentally or otherwise, careful assessment of the family history will reveal the presence of a parent or other family member with thrombocytopenia. In such instances, identifying the condition in the family member should result in directed laboratory assessment to identify the same condition in the patient. It should be noted that in many instances a family history of thrombocytopenia will be present, but the family member will not know the cause of his/her condition. In this situation, it would be appropriate to perform an evaluation in the family member, thus sparing the newborn from venipuncture.

Diagnosis

As previously discussed, whether or not to embark on a detailed diagnostic evaluation of neonatal thrombocytopenia depends in part on whether the cause is believed to be primary or secondary. Primary thrombocytopenia always warrants an evaluation aimed at arriving at the correct diagnosis. If secondary thrombocytopenia is present, then a detailed evaluation may not be warranted, and identifying and treating the underlying cause should suffice to restore the platelet count to normal.

Before launching a laboratory investigation, it is paramount to obtain not only a detailed history of the newborn, but, as is often the case with neonates, a history of the mother's overall health as well as her pregnancy. In addition, obtaining the family history may yield important clues, particularly the presence of thrombocytopenia in previous children, especially if that thrombocytopenia occurred in the newborn period. Among the most important pieces of information to obtain would be the mother's platelet count: Thrombocytopenia in the mother is often due to ITP (which can be acquired during pregnancy), which will often lead to neonatal thrombocytopenia. In addition, pregnancy complications such as pregnancy-induced hypertension, preeclampsia/eclampsia, and the HELLP syndrome may result in neonatal thrombocytopenia. The presence of neonatal thrombocytopenia in a previous pregnancy strongly suggests the possibility of NAIT, especially if the thrombocytopenia in the previous newborn resolved during infancy. The presence of chronic thrombocytopenia in family members, particularly first-degree relatives, suggests the presence of a congenital thrombocytopenia—in particular, the myosin heavy chain-9 (MYH-9) related disorders (Althaus and Greinacher, 2009) (see Table 76-1), because these are inherited in an autosomal dominant fashion. In addition to maternal and other family history, the history of the neonatal course is crucial. Perinatal hypoxia, for example, often results in temporary thrombocytopenia, as does the presence of sepsis or other infections. Furthermore, identifying the presence of any of the many causes of acquired thrombocytopenia is important (see Table 76-2).

A thorough physical examination is another crucial aspect not only in determining the cause of the thrombocytopenia

TABLE 76-3 Laboratory and Imaging Evaluation of Thrombocytopenia

Maternal Platelet Count Normal	Maternal Thrombocytopenia	Congenital Anomalies Present
Blood culture TORCH evaluation DIC panel (PT, PTT, fibrinogen, D-dimer) Karyotype (mosaicism for trisomies, other chromosomal abnormalities) Bone marrow aspiration (CAMT)	Neonatal alloimmune thrombocytopenia panel (maternal platelet genotype, paternal platelet genotype, maternal antiplatelet antibodies)	Karyotype Radial imaging (confirming TAR syndrome) Bone marrow aspiration (CAMT with anomalies)

CAMT, Congenital amegakaryocytic thrombocytopenia; *DIC*, disseminated intravascular coagulation; *PT*, prothrombin time; *PTT*, partial thromboplastin time; *TAR*, thrombocytopenia–absent radius; *TORCH*, toxoplasmosis, other infections, rubella, cytomegalovirus, herpes simplex.

but also to assess the potential for bleeding complications. The presence of physical stigmata associated with thrombocytopenic disorders can at times reveal the diagnosis without much additional testing, as in the TAR syndrome wherein a plain film of the forearm is diagnostic. The presence of findings suggestive of TORCH infections (small for gestational age, hepatosplenomegaly) or chromosomal disorders (trisomy 13, 18, and 21) may also be revealing and lead to the performance of specific laboratory tests (see later discussion). The presence of a vascular malformation suggests that thrombocytopenia may be due to consumption of platelets by the mass. Occasionally, thrombocytopenia may be the only laboratory manifestation of a secondary cause; for example, this finding in association with hepatosplenomegaly suggests the possibility of a storage disease. The laboratory assessment for conditions that are known to cause thrombocytopenia in the neonate should be tailored to the findings on history and physical examination (Table 76-3 summarizes laboratory assessment for specific conditions). In most cases, thrombocytopenia is due to secondary causes, is mild to moderate, and does not cause bleeding, and thus, a laboratory investigation may not be necessary. If the thrombocytopenia may be due to the presence of easily assayed secondary causes or if it is due to a primary cause, laboratory assessment is warranted and may include any of the following: laboratory testing for NAIT (see later discussion), TORCH evaluation, chromosomal analysis (e.g., karyotype, fluorescence in situ hybridization), evaluation for metabolic disorders, or evaluation for genetic thrombocytopenias (MYH-9 disorders, congenital amegakaryocytic thrombocytopenia). Testing for NAIT is crucial not so much for the newborn in question but for subsequent pregnancies, because invariably the condition will be repeated, and often with worse thrombocytopenia and perhaps a worse outcome (Bussel and Sola-Visner, 2009). This testing does not require blood from the newborn, but rather, blood from both parents, and testing should be done in a reputable laboratory equipped to perform this analysis. If the laboratory test result is abnormal, a specific diagnosis can be made, and then any necessary treatment plans can be undertaken.

Treatment

The management of thrombocytopenia in neonates is dependent more on the diagnosis and presence of bleeding than on the platelet count. For example, for the same platelet count, patients with NAIT generally have worse bleeding and worse outcomes than patients with passive transfer ITP. Because patients with NAIT have a much higher rate of ICH, treatment of such patients should be much more aggressive. Similarly, neonates with thrombocytopenia due to DIC will likely bleed at higher platelet counts than patients with congenital thrombocytopenias. The management approaches can be divided into *therapeutic*, defined as treatment given for the management of bleeding, and *prophylactic*, wherein treatment is only given for a low platelet count, in the absence of bleeding. Treatment decisions would be simplified if bleeding could be expected to occur at a specific platelet count threshold; however, unfortunately, there are no data to suggest a specific platelet count below which prophylactic treatment should be instituted for any of the causes of thrombocytopenia. Thus, it is incumbent on the treating physician to weigh the risks and benefits of therapy before instituting any specific treatment.

With this in mind, the following are the major potential therapeutic options for managing thrombocytopenia (assuming treatment is under way for the underlying disorder of secondary thrombocytopenias):

- Observation
- Platelet transfusion
- Intravenous immunoglobulin (IVIG)
- Corticosteroids

In addition, adjuvant treatments to manage bleeding include antifibrinolytic agents, topical agents, and direct pressure.

The management of immune thrombocytopenia (passive transfer ITP and NAIT) may include IVIG, corticosteroids, and platelet transfusions (Bussel and Sola-Visner, 2009). For patients in whom treatment is warranted, IVIG has been shown to be effective at raising the platelet count in both conditions, although this increase in platelet count takes 24–48 hours, making this approach reasonable only for patients in whom treatment is given either for mild bleeding symptoms (mucocutaneous bleeding) or prophylactically. Although data are lacking regarding specific platelet count thresholds, most neonatologists and hematologists would recommend treating patients with passive transfer ITP who have platelet counts $<10 \times 10^9$/L and withholding treatment for platelet counts $>30 \times 10^9$/L. For platelet counts in between, either observation or treatment is reasonable. Conversely, because of the high risk of ICH in patients with NAIT, it is suggested that all such patients with platelet counts less than 50×10^9/L receive treatment with IVIG and additionally, receive a platelet transfusion if ICH has occurred or if it occurred in previously affected siblings. If the antibody specificity is known (from a previously affected newborn), then it is important to make an effort to obtain antigen-negative platelets, but only if this will not result in a delay in platelet administration.

Random-donor (i.e., antigen-untested) platelets will often result in a rise in the platelet count, although this rise may be more short-lived than for antigen-negative platelets. One strategy is to administer antigen-untested platelets and simultaneously collect platelets from the mother (by definition she is antigen-negative), if feasible, for subsequent use. It is not common to confirm the diagnosis of NAIT in first-borns; however, if the clinical suspicion is high, aggressive treatment is warranted. Although NAIT will resolve over a period of days to weeks, it is recommended that the platelet count be followed closely and transfusions administered for platelet counts of $<50 \times 10^9$/L, at least in the 1st week of life, as this is the highest-risk period for ICH in the postnatal period. If therapy with IVIG is effective, the platelet count may rise and remain elevated for several weeks, obviating the need for further platelet transfusions.

Newborns with congenital thrombocytopenia can present with a wide range of platelet counts, and in these disorders, the risk for bleeding *does* relate to the degree of thrombocytopenia. Fortunately, most patients with these disorders do not have severe thrombocytopenia (platelet count $<10 \times 10^9$/L); thus, the risk for bleeding is low, and observation is the recommended approach. For bleeding that occurs in these conditions, the only treatment that can raise the platelet count is a platelet transfusion; thus, it is important to weigh the risks and benefits of therapy.

For newborns with secondary thrombocytopenia, the emphasis of treatment should be on managing the underlying condition. Normalization of the platelet count is expected once the underlying condition resolves. If bleeding occurs, platelet transfusions should raise the platelet count in most instances and will be effective at controlling the bleeding so long as the bleeding was not due to other causes such as abnormal coagulation factor levels. The decision to give platelet transfusions depends on multiple factors including the platelet count, presence of other risk factors for bleeding, the underlying medical condition, recent invasive procedures, and the need for ongoing platelet-inhibiting medications. Last, the effectiveness of nonspecific methods for managing bleeding should not be underestimated. The use of direct pressure or topical agents is an effective way to arrest bleeding if the source of bleeding is easily accessible. Both topical thrombin (bovine or human) and fibrin sealant can be applied directly to sites of bleeding and are generally safe and often effective. Antifibrinolytic agents (ε-aminocaproic acid and tranexamic acid) are also quite safe and can be effective, particularly for mucous membrane bleeding. These agents inhibit plasmin-mediated thrombolysis and presumably exert their effect by stabilizing the less-than-ideal clots that are formed in patients with bleeding disorders in general, including platelet function defects. Thus, one can think of these agents as effective at preventing rebleeding, a common problem in bleeding disorders. These agents can be given intravenously or orally and can be used either therapeutically after bleeding has occurred or prophylactically as part of perioperative management. Regarding adverse effects, topical thrombin use can rarely result in the development of antibodies against FV which can result in severe bleeding (it is believed, though not clinically proved, that the use of the human protein will result in a lower risk for antibody development than the bovine version). Antifibrinolytics can increase the risk for thrombosis; however, in general the benefits for managing bleeding far outweigh this relatively small risk. Otherwise, these agents do not appear to have side effects in neonates.

Outcomes

The outcome of neonates with thrombocytopenia depends almost exclusively on the occurrence of serious bleeding. For neonates with NAIT who have suffered an ICH, there may be permanent sequelae, whereas for those without serious bleeding, the prognosis is excellent because the thrombocytopenia will fully resolve. The same can be said for patients with passive transfer ITP. For neonates with secondary thrombocytopenia, the outcome largely depends on the condition that led to the thrombocytopenia in the first place. Once the underlying condition resolves, the thrombocytopenia resolves.

For patients with congenital thrombocytopenia, there are variable outcomes related to the specific disorders. For example, patients with CAMT often go on to develop aplastic anemia and rarely, leukemia—usually when they are several years old. In fact, these patients may not even be diagnosed in the newborn period unless they develop bleeding or a CBC is performed. Ultimately, the prognosis of these patients depends on their response to treatment of the aplastic anemia or leukemia. For the other congenital thrombocytopenias, the outcome is more favorable and, similar to CAMT, some may not be diagnosed in the newborn period. Patients with TAR syndrome will, of course, be diagnosed immediately because of their obvious deformity. They have a very favorable hematologic outcome: The platelet count tends to improve over time, with many patients achieving platelet counts >100 × 10⁹/L. For the various *MYH9* gene mutations, the hematologic outcome is excellent; many of these patients do not bleed despite their thrombocytopenia, because their larger than normal platelets exert increased functionality compared to normal-sized platelets. Some patients with these disorders will develop renal failure, deafness, and/or cataracts; however, this will occur many years after the newborn period and often not until the second or third decade of life.

PLATELET FUNCTION DISORDERS

Etiology/Pathophysiology

As discussed earlier, platelets play a major role in hemostasis both by supporting the cellular structure for the primary platelet plug and by providing a phospholipid surface on which the plasma elements involved in coagulation can bind. Thus, a decrease in the platelet count and/or poor platelet function can result in bleeding symptoms. Abnormalities in platelet function can occur in any of the multitude of components (functional, structural, and regulatory proteins) required for normal platelet function. For example, defects in glycoprotein Ib or IIb/IIIa result in Bernard-Soulier disease or Glanzmann's thrombasthenia (the most severe platelet function defect), respectively (Nurden and Nurden, 2008). The most common platelet function defect, the δ-storage pool defect, results in reduced

secretion of ADP. However, the degree of bleeding associated with this condition rarely leads to manifestation in the neonatal period.

The differential diagnosis of platelet function defects can be divided into congenital and acquired defects and can be thought of in terms of the structural components of the platelets. As mentioned, congenital disorders of platelet receptors such as glycoprotein Ib and IIb/IIIa result in Bernard-Soulier disease and Glanzmann's thrombasthenia, respectively. There are genetic defects resulting in δ-storage pool defect (including the common ADP secretion defect and the less common absence of dense bodies associated with Hermansky-Pudlak syndrome) and α-granules (gray platelet syndrome). Although there are likely many more genetic defects as yet unidentified in the various steps involved in normal platelet function, a platelet function defect can often be determined from laboratory testing. However, further delineating the defect is difficult, because the types of assays required to uncover the specific defect are not available in commercial laboratories.

Acquired platelet defects are most commonly due to medications, chronic medical conditions (uremia being the prime example), or medical interventions such as ECMO. The list of medications resulting in platelet dysfunction is vast, and it is suggested that in the evaluation of a patient with a bleeding disorder who is receiving medication, a reference manual be consulted to assess the possibility that this medication leads to platelet dysfunction. The most common medications resulting in platelet dysfunction include aspirin and other nonsteroidal antiinflammatory drugs (indomethacin), prostacyclin, certain anticonvulsants (valproic acid in particular), and some antibiotics.

Among the medical disorders associated with platelet dysfunction, the most common and best described is uremia. Although the exact mechanism by which the platelets are affected is not clear, a prevailing theory is that the accumulation of certain substances associated with uremia disrupts the platelet phospholipid surface. Last, other than prescribed medications, certain medical procedures are associated with platelet dysfunction, with the most common being the use of extracorporeal circuits (ECMO and cardiopulmonary bypass). There are probably a number of mechanisms involved in this process; however, clearly the passage of platelets through an artificial surface affects the ability of platelets to adhere and aggregate. A detailed review of platelet function defects is beyond the scope of this chapter; there are a number of excellent review articles that address the topic of platelet function defects.

Clinical Presentation

Patients with platelet function disorders present with bleeding signs similar to thrombocytopenia. In essence, this includes mucocutaneous bleeding (nose, mouth, gastrointestinal tract, genitourinary tract) and bruising. The extent, location, and nature of the bruises are generally related to birth trauma and invasive procedures. Rarely, some patients may present as a result of a family history of bleeding without having bleeding themselves. Last, patients may present as the result of an abnormal screening test (bleeding time, PFA) ordered by a surgeon before undergoing a medical procedure. In such situations, it is critical to take a detailed medical history, because it is possible that such patients do not have a bleeding disorder.

Diagnosis

The diagnosis of platelet function disorders in neonates is problematic, because the tests either are difficult to perform (the bleeding time) or require a large amount of blood (platelet aggregation studies) (Israels, 2009). Although the PFA has been used in the neonatal population, there are few studies establishing normal ranges, and the test should not be performed in patients with thrombocytopenia and anemia, a common finding in the neonatal intensive care unit. Importantly, the first step in evaluating a patient for a platelet function disorder is ensuring that the platelet count is normal, because the assays of platelet function will be abnormal if the platelet count is low, thereby rendering the results useless. In addition, some assays such as the PFA will also be abnormal if there is significant anemia. A CBC is thus the first laboratory test that should be performed, and it should be done before embarking on platelet-specific assays.

There are two tests that can screen for platelet function disorders; however, both have significant limitations. The original screening test is the bleeding time, a test that is notoriously difficult to perform, particularly in neonates, and as a result has fallen out of favor and is no longer recommended. The PFA is a widely used laboratory assay available in most coagulation laboratories and is a useful screening assay to evaluate for disorders of primary hemostasis. Normal ranges for the PFA have been established in neonates (Israels et al, 2009). Patients with severe platelet function defects such as Bernard-Soulier and Glanzmann's thrombasthenia always have significantly abnormal results. The PFA is often abnormal in the milder disorders such as the common ADP secretion defects; however, its sensitivity for these disorders is not sufficient to allow such defects to be ruled out if the results are normal. The PFA is also abnormal in patients on aspirin (both cartridges) and clopidogrel and ticlopidine (the collagen/ADP cartridge). The effects of other medications known to affect platelet function (e.g., valproic acid) are not clear. Thus, the PFA is a useful screen for the platelet function defects. However, it cannot rule out milder defects. Thus, if a bleeding disorder is suspected based on history, further testing is required even if the PFA result is normal.

The major specific assay of platelet function is platelet aggregometry. This assay uses a set concentration of platelet-rich plasma and assesses platelet aggregation via light transmission after addition of a variety of platelet agonists (ADP, epinephrine, ristocetin, arachidonic acid, collagen, and thrombin-related activation peptide). Neonates have reduced aggregation compared to older children and adults; however, the clinical utility of testing in newborns is questionable and as stated in the PFA-100 assay, the clotting time for newborns is actually shorter than those for older children and adults, suggesting better platelet function. Thus it remains unclear whether neonatal platelets are hyper- or hyporesponsive. The major limitation of platelet aggregometry in neonates is the large amount of blood required (20–30 mL depending on the platelet count and how many agonists will be tested). Furthermore, as with the PFA, many medications and supplements affect platelet aggregation studies, and thus, if possible, the assay should be done when patients are no longer receiving these medications or supplements. A more detailed discussion of platelet aggregation can be found in the reviews of platelet function disorders. Some platelet function defects lead to easily identifiable ultrastructural changes in the platelets that can be visualized by electron microscopy. In particular, patients with a deficiency or absence of dense bodies (δ-storage pool deficiency) or α-granules (gray platelet syndrome) can be demonstrated by electron microscopy. Last, flow cytometry can quantify the levels of platelet surface receptors and can confirm the diagnosis of Bernard-Soulier and Glanzmann's thrombasthenia if the diagnosis is in doubt after platelet aggregation studies.

Treatment

The management of congenital platelet function defects relies on several medications and platelet transfusions in dire situations when the medications or local measures are ineffective. In acquired conditions, reversal of the condition that led to the platelet dysfunction will reverse the platelet defect, but this is not always possible. In such situations, the approach to management of bleeding is similar to that for congenital disorders—for example, platelet transfusions or the medications described later. Several medications have nonspecific mechanisms whereby they can enhance hemostasis when platelet function is abnormal. These include desmopressin, antifibrinolytic agents, and recombinant activated FVII (rFVIIa). Desmopressin has been demonstrated to improve platelet function in many congenital disorders, in uremia, and during cardiopulmonary bypass. The mechanism whereby it exerts its effect is not clear, although it is known that this agent increases circulating levels of VWF and FVIII. This medication can be given intravenously or subcutaneously. Desmopressin is generally a very safe agent, although it can lead to vasodilatation, resulting in reductions in blood pressure sufficient to lead to clinical signs, and because it is an analogue of antidiuretic hormone, it can lead to water retention and hyponatremia, which can result in seizures. Neonates are at particularly high risk for this complication; thus, if desmopressin is employed, monitoring of serum sodium levels is essential. As discussed previously for thrombocytopenia, antifibrinolytic agents are excellent adjunctive therapies.

Recombinant FVIIa was developed for the management of bleeding in patients with hemophilia and inhibitors; however, it has been shown to also be effective for managing severe bleeding in patients with severe platelet function defects. It is licensed in Europe for the management of bleeding in patients with Glanzmann's thrombasthenia who are refractory to platelet transfusions. Although there are some reports touting the effectiveness of this agent in platelet function defects, other reports are less complimentary. The drawbacks of this agent are the expense and the risk for thrombosis. Thus, it is suggested that rFVIIa be used only for patients with severe bleeding in whom standard therapeutic measures have failed. The use of this

TABLE 76-4 Classification and Diagnosis of von Willebrand's Disease

Subtype	Defect	VWF Ag	RCof	FVIII	VW Multimers
1	Partial quantitative	↓	↓	↓	Normal distribution
2A	Multimerization	↓	↓↓	↓	Decreased high- and intermediate-weight multimers
2B	Increased binding of high-molecular-weight multimers to platelets	↓	↓↓	↓	Decreased high-molecular-weight multimers
2M	Decreased binding to platelets	Normal	↓↓	Normal	Normal distribution
2N*	Decreased binding to FVIII	↓	↓	↓↓	Normal distribution
3	Complete deficiency	↓↓↓	↓↓↓	↓↓↓	Absent
Platelet type	Increased binding of high-molecular-weight multimers to platelets	↓	↓↓	↓	Decreased high-molecular-weight multimers

RCof, Ristocetin cofactor activity; *VWF Ag*, von Willebrand factor antigen.
*Patients with type 2N are usually compound heterozygotes for a type 1 mutation and therefore have low VWF Ag and RCof.

agent in neonates has been reported, and it appears that neonates are at increased risk for thrombosis from this agent compared with older children when it is employed for unlicensed uses (Young et al, 2009).

For severe bleeding that has not responded to the measures just described, a platelet transfusion should be given in order to provide normally functioning platelets. Although most platelet function defects are mild enough that this will never be required, for the more severe disorders such as Bernard-Soulier and Glanzmann's thrombasthenia, a platelet transfusion may be life-saving. The risks associated with a platelet transfusion are no different from those for other patients, with one important exception: Patients with Bernard-Soulier and Glanzmann's thrombasthenia are at risk for alloimmunization, resulting in the formation of antibodies to GPIb and IIb/IIIa, respectively. Once these antibodies develop, future platelet transfusions are likely to be ineffective. Thus, it is *imperative to withhold platelet transfusions for these patients except in life-threatening hemorrhage, because it may be possible to use this therapy only once in a patient's lifetime.* Last, as described earlier, the benefits of local measures cannot be overstated in the management of bleeding.

Prognosis and Outcomes

Most platelet function disorders are mild and easily managed with the aforementioned approaches. For most patients, these disorders rarely lead to serious bleeding complications. Among the more serious conditions, Glanzmann's thrombasthenia is the most severe and is the one most likely to result in neonatal bleeding, although most patients will not present during this time unless they undergo a hemostatic challenge. After discharge from the neonatal intensive care unit or newborn nursery, patients with platelet function disorders largely lead normal lives with easily manageable and rarely serious bleeding. Patients with Glanzmann's thrombasthenia have the worst outcomes, but even these patients manage to lead relatively normal lives, although they are more likely to require treatment and have interruptions in their daily lives due to bleeding symptoms.

VON WILLEBRAND'S DISEASE

Etiology/Pathophysiology

As discussed previously, VWF is the primary plasma protein required for platelet adhesion, and it also plays an important role in platelet aggregation. The absence (or reduced amount) of VWF or abnormal VWF function leads to defects in platelet adhesion and aggregation resulting in increased bleeding. In addition, VWF is the carrier protein for FVIII, and patients with VWF may have reduced levels of circulating FVIII, further affecting the quality of hemostasis. The effectiveness of VWF as an adhesive protein relies on multimerization of the protein, resulting in very large molecules (among the largest made in the body) that comprise what are known as high-molecular-weight multimers.

Similar to platelet disorders, VWD can be either congenital or acquired, although the congenital form is by far the most common (Nichols et al, 2008). Many mutations have been identified in the various structural components, which can lead either to reduced production or secretion of normally structured VWF or to the production of a dysfunctional protein. As a result of the variety of mutations, VWD has been subcategorized into two basic types: a quantitative defect that can be partial (type 1) or complete (type 3), and qualitative defects (type 2). Table 76-4 describes this classification and diagnosis of VWD in detail. Type 1 is due to reduced amounts of plasma VWF that can result from either decreased production/secretion of VWF or increased clearance of circulating VWF (Vicenza type). Type 3 is due to a complete absence of protein in the plasma and is likely due to severe mutations in the VWF gene. There are four recognized type 2 defects. Type 2A is due to defects in multimerization and results in an absence of large and medium-sized multimers, required for normal platelet adhesion. Type 2B is due to a gain-of-function mutation (similar to platelet type VWD) in VWF leading to increased binding of the high-molecular-weight multimers to circulating platelets, effectively removing these from the available pool in the plasma. Type 2M is due to a mutation resulting in the loss of the ability of

VWF to bind to platelets. Type 2N is due to a defect in the binding of VWF to FVIII resulting in a reduction in circulating FVIII. In general, patients presenting with this subtype are compound heterozygotes for a type 1 defect and the type 2N mutation. These patients are often difficult to distinguish from those with mild hemophilia without the performance of an assay specific to the condition (see Diagnosis section, later).

Acquired von Willebrand's syndrome (AVWS) is a rare condition that has been reported in a variety of unrelated medical conditions. In children, it has been associated with Wilms' tumor, congenital heart disease, and systemic lupus erythematosus. The pathophysiology of the acquired von Willebrand's syndrome is heterogeneous and depends on the associated condition. Some of the described mechanisms are antibody formation, decreased production, proteolysis, and adsorption of VWF onto malignant cells.

Clinical Presentation

The clinical presentation of VWD rarely occurs in the newborn period and is essentially identical to that of platelet function disorders described earlier, with the following exceptions. First, VWD is more common and better described than platelet function defects such that some patients will present based on a known family history in the mother or father. Second, there are relatively few medications that affect production or function of VWF, although valproic acid has been implicated as one of the medications that can lead to AVWS. Third, the disorders that lead to AVWS are different from those that lead to platelet dysfunction.

Diagnosis

The diagnosis of VWD relies on testing for the presence and the two functions of VWF (see Table 76-4). The initial assays for VWD include measurement of the amount of VWF (the VWF antigen assay), the platelet binding function (ristocetin cofactor assay), and the FVIII binding function (FVIII activity). Based on these results, additional testing can be ordered in consultation with a pediatric hematologist.

Treatment

The principles of managing VWD are similar to those for managing platelet dysfunction, with the major exception that replacement therapy rather than platelet transfusion is accomplished with VWF-containing concentrates derived from human plasma. Mild to moderate bleeding associated with type 1 VWD is best managed with desmopressin and, if necessary, antifibrinolytic agents. As noted previously, desmopressin may lead to hypotension and hyponatremia, particularly in neonates. In the case of VWD, the mechanism of action of desmopressin has been well described and is the result of secretion of stored VWF from the Weibel-Palade bodies in endothelial cells. More than 90% of patients with type 1 disease will respond with often dramatic increases in VWF. It should be noted that repeated administration of desmopressin will lead to tachyphylaxis,

presumably from exhaustion of the storage pool of VWF. Thus it is best to administer desmopressin no more than once daily and no more than 2 days in a row, although exceptions can be made. Desmopressin in general should not be used for patients with type 2 disease and is ineffective in type 3 disease. There are some reports of the benefits of desmopressin in all type 2 subtypes, although it should be used with caution in patients with type 2B because it could lead to significant thrombocytopenia as a result of in vivo platelet aggregation (Peyvandi et al, 2008).

For patients with types 2 and 3 disease who develop significant bleeding, replacement therapy with a VWF-containing concentrate should be given. There are currently four products available in the United States (Humate P, Alphanate, Wilate and Koate DVI), with similar products available in other countries. All of these concentrates contain VWF and FVIII in varying ratios and with variable amounts of the different-sized multimers. Although there are theoretical advantages to having a higher (or lower) ratio of VWF to FVIII, the fact is that all of these products have been demonstrated to be effective for the management of bleeding and for the prevention of bleeding in patients requiring invasive procedures. The choice of which product to use is at the discretion of the treating physician in consultation with the hematologist. Often, hospital formularies carry only one of the products, simplifying the choice for inpatient use. All the products are safe, although it should be pointed out that they are all derived from human plasma (all undergo viral inactivation methods and there is no known transmission of infectious agents with any of the products). As with all human plasma products, there is a possibility of allergic reactions, but these have been infrequently reported.

Antifibrinolytic agents and topical agents are useful adjunctive therapies and can be used as described earlier. The benefits and risks of these agents are the same as previously described. Management of bleeding in AVWS is the same as for congenital VWD. However, because this is an acquired condition, treatment of the underlying disorder leading to AVWS should be undertaken in order to resolve the VWF defect.

Prognosis and Outcomes

Patients with most forms of VWD largely lead live normal lives with easily manageable and rarely serious bleeding. Only patients with type 3 VWD, the rarest subtype, suffer from recurrent and serious bleeding leading to complications such as chronic joint disease.

HEMOPHILIA A AND B (FACTOR VIII AND IX FACTOR DEFICIENCY)

Etiology/Pathophysiology

The physiology of hemostasis described earlier demonstrates the critical roles that FVIII and FIX play in ensuring proper thrombin generation and ultimately fibrin clot formation. The absence of either FVIII or FIX results in reduced thrombin generation on the surface of the activated platelets at the site of bleeding. This results in a clot with poor structural integrity, which can be seen on electron microscopy with the formation of large, coarse fibrin strands, rather than the thinner strands that form a much tighter network. In addition, reduced thrombin generation results in decreased generation of activated FXIII, which is required for crosslinking the fibrin monomers and decreased generation of TAFI, both of which result in a clot that is less resistant to thrombolysis. Thus, deficiencies of FVIII or FIX result in less well formed clots that are more susceptible to fibrinolysis. This results in the bleeding manifestations seen in patients with hemophilia.

Deficiencies of FVIII and FIX most commonly occur as a result of genetic mutations on the X chromosome where both genes reside. These deficiencies therefore occur much more commonly in males as a result of the hemizygosity state. Heterozygous females may have mild hemophilia as a result of nonrandom X-chromosome inactivation with resultant FVIII or FIX levels in the range of mild hemophilia described later. In the past, these women were called symptomatic carriers; however, they are now more appropriately classified as having mild hemophilia. There are a variety of mutations that can result in hemophilia. The type of mutation (deletion, inversion, missense, nonsense) and the part of the protein that is affected will determine the severity of the disease. Although hemophilia is an X-linked disorder, in approximately 25% of cases, no family history is identified. In such cases, either there were no affected males (or symptomatic females) in the pedigree, or a new mutation arose in either the patient or more often the mother or the maternal grandfather's germ cells, as has been demonstrated for one particular mutation in FVIII known as the intron 22 inversion.

Acquired hemophilia is a very rare condition and can present during pregnancy. Because the antibodies are most often of the IgG subtype, it is possible for these antibodies to be transplacentally transferred, resulting in the same condition in the fetus and newborn. The symptoms of acquired hemophilia are similar to those of congenital hemophilia; however, there seems to be a higher predilection for mucocutaneous bleeding. Otherwise, there is no specific bleeding pattern, although it is rare for there not to be significant cutaneous bleeding.

Clinical Presentation

The clinical presentation of congenital hemophilia is highly variable and depends on the severity of the disease and on whether or not a family history is present (Kulkarni et al, 2006). For patients with a known family history (particularly if the mother is an obligate carrier, e.g., the daughter of a hemophiliac), the diagnosis can be made shortly after birth by assaying FVIII or FIX from umbilical cord blood. Prenatal testing can be performed; however, it is not generally recommended, because it should not alter the course of the pregnancy or the planned mode of delivery (the mode of delivery of a known hemophiliac remains somewhat controversial). For patients in whom there is no family history or for whom testing was not done after birth, symptoms can develop at any time and more or less correlate with the severity of disease.

Severe hemophilia (defined as a factor level below 1%) can manifest in the newborn period with any of the following: intra- or extracranial bleeding, prolonged bleeding from venipuncture or heelstick puncture, prolonged bleeding after circumcision, excessive bruising, muscle hematomas after intramuscular injections such as vaccinations, or bleeding after surgery. For patients in whom none of these symptoms develop, the presentation will occur later in life and thus not under the purview of a neonatologist.

Diagnosis

The laboratory diagnosis of hemophilia is fairly straightforward. A clinical suspicion for a bleeding disorder should trigger the ordering of a PT and PTT, and the PTT is nearly always abnormal. There are rare instances where the PTT may not be abnormal. After the identification of a prolonged PTT, factor levels will elucidate the type (FVIII or FIX) and the severity of hemophilia. There are several caveats to the measurement of factor levels. First, proper specimen procurement and handling is critical; otherwise, results may be falsely low. Second, testing of cord blood specimens may result in levels that may be somewhat above what they would be on repeat testing; thus, although cord blood factor levels are useful in determining the presence of hemophilia, it is recommended that additional testing be done at a later date in order to ascertain more accurately the severity of hemophilia. Third, the normal range for FVIII in the newborn is at or slightly higher than adult normal values. However, FIX levels are significantly lower in newborns than in adults (consult a table for the exact levels at different ages in the 1st month of life). Of note, preterm neonates have even lower FIX levels. Fourth, the factor assays at very low levels (1–2%) are less reliable, and thus repeated testing is recommended in order to differentiate patients with severe and moderate hemophilia. Fifth, there are rare occasions when a patient may have a normal factor level on the one-stage clotting assay (the one most commonly used in the United States), whereas an abnormal result will be obtained on the two-stage chromogenic assay. Last, inflammation may increase FVIII levels for patients with mild hemophilia, and thus it is best to measure levels while patients are in their usual state of health.

Treatment

The mainstay of hemophilia treatment is factor replacement therapy. A number of factor concentrates are commercially available for both FVIII and FIX deficiency. The choice of which specific product to use is complicated by issues such as the availability and cost of each agent as well as real and perceived benefits of plasma-derived versus recombinant products and among different generations of recombinant FVIII products, of which there are currently four agents and five products (one agent is marketed and sold under two names by two pharmaceutical companies). Ultimately, the choice of factor concentrate should be made in consultation with a pediatric hematologist.

Many neonates will not require treatment during the newborn period because they will not manifest bleeding symptoms (or the diagnosis will not have been made). For those in whom bleeding has occurred, factor replacement therapy is indicated, and the specific dosing regimen should be determined in consultation with a pediatric hematologist. For those with a known prenatal or early postnatal diagnosis in whom circumcision (or any other surgical procedure) is to be performed, treatment with factor replacement is mandatory in order to prevent bleeding and improve the outcome of the procedure. On rare occasions, neonates will present with severe bleeding symptoms such as ICH. In such cases, factor replacement therapy should be initiated as soon as possible, and therapy should be continued for at least several days if not several weeks. The duration and intensity of therapy depends on the location and severity of bleeding. Again, dosing regimens can be determined in consultation with a pediatric hematologist.

Adjuvant therapies for hemophilia exist that are similar to those for platelet defects and VWD. For patients with mild FVIII deficiency, desmopressin can increase factor levels to hemostatic levels and can be useful for the management of minor bleeding. The use of antifibrinolytic agents for mucous membrane bleeding is also effective and can be used as an adjunct to desmopressin or factor replacement.

The most important complication of factor therapy in hemophilia is the development of neutralizing antibodies termed inhibitors. Inhibitors render standard factor replacement therapy ineffective, resulting in bleeds that are more difficult to control, which leads to increased morbidity and mortality (Young, 2006). The incidence of inhibitors in previously untreated FVIII-deficient patients is between 20% and 35%, whereas for FIX-deficient patients it is approximately 5%. The prevalence of inhibitors is approximately 10% in FVIII deficiency and 3% to 5% in FIX deficiency. Inhibitors will rarely manifest in the newborn period, because in general it takes 10 to 20 doses of factor before an inhibitor develops, and most neonates will not receive this many doses of factor except for those with major bleeding symptoms. For those in whom multiple doses have been administered, the possibility for the development of an inhibitor should be considered if bleeding occurs despite factor replacement therapy.

The management of bleeding episodes in patients with inhibitors can be a significant challenge, and much of the morbidity from hemophilia in the United States occurs in patients with high-titer inhibitors. Presently, there are only two agents available for the management of bleeding in inhibitor patients, activated prothrombin complex concentrate (APCC) (FEIBA, Baxter, Westlake Village, CA) and recombinant activated factor VII (rFVIIa; Novoseven, Novo Nordisk, Bagsvaerd, Denmark). Activated prothrombin complex concentrate is a plasma-derived mixture of clotting factors, some of which are activated. The mechanism of action is felt to be due to the presence and action of activated FX and prothrombin, although this product also contains activated FIX and FVII as well as a small amount of nonactivated FVIII. Recombinant activated FVII is (as its name implies) a recombinant form of activated FVII and contains no other human proteins. The mechanism of action of rFVIIa involves the generation of thrombin on the surface of activated platelets through tissue-factor-dependent and -independent mechanisms. Both products have been demonstrated to be safe and effective, with variable response rates generally between 70% and 90%, depending on the study. Both products have a long

track record of safety (more than 30 years for APCC and 10 years for rFVIIa), with few reported thrombotic events in patients with hemophilia and inhibitors. In addition, from an infectious disease standpoint, the APCC has an excellent safety record with no documented transmission of viral infections, whereas rFVIIa has, as expected, no known transmission of any infections. Because APCC contains small amounts of FVIII, it could in theory lead to an increase in the inhibitor titer (anamnesis); thus, it is recommended to avoid APCC if possible in the newborn period. Again, management of bleeding is critical, so this is not a contraindication to using APCC during this time, and if a bleeding episode does not respond to rFVIIa, then APCC should be used without hesitation. Dosing for these agents should be done in consultation with a pediatric hematologist. For patients receiving inhibitors in whom invasive procedures are required, rFVIIa can be used perioperatively to prevent bleeding (APCC can be used as well if rFVIIa is not effective). In the extraordinarily rare circumstance of acquired hemophilia antibodies passively transferred to a newborn, the management of bleeding is similar to that of congenital hemophilia with inhibitors.

Prognosis and Outcomes

Currently, patients with severe hemophilia in whom inhibitors do not develop and who are on prophylaxis have an excellent prognosis and often lead normal lives free of debilitating hemophilic arthropathy. This has been documented well by the Swedish cohort for almost the past 40 years. For patients with inhibitors, the prognosis is more guarded. For those in whom ITT is effective, their outcome can be as good as for those who never developed an inhibitor, provided they did not develop joint damage before tolerization. It is likely, however, that many of these patients will have had a number of bleeding episodes in joints, muscles, or, rarely, in the brain, and that some of these patients will have permanent deficits. For inhibitor patients in whom ITT was not successful, significant joint morbidity is very common, often leading to permanent disability and relatively poor quality of life. Nevertheless, with the reduced reluctance to perform surgery in inhibitor patients combined with the increased use of prophylaxis, it is possible to intervene and ameliorate the effects of joint damage and allow patients to lead more productive lives.

RARE FACTOR DEFICIENCIES

Etiology/Pathophysiology

As with deficiencies of FVIII and FIX, deficiencies in other important hemostatic clotting factors result in reduced thrombin generation or, particular to FXIII, reduced fibrin cross-linking resulting in poor clot formation and reduced resistance to fibrinolysis. Deficiencies of fibrinogen and FII, FV, FVII, FX, FXI, and FXIII all result in variable bleeding diatheses (Peyvandi et al, 2008). In general, the severity of the bleeding is related to the factor levels (although this is less clear for FXI deficiency).

Rare factor deficiencies can be the result of genetic defects or acquired conditions. The genes for all of the

TABLE 76-5 Classification of Vitamin K Deficiency Bleeding (VKBD)

Feature	Early	Classical	Late
Age	<24 hours of age	1–7 days	2 weeks and older
Risk factors	Maternal medications (vitamin K antagonists, anticonvulsants, antituberculin drugs)	Lack of prophylactic vitamin K treatment, poor feeding (particularly if breastfed)	Exclusive breastfeeding, poor feeding, gastrointestinal disorders, liver disease, pancreatic disease, antibiotic therapy
Sites of bleeding	Cephalhematoma, umbilical stump, intracranial	Gastroinestinal, umbilicus, mucocutaneous, circumcision, intracranial	Intracranial, mucocutaneous, gastrointestinal
Frequency	Less than 5% in at-risk population	With prophylactic vitamin K—extremely rare, Without prophylactic vitamin K (0.01% to 1%)	Variable depending on age and conditions listed above
Treatment	Prothrombin complex concentrates, vitamin K (may not be effective)	Parenteral vitamin K (intravenous preferred) Prothrombin complex concentrates for active bleeding	Vitamin K, prothrombin complex concentrates for active bleeding, recombinant factor VIIa (for mild cases in which only the PT is prolonged)
Prevention	Avoidance of above medications during pregnancy	Vitamin K prophylaxis at birth	Adequate vitamin K replacement (in many cases will need to be parenteral)

PT, Prothrombin time.

foregoing factors are located on somatic chromosomes and thus affect males and females equally. The specific defect will dictate the resultant factor activity level and thus the phenotypic severity. In neonates, acquired rare factor deficiencies are more common and can result from a variety of conditions, including vitamin K deficiency, liver disease, and Kasabach-Merritt syndrome.

Vitamin K is required for the gamma-carboxylation of FII, FVII, FIX, and FX, and the absence of gamma-carboxylation renders these proteins nonfunctional. Vitamin K deficiency still occurs in newborns, particularly in those born at home where vitamin K administration is less likely to occur or in those children whose parents refuse vitamin K administration for their child. Vitamin K deficiency bleeding (VKDB) is classified as early, classical or late (Table 76-5) (Shearer, 2009). Early onset occurs in the first 24 hours of life and is due to the cross-placental transfer of compounds that interfere with vitamin K metabolism or function including some anticonvulsants, antibiotics, antituberculin agents and vitamin K antagonists e.g., warfarin. Classical VKDB occurs in the 1st week of life and is due to a physiologic deficiency in vitamin K at birth combined with a lack of vitamin K in breast milk or due to inadequate feeding. Vitamin K prophylaxis has its biggest impact on preventing this type of VKDB. Late-onset VKDB can occur at any age, although it is classically described as occurring between 2 weeks and 6 months of age. Almost all infants with the disorder are exclusively breastfed because it is believed to be caused by inadequate vitamin K content in breast milk. In late-onset vitamin K deficiency, additional risk factors for vitamin K deficiency must be present that intuitively have in common reduced vitamin K intake and absorption. Some examples of conditions that lead to late-onset vitamin K deficiency are liver or pancreatic disease, both leading to an inability to absorb fat-soluble vitamins; gastrointestinal disorders that affect intestinal flora, because a secondary source of vitamin K is production by intestinal microorganisms; prolonged antibiotic use, again due to an alteration of

intestinal flora; and ingestion (accidental or otherwise) of vitamin K antagonists, which, although perhaps not technically vitamin K deficiency, can be overcome with vitamin K.

Before the widespread use of vitamin K prophylaxis, the incidence of classical VKDB was reported to be as high as 1.5%; however, the condition now is considered rare. A recent comprehensive survey from Great Britain and Ireland demonstrated a rate of 0.14 per 100,000 live births in a population with a high rate of prophylactic vitamin K administration. The incidence for early- and late-onset VKDB is not known. However, early-onset VKDB occurs in only a small proportion (probably <5%) of at-risk births. The variety of conditions that lead to late-onset VKDB make defining the incidence challenging.

Regarding the other rare factor deficiencies, all are known to occur in association with specific medical conditions. Specifically, hypofibrinogenemia can result from liver disease, the Kasabach-Merrit syndrome (hemangioma with consumptive coagulopathy), and DIC. Factors II, VII, and X are vitamin K dependent (as is FIX, which was covered in the preceding section) and synthesized in the liver, and thus they become deficient in liver failure and vitamin K deficiency as described earlier. In addition, FII deficiency can rarely occur as part of the antiphospholipid syndrome, which, although uncommon in newborns, can result from transplacental transfer of maternal antibodies. Deficiency of FV has been reported after exposure to topical thrombin (commonly used in cardiac surgery) as a result of autoantibody formation. DIC is a serious disorder resulting from a variety of medical conditions which leads to consumption of clotting factors and thus can result in bleeding. In DIC, multiple factors are often deficient.

Finally, there are two inherited multifactor deficiency disorders. One results in deficiencies of FV and FVIII and is the result of a mutation in a protein (endoplasmic reticulum Golgi intermediate compartment [ERGIC]-53) required for assembly and secretion of these two similarly

TABLE 76-6   Bleeding Sites/Symptoms and Factor Replacement Choices for Rare Factor Deficiencies

Factor Deficiency	Bleeding Sites	Other Symptoms	Factor Replacement	Causes for Acquired Deficiency
Fibrinogen	No typical sites	Splenic rupture Miscarriage Thrombosis	Fibrinogen concentrate (RiaStap) Cryoprecipitate	Liver disease Asparaginase therapy DIC
FII (prothrombin)	No typical sites	None	PCC	Vitamin K deficiency Liver disease Vitamin K antagonists Antiphospholipid syndrome
FV	No typical sites	None	FFP Platelet transfusion	Exposure to topical bovine thrombin
FVII	Intracranial	Thrombosis	rFVIIa	Vitamin K deficiency Liver disease Vitamin K antagonists
FX	Intracranial	None	PCC	Vitamin K deficiency Liver disease Vitamin K antagonists Amyloidosis
FXI	Postoperative or trauma-related	None	FFP (FXI concentrates are available in some countries)	Autoantibodies (rare)
FXIII	Intracranial Umbilical stump	Poor wound healing Miscarriage	Cryoprecipitate pdFXIII concentrate is available in the US as part of a clinical trial	Cardiopulmonary bypass Inflammatory bowel disease

FFP, Fresh frozen plasma
RiaStap (fibrinogen concentrate) is licensed only for congenital afibrinogenemia.
Recombinant FVIIa is licensed for the treatment of congenital FVII deficiency.
Prothrombin complex concentrates (PCC) are not licensed for the treatment of rare factor deficiencies and contain variable amounts of FII, FVII, and FX (the amounts are in the prescribing information). Dosing is based on FIX units.

structured proteins. A second disorder results in deficiency of all of the vitamin K–dependent proteins and is due to a number of mutations in enzymes in the vitamin K pathway. Both conditions are very rare and have mostly been reported in consanguineous families. Both can lead to significant bleeding symptoms.

Clinical Presentation

The clinical presentation of the congenital rare factor deficiencies is similar to that for hemophilia and can be discovered as a result of a known family history, although this is far less common for these deficiencies because their mode of inheritance is autosomal recessive. More likely, they present with excessive bleeding, which ranges from mild mucocutaneous bleeding to catastrophic ICH. Unique features for each factor deficiency can be found in Table 76-6. Several conditions leading to rare factor deficiencies can present in the newborn period. As mentioned, DIC can be the result of a variety of clinical conditions, most commonly sepsis, and often the coagulation problems (bleeding or thrombosis) present after the onset and even the diagnosis of the underlying condition. Patients with the Kasabach-Merritt syndrome will usually (although not always) have an easily visible mass, which can occur anywhere. Occasionally, the lesion leading to Kasabach-Merritt syndrome is deep-seated and not obvious on physical examination, in which case it may be diagnosed by diagnostic imaging. Patients with coagulopathy associated with liver failure should (although again this is not universal) have clear signs of liver dysfunction.

Diagnosis

Once suspected, the diagnosis of rare factor deficiencies is relatively straightforward. In many patients, the presentation may be obvious, such as those with signs of liver failure, a lesion suspicious for Kasabach-Merritt syndrome, conditions associated with DIC, or a history of a lack of vitamin K administration. Regarding the laboratory diagnosis, all of the described deficiencies with the exception of FXIII deficiency result in a prolonged PT, PTT, or both. Depending on the results of these screening tests, specific factor assays can be performed, leading to the correct diagnosis. For example, deficiencies of FII, FVII, FIX, and FX suggest either vitamin K deficiency or liver disease, whereas significant hypofibrinogenemia is associated with DIC or Kasabach-Merritt syndrome (other factor deficiencies are associated with these conditions, but a low fibrinogen is a hallmark of these conditions). FXIII deficiency can be diagnosed via a qualitative assay (clot solubility assay) or a quantitative assay. The clot solubility assay is abnormal only if the FXIII level is less than about 5%; thus, it is not sensitive for milder deficiencies, although it is not clear that mild FXIII deficiency results in a bleeding diathesis.

Treatment

In neonates with rare factor deficiencies, there is nearly always an acquired cause; therefore, treatment of that condition should result in resolution or improvement of the factor deficiencies. For vitamin K deficiency, treatment with vitamin K will result in complete resolution of the factor deficiencies. Importantly, however, if patients have active bleeding, it should be noted that the correction of the deficiencies will take as long as 24 hours, thus necessitating immediate factor replacement therapy to control the bleeding. Products referred to as prothrombin complex concentrates contain all the vitamin K–dependent factors and should be administered immediately if vitamin K–deficient bleeding is occurring. Consultation with a hematologist is recommended to assist in selection of the correct product and dose.

For patients with DIC or liver disease, correction of those conditions will result in correction of the factor deficiencies. For patients with active bleeding, fresh frozen plasma and cryoprecipitate are the treatment of choice to correct the factor deficiencies of DIC, whereas for liver failure, the prothrombin complex concentrates and cryoprecipitate (if the fibrinogen is low) are the treatment of choice. In patients with Kasabach-Merritt syndrome, treatment of the lesion will result in correction of the factor deficiencies, and because hypofibrinogenemia and thrombocytopenia are likely the main causes for bleeding, treatment with cryoprecipitate and platelet transfusions may be effective. It should be emphasized that the foregoing therapies are recommended only if bleeding is occurring and not simply for abnormal laboratory test results.

For the rare patient with congenital factor deficiencies, the hallmark of therapy is replacement of the deficient factor either after bleeding occurs or prophylactically as described for FVIII and FIX earlier. Table 76-6 lists the available therapies for factor replacement. For the most part, patients with these factor deficiencies are treated only when they bleed; however, there are some notable exceptions. Because severe deficiencies of FX and FXIII frequently result in catastrophic ICH, such patients should receive lifelong prophylaxis. For FX deficiency, this is accomplished by twice-weekly infusions of prothrombin complex concentrate (PCC), whereas for FXIII, this is accomplished via monthly infusions of cryoprecipitate or plasma-derived FXIII concentrate (Corifact, CSL Behring, King of Prussia, Penn.). Severe FVII deficiency can also result in ICH, although less so than for FX and FXIII deficiencies, and prophylactic therapy with rFVIIa should be considered.

Prognosis and Outcomes

The congenital rare factor disorders are highly variable conditions both within each specific deficiency and among the deficiencies. Furthermore, not only are the acquired conditions leading to rare factor deficiencies variable, but some may spontaneously remit (FV antibodies secondary to topical thrombin), whereas others have significant morbidity and mortality (liver failure). Thus, it is difficult to discuss prognosis and outcome in general for these disorders. Suffice it to say that mild or moderate congenital rare factor deficiencies do not generally lead to major health problems, and the bleeding associated with these conditions can be easily managed. For severe congenital deficiencies, particularly those associated with serious bleeding complications, prophylactic therapy is an effective approach, and for such patients, outcomes are excellent so long as they have not yet suffered permanent sequelae as the result of a bleed. For patients with acquired rare factor deficiencies, outcomes are excellent for those who recover from their underlying condition that led to the coagulopathy—again, so long as they have not suffered a catastrophic bleed. For those whose underlying condition cannot be readily treated, their prognosis is generally poor and more often related to consequences of the underlying condition rather than bleeding, although occasionally the bleeding in and of itself leads to severe sequelae.

THROMBOTIC DISORDERS

PHYSIOLOGY OF THROMBOSIS

The pathophysiology of thrombosis in neonates fits well within the concepts of Virchow's triad, which includes hypercoagulability, disturbances in blood flow, and endothelial damage or disruption (Bagot and Arya, 2008). When this paradigm is applied to neonates, patients with thrombosis will have at least one, if not two or three, of these abnormalities ongoing. With respect to hypercoagulability, neonates physiologically are all deficient in proteins important in inhibiting coagulation (proteins C and S and antithrombin), with premature neonates being even more deficient than full-term ones. Although neonates are also deficient in procoagulant proteins, the combination of the physiologic deficiency along with other disturbances pointed out by Virchow will tilt the precarious hemostatic balance in favor of thrombosis. In addition, neonates who develop thrombotic complications may have inherited abnormalities that predispose to thrombosis (so-called inherited thrombophilia). The most striking example is that of the neonate with severe (usually homozygous) protein C deficiency who presents with purpura fulminans immediately after delivery with thrombotic complications occurring in utero (Thornburg and Pipe, 2006). Another example is that of the newborn with homocystinuria resulting in very high homocysteine levels, which is associated with arterial and venous thrombosis. The second aspect of Virchow's triad is disturbances in blood flow, such as the stasis or hemodynamic compromise that is associated with hypotension. There are a variety of situations in neonates where this may occur. Perhaps the most obvious example would be in the neonate presenting with shock (for any reason) in whom sluggish blood flow may result in the formation of thrombi. Other examples are congenital heart disease with anomalous blood flow; polycythemia in, for example, infants of diabetic mothers; and cyanotic heart lesions. Last, endothelial damage or disruption is another important aspect of the pathophysiology of thrombosis, and by the far the most common reason for this is vascular catheterization, which could be temporary, that is, diagnostic cardiac catheterization, or of much longer duration, such as the use of central venous catheters. In fact, the vast majority of neonates with thrombosis have catheter-related thrombosis. Taking all of the foregoing into consideration, it should not be surprising that neonates have the highest rate of thrombosis of all the pediatric age groups.

TABLE 76-7 Risk Factors for Deep Vein Thrombosis

Inherited	Acquired
Protein C deficiency	Intravascular catheters
Protein S deficiency	Congenital heart disease
Antithrombin deficiency	Infection
Factor V Leiden	Immobilization
Prothrombin mutation	Artificial heart valves
Hyperhomocysteinemia	Dehydration
Lipoprotein(a) elevation	Surgery
	Trauma
	Malignancy
	Antiphospholipid antibody
	syndrome

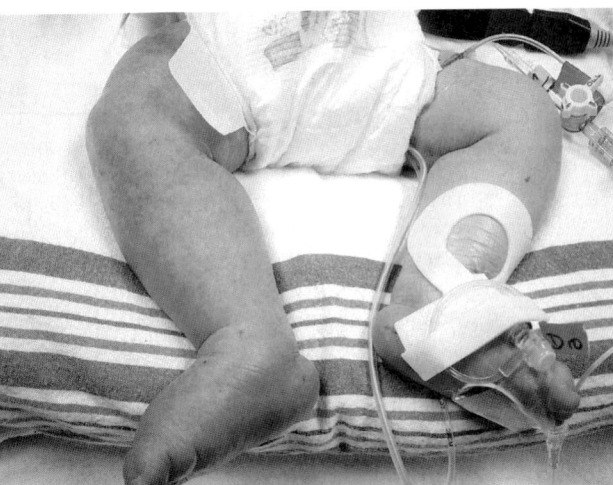

FIGURE 76-2 **Femoral deep vein thrombosis.** Note the swollen leg with venous congestion pattern on the skin.

VENOUS THROMBOSIS

Epidemiology

As stated earlier, neonates have the highest rate of thrombosis (including DVT) of all the pediatric age groups. A variety of studies have reported an incidence rate for neonatal thrombosis of between 13% and 65% (Veldman et al, 2008). A 1995 study determined that 2.4 of 1000 newborns admitted to the neonatal intensive care unit develop a thrombotic event; however, that number is surely higher today, given the increased use of central venous catheters and improved survival of critically ill neonates (Veldman et al, 2008). There are numerous risk factors associated with DVT in newborns (Table 76-7). The most common cause for thrombosis is the presence of central venous catheters, although the precise incidence is unknown. Some studies have shown rates as high as approximately 60% (Veldman et al, 2008; Hermansen and Hermansen, 2005). As can be expected, these events occur in the region of the catheter tip or insertion point. All types of venous catheters, from umbilical venous catheters to centrally inserted tunneled catheters to peripherally inserted central catheters, can lead to thrombosis (Hermansen and Hermansen, 2005).

Other important causes of venous thrombosis in newborns include congenital heart disease, sepsis (particularly with DIC), dehydration, perinatal asphyxia; although rare, genetic disorders should also always be considered. Patients with congenital heart disease, although at risk for developing catheter-related thrombosis, are also at risk for a variety of non-catheter-related thrombotic events. In such cases, thrombotic events occur either in the heart with atrial or, more rarely, ventricular thrombi or in surgically created shunts such as Blalock-Taussig shunts. Pulmonary emboli may also occur as a result of thrombi presenting in the pulmonary artery. In patients with sepsis, most thrombotic events are associated with catheters; however, when accompanied by hemodynamic instability or DIC, venous thrombosis can occur in any of the deep veins. Perinatal asphyxia with or without therapeutic hypothermia and dehydration can result in cerebralsinus thrombosis, although patients may have clots elsewhere. Patients with perinatal asphyxia can also develop non–catheter-related DVT as a result of prolonged reduced blood flow. Last, newborns apart from older children have a predilection for developing renal vein thrombosis for reasons which are not clear. It typically occurs in patients with inferior vena cava thrombosis secondary to catheters as a result of extension but idiopathic cases are not unusual. In some registries, renal vein thrombosis accounted for as much as 58% of all neonatal thrombosis although in other thrombosis registries, it occurred in just 2% of affected patients (Chalmers, 2006). This is likely due to differences in definitions. Regardless, renal vein thrombosis is an important manifestation of venous thrombosis in the neonatal population (Lau et al, 2007).

Clinical Presentation

As stated, DVT is most often associated with the presence of central venous catheters, and when considering the clinical presentation, the mere presence of a catheter should trigger an assessment by history and examination, including catheter location. The typical signs of venous thrombosis are related to decreased venous drainage of the area distal to the thrombus. Thus, thrombosis affecting the limbs will initially result in swelling and pain (difficult to assess in neonates) of the affected extremity (Figure 76-2). Occlusion of the central veins is often asymptomatic and discovered as an incidental finding on an imaging study, or it can result in dramatic physical signs such as in superior vena cava syndrome. Occasionally, the presentation may be more subtle, such as ascites (secondary to portal vein thrombosis) or organomegaly (typically associated with renal or splenic vein thrombosis). The same physiologic principle applies, however, which is decreased venous drainage of an affected organ or location. In superior vena cava syndrome, the onset of symptoms is fairly acute, with an often dramatic swelling of the head and neck associated with significant headache and discomfort. Thrombosis affecting particular organs will often result in nonspecific signs and symptoms such as ascites (portal vein), splenomegaly with or without hypersplenism (splenic vein), hematuria (renal vein), abdominal pain (mesenteric vein), or hepatomegaly and hyperbilirubinemia (hepatic vein). Another manifestation of venous thrombosis is cerebral sinus thrombosis. It most often presents in neonates suffering from dehydration or those with head and neck infections. Occasionally, no cause is identified. The symptoms again are related to decreased venous drainage, with the brain being the affected organ. Clinical manifestations are often nonspecific and include signs of raised intracranial pressure such as a bulging fontanel, irritability, and rarely neurologic disturbances such as seizures or focal neurologic signs, particularly if venous infarcts have occurred. Early diagnosis of the thrombosis as well as its underlying cause is important in order for treatment to be effective at preventing permanent neurologic sequelae.

Last, pulmonary embolism is an important and often undiagnosed event in children and particularly difficult to diagnose in sick neonates, who often already have reduced pulmonary capacity. In otherwise well neonates, the symptoms are usually subtle because of the inherent ability of patients of this age to compensate for hypoxemia, and the symptoms when they do occur are nonspecific and include tachypnea, cough, chest pain, and rarely respiratory distress. Hypoxemia is not always present. Pulmonary embolism should be in the differential diagnosis for newborns with a known thrombus and unusual or unexpected pulmonary symptoms when alternative diagnoses have been eliminated.

Unique to newborns, thrombocytopenia not infrequently occurs as a manifestation of thrombosis. For reasons that are unclear, although thrombocytopenia in and of itself is not a manifestation of DVT in older children, newborns with thrombosis may have thrombocytopenia solely as a clinical manifestation of the clot itself, and this in fact may be the presentation of thrombosis. Thus, in a newborn with unexplained thrombocytopenia, thrombosis must be considered in the differential diagnosis.

Diagnosis

There are two important points of discussion when it comes to the diagnosis of DVT in newborns: the identification of the location and extent of the thrombus, and the underlying conditions and risk factors that may have caused the thrombus to occur in the first place.

Once a thrombus is suspected, the appropriate diagnostic imaging study should be performed to confirm the clinical suspicion (Veldman et al, 2008). The most common imaging approach for venous thrombosis is Doppler ultrasonography. This method assesses the veins by direct visualization for thrombosis, detection of flow via the Doppler effect, and compressibility. Other imaging modalities include computed tomography (CT), CT venography, magnetic resonance imaging (MRI) or MR venography, and echocardiography. It is important to note that none of the listed approaches has been formally studied in newborns, and it is difficult to determine which methods would be most suitable for any given situation. The "gold standard" for diagnosing venous thrombosis is venography. However, despite its high sensitivity and specificity, it is not frequently used because of the need to place a peripheral intravenous line, the availability and relative ease of Doppler ultrasonography, and the reluctance of many radiologists to perform the test. Venography is nonetheless the most reliable diagnostic method. In clinical practice, the general approach is to order the simplest and least invasive imaging study first (Doppler ultrasonography), followed by the more logistically complicated and/or expensive

studies (MRI, CT, venography) if the first approach is not adequate.

Although Doppler ultrasonography is sensitive for the lower extremities, it has very poor sensitivity (approximately 30% in a study of young children) for veins proximal to the distal subclavian vein because of the presence of the clavicle overlying the subclavian vein, the inability to compress the veins, and the depth of the veins in the chest (Male et al, 2003). Of note, venography is not sensitive for thrombosis in the internal jugular veins, because the injected dye will not flow in a retrograde fashion. Thus both ultrasonography and venography (or an alternative) are required for a complete assessment of the upper venous system. Cerebral sinus thrombosis is most effectively diagnosed via MRI/MRV of the brain, and although a CT scan may reveal the abnormality, a normal study does not exclude the diagnosis. Pulmonary embolism when suspected is best diagnosed via CT venography.

The second aspect of the diagnostic evaluation in neonates with thrombosis is the identification of specific risk factors and underlying conditions that led to the DVT (Kenet and Nowak-Gottl, 2006; Veldman et al, 2008). This has important implications regarding management of the patient, including the decision to anticoagulate and, if so, with which agent, at what intensity, and for what duration, as well as decisions regarding vascular access, such as removing a central venous catheter. In addition, the diagnosis of a thrombotic event may lead to an explanation of clinical findings such as thrombocytopenia or cardiac dysfunction that will have implications for the management of these disorders. Nearly all newborns with DVT have multiple risk factors leading to the development of the thrombotic event.

The risk factors associated with pediatric thrombosis can be separated into two main groups: inherited and acquired (see Table 76-7). For each individual patient, it is important to document all of the potential risk factors that may have been associated with the induction of the thrombotic event. If acquired risk factors are identified that can be eliminated or ameliorated, this may be helpful in the management of the thrombosis (see Treatment section, later). For example, a dehydrated infant with cerebral sinus thrombosis would obviously benefit from rehydration. The decision to treat or remove other risk factors is less straightforward. For example, although it may be beneficial from the standpoint of the clot to remove a catheter that led to a thrombosis, when evaluating the patient's situation as a whole, it may be prudent to leave the catheter in place and treat with anticoagulation. Removing a central venous catheter from one location where a clot developed only to place a new catheter in a new location where another clot could develop may not be the best approach. If, on the other hand, the patient can be managed without a central venous catheter, it then would be appropriate to remove this catheter.

Genetic risk factors obviously cannot be modified, and whether or not testing for these risk factors should be done is controversial (Kenet and Nowak-Gottl, 2006). On the one hand, identification of a genetic risk factor may provide insight into why a thrombotic event occurred. On the other hand, in a neonate with multiple risk factors (especially those with a central venous catheter) what, if any, role the genetic risk factor played cannot be ascertained.

TABLE 76-8 Laboratory Evaluation for Thrombophilia

Inherited Causes	Acquired Causes
Protein C activity	Antiphospholipid antibodies
Protein C antigen	(anticardiolopin antibodies,
Protein S activity	anti-β2 glycoprotein I
Protein S activity, free	antibodies, lupus anticoagu-
Protein S activity, total	lant)
Antithrombin activity	
Antithrombin antigen	
Factor V Leiden (DNA assay)	
Prothrombin mutation (DNA assay)	
Homocysteine level	
Lipoprotein(a) level	

A second argument in favor of testing is that on occasion, identifying a genetic abnormality may lead to changes in the treatment approach. For example, an elevated homocysteine level may lead to identification of an inherited disorder of metabolism, which would lead to therapy aimed at lowering the homocysteine level or, if that were not possible, anticoagulation therapy, which would be continued perhaps indefinitely. An additional argument against testing is that in approximately 10% of whites (less so in nonwhites), a genetic defect will be identified, and yet the attribution of the genetic defect (e.g., factor V Leiden) to the causation of the thrombosis in a neonate with multiple acquired risk factors is not clear. Furthermore, even if a genetic defect is identified, how (if at all) it should change the management approach is not clear because of a lack of evidence-based studies in children in general and in neonates in particular. Thus, it is important to consider the pros and cons of performing a thrombophilia laboratory evaluation before embarking on such an evaluation, and in particular, the physician ordering such tests should have a clear idea of how the results would affect ongoing management. Under some rare circumstances, testing is warranted. These circumstances would include those in which a neonate with purpura fulminans may have severe protein C deficiency (or rarely severe protein S deficiency) and a newborn has an idiopathic DVT, which, as mentioned is a very rare event. It is suggested that a pediatric hematologist with expertise in coagulation disorders in neonates be consulted before testing in order to be sure that testing is necessary in the first place, and second, that the appropriate tests are in fact ordered.

Table 76-8 provides a general overview of the tests.

The extent of the laboratory investigation for thrombophilia is controversial. In general, the following first-line tests should be included: genetic analysis for factor V Leiden and the prothrombin G20210A mutation; assays for proteins C and S and antithrombin; measurement of homocysteine and lipoprotein(a) level; and evaluation for antiphospholipid antibodies, including lupus anticoagulant, anti-cardiolipin, and anti-β2 glycoprotein I antibodies. Additional conditions and the tests to assess them that are not usually part of the first line of tests include elevated FVIII (FVIII activity), dysfibrinogenemia (thrombin time, reptilase time, functional fibrinogen), and disorders of fibrinolysis (euglobulin clot lysis time). Finally, it should be noted that children (particularly infants) have different

normal ranges for many of the mentioned tests compared to adults, yet most laboratories will only report a reference range for adults; thus at first glance it appears that all neonates are deficient in antithrombin, protein C, and protein S (Andrew, 1995, 1997). Furthermore, some tests performed during the acute phase may be abnormal simply as a result of consumption of proteins. Thus, pediatric laboratory results should be interpreted with these caveats.

The most common genetic condition associated with thrombosis is the factor V Leiden mutation. It occurs in approximately 5% of whites or those of mixed race with white ancestry. The diagnosis is based on identifying the mutation in a simple DNA-based assay. This mutation does not alter the procoagulant function of factor V but results in resistance to deactivation such that the molecule remains in the active state. Therefore, it is referred to as a "gain-of-function" mutation. The relative risk of venous thrombosis in heterozygotes is approximately 8, whereas the relative risk in the homozygous state is approximately 80.

The second most common mutation associated with thrombosis is the prothrombin G20210 mutation (generally referred to as the prothrombin mutation). It also occurs solely in whites and affects about 2% to 3% of individuals in this group. The diagnosis is based on identifying the mutation in a simple DNA-based assay. The relative risk of DVT in adults is approximately 2 to 3. Unlike factor V Leiden, the prothrombin mutation has been associated with arterial thrombosis in adults and children, with a predilection for venous and arterial thrombosis in the central nervous system.

The next section describes three related disorders that are referred to as the classical thrombophilic defects. As described in the first section, the coagulation system is composed of procoagulants as well as natural inhibitors. These natural inhibitors are proteins C and S and antithrombin (previously referred to as antithrombin III). Protein C is activated by thrombin via a cell surface receptor known as thrombomodulin and, along with its cofactor, protein S, deactivates factors VIII and V (the main catalysts required for thrombin generation). Deficiencies of proteins C or S result in an inability to deactivate the coagulation system, thus resulting in hypercoagulability (Knoebl, 2008; ten Kate and van der Meer, 2008). Heterozygous protein C deficiency occurs in about 1 in 300 individuals, and heterozygous protein S deficiency occurs in about 1 in 5000 individuals (Petaja and Manco-Johnson, 2003; ten Kate and van der Meer, 2008). In general, these conditions are associated with venous thrombosis, and the first thrombotic event occurs between the 2nd and 4th decade of life. The relative risk for a first venous thrombosis in children is around 8 for protein C deficiency and 6 for protein S deficiency (Young et al, 2008). Conversely, homozygous individuals will present in the immediate newborn period with purpura fulminans and often have central nervous system thrombosis, including thrombosis in the retinal vessels resulting in retinal detachment and resultant loss of vision (Petaja and Manco-Johnson, 2003). Although newborns presenting with purpura fulminans will usually have other conditions such as sepsis and DIC, any neonate presenting with purpura fulminans should be evaluated for deficiencies of protein C and S as rapidly as possible, because treatment could be life-saving and will prevent complications such as brain injury, vision loss, and skin necrosis. Homozygous protein C deficiency occurs in about 1 in 500,000 individuals, whereas homozygous protein S deficiency occurs in about 1 in 1 million individuals (Petaja and Manco-Johnson, 2003). The diagnosis is based on laboratory assays that can assess the presence and activity of these proteins. The presence of the proteins is measured by immunologically based assays called protein C and S antigen. The function of the proteins can be assayed by tests referred to as either protein C (or S) activity or function. Ultimately, it is the protein function that is the most important to measure; thus, if only one test is ordered it should be the functional assay. It is critical to understand that neonates are physiologically deficient in both proteins C and S, and their levels in the first few days of life are normally about 25% of adult norms. Few laboratories have normative values for neonates; thus, in interpreting the results, the normal ranges provided by the laboratory should be ignored. If the laboratory does not provide normative values for neonates, then one should refer to published reference values from previous studies. For the rare infant with purpura fulminans, assessing proteins C and S is critical, because the homozygous state can be identified by demonstrating unmeasurable levels of the proteins.

Congenital antithrombin deficiency occurs less commonly than deficiencies of proteins C and S, with an incidence of about 1 in 500 to 1 in 5000 (Patnaik and Moll, 2008). The relative risk for a first venous thrombosis in children is approximately 9 (Young et al, 2008). Antithrombin downregulates the thrombotic process by directly binding to and inactivating thrombin, and a deficiency of antithrombin results in hypercoagulability due to the excess thrombin. Although antithrombin deficiency most often is associated with venous thrombosis, it can also result in arterial thrombosis. Homozygous antithrombin deficiency has never been identified and is known to be lethal in animal knockout models; thus it is felt to be incompatible with life. Heterozygous deficiency usually manifests in later childhood or young adulthood and not in the neonatal period. The diagnosis is based on measuring antithrombin levels as described earlier for proteins C and S; as stated previously, measuring the function of antithrombin is the most important laboratory assay, and as with proteins C and S, antithrombin levels are physiologically low in newborns. Unlike protein C or S deficiency, acquired isolated antithrombin deficiency is not uncommon and most often occurs in patients with protein-losing syndromes such as protein-losing enteropathy, nephrosis, or chronic chylothorax. In addition, patients on extracorporeal circulation often have consumption of antithrombin. In patients with such disorders, antithrombin levels should be monitored.

Homocysteine is a naturally occurring amino acid that in high levels leads to damage to the endothelium, resulting in arterial and venous thrombosis (Cattaneo, 1999). A number of genetic and acquired conditions can result in hyperhomocysteinemia. There are a number of inborn errors of metabolism that result in elevated homocysteine levels and occasionally extremely elevated levels as in homocystinuria, a mutation in cystathione β-synthase. Other inborn errors of metabolism in the same metabolic pathway can result in mild to moderate elevations in homocysteine (for details, see Chapter 22). Importantly, a

thrombotic event including stroke may be the presenting feature for these inborn errors of metabolism, and measurement of homocysteine can thus lead to the diagnosis.

Lipoprotein(a) is one of the many lipoproteins such as cholesterol present naturally in the plasma. Its function is unknown, but its structure, which is similar to that of plasminogen, results in competition with binding sites on tissue plasminogen activator, thereby inhibiting fibrinolysis. This is felt to be the mechanism by which elevated lipoprotein(a) results in thrombosis. There have been a number of epidemiologic studies of lipoprotein(a) in children, although not specifically neonates, and the results demonstrate an association with both venous thrombosis and stroke (Young et al, 2008).

An important acquired risk factor for thrombosis in neonates is passive transfer of maternal antiphospholipid antibodies (Boffa and Lachassinne, 2007). This may occur from a mother known to have this condition or from an asymptomatic mother. There are reports of venous thrombosis occurring in newborns in association with the presence of antiphospholipid antibodies, which are presumed to have been transferred from the mother. De novo antiphospholipid antibodies have also been reported; however, the incidence of this condition is unknown.

Treatment

It should be noted that there is a near-complete lack of evidence-based medicine when it comes to treatment-related decisions in the management of neonatal thrombosis. This must be tempered with the knowledge that despite the lack of information, patients must still be treated. There are published treatment guidelines for the management of pediatric (including neonatal) thrombosis, but these are based largely on the opinions of a small group of experts, and most recommendations are based on the lowest level of evidence (i.e., case reports, case series, and small cohort studies) (Monagle et al, 2008). The following discussion should be interpreted in light of this caution, and the most important recommendation is to solicit the consultation of a pediatric hematologist with a specific interest in pediatric thrombosis.

There are two principles that need to be taken into consideration in managing DVT in neonates. First is the need to prevent an embolic event. This is of particular importance in neonates because a venous thrombus will likely embolize to the central nervous system because of the patent foramen ovale. Second, treatment of the thrombus itself is important in order to prevent the postthrombotic syndrome (PTS). PTS is caused by venous insufficiency secondary to valvular damage caused by the thrombus and results in an inability to drain the affected area. This results in swelling and pain in the area distal to the damaged vein. PTS is largely confined to the extremities and mostly to the lower extremities, but similar events can occur elsewhere. For example, ascites resulting from a portal vein thrombosis is essentially due to the same physiologic problem. Prevention of PTS is the most important reason to treat DVT. Although embolic events could be catastrophic, they are uncommon. PTS has been demonstrated in 10% to 60% of children with DVT (the widely varying outcomes result from the lack of a single definition or scoring system for PTS). Although PTS will rarely manifest in the neonatal period, early treatment of DVT in the neonatal unit is an important factor in prevention.

After the diagnosis of DVT is made, treatment should begin immediately, because delays could result in treatment failure. Unless there is a contraindication to anticoagulation, therapy should not be withheld. Once a thrombus is identified, an assessment for acquired risk factors should be performed in order to determine whether any of these factors can be eliminated, such as removing a central line that is no longer needed, or treating dehydration, infections, or an elevated homocysteine level. Regardless of whether such risk factors can be removed or ameliorated, that treatment step is not a substitute for anticoagulation.

With respect to medical therapy, anticoagulation is always necessary. If there is a temporary contraindication to anticoagulation (planned invasive procedure in the next 1 to 2 days), then therapy can be withheld until the contraindication no longer exists. Currently, the anticoagulants that can be used in newborns are limited to unfractionated heparin (hereafter referred to as heparin), low-molecular-weight heparin (LMWH), and warfarin. All three have significant limitations that have been reviewed elsewhere (Young, 2004), and a detailed discussion is beyond the scope of this chapter. Suffice it to say that heparin has a rapid onset of action (after a bolus) and has a short half-life such that it is given via continuous infusion, whereas LMWH (mostly enoxaparin) has somewhat longer onset of action (several hours) and a longer half-life such that it is dosed twice daily and is administered via subcutaneous injection. Intravenous LMWH should not be administered outside the context of a clinical trial. Warfarin is the only orally available anticoagulant; however, its numerous drug and food interactions as well as the fact that it cannot be compounded into a liquid reduce its utility in neonates. Furthermore, achieving a therapeutic international normalized ratio (INR) in infants occurs only about 50% of the time, such that the safety of this agent in neonates from both the bleeding perspective (increased INRs) or thrombotic standpoint (decreased INRs) is questionable. It is best to avoid warfarin in the newborn period unless there is a clear reason why it would be a better option than LWMH (artificial heart valves, for example). Although there are published therapeutic ranges for both heparin (PTT level) and LMWH (anti-Xa level), the evidence that these specific intensities are related to a clinical outcome is not available. There is also no available evidence regarding the duration of therapy, although the general recommendation is 3 to 6 months based on extrapolation from adult data. Again, it is recommended that decisions regarding choice of anticoagulant and intensity and duration of therapy be discussed in consultation with a pediatric hematologist with specific expertise in pediatric thrombosis. Furthermore, because many newborns with DVT are discharged before reaching these time points, such consultation would help facilitate outpatient follow-up. Of note, other than rare situations, thrombolysis is not recommended for the management of DVT in newborns because of the increased risk for ICH, particularly in preterm neonates. In selected and severe situations such as superior vena cava syndrome and pulmonary embolism, thrombolysis could be considered, but such therapy should only be performed under the direct supervision of a hematologist (or other physician) with expertise on its use and only after a discussion with the parents regarding the risks and benefits of this approach.

With rare exceptions, the results of the thrombophilia evaluation (if it is performed) will not affect the approach to management. First, therapy will need to be initiated before results are generally available, and second, the presence of most of the thrombophilias discussed earlier will not influence the choice, intensity, or duration of anticoagulation. Although two recent studies suggested that there is an increased risk for thrombosis recurrence with deficiencies of proteins C and S and antithrombin and with the prothrombin mutation, it is not clear how this evidence should be translated to treatment (Young et al, 2008). In some circumstances, the results of the thrombophilia evaluation will affect therapy. The most obvious example is that of homozygous protein C or protein S deficiency, in which replacement therapy is mandatory (Thornburg and Pipe, 2006). Historically, replacement therapy was accomplished via frequent infusions of fresh frozen plasma; however, the availability of a protein C concentrate (Ceprotin, Baxter, Westlake Village, Calif.) currently makes protein C replacement significantly simpler. Unfortunately, protein S replacement still relies on frequent plasma infusions. For patients with homozygous protein C deficiency, replacement therapy is required lifelong with infusions administered three times per week. For those with homozygous protein S deficiency, there is no standard approach because there are so few cases reported, and prophylactic replacement with fresh frozen plasma, although feasible, is logistically difficult. Once the initial purpura fulminans is treated, ongoing therapy with anticoagulation can be considered. Replacement therapy is not indicated for heterozygotes. In addition to the foregoing, patients with low antithrombin levels may have heparin (and LMWH) resistance because these medications require antithrombin to exert their effects. Antithrombin replacement can be achieved via both a plasma-derived (Thrombate III, Talecris, Research Triangle Park, NC) and more recently a recombinant product (Atryn, GTC Biotherapeutics, Framingham, Mass.). Although a low antithrombin level in the newborn period may not be diagnostic of a genetic deficiency, the low levels nevertheless could result in heparin resistance such that replacement therapy may be indicated. Last, identification of elevated homocysteine levels, whether moderate or severe, will result in therapy aimed at lowering the levels via vitamin B therapy. In summary, treatment of DVT relies on removing or ameliorating acquired risk factors, anticoagulation, and management of a thrombophilic defect in the rare instances when these are found and can be treated.

Outcomes

There is little to no reported research on the outcome of neonates with DVT. Although there is little doubt that PTS occurs, its incidence and severity as a result of neonatal DVT are unknown. Even less is known regarding the outcomes of pulmonary embolism, cerebral sinus thrombosis, portal or renal vein thrombosis, and superior vena cava syndrome. Outcome after neonatal venous thromboembolism is one of the many needed areas for future pediatric thrombosis research.

STROKE

Epidemiology

The term *stroke* is quite ill defined in pediatrics, necessitating a few comments. For the purposes of this chapter, stroke is defined as ischemic brain injury resulting from occlusion of the arterial blood supply to or within the brain. In some publications (Kirton and de Veber, 2009), cerebral sinus thrombosis has been included in the stroke definition; however, although brain infarction can occur in this condition, cerebral sinus thrombosis is more appropriately included with DVT because it shares all the same features as other DVT and is treated similarly. In addition to strokes resulting from vascular occlusion, there are a number of metabolic disorders that can result in a clinical scenario similar to stroke and that result from a lack of required nutrients, toxic effects or other mechanisms; however, because these conditions are metabolic in nature, they are covered in other chapters.

The neonatal period is one of the most common times for a pediatric patient to present with stroke. It is estimated that from 18 to 43 per 100,000 neonates will have acute ischemic stroke (Bernard and Goldenberg, 2008; Kirton and de Veber, 2009). A number of risk factors have been identified that are associated with stroke in the newborn period. These include placental disorders (especially those associated with placental thrombosis), perinatal asphyxia, congenital heart disease, anomalous vasculature, vascular malformations, and perinatal infections including TORCH infections (Bernard and Goldenberg, 2008). Other risk factors include some thrombophilias such as homozygous protein C deficiency, elevated lipoprotein(a), and hyperhomocysteinemia (Bernard and Goldenberg, 2008). Despite detailed investigations, in many instances no clear cause for stroke is identified. There is a notion that many of these events occur as a result of a perinatal embolic event in which tissue such as amniotic fluid or placental thrombi enter the neonatal venous system, resulting in a paradoxic embolus. Unfortunately, it is currently not possible to prove this by any diagnostic test.

Clinical Presentation

The clinical presentation of neonatal stroke ranges from the dramatic (seizures) to the subtle (poor feeding) to an asymptomatic incidental imaging finding. Approximately half of patients with acute ischemic stroke present with seizures within hours up to a day or two after delivery. Other presenting manifestations include nonspecific respiratory abnormalities such as apnea or grunting and occasionally feeding difficulties. Focal neurologic signs are rare, although occasionally seizures will be focal, at least initially, before becoming generalized. On occasion, central nervous system imaging is obtained for reasons unrelated to the foregoing symptoms, and an infarct is found incidentally with no symptoms. Not infrequently, patients may present months later with what is presumed to be neonatal stroke when they have focal neurologic signs or even seizures without a precipitating event, and imaging demonstrates an old infarct. Such infants will obviously not present in the newborn period.

Diagnosis

The diagnosis of acute ischemic stroke requires imaging of the brain with either CT or MRI. Although CT imaging may be easier to obtain, MRI is more sensitive, and its higher resolution as well as the ability to obtain a variety of image types (T1, T2, and diffusion weighting) allows for better characterization of the lesion. Occasionally, a stroke may be suspected based on head ultrasound; however, in such cases obtaining an MRI is recommended. After identification of the lesion by diagnostic imaging, a full and detailed evaluation for the determination of risk factors is warranted (as discussed with DVT). It is critical to identify, if possible, the risk factors that led to the stroke, because this will dictate the treatment and assist in formulating a prognosis. For example, the presence of a stroke may unmask a previously undiagnosed heart lesion, a vascular malformation, or a severe thrombophilia. In many instances, no risk factors will be found, making decisions regarding treatment and discussion of prognosis vis-à-vis a second stroke difficult. For situations in which risk factors are identified, management of such conditions is an important step toward preventing a second event.

One approach to an evaluation for risk factors is first to obtain a detailed history from the parents regarding the pregnancy and family history of thrombotic events. Second is to rule out important causes for stroke such as congenital heart disease and vascular malformations. This evaluation would include an echocardiogram and possibly a cerebral angiogram or cardiac catheterization. If a venous catheter is present either in the umbilical vein or elsewhere, evaluation for DVT is required, because the stroke may have resulted from a paradoxical venous embolus. The likelihood of a venous thrombus in the absence of a catheter is so remote that such an evaluation is unnecessary unless a venous catheter is present or there is a suspicion for a venous thrombosis based on clinical grounds.

From the standpoint of a laboratory evaluation, obtaining a thrombophilia evaluation as described previously remains controversial, especially if other risk factors are identified. In the absence of any identifiable risk factors, a thrombophilia evaluation would be a reasonable course of action. The question is which assays to perform and, importantly, when to perform them, either in the neonatal period or at the age of 6 months or beyond. The advantage of obtaining an evaluation in the newborn period is the possibility of identifying an abnormality that requires treatment such as severe protein C or S deficiency or hyperhomocysteinemia. The disadvantage is that because levels of proteins C and S and antithrombin are physiologically low in the newborn period, it will be necessary to repeat these tests after 6 months of age in order to be sure that normal adult levels have been achieved. Thus, the most prudent approach if one elects to perform a thrombophilia evaluation is to at least obtain protein C and S activity levels, an antithrombin level, and a homocysteine level initially, and to perform the rest of the evaluation when repeating the protein C and S and antithrombin levels at 6 months of age. In addition to the genetic defects described earlier, it is important to evaluate for the antiphospholipid syndrome, because it is possible for the antibodies to be transplacentally transferred from an asymptomatic mother.

Abnormal results in the newborn should prompt an evaluation of the mother.

Other laboratory tests that could be considered are an erythrocyte sedimentation rate, C-reactive protein, and TORCH screen if indicated. Last, if at all possible, pathologic examination of the placenta may reveal the presence of thrombi, which could indicate that the stroke was the result of embolization from placental thrombi.

Treatment

The management of acute ischemic stroke depends largely on the etiology if it can be identified. Obviously, a heart lesion resulting in embolization of thrombi requires rapid correction, as do vascular lesions resulting in ischemia. Severe thrombophilia such as hyperhomocysteinemia or protein C and S deficiency requires specific therapies as previously described. In the more typical situation, however, either no risk factors or more subtle nonspecific risk factors such as infection are present. In such situations, management is much less straightforward. There are no clinical trials that have evaluated anticoagulation or antiplatelet therapy in a prospective or controlled fashion. Although treatment guidelines have been published, these are based on very low-level evidence, as is the case for DVT (Monagle et al, 2008). Although anticoagulation therapy is clearly required for management of DVT and often for acute ischemic stroke in older children, the appropriateness of such therapy for neonates is questionable. If the stroke was felt to be the result of a perinatal embolic event, then the likelihood of a second stroke is essentially zero because, clearly, the risk factor (the birth process and fetal circulation) will never recur. Thus, secondary prevention with anticoagulation or antiplatelet therapy is not required. For those neonates with clear ongoing risk factors such as congenital heart disease or thrombophilia, anticoagulation/antiplatelet therapy should be considered. Unfortunately, data do not exist to support decisions such as which agent to use, at what intensity, and for what duration. For lesions that are clearly arterial, antiplatelet therapy with aspirin is the most appropriate approach, whereas for venous emboli, anticoagulation is more appropriate. Combining these two therapies is another approach although the risk for bleeding certainly rises in this situation. Antiplatelet therapy with aspirin appears to be safe; non–weight-based dosing at 40 mg will result in a significant antiplatelet effect. Anticoagulation therapy as for DVT can be used (see DVT section for details). It is suggested that consultation with a pediatric hematologist and/or neurologist with specific expertise in childhood stroke be sought to assist with therapeutic decisions and for ongoing follow-up after discharge.

Outcomes

Neonates who suffer an overt symptomatic stroke have quite variable and rather unpredictable outcomes. Even those in whom a large area of infarction occurs may have an excellent neurologic outcome, demonstrating the known plasticity of the newborn brain. On average, about 50% to 75% of patients with acute ischemic stroke will have neurologic sequelae, most commonly hemiplegia

and epilepsy (Kirton and de Veber, 2009). Other defects such as vision loss, language deficits, and general cognitive impairment may also be noted. It is important to note that the outcomes do not necessarily correlate with the severity of the lesion, making it hard to predict the outcome in any individual patient. It is suggested that the prognosis be discussed in general and broad terms and that parents be made aware that although neurologic sequelae are common, they are not universal, and that their child should have careful monitoring of development such that specific interventions (physical, occupational and speech therapy, for example) begin as early as possible.

Fortunately, recurrence is rare in neonatal stroke, except for patients with the specific disorders discussed earlier, and in such cases preventive therapy with antiplatelet or anticoagulant medications presumably reduces the risk of recurrence, although there are no data to support this.

ARTERIAL THROMBOSIS (NOT RELATED TO THE CENTRAL NERVOUS SYSTEM)

Epidemiology

Peripheral and central arterial thrombosis is not common, although the incidence is not known. It occurs almost exclusively in association with either arterial catheterization or an inadvertent arterial injury during venous catheterization (Aslam et al, 2008). Arterial thrombosis can occur in any vessel that is catheterized; however, because the most common sites for catheterization are the femoral arteries and aorta (umbilical catheters), these would be the most common sites affected. Patients at highest risk are those with congenital heart disease who may undergo multiple catheterizations of the femoral artery, and premature patients in whom umbilical artery catheters are commonly used. On rare occasion, patients my develop thrombosis of the arteries feeding a visceral organ, with renal artery thrombosis being the most common. Even in this setting, it may have resulted from the presence of an umbilical artery catheter.

Clinical Presentation

Patients with femoral or subclavian/brachial artery thrombosis present with signs of decreased perfusion and ischemia distal to the occlusion. This may include color changes such as pallor or cyanosis, decreased pulses, and eventually tissue necrosis. The signs and symptoms are generally quite obvious (Figure 76-3) and may develop suddenly or may occur incrementally, that is, first loss of pulses followed by color changes followed by necrosis. The presentation of thrombosis in the aorta is usually an incidental finding determined by diagnostic imaging of the abdomen or chest for other reasons. When symptoms are present, they may be subtle, such as differential blood pressures between the upper and lower extremities. Rarely, there may be signs of decreased perfusion distal to the occlusion with symptoms similar to the foregoing. Renal artery thrombosis manifests with hypertension due to disruption of the renin-angiotensin-aldosterone system. Thrombosis of arteries to other organs is extremely rare and will manifests with organ dysfunction.

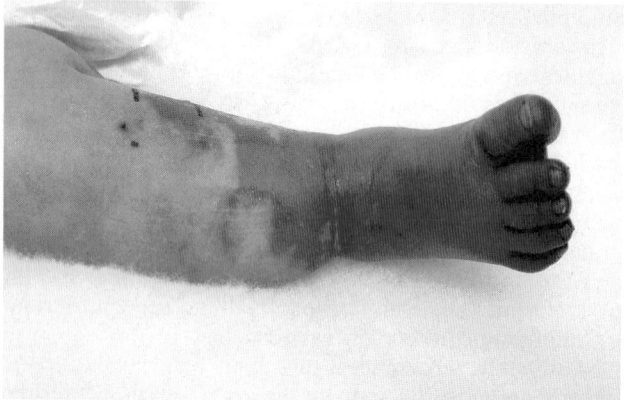

FIGURE 76-3 *(See also Color Plate 34.)* Arterial thrombosis with skin necrosis.

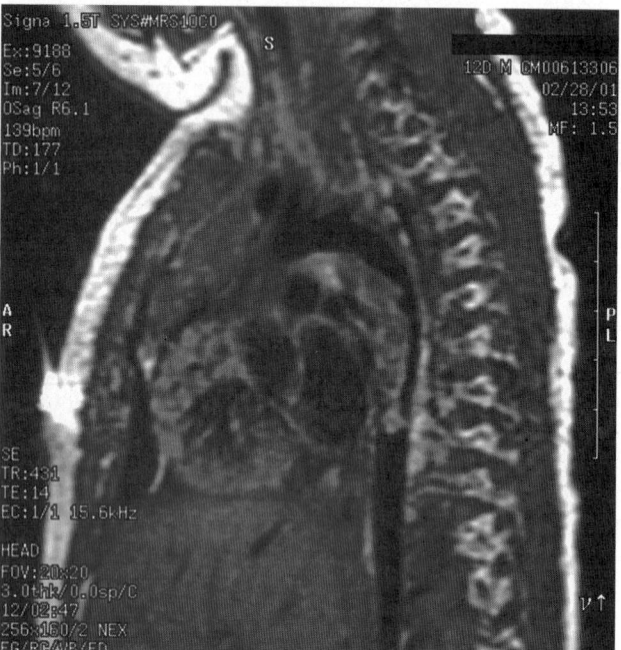

FIGURE 76-4 Aortic thrombus diagnosed by magnetic resonance imaging.

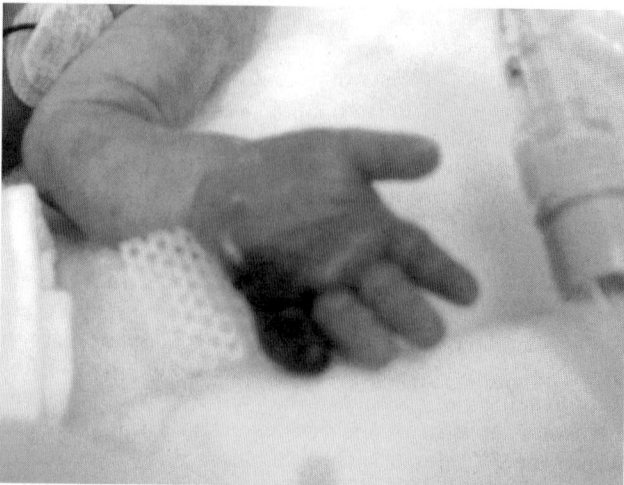

FIGURE 76-5 Arterial thrombosis of digital artery before treatment with tPA. See Figure 76-6.

Diagnosis

The diagnosis is based on demonstrating arterial occlusion by diagnostic imaging. The most commonly used imaging modality is Doppler ultrasonography, which is sensitive for peripheral arteries as well as the femoral and subclavian arteries and the abdominal aorta. The proximal portion of the thoracic aorta can be visualized by echocardiography. Large visceral arteries can also be assessed by ultrasonography. When ultrasonography is not diagnostic, CT/CT angiography or MRI/MR angiography can often demonstrate the thrombus (Figure 76-4). Occasionally, treatment involves catheter-directed thrombolysis (see later discussion), and in such instances, an angiogram is performed before the procedure, which can further define the occlusive lesion.

As in the previous sections, an assessment of the risk factors that led to the thrombosis is crucial only in this instance, the cause is usually obvious because, again, catheterization is nearly always the cause of arterial thrombosis

in neonates. With this in mind, it is difficult to justify a thrombophilia evaluation in this group of patients, with the exception being the rare patient in whom no cause for the thrombosis can be identified.

Treatment

The first and most important aspect of therapy is to remove the arterial catheter if it is still in place. This is in contradistinction to the recommendation for venous catheters and DVT. Second, determining the degree of obstruction and ischemia is crucial, because this will dictate the aggressiveness of the therapeutic approach. For patients in whom perfusion is relatively maintained, simply removing the catheter may be sufficient. For those with more significant perfusion deficits, such as absent pulses and signs of diminished perfusion (pallor, prolonged capillary refill), anticoagulation therapy with unfractionated heparin is recommended. For those with a complete occlusion or with significant ischemia or signs of necrosis, thrombolysis should be attempted so long as there are no contraindications (Raffini, 2009). This can be achieved via systemic infusion or local infusion. The advantages of a systemic infusion are that it does not require an interventional radiologist or other specialist, can be initiated almost immediately, and is often very effective (Figures 76-5 and 76-6). If local thrombolysis is feasible, then this has the advantage of using lower doses and directing the thrombolysis at the thrombus. This results in improved safety due to the lower doses used as well as the potential for more rapid resolution. For systemic thrombolysis with alteplase (tPA)—the only currently available agent studied in neonates—the recommended dose is 0.1 to 0.5 mg/kg/hour with no bolus. Systemic tPA should be administered only under the supervision of a physician (often a hematologist) experienced with the use of this agent, because it carries with it a significant risk for bleeding. This risk is significantly increased in premature infants. In general, tPA is contraindicated in patients who have had recent (approximately 7 days) surgery or other invasive procedures. Some guidelines recommend administering low-dose heparin (10 units/kg/hour) in conjunction with tPA,

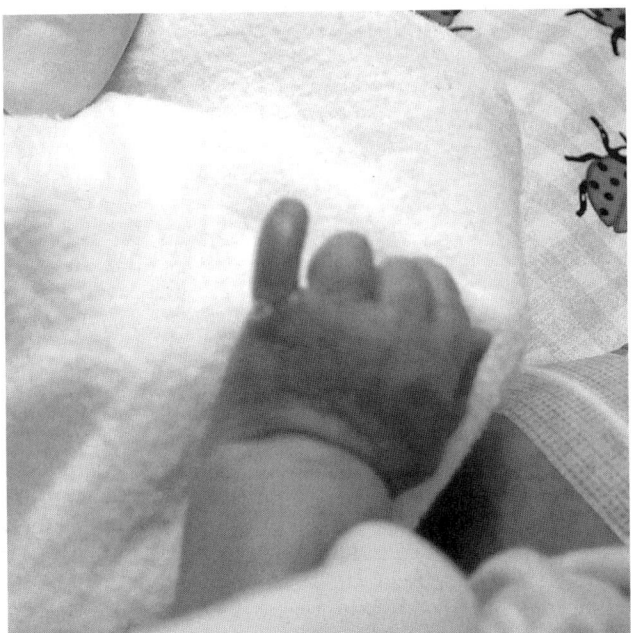

FIGURE 76-6 Arterial thrombosis of digital artery after treatment with tPA.

although the utility of this approach is not clear. Full-dose anticoagulation should not be given in conjunction with tPA.

Once the thrombus resolves and blood flow is restored, anticoagulation is recommended for at least several weeks until the endothelium of the vessel heals. Again, there are no studies supporting such an approach, but it is reasonable from a physiologic point of view. How long to treat depends on the extent and severity of the thrombus, and this decision should be made in conjunction with a pediatric hematologist familiar with neonatal thrombosis. The management of asymptomatic thrombi is unclear. On the one hand, blood flow is probably not normal in that segment, suggesting that the thrombus may worsen; however, because these are incidental findings, it is possible that the thrombus may resolve without any treatment. What is clear, though, is that aggressive therapy is not warranted. Clearly, more research in the management of neonatal arterial (and venous) thrombosis is needed.

Outcomes

The outcome for peripheral arterial thrombosis is fairly straightforward. If tissue perfusion is restored before permanent injury, then the outcome is excellent in general; however, leg length discrepancy can occur if there is a significant enough residual decrease in blood flow to the affected leg. Poor outcomes can range from loss of skin requiring plastic surgery to amputation of digits and even limbs. The long-term outcome of asymptomatic aortic thrombi is unknown. The outcome of visceral artery thrombosis is dependent on survival of the organ. Unilateral renal atrophy due to renal artery thrombosis can result in severe hypertension, which can be difficult to manage.

SUGGESTED READINGS

Andrew M: Developmental hemostasis: relevance to thrombembolic complications in pediatric patients, *Thromb Haemost* 74:415-425, 1995.

Andrew M: The relevance of developmental hemostasis to hemorrhagic disorders of newborns, *Semin Perinatol* 21:70-85, 1997.

Bernard TJ, Goldenberg NA: Pediatric arterial ischemic stroke, *Pediatr Clin North Am* 55:323-338, 2008.

Bussel JB, Sola-Visner M: Current approaches to the evaluation and management of the fetus and neonate with immune thrombocytopenia, *Semin Perinatol* 33:35-42, 2009.

Kenet G, Nowak-Gottl U: Fetal and neonatal thrombophilia, *Obstet Gynecol Clin North Am* 33:457-466, 2006.

Kulkarni R, Ponder KP, James AH, et al: Unresolved issues in the diagnosis and management of inherited bleeding disorders in the perinatal period: a White Paper of the Perinatal Task Force of The Medical and Scientific Advisory Council of the National Hemophilia Foundation, USA, *Haemophilia* 12:205-211, 2006.

Monagle P, Chalmers E, Chan A, et al: Antithrombotic therapy in neonates and children: American College of Chest Physicians Evidence-Based Clinical Practice Guidelines, ed 8, *Chest* 133:887-968, 2008.

Roberts HR, Hoffman M, Monroe DM: A cell-based model of thrombin generation, *Semin Thromb Hemost* 32(Suppl 1):32-38, 2006.

Shearer MJ: Vitamin K deficiency bleeding (VKDB) in early infancy, *Blood Rev* 23:49-59, 2009.

Sola-Visner M, Sallmon H, Brown R: New insights into the mechanisms of nonimmune thrombocytopenia in neonates, *Semin Perinatol* 33:43-51, 2009.

Thornburg C, Pipe S: Neonatal thrombembolic emergencies, *Semin Fetal Neonatal Med* 11:198-206, 2006.

Veldman A, Nold MF, Michel-Benke I: Thrombosis in the critically ill neonate: incidence, diagnosis, and management, *Vasc Health Risk Manag* 4:1337-1348, 2008.

Complete references and supplemental color images used in this text can be found online at www.expertconsult.com

CHAPTER 77

ERYTHROCYTE DISORDERS IN INFANCY

Dana C. Matthews and Bertil Glader

NORMAL ERYTHROCYTE PHYSIOLOGY IN THE FETUS AND NEWBORN

FETAL ERYTHROPOIESIS

Fetal erythropoiesis occurs sequentially during embryonic development in three different sites: yolk sac, liver, and bone marrow (Brugnara and Platt, 2009). The growth factors and cytokines that regulate embryonic hematopoiesis are the subject of active study (Orkin and Zon, 2008), and animal work suggests that they are different from those that regulate proliferation and differentiation of stem cells in later life (Zon, 1995). Yolk sac formation of red blood cells (RBCs) is maximal between 2 and 10 weeks' gestation. Myeloid, or bone marrow, production of RBCs begins around week 18, and by the 30th week of fetal life, bone marrow is the major erythropoietic organ. At birth, almost all RBCs are produced in the bone marrow, although a low level of hepatic erythropoiesis persists through the first few days of life. Sites of fetal erythropoiesis occasionally are reactivated in older patients with hematologic disorders such as myelofibrosis, aplastic anemia, and severe hemolytic anemia.

RBC production in extrauterine life is controlled in part by erythropoietin, a humoral erythropoietic-stimulating factor (ESF) produced by the kidney. The role of erythropoietin in the developing fetus has not been completely defined, but ESF is not thought to influence yolk sac erythropoiesis. It may have a role in hepatic erythropoiesis and may partially regulate RBC production by the bone marrow (Finne and Halvorsen, 1972). ESF is detected in fetal blood and amniotic fluid during the last trimester of pregnancy. The concentration of this hormone increases directly with the period of gestation, and thus, erythropoietin levels in term newborns are significantly higher than in premature infants. This difference may reflect some degree of fetal hypoxia during late intrauterine life. Increased ESF titers also are seen in placental dysfunction, fetal anemia, and maternal hypoxia (Finne, 1966). Fetal RBC formation is not influenced by maternal erythropoietin, because transfusion-induced maternal polycythemia (decreased maternal ESF levels) has no effect on fetal erythropoiesis (Jacobson et al, 1959). Maternal nutritional status also is not a significant factor in the regulation of fetal erythropoiesis, because iron, folate, and vitamin B_{12} are trapped by the fetus irrespective of maternal stores. Most studies have demonstrated that women with severe iron deficiency bear children with normal total body hemoglobin content (Lanzkowsky, 1961). However, a recent study of the correlation between severe maternal iron deficiency anemia and lower cord blood hemoglobin and ferritin levels in cord blood recently reported (Kumar et al, 2008) suggests that placental iron transport mechanisms may not always be adequate in severe maternal iron deficiency.

Hemoglobin, hematocrit, and RBC count increase throughout fetal life (Table 77-1). Extremely large RBCs (mean corpuscular volume [MCV] of 180 fL) with an increased hemoglobin content (mean corpuscular hemoglobin [MCH] of 60 pg/cell) are produced early in fetal life. The size and hemoglobin content of these cells decrease throughout gestation, but the mean corpuscular hemoglobin concentration (MCHC) does not change significantly. Even at birth, the MCV and MCH are greater than those in older children and adults. Many nucleated RBCs and reticulocytes are present early in gestation, and the percentage of these cells also decreases as the fetus ages.

Hemoglobin production increases markedly during the last trimester of pregnancy. The actual hemoglobin concentration increases, but, more important, body weight, blood volume, and total body hemoglobin triple during this period. Fetal iron accumulation parallels the increase in total body hemoglobin content. The neonatal iron endowment at birth, therefore, is directly related to total body hemoglobin content and length of gestation. Term infants have more iron than premature infants.

RBC PHYSIOLOGY AT BIRTH

In utero, the Po_2 in blood delivered to the tissues is only one third to one fourth the value in adults. This relative hypoxia may be responsible for the increased content of erythropoietin and signs of active erythropoiesis (nucleated RBCs, increased reticulocytes) seen in newborns at birth. When lungs become the source of oxygen, hemoglobin-oxygen saturation increases to 95% and erythropoiesis decreases. Within 72 hours, erythropoietin is undetectable, nucleated RBCs disappear, and by 7 days, reticulocytes decrease to less than 1%.

The concentration of hemoglobin during the first few hours of life increases to values greater than those in cord blood. This is both a relative increase caused by a reduction in plasma volume (Gairdner et al, 1958) and an absolute increase caused by placental blood transfusion (Usher et al, 1963). The umbilical vein remains patent long after umbilical arteries have constricted, and thus transfusion of placental blood occurs when newborns are placed at a level below the placenta. The placenta contains approximately 100 mL of fetal blood (30% of the infant's blood volume). Approximately 25% of placental blood enters the newborn within 15 seconds of birth, and by 1 minute, 50% is transfused. The time of cord clamping is thus a direct determinant of neonatal blood volume. The blood volume in term infants (mean of 85 mL/kg) varies considerably (50 to 100 mL/kg) because of different degrees of placental transfusion (Usher et al, 1963). These differences are readily apparent when the effects of early versus delayed cord clamping are compared at 72 hours of age: 82.3 mL/kg (early clamping) versus 92.6 mL/kg (delayed clamping).

TABLE 77-1 Mean Red Blood Cell (RBC) Values During Gestation

Age (wk)	Hb (g/dL)	Hematocrit (%)	RBC (10⁶/mm³)	Mean Corpuscular Volume (fL)	Mean Corpuscular Hb (pg)	Mean Corpuscular Hb Concentration (g/dL)	Nucleated RBCs (% of RBCs)	Reticulocytes (%)	Diameter (μm)
12	8.0–10.0	33	1.5	180	60	34	5.0–8.0	40	10.5
16	10.0	35	2.0	140	45	33	2.0–4.0	10–25	9.5
20	11.0	37	2.5	135	44	33	1.0	10–20	9.0
24	14.0	40	3.5	123	38	31	1.0	5–10	8.8
28	14.5	45	4.0	120	40	31	0.5	5–10	8.7
34	15.0	47	4.4	118	38	32	0.2	3–10	8.5

Data from Oski FA, Naiman JL: *Hematologic problems in the newborn*, ed 3, Philadelphia, 1982, WB Saunders.
Hb, Hemoglobin.

These changes are largely the result of differences in RBC mass (early clamping, 31 mL/kg; delayed clamping, 49 mL/kg). The blood volume in premature infants (89 to 105 mL/kg) is slightly greater than that in term infants, but this difference is due in large part to an increased plasma volume (Usher and Lind, 1965). The RBC mass in premature infants, expressed in milliliters per kilogram, is the same as in term newborns.

FETAL AND NEONATAL HEMOGLOBIN FUNCTION

A variety of hemoglobins are present during fetal and neonatal life (see Hemolysis Due to Hemoglobin Disorders, later). Fetal hemoglobin is the major hemoglobin in utero, whereas hemoglobin A is the normal hemoglobin of extrauterine life. A single RBC may contain both hemoglobin F and hemoglobin A in varying proportions, depending on gestational and postnatal age. One major difference between hemoglobins A and F is related to oxygen transport.

The transport of oxygen to peripheral tissues is regulated by several factors, including blood oxygen capacity, cardiac output, and hemoglobin-oxygen affinity. (1) Oxygen capacity is a direct function of hemoglobin concentration (1 g hemoglobin combines with 1.34 mL oxygen). (2) Compensatory changes in cardiac output can maintain normal oxygen delivery under conditions in which oxygen capacity is significantly reduced. (3) The oxygen affinity of hemoglobin also influences oxygen delivery to tissues. Hemoglobin A is 95% saturated at an arterial Po_2 of 100 mm Hg, but this decreases to 70% to 75% saturation at a venous Po_2 of 40 mm Hg. The difference in O_2 content at arterial and venous oxygen tensions reflects the amount of oxygen that can be released. Changes in hemoglobin affinity for oxygen can influence oxygen delivery (Oski and Delivoria-Papadopoulos, 1970) (Figure 77-1). At any given Po_2, more oxygen is bound to hemoglobin when oxygen affinity is increased. Stated in physiologic terms, increased hemoglobin-oxygen affinity reduces oxygen delivery, whereas decreased hemoglobin-oxygen affinity increases oxygen release to peripheral tissues.

The oxygen affinity of hemoglobin A in solution is greater than that of hemoglobin F. Paradoxically, however,

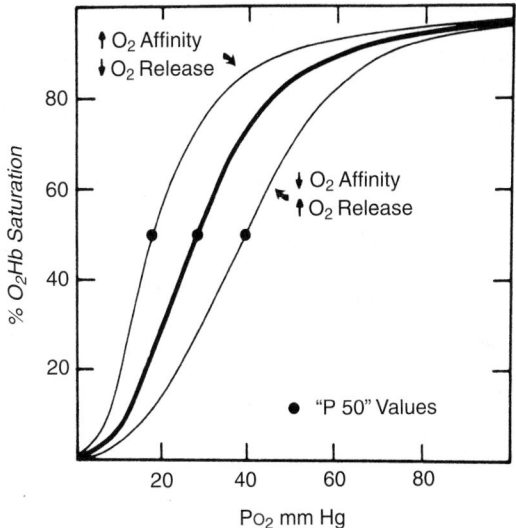

FIGURE 77-1 The oxygen dissociation curve for normal adult hemoglobin (*bold line*). The percent oxygen saturation (ordinate) is plotted for arterial oxygen tensions between 0 and 100 mm Hg (abscissa). As the curve shifts to the right, more oxygen is released at any given Po_2. Conversely, as the curve shifts to the left, more oxygen is retained on hemoglobin at any given Po_2. The "P 50" refers to that Po_2 in which hemoglobin is 50% saturated with oxygen. This term is useful in comparing the oxygen affinities of different hemoglobins. (*From Oski FA, Delivoria-Papadopoulos M: The red cell, 2,3-diphosphoglycerate, and tissue oxygen release*, J Pediatr 77:941-956, 1970.)

whole blood from normal children (hemoglobin A) has a lower oxygen affinity than that of neonatal blood (hemoglobin F) (Allen et al, 1953). This difference is related to an intermediate of RBC metabolism, 2,3-diphosphoglycerate (2,3-DPG). This organic phosphate compound interacts with hemoglobin A to decrease its affinity for oxygen, thereby enhancing O_2 release. Fetal hemoglobin does not interact with 2,3-DPG to any significant extent (Bauer et al, 1968); consequently, cells containing hemoglobin F have a higher oxygen affinity than those containing hemoglobin A. The increased oxygen affinity of fetal RBCs is advantageous for extracting oxygen from maternal blood within the placenta.

A few months after birth, infant blood acquires the same oxygen affinity as that of older children (Figure 77-2). The postnatal decrease in oxygen affinity is due to a reduction in hemoglobin F and an increase in hemoglobin A (which interacts with 2,3-DPG). Oxygen delivery (the difference in arterial and venous O$_2$ content) actually increases while oxygen capacity (hemoglobin concentration) decreases during the 1st week of life (Figure 77-3). This enhanced delivery is largely a reflection of the decreased oxygen affinity of infant blood (Delivoria-Papadopoulos et al, 1971). The oxygen affinity of blood from premature infants is higher than that of term infants, and the normal postnatal changes (decrease in oxygen affinity, increase in oxygen delivery) occur much more gradually in premature infants (see Figure 77-3).

GENERAL APPROACH TO ANEMIC INFANTS

MEDICAL HISTORY AND PHYSICAL EXAMINATION

The cause of anemia frequently can be ascertained by medical history and physical examination. Particular importance is given to family history (anemia, cholelithiasis, unexplained jaundice, splenomegaly), maternal medical history (especially infections), and obstetric history (previous pregnancies, length of gestation, method and difficulty of delivery). The age at which anemia becomes manifest also is of diagnostic importance. Significant anemia at birth is generally due to blood loss or alloimmune hemolysis. After 24 hours, internal hemorrhages and other causes of hemolysis become evident. Anemia that appears several weeks after birth can be caused by a variety of conditions, including abnormalities in the synthesis of hemoglobin beta chains, hypoplastic RBC disorders, and the physiologic anemia of infancy or prematurity.

Infants with anemia resulting from chronic blood loss may appear pale, without other evidence of clinical distress. Acute blood loss can produce hypovolemic shock and a clinical state similar to severe neonatal asphyxia. Newborns with hemolytic anemia frequently show a greater-than-expected degree of icterus. In addition, hemolysis often is associated with hepatosplenomegaly, and in cases resulting from congenital infection, other stigmata may be present.

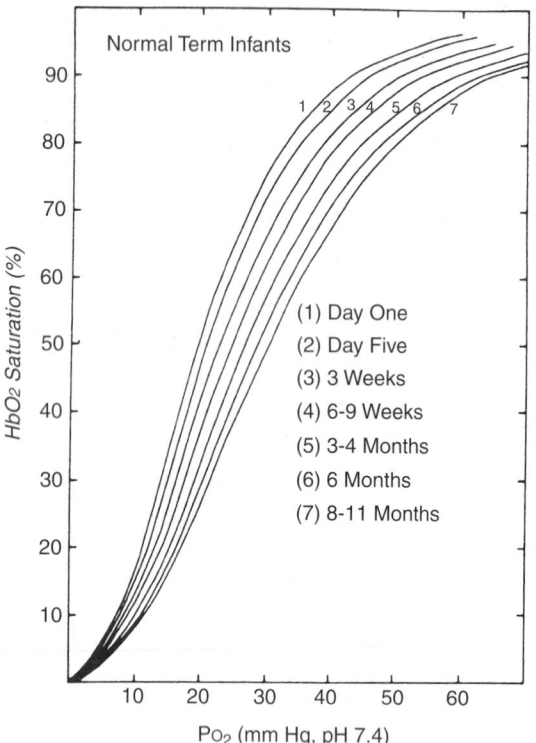

FIGURE 77-2 **The oxygen affinity of blood from term infants at birth and at different postnatal ages.** The gradual rightward shift of the oxygen saturation curve indicates increased oxygen release from hemoglobin as infants get older. This decreased oxygen affinity is due to a decrease in hemoglobin F and an increase in hemoglobin A. *(From Oski FA, Delivoria-Papadopoulos M: The red cell, 2,3-diphosphoglycerate, and tissue oxygen release, J Pediatr 77:941-956, 1970.)*

FIGURE 77-3 Oxygen delivery in normal term and premature infants. Oxygen content (a function of total hemoglobin) is on the ordinate. Oxygen tension is on the abscissa. Oxygen delivery is measured by the difference in oxygen content at arterial (100 mm Hg) and venous (40 mm Hg) oxygen tensions. For both term and premature infants, oxygen delivery *(shaded areas)* increases with age. This occurs despite a decrease in oxygen content. *(From Delivoria-Papadopoulos M, Roncevic NP, Oski FA: Postnatal changes in oxygen transport of term, premature, and sick infants: the role of red cell 2,3-diphosphoglycerate and adult hemoglobin, Pediatr Res 5:235-245, 1971.)*

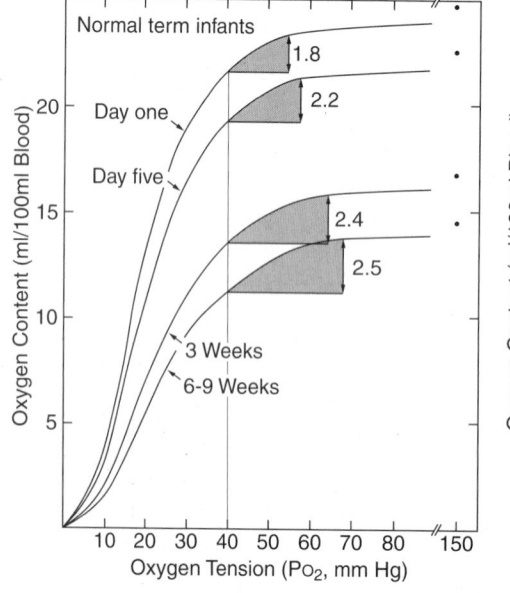

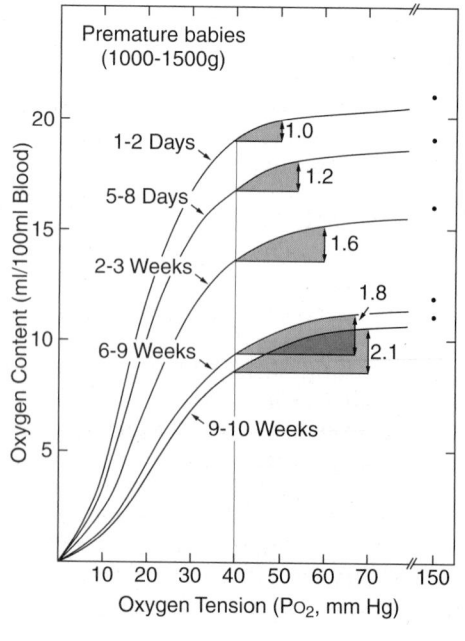

TABLE 77-2 Differential Approach to Anemia in the Newborn Period

Hemoglobin	Reticulocytes	Bilirubin	DAT	Clinical Considerations
Decreased	Normal/decreased	Normal	Negative	Physiologic anemia of infancy and prematurity Hypoplastic anemia
Decreased	Normal/increased	Normal	Negative	Hemorrhagic anemia
Decreased	Normal/increased	Increased	Positive	Immune-mediated hemolysis
Decreased	Normal/increased	Increased	Negative	Acquired or hereditary red blood cell defects Enclosed hemorrhage with resorption of blood DAT-negative ABO incompatibility

DAT, Direct antiglobulin test (previously known as direct Coombs' test).

TABLE 77-3 RBC Values in Term and Premature Infants During the First Week of Life

	Hb (g/100 mL)	Hct (%)	Reticulocytes (%)	Nucleated RBCs (cells/1000 RBCs)
Term				
Cord blood	17.0 (14–20)	53.0 (45–61)	<7	<1.00
Day 1	18.4	58.0	<7	<0.40
Day 3	17.8	55.0	<3	<0.01
Day 7	17.0	54.0	<1	0
Premature (Birthweight <1500 g)				
Cord blood	16.0 (13.0–18.5)	49	<10	<3.00
Day 7	14.8	45	<3	<0.01

Hct, Hematocrit; *Hb,* hemoglobin; *RBCs,* red blood cells.

LABORATORY EVALUATION OF ANEMIA

A simple classification of neonatal anemia based on physical examination and basic laboratory tests is presented in Table 77-2. More extensive RBC testing is discussed elsewhere (de Alarcón et al, 2005).

Red Blood Cell Count, Hemoglobin, Hematocrit, and Red Blood Cell Indices

RBC values during the neonatal period are more variable than at any other time of life. The diagnosis of anemia must therefore be made in terms of "normal" values appropriate for gestational and postnatal ages. The mean cord blood hemoglobin of healthy term infants ranges between 14 and 20 g/100 mL (Table 77-3). Shortly after birth, however, hemoglobin concentration increases. This increase is both relative (owing to a reduction of plasma volume) and absolute (owing to placental RBC transfusion). Failure of hemoglobin to increase during the first few hours of life may be the initial sign of hemorrhagic anemia. RBC values at the end of the 1st week are virtually identical to those seen at birth. Anemia during the 1st week of life is thus defined as any hemoglobin value less than 14 g/100 mL. A significant hemoglobin decrease during this time, although within the normal range, is suggestive of hemorrhage or hemolysis. For example, 14.5 g hemoglobin at 7 days of age is abnormal for a term infant whose hemoglobin was 18.5 g at birth. A slight hemoglobin reduction normally occurs in premature infants during the 1st week of life. Beyond the 1st week, however, the hemoglobin concentration decreases in both term and premature infants (see Physiologic Anemia of Infancy and Prematurity, later).

The electronic equipment used for blood counts also gives statistical information regarding erythrocyte size (MCV) and hemoglobin content (MCH). The normal MCV in older children ranges from 75 to 90 fL. MCV values of less than 75 fL are considered microcytic, whereas those over 100 fL indicate macrocytosis. Normal infant RBCs are large (MCV 105 to 125 fL), and not until 8 to 10 weeks of age does cell size approach that in older children. Neonatal microcytosis is defined as an MCV of less than 95 fL at birth. The RBC hemoglobin content of neonatal cells (MCH 35 to 38 pg/cell) is greater than that seen in older children (MCH 30 to 33 pg/cell). Neonatal hypochromia is defined as an MCH of less than 34 pg/cell. Hypochromia and microcytosis generally occur together, and invariably these abnormalities are due to hemoglobin production defects. Neonatal hypochromic microcytosis is seen with iron deficiency (chronic blood loss) and thalassemia disorders (α- and γ-thalassemias). Both the MCV and MCH are higher in preterm infants as shown in Figure 77-4 (Christensen et al, 2009).

The site from which blood is obtained is important, because hemoglobin and hematocrit are higher in capillary blood than in simultaneously obtained central venous samples (up to 20%). This difference can be minimized by warming an extremity to obtain "arterialized capillary blood" (Oh and Lind, 1966). In the face of acute hemorrhage, however, central venous samples must be obtained because of marked peripheral vasoconstriction.

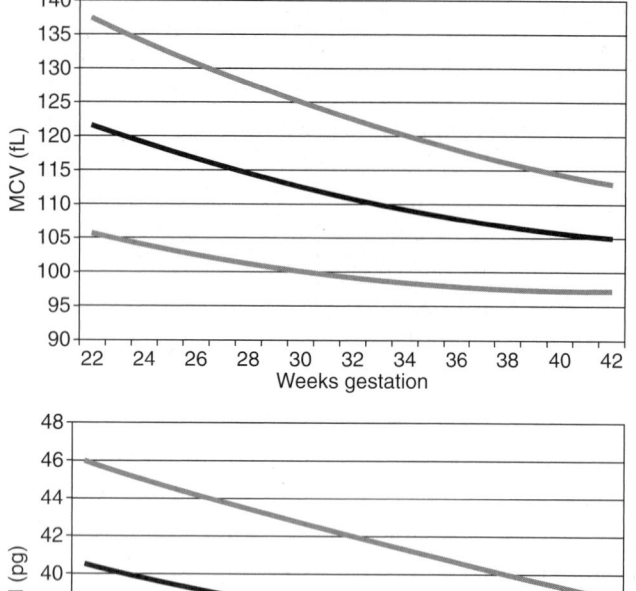

FIGURE 77-4 Reference ranges for MCV *(upper panel)* and MCH *(lower panel)* for neonates on the first day after birth. The lower line shows the 5th percentile values, the middle line shows the mean values, and the upper line shows the 95th percentile values. *From Christensen RD, Henry E, Jopling J, Wiedmeier SE: The CBC: reference ranges for neonates, Semin Perinatol 33:3-11, 2009.*

Reticulocyte Count

The normal reticulocyte count in children and older infants is 1% to 2% of the circulating red cells. The reticulocyte count in term infants ranges between 3% and 7% at birth, but this decreases to less than 1% by 7 days of age (see Table 77-3). In premature infants, reticulocyte values at birth are higher (6% to 10%) and may remain elevated for a longer period of time. Nucleated RBCs are seen in newborn infants, but they generally disappear by the 3rd day of life in term infants and in 7 to 10 days in premature infants. The persistence of reticulocytosis or nucleated RBCs suggests the possibility of hemorrhage or hemolysis. Hypoxia, in the absence of anemia, also can be associated with increased release of reticulocytes and nucleated RBCs.

Peripheral Blood Smear

Examination of the peripheral blood smear is an invaluable aid in the diagnosis of anemia. The smear is evaluated for alterations in the size and shape of RBCs as well as abnormalities in leukocytes and platelets. Erythrocytes of older children are approximately the size of a small lymphocyte nucleus, whereas those of newborns are slightly larger. RBC hemoglobinization (e.g., hypochromia) is estimated by observing the area of central pallor, which is one third

the diameter of normal RBCs and more than one half the diameter of hypochromic cells. Spherocytes are detected by the complete absence of central pallor. The degree of reticulocytosis can be estimated, because these cells are larger and have a bluish coloration.

Direct Antiglobulin Test

Most cases of neonatal hemolytic anemia are due to isoimmunization. The direct antiglobulin test (DAT), previously known as the direct Coombs' test, detects the presence of antibody on RBCs The indirect antiglobulin test, previously known as indirect Coombs' test, detects anti-RBC antibodies in the plasma.

BLOOD TRANSFUSIONS IN THE TREATMENT OF ANEMIA

A hemoglobin of 14 g/100 mL corresponds to an RBC mass of 31 mL/kg. Thus, an RBC transfusion of 2 mL/kg will increase the hemoglobin concentration by approximately 1 g/100 mL. Packed RBCs (hematocrit approximately 67%) contain 2 mL of RBCs/3 mL of packed RBCs. Whole blood (hematocrit approximately 33%) contains 2 mL of RBCs/6 mL whole blood. Thus, the transfusion of 3 mL of packed RBCs/kg or 6 mL of whole blood/kg increases hemoglobin concentration by approximately 1 g/100 mL.

Packed RBCs are the product of choice when transfusion is necessary for simple anemia, as occurs in hemolysis. If anemia is accompanied by hypovolemia from acute blood loss, volume expansion must be achieved promptly, using either whole blood, or packed RBCs and normal saline or a colloid such as 5% serum albumin (infused separately). Because of the reduced availability of whole blood, owing to the demand for its components, in most medical centers the usual choice is packed RBCs and crystalloid or colloid. The previously common practice of reconstituting RBCs with fresh frozen plasma to make "whole blood" is no longer acceptable, because the increased donor exposure increases the risk of transmitting infectious disease. When packed RBCs need to be diluted to facilitate nonurgent transfusion, isotonic saline is the preferred diluent. If exchange transfusion is needed to treat hyperbilirubinemia, the capability of albumin to improve bilirubin binding and removal is ample reason to request whole blood. Although fresh blood less than 2 days old is ideal because there is a reduced risk of hyperkalemia, this is not usually available. An acceptable substitute is packed RBCs less than 4 to 5 days old. These packed RBCs provide adequate oxygen delivery; hyperkalemia can be prevented by washing the RBCs once in saline and then reconstituting with normal saline. Washing is not required for the usually small, simple transfusions of packed RBCs, because the small volume of plasma minimizes any toxic effect of increased concentration of potassium in the plasma.

Blood currently available in most blood banks is anticoagulated with citrate-phosphate-dextrose (CPD), CPD-adenine (CPDA-1), or adenine-saline (AS-3), with a shelf life of 21, 35, or 42 days, respectively. Hematocrit usually ranges between 65% and 80% for packed RBCs. Near-normal 2,3-DPG levels are maintained for up to 12 to 14 days, which is advantageous in transfusing infants with acute hypoxia or those receiving large volumes of blood. Hematocrits range from 55% to 65%, thus facilitating flow during infusion. The newest of these preparations, AS-3, is well tolerated by newborns even after up to 42 days of storage, so long as only small-volume transfusions are given at any one time (Strauss, 2000). Designation of a single AS-3–preserved red cell donation for use by one neonate is an effective way to limit donor exposures and reduce the risk of transfusion-associated infections (Goldman, 2001).

Preterm infants born weighing less than 1250 g are uniquely susceptible to potentially serious cytomegalovirus (CMV) infection from transfused blood, particularly if they lack immunity because their mothers are seronegative. CMV infection can be prevented by using blood products only from seronegative donors (Yeager et al, 1981). Because approximately 40% to 60% of adults are seropositive, this limits the availability of seronegative donors. Reserving seronegative blood for the minority of infants who are seronegative can reduce the demand for such donors. Alternatively, because CMV resides mainly in leukocytes, removal of such cells also can prevent transmission of the virus, and the use of high-efficiency leukocyte depletion filters (Gilbert et al, 1989) has proven effective. A potential disadvantage of using CMV-seronegative blood in CMV-positive infants receiving large amounts of blood is dilution of infant's antibody level, resulting in increased susceptibility to nursery-acquired CMV infection. Currently, a majority of neonatal services utilize leukocyte-reduced red cell products rather than relying on CMV-negative products to prevent CMV infection (Engelfreit and Reesink, 2001).

Graft-versus-host (GVH) reaction rarely follows transfusion and occurs mainly in certain newborns at risk. For this to occur, viable lymphocytes in cellular blood products must be able to engraft and react against foreign antigens on tissues of the recipient. Infants at risk include those with congenital or acquired defects of cellular immunity, those who as fetuses received intrauterine transfusion of RBCs or platelets, newborns receiving exchange transfusion following intrauterine transfusion (Naiman et al, 1969; Parkman et al, 1974), and infants receiving directed blood donations from first-degree relatives (whose genetic similarity may increase the likelihood of engraftment). Irradiation of RBCs, whole blood, platelets, and granulocytes with a minimum of 1500 rads has proved effective in preventing GVH reaction. Reports of GVH reaction after RBC transfusion in very premature infants without known risk factors (Enoki et al, 1985; Sanders et al, 1989) have prompted most neonatal services to irradiate all RBC blood products (Engelfreit and Reesink, 2001).

HEMORRHAGIC ANEMIA

Anemia frequently follows fetal blood loss, bleeding from obstetric complications, and internal hemorrhages associated with birth trauma (Box 77-1). Iatrogenic anemia due to repeated removal of blood for laboratory testing is common in premature infants. The clinical presentation of anemia depends on the magnitude and acuteness of blood loss.

Infants with anemia subsequent to moderate hemorrhage or chronic blood loss are generally asymptomatic.

BOX 77-1   Causes of Hemorrhagic Anemia in Newborns

FETAL HEMORRHAGE

Spontaneous fetomaternal hemorrhage
Hemorrhage following amniocentesis
Twin-twin transfusion
Nuchal cord

PLACENTAL HEMORRHAGE

Placenta previa
Abruptio placentae
Multilobed placenta (vasa previa)
Velamentous insertion of cord
Placental incision during cesarean section

UMBILICAL CORD BLEEDING

Rupture of umbilical cord with precipitous delivery
Rupture of short or entangled cord

POSTPARTUM NEONATAL HEMORRHAGE

Bleeding from umbilicus
Cephalhematomas, scalp hemorrhages
Hepatic rupture, splenic rupture
Retroperitoneal hemorrhages

The only physical finding is pallor of the skin and mucous membranes. Laboratory studies can range from a mild normochromic normocytic anemia (hemoglobin 9 to 12 g/100 mL) to a more severe hypochromic microcytic anemia (hemoglobin 5 to 7 g/100 mL). The only therapy required for asymptomatic children is iron (2 mg elemental iron/kg three times a day for 3 months). RBC replacement is indicated only if there is evidence of clinical distress (tachycardia, tachypnea, irritability, feeding difficulties). In most cases, increasing the hemoglobin to 10 to 12 g/100 mL removes all signs and symptoms associated with anemia. Because severely anemic infants are frequently in incipient heart failure, however, these children should be transfused very slowly (2 mL/kg/hour). If signs of congestive heart failure appear, a rapid-acting diuretic (furosemide, 1 mg/kg intravenously) should be given before proceeding with the transfusion. An alternative approach is to administer a partial exchange transfusion with packed RBCs to severely anemic infants. This approach increases the hemoglobin concentration without the danger of increasing blood volume and precipitating congestive heart failure.

Infants who rapidly lose large volumes of blood appear to be in acute distress (pallor, tachycardia, tachypnea, weak pulses, hypotension, and shock). This presentation is distinct from that seen in neonatal respiratory asphyxia (slow respirations with intercostal retractions, bradycardia, and pallor with cyanosis) (Table 77-4). Infants with respiratory problems demonstrate a marked improvement with assisted ventilation and oxygen, whereas there is little change in anemic newborns. Cyanosis is not a feature of severe anemia because the hemoglobin concentration is too low (for clinical cyanosis to be apparent, there must be at least 5 g/100 mL of deoxygenated hemoglobin). The hemoglobin concentration immediately after an acute hemorrhage may be normal, and a decreased hemoglobin may not be seen until the plasma volume has reexpanded several hours later. Thus, the diagnosis of acute hemorrhagic anemia is based

TABLE 77-4 Comparative Clinical Findings in Neonatal Asphyxia and Acute Hemorrhage

	Neonatal Asphyxia	Acute Blood Loss
Heart rate	Decreased	Increased
Respiratory rate	Decreased	Increased
Intercostal retractions	Present	Absent
Skin color	Pallor with cyanosis	Pallor without cyanosis
Response to oxygen and assisted ventilation	Marked improvement	No significant change

largely on physical findings and evidence of blood loss. It is important to recognize these clinical features because immediate therapy is required. Treatment is directed at rapid expansion of the vascular space (20 mL fluid/kg) by rapid infusion of either isotonic saline or 5% albumin, followed by either type-specific, cross-matched whole blood or packed RBCs resuspended with saline, depending on availability. In infants in whom anemia and hypoxia are severe, non-cross-matched group O, Rh-negative RBCs are an acceptable alternative to cross-matched RBCs. Infants with hypovolemic shock caused by acute external blood loss usually show marked clinical improvement after this treatment. A poor response is seen in newborns with severe internal hemorrhage.

FETAL HEMORRHAGE

Fetomaternal Hemorrhage

Significant bleeding into the maternal circulation occurs in approximately 8% of all pregnancies and thus represents one of the most common forms of fetal bleeding. Small amounts of fetal blood are lost in most cases, but in 1% of pregnancies, fetal blood loss may exceed 40 mL (Cohen et al, 1964). Fetomaternal hemorrhage occasionally follows amniocentesis and placental injury (Zipursky et al, 1963), although anemia is seen only after unsuccessful amniocentesis or when there is evidence of a bloody tap (Woo Wang et al, 1967). For this reason, infants born to mothers who have had amniocentesis should be observed closely for signs of anemia. The effects of anemia resulting from fetomaternal hemorrhage are variable. Large acute hemorrhages can produce hypovolemic shock, whereas slower, more chronic blood loss results in hypochromic microcytic anemia resulting from iron deficiency. Some newborns with severe chronic fetal anemia (hemoglobin levels as low as 4 to 6 g/100 mL) may have minimal symptoms.

An examination of maternal blood for the presence of fetal cells is necessary in any infant with suspected fetomaternal hemorrhage. Two techniques are available. The Kleihauer-Betke preparation involves examination of a stained specimen of maternal blood by microscopy following differential elution of hemoglobin A but not hemoglobin F from the red cells. Alternative, flow cytometry–based techniques are probably more accurate but are less widely available. These approaches use antibodies against fetal hemoglobin (sometimes combined with antibodies against carbonic anhydrase) or against the D antigen to distinguish fetal RBCs from adult cells (Little et al, 2005; Porra et al, 2007; Savithrisowmya et al, 2008).

Approximately 50 mL of fetal blood must be lost to produce significant neonatal anemia. This volume is greater than 1% of the maternal blood volume, and therefore fetal cells within the maternal circulation may be detected readily. Tests that depend on the presence of fetal hemoglobin are not valid when a maternal hemoglobinopathy with increased hemoglobin F levels coexists. In addition, fetomaternal ABO incompatibility may cause rapid removal of fetal RBCs, thus obscuring any significant hemorrhage. For this reason, it is important to examine maternal blood as soon as anemia from fetal hemorrhage is suspected.

TWIN-TWIN TRANSFUSION

Transfusion of blood from one monozygous twin to another can result in anemia in the donor twin and polycythemia in the recipient. Significant hemorrhage is seen only in monochorionic monozygous twins (approximately 70% of all monozygous twins). The most common form, chronic twin-to-twin transfusion (TTTS), is seen in 10% to 15% of monochorionic pregnancies (Huber and Hecher, 2004; Lopriore and Oepkes, 2008). Bleeding occurs because of vascular anastomosis in monochorionic placentas. The anemic donor twin is usually smaller than the polycythemic recipient, with a greater than 20% difference in birthweight. Polyhydramnios is frequently seen in the recipient twin and oligohydramnios is seen in the donor, and current diagnostic criteria for chronic TTTS include the demonstration by prenatal ultrasound of the twin oligopolyhydramnios sequence (TOPS). The high rate of intrauterine mortality (approximately 63% with conservative management) has spurred attempts at fetal therapy, including decompression amniocentesis, laser coagulation of vascular anastomoses, interfetal septal disruptions, and selective feticide (Seng and Rajadurai, 2000; van Gemert et al, 2001). A prospective randomized trial demonstrated that fetoscopic laser surgery had better overall survival (57%) as compared to serial amnioreduction (41%) (Senat et al, 2004). Many centers are now achieving survival rates of at least 70%, but residual vascular anastomoses can still result in polycythemia-hyperviscosity syndrome in the recipient and chronic anemia in the donor (Lopriore and Oepkes, 2008). Twin-twin transfusions should be suspected when the hemoglobin concentration of identical twins differs by more than 5 g/100 mL. However, such a difference in hemoglobin concentration does not prove there has been a twin-twin transfusion, because such a hemoglobin difference has been observed in some dichorionic twins, in whom there are no vascular anastomoses and therefore no possibility for twin-twin transfusion (Danskin and Neilson, 1989).

PLACENTAL BLOOD LOSS

Placental bleeding during pregnancy is common, but in most cases hemorrhage is from the maternal aspect of the placenta. In placenta previa, however, the thinness of the placenta overlying the cervical os frequently results in fetal blood loss. The vascular communications between multi-lobular placental lobes also are very fragile and are easily subjected to trauma during delivery. Vasa previa is the condition in which one of these connecting vessels overlies the cervical os and thus is prone to rupture during delivery. Abruptio placentae generally causes fetal anoxia and death, although some infants survive but can be severely anemic. Bleeding also follows inadvertent placental incision during cesarean section (Montague and Krevans, 1966), and thus the placenta should be inspected for injury following all cesarean sections.

UMBILICAL CORD BLEEDING

The normal umbilical cord is resistant to minor trauma and does not bleed. The umbilical cord of dysmature infants, however, is weak and thus vulnerable to rupture and hemorrhage (Raye et al, 1970). In cases of precipitous delivery, a rapid increase in cord tension can rupture the fetal aspect of the cord, causing serious acute blood loss. Short or entangled umbilical cords and abnormalities of umbilical blood vessels (velamentous insertions into the placenta) are also vulnerable to rupture and hemorrhage. Bleeding from injured umbilical cords is rapid but generally ceases after a short period of time, owing to arterial constriction. The umbilical cord should always be inspected for abnormalities or signs of injury, particularly after unattended, precipitous deliveries.

HEMORRHAGE AFTER DELIVERY

Hemorrhagic anemia due to internal bleeding is occasionally associated with birth trauma. Characteristically, internal hemorrhages are asymptomatic during the first 24 to 48 hours of life, with signs and symptoms of anemia developing after this time. Cephalhematomas can be sufficiently large to cause anemia and hyperbilirubinemia, secondary to the resorption of blood. Subgaleal hemorrhages are seen infrequently, sometimes occurring after vacuum extraction is used during delivery. In contrast to cephalhematomas, subgaleal bleeding can be extensive because hemorrhage is not limited by the periosteum. Adrenal and kidney hemorrhages occasionally follow difficult breech deliveries. Splenic rupture and hemorrhage occur most commonly in association with splenomegaly, as in erythroblastosis fetalis. Hepatic hemorrhages are generally subcapsular and may be asymptomatic. Rupture of the hepatic capsule results in hemoperitoneum and hypovolemic shock. Hepatic hemorrhages are suspected when a previously healthy infant goes into shock with clinical manifestations of an increasing right upper quadrant abdominal mass, shifting dullness on percussion, and evidence of free fluid on abdominal radiographs. In contrast with newborns with acute blood loss from fetomaternal or umbilical vessel bleeding, infants with hepatic hemorrhage generally demonstrate a poor clinical response to blood replacement.

HEMOLYTIC ANEMIA

RBCs from children and adults normally circulate for 100 to 120 days. Erythrocyte survival in newborns is somewhat shorter: 70 to 90 days in term infants, 50 to 80 days

> **BOX 77-2** Causes of Hemolytic Anemia During the Newborn Period
>
> **IMMUNE DISORDERS**
> Isoimmune: Rh and ABO incompatibility
> Maternal immune disease: autoimmune hemolytic anemia, systemic lupus erythematosus
> Drug-induced: penicillin
>
> **ACQUIRED RED BLOOD CELL (RBC) DISORDERS**
> Infection: cytomegalovirus, toxoplasmosis, syphilis, bacterial sepsis
> Disseminated and localized intravascular coagulation, respiratory distress syndrome
>
> **HEREDITARY RBC DISORDERS**
> Membrane defects: hereditary spherocytosis, hereditary elliptocytosis
> Enzyme abnormalities: glucose-6-phosphate dehydrogenase, pyruvate kinase
> Hemoglobinopathies: α-thalassemia syndromes, γ/β-thalassemia

in premature infants (Pearson, 1967). Hemolytic anemia, which further shortens RBC survival, may arise for many reasons (Box 77-2). Red cell destruction can occur by macrophage recognition of abnormal RBC membrane properties (extravascular hemolysis) or, alternatively, RBC destruction can occur by direct damage of the RBC in the circulation with the resultant release of hemoglobin (intravascular hemolysis). In most cases some degree of both types of hemolysis occurs.

In older infants and children, the usual response to increased RBC destruction is enhanced erythropoiesis, and there may be little or no anemia if the rate of production matches the accelerated rate of destruction. In these cases of well-compensated hemolysis, the major manifestations are due to increased erythrocyte destruction (hyperbilirubinemia) and augmented erythropoiesis (reticulocytosis). During the early neonatal period, however, the increased oxygen-carrying capacity of blood (see Physiologic Anemia of Infancy and Prematurity, later) may blunt any compensatory erythropoietic activity in cases of mild hemolysis. Consequently, hyperbilirubinemia in excess of normal neonatal levels may be the only apparent manifestation of hemolysis. In most cases of significant hemolysis, however, some degree of reticulocytosis is usually present.

IMMUNE HEMOLYSIS

Placental transfer of maternal antibodies directed against fetal RBC antigens is the most common cause of neonatal hemolysis. This phenomenon is a consequence of maternal sensitization to fetal RBC antigens inherited from the father. Hemolysis occurs only in the fetus. The spectrum of clinical problems ranges from minimal anemia and hyperbilirubinemia to severe anemia with hydrops fetalis. At one time, before effective prevention of Rh sensitization was available, hemolytic disease of the newborn was responsible for more than 10,000 deaths annually in the United States (Freda et al, 1975). Since the development of immunoprophylaxis against Rh(D) sensitization, the overall incidence of alloimmune hemolysis has decreased dramatically in developed countries of the world (Figure 77-5).

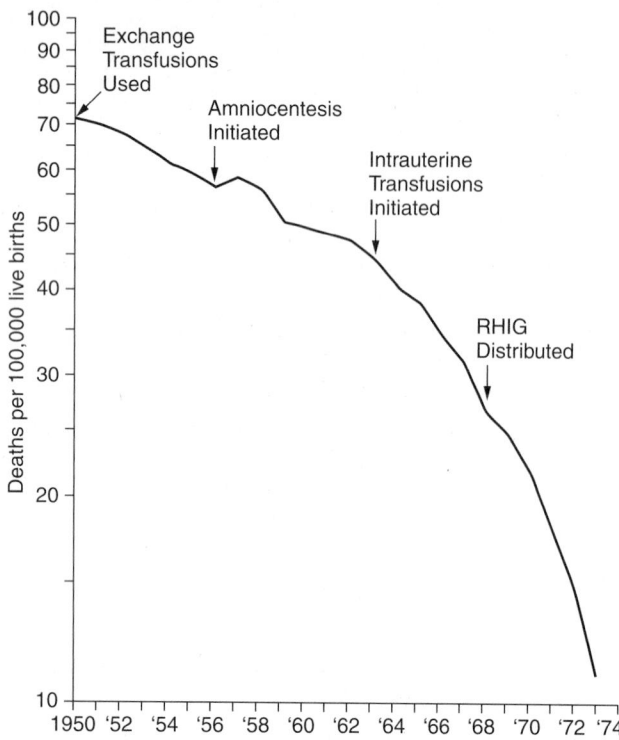

FIGURE 77-5 Infant death rates from hemolytic disease of the newborn, United States, 1950 to 1973. *(From Centers for Disease Control:* Rh hemolytic disease surveillance annual report, *Atlanta, Ga., June 1975.)*

Nevertheless, Rh incompatibility still occurs in areas where immune prophylaxis is not readily available. In the United States, most cases of alloimmune hemolysis are due to ABO maternal-fetal incompatibility with a smaller fraction resulting from sensitization to Kell, Duffy, Kidd, and other Rh antigens such as c and E.

Rh Hemolytic Disease: Erythroblastosis Fetalis

The role of Rh antibody in classic erythroblastosis fetalis was first elucidated by Levine and Katzen in 1941 (Levine et al, 1941). Several Rh antigens are recognized, each of which is detected by specific antibodies. It is known that Rh blood group antigens are determined by at least two homologous but distinct membrane-associated proteins. Two of these membrane proteins have separate isoforms (C and c; E and e), which are detected by specific antibodies (anti-C and anti-c; anti-E and anti-e). The most important of the membrane Rh proteins is the D antigen. Rh-positive RBCs are those that possess this antigen. A lowercase d is used to denote the absence of D, or Rh-negative status; it is not related to a specific antigen—no "anti-d" serum has been identified. Rh proteins are encoded by two separate genes located on chromosome 1; they are designated *RHCE* and *RHD* (Mouro et al, 1993). The *RHCE* gene encodes both the C/c and E/e proteins. The *RHD* gene encodes the Rh D proteins. The Rh-negative phenotype results from deletion of the *RHD* gene on both chromosomes. In most cases, the Rh-negative phenotype also is associated with Rh c and Rh e (i.e., Rh cde). The frequency of Rh negativity varies in different racial groups. It is high

in whites (15%), lower in blacks (5%), and virtually non-existent in Asians. The Rh-positive phenotype may result from homozygosity (DD) or heterozygosity (Dd) for the D antigen. In Rh-positive whites, approximately 44% are homozygous (DD) and 56% are heterozygous (Dd). Knowledge of differences in *RHD* genotype is important because approximately 25% of fetuses of couples with an Rh(D)-negative mother and an Rh(D)-positive father will be Rh(D)-negative.

Current understanding of the natural history of Rh sensitization is derived largely from clinical experience gained before the immunologic prevention of neonatal hemolysis was readily available. The pathophysiology of alloimmune hemolysis resulting from Rh incompatibility includes the following: an Rh-negative mother, an Rh-positive fetus, leakage of fetal RBCs into maternal circulation, maternal sensitization to D antigen on fetal RBCs, production and transplacental passage of maternal anti-D antibodies into fetal circulation, attachment of maternal antibodies to Rh-positive fetal RBCs, and destruction of antibody-coated fetal RBCs. Historically, Rh hemolytic disease was rare (occurring in 1% of cases) during the first pregnancy involving an Rh-positive fetus but increased significantly with each subsequent pregnancy. Small volumes of fetal RBCs enter the maternal circulation throughout gestation, although the major fetomaternal bleeding responsible for sensitization occurs during delivery (Zipursky et al, 1963). Once sensitization has occurred, reexposure to Rh(D) RBCs in subsequent pregnancies leads to an anamnestic response, with an increase in the maternal anti-D titer. Currently, significant hemolysis occurring in the first pregnancy indicates prior maternal exposure to Rh-positive RBCs, a consequence of fetal bleeding associated with a previous spontaneous or therapeutic abortion, ectopic pregnancy, or a variety of different prenatal procedures. On occasion the sensitization may be a consequence of an earlier transfusion in which Rh-positive RBCs were administered by mistake or in which some other blood component (e.g., platelets) containing Rh(D) RBCs was transfused.

The major factor responsible for the reduced death rate is the development of Rh immune globulin to prevent maternal sensitization. Important early observations were that fetomaternal RBC transfer (and thereby sensitization) occurs primarily during delivery and that the frequency of Rh immune hemolytic disease was much lower in ABO-incompatible pregnancies (maternal RBC type O, fetal RBC type A or B). The apparent beneficial effect of ABO incompatibility is due to the fact that maternal anti-A and anti-B antibodies recognize the corresponding A and B fetal RBCs, leading to their destruction before sensitization can occur. The practice of administering a single intramuscular dose of Rh immune globulin (300 μg) to unsensitized Rh-negative mothers within 72 hours of delivering an Rh-positive infant led to the virtual elimination of Rh(D) sensitization as a major cause of hemolytic disease in newborns (Freda et al, 1975). The few treatment failures seen were attributed to fetomaternal bleeding of greater than 30 mL at delivery or bleeding that occurred antenatally. This led to the current standard of practice of administering a full dose of Rh immune globulin to all unsensitized Rh-negative women at 28 weeks' gestation, with an additional dose given at birth if the infant is Rh-positive. Moreover, the dose of Rh immune globulin should be increased proportionately when there is evidence of larger-than-normal fetomaternal bleeding at delivery. All women should be screened at the time of delivery using the rosette test to screen for fetal red cells (Brecher, 2002). Positive results should be followed by a quantitative test such as the Kleihauer-Betke test (Judd, 2001). In suspicious cases (e.g., with placental abruption or neonatal anemia), the volume of fetal hemorrhage can be quantified using the Kleihauer-Betke procedure. Rh immune globulin also should be administered to unsensitized Rh-negative women after any event known to be associated with increased risk of fetomaternal hemorrhage (e.g., spontaneous or therapeutic abortion, amniocentesis, chorionic villus biopsy). The risk of anti-Rh desensitization ranges from 0.6% to 5.4% when nonsensitized Rh-negative women undergo amniocentesis (Spinnato, 1992). Despite the use of antenatal and postnatal prophylaxis with Rh immune globulin, 0.1% to 0.3% of Rh-negative women with Rh-positive pregnancies develop Rh sensitization (Engelfriet et al, 2003; Koelewijn et al, 2008). A recent case-control study (Koelewijn et al, 2009) demonstrated several independent risk factors for sensitization, including nonspontaneous delivery (i.e., caesarean section or assisted vaginal delivery), pregnancy-related red cell transfusion, postmaturity (>42 weeks' gestation), and younger age at first delivery. However, in almost half of the failures, none of these risk factors could be identified.

In pregnant Rh-negative women previously sensitized to Rh(D), the transplacental passage of maternal anti-D leads to a positive DAT on Rh(D) fetal RBCs. Depending on the amount of anti-D absorbed, a variable degree of fetal hemolysis occurs, thereby leading to anemia, hepatosplenomegaly, and increased bilirubin formation. In utero, bilirubin is removed by transfer across the placenta into the maternal circulation; therefore, hyperbilirubinemia is not a problem until after delivery, when levels may increase because of immaturity of hepatic conjugating enzymes. The major threat to the fetus is severe anemia leading to hydrops fetalis and intrauterine death. The clinical severity of neonatal hemolytic disease varies.

Mild hemolytic disease is most common, manifested by a positive DAT with minimal hemolysis, little or no anemia (cord blood hemoglobin greater than 14 g/dL), and minimal hyperbilirubinemia (cord blood bilirubin less than 4 mg/dL). Aside from early phototherapy, these newborns generally require no therapy unless the postnatal rate of rise in bilirubin is greater than expected. Infants who do not become sufficiently jaundiced to require exchange transfusion are at risk of development of severe late anemia associated with a low reticulocyte count, usually at 3 to 6 weeks of age; thus, it is important to closely monitor hemoglobin levels after hospital discharge.

Moderate hemolytic disease is found in a smaller fraction of affected infants. This form is characterized by hemolysis, moderate anemia (cord blood hemoglobin less than 14 g/dL), and increased cord blood bilirubin levels (greater than 4 mg/dL). The peripheral blood may reveal numerous nucleated RBCs, decreased numbers of platelets, and occasionally a leukemoid reaction with large numbers of immature granulocytes. Infants with Rh disease also may exhibit marked hepatosplenomegaly, a consequence of

extramedullary hematopoiesis and sequestration of antibody-coated RBCs. The risk of development of bilirubin encephalopathy is high if these neonates do not receive treatment. Thus, early exchange transfusion with type O Rh-negative fresh RBCs (less than 5 days old) is usually necessary, in conjunction with intensive phototherapy. This approach has been responsible for the favorable outcome for most infants with moderate alloimmune hemolysis. It is common for newborns who receive exchange transfusion to demonstrate a lower-than-normal hemoglobin concentration at the nadir of their "physiologic" anemia. Therefore, follow-up evaluation of hemoglobin for at least 2 months is important. The decrease in hemoglobin may be due in part to persistence of some anti-D antibody and destruction of the patient's own Rh(D)-positive RBCs. Also, this low hemoglobin measurement may reflect the decreased oxygen affinity and enhanced oxygen delivery of adult RBCs used for the exchange process, thereby blunting the expected erythropoietic response to hypoxia. Some studies suggest that the administration of recombinant human erythropoietin (rHuEPO) may minimize this late anemia of Rh hemolytic disease (Ovali et al, 1996; Scaradavou et al, 1993), although it is not always effective (Pessler and Hart, 2002).

Severe hemolytic disease is seen in approximately 25% of affected infants, who are either stillborn or hydropic at birth. Understanding of hydrops fetalis, originally attributed to high-output cardiac failure secondary to severe anemia, is incomplete. Two other consequences of anemia also may contribute to the edema of hydrops. One of these is low colloid osmotic pressure resulting from hypoalbuminemia, a consequence of hepatic dysfunction. The second is a capillary leak syndrome secondary to tissue hypoxia. Management of seriously affected fetuses is directed at the prevention of severe anemia and death. To accomplish this, it first is necessary to identify those fetuses at risk. An increase in the maternal anti-D titer in a previously sensitized Rh-negative woman is a good serologic measure of a fetus in potential jeopardy. Moreover, a previous history of neonatal hemolytic disease resulting from anti-D antibodies suggests that the current fetus also may be at risk. In this regard it may be useful to know the fetal Rh blood type because this identifies those Rh-negative infants who are not at risk. In many cases this can be accomplished by direct Rh typing of fetal RBCs obtained via cordocentesis. Alternatively, molecular biologic techniques can be used to determine the Rh genotype in DNA obtained from amniocytes or chorionic villus samples (Bennett et al, 1993; Fisk et al, 1994). Recently, methods have been developed to perform such analysis of free fetal DNA in maternal blood (Daniels et al, 2009). When the fetus is found to be Rh-negative, no further maternal monitoring or fetal blood studies are necessary.

An increase in the maternal titer of immunoglobulin G (IgG) anti-D indicates maternal sensitization but does not accurately predict the potential severity of fetal hemolysis. Previously, when the indirect antiglobulin test exceeded a critical threshold level (1:16 to 1:32), amniocentesis was done to perform spectrophotometric estimation of bile pigment in amniotic fluid as measured by the deviation in optical density (OD) at 450 nm. Plotting the "ΔOD_{450nm}" against fetal age provided a good correlation with the

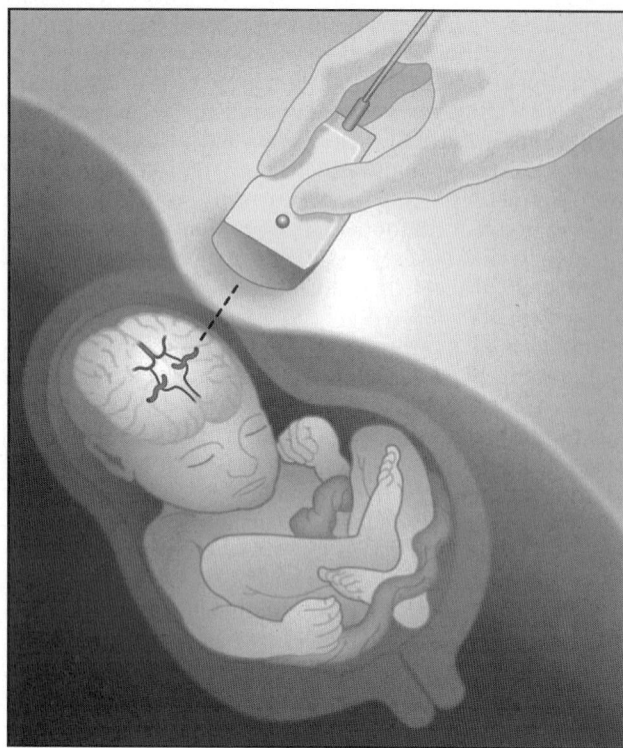

FIGURE 77-6 Obtaining a middle cerebral artery Doppler peak systolic velocity. *(From Moise KJ: Management of Rhesus alloimmunization in pregnancy,* Obstet Gynecol *112:164-176, 2008b.)*

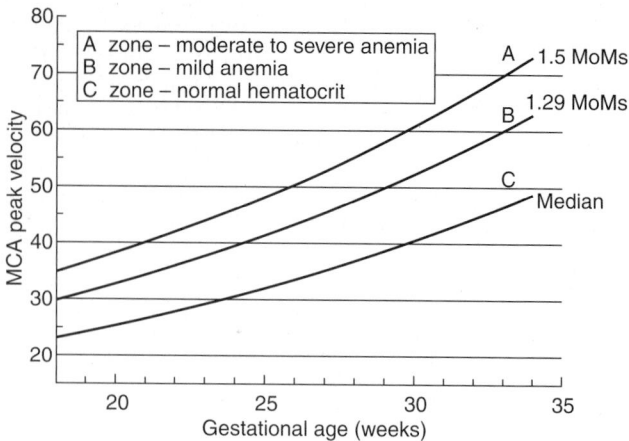

FIGURE 77-7 Middle cerebral artery (MCA) Doppler graph based on gestational age. *(From Moise KJ: Management of Rhesus alloimmunization in pregnancy,* Obstet Gynecol *112:164-176, 2008b.)*

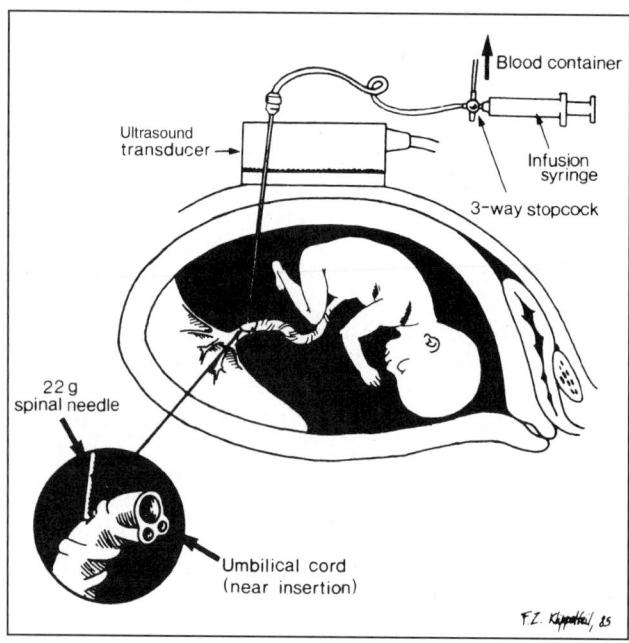

FIGURE 77-8 Diagrammatic view of in utero direct intravascular transfusion. *(From Grannum PA, Copel JA, Plaxe SC, et al: In utero exchange transfusion by direct intravascular injection in severe erythroblastosis fetalis,* N Engl J Med *314:1431, 1986. Reprinted by permission of the* New England Journal of Medicine.)

severity of fetal hemolysis during the third trimester, and the trend of two or more values is a more reliable predictor of severity of fetal disease (Liley, 1961).

More recently, efforts have been made to use noninvasive detection of fetal anemia. Ultrasonography signs of hydrops fetalis represent a relatively late sign of fetal anemia, often not developing until Hgb values are more than 7 gm/dL below gestational age norm. However, Doppler assessment of peak velocity in the fetal middle cerebral artery (MCA), reflecting the lower viscosity associated with more severe anemia, has become the standard of care at most centers (Figure 77-6). MCA Doppler has been compared to the previous gold standard of the amniocentesis for "ΔOD_{450nm}" (Oepkes et al, 2006). In this study, 45% of infants had severe anemia at cordocentesis, defined as a hemoglobin level at least 5 standard deviations below the mean for gestational age. The MCA Doppler was both more accurate than the ΔOD_{450nm} (85% as compared with 76%) and more sensitive (88% as compared with 76%). It was suggested by the authors that more than 50% of invasive procedures might be avoided using this technique.

In severely affected fetuses, hydrops may occur as early as 20 to 22 weeks' gestation. Measurement of the peak MCA Doppler can begin as early as 18 weeks but more commonly is initiated at approximately 24 weeks, then repeated every 1 to 2 weeks, with adjustment in normal velocity with advancing gestation age to define the risk of severe anemia (Figure 77-7). When the MCA Doppler exceeds 1.5 MoM (A Zone) between 24 and 35 weeks' gestation, cordocentesis is required for direct determination of hematocrit as well as fetal blood type, DAT, reticulocyte count, and total bilirubin (Figure 77-8) (Moise,

2008b). The rate of fetal trauma and morbidity associated with cordocentesis is less than 2% (Parer, 1988; van Kamp et al, 2005). Cordocentesis should be performed with blood available for intravascular intrauterine transfusion if necessary. Such blood should be type O, RhD negative, cytomegalovirus negative, and less than 72 hours from collection; extended crossmatch is often performed with maternal blood type. Irradiation is mandatory, and many centers also perform leukoreduction. The transfusion is generally administered at approximately 20 mL per kg estimated fetal weight with a target of 40 to 50% hematocrit. Beyond 35 weeks, amniocentesis to determine both fetal lung maturity and the ΔOD_{450nm} should be performed. Induction of delivery should be considered if lungs are mature in order to decrease the risk of needing subsequent intrauterine transfusion with their attendant risks, or postnatal exchange transfusion for hyperbilirubinemia. For a full discussion and algorithm for management of pregnant patients with RhD alloimmunization, see Moise, 2008b.

Hyperbilirubinemia (with elevation of the conjugated fraction) often develops in newborns who have received intrauterine RBC transfusions and often predicts the need for exchange transfusions. This hyperbilirubinemia reflects the severity of hemolysis and its effects on the fetal liver. In some cases, anemia may be minimal or absent, and the DAT may be negative if the Rh-negative RBCs transfused prenatally still predominate. In such cases the infant may not require exchange transfusion. Neonatal exchange transfusion, amniocentesis, selective early induction of delivery, and intrauterine fetal blood transfusions all have contributed to the declining neonatal death rate from Rh incompatibility.

ABO Incompatibility

Hemolysis associated with ABO incompatibility is similar to Rh hemolytic disease in that maternal anti-A or anti-B antibodies enter the fetal circulation and react with A or B antigens on the erythrocyte surface (Table 77-5). In persons with type A and type B blood, naturally occurring anti-B and anti-A isoantibodies largely are IgM molecules that do not cross the placenta. In contrast, the alloantibodies present in persons with type O blood also include IgG antibodies that can traverse the placenta (Abelson and Rawson, 1961). For this reason, ABO incompatibility is largely limited to type O mothers with type A or B fetuses. The presence of IgG anti-A or anti-B antibodies in type O mothers also explains why hemolysis caused by ABO incompatibility frequently occurs during the first pregnancy without prior "sensitization." ABO incompatibility is present in approximately 12% of pregnancies, although evidence of fetal RBC sensitization (i.e., positive result on DAT) is found in only 3% of births, and less than 1% of live births are associated with significant hemolysis (Kaplan et al, 1976; Zipursky et al, 1963). The relative mildness of neonatal ABO hemolytic disease contrasts sharply with the findings in Rh incompatibility. In large part, this is because A and B antigens are present in many tissues besides RBCs; consequently, only a small fraction of anti-A or anti-B antibody that crosses the placenta actually binds to erythrocytes, the remainder being absorbed by other tissues and soluble A and B substances in plasma.

Although hemolytic disease resulting from ABO incompatibility is milder than Rh disease, severe hemolysis occasionally occurs. In suspected cases of ABO incompatibility, it is essential to exclude other antibodies and other nonimmune causes of hemolysis such as glucose-6-phosphate dehydrogenase (G6PD) deficiency or hereditary spherocytosis. In most cases, pallor and jaundice are minimal (see Table 77-5). Hepatosplenomegaly is uncommon. Laboratory features include evidence of minimal to moderate hyperbilirubinemia and, occasionally, some degree of anemia. The DAT sometimes is negative, although the indirect antiglobulin test (neonatal serum plus adult group A or B RBCs) more commonly is positive. This paradox is related to the fact that fetal

TABLE 77-5   Clinical and Laboratory Features of Immune Hemolysis Due to Rh Disease and ABO Incompatibility

	Rh Disease	ABO Incompatibility
Clinical Features		
Frequency	Unusual	Common
Pallor	Marked	Minimal
Jaundice	Marked	Minimal to moderate
Hydrops	Common	Rare
Hepatosplenomegaly	Marked	Minimal
Laboratory Features		
Blood type		
Mother	Rh(−)	O
Infant	Rh(+)	A or B
Anemia	Marked	Minimal
Direct antiglobulin test	Positive	Frequently negative
Indirect antiglobulin test	Positive	Usually positive
Hyperbilirubinemia	Marked	Variable
RBC morphology	Nucleated RBCs	Spherocytes

RBC, Red blood cell.

RBCs, compared with adult erythrocytes, have less type-specific antigen on their surface (Voak and Williams, 1971). The peripheral blood smear is characterized by marked spherocytosis that is indistinguishable from that seen in hereditary spherocytosis (see Hereditary Spherocytosis, later).

Hemolysis in ABO incompatibility is usually mild, presenting with some degree of hyperbilirubinemia. Of major concern in the current cost-conscious health care environment is that some infants with ABO incompatibility may be discharged home from medical establishments before significant clinical jaundice is evident. It is critical that infants with ABO incompatibility be monitored closely for evolving jaundice and hyperbilirubinemia in the first few days of life. In most cases, hyperbilirubinemia is readily controlled by phototherapy. In the minority of cases not controlled by phototherapy, exchange transfusion with group O Rh-compatible RBCs is utilized. Additional follow-up at 2 to 3 weeks of age to check for anemia in these infants is essential.

Minor Blood Group Incompatibility

With the sharp decline of hemolytic disease caused by Rh incompatibility, the proportion of cases caused by Rh c, Rh E, Kell, Duffy, and Kidd incompatibility has increased from the previous estimates of 1% to 3%, to as high as 20% (for Kell sensitization) (Geifman-Holtzman et al, 1997; Moise, 2008a). The pathophysiology of these disorders is similar to that of Rh and ABO incompatibility. The infrequency of minor group incompatibility is primarily a reflection of the lower antigenicity of these RBC antigens. Diagnosis of minor group incompatibility is suggested by hemolytic anemia with a positive DAT in the absence of

ABO or Rh incompatibility and with a negative maternal DAT. Definitive diagnosis requires identification of the specific antibody in neonatal serum or an eluate from neonatal RBCs. This is readily accomplished by testing maternal serum against a variety of known RBC antigens. With some antibodies such as Kell, antibody titer and amniocentesis findings may underestimate the severity of fetal hemolysis.

Immune Hemolytic Anemia Due to Maternal Disease

Maternal autoimmune hemolytic anemia or lupus erythematosus during pregnancy may be associated with passive transfer of IgG antibody to the fetus. The diagnosis is suggested by the presence of neonatal hemolytic disease, a positive DAT, absence of Rh or ABO incompatibility, and antiglobulin-positive hemolysis in the mother. Treatment with prednisone in the mother may reduce both maternal hemolysis and the risk of neonatal morbidity. As in other cases of neonatal hemolysis, treatment is focused on prevention of severe hyperbilirubinemia and kernicterus.

NONIMMUNE ACQUIRED HEMOLYTIC DISEASE

Infection

Cytomegalic inclusion disease, toxoplasmosis, syphilis, and bacterial sepsis all can be associated with hemolytic anemia. In most of these conditions, some degree of thrombocytopenia also exists. Generally, hepatosplenomegaly is present. In cases of bacterial sepsis, both the direct and indirect bilirubin levels may be elevated. The mechanism of hemolysis associated with infection is not clearly defined. Documentation of infection as the cause of hemolysis is made by the presence of other clinical and laboratory evidence of neonatal infections. Hemolysis caused by infections may present early in the neonatal period, or it can be delayed for several weeks.

Schistocytic Anemias

Disseminated intravascular coagulation (DIC) is discussed in Chapter 76. The hemolytic component of this disorder is secondary to the deposition of fibrin within the vascular walls. When erythrocytes interact with fibrin, fragments of RBCs are broken off, producing fragile, deformed RBCs, or schistocytes. Abnormalities of the placental microcirculation or macrovascular anomalies such as an umbilical vein varix are rare causes of congenital schistocytic anemia (Batton et al, 2000).

HEREDITARY RED BLOOD CELL DISORDERS

Membrane Defects

The customary findings in RBC membrane disorders are the presence of dominant inheritance and abnormal RBC morphology (Figure 77-9). Aside from hereditary spherocytosis, these disorders are uncommon.

Hereditary Spherocytosis

The hallmark of hereditary spherocytosis (HS) is the presence of spherocytes in the peripheral blood smear. Inherited mutations in components of the membrane cytoskeleton (spectrin, ankyrin, or band 3) weaken the stability of the interactions between the cytoskeleton and the membrane lipid bilayer, promoting vesiculation and loss of bits of the bilayer, thus leading to progressive loss of membrane surface area (Gallagher and Glader, 2009). As RBCs become more spherical, they lose flexibility and become vulnerable to entrapment in the spleen and attack by macrophages, leading to hemolysis. Removal of the spleen after 5 years of age allows spherocytes to have a near-normal life span despite their cytoskeletal defects and abnormal shape.

The clinical manifestations of HS in neonates range from the very rare presentation of hydrops fetalis with fetal death (Gallagher et al, 1997) to fully compensated, lifelong hemolysis marked by reticulocytosis but no anemia (Gallagher and Glader, 2009). Twenty-eight percent to 43% of infants are anemic at birth (Hgb <15 gm/dL) (Perrotta et al, 2008). Neonatal hemolysis or hyperbilirubinemia appears in approximately half of all affected infants (Stamey and Diamond, 1957). In fact it is often the exaggerated neonatal hyperbilirubinemia that raises the suspicion of an underlying hemolytic disorder. In many cases, other family members are affected in a pattern consistent with autosomal dominant inheritance. In 20% to 30% of cases, recessive inheritance is noted, but only homozygotes express the clinical features of spherocytosis. Occasionally, the appearance of a new case of spherocytosis in a previously unaffected family is due to spontaneous mutation.

The diagnosis of HS is suspected when spherocytes are seen on the blood smear of an infant with hyperbilirubinemia or other laboratory evidence of hemolysis. Spherocytes also are seen in ABO incompatibility. Blood typing and a DAT may support the diagnosis of ABO incompatibility, but the DAT occasionally can be negative and thus misleading. In this situation, evaluation of the family for other persons affected with spherocytosis may point to a hereditary rather than an acquired cause. Sometimes it is necessary to wait until the infant is 3 months of age or so to obtain a definitive laboratory diagnosis of hereditary spherocytosis, because, by this age, the confounding effects of maternal antibody and fetal RBCs are no longer present. Supporting evidence of HS may be the "gold standard" of an abnormal osmotic fragility test or a newer method that uses flow cytometric analysis of eosin-5'-maleimide-labeled red blood cells, with lower fluorescence levels in spherocytosis patients reflecting lower total amounts of RBC band 3 protein (Girodon et al, 2008; King et al, 2000).

The mainstay of treatment during the newborn period is directed toward management of hyperbilirubinemia, which often is present and may not peak until the infant is several days of age. Occasionally, RBC transfusions are required in the neonatal period for management of symptomatic anemia (Gallagher et al, 1997). A common occurrence is the appearance of a transient but severe anemia during the first 20 days of life due to underproduction of

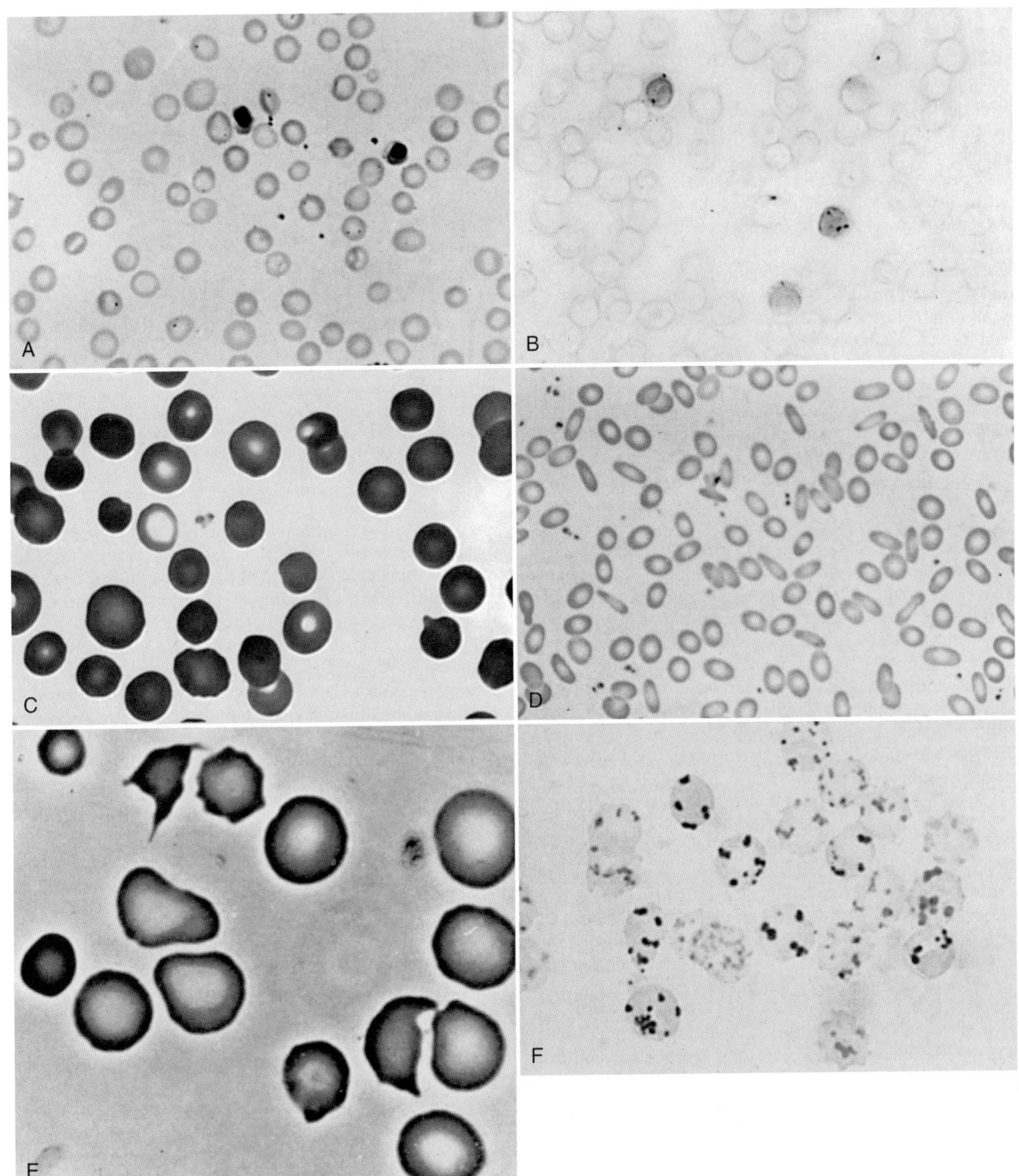

FIGURE 77-9 **A,** Hypochromic-microcytic red blood cells (RBCs) secondary to chronic fetal blood loss. **B,** Fetal RBCs in the maternal blood after a fetomaternal hemorrhage (acid-elution technique). **C,** Hereditary spherocytosis. **D,** Hereditary elliptocytosis. **E,** Glucose-6-phosphate dehydrogenase (G6PD)-deficient RBCs during acute hemolytic episode. **F,** Heinz bodies from a patient with G6PD-deficient hemolysis (stained with supravital dye).

erythropoietin in the face of continuing hemolysis (Delhommeau et al, 2000). Careful monitoring of affected infants after discharge from the nursery is warranted. Splenectomy is the definitive treatment for hereditary spherocytosis, but this is not recommended before 5 years of age because of the increased risk of overwhelming sepsis with encapsulated organisms such as *Streptococcus pneumoniae* (Diamond, 1969) that occurs following splenectomy in infants and young children. Guidelines regarding the indications for total or partial splenectomy have been reviewed (Bader-Meunier et al, 2001; Bolton-Maggs et al, 2004).

Hereditary Elliptocytosis

Hereditary elliptocytosis is an autosomal dominant, clinically heterogeneous group of disorders that are caused by mutations of the RBC membrane cytoskeletal proteins (usually spectrin or protein 4.1) that weaken skeletal protein interactions and increase RBC mechanical fragility (reviewed in Gallagher and Glader, 2009). Heterozygotes usually exhibit elliptocytes on the blood smear, but in the vast majority of instances hemolysis is absent. Homozygotes or compound heterozygotes may have sufficient weakening of the cytoskeleton to cause significant hemolysis accompanied by striking abnormalities in RBC morphology (homozygous hereditary elliptocytosis or hereditary pyropoikilocytosis).

Transient poikilocytosis and hemolysis may occur during the newborn period in infants destined ultimately to have asymptomatic elliptocytosis (Austin and Desforges, 1969). RBC membrane mechanical fragility is strikingly abnormal in these infants, probably as a consequence of the destabilizing influence of large amounts of free intraerythrocytic 2,3-DPG, a by product of the presence of fetal hemoglobin (Mentzer et al, 1987). As fetal hemoglobin levels decline postnatally in affected infants, membrane mechanical fragility lessens, hemolysis disappears, and RBC morphology undergoes a transition from poikilocytosis to elliptocytosis. Without knowledge of the membrane protein mutations present in the infant and the infant's family, it is difficult to predict at birth who will have transient poikilocytosis with ultimate recovery and who is destined to have lifelong pyropoikilocytosis with hemolysis. A practical approach to this problem is to wait 4 to 6 months to see if common HE evolves or chronic hemolysis with abnormally shaped RBCs persists.

Red Blood Cell Enzyme Abnormalities

Hyperbilirubinemia, anemia, and even hydrops fetalis can be the result of inherited RBC enzymopathies. The two most commonly encountered red cell enzyme disorders are glucose-6–phosphate dehydrogenase (G6PD) deficiency and pyruvate kinase (PK) deficiency. Overviews of these two disorders, as well as other more esoteric enzyme deficiencies, are available elsewhere (Glader 2009; Luzzato and Poggi, 2009; Mentzer, 2009) and the special features of RBC enzymopathies in the newborn period have also been summarized (Matthay and Mentzer, 1981).

Glucose-6-Phosphate Dehydrogenase Deficiency

G6PD deficiency is a sex-linked disorder that affects millions of people throughout the world, particularly in Mediterranean countries, the Middle East, Africa, and Asia. Like sickle cell trait and thalassemia, G6PD deficiency is thought to have become common because it provides a measure of protection against malaria. In most G6PD-deficient persons, hemolysis and anemia are present only episodically. Precipitating factors can include infection, exposure to medications that are potent oxidants, or to other agents such as fava beans, naphthalene, or certain petrochemical-derived substances. Rarely, hemolytic

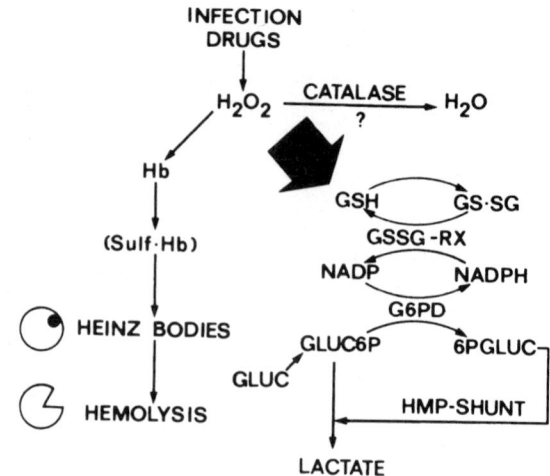

FIGURE 77-10 Glucose-6-phosphate hemolysis pathophysiology. *GSH,* Reduced glutathione; *GS-SG,* oxidized glutathione; *GSSG-RX,* glutathione reductase; *GLUC6P,* glucose-6-phosphate; *6PGLUC,* 6-phosphogluconate; *G6PD,* glucose-6-phosphate dehydrogenase; *HMP-SHUNT,* hexose monophosphate shunt.

anemia is chronic rather than episodic and is present even in the absence of obvious exposure to oxidant stress. The clinical heterogeneity of G6PD deficiency is due to the different mutations, usually single amino acid substitutions, that lead to altered enzyme function (Beutler et al, 1996; Miwa and Fujii, 1996). Normal RBCs contain abundant amounts of reduced glutathione (GSH), a sulfhydryl-containing tripeptide that serves as an intracellular antioxidant, neutralizing oxidant drug metabolites and activated oxygen species released during phagocyte activation. Because of the enzyme deficiency, G6PD-deficient RBCs have a limited capacity to regenerate GSH from oxidized glutathione (Figure 77-10). In the absence of GSH, RBCs are vulnerable to oxidant injury of hemoglobin. Denatured globin precipitates termed *Heinz bodies* bind to the cell membrane, unfavorably altering its structure and function. Membrane lipid peroxidation may contribute to altered function. The ultimate result of these insults is hemolysis.

The variant G6PD A– is responsible for nearly all of the G6PD deficiency seen in Africans (and is present in approximately 10% of African Americans). It previously was considered to be a single biochemical disorder, but is now known to be due to three different genotypes. G6PD A– affects the stability of the enzyme, causing an accelerated decline in activity during the life span of the RBC. Only in the oldest RBCs does enzyme activity reach low enough levels to create vulnerability to oxidant hemolysis. For this reason, hemolysis, if it occurs, is usually mild and self-limited. In contrast, in Asians and persons of Mediterranean or Middle Eastern descent, G6PD deficiency decreases the enzyme activity in young and old RBCs alike. Hemolysis is usually more severe and can be life threatening. It is of interest that the G6PD variants found throughout the Mediterranean and Middle East, once thought to be biochemically different, are now recognized to be due to one common single genotype. In these ethnic groups, inheritance of an as-yet-unidentified factor renders some G6PD-deficient persons susceptible to severe and even fatal episodes of hemolysis following exposure to fava beans (favism). The hemolytic factor can be transmitted to neonates via breast milk (Kaplan et al, 1998). Favism is not seen in African-Americans with G6PD A−.

The gene for G6PD is located on the X chromosome. All of the RBCs of G6PD-deficient males are affected by the enzyme deficiency, whereas a variable fraction of RBCs of G6PD-deficient females are enzyme deficient, depending on the degree of lyonization (Lyon, 1961). Because of these differences, hemolysis due to G6PD deficiency occurs mainly in males and is much less common in females.

The diagnosis of G6PD deficiency is suggested by the appearance of a DAT-negative hemolytic anemia in association with infection or the administration of drugs. Cells that appear as if a bite had been taken from them (as a result of splenic removal of Heinz bodies) are occasionally seen on the peripheral blood smear. Supravital stains of the peripheral blood with crystal violet may reveal Heinz bodies during hemolytic episodes. Although screening tests are available, they are not as sensitive as direct assay of RBC G6PD activity. Measurement of enzyme activity may not reveal the deficiency in African Americans immediately after a hemolytic episode, because the population of enzyme-deficient cells has been eliminated. Repeating the assay at a later date is often necessary. Identification of specific G6PD mutations by DNA analysis is available, but rarely used for diagnostic purposes (Beutler, 1996; Miwa and Fujii, 1996).

In the neonatal period the major manifestation of G6PD deficiency is hyperbilirubinemia. There usually is more jaundice than anemia, and the anemia is rarely severe. Also, in contrast to classic Rh-related neonatal hyperbilirubinemia, neonatal jaundice due to G6PD deficiency rarely is present at birth, with clinical onset usually occurring between days 2 and 3 (Kaplan and Hammerman, 2004). Most infants with hyperbilirubinemia due to G6PD deficiency are of Mediterranean, Middle Eastern, or Asian descent.

In the majority of cases of neonatal hyperbilirubinemia due to G6PD deficiency, there is no obvious exposure to external oxidants. The degree of hyperbilirubinemia reflects both the increased bilirubin load presented to the liver by hemolysis of G6PD-deficient RBCs and the presence or absence of the variant form of UGT responsible for Gilbert syndrome (Kaplan et al, 2001). The relative importance of the latter is underscored by the observations that most jaundiced G6PD-deficient neonates are not anemic and that often, evidence for increased bilirubin production secondary to hemolysis is lacking (Kaplan et al, 1996, 1999).

The severity of jaundice varies widely, from being subclinical to imposing the threat of kernicterus if not treated (Johnson et al, 2009). Data from the USA Kernicterus Registry from 1992 to 2004 indicate that more than 30% of kernicterus cases are associated with G6PD deficiency. These observations have raised the question of whether testing for G6PD deficiency should be included in newborn screening programs worldwide (Kaplan and Hammerman, 2009). Neonatal screening for G6PD deficiency has been very effective in reducing the incidence of favism later in life in Sardinia (Meloni et al, 1992) and in other regions where this potentially fatal complication is common. Currently, only the District of Columbia in the United States requires such newborn screening.

Therapy for neonatal hemolysis and hyperbilirubinemia resulting from G6PD deficiency includes (1) phototherapy or exchange transfusion to prevent kernicterus, (2) RBC transfusion for symptomatic anemia, (3) removal of potential oxidants that may be contributing to hemolysis, and (4) treatment of infections using agents that do not themselves initiate hemolysis. In infants known to be G6PD deficient, prevention of severe hyperbilirubinemia by administration of a single intramuscular dose of tin-mesoporphyrin, an inhibitor of heme oxygenase, has been advocated (Kappas et al, 2001; Stevenson and Wong, 2010).

Pyruvate Kinase Deficiency

Pyruvate kinase (PK) deficiency is an autosomal recessive disorder that occurs in all ethnic groups. Although it is the most common of the Embden-Meyerhof glycolytic pathway defects, it is rare in comparison with G6PD deficiency. Hundreds of cases, mostly in northern Europeans, have been described in the literature, although many more unpublished cases also occur (Zanella and Bianchi, 2000). PK is one of the two enzymes that generate adenosine triphosphate (ATP) in RBCs. Because nonerythroid tissues have alternative means of generating ATP, clinical abnormalities in PK deficiency are limited to RBCs. More than 180 PK mutations have been defined at the nucleic acid level and many more in terms of abnormalities of the PK protein (Pissard et al, 2006; Zanella and Bianchi, 2000). Reflecting this genetic diversity, the hemolytic anemia that characterizes PK deficiency varies considerably in severity from family to family. Approximately one third of PK-deficient babies experience hyperbilirubinemia during the newborn period. Death or kernicterus may occur. Severe intrauterine anemia and hydrops fetalis have been reported (Zanella and Bianchi, 2000). In two recent cases, newborns with PK deficiency presented with neonatal cholestasis and developed progressive liver dysfunction leading to fatal hepatic failure (Raphaël et al, 2007).

The diagnosis of PK deficiency should be considered in a jaundiced newborn with evidence of nonimmune hemolysis in the absence of infection or exposure to hemolytic agents. Hemoglobinopathies and membrane disorders should be ruled out by examination of the blood smear and other appropriate diagnostic tests before proceeding to assay of RBC PK activity. RBC morphology is normal in PK deficiency, although a few dense cells with irregular margins (echinocytes) are occasionally seen. PK heterozygotes are clinically and hematologically normal but usually have roughly half the normal amount of RBC PK activity. When infants have been transfused before confirmation of diagnosis, the determination of RBC PK activity in parents may detect the heterozygous state and help lead to the diagnosis (Pissard et al, 2007).

Treatment of hyperbilirubinemia by phototherapy and exchange transfusion if necessary is usually the only therapy necessary in the newborn period. RBC transfusions for anemia occasionally are required. Splenectomy may reduce the rate of hemolysis but should be avoided in infancy and early childhood because of the high risk of infection after splenectomy.

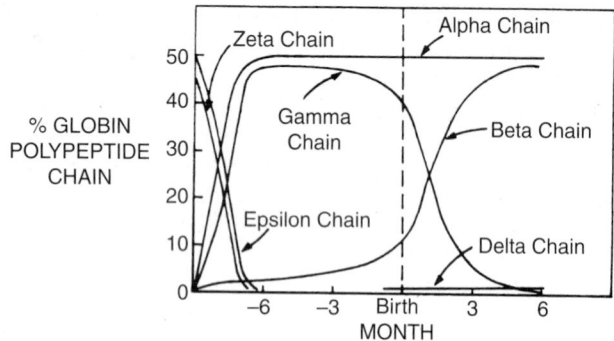

FIGURE 77-11 Fetal and neonatal hemoglobin production.

	HEMOGLOBIN	GLOBIN POLYPEPTIDES	% IN CORD BLOOD
EMBRYONIC	GOWER - 1	Zeta-2, Epsilon-2 ($\zeta_2\epsilon_2$)	0
	GOWER -2	Alpha-2, Epsilon-2 ($\alpha_2\epsilon_2$)	0
	PORTLAND	Zeta-2, Gamma-2 ($\zeta_2\gamma_2$)	0
FETAL	BARTS	Gamma-4 (γ_4)	<1%
	Hgb F	Alpha-2, Gamma-2 ($\alpha_2\gamma_2$)	60-85%
ADULT	Hgb A	Alpha-2, Beta-2 ($\alpha_2\beta_2$)	15-40%
	Hgb A$_2$	Alpha-2, Delta-2 ($\alpha_2\delta_2$)	<1%

FIGURE 77-12 Hemoglobin composition of cord blood.

HEMOLYSIS DUE TO HEMOGLOBIN DISORDERS

Beyond infancy the predominant hemoglobin tetramer is hemoglobin A (HbA), composed of two alpha globin chains and two beta globin chains ($\alpha_2\beta_2$). To appreciate the hemoglobinopathies that occur in newborns, however, it is necessary to understand the normal developmental changes that occur in globin synthesis during fetal and neonatal life. Embryonic hemoglobins are composed of zeta and epsilon chains. The transition from zeta to alpha globin chains is complete by the end of the first trimester. Epsilon chains disappear more slowly and are replaced first by gamma chains to form fetal hemoglobin (Hb F, $\alpha_2\gamma_2$) and next by beta chains to form hemoglobin A (Figure 77-11). The various possible combinations of these different globin chains form a number of different hemoglobin tetramers that are characteristically found in embryonic, fetal, and postnatal life (Figure 77-12).

Fetal hemoglobin is the major hemoglobin found in fetuses after the first trimester. Its replacement by adult hemoglobin A begins before birth, such that 60% to 90% of the hemoglobin found in the normal term infant is hemoglobin F. After birth, gamma chain synthesis declines rapidly as beta chain synthesis increases (see Figure 77-11) so that most newly formed hemoglobin is hemoglobin A. As RBCs made before birth are replaced postnatally, the percentage of hemoglobin F declines rapidly, reaching a level of approximately 5% by 6 months of age (Figure 77-13). Only trace amounts of the minor adult hemoglobin, hemoglobin A$_2$ ($\alpha_2\delta_2$), and hemoglobin Barts (γ_4) are present in cord blood. Hemoglobin Barts quickly disappears, whereas the hemoglobin A$_2$ level increases gradually to the adult level of 2% to 3% by 1 year of age.

Beta globin disorders such as sickle cell disease or beta-thalassemia major are not clinically apparent until several months of age, when the switch from hemoglobin F to

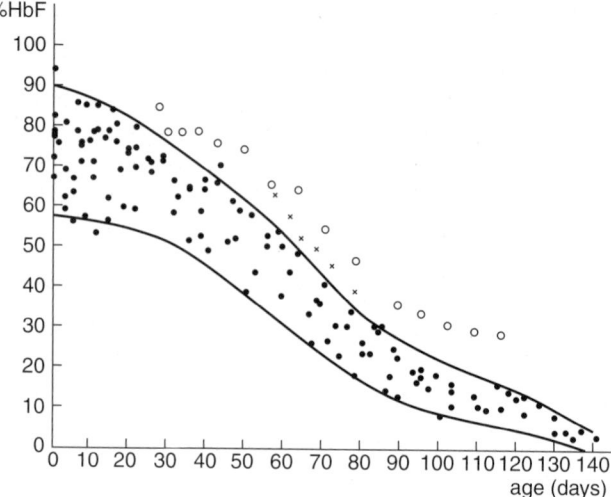

FIGURE 77-13 Decreasing concentration of fetal hemoglobin after birth. *(From Garby L, Sjöhn S, Vuille JC: Studies of erythro-kinetics in infancy. II. The relative rates of synthesis of haemoglobin F and haemoglobin A during the first months of life,* Acta Paediatr *51:245-254, 1962.)*

hemoglobin A synthesis reveals the defect. In contrast, gamma globin mutations are most evident in fetal and neonatal life and then disappear by approximately 3 months of age as gamma globin synthesis wanes. Alpha globin disorders are evident at all stages of development from fetal to adult.

Thalassemia Syndromes

Thalassemias are due to absent or deficient synthesis of one normal globin chain, leading to a relative excess of the complementary or partner chain. For example, alpha-thalassemias are due to diminished synthesis of alpha globin chains, leading to an excess of beta chains (or, in the fetus, of gamma chains). The excess beta chains form tetramers (β_4 or hemoglobin H) that are unstable and can lead to hemolysis beyond infancy. The excess gamma chains also form tetramers (γ_4 or hemoglobin Barts) that have an increased affinity for oxygen but do not cause hemolysis. In beta-thalassemia, excess alpha globin chains accumulate, forming aggregates that injure the cell membrane, leading to hemolysis. In addition, the decrease in overall production of hemoglobin produces small RBCs (microcytosis) that are often filled with less than the normal amount of hemoglobin (hypochromia).

In the United States, changing immigration patterns have markedly increased the numbers of infants born with significant hemoglobinopathies. In California, analysis of newborn screening results between 1998 and 2006 demonstrated clinically significant hemoglobin genotypes in 0.05% of newborns; of these, the prevalence of alpha- and beta-thalassemia syndromes combined (28%) was almost as high as the prevalence of sickle cell disease (32%) (Michlitsch et al, 2009).

Alpha-Thalassemia

Alpha-thalassemia is of particular importance to neonatologists because its clinical manifestations are present in utero and at birth. The more severe forms of alpha-thalassemia are found in Southeast Asians (Glader and Look, 1996) and

TABLE 77-6 Alpha-Thalassemia Syndromes

		Anemia	Hemolysis	α:β Chain Synthesis	Abnormal Hemoglobins	
					Cord Blood	Adult Blood
Normal	$\dfrac{\alpha/\alpha}{\alpha/\alpha}$	None	None	0.95–1.10	0%–1% γ_4	—
Silent carrier	$\dfrac{\alpha/-}{\alpha/\alpha}$	None	None	0.85–0.95	1%–2% γ_4	—
Alpha-thalassemia trait	$\dfrac{-/-}{\alpha/\alpha}$	Mild hypochromic Microcytic	None	0.72–0.82	5%–6% γ_4	—
Hemoglobin "H" disease	$\dfrac{-/-}{\alpha/-}$	Moderate hypochromic Microcytic	Moderate	0.30–0.52	20%–40% γ_4 0%–5% β_4	20%–40% β_4
Homozygous alpha-thalassemia ("hydrops")	$\dfrac{-/-}{-/-}$	Severe hypochromic Microcytic	Severe	0	70%–80% γ_4 15%–20% β_4 0%–10% $\zeta_2\gamma$	

less commonly in infants of Mediterranean origin, and are rare in Africans. The molecular basis for alpha-thalassemia is usually deletion of one or more of the four alpha globin genes. A thalassemic hemoglobinopathy involving the abnormal hemoglobin Constant Spring also may behave functionally as a mild form of alpha-thalassemia. Clinical severity is dictated by how many alpha globin genes are absent or nonfunctional. An infant can inherit no, one, or two alpha-thalassemia genes from each parent, giving rise to the following four clinical syndromes:

1. *Silent carrier state.* Deletion or nonfunction of a single alpha globin gene is not accompanied by any clinical or hematologic abnormalities.
2. *Alpha-thalassemia trait.* Deletion or nonfunction of two alpha globin genes, in *cis* (Asians) or *trans* (Africans), is associated with mild microcytic anemia, without hemolysis or reticulocytosis.
3. *Hemoglobin H disease.* When three of four alpha globin genes are deleted or nonfunctional, a mild to moderate hemolytic anemia is found, often aggravated by oxidant stresses just as in G6PD deficiency. The RBCs are hypochromic and microcytic and contain inclusions of hemoglobin H when appropriate staining is performed. Hemoglobin H Constant Spring can be a particularly severe syndrome with up to one third requiring regular transfusions (Vichinsky et al, 2005)
4. *Homozygous alpha-thalassemia.* Lack of all four alpha globin genes is associated with a severe intrauterine hemolytic anemia and hydrops fetalis, with massive hepatosplenomegaly, and, in most instances, fetal demise. The RBCs are very hypochromic, fragmented, and bizarre in shape. Erythroblastosis is present (Chui and Waye, 1998).

The diagnosis of the alpha-thalassemia syndromes is easily made during the newborn period by correlation of the clinical and hematologic appearance of the child with the amount of hemoglobin Barts (γ_4) present in the RBCs (Lorey et al, 2000) (Table 77-6). Screening of all newborns for hemoglobin H disease is justified in populations with a substantial number of at-risk pregnancies (Lorey et al, 2000; Michlitsch et al, 2009). The large amount of

hemoglobin Barts found in the RBCs of homozygotes for alpha-thalassemia contributes to the clinical severity of the syndrome, because the increased oxygen affinity of this hemoglobin impairs oxygen release to the tissues. DNA-based diagnostic tests are available for prenatal diagnosis, which is often carried out when a pregnancy at risk for a fetus with homozygous alpha-thalassemia is identified (Chui and Waye, 1998). The increased risk of eclampsia in mothers of such fetuses is an important justification for early identification and termination of the pregnancy.

No treatment is needed for the silent carrier state or for alpha-thalassemia trait, but studies to determine the thalassemia status of other family members, particularly those in their reproductive years, are recommended so that genetic counseling (and prenatal diagnosis if indicated) can be provided. Parents of infants who have hemoglobin H disease should be instructed to avoid oxidant agents that can cause hemolysis (the same list that is given to patients with G6PD deficiency). Although these infants are usually only mildly anemic, they may experience severe episodes of hemolysis during infections or with exposure to oxidant agents. Fetuses with homozygous alpha-thalassemia that are not aborted are usually stillborn. A few affected children have been born alive and resuscitated (Lee et al, 2007), or supported with in utero transfusion before delivery (Sohan et al, 2002). Although such infants can subsequently receive chronic RBC transfusions, and a small number have undergone bone marrow transplantation (Yi et al, 2009), the long-term outcome for such infants is uncertain.

Beta-Thalassemia

Like alpha-thalassemia, beta-thalassemia is found in regions of the world where malaria was formerly endemic: Southeast Asia, India, Africa, and the Mediterranean basin. Although deletion of the beta globin locus is an occasional cause of beta-thalassemia, most cases are caused by point mutations that affect transcription, messenger RNA (mRNA) processing, or translation (Cunningham et al, 2009; Galanello, 1995; Olivieri, 1999). Two general types of beta-thalassemia are recognized. In beta^0-thalassemia, no beta globin at all is produced by the thalassemic locus, whereas in beta$^+$-thalassemia, there is reduced but measurable output of beta globin. The severity of homozygous beta-thalassemia (or beta-thalassemia major) is greatest when two beta^0-thalassemia genes are inherited; clinical disease usually is much milder when two beta$^+$-thalassemia genes are inherited. By contrast, the inheritance of one thalassemia gene (beta thalassemia trait) is characterized by a mild microcytic anemia that needs to be distinguished from alpha thalassemia and iron deficiency. Severe beta-thalassemia is associated with lifelong hemolytic anemia, dependence on regular RBC transfusions for survival, and the gradual development of transfusion-associated hemosiderosis (Olivieri, 1999). Survival has improved, however, with improvements in iron chelation and with the use of hematopoietic stem cell transplantation for patients with available matched donors (Cunningham, 2008, Rund and Rachmilewitz, 2005).

The clinical abnormalities of beta-thalassemia are not evident at birth but first manifest only after 3 months of age, when beta globin normally becomes the dominant form of non-alpha globin synthesized. Although affected newborns appear clinically normal, the diagnosis of beta^0-thalassemia can be made at birth by detecting a complete absence of hemoglobin A, using hemoglobin electrophoresis or similar techniques. Definitive diagnosis of beta$^+$-thalassemia by these techniques, however, is not possible in the newborn period, because the reduced amount of hemoglobin A produced overlaps the range for normal babies. Direct identification of beta-thalassemia mutations by DNA diagnostic techniques is increasingly available and allows the identification at birth of all infants with beta-thalassemia major. These techniques, however, are more commonly used for prenatal diagnosis of beta-thalassemia syndromes. DNA can be obtained during midtrimester from fetal amniocytes (15 to 17 weeks) or during the first trimester from chorionic villi (9 to 11 weeks), and the assay is completed within a few days, allowing families to make informed decisions regarding termination of pregnancy (Kazazian and Boehm, 1988). The implementation of a strategy of carrier detection, genetic counseling, and prenatal diagnosis in countries where beta-thalassemia is common has led to a striking reduction in the number of births of infants with beta-thalassemia major (Cao et al, 1996). More recent advances have included preimplantation genetic diagnosis (Harteveld et al, 2009).

Hemoglobin E/Beta-Thalassemia

Hemoglobin E is a structurally abnormal hemoglobin that results from an amino acid substitution (lysine for glutamine) at the number 26 amino acid of beta globin, counting from the N terminus. Because this mutation also adversely affects mRNA processing, there is reduced output of beta globin mRNA. Hemoglobin E trait is therefore an example of a thalassemic hemoglobinopathy. Hemoglobin E carriers are microcytic but not anemic. Even hemoglobin E homozygotes have little or no anemia. However, coinheritance of hemoglobin E trait and beta^0-thalassemia trait can give rise to a transfusion-dependent form of beta-thalassemia major (Oliveri et al, 2008). As with other types of beta-thalassemia major, clinical abnormalities are not seen until the infant is 3 to 6 months of age. However, the presence of hemoglobin E is easily detected at birth by hemoglobin electrophoresis or related techniques. Infants found to have hemoglobin E need careful follow-up evaluation to exclude the possibility of hemoglobin E beta-thalassemia. DNA-based detection of the hemoglobin E mutation is feasible (Embury et al, 1990) and has been applied to both prenatal and neonatal diagnosis. Infants born to mothers with hemoglobin E beta-thalassemia have a higher risk of preterm birth, low birthweight, and fetal growth restriction (Luewan et al, 2009).

Gamma-Thalassemia

Large deletions within the beta globin gene cluster may remove both gamma globin genes ($^A\gamma$ and $^G\gamma$) as well as the delta and beta globin genes. The resulting gamma-delta-beta-thalassemia is lethal in the homozygous state but in the heterozygote produces a transient but moderately severe microcytic anemia in the newborn. Over the first few months of life, the anemia resolves to a variable extent without specific therapy, and eventually the hematologic picture is that of beta-thalassemia trait. Several different gamma-delta-beta deletions have been reported, all but one in families of European origin (Cunningham et al, 2009).

Sickle Cell Disease

The sickling hemoglobinopathies are beta globin mutations that, as with beta-thalassemia, do not become clinically evident until the infant reaches several months of age. Sickle cell anemia, the most severe of the disorders, is the result of inheritance of two beta^S mutations (substitution of valine for glutamic acid at the sixth amino acid on the beta globin chain), one from each parent. Sickle-beta^0-thalassemia, phenotypically identical to sickle cell anemia, is caused by inheritance of one beta^S and one beta-thalassemia mutation. The third common form of sickle cell disease, hemoglobin S-C disease, is somewhat milder than sickle cell anemia or sickle-beta^0-thalassemia. It is the consequence of inheritance of one beta^S mutation and one beta^C mutation (the substitution of lysine for glutamic acid at the sixth amino acid on the beta globin chain). Although no clinical abnormalities are present at birth, early diagnosis is important, because two potentially fatal but largely preventable complications may occur during the 1st year of life (Lenfant, 2002). The first is the splenic sequestration crisis, an unpredictable pooling of large numbers of RBCs in the spleen, which leads to a rapid decrease in hematocrit and, in the most severe cases, cardiovascular collapse and death. The second is overwhelming septicemia, usually caused by *S. pneumoniae*. The unusually high susceptibility to infection with encapsulated organisms such as *S. pneumoniae* is the consequence of functional asplenia, which commonly appears by 1 year of age in infants with sickle cell anemia or sickle-beta^0-thalassemia (but not until later in persons with hemoglobin S-C disease). Prompt treatment of splenic sequestration with RBC transfusions is life saving, so parents are taught to recognize early manifestations such as splenic enlargement, lethargy, or pallor.

Overwhelming sepsis can be prevented in most instances by early immunization with *Haemophilus influenzae* and conjugated pneumococcal vaccines, beginning at 2 months of age, and by institution of daily prophylactic penicillin at a dose of 125 mg twice daily (Gaston et al, 1986). It is the need to institute these prophylactic measures within the first 1 to 2 months of life that provides a compelling rationale for neonatal diagnosis of the sickling disorders. Recent data regarding the impact of these interventions have confirmed a 68% reduction in mortality from sickle cell disease for children ages 0 to 3, between 1983 and 1986 and between 1999 and 2002 (Yanni et al, 2009). In many states, all newborns are screened for these disorders, whereas in others, only high-risk ethnic groups are targeted. Usually a dried sample of blood on filter paper, collected at the same time as for other screening tests for inherited metabolic disorders, is used, but cord blood also is satisfactory. Tests that quantitate the amount of hemoglobin S, such as high-performance liquid chromatography, thin-layer isoelectric focusing, or electrophoresis on both cellulose acetate (in an alkaline buffer) and citrate agar (in an acid buffer), are valid. However, sickle solubility tests or the sodium metabisulfate "sickle prep" are not good tests because they do not clearly distinguish sickle cell disease from sickle cell trait; also, the tests are not sensitive enough to detect reliably the small percentage of hemoglobin S present in the RBCs of the newborn.

An excellent overview of issues related to newborn screening for sickle cell disease has been published by Wethers et al (1989). Extensive experience with mandatory statewide screening for all infants has been accumulated in New York (Diaz-Barrios, 1989), California (Lorey et al, 1996), and elsewhere (Wethers et al, 1989). Today, all 50 states screen for sickle cell disease (Michlitsch et al, 2009).

Infants without a hemoglobinopathy born to mothers with sickle cell disease present more of a clinical problem during gestation and the neonatal period than is the case with infants who actually have sickle cell disease. Low birthweight occurs in 28% to 42% of pregnancies (Smith et al, 1996; Thame et al, 2007) and has been correlated with gestational age and placental weight. Asymmetric growth restriction is frequent, as is intrauterine growth restriction (present in approximately 15% of cases). Spontaneous abortion, stillbirth (in 6% to 10%), preterm labor and delivery, and perinatal mortality (in approximately 15%) all are more frequent in the infants of mothers with sickle cell anemia. These problems may be traced to abnormalities of the placenta such as small size, infarction, and an increased incidence of placenta previa and abruptio placentae, which appears to be the consequence of sickle vaso-occlusive events within the maternal side of the placental circulation. They are not caused by the presence of the sickle trait, beta-thalassemia trait, or hemoglobin C trait in the infant, because no hematologic disease is associated with the carrier state for these mutations, even in adult life when they are fully expressed, except under conditions of extreme hypoxia.

One caveat regarding sickle trait blood is that blood from an adult donor who has sickle trait should not be used for exchange transfusions in the newborn, particularly if hypoxemia is present, because use of sickle trait RBCs in this setting may contribute to a fatal outcome (Veiga and Vaithianathan, 1963).

HYPOPLASTIC ANEMIA

Diamond-Blackfan Anemia

The two major causes of RBC aplasia in children are Diamond-Blackfan anemia (DBA) and transient erythroblastopenia of childhood (TEC). The latter condition, TEC, is a disease that rarely occurs before 6 months of age (Miller and Berman, 1994; Ware and Kinney, 1991), and most children with this disorder are older infants or young children. In contrast, many infants with DBA are anemic at birth or become so in the first months of life.

Also known as *congenital hypoplastic anemia*, DBA is a red cell aplasia characterized by the absence of recognizable erythroid precursor cells in the bone marrow (Lipton and Ellis, 2009). It is now considered to be a disorder of ribosome biogenesis (Dianzani and Loreni, 2008) that results in profound erythroid hypoplasia because erythroid progenitors and precursors are highly sensitive to apoptotic cell death. Although many cases are sporadic, familial, autosomal-dominant DBA has recently been estimated to account for up to 45% of cases (Orfali et al, 2004). At least 11 different ribosomal protein gene mutations have been identified in DBA patients. Approximately 25% of these are due to mutations in RPS19 on chromosome 19q (Gustavsson et al, 1997). Recent studies have identified that a significant fraction of DBA cases are linked to genes on chromosome 8p (Gazda et al, 2001). Work is ongoing to fully elucidate the relationship of these abnormalities to the pathophysiology of DBA. A working ribosomal stress hypothesis proposes that p53 is activated because of decreased ribosome protein synthesis, which leads to cell cycle arrest or apoptosis and ultimately anemia, poor growth, and congenital malformations.

Anemia is lifelong, but the onset of the disease is variable. Many affected infants are severely anemic in the newborn period, and pallor at birth or soon thereafter has been a feature of the disease in most cases. Fetal growth restriction, skeletal abnormalities, or other congenital anomalies are seen in almost one third of patients. The diagnosis of DBA is suggested by anemia and reticulocytopenia appearing in the first 6 months of life. Certain unusual features of the RBCs (macrocytosis, elevated fetal hemoglobin, increased adenosine deaminase activity) may assist in diagnosis. Also, tests for many of the DBA gene mutations are available in commercial gene diagnostic laboratories.

Many patients achieve durable remissions from anemia when treated with corticosteroids. Those who do not respond to corticosteroids require chronic RBC transfusions and are at risk of transfusion hemosiderosis. Transfusion-dependent DBA can be cured by allogeneic bone marrow transplantation from HLA-compatible siblings (Lipton et al 2006; Roy et al, 2005). The incidence of cancer is probably increased in DBA patients, based on cases reported to the Diamond Blackfan Anemia Registry (Lipton and Ellis, 2009). Although a variety of solid tumors, in particular an increased incidence of osteogenic sarcoma, have been reported, the most common malignancy

TABLE 77-7   Hemoglobin Changes During the First Year of Life

Week	Term	Premature (1.2–2.5 kg)	Premature (<1.2 kg)
0	17.0 (14.0–20.0)*	16.4 (13.5–19.0)	16.0 (13.0–18.0)
1	18.8	16.0	14.8
3	15.9	13.5	13.4
6	12.7	10.7	9.7
10	11.4	9.8	8.5
20	12.0	10.4	9.0
50	12.0	11.5	11.0
Lowest hemoglobin: mean (range)	10.3 (9.5–11.0)	9.0 (8.0–10.0)	7.1 (6.5–9.0)
Time of nadir	6–12 wk	5–10 wk	4–8 wk

*Hemoglobin concentration (g/100 mL).

reported in the registry and the published medical literature has been acute myeloid leukemia.

PHYSIOLOGIC ANEMIA OF INFANCY AND PREMATURITY

At birth, the mean hemoglobin of term infants (17 g/100 mL) is slightly greater than in premature infants (16 g/100 mL). The hemoglobin concentration in term infants subsequently decreases to a plateau at which it remains throughout the first year of life (Table 77-7). Termed *physiologic anemia of infancy*, this anemia characterized by low (relative to adult values) hemoglobin is a normal part of development and has no adverse clinical effects. A similar process (*anemia of prematurity*) occurs in premature infants, but the hemoglobin decreases more rapidly and reaches a lower nadir. After 1 year of age, there is little difference between the hemoglobin values of term and premature infants.

Physiologic Anemia of Infancy

With the onset of respirations at birth, considerably more oxygen is available for binding to hemoglobin, and the hemoglobin-oxygen saturation increases from approximately 50% to 95% or more. Furthermore, the normal developmental switch from fetal to adult hemoglobin synthesis actively replaces high-oxygen-affinity fetal hemoglobin with lower-oxygen-affinity adult hemoglobin, which can deliver a greater fraction of hemoglobin-bound oxygen to the tissues. Therefore, immediately after birth the increase in blood oxygen content and tissue oxygen delivery downregulates erythropoietin production; as a consequence, erythropoiesis is suppressed. In the absence of erythropoiesis, hemoglobin levels decrease because there is no replacement of aged RBCs as they are normally removed from the circulation. Iron from degraded RBCs is stored for future hemoglobin synthesis. The hemoglobin concentration continues to decrease until tissue oxygen needs are greater than oxygen delivery. Normally, this point is reached between 6 and 12 weeks of age, when the hemoglobin concentration is 9.5 to 11 g/dL. This physiologic hemoglobin decrease does not represent anemia in the true sense of the term; rather, it is a normal adjustment reflecting the presence of excess capability for oxygen delivery relative to tissue oxygen requirements. It is

unnecessary to administer iron during this period, because it does not prevent the physiologic decrease in hemoglobin, and any iron administered is added to stores for future use. As hypoxia is detected by renal or hepatic oxygen sensors, erythropoietin production increases and erythropoiesis resumes. The iron previously stored in reticuloendothelial tissues can then be used for hemoglobin synthesis and is typically sufficient for hemoglobin synthesis, even in the absence of dietary iron intake, until approximately 20 weeks of age. In fact, the American Academy of Pediatrics recommendation that any cow milk or soy formula used to supplement breast milk be iron-fortified has the goal of preventing the late iron deficiency that can occur when the shift is made to the typical cow's-milk–based, iron-poor diet of later infancy and toddlerhood (American Academy of Pediatrics, 1999).

Anemia of Prematurity

The physiologic anemia seen in preterm infants is more profound and occurs earlier (see Table 77-7). Because symptoms may occur, the anemia of prematurity is considered nonphysiologic. The cause of anemia is multifaceted. The lower hemoglobin may be in part a physiologic response to the lower oxygen consumption in premature infants compared with that in term infants, a consequence of their diminished metabolic oxygen needs (Mestyan et al, 1964). An important component in the first few weeks of life is blood loss due to sampling for the many laboratory tests necessary to stabilize the clinical status of these infants, particularly those with cardiorespiratory problems. The erythropoietic response to anemia also is suboptimal, a significant problem because demands on erythropoiesis are heightened by the short survival of the RBCs of premature infants (approximately 40 to 60 days instead of 120 days as in adults) and the rapid expansion of the RBC mass that accompanies growth. The basis for suboptimal erythropoiesis in prematurity appears to be inadequate synthesis of erythropoietin in response to hypoxia. Figure 77-14 illustrates the magnitude of the deficiency, which, as shown by Stockman et al (1984), is greatest in the smallest, least mature infants. Because the liver is the predominant source of erythropoietin during fetal life, it has been proposed that relative insensitivity of the hepatic oxygen sensor to hypoxia explains the blunted

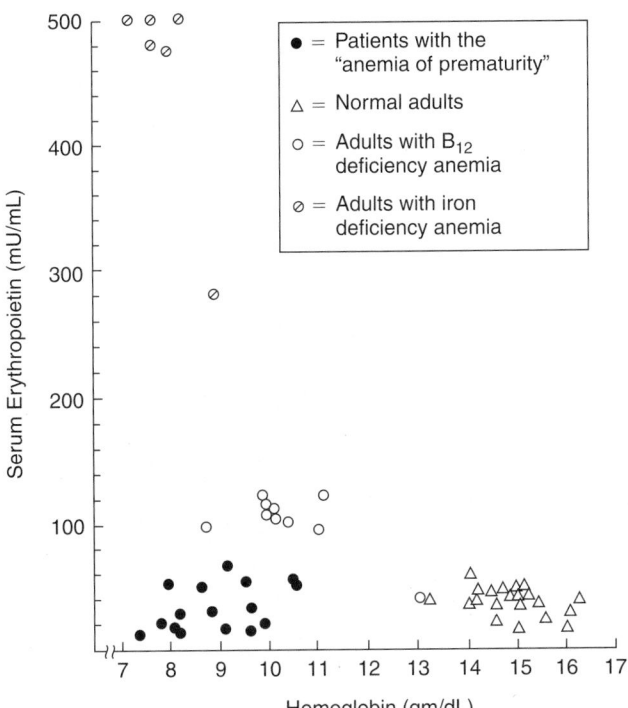

FIGURE 77-14 **Hemoglobin levels and corresponding serum erythropoietin levels are shown.** Values are from infants with the anemia of prematurity, normal adults, adults with vitamin B_{12} deficiency anemia, and adults with iron deficiency anemia. *(From Ross MP, Christensen RD, Rothstein G, et al: A randomized trial to develop criteria for administering erythrocyte transfusions to anemic preterm infants 1 to 3 months of age,* J Perinatol *9:246-253, 1989. Reprinted by permission of Appleton & Lange, Inc.)*

erythropoietin response seen in premature infants (Dallman, 1993). The spontaneous resolution of the anemia that occurs by approximately 40 weeks' gestational age is in keeping with a developmental switch from the relatively insensitive hepatic oxygen sensor to the renal oxygen sensor, which is exquisitely sensitive to hypoxia, because by this time the predominant site of erythropoietin synthesis has shifted to the kidneys. The problem does not lie with altered sensitivity of erythroid progenitors to erythropoietin because this has been shown to be normal (Shannon et al, 1987).

The anemia of prematurity occurs even in nutritionally replete infants, but it may be heightened by deficiencies of folate, vitamin B_{12}, or vitamin E (Worthington-White et al, 1994). Premature infants are endowed at birth with significantly less vitamin E than is present in term infants, and unless supplemental vitamin E is provided, this deficiency state persists for 2 to 3 months. Vitamin E is an antioxidant compound vital to the integrity of erythrocytes, and in its absence, these cells are susceptible to lipid peroxidation and membrane injury. One clinical consequence of vitamin E deficiency is that hemolytic anemia can occur in small premature infants (weighing less than 1500 g) at 6 to 10 weeks of age (Oski and Barness, 1967; Ritchie et al, 1968). This hemolytic anemia, which is characterized by reduced vitamin E levels and increased RBC peroxide hemolysis, rapidly disappears following vitamin E administration. A logical conclusion is that vitamin E deficiency might contribute to the anemia of prematurity in a more general sense. In fact, premature infants given

daily vitamin E (15 IU/day) had higher hemoglobin levels and lower reticulocyte levels than a control group not given the vitamin (Oski and Barness, 1967). However, more recent studies found no hematologic benefit for the administration of 25 IU or 50 IU of vitamin E daily to premature infants (Pathak et al, 2003; Zipursky et al, 1987). A recent Cochrane review of the use of vitamin E in preterm infants suggested that routine vitamin E supplementation increased the hemoglobin concentration by a significant but small amount (Brion et al, 2003). In very low-birthweight infants, there was a decreased risk of retinopathy and blindness but increased risk of sepsis. This review concludes that the routine use of high-dose intravenous vitamin E, or to achieve tocopherol levels greater than 3.5 mg/dL, is not supported by evidence. Although it has become standard practice to administer vitamin E to all premature infants, the hemoglobin nadir in these babies is still lower than that in term newborns, indicating that anemia is largely caused by other factors such as erythropoietin deficiency.

The optimum management of anemia of prematurity requiring intervention beyond nutritional and vitamin support remains controversial (Bishara and Ohls, 2009; Strauss, 2006; Von Kohorn and Ehrenhranz, 2009). Primary questions include the role of erythropoietin and the application of liberal versus restrictive transfusion thresholds.

TREATMENT OF ANEMIA OF PREMATURITY WITH RECOMBINANT HUMAN ERYTHROPOIETIN

Because a relative deficiency of erythropoietin is present in the anemia of prematurity, a number of studies have evaluated the safety and efficacy of rHuEPO therapy in this setting. The optimal timing for initiation of rHuEPO therapy and the optimal dose have yet to be determined. Trials have used two different timing strategies: early treatment (before 8 days of age) and "late" treatment. The former has the goal of preventing anemia of prematurity, whereas the latter aims to treat anemia of prematurity and decrease transfusions after the acute stage. Although many studies have shown a modest decrease in RBC transfusion with either approach, there have not been significant differences between these two practices (Aher and Ohlsson, 2006; Kotto-Kome et al, 2004). Although infants require relatively high doses of rHuEPO/kg compared to adults because of more rapid clearance and higher volume of distribution, a trial of high dose (1500 unit/kg/wk) as compared to low dose (750 u/kg/wk) resulted in no difference in transfusion requirement (Maier et al, 1998). Even in very small premature infants (less than 1300 g birthweight) with the highest likelihood of needing a transfusion, the effects are minimal, except in infants with birthweight <1000 g. (Meyer et al, 2003). To optimize response to rHuEPO, infants must have adequate protein intake, receive vitamin E, and receive iron supplementation. To achieve the best results, supplemental oral iron at a dose of at least 6 to 9 mg/kg per day needs to be administered. It may be possible to use parenteral iron supplements, particularly in young very low-birthweight infants who are not able to take oral iron (Heese et al, 1990) or as a supplement to oral iron (Pollak et al, 2001).

A metaanalysis of 21 prospective controlled trials of rHuEPO treatment of the anemia of prematurity was published (Vamvakas and Strauss, 2001). Although there was considerable variation between studies, in general the efficacy of rHuEPO in reducing the need for red cell transfusions was modest. The authors concluded that it was premature to recommend rHuEPO for standard therapy for the anemia of prematurity. Given the current standard of using dedicated RBC-unit transfusion strategies, a modest rHuEPO effect is less likely to decrease the chance of exposure to multiple blood donors; in that case, the reduction of mL/kg/patient transfused or number of transfusions is less important. At this point, there is wide variation in the use of rHuEPO for very low-birthweight infants in the United States (Von Kohorn and Ehrenkranz, 2009). There is disagreement regarding the cost-benefit ratio of rHuEPO therapy (Maier et al, 1994; Shireman et al, 1994; Wandstrat and Kaplan, 1995; Zipursky, 2000).

Although recent studies in adults have raised questions about the safety of rHuEPO and have led to reductions in its use in patients with malignancy and with renal insufficiency, there are no definitive data supporting safety concerns in premature infants. Previous questions regarding neutropenia and retinopathy of prematurity have not been borne out as significant. In fact, recent interest in potential neuroprotective effects of rHuEPO has led to careful testing of three different high doses of rHuEPO in extremely low-birthweight infants ≤1000 g and ≤28 weeks of age (Juul et al, 2008). Erythropoietin treatment may have a particularly important role to play in the management of infants whose parents refuse to allow blood transfusions on religious grounds (Davis et al, 1991).

RED BLOOD CELL TRANSFUSION THERAPY IN PREMATURE INFANTS

As recently as 1991, it was estimated that of the approximately 38,000 infants born weighing less than 1500 g in the United States each year, 80% received multiple RBC transfusions (Strauss, 1991). Most transfusions given in the first several weeks of life are to replace losses from phlebotomy required for laboratory monitoring during ventilator support and other intensive care measures. After the first few weeks of life, most transfusions are given to treat the symptoms of anemia of prematurity. The risks associated with use of allogeneic RBC transfusion in premature infants include exposure to viral infections, graft-versus-host disease, electrolyte and acid-base imbalances, exposure to plasticizers, hemolysis when T antigen activation of RBCs has occurred, and immunosuppression (Strauss, 1991).

Many strategies to reduce the need for allogeneic RBC transfusion in premature infants have been developed and have resulted in a marked decrease in the number of transfusions and number of donor exposures for most premature infants. Reducing phlebotomy losses by use of noninvasive monitoring techniques has been of only limited usefulness (Strauss, 1991). Donor exposures can be reduced by assigning a specified bag of adult donor blood to a sick neonate for multiple transfusions (Cook et al, 1993), particularly because it has been shown that blood stored for up to 35 days in CPDA-1 (Liu et al, 1994) or AS-3 (Goldman et al, 2001; Strauss et al, 2000) is safe for

use in this setting. Defining strict criteria for RBC transfusions also can reduce the number of donor exposures in routine nursery practice (Batton et al, 1992; Maier et al, 2000). Traditionally, RBC transfusions have been given to replace phlebotomy losses or in the presence of symptoms thought to reflect hypoxia (e.g., tachycardia, tachypnea, dyspnea, apneic spells, poor feeding) (Oski and Naiman, 1982; Wardrop et al, 1978). However, studies to validate such practices have yielded conflicting results. Stockman and Clark (1984) showed a beneficial effect of transfusion on weight gain, but no benefit was found by Blank et al (1984). Similarly, apneic spells were reduced in frequency following RBC transfusion in some studies (Joshi et al, 1987; Ross et al, 1989) but not others (Bifano et al, 1992; Blank et al, 1984; Keyes et al, 1989). Lachance et al (1994) measured oxygen consumption, myocardial function, resting energy expenditure, and other physiologic variables before and after RBC transfusions. They concluded that in asymptomatic anemic premature infants, oxygenation was well maintained without RBC transfusions when the hemoglobin level was 6.5 g/dL or more. Nelle et al (1994) studied a similar group of asymptomatic anemic premature infants and found that RBC transfusion improved systemic oxygen transport as well as transport in the cerebral and gastrointestinal arteries. When clinical features of hypoxia are absent or findings are equivocal, an elevated blood lactate level may predict a need for transfusion (Izraeli et al, 1993) but in the experience of Frey and Losa (2001) adds little value to the decision-making process in the individual patient. At present, most neonatal intensive care units have abandoned earlier practices of automatically replacing phlebotomy losses in favor of transfusing for clear-cut symptoms of hypoxia or for significant anemia unaccompanied by evidence of an adequate erythropoietic response (Alagappan et al, 1998; Engelfriet and Reesink, 2001).

The question of optimum guidelines for transfusion in preterm infants has been studied in two important prospective randomized clinical trials comparing liberal (high) and restrictive (low) transfusion thresholds (Table 77-8). The Iowa study enrolled 100 infants with birthweights of 500 to 1300 g, using either liberal or restricted transfusion thresholds, with thresholds depending on need for respiratory support (Bell et al, 2005). The PINT Canadian study enrolled 451 infants under 1000 g; transfusion thresholds were different for infants requiring respiratory support or not, and changed for 1st, 2nd, and 3rd to 4th weeks of life (Kirpalani et al, 2005).

In the Iowa study, only 10% to 12% of patients required transfusions. The restrictive group received fewer transfusions (3.3±2.9) as compared to the liberal group (5.2±4.5), but the number of donor exposures was similar (2.8±2.5 for liberal group, 2.2±2.0 for restrictive group). There was more apnea in the restricted transfusion group. In addition, although the study was not designed to detect a difference in CNS outcome, there was a higher rate of grade IV intraventricular hemorrhage (IVH) and periventricular leukomalacia in the restricted group.

In the Canadian study, 89% to 95% of infants received at least one transfusion, and the number of transfusions per infant was not significantly different, 4.9 versus 5.7. There was no difference between groups for primary endpoint for the PINT study, which was a composite of death before discharge or survival with bronchopulmonary dysplasia, severe retinopathy, or brain injury on cranial ultrasound. This study had smaller, sicker infants with 70% to 74% suffering the composite primary endpoint, so it was difficult to discern possible differences between the liberal and restrictive groups. In a follow-up report (Whyte et al, 2009), an assessment of preplanned secondary neurologic outcomes did not show a difference between groups, though the liberal transfusion group had a lower rate of cognitive delay when redefined as a Mental Development Index <85 in post hoc analysis.

A recent analysis of these two studies (Strauss, 2008) noted that the lack of difference in number of RBC transfusions in the Canadian trial likely reflected the relatively small differences in transfusion triggers between the two groups, and also that transfusions for clinical indications, rather than hematocrit thresholds, made up 16% of all transfusions in that study. However, the apparent higher rate of IVH and periventricular leukomalacia in the restrictive group in the Iowa study certainly raises the potential impact of a low transfusion threshold and resulting low hematocrit on the immature central nervous system. In a study of 25 preterm infants (Kissack, 2004), high cerebral fractional oxygen extraction was associated with intraventricular hemorrhage and/or hemorrhagic parenchymal infarction. The potential for a higher blood hemoglobin content and/or blood volume and cardiovascular stability to improve oxygen delivery to tissues and decrease rates of IVH is supported by the lower rate of IVH (14%) in infants <32 weeks undergoing delayed umbilical cord clamping as compared with 35% in those undergoing immediate clamping (Mercer et al, 2006).

Thus, the optimum transfusion threshold for preterm infants remains uncertain, especially with respect to neurologic sequelae. Strauss concludes that the potential risk of using very restrictive transfusion guidelines may be greater than the risk of more frequent transfusions, especially given the availability of "single-donor" transfusion practices that limit exposures to multiple blood donors (Strauss, 2008). He thus recommends following conventional transfusion guidelines, which are generally liberal, while stressing the need to continue to study these questions. In particular, there is a need for a prospective clinical trial of transfusion thresholds that is designed to determine whether liberal RBC transfusions may have a neuroprotective effect.

Despite controversies, there is agreement that the optimum approach to the anemia of prematurity includes delayed clamping of the umbilical cord (at least 30 seconds) (Rabe et al, 2009); limiting blood loss by phlebotomy; use of dedicated red blood cell units to minimize donor exposure; optimizing nutrition including protein, iron, folate, vitamin B_{12}, and vitamin E; and use of standardized transfusion guidelines.

POLYCYTHEMIA

Neonatal polycythemia usually is caused by one of two conditions: increased intrauterine erythropoiesis or fetal hypertransfusion (Table 77-9). Other causes seen in older children, such as arterial hypoxemia (cyanotic heart disease, pulmonary disease), abnormal hemoglobins, or hypersecretion of erythropoietin by tumors, are rare, and primary polycythemia or polycythemia vera is virtually nonexistent. In normal term infants, delayed clamping of the cord leading to an increased transfer of placental blood to the infant is the most common cause of polycythemia. In the setting of acute intrapartum hypoxia, increased placental transfusion also may account for the observed increase in fetal RBC mass, according to animal studies by Oh et al (1975). Placental insufficiency and chronic intrauterine hypoxia, as seen typically in small-for-gestational-age infants, most commonly underlie increased intrauterine erythropoiesis.

As the hematocrit increases, blood viscosity increases exponentially (Figure 77-15). Blood flow is impaired by hyperviscosity at hematocrits of 60% or more. Oxygen transport, which is determined by both hemoglobin levels (i.e., oxygen-binding capacity) and blood flow, is maximal in the normal hematocrit range. At low hematocrits, oxygen transport is limited by reduced oxygen-binding

TABLE 77-8 Comparison of Iowa and Canadian Prospective Randomized Trials for Premature Infants: Transfusion Thresholds (Triggers)

		Iowa Trial		Canadian Trial (PINT)	
		Liberal*	Restrictive*	Liberal†	Restrictive†
Mechanical ventilation	≤7 days	46%	34%	41%	35%
	8–14 days			36%	30%
	≥15 days			30%	26%
CPAP or nasal O_2	≤7 days	38%	28%	41%	35%
	8–14 days			36%	30%
	≥15 days			30%	26%
No respiratory support	≤7 days	30%	22%	36%	30%
	8–14 days			30%	26%
	≥15 days			26%	23%

CPAP, Continuous positive airway pressure; *Hct*, hematocrit; *RBC*, red blood cell.
*Hct threshold prompting RBC transfusion.
†Hct threshold, calculated as 3 × the hemoglobin in g/dL, prompting RBC transfusion.
Adapted from Strauss RG: Commentary: is it safe to limit allogeneic red blood cell transfusions to neonates? *Neonatology* 93:217-222, 2008.

capacity, whereas at higher hematocrits, reduction in blood flow secondary to hyperviscosity may similarly limit oxygen transport. At any given hematocrit, expansion of the blood volume beyond the normal level (hypervolemia) distends the vasculature, decreases peripheral resistance, and increases blood flow and, ultimately, oxygen transport. These physiologic observations have implications for therapy of polycythemia.

Most polycythemic infants have no symptoms, particularly if the polycythemia becomes apparent only on routine neonatal screening. Symptoms, when present, usually are attributable to hyperviscosity and poor tissue perfusion or to associated metabolic abnormalities such as hypoglycemia and hypocalcemia. Common early signs and symptoms include plethora, cyanosis (resulting from peripheral stasis), lethargy, hypotonia, poor suck and feeding, and tremulousness. Serious complications include cardiorespiratory distress (with or without congestive heart failure),

seizures, peripheral gangrene, necrotizing enterocolitis, renal failure (occasionally resulting from renal vein thrombosis), and priapism. Because the elevated RBC mass increases the catabolism of hemoglobin, hyperbilirubinemia is common and gallstones occasionally occur.

In the symptomatic infant, a venous hematocrit of 65% or more (or a hemoglobin greater than 22 g/dL) confirms the presence of polycythemia. In screening apparently healthy newborns for polycythemia, however, account must be taken of a number of physiologic variables that influence the hematocrit during the first 12 hours of life:

1. Time of cord clamping—immediate clamping (within 30 seconds) minimizes placental transfusion.
2. Age at sampling—values increase from birth to a peak at 2 hours, gradually decreasing to cord levels around 12 to 18 hours (Ramamurthy and Berlanga, 1987; Shohat et al, 1984).
3. Site of sampling—values from blood extracted by the heelstick method exceed those from venous blood (the difference can be minimized by prewarming the heel).
4. Method of hematocrit determination—spun values are higher than those obtained by electronic cell counter and show better correlation with blood viscosity (Villalta et al, 1989).

One way to standardize and simplify screening for polycythemia is as follows: At birth, clamp the cord at about 30 to 45 seconds; at 4 to 6 hours of age, obtain a blood sample from a warmed heelstick and perform a spun hematocrit determination. If the result is greater than 70%, repeat the test on a venous sample. A venous hematocrit of 65% or more indicates polycythemia. By this approach, 1% to 5% of newborns are polycythemic; the range largely reflects differences in altitude at which the study population resides. Because the hematocrit is lower with increasing prematurity, polycythemia is seen less frequently in preterm infants than in term babies.

Following diagnosis, an attempt should be made to determine the cause of polycythemia (see Table 77-9). The condition is particularly common in infants of diabetic mothers or those with Down syndrome (Mentzer, 1978) and may also occur in the setting of maternal hypertension (Kurlat and Sola, 1992) or, rarely, fumaric aciduria (Kerrigan et al, 2000). However, no apparent cause is found in most cases. Studies to determine the effects of polycythemia are dictated by the clinical findings but should usually

TABLE 77-9 Etiology of Neonatal Polycythemia

Active (Increased Intrauterine Erythropoiesis)	Passive (Secondary to Erythrocyte Transfusions)
Intrauterine hypoxia	Delayed cord clamping
Placental insufficiency	Intentional
Small-for-gestational-age infant	Unassisted delivery
Postmaturity	Maternofetal transfusion
Toxemia of pregnancy	Twin-twin transfusion
Drugs (propranolol)	
Severe maternal heart disease	
Maternal smoking	
Maternal diabetes	
Neonatal hyperthyroidism or hypothyroidism	
Congenital adrenal hyperplasia	
Chromosome abnormalities	
Trisomy 13	
Trisomy 18	
Trisomy 21 (Down syndrome)	
Hyperplastic visceromegaly (Beckwith syndrome)	
Decreased fetal erythrocyte deformability	

Data from Oski FA, Naiman JL: *Hematologic problems in the newborn*, ed 3, Philadelphia, 1982, WB Saunders.

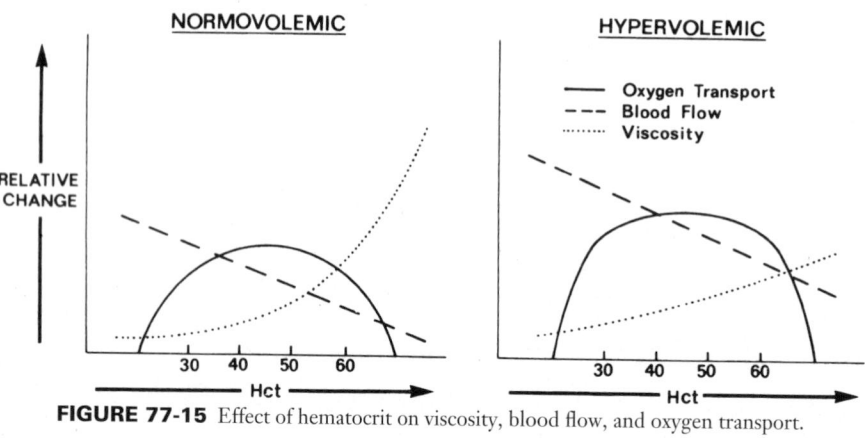

FIGURE 77-15 Effect of hematocrit on viscosity, blood flow, and oxygen transport.

include serum bilirubin, glucose, calcium, urea nitrogen, and creatinine levels.

Treatment by isovolumetric partial exchange transfusion (PET) is recommended to reduce the RBC mass without inducing hypovolemia. However, the precise indications for PET and the impact of the procedure on outcome have been questioned. In a review of randomized or quasirandomized studies of infants with symptomatic or asymptomatic polycythemia (Dempsey and Barrington, 2006), there was no evidence of difference in either long-term neurodevelopmental outcome or short-term neurobehavioral scores. There was a trend toward an earlier improvement in symptoms, but an apparent increase in risk of necrotizing enterocolitis (relative risk 8.68, 95% confidence interval 1.06 to 71.1), although several of the studies used fresh frozen plasma. The general finding that polycythemic infants have a poorer outcome than concurrent infants without polycythemia has been thought to be related to the underlying cause of the polycythemia; in one study, perinatal risk factors other than polycythemia were best correlated with outcome and thought to underlie both the polycythemia and the developmental delay (Bada et al, 1992).

Many neonatal intensive care units use PET for symptomatic infants with hematocrits greater than 60% to 65%, and for asymptomatic infants with hematocrits greater than 65% to 70%. However, the Committee on the Fetus and Newborn of the American Academy of Pediatrics acknowledged in their 1993 statement that "there is no evidence that exchange transfusion affects long term outcome. ... Universal screening for polycythemia fails to meet the methodology and treatment criteria and also, possibly the natural history criterion." Thus, Schimmel et al (2004) made the following recommendations based on the available evidence, until such time as systematic studies can be conducted directly measuring blood viscosity to allow development of objective criteria for PET in polycythemia:

- In symptomatic patients with hematocrit >65%, PET with normal saline should be used to reduce possible ongoing injury to tissues by enhancing blood flow.
- In asymptomatic polycythemic infants with presumed normal or increased blood volume, careful monitoring (glucose, cardiorespiratory) is adequate.
- In infants with presumed reduced plasma or blood volume status, treat with early feeding or intravenous fluids.
- For asymptomatic polycythemic infants with presumed normal blood and plasma volume, consider PET only if repeated venous hematocrits are >75%.

Systematic reviews of several studies comparing the use of crystalloid or colloid for PET have concluded that crystalloid solutions are as effective as colloid solutions (Dempsey and Barrington, 2005; de Waal et al, 2006). Thus, normal saline, as an inexpensive product that carries no risk of transfusion-associated infection or reaction to plasma proteins, should be used. Withdrawal of blood for a partial exchange transfusion is most easily done using an umbilical artery catheter. Any vessel may be used for blood withdrawal, and all but arterial lines can be used to infuse volume. An umbilical venous catheter inserted into the right atrium also provides acceptable access, but if correct placement cannot be achieved, the catheter should be inserted just far enough into the vessel to allow blood to be withdrawn. Calculation of the total volume of blood to be exchanged for diluent uses the following formula (Oski and Naiman, 1982):

$$\text{Exchange volume} = \frac{\substack{\text{observed Hct} - \text{desired Hct} \times \\ \text{BV (mL/kg)} \times \text{weight (kg)}}}{\text{observed Hct}}$$

where blood volume (BV) usually is 100 mL/kg but in infants of diabetic mothers may be lower (80 to 85 mL/kg).

Example: A 3-kg dyspneic infant with an 80% hematocrit requires a partial exchange transfusion.

$$\text{Blood volume} = 3 \text{ kg} \times 100 \text{ mL/kg} = 300 \text{ mL}$$

$$\frac{\text{observed Hct} - \text{desired Hct}}{\text{observed Hct}} = \frac{80 - 55}{80} = 0.31$$

Therefore, volume of exchange = 300 mL × 0.31 = 93 mL.

Because coexisting hypoglycemia is an important determinant of adverse neurologic outcome, careful monitoring and maintenance of adequate glucose levels and hydration are essential.

METHEMOGLOBINEMIA

Methemoglobin (metHb) is an oxidized derivative of hemoglobin in which heme iron is in the ferric (Fe^{3+}) or oxidized state rather than the ferrous (Fe^{2+}) or reduced state. Because methemoglobin is unable to bind (or release) oxygen, the presence of significant amounts of metHb adversely affects oxygen transport. Small amounts of methemoglobin normally are formed daily, associated with the release of oxygen from hemoglobin (auto-oxidation). The metHb that is formed rapidly is reduced through the action of RBC NADH-methemoglobin reductase (also known as cytochrome b_5 reductase), so that in normal persons, levels of metHb seldom exceed 1%. A second methemoglobin reductase, dependent on NADPH as cofactor, also is present in RBCs. This enzyme has little function under normal physiologic conditions, but it is greatly activated by the presence of certain redox compounds such as methylene blue, forming the basis for the clinical treatment of methemoglobinemia.

Acquired methemoglobinemia can occur in normal individuals following exposure to chemicals that oxidize hemoglobin iron. Newborns are particularly susceptible because fetal hemoglobin is more readily oxidized to the ferric state than is hemoglobin A and because RBC NADH-methemoglobin reductase activity is low during the first few months of life. Merely marking the diapers of newborns with aniline dyes has caused methemoglobinemia. Drugs such as prilocaine, administered before birth to provide local anesthesia, can produce methemoglobinemia in both mother and infant. Although in most infants, no increase in methemoglobin levels follows the use of lidocaine-prilocaine cream (Emla Cream) to provide analgesia during circumcision (Taddio et al, 1997), a few case reports of visible cyanosis due to methemoglobinemia in infants treated with this cream have appeared (Couper, 2000; Tse et al, 1995). Perhaps the best-known agent that may cause methemoglobinemia is nitrite, either present de novo in ingested material or generated by administering nitric oxide to term babies in high concentrations for treatment of persistent pulmonary hypertension (Davidson et al, 1998). Nitrates can be converted to nitrite by the action of intestinal bacteria. It is for this reason that well water or foods with a high nitrate content (e.g., cabbage, spinach, beets, carrots) can produce methemoglobinemia in infants (Keating et al, 1973). Accumulation of nitrate in the intestinal tracts of infants with diarrhea and acidosis (Kay et al, 1990; Yano et al, 1982) or symptomatic dietary protein intolerance (Murray and Christie, 1993) is thought to underlie the transient methemoglobinemia that occurs in these conditions.

Congenital methemoglobinemia is due to inherited disorders of hemoglobin structure or to a severe deficiency of NADH methemoglobin reductase activity. The inherited abnormalities of hemoglobin structure that give rise to methemoglobinemia, known collectively as the hemoglobin M disorders, are rare autosomal-dominant defects caused by point mutations that alter a single amino acid in the structure of normal globin. The altered conformation that ensues favors the persistence of the ferric rather than the ferrous form of heme iron. The normal methemoglobin reductive capacity of the RBC cannot compensate for such instability of ferrous heme. Two of the mutations affect the alpha globin chain, three affect the beta globin chain, and two affect the gamma chain. Only the alpha and gamma globin chain mutations are associated with neonatal methemoglobinemia, because these are the globins that form hemoglobin F. Neonatal methemoglobinemia is transient when produced by one of the two gamma chain mutations, hemoglobin FM–Osaka (Hayashi et al, 1980) or hemoglobin FM–Fort Ripley (Priest et al, 1989), because the normal developmental switch from fetal to adult hemoglobin eliminates all but a trace of the mutant hemoglobin. Hemoglobin M heterozygotes inheriting alpha or beta globin mutations have lifelong cyanosis, but they are usually asymptomatic. No therapy is needed (and none is possible). The homozygous state is incompatible with life. Diagnosis of the hemoglobin M disorders is made by special tests in RBC diagnostic laboratories.

NADH-methemoglobin reductase deficiency is a rare autosomal recessive disorder. Heterozygotes are asymptomatic and do not have methemoglobinemia under normal circumstances. However, if challenged by drugs or chemicals that cause methemoglobinemia, heterozygous deficient patients may become cyanotic and symptomatic at doses that have no effect in normal persons. Homozygotes have lifelong methemoglobin levels of 15% to 40% and are cyanotic but otherwise asymptomatic unless exposed to toxic agents. Diagnosis of NADH-methemoglobin reductase deficiency is by assay of RBC enzyme activity, a procedure available only in specialized hematology laboratories.

The cardinal clinical manifestation of methemoglobinemia is cyanosis not resulting from cardiac or respiratory disease. Cyanosis present at birth suggests hereditary methemoglobinemia, whereas that appearing suddenly in an otherwise asymptomatic infant is more consistent with acquired methemoglobinemia (Box 77-3). The blood is

---

BOX 77-3 Approach to Infants With Cyanosis and Methemoglobinemia

CYANOSIS WITH RESPIRATORY AND CARDIAC ABNORMALITIES:

Blood turns red when mixed with air
Decreased arterial P_{O_2}
Consider pulmonary, cardiac, or central nervous system disease

CYANOSIS WITH OR WITHOUT RESPIRATORY OR CARDIAC ABNORMALITIES:

Blood turns red when mixed with air
Normal arterial P_{O_2}
Consider polycythemia syndromes

CYANOSIS WITHOUT RESPIRATORY OR CARDIAC ABNORMALITIES:

Blood remains dark after mixing with air
Normal arterial P_{O_2}
Consider methemoglobinemia syndromes
1. With rapid clearing of methemoglobin following methylene blue:
   a. Consider toxic methemoglobinemia (look for environmental oxidants)
   b. Consider NADH-methemoglobin reductase deficiency (perform enzyme assay)
2. With reappearance of methemoglobinemia after initial response to methylene blue:
   a. Consider NADH-methemoglobin reductase deficiency
3. With no change in methemoglobin following methylene blue:
   a. Consider hemoglobin M disorders (perform hemoglobin electrophoresis)
   b. Consider associated glucose-6-phosphate dehydrogenase deficiency (perform enzyme assay)

---

dark and, unlike deoxygenated venous blood, does not turn red when exposed to air. Rapid screening for methemoglobinemia can be done by placing a drop of blood on filter paper and then waving the filter paper in air to allow the blood to dry. Deoxygenated normal hemoglobin turns red, whereas methemoglobin remains brown. Methemoglobin levels of 10% or more can be detected (Harley and Celermajer, 1970). More accurate determination of methemoglobin levels is accomplished in the blood gas laboratory by co-oximetry or in the clinical laboratory using a spectrophotometer. Cyanosis is first clinically evident when methemoglobin levels reach approximately 10% (1.5 g/dL), but symptoms attributable to hypoxemia and diminished oxygen transport do not appear until levels increase to 30% to 40% of total hemoglobin. Death occurs at levels of 70% or greater. Methemoglobinemia is not associated with anemia, hemolysis, or other hematologic abnormalities.

Treatment with intravenous methylene blue (1 mg/kg as a 1% solution in normal saline) is indicated when methemoglobin levels are greater than 15% to 20%. Doses greater than 1 mg/kg should be avoided, because they may be toxic (Porat et al, 1996). The response to methylene blue is both therapeutic and diagnostic. Methemoglobin levels decrease rapidly, within 1 to 2 hours, if methemoglobinemia is caused by a toxic agent or by a deficiency of NADH-methemoglobin reductase. In contrast, the hemoglobin M disorders do not respond to methylene blue. Reappearance of methemoglobinemia after an initial response to methylene blue suggests a deficiency of

NADH-methemoglobin reductase or the persistence of an occult oxidant. A poor response to methylene blue also is seen in G6PD-deficient persons because this disorder is characterized by suboptimal generation of NADPH, a required cofactor in the reduction of methemoglobin by methylene blue in deficient persons. In general, most infants with hereditary methemoglobinemia are asymptomatic and require no therapy.

Controversy Box

1. The use of erythropoietin in premature infants. Given the use of dedicated RBC-unit strategies, a modest rHuEPO effect is less likely to decrease the chance of exposure to multiple blood donors. There is wide variation in the use of rHuEPO for very low-birthweight infants in the United States, and disagreement regarding the cost-benefit ratio of rHuEPO therapy.

2. The optimum transfusion threshold for premature infants. Recent prospective randomized studies comparing liberal (high) and restrictive (low) transfusion thresholds were designed differently and came to different conclusions regarding outcomes. However, concerns were raised regarding the potential impact of a restrictive threshold and low hematocrit on the developing central nervous system.

3. The appropriate indications for partial exchange transfusion for infants with polycythemia. In a review of randomized or quasirandomized studies of infants with symptomatic or asymptomatic polycythemia, there was no difference in either long-term neurodevelopmental outcome or short-term neurobehavioral scores.

SUGGESTED READINGS

Bell EF, Strauss RG, Widness JA, et al: Randomized trial of liberal versus restrictive guidelines for red blood cell transfusion in preterm infants, *Pediatrics* 115:1685-1691, 2005.

Dempsey EM, Barrington K: Crystalloid or colloid for partial exchange transfusion in neonatal polycythemia: a systematic review and meta-analysis, *Acta Paediatr* 94:1650-1655, 2005.

Kirpalani H, Whyte RK, Andersen C, et al: The Premature Infants in Need of Transfusion (PINT) study: a randomized, controlled trial of a restrictive (low) versus liberal (high) transfusion threshold for extremely low birth weight infants, *J Pediatr* 149:310-317, 2006.

Lopriore E, Oepkes D: Fetal and neonatal haematological complications in monochorionic twins, *Semin Fetal Neonatal Med* 13:231-238, 2008.

Mercer JS, Vohn BR, McGrath MM, et al: Delayed cord clamping in very preterm infants reduces the incidence of intraventricular hemorrhage and late-onset sepsis: a randomized, controlled trial, *Pediatrics* 111:1235-1242, 2006.

Moise KJ: Management of Rhesus alloimmunization in pregnancy, *Obstet Gynecol* 112:164-176, 2008.

Orkin SH, Zon LI: Hematopoiesis: an evolving paradigm for stem cell biology, *Cell* 132:631-644, 2008.

Strauss RG: Controversies in the management of the anemia of prematurity using single-donor red blood cell transfusions and/or recombinant human erythropoietin, *Transfus Med Rev* 20:34-44, 2006.

Von Kohorn I, Ehrenkranz RA: Anemia in the preterm infant: erythropoietin versus erythrocyte transfusion: it's not that simple, *Clin Perinatol* 36:111-123, 2009.

Complete references and supplemental color images used in this text can be found online at www.expertconsult.com

NEONATAL LEUKOCYTE PHYSIOLOGY AND DISORDERS

Evan B. Shereck, Carmella van de Ven, and Mitchell S. Cairo

This chapter presents an overview of neonatal leukocyte physiology and quantitative and qualitative disorders of leukocytes. Topics include the normal physiology and defects associated with neonatal hematopoiesis, neutrophils, lymphocytes, monocytes, dendritic cells, and natural killer cells. Novel therapeutic approaches also are discussed.

HEMATOPOIESIS

Hematopoiesis is a complex process that begins with an uncommitted pluripotent hematopoietic stem cell that progresses through a series of steps to development of a single-lineage progenitor cell. The final result of this physiologic process is a mature, lineage-restricted effector cell that circulates either in the bloodstream or within tissue. In 1961, Till and McCulloch demonstrated that when bone marrow cells were transfused into lethally irradiated mice, separate colonies of hematopoietic cells could be identified in the spleen of the recipient. Each colony, containing neutrophils, monocytes, erythrocytes, megakaryocytes, eosinophils, and basophils, was derived from an individual cell, and many of the colonies contained cells that were capable of such colony formation when transplanted into a second irradiated animal. Such cells, which are capable of unlimited self-renewal, have been referred to as *pluripotent stem cells*.

FETAL AND NEONATAL HEMATOPOIESIS

In human ontogeny, the process of hematopoietic maturation involves the orderly shift of hematopoiesis from extramedullary organs to the bone marrow (Nathan, 1989). Hematopoietic cells are derived from the mesodermal layer of the blastula in embryogenesis. This layer contains undifferentiated, self-renewing cells that will migrate to different tissues, including blood. The first step towards hematopoietic maturation occurs when these hematopoietic cells migrate to the blood islands formed by the yolk sac by embryo day 15 (Zon, 1995). The erythrocytes are the predominant lineage during this time. Yolk sac erythrocytes are large nucleated cells, expressing the products of certain genes that are unique to this phase of development. Shortly after, the yolk sac develops single and multilineage myeloerythroid progenitor cells (Gekas, 2005). Although the yolk sac greatly expands the hematopoietic progenitor pool, these cells do not differentiate into mature blood cells (Palis et al, 1999). These progenitor cells then migrate from the yolk sac to the fetal liver (Zon, 1995). There are studies suggesting that hematopoietic progenitor cells from the aorto-gonado-mesonephron and placenta also contribute to fetal liver seeding (Gekas, 2005;

Zon, 1995). The fetal liver then becomes the main site of hematopoiesis until hematopoiesis relocates to the bone marrow perinatally (Ema and Nakauchi, 2000).

Granulocyte-macrophage colony-forming units (CFU-GMs) have been identified in the fetal liver as early as 5 weeks' gestation. However, their number is low compared with that of cells of the erythroid lineage. Myelopoiesis increases fourfold once hematopoiesis relocates to the bone marrow of the fetus at 14 weeks' gestation, but the myeloid cells remain comparatively limited (Kelemen et al, 1979). Myeloid cells (neutrophil progenitor cells) constitute less than 5% of nucleated marrow cells in the fetus, compared with 31% to 69% in term neonates and 25% to 52% in adults.

HEMATOPOIETIC GROWTH FACTORS

The regulation of hematopoiesis is a complex biologic process involving multifactorial mechanisms. As reported by our group (Abu-Ghosh et al, 2000), in vitro culture of hematopoietic progenitor cells has enabled the categorization, functional analysis, and definition of the growth factor requirements of the various committed progenitor cells (Figure 78-1).

The hematopoietic pluripotent stem cell (PPSC) that expresses CD34 represents an early and primitive hematopoietic stem cell that can be identified by immunophenotyping. This cell can either undergo self-renewal or proliferate and differentiate into any of the hematopoietic blood lineages depending on its exposure to individual and combinations of hematopoietic growth factors (HGFs). Primitive progenitor cells maintain their multipotent potential, whereas more mature progenitor cells become committed as they differentiate into specific lineages. A relatively small and common set of pluripotent stem cells gives rise to large numbers of functionally diverse mature cells.

Cell proliferation and differentiation is regulated and controlled by highly specific protein factors, affecting single- and multiple-lineage hematopoiesis. These growth-promoting factors are named colony-stimulating factors (CSFs). CSFs are a group of glycoproteins with molecular masses of 18 to 90 kDa, defined by their abilities to support proliferation and differentiation of hematopoietic cells of various lineages (see Figure 78-1).

GRANULOCYTE COLONY-STIMULATING FACTOR

Human granulocyte colony-stimulating factor (G-CSF) was first purified to homogeneity from a medium conditioned by the bladder carcinoma cell line 5637 (Welte

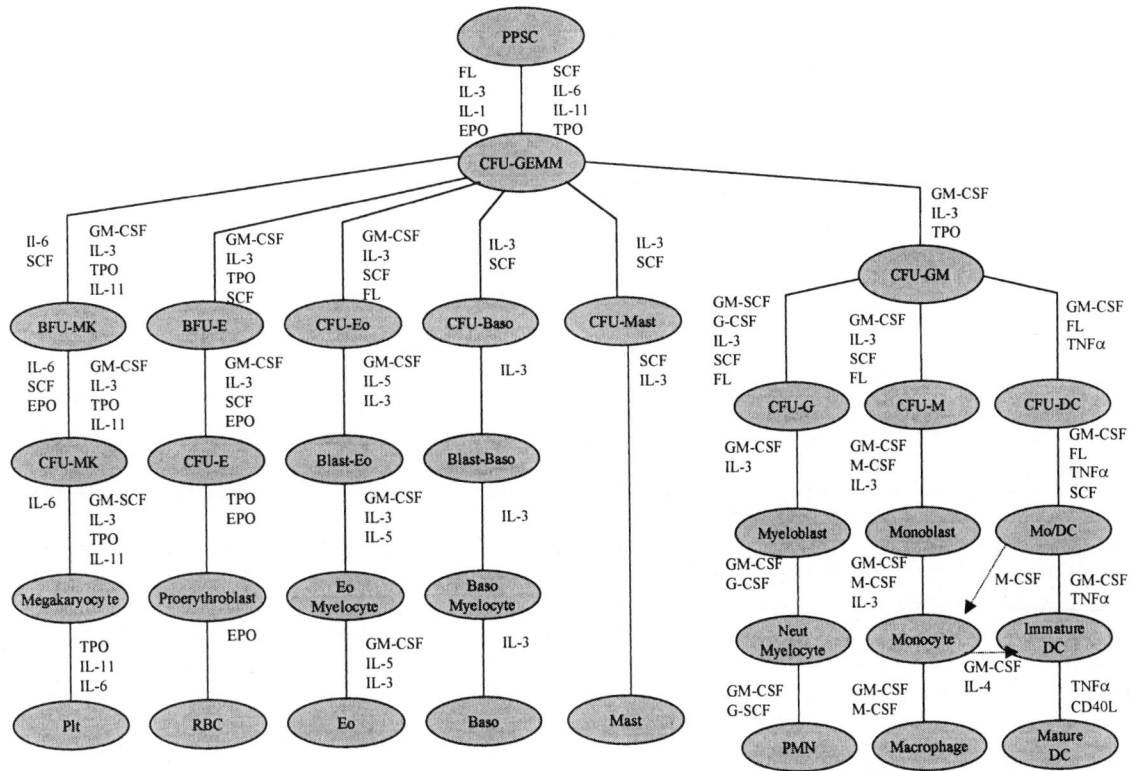

FIGURE 78-1 **Hematopoiesis and hematopoietic growth factors.** *Baso,* Basophil; *BFU,* burst-forming unit; *CFU,* colony-forming unit; *CSF,* colony-stimulating factor; *DC,* dendritic cell; *E,* erythroid; *Eo,* eosinophil; *EPO,* erythropoietin; *FL,* Flt 3 ligand; *G,* granulocyte; *GEMM,* granulocyte, erythrocyte, macrophage, and megakaryocyte; *GM,* granulocyte-macrophage; *IL,* interleukin; *M,* macrophage; *MK,* megakaryocyte; *Mo,* monocyte; *Neut,* neutrophil; *Plt,* platelet; *PMN,* polymorphonuclear neutrophil leukocyte; *PPSC,* pluripotent stem cell; *RBC,* red blood cell; *SCF,* stem cell factor; *TNFα,* tumor necrosis factor-α; *TPO,* thrombopoietin.

et al, 1985). The molecular mass of this glycoprotein is between 18 and 20 kDa, and the gene has been localized to chromosome 17q11-21. It has been identified in the 15-to-17 chromosomal translocation commonly found in acute promyelocytic leukemia. G-CSF is produced primarily by mature macrophages, endothelial cells, fibroblasts, and mesothelial cells. Its production can be stimulated in these cells by tumor necrosis factor, lipopolysaccharide (LPS), and the interleukins IL-1, IL-3, and IL-6 and also stem cell factor (SCF) (Lieschke and Burgess, 1992). G-CSF stimulates the proliferation of committed myeloid progenitor cells and has specific activity toward granulocyte colony formation with pure neutrophil colony proliferation. G-CSF affects mature neutrophil effector function in that it primes neutrophils to increase expression of chemotactic receptors and to enhance bactericidal and phagocytic activity, superoxide generation, antibody-dependent cellular cytotoxicity, and antiapoptotic prosurvival (Molloy et al, 2005).

Clinical studies have shown that G-CSF therapy results in a dose-dependent increase in the circulating neutrophil count in children and adults with congenital and acquired neutropenia syndromes as well as chemotherapy-induced neutropenia (Bonilla et al, 1989; Hammond et al, 1989). Significant differences in G-CSF production, G-CSF gene expression, and circulating G-CSF level exist between adults and newborns (Cairo et al, 1993). Gessler et al (1995) reported G-CSF serum levels at birth with respect to neutrophil count, infection, and gestational age. Serum concentrations of G-CSF in term and preterm neonates without infection reached peak levels within the first 7 hours of life (mean values of 261 pg/mL and 126 pg/mL in term and preterm infants, respectively). Levels decreased to normal adult range (<50 pg/mL) between 4 and 7 days of age and were unchanged at 2 to 3 weeks of age.

From neonatal animal model studies, it appears that the administration of recombinant human G-CSF (rhG-CSF) has significant effects on neonatal rat hematopoiesis, with a marked increase in the circulating neutrophil count, bone marrow myeloid progenitor pool, and neutrophil storage pool (NSP) (Cairo et al, 1990a). Combining G-CSF with earlier-acting cytokines such as SCF, IL-6, and IL-11 further enhances these effects on neonatal rat hematopoiesis (Cairo et al, 1991a, 1992a, 1993, 1994).

G-CSF acts synergistically with antibiotics to improve survival during neonatal sepsis, but only if given before or at the start of experimental sepsis (Cairo et al, 1990a, 1992b). Additionally, improved survival during experimental sepsis in neonatal rats has been demonstrated following prophylactic use of G-CSF in combination with antibiotics and either SCF or IL-11 (Cairo et al, 1992a, 1994; Chang et al, 1994).

G-CSF has been used in clinical trials for both prevention and therapy of neonatal sepsis. One study investigated the safety, pharmacokinetics, and biologic efficacy of administration of G-CSF to newborn infants with sepsis (Gillan et al, 1994). Forty-two newborn infants, both term and preterm, with presumed sepsis during the first 3 days of life were randomized to receive either placebo or varying doses of rhG-CSF. The growth factor was given for 3 days at doses of 1, 5, or 10 μg/kg every day or 5 or 10 μg/kg twice a day. The half-life of rhG-CSF was 4.4 ± 0.4 hours. Intravenous rhG-CSF was well tolerated at all gestational ages and was not associated with any recognized acute toxicity. RhG-CSF induced a significant increase in the absolute neutrophil count (ANC) within 24 hours following doses of 5 and 10 μg/kg given either every 24 hours or divided every 12 hours. The increased neutrophil count was maintained for 96 hours, 48 hours after the last rhG-CSF dose. Bone marrow aspirates demonstrated a dose-dependent increase in NSP following treatment with rhG-CSF. In addition, polymorphonuclear neutrophil (PMN) C3bi expression was significantly increased at 24 hours following administration of 10 μg/kg of rhG-CSF every 24 hours. The enhancement of neonatal neutrophil C3bi expression indicates that rhG-CSF may induce functional maturation of neonatal neutrophils. A 2-year follow-up analysis in these patients has shown that rhG-CSF therapy for presumed neonatal sepsis was not associated with long-term hematologic, immunologic, or developmental adverse effects (Rosenthal et al, 1996).

Several other clinical studies have evaluated the efficacy of G-CSF in neonates with presumed sepsis or neutropenia. A randomized, placebo-controlled trial of G-CSF administration to infants with neutropenia and clinical signs of early-onset sepsis was recently reported (Schibler et al, 1998). Twenty infants, term and preterm, were given G-CSF (10 μg/kg/day) or placebo for 3 days. Absolute neutrophil count (ANC), ratio of immature to total neutrophils (I/T ratio), bone marrow NSP, bone marrow neutrophil proliferative pool (NPP), and plasma concentration of G-CSF were evaluated and found to be similar in treated and control infants. No significant differences were found in outcome measures such as severity of illness and mortality.

Ahmad et al (2004) studied the outcome of 14 neutropenic very low-birthweight (VLBW) and preeclamptic neutropenic versus nonseptic neonates (gestational ages 24 to 30 weeks) similarly treated with G-CSF (10 μg/kg/day) for 3 days. They also assessed phagocytic and oxidative burst activity before and after treatment with rhG-CSF. Following rhG-CSF treatment the neutropenic neonates increased their ANC by >12-fold, whereas the nonneutropenic group increased their ANC by 2.6-fold. Further, septic neutropenic neonates showed greater oxidative burst activity but a lower phagocytic response compared to nonseptic neutropenic neonates (Ahmad et al, 2004).

A recent multicenter randomized placebo-controlled study evaluated prophylactic rG-CSF treatment of neutropenic premature neonates with recombinant G-CSF (Kuhn et al, 2009). Twenty-five neonatal intensive care units participated, treating neutropenic (<1500 neutrophils/mm^3) premature infants (≤32 weeks' gestation). The results of the study confirm that prophylactic rG-CSF had a modest effect on the reduction of the incidence of nosocomial infections. Although survival free of confirmed infection did not differ significantly between the rG-CSF and control groups, rG-CSF treated neonates had significantly greater survival without confirmed infection (84%

vs. 71%, p = 0.028, respectively), and survival free of any type of infection was also significantly greater in the rG-CSF treated group (69%) versus placebo controls (55%), p=0.049 (Kuhn et al, 2009).

GRANULOCYTE-MACROPHAGE COLONY-STIMULATING FACTOR

Granulocyte-macrophage colony-stimulating factor (GM-CSF) was purified from a medium conditioned by the human T-cell lymphotropic virus-II (HTLV-II)-infected T-lymphoblast cell line MO. Characterization of the purified material showed that GM-CSF is a glycoprotein of 22 kDa, and the gene is located on chromosome 5q21-32 (Huebner et al, 1985). Potential physiologic sources for GM-CSF are T and B lymphocytes, macrophages, fibroblasts, mast cells, endothelial cells, mesothelial cells, and osteoblasts.

GM-CSF acts as a potent growth factor both ex vivo and in vivo by stimulating proliferation and maturation of myeloid progenitor cells, subsequently giving rise to neutrophils, eosinophils, and monocytes. GM-CSF has direct and indirect effects on human neutrophils. Direct effects include inhibition of neutrophil migration, enhanced degranulation, induction of adhesion, and changes in cytoskeleton and cell shape. Indirect actions enhance the ability of the neutrophil to respond to triggering stimuli. Among these effects are increased superoxide generation, Ca^{2+} fluxes, and production of inflammatory mediators such as leukotriene B_4.

Administration of GM-CSF in clinical trials results in an immediate and transient decrease in circulating neutrophils, eosinophils, and monocytes, followed by a recovery to baseline within 2 hours. A second phase follows in which the number of leukocytes increases, with a marked "shift to the left" as a result of demargination from the bone marrow NSP and increased myeloid production in the marrow.

The effect of GM-CSF on the incidence of sepsis in human neonates has also been evaluated. A phase I/II trial determined the feasibility, safety, and biologic response of GM-CSF in VLBW (≤1500 g) neonates. Twenty neonates (500 to 1500 g) were randomized in the first 3 days of life to receive GM-CSF at 5 μg/kg/day, 5 μg/kg/twice a day (or 10 μg/kg/day) or placebo. The study demonstrated that GM-CSF was well tolerated with no toxic acute effects. GM-CSF induced a significant increase in ANC, absolute monocyte count (AMC), bone marrow NSP, and neutrophil C3bi expression (Cairo et al, 1995).

A phase III multicentric, randomized, prospective, double-blind, placebo-controlled trial was performed to determine whether prophylactic administration of GM-CSF would reduce nosocomial infections in VLBW neonates. Infants (264, weighing 500 to 1500 g) were randomized in the first 3 days of life to receive either GM-CSF (8 μg/kg/day) for 7 days and then every other day for 21 days or placebo. No toxicity was recorded. The ANC was significantly elevated in the GM-CSF group on days 7, 14, and 21, and the absolute eosinophil count (AEC) on days 7 and 28. However, there was no difference in the incidence of confirmed nosocomial infections between the two groups (Cairo et al, 1999).

A recent single-blind, multicenter, randomized controlled trial was conducted in 26 centers in the United Kingdom (Carr et al, 2009). Infants (≤31 weeks, <10th percentile birthweight) were randomized to receive either GM-CSF (10 µg/kg/day) for 5 days or standard management and monitored for 28 days. Neutrophil counts after treatment were significantly higher in infants treated with GM-CSF than in control infants in the first 11 days. However, there was no significant difference in sepsis-free survival between the groups (Carr et al, 2009).

NEONATAL NEUTROPENIA

Manroe et al (1979) established reference values for ANCs in term and preterm infants during the first 28 days of life for both healthy infants and those with perinatal complications. Mouzinho et al (1994) studied serial white blood cells counts in healthy preterm VLBW infants to investigate whether this patient cohort had different neutrophil counts from those found in previous studies in which cohorts consisted mostly of term infants. They found that there was a wider range of the absolute total neutrophil count, mostly resulting from a downward shift of the lower boundary, especially during the first 60 hours of life. However, there was no difference in absolute total immature neutrophil counts or in I/T ratio. Schmutz et al (2008) demonstrated that the ANC reached its peak value at 6 to 8 hours for those neonates born at ≥28 weeks' gestation, but at 24 hours for those delivered at <28 weeks. The 5th and 95th percentiles for ANCs at 72 to 240 hours among neonates born at >36 weeks were 2700/µL and 13,000/µL, respectively; for neonates born at 28 to 36 weeks were 1000/µL and 12,500/µL, respectively; and for neonates born at <28 weeks were 1300/µL and 15,300/µL, respectively (Christensen et al, 2009). Another factor that contributes to the ANC at birth is the amount of labor the mother experienced. There are higher ANCs in neonates whose mothers had labored significantly versus those whose mothers who had not. Also, female newborns' ANC averages about 2000 cells/µL more than their male counterparts (Christensen et al, 2009).

The pathophysiologic mechanism responsible for neonatal neutropenia may be exhaustion of myeloid committed progenitor cells, inadequate response of progenitor cells to proliferative or maturational signals, and increased usage and destruction. In a series of studies, Christensen and Rothstein (1984) documented significant differences in myeloid progenitor pools and cell kinetics in fetal and neonatal rats compared with adult rats. In the newborn rat, the myeloid progenitor pool, consisting of CFU-GMs in the bone marrow, is only 25% of that of adult animals and requires 4 weeks of maturation to reach adult levels. Additionally, despite a lower number, the CFU-GM of the newborn rat is in a state of near-maximal proliferative capacity, the maximal rate of proliferation being 75% to 80%, whereas that of the adult CFU-GM is only 25% (Christensen and Rothstein, 1984). Concomitantly with reduced numbers of myeloid progenitor cells (lower numbers of CFU-GMs) and lower expansion capacity (already near maximal proliferative rate), the neonatal rat also possesses reduced numbers (25% of adult) of NSP, defined as the percentage of metamyelocytes, bands, and mature neutrophils in the bone marrow. The NSP reaches adult levels in the neonate rat at 4 weeks of age. These factors make it difficult for the neonatal rat to compensate when there is an increased demand.

SEPSIS-INDUCED NEUTROPENIA

Neonates with overwhelming sepsis often develop neutropenia, which illustrates some of the differences between adult and neonatal neutrophils. Neonates have fewer neutrophil progenitors and a diminished precursor storage pool so that neutrophils are easily depleted in stress conditions (Levy, 2007). Following experimental sepsis with group B streptococci (GBS), adult rats respond with a transient decrease in circulating neutrophil counts followed by significant neutrophilia associated with a two- to threefold increase in the progenitor pool (CFU-Meg) and an increase in the proliferative rate to 75% of the maximal capacity (Christensen et al, 1982, 1983). In contrast, neonatal rats under the same conditions had a decrease of 50% of their progenitor pool and failed to increase their myeloid proliferative rate, which, as discussed previously, was already at near-maximal levels. Most important, during experimental sepsis, neonatal rats had further depletion of their already reduced NSP reserves by almost 80%, compared with a decline of 33% in adult rats.

ALLOIMMUNE NEONATAL NEUTROPENIA

Alloimmune neonatal neutropenia occurs as a result of maternal sensitization to neutrophil antigens present on the infant's neutrophils (paternally acquired) that are not present on the maternal neutrophils, with subsequent production of immunoglobulin G (IgG). Neutrophil-specific antibodies are found in the maternal and infant sera, but the mother has a normal neutrophil count. It is estimated to occur at a frequency of 3% of live births (Curnette, 1993). The most common antigens involved in the United States are HNA-1a, HNA-1b, and HNA-2a. Because the antibodies are IgG, which crosses the placenta, peripheral blood counts show profound neutropenia and often demonstrate a monocytosis and eosinophilia. The condition is self-limiting and typically lasts for 6 to 7 weeks, during which time the neonate is susceptible to infections, mostly cutaneous in nature. Although most infections are typically mild, occasionally life-threatening infections may occur necessitating intensive support. Therapeutic interventions that have been attempted include antimicrobials, granulocyte colony stimulating factor, intravenous immune globulin (IVIG) infusions, and granulocyte transfusions that lack the disparate antigen (Maheshwari et al, 2002).

AUTOIMMUNE NEUTROPENIA OF INFANCY

This disorder is analogous to autoimmune hemolytic anemia or immune thrombocytopenic purpura. In this case, however, the infant develops antibodies directed toward its own neutrophils. The etiological mechanism is not yet understood. The incidence is estimated at 1 in 100,000 in children between infancy and 10 years of age (Hartman et al, 1994), though there may be many more children who remain undiagnosed because they lack any clinical characteristics to prompt a complete blood count to be drawn. Although it is most commonly diagnosed from 3 to 30 months, it can occur during the neonatal period (Maheshwari et al, 2002). The most common antigenic targets include HNA-1a,-1b,-2a, FCγ receptor IIB, leukocyte adhesion molecule b, and the C3b complement receptor CR1 (Bux et al, 1997; Rios et al, 1991). If an infection does occur, it is typically mild, although there are some cases of pneumonia, sepsis or meningitis. The vast majority of children will recover by 4 years of age (Bux et al, 1998; Conway et al, 1987).

NEONATAL AUTOIMMUNE NEUTROPENIA

This is a disorder where antineutrophil antibodies are passively transferred to the fetus from a mother with autoimmune disease. Unlike autoimmune neutropenia of infancy, both mother and neonate have neutropenia. The neutropenia is transient and depends on the time needed to clear the maternal IgG antibody, but typically lasts a few weeks to a few months. The majority of neonates will be asymptomatic (Maheshwari et al, 2002).

Rh HEMOLYTIC DISEASE OF THE NEWBORN

Neutropenia has been demonstrated in neonates with Rh hemolytic disease of the newborn and seems to correlate with the severity of disease. This phenomenon can be explained by decreased production of neutrophil progenitors in the bone marrow. Koenig and Christensen (1989a) demonstrated that patients with severe hemolytic disease of the newborn had lower concentrations of granulocyte-macrophage progenitors and decreased proliferative rates of these progenitors, and they lacked a left shift as would be expected if the decrease was due to neutrophil consumption.

MATERNAL HYPERTENSION-ASSOCIATED NEUTROPENIA

One of the most common and well-described causes of transient neonatal neutropenia is maternal hypertension. Infants of hypertensive mothers seem to have decreased production of neutrophils, but the cause is uncertain. Several studies have demonstrated a decrease in neutrophil progenitor cells, decreased cycling of these cells, a relatively normal NPP and NSP, and the absence of a "left shift" (Koenig and Christensen, 1989b). In fact, many investigators have documented an increased incidence of nosocomial infections if neutropenia is associated with maternal hypertension (Doron et al, 1994). In a prospective study, Mouzinho et al (1994) analyzed the incidence of neonatal neutropenia in relation to birthweight, gestational age, and severity of maternal hypertension. They concluded that the neonatal neutropenia was inversely related to the birthweight and gestational age and directly related to the severity of the hypertension. The incidence was nearly 80% among neonates born at less than 30 weeks' gestation and was statistically different from that in similar infants born to normotensive mothers. In most cases, the neutropenia resolves within 72 hours; it almost always resolves by day 5 of life,

but may persist even longer (Koenig and Christensen, 1991; Tsao et al, 1999).

DRUG- OR CHEMICAL-INDUCED NEUTROPENIA

Drug (nonchemotherapy)-induced neutropenia is one of the most common causes for neutropenia in the newborn period and may result in a high rate of infectious complications. There are several mechanisms by which this can occur. Some cases are immune mediated with antineutrophil antibodies present, as is seen with penicillin (Salama et al, 1989). In some cases, the drugs can damage the myeloid precursors directly, as is seen with ibuprofen and indomethacin. Other cases may be due to hypersensitivity that leads to direct damage of the precursors, as is seen with phenothiazines and sulfasalazine. It is also important to evaluate not only the newborn's drug history, but the mother's as well. Some drugs are capable of crossing the placenta and causing neutropenia in the neonate. The management for drug-induced neutropenia includes removing the offending agent and possibly starting G-CSF, especially if the patient develops a severe infection (Andres et al, 2002).

CONGENITAL DISORDERS ASSOCIATED WITH NEONATAL NEUTROPENIA

There are several congenital disorders associated with neutropenia. Please see Table 78-1 for a summary.

Severe Congenital Neutropenia

Severe congenital neutropenia (SCN) is a group of heterogenous disorders that characteristically manifest within the first few months of life with severe, persistent neutropenia, with ANCs of less than 500/mm^3 and often less than 200/mm^3. Bone marrow examination typically demonstrates a maturational arrest at the promyelocyte stage (Kostmann, 1956). Affected children have frequent infections, especially of the skin and oral mucosa, as well as recurrent fevers and early life-threatening infections. Until recently, these were all grouped under the name of Kostmann's syndrome, but they are now believed to be separate entities.

Dale et al (2000) described the occurrence of mutations of the gene encoding neutrophil elastase (ELA2) in 22 patients with severe congenital neutropenia. Autosomal dominant mutations of this same gene are responsible for cyclic neutropenia (Horwitz et al, 1999), which is typically diagnosed in later infancy. Eighty percent of patients with severe congenital neutropenia have autosomal dominant heterozygous mutations, and of these, 50% to 60% are caused by mutations of ELA2 (Bellanne-Chantelot et al, 2004; Boxer et al, 2006; Skokowa et al, 2007). Neutrophil elastase is a serine protease exclusively found in the neutrophil and monocyte that is synthesized and packaged in promyelocytes at early stages of development. The pathogenic role of the elastase mutation in causing neutropenia, in both congenital and cyclic neutropenia, may be linked to the poor survival of early myeloid precursor cells and/or aberrant differentiation.

TABLE 78-1 Selected Neutropenic Syndromes

Syndrome	Inheritance	Gene	Clinical Features
Severe congenital neutropenia	Autosomal dominant	ELA2	Static neutropenia MDS and AML
	Autosomal dominant	GFI1	Static neutropenia Lymphopenia
	X-Linked	WASP	Neutropenia No Wiskott-Aldrich syndrome
Kostmann's syndrome	Autosomal recessive	HAX1	Neutropenia No MDS or AML
Cyclic neutropenia	Autosomal dominant	ELA2	Periodic oscillations (typically every 21 days) of neutrophil count
Shwachman-Diamond syndrome	Autosomal recessive	SBDS	Neutropenia Exocrine pancreatic insufficiency Metaphyseal chondrodysplasia Bone marrow failure
Barth syndrome	X-linked	TAZ	Neutropenia Cardiomyopathy Growth deficiency 3-Methylglutaconic aciduria
WHIM syndrome	Autosomal dominant Autosomal recessive	CXCR4	Warts Hypogammaglobulinemia Immunodeficiency Myelokathexis

AML, Acute myeloid leukemia; *MDS*, myelodysplastic syndromes.

Other mutations have been implicated in SCN. Klein et al (2007) recently discovered the gene responsible for classical autosomal recessive severe congenital neutropenia, first described by Kostmann (1956). The defect is in a gene responsible for an antiapoptotic molecule called HCLS1-associated protein X-1 (HAX1) (Klein et al, 2007).

There have been a few patients with mutations in the WAS gene, which is the same gene that is responsible for Wiskott-Aldrich syndrome, who have developed Kostmann's syndrome, which is distinctive from Wiskott-Aldrich. Recently the growth factor-independent protein 1 (GFI1) gene has been implicated in some cases of SCN (Person et al, 2003). There are still some patients with SCN who do not have any one of the known mutations.

It had been known for some time that patients with SCN are at high risk for leukemic transformation. Recently, this risk has been linked to acquired mutations for the CSF3R gene, responsible for the intracytoplasmic domain of the G-CSF receptor, that are not present from birth (Ancliff et al, 2003). The mechanism for how these mutations are acquired and how they predispose to leukemia is still under investigation.

G-CSF has been used with success for increasing the ANC and decreasing the number of infections in patients with severe congenital neutropenia (Bonilla et al, 1989; Welte et al, 1990). Dale et al (1993) have described the successful use of G-CSF in the treatment of infants, children, and adults with either congenital neutropenia or cyclic neutropenia, with significant laboratory and clinical responses. Although there is great benefit from G-CSF in that children with SCN can now live into adulthood, it must be used with caution. There is an 8% risk per year of developing leukemia after G-CSF has been used for 12 consecutive years (Rosenberg et al, 2006). Also, despite having the neutrophil count increased by G-CSF, there remains a 0.9% risk per year of dying from a serious infection (Rosenberg et al, 2006). Bone marrow transplantation has been used for those patients in whom medical therapy fails and who have a human leukocyte antigen (HLA)-identical unaffected sibling.

Glycogen Storage Disease Type Ib

Glycogen storage disease type Ib (GSD Ib) is a rare autosomal recessive disorder caused by a deficiency of glucose-6-phosphate translocase, which plays a pivotal role in converting glucose 6-phosphate to glucose. This deficiency results in accumulation of glycogen in the liver, kidneys, and intestines. Patients also have severe fasting hypoglycemia. In addition, these patients may also have neutropenia and neutrophil dysfunction that may lead to severe infections and inflammatory bowel disease (IBD). Although patients with GSD Ib typically present at a median of 4 months, there have been patients identified as early as 1 day of life. Presenting features may consist of any of the following: acute metabolic derangement, failure to thrive, recurrent infections, muscular hypotonia, and delayed psychomotor development (Rake et al, 2002). Lack of transport of glucose 6-phosphate may impair cellular function and lead to apoptosis (Hiraiwa et al, 1999; Kilpatrick et al, 1990). GSD Ib patients have been successfully maintained on GCSF with doses anywhere between 0.5 and 10 μg/kg given on varied schedules from daily to 2 to 4 times per week to intermittent with reduction in infections and IBD (Visser et al, 2002).

Cartilage-Hair Hypoplasia

Cartilage-hair hypoplasia (CHH), inherited as an autosomal recessive trait common among Amish populations, is characterized by short-limbed dwarfism, fine hair, and increased susceptibility to infections. Immunologic and hematologic investigations in patients with recurrent infections revealed the presence of chronic noncyclic neutropenia and lymphopenia. Neutropenia may be due to an arrest of myeloid maturation, with underproduction of mature neutrophils and diminished bone marrow storage pools. Lymphopenia, decreased delayed hypersensitivity, and impaired in vitro responsiveness of lymphocytes to mitogens suggest functional dysfunction of small lymphocytes (Lux et al, 1970).

Shwachman-Diamond Syndrome

Shwachman-Diamond syndrome (SDS) is a rare multiorgan disease characterized by metaphyseal chondrodysplasia, dwarfism, pancreatic exocrine insufficiency, neutropenia, and bone marrow failure. Clinical manifestations begin in neonates with diarrhea, weight loss, failure to thrive, eczema, otitis media, and pneumonia. By 2 years of age, dwarfism is evident; later, gait disturbances result from metaphyseal chondrodysplasia. Neutropenia is severe (ANC of 200 to 400/mm^3) and leads to recurrent infections. Aplastic anemia occurs in about 25% of the cases, and leukemic transformation has been described. Homozygous mutations in a novel gene, the *SBDS* gene, appear to be responsible for SDS (Boocock et al, 2003; Lai et al, 2000). The exact function of the *SBDS* gene is not known, but studies suggest that it may have a role in ribosome biogenesis and RNA processing (Koonin et al, 2001; Rujkijyanont et al, 2009; Wu et al, 2002). In vivo administration of G-CSF has been reported to increase the neutrophil count to normal levels. Allogeneic bone marrow transplantation is the only cure for this bone marrow failure syndrome.

Reticular Dysgenesis

Reticular dysgenesis is characterized by extremely severe neutropenia, leukopenia, agammaglobulinemia, and presence of rudimentary thymic, lymphoid, and splenic tissue. In the bone marrow, erythroid and megakaryocyte elements are normal, but myeloid cells are absent or sparse, possibly owing to a maturation defect in a progenitor cell (Roper et al, 1985). Use of GM-CSF or G-CSF has been ineffective. Allogeneic bone marrow transplantation remains the only available curative option.

Barth Syndrome

Barth syndrome is an X-linked recessive disorder characterized by neutropenia, cardiomyopathy, skeletal myopathy, growth deficiency, and 3-methylglutaconic aciduria. The disorder has been linked to a mutation in taffazin gene (TAZ) at Xq28 that leads to severe cardiolipin deficiency in the mitochondrial membrane. A recent study demonstrated neutropenia in 25% of patients, but normal hematocrit and platelets (Spencer et al, 2006).

WHIM Syndrome

WHIM syndrome is characterized by warts, hypogammaglobulinemia, immunodeficiency, and myelokathexis. Myelokathexis is identified by hypersegmented neutrophils with increased apoptosis (Zuelzer, 1964). Heterozygous mutations in CXCR4, a chemokine receptor gene, have been implicated as the cause of WHIM syndrome (Hernandez et al, 2003; Kawai et al, 2007; Sanmun et al, 2006).

QUALITATIVE DEFECTS (DYSFUNCTION) OF NEONATAL PHAGOCYTIC IMMUNITY

The immaturity of the neonatal phagocytic immune system in both humans and animals predisposes the neonate to greatly increased morbidity and mortality during bacterial sepsis. This impairment is attributed to both the inadequacies of the neonatal adaptive immune response characterized by the lack of established memory cell mechanisms and decreased Th1-type responses and also the impairment of the innate immune system (Figure 78-2). Neutrophils and macrophages play vital roles as effector cells in the phagocytic system. The efficient function of the phagocyte system depends on several factors, including the presence of adequate numbers of phagocytes in the peripheral blood, the ability to respond to signals from the sites of inflammation, the ability to migrate to these sites, and the capability to ingest and kill invading microorganisms.

Toll-like receptors (TLRs) play a critical role in the detection and recognition of microbes in the innate immune response. TLRs are highly conserved components of the innate immune system and are involved in the recognition of microbial pathogen antigen molecular patterns. These receptors are essential in initiating and orchestrating the immune response. TLR activation triggers intracellular signaling cascades resulting in production of inflammatory mediators that modulate the primary immune response and instruct the adaptive immune system (Belderbos et al, 2009). Humans express 10 TLR proteins that facilitate the recognition of microbial products and initiate intercellular signaling resulting in the nuclear translocation of nuclear factor (NF)-κB and consequent expression of genes mediating the inflammatory response. Some TLRs are positioned at the cell surface, and others are located in the endoplasmic reticulum. TLR2 and TLR4 are expressed at the cell surface and are involved in recognition of the cell wall components of gram-positive and gram-negative bacteria, respectively. TLR2 recognizes the receptor of gram-positive peptidoglycan and bacterial lipopeptides, and TLR4 is part of a receptor complex recognizing gram-negative bacteria LPS and lipoteichoic acid. Cytoplasmic TLRs (TLR3, 7 8, 9) recognize nucleic acids, with TLR3 sensing dsRNA, TLR7 and 9 sensing ssRNA, and TLR9 unmethylated DNA (Marodi, 2006).

TLRs mediate intracellular signals that trigger inflammatory gene responses through an IL-1 receptor–like pathway that uses the MyD88 protein, IL-1 receptor associated kinase (IRAK), and tumor necrosis factor receptor-associated factor (TRAF)-6 signaling to activate NF-κB and mitogen-activated protein kinase dependent signaling pathways (Viemann et al, 2005).

Several studies have reported differences in the expression of TLRs on granulocytes and monocytes in neonates and adults. Results have shown that the levels of TLR2 and TLR4 expression in healthy adult and full-term neonate phagocytes appeared to be similar (Levy, 2007). However,

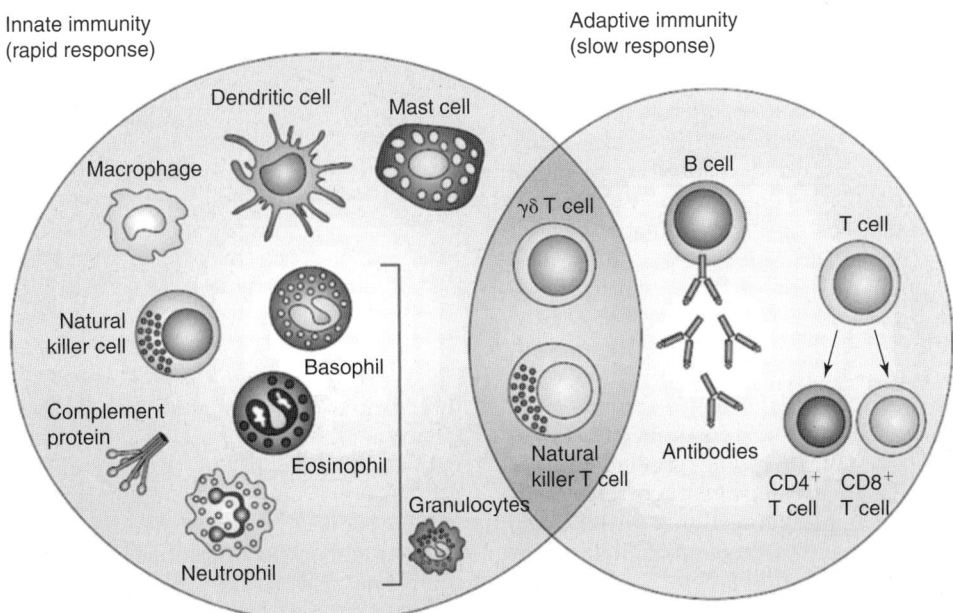

FIGURE 78-2 The innate and adaptive immune response. The innate immune response functions as the first line of defense against infection. It consists of soluble factors, such as complement proteins, and diverse cellular components, including granulocytes (basophils, eosinophils, and neutrophils), mast cells, macrophages, dendritic cells, and natural killer cells. The adaptive immune response is slower to develop but manifests as increased antigenic specificity and memory. It consists of antibodies, B cells, and CD4+ and CD8+ T lymphocytes. Natural killer T cells and γδ T cells are cytotoxic lymphocytes that straddle the interface of innate and adaptive immunity. *(Reprinted with permission from Macmillan Publishers Ltd: Nature Reviews Cancer. Dranoff, G. 4:11-22, copyright 2004.)*

neonates with clinical sepsis showed a significant increase of TLR2 expression on granulocytes and monocytes compared to healthy controls. During the course of sepsis, the expression of TLR4 on granulocytes remained low with no significant changes, but on monocytes the expression level was higher compared to granulocytes (Viemann et al, 2005). Age-related monocyte TLR4 expression and LPS-induced cytokine secretion was compared in VLBW infants, newborns (>30 weeks), and healthy adults. In the VLBW group, expression of TLR4 surface protein and TLR4-specific messenger RNA (mRNA) was significantly reduced in comparison to mature infants and adults. TLR4 expression was accompanied by significantly diminished ex vivo LPS stimulated IL-1β, IL-6, and tumor necrosis factor (TNF)-α release (Forster-Waldl et al, 2005). Other studies have shown that stimulation of newborn monocytes with LPS produced a significant decrease in the expression of MyD88, supporting the premise of impaired TLR4-mediated signaling (Marodi, 2006). Recent studies compared TLR agonist-induced cytokine production from cord blood (CB) from healthy neonates, neonatal venous blood at the age of 1 month, and adult venous blood. CB demonstrated similar TLR3 and TLR7 or increased TLR4 and TLR9 levels of agonist-induced IL-10. However, CB production of IL-12p70 and interferon (IFN)-α in response to TLR3, TLR4, and TLR7 was decreased compared to adults. Neonatal responses to TLR3, TLR7, and TLR9 producing IL-12p70 and IFN-α rapidly increased to adult levels within the 1st month of life, although TLR4-mediated production of IL-12p70 and IFN-α remained significantly decreased compared to adults (Belderbos et al, 2009).

The immaturity of neonatal host defense is also characterized by profound deficiencies in quantitative and qualitative phagocytic effector cell function. Stressed and septic neonates exhibit significant dysfunction of the phagocytic process. Chemotaxis is the initial step in the inflammatory response. Chemotaxis is a process that involves numerous changes in cellular motility and mobility, followed by intracellular biochemical changes. It begins with stimuli from the invading microorganism and continues with the directed migration of neutrophils to the site of invasion, ingestion of the pathogen, and killing by oxygen-dependent and -independent mechanisms. Qualitative abnormalities of neonatal neutrophils include decreased deformability and impaired functions including chemotaxis, phagocytosis, adherence, bacterial killing, aggregation, and oxidative metabolism (Cairo et al, 1990b).

GM-CSF increases adult neutrophil oxidative metabolism by augmenting N-formyl-L-methionyl-L-leucylphenylalanine (FMLP)-, C5a–, and leukotriene B4–induced superoxide anion production. Additionally, GM-CSF increases FMLP-stimulated chemotaxis, promotes phagocytosis of *Staphylococcus aureus*, and augments neutrophil aggregation by the increased expression of surface adhesion (Gasson et al, 1984; Weisbart et al, 1985). Our laboratory investigated the biologic effects of GM-CSF on CB neutrophil oxidative metabolism, bacterial killing, and chemotaxis (Cairo et al, 1989). We determined that GM-CSF is not a direct stimulant of in vitro neonatal neutrophil function; however, when CB was preincubated with GM-CSF and stimulated with FMLP or opsonized zymosan particles, a significant increase in superoxide production was observed. Priming with GM-CSF and subsequent stimulation with phorbol myristate acetate (PMA) did not evoke a significant difference in superoxide release when CB neutrophils were compared with unprimed controls. Furthermore, when CB was compared with adult neutrophils, an earlier but less maximal superoxide generation was seen in CB.

The diminished inflammatory response of CB neutrophils results in a high incidence of microbial invasion. Significant defects in the upregulation of surface-active glycoprotein receptors (C3bi) and reduced aggregation also predispose the neonate to impaired response to bacterial infection. C3bi expression has been compared in adult blood and CB neutrophils and found to be significantly less in CB when stimulated by FMLP- or zymosan-activated serum (Cairo et al, 1990b). However, CB neutrophils incubated with GM-CSF demonstrated a significant induction of C3bi expression. Also, a significant increase in C3bi expression was seen when CB neutrophils were pretreated with GM-CSF and subsequently stimulated with calcium ionophore A23187. The upregulation of C3bi receptor by GM-CSF also appears to correlate with enhancement of CB neutrophil aggregation. GM-CSF also primes CB neutrophils for increased neutrophil aggregation following agonist (FMLP) stimulation.

G-CSF and TNF-α also have been reported to modulate the function of adult and CB neutrophils in a manner similar to that for GM-CSF. Priming CB neutrophils with G-CSF or TNF-α and subsequent stimulation with FMLP induces the expression of C3bi receptors and enhances bacterial and phagocytic activity and superoxide generation.

MONOCYTE PHYSIOLOGY AND DYSFUNCTION

GRANULOCYTE COLONY-STIMULATING FACTOR

Our laboratory has demonstrated a significant reduction in G-CSF mRNA transcript expression as well as decreased production of G-CSF protein in stimulated CB versus adult peripheral blood (APB) mononuclear cells (MNCs) (Cairo et al, 1992b). Furthermore, we have determined that circulating serum G-CSF levels, measured by enzyme-linked immunosorbent assay (ELISA), in CB from term infants are low but similar to healthy adult levels (50 pg/mL). However, we found that G-CSF levels are approximately threefold higher in CB from healthy preterm infants than in CB from 1- to 3-day-old term infants. G-CSF production in the first days of life is associated with peak values at 7 hours of life, followed by a peak neutrophil count approximately 6 hours later.

GRANULOCYTE-MACROPHAGE COLONY-STIMULATING FACTOR

On stimulation of mononuclear cells with phytohemagglutinin and phorbol-12-myristate-6-acetate (PMA), we have observed a sevenfold decrease of GM-CSF protein production in CB versus APB (Table 78-2). Additionally, a fourfold decrease in the expression of GM-CSF mRNA and a threefold lower GM-CSF half-life were measured in CB versus APB stimulated MNCs. Although no difference in rate of transcriptional activation from activated CB and APB MNCs was noted, actinomycin D transcriptional decay studies demonstrated reduced GM-CSF half-life

TABLE 78-2 Cytokine Production in Stimulated Adult versus Neonatal Mononuclear Cells

Cytokine	Adult	Neonate
G-CSF	↑	↓
GM-CSF	↑	↓
M-CSF	↑	↓
IL-12	↑	↓
IL-15	↑	↓
IL18	↑	↓

in activated CB compared with APB mononuclear cells (Cairo et al, 1991).

We thus established that the decrease in GM-CSF mRNA expression and protein in activated CB versus APB MNCs is due to a decrease in posttranscriptional mRNA stability and not to alterations in GM-CSF gene transcription. The cytoplasmic instability of GM-CSF mRNA is regulated in part by adenosine + uridine-rich elements in the 3'-untranslated region of the cytokine transcript. We have previously investigated the molecular basis for the differential stability of GM-CSF mRNA in CB and APB MNCs using electrophoretic mobility-shift assays. We demonstrated that the destabilization of GM-CSF mRNA in CB MNC is translation dependent and that increased levels of the specific RNA binding protein AUF-1 isoforms in the CB MNC may target transcripts for increased degradation and contribute to the dysregulation of phagocytic immunity (Buzby et al, 1996).

MACROPHAGE COLONY-STIMULATING FACTOR

Macrophage colony-stimulating factor (M-CSF) is a hematopoietic growth factor that regulates the proliferation, differentiation, and functional activation of monocytes. Normally detected in human serum, M-CSF plays an important role in enhancing the effector functions of mature monocytes and macrophages. M-CSF serum levels are increased in CB and further increased in the neonate. Our laboratory studied the regulation of the M-CSF gene expression under basal and activated conditions and the transcriptional and posttranscriptional regulation of M-CSF in CB versus APB. Both CB and adult blood MNCs constitutively express M-CSF mRNA on adhesion to tissue culture flasks. However, when GM-CSF was added as a costimulator, CB MNCs produced two- to threefold less M-CSF protein compared with APB MNCs, and a fourfold decrease in M-CSF mRNA expression was shown in both unstimulated and GM-CSF-induced CB versus APB MNCs (see Table 78-2). Furthermore, we determined that M-CSF mRNA expression peaked between 16 and 24 hours after stimulation and fell to normal levels by 48 hours in both CB and APB (Suen et al, 1994). This study also demonstrated that the transcriptional rates of the M-CSF gene were similar in CB and APB even after stimulation with rhGM-CSF. However, actinomycin D decay studies showed that the half-life of M-CSF mRNA in CB MNCs was significantly lower, and the induction of M-CSF mRNA after cycloheximide administration in CB compared with APB MNCs was significantly increased, suggesting that one or more labile proteins may be involved in regulating M-CSF transcript stability (Suen et al, 1994).

INTERLEUKIN-12 AND INTERLEUKIN-15

IL-12 is a critical cytokine regulating many of the biological functions of natural killer (NK) and T cells. IL-12 is a heterodimer of 70 kDa (p70) formed by two covalently linked glycolated chains of 40 kDa (p40) and 35 kDa (p35). The heterodimeric form of IL-12 is produced by activated monocytes, B cells, and macrophages in response to TLR signaling from bacteria or parasites or their products (Lee et al, 1996). IL-12 enhances Th1 development and suppresses Th2 development in humans. IL-12 is a potent inducer of IFN-γ production but also stimulates the production of other inflammatory agonists, including TNF-α, GM-CSF, MCSF, IL-3, IL-8, and IL-2 from NK and T cells. In addition, IL-12 enhances the cytolytic activity of resting and activated NK and lymphocyte activated killer (LAK) cells (Satwani et al, 2005a). IL-15 is a cytokine that has biological properties similar to IL-2. IL-15 induces the proliferation of T cells, B cells, and notably NK cells. IL-15 enhances nonspecific NK and LAK cytotoxic activity and induces NK cell production of IFN-γ, TNF-α, TNF-β, and GM-CSF.

Our laboratory compared the expression and production of IL-12, the regulatory mechanisms associated with IL-12 expression in CB MNC. We reported a three- to fourfold decrease in IL-12 mRNA and protein production in activated CB versus APB MNC, but no differences in the basal levels of transcription or transcriptional activation of the IL-12 gene (see Table 78-2). Further, we demonstrated that IL-12 is a significant inducer of IFN-γ in CB and APB MNCs, although levels of IFN-γ were lower in stimulated CB versus APB. Our studies show that IL-12 can significantly enhance CB NK cytotoxicity to comparable levels of APB and in combination with low doses of IL-2 can further enhance NK CB cytotoxicity (Lee et al, 1996). Additionally, IL-12 significantly enhanced CB NK and LAK in vitro activity against a broad range of tumor cell lines (Lee et al, 1998).

Similar to IL-12, we demonstrated that IL-15 mRNA and protein production is significantly decreased in activated CB MNCs compared to APB MNCs (see Table 78-2). The discrepancy in IL-15 production is secondary, in part, to altered posttranscriptional regulation. IL-15 also significantly enhanced CB NK and LAK activity in vitro against several tumor lines and also induced the production of IFN-γ and TNF-α in CB MNC. Further, the combination of IL-12 and IL-15 produced additive and synergistic augmentation in CB NK and LAK cytotoxic activity (Qian et al, 1997).

INTERLEUKIN-18

IL-18 has a similar structure to IL-1 and is considered to be a member of the IL-1 superfamily because it binds to the IL-1 receptor. IL-18 induces the production of multiple cytokines including IFN-γ, IL-13, IL-4, IL-8, and GM-CSF and both Th1 and Th2 lymphokines. Additionally,

IL-18 upregulates the expression of Fas ligand on both NK and T cells and facilitates target cell killing (Satwani et al, 2005b).

Our laboratory compared the regulation of IL-18 gene expression and protein production in activated CB and APB MNCs. Constitutive levels of IL-18 produced by APB MNCs were significantly higher compared with CB MNCs (see Table 78-2). Upon stimulation with Staphylococcus endotoxin, IL-18 production was increased in both CB and APB MNCs; however, IL-18 levels were significantly higher in APB versus CB MNCs. Further, IL-18 mRNA expression in both activated MNCs was seen, but mRNA expression was significantly lower in CB compared to APB MNCs. IL-18 stimulation of CB MNCs showed no significant increase in IFN-γ production; however, IFN-γ secretion was significantly induced in similarly stimulated APB MNCs. Interestingly, the combination of IL-18 + IL-12 for stimulation of APB and CB MNCs induced a significant increase in IFN-γ production. However, IFN-γ production from CB stimulated with IL-18 or IL-18 + IL-12 was significantly less than from APB stimulated cells (Satwani et al, 2005b).

NEGATIVE REGULATORS OF HEMATOPOIESIS

Cytokines also play a predominant role as negative regulators of hematopoiesis. These negative growth factors regulate early hematopoiesis with suppressive effects on the proliferation of early myeloid and lymphoid progenitors. The most notable negative regulators of hematopoiesis are transforming growth factor-β1 (TGF-β1), macrophage inflammatory protein-1α (MIP-1α), and IL-8. TGF-β1 induces a wide range of responses, including the inhibition of lymphocyte, thymocyte, and epithelial cell proliferation as well as the suppression and proliferation of early progenitor cells. MIP-1α and IL-8 also have suppressive effects on early progenitors, similar to TGF-β1. Our laboratory measured the protein levels of TGF-β1 and MIP-1α in the conditioned media of phytohemagglutinin and PMA-stimulated CB and APB MNCs. Both TGF-β1 and MIP-1α levels were significantly less in CB supernatants compared with APB supernatants. Furthermore, the mRNA expression of TGF-β1, MIP-1α, and IL-8 in stimulated CB and APB MNCs was found to be significantly less in CB MNCs; yet no significant difference was seen in the transcription rate of either the TGF-β1 or MIP-1α genes in CB compared with APB. These results suggested that the reduced mRNA of the negative regulators, TGF-β1 and MIP-1α, may be secondary to alterations in posttranscriptional regulation, and that the altered expression of both positive and negative regulators may be involved in the immaturity of host defense in the neonate (Chang et al, 1994).

MONOCYTES

Ontogeny

Embryonic macrophages are found among hematopoietic cells in the yolk sac at 3 to 6 weeks' gestation. After 6 weeks, the fetal liver becomes the primary site of hematopoiesis for the next 6 to 22 weeks of gestation, when the bone marrow becomes the lifelong center of blood cell production (Palis et al, 2001). Monocytes are present in high proportions in the early hematopoietic tissues, with approximately 70% of hematopoietic cells at 4.5 weeks' gestation morphologically identifiable as monocytes. This proportion decreases to 1% to 2% over the next 6 weeks as erythroid cells become predominant. The precursors of monocytes, monoblasts, and promonocytes continue to be present in the fetal liver; however, intravascular monocytes are not observed until the 5th month of gestation. Circulating monocytes do not appear with regularity until hematopoiesis is first established in the bone marrow after the 10th week of gestation.

At birth, the number of circulating granulocyte-monocyte progenitor cells (CFU-GMs), the committed progenitor precursor to monocytes, are increased in CB before 32 weeks, but levels fall shortly after birth. The estimated total bone marrow cellularity of the term neonate at birth is approximately 1.36×10^{11} cells/L, and the total cell numbers decline over the first 1 to 2 weeks to 3.5×10^{10}/L. These levels remain low through the neonatal period, in which circulating monocyte counts are highest in the 1st week of life, ranging from 1340 to 2200 cells/μL, and gradually fall in successive weeks to 700 cells/mm^3 at 3 weeks and 450 cells/mm^3 by 6 years of age.

Morphology

Immunophenotyping using fluorescent conjugated monoclonal antibodies also has been used to identify monocyte cell subpopulations and give insight to cell activation and function. During ontogeny, macrophages in the fetal liver express CD11b as early as 12 weeks' gestation. The classic monocyte marker, CD14, does not appear until about 15 to 21 weeks' gestation. CD14 expression on circulating MNCs is equivalent in CB and APB. CD11a, CD11b, and CD11c are expressed in lower densities on CB monocytes than on adult cells. There is also lower expression of class II major histocompatibility complex (MHC) antigens HLA-DR, HLA-DP, and HLA-DQ on neonatal monocytes compared with adult monocytes. HLA-DR expression also is significantly lower in CD14$^+$ populations in CB compared with APB CD14$^+$. The density of these class II MHC antigens has been correlated with antigen-presenting capacity of monocytes in vitro; however, it has not been determined whether this deficiency affects neonatal host defense. Other important monocyte markers are the receptors for the Fc moiety of IgG (FcγR) and the TLRs. FcγR receptors are important in the process of monocyte and macrophage phagocytosis of microbes and antibody-dependent cytotoxicity. Monocytes constitutively express the high- affinity receptor FcγRI (CD64) and FcγRII (CD32). FcγR-III$^+$ monocytes in adult blood are significantly higher compared with CB samples. Despite the difference in the FcγR-III$^+$ populations, the intensity of FcγR-III expression is higher in CB than in APB. TLRs play a critical role in the recognition of microbial pathogens. Full-term neonatal monocytes express normal basal levels of TLR2 and TLR4 at both the protein and mRNA levels, but reduced TNF-α release in response to stimulation to a range of TLRs (Levy, 2005; Sadeghi et al, 2007;

TABLE 78-3 Characteristic Function and Phenotype of Adult versus Neonatal Mononuclear Cells

Cell	Function/Phenotype	Adult	Neonate
Monocyte	Chemotaxis	↑	↓
	Phagocytosis	↑	↓
	Adhesion	≈	≈
	Respiratory burst	≈	≈
Dendritic cells	Expression CD83, CD86	↑	↓
	Mixed lymphocyte reaction	↑	↓
	IL-12 (p40) production	↑	↓
	IL-12	↑	↓
	IL-10	↓	↑
Natural killer cells	Expression CD8, CD57	↑	↓
	Expression ICAM-1, CD161	↑	↓
	Cytolytic activity	↑	↓

↑, Increased; ↓, decreased; ≈, similar.

Viemann et al, 2005). CB monocytes of preterm neonates, however, have diminished basal TLR4 expression but normal TLR2 expression compared with APB monocytes (Forster-Waldl et al, 2005).

Function

Monocytes exhibit the characteristic properties of phagocytosis—namely, movement, adherence, endocytosis, and microbial activity. Monocytes are capable of directed movement (chemotaxis) in response to substances (chemokines) produced by bacteria or by accessory cells at the site of injury or invasion. Chemotactic capabilities of neonatal and adult peripheral blood monocytes have been compared, and chemotaxis was found to be less pronounced in neonates than in adults (Table 78-3).

The cascade of reactions within the immune response to infection involves monocyte upregulation and adherence via CD11b/CD18 receptors followed by cell activation and the release of cytokines (TNF, IL-1, and IL-6) and bactericidal products—superoxide radicals, nitric oxide, and granule contents released in the process of degranulation. Adherence requires the interaction of monocytes and the endothelium. Activated monocytes migrate from circulation into the tissues by firmly adhering to endothelial surfaces through the interaction of the integrins (CD11a-c and CD18) expressed on the monocyte cell membrane and the intercellular adhesion molecule-1 (ICAM-1) or ICAM-2 on the endothelial surface. Finally, the activated monocyte moves through the endothelium to the site of inflammation or infection. Preliminary studies demonstrate that levels of monocyte adhesion molecule expression are comparable in neonate and adult peripheral blood (Schibler, 2000). The β-2 integrin, CR3, plays a major role in the migration to sites of infection by mediating the binding to ICAM-1 and also is responsible for mediating the recognition of opsonized microbial pathogens. Neonatal monocytes express approximately 85% as much CR3 as is expressed by adult monocytes.

Antimicrobial activity of monocytes includes oxygen-dependent mechanisms such as the respiratory burst, which through a complex series of reactions forms highly reactive hydroxyl radicals that damage host and microbial membranes. The ability of monocytes of fetal and neonatal monocytes to kill pathogens (*Staphylococcus aureus*, *S. epidermidis*, *Escherichia coli*, and *Candida albicans*) is shown to be equivalent to that of APB monocytes (see Table 78-3). However, a recent study of isolated CB plastic adherent monocytes from preterm and full-term infants revealed a significant decrease in superoxide production and degranulation in preterm compared with full-term monocytes.

Activated monocytes and macrophages in response to the recognition of microbial antigens by collaborative actions of soluble recognition proteins including CD14, bacterial lipopeptides and TLRs produce several cytokines and chemokines contributing to the inflammatory process. IL-1, IFN-α, and TNF-α are synthesized at similar levels in adults and neonates. Kaufman et al (1999) found a significant decrease in the secretion of TNF-α by LPS-stimulated adherent monocytes from preterm infants compared with full-term infants; however, no difference was seen in the production of IL-1β or IL-6. They showed a significant decrease in the expression of CD11b and CD18 adhesion receptor subunits in monocytes collected from preterm infants compared with that in full-term infants. Further, whereas TLR expression of full-term neonatal monocytes is similar to that in adult monocytes, the functional response is quite different. Levy et al reported a 1–3 log decrease in sensitivity to the induction of TNF-α by multiple TLR ligands in CB monocytes compared to APB, and the differences in TNF-α release correlated with the ligand-induced changes in monocyte TNF-α mRNA levels (Levy et al, 2004). A more recent study reported that the innate immune responses of neonatal monocytes to microbial TLR agonists are biased toward a high IL-6 but low TNF-α levels in vitro due to distinct neonatal cellular (monocyte) and humoral (serum) factors, and such a pattern was also evident postnatally in vivo (see Figure 78-2) (Angelone et al, 2006).

Our laboratory has compared the differential gene expression basal and LPS (TLR4)-stimulated profiles of APB versus CB monocytes. Genes whose basal expression were significantly higher in APB versus CB monocytes included cytokines/cytokine receptors, chemokines, immunoregulators, genes for signal transduction, and cytoskeleton/cell structure regulatory genes. Genes with expression higher in CB compared to APB monocytes include several adhesion molecules (CD9, integrin-αM, cyclin-dependent kinase inhibitor 1C). Following stimulation with LPS (TLR4), CB monocytes exhibited increases in cytokine/cytokine receptor, chemokine, immunoregulatory, apoptosis, signal transduction, and cytoskeleton/cell structure regulation genes. Further analysis revealed 82 genes whose expression was significantly increased in LPS-activated APB versus CB monocytes, including cytokine/cytokine receptor, chemokine, and immunoregulatory genes. Conversely, gene expression increased in CB versus APB monocytes including genes regulating apoptosis/cell cycle regulation, growth factor/ligand/receptor, and cytoskeleton structure regulation (Jiang et al, 2004).

DENDRITIC CELLS

Dendritic cells (DCs) are specialized mononuclear cells with highly developed antigen-presenting capabilities that play a pivotal role in humoral and cellular immunity by initiating primary and secondary T cell responses. DCs can be categorized into several types: follicular, lymphoid, and circulating blood DCs. Follicular DCs are located in the paracortical areas of the spleen and lymph nodes and express receptors for immunoglobulin and complement. Their role is to present antigen to B lymphocytes. Lymphoid DCs are highly motile, low-density cells found in several locations. These DCs express high levels of costimulatory molecules and class II MHC and function to present antigen to T cells. Circulating blood DCs constitute from 0.1% to 1.0% of peripheral blood mononuclear cells and migrate to the lymph nodes. The function of circulating DCs is similar to that of the lymphoid DCs—stimulating T cells by the presentation of antigen. DCs are derived from pluripotent hematopoietic stem cells (CD34+) that differentiate along myeloid or lymphoid lineages. Recent studies have suggested that DCs derived from a novel population of progenitors (CD34+/CD7+/CD45RA+) in CB represent an original lymphoid DC population. These DCs produce two- to fourfold higher levels of IL-6, IL-12, and TNF-α on stimulation with CD40L and demonstrate a higher allogeneic T-lymphocyte reactivity. Two classes of dendritic cells have been characterized on the basis of expression of CD8a. CD8a+ DCs are derived from lymphoid tissue, and CD8a− DCs are derived from myeloid tissue.

Caux et al (1997) generated DCs in vitro from CB D34+ hematopoietic stem cells stimulated with GM-CSF plus TNF-α. Two subsets of DCs were generated: one expressing CD1a and the other, CD14 surface antigens. These subsets further differentiated along two independent DC pathways, with cells expressing either the CD1a+ or CD14+ membrane antigen. CD1a+ cells differentiated into Langerhans cells, characterized by Birbeck granules, the Lag antigen, and E-cadherin. CD14+ progenitors matured into CD1a+DCs that expressed CD2, CD9, and CD 68 and could be induced to differentiate into circulating blood DCs. CD40 activates CB CD34+ cells to proliferate and differentiate independently of GM-CSF into a cell population with prominent DC characteristics. DCs generated with CD40 are able to prime allogeneic T cells and express high levels of HLA-DR but lack the characteristic CD1a and CD40 surface molecules (Flores-Romo et al, 1997).

Mature DCs express high levels of CD80 and CD83 on the cell membrane. Several agents have been shown to increase CD80 and CD83 expression on DCs, including TNF-α, bacterial LPS, and monocyte-conditioned media. Interactions with other cells also can induce activation and maturation of DCs, as demonstrated by the crosslinking of CD40 that is mediated by T cells.

We have demonstrated the ability to generate CB DCs ex vivo in serum-free media with GM-CSF, IL-4, Flt-3 ligand, TGF-β, and TNF-α. We found that the ex vivo–generated CB DCs from plastic adherent MNCs exhibit morphology and immunophenotypic characteristics similar to those of APB DCs; however, CB adherent MNC-derived DCs have differential potency in stimulating allogeneic mixed leukocyte reaction when compared with adult adherent MNC-derived DCs (Bracho et al, 2000).

Morphology

The cardinal properties of DCs include the ability to take in, process, and present antigen and the ability to migrate selectively through tissues and interact with, stimulate, and direct T-cell responses. DCs have a distinct morphology and are noted for their irregular shape with veil-like ruffled cell membranes (lamellipodia) that include many pseudopods and numerous membrane processes. Microscopic examination of DCs reveals prominent mitochondria and endosomes and lysosomes within the cytoplasm, which are necessary for the processing of antigen. The morphology of DCs in CB and APB is identical; however, the mean percentage of DCs is lower in CB (0.5%) than in adult blood (1%).

Immunophenotyping studies have shown that DCs express numerous surface molecules commonly found on mononuclear cells, MHC molecules, CD4, CD45 isoforms, adhesion molecules (ICAM-1, -2, -3 and leukocyte function-associated antigen-1 [LFA-1]), and Fc receptors (FcγI [CD64], FcγII [CD3]). Maturation of DCs is commonly associated with high expression of CD80 and CD83. On stimulation, DCs upregulate costimulatory molecules CD40, CD80, and CD86. Flow cytometric studies, however, show levels of ICAM-1 (CD54), MHC class I (HLA-ABC) and II (HLA-DR), CD80, and CD40 antigens to be significantly lower on CB DCs (Goriely et al, 2001; Hunt et al, 1994). Liu et al (2001) compared the phenotypic and functional characteristics of monocyte-derived DCs in CB versus APB. After 7 days of culture with GM-CSF plus IL-4, CB monocytes generated fewer CD1a+ cells than those generated by APB monocytes, and the cultured CB DCs had a reduced intensity of CD1a expression and MHC class II molecules. These investigators further reported that both the endocytotic ability and ability to stimulate CD3+ T cells was reduced in CB DCs compared with APB DCs.

Function

The activation of TLR pathways are shown to mediate DC maturation. Krutzik et al (2005) demonstrated that TLR activation of monocytes induces rapid differentiation to CD1b+ DCs that could be expanded by TLR-mediated upregulation of GM-CSF, promoted T cell activation and secreted proinflammatory cytokines (IFN-γ). A more recent study found that exposure to TLR4 or TLR8 alone induced upregulated expression of CD80, CD83, and CD86 in APB monocyte-derived dendritic cells (MoDCs), whereas CB MoDC showed lower expression of CD83 and CD86 (see Table 78-3). When TLR3-ligand was combined with TLR8 ligand, CB MoDC showed a synergistic increase in the expression of CD83 and CD86, but no further upregulation of CD80, CD83, and CD86 in APB MoDC (Krumbiegel et al, 2007).

Our laboratory compared gene expression between APB and CB immature (iDC) and mature DC (mDC) populations. Surface molecules, transcription regulator genes, cell adhesion, and structure regulators were more significantly expressed (twofold or more) in APB versus CB iDCs. Following maturation induced by LPS (TLR4) and comparing APB to CB mDCs, significantly higher expression of chemokine genes, cytokine and cytokine receptor genes, IFN-inducible genes, TNF-α-induced protein, and expression of cell surface MHC class II molecules. Additionally, apoptotic regulator genes were significantly amplified, as well as the expression of several signaling genes, TLR signaling pathway family genes, and transcription and structure regulator genes. Conversely, a group of cell cycle regulator and transcription factor genes were significantly decreased in APB versus CB mDCs (Jiang et al, 2009).

Cytokine production by stimulated neonatal DCs can provide insight into the defect of their impaired immune response. IL-12 plays a critical role in the stimulation of T cells by mature DCs. Goriely et al (2001) reported comparable levels of IL-6, IL-8, TNF-α, and IL-10 in newborn and adult DCs after stimulation with LPS or CD40 ligand. However, IL-12 (p40) levels secreted by neonatal DCs were significantly lower on stimulation with LPS but not with CD40 ligand. Also, after either LPS or CD40 ligand stimulation, neonatal DCs produced lower levels of IL-12 (p70) than adult DCs. CB DCs stimulated with LPS, CD40 ligand, or poly(I;C) showed a selective defect in the synthesis of IL-12. Furthermore, when stimulated with poly(I;C), neonatal DCs produced deficient levels of IL-12 (p70), but their production of IL-12 (p40) was similar to that of adult DCs. Neonatal DCs were also placed in mixed leukocyte culture with adult CD4+ T cells, and neonatal DCs induced significantly lower levels of IFN-γ but higher levels of IL-10 than did adult DCs (see Table 78-3). Analysis of IL-12 (p35) mRNA from LPS stimulated neonatal and adult DCs by real-time polymerase chain reaction assay revealed significantly lower levels in neonatal versus adult DCs; however, the addition of rIFN-γ to LPS-stimulated newborn DCs restored the expression of and synthesis of IL-12 to adult levels.

TLRs are also integral in initiating and directing the response of MoDCs. Several studies have demonstrated TLR-mediated responses in human cord blood dendritic cells to be impaired. A recent study reported the significant increase of IL-12p70 production in APB but not CB MoDC on simultaneous stimulation with TLR3 and TLR8. However, stimulation with TLR4/TLR8-ligands in CB DC induced adult-like levels of IL-12p40 and upregulation of IL-12p70, but not to the levels seen in APB DC (Krumbiegel et al, 2007). Another study demonstrated a skewed pattern of cytokine production in CB MoDCs in response to TLR4. MoDC stimulated in vitro with TLR4 showed a significantly lower expression of activation markers CD40 and CD80 and decreased production of IL-12 p70 and IFN-β compared to adult MoDCs (Belderbos et al, 2009).

Functional differences between neonatal and adult DCs have been examined by several investigators. CB DCs have been found to be poor stimulators of T cells in a mixed leukocyte reaction when either adult-blood or CB mononuclear cells or T cells were used as responder cells (Bracho et al, 2001) (see Table 78-3). In contrast, CB T cells and mononuclear cells responded normally to allogeneic adult DCs. Furthermore, CB DCs performed poorly as accessory cells for T-cell mitogenic responses (Hunt et al,

1994). Recent studies of the ontogeny of DCs have shown that DCs from 3- and 7-day-old mice were severely defective in presenting tetanus toxoid to antigen-specific T-cell clones. However, the ability of the neonatal DCs to present antigen improved with age, reaching adult levels by 4 weeks of age.

NATURAL KILLER CELLS

NK cells are an essential part of the innate immune system. They have the ability to lyse target cells and secrete immunomodulatory cytokines (Robertson and Ritz, 1990). NK cells make up 10% of peripheral blood lymphocytes and are characterized by lack of CD3, but expression of CD56 (Farag et al, 2002). NK cells can be further divided based on the surface density of CD56 into CD56^{bright} (high density) and CD56^{dim} (low density). The CD56^{dim}, which are the more cytotoxic NK cells, usually represent 90% of the NK population. The CD56^{dim} have high expression of CD16, which is the Fcγ receptor III responsible for antibody-dependent cellular cytotoxicity (Leibson, 1997). The CD56^{bright} have less expression of CD16 and are known to produce immunoregulatory cytokines.

NK cells develop from the HSCs that are found in the aorto-gonado-mesonephron and later within the fetal liver (Godin and Cumano, 2002). However, committed NK cell lineage cells are first identified in the fetal thymus by embryonic day 15.5 (Carlyle and Zuniga-Pflucker, 1998). As the bone marrow starts to develop, NK cell development eventually relocates there. The bone marrow then remains the primary site of maturation (Miller et al, 1992; Shibuya et al, 1993). Human NK cell development occurs in two phases. First, after exposure to early growth factors (flt-3 ligand or kit ligand),the NK progenitor cell (CD34$^+$Lin$^-$) develops into the NK precursor intermediate with the phenotype of CD34$^+$IL-15R$^+$. On exposure to IL-15, the NK cell becomes a mature NK cell that is CD56^{bright}. This cell can then undergo further differentiation to become a CD56^{dim} NK cell.

NK cells express a repertoire of classes of receptors (NKRs) that bind to MHC class I or class I–like molecules or targets that regulate whether NK cells will be activated or inhibited (Farag et al, 2002; Moretta et al, 2001). When NK cells fail to interact with the MHC class I molecule and the activating receptor is activated, NK-mediated cell lysis will ensue, as occurs in the case of infection. Viral infections, such as with cytomegalovirus, downregulate the MHC class I molecule, which when expressed would inhibit cell lysis (Moretta et al, 2005). After activation, lysosome-like vesicles containing perforin, serine esterases, and sulfated proteoglycans are secreted toward the target cell. Perforin forms pores in the target cell, leading to osmotic lysis. The serine esterases, including granzymes, induces apoptosis. TNF-α activates a target cell endonuclease which degrades genomic DNA. Proteoglycans protect the granzymes from inactivation by protease inhibitors (Berthou et al, 1995; Moretta et al, 2005; Pao et al, 2005; Robertson and Ritz, 1990; Spaeny-Dekking et al, 2000). After stimulation with cytokines, the CD56^{bright} NK cells are able to produce positive feedback by secreting IFN-γ, TNF-α, and granulocyte macrophage stimulating factor. These cytokines help to recruit macrophages and

other antigen-presenting cells for more efficient control of the infection (Cooper et al, 2001a, 2001b).

Neonates appear to have immature NK cells, which leads to an impaired immune system. Cord-blood NK cells have lower expression of CD8 and CD57, which are surface markers that confer maturity (Dalle et al, 2005) (see Table 78-3). Cord-blood NK cells also had lower expression of ICAM-1 and CD161, adhesion and activating molecules, respectively, when compared to their adult counterparts (Dalle et al, 2005). Cord-blood NK cells have been demonstrated to have less spontaneous cytolytic activity when compared to adult NK cells (Dalle et al, 2005). This leads to impaired clearance of intracellular pathogens (Wynn et al, 2009). Interestingly, the cytolytic potential of NK cells can be increased to adult levels after exposure to IL-15 (Dalle et al, 2005).

HEMOPHAGOCYTIC LYMPHOHISTIOCYTOSIS

Hemophagocytic lymphohistiocytosis (HLH) can appear anytime between fetal life and adulthood. NK cell dysfunction can result in HLH. HLH presents as a multisystem disorder characterized by prolonged fever, hepatosplenomegaly, and occasional neurologic symptoms. Laboratory analysis reveals cytopenias, liver dysfunction, hypofibrinogenemia, hypertriglyceridemia, hypoalbuminemia, and hyponatremia. Several genes have been linked to this disorder. The first gene linked was that for perforin and accounts for 15% to 20% of HLH cases. Another cause is a mutation in MUNC13-4, which is necessary for cytolytic granule fusion with the cytoplasmic membrane during the process of degranulation. MUNC 13-4 mutations account for another 15% to 20% of HLH cases. In Turkish families, a mutation in syntaxin 11 has been demonstrated to cause HLH. Syntaxin 11 is important in facilitating membrane trafficking events. Untreated HLH is almost uniformly fatal. Treatment may include chemotherapy and/or hematopoietic stem cell transplant (Filipovich, 2008).

HERMANSKY-PUDLAK SYNDROME TYPE 2

Although Hermansky-Pudlak syndrome (HPS2) is characterized by congenital neutropenia, oculocutaneous albinism, and prolonged bleeding, it is also associated with defects in NK cells. Unlike other severe inherited neutropenias, there are mature neutrophils present in the bone marrow. The defect caused by a mutation in the AP3B1 gene, prevents trafficking proteins to transport to the lysosomes. Recent studies have demonstrated that HPS2 also causes decreased NK cytotoxicity and reduced perforin expression (Fontana et al, 2006).

SUMMARY

Immaturity of neonatal neutrophils, monocytes, lymphocytes, dendritic cells, and NK cells predisposes the newborn to an increased incidence and/or severity of infectious complications. An increased understanding of the genetic mechanisms responsible for these defects will provide insight regarding future treatment strategies to prevent and/or treat serious or overwhelming infection in the newborn.

ACKNOWLEDGMENT

We thank Linda Rahl and Erin Morris, RN, for their expert editorial assistance in the preparation of this chapter. This chapter is based on work supported in part by a grant from the Pediatric Cancer Research Foundation.

SUGGESTED READINGS

Christensen RD, Henry E, Jopling J, et al: The CBC: reference ranges for neonates, *Semin Perinatol* 33:3-11, 2009.

Dale DC, Bonilla MA, Davis MW, et al: A randomized controlled phase III trial of recombinant human granulocyte colony-stimulating factor (filgrastim) for treatment of severe chronic neutropenia, *Blood* 81:2496-2502, 1993.

Farag SS, Fehniger TA, Ruggeri L, et al: Natural killer cell receptors: new biology and insights into the graft-versus-leukemia effect, *Blood* 100:1935-1947, 2002.

Klein C, Grudzien M, Appaswamy G, et al: HAX1 deficiency causes autosomal recessive severe congenital neutropenia (Kostmann disease), *Nat Genet* 39:86-92, 2007.

Kostmann R: Infantile genetic agranulocytosis; agranulocytosis infantilis hereditaria, *Acta Paediatr Suppl* 45(S105):1-78, 1956.

Maheshwari A, Christensen RD, Calhoun DA: Immune-mediated neutropenia in the neonate, *Acta Paediatr Suppl* 91:98-103, 2002.

Robertson MJ, Ritz J: Biology and clinical relevance of human natural killer cells, *Blood* 76:2421-2438, 1990.

Zon LI: Developmental biology of hematopoiesis, *Blood* 86:2876-2891, 1995.

Complete references and supplemental color images used in this text can be found online at www.expertconsult.com

NEONATAL INDIRECT HYPERBILIRUBINEMIA AND KERNICTERUS

Jon F. Watchko

Hyperbilirubinemia is the most common clinical condition requiring evaluation and management in the newborn. Bilirubin is a breakdown product of hemoglobin and other heme proteins. Heme oxygenase converts heme to biliverdin, producing an equimolar amount of carbon monoxide with biliverdin subsequently reduced to bilirubin by biliverdin reductase. Bilirubin is transported in plasma bound to albumin and there is rapid and selective uptake of bilirubin from blood into hepatocytes where it is conjugated with glucuronic acid by the uridine diphosphate glucuronosyl transferase 1A1 (*UGT1A1*) isoenzyme. Conjugated bilirubin is actively transported into bile and bilirubin eliminated via stool passage.

Neonatal hyperbilirubinemia reflects the interplay of developmentally modulated changes in bilirubin production, metabolism, and excretion characterized by (1) an increased bilirubin load on hepatocytes and (2) decreased hepatic and enteric bilirubin clearance. The increased hepatic bilirubin load is the result of bilirubin overproduction reflective of the newborn's large red cell mass, an overall reduced red cell life span, and in a subset of neonates, hemolytic conditions known to accelerate red cell turnover. Decreased neonatal bilirubin clearance results primarily from limited hepatic bilirubin uptake and conjugation. In addition, an increased reabsorption of bilirubin from the intestinal tract (i.e., enterohepatic bilirubin circulation) limits bilirubin clearance and thereby enhances the hepatic bilirubin load. The following equation reflects the complexity of interactions among the rates of bilirubin production (a), the enterohepatic circulation of bilirubin (b), and bilirubin elimination (c) in determining the total serum bilirubin (TSB) levels at any postnatal time point t, where TSB_0 is the cord blood TSB (Valaes, 2001).

$$TSB_t = TSB_0 + \sum [a(t) + b(t) - c(t)^{\Delta t}]$$

A variety of specific clinical factors can increase bilirubin load and/or decrease bilirubin clearance and thereby contribute to neonatal indirect hyperbilirubinemia in any given infant (Box 79-1), although quantifying the individual contribution of each may not be possible. In a small fraction of neonates, a constellation of conditions may lead to hazardous levels of hyperbilirubinemia that pose a neurotoxic risk.

INCREASED HEPATIC BILIRUBIN LOAD: ENHANCED ENTEROHEPATIC CIRCULATION

Intestinal absorption of bilirubin excreted into the intestine is enhanced by several features of newborn physiology, thereby adding to the tendency for newborns to become jaundiced. Conjugated bilirubin, as either the mono- or diglucuronide, is unstable and can be spontaneously or enzymatically (via β-glucuronidase) hydrolyzed back to unconjugated bilirubin, which is easily reabsorbed through the intestinal mucosa. In addition, absorption is enhanced by the sterility of the intestinal contents. Older children and adults have intestinal flora, which can metabolize conjugated bilirubin to the water-soluble and readily excretable breakdown products urobilin and stercobilin. Newborns have no such advantage; instead, the neonatal intestinal mucosa has a greater concentration of β-glucuronidase than is found in the adult. This enzyme can deconjugate bilirubin to form more unconjugated bilirubin, which can be absorbed via the enterohepatic circulation, adding further to the hepatic unconjugated bilirubin load. Two other factors accelerating the deconjugation of bilirubin glucuronides in the newborn intestine are the mildly alkaline pH of the proximal intestine, which facilitates nonenzymatic hydrolysis, and the predominance of monoglucuronides as the main excretion form of bilirubin in the first few days of life.

INCREASED HEPATIC BILIRUBIN LOAD: HEMOLYTIC DISEASE

The reduced erythrocyte life span of normal newborn red cells (70 to 90 days as opposed to 120 days in the adult) (Pearson, 1967; Vest et al, 1961) contributes to an enhanced level of bilirubin production. It follows that an increase in red cell mass, that is, polycythemia, and factors known to accelerate red cell turnover, that is, hemolytic disorders, are clinically important conditions that increase the risk for developing neonatal hyperbilirubinemia. Of these, hemolysis is the most potent contributor to the genesis of marked hyperbilirubinemia and merits special consideration. The causes of hemolysis in the neonatal period are many but can be broadly grouped into three major categories: (1) heritable defects in red cell metabolism, membrane structure, or hemoglobin; (2) acquired disorders; and (3) immune mediated mechanisms (see Box 79-1).

HERITABLE CAUSES OF HEMOLYSIS: RED CELL MEMBRANE DEFECTS

Of the many red cell membrane defects that lead to hemolysis, only hereditary spherocytosis, elliptocytosis, stomatocytosis, and infantile pyknocytosis manifest themselves in the newborn period (Caprari et al, 1997; Oski, 1993a; Tuffy et al, 1959). Establishing a diagnosis of these disorders is often difficult because newborns normally exhibit a marked variation in red cell membrane size and shape (Oski, 1982, 1993a; Stockman, 1988; Zipursky et al, 1983). Spherocytes, however, are not often seen

BOX 79-1   Causes of Indirect Hyperbilirubinemia in Neonates

A. INCREASED HEPATIC BILIRUBIN LOAD

1. Hemolytic disease—red blood cell membrane defects
   a. Hereditary spherocytosis
   b. Elliptocytosis
   c. Stomatocytosis
   d. Pyknocytosis
2. Hemolytic disease—red blood cell enzyme abnormalities
   a. Glucose-6-phosphate dehydrogenase deficiency
   b. Pyruvate kinase deficiency
3. Hemolytic disease—hemoglobinopathies
   a. Alpha-thalassemia
   b. Gamma-thalassemia
4. Hemolytic disease—immune mediated (positive direct Coombs' test)
   a. Rh isoimmunization
   b. ABO incompatibility
   c. Minor blood group incompatibility
5. Enhanced enterohepatic bilirubin circulation
   a. Intestinal obstruction, pyloric stenosis
   b. Ileus, meconium plugging, cystic fibrosis
   c. Breast milk feeding
6. Extravascular blood (e.g., cephalhematoma)
7. Polycythemia

B. DECREASED HEPATIC BILIRUBIN CLEARANCE

1. Prematurity including late-preterm gestation
2. Hormonal deficiency
   a. Hypothyroidism
   b. Hypopituitarism
3. Impaired hepatic bilirubin uptake
   a. Patent ductus venosus
   b. *SLCO1B1* gene polymorphisms
4. Disorders of bilirubin conjugation—*UGT1A1* gene variants
   a. Crigler-Najjar syndrome type I
   b. Crigler-Najjar syndrome type II (Arias disease)
   c. Gilbert disease
5. Enhanced enterohepatic circulation
   a. Intestinal obstruction, pyloric stenosis
   b. Ileus, meconium plugging, cystic fibrosis
   c. Breast milk feeding

SLCO1B1, Solute carrier organic anion transporter 1B1; *UGT1A1,* uridine diphosphate glucuronosyltransferase 1A1.

on red cell smears of hematologically normal newborns, and this morphologic abnormality, when prominent, may yield a diagnosis of hereditary spherocytosis in the immediate neonatal period. A mean corpuscular hemoglobin concentration of ≥36.0 g/dL can also be used to alert neonatal caregivers to the possible presence of hereditary spherocytosis (Christensen and Henry, 2010). Given that approximately 75% of families affected with hereditary spherocytosis manifest an autosomal-dominant phenotype, a positive family history can often be elicited and provide further support for this diagnosis. The diagnosis of hereditary spherocytosis can be confirmed using the incubated osmotic fragility test, which is a reliable diagnostic tool in neonates after the first weeks of life when coupled with fetal red cell controls. One must rule out symptomatic ABO hemolytic disease by performing a direct Coombs' test, because infants so affected may also manifest prominent microspherocytosis (Becker et al, 1993). Moreover, hereditary spherocytosis and symptomatic

ABO hemolytic disease can occur in the same infant and result in severe anemia and hyperbilirubinemia (Trucco et al, 1967).

Hereditary elliptocytosis and stomatocytosis are rare but reported causes of hemolysis in the newborn period (Oski, 1993a). Infantile pyknocytosis, a transient red cell membrane abnormality manifesting itself during the first few months of life, is more common. The pyknocyte, an irregularly contracted red cell with multiple spines, can normally be observed in newborns, particularly premature infants where up to approximately 5% of red cells may manifest this morphologic variant (Tuffy et al, 1959). In newborns affected with infantile pyknocytosis, up to 50% of red cells exhibit the morphologic abnormality, and this degree of pyknocytosis is associated with jaundice, anemia, and a reticulocytosis. Infantile pyknocytosis can cause hyperbilirubinemia that is severe enough to require control by exchange transfusion (Tuffy et al, 1959). Red cells transfused into affected infants become pyknocytic and have a shortened life span, suggesting that an extracorpuscular factor mediates the morphologic alteration (Ackerman, 1969; Keimowitz et al, 1965; Tuffy et al, 1959). Whatever the mechanism underlying infantile pyknocytosis, the disorder tends to resolve after several months of life. Pyknocytosis may also occur in other conditions including glucose-6-phosphate dehydrogenase (G6PD) deficiency and hereditary elliptocytosis, and these must be excluded before a diagnosis of infantile pyknocytosis is made.

HERITABLE CAUSES OF HEMOLYSIS: RED CELL ENZYME DEFICIENCIES

The two most common red cell enzyme defects that can lead to hyperbilirubinemia in the neonatal period are G6PD (Beutler, 1994; Kaplan et al, 1998, 2004; Luzzatto, 1993; MacDonald, 1995; Valaes, 1994) and pyruvate kinase deficiency (Luzzatto, 1993). G6PD deficiency is an X-linked enzymopathy affecting hemizygous males, homozygous females, and a subset of heterozygous females (via X chromosome inactivation) and remains a noteworthy cause of hazardous hyperbilirubinemia and kernicterus worldwide including the United States. G6PD is critical to the redox metabolism of red blood cells, and G6PD deficiency may be associated with acute hemolysis in newborns following exposure to oxidative stress. Reported hemolytic triggers in G6PD deficiency are outlined in Box 79-2. Severe hemolysis and marked hyperbilirubinemia may occur in this context and result in kernicterus (Kaplan et al, 1998, 2004; Valaes, 1994). Another important hemolytic trigger in G6PD-deficient newborns is infection. Hemolysis in G6PD-deficient neonates, however, is often self-limited and overt anemia not necessarily noted, masked by other factors that modulate hemoglobin concentration in the immediate newborn period (Valaes, 1994). Indeed, severe jaundice rather than anemia may predominate in the clinical presentation. Moreover, severe neonatal jaundice can develop in the absence of significant hemolysis in some G6PD-deficient babies (Kaplan et al, 2008). In other neonates, the combination of G6PD deficiency with the hepatic bilirubin conjugation defects of Gilbert syndrome significantly increases

Box 79-2 Agents Triggering Hemolysis in Patients With Glucose-6-Phosphate Dehydrogenase Deficiency

ANTIMALARIALS
Pamaquine
Pentaquine
Plasmoquine
Primaquine
Quinacrine
Quinine
Quinocide
Sulfonamides
Sulfacetamide
Sulfamethoxazole

SULFANILAMIDE
Sulfamethoxypyridazine
Sulfapyridine
Sulfisoxazole
Trisulfapyrimidine

SULFONES
Nitrofurans
Furaltadone
Furazolidone
Nitrofurantoin
Nitrofurazone
Thiazolesulfone

ANTIPYRETICS AND ANALGESICS
Acetophenetidin
Acetylsalicylic acid
Aminopyrine
Antipyrone
p-Aminosalicylic acid

OTHERS
Ascorbic acid
Chloramphenicol
Chloroquine
Aniline dyes
Dimercaprol (BAL)
Fava beans
Methylene blue

NALIDIXIC ACID
Naphthalene* (used in mothballs)
Naphthoquinones* (used in mothballs)
Paradichlorobenzenes (moth repellent, car freshener, bathroom deodorizer)
Phenylhydrazine
Probenecid
Quinidine

TOLBUTAMIDE
Vitamin K, water-soluble analogues
Menadione diphosphate
Menadione sodium disulfate

Adapted from Oski FA, Naiman JL: *Hematologic problems in the newborn*, ed 2, Philadelphia, 1972, WB Saunders; and from Valaes F: Severe neonatal jaundice associated with glucose-6-phosphate dehydrogenase deficiency: pathogenesis and global epidemiology, *Acta Paediatr Suppl* 394:58-76, 1994.
*Associated with most severe and numerous hemolytic episodes.

the risk of hyperbilirubinemia (Kaplan et al, 1997). Details regarding this icterogenic genetic interaction and other aspects of G6PD deficiency in neonates are described later under hyperbilirubinemia risk factors.

Pyruvate kinase deficiency is an autosomal recessive disorder that is less prevalent than G6PD deficiency and typically presents with jaundice, anemia, and reticulocytosis (Mentzer, 1993; Oski, 1982). Such jaundice may be severe; in one historical series, a full third of affected infants required exchange transfusion to control their hyperbilirubinemia (Matthay et al, 1981), and kernicterus in the context of pyruvate kinase deficiency has been described (Oski et al, 1964). The diagnosis of pyruvate kinase deficiency is often difficult because the enzymatic abnormality is frequently not simply a quantitative defect, but in many cases involves abnormal enzyme kinetics or an unstable enzyme that decreases in activity as the red cell ages. The diagnosis of pyruvate kinase deficiency should be considered whenever jaundice and a picture of nonspherocytic, Coombs'-negative hemolytic anemia is observed, particularly in newborns from tightly inbred communities as in the case of the Amish and Mennonites.

HERITABLE CAUSES OF HEMOLYSIS: HEMOGLOBINOPATHIES

Defects in hemoglobin structure or synthesis are disorders that infrequently manifest themselves in the neonatal period. Of these, the alpha-thalassemia syndromes are the most likely to be clinically apparent in newborns. Each human diploid cell contains four copies of the alpha-globin gene, and thus, four alpha-thalassemia syndromes have been described reflecting the presence of defects in 1, 2, 3, or 4 alpha-globin genes. Silent carriers have one abnormal alpha-globin chain and are asymptomatic. Alpha-thalassemia trait is associated with two alpha-thalassemia mutations and in neonates is not associated with hemolysis. Alpha-thalassemia trait, however, is common in African American populations and can be detected by a low mean corpuscular volume of <95 μm^3 (normal infants 100 to 120 μm^3) (Schmaier et al, 1973). Hemoglobin H disease results from the presence of three thalassemia mutations and can cause hemolysis and anemia in neonates (Pearson, 1982). Homozygous alpha-thalassemia (total absence of alpha chain synthesis) results in profound hemolysis, anemia, hydrops fetalis, and almost always stillbirth or death in the immediate neonatal period.

The pure beta thalassemias do not manifest themselves in the newborn period and the gamma thalassemias are (1) incompatible with life (homozygous form), (2) associated with transient mild to moderate neonatal anemia (if one or two genes are involved) that resolves when beta chain synthesis begins, or (3) in combination with impaired beta chain synthesis, associated with severe hemolytic anemia and marked hyperbilirubinemia (Oort et al, 1981).

ACQUIRED CAUSES OF HEMOLYSIS

Acquired causes of hemolysis comprise a miscellaneous group of disorders that include among others (1) the microangiopathic hemolysis associated with disseminated intravascular coagulation or hemangiomas and (2) infection (bacterial sepsis or congenital infections) (Oski, 1982). The mechanism(s) underlying the hemolytic process in the latter is not fully understood but may also serve as a hemolytic trigger in the context of G6PD deficiency.

IMMUNE-MEDIATED HEMOLYTIC DISEASE

Immune-mediated hemolysis encompasses the fetomaternal incompatibilities of the Rhesus (Rh), ABO (major), and minor blood group systems. Historically Rh incompatibility has been viewed as the most clinically important immune-mediated hemolytic disorder. The incidence of isoimmunization to the Rh D antigen, however, has declined since the introduction of $Rh_0(D)$ immune globulin in 1968 and is now estimated at approximately 1 case per 1000 live births (Bowman, 2000; Chavez et al, 1991). Most instances of Rh isoimmunization are due to the Rh D antigen (Bowman, 2000; Gottvall et al, 1994). The severity of hemolysis varies in the context of Rh isoimmunization, but almost half of Rh-positive infants born to Rh-sensitized mothers will have moderate or severe disease. Affected infants develop significant hyperbilirubinemia that frequently requires exchange transfusion, in addition to intensive phototherapy. Isoimmunization secondary to minor blood group antigens, such as Kell, Duffy, and Kidd, can also lead to significant hemolysis in utero and postnatal hyperbilirubinemia, although these antigens are far less potent in inducing antibodies than Rh D. The incidence of clinically significant sensitization to the minor blood group antigens as determined by metaanalysis approximates 1 in 330 pregnancies (Solola et al, 1983).

Hemolytic disease related to ABO incompatibility is generally limited to infants of blood group A or B whose mothers are blood group O (Naiman, 1982; Ozolek et al, 1994). Although this association exists in approximately 15% of pregnancies, only a fraction of infants born in this context will develop significant hyperbilirubinemia (Naiman, 1982; Ozolek et al, 1994). Defining which infants will become so affected is difficult to predict using laboratory screening tests. Ozolek et al observed that of type A or B infants born to mothers who are blood group O, only one third had a positive direct Coombs' test, and of those with a positive direct Coombs' test, only approximately 15% had peak serum bilirubin levels ≥12.8 mg/dL (Ozolek et al, 1994). Thus, evidence of symptomatic ABO hemolytic disease was found in only 4% of such incompatible mother-infant pairs and was not strongly predicted by the Coombs' test. Similarly, group A or B infants born to respectively incompatible group B or A mothers are not likely to manifest symptomatic ABO hemolytic disease or have a positive direct Coombs' test (<1%) (Ozolek et al, 1994). Infants born of ABO-incompatible mother-infant pairs who have a negative direct Coombs' test as a group appear to be at no greater risk for developing hyperbilirubinemia than their ABO-compatible counterparts, regardless of the indirect Coombs' test status (Ozolek et al, 1994).

Despite the difficulty in predicting its development, symptomatic ABO hemolytic disease does occur and in individual instances may develop even in the absence of a positive direct Coombs' test (Naiman, 1982; Voak et al, 1969). The latter may reflect a paucity of A and B antigens on newborn red cells and/or the absorption of serum antibody by A and B antigen epitopes throughout the body tissues and fluids (Naiman, 1982). The diagnosis of symptomatic ABO hemolytic disease should be considered in infants who develop marked jaundice in the context of ABO incompatibility that is generally accompanied by a positive direct Coombs' test and prominent microspherocytosis on red cell smear (Naiman, 1982). The hyperbilirubinemia seen with symptomatic ABO hemolytic disease is often detected within the first 12 to 24 hours of life (i.e., icterus praecox) (Halbrecht, 1944) and is usually controlled by using intensive phototherapy alone (Naiman, 1982). Only a few affected infants develop hyperbilirubinemia to levels requiring exchange transfusion (Mollison, 1983). Nevertheless, in hyperbilirubinemic newborns with ABO hemolytic disease, TSB should be followed during phototherapy to ensure that the TSB does not rise to levels that merit exchange transfusion. Routine screening of all ABO-incompatible cord blood has been recommended in the past (Hubinont, 1960) and remains common practice in many nurseries (Leistikow et al, 1995). More current literature (Leistikow et al, 1995; Quinn et al, 1988; Ozolek et al, 1994), however, suggests that such routine screening is not warranted given the low yield and cost, consistent with the tenor of recommendations of the American Association of Blood Banks (Judd et al, 1990). A blood type and Coombs' test are indicated, however, in the evaluation of any newborn with early and/or clinically significant jaundice.

DECREASED HEPATIC BILIRUBIN CLEARANCE

HEPATIC BILIRUBIN UPTAKE

During intrauterine life, fetal bilirubin is removed by the placenta, metabolized, and excreted by the maternal liver, and thus the bilirubin in cord blood is virtually entirely unconjugated. At birth, blood supply to the newborn right liver lobe changes from the high oxygen content of the umbilical vein to the low oxygen content of the portal vein. Blood flow through the hepatic arteries develops only in the 1st week of extrauterine life, and the ductus venosus may remain partially patent for several days, allowing blood to bypass the liver. These factors can contribute to a delay in the plasma clearance of bilirubin. In addition, recent evidence suggests that unconjugated bilirubin may be a substrate for the solute carrier organic anion transporter *SLCO1B1*, a sinusoidal transporter that facilitates the hepatic uptake of a broad range of endogenous substrates and xenobiotics in an ATP-independent fashion (Cui et al, 2001). It follows that the developmental expression of *SLCO1B1* (Daood et al, 2006) and nonsynonymous *SLCO1B1* gene variants may affect hepatic bilirubin uptake kinetics and bilirubin metabolism of neonates (Huang et al, 2004).

HEPATIC BILIRUBIN CONJUGATION

The bilirubin conjugating capacity of infants is dependent on the activity of hepatic uridine diphosphate-glucuronosyltransferase 1A1 (*UGT1A1*). UGT1A1 isoenzyme expression is modulated in a developmental manner such that its activity is 0.1% of adult levels at 17 to 30 weeks' gestation, increasing to 1% of adult values between 30 and 40 weeks' gestation and reaching adult levels by 14 weeks of postnatal life (Coughtrie et al, 1988; Kawade et al, 1981). This graded upregulation of hepatic UGT1A1 activity over the first few days of life may be induced by the TSB itself and is noted following birth regardless of the newborn's gestational age. Induction of *UGT1A1* is also enhanced by certain drugs. Phenobarbital is known to have this effect, and a phenobarbital responsive enhancer module (PBREM) in the *UGT1A1* gene promoter element has been identified. Indeed, a polymorphism of the *UGT1A1* PBREM (T-3279G) is associated with an increased risk of hyperbilirubinemia (Sugatani et al, 2002).

In addition to the developmentally modulated postnatal transition in hepatic bilirubin *UGT1A1* activity, there are congenital inborn errors of *UGT1A1* expression, commonly referred to as the indirect hyperbilirubinemia syndromes (Valaes, 1976). These include the Crigler-Najjar type I and II (Arias) syndromes, and Gilbert syndrome

TABLE 79-1 Congenital Nonhemolytic Unconjugated Hyperbilirubinemia: Clinical Syndromes

Characteristic	Severity		
	Marked (Crigler-Najjar Type I)	Moderate (Crigler-Najjar Type II, Arias)	Mild (Gilbert Syndrome)
Steady-state total serum bilirubin	>20 mg/dL	<20 mg/dL	<5 mg/dL
Range of bilirubin values	14–50 mg/dL	5.3–37.6 mg/dL	0.8–10 mg/dL
Total bilirubin in bile	<10 mg/dL (increased with phototherapy)	50–100 mg/dL	Normal
Conjugated bilirubin in bile	Absent	Present (only monoglucuronide)	Present (50% monoglucuronide)
Bilirubin clearance	Extremely decreased	Markedly decreased	20–30% of normal
Hepatic bilirubin uptake	Normal	Normal	Reduced
Bilirubin *UGT1A1* activity	None detected	None detected	Decreased
Genetics	Autosomal recessive	Heterogeneity of defect distinctly possible	Genetic polymorphisms: 1. Thymine-adenine $(TA)_7$ and $(TA)_8$ repeats in the *UGT1A1* promoter region 2. G211A (Gly71Arg) *UGT1A1* coding sequence mutation identified in Asian populations 3. Linkage disequilibrium between $(TA)_7$/ $(TA)_7$ and T-3279G PBREM *UGT1A1* promoter polymorphisms

Adapted, updated, and modified from Valaes T: Bilirubin metabolism: review and discussion of inborn errors, *Clin Perinatol* 3:177, 1976.
UGT1A1, Uridine diphosphate glucuronosyltransferase 1A1 isoenzyme.

(Table 79-1). Crigler and Najjar first described a clinical syndrome of severe chronic nonhemolytic unconjugated hyperbilirubinemia in 1952 (Crigler et al, 1952). Affected infants have complete absence of bilirubin *UGT1A1* activity and are at significant risk for hyperbilirubinemic encephalopathy and its neurodevelopmental sequelae. Although inherited in an autosomal recessive pattern, the type I syndrome has marked genetic heterogeneity (Clarke et al, 1997). Currently, more than 30 different genetic mutations have been identified in Crigler-Najjar type I syndrome, and defects common to both the *UGT1A1* exon and those comprising the constant domain (exons 2 to 5) (Clarke et al, 1997) underlie most cases. Such gene defects are typically nonsense or "stop" mutations in nature.

Phototherapy is the mainstay of treatment for infants and children with Crigler-Najjar type 1 syndrome, although neonates may develop hazardous levels of hyperbilirubinemia necessitating exchange transfusion. Liver transplantation is the only current definitive therapeutic intervention for this disorder (Shevell et al, 1987). Human hepatocyte transplantation holds promise to enhance hepatic *UGT1A1* activity as an alternative approach that could obviate the need for liver transplantation. The ultimate treatment for this inborn error of bilirubin *UGT1A1* expression will reside in the development of an effective gene therapy strategy (Roy-Chowdhury et al, 2001).

In contrast, the Arias syndrome, typified by more moderate levels of indirect hyperbilirubinemia as well as low but detectable hepatic bilirubin *UGT1A1* activity, appears in the majority of cases to be mediated by missense mutations in the *UGT1A1* gene (Clarke et al, 1997). Phenobarbital can be trialed to induce residual *UGT1A1* activity. These rare but important clinical syndromes must be included in the differential diagnosis of prolonged marked indirect hyperbilirubinemia.

Gilbert syndrome, originally described at the turn of the previous century (Gilbert et al, 1901), is far more common and characterized by mild, chronic, or recurrent unconjugated hyperbilirubinemia in the absence of liver disease or overt hemolysis (Gourley, 1994). Hepatic *UGT1A1* activity is reduced at least 50% in affected subjects and more than 95% of their total serum bilirubin is unconjugated (Gourley, 1994). Typically, the indirect hyperbilirubinemia associated with Gilbert syndrome is seen during fasting associated with an intercurrent illness. Interestingly, in about half of patients there is also an unexplained, shortened red cell life span and increased bilirubin production (Powell et al, 1967).

Gilbert syndrome affects ~9% of the population and a genetic basis for this disorder has been defined (Bosma et al, 1995). The start site on the *UGT1A1* gene where transcription of messenger RNA begins, that is, the promoter element is abnormal. More specifically, the variant promoter for the gene encoding *UGT1A1* contains a two base-pair addition (TA) in the TATAA promoter element giving rise to 7 ($A[TA]_7TAA$) rather than the more usual 6 ($A[TA]_6TAA$) repeats and is known as *UGT1A1*28*. This extra TA repeat ($A[TA]_7TAA$) impairs proper message transcription and accounts for a reduced *UGT1A1* activity (Bosma et al, 1995). Indeed, as the repeat number increases, *UGT1A1* activity decreases (Beutler et al, 1998). Subjects with Gilbert syndrome are homozygous for the *UGT1A1*28* variant promoter providing a genetic marker for this disorder. The expanded $A[TA]_7TAA$ promoter motif is expressed in the heterozygous form in 40% of the population (Bosma et al, 1995).

Although Gilbert syndrome is most commonly diagnosed in young adulthood, investigators have long speculated that this disorder might contribute to indirect hyperbilirubinemia in the newborn period (Odell, 1980; Oski, 1984; Valaes, 1976). Identification of a molecular marker for Gilbert syndrome has provided investigators with an important tool to study the role of Gilbert syndrome in the pathogenesis of neonatal jaundice. Bancroft et al reported that newborn infants with the A(TA)$_7$TAA *UGT1A1* promoter polymorphism have accelerated jaundice and decreased fecal excretion of bilirubin mono- and diglucuronides. Roy-Chowdhury et al 2002 in an analogous study demonstrated that the A(TA)$_7$TAA variant is associated with modestly higher postnatal TSB levels. Others have failed to demonstrate a clinically significant effect of A(TA)$_7$TAA alone on peak TSB. However, the coupling of A(TA)$_7$TAA with icterogenic conditions such as G6PD deficiency and hereditary spherocytosis markedly increases a newborn's risk for hyperbilirubinemia (Iolascon et al, 1998; Kaplan et al, 1997). Others have clearly demonstrated that the A(TA)$_7$TAA promoter variant is prevalent in breastfed infants who develop prolonged neonatal indirect hyperbilirubinemia (Maruo et al, 1999; Monaghan et al, 1999; Roy-Chowdhury et al, 2002). In Asian populations, the nucleotide 211 guanine-to-adenine mutation (G71R) in the coding sequence of *UGT1A1* (*UGT1A1*6*) appears to underlie the Gilbert phenotype and contribute to neonatal hyperbilirubinemia risk (Huang, 2005; Huang et al, 2002a, 2004). Taken together, these studies demonstrate that Gilbert syndrome is a significant contributing factor to neonatal jaundice. The role of Gilbert syndrome in the genesis of extreme hyperbilirubinemia remains unclear, although (1) the low direct bilirubin fractions and (2) evidence of poor feeding and prominent weight loss (i.e., a state resembling fasting) reported in several of the published cases of extreme neonatal hyperbilirubinemia (Bhutani et al, 2004; Maisels et al, 1995) suggest that Gilbert syndrome might contribute to some cases of marked jaundice.

CLINICAL RELEVANCE

All of the aforementioned physiologic phenomena have the combined effect of increasing TSB levels in the healthy term newborn. The late-preterm and premature newborn are even more susceptible to these influences. Because individual variation in the maturation of these systems is great, TSB levels in a normal neonatal population vary widely. Slight perturbations in any of these processes can result in increased TSB levels. For example, through studies of production of carbon monoxide (CO), an index of heme breakdown produced in equimolar amounts to biliverdin by heme oxygenase, it has been determined that the infant of a diabetic mother has an increased propensity for jaundice because of enhanced production as well as impaired elimination of bilirubin. Any pathologic process that increases the production or impairs the elimination of bilirubin can exacerbate the normally occurring physiologic jaundice in newborns.

Certain demographic, environmental, and genetic risk factors, among a myriad of icterogenic contributors, merit special clinical attention. These are characterized as major risk factors for the development of severe hyperbilirubinemia in the 2004 American Academy of Pediatrics (AAP) clinical practice guideline on hyperbilirubinemia management in infants of 35 or more weeks' gestation (Box 79-3) (AAP, 2004). Although each holds the potential

---

BOX 79-3 Major Risk Factors for Development of Severe Hyperbilirubinemia in Infants of 35 or More Weeks' Gestation

Gestational age 35–36 weeks

Exclusive breastfeeding, particularly if nursing is not going well and weight loss is excessive

Blood group incompatibility with positive direct antiglobulin test, other known hemolytic disease (e.g., G6PD deficiency)

East Asian race

Jaundice observed in the first 24 hours

Cephalhematoma or significant bruising

Previous sibling received phototherapy

Predischarge TSB or TcB level in the high-risk zone

Adapted from: American Academy of Pediatrics: Management of hyperbilirubinemia in the newborn infant 35 or more weeks of gestation, *Pediatrics* 114:297-316, 2004.

---

to be a singularly important, even sole, contributor to an infant's hyperbilirubinemia, more often one risk factor is observed in combination with others (Huang et al, 2004; Newman et al, 2000; Watchko et al, 2009), particularly in the genesis of marked hyperbilirubinemia. Indeed, in infants with peak TSB levels ≥25 mg/dL (428 μmol/L), 88% had a least two and 43% had three or more identified risk factors in one recent report (Newman et al, 2000), and 58% with peak TSB ≥20 mg/dL (342 μmol/L) had at least two risk factors in another (Huang et al, 2004). Data derived from risk instruments that incorporate several factors support the potential multifactorial etiopathogenesis of marked hyperbilirubinemia; albeit genetic contributors may go undetected and individual factors confer different degrees of risk (Newman et al, 2000, 2005). These instruments further highlight the clinical importance of two specific risk factors in particular, namely (1) late preterm gestational age and (2) exclusive breastfeeding (Keren et al, 2008; Newman et al, 2000, 2005). These two contributors and six others of notable clinical impact—(1) glucose-6-phosphate dehydrogenase (G6PD) deficiency, (2) ABO hemolytic disease, (3) East Asian ethnicity, (4) jaundice observed in the first 24 hours of life, (5) cephalhematoma or significant bruising, and (6) history of previous sibling treated with phototherapy—are reviewed in further detail.

LATE-PRETERM GESTATION

Late preterm (34$^{0/7}$ to 36$^{6/7}$ weeks' gestation) and full-term infants become jaundiced by similar mechanisms, including (1) an increased bilirubin load on the hepatocyte as a result of decreased erythrocyte survival, increased erythrocyte volume, and the enterohepatic circulation of bilirubin and (2) defective hepatic bilirubin conjugation (Watchko, 2006b). Late preterm infants evidence a similar degree of red blood cell turnover and heme degradation as their term counterparts, but demonstrate lower *UGT1A1* enzyme activity as compared to their term counterparts (Kaplan et al, 2005; Kawade et al, 1981). Moreover, although there is a marked postnatal increase in *UGT1A1* enzyme activity in newborns, such maturation appears to be slower in late preterm neonates during the 1st week of life (Kawade et al,

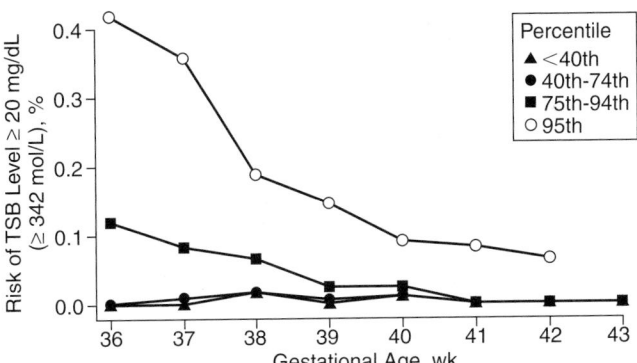

FIGURE 79-1 Risk of developing a TSB ≥20 mg/dL (342 μmol/L) as a function of gestational age (weeks) and percentile-based TSB measured at <48 hours using the Bhutani nomogram. *(Modified from Arch Pediatr Adolesc Med 159:117, Copyright 2005, American Medical Association. All rights reserved.)*

1981). This exaggerated hepatic immaturity contributes to the greater prevalence, severity, and duration of neonatal jaundice in late preterm infants.

Underscoring the importance of late preterm gestational age is the ≈8-fold increased risk of developing a TSB of ≥20 mg/dL (342 μmol/L) in infants born at 36 weeks' gestation (5.2%) as compared to those born at 41 or ≥42 weeks' gestation (0.7% and 0.6%, respectively) (Newman et al, 1999). This gestational age effect is even more evident when examined as a function of hour-specific TSB risk zones using the percentile-based nomogram described by Bhutani et al (1999) as shown in Figure 79-1 (Newman et al, 2005). It can be seen, for example, that coupling 36 weeks' gestation with a high risk zone (≥95%) TSB is associated with a >40% chance of developing a TSB of ≥20 mg/dL (342 μmol/L) (Newman et al, 2005). Even a high intermediate risk zone (75% to 94%) TSB in a 36-week-gestation late preterm neonate is associated with >10% chance of developing a TSB ≥20 mg/dL (342 μmol/L), a risk greater than that for a full-term newborn with a TSB level ≥95% (Newman et al, 2005). The reported difficulty in visually assessing the degree of jaundice in late preterm newborns (Keren et al, 2009) suggests that birth hospitalization TSB or transcutaneous bilirubin screening before discharge is warranted to more fully ascertain hyperbilirubinemia risk as recently recommended (Maisels et al, 2009b).

Late preterm infants are disproportionately overrepresented in the U.S. Pilot Kernicterus registry, a database of voluntarily reported cases of kernicterus (Bhutani et al, 2004, 2006). Moreover, the registry demonstrates that late preterm neonates show signs of bilirubin neurotoxicity at an earlier postnatal age than term newborns, indirectly suggesting a greater vulnerability to bilirubin-induced brain injury (Bhutani et al, 2006). Clinical hyperbilirubinemia management guidelines for late preterm infants therefore recommend treatment at lower TSB thresholds than term newborns, a distinction that is an important component of the 2004 American Academy of Pediatrics practice guideline on neonatal jaundice (AAP, 2004). In this regard it is important to note that (1) the management of late preterm newborns born between 34⁰ᐟ⁷ and 34⁶ᐟ⁷ weeks' gestation is not addressed

by the 2004 AAP guideline, and (2) infants born between 37⁰ᐟ⁷ and 37⁶ᐟ⁷ weeks' gestation, although strictly defined as term, are characterized in the 2004 AAP guideline as medium to higher risk and are to be managed as "late preterm" regarding phototherapy and exchange transfusion thresholds (AAP, 2004).

Of the other clinical factors observed in conjunction with late preterm gestation hyperbilirubinemia risk, breast milk feeding has been identified most consistently, indeed almost uniformly, and therefore appears to be of paramount importance (Bhutani et al, 2004, 2006). Late preterm neonates, because of their immaturity, often demonstrate less effective sucking and swallowing and may have difficulties achieving consistent nutritive breastfeeding (Wang et al, 2004), phenomena that may predispose to varying degrees of lactation failure. Suboptimal feeding was the leading reason for discharge delay during birth hospitalization in late preterm neonates in one recent study (Wang et al, 2004). Pediatricians, therefore, need to be alert to the potential of suboptimal breast-milk feeding in late preterm neonates and not be misled by the seemingly satisfactory breastfeeding efforts of late preterm newborns during the birth hospitalization when limited colostrum volumes make it a challenge to adequately assess the effectiveness of breast-milk transfer (Neifert, 2001). Late preterm infants who are breastfed merit timely post birth-hospitalization discharge follow-up and lactation support (Bhutani et al, 2006; Watchko, 2006b). Lactation support coupled with regular neonatal weight checks is helpful in averting lactation difficulties and in the early identification of those mother-infant pairs prone to lactation failure. Parental education (written and verbal) about neonatal jaundice and when to call the pediatrician are also important (AAP, 2004). A shortened hospital stay (<48 hours after delivery), although permitted for selected healthy term neonates, is not recommended for late-preterm neonates (AAP, 2007).

EXCLUSIVE BREAST MILK FEEDING

It is likely no coincidence that almost all reported cases of kernicterus over the past two and one-half decades have occurred in breastfed infants (Bhutani et al, 2004). As such, exclusive breast milk feeding, particularly if nursing is not going well and weight loss is excessive, is listed as a major hyperbilirubinemia risk factor in the 2004 AAP practice guideline. What does the association between exclusive breast milk feeding and kernicterus imply with respect to the etiopathogenesis of marked neonatal jaundice? Numerous studies have reported an association between breastfeeding and an increased incidence and severity of hyperbilirubinemia, both during the first few days of life and in the genesis of prolonged neonatal jaundice (Hansen, 2001; Kivlahan et al, 1984; Linn et al, 1985; Maisels et al, 1986; Schneider, 1986). A pooled analysis of 12 studies comprising more than 8000 neonates showed a threefold greater incidence in TSB of ≥12.0 mg/dL (205 μmol), and a sixfold greater incidence in levels of ≥15 mg/dL (257 μmol) in breastfed infants as compared with their formula-fed counterparts (Schneider, 1986). Others, however, report that if adequate breastfeeding is established and sufficient lactation support is in place, breastfed infants should be at no greater risk for hyperbilirubinemia than their formula-fed counterparts (De Carvalho et al, 1982; Nielsen et al, 1987; Rubaltelli, 1993; Yamauchi et al, 1990). The latter studies suggest that many breastfed infants who develop marked neonatal jaundice do so in the context of a delay in lactation or varying degrees of lactation failure. Indeed, an appreciable percentage of the breastfed infants who develop kernicterus have been noted to have inadequate intake, and variable but substantial degrees of dehydration and weight loss (Bhutani et al, 2004; Johnson et al, 2002; Maisels et al, 1995).

Inadequate breast milk intake, in addition to contributing to dehydration, can further enhance hyperbilirubinemia by increasing the enterohepatic circulation of bilirubin and resultant hepatic bilirubin load. The enterohepatic circulation of bilirubin is already exaggerated in the neonatal period, in part because the newborn intestinal tract is not yet colonized with bacteria that convert conjugated bilirubin to urobilinogen, and because intestinal β-glucuronidase activity is high. Earlier studies in newborn humans and primates suggest that the enterohepatic circulation of bilirubin may account for up to 50% of the hepatic bilirubin load in neonates (Gartner et al, 1977; Poland et al, 1971). Moreover, fasting hyperbilirubinemia is largely due to intestinal reabsorption of unconjugated bilirubin, an additional mechanism by which inadequate lactation and/or poor enteral intake may contribute to marked hyperbilirubinemia in some newborns. In the context of limited hepatic conjugation capacity in the immediate postnatal period, any further increase in hepatic bilirubin load will likely result in more hyperbilirubinemia. Recent studies confirm that early breastfeeding jaundice is associated with a state of relative caloric deprivation (Bertini et al, 2001) and resultant enhanced enterohepatic circulation of bilirubin (Bertini et al, 2001; Maisels, 2000a). Breastfeeding-associated jaundice, however, is not associated with increased bilirubin production (Stevenson et al, 1980).

Lactation failure is not uniformly present in affected infants, suggesting that other mechanism(s) may be operative in breastfeeding-associated jaundice, a finding that merits further clinical study. Breast-milk feeding may act as an environmental modifier for selected genotypes and thereby potentially predispose to the development of marked neonatal jaundice (Watchko, 2005, 2004). A recent report lends credence to this possibility, demonstrating that the risk of developing a TSB ≥20 mg/dL (342 µmol/L) associated with breast-milk feeding was enhanced 22-fold when combined with expression of either a coding sequence gene polymorphism of (1) the bilirubin conjugating enzyme *UGT1A1* (the nucleotide 211 guanine to adenine [G211A] missense mutation *UGT1A1*6*) or (2) the solute carrier organic anion transporter 1B1 (*SLCO1B1*; also known as organic anion transporter polypeptide 2 [*OATP-2*]; the A388G missense variant *SLCO1B1*1b*) (Huang et al, 2004). SLCO1B1 is a sinusoidal membrane protein putatively involved in facilitating the hepatic uptake of unconjugated bilirubin (Cui et al, 2001). This hyperbilirubinemia risk increased to 88-fold when breast-milk feedings were combined with *both UGT1A1* and *SLCO1B1* variants (Huang et al, 2004). Others have previously reported an association between prolonged (>14 days) breast-milk jaundice and expression

of the *UGT1A1* gene promoter variant allele A(TA)₇TAA (*UGT1A1*28*) (Maruo et al, 1999; Monaghan et al, 1999). Although the relationship between breast-milk feeding and jaundice must be recognized, the benefits of breast-milk feeds far outweigh the related risk of hyperbilirubinemia. Cases of severe neonatal hyperbilirubinemia with suboptimal breast-milk feedings underscore the need for effective lactation support and timely follow-up exams.

G6PD DEFICIENCY

G6PD deficiency is an X-linked enzymopathy affecting hemizygous males, homozygous females, and a subset of heterozygous females (via nonrandom X chromosome inactivation); it is an important cause of severe neonatal hyperbilirubinemia and kernicterus worldwide (Beutler, 1994; Kaplan et al, 1998, 2004; Valaes, 1994, 2000). Although most prevalent in Africa, the Middle East, East Asia, and the Mediterranean, G6PD deficiency has evolved into a global problem as a result of centuries of immigration and intermarriage (Beutler, 1994; Kaplan et al, 1998, 2004; Valaes, 1994, 2000). It is a noteworthy contributor to endemic rates of bilirubin encephalopathy in several developing countries (e.g., Nigeria where approximately 3% of neonatal hospital admissions evidence bilirubin encephalopathy) (Oguniesi et al, 2007) and accounts for a substantial and disproportionate number of neonates with kernicterus in the U.S. Pilot Kernicterus registry (20.8% of all reported cases) (Bhutani et al, 2004). Although the majority of the latter cases are African American males, other U.S. population subgroups at risk for G6PD deficiency include African American females and newborns of East Asian, Greek, Italian (especially Sardinia and Sicily), and Middle Eastern descent (Kaplan et al, 2004).

Current G6PD deficiency prevalence rates in the United States are 12.2% for African American males, 4.1% for African American females, 4.3% for Asian males, and 2.0% for Hispanic males (Table 79-2) (Chinevere et al, 2006). Even the ethnicity subset characterized as unknown or other in this large U.S.-based cohort showed a G6PD deficiency prevalence of 3.0% in males and 1.8% in females (Chinevere et al, 2006). In this regard, *G6PD* is remarkable for its genetic diversity (more than 370 variants have

TABLE 79-2 Presence of G6PD Deficiency in United States Military Personnel by Sex and Self-Reported Ethnicity

Ethnicity	Deficient* Female	Deficient* Male	Total
American Indian/Alaskan	112 (0.9)	492 (0.8)	604 (0.8)
Asian	465 (0.9)	1,658 (4.30)	2,123 (3.6)
African American	2,763 (4.1)	8,513 (12.2)	11,276 (10.2)
Hispanic	842 (1.2)	4,462 (2.0)	5,304 (1.9)
White	4,018 (0.0)	38,108 (0.3)	42,126 (1.3)
Unknown/other	228 (1.8)	1,641 (3.0)	1,869 (2.9)

Adapted from Chinevere TD, Murray CK, Grant E, et al: Prevalence of glucose-6-phosphate dehydrogenase deficiency in U.S. Army personnel, *Milit Med Int J AMSUS* 171:906, 2006.
*Number tested (percent deficient).

been described) (Beutler, 2008) and those mutations seen in the United States include, among numerous others, (1) the *African A*-variants, a group of double site mutations, all of which share the A376G variant (also known as G6PD A+ when expressed alone; a nondeficient variant), coupled most commonly with the G202A mutation (G202A;A376G), but on occasion with the T968C variant (T968C;A376G; also known as G6PD Betica) or the G680T mutation (G680T;A376G); (2) the *Mediterranean* (C563T) mutation; (3) the *Canton* (G1376T) mutation; and (4) the *Kaiping* (G1388A) variant (Beutler, 1994; Lin et al, 2005).

Two modes of hyperbilirubinemia presentation have classically been reported in *G6PD*-deficient neonates (with overlap between the two on occasion): (1) an acute, often sudden, unpredictable rise in TSB to potentially hazardous levels precipitated by an environmental trigger (e.g., naphthalene in mothballs or infection) (Beutler, 1994; Kaplan and Hammerman, 2004a; Kaplan et al, 1998; Valaes, 1994, 2000); this mode is difficult to foretell and therefore anticipate or prevent, and it is often a challenge to ascertain the trigger; and (2) low-grade hemolysis coupled with genetic polymorphisms of the *UGT1A1* gene that reduce *UGT1A1* expression and thereby limit hepatic bilirubin conjugation. These include the $(TA)_7$ dinucleotide repeat TATAA box promoter element (*UGT1A1*28*) (Kaplan et al, 1997, 2004a; Valaes, 1994, 2000) and the G211A coding sequence (UGT1A1*6) (Huang et al, 2002b) variants; the former underlies the Gilbert's syndrome phenotype in Caucasians (Bosma et al, 1995), whereas the latter underlies the Gilbert's syndrome phenotype in East Asians (Huang et al, 2002a, 2005). Kaplan et al were the first to demonstrate dose-dependent genetic interactions between the *UGT1A1*28* promoter variant and G6PD deficiency that enhance neonatal hyperbilirubinemia risk (1997). Others have subsequently confirmed that coupling of (1) G6PD deficiency and (2) other genetically determined hemolytic conditions (e.g., hereditary spherocytosis) *with* hepatic gene variants that adversely affect bilirubin clearance (i.e., hepatic bilirubin uptake [*SLCO1B1*] and/or conjugation [*UGT1A1*]) increases the risk of significant neonatal hyperbilirubinemia) (Huang et al, 2002b, 2005; Iolascon et al, 1998; Watchko et al, 2009). Coexistent nongenetic factors may also impact hyperbilirubinemia) risk in G6PD-deficient African American male neonates as shown in those who are also late preterm and breastfed (Kaplan et al, 2006). Sixty percent of this subgroup demonstrate bilirubin levels >95% (high risk zone) on the bilirubin nomogram of Bhutani et al (odds ratio 10.2 [1.35 to 76.93 95% confidence interval]) (Kaplan et al, 2006).

African Americans as a group have a lower incidence of neonatal hyperbilirubinemia: odds ratio 0.43 for bilirubin level that exceeded or was within 1 mg/dL [17 µmol/L] of 2004 AAP hour-specific phototherapy treatment threshold (Keren et al, 2008) and odds ratio 0.56 for TSB ≥20 mg/dL [342 µmol/L] (Newman et al, 1999) than the rest of the population; as a result, numeric instruments designed to predict hyperbilirubinemia risk in newborns deduct points for African American race (Newman et al, 2000, 2005). This lower overall hyperbilirubinemia incidence, however, may belie the hyperbilirubinemia risk for G6PD-deficient

African American newborns, leading some to caution that African American neonates with overt jaundice (male or female) merit special attention and follow-up because such infants represent exceptions to this general pattern, a subset of which might be G6PD deficient. It may be that once an African American infant develops notable jaundice, he/she is at equal or perhaps even greater risk, if G6PD deficient, for marked hyperbilirubinemia. Consistent with this assertion, Kaplan and Hammerman, (2004a) have reported that 48.4% of G6PD-deficient African American neonates developed a TSB level ≥75% and 21.9% a TSB level ≥95%. In contrast, Keren et al (2008) report that neither the presence of a G6PD mutation nor overt clinical jaundice was associated with the development of significant hyperbilirubinemia in African American infants or African American male infant cohorts. This matter merits further clinical study and clarification (Watchko, 2010).

Although there has been discussion on the potential utility of screening for G6PD deficiency in the United States, no consensus has emerged on whether or how best to screen for this condition in America, and point-of-care testing during birth hospitalization is not routinely practiced. Reports from abroad (e.g., Israel, Singapore, Taiwan) (Kaplan et al, 2008; Padilla et al, 2007) show that various point-of-care G6PD screening strategies, some that target specific at-risk population subgroups, others that screen population-wide, are associated with reductions in the prevalence of severe hyperbilirubinemia and kernicterus.

ABO HEMOLYTIC DISEASE

Hemolytic disease related to ABO incompatibility is noted to be a major risk factor for severe hyperbilirubinemia in the 2004 AAP practice guideline and for all intents and purposes is limited to infants of blood group A or B born to mothers who are blood group O as detailed earlier in this chapter. Although this association exists in approximately 15% of pregnancies, only a small fraction of such infants will develop significant hyperbilirubinemia. The diagnosis of symptomatic ABO hemolytic disease should be considered in infants who develop marked jaundice in the context of ABO incompatibility with a positive direct Coombs' test, often accompanied by microspherocytosis on red cell smear (Hershel et al, (2002); Naiman, 1982; Ozolek et al, 1994). Underscoring the importance of a positive direct Coombs' test in support of the diagnosis of ABO hemolytic disease, Herschel et al (2002) recently concluded that in direct Coombs'-negative newborns of ABO incompatible mother-infant pairs with significant hyperbilirubinemia, a cause other than isoimmunization should be sought.

Despite the difficulty in predicting its development, symptomatic ABO hemolytic disease does occur, often with clinical jaundice detected within the first 12 to 24 hours of life. The early rapid rise in TSB during the first 24 hours of life to the 10 to 15 mg/dL range or slightly higher is typically followed by a plateau at 15 to 20 mg/dL on the 2nd day of life (Cashore, 1990; Naiman, 1982). Hyperbilirubinemia secondary to ABO hemolytic disease was recognized decades ago to be controllable with phototherapy in most cases (Cashore,

1990; Naiman, 1982), and even more so using current intensive phototherapy strategies with special blue fluorescent lamps (Maisels et al, 2008). The addition of intravenous immune globulin (IVIG) to the therapeutic armamentarium against immune-mediated (positive direct Coombs') hyperbilirubinemia has proven effective in reducing hemolysis and the need for exchange transfusion in ABO hemolytic disease (number needed to treat 2.7) (Gottstein et al, 2003; Hammerman et al, 1996). The mechanism of IVIG action is not clear but is thought to inhibit hemolysis by blocking antibody receptor sites on red blood cells. Few affected infants with ABO hemolytic disease ever develop hyperbilirubinemia to levels requiring exchange transfusion (Naiman, 1982), although preparations for possible double volume exchange should be made when exchange thresholds are approached (AAP, 2004).

EAST ASIAN ETHNICITY

Neonates of East Asian ethnicity encompassing the populations of mainland China, Hong Kong, Japan, Macau, Korea, and Taiwan evidence a higher incidence of hyperbilirubinemia than others and an overall increased risk for a TSB of ≥20 mg/dL (342 μmol/L) (odds ratio 3.1 [1.5 to 6.3 confidence interval]) (Newman et al, 2000). Therefore, East Asian ancestry is listed as a major risk factor for severe hyperbilirubinemia in the 2004 AAP clinical practice guideline. Investigators have speculated as to the nature of this phenomenon invoking potential population differences in the incidence of ABO hemolytic disease and G6PD deficiency as well as environmental exposures to Chinese materia medica, among others (Ho, 1992). There is little doubt that G6PD deficiency is an important contributor to hyperbilirubinemia risk in East Asian newborns. Innate ethnic variation in hepatic bilirubin clearance (Ho, 1992) also contributes to the biologic basis of hyperbilirubinemia risk in Asian newborns as revealed by genetic analysis of enzymatic variants that modulate bilirubin metabolism. Four different *UGT1A1* coding sequence variants—G211A (*UGT1A1*6*), C686A (*UGT1A1*27*), C1091T (*UGT1A1*73*), and T1456G (*UGT1A1*7*)—have been described in East Asian populations, each associated with a Gilbert's syndrome phenotype (Huang et al, 2000, 2004). Of these, the *UGT1A1*6* variant is predominant, with an allele frequency of 11% to 13% in East Asians (Huang et al, 2000) (as high as 30% in neonates with hyperbilirubinemia ≥15 mg/dL [257 μmol/L]) (Huang et al, 2002a) and an associated significant decrease in UGT1A1 enzyme activity (Yamamoto et al, 1998). Hepatic *SLCO1B1* gene variants are also prevalent in East Asian populations (Huang et al, 2004; Kim et al, 2008), and the *SLCO1B1*1b* variant has been demonstrated to enhance neonatal hyperbilirubinemia risk (Huang et al, 2004). As noted in the section on breastmilk feeding, coupling *UGT1A1* and *SLCO1B1* variants together enhances hyperbilirubinemia risk, which is further increased when that infant is also exclusively breastfed (Huang et al, 2004). The high incidence of neonatal hyperbilirubinemia in East Asian populations appears to be at least partly attributable to the prevalence of these hepatic gene polymorphisms.

JAUNDICE OBSERVED IN THE FIRST 24 HOURS OF LIFE

Jaundice appearing in the first 24 hours of life has long been regarded as an abnormal clinical finding and an indication for obtaining a serum bilirubin measurement (AAP, 2004). Approximately 2.8% of newborns will evidence jaundice within 18 hours and 6.7% within 24 hours of age (Newman et al, 2002). As contrasted with nonjaundiced newborns on the first postnatal day, newborns with overt jaundice in the first 24 postnatal hours are more likely to receive phototherapy (18.9% vs. 1.7%; relative risk, 10.1; 95% confidence interval 4.2 to 24.4) and to develop a TSB ≥25 mg/dL (428 μmol/L) (odds ratio 2.9; 95% confidence interval 1.6 to 5.2) (Newman et al, 2002). Hemolytic disease, immune mediated and otherwise, should be a diagnostic consideration in any infant with early clinical jaundice.

CEPHALHEMATOMA OR SIGNIFICANT BRUISING

Internal hemorrhage, ecchymoses, and other extravascular blood collections will enhance the bilirubin load on the liver. Extravascular red cells have a markedly shortened life span, and their heme fraction is quickly catabolized to bilirubin by tissue macrophages that contain heme oxygenase and biliverdin reductase (Odell, 1980). Thus, cephalhematoma, subdural hemorrhage, massive adrenal hemorrhage, and marked bruising can be associated with increased serum bilirubin levels, typically manifest 48 to 72 hours after the extravasation of blood (Odell, 1980). This temporal pattern is consistent with the evolution of ecchymoses and bilirubin formation in situ and also accounts for why extravascular blood can cause prolonged indirect hyperbilirubinemia (Odell, 1980). An unusual but dramatic example of how extravascular blood can contribute to the genesis of hyperbilirubinemia is found in reports of marked jaundice associated with the delayed absorption of intraperitoneal blood in infants who received fetal intraperitoneal red cell transfusions (Rajagopalan et al, 1984; Wright et al, 1982). In one such case, 13 exchange transfusions were necessary to control the hyperbilirubinemia that resolved only when approximately 87 mL of packed red cells were evacuated from the intraperitoneal cavity (Wright et al, 1982). In this instance, the intraperitoneal blood hematocrit of 60% had the potential to contribute up to approximately 600 mg of bilirubin to the infant's bilirubin load over time. Although other causes of extravasation generally are not associated with such large amounts of sequestered blood and resultant bilirubin load, they can nevertheless contribute to the development of jaundice.

PREVIOUS SIBLING TREATED WITH PHOTOTHERAPY

A history of a previous sibling treated with phototherapy is an identified risk factor for hyperbilirubinemia (Gale et al, 1990; Newman et al, 2000) and most notable with a higher TSB in the index case (>15 mg/dL [257 μmol/L]) (Khoury et al, 1988). This relationship may reflect recurrent ABO or Rh hemolytic disease (Maisels,

1982) or exposure to a common environmental factor in addition to a shared genetic background (Gale et al, 1990). It is known that the recurrence rate of ABO hemolytic disease is high—88% in infants of the same blood type as their index sibling, with almost two thirds of the affected infants requiring treatment (Katz et al, 1982). However, an excess risk in siblings independent of other hyperbilirubinemia risk factors expected to recur in sibships (including breastfeeding, lower gestational age, and hemolytic disease) suggests that genetic rather than environmental effects are responsible (Gale et al, 1990; Khoury et al, 1988). Consistent with this hypothesis, there is a higher concordance level in TSB between monozygotic (identical) as opposed to dizygotic (fraternal) twins when controlled for confounders known to modulate neonatal bilirubinemia (Ebbesen et al, 2003). Regardless of the etiopathogenesis, a previous sibling treated with phototherapy is a risk factor for neonatal hyperbilirubinemia (AAP, 2004).

COMBINING CLINICAL RISK FACTOR ASSESSMENT WITH PREDISCHARGE BILIRUBIN MEASUREMENT

Several clinical studies suggest that combining clinical risk factor analysis with a birth hospitalization predischarge measurement of TSB or TcB improves the prediction of subsequent hyperbilirubinemia risk (Keren et al, 2008; Maisels et al, 2009a; Newman et al, 2005). Indeed, an hour-specific predischarge TSB or TcB level in the high risk zone (>95%) using the percentile-based bilirubin nomogram described by Bhutani et al (1999) (Figure 79-2) is itself a major risk factor for severe hyperbilirubinemia (Bhutani et al, 1999, 2000) (see Box 79-3). Not surprisingly, the clinical factors most predictive of hyperbilirubinemia

risk when combined with the risk zone characterization are lower gestational age and exclusive breastfeeding (Keren et al, 2008; Maisels et al, 2009a; Newman et al, 2000, 2005). On the basis of these recent reports, the authors of a commentary that provides clarifications on the 2004 American Academy of Pediatrics clinical practice guideline on the management of hyperbilirubinemia in the newborn infant 35 or more weeks' gestation recommend universal predischarge bilirubin screening to help assess the risk of subsequent severe hyperbilirubinemia (Maisels et al, 2009b). Recently published data further suggest that predischarge bilirubin screening is associated with a reduction in the incidence of TSB ≥25 mg/dL (428 µmol/L) (Eggert et al, 2006; Kuzniewicz et al, 2009), possibly by increasing the use of phototherapy (Kuzniewicz et al, 2009). The efficacy and cost effectiveness of a combined percentile based risk zone–clinical risk factor analysis in preventing bilirubin encephalopathy is unknown (Maisels et al, 2009b).

CLINICAL EVALUATION OF JAUNDICE

Jaundice is the visible manifestation in the skin of elevated serum concentrations of bilirubin. Although most adults are jaundiced when total serum bilirubin (TSB) levels exceed 2.0 mg/dL (34 µmol/L), neonates characteristically do not appear jaundiced until the TSB exceeds 5.0 to 7.0 mg/dL (86 to 120 µmol/L). Some degree of jaundice develops in approximately 60% of neonates, and chemical hyperbilirubinemia, defined as a TSB ≥2.0 mg/dL (34 µmol/L), is virtually universal in newborns during the 1st week of life. Jaundice in neonates becomes evident first on the face and progresses in a cephalocaudal fashion with increasing hyperbilirubinemia as classically characterized by Kramer (1969). Recent studies, however,

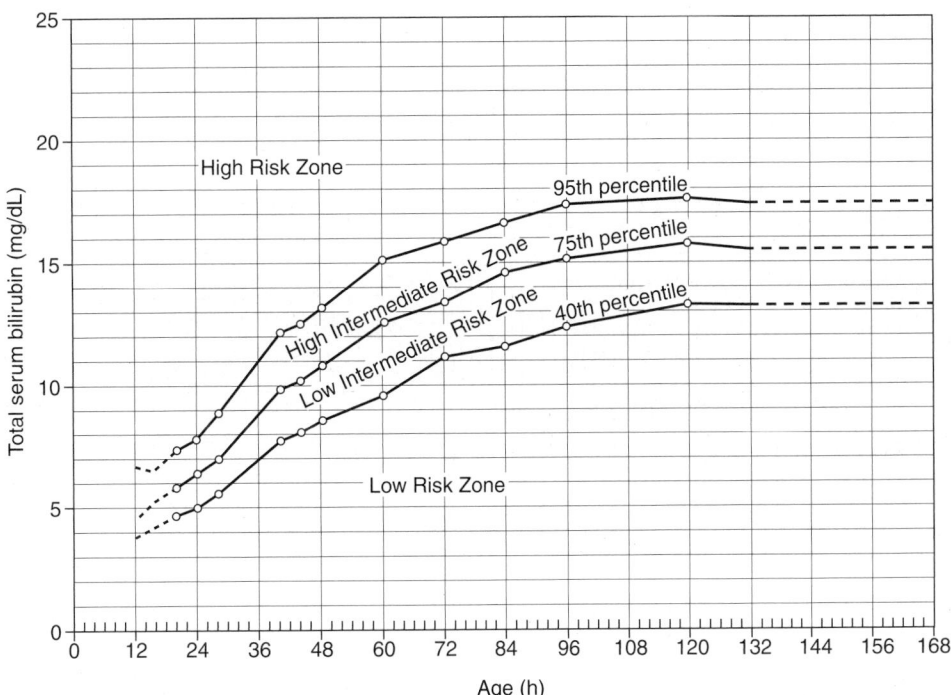

FIGURE 79-2 Nomogram for designation of hyperbilirubinemia risk based on hour-specific bilirubin value. (*Adapted from Bhutani V, Johnson L, Sivieri EM, et al: Predictive ability of a predischarge hour-specific serum bilirubin for subsequent significant hyperbilirubinemia in healthy term and near-term newborns, Pediatrics 103:6-14, 1999.*)

suggest that the pattern and intensity of jaundice during the birth hospitalization may not be as reliable an indicator of degree of hyperbilirubinemia as previously thought (Keren et al, 2009; Moyer et al, 2000). Therefore, the AAP (2004) cautions that "visual estimation of bilirubin levels can lead to errors". Nevertheless, the absence of jaundice has excellent negative predictive value (99%) for developing a TSB that merits phototherapy (Keren et al, 2009); also, jaundice limited to the face and upper chest likely predicts a TSB <12.0 mg/dL (Moyer, 2000). It is currently recommended that a transcutaneous (TcB) or TSB measurement complement the clinical assessment for jaundice in every neonate during the birth hospitalization to assist in hyperbilirubinemia detection and neonatal management (Maisels et al, 2009b).

KERNICTERUS: CHRONIC BILIRUBIN ENCEPHALOPATHY

The clinical focus on neonatal hyperbilirubinemia derives from the neurotoxic risk hazardous bilirubin levels pose. Acute bilirubin encephalopathy may develop during hazardous hyperbilirubinemia and evolve into the chronic adverse neurodevelopmental sequelae of kernicterus. Kernicterus is a devastating, disabling neurologic disorder classically characterized by the clinical tetrad of (1) choreoathetoid cerebral palsy, (2) high-frequency central neural hearing loss, (3) palsy of vertical gaze, and (4) dental enamel hypoplasia, the result of bilirubin-induced cell toxicity (Perlstein, 1960). The central nervous system (CNS) sequelae reflect both a predilection of bilirubin toxicity for neurons (rather than glial cells) (Notter and Kendig, 1986), and the regional topography of bilirubin-induced neuronal injury that is characterized by prominent basal ganglia, cochlear, and oculomotor nuclei involvement (Ahdab-Barmada, 1983, 2000; Ahdab-Barmada and Moossy, 1984). Originally described in the context of severe hyperbilirubinemia secondary to Rh hemolytic disease (Evans and Polani, 1950; Vaughan et al, 1950), kernicterus has also been reported in other hemolytic conditions (e.g., hereditary spherocytosis and pyruvate kinase deficiency) (Watchko, 2000b), G6PD deficiency (MacDonald, 1995; Valaes, 1994, 2000), premature neonates (Ahdab-Barmada et al, 1984; Watchko et al, 1994) and in otherwise healthy term ($\geq37^{0/7}$ weeks) and late preterm ($34^{0/7}$ to $36^{6/7}$ weeks) gestation breastfed infants without hemolysis (Bhutani et al, 2004; Maisels et al, 1995). The pediatric community's recent decades' experience with kernicterus is notable for the number of reported cases in the United States (Bhutani et al, 2004; Johnson et al, 2009; Maisels and Newman, 1995) and abroad (Ebbesen, 2000; Hansen, 2002; Kaplan and Hammerman, 2004b), a phenomenon that arose during the mid-to-late 1980s in conjunction with a striking sustained increase in breastfeeding initiation at birth (Ryan et al, 2002) and concurrent progressive decline in birth hospitalization length of stay (Curtin and Kozak, 1998) (Figure 79-3). These factors have combined to unmask a previously underappreciated potential to develop extreme hyperbilirubinemia among a select number of neonates, the biological basis of which appears to be in part genetically determined. Recent population-based kernicterus incidence estimates for term neonates in developed countries range from approximately 1 per 30,000 (Sgro et al, 2006) to 1 per 100,000 (Manning et al, 2006); higher rates have been reported for (1) preterm newborns (Watchko, 1994) and (2) infants born in developing countries where kernicterus is a serious endemic problem (e.g., Nigeria, where approximately 3% of neonatal hospital admissions evidence bilirubin encephalopathy) (Oguniesi et al, 2007; Zipursky, 2009).

Bilirubin toxicity usually does not become overt until high TSB levels have been established for several hours. Acute bilirubin encephalopathy typically progresses through three stages. Stage 1 occurs during the first few days, with the infant having decreased activity, poor sucking, hypotonia, and a slightly high-pitched cry. If the TSB level is rapidly decreased (e.g., by way of exchange transfusion), these nonspecific abnormalities can be reversed.

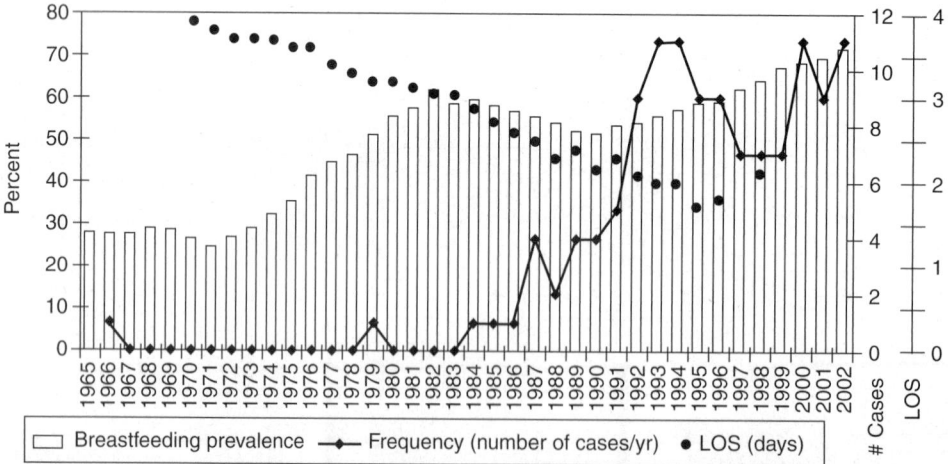

FIGURE 79-3 Number of reported kernicterus cases by birth year from 1965 to 2002 (*solid diamonds*) (Bhutani et al, 2004) shown in relation to annual prevalence of breastfeeding at birth hospitalization (*open bars as percentage*) (Ryan et al, 2002) and birth hospitalization length of stay (*solid circles in days*) (Curtin et al, 1998). An increase in reported cases of kernicterus is seen in conjunction with a sustained resurgence of breastfeeding initiation prevalence during birth hospitalization and concurrent decreased birth hospitalization length of stay (LOS). (*Adapted from Springer Science+Business Media:* Neuromolecular Medicine, *Volume 8, 2006: Kernicterus and the molecular mechanisms of bilirubin-induced CNS injury in newborns, Jon F. Watchko, page 515, Figure 1.*)

In stage 2, the infant demonstrates the features of stage 1 and also rigid extension of all four extremities, tight-fisted posturing of the arms, crossed extension of the legs, and a high-pitched, irritable cry. Sometimes these changes are accompanied with seizure activity, backward arching of the neck (retrocollis) and trunk (opisthotonos), and fever. Stage 3 is evidenced by hypertonia with marked retrocollis and opisthotonos, stupor, coma, and a shrill cry. The preponderance of evidence in the medical literature suggests that once an infant demonstrates signs of opisthotonos, some damage to the central nervous system has occurred. Van Praagh (1961) reported that all infants with definite opisthotonos (20 of 20 infants in his review) proved to have kernicteric sequelae on follow-up, although he did not comment on the extent of the adverse neurodevelopmental findings. Jones et al (1954) reported that the presence of definite abnormal signs, such as opisthotonos, in the neonatal period was associated with the development of handicap(s) but was not necessarily predictive of the severity of that handicap(s) (although most infants experienced moderate to severe neurodevelopmental sequelae). In contrast to these earlier reports, Harris et al (2001) follow-up experience in six neonates with marked hyperbilirubinemia showed that transient neurologic abnormalities may not correlate with long-term prognosis. In their study, however, only two infants demonstrated opisthotonos; one recovered without sequelae (peak serum bilirubin 30.6 mg/dL [523 µmol/L] on readmission on day 5 of life), whereas the other (peak serum bilirubin 36.9 [631 µmol/L] on readmission on day 6 of life) had profound long-term adverse neurodevelopmental deficits despite aggressive treatment with phototherapy and exchange transfusion. Most recently, Hansen et al (2009) reported a cohort of six extremely jaundiced neonates (TSB range 27.9 to 46.3 mg/dL [477 to 792 µmol/L]) with signs of intermediate

to advanced phase acute bilirubin encephalopathy (e.g., seizures, opisthotonos, retrocollis) who were treated with rapid and aggressive intervention and demonstrated normal neurologic development. These more recent findings support the potential clinical utility of the AAP recommendation for immediate exchange transfusion in any infant who is jaundiced and manifests the signs of intermediate to advanced stages of acute bilirubin encephalopathy (hypertonia, arching, retrocollis, opisthotonos, fever) even if the TSB level is falling (AAP, 2004).

Magnetic resonance imaging (MRI) offers a tool by which to assess possible bilirubin-induced brain damage in neonates with marked hyperbilirubinemia (Figure 79-4). The first MRI showing such damage was done in a full-term neonate with G6PD deficiency (Penn et al, 1994). The MRI at 8 days of age showed abnormally high signal intensity on T1-weighted images of the basal ganglia, thalamus, and internal capsule. A similar but less intense signal was seen on T2-weighted images. Subsequently there have been several reports of abnormalities seen in the globus pallidus on MRI in infants with bilirubin encephalopathy, typically with increased signal intensity of T1-weighted images early and that of T2-weighted images later. Although these findings often correlate with adverse long-term neurologic outcome, there have been reports of exceptions to this rule, including both infants with abnormal MRI who are subsequently normal on follow-up and infants with normal MRI who evidence long-term neuromotor sequelae characteristic of bilirubin-induced brain damage.

The ongoing occurrence of kernicterus has rekindled an interest in its molecular pathogenesis (Tiribelli and Ostrow, 2005; Watchko, 2006a) and in efforts to identify potential novel strategies to protect the CNS against bilirubin-induced injury. Although no one disputes the

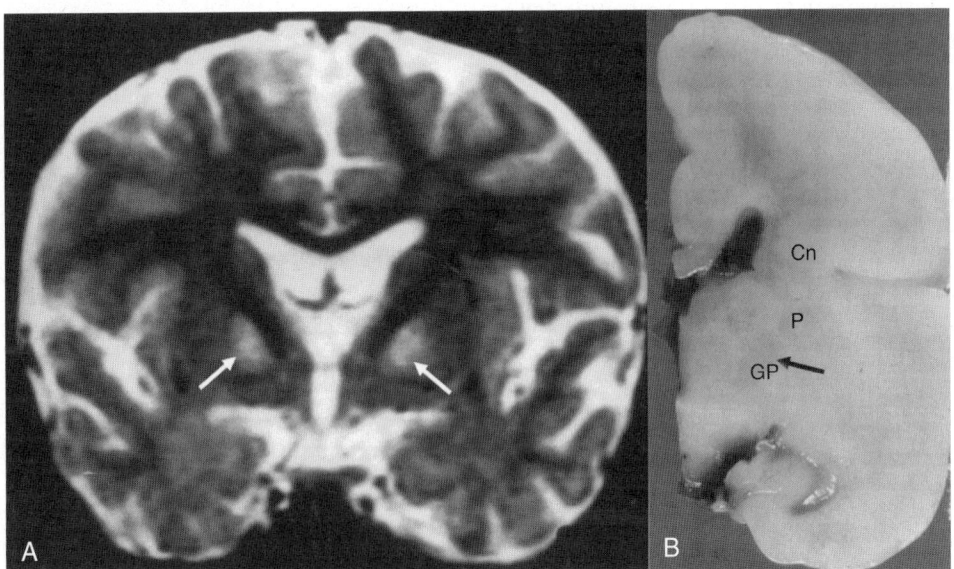

FIGURE 79-4 *(See also Color Plate 35.)* **A,** Coronal T1-weighted magnetic resonance image at the level of the basal ganglia in one infant is shown on the left, demonstrating bilateral, symmetric high-intensity globus pallidus *(GP)* signals *(arrows).* **B,** Deep orange-yellow staining of the globus pallidus (GP) of the coronal section at postmortem in another neonate. Note unstained putamen *(P)* and caudate nucleus *(Cn)*. These findings illustrate the selective vulnerability and regional nature of kernicterus and concordancy of neuroimaging and neuropathology in this disorder. (**A,** *Reprinted with permission from Coskun A, Yikilmaz A, Kumandas S, et al: Hyperintense globus pallidus on T1-weighted MR imaging in acute kernicterus: is it common or rare? Eur Radiol 15:1263-1267, 2005;* **B,** *reprinted with permission from* Monographs in Clinical Pediatrics *11:78, 2000. Available at www.tandf.co.uk.)*

neurotoxic potential of bilirubin, the cellular and molecular events attendant on bilirubin-induced neurotoxicity have been only partially characterized, and there is little agreement as to which, from a mechanistic standpoint, may be the most clinically relevant. Almost without exception, kernicterus has occurred during extreme unconjugated hyperbilirubinemia (UCB), and it is the UCB fraction not bound to albumin, that is, free bilirubin (B_F), that can cross the blood-brain barrier and prove neurotoxic. The concentration of this unbound bilirubin fraction is believed to dictate the biologic effects of bilirubin in jaundiced newborns, including its potential neurotoxicity. The full-term newborn infant has a significantly lower plasma albumin level than the adult and, correspondingly, fewer bilirubin binding sites. The albumin level is inversely correlated with gestational age, so this lack of binding sites is more pronounced in preterm infants. Bilirubin-albumin binding may also be modified by clinical conditions and the presence of competing compounds. It is notable that susceptibility for bilirubin-induced neurotoxicity is enhanced by prematurity (Gartner et al, 1970; Govaert et al, 2003); by drugs that displace bilirubin from albumin, thereby increasing B_F (Silverman et al, 1956); and possibly by concurrent marked conjugated bilirubinemia (Ebbesen, 1982; Grobler et al, 1997; Merhar et al, 2005).

BILIRUBIN-INDUCED CNS INJURY IN NEONATES LESS THAN 35 WEEKS' GESTATION

Hyperbilirubinemia in preterm infants is more prevalent and its course more protracted than in term neonates as a result of exaggerated neonatal red cell, hepatic, and gastrointestinal immaturity. The postnatal maturation of hepatic bilirubin uptake and bilirubin conjugation may also be slower in premature infants (Cashore, 2000). In addition, the delay in the initiation of enteral feedings that is so common in the clinical management of sick premature newborns may limit intestinal flow and bacterial colonization, resulting in a further enhancement of bilirubin enterohepatic circulation (Cashore, 2000). These developmental and clinical phenomena contribute to the greater degree and duration of neonatal jaundice in premature infants.

Despite the near-universal finding of clinical jaundice in the very low-birthweight infant, kernicterus has virtually disappeared in postmortem series of premature neonates (Jardine, 1989; Perlman, 1978; Watchko, 1994), and postkernicteric bilirubin encephalopathy and central neural hearing loss related to neonatal hyperbilirubinemia have not emerged as important clinical sequelae in neurodevelopmental follow-up of premature infants (Cashore, 2000). Yet kernicterus has occurred in preterm infants at low bilirubin levels and in the absence of acute neurologic signs (Gartner et al, 1970; Harris et al, 1958; Okumura et al, 2009; Sugama et al, 2001), and investigators have suggested that moderate hyperbilirubinemia (total serum bilirubin levels higher than 10 to 14 mg/dL [170–239 μmol/L]) may be associated with milder forms of central nervous system dysfunction and sequelae (Naeye, 1978; Scheidt et al, 1977; van de Bor et al, 1989). Recent studies report that hyperbilirubinemic extremely low-birthweight premature neonates may evidence athetotic cerebral palsy

with features similar to term infants with kernicterus (Okumura et al, 2009) and further suggest an association between peak total serum bilirubin and long-term adverse neurodevelopmental sequelae in this high-risk group (Oh et al, 2003). However, there remains considerable debate regarding the risk that neonatal hyperbilirubinemia poses for neuronal injury in the premature neonate, how to quantify that risk, and when to intervene with phototherapy or exchange transfusion (Hansen, 1996; Maisels and Watchko, 2003; NICHD, 1985). As a result, the framing of guidelines for the use of phototherapy and exchange transfusion in these infants is a capricious exercise at best and one for which no claim of an evidence base can be made (Maisels et al, 2003). Tables 79-3 to 79-5 illustrate a range of TSB levels for intervention in varying circumstances. These guidelines are provided by various experts, none of whom would likely make any claim for the greater validity of one approach versus another. A recent report from the United Kingdom showing a wide range of treatment

---

TABLE 79-3   Guidelines for the Use of Phototherapy and Exchange Transfusion in Low-Birthweight Infants Based on Birthweight*

Birthweight (g)	Total Bilirubin Level (mg/dL [μmol/L])[†]	
	Phototherapy[‡]	Exchange Transfusion[§]
≤1500	5–8 (85–140)	13–16 (220–275)
1500–1999	8–12 (140–200)	16–18 (275–300)
2000–2499	11–14 (190–240)	18–20 (300–340)

From: Maisels MJ. Jaundice. In Avery GB, Fletcher MA, MacDonald MG, editors: *Neonatology: pathophysiology and management of the newborn*, Philadelphia, 1999, JB Lippincott, pp 765-819.
*Note that these guidelines reflect ranges used in neonatal intensive care units. They cannot take into account all possible situations. Lower bilirubin levels should be used for infants who are sick (e.g., presence of sepsis, acidosis, hypoalbuminemia) or have hemolytic disease.
[†]Consider initiating therapy at these levels. Range allows discretion based on clinical conditions or other circumstances. Note that bilirubin levels refer to total serum bilirubin concentrations. Direct reacting or conjugated bilirubin levels should not be subtracted from the total.
[‡]Used at these levels and in therapeutic doses, phototherapy should, with few exceptions, eliminate the need for exchange transfusions.
[§]Levels for exchange transfusion assume that bilirubin continues to rise or remains at these levels despite intensive phototherapy.

TABLE 79-4   Guidelines for Use of Phototherapy and Exchange Transfusion in Preterm Infants Based on Gestational Age[a]

Gestational Age (weeks)	Total Bilirubin Level (mg/dL [μmol/L])		
	Phototherapy	Exchange Transfusion	
		Sick*	Well
36	14.6 (250)	17.5 (300)	20.5 (350)
32	8.8 (150)	14.6 (250)	17.5 (300)
28	5.8 (100)	11.7 (200)	14.6 (250)
24	4.7 (80)	8.8 (150)	11.7 (200)

*Rhesus disease, perinatal asphyxia, hypoxia, acidosis, hypercapnia; a, From Ives NK: Neonatal jaundice. In Rennie JM, Robertson NRC, editors: *Textbook of neonatology*, New York, 1999, Churchill Livingstone, pp 715-732.

thresholds for phototherapy and exchange transfusion in premature neonates further underscores this uncertainty (Rennie et al, 2009).

The recent NICHD Neonatal Network study on aggressive versus conservative phototherapy for infants with extremely low birthweight (<1000 g) has shed some new insight on hyperbilirubinemia risk and treatment options in the tiniest of preterm neonates but has also raised important new questions (Morris et al, 2008). Table 79-6 outlines the aggressive and conservative phototherapy treatment guidelines and exchange transfusion thresholds used in the Network study. Their data suggest that aggressive phototherapy may be preferred for infants of 751 to 1000 g birthweight because of significant neurodevelopmental benefit including a reduction in athetosis and severe hearing loss (Morris et al, 2008). However, their findings also raised concerns for aggressive phototherapy use in infants with birthweight of 501 to 750 g because of a higher mortality rate in that subgroup—that is, increased mortality may offset any potential neurologic benefits of aggressive treatment in these smallest of infants (Morris et al, 2008). Although it is unclear why phototherapy might increase mortality in this birthweight cohort, speculation focuses on greater light penetration deep into subcutaneous tissues via thin gelatinous skin and possible oxidative injury to cell membranes (Maisels, 2009; Vreman et al, 2004). Few neonates required exchange transfusion, confirming again the broad efficacy of phototherapy in preterm neonates. However, additional clinical study is needed to further clarify the hyperbilirubinemia risk of premature neonates and frame guidelines for

phototherapy and exchange transfusion in preterm infants that are evidence based (Maisels et al, 2003).

CLINICAL EFFORTS AT KERNICTERUS PREVENTION

The key elements to preventing kernicterus in term and late preterm neonates are (1) hyperbilirubinemia risk assessment, (2) appropriate and timely birth-hospitalization follow-up, and (3) timely and effective treatment of marked hyperbilirubinemia with phototherapy and/or exchange transfusion when it occurs. Support of successful breastfeeding is also an important part of hyperbilirubinemia control. Recent clinical evidence suggests that a TSB or TcB measured ≥18 hours after birth combined with assessment of hyperbilirubinemia risk factors significantly improves the prediction of subsequent hyperbilirubinemia (Keren, 2008; Maisels, 2009; Newman, 2005), and a group of experts now recommends the approach outlined in Figure 79-5 (Maisels et al, 2009b). In this approach, the predischarge TSB or TcB is plotted according to the infant's age in hours using the Bhutani hour-specific nomogram (see Figure 79-2). The bilirubin risk zone, gestational age at birth, and hyperbilirubinemia risk factors (see Box 79-3) are then combined to assess the risk of subsequent hyperbilirubinemia and formulate a plan for management and timely post–birth-hospitalization follow-up (see Figure 79-5). Critical in the effort are the characterization of the birth-hospitalization TSB/TcB bilirubin risk zone (Bhutani et al, 1999), accurate knowledge of the infant's gestational age in weeks, and details regarding the presence of other hyperbilirubinemia risk factors. Coupling the gestational age with knowledge of hyperbilirubinemia risk factors will determine which portion of the algorithm is operative for a given neonate. Using the predischarge TcB/TSB determined risk zone, the algorithm will provide direction regarding further evaluation and management, including timing of post-discharge follow-up and whether additional TSB/TcB measurements are indicated. The AAP has developed a resource kit for hospitals and clinicians to help provide breastfeeding support and manage the jaundiced newborn (www.aap.org/bookstore) and a Web-based program developed at Stanford, accessible at www.bilitool.org, is a practical instrument for plotting hour-specific TSB/TcB measurements.

TREATMENT CONSIDERATIONS

Phototherapy and exchange transfusion are the staples of intervention for the hyperbilirubinemic newborn, and current AAP phototherapy and exchange transfusion treatment

TABLE 79-5 Guidelines for Exchange Transfusion in Low-Birthweight Infants Based on Total Bilirubin (mg/dL) and Bilirubin/Albumin Ratio (mg/g)*

	Birthweight (g)			
	<1250	1250–1499	1500–1999	2000–2499
Standard risk	13	15	17	18
Or bilirubin/ albumin ratio	5.2	6.0	6.8	7.2
High risk[†]	10	13	15	17
Or bilirubin/ albumin ratio	4.0	5.2	6.0	6.8

From: Ahlfors CE: Criteria for exchange transfusion in jaundiced newborns, *Pediatrics* 93:488-494, 1994.
*Exchange transfusion at whichever comes first.
†Risk factors: Apgar <3 at 5 minutes; PaO_2 < 40 mm Hg ≥ 2 h, pH ≤ 7.15 > 1 h; birthweight <1000 g; hemolysis; clinical or central nervous system deterioration; total protein <4 g/dL or albumin ≤2.5 g/dL.

TABLE 79-6 Guidelines for Initiating Phototherapy and Exchange Transfusions—NICHD Neonatal Research Network Trial*

Birthweight	Aggressive Management		Conservative Management	
	Phototx Begins	Exchange Transfusion	Phototx Begins	Exchange Transfusion
501–750 g	ASAP after enrollment	≥13.0 mg/dL	≥8.0 mg/dL	≥3.0 mg/dL
751–1000 g	ASAP after enrollment	≥15.0 mg/dL	≥0.0 mg/dL	≥15.0 mg/dL

From Morris BH, Oh W, Tyson JE, et al: Aggressive vs. conservative phototherapy for infants with extremely low birth weight, *N Engl J Med* 359:1885-1896, 2008.
*Enrollment is expected within the period 12 to 36 hours after birth, preferably between 12 and 24 hours.

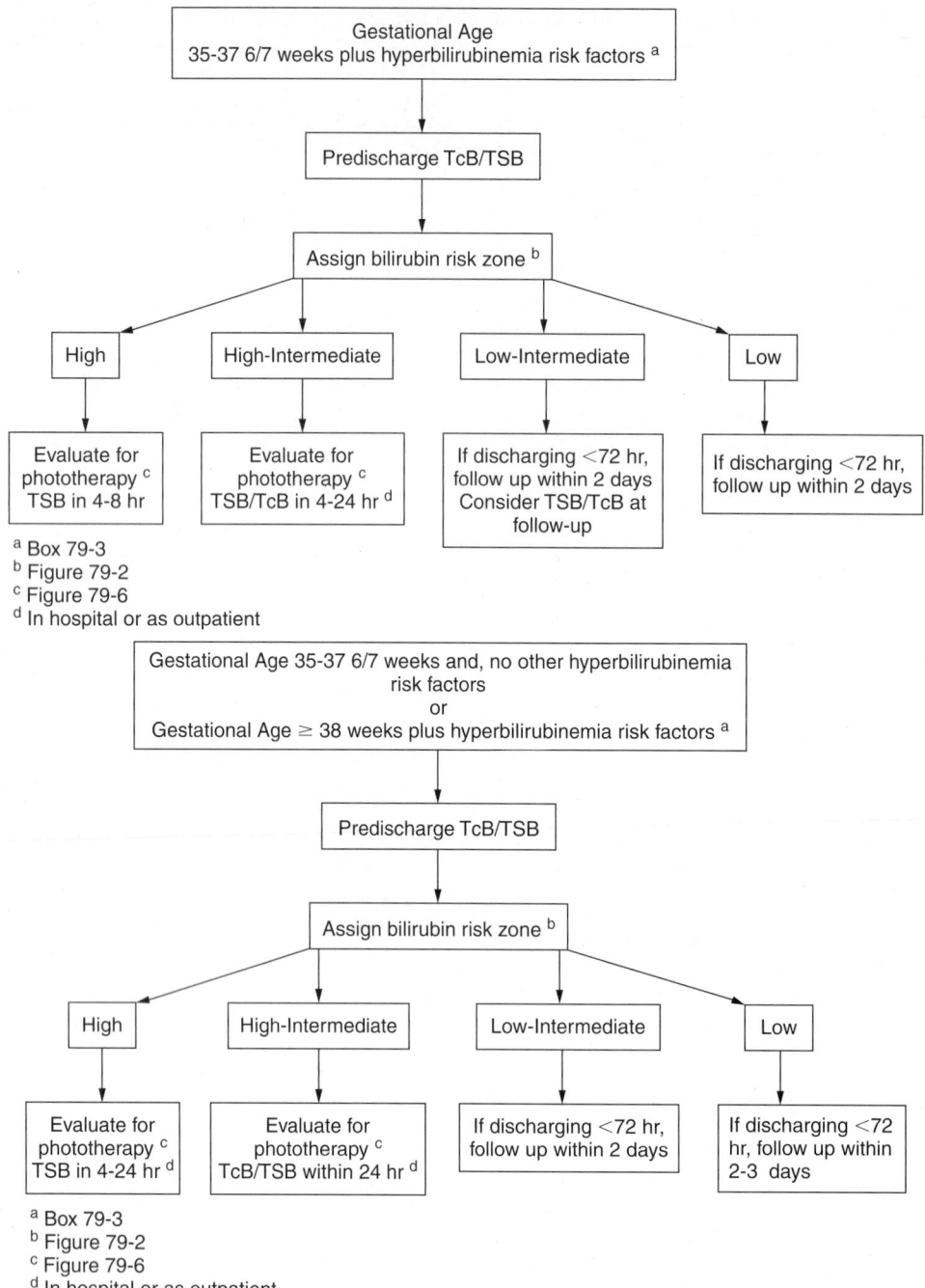

FIGURE 79-5 Algorithm providing recommendations for management and follow-up according to predischarge bilirubin measurements, gestational age at birth, and other risk factors for subsequent hyperbilirubinemia.

thresholds for infants ≥35 weeks' gestation are shown in Figures 79-6 and 79-7, respectively (AAP, 2004). Tables 79-4 to 79-6 illustrate a range of TSB levels for intervention in varying circumstances for preterm neonates. Phototherapy was first introduced at the Rochford (Essex) General Hospital by Cremer et al (1958) and has proven to be exceedingly successful. Just how effective phototherapy has been can be gauged by the impact it has had on the number of exchange transfusions performed for hyperbilirubinemia (Maisels, 2001; O'Shea et al, 1992), particularly in the neonatal intensive care unit population of infants weighing <1500 g. Certainly phototherapy, if used

appropriately (Maisels, 1996), is capable of controlling the bilirubin levels in almost all low-birthweight infants, with the possible exception of the occasional infant with severe erythroblastosis fetalis or marked bruising. In a similar fashion, phototherapy has proven effective in controlling bilirubin levels and preventing the need for exchange transfusion in most term and late-preterm neonates as well— exceptions on occasion being infants with severe hemolysis. Indeed, a rising TSB on phototherapy should raise the concern that the neonate has significant hemolysis, and preparations for exchange should be made in anticipation of the TSB possibly rising to the exchange threshold.

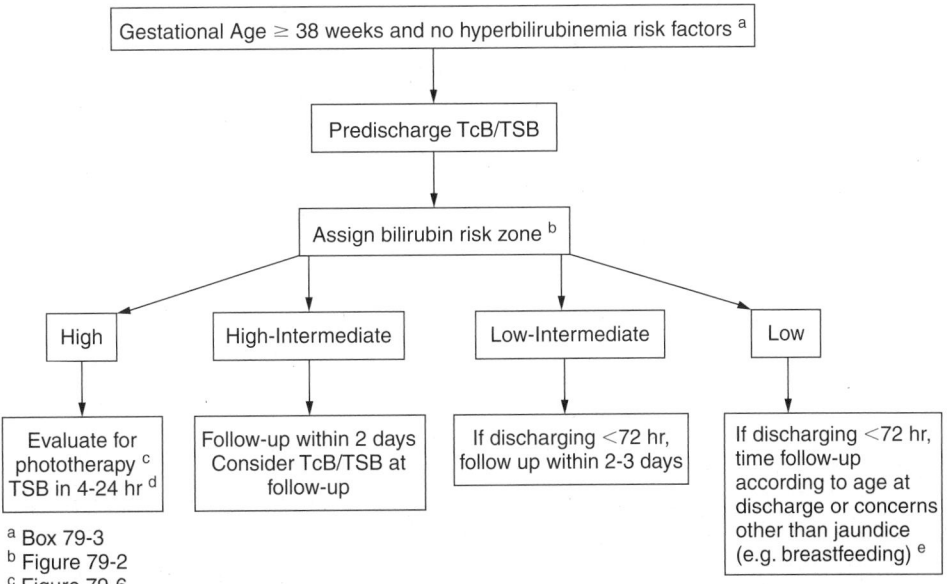

ᵃ Box 79-3
ᵇ Figure 79-2
ᶜ Figure 79-6
ᵈ In hospital or as outpatient
ᵉ Follow-up recommendations can be modified according to level of risk for hyperbilirubinemia.
  Depending on the circumstances, in infants at low risk, later follow-up can be considered

FIGURE 79-5—cont'd For legend see facing page.

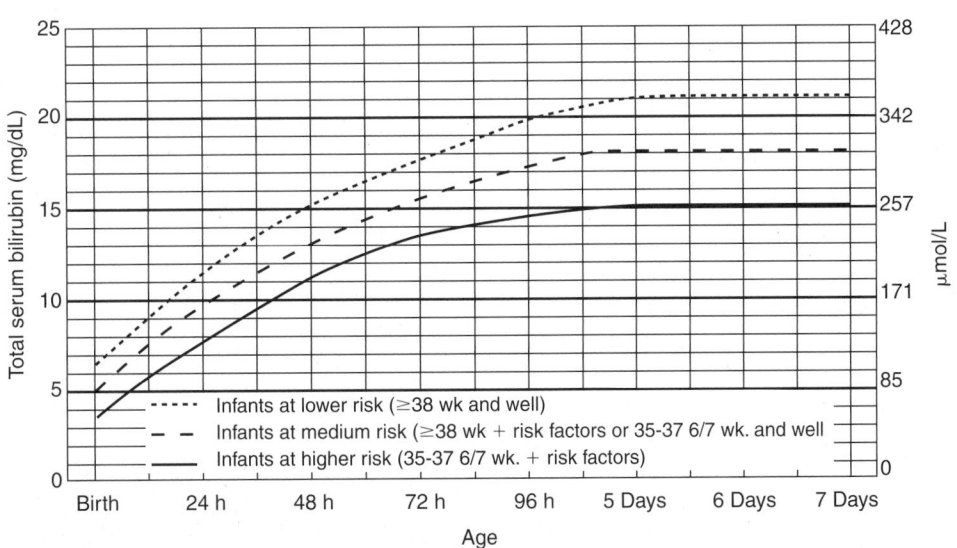

FIGURE 79-6 Guidelines for phototherapy in hospitalized infants ≥35 weeks' gestation.
- Use total bilirubin. Do not subtract direct reading or conjugated bilirubin.
- The lines for lower, medium, and higher risk refer to risk for neurotoxicity.
- Risk factors for neurotoxicity—isoimmune hemolytic disease, G6PD deficiency, asphyxia, significant lethargy, temperature instability, sepsis, acidosis or albumin <3.0 g/dL (if measured).
- For well infants 35 to 37⁶ᐟ⁷ wk can adjust TSB levels for intervention around the medium risk line. It is an option to intervene at lower TSB levels for infants closer to 35 wk and at higher TSB levels for those closer to 37⁶ᐟ⁷ wk.
- It is an option to provide conventional phototherapy in hospital or at home at TSB levels 2 to 3 mg/dL (35 to 50 mmol/L) below those shown, but home phototherapy should not be used in any infant with risk factors.

These guidelines refer to the use of intensive phototherapy, which should be used when the TSB exceeds the line indicated for each category. Infants are designated as "higher risk" because of the potential negative effects of the conditions listed on albumin binding of bilirubin, the blood-brain barrier, and the susceptibility of the brain cells to damage by bilirubin.

"Intensive phototherapy" implies irradiance in the blue-green spectrum (wavelengths of approximately 430 to 490 nm) of at least 30 μW/cm2 per nm (measured at the infant's skin directly below the center of the phototherapy unit) and delivered to as much of the infant's surface area as possible. Note that irradiance measured below the center of the light source is much greater than that measured at the periphery. Measurements should be made with a spectroradiometer specified by the manufacturer of the phototherapy system.

If the total serum bilirubin does not decrease or continues to rise in an infant who is receiving intensive phototherapy, this strongly suggests the presence of hemolysis. (*Adapted from American Academy of Pediatrics: Management of hyperbilirubinemia in the newborn infant 35 or more weeks of gestation,* Pediatrics *114:297-316, 2004.*)

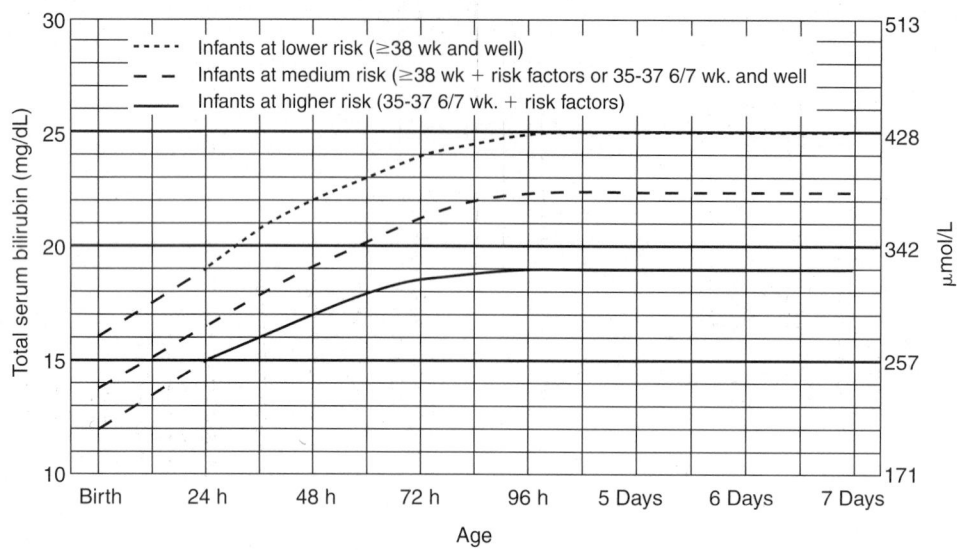

FIGURE 79-7 Guidelines for exchange transfusion in infants ≥35 weeks' gestation.

- The *dashed lines* for the first 24 hours indicate uncertainty due to a wide range of clinical circumstances and a range of responses to phototherapy.
- Immediate exchange transfusion is recommended if infant shows signs of acute bilirubin encephalopathy (hypertonia, arching, retrocollis, opisthotonos, fever, high-pitched cry) or if TSB is ≥5 mg/dL (85 μmol/L) above these lines.
- The lines for lower, medium, and higher risk refer to risk for neurotoxicity.
- Risk factors for neurotoxicity: isoimmune hemolytic disease, G6PD deficiency, asphyxia, significant lethargy, temperature instability, sepsis, acidosis.
- Measure serum albumin and calculate B/A ratio (see legend).
- Use total bilirubin. Do not subtract direct reacting or conjugated bilirubin.
- If infant is well and 35 to 37⁶ᐟ⁷ wk (median risk), can individualize TSB levels for exchange based on actual gestational age.
- During birth hospitalization, exchange transfusion is recommended if the TSB rises to these levels despite intensive phototherapy. For readmitted infants, if the TSB level is above the exchange level, repeat TSB measurement every 2 to 3 hours and consider exchange if the TSB remains above the levels indicated after intensive phototherapy for 6 hours.
- The following B/A ratios can be used together with but in not in lieu of the TSB level as an additional factor in determining the need for exchange transfusion (Ahlfors, 1994).

Risk Category	B/A Ratio at Which Exchange Transfusion Should Be Considered	
	TSB mg/dL/Alb, g/dL	TSB μmol/L/Alb, μmol/L
Infants ≥38⁰ᐟ⁷ wk	8.0	0.94
Infants 35⁰ᐟ⁷–36⁶ᐟ⁷ wk and well or ≥38⁰ᐟ⁷ wk if higher risk or isoimmune hemolytic disease or G6PD deficiency	7.2	0.84
Infants 35⁰ᐟ⁷–37⁶ᐟ⁷ wk if higher risk or isoimmune hemolytic disease or G6PD deficiency	6.8	0.80

If the TSB is at or approaching the exchange level, send blood for immediate type and crossmatch. Blood for exchange transfusion is modified whole blood (red cells and plasma) crossmatched against the mother and compatible with the infant. (*Adapted from American Academy of Pediatrics: Management of hyperbilirubinemia in the newborn infant 35 or more weeks of gestation,* Pediatrics 114:297-316, 2004.)

PHOTOTHERAPY

The most effective phototherapy units deliver output in the blue-green region of the visible spectrum including the commercially available special blue fluorescent tubes (Ennever, 1990). These tubes are labeled F20 T12/BB or PL52/20W, and they provide much greater irradiance than regular blue tubes (labeled F20T12/B). Special blue tubes are particularly effective because they provide light with wavelengths that penetrate the skin well and are absorbed maximally by bilirubin (Ennever, 1990). Phototherapy effectiveness can be further enhanced by increasing the irradiance and the surface area exposed (Maisels, 1996, 2001; Maisels et al, 2008). Irradiance increases dramatically as the distance between the light source and the infant decreases, and this effect is most significant when special blue tubes are used (Maisels et al, 2003). If bilirubin levels are rising in spite of conventional phototherapy (e.g., severely bruised infants or those with hemolytic disease), a free-standing bank of special blue fluorescent tubes may be placed about 10 cm above the infant (Maisels et al, 2003). This proximity is accomplished by placing the fluorescent bank of lights between the radiant warmer and the infant and cannot be achieved when the infant is in an incubator. If halogen spot phototherapy lamps are used, they must not be positioned closer to the infant than recommended by the manufacturer because of the risk of a burn (Maisels et al, 2003). In addition, if two or more halogen lamps are used, they should never be focused on the same area of the infant's skin, as this might also cause a burn. The efficacy of phototherapy is also closely related to the surface area of the infant exposed to the phototherapy lights, and the simplest way of increasing the surface area exposed is to place fiberoptic pads below the infant with phototherapy lamps above (Maisels et al, 2003). Clinical studies comparing intermittent vs. continuous phototherapy have produced conflicting results, but in many circumstances, phototherapy does not need to be continuous. As long as

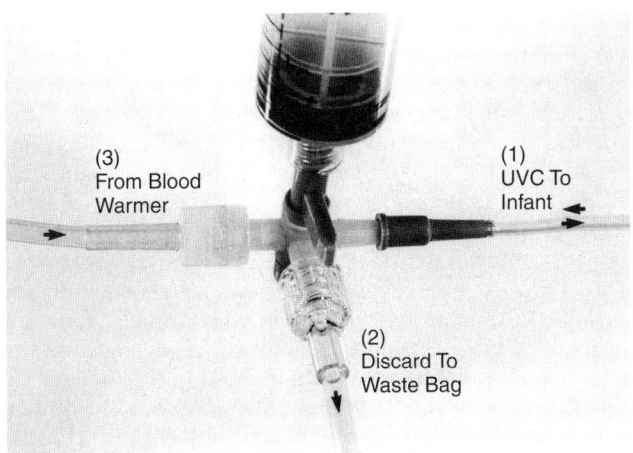

FIGURE 79-8 Special four-way stopcock assembly. *(1)* Male adapter to umbilical venous line; *(2)* female adapter to waste container; and *(3)* attachment to blood bag and warmer. The stopcock handle points to the port that is open to the syringe, and stopcock handle is rotated in a clockwise fashion when correctly assembled (e.g., first, withdraw aliquot from infant; second, discard to waste container; third, draw fresh blood from bag; and then fourth, infuse into infant to complete one cycle). *(From Watchko JF: Exchange transfusion in the management of neonatal hyperbilirubinemia. In Maisels MJ, Watchko JF, editors:* Neonatal jaundice, *Amsterdam, 2000c, Harwood Academic, pp 169-176.)*

the serum bilirubin level is being controlled, phototherapy can be interrupted during feeding or short parental visits.

Some studies suggest that phototherapy significantly increases insensible water loss, particularly in preterm infants (Kjartansson et al, 1992; Wu and Hodgman, 1974), but more recently it has been shown that as long as skin temperature is kept constant (by servo-control) and infants are not subjected to heat stress, phototherapy does not lead to an increase in oxygen consumption or insensible water loss through the skin or the respiratory tract (Fok et al, 2001; Kjartansson et al, 1992). Because we have effective means of monitoring newborn hydration (such as a daily weight and measurements of serum electrolytes), there is no reason to provide additional fluids routinely to infants who are receiving phototherapy. They should, of course, be kept adequately hydrated, not because phototherapy produces dehydration but because adequate urine output is important for effective phototherapy. The bilirubin isomer, lumirubin, is excreted in the bile and the urine, and lumirubin excretion appears to be an important element in the bilirubin-lowering function of phototherapy (Ennever, 1990).

Significant complications associated with phototherapy are exceptionally rare. Perhaps the most important clinical complication encountered during the use of phototherapy is that associated with the presence of direct hyperbilirubinemia or cholestatic jaundice. When infants with direct hyperbilirubinemia are exposed to phototherapy, they may develop a dark, grayish-brown discoloration of the skin, serum, and urine (i.e., bronze baby syndrome) (Rubaltelli et al, 1983, 1996). The pathogenesis of this syndrome is unknown but is possibly related to the accumulation of porphyrins or other pigments in the plasma in the presence of cholestasis (Onishi et al, 1982; Rubaltelli et al, 1983, 1996). Although few deleterious consequences of the bronze baby syndrome have been described, two infants with this syndrome who died were shown to have

kernicterus at autopsy (Clark et al, 1976; Rubaltelli et al, 1996). With the exception of these case reports, there are no other reports of significant complications in infants who develop the bronze baby syndrome, although impaired binding of bilirubin to albumin has been detected in three infants with this syndrome and in infants with cholestasis (Ebbessen, 1982; Kopelman et al, 1972). If there is a need for phototherapy, the presence of direct hyperbilirubinemia should not be considered a contraindication to its use, particularly in the sick newborn, and, as a rule, the direct serum bilirubin level should not be subtracted from the total bilirubin concentration when decisions are made about initiating phototherapy or an exchange transfusion. In infants who develop the bronze baby syndrome, exchange transfusion should be considered if phototherapy does not lower the total serum bilirubin. Because of the paucity of data, however, firm recommendations cannot be made. Rarely, purpuric bullous eruptions have also been described in infants with severe cholestatic jaundice receiving phototherapy.

EXCHANGE TRANSFUSION

Exchange transfusion occupies a unique place in the history of neonatal jaundice because it was the first intervention to permit effective control of severe hyperbilirubinemia and to have the potential to prevent kernicterus. In addition to immediate control of hyperbilirubinemia, an exchange transfusion in immune-mediated hemolytic disease also achieves: (1) the removal of antibody-coated red blood cells (a source of "potential" bilirubin), (2) the correction of anemia (if present), and (3) the removal of maternal antibody. A "double volume" exchange refers to an exchange of twice the neonate's blood volume or approximately 170 to 200 mL/kg and removes approximately 110% of circulating bilirubin (extravascular bilirubin enters the blood during the exchange), but only 25% of total body bilirubin. The exchange transfusion is much less efficient in the removal of total body bilirubin compared to circulating bilirubin because the majority of the infant's bilirubin is in the extravascular compartment (Valaes, 1963). Postexchange bilirubin levels are approximately 60% of preexchange levels, but the rapid (approximately 30 min) reequilibration of bilirubin between the vascular and extravascular compartments produces a rebound of serum bilirubin levels to 70% to 80% of preexchange levels (Brown, 1957).

Exchange transfusions are most readily performed via the umbilical vein using a 5 or 8 French umbilical catheter inserted just far enough to obtain free flow of blood (usually no more than the distance between the xiphoid process and umbilicus). The push-pull method with a single syringe and special four-way stopcock assembly permits a single operator to complete the procedure (Figure 79-8) (Watchko, 2000c). Fresh citrate-phosphate-dextrose preserved blood (<72 hours old, and devoid of the offending antigen in the case of immune-mediated hemolytic disease) crossmatched to the infant should be used. Although the risk for graft-versus-host disease following an exchange transfusion is extremely rare, blood for exchange transfusion should be irradiated if possible. The blood should be warmed to body temperature by a blood/fluid warmer. The actual exchange should be performed slowly in aliquots of 5 to 10 mL/kg body weight with each withdrawal-infusion cycle approximating 3 minutes' duration (Aranda, 1977). Using this approach, a double volume exchange should take approximately 1.5±0.5 hours. This rate has been demonstrated to be both safe and efficient (Forfar, 1958) and avoids deleterious hemodynamic changes (Aranda, 1977).

During the exchange, the infant's vital signs should be monitored closely, including heart rate/rhythm respiration, oxygen saturation, temperature, and blood pressure. Symptomatic hypocalcemia in early studies was reported in up to 5% of healthy infants, but supplemental calcium gluconate administration during the exchange transfusion has little effect on serum ionized calcium (Ellis, 1979; Maisels, 1974; Wieland, 1979), and too rapid infusion of calcium may cause bradyarrhythmias or cardiac arrest. If symptomatic hypocalcemia develops, temporary cessation of the procedure will allow recovery toward normal calcium levels as the citrate (which binds calcium) is metabolized by the liver. Postexchange studies should include bilirubin, hemoglobin, platelet count, ionized calcium, serum electrolytes, and serum glucose.

The unintended consequences of exchange transfusion include cardiovascular, hematologic, gastrointestinal, biochemical, and infectious hazards, among others (Watchko, 2000c). Previously reported overall mortality rates associated with exchange transfusion ranged from 0.3 to 0.95 per 100 procedures (Hovi et al, 1985; Keenan et al, 1985), and significant morbidity (apnea, bradycardia, cyanosis, vasospasm, thrombosis) was observed in 6.7% of infants who received exchange transfusion in the NICHD collaborative phototherapy study (Keenan et al, 1985). These rates, however, may not be generalizable to the current era if, as with most procedures, frequency of performance is an important determinant of risk and experience with exchange transfusion is decreasing (Newman e al, 1992). It is quite possible that the mortality (and morbidity) for this now infrequently performed procedure might be considerably higher than previously reported. On the other hand, none of the reports before 1986 included contemporary monitoring capabilities such as pulse oximetry. Jackson (1997) reported a 2% overall mortality rate (2 of 106) associated with exchange transfusions between 1980 and 1995 and a 12% risk of serious complications attributable to exchange transfusion in ill infants. Moreover, in infants classified as ill with medical problems in addition to hyperbilirubinemia, the incidence of exchange transfusion related complication leading to death was 8%. There were no procedure-related deaths in 81 healthy infants. Symptomatic hypocalcemia, bleeding related to

thrombocytopenia, catheter-related complications, and apnea-bradycardia requiring resuscitation were common serious morbidities observed in this study, suggesting that exchange transfusion should be performed by experienced individuals in a neonatal intensive care unit with continuous monitoring (including pulse oximetry) prepared to respond to these adverse events (Jackson, 1997). Finally, although the risk of blood transfusion is now very low, transfusion always carries some infection risk (Schreiber et al, 1996). The risk estimates (risk per tested unit) for transfusion-transmitted viruses in the United States for the period 1991 through 1993 were as follows: for the human immunodeficiency virus (HIV), 1:493,000 (95% confidence interval, 202,000 to 2,778,000); for the human T cell lymphotropic virus (HTLV), 1:641,000 (256,000 to 2,000,000); for the hepatitis C virus (HCV), 1:103,000 (28,000 to 288,000); and for the hepatitis B virus (HBV), 1:63,000 (31,000 to 147,000) (Schreiber et al, 1996).

ACKNOWLEDGMENTS

The contributions of Dr. Frank A. Oski, who authored the original chapter, and Drs. Ashima Madan, James R. MacMahon, and David K. Stevenson, who coauthored recent editions, are gratefully acknowledged. Their work has been invaluable in preparing the current chapter.

SUGGESTED READINGS

American Academy of Pediatrics: Subcommittee on Neonatal Hyperbilirubinemia: Neonatal jaundice and kernicterus, *Pediatrics* 108:763-765, 2001.
Bhutani VK, Johnson LH, Maisels MJ, et al: Kernicterus: epidemiological strategies for its prevention through systems-based approaches, *J Perinatol* 24: 650-662, 2004.
Kaplan M, Hammerman C: Bilirubin and the genome: the hereditary basis of unconjugated neonatal hyperbilirubinemia, *Curr Pharmacogenomics* 3:21-42, 2005.
Maisels MJ, Bhutani VK, Bogen D, et al: Management of hyperbilirubinemia in the newborn infant 35 or more weeks of gestation—an update with clarifications, *Pediatrics* 124:1193-1198, 2009.
Maisels MJ, McDonagh AF: Phototherapy for neonatal jaundice, *N Engl J Med* 358:920-928, 2008.
Maisels MJ, Watchko JF, editors: *Neonatal jaundice*, Amsterdam, 2000, Harwood Academic.
Odell GB: *Neonatal hyperbilirubinemia*, New York, 1980, Grune & Stratton.
Subcommittee on Hyperbilirubinemia: Management of hyperbilirubinemia in the newborn infant 35 or more weeks of gestation, *Pediatrics* 114:297-316, 2004.
Valaes T: Problems with prediction of neonatal hyperbilirubinemia, *Pediatrics* 108:175-177, 2001.
Watchko JF: Vigintiphobia revisited, *Pediatrics* 115:1747-1753, 2005.
Watchko JF: Kernicterus and the molecular mechanisms of bilirubin-induced CNS injury in newborns, *Neuromolecular Medicine* 8:513-529, 2006a.
Watchko JF, Lin Z: Exploring the genetic architecture of neonatal hyperbilirubinemia, *Semin Fetal Neonatal Med* 15:169-175, 2010.

Complete references and supplemental color images used in this text can be found online at www.expertconsult.com

CONGENITAL MALIGNANT DISORDERS

Elizabeth Robbins, Mignon L. Loh, and Katherine K. Matthay

Neonatal malignancies differ in incidence, clinical behavior, and heritable features from cancers seen in older children. Whereas acute leukemia is the most common malignancy in young children, the majority of neonatal tumors are solid tumors, many of which are detected prenatally during routine ultrasonography. Some childhood malignancies that carry excellent prognoses, such as acute lymphoblastic leukemia, are often fatal in neonates. In contrast, neuroblastoma, which responds poorly to treatment in older children, often spontaneously regresses in newborns.

Treatment of cancer in the neonatal period presents special challenges. Among these are differences in drug metabolism in newborns, the sensitivity of rapidly growing normal tissues to chemotherapeutic agents and radiation, and the increased possibility of late effects including neurocognitive sequelae, impaired reproductive capacity, growth disturbances, and secondary malignancies. The epidemiology, etiology, and diagnosis of neonatal malignancy are reviewed here, followed by a discussion of commonly encountered malignancies.

EPIDEMIOLOGY, ETIOLOGY, AND DIAGNOSIS OF NEONATAL MALIGNANCY

EPIDEMIOLOGY: INCIDENCE AND MORTALITY

Neonatal tumors are rare, with an incidence of approximately 1 per 12,500 to 27,500 live births; they make up 2% of childhood malignancies (Gurney et al, 1997; Moore et al, 2003). Although trend analyses suggest that the incidence of malignancy in the pediatric population may be increasing (Linabery and Ross, 2008), a number of factors affect incidence rates, including improvements in molecular methods of diagnosis, changes in population characteristics, screening fetal ultrasound practices, and case ascertainment by cancer registries (Spector and Linabery, 2009).

The most common malignancy in infants is neuroblastoma, followed by leukemia, central nervous system tumors, retinoblastoma, and germ cell tumors (Linabery and Ross, 2008). Female and male infants have similar cancer incidence rates, but white infants have significantly higher rates than those reported in African American infants for all histologic types. The distribution of the major types of cancers in newborns, infants, and children is depicted in

Table 80-1. Incidence rates for the most common types of malignancy in infants are shown in Table 80-2.

The mortality rates for infants with cancer exceed those for older children, even among similar histologic groups (Ries et al, 1999). Despite cure rates exceeding 75% for children older than 1 year who are diagnosed with acute lymphoblastic leukemia (ALL), newborns with ALL experience cure rates of less than 25% (Bresters et al, 2002). This is likely due to biologic differences in the leukemias afflicting infants: infants with leukemia, but not older children, often harbor rearrangements of the *MLL* (mixed lineage leukemia) gene, which confer a poor prognosis. Poorer survival patterns for infants are also seen with rhabdomyosarcoma and central nervous system (CNS) tumors, including primitive neuroectodermal tumor (PNET) and ependymoma (Ries et al, 1999). Two notable exceptions are neuroblastoma, for which 5-year survival in newborns with disseminated disease is >90%, and infantile fibrosarcoma, for which cure rates often exceed those achieved in older children or adults.

ETIOLOGY

Genetic Predisposition Syndromes and Congenital Defects

The etiology of cancer in children is multifactorial, involving both genetic and environmental factors; in neonates, predisposing genetic factors frequently play an important role. An acquired or inherited abnormality of a cancer-predisposing gene that is critical during embryogenesis underlies many cases of neonatal cancer. Malignant transformation of normal cells results from the activation or suppression of these cancer-predisposing genes. The retinoblastoma gene at 13q is an example of a constitutional chromosomal abnormality that results in a high risk of malignancy.

A number of well-defined hereditary conditions are associated with an increased incidence of specific neoplasms; these are listed in Table 80-3. Except for retinoblastoma, hepatoblastoma, and Wilms' tumor, the neoplasms associated with these syndromes seldom manifest in the neonatal period, but the associated abnormalities may be recognized early, allowing for regular screening. A lack of family history should not dissuade the clinician from investigating these syndromes, because both spontaneous germline mutations and parental mosaicism occur. The genetic

TABLE 80-1 Percent Distribution of the Major Types of Cancer in Newborns, Infants, and Children

Malignancy	Newborns <30 d (%)	Infants <1 yr (%)	Children <15 yr (%)
Leukemia	13	14	31
Central nervous system tumors	3	15	18
Neuroblastoma	54	27	8
Lymphoma	0.3	1	14
Renal tumors	13	11	6
Sarcoma	11	5	11
Hepatic tumors	0	3	1.3
Teratoma	0	6	0.4
Retinoblastoma	0	13	4
Other	5.7	5	6.3

From Reaman GH, Bleyer WA, in *Principles and practice of pediatric oncology*, Philadelphia, 2006, Lippincott Williams & Wilkins.

TABLE 80-2 Incidence of Malignant Tumors in U.S. Infants <1 Year

Malignancy	Number	% of Total	Incidence Rate*
Neuroblastoma	402	24	54.1
Leukemia	296	18	39.9
CNS tumors	225	13	30.3
Retinoblastoma	196	12	26.4
Germ cell tumors	156	9	21.5
Wilms' tumor	107	6	14.4
Hepatoblastoma	78	5	10.5
Soft tissue sarcoma (nonrhabdomyo-sarcoma)	76	5	10.2
Rhabdomyosarcoma	39	2	5.3

From Linabery AM, Ross JA: Trends in childhood cancer incidence in the U.S. (1992-2004), *Cancer* 112:416-432, 2008.
*Incidence rate per 1 million person-years, age-adjusted to the 2000 U.S. Standard population.

defect in many of these neoplasms has been identified. For example, the NF1 gene, located at 17q11.2, encodes a protein, neurofibromin, that normally acts as a guanosine triphosphatase activating protein that downregulates the Ras signaling pathway. Children with NF1 are at increased risk of developing juvenile myelomonocytic leukemia (JMML), a rare but aggressive myeloproliferative neoplasm that is currently only cured with hematopoietic stem cell transplant (Niemeyer and Kratz, 2008). In children with NF1 and JMML, the hematopoietic cells display loss of the wild type *NF1* gene and duplication of the mutant allele, thus resulting in the complete loss of the normal neurofibromin protein in the leukemia cells (Stephens et al, 2006). This promotes cell growth because there is no functional off switch.

A large number of childhood tumors occur in association with congenital defects. For instance, children with congenital aniridia have an increased incidence of Wilms' tumor. Although aniridia is found in only 1 of 75,000 persons, it is found in as many as 1 in 75 children with Wilms' tumor. Children with abnormalities of the Wilms' tumor 1 gene (*WT1*), located on chromosome 11p13, also have an increased risk of developing Wilms' tumor (Scott et al, 2006). Most patients with constitutional *WT1* defects have associated phenotypic syndromes that include combinations of genitourinary abnormalities, renal dysfunction, and mental retardation. The Beckwith-Wiedemann syndrome (BWS) and hemihypertrophy syndromes are associated with Wilms' tumor as well as several other childhood neoplasms. These syndromes are typified by macroglossia, gigantism, and abdominal wall defects; patients may also have visceromegaly, flame nevus, neonatal hypoglycemia, microcephaly, and retardation (Scott et al, 2006). Approximately 8% of infants with either the complete or partial syndrome develop neoplasms including Wilms' tumor, adrenal cortical carcinoma, and hepatoblastoma—tumors of the same organs in which visceromegaly develops. Also reported are rhabdomyosarcoma, neuroblastoma, ganglioneuroma, and adenomas and hamartomas. BWS is linked with abnormalities of 11p15; this is the location of the

insulin-like growth factor II gene (*IGF-2*) and the tumor suppressor gene *H19* (Rahma, 2005).

Transplacental Tumor Passage

A rare cause of cancer in neonates and infants is the transplacental passage of tumor cells from the mother. Fewer than 20 cases of transplacentally transmitted cancer have been reported (Walker et al, 2002). Malignancies transmitted include leukemia, melanoma, lymphoma, hepatic carcinoma, and lung cancer. Transplacentally acquired neoplasm is usually apparent at birth or shortly thereafter, but diagnosis has been reported as late as age 8 months (Maruko et al, 2002).

The frequency of malignancy in pregnant women is estimated at 1 per 1000 pregnancies (Greenlund et al, 2001; Maruko et al, 2004; Pavlidis, 2002). That transplacental transmission is so rare is attributed to the protective function of the placenta.

Twin-to-Twin Transmission

The risk of development of leukemia is increased in a monozygotic twin. If one monozygotic twin has leukemia, the co-twin has an approximately 25% chance of developing leukemia, usually within weeks or months of the diagnosis of the sibling. A dizygotic twin has only a slightly increased risk of developing leukemia. Growing evidence suggests that this increased incidence is likely due to in utero twin-to-twin transmission of a preleukemic clone rather than to the simultaneous development of a shared germline mutation facilitating the later development of leukemia (Greaves et al, 2003; Mahmoud et al, 1995).

Environmental Factors

Environmental factors are probably less important in the development of neonatal cancer compared with their role in the development of cancer in older children and adults. Nonetheless, there is evidence that environmental

TABLE 80-3 Hereditary Conditions With Associated Tumors

Syndrome	Gene	Locus	Inheritance Pattern	Most Common Tumors
Ataxia-telangiectasia	*ATM*	11q22-q23	Recessive	Leukemia Lymphoma
Beckwith-Wiedemann syndrome	IGF2	11p15	Some auto dominant imprinting	Wilms' tumor Hepatoblastoma Adrenal cortical carcinoma Rhabdomyosarcoma
Bloom syndrome	*BLM*	15q26	Auto recessive	Leukemia
Denys-Drash syndrome	*WT1*	11p13	Auto dominant	Familial Wilms' tumor
Down syndrome		Trisomy 21	Sporadic	Leukemia
Fanconi's anemia		Many	Auto recessive	Leukemia
Gonadal dysgenesis		45X/46XY	?X-linked	Gonadoblastoma Germinoma
Gorlin's syndrome	*PTCH2*	1p33	Auto dominant	Medulloblastoma Basal cell carcinoma
Klinefelter's syndrome	?	XXY	Sporadic	Teratoma Leukemia Breast cancer
Li-Fraumeni syndrome	*TP53*		Auto dominant	Sarcoma CNS Breast cancer
Neurofibromatosis	*NF1*	17q11.2	Auto dominant	Glioma Leukemia (JMML) Sarcoma
Retinoblastoma	*RB*	13q14	Auto dominant	Retinoblastoma Osteosarcoma Rhabdomyosarcoma
Trisomy 18	?	Trisomy 18	Sporadic	Wilms' tumor
Turner's syndrome		XO	Sporadic	?Neuroblastoma
Von Hippel-Lindau syndrome	*VHL*	3p26	Auto dominant	Hemangioblastoma
WAGR syndrome	*WT1*	11p13		Wilms' tumor
Wiskott-Aldrich syndrome	*WAS*	Xp11.23	X-linked	Non-Hodgkin's lymphoma
X-linked lymphoproliferative disorders	*SAP*	Xq25	X-linked	EBV lymphomas

Auto, Autosomal; *CNS,* central nervous system; *EBV,* Epstein-Barr virus; *JMML,* juvenile myelomonocytic leukemia; *WAGR,* Wilms' tumors, *a*niridia, genitourinary abnormalities, mental *r*etardation.

influences including radiation exposure, maternal medication use, and various environmental exposures may affect the incidence of neonatal cancer (Moore et al, 2003).

Exposure to ionizing radiation during pregnancy is known to increase the risk of a number of tumors, including acute leukemia, in exposed offspring. There appears to be a dose-response relationship between the dose of ionizing radiation received by the fetus in utero and the subsequent development of cancer in childhood, with doses on the order of 10 mGy sufficient to produce an increase in risk (Doll and Wakeford, 1997).

Maternal exposure to drugs during pregnancy has been associated with the subsequent development of cancer in offspring. Maternal use of diethylstilbestrol has been strongly associated with the development of clear cell adenocarcinoma of the vagina and cervix in daughters born from those pregnancies (Herbst et al, 1971). A number of substances known to be teratogenic also may be carcinogenic to offspring. In utero exposure to phenytoin or other antiepileptic drugs can result in the fetal hydantoin syndrome; some infants with this syndrome have developed neuroblastoma (Ehrenbard and Chaganti, 1981). Excessive maternal

alcohol consumption may be linked to an increased risk of developing cancer in the newborn period, particularly acute myeloid leukemia (Shu et al, 1996). The use of fertility drugs does not appear to increase the risk of cancer in the exposed offspring (Basatemur and Sutcliffe, 2008).

Environmental exposures of the mother or father to hydrocarbons, dyes, and other chemicals and solvents may be related to the development of neonatal tumors, but there is only a weak association for most of the risk factors identified. The association of neoplasms with other environmental factors, such as maternal use of tobacco, has not been conclusively proven (Shu et al, 1996).

DIAGNOSIS AND EVALUATION

The diagnostic evaluation of a newborn infant suspected to have cancer is guided by the signs and symptoms of the disease. Symptoms of malignancy in neonates can be nonspecific, such as irritability, poor feeding, failure to thrive, and fever. Table 80-4 lists clinical features associated with the more common malignancies found in the neonatal period. Most neonatal tumors present as a mass at birth; often the mass has previously been identified by prenatal ultrasonography. Postnatal imaging with magnetic resonance imaging (MRI) or computed tomography (CT) is usually required to better delineate the lesion.

Laboratory and pathologic evaluations should be directed at making the diagnosis efficiently, sparing the newborn unnecessary procedures that can result in acute and chronic morbidity. Routine laboratory studies including a complete blood cell count (CBC) and liver and renal function tests should be obtained. Urine catecholamine excretion should be measured when neuroblastoma is being considered.

TABLE 80-4 Differential Diagnosis of Malignant and Nonmalignant Conditions in Infancy

Feature	Malignancy	Nonmalignant Condition
Skin nodules	Neuroblastoma Acute leukemia Reticuloendothe-lioses	Congenital viral infections Vasculitis Fibromatosis Neurofibromatosis Xanthoma
Head and neck masses	Rhabdomyosar-coma Orbital Cervical Nasopharyngeal Neuroblastoma Lymphoma Infantile fibrosar-coma	Brachial cleft cyst Thyroglossal duct cyst Cystic hygroma Fibromatosis Hemangioma Abscess Cellulitis Reactive hyperplasia of cervical nodes Granulomatous lesions (e.g., atypical tuberculosis)
Abdominal or pelvic masses	Neuroblastoma Wilms' tumor Sarcoma Malignant tera-toma Lymphoma Germ cell tumor	Polycystic kidneys Hydronephrosis Benign teratoma Urinary retention Gastrointestinal duplication Intussusception Chordoma Meningomyelocele Horseshoe kidney Splenomegaly Hepatomegaly
Hepato-megaly	Neuroblastoma Acute leukemia Hepatoblastoma Reticuloendothe-lioses	Congenital viral infections Storage diseases Cavernous hemangioma Hemangioendothelioma
Signs/symp-toms of increased intracranial pressure	Brain tumors Acute leukemia Retinoblastoma	Intracranial hemorrhage Communicating hydro-cephalus Dandy-Walker malformation Vascular malformations
Anemia	Acute leukemia Neuroblastoma	Acute or chronic blood loss Hypoproliferative anemia (nutritional, congenital) Dyserythropoietic anemias Hemolytic anemia Transient erythroblastopenia
Pancytopenia	Acute leukemia Neuroblastoma Retinoblastoma (disseminated)	Congenital viral infections Immune-mediated neutrope-nia and thrombocytopenia Congenital and acquired aplastic anemias

Adapted from Reaman GH, Bleyer WA, in *Principles and practice of pediatric oncology*, Philadelphia, 2006, Lippincott Williams & Wilkins.

Serum alpha-fetoprotein (AFP) and beta human chorionic gonadotrophin (hCG) levels should be obtained in infants suspected of having a germ cell tumor or teratoma; these can serve as tumor markers, although the normally elevated levels in infancy can complicate the interpretation of these values. Consultation with a pediatric oncologist should be obtained for help in making the initial diagnosis. Surgeons and pathologists should submit biopsy tissue for histologic examination, immunoperoxidase staining, flow cytometry, cytogenetic analysis, and tumor banking.

SPECIFIC NEOPLASMS

NEUROBLASTOMA

Neuroblastoma is the most common malignant tumor in infants, accounting for about 27% of cancers diagnosed in infants less than age 1, and about 54% of cancers diagnosed in neonates less than 1 month of age. The small round blue cell neoplasm originates from neural crest cells that normally give rise to the adrenal medulla and sympathetic ganglia (Figure 80-1). In infants, the first clinical manifestations in more than half of cases result from the presence of metastatic disease rather than the primary tumor. However, despite the occurrence of widespread disease, neuroblastoma in newborn infants is almost always associated with biologically favorable features and carries a remarkably good prognosis.

Etiology

The etiology of neuroblastoma is largely unknown. Neuroblastoma usually occurs sporadically, likely following random genetic mutations; environmental factors do not appear to play a significant role. There are rare familial cases, accounting for 1% to 2% of patients. These cases may result from a hereditary-predisposition locus now attributed to multiple different genetic aberrations. Chromosome 16p12-13 was identified as a likely predisposition locus, though no causal gene has been identified (Kushner et al, 2005; Maris et al, 2002). More recently, multiple groups have identified the anaplastic lymphocyte kinase gene (*ALK*) as a predisposition gene in familial neuroblastoma (Janoueix-Lerosey et al, 2008). Familial neuroblastoma is inherited in an autosomal dominant mendelian fashion with incomplete penetrance. Affected children

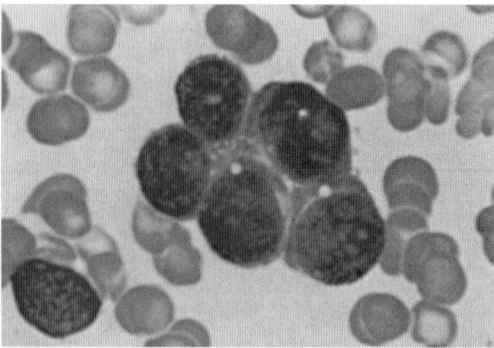

FIGURE 80-1 Clump of neuroblastoma cells found in bone marrow aspirate.

differ from those with sporadic disease in that they are often diagnosed at an earlier age (usually infancy) and/or they have multiple primary tumors.

Neuroblastoma has also been seen in several patients with constitutional chromosomal rearrangements, including deletions overlapping putative tumor suppressor loci at chromosome bands 1p36 and 11q14-23. Additionally, neuroblastoma has been reported in patients with other neural-crest disorders such as Hirschsprung's disease and central hypoventilation syndrome; these cases are associated with a germline mutation at chromosome band 4p12 (the *PHOX2B* gene) (Raabe et al, 2008).

Clinical Manifestations

Neuroblastoma may manifest as a tumor mass anywhere sympathetic neural tissue normally occurs. The clinical presentation can range from an asymptomatic newborn with an incidentally noted mass on prenatal ultrasound to a critically ill infant with massive hepatomegaly and respiratory distress. In the newborn, neuroblastoma most commonly manifests by enlargement of the liver alone, seen in 65% of cases, followed with subcutaneous metastases, seen in 32%. These percentages differ strikingly from those for older infants and children (Table 80-5). Metastases to lungs, bones, skull, and orbit are rare in the newborn, although clumps of tumor cells are often found in the bone marrow.

The most common site for the primary tumor is within the abdomen, arising in the adrenal medulla or a sympathetic ganglion. The tumor may also arise in the posterior mediastinum with resultant bronchial obstruction or invasion of the neural foramina, with neurologic symptoms. Increasing dyspnea, cough, wheezing, or pulmonary infection may be the presenting sign or symptom. Metastatic lesions, especially of the skin and liver, are common presenting features in the neonatal period; in the newborn, the primary site often cannot be discovered. Rapidly progressive hepatic involvement from multiple foci of neuroblastoma can cause abdominal distention, coagulopathy, and life-threatening respiratory distress (Figure 80-2). In some cases hepatomegaly at birth causes dystocia. Massive liver involvement in newborns with disseminated neuroblastoma is responsible for the higher mortality rate in newborns compared with older infants (Nickerson et al, 2000). Subcutaneous skin nodules, which may be present at birth, are typically bluish in color. On palpation, the skin nodules may become erythematous for 2 to 3 minutes, followed by blanching of the lesion. The blanching is presumably due to vasoconstriction caused by release of catecholamines from the tumor cell and may be a diagnostic sign of subcutaneous neuroblastoma.

The neoplasm may also arise in the neck or pelvis. Involvement of the stellate ganglion may result in Horner's syndrome, which includes ptosis of the upper eyelid, slight elevation of the lower lid, miosis, narrowing of the palpebral fissure, anhidrosis, and enophthalmos (Figure 80-3). Neuroblastoma arising from a paravertebral sympathetic ganglion has a tendency to grow into the intervertebral foramina, causing spinal cord compression and resultant paralysis. Careful periodic neurologic evaluation should be performed on a child with a neuroblastoma arising in this location, because the onset of cord compression may necessitate emergency intervention with chemotherapy, surgery, or irradiation.

Unusual Presentations

Intractable diarrhea can be the sole presenting manifestation of neuroblastoma. Secretion of vasoactive intestinal peptide by the tumor has been postulated to be the cause of the diarrhea, which resolves following surgical removal of the tumor (Bourdeaut et al, 2009).

Opsoclonus and myoclonus (i.e., dancing eyes, dancing feet) is associated with neuroblastoma, although this presentation is only rarely seen in the neonatal period (Rudnick et al, 2001). Patients have rapid multidirectional eye

TABLE 80-5   Sites of Metastatic Disease at Diagnosis for 81 Patients With Stage IVS, 133 Patients With Stage IV <1 Year, and 434 Patients With Stage IV ≥1 Year

Sites of Metastases	Stage IVS	Stage IV <1 year	Stage IV ≥1 year	Total (%)
Bone marrow*,†	28 (34.6)	76 (57.1)	353 (81.3)	70.5
Bone†	0 (0.0)	65 (48.9)	296 (68.2)	55.7
Lymph node	7 (8.6)	38 (28.6)	155 (35.7)	30.9
Liver*,†	65 (80.2)	71 (53.4)	56 (12.9)	29.6
Intracranial/Orbit	0 (0.0)	34 (25.6)	84 (19.6)	18.2
Adrenal†	5 (6.2)	18 (13.5)	26 (6.0)	7.6
Skin†	11 (13.6)	11 (8.3)	4 (0.9)	4.0
Pleura	0 (0.0)	6 (4.5)	16 (3.7)	3.4
Lung	0 (0.0)	3 (2.3)	18 (4.1)	3.2
Peritoneum	0 (0.0)	5 (3.8)	9 (2.1)	2.2
Other	0 (0.0)	5 (3.8)	7 (1.6)	1.9
CNS	0 (0.0)	0 (0.0)	4 (0.9)	0.6

From Dubois S, Kalika Y, Lukens J, et al: Metastatic sites in stage IV and IVA neuroblastoma correlate with age, tumor biology, and survival, *J Pediatr Hematol Oncol* 21:181-189, 1999.
*Indicates a significant difference between the proportion of patients with stage IVS with the site and the proportion of patients with stage IV <1 year with the site (p < 0.01), only for those sites that are included in the definition of stage IVS.
†Indicates a significant difference between the proportion of patients with stage IV <1 year with the site and the proportion of patients with stage IV ≥1 year with the site (p < 0.02).

movements (opsoclonus), myoclonus, and truncal ataxia (OMA) in the absence of increased intracranial pressure. The condition may be due to an autoimmune reaction, because the presence of antineuronal antibodies has been shown to be significantly more common in children with neuroblastoma and OMA than in case-control neuroblastoma patients (Antunes et al, 2000). Removal of the tumor usually results in a decrease in neurologic signs and symptoms, but the use of steroids is frequently required for complete resolution. In general, the prognosis for survival of children with opsomyoclonus is excellent, although long-term neurologic deficits and learning delays are common and can be quite debilitating.

Maternal symptoms such as sweating, pallor, headaches, palpitations, hypertension, and tingling in the feet and hands during the 8th and 9th months of pregnancy may be a sign of neuroblastoma in the fetus (Newton et al, 1985). The symptoms, which disappear postpartum, are likely caused by fetal catecholamines entering the maternal circulation. Newborns with neuroblastoma whose mothers have experienced these symptoms are typically diagnosed with neuroblastoma shortly after birth or during the first few months of life.

Erythroblastosis with hepatosplenomegaly, severe jaundice, and an increase in nucleated red blood cells is occasionally seen in newborns with neuroblastoma. Congenital neuroblastoma with metastases to the liver and placenta can be clinically indistinguishable from hydrops fetalis.

Catecholamine Secretion

A hallmark of neuroblastoma cells is the ability to store and secrete catecholamines. Patients with neuroblastoma usually have elevated urinary levels of norepinephrine as well as its biochemical precursors and their metabolites. More than 90% of patients have an elevated urinary excretion of vanillylmandelic acid (VMA) or homovanillic acid (HVA), or both. VMA and HVA determinations can be made on random urine samples when values are normalized for creatinine concentration. In the occasional case with no elevation of catecholamines, a 24-hour urine collection is necessary. Urine catecholamines must be measured before surgical removal of the tumor or before initiation of therapy. Catecholamine secretion can be used not only as a diagnostic aid but also as a means to assess the response to therapy and to detect tumor recurrence.

Diagnosis

Clinical evaluation should include a physical examination with particular attention paid to detecting an abdominal mass, hepatomegaly, lymphadenopathy, Horner's syndrome, and skin lesions; a baseline neurologic exam is also performed. Laboratory evaluation should include a CBC, urine for VMA and HVA, and serum ferritin and lactate dehydrogenase. Although the initial imaging study in an infant is often an abdominal ultrasound, additional imaging to better delineate the tumor and to evaluate for metastatic disease is needed; this should include CT or MRI of the primary lesion. MRI of the spine should be obtained for paraspinal and posterior mediastinal lesions: An ^{123}I-metaiodobenzylguanidine (MIBG) scan is particularly important for diagnosis and follow-up. MIBG, a norepinephrine analogue specifically taken up by neuroblastoma in bone and soft tissue, serves as a sensitive modality for disease localization (Taggart et al, 2008). Bilateral bone marrow aspiration (along with bilateral bone marrow biopsy in patients over age 6 months) is also part of the initial evaluation.

Histologic evidence provides confirmation of the diagnosis of neuroblastoma. Tissue may be obtained from a primary lesion or a metastatic site. Because tumor-specific biologic information plays a critical role in risk classification and treatment recommendations, obtaining adequate tissue for biologic studies is essential.

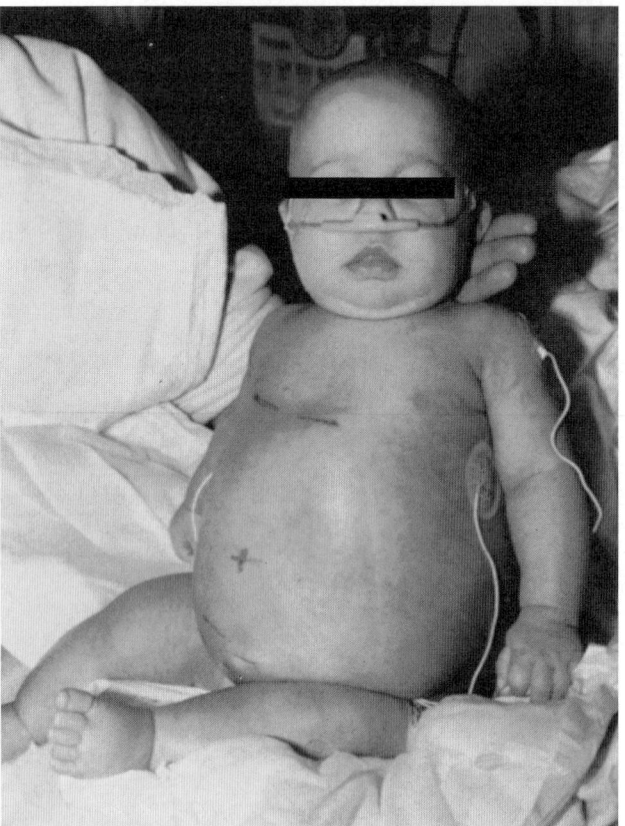

FIGURE 80-2 Stage 4S neuroblastoma causing abdominal distention and respiratory distress secondary to hepatic infiltration.

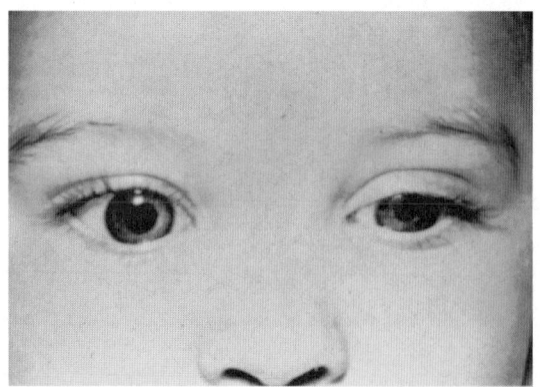

FIGURE 80-3 Horner's syndrome in an infant with neuroblastoma arising from the left cervical sympathetic ganglion.

Pathologic Classification

The histopathologic appearance of neuroblastoma ranges from undifferentiated neuroblasts, to more mature ganglioneuroblastoma, to fully differentiated and benign ganglioneuroma. The most widely used morphologic classification system is based on that proposed by Shimada, in which tumors are classified as favorable or unfavorable (Sano et al, 2006; Shimada et al, 1999). Classification is dependent on age, the degree of differentiation of the neuroblasts, the cellular turnover (mitosis-karyorrhexis) index, and the presence or absence of Schwannian stromal development.

Genetic Prognostic Factors: Tumor Biology

In addition to clinical factors and histology, a number of biologic factors have been shown to correlate with prognosis (Table 80-6). Genomic data currently used in risk classification schemes includes status of the *MYCN* oncogene; tumor cell DNA content (ploidy); and the allelic status of chromosomes 1p, 11q, 14q, and 17q (Ambros et al, 2009).

Amplification of the *MYCN* oncogene is present in 25% of primary neuroblastomas and has been shown to correlate with poor prognosis independent of age, stage, and other genetic alterations (Schneiderman et al, 2008). Patients with stage 1, 2, or 4S disease demonstrate *MYCN* amplification only rarely; when present, it has been associated with rapid disease progression in these usually favorable stages (Perez et al, 2000). In a Children's Cancer Group study of stage 4 neuroblastoma in infants, the progression-free survival rate after 3 years was less than 10% in infants with tumors that demonstrate *MYCN* amplification, compared with 93% for those with single-copy tumors (Schmidt et al, 2000).

Total cellular DNA content also predicts response to therapy in infants with neuroblastoma (Look et al, 1991). Diploid DNA content is an unfavorable prognostic factor, particularly in infants less than 12 months of age. Infants with hyperdiploid tumors have a significantly better response to therapy than those with diploid tumors (Bourhis, 1991). Diploidy often correlates with tumor *MYCN* amplification, although in rare cases of hyperdiploidy with *MYCN* amplification, the *MYCN* amplification portends an unfavorable outcome.

Tumor karyotype also influences outcome. Common genomic aberrations found in neuroblastoma include deletion at the chromosomal region 1p36.3 or 11q23; deletion of 14q32; and unbalanced gain of the long arm of chromosome 17 (17q21 to 17qter) (Ambros et al, 2009). Loss of heterozygosity (LOH) of 1p occurs in up to 36% of primary tumors, and is associated with *MYCN* amplification. LOH at 11q23 is seen in 44% of primary neuroblastomas, and rarely is associated with *MYCN* amplification (Guo et al, 1999). Comprehensive genome-wide approaches such as comparative genomic hybridization are becoming increasingly useful in refining the prognostic accuracy of chromosomal alterations (Schleiermacher et al, 2007).

Staging

Neuroblastoma has traditionally been staged according to the International Neuroblastoma Staging System (INSS) summarized in Table 80-7 (Brodeur et al, 1993). Staging is based on age, disease site(s), and degree of surgical resection. New guidelines for a pretreatment risk classification system have been developed by the International Neuroblastoma Risk Group (INRG) Task Force and are being used in addition to the INSS system (Montclair et al, 2009); this system will facilitate the comparison of risk-based clinical trials. INRG stages include L1, localized tumor not involving vital structures (corresponds to INSS stages 1 and 2); L2, locoregional tumor with one or more image-defined risk factors (corresponds to INSS stage 3); M, metastatic disease (corresponds to INSS stage 4); and MS, metastatic disease in children younger than 18 months with metastases confined to skin, liver, or

TABLE 80-6 Features That Affect Prognosis in Neuroblastoma

Feature	Favorable	Unfavorable
Age at diagnosis	<1.5 years	>1.5 years
INSS stage	Stage 1, 2, or 4S	Stage 3, 4
MYCN status	Nonamplified	Amplified
Shimada histology	Favorable	Unfavorable
DNA ploidy (DNA index)	DI >1 or <1	DI = 1
Allelic status of 11q	Normal	11q deletion or LOH at 11q

INSS, International Neuroblastoma Staging System.

TABLE 80-7 International Staging System for Neuroblastoma

Stage	Definition
Stage 1	Localized tumor confined to the area of origin; complete gross excision, with or without microscopic residual disease; identifiable ipsilateral and contralateral lymph nodes negative microscopically (adherent nodes may be positive)
Stage 2A	Localized tumor with incomplete gross excision; identifiable ipsilateral and contralateral lymph nodes negative microscopically
Stage 2B	Localized tumor with complete or incomplete gross excision, with positive ipsilateral nonadherent regional lymph nodes; identifiable contralateral lymph nodes negative microscopically
Stage 3	Unresectable tumor initiating across the midline with or without regional lymph node involvement; or unilateral tumor with contralateral regional lymph node involvement; or midline tumor with bilateral regional lymph node involvement; bilateral extension by infiltration
Stage 4	Dissemination of tumor to distant lymph nodes, bone, bone marrow, and liver and/or other organs (except as defined in stage 4S)
Stage 4S	Localized primary tumor as defined for stage 1 or 2 with dissemination limited to liver, skin, and bone marrow in infant <1 year of age

Data from Brodeur GM, Pritchard J, Berthold F, et al: Revisions of the international criteria for neuroblastoma diagnosis, staging and response to treatment, *J Clin Oncol* 11:1466, 1993.

bone marrow (corresponds to INSS stage 4S). Two important differences in the INRG system compared to the INSS are that it is a radiologic rather than a surgical staging system, and that the upper age limit for stage MS has been extended from 12 to 18 months.

Stage 4S (MS) comprises a unique group of patients with disseminated disease but a good prognosis, a combination that occurs exclusively in infants younger than 12 months of age. In this special group of children, typical findings include a small primary tumor that does not cross the midline and remote spread involving the liver, skin, or bone marrow (less than 15% of marrow replacement by tumor), without roentgenographic evidence of skeletal metastases. The primary tumor may be unidentifiable. There is lack of *MYCN* oncogene amplification in stage 4S tumors, in contrast to stage 4 tumors (Seeger et al, 1985). Infants with stage 4S disease have a very good prognosis despite having disseminated disease; spontaneous regression occurs without cytotoxic therapy in approximately 50% of cases.

Treatment

Treatment modalities for neuroblastoma include observation alone, surgery, chemotherapy, and radiation therapy. Factors that affect outcome include the age at diagnosis, stage of disease, histology, and tumor biology (see Table 80-6). Patients with stage 1 and stage 2 neuroblastoma have a 96% to 100% survival rate with surgery alone (Perez et al, 2000). Observation alone is justified in well infants with congenital, small, localized neuroblastoma without *MYCN* amplification; in these infants spontaneous regression occurs in about half the cases (Hero et al, 2008). Infants with stage 3 and stage 4 disease have a poorer survival, even with aggressive chemotherapy, although the outcome, with better than 70% surviving overall, is far better than the 10% to 20% reported for older children with these stages (Schmidt et al, 2000). Infants with stage 4S disease have a very good prognosis, with a 5-year survival >90%, despite having disseminated disease.

The unpredictable course of neuroblastoma, with its occasional spontaneous maturation or regression, not only makes this tumor unusual but also causes difficulty in planning therapy. The type and intensity of treatment is determined by identifying infants with relatively good, intermediate, and poor prognoses based on stage, international pathology classification, Shimada histology, ploidy, and *MYCN* amplification. Patients who have localized disease (stage 1 or 2) without amplification of *MYCN* have a 90% to 100% survival with surgery alone, even if the tumor is not completely resected. Such patients should undergo surgical resection or partial resection, but they likely will not derive any additional benefits from postoperative chemotherapy or radiation therapy. An exception to this rule is in the case of spinal cord compression, in which prompt decompression with chemotherapy, laminectomy, or local irradiation may be used to preserve function. There is an increasing trend to use chemotherapy first, given the exquisite sensitivity of the tumor to chemotherapeutic agents, but a rapid deterioration in neurologic function should prompt alternative interventions. A neurosurgeon should be consulted early in the diagnosis. The combination of extensive laminectomy with postoperative irradiation should be avoided because later spinal deformity is almost inevitable. Infants with stage 3 and stage 4 disease usually are treated with combination chemotherapy and local surgery, with radiation therapy given only as necessary to eradicate residual disease. Active drugs that are most commonly used include cisplatin, etoposide, doxorubicin, cyclophosphamide, vincristine, and ifosfamide. Infants with stage 4 disease with amplification of the *MYCN* oncogene have a very unfavorable prognosis; standard chemotherapy regimens are not usually sufficient for cure. In these high-risk patients, intensive chemotherapy followed by myeloablative therapy and stem cell support may offer additional benefit (Canete et al, 2009). In addition, the use of the differentiation agent *cis*-retinoic acid has been shown to improve survival in patients with advanced-stage, high-risk neuroblastoma (Matthay et al, 2009).

Infants with stage 4S disease have a highly favorable prognosis and may require minimal or no therapy. Because many patients undergo spontaneous regression without chemotherapy and the overall disease-free survival rate is 85% to 90%, therapy should be directed toward supportive care, with use of chemotherapy and surgery restricted to relieving symptoms (De Bernardi et al, 2009). The main cause of death in these patients is massive hepatic involvement resulting in respiratory insufficiency or compromise of renal or gastrointestinal function. Symptomatic patients are treated with chemotherapy. When there is a risk of organ impairment due to tumor bulk not responding to initial chemotherapy, low-dose radiotherapy can be administered (450 cGy given in three fractions). No benefit has been shown to result from resection of the primary tumor.

Prenatal Diagnosis

Neuroblastoma is increasingly being detected prenatally by screening ultrasonography. Newborns with adrenal or other mass lesions detected prenatally should be evaluated with urine catecholamines and follow-up ultrasonography. Careful observation may be adequate for infants with localized tumors, which frequently regress.

Newborn Screening

Newborn screening for neuroblastoma by measuring urine catecholamines has been studied in Japan and a number of other countries (Hiyama et al, 2008). It was hoped that early diagnosis of neuroblastoma would reduce the frequency of cases with poor prognosis from advanced-stage disease. Screening, however, has shown no impact on survival; neuroblastomas detected by screening almost always have favorable biologic features (Schilling et al, 2002). Thus, routine screening of infants for neuroblastoma is not currently recommended.

CONGENITAL LEUKEMIA

Epidemiology

Although leukemia is the second most common malignancy in infants, congenital leukemia, defined as leukemia diagnosed in the first 4 weeks of life, is quite rare. The incidence of leukemia in the first 3 months is approximately

5 cases per million (Bajwa et al, 2004). Two thirds of congenital leukemia cases arise from the myeloid lineage, in contrast to older infants and children in whom acute lymphoblastic leukemia predominates. Congenital leukemia is associated with a high mortality with an overall survival at 24 months of only 23% (Bresters et al, 2002); this is due to the aggressive biology of these leukemias and to treatment complications.

The etiology of leukemia is unclear. In infants and older children, a number of factors are associated with the development of leukemia; these include genetic factors, environmental influences, viral infections, and immunodeficiency. Genetic epidemiologic studies of infant leukemia indicate that many cases, if not all, are initiated in utero and involve genetic rearrangements; chromosome 11q23 (*MLL* rearrangement) is frequently involved (Greaves et al, 2003). Leukemia-associated gene rearrangements have been retrospectively identified in archived newborn blood spots of children who subsequently developed leukemia (Hjalgrim et al, 2002; Taub et al, 2002; Wiemels et al, 2002). Intrauterine exposure to topoisomerase 2 inhibitors may be responsible for some cases of infant leukemia (Pui and Evans, 1999; Ross, 2000). The Children's Cancer Group has reported a higher incidence of acute myeloid, but not lymphoid, leukemia in infants of mothers who consumed larger amounts of naturally occurring topoisomerase 2 inhibitors, such as those in foods high in flavonoids and phytates (Ross et al, 1996). Nucleotides involved in the breakpoint of the 11q23 locus may be particularly susceptible to topoisomerase 2–induced breaks (Strick et al, 2000).

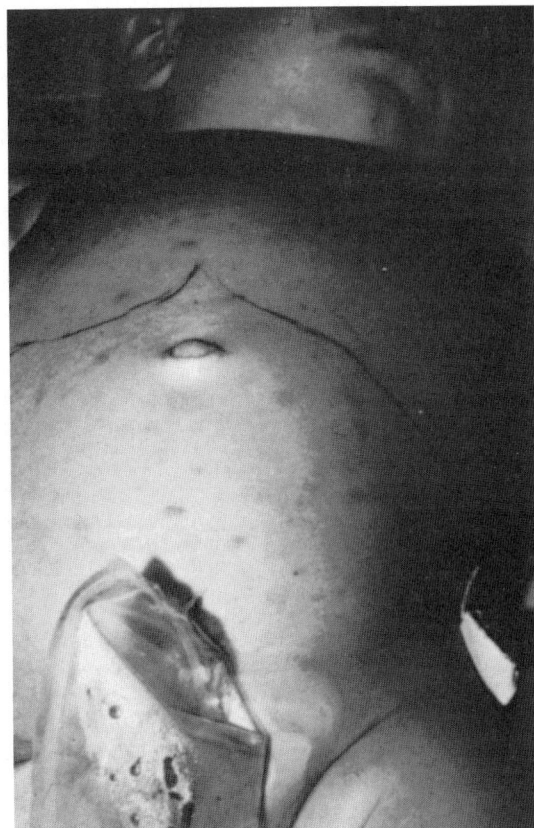

FIGURE 80-4 Leukemia cutis in a newborn infant.

Clinical Manifestations

Clinical signs of leukemia may be evident at birth and include hepatosplenomegaly, petechiae, and ecchymoses. Myeloid leukemic cell infiltration of the skin (i.e., leukemia cutis) is present in 25% to 30% of patients with congenital leukemia; a skin nodule may be the first clinical sign of leukemia (Figure 80-4). Patients typically have multiple nodules that are freely movable over the subcutaneous tissue (Resnik and Brod, 1993). There is usually a greenish-blue discoloration of the overlying skin due to the abundance of myeloperoxidase—hence the name *chloroma*. Lesions can also be pink or bluish. It is important to perform cytogenetic studies, in addition to flow cytometry, on the skin biopsy specimen; infants found to have an 11q23 rearrangement have a poor prognosis even in the absence of marrow involvement and should be treated aggressively (Zhang et al, 2006). When chloromas are present on the head or neck, imaging studies should be obtained to assess for the presence of intracranial or skull involvement. At birth, many infants have respiratory distress from leukemic infiltration in the lungs. Severe respiratory difficulty may develop soon after birth from pulmonary hemorrhage secondary to thrombocytopenia. Some infants with leukemia may appear somnolent or have periodic apnea as a result of CNS leukostasis, caused by sludging of leukemic cells in blood vessels.

In those infants in whom signs of the disease develop within the 1st month but in whom no detectable signs of leukemia were noted at birth, presenting symptoms and signs are nonspecific, including lethargy, diarrhea, hepatomegaly, and poor feeding with failure to gain weight. In addition, affected infants can present with fever due to bacterial infections or hemorrhagic manifestations due to thrombocytopenia.

Laboratory Manifestations

Hemoglobin levels may be normal initially, but anemia soon develops as the normal postnatal decrease in red cell production is combined with the expansion of the leukemic clone in the marrow. Total white blood cell count may be normal or decreased, but leukocytosis is more often present. White blood cell counts of 150,000 to 250,000/mm^3 or higher are common, and counts as high as 1.3 million/mm^3 have been recorded. There is usually a predominance of blast cells and immature granulocytes. Auer rods, intracellular inclusions composed of lysosomes, may be present; they are pathognomonic of acute myelogenous leukemia (AML) (Figure 80-5).

Differential Diagnosis

A number of conditions can mimic congenital leukemia. Leukocytosis, organomegaly, and thrombocytopenia can be seen in congenital infections caused by syphilis, cytomegalovirus (CMV), herpes simplex, toxoplasmosis, and bacteria. Thrombocytopenia and a leukemoid reaction can be seen in infants with congenital amegakaryocytic thrombocytopenia; the absence of radii, commonly seen in these

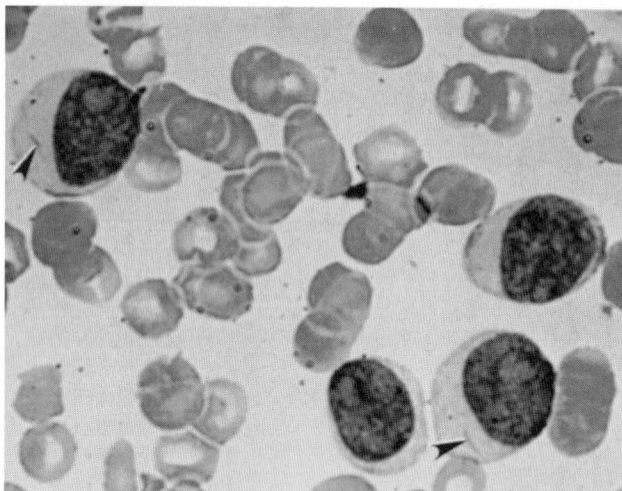

FIGURE 80-5 Malignant blast cells with Auer rods (*arrowheads*) present in cytoplasm. This finding is diagnostic of acute myelogenous leukemia.

TABLE 80-8 Morphologic and Immunophenotypic Classification of Childhood Acute Leukemia

FAB System	Morphology	Antigen Expression*
ALL		
L₁	Small cells, homogeneous Regular nuclei, scant cytoplasm Inconspicuous nucleoli	Pre=B: HLA-DR, CD10, CD19, CD20, CD24
L₂	Large cells, heterogeneous, irregular or cleft nuclei May be multiple large nucleoli Moderate cytoplasm	T: CD2, CD5, CD7
L₃	Large cells, homogeneous Regular nuclear shape Prominent nucleoli Moderately abundant, deeply basophilic cytoplasm with vacuolation	B: HLA-DR, CD10, CD19, CD20, CD24, SIg*
ANLL System		
M0	Minimal myeloid differentiation (MPO⁻)	CD13, CD33, CD34
M1	Poorly differentiated myeloblasts (MPO⁺)	CD13, CD33, CD34
M2	Myeloblastic with differentiation (MPO⁺)	CD13, CD33, CD34
M3	Promyelocytic (MPO⁺)	CD11b, CD13, CD33, CD34
M4	Myelomonoblastic (MPO⁺, NSE⁺)	CD11b, CD13, CD14, CD15, CD33, CD34
M5	Monoblastic (NSE⁺)	CD11b, CD13, CD14, CD15, CD33, CD34
M6	Erythroleukemic (MPO⁺, PAS⁺)	Glycophorin CD34
M7	Megakaryoblastic (PPO⁺)	CD41, CD42, CD34, CD61

ALL, Acute lymphocytic leukemia; *ANLL*, acute nonlymphocytic leukemia; *FAB*, French-American-British; *MPO*, myeloperoxidase; *NSE*, nonspecific esterase; *PPO*, platelet peroxidase; *SIg*, surface immune globulin.
L₁ or L₂ may show either pre-B or T antigens.
*The indicated FAB type may express some or all of the indicated antigens.

children, provides a clue to the correct diagnosis. A transient leukemoid reaction (i.e., transient myeloproliferative disorder [TMD]) occurs in many infants with trisomy 21. The leukemoid reaction usually resolves, but these infants are at higher risk for the subsequent development of acute leukemia (see later discussion).

Severe erythroblastosis fetalis can mimic leukemia. Affected infants usually have hepatosplenomegaly, large numbers of nucleated erythroblasts in the peripheral blood, and occasionally, thrombocytopenia. Small infiltrates of extramedullary erythropoiesis may appear in the skin, resembling leukemia cutis. Infants with neonatal neuroblastoma may have symptoms similar to those of congenital leukemia, with hepatomegaly and discolored tumor nodules in the subcutaneous tissue. Blood counts are usually normal, without circulating blasts. Bone marrow aspirate sometimes shows clusters of neuroblastoma cells (see Figure 80-1). Increased excretion of catecholamine metabolites, the presence of an abdominal mass or other primary lesion, and the presence of neuroblastoma cells in the bone marrow are clues to the diagnosis of neuroblastoma.

Congenital human immunodeficiency virus (HIV) infection may rarely be confused with leukemia. Clonal B-cell expansions in such patients may cause lymphadenopathy. Thrombocytopenia, usually immune-mediated in HIV, has been reported (Voelkerding et al, 1988). A marked but transient leukemoid reaction may occur in the newborn following in utero exposure to betamethasone (Calhoun et al, 1996). History of prenatal exposure to corticosteroids and lack of the usual clinical and laboratory findings of leukemia usually excludes the diagnosis of leukemia.

Cellular Morphology and Immunophenotype

The bone marrow of a newborn with leukemia shows extreme hypercellularity and a marked predominance of immature cells, either myeloid or lymphoid. AML and ALL are differentiated on the basis of typical morphologic characteristics, such as the presence of granules or

Auer rods (in AML) and nuclear and cytoplasmic morphology, cytochemical stains, immunophenotyping, and chromosome analysis. Terminal deoxynucleotidyl transferase, a DNA polymerase that catalyzes the polymerization of deoxynucleotides in thymocytes, is usually present in lymphoblasts, but is only rarely present in myeloblasts. Myeloblasts are usually positive for myeloperoxidase, whereas lymphoblasts are not. Both types of leukemia are subclassified according to an international French-American-British (FAB) classification based on morphology and histochemistry (Table 80-8). The most common FAB morphology in neonatal and infant AML is monocytic (FAB M5) or myelomonocytic (FAB M4), whereas the most common subtype in ALL is the FAB L1 variety (Sande et al, 1999). The traditional FAB classification system is being replaced by the World Health Organization classification system, which incorporates additional information including genetics, immunophenotype, and clinical features (Vardiman et al, 2009).

The immunophenotype, determined using a panel of fluorescent-labeled monoclonal antibodies against cluster differentiation (CD) antigens, is critical for differentiating myeloid from lymphoid leukemia (Craig and Foon, 2008). Myeloid leukemia cells usually react with antibodies to the CD13/CD33 antigens, present on cells of myeloid and monocytic lineage. The only exception is the FAB M7 category, acute megakaryoblastic leukemia, which expresses the CD41/CD42 platelet glycoprotein and CD61. Acute megakaryoblastic leukemia is most commonly seen in patients with trisomy 21. Most neonatal and infant acute lymphoblastic leukemia cells exhibit an early precursor B-cell phenotype and often are CD1a, CD19, CD24, and CD15 positive and CD10 negative (Pui et al, 1995; Pui and Evans, 1999). In addition, coexpression of myeloid antigens is often present. Frequently there are rearrangements of the immune globulin heavy-chain gene and occasionally the light-chain gene, but almost never the T-cell receptor gene (Felix et al, 1987; Ludwig et al, 1989). Surface antigen expression in acute leukemia is summarized in Table 80-8.

Genetics and Prognosis

A number of cytogenetic abnormalities have been found in association with congenital leukemia; many of these abnormalities are independent prognostic indicators. The most frequent abnormalities involve disruptions of the mixed lineage leukemia (MLL) gene at 11q23. Abnormalities of 11q23 are found in approximately 65% of infant AML and 93% of infant ALL cases (Chowdhury and Brady, 2008; Pui et al, 2003; Van der Linden, 2009). These are nonhereditary, nonconstitutional abnormalities that occur in utero (Ford et al, 1993). The MLL gene is the human homologue of the trithorax gene in Drosophila melanogaster (Ziemin-van der Poel et al, 1991). In mice and in humans, the MLL protein positively regulates HOX genes, which are critical for hematopoietic development (Armstrong et al, 2002). Rearrangements in the MLL gene confer a poor prognosis, which worsens with decreasing age (Chen et al, 1993).

The t(4;11)(q21;q23) gene rearrangement, detected in up to 48% of infants with acute lymphoblastic leukemia, is the most prevalent subtype of 11q23/MLL rearrangements (Van der Linden, 2009). It confers a particularly poor prognosis in infants younger than 6 months of age (Heerema et al, 1999; Pui et al, 2003). It is usually associated with hyperleukocytosis, CNS leukemia, and a precursor B-cell immunophenotype with CD19+/CD15+/CD10-. Interestingly, older children harboring this same rearrangement do not have the same dismal prognosis as infants. Studies in gene expression analysis demonstrate unique genetic signatures that distinguish infant ALL with MLL rearrangements from ALL and AML in older children (Armstrong et al, 2002).

Approximately 35% of infants with AML have 11q23 rearrangements. Half of the patients have t(9;11) abnormalities; t(11;19) and t(10;11) are also common (Chowdhury and Brady, 2008). AML in infants is commonly associated with hyperleukocytosis and extramedullary involvement. Spontaneous resolution without chemotherapy has occasionally occurred in leukemia cutis and rarely in infant leukemia without bone marrow involvement; in general, these leukemias lack 11q23 rearrangements (Mora et al, 2000). When 11q23 rearrangements are present, systemic disease usually develops.

Treatment

The course of congenital leukemia is usually characterized by rapid deterioration and death from hemorrhage or infection. Although survival has been significantly prolonged in older children with leukemia, success has been limited in newborns; survival at 2 years is only 23% (Bresters et al, 2002). Infants with leukemia frequently present with hyperleukocytosis (blast cell count in excess of 100,000/mm^3), which may result in sludging of blast cells in capillaries with resultant intracranial hemorrhage, respiratory distress, or tumor lysis syndrome (hyperkalemia, hyperphosphatemia, hypocalcemia, hyperuricemia, and renal failure). Disseminated intravascular coagulation is another common complication, especially when monocytic subtypes are suspected. Monoblasts release procoagulants, causing a consumptive coagulopathy; this may be exacerbated by further cell lysis induced with chemotherapy.

Initial supportive care includes correction of metabolic and hemorrhagic complications. Transfusion of platelets and fresh frozen plasma is frequently required. Exchange transfusion is sometimes undertaken in infants to lower the white blood cell count and to correct metabolic abnormalities. Rasburicase, a recombinant urate oxidase enzyme, has been safely used in infants with hyperuricemia (McNutt et al, 2006).

In infants with AML, intensive chemotherapy regimens have resulted in an improved rate of remission induction (Bresters et al, 2002; Chessells et al, 2002; Kawasaki et al, 2001). More than half of infants with myelomonocytic or monocytic subtypes obtain complete remission with chemotherapy. Chemotherapy regimens used in infants with myeloid leukemia are identical to those used in older children and usually include daunomycin, cytosine arabinoside, and etoposide. Because CNS involvement is common in infants with AML and ALL, intrathecal chemotherapy is a routine part of treatment. Radiation therapy, indicated in older children with CNS leukemia, is deferred in most instances until 1 year after diagnosis to limit potential late effects (which include neurocognitive sequelae and secondary malignancies).

Young infants with ALL fare significantly worse than do older children with ALL, in whom chemotherapy produces disease-free survival in more than 80%. Studies of infant leukemia have reported only 5% to 20% survival for infants younger than 6 months of age at diagnosis (Chessells et al, 1994; Heerema et al, 1994; Pui et al, 2003). However, outcomes for infants may be improving with the addition of high-dose cytarabine and high-dose methotrexate (Silverman et al, 1997). The use of cytarabine, which is used in the treatment of AML, may address the more primitive nature of the MLL-rearranged ALL cell, with its frequent coexpression of myeloid antigens and lack of CD10 positivity. The use of stem cell transplantation has not been shown to be of benefit in the treatment of congenital leukemia (Pui et al, 2003).

Transient Myeloproliferative Disorders and Leukemia in Patients with Down Syndrome

The incidence of acute leukemia in children with Down syndrome (DS) is 20-fold higher than in the general population. In DS children younger than 3 years, the rare megakaryoblastic subtype (M7) predominates and the prognosis is usually favorable (Pui, 1995). In older DS children, both AML and ALL occur; about one third of cases are AML. Neonates with DS frequently present with a TMD that mimics acute leukemia. Although it usually resolves without treatment, it is considered to be a pre-leukemic syndrome: approximately 20% of neonates with TMD develop acute megakaryoblastic leukemia within 4 years (Malinge et al, 2009). Neonates with DS and TMD should have careful follow-up.

Transient Myeloproliferative Disorder

TMD, which occurs in 4% to 10% of neonates with DS, is clinically indistinguishable from acute myelocytic leukemia (Malinge et al, 2009). Although the majority of cases of TMD occur in DS patients, TMD rarely can be seen in patients with no constitutional chromosomal abnormalities or with trisomy mosaicism. TMD is a clonal disorder typically manifested by hepatomegaly, splenomegaly, and circulating myeloblasts. There may or may not be associated anemia and thrombocytopenia. In general, the blast count of the peripheral blood exceeds that of the marrow. Blast cells often have cell surface antigens characteristic of megakaryoblasts (Zipursky et al, 1997). Somatic mutations in the *GATA1* transcription factor have been detected in nearly all cases of TMD and acute megakaryoblastic leukemia in patients with DS (Mundschau et al, 2003; Wechsler et al, 2002).

Most neonates with DS and TMD experience complete clinical and hematologic recovery without systemic therapy, usually within 3 months. The blast count slowly decreases over 2 to 3 weeks, and the hemoglobin and platelet counts normalize. In some cases, however, spontaneous resolution does not occur, and the neonate may experience clinical deterioration manifested by progressive hepato-splenomegaly, hepatic dysfunction, coagulation disorder, ascites, and pleural or pericardial effusions. Approximately 20% of DS patients with TMD die, usually from hepatic or cardiopulmonary failure (Muramatsu et al, 2008). Treatment with low-dose cytarabine can benefit high-risk neonates with TMD. Indications for starting treatment vary, but generally include WBC >50,000, platelet count <100,000, or signs of cholestasis or liver dysfunction (conjugated bilirubin ≥15, increase of transaminases >2 times the standard deviation of normal, or hepatomegaly with liver size >3 cm above normal, as measured by ultrasound) (Klusmann et al, 2008). In some instances, complications from TMD occur in utero, and varying degrees of hydrops fetalis can result. CNS involvement is rare in neonates with TMD.

GERM CELL TUMORS

Germ cell tumors are neoplasms derived from primordial germ cells. They are a heterogeneous group of tumors, varying in site, age at presentation, histopathology, and malignant potential. They can occur in both gonadal and extragonadal sites. The etiology is unknown; they are thought to arise from sporadic genetic mutations (Horton et al, 2007).

Most germ cell tumors in the fetus and newborn are benign and are classified as either mature or immature teratomas (Isaacs, 2004). However, one or more of the germ-layer derivatives may develop malignant characteristics. Extragonadal germ cell tumors may arise in a variety of locations in the body, usually along the axial midline. Common sites in children include the pineal gland, neck, mediastinum, retroperitoneum, and sacrococcygeal region. In the neonatal period, a majority of teratomas occur in the sacrococcygeal region, followed next by tumors in the neck. After puberty, teratomas most frequently occur in the gonads, particularly the ovary.

Yolk sac tumor (endodermal sinus tumor) is the most common malignant germ cell tumor in neonates and young children. In the neonate it most often occurs with a teratoma, often in the sacrococcygeal region (see later discussion).

Pathology

Teratomas are composed of tissues arising from all three layers of the embryonic disk. Ectodermal components, including glial tissue, are a major component of teratomas presenting at birth—in particular, sacrococcygeal tumors. There are often skin, hair, and teeth elements. Mesodermal components, including fat, bone, and muscle, also are present. Less commonly seen are endodermal components such as digestive tract tissue. Occasionally, less mature elements coexist within the teratoma and are typified by higher grade histologic features including nuclear atypia, mitotic activity, and hypercellularity. Hormonal markers, including serum AFP and hCG, often are elevated in the presence of malignant tissue within the teratoma and are useful to follow as therapy progresses. Elevated serum AFP indicates the presence of immature endodermal sinus tissue or yolk sac elements, whereas elevated hCG indicates the presence of embryonal carcinoma. Choriocarcinoma, which is rarely seen in newborns, manifests with an elevated hCG.

Evaluation

MRI or CT imaging of the primary tumor is indicated to evaluate the extent of disease. Sacrococcygeal tumors should be imaged using MRI because of the possible involvement of the spinal cord. The entire abdomen is included in the imaging study to assess the extent of any local invasion, particularly involvement of the rectal wall. A CT scan of the chest is performed to rule out metastasis. Baseline levels of serum AFP and hCG, which are normally elevated in newborns, are measured. Because of the variation in levels at birth and the variation in rates at which levels decline to normal, these tumor markers can be difficult to interpret as measures of residual disease or recurrence. The half-life of AFP is 5 to 7 days; that of hCG is 24 to 36 hours.

Sacrococcygeal Teratomas

Sacrococcygeal teratomas are the most common solid tumors in newborns. The estimated incidence is 1 in 27,000 live births (Swamy et al, 2008). A minority are malignant: 10% to 17% of sacrococcygeal teratomas contain yolk sac tumor (Isaacs, 2007). Females are affected 2 to 4 times more frequently than males. Half of sacrococcygeal teratomas are diagnosed prenatally by ultrasonography. Polyhydramnios, nonimmune fetal hydrops, and dystocia have all been described in association with sacrococcygeal teratomas. Congenital anomalies, including genitourinary, hindgut, and lower vertebral malformations, are present in 15% of patients (Isaacs, 2007). In most cases, the tumor manifests as a mass protruding between the coccyx and rectum; the mass may be quite large (Figure 80-6). About 10% of these tumors are only found by rectal examination. Nearly all arise at the tip or inner surface of the coccyx.

Differential Diagnosis

Sacrococcygeal teratomas may be confused with meningomyelocele, rectal abscess, pelvic neuroblastoma, pilonidal cyst, and a variety of very rare neoplasms that may occur in the sacral region. Most benign teratomas in this area produce no functional difficulties, even when marked intrapelvic extension is present. Bowel or bladder dysfunction, painful defecation, and vascular or lymphatic obstruction suggest that the lesion is malignant.

Treatment

Treatment of sacrococcygeal tumors is primarily surgical if age-adjusted AFP and hCG levels are normal (Horton et al, 2007). The tumor should be radically excised as soon as possible because small, undifferentiated foci may proliferate and become aggressive. Removal of the entire coccyx is required. Failure to remove the coccyx carries a 30% to 40% risk of local recurrence, which is sometimes accompanied by malignant elements. The survival rate for neonates with sacrococcygeal teratoma is 85% (Isaacs, 2007).

Sacrococcygeal teratomas diagnosed prenatally by ultrasound (approximately 50% of cases) are associated with a worse outcome; the survival rate is only 53% (Isaacs, 2004).

Fetal hydrops and prematurity are the main factors contributing to the poor survival rate. If hydrops occurs before fetal pulmonary maturity, fetal surgical intervention to debulk and devascularize the tumor may be an option (Adzick, 2010).

Infants with sacrococcygeal teratoma containing malignant yolk sac elements are treated with surgery followed by chemotherapy with cisplatin, etoposide, and bleomycin. Acute and late complications of this regimen can be significant and include hearing loss, pulmonary fibrosis, and secondary malignancy.

RENAL NEOPLASMS

Approximately two thirds of intraabdominal masses in the neonatal period arise from the kidney. The vast majority of these neoplasms are nonmalignant and are generally due to congenital defects such as polycystic or dysplastic kidneys or other conditions causing hydronephrosis. The most common intrarenal neoplasm manifesting at birth is congenital mesoblastic nephroma, followed by Wilms' tumor. Less common intrarenal neoplasms seen in the newborn period are rhabdoid tumor, nephroblastomatosis, clear cell sarcoma of the kidney, cystic renal tumors, renal cell carcinoma, rhabdomyosarcoma, hemangiopericytoma, and lymphoma. The typical clinical manifestation is an asymptomatic abdominal mass detected on physical examination or by ultrasonography.

Congenital Mesoblastic Nephroma

Congenital mesoblastic nephroma (CMN), or fetal mesenchymal hamartoma, is the most common intrarenal neoplasm in the neonate. It usually behaves as a benign neoplasm, but the histopathologic subset, cellular CMN, is associated with an increased incidence of recurrence and metastases. The typical clinical presentation is an asymptomatic abdominal mass detected on physical examination or by ultrasonography. Occasionally patients present with complications including respiratory distress, fetal hydrops, and circulatory problems caused by the size of the mass. The tumor infiltrates into normal renal parenchyma and is not encapsulated (Figure 80-7). Specific sonographic features can help to differentiate CMN from Wilms' tumor

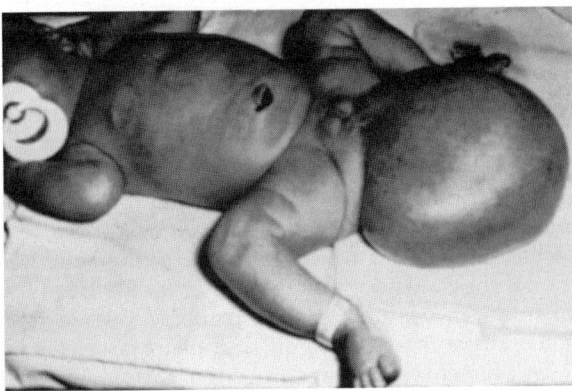

FIGURE 80-6 Large sacrococcygeal teratoma in a newborn girl.

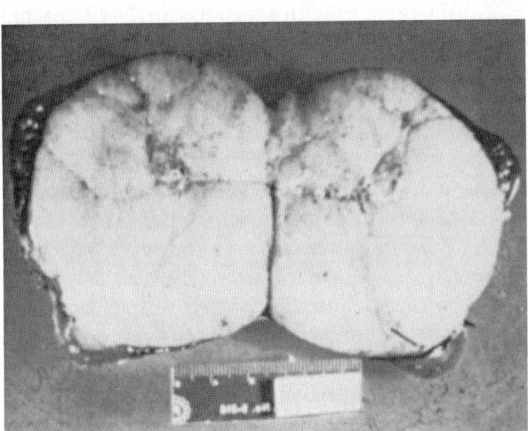

FIGURE 80-7 Congenital mesoblastic nephroma compressing and nearly totally replacing the kidney.

(Chan et al, 1987). The tumor may be diagnosed prenatally with ultrasonography, which reveals a greatly enlarged kidney distorted by the tumor. There is an increased incidence of polyhydramnios (71%) and premature labor (Glick et al, 2004).

Two histologic subtypes of congenital mesoblastic nephroma have been identified: the "classic" subtype and the cellular variant. The classic histologic subtype, which represents about one third of cases, has a preponderance of interlacing bundles of spindle-shaped cells, within which dysplastic tubules and glomeruli are irregularly scattered. Extrarenal infiltration is common. The cellular or atypical variant demonstrates increased cellularity, focal hemorrhage, necrosis, and a high mitotic index. The cellular variant usually manifests at an older age (3 months) than the classic type (mean age at presentation 1 month). Cytogenetic analysis of the cellular variant shows a translocation t(12;15)(p13;q25) that results in a ETV6-NTRK3 fusion protein that is identical to that found in infantile fibrosarcoma (Bavindir et al, 2009; Glick et al, 2004).

Complete surgical resection is usually an effective treatment for the classic form of CMN. Patients with the cellular variant are also treated with complete resection, but local and distant recurrences, for example to lung or brain, can be problematic. Positive surgical margins or tumor rupture during resection are risk factors for recurrence, which usually occurs within the 1st year following surgery. Resection and chemotherapy can successfully treat recurrent disease (Glick et al, 2004). Overall survival for CMN is 95% to 98% (Isaacs, 2008).

Wilms' Tumor

Wilms' tumor, or nephroblastoma, is the most common intraabdominal tumor of childhood, affecting 1 in 8000 children, but it is relatively rare in the neonatal period. In subsets of children with aniridia, the incidence is much higher.

Clinical Manifestations

The tumor lies deep in the flank, is attached to the kidney or is part of it, and is usually firm and smooth. It seldom extends beyond the midline, even though it may grow downward beyond the iliac crest. In 5% to 10% of all cases, tumors involve both kidneys. Most children with Wilms' tumor present with an abdominal or flank mass or an increase in abdominal size. Gross hematuria is a rare presenting symptom, but microscopic hematuria is found in approximately 25% of cases. Hypertension, occasionally noted in older infants and children, has not been observed in the newborn. The tumor may sometimes manifest with abdominal pain and be discovered at laparotomy, and occasionally acute hemorrhage into the tumor may result in a rapidly enlarging mass, usually associated with anemia and fever.

Wilms' tumor is seldom diagnosed at birth or during the neonatal period. Characteristics associated with an earlier presentation include bilaterality and associated aniridia or hypospadias (Pastore et al, 1988) and a positive family history. Rare cases of Wilms' tumor associated with polycythemia have been reported; this finding is secondary to an increased production of erythropoietin by the neoplasm.

Hereditary Associations and Congenital Anomalies

Although most cases of Wilms' tumor are sporadic, a number of conditions are associated with an increased risk of developing the tumor. These include *WT1*-associated phenotypes caused by deletions and mutations of the *WT1* gene (11p13), familial Wilms' tumor, overgrowth syndromes, and constitutional chromosomal disorders (Scott et al, 2006). The WAGR syndrome (*W*ilms' tumor, *a*niridia, *g*enitourinary abnormalities, mental *r*etardation) is found in approximately 0.8% of individuals with Wilms' tumor; the Wilms' tumor predisposition is due to a deletion in *WT1*, and the aniridia is due to a deletion of *PAX6* (Breslow et al, 2003). From a clinical perspective, if an infant has aniridia, chromosome analysis should be undertaken. If a deletion of chromosome band 11p13 is found, the child should be monitored for the development of Wilms' tumor with serial ultrasonographic studies of the kidneys. Wilms' tumor develops in approximately half of these patients. Hemihypertrophy, which either can be isolated or associated with various genetic syndromes, is associated with an increased risk of the development of Wilms' tumor. Beckwith-Wiedemann syndrome (BWS), an overgrowth disorder caused by dysregulation of imprinted genes at chromosome 11p15, is also associated with an increased risk of Wilms' tumor, particularly bilateral disease. Between 1% and 8% of individuals with BWS develop Wilms' tumor (Scott et al, 2006). Other heritable disorders may predispose a patient to Wilms' tumor. Denys-Drash syndrome, caused by a variant mutation at 11p13, includes Wilms' tumor, genital anomalies, and nephropathy. Bloom syndrome, an autosomal recessive disease, and Li-Fraumeni syndrome, an autosomal dominant tumor predisposition syndrome, are both associated with an increased incidence of Wilms' tumor. Patients with Fanconi anemia with biallelic *BRCA2* mutations are also at higher risk of developing Wilms' tumor. Between 1% and 2% of Wilms' tumor cases occur within families, but the underlying cause of familial Wilms' tumor is currently unknown (Scott et al, 2006).

Prognostic Factors

Important prognostic factors include the histologic pattern, the extent of disease, and chromosomal abnormalities. Well-differentiated tumors with glomeruloid and tubular formation have a better prognosis than those with anaplastic and sarcomatous morphology. Absence of tumor-specific loss of heterozygosity for chromosomes 1p and 16q is associated with a better prognosis (Grundy et al, 2005). Patients younger than 2 years of age have fewer relapses, especially to distant sites, than older children.

Evaluation and Staging

The most common staging system in use is that of the National Wilms Tumor Study (NWTS) (Table 80-9). Clinical staging, which includes a CT scan of the abdomen and chest, is an important factor in predicting survival; tumors with more extensive spread carry a poorer prognosis. The most common sites of metastasis are the liver and lungs (Figure 80-8). Tumor thrombus is occasionally noted in the inferior vena cava. Other sites of

TABLE 80-9 Wilms' Tumor Staging

Stage I	Tumor limited to kidney, completely resected. Renal capsule is intact. No evidence of tumor at or beyond the margins of resection. No rupture or prior biopsy.
Stage II	Tumor is completely resected. No evidence of tumor at or beyond the margins of resection. The tumor extends beyond the kidney, for example, penetration of the renal capsule, presence of tumor cells within blood vessels of the renal sinus. No rupture or prior biopsy.
Stage III	Residual nonhematogenous tumor present following surgery, including peritoneal implants or tumor spillage before or during surgery.
Stave IV	Hematogenous metastases (lung, liver, bone, brain, etc.), or lymph node metastases outside the abdominopelvic region.
Stage V	Bilateral renal involvement.

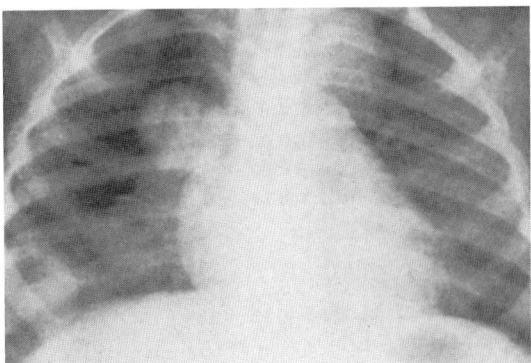

FIGURE 80-8 Pulmonary metastases from Wilms' tumor.

metastatic spread are the retroperitoneum, peritoneum, mediastinum, and pleurae. Approximately 10% of patients will have disease in both kidneys. A bone scan is necessary if histologic studies show clear cell sarcoma because of the possibility of bone metastases. CT or MRI of the brain is necessary in patients with rhabdoid tumors (which may be confused radiologically with Wilms' tumor) because they frequently metastasize to brain.

Treatment

Patients with low-stage Wilms' tumor have a cure rate of >90%. Patients with small tumors limited to the kidney can be cured with surgery alone. Follow-up involves periodic screening with abdominal ultrasonography, chest x-ray, and urinalysis. Patients with intermediate-stage Wilms' tumor are treated with a short course (12 weeks) of chemotherapy with vincristine and dactinomycin. More extensive disease requires the addition of doxorubicin. Radiation therapy is indicated in children with diffuse abdominal disease or nonresponsive pulmonary metastases. Even patients with metastatic disease have a good prognosis, with 70% long-term survival. Recurrent disease, which can be local or may involve metastases to the lungs or brain, is treated, often successfully, with additional chemotherapy and radiation.

Infants younger than 12 months of age have experienced significant toxicities to the hematopoietic system, liver, and lungs from dactinomycin, vincristine, and doxorubicin. Drug doses for infants are approximately 50% of the usual per kilogram dose for older children; this has not affected the very favorable cure rate.

Rhabdoid Tumor of the Kidney

Rhabdoid tumor of the kidney (RTK) is an uncommon tumor of children that is one of the most lethal neoplasms of early neonatal life, with a mortality rate exceeding 80%. RTK is the second most common malignant neoplasm of the kidney in neonates, after Wilms' tumor. It has a predilection for males, with a male-to-female ratio of 1.5:1, and for infants, with median age at diagnosis of 11 months. It is often widely metastatic at diagnosis; metastatic sites include lung, abdomen, lymph nodes, liver, bone, skin, and brain. Renal rhabdoid tumors occasionally manifest simultaneously with brain tumors, which are usually in the midline cerebellum. Although the brain tumors have been classified histologically as medulloblastoma or primitive neuroectodermal tumors, they show the same chromosome 22 abnormalities seen in RTK. Homozygous inactivating deletions or mutations of the *INI1* gene, located in chromosome band 22q11.2, are responsible for a majority of rhabdoid tumors (Jackson et al, 2007). *INI1* functions as a tumor suppressor gene; loss of expression in RTK can be detected immunohistochemically.

The prognosis for infants with RTK is extremely poor. Survival at 4 years for infants diagnosed before 6 months of age is less than 10% (Tomlinson et al, 2005). Virtually all patients with distant metastases will have a fatal outcome. Treatment modalities have included surgical resection, chemotherapy, and radiation therapy.

Persistent Renal Blastema and Nephroblastomatosis

Accumulations of immature renal tissue are not normally found beyond 36 weeks' gestation, the time at which nephrogenesis normally ceases. Nodular renal blastema is characterized by microscopic nests of primitive cells in the subcapsular renal cortex; these cells resemble the blastemal cells of Wilms' tumor but lack mitoses. Although benign, these nodules are believed to have the potential for neoplastic transformation. They are found in 1 of every 200 to 400 postmortem examinations of infants dying from other causes before 4 months of age. When nodular renal blastema becomes massive and confluent and replaces the cortex, it is referred to as *nephroblastomatosis*. Children with massive bilateral involvement often respond to therapies used for Wilms' tumor. Although persistent renal blastema is not a true malignancy, it probably has been confused with Wilms' tumor in the past, and it appears in many instances to be a precursor of this malignancy (Beckwith, 1993).

Cystic Partially Differentiated Nephroblastoma

This renal neoplasm is known by a variety of names: polycystic nephroblastoma, benign multilocular cystic nephroma, well-differentiated polycystic Wilms' tumor, and cystic partially differentiated nephroblastoma. It is a cystic encapsulated tumor occurring before 2 years of age.

The cysts are lined by epithelium and show a mixture of partially differentiated and undifferentiated metanephrogenic blastemas, a finding that differentiates this lesion from multilocular cysts of the kidney. The tumor appears to have a benign course, and nephrectomy is the treatment of choice. These neoplasms probably represent a differentiated form of nephroblastoma (van den Hoek et al, 2009).

RETINOBLASTOMA

Retinoblastoma is a malignant ocular tumor that arises from embryonic retinal cells. It occurs in the setting of hereditary and nonhereditary disease. The incidence of retinoblastoma is approximately 1 in 18,000 live births; between 250 and 350 cases are diagnosed in the United States each year (Kiss, 2008). Bilateral involvement, which occurs in the setting of heritable disease, is observed in 20% to 35% of patients. Whereas the incidence of heritable retinoblastoma is constant among various population groups, the incidence of sporadic, nonheritable, unilateral retinoblastoma is increased in poorer, tropical, and subtropical regions (Kiss, 2008).

Genetics

Approximately one third of patients have hereditary disease, which is often bilateral. Patients with hereditary disease have a germline mutation in the retinoblastoma gene, *RB1*, a tumor suppressor gene located on chromosome band 13q14. The mutation either is inherited from a parent or occurs during embryonic development. There is autosomal transmission with high penetrance, approximately 90%. Patients with nonhereditary disease, about 60% of cases, have unilateral retinoblastoma. Their disease is the result of acquired somatic mutations in both *RB1* alleles.

Approximately 5% of retinoblastoma patients are born with a constitutional deletion of chromosome 13, 13q–. These patients have associated constitutional anomalies including micrencephaly, macrognathia, malformed ears and thumbs, hypertelorism, microphthalmia, ptosis, short stature, cleft palate, and developmental delay.

Children with the bilateral and hereditary form often are diagnosed at an earlier age, in part because the family history leads to screening starting early in the postnatal period. In rare instances, family history of the disorder may be lacking; hereditary bilateral retinoblastoma may be the result of germline mosaicism in the parent.

Clinical Manifestations

Patients with retinoblastoma commonly present with leukocoria (i.e., cat's eye), with squinting, or with strabismus caused by loss of vision in the affected eye. Multifocal retinal involvement is common, occurring in 84% of the cases. Intraocular spread may fill the vitreous body by extension or seeding, whereas exophytic tumors arise from the outer retinal layer and cause retinal detachment. Extraocular spread is seen in less than 15% of patients, usually occurring by direct invasion of the optic nerve and eventually leading to subarachnoid involvement and intracranial spread. In such cases the cerebrospinal fluid may contain tumor cells. Rarely, tumors may spread by invasion of the orbit or by hematogenous dissemination to bone and bone marrow. Children with bilateral retinoblastoma are at risk for tumor dissemination to the pineal gland, a condition known as trilateral retinoblastoma; these children should be evaluated periodically by brain MRI.

The diagnosis is made by funduscopic examination performed with the patient under general anesthesia. CT or MRI of the eye is useful to determine tumor extent and optic nerve involvement. A lumbar puncture for cerebrospinal fluid cytology is performed if there is optic nerve invasion, but more extensive evaluation with bone marrow biopsy or bone scan is not usually necessary. Tumors are staged according to the International Classification of Retinoblastoma, based on tumor size and location and the extent of vitreous and subretinal seeding (Kiss, 2008).

Treatment

Because extraocular spread and death from dissemination are rare, the main goal of treatment is local control and preservation of vision. Surgical enucleation is used only when there is no chance for useful vision, if glaucoma is present, or if conservative measures fail to control the tumor. Small tumors confined to the retina often can be controlled with focal consolidative therapies such as cryotherapy and laser photocoagulation. Systemic chemotherapy with agents such as carboplatin, vincristine, and etoposide is frequently used concurrently with cryotherapy and laser therapy. External beam radiation therapy is an effective treatment, but because of the late effects of radiation on bone growth and the potential for second tumor induction, aggressive local therapy and chemotherapy are preferable.

Prognosis

The prognosis for children with unilateral retinoblastoma is excellent, with cure rates of 85% to 90%. However, patients with bilateral disease have a much lower long-term survival rate because of the high incidence of second malignancies, which may occur at any point in the life span. Patients with hereditary disease can develop secondary sarcomas in the area treated with radiation therapy; they are also at increased risk of developing sarcomas in other, nonirradiated areas. Local extension of retinoblastoma confers a poor prognosis, with survival rates of less than 10% with orbital extension or distant dissemination.

CENTRAL NERVOUS SYSTEM TUMORS

Incidence and Epidemiology

Congenital brain tumors are rare, with an incidence of approximately 1 to 3 per million live births (Lasky, 2008). Most brain tumors in infants are supratentorial. Half are gliomas, including astrocytomas. PNETs and medulloblastomas also occur. Atypical teratoid or rhabdoid tumor of the CNS is associated with a high mortality rate (Packer et al, 2002). In general, brain tumors manifesting in the perinatal period carry a very poor prognosis.

Clinical Manifestations

Macrocephaly is often the first sign of a congenital CNS tumor. Signs and symptoms of increased intracranial pressure (ICP) may be present. In infants these include a bulging fontanel, split sutures, or rapidly enlarging head size. Poor feeding, vomiting, lethargy, and irritability also can be symptoms of increased ICP. Funduscopic examination may or may not show papilledema. Loss of developmental milestones may be detected in older infants and children. Specific neurologic abnormalities include Parinaud's syndrome (impaired upward gaze secondary to increased pressure in the dorsal midbrain), cranial nerve palsies, and nystagmus. Head tilting can occur in patients with posterior cerebellar masses secondary to cervical root irritation.

Congenital brain tumors are sometimes detected prenatally by ultrasound. CT scan is often the initial imaging study performed, but MRI provides more detailed information.

Treatment

The optimal therapy is surgical resection of the tumor. The degree of surgical resection is the single most important predictor of survival (Lasky, 2008). Complete resection is often not possible. Tumors in infants tend to be large, highly malignant, and invasive. They are also highly vascular, making it difficult to remove the tissue without significant morbidity.

Radiation therapy, a backbone of treatment for older children with malignant brain tumors, is avoided if possible in young infants because they experience devastating late effects including neurocognitive deficits and growth impairment. Adjuvant chemotherapy can play a role in treatment; this may allow necessary radiation therapy to be delayed until the child is older. Conformal stereotactic techniques that target the tumor and minimize radiation to normal brain structures may help lessen late complications.

SARCOMAS

Soft tissue sarcomas are rarely seen in newborns. The most commonly diagnosed soft tissue sarcoma in the neonatal age group is infantile or congenital fibrosarcoma, which is classified as a low-grade nonrhabdomyosarcoma soft tissue sarcoma. The incidence in infants between age 1 and 12 months is 5 cases per 1 million infants (Ries et al, 1999). In general, infantile fibrosarcoma is treated by complete surgical excision, although neoadjuvant chemotherapy with a variety of agents has been successfully used for tumor shrinkage, with subsequent reduction in the morbidity related to radical surgical procedures (Russell et al, 2009). The cure rates for infantile fibrosarcoma, with surgery alone or with chemotherapy and surgery, approach 100% (Kurkchubasche et al, 2000; Loh et al, 2002).

The initial evaluation of a patient with a congenital fibrosarcoma includes imaging of the primary tumor by MRI or CT, and a chest CT scan. Diagnosis is made by biopsy of the lesion. Chemotherapy regimens used successfully for treatment of this tumor include vincristine, actinomycin D, and cyclophosphamide, as well as etoposide and ifosfamide. Doxorubicin, although efficacious, is generally avoided because of the risk of cardiac toxicity. Duration of therapy depends on the size, location, and response of the tumor, but the general goal is to reduce the tumor size to maximize chances of surgical local control. Radiation therapy is usually avoided to spare the infant the associated late effects of poor growth and secondary cancers.

Rhabdomyosarcoma (RMS), the most common soft-tissue sarcoma in children, is rarely seen in neonates: fewer than 1% of RMS cases are diagnosed in the 1st month of life (Lobe et al, 1994). Congenital rhabdomyosarcoma often involves the genitourinary tract and is frequently of the embryonal subtype. Congenital embryonal rhabdomyosarcoma appears to be associated with a specific translocation, t(2;8)(q35;q13) (Meloni-Ehrig et al, 2009).

HISTIOCYTOSIS

The histiocytoses are a diverse group of disorders characterized by the accumulation and proliferation of cells derived from the monophagocytic system (Isaacs, 2006). These disorders have been categorized into three classes (Table 80-10). Class I disorders, which are dendritic cell–related, include Langerhans cell histiocytosis (LCH) (formerly known as histiocytosis X), Letterer-Siwe disease, Hand-Schüller-Christian disease, eosinophilic granuloma, and pure cutaneous histiocytosis. Class II disorders, which involve macrophage-derived cells, include familial hemophagocytic lymphohistiocytosis (FHL) and infection-associated hemophagocytic syndrome (IAHS). Class III disorders are malignant disorders of mononuclear phagocytes and include acute monocytic leukemia, malignant histiocytosis, and histiocytic lymphoma. In addition to these three classes, other rare, noncategorized histiocytoses can occur in newborns, in particular, juvenile xanthogranuloma (JXG). The pathophysiology of the histiocytic disorders appears to be related to abnormal regulation of histiocyte activation resulting in cell proliferation and cytokine production (Isaacs, 2006).

The most common histiocytic disease seen in the fetus and neonate is LCH. About half of newborns with LCH have disease confined to the skin; the other half have disseminated disease with resultant organ dysfunction, usually involving bone marrow, liver, or lung. Presenting symptoms of LCH in neonates include skin lesions, hepatosplenomegaly, lymphadenopathy, and respiratory distress. Histologically, both cutaneous and disseminated LCH are characterized by granuloma-like lesions. Diagnosis is made by biopsy; Langerhans cells are positive by immunohistochemistry for CD1A.

The course of LCH is unpredictable. The pure cutaneous form of LCH usually resolves spontaneously in 2 to 3 months, whereas disseminated LCH, which can also manifest with skin lesions, carries a poor prognosis with 52% mortality (Isaacs, 2006). Newborns presenting with skin lesions may not develop the symptoms of disseminated disease for several weeks to months. Disseminated LCH is usually treated with chemotherapeutic drugs including vinblastine and prednisone.

FHL and IAHS are also seen in the newborn period. FHL has an incidence of approximately 1 in 50,000 liveborn children (Henter et al, 2007). The overall survival for newborns with FHL is only 9% unless stem cell transplant

TABLE 80-10   Classification of Childhood Histiocytoses

Feature	Class I	Class II	Class III
Diseases included	Langerhans cell histiocytosis Pure cutaneous histiocytosis	IAHS; FEL; grouped together as the hemophagocytic lymphohistiocytoses (HLHs)	Malignant histiocytosis; acute monocytic leukemia; true histiocytic lymphoma
Cellular characteristics	Langerhans cells with cleaved nuclei and Birbeck granules seen by electron microscopy; cell surface antigens include S100 and CD1a; cells mixed with varying proportions of eosinophils; multinucleated giant cells sometimes seen	Morphologically normal, reactive macrophages with prominent erythrophagocytosis; process involves entire reticuloendothelial system	Neoplastic cellular proliferation of cells exhibiting characteristics of macrophages or dendritic cells or their precursors; localized or systemic
Proposed pathophysiologic mechanisms	Immunologic stimulation of a normal antigen-presenting cell—the Langerhans cell—in an uncontrolled manner	Histiocytic reaction secondary to an unknown antigenic stimulation (FEL) or to an infectious agent (IAHS), with erythrophagocytosis possibly reflecting foreign antigens absorbed on erythrocytes or activation of macrophages by excess lymphokine production due to abnormal immunoregulation	Neoplasm; clonal autonomous uncontrolled proliferative process

From Ladisch S, Jaffe ES, in *Principles and practice of pediatric oncology*, Philadelphia, 2006, Lippincott Williams & Wilkins.
FEL, Familial erythrophagocytic lymphohistiocytosis; *IAHS*, infection-associated hemophagocytic syndrome.
Note: Previously known as histiocytosis X and its related syndromes of eosinophilic granuloma, Hand-Schüller-Christian disease, and Letterer-Siwe disease.

is performed; survival for IAHS is 59% (Isaacs, 2006). Newborns with these disorders commonly present with fever, hepatosplenomegaly, and cytopenias. Other symptoms include liver dysfunction, neurologic symptoms, hypertriglyceridemia, elevated serum ferritin levels, and hypofibrinogenemia. Diagnostic criteria are listed in Box 80-1. Hemophagocytosis is found in the bone marrow in 76% of patients. Natural killer cell and cytotoxic T cell activity is reduced or absent. Thirty percent of patients with FHL harbor constitutional mutations in the perforin gene, which encodes an essential protein for cellular immune activation (Stepp et al, 1999). Several additional mutations can also cause FHL, including mutations in *UNC13D* on chromosome 17q25 and mutations in *STX11* on chromosome 6q24 (Trizzino et al, 2008). Patients with FHL are usually well at birth, then develop clinical symptoms by age 2 to 6 months. Constant fever, cytopenias, marked hepatosplenomegaly, and progressive cerebromeningeal symptoms characterize the disease course. Progressive disease usually leads to death within 4 months of diagnosis, but hematopoietic cell transplantation can increase 3-year survival to 64% (Jordan and Filipovich, 2008).

Patients with IAHS, whose symptoms are similar to those of patients with FHL, experience a high recovery rate (59%) when appropriate antibiotic treatment is promptly administered (Isaacs, 2006). Leukocytosis is common in IAHS, possibly reflecting the underlying infectious etiology.

JXG, a disorder of dendritic-related cells, is less common in neonates than LCH. Two forms are recognized, cutaneous and extracutaneous. Patients present with one or multiple cutaneous nodules, which are reddish to yellow-brown papules on the head, neck, and extremities. Three fourths of neonates with cutaneous JXG present with a solitary nodule; one fourth present with multiple nodules. Nodules typically resolve spontaneously over approximately 2 years. Survival is excellent for neonates with JXG limited to the skin and subcutaneous tissue, with

no deaths reported in one series (Isaacs, 2006). Treatment is not generally indicated. Extracutaneous or disseminated JXG can involve the subcutaneous and soft tissues, liver, lung, spleen, eye, lymph nodes, and brain. Twenty-five percent of neonates with disseminated JXG do not have cutaneous lesions. Jaundice, hepatosplenomegaly, and thrombocytopenia can be seen. Although most cutaneous and extracutaneous lesions resolve spontaneously without treatment, disseminated JXG has an 11% death rate (Isaacs, 2006). Ocular and CNS involvement can cause significant morbidity. Systemic JXG is usually treated with chemotherapy and/or corticosteroids.

HEPATOBLASTOMA

Hepatoblastoma is an embryonal neoplasm composed of malignant epithelial tissue. The incidence in infants is 11.2 cases per million; the incidence is increased as much as 15-fold in premature infants with low birthweights (Feusner and Plaschkes, 2002). The female-male ratio in neonates is 1:6 (Isaacs, 2007). Histologic subtype is associated with outcome, with pure fetal histology having the best prognosis. Hepatoblastoma is associated with a number of genetic abnormalities and malformation syndromes, including Beckwith-Wiedemann syndrome and trisomy 18 (Von Schweinitz, 2003).

Chromosome abnormalities in tumor tissue include trisomy of chromosomes 2 and 20. Chromosomal gains at chromosome 8 and 20 may be associated with an adverse prognosis. Patients with Beckwith-Wiedemann syndrome demonstrate loss of heterozygosity at 11p15.5, the Beckwith-Wiedemann locus.

The most common presenting symptom in neonates is abdominal distention. Even in the absence of distention an abdominal mass can sometimes be palpated. Anemia, fetal hydrops, and respiratory distress are other initial findings. Serum alpha-fetoprotein is elevated in half of patients. Hepatoblastoma is occasionally diagnosed prenatally by screening ultrasound. Tumor rupture can occur during birth, resulting in massive hemorrhage.

Ultrasonography is useful to distinguish cystic and solid masses from diffuse hepatic enlargement. CT scan of the abdomen demonstrates the extent of tumor involvement, anatomic landmarks, and operability; MRI most accurately shows tumor margins and vessel involvement.

The goal of therapy is complete surgical resection. Infants with pure fetal histology whose tumors are completely resected have a 92% 24-month survival rate. A lobectomy of the involved portion of the liver is performed if one lobe is free of malignancy and there is no evidence of distant metastases. For unresectable but nonmetastatic tumors, initial treatment consists of chemotherapy with cisplatin and vincristine. If adequate tumor shrinkage results, the tumor is then resected. Orthotopic liver transplant is curative in patients with unresectable, nonmetastatic hepatoblastomas.

HEPATIC HEMANGIOENDOTHELIOMA

Hepatic hemangioendothelioma, also referred to as hepatic hemangioma, is a benign vascular tumor of the liver; it is the most frequent liver tumor of infants (Warmann, 2003). The disease is classified into three subtypes: focal, multiple, and diffuse hepatic lesions. Some patients also present with cutaneous hemangiomas. Although some infants with small tumors are asymptomatic, infants with larger tumors can present with multiple symptoms including abdominal distention, respiratory distress, high-output cardiac failure, and consumptive coagulopathy. The diagnosis is often suspected prenatally when a hepatic mass is detected by ultrasonography. The diagnostic evaluation usually includes an abdominal ultrasound examination and CT or MRI. If imaging studies fail to reveal a diagnosis,

then a biopsy is performed. Infants with focal or multifocal disease without evidence of cardiac failure can usually be carefully observed with periodic physical exams and ultrasound examinations. Symptomatic infants are usually treated with corticosteroids. Infants with diffuse hepatic hemangiomas, who are at the greatest risk of morbidity or death, are treated with vincristine in addition to corticosteroids. Embolization or hepatic artery ligation can be considered if pharmacologic intervention is unsuccessful (van der Meijs, 2008). Overall survival in fetal and neonatal focal hemangioma is 86%; overall survival in fetal and neonatal multifocal disease is 71% (Isaacs, 2007).

TREATMENT CONSIDERATIONS IN INFANTS

CHEMOTHERAPY DOSING

Neonates and infants experience more frequent and more severe side effects and late effects from chemotherapy compared to older children and adults. This is likely due to age-related differences in body composition, drug bioavailability, and drug metabolism. Infants have increased total body water; decreased activity of drug-metabolizing enzymes, particularly P450 enzymes; and less efficient renal function. To compensate for these differences, specific chemotherapy dosing protocols have been developed for neonates and infants. Doses for systemic chemotherapy are reduced overall and are frequently calculated by weight instead of by body surface area. Interestingly, the volume of the CSF in relation to body surface area is much greater in young children than in adults; accordingly, doses of intrathecal chemotherapy are adjusted for age to avoid underdosing young infants with leukemia.

RADIATION EFFECTS

The use of radiation therapy in newborn infants is reserved for acute life-threatening situations in which the benefits of radiation clearly outweigh the risks of adverse late effects, which include growth impairment, cognitive impairment, and secondary malignancies. The goal is to use as little radiation as possible to spare the infant potentially morbid side effects.

PAIN MANAGEMENT

Infants experience pain and should be treated with adequate pain medication. Signs of pain in the neonate can be subtle and can include crying, grimacing, poor feeding, tachycardia, and high blood pressure. Acetaminophen can be an effective analgesic in infants, but it must be used judiciously to avoid masking a fever that could signify an infection, particularly if a central line is in place or in the setting of neutropenia. Nonsteroidal antiinflammatory medications are usually avoided in patients with cancer because of the risks of interfering with platelet function. Narcotics can be used as needed provided that adequate monitoring of side effects such as respiratory depression is in place. Narcotics can produce physical dependence when used for more than 1 week, and doses may need to be tapered to avoid symptoms of withdrawal.

NUTRITION

Adequate nutrition is particularly important for neonates and infants. Patients might require supplemental nutrition via nasogastric tube or intravenous parenteral nutrition. A nutritionist should be consulted to help assess the infant's nutritional needs. Breastfeeding can usually be continued in neonates with malignancy.

INTRAVENOUS ACCESS

Most neonates and infants diagnosed with cancer will require a central venous catheter in order to facilitate delivery of chemotherapy, blood product support, and parenteral nutrition. Some chemotherapy agents, such as vincristine and doxorubicin, are vesicants and can cause severe skin and subcutaneous burns if inadvertently infiltrated underneath the skin. The type of central line inserted depends on the size of the infant and the specific needs associated with the chemotherapy regimen.

TRANSFUSIONS

Cancer patients frequently require blood product support for correction of life-threatening cytopenias and coagulopathies. To minimize the risk of transfusion-associated infections and complications, a number of guidelines exist. These include the use of CMV-negative blood to prevent transmission of CMV, which is potentially life-threatening; the use of irradiated blood products to prevent the possibility of graft-versus-host disease in the immunocompromised recipient; and the use of leukocyte-depleted blood products to minimize febrile or allergic reactions. Donor-designated blood is usually discouraged in infants with congenital leukemia, given the possibility of future bone marrow transplantation.

IMMUNIZATIONS

Immunizations generally are avoided until the patient has been off chemotherapy for at least 6 months. In addition, close contacts of the patient should receive the inactivated polio vaccine rather than the live oral polio vaccine. There is no contraindication to immunizing first-degree relatives with the varicella vaccine. However, any person in whom a rash develops after the vaccination should be kept away from the patient.

PSYCHOSOCIAL CONSIDERATIONS

Social services and psychological support are essential for families. These services are usually best coordinated through the efforts of a multidisciplinary team composed of nurses, social workers, and the pediatric oncologist.

LATE EFFECTS

Infants who receive treatment for cancer during the 1st year of life are at risk for many late effects directly related to chemotherapy, surgery, and radiation therapy. Infants in the neonatal period will be particularly susceptible to therapies affecting normal growth and development.

Information about late effects of treatment and suggested screening after childhood cancer may be found on the Children's Oncology Group website (www.childrensoncologygroup.org). Infants require follow-up evaluations at routine intervals by a pediatric oncologist (or multidisciplinary cancer survivor team) who can help identify appropriate screening tests and appropriate support.

CONCLUSION

Cancer in the neonatal period is rare, but must be diagnosed and treated promptly, with careful attention to the epidemiologic and clinical features that differ from those in older children with similar malignancies. There are special challenges in treating the neonate with cancer, including the newborn's unique physiologic status, which results in marked susceptibility to acute and late toxicities of treatment. Careful teamwork is necessary among the neonatologist, pediatric oncologist, surgeon, radiation therapist, nurse, and social worker in order to support and treat the patient and family.

SUGGESTED READINGS

Ambros PF, Ambros IM, Brodeur GM, et al: International consensus for neuroblastoma molecular diagnostics: report from the International Neuroblastoma Risk Group (INRG) Biology Committee, Br J Cancer 100:1471-1482, 2009.

Bruinsma F, Venn A, Lancaster P, et al: Incidence of cancer in children born after in vitro fertilization, Hum Reprod 15:604-607, 2000.

Chessells JM, Harrison CJ, Kempski H, et al: Clinical features, cytogenetics and outcome in acute lymphoblastic and myeloid leukaemia of infancy: report from the MRC Childhood Leukaemia working party, Leukemia 16:776-784, 2002.

De Bernardi B, Gerrard M, Boni L, et al: Excellent outcome with reduced treatment for infants with disseminated neuroblastoma without MYCN gene amplification, J Clin Oncol 27:1034-1040, 2009.

De Bernardi B, Pianca C, Pistamiglio P, et al: Neuroblastoma with symptomatic spinal cord compression at diagnosis: treatment and results with 76 cases, J Clin Oncol 19:183-190, 2001.

Fuchs J, Rydzynski J, Von Schweinitz D, et al: Pretreatment prognostic factors and treatment results in children with hepatoblastoma: a report from the German Cooperative Pediatric Liver Tumor Study HB 94, Cancer 95:172-182, 2002.

Glick RD, Hicks J, Nuchtern JG, et al: Renal tumors in infants less than 6 months of age, J Pediatr Surg 39:522-525, 2004.

Greaves MF, Maia AT, Wiemels JL, et al: Leukemia in twins: lessons in natural history, Blood 102:2321-2333, 2003.

Henter J-I, Horne A, Arico M, et al: HLH-2004: diagnostic and therapeutic guidelines for hemophagocytic lymphohistiocytosis, Pediatr Blood Cancer 48:124-131, 2007.

Hero B, Simon T, Spitz R, et al: Localized infant neuroblastomas often show spontaneous regression: results of the prospective trials NB95-S and NB97, J Clin Oncol 26:1504-1510, 2008.

Horton Z, Schlatter M, Schultz S: Pediatric germ cell tumors, Surg Oncol 16:205-213, 2007.

Isaacs H: Fetal and neonatal renal tumors, J Pediatr Surg 43:1587-1595, 2008.

Kiss S, Leiderman YI, Mukai S: Diagnosis, classification, and treatment of retinoblastoma, Int Ophthalmol Clin 48:135-147, 2008.

Klusmann J-H, Creutzig U, Zimmermann M, et al: Treatment and prognostic impact of transient leukemia in neonates with Down syndrome, Blood 111:2991-2998, 2008.

Lasky JL, Choi EJ, Johnston S: Congenital brain tumors, J Pediatr Hematol Oncol 30:326-331, 2008.

Leiderman YI, Kiss S, Mukai S: Molecular genetics of RB1—the retinoblastoma gene, Semin Ophthalmol 22:247-254, 2007.

Lin P, O'Brien J: Frontiers in the management of retinoblastoma, Am J Ophthalmol 148:192-198, 2009.

Loh ML, Ahn P, Perez-Atayde AR, et al: Treatment of infantile fibrosarcoma with chemotherapy and surgery: results from the Dana-Farber Cancer Institute and Children's Hospital, Boston, J Pediatr Hematol Oncol 24:722-726, 2002.

Montclair T, Brodeur GM, Ambros PF, et al: The International Neuroblastoma Risk Group (INRG) staging system: an INRG Task Force report, J Clin Oncol 27:298-303, 2009.

Moore SW, Satgé D, Sasco AJ, et al: The epidemiology of neonatal tumours, Pediatr Surg Int 19:509-519, 2003.

Pizzo PA, Poplack DG: Principles and practice of pediatric oncology, ed 5, Philadelphia, 2006, Lippincott Williams & Wilkins.

Pui CH, Relling MV, Downing JR: Acute lymphoblastic leukemia, *N Engl J Med* 350:1535-1548, 2004.

Schneiderman J, London WB, Brodeur GM, et al: Clinical significance of *MCYN* amplification and ploidy in favorable-stage neuroblastoma: a report from the Children's Oncology Group, *J Clin Oncol* 26:913-918, 2008.

Scott RH, Stiller CA, Walker L, et al: Syndromes and constitutional chromosomal abnormalities associated with Wilms tumour, *J Med Genet* 43:705-715, 2006.

Spector LG, Feusner JH, Ross JA: Hepatoblastoma and low birth weight, *Pediatr Blood Cancer* 43:706, 2004.

Van der Linden MH, Valsecchi MG, De Lorenzo P, et al: Outcome of congenital acute lymphoblastic leukemia treated on the Interfant-99 protocol, *Blood* 29:3764-3768, 2009.

Vardiman JW, Thiele J, Arber DA, et al: The 2008 revision of the World Health Organization (WHO) classification of myeloid neoplasms and acute leukemia: rationale and important changes, *Blood* 114:937-951, 2009.

Von Schweinitz D: Neonatal liver tumors, *Semin Neonatol* 8:403-410, 2003.

Complete references used in this text can be found online at www.expertconsult.com

PART XVII

RENAL AND GENITOURINARY SYSTEMS

RENAL MORPHOGENESIS AND DEVELOPMENT OF RENAL FUNCTION

Jean-Pierre Guignard and Endre Sulyok

RENAL MORPHOGENESIS

The fetal kidney develops from three successive mesodermic structures: the pronephros, the mesonephros, and the metanephros. The pronephric tubule extends into the intermediate mesoderm of the mesonephros to form the wolffian duct. The metanephros develops from an outbranch of the wolffian duct called the *ureteric bud* that extends into a mass of undifferentiated metanephric mesenchyme. Reciprocal inductive interactions between the ureteric bud epithelium and the metanephric mesenchyme result in the formation of both the collecting duct system and the nephrons of the permanent kidney. Cells of the metanephric mesenchyme adjacent to the tip of the ureteric bud are induced to aggregate and signal the ureteric bud to grow and branch repeatedly (branching morphogenesis), eventually leading to the formation of the renal collecting system. The ureteric bud also induces the mesenchyme to undergo a mesenchymal-epithelial transformation resulting in the formation of the glomeruli and renal tubules. Ureteric bud outgrowth requires inductive signals derived from the metanephric mesenchyme under the control of transcription factors and signaling molecules including Wilms' tumor gene 1 (WT1) protein and glial cell line–derived neurotrophic factor (GDNF). Normal ureteric bud response to these inductive signals is under the control of several transcription factors such as Pax2 and Lim1 and the *Formin* gene.

Differentiation of the metanephros starts around 5 weeks' gestation, and the first nephrons are formed by week 8. Nephrogenesis continues up to weeks 34 to 35, with the deep nephrons being formed first. From the completion of nephrogenesis around week 35 until birth, the nephrons grow only in size. At birth, juxtamedullary nephrons are more mature than superficial nephrons. The total number of nephrons varies widely ranging from 600,000 to 1.2 million per kidney. Fetal growth retardation and premature delivery are associated with a low number of nephrons, so that a positive correlation exists between birthweight and the final number of nephrons (Merlet-Bénichou et al, 1999). Exposure to drugs (gentamicin, β-lactam antibiotics, cyclosporin, excess glucocorticoid), vitamin A deficiency, hyperglycemia, obstruction in the urinary tract, and deletion of an allele of the *GDNF* gene can also impair nephrogenesis, leading to a permanent nephron deficit (Gilbert and Merlet-Bénichou, 2000).

Mutations in any one of the genes controlling renal morphogenesis result in severe renal developmental defects. The angiotensinogen and angiotensin receptor genes, best known for controlling renal hemodynamics, also play a role in the development of calyces and pelvis. Mutational inactivation of the angiotensin receptor 2 (Agtr2), encoded on the X chromosome, results in a range of anomalies including vesicoureteral reflux, duplex kidney, renal ectopia, ureteropelvic junction stenosis, ureterovesical junction stenosis, renal dysplasia, renal hypoplasia, multicystic dysplastic kidney, and renal agenesis (the CAKUT sequence—*c*ongenital *a*nomalies of the *k*idney and *u*rinary *t*ract) (Winyard and Chitty, 2008; Woolf, 2006).

Major renal malformations resulting from mutations in transcription factors, signaling molecules and gene products are discussed in various reviews (Burrow, 2000; Cooper et al, 2006; Pohl et al, 2002).

The glomerular diameter approximates 110 μm at birth (200 μm in the adult), and the average proximal tubular length reaches 2 mm (20 mm in the adult). Postnatal growth is characterized by accelerated growth of the proximal tubular volume compared with the glomerular filtering area. The glomerular basement membrane, which behaves as a filtration barrier, is thinner in neonates (100 nm) than in adults (300 nm). The size of the apertures in this "barrier" limits the passage of compounds through the capillary wall. In addition, an electrostatic barrier, resulting from the presence of negatively charged glycosialoproteins in the glomerular capillary wall, further restricts the filtration of negatively charged molecules. In the adult, the molecular weight cutoff for the filter is about 70,000. Molecules with a radius less than 1.8 nm are filtered freely. Molecules larger than 3.6 nm are not freely filtered. The permeability of the glomerular basement membrane is greater in newborn animals than in more mature animals.

During the second half of gestation, kidney weight increases proportionally to gestational age, body weight, and body surface area. The kidney and bladder can be visualized by ultrasonography from week 15 of gestation; the precise renal architecture is clearly defined only by week 20. Kidney size as measured by ultrasonography increases proportionally to gestational age (Shin et al, 2007). The ratio between the renal and the abdominal circumferences at the level of the umbilical vein remains constant during gestation, with values ranging from 0.27 to 0.30 (Grannum et al, 1980). At birth, renal volume approximates 10 mL, and it reaches 23 mL by the third week of life. Each kidney weighs about 12.5 g (approximately 150 g in the adult) and has a length of about 4.5 cm (11.5 cm in the adult) at term birth. The surface of the kidney is lobulated and remains so for months after birth. Fetal bladder volume can also be assessed by ultrasonography. With a maximal capacity of 10 mL at 32 weeks, the bladder can contain up to 40 mL near term.

RENAL FUNCTION IN UTERO

The placenta is the major regulatory organ of the fetus, so that renal growth does not appear to be governed by functional requirements. Urine formation starts around 10 to 12 weeks' gestation. Fetal urine is a major constituent of amniotic fluid, and its production increases with age. Mean hourly urine flow rate is high and approximates 5 mL at 20 weeks, 10 mL at 30 weeks, and 30 mL at 40 weeks of postconceptional age (Chevalier, 2008). Fetal oliguria with a consequent decrease in amniotic fluid results in the oligohydramnios sequence, which includes facial compression (loose skin folds, flattened or beaked nose, large flat ears), positional deformities (asymmetric club feet, major contractures, broad flat hands), and pulmonary hypoplasia.

The fetal urine is hypotonic throughout gestation, with sodium as the major osmotic component. The kidney actively reabsorbs electrolytes and solutes from the glomerular ultrafiltrate. Elevated concentrations of sodium (>100 mmol/L), chloride (>90 mmol/L), and osmolality (>210 mOsm/L) in the urine of a dilated kidney have been considered to be indicators of poor renal prognosis during the postnatal period. However, the sensitivity (40% to 80%) and the specificity (<80%) of these parameters are not ideal.

Fetal renal blood flow (RBF), as measured by Doppler ultrasonography, reaches 20 mL/min at 25 weeks' gestation and 60 mL/min near term (Veille et al, 1993). The low rate of RBF in the fetus is associated with an elevated renal vascular resistance (RVR). Of interest, the fetus appears able to autoregulate RBF within modest limits.

Fetal glomerular filtration rate (GFR) increases rapidly as the number and size of nephrons increase. When the full complement of nephrons is attained, GFR increases in parallel with renal mass, and hence with body weight and body surface area. From 28 to 35 weeks' gestation, GFR (measured by inulin clearance in 1- to 2-day-old neonates) increases proportionally to gestational age and then levels off up to the time of birth (Figure 81-1).

Several vasoactive agents and hormones play a major role in modulating the fetal RBF and GFR, including the renin-angiotensin system, the catecholamines, the prostaglandins, the kallikrein-kinin system, endothelin, nitric oxide, and atrial natriuretic peptide (Table 81-1). Interference with these systems can lead to severe renal dysfunction in the fetus. A clinical example is fetal renal failure after maternal administration of inhibitors of angiotensin-converting enzyme (ACE) or prostaglandin synthesis. In response to ACE inhibition, the decrease in GFR probably results from the attenuated vasoconstriction of the efferent artery by angiotensin II inhibition. Reduced prostaglandin-dependent afferent vasodilation

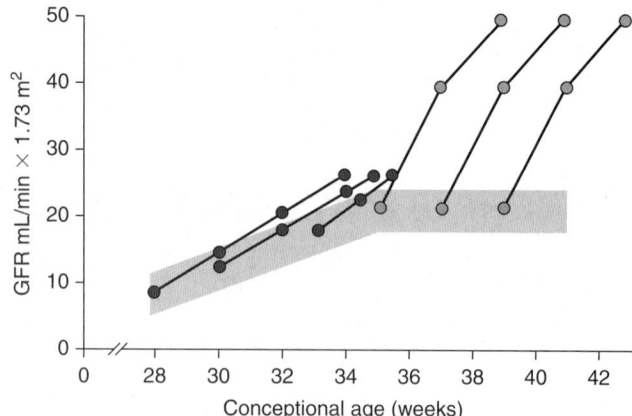

FIGURE 81-1 Maturation of GFR (C_{inulin}) in relation to conceptional age during the last 3 months of gestation and during the 1st month of postnatal life. The *shaded area* represents the range of normal values. The postnatal increase in GFR observed in preterm (•–•) and term neonates (•–•) is schematically represented. *(Adapted from Guignard JP, John EG: Renal function in the tiny, premature infant, Clin Perinatol 13:377-401, 1986.)*

TABLE 81-1   Vasoactive Factors Regulating the Glomerular Microcirculation

Constrictors	Vasodilators
Circulating hormones	Circulating hormones
• Catecholamines	• Dopamine
• Angiotensin II	
• Vasopressin	
• Glucocorticoids	
Paracrine + autacoids	Paracrine + autacoids
• Endothelin	• Nitric oxide
• Thromboxane A$_2$	• Acetylcholine
• Leukotrienes	• Prostaglandins PGI$_2$ + PGE$_2$
• Adenosine	• Bradykinin
	• Adenosine

and the unopposed vasoconstrictive effects of angiotensin II and catecholamines may explain the drop in GFR observed in fetuses of mothers given nonselective or cyclooxygenase type 2 (COX-2)-selective nonsteroidal antiinflammatory drugs (NSAIDs) (Guignard, 2002).

POSTNATAL MATURATION OF RENAL BLOOD FLOW

RBF is determined primarily by the mean arterial pressure and the resistance at the level of the renal arterioles. In the adult, physiologic intrinsic autoregulation maintains a constant RBF at varying perfusion pressures ranging from 80 to 200 mm Hg. This means that as perfusion pressure increases, the resistance to flow also increases. Both afferent and efferent arterioles participate in the vasoconstriction. In children and adults, RBF approximates 20% to 25% of cardiac output, and it is around 1200 mL/min × 1.73 m^2 of body surface area. A major part of the blood flow supplies the cortex, with medullary blood flow representing only 10% of the total RBF.

During fetal life, RBF is low, representing only 2% to 4% of the total cardiac output. This proportion increases after birth, from a value of 5% in the first 12 hours of life to 10%

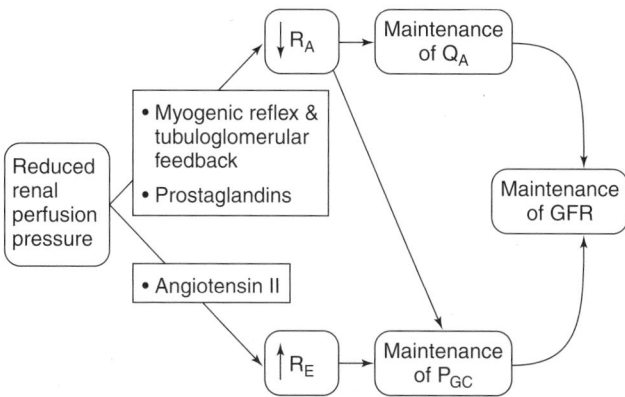

FIGURE 81-2 Mechanisms contributing to the autoregulation of renal blood flow and glomerular filtration rate (GFR). P_{GC}, Glomerular capillary hydraulic pressure; Q_A, glomerular plasma flow rate; R_A, afferent arteriolar resistance; R_E, efferent arteriolar resistance.

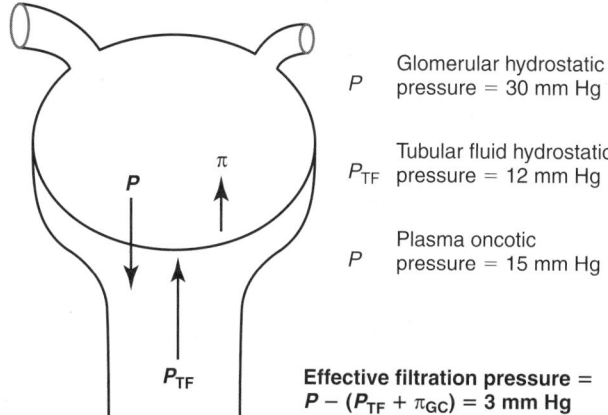

FIGURE 81-3 Starling forces modulating effective filtration pressure in the neonate. The given values of hydrostatic and oncotic pressures are estimates from experimental animal data. P, Glomerular hydrostatic pressure; P_{TF}, tubular fluid hydrostatic pressure; π_{GC}, plasma oncotic pressure.

at the end of the first week. During the first 5 months, RBF increases rapidly from a value of 250 mL/min × 1.73 m² at 8 days of age to approximately 770 mL/min × 1.73 m² by 5 months of age. The postnatal maturation of RBF is associated with a striking decrease in RVR and a marked increase in systemic blood pressure. The decrease in RVR occurs along with a decrease in the resistance of both the afferent and the efferent arterioles. Animal studies suggest that autoregulation of RBF is present in the immature kidney but is set at a lower range of blood pressure (Chevalier et al, 1987).

Several autocrine, paracrine, and endocrine factors regulate RBF, intrarenal hemodynamics, and GFR (Seri, 1995) (Figure 81-2; see also Table 81-1). Overactivation of the vasoconstrictive forces that regulate renal hemodynamics in the neonatal period may impair the maturation of RBF and induce renal hypoperfusion. Such activation is seen during respiratory distress, hypoxemia, asphyxia, metabolic acidosis, hypercapnia, hyper- and hypothermia, and positive-pressure ventilation as well as in response to the administration of various medications (Guignard and John, 1986; Tøth-Heyn et al, 2000).

POSTNATAL MATURATION OF GLOMERULAR FILTRATION RATE

DETERMINANTS OF GLOMERULAR FILTRATION RATE

The rate of filtration is governed by the rate at which plasma flows through the glomerular capillaries, the balance of Starling forces across the glomerular capillary walls, the permeability of the basement membrane of the glomerular capillary wall to water and small solutes, and the total surface area of the capillaries. The ultrafiltration coefficient (K_f) represents the product of the permeability of the glomerular membrane and the glomerular filtering area. GFR is proportional to the Starling forces across the glomerular capillaries times the K_f:

$$GFR = K_f \times [P_{GC} - (P_{IT} + \pi_{GC})]$$

where P_{GC} is the hydrostatic pressure in the glomerular capillary, P_{IT} is the proximal intratubular hydrostatic pressure, and π_{GC} is the oncotic pressure in the glomerular

capillary. In adults, the average value of P_{GC} probably approximates 60 mm Hg, the pressure in Bowman's capsule 15 mm Hg, and the oncotic glomerular capillary pressure 25 mm Hg. Thus, the average net filtration pressure is probably close to 20 mm Hg at the afferent end of the glomerular capillaries. It decreases to 10 mm Hg at the end of the efferent glomerular capillaries. Because of the very low mean arterial pressure present in neonates, the net transglomerular filtration pressure is probably not greater than 3 to 5 mm Hg (Figure 81-3). The relative state of vasoconstriction of the afferent and efferent arterioles plays a major role in regulating the intracapillary hydrostatic pressure. The factors modulating the state of vascular contraction are listed in Table 81-1.

During the early neonatal period, the factors regulating GFR mature rapidly. Systemic blood pressure and mean transcapillary hydraulic pressure increase, followed by a parallel increase in GFR (Guignard and Gouyon, 2008; Guignard and John, 1986). The plasma oncotic pressure also increases, but at a lower rate than for the transcapillary hydraulic pressure, so that the net ultrafiltration pressure increases. The low glomerular plasma flow rate present at birth is due to elevated afferent and efferent arteriolar resistances. A systemic increase in the ultrafiltration coefficient also occurs during maturation and may be attributed to an increase in both the hydraulic permeability and the glomerular capillary area.

In the fetus and neonate, the low systemic blood pressure and hence the low glomerular capillary hydrostatic pressure are the main factors limiting the rate of filtration. Vasoactive factors modulating the intraglomerular filtration pressure thus play a key role in maintaining filtration (Guignard and Gouyon, 2008). Vasodilatory prostaglandins, the concentration of which is elevated during fetal and early postnatal life, improve filtration by dilating the afferent arteriole. Angiotensin II also increases filtration by preferentially constricting the efferent arteriole (Figure 81-4). Minute-to-minute regulation of the contractile tone also depends on endothelium-released vasoactive factors such as nitric oxide and endothelin. Although endogenous endothelin behaves as a potent constrictor in the adult, it may actually vasodilate the afferent artery in the immature

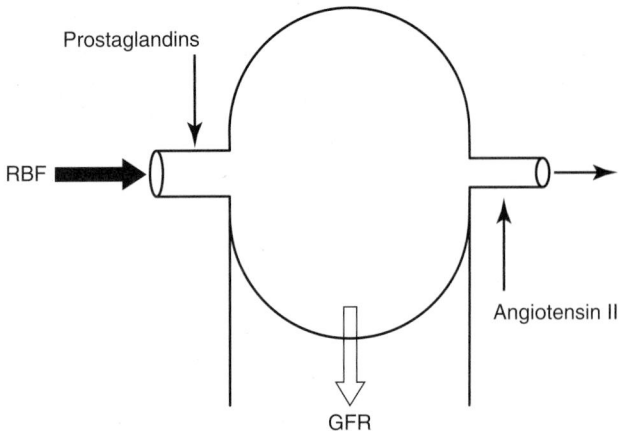

FIGURE 81-4 The physiologic regulation of GFR depends on two main factors: the afferent vasodilator prostaglandins and the efferent vasoconstrictor angiotensin II. *GFR*, Glomerular filtration rate; *RBF*, renal blood flow.

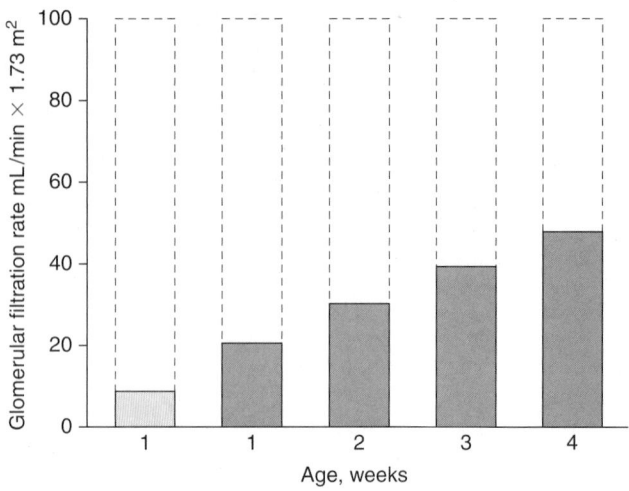

FIGURE 81-5 Glomerular filtration rate during the 1st month of life of preterm and term neonates, compared with adult values (*open columns*). Note that at the end of the 1st month of life, the human neonate is in a state of relative renal insufficiency. (*Adapted from Guignard JP, Torrado A, Da Cunha O, et al: Glomerular filtration rate in the first three weeks of life, J Pediatr 87:268-272, 1975.*)

kidney (Semama et al, 1993). Atrial natriuretic peptide, the concentration of which also is elevated in the fetus, vasodilates the afferent arteriole (Robillard et al, 1992). Adenosine, a regulator of the tubuloglomerular feedback mechanism, is an efferent vasodilator. When acting in conjunction with elevated levels of angiotensin II, adenosine also vasoconstricts the afferent arteriole (Vallon and Osswald, 2009). Although the overactivation of adenosine plays a critical role in the pathogenesis of the hypoxemia-induced vasomotor insufficiency (Gouyon and Guignard, 1988), the exact physiologic role of intrarenal adenosine in the fetus and neonate is still ill defined.

ASSESSMENT OF GLOMERULAR FILTRATION RATE

Measurement of inulin clearance is the gold standard for assessing GFR in both the immature and the mature kidney. Inulin is freely filtered even in the preterm neonate with a very low gestational age. The postnatal development of GFR has been assessed in premature neonates at different gestational ages and in term neonates. From a value of 20 mL/minute × 1.73 m² at birth, GFR doubles in the first 2 weeks of life in term neonates (Guignard et al, 1975; Guignard, 2008) (Figure 81-5). GFR is lower in premature infants and, because of incomplete nephrogenesis, also develops at a lower velocity. GFR reaches mature levels by the first year of life (Figure 81-6).

Creatinine, the most commonly used glomerular marker in mature persons, also is frequently used to assess GFR in neonates. However, the use of creatinine presents several drawbacks. The concentration of creatinine is elevated at birth, reflecting maternal levels. A complete equilibration between the maternal and fetal plasma creatinine levels is achieved throughout pregnancy (Guignard and Drukker, 1999). During the first postnatal week, the highest levels are observed in the most premature neonates (Bueva and Guignard, 1994). In term neonates, serum creatinine decreases rapidly to reach stable neonatal levels close to 0.40 mg/dL (35 μmol/L) by 1 to 2 weeks postnatally. In very premature infants, there is a transient increase in serum creatinine, peaking on postnatal day 4 (Gallini et al,

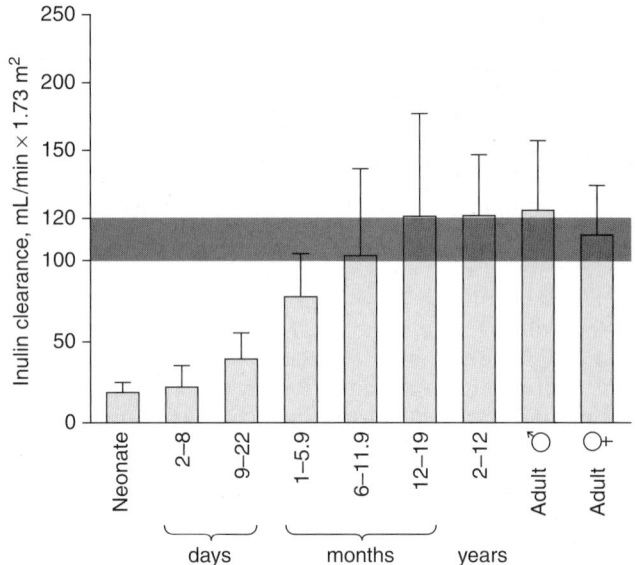

FIGURE 81-6 Maturation of GFR (C_{inulin}) throughout the first year of life.

2000; Miall et al, 1999) (Table 81-2; see also Figure 81-6), followed by a progressive decline toward normal neonatal levels by 3 to 4 weeks of life. The transient increase in plasma creatinine is caused in part by passive reabsorption (back-diffusion) of creatinine across leaky tubules (Matos et al, 1998). The reabsorption of creatinine by the premature infant accounts for the negative correlation between gestational age and the plasma creatinine during the first postnatal week (Bueva and Guignard, 1994), and in very premature neonates, creatinine clearance frequently underestimates inulin clearance. In spite of these drawbacks, creatinine clearance correlates with inulin clearance (Van den Anker et al, 1995), and creatinine clearance studies in neonates have confirmed the rapid development of GFR during the first postnatal week and that GFR develops

TABLE 81-2   Changes in Plasma Creatinine Over Time for Different Gestational Ages.

Gestational Age (weeks)	Birth Creatinine (µmol/L)	Peak Plasma Creatinine (µmol/L)	Time to Peak Plasma Creatinine (hours)*
23–26	67–92	195–247	40–78
27–29	65–89	158–200	28–51
30–32	60–69	120–158	25–40
33–45	67–79	99–140	8–23

Range intervals.
After Miall LS, Henderson MJ, Turner AJ, et al: Plasma creatinine rises dramatically in the first 48 hours of life in preterm infants, *Pediatrics* 104:e76, 1999.

at a lower velocity in premature infants (Bueva and Guignard, 1994). The differences in GFR among infants with different gestational and postnatal ages explain why the specific dosage recommendations are tailored to the given gestational and postnatal ages for medications eliminated primarily via glomerular filtration (e.g., aminoglycosides, vancomycin, digoxin).

REGULATION OF BODY FLUID TONICITY AND VOLUME

The kidney is responsible for maintaining the extracellular fluid (ECF) volume and osmolality despite large variations in salt and water intake (Ranadive and Rosenthal, 2009). By modulating the renal conservation of water, the antidiuretic hormone (ADH) system plays a central role in the regulation of body fluid tonicity. Sodium chloride, the major osmotically active solute in ECF, determines its volume. The balance between the intake and the renal excretion of sodium thus regulates ECF volume.

SODIUM, CHLORIDE, AND WATER REABSORPTION

Active sodium reabsorption occurs throughout the nephron, driven by the Na^+,K^+-ATPase localized at the basolateral membrane. Two thirds of the filtered Na^+ load is reabsorbed in the proximal tubule via the Na^+-glucose, Na^+-amino acid, Na^+-P_i, and Na^+-lactate cotransporters, and by the Na^+-H^+ antiporter. Because water passively follows Na^+ across the highly water-permeable proximal tubule, the osmolality of the proximal tubule fluid remains isotonic. Twenty percent of the filtered sodium load is reabsorbed in the ascending limb of the loop of Henle, which is relatively impermeable to water. Accumulation of NaCl and recycling of urea into the medullary interstitium lead to the formation of a hyperosmotic medulla. The thick ascending limb also reabsorbs calcium, magnesium, and potassium. The distal tubule and collecting duct reabsorb 10% of the filtered Na^+ and Cl^- load. In the distal tubule, the continuing NaCl reabsorption in the absence of water reabsorption further decreases the osmolality of the tubular fluid, allowing the formation of hypotonic urine. Excretion of solute-free water thus is dependent on Na^+ delivery to and reabsorption at the distal diluting site. The permeability of the collecting duct to water depends on the presence of ADH or arginine vasopressin (AVP).

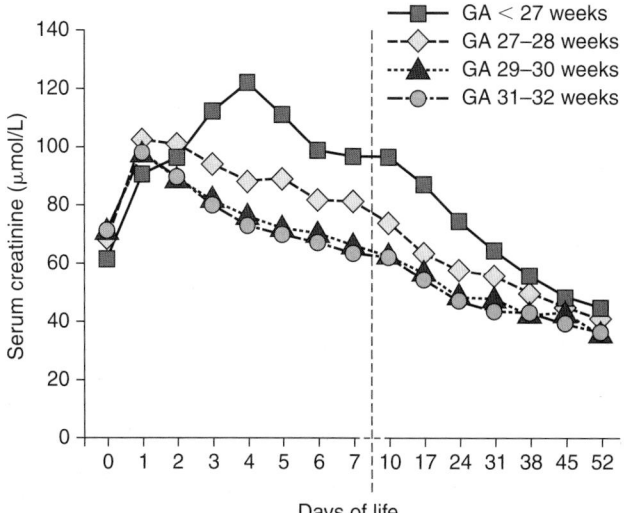

FIGURE 81-7   Changes in serum creatinine concentration (µmol/L) in the first 52 hours of life in premature infants. *GA,* Gestational age. *(Adapted from Gallini F, Maggio L, Romagnoli C, et al: Progression of renal function in premature neonates with gestational age ≤32 weeks, Pediatr Nephrol 15:119-124, 2000.)*

The release of AVP by the posterior pituitary gland is regulated by osmoreceptors located in the supraoptic nucleus of the hypothalamus. By binding to its cell membrane receptors and activating adenylate cyclase, AVP increases the intracellular levels of cyclic adenosine monophosphate (cAMP). This increase ultimately leads to phosphorylation of the aquaporin water channels, which in turn results in insertion of these channels into the luminal membrane of the collecting duct cells, rendering the collecting duct permeable to water. In the absence of AVP, a large volume of hypotonic urine is excreted. In contrast, when elevated levels of AVP are present, water passively diffuses out of the collecting duct into the hyperosmotic interstitium, and a small volume of concentrated urine is excreted.

Water transport depends on the intact function of the aquaporin water channels (AQPs). AQPs, a family of integral plasma membrane proteins, facilitate water permeation across biologic membranes (Nielsen et al, 2000). To date 13 members of the AQP family (AQP0–AQP12) have been identified in mammals with specific expression patterns and distinct roles in given cells and tissues. At least seven AQP isoforms are expressed in different nephron segments (AQP1, 2, 3, 4, 6, 7, 11), where they provide pathways for constitutive- or vasopressin-stimulated water flow (King et al, 2004). AQP2 is the vasopressin-responsive AQP in collecting principal duct cells. Mutations in the AVP V2 receptor gene located at Xq28 are responsible for *X-linked recessive diabetes insipidus.* When inherited as an autosomal recessive or dominant trait, diabetes insipidus usually is caused by various mutations in the *AQP2* gene, located at 12q13.

Sodium

During development, proximal active Na^+ reabsorption increases three- to fourfold, this increase being associated with a threefold increase in Na^+,K^+-ATPase activity in the corresponding segment (Celsi et al, 1986), and with an increase in the number of cotransporters for glucose and bicarbonate reabsorption (Schwartz and Evan, 1983). The immature proximal tubule has a lower reflection coefficient for mannitol, indicating increased permeability of the proximal tubule to various solutes. The low capacity of the immature thick ascending limb of the loop of Henle to reabsorb Na^+ is associated with a low activity of the tubular Na^+,K^+-ATPase. As a consequence of the reduced Na^+ reabsorption in the loop of Henle, immature nephrons deliver a greater fraction of filtered Na^+ to the distal nephrons. The activity of the Na^+,K^+-ATPase also increases in this segment during development. As a result of the maturational process, the fractional excretion of Na^+ decreases during development, from a value of 13% in the fetus to 3% in premature neonates less than 30 weeks' gestation, and to 1% in term neonates (Bueva and Guignard, 1994). Very low-birthweight (VLBW) infants may be at risk for negative sodium balance around postnatal weeks 2 to 3, when Na^+ retention is required for growth. Partial resistance to aldosterone has been described and ascribed to the low renal mineralocorticoid receptor expression at birth (Martinerie, et al 2009).

The study of the developmental changes in the various tubular epithelial transport mechanisms, the delineation of the molecular basis of such mechanisms, and associated genetic defects have shed new light on a number of rare pediatric renal tubular disorders (Zelikovic, 2001) related to abnormal sodium and water homeostasis. Constitutive activation of the amiloride-sensitive epithelial Na^+ channel (ENaC) is seen in Liddle's syndrome, characterized by salt retention, early-onset hypertension, metabolic alkalosis, and hypokalemia. Autosomal recessive pseudohypoaldosteronism, characterized by renal salt wasting and end-organ unresponsiveness to mineralocorticoids, is due to decreased activity of ENaC. The activity of ENaC is under the tight control of aldosterone and vasopressin (Rossier et al, 2002). ENaC is composed of three subunits: α, β, and γ. The α subunit of ENaC is the most important and is also expressed in other organs such as the lungs. Thus, the α subunit of ENaC is required not only for channel function in the collecting duct of the kidney but also for active lung fluid clearance. Developmental studies on α-ENaC expression in human kidney homogenates from fetuses of 20–36 weeks' gestation have revealed a progressive increase of about 25% in this channel protein abundance during the observational period that corresponds to the improvement in sodium renal conservation (Delgado, et al. 2003).

Experimental evidence suggests that intrauterine growth retardation is associated with upregulation of renal sodium transporters with subsequent sodium retention, suppression of the renin-angiotensin system, and reduction in the number of nephrons. All these changes may contribute to the prenatally programmed hypertension observed later in life. Furthermore, a maternal diet high in sodium is also implicated in fetal programming by inducing oxidative stress, endothelial dysfunction, and restricted nephron number in the offspring (Koleganova et al, 2009).

Chloride

A major fraction of chloride reabsorption in the proximal tubule occurs by paracellular diffusion. Active chloride countertransport with organic anions (formate, oxalate) also takes place in the proximal tubule. In the ascending limb of Henle, the Na^+,K^+-ATPase is the driving force for active NaCl reabsorption and accumulation in the medullary interstitium. Here, Na^+-K^+-$2Cl^-$ cotransporters and Cl^- channels are involved in the transport of chloride. Renal salt wasting with hypokalemic metabolic alkalosis, hyperreninemic hyperaldesteronism, and normal blood pressure are the features of *Bartter's syndrome*. Antenatal Bartter's syndrome, sometimes called hyperprostaglandin E syndrome, is the most severe form of the disease. Congenital defects in genes encoding various chloride transporters, cotransporters, and channels in the thick ascending limb and distal tubule are responsible for the various forms of Bartter's syndrome and Gitelman's syndrome (Rodriguez-Soriano, 1998; Zekikovic, 2001).

Mutations of the chloride channel with gain in function are also associated with Dent's disease, an X-linked renal tubular disorder characterized by low-molecular-weight proteinuria, renal Fanconi syndrome, hypercalciuria, nephrocalcinosis, and nephrolithiasis. Neonatal variants of the disease suggest that the expression and segmental distribution of Cl^- channel proteins is achieved before birth (Ludwig et al, 2006). In fact, during human nephrogenesis, Cl^- channel proteins are identified early in the second trimester, followed by subsequent progressive maturation. It is first distributed in the proximal tubule and appears some weeks later in the principal cells of the collecting duct (Jouret et al, 2004).

BODY FLUID TONICITY

Although the volume of body fluids varies during growth, the tonicity of ECF is maintained constant by the kidneys, which excrete or retain appropriate amounts of water.

Excretion of Free Water

When plasma osmolality decreases, the release of ADH also diminishes, leading to the excretion of dilute urine. The newborn infant, preterm or term, is able to decrease urine osmolality to values as low as 40 mOsm/kg H_2O (Guignard and John, 1986). Because GFR is low in the newborn infant, ability to excrete large amounts of free water and consequently to cope with a hypotonic fluid load is limited. Excessive hypotonic fluid loading leads to hyponatremia.

Hyponatremia also may occur in the syndrome of inappropriate secretion of antidiuretic hormone (SIADH), when the excretion of free water is impaired. This syndrome can occur in term as well as in preterm infants presenting with various cerebral injuries or pulmonary disorders, in infants undergoing mechanical ventilation, and in response to some drugs. Because the renal response to AVP is maturation dependent, the more immature the neonate, the less severe the clinical presentation of the SIADH. Gain-of-function mutation of the AVP V2 receptor gene results in symptoms mimicking SIADH, but with a marked reduction in AVP secretion (Gitelman and Feldman, 2006).

Concentration of Urine

By comparison with adults, who can concentrate urine up to 1400 mOsm/kg H_2O, the concentrating ability is limited in the neonate and matures during the 1st

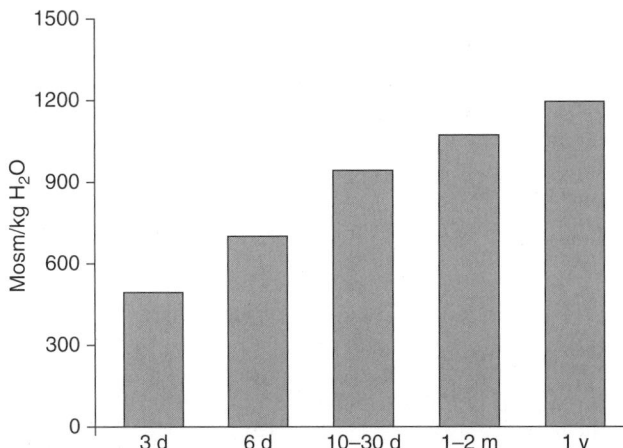

FIGURE 81-8 Maturation of the concentrating ability during the first year of life in term infants. (*Adapted from Polácek E, Vocel J, Neugebauerová L, et al: The osmotic concentrating ability in healthy infants and children,* Arch Dis Child *40:291-295, 1965.*)

year of life (Figure 81-8). The maximal urine osmolality achieved with dehydration or after exogenous vasopressin (DDAVP) administration (10 μg) remains below 430 mOsm/kg H_2O and 630 mOsm/kg H_2O in 1- to 3-week-old and 4- to 6-week-old term infants, respectively. Osmolalities achieved by preterm neonates are slightly lower (Svenningssen and Aronson, 1974). The relative ineffectiveness of the concentrating ability of the neonate is related to several factors including the low corticomedullary solute gradient associated with a limited accumulation of sodium chloride and urea in the medullary interstitium, the decreased formation of cAMP in response to ADH, the shortness of the loops of Henle, and the interference of prostaglandins with the vasopressin-stimulated cAMP synthesis. Low expression of AQP2 mRNA and protein is an additional limiting factor that impairs concentrating ability. The postnatal increase in AQP2 expression parallels that of AVPR2 along with improving concentrating capacity. Of interest, the developmental expression pattern of proximal (AQP1-7-11) and distal (AQP2-3-4) renal AQPs is different. AQP1, AQP3, and AQP4 exhibit a later and more abrupt increase with transient postnatal overexpression. These distinct expression patterns of renal AQPs can be ascribed to structural kidney maturation and vasopressin regulation (Parreira et al, 2009). An additional mechanism for impaired concentrating ability of the immature kidney is the markedly elevated interstitial hyaluronan in the inner medulla/papilla that can antagonize renal tubular water reabsorption (Sulyok, 2008).

NEONATAL REDISTRIBUTION OF BODY WATER COMPARTMENTS

Redistribution of body fluid compartments occurs soon after birth. The early postnatal weight loss observed in the first days of life is usually ascribed to the isotonic contraction of ECW volume and the elimination of excess sodium and water by the kidney. According to a recent hypothesis, cell water rather than extracellular water may be the source of significant neonatal water losses (Sulyok, 2008).

The physical compartmentalization and mobility of tissue water could play a significant role in neonatal body fluid redistribution. The term *physical water compartments* designates the physical states of tissue water and assumes interactions between dipole water molecules and tissue biopolymers, including proteins and glycosaminoglycans. Two distinct water fractions should be considered: the free "bulky" water and the relatively slow-motion bound water. Water can be liberated from this latter bound fraction in a regulated manner irrespective of its location in the cellular or extracellular space. The bound water fraction appears to be related to the osmotically inactive body sodium mainly stored in glycosaminoglycan-rich tissues (Titze et al, 2003), which provides a buffer system in the control of physiologic dehydration.

EXTRACELLULAR FLUID VOLUME

The ECF volume is a function of the ECF sodium content. Under normal conditions, plasma volume is closely related to ECF volume. Volume receptors distributed both on the venous (low-pressure receptors) and the arterial (high-pressure receptors) sides of the circulation sense the changes in plasma volume. Arterial sensors perceive the "effective arterial volume." Atrial filling volume is monitored by stretch receptors, which mediate the release of natriuretic peptide (Semmekrot and Guignard, 1991) that promotes diuresis and natriuresis. Effective renal arterial volume also is sensed by baroreceptors located in the juxtamedullary apparatus of the kidney. A decrease in renal perfusion pressure activates the renin-angiotensin-aldosterone system (see Figure 81-2). Angiotensin II, a potent renal and peripheral vasoconstrictor, promotes sodium reabsorption, stimulates thirst, and favors the renal production of prostaglandins and bradykinin, hormones that play a role in sodium homeostasis. Aldosterone increases sodium reabsorption in the distal tubule, leading to further conservation of ECF volume.

The neonatal period is characterized by the rapid physiologic constriction of the expanded ECF volume, as well as by elevated levels of several hormonal systems participating in the regulation of sodium balance. Although angiotensin II induces sodium retention by direct action on the proximal tubule and stimulation of aldosterone secretion, the role of atrial natriuretic peptide in defending the plasma volume is still unclear. The elevated levels of plasma renin activity, which are inversely correlated with gestational age, may be important in maintaining and distributing blood flow to various organs. The integrity of the renin-angiotensin system also appears to be crucial for maintaining renal blood flow and GFR at low perfusion pressure in the neonate (Guignard and Gouyon, 2008). Other factors that may be involved in regulating sodium excretion include atrial natriuretic peptide, bradykinin, dopamine, nitric oxide, endothelin, and adrenomedullin. Dopamine, synthesized by the renal proximal tubule cells, reduces sodium reabsorption by inhibiting the Na^+,K^+-ATPase and decreasing Na^+-H^+ antiporter and sodium-inorganic phosphate (Na^+-P_i) cotransporter activity (Seri, 1995). Agents such as nitric oxide, endothelin, and adrenomedullin can all increase sodium excretion and may participate in sodium homeostasis.

REGULATION OF ACID-BASE BALANCE

The kidneys maintain the acid-base balance by preventing loss of bicarbonate in urine and excreting the daily production of fixed acids. Bicarbonate reabsorption occurs mainly in the proximal tubule (80%) and to a lesser extent in the thick ascending limb of Henle (10%) and the distal nephron (9%). It is mediated by active secretion of hydrogen ions and is closely linked to the tubular reabsorption of sodium. Hydrogen ion secretion occurs through the Na^+-H^+ antiporter (NHE-3) but is also mediated in part by H^+-ATPase. In the tubular lumen, secreted H^+ reacts with filtered HCO_3^- to form H_2CO_3, which quickly dissociates under the influence of the brush border carbonic anhydrase enzyme (CAIV). Luminal CO_2 freely diffuses back into the tubular cells. H_2CO_3 is then formed within the cell by hydration of CO_2, a reaction catalyzed by carbonic anhydrase type 2 (CAII). After crossing the luminal membrane as CO_2, most HCO_3^- exits the tubular cells via a Na^+-HCO_3^- cotransporter (NBC I, II, and III), which couples the transport of 1 Na^+ with 3 HCO_3^-, or in exchange for Cl^- via a Cl^--HCO_3^- antiporter.

The excretion of fixed acids occurs mainly in the distal tubule, where secreted H^+ is buffered by NH_3 and HPO_4^{2-} and excreted as NH_4^+ and $H_2PO_4^-$ (titratable acid). Free H^+ concentration determines the urine pH. The ability of the collecting duct to lower the urine pH is critically important for the excretion of urinary buffers and ammonium. NH_3 is produced by the kidneys; its synthesis and subsequent excretion can be regulated in response to acid-base requirements of the body. To produce NH_3, the kidneys metabolize glutamine, excrete NH_4^+ with the acid salts, and return the generated HCO_3^- to the blood. NH_3 synthesis is upregulated by metabolic acidosis and hypokalemia.

During fetal life, the placenta is responsible for the excretion of H^+. In experimental studies, the fetus responds to an acid load by increasing the excretion of NH_4^+ and titratable acid, and decreasing the urine pH. In early postnatal life, several transporters and enzymes involved in bicarbonate reabsorption are weakly expressed, so that the functioning of the Na^+-H^+ antiporter is clearly impaired (Rodriguez-Soriano, 2000). Consequently, the limited capacity of the immature kidney to excrete H^+ is associated with an obligatory loss of sodium. The maturation of renal acidifying processes with increasing gestational and postnatal ages results in a progressive increase in renal Na^+-H^+ exchange and in a steady decline in urinary sodium excretion (Kerpel-Fronius et al, 1970). The proximal reabsorption of bicarbonate is reduced, resulting in low bicarbonate threshold. This low threshold accounts for the low "physiologic" plasma bicarbonate concentration in neonates: 16 to 20 mmol/L in extremely immature infants and 19 to 21 mmol/L in term infants. In addition to immature carbonic anhydrase activity, the relative expansion of ECF volume at birth may account for the reduced bicarbonate threshold. Immature carbonic anhydrase (CAII and CAIV) enzyme activities may also play an important role in the low bicarbonate proximal reabsorption rate. Maturation of HCO_3^- reabsorption increases proportionally to the increase in proximal tubular basolateral area and Na^+,K^+-ATPase

activity (Rodriguez-Soriano, 2000). However, the age-dependent renal expression and segmental distribution of some individual acid-base transporters may be markedly different—for example, the progressive increase of H^+-ATPase expression during fetal development contrasts with the postnatal upregulation of CAII (Jouret et al, 2004; Wang et al, 2009). The functional maturation of renal acidification can be accelerated by glucocorticoids, angiotensin II, catecholamines, thyroid hormones, and metabolic acidosis. The administration of glucocorticoids stimulates the maturation of both the Na^+-H^+ antiporter messenger RNA (mRNA) and activity (Shah et al, 1999). On the other hand, dopamine inhibits NHE-mediated sodium uptake, leading to urinary sodium loss and H^+ accumulation (Gesek and Schoolwerth, 1990).

Distal tubular acidification is more mature than proximal tubular bicarbonate reabsorption. The ability of the neonate to excrete an acid load is fairly well developed. Deficient ammoniagenesis results, however, in low glutamine uptake, decreased NH_3 production and excretion, and, ultimately, impaired ability to excrete an acid load.

Mutations in the various genes encoding the Na^+-HCO_3^- cotransporter (NBC-I), the Cl^--HCO_3^- exchanger (AE1), the H^+-ATPase, and CAII are responsible for the various forms of renal tubular acidosis (Rodriguez-Soriano, 2000, 2002).

Under normal conditions, very little bicarbonate is lost in the urine. The reabsorption of bicarbonate is increased by extracellular volume contraction, hypercapnia, hypokalemia, chloride deficiency, glucocorticoids, angiotensin, aldosterone and alpha-adrenergic stimulation; it is depressed by volume expansion and parathyroid hormone (PTH) (Rodriguez-Soriano, 2000, 2002). The postnatal renal compensation for hypercapnia involves increased bicarbonate reabsorption and excretion of fixed acids, to reduce the decrease in plasma pH. Animal studies and clinical observations indicate that this compensating mechanism is functional in the neonate (van der Heijden and Guignard, 1989).

REGULATION OF POTASSIUM HOMEOSTASIS

Ninety-eight percent of potassium in the body is intracellular, resulting in a high intracellular concentration of potassium. High intracellular concentration of potassium also is required for cell growth and division. Potassium homeostasis depends on an internal balance that maintains a constant potassium concentration in the intracellular and extracellular fluid space. An external balance requires that potassium be absorbed by the gastrointestinal tract in excess of the amount needed for growth that is eventually excreted by the kidneys.

In the proximal tubule, some 70% of filtered potassium is predominantly reabsorbed passively, although active reabsorption against a concentration gradient also occurs. About 20% of filtered potassium is reabsorbed in the ascending limb of the loop of Henle, where reabsorption occurs via both a passive paracellular route and a transcellular route that exploits secondary active Na^+-K^+-Cl^- cotransport. In the cortical collecting duct, K^+ is both reabsorbed by the intercalated cells and secreted by the principal cells. The overall rate of potassium excretion is determined by the function of the distal tubule and collecting duct (Lorenz, 2008). Plasma potassium concentration and aldosterone are the major physiologic regulators of potassium secretion. Hyperkalemia stimulates the Na^+,K^+-ATPase activity, increases the permeability of the luminal membrane to potassium, and stimulates the secretion of aldosterone by the adrenal cortex. Aldosterone in turn stimulates sodium reabsorption and enhances potassium secretion by stimulating the basolateral Na^+,K^+-ATPase. Elevation of intracellular potassium occurs by increasing the permeability of the luminal membrane to potassium. Aldosterone probably plays a more important role in determining potassium balance than in regulating sodium excretion. The aldosterone-sensitive transport mechanisms for sodium and potassium are largely independent of each other. Other factors favoring potassium secretion by the distal tubule and collecting duct include a rise in tubular flow rate, alkalosis, and an increase in the tubular fluid sodium concentration.

Potassium excretion remains low throughout gestation, and the fetal potassium concentration is maintained at levels exceeding 5 mmol/L. Postnatal growth is associated with an increase in total body potassium from approximately 8 mmol/cm body height at birth to more than 14 mmol/cm body height by 18 years of age (Butte et al, 2000).

In neonatal tissues, K^+ content is significantly higher than in adult tissues. The plasma K^+ concentration is also elevated during the first 3 to 4 postnatal months. The intracellular versus extracellular potassium distribution in infancy may be influenced not only by the expression of the Na^+,K^+-ATPase, potassium transporters, and channels but also by the expression of hormone receptors and intracellular messengers.

Clinical and experimental studies in the newborn demonstrate low rates of urinary K^+ excretion under basal conditions and an inability to efficiently excrete an exogenous potassium load. With advancing gestational and postnatal ages, there is a steady rise in the renal excretory capacity (Aizman et al, 1998). The major cause of impaired potassium excretion by the immature kidney is the low rate of potassium secretion by the principal cells in the collecting duct. It is attributed to the low Na^+,K^+-ATPase activity, low cellular K^+ concentration, and unfavorable electrochemical gradient. Potassium permeability of the apical membrane is also reduced because of low number, low open probability, and low conductivity of the K^+-channel protein. Potassium excretion is further compromised by impaired aldosterone reactivity and limited flow-mediated activation of the K^+ channel. In addition to decreased K^+ secretion, K^+ retention needed for growth can also be ascribed to enhanced apical absorption by Na^+,K^+-ATPase in the intercalated cells of the developing cortical collecting duct (Lorenz, 2008; Sulyok et al, 1979).

In clinical settings, the transtubular potassium gradient (TTKG) is a reliable estimate of distal tubular K^+ secretion, provided that the urine is at least isoosmolar to plasma and the final urine K^+ concentration is equal to or greater than the plasma K^+ concentration. The TTKG is expressed by the following ratio: TTKG = {K^+_{urine}/$(U/P)_{osm}$}/K^+_{plasma} (Kamel et al, 1994), and it has a normal value close to 10. The values observed in healthy neonates

are well below the normal range for infants and children, confirming the state of renal unresponsiveness to aldosterone in the neonate.

Transient hyperkalemia sometimes occurs in the early neonatal period in VLBW infants. A lower renal K^+ excretory capacity and a low tissue K^+ uptake due to low Na^+,K^+-ATPase activity are thought to be responsible for this nonoliguric hyperkalemia (Lorenz et al, 1997). In contrast with healthy premature infants, critically ill and stressed premature neonates may develop a negative potassium balance. In sick neonates, potassium losses can be exaggerated by the use of diuretics and volume expansion.

REGULATION OF CALCIUM, PHOSPHATE, AND MAGNESIUM HOMEOSTASIS

The kidney, in conjunction with the gastrointestinal tract and bone, plays a major role in maintaining calcium, phosphate, and magnesium homeostasis.

REGULATION OF CALCIUM HOMEOSTASIS

The blood ionic calcium concentration in plasma is maintained within narrow limits at approximately 1.10 to 1.30 mmol/L. The distribution of calcium between the intracellular (bone) and extracellular compartment is regulated mainly by PTH. The parathyroid gland has the ability to determine the level of blood-ionized calcium by a calcium sensor (CaSR) located on the extracellular site of membrane. The CaSR appears to act via a G protein–coupled signaling system, and its gene has been cloned (Brown, 1999). Loss-of-function and gain-of-function mutations in the CaSR gene are responsible for autosomal dominant familial hypercalcemia with hypocalciuria and autosomal dominant hypoparathyroidism with hypocalcemia (Langman, 2000).

PTH increases plasma calcium concentration by stimulating bone resorption, by activating the synthesis of 1,25-dihydroxyvitamin D_3 ($1,25(OH)_2D_3$ or calcitriol), and by increasing calcium reabsorption by the kidney. Normally, 99% of the filtered calcium is reabsorbed by the nephron, mainly by the proximal tubule and the loop of Henle. In the proximal tubule and the thick ascending limb, calcium reabsorption is passive and closely linked to sodium reabsorption. By contrast, in the distal tubule and collecting duct, calcium reabsorption is active and independent of sodium transport, so that net calcium and sodium excretions do not always change in parallel. PTH is the main regulator of the renal excretion of calcium, and it strongly stimulates calcium reabsorption in the distal tubule and collecting duct, resulting in reduced calcium excretion. Volume expansion depresses both sodium and passive calcium reabsorption in the proximal tubule and thus increases calcium excretion. Calcium excretion is increased by acidosis and decreased by alkalosis. Finally, $1,25(OH)_2D_3$ stimulates distal calcium reabsorption and thus decreases its excretion. Whereas the single most important action of PTH is on bone, that of vitamin D_3 is in the intestine.

During weeks 26 to 36 of gestation, the mean intrauterine accumulation of calcium is about 130 mg/kg/day (Forbes, 1976; Wharton et al, 1987). The calcium levels in fetal plasma are higher than maternal levels (Delivoria et al, 1967), averaging 1.40 to 1.60 mmol/L. Of interest, the fetal kidney also is able to effectively produce $1,25(OH)_2D_3$. The 25-hydroxyvitamin D_3-1α hydroxylase is produced by the renal proximal tubule mitochondria. The $1,25(OH)_2D_3$ binds to an intracellular receptor to stimulate intestinal calcium reabsorption. During the neonatal period, the urinary calcium-to-creatinine ratio is higher in neonates than later in infancy (2.5 vs. 0.7) (Matos et al, 1997). Loop diuretics are potent calciuric agents that may lead to neonatal nephrocalcinosis.

The relatively low efficacy of calcium reabsorption by the developing kidney may be the result of low expression and activity of the epithelial Ca^{2+} channel in the apical membrane and the Ca^{2+}-ATPase and Na^+-Ca^{2+} exchanger in the basolateral membrane of the distal nephron. Maturity-related defective function of the Cl^- channel may also contribute, because gene mutations of this membrane protein are associated with hypercalciuria (Bartter's syndrome, Dent's disease, knockout animals) (Chadha and Alon, 2009; Scheinman, 1998).

REGULATION OF PHOSPHATE HOMEOSTASIS

Plasma phosphate concentration is regulated by the kidney. In the urine, phosphate binds H^+ ions and is eliminated as acid phosphate (a component of titratable acid). Phosphate release from the intracellular stores (mainly bone) is increased by PTH and $1,25(OH)_2D_3$. The proximal tubule reabsorbs approximately 80% of the filtered phosphate load; 10% is reabsorbed by the distal tubule; and 10% is excreted in the urine. Factors that increase the excretion of phosphate include PTH, glucocorticoids, calcitonin, glucagon, volume expansion, dopamine administration, and acidosis. PTH is the main physiologic hormone regulating renal phosphate excretion, and it exerts this effect mainly by the inhibition of the Na^+-P_i cotransporter in the proximal tubule. There are three Na^+-P_i cotransporters: types I, IIa, and IIb. The type IIa cotransporter plays a key role in determining brush border Na^+-P_i cotransport, and thus the overall P_i homeostasis (Mürer et al, 2000). Several genetic defects resulting in isolated renal phosphate wasting include X-linked hypophosphatemic rickets, the autosomal dominant hypophosphatemic rickets without hypercalciuria, and the hereditary hypophosphatemic rickets with hypercalciuria. The X-linked syndrome is caused by mutations in the PHEX gene that indirectly affects the Na^+-P_i cotransporter. Phosphate renal transport is also modulated by changes in dietary intake.

During weeks 26 to 36 of gestation, the mean intrauterine accumulation of inorganic phosphate is close to 75 mg/kg/day (Wharton et al, 1987). At birth, approximately 80% of the phosphorus is in bones (Royer, 1981). During early postnatal life, because of the efficient intestinal absorption and renal retention of phosphate, the neonate is in a positive phosphate balance and presents with elevated plasma concentrations of this anion. The transport rate of Na-Pi is substantially higher in brush-border membrane vesicles obtained from neonates than in those from adults. The high transport capacity is however associated with low adaptability to changes in dietary Pi intake. Of interest, the expression of Na-Pi mRNA in the newborn is similar to or lower than that in the adult, suggesting that the increased protein levels and activity of this cotransporter early in life may be due to posttranscriptional regulation (Spitzer and Barac-Nieto, 2001).

Although fetuses and neonates appear to synthesize PTH in response to hypocalcemia, the phosphaturic response to PTH is attenuated. This phenomenon may be due to decreased sensitivity of the proximal tubule to the hormone. This may reflect homeostatic regulation at a time when phosphate retention is essential for growth. Growth hormone stimulates renal phosphate retention and increases the plasma concentration of phosphate.

REGULATION OF MAGNESIUM HOMEOSTASIS

Magnesium is the second most abundant intracellular cation. It plays a major role in the regulation of protein synthesis and bone formation and regulates potassium and calcium channels in cell membranes. The kidney maintains magnesium balance by excreting in urine the amount of magnesium that is absorbed by the gastrointestinal tract and exceeds that retained for growth. In normal conditions, approximately 3% of the filtered magnesium load is excreted in urine. Magnesium is passively reabsorbed by the proximal tubule and the thick ascending limb. Regulation of magnesium excretion takes place in the thick ascending limb, where approximately 65% of the filtered load is reabsorbed. In this segment, claudin 16, a specific tight junction protein, is necessary for paracellular Mg^{2+} reabsorption. Magnesium reabsorption along the distal convoluted tubule and collecting duct accounts for approximately 10% of the filtered load. Factors that increase magnesium excretion include ECF volume expansion, acidosis, hypercalcemia, and hypermagnesemia. PTH decreases the excretion of magnesium. Most diuretics increase magnesium excretion.

During weeks 26 to 36 of gestation, the mean intrauterine accumulation of magnesium approximates 3.5 mg/kg/day (Wharton et al, 1987). At birth, the urinary excretion of magnesium is low (Chan et al, 1984). Magnesium excretion increases 10-fold during the 1st month of life, reaching values close to 2 mg/kg/day (De Santo et al, 1988). Plasma magnesium levels follow a circadian rhythm, being higher at night (De Santo et al, 1988). Neonatal hypomagnesemia is associated with intrauterine growth restriction, whereas neonatal hypermagnesemia frequently occurs following maternal magnesium administration in the immediate prenatal period. Mutations in the gene encoding the Na^+,K^+-ATPase γ subunit, localized on the basolateral membrane of the distal convoluted tubule, result in magnesium wasting of the so-called isolated renal magnesium wasting syndrome, a rare autosomal dominant disorder.

SUMMARY

Normal renal maturation and adaptive responses at birth play an essential role in the neonate and contribute to the establishment of an intracellular and extracellular milieu necessary for survival and appropriate growth. Renal development and function are regulated by numerous hormones, paracrine factors, and signaling molecules. Recent advances in the understanding of the molecular basis of renal development and function have provided invaluable insights into the pathophysiology of inherited and acquired renal conditions during development. An understanding of basic principles in renal developmental physiology is essential for successful clinical management of sick preterm and term neonates.

SUGGESTED READINGS

Burrow CR: Regulatory molecules in kidney development, *Pediatr Nephrol* 14: 240-253, 2000.

Chadha V, Alon US: Hereditary tubular disorders, *Semin Nephrol* 29:399-411, 2009.

Chevalier RL: Obstructive uropathy: assessment of renal function in the fetus. In Oh W, Guignard J-P, Baumgart S, editors: *Nephrology and fluid/electrolyte physiology: neonatology questions and controversies*, Philadelphia, 2008, Saunders Elsevier, pp 225-250.

Guignard JP: Glomerular filtration rate in neonates. In Oh W, Guignard J-P, Baumgart S, editors: *Nephrology and fluid/electrolyte physiology: neonatology questions and controversies*, Philadelphia, 2008, Saunders Elsevier, pp 79-96.

Guignard JP, Torrado A, Mazouni SM, et al: Renal function in respiratory distress syndrome, *J Pediatr* 88:845-850, 1976.

Pohl M, Bhatnagar V, Mendoza SA, Nigam SK: Toward an etiological classification of developmental disorders of the kidney and upper urinary tract, *Kidney Int* 61:10-19, 2002.

Rodriguez-Soriano J: Renal tubular acidosis: the clinical entity, *J Am Soc Nephrol* 13:2160-2170, 2002.

Rossier B, Pradervand S, Schild L, et al: Epithelial sodium channel and the control of sodium balance: interaction between genetic and environmental factors, *Annu Rev Physiol* 64:877-897, 2002.

Sulyok E: Physical water compartments: a revised concept of perinatal body water physiology, *Physiol Res* 55:133-138, 2005.

Tøth-Heyn P, Drukker A, Guignard JP: The stressed neonatal kidney: from pathophysiology to clinical management of neonatal vasomotor nephropathy, *Pediatr Nephrol* 14:227-239, 2000.

Zelikovic I: Molecular pathophysiology of tubular transport disorders, *Pediatr Nephrol* 16:919-935, 2001.

Complete references and supplemental color images used in this text can be found online at www.expertconsult.com

CLINICAL EVALUATION OF RENAL AND URINARY TRACT DISEASE

Carlton M. Bates and Andrew L. Schwaderer

PRENATAL EVALUATION OF RENAL AND URINARY TRACT DISEASE

PRENATAL DIAGNOSIS

Renal anomalies will be frequently encountered in neonatal practice, because they are identified in 0.5% of pregnancies and account for 20% of all anomalies diagnosed with prenatal imaging (Scott, 2002; Scott and Renwick, 1988). Disorders of the renal and urinary tract include a broad spectrum of clinical entities with a wide variation of severity. This variation may result in challenging clinical diagnosis and management scenarios. Thus, an understanding of the clinical evaluation in the prenatal and neonatal periods is an essential component of neonatal clinical practice.

PRENATAL RENAL ULTRASOUND

The primary tool utilized in the diagnosis of disorders of the renal and urinary tract is the prenatal ultrasound. Although the kidneys may be visualized at 10 weeks' gestation, accurate determination of renal anatomy is usually not possible until 16 weeks (Stamilio and Morgan, 1998). Findings on a prenatal ultrasound that suggest renal or urinary tract disease include hydronephrosis, renal cysts, hyperechoic kidneys, renal mass, oligohydramnios, and polyhydramnios. Hydronephrosis (dilation of the renal pelvis) is the most common identified renal anomaly (Dicke et al, 2006). The presence of prenatal hydronephrosis may indicate a variety of renal disorders, including vesicoureteral reflux, upper urinary tract obstruction (ureteropelvic junction obstruction, ureterovesical junction obstruction, and obstructive megaureter), and lower urinary tract obstruction (posterior urethral valves and prune-belly syndrome) (Stamilio and Morgan, 1998; Yiee and Wilcox, 2008). Increasing hydronephrosis is associated with more severe disease, and bilateral hydronephrosis suggests lower urinary tract obstruction, particularly in male fetuses (Yiee and Wilcox, 2008). Prenatal renal cysts can be seen with autosomal dominant polycystic kidney disease (ADPKD), multicystic dysplastic kidneys, and cystic renal dysplasia (Stamilio and Morgan, 1998). Hyperechoic kidneys can result from tubular dilations (autosomal recessive polycystic kidney disease or ARPKD), dysplasia, or multiple microscopic cysts (Bardet-Biedel syndrome, Meckel-Gruber syndrome, and nephrotic syndrome) (Chaumoitre et al, 2006). The etiology of oligohydramnios is not limited to renal disorders; however, its presence can indicate decreased fetal output and renal function (Kemper and Mueller-Wiefel, 2007). Oligohydramnios should prompt an evaluation for severe, bilateral, poorly functioning or absent kidneys as can be seen with renal agenesis, renal dysplasia, ARPKD, and lower urinary tract obstruction

(Deshpande and Hennekam, 2008; Kemper and Mueller-Wiefel, 2007). Polyhydramnios is caused by renal anomalies in a small percentage of cases, but can indicate the presence of a renal concentrating defect associated with renal dysplasia, nephrotic syndrome, or inherited renal tubular defects (Cole and Quamme, 2000; Deshpande and Hennekam, 2008; van Eijk et al, 2002). Congenital renal tumors are rare. The most common tumor is the mesoblastic nephroma, which appears as a unilateral, single, solid mass on prenatal ultrasound (Giulian, 1984).

FETAL MAGNETIC RESONANCE IMAGING

An emerging adjunct therapy to ultrasound is fetal magnetic resonance imaging (MRI). The typical indication for fetal urinary tract MRI evaluation is a second- or third-trimester pregnancy with oligohydramnios and an inconclusive prenatal renal ultrasound examination (Poutamo et al, 2000). Fetal MRI lends insight into the evaluation of renal cysts and renal agenesis. Differentiating renal cysts from dilated collecting system is often problematic; the detailed anatomy provided by MRI can help determine if the apparent cysts are limited to the periphery (consistent with cyst) (Figure 82-1) or central in location (consistent with a dilated collecting system) (Hormann et al, 2006). An increase in signal intensity in the renal cortex can differentiate between ARPKD and other polycystic diseases, which have a similar hyperechoic appearance on ultrasound imaging (Liu et al, 2006). When oligohydramnios is present and the kidneys cannot be conclusively identified on ultrasound, MRI is effective at identifying an empty renal pouch, underlying changes (renal dysplasia), or ectopic kidneys (Hormann et al, 2006). In addition to providing more detail of the renal anatomy, MRI studies are also useful in measuring the amniotic fluid, evaluating bladder filling, and assessing lung maturation (Hormann et al, 2006). The aforementioned findings are indirect measures of kidney function that can help define the degree of renal impairment.

AMNIOTIC FLUID AND CHORIONIC VILLUS SAMPLING

The diagnosis of most genetic disease with renal and urinary tract manifestations is based on the characteristic multiorgan findings on imaging. With an increasing number of conditions, analysis of DNA or tissue from amniocentesis or chorionic villus biopsy can be used to confirm a suspected disorder or determine prognosis. Examples are:
1. Molecular testing for the Lamb2 gene, which causes a severe form of infantile nephrotic syndrome, is possible by chorionic villus sampling in fetuses with polyhydramnios and hyperechoic kidneys (Deshpande and Hennekam, 2008).

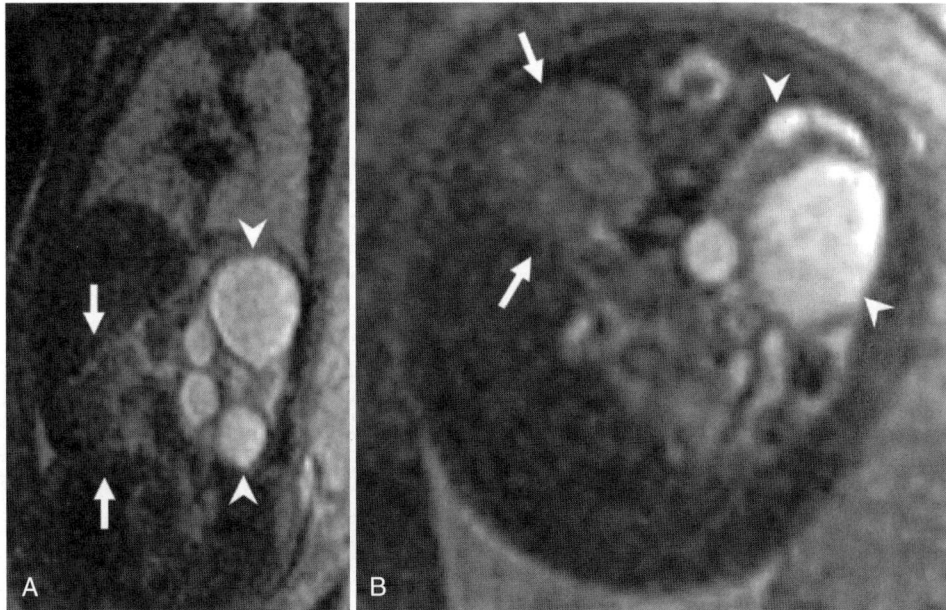

FIGURE 82-1 Coronal (**A**) and axial (**B**) images of the fetal kidneys on T2-weighted MRI. Note the normal right kidney (*arrows*) and large multi-cystic dysplastic left kidney (*arrowheads*) with the hyperintense peripheral cyst.

2. Fetal karyotyping by amniocentesis or chorionic villus sampling performed when kidney defects occur with anomalies of other organ systems can help identify the precise chromosome anomaly present (Deshpande and Hennekam, 2008).
3. Beckwith-Wiedemann syndrome, which can be associated with Wilms' tumor and other renal anomalies, can be diagnosed by specific 11p methylation studies in amniotic fluid (Deshpande and Hennekam, 2008).
4. Hypotonic fetal urine characterized by a sodium <90 mEq/L, chloride concentration <80 mEq/L, and osmolarity <180 mOsm/L in patients with bilateral hydronephrosis and no evidence of renal dysplasia is associated with a good prognosis, particularly if present on sequential samples taken 48 to 72 hours apart (Johnson et al, 1995; Wu and Johnson, 2009).

PRENATAL MANAGEMENT OF RENAL AND URINARY TRACT DISEASE

GOALS OF MANAGEMENT AND PROGNOSTIC FACTORS

Identification of renal and urinary tract disease on prenatal screening provides the basis for formulating a differential diagnosis, determining prenatal and postnatal risks, and screening for other anomalies. The goals of prenatal intervention include the preservation of renal function and the promotion of lung maturation (Yiee and Wilcox, 2008). Potential management options include parental counseling, follow-up or serial prenatal imaging, postnatal imaging, fetal interventions, and early multispecialty collaboration (Pates and Dashe, 2006; Yiee and Wilcox, 2008). Factors associated with a poor outcome include bilateral involvement of the kidneys and oligohydramnios. If oligohydramnios is severe, the oligohydramnios sequence can occur. This is characterized by pulmonary hypoplasia, "flattened" face, "squashed" nose, and positional limb

abnormalities (Deshpande and Hennekam, 2008). When oligohydramnios is present, the prognosis may vary based on the underlying renal diagnosis. Bilateral renal agenesis is considered a lethal disorder, whereas the prognosis is potentially more favorable if the oligohydramnios is secondary to obstruction (Cendron et al, 1994; Kemper and Mueller-Wiefel, 2007; Schwaderer et al, 2007).

INTERVENTIONS

The effectiveness of fetal intervention for hydronephrosis is controversial (Hubert and Palmer, 2007). The primary procedure is placement of a vesicoamniotic shunt with the goal of relieving obstruction (potentially preventing further renal damage) and decreasing oligohydramnios (Wu and Johnson, 2009). This procedure may be considered when bladder outlet obstruction is present, the life of the neonate is at risk, the fetus will likely benefit from bladder decompression, the pregnancy is singleton, and the fetus has a normal karyotype (Hubert and Palmer, 2007). It is a matter of debate whether amnioinfusion prevents or decreases pulmonary hypoplasia. Although some reports have suggested a benefit for oligohydramnios secondary to premature rupture of membranes, prospective data regarding oligohydramnios of renal origin are not yet available (De Carolis et al, 2004; Klaassen et al, 2007).

POSTNATAL EVALUATION OF RENAL AND URINARY TRACT DISEASE

PRENATAL AND PERINATAL HISTORY

As noted earlier, a history of oligohydramnios is often associated with poor urine flow and poor kidney function. Forms that occur in the first trimester (e.g., bilateral renal agenesis or severe dysgenesis) are often associated with poor prognoses, in part from poor pulmonary development. Other causes, such as obstructive nephropathy, may have a more favorable outcome (Kemper and Mueller-Wiefel, 2007). As noted earlier, polyhydramnios is often idiopathic or secondary to nonrenal problems such as gastrointestinal or central nervous system abnormalities (Deshpande and Hennekam, 2008), but is associated with renal anomalies such as infantile Bartter's syndrome or nephrogenic diabetes insipidus. A large placenta (>25% of birthweight) can be a sign of congenital nephrotic syndrome (Holmberg et al, 1996). Hypoxia/ischemia (e.g., perinatal anoxia, placental abruption), toxin exposure (e.g., pre- or perinatal use of nonsteroidal antiinflammatory agents, aminoglycosides), and shock (e.g., blood loss, sepsis) increase the risk of acute kidney injury (which has an incidence of more than 20 per 100,000 neonatal patients) (Andreoli, 2004; Askenazi et al, 2009).

FAMILY HISTORY

Renal agenesis or severe dysgenesis in parents or siblings increases the risks of congenital kidney disease in newborn patients (Roodhooft et al, 1984; Schwaderer et al, 2007). Some forms of polycystic kidney disease (PKD), vesicoureteral reflux, and medullary cystic kidney disease follow autosomal dominant inheritance patterns; thus, screening should be considered in neonates whose parents have these disorders. Appropriate screening would be indicated in neonates whose siblings have autosomal recessive diseases (e.g., autosomal recessive PKD, cystinosis) or X-linked diseases (e.g., Alport's disease or Lowe syndrome).

PHYSICAL EXAM

Hypertension

As discussed in Chapters 86 and 88, increased blood pressure in the neonatal period is frequently secondary to renovascular and/or parenchymal disorders and should receive appropriate evaluation.

Micturition

Frequently, healthy neonates will not void until 12 hours or later after birth, although nearly all will produce some urine by 24 hours (Clark, 1977). Once voiding commences, it almost never occurs during sleep in term infants, whereas 60% of preterm infants will void when asleep; furthermore, both term and preterm neonates tend to void frequently (often hourly) with quite variable volumes (Sillen, 2001; Sillen and Hjalmas, 2004). Delayed voiding (beyond 24 hours after birth) is often seen after stressful deliveries and has been correlated with enhanced arginine vasopressin and aldosterone secretion (Vuohelainen et al, 2008). Prolonged absence of urine formation should prompt evaluation for acute kidney injury or structural kidney or urinary tract disease.

Abdominal Masses

Palpation of the abdomen for masses is best performed within the first few days after birth, during which there is relative hypotonia of the abdominal musculature

(Perlman and Williams, 1976). Palpable abdominal masses, particularly flank masses, in neonates most often originate from the urinary tract (Chandler and Gauderer, 2004). Among three studies that each enrolled more than 10,000 newborn infants, the incidence of renal/urinary tract anomalies detected by deep palpation ranged from 0.2% to 0.6%. The most common urinary tract anomalies detected as abdominal masses are hydronephrotic kidneys, followed by multicystic dysplastic kidneys (Chandler and Gauderer, 2004). Bilateral flank masses may be palpated in patients with ARPKD. Although less common, tumors of renal origin are most often congenital mesoblastic nephromas (usually benign) as opposed to Wilms' tumors, which are most often diagnosed after 6 months of age (Chandler and Gauderer, 2004; Glick et al, 2004). Once an abdominal mass is palpated, imaging such as an abdominal ultrasound or MRI should be obtained (see Imaging, later).

Edema

Edema occurs when there is an imbalance between capillary hydrostatic and interstitial oncotic forces. Neonatal edema is more commonly seen in preterm infants than in term infants and is often transient, resolving a few days after birth (Cartlidge and Rutter, 1986; Griffiths, 1959; Hahn et al, 1997). Most cases of persistent, pathologic edema are extrarenal in origin. The major renal causes include total body fluid overload secondary to a decrease in glomerular filtration rate (GFR) (from acute or chronic renal injury) and low intravascular oncotic pressure from urinary protein losses (from congenital nephrotic syndrome—see Proteinuria, later).

Ascites

As with edema, ascites can arise as an imbalance between hydrostatic and oncotic pressures, but it can also occur secondary to decreased lymphatic drainage. Although neonatal ascites is somewhat rare, urinary tract abnormalities account for a significant number of cases (Aslam et al, 2007; Griscom et al, 1977). The most common urinary tract cause is urinary ascites from perforation of the ureter, renal pelvis, or bladder from obstruction (e.g., posterior urethral valves). Less common conditions leading to ascites are congenital nephrotic syndrome and renal vein thrombosis.

LABORATORY TESTS

Serum Estimates of Glomerular Filtration Rate

Absolute and relative (corrected for body surface area) GFR is much lower in newborns than older children and adults; at day 1 of life, GFR may be as low as 30 mL/min/1.73 m^2 in term infants (and even lower in preterm infants), rising to about 50 mL/min/1.73 m^2 by 1 month of life and 75 mL/min/1.73m^2 by 2 months of life (Arant, 1987; Chevalier, 1996). Because of technical difficulties with 24-hour urine collections for clearance measurements and/or the use of exogenous agents that are freely filtered at the glomerulus, most often assays of endogenous serum molecules are used to estimate GFR in neonates. Although concentration of cystatin C has been proposed in more recent times as a good way to approximate kidney function (Finney et al, 2000), serum creatinine still remains the most widely used assay. As in adults, serum creatinine is both filtered and secreted in the kidney; however, creatinine also appears to be reabsorbed within the tubules of immature kidneys (with more reabsorption in preterm infants) (Guignard and Drukker, 1999). This likely accounts for the delay in the drop in creatinine level that occurs from the time of birth (at which time serum creatinine reflects the mother's level) until about 7 to 10 days after birth in term infants and which may extend to 3 weeks in preterm infants (tubular reabsorption may also explain creatinine levels slightly greater than the mother's in many preterm infants just after birth). In one study, term infants had a mean serum creatinine of 0.85 ± 0.43 mg/dL at 2 days of age, 0.57 ± 0.40 mg/dL at 7 days of age, and 0.42 ± 0.23 mg/dL at 14 days of age (Rudd et al, 1983). In 28 weeks' gestation preterm infants, the same study reported serum creatinine measurements of 1.31 ± 0.45 mg/dL at 2 days of age, 0.95 ± 0.36 mg/dL at 7 days of age, and 0.81 ± 0.36 mg/dL at 14 days of age. Blood urea nitrogen concentration is also often used as another indirect measure of kidney function, but is less reliable than creatinine because of alterations based on protein intake and hydration status.

Other Serum Chemistry Studies

In addition to GFR, renal tubular function often differs in the neonatal kidney from that of adults, and recently, many of the reasons for the differences between neonatal and adult tubular function have been further clarified. Acidification differs with normal serum bicarbonate levels in the term neonate ranging from 19 to 21 mEq/L and in the preterm infant ranging from 16 to 20 mEq/L (Shaw, 2008). The lower serum bicarbonate is due to a lower threshold at the proximal tubule; the lowered threshold is likely due to the presence of different acid transporter isoforms in maturing kidneys versus adult kidneys as well as to hormonal influences on the abundance and activity of these transporters (Baum, 2008; Baum and Quigley, 1995). Serum potassium is less well excreted in the collecting ducts of neonates compared to older children and adults, with normal newborn levels up to 6.7 mmol/L (Lorenz, 1997). This physiologic increase in potassium (to accommodate vigorous growth over the 1st year of life) is due to a paucity of aldosterone-sensitive secretory potassium channels and an abundance of potassium-reabsorbing transporters on the luminal surface of collecting ducts (Gurkan et al, 2007). Sodium must remain in positive balance for rapidly growing neonates (despite a diet that is typically low in sodium). The ability to excrete less sodium chloride appears to be due to differences in expression of sodium/proton antiporter isoforms and tight junction proteins, called claudins, in neonates versus adults and older children (Baum, 2008; Baum and Quigley, 2004). Serum phosphate levels are also typically higher in newborn infants with serum levels ranging from 5.8 to 9.3 mg/dL on the 1st day of life (with the higher levels typically in preterm infants (Barac-Nieto, 2001; Hellstern et al, 2003;

Spitzer and Barac-Nieto, 2001). This physiologic increase in serum phosphate levels compared with older humans (again, to accommodate rapid growth) is due to enhanced capacity of sodium phosphate transport at the proximal tubule in neonates (Spitzer and Barac-Nieto, 2001).

Urine

Urinary Tract Infection

Most frequently urine collections in newborn infants are performed because of suspected urinary tract infection (UTI). Evidence-based guidelines were published regarding evaluation for UTI in patients from 2 months to 2 years of age (American Academy of Pediatrics, 1999). Some of these guidelines indicated that UTI should be considered in all patients with unexplained fever, which is best assessed with a urine culture. Although suprapubic aspiration (SPA) or transurethral catheterization (TUC) is highly recommended, for patients who do not appear to be "so ill as to require immediate antimicrobial therapy" one could consider using a bagged urine collection for a urine analysis and then following up with an SPA or TUC urine culture if the urine analysis or clinical course suggests UTI. For patients under 2 months of age with suspected UTI, one should always collect urine via SPA or TUC for culture.

Concentrating/Diluting

Compared with adults, newborn infants also have a diminished capacity to concentrate their urine based on relative insensitivity to antidiuretic hormone and a less hypertonic medulla due to less sodium chloride and urea transport (Bonilla-Felix, 2004; Quigley et al, 2001). Neonates have less ability to dilute their urine compared with adults and older children, although they can handle the typically hypotonic fluids they receive for nutrition.

Proteinuria

Physiologic and pathologic proteinuria can be seen in newborn infants, particularly in preterm and/or low birthweight infants. Normal preterm and term infants have an average 182 mg/m^2/day and 145 mg/m^2/day of total urine protein, respectively, compared with 91 mg/m^2/day in children 2 to 4 years of age (Loghman-Adham, 1998). A recent study also found that very low birthweight infants had a higher risk of pathologic albuminuria (albumin/creatinine ratio >20 mg/g) than normal infants, particularly in those who developed hypotension after birth (Iacobelli et al, 2007). Another study showed that preterm infants were more likely to develop pathologic tubular proteinuria (α1 microglobulin/creatinine ratio >10 mg/mmol) than term infants (Ojala et al, 2006). Low gestational age enhanced the risk of early tubular proteinuria, the highest α1 microglobulin/creatinine ratios, and delayed normalization of proteinuria.

A more rare but serious pathologic finding is congenital nephrotic syndrome, defined as high-grade proteinuria, low serum albumin, and edema within the 1st year of life. The differential diagnosis includes primary/genetic causes (e.g., Finnish type nephrotic syndrome and diffuse mesangial sclerosis) and secondary causes such as infections (e.g., cytomegalovirus, syphilis, hepatitis), genetic syndromes (e.g., Denys-Drash, Frasier syndrome), toxins/drugs, hemolytic uremic syndrome, systemic lupus erythematosus, and nephroblastoma (Papez and Smoyer, 2004). Unlike nephrotic syndrome in later childhood, congenital nephrotic syndrome usually portends a poor prognosis, including end-stage renal failure (with the exception of some infectious forms that respond to appropriate therapy). Interestingly, a recent study found that two thirds of all cases of primary/genetic congenital nephrotic syndrome were caused by mutations in 1 of 4 genes, encoding for nephrin (major cause of Finnish type), podocin, Wilms' tumor suppressor gene 1 (found in Denys-Drash, Frasier syndrome), and laminin β2 (a cause of diffuse mesangial sclerosis) (Hinkes et al, 2007).

Other Urinary Findings (Hematuria, Hemoglobinuria, Myoglobinuria, Uricosuria)

Hematuria is a rare finding in neonates and, when present, has a wide differential diagnosis including renal vein thrombosis, polycystic kidney disease, obstructive nephropathy, tumor, congenital malformations, UTI, and acute kidney injury (Emanuel and Aronson, 1974). Hemoglobinuria, another rare finding in newborn infants, occurs secondary to intravascular hemolysis, of which the most common etiology is ABO blood group incompatibility (Murray and Roberts, 2007). Myoglobinuria is even more rarely detected in neonates, but has been reported secondary to rhabdomyolysis from asphyxia and shock (Sirota et al, 1988). Finally, pink or red uric acid crystals are often seen in diapers of otherwise healthy newborn infants; although this has been reported to be a consequence of high urine uric acid levels in normal newborn infants, a recent study challenges that contention (Kupeli et al, 2005).

IMAGING

Renal Ultrasound Examination

The primary indications for renal ultrasound imaging in the neonatal period include a palpable abdominal mass, hypertension, renal failure, and suspected malformations of the renal and urinary tract (McInnis et al, 1982). The neonatal presentation of a renal mass or renal failure is often suggested by the prenatal evaluation (Riccabona, 2006). An abdominal mass of renal etiology might appear as large kidneys, hydronephrotic kidneys, or a renal tumor. Renal ultrasound can be useful to distinguish among intrinsic, prerenal, and postrenal failure. Regarding intrinsic causes of renal failure, neonatal nephrotic syndrome and glomerulonephritis will manifest as large echogenic kidneys; renal vein thrombosis will present as large echogenic kidneys with renal vein color signal missing on veins with thrombosis and increased resistive indices on a duplex exam; and congenital dysplasia will present as small echogenic kidneys (Riccabona, 2006). Postrenal failure is characterized by hydronephrosis, and prerenal failure by echogenic kidneys with decreased flow velocities with elevated resistive index values on duplex exam (Riccabona, 2006). Ultrasound imaging has been recommended as a noninvasive study that should be obtained in all hypertensive infants because it may potentially identify correctable causes of the hypertension, including renal vein thrombosis, aortic/renal artery

thrombi, or anatomic renal abnormalities (Flynn, 2000). If a renal ultrasound is planned for follow-up evaluation of prenatal hydronephrosis, it is advantageous to wait until day 3 of life because the initial period of neonatal oliguria might mask renal collecting system dilation (Kennedy, 2002).

Computed Tomography Scan

The risk of ionizing radiation injury from CT is higher in neonates secondary to more radiosensitive tissues and longer life expectancies (Brenner et al, 2001). Further, the CT evaluation of the kidney is limited by reduced contrast uptake by the renal parenchyma (Olsen and Gunny, 2006). Because of the aforementioned factors, CT has limited use in the evaluation of the renal and urinary tract during the neonatal period. Nonetheless, CT does have a role when ultrasound results are inconclusive for complex anomalies of the kidney, abdominal masses, and suspected renal vascular anomalies and when MRI would be problematic because of sedation risk or in the presence of a contraindication to MRI contrast (Gnanasambandam and Olsen, 2006; Grobner and Prischl, 2007; Olsen and Gunny, 2006;).

Magnetic Resonance Imaging

MRI has several advantages in imaging the neonatal kidney and urinary tract. The absence of radiation and detailed anatomy of soft tissue with MRI make it an attractive tool to clearly define normal and abnormal renal anatomy when ultrasound is insufficient. However, MRI has disadvantages because sedation is necessary for infants (Michael, 2008). The risk of MRI contrast (gadolinium)-associated nephrogenic systemic fibrosis in the immature neonatal kidney and gadolinium depositions in the bone marrow are concerns (Michael, 2008). Applications in which MRI is particularly useful include the identification of a suspected ectopic or dysplastic kidney and the identification of renal vascular causes of hypertension in neonates unable to tolerate angiography (Michael, 2008; Mustafa et al, 2006).

Voiding Cystourethrography

Voiding cystourethrography (VCUG) is utilized to evaluate for lower urinary tract obstruction and vesicoureteral reflux. In males, a fluoroscopic as opposed to a nuclear medicine VCUG should be used, because the anatomic details of the male urethra warrant a complete evaluation (Kennedy, 2002).

Nuclear Medicine

The use of nuclear medicine is limited in neonatal practice. Two studies that might be occasionally used include DMSA cortical scintigraphy and the DTPA or MAG3 diuretic renogram. Cortical DMSA cortical scintigraphy can be used to evaluate left and right relative renal function and for evaluation of acute pyelonephritis (Piepsz and Ham, 2006). The diuretic renogram is indicated to evaluate for upper urinary tract obstruction when fetal hydronephrosis has persisted and vesicoureteral reflux has been excluded (Kennedy, 2002; Piepsz and Ham, 2006). It may also be used to identify ectopic renal tissue (Piepsz and Ham, 2006).

SUMMARY

Structural abnormalities are common causes of kidney and urinary tract disorders in the perinatal period of life. Thus, imaging modalities such as renal ultrasonography remain very useful tools in evaluating patients with suspected kidney and/or urinary tract disease. A careful history and physical exam will also offer insights into the underlying causes of kidney and urinary tract disorders. Finally, compared with older children and adults, the neonatal kidney is less efficient at clearance and has reduced tubular function (acidification, potassium secretion, sodium transport), except for phosphate, which is reabsorbed more efficiently in the very young.

SUGGESTED READINGS

Baum M: Developmental changes in proximal tubule NaCl transport, *Pediatr Nephrol* 23:185-194, 2008.

Bonilla-Felix M: Development of water transport in the collecting duct, *Am J Physiol Renal Physiol* 287:F1093-F1101, 2004.

Chandler JC, Gauderer MW: The neonate with an abdominal mass,. *Pediatr Clin North Am* 51:979-997, 2004ix.

Deshpande C, Hennekam RC: Genetic syndromes and prenatally detected renal anomalies, *Semin Fetal Neonatal Med* 13:171-180, 2008.

Gurkan S, Estilo GK, Wei Y, Satlin LM: Potassium transport in the maturing kidney, *Pediatr Nephrol* 22:915-925, 2007.

Hellstern G, Poschl J, Linderkamp O: Renal phosphate handling of premature infants of 23-25 weeks gestational age, *Pediatr Nephrol* 18:756-758, 2003.

Hinkes BG, Mucha B, Vlangos CN, et al: Nephrotic syndrome in the first year of life: two thirds of cases are caused by mutations in 4 genes (NPHS1, NPHS2, WT1, and LAMB2), *Pediatrics* 119:e907-e919, 2007.

Hormann M, Brugger PC, Balassy C, et al: Fetal MRI of the urinary system, *Eur J Radiol* 57:303-311, 2006.

Kennedy W: Assessment and management of fetal hydronephrosis, *NeoReviews* 3(10):e214-e219, 2002.

Papez KE, Smoyer WE: Recent advances in congenital nephrotic syndrome, *Curr Opin Pediatr* 16:165-170, 2004.

Piepsz A, Ham HR: Pediatric applications of renal nuclear medicine, *Semin Nucl Med* 36:16-35, 2006.

Riccabona M: Renal failure in neonates, infants and children: the role of ultrasound, *Ultrasound Clin* 1:457-469, 2006.

Complete references used in this text can be found online at www.expertconsult.com

DEVELOPMENTAL ABNORMALITIES OF THE KIDNEYS

Lawrence Copelovitch and Bernard S. Kaplan

The increasing use of prenatal ultrasonography, continuing improvements in ventilator and nutritional support, and progress in dialysis techniques for newborns and in renal transplantation for young children have changed the natural history of cystic and dysplastic kidney diseases. Information gathered from many sources must be evaluated carefully to manage optimally a newborn with a genetic or developmental disorder of the kidneys. Clearly a team approach is needed. Errors occur with insufficient data, inadequate communication, and poor understanding of the natural history of these disorders. Renal tract malformations are, collectively, the major cause of childhood end-stage renal disease, and their contribution to the number of adults on renal replacement therapy is less clear and has possibly been underestimated (Kerecuk et al, 2008). Many newborns who might have died in the past can now be dialyzed from birth and then transplanted when they reach about 10 kg. A precise diagnosis must be made before starting dialysis because some of these problems impose enormous emotional and financial burdens on families. The diagnosis depends on the evaluation of the prenatal history, results of fetal ultrasonography, family history, clinical examination, imaging studies of infants and parents when indicated, laboratory studies (including DNA tests if available), and interpretation of pathology. Several guiding principles are worth keeping in mind. Few genetic renal disorders are confined to kidneys, and many syndromes have renal involvement. Therefore, ultrasonography of kidneys and urinary tract should be done in all newborns with multiple defects. Also, ultrasonographic features can change over time, and in some cases may give erroneous information (Mashiach et al, 2005). Variable expression of congenital renal defects may occur within and among kindreds; this is particularly true in autosomal recessive polycystic kidney disease. There are many classifications of cystic and dysplastic kidneys, but the one shown in Box 83-1 lists conditions that can be seen in newborns.

ECTOPIC KIDNEY, HORSESHOE KIDNEY, AND CROSSED FUSED ECTOPIA

Ectopic kidney, horseshoe kidney, and crossed fused ectopia are abnormalities in the position of the kidney(s), They do not have important long-term effects unless associated with lower urinary tract anomalies, such as reflux or obstruction. In essence, these kidneys are at risk for the same problems as those in normal positions. Horseshoe kidney, however, does occur with increased frequency in Turner and other syndromes. A voiding cystourethrogram should be done to exclude the possibility of reflux, and a technetium-99m–labeled diethylenetriaminepentaacetic acid (DTPA) scan should be done if there is evidence on ultrasonography of an obstruction.

MULTICYSTIC KIDNEY

Multicystic kidney is the second most common cause of a flank mass in the newborn with a prevalence rate of 1 in 4300. Multicystic kidney is almost always a sporadic, nonsyndromal, congenital anomaly. The diagnosis is made by in utero ultrasonography or by detection of an abdominal

---

BOX 83-1 Cystic and Dysplastic Kidneys in Newborns

Ectopic kidney, horseshoe kidney, crossed fused ectopia
Multicystic kidney
Unilateral renal agenesis
Bilateral renal agenesis
Renal adysplasia/dysplasia
    Isolated adysplasia/dysplasia
    Hypoplastic kidneys
   Dysplasia/adysplasia in regional defects
    Prune-belly syndrome (PBS) [McKusick #100100]
    Posterior urethral valves (PUV) [McKusick #100100]
   Adysplasia/dysplasia with multiple-congenital-abnormalities syndromes
    Branchio-oto-renal dysplasia (BOR syndrome) [McKusick #113650]
    Mayer-Rokitansky-Küster-Hauser syndrome
    Kallmann's syndrome (KAL1) [McKusick #308700]
  Acrorenal syndromes
  Ectodermal dysplasia, ectrodactyly, cleft lip/palate syndrome
    Fanconi's pancytopenia syndrome
    Thrombocytopenia-absent radius syndrome
    Townes-Brocks syndrome (TBS) [McKusick #107480]
    Fraser syndrome [McKusick #219000]
    Fryns syndrome
    Pallister-Hall syndrome [McKusick #146510]
  Polycystic kidneys
    Autosomal recessive polycystic kidney disease [McKusick #263200]
    Autosomal dominant polycystic kidney disease [McKusick #179300]
    Tuberous sclerosis (TS) [McKusick #191100]
Cystic kidneys with autosomal recessive inheritance
    Meckel's syndrome (MKS 1, MKS 2) [McKusick #249000]
    Jeune asphyxiating thoracic dystrophy syndrome [McKusick #208500]
    Renal-hepatic-pancreatic dysplasia (Ivemark's syndrome)
Glomerulocystic kidneys
Dysgenetic kidneys
    Congenital hypernephronic nephromegaly with tubular dysgenesis [McKusick #267430]
Overgrowth syndromes
    Beckwith-Wiedemann syndrome [McKusick #130650]
    Perlman syndrome [McKusick #267000]
    Simpson-Golabi-Behmel syndrome type 1 (SGBS1) [McKusick #312870]
In utero exposure to teratogens
    Anticonvulsants; cocaine; indomethacin; lead; phenacetin; salicylate; warfarin; gentamicin
Inborn errors of metabolism
    Glutaric aciduria type II (multiple acyl-CoA dehydrogenase deficiencies)
    Zellweger cerebrohepatorenal syndrome [McKusick #214100]
    Carbohydrate-deficient glycoprotein syndrome

CoA, coenzyme A.

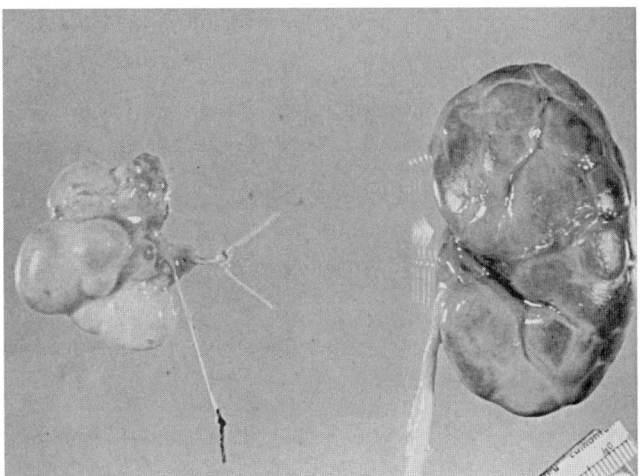

FIGURE 83-1 Multicystic kidney with atretic ureter (*right*). Large cysts with no normal renal tissue.

mass. Multicystic kidney is rarely the cause of symptoms in the newborn. Pathologic findings are ureteropelvic dysplasia or atresia, enlarged kidney, cysts of varying size that do not communicate, and no demonstrable pelvis or calyces (Figure 83-1) (Bernstein, 1991). Multicystic kidney must be differentiated from obstructive cystic renal dysplasia associated with hydronephrosis and other causes of obstructive uropathy by doing a DTPA scan. The multicystic kidney does not function. The contralateral kidney is usually normal, but in up to 33% to 50% of cases it may be absent, hydronephrotic, ectopic, refluxing, and occasionally dysplastic (Ativeh et al, 1992; Schreuder et al, 2009). Reflux may be present in up to 20% of contralateral kidneys, 40% of which are grade 3 or higher. Compensatory hypertrophy of the contralateral kidney is a common finding in childhood (Schreuder et al, 2009). Nephrectomy of the multicystic dysplastic kidney in typical cases is unnecessary (Kuwertz-Broeking et al, 2004). There may be a spectrum, within and among kindreds, of calyceal diverticulum, pyelogenous cyst, ureteropelvic junction stenosis, infundibular stenosis, pelvic stenosis, and multicystic kidney (Kelalis and Malek, 1981). Most patients are followed by ultrasonography, and spontaneous involution often occurs without complications of infection, bleeding, hypertension, or malignancy (Wacksman and Phipps, 1993).

RENAL ADYSPLASIA AND DYSPLASIA

The term *adysplasia* encompasses a spectrum of renal anomalies that include renal agenesis, hypoplasia, dysplasia, and hypodysplasia that occur in a patient (such as unilateral agenesis with contralateral dysplasia) or within a kindred (Buchta et al, 1973). Dysplastic kidneys can be unilateral or bilateral, often contain cysts, are disorganized, and may also contain ectopic cartilage and muscle. They may or may not function. The clinical picture depends on the severity of the renal anomaly, whether it is unilateral or bilateral, and the presence of associated anomalies (Fitch, 1977). The newborn may look normal or may have features of the oligohydramnios sequence, prune-belly syndrome, or malformation syndromes.

Adysplasia and dysplasia can be the result of a single autosomal recessive (Cole et al, 1976) or dominant gene disorder (McPherson et al, 1981). Absent or dysplastic kidneys can also occur by multifactorial inheritance (Holmes, 1989), in chromosomal disorders (Egli and Stalder, 1973), and as a consequence of in utero infections or exposure to toxins. The precise genetics of isolated renal adysplasia remain elusive. Mutations in the SIX6 and BMP4 genes are associated with hypodysplasia (Weber, 2008). Occasionally, PAX2, TCF2, and SALL1 mutations result in isolated adysplasia (Weber, 2006), although they usually occur as part of a global syndrome (see later discussion). Prenatal diagnosis by ultrasonography is possible, especially if there is oligohydramnios or associated anomalies such as limb defects.

UNILATERAL RENAL AGENESIS

Unilateral renal agenesis is usually an isolated (nonsyndromic), sporadic abnormality that is detected during prenatal ultrasonography. Unilateral renal agenesis is an important finding if the solitary kidney is abnormal, is part of a syndrome, or is an expression of hereditary renal dysplasia (Moerman et al, 1994). The incidence is between 1 in 500 and 1 in 800 live births. If the solitary kidney is normal, there is little risk of chronic renal failure in adulthood. The newborn must be examined carefully for additional anomalies—cleft palate, ocular abnormalities, preauricular pits, abnormalities of digits, cardiac and vertebral defects, and mullerian duct aplasia (Tarry et al, 1986). A voiding cystourethrogram should be done to exclude reflux. No further evaluations are needed beyond 1 year of age if renal ultrasonography shows that the kidney is growing normally with appropriate compensatory hypertrophy.

BILATERAL RENAL AGENESIS

Bilateral renal agenesis can occur as an isolated (nonsyndromal), sporadic abnormality detected during prenatal ultrasonography. It can also be a component of a syndrome such as the branchio-oto–renal dysplasia (BOR) syndrome, or an expression of hereditary renal adysplasia. There can be variable expression within a family, and both autosomal recessive and dominant inheritance occur. The incidence is about 1 in 3000 births. Bilateral renal agenesis is an important cause of the oligohydramnios sequence (Potter's syndrome), in which decreased amniotic fluid causes uterine compression of the fetus. This produces the Potter facies with wide-set eyes, a prominent skin fold that extends from medial canthus to cheek, a parrot-beak nose, pliable low-set ears, and receding chin. There are also lower limb deformations and, most importantly, a narrow, small chest with pulmonary hypoplasia. The infant is anuric and dies from pulmonary insufficiency. Bilateral renal agenesis is the most important cause of oligohydramnios, and the diagnosis can be confirmed by prenatal ultrasonography.

ISOLATED DYSPLASIA AND ADYSPLASIA

The incidence of isolated (nonsyndromic) bilateral renal dysplasia is about 15 per 100,000 newborns (Holmes, 1989). Modes of transmission are autosomal dominant

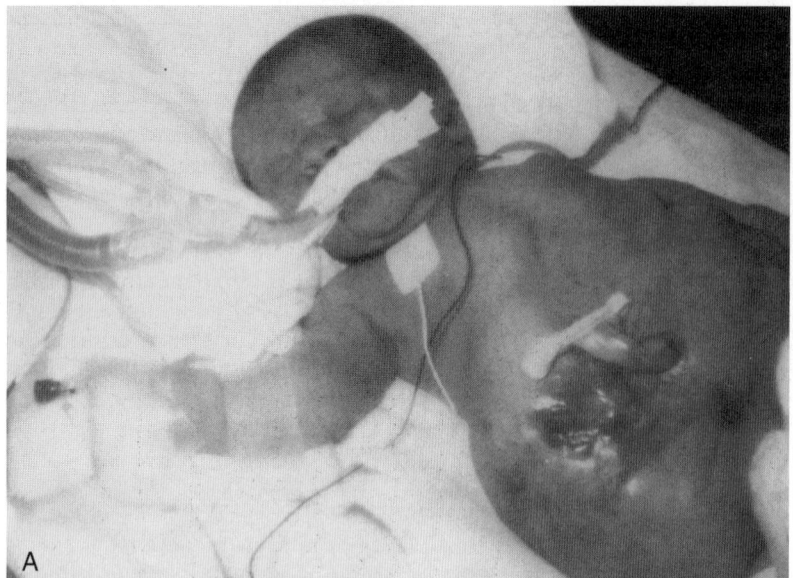
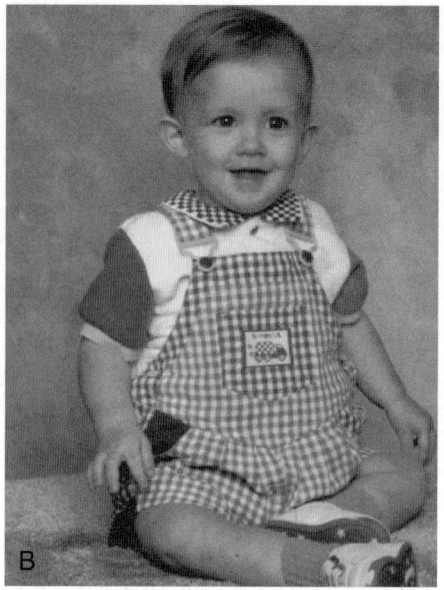

FIGURE 83-2 A, Newborn with prune-belly syndrome. The abdomen is protuberant, and the outlines of intestines can be seen. The right ureter ruptured into the amniotic sac, thereby preventing development of features of the oligohydramnios sequence. **B,** The same patient at age 19 months.

inheritance with reduced penetrance and multifactorial inheritance. A parent and/or siblings may be unaffected, have unilateral dysplasia, or have unilateral agenesis. Sporadic adysplasia may be caused by a new mutation or inheritance of gene(s) from a nonmanifesting parent. First-degree relatives should be screened by ultrasonography to provide genetic counseling. The empiric risk of bilateral renal adysplasia for future siblings is 3.5% (Carter, 1970). The recurrence risk increases if two siblings are affected.

HYPODYSPLASIA

Hypoplastic kidneys are small, have fewer calyces, and may be dysplastic. Simple hypoplasia, oligomeganephronia, and renal dysplasia are the types of small kidneys that are seen in newborns. In older children, small kidneys may also be the result of chronic pyelonephritis, chronic glomerulonephritis, renovascular accident, or nephronophthisis. In simple hypoplasia, the renal architecture is normal, but there are a decreased number of reniculi and small nephrons. Oligomeganephronic kidneys are small and have a decreased number of enlarged glomeruli (Royer et al, 1974). This is probably not a specific clinicopathologic entity. Some patients with oligomeganephronic kidneys have chromosome 4 abnormalities (Anderson et al; 1997), and others have heterozygous PAX2 mutations (Salomon et al, 2001).

DYSPLASIA AND ADYSPLASIA IN REGIONAL DEFECTS: PRUNE-BELLY SYNDROME [McKUSICK #100100] AND POSTERIOR URETHRAL VALVES [McKUSICK #100100]

Renal adysplasia occurs in prune belly syndrome (PBS) and posterior urethral valves (PUV), possibly as a result of obstructive uropathy (Bernstein, 1991). The renal pathology ranges from minor anomalies to severe dysplasia

with and without cysts. The features of PBS are deficient abdominal wall muscles (Figure 83-2), unilateral or bilateral undescended testes, and urinary tract abnormalities. Females are rarely affected but may have uterine or vaginal anomalies. PBS is also associated with lower intestinal tract malrotation and atresias, lower limb deformations, and cardiovascular defects.

PUV are characterized by urethral valves (either a flap valve or a diaphragm in the prostatic urethra) and features of obstructive uropathy. A dilated prostatic urethra, megacystis, and megaureters can occur in both conditions. The most frequent clinical presentation in the newborn of both conditions consists of features of the oligohydramnios sequence. The survival of newborns with PBS or PUV depends on the severity of pulmonary hypoplasia and severity of renal dysplasia. Both conditions are usually isolated occurrences, although PUV may occur rarely in families and in malformation syndromes.

DYSPLASIA AND ADYSPLASIA WITH MULTIPLE CONGENITAL ANOMALIES

Branchio-oto–renal Dysplasia [McKusick #113650]

The spectrum of renal anomalies in BOR syndrome ranges from unilateral dysplasia to bilateral agenesis. The kidneys may even be normal. Renal function ranges from normal to severe reduction in glomerular filtration rate. Extrarenal manifestations include preauricular pits, branchial clefts, sensorineural deafness, and lacrimal duct atresia. The incidence is 1 in 40,000 newborns. Inheritance is autosomal dominant with high penetrance and variable expression. Mutations in the EYA1 (chromosomal locus 8q13.3), SIX1 (chromosomal locus 14q23.1), and SIX5 (chromosomal locus 19q13.32) genes have been found to be causative (Abdelhak et al, 1997; Hoskins et al, 2007; Kumar et al, 1997; Ruf et al, 2004). The prognosis depends on the severity of the renal disorder.

Renal-Coloboma Syndrome [OMIM 120330]

Renal anomalies in this syndrome include hypoplasia, dysplasia, oligomeganephronia, agenesis, and vesicoureteral reflux. Renal hypoplasia is the most common abnormality. The degree of renal insufficiency is highly variable. Extrarenal manifestations include optic nerve coloboma, sensorineural deafness, joint laxity, mental retardation, and skin anomalies. Heterozygous mutations in the PAX2 gene located on 10q24-25 arising either sporadically or inherited in an autosomal dominant fashion are known to be causative (Sanyanusin, 1995). The PAX2 gene encodes a transcriptional factor that is a member of the paired-box family of homeotic genes that is central to urogenital development.

Hypoparathyroidism-Deafness–Renal Dysplasia Syndrome [OMIM 146255]

Renal manifestations include renal agenesis, renal hypoplasia, renal dysplasia, and vesicoureteral reflux. Extrarenal manifestations include hypoparathyroidism and sensorineural deafness. The degree of hypocalcemia, hearing loss, and renal abnormalities varies. Mutations in the *GATA3* gene on chromosome 10p15 encoding the trans-acting T-cell-specific transcription factor GATA-3 are causative (Van Esch, 2001). A contiguous gene syndrome with features of a DiGeorge-like phenotype (heart defects and immunodeficiency) and the hypoparathyroidism-deafness–renal dysplasia triad has been reported with terminal chromosome 10p deletions (Daw, 1996).

Mayer-Rokitansky-Kuster-Hauser Syndrome

Females with this syndrome have renal adysplasia and mullerian anomalies of vaginal atresia and bicornuate or septated uterus (Tarry et al, 1986). The fallopian tubes, ovaries, and broad and round ligaments are normal. There is a normal female karyotype and normal secondary sexual development. Rarely, this genetically heterogeneous condition has been associated with mutations in the *WNT4* gene located on chromosome 1p36.12 encoding a member of the frizzled family of seven transmembrane receptors (Philibert et al, 2008).

Kallmann's Syndrome (KAL1) (Hypogonadotropic Hypogonadism and Anosmia) [McKusick #308700]

Males with KAL1 have hypogonadotropic hypogonadism that manifests with delayed puberty and infertility; anosmia caused by agenesis of the olfactory lobes; and renal abnormalities (Colquhoun-Kerr et al, 1999; Deeb et al, 2001; Dissaneevate et al, 1998; Hardelin et al, 1992). Urogenital abnormalities include unilateral renal agenesis, bilateral renal agenesis, multicystic dysplastic kidney, cryptorchidism, testicular atrophy, and micropenis. Males may die at birth as a result of bilateral renal agenesis. Additional features include coloboma of iris, deafness, midline anomalies, oculomotor apraxia (bimanual synkinesis), and Moebius anomalad. The X-linked form is the result of a mutation in the *KAL-1* gene on Xp22.3 encoding the extracellular matrix glycoprotein anosmin-1. The autosomal recessive and dominant forms of Kallman's syndrome are not associated with renal adysplasia. Treatment with testosterone or estrogen for induction of puberty induces appropriate pubertal development.

Acrorenal Syndromes

Radial and renal anomalies occur in many syndromes. In the ectodermal dysplasia-ectrodactyly-cleft lip and/or palate (EEC 1) syndrome [McKusick #128930] there are combinations of urogenital defects, ectrodactyly, ectodermal dysplasia, clefting, lacrimal duct anomalies, and conductive hearing loss (Maas et al, 1996; Roelfsema and Cobben, 1996). Inheritance is autosomal dominant, with variable penetrance and expression. In the VACTERL /VATER association [McKusick #192350] there is variable occurrence of vertebral anomalies, anal atresia, congenital cardiac disease, tracheoesophageal fistula, renal abnormalities, and radial-limb dysplasia. VACTERL is usually sporadic. Neonates with features of VACTERL must be tested for Fanconi's anemia. Congenital malformations occur in 60% of cases of Fanconi anemia (pancytopenia) syndrome (FA). Affected patients may have renal malformations, short stature, café-au-lait spots, radial-ray abnormalities, gastrointestinal, microcephaly, skeletal abnormalities, and, in males, genital anomalies, hypogonadism, and infertility (Giampietro et al, 1993). There is chromosomal instability and mutagen hypersensitivity in cells. Inheritance is autosomal recessive with variable expression and mutations in one of at least seven different genes (Joenje and Patel, 2001). Renal anomalies may occur in thrombocytopenia absent radius syndrome (TAR) [McKusick #274000] and the omphalocele, exstrophy of the cloaca, imperforate anus, and spinal defects (OEIS) complex [OMIM 258040] (Lizcano-Gil, 1995).

The clinical features of Townes-Brocks radial-ear-anal-renal syndrome (TBS) [McKusick #107480] include broad, bifid, or triphalangeal thumb; flat thenar eminences; small, "lop," or "satyr" external ear; preauricular pits or tags; sensorineural hearing loss; and imperforate or stenotic or anteriorly placed anus. Renal and urological anomalies encompass renal hypoplasia, renal dysplasia, unilateral renal agenesis, horseshoe kidney, posterior urethral valves, ureterovesical reflux, and meatal stenosis (Salerno et al, 2000). Inheritance is dominant with a defect in the gene encoding SALL-1 on chromosome 16q12.1. Renal anomalies can occur in association with numerous other abnormalities in Wolf-Hirschhorn syndrome (4p- syndrome) [McKusick #194190] (Grisaru et al, 2000), Fraser syndrome [McKusick #219000] (Schauer et al, 1990), Fryns syndrome [McKusick #229850] (Moerman et al, 1988), De Lange syndrome (Kroes, 2004), Goldenhar syndrome (Kroes, 2004), and Pallister-Hall congenital hypothalamic hamartoblastoma syndrome (PHS) [McKusick #146510] (Killoran et al, 2000).

CILIOPATHIES

The term *ciliopathy* describes a group of genetic conditions with defective cilia. A number of syndromes that had been previously loosely associated due to shared clinical features

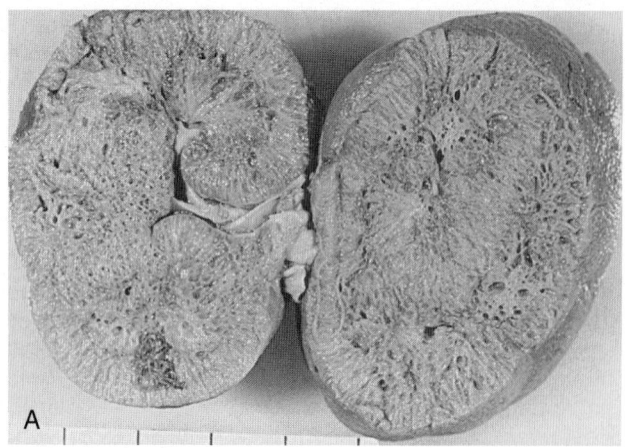
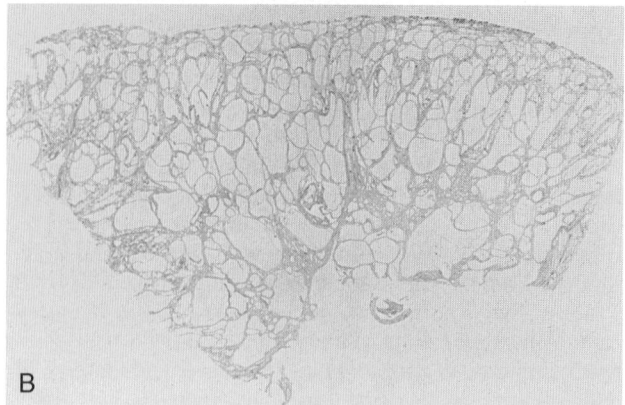

FIGURE 83-3 **A,** Large spongy kidneys (autosomal recessive kidneys). **B,** Photomicrograph of autosomal recessive kidneys with dilated tubules and paucity of glomeruli.

are now grouped under this classification. Most of these conditions display renal cystic and hepatobiliary disease, some have laterality defects and retinal degeneration, and several have polydactyly. The ciliopathies include autosomal recessive and dominant polycystic kidney disease, Bardet-Biedl syndrome, Meckel syndrome (MKS), Joubert's syndrome, nephrophthisis, Senior-Loken syndrome, Jeune's syndrome, oro-facial-digital syndrome type, Ellis-van Creveld syndrome, and Alstrom syndrome. Several of the ciliopathies account for the majority of conditions associated with large fetal echogenic kidneys with or without cysts. Autosomal dominant polycystic kidney disease (ADPKD), autosomal recessive polycystic kidney disease (ARPKD), Bardet-Biedl syndrome, and Meckel-Gruber syndrome are most commonly associated (Chaumoitre et al, 2006). Identifying the primary ciliary defect has contributed to understanding defective cellular processes and potential therapeutic targets. Several agents show promise preclinically and provide hope for effective treatments of the ciliopathies in the future (Harris, 2009).

POLYCYSTIC KIDNEYS

The term *polycystic kidneys* should be applied only to autosomal recessive polycystic kidneys and autosomal dominant polycystic kidneys. In these conditions, there are cysts in both kidneys, there is no evidence of renal dysplasia, and there is continuity of the lumen of the nephron from the uriniferous space to the urinary bladder. Patients with tuberous sclerosis can have cystic kidneys that appear identical by ultrasonography to autosomal dominant polycystic kidneys.

Autosomal Recessive Polycystic Kidney Disease [McKusick # 263200]

The incidence of ARPKD is 1 in 16,000 newborns, inheritance is autosomal recessive, there may be variable expression within a sibship (Kaplan et al, 1988), and the parents are unaffected. Mutations in the PKHD1 gene located on chromosome 6p21 (Guay-Woodford et al, 1995; Ward et al, 2001; Zerres et al, 1998) are causative. The gene encodes for fibrocystin, a hepatocyte growth factor receptor-like protein that functions in the primary cilia of renal

and biliary epithelial cells. In the newborn, the kidneys are much more severely affected than the liver, whereas liver disease is more prominent when the disorder is diagnosed in older children. Features of the oligohydramnios sequence occur if there is severe oliguria or anuria in utero. The abdomen is protuberant, and the kidneys are large and easily palpable. Hypertension is often severe, may be caused by volume expansion, and can be difficult to control. Peripheral renin activity and aldosterone excretion are reduced (Kaplan et al, 1989), although intrarenal angiotensin II levels may be high (Loghman-Adham et al, 2005). Hyponatremia is often induced iatrogenically as a result of inappropriate administration of free water and is not associated with increased urinary losses of sodium (Kaplan et al, 1989). Furosemide or metolazone may correct hyponatremia, but additional sodium chloride may be needed. The hypertension often responds to treatment with an angiotensin-converting enzyme inhibitor and a loop diuretic. Renal sonography has superseded excretory urography and histology as the main diagnostic procedure. The sonographic appearances in the newborn are large kidneys, increased echogenicity of the parenchyma, loss of corticomedullary differentiation, and loss of central echo complex (Metreweli and Garel, 1980). Dilated collecting tubules are seen on ultrasonography. The cortex is preserved, and the papillae are echogenic. There may be macrocysts that are less than 2 cm in diameter. The liver is echodense, and biliary ducts are dilated. It is important to note that renal ultrasonography does not always distinguish between autosomal recessive polycystic kidneys and autosomal dominant polycystic kidneys, or between autosomal recessive polycystic kidneys and transient nephromegaly (Stapelton et al, 1981), or between autosomal recessive polycystic kidneys and glomerulocystic kidneys (Fitch and Stapleton, 1986). At postmortem, the kidneys are enlarged, are spongy, and maintain their renal contours (Figure 83-3, *A*). The dilated collecting ducts are arranged perpendicular to the surface of the kidney (Figure 83-3, *B*). There are no dysplastic elements. The liver is always involved; portal areas are expanded by increased numbers of dilated bile ductules surrounded by fibrous tissue. The dilated ductules may become cystic. The liver cells are normal. Autosomal recessive polycystic kidneys can be diagnosed after 24 weeks' gestation by ultrasonographic demonstration of large hyperechogenic kidneys, oligo-hydramnios, and an empty bladder (Romero et al, 1984). Most infants who are symptomatic at birth die from respiratory or renal causes. Respiratory and renal function can improve in some cases, and a small number of patients who survive the neonatal period may maintain adequate renal function into adolescence. Massively enlarged kidneys may cause feeding difficulties and respiratory distress by restricting diaphragmatic excursion, and therefore bilateral nephrectomies may improve both ventilation and feeding tolerance (Beaunoyer et al, 2007). Peritoneal dialysis may then be performed until the infant can have a kidney transplant (Sumfest et al, 1993). Seventy-five percent of infants with ARPKD who survive to 1 year of age can live for more than 15 years (Kaplan et al, 1989).

Autosomal Dominant Polycystic Kidney Disease [McKusick #179300]

The incidence of ADPKD in live-born infants is 1 to 3 per 100,000. Although this is the second most common autosomal dominant mutation in humans, with an estimated prevalence in the population of between 1 in 200 and 1 in 1000, ADPKD rarely presents with clinical findings at birth (Fick et al, 1993). The prognosis is favorable in most children with prenatal or neonatal ADPKD throughout childhood (Boyer et al, 2007). The inheritance is autosomal dominant with variable expression. At ages above 10 years, and especially over 30 years, a negative ultrasound examination provides reassurance for persons at 50% risk (Bear et al, 1992). Occasionally an infant may have symptoms before the parent. Prediction by DNA analysis complements ultrasonography for detection, is not age-dependent, and may not be informative in every family. Mutations in at least three genes cause ADPKD. *PKD1*, in 85% of families, is caused by a mutation on chromosome 16p13.3 (Breuning et al, 1987). Patients with *PKD2*, in about 5% of families, have the same phenotype as *PKD1*, and the mutation is at chromosomal locus 4q21 (Peters et al, 1993). Intrafamilial phenotypic variability indicates that both genetic background and environmental factors are important. The specific gene involved is an important factor with end-stage renal disease occurring on average 20 years later in *PKD2* (Rossetti et al, 2007). The location of the third gene *(PKD3)* is unknown. Polycystin-1, the *PKD1* gene product, is a matrix receptor that links the extracellular matrix to the actin cytoskeleton via focal adhesion proteins (Wilson, 2001). The *PKD2* gene encodes polycystin-2, a member of the transient receptor protein polycystin family of calcium-channel proteins (Mochizuki et al, 1996). The two gene products, polycystin-1 and polycystin-2, are thought to form a receptor channel complex that localizes to the primary cilium (Nauli, 2003). The mean age at onset of end-stage renal disease in individuals with *PKD1* is 56.7 ± 1.9 years, as compared with 69.4 ± 1.7 years in those with *PKD2*. Hypertension and renal impairment are less frequent and occur later in the *PKD2* families. The kidneys are enlarged and lobular, and the calyces are stretched and distorted by cysts, which produce smooth or irregular indentations. Numerous cysts of various sizes are seen in the parenchyma of severely affected

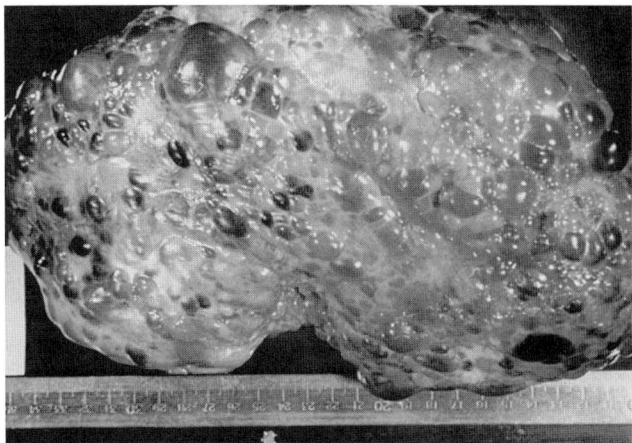

FIGURE 83-4 **Autosomal dominant polycystic kidney.** The kidney is large, and there are numerous cysts on the surface.

patients. Post mortem, the kidneys are large with numerous round protuberances on their surfaces (Figure 83-4). Cysts are irregularly dispersed through the parenchyma and arise from many nephron segments. Ultrasonography and computed tomography (CT) scans are more sensitive methods for detecting cysts than intravenous urography. Cysts may be seen in liver, pancreas, and spleen.

ADPKD may be detected prenatally by ultrasonography (Sedman et al, 1987). Some patients have the oligohydramnios sequence, enlarged kidneys, and hematuria. Associated abnormalities reported in infants with ADPKD are endocardial fibroelastosis, an intracerebral vascular anomaly, pyloric stenosis, and hepatic fibrosis (Cobben et al, 1990). The finding of hepatic fibrosis in some patients can make differentiation between ARPKD and ADPKD difficult. In the past, about half the reported patients with ADPKD presenting in utero or in the first few months of life died before 1 year, but more recent studies of larger numbers of patients show a much more optimistic prognosis (Fick et al, 1993). Adult males are also at increased risk for fertility problems including necrospermia, immotile sperm, seminal vesicle cysts, and ejaculatory duct cysts (Vora et al, 2008).

Tuberous Sclerosis [McKusick #191100]

Tuberous sclerosis (TS) is characterized by hamartomata in numerous organs. Rarely, polycystic or unilateral cystic disease is found in a newborn in which a diagnosis of TS is made later (Brook-Carter et al, 1994; Sampson et al, 1997). Renal cysts or polycystic disease in TS are identical to simple cysts or ADPKD in their ultrasonographic, intravenous urogram, and CT scan appearances. Nonsymptomatic renal lesions (cysts and/or angiomyolipomas) occur in about 60% of individuals with TS (Cook, 1996). Other features include skin lesions in 96%, epilepsy, learning difficulties, and behavioral problems. Cardiac rhabdomyoma(s) detected on routine antenatal sonography, cerebral lesions, hydrops, and stillbirth are the major presenting findings in the fetus, whereas respiratory distress, arrhythmias, murmurs, and cardiomegaly are the main signs initially in the neonate. Skin lesions and retinal hamartomas are rarely noted at birth (Isaacs et al,

2009). Ash leaf hypopigmented nevi may be the only skin manifestation of TS in infancy, and babies with polycystic kidneys must be examined for the nevi under ultraviolet light. Shagreen patches and adenoma sebaceum develop before 14 years; nail fibromas appear after 5 years and increase with age. Ventricular rhabdomyomas and seizures may occur in infancy. Patients usually survive to adolescence and adulthood, but those with early-onset polycystic kidneys may develop end-stage renal failure. Inheritance is autosomal dominant with variable expression within a family, nonpenetrance of the gene, or germinal mosaicism. A parent with the gene may appear unaffected, so the parents must also be examined clinically and radiologically for stigmata of TS. TS is linked in half the cases to a gene TSC1 (hamartin) on 9q34. In other patients TS is linked to a marker gene, *TSC2* (tuberin), near the locus for *PKD1* on 16p13.3 (van Slegtenhorst et al, 1998; Kandt et al, 1992). Large deletions can result in *PKD1/TSC2* contiguous gene deletion syndrome.

CYSTIC KIDNEYS WITH AUTOSOMAL RECESSIVE INHERITANCE

Meckel Syndrome (Meckel-Gruber Syndrome) [McKusick #249000]

Polycystic kidneys are an obligatory feature; a consistent feature is hepatic fibrosis with variable reactive ductule proliferation, dilatation, and portal fibrosis. Other features include a sloping forehead, posterior encephalocele, microphthalmia, postaxial polydactyly, ambiguous genitalia, and cleft lip and palate. Complete or partial situs inversus has been reported. Fifty percent of the cases feature oligohydramnios with perinatal death. In Goldston syndrome there are cystic kidneys, hepatic fibrosis, and Dandy-Walker malformation. This, and other syndromes, may be part of the spectrum of MKS or discrete entities (Gloeb et al, 1989). The incidence of MKS is 1 in 9000 newborns. Inheritance is autosomal recessive with variable expression within and among families (Fraser and Lytwyn, 1981). Six gene loci on 17q22-q23 (*MKS 1*), 11q13, (*MKS 2*), 8q24 (*MKS3/TMEM67*), 12q21 (*CEP290/NPHP6*), 16q21 (*RPGRIP1L*), and 4p15 (*CC2D2A/MKS6*) have been associated with MKS (Baala et al, 2007; Delous et al, 2007; Morgan et al, 2002; Roume et al, 1998; Tallila et al, 2008). The *MKS1* and *MKS3* genes encoding the Meckel's syndrome type 1and 3 proteins have recently been identified and appear to affect ciliary function. There is considerable phenotypic overlap among several of the ciliopathies in MKS. *MKS3, RPGRIP1L,* and *CC2D2A* gene mutations have also been reported in patients with Joubert's syndrome (Arts et al, 2007; Brancati et al, 2009; Gorden et al, 2008), MKS1 mutations have been seen in patients with Bardet-Biedl syndrome (Leitch et al, 2008), and *CEP290/NPHP6* mutations have been reported in patients with Bardet-Biedl syndrome, Joubert's syndrome, and Senior-Loken syndrome (Brancati et al, 2009; Helou et al, 2007; Leitch et al, 2008). Prenatal diagnosis is possible by ultrasonography and by detection of increased alpha-fetoprotein levels in amniotic fluid.

TABLE 83-1 Genetics of Bardet-Biedl Syndrome

Gene	Chromosome	Protein
BS1	11q13	BBS protein 1
BBS2	16q21	BBS protein 2
ARL6/BBS3	3p12-q13	ADP-ribosylation factor-like protein 6; BBS protein 3
BBS4	15q22.3	BBS protein 4
BBS5	2q31	BBS protein 5
MKKS/BBS6	20p12	McKusick-Kaufman/Bardet-Biedl syndromes putative chaperonin; BBS protein 6
BBS7	4q27	BBS protein 7
TTC8/BBS8	14q32.11	Tetratricopeptide repeat protein 8; BBS protein 8
PTHB1/BBS9	7p14	Parathyroid hormone-responsive B1 gene protein; BBS protein 9
BBS10	12q	BBS protein 10
TRIM32/BBS11	9p33.1	Tripartite motif-containing protein 32; BBS protein 11

Bardet-Biedl Syndrome (Laurence-Moon-Bardet-Biedl Syndrome) [McKusick #209900]

Bardet-Biedl syndrome (BBS) is a multisystemic disorder characterized by renal disease, mental retardation, obesity, postaxial polydactyly, hypogenitalism, and retinal degeneration. All patients have some abnormalities in renal structure, function, or both. Most have minor functional abnormalities and radiological appearances of calyceal clubbing, calyceal cysts, and medullary or cortical cysts. Other manifestations include diabetes mellitus, heart disease, dental malformations, situs inversus, and hepatic fibrosis. Because of the late onset of symptoms, the diagnosis of BBS is usually made during childhood. Obesity appears around age 2 to 3 years, and retinal degeneration becomes clinically apparent only at age 8 years. The only features that may be present at birth are polydactyly, kidney anomaly, hepatic fibrosis, and genital or heart malformations (Beales et al, 1999). Occasionally, the syndrome manifests in utero with large echogenic or cystic kidneys (Karmous-Benailly et al, 2005). Most cases are autosomal recessive, although triallelic inheritance has been described. Currently, 14 genes (*BBS1 to BBS14*) have been identified (Table 83-1) (Quinlan et al, 2008).

Jeune Asphyxiating Thoracic Dystrophy Syndrome [McKusick #208500]

Jeune asphyxiating thoracic dystrophy syndrome has autosomal recessive inheritance and variable expression. Respiratory distress, dysostoses, renal cystic disease, and congenital hepatic fibrosis characterize the disorder. Dysostoses include short ribs, small and long thoracic cage, small pelvis, trident acetabular margins, short and thick second and third phalanges, cone-shaped epiphyses, handlebar clavicle, and mesomelic shortening of the limbs (Donaldson et al, 1985). Three different morphologic lesions of the kidneys have been described: (1) dilated proximal and distal tubules and Bowman capsule with interstitial fibrosis, (2) cystic dysplasia and disorganized renal architecture, and (3) chronic tubulointerstitial disease resembling juvenile nephronophthisis. At least three genetic loci have been associated with this genetically heterogeneous condition. One locus has been mapped to 15q13 (Morgan et al, 2003), a second on 3q26.1 in the region encoding the intraflagellar transport protein 80 (IFT80) gene (Beales et al, 2007), and the third on chromosome 11q22.3 in the region of dynein cytoplasmic heavy chain 2 (DNCH2) gene (Dagoneau et al, 2009). The differential diagnosis includes Ellis-van Creveld syndrome, Saldino-Noonan short rib–polydactyly syndrome (type II), and Majewski short rib–polydactyly syndrome, and Naumoff syndrome (type III). Survivors develop metaphyseal dysplasia with short-limb dwarfism. Treatment of renal failure may require dialysis and transplantation. Prenatal diagnosis by ultrasonography is possible by 18 weeks (Elejade et al, 1985).

Renal-Hepatic-Pancreatic Dysplasia (Ivemark's Syndrome)

Inheritance of Ivemark's syndrome is autosomal recessive. Patients may have the oligohydramnios sequence. The kidneys may be dysplastic with peripheral cortical cysts, primitive collecting ducts, glomerular cysts, and metaplastic cartilage (Bernstein et al, 1987). There is fibrosis of the liver and pancreas. Most patients die from respiratory insufficiency in the newborn period. Inheritance is autosomal recessive.

GLOMERULOCYSTIC KIDNEYS

In the purest form of glomerulocystic kidney, there are dilated Bowman spaces, with few or no cysts in the tubule (Bernstein, 1993). The rest of the renal architecture is normal. The kidneys may be large or small. The liver is normal. Glomerular cysts are also seen in obstructive uropathy, in autosomal dominant polycystic kidneys, in association with malformations of other organs, in dysplastic kidneys, and in infants whose mothers received phenacetin or indomethacin during pregnancy. Glomerular cysts are often subcapsular and may contain more than one glomeruloid structure (Figure 83-5). Glomerulocystic kidneys may occur sporadically. Autosomal dominant inheritance of the hypoplastic subtype is found in some kindreds in association with mutations in the gene encoding hepatocyte nuclear factor (HNF)-1β and early-onset diabetes (Bingham et al, 2001).

DYSGENETIC KIDNEYS

Renal Tubular Dysgenesis (Congenital Hypernephronic Nephromegaly With Tubular Dysgenesis) [McKusick #267430]

Clinical features of congenital hypernephronic nephromegaly with tubular dysgenesis, an autosomal recessive condition, include late-onset oligohydramnios after

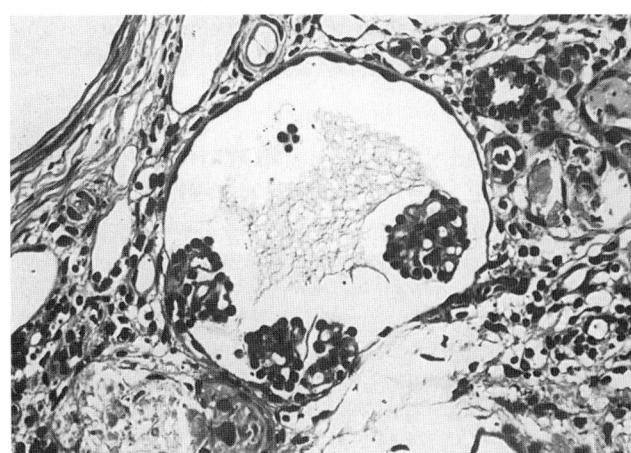

FIGURE 83-5 Glomerulocystic kidneys. Photomicrograph of glomerulus with three glomeruloid structures in a dilated Bowman capsule.

24 weeks of gestation and large nonfunctioning kidneys (Allanson et al, 1992). The calvaria may be underdeveloped with wide sutures. Similar calvarial anomalies occur in patients with the Finnish-type congenital nephrotic syndrome and in infants exposed in utero to angiotensin-converting enzyme inhibitors. The kidneys are enlarged symmetrically by ultrasonography, and the corticomedullary junction is poorly defined. There is an apparent increase in the number of glomeruli and there are immature tubules without proximal convolutions. Prenatal diagnosis is not possible before 20 weeks. Mutations in genes encoding renin, angiotensinogen, angiotensin-converting enzyme, and angiotensin II receptor type 1 have been found (Gribouval et al, 2005). Most patients die in the neonatal period.

OVERGROWTH SYNDROMES

Beckwith-Wiedemann syndrome, Simpson-Golabi-Behmel syndrome, and Perlman syndrome are overgrowth syndromes, with overlapping features including kidneys that may be abnormal at birth (Coppin et al, 1997).

Beckwith-Wiedemann Syndrome [McKusick #130650]

Patients may have nephromegaly, Wilms' tumor, medullary renal cysts, calyceal diverticula, hydronephrosis, and nephrolithiasis (Choyke et al, 1998). The syndrome is caused by mutation of a gene encoding human cyclin-dependent kinase inhibitor p57 (KIP2) at chromosomal locus 11p15.5 (Matsuoka et al, 1996). Patients should be screened by renal ultrasound for Wilms' tumor every 3 months for the first 7 years.

Perlman Syndrome With Renal Hamartomas, Nephroblastomatosis, and Fetal Gigantism [McKusick #267000]

Features include polyhydramnios, macrosomia and bilateral nephromegaly with nephroblastomatosis, visceromegaly, cryptorchidism, diaphragmatic hernia, interrupted aortic arch, hypospadias, polysplenia and renal findings of dysplasia, microcysts, and nephrogenic rests (Greenberg et al, 1988; Schilke et al, 2000). Inheritance is autosomal recessive.

Simpson-Golabi-Behmel Syndrome, Type 1; SGBS1 [McKusick #312870]

Features include pre- and postnatal overgrowth, "coarse" face, hypertelorism, broad nasal root, cleft palate, full lips with a midline groove of the lower lip, grooved tongue with tongue tie, prominent mandible, congenital heart defects, arrhythmias, supernumerary nipples, splenomegaly, large dysplastic kidneys, cryptorchidism, hypospadias, skeletal abnormalities, and postaxial hexadactyly. Inheritance is X-linked. Some cases are caused by mutation in the gene for glypican-3, which maps to Xq26 (Pilia et al, 1996). A second SGB syndrome locus, SGBS2, is located on Xp22 (Brzustowicz et al, 1999).

IN UTERO EXPOSURE TO TERATOGENS

No convincing proof of a cause-and-effect relationship has been provided for associations of in utero exposure to teratogens. Urogenital anomalies are found occasionally in infants exposed in utero to valproic acid and other anticonvulsant agents (Ardinger et al, 1988). Maternal cocaine (and polydrug) use may produce genitourinary abnormalities (Chasnoff et al, 1988). Indomethacin may cause renal dysgenesis in fetal monkeys and possibly in humans exposed early in utero to prolonged high doses (Kaplan et al, 1994). Prenatal lead exposure is incriminated as a possible cause of the VACTERL association (Levine and Muenke, 1991). Glomerulocystic disease was reported in an infant exposed to phenacetin and salicylate in utero (Krous et al, 1977). Unilateral renal agenesis and abnormalities of position were noted in three infants exposed prenatally to warfarin (Hall, 1989).

INBORN ERRORS OF METABOLISM

Several inborn errors of energy metabolism that manifest in the newborn period have morphologic and functional abnormalities of the kidneys. These are all rare conditions.

Glutaric Aciduria Type II (Multiple Acyl-CoA Dehydrogenase Deficiencies)

The clinical features of type IIa neonatal onset form include prematurity, hypotonia, hepatomegaly, nephromegaly, craniofacial anomalies, rocker-bottom feet, anterior abdominal wall defects, and external genital anomalies. An odor of sweaty feet may be present. In affected children there is a high degree of phenotypic variability ranging from milder forms susceptible to decompensation only at times of metabolic stress, to severe forms resulting in congenital anomalies and perinatal death. Within 24 hours there is severe hypoglycemia but no ketosis, a metabolic acidosis with an increased undetermined anion gap, lactic acidosis, and mild hyperammonemia. Elevated levels of organic acids are found in body fluids. Renal cystic dysplasia occurs in many cases (Wilson et al, 1989). The deficiencies in electron transfer flavoprotein or electron transfer ubiquinone oxidoreductase are inherited as autosomal recessive traits. Prenatal diagnosis may be possible by assaying enzyme in amniocytes and/or elevated glutaric acid in amniotic fluid. Ultrasonography in utero may show enlarged cystic kidneys. Treatment with a high-calorie, low-fat, low-protein diet has been tried. Oral supplements of L-carnitine and riboflavin may result in significant improvement.

Zellweger Cerebro-hepato–renal Syndrome [McKusick #214100]

Clinical features are similar to glutaric aciduria type II with profound hypotonia, nystagmus, cataracts (oil droplets), pigmentary retinopathy, optic disc pallor, and stippled epiphyses of patella and acetabulum. Odor is not abnormal. Most cases are associated with mutations in members of the peroxisomal AAA-type ATPase family (PEX gene). All peroxisomal functions are abnormal: elevated plasma very long-chain fatty acids, bile acids, pipecolic acid, phytanic acid, and urine dicarboxylic acids, and low cholesterol and triglycerides. Pathologic features are cortical renal cysts, micronodular cirrhosis, brain heterotopias, abnormal brain gyri, and absence of the corpus callosum. Inheritance is autosomal recessive. Prenatal diagnosis is possible by enzyme assays in amniocytes or chorionic villus cells. Most patients die within 6 months, but those with a milder form can survive into adolescence with retardation, deafness, and seizures.

Carbohydrate-Deficient Glycoprotein Syndrome/Congenital Disorders of Glycosylation

Multiple renal microcysts are found in the carbohydrate-deficient glycoprotein syndrome (Strom et al, 1993). There is multisystem involvement with olivopontocerebellar atrophy, retinitis pigmentosa, testicular atrophy, hypothyroidism, and immune deficiency. This is a heterogeneous group of autosomal recessive genetic conditions caused by the abnormal synthesis of glycan moieties or their attachment to glycoconjugates. Several glycoproteins are deficient in their carbohydrate moieties. The prognosis is highly variable.

Complete references used in this text can be found online at www.expertconsult.com

DEVELOPMENTAL ABNORMALITIES OF THE GENITOURINARY SYSTEM

Stephen A. Zderic and Sarah M. Lambert

This chapter reviews the most common clinical presentations that prompt urologic consultation during the neonatal period. Anomalies of the urinary tract and disorders of the external genitalia are reviewed respectively. Advances in imaging technology and the widespread use of screening prenatal sonography have resulted in antenatal detection of many urinary tract anomalies and disorders of the external genitalia. This early detection results in earlier management and intervention, thereby decreasing the number of neonates presenting with urosepsis in the postnatal period. These benefits are tempered by the heightened concern raised and often excessive evaluation that is initiated when anatomic variants or incidental findings are discovered (Thomas, 2008). It must also be remembered that not all urologic conditions will be revealed by prenatal sonography. Additionally, these technologic advances only benefit expectant mothers with access to medical care.

PRENATAL DIAGNOSIS

The widespread use of ultrasonography in screening for fetal anomalies has profoundly changed neonatal urology within the past two decades. In optimal circumstances, prenatal consultation was obtained and the urologist and family have already discussed the relevant urologic issues affecting the fetus. These families have the potential for a greater understanding of the clinical parameters and are able to plan for evaluation and management in the postnatal period. Two decades ago, most children with congenital anomalies of the urinary tract presented with urosepsis. In contrast, prenatal ultrasonography now identifies patients at risk; if indicated, in utero decompression of an obstructed urinary tract (i.e., from posterior urethral valves or ureterocele) may be performed, or antibiotic prophylaxis may be initiated in the immediate postnatal period. Additionally, intervention can occur at an earlier date. Prenatal diagnosis has also led to a decrease in the incidence of several severe congenital anomalies, such as prune-belly syndrome, posterior urethral valves, and spina bifida, because some parents decide to terminate the pregnancy (Cromie et al, 2001).

Primarily because of the high fetal urine output, most prenatally discovered cases of hydronephrosis will be benign and self-limiting in nature. Therefore, it is important to give realistic advice and reassurance in cases of functional hydronephrosis. With severe congenital anatomic obstructions, fetal intervention may be considered (Biard et al, 2005). Recent studies suggest that such interventions offer little benefit to renal function (Coplen et al, 1996) but may serve to facilitate pulmonary development. In addition to the obstructive uropathies, disorders of sexual differentiation and other disorders of the external genitalia are being detected with prenatal sonography (Rintoul and Crombleholme, 2002).

HYDRONEPHROSIS

As mentioned earlier, most patients with prenatally diagnosed hydronephrosis have transient dilatations of the urinary tract that may reflect a more distensible fetal urinary tract and large volumes of dilute fetal urine. With the cardiovascular and hormonal changes in the immediate postnatal period, urine output per kilogram of body weight decreases, resulting in the resolution of prenatally detected "functional" renal and ureteral dilatation. In addition, the ureter may contain small kinks or folds that normalize with time. The potential explanations for spontaneous improvement in these systems is seemingly endless. Even though most dilatations of the fetal urinary tract prove to be of no long-term significance, a small subset of affected patients will prove to have anatomic obstructions requiring surgical correction (Lee et al, 2006).

The neonatal evaluation of antenatal hydronephrosis is influenced by gender, the presence or absence of hydronephrosis, and laterality of hydronephrosis. The rigor of the initial evaluation varies considerably (Estrada, 2008; Estrada et al, 2009; Yerkes et al, 1999) (Figure 84-1). Bilateral hydroureteronephrosis in a boy should raise concerns regarding the presence of posterior urethral valves (PUVs). PUVs can be diagnosed by performing an ultrasound examination and voiding cystourethrogram (VCUG) within 24 hours of birth. Unilateral hydronephrosis in a boy or girl can be evaluated by performing an ultrasound of the kidneys and bladder at 2 to 5 days of age. Performing an ultrasound study too early in the first postnatal hours may show minimal to no hydronephrosis, resulting from the significant and physiologic decrease in urine output during the period of transition to extrauterine life. In these cases, a follow-up study should be performed to ensure that, with the ensuing increase in the urine output over the first few days, the collecting system remains unobstructed (Dejter and Gibbons, 1989). For patients with persisting unilateral hydronephrosis, a VCUG and mercaptoacetyltriglycine (MAG3) or renal diethylenetriaminepentaacetic acid (DTPA) renal scan should be performed at about 1 month of age. In the interim, antimicrobial prophylaxis is essential, usually one dose of amoxicillin (12.5 mg/kg) at bedtime. The algorithm presented in Figure 84-1 represents one such approach to the management of neonatal hydronephrosis, which seeks to maximize safety while avoiding exposures to invasive studies and radiation exposures in situations that are deemed to be low yield.

Ample controversy exists concerning some of the fine points of this management algorithm. Because 20% of children with prenatal hydronephrosis have reflux, should all children get a VCUG irrespective of their first ultrasound findings? If results on their initial ultrasound examination are negative, should these children then be placed on antimicrobial prophylaxis until their next ultrasound study is done and judged to be normal? Yerkes et al (1999) have suggested that for patients with mild pelviectasis and no caliectasis or hydroureter, the diagnostic yield of the VCUG is low, and the study may be deferred. Other authors argue in favor of a VCUG for all patients with a prenatal diagnosis of hydronephrosis (Estrada et al, 2009; Herndon et al, 1999). In support of more aggressive screening for these patients, Walsh et al (2007), using a Washington state registry, have shown that infants with an antenatal diagnosis of hydronephrosis have a 12-fold higher risk of being hospitalized for pyelonephritis within the 1st year of life. Further outcome studies are essential to help drive refinement of such algorithms (Estrada, 2008). It is important to remember that while the urologic

issues are being sorted out, antibiotic prophylaxis is cost-effective and protects against urosepsis. Therefore, when the diagnosis is unclear, the clinician should provide empiric antibiotic prophylaxis.

OBSTRUCTIVE UROPATHY

URETEROPELVIC JUNCTION OBSTRUCTION

Ureteropelvic junction (UPJ) obstruction is the most common obstructive uropathy in children. Ultrasonography will reveal a dilated renal pelvis with or without caliectasis, and the absence of ureteral dilatation (Figure 84-2). Conversely, a dilated distal ureter can be observed with uretero-vesical junction obstruction, megaureter, vesicoureteral reflux, or ureteral ectopia. The sonographic appearance of a UPJ obstruction is not always predictive of function. Many infants with fairly impressive dilatation of the renal pelvis in the neonatal period demonstrate partial or complete resolution of their hydronephrosis with preservation of renal function (see Figure 84-2). Functional imaging is often obtained before any surgical repair. Although any kidney with an anteroposterior diameter greater than 2 cm has a greater risk of functional compromise (Ransley et al, 1990), many patients demonstrate stable renal function over time (Ulman et al, 2000). DTPA or MAG-3 renal scans allow for careful selection of those patients with a loss of function as defined by a decrease in glomerular filtration rate. The degree of functional impairment necessary to prompt surgical intervention remains controversial. Some authorities advocate intervention only if the differential function in the affected kidney falls below 35% (Cartwright et al, 1992), whereas others recommend intervention at 40% differential function (Chertin et al, 2006). Magnetic resonance imaging (MRI) urogram represents a newer imaging modality that provided functional and anatomic information in one study. Although many centers still rely on the use of a carefully performed diuretic renogram with furosemide washout curves to identify those patients whose urinary tract is truly obstructed or wide open (Conway and Maizels, 1992), there is a tendency toward the use of the MRI urogram in situations that are equivocal or complex (McMann et al, 2006). Given the expense of MRI as well as the need for sedation, this may be a reasonable approach.

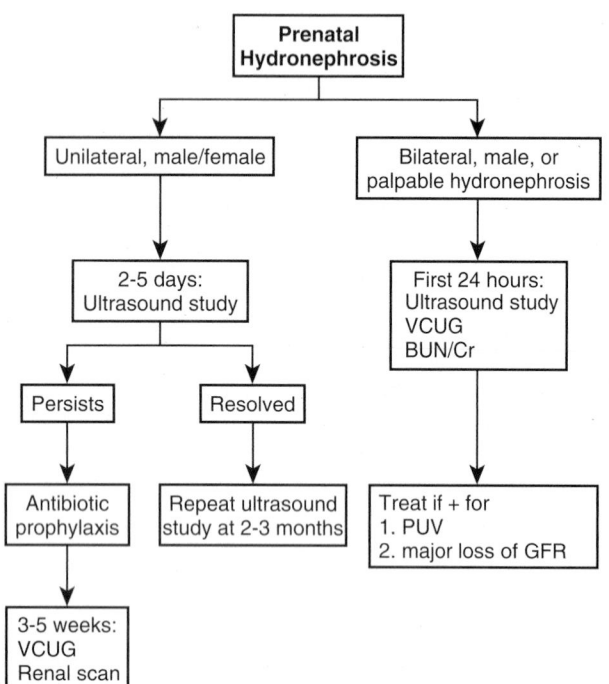

FIGURE 84-1 **An algorithm for the approach to the work-up of a patient with antenatally diagnosed hydronephrosis.** With further experience and clinical outcome studies, it may be possible to better select which patients require a voiding cystourethrogram *(VCUG)* and renal MAG3 on DTPA scan. *BUN,* Blood urea nitrogen; *Cr,* serum creatinine; *GFR,* glomerular filtration rate; *PUV,* posterior urethral valve.

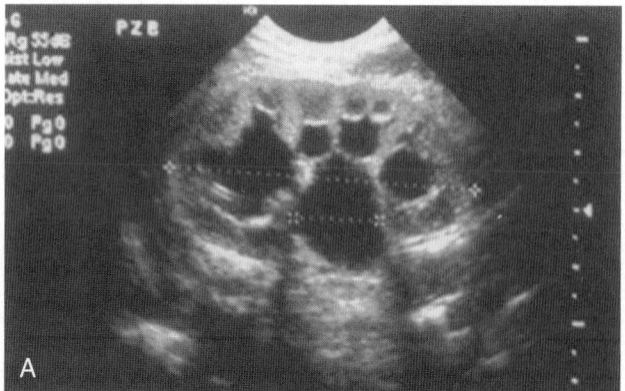
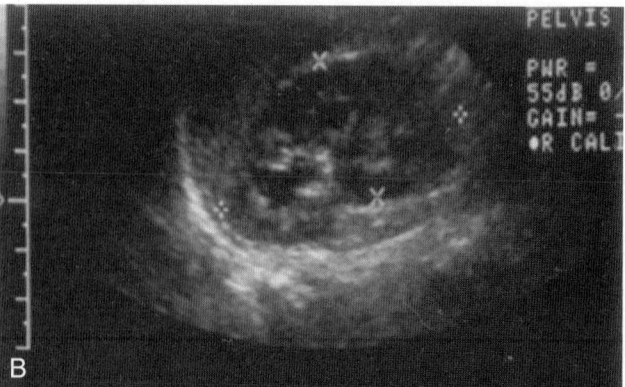

FIGURE 84-2 An example of antenatal hydronephrosis consistent with a partial ureteropelvic junction obstruction **(A)** that spontaneously resolved over a 6-month interval **(B).**

Many patients will demonstrate good function and rapid washout curves despite a significant degree of hydronephrosis (Figure 84-3). For those patients in whom a UPJ obstruction is diagnosed by sonography, and in whom the renal scan shows diminished function, pyeloplasty is indicated. Antimicrobial prophylaxis is not effective in children with a poorly functioning kidney because the affected kidney will not deliver enough antibiotic into the collecting system. As a result, the child remains at risk for urosepsis. It is important to note that with most severe UPJ obstructions, the kidney does not recover normal function following surgical correction. In addition, infection in the presence of a UPJ obstruction further increases the risk of permanent renal damage. Unfortunately, no preoperative test will predict recovery of renal function following relief of obstructive uropathy.

Finally, few prenatally diagnosed cases of UPJ obstruction require immediate repair. These cases rarely result in palpable hydronephrosis, and most affected infants will have good renal function. Therefore, a nonemergent evaluation and surgical repair if necessary can be performed at 3 to 6 weeks of life. This group of patients may be divided into three subgroups (Homsy et al, 1990). One third will demonstrate severe obstruction and require intervention, one third will have a normal postnatal evaluation, and the remaining one third may be observed with serial sonograms and renal scans. Of this observed group, up to one third of the patients may ultimately need surgical correction. The postnatal evaluation and treatment of prenatally diagnosed hydronephrosis must contain two key elements: (1) antimicrobial prophylaxis and (2) thorough follow-up evaluation. Although expectant management may eliminate unnecessary surgical procedures that may offer little benefit, this advantage mandates careful follow-up evaluation (Cordero et al, 2009). This aspect of management must be made clear to the family in no uncertain terms.

MULTICYSTIC DYSPLASTIC KIDNEY

The diagnosis of multicystic dysplastic kidney (MCDK) is applied to a kidney that on ultrasound examination consists of multiple cysts of roughly equal size, which results in a classic "bunch of grapes" pattern and no function on a DTPA renal scan (Figure 84-4). The contralateral kidney is often hypertrophied with an increased length and width. If the MCDK has one large, centrally located cyst, it may appear similar to a severe UPJ obstruction. In these rare instances it may prove necessary to explore the kidney to see if there is any salvageable renal function that might be amenable to relief of the obstruction. In most cases of MCDK, the cysts will involute completely without intervention. There is considerable debate regarding the follow-up and indication for surgical intervention in patients with MCDK. Ultrasound imaging of the contralateral kidney is also recommended because metachronous contralateral obstruction has been reported (Weiser et al, 2002). Concerns have been raised about the occasional case reports of malignancy in MCDK. It has been estimated that 80,000 nephrectomies would have to be performed to save one patient with MCDK from developing a malignancy. In practice, if involution fails to occur by 1 to 2 years of age, simple nephrectomy is often recommended. Increasingly, surgical extirpation is performed using the techniques of modern minimally invasive surgery.

URETEROVESICAL JUNCTION OBSTRUCTION: MEGAURETER

Primary megaureters account for 15% of prenatally diagnosed cases of hydronephrosis and are characterized by pelviectasis, caliectasis, and ureteral dilatation. Ureteral dilatation is usually visualized posterior to a distended bladder. A VCUG is indicated to eliminate concomitant vesicoureteral reflux. Reflux into a partially obstructed system can occur, creating the paradoxical refluxing obstructed megaureter. Often times a VCUG reveals a

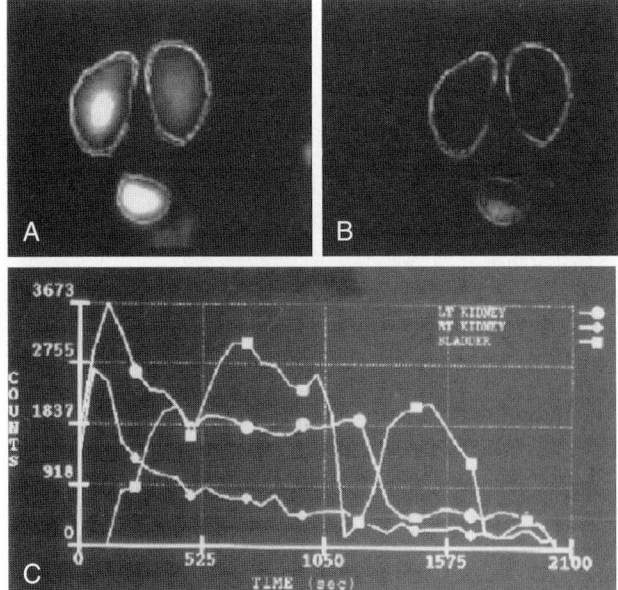

FIGURE 84-3 A, This renal MAG3 scan demonstrates equal function in the right and left kidneys but marked stasis in the left kidney. **B** and **C,** Following administration of furosemide, stasis in the left renal pelvis cleared quickly.

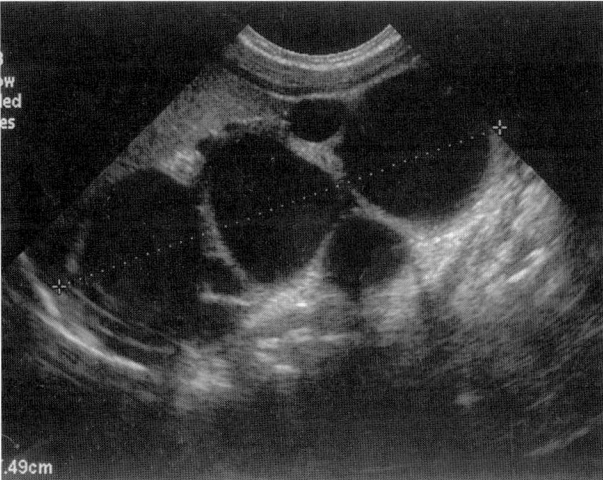

FIGURE 84-4 Sonographic view of a multicystic dysplastic kidney in which multiple cysts that do not communicate with one another are grouped together, giving the typical "bunch of grapes" appearance. No function was noted on the patient's renal scan, confirming this diagnosis.

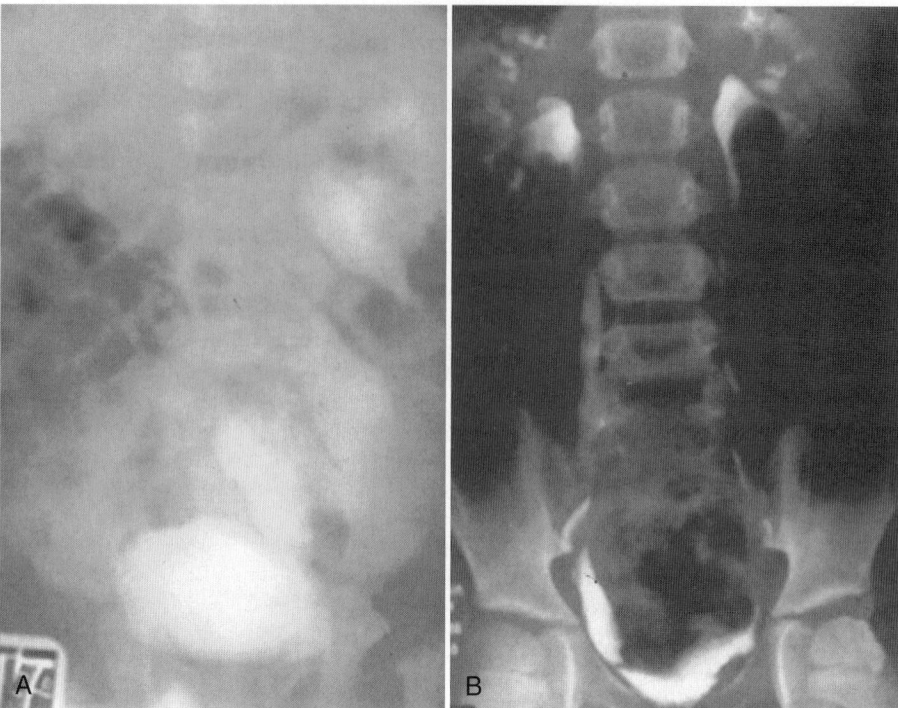

FIGURE 84-5 A, This radiograph shows significant hydroureteronephrosis that was diagnosed by antenatal sonography and was shown to be consistent with bilateral primary megaureters. Renal function was normal despite the abnormal morphologic appearance. **B,** With time, the radiographic findings showed marked improvement.

dilutional effect due to urinary stasis within the dilated ureter in comparison with the bladder. Furthermore, on the postvoid images, the contrast will often be retained within the ureter. Some investigators believe that refluxing primary megaureter should be repaired to prevent an infection in a partially obstructed system. Functional imaging such as a MAG3 renal scan or MRI urography is critical for assessing upper tract drainage (Figure 84-5). In systems with good renal function, patients may be safely managed with antimicrobial prophylaxis because of the potential for spontaneous resolution. In a longitudinal study, Shukla et al (2005) demonstrated that renal function is well preserved, and in many instances, the morphologic appearance of the system is substantially improved. However, this series also presented the rare occurrence of late-stage decompensation in a patient who required surgical intervention. It is the potential for later decompensation that prompts long-term surveillance in patients with a megaureter. Certainly if, based on poor function, surgical correction is indicated, excellent results can be obtained (Peters et al, 1989). More recent studies suggest that risk factors for decompensation and loss of function over time include a differential function <30% and ureteral diameters in excess of 1.2 cm (Chertin et al, 2008).

POSTERIOR URETHRAL VALVES

Although most PUVs are detected on prenatal sonography, the clinical manifestations vary across a wide spectrum of disease states. For example, oligohydramnios, pulmonary hypoplasia, and chronic renal insufficiency in a neonate represent a severe manifestation of PUV. In highly selected cases, extracorporeal membrane oxygenation (ECMO) has been used, and long-term survivors have been reported. Most of these survivors, however, ultimately require renal transplantation. At the other end

of the spectrum, some PUVs result in minimal functional disturbance. If the abnormality is not detected in utero, patients with PUVs may present with urosepsis. The prenatal diagnosis by ultrasound examination offers the pediatric urologist an opportunity to intervene before the obstructive uropathy is further compromised by the additional burden of infection.

The postnatal evaluation of a child with suspected PUV should begin with a renal and bladder ultrasound (Strand, 2004; Zderic, 2007). The examination should be performed before placement of a urinary catheter to reveal the anatomy of the urinary tract and the degree of distention. There will usually be severe bilateral hydroureteronephrosis. In severe cases, the renal parenchyma will be of extremely poor quality, comprising a thin rim with a highly echogenic appearance. When these findings are associated with a thick-walled bladder in a male infant, the suspected diagnosis is PUV until proven otherwise. Ultrasound examination of the bladder also may reveal a dilated posterior urethra resulting in the classic "keyhole" appearance (Figure 84-6). A catheter should be passed into the bladder and the sonographic examination repeated to document proper placement and decompression of the urinary tract. In some instances, the posterior urethra and bladder are so severely distorted that the catheter cannot pass into the bladder without extensive manipulation.

A fluoroscopic VCUG provides the definitive diagnosis of PUV. This study will demonstrate a dilated posterior urethra, valve cusps at the distal aspect of the prostatic fossa (see Figure 84-6), a heavily trabeculated bladder, and associated high-grade vesicoureteral reflux in many cases. Once the diagnosis is established, endoscopic valve ablation is indicated (Zderic, 2006). In rare instances, the pediatric urologist may opt for a temporizing vesicostomy if the neonate is premature or small for gestational age. A circumcision should be performed at the time of valve

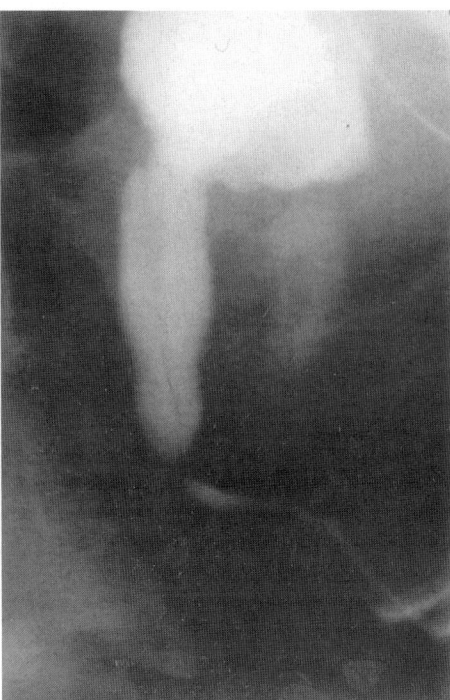

FIGURE 84-6 This voiding cystourethrogram shows a classic posterior urethral valve, with narrowing of the urethra at the most distal end of the prostate. This area corresponds to a flap of tissue that serves as an obstructing valve leaflet.

resection, to minimize the risk of urinary tract infection (Wiswell and Geschke, 1989), because these patients are at high risk.

In severe cases of PUV, decompression may result in postobstructive diuresis. For this reason, neonates with PUVs should remain in the neonatal intensive care unit (NICU) for fluid and electrolyte monitoring after catheter placement. The diuresis may be severe, necessitating hourly records of urine output with appropriate replacement of fluids and electrolytes. Failure to replace fluids and electrolytes may result in hypotension and electrolyte disturbances, thereby further aggravating renal insufficiency. Once the bladder has been decompressed with a catheter, antibiotics should be administered, and the child's medical condition must be optimized before any operative intervention is pursued.

Up to 30% of these patients may require renal replacement therapy during their lifetimes (Smith et al, 1996). In the neonatal period, renal function should be optimized and sterile urine maintained with antibiotic prophylaxis. A subset of patients with PUV present with unilateral reflux and dysplasia. This laterality acts as a "pop-off" valve to lower bladder pressure, sparing the contralateral kidney. Many such pop-off mechanisms have been described and are associated with better long-term renal (Rittenberg et al, 1988) and bladder (Kaefer et al, 1995) function. When bringing the infant home, families must be cautioned that these infants have poor urinary concentrating ability; their additional fluid requirements result in increased susceptibility to dehydration with even mild diarrhea or emesis. The initial follow-up evaluation within 1 month should include a physical examination, renal and bladder ultrasound, and serum creatinine measurement. Antibiotic prophylaxis should be maintained for a long period in these patients.

URETEROCELE

A ureterocele is a cystic dilatation of the distal ureter that protrudes into the urinary bladder and may extend past the bladder neck into the urethra. Ureteroceles are found primarily in duplex systems and are associated with the upper pole renal parenchyma. In a duplex system, the upper pole parenchyma associated with a ureterocele is usually of low volume and may even contain dysplastic elements. The ureterocele creates an obstructed system; accordingly, the prevention of urosepsis in the obstructed system is paramount. Renal-bladder ultrasound examination of a ureterocele demonstrates three characteristic findings (Figure 84-7). First, the upper pole of the duplex system will be dilated and hydronephrotic (although single systems also may contain ureteroceles). Second, significant ureteral dilatation to the level of the bladder will be present. Third, a cystic lesion within the lumen of the bladder adjacent to the bladder base will be demonstrated. A VCUG will complete the evaluation and determine whether vesicoureteral reflux is present in the ipsilateral or contralateral ureter(s). Ureteroceles may prolapse into the urethra and constitute the most common form of bladder outlet obstruction in female neonates. A prolapsed ureterocele appears as a cystic bulge within the labia and must be considered in the differential diagnosis of an introital mass.

Several surgical options exist for the management of the newborn with a ureterocele, including endoscopic puncture (Hagg et al, 2000), ureteroureterostomy (Prieto et al, 2009), upper pole partial nephrectomy, and excision of the ureterocele with ureteral reimplantation. Finally, an additional surgical approach is to perform a cutaneous ureterostomy and defer definitive lower tract reconstruction until the child is 1 to 2 years of age.

ECTOPIC URETERS

Most ectopic ureters today will be detected with prenatal sonography. This prenatal imaging ultimately results in a neonatal evaluation. Physical examination in these patients will often be unremarkable. A boy will never present with incontinence secondary to an ectopic ureter because the ureter enters the urethra proximal to the level of the external sphincter. Girls, in contrast, may present with urinary incontinence because the ureter may be ectopic to the urethra or vaginal vault. In these cases, urinary incontinence is continuous and detectable on physical examination. Addressing ectopic ureters early in life prevents the potential for urosepsis in an obstructed system and allows for normal toilet training in young girls. Historically, ectopic ureters were often diagnosed in young women with refractory and continuous urinary incontinence. The incidence of this delayed presentation has declined as a result of antenatal screening.

Most ectopic ureters occur in duplex systems and are associated with the upper pole moiety. The ultrasound findings in ectopic ureter include the presence of hydronephrosis, usually of an upper pole of a duplex system (although single systems may also be involved); a dilated distal ureter that lies behind the bladder; and extension of this dilated distal ureter distal to the bladder neck. Ultrasonography of an ectopic ureter will not demonstrate a

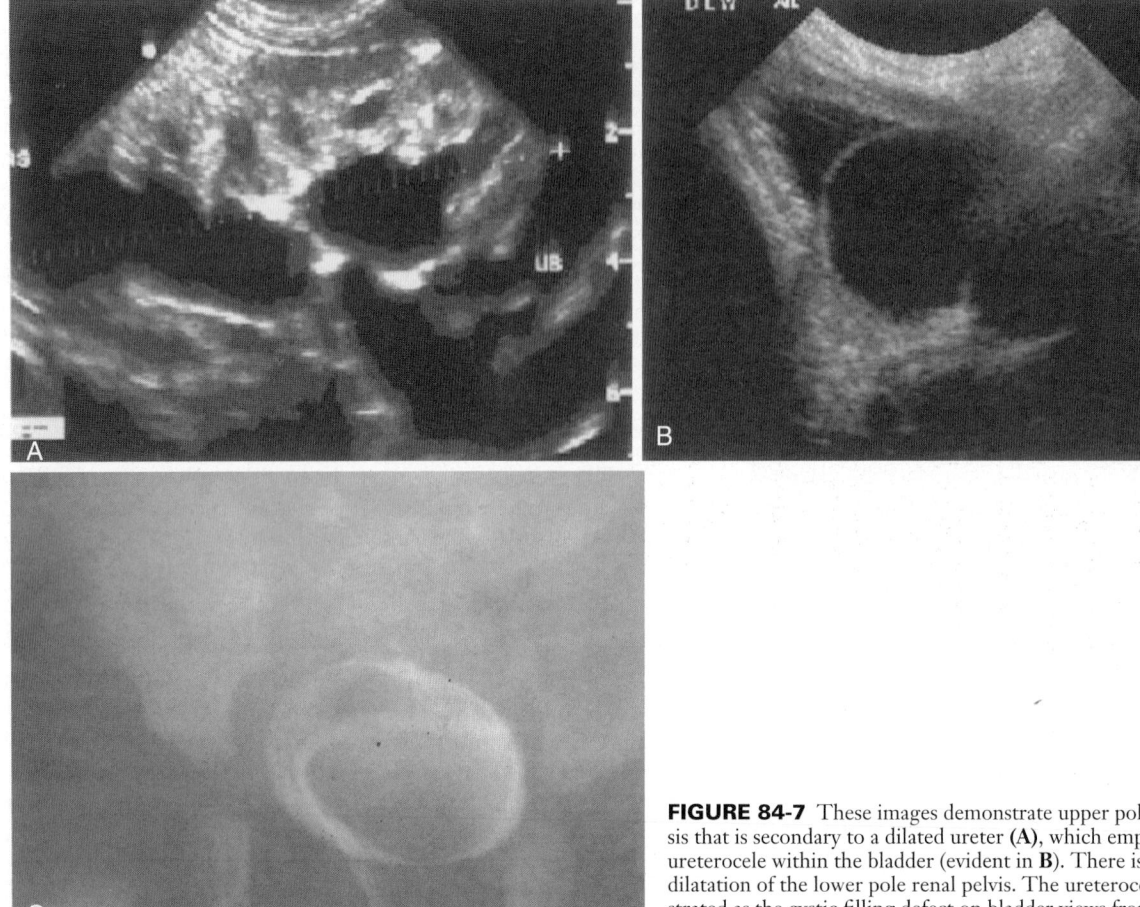

FIGURE 84-7 These images demonstrate upper pole hydronephrosis that is secondary to a dilated ureter (**A**), which empties into a larger ureterocele within the bladder (evident in **B**). There is also secondary dilatation of the lower pole renal pelvis. The ureterocele is demonstrated as the cystic filling defect on bladder views from the ultrasound study (**B**) as well as the voiding cystourethrogram (**C**).

cystic lesion within the bladder itself, as is seen with a ureterocele. The VCUG should be included in the evaluation of these patients because 70% of cases may demonstrate reflux into the ectopic ureter. It is important to note that reflux may not be apparent on the first void. Instead, it may be necessary to "cycle" the bladder several times before reflux may be demonstrated. If the ultrasound suggests an ectopic ureter, MRI urography assists in confirming the diagnosis and further evaluating the associated renal function and anatomy (Hanson et al, 2007).

An endoscopic option does not exist for repairing an ectopic ureter. The surgical options include a partial nephrectomy of the upper pole with or without excision of the distal ureter, simple nephrectomy in a nonfunctioning kidney, a cutaneous ureterostomy with delayed reimplantation and excision of the distal stump, and an immediate complete reconstruction with reimplantation and excision of the ectopic stump. The surgical management plan is usually dictated by the amount of renal function in the upper pole segment.

PRUNE-BELLY SYNDROME

Prune-belly syndrome is characterized by a triad of abdominal wall laxity, bilateral undescended testes, and a massively dilated upper urinary tract and bladder (Figure 84-8). The abdominal wall defects impact pulmonary function and development of the diaphragm as well. In severe

cases, respiratory insufficiency may mandate temporary mechanical ventilation. Historically, pulmonary complications were a common source of neonatal demise. Currently, the advent of prenatal sonography allows for earlier detection and planned neonatal interventions. These neonates are often born with significant renal dysplasia and ultimately develop end-stage renal disease. Indeed, if the nadir serum creatinine remains above 1.0 mg/dL by 1 year of age, the infant with prune-belly syndrome is more likely to develop end-stage renal disease (Noh et al, 1999). However, this disease manifests across a wide spectrum; some patients may not develop renal insufficiency until adulthood, if at all, despite the massively dilated urinary tracts.

Prune-belly syndrome is a clinical diagnosis that should prompt the initiation of prophylactic antibiotics (Strand, 2004). An ultrasound study to assess the renal parenchyma also is warranted. In contrast, a VCUG is contraindicated because of increased risk of urinary tract infections. Instrumenting a neonate with prune-belly syndrome who is voiding satisfactorily should be avoided. Catheterization procedures increase the risk of urosepsis owing to the presence of the large, distended, and poorly emptying bladder. Furthermore, the diagnosis of vesicoureteral reflux does not affect neonatal management; these infants require antibiotic prophylaxis regardless of the presence or absence of vesicoureteral reflux. The essential tenet of management in boys with prune-belly syndrome is to maintain sterile urine and institute careful follow-up evaluation

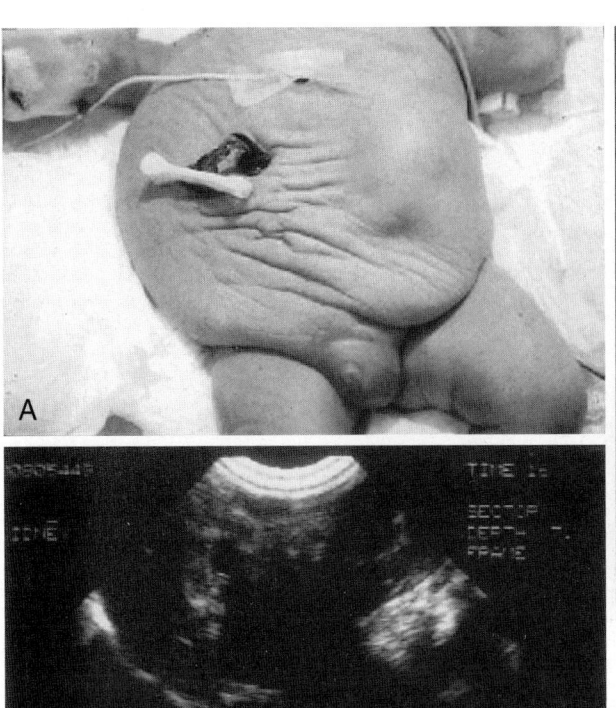

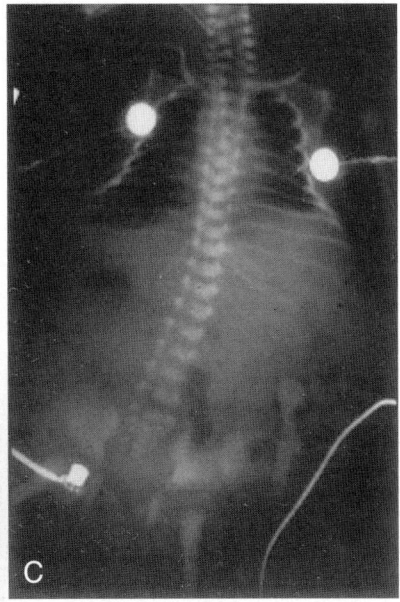

FIGURE 84-8 *(See also Color Plate 36.)* The classic wrinkled abdominal wall seen in the prune-belly syndrome is accompanied by bilateral undescended testes **(A)**. Affected patients will have marked hydronephrosis. In severe cases as illustrated here, these small kidneys may have a markedly dysmorphic sonographic appearance **(B)**, and renal insufficiency may be present from the beginning. In cases with severe renal insufficiency, pulmonary development may be compromised, as evident on the radiograph **(C)**; the patient required prolonged mechanical ventilation in the neonatal period.

(Noh et al, 1999). If the voiding dynamics in the neonatal period are significantly altered, a vesicostomy may safely decompress the urinary tract. Despite tremendous distortions of the urinary tract, the bladder may empty quite adequately, and improvement may occur over time in the quality of the upper tracts. In very rare instances where geography separates patients from specialty care, consideration is given to an aggressive reconstruction of the urinary tract (Denes et al, 2004). In general, reconstructive procedures for these children are limited to bilateral orchiopexies and abdominal wall plication.

THE EXSTROPHIES

Bladder Exstrophy

Classic bladder exstrophy manifests with a bladder plate that protrudes from the abdominal wall in the suprapubic area and extends up to just below the umbilicus (Figure 84-9). In boys, complete epispadias also results. In both male and female neonates, absence of the bladder neck results in urinary incontinence. The prenatal diagnosis of bladder exstrophy is increasingly common; failure to visualize a full bladder on several prenatal sonograms raises the suspicion of exstrophy. Classic bladder exstrophy is not associated with any other anomalies. As a result, many families decide to continue the pregnancy. Children with bladder exstrophy have an excellent prognosis and with proper management can lead nearly normal lives.

The traditional approach to the patient with classic bladder exstrophy included a staged reconstruction beginning with tubularization of the bladder plate within the first 24 hours of life (Kiddoo et al, 2004). These children were left incontinent until the age of 5 to 7 years. At that time, a surgical reconstruction of the bladder neck was performed. This repair was done at 5 to 7 years of age to facilitate self-catheterization, should catheterization be required to empty the bladder and maintain safe storage pressures. In some series, 90% of these children required long-term clean intermittent catheterization (CIC) to achieve continence and maintain stable renal function.

These adverse outcomes associated with staged exstrophy reconstruction led Mitchell and Bagli (1996) to propose a one-stage reconstruction during the 1st month of life. In boys, this procedure includes a deconstruction of the penis with separation of the corporal bodies and urethral realignment. With this method, the bladder neck is reapproximated in an attempt to provide an anatomic closure, thus creating a resistance that stimulates bladder growth; ideally, the one-stage approach will increase the percentage of patients who void spontaneously while maintaining continence.

Cloacal Exstrophy

Cloacal exstrophy manifests with several distinct clinical features (see Figure 84-9), including the presence of two bladder halves fully exposed on the anterior abdominal wall and an abdominal midline that consists of the entire cecal plate allowing for egress of stool. Commonly, a protruding loop of prolapsed distal ileum is visualized within the cecal plate. An omphalocele of variable size is located directly above these structures (Zderic et al, 2002). In addition to these obvious malformations, 50% of these children will

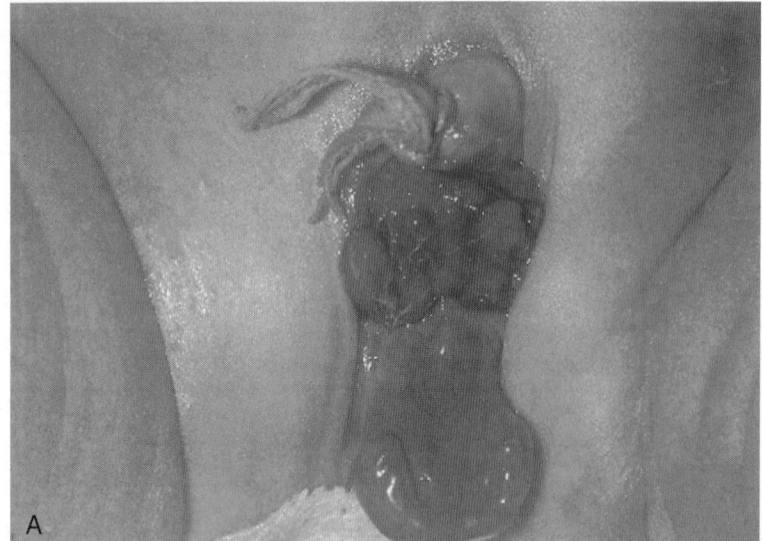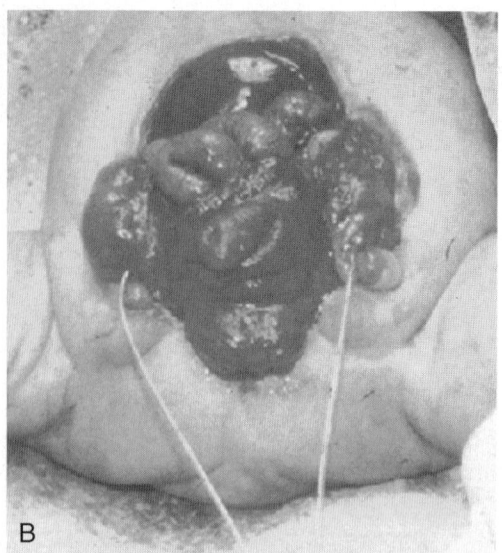

FIGURE 84-9 *(See also Color Plate 37.)* The appearance of classic bladder exstrophy **(A)**, in contrast with the dramatic appearance of cloacal exstrophy **(B)**. In cloacal exstrophy, the bladder halves are separated by the presence of a large cecal plate and a protruding ileal stump. **B,** In this intraoperative photograph, the omphalocele has been removed to expose the small bowel and liver.

have associated spinal dysraphism of various degrees. The risks of fluid loss, hypothermia, and infection from the exposed viscera mandate covering the exposed viscera with plastic wrap and immediately transferring the patient to a NICU with pediatric surgical coverage.

The first stage of reconstruction should be undertaken as soon as the child's condition has stabilized. A central line should be placed, because all of these children will have some degree of short bowel syndrome and require hyperalimentation for varying periods postoperatively. The goals of the initial surgical intervention are to tubularize the cecal plate, create a colostomy, and reapproximate the two bladder halves. In some instances, the limited size of the abdominal cavity requires a staged closure of the cecal plate followed by a closure of the omphalocele. In such an instance, the bladder halves are addressed during a second-stage repair 6 to 12 months later. For most of these children, attainment of urinary continence will require intermittent catheterization because 50% or more have a neural tube deficit.

Male infants with cloacal exstrophy will present with testes and rudimentary corporal bodies. The traditional management of these patients included gender reassignment given the minimal success of reconstructive phalloplasty. Currently, the impact of testosterone imprinting on the fetal brain is recognized and gender reassignment is avoided. These basic science data are corroborated by several reassigned patients reverting to a male role (Reiner and Gearhart, 2004). Indeed, patient dissatisfaction with gender reassignment and the newer surgical techniques available (Mitchell and Bagli, 1996) result in the maintenance of male sex of rearing.

SPINA BIFIDA

The primary goal of the urologist in management of the neonatal patient with spina bifida is the preservation of renal function. In such cases, the main detriment to renal function results from abnormal bladder function.

Traditionally, spinal closure occurs in the immediate neonatal period. However, prenatal diagnosis of spina bifida allows for fetal surgical repair in certain patients (Farmer et al, 2003). Evaluating the effects of fetal intervention on bladder function, early urodynamic outcome studies from two centers suggested no improvement in urologic outcomes between the traditional postnatal closure and the fetal repair groups (Holmes et al, 2001; Holzbeierlein et al, 2000). The difficulties encountered in interpreting data from several centers performing a complex surgical procedure under different conditions (Fichter et al, 2008) led to the establishment of an NIH-funded randomized clinical trial comparing outcomes of fetal versus neonatal spina bifida repair. With the impending completion of the MOMS trial, definitive data regarding the long-term outcome for these patients after in utero repair will be available.

Most neonates experience urinary retention after spinal closure. Clean intermittent catheterization in the immediate postclosure period prevents bladder wall overdistention. If the neonate is able to empty his or her bladder, the use of CIC allows for determination of the residual urine. If the urinary volumes on serial catheterizations remain consistently low, clean intermittent catheterization can be discontinued. A baseline renal bladder ultrasound study should be obtained within 1 week of closure to evaluate for hydronephrosis. After discharge from the NICU, a video-urodynamic assessment is performed at 4 to 8 weeks of age. The video-urodynamic studies are then repeated at 6 months of age and thereafter on a yearly basis until 5 years of age. This follow-up is necessary because up to 32% of patients with an initially favorable urodynamic profile demonstrate evidence of deterioration (Bauer et al, 1984). The purpose of the urodynamic studies is to identify early evidence of a hostile bladder. A hostile bladder has poor function that results in compromised renal function if not addressed. Grading scales have been designed to predict those infants at risk of upper urinary tract damage (Bauer et al, 1984). If there is evidence of a hostile bladder, many pediatric urologists favor the immediate institution of CIC in conjunction with antimicrobial prophylaxis and anticholinergic medications (de Jong et al, 2008; Edelstein et al, 1995; Joseph, 2008). In addition to the known benefits regarding preservation of renal function, recent studies suggest that early institution of CIC and anticholinergic therapy may also improve long-term bladder compliance and decrease the likelihood of bladder augmentation surgery (Kaefer et al, 1999b). Yearly ultrasound examinations must also be performed to ensure that the upper tracts continue to be protected. If the initial ultrasound findings are abnormal, video-urodynamic studies are performed sooner.

An additional option for treatment of a hostile neurogenic bladder is the surgical creation of a vesicostomy. Although CIC offers many benefits, compliance may be difficult with the strict regimen required to maintain safe storage pressures. Vesicostomy is a valid option because the low-pressure drainage preserves the upper urinary tract (Snyder et al, 1983) and can dramatically diminish admission rates for urosepsis. A vesicostomy is especially important in the child with spina bifida and vesicoureteral reflux because it is impossible to maintain sterile urine with use of CIC. Indeed, a child with spina bifida and vesicoureteral reflux who is maintained on CIC is at greater risk of developing pyelonephritis.

The child without evidence of a hostile bladder may be followed with ultrasound examinations every 6 to 12 months. Such children must, however, be evaluated with at least one examination annually, because the bladder may undergo degenerative changes over time, especially within the first 3 years of life. At 3 to 4 years of age, the issues of fecal and urinary continence must be addressed. These children will require fecal training and in most cases a daily enema followed by planned timed evacuation. Urinary continence is rare in these patients; most large series report that fewer than 5% to 10% of patients void to completion without incontinence. For this reason, these children must master the process of CIC. Once compliance with a CIC regimen has been established, further surgical reconstruction of the lower urinary tract may be required in order to achieve complete urinary continence.

IMPERFORATE ANUS

The diagnosis of imperforate anus prompts an immediate general surgical consultation and usually results in a diverting colostomy. It is important to recognize that affected infants often have associated urologic findings. Urologic abnormalities are more common in patients in whom the rectum ends in the supralevator position (30%) as opposed to the infralevator position (15%). Up to 40% of these patients may have an associated lumbosacral lesion such as spina bifida occulta or a tethered cord (Pena and Hong, 2000). These patients must be identified because their bladders are at risk for neurogenic voiding dysfunction even before the rectal pull-through (De Filippo et al, 1999). These patients often require intermittent catheterization to achieve continence.

The urological radiographic evaluation of these patients should include a renal-bladder ultrasound study and VCUG. The renal sonogram will identify those patients with renal

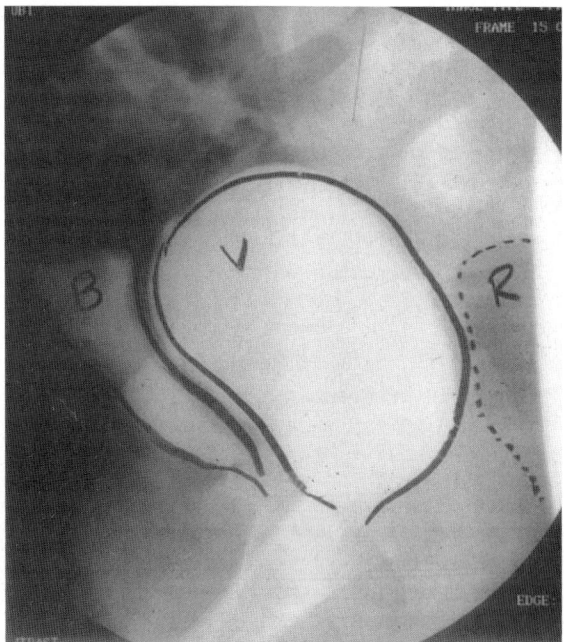

FIGURE 84-10 This genitogram, performed by retrograde injection of contrast into a single sinus anterior to the patient's rectum, demonstrates the anteriorly placed bladder *(B)* and posteriorly placed vagina *(V)*. The vagina and urethra merged into a common sinus, which then traveled a distance of 2 cm before emerging on the perineal body. The rectum *(R)* was normally placed. The vagina distended as a result of urinary entrapment, and the patient presented with a lower abdominal mass.

agenesis, anomalies of renal fusion, or occasional obstructive uropathy. If the VCUG identifies vesicoureteral reflux, antibiotic prophylaxis should be initiated. In addition, the VCUG may identify signs of a coloprostatic or colovaginal fistula and aid in subsequent anorectal reconstruction. Finally, an MRI study of the lumbosacral spine will identify that subset of patients with a tethered cord or spinal dysraphism. Patients who require detethering should undergo a video-urodynamic assessment postoperatively.

CLOACAL ANOMALIES

Cloacal anomalies associated with incomplete caudal differentiation manifest as a wide spectrum of clinical abnormalities. The urogenital sinus is a common variant in the female neonate. The term *urogenital sinus* in the setting of cloacal anomalies describes a completely "normal" although anteriorly placed rectum and a common urogenital channel or sinus into which the vagina and urethra merge (Figure 84-10). Such neonates may present with a pelvic mass that is cystic and posterior to the bladder on pelvic sonography. Close inspection of the genitalia reveals one common sinus, which is narrow and offers high resistance to urinary flow. As a consequence, the bladder empties into the vaginal vault, which progressively expands. In severe cases, this dilated vagina may even produce ureteral obstruction and hydronephrosis. The definitive diagnosis is made by a fluoroscopic genitogram or MRI genitogram. The term *cloaca* describes complete fusion of colonic, urinary, and genital systems; urethra, vagina, and rectum empty into the perineum via one common channel. The embryology, anatomy, and complex management of

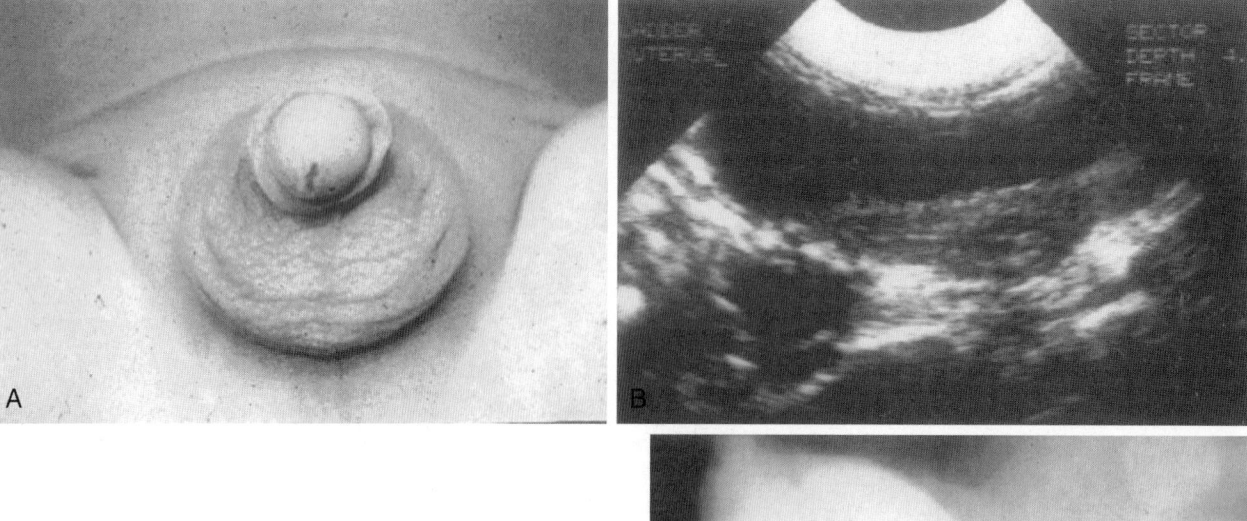

FIGURE 84-11 A, The patient presented clinically with "bilateral impalpable undescended testes." **B,** An ultrasound examination revealed the presence of a uterus behind the bladder, confirming that the underlying diagnosis was congenital adrenal hyperplasia manifesting in a genetic female. **C,** A genitogram confirmed the presence of a vagina, and a cervical imprint was also noted.

these rare cases have been reviewed in great detail by Pena et al (2004). These anomalies constitute neonatal surgical emergencies, in which management decisions are highly individualized.

DISORDERS OF THE GENITALIA

UNDESCENDED TESTES

Three percent of full-term boys have an undescended testicle. By 1 year of age, this percentage decreases to approximately 0.8%. Most spontaneous testicular descent will occur by 6 to 9 months of life (Wenzler et al, 2004). Up to 30% of patients with undescended testes present with bilateral undescended testes. The presence of bilateral impalpable undescended testes in a newborn boy warrants a genetic and endocrine evaluation for a disorder of sexual differentiation. In addition, failure to appreciate the significance of bilateral and impalpable undescended testes in the NICU could result in missed diagnosis of congenital adrenal hyperplasia in a virilized female neonate (Figure 84-11). Although in most cases of bilateral impalpable testes the infant proves to be a normal boy, neonates with congenital adrenal hyperplasia often have inadequate cortisol and mineralocorticoid function, leaving the child susceptible to electrolyte imbalances and dehydration. Furthermore, failure to diagnosis a disorder of sexual differentiation delays a decision regarding the sex of rearing. Similar concerns arise if undescended testes are found in

the presence of a hypospadias (see later section on ambiguous genitalia).

The neonate with a unilateral undescended testis and a normal phallus may be referred for a urologic follow-up evaluation at 3 to 6 months of age. If at 6 months of age the testis remains out of position, surgical intervention should be undertaken to reposition the testis within the scrotum. The impalpable testis may be a true intraabdominal gonad or a testis that is intermittently in and out of a large patent processus vaginalis; or the testis may be completely absent secondary to an antenatal torsion. If testicular agenesis is present, the contralateral testis usually demonstrates some degree of compensatory hypertrophy. This hypertrophy is recognized on physical examination or manifests with an increased volume by sonographic measurements. The increased contralateral testis volume, however, does not preclude the need for exploration. Parents need to be reminded that in 80% of cases of inguinal exploration for an impalpable testis, the testis is located and a successful orchiopexy is performed. The child who presents at 6 months of age with an undescended testis high in the inguinal canal is also a candidate for surgical intervention, because the testis is unlikely to descend spontaneously. If the testis is near the scrotum, a repeat examination is prudent before pursuing surgical repair.

Long-term issues associated with cryptorchidism include an increased risk of infertility and testicular malignancy. Fertility rates vary greatly depending on whether cryptorchidism is unilateral or bilateral. Long-term follow-up studies evaluating paternity suggest that 90% of boys with unilateral cryptorchidism report paternity in later years (Cendron et al, 1989; Lee et al, 1996). Furthermore, paternity was not affected by the age at the time of surgery (Lee et al, 1995). However, paternity rate decreased to 50% for patients with bilateral undescended testes who underwent orchiopexy in the first 3 years of life. As age at the time of bilateral orchiopexy increases, the paternity rates decline (Lee et al, 1997). A number of studies have demonstrated that cryptorchidism results in lower sperm counts despite surgical correction, and that the lowest counts are observed in patients with bilateral cryptorchidism. Testicular biopsy at the time of orchiopexy may offer a potential to identify those patients at the greatest risk of infertility 20 and 30 years later; a histologic scoring system allowing the prediction of a high-risk cohort of patients was recently validated with long-term follow-up semen analyses (Rusnack et al, 2003). The ability to predict low sperm counts using biopsy criteria also may allow for early hormonal treatment to enhance future fertility prospects in this select group of patients.

The etiology of cryptorchidism remains poorly understood. A genetic contribution is suggested by the presence of a family history in 5% to 10% of cases (Chacko and Barthold, 2009). Antiandrogen treatment increased the likelihood of cryptorchidism in a rat model offering support for an environmental exposure hypothesis (Spencer et al, 1991). Deletion of the insulin 3 gene in mice results in cryptorchidism that, if untreated, results in infertility; however, microsurgical orchiopexies in this population of mice improved testicular histology and enhanced fertility (Nguyen et al, 2002). This work offers a scientific basis for orchiopexy, which remains one of the more commonly performed pediatric surgical procedures. In human studies of cryptorchidism, mutations in the insulin-3 gene are rare (Baker et al, 2002), suggesting that other pathways or mutations downstream of insulin-3 are responsible for this phenotype.

The relative risk for testicular cancer in patients with an undescended testis increases approximately eightfold over that in the normal population, yet this observation is tempered by the rarity of testicular cancer. Thus, the overall lifetime risk of developing testicular cancer remains low for the individual patient, and in a large Scandinavian series, the incidence of malignancy was further diminished if surgical intervention was performed before puberty (Pettersson et al, 2007). Therefore, orchiopexy is recommended to place the testes in the proper scrotal position and to allow for monthly self-examination once the patient enters puberty.

TESTICULAR TORSION

Torsion of the testes is a rare event in the neonatal period, and its management remains controversial. In determining the proper intervention, it is essential to document the appearance of the scrotum and testes at birth. The newborn who presents in the delivery room with a painless, blue, and edematous hemiscrotum will likely have had an antenatal torsion. In this type of torsion, the entire tunica vaginalis and spermatic vessels twist at the level of the gonadal vessels and occlude the vascular pedicle, thus resulting in testicular ischemia. This event often occurs during the last trimester, and thus the indurated hemiscrotum observed in the delivery room is a late presentation of a terminal process. If the antenatal torsion occurs early in gestation, all inflammation will have resolved, and the neonate presents with an impalpable testis. Surgical findings include blood vessels and a vas deferens that end blindly at a common point where a small nubbin is occasionally located.

Little controversy exists over management of the neonate who was born with a normal scrotal exam but subsequently develops scrotal swelling and erythema; these patients should undergo a Doppler ultrasound and surgical exploration if blood flow cannot be confirmed (Guerra et al, 2008). The persisting controversy surrounds the management of the infant who is born with a clinically apparent torsion. In this setting, immediate exploration in the hours after birth rarely results in testicular salvage, and the risks of anesthesia are elevated. However, multiple case reports have documented bilateral metachronous torsions (Baglaj and Carachi, 2007). Although rare, the potential for bilateral anorchia is devastating given the long-term sequelae of infertility and need for testosterone replacement therapy in puberty and beyond. As the risks of neonatal anesthesia have declined over the years, a growing number of urologists are advocating early exploration with removal of the torsed testes that cannot be salvaged and contralateral orchiopexy to protect the remaining gonad (Guerra et al, 2008). Testes with antenatal torsion may also present as a firm mass in the neonatal period. The use of Doppler ultrasonography will help differentiate testicular torsion from the more rare neonatal yolk sac tumor where testicular blood flow will be demonstrated.

HYDROCELE

A hydrocele is a collection of fluid between the tunica vaginalis and tunica albuginea, which covers the surface of the testes. In the neonate, this fluid originates in the peritoneal cavity that communicates with the scrotum via an evagination or extension of the peritoneum termed a patent processus vaginalis. If the patency is small, peritoneal fluid may become trapped in the scrotum. This unidirectional fluid flow explains the slow and progressive increase in scrotal size that may be observed in some cases. In other cases with a large patency, the fluid may move in and out of the scrotum with ease such that when the urologist arrives to examine the child, the swelling is absent. It is important to reassure families that communicating hydroceles often improve over time. Indeed, the frequency of a patent processus vaginalis in autopsy series of men with no history of hernias or hydroceles was 20%. In addition, hydroceles may present acutely following the placement of ventriculoperitoneal shunts or peritoneal dialysis catheters. In these instances, both sides should be repaired because there is a 30% chance that the contralateral side will also become symptomatic. However, overly aggressive therapy of the neonatal hydrocele should be avoided, because many of these hydroceles will resolve spontaneously, and surgical intervention may damage the vas deferens or testicular vessels, resulting in testicular atrophy. The likelihood of such an iatrogenic injury is increased in the small neonate.

HERNIA

In cases where the patency of the processus vaginalis is large enough, intestines and other viscera (including the bladder) may migrate into the scrotum (Lau et al, 2007). This, by definition, is a hernia, which is often easily reducible and not a surgical emergency. In contrast, a difficult-to-reduce or incarcerated hernia requires urgent repair to preserve the herniated structure. If the hernia becomes strangulated, blood supply to the intestine will be compromised. This represents a surgical emergency.

HYPOSPADIAS

The diagnosis of hypospadias is established when the urethral meatus is not present in the normal glanular position; the meatus may be present anywhere along the ventral penile surface from the glans to the perineum. In addition, there is an asymmetrical or dorsally hooded foreskin, and the penis may be tethered, creating a significant bend (chordee). The etiology of hypospadias remains uncertain, although a genetic contribution is postulated, because a family history is reported in 5% to 10% of cases. More recently, investigators have postulated that environmental exposures to endocrine disruptors provide a significant contribution (Wang and Baskin, 2008). Experimental studies in mice suggest that exposures to high doses of estrogens lead to malformation of the urethral seam in the developing genital tubercle (Yucel et al, 2003), which would provide a mechanism by which endocrine disruptors could lead to hypospadias. Proponents of the endocrine disruptor theory note that the incidence of hypospadias has increased over the past 30 years (Paulozzi et al, 1997); however, other studies have failed to demonstrate such an increase (Fisch et al, 2009).

These infants must not undergo neonatal circumcision; the foreskin is crucial for use in the urethral reconstruction and correction of the chordee. However, up to 10% of patients with a hypospadias may have an intact foreskin, and the diagnosis is determined only after circumcision. These cases constitute the megameatus–intact prepuce variants. In such cases, the loss of foreskin does not compromise the hypospadias repair, which is completed at approximately 6 months of age (Snodgrass and Khavari, 2006). It is important to confirm that both testes are properly descended; hypospadias in conjunction with an undescended testis should raise the possibility of disorder of sexual differentiation (Cox et al, 2008; Kaefer et al, 1999a). This evaluation is critical if both testes are undescended and impalpable, because this phenotype may represent a diagnosis of congenital adrenal hyperplasia in a female neonate (see later section on ambiguous genitalia).

For an infant with hypospadias and bilaterally descended testes, an outpatient urological evaluation should be arranged within 2 to 6 months of age. The greatest chance for an underlying disorder of sexual differentiation being present is seen in proximal hypospadias associated with one or two impalpable testes (Kaefer et al, 1999a). In that setting, urologic consultation should be obtained in the NICU before discharge.

Hypospadias presents with a wide spectrum of severity. The best functional and cosmetic results are obtained in 90% of cases in which the meatus is present anywhere along the penile shaft. Snodgrass and Yucel (2007) have developed a versatile repair that offers high success rates for hypospadias when the meatus is present along the penile shaft. Current hypospadias repairs offer functional improvement in terms of the quality of stream and cosmetic results that are increasingly approaching those seen in normal males. Even the 10% of cases that constitute the most severe penoscrotal hypospadias may be reconstructed with good cosmetic and functional results. The key in all of these cases is the preservation of all genital skin that is to be used in reconstruction—hence the need to avoid circumcision.

CIRCUMCISION

Few topics arouse as much controversy, office visits, phone calls, and annoyance for families, pediatricians, and urologists as the issue of routine circumcision in the newborn boy. Circumcision has been practiced for centuries, and despite efforts to discourage the practice, families have continued to request this surgical procedure. In many parts of the United States, nearly 80% of the male population is circumcised. In fact, the incidence of circumcision appears to be rising in the United States (Nelson et al, 2005). In patients with poor hygiene, a nonretractile foreskin may increase the risk of penile cancer and mask the onset of carcinoma of the penis. Yet, penile carcinoma is a rare malignancy in the United States and a common malignancy in underdeveloped nations where circumcision is not practiced. The risk for penile cancer is associated with limited access to regular bathing, basic hygiene, and the ability to retract the foreskin when sexual activity begins. The etiology of carcinoma of the penis is polyfactorial, and the threat of malignancy is not a mandate for circumcision. Based on recent clinical trials in Africa, it has been demonstrated that circumcision is associated with a significantly lower rate of HIV seroconversion (Siegfried et al, 2009; Tobian et al, 2009). Although the role of circumcision in Africa is expected to increase given these data, educational efforts on behalf of diminished promiscuity, condom use, and basic hygiene are essential to public health.

Parents may cite a significant study reported by Wiswell and Geschke (Wiswell, 1997; Wiswell and Geschke, 1989), that identified a small but very real medical benefit to circumcision. By evaluating discharge data from U.S. Army hospitals worldwide, these investigators correlated the status of the foreskin with subsequent urinary tract infections. Their findings reveal that, within the 1st year of life, although only 20% of males were not circumcised, this 20% accounted for 80% of all urinary tract infections. In other words, these investigators demonstrated that the presence of foreskin increased the risk of a urinary tract infection by approximately fourfold during the 1st year of life. Therefore, circumcision is to be encouraged for any neonate with an underlying congenital anomaly of the urinary tract such as reflux, posterior urethral valves, or megaureters, where the added burden of a urinary tract infection has serious consequences.

The three main techniques for circumcision are those using the Plastibell, the Gomco clamp, and the Mogen clamp. Each has benefits and drawbacks; each physician

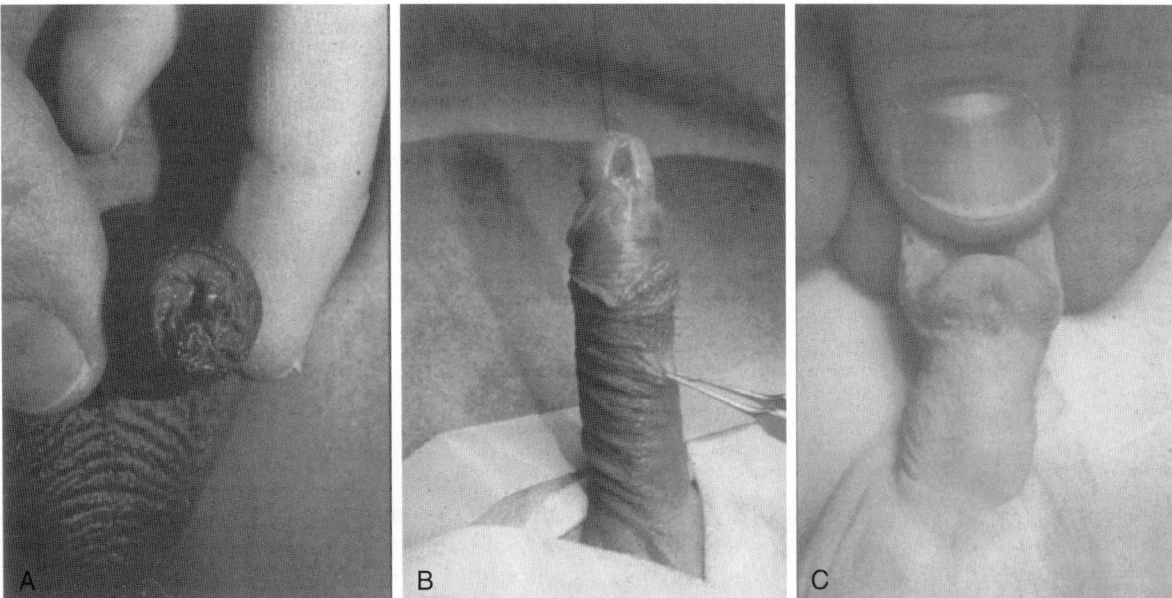

FIGURE 84-12 Hypospadias may not be discovered until the time of circumcision, because the foreskin has such a normal appearance, as in **A** and **B**. These cases represent the megameatus–intact prepuce variant, in which circumcision is not at all detrimental to future reconstruction. **C,** This photograph shows a more typical hypospadias with an asymmetric foreskin and a meatus that is present at the glanular margin. In such cases, circumcision should be deferred because the hooded preputial skin may be required for subsequent reconstruction.

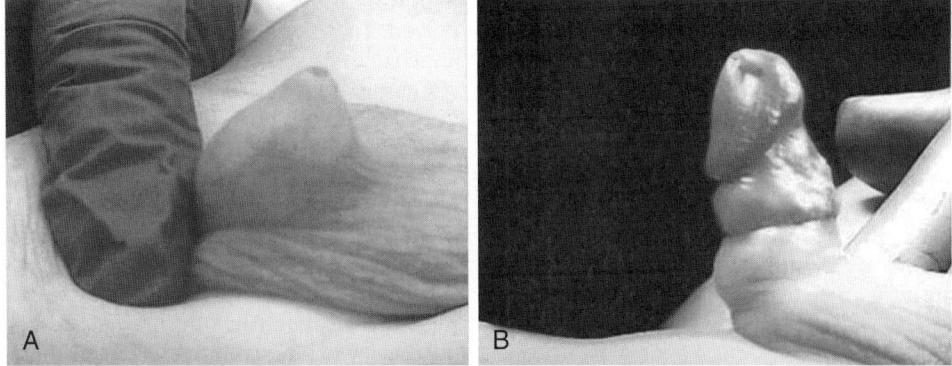

FIGURE 84-13 **A,** This is an example of true penile webbing in which the penile shaft is attached to the scrotal skin for more than 50% of the length of the shaft. This webbing or tethering can only be repaired by a surgical approach **(B)**; such a patient is not a candidate for circumcision done in the neonatal unit.

performing circumcisions will find the method with which he or she feels most comfortable and should use it repetitively. If there is doubt about the penile articular anatomy, the procedure should be terminated and urologic consultation obtained. The use of topical EMLA cream followed by a circumferential penile block is highly effective in minimizing pain associated with the procedure and offers a cost-effective means of providing this service (Jayanthi et al, 1999). Every effort should be made to perform circumcision in the newborn period and thus avoid the use of a general anesthetic in the older child. A study within the Kaiser health plan considered the issue of circumcision from a cost-effectiveness standpoint and came to the conclusion that the system could demonstrate a cost savings of $183 per patient even if routine neonatal circumcision was performed at an average cost of $200 (Schoen et al, 2006).

The leading contraindication to circumcision is medical fragility of the infant. Circumcision in a premature baby may present a technical challenge related to the infant's smaller size. In such instances, circumcision should be deferred until just before discharge from the NICU. In the child with a complex medical course, this timing also offers the physician a chance to perform a circumcision with full cardiovascular and respiratory monitoring that is not available in an office-based setting. Circumcision must never be performed in any child with hypospadias or epispadias (Figure 84-12), because as mentioned earlier, this skin is essential to the urethral reconstruction. In recent years there has been an increase in the diagnosis of penile webbing, which often results in circumcision being deferred to specialty care and performed under a general anesthetic. A case of significant penile webbing is shown in Figure 84-13, and in this instance an operative repair was indicated.

Bleeding after a routine circumcision may be observed in 10% to 20% of cases, and minor bleeding is not cause for alarm. If the bleeding has saturated the dressing and repositioning of the pressure dressing fails to stop the bleeding, the frenulum should be inspected because most bleeding vessels are found in this area. If the bleeding persists, the clinician should not hesitate to obtain coagulation studies; hemophilia and von Willebrand's disease may manifest in this manner. Rarely, there is injury to the glans and urethra that requires urological intervention. Typically, the most common problem arising after circumcision is the formation of penile adhesions. This complication may be prevented by teaching parents to retract the penile shaft skin and apply petrolatum over the glans. Parents also should be warned that despite a nice skin fit in the neonatal period, the cosmetic appearance of the penis may change as the prepubic fat pad grows. The result may be that a perfect circumcision is obscured as the penis is pulled back into the fat pad; in such cases, reassurance, and not surgical revision, is indicated.

AMBIGUOUS GENITALIA

The diagnosis and management of the child with ambiguous genitalia remain a medical and social emergency; a complete discussion of this topic is beyond the scope of this section. Currently, prenatal diagnosis has allowed discussions about genital ambiguity to begin before delivery (Rintoul and Crombleholme, 2002). The widespread use of ultrasonography and increasing use of amniocentesis have allowed the in utero diagnosis of virilizing congenital adrenal hyperplasia and androgen resistance syndromes. Such diagnosis is possible because the sonographic appearance of genitalia at birth does not correspond to the karyotype obtained at amniocentesis.

The most common presentation is the female neonate with congenital adrenal hyperplasia. Findings on physical examination range from severe clitoromegaly with hypospadias to a fully developed phallus with no palpable gonads (see Figure 84-11). This virilization is caused by enzymatic deficiencies in the pathways of cortisol synthesis, leading to shunting into the androgen biosynthetic pathways (Speiser and White, 2003). Family history is useful, because an older sibling or relative may have been diagnosed with this condition. It is also useful to know if a karyotype was performed during gestation. If a karyotype was not performed or the results are not available, an ultrasound examination of the pelvis should be ordered to evaluate for mullerian structures (see Figure 84-11), and a karyotype should be ordered. Virilizing congenital adrenal hyperplasia is a rare diagnosis, and most neonates with bilateral impalpable testes will prove to be normal males. However, a delay in establishing this diagnosis is dangerous because replacement therapy with cortisol must be initiated. A genitogram (see Figure 84-11) will delineate the extent of surgery required. Whereas 20 years ago, surgery was encouraged in the neonatal period with the idea that it would enable better acceptance of a female gender role by the parents and child, today the timing of surgery is controversial; these issues are addressed in the final paragraph.

Another common presentation is that of the child with androgen insensitivity who is presents as a phenotypic female despite an XY karyotype from an amniocentesis.

Mutations in the androgen receptor or in the downstream pathway result in a phenotypic female with bilateral testes. These testes produce the mullerian inhibitory substance—hence, the uterus and the upper two thirds of the vaginal vault will be absent. There are no surgical management or gender assignment issues for these patients in the neonatal period.

Mixed gonadal dysgenesis is diagnosed in the NICU or newborn nursery when neonates present with severe hypospadias and unilateral undescended testis (Rajfer and Walsh, 1976). These patients may have a normal XY karyotype or a mosaic presentation. At exploratory laparotomy, the gonads are biopsied; a testis will be found on one side and a primitive streak on the opposite side. Rudimentary mullerian structures may be seen on the side of the streak gonad and may include a hypoplastic uterus. Streak gonads are removed because of their malignant potential. Historically, female gender assignment was considered, but currently, maintaining a male gender of rearing with advanced hypospadias reconstruction is recommended.

The traditional approach to the diagnosis and management of genital ambiguity has undergone a great deal of criticism and increasing scrutiny over the past decade. With the traditional approach, a heavy emphasis was placed on assigning a sex of rearing as soon as possible and initiating any surgical reconstructions in the neonatal period. In recent years, it has become apparent that this approach is problematic. Physicians and parents assign a sex and gender role to a neonate. However, the long-term question arises as to whether a child's own gender identity will be congruent with the assigned gender role. For years it was believed that gender identity was not fixed until 2 years of age. Given the technical problems encountered in phallic reconstruction, it was believed that if a satisfactory phallus could not be reconstructed, a female sex should be assigned. The recent reports of several patients who, on reaching teenage years, have reverted back to a male gender after early female gender assignment have challenged this practice (Diamond and Sigmundson, 1997; Reiner, 2002). In light of these scientific and clinical concerns, some authors and patients have called for a moratorium on surgery in infancy for patients with genital ambiguity (Diamond, 1999). They propose that all diagnostic tests be performed to allow for a determination of what the appropriate gender assignment will be for the child. However, no irreversible surgery would be performed until the child determines his or her gender identity and pediatric assent is obtained. It is important to note that many patients with an XY karyotype assigned to a female gender have adjusted to their situation (Schober et al, 2002). However, because the brain is a sexually dimorphic organ, many of the structural differences between the two genders exist because of hormonal imprinting in utero (Gorski, 2002; Swaab et al, 2002), and hence such compensatory findings will be variable.

Complete references used in this text can be found online at www.expertconsult.com

ACUTE KIDNEY INJURY AND CHRONIC KIDNEY DISEASE

David Askenazi, Lorie B. Smith, Susan Furth, and Bradley A. Warady

ACUTE KIDNEY INJURY

DEFINITION

Previously referred to as *acute renal failure*, acute kidney injury (AKI) is characterized by a sudden impairment in kidney function, that results in the retention of nitrogenous waste products (e.g., urea) and alters the regulation of extracellular fluid volume, electrolytes, and acid-base homeostasis. The term *acute kidney injury* has replaced *acute renal failure* by most critical care and nephrology societies, primarily to highlight the importance of recognizing this process at the time of injury as opposed to waiting until failure has occurred (Mehta, 2007). Despite its limitations, serum creatinine (SCr) is the most commonly used measure to evaluate glomerular filtration in the clinical setting and is more specific than blood urea nitrogen (BUN). BUN is an insensitive measure of glomerular filtration rate (GFR) because it can be increased out of proportion to changes in GFR with high dietary protein intake, gastrointestinal bleeding, use of steroids, and hypercatabolic states. If the BUN-to-SCr ratio exceeds 20, increased urea production or increased renal urea reabsorption that occurs in prerenal azotemia should be suspected (Feld et al, 1986).

In the neonatal population, the most common SCr cut-point used to define AKI has arbitrarily been set at 1.5 mg/dL or greater, independent of day of life and regardless of the rate of urine output. Although SCr is the most common method to diagnose AKI, it has significant shortcomings, including

- SCr concentrations may not change until 25% to 50% of the kidney function has already been lost; therefore it may be days after an injury before a significant rise in SCr is seen (Brion, 1986).
- At a lower GFR, SCr will overestimate renal function because of tubular secretion of creatinine (Brion, 1986).
- SCr varies by muscle mass, hydration status, sex, age, and gender.
- Different methods (Jaffe reaction versus enzymatic) produce different values, and medications and bilirubin can affect SCr measured by the Jaffe method (Lolekha, 2001; Rajs and Mayer, 1992).
- Once a patient receives dialysis, SCr can no longer be used to assess kidney function because SCr is easily dialyzed.

Additional problems with using SCr as a measure of AKI specific to neonates include

- SCr in the first few days of life reflects the mother's SCr; thereafter, the normal distribution of SCr values demonstrates variation that is greatly dependent on the level of prematurity and age (Gallini, 2000) (Figure 85-1)

- Normal nephronogenesis in healthy term infants begins at 8 weeks' gestation and continues until 34 weeks' gestation, at which time the number of nephrons (1.6 to 2.4 million) approximates that of an adult (Abrahamson, 1991). Depending on the degree of prematurity, GFR steadily improves from 10 to 20 mL/min per 1.73 m² during the first week of life to 30 to 40 mL/min per 1.73 m² by 2 weeks after birth, concomitant with alterations in renal blood flow. GFR improves steadily over the first few months of life (Brion, 1986) (Table 85-1).
- Bilirubin levels in premature infants are normal at birth, rise in the first several days, and return to normal after a few weeks; this can have an impact if the Jaffee method of SCr determination is used (Lolekha, 2001).

Other problems with using a threshold cutoff to define AKI is that this approach fails to delineate the severity, timing, and cause of the injury. In the adult and pediatric populations, classification definitions of AKI based on SCr and urine output have gained acceptance. The two most common classification schemes that delineate different severities of AKI are the Risk, Injury, Failure, Loss, and End-Stage Renal Disease (RIFLE) (Bellomo et al, 2004) and the Acute Kidney Injury Network (AKIN) (Mehta, 2007) classifications. These AKIN classification definitions have created commonality in defining AKI, and they clearly show that incremental degrees of AKI independently affect survival after correcting for comorbidities, complications, and severity of illness in pediatric and adult studies (Abosaif et al, 2005; Chertow et al, 1998; Hoste et al, 2006). These data suggest that patients may not only die with kidney failure, but that this dysfunction causes functional and transcriptional changes in the lungs and other organs that ultimately lead to poor outcomes (Bellomo et al, 2004; Elapavaluru and Kellum, 2007; Hoste et al, 2006). These studies have not been reproduced in critically ill neonatal populations.

In children, Akcan-Arikan et al (2007) proposed a modified pediatric RIFLE (pRIFLE) classification that is similar to the adult RIFLE classification except for a lower cutoff of SCr to achieve the F category, thereby reflecting the fact that children have a lower baseline SCr. An SCr of 4.0 mg/dL is not needed to have severe dysfunction. Similar classification definitions of AKI are greatly needed to better describe the incidence and outcomes of AKI in different populations of critically ill neonates. Delineation between the 1st week of life (when the infant has a high SCr level that will slowly fall) and changes in SCr level after the 1st week will be needed in a neonatal AKI classification system.

Despite these working classification systems, the diagnosis of AKI is problematic, because current diagnosis relies on two functional abnormalities: functional changes in SCr (marker of GFR) and oliguria. Both of these

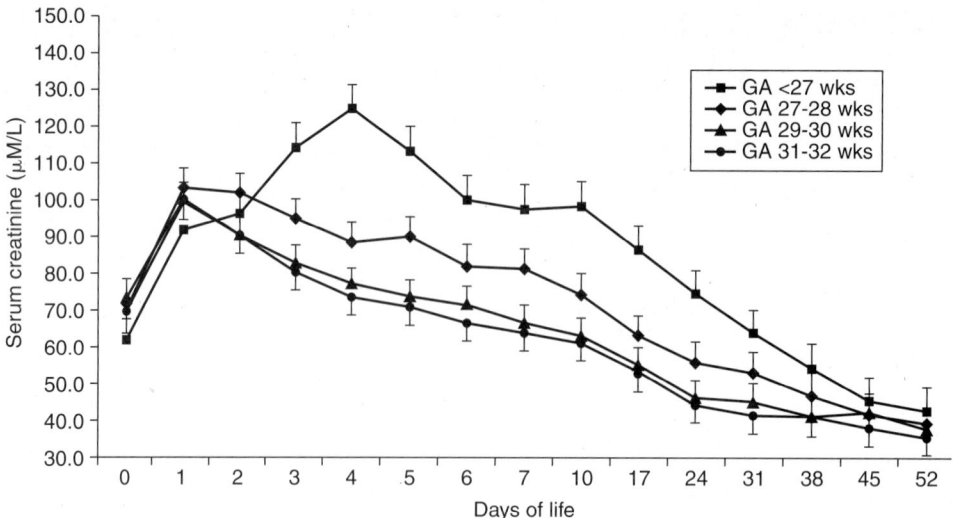

FIGURE 85-1 Serum creatinine concentrations (μM/L) during the first days of life, with values given as means and standard error for infants born at different gestational ages.

TABLE 85-1 Insulin Clearance GFR in Healthy Premature Infants

Age	GFR (mL/min per 1.73 m²)
1-3 days	14.0 ± 5
1-7 days	18.7 ± 5.5
4-8 days	44.3 ± 9.3
3-13 days	47.8 ± 10.7
1.5-4 months	67.4 ± 16.6
8 years	103 ± 12

Adapted from Schwartz GJ, Furth SL: Glomerular filtration rate measurement and estimation in chronic kidney disease, *Pediatr Nephrol* 22:1839-1848, 2007. *GFR,* Glomerular filtration rate.

measures are late consequences of injury and not markers of the injury itself. The ideal marker to detect AKI should be upregulated shortly after an injury and be independent of the GFR (Askenazi, 2009a). Current studies of urinary and serum biomarkers of AKI promise to improve our ability to diagnose AKI early in its disease process. For example, urine and serum neutrophil gelatinase-associated lipocalin, urine interleukin-18, kidney injury marker 1, and others have been shown to predict which neonates undergoing cardiopulmonary bypass will develop a rise in SCr level by greater than 0.5 mg/dL (Mishra et al, 2005; Parekh et al, 2006) (Figure 85-2). Creating AKI definitions using early injury biomarkers, which can ultimately predict morbidity and mortality, is of paramount importance. In addition, well-designed clinical research studies on early noninvasive biomarkers of AKI in different neonatal populations are needed to better characterize AKI and predict outcomes. Once we can reliably identify AKI early in the disease process, preventive and therapeutic interventions can be studied to improve outcomes in neonates with AKI.

EPIDEMIOLOGY

Critically ill neonates are at risk of AKI because they are commonly exposed to nephrotoxic medications and have frequent infections that lead to multiple organ failure (Andreoli, 2004). The exact incidence of neonatal AKI is difficult to quantify because infants commonly

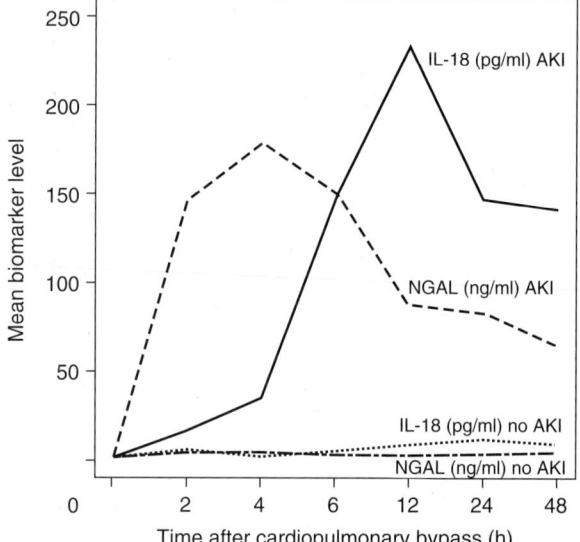

FIGURE 85-2 Mean values of urine interleukin-18 (pg/mL) and neutrophil gelatinase-associated lipocalin (ng/ml) over the first hours after cardiopulmonary bypass in infants who develop acute kidney injury (50% increase in serum creatinine) compared with those who did not develop acute kidney injury.

have nonoliguric renal failure and may therefore not be screened with SCr for AKI. Additionally, most reports define only severe cases of AKI (usually SCr >1.5 mg/dL or need for renal replacement therapy [RRT]) (Agras et al, 2004; Stapleton et al, 1987). Published studies estimate the incidence of neonatal AKI in critically ill neonates between 8% to 24% and mortality rates between 10% to 61% (Andreoli, 2004). Moghal et al (1998) suggested that relative to adult and pediatric critically ill populations, neonates have the highest incidence of AKI.

Infants With Perinatal Hypoxia

Most studies of neonatal AKI describe term infants with asphyxia at the time of birth. Hypoxic-ischemic encephalopathy accounts for 23% of the 4 million neonatal deaths globally and high rates of disability (Lawn et al, 2005).

Three different observational studies describe the incidence of AKI (defined as SCr >1.5 mg/dL) in asphyxiated critically ill newborns. Karlowicz and Adelman (1995) compared term infants with severe asphyxia (according to Portman's asphyxia morbidity scoring system) (Portman et al, 1990) to similar infants with moderate asphyxia scores. They found that AKI occurred in 20 of 33 (66%) of infants with severe asphyxia compared to 0 of 33 (0%) in those with moderate asphyxia. In a case control analysis (matching for gestational age and birthweight in otherwise healthy newborns), Aggarwal et al (2005) observed the incidence of AKI in infants with 5-minute Apgar scores of 6 or less to be 56% versus 4% in controls. Similarly, Gupta et al (2005) found a 47% incidence of AKI and 14.1% mortality in infants with Apgar scores of 6 or less. All these studies report more than 50% of AKI cases to be nonoliguric, which highlights the insensitivity of oliguria in predicting AKI in neonates.

General Neonatal Population

Three recent studies have explored AKI in the general critically ill neonatal population and confirmed the high incidence of AKI and mortality in these infants. In a retrospective analysis, Agras et al (2004) found 25% hospital mortality in neonates with AKI. Many (47%) of their patients had nonoliguric renal failure, and premature infants constituted 31% of the cases. Mathur et al (2006) prospectively studied mostly term neonates with sepsis and found a 26% incidence of AKI. The mortality rate was significantly higher in those with AKI versus those without AKI (70.2% versus 25%; p <0.001). Although this study gives insight into the incidence of AKI in neonates, this study is limited by their choice of the definition of AKI (BUN >20) and their inability to control for gestational age, birthweight, comorbidity, and severity of illness.

To better ascertain the independent role of AKI on survival in premature infants, a recent case-control study (Askenazi et al, 2009b) matching premature infants by gestational age and birthweight found that for every 1 mg/dL increase in SCr, the odds ratio for death increased by a factor of almost 2 (odds ratio [OR], 1.94; 95% confidence interval [CI], 1.13 to 3.32). The OR for death increased even when confounding variables were adjusted (adjusted OR, 3.44; 95% CI, 1.23 to 9.61). Because of study design limitations, caution must be exercised in making inferences about the true incidence and outcomes of neonatal AKI based on these studies. Additional prospective, multicenter studies are needed to determine whether this association exists.

Infants Requiring Cardiopulmonary Bypass

The incidence and outcome data for neonates who require cardiopulmonary bypass are based on single-center experiences, most of which define AKI as a requirement of RRT. Reported incidence of AKI in this population is between 2.7% and 24.6% (Bailey et al, 2007; Picca et al, 1995), with survival rates ranging from 21% to 80% (Picca et al, 1995; Sorof et al, 1999). The causes of AKI in this group are based on preoperative factors, intraoperative changes, and postoperative events. Preoperative risk factors for AKI include hypotension, use of diuretics, angiotensin-converting enzyme inhibitors [ACE-I], indomethacin, hypoxemia, hypothermia, infection, positive pressure ventilation, nephrotoxic medications, and intravenous contrast. Intraoperative changes including hemodynamic changes, aortic clamp time, and inflammatory response to cardiopulmonary bypass influence postoperative AKI. The most important factors that influence the development of postoperative AKI are cardiac performance and sepsis (Picca et al, 2008).

Infants Requiring Extracorporeal Membrane Oxygenation

Several studies of infants and children (Cavagnaro et al, 2007; Meyer et al, 2001; Sell et al, 1987; Shaheen et al, 2007; Weber et al, 1990) who receive extracorporeal membrane oxygenation suggest both AKI and RRT are associated with mortality. To explore the independent role of AKI and receipt of RRT on outcomes, Askenazi et al (2011) performed a retrospective cohort study of 7941 neonates enrolled between 1998 and 2008 in the extracorporeal life-support organization registry. AKI was defined as infants in the registry who had an SCr level greater than 1.5 mg/dL or an International Classification of Diseases code for acute renal failure. Neonatal mortality was 2175 in 7941 (27.4%). Nonsurvivors experienced more AKI (413/2175 [19%] versus 225/5766 [3.9%]; p <0.0001) and more of them received RRT (863/2175 [39.7%] versus 923/5766 [16.0%]; p <0.0001) than survivors. After adjusting for confounding variables, the adjusted OR for the neonatal group was 3.2 (p <0.0001) after AKI and 1.9 (p <0.0001) with RRT. Additional studies to ascertain AKI risk factors, test novel therapies, and optimizing the timing and delivery of RRT can positively affect survival.

One of the most common morbidities of prematurity is the propensity to develop bronchopulmonary dysplasia; it affects 10% and 40% of surviving very low-birthweight and extremely low-birthweight infants, respectively (Eichenwald and Stark, 2008). The pathophysiology of this chronic lung condition involves elevated levels of proinflammatory interleukins, tumor necrosis factor-α, leukotrienes, and increased pulmonary vasculature permeability, which culminate in abnormal lung development and fibrosis. Not only does AKI cause pulmonary edema secondary to volume overload, but evidence in ischemic, nephrotoxic, and bilaterally nephrectomized animal models shows that AKI induces a proinflammatory process highlighted by increase in neutrophils, tumor necrosis factor-α, interleukins, free radicals, endothelial growth factors, and granulocyte colony-stimulating factor (Faubel, 2008; Hoke et al, 2007; Kim do et al, 2006). Clinically it has been recognized that critically ill adults receiving mechanical ventilation with AKI have a dismal prognosis (80% mortality), and they have an impaired ability to wean from mechanical ventilation (Vieira et al, 2007). To date, little is known about the lung-kidney interactions in premature infants, nor the role of AKI on chronic lung disease.

A large prospective cohort study with classification definitions of AKI is greatly needed to better understand the incidence and independent effect of AKI in asphyxiated infants, premature infants, infants undergoing cardiopulmonary bypass, and the general critically ill newborn population. The role of the kidney in acute and chronic pulmonary disease in premature infants needs to be explored.

PATHOPHYSIOLOGY

Prerenal Azotemia

Prerenal azotemia (sometimes referred to as *pre–kidney failure*, but perhaps better termed *acute kidney success*) occurs in response to decreased renal blood flow (RBF). Causes of prerenal azotemia in neonates include loss of effective circulating blood volume (perinatal blood loss, hemorrhage), dehydration (diarrhea, transepidermal free water losses, poor intake, gastric or chest tube losses), capillary leak (hydrops, infection, or hypoalbuminemia), increased abdominal pressure (necrotizing enterocolitis, ascites, repair or reduction of gastroschisis, omphalocele, or congenital diaphragmatic hernia), and decreased cardiac output (cardiac surgery, heart failure, or the use of extracorporeal membrane oxygenation, which results in a lack of pulsatile flow) (Liem et al, 1995a, 1995b). Nonsteroidal antiinflammatory drugs (NSAIDs), such as indomethacin and angiotensin-converting enzyme inhibitors (ACE-Is), can decrease RBF (Box 85-1).

When low RBF occurs, renal autoregulation preserves GFR by increasing renal sympathetic tone, activating the renin-angiotensin-aldosterone system, and increasing activation of hormones such as vasopressin and endothelin. An increase in filtration fraction (GFR/RBF × 100) increases peritubular oncotic pressure, resulting in enhanced proximal tubular sodium and water reabsorption (Feld et al, 1986) in those with intact tubular function. These renal hemodynamic changes lead to decreased water and sodium losses, so as to maintain systemic volume expansion and blood pressure. Oliguria does not develop in some newborns because of poor vasopressin secretion, weak renal responsiveness to vasopressin (Dixon and Anderson, 1985), poor tubular function in underdeveloped tubular cells, or after prolonged or severe hypoperfusion. In the context of renal hypoperfusion, correction of the underlying condition restores normal renal function unless renal hypoperfusion has been sufficiently severe or prolonged that renal parenchymal damage has already developed. Once parenchymal damage occurs, renal tubular cell damage (acute tubular necrosis) occurs even if renal perfusion is restored.

Intrinsic Acute Kidney Injury

Prolonged or severe hypoperfusion is the most common cause of intrinsic AKI. Other causes of intrinsic AKI include nephrotoxic medications and sepsis, which can cause AKI in both hypodynamic and hyperdynamic blood flow. Approximately 6% to 8% of newborns admitted to NICUs have intrinsic AKI, with severe perinatal asphyxia being the most common cause (Stapleton et al, 1987). Other rare causes of AKI include renal vein thrombosis, renal artery thrombosis, uric acid nephropathy, hemoglobinuria, and myoglobinuria (see Box 85-1). Congenital abnormalities of the kidneys and urinary tract (CAKUT) are discussed further in the section under chronic kidney disease (CKD) of the newborn.

BOX 85-1 Causes of Acute Kidney Injury in the Newborn*

Prerenal Azotemia	Intrinsic Acute Kidney Injury	Obstructive Renal Failure
Loss of effective blood volume	Acute tubular necrosis	Congenital malformations
Absolute loss	Severe renal ischemia	Imperforate prepuce
Hemorrhage	Nephrotoxins	Urethral stricture
Dehydration	Infections	PUV
Relative loss	Congenital infections	Urethral diverticulum
↑ Capillary leak	Pyelonephritis	Ureterocele
Sepsis	Bacterial endocarditis	Megaureter
NEC	Renal vascular causes	UPJ obstruction
RDS	Renal artery thrombosis	Extrinsic compression
ECMO	Renal vein thrombosis	Sacrococcygeal teratoma
Hypoalbuminemia	DIC	Hematocolpos
Renal hypoperfusion	Nephrotoxins	Intrinsic obstruction
Congestive heart failure	Aminoglycosides	Renal calculi
Pharmacologic agents	Indomethacin	Fungus balls
Indomethacin	Amphotericin B	Neurogenic bladder
Tolazoline	Radiocontrast dyes	
ACE inhibitors	Acyclovir	
	Intrarenal obstruction	
	Uric acid nephropathy	
	Myoglobinuria	
	Hemoglobinuria	
	Congenital malformations	
	Bilateral renal agenesis	
	Renal dysplasia	
	Polycystic kidneys	

ACE, Angiotensin-converting enzyme; *DIC*, disseminated intravascular coagulation; *ECMO*, extracorporeal membrane oxygenation; *NEC*, necrotizing enterocolitis; *PUV*, posterior urethral valve; *UPJ*, ureteropelvic junction.
*In many cases, a combination of several causative factors contributes to the development of acute renal failure. For example, absolute hypovolemia, increased capillary leak–induced loss of effective circulating blood volume, and reflex renal vasoconstriction—all can contribute to renal hypoperfusion and ensuing renal injury in newborns with severe forms of shock.

Ischemic Acute Kidney Injury

Despite being the best-oxygenated organ, the kidney is susceptible to hypoxic-ischemic injury because of the redistribution of its blood flow under pathologic circumstances to the vital organs, and because of the unique vascular supply of the renal medulla. The presentation and course of renal damage depend on the severity and duration of the insult. In contrast to prerenal azotemia, renal function abnormalities in intrinsic AKI are not immediately reversible. The severity of intrinsic AKI ranges from mild tubular dysfunction, to acute tubular necrosis, to renal infarction and corticomedullary necrosis with irreversible renal damage (Feld et al, 1986).

Prerenal azotemia and ischemic AKI represent extremes on a continuum of physiologic responses. The main difference between prerenal AKI and ischemic AKI is that in the latter, hypoperfusion induces injury to renal parenchymal cells, particularly to tubular epithelium of the terminal medullary portion of the proximal tubule (S3 segment) and of the medullary portion of the thick ascending limb of the loop of Henle.

The course of ischemic AKI can be subdivided into prerenal, initiation, extension, maintenance, and recovery phases (Sutton et al, 2002) (Figure 85-3). If during prerenal azotemia, restoration of renal blood flow occurs, GFR can return promptly to normal. The initiation phase includes the original insult and the associated events resulting in a

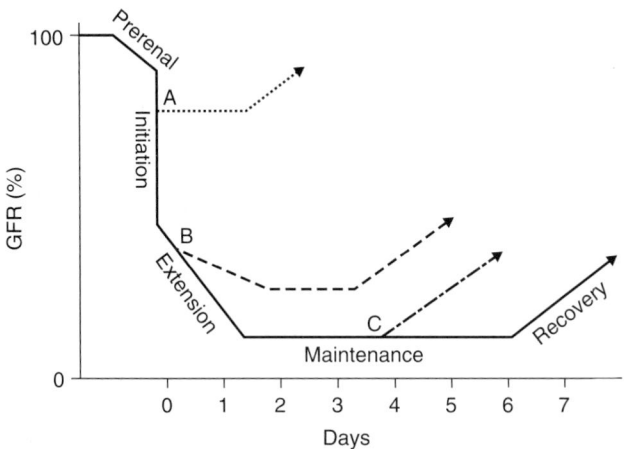

FIGURE 85-3 Schematic representation of stages of the progression in acute kidney injury.

drop in GFR. Tubular dysfunction with low GFR represents the maintenance phase. The duration of the maintenance phase depends, at least in part, on the severity and duration of the initial insult. The recovery phase is characterized by the gradual restoration of GFR and tubular function, which can take months to occur. During the maintenance and recovery phases of AKI, the kidney is susceptible to further damage from additional insults. Recognition of the different phases of intrinsic AKI is helpful in the diagnosis, clinical management, and prognostication of the disorder.

The histologic hallmark of severe ischemic AKI is damage to epithelial tubular cells with a characteristic bleb formation and loss of brush border in the apical portion of the cell, cytoskeleton disruption, and loss of tight junctions between cells. If injury is severe enough, apoptosis and necrosis will occur with resultant desquamation of cells, which lead to tubular obstruction. Tubular epithelial cells are critical in the pathophysiology of ischemic AKI, and damage to the innermost lining of the renal vascular system, endothelial cells, has a critical role in the initiation, extension, maintenance, and recovery phases of ischemic AKI (Basile, 2007; Basile et al, 2001; Molitoris and Sutton, 2004).

When endothelial cell damage occurs, activation of vasoconstriction, impaired vasodilation, and impaired leukocyte adhesion result in capillary obstruction and distorted peritubular capillary morphology. Capillary obstruction and impaired morphology lead to a cycle of increasing ischemia and vascular inflammation. The loss of endothelial cell function may represent an important therapeutic target in which vascular support or endothelial regeneration by progenitor cells can affect the short- and long-term consequences of AKI (Liu and Brakeman, 2008).

Damaged endothelial and tubular cells do not only lead to dysfunction within the kidney; they produce a systemic inflammatory response that has been shown to lead to significant distant organ dysfunction. The inflammatory dysregulation is due, at least in part, to dysfunctional immune, inflammatory, and soluble mediator metabolism. AKI has also been shown to directly affect the brain, lung, heart, liver, bone marrow, and gastrointestinal tract (Awad and Okusa, 2007; Sorof et al, 1999). Mice with AKI (induced by bilateral renal ischemia for 60 minutes) had increased levels of proinflammatory chemokines, keratinocyte-derived chemoattractant, and granulocyte colony-stimulating factor in the cerebral cortex and hippocampus, which results in increased neuronal pyknosis and microgliosis in brain (Liu and Brakeman, 2008). In the lung, mechanistic studies demonstrate that AKI induces increased pulmonary vascular permeability, soluble and cellular inflammation, and dysregulated salt and water channels. Because neurologic and pulmonary morbidity is high in the critically ill neonatal population, the potentially deleterious effects of AKI on these organs need to be explored.

Nephrotoxic Acute Kidney Injury

Pharmacologic agents are the most common cause of nephrotoxic AKI in neonates, although endogenous substances (hemoglobin and myoglobin) may also be toxic to the kidney. These toxins can cause neonatal AKI by decreasing renal perfusion (NSAIDs, diuretics, ACE-Is), direct tubular injury (aminglycosides, cephalosporins, amphotericin B, rifampin, vancomycin, NSAIDs, contrast media, myoglobin–hemoglobin), interstitial nephritis, and tubular obstruction (acyclovir). Although the following discussion is not a comprehensive review, some of the most common nephrotoxic medications in neonates are described.

Indomethacin, a prostaglandin inhibitor used to treat patent ductus arteriosus in premature infants, is one of the most commonly used medications in the neonatal intensive care unit. Severe, although usually transient, nephrotoxicity can occur with indomethacin administration. The primary mechanism of renal action of these drugs is the potentiation of vasoconstrictive and sodium- and water-retaining effects of angiotensin II, norepinephrine, and vasopressin by the indomethacin-induced inhibition of renal prostaglandin production. Because neonatal renal function is more dependent on local prostaglandin production than that of the euvolemic adult—especially when intravascular volume is decreased as a result of fluid restriction, increased capillary leak, and transepidermal water losses in the preterm infant with patent ductus arteriosus—indomethacin administration is commonly associated with elevated SCr concentrations, decreased urine output, and hyponatremia (Cifuentes et al, 1979).

Amphotericin B alters renal function by directly affecting tubular function, resulting in renal tubular acidosis and increasing urinary potassium excretion. Although these nephrotoxic effects are most often reversible, cases of fatal neonatal renal failure caused by amphotericin B toxicity have been reported (Baley et al, 1984). Amphotericin B lipid complex (ABLC), liposomal amphotericin and other lipid formulations of this drug consist of nonliposomal lipid bilayers complexed with amphotericin B. This lipid bilayer causes a higher affinity to fungal rather than mammalian cellular membranes and therefore is less nephrotoxic (Wurthwein et al, 2005). Auron et al (2007) recently showed no differences in blood urea nitrogen or SCr, serum sodium, and serum potassium in 35 premature infants (average birthweight, 764 ± 196 g) compared with similar infants (controlling for gestational age and birthweight). Therefore a 2-week course of amphotericin B complex is likely to be safe in premature infants, although studies to explore longer use of ABLC are needed.

Aminoglycosides are one of the most commonly used medications in the treatment of suspected or proven neonatal sepsis. Aminoglycosides inhibit lysosomal phospholipases, leading primarily to proximal tubule cell damage (Giuliano et al, 1984), although changes in the ultrastructure of the glomerulus also occur (Ojala et al, 2001). A metaanalysis of 11 studies in septic neonates demonstrated that both once-a-day and multiple-dose regimens led to adequate clearance of sepsis. Although rates of ototoxicity or nephrotoxicity were not different among the two groups, pharmacokinetic studies reveal that once-a-day dosing causes less drug accumulation in the kidney's proximal cells, and it usually achieved adequate peak concentrations (>5.0 μg/dL) while avoiding toxic trough levels (<2 μg/dL) (Rao et al, 2006).

Aminoglycosides should be used with caution in any patient with renal dysfunction, concomitant nephrotoxic medication use, or poor renal perfusion owing to volume, hypoalbuminuria, or heart failure. In patients with poor renal dysfunction or risk for impaired aminoglycoside clearance, serial monitoring to assure proper clearance of medication is needed to prevent AKI. Because aminoglycoside toxicity is usually nonoliguric, serial monitoring of SCr values is necessary, especially during prolonged administration of these antibiotics, to detect their potential nephrotoxicity in the newborn.

Acyclovir has replaced vidarabine for treatment of herpes simplex disease because of its ease of use and more favorable side effect profile. High-dose acyclovir (60 mg/kg/day for 21 days) decreased the mortality and CNS disease from sepsis and meningitis associated with herpes simplex virus to 29% and 4%, respectively (Kimberlin et al, 2001). Acyclovir is an antiviral agent that is eliminated rapidly in urine through glomerular filtration and tubular secretion. It is nearly insoluble in urine and may precipitate, particularly in the distal tubular lumen. Intravenous high-dose acyclovir treatment can lead to intratubular crystal precipitation and renal failure. Acyclovir-related nephrotoxicity can be limited by avoiding its use in those with renal insufficiency or intravascular volume depletion, infusing the drug slowly (over several hours), and by assuring adequate hydration to maintain high urinary flow rate, which will reduce the likelihood of crystal deposition in tubules (Izzedine et al, 2005).

Finally, medications given to pregnant women can cause combined ischemic and nephrotoxic renal injury in the fetus, resulting in the clinical presentation of AKI after birth. A frequently used class of medications that fall into this category are the NSAIDs prescribed for tocolysis—both nonselective and selective cyclooxygenase inhibitors such as indomethacin or ketoprofen (Bannwarth et al, 1999; Peruzzi et al, 1999)—which can lead to severe AKI in the newborn.

Acute Obstruction

The most common cause for obstruction induced kidney dysfunction in the newborn is congenital malformations, including imperforate prepuce, urethral stricture, prunebelly syndrome, and posterior urethral valves. Other causes of acute obstruction include neurogenic bladder, extrinsic compression (e.g., hematocolpos, sacrococcygeal teratoma), and intrinsic obstruction from renal calculi or

fungal balls. Depending on the cause and associated damage to the kidneys, relieving the obstruction will markedly improve renal function.

EVALUATION

The pregnancy history, findings on prenatal tests, vital signs, changes in neonatal body weight, physical examination, interventions, and medications prescribed provide important clues about the cause of neonatal AKI. Serum laboratory values to be monitored in the infant with AKI include serum sodium, potassium, chloride, bicarbonate, calcium, phosphorus, magnesium, urea, creatinine, uric acid, glucose, blood gases, hemoglobin, and platelets. As discussed in the section defining AKI, SCr often does not rise for days after an injury, thus monitoring these values for several days after the inciting event is necessary to determine if AKI occurred. If urine is available, then urinalysis, urine culture, and a spot urine sample for sodium, creatinine, and osmolality can help to differentiate the cause.

One of the major goals in the initial evaluation of neonatal AKI is to determine whether the kidney is hypoperfused. Several laboratory, clinical, and therapeutic interventions can help to delineate prerenal azotemia from intrinsic AKI (Table 85-2). Decreased body weight, tachycardia, dry mucous membranes, poor skin turgor, flattened anterior fontanel, and elevated serum sodium levels can be seen in infants with low intravascular volumes. Measurement of serum albumin will alert the physician if appropriate oncotic pressure is present (serum albumin >2.0, but preferable at 2.5 mg/dL). When the kidney is hypoperfused, it will avidly retain sodium and water to preserve overall intravascular volume. Preservation of urine sodium

TABLE 85-2 Diagnostic Indices Suggestive of Prerenal Azotemia versus Intrinsic Acute Kidney Injury in the Newborn

	Prerenal Azotemia	Intrinsic Acute Kidney Injury
Urine flow rate (mL/kg/h)	Variable	Variable
Urine osmolality (mOsm/L)	>400	≤400
Urine-to-plasma osmolal ratio	>1.3	≤1.0
Urine-to-plasma creatinine ratio	29.2 ± 1.6*	9.7 ± 3.6*
Urine [Na+] (mEq/L)	10-50	30-90
FENa† (%)	<0.3 (0.9 ± 0.6)*	>3.0 (4.3 ± 2.2)*
Renal failure index‡	<3.0 (1.3 ± 0.8)*	>3.0 (11.6 ± 9.5)*
Response to fluid challenge	Improved tachycardia, increased UOP	No effect on tachycardia or UOP

Data from Feld LG, Springate JE, Fildes RD: Acute renal failure. I. Pathophysiology and diagnosis. *J Pediatr* 109:401-408, 1986; Karlowicz MG, Adelman RD: Acute renal failure in the neonate, *Clin Perinatol* 19:139-158, 1992; and Mathew OP, Jones AS, James E, et al: Neonatal renal failure: usefulness of diagnostic indices, *Pediatrics* 65: 57-60, 1980.

UOP, Urine output.

*Mean ± SD.

†Fractional excretion of sodium (FENa) = (Urine [Na+]/Serum [Na+])/(Urine [Cr]/Serum [Cr]) × 100.

‡Renal failure index (RFI) = Urine [Na+]/(Urine [Cr]/Serum [Cr]).

and water is dependent on intact tubular function. Disturbances of tubular function can occur with diuretic use, ischemic or nephrotoxic tubular injury, or primary tubular diseases. Laboratory markers of prerenal azotemia include low urinary sodium excretion, low fractional excretion of sodium, low renal failure index, and high BUN:SCr ratio. These laboratory studies have important limitations in premature infants. Unfortunately, laboratory tests to determine whether elevated SCr is from prerenal azotemia versus intrinsic AKI are insensitive and nonspecific in premature infants because of underdeveloped tubular function. Normal fractional sodium excretion in preterm infants born before 32 weeks' gestation is usually higher than 3% (Ellis and Arnold, 1982). In addition, because of the developmentally regulated limitation of their concentrating capacity and the effects of low protein intake and urea excretion on urine osmolality, the urine-to-plasma creatinine ratio instead of the urine-to-plasma osmolality ratio should be used in newborns to evaluate their renal tubular reabsorptive capacity (Feld et al, 1986).

If suspicion of renal hypoperfusion is high, an appropriate fluid challenge with 10 to 20 mL/kg of isotonic fluids (usually normal saline) over 30 minutes should be given. Close observation to vital signs and urine output may serve to delineate the presence of intravascular hypoperfusion. Several boluses may be necessary with careful prescription of fluid volume for the next 24 hours. Care to avoid fluid challenges is advised in those with suspected urinary outlet obstruction or congestive heart failure.

A second major goal of AKI evaluation is to detect anatomic causes of AKI, if present. A renal and bladder ultrasound examination should be performed without delay if an obstructive process is suspected and to detect congenital renal abnormalities if present. If hematuria, hypertension, or both are present, the possibility of renal vascular disease should also be considered. Doppler ultrasound examination of renal vessels can be performed if renal vascular thrombosis is suggested.

MANAGEMENT

The approach using fluid boluses (if appropriate) as part of the evaluation of prerenal azotemia also serves as the initial management of this condition. If obstruction of the urinary outflow is discovered, then interventions to eliminate the obstruction should be undertaken followed by plans for surgical correction. Polyuria with electrolyte losses can occur after relief of the obstruction; therefore close monitoring of serum electrolytes, especially bicarbonate, and appropriate replacement of these losses are necessary. Besides these specific management options, there are currently no specific medical therapies to treat AKI. To maximize the chance for survival, the clinician must support the cardiorespiratory system, maintain maximal nutrition, balance homeostasis, and manage the consequences of AKI. Dialysis can provide renal suppport to achieve goal-oriented therapies.

Despite numerous promising therapies in animal studies and many clinical pharmacologic trials, no approved therapies are available to treat AKI in neonates, children, or adults. Only supportive care of the patient (with medications, renal support therapies, or both) is currently

available for the care of the infant with AKI (Walters et al, 2009). Several therapies are commonly used in patients with AKI; however, few data are available to support the use of low-dose dopamine, fenoldopam (a selective dopamine-1 receptor agonist), or diuretics for the treatment or prevention of AKI.

Dopamine can increase renal perfusion in the sick preterm and term infant with prerenal azotemia caused by hypoxemia, acidosis, or indomethacin administration (Seri, 1995; Seri et al, 1998, 2002). Although low dose dopamine increases renal perfusion, well-powered randomized controlled studies in adults with AKI have reached the same conclusion (Bellomo et al, 2000; Friedrich et al, 2005; Hoste et al, 2006; Marik, 2002). Compared with placebo, low-dose dopamine does not improve survival, shorten hospital stay, or limit dialysis use. These studies have not been performed in children or neonates.

Diuretics are commonly used to induce diuresis in critically ill neonates; however, no studies in neonates, children, or adults have shown that diuretics are effective in preventing AKI or improving outcomes once AKI occurs (Bellomo et al, 2000). If loop diuretics are to be used in neonates, continuous doses of furosemide may be superior to larger intermittent doses. In neonates with cardiac surgery, continuous doses were shown to be as effective despite smaller total quantities of medications. The authors conclude that those with continuous dosing may have less risk for nephrotoxicity or ototoxicity than occurs with large intermittent doses of this drug (Luciani et al, 1997). The potential toxicity of long-term and aggressive furosemide therapy—including ototoxicity, interstitial nephritis, osteopenia, nephrocalcinosis, hypotension, and persistence of patent ductus arteriosus—should be considered, especially in the preterm newborn (Karlowicz and Adelman, 1992). The mannitol test (used to test whether a patient has renal hypoperfusion) is contraindicated in newborns with a predisposition for intraventricular hemorrhage or periventricular leukomalacia because of a drug-induced, sudden increase in serum osmolality.

Fenoldopam is a selective dopamine-1 receptor agonist whose effects include vasodilation of renal and splanchnic vasculature, increased renal blood flow, and increased GFR. Fenoldopam is approved to treat severe hypertension in adults, but is not clinically approved for the treatment of AKI. Nonetheless, its use in neonates with AKI has been explored in several single-center analyses. Although two separate retrospective single-center analyses (Moffett et al, 2008; Yoder and Yoder, 2009) found increased urine output in a select group of neonates with oliguria, Ricci et al (2008) performed a prospective controlled trial of low-dose fenoldopam (0.1 µg/kg/min) in infants undergoing cardiac surgery with cardiopulmonary bypass. Compared with placebo, low-dose fenoldopam did not show beneficial effects on AKI incidence, fluid balance control, time to sternal closure, time to extubation, or time to intensive care discharge. Because low-dose dopamine, diuretics, and fenoldopam are unlikely to positively affect the outcomes of infants with AKI, efforts should be maximized to support the infant's cardiorespiratory system and to manage and prevent the ill effects of AKI.

If systemic hypotension develops despite adequate volume administration, early initiation of blood pressure support often establishes appropriate renal perfusion (Seri et al, 1993, 1998). In cases of pressor-inotrope–resistant hypotension and shock, a brief course of low-dose hydrocortisone has been demonstrated to be effective in restoring systemic perfusion and renal function in preterm neonates (Seri, 2001). Other management goals include maintaining blood oxygen content, providing blood products for specific indices, limiting severe acidosis, and maintaining normal serum albuminemia (at least 2.0 mg/dL, but preferably 2.5 mg/dL).

Hypertension is common in neonates with AKI. It can be caused by increased renin release in malformed or damaged kidneys or secondary to increased intravascular volume from a lack of free water clearance. If hypertension is due to fluid overload, inducing free water clearance with diuretics or fluid removal with dialysis will address its cause. Calcium-channel blockers work by selectively causing vasodilatation of the venous system. Short-acting calcium-channel blockers (e.g., isradipine) are reliable, have a quick onset of response, and are well tolerated. Long-acting calcium-channel blockers (e.g., amlodipine) take longer to take effect, but they provide less lability with longer dosing intervals. β-Blockers (propranolol or labetolol) are also commonly used to treat hypertension in neonates. Use of ACE-I in children with ischemic AKI should be avoided, because it can produce further renal hypoperfusion and can alter intrarenal hemodynamics in an already injured kidney. See Chapter 88 for more information on neonatal hypertension.

Managing fluids in the critically ill neonate with AKI can be difficult. These infants may require large volumes of fluid to maintain adequate nutrition and hematologic indices and to provide appropriate medications. However, these fluids can be detrimental in a child with oliguria or anuria, because they can cause congestive heart failure, chest wall edema, and pulmonary failure. Therefore, once adequate intravascular volume has been restored, prevent severe fluid overload (by limiting crystalloid infusions) and maximize nutritional supplements concentration. Severe fluid restriction limiting intake to insensible and gastrointestinal and renal losses is sometimes required, but at a heavy price (inadequate nutrition). Decisions regarding placement of dialysis access should be made early in the course of AKI before severe fluid overload has occurred, because once severe fluid overload occurs, placement of a peritoneal dialysis or a hemodialysis catheter can be significantly more difficult, as is support of the infant with severe pulmonary edema.

Electrolyte abnormalities can vary depending on the cause of AKI. For example, aminoglycoside toxicity is commonly nonoliguric with ongoing potassium and magnesium losses. Alternatively, ischemic AKI causes oliguria–anuria, hyponatremia, hyperkalemia, hyperphosphatemia, and hypocalcemia. Management of electrolyte disorders can usually be managed by attention to electrolyte intake during the initial course of AKI with frequent evaluation and specific therapies.

Most cases of hyponatremia are due to water overload and less commonly due to low total body sodium content. Attention to fluid status is critical to determine the cause and proper therapy of hyponatremia. In cases of nonsymptomatic hypervolemic hyponatremia (serum sodium

concentrations usually between 120 and 130 mEq/L), restriction of free water intake is recommended. If hyponatremia at this level results in clinical signs and symptoms (e.g., lethargy, seizures) or serum sodium concentration falls to less than 120 mEq/L, use of 3% sodium chloride over 2 hours according to the following formula should be considered:

$$Na^+_{Required} (mEq) = ([Na^+]_{Desired} - [Na^+]_{Actual}) \times Body\ weight\ (kg) \times 0.7$$

Possible complications of hypertonic saline administration include congestive heart failure, pulmonary edema, hypertension, intraventricular hemorrhage, and periventricular leukomalacia. Care should be taken not to increase serum sodium concentration more rapidly than 0.5 mEq/h.

Severe hyperkalemia is a life-threatening medical emergency. Hyperkalemia that is unresponsive to medical management is one of the most common indications for peritoneal and hemodialysis in the newborn (Coulthard and Vernon, 1995; Karlowicz and Adelman, 1992). Signs of progressive hyperkalemia on the electrocardiogram, in order of severity, consist of tall peaked T waves, heart block with widened QRS complexes, U wave formation, the development of sine waves, and finally cardiac arrest. Measures to remove potassium from the body include oral or rectal sodium polystyrene (Kayexalate), loop diuretics to enhance potassium excretion (if not anuric), and dialysis. Several methods to move potassium from the extracellular to the intracellular compartment are available, including albuterol inhalation, sodium bicarbonate, and insulin plus glucose. Adequate ionized calcium levels for cardioprotection should be sought in the context of hyperkalemia (Table 85-3). Vemgal and Olhson (2007) performed a metaanalysis of studies on the management of hyperkalemia in premature infants. Given the limited data available, no firm clinical practice recommendations on which treatment modality was best to treat infants with hyperkalemia are available, except that insulin plus glucose may be better in premature infants.

Hyperphosphatemia is common in AKI and should be treated with low phosphorus intake. Breastmilk and Similac 60/40 both contain low phosphorous and low potassium compared with other neonatal infant formulas. Significant elevations in serum phosphate represent a risk of development of extraskeletal calcifications of the heart, blood vessels, and kidneys in the newborn, especially when the calcium-phosphorus product exceeds 70 (Sell et al, 1987). Calcium carbonate may be used as a phosphate-binding agent in infants whose phosphorous intake exceeds excretion. Although rarely an indication for dialysis without fluid overload or hyperkalemia, severe hyperphosphatemia is best treated with dialysis.

The incidence of hypocalcemia is low in neonates with severe and prolonged AKI, especially in those who develop an inability to convert 25-hydroxy–vitamin D to 1,25-hydroxy–vitamin D. Ionized calcium should be measured when low total calcium levels and concomitant hypoalbuminemia are encountered, because the latter can affect total calcium levels. If ionized calcium is decreased and the newborn is symptomatic, 100 to 200 mg/kg of calcium gluconate should be infused over 10 to 20 minutes and repeated every 4 to 8 hours as necessary. If hypocalcemia

TABLE 85-3 Medical Management of Hyperkalemia in the Newborn

Drug	Dose	Onset of Action	Duration of Action
Calcium gluconate (10%)	0.5-1 mL/kg (IV over 10 min)	1-5 min	15-60 min
Sodium bicarbonate (3.75% solution)	1-2 mEq/kg (IV over 10 min)	5-10 min	2-6 h
Insulin	1 IU/5 g glucose (IV bolus or continuous infusion)	15-30 min	4-6 h
Glucose	≤14 mg/kg/min (IV bolus or continuous infusion)	15-30 min	4-6 h
Furosemide	1 mg/kg dose or as continuous infusion	5-10 min	2-3 h
Sodium polystyrene sulfonate	1 g/kg dose every 6 h as needed (orally/rectally)	1-2 h*	4-6 h
Dialysis	Nephrology will prescribe dialysis treatment	Immediate	Duration of therapy

*Onset of action may take up to 6 hours, and the drug may be ineffective in preterm infants born at less than 29 weeks' gestation.
IV, Intravenous.

is severe, oral or intravenous calcitriol can be administered to increase intestinal reabsorption of calcium.

Normal acid–base homeostasis depends on the kidneys' ability to reabsorb bicarbonate; therefore infants with AKI commonly have a non–anion gap metabolic acidosis. Replacement with bicarbonate or acetate as a base is indicated in infants with AKI to avoid or treat metabolic acidosis. In infants with severe respiratory failure, large doses of bicarbonate should be avoided because they can culminate in increased carbon dioxide retention. Metabolic acidosis should be treated aggressively in infants with severe pulmonary hypertension, because an acidic environment can worsen this condition.

Nutritional goals in infants with AKI are similar to those of infants without AKI. Commonly parenteral nutrition, feeds, or both will need to be concentrated to avoid excessive fluid gains. If nutritional goals are unable to be achieved because of oliguria or ongoing fluid overload, the potential risks of dialysis therapy versus the potential risks associated with inadequate calorie and protein administration should be discussed with the parents. If a neonate is receiving continuous peritoneal dialysis or hemodialysis, an additional 1 g/kg/day of protein is needed to supplement the protein losses that occur with these forms of dialysis (Zappitelli et al, 2008, 2009).

In a neonate with AKI, careful assessment of medication dosing is imperative. Because many drugs are excreted in the urine, impaired metabolism or clearance from the kidneys can cause drug accumulation and adverse side effects. In infants receiving dialysis, pharmacokinetic properties of drugs (e.g., volume of distribution, protein binding, size, charge), dialysis modality (peritoneal dialysis versus hemodialysis), interval of dialysis (intermittent versus continuous) will affect drug availability (Churchwell and Mueller, 2009). Consultation with pharmacists and a nephrologist familiar with drug dosing in renal failure is invaluable.

Dialysis

Decisions to initiate dialysis (especially in infants with severe congenital malformations of the kidney and urinary tract) is a complex decision that requires a multidisciplinary approach to guide the family as they consider very difficult decisions. Access placement and some technical challenges make infant dialysis more difficult than in older children, but this therapy is feasible in experienced programs with dedicated pediatric neonatologists, dialysis nurses, and surgeons.

Indications for Dialysis Initiation

Absolute indications to initiate dialysis include: severe electrolyte abnormalities that are not correctable with medical interventions, life-threatening intoxication by medications that can be cleared with dialysis, inborn errors of metabolism, fluid overload, inability to provide adequate nutritional requirements, and uremia. If renal dysfunction, fluid overload, or both occur, then discussions about dialysis initiation should occur early in the disease process, because prolonged fluid overload or uremia can create worse pulmonary edema and cardiopulmonary instability and make placement of access for dialysis difficult.

The timing of dialysis initiation in infants with AKI is controversial. Several observational studies show a clear advantage in adults receiving dialysis early versus late (Liu et al, 2006; Ronco et al, 1986). In addition, multicenter data show that the degree of fluid overload at the initiation of dialysis is an independent risk factor for survival in critically ill children (Gillespie et al, 2004; Goldstein et al, 2001; Symons et al, 2007) and adults (Gibney et al, 2008; Mehta, 2009). Similar studies in neonates need to be performed. Over the last decade, advocates for early initiation of renal support argue that critically ill patients benefit from early dialysis. Metabolic control is gained faster because of earlier removal of excess fluid, and provision of renal support allows maximal nutrition without progressive fluid overload. Because technical access and machine advances have made neonatal dialysis safer and technically possible, early initiation of dialysis can improve outcomes in critically ill neonates with AKI. Further study is needed before recommendations on the timing of dialysis can be made.

Access

The limiting factor in performing dialysis in the smallest of babies is access to the peritoneal or vascular space for dialysis. Peritoneal dialysis access can be performed with either a straight uncuffed catheter or a curved and tunneled cuffed catheter. The advantage of the straight uncuffed catheter is that it can be placed at the bedside and can be used soon after insertion. However, these catheters are more likely to become infected or leak fluids around the insertion site. The ideal peritoneal dialysis catheter is one with two subcutaneous cuffs and a downward-facing exit site away from the diaper area and away from a gastrostomy tube (Auron et al, 2007). As with all pediatric surgical procedures, the exact catheter, timing, and location of catheter insertion needs to be tailored to the individual patient (Shaheen et al, 2007). If a hernia is present, it should be repaired at the time of catheter insertion.

Vascular access for hemodialysis requires a large (at least 7F, but preferably 8F) double-lumen catheter that can be placed in the femoral or internal jugular vein. Double-lumen catheters that are smaller than 7F have a much higher chance of developing problems during the dialysis procedure (Symons et al, 2007). Catheterization of the umbilical vessels does not provide sufficient blood flow necessary for conducting hemodialysis. If 7F catheter cannot be placed, two 5F catheters in different sites can be life-saving. If the need for dialysis is likely to last more than 1 week, a cuffed catheter is preferred to decrease the likelihood of infection. The length of the catheter should be chosen such that the tip of the catheter resides in the superior vena cava–right atrium (for internal jugular catheters) and the inferior vena cava for femoral catheters. Unless no other choice is available, use of the subclavian artery should be avoided in infants who are likely to require long-term renal replacement therapy, because in the future the forearm fistula of the ipsilateral arm can fail with mild stenosis of the subclavian vein.

Peritoneal Dialysis

Once a peritoneal dialysis access catheter is placed and the decision to start dialysis has occurred, small-volume continuous cycles (10 mL/kg) are performed. Fluid is filled with dialysate solution, left in the peritoneal cavity to dwell, and drained. Continuous cycles are performed, with each cycle lasting approximately 1 hour. The dextrose concentration in the fluid will determine the amount of net water losses (ultrafiltration). Complications associated with peritoneal dialysis include peritonitis, leakage around the catheter exit site rendering the dialysis virtually impossible, tunnel infection, catheter malfunction, and obstruction by omentum (Coulthard and Vernon, 1995). Fluid leakage into other compartments (including the chest in patients without an intact diaphragm) can occur and if suspected, the fluid composition will reveal high glucose levels if a leak is present. Absolute or relative contraindications to peritoneal dialysis include necrotizing enterocolitis, abdominal wall defects, and the presence of an intraabdominal foreign body, such as a ventriculoperitoneal shunt or diaphragmatic patch.

Hemodialysis

Once reliable access to the vascular space is achieved, the hemodialysis procedure can be performed in neonates. The two types of hemodialysis, intermittent hemodialysis and continuous renal replacement therapy (CRRT), differ mainly on the duration of the procedure. Intermittent hemodialysis is significantly more efficient than CRRT. Because much larger volumes of dialysis are used, the blood flow becomes the limiting factor in the amount of clearance that can be achieved. Even with the

smallest dialyzers and neonatal tubing, most infants need blood priming of the extracorporeal circuit for therapy. Skilled pediatric hemodialysis nurses are required at the bedside during the entire procedure, which typically lasts 3 to 4 hours. Achieving adequate fluid removal is sometimes difficult, especially in hemodynamically unstable infants. This approach usually requires systemic heparinization, with activated clotting time usually maintained at 180 to 200 seconds, rendering this approach risky in preterm newborns and others at high risk for intracranial bleeding.

Ronco et al (1986) described the use of CRRT in a critically ill newborn. Before the recent roller pump technology, CRRT used the patient's arterial blood pressure as a pump for the dialysis machine. The advent of newer roller pump technology improved the accuracy of small flows as low as 10 mL/min and provided the option of using the machine to pump blood via a double lumen catheter placed in a major vein. The main advantage of a continuous modality is that lower blood flow and fluid removal rates can be used to accomplish the desired ultrafiltration and clearance goals. Anticoagulation with CRRT is achieved with either systemic heparin or citrate regional anticoagulation. The advantage of regional citrate anticoagulation is that the patient is not anticoagulated; however, this method of anticoagulation has the added risk of hypocalcemia caused from citrate excess (especially in those infants with impaired liver metabolism) and metabolic alkalosis (Tolwani and Willie, 2009).

Outcome data in neonates who require CRRT are scarce. Symons et al (2003) reported a survival rate of 32 in 85 (37.6%) in neonates who received CRRT in five large children's hospitals in the United States. Between 2001 and 2007, the prospective pediatric CRRT group, a multicenter registry of 14 pediatric CRRT programs, reported outcomes for infants in whom CRRT was initiated before 1 month of age (Symons et al, 2007). Approximately 8% (35 neonates) in the registry were dialyzed in the 1st month of life. In this group, the median age was 8 days; the median weight was 3.2 kg, with the smallest infant weighing 1.3 kg. Of the 35 infants in the registry, 24 received dialysis for fluid overload, electrolyte imbalance, or both, and 11 of 35 received dialysis for inborn errors of metabolism. Overall survival was 43%. Infants receiving dialysis for inborn errors had a better survival rate (73%) compared with others (30%).

Several technical issues specific to infants arise when using CRRT for dialysis. The extracorporeal volume can incorporate greater than 50% of the infant's blood volume. For example, a 2.3-kg infant has a blood volume of approximately 184 mL; the Prisma circuit requires 90 mL, which is approximately 50% of the infant's blood volume. Priming the blood circuit with blood will effectively limit this problem. In addition, because standard protocols on citrate regional anticoagulation anticipate normal liver metabolism of citrate, caution must be exercised when performing dialysis in premature infants or newborns with multiple organ failure who may have impaired liver function. Risk for bradykinin reaction that can occur at the initiation of CRRT with AN69 dialyzer membranes can be reduced using several techniques (Brophy et al, 2001; Hackbarth et al, 2005).

ACUTE KIDNEY INJURY AS A CAUSE OF LONG-TERM CHRONIC KIDNEY DISEASE

Total GFR is determined by the filtration rate of a single nephron and the number of nephrons present. When the number of nephrons is diminished, single nephron GFR increases as the kidney works to compensate for low nephron numbers. This compensatory hypertrophy causes glomeruli to function under increased intracapillary hydraulic pressure, which over time causes damage to capillary walls. This abnormal process leads to progressive glomerulosclerosis, proteinuria, hypertension, and CKD (Brenner et al, 1996). The hyperfiltration hypothesis has been applied and confirmed in autopsy data of patients with hypertension (Keller et al, 2003; Ohishi et al, 1995) and has been reported at length in infants with intrauterine growth retardation (Barker and Osmond, 1988; Barker et al, 1989; Manalich et al, 2000; Wadsworth et al, 1985; White et al, 2009). A systematic review and metaanalysis in 2009 concluded that low-birthweight infants (5.5 lb [2.5 kg]) were 70% more likely to develop CKD later in life compared to individuals with normal birthweight (White et al, 2009).

Premature infants (even those born appropriate for gestational age) are born with low nephron numbers. Using computer-assisted morphometry, Rodriguez et al (2004) showed that premature infants have lower numbers of nephrons compared with term infants. Premature infants who had long survival (to at least 36 weeks after conception) had nephron numbers similar to those in premature infants with short survival, suggesting that the extrauterine environment does not allow for proper neoglomerulogenesis. In addition, preterm infants with AKI had fewer nephrons than did similar infants without AKI (Rodriguez et al, 2004).

Animal and epidemiology data suggest that AKI leads to CKD. As discussed in the section on ischemic AKI, tubular and vascular endothelial cellular damage occurs with prolonged hypoperfusion. Animal models suggest that although tubular recovery occurs, damage to vascular endothelial cells remains and leads to interstitial fibrosis and progressive kidney dysfunction (Basile et al, 2001).

Studies on children with AKI show that more than 50% of those with AKI have at least one sign of CKD 3 to 5 years after the inciting event. Large adult studies suggest that after AKI, rates of CKD (low GFR) are 5% to 10%, with approximately 3% to 5% developing end-stage renal disease (ESRD).

The exact prevalence of CKD after neonatal AKI is not known. Stapleton (1987) reviewed the published single-center data and reported a 40% to 88% prevalence of long-term CKD after oliguric renal failure. Since then, other retrospective, small, single-center retrospective studies describe similar tubular and glomerular dysfunction and hypertension in survivors of neonatal AKI (Abitbol et al, 2003; Chevalier et al, 1984; Polito et al, 1998). Data on outcomes of premature infants after AKI are scarce. Rodriguez et al (2004) performed a cross-sectional study on premature infants (birthweight <1000 g) during childhood and found that estimated GFR and tubular function were lower than in similar term children. Despite the limitations of these single-center studies,

these data suggest that prematurity, intrauterine growth retardation and AKI lead to a lower number of nephrons, endothelium dysfunction, or both, and an increased risk of long-term renal dysfunction. To further delineate the likelihood and extent of AKI causing CKD, a prospective study is greatly needed to provide guidelines for long-term follow-up. Future studies on interventions (e.g., angiotensin-converting enzyme inhibitors) to decrease the rate of CKD progression in this growing population should be explored.

CHRONIC KIDNEY DISEASE

Neonatal CKD is diagnosed when sustained derangements of glomerular filtration or tubular function occur with minimal to no resolution over time. In many cases CKD follows AKI, and in others the acute phase of the renal compromise has not been detected or has occurred in utero often as a result of anatomic abnormalities (e.g., hypoplasia, dysplasia, malformations), and the diagnosis of CKD is established without documented evidence of preexisting AKI. According to guidelines published by the Kidney Disease Outcomes Quality Initiative, CKD is present if there is evidence of kidney damage for more than 3 months, as defined by structural or functional abnormalities, with or without decreased GFR, or a GFR less than 60 mL/min per 1.73 m^2 for more than 3 months in children older than 2 years with or without kidney damage. GFR increases with maturation from infancy and approaches the adult mean value by 2 years of age. Thus it is important to note that the ranges of GFR that define the stages of CKD apply only to children 2 years and older. The GFR ranges defining CKD do not apply to infants, because they will normally have a lower GFR even when corrected for body surface area. ESRD, the point at which dialysis or kidney transplantation is necessary to ameliorate the physiologic complications of uremia owing to kidney failure, represents the most severe stage of CKD. The pathophysiologic mechanisms leading to the progression of AKI to CKD and ESRD are discussed earlier in this chapter.

EPIDEMIOLOGY

Reports of the regional incidence of neonatal ESRD differ greatly, and the worldwide incidence is unknown. In one study, the estimated incidence of neonatal ESRD in the United States and Canada was 0.32 in 100,000 live births (Carey et al, 2007). Rees (2008) reported that six new infants per 1 million population initiate dialysis per year compared to three per 1 million in the United Kingdom. In a German study, Wedekin et al (2008) estimated the incidence of CKD in infants to be 1 in 10,000 live births and found a male-to-female ratio of 2.8:1. They also found that 53% of these infants were premature, a figure significantly higher than in the total infant population of Germany. The most common causes of renal failure in most studies of neonates are renal dysplasia or obstructive uropathy (Carey et al, 2007; Ledermann et al, 1999; Rees, 2008; Shroff et al, 2003; Wedekin et al, 2008)—specifically, posterior urethral valves (Ledermann et al, 1999).

SEQUELAE AND TREATMENT

Anemia

Anemia is a frequent complication of CKD in infants and children, and there is evidence to suggest that it is an important predictor of patient morbidity and mortality. The anemia of CKD is associated with a number of physiologic abnormalities, including decreased tissue oxygen delivery, increased cardiac output, cardiac enlargement, ventricular hypertrophy, congestive heart failure, and impaired immune responsiveness (Gafter et al, 1994; Mitsnefes et al, 2000). There is also evidence to suggest that the presence of anemia is associated with an increased risk of hospitalization in children with CKD (Staples et al, 2009).

The prevalence of anemia increases with worsening stages of CKD. In a study of the North American Pediatric Renal Trials and Collaborative Studies (NAPRTCS), Staples et al (2009) found that the prevalence of anemia increased from 18.5% in CKD stage II to 68% in CKD stage V (Staples et al, 2009).

Guidelines for the evaluation and treatment of anemia in the pediatric patient with CKD have been published as the *KDOQI Clinical Practice Guidelines and Clinical Practice Recommendations for Anemia in Chronic Kidney Disease* by the National Kidney Foundation (National Kidney Foundation, 2006, 2007). According to the guidelines, *anemia* is defined as a hemoglobin (Hgb) concentration less than the 5th percentile of normal for age and sex (Table 85-4). The normative values used to define anemia in children older than 1 year are taken from the third National Health and Nutrition Examination Survey (Astor et al, 2002) database, whereas the norms for infants younger than 1 year are derived from other reference sources (Nathan and Orkin, 2003).

The pathophysiology of anemia in infants and young children with CKD is primarily the result of a decrease in renal production of erythropoietin, iron deficiency, or both (Koshy and Geary, 2008). Other potential contributing factors include a shortened red blood cell life span, secondary hyperparathyroidism, hypothyroidism, folate and vitamin B_{12} deficiency, chronic inflammation and hemoglobinopathies. The etiology of absolute iron deficiency is multifactorial and can be related to poor intake, gastrointestinal blood loss, and repeated phlebotomies for laboratory tests. Functional iron deficiency, defined as occurring when there is a greater need for iron to support Hgb synthesis than can be released from iron stores, may in part be related to the presence of elevated levels of the liver-derived peptide hepcidin—a subject about which further study is needed in the pediatric CKD population (Zaritsky et al, 2009).

The KDOQI guidelines recommend that the initial workup for anemia in children with CKD should include red blood cell indices, reticulocyte count, white blood cell count with differential and platelet count, and iron parameters (serum iron, total iron binding capacity, and serum ferritin) (National Kidney Foundation, 2006, 2007).

Erythropoiesis-stimulating agents (ESAs) such as erythropoietin-alfa (EPO), along with iron supplements, are the key elements of anemia management in CKD. Whereas the average dose of EPO for children with CKD is 150 to 200 units/kg/week given by the subcutaneous route, younger children (<1 year) often require doses as high as

TABLE 85-4 Hemoglobin Levels (g/dL) in Children between Birth and 24 Months Old for Initiation of Anemia Workup

Age	Mean Hemoglobin	−2 SD
Term (cord blood)	16.5*	13.5†
1-3 d	18.5	14.5
1 wk	17.5	13.5
2 wk	16.5	12.5
1 mo	14.0	10.0
2 mo	11.5	9.0
3-6 mo	11.5	9.5
6-24 mo	12.0	10.5

From National Kidney Foundation: KDOQI clinical practice guidelines and clinical practice recommendations for anemia in chronic kidney disease, *Am J Kidney Dis* 47(Suppl 3):S88, 2006.
*Data taken from normal reference values.
†Values 2 standard deviations (SD) below the mean are equivalent to <2.5th percentile.

350 units/kg/week. The difference is possibly related to an increased presence of nonhematopoietic binding sites for EPO in younger children that lead to increased clearance (NAPRTCS, 2008; Port et al, 2004). Children receiving peritoneal dialysis (PD) typically require less EPO than patients receiving hemodialysis (HD) as a result of the blood loss that occurs with HD. A recent report on the use of darbepoetin-alfa, an analogue of erythropoietin with a longer half-life, has been conducted in infants with CKD and revealed that the therapy was effective when dosing regimens were individualized (12).

Iron therapy typically consists of the provision of oral elemental iron in doses ranging from 2 to 3 mg/kg/day up to 6 mg/kg/day in two to three divided doses (National Kidney Foundation, 2006). Iron should be taken 2 hours before or 1 hour after all calcium containing phosphate binders to maximize gastrointestinal absorption. Levels of serum ferritin greater than 100 ng/mL and transferrin saturation greater than 20% are believed to reflect adequate iron stores in patients with CKD (National Kidney Foundation, 2006).

In the absence of definitive evidence in pediatrics to support the association of benefit or harm to any given level of Hgb for an individual child, the target Hgb is 10 to 12 g/dL for patients receiving ESAs and iron therapy (National Kidney Foundation, 2006, 2007; Staples et al, 2009). In turn, the rate of rise of the Hgb level should be no more than 1 to 2 g/dL per month. At the initiation of ESA therapy, monitoring of the Hgb level should occur every 1 to 2 weeks; the frequency of monitoring can be decreased once the target Hgb level has been achieved and the patient is receiving a stable dose of ESA.

Acid-Base and Electrolytes

Fluid and electrolyte requirements of individual children with CKD vary according to their primary kidney disease and the degree of residual kidney function. Infants and children normally have a relatively larger endogenous hydrogen ion load (2 to 3 mEq/kg) than do adults, resulting in metabolic acidosis as a common manifestation of CKD in

TABLE 85-5 Recommended Parameters and Frequency of Nutritional Assessment for Children With CKD Stages 2 to 5 and 5D

	Minimum Interval (mo)					
	Age 0 to <1 y			Age 1-3 yr		
Measure	**CKD 2-3**	**CKD 4-5**	**CKD 5D**	**CKD 2-3**	**CKD 4-5**	**CKD 5D**
Dietary intake	0.5-3	0.5-3	0.5-2	1-3	1-3	1-3
Height or length-for-age percentile or SDS	0.5-1.5	0.5-1.5	0.5-1	1-3	1-2	1
Height or length velocity-for-age percentile or SDS	0.5-2	0.5-2	0.5-1	1-6	1-3	1-2
Estimated dry weight and weight-for-age percentile or SDS	0.5-1.5	0.5-1.5	0.25-1	1-3	1-2	0.5-1
BMI-for-height-age percentile or SDS	0.5-1.5	0.5-1.5	0.5-1	1-3	1-2	1
Head circumference–for–age percentile or SDS	0.5-1.5	0.5-1.5	0.5-1	1-3	1-2	1-2

Modified from National Kidney Foundation: KDOQI clinical practice guideline for nutrition in children with CKD: 2008 update, *Am J Kidney Dis* 53(Suppl 2):S16, 2009.
BMI, Body mass index.

children and an important negative influence on growth. Metabolic acidosis leads to both endogenous growth hormone and recombinant growth hormone resistance. Based on the experience of successfully enhancing the growth of infants and children with isolated renal tubular acidosis with alkalai therapy, it is recommended that children with CKD be treated to achieve a serum bicarbonate level of at least 22 mmol/L (National Kidney Foundation, 2009).

Nutrition

Protein energy malnutrition is a common problem in patients with CKD and is one of the major contributors to poor growth in the first few years of life. The origin of malnutrition in children with CKD is multifactorial; however, an inadequate voluntary intake is considered a major contributing factor, especially in infants. Nausea and vomiting are common in infants and children with CKD, with delayed gastric emptying and gastroesophageal reflux being detected in as many as 75% of patients with these problems (Ruely et al, 1989). In view of the importance of the nutritional status to the outcome of the infant and young child with CKD, frequent monitoring of the patient is mandatory. An age-related schema for parameters and frequency of nutritional assessment for patients with CKD has recently been published (Table 85-5) (National Kidney Foundation, 2009). The World Health Organization Growth Standards of length-for-age, weight-for-age, weight-for-length, body mass index–for-age and head circumference–for-age should be used as the reference for children from birth to 2 years (World Health Organization, 2006). Whereas nutritional intervention is indicated in children with CKD for findings that include an impaired ability to ingest or tolerate oral feedings, a body mass index value less than the 5th percentile of height-for-age, an acute weight loss of 10% or more or a length/height ratio more than 2 standard deviations (SD) less than the mean, neonates with CKD should be considered to be at nutritional risk if they are preterm or have any of the following:

- Low birth weight (<2500 g)
- A birth weight z score less than –2 SD for gestational age
- Polyuria and an inability to concentrate urine

TABLE 85-6 Equations to Estimate Energy Requirements for Children at Healthy Weights

Age (mo)	EER (kcal/d) = Total energy expenditure + Energy deposition
0-3	EER = 89 × Weight (kg) – 100 + 175
4-6	EER = 89 × Weight (kg) – 100 + 56
7-12	EER = 89 × Weight (kg) – 100 + 22
13-35	EER = 89 × Weight (kg) – 100 + 20

Modified from National Kidney Foundation: KDOQI clinical practice guideline for nutrition in children with CKD: 2008 update, *Am J Kidney Dis* 53(Suppl 2):S36, 2009.
EER, Estimated energy requirement.

In children with CKD, the spontaneous energy intake decreases with deteriorating kidney function. Energy requirements should, however, be considered to be 100% of the estimated energy requirement for chronologic age (Table 85-6) (Food and Nutrition Board, 2002; Ruely et al, 1989). Because energy intake is the principal determinate of growth during infancy, malnutrition has the most marked negative effect on the growth of children with congenital disorders leading to CKD (Betts et al, 1977). Supplemental nutritional support is indicated when the voluntary intake by the child fails to meet energy requirements and the child is not achieving expected rates of weight gain or growth for age. In infants requiring fluid restriction because of their impaired kidney function, oral intake of an energy-dense diet with a milk formula that has a caloric density greater than 20 kcal/oz, and the appropriate phosphorus content for CKD stage is preferred. If poor appetite or vomiting preclude an adequate oral intake, tube feedings (e.g., nasogastric, gastrostomy, gastrojejunostomy) should be considered and provided by either bolus or continuous infusion. The development of repeated emesis in children fed per nasogastric tube has prompted the use of gastrostomy as the preferred route of therapy (Warady et al, 1996). In infants younger than 1 year, an initial infusion rate of 10 to 20 mL/h or 1 to 2 mL/kg/h is generally well tolerated, to be followed by a daily increase of 5 to 10 mL per 8 hours or 1 mL/kg/h toward achieving the treatment goal. It is imperative that tube-fed

TABLE 85-7   Recommended Dietary Protein Intake in Children with CKD Stages 3 to 5 and 5D

Age	Dietary Reference Intake (DRI)				
	DRI (g/kg/d)	Recommended for CKD Stage 3 (g/kg/d) (100%-140% DRI)	Recommended for CKD Stages 4-5 (g/kg/d) (100%-120% DRI)	Recommended for HD (g/kg/d)*	Recommended for PD (g/kg/d)†
0-6 mo	1.5	1.5-2.1	1.5-1.8	1.6	1.8
7-12 mo	1.2	1.2-1.7	1.2-1.5	1.3	1.5
1-3 y	1.05	1.05-1.5	1.05-1.25	1.15	1.3

Modified from National Kidney Foundation: KDOQI clinical practice guideline for nutrition in children with CKD: 2008 update, *Am J Kidney Dis* 53(Suppl 2):S49, 2009.
*DRI + 0.1 g/kg/d to compensate for dialytic losses.
†DRI + 0.15 – 0.3 g/kg/d depending on patient age to compensate for peritoneal losses.

TABLE 85-8   Dietary Reference Intake for Healthy Children for Sodium, Chloride, and Potassium

Age	Sodium (mg/d)		Chloride (mg/d)		Potassium (mg/d)	
	AI	Upper Limit	AI	Upper Limit	AI	Upper Limit
0-6 mo	120	ND	180	ND	400	ND
7-12 mo	370	ND	570	ND	700	ND
1-3 y	1000	1500	1500	2300	3000	ND

Modified from National Kidney Foundation: KDOQI clinical practice guideline for nutrition in children with CKD: 2008 update, *Am J Kidney Dis* 53(Suppl 2):S49, 2009.
AI, Adequate intake; *ND,* not determined.

infants be encouraged to continue some oral intake or have oral stimulation (e.g., pacifier) if persistent feeding dysfunction is to be prevented.

Whereas the spontaneous dietary protein intake (DPI) is reduced in progressive CKD in a manner similar to that of energy intake, the DPI is typically far in excess of the average requirements. At the same time, there is no evidence that strict dietary protein restriction (120% recommended daily allowance) has any nephroprotective effect, nor does this level of intake compromise growth. Because moderate protein restriction reduces the accumulation of nitrogenous waste products and helps to lower dietary phosphorus intake, it is appropriate to gradually lower the DPI toward 100% of the dietary reference intake (DRI) as CKD progresses toward the need for dialysis (Ruely et al, 1989). More specifically, a DPI of 100% to 140% DRI for CKD stage 3, 100% to 120% DRI for CKD stage 4 to 5, and 100% DRI for CKD stage 5D (dialysis) has been proposed (Table 85-7). In patients receiving dialysis, the protein requirements are increased to account for dialysis-related protein losses.

Whereas restriction of sodium and water is often indicated in children with CKD complicated by sodium and fluid retention and systemic hypertension, infants and children with CKD secondary to obstructive uropathy or renal dysplasia often have polyuria and may experience substantial urinary sodium losses despite advanced stages of CKD. This scenario can result in contraction of the extracellular volume, in addition to having an adverse effect on growth and nitrogen retention (Wassner and Kulin, 1990). Infants and children with salt-wasting forms of CKD who do not receive salt supplementation may in turn experience vomiting, constipation, and significant growth retardation (Parekh et al, 2001). The same holds true for infants receiving peritoneal dialysis even if they are anuric, because most patients lose significant quantities of sodium in the

dialysate. Sodium depletion in the PD population has resulted in cerebral edema and blindness (Lapeyraque et al, 2003). Individualized therapy can be achieved by first prescribing at least the age-related DRI of sodium and chloride (Table 85-8), with subsequent modification of therapy based on regular assessment of clinical and laboratory data.

Potassium homeostasis in children with CKD is usually unaffected until the GFR falls to less than 10% of normal. However, infants and children with disorders such as renal dysplasia and reflux nephropathy often demonstrate resistance to aldosterone and may experience hyperkalemia, even when the GFR is preserved. The hyperkalemia can be exacerbated by volume contraction, as can be seen in patients with salt-wasting forms of CKD. In patients who remain hyperkalemic despite repletion of salt and water, restriction of dietary potassium intake is critical. For infants and young children, 40 to 120 mg (1 to 3 mmol/kg/d) of potassium may be a reasonable start. Breast milk has a lower potassium content (546 mg/L; 14 mmol/L) than commercial milk–based infant formula (700 to 740 mg/L; 18 to 19 mmol/L) (National Kidney Foundation, 2009). Pretreatment of infant formula with a potassium binder, treatment of constipation, and attention to medications that can exacerbate hyperkalemia (e.g., potassium-sparing diuretics, angiotensin-converting enzyme inhibitors, angiotensin-receptor blockers) may also be necessary in many patients (Bunchman et al, 1991; Fassinger et al, 1998).

Ethics of Initiating or Withdrawing Renal Replacement Therapy

Decisions to withdraw or withhold treatment have to be made for many patients in neonatology units, and for as many as 30% to 58% of patients in pediatric intensive care units. On rare occasions, such decisions pertain to the infant with ESRD confronted with the prospect of a lifetime of dialysis and transplantation. With the advent of advanced technology in the 1980s that made possible the provision of safe and effective peritoneal dialysis to even the smallest infant came increasing ethical dilemmas and significant variations in practice (Fauriel et al, 2004; Shooter and Watson, 2000; Watson and Shooter, 2004).

In one of the most interesting studies on the topic, Geary (1998) conducted an international survey on the attitudes of pediatric nephrologists regarding the management of ESRD during infancy (Geary, 1998). More than 200 physicians from eight countries replied to a series of questions pertaining to the provision of RRT to infants younger than 1 month of age versus those 1 to 12 months old. The factors that most often influence the decision to initiate or withhold RRT were found to be the presence of coexistent serious medical disorders and the anticipation of significant morbidity for the child. Only 25% of respondents believed it was usually ethically acceptable for parents to refuse RRT in infants beyond the 1st month of life compared with 50% with the same opinion concerning younger infants. Overall, only 41% of respondents offered RRT to all infants younger than 1 month, and 53% offered this therapy to all infants 1 to 12 months old, despite recent evidence supporting the use of this therapy as a reasonable treatment option (Carey et al, 2007). Evidence for this variation in practice has been seen in other surveys as well (Fauriel et al, 2004).

Most clinicians agree that there is more to their skill than the indiscriminant application of technology. Factors to consider when making the decision regarding initiation or withdrawal of RRT during infancy include quality of life concerns, allocation of resources, legal issues, and most importantly the opinions of the hospital team and the parents. The role of hospital ethics committees in the process remains extremely variable. In the end, clinicians and parents often struggle bravely to reach a compassionate decision with as much agreement as possible. Principles of practice that may provide valuable assistance in this process have been published previously (Watson and Shooter, 2004).

Renal Replacement Therapy

End-stage renal disease is an uncommon disorder in children, with an incidence in the United States of approximately 14 patients per 1 million children of a similar age (U.S. Renal Data System, 2008). The incidence varies within the pediatric population with a rate of 29 per 1 million for children 15 to 19 years old, in contrast to a rate of 9 per 1 million for children 0 to 4 years old. In a recent study by the NAPRTCS, Carey et al (2007) estimated the incidence of dialysis-treated neonatal ESRD as 0.045 cases per 1 million population per year (Carey et al, 2007). Although kidney transplantation is the nearly universal goal for children who develop ESRD, approximately 75% of pediatric patients initially receive chronic peritoneal dialysis or hemodialysis before a kidney transplant.

Peritoneal Dialysis

Peritoneal dialysis is the preferred chronic dialysis modality for infants with ESRD. Subsequent to the development of continuous ambulatory PD in 1976, the availability of small dialysate bags resulted in a number of reports of infants receiving continuous ambulatory PD in the middle 1980s. The later emergence of automated cycling machines that were able to deliver fill volumes as low as 50 mL, with incremental adjustments of 10 mL, allowed for the provision of safe and effective PD in neonates and infants. The preference for PD, and specifically automated PD as the chronic dialysis modality in infants and young children, is reflected by data from NAPRTCS in which 93% of patients 0 to 1 year old and receiving dialysis were receiving PD at dialysis initiation (Carey et al, 2007; NAPRTCS, 2008).

Peritoneal dialysis makes use of the peritoneal membrane as a natural dialyzing membrane. Dialysis solution is instilled and dwells within the peritoneal cavity, during which time bloodstream-derived solutes move down a concentration gradient based on diffusion, and fluid is removed as a result of the osmotic gradient created by the dextrose component of the dialysis fluid. The inflow, dwell, and drainage of dialysate characterize a single dialysis cycle or exchange. The peritoneal catheter is the cornerstone of successful PD, and the PD prescription accounts for the dextrose concentration and amount of dialysis solution (initially 600 to 800 mL/m^2 body surface area in infants) during each exchange and the length of the exchange (National Kidney Foundation, 2006).

The infant with ESRD who receives chronic PD is at risk for a variety of treatment-related complications that are ideally either prevented or identified early and treated aggressively if morbidity and mortality are to be minimized. The single most serious complication is peritonitis. The incidence of this infection is greatest during infancy, with a rate of 1 infection every 14.2 patient months reported by the NAPRTCS (2008). Whereas gram-positive organisms account for the majority of infections, gram-negative episodes of peritonitis are common in infants and young children (Zurowska et al, 2008). In turn, when peritonitis is suggested, empiric antibiotic therapy should provide coverage for gram-positive and gram-negative organisms (Warady et al, 2000). In some cases, infants may experience hypogammaglobulinemia in this situation and may benefit from replacement therapy (Neu et al, 1998). Other treatment-related complications that occur most frequently during infancy include anterior ischemic optic neuropathy and sudden blindness secondary to hypovolemia, excessive loss of protein across the peritoneal membrane and hernia formation (Lapeyraque et al, 2003; Quan and Baum, 1996; Warady et al, 2009).

Hemodialysis

The use of HD during infancy is dictated often by the presence of a medical condition that contraindicates use of the peritoneal membrane (e.g., omphalocele, gastroschisis, diaphragmatic hernia, bladder exstrophy). The procedure is complicated, and limited clinical experience has revealed a high incidence of patient morbidity (Al-Hermi et al, 1999; Kovalski et al, 2007; Shroff et al, 2007). Whereas the infrequent use of HD in infants precludes the generation of an evidence base upon which to guide maintenance therapy, there are some key treatment-related principles to consider when conducting the procedure. Despite the availability of neonatal-sized tubing, the extracorporeal volume usually comprises more than 10% of the patient's blood volume in infants weighing less than 8 kg; this necessitates circuit priming with 5% albumin or packed red blood cells diluted to a hematocrit of 35% (Warady et al, 2009). Blood access is typically in the form of a 7F or 8F dual-lumen catheter, which allows blood pump flow rates of 30 to 50 mL/min. Despite the use of HD machines with volumetric control capability, the accuracy is only to 50 to 100 mL, thus mandating the use of continuous monitoring of the patient's weight with a digital scale when conducting HD on neonates. The complicated nature of the procedure mandates that it be performed only in highly qualified centers.

Transplantation

The topic of kidney transplantation in patients who develop ESRD as neonates or young infants is complicated, and a lengthy discussion is beyond the scope of this chapter. In short, transplantation is a viable alternative for these young patients and is their best hope for long-term survival. In a review of NAPRTCS data, Carey et al (2007) found that 3 years after dialysis initiation, 80% of 63 neonates had undergone transplantation. What is often most important for the neonatologist is recognizing the need to develop a collaborative strategy with members of the pediatric nephrology and urology team for management of congenital structural abnormalities of the urinary tract that are present in the patient with severe CKD/ESRD, the majority of which will ultimately require transplantation (Sarwal and Salvatierra, 2004). Minimizing the use of interventions that greatly increase the risk of central venous thrombosis should also be encouraged. The most recent report of the U.S. Renal Data System reveals that 51 infants younger than 1 year and 89 children aged 1 to 4 years received a kidney transplant in 2006 (U.S. Renal Data System, 2008). The 3-year graft survival for patients who received a living donor transplant in 2003 was 83.9% and 94.6% for patients who were less than 1 and 1 to 4 years old, respectively, at the time of transplant. In the case of deceased donor transplants, the graft survival for those aged 1 to 4 years was 89.7%, while the number of deceased donor transplants performed during infancy was exceptionally small.

OUTCOMES

Growth and Development

Children with CKD often experience some degree of growth failure. This failure is especially concerning when CKD occurs in infancy, a time of rapid growth. By 2 years of age, approximately one third of postnatal growth has occurred (Haffner, 2008); therefore early intervention to address treatable causes of CKD-associated growth failure is essential to maximize the growth of these infants. The disordered growth in patients with CKD is a multifactorial process. Protein-calorie malnutrition, metabolic acidosis, electrolyte disarray, renal osteodystrophy, and changes in the gonadotropic hormone axis in the face of uremia, corticosteroid treatment, or both are factors that contribute to this challenging problem (Geary, 1998; Haffner, 2008).

Infants with CKD are especially susceptible to protein-calorie malnutrition because of the high energy demands in this age group.

Several studies have shown that infants have impaired growth at initiation of chronic dialysis. There are conflicting reports regarding improvement in growth with renal replacement therapy. Most studies suggest that young children on dialysis fail to grow well, despite meeting 100% of the recommended daily allowance of caloric intake (Shroff et al, 2003). Growth outcomes may be better after transplantation (Ledermann et al, 1999), and Hijazi et al (2009) report that current growth outcomes of infants with ESRD have improved over time, possibly because of advances in medical and surgical therapies. To continue this trend of improvement, clinicians must address comorbidities including protein-calorie malnutrition in these infants with CKD. Recent reports have described improved longitudinal growth and sustained catch-up growth in infants with chronic renal failure in whom growth hormone treatment was initiated in the 1st year of life. Mencarelli et al (2009) reported 12 infants initiated on recombinant human growth hormone at a median age of 0.5 years had significantly better height SDS scores and change-in-height SDS scores versus a control group not treated with growth hormone, despite similar nutritional intake.

In addition to growth impairments, neurodevelopmental impairments may also be present in children with CKD during infancy and early childhood. Like many children with chronic illnesses, children with CKD may have delayed achievement of many developmental milestones. In addition, delayed cognitive performance especially in regard to general intelligence, attention, executive function, language, visual-spatial abilities, and memory, has been repeatedly reported in children with CKD (Geary, 1998; Gipson, 2008). Whereas some children have renal involvement as part of a larger syndrome that may involve structural or functional abnormalities of the central nervous system, other comorbidities of CKD (e.g., anemia, hypertension, cerebral vascular accidents, adverse effects of therapy) have been implicated in the neurodevelopmental impairments in many patients (Geary, 1998). The brain undergoes rapid growth during infancy, reaching half of its adult weight by 6 months of age (Harris, 2006). Postnatal brain growth includes neuronal differentiation, dendritic branching, and axonal myelination (Gipson, 2008). Renal impairment in infancy, a crucial time of neural development, raises concerns regarding the neurodevelopmental outcomes in these children. In one study, 28 patients initiating chronic peritoneal dialysis by 3 months of age underwent formal neurodevelopmental testing. Only 6 of the 28 patients were functioning below the average level. Nineteen of these patients were retested after their fourth birthday. Fifteen of the 16 school-aged patients were full-time students in age-appropriate classrooms, and all of the children younger than 5 years were in preschool (Warady, 1999). In another longitudinal study of 31 patients with ESRD diagnosed in infancy, 18 were attending regular school, 13 had significant neuropsychologic impairments, 9 required special education classes, and 4 were severely impaired (Hijazi et al, 2009). Eleven patients with ESRD diagnosed before 2 years of age were followed; six had appropriate milestones, whereas five had special education needs (Shroff et al, 2003). Yet another study followed 16 patients with ESRD diagnosed in infancy and found that 14 achieved age-appropriate developmental milestones (Ledermann et al, 1999). Most recently, Madden et al (2003) reported on the cognitive and psychosocial outcome of 16 infants who began PD during the 1st year of life; a majority (75%) had a functioning transplant at the time of their reassessment at a mean age of 5.8 years. Ten (67%) children had an intelligence quotient in the normal range, whereas 13 of 15 (87%) were within 2 standard deviations of the mean (Madden et al, 2003). Thus, although existing reports are largely case series with relatively small sample sizes, more recent literature suggests improved neurodevelopmental outcomes for children with CKD and ESRD in infancy compared with reports before 2000. It appears that at least 25% of infants and toddlers who have severe renal insufficiency are reported to have developmental delay, whereas the effects of milder forms of CKD on the neurodevelopment of infants remains less clear. Large multicenter longitudinal studies may provide more insight into the developmental outcomes of infants with CKD.

Hospitalization

There is emerging evidence to support the clinical expectation that a majority of neonates and infants with CKD or ESRD require frequent hospitalization throughout childhood. In one study of 18 children requiring chronic hemodialysis by 2 years of age, the median number of hospital admissions while receiving dialysis was 6 (range 3 to 16). Of those hospitalized, the median hospitalization rate per patient was 8.2 admissions per year with the duration ranging from 63 to 399 days (Shroff et al, 2003). Another study divided 698 children requiring chronic dialysis by 2 years old into those initiating dialysis by 1 month of age and those initiating dialysis between 1 month and 24 months of age. Approximately 80% of children in both groups required hospitalization at some point in the 13-year follow-up period. Among children ever hospitalized, those initiating dialysis as neonates were hospitalized more frequently than were children starting dialysis later (mean number of hospitalizations, 54 versus 39; p <0.001) and had longer hospital stays (Carey et al, 2007).

Renal Osteodystrophy

There is a paucity of outcome data in the neonatal and infant populations regarding many of the other comorbidities associated with CKD. There is evidence suggesting that infants with secondary hyperparathyroidism from CKD have improvement with chronic renal replacement therapy. One study followed 17 patients initiating hemodialysis between birth and 2 years of age and found that the percentage of patients with intact parathyroid hormone concentrations less than twice the upper limit of normal increased after 3 months of hemodialysis (41% at initiation versus 69% after 3 months; Shroff et al, 2003). Another study of 20 infants on long-term PD revealed similar results (58% after 6 months of PD versus 100% after 1 year of PD) (Ledermann, 2000). Further study regarding the prevalence of renal osteodystrophy in this population is needed.

Survival

Long-term survival of neonates with CKD or ESRD appears to be similar to that of older infants and young children (Carey et al, 2007, Hijazi et al, 2009, Wedekin et al, 2008). Factors reportedly associated with mortality include African American race, presence of comorbidities such as chronic lung disease, multiorgan dysfunction, diagnosis of a syndrome, and oliguria or anuria (Hijazi et al, 2009). Approximately 25% of neonates died over 18 months of follow-up in one study, which was similar to the mortality rate of older children (Carey et al, 2007). Another study found 22% mortality (Shroff et al, 2003). Yet another study following infants with CKD for 25 years reported 54% mortality, but found a 5-year survival rate of 87% among patients surviving the 1st year (Hijazi et al, 2009). In addition, Wedekin et al (2008) followed 119 infants with CKD and estimated the 1-, 2-, and 5-year survival rates to be 78%, 68%, and 63%, respectively. However, if the patients were receiving renal replacement therapy, survival improved to 91%, 83%, and 83% for 1, 2, and 5 years, respectively. Among the patients who received renal transplants, the 1-, 2-, and 5-year survival rates were greater than 95% (Wedekin et al, 2008). A majority of children with ESRD diagnosed as neonates undergo renal transplantation in the first few years of life. In a study by Carey et al (2007) 80% of neonates with ESRD diagnosed in the neonatal period received a kidney transplant within 5 years of initiating dialysis (Carey). It appears that younger children are receiving transplants more readily in recent years (Carey), which is encouraging in the face of more favorable survival.

SUGGESTED READINGS

Andreoli SP: Acute renal failure in the newborn, *Semin Perinatol* 28:112-123, 2004.

Askenazi DJ, Ambalavanan N, Goldstein SL: Acute kidney injury in critically ill newborns: what do we know? What do we need to learn? *Pediatr Nephrol* 24:265-274, 2009.

Basile DP: The endothelial cell in ischemic acute kidney injury: implications for acute and chronic kidney function, *Kidney Int* 72:151-156, 2007.

Brenner BM, Lawler EV, Mackenzie HS: The hyperfiltration theory: a paradigm shift in nephrology, *Kidney Int* 49:1774-1777, 1996.

Carey WA, Talley LI, Sehring SA, et al: Outcomes of dialysis initiated during the neonatal period for treatment of end-stage renal disease: a North American Pediatric Renal Trials and Collaborative Studies Special Analysis, *Pediatrics* 119:e468-e473, 2007.

Geary DF: Attitudes of pediatric nephrologists to management of end-stage renal disease in infants, *J Pediatr* 133:154-156, 1998.

Hijazi R, Abitbol C, Chandar J, et al: Twenty-five years of infant dialysis: a single center experience, *J Pediatr* 155:111-117, 2009.

Mehta RL, Kellum JA, Shah SV, et al: Acute Kidney Injury Network (AKIN): report of an initiative to improve outcomes in acute kidney injury, *Crit Care* 11:R31, 2007.

National Kidney Foundation: KDOQI clinical practice guideline for nutrition in children with CKD: 2008 update, *Am J Kidney Dis* 53(Suppl 2):S1-S124, 2009.

Rees L: Management of the neonate with chronic renal failure, *Semin Fetal Neonat Med* 13:181-188, 2008.

Shooter M, Watson A: The ethics of withholding and withdrawing dialysis therapy in infants, *Pediatr Nephrol* 14:347-351, 2000.

Symons JM, Chua AN, Somers MJ, et al: Demographic characteristics of pediatric continuous renal replacement therapy: a report of the prospective pediatric continuous renal replacement therapy registry, *Clin J Am Soc Nephrol* 2:732-738, 2007.

Watson AR, Shooter M: The ethics of withholding and withdrawing dialysis in children. In Warady BA, Schaefer FS, Fine RN, Alexander SR, editors: *Pediatric dialysis*, Dordrecht, the Netherlands, 2004, Kluwer Academic Publishers, p 501.

Wedekin M, Ehrich J, Offner G, Pape L: Aetiology and outcome of acute and chronic renal failure in infants, *Nephrol Dial Transplant* 23:1575-1580, 2008.

White SL, Perkovic V, Cass A, et al: Is low birth weight an antecedent of CKD in later life? A systematic review of observational studies, *Am J Kidney Dis* 54:248-261, 2009.

Complete references used in this text can be found online at www.expertconsult.com

GLOMERULONEPHROPATHIES AND DISORDERS OF TUBULAR FUNCTION

Lawrence Copelovitch and Bernard S. Kaplan

GLOMERULONEPHROPATHIES

Glomerulonephropathies generally present with features of the nephrotic syndrome and less often with nephritic syndrome. Massive proteinuria, hypoalbuminemia, hyperlipidemia, and edema characterize the nephrotic syndrome. Newborns may have transient proteinuria without apparent glomerular injury, and serum albumin levels can be in the nephrotic range in normal premature infants. Therefore, the diagnosis of nephrotic syndrome should be made only in patients with persistent, massive proteinuria; severe hypoalbuminemia; hyperlipidemia not caused by hyperalimentation; and edema that is not the result of fluid overload, capillary leak, or both. Nephrotic range proteinuria is defined as greater than 4 mg/kg/hour in the neonatal period. Nephritis (hematuria, red blood cell casts, oliguria or anuria, hypertension, and azotemia) is uncommon in newborns.

The nephrotic syndrome can be inherited as an entity isolated to the kidneys (congenital nephrotic syndrome of the Finnish type [CNF] and as isolated diffuse mesangial sclerosis) or as part of a defined malformation syndrome (Denys-Drash syndrome, Galloway-Mowat syndrome, Pierson syndrome, Frasier syndrome, and nail-patella syndrome). Glomerulopathies that occur in newborns and infants can also be divided into primary glomerular conditions with nephrotic syndrome (e.g., CNF) and secondary glomerular conditions (e.g., congenital syphilis). Only CNF and congenital syphilis typically manifest with nephrotic syndrome at birth. Diffuse mesangial sclerosis (DMS), Denys-Drash syndrome, Pierson syndrome, and Galloway-Mowat syndrome infrequently manifest in the neonatal period. Rarely, maternal transmission of anti-glomerular antibodies can result in neonatal membranous glomerulonephritis (Debiec et al, 2002). Minimal change nephrotic syndrome, focal segmental glomerulosclerosis (FSGS), primary membranous glomerulonephritis, collagen type III glomerulopathy, and mercury toxicity do not occur in newborns but occasionally are seen in infants. Lupus nephritis and congenital toxoplasmosis have been reported in a neonate (Lam et al, 1999). Renal vein thrombosis can be a consequence of the nephrotic syndrome but is not a cause of the syndrome. There is no convincing evidence that intrauterine infections with cytomegalovirus (Batisky et al, 1993), rubella (Beale et al, 1979), or toxoplasmosis (Shahin et al, 1974) are causes of neonatal nephrotic syndrome. There are reports of *unique* family syndromes in which congenital nephrotic syndrome occurred in association with congenital anomalies, such as buphthalmos. There are reports of congenital glomerular injury that elude classification and reports of spontaneous remission of apparent congenital nephrotic syndrome (Haws et al, 1992).

CONGENITAL NEPHROTIC SYNDROME OF THE FINNISH TYPE (NPHS1) [McKUSICK #256300]

Inheritance is autosomal recessive and the locus is assigned on 19q12-q13.1 (Kestila et al, 1994). The *NPHS1* gene that is mutated in *NPHS1* codes for nephrin, a cell-surface podocyte protein. Two mutations, Fin-major and Fin-minor, are found in more than 90% of Finnish patients (Patrakka et al, 2000). CNF occurs in all population groups, but the highest prevalence is in Finland with an incidence of 12.2 per 100,000 newborns (Huttunen, 1976). There is minor intrafamilial and interfamilial variability in the severity and age of onset of the nephrotic syndrome. Absence of a history of Finnish ancestry does not exclude the diagnosis. Proteinuria is detected within the 1st week of life in 71% of cases and by 2 months in all affected infants (Huttunen, 1976). Early onset of hypertension and renal failure are uncommon. Infants are often premature and small for gestational age. Although there are no typical dysmorphic features, large anterior fontanel, limb deformations, and pyloric stenosis do occur (Sibley et al, 1986). Maternal serum and amniotic fluid alpha-fetoprotein levels are elevated (Seppala et al, 1976), and increased concentrations of albumin are detected in the amniotic fluid of some patients. The diagnosis may be made coincidentally by the finding of a low thyroxine level during screening for hypothyroidism (Finnegan et al, 1980). Most of these patients have a primary form of hypothyroidism characterized by low thyroxine and high thyroid-stimulating hormone levels caused by urinary losses of thyroxine and iodine (McLean et al, 1982). The placenta is large, with a mean placenta–neonatal weight ratio of 0.43 (normal ratio is 0.18).

Echodense kidneys are symmetrically enlarged on ultrasonography. Histologically the glomeruli initially appear normal; proximal tubules are dilated in 74% of cases. Ultrastructural studies show the effacement (*fusion*) of epithelial cell foot processes and, later in the course, interstitial fibrosis, lymphocytic and plasma cell infiltration, periglomerular fibrosis, and glomerular sclerosis (Habib, 1993).

The course is characterized by nephrotic syndrome complicated by failure to thrive, recurrent infections, and eventual chronic renal failure. Renal vein thrombosis may occur in utero and postpartum. The nephrotic syndrome is resistant to treatment. Aggressive feeding by nasogastric or gastrostomy tubes can ensure weight gain. Massive edema is treated with intravenous albumin. Furosemide is added if the patient is not volume-depleted. Hypothyroidism is treated with thyroxine. Bilateral nephrectomies and dialysis are indicated if edema, volume depletion, and inanition cannot be controlled. Long-term peritoneal dialysis is difficult, but feasible, in small infants. The results of living-relate renal transplantation are encouraging; however, a subset of patients will have recurrence due to the development of anti-nephrin antibodies in response to novel antigen exposure (Patrakka, 2002).

DENYS-DRASH SYNDROME

Early onset of nephrotic syndrome with DMS can occur in the Denys-Drash syndrome. The syndrome consists of overlapping features of ambiguous genitalia in males, nephrotic syndrome with DMS (Habib, 1993), and Wilms' tumor. All 46XY patients have either ambiguous genitalia or female phenotype. Phenotypic females (XX or XY) may go unrecognized. Heterozygous zinc finger mutations in either exon 8 or exon 9 of the *WT1* gene on chromosome 11p are causative (Niaudet et al, 2006; Schumacher et al, 1998). Occasional patients present with nephrotic syndrome in the neonatal period (Gertner et al, 1980). Patients should undergo frequent ultrasound screening to monitor the possible development of Wilms' tumor. Siblings are not affected. Most patients die by 4 years of age unless transplanted. In such cases, bilateral native nephrectomies are performed as soon as possible.

A related condition, Frasier syndrome, is caused exclusively by mutations in the donor splice site in intron 9 of the *WT1* gene. The syndrome is characterized by nephrotic syndrome (FSGS), male pseudohermaphroditism, and gonadal dysgenesis with increased risk of gonadoblastoma and malignant germ-cell tumors. As in DDS, phenotypic females may go unrecognized. Onset of nephrotic syndrome is usually in adolescence but has been described in children as young as 6 months of age (Gwin et al, 2008).

DIFFUSE MESANGIAL SCLEROSIS

DMS can be inherited as an autosomal recessive condition, occur sporadically, or be a component of Denys-Drash (Habib, 1993) or Pierson syndromes (Zenker et al, 2004). DMS has been reported in an 18-week fetus (Spear et al, 1991) and occasionally can present in the neonatal period (Scott and Rochefort, 1992). Recessively inherited DMS can be caused by mutations mapped to 10q23 in the region encoding the phospholipase C epsilon 1 (PLCE1) gene. This phospholipase is a key component in the second messenger pathway and is thought to be involved in growth and development of the podocyte (Hinkes, 2006). Maternal and fetal alpha-fetoprotein concentrations and placental size are usually normal (Scott and Rochefort, 1992). Most patients present with nephrotic syndrome and chronic renal failure between 3 and 6 months and are hypertensive. There are no dysmorphic features. The kidneys are enlarged and echodense by ultrasound examination. The fully developed renal lesion consists of mesangial sclerosis, collapsed tufts, embedded mesangial cells, thick glomerular basement membranes, and tubulointerstitial lesions (Habib, 1993).

There is no specific treatment. Hypertension is treated with angiotensin-converting enzyme inhibitors but often requires several additional agents. Treatment of DMS includes optimal calories, peritoneal dialysis, and transplantation.

DMS does not recur after transplantation. All female patients with isolated DMS should undergo karyotype analysis, because Denys-Drash syndrome may go unrecognized in phenotypic females. It is important to determine whether there is a mutation in the *WT1* gene at chromosomal locus 11p to rule out Denys-Drash syndrome. If that cannot be done, renal ultrasound examinations may be warranted every few months to monitor for Wilms' tumor.

GALLOWAY-MOWAT SYNDROME

This rare condition consists of abnormal central nervous system development and nephrotic syndrome (Cooperstone et al, 1993). Inheritance is autosomal recessive, and there may be variable expression in a family (Cohen et al, 1994). Patients may be small for gestational age. The nephrotic syndrome usually manifests before the age of 3 years and often before 3 months of age. There are no consistent glomerular histopathologic changes. The pathogenesis has not been determined. Neurologic findings are microcephaly, wide sulci, abnormal gyral patterns, developmental retardation, and seizures (Kucharczuk et al, 2000). Large floppy ears, a receding forehead, and hiatal hernia are features in some cases (Cooperstone et al, 1993). Death usually occurs before 6 months of age. The nephrotic syndrome does not respond to treatment. Renal transplantation is not encouraged because of the progressive nature of the severe neurologic disorder. Increased maternal serum and amniotic fluid alpha-fetoprotein assays and abnormal renal ultrasonographic findings may prove useful for prenatal diagnosis (Palm et al, 1986).

PIERSON SYNDROME

This syndrome is characterized by microcoria and congenital nephrotic syndrome. Mutations at chromosomal locus 3p21 in the Laminin Beta 2 *(LAMB2)* gene, which encodes an essential glomerular basement membrane protein, have been associated with this condition (Zenker et al, 2004). Inheritance is autosomal recessive. Edema in the newborn period, progressive renal failure within the 1st year of life, and neurocognitive deficits, with ocular maldevelopment, abnormal lens shape, cataracts, retinal abnormalities, and microcoria, are the phenotypic features. The kidneys are enlarged and echodense by ultrasound examination. Diffuse mesangial sclerosis is the hallmark lesion seen on renal biopsy (Zenker et al, 2004), although focal segmental glomerulosclerosis and minor glomerular changes have been described. Occasionally, *LAMB2* mutations are associated with milder clinical involvement of kidneys and/or eyes (Kagan et al, 2008).

CONGENITAL SYPHILIS

Clinical features of nephrotic syndrome predominate over those of nephritis. The diagnosis must be suspected in an infant who has edema, proteinuria, and signs of congenital syphilis (McDonald et al, 1971). The glomerular findings implicate an immune pathogenesis with subepithelial deposits that contain imunoglobulin G (IgG) and *Treponema* antigen (O'Regan et al, 1976). Treatment with penicillin results in permanent remission of the glomerulopathy.

DISORDERS OF RENAL TUBULAR FUNCTION

A diagnosis of a renal tubular disorder cannot be made without an appreciation of normal renal maturation. Premature newborns (and even full-term newborns) can waste sodium and chloride and have variable combinations of aminoaciduria, glucosuria, phosphaturia, impaired potassium excretion, reduced reabsorptive capacity for sodium bicarbonate, and inability to concentrate urine maximally. In healthy newborns, these are transient aberrations that tend to be isolated and do not cause problems except for the low bicarbonate threshold in preterm infants. This can lead to mild metabolic acidosis during the first few months of life. Very low-birthweight newborns may have nonoliguric hyperkalemia, in part secondary to decreased Na^+,K^+-ATPase activity, which increases with maturation. Therefore, except in specific circumstances, it is not necessary to embark on a full-scale evaluation.

Some renal tubular disorders may be suspected and confirmed in utero. A prenatal diagnosis, however, requiring chorionic villus sampling or amniocentesis can be made only after diagnosis of a condition in an older sibling. Postnatally, the possibility of a tubular disorder may arise when abnormal blood gas and electrolyte results are obtained. The initial manifestations of a renal tubular disorder may not include all the findings associated with the disorder.

Three constellations of fluid and electrolyte imbalances should alert a neonatologist to the possibility of a disorder of renal tubular function. The combination of metabolic acidosis, hyperkalemia, and hyponatremia is seen in renal dysplasias, obstructive uropathy (especially if complicated by a urinary tract infection), and pseudohypoaldosteronism. Furthermore, congenital adrenal hyperplasia can present with these abnormalities. Metabolic acidosis, hypokalemia, and hypophosphatemia are the characteristic findings seen in patients with proximal renal tubular dysfunction, the so-called Fanconi's syndrome. Metabolic alkalosis, hypokalemia, and hyponatremia occur in Bartter's syndrome.

Important clinical clues to the presence of a renal tubular disorder are poor feeding, unexplained vomiting, dehydration, failure to thrive, drowsiness, irritability, tetany, seizures, and unexplained icterus. Isolated proximal renal tubular acidosis (RTA) is uncommon, and the need for large quantities of bicarbonate to correct a hyperchloremic metabolic acidosis is a clue to the diagnosis. Fructose intolerance and galactosemia must be considered in a jaundiced newborn with Fanconi's syndrome. Hypophosphatemia and renal phosphate wasting are manifestations of X-linked hypophosphatemic rickets, but it is uncommon for this condition to be diagnosed in a newborn. Hyperchloremic metabolic acidosis with a decrease in the unmeasured anion gap and in the absence of diarrhea raises the possibility of distal RTA. Distal RTA rarely manifests in the neonatal period, however. More commonly, diarrhea with resultant loss of bicarbonate in stool and an inappropriate increase in urine pH may mimic distal RTA. This occurs as a result of decreased sodium delivery to the distal nephron, which is required for normal hydrogen ion excretion (Izraeli et al, 1990). Pseudohypoaldosteronism, Bartter's syndrome, and renal dysplasias must be considered in newborns with severe hyponatremia and renal salt wasting.

Infants with Bartter's syndrome are hypokalemic, whereas those with renal adysplasia, pseudohypoaldosteronism, and the renal tubular hyperkalemia syndromes are hyperkalemic. Hematuria, renal calculi, and nephrocalcinosis with hypercalciuria can occur in newborns with prolonged use of furosemide (see Chapter 34). Primary hyperoxaluria type 1 may present in the newborn period with acute renal failure and nephrocalcinosis (Ellis et al, 2001). Nephrocalcinosis in neonates and early infancy is also associated with prematurity, distal RTA, Bartter's syndrome, hypercalcemia, vitamin D intoxication, X-linked hypophosphatemic rickets, and familial hypomagnesemia with hypercalciuria and nephrocalcinosis.

RENAL FANCONI SYNDROME OF PROXIMAL TUBULAR DYSFUNCTION

The renal Fanconi syndrome is characterized by generalized proximal renal tubular dysfunction with impaired net reabsorption of amino acids, bicarbonate, glucose, phosphate, urate, sodium, potassium, and low-molecular-weight proteins. Renal excretion of these solutes and water is increased, and the serum concentrations of some are variably reduced. Hypophosphatemia results in vitamin D–resistant rickets, and bicarbonaturia causes a hyperchloremic metabolic acidosis. In newborns, the clinical manifestations of renal Fanconi syndrome may include polyuria, dehydration, metabolic acidosis, and glycosuria. These features are often asynchronous. Growth retardation and rickets mostly occur later in infancy.

HEREDITARY FRUCTOSE INTOLERANCE [McKUSICK #229600]

Hereditary fructose intolerance presents only in newborns fed sucrose or fructose in formula, antibiotics, fruit juices, or honey. The symptoms are poor feeding, vomiting, and failure to thrive (Gitzelman et al, 1989). The diagnosis can be made by molecular analysis of the aldolase-B gene in blood (Brooks and Tolan, 1993). Inheritance is autosomal recessive. Fructose-containing foods must be withdrawn from the diet as soon as the condition is suspected.

GALACTOSEMIA [MCKUSICK #230400]

Classic galactosemia deficiency can manifest in neonates with vomiting, diarrhea, hyperbilirubinemia with jaundice, hepatomegaly, ascites, and *Escherichia coli* sepsis a few days after starting milk ingestion. Cataracts are occasionally detectable by slit-lamp examination in neonates. This autosomal recessive disease is caused by deficient activity of galactose-1-phosphate uridyl transferase (GALT) as a result of mutations in the *GALT* gene at chromosomal locus 17q (Tyfield et al, 1999). Two other autosomal recessively inherited disorders of galactose metabolism (transferase and epimerase deficiency) occur more rarely. Newborn screening programs include tests for detection of galactosemia. The diagnosis is suggested by demonstrating increased concentrations of galactose in blood and urine and confirmed by demonstrating deficient red blood cell galactose-1-phosphate uridyl transferase (or galactokinase). Milk and milk-containing products must be withdrawn from the diet.

CYTOCHROME *c* OXIDASE DEFICIENCY

A fatal infantile cytopathy with variable manifestations in brain, skeletal and cardiac muscle, liver, and occasionally renal Fanconi syndrome is one of the mitochondrial cytopathy syndromes associated with defects in complex IV of the respiratory chain (cytochrome *c* oxidase) (EC 1.9.3.1). Inheritance appears to be autosomal recessive. Clinical features include neonatal onset of hypotonia; hyporeflexia; respiratory failure; elevated levels of lactic and pyruvic acids in blood, cerebrospinal fluid, or urine; and renal Fanconi syndrome (Lombes et al, 1996). There is no treatment, prognosis is dismal, and most neonates die in infancy.

CYSTINOSIS [McKUSICK #219800]

Affected individuals appear normal at birth and develop manifestations of the renal Fanconi syndrome between 6 and 12 months. The diagnosis should be considered if there are features of the renal Fanconi syndrome in a neonate. Inheritance is autosomal recessive, and there is defective lysosomal transport of cystine. The cystinosis gene, *CTNS*, maps to chromosome 17p13 and encodes an integral membrane protein, cystinosin (Town et al, 1998). Cystinosis can be diagnosed in utero by cystine measurements in chorionic villi by 9 weeks (Smith et al, 1987). Early and adequate treatment with oral cysteamine retards progression to end-stage renal failure (Markello et al, 1993), and administration of 0.55% cysteamine eyedrops from 1 year of age dissolves the corneal cystine crystals (Gahl et al, 2000).

TYROSINEMIA TYPE 1 [McKUSICK #276700]

Type 1 tyrosinemia is caused by deficiency in the gene for fumarylacetoacetate hydrolase at chromosomal locus 15q23-q25. Although type 1 tyrosinemia is an important cause of renal Fanconi syndrome and hepatocellular carcinoma, this rarely manifests in the neonate (Vanden Eijnden et al, 2000).

FANCONI-BICKEL SYNDROME

Fanconi-Bickel syndrome is caused by a homozygous deficiency in the gene for the glucose transporter 2 (GLUT 2) on chromosome 3q26. It is characterized by hepatorenal glycogen accumulation, fasting hypoglycemia, hepatomegaly, proximal tubular dysfunction, rickets, and short stature. The first manifestations usually appear between 3 and 10 months of age but are occasionally present in the newborn period (Riva, 2004).

RENAL GLYCOSURIA

Isolated forms of renal glycosuria rarely manifest in the newborn and are benign. Intermittent or constant renal glycosuria can also be detected in newborns who have the rare, autosomal recessive condition of glucose and galactose malabsorption (Markello et al, 1993).

RENAL TUBULAR ACIDOSIS

Primary RTA is characterized by chronic hyperchloremic metabolic acidosis associated with an inability to either acidify urine or reabsorb bicarbonate. It may be a primary disorder or secondary to acquired renal injury. Primary RTA is not associated with the renal Fanconi syndrome. Primary RTA is separated into three main types: proximal RTA (pRTA or type 2 RTA); distal RTA or *classic* RTA (type 1) and hyperkalemic RTA (type 4).

Primary Proximal Renal Tubular Acidosis

Proximal renal tubular acidosis (pRTA) is an integral feature of the renal Fanconi syndrome, and primary pRTA is extremely uncommon. The primary form may be inherited in autosomal dominant, recessive, or sporadic fashion. The recessive form may be associated with ocular abnormalities such as band keratopathy, glaucoma, and cataracts and is caused by a mutation in 4q21 encoding the apically located Na^+-HCO_3 cotransporter (NBC-1) (Usui et al, 2001). The underlying defect in pRTA is an inability to reabsorb filtered bicarbonate in the proximal tubule with bicarbonate wasting and hyperchloremic metabolic acidosis but normal distal tubular acidification. Therefore, when filtered bicarbonate is reclaimed to maximal renal tubular reabsorptive capacity for a patient with pRTA, the urine pH is appropriate for the severity of metabolic acidosis, with values below 5.3. When pRTA occurs as an isolated defect, it is usually transient (Nash et al, 1972).

Distal Renal Tubular Acidosis

Clinical manifestations of distal RTA (dRTA) are anorexia, failure to thrive, hypotonia, persistently low serum bicarbonate, elevated serum chloride, inappropriately high urine pH, and, in some cases, nephrocalcinosis. Additional findings are decreased urinary excretion of titratable acid, NH_4^+ (ammonium), and citrate. Some patients have congenital high-frequency nerve deafness. Untreated patients develop rickets (Caldas et al, 1992). dRTA is often considered in the differential diagnosis of a neonate with a non-anion-gap acidosis, but there are few reports of dRTA in neonates (Caldas et al, 1992; McSherry et al, 1978). The possibility of dRTA can be inferred from calculating the rate of excretion of NH_4^+. This can be determined indirectly by calculating the urinary net charge or urine anion gap (Goldstein et al, 1986): $Na^+ + K^+ + NH_4^+ = Cl^- + 80$. The kidney is not the cause of acidosis if the Cl^- (chloride) is greater than the sum of Na^+ (sodium) + K^+ (potassium). If $Na^+ + K^+$ is greater than Cl^- (chloride), then the urinary NH_4^+ may be less than 80 mmol per day, in keeping with dRTA (Carlisle et al, 1991). The diagnosis of dRTA is often made erroneously in patients with diarrhea who develop a hyperchloremic metabolic acidosis and have an *inappropriate* urine pH over 6 (Izraeli et al, 1990).

Regardless of whether a transient or permanent form of distal RTA is suspected, adequate amounts of alkali, either as bicarbonate or citrate, in doses of 2 to 3 mEq/kg/day are required to maintain a normal serum bicarbonate concentration (Igarashi et al, 1992). This can be withdrawn after several months to challenge the diagnosis, or the infant can be allowed to outgrow the dose. Challenging with an ammonium chloride loading test is not necessary because the diagnosis can be inferred from indirect tests such as the urine anion gap.

There are at least three autosomal recessively inherited forms of dRTA. In dRTA *without* nerve deafness, a mutation in the gene is located on chromosome 7q33-34; the gene product is the 116-kDa B-subunit of the apical pump (ATP6N1B) (Smith et al, 2000). dRTA *with* nerve deafness (Karet et al, 1999) is caused by mutations in ATP6B1, located on chromosome 2p13, and encoding the B-subunit of the apical proton pump mediating distal nephron acid secretion. Autosomal recessive dRTA without deafness in Asians and autosomal dominant dRTA without deafness in whites are caused by a mutation located on chromosome 17q21-22, which encodes the anion exchanger-1 (AE-1) located in the basolateral membrane of the cortical collecting duct (Sritippayawan, 2004).

Renal Tubular Acidosis Caused by Maternal Sniffing of Toluene

Maternal toluene abuse from paint or glue sniffing during pregnancy causes severe renal tubular acidosis in mother and neonate (Lindemann, 1991).

BARTTER'S SYNDROMES (INHERITED HYPOKALEMIC RENAL TUBULAR DISORDERS)

Bartter's syndrome is a congenital chronic tubular disorder characterized by hypokalemic metabolic alkalosis, polyuria, salt wasting, hyperkaliuria, hyperaldosteronism, resistance to the pressor effect of angiotensin, juxtaglomerular apparatus hyperplasia, increased renal renin production, and, in some patients, hypercalciuria and nephrocalcinosis. Similar features occur with loop diuretic treatment and congenital chloride diarrhea. There are at least three clinical subtypes of Bartter's syndromes with marked phenotypic variations within each subtype. These include *antenatal hypercalciuric variant* (hyperprostaglandin E syndrome, HPS/aBS); *classic Bartter's syndrome* (cBS); and the *Gitelman variant of Bartter's syndrome* (GS). The common characteristics of each subtype are hypokalemic metabolic alkalosis and renal salt wasting.

Antenatal Hypercalciuric Variant (Hyperprostaglandin E Syndrome, HPS/aBS)

This is a life-threatening neonatal disorder. Features include polyhydramnios, premature delivery, hypokalemia, hypercalciuria, metabolic alkalosis, fever, vomiting, diarrhea and failure to thrive, hyposthenuria, and nephrocalcinosis. The inheritance is autosomal recessive with mutations in the gene for either furosemide-sensitive NaK-2Cl cotransporter NKCC2 (*SLC12A1*) on 15q21.1 (Simon, 1996), inwardly rectifying potassium channel, subfamily J, member 1, ROMK (*KCNJ1*) on 11q24 (Jeck et al, 2001), or an essential B-subunit of the CLCNKB channel, Barttin, encoded by the *BSND* gene on chromosome 1p32.3 (Estevez, 2001). Classic Bartter's syndrome may also be caused by mutations in *NKCC2* or *ROMK* genes, suggesting that antenatal and classic forms are different manifestations of severity of the same disorder. Barttin mutations are associated with sensorineural deafness, because the protein is also expressed in stria

vascularis of the ear (Estevez, 2001). There is no cure for Bartter's syndrome, but treatment with inhibitors of prostaglandin synthesis improve polyuria, correct biochemical abnormalities, and permit satisfactory growth and development. The nephrocalcinosis, however, may not improve (Mourani et al, 2000).

Classic Bartter's Syndrome [McKusick #241200]

The clinical phenotype varies ranging from episodes of neonatal severe volume depletion with hypotension and hypokalemia to mildly symptomatic patients diagnosed in adolescence. Serum magnesium concentrations are normal. There are several cases involving mutations in one of three genes encoding ascending limb of Henle transporters such as (1) the basolateral chloride channel, CLCNKB, on 1p36; (2) the Na-K-2Cl cotransporter gene, SLC12A1/NKCC2, on 15q13; or (3) the K+ inwardly-rectifying channel, subfamily J, member 1, ROMK (ROMK1/KCNJ1) on chromosome 11q24. CLCNKB mutations may occasionally manifest with a congenital Bartter's (HPS/aBS) or a Gitelman-like phenotype.

Gitelman Variant of Bartter's Syndrome [McKusick# 263800]

This syndrome usually does not manifest in neonates (Bettinelli et al, 2000). Hypocalciuria and hypomagnesemia are specific clinical features of Gitelman's syndrome. The Gitelman variant is caused by mutations in the gene for the thiazide-sensitive NaCl cotransporter NCCT (SLC12A3) of the distal tubule, located on 16q13.

RENAL TUBULAR HYPERKALEMIA

The causes of neonatal renal tubular hyperkalemia (RTH) are marked prematurity, renal adysplasia, urinary tract obstruction, urinary tract infection, pseudohypoaldosteronism, and congenital adrenal hyperplasia (Rodriguez-Soriano et al, 1995). In RTH, there are inappropriately low urine potassium concentration, renal salt wasting, and metabolic acidosis. The serum creatinine concentration is often increased because of volume depletion (pseudohypoaldosteronism, congenital adrenal hyperplasia), reduced nephron mass (renal adysplasia), and/or obstruction (posterior urethral valves).

PSEUDOHYPOALDOSTERONISM

There are two syndromes of aldosterone resistance: pseudohypoaldosteronism type I and pseudohypoaldosteronism type II (Hanukoglu, 1991). Furthermore, there are two clinically and genetically distinct forms of type I pseudohypoaldosteronism: renal pseudohypoaldosteronism and multiple-organ pseudohypoaldosteronism. Pseudohypoaldosteronism may be inherited as an autosomal dominant or autosomal recessive trait. In the dominant form of pseudohypoaldosteronism type I there are mutations in the gene *MLR*, encoding the mineralocorticoid receptor. In the recessive form of pseudohypoaldosteronism type I, there are mutations in genes *SNCC1A*,

SNCC1B, and *SCNN1G*, which encode subunits of the epithelial Na⁺ channel (ENaC) (Rodriguez-Soriano, 2000).

Pseudohypoaldosteronism Type I

Renal pseudohypoaldosteronism usually starts in early infancy and is characterized by diminished renal tubular responsiveness to aldosterone with hyponatremia, hyperkalemia, markedly elevated plasma aldosterone, and hyperreninemia. The clinical expression ranges from severe, with death occurring in infancy, to asymptomatic. Symptomatic patients are treated with sodium supplementation, which they usually outgrow by 2 years of age.

Multiple-Organ Pseudohypoaldosteronism

There is impaired responsiveness to aldosterone in salivary and sweat glands, renal tubules, alveoli, and colonic mucosal cells. The course is protracted, with life-threatening episodes of salt wasting.

Pseudohypoaldosteronism Type II (Gordon Hyperkalemia-Hypertension Syndrome, Familial Hyperkalemic Hypertension)

The features are hyperkalemia, despite a normal glomerular filtration rate, hypertension variable mild hyperchloremia, metabolic acidosis, and suppressed plasma renin activity (Schambelan, 1981). The metabolic abnormalities are corrected by treatment with thiazide diuretics. Mutations in *WNK* (with no lysine kinase) 1 and 4 genes resulting in functional hyperactivity of the thiazide-sensitive Na-Cl cotransporter (NCCT) have been found to be causative (Wilson, 2001). There are no reports of neonatal presentation.

CONGENITAL NEPHROGENIC DIABETES INSIPIDUS

Nephrogenic diabetes insipidus (NDI) can result from congenital or acquired insults to kidneys including electrolyte abnormalities (hypokalemia, hypocalcemia), drugs (aminoglycosides), tubular interstitial inflammation, obstruction, and dysplasia. In congenital or inherited forms of NDI, insensitivity of the distal nephron to the antidiuretic effect of vasopressin results in an inability to concentrate urine, leading to large quantities of hypotonic urine (Bichet et al, 1997; van Lieburg et al, 1999). Affected neonates may be irritable, feed poorly, fail to gain weight, and have unexplained dehydration and fevers. Serum concentrations of sodium, chloride, creatinine, and blood urea nitrogen are elevated, and serum concentrations of vasopressin are normal or increased. There is a blunted response of plasma factor VIII, von Willebrand factor, and plasminogen activator after administration of 1-desamino-8-ᴅ-arginine vasopressin. Treatment with hydrochlorothiazide (3 mg/kg/day) and amiloride (0.3 mg/kg/day three times a day) may be preferable to hydrochlorothiazide and indomethacin because indomethacin can cause bleeding. Treatment can prevent dehydration, electrolyte imbalances, cerebral calcification, and seizures and result in normal growth, but patients continue to have polydipsia and polyuria.

About 90% of patients with inherited NDI are males with the X-linked form caused by mutations in the arginine vasopressin receptor 2 gene (*AVPR2*) that codes for the V2 receptor located in chromosomal region Xq28 (Morello and Bichet, 2001). In fewer than 10% of families, the inheritance of NDI is autosomal recessive or autosomal dominant. Mutations have been identified in the aquaporin-2 gene (*AQP2*) on 12q13 that codes for the vasopressin-sensitive water channel (Goji et al, 1998). The reliability of prenatal diagnosis of the X-linked form of NDI is about 96%.

Complete references used in this text can be found online at www.expertconsult.com

URINARY TRACT INFECTIONS AND VESICOURETERAL REFLUX

Stephen A. Zderic

This chapter provides an overview of the epidemiology, pathophysiology, radiographic evaluation, and management of urinary tract infections (UTIs) in the neonate. Although the focus is on the management of vesicoureteral reflux as one of the congenital conditions frequently associated with UTI, it can also be the mode of presentation for other congenital urologic anomalies. Of the several key points emphasized in this chapter, one of the most important is that reflux itself does not cause UTI. Many children may have reflux without any symptoms, which has become increasingly apparent during the past 20 years as many newborns with prenatal hydronephrosis were subjected to a voiding cystourethrogram (VCUG). Neonates who develop bladder infections and have reflux will be more likely to present clinically with a febrile UTI. It also is important to remember that biologic susceptibility has a major role in the cause of neonatal UTIs. Finally, it has been recognized that not all damage to kidneys associated with reflux reflects scarring from infection. Some kidneys with high-grade reflux have elements of dysplasia and scarring at the time of initial presentation and in the absence of infection.

URINARY TRACT INFECTIONS

EPIDEMIOLOGY

Within the first several months of postnatal life, UTIs are more common in boys. After the first 6 months, the incidence in girls increases steadily as it declines in boys (Chang and Shortliffe, 2006), such that from 1 to 3 years of age females have a 10- to 15-fold greater risk. Wiswell observed that although only 20% of males were uncircumcised, this group accounted for 80% of all UTIs in boys, thus identifying phimosis as a significant risk factor (Wiswell, 1997; Wiswell and Geschke, 1989). These data suggest that circumcision offers protection against UTIs in the 1st year of life and in particular offers support for encouraging circumcision in males with congenital structural or functional abnormalities that place them at high risk for pyelonephritis and sepsis, such as patients with posterior urethral valves or reflux.

DIAGNOSIS

The diagnosis of a UTI in a young infant is not always straightforward, and a high index of suspicion is required because the symptoms are generalized. Many of the patients will have confounding signs: up to 60% are irritable, 50% show signs of feeding poorly, and up to 40% may have vomiting or diarrhea. In a more recent study of infants with UTI, the best correlates proved to be a body

temperature greater than 38° C and uncircumcised males (Shaikh et al, 2007; Zorc et al, 2005). The index of suspicion must rise when these aforementioned symptoms are present with no localizing source. In such instances, obtaining a urine specimen for analysis and culture must be included in the evaluation.

Much has been said and written about the procurement of specimens by the techniques of clean catch (not applicable in neonates), use of a bag, catheterization, or suprapubic puncture (Stamey, 1980). Results of studies on bag or clean-catch specimens are valid only if cultures are truly negative. These collection methods are susceptible to contamination in girls and especially in uncircumcised males (Figure 87-1). Knowledge of the composition of preputial or vaginal flora is of little use in managing the febrile child. What matters most is the composition of urine within the bladder itself. This problem is compounded when bagged specimens are obtained at home and arrive "fresh" at the office to be sent to a central laboratory before plating. Another problem arises with the definition of what a negative urine culture means. In many instances, the reports state that the results are negative only because the presence of 100,000 colony-forming units (CFUs) is used as a cutoff to define a positive culture. Hoberman et al (1994) examined the frequency distribution of voided or bag specimens and compared the findings with those obtained as post-void specimens by catheterization of febrile infants. The authors found that 10,000 to 49,000 CFUs/mL usually represented contamination, whereas counts in excess of 50,000 CFUs/mL were more characteristic of a true positive. Still, there was overlap between these groups; thus numeric quantitation remains an inexact tool.

The standard for specimen collection remains suprapubic aspiration, which is accurate and can be safely performed in a neonate because the bladder is a pelvic organ. A 21-gauge needle can be inserted into the palpable bladder just above the pubic symphysis in the midline to collect an aspirate; however, urologists rarely use this method of collection. A catheterized specimen is easy to obtain and provides accurate results, especially if the first 2 to 3 mL of urine, which can contain urethral contaminants, is discarded. For a febrile child with possible urosepsis in an emergency department, or requiring hospital admission, documentation of a UTI should be established on the basis of a catheterized specimen or a suprapubic aspirate. Voided clean-catch or bag methods can be used early in an evaluation before the urinary tract is considered a source. However, the increased incidence of false-positive findings seen with these collection methods leads to more patients being subjected to antibiotic therapy and a costly and invasive radiographic workup. The greatest diagnostic yield from doing these expensive and invasive studies

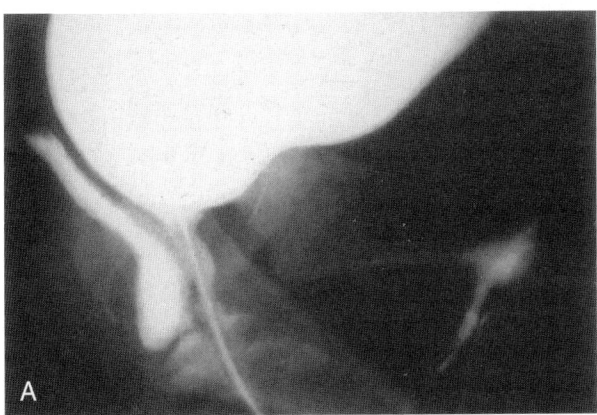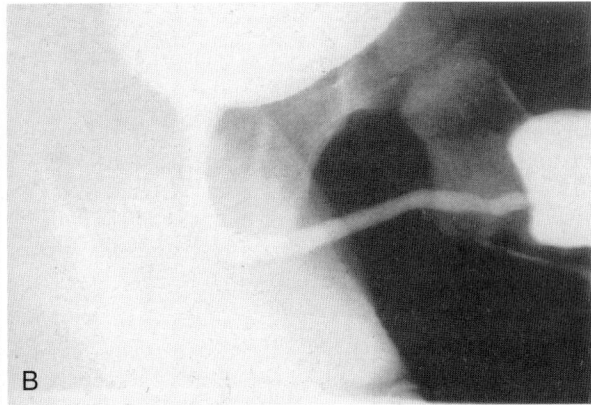

FIGURE 87-1 These voiding cystourethrogram images demonstrate how bagged specimens may lead to false-positive results in infant females or uncircumcised males. Vaginal reflux allows for contaminants in the bagged specimen from an infant female **(A)**. In the uncircumcised male, urine may pool underneath the foreskin and acquire contaminating flora **(B)**.

will be in the population of patients whose UTI was most accurately diagnosed by using catheterized or suprapubic specimens.

TREATMENT

The neonate with suspected urosepsis should receive broad-spectrum antibiotic coverage until the results of sensitivity testing dictate a shift to single-antibiotic coverage. Ampicillin and gentamicin provide excellent treatment for the most common pathogens that are likely to be present. The most likely pathogen is *Escherichia coli*, but there is always a possibility of *Pseudomonas* spp., especially in an infant who was just discharged home after a stay in the neonatal intensive care unit. The duration of intravenous antibiotic therapy for pyelonephritis can be debated, but parenteral therapy at least avoids the concern of compliance issues. Experimental evidence demonstrates that reflux-associated pyelonephritis in piglets confirmed by ^{99m}Tc dimercaptosuccinic acid (DMSA) scan can be successfully treated only with oral nitrofurantoin (Macrodantin; Risdon et al, 1994). In view of given the expense of hospitalization or home-based intravenous antibiotic therapy, the mandatory duration of parenteral therapy will continue to be debated, especially in older children (Hoberman and Wald, 1999). However, in the more susceptible neonate, parenteral therapy should be instituted in a hospital setting and continued until results of a follow-up urine culture become negative (American Academy of Pediatrics, 1999). At that point, oral antibiotic therapy can be started for a total course of 10 to 14 days.

Once the acute infection has been treated, antibiotic prophylaxis should be instituted until the child is ready for radiographic imaging studies. The use of amoxicillin (12.5 mg/kg) in neonates, or trimethoprim-sulfamethoxazole in infants, is acceptable prophylaxis. The use of trimethoprim-sulfamethoxazole in urology patients for suppression is based on the work of Stamey (1980), who demonstrated that low-dose antibiotic treatment does not produce shifts in fecal flora. In contrast, high doses of trimethoprim-sulfamethoxazole, and especially of broad-spectrum antibiotics, have been shown to produce greater and more concerning shifts in fecal flora. This finding is especially significant because feces serve as the origin for most (>90%) bacteria that colonize the perineum and vagina and thus ultimately produce a UTI.

RADIOGRAPHIC WORK-UP

Once a diagnosis of UTI has been established and treated, it is important to initiate a radiographic workup to look for any underlying structural anomalies (American Academy of Pediatrics, 1999). It has been stated that up to 30% of children with a UTI have aberrant urinary tract anatomy or function (Lebowitz and Mandell, 1987). For this reason, a radiographic evaluation of the urinary tract should be undertaken, consisting of an ultrasound study of *kidneys and bladder*, followed by a VCUG. A more contemporary study shows that 15% of hospitalized neonates and infants with a UTI prove to have an underlying anatomic diagnosis (Hsieh et al, 2009). The traditional standard of care has been to obtain a renal bladder ultrasound at the time of hospitalization for a pediatric UTI. Typically, a 2- to 4-week period has been recommended between the infection and the VCUG, but this interval is arbitrary. It is more important to ensure that the urine is sterile before performance of the VCUG. A patient should be maintained on antimicrobial prophylaxis until imaging rules out any urinary tract pathology. On sonography, it is important to obtain both kidney and bladder views, because sometimes the kidneys alone are imaged and shown to be normal and the workup is terminated; several infections later, a bladder ultrasound study shows a stone, ureterocele, or diverticulum. Even if a VCUG is being done on the same day of the renal ultrasound examination, a small ureterocele may be missed at fluoroscopy that would be seen on bladder sonogram.

The VCUG must be done carefully and requires patience on the part of all concerned. Because the act of voiding is required to demonstrate reflux in 20% to 30% of reflux cases, such cases would be missed if the child were anesthetized for a static cystogram. The standard approach is to obtain a classic fluoroscopic study first, define the anatomy, and accurately grade the reflux if it is present. Some groups have advocated that a radionuclide VCUG be used as the initial screening study. However, to appropriately define the anatomy, the contrast VCUG remains the "gold standard". As discussed later in the section on reflux, the cornerstone of accurate management is grading

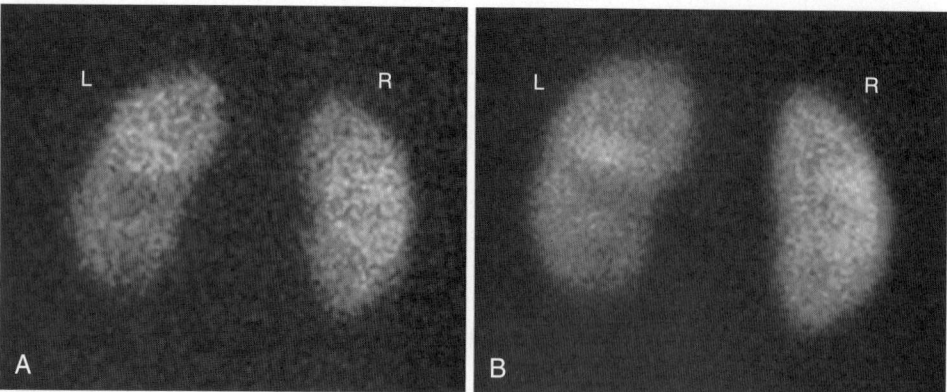

FIGURE 87-2 An example of an acute positive dimercaptosuccinic acid (DMSA) scan taken at the time of hospitalization for a febrile urinary tract infection showing multiple cold spots within a kidney **(A)**. A follow-up DMSA scan done almost 1 year later shows chronic changes after this episode of febrile urinary tract infection **(B)**.

of the reflux, which can be provided only by a well-executed VCUG study.

Within the past 5 years, there has been a growing movement toward limiting the anatomic workup for children with UTIs. There is a growing consensus that many of the radiographic workups done for UTI might be avoided with minimal risk. For example, Hoberman et al (2003) demonstrated that an ultrasound examination done at the time of hospitalization for a febrile UTI had a diagnostic yield of less than 1%. However, it is crucial to note that this study was limited to patients older than 2 months who had all been screened with antenatal sonograms and who had no comorbidities. Understanding these study limitations is critical before trying to apply these criteria to fragile neonates who often have comorbidities. These principles are further illustrated in clinical scenarios presented in this chapter.

In recent years there has been growing support in the literature for the use of DMSA scanning to identify patients with acute pyelonephritis. Hoberman's study demonstrated that only 50% of children with a febrile UTI proved to have a positive DMSA scan (Figure 87-2; Hoberman et al, 2003). Of this subset, 80% had a normal DMSA scan at a follow-up evaluation 6 months later, suggesting that most pediatric patients with a febrile UTI are not prone to renal scarring. Surprisingly, Hoberman's data did not suggest that age (stratified into groups of patients older or younger than 1 year of life) was a risk factor for a positive follow-up scan. It is important to note that other studies based on patients referred to a pediatric urology or nephrology specialty practice reported residual positive DMSA scans in as many as 32% of patients (Biggi et al, 2001; Rushton and Majd, 1992). This finding would suggest that there are critical differences between studies done on a patient population that is drawn on the "first pass" from primary care settings, as opposed to those originating from tertiary care settings. Several studies in the 1990s advocated the use of DMSA scanning to stratify patients into high-risk (positive DMSA scan) or low-risk (negative DMSA scan) groups (Rushton and Majd, 1992), and some have begun to advocate limiting VCUG to the high-risk group alone (Hardy and Austin, 2008; Tseng et al, 2007). However, these studies are all based on older patients and should not be applied to fragile neonates.

PATHOPHYSIOLOGY

UTI has a multifactorial etiology and represents an altered balance between host and pathogen. Abnormal anatomy serves to exacerbate the effects of a UTI (Lebowitz and Mandell, 1987; Shortliffe, 2007). Hematogenous spread of bacteria to the urinary tract can occur but is rare. Most UTIs will start in the bladder and then ascend to produce pyelonephritis. This ascent of infected urine from the bladder to the kidney can take place via two major mechanisms: (1) the bacteria are extremely virulent and produce pili that allow the bacteria to attach themselves to the ureter and migrate upstream or (2) the patient has reflux that showers the renal pelvis, allowing for intrarenal reflux and seeding of the renal parenchyma (Figure 87-3). Once bacteria are injected into the renal parenchyma under high pressures, areas of focal infection and inflammation develop (Figure 87-4), and a series of complex steps in the inflammatory cascade occur. If this process is not interrupted by treatment, it can produce severe renal injury or scarring. Furthermore, if repeated infectious insults such as these continue without adequate therapy, the long-term result is significant renal scarring, which in its extreme produces reflux nephropathy that in turn can lead to end-stage renal disease (ESRD). However, recent advances in understanding embryonic development of the ureter and kidney suggest that infection-induced scarring is a rare mechanism of ESRD in patients with reflux, given today's heightened awareness of urine as a source of fever in pediatric patients (Sreenarasimhaiah and Hellerstein, 1998). As mentioned previously, Hoberman's study suggested that only 50% of patients with a well-documented febrile UTI had a positive DMSA scan, and the positive scans done at the time of acute infection reverted to normal within 6 months in 80% of this subset of patients (Hoberman et al, 2003).

Equally important in the pathogenesis of UTIs is the biology of the patient. Many patients are more susceptible to bacterial UTIs because their bladder mucosa expresses cell surface proteins that have a high affinity for cell surface antigens on the bacterial cell wall. A great deal is known about the bladder mucosal expression of these complex glycoproteins, with some being mannose-sensitive. In these cases, the receptor-ligand interaction between pathogen and host is based on molecular recognition of

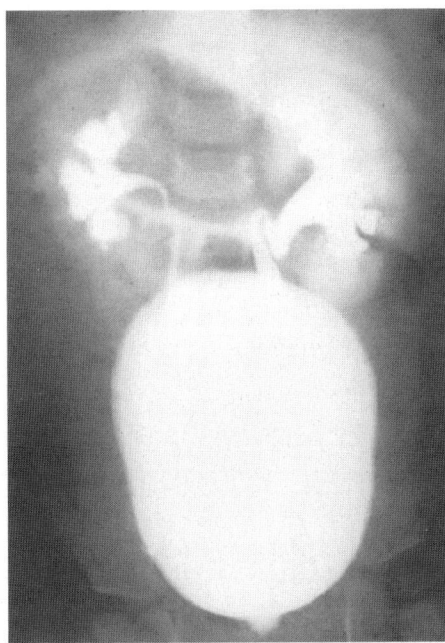

FIGURE 87-3 High-grade bilateral vesicoureteral reflux with evidence of pyelotubular backflow within the left kidney is demonstrated on this voiding cystourethrogram in a neonate.

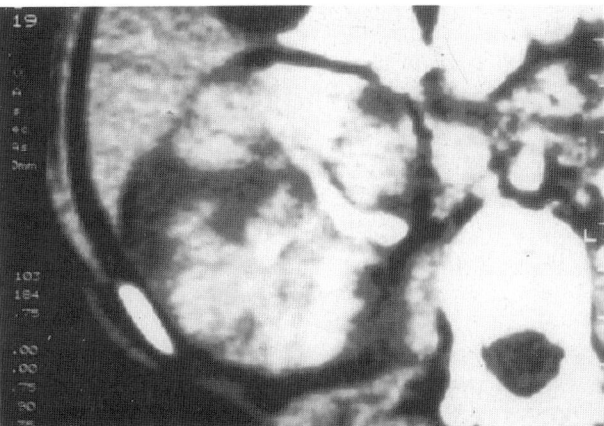

FIGURE 87-4 This computed tomography scan of an infant with right pyelonephritis and associated grade II reflux shows signs of lobar nephronia. Areas within the right kidney function well and excrete contrast, whereas other lobes show signs of poor perfusion.

mannose-6-phosphate. In addition to genetic alterations that increase a patient's susceptibility to bacterial colonization and infection, there may be other differences in a patient's immune system response that affect the individual's propensity for scarring.

URINARY TRACT INFECTIONS COMPLICATED BY OBSTRUCTIVE UROPATHY

An important consideration is what happens when UTIs develop in a newborn with an abnormal urinary tract. It used to be extremely common for obstructive uropathies to manifest after urosepsis had developed. With the widespread use of prenatal sonography, however, most neonates with an obstructive uropathy are identified at birth, and antibiotic prophylaxis is initiated. However, a neonate may still exhibit urosepsis secondary to an obstructive uropathy. In such cases, the obstructive uropathy might have developed after the initial early normal prenatal ultrasound examination, or the problem went undiscovered because of a lack of access to prenatal care, as illustrated in Figure 87-5.

The most common anatomic factor associated with a febrile UTI in a neonate or infant is vesicoureteral reflux. Occasionally an obstructed system will be discovered during the workup. The presence of an obstruction produces a dangerous combination of bacteria, urinary stasis, and a warm environment with a near-ideal culture broth. As a result there is always the possibility of an infection developing in an obstructed system. Keeping this possibility in mind is important because the management may be altered by the use of surgical drainage by either ureterostomy or percutaneous nephrostomy. During treatment for acute pyelonephritis, the patient may not defervesce for 48 to 72 hours; however, beyond 72 hours, underlying obstruction must be suspected if fever persists or the neonate's

condition worsens. Under these circumstances, an ultrasound examination to rule out obstruction is warranted. Infections can become established in primary megaureters, ureteroceles, or ectopic ureters (see Figure 87-5) and, on rare occasions, in ureteropelvic junction obstructions. Urine production allows for some antibiotic to reach these bacteria, and a good response may be seen if the patient receives treatment early in the course of infection. In advanced cases, especially in those associated with poor renal function, temporary drainage procedures, such as percutaneous nephrostomy or a cutaneous ureterostomy, will allow for eradication of infection and stabilization of the patient's condition before undertaking definitive surgical repair.

VESICOURETERAL REFLUX

Vesicoureteral reflux exists when urine flows from the bladder back toward the kidney; this reverse flow can occur during bladder filling or emptying (voiding). The etiology of reflux remains debated, but there is growing agreement that reflux constitutes a syndrome. Some patients with reflux have a congenital anatomic basis for the reflux. The normal course of the ureter travels through the bladder wall and underneath the mucosal layer to create a flap valve mechanism, which prevents vesicoureteral reflux. Reflux caused by anatomic malposition of the ureteral insertion into the bladder is referred to as *primary reflux*. In other patients, reflux occurs secondary to increases in bladder pressure, a condition referred to as *secondary reflux*. For example, many patients with posterior urethral valves may have reflux that disappears once the valves are resected. This distinction is important because the rules for primary reflux resolution do not apply to cases of reflux secondary to obstructing lesions, such as posterior urethral valves or the neurogenic bladder seen with spina bifida.

Using contrast VCUG, it is possible to grade primary reflux from I through V (Figure 87-6). Grading reflux allows physicians to communicate findings quickly and to understand what the chances are for the natural resolution of primary reflux. Many additional findings appear on the VCUG images, such as whether there was reflux on filling,

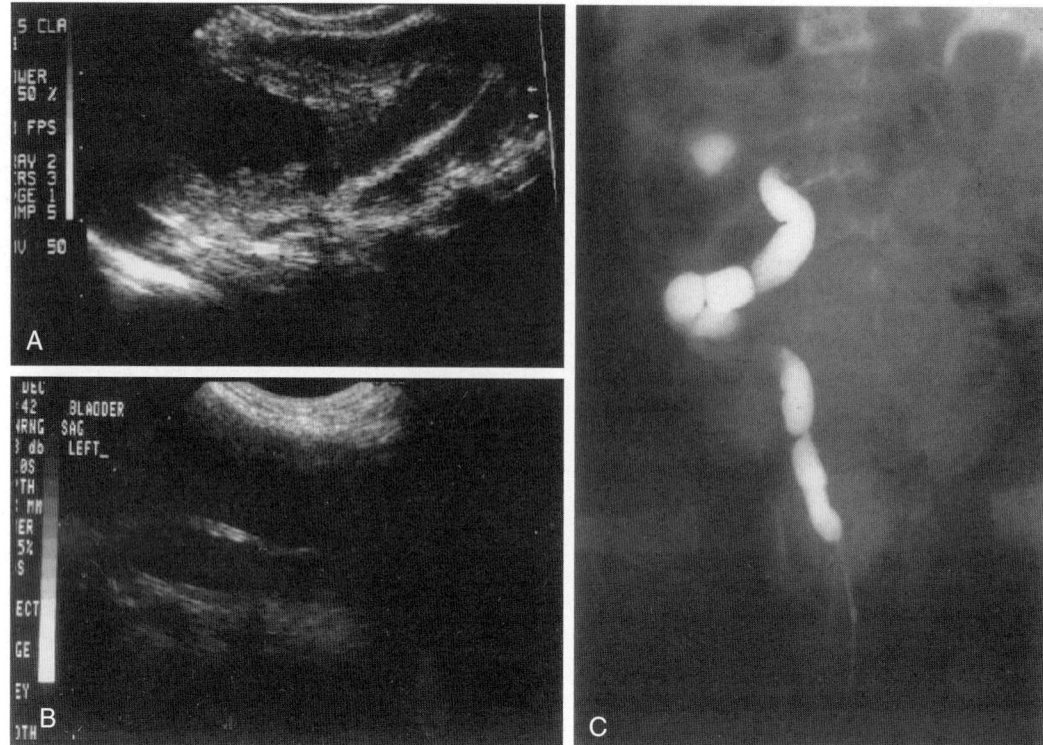

FIGURE 87-5 Ectopic ureter and urosepsis. This 3-month-old infant had a high fever and a positive urine culture that failed to respond to parenteral antibiotic therapy. **A** and **B,** The ultrasound examination showed signs of right hydronephrosis and hydroureter. **C,** A retrograde pyelogram confirmed a diagnosis of ectopic ureter. Most cases are identified by fetal sonography; however, in this instance, the young parents did not seek prenatal care. After cutaneous diversion of this ectopic ureter, the infant became afebrile, and ureteral reimplantation was performed successfully 6 months later.

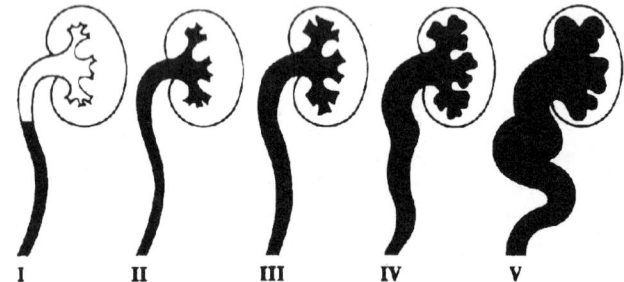

FIGURE 87-6 Grading scale for reflux. The International Reflux Study used this grading scale, which is based on findings of a conventional fluoroscopic voiding cystourethrogram.

whether it started at the beginning or at the end of the filling phase, how much contrast was added to the bladder prior to the initiation of voiding, and whether there was evidence of a pyelotubular backflow (see Figure 87-2). By evaluating the findings in detail, a better understanding of the severity, potential treatment modalities, and outcome can be achieved and used for the benefit of the patient. It is essential to remember that reflux grading for the purposes of calculating the spontaneous resolution applies only to primary reflux; this scale does not apply to secondary reflux such as that seen with posterior urethral valves, or to complex anatomic situations such as ectopic ureters (Figure 87-7). In fact, contrast VCUG is essential in making the diagnosis of an ectopic ureter, because for these patients spontaneous resolution will never occur, and surgery is indicated.

Growing clinical evidence (Sillen et al, 1992, 1996a, 1996b) suggests that voiding pressures are dramatically increased in infants with reflux, especially in boys. These studies have shown that, even in normal males, voiding pressures are elevated in the neonatal period and decline dramatically during the first 2 years of life. The data demonstrate that voiding pressures in boys with high-grade reflux are often threefold to fourfold higher than those seen in older children. In these boys, reflux often resolves in a surprisingly short period of time, implying that the pressures drop with maturation of bladder function. Of interest, female newborns do not fare as well with resolution of neonatal reflux on a grade-for-grade basis, nor are their voiding pressures as elevated. These clinical observations are supported by experimental findings suggesting that there are gender-related differences in bladder neck function. The key concept is that voiding pressures are elevated, especially in male neonates with reflux, and that these pressures diminish over time. These observations have great bearing on how reflux resolution rates should be interpreted in newborns.

Outcomes for reflux resolution in neonates have been studied more extensively over the past 15 years (Sjöström et al, 2004); this was made possible by the increased number of cases detected by prenatal ultrasonography. Evidence from a multicenter study suggests that reflux detected in the first months of life as part of a workup for prenatal hydronephrosis has a better chance for spontaneous resolution, grade for grade, than that diagnosed in the child at 2 to 4 years of age (Herndon et al, 1999). Given this

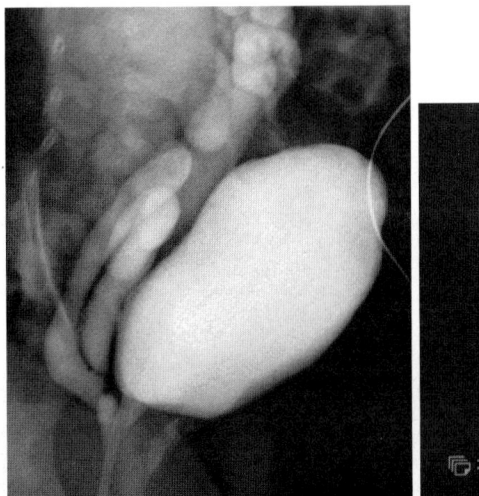
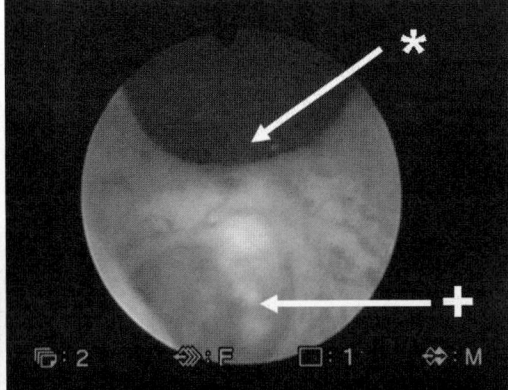

FIGURE 87-7 This voiding phase of the voiding cystourethrogram demonstrates reflux into a Y-type duplex right-sided ureter that has a single opening into an ectopic location within the proximal urethra just below the bladder neck. This radiographic finding was also confirmed at cystoscopy, where the ectopic ureter (+) clearly enters the proximal urethra below the bladder neck (*).

information, recommendations that can be made about neonatal reflux management will be altered by the mode of presentation and social circumstances (compliance issues). For a newborn with prenatally diagnosed grade IV or V reflux, expectant observation with antibiotic prophylaxis seems most reasonable (Sillen, 1999). However, this course of action demands that parents comply with antibiotic prophylaxis and understand that a breakthrough infection rate as high as 20% is possible (Herndon et al, 1999). This series also indicated the benefit of circumcision in males with known reflux (Herndon et al, 1999). The case can be made for a more aggressive surgical approach if a neonate has urosepsis and high-grade (IV or V) reflux; follow-up studies continue to demonstrate that it is in this cohort of patients that the risk of acquired scarring remains high (Sjöström et al, 2009). It is absolutely crucial for any parent and referring physician to understand that successful reimplantation surgery diminishes but does not eradicate the likelihood of pyelonephritis. A child with innate susceptibility will still experience bladder infections despite the absence of reflux.

Several studies have shown that siblings of patients with reflux also have a higher likelihood of having reflux, with an incidence that declines in older siblings. Sibling screening studies in the 1st year of life have shown that 20% to 50% of the siblings will have a VCUG that is positive for reflux (Noe, 1995; Parekh et al, 2002) up to the age of 9 years. Several studies have shown an increased incidence of renal scarring in siblings whose reflux was discovered by screening (Sweeney et al, 2001; Wan et al, 1996). However, Parekh et al (2002) suggest that sibling reflux follows a more benign course, and they noted no renal scarring after antibiotic prophylaxis. On the other hand, would the cohort of patients in this study have done as well without a diagnosis and antibiotic prophylaxis? It is important to remember that many asymptomatic infants have undiagnosed reflux, never develop UTIs, resolve their reflux, and live normal lives. In one metaanalysis of the world literature on screening studies for reflux in asymptomatic

siblings, Hollowell and Greenfield (2002) concluded that there was no evidence to support this practice. The extent to which screening averts renal complications or hospital admissions for pyelonephritis will be best answered by prospective trials.

The traditional view was that identifying the pediatric patient with reflux was crucial to allow for antibiotic prophylaxis to be administered to prevent recurrent pyelonephritis and renal scarring. This traditional view has come under closer scrutiny in recent years. The embryologic studies of Mackie and Stephens (1975) suggested that much of the focal hypoplasia seen in kidneys with reflux is present at birth and have been borne out in clinical practice by a 20-year experience of neonatal evaluations for antenatally diagnosed hydronephrosis. Further support has come from newer molecular studies of ureteral bud development in knockout and transgenic mice, showing that aberrant ureteric bud development is associated with abnormal renal morphology. It is becoming clear that most of the renal insufficiency in patients with reflux reflects aberrant embryogenesis and not damage secondary to infection. This case is demonstrated in Figure 87-8, in which a VCUG was done for antenatal reflux and demonstrated massive grade V reflux. In this 3-day-old neonate, there was never a history of UTI, yet serum creatinine was already abnormal and ultrasound examination findings demonstrated increased echogenicity with a loss of corticomedullary differentiation. In this setting, the high-grade reflux was associated with renal dysplasia at the onset, and renal failure was progressive.

Clearly, episodes of pyelonephritis and the resulting renal inflammation (see Figure 87-3) can do harm if left untreated. It is estimated that each episode of febrile UTI can lead to a 5% risk of new renal scar formation per episode, and it is generally agreed that repeated and untreated infection harms the kidney. What is currently being debated is the role of long-term antibiotic prophylaxis in the management of these patients. One recent randomized trial suggested that there is no measurable benefit to prophylaxis (Garin et al, 2006); however, this study was

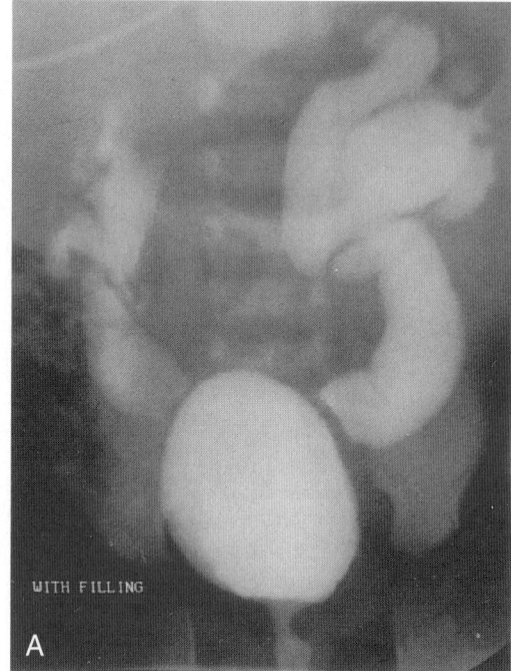
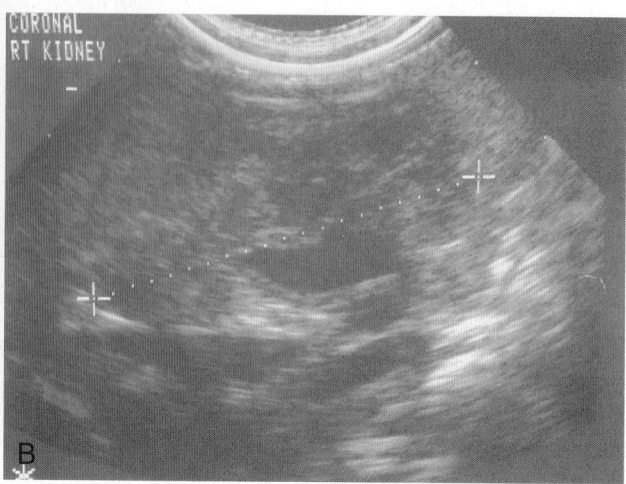

FIGURE 87-8 Dysplasia and high-grade reflux. This case demonstrates the association of bilateral grade V reflux with renal dysplasia. The voiding cystourethrogram **(A)** and ultrasound scan **(B)** shown here were performed within the first 2 weeks of life, and the child had never had a diagnosed urinary tract infection during this interval. Despite sterile urine, the serum creatinine level was elevated, and the renal sonogram showed increased echogenicity and poor corticomedullary differentiation. This case indicates that renal insufficiency associated with reflux often is present at the outset and is not always secondary to infection.

limited by a small sample size and a wide distribution of ages and reflux grades. The National Institutes of Health has currently funded the multicenter Randomized Intervention Vesicoureteral Reflux trial (Mathews et al, 2009) with the goal of obtaining the best data to help settle this debate. However, these studies do not enroll patients younger than 2 months, and they exclude patients with comorbidities. The current standard of care continues to be a full radiographic workup and antibiotic prophylaxis for the neonate with febrile UTI and reflux.

SUGGESTED READINGS

Herndon CD, Mckenna PH, Kolon TF, et al: A multicenter outcomes analysis of patients with neonatal reflux presenting with prenatal hydronephrosis, *J Urol* 162:1203-1208, 1999.

Hoberman A, Charron M, Hickey RW, et al: Imaging studies after a first febrile urinary tract infection in young children, *N Engl J Med* 348:195-202, 2003.

Hoberman A, Wald ER: Treatment of urinary tract infections, *Pediatr Infect Dis J* 18:1020-1021, 1999.

Hoberman A, Wald ER, Reynolds EA, et al: Pyuria and bacteriuria in urine specimens obtained by catheter from young children with fever, *J Pediatr* 124:513-519, 1994.

Mackie GG, Stephens FD: Duplex kidneys: a correlation of renal dysplasia with position of the ureteral orifice, *J Urol* 114:274-280, 1975.

Shortliffe LD, editor: Infection and inflammation of the pediatric genitourinary tract. In *Campbell Walsh textbook of urology*, Philadelphia, 2007, Elsevier.

Sillen U, Bachelard M, Hansson S, et al: Video cystometric recording of dilating reflux in infancy, *J Urol* 155:1711-1715, 1996a.

Sjöström S, Jodal U, Sixt R, et al: Longitudinal development of renal damage and renal function in infants with high grade vesicoureteral reflux, *J Urol* 181:2277-2283, 2009.

Stamey TA: *Pathogenesis and treatment of urinary tract infections*, Baltimore, 1980, Williams and Wilkins.

Wiswell TE, Geschke DW: Risks from circumcision during the first month of life compared with those for uncircumcised boys, *Pediatrics* 83:1011-1015, 1989.

Complete references used in this text can be found online at www.expertconsult.com

RENAL VASCULAR DISEASE IN THE NEWBORN

Halima Saadia Janjua and Donald L. Batisky

There is a significant risk of neonates developing complications related to thromboembolic phenomena, and the issues related to vessels supplying and draining renal vasculature will be discussed in this chapter. Clearly there are a number of conditions that can result in an imbalance of the delicate homeostasis between bleeding and thrombosis. Some may be genetic, some may relate to underlying stresses during pathologic processes, and some may relate to treatments for the pathologic processes.

RENAL ARTERIAL OBSTRUCTION

INCIDENCE AND ETIOLOGY

Renal artery thrombosis in the neonate is far less common than renal vein thrombosis. A major risk factor for renal arterial obstruction is umbilical artery catheterization. Before the advent of umbilical artery catheterization, only a few cases of renal artery thrombosis were seen. Other significant risk factors are shock, coagulopathy, and congestive heart failure. The reported incidence of umbilical artery–related thromboembolism reflects, in large part, the diagnostic test chosen. Doppler ultrasonography underestimates this incidence. Studies using ultrasound report an incidence of umbilical artery–related thromboembolism from 14% to 35%, whereas studies using angiography document incidences up to 64%. Autopsy studies have shown an incidence of umbilical artery–related thromboembolism between 9% and 28%, although major clinical symptoms of umbilical artery–related thromboembolism occur in 1% to 3% of infants (Andrew et al, 2001). Trauma at the time of insertion of umbilical artery catheter by endothelial injury is postulated to be the cause of aortic thrombus formation which then leads to thrombosis of one or both renal arteries (Box 88-1).

High umbilical artery catheters, placed at the T6 to T10 vertebral level, have been associated with a decreased incidence of clinical vascular complications without a statistically significant increase in any adverse effects (Barrington, 2000b). The chances of umbilical artery catheter occlusion can be decreased by adding heparin to the infusing fluid at a concentration as low as 0.25 unit/mL (Barrington, 2000a).

CLINICAL PRESENTATION

Clinical presentation varies with the extent and severity of thrombosis. Thrombosis of the abdominal aorta or renal arteries can manifest in any of the following ways: signs of congestive heart failure, hypertension, oliguria, renal failure, bowel ischemia or frank necrotizing enterocolitis secondary to superior or inferior mesenteric artery, and decreased femoral pulses with lower limb ischemia. Symptoms of renal arterial thrombosis manifest within the first few postnatal days in a term infant compared with a median age of 8 days in a preterm infant. The symptoms can be classified based on clinical severity; minor thrombosis with mildly decreased limb perfusion, hypertension, and hematuria; moderate thrombosis with decreased limb perfusion, hypertension, oliguria, and congestive heart failure; and major thrombosis with hypertension and multiorgan failure (Box 88-2).

Laboratory findings associated with renal arterial thrombosis are thrombocytopenia, hypofibrinogenemia, elevated fibrin split products, variable prothrombin and thromboplastin times, conjugated hyperbilirubinemia, elevated blood urea nitrogen and creatinine, hyperreninemia, and hematuria.

DIAGNOSIS

Doppler ultrasonography is used as the first line of imaging for diagnosing neonatal thrombosis although it usually fails to detect smaller intraarterial thrombi and some larger asymptomatic venous thrombi (Roy et al, 2002). If ultrasonography is inconclusive, radionuclide imaging could also be used. Angiography is the standard diagnostic modality and should be performed through the umbilical artery line if surgical intervention or intrathrombotic fibrinolytic therapy is being considered.

TREATMENT

For asymptomatic or minimally symptomatic newborns, only supportive care is recommended, such as removal of the umbilical artery catheter and close ultrasonographic monitoring. Most of these thrombi resolve spontaneously.

In newborns with mild signs of organ dysfunction and stable aortic and renal arterial thrombosis, management of hypertension, transient renal insufficiency, and mild congestive heart failure is recommended. Systemic heparin is given for anticoagulation. Close laboratory monitoring is done to avoid excessive heparinization, and clinical response is monitored by Doppler ultrasonography. However, there are age-dependent variations in the mechanism of action of heparin, and activated partial thromboplastin time (APTT) monitoring might not be a reliable marker for therapeutic heparin levels in infants (Ignjatovic et al, 2006; Monagle et al, 2008; Newall et al, 2009). If only APTT is used to titrate the heparin dose in infants, it can result in subtherapeutic levels of heparin; therefore heparin dose should be titrated to both APTT and heparin levels, accounting for the size of the clot and risk of bleeding associated with anticoagulation (Monagle et al, 2008; Newall et al, 2009). Heparin is dosed as an initial loading dose followed by a continuous infusion. The loading dose is 75 to 100 IU/kg over 10 minutes followed by 28 IU/kg/h. Heparin has a larger volume of distribution

---

BOX 88-1 Risk Factors for Aortic and Renal Arterial Thrombosis

- Systemic infection
- Birthweight <1500 g
- Perinatal asphyxia
- Polycythemia
- Intrauterine cocaine exposure
- Maternal diabetes mellitus
- Maternal lupus
- Congenital heart disease
- Hypercoagulability
- Dehydration
- Infusion of calcium salts
- Hyperalimentation
- Intravenous fat preparation
- Resistance to activated protein C (secondary to mutation of coagulation factor V gene in more than 90% of the cases)
- Homozygous congenital protein C deficiency

BOX 88-2 Clinical Presentation of Aortic and Renal Arterial Thrombosis

- Signs of congestive heart failure
- Hypertension
- Oliguria
- Renal failure
- Bowel ischemia or frank necrotizing enterocolitis secondary to superior or inferior mesenteric artery
- Decreased femoral pulses with lower limb ischemia
- Thrombocytopenia, hypofibrinogenemia, elevated fibrin split products, variable prothrombin and thromboplastin times
- Conjugated hyperbilirubinemia
- Elevated blood urea nitrogen and creatinine
- Hyperreninemia
- Hematuria

---

in infants and is cleared faster, which leads to higher dose requirements. Bleeding can occur in newborns secondary to heparin, in which case heparin infusion should be stopped. If bleeding is life threatening or needs to be stopped immediately, protamine sulfate is given, 1 mg for every 100 units of heparin given over the last 2 hours (McDonald et al, 1981).

Low-molecular-weight heparins (LMWHs) have some advantages over unfractionated heparin, thereby making them safe and efficacious alternatives to unfractionated heparin therapy. LMWHs have superior bioavailability, a longer half-life, and dose-independent clearance, which gives a more predictable anticoagulant response. The incidences of heparin-induced thrombocytopenia and osteoporosis are rare with LMWHs; they can be used in neonates with poor venous access because they are administered subcutaneously. LMWHs also do not need frequent laboratory monitoring and dose adjustment. Use of subcutaneous catheters for administration, which can remain in place for 7 days, can reduce the number of injections to as few as one per week (Albisetti and Andrew, 2002). In case of clinically significant bleeding, protamine sulfate should be administered intravenously. The dose is based on the amount of LMWH received in the previous 3 to 4 hours;

1 mg protamine sulfate can inactivate 100 units of LMWH (Hirsh et al, 2008).

In case of potential life-threatening complications of aortic or renal thrombosis, fibrinolytic therapy (systemic or intrathrombotic) along with supportive care is indicated. There are limited data on efficacy, dose, and safety of fibrinolytic agents in infants (Manco-Johnson et al, 2002; Monagle et al, 2008). The intrathrombotic infusion of fibrinolytic agent reduces the cumulative dose and possible systemic adverse effects. Close monitoring by ultrasonography or angiography should be done to evaluate the response to this therapy. Fibrinolytic agents act by catalyzing the conversion of endogenous plasminogen to plasmin. The most commonly used agent is recombinant tissue plasminogen activator (tPA).

There are limited data on efficacy, dose, and safety of fibrinolytic agents in infants (Manco-Johnson et al, 2002; Monagle et al, 2008). The tPA is usually administered systemically as a continuous infusion or directly administered into the catheter. For systemic infusion, it can be given with a bolus at its initiation or without it (Gupta et al, 2001; Goldenberg et al, 2007; Wang et al, 2003). The dose for recombinant tPA varies between 0.1 and 0.6 mg/kg/h over a duration of 6 hours (Monagle et al, 2008). A lower dose of recombinant tPA at 0.01 to 0.06 mg/kg/h is associated with decreased incidence of major bleeding (Goldenberg et al, 2007; Wang et al, 2003). Catheter-directed fibrinolysis can be considered, especially if the catheter is already close to the thrombus, in which case a low-dose infusion of recombinant tPA is given (0.01 to 0.2 mg/kg/h for 24 hours). This dosing has advantages such as higher response rate and decreased major bleeding complications. After leaving tPA in the catheter for 2 to 4 hours, catheter patency should be checked by drawing blood. If this dosing level is unsuccessful, a second round of therapy should be started. When fibrinolytic therapy is done for more than 24 hours, its efficacy is reduced because of depleted endogenous plasminogen. This phenomenon is called *plasminogen steal*; it can be overcome by giving supplementary plasminogen if plasminogen levels are low. The major complication of tPA therapy is bleeding. Thrombocytopenia and vitamin K deficiency, if present, should be corrected before the start of treatment. Development of intraventricular hemorrhage or cerebral edema should be monitored closely. Mild bleeding secondary to fibrinolytic therapy can be stopped with local pressure. In the event of major bleeding, tPA should be stopped and intravenous fresh frozen plasma (FFP) or cryoprecipitate should be given. The antifibrinolytic agent aminocaproic acid (Amicar) should be considered if the bleeding is life threatening.

PROGNOSIS

The overall mortality rate with aortic and renal arterial thrombosis is between 9% and 20%, with mortality being higher with major aortic and renal arterial thrombosis (Nowak-Gottl et al, 1997). Renovascular hypertension is the most common long-term complication of renal arterial thrombosis. In most cases, these infants eventually are weaned from antihypertensive medications and remain normotensive. Another consequence of renal arterial thrombosis is chronic renal insufficiency caused by irreversible renal parenchymal damage; this is seen less frequently but always in cases with severe aortic and bilateral renal arterial thrombosis.

RENAL VEIN OBSTRUCTION

INCIDENCE AND ETIOLOGY

Renal vein thrombosis (RVT) is the most common thrombosis in infancy and occurs primarily in the newborn period. It has an incidence of 2.2 cases per 100,000 live births (Bokenkamp et al, 2000). Renal vein thrombosis has a male predominance of approximately 67%; it is unilateral in more than 70% of patients and more prevalent on the left side (approximately 63%). The thrombus also involved the inferior vena cava in approximately 43% of the cases, and it was associated with adrenal hemorrhage in approximately 15% (Dauger et al, 2009; Lau et al, 2007).

The cause of renal vein thrombosis is unknown, although a number of factors are associated with this disorder. Prothrombotic factors—including lupus anticoagulant, protein C, protein S, plasma antithrombin III activity, lipoprotein(a), factor V Leiden mutation, prothrombin gene mutation, and methylenetetrahydrofolate (*MTHFR*) thermolabile mutation—have a significant role in the pathogenesis of neonatal RVT (Kosch et al, 2004; Lau et al, 2007; Marks et al, 2005). Other associated factors are maternal diabetes, traumatic delivery, prematurity, hyperviscosity, hypovolemia, hemoconcentration, sepsis, birth asphyxia, cyanotic congenital cardiac disease, congenital renal vein defects, and an indwelling umbilical venous catheter (Bokenkamp et al, 2000; Lau et al, 2007; Nowak-Gottl et al, 1997; Proesmans et al, 2005) (Box 88-3).

CLINICAL PRESENTATION

There are three cardinal signs of renal vein thrombosis: macroscopic hematuria, palpable abdominal mass, and thrombocytopenia; these signs have been found in approximately 56%, 45%, and 47% of cases, respectively (Lau et al, 2007). Other signs and laboratory findings associated with renal vein thrombosis are oliguria or anuria, hemolytic anemia, metabolic acidosis, azotemia, and variable prothrombin and partial thromboplastin times (Box 88-4).

DIAGNOSIS

Renal ultrasonography is a useful and convenient way of diagnosing RVT. It shows unilaterally or bilaterally enlarged and echogenic kidneys with attenuation or loss of corticomedullary differentiation and little blood flow. In many cases, calcification and thrombus may be seen extending into the inferior vena cava (Proesmans et al, 2005). Doppler studies are useful for detecting resistance or absence of flow in renal venous branches and collateral vessels. Thrombosis in small intrarenal veins can cause increased resistance in renal arteries, even when blood flow in the main renal vein and its branches is normal (Lau et al, 2007). Length of the kidney has been reported to correlate negatively with renal outcomes (Winyard et al, 2006). Ultrasonography may also be used as a prognostic tool.

Although renal ultrasonography is the most commonly used imaging modality for diagnosing renal vein

BOX 88-3 Risk Factors for Renal Vein Thrombosis

INHERITED
- Lupus anticoagulant
- Protein C and protein S deficiency
- Plasma antithrombin III activity
- Elevated lipoprotein (a)
- Factor V Leiden mutation
- Prothrombin gene mutation
- Methylenetetrahydrofolate (*MTHFR*) thermolabile mutation

ACQUIRED
- Maternal diabetes
- Traumatic delivery
- Prematurity
- Hyperviscosity
- Hypovolemia
- Hemoconcentration
- Sepsis
- Birth asphyxia
- Cyanotic congenital cardiac disease
- Congenital renal vein defects
- An indwelling umbilical venous catheter

BOX 88-4 Clinical Presentation of Renal Vein Thrombosis

- Macroscopic hematuria
- Palpable abdominal mass
- Thrombocytopenia
- Oliguria/anuria
- Hemolytic anemia
- Metabolic acidosis
- Azotemia
- Variable prothrombin and partial thromboplastin times

thrombosis, contrast angiography is considered the gold standard. Angiography, however, is invasive and requires exposure to ionizing radiation and can be performed only in a neonate in stable condition. Magnetic resonance imaging has also been reported to give excellent diagnostic findings in RVT, although it should be reserved for those cases in which Doppler findings are inconclusive (Basterrechea Iriarte et al, 2008).

TREATMENT

Treatment of neonatal RVT remains controversial because there is not enough literature to compare supportive therapy with anticoagulation, fibrinolysis, or both. Supportive therapy should be provided to all affected infants in an attempt to correct any abnormalities in fluid, electrolyte, and acid-base balance. Hypertonic solutions, nephrotoxic medications, hyperosmotic radiographic contrast agents, and unnecessary use of diuretics should be avoided. Prophylactic heparin therapy has been recommended in a majority of cases to prevent thrombus extension by some authors (Dauger et al, 2009), whereas others advocate similar renal outcomes between supportive treatment and heparin therapies, including a similar proportion of atrophic kidneys secondary to RVT in neonates whether they were managed supportively or with heparin (Lau et al, 2007). LMWH is being used more frequently than unfractionated heparin for anticoagulation. Fibrinolysis is usually reserved for more severe cases, such as bilateral thrombosis and systemic effects (Dauger et al, 2009). Whichever the treatment approach, affected neonates must be followed closely for renal complications such as hypertension, chronic renal insufficiency, and renal atrophy.

Surgical interventions such as thrombectomy or nephrectomy have not shown any benefit. Thrombectomy prevents the main thrombus from extending into inferior vena cava or the contralateral kidney, but it does not prevent renal infarction because smaller intrarenal veins are almost always involved.

PROGNOSIS

Renal scarring and atrophy are well-recognized complications of RVT in the affected kidney, which can be assessed with a radionuclide scan. Approximately 19% of patients have persistent elevation of blood pressure (BP), which has been shown to be slightly higher—at 21% for those with bilateral RVT. The mortality rate for neonates with RVT is approximately 3% (Lau et al, 2007). Most of the deaths are due to underlying disease and not RVT or secondary renal dysfunction. Because more than 80% of neonates with RVT have shown persistent abnormalities on renal imaging and there are not enough data on long-term outcome of such neonates, continued follow-up is strongly recommended.

RENAL CORTICAL AND MEDULLARY NECROSIS

INCIDENCE AND ETIOLOGY

Renal cortical and medullary necrosis are uncommon in newborns and are usually encountered in critically ill newborns as a manifestation of perinatal and postnatal stress leading to end-organ injury. It is usually diagnosed on autopsy. The incidence is 5% in infants who die at less than 3 months of age (Lerner et al, 1992). Risk factors associated with renal cortical and medullary necrosis are congenital heart disease, perinatal anoxia, placenta abruption, twin-twin or twin-maternal transfusions, sepsis, infectious myocarditis, vascular malformations, dehydration, prematurity, respiratory distress syndrome, bleeding diathesis, cardiac catheterization, and intravenous contrast agents (Lerner et al, 1992; Nygren et al, 1988).

PATHOPHYSIOLOGY

Medication administration can interfere with compensatory mechanisms to maintain renal perfusion and can lead to acute tubular necrosis that, depending on the severity of the insult, then may lead to vasculature injury and microthrombi formation with subsequent renal cortical and medullary necrosis. Antiinflammatory medications like indomethacin, which are used to close a patent ductus arteriosus, have been shown to worsen renal ischemia in the setting of hypoperfusion, potentially leading to

renal cortical and medullary necrosis. When renal perfusion is decreased, it results in increased catecholamine secretion, activation of the renin-angiotensin system and the generation of prostaglandins. The intrarenal generation of vasodilatory prostaglandins mediates vasodilation of renal microvasculature to maintain renal perfusion. In this scenario, nonsteroidal antiinflammatory drugs can inhibit this compensatory mechanism and cause acute renal insufficiency during renal hypoperfusion, leading to renal cortical and medullary necrosis (Andreoli, 2004; Badr and Ichikawa, 1988).

In the same way that renal perfusion pressure is low as in renal artery stenosis, increased intrarenal generation of angiotensin II works to increase efferent arteriolar resistance in order to provide the necessary intraglomerular pressure for filtration (Badr and Ichikawa, 1988). Administration of angiotensin-converting enzyme inhibitors in this setting can precipitate acute renal failure and eventually renal cortical necrosis.

CLINICAL PRESENTATION

The clinical manifestations include hematuria, oliguria, and renal enlargement, which are nondiagnostic and associated with many other common neonatal renal abnormalities. Because renal cortical and medullary necrosis usually develops in critically ill newborns in the setting of shock, diagnosis of renal cortical and medullary necrosis is usually delayed or never considered.

DIAGNOSIS

In renal cortical and medullary necrosis, laboratory features may be present, such as hematuria, elevated blood urea nitrogen and creatinine, and thrombocytopenia. Renal ultrasound examination results are normal initially, but may show renal atrophy with substantially decreased size of kidneys later in the course. A radionucleotide renal scan shows decreased to no perfusion with delayed or no function (Andreoli, 2004).

MANAGEMENT AND PROGNOSIS

Infants with cortical necrosis may have partial recovery or no recovery at all. Typically they need renal replacement therapy, short-term or long-term, but those who recover enough renal function to be managed without dialysis are at risk for late development of chronic renal failure.

ADRENAL HEMORRHAGE

INCIDENCE AND ETIOLOGY

The incidence of neonatal adrenal hemorrhage is approximately 0.2% (Avolio et al, 2002). The actual incidence is difficult to ascertain because most cases are asymptomatic. Bilateral hemorrhages are seen in 5% to 15% of cases (Khuri et al, 1980). The right side is involved in 70% of unilateral cases (Fang et al, 1999). Factors involved in neonatal adrenal hemorrhage include anoxia or hypoxia during delivery, being large for gestational age, prolonged labor, trauma during delivery, shock or sepsis, bleeding disorders, and renal vein thrombosis (Fang et al, 1999; Velaphi and Perlman, 2001).

PATHOPHYSIOLOGY

The adrenal gland in an infant is significantly larger than that in an adult and regresses in size during the 1st year of life. The cortex of the gland loses approximately one third of its weight in the first 3 weeks of life. Mechanical trauma and changes in BP easily cause hemorrhage in the adrenal gland, which is more susceptible because of its large size, vascularity, and relative hyperemia. The right adrenal gland is trapped between the liver and spine, which makes it an easy target for mechanical trauma (Velaphi and Perlman, 2001), and its direct venous drainage into the inferior vena cava makes it more susceptible to changes in central venous pressure.

CLINICAL PRESENTATION

Clinical signs and symptoms are usually nonspecific and depend on the volume of bleeding. Smaller bleeds may be asymptomatic or result in unexplained persistent jaundice or mild anemia (Adorisio et al, 2007). Larger bleeds can cause abdominal distention associated with an abdominal mass. Adrenal hemorrhage can also manifest with a scrotal mass that could be confused with testicular torsion (Avolio et al, 2002). Severe hypovolemic shock and hypoglycemia can occur with larger or bilateral bleeds.

DIAGNOSIS

The differential diagnosis of prolonged anemia and jaundice will include hemolysis, liver dysfunction, inborn errors of metabolism, and other forms of jaundice. In case of an abdominal mass, neuroblastoma, mesoblastic nephroma, teratoma, or other masses such as adrenal, hepatic, ovarian, pancreatic, and choledochal cysts should be considered (Fang et al, 1999). Testicular torsion, incarcerated hernia, epididymitis, hematocele, tumor, or orchitis should be considered in patients with a scrotal mass (Bor et al, 2000). In case of shock, sepsis should be evaluated and empirically treated along with BP support and volume replacement.

Laboratory tests that help in the diagnosis are complete blood cell count, serum bilirubin, serum glucose, urinary catecholamines, and their metabolites. Ultrasonography is the most commonly used diagnostic modality (Perl et al, 2007); it can also identify features of evolution of adrenal hemorrhage that follows hemorrhage, such as fibrosis and calcification. Calcification is usually identified 2 weeks after adrenal hemorrhage. Computed tomography scans and magnetic resonance imaging have also been used to identify adrenal hemorrhages, although the former is associated with concerns about radiation exposure and the latter is more accurate than other modalities for identifying adrenal hemorrhages but is not readily available and is time-consuming (Abdu et al, 2009). Laparotomy is needed only rarely for diagnosis.

MANAGEMENT AND PROGNOSIS

Adrenal hemorrhage is usually managed with supportive care, such as volume expansion, administration of blood products, and BP support. Serial imaging can guide

changes in the adrenal size and consistency, which can be helpful in identifying certain tumors. Most infants recover completely. Adrenal insufficiency can occur but is rare and usually occurs with bilateral adrenal involvement (Perl et al, 2007; Ruminska et al, 2008).

HYPERTENSION IN THE NEWBORN

DEFINITION

BP measurements in the newborn infant are an important indicator of appropriate circulation. Determining whether a neonate is hypotensive or hypertensive requires normative BP values. In the pediatric population, *hypertension* is defined as systolic or diastolic BP in the 95th percentile or higher (or more than two standard deviations above the mean values). Hypertension is considered stage 1 if the BP is at the 95th percentile to less than the 99th percentile, and stage 2 if the BP is 99th percentile or greater plus 5 mm Hg (National High Blood Pressure Education Program Working Group on High Blood Pressure in Children and Adolescents, 2004).

NORMAL BLOOD PRESSURE IN NEWBORN

An Australian study of 406 term infants showed a median systolic BP of 65 mm Hg (range, 46 to 94 mm Hg), diastolic BP of 45 mm Hg (range, 24 to 57 mm Hg), and a mean BP of 48 mm Hg (range, 31 to 63 mm Hg) at 12 to 24 hours of life. Blood pressure was seen to increase over the next four days by 1 to 2 mm Hg per day. This study did not show any significant difference in BP depending on birthweight or length (Kent et al, 2007), although in another larger study there was a significant difference in gestational age, birthweight, and length between infants with and without systemic hypertension (Seliem et al, 2007) (Figures 88-1 to 88-3).

EPIDEMIOLOGY

In an Australian study of 2572 newborn infants born between 2001 and 2005, the incidence of hypertension was 1.3% (Seliem et al, 2007). In another study of 3179 infants admitted to the neonatal intensive care unit over a 6-year period, the incidence of hypertension was reported as 0.81% (Singh et al, 1992). Factors associated with hypertension included lower gestational age, lower birthweight, decreased length, maternal antenatal steroid administration, maternal hypertension, umbilical arterial catheterization, postnatal acute renal failure, patent ductus arteriosus, and bronchopulmonary dysplasia (Seliem et al, 2007; Singh et al, 1992).

BLOOD PRESSURE MEASUREMENT

Invasive (Direct) Measurement

Invasive measurement of BP is used in critically ill newborns and is the preferred method of measurement in severely ill and preterm neonates. Direct intraarterial measurement through a catheter placed in the aorta or radial artery is the most accurate technique and provides continuous readings. The degree to which radial measurements correlate with aortic pressures is uncertain. In

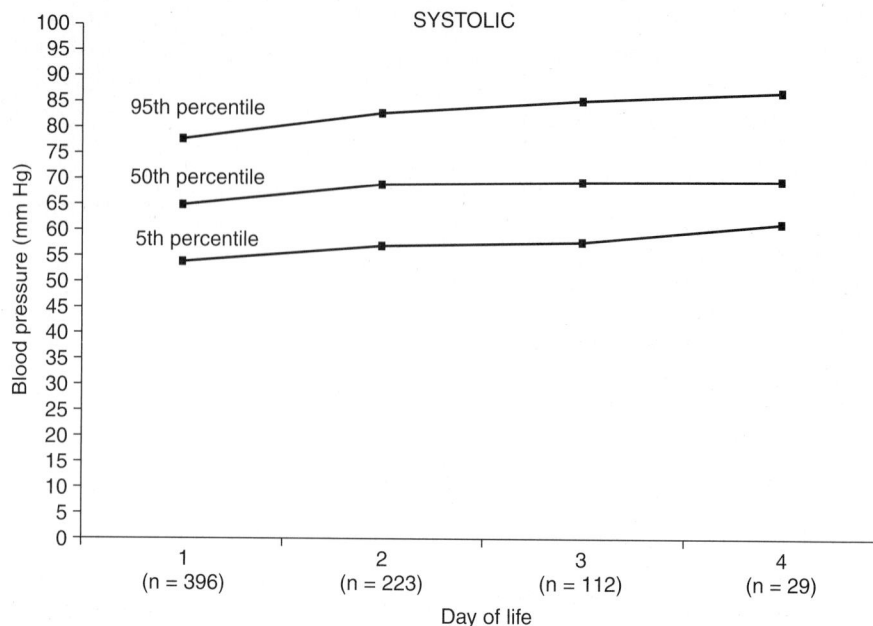

FIGURE 88-1 Systolic blood pressure percentiles (5th, 50th, and 95th) at 1 to 4 days old. *(Reproduced with permission from Kent AL, Kecskes Z, Shadbolt B, et al: Normative blood pressure data in the early neonatal period. In* Pediatric nephrology, *vol 22, New York, 2007, Springer Science+Business Media, p 1336.)*

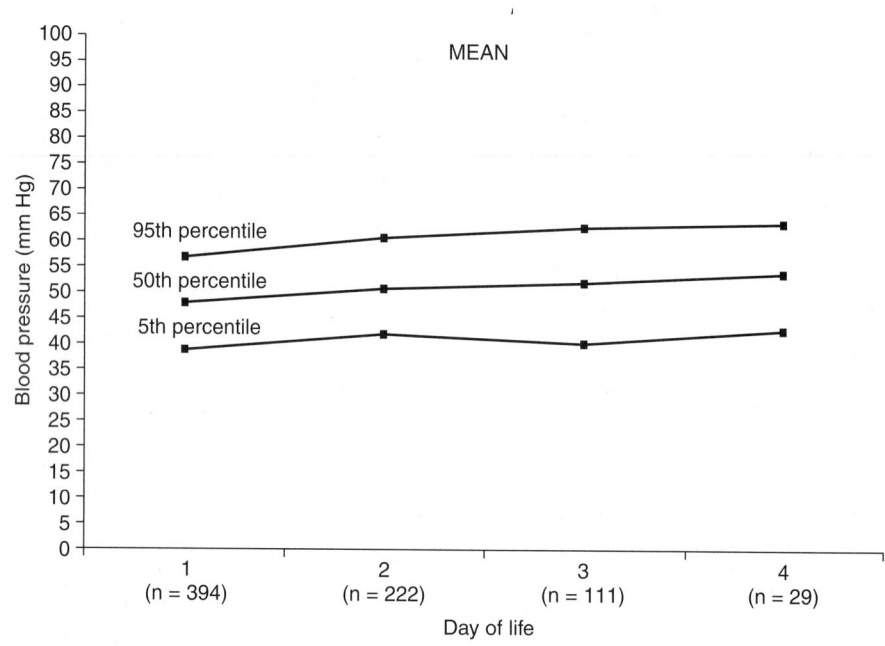

FIGURE 88-2 Mean blood pressure percentiles (5th, 50th, and 95th) at 1 to 4 days old. *(Reproduced with permission from Kent AL, Kecskes Z, Shadbolt B, et al: Normative blood pressure data in the early neonatal period. In* Pediatric nephrology, *volume 22, New York, 2007, Springer Science+Business Media, p 1337.)*

adults, radial artery systolic BP measurements can be 20% to 30% higher than central values, although mean and diastolic measurements are comparable (Pauca et al, 1992). However, radial pressures may more closely mimic aortic pressures in newborns (Gevers et al, 1993). Complications associated with intraarterial catheters include thrombosis and infection; therefore they should be used to monitor BP only when the catheter is needed for another indication, such as frequent arterial blood sampling.

Noninvasive (Indirect) Measurement

Noninvasive BP measurement commonly involves three methods: auscultation, Doppler ultrasound, and automatic oscillometry. Blood pressure measurement by auscultation is usually insensitive in the setting of low stroke volume,

although it is recommended to recheck a high BP reading by auscultation (National High Blood Pressure Education Program Working Group on High Blood Pressure in Children and Adolescents, 2004). Doppler ultrasound does not accurately detect diastolic BP but measures systolic BP reliably. Oscillometry is the most commonly used noninvasive method. It gives an accurate and reproducible estimate of BP. It also measures mean arterial pressure instead of calculating it. For small infants, noninvasively measured BP readings tend to be too high, whereas larger infants tend to have falsely low BP readings (Dannevig et al, 2005). There may also be significant differences between oscillometer BP monitoring systems (Dannevig et al, 2005).

To get an accurate estimate of BP by noninvasive methods, it is important that an appropriate arm cuff is chosen and that the monitor is calibrated according to manufacturer's

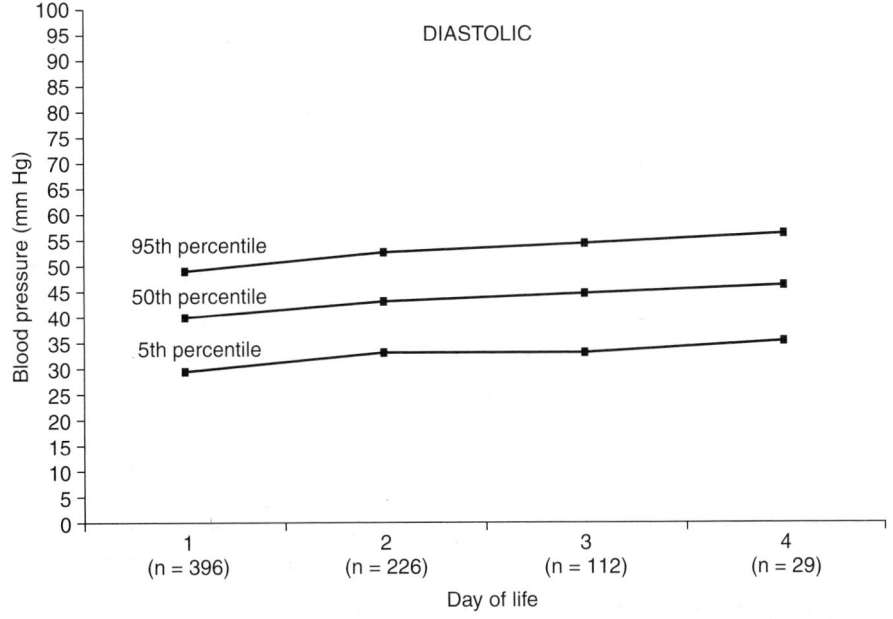

FIGURE 88-3 Diastolic blood pressure percentiles (5th, 50th, and 95th) at 1 to 4 days old. *(Reproduced with permission from Kent AL, Kecskes Z, Shadbolt B, et al: Normative blood pressure data in the early neonatal period. In* Pediatric nephrology, *volume 22,* New York, 2007, *Springer Science+Business Media, p 1337.)*

specifications. An appropriate cuff size has an inflatable bladder width that is at least 40% of the arm circumference at a point midway between the olecranon and acromion. For such a cuff to be optimal for an arm, the cuff bladder length should cover 80% to 100% of the arm circumference. This translates into bladder width-to-length ratio of at least 1:2. Blood pressure estimation is higher to a greater extent with a cuff that is too small and lower by a cuff that is too large. If a cuff is too small, the next largest size should be used, even if it appears large (Adelman, 1988).

In neonates the BP is significantly lower while prone than while supine. Blood pressure tends to decrease with repeated measurements. First BP reading by oscillometry is significantly higher than the second or third reading (Nwankwo et al, 1997).

ETIOLOGY

Infants with hypertension and a history of umbilical arterial catheter do not always demonstrate thrombi in renal arteries (Flynn, 2000). Thromboembolic events related to umbilical arterial catheter are postulated to occur because of endothelial injury at the time of line placement. The suggested mechanism for hypertension is that thromboemboli decrease perfusion to the kidney, resulting in increased renin and aldosterone production with subsequent sodium and water retention (Kilian, 2003).

Neonatal hypertension usually occurs as a result of renal vein thrombosis, which is usually a result of perinatal hypoxia; this can result in persistent hypertension in up to 30% of cases (Mocan et al, 1991). Hypertension in the 1st month of life can also occur as a consequence of acute tubular necrosis and cortical necrosis, which may follow perinatal hypoxia or severe sepsis in extremely premature infants (Buchi and Siegler, 1986). Fluid overload in these circumstances is usually the cause of hypertension.

Antenatal steroids, administered to accelerate lung maturity, have been associated with an eightfold increase in the risk of developing neonatal systemic hypertension

(Seliem et al, 2007), which supports the hypothesis of prenatal glucocorticoids and long-term programming (Seckl, 2004). Many animal experiments have also suggested that exposure to steroids in utero is associated with elevated BP (Koenen et al, 2002). Contrary to these studies, a 30-year follow-up of a randomized controlled trial after exposure to betamethasone showed no increased risk of hypertension (Dalziel et al, 2005).

Chronic lung disease in prematurity is a significant risk factor for developing systemic hypertension (Flynn, 2000). The underlying mechanism—whether related to altered neurohumoral regulation or increased catecholamines, angiotensin, or antidiuretic hormone concentrations—remains unknown (Abman, 2002).

Patent ductus arteriosus is a risk factor for neonatal hypertension (Seliem et al, 2007). It is difficult to discern whether the hypertension is a result of fluid retention or renal hypoperfusion, because many of these infants are treated with indomethacin (Box 88-5).

CLINICAL SIGNS

The magnitude of hypertension does not correlate with the presence of signs and symptoms or their severity. Some patients with severe hypertension manifest few or no symptoms. In many neonates, hypertension will be discovered on routine monitoring of vital signs, particularly in the most acutely ill neonates. In less acutely ill infants, hypertension can manifest with feeding difficulties, unexplained tachypnea, apnea, lethargy, irritability, or seizures. In older infants, unexplained irritability or failure to thrive may be the only manifestation of hypertension (Flynn, 2000) (Box 88-6).

EVALUATION

To diagnose the cause of hypertension, attention should be paid to a history that includes pertinent prenatal exposures, exposure to procedures such as umbilical catheter placement, and current medications. The physical examination

BOX 88-5   Causes of Neonatal Hypertension

VASCULAR

- Renal artery thrombosis
- Aortic thrombosis
- Coarctation of aorta
- Hypoplastic aorta
- Renal vein thrombosis
- Thrombosis of the ductus arteriosus
- Renal artery stenosis
- Intimal hyperplasia
- Idiopathic arterial calcification

RENAL PARENCHYMAL

- Acute renal failure
- Polycyctic kidney disease
- Renal cortical and medullary necrosis
- Hypoplastic/dysplastic kidney
- Acute renal infection
- Pyelonephritis with scarring
- Obstructive uropathy
- Constrictive perirenal hematoma or urinoma
- Congenital mesoblastic nephroma
- Nephrolithiasis
- After pyeloplasty of a hydronephrotic kidney
- Multicystic kidney

ENDOCRINE

- Pheochromocytoma
- Neuroblastoma
- Adrenal disorders (hyperplasia, hyperaldosteronism, carcinoma, hematoma)
- Hyperthyroidism

IATROGENIC

- Corticosteroids
- Theophylline
- Pancuronium
- Intrauterine cocaine exposure
- Phenylephrine eye drops

OTHER

- Extracorporeal membrane oxygenation
- Bronchopulmonary dysplasia
- Increased intarcranial pressure/seizures
- Fluid and electrolyte overload
- After closure of abdominal wall defect

BOX 88-6   Clinical Signs of Neonatal Hypertension

ASYMPTOMATIC
Cardiovascular

- Congestive heart failure
- Decreased or unequal pulses
- Cardiomegaly
- Hepatomegaly
- Vasomotor instability
- Mottling

Respiratory

- Tachypnea
- Cyanosis

Neurologic

- Tremors
- Lethargy
- Seizures
- Coma
- Apnea
- Hypertonicity
- Asymmetric reflexes
- Hemiparesis
- Facial palsy
- Hypertensive retinopathy
- Cerebral edema
- Intracranial hemorrhage

Renal

- Dehydration
- Sodium wasting
- Oliguria/anuria
- Polyuria
- Renal enlargement

NONSPECIFIC

- Abdominal distention
- Edema
- Fever
- Failure to thrive
- Adrenal mass

should include BP readings in all four extremities to rule out coarctation of the thoracic aorta. A thorough cardiac and abdominal examination should be performed. The presence of a flank mass may indicate ureteropelvic junction obstruction, and an epigastric bruit may indicate renal arterial stenosis. Pain or agitation should also be evaluated as a potential cause of hypertension. It is important to assess serum electrolytes, creatinine, and blood urea nitrogen and to perform a urinalysis (Flynn, 2000).

Ultrasound imaging, including Doppler ultrasound of the genitourinary tract, should be done in all hypertensive infants. Ultrasound can help to diagnose causes of hypertension such as renal venous thrombosis, aortic or renal arterial thrombosis, and anatomic or congenital renal abnormalities. An echocardiogram should be done to evaluate the effects of hypertension, such as concentric left ventricular hypertrophy, left ventricular systolic dysfunction, or left atrial dilation and aortomegaly (Peterson et al, 2006).

Radionuclide imaging should be performed in neonates with extremely severe BP elevation when ultrasonography is not diagnostic. An abnormal kidney typically shows decreased effective renal plasma flow, decreased urine flow rate, and increased isotope concentration. These findings may be present when the ultrasound appearance and serum creatinine concentration are normal. If radionuclide imaging is also inconclusive in neonates with severe hypertension, angiography should be considered. Angiography, though invasive, is the standard modality for diagnosis of renovascular hypertension. But angiography should be deferred in a small infant until the body weight is more than 3 kg. Magnetic resonance angiography has also been used as a less invasive way to detect a vascular lesion by some (Cachat et al, 2004).

TREATMENT

The threshold for starting antihypertensive therapy has not been well defined, therefore the optimal management of neonatal hypertension is uncertain. An asymptomatic

TABLE 88-1 Oral Antihypertensive Agents Used for Neonatal Hypertension

Drug	Class	Dose	Comments
Isradipine	Ca²⁺ channel blocker	0.05-0.15 mg/kg divided four times per day	Used in both acute and chronic HTN
Captopril	ACE inhibitor	0.05-0.5 mg/kg per day divided three times per day	Monitor serum potassium and creatinine
Chlorothiazide	Thiazide diuretic	10-40 mg/kg per day divided twice per day	Monitor serum electrolytes
Hydrochlorothiazide	Thiazide diuretic	2-4 mg/kg per day divided twice per day	Monitor serum electrolytes
Spironolactone	Aldosterone antagonist	1-3 mg/kg per day divided two to four times per day	Can cause hyperkalemia
Hydralazine	Vasodilator	0.75-7.5 mg/kg per day divided three or four times per day	Tachycardia, fluid retention, SLE-like syndrome in slow acetylators
Propranolol	β-Blocker	1.0-8.0 mg/kg per day divided three times per day	Can precipitate heart failure, bronchospasm, and hypoglycemia; avoid in infants with BPD
Labetalol	α- and β-blocker	4.0-40 mg/kg per day divided two or three times per day	Monitor heart rate. Avoid in infants with BPD
Minoxidil	Vasodilator	0.2-5 mg/kg per day divided two or three times per day	Most potent vasodilator. Used for refractory HTN
Amlodipine	Ca²⁺ channel blocker	0.05-0.17 mg/kg per dose divided once or twice per day	Longer duration of action than isradipine, useful for chronic HTN

ACE, Angiotensin-converting enzyme; *BPD,* bronchopulmonary dysplasia; *HTN,* hypertension; *SLE,* systemic lupus erythematosus.

neonate with a systolic pressure consistently between the 95th and 99th percentiles and with no end organ involvement should be observed but not treated. The hypertension resolves over time in most cases. If the systolic pressure is above the 99th percentile or if there is end organ involvement with a systolic pressure above the 95th percentile, the neonate should be treated. There is little if any evidence for a precise, single starting point of treatment. Treatment should be directed at the primary cause. If the neonate is receiving any treatment that could raise BP, attempts should be made to reduce or withdraw that treatment. Salt or fluid overload should be corrected as well (Watkinson, 2002).

If an antihypertensive agent is needed, the group of drugs chosen should depend on the cause of hypertension, routes available for administration, and possibility of impending hypertensive crisis. Treatment is difficult because of idiosyncratic responses to drugs in neonates with varying renal and hepatic function. All drugs should be started at their lowest doses. When an antihypertensive agent is started, the BP should be monitored closely. Neonatal hypertension can be treated with any of these five classes: diuretics, angiotensin-converting enzyme inhibitors, β-blockers, calcium channel blockers, and direct peripheral vasodilators. Diuretics increase salt and water excretion, which results in decreased extracellular and plasma volumes. Compensatory mechanisms then begin to maintain sodium homoeostasis, and plasma volume may return to normal. Despite these compensatory mechanisms, there is a sustained reduction in volume and BP (Sinaiko, 1993). Diuretics can contribute to a hypotensive crisis if used with other antihypertensive drugs in the absence of volume overload. Propranolol is the most extensively used β-blocker in neonates with hypertension; it has a low incidence of side effects. Labetalol blocks both β and α receptors, although it is much more potent than propranolol. Calcium channel blockers, such as isradipine and amlodipine, have vasodilator action that lowers peripheral vascular resistance.

Direct vasodilators, such as hydralazine and minoxidil, reduce peripheral vascular resistance by directly acting on vascular smooth muscle. Minoxidil is more potent and has a number of side effects; therefore it is reserved only for refractory hypertension. Both hydralazine and minoxidil can initially cause an increase in heart rate and cardiac output with flushing. Angiotensin-converting enzyme inhibitors are more effective in neonates because renal vascular resistance is high in this population; however, if renal vascular disease is suspected, this latter class of drugs should be avoided until normal vasculature is confirmed. Captopril is a commonly used drug in this class (Watkinson, 2002) (Table 88-1).

In a hypertensive crisis, the drug of choice in this population is a calcium channel blocker—nicardipine. Other agents have also been used, such as esmolol, labetalol, hydralazine, sodium nitroprusside, and enalapril. Regardless of the drug used, BP should be monitored preferably continuously via an indwelling arterial catheter; if this is not an option, then monitoring by cuff readings should be done every 10 to 15 minutes. As a result, the drug can be titrated to achieve the desired degree of BP control. Intermittently administered intravenous agents, such as hydralazine and labetalol, can be used in infants. Intravenous sodium nitroprusside, a potent vasodilator, acts rapidly but has a short duration of action. Sodium nitroprusside can cause renal insufficiency or thiocyanate toxicity with greater than 72 hours of administration; therefore thiocyanate levels should be monitored with this drug if it is used for a prolonged period. Enalaprilat, the intravenous angiotensin-converting enzyme inhibitor, has also been reported to be useful in the treatment of neonatal renovascular hypertension. This drug should be used cautiously because its use, even in doses at the lower end of published ranges, can lead to significant and prolonged hypotension and oliguric acute renal failure (Flynn, 2000) (Table 88-2).

Neonatal hypertension caused by ureteral obstruction or aortic coarctation is best managed surgically. Balloon

TABLE 88-2 Intravenous Antihypertensive Agents Used for Hypertensive Emergency

Drug	Class	Dose	Comments
Nicardipine	Ca²⁺ channel blocker	0.5-3.0 μg/kg per min by IV infusion	Monitor for tachycardia
Esmolol	β-Blocker	100-300 μg/kg per min by IV infusion	Very short acting
Labetalol	α- and β-Blocker	0.20-1.0 mg/kg by IV bolus; 0.25-3.0 mg/kg/h by IV infusion	Relatively contraindicated in BPD and heart failure
Hydralazine	Vasodilator	0.15-0.6 mg/kg	Monitor for tachycardia
Sodium nitroprusside	Vasodilator	0.5-10 μg/kg per min by IV infusion	Thiocyanate toxicity with >72 hr use or in renal failure
Enalaprilat	ACE inhibitor	5-10 μg/kg by IV bolus	Monitor for acute renal failure, prolonged hypotension

ACE, Angiotensin-converting enzyme; *BPD*, bronchopulmonary dysplasia; *IV*, intravenous.

angioplasty or surgical reconstruction can be used in infants with renal arterial stenosis. These infants are usually managed medically until they have grown sufficiently. Hypertension secondary to Wilms' tumor or neuroblastoma requires surgical tumor resection.

PROGNOSIS

In most cases of neonatal hypertension, BP can be controlled adequately with pharmacotherapy. Hypertension resulting from acute tubular necrosis resolves when renal function improves, as is the case with other reversible causes. In bronchopulmonary dysplasia, if hypertension is due to steroid intake (rarely used), it improves once the treatment is stopped. In hypertension secondary to renal artery or aortic thrombosis, the usual duration of drug therapy is a few weeks to several months. The infant can be weaned from medications once the BP is stable for 4 to 8 weeks, and ultrasonography is used to confirm resolution of thrombus (Adelman, 1987; Caplan et al, 1989). Because there is not enough information about the outcome of neonatal hypertension in early adulthood and beyond, close long-term follow-up with regular monitoring of BP and renal function is recommended.

SUGGESTED READINGS

Abdu AT, Kriss VM, Bada HS, Reynolds EW: Adrenal hemorrhage in a newborn, *Am J Perinatol* 26:553-557, 2009.

Andreoli SP: Acute renal failure in the newborn, *Semin Perinatol* 28:112-123, 2004.

Andrew ME, Monagle P, deVeber G, Chan AK: Thromboembolic disease and antithrombotic therapy in newborns, *Hematology Am Soc Hematol Educ Program* 358-374, 2001.

Barrington KJ: Umbilical artery catheters in the newborn: effects of heparin, *Cochrane Database Syst Rev* 2:CD000507, 2000.

Flynn JT: Neonatal hypertension: diagnosis and management, *Pediatr Nephrol* 14:332-341, 2000.

Kent AL, Kecskes Z, Shadbolt B, Falk MC: Normative blood pressure data in the early neonatal period, *Pediatr Nephrol* 22:1335-1341, 2007.

Lau KK, Stoffman JM, Williams S, et al: Neonatal renal vein thrombosis: review of the English-language literature between 1992 and 2006, *Pediatrics* 120:e1278-e1284, 2007.

Monagle P, Chalmers E, Chan A, et al: Antithrombotic therapy in neonates and children: American College of Chest Physicians Evidence-Based Clinical Practice Guidelines (8th Edition), *Chest* 133(Suppl 6):887S-968S, 2008.

Proesmans W, van de Wijdeven P, Van Geet C: Thrombophilia in neonatal renal venous and arterial thrombosis, *Pediatr Nephrol* 20:241-242, 2005.

Seliem WA, Falk MC, Shadbolt B, Kent AL: Antenatal and postnatal risk factors for neonatal hypertension and infant follow-up, *Pediatr Nephrol* 22:2081-2087, 2007.

Complete references used in this text can be found online at www.expertconsult.com

PART XVIII

ENDOCRINE DISORDERS

EMBRYOLOGY, DEVELOPMENTAL BIOLOGY, AND ANATOMY OF THE ENDOCRINE SYSTEM

Lewis P. Rubin

ENDOCRINE AND NEUROENDOCRINE DEVELOPMENT IN THE FETUS AND PERINATAL TRANSITION

The endocrine system consists of interacting effector-target organ feedback pathways. This chapter reviews several developmental themes, many of which are explored further in the following chapters in Endocrine Disorders and other parts of this text. In addition, lessons learned from development of critical endocrine interactions and intracellular regulatory events, such as the endocrine pancreas (Puri and Hebrok, 2010), are being applied to regenerative medicine and modulating cell fate determination in the adult.

The placental-fetal unit sustains "the unique endocrine milieu of the fetus" (Fisher, 1986) and promotes adaptation for postnatal life. During fetal development into the perinatal transition, the organism shifts from dependence on placenta to independent homeostatic regulation. The functional development of fetal endocrine glands and hormonal responsiveness of target tissues are influenced by fetal genotype, maternal genotype, maternal pre-pregnancy and pregnancy health and nutrition, and pregnancy-associated and preexisting maternal conditions. This complex interplay of genotype and environment is emerging as a central thesis in translational research. By modifying placental and fetal growth and metabolism, hormones play a central role in programming development in utero and adjusting phenotype, especially in response to adverse intrauterine conditions (Fowden and Forhead, 2009).

Of note, much understanding about endocrine developmental biology has been derived from large animal fetal physiology models and gene manipulation in mice. When comparing ontogenic studies performed in different species, one must consider similarities and differences from human fetuses and newborns. A critical point for interspecies comparisons is the maturational state at birth. Different species (and different organ systems in the same species) may be classified either as immature (altricial) or more developed (precocial). In particular, the human term newborn has a relatively mature (precocial) brain and respiratory, neuroendocrine and parathyroid-renal pathways but is relatively clumsy, that is, is motorically immature (altricial).

A second principle is that the human fetal endocrine system begins development more or less independent from maternal endocrine influence. This separation is possible because the placenta is an efficient barrier to fetal access to most maternal hormones, including steroids, sterols, peptides, glycoproteins, and catechols. Nevertheless, transplacental passage of even minute amounts of several maternal hormones can be essential for normal fetal development. For example, in human fetuses with congenital hypothyroidism (Chapter 93), maternal-fetal transfer of thyroid hormone (T_4) may result in neonatal plasma levels 25% to 50% of those in normal newborns (Vulsma et al, 1989). Therefore, neurodevelopmental outcome in congenital hypothyroidism is generally good when T_4 replacement is initiated within the first 2 weeks after birth. In contrast, maternal hypothyroidism during pregnancy adversely affects neurodevelopmental outcome in the offspring (Haddow et al, 1999), and the combination of severe maternal and fetal hypothyroxinemia results in profound neurodevelopmental disability (Yasuda et al, 1999).

A third principle is that disturbances in transplacental substrate transfer—for example, calcium (Chapter 90) or glucose (Chapter 94)—can modify development of fetal and neonatal hormonal pathways. Maternal immunoglobins and certain therapeutic agents also are transported to the fetus. In the example of Graves' disease (autoimmune hyperthyroidism), transplacental transfer of maternal thyroid-stimulating antibodies may cause fetal hyperthyroidism, and maternal antithyroid medications (e.g., propylthiouracil, methimazole) in sufficient doses suppress fetal thyroid function (Chapter 93).

MOLECULAR DETERMINANTS OF ENDOCRINE DEVELOPMENT

Genotyping studies show that functional mutations in a single gene, usually one encoding a transcription factor (TF), can produce endocrine organ hypoplasia or aplasia. Important clinical instances include isolated growth hormone (GH) deficiency or combined pituitary hormone deficiencies associated with mutations in TFs encoding genes that control organogenesis or cell differentiation. Hesx1, a "master switch" essential for normal optic nerve and pituitary development, orchestrates expression or activation of other factors involved in pituitary organogenesis (Corneli et al, 2008). Mutations in HESX1 are reported in patients with hypopituitarism either with typical septo-optic dysplasia (SOD) or with neuromorphologic abnormalities not included in classic SOD. At least nine mutated pituitary transcription factors have been identified that alter hypothalamic-pituitary development and structure (Table 89-1). More recently, mutations in OTX2, a pituitary HESX1-regulated TF, has been shown to produce a variety of pituitary phenotypes (Dateki et al, 2010). Genetic causes of other endocrine glandular development occur with IPF1 (insulin promoter factor 1) in pancreatic agenesis (Schwitzgebel et al, 2003; Stoffers et al, 1997) and neonatal diabetes mellitus, PAX8 in congenital hypothyroidism associated with thyroid hypoplasia (Tonacchera et al, 2007), or DAX1 in X-linked adrenal hypoplasia congenita and hypogonadotropic hypogonadism (McCabe, 2007).

Congenital (nonneoplastic) endocrine hyperfunction also often is caused by single gene mutations that lead to gene inactivation (CaSR, SUR1, Kir6.2) or activation (TSHR, LHR, GK, GLUD1) (Table 89-2). Proteins currently known to cause fetal and neonatal nonneoplastic endocrine hyperfunction disrupt hormone exocytosis or cell sensing of an extracellular regulator of hormone exocytosis (Marx, 1999).

A second important genetic mechanism for developmental endocrinopathies involves genomic imprinting. In mammals, some (imprinted) genes are expressed solely from either the paternally or maternally inherited allele. Maternal and paternal imprints are established, respectively, in dividing diplotene oocytes and prospermatogonia. Lack of imprinting of specific chromosomes or chromosome segments occurs as a result of uniparental disomy or deletions of imprinted centers. Imprinting defects can cause distinct developmental abnormalities according to the chromosome involved (Tilghman, 1999). The chief mechanism involves differential methylation of specific sites in or near imprinted genes. These methylation marks are maintained

TABLE 89-1 Human Mutations Causing Abnormal Hypothalamopituitary Development

Gene	Syndrome	Phenotype	Inheritance
POU1F1	Combined pituitary hormone deficiency (CPHD)	GH, TSH, PRL deficiencies; usually severe; small to normal AP	Recessive, dominant
PROP1	CPHD	GH, TSH, LH, PRL deficiency; evolving ACTH deficiency; small, normal or enlarged AP	Recessive
HESX1	Specific syndrome	IGHD, CPHD, septo-optic dysplasia; APH, EPP, absent infundibulum, ACC	Recessive, dominant
LHX3	Specific syndrome	CPHD (GH, TSH, LH, FSH, PRL deficiencies), short neck, limited rotation; small, normal or enlarged AP, short cervical spine	Dominant
LHX4	Specific syndrome	CPHD (GH < TSH < ACTH defs.); small AP, EPP, cerebellar abnormalities	Dominant
SOX3	Specific syndrome	IGHD, mental retardation, panhypopituitarism; APH, infundibular hypoplasia, EPP	X-linked
SOX2	Specific syndrome	Hypogonadotrophic hypogonadism; APH, bilateral anophthalmia/microphthalmia, abnormal corpus callosum, learning difficulties, esophageal atresia, sensorineural hearing loss	De novo
TBX19	Specific syndrome	Neonatal ACTH deficiency	Recessive

Adapted from Kelberman D, Dattani MT: Hypothalamic and pituitary development: novel insights into the aetiology, *Eur J Endocrinol* 157:S3-S14, 2007.
ACC, Agenesis of the corpus callosum; *ACTH*, adrenocorticotropic hormone; *AP(H)*, anterior pituitary (hypoplasia); *EPP*, ectopic posterior pituitary; *GH*, growth hormone; *IGHD*, isolated GH deficiency; *LH*, luteinizing hormone; *PRL*, prolactin; *TSH*, thyroid-stimulating hormone.

TABLE 89-2 Features of Nonneoplastic Endocrine Hyperfunction Disorders

Tissue Expressing Hyperfunction	Syndrome	Gene Mutated	Typical Onset Age (years)	Treatment
Parathyroid cells	FHH	**CaSR**	0	None
	NSHPT	*CaSR*	0	Total excision
Pancreatic islet β-cells	PHHI-1	*SUR1*	0	Near total excision
	PHHI-2	*Kir6.2*	0	Near total excision
	PHHI-3	*GK*	15	Diazoxide
	PHHI-4	*GLUD1*	0	Diazoxide
Thyrocytes	Congenital thyrotoxicosis	*TSHR*	0-10	Medical or ablate
Leydig cells	Testotoxicosis	*LHR*	3	Medical

Adapted from Marx SJ: Contrasting paradigms for hereditary hyperfunction of endocrine cells, *J Clin Endocrinol Metab* 84:3001-3009, 1999.
CaSR, Gene for calcium sensing receptor; *FHH*, familial hypocalciuric hypercalcemia; *GK*, gene for glucokinase; *GLUD1*, gene for glutamate dehydrogenase type 1; *Kir6.2*, gene for β-cell ATP-binding subunit of inward rectifying potassium channel; *LHR*, gene for luteinizing hormone receptor; *NSPHT*, neonatal severe hyperparathyroidism; *PHHI*, persistent hyperinsulinemic hypoglycemia of infancy; *SUR1*, gene for β-cell specific sulfonylurea receptor (component of potassium channel); *TSHR*, gene for thyroid stimulating hormone receptor.

throughout development and are only erased and reestablished in the germ line. Human endocrinopathies caused by imprinting defects include transient neonatal diabetes mellitus (Chapter 94) and Albright's hereditary osteodystrophy (*GNAS1* imprinting defect) (Chapter 90).

STEROIDOGENESIS AND THE MATERNAL-PLACENTAL-FETAL UNIT

During pregnancy, the mother, fetus, and placenta function in concert as a steroidogenic unit for estrogen and progesterone production. Maternal cholesterol is the principal substrate for placental synthesis of progesterone precursors in fetal androgen production. Although the placenta lacks 17-hydroxylase and 17,20-desmolase (CYP17) activities for estrogen synthesis, the human fetal adrenal compensates with a considerable output of Δ5-steroids (17-hydroxylated precursors), particularly dihydroepiandrosterone sulfate (DHEAS) (Figure 89-1). In primates, estrogen plays an integrative role in modulating placental-fetal communication and in intrauterine development (Albrecht and Pepe, 1999). Estrogen promotes placental trophoblast differentiation into syncytiotrophoblast and upregulates key enzymes in progesterone biosynthesis and cortisol-cortisone conversion.

Throughout most of gestation, protection from hypercortisolism is critical for normal neuroendocrine development. Late in gestation, with activation of the fetal hypothalamic-pituitary-adrenal (HPA) axis, fetal cortisol triggers parturition; lung, gastrointestinal, brain and adrenal medullary maturation; induction of numerous metabolic pathways; and increased β-adrenergic receptor density in heart, lung, and brown fat. Studies on the role of glucocorticoids in preterm labor and fetal maturation have led to the successful, widespread use of antenatal glucocorticoids to accelerate fetal, especially lung, maturation (Liggins and Howie, 1972) (Chapter 42). On the other hand, chronic or repetitive fetal exposure to antenatal glucocorticoid has a profound, sometimes deleterious,

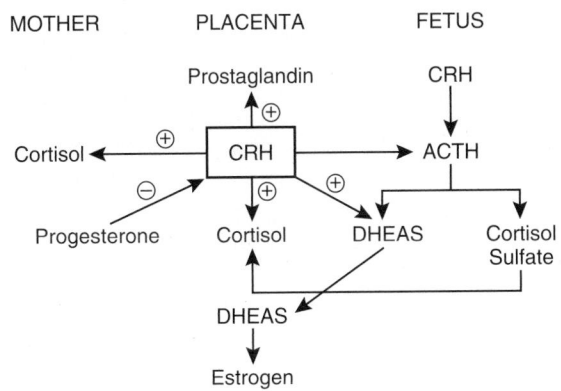

FIGURE 89-1 Schematic representation of the interrelationships among the mother, placenta, and fetus in the upregulation of placental CRH production in response to stress. Maternal and/or fetal cortisol stimulates placental CRH expression. Placental CRH, in turn, stimulates the fetal HPA axis and secretion of DHEAS from the fetal zone of adrenal cortex. *CRH,* Corticotropin-releasing hormone; *DHEAS,* dihydroepiandrosterone sulfate. *(Adapted from Challis JRG, Sloboda D, Matthews SG, et al: The fetal placental hypothalamic-pituitary-adrenal [HPA] axis, parturition and post natal health,* Mol Cell Endocrinol *185:135-144, 2001.)*

influence on postnatal adaptation and activity of the endocrine pancreas, pituitary-adrenal axis, and cardiovascular activity (see Developmental Origins of Health and Disease Hypothesis, later) (Challis et al, 2001).

It is not surprising that in all placental species studied, including humans (Beitins et al, 1973), fetal access to maternal glucocorticoid is restricted and fetal glucocorticoid levels (cortisol or corticosterone) are low. This maternal-fetal gradient is maintained by the enzyme 11β-hydroxysteroid dehydrogenase (11β-HSD). The type 1 isoform is bidirectional. The type 2 isoform (11β-HSD2) unidirectionally converts cortisol and corticosterone to inactive cortisone and 11-dehydrocorticosterone, respectively. The low cortisol:cortisone ratio in fetal circulation (approximately 0.3) reflects low fetal cortisol production and high placental 11β-HSD2 activity. After birth, the cortisol-cortisone ratio rises.

As pregnancy progresses into the third trimester, the maternal-placental-fetal steroidogenic unit activates the fetal HPA axis. This is a central mechanism for the fetus to exert an influence on pregnancy duration. Placental production of corticotropin-releasing hormone (CRH) is correlated with the length of gestation so that maternal plasma levels of CRH rise exponentially as pregnancy progresses toward term and peak during labor (Grammatopoulos, 2008). A CRH/ACTH (adrenocorticotropic hormone)/cortisol surge near term induces involution of the fetal adrenal cortex, increased adrenal 3β-hydroxysteroid dehydrogenase (3β-HSD) activity, and a relative reduction in the placental 11β-HSD2-11βHSD1 ratio. In humans, the fall in placental 11β-HSD2 mRNA expression and the rise in fetoplacental cortisol levels lead to a rise in placental prostaglandin (PGE_2 and $PGF_{2\alpha}$) synthesis that, in turn, stimulates uterine contractility and further CRH expression (see Figure 89-1). The increased fetal adrenal cortisol production and decreased placental cortisol clearance synchronize maturation of critical organs (lung, liver, intestine, adrenal, brain). In effect, term birth may be viewed as an escape mechanism from this intrauterine environment of increasing hypercortisolemia. The postnatal transition is promoted by the newborn's disconnection from this robust placental steroid production.

A critical aspect of intrauterine endocrinology is the opposite effect of the increase in late fetal cortisol levels on hypothalamic and placental CRH expression. Cortisol inhibits hypothalamic CRH production via the HPA negative feedback loop but stimulates placental CRH production, an effect mediated via the cAMP response element in the CRH promoter (Cheng et al, 2000). Positive feedback loops are intrinsically unstable and, in this instance, terminate in birth.

Human placental CRH production may have evolved to stimulate fetal ACTH release and adrenal steroidogenesis, thus satisfying the high demand for synthesis of dehydroepiandrosterone (DHEA), the predominant source of placental estradiol (E_2). Placental CRH stimulates the fetal adrenal zone, an adrenal structure unique to primates (see later discussion), to produce DHEA sulfate (DHEAS), which is converted to E_2 by the placenta (Power and Schulkin, 2006). Placental CRH-induced cortisol output from the fetal and maternal adrenal glands induces further placental CRH expression, forming a positive feedback system that results in increasing placental production of E_2. Concomitant CRH stimulation by placental CRH of fetal cortisol and DHEA would couple the glucocorticoid effects on fetal organ maturation with the timing of parturition, as Majzoub et al (1999) have pointed out, an obvious benefit in postnatal survival. Umbilical plasma E_2 and progesterone levels are quite high and fall by approximately 100-fold during the 1st day after birth.

From this perspective, preterm birth may have adverse endocrine consequences for the newborn. Current evidence suggests that relative adrenal insufficiency in extremely low-birthweight (ELBW) infants may be inadequate for systemic response to stress. Low cortisol concentrations in these infants have been correlated with increased severity of illness, hypotension, mortality, and development of bronchopulmonary dysplasia (Aucott et al, 2008; Watterberg et al, 2007). Selective hydrocortisone supplementation may be a promising strategy for care of these infants.

Similarly, the consequences of E_2 and progesterone withdrawal so early in development remain largely unknown. Pilot studies of E_2 and progesterone supplementation in ELBW infants have shown trends toward increased bone mineralization and a decrease in chronic lung disease (Trotter et al, 2001, 2007). Further clinical trials of "physiologic replacement" in extremely preterm newborns may answer some of these important clinical questions.

HYPOTHALAMIC-PITUITARY-ADRENAL AXIS

The hypothalamus forms an interface between the endocrine and autonomic systems and regulates thermoregulation, blood pressure, energy balance, and behavioral responses. Advancing pregnancy is associated with HPA axis maturation. In utero and at birth, this neuroendocrine network facilitates adaptation to environmental stresses and regulates somatic growth, reproduction, and lactation.

Early specification signals for forebrain induction are required before or during gastrulation. Later in embryogenesis, ventralizing and rostralizing signals from the axial mesoderm (e.g., Sonic hedgehog) are required to induce the cell types of the presumptive hypothalamus (Michaud, 2001). The fetal hypothalamus begins to form soon after the appearance of the hypothalamic sulcus in the 32-day embryo. Classic dating studies have established that the hypothalamus follows an "outside-in" pattern of neurogenesis, with neurons of the lateral hypothalamus being born before the medial ones. The developmental program for neurons of the anterior hypothalamus requires function of the TF Sim1 (Caqueret et al, 2006). Between 6 and 12 weeks, the basal hypothalamus differentiates into distinct nuclei and fiber tracts and produces hormones detectable by immunohistochemistry or immunoassay. Portal vascular connections to the anterior pituitary are established by about 12 weeks (Thliveris and Currie, 1980), although the definitive hypothalamo-hypophyseal portal system develops primarily in the third trimester. Failure of ventral forebrain induction causes holoprosencephaly (see Chapter 60). Endocrine deficiencies caused by hypothalamic and/or pituitary dysfunction may be the only clinical sign in milder forms of (lobar) holoprosencephaly.

Neuropeptide secretion from hypothalamic neurons and negative and positive feedback loops from target organs regulate the synthesis and secretion of distinct pituitary hormones. The anterior pituitary gland (adenohypophysis) derives from ectodermal thickening of the diencephalon and roof of the oral pit. The pituitary diverticulum (Rathke's pouch) bulges into the floor of the prosencephalon by week 4. In week 6, sphenoidal mesenchyme pinches off the pituitary diverticulum from the oral pit. The precursor cells of the anterior pituitary begin to differentiate by week 8. These distinct pituitary cell types arise in a temporally and spatially specific pattern and in tandem with their inputs from hypothalamic nuclei. Development of the hypothalamo-hypophyseal portal veins permits the local circulation of releasing hormones, including thyrotropin-releasing hormone (TRH), growth hormone–releasing hormone (GHRH), CRH, and somatostatin (SS).

During the second trimester, the anterior pituitary differentiates into the five endocrine cell types that secrete six hormones: (1) proopiomelanocortin (POMC) (which is proteolytically cleaved to adrenocorticotropic hormone [ACTH] in corticotropes and melanocyte-stimulating hormone [MSHα] in melanotropes), (2) thyroid-stimulating hormone (TSH) in thyrotropes, (3) growth hormone (GH) in somatotropes, (4) prolactin (PRL) in lactotropes, and (5) follicle-stimulating hormone (FSH) and (6) luteinizing hormone (LH) in gonadotropes (Figure 89-2). Serum GH concentrations peak at 20 to 24 weeks (Suganuma et al, 1989) and decline steadily thereafter, perhaps as a result of hypothalamic-pituitary maturation and increased interaction between GHRH and somatotropin release-inhibiting hormone (SRIH).

Anterior pituitary organogenesis illustrates how mutation of a single regulatory gene can cause multiple hormone deficiencies (MPHDs or panhypopituitarism) (Romero et al, 2009), even though the genes encoding those hormones are dispersed throughout the genome. Transient embryonic morphogenetic signaling gradients induce overlapping expression patterns of transcription factors (repressors, activators) and co-regulators and direct positional cell fates. These pituitary and hypothalamic transcription factors coordinate gland formation, differentiation, expansion, and definitive function of the distinct pituitary cell types. Pituitary development and hormone expression require Pit-1, a pituitary-specific transcription factor. Pit-1 gene expression directs differentiation and proliferation of somatotrophs, lactotrophs, and thyrotrophs and transactivation of the GH, PRL, and TSHα genes. Several Pit-1 mutations have been shown to be responsible for a phenotype of multiple congenital pituitary hormone deficiency involving GH, PRL, and TSH (Kelberman and Dattani, 2007). The repressor Hesx1 (homeobox gene expressed in embryonic stem cells) is expressed early in the anterior region of the embryo and is involved in the initial determination of optic nerves and anterior pituitary (see Figure 89-2). Hesx1 mutations can cause recessive and autosomal forms of hypopituitarism and septo-optic dysplasia.

The neural component of the pituitary, the posterior pituitary gland or neurohypophysis, grows from an

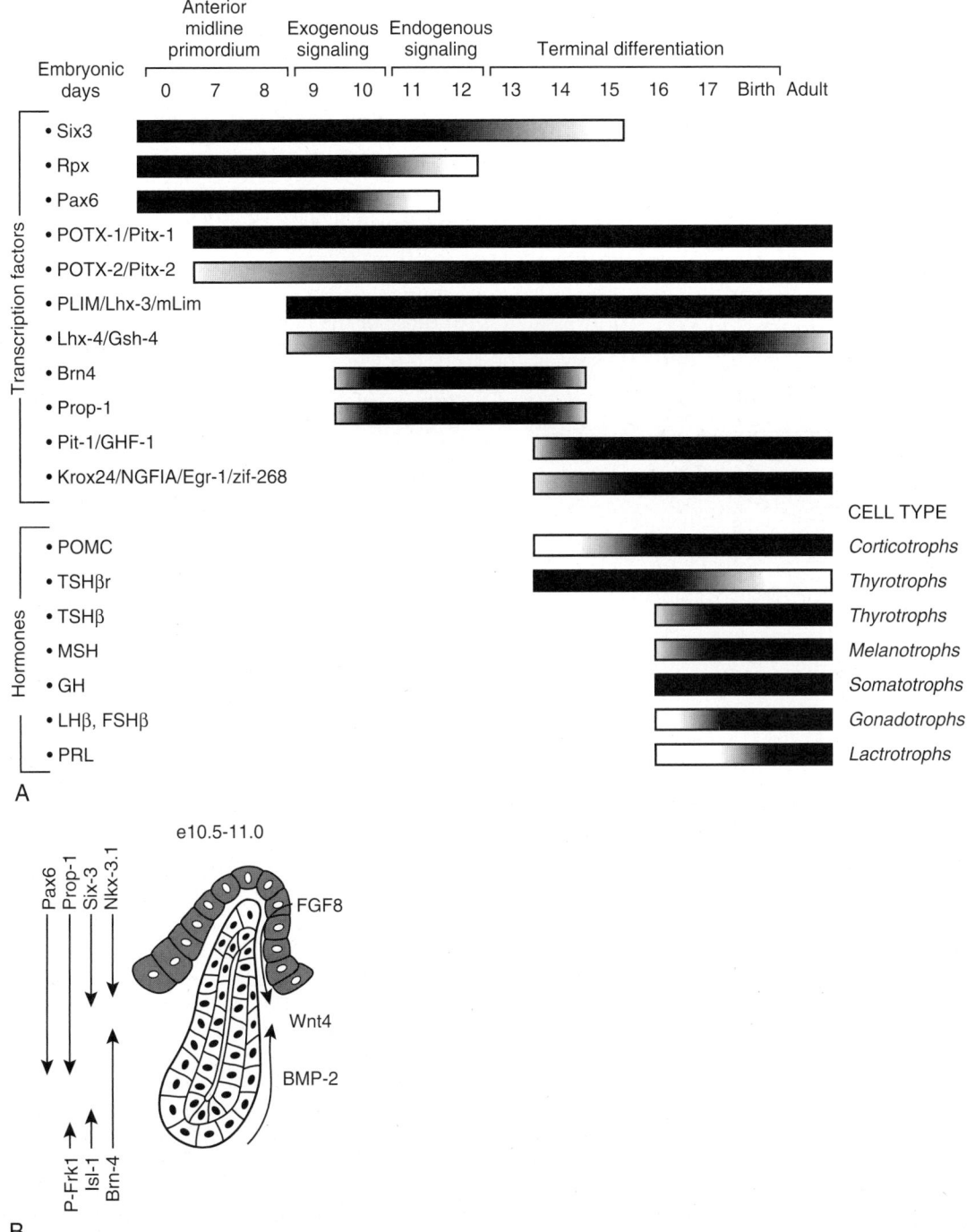

FIGURE 89-2 Modified overview of pituitary development adapted from embryologic studies performed in murine species. The development of the mature pituitary gland is dependent on contact of the oral ectoderm with the ventral diencephalon (neural ectoderm) followed by a cascade of events consisting of both signaling molecules and transcription factors expressed in a specific temporal and spatial manner. At approximately embryologic day 9.5 (e9.5), BMP-4 and Nkx2.1 along with Sonic hedgehog (Shh) participate with the initial evagination of ventral diencephalon and invagination of oral ectoderm to form the primordial Rathke's pouch (RP). In addition, expression of Gli 1,2, Lhx3, and Pitx 1,2 plays an important role in the development of progenitor pituitary cell types. This is closely followed by the expression of Hesx1, Isl1, Pax6, and Six3, 6, which are also implicated in cellular development, proliferation, and migration. Interactions between factors is illustrated by the attenuation of Hesx1 (*hashed arrows*) at approximately e12.5 that is required for the expression of Prop1. By e12.5, RP has formed, and by e17.5, differentiation of specific pituitary cell types has been completed. The expression of Pit1 is also marked with the attenuation of Prop1 expression (*hashed arrows*). The mature pituitary gland is marked by the differentiated cell types: somatotrophs (S), lactotrophs (L), thyrotrophs (T), gonadotrophs (G), and corticotrophs (C). Also shown are the posterior and intermediate lobe of the pituitary and the location of melanotropes (M). (*From Kioussi C, Carriere C, Rosenfeld MG: A model for the development of the hypothalamic-pituitary axis: transcribing the hypophysis,* Mech Dev *81:23-35, 1999.*)

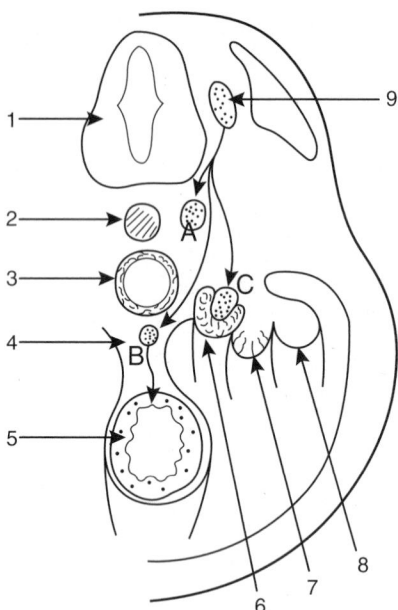

FIGURE 89-3 Transverse cross-section of human adrenal development: neural tube *(1)*, chorda *(2)*, aorta *(3)*, base of the mesentery *(4)*, digestive tube *(5)*, adrenal cortex *(6)*, undifferentiated gonad *(7)*, mesonephros *(8)*. Migration of neuronal cells *(arrows)* from the neural crest *(9)* forms the sympathetic trunk ganglia *(A)*, sympathetic plexuses *(B)*, and the medulla and paraganglia *(C)*. *(From Avisse C, Marcus C, Patey M, et al: Surgical anatomy and embryology of the adrenal glands,* Surg Clin North Am *80:403-415, 2000.)*

infundibular sac projecting from the floor of the diencephalon (5 to 8 weeks). Magnocellular neurons from the hypothalamus synapse with posterior lobe neurosecretory cells. Two hormones, oxytocin and vasopressin, are secreted directly into the general circulation.

The adrenal (or suprarenal) glands develop as a fusion of two distinct embryologic tissues, the cortex and the medulla (Figure 89-3). The adrenal cortex arises bilaterally from coelomic mesothelium between the base of the mesentery (mesogastrium) medially and the mesonephros and undifferentiated gonad (urogenital ridge) laterally. The close proximity of these embryonic structures explains why ectopic cortical tissue may be located inferior to kidneys and sometimes associated with ovaries or testes. In week 6, coelomic cells become embedded in the underlying mesoderm, where they meet and envelop neural crest cells migrating from the sympathetic chain.

This migration of neuroblasts (neuroectoderm) forms the ganglia of the sympathetic trunk and sympathetic plexuses as well as the catecholamine-secreting paraganglia. In the human embryo, the sympathetic trunk arises by about week 7. After weeks 10 to 12, chromaffin tissue (stains brown with chromium salts) develops along the aorta and subsequently differentiates into paraganglia and the adrenal medulla. Most of the paraganglia reach maximal size by about 28 weeks. However, ventral to the aortic bifurcation, the organ of Zuckerkandl continues to enlarge until term (Lagerkrantz, 2003). Usually, paraganglionic chromaffin tissues involute with age, but they may develop into extraadrenal pheochromocytomas.

The adrenal medulla functions as a classic endocrine (ductless) gland, that is, it secretes hormones directly into

the bloodstream. It also participates in sympathetic control via preganglionic sympathetic nerve fibers. Pheochromocytoblasts give rise to the medullary pheochromocytes, which are epinephrine- and norepinephrine-secreting homologues of sympathetic postganglionic cells. Histologically, medullary cells are chromaffin and argyrophilic (stain with silver salts). By 3 months in utero, adrenal pheochromocytes secrete epinephrine and norepinephrine into the medullary sinusoids and then into the systemic circulation. In humans, the hypothalamic-pituitary-*medullary* adrenal axis becomes sufficiently functional by mid-gestation so that fetal stress responses can be independent of those of the mother (Gitau et al, 2001). This fetal catecholamine stress response contrasts with the fetal cortisol output capacity. The fetal adrenal *cortex* minimally secretes cortisol before mid-gestation, and fetal cortisol surges are determined by placental transfer from the mother.

From the 3rd month, the superficial shell of adrenal cortical cells forms the precursor of the postnatal zona glomerulosa and zona fasciculata, that is, the definitive or adult cortex. The more superficial zona glomerulosa has a pseudoglomerular histology and secretes the mineralocorticoid aldosterone. The zona fasciculata contains large cells packed in columns alternating with sinusoids and arterioles and secretes cortisol. The third definitive cortical layer, a network of cell cords called the zona reticularis, is absent at birth and develops from 3 years onward. It is an extragonadal source of sex steroids.

Deep to the presumptive definitive layer, cells proliferate inward, forming a "fetal cortex" that is unique to primate gestation. The outer (transitional) zone of the fetal cortex contains smaller (10- to 20-μm) basophilic cells. This transitional zone, between the inner (fetal) and outer (definitive) zones, expresses CYP17 and 3βHSD relatively late in gestation, contributing to increased fetal adrenal cortisol production which also increases only relatively late in normal gestation. Most of the inner fetal zone consists of large (20- to 50-μm) eosinophilic cells that are the primary site for steroidogenesis, including abundant secretion of Δ5 steroid substrates for placental estrogen production (see Steroidogenesis and the Maternal-Placental-Fetal Unit, earlier). The fetal zone accounts for about 80% of fetal adrenal mass, or about 8 g at birth. During the 1st year, the fetal cortex regresses and adrenal mass diminishes to 2 to 3 g.

Evaluation of the HPA axis in infants is used to test for primary adrenal suppression as well as for secondary adrenal insufficiency, either in preterm neonates who are thought to be cortisol deficient (Watterberg et al, 2005) or following dexamethasone treatment. Short CRH tests may more reliably assess HPA insufficiency than ACTH(1-24) testing for various neonatal indications (Bolt et al, 2002; Karlsson et al, 2000; van Tijn et al, 2008). It remains controversial whether the low circulating cortisol levels in ELBW infants reflect clinically relevant glucocorticoid deficiency.

HYPOTHALAMIC-PITUITARY-THYROID AXIS

Throughout gestation, maternal transfer of thyroid hormone (T$_4$), detectable in embryonic fluids by 4 weeks, protects fetal brain development (Obregon et al, 2007). Maturation of the fetal thyroid axis occurs in three phases: hypothalamic, pituitary, and thyroidal (Raymond and LaFranchi, 2010). At 10 to 20 weeks' gestation, secretory granules can be identified in differentiating pituitary thyrotropes, and TSH is detectable by bio- and immunoassay.

The thyroid is the first endocrine gland to develop in the embryo. It forms at about 24 days from a pharyngeal outpouching, the thyroid diverticulum, and, as the anterior embryo grows, it migrates ventrally to the developing hyoid bone and laryngeal cartilages. By 7 weeks, the thyroid gland assumes its definitive lobar shape and final location in the neck. By 10 to 11 weeks, clusters of endodermal epithelial cells form single layers around lumens, the thyroid follicles, in which colloid begins to appear. Umbilical blood sampling has demonstrated that fetal TSH and T_4 are already detectable by 12 weeks and increase gradually through pregnancy to about 7 mU/L TSH and 19.9 pmol/L T_4 by term (Thorpe-Beeston et al, 1991). The fetal pituitary-thyroid feedback mechanism appears to be fully responsive by 18 to 20 weeks. By that time, in pregnant women with Graves' disease, transplacental passage of maternal thyroid-stimulating autoantibodies can induce fetal hyperthyroidism (Rakover et al, 1999). Biochemical hypothyroidism often occurs in extremely preterm newborns. It remains uncertain whether this phenomenon is largely a biomarker for immaturity or has clinical consequences. Currently, trials of thyroid supplementation in prematurity are in progress or being planned (La Gamma et al, 2009).

Because pituitary and thyroid differentiation is contemporaneous, it has been suggested that the controlling events are independent. During the second half of gestation, fetal thyroid gland function is believed to mature under the influence of increased hypothalamic TRH secretion, pituitary TSH secretion, thyroid cell sensitivity to TSH, and pituitary sensitivity to negative feedback by T_4 (Chapter 93). However, as described earlier (Endocrine and Neuroendocrine Development in the Fetus and Perinatal Transition), small amounts of maternal thyroid hormones cross the placenta, and adequate functioning of both maternal and fetal thyroid glands is important for normal fetal development. In congenital hypothyroidism due to defects in glandular ontogenesis (athyreosis), maternal thyroid hormones lessen the impact on fetal neurologic development. Early neonatal diagnosis and T_4 treatment permit normalized growth and development. In contrast, when the mother is hypothyroid throughout gestation, the consequences for the conceptus are more severe (Glinoer and Delange, 2000).

ENDOCRINE PANCREAS

During the first 4 weeks of gestation, the ventral and dorsal pancreatic anlage arises from evaginations of the embryonic foregut. After rotation of the stomach and duodenum, the ventral pancreatic bud migrates and fuses with the dorsal bud. Branching morphogenesis of the ductal pluripotential epithelial cells gives rise to endocrine and acinar cells under the influence of locally acting signals and activation of lineage-specific transcription factors (Peters, 2000; Puri and Hebrok, 2010). Figure 89-4 indicates early pancreatic cell specification in mouse studies. Beginning by week 7 of human gestation, scattered endocrine cells produce somatostatin, pancreatic polypeptide

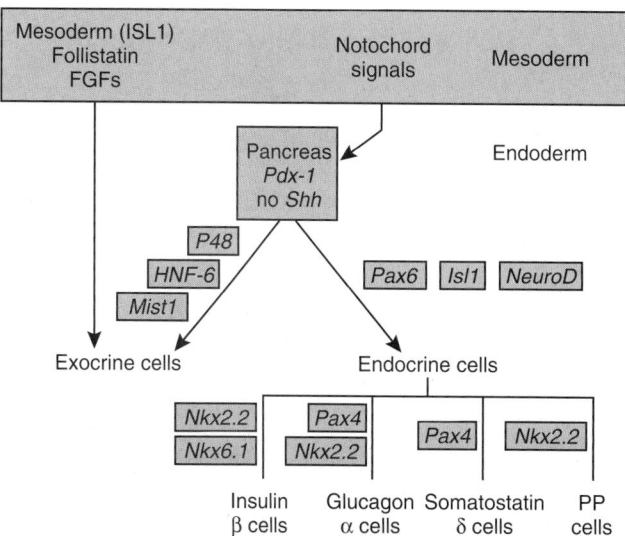

FIGURE 89-4 Molecular control of cell fate choices in the pancreas. *Pax6 and Isl1* are expressed early, and their disruption leads to the reduction or absence of endocrine differentiation which suggests that they could be expressed in endocrine progenitors able to give rise to all cell types. In *Isl1* mutant mice, *Pax6* is not expressed, which suggests *Pax6* is downstream of *Isl1*. Although *Pax4, NeuroD, Ndx2.2,* and *Ndx6.1* are expressed as early as *Pax6* and *Isl1,* they affect the differentiation of only a subset of lineages. *Pax4* is required for glucagon- and somatostatin-producing cell differentiation. *Ndx2.2* is expressed in all islet cells, except somatostatin-producing cells, and its inactivation leads to the absence of the cell types where it is expressed. *Ndx6.1* is itself required for insulin cell differentiation. Although *Mist1* and *HNF-6* are expressed in endocrine cell lineages, their function has not yet been assessed by inactivation experiments. *FGFs,* Fibroblast growth factors; *PP,* pancreatic peptide. *(From Grapin-Botton A, Melton DA: Endoderm development: from patterning to organogenesis,* Trends Genet *16:124-130, 2000.)*

(PP) and glucagon and, by week 9, insulin. Pax and Ndx family transcription factors control the further fate determination of α, β, γ, and PP endocrine cells. Ongoing β-cell proliferation and differentiation are dependent on IGF-II gene expression in islets.

In the human, islet formation begins by week 12. Polyclonal clusters of endocrine cells aggregate in response to developmental expression of cell adhesion molecules. In 24-week fetuses, islets generally remain in direct contact with the ducts, whereas by term, the islets have separated from the ducts. In adults, the islets are dispersed throughout the lobule (Watanabe et al, 1999). Islet volume also increases from about 4% to 13% of total pancreatic tissue by term (Peters, 2000). Endodermal differentiation into pancreatic endocrine cells, like other epithelial differentiation, depends on inductive signals derived from surrounding mesenchyme. Targeted gene deletion studies in mice have demonstrated critical roles for several transcription factors in pancreatic endocrine development.

Neonatal insulin kinetics and end-organ sensitivity to insulin appear to be established during the third trimester in preparation for extrauterine fuel metabolism. The maternal environment and fetal genome appear to influence the number and/or function of pancreatic β-cells in early life, with lifelong implications for postnatal diabetes. In contrast, insulin gene–knockout mice and human newborns with pancreatic agenesis suffer severe intrauterine growth restriction (IUGR), consistent with insulin's role in mitogenesis and growth.

PARATHYROID-RENAL AXIS

The parathyroid-renal (PTH–vitamin D) axis is the principal regulatory pathway in mammalian mineral and bone homeostasis (Chapter 90). The parathyroid glands arise from the dorsal parts of pharyngeal or branchial ("gill") pouches 3 and 4. These paired endodermal cell masses migrate ventrally and come to rest and differentiate in the back of the thyroid lobes as the superior (fourth pouch) and inferior (third pouch) parathyroid glands. The presence of immunoreactive PTH-containing cells can be detected in the human fetal parathyroids at 10 weeks. Defects in neural crest cell migration, such as DiGeorge syndrome (Chapter 90), result in embryonic field defects including parathyroid aplasia or hypoplasia. The caudal pharyngeal complex (pouches 4 and 5) develops into the calcitonin-secreting C cells embedded in the thyroid gland. Calcitonin is detectable in fetal thyroidal C cells as early as 14 weeks. The fetal renal tubules can synthesize the active hormonal form of vitamin D, $1,25(OH)_2$-vitamin D, at least as early as the second half of gestation. Fetal plasma $1,25(OH)_2$-vitamin D levels remain low, however, as a result of high placental clearance.

GONADAL AXES

Human reproductive system development is regulated by complex genetic, endocrine, and environmental signals. The gonadal primordium is the only tissue in mammals that has two divergent developmental fates, leading ultimately to the formation of either a testis or an ovary (Cederroth et al, 2007). Sex-specific organogenesis begins in the early embryo, and sexual dimorphism results in the development of either ovaries or testes by birth. Further sexual maturation occurs in the perinatal period and at puberty (Chapter 92).

In mammals, genetic sex is determined by inheritance of either an X or Y chromosome from the male gamete. The initial stages of gonadal and genital development in male and female embryos are morphologically indistinguishable. The gonads arise from thickening of the ventrolateral surface of the embryonic mesonephros (the genital ridge). Several genes are required for testicular induction of the bipotential gonads, including the orphan nuclear receptor Steroidogenic Factor-1 (SF-1), the Wilms' tumor-associated gene (WT1), and the homeobox genes Lhx1 (Lim1) and Lhx9. The two pituitary gonadotropins, LH and FSH, play a key role in cell fate determination and maturation of the sexual organs. Mutations in gonadotropin-subunit or gonadotropin-receptor genes have been associated with various types of hypogonadism in males and females.

In females, the müllerian ducts give rise to the uterus, fallopian tubes, and proximal vagina. The fetal ovarian germ cells are maintained in early meiotic arrest. The fetal ovary has late expression of the LH receptor (compared to the testis), late onset of aromatase activity, and low estradiol (E_2) content. Postnatally, ovarian follicles are prominent, and serum E_2 levels in female neonates remain low.

In males, wolffian ducts develop into the epididymis, vas deferens, seminal vesicles, and prostate. Divergence from the female developmental pathway toward male sexual differentiation requires secretion of several testicular hormones. After gonad formation, expression of the SRY (sex-determining region of the Y chromosome) gene initiates the male developmental cascade. SRY contains a high-mobility group (HMG) box, a conserved transcription factor motif that, in this instance, targets testicular Sertoli cell differentiation. Mutations in the HMG box are associated with 46,XY pure gonadal dysgenesis and sex reversal. Early events in testis development are differentiation of Sertoli cells and androgen-producing Leydig cells, LH receptor and steroid enzyme expression, autonomous steroid secretion, and high testosterone content. In contrast, germ-cell maturation occurs later in gestation. Postnatally, testicular Leydig and Sertoli cells are prominent and serum testosterone levels are high.

Müllerian inhibiting substance (MIS) produced by Sertoli cells induces müllerian duct regression. LH and placental human chorionic gonadotropin induce Leydig cell androgen synthesis. In turn, testosterone and dihydrotestosterone promote development of the wolffian duct derivatives (male internal reproductive tract) and the virilization of external genitalia. Therefore, inadequate fetal and neonatal testosterone secretion (e.g., due to hypogonadotropic hypogonadism or panhypopituitarism) impairs normal phallus and scrotum development. Leydig cell insulin-like hormone 3 (INSL3) with androgen mediate transabdominal testicular descent into the scrotum (Nation et al, 2009). Female embryonic differentiation continues when the absence of MIS permits persistence of müllerian structures, a lack of androgens permits wolffian duct degeneration, and the absence of INSL3 maintains gonads in the abdomen.

FETAL AND NEONATAL CIRCADIAN RHYTHMS

Neuroendocrine rhythmicity is an essential aspect of normal physiology and behavior. Certain rhythms occur in response to light:dark cycles. Ultradian rhythms have a periodicity shorter than 1 day but longer than 1 hour. Others, termed circadian rhythms, occur with a periodicity roughly matching the earth's rotation (24 hours) and persist even in the absence of environmental stimuli. As yet, there are few data on the maturational onset of ultradian or circadian hormonal secretion in the face of perturbing factors such as prematurity or intrauterine and neonatal hormone treatment.

The master clock or pacemaker that controls circadian rhythms is located in oscillating neurons of the hypothalamic suprachiasmatic nuclei (SCN). The molecular mechanisms of SCN rhythmogenicity involve pulsed expression of specific transcription factors that induce the oscillatory secretion of neuropeptides including somatostatin, vasoactive intestinal peptide (VIP), vasopressin (AVP), and neurotensin. Efferent pathways project from the SCN to other nuclei, such as the paraventricular nucleus (PVN). SCN efferents to the PVN stimulate secretion of CRH, which results in circadian adrenal cortisol secretion (see Hypothalamic-Pituitary-Adrenal Axis, earlier), and pineal gland expression of melatonin.

Regulation and entrainment of the circadian clock(s) occur by transcriptional negative feedback loops and posttranscriptional controls. In the human fetus, heart rate, fetal movements, and some other outputs may be entrained to maternal rhythms. However, by late pregnancy the fetus establishes a circadian rhythm of cortisol secretion, presumably controlled by the fetal hypothalamic pacemaker. The adult pattern of circadian cortisol secretion is established by 2 to 4 months after birth (Rivkees, 2003). Importantly, adult-type salivary cortisol circadian rhythm is rarely evident in hospitalized preterm infants born before 30 weeks' gestation (Kidd et al, 2005). The onset of salivary cortisol circadian rhythm appears at the same postnatal age in mono- and dizygotic twin infants, suggesting less genetic than environmental impact on this phenomenon; additionally, each twin pair in this study showed synchrony, implying the importance of shared prenatal and postnatal environmental synchronizers (Custodio et al, 2007). The onset of circadian melatonin secretion is related to postconceptional, not postnatal, age. Understandably, exploration of environmental influences on biologic rhythms of preterm infants is an emerging area of emphasis in neonatal care.

DEVELOPMENTAL ORIGINS OF HEALTH AND DISEASE HYPOTHESIS

Research from a wide range of disciplines has shown that endocrine function in adult life is influenced, sometimes profoundly, by environmental influences acting at different stages of development spanning conception into infancy. Initially called the "fetal origins of adult disease" hypothesis, this emerging theme in development is more appropriately referred to as the developmental origins of health and disease (Godfrey, 2010; Wadhwa et al, 2009). Programming is a process by which environmental stimuli during critical periods of growth and development have lasting effects on the structure or function of tissues and physiologic systems. For example, intrauterine stresses can affect HPA axis development and program distinct autonomic, neuroendocrine, and behavioral responses into adulthood.

The developmental origins hypothesis proposes that the fetus adapts to a limited supply of nutrients, yielding a fetal/neonatal "thrifty phenotype" adapted for survival, but in a manner that permanently alters its physiology and metabolism and increases risk of disease in later life (Hales and Barker, 1992). The Dutch famine of 1944–1945 provided a unique opportunity to examine the long-term effects of intrauterine malnutrition in humans. The famine was imposed for a defined period on a previously well-nourished population. Extensive and reliable records have permitted unprecedented analysis of a birth cohort exposed to this discrete intrauterine insult (Heijmans et al, 2008). Additionally, David Barker and colleagues in Southampton, UK, have exploited detailed obstetric records in British hospitals to establish that IUGR is a strong predictor of adult metabolic and cardiovascular disease (e.g., Barker, 1998). For example, the relative risk for insulin resistance, obesity, and the metabolic syndrome (including type 2 diabetes, hypertension, and hyperlipidemia) is significantly higher in individuals who were thin at birth with a low ponderal index. Clinical studies also uphold the association of maternal psychosocial state or stress in pregnancy with qualitative and quantitative changes in birth outcome

and fetal and neonatal neuroendocrine activity (Wadhwa et al, 2005).

Increased fetal access to glucocorticoids during critical developmental periods may be a common mechanism explaining how diverse maternal and uteroplacental stresses, including maternal undernutrition, psychosocial stress, and uteroplacental hypoxemia, induce fetal programming. Increased fetal glucocorticoids and stress both program specific effects in the brain, notably the HPA axis and dopaminergic-motor systems (Challis and Connor, 2009; Welberg et al, 2005) and can induce IUGR. The principal stress-mediated catecholamines (norepinephrine, epinephrine) transcriptionally repress placental trophoblast 11β-HSD2 expression via α-adrenergic pathways (Sarkar et al, 2001), thereby increasing transplacental transfer of maternal cortisol to the developing fetus.

IUGR and metabolic programming in girls interact with the genotype to influence the onset of endocrine, metabolic, and cardiovascular disease in later life (Ibáñez et al, 2001, 2007). Intrauterine stress producing low birthweight is associated with altered basal and stimulated cortisol levels as an early marker of HPA responsiveness, followed by glucose intolerance (insulin resistance) and hypertension (Levitt et al, 2000). Similarly, some nutritional practices in the neonatal intensive care unit may promote excessive adiposity in ELBW infants as they recover over time (Rubin, 2009).

IUGR also results in a reduced β-cell population at birth (van Assche et al, 1977). Fetal β-cell growth and development may be more sensitive to ambient amino acid than to glucose concentrations, suggesting a role for intrauterine protein availability in normal insulin homeostasis. In IUGR due to fetal malnutrition, altered expression of IGF-II (an islet cell survival factor) or IGF binding proteins may severely alter β-cell ontogeny and result in a β-cell population poorly suited for responding to subsequent metabolic stress (Hill and Duvillie, 2000).

ENVIRONMENTAL ENDOCRINE HYPOTHESIS

Recent environmental changes may have potentially important effects on the development of the endocrine system. Specifically, industrial and agricultural chemicals, through their actions on endocrine function, may be responsible for a number of reproductive and developmental abnormalities in a wide range of species, including humans (Cooper and Kavlock, 1997; Krimsky, 2000). These exogenous agents, or "endocrine disruptors," can interfere with the synthesis, storage/release, transport, metabolism, binding, action, or elimination of natural hormones. This importance of environmental endocrine-disrupting chemicals for public health and ecology, first stressed by Theo Colborn in the late 1980s, prompted passage in the United States of the Food Quality Protection Act and the Safe Drinking Water Estrogenic Substances Screening Act of 1996.

Three independent lines of research have provided the initial evidence for the importance of environmental agents on human endocrine development: recognition of the adverse effects of the potent synthetic estrogens and endocrine disrupters, that is, diethylstilbestrol (DES), bisphenol A, and related compounds, on female and male reproductive tract development; field and laboratory studies associating wildlife reproductive malformations to chemical pollutants; and research linking xenoestrogens to declines in human sperm counts (Krimsky, 2000). Some structural abnormalities of the reproductive tract, including hypospadias and cryptorchidism, which have potential hormone-mediated origin and a critical developmental component, may show upward secular trending.

During development, reproductive tract tissues are especially sensitive to low concentrations of sex steroids. Androgens secreted by a maternal adrenal tumor can virilize a female fetus (Kirk et al, 1992). Increased placental estradiol production has been associated with cryptorchidism in male newborns (Hadziselimovic et al, 2000). A mechanism is estrogenic downregulation of Insl3 expression by embryonic Leydig cells. Similarly, endocrine disruptors with antiandrogenic or estrogenic activity can have feminizing effects in the developing male fetus. Estrogens may induce adverse reproductive changes in female fetuses, but antiandrogens have little effect (Toppari and Skakkebaek, 1998). Changes induced by intrauterine exposure to endocrine disruptors may be irreversible, in contrast with the reversible changes induced by transient hormone exposure in the adult.

Endocrine disruptors such as organochlorines—for example, the pesticide DDT—can alter normal gonadal ontogeny. Prenatal exposure to the estrogenic agent DES increases risk of reproductive teratogenicity in female and male offspring. Exposure of the conceptus to antiandrogenic pharmaceuticals such as the androgen receptor antagonist flutamide and the 5α-reductase inhibitor finasteride generally affects males, causing hypospadias, cryptorchidism, reduced testicular mass, or decreased sperm production. Exposure to polychlorinated biphenyl (PCB) congeners, either in utero or via breastfeeding, has structural, functional, and behavioral effects, particularly on thyroidal axis development and differentiation of the male reproductive tract (Brouwer et al, 1998). It is evident that the endocrine system presents a number of target sites for adverse effects of environmental agents. Much more information is needed about these specific ecologic and public health risks.

SUGGESTED READINGS

Barker DJP, editor: *Mothers, babies and health in later life*, ed 2, Edinburgh, 1998, Churchill Livingstone.

Cederroth CR, Pitetti JL, Papaioannou MD, Nef S: Genetic programs that regulate testicular and ovarian development, *Mol Cell Endocrinol* 265-266:3-9, 2007.

Challis JRG, Connor K: Glucocorticoids, 11β-Hydroxysteroid dehydrogenase: mother, fetus, or both? *Endocrinology* 150:1073-1074, 2009.

Challis JRG, Matthews SG, Gibb W, Lye SJ: Endocrine and paracrine regulation of birth at term and preterm, *Endocr Rev* 21:514-550, 2000.

de Escobar GM, Obregón MJ, del Rey FE: Iodine deficiency and brain development in the first half of pregnancy, *Public Health Nutr* 10:1554-1570, 2007.

Fisher DA: The unique endocrine milieu of the fetus, *J Clin Invest* 78:603-611, 1986.

Fowden AL, Forhead AJ: Endocrine regulation of feto-placental growth, *Horm Res* 72:257-265, 2009.

Godfrey KM, Gluckman PD, Hanson MA: Developmental origins of metabolic disease: life course and intergenerational perspectives, *Trends Endocrinol Metab* 21:199-205, 2010.

Krimsky S: *Hormonal chaos: the scientific and social origins of the environmental endocrine hypothesis*, Baltimore, 2000, Johns Hopkins University Press.

Rivkees SA: Developing circadian rhythmicity in infants, *Pediatrics* 112:373-381, 2003.

Romero CJ, Nesi-França S, Radovick S: The molecular basis of hypopituitarism, *Trends Endocrinol Metab* 20:506-516, 2009.

Tilghman SM: The sins of the fathers and mothers: genomic imprinting in mammalian development, *Cell* 96:185-193, 1999.

Wadhwa PD, Buss C, Entringer S, Swanson JM: Developmental origins of health and disease: brief history of the approach and current focus on epigenetic mechanisms, *Semin Reprod Med* 27:358-368, 2009.

Complete references used in this text can be found online at www.expertconsult.com

DISORDERS OF CALCIUM AND PHOSPHORUS METABOLISM

Lewis P. Rubin

HOMEOSTATIC CONTROL OF CALCIUM AND MAGNESIUM

Calcium plays two important physiologic roles. Calcium salts in bone provide structural integrity. Calcium ions present in the cytosol and extracellular fluid (ECF) are essential for maintenance and control of many biologic processes, including cell-cell communication, cell aggregation and division, coagulation, neuromuscular excitability, membrane integrity and permeability, enzyme activity, and secretion. This functional diversity is made possible by the maintenance of a large electrochemical gradient between the ECF Ca^{2+} concentration, which is in the 1 mmol/L range, and resting intracellular (cytosolic) Ca^{2+} concentration, which is about 0.1 μmol/L.

Significant alterations in serum calcium concentration occur frequently in the neonatal period. It is important to evaluate these potential derangements in light of normal dynamic changes that take place during the perinatal transition. After the first 2 to 3 extrauterine days, normal serum calcium concentrations vary only slightly with age, range between 8.8 and 10.6 mg/dL, and average about 10 mg/dL. In the United States, serum or plasma calcium levels usually are reported as mg/dL, which may be converted to molar units by dividing by 4 (e.g., 10 mg/dL is equivalent to 2.5 mmol/L).

Approximately 55% to 60% of the total plasma calcium is diffusible (or ultrafilterable), the remainder being protein bound. Most diffusible calcium is ionized, but about 5% of total circulating calcium is complexed to plasma anions, such as phosphates, citrate, and bicarbonate. Ionized calcium (Ca^{2+}) is the only biologically available fraction of ECF calcium. It is subject to precise metabolic control based on the integrated regulation of calcium fluxes with respect to the intestine, kidneys, and bone. The precise regulation of circulating Ca^{2+} is controlled by calcium itself, through a calcium receptor and several hormones, the most important of which are parathyroid hormone and 1,25(OH)$_2$-vitamin D (Allgrove and Shaw, 2009; Carmeliet et al, 2003; Ramasamy, 2008).

Hypoalbuminemia leads to a decline in total serum calcium, but proportionate increases in the ionized fraction usually maintain serum Ca^{2+} within the normal range. Acute alkalosis (e.g., hyperventilation or bicarbonate infusion) or rapid administration of citrate-buffered blood (e.g., during exchange transfusion, initiation of extracorporeal membrane oxygenation [ECMO], cardioplegia, or organ transplantation) may acutely lower serum Ca^{2+} by increasing albumin binding or citrate chelation. These conditions can produce transient clinical manifestations of hypocalcemia but do not lower the total serum calcium concentration. Electrocardiogram Q-Tc intervals and

algorithms for correcting serum total calcium for alterations in serum albumin concentration and/or pH or for calculating "free" calcium concentration have not proved to be reliable compared with actual measurement of Ca^{2+} using ion-selective electrodes (Clase et al, 2000). Generally, for routine clinical purposes, measuring total serum calcium often suffices.

Bulk calcium exchange takes place in kidney, bone, and intestine. Although the intestine has considerable calcium absorptive capacity, renal tubular calcium reabsorption usually exceeds intestinal absorption by at least 40-fold. Most of the tubular Ca^{2+} load is reabsorbed in the proximal tubule and thick ascending limb of the loop of Henle via paracellular, passive flux (coupled with sodium reabsorption) driven by the existing electrochemical gradient. A transcellular pathway in the distal nephron tightly regulates the rest of urinary Ca^{2+} reabsorption. Calcitropic hormones regulate the distal Ca^{2+}-selective, Na^+-independent channels. More than 98% of total body calcium is deposited in the skeleton as hydroxyapatite [$Ca_5(OH)(PO_4)_3$]; the ECF and soft tissues contain the remainder. A small fraction of skeletal calcium freely exchanges with the ECF and serves as an important buffer of circulating calcium. Consequently, decreased skeletal calcium is a hallmark of most metabolic bone diseases.

Magnesium homeostasis also is largely renally mediated. Approximately 80% of total plasma magnesium is filtered through the glomerulus and is reabsorbed mainly in cortical segments of the thick ascending limb of the loop of Henle. Once the maximal tubular reabsorption is exceeded, filtered magnesium is excreted into the urine. Hormones regulate magnesium reabsorption by changing the transepithelial voltage and paracellular permeability of tubular cells.

HOMEOSTATIC CONTROL OF PHOSPHORUS

Blood inorganic phosphate (P_i) concentration varies with age. It is highest during infancy and gradually declines to adulthood. Approximately 10% of plasma P_i is noncovalently bound to protein, whereas 90% circulates as ions or as complexes with sodium, calcium, or magnesium. About 80% to 85% of total body phosphorus contributes to mechanical support as part of the hydroxyapatite lattice of bone. The remainder is distributed in the ECF, largely as inorganic ions or complexes, and in soft tissues as phosphate esters. Intracellular phosphate esters and phosphorylated intermediates regulate cell metabolism and gene expression (via phosphorylase, kinase, and phosphatase activities) and generate and transfer cellular energy

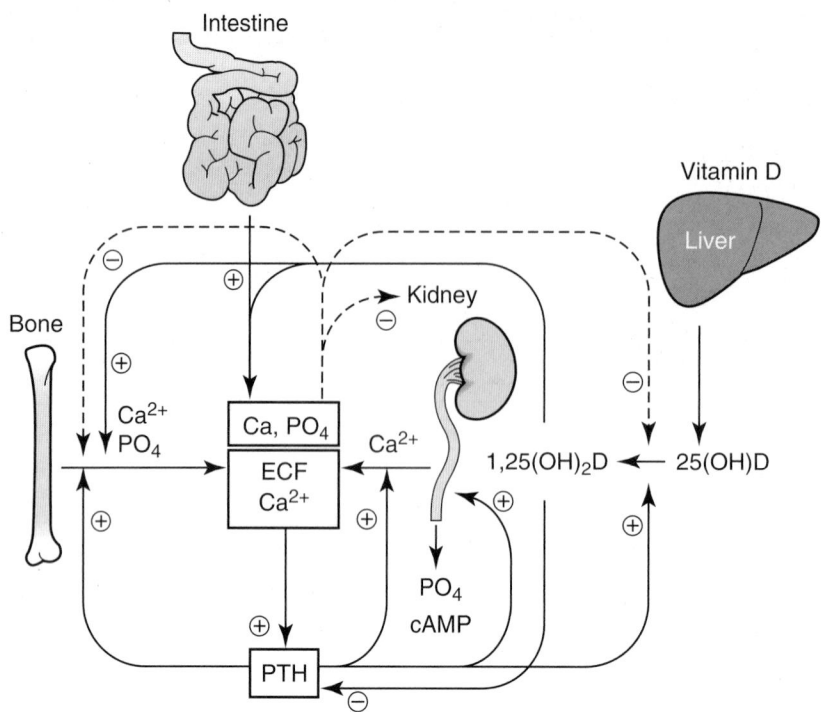

FIGURE 90-1 Hormonal regulation of calcium and phosphate by PTH and 1,25(OH)₂D. Decreased Ca^{2+} stimulates PTH and 1,25(OH)₂D secretion. Renal, gastrointestinal, and skeletal mechanisms increase Ca^{2+}, inhibiting PTH secretion and closing the negative feedback loop. Ca^{2+}, Ionized calcium; *cAMP*, cyclic adenosine monophosphate; *ECF*, extracellular fluid; *25(OH)D*, 25-hydroxyvitamin D; *1,25(OH)₂D*, 1,25-dihydroxyvitamin D; *PO₄*, inorganic phosphate; *PTH*, parathyroid hormone. *(From Brown EM, MacLeod RJ: Extracellular calcium sensing and extracellular calcium signaling, Physiol Rev 81:239-297, 2001.)*

(i.e., via adenosine triphosphate [ATP]). Cytosolic and ECF phosphorus levels (approximately 0.1 mmol/L and 0.2 mmol/L, respectively) are less stringently regulated than are levels of Ca^{2+} and Mg^{2+}.

Dietary phosphate generally is absorbed in proportion to its content in food. Although phosphorus and calcium can be absorbed along the entire length of the small intestine, most phosphate transport takes place in the jejunum and ileum, whereas most calcium absorption occurs in the duodenum. The renal proximal tubule is the principal regulatory site for phosphorus homeostasis (Silver and Naveh-Maney, 2009). Renal regulation is accomplished primarily by varying the threshold for phosphate reabsorption (the tubular maximum for P_i/glomerular filtration rate, or TmP/GFR). Hormones (parathyroid hormone [PTH], parathyroid hormone–related protein [PTHrP], growth hormone) and dietary phosphate reset this theoretical threshold by regulating apical tubular Na^+-P_i cotransporters (Murer and Biber, 1995). Essentially, the TmP/GFR is the "set point" that defines the fasting serum phosphorus concentration. At lower serum phosphorus levels, most filtered phosphorus is reabsorbed; at higher levels, most filtered phosphorus is excreted. To assess the TmP/GFR, a fasting urine specimen is obtained for measurement of phosphorus and creatinine along with simultaneous determination of serum phosphorus and creatinine. A nomogram has been constructed so that TmP/GFR can easily be derived from these values (Walton and Bijvoet, 1975).

The higher serum phosphate levels in infants (e.g., 4.5 to 9.3 mg/dL) compared with those in adults (3.0 to 4.5 mg/dL) reflect infants' greater tubular phosphate resorption. This adaptation permits avid tubular phosphate

conservation despite high ambient serum phosphate levels. For this reason, neonatal disorders of chronic hypophosphatemia and/or phosphorus depletion usually result from inadequate dietary supply (as in preterm infants) or intrinsic (e.g., familial hypophosphatemic rickets) or extrinsic (e.g., hyperparathyroidism) alterations in TmP/GFR. Similarly, chronic hyperphosphatemia usually implies either intrinsic (e.g., renal insufficiency) or extrinsic (e.g., hypoparathyroidism) abnormalities in TmP/GFR.

PARATHYROID-RENAL HORMONAL AXIS

In mammals, calcium and phosphate homeostasis is controlled by a parathyroid-renal hormonal axis involving PTH and 1,25-dihydroxyvitamin D [1,25(OH)₂D]. The influence of these two hormones on bone deposition, mobilization of mineral, and regulation of intestinal and renal absorption is depicted in Figure 90-1. Deficiency or excess of either hormone causes hypocalcemia or hypercalcemia, respectively.

PARATHYROID HORMONES

PTH is a 9500-Da, single-chain polypeptide. PTH is synthesized by the four parathyroid glands, which are derived from the embryonic third and fourth pharyngeal pouches. The messenger RNA (mRNA) for PTH (preproPTH) encodes the 84 amino acids of the mature peptide, an amino-terminal (N-terminal) "pre" sequence of 25 amino acids, and a basic "pro" hexapeptide, which is clipped intracellularly. After secretion, the intact PTH molecule

[PTH(1-84)] is further metabolized and rapidly cleared from the circulation, with a half-life of less than 4 minutes. The N-terminal region of the PTH molecule [PTH(1-34)] binds the PTH receptor and shows full biologic activity, whereas the C terminus has specific, albeit poorly understood, activities in osteoclasts and osteoclastic precursors.

Secretion of PTH fragments by the parathyroid glands and prolonged clearance of carboxyl-terminal (C-terminal) PTH metabolites add considerable immunoheterogeneity to circulating PTH. The numerous inconsistencies found in reports on PTH pathophysiology until the late 1980s are due to use of earlier-generation "C-terminal" and "mid-molecule" PTH assays. In contrast, current two-site "intact PTH" assays are sufficiently sensitive and specific to detect physiologic levels of biologically active PTH(1-84) and to distinguish hypoparathyroid from euparathyroid states. The normal circulating levels of intact PTH range from approximately 10 to 60 pg/mL; the maximally stimulated (hypocalcemic) and maximally suppressed (hypercalcemic) levels for normal parathyroid function are about 100 to 150 pg/mL and 2 to 5 pg/mL, respectively.

Parathyroid cells are exquisitely responsive to changes in ambient Ca^{2+}. PTH secretion may be described as an inverse sigmoid hysteretic relationship between serum PTH and Ca^{2+} with a parathyroid cell set point (the Ca^{2+} at which PTH secretion is half-maximal) of 1.2 to 1.25 mmol/L. The parathyroid "calcistat" detects perturbations of blood Ca^{2+} as small as 0.025 to 0.05 mmol/L and promptly adjusts PTH secretion. The molecular mechanism that enables specific cells (e.g., parathyroid cells, thyroidal C cells, renal tubular cells, osteoblasts) to sense these minute changes in ECF Ca^{2+} involves a member of the family C of G protein–coupled receptors (GPCRs), the Ca^{2+}-sensing receptor (CaSR). ECF Ca^{2+} (and, at lower affinity, Mg^{2+}) binds the CaSR, activates several intracellular effector pathways, and ultimately leads to oppositely directed changes in PTH secretion and altered renal cation handling (Gamba and Friedman, 2009). CaSR activation inhibits renal cellular Ca^{2+} absorption induced by PTH, as well as passive paracellular Ca^{2+} transport. As described later, loss-of-function (or inactivating) mutations in the *CaSR* gene are responsible for neonatal hyperparathyroidism and familial hypocalciuric hypercalcemia, whereas gain-of-function *CaSR* mutations result in autosomal dominant neonatal hypocalcemia (Brown, 2007).

PTH mobilizes calcium and phosphorus from bone, stimulates calcium reabsorption, inhibits phosphorus reabsorption by reducing TmP/GFR, and stimulates the renal synthesis of $1,25(OH)_2D$, which participates with PTH in reabsorbing bone mineral and also increases efficiency of intestinal absorption of calcium and phosphorus. Therefore, PTH secretion causes the serum calcium concentration to rise and the serum phosphorus concentration to be maintained or decline.

PTH-related protein (PTHrP) is a second member of the PTH family, first identified as the cause of humoral hypercalcemia of malignancy. The amino acid sequences of PTHrP and PTH are homologous at the N terminus, and 8 of the first 13 amino acids are identical. Beyond this region, the sequences have little in common. PTHrP is a multifunctional molecule, like neuropeptides such as pro-opiomelanocortin (the precursor of corticotropin, endorphins, and melanocyte-simulating hormones). The three PTHrP isoforms (139, 141, and 173 amino acids) give rise to several secreted peptide fragments. PTHrP is widely expressed, especially in fetal tissues, and has important local functions in morphogenesis and differentiation. The normal circulating levels of PTHrP are considerably lower than the levels of PTH, and it is doubtful that PTHrP has a major role in calcium homeostasis. Two important exceptions are in the fetus and lactating woman, for whom PTHrP appears to be an important calcitropic hormone (Mitchell and Jüppner, 2010).

The actions of PTH on its two major target organs, kidney and bone, are mediated through the type 1 PTH/PTHrP receptor (PTHR1) (Kronenberg, 2003), a GPCR belonging to a receptor subfamily that includes receptors for calcitonin, secretin, and corticotropin-releasing hormone. This versatile receptor mediates actions of its two physiologic ligands in multiple tissues and signals through several second messenger pathways. The best-characterized effector of PTH action is cyclic adenosine monophosphate (cAMP).

VITAMIN D

Vitamin D is a secosteroid synthesized in the skin or absorbed from the diet (Holick et al, 2007; Kimball et al, 2008). Exposure to sunlight (290–320 nm) cleaves the B ring of 7-dehydrocholesterol (7-DHC), or provitamin D, the immediate precursor of cholesterol, to form a sterol, previtamin D. Previtamin D in the skin undergoes isomerization to the biologically inert vitamin D. Vitamin D enters the circulation bound to vitamin D–binding protein and is transported to the liver, where a mitochondrial cytochrome P450 vitamin D-25-hydroxylase produces 25-hydroxyvitamin D [25(OH)D]. 25(OH)D (provitamin D) is the major circulating vitamin D metabolite. Because activity of hepatic 25-hydroxylase is not tightly regulated, measurement of serum 25(OH)D is a useful assessment of vitamin D stores. In renal proximal tubule cells, mitochondrial cytochrome P450 25(OH)D–1α-hydroxylase metabolizes 25(OH)D to the biologically active hormone, $1,25(OH)_2D$. The normal circulating level of 25(OH)D is approximately 10 to 50 ng/mL. The normal circulating concentration of $1,25(OH)_2D$ ranges from 30 to 75 pg/mL, or about 1/1000 that of 25(OH)D.

Serum 25(OH)D levels are increased by sunlight exposure and by vitamin D ingestion and are decreased in vitamin D deficiency and in hepatobiliary disorders. Circulating $1,25(OH)_2D$ levels are increased by hyperparathyroidism and phosphate depletion and are reduced in hypoparathyroidism. $1,25(OH)_2D$ is biologically inactivated through a series of reactions beginning with 24-hydroxylation. $1,25(OH)_2D$ induces the 24-hydroxylase in vitamin D target cells. Hypocalcemia, by increasing PTH levels, suppresses this enzyme. 24-Hydroxylase metabolizes 25(OH)D as well as $1,25(OH)_2D$. In vitamin D–sufficient states, the kidney preferentially 24-hydroxylates the prohormone, 25(OH)D, to $24,25(OH)_2D$. In contrast, when vitamin D action is required, 25(OH)D–1α-hydroxylase is preferentially activated for $1,25(OH)_2D$ synthesis.

A chief biologic function of $1,25(OH)_2D$ is to increase intestinal absorption of calcium and phosphorus. During low calcium intake, increased PTH levels stimulate the renal conversion of 25(OH)D to 1,25(OH)$_2$D, which in turn stimulates osteoclast differentiation and bone resorption. Most of the identified biologic actions of 1,25(OH)$_2$D are mediated via binding to the vitamin D receptor (VDR), a member of the intracellular receptor superfamily. VDR interacts with specific response elements (VDREs) in promoters of vitamin D–responsive genes.

The parathyroid-renal [PTH-1,25(OH)$_2$D] axis, reminiscent of the hypothalamic-pituitary-adrenal axis, is the principal means for systemic response to a sustained or major hypocalcemic challenge. In this long-loop feedback system, 1,25(OH)$_2$D-mediated calcium absorption provides the ultimate feedback on PTH secretion. PTH secreted in response to hypocalcemia is the principal regulator of renal production of 1,25(OH)$_2$D that, in turn, feeds back to suppress PTH gene expression (see Figure 90-1). PTH regulates minute-to-minute perturbations of ECF [Ca^{2+}]. Maximal adjustments of intestinal calcium absorption via the PTH-1,25(OH)$_2$D axis require 1 to 2 days to become fully operative, so 1,25(OH)$_2$D effects come into play only when a hypocalcemic stress persists.

CALCITONIN

Calcitonin, a peptide hormone synthesized by thyroid parafollicular C cells, has an antihypercalcemic effect, that is, opposite that of PTH. Human calcitonin is a 32-amino-acid chain with a 1,7-disulfide bridge and a C-terminal prolinamide. Alternative splicing of several transcripts from the calcitonin gene produces several polypeptide products, some of which have uncertain calcitropic importance. The primary stimulus for calcitonin secretion is a rise in circulating calcium concentration. Calcitonin lowers serum calcium and phosphorus chiefly by inhibiting bone resorption.

Currently, there is no compelling evidence that the calcitonin-like calcium-lowering hormones are critical regulators of calcium homeostasis in nonpregnant adult humans, perhaps because the low prevailing rate of bone turnover blunts the impact of the antiresorptive actions. However, calcitonin may have important calcitropic functions in pregnant and lactating women and in the fetus and neonate, and in other mammals, particularly rodents, whose bones are constantly growing. In human newborns, the C cell population and serum calcitonin concentrations are much greater than in adults.

PERINATAL MINERAL METABOLISM

During human pregnancy, approximately 30 g of calcium and more than 16 g of phosphorus are transferred transplacentally from the maternal circulation to the growing fetus, the bulk during the third trimester when fetal calcium accretion is approximately 140 to 150 mg/kg per day. In humans, a doubling of maternal intestinal calcium absorption and a net increase of calcium accretion into bone compensate for the formidable demand on maternal calcium (Prentice, 2000). A mid-molecule PTHrP hormone (Kovacs et al, 1996) expressed principally by placenta regulates this transplacental calcium pump. TRPV6, a member of the transient receptor potential channel

superfamily, may be the primary calcium channel at the trophoblast apical membrane. Calcium flux across the placenta in TRPV6-null mice is reduced by approximately 40% (Suzuki et al, 2008).

PREGNANCY

Pregnancy constitutes a unique hormonal milieu that promotes a state of "physiologic absorptive hypercalciuria" (Gertner et al, 1986). Maternal total serum calcium declines slightly during pregnancy, reaches a nadir in the mid-third trimester, and then increases slightly toward term. The maternal serum phosphorus and magnesium profiles are similar to that of calcium. Maternal serum 25(OH)D varies seasonally and with vitamin D intake, but the vitamin D transport protein (DBP) increases during pregnancy. Serum 1,25(OH)$_2$D concentrations increase early in pregnancy and continue to rise through gestation (Seely et al, 1997). The calculated concentration of free 1,25(OH)$_2$D also rises. For many years, it was believed that PTH levels also increased steadily through pregnancy. However, use of newer immunometric "sandwich" assays indicates that PTH actually declines during the course of pregnancy (Davis et al, 1988; Saggese et al, 1991; Seely et al, 1997). PTHrP levels, in contrast, may be higher in pregnant than in nonpregnant women (Bertelloni et al, 1994). The role of circulating calcitonin in pregnancy is uncertain.

1,25(OH)$_2$D drives enhanced maternal intestinal mineral absorption (reviewed in Kovacs, 2008). After parturition, 1,25(OH)$_2$D concentrations and calcium absorption rates (Kent et al, 1991) fall to prepregnancy levels. The interplay of calcitropic and progestational hormones in pregnancy protects the maternal skeleton from demineralization. In contrast, during the relatively low estrogen state of lactation, calcium is mobilized from bone stores, possibly under the influence of PTHrP (Dobnig et al, 1995).

In the third trimester, fetal plasma total and ionized calcium and phosphorus levels are higher than maternal levels, producing a state of "physiologic fetal hypercalcemia" (Rubin et al, 1991). Fetal plasma PTH is low, and calcitonin and PTHrP levels are relatively high. Even these low circulating PTH levels may be functionally important in fetal calcium and magnesium metabolism. There also is a close correlation between maternal and fetal serum 25(OH)D levels, consistent with transplacental transfer of this metabolite. Low levels may be found in infants born to women with low circulating 25(OH)D resulting from poor dietary intake of vitamin D and lack of sunlight exposure. Fetal plasma 1,25(OH)$_2$D also is relatively low, despite robust renal 25(OH)D–1α-hydroxylase activity, whereas concentrations of 24,25(OH)$_2$D are high. In fact, the major function of the fetal kidneys in calcium homeostasis may be production of 1,25(OH)$_2$D, rather than renal tubular regulation of calcium excretion. The high circulating concentrations of calcitonin may support this stimulated fetal 25(OH)D–1α-hydroxylase activity. In contrast, the relatively low circulating fetal 1,25(OH)$_2$D concentrations are a consequence of enhanced placental clearance (Ross et al, 1989). Constitutively activated placental 24-hydroxylase activity (Rubin et al, 1993) also preferentially hydroxylates maternally derived 25(OH)D to 24,25(OH)$_2$D. This placental capacity to metabolize 25(OH)D and 1,25(OH)$_2$D accounts for the enhanced clearance of fetal 1,25(OH)$_2$D, limits access of placentally synthesized 1,25(OH)$_2$D to the fetal and maternal circulations, and, in effect, partitions the maternal and fetal vitamin D pools.

THE NEONATE

Placental transfer of calcium ceases abruptly at birth. In healthy term newborns, total calcium concentration and Ca^{2+} decline from nearly 11 mg/dL and 6 mg/dL, respectively, in umbilical cord blood to serum levels of 8 to 9 mg/dL and 5 mg/dL by 24 to 48 hours. The nadir of Ca^{2+} may range from 4.4 to 5.4 mg/dL. Concomitant rises in PTH and 1,25(OH)$_2$D stabilize serum calcium as the newborn adapts to extrauterine mineral homeostasis and dietary calcium intake. In preterm infants, calcium absorption from the intestine is nonsaturable and may be vitamin D–independent (Bronner et al, 1992). Serum calcitonin levels increase sharply during the 1st day and remain elevated compared with those in adults. In the mother, prolactin helps stimulate PTHrP expression in lactating breast tissue. PTHrP is secreted into milk at concentrations 10,000-fold higher than in serum. It is likely that the abundant milk PTHrP content ingested by the neonate also is important for mineral regulation. By 2 weeks of life, serum calcium rises to the mean values observed in older children and adults.

During the 1st week of life, urinary phosphate excretion is significantly higher in preterm than in term infants but then approximates that of term infants, possibly owing to accelerated postnatal renal maturation. Calcium excretion is low during the 1st week, when the newborn must compensate for the postpartum fall in serum calcium. After the first several days, calcium excretion increases with a magnitude inversely proportional to gestation. The high urinary calcium-to-creatinine ratio (UCa/Cr) of young infants then steadily declines with age (Sargent et al, 1993). However, in preterm breastfed infants who are more than 2 weeks old, the UCa/Cr can exceed 2.0 (Karlen et al, 1985). These changes may reflect the relative phosphate deficiency in many preterm infants, which results in an adaptively low urinary phosphate excretion, decreased bone mineralization, and, consequently, relatively high urinary calcium excretion.

CALCIUM METABOLISM IN THE NEWBORN

NEONATAL HYPOCALCEMIA

Neonatal hypocalcemia has been variously defined as a serum calcium level of less than 8 mg/dL, less than 7.5 mg/dL, or less than 7.0 mg/dL and as a Ca^{2+} level of less than 4.0 mg/dL. Under conditions of normal acid-base status and normal serum albumin, serum total calcium and Ca^{2+} levels are linearly correlated, so total serum calcium measurements remain useful as a screening test. However, because Ca^{2+} is the physiologically relevant fraction, in sick infants it may be preferable to assay [Ca^{2+}] directly in freshly obtained blood samples. A precise definition of hypocalcemia, like hypoglycemia, in preterm infants is particularly difficult to formulate. Preterm hypocalcemia is probably best defined with reference to Ca^{2+}.

A useful approach to the classification of neonatal hypocalcemia is by time of onset. "Early" and "late" occurring hypocalcemia (Box 90-1) have different causes, usually

---

BOX 90-1   Causes of Neonatal Hypocalcemia

Early-onset hypocalcemia (<48 hours of age)
  Prematurity
  Perinatal distress/asphyxia
  Infants of diabetic mothers
  Intrauterine growth restriction
Late-onset hypocalcemia (1st week of life)
  High phosphate load ± hypoparathyroidism or vitamin D deficiency
Neonatal hypoparathyroid syndromes
  Parathyroid agenesis
  DiGeorge syndrome (22q11.2 deletions)
  Familial isolated hypoparathyroidism
    PTH gene mutations
  Autosomal dominant hypocalcemic hypocalciuria (ADHH)
    Activating mutations of the Ca^{2+}-sensing receptor
  Neonatal hypoparathyroidism secondary to maternal hyperparathyroidism
  Autoimmune-candidiasis-ectodermal dystrophy (APECED or APS1)
  Hypoparathyroidism associated with skeletal dysplasias
    Kenny-Caffey syndrome
    Sanjad-Sakati (hypoparathyroidism-retardation-dysmorphism [HRD]) syndrome
    Osteogenesis imperfecta type II
  PTH resistance (transient neonatal pseudohypoparathyroidism)
  Hypomagnesemia ± distal renal tubular acidosis
    Primary hypomagnesemia
    Renal tubular acidosis type 1

Abnormal vitamin D [1,25(OH)$_2$D] production or action ("hypocalcemic rickets")
  Vitamin D deficiency (secondary to maternal vitamin D deficiency)
  Acquired or inherited disorders of vitamin D metabolism
  Resistance to the actions of vitamin D
Hyperphosphatemia
  Excessive dietary phosphate
  Phosphate-containing enemas
  Rhabdomyolysis-induced acute renal failure
  Hyperphosphatemic renal insufficiency
"Hungry bones syndrome" (mineralization outpacing osteoclastic bone resorption)
Other causes
  Metabolic or respiratory alkalosis
  Phototherapy
  Long chain 3-hydroxyacyl-CoA dehydrogenase deficiency (LCHAD)
  Pancreatitis
  Sepsis, septic shock
  Rotavirus gastroenteritis
  Osteopetrosis and other skeletal dysplasias
  Pseudohypocalcemia (hypoalbuminemia)
  Medications
    Bicarbonate
    Rapid transfusion or plasmapheresis with citrated blood
    Furosemide-induced
    Lipid infusions

CoA, Coenzyme A; *1,25(OH)$_2$D*, 1,25-dihydroxyvitamin D.

occur in different clinical settings, and should prompt different approaches to evaluation and management.

Clinical Findings

Because Ca^{2+} couples excitation and contraction in skeletal and cardiac muscle, increased neuromuscular excitability (tetany) is a cardinal feature of hypocalcemia. However, hypocalcemic signs in neonates are variable and may not correlate with the magnitude of the decline in Ca^{2+}. Although some infants are severely affected, others having equally depressed serum calcium levels may be asymptomatic.

Tetanic infants are jittery and hyperactive, frequently exhibit muscle jerks and twitches, and may have generalized or focal clonic seizures. Exaggerated responses to environmental noises (e.g., "spontaneous" Moro reflex) can indicate hyperacusis. Occasionally, respiratory or gastrointestinal rather than neurologic signs predominate. Laryngospasm with inspiratory stridor, sometimes severe enough to cause cyanosis or anoxia, or wheezing due to bronchospasm may be a presenting manifestation. Vomiting, possibly related to pylorospasm, sometimes causes hematemesis or melena. At times, the gastrointestinal signs are severe enough to mimic those of intestinal obstruction. Other signs of neonatal tetany include extensor hypertonia, apnea, tachycardia, tachypnea, and edema. Carpopedal spasm and Chvostek's sign are not as reliably elicited in hypocalcemic newborns as in older children or adults.

Early Neonatal Hypocalcemia

Hypocalcemia occurring during the first 3 days of life, usually between 24 and 48 hours postpartum, is termed *early neonatal hypocalcemia*. It is a pathologic exaggeration of the normal decline in circulating calcium. Early neonatal hypocalcemia typically is seen in any of four circumstances: prematurity, severe stress or asphyxia, maternal diabetes, or significant intrauterine growth restriction (IUGR). In preterm infants, there is a steeper and more rapid postnatal decline in serum calcium; the magnitude of depression is inversely proportional to gestational age. Untreated, many low-birthweight (LBW) infants and essentially all extremely low-birthweight (ELBW) infants exhibit total calcium levels of less than 7.0 mg/dL by day 2. However, the fall in Ca^{2+} is not proportional to the fall in total calcium concentration, and the ratio of ionized to total calcium in these newborns is higher than at term. This "sparing" of Ca^{2+} may be related to the lower serum protein concentration and pH in prematurity. The sparing effect on Ca^{2+} also, in part, explains the frequent absence of hypocalcemic signs in preterm infants.

The neonatal parathyroid glands, regardless of degree of prematurity, can mount an appropriate PTH response to hypocalcemia. In fact, hypocalcemia in extremely preterm newborns (Rubin et al, 1991) or infants undergoing cardiac bypass (Robertie et al, 1992) stimulates increases in serum PTH at least as great as those seen in adults during citrate-induced hypocalcemia (Grant et al, 1990). PTH resistance plays an uncertain role in early neonatal hypocalcemia. A several-day delay in the phosphaturic and renal cAMP responses to PTH has inconsistently been reported, suggesting that there might be a maturational delay in renal responses to PTH. High renal sodium excretion in preterm infants also probably aggravates calciuric losses. In addition, the preterm infant's exaggerated rise in calcitonin may promote hypocalcemia. Currently, there is no convincing evidence that abnormalities in vitamin D metabolism are involved in the etiopathogenesis of hypocalcemia in preterm infants. Like fetuses, even ELBW newborns efficiently synthesize $1,25(OH)_2D$ when vitamin D stores are adequate.

Early neonatal hypocalcemia with hyperphosphatemia is frequently observed in severely stressed or asphyxiated infants. The causes are probably multifactorial and include, to varying degrees, renal insufficiency, tissue catabolism, and acidosis. There is an exaggerated serum calcitonin response and elevated PTH levels. Low serum Ca^{2+} and elevated serum magnesium levels have been correlated with severity of hypoxic-ischemic encephalopathy and poor outcome (Ilves et al, 2000).

Infants of diabetic mothers (IDMs) show an exaggerated postnatal drop in circulating calcium levels compared to gestational-age controls. The course usually is similar to that of early neonatal hypocalcemia in preterm infants, although hypocalcemia sometimes persists for several additional days. Maternal and neonatal hypomagnesemia (Banerjee et al, 2003) and low fetal PTH/PTHrP biologic activity (Rubin et al, 1991) may be causative factors. The greater bone mass and relative undermineralization typical of macrosomic IDMs also may increase the neonatal demand for calcium, producing a deeper and prolonged decline in postnatal serum calcium levels. Similar mechanisms may come into play in the transient hypocalcemia often observed in small-for-gestational-age (SGA) infants. Hypercalcitonemia, hypoparathyroidism, abnormalities in vitamin D metabolism, and hyperphosphatemia all have been implicated, but none has been consistently found.

Historically, symptomatic neonatal hypocalcemia in IDMs has been associated with the severity of maternal diabetes (e.g., White classification) and inadequate glycemic control. Not surprisingly, preterm IDMs who have sustained IUGR and asphyxia as a result of uteroplacental insufficiency invariably become quite hypocalcemic. In recent years, improved metabolic control for pregnant diabetic women has markedly diminished the occurrence and severity of early neonatal hypocalcemia in IDMs (Demarini et al, 1994). Healthy IDMs who are able to begin milk feedings on the 1st day do not require serum calcium monitoring unless suspicious signs (e.g., jitteriness, stridor) are noted.

Late Neonatal Hypocalcemia

Late neonatal hypocalcemia, or hypocalcemia developing after 3 to 5 days of life, occurs more frequently in term than in preterm newborns and is not usually associated with maternal diabetes, birth trauma, or asphyxia. Historically associated with cow's-milk or cow's-milk formula feedings, it also occasionally occurs in breastfed infants. The entity of "late infantile tetany" seen in infants fed whole cow's milk has become a rarity with adjustment of phosphorus content in humanized cow's-milk and soy infant formulas.

The hyperphosphatemia that is a prominent feature of late neonatal hypocalcemia may result from varying combinations of dietary phosphate load, immature renal tubular phosphate excretion, transiently low levels of circulating PTH, hypomagnesemia, and marginal maternal vitamin D intake. A relatively high dietary phosphate load coupled with a low GFR leads to an increase in serum phosphate levels and a reciprocal decline in serum calcium levels. The physiologic response to hypocalcemia is an increase in PTH secretion, leading to increased urinary phosphate excretion and tubular calcium resorption. It is relevant, therefore, that low circulating PTH levels are sometimes observed in infants with late neonatal hypocalcemia. Serum calcium levels frequently increase when these infants are placed on a low-phosphate formula and supplemental calcium. After several days to weeks, serum PTH usually increases, and the infants then can tolerate more dietary phosphate. The pathogenesis of this "transient hypoparathyroidism" in late neonatal hypocalcemia is not readily apparent. Some of these infants show a persistent or recurrent inability to mount an adequate PTH response to a hypocalcemic challenge, indicating partial hypoparathyroidism.

In other infants, maternal vitamin D deficiency can cause late (or occasionally "early") neonatal hypocalcemia. This possibility is checked by measuring maternal and neonatal serum 25(OH)D levels. Maternal vitamin D deficiency also is implicated by the increased incidence of late neonatal hypocalcemia in winter. The high prevalence of enamel hypoplasia of incisor teeth reported in affected infants indicates that the mineralization defect begins during the third trimester of pregnancy.

Hypocalcemia and hyperphosphatemia after the first 2 to 3 days always should prompt a thorough investigation for underlying cause(s) (see Box 90-1). Hypocalcemia in this setting usually implies primary or secondary dysregulation of (1) the parathyroid-renal [PTH-1,25(OH)$_2$D] axis, (2) hypomagnesemia, or (3) renal insufficiency. The primary hormonal and end-organ disturbances that cause neonatal hypocalcemic syndromes are described in a later section. As a cautionary note, earlier observations of generally favorable neurologic outcomes in newborns with hypocalcemic or hypomagnesemic seizures (which may have been related to a nutritional metabolic disturbance) may be less relevant to the current neonatal population, in which hypocalcemia or hypomagnesemia due to dietary phosphate overload seldom is observed. In this group, neurologic prognosis may be more closely related to the causative disorder (Lynch and Rust, 1994).

Hypocalcemia Caused by Hypoparathyroid Syndromes

The biochemical hallmarks of hypoparathyroidism are hypocalcemia and hyperphosphatemia in the presence of normal renal function. Serum PTH concentrations are inappropriately low or undetectable. Cytogenetic and molecular genetic diagnosis also permits characterization of several types of congenital hypoparathyroidism. Isolated hypoparathyroidism is usually sporadic but may show X-linked, autosomal recessive, or autosomal dominant inheritance.

Congenital hypoparathyroidism is a common feature of the DiGeorge syndrome (DGS). Fully expressed DGS comprises hypoparathyroid hypocalcemia, thymic hypoplasia with defects in T-cell immunity, conotruncal cardiac defects, palatal insufficiency, characteristic facies, and neurobehavioral and psychiatric features. The phenotypes result from defects in cervical neural crest cell migration into the derivatives of the third and fourth pharyngeal (branchial) pouches. DiGeorge, velocardiofacial (Shprintzen), and conotruncal face anomaly (Takao) syndromes commonly result from contiguous gene deletions in the same chromosomal region. That also is true for some isolated cardiac outflow tract defects and transient congenital hypoparathyroidism in the absence of a DGS phenotype. These infants should be evaluated and monitored for recurrence of hypocalcemia.

Most persons having a clinical diagnosis of DGS share a common 1.5- to 3-Mb deletion (monosomy or partial monosomy) of chromosome region 22q11.2, but there is molecular heterogeneity and rearrangement within this region (Emanuel, 2008). Haploinsufficiency of the TBX1 transcription factor gene may be responsible for most features. Fluorescence in situ hybridization (FISH) using 22q11 probes had a higher detection rate than that for high-resolution G band karyotyping. However, the most sensitive (and preferred) laboratory assay is array-comparative genomic hybridization (aCGH). Additionally, rarer identification of other cytogenetic abnormalities suggests that several distinct molecular defects (Rope et al, 2009) can lead to disturbed cranial neural crest cell migration and DGS phenotypes.

The incidence of DGS may be at least 1 case per 5000 live births (Ryan et al, 1997). Sporadic loss in the DGS region is more common than parental transmission. In members of the same family, DGS may be associated with different phenotypic features, depending on whether endocrinologic, cardiac, craniofacial, or palatal abnormalities are the initial focus of attention.

DGS often manifests in the 1st week of life with hypocalcemic tetany or seizures. Craniofacial features include microretrognathia, submucous cleft palate, low-set and abnormal pinnae, telecanthus with short palpebral fissures, short philtrum, and a relatively small mouth. The presence of cardiac outflow tract or aortic arch abnormalities (especially pulmonary atresia/tetralogy of Fallot, type B interrupted aortic arch, truncus arteriosus, anomalies of aortic arch laterality, or abnormal branching of the brachiocephalic vessels), even in the absence of other DGS features, should prompt genetic investigation. Parents of an infant with DGS should be screened for carrier status. These neonates require close anticipatory monitoring for the onset of hypocalcemia. Absence of a thymic shadow on chest radiograph is not a reliable indicator. Because of the potential for inducing graft-versus-host disease, until T cell competence has been demonstrated, irradiated red blood cell transfusions may be preferred.

A normal serum PTH obtained when an infant is relatively normocalcemic also does not exclude the diagnosis of DGS. Infants with DGS may show resolution of hypoparathyroidism by early childhood, although PTH reserves may remain inadequate for defense against hypocalcemic stresses.

Hypoparathyroidism is a prominent feature of several rare skeletal dysplasias. Kenny-Caffey syndrome is a rare osteosclerotic bony dysplasia associated with hypocalcemia and ocular abnormalities. Autosomal recessive and autosomal dominant inheritance patterns have been described. Features include IUGR, transient neonatal hypoparathyroidism, short stature, macrocephaly, delayed fontanel closure, dysmorphic facies, and cortical thickening of tubular bones. In hypoparathyroidism-retardation-dysmorphism (HRD) syndrome (Sanjad-Sakati syndrome), hypoparathyroidism also is associated with IUGR, poor postnatal growth, characteristic facies (deep-set eyes, depressed nasal bridge, beaked nose, long philtrum, thin upper lip, micrognathia, large and floppy earlobes), small hands and feet, skeletal defects, and developmental delay (Sanjad et al, 1991). This autosomal recessive disorder has been described in persons of Gulf Arab and Bedouin ancestry. The loci for HRD syndrome and recessive Kenny-Caffey syndrome and HRD syndrome are allelic on chromosome 1q42-q43. Parvari et al (2002) have identified mutations in the gene encoding tubulin-specific chaperone E (*TBCE*) in both disorders.

Although osteogenesis imperfecta (OI) type II usually is perinatally lethal, some infants have prolonged survival. Knisely et al (1988) showed that acute parathyroid hemorrhage ("parathyroid apoplexy") is a common event in OI II and may contribute to early death.

The parathyroid glands are an infrequent target for autoimmunity, the exception being autoimmune polyglandular syndrome type 1 (APS 1), also known as autoimmune-candidiasis-ectodermal dystrophy (APECED), in which autoimmune hypoparathyroidism is the rule (Brown, 2009). APS 1 is a rare autosomal recessive disorder characterized by hypoparathyroidism, adrenal insufficiency, and chronic mucocutaneous candidiasis. Afflicted persons often eventually develop chronic hepatitis, malabsorption, juvenile-onset pernicious anemia, alopecia, and primary hypogonadism. APS 1 results from inheritance of mutations in an autoimmune regulator gene (*AIRE*). When this disorder is diagnosed in early infancy, which is rare, hypocalcemia (with or without candidiasis) typically is the presenting sign.

The association of several forms of autosomal dominant and autosomal recessive congenital hypoparathyroidism with allelic variants of the *preproPTH* and calcium-sensing receptor (*CaSR*) genes has advanced diagnosis and therapy for these disorders. Affected infants have subnormal or undetectable serum PTH levels but do not have congenital anomalies or developmental field defects, DGS locus deletions, candidiasis or autoimmune polyglandular failure, or anti-endocrine antibodies. Autosomal dominant and autosomal recessive forms of familial isolated hypoparathyroidism have been related to mutations in the *preproPTH* gene (Sunthornthevarakul et al, 1999). Activating *CaSR* gene mutations cause autosomal dominant hypocalcemic hypocalciuria (ADHH) or "CaSR hyperfunction." The parathyroid and renal calcistat is reset downward, so that hypocalcemia does not elicit normal compensatory PTH secretion or renal calcium reabsorption. Because de novo *CaSR* mutations producing CaSR hyperfunction may account for many cases of so-called sporadic idiopathic hypoparathyroidism (Egbuna and Brown, 2008),

mutational analysis of the *CaSR* gene should be considered in the work-up of isolated hypoparathyroidism in infants, especially when hypocalcemia manifests with inappropriately normal urinary calcium excretion (relative hypercalciuria). In fact, hypercalciuria and nephrocalcinosis can develop even when serum calcium remains below the normal range. Therefore, these patients require close monitoring of urinary calcium excretion for adjusting therapy with $1,25(OH)_2D$ analogues.

There are three principal forms of hormone resistance to PTH. Deletion of the PTH/PTHrP receptor is embryologically or perinatally lethal. Loss of one allele for *GNAS1*, which encodes $G_s\alpha$, the G protein α subunit required for receptor-stimulated cAMP generation, produces pseudohypoparathyroidism type 1A (PHP1A). PHP1A is characterized by PTH-resistant (pseudo)hypoparathyroidism and characteristic somatic features (short stature, brachydactyly, and subcutaneous ossification), which collectively are known as Albright hereditary osteodystrophy. Isolated PTH resistance in the absence of this somatic phenotype is called pseudohypoparathyroidism type 1B (PHP1B). This disorder is an imprinting defect in which both *GNAS1* alleles have an unmethylated (paternal) pattern (Liu et al, 2000). Although most persons eventually diagnosed with a PTH resistance syndrome usually are not hypocalcemic during the 1st month of life, transient neonatal pseudohypoparathyroidism occasionally has been reported (Minagawa et al, 1995). Neonatal PTH resistance, which has an unknown frequency, can manifest as hypocalcemic seizures with hyperphosphatemia and an elevated PTH.

Neonatal Hypocalcemia Associated With Maternal Hyperparathyroidism

Hypocalcemia is commonly observed in newborns of hyperparathyroid mothers. These infants may show increased neuromuscular irritability during the first 3 weeks of life but, occasionally, do so much later as limited PTH reserve and latent hypoparathyroidism emerge under stress or with time. The serum calcium levels usually range from 5.0 to 7.5 mg/dL, and the serum phosphate levels are often greater than 8.0 mg/dL. Hypocalcemic signs may be exacerbated by high-phosphate diets or maternal vitamin D deficiency. In some instances, signs of hypocalcemia can be quite severe and resistant to therapy. Calcium supplementation, which in some instances must be continued for several weeks, produces eventual improvement.

In maternal hyperparathyroidism, the increased maternal serum calcium facilitates transplacental calcium transport, producing fetal hypercalcemia greater than the moderate elevations of serum calcium normally observed in the third trimester. As a result, fetal PTH secretion is suppressed more than it is in normal pregnancy. The suppressed parathyroids are unable to maintain normal serum calcium levels postpartum. The reason for the hypomagnesemia observed in some infants born to hyperparathyroid mothers is uncertain, but this derangement may be due to (1) maternal magnesium depletion as a complication of hyperparathyroidism; (2) transient neonatal hypoparathyroidism; or (3) hyperphosphatemia, which may result from transient hypoparathyroidism or high dietary phosphate intake, or both.

Maternal serum calcium and phosphorus should be assayed whenever this diagnosis is suspected. Hypocalcemic tetany occurring in the infant may lead to diagnosis of hyperparathyroidism in an asymptomatic mother. Maternal serum calcium values in the upper normal range may be falsely reassuring if the samples were obtained during pregnancy, a time when serum calcium levels normally decline.

Neonatal Hypocalcemia Associated With Hypomagnesemia or Renal Tubular Acidosis

Hypomagnesemia causes hypocalcemia by interfering with the parathyroid cell CaSR-mediated release of PTH and by blunting end-organ PTH response. Depression of serum magnesium levels in newborns may be chronic, sometimes as primary hypomagnesemia with secondary hypocalcemia, or transient.

Hypomagnesemia with secondary hypocalcemia (HOMG1), also known as hypomagnesemia with secondary hypocalcemia (HSH), can present in the first weeks of life as persistent hypocalcemia, tetany, and seizures uncontrolled by anticonvulsants or calcium therapy. Delay in establishing the diagnosis may lead to permanent neurologic impairment. This rare autosomal recessive disorder results from defective intestinal magnesium absorption and renal magnesium leak. HOMG1 is caused by mutations in the TRPM6 gene, a member of the transient receptor potential channel family expressed in intestinal epithelia and renal tubules (Schlingmann et al, 2005).

Several forms of primary renal hypomagnesemia have been described, including autosomal recessive familial hypomagnesemia with hypercalciuria and nephrocalcinosis caused by mutations in the claudin-16 (paracellin-1) gene (Simon et al, 1999) and a genetically heterogeneous autosomal dominant "isolated renal magnesium wasting" (Kantorovich et al, 2002). The clinical spectrum includes polyuria, hyposthenuria, moderate metabolic acidosis with an inappropriately high urine pH and a positive urine anion gap, low citrate excretion, renal magnesium and calcium wasting, secondary renal potassium wasting, nephrocalcinosis, muscle weakness, persistent tetany, seizures, and sometimes abnormal facies and sensorineural hearing loss. The partial distal acidification defect, which is probably secondary to a medullary interstitial nephropathy, can be functionally distinguished from primary distal renal tubular acidosis (RTA1) (Rodriguez-Soriano and Vallo, 1994). In primary hypomagnesemia, the serum magnesium is frequently less than 0.8 mg/dL (normal 1.6 to 2.8 mg/dL), and the magnesium deficiency leads to parathyroid failure and peripheral PTH resistance, despite hypocalcemia. High-dose enteral magnesium leads to spontaneous parallel increases in serum PTH and calcium levels and renal phosphate clearance. Renal transplantation normalizes serum magnesium and urinary calcium.

A transient hypomagnesemia in newborns often occurs in association with hypocalcemia. Less commonly, the serum calcium level may be normal. In transient hypomagnesemia, the decrease in serum magnesium level typically is less severe (0.8 to 1.4 mg/dL) than in magnesium transport defects. In many infants with transient hypomagnesemia, the serum magnesium level increases spontaneously as the serum calcium level normalizes following the administration of calcium supplements. However, in other cases, hypocalcemia responds poorly to calcium therapy, but when magnesium salts are given, both serum calcium and magnesium levels rise.

Secondary hypomagnesemia from renal magnesium wasting can result from drug administration (loop diuretics, aminoglycosides, amphotericin B) or by urinary tract obstruction. It also may occur during the diuretic phase of acute renal failure. The disorder may be mistaken for neonatal hypoparathyroidism because of tetany and hypocalcemia, or for Bartter's syndrome (hypokalemic alkalosis with hypercalciuria) because of secondary potassium wasting. An index of suspicion should be raised whenever hypomagnesemia occurs in one of these situations. Finding low serum magnesium levels with inappropriately high urinary magnesium excretion confirms a diagnosis of renal magnesium wasting. Regardless of cause, hypokalemia is a common laboratory feature of magnesium depletion. Attempts to replace the potassium deficit with potassium alone usually are unsuccessful unless magnesium is given concurrently.

Distal renal tubular acidosis (i.e., RTA1) is characterized by hypocalcemia, hypercalciuria, varying degrees of hypomagnesemia, hyperchloremia, low serum bicarbonate, and a fixed urinary specific gravity and urinary pH (about 5.0). The mineral excretion defect leads to nephrocalcinosis and metabolic bone disease. RTA1 sometimes manifests during early infancy, when hypocalcemia may precede the RTA. Lewis (1992) proposed that Tiny Tim in Dickens' *A Christmas Carol* had RTA1, which would account for Tim's growth failure, osteomalacia, fractures, and neuromuscular weakness.

Hypocalcemia Resulting from Vitamin D Disorders

In older children and adults, disorders of vitamin D intake or metabolism rarely present as isolated hypocalcemia. Instead, most persons having abnormalities in either production or action of $1,25(OH)_2D$ manifest with rickets or osteomalacia. In sharp contrast, young infants may exhibit hypocalcemic tetany before rachitic features become conspicuous. Abnormalities in vitamin D metabolism can be divided into three broad categories: vitamin D deficiency, acquired or inherited disorders of vitamin D metabolism, and resistance to vitamin D actions.

Maternal vitamin D deficiency is the major risk factor for neonatal vitamin D deficiency manifesting as hypocalcemia. Maternal vitamin D deficiency is becoming less common in countries where dairy products and other foods are supplemented with vitamin D. It is still a common and serious health problem of women of reproductive age and their infants in developing countries. Female immigrants from the Middle East or South Asia who wear traditional concealing dress, have inadequate dietary vitamin D intake, or are dark-skinned are at particularly high risk (Dijkstra et al, 2007; Hobbs et al, 2009), especially during pregnancy. Breastfed infants of lactovegetarian mothers also are susceptible to early-onset hypocalcemic rickets. Nutritional rickets in newborns can be prevented by daily supplementation of 400 IU for infants and 400 IU daily for mothers during pregnancy and lactation or 1000 IU daily if begun in the third trimester.

Intestinal absorption of fat-soluble vitamin D requires a functioning exocrine pancreas, biliary tract, and bowel mucosa. Consequently, pregnant women with malabsorption syndromes may be vitamin D deficient. Anticonvulsant therapy (e.g., with phenobarbital or diphenylhydantoin) during pregnancy, which increases hepatic catabolism of 25(OH)D, also can induce maternal and fetal vitamin D deficiency. Pregnant women who take anticonvulsants should receive vitamin D supplementation (800 to 1000 IU/day).

Phosphate-Induced Hypocalcemia

Hypocalcemia is the systemic response to hyperphosphatemia. Conditions conducive to phosphate-induced neonatal hypocalcemia are excessive phosphate intake, rhabdomyolysis-induced acute renal failure, and hyperphosphatemic renal insufficiency. In the instance of excess intake, phosphate-containing enemas can produce significant phosphate absorption. Their use is hazardous and contraindicated for infants. Chronic renal failure is the primary cause of secondary hyperparathyroidism. Patients with mineral metabolism disorders commonly present with low serum calcium levels, hyperphosphatemia, and calcitriol deficiency. In uremic conditions, however, parathyroid glands become hyperplastic and leave quiescence. In recent years, there has been identification of important molecular mediators including the CaR, parathyroid expression of the vitamin D receptor (VDR), and a central role of the fibroblast growth factor 23 (FGF-23) (Cozzolino et al, 2009).

Other Causes of Neonatal Hypocalcemia

It is important to recognize that hypocalcemia may occur whenever skeletal mineralization significantly outpaces the rate of osteoclastic bone resorption. Examples of this type of hypocalcemia occur with overzealous vitamin D replacement in infants with rickets or hypoparathyroidism. Pancreatitis can cause hypocalcemia and tetany through the action of pancreatic lipase on retroperitoneal and omental fat to release free fatty acids (FFAs). FFAs avidly chelate calcium and remove it from the ECF. Pancreatitis also may release pancreatic calcium-lowering factors (Tomomura et al, 1995). Sepsis and septic shock cause hypocalcemia by unknown mechanisms. Neonatal or infantile hypocalcemia and hypocalcemic seizures may accompany long-chain 3-hydroxyacyl-coenzyme A (CoA) dehydrogenase deficiency (LCHAD) (Ibdah et al, 1999) and severe cases of rotavirus gastroenteritis (Foldenauer et al, 1998). Hypocalcemic jitteriness or seizures can be the presenting sign of infantile osteopetrosis (Srinivasan et al, 2000). Prompt recognition permits early referral for bone marrow or hematopoietic stem cell transplantation. Certain other skeletal dysplasia syndromes are associated with neonatal hypocalcemia, which may be severe.

Several common therapeutic interventions can induce hypocalcemia. Bicarbonate therapy, as well as any form of metabolic or respiratory alkalinization, decrease both

Ca^{2+} levels and bone turnover. Rapid blood transfusion or plasmapheresis can promote calcium complexes with the infused citrate, decreasing Ca^{2+}. Hypocalcemia after initiation of ECMO is related to composition of the circuit-priming solution and to acute citrate loading and may lead to hemodynamic instability (Meliones et al, 1995). Furosemide therapy promotes calciuresis and nephrolithiasis. Phototherapy for hyperbilirubinemia may be associated with mild hypocalcemia. This effect has been attributed to decreased melatonin secretion, which potentiates glucocorticoid actions on bone metabolism. Lipid infusions may elevate serum FFAs, which form insoluble complexes with calcium. Most of these effects are transient, and cessation of therapy is followed by a return to normal serum calcium levels. The major exception is aggressive furosemide therapy, which, when prolonged, may lead to bone demineralization and renal dysfunction (Downing et al, 1992).

Treatment

The decision to treat hypocalcemia in an infant depends on the severity of the hypocalcemia and the presence of clinical signs and symptoms. The morbidity associated with calcium treatment must be weighed against the potential benefits. Hypocalcemic preterm infants who have no symptoms and are not ill from any other cause probably do not need specific treatment. Early neonatal hypocalcemia should resolve by day 3. Some clinicians begin treatment in preterm newborns once serum calcium levels have dropped to 6.0 to 6.5 mg/dL or after Ca^{2+} has decreased to 2.5 to 3.0 mg/dL. Another reasonable approach is to initiate prophylactic calcium infusions (or calcium-containing parenteral nutrition) for all ELBW infants within the first 24 hours. There is no role for prophylaxis or treatment with pharmacologic doses of vitamin D. For newborns who exhibit cardiovascular compromise (e.g., severe respiratory distress, pulmonary hypertension, asphyxia, sepsis) or who require cardiotonic drugs or blood pressure support, monitoring blood $[Ca^{2+}]$ is particularly helpful, with the aim of preventing the onset of significant hypocalcemia.

The mainstay of treatment for neonatal hypocalcemia is intravenous administration of calcium salts. Calcium gluconate is preferred over calcium chloride (which, in sufficient doses, produces hyperchloremic acidosis) or calcium lactate. A 10% solution of calcium gluconate contains 9.4 mg Ca/mL. A constant infusion of approximately 45 to 75 mg/kg/day usually produces a sustained increase in serum calcium level (7 to 8 mg/dL). Bolus infusions are hazardous and only transiently effective.

Risks associated with calcium infusions are minimized by attention to detail. Rapid intravenous infusion of calcium can cause sudden elevation in serum calcium, leading to bradyarrhythmias. Bolus infusion of calcium should be reserved for treating hypocalcemic tetany and seizures. Extravasation of calcium solutions into subcutaneous tissues may cause necrosis and subcutaneous calcification. Therefore, meticulous care of peripheral intravenous catheter sites is particularly important when calcium-containing solutions are infused. Inadvertent intrahepatic infusion of calcium through an umbilical vein catheter (due to failure to reach the inferior vena cava) can cause hepatic necrosis. Rapid intraaortic infusion via an umbilical artery can cause arterial spasm and, at least experimentally, intestinal necrosis.

Hypocalcemic Crisis

For emergency treatment of hypocalcemic crisis with seizures, tetany, or apnea, 1 to 2 mL/kg of a 10% solution of calcium gluconate should be given over 5 to 10 minutes. The initial serum calcium level may be less than 5.0 mg/dL. Careful observation of the infant and infusion site is essential, and the infusion should be discontinued if there is bradycardia or when the desired clinical result is obtained. The intravenous dose of calcium gluconate necessary to stop convulsions is usually 1 to 3 mL/kg. Toxic reactions are avoided if the maximum intravenous dose of calcium gluconate given at any one time does not exceed 2 mL/kg; doses above 3 mL/kg should be administered with caution. If necessary, intravenous calcium therapy may be repeated 3 or 4 times in 24 hours to help control acute symptoms.

Nonemergency Treatment

After acute symptoms have been controlled, calcium therapy should be continued as needed to maintain serum calcium above 7.0 mg/dL. In part, the level of serum calcium to be achieved depends on serum total protein, particularly albumin. In hypoalbuminemic infants, lower levels of total serum calcium are normally present. In preterm and sick infants for whom oral intake is limited, 5 to 8 mL/kg of 10% calcium gluconate (45 to 75 mg Ca/kg) may be infused with intravenous fluids over a 24-hour period. The lower dose range is preferred whenever there is hyperphosphatemia. If oral feedings are tolerated, 10% calcium gluconate may be given in the same daily dose divided into 4 to 6 feedings. Alternatively, calcium glubionate (Neo-Calglucon), which contains 23.6 mg Ca/mL, may be given in a dose of 2 mL/kg/day divided into feedings. Oral calcium gluconate is better tolerated by young infants because the high sugar content and osmolality of calcium glubionate may cause gastrointestinal irritation or diarrhea. Intravenous or oral calcium supplements should be continued until the serum calcium level stabilizes.

Dietary factors and hypoparathyroidism are important in the pathogenesis of late neonatal hypocalcemia. Therefore, therapy is often directed at reducing the phosphate load and increasing the calcium-to-phosphorus ratio of feedings to 4:1. This can be accomplished by the use of low-phosphorus feedings such as human milk or Similac PM 60/40 in conjunction with calcium supplements. These interventions inhibit intestinal absorption of phosphorus. Phosphate binders are not generally necessary. Serum calcium and phosphorus levels should be monitored at least once to twice weekly and the calcium supplements discontinued in a stepwise fashion after several weeks.

Magnesium Administration

When hypomagnesemia contributes to (or causes) hypocalcemia, administration of magnesium salts is indicated. Magnesium may be given intramuscularly as a 50% solution of magnesium sulfate (50% $MgSO_4 \cdot 7H_2O$ contains 4 mEq/mL of magnesium). The suggested intramuscular or intravenous dose of 50% magnesium sulfate is 0.1 to 0.2 mL/kg. Intravenous infusions should be administered slowly using electrocardiographic monitoring to detect rhythm disturbances, which may include prolonged atrioventricular conduction time and sinoatrial or atrioventricular block. The magnesium dose may be repeated every 12 to 24 hours, depending on the clinical and serum magnesium response. Many infants with transient hypomagnesemia will respond sufficiently to one or two magnesium injections. Infants with primary hypomagnesemia have permanent magnesium wasting. The low serum magnesium levels may require lifelong treatment with magnesium supplements.

Vitamin D Treatment

Infants with normal intestinal absorption who develop late hypocalcemia with vitamin D deficiency rickets usually respond within 4 weeks to 1000 to 2000 IU/day of oral vitamin D. These infants should receive at least 40 mg/kg/day of elemental calcium in order to prevent hypocalcemia because the unmineralized osteoid may avidly incorporate calcium once vitamin D is provided ("hungry bones" syndrome). PTH-dependent renal production of $1,25(OH)_2D$ is deficient in all hypoparathyroid states. Therefore, in persistent congenital hypoparathyroidism, long-term treatment with vitamin D or a shorter-acting vitamin D analogue is indicated.

NEONATAL HYPERCALCEMIA

Hypercalcemia usually is defined as total serum calcium concentration greater than 11.0 mg/dL and $[Ca^{2+}]$ greater than 5.0 mg/dL. Neonatal hypercalcemia is associated with several clinical entities (Box 90-2). It may be asymptomatic and discovered incidentally or may manifest dramatically (especially if serum calcium is 14.0 mg/dL or greater) and be life-threatening, requiring immediate intervention. The clinical findings may include poor feeding, vomiting, constipation, polyuria, hypertension, tachypnea, dyspnea, hypotonia, lethargy, and seizures. Polyuria is due to an impaired renal response to vasopressin (nephrogenic diabetes insipidus) and may lead to dehydration. The hypertension is probably due to a direct vasoconstrictive effect of the elevated ECF calcium as well as to increased activity of the renin-angiotensin system resulting from renal arteriolar constriction. The central nervous manifestations result from direct neuronal effects of calcium, hypertensive encephalopathy, and cerebral ischemia. Persistent hypercalcemia may produce extraskeletal calcification in the kidney, skin, subcutaneous tissue, falx cerebri, arteries, myocardium, lung, or gastric mucosa. Nephrocalcinosis, nephrolithiasis, diffuse bone undermineralization (and occasionally osteitis fibrosa) are well-recognized hypercalcemic complications. In infants, the predominant manifestation of chronic, moderate elevations of serum calcium may be failure to thrive. The physical examination usually is otherwise normal, except in those infants who have subcutaneous fat necrosis, Williams syndrome, or skeletal dysplasias.

Normally, the parathyroid-renal axis prevents hypercalcemia via inhibition of PTH secretion and $1,25(OH)_2D$ synthesis, which reduces calcium absorption from the intestine, mobilization from bone, and reabsorption from the kidney. (The physiologic role of calcitonin is uncertain.) An elevated serum calcium, therefore, indicates an inappropriate calcium influx to the ECF from one or more of these pools. Because the kidney is the principal organ for stoichiometric calcium balance, hypercalcemia usually means that the renal capacity to excrete calcium has been exceeded. In fact, abnormalities in distal tubular resorption are involved in the pathogenesis of many hypercalcemic conditions (e.g., hyperparathyroidism), and renal impairment frequently accompanies many hypercalcemic syndromes.

Neonatal Hyperparathyroid Syndromes and Familial Hypocalciuric Hypercalcemia

Neonatal severe primary hyperparathyroidism (NSPHP) is a rare, life-threatening disorder (Egbuna and Brown, 2008). The enlarged (hyperplastic) parathyroid glands are resistant to regulation by Ca²⁺, resulting in marked hypercalcemia, although milder clinical expression also occurs. These infants may appear normal at birth or have a narrow thorax, depressed sternum, or thoracolumbar kyphosis. Signs of hypercalcemia usually develop during the first days of life. Serum calcium levels may range between 15 and 30 mg/dL, serum phosphorus concentration is frequently less than 3.5 mg/dL with significant hyperphosphaturia, and PTH levels are very elevated. Anemia, hepatomegaly, and splenomegaly have been reported. Skeletal radiographs may show generalized undermineralization, irregular metaphyses (subperiosteal erosions), and

multiple pathologic fractures of the long bones and ribs (Nyweide et al, 2006). Nephrocalcinosis is common. The bone findings initially may be mistaken for osteogenesis imperfecta or abuse.

Inheritance studies have long suggested a connection between NSPHP and a milder disease, familial (benign) hypocalciuric hypercalcemia (FBHH), as well as a relationship of both to PTH-independent "resetting" of parathyroid Ca²⁺ sensing and renal calcium handling. Sequencing of the parathyroid and renal CaSR has clarified these relationships. Partial or total inactivating CaSR mutations cause increased renal tubular calcium reabsorption (hypercalciuria) and persistent PTH secretion despite hypercalcemia. Homozygosity for inactivating CaSR mutations causes NSPHP, whereas heterozygosity results in the autosomal dominant FBHH. FBHH is genetically heterogeneous and includes at least three types, FBHH1, FBHH2, and FBHH3, whose chromosomal locations are 3q21.1, 19p, and 19q13, respectively. FBHH1, related to NSPHP, is caused by mutations of CaSR, but the abnormalities underlying FBHH2 and FBHH3 are unknown. Additionally, certain de novo or inherited heterozygous CaSR mutations account for some cases of NSPHP (Gunn and Gaffney, 2004).

Newborns (and older children and adults) with FBHH have mild (often asymptomatic) intermittent hypercalcemia without hypercalciuria. In distinction to neonatal hyperparathyroidism, circulating levels of PTH, phosphorus, and 1,25(OH)₂D tend to be normal. Persons who have FBHH are at risk for having a child with NSPHP. Conversely, parents of an infant with hyperparathyroidism should be screened with serum calcium and phosphorus levels and a urinary UCa/Cr. A UCa/Cr below 0.01 supports the diagnosis. Early diagnosis and parathyroidectomy have been necessary for survival in fulminant NSHPT. Recently, bisphosphonate (pamidronate) therapy has been used in term (Waller et al, 2004) and preterm (Fox et al, 2007) infants having NSHPT in order to reverse the severe hypercalcemia and postpone parathyroidectomy until the infants were clinically stable. In less severe cases, which can be self-limiting and are often due to heterozygous CaSR mutations, conservative management may be warranted.

Neonatal hyperparathyroidism occasionally occurs as part of the syndrome of multiple endocrine adenomatosis. There also have been reports of sporadic and familial forms of renal tubular acidosis with secondary hyperparathyroidism manifesting as hyperchloremia, hypercalcemia, elevated serum PTH, and severe metabolic acidosis (Igarashi et al, 1992; Savani et al, 1993). Serum calcium and PTH may promptly revert to normal values after initiation of alkali therapy. Often, the acidification defect is transient (Igarashi et al, 1992). As the hyperparathyroidism and ECF volume contraction are corrected, serum calcium normalizes.

Neonatal Hyperparathyroidism Associated With Maternal Hypoparathyroidism

Fetal and neonatal hyperparathyroidism may occur in infants born to mothers with poorly controlled (hypocalcemic) hypoparathyroidism. Maternal hypocalcemia leads to impaired transplacental calcium transfer and causes chronic stimulation of the fetal parathyroid glands. In contrast to infants with NSPHP, these newborns are frequently of low birthweight and have depressed or normal (rather than elevated) serum calcium levels and normal to mildly elevated (rather than depressed) serum phosphorus levels. The reasons for these differences between the two groups are unknown.

Mortality rates are high in infants born to poorly or untreated hyperparathyroid mothers, especially if there is significant IUGR. In survivors, the skeletal abnormalities usually regress and bone radiographs normalize by 4 to 7 months. In hypoparathyroid pregnant women, correction of hypocalcemia with calcium and vitamin D supplements can prevent fetal hyperparathyroidism.

Williams Syndrome and Idiopathic Infantile Hypercalcemia

Williams syndrome (WS) (or Williams-Beuren syndrome) is an autosomal dominant, multisystemic neurodevelopmental disorder caused by a hemizygous deletion of 1.55 Mb on chromosome 7q11.23 spanning 28 genes (Ferrero et al, 2010). It is one of the better described human microdeletion syndromes. Fully expressed WS includes transient hypercalcemia in infancy and cardiac defects, especially supravalvular aortic stenosis and multiple peripheral pulmonary arterial stenoses (Collins et al, 2010). Haploinsufficiency of the elastin (*ELN*) gene is responsible for these defects. Other common features are elfin facies, mental and height deficiency, and dental malformations. The specific facial features include supraorbital fullness with a broad forehead, short palpebral fissures with a medial flare to the eyebrows, a flat nasal bridge with a full tip and anteverted nostrils, ocular hypertelorism, strabismus, stellate iris, malar hypoplasia with a wide mouth and a full lower lip, and hypoplastic teeth with malocclusion. Hallux valgus with a small curved fifth digit is common. Pectus excavatum and umbilical or inguinal hernia are less commonly noted.

Two thirds of newborns with WS are small for gestational age, and many are born post-dates. The frequency of WS is estimated to be about 1 in 10,000 to 1 in 20,000. Expression of the full WS phenotype may be related to the size of the deletion. FISH for the detection of deleted WS gene markers is an appropriate initial diagnostic assay.

Although the hypercalcemia is often diagnosed after the 1st month, the child with WS sometimes comes to clinical attention in the neonatal period (Shimizu et al, 1994). The hypercalcemia rarely persists beyond several months and generally resolves spontaneously, but hypercalciuria may persist. The pathogenesis of hypercalcemia in WS is not well established. Elevated serum calcium associated with normal or increased serum phosphorus levels and characteristic radiographic findings differentiate WS from primary hyperparathyroidism. In some older infants, the serum calcium level is normal, but the presence of nephrocalcinosis and other soft tissue calcifications suggests that hypercalcemia occurred earlier. Increased calcium absorption has been demonstrated, but enhanced vitamin D sensitivity or other disorders of specific calcitropic hormones have not been consistently found. A cautionary note is that many of these children were studied after their hypercalcemia had resolved. A low-calcium diet usually controls the hypercalcemia.

In the early 1950s in England, Lightwood (1952) reported a series of infants with severe hypercalcemia. Hypervitaminosis D was suggested by the findings of osteoporosis and dense bands of mineralization at the metaphyseal ends of long bones. Epidemiologic investigations revealed that a majority of these infants were born to mothers who ingested foods heavily fortified with vitamin D. Some infants also had received 3000 to 4000 IU of vitamin D daily in an effort to prevent nutritional deficiencies. With reduction of vitamin D supplementation, the incidence of infantile hypercalcemia has declined dramatically. However, in other instances, no known previous exposure to excessive maternal vitamin D intake has occurred. The incidence of this milder (Lightwood-type) "idiopathic" infantile hypercalcemia (IIH) without WS phenotypic features has remained relatively fixed over time. Further distinction between these conditions probably awaits more extensive genetic analysis and definition of the mineral metabolic derangement(s). In contrast to WS, serum calcium levels remain elevated for a prolonged period in severely affected infants having IIH. There may be an exaggerated increase in serum $1,25(OH)_2D$ in response to exogenous PTH administration. Therefore, in addition to dietary calcium restriction and avoidance of vitamin D, glucocorticoid therapy to reduce gastrointestinal calcium absorption sometimes is helpful.

Neonatal Hypercalcemia Associated With Subcutaneous Fat Necrosis

Hypercalcemia is an occasional, severe complication of subcutaneous fat necrosis of the newborn (SFN) (Mahé et al, 2007). SFN is a rare, self-limited disorder that may appear up to several weeks after delivery in term or post-term neonates. Frequently, there is a history of difficult delivery, trauma, hypothermia, or asphyxia. Erythematous to violaceous, indurated subcutaneous nodules and plaques often overlie bony prominences on the buttocks, thighs, trunk, cheeks, or arms. Lesions may resemble those of sclerema neonatorum.

Hypercalcemic infants may present with poor weight gain despite adequate energy intake or with nephrocalcinosis. Hypercalcemia should be sought for in all infants with subcutaneous fat necrosis. Laboratory evaluation shows high blood $1,25(OH)_2D$ levels and usually normal phosphorus and alkaline phosphatase. Radiographs of the long bones also are usually normal, although periosteal elevation, features similar to those of WS, or ectopic calcification may be present. Lesion punch biopsy or aspirate specimens show lobular panniculitis with necrotic adipocytes, abundant histiocytes, and giant cells with radial crystals. Magnetic resonance imaging (MRI) may point to the correct diagnosis without biopsy.

Hypercalcemia in SFN, like in other granulomatous disorders, is caused by unregulated production of $1,25(OH)_2D$ by activated macrophages. Lesion prostaglandin E release also may contribute to hypercalcemia and osteoclastic bone resorption. Hypercalcemia associated with SFN may persist for days to weeks. Treatment consists of intravascular volume expansion, furosemide, prednisone, a low-calcium, low-vitamin D diet, and, increasingly, bisphosphonates (pamidronate).

Blue Diaper Syndrome

Blue diaper syndrome is a rare familial disease in which hypercalcemia and nephrocalcinosis are associated with a defect in the intestinal transport of tryptophan (Drummond et al, 1964). Current speculations focus on causal defects in L-type (e.g., LAT2) and T-type (e.g., TAT1) amino acid transporters. Bacterial degradation of tryptophan in the intestine leads to excessive indole production, which is converted to indican in the liver. Oxidative conjugation of indican in the urine forms the water-insoluble dye indigo blue (indigotin), with a consequent peculiar bluish discoloration of the diaper. The clinical course is characterized by failure to thrive, recurrent unexplained fever, infections, marked irritability, and constipation. The mechanism of hypercalcemia is uncertain, although oral tryptophan loading in human subjects and experimental animals also elevates serum calcium. Treatment consists of glucocorticoids and a low-calcium, low–vitamin D diet.

Hypercalcemia Associated With Skeletal Dysplasias

Several skeletal dysplasia syndromes are associated with hypercalcemia. The distinctive phenotypes point to the appropriate diagnosis.

Hypophosphatasia (Mornet, 2007) is a rare autosomal recessive condition caused by mutations in the liver/bone/kidney alkaline phosphatase gene (ALPL) leading to deficiency of the tissue-nonspecific alkaline phosphatase. The perinatal and early infantile onsets are characterized by defective bone (and tooth) mineralization. Depending on the age at diagnosis, six clinical forms are currently recognized: perinatal (lethal), perinatal benign, infantile, childhood, adult, and odontohypophosphatasia. Prominent features of the early-onset, severe forms are respiratory complications, premature craniosynostosis, widespread undermineralization, rickets, and hypercalcemia. Attempts to control the hypercalcemia, hypercalciuria, and chronic bone demineralization using chlorothiazide, calcitonin, and bisphosphonates have been disappointing.

Jansen metaphyseal chrondrodysplasia in newborns is characterized by hypercalcemia and skeletal radiographs that mimic rachitic changes. This severe autosomal recessive disorder results from gain-of-function mutations in the PTHR1 receptor that result in ligand-independent receptor activation (Schipani and Provot, 2003). PTH and PTHrP levels are low or undetectable. The functional consequences are premature chondrocyte maturation, accelerated endochondral bone formation, and hypercalcemia.

Hypercalcemia Associated With Phosphate Depletion

Neonatal hypercalcemia due to phosphate depletion is most often seen in very-low-birthweight (VLBW) infants who are fed unsupplemented human milk. The low phosphate content of human milk leads to hypophosphatemia,

which stimulates renal $1,25(OH)_2D$ synthesis and intestinal calcium absorption. When phosphate is limited, little calcium can be deposited in bone, leading to osteopenia, hypercalcemia, and hypercalciuria. Extremely high serum calcium levels (greater than 15 mg/dL), serum phosphorus less than 2 mg/dL, and suppressed PTH may be observed in VLBW infants in this setting. These infants respond to cautious phosphate replenishment. The condition is preventable by anticipatory monitoring of serum calcium and phosphorus levels in high-risk infants. Hypophosphatemic bone disease in VLBW infants is discussed later (see section Osteopathy of Prematurity).

Vitamin D Toxicity

Excessive supplementation with vitamin D will cause hypercalcemia in newborns and infants. In preterm infants, prolonged feeding with preterm formula or mineral- and vitamin D–supplemented human milk fortifiers also has led to mild to significant hypercalcemia. Infants respond to discontinuation of vitamin D supplements. These occurrences have prompted vitamin reformulation of preterm nutritional products. Laboratory studies in hypervitaminosis D typically show elevated 25(OH)D but not $1,25(OH)_2D$. Serum PTH usually is suppressed by the hypercalcemia. Biochemical resolution may be protracted because vitamin D accumulates in body fat.

Other Causes of Neonatal Hypercalcemia

Hypervitaminosis A and thyrotoxicosis also accelerate bone turnover and can induce hypercalcemia. Tumor-associated hypercalcemia in neonates is extremely rare. Most cases have been associated with congenital mesoblastic nephroma, the most common renal tumor of early infancy. Hypercalcemia in the presence of chronic diarrhea should suggest hereditary disaccharide intolerance type I (congenital sucrase-isomaltase deficiency) or type II (congenital lactase deficiency) (Belmont et al, 2002). Modest hypercalcemia also may occur in acute adrenal insufficiency. The pathogenesis is uncertain. ECMO initiation and prolonged support have been associated with hypercalcemia (greater than 11 mg/dL) (Fridriksson et al, 2001; Hak et al, 2005). The causes appear to be multifactorial.

Treatment

The first principle of the medical management of hypercalcemia is to increase urinary calcium excretion by maximizing glomerular filtration rate (GFR) and urinary sodium excretion. In the normal kidney, sodium and calcium clearances are very closely linked during water or osmotic diuresis. Two-thirds normal to isotonic saline containing 20 to 30 mEq of potassium chloride per liter may be infused intravenously at a rate to correct dehydration and maximize GFR. After rehydration, furosemide (1 mg/kg) may be given intravenously at 6- to 8-hour intervals to inhibit tubular reabsorption of calcium.

When severe hypercalcemia is associated with hypophosphatemia, 30 to 50 mg/kg/day of oral or intravenous phosphorus as a phosphate salt may be given. Unlike sodium, phosphate does not remove calcium from the body but causes a redistribution of calcium. The goal of phosphate therapy is to maintain serum phosphorus levels in a range of 3 to 5 mg/dL. The oral route is preferable because of the potential for serious complications with intravenous phosphate treatment. Therapy usually results in a significant reduction in serum calcium concentration over 1 to 2 days. In more severe and resistant cases, glucocorticoids (e.g., prednisone, 2 mg/kg per day) may be added. Glucocorticoids suppress intestinal calcium absorption and increase renal excretion. Although glucocorticoids are effective in several types of hypercalcemia, they are relatively ineffective for the treatment of hypercalcemia associated with primary hyperparathyroidism. Clinical experience with use of other antihypercalcemic agents has been limited, although bisphosphonates are assuming an increasing role in management of neonatal hypercalcemia and calcium wasting from bone (e.g., Zeitlin et al, 2003).

The mainstays of the *nonacute* treatment of milder neonatal hypercalcemia are restriction of dietary calcium, elimination of vitamin D supplements, and limiting sunlight exposure.

NEONATAL DISORDERS OF SERUM MAGNESIUM

Neonatal hypomagnesemia is discussed in a preceding section (Neonatal Hypocalcemia Associated with Hypomagnesemia or Renal Tubular Necrosis).

Neonatal hypermagnesemia usually is due to maternal magnesium sulfate administration or magnesium in neonatal parenteral nutrition solutions that exceeds magnesium clearance. Later-onset neonatal hypermagnesemia can result from use of magnesium hydroxide–containing antacids (e.g., "milk of magnesia"). The hypermagnesemic newborn may exhibit varying degrees of flaccidity, unresponsiveness, respiratory insufficiency and apnea, ileus, or delayed passage of meconium. These signs may be mistaken for those of perinatal asphyxia. Occasionally, short-term endotracheal intubation and mechanical ventilation are required. Feedings should be deferred until normalization of bowel function occurs. Prolonged fetal hypermagnesemia also increases the risk of meconium obstruction. Aside from this latter possibility, the neonatal effects of hypermagnesemia are usually transient. Generally, newborns effectively excrete a magnesium load, and serial monitoring of serum levels may not be necessary. However, in preterm newborns, who have limited renal magnesium excretory capacity, hypermagnesemia may persist for more than 48 hours. No magnesium should be added to parenteral nutrition solutions until serum magnesium falls. Early hypermagnesemia in preterm infants also may suppress PTH secretion (Rantonen et al, 2001). Finally, infusion of calcium salts may antagonize some of the adverse effects of excess magnesium.

METABOLIC BONE DISEASE IN NEWBORNS AND INFANTS

Forms of metabolic bone disease manifesting in infants and children are listed in Box 90-3. The following are commonly used definitions:

> **BOX 90-3   Forms of Metabolic Bone Disease Manifesting in Newborns and Infants**
>
> Vitamin D deficiency
>   Maternal vitamin D deficiency (congenital rickets)
>   Inadequate intake of dietary vitamin D
>   Lack of adequate sunlight exposure + dietary inadequacy
> Vitamin D malabsorption
>   Hepatic disease (steatorrhea)
>   Short bowel syndrome
>   Pancreatic insufficiency
> Vitamin D metabolic defects
>   Hepatic rickets (inadequate vitamin D 25-hydroxylation)
>   Vitamin D-dependent rickets (VDDR1) defects in 1α-hydroxylation
>   Renal insufficiency (renal osteodystrophy)
>   Anticonvulsants [increased 25(OH)D metabolism]
> Vitamin D receptor defects
>   Vitamin D–resistant rickets (VDRR2)
> Phosphate deficiency rickets
>   Osteopathy of prematurity
>   X-linked hypophosphatemic rickets
>   Fanconi's syndrome
>   Antacid-induced osteopathy (aluminum hydroxide)
>   Tumor (including hemangioma)-associated rickets
> Calcium deficiency rickets
>   Osteopathy of prematurity
>   Inadequate intake of dietary calcium after weaning
>   Inadequate calcium in TPN solution

TPN, Total parenteral nutrition; *25(OH)D*, 25-hydroxyvitamin D.

Osteopenia is defined as radiographic evidence of diminished bone density. Osteopenia is present in rickets, osteomalacia, and osteoporosis.

Rickets is a disorder of the bone matrix, or osteoid, in growing bone resulting from undermineralization of cartilage; it involves both the growth plate (physis) and newly formed trabecular and cortical bone. In infancy, the most rapidly growing bones are the skull, upper limbs, and ribs. Early development of rickets, therefore, leads to craniotabes ("ping-pong ball" sign), widened cranial sutures, frontal bossing, swollen epiphyses of wrists, costochondral beading ("rachitic rosary"), and Harrison's sulcus (caused by diaphragmatic depression of the lower thorax on inspiration). The thoracic osteochondrodystrophy increases risk of pneumonia. Manifestations of muscle weakness (myopathy) may include dilated cardiomyopathy and ventricular dysfunction, which respond to vitamin D therapy (Brown et al, 2009). Radiographic features in rickets result from expansion of the cartilaginous growth plate and delayed mineralization. They include lucency and widening of the gap between metaphysis and epiphysis (the zone of provisional calcification), that is, irregularity, cupping, or fraying of the metaphyseal margin and osteopenia. Serum phosphorus or calcium or both characteristically are depressed and serum alkaline phosphatase is elevated. An exception is the hyperphosphatemia of renal osteodystrophy.

Osteomalacia is rickets that occurs in the absence of linear growth. This is the typical pattern in adults, but it also may occur in poorly nourished preterm infants. In osteomalacia, the radiographic features of rickets at the cartilage-shaft junction are generally absent.

Osteoporosis in adults is defined as a state of reduced bone mass per unit volume with a normal ratio of mineral to matrix. Unlike in rickets and osteomalacia, where mineralization defects predominate, the primary abnormality in osteoporosis is either a decrease in matrix formation or an increase in matrix and mineral resorption. There is no generally accepted pediatric definition for osteoporosis.

OSTEOPATHY OF PREMATURITY

In preterm infants, osteopenia with or without rachitic changes at the cartilage-shaft junction usually appears between 3 and 12 weeks of age. This metabolic bone disorder, which remains very common, has also been called "rickets of prematurity" or "osteopenia of prematurity." "Osteopathy" is probably the most accurate term. The incidence and severity increase with decreasing gestational age and birthweight and are more common in preterm infants having a complicated medical course and delayed nutrition. On the other hand, osteopathy usually is not a problem for healthier, larger preterm infants. In VLBW babies, postnatal bone mineralization significantly lags behind the expected intrauterine bone mineralization rate. The pathogenesis involves increased endosteal resorption more than decreased bone formation—that is, it is a high-turnover osteopathy (Beyers et al, 1994).

The clinical findings in VLBW infants having severe osteopathy, as in older, term infants with rickets, include a widened anterior fontanel, craniotabes, bony expansion of wrists, costochondral beading, and rib or long-bone fractures. Rib undermineralization, softening, and fractures can lead to respiratory distress (especially tachypnea), atelectasis, or pneumonia. However, long-term effects of osteopathy of prematurity may include delayed dental maturation (Seow, 1996) and reduced height and bone mineral density in adulthood (Hovi et al, 2009). Bone mineral density later in childhood and adulthood is also probably influenced by polymorphisms in multiple bone regulatory genes.

Although the clinical features of nutritional rickets in term infants and osteopathy of prematurity are similar, the latter has a distinctive pathogenesis. Preterm osteopathy is caused chiefly by deficiencies in dietary phosphate and calcium, rather than by vitamin D deficiency. Eighty percent of bone mineralization in the fetus occurs during the third trimester, when fetal calcium and phosphorus requirements are at least 100 to 120 mg/kg/day and 60 to 75 mg/kg/day, respectively. Low mineral (especially phosphorus)-content diets predispose preterm infants to osteopathy. The greatest risks for phosphate deficiency result from (1) feeding unsupplemented human milk, (2) milk formulas not designed for use in preterm infants, or (3) prolonged parenteral nutrition. Even close attention to nutrition support does not prevent a high prevalence of bone disease in ELBW infants (Mitchell et al, 2009).

Most often, neither hyperparathyroidism nor vitamin D deficiency is present in phosphate-deficient osteopathy of prematurity. In contrast, the pathogenesis of calcium-deficiency rickets and that of vitamin D deficiency are similar in that hypocalcemia causes hyperparathyroidism. The elevated PTH increases bone resorption and enhances renal 1,25(OH)$_2$D synthesis, which, in turn, increases intestinal calcium and phosphorus absorption. Individual preterm babies may have predominant phosphate depletion, but mixed phosphate and calcium deficiency is more common; isolated calcium deficiency is rare. In dual mineral deficiency, laboratory values may show low, normal, or slightly elevated serum calcium and low to low-normal phosphorus. In cases of severe or complicated bone disease, serum 25(OH)D is a useful screen for evaluating sufficiency of vitamin D stores; levels less than 6 ng/mL indicate *severe* vitamin D deficiency. For evaluating bone mineral status in preterm neonates, measurement of bone cortical thickness and visual inspection of the proximal humerus on a chest radiograph are a simple and effective screen (Figure 90-2).

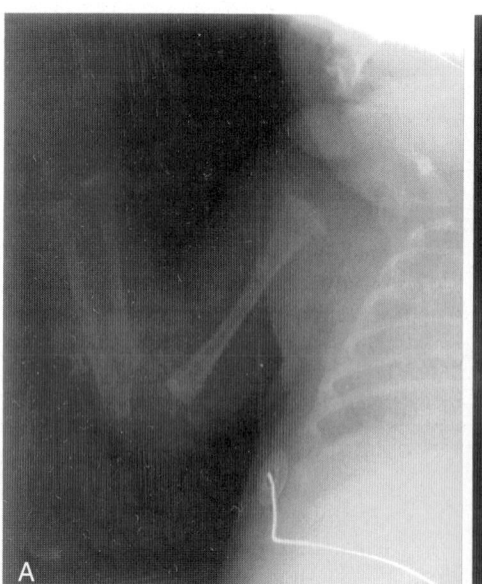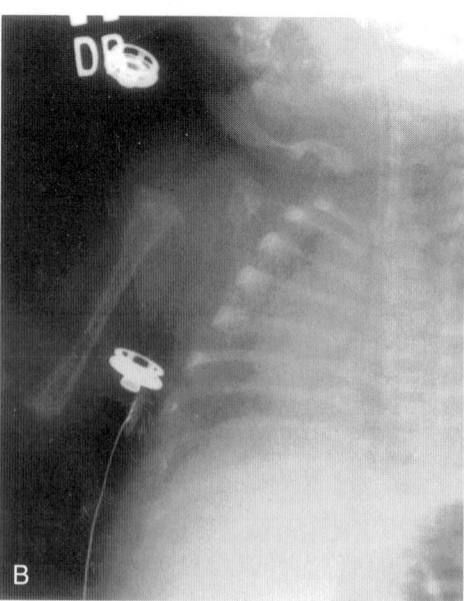

FIGURE 90-2 Chest radiographs from a 700-g-birthweight, 25-week-gestation infant with bronchopulmonary dysplasia and osteopathy of prematurity. **A,** At 34 weeks of postconceptional age, mild osteopenia and metaphyseal changes (especially in right arm and wrist) are evident. **B,** Two weeks later, signs of rachitic healing can be seen in ribs and long bones.

Serum alkaline phosphatase, a marker of osteoblastic bone formation, is frequently used to monitor skeletal metabolism in preterm infants. However, the magnitude of elevations in alkaline phosphatase (or osteocalcin) concentrations is not a good predictor of the extent of bone mineral deficits. Serial urinary biomarkers of bone metabolism (e.g., pyridinoline, deoxypyridinoline) have not yet been shown useful in predicting severe osteopathy, because levels are related to bone volume and normative data for growing preterm infants are lacking. Longitudinal quantitative ultrasound measurement of the speed of sound in long bones, combined with serum bone markers, is a promising assessment tool (Ashmeade et al, 2007). Longitudinal assessment of bone mineral content by dual x-ray absorptiometry is not widely available.

Phosphate depletion and osteopathy occur in rapidly growing preterm infants fed unsupplemented human milk, which has low phosphate content. Characteristically, these infants develop hypophosphatemia, hypophosphaturia, hypercalcemia, and hypercalciuria. Serum PTH may be low or normal, 25(OH)D is normal, and 1,25(OH)$_2$D is elevated. The hypophosphatemia stimulates production of 1,25(OH)$_2$D, which in turn increases intestinal calcium absorption. However, in the presence of hypophosphatemia, only limited amounts of calcium can be deposited in bone, leading to hypercalcemia and hypercalciuria. The hypercalcemia inhibits PTH secretion.

This form of osteopathy does not respond to vitamin D therapy unless vitamin D deficiency also is present. In fact, vitamin D supplementation without prior correction of the underlying dietary phosphate deficiency may aggravate hypercalcemia and hypercalciuria by enhancing intestinal calcium absorption. The bone disease in these infants does respond to increased dietary phosphate, accomplished by adding a human milk supplement designed for preterm infants or switching to a preterm milk formula; both diets provide additional calcium as well as phosphorus. Addition of 20 to 25 mg/kg/day of potassium phosphate also will increase serum phosphorus levels. However, because phosphate repletion promotes bone mineralization, serum calcium may fall to subnormal levels ("hungry bones" syndrome) unless supplemental calcium (e.g., 30 mg/kg/day) also is provided. Recommended intakes of calcium and phosphorus (Demarini, 2005) have benefits of improved bone growth, less severe dolichocephaly, and avoidance of fractures. For infants having a history of osteopathy of prematurity, it is important that after hospital discharge a mineral-enriched diet and serial laboratory monitoring be maintained for several weeks to months.

Human milk has a total antirachitic sterol activity of only 25 to 50 IU/L (Reeve et al, 1982), which may be insufficient for maintaining normal 25(OH)D levels in preterm infants. Therefore, preterm infants fed unsupplemented human milk also should receive 400 to 600 IU daily of vitamin D. Current recommendations are that preterm infants who are feeding fortified human milk or standard high-calcium, high-phosphorus preterm formulas also receive vitamin D supplementation of 400 to 600 IU daily.

Additional, nonnutritional risk factors for osteopathy in ill preterm infants are the early withdrawal of placental estradiol and progesterone, lack of mobility, and therapy with dexamethasone, methylxanthines, or aminoglycosides, any of which can increase urinary calcium excretion and contribute to serum mineral imbalance, nephrocalcinosis, and osteopenia. Mechanical stimulation in preterm and term newborns with musculoskeletal problems is becoming an important therapeutic option (Moyer-Mileur et al, 2008). Glucocorticoids decrease bone formation by inhibiting osteoblast growth and increasing cell death of osteoblasts and osteocytes and, at least over several months, increasing osteoclastogenesis and bone resorption. Copper deficiency is a rare contributor to osteopenia in preterm infants (Olivares and Uauy, 1996).

NUTRITIONAL (VITAMIN D DEFICIENCY) RICKETS

Rickets most often occurs in exclusively breastfed infants who also have little exposure to sunlight and are dark-skinned. Historically, a marked rise in prevalence in nutritional rickets has accompanied industrialization and urban crowding. Clinical rickets often manifests at 3 months of age or later, but onset in early infancy is not uncommon. In developed countries, nutritional rickets has never been eradicated, and there is a resurgence of vitamin D deficiency in North America and Europe (Rovner and O'Brien, 2008). As reviewed (see Hypocalcemia Resulting from Vitamin D Deficiency, earlier), maternal vitamin D deficiency during pregnancy and lactation puts the newborn at high risk. There are long-term deleterious effects on musculoskeletal health (Nabulsi et al, 2008). The 2008 American Academy of Pediatrics (AAP) statement for Prevention of Rickets and Vitamin D Deficiency (Wagner et al, 2008) doubles the previous AAP vitamin D intake recommendation. These new guidelines state that breastfed and partially breastfed infants should be supplemented with 400 IU/day of vitamin D beginning in the first few days of life. All infant formulas available in the United States must contain at least 400 IU/L of vitamin D. Consequently, the guidelines also state all nonbreastfed infants who are ingesting less than 1 L/day of formula should receive a vitamin D supplement of 400 IU/day. Higher doses of vitamin D may be necessary for infants having fat malabsorption or those taking anticonvulsant medications. Vitamin D status should be assessed using 25(OH)D and PTH concentrations and measures of bone mineral status. Stoss therapy, which occasionally is used to treat rickets, consists of a single intramuscular large dose (150,000 to 500,000 IU) of vitamin D.

Nutritional rickets worldwide can be due to degrees of vitamin D deficiency or calcium deficiency. Calcium deficiency is the major cause of rickets in Africa and some parts of tropical Asia, but is being recognized increasingly in other parts of the world (Thacher et al, 2006). As a consequence, in tropical populations, rickets may occur later than at higher latitudes, between 1 and 2 years of age, after weaning and with introduction of a low-calcium diet. A recent study showed, for example, that in Turkey most rachitic children had vitamin D deficiency, whereas in Egypt they had mostly calcium insufficiency combined with vitamin D deficiency (Baroncelli et al, 2008). It is likely that relative deficiencies of calcium and vitamin D interact with genetic (e.g., vitamin D receptor genotypes) and/or environmental factors to stimulate the development of rickets. Therefore, the current North American and European recommendations for vitamin D supplementation may need adjustments for other pediatric populations with limited calcium intake.

Congenital rickets should always prompt an investigation for maternal vitamin D deficiency. Rickets, hypercalciuria, and hypophosphatemia also occur in Fanconi renotubular syndrome. Prolonged treatment with aluminum-containing antacids can induce hypophosphatemia and rickets (Pattaragarn and Alon, 2001). These antacids should be avoided or used with caution during infancy.

RENAL OSTEODYSTROPHY

Because normal renal function is essential for physiologic mineral and bone metabolism, renal insufficiency induces hyperphosphatemia and bone disease. Renal osteodystrophy can be predominantly high or low bone turnover, or the two types may alternate during the clinical course in an individual infant. High bone turnover or osteitis fibrosa is a manifestation of secondary hyperparathyroidism. Parathyroid hyperfunction often occurs early in the course of renal failure. Contributing factors include phosphate retention, impaired renal $1,25(OH)_2D$ synthesis, hypocalcemia, parathyroid gland hyperplasia, and skeletal resistance to PTH actions. Low-turnover osteodystrophy (adynamic bone or osteomalacia) results from suppressed bone formation; it is a major concern in management of dialyzed infants. The relative incidences of renal osteodystrophy in newborns have not been explored.

A principal goal of therapy is to lower serum phosphate in order to prevent hypocalcemia and severe hyperparathyroidism. Phosphate restriction is accomplished with feeding breast milk or Similac PM 60/40. Hypocalcemia and metabolic acidosis should be treated with appropriate supplements. If serum $1,25(OH)_2D$ is low, $1,25(OH)_2D$ therapy will increase intestinal calcium absorption, transcriptionally suppress PTH gene expression, and decrease parathyroid hyperplasia. Serum calcium, phosphorus, and PTH levels, as well as linear growth and bone radiographs, should be serially monitored. Management of severe renal osteodystrophy in neonates is particularly complicated by increased phosphate requirements for growth. Calcium supplementation and use of potent vitamin D metabolites also may produce an "oversuppression" of PTH. As with any complex disorder, effective clinical management requires close monitoring and an integrated team approach.

INHERITED METABOLIC BONE DISEASE IN INFANCY

Several forms of metabolic bone disease or rickets have been described that can present in newborns and infants (DiMeglio and Econs, 2001). Vitamin D–dependent rickets type 1A (VDDR1A) is caused by mutations in the gene encoding 25(OH)D–1α-hydroxylase (CYP27B1). This autosomal recessive disorder is most common in French Canadian kindreds. Muscle weakness and rickets appear shortly after birth. Treatment with 1α-hydroxylated vitamin D analogues induces remission.

Vitamin D–dependent rickets type 2A (VDDR2A) is caused by mutations in the vitamin D receptor (VDR) gene. Affected infants show early-onset rickets, hypocalcemia, elevated serum $1,25(OH)_2D$ levels, secondary hyperparathyroidism, and alopecia. Depending on the genotype, there is a variable response to supraphysiologic doses of $1,25(OH)_2D$ analogues and calcium.

X-linked dominant hypophosphatemia (XLH), also known as familial hypophosphatemic rickets or vitamin D–resistant rickets, is a disorder of phosphate homeostasis. Its prevalence is 1 in 20,000. XLH is characterized by poor linear growth, rickets, and hypophosphatemia associated with a low TmP and renal tubular phosphate leak. Defective regulation of vitamin D metabolism results in inappropriately normal $1,25(OH)_2D$ concentrations in the face of hypophosphatemia. XLH is caused by mutations in the phosphate-regulating endopeptidase homologue, X-linked gene (PHEX). The phenotypes and responses to therapy are highly variable. Autosomal recessive hypophosphatemic rickets (ARHR1 and ARHR2) are caused, respectively, by mutations in the dentin matrix acidic phosphoprotein (DMP1) and ectonucleotide pyrophosphatase/phosphodiesterase 1 (ENPP1) genes that interfere with bone mineralization and renal phosphate handling.

Neonatal rickets with increased bone density rather than osteopenia can occur in infantile osteopetrosis, a rare autosomal recessive disorder of osteoclast formation. Diagnosis may be obscured by concurrent maternal vitamin D deficiency (Popp et al, 2000).

SUGGESTED READINGS

Allgrove J, Shaw NJ, editors: *Calcium and bone disorders in children and adolescents*, Endocr Dev, Basel, 2009, Karger.
Carmeliet G, Van Cromphaut S, Daci E, et al: Disorders of calcium homeostasis, *Best Pract Res Clin Endocrinol Metab* 17:529-546, 2003.
DiMeglio LA, Econs MJ: Hypophosphatemic rickets, *Rev Endocr Metab Disord* 2:165-173, 2001.
Holick MF, Chen TC, Lu Z, Sauter E: Vitamin D and skin physiology: a D-lightful story, *J Bone Miner Res* 22(Suppl 2):V28-V33, 2007.
Kimball S, Fuleihan Gel H, Vieth R: Vitamin D: a growing perspective, *Crit Rev Clin Lab Sci* 45:339-414, 2008.
Kovacs CS: Vitamin D in pregnancy and lactation: maternal, fetal, and neonatal outcomes from human and animal studies, *Am J Clin Nutr* 88:520S-528S, 2008.
Mitchell DM, Jüppner H: Regulation of calcium homeostasis and bone metabolism in the fetus and neonate, *Curr Opin Endocrinol Diabetes Obes* 17:25-30, 2010.
Mustafa A, Bigras JL, McCrindle BW: Dilated cardiomyopathy as a first sign of nutritional vitamin D deficiency in infancy, *Can J Cardiol* 16:699-701, 1999.
Pittard WB 3rd, Geddes KM, Hulsey TC, Hollis BW: Osteocalcin, skeletal alkaline phosphatase, and bone mineral content in very low-birth-weight infants: a longitudinal assessment, *Pediatr Res* 31:181-185, 1992.
Prentice A: Calcium in pregnancy and lactation, *Annu Rev Nutr* 20:249-272, 2000.
Ramasamy I: Inherited disorders of calcium homeostasis, *Clin Chim Acta* 394:22-41, 2008.
Rauch F, Schoenau E: Skeletal development in premature infants: a review of bone physiology beyond nutritional aspects, *Arch Dis Child* 86:F82-F85, 2002.
Rovner AJ, O'Brien KO: Hypovitaminosis D among healthy children in the United States: a review of the current evidence, *Arch Pediatr Adolesc Med* 162:513-519, 2008.
Silver J, Naveh-Many T: Phosphate and the parathyroid, *Kidney Int* 75:898-905, 2009.
Ryan SW, Truscott J, Simpson M, James J: Phosphate, alkaline phosphatase and bone mineralization in preterm infants, *Acta Paediatr* 82:518-521, 1993.

Shalev H, Phillip M, Galil A, et al: Clinical presentation and outcome in primary familial hypomagnesaemia, *Arch Dis Child* 78:127-130, 1998.

Sharma S, Khan N, Khadri A, et al: Vitamin D in pregnancy—time for action: a paediatric audit, *BJOG* 116:1678-1682, 2009.

Stuart AF: Translational implications of the parathyroid calcium receptor, *N Engl J Med* 351:324-326, 2004.

Taylor JA, Geyer LJ, Feldman KW: Use of supplemental vitamin D among infants breastfed for prolonged periods, *Pediatrics* 125:105-111, 2010.

Complete references used in this text can be found online at www.expertconsult.com

DISORDERS OF THE ADRENAL GLAND

Saroj Nimkarn and Maria I. New

THE ADRENAL GLAND

EMBRYOLOGY

The dual embryologic origin of the human adrenal gland results in two distinct parts of the gland, an outer adrenal cortex and an inner adrenal medulla. Each part secretes different vital hormones; therefore normal adrenal function is critically important for maintenance of intrauterine homeostasis, promotion of organ maturation, and adaptation to extrauterine life. Embryologically, the adrenal cortex develops from the coelomic mesoderm of the urogenital ridge, whereas the medulla arises from neural crest tissue in the adjacent sympathetic ganglion at celiac plexus level. During the 5th week of fetal development, mesothelial cells from the posterior abdominal wall, between the root of the bowel mesentery and developing mesonephros, proliferate and form the primitive adrenal cortex. In the 6th week, a second wave of mesothelial cells surrounds the primitive cortex and later forms the adult or definitive cortex. By 8 weeks' gestation, the cortical mass separates from the rest of mesothelial tissue and becomes surrounded by connective tissue (Sadler, 2000). This separation divides adrenocortical and gonadal primodium (Mesiano and Jaffe, 1997). Chromaffin cells, which originate from neural crest, migrate toward the adrenal cortex around this time and gradually invade the medial aspect of the cortical tissue along its central vein to gain central position, forming the adrenal medulla. However, encapsulation of the adrenal medulla does not occur until late fetal development. Postnatally, the fetal or primitive zone of the adrenal gland rapidly involutes to disappear by approximately 6 months of age (Kempna and Fluck, 2008). Zonation of the cortex, zona glomerulosa, and fasciculata is present at birth, but full differentiation into three separate zones occurs much later, at approximately 3 years of age, when zona reticularis development takes place (Barwick et al, 2005). This chapter focuses on the development, function, and pathophysiology of the steroidogenic adrenal cortex.

MORPHOLOGY

The adrenal glands are bilateral structures, located above the kidneys in the retroperitoneum area. At birth, the adrenals are 10- to 20-fold larger than the adult glands relative to body weight, thereby approximating one third the size of neonatal kidneys (Moore and Persaud, 1998). In late fetal and neonatal phases, the glands predominantly consist of cortex, where active production of glucocorticoids, steroid precursors, estrogens, and progesterone occurs during the third trimester and the first 3 months after birth. Ultrasonographically, the neonatal adrenal gland characteristically has a thin reflective core surrounded by a thick transonic zone. The gland subsequently decreases in size

as the active fetal cortex regresses to reach approximately 8% of the kidney size in adulthood (Barwick et al, 2005).

Histologically, the fetal adrenal cortex consists of a small outer definitive zone, which appears to produce few adrenal steroid hormones until late gestation, and a larger inner fetal zone that produces adrenal steroid hormones throughout gestation. In addition, there is a transitional zone where cortisol production takes place toward the end of fetal development (Mesiano and Jaffe, 1997). At birth, the large fetal zone of the fetal adrenal involutes and disappears by 6 months of age. Concurrently, the definitive zone together with the transitional zone develops into the fully differentiated zona glomerulosa and fasciculata by the age of 3 years. The zona reticularis begins to develop only after 4 years of age and may not be fully differentiated before the age of 15 years. In an adult adrenal gland, these three distinctive zones lie adjacent to one another. The zona glomerulosa is located immediately below the capsule, the zona fasciculata being in the middle, and the innermost zone next to the medulla is the zona reticularis.

FETAL AND ADULT ADRENAL FUNCTIONS

A cascade of adrenal steroidogenesis in adult is shown in Figure 91-1. Three major pathways of mineralocorticoid, glucocorticoid, and androgen synthesis take place mainly in the glomerulosa, fasciculata, and reticularis zones of the cortex, respectively. Aldosterone is the main mineralocorticoid regulating sodium and fluid volume homeostasis; it is under the control of the renin-angiotensin system and blood potassium concentrations (Kuhnle et al, 1981). The principal glucocorticoid in humans is cortisol, with a wide range of roles in regulating body functions, from carbohydrate metabolism, immune system, and acute and chronic stress response to musculoskeletal metabolism. Cortisol production is regulated through a negative feedback loop involving hypothalamic corticotropin-releasing hormone (CRH) and pituitary adrenocorticotropic hormone (ACTH) (New and Wilson, 1999). Adrenal androgens have an age-specific secretion profile from adrenarche around the time of puberty and a gradual decrease with aging until andropause (Orentreich et al, 1984). The regulatory mechanism behind normal adrenal androgen production is largely unknown, but involves ACTH to some extent (Hanley and Arlt, 2006).

In the fetal adrenal gland, steroidogenic enzymes are found as early as 7 weeks' gestation (Goto et al, 2006; Hanley and Arlt, 2006). At 8 weeks' gestation, the fetal adrenal gland produces cortisol under ACTH control. A transient expression of 3β-hydroxysteroid dehydrogenase type 2 (3β-HSD2) during this critical time from 7 to 12 weeks' gestation allows the fetal adrenal gland to produce cortisol. Activation of 3β-HSD2 serves principally to prevent

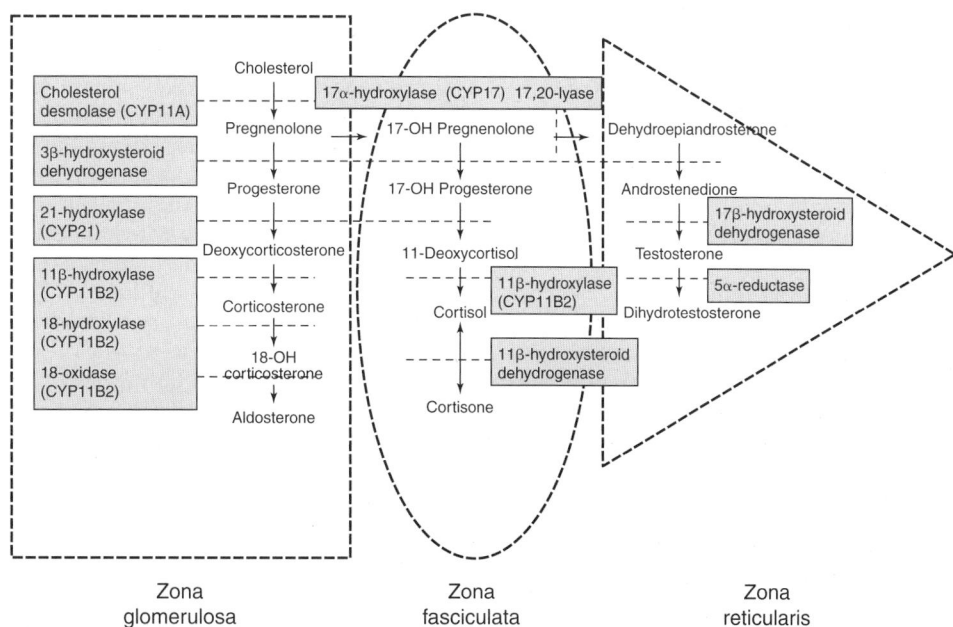

FIGURE 91-1 Steroidogenesis of the adult adrenal gland. Each of the three biosynthetic pathways take place in different zones: aldosterone biosynthesis in zona glomerulosa, cortisol biosynthesis in zona fasciculata, and androgen production in zona reticularis. The enzymes that catalyze the reactions are indicated in *boxes*.

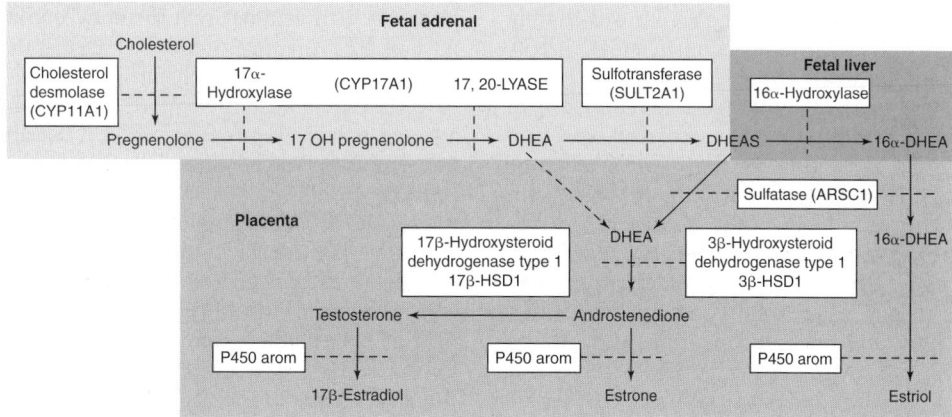

FIGURE 91-2 Steroidogenesis of the fetal adrenal gland and fetoplacental unit. Predominant DHEA and DHEAS production occurs after 12 weeks' gestation.

virilization of the female genital enlage because of overwhelming amounts of DHEAS and its downstream androgen metabolites. It is believed that a transient peak of cortisol during this time suppresses the fetal hypothalamic-pituitary-adrenal (HPA) axis, keeping DHEAS production at a low level (Goto et al, 2006; White, 2006). By the end of the first trimester, cortisol secretion from the fetal adrenal gland begins to wane as a result of decrease in 3β-HSD2 expression, thus decreasing HPA axis suppression with resultant increased DHEAS secretion. During the second and third trimesters, the fetal adrenal gland secretes abundant amounts of DHEA and its sulfated derivative DHEAS, earning the term *androgen factory* (Kempna and Fluck, 2008). The rate of steroid secretion by the fetal adrenal glands may be fivefold that of the adult adrenal glands at rest (Carr and Simpson, 1981). Placenta can also convert DHEAS back to DHEA by a sulfatase enzyme (i.e., arylsulfatase). These adrenal steroids serve as precursors for P450C17 and 17,20

lyase enzymes for androgen production and subsequent estrogen production (Figure 91-2). In addition, DHEAS is oxidized in the fetal liver to a 16α-hydroxylated derivative, which is converted by the placenta to estriol by the same set of enzymes as in estradiol synthesis.

The physiology of human pregnancy involves a continuous supply of relatively increased amount of estrogens. In near term human pregnancy, the rate of estrogen production increases strikingly, reaching concentrations 1000-fold greater than that of nonpregnant women (Carr and Simpson, 1981). During early gestation, the estradiol required to maintain pregnancy is provided by the corpus luteum of the maternal ovary. But after 8 weeks' gestation, most of the estradiol is synthesized by the fetoplacental unit (Simpson and MacDonald, 1981).

As mentioned earlier, DHEAS is the main steroid secreted by the fetal adrenal cortex from mid-gestation onward. The activity of 3β-HSD2 controls the fetal cortisol synthesis. By the end of pregancy, fetal cortisol is required in preparation for parturition (i.e., lung maturation or surfactant production) and could have a role in triggering parturition, as shown in other species (Gross et al, 2000). Maternal cortisol cannot normally reach the fetus because it is oxidized to cortisone, an inactive steroid, by placental 11β-hydroxysteroid dehydrogenase type 2 (Wilson et al, 2001). When pregnancy approaches term, *HSD3B2* expression increases again and remains high, allowing increased cortisol secretion. In a child, 3β-HSD2 secretion is high in the adrenal gland until adrenarche, when 3β-HSD2 activity decreases again to allow an increase in DHEA (Gell et al, 1998) and its downstream androgen metabolite secretion, which gives rise to the development of pubic and axillary hair.

CONTROL OF GLUCOCORTICOID AND MINERALOCORTICOID PRODUCTION

Two distinct regulatory circuits control adrenal glucocorticoid and mineralocorticoid secretion. The HPA axis determines the set point for circulating glucocorticoid (cortisol) concentration. The neuropeptide CRH and arginine vasopressin are synthesized in the hypothalamic paraventricular nucleus and released into the hypophysial portal circulation at the median eminence in response to stress (Aguilera, 1994) and, beginning at approximately 6 months of age, to circadian cues (Onishi et al, 1983). These neuropeptides stimulate the release of ACTH from the anterior pituitary corticotrophs. ACTH released into the systemic circulation augments adrenocortical secretion of DHEA and cortisol by acting on the ACTH receptor (Clark and Cammas, 1996), a member of the melanocortin receptor family. The ACTH receptor is present on steroidogenic cells of the fetal zone and transitional zone of the fetal adrenal as well as the adult adrenal cortex. The resulting increase in plasma cortisol concentration limits further release of hypothalamic neuropeptides and ACTH by negative feedback through glucocorticoid receptors at the central nervous system and pituitary sites. As a corollary, if glucocorticoid production is impaired by intrinsic adrenal dysfunction, then neuropeptide and ACTH release are augmented.

The components of the HPA axis are present early in human development (Mesiano and Jaffe, 1997). As detailed earlier, the fetal adrenal gland begins to develop at 4 weeks' gestation, when initial evagination of the pituitary primordium occurs (Conklin, 1968). ACTH-producing pituitary cells can be detected at 7 weeks' gestation, and an intact hypophysial portal vascular system is present by 12 weeks' gestation (Baker and Jaffe, 1975; Thliveris and Currie, 1980). Nerve terminals containing CRH can be detected in the hypothalamus by approximately 16 weeks' gestation. Virilization caused by increased production of adrenal androgens in females with congenital adrenal hyperplasia occurs before 12 weeks' gestation; therefore ACTH-producing corticotrophs must undergo cortisol-mediated feedback modulation at the initial stages of hypothalamic-pituitary development (White, 2006).

Mineralocorticoid (aldosterone) release by the zona glomerulosa of the adrenal cortex is determined by the renin-angiotensin system, with acute modulation to a lower extent by ACTH as well (Dzau, 1988). Decreases in vascular volume result in increased secretion of renin by the renal juxtaglomerular apparatus. Renin, a proteolytic enzyme, cleaves angiotensinogen to angiotensin I. Angiotensin I is then cleaved and activated by angiotensin-converting enzyme in the lung and other peripheral sites to angiotensin II. Angiotensin II and its metabolite angiotensin III possess vasopressor and potent aldosterone secretory activity. Although angiotensin II receptors are present on cells of the definitive zone at 16 weeks' gestation, significant aldosterone production by the fetal adrenal gland does not occur until the third trimester of pregnancy (Mesiano and Jaffe, 1997).

MOLECULAR BASIS OF ADRENAL DEVELOPMENT

Several transcription factors are critically important for normal adrenal development. Two related transcription factors have emerged as key regulators of adrenal development: the nuclear receptors DAX1 (dosage-sensitive sex reversal, adrenal hypoplasia congenita [AHC], critical region on the X chromosome, gene-1, NR0B1/*AHC*) and steroidogenic factor-1 (SF1, *NR5A1*, also known as Ad4BP). SF1 knockout mice lack adrenal glands and gonads, and subsequent identification of SF1 mutations in humans with adrenal insufficiency confirms the essential role of SF1 in development (Parker, 1998). SF1 expression is found in the early urogenital ridge of the mouse in cells that give rise to both the bipotential gonad and adrenal cortex. Expression of SF1 remains high throughout embryogenesis, the postnatal period, and adult life (Parker, 1998).

DAX1 (dosage-sensitive sex reversal–adrenal hypoplasia congenita critical region on the X chromosome) is an orphan nuclear receptor that colocalizes with SF1 in the cells of adrenal glands, gonads, gonadotropes, and ventral-medial lateral nucleus of the hypothalamus. Deletion of DAX1 results in adrenal hypoplasia congenita. Although the exact role of DAX1 in adrenal development is not known, it has been shown to interact with SF1 (Ikeda et al, 2001). Normally, DAX1 recruits the nuclear corepressor N-CoR to SF1 and represses SF1 (Crawford et al, 1998)

Similarly, the WT1 (Wilms' tumor gene) protein has been shown to interact with SF1. *WT1* encodes 24 different protein isoforms that act as transcription factors. WT1 is detected in the urogenital ridge of the mouse embryo, but is not detected in adult or fetal adrenals. Mutations in *WT1* have resulted in abnormal development of the adrenal in the mouse, but have not been clearly correlated with abnormal human adrenal development (Vidal and Schedl, 2000).

ASSESSING ADRENAL FUNCTION IN THE NEWBORN

Significant evolution of adrenal steroid production occurs over the first days and months of life as the adrenal cortex plays a major role in the newborn infant's postnatal adaptation. During interpretation of the newborn adrenal steroidogenic function, special attention must be paid to age-related changes in adrenal steroid intermediates, circulating cortisol, and aldosterone concentrations that reflect ongoing adrenal maturation (Lashansky et al, 1991; Sippell et al, 1978, 1980). For example, until at least 1 month postnatally, a large proportion of cortisol and its metabolites are excreted as sulfate esters. This sulfation may serve to inactivate a number of circulating cortisol metabolites during fetal and neonatal life (Ducharme et al, 1970).

As mentioned previously, immediately after birth the third-trimester fetal zone that once was the predominant component of the adrenal cortex in the fetus and preferentially produced DHEA and DHEAS, starts to reduce in size. This rapid loss of the fetal zone during this period results in a dramatic fall of the circulating DHEA concentration over the 1st week to 1 month postnatally. The variable pattern of decline in the ensuing weeks probably reflects variation in remodeling of the fetal zone and emergence of the zona fasciculata of the definitive zone, the latter being feature of an adult cortex. In addition to diminished 3β-HSD2 activity, preterm infants have sustained elevations in 17-hydroxyprogesterone and the 17-hydroxyprogesterone-to-cortisol ratio, suggesting a reduction in 21-hydroxylase activity (al Saedi et al, 1995; Lee et al, 1989). Because blood-spot 17-hydroxyprogesterone concentration is used for newborn screening of congenital adrenal hyperplasia (CAH) in many states (White, 2009), many preterm infants initially have an abnormal test result. Subsequent follow-up testing is then required to determine whether CAH is present. Plasma aldosterone concentrations tend to be higher in preterm infants than in term infants, both of which in turn are higher than in older children and adults (Doerr et al, 1988; Kotchen et al, 1972).

Cortisol has a critical role in maintaining homeostasis in response to stress. Relative adrenal insufficiency occurs when the hypothalamic-pituitary-adrenal axis produces less than adequate cortisol for the degree of illness or stress. Immaturity of the adrenal gland and the HPA axis of the premature newborn infant suggests a rationale for why preterm infants are at increased risk of cortisol insufficiency (Fernandez and Watterberg, 2009). Clinicians are commonly faced with critically ill infants who have cardiovascular insufficiency with hypotension, a condition that has also been associated with adverse consequences. The question often arises as to whether these manifestations reflect underlying glucocorticoid insufficiency. There is increasing evidence that relative adrenal insufficiency may be a cause of hemodynamic instability and hypotension in the crtically ill newborn, but there is definitely a paucity of data in this population.

Random plasma cortisol measurement is often inadequate to answer this question, because the majority of critically ill newborns have low cortisol and ACTH values, without the expected increase in response to critical illness. However, response to exogenous ACTH (cosyntropin) is usually normal, suggesting that the inadquate response to critical illness in these newborns does not result from adrenal dysfunction, but arises from some other components of the HPA axis (Fernandez et al, 2008). Interestingly, in extremely low-birthweight infants (500 to 999 g) low cortisol concentrations were not predictive of adverse short-term mortality and morbidity. In contrast, high basal cortisols were associated with severe intraventricular hemorrhage, and extremely elevated values were associated with morbidity and death (Aucott et al, 2008).

Data associating treatment of adrenal insufficiency with outcomes in the term newborn are limited, and there have been no studies on outcomes beyond the immediate neonatal period. Nonetheless, no adverse events have been attributed to glucocorticoid treatment based on a relatively small number of study subjects. A multicenter, randomized trial of hydrocortisone treatment for prophylaxis of relative adrenal insufficiency is currently underway (Aucott et al, 2008). Currently there is insufficient evidence to support the routine use of glucocorticoids in critically ill newborns. On encountering an infant with vasopressor-resistant hypotension, accompanied by signs of cardiac hypofunction, the clinician must consider the risk-to-benefit ratio before arriving at the appropiate management. Therapeutic trials with hydrocortisone at the dose of 1 mg per kilogram of body weight have been suggested (Fernandez and Watterberg, 2009) and can be discontinued if there is no clinical improvement or if the pretreatment cortisol level is later observed to be greater than 15 µg/dL. Special attention should be paid to the premature newborn who concurrently is receiving indomethacin, because this combination is associated with spontaneous gastrointestinal perforation (Peltoniemi et al, 2005).

PRIMARY ADRENAL DISORDERS

STEROIDOGENIC DEFECTS CAUSED BY ADRENAL ENZYME DEFICIENCY

Congenital adrenal hyperplasia refers to a family of inherited disorders in which defects occur in one of the enzymatic steps required to synthesize cortisol from cholesterol in the adrenal gland; therefore impaired cortisol synthesis is the cornerstone shared by all forms of CAH. The pathway of steroidogenesis in the adrenal cortex is illustrated in Figure 91-1. Five forms of CAH with autosomal recessive mode of inheritance are summarized in this section.

Disorders That Lead to Virilization in Females

21-Hydroxylase Deficiency

Pathophysiology

In 21-hydroxylase deficiency (21-OHD), responsible for 90% to 95% of all CAH cases, the conversion of 17α-hydroxyprogesterone (17-OHP), the main substrate of the 21-hydroxylase enzyme, to 11-deoxycortisol in the pathway of cortisol synthesis is impaired and precursors are shunted through the androgen pathway. The enzyme defect also impairs the conversion of progesterone to aldosterone, causing abnormal salt loss (New and Seaman, 1970; New et al, 1966). There are two forms of classic 21-OHD: simple virilizing and salt wasting, distinguished by the adrenal gland's ability to produce adequate aldosterone. In both forms, severe 21-OHD results in elevated levels of adrenal androgens that cause ambiguous genitalia in the genetic female fetus. Diagnosis is made by the detection of extremely high concentrations of basal and stimulated 17-OHP after performing an ACTH stimulation test. The diagnosis is confirmed by molecular genetic analysis of the *CYP21* gene.

Clinical Signs and Symptoms

Females with simple virilizing CAH can be diagnosed at birth immediately because of the apparent genital ambiguity (Prader, 1958). For newborn males, however, differentiation of the external genitalia is not affected, because the main source of testosterone is the testes and not the adrenal gland. Postnatally, genitalia may continue to virilize because of an excess of adrenal androgens, and pseudoprecocious puberty can occur. In affected adolescent females, signs of hyperandrogenism include facial, axillary, and pubic hair, adult body odor, temporal balding, severe acne, irregular menses, and reduced fertility. Poor control of adrenal androgens in males has been associated with small testes, infertility, and short stature. Infertility occurs because the excess androgens are aromatized peripherally to estrogens, which suppress pituitary gonadotropins and function of the gonads. The high estrogens also advance bone age. The high levels of androgens can also accelerate growth in early childhood, producing an unusually tall and muscular child. Thus, the patients are tall children but short adults. The salt-wasting phenotype, which occurs in approximately 75% of CAH cases (New and White, 1995), is biochemically distinct from the simple virilizing form because of a deficiency of aldosterone, the salt-retaining hormone (New et al, 1966; Nimkarn et al, 2007). Resulting hyponatremia, hyperkalemia, high plasma renin activity, and fluid volume depletion are potentially fatal.

Epidemiology

Newborn screening worldwide of almost 6.5 million babies has demonstrated an overall incidence of 1:15,000 live births for the classic form of 21 OHD (Pang and Clark, 1990, 1993; Pang et al, 1988). The incidence of classic CAH in either homogeneous or heterogeneous general populations is as high as 1 case per 7500 live births (Speiser et al, 1985).

Molecular Genetics

Hormonally and clinically defined forms of 21 OHD CAH are associated with distinct genotypes characterized by varying enzyme activity demonstrated by in vitro expression studies. The gene encoding 21 hydroxylase is a microsomal cytochrome P450, family 21, subfamily A, polypeptide 21 (*CYP21A2*) located on the short arm of chromosome 6, within the human leukocyte antigen complex (Dupont et al, 1977; Nebert et al, 1991). *CYP21A2* and its homolog the pseudogene *CYP21A1P* alternate with two genes, *C4B* and *C4A*, that encode two isoforms of the fourth component of the serum complement system (White et al, 1986). More than 100 mutations have been described to date. These mutations include point mutations, small deletions, small insertions, and complex rearrangements of the gene (Stenson et al, 2003). The most common mutations appear to be the result of two types of meiotic recombination between *CYP21A2* and *CYP21A1P*: (1) misalignment and unequal crossing over, resulting in large-scale DNA deletions, and (2) apparent gene conversion events that result in the transfer to *CYP21A2* of smaller-scale deleterious mutations present in the *CYP21A1P* pseudogene. It is not always possible to accurately predict the phenotype on the basis of the genotype; such predictions have been shown to be 79% to 88% accurate (Speiser et al, 1992; Wedell et al, 1992; Wilson et al, 1995) with some nonconcordance. Studies have demonstrated that there is often a divergence in phenotypes within mutation-identical groups, the reason for which requires further investigation (Chemaitilly et al, 2005; Krone et al, 2000).

Management Issues

Hormonal replacement therapy with corticosteroids is used to correct the deficiency in cortisol secretion, which will in turn suppress ACTH overproduction and subsequent stimulation of the androgen pathway (New and Wilson, 1999). Thus, further virilization is prevented, allowing normal growth and onset of puberty. The dose of cortisol required is usually 15 to 20 mg/m^2/day divided into two to three doses per day (Clayton et al, 2002; New et al, 2006). It is important that the appropriate balance must be maintained to avoid hypercortisolism, which can result in Cushing's syndrome and suppression of linear growth. Attempts to suppress 17OHP levels to normal will inevitably result in iatrogenic Cushing's syndrome. Hormonal control can be difficult to achieve in many cases, and adrenalectomy may be offered as an alternative therapeutic option in select patients (Gmyrek et al, 2002; New, 1996; Van Wyk et al, 1996). Patients with salt-losing CAH have elevated plasma renin activity and require mineralocorticoid replacement with 0.05 to 0.2 mg per day of fludrocortisone. In infancy, patients also require oral salt supplement as in other forms of primary adrenal insufficiency. Because females with classic 21 OHD CAH are born with ambiguous genitalia caused by the production of excess androgens in utero, corrective surgery is contemplated. However, before surgical correction is considered as a form of treatment in patients with ambiguous genitalia, consultation with the patient's parents, psychoendocrinologists, pediatric endocrinologists, and pediatric urologists is essential. Prevention of antenatal virilization in affected females is possible with proper prenatal diagnosis and treatment program. The disease can be diagnosed prenatally through molecular genetic analysis of fetal DNA. Appropiate prenatal treatment by dexamethasone administration before the 9 weeks' gestation to the pregnant mother carrying an at-risk fetus is effective in reducing virilization in the genetic female, making postnatal genitoplasty unnecessary and thereby avoiding potential impairment of sexual function. After diagnosis is made by fetal DNA analysis obtained from chorionic villus sampling at 8 to 12 weeks' gestation, therapy in unaffected or male fetuses is discontinued (Nimkarn and New, 2006). There are accurate, compelling data from the largest human studies (Forest et al, 1989; Mercado et al, 1995; New et al, 2001) indicating the benefit of prenatal treatment and that it is safe in the short term for both the fetus and the mother. Preliminary data from long-term studies also support these results (Nimkarn and New, 2009), although long-term follow-up studies are still underway.

11β-Hydroxylase Deficiency

Pathophysiology

The 11β-hydroxylase deficiency (11β-OHD) form of congenital adrenal hyperplasia represents 5% to 8% of all cases in the general population (White et al, 1994).

Deficiency of this enzyme results in an accumulation of 11-deoxysteroid precursors, which are shunted into the androgen pathway. Excess adrenal androgen secretion results in ambiguous genitalia in the affected female fetus. Hypertension in patients with this disorder is commonly attributed to deoxycorticosterone (DOC)-induced sodium retention (Nimkarn and New, 2008b). The hallmark serum abnormality in patients with 11β-OHD is suppressed renin, because hypokalemia is not uniformly present in all cases. Diagnosis is made by extremely high basal and stimulated levels of DOC and compound S after performing an ACTH stimulation test. The diagnosis can be confirmed by molecular genetic analysis of the *CYP11B1* gene.

Clinical Signs and Symptoms

Hypertension occurs in approximately two thirds of patients with 11β-OHD and distinguishes 11β-OHD from the more common 21 OHD in cases of virilizing CAH (Nimkarn and New, 2008b; Rosler et al, 1982). However, hypertension correlates variably with the presence of hypokalemia or with the extent of virilization (Rosler et al, 1982). Patients can present with or without hypokalemic alkalosis. It is usually not identified until later in childhood or in adolescence, although its appearance in early childhood has been documented. A patient was positively identified by the newborn screening program aiming for 21 OHD CAH (Peter et al, 2008).

Epidemiology

Classic 11β-OHD CAH occurs in approximately 1 in 100,000 births in the general white population (Zachmann et al, 1983). A large number of cases have been reported in Israel, where the incidence was estimated to be 1 in 5000 to 1 in 7000 births, with a gene frequency of 1 in 71 to 1 in 83. Subsequent study showed that 11β-OHD CAH occurred in a lower frequency (Paperna et al, 2005), yet remains more common in this population than in others. This unexpected clustering of cases was traced to Jewish families of North African origin, particularly from Morocco and Tunisia (Rosler et al, 1992).

Molecular Genetics

Two 11β-hydroxylase genes have been identified within the human adrenal cortex, each encoding for a different enzyme with distinct enzymatic ability. The two genes *CYP11B1* and *CYP11B2* are located 30 to 40 kilobases apart on chromosome 8q (Chua et al, 1987; Taymans et al, 1998). Although gene conversions occur between *CYP11B1* and *CYP11B2* (Merke et al, 1998; Mulatero et al, 1998), the majority of the mutations found in *CYP11B1* are random point mutations (Curnow et al, 1993; Rosler et al, 1982; White et al, 1991; Zachmann et al, 1983), unlike what was found in 21 OHD CAH. To date, approximately 41 mutations in *CYP11B1* from individuals of diverse ethnic backgrounds have been identified (Krawczak and Cooper, 2003).

Management Issues

Similar to 21-OHD CAH, glucocorticoid therapy is the most effective means of regaining hormonal control in patients with 11β-OHD. Corticosteroids at the same dose range as for 21-OHD CAH provide feedback inhibition of ACTH, reduce stimulation of the androgen pathway, and allow normal growth and the onset of puberty. Treatment with corticosteroids also contributes to the reduction of DOC and thus controls hypertension. Through careful clinical monitoring, doses can be continuously adjusted to match patients' needs while avoiding suppression of linear growth caused by overdosing. In addition to hormonal therapy, reduced salt intake is often used to reduce fluid volume and hypertension. Maintaining fluid balance in children, however, is often difficult and poses an ongoing challenge to treatment. Affected females suffer from genital ambiguity and may require genital reconstructive surgery after multidisciplinary consultations. To prevent antenatal virilization, a similar protocol to 21 OHD CAH for prenatal diagnosis and treatment can be performed (Cerame et al, 1999).

Disorders That Lead to Undervirilized Males

17-Hydroxylase (CYP 17) Deficiency

Pathophysiology

This form of CAH involves an enzyme that catalyzes more than one reaction—namely both the 17α-hydroxylation and 17,20-lyase reactions—and both reactions are commonly impaired in the disorder. Affected individuals cannot produce cortisol but synthesize large amounts of corticosterone (a weak glucocorticoid that mitigates the adrenal insufficiency) and deoxycorticosteroid, which causes hypertension and hypokalemia. Deficiency of 17,20-lyase impairs the ability to synthesize androgens and estrogens and cause male pseudohermaphroditism, the new term being 46,XY disorder of sex development (DSD) (Hughes et al, 2006), at birth and results in failure to virilize at puberty. Affected females have primary amenorrhea and clinical hypogonadism (Auchus, 2001; Yanase et al, 1991).

Clinical Features

The typical features of complete deficiency include hypertension and hypokalemia with associated sexual infantilism in genetic females and pseudohermaphroditism and sexual infantilism in genetic males. Nevertheless, there is considerable variability in the clinical and biochemical features, including a few mutations that cause isolated 17,20-lyase deficiency (Auchus, 2001). The age of onset of hypertension and the severity of hypokalemia are highly variable, even among individuals with the same mutations (Costa-Santos et al, 2004). Sexual infantilism is more consistent.

Epidemiology

This disorder has an estimated frequency in most countries of approximately 1 case per 50,000 newborns and accounts worldwide for approximately 1% of all cases of congenital adrenal hyperplasia (Yanase et al, 1991). However, CYP17 deficiency is the second most common cause of CAH in Brazil (Costa-Santos et al, 2004; Santos et al, 1998), and this remarkable frequency is the result of two founder effects in areas with high coefficients of inbreeding so that two mutations account for more than 80% of cases in that country (Costa-Santos et al, 2004).

Molecular Genetics

Since the cloning of the gene (Picado-Leonard and Miller, 1987) nearly 50 different mutations have been described in *CYP17* (Krawczak and Cooper, 1997). Founder effects probably explain the high incidence of the disease in other patient populations in the Netherlands and Japan (Costa-Santos et al, 2004). Severity of disease tends to be milder with mutations that retain partial catalytic activity, but the nature of the variability in hypertension and hypokalemia is unclear.

Management Issues

Adequate glucocorticoid administration suppresses ACTH and the excessive mineralocorticoid secretion and generally normalizes the blood pressure. Adult females and males reared as females require estrogen therapy. Abdominal testes should be removed because of the risk of malignancy. Adult genetic males reared as males need surgical correction of the external genitalia and androgen replacement.

3β-Hydroxysteroid Dehydrogenase Type II Deficiency

Pathophysiology

3β-Hydroxysteroid dehydrogenase converts 3β-hydroxy $^5\Delta$ steroids to 3-keto $^4\Delta$ steroids and is essential for the biosynthesis of mineralocorticoids, glucocorticoids, and sex steroids (Mebarki et al, 1995). Two forms of the enzyme have been described in humans: type 1 enzyme expressed in placenta and skin, and type 2 expressed in adrenal glands and gonads. The type 1 and 2 genes are known to be closely linked on chromosomal region 1p13.1. The two forms are closely related in structure and substrate specificity, although the type 1 enzyme has higher substrate affinity and a fivefold greater enzymatic activity than for type 2 (Simard et al, 2005).

Clinical Signs and Symptoms

3β-HSD2 enzyme is essential for the formation of progesterone, the precursor for aldosterone, 17-OHP, the precursor for cortisol in the adrenal cortex, androstenedione, testosterone, and estrogen. Simultaneous 3β-HSD2 deficiency in both gonads and adrenal glands result in incomplete virilization of the external genitalia in males. Male patients with 3β-HSD2 deficiency present with ambiguous external genitalia, characterized by micropenis, perineal hypospadias, bifid scrotum, and blind vaginal pouch (Simard et al, 1994) with or without salt loss (Mebarki et al, 1995). Gynecomastia is common at pubertal stage in affected males. In females, virilization of external genitalia occurs as a result of the androgen effect from the peripheral conversion of circulating $^5\Delta$ precursors to active $^4\Delta$ steroids; therefore genital ambiguity can result in both sexes. Clinical presentations also include salt wasting crisis, premature pubic hair development, hirsutism, and menstrual disorders (Lutfallah et al, 2002).

Epidemiology

The exact frequency of this rare disorder remains unknown.

Molecular Genetics

The disorder has an autosomal recessive inheritance. *HSD3B2* is the gene responsible for 3β-HSD2 deficiency CAH. There are approximately 40 mutations in the *HSD3B2* gene already described (Krawczak and Cooper, 2003). Mutations that lead to the abolition of 3β-HSD2 activity lead to the salt-wasting form (Alos et al, 2000; Chang et al, 1993; Lutfallah et al, 2002; Rheaume et al, 1992). Mutations that reduce but do not abolish type II activity lead to CAH with mild or no salt loss, which in males is associated with pseudohermaphroditism (46,XY DSD) as a result of the reduction in androgen synthesis (Lutfallah et al, 2002). Mild mutations were also associated with hyperandrogenic symptoms of premature pubic hair development and hirsutism (Mermejo et al, 2005; Pang et al, 2002).

Management Issues

Similar to other forms of CAH, corticosteroid is the mainstay therapy. Salt-wasting phenotypes in some patients can be managed the same way as the salt-wasting form of 21 OHD CAH. Male patients with 3β-HSD2 deficiency have ambiguous external genitalia. Although most males are raised as males and retain the male social sex at puberty (Mendonca et al, 2008), gender identity is an important management issue. In one Brazilian family, two cousins with 46,XY DSD caused by 3β-HSD2 deficiency were reared as females; one of them was castrated in childhood and retained the female social sex; the other was not castrated in childhood and changed to male social sex at puberty (Mendonca et al, 1987).

Male patients may require testosterone replacement therapy during puberty and adulthood. The aim of the surgical treatment in this condition is to allow development of adequate external genitalia and remove internal structures that are inappropriate for the social sex. Patients must undergo surgical sex reversal procedure preferably before 2 years of age, which is the time when the child becomes aware of his or her genitals and social sex. Only skilled surgeons with specific training in the surgery of DSD should perform these procedures (Hughes et al, 2006).

Lipoid Congenital Adrenal Hyperplasia

Lipoid CAH is a severe form of congenital adrenal insufficiency. Affected patients exhibit glucocorticoid and mineralocorticoid deficiencies early in life, and males exhibit undervirilization. The reduced synthesis of steroids in patients with lipoid CAH results from an inability to transfer cholesterol to the inner mitochondrial membrane where the cholesterol side-chain cleavage complex is located (Lin et al, 1995). It is characterized by lipid droplet accumulation in the cytoplasm of the adrenocortical cells. Most cases of lipoid CAH are caused by recessive mutations in the gene encoding steroidogenic acute regulatory protein (StAR). StAR locus is in the 8p11.2 region and is a protein with an essential role in cholesterol transfer from the outer to the inner mitochondrial membrane, thus providing the substrate for steroid hormone biosynthesis (Bose et al, 1996). Once in the mitochondria, cholesterol is converted to pregnenolone by the cytochrome P450 side-chain cleavage (CYP11A1) enzyme, and then steroid biosynthesis is initiated. Karyotypic 46,XY persons are phenotypically female because of Leydig cell destruction and impaired testosterone production. The ovary in XX subjects is initially spared damage because steroidogenesis is delayed until the time of puberty, after which stimulation of steroidogenesis by the tropic hormones (i.e., luteinizing and follicle-stimulating hormones) causes progressive damage to the ovary (Fujieda et al, 1997). StAR mutations have been described most frequently in Japanese and Palestinian populations, in part because certain mutations occur repeatedly, probably reflecting a founder effect (Bose et al, 1996; Nakae et al, 1997). Although less common than mutations in StAR, mutations in CYP11A1 can also cause lipoid CAH (Hiort et al, 2005; Katsumata et al, 2002).

Rare Form of Congenital Adrenal Hyperplasia With Variable Phenotypes

Cytochrome P450 oxidoreductase deficiency is a disorder of steroidogenesis with a phenotypic spectrum ranging from cortisol deficiency at the milder end to classic Antley-Bixler syndrome (ABS) at the severe end, and the phenotype of cortisol deficiency can range from clinically insignificant to life threatening. Manifestations can include ambiguous genitalia in both males and females, primary amenorrhea and enlarged cystic ovaries in females, poor masculinization during puberty in males, and maternal virilization during pregnancy if the fetus is affected. Manifestations of Antley-Bixler syndrome include craniosynostosis; hydrocephalus; distinctive facies; choanal stenosis or atresia; low-set, dysplastic ears with stenotic external auditory canals; skeletal anomalies (radiohumeral synostosis, neonatal fractures, congenital bowing of the long bones, joint contractures, arachnodactyly, clubfeet); renal anomalies (ectopic kidneys, duplication of kidneys, renal hypoplasia, horseshoe kidney, hydronephrosis); and reduction of cognitive function and developmental delay. In moderate cytochrome P450 oxidoreductase deficiency, craniofacial and skeletal anomalies are less severe than in Antley-Bixler syndrome (Scott and Miller, 2008).

Familial Glucocorticoid Deficiency

Familial glucocorticoid deficiency (FGD) is an autosomal recessive disorder resulting from defects in the action of adrenocorticotropic hormone (ACTH) to stimulate glucocorticoid synthesis in the adrenal. It is also known as isolated glucocorticoid deficiency or hereditary unresponsiveness to ACTH. The majority of patients with FGD have episodes of hypoglycemia in the neonatal period. These episodes will often respond quickly to more frequent feeding regimens. In a few cases, excessive skin pigmentation is recognized at this early stage. Biochemically, patients with FGD have low or undetectable cortisol levels and—because of the failure of the negative feedback loop to the pituitary and hypothalamus—grossly elevated ACTH levels are seen. Mineralocorticoid deficiency usually is not a presentation; therefore aldosterone levels, plasma renin measurements, and serum electrolytes are normal. A clinical feature sometimes observed in patients with FGD is tall stature that is identified later in life (Elias et al, 2000). Approximately half of all cases result from mutations in the ACTH receptor (melanocortin 2 receptor) FGD type 1 or from mutations in the melanocortin 2 receptor accessory protein (MRAP), FGD type 2, but other genetic causes of this potentially lethal disorder remain to be discovered. (Clark et al, 2009).

Allgrove Syndrome

Allgrove, or triple A, syndrome is a similar disorder to FGD, with additional features of alacrima and achalasia. Presenting in the first decade of life, it is frequently associated with progressive neurologic dysfunction, polyneuropathy, deafness, mental retardation, and hyperkeratosis of palms and soles (Houlden et al, 2002). Some of these families have a defect in the alacrima–achalasia–adrenal insufficiency syndrome gene encoding a protein named ALADIN, which is postulated to be involved in either cytoplasmic trafficking or peroxisomal activities (Tullio-Pelet et al, 2000). ALADIN belongs to a WD-repeat family of regulatory proteins that shares a common made up of highly conserved repeating units usually ending with Trp-Asp (WD) (Neer et al, 1994).

Neonatal Adrenoleukodystrophy

Neonatal adrenoleukodystrophy (NALD) is a fatal autosomal recessive disease of impaired peroxisome biogenesis. NALD belongs to a class of disorders involving peroxisomal biogenesis that includes Zellweger syndrome and infantile Refsum's disease. NALD is the only one of the three diseases that often involves adrenal insufficiency. Mutations in seven different peroxisome biogenesis factors have been shown to cause NALD (Moser, 1999). Mutations in PEX1 (peroxisome biogenesis factor 1), are the most common cause of NALD (Tamura et al, 2001). As in X-linked adrenoleukodystrophy (X-ALD), patients with NALD accumulate very long-chain fatty acids and develop degenerative changes of the white matter of the nervous system and adrenal atrophy. Infants with NALD characteristically demonstrate dolichocephaly, prominent and high forehead, esotropia, epicanthic folds, broad nasal bridge, high-arched palate, low-set ears, and anteverted nostrils. Affected patients usually die in early childhood (Walter et al, 2001). X-ALD is a recessively inherited X-linked defect of the adrenoleukodystrophy protein. It is also a peroxisomal defect that usually results in adrenal insufficiency and CNS deterioration. However, X-ALD does not usually appear before early childhood but manifest later in adulthood (Moser et al, 1984).

Defective Cholesterol Metabolism: Smith-Lemli-Opitz Syndrome

The clinical picture of adrenal insufficiency and 46,XY gonadal dysgenesis may be caused by a deficiency of 7-dehydrocholesterol C-7 reductase enzyme that catalyzes the final step in cholesterol biosynthesis leading to primary adrenal insufficiency. The syndrome results from mutations in the sterol Δ-7-reductase gene (DHCR7) located at 11q12-q13. Smith-Lemli-Opitz (SLO) syndrome can manifest with typical facial appearance, mental retardation, microcephaly, proximally placed thumbs, congenital cardiac abnormalities, syndactyly of the second and third toes, incomplete development of the male genitalia, and photosensitivity. The biochemical abnormalities of SLO syndrome include low cholesterol and high 7-dehydrocholesterol (Tint et al, 1994) In utero, the primary defect in fetal adrenal glands results in a combination of low maternal estriol levels, sex reversal, and large adrenal glands in the fetus with SLO syndrome. Preliminary studies suggest that cholesterol supplementation may be of benefit to patients with the SLO syndrome (Andersson et al, 1999). The birth prevalence of SLO syndrome is estimated to be approximately 1:20,000 to 1:40,000 live births (Tint et al, 1994). Among persons of northern or central European ancestry, it has been estimated to range from 1:10,000 to 1:60,000 (Porter, 2000). SLO syndrome is less common in those of Asian or African ancestry.

Adrenal Insufficiency Associated With Other Syndromic Disorders
Lysosomal Storage Disorders
Complete deficiency of lysosomal esterase can also result in adrenal insufficiency in Wolman disease, a rare autosomal recessive disease. Wolman disease is rare, with only 50 reports of the disease published in the worldwide medical literature. Wolman disease usually is fatal in the 1st year of life. Affected infants exhibit mild mental retardation, hepatosplenomegaly, vomiting, diarrhea, growth failure, and adrenal calcifications. Calcifications that delineate the outline of both adrenals are pathognomonic of this condition (Wolman, 1995).

Mitochondrial Disorders
Adrenal insufficiency can result from mitochondrial disorders, characterized by chronic lactic acidosis, myopathy, cataracts, and nerve deafness (Bruno et al, 1998; Nicolino et al, 1997). Cases with the Kearns-Sayre syndrome form of mitochondrial myopathy, deafness, with large-scale deletions in mitochondrial DNA are often associated with endocrine dysfunction, particularly short stature, hypogonadism, diabetes, hypoparathyroidism, hypothyroidism, and adrenal insufficiency (Artuch et al, 1998; Boles et al, 1998).

Intrauterine Growth Retardation, Metaphyseal Dysplasia, AHC and Genital Anomalies
Three patients with adrenal hypoplasia congenita and additional findings that represent a new syndrome known as *IMAGe* (i.e., intrauterine growth retardation, metaphyseal dysplasia, AHC and genital anomalies) were reported. Genital abnormality was described as bilateral cryptorchidism, small penis, and hypogonadotropic hypogonadism. The patients also had hypercalciuria with or without hypercalcemia resulting in abnormal calcium deposits in vital organs. They all had no evidence of glycerol kinase deficiency and no alteration of either the *SF1* or *DAX1* gene (Vilain, 1999).

Adrenal Hypoplasia Congenita
AHC, a rare familial condition in which the adrenal cortex has arrested development, occurs in approximately 1 in 12,500 births (Jones et al, 1995; Laverty et al, 1973). The disorder can manifest as four clinical forms of primary adrenal insufficiency: (1) a sporadic form associated with pituitary hypoplasia; (2) an autosomal recessive form with a distinct miniature adult adrenal morphology, characterized by small glands with a permanent cortical zone but a diminished fetal zone (the genetic basis of the recessive form of AHC is unknown); (3) an X-linked cytomegalic form associated with hypogonadotropic hypogonadism;

and (4) an X-linked form associated with glycerol kinase deficiency and Duchenne muscular dystrophy (Bartley et al, 1982). Mutations in *DAX1* are responsible for both X-linked forms.

The X-linked or cytomegalic form of AHC is characterized by the absence or near absence of the permanent or adult zone of the adrenal cortex and by structural disorganization of the fetal cortex with abnormally large cells. It differs from the autosomal recessive miniature adult form of AHC, in which the adrenal cortex has the normal adult structure but is small. X-linked AHC results in severe primary adrenal insufficiency involving glucocorticoids and mineralocorticoids and failure to respond to elevated levels of ACTH with usual age at onset in the neonatal period or during infancy. However, in some patients, age of onset is later, up to several years of age and presumably caused by residual functional cortex (Achermann et al, 2001; McCabe, 2000). The secretion of other pituitary hormones is not impaired. Hypogonadotropic hypogonadism can manifest with cryptorchidism or delayed puberty (Golden et al, 1977). Whereas presentation of adrenal insufficiency can occur from birth, there is great variability of presentations. Isolated adrenal insufficiency in infancy, isolated adrenal insufficiency later in life, isolated hypogonadotropic hypogonadism, adrenal insufficiency and hypogonadotropic hypogonadism, delayed-onset adrenal insufficiency from 2 to 9 years of age with incomplete hypogonadotropic hypogonadism, and delayed puberty in females all may result (Ten et al, 2001). The phenotypical variation does not correlate well with genotype.

Adrenal Hypoplasia as Part of Contiguous Gene Deletion Syndrome
An X-linked form of adrenal insufficiency, associated with glycerol kinase deficiency is characterized by psychomotor retardation, muscular dystrophy, characteristic facies with hypertelorism, alternating strabismus, and drooping mouth. Additional phenotypic features can include testicular abnormalities (anorchia or cryptorchidism), short stature, and osteoporosis. Time of presentation can vary from birth through childhood. Nearly all patients reported were male. The genetic locus was mapped to Xp21.3-21.2 and variants of contiguous gene deletion syndrome (glycerol kinase deficiency, Duchenne muscular dystrophy, ornithine transcarbamylase deficiency, and mental retardation) can be seen.

ABNORMALITIES OF DEVELOPMENT: DAX1 AND SF1 DEFICIENCY
The nuclear receptors DAX1 (dosage-sensitive sex reversal, AHC, critical region on the X chromosome, gene-1, NR0B1/*AHC*) and SF1 (*NR5A1*, also known as Ad4BP) (Phelan and McCabe, 2001) have an important role in adrenal development and function, and mutations in these transcription factors have been found in patients with adrenal hypoplasia (see Molecular Basis of Adrenal Development, earlier). Both SF1 and DAX1 belong to the family of nuclear hormone receptors. DAX1 protein is expressed in the developing urogenital ridge, ovary, testis, all zones of the fetal adrenal cortex, hypothalamus, and anterior pituitary gland—sites in which it colocalizes with

SF1 (Guo et al, 1995; Parker et al, 2002). SF1 is essential for the development of the adrenal cortex, gonads, and ventromedial nucleus of the hypothalamus because it interacts with the genes for the α-subunits of the pituitary glycoprotein hormones, müllerian-inhibiting hormone, and the promoter of the *DAX1* gene (Kawabe et al, 1999). Furthermore, SF1 is a transcription factor that regulates gene expression of the CYP steroid hydroxylases (21-hydroxylase, the aldosterone synthase isoenzyme of steroid 11β-hydroxylase, CYP11A), 3-β-hydrosteroid dehydrogenase, aromatase, and StAR in the adrenal gland; therefore it is essential for development of the adrenal cortex.

In one large study of this relatively rare disease, *DAX1* mutations were found in 58% of 46,XY phenotypic boys referred with adrenal hypoplasia and in all boys with hypogonadotropic hypogonadism and a family history suggestive of adrenal failure in males. *SF1* mutations causing adrenal failure were found in only two patients with 46,XY gonadal dysgenesis. No *DAX1* or *SF1* mutations were identified in the adult-onset group (Lin et al, 2006).

Human mutations in SF1 are even rarer and have been described in a few patients with primary adrenal failure. Two individuals with a 46,XY genotype, female phenotype, and müllerian structures harbor missense mutations that affect DNA binding (Achermann et al, 1999, 2002), whereas a 46,XX girl with an SF1 mutation had primary adrenal failure and apparently normal ovarian development (Biason-Lauber and Schoenle, 2000). In addition, it is now emerging that heterozygous nonsense or frameshift mutations associated with haploinsufficiency of SF1 can cause 46,XY gonadal dysgenesis in patients with normal adrenal function (Correa et al, 2004; Hasegawa et al, 2004; Mallet et al, 2004). Therefore it is possible that a range of different endocrine phenotypes are associated with mutations in different domains of SF1.

Adrenal Hemorrhage

Adrenal hemorrhage is not uncommon at birth. At birth, adrenal hemorrhage from anoxia or sepsis is most common, and adrenal insufficiency from CAH usually manifests in neonates (Ten et al, 2001). The incidence in the neonate is reported to be 1.7 cases per 1000 autopsied infants and as many as 3% of infants screened by abdominal ultrasound examination. The etiology of neonatal adrenal hemorrhage is largely unknown, but it has been associated with birth trauma related to difficult deliveries, sepsis, coagulopathies, traumatic shock, and ischemic disorders. Infants with minimal hemorrhage may be asymptomatic and be discovered incidentally to have adrenal calcifications, indicating an earlier hemorrhage. Major adrenal hemorrhage can manifest as an abdominal mass, anemia from blood loss, or jaundice from reabsorption of the hematoma. Hemorrhage can also lead to adrenal insufficiency, which can manifest as neonatal hypoglycemia, hypotension, hypothermia, apnea, or shock. Because of the location of the right adrenal gland between the liver and spine, it is the one most often affected by hemorrhage (Velaphi and Perlman, 2001).

In meningococcal septicemias, hemorrhage into the adrenal glands can complicate the clinical picture, leading to circulatory collapse (Waterhouse-Friderichsen syndrome or adrenal hemorrhage in association with fulminant septicemia; Enriquez et al, 1990). Other infections in the neonate that have been associated with adrenal hemorrhage and insufficiency include those caused by herpesvirus, *Pseudomonas aeruginosa*, *Bacteroides* spp., herpes simplex virus type 6, echovirus types 11 and 6 (Bekdash and Slim, 1981; Jain et al, 1996; Margaretten et al, 1963; Ohta et al, 1978; Schmitt et al, 1996). Septic shock in newborns, especially in those who are small for age, can result in adrenal hemorrhage with rhabdomyolysis and renal insufficiency (Ten et al, 2001).

Secondary and Tertiary Adrenal Insufficiency

Iatrogenic Adrenal Insufficiency

Secondary and tertiary forms of adrenal insufficiency result from defects in pituitary corticotroph and hypothalamic function, respectively. Supraphysiologic doses of glucocorticoids often are used for the treatment of bronchopulmonary dysplasia. With prolonged use of supraphysiologic doses of glucocorticoids, these neonates are at risk for iatrogenic suppression of corticotroph ACTH release, with secondary adrenocortical atrophy and adrenal insufficiency (Axelrod, 1992). Evidently, even a single course of antenatal betamethasone treatment induces a suppression of stress reactivity in healthy newborns (Schaffer et al, 2009). The duration of recovery of corticotroph function from adrenal suppression, once administration of glucocorticoids is discontinued, is highly variable with evidence of suppression of the HPA axis evident in some patients for more than 1 year (Livanou et al, 1967). Even in preterm infants, the HPA axis behaves in a similar manner as in adult subjects, and the pituitary function recovers earlier than that of hypothalamus and adrenals (Ng et al, 2008).

Developmental Adrenal Insufficiency

Secondary or tertiary adrenal insufficiency in the neonate often is a consequence of abnormalities in development of the hypothalamus and pituitary associated with adrenal insufficiency, including de Morsier syndrome (septo-optic dysplasia; De Morsier, 1956), hydrancephaly or anencephaly, and pituitary hypoplasia or aplasia. If these infants have concomitant diabetes insipidus, they have an increased risk of sudden death during childhood (Dattani et al, 1998; Kelberman et al, 2006). Patients with developmental abnormalities of the pituitary or hypothalamus often have deficiencies of other hormones. ACTH deficiency can be part of mutiple pituitary hormone deficiency syndrome caused by abnormal expression of transcription factors such as HESX1, LHX4, SOX3, or PROP1 (Mullis, 2001). Isolated ACTH insufficiency is a rare condition that can be caused by mutations in TPIT, a T-box factor that controls transcription of the proopiomelanocortin gene in corticotrophes only, thereby resulting in an adrenal-only phenotype (Vallette-Kasic et al, 2005). However, approximately 50% of patients do not carry mutations in TPIT, suggesting that other unknown factors exist (Metherell et al, 2004; Vallette-Kasic et al, 2004). Septooptic dysplasia can be caused by mutations in HESX1 and SOX2 (Dattani et al, 1998; Kelberman et al, 2006). Signs of hypopituitarism in a neonate include hypoglycemia, prolonged jaundice, shock, and microphallus in males. Trauma to the hypothalamus, pituitary, or hypophysial portal circulation from significant head injury, cerebrovascular accident, Sheehan syndrome, or hydrocephalus may be a cause of central adrenal insufficiency. Historical factors associated with increased risk for central adrenal insufficiency include maternal drug use and traumatic delivery.

There have been rare case reports of families with inherited abnormalities of neuropeptides involved in HPA axis regulation. Adrenal insufficiency, pigmentary abnormalities, and obesity have been described in families with a defect in POMC (Krude et al, 1998). One kindred has been reported with Arnold-Chiari type I malformation and suspected *CRH* deficiency. The mutation in this kindred is linked to the *CRH* locus; however, a specific mutation in the *CRH* gene has not yet been defined (Kyllo et al, 1996).

MANAGEMENT

Adrenal crisis is a potentially life-threatening disorder that can manifest with a salt-losing crisis or profound hypoglycemia in infancy or childhood and requires immediate resuscitation and appropriate steroid replacement. Determining the exact cause of this condition can be challenging once the child has started treatment, but defining a precise etiology has important implications for long-term management, for identifying associated features, and for appropriate counseling regarding inheritance and the risks of other family members being affected (Lin et al, 2006). Detailed questioning about family history that could reveal any insight into possible adrenal disease is important.

Initial Management

In the event of a suspected adrenal crisis, blood for determination of electrolytes, aldosterone, plasma renin activity, cortisol, and ACTH should be drawn and treatment started before the results are obtained. Fluid resuscitation with normal saline containing 5% dextrose should be given as a bolus to restore cardiovascular stability. Plasma sodium should be monitored closely, as rapid correction of hyponatremia with sodium repletion of more than 0.5 to 1 mEq/L/h increases the risk of central pontine myelinolysis. The sodium deficit may be calculated by subtracting the infant's sodium from a customarily normal sodium of 140 mEq/L and then multiplying this value by 0.6 × weight (in kg). The rate of replacement should occur over an initial rate such that the sodium increase does not exceed 0.5 mEq/L/h. Intravenous hydrocortisone should be given initially at 100 mg/m^2 and then continued at 100 mg/m^2/day, divided every 6 to 8 hours, until the infant's condition is stable.

Maintenance Therapy

Corticosteroid and mineralocorticoid replacement therapies should suppress the excessive secretion of CRH, ACTH, and resting renin levels. The normal daily cortisol production rate has been shown to be 6 to 7 mg/m^2/day

in children and adolescents (Kerrigan et al, 1993; Linder et al, 1990). This rate translates to approximately 10 to 12 mg/m^2/day of oral hydrocortisone, to allow for step-down losses from absorption, hepatic processing, and metabolic bioavailability. Because the bioavailability of oral steroids varies from person to person (Bright and Darmaun, 1995), infants should be monitored closely for signs of either inadequate cortisol replacement or cortisol excess (Heazelwood et al, 1984). Although adults and older children may be able to take hydrocortisone twice daily, most infants should be dosed three times daily to avoid hypoglycemia associated with low cortisol on a twice-daily regimen (DeVile and Stanhope, 1997; Groves et al, 1988). It is conceivable to say that other steroids can be used; hydrocortisone is preferred in infants because it has fewer growth-suppressive effects than those associated with use of synthetic steroids (Allen, 1996; Allen et al, 1998; Punthakee et al, 2003). The U.S. Food and Drug Administration withdrew oral hydrocortisone suspension from the market because of poor absorption and undertreatment of children (Ten et al, 2001).

In primary adrenal insufficiency, aldosterone production is usually decreased. Physiologic doses of hydrocortisone do not provide enough mineralocorticoid activity to prevent salt wasting (New et al, 1966); therefore these infants often require 0.05 to 0.2 mg/day of fludrocortisone acetate (Florinef) (Ten et al, 2001) and added salt. Because after the 1st month of life aldosterone production does not vary, the dose of fludrocortisone does not change with growth and aging (Sippell et al, 1978; Weldon et al, 1967). Infants with mineralocorticoid deficiency require 1 to 2 g of NaCl (1 g contains 17 mEq of sodium) added to their diet, because formula and breast milk are low in sodium content (approximately 8 mEq/L) (Mullis et al, 1990).

Stress Replacement

The normal response to surgery, trauma, or critical illness is to increase plasma ACTH and cortisol levels (Lamberts et al, 1997). The secretion rate of cortisol has been found to be proportional to the degree of stress and ranges from 60 to 167 mg/day in adults after surgery (Chernow et al, 1987; Hume et al, 1962). Based on data from adults, it is recommended that infants with adrenal insufficiency receive 30 to 100 mg/m^2/day divided every 6 to 8 hours of hydrocortisone when stressed. Stress doses of hydrocortisone should be given with the onset of fever and gastrointestinal or other significant illness, and continued for 24 hours after the symptoms resolve (Nimkarn and New, 2008). Usually this treatment translates to the routine steroid dose being tripled and administered over three divided daily doses. If oral steroids are not tolerated, an intramuscular or intravenous dose should be given. For surgery, infants should be given 30 to 100 mg/m^2 of intravenous hydrocortisone on call to the operating room before the administration of anesthesia. Stress dosing of hydrocortisone (30 to 100 mg/m^2/day divided every 6 to 8 hours) should be continued postoperatively for the next 24 to 48 hours. It is unnecessary to give mineralocorticoids over such periods if the patient begins the operative period in adequate salt balance.

The patients and their families should have instructions for such instances. Every patient should wear a medical identification (e.g., MedicAlert) bracelet or necklace and carry the emergency medical information card that is supplied with it. Both should indicate the diagnosis, the daily medications and doses, and the physician to call in the event of an emergency.

Secondary or Tertiary Adrenal Insufficiency

Cortisol replacement for patients with secondary or tertiary adrenal insufficiency is the same as described for patients with primary adrenal insufficiency. To minimize growth suppression, these children can be treated with doses of hydrocortisone that are slightly less than physiologic replacement doses. Furthermore, because mineralocorticoid production is under the control of the renin-angiotensin system, patients with secondary or tertiary adrenal insufficiency do not require mineralocorticoid replacement. However, these infants require evaluation for deficiencies of other pituitary hormones.

Case Study 1

A 3-week-old phenotypic male infant presented with lethargy, poor oral intake, and progressive vomiting for 1 week. He refused to eat over the previous 7 hours. There was no history of fever. Prenatal history was unremarkable. Birth history: normal vaginal delivery, Apgar scores of 8 and 9 with a birthweight of 8 pounds, 14 ounces (4.03 kg). The newborn examination performed in the nursery identified perineal hypospadias, but the infant was discharged home on day 2 of life. Over the first 2 weeks of life, weight gain was poor, and appetite was markedly decreased over the 1 to 2 days before evaluation in the emergency department. Family history revealed that he was the second child of the family, from a nonconsanguineous marriage of Chinese background. (The first boy died at 1 month of age in China because of gastroenteritis.) On examination, vital signs were body temperature, 36.5° C; blood pressure, 52/32 mm Hg; pulse, 160 beats/min. He was severely dehydrated. There was no hyperpigmentation. The physical examination was notable for a weight of 3.1 kg and a phallus with a length of 2.5 cm, a midshaft diameter of 1.5 cm with hypospadias near the perineum, a hyperpigmented and rugated shawl scrotum, and no palpable testes. Initial blood glucose level was 40 mg/dL. The infant's mental status was improved after administration of 25% dextrose via an intraosseous line. Resuscitation was continued with dextrose containing normal saline. Initial laboratory values showed sodium of 107 mmol/L, potassium of 7.1 mmol/L, chloride of 87 mmol/L, total CO_2 of 5.0 mmol/L. Blood urea nitrogen was 40.5 mg/dL, creatinine was 0.6 mg/dL. After the critical blood sample was obtained, the infant was given 100 mg/m² of intravenous hydrocortisone. Additional evaluation revealed 46,XX chromosomes and enlarged adrenals, as well as a small uterus on ultrasound examination. The clinical course was complicated by necrotizing enterocolitis that led to a stay in the hospital for 3 weeks with conservative management including administration of antibiotics. Initial laboratory results noted 17 OHP of 111,000 ng/dL, ACTH of 4755 pg/mL, and cortisol 3.9 of μg/dL before hydrocortisone (no ACTH stimulation performed). Aldosterone and renin

analyses were not performed because of difficulty obtaining adequate blood. CYP21A2 analysis revealed a genotype as follows: exon1, intron2, and exon3/intron2 mutations (<1% of enzyme activity in vitro for both mutations). This case is a classic presentation of the salt-wasting form of 21 OHD CAH. Family pedigree is shown below:

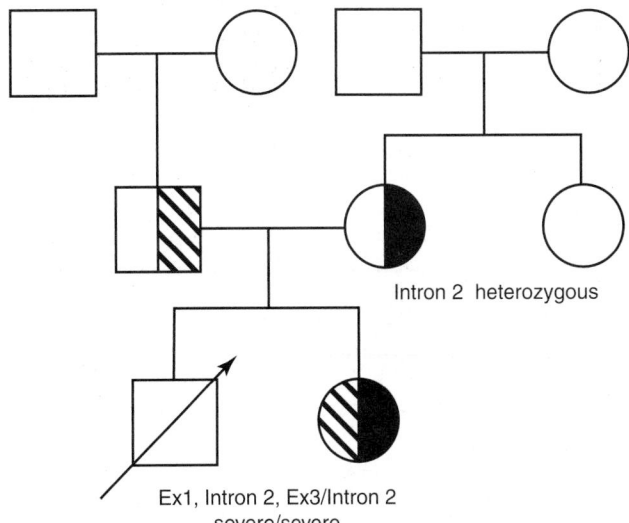

Intron 2 heterozygous

Ex1, Intron 2, Ex3/Intron 2
severe/severe

Comment

The lesson learned from this case is that in a phenotypic male without palpable testes, the genitourinary anomalies should be considered ambiguous genitalia. Further work-up is merited in the immediate perinatal period. Family history suggests a severe recessive disorder. Genetic analysis is available and can be used to confirm the diagnosis before lifetime therapy and is of value in genetic counselling. In addition, the institution of newborn screening for elevated 17-OHP allows earlier detection of salt-wasting 21 OHD, before the occurrence of a life-threatening event.

SUGGESTED READINGS

Bornstein SR: Predisposing factors for adrenal insufficiency, *N Engl J Med* 360:2328-2339, 2009.

Coulter CL: Fetal adrenal development: insight gained from adrenal tumors, *Trends Endocrinol Metab* 16:235-242, 2005.

El-Khairi R, Martinez-Aguayo A, Ferraz-de-Souza B, et al: Role of DAX-1 (NR0B1) and steroidogenic factor-1 (NR5A1) in human adrenal function, *Endocr Dev* 20:38-46, 2011.

Hanley NA, Arlt W: The human fetal adrenal cortex and the window of sexual differentiation, *Trends Endocrinol Metab* 17:391-397, 2006.

Krone N, Hanley NA, Arlt W: Age-specific changes in sex steroid biosynthesis and sex development, *Best Pract Res Clin Endocrinol Metab* 21:393-401, 2007.

Miller WL, Auchus RJ: The molecular biology, biochemistry, and physiology of human steroidogenesis and its disorders, *Endocr Rev* 32:81-151, 2011.

Nimkarn S, Lin-Su K, New MI: Steroid 21 hydroxylase deficiency congenital adrenal hyperplasia, *Endocrinol Metab Clin North Am* 38:699-718, 2009.

Speiser PW, Azziz R, Baskin LS, et al: Congenital adrenal hyperplasia due to steroid 21-hydroxylase deficiency: an Endocrine Society clinical practice guideline, *J Clin Endocrinol Metab* 95:4133-4160, 2010.

Stewart P, Krone N: The adrenal cortex. In Melmed S, Polonsky K, Larsen P, et al: *Williams textbook of endocrinology*, ed 12, Philadelphia, 2011, WB Saunders.

White PC: Adrenocortical insufficiency. In Kliegman R, Behrman R, Jenson H, et al, editors: *Nelson textbook of pediatrics*, ed 18, Philadelphia, 2007, WB Saunders.

Complete references used in this text can be found online at www.expertconsult.com

AMBIGUOUS GENITALIA IN THE NEWBORN

Karen Lin-Su and Maria I. New

"Is it a boy or a girl?" is often one of the first questions asked when a baby is born. For parents of a newborn infant with genitalia that are not clearly male or female, the ambiguity can be a distressing matter that needs to be addressed with sensitivity and with some urgency. There are four general classifications that can cause disorders of sexual differentiation: (1) masculinization of the 46,XX female, (2) incomplete masculinization of the 46,XY male, (3) gonadal differentiation and chromosomal disorders, including ovotesticular disorder of sexual differentiation, or (4) syndromes associated with incomplete genital development (Box 92-1). The first two categories comprise a majority of definable cases of ambiguous genitalia.

This chapter presents an overview of the pathophysiology of disorders of sexual differentiation (DSDs), including a discussion of the practical aspects of diagnosis and management. An overview of the traditional surgical methods used in the management of infants with DSDs, including the risks and benefits of these procedures, is included at the end of the chapter.

GENERAL CONSIDERATIONS IN THE APPROACH TO THE NEWBORN WITH AMBIGUOUS GENITALIA

The medical evaluation of a newborn with ambiguous genitalia is necessarily time-consuming. Open and honest discussions with the parents are invaluable in allaying anxiety and establishing a trusting relationship. Full disclosure of available information is essential in this regard.

Care must be taken to avoid premature gender assignment for the infant. Proper evaluation of the infant with ambiguous genitalia requires a multidisciplinary team that should include the primary care physician, neonatologist, pediatric endocrinologist, psychologist, pediatric urologist, and pediatric geneticist. Psychological assessment and support of the family are essential in the newborn period, along with long-term psychological follow-up evaluation (Guerra-Junior, 2007; Hines, 2004; Slijper et al, 1998). Decisions regarding the gender of rearing should be made collaboratively between the multidisciplinary team and the parents, with the recognition that cultural and psychosocial factors are likely to be influential (Grumbach and Conte, 1998, Kuhnle and Krahl, 2002).

In the past, gender assignment was based largely on phallus size, relative ease of surgical reconstruction, or the potential for fertility. This approach has come under criticism as dissatisfaction with gender assignment based on these criteria has been reported in several case studies (Diamond and Sigmundson, 1997b; Hughes et al, 2007; Phornphutkul et al, 2000; Reiner, 1997). The importance of prenatal androgen imprinting has been implicated

as an important variable in some of these cases (Reiner, 1997). Studies in undervirilized 46,XY males indicate that a small phallus can be associated with a satisfying adult sex life (Reilly and Woodhouse, 1989). Other studies have found that gender role tends to increasingly correspond with assigned sex as individuals with DSD proceed into adulthood (Pappas et al, 2008); therefore female gender assignment might not be necessarily warranted for intermediately undervirilized 46,XY males.

The degree of genital virilization is still an important determinant of gender assignment in the infant with ambiguous genitalia; however, other, incompletely understood factors appear to be involved. The formation of a healthy gender identity seems to involve a complex interplay between psychobiologic and environmental factors (Meyer-Bahlburg et al, 1996, 2006; Money and Ehrhardt, 1972; Singh et al, 2009; Slijper et al, 1998).

EMBRYOLOGY OF SEXUAL DIFFERENTIATION

Normal and abnormal sexual differentiation constitute superb examples of how an understanding of embryology is critical to the approach and management of a group of complex and intriguing clinical disorders.

Sexual differentiation is a sequential process that can be divided into three stages. Jost (1970) established the sequence as follows: chromosomal sex is determined at fertilization and dictates the differentiation of the gonad, which in turn dictates the phenotypic sex, or the differentiation of the internal ductal system and external genitalia (Grumbach and Conte, 1998).

Chromosomal sex is determined at the moment of conception by the sex chromosome complement of the fertilizing sperm. If this sperm carries an X chromosome, a 46,XX (normal female) complement results. If the sex chromosome is Y, a 46,XY (normal male) genotype results. The *SRY* (i.e., sex-determining region of the Y chromosome) gene is necessary but not sufficient for testicular differentiation. *SRY* causes the medullary region of the gonad to develop into Sertoli cells and later into testis cords and seminiferous tubules.

In addition to X chromosome genes, autosomal genes also may influence sexual differentiation, insofar as mutations to these genes result in disorders of sexual differentiation. Some of these genes include *WT1* (Wilms' tumor gene 1), associated with Denys-Drash syndrome and WAGR (*W*ilms' tumor, *a*niridia, *g*enitourinary abnormalities, mental *r*etardation) syndrome; the steroidogenic factor 1 gene; and *SOX9*, which has been associated with camptomelic dysplasia (Grumbach and Conte, 1998). The *DMRT1* and *DMRT3* genes, when deleted, are associated with male-to-female sex reversal. The *BPESC1* gene exhibits testis-specific expression and is located within the

BOX 92-1   Differential Diagnosis for Ambiguous Genitalia

46,XX VIRILIZED FEMALE

- Congenital adrenal hyperplasia
  - 21-Hydroxylase deficiency
  - 11-Hydroxylase deficiency
  - 3β-Hydroxysteroid dehydrogenase deficiency
  - Aromatase deficiency (fetal and maternal virilization)
- Virilizing maternal conditions
  - Congenital adrenal hyperplasia
  - Adrenal/ovarian tumors/luteoma of pregnancy
  - Maternal ingestion of progestins, androgens

46,XY UNDERVIRILIZED MALE

- Androgen insensitivity
  - Partial
  - Complete
- 5α-Reductase-2 deficiency
- Testosterone biosynthetic defects
  - 17β-Hydroxysteroid hydrogenase 3 deficiency
  - 3β-Hydroxysteroid dehydrogenase deficiency
  - 17α-Hydroxylase/17,20-lyase deficiency
  - Congenital lipoid adrenal hyperplasia
- Leydig cell hypoplasia
- Idiopathic, undetermined
- Drug ingestion: progestins, spironolactone, cimetidine, phenytoin
- Persistent müllerian duct syndrome

GONADAL DIFFERENTIATION AND CHROMOSOMAL DISORDERS

- 46,XY gonadal dysgenesis
  - Complete (Swyer syndrome)
  - Partial
  - Mixed (45,X/46,XY)
- True hermaphroditism
  - 46,XX, 46,XY, 46,XX/46,XY

SYNDROMES ASSOCIATED WITH AMBIGUOUS GENITALIA

- Gonadal dysgenesis
  - 46,XY partial gonadal dysgenesis (Turner syndrome features)
  - Camptomelic dysplasia
- Renal degenerative diseases and gonadal dysgenesis
  - Denys-Drash syndrome
  - Frasier syndrome
  - WAGR (Wilms' tumor, aniridia, genitourinary abnormalities, mental retardation) syndrome
- Smith-Lemli-Opitz syndrome (7-dehydrocholesterol reductase deficiency)
- Robinow syndrome

in mice (Ketola et al, 2000; Tevosian et al, 2002; Viger et al, 1998).

The gonad develops from both somatic and germ cells. The somatic cells are located at the ventral region of the mesonephros and arise from the mesonephric cells and the coelomic epithelium. Somatic cells become the Sertoli cells of the testis and the granulosa cells of the ovary. The germ cells migrate from a more inferior position on the yolk sac to the genital ridge, just medial to the mesonephros on each side (Figure 92-1, *upper left*). This migration occurs between 4 and 6 weeks' gestation. Once the germ cells reach the gonadal ridge, they become surrounded by the somatic cells, which appear to regulate germ cell differentiation.

Gonadal sex is established by 7 weeks' gestation. At this stage the fetus contains two internal ductal systems—wolffian and müllerian—and undifferentiated external genital primordia. The wolffian or mesonephric duct is a tubular structure that connects the capillary network of the mesonephros to the urogenital sinus. Evagination of the coelomic epithelium leads to formation of a second tubular structure adjacent to the mesonephric duct—the paramesonephric, or müllerian, duct. The distal ends of these two ducts are joined. That portion of the urogenital sinus distal to the termination of these ducts contributes to external genital development, whereas the proximal portion develops into the bladder, trigone, and posterior urethra.

Phenotypic sexual differentiation is predicated on establishing gonadal sex. If an ovary develops, the wolffian ducts involute because of a lack of testosterone, and only its terminal portion persists as Gartner's duct. The müllerian ducts develop into the proximal vagina, uterus, and fallopian tubes (see Figure 92-1). The unfused cephalic portions of the müllerian ducts form the fallopian tubes, whereas the caudal ends fuse to form the ureterovaginal canal (see Figure 92-1). The union of the fused caudal ends of the müllerian ducts and urogenital sinus forms the vagina. The proximal two thirds of the vagina is of müllerian duct origin, and the distal third is of urogenital sinus origin.

Male phenotypic differentiation is the result of the elaboration of two distinct testicular hormones: testosterone and müllerian-inhibiting factor (MIF). These factors are produced and secreted by the 8-week stage of development, and they are essential for normal male differentiation. Involution of the müllerian ducts is caused by MIF, which is a glycoprotein secreted by the fetal Sertoli cells. The remnants of the müllerian ducts persist caudally as the prostatic utricle and cephalically as the appendix testis. MIF exerts its action unilaterally and locally (exocrine secretion) rather than bilaterally via the systemic circulation.

Immediately after müllerian duct regression, the wolffian ducts develop under the influence of testosterone secreted by the fetal Leydig cells. The Leydig cells, like the Sertoli cells, differentiate from the mesenchymal cells within the gonadal ridges; this occurs at 9 to 10 weeks' of gestation. Under the influence of testosterone, the wolffian ducts evolve into the epididymis, vas deferens, and seminal vesicles (see Figure 92-1). The mesonephric tubules develop into the ductuli efferentes, which will provide continuity between the seminiferous tubules and rete

homologous region in the human at 3q23 (Crisponi et al, 2001). The *DAX1* gene is located on Xp22 and appears to be necessary for correct testis determination and, in the mouse at least, necessary for the upregulation of *Sox9* expression (Bouma et al, 2005). The gene *WNT4* is critical for normal ovarian and female sexual development. A mutation in *WNT4* leads to müllerian duct regression and virilization in a 46,XX female (MacLaughlin and Donahoe, 2004), whereas duplication of the locus containing WNT4 leads to 46,XY sex reversal (Jordan et al, 2001). The Desert hedgehog gene (*Dhh*) is a member of a family of signaling genes with an important role in regulating morphogenesis. The *follistatin* (*Fst*) and the *bone morphogenetic protein 2* (*Bmp2*) genes appear to be important for ovary organogenesis (Menke et al, 2003; Yao et al, 2004). Mutations in *Gata4* or *Fog2* can cause sex reversal

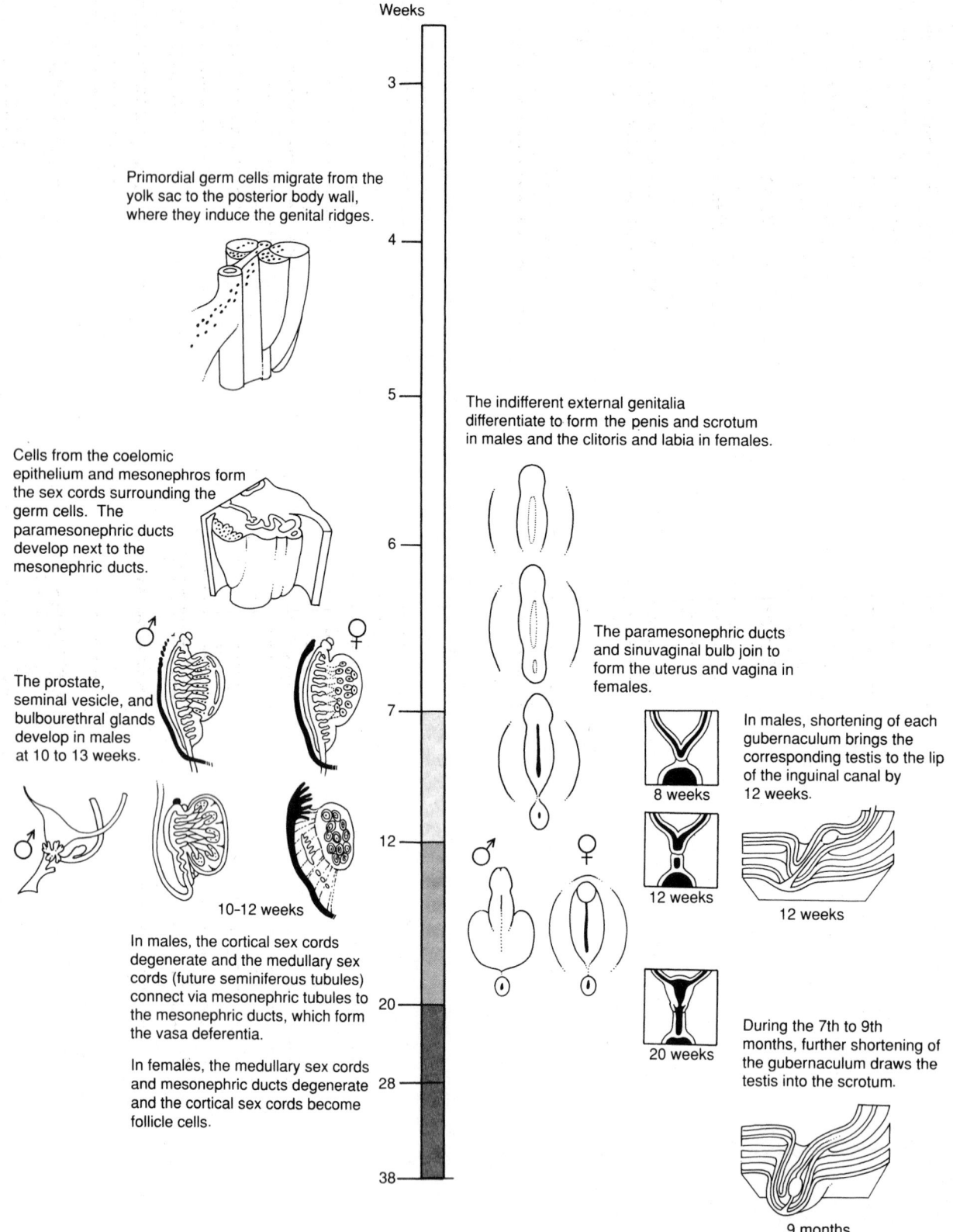

FIGURE 92-1 Embryologic time line for gonadal and internal and external genitalia development. *(From Larsen WJ: Human embryology, New York, 1993, Churchill Livingstone, p 237.)*

testis to the vas deferens. This process occurs as a direct action of testosterone on the ductal structures.

Virilization of the male external genitalia, starting at approximately 8 weeks' gestation (see Figure 92-1), relies on the ability of the tissues involved to convert testosterone into a more potent androgen—dihydrotestosterone. The target cells possess the enzyme 5α-reductase, which is necessary for this conversion. By 12 to 14 weeks' gestation, formation of the male external genitalia is nearly complete. Androgen exposure after this time results in further phallic enlargement.

CLINICAL ASSESSMENT OF DISORDERS OF SEX DIFFERENTIATION

HISTORY

A detailed family history is important in the evaluation of ambiguous genitalia. Information on early neonatal deaths, consanguinity, or urogenital anomalies should be obtained. A family history of female infertility or amenorrhea can be suggestive of a DSD. In one study of androgen insensitivity disorders, a positive family history of a sex differentiation disorder was often overlooked (Viner et al, 1977).

The presence of maternal virilization is suggestive of a variety of disorders that can affect fetal masculinization. Features of maternal virilization include hirsutism, severe acne, deepening of the voice, and clitoromegaly on examination.

The ingestion of any recreational drugs, alcohol, or medications by the mother during pregnancy should be noted. Particular attention to medications with androgenic or progestational activity is indicated. Medications that affect fetal genital development include cimetidine, spironolactone, hydantoin, and progestational agents (Grumbach and Conte, 1998).

PHYSICAL EXAMINATION

There is significant overlap of the genital anatomy among the various sex differentiation disorders. The physical examination, however, can provide the first clues to the underlying pathology. In addition, the physical examination will provide important information about the degree of virilization of the external genitalia and the presence or absence of palpable gonads.

Clitoris

Significant clitoral enlargement deserves a careful evaluation. A point to keep in mind is that premature infants have relatively underdeveloped labia majora, so that the clitoris may appear enlarged. A truly enlarged clitoris can be distinguished from a generous clitoral hood by the presence of palpable corporal or erectile tissue.

Penis (Phallus)

Measurements of the phallic stretch length and middle shaft diameter are important in determining the degree of virilization. The phallus should be stretched and measured from the pubic ramus to the tip of the glans. Gestational age–corrected phallic stretch lengths are shown in Figure 92-2. The presence of a chordee structure on the ventral surface of the phallus can impair measurement of the true phallic length (Feldman, and Smith 1975) (Figure 92-3). A chordee is residual urethral tissue that tethers the phallus to the perineum. Measurement of the middle shaft diameter is particularly useful in this circumstance. For term male infants, a normal middle shaft diameter is approximately 1 cm (Feldman and Smith, 1975).

A microphallus warrants careful evaluation for the presence of hypopituitarism or growth hormone deficiency, particularly in the presence of hypoglycemia or unexplained

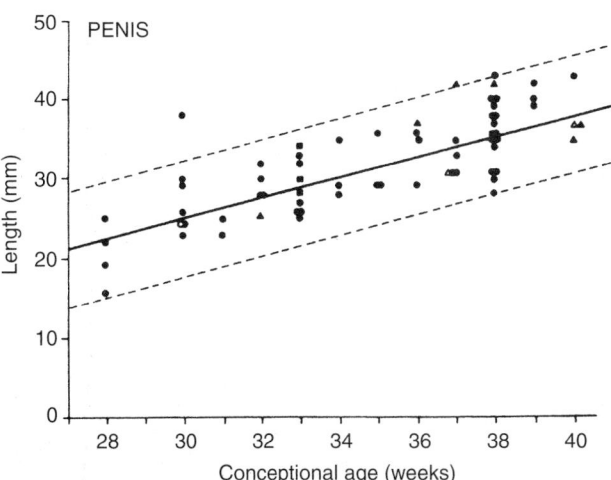

FIGURE 92-2 Penis stretch length in 63 normal premature and full-term male infants (•), showing lines of mean ±2 SD. Superimposed are data for two small-for-gestational age infants (∆), seven large-for-gestational age infants (▲), and twins (■). *(Reproduced with permission from Feldman KW, Smith DW: Fetal phallic growth and penile standards for newborn male infants,* J Pediatr *86:395-398, 1975.)*

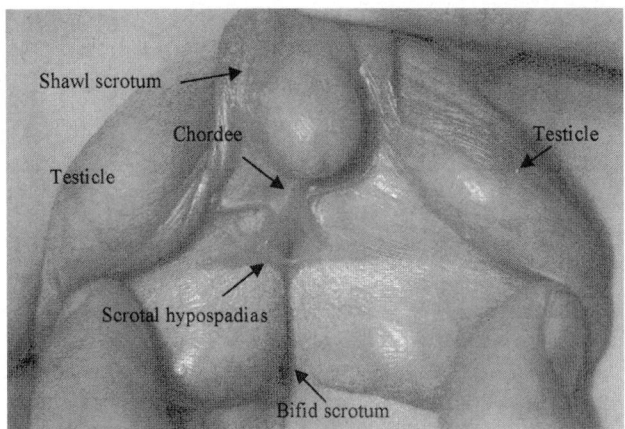

FIGURE 92-3 Undervirilized male demonstrating bifid scrotum, scrotal hypospadias, chordee, and bilateral descended testes.

jaundice. Microphallus and undescended testes may occasionally be the presenting phenotype for a DSD.

Labioscrotal Folds

Assessment of the degree of fusion of the labioscrotal folds should be performed. When the infant is exposed to androgens during embryogenesis, fusion of the labioscrotal folds progresses from a posterior to an anterior direction. The spectrum of labial fusion can vary from mild posterior fusion to complete labial fusion (Figure 92-4). The examiner should note whether the folds are rugate or hyperpigmented. Is the phallus positioned in the normal superior position relative to the scrotum, or is there a shawl scrotum? Is the scrotum fused normally in the midline or is the scrotum bifid? (See Figure 92-3.)

Gonads

Careful examination for the presence of gonads should be performed in all infants with ambiguous genitalia. The presence of bilateral gonads in the labial folds is highly

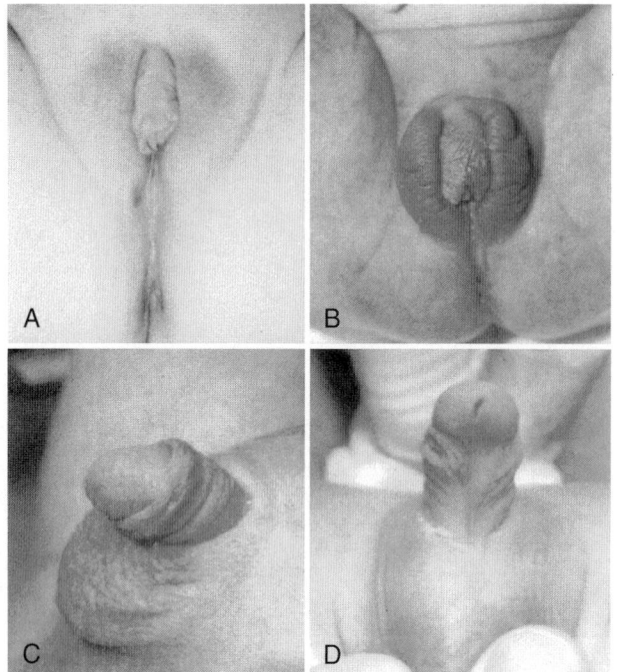

FIGURE 92-4 Virilization of external genitalia in 46,XX congenital adrenal hyplasia (21-hydroxylase deficiency). **A,** There is a mild to moderate degree of virilization, with primarily clitoral hypertrophy and significant fusion of the labia. **B,** Virilization is moderate, with clitoromegaly, labial fusion, and rugation of labial folds. **C** and **D,** Complete masculinization is evident.

suggestive of an undermasculinized genetic male (see Figure 92-3). A unilaterally palpable gonad is often seen in infants with mixed gonad dysgenesis or hermaphroditism (Figure 92-5), although other disorders such as androgen insensitivity can manifest similarly. When cryptorchidism and hypospadias occur simultaneously, there is a greater than 25% chance of a DSD (Albers et al, 1997; Rajfer and Walsh, 1976).

Hypospadias, Perineum

The severity of hypospadias can vary, with the condition ranging from mild glandular to penoscrotal, although most disorders of sexual differentiation manifest with severe penoscrotal or scrotal hypospadias (see Figures 92-3 and 92-3). Examination for the presence of separate urethral and vaginal openings versus a single perineal opening (urogenital sinus) conveys important anatomic information. The vagina may be blind-ending or completely formed. A urogenital sinus results from failure of the urologic and genital tracts to differentiate completely. In virilized females, the level at which the vagina enters the sinus (low- versus high-level vaginal entry) has important implications for determining the ease of subsequent surgical exteriorization of the vagina (Figure 92-6). In addition, when the urethra enters a urogenital sinus, there is potential for urinary stasis and therefore urinary tract infections. Excessive pigmentation of the genitals or signs of dehydration should alert the examiner to the possibility of congenital adrenal hyperplasia (CAH).

Dysmorphic features suggestive of Turner syndrome indicate the possibility of gonadal dysgenesis or mixed

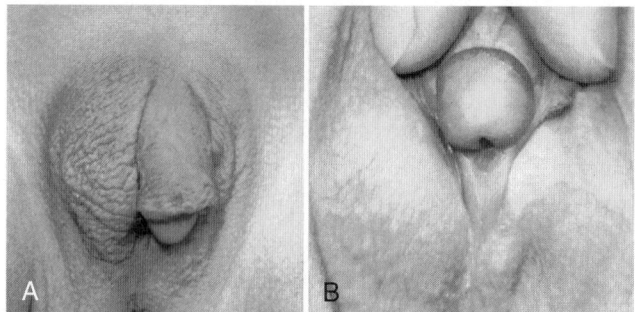

FIGURE 92-5 Asymmetric external genitals with left unilateral descended testis **(A)**, penoscrotal hypospadias, and chordee **(B)**. Asymmetrical external genital development or gonadal descent would be characteristic of mixed gonadal dysgenesis or hermaphroditism.

gonadal dysgenesis. Such abnormalities or multiple congenital anomalies could indicate any of a variety of syndromes associated with ambiguous genitalia (see Box 92-1).

RADIOLOGIC INVESTIGATIONS

Pelvic Ultrasonography

Pelvic ultrasonography reveals vital information in the evaluation of DSDs. The presence or absence of a uterus is a critically important determinant in the initial evaluation (Figures 92-7 to 92-9). The newborn period is a time when the uterus, ovaries, and adrenal glands are optimally visualized (Wright et al, 1995). The presence of a well-developed uterus will direct the differential diagnosis toward virilization of a genetic female, true hermaphroditism, or persistent müllerian duct syndrome (PMDS); however, a rudimentary uterus may be seen in gonadal dysgenesis or hermaphroditism. Ultrasonography can locate undescended testes and determine gonadal size or irregularity, such as an oblong ovotestis. Gonads in the newborn are not always well visualized by ultrasound examination, but that does not necessarily mean they are absent or abnormal. In ovotesticular DSD, loss of the uniform testicular echotexture suggests the presence of an ovotestis. Ultrasound examination can determine whether the adrenal glands appear enlarged, as in CAH; however, normal adrenal size does not rule out CAH.

Genitourethrogram

A genitourethrogram is a fluoroscopically guided genital dye study that can provide important information on the urethra and internal genital ducts (Wright et al, 1995). An experienced radiologist should perform this study. It is important to ensure that all perineal orifices are examined. The main features to be noted are the presence or absence of a vagina (or prostatic utricle) and the relationship between the vagina and the urethra (see Figure 92-6). Demonstration of the level at which the vagina opens into the urogenital sinus and its relationship to the external sphincter has important surgical implications. Recognition of male or female urethral configurations also may be possible during genitourethrography.

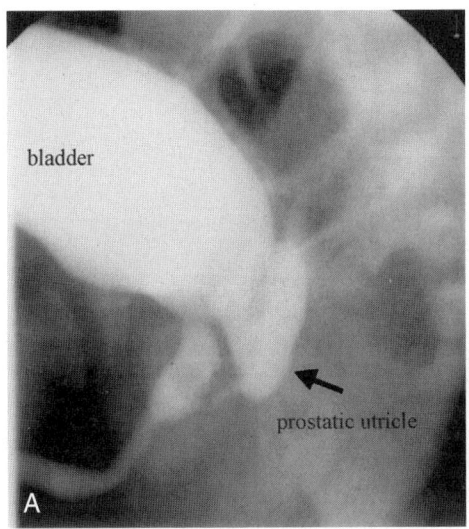
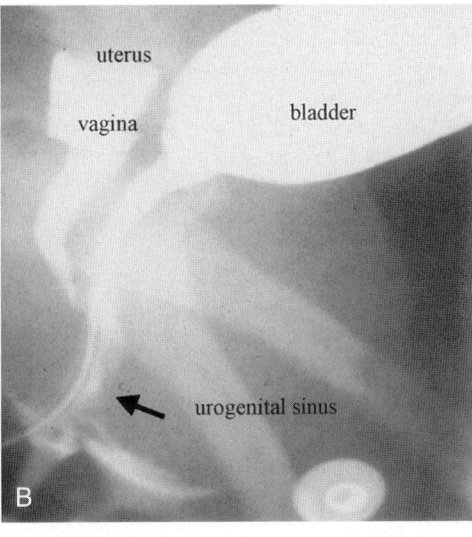

FIGURE 92-6 Genitourethrograms. A, Genitogram from a 46,XY infant with microphallus and undescended testes with a clearly delineated prostatic utricle (see Case Study 2). **B,** Genitogram from a 46,XX infant with congenital adrenal hyperplasia and severe masculinization of external genitals. The confluence of the vagina with the urogenital sinus is of intermediate severity.

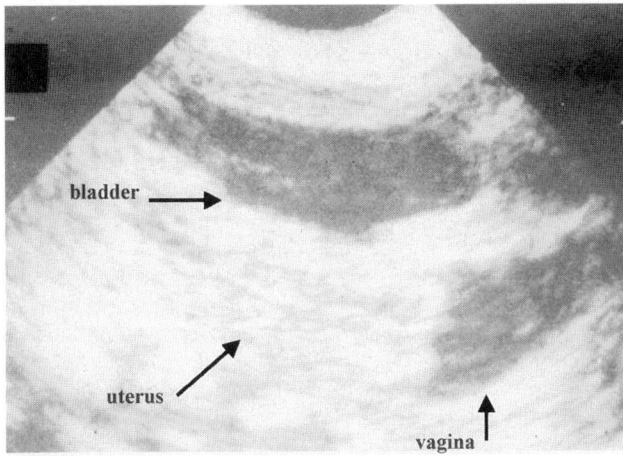

FIGURE 92-7 Ultrasound image from a 46,XX infant with ambiguous genitalia. Note the presence of a well-developed uterus with an endometrial stripe.

Magnetic Resonance Imaging

Magnetic resonance imaging (MRI) has been used to assess the internal genitalia of a limited number of infants and children with genital differentiation disorders. The strength of MRI lies in its ability to image large areas in multiple planes and characterize soft tissues. Detailed information about müllerian and wolffian structures and the position of the gonads can be obtained; however, thin sections (3 to 5 mm) are required for an adequate study. Streak gonads remain difficult to visualize. MRI has the capability to differentiate between an enlarged clitoris and a penis, because the bulbospongiosus muscle and transverse perineal muscle are absent or poorly visualized in the virilized female (Wright et al, 1995). MRI is a promising modality for the evaluation of ambiguous genitalia; however, further study is needed to demonstrate efficacy over other imaging modalities.

Laboratory Investigations

Endocrine and genetic laboratory studies are germane in the evaluation of ambiguous genitalia in the newborn. Day 1 of life is an ideal time to obtain serum testosterone and

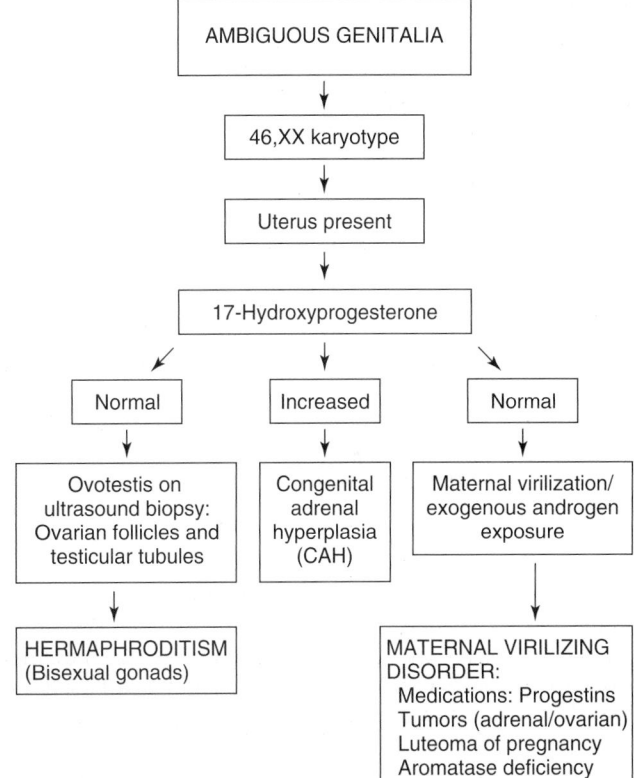

FIGURE 92-8 Algorithm for evaluation of the 46,XX infant with ambiguous genitalia. The presence of a uterus would be determined radiographically by ultrasound examination, genitourethrogram, or magnetic resonance imaging.

dihydrotestosterone (DHT) levels, as testosterone levels fall rapidly in the first several days of life (Forest et al, 1980). Material for chromosomal studies should optimally be obtained on day 1, as at least 48 to 72 hours are required to complete the study. On days 2 or 3 of life, determinations of serum 17-hydroxyprogesterone, 17-hydroxypregnenolone, 11-deoxycortisol, dehydroepiandrosterone (DHEA), androstenedione, and plasma renin activity are performed if CAH is suggested. Some clinicians perform an adrenocorticotropic hormone (ACTH) stimulation test at this time to

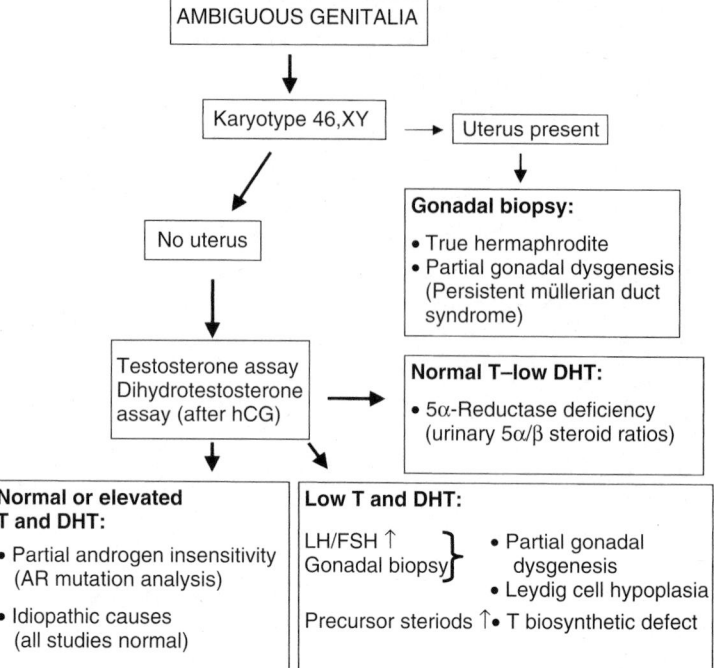

FIGURE 92-9 Algorithm for evaluation of the infant with ambiguous genitalia and 46,XY karyotype. The presence or absence of a uterus would be determined by radiographic imaging including ultrasound examination, genitourethrogram, or magnetic resonance imaging, as appropriate. Testosterone (T) and dihydrotestosterone (DHT) levels ideally should be obtained after human chorionic gonadotrophin (hCG) stimulation. AR, Androgen receptor; FSH, follicle-stimulating hormone; LH, luteinizing hormone.

more clearly demonstrate a block in steroid biosynthesis. Results of these studies should be sent immediately to the appropriate reference laboratory for analysis. Alerting the reference laboratory to the urgent nature of the studies performed will facilitate rapid processing. 17-Hydroxyprogesterone levels are physiologically elevated in the 1st day of life, and screening for congenital adrenal hyperplasia should preferably not be done at this time. Serum gonadotropins are often suppressed in the immediate newborn period, so they should be measured after 1 week of life. Luteinizing hormone (LH) and follicle-stimulating hormone (FSH) levels are helpful in assessing for androgen insensitivity, gonadal dysgenesis, and LH receptor abnormalities. Repeated LH, FSH, testosterone, and DHT testing should be done between 2 and 8 weeks of life in the evaluation of undervirilized males. This time period coincides with the physiologic testosterone surge seen in healthy male infants (Forest et al, 1980). When congenital adrenal hyperplasia is suggested, it is important to check sodium and potassium levels on a daily basis to prevent a salt-wasting crisis.

A human chorionic gonadotrophin (hCG) test will be useful in the evaluation of suspected incomplete masculinization of the genetic male. HCG binds the LH receptor and stimulates the testes to synthesize sex steroids. An adequate testosterone response rules out a testosterone biosynthetic defect, and a normal testosterone-to-DHT ratio argues against 5α-reductase-2 deficiency. In addition, the test can result in phallic enlargement. Almaguer et al (1993) reported an increase in phallic length of 0.25 to 0.75 cm in six 46,XY males with idiopathic microphallus within 5 days of beginning injections. A bolus of 1500 IU of hCG was given intramuscularly on 3 consecutive days, with steroids and phallic length measured on the 5th day. Growth of the phallus in response to hCG suggests that the phallus will further virilize at puberty, although no longitudinal study has documented this assumption.

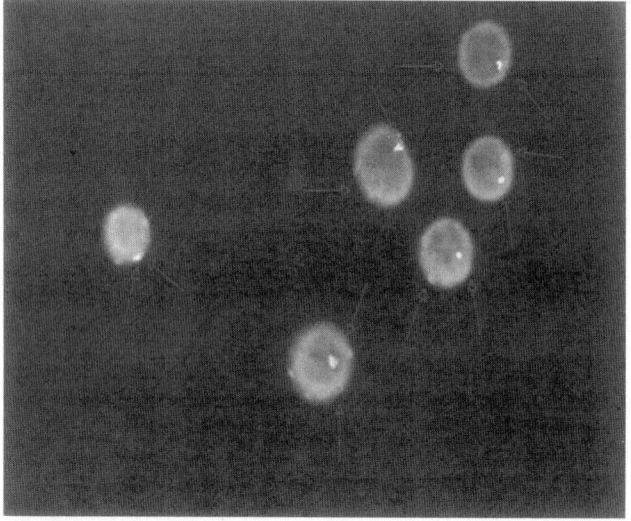

FIGURE 92-10 Fluorescence in situ hybridization (FISH) technique demonstrating the sex chromosome constitution of peripheral blood leukocytes.

A testosterone level greater than 200 ng/dL with a testosterone-to-DHT ratio of less than 8:1 is considered a normal response to hCG.

Fluorescence in situ hybridization (FISH) can rapidly determine the sex chromosome complement of the newborn by using X chromosome– and Y chromosome–specific centromeric probes (Schwartz et al, 1997) (Figure 92-10). In addition, this methodology allows for the detection of low levels of chromosomal mosaicism, because hundreds of cells can be analyzed rapidly. FISH is also useful in identifying a translocated SRY to an X chromosome (Wang et al, 2009). FISH analysis for determination of sex chromosome constitution has been shown to be highly reliable, although this methodology has not been used extensively in the evaluation of ambiguous genitalia of the newborn. As a result, results should be interpreted with some degree of caution until confirmation by karyotypic analysis is available.

In a small percentage of ambiguous genitalia cases, laparoscopy with gonadal biopsy is necessary to confirm the diagnosis of true hermaphroditism, gonadal dysgenesis, or Leydig cell aplasia. Obtaining a karyotype from gonadal tissue may be helpful when sex chromosome mosaicism is suggested.

DISORDERS RESULTING IN AMBIGUOUS GENITALIA

VIRILIZATION OF THE FEMALE

Virilization of an XX infant is most commonly caused by CAH, although other virilizing conditions can be involved (see Figure 92-8). CAH encompasses a group of disorders of adrenal steroid hormone biosynthesis, of which more than 95% are due to 21-hydroxylase deficiency (New, 1992) (Figure 92-11).

Occasionally, the presence of excess androgens of maternal origin can result in virilization of the female fetus (Grumbach and Conte, 1998). A unique cause of both maternal and fetal masculinization is placental aromatase deficiency (Conte et al, 1994). 46,XX male sex reversal syndrome can occur when the SRY gene is translocated from the Y to an X chromosome. Most patients with SRY-positive 46,XX male sex reversal syndrome have normal male external genitalia, but occasionally the genitalia are ambiguous (Ergun-Longmire et al, 2005; Wang et al, 2009).

CONGENITAL ADRENAL HYPERPLASIA

21-Hydroxylase deficiency is the most common cause of ambiguous genitalia in the newborn female (New, 1992). 21-Hydroxylase deficiency has a population frequency of approximately 1 in 15,000, and the disorder is inherited in an autosomal recessive fashion. Males and females are equally affected; however, in classic cases, females usually

are virilized at birth, resulting in the clinical presentation of ambiguous genitalia.

Deficiency of the 21-hydroxylase enzyme results in excess accumulation of the substrate 17-hydroxyprogesterone, which is shunted into the androgen synthesizing pathway and results in excess levels of androstenedione (see Figure 92-11). Androstenedione is then converted peripherally to testosterone. The excess production of androgens results in masculinization of the external genitalia of the female fetus, whereas a male infant with 21-hydroxylase deficiency is phenotypically normal. The degree of masculinization in the female is variable and can range from mild enlargement of the clitoris to complete closure of the urethra at the tip of the phallus (see Figure 92-4). The degree of virilization can be classified by Prader stages, ranging from I to V (Figure 92-12). Stage I represents mild enlargement of the clitoris only. Stage V

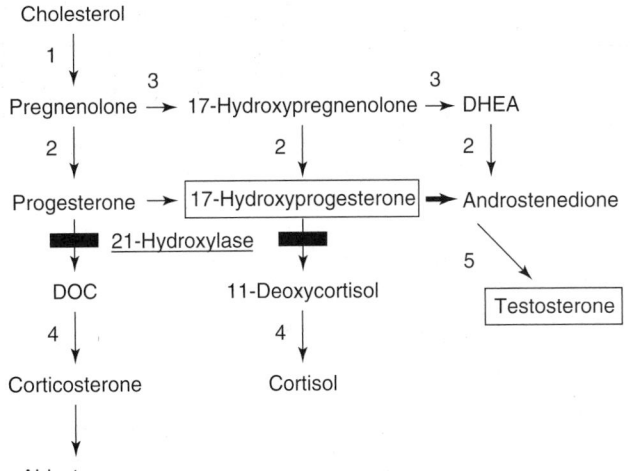

FIGURE 92-11 Steroid biosynthetic pathway demonstrating the defect in 21-hydroxylase deficiency (*solid bars*) and accumulated precursor 17-hydroxyprogesterone. Note the increased shunting into androgen-producing pathways. Steroidogenic enzymes are indicated as follows: (1) steroidogenic acute regulatory protein and side chain cleavage, (2) 3β-hydroxysteroid dehydrogenase, (3) 17α-hydroxylase/17,20-lyase, (4) 11β-hydroxylase, and (5) 17β-hydroxysteroid dehydrogenase. *DHEA,* Dehydroxyepiandrosterone; *DOC,* deoxycorticosterone.

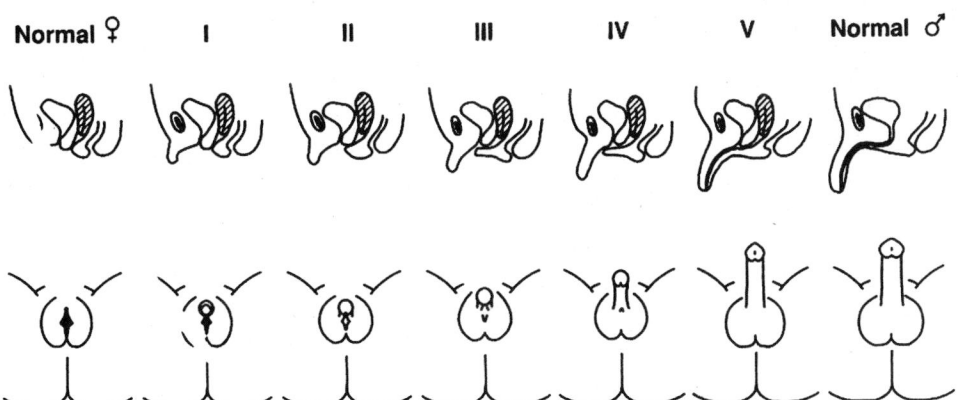

FIGURE 92-12 The stages of virilization of the female with congenital adrenal hyperplasia as developed by Prader. Stage I indicates mild clitoromegaly only; stage V indicates complete masculinization. (*Reproduced with permission from Migeon CJ, Berkovitz G, Brown T: Sexual differentiation and ambiguity. In Kappy MS, Blizzard RM, Migeon CJ, editors: Wilkens' diagnosis and treatment of endocrine disorders in childhood and adolescence, ed 4, Springfield, Ill, 1994, Charles C. Thomas, p 573.*)

represents complete masculinization of the external genitalia, with intermediate stages designating lesser degrees of involvement. The internal genitalia (ovaries, uterus, and fallopian tubes) of virilized females are normal, however, and wolffian duct–derived structures are absent.

The degree of masculinization of the external genitalia of 46,XX fetuses is dependent on the timing and magnitude of androgen exposure of the fetus. Exposure of the female fetus to high androgen levels earlier then 12 weeks' gestation results in fusion of the labial folds with formation of a urogenital sinus. In severely masculinized cases, the external genitalia may appear completely male (see Figure 92-4, *C* and *D*). High-level androgen exposure after 12 weeks' gestation will result in mainly clitoral hypertrophy (see Figure 92-4, *A*).

CAH with 21-hydroxylase deficiency will result in mineralocorticoid deficiency and salt loss in up to 75% of cases (New, 1992; Therrell et al, 1998). However, clinical manifestations of salt loss typically will not become apparent until several days or weeks after birth; therefore all infants with suspected salt-losing CAH need to be followed carefully during this time. Of note a male infant with salt-losing CAH will be phenotypically normal, and he is at great risk for salt-losing crisis after discharge from the newborn nursery. Fortunately, all 50 states within the United States now screen for CAH to prevent males from developing salt-losing crisis, and to prevent incorrect gender assignment of profoundly virilized female infants.

NEWBORN SCREENING

Diagnosis of 21-hydroxylase deficiency can be made by microfilter paper radioimmunoassay for 17-hydroxyprogesterone; this has been useful as a rapid screening test for congenital adrenal hyperplasia in newborns (Pang et al, 1977). This convenient test requires only 20 µL of blood, obtained by heel stick and blotted on microfilter paper, to provide a reliable diagnostic measurement of l7-hydroxyprogesterone, a cortisol precursor that accumulates in elevated concentrations in 21-hydroxylase deficiency. The simplicity of the test and the ease of transporting the microfilter paper specimens through the mail have facilitated the implementation of many congenital adrenal hyperplasia newborn screening programs in the United States and worldwide (Therrell et al, 1998).

There are, however, certain limitations to the screen (Gruneiro-Papendieck et al, 2001; Olgemoller et al, 2003; Therrell et al, 1998; van der Kamp et al, 2005). First, it is not always possible to determine the subtype of CAH solely through the screening of 17-hydroxyprogesterone; therefore, once a diagnosis of CAH has been made, genotyping is recommended to aid in classifying the subtype. Second, to maintain good specificity, many cases of the mild nonclassic form will be missed. Third, the cutoff values for a positive screen vary among different countries and among the different states within the United States. Fourth, preterm infants have higher 17-hydroxyprogesterone levels because of immaturity of the adrenal cortex (Hingre et al, 1994), which may present a challenge in determining what is normal. Cutoff values in the United States, Canada, and New Zealand are typically based on birthweight, although reports from

screening programs in other countries indicate that gestational age, despite being less reliable than birthweight, may be a better predictor (Gruneiro-Papendieck et al, 2001; van der Kamp et al, 2005).

Finally, 17-hydroxyprogesterone levels rapidly decline after birth, and interpretation of the screening value depends on when the sample was drawn. It has been suggested that using a multitiered method using both birthweight and postnatal age can improve the positive predictive value of the screen (Olgemoller et al, 2003). Despite some issues that still need to be resolved, overall the newborn screening program for CAH has been widely successful in achieving the goals of an ideal screen: a relatively easy and efficient test, high morbidity and mortality if the screened disorder is untreated, relatively high disease incidence, and established effective treatment to minimize life-threatening complications after diagnosis.

The diagnosis of 21-hydroxylase deficiency should be suspected in all newborns with ambiguous genitalia (or clitoral hypertrophy) and absent gonads in the labial or scrotal folds. A serum 17-hydroxyprogesterone level obtained after the 1st day of life will often be diagnostic. 17-Hydroxyprogesterone levels are usually 50- to 100-fold above the normal range in classic cases, with typical random levels of 10,000 ng/dL or higher (New, 1992). In

Case Study 1
History
- A 3.5-kg term infant born after uncomplicated pregnancy
- Cryptorchidism and hypospadias noted, so infant discharged home as a male with plan for outpatient surgical evaluation
- Infant fed poorly at home, with intake of approximately 4 oz/day, no vomiting
- On day 5 of life, notification of abnormal newborn screen for congenital adrenal hyperplasia by health department; referred to emergency department

Evaluation
- On presentation to emergency department: infant was well-appearing, weight 2.9 kg (representing a loss of 0.6 kg)
- Genital examination: 2.3 × 1.1 cm phallus, severe hypospadias, marked labial fusion, no palpable gonads, marked hyperpigmentation of genitalia
- Electrolytes: sodium 140 mEq/L, potassium 5.8 mEq/L, chloride 107 mEq/L, CO_2 19 mEq/L, BUN 15 mg/dL, Cr 1.0 mg/dL
- Glucose 94 mg/dL
- Ultrasound examination: uterus present, enlarged adrenals, no gonads seen
- Karyotype 46,XX
- 17-Hydroxyprogesterone 20,000 ng/dL (normal < less than 200—unstimulated)
- Plasma renin activity 201 ng/mL/h (normal < less than 26)

Management and Outcome
- Gender was reassigned female
- Hydrocortisone (Cortef) and fludrocortisone acetate (Florinef) started along with NaCl supplements
- On day 10 of life, weight 3.2 kg, feeding 4 oz/4 hours
- By 4 months of age, significant reduction in clitoral and labial enlargement as well as resolution of hyperpigmentation
- By 3 years of age, the clitoral size had not normalized and the mother became very concerned about the child showing signs of gender "confusion," and hence clitoral reduction surgery was performed

some cases of 21-hydroxylase deficiency, ACTH stimulation testing may be necessary to establish the diagnosis.

Levels of androstenedione, testosterone, electrolytes, and plasma renin activity should also be determined. Plasma renin activity is a sensitive indicator of the intravascular volume status of the infant. Impaired sodium-potassium and sodium-hydrogen exchange owing to aldosterone deficiency in the distal tubule of the kidney results in hyponatremic dehydration, hyperkalemia, and metabolic acidosis.

Assessment for the less common forms of CAH resulting in ambiguous genitalia—11β-hydroxylase deficiency and 3β-hydroxysteroid dehydrogenase deficiency (3β-HSD)—include measuring 11-deoxycortisol, deoxycorticosterone (DOC), and 17-hydroxypregnenolone. (Use of a comprehensive steroid panel from a reliable reference laboratory will limit the amount of required blood to 3 to 5 mL.)

11β-Hydroxylase deficiency accounts for approximately 5% of CAH cases worldwide, and this disorder will result in masculinization of the female fetus (see Figure 92-11). However, the presence of volume overload and hypertension distinguishes this disorder from 21-hydroxylase deficiency (New, 1992). Presumably the hypertension is caused by the excess mineralocorticoid activity of the DOC metabolite. Typically, 11-deoxycortisol (compound S) is elevated and plasma renin activity is suppressed in this disorder.

3β-HSD may result in ambiguous genitalia in the newborn period (see Figure 92-11). Unlike 21-hydroxylase deficiency, this enzyme is present in the gonads as well as the adrenal glands, and deficiency of 3β-HSD can result in undermasculinization of the male infant or mild masculinization of the female infant. The 3β-HSD enzyme is needed for testosterone biosynthesis; therefore the male fetus may be inadequately masculinized. This enzyme deficiency results in excess production of the steroid DHEA, which can be converted to more potent androgens peripherally. The female infant with this disorder can have clitoromegaly, although such children often are phenotypically normal. A marked increase in the ratios of 17-hydroxypregnenolone or 17-hydroxyprogesterone and of DHEA or androstenedione is diagnostic in mutation-positive forms of this disorder (Sakkal-Alkaddour et al, 1996).

Treatment of CAH in the newborn period consists of glucocorticoid and mineralocorticoid replacement. Hydrocortisone is the most physiologic form of synthetic glucocorticoids and is less likely to result in unwanted side effects. Hydrocortisone is administered orally at a dose of approximately 25 mg/m²/day (divided into three doses) in the newborn period. No liquid preparation of hydrocortisone is currently available, so tablets must be crushed and administered carefully with formula or food. Mineralocorticoid replacement (fludrocortisone acetate [Florinef]) at a starting dose of 0.1 mg/day in the newborn is recommended. Sodium chloride supplements (approximately 1 to 2 g/day) may be a useful adjunctive therapy in salt-losing CAH, because formula and human milk have low salt contents. Once therapy is initiated, careful monitoring of the infant's growth and determination of serum 17-hydroxyprogesterone, androstenedione, testosterone, aldosterone and plasma renin activity are recommended.

Salt-losing crisis and acute adrenal insufficiency should be treated with stress doses of hydrocortisone (100 mg/m²/day), which can be given either continuously as a drip or divided into equal doses every 6 hours. Intravenous fluids with ample sodium chloride (normal saline for boluses and one-half normal saline for maintenance fluids) are an essential component of treating salt-losing crisis. Care should be taken not to overhydrate or underhydrate the infant. Hyperkalemia often decreases after sodium chloride and hydrocortisone are provided intravenously, although severe cases of hyperkalemia may require additional therapies.

Gender assignment for 46,XX infants with 21-hydroxylase deficiency has traditionally been female (American Academy of Pediatrics Committee on Genetics, 2000; Donahoe, 1991; Forest, 2001; Migeon et al, 1994; New, 1992;). Gender identity of 46,XX adults with CAH typically is female, with various degrees of masculinized behavior (Money and Ehrhardt, 1972; Reiner, 1997). Prenatal androgenization affects gender-related behavior, but not gender identity, in girls with CAH aged 5 to 12 years (Meyer-Bahlburg et al, 2004a). Cases of gender identity disorder have been reported in treated females with CAH (Slijper et al, 1998), and cases of gender reassignment from female to male have been reported (Meyer-Bahlburg et al, 1996). Persons with undiagnosed 46,XX CAH who are profoundly virilized have functioned successfully as males (Blizzard, 1999; Meyer-Bahlburg, 2009). Diamond and Sigmundson (1997a) have suggested male gender assignment in profoundly virilized 46,XX individuals, although female gender assignment is likely to prevail in current practice until evidence is obtained to indicate otherwise (Crouch et al, 2008; Lee, 2001).

In addition to medical therapies for CAH, efforts to normalize the appearance of the external genitalia may be pursued. It should be kept in mind that hypertrophy of the clitoris will gradually lessen after medical therapy is instituted; however, complete normalization in the more virilized cases is not likely to occur. In severe cases of clitoral enlargement, clitoral reduction surgery is a treatment option, although suboptimal cosmetic results have been reported in long-term outcome studies. Atrophy or loss of the clitoris or excessive regrowth of clitoral tissue has been described in examinations of adolescent and adult patients who underwent genital surgery in early childhood (Alizai et al, 1999; Creighton et al, 2001). The risk of surgery needs to be balanced against the potential detrimental effects of masculinized genitalia on the development of a poor body image (Meyer-Bahlburg et al, 1996) and of social stigmatization by family or community members (Money et al, 1986). Recently, nerve-sparing ventral clitoroplasty in virilized females has been shown to preserve dorsal nerves for better sensitivity after surgery (Poppas et al, 2007).

Surgical correction of the vagina in CAH is performed to exteriorize the vagina and to enlarge the vaginal opening so that successful intercourse can occur later in life (see later section on surgery). There is considerable debate about when to perform vaginal exteriorization surgery. A number of studies have demonstrated the development of vaginal stenosis when vaginoplasties are performed in the prepubertal period (Alizai et al, 1999;

Creighton et al, 2001; Krege et al, 2000). The investigators advocate delaying vaginoplasty until puberty or later, when manual dilation can be undertaken by the patient and estrogenization of the vaginal mucosa can help to prevent stricture formation. Others recommend that vaginoplasties be undertaken early in life, because the procedure is technically easier in the first several years of life and the emotional trauma of a major surgery at adolescence is avoided (Donahoe, 1991; Schnitzer, 2001). Recent reports of long-term outcome of genitoplasty by patient advocate groups such as the Intersex Society of North America (ISNA) and others have called for a general moratorium on all nonessential genital surgery in infancy, until affected persons are old enough to express their wishes and give consent (Diamond and Sigmundson, 1997a). Problems with loss of sexual sensation and pleasure have been reported in adult patients as a consequence of genital surgery in early life. However, in cases of severe discordance between assigned sex and genital appearance, the psychosocial consequences of uncorrected genital anomalies can be damaging (Money and Ehrhardt, 1972; Money et al, 1986). Participation of the parents in the decision to pursue genital surgery after they have been fully informed of the benefits and risks is perhaps the most judicious approach at this time (Daaboul and Frader, 2001; Lee, 2001; Reiner, 1997).

Significant reductions in fertility have been reported in women with salt-losing CAH (Kuhnle et al, 1995; Mulaikal et al, 1987). Suggested explanations for reduced fertility included increased anovulatory cycles, low rates of heterosexual activity, inadequate vaginal introitus, and poor compliance with medical treatment (Mulaikal et al, 1987). Problems with a disturbed body image and feeling less feminine were associated with a lower rate of success among women with CAH in terms of the ability to establish a partnership or marry (Kuhnle et al, 1995). Overall quality of life for female patients with CAH was comparable with that for controls, suggesting that affected women may develop coping strategies and cognitive appraisals that enable them to accept their life and view it as satisfying (Kuhnle et al, 1995).

PRENATAL DIAGNOSIS AND TREATMENT

DIAGNOSIS

Since the report by Jeffcoate et al (1965) of the successful identification of an affected fetus by elevated concentrations of 17-ketosteroids and pregnanetriol in the amniotic fluid, investigators in the past have performed prenatal diagnosis for congenital adrenal hyperplasia by measurements of hormone levels in pregnancy (Jeffcoate et al, 1965; Levine et al, 1986; New and Levine, 1973). The most specific hormonal diagnostic test for 21-hydroxylase deficiency is elevated 17-OHP in the amniotic fluid (Frasier et al, 1974; Hughes and Laurence, 1979, 1982; Nagamani et al, 1978; Pang et al, 1980); Δ4-androstenedione can be used as an adjunctive diagnostic assay (Pang et al, 1980). Amniotic fluid testosterone levels might not be outside the normal range in an affected male (Wilson et al, 1995). Measuring hormone levels in amniotic fluid detects only

severe cases, and for the most part it has been replaced by molecular diagnosis.

HLA genotyping of amniotic fluid cells is another possible means of diagnosis, but it has been superseded by direct molecular analysis of the 21-hydroxylase locus. With the advent of chorionic villus sampling, evaluation of the at-risk fetus is currently possible in the first trimester at 9 to 11 weeks' gestation. The fetal DNA is used for specific amplification of the *CYP21A2* gene using polymerase chain reaction and Southern blotting, which has the advantage of requiring small amounts of DNA (Speiser et al, 1990). Because of improved accuracy and earlier diagnosis, molecular analysis of fetal DNA is now the method of choice for prenatal diagnosis. See Chapter 91 for more details.

TREATMENT

Treatment with dexamethasone can be used in pregnancies at risk for 21-hydroxylase deficiency (Dorr et al, 1986; Evans et al, 1985; Forest and David, 1991; Mercado et al, 1995; Speiser et al, 1990). When properly administered, dexamethasone is effective in preventing ambiguous genitalia in the affected female. The current recommendation is to treat the mother with a pregnancy at risk for 21-hydroxylase deficiency with dexamethasone in a dose of 20 μg/kg divided into two or three doses daily (Mercado et al, 1995).

Adrenocortical steroidogenesis begins at approximately 6 weeks' gestation, and differentiation of the external genitalia and urogenital sinus begins at approximately 9 weeks' gestation (New et al, 1989). The institution of dexamethasone therapy is recommended as soon as pregnancy is confirmed and no later than 9 weeks after the last menstrual period; this will effectively suppress adrenal androgen production, allow normal separation of the vaginal and urethral orifices, and prevent clitoromegaly. The need to initiate at such an early date means that treatment is blind to the sex of the fetus. If the fetus is determined to be a male upon karyotyping or an unaffected female upon DNA analysis, treatment is discontinued. Otherwise, treatment is continued to term.

Between 1978 and 2002, prenatal diagnosis and treatment of CAH caused by 21-OHD was performed in 595 pregnancies at The New York–Presbyterian Hospital–Weill Medical College of Cornell University, of which 108 infants were affected with classic 21-OHD. Of these, 64 were females, 51 of whom were treated prenatally with dexamethasone. Dexamethasone administered at or before 9 weeks' gestation was effective in reducing virilization, thus avoiding postnatal genitoplasty (Carlson et al, 1999; New et al, 2003). No significant or enduring side effects were noted in the mothers (other than greater weight gain and a higher incidence of striae and edema than untreated mothers) or the fetuses. There was no statistically significant difference in hypertension or gestational diabetes between treated and untreated mothers. All mothers who took partial or full treatment stated they would take dexamethasone again in the event of a future pregnancy. In our report and in others, no cases have been reported of cleft palate, placental degeneration, or fetal death, which have been observed in a rodent model of in utero exposure to high-dose glucocorticoids (Goldman, 1978; Nimkarn, 2005). In contrast, another study noted some significant maternal side effects, including excessive weight gain, cushingoid facial features, severe striae resulting in permanent scarring, and hyperglycemic response to oral glucose administration (Pang et al, 1992).

A long-term follow-up study of 44 children treated prenatally in Scandinavia demonstrated normal prenatal and postnatal growth compared with matched controls (Lajic et al, 1998). Prenatally treated newborns also did not differ in weight, length, or head circumference from untreated, unaffected newborns (Carlson et al, 1999; New et al, 2003). Moreover, a survey of 174 children aged 1 month to 12 years and exposed prenatally to dexamethasone (including 48 with CAH) compared with 313 unexposed children (including 195 with CAH) found no differences in cognitive or motor development between the two groups (Meyer-Bahlburg et al, 2004b). Therefore we believe that proper prenatal treatment of fetuses at risk for CAH can be considered effective and safe. Long-term studies on the psychological development of patients treated prenatally are currently under way. This therapy may be controversial in other centers.

The efficacy of prenatal treatment in 11β-OHD CAH has been shown as well. In 1999 Cerame et al (1999) reported the first prenatal diagnosis and treatment of an affected female with 11β-OHD CAH. As an indication of the treatment's success, the prenatally treated newborn had normal female external genitalia.

INCREASED MATERNAL ANDROGENS AND PROGESTINS

Masculinization of the female fetus has been reported in pregnant mothers taking various progestational agents to prevent miscarriage. These agents include norethindrone, ethisterone, and medroxyprogesterone. Danazol, which has been used in the treatment of endometriosis, has been associated with fetal masculinization (Grumbach and Conte, 1998). Masculinization of the female fetus due to maternal virilizing ovarian or adrenal tumors or luteomas of pregnancy has been reported. In such cases, virilization beyond the time of birth does not occur, and the prognosis is good (Grumbach and Conte, 1998).

PLACENTAL AROMATASE DEFICIENCY

Placental aromatase deficiency has been associated with masculinization of the female fetus. Aromatase is a cytochrome P450 enzyme that is responsible for the conversion of testosterone to estradiol and of androstenedione to estrone. Autosomal recessive inheritance of aromatase deficiency causes virilization of the female because of a failure to metabolize the large amounts of androstenedione and testosterone produced by the placenta. This disorder also will cause significant virilization of the mother. The affected infant will be virilized with normal müllerian structures. Gonadotropins are elevated in infancy, and ovarian cysts may develop. At puberty, females have hypergonadotropic hypogonadism with failure to feminize and progressive virilization. Plasma androstenedione and testosterone levels are elevated, whereas estrone and estradiol

levels are low. Postpubertal patients have delayed bone maturation, tall stature, and osteopenia (Conte et al, 1994).

INCOMPLETELY MASCULINIZED MALES

Incomplete masculinization refers to absence of or incomplete masculinization of the external and internal genitalia in a person with a 46,XY karyotype and normal testes. Disorders leading to incomplete masculinization of the male include androgen receptor defects, testosterone biosynthetic defects, 5α-reductase deficiency, Leydig cell hypoplasia, and effects of maternal medications (see Figure 92-9).

It should be noted that in 25% to 50% of undermasculinized males, a specific cause cannot be found (Al-Agha et al, 2001; Eil et al, 1984). Other factors such as medications and placental insufficiency may potentially interfere with genital masculinization. Placental insufficiency may be related to genital underdevelopment through the presumed mechanism of inadequate hCG production. Placental hCG is required for early fetal testosterone production and therefore early fetal genital development.

Medications such as cimetidine, spironolactone, phenytoin (Dilantin), phenobarbital, medroxyprogesterone, and cyproterone acetate have been associated with altered androgen action or metabolism. Their use during pregnancy may be detrimental to male genital development (Donahoe, 1991; Grumbach and Conte, 1998). Furthermore, various xenobiotics can bind the androgen receptor; therefore there has been speculation regarding the role of environmental factors in abnormal sex differentiation (Danzol, 1998).

ANDROGEN RECEPTOR DEFECTS (ANDROGEN INSENSITIVITY)

Disorders of the androgen receptor are the most common definable cause of incomplete masculinization of the genetic male (Quigley et al, 1995). Disorders of the androgen receptor can be divided into complete androgen insensitivity and partial androgen insensitivity (PAIS) syndromes. The gene for the androgen receptor (*AR*) is located on the X chromosome, and more than 300 mutations have been found (Griffin et al, 2001). Mutations have been found throughout the *AR* gene, with most mutations occurring in the DNA or steroid-binding domains. Despite extensive characterization of the molecular genetics of *AR* mutations, no genotype–phenotype correlation has been found (Quigley et al, 1995).

The sex-differentiating actions of testosterone and DHT are mediated by the androgen receptor. DHT is important in the differentiation of the male external genitalia and prostate, whereas testosterone is important in the differentiation of internal wolffian ducts to epididymis, vas deferens, and seminal vesicles.

Complete Androgen Insensitivity

Complete androgen insensitivity syndrome in a 46,XY individual is characterized by phenotypically normal female external genitalia (Figure 92-13). Affected

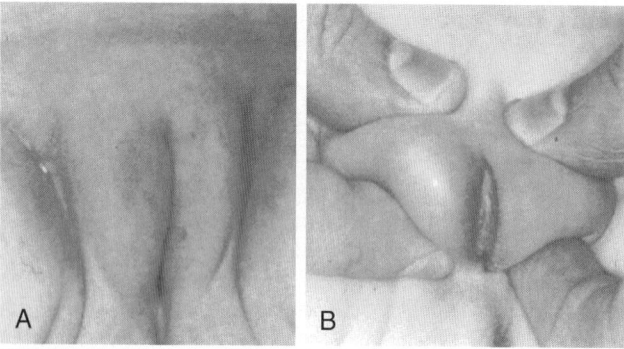

FIGURE 92-13 **A,** Appearance of external genitalia of a 46,XY infant with complete androgen insensitivity syndrome. **B,** Note presence of bilateral palpable gonads.

children will have an inguinal hernia before puberty or primary amenorrhea after puberty onset. Robust breast development occurs at puberty that is due to peripheral aromatization of testosterone to estrogen. There is usually scant or absent pubic and axillary hair with some vulvar hair. The vagina is short and blind-ending, and müllerian structures (cervix, uterus, fallopian tubes) are absent. There are only vestigial or no wolffian duct–derived internal structures. The testes are located in the abdomen or inguinal canal or in the labia majora. Gender identity and role behaviors are typically female. Removal of the testes is recommended because of risk for development of gonadoblastoma, although there is no consensus on the timing of orchidectomy (Forest, 2001; Migeon et al, 1994).

Partial Androgen Insensitivity

PAIS is characterized by varying degrees of ambiguity of the external genitalia. The term *Reifenstein syndrome* formerly was used to describe partial androgen insensitivity with intermediate degrees of masculinization. Affected infants have a small phallus and a ventral chordee that tethers the phallus to the perineum. There is often a penoscrotal hypospadias and a bifid scrotum, which may or may not contain gonads (see Figure 92-3). Cryptorchidism is a common finding. Müllerian structures are absent, and the wolffian duct–derived structures are absent or poorly developed. A genitourethrogram may demonstrate a urogenital sinus.

The diagnosis of partial androgen insensitivity is complex. A family history of ambiguous genitalia in male relatives would be suggestive of this diagnosis. However, Viner et al (1977) reported a positive family history in only 25% of patients with PAIS. 5α-Reductase deficiency and testosterone biosynthetic defects should be ruled out by appropriate steroid analysis. This can be accomplished by measuring intermediates in testosterone biosynthesis and by measuring the ratio of testosterone to DHT. It should be noted that abnormal testosterone-to-DHT ratios can be seen in PAIS (Ahmed et al, 1999); this could be caused by poor development of tissues, which express 5α-reductase-2 in PAIS (Griffin et al, 2001).

Androgen levels in normal newborns are highest at birth and then decline rapidly during the 1st week. A second testosterone surge occurs between 15 and 60 days of life (Forest et al, 1980). Androgen and LH levels should be obtained at these peak production times. Alternatively, an hCG stimulation test may be performed as follows: a dose of 1500 IU of hCG is given intramuscularly daily for 3 days; androgen and gonadotropin levels are measured at baseline and then 24 hours after the third dose. Abnormally elevated levels of LH, testosterone, or both in the first several months of life are suggestive of androgen insensitivity. However, a recent report of five neonatal cases of PAIS showed testosterone values in the high-normal range on days 2 to 7 of life (mean, 107 ± 27 ng/dL) and on day 30 (mean, 411 ± 154 ng/dL; Bouvattier et al, 2002). LH levels were elevated in comparison with historic controls (mean LH levels on days 7 to 15 of life were 5.2 IU/L ± 4.0 ng/dL; on day 30 of life mean levels were 8.7 IU/L ± 2.5 ng/dL). Testosterone response to hCG and LH response to gonadotropin-releasing hormone were exaggerated (Bouvattier et al, 2002).

The androgen receptor binding assay was considered standard for defining this disorder in the past. However, normal ligand binding does not rule out androgen insensitivity, because there may be mutations in domains of the androgen receptor not involved in ligand binding. Direct sequencing of the androgen receptor for mutation analysis is commercially available (GeneTest) and can detect up to 95% of mutations associated with complete androgen insensitivity. Androgen receptor mutations, however, are not always found in cases of possible partial androgen insensitivity, and it is speculated that defects in androgen receptor–interacting proteins may be involved.

Determining the gender of rearing in partial androgen insensitivity is a difficult task, and multiple factors must be considered. If there is a significant degree of virilization (Prader stages 4 and 5; see Figure 92-12), then male sex assignment is made (Diamond and Sigmundson, 1997b; Reiner, 1997). If masculinization is severely limited (Prader stages 1 and 2), then female sex assignment is recommended. In intermediate forms (Prader stage 3), responsiveness to exogenously administered hCG or testosterone may be of help in the decision-making process (Daaboul and Frader, 2001; Grumbach and Conte, 1998). However, adult males with a small phallus have reported satisfactory sex lives (Reilly and Woodhouse, 1989). These cases perhaps deemphasize the importance of phallic size in male sex assignment. Slijper et al (1998) reported the absence of serious gender identity disorder in five undervirilized 46,XY males, although these boys were "more fearful and bothered about the smallness of their penises." Money and Ehrhardt (1972) cautioned about the devastating psychosocial effects of male sex assignment when the phallus is only slightly larger than a clitoris and does not respond to testosterone.

In a study of 32 undervirilized males who were assigned female gender for rearing, significant gender transposition (i.e., gender change and homosexual orientation) correlated with the presence of childhood stigmatization and a relatively late age at feminizing surgery (Money et al, 1986). Stigmatization in the home was reflected by treating the child differently from other children, including elaborate efforts at maintaining the privacy of the genital anomaly, keeping the child at home and forbidding play with neighborhood children, and refusal of open communication within the family about the medical condition. Stigmatization in the community was reflected by teasing, such as about the genital anomaly, body habitus, and mannerisms. Stigmatization by parents or the community also was found to be associated with gender transposition in undervirilized males who were assigned male gender for rearing; cosmetic inadequacy of the external genitalia was less important (Money and Norman, 1987).

These studies indicate the importance of a nurturing, supportive environment to a successful long-term outcome for these children. More comprehensive long-term outcome studies of partial androgen insensitivity are greatly needed.

5α-REDUCTASE-2 DEFICIENCY

5α-Reductase-2 deficiency is an autosomal recessive disorder that results in an inability to convert testosterone to DHT. DHT is required for the development of the male external genitalia.

At birth, these 46,XY infants typically have a very small phallus that appears to be a normal or slightly enlarged clitoris. However, more significant virilization of the phallus may occur, and the affected child will then be identified as a male with hypospadias. There is usually severe penoscrotal hypospadias. The scrotum is bifid, with slight posterior fusion. The testes are usually in the inguinal canals or labial folds. Approximately half of these patients have a penoscrotal urethra with a separate blind-ending vagina; a smaller percentage have a single urogenital sinus opening on the perineum (Griffin et al, 2001). Müllerian structures are absent, and wolffian duct–derived structures (vas deferens, epididymis, seminal vesicles) are well developed. The prostate is poorly developed.

At the time of puberty, individuals with this disorder will characteristically virilize. The phallus will typically increase to a length of 4 to 8 cm (Migeon et al, 1994). In affected persons who were raised as females, a change to the male gender role after puberty is commonly seen (Griffin et al, 2001; Imperato-McGinley, 1997). Unlike in partial androgen insensitivity, gynecomastia does not occur in the pubertal period.

5α-Reductase-2 deficiency has been diagnosed in the postpubertal period in most cases, although diagnosis in the newborn period has been reported (Imperato-McGinley et al, 1986; Odame et al, 1992). The disorder is diagnosed by assessing the ratio of testosterone to DHT in blood (Peterson et al, 1977). The normal testosterone-to-DHT ratio in the newborn period is 4:1, whereas the ratio in infants and children with this disorder is often greater than 14:1. An hCG stimulation test usually is needed to obtain a more definitive diagnosis in the prepubertal period. A positive response to hCG rules out Leydig cell aplasia or a testosterone biosynthetic defect. Measurement of normal androstenedione levels will rule out the testosterone biosynthetic defect—17β-HSD dehydrogenase deficiency. This enzyme is responsible for the conversion of androstenedione to testosterone, and the clinical presentation in infancy can be similar to that of 5α-reductase deficiency.

In addition, abnormal ratios of 5β- to 5α-urinary steroids can establish a definitive diagnosis of 5α-reductase deficiency-2 (Imperato-McGinley et al, 1986). Distinguishing 5α-reductase deficiency from partial androgen insensitivity is important, because androgen insensitivity can cause a secondary DHT deficiency owing to the incomplete development of tissues that express 5α-reductase activity (Griffin et al, 2001). Measurement of urinary 5β- and 5α-glucocorticoids will help to make this distinction, because only 5α-reductase deficiency will also affect glucocorticoid metabolism. Analysis of 5α-reductase-2 activity in genital fibroblasts also can be determined. Finally, analysis for mutations in the *SRD5A2* gene is diagnostic; however, this test is not commercially available.

Sex assignment in cases of 5α-reductase deficiency is a complicated issue, but there is long-term outcome information available. As in androgen insensitivity disorders, sex assignment is often significantly influenced by the degree of masculinization at birth, and because infants with this disorder usually are markedly undervirilized, female sex assignment has been advocated (Grumbach and Conte, 1998; Migeon et al, 1994). However, if the disorder is diagnosed early, topical DHT treatment has been shown to enlarge the phallus (Odame et al, 1992). In addition, the natural history of the disorder is for masculinization of the phallus to occur at puberty. Testicular histopathologic analysis in of males with this disorder has shown that, unlike in isolated bilateral cryptorchidism, their testes display type Ad (i.e., dark) spermatogonia and a normal germ cell count. These patients are largely infertile because of defective transformation of spermatogonia into spermatocytes (Hadziselimovic and Dessouky, 2008).

There are frequent reports of reversal from female to male gender behavior after puberty (Wilson, 2001; Wilson et al, 1993). The accumulated evidence would support male sex assignment in this disorder (Imperato-McGinley, 1997), although female sex assignment is likely in the newborn period if the diagnosis is overlooked.

TESTOSTERONE BIOSYNTHETIC DEFECTS

Five enzymes are necessary for the synthesis of testosterone. A defect at any step will result in inadequate testosterone synthesis (see Figure 92-11). Defects in the first three enzymes of the testosterone synthesis pathway will also affect adrenal steroid production, resulting in both an undervirilized male and CAH. Because testosterone production is impaired in these disorders, wolffian duct structures are likely to be underdeveloped, whereas müllerian structures are absent because of normal testicular MIF production. These enzyme deficiencies are rare; therefore these disorders are discussed only briefly.

17β-Hydroxysteroid Dehydrogenase-3 Deficiency (17-Ketosteroid Reductase Deficiency)

The final step in testosterone biosynthesis involves the conversion of androstenedione to testosterone by the enzyme 17β-HSD in the testicle. Mutations that impair the function of 17β-HSD are the cause of this relatively rare autosomal recessive disorder (Wilson, 2001).

The clinical presentation externally is that of a female at birth with perhaps a mild degree of clitoral enlargement. The phenotype is female; therefore these infants typically are raised as females. At puberty, there is progressive masculinization, with enlargement of the phallus to 4 to 6 cm with labial enlargement and rugation. By late puberty, the testes are found at the lower ring of the inguinal canal, and they are of normal size and consistency. Internal wolffian duct–derived structures are found. In addition, a male body habitus develops, with deepening of the voice and appearance of male body hair, including mustache and beard (Migeon et al, 1994).

Most patients receive a diagnosis at puberty or as adults. Endocrine studies reveal markedly elevated androstenedione levels, whereas testosterone levels are in the low-normal range (Mendonca et al, 2000). Plasma LH levels are consistently high. In infancy or childhood, the presence of inguinal hernias may bring the child to medical attention. Androstenedione levels in the prepubertal patient may be normal, and the hCG stimulation test is required to elucidate the defect.

Gender of rearing often is influenced by the cultural context. In societies in which a high priority is given to the male gender, gender reassignment at puberty has been successful (Forest, 2001). Mendonca et al (2000) have observed changes in gender role (female to male) in 3 of 10 affected individuals. Despite virilization in some affected persons, the female gender role was maintained.

Congenital Lipoid Adrenal Hyperplasia

Lipid accumulation in both the adrenal glands and gonads is characteristic of this disorder pathologically—hence the name *congenital lipoid adrenal hyperplasia*. Because all adrenal and gonadal steroid synthesis is affected by this disorder, infants are likely to exhibit complete adrenal insufficiency, characterized by vomiting, weight loss, and hypotension. The phenotype is likely to be female, although there is clinical variability. In the 35 cases reported in the medical literature, only 11 patients have survived beyond infancy (Forest, 2001).

Endocrinologic findings include elevation of ACTH and plasma renin activity, but low or immeasurable levels of all steroid hormones. The main consideration in the differential diagnosis is CAH. The presence of markedly enlarged lipid-laden adrenals on ultrasound, computed tomography, or MRI studies is highly suggestive of the disorder. Successful treatment has occurred and requires replacement of both glucocorticoids and mineralocorticoids. All persons with this diagnosis have been raised as females (Grumbach and Conte, 1998).

In vitro studies performed on either adrenal or testicular tissue demonstrated an inability to convert cholesterol to pregnenolone in these patients. A defect in the first step of adrenal and gonadal steroid biosynthesis mediated by the cytochrome P450 side chain cleavage (P450scc) enzyme was suspected. However, subsequent molecular studies demonstrated mutations in the steroidogenic acute regulatory protein (StAR) (Grumbach and Conte, 1998). StAR acts to promote sterol translocation to the P450scc enzyme in mitochondria (see Figure 92-11 and Case Study 2).

Case Study 2

History

- The infant was born at 41 weeks' gestation, weighing 3.2 kg.
- Pregnancy was complicated by preterm contractions from 29 to 34 weeks requiring bed rest.
- Triple screen was abnormal and amniocentesis was performed, revealing a 46,XY karyotype with no mosaicism. The parents did not want to know the karyotype because they did not wish to know the sex of the baby.
- At birth the infant was thought to have normal female genitalia and was assigned to the female sex.
- On careful physical examination the infant was found to have mildly virilized genitalia.

Physical Examination and Laboratory Studies

- Genital examination: mild clitoromegaly, mild posterior labial fusion, a single urogenital sinus, and bilateral inguinal hernias with gonads present
- Ultrasound examination: testicle like structures in the upper portion of the inguinal canal without evidence of a uterus or ovaries
- Karyotype and FISH: confirmed 46,XY, no mosaicism
- Endocrine studies

6 Weeks of age
- Testosterone, 20 ng/dL; DHT, 11 ng/dL
- FSH, 4.3 mIU/mL; LH, 9.0 mIU/mL
- No mutations identified in the androgen receptor

3 Months of age
- Patient underwent a bilateral orchiectomy, inguinal hernia repair, and vaginoplasty.
- Testicular pathology was consistent with prepubertal seminiferous tubules, spermatic cord with vas deferens, epididymis, and hernia sac.

Further clinical course: 6 months of age
- The patient had 2-week history of irritability and, several days of intermittent vomiting, and was admitted to the hospital with dehydration and in adrenal crisis.
- Serum sodium (Na^+) was 124 meq/mL.
- Serum potassium (K^+) was 7.7 meq/mL.
- There were low levels of all adrenal hormones, including testosterone, with no response to ACTH stimulation; baseline cortisol was 10 μg/dL, stimulating to only 12 μg/dL 60 minutes after ACTH was administered.
- Plasma renin activity was 14,345 ng/dL/h.
- Baseline ACTH level was 4781 pg/mL.
- Genetic analysis revealed c.178+1G>C intron 2 homozygous splicing mutation of the *StAR* gene.

Diagnosis

- Congenital lipoid adrenal hyperplasia owing to StAR protein gene mutation

Management and Outcome

- Glucocorticoid supplementation with hydrocortisone and mineralocorticoid supplementation with fludrocortisone initiated
- Female gender assignment maintained

3β-Hydroxysteroid Dehydrogenase Deficiency II

3β-HSD deficiency was first reported by Bongiovanni (1962). 3β-HSD is an important enzyme required for the conversion of Δ-5 to Δ-4 steroids in the adrenal glands and gonads (see Figure 92-11). There is marked heterogeneity in clinical presentation, and both genders are affected (Forest, 2001). With severe deficiency of 3β-HSD, salt-losing crisis can occur. Male infants may have ambiguous or completely feminine external genitalia, whereas female infants may be mildly virilized. Severely undervirilized males may have normal mineralocorticoid activity; fully masculinized males may display salt loss.

Diagnosis of this disorder in the newborn period can be difficult because of relatively high levels of Δ-5 steroids physiologically. The diagnosis is based on the ratio of 17-hydroxyprogesterone to 17-hydroxypregnenolone and of DHEA to androstenedione in the basal and stimulated states (Sakkal-Alkaddour et al, 1996).

17α-Hydroxylase/17,20-Lyase Deficiency

A single enzyme encoded on the P450c17 (*CYP17A1*) gene mediates the 17-hydroxylation of pregnenolone and progesterone and the conversion of 17-hydroxypregnenolone and 17-hydroxyprogesterone to DHEA and androstenedione. Specific mutations can cause partial loss of 17α-hydroxylase/17,20-lyase activites or dissociation between the 17α-hydroxylase and 17,20-lyase function (Dhir et al, 2009). Clinical disorders of this enzyme affect primarily either the hydroxylation or the lyase reaction, although there have been reports of combined 17α-hydroxylase and 17,20-lyase deficiency (Sahakitrungruang et al, 2009). Cases of primarily 17-hydroxylase deficiency should be considered in undervirilized males or females with low renin hypertension and hypokalemic alkalosis. The hypertension is presumably due to elevated levels of DOC and corticosterone (see Figure 92-11). Most cases are diagnosed in the pubertal period because the 46,XY phenotype is largely female. Of interest, although cortisol synthesis is blocked, the overproduction of DOC and corticosterone is protective against adrenal insufficiency. This disorder is treated with glucocorticoid, which suppresses ACTH overproduction and subsequently suppresses DOC and corticosterone overproduction (Grumbach and Conte, 1998). Sex steroid replacement is needed at puberty.

17,20-Lyase deficiency results in various degrees of undermasculinization of the 46,XY infant. The phenotype ranges from complete female external genitalia to ambiguous genitalia to a mildly undervirilized male. 46,XX females will fail to enter puberty. Gonadotropins will be elevated, along with impaired formation of DHEA and androstenedione (see Figure 92-11). DOC and corticosterone are normal in this form of the disorder. HCG and ACTH stimulation tests may be helpful to more fully reveal the steroid biosynthetic block.

LEYDIG CELL HYPOPLASIA

Failure of the testicles to produce testosterone in response to hCG is characteristic of this disorder. Histologic examination of the testes reveals absent or low numbers of Leydig cells, normal-appearing Sertoli cells, and seminiferous tubules with spermatogenic arrest (Grumbach and Conte, 1998). LH receptor mutations have been described in this disorder. Phenotypically, the external genitalia range from those of a normal female to those of a male with microphallus. Müllerian-derived structures are absent in all patients, whereas wolffian structures may be present. LH and FSH levels are elevated in postpubertal patients, and LH levels decrease after testosterone administration. In less severe forms of the disorder, testosterone therapy augments phallic growth. In severe forms of testicular unresponsiveness to hCG/LH, gender assignment has been female. The gonads are removed, and estrogen replacement therapy is instituted at the time of expected puberty (Grumbach and Conte, 1998).

PERSISTENT MULLERIAN DUCT SYNDROME

The diagnosis of PMDS often is made in otherwise phenotypically normal 46,XY males at the time of surgery for an inguinal hernia or orchidopexy. In the case of hernia repair, a fallopian tube and uterus are often found along with a partially descended testis. In other cases, testes, uterus, and fallopian tubes are found in the pelvis. Inheritance of PMDS is autosomal recessive, although the female phenotype is completely normal. The disorder has been found to be due to a mutation in the antimüllerian hormone or receptor (Grumbach and Conte, 1998). Therapy involves orchidopexy and partial hysterectomy, with care taken to avoid injuring the vas deferens that is embedded in the uterine wall.

GONADAL DIFFERENTIATION AND CHROMOSOMAL DISORDERS

46,XY Complete Gonadal Dysgenesis

46,XY complete gonadal dysgenesis was first described by Swyer in 1955 (Grumbach and Conte, 1998). The phenotype of the external genitalia was female with normal development of müllerian-derived internal structures. Streak gonads are found that are completely nonfunctional; therefore müllerian structures do not regress, and wolffian structures are poorly developed or absent (Figure 92-14). Most affected persons are seen in the teenage years with lack of pubertal development. Serum gonadotropin levels are elevated. Mutations in the *SRY* gene account for only a small proportion of these cases (Forest, 2001). Familial cases have been reported. There has been report of a 46,XY mother who developed as a normal woman and gave birth to a 46,XY daughter with complete gonadal dysgenesis in a family with multiple disorders of sexual development, suggesting an unidentified sex-determining gene (Dumic et al, 2008). In up to 30% of affected persons, gonadoblastomas will develop in the streak gonad; therefore removal of the streak gonad is recommended (Migeon et al, 1994) (see Figure 92-14). Estrogen replacement therapy will provide appropriate feminization.

46,XY Partial Gonadal Dysgenesis

Patients with 46,XY partial gonadal dysgenesis will typically be seen in the newborn period for evaluation of ambiguous genitalia (Berkovitz et al, 1991). The extent of masculinization of the external genitalia depends on the extent of testicular differentiation. Gonadal tissue is usually intraabdominal, but testes can be found in the scrotum. One quarter of these patients will have phenotypic features of Turner's syndrome (Migeon et al, 1994). Testosterone response to hCG is variable but usually low. In most cases, there is a mix of müllerian and wolffian structures. The presence of müllerian structures on genitourethrogram or ultrasound

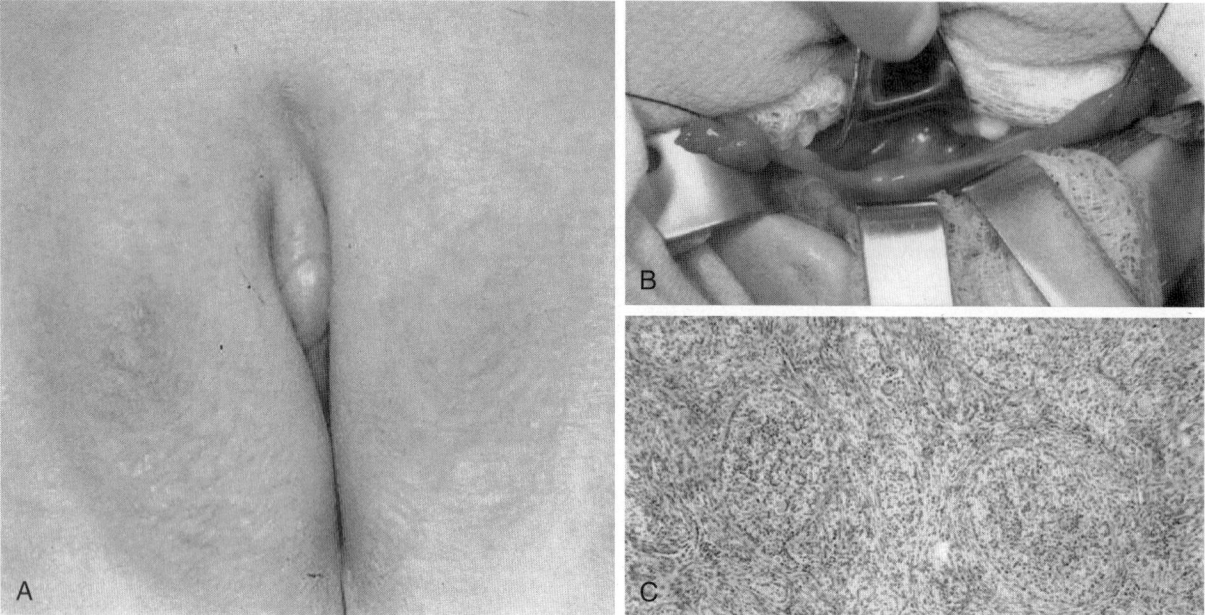

FIGURE 92-14 A, Appearance of external genitalia in complete gonadal dysgenesis in a 46,XY infant with features of Turner's syndrome. **B,** Uterus and fallopian tubes were found at surgery, along with a gonadoblastoma, at 1 year of age. **C,** Micrograph of tumor cells.

examination increases the index of suspicion for this disorder. The diagnosis is confirmed by gonadal biopsy. Some affected children are found to have one dysgenetic gonad on one side and a streak gonad on the other; others have bilateral dysgenetic gonads. Dysgenetic gonads are histologically defined by poorly formed and disorganized seminiferous tubules surrounded by wavy ovarian stroma. In many cases, the dysgenetic gonads resemble ovotestes, except that primordial ovarian follicles are lacking (Berkovitz et al, 1991).

MIXED GONADAL DYSGENESIS

Mixed gonadal dysgenesis (MGD) refers to asymmetric gonadal dysgenesis with ambiguous genitalia (see Figure 92-5) and a mosaic karyotype with an XY cell line. The most common karyotype is 45,XO/46,XY. There is a wide spectrum of phenotypes, ranging from a female with clitoral enlargement to a male with hypospadias. Asymmetric external and internal genital development has been classically described in this syndrome (Forest, 2001). Considerable phallic development was reported in a majority of patients in one study, and there was often penoscrotal hypospadias (Davidoff and Federman, 1973). The phenotypic features of Turner's syndrome are described in a significant percentage of patients, although these features may not be readily apparent in the newborn period. An incompletely formed uterus is found in almost all patients. Fallopian tubes are always found on the side of the streak gonad and often on the side with the dysgenetic gonad. Wolffian structures may be developed on the side with the dysgenetic gonad.

A genitourethrogram is likely to demonstrate internal müllerian structures that can be confirmed at laparoscopy. Demonstration of abnormal gonadal histopathologic features will confirm the diagnosis. It should be noted that mixed gonadal dysgenesis shares many features with partial gonadal dysgenesis, and some authors view these disorders as representing a continuum of gonadal dysgenesis (Berkovitz et al, 1991). Histologic analysis will also differentiate this disorder from true hermaphroditism. Although the characteristic karyotype is 45,XO/46,XY, it should be noted that this genotype has been associated with normal male differentiation in a majority of cases diagnosed by prenatal amniocentesis (Wheeler et al, 1988).

Some authors advocate female sex assignment in mixed gonadal dysgenesis, because surgical repair of the vagina is usually easy and a uterus or hemiuterus is present. In addition, the dysgenetic gonad is at risk for development of a tumor and should be removed, particularly if the gonad cannot be brought down into the scrotum (Forest, 2001). However, sex assignment is likely to be guided by the degree of virilization, with the more virilized cases being assigned as males. The capacity for near-normal androgen production in this disorder has been described (Davidoff and Federman, 1973). In all cases, the streak gonads should be removed because of the risk for malignancy.

TESTICULAR REGRESSION SYNDROME

Testicular regression syndrome refers to the spectrum of disorders affecting persons with 46,XY karyotype who demonstrate evidence of prior testicular function, followed by usually symmetric gonadal regression. Loss of testicular function between weeks 8 and 10 of gestation would result in ambiguous genitalia and variable internal genitalia. Loss of testicular function after 12 to 14 weeks' gestation would result in normal male genital differentiation with a small phallus. When the male external and internal ducts are completely normal, the term *vanishing testis syndrome* is used by some authors. Presumably the testes were lost during the second half of pregnancy. Testicular torsion has been invoked as a possible explanation in this syndrome.

FSH levels are elevated in infancy, and an exaggerated response to gonadotropin-releasing hormone in the prepubertal period typically is seen (Grumbach and Conte, 1998). Antimüllerian hormone levels in infancy and childhood are very low in anorchia and intermediately low with abnormal testes (Lee, 2001).

OVOTESTICULAR DISORDER OF SEX DIFFERENTIATION

Ovotesticular DSD is defined as the presence of both testicular tissue with distinct seminiferous tubules and ovarian tissue containing mature graafian follicles in a single individual. Both testicular and ovarian elements may be found in the same gonad, or one testicle and one ovary may be found in the same individual. In a majority of cases the karyotype is 46,XX; 46,XX/46,XY chimerism and 46,XY karyotypes also can be found. Clinically the external genitalia are often ambiguous, but predominantly male or female phenotypes have been described (Grumbach and Conte, 1998; Hadjiathanasiou et al, 1994). In ambiguous cases, a relatively marked degree of virilization can be found. Almost all have some degree of hypospadias and incomplete labioscrotal fold fusion. The labioscrotal folds are asymmetric, with an appearance of a hemiscrotum on one side and labium majus on the other being seen in 10 of 22 cases (Hadjiathanasiou et al, 1994). At least one gonad is usually palpable. A vagina and uterus are present in most patients, and a genitourethrogram may be required for elucidation. Internal duct development is consistent with the associated gonad, although müllerian ducts predominate with an ovotestis. Breast development is common during puberty, and menses can occur in up to 50%.

The diagnosis should be suggested in 46,XX/46,XY individuals with ambiguous genitalia. Palpation of a polarized gonad should also lead the clinician to suggest the diagnosis. In one study, 11 of 12 46,XX true hermaphrodites examined before 6 months of age had baseline testosterone levels greater than 40 ng/dL; normal levels for females of this age would be less than 15 ng/dL (Hadjiathanasiou et al, 1994).

Gender assignment depends on the degree of masculinization, capacity of testicular tissue to secrete testosterone, and the presence or absence of a uterus and tubes. In general, a female gender assignment is favored because of the presence of ovarian tissue and external genitalia that can more easily be reconstructed as female. Male gender assignment is more likely if there is significant virilization. Removal of ductal or gonadal structures not consonant with the gender of rearing is recommended. Testes are usually dysgenetic, which carries an increased risk of gonadoblastoma formation; therefore careful follow-up evaluation is indicated. As in all cases of DSD, gender identity and behavior issues, along with general psychological well-being, should be evaluated longitudinally.

SYNDROMES ASSOCIATED WITH AMBIGUOUS GENITALIA

Denys-Drash syndrome is a rare syndrome consisting of the classic triad of congenital nephrotic syndrome leading to end-stage renal failure, XY ambiguous genitalia, and Wilms' tumor. The external genitalia of 46,XY individuals are either ambiguous or female. Gonadal development encompasses a spectrum from streak gonads to dysgenetic testes. Nephropathy and proteinuria are noted at an early age, and renal biopsy will demonstrate mesangial sclerosis. Greater than 90% of cases will have a mutation in the *WT1* gene, which is a critical gene for the development of the normal genital tract. *WT1* also is associated with the WAGR syndrome. Large deletions of chromosome 11p13 that encompass the *WT1* gene are responsible for this disorder. Frasier syndrome also involves the *WT1* gene. This syndrome manifests in 46,XY females with gonadal dysgenesis and progressive glomerulopathy.

Camptomelic dysplasia is a rare autosomal dominant disorder associated with often lethal skeletal dysplasia, in which 75% of affected 46,XY males have dysgenetic testes associated with undervirilization (Grumbach and Conte, 1998). Manifestations of this disorder include bowing of the femora and tibiae, hypoplastic scapulae, 11 rib pairs, pelvic malformations, bilateral clubfoot, cleft palate, macrocephaly, micrognathia, hypertelorism, and a variety of cardiac and renal defects. The disorder is caused by heterozygous mutations in the *SOX9* gene (Grumbach and Conte, 1998). Most patients die in the neonatal period from respiratory distress.

Smith-Lemli-Opitz syndrome is an autosomal recessive disorder with an estimated frequency of 1 in 20,000 to 1 in 40,000. The disorder is caused by 7-dehydrocholesterol reductase deficiency (Forest, 2001). This enzyme catalyzes the final step in cholesterol biosynthesis; therefore the combination of low serum cholesterol and a high serum 7-dehydrocholesterol is suggestive of the diagnosis. Growth and developmental delay and multiple congenital anomalies characterize this disorder. Genital anomalies may include hypospadias, cryptorchidism, micropenis, and hypoplastic scrotum. Craniofacial abnormalities may include microcephaly, narrow bifrontal diameter, broad maxillary ridges, ptosis of the eyelids, micrognathia, and anteverted nostrils (Jones, 1997). Syndactyly of the second or third toes is a common feature. Adrenal insufficiency has been reported in this condition. Treatment with cholesterol improves growth and neurodevelopmental status.

Robinow syndrome is an autosomal dominant disorder characterized by a flat facial profile, short forearms, and hypoplastic genitals (Jones, 1997). Sporadic cases have been reported. Microphallus may be severe in males, although normal virilization at the time of puberty has been reported (Jones, 1997). Undescended testes have been reported in 65% of affected boys. Females have characteristic hypoplastic labia and clitoris. Other features include small size at birth, macrocephaly, frontal bossing, hypertelorism, prominent eyes, small upturned nose, micrognathia, and posteriorly rotated ears. Short forearms are seen in 100% of described cases. Other skeletal abnormalities include thoracic hemivertebrae, fusion or absence of ribs, and scoliosis. The abnormal facial features become less pronounced as the child grows, and cognitive performance has been normal in most affected persons.

OTHER DISORDERS OF GENITAL DIFFERENTIATION

Hypospadias is one of the most common anomalies of male genital development, with an estimated incidence of 4 to 8 cases per 1000 male births (Grumbach and

Conte, 1998). Hypospadias can be classified as glandular, penile, penoscrotal, scrotal, and perineal. Typically the more severe forms of hypospadias have been associated with DSDs, although the phenotypic spectrum of DSDs is wide. In a study of 33 patients with severe (scrotal or penoscrotal) hypospadias, 12 were found to have a DSD, which included Denys-Drash syndrome (in 3 of the 12), partial androgen insensitivity (in 2), true hermaphroditism (in 2), chromosomal abnormality (in 1), MIF abnormality (in 1), gonadal dysgenesis (in 1), 5α-reductase deficiency (in 1), and 46,XX male karyotype (in 1, *SRY* positive) (Albers et al, 1997). It should be noted that the testes were undescended in 11 of the 12 patients. Aarskog (1970) found an approximately 15% prevalence of DSDs in association with hypospadias, in addition to a significant role for maternal progestins.

Thus, severe cases of hypospadias require a thorough evaluation including karyotype and hCG stimulation testing, along with examination of the genitourinary tract, particularly if accompanied by undescended testes.

OVERVIEW OF THE SURGICAL MANAGEMENT OF DISORDERS OF SEXUAL DIFFERENTIATION

Surgery for DSD conditions has been criticized recently. The criticism has focused not only on the timing of surgery but on whether reconstructive surgery should be done at all. Some authorities have advised that surgery be postponed until the affected person is of an age to make his or her own decision regarding the advisability of surgical correction (Diamond and Sigmundson, 1997a). Others have found that delay in surgery may be associated with problematic outcomes (Meyer-Bahlburg et al, 1996; Money et al, 1986; Reiner, 1997). It is imperative that these divergent viewpoints be discussed with the parents of an infant with a DSD condition.

These issues must be kept in mind in any decision regarding surgery for management of DSDs. Current surgical techniques that are available for correction of ambiguous genitalia and DSDs are presented next.

FEMINIZING GENITOPLASTY

Feminizing genitoplasty is one of the more common procedures done for correction of ambiguous genitalia. Feminizing genitoplasty is indicated in the genetic female who is externally virilized, most commonly as the result of CAH. The degree of virilization can be highly variable (see Figure 92-4). The degree of virilization will have a significant influence on the type of procedure done, especially the vaginoplasty portion of the operation. Reconstruction in this group of patients has three components: clitoral reduction, vaginoplasty, and labial reconstruction. The timing of surgical correction also has undergone some changes over the years. The current thinking is that once a decision is made to proceed with genital reconstruction, performing this type of surgery at a younger age will have distinct advantages, including easier mobilization of the urogenital sinus and a more benign postoperative course.

Clitoral Reduction

Attempts at managing the enlarged clitoris in genetic females with clitoral hypertrophy started with total clitorectomy. Young (1937) originally advocated this procedure. Later, Lattimer (1961) suggested a recession rather than a resection of the clitoris, and he hoped to be able to preserve the arousal function of the clitoris. This led to cases in which painful clitoral erections occurred later in life; therefore further modification was needed. Spence and Allen (1973) advocated the preservation of the glands with reduction in the size of the clitoris. Since then, several reports have examined preservation of the neurovascular bundle using a clitoral reduction and recession type of approach. Kogan (1987) and Snyder (1983) and their colleagues separately described a similar approach in which the erectile tissue of the clitoris is removed, but preservation of the neurovascular bundle and the glands is afforded to preserve the neurologic and arousal functions of the clitoris. If the gland is unusually large in size, then a reduction of the gland size may be indicated as well.

Vaginoplasty

Reconstruction of the vagina in cases of virilization in females requires an understanding of the anatomy. One may consider the anatomic abnormality an embryologic arrest of maturation with a persistence of an early embryologic stage. The anatomic issue that is important to the surgical management of the common urogenital sinus is the site of confluence of the genital tract and urethra. This site varies considerably but is somewhat predictable from the appearance of the degree of external virilization. Children with severe degrees of external virilization are more likely to have a higher confluence of the urethral and vaginal channels, leading to a longer urogenital sinus or a more masculinized urogenital sinus. In the classic article on urogenital sinus abnormalities, Hendren and Crawford (1969) described the variable anatomy that can be seen in these children and noted that the operative procedures needed to be tailored toward the location of the confluence of the urinary and genital tracts. One may describe the confluence anatomically as it relates to the external sphincter, with confluences distal to the external sphincter being considered *low* and those proximal to the external sphincter being referred to as *high*. One also may describe the variable anatomy according to the length of the urethra from the bladder neck to the point of confluence. If that length of urethra were long, then one would consider this a low confluence. Conversely, if the length of the urethra were short and therefore close to the bladder neck, then a high confluence would be present (see Figure 92-6, *B*).

The low confluence cases can generally be repaired either by a cutback procedure on the fused labioscrotal folds or by a flap vaginoplasty. A cutback procedure would be indicated in cases with a minor degree of fusion of the labioscrotal folds. The middle to high vaginal confluence, however, generally requires either a pull-through vaginoplasty or a total urogenital mobilization to bring the vagina down to the perineum.

Flap Vaginoplasty

The flap vaginoplasty should be used for a low confluence of the urogenital sinus. The procedure entails mobilization of a perineum-based flap with its apex at the meatus of the urogenital sinus. Dissection then proceeds along the posterior wall of the urogenital sinus until the vaginal opening is identified. The perineum-based flap is then inserted into the posterior wall of the vagina, thereby exteriorizing the vagina to the perineum.

Total Urethral Mobilization

Total urogenital mobilization can be used for the high urogenital sinus, which has been advocated by Pena (1997) and subsequently substantiated by reports from Rink et al (1997). This approach has been shown to have a superior cosmetic result, compared with that obtained with a flap vaginoplasty, for a middle to high confluence. In addition, there has been a reduced incidence of urethral vaginal fistula and vaginal stenosis. The mobilization occurs in a plane both anterior to the urogenital sinus and up to the bladder neck under the pubic symphysis and posteriorly along the urogenital sinus, and then along the posterior wall of the vagina.

Pull-Through Vaginoplasty

The pull-through vaginoplasty is reserved for use in severely masculinized genetic females, whose surgical management continues to present a major challenge. Initially, the approach was a combined perineal and abdominal approach with complete mobilization of the vagina and uterus and separation of the vagina from the urethra at the confluence. The abdominal mobilization will then allow the vagina to be brought down to the perineum. A modification of this approach was described by Passerini-Glazel (1989) in which the more distal urogenital sinus tissue was used to provide an anterior vaginal wall flap, which will then connect to the true vagina and allow for a complete perineal approach to the procedure.

VAGINAL AGENESIS

Vaginal replacement has a role in certain DSDs or structural abnormalities of the genital urinary tract. The DSDs in which vaginal replacement may be indicated are 46,XX vaginal agenesis, 46,XY male karyotype with severely inadequate virilization or complete androgen insensitivity syndrome, structural urogenital defects such as cloacal exstrophy or persistent cloaca, or after a pelvic exenteration for malignancy. There are a variety of tissues and techniques used for vaginal reconstruction: skin grafting, progressive perineal indentation, and split-thickness or fold thickness tissue grafts with expanders, myocutaneous flaps, and bowel. The critical point in creating a vagina is to maintain an adequate perineal opening, an adequate-length tunnel, and good fixation to pelvic structures. This area is highly controversial in terms of the best management. Overall, the most popular tissue for vaginal plate replacement has been the split-thickness skin graft as described by McIndoe (1950). The major disadvantage of

this technique has proved to be the need for long-term dilatation to maintain patency and to avoid vaginal stenosis. The use of bowel segments for vaginal replacement was first described by Baldwin (1904). Because of an extraordinarily high mortality rate associated with this approach, earlier attempts using this technique were abandoned. Since then, this approach has been adopted by many groups and has been shown to be highly successful, with minimal complication rates. A major advantage of a bowel-segment vagina over a skin graft is the minimal risk of "poor take" because of the vascularized pedicle to the segment of bowel that is used. Length and patency of the bowel are not issues for similar reasons, because it maintains its blood supply. No dilatation is needed. Early on, intestinal mucus production can be a problem, but this lessens over time, and mucus may act as a natural lubricant. Minimal perineal scarring is associated with this approach as well, and it can be done at a very young age (Hensle and Dean, 1992).

UNDERVIRILIZED MALES

Inadequate virilization results in hypospadias with or without cryptorchidism. In more severe cases, such as a complete form of androgen insensitivity, these children may appear as phenotypically normal females and present at the time of puberty with primary amenorrhea. Vaginoplasty is frequently needed after puberty in that population. Children with varying degrees of hypospadias, with or without cryptorchidism, will usually require a repair following the usual principles of hypospadias and cryptorchidism repair. These repairs are generally done at 6 months of age and are tolerated well as outpatient procedures.

GONADECTOMY

Gonadectomy is required under two circumstances in DSDs. Gonadectomy would be recommended when the gonads are inconsistent with the sex of rearing. This is most commonly seen in androgen insensitivity syndrome (46,XY karyotype) in which normal testes are present, but a female gender assignment has been made. The timing of the gonadectomy is controversial; however, it is currently thought to be best managed once the diagnosis has been made, because the role of postnatal testosterone imprinting in a child's psychosocial development is uncertain.

The other circumstance in which gonadectomy is recommended is in DSDs in which gonadal malignancy is a significant risk. This is most likely to occur in cases in which dysgenetic gonads and a Y chromosome are present. An example is shown in Figure 92-14, in which a 1-year-old infant with pure XY gonadal dysgenesis was found to have a gonadoblastoma on gonadectomy. Other syndromes in which gonadal malignancy is a concern include mixed gonadal dysgenesis and the presence of a dysplastic testis in a dysgenetic XY male.

CONCLUSIONS

Significant advances have been made in our understanding of the pathophysiology and molecular genetics of DSD. A systematic diagnostic approach to the infant with ambiguous genitalia should be undertaken to identify the underlying disorder. Establishing the diagnosis will often provide a better understanding of the natural history of the disorder.

The need for surgical intervention in DSDs should be assessed on a case-by-case basis. The parents need to be informed about the risks and benefits of surgery. Surgery on the external genitalia should perhaps be reserved for individuals with significant discord between the sex of rearing and the appearance of the external genitalia.

The infant with a DSD and the family will have to cope with difficult psychosocial challenges throughout life. Physicians caring for these patients should try to ensure the integration of well-trained mental health professionals into the longitudinal care of these complex infants and children.

ACKNOWLEDGMENT

This chapter was originally written by Gregory Goodwin and Anthony Caldamone. It has been modified and updated to its current form by Karen Lin-Su and Maria I. New.

SUGGESTED READINGS

American Academy of Pediatrics Committee on Genetics: Section on Endocrinology/Section on Urology: Evaluation of the newborn with developmental anomalies of the external genitalia, *Pediatrics* 106:138-142, 2000.

Ergun-Longmire B, Vinci G, Alonso L, et al: Clinical, hormonal and cytogenetic evaluation of 46, XX males and review of the literature, *J Pediatr Endocrinol Metab* 18:739-748, 2005.

Forest MG: Diagnosis and treatment of disorders of sexual development, In Degroot LJ, Jameson JL, editors: *Endocrinology*, ed 4, Philadelphia, 2001, WB Saunders.

Grumbach MM, Conte FA: Disorders of sex differentiation, In Wilson JD, Foster DW, Kronenberg HM, Larsen PR, editors: *Williams textbook of endocrinology*, ed 9, Philadelphia, 1998, WB Saunders, pp 1303-1426.

Hughes IA, Nihoul-Fekete C, Thomas B, Cohen-Kettenis PT: Consequences of the ESPE/LWPES guidelines for diagnosis and treatment of disorders of sex development, *Best Pract Res Clin Endocrinol Metab* 21:351-365, 2007.

Jost A, Price D, Edwards RG: Hormonal factors in the sex differentiation of the mammalian foetus, *Biological Sciences* 259:119-131, 1970.

MacLaughlin DT, Donahoe PK: Sex determination and differentiation, *N Engl J Med* 350:367-378, 2004.

Meyer-Bahlburg H, Dolezal C, Baker S, et al: Prenatal androgenization affects gender-related behavior but not gender identity in 5-12-year-old girls with congenital adrenal hyperplasia, *Arch Sex Behav* 33:97-104, 2004a.

Migeon CJ, Berkovitz G, Brown T: Sexual differentiation and ambiguity. In Kappy MS, Blizzard RM, Migeon CJ, editors: *Wilkens' diagnosis and treatment of endocrine disorders in childhood and adolescence*, ed 4, Springfield, Ill, 1994, Charles C Thomas. p 573.

Money J, Devore H, Norman BF: Gender identity and gender transposition: longitudinal outcome study of 32 male hermaphrodites assigned as girls, *J Sex Marital Ther* 12:165-181, 1986.

New MI, Carlson A, Obeid J, et al: Prenatal diagnosis for congenital adrenal hyperplasia in 532 pregnancies, *J Clin Endocrinol Metab* 86:5651-5657, 2001.

New MI, Levine LS: Congenital adrenal hyperplasia, In Harris H, Hirschhorn K, editors: *Adv Hum Genet*, vol 4, New York, 1973, Plenum Publishing, pp 251-326.

Complete references used in this text can be found online at www.expertconsult.com

DISORDERS OF THE THYROID GLAND

Sureka Bollepalli and Susan R. Rose

Thyroid hormone is an integral requirement for normal fetal brain development and for growth and regulation of energy metabolism throughout infancy and childhood. An understanding of thyroid physiology and embryogenesis of the thyroid gland in the perinatal period is important for proper interpretation of abnormal laboratory results and initiation of appropriate treatment. Currently, in the United States and in most other countries, newborn screening is available for early recognition of abnormal thyroid function and to aid in early intervention. However, certain conditions such as hyperthyroidism and central hypothyroidism may be missed by newborn screening. Thyroid hormone abbreviations are defined in Table 93-1.

EMBRYOGENESIS OF HYPOTHALAMIC-PITUITARY-THYROID AXIS

The human thyroid gland is a derivative of the primitive buccopharyngeal cavity. It develops from contributions of two anlagen: a midline thickening of the pharyngeal floor (median anlage) and paired caudal extensions of the fourth pharyngobranchial pouch (lateral anlagen). All of these structures are visible by days 16 to 17 of gestation. The median anlage is initially in close contact with the endothelial tubes of the embryonic heart. A pair of ultimobranchial bodies arise from the lateral anlagen. The parafollicular or C cells arise from the ultimobranchial bodies in mammals and are the source of calcitonin. By 40–50 days' gestation, the median and lateral anlagen have fused and the buccal stalk has ruptured. During this period, the thyroid gland migrates caudally to its definitive location in front of the second to sixth tracheal ring, helped in part by its relationship with developing cardiac structures. The pharyngeal region contracts to become a narrow stalk called the thyroglossal duct, which subsequently atrophies. An ectopic thyroid gland or persistent thyroglossal duct or cyst results from abnormalities of thyroid descent (Brown et al, 2005; Santisteban, 2005).

By the latter part of the 10th week of gestation, the histogenesis of the thyroid is virtually complete, although the follicles do not contain colloid until 13 weeks' gestation (Santisteban, 2005). A single layer of endothelial cells surrounds the follicular lumen. Thyroxine (T_4) has been detected in the serum of a 78-day-old fetus. At this age, the fetal thyroid is capable of trapping and oxidizing iodide (Foley, 1994). Then fetal thyroid begins to secrete thyroid hormone and contributes to the fetal circulation of thyroid hormone by the beginning of the second trimester.

At the same time as the development of the thyroid gland, the fetal pituitary and hypothalamus are also forming and beginning to function. The anterior pituitary gland is derived from Rathke's pouch, which originates at the roof of the pharynx. Histologic differentiation of pituitary cells can be observed by 7 to 10 weeks' gestation, and thyroid-stimulating hormone (TSH) can be detected in fetal blood by 10 to 12 weeks (Kratzsch and Pulzer, 2008). The hypothalamus develops from the ventral portion of the diencephalon (Santisteban, 2005). Thyroid hormone–releasing hormone (TRH) has been found in fetal whole-brain extracts by 62 days and in the hypothalamus by 9 weeks of gestation (Polk et al, 1991).

FETAL-PLACENTAL-MATERNAL THYROID INTERACTION

In considering the fetal-maternal relationship, the placenta is of major importance (Figure 93-1). The fetus requires thyroid hormone throughout pregnancy for optimal neurodevelopment. TSH does not cross the placental barrier, whereas TRH does. Maternal to fetal transport of T_4 during the first trimester is critical because the fetal thyroid axis is not independently functional until mid-gestation. The importance of sufficient maternal thyroid hormone supply, during the first half of pregnancy, is evidenced by poor neurodevelopmental outcomes in offspring of mothers with iodine deficiency or maternal hypothyroidism that was untreated (Kooistra et al, 2006; Morreale de Escobar et al, 2004).

Placental T_4 transfer in a fetus with a total inability to synthesize T_4 results in a fetal T_4 concentration that is 25% to 50% of that found in normal neonates. As a result, in a mother with normal thyroid function, the hypothyroid fetus is somewhat protected. The mother with hypothyroidism and a normal fetus may have a relative thyroid deficit in the first trimester of gestation, whereas the mother with hypothyroidism and a hypothyroid fetus may experience a more significant deficit (Glinoer, 2001).

Triiodothyronine (T_3) is not transferred across the placenta from the mother. Fetal serum T_3 results from metabolism of maternal T_4 that reaches fetal tissues (Calvo et al, 2002). Cerebral T_3 is necessary for normal development of the neocortex; however, T_3 in serum only minimally contributes to cerebral T_3. Therefore, fetal cerebral T_3 levels are dependent on maternal T_4, not serum T_3 (Morreale de Escobar et al, 1992). The astrocytes take up maternal T_4; the T_4 is then converted to T_3 by type II monodeiodinase (MDI) within astrocytes that deliver T_3 to neurons (Bernal, 1999).

Iodides cross the placenta readily. Iodides and iodine, when given in large quantities, produce a transient inhibition of T_4 synthesis by diminishing iodination, probably through effects on thyroidal autoregulation. Therefore, excess iodine given to the mother causes goiter in the offspring; however, pregnant women should be taking 250 µg of iodine daily (Abalovich et al, 2007).

Other clinically important compounds that can affect fetal thyroid function by crossing the placenta from the mother to the fetus are antithyroid drugs, environmental goitrogens, endocrine disruptors, and thyroid antibodies (Foley, 1994; Mastorakos et al, 2007). Antithyroid drugs include

TABLE 93-1 Abbreviation List

CH	Congenital hypothyroidism
FT₃	Free T₃
FT₄	Free T₄
hCG	Human chorionic gonadotropin
MTZ	Methimazole
PTU	Propylthiouracil
RI	Radioactive iodine
RIA	Radioimmunoassay
rT₃	Reverse T₃ (3,3′,5′-L-triiodothyronine)
TBG	Thyroid (thyroxine)-binding globulin
TBII	Thyrotropin binding inhibiting immunoglobulin
TBPA	Thyroxine-binding prealbumin
TG	Thyroglobulin
TPO	Thyroid peroxidase
TRBAb	TSH receptor–blocking antibodies
TRH	Thyroid–releasing hormone
TSA	TSH receptor stimulating antibodies
TSH	Thyroid-stimulating hormone (thyrotropin)
TSH-R	Thyroid-stimulating hormone Receptor
TSI	Thyroid-stimulating immunoglobulin
T₂	Diiodothyronine
T₃	Triiodothyronine (3,5,3′-L-triiodothyronine)
T₃U (T₃RU)	T₃ resin uptake to estimate thyroid binding
T₄	Thyroxine (tetraiodothyronine)
Type I MDI	Type I monodeiodinase
Type II MDI	Type II monodeiodinase
Type III MDI	Type III monodeiodinase

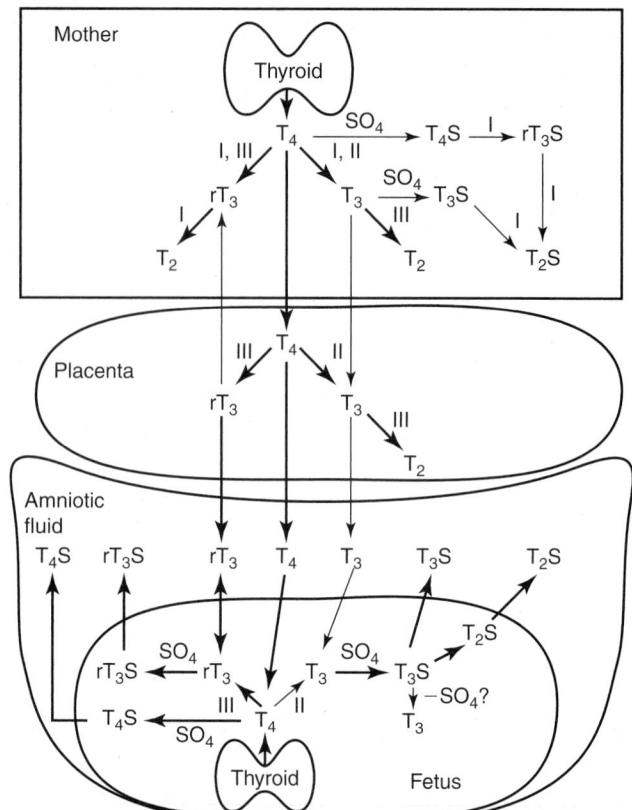

FIGURE 93-1 Interrelations of maternal, placental, and fetal thyroid metabolism. *(From Burrow GN, Fisher DA, Larsen PR: Maternal and fetal thyroid function, N Engl J Med 331:1072-1078, 1994. Copyright 1994, Massachusetts Medical Society. All rights reserved.)*

perchlorates and thionamide compounds such as thiourea, thiouracil, propylthiouracil (PTU), methimazole, and carbimazole. Transplacental transfer of these drugs can result in fetal goiter with or without hypothyroidism (Laurberg et al, 2009). Transfer of thyroid-stimulating immunoglobulin (TSI) across the placenta to the fetus can lead to transient neonatal thyrotoxicosis (Polak, 1998) (see Hyperthyroidism, later); the placental transfer of TSH receptor blocking antibodies (TRBAb) can cause transient neonatal hypothyroidism (Brown et al, 1996).

In summary, placental permeability to maternal molecules may affect fetal thyroid function as a result of maternal pathophysiologic states (acute iodide administration, autoimmune thyroid disease, or pharmacotherapy of thyrotoxicosis). Maternal-to-fetal transplacental transfer of thyroid hormone continues throughout pregnancy and preserves normal fetal central nervous system maturation in fetuses with hypothyroidism. However, the fetal hypothalamic-pituitary-thyroid axis normally develops independent of the maternal thyroid axis influence.

THYROID SYSTEM MATURATION

The fetal thyroid gland is able to concentrate iodine for synthesis of iodothyronines by 12 weeks' gestation. Therefore, T₄ is detectable in fetal serum by the 12th week of gestation (Singh et al, 2003). Subsequently, both T₄ and free T₄ (FT₄) increase linearly in relation to gestational age. Mean cord concentration of T₄ between 20 and 30 weeks' gestation is 5.5 ± 1.6 µg/dL. Normal ranges have been published for thyroid hormone concentrations in third-trimester amniotic fluid (Singh et al, 2003). At term, T₄ reaches 10 µg/dL in umbilical cord serum, 10% to 20% lower than the corresponding value in maternal serum. FT₄ in cord blood is equal to or higher than that in maternal blood. Fetal T₄ metabolism differs markedly from that in postnatal life (LaFranchi, 1999).

In the fetus, T₄ is metabolized predominantly to reverse T₃ (rT₃) rather than to T₃ by type III MDI in placenta. Type III placental MDI converts T₄ to rT₃ and T₃ to diiodothyronine (T₂) (Huang, 2005). Therefore, the concentration of rT₃ in the fetus exceeds 250 ng/dL early in the third trimester and progressively decreases to 150 to 200 ng/dL at term (Kratzsch and Pulzer, 2008). Fetal serum T₃ concentration remains low (less than 15 µg/dL) until 30 weeks' gestation, then rises slowly related to an increase in hepatic type I MDI activity. Type I MDI increases hepatic conversion of T₄ to T₃ and decreases placental degradation of T₃ by type III MDI (Kuiper et al, 2005). T₃ levels reach approximately 50 ng/dL in term cord blood (Kratzsch and Pulzer, 2008). TSH is also present in the 12-week-old fetus and rapidly rises thereafter, in parallel with the increasing FT₄ (LaFranchi, 1999). At term, the fetal value of TSH is more than twice that found in the mother, suggesting

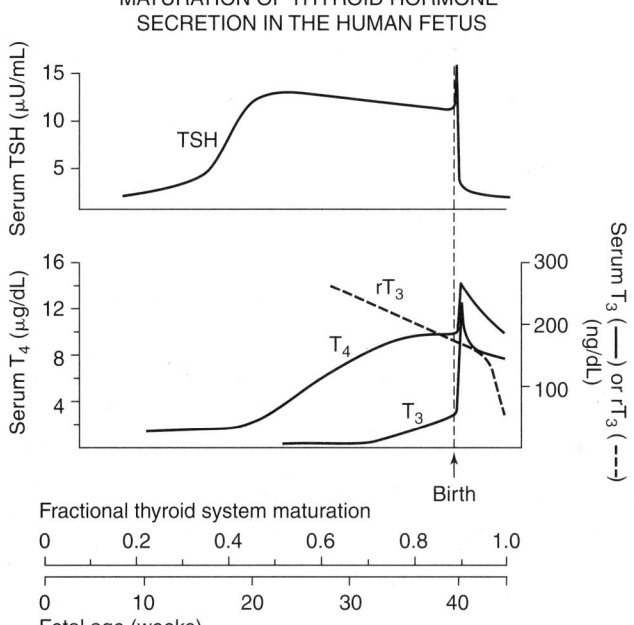

FIGURE 93-2 Patterns of circulating levels of TSH, rT$_3$, T$_4$, and T$_3$ in the fetus and newborn.

that fetal TSH regulates fetal thyroid function (LaFranchi, 1999; Thorpe-Beeston et al, 1992). Hypothalamic TRH levels coincide with this increase in TSH. Extrahypothalamic sources of TRH include the placenta and pancreas; however, their role in thyroid system maturation is unclear (Polk et al, 1991). The pattern of thyroid hormone secretion in the perinatal period is shown in Figure 93-2.

REGULATION OF THYROID FUNCTION

Control of thyroid function by the hypothalamic-pituitary axis matures in the latter half of gestation and continues during the early weeks of postnatal life (Fisher and Polk, 1989). Therefore, maternal hypothyroxinemia in the first half of gestation can contribute to a decreased IQ in offspring, because the fetus is dependent on maternal thyroid hormone concentrations in the first half of gestation as discussed earlier.

Basophilic cells of the anterior pituitary gland synthesize and store TSH (Kurosumi, 1991), a glycoprotein capable of rapidly increasing intrathyroidal cAMP. TSH release from the pituitary causes an increased uptake of iodine by the thyroid, accelerates virtually all steps of iodothyronine synthesis and release, and increases the size and vascularity of the thyroid. These changes are mediated by activation of adenylate cyclase and tyrosine kinase (Kohrle et al, 1990). Human chorionic gonadotropin (hCG) weakly competes with TSH for receptors on thyroid follicular cells. The mild TSH-like activity of hCG contributes to the elevation in maternal T$_4$ seen during pregnancy, along with the effects of increased concentrations of thyroid (thyroxine)-binding globulin (TBG) associated with higher amounts of estrogen during pregnancy (Yoshimura and Hershman, 1995).

Secretion and plasma levels of TSH are inversely related to circulating levels of free T$_3$ (FT$_3$) and FT$_4$. Inhibitory feedback action of FT$_3$ and FT$_4$ involves a direct action of these hormones on the pituitary gland without involving the hypothalamus. Secretion of TSH is regulated directly by the ambient intrapituitary T$_3$ concentration and intrapituitary deiodination of T$_4$ to T$_3$ by type II MDI activity (Kuiper et al, 2005). A progressive decline in the T$_4$ secretion rate with increasing age partially reflects maturational changes in TRH and TSH secretion (Elmlinger et al, 2001; Fisher et al, 2000).

A circadian variation of circulating TSH has been found in normal children and adults. A peak TSH concentration (about 3 to 4 µU/L) develops between 10:00 PM and 4:00 AM and is about twofold higher (50% to 300% higher) than the afternoon (2:00 PM to 6:00 PM) nadir values (Rose and Nisula, 1989). This nocturnal TSH surge is not directly related to sleep; it is blunted or absent in central (secondary or tertiary) hypothyroidism but maintained in primary hypothyroidism (Rose et al, 1990). The circadian pattern of TSH is not yet present in neonates but is established in infants as young as 4 months of age (Mantagos et al, 1992).

THYROID HORMONE SYNTHESIS

Circulating plasma iodide enters the thyroid follicular cells and is combined with tyrosine through a series of enzymatically mediated reactions to form the active thyroid hormones 3,5,3′-triiodothyronine (T$_3$) and thyroxine (T$_4$). The steps in synthesis and release of thyroid hormones include (1) active transport of inorganic iodide from plasma to thyroid cell; (2) synthesis of tyrosine-rich thyroglobulin, which acts as the intermediate iodine acceptor; (3) organification of trapped iodide as iodotyrosines; (4) coupling of monoiodotyrosines (MITs) and diiodotyrosines (DITs) to form the iodothyronines, T$_3$ and T$_4$, with storage of iodotyrosines and iodothyronines in follicular colloid; (5) endocytosis and proteolysis of colloid thyroglobulin to release MIT, DIT, T$_3$, and T$_4$; and, (6) deiodination of released iodotyrosines within the thyroid cell with reutilization of iodine. Defects in these biochemical processes can result in hypothyroidism.

SERUM PROTEIN BINDING OR TRANSPORT

Blood concentration of T$_4$ is 50 to 100 times greater than that of T$_3$. T$_4$ and T$_3$ secreted into the circulation are transported by loose attachment, through noncovalent bonds, to various plasma proteins including TBG, thyroxine-binding prealbumin (TBPA), and albumin. TBG serves as the primary transport protein for 75% of serum T$_3$ and T$_4$. The rest of the thyroid hormone is distributed almost equally between TBPA and albumin. The FT$_4$ concentration more accurately indicates the metabolic status of the individual than does either total T$_4$ or T$_3$, because only free hormones can enter cells to exert their effects. The binding affinities of these proteins are such that adult free T$_4$ and free T$_3$ concentrations are about 0.03% and 0.3%, respectively, of the total hormone concentration (Benvenga, 2005).

TBG, TBPA, and albumin are produced by the liver, and production of these proteins increases progressively

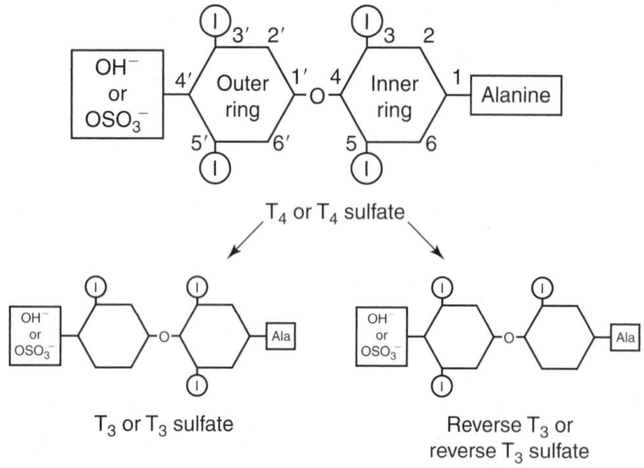

FIGURE 93-3 Structures of T_4, T_3, and reverse T_3. Sulfation at the 4'-hydroxyl position produces the sulfate conjugates of T_4, T_3, and reverse T_3. *(From Burrow GN, Fisher DA, Larsen PR: Maternal and fetal thyroid function, N Engl J Med 331:1072-1078, 1994. Copyright 1994, Massachusetts Medical Society. All rights reserved.)*

during the second half of gestation. Hepatic TBG production is stimulated by estrogen, and the increasing levels of estrogens during pregnancy account, at least in part, for the progressive increase in total plasma T_4 concentration, from mid-gestation until 34 to 35 weeks' gestation (Ain et al, 1987). Although a rise in concentration of T_4 and T_3 follows an increase in TBG levels, the fetal concentration of FT_4 and FT_3 remains more stable.

FETAL THYROID HORMONE METABOLISM

Thyroid hormone metabolism results from enzymatic deiodination (Figure 93-3). Monodeiodination can occur at either the outer (phenolic) ring or at the inner (tyrosyl) ring of the iodothyronine molecule. Deiodination of T_4 at the outer ring produces T_3. T_3 is the active form of thyroid hormone with greatest affinity for the thyroid receptor. Deiodination at the inner ring of T_4 produces rT_3 and at the inner ring of T_3 produces T_2. Both rT_3 and T_2 are inactive metabolites (Kuiper et al, 2005).

There are three enzymes involved in deiodination: types I, II and III monodeiodinases (MDI). Type I MDI (an outer-ring and inner-ring deiodinase) is expressed predominantly in liver, kidney and thyroid. It is inhibited by PTU and stimulated by thyroid hormone. Outer-ring monodeiodination by type I MDI converts T_4 to T_3, and inner-ring monodeiodination converts T_4 sulfate to rT_3 sulfate and T_3 sulfate to T_2 sulfate. Type II MDI (an outer-ring deiodinase), located in brain, pituitary, placenta, skeletal muscle, heart, thyroid, and brown adipose tissue, is insensitive to PTU and inhibited by thyroid hormone. Outer-ring monodeiodination by type II MDI converts T_4 to T_3, contributing to both local and peripheral levels of T_3, including intraneuronal T_3 (Kuiper et al, 2005). Type III MDI (an inner-ring deiodinase) is located in most fetal tissues, including the brain, placenta, uterus, and fetal skin. This enzyme system catalyzes the conversion of T_4 to rT_3 and of T_3 to T_2 (Huang, 2005).

In the fetus, levels of three MDI enzymes vary throughout gestation and reflect changes in thyroid hormone values. Hepatic type I MDI activity is low throughout gestation until the final weeks of gestation (Fisher et al, 1994). Type II MDI activity in the fetal cerebral cortex increases between 13 and 20 weeks; levels increase in the cerebellum after mid-gestation (Kester et al, 2004). The predominance of type III MDI activity in the fetus accounts for increased levels of rT_3 in the fetus. Both type I and type II MDI enzymes are thyroid hormone–responsive. Therefore, a hypothyroid fetus has elevated levels of type II MDI in brain tissue and decreased levels of hepatic type I MDI. This allows for shunting of T_4 to the brain where it is preferentially deiodinated to T_3 by type II MDI, preserving normal central nervous system development (Fisher et al, 1994).

EXTRAUTERINE THYROID ADAPTATION

At the time of parturition, partly in response to cold and stress, an acute release of TSH occurs, resulting in a peak TSH level of 70–100 mU/L at 30 minutes of age (Figure 93-4). This hypersecretion of TSH persists during the next 6 to 24 hours (LaFranchi, 1999). Both T_3 and T_4 serum concentrations also increase four- to sixfold within the first few hours of life, peaking at 24 to 36 hours after birth. These levels then gradually decline to slightly higher than normal childhood values over the first 4 to 5 weeks of life. TSH has usually declined to less than 5 mU/L by 1 month of age (LaFranchi, 1979). By 2 months of age, most normal infants have a TSH of 0.5 to 4 mU/L, similar to adults (Baloch et al, 2003). It is important to recognize this gradual decline in interpreting TSH values during the first few months of life.

The increases in thyroid hormone that occur immediately after birth are not totally dependent on TSH and may represent other influences on the thyroid gland at the time of parturition. The high postnatal T_3 levels in days following birth are due both to TSH stimulation of thyroidal T_3 secretion and to rapid maturation of tissue outer-ring monodeiodinase activity (Santini et al, 1999).

Preterm infants qualitatively have a similar TSH surge, but it is blunted compared to that of the term infant as a result of immaturity of the hypothalamic pituitary thyroid axis (see Figure 93-4). TSH peaks to 40 mU/L at 30 minutes. The rise in T_4 and T_3 is also of a lesser magnitude (LaFranchi, 1999).

CONGENITAL HYPOTHYROIDISM

Congenital hypothyroidism (CH) is a common cause of mental retardation if not treated promptly. The overall incidence is 1 in 2500 to 1 in 3000 newborns (Harris and Pass, 2007; Waller et al, 2000). Higher rates of incidence have been reported in certain populations. A Dutch study reported an overall CH incidence of 1 in 1800 (Kempers et al, 2006). A retrospective study of an Italian population reported a higher incidence of CH, 1 in 1446, 32% with thyroid dysgenesis; of those with gland in situ, 78% had permanent thyroid dysfunction when evaluated 3 to 5 years later (Corbetta et al, 2009). The prevalence rates of

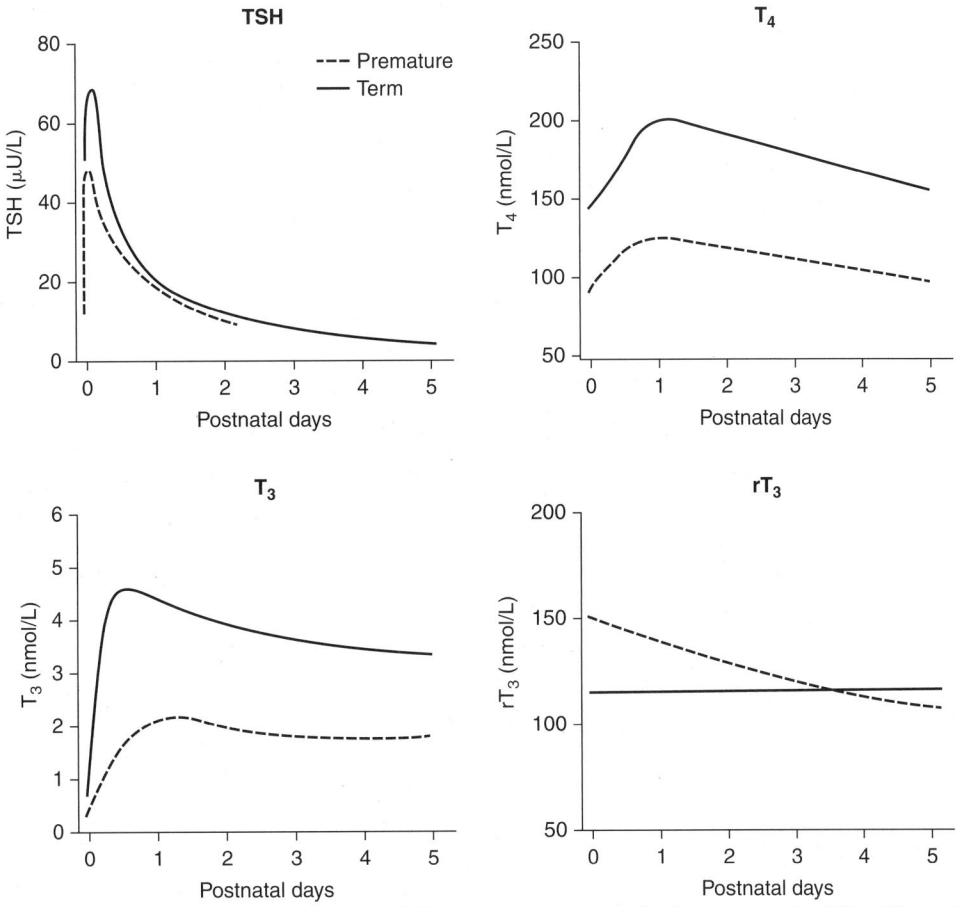

FIGURE 93-4 Postnatal TSH, T_4, T_3, and rT_3 secretion in the full-term and premature infant in the 1st week of life. (*Adapted from* www.thyroid manager.org, *the free online thyroid textbook. In Brown R, Larsen PR, De Groot LJ, editors:* Thyroid gland development and disease in infants and children, *South Dartmouth, Mass., 2009, Endocrine Education, Inc, Chapter 15, Figure 15-4, p 9.*)

CH can vary with sex, ethnicity, and birthweight. Twice as many female as male infants are affected. Compared to whites, the prevalence of CH is higher in Asians and Hispanics and lower in blacks. A recent study noted an increased risk of CH in macrosomic (>4500 g) and low-birthweight (<2000 g) infants (Waller et al, 2000).

The underlying etiology of hypothyroidism may be transient or permanent. Potential causes are listed in Table 93-2. Regardless of duration of the thyroid dysfunction, immediate treatment with levothyroxine (T_4) in the newborn period is needed to prevent cognitive or neurodevelopmental decline. The developing fetal brain is protected in utero by an adequate source of T_3, supplied by local deiodination of maternal T_4 in the fetal brain.

CLINICAL MANIFESTATIONS

The diagnosis of hypothyroidism should be considered in any infant with prolonged jaundice, transient hypothermia, an enlarged (greater than 1 cm) posterior fontanel, failure to feed properly, or respiratory distress with feeding (Pezzuti et al, 2009). The classic signs evolve during the first weeks after birth. Fetal growth is normal; however, there is delay in bone maturation and a rapid reduction in growth rate after birth (Van Vliet, 2005), with progressively worsening myxedema in subcutaneous

TABLE 93-2   Thyroid Disorders and Their Approximate Incidence in the Neonatal Period

Disorder	Incidence
Thyroid dysgenesis	1/2500 to 1/4000
Agenesis	
Hypogenesis	
Ectopia	
Thyroid dyshormonogenesis	1/30,000
TSH receptor defect	
Iodide-trapping defect	
Organification defect	
Iodotyrosine deiodinase deficiency	
Defect in thyroglobulin	
Transient hypothyroidism	1/12,000 to 1/30,000
Drug-induced	
Maternal antibody–induced	
Idiopathic	
Hypothalamic-pituitary hypothyroidism	1/21,000 to 1/100,000
Hypothalamic-pituitary anomaly	
Panhypopituitarism	
Isolated TSH deficiency	

tissues and tongue. The thickened tongue becomes protuberant, and increasing difficulty in nursing and handling salivary secretions is noted. The cry is hoarse because of myxedema of vocal cords. Additional signs and symptoms include marked muscular hypotonia; constipation; thick, dry, cold skin; long and abundant coarse hair; large tongue; abdominal distention; umbilical hernia; hyporeflexia; bradycardia; hypotension with narrow pulse pressure; anemia; and widely patent cranial sutures. The typical facies are characterized by a depressed nasal bridge, a relatively narrow forehead, and puffy eyelids (Foley, 1994). The cardiac silhouette may be enlarged, and the electrocardiogram shows low voltage and a prolonged conduction time. Some of the signs and symptoms are present by 6 to 12 weeks postnatally, especially lethargy, constipation, and the umbilical hernia. The cretinoid facies and growth retardation become increasingly obvious during the first several months of life.

Nonspecific symptoms and signs associated with hypothyroidism are listed in Table 93-3. Of note, clinical manifestations of hypothyroidism may not appear until weeks after birth, even in athyreotic infants. Newborn screening has enabled pediatricians to identify newborns with low thyroid hormone production and to initiate therapy within the first 2 weeks of life, before the development of signs and symptoms (Rose et al, 2006).

NEONATAL SCREENING FOR HYPOTHYROIDISM

Newborn screening programs for CH avoid delay in its diagnosis, because signs and symptoms of CH may not manifest for several weeks. The screening programs are designed to detect elevated serum TSH levels in blood samples collected on filter paper. Some programs measure TSH directly, and others measure TSH in those samples with low or low-normal T_4 concentrations. Screening programs have been established in the United States, western Europe, parts of eastern Europe, Japan, Australia, and parts of Asia, South America, and Central America. However, many countries still do not have a nationwide program for neonatal thyroid screening.

Both methods of screening (primary TSH and primary T_4 + TSH) appear to be capable of detecting almost all infants with primary CH. Primary CH is the only form of CH that carries a high risk of mental retardation if not detected early and treated adequately (Gruters and Krude, 2007; Rose et al, 2006). Primary CH is associated with a low serum T_4 and FT_4 and a high TSH concentration in cord blood or neonatal blood samples. It is estimated that 5% to 8% of affected infants can escape detection by newborn screening because of a delayed elevation in serum TSH or because of errors in sample collection or laboratory routine. Also, infants with TSH deficiency who have normal TSH levels are not detected, because most newborn screening programs report only those infants with elevated TSH levels. Infants who present with signs or symptoms suggestive of thyroid dysfunction (see Table 93-3) should be investigated regardless of previous screening results. A determination of serum FT_4, T_4, and TSH values is necessary in any infant with suspicious clinical or laboratory findings.

TABLE 93-3 Clinical Signs and Symptoms of Congenital Hypothyroidism in Infancy

Age/Manifestation	Frequency (%)
0 to 7 Days	
Prolonged jaundice >3 days	73
Birthweight >4 kg	40
Poor feeding	40
Transient hypothermia	38
Large posterior fontanel (>5 mm)	32
1 to 4 Weeks	
Failure to gain weight	45
Constipation	35
Hypoactivity	33
1 to 3 Months	
Failure to thrive	90
Umbilical hernia	49
Macroglossia	43
Myxedema	40
Hoarse cry	30

The practice of early hospital discharge (before 48 hours of age) has led to an increased frequency of false positive results because of the normal physiologic TSH surge that occurs after birth. Infants screened before 48 hours of age require recheck of the newborn screen by the primary care physician at 2 weeks of life.

THYROID FUNCTION TESTS

When the diagnosis of CH is suspected, thyroid function tests should be performed. It is advisable to assess FT_4, T_4, TSH, and thyroglobulin (TG) levels. Measurements of T_3, rT_3, FT_3, and T_3 resin uptake (T_3U) are not indicated (Rose et al, 2006). Elevated serum TSH value is the most sensitive and specific test to confirm the diagnosis of primary hypothyroidism. Typical laboratory findings for primary hypothyroidism include elevated TSH, with T_4 and FT_4 values in the low or low-normal range. A low or undetectable TG concentration (Sobrero et al, 2007) with TSH elevation confirms a dysgenetic or absent thyroid gland (Djemli et al, 2004), whereas a high TG with TSH elevation suggests an organification defect (Vulsma et al, 1991). In central hypothyroidism, TSH is usually normal, T_4 is low normal, and FT_4 is in the lowest third of normal (van Tijn et al, 2008).

INTERPRETING THYROID FUNCTION TESTS

In interpreting thyroid function tests, it is critically important to take into account the day of life the laboratory tests were drawn. Recommended time period for newborn screening of thyroid function is at 2 to 4 days of life. If screening is done at less than 24 hours of life, it must be rechecked, regardless of the results. After 24 hours of life, a TSH value >40 µU/L is highly suggestive of hypothyroidism but confirmatory testing is required. A TSH value above the normal limit for hours of life and gestational age

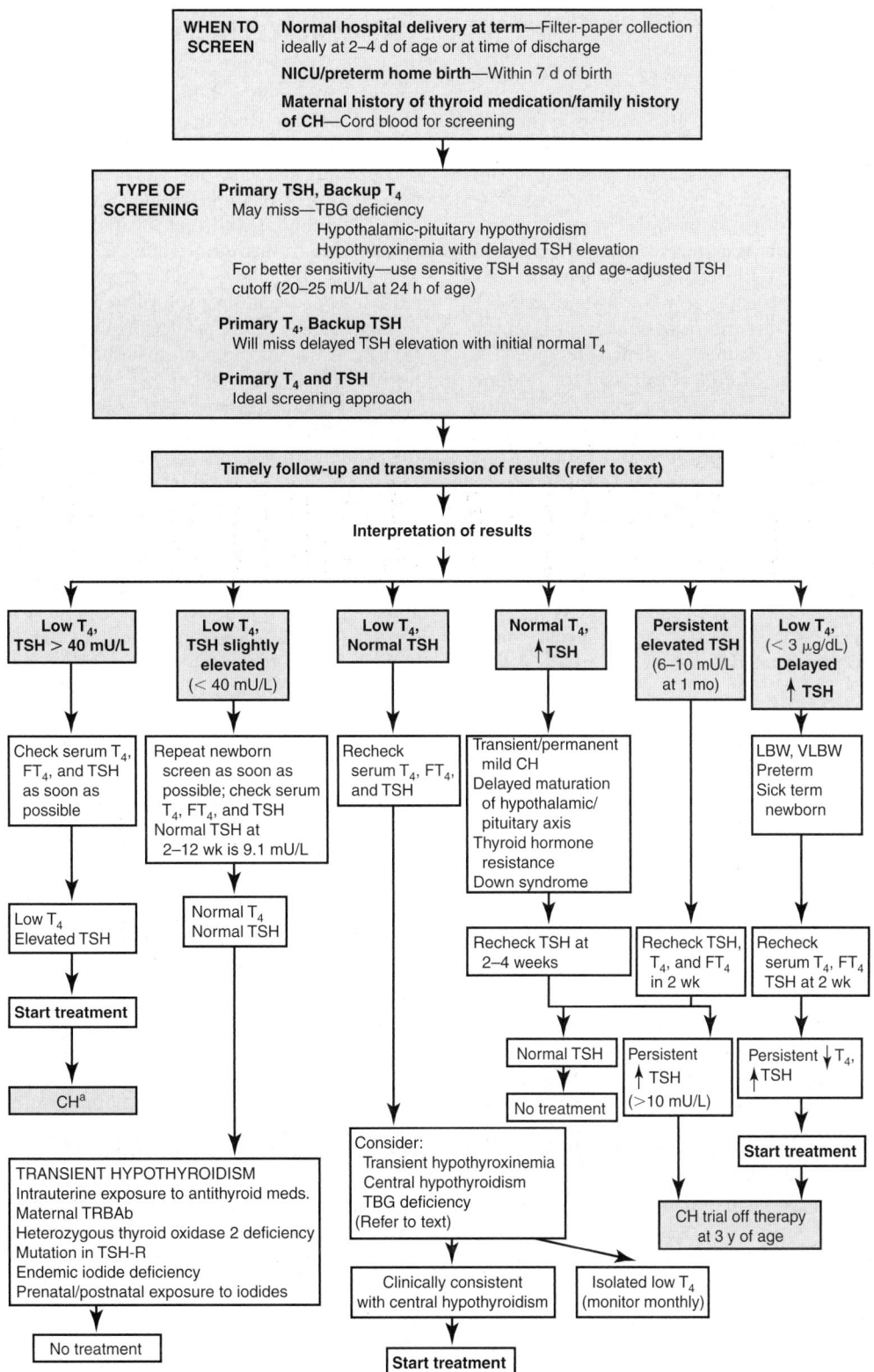

FIGURE 93-5 Algorithm for evaluating CH based on newborn screening results. (*Adapted from Rose SR, Brown RS, Foley T, et al: Update of newborn screening and therapy for congenital hypothyroidism, Pediatrics 117:2290-2303, 2006. Copyright 2006 by the American Academy of Pediatrics.*)

but <40 mU/L is indeterminate. Therefore, repeat testing is necessary and the primary care physician is informed of the need to obtain a second screen (Figure 93-5). The practice of early hospital discharge (before 48 hours of age) has led to a higher rate of indeterminate results.

Eight percent to 10% of infants with CH have screening TSH values of less than 50 mU/L. One in 12 to 24 hypothyroid infants (1 in 50,000 to 1 in 100,000 newborns) will have a screening TSH level of less than 20 mU/L, with a delayed postnatal increase to hypothyroid levels (Hyman et al, 2007). Therefore, any infant with suspicious screening or neonatal sampling results requires confirmatory testing with measurement of serum FT_4, T_4, and TSH concentrations (Rose et al, 2006).

The biochemical profile of hypothalamic-pituitary hypothyroidism comprises low serum T_4 concentration with a normal TSH value. A similar biochemical profile characterizes TBG deficiency. However, the two states can be differentiated by further assessment of TBG and FT_4 levels. Measurement of a low serum TBG concentration and a normal FT_4 level identifies patients with TBG deficiency. In contrast, a low or low-normal FT_4 and normal TBG levels identify a patient with hypothalamic-pituitary hypothyroidism. An infant with a low FT_4 concentration needs to be carefully examined for evidence of hypothyroidism, and other tests of pituitary function should be conducted. TRH stimulation testing can be used to differentiate between primary and central hypothyroidism. TRH, however, is not available in the United States. A subnormal TSH response to TRH or a normal but delayed and prolonged TSH response to TRH is indicative of central hypothyroidism (van Tijn et al, 2008). TSH deficiency may be isolated or associated with other pituitary hormone deficiencies. Frequently it is not possible to discriminate between secondary and tertiary hypothyroidism, so the most useful diagnostic term is central hypothyroidism.

THYROID DYSGENESIS

Among cases of permanent congenital hypothyroidism, 85% are associated with abnormal development of the thyroid gland, which includes agenesis (35%), ectopy (65%) or hypoplasia (<5%) of the gland (Topaloglu, 2006). There is female predominance associated with ectopic glands. Ectopic locations of the thyroid gland include lingual, neck, and substernal. Most cases are sporadic; however, more recent studies show evidence for genetic factors being involved in the pathogenesis. Studies in mice and fetal tissues show that congenital defects in thyroid gland development can be associated with mutations in transcription factors such as NKX2.1 (TTF-1), PAX-8, thyroid-stimulating hormone receptor (TSH-R), and FOXE-1 (TTF-2), which are involved in thyroid organogenesis (Deladoey et al, 2007; Trueba et al, 2005). Mutation in NKX2.5, a transcription factor involved in heart morphogenesis, has also been reported to be associated with thyroid dysgenesis (Dentice et al, 2006).

Extrathyroidal abnormalities occur at a higher frequency in children with congenital hypothyroidism. The most frequent malformations associated with thyroid dysgenesis are cardiac, largely septation defects (Devos et al, 1999). Other relatively common malformations include anomalies of the gastrointestinal tract, nervous system, and eyes (Gu et al, 2009; Kreisner et al, 2005; Olivieri et al, 2002).

The biochemical picture can vary depending on the amount of thyroid tissue remaining. The presence of residual thyroid tissue is evident by detectable thyroglobulin levels and normal or near-normal T_3 with low T_4 and elevated TSH values. The presence of residual thyroid tissue can be confirmed with a thyroid scan.

THYROID DYSHORMONOGENESIS

The remaining 10% to 20% of cases of congenital hypothyroidism involve defects in synthesis of thyroid hormone. These patients often present with a normally located and normal-sized gland. Thyroid enlargement can present at birth, but more commonly a goiter develops later in life. Inheritance pattern is autosomal recessive (Topaloglu, 2006). Elevated thyroglobulin is often observed in dyshormonogenesis.

Defects associated with trapping of iodide or in the oxidation or organification of iodide can result in dyshormonogenesis. These mutations include (1) point mutation in SLC5A5, the sodium-iodide symporter; (2) thyroid peroxidase (TPO) deficiency or a defective TPO, or defective cofactors that are required for activation of the TPO enzyme or for the hydrogen peroxide generating system (mutations THOX1 or THOX2) (de Vijlder, 2003; Moreno et al, 2002) usually associated with more severe hypothyroidism; (3) TG defect; and (4) biallelic mutations in the SLC264A4 gene (Pendred's syndrome). Pendred's syndrome is an autosomal recessive disorder associated with a partial defect in iodine organification and sensorineural hearing loss. The anion transporter gene, SLC264A4, encodes pendrin. Pendrin functions to maintain the endocochlear potential and is involved in the apical efflux of iodide in the thyroid follicular cells (Kopp et al, 2008). A white forelock may be observed in patients with Pendred's syndrome.

CENTRAL HYPOTHYROIDISM

In the United States, combined incidence of secondary and tertiary hypothyroidism is about 1 in 80,000 to 1 in 100,000 births. Studies in the Netherlands suggest a higher incidence at 1 in 21,000 (Kempers et al, 2006; van Tijn et al, 2005). Congenital central hypothyroidism is often associated with mutations in transcription factors involved with pituitary development, including *Pit-1*, *LHX3*, *PROP1*, *HESX1*, and others and can also be associated with other hormone deficiencies.

Other midline facial, cranial, or intracranial defects should suggest the possibility of hypopituitarism, including altered functioning of the hypothalamic-pituitary-thyroid axis. Septo-optic dysplasia, often associated with pituitary hormone deficiencies, can be manifested as secondary or (more commonly) tertiary hypothyroidism. Clinical symptoms of hypopituitarism, such as neonatal hypoglycemia (from growth hormone and adrenocorticotropic hormone deficiencies), polyuria (from antidiuretic hormone deficiency), or a small phallus in boys (from gonadotropin deficiency), whether or not accompanied by the presence of blindness, congenital nystagmus, or midline defects of the brain, should alert the physician to suspect septo-optic dysplasia.

The consequences of central hypothyroidism are as neurologically devastating as those of primary hypothyroidism and therefore also require prompt treatment (van Tijn et al, 2005). However, many newborn screening programs that use elevated TSH values to recognize thyroid dysfunction are inadequate in identifying newborns with central hypothyroidism.

Central hypothyroidism may be acquired during difficult or breech delivery; however, the FT_4 may not become abnormal until 2 weeks of age. The biochemical picture comprises normal or low TSH with low or low-normal T_4 levels and low FT_4. Other laboratory evidence includes an abnormal TSH surge of less than 50% and a subnormal TSH response to a TRH stimulation test. Attention to other clinical features such as hypoglycemia, microphallus, and midline facial defects can lead to earlier identification of central hypothyroidism.

HYPERTHYROTROPINEMIA: DOWN SYNDROME

Incidence of CH (including dyshormonogenesis) is greatly increased in Down syndrome, as are acquired autoimmune diseases of the thyroid gland, pancreas, stomach, and adrenal gland (Hasanhodzic et al, 2006). Obvious CH occurs in 1 of about 140 subjects with Down syndrome. T_4 concentrations in 284 newborns with Down syndrome were significantly decreased compared with those in controls (van Trotsenburg et al, 2003). Many additional children with Down syndrome have mildly elevated TSH (5 to 15 mU/L) and low-normal FT_4 values. TSH bioactivity appears to be normal, suggesting that these children with Down syndrome and mild TSH elevation have mild tissue hypothyroidism. If TSH elevation persists up to 4 weeks of age, the child's mental development may be best protected by initiating thyroid hormone replacement, as in transient hypothyroidism (Rose et al, 2006).

CONSUMPTIVE HYPOTHYROIDISM

Consumptive hypothyroidism may occur in infants with hepatic hemangiomas (Huang et al, 2000). Hemangiomas occur at a high frequency in infancy, with rapid growth during the 1st year of life, followed by involution and gradual regression by adolescence. Because the period of growth of the hemangioma coincides with the critical period of growth and intellectual development, the infant is at risk for permanent neurological damage.

The mechanism involves increased expression of type III MDI mRNA in the tumor that accelerates the rate of degradation of thyroid hormone (Bessho et al, 2010; Huang et al, 2000). As previously discussed, type III MDI catalyzes the conversion of T_4 to rT_3 and T_3 to T_2, both of which are inactive metabolites. Because of the rapid rate of thyroid hormone breakdown, the degree of hypothyroidism is refractory to thyroid hormone replacement. Therefore, unusually high doses, up to 8 to 9 times more than usual doses of oral or intravenous liothyronine (T_3) and levothyroxine (T_4) are required to normalize TSH levels. T_4 must be given for neurologic benefit. The biochemical profile comprises low T_3 and T_4, elevated TSH and elevated serum rT_3 levels. The thyroid hormone levels normalize with regression of the hemangioma (Huang et al, 2000).

TRANSIENT PRIMARY HYPOTHYROIDISM

Hypothyroidism in the newborn period can be transient in 10% of cases (Rose et al, 2006). Studies in the Netherlands report an incidence of 1 in 12,000 (Kempers et al, 2006).

The newborn screen is initially abnormal with a low T_4 and slightly elevated TSH. However, repeated laboratory evaluation may demonstrate normalization of thyroid function tests indicating a transient state of thyroid dysfunction. Because normalization may not occur for several months, thyroid hormone therapy should be initiated for protection of the infant's brain development if TSH remains elevated at 2 weeks of life. Therapy should be continued until age 3 years, when the child should be reevaluated. Transient hypothyroidism is more common in preterm infants. It may result from intrauterine exposure to maternal antithyroid medications, maternal TRBAb, heterozygous thyroid oxidase 2 deficiency, mutation in TSH-R, endemic iodide deficiency, or prenatal/postnatal exposure to iodides (Rose et al, 2006).

Transplacental passage of maternal TRBAb (also known as thyrotropin binding inhibiting immunoglobulin, or TBII) is estimated to cause transient thyroid dysfunction in 2% of newborns with congenital hypothyroidism (Brown et al, 1996). This transient thyroid dysfunction is often difficult to differentiate from permanent forms of hypothyroidism in the newborn period. These babies should be treated but will not require lifelong treatment.

Although many women with autoimmune disease are receiving thyroid replacement therapy, some may be clinically euthyroid and not on medications. Some of these women actually have hyperthyroidism or a history of Graves' disease but may not currently be on medication. Therefore, diagnosis of thyroid dysfunction may be delayed until the postpartum period (Brown et al, 1996).

TRBAb, like other IgGs, do not cross the placenta until after 16 weeks' gestation. Therefore, the TRBAb do not affect thyroid embryogenesis and infants do not develop permanent abnormalities in thyroid function (McKenzie and Zakarija, 1992). The severity and duration of the hypothyroid state in these newborns correlates with the initial titer of the blocking antibody and duration of its presence in the infant's blood (Brown et al, 1996).

If TSH remains elevated at 2 weeks of age, thyroid hormone therapy should be initiated for protection of the infant's brain development. Thyroid status should be reevaluated off therapy at age 3 years, or sooner if the diagnosis is known. Subsequent offspring remain at risk, because the antibodies can persist up to 7 years in maternal sera (Brown et al, 1996).

The biochemical profile is that of congenital hypothyroidism, comprising low T_4 with elevated TSH that subsequently normalize. A thyroid scan is not helpful because the TRBAb are sufficiently potent to block TSH-induced uptake of radioactive iodine, which can be misleading and suggestive of thyroid agenesis. The distinguishing feature is the presence of TRBAb in newborn and maternal sera. However, routine screening for TRBAb is not currently indicated. This diagnosis should be suspected in any infant with congenital hypothyroidism born to a woman who has history of autoimmune disease, or if previous offspring had thyroid disease (Brown et al, 1996).

EUTHYROID SICK SYNDROME

In acutely ill patients, serum T_3 is decreased. Current hypothesis is that alterations in thyroid hormone occur as an adaptive response to decreased basal metabolic rates in severely ill patients. The syndrome has been recognized in sick infants and children (Carrascosa et al, 2008). These patients may have severe nonthyroidal illnesses that are either acute or chronic. The consistent finding is an abnormally low serum T_3 level, accompanied by an increase in the rT_3 level. T_4 may be low or normal and FT_4 may be normal, depending on metabolic clearance rate of T_4. Serum TBG may be low or normal, and TSH is normal. In preterm infants, T_4, FT_4, and T_3 levels are naturally lower than those in term infants, and rT_3 is high (Fisher, 2007). Therefore, thyroid tests in preterm infants may present a confusing situation when the infants are ill from nonthyroidal diseases.

In the neonatal period, preterm infants with respiratory distress syndrome are the most frequently encountered patients with euthyroid sick syndrome (Fisher, 2007; Tanaka et al, 2007). In children, a variety of nonthyroidal illnesses have been associated with this syndrome, including severe gastroenteritis, acute leukemia, anorexia nervosa, renal disease, burns, and surgical stress. An alteration in T_4 metabolism to favor production of rT_3 over T_3 occurs rapidly. Euthyroid sick syndrome is found in patients with acute metabolic stress (e.g., diabetic ketoacidosis) and occurs in all pediatric patients who underwent cardiac surgery. There is a sharp rise in rT_3 and a less dramatic fall in T_3 by 2 hours after cardiac surgery. Reverse T_3 returns to normal before T_3, and there is an inverse relationship between the severity of illness and the T_3 level. In euthyroid sick syndrome, abnormal thyroid function gradually reverts to normal function as the patient's primary illness improves (Foley, 1994). During recovery, TSH may be transiently elevated (up to 15 mU/L). Treatment with thyroid hormone is not indicated in these patients.

TRANSIENT HYPOTHYROXINEMIA OF PREMATURITY

Postnatal thyroid hormone concentrations in preterm infants differ from those of term infants, as reflected by changes in thyroid hormone production in utero, as discussed previously. The levels differ across the range of prematurity and are associated with multiple etiologies, including loss of maternal transfer of T_4 (Morreale de Escobar and Ares, 1998), immaturity of hypothalamic-pituitary-thyroid axis (Murphy et al, 2004) and peripheral metabolism of iodothyronines (Pavelka et al, 1997), iodine deficiency (Ares et al, 1997), nonthyroidal illness (Fisher, 2007), and decreased TBG concentrations secondary to compromised nutrition or hepatic dysfunction (Klein et al, 1997). Other factors that interfere with thyroid metabolism in the preterm infant include exogenous sources of iodine (antiseptic), dopamine infusions, blood transfusions, and glucocorticoid treatment.

In preterm infants, hypothalamic-pituitary-thyroid immaturity is evidenced by a limited neonatal TSH surge, decline in T_4 in the 1st week of life, limited TSH response to hypothyroxinemia, and a prolonged TSH response to TRH. Hypothalamic TRH production begins to increase markedly only in the third trimester (Fisher and Polk, 1989; LaFranchi, 1999).

The biochemical profile of transient hypothyroxinemia in premature infants (before 30 to 32 weeks' gestation) comprises low T_4 and FT_4 levels with normal or low

TSH levels. Therapy has not been consistently effective in improving neurologic outcomes or reducing morbidity (Osborn, 2001; Valerio et al, 2004). Research efforts continue to evaluate this. At the current time, therapy is only recommended when low T_4 is accompanied by TSH elevation (Fisher, 2007; Osborn, 2001).

As mentioned previously, abnormalities in thyroid levels in preterm infants can be difficult to interpret when the infants are ill from nonthyroidal diseases. Therefore, preterm infants at risk should be monitored by serial determinations of FT_4 and TSH, and T_4 treatment should be initiated if there is a progressive increase in serum TSH and decrease in FT_4 (Fisher, 2007). Probably T_4 treatment should be initiated if the illness state is expected to be persistent and TSH remains elevated for a month or longer.

LOW TRIIODOTHYRONINE SYNDROME IN PREMATURE INFANTS

In the preterm infant, changes in thyroid function parameters during neonatal adaptation are qualitatively similar to those in term infants but at lower concentrations. The neonatal TSH surge and T_4 and T_3 peak responses diminish with decreasing gestational age (see Figure 93-4) (LaFranchi, 1999). Premature infants have an increased susceptibility to neonatal morbidity, including birth trauma, acidosis, hypoxia, hypoglycemia, hypocalcemia, and infection, all superimposed on feeding disorders and relative malnutrition. All of these factors tend to inhibit peripheral T_4-to-T_3 conversion, thereby aggravating the low-T_3 state characteristic of prematurity. Serum T_3 values may remain low in these infants for 1 to 2 months.

Features of the low-T_3 syndrome in premature infants include a low serum T_3 concentration secondary to a decreased rate of conversion of T_4 to T_3, variable but usually elevated serum rT_3 levels, and normal or low total serum T_4 concentrations. Free T_4 levels usually are in the range of values for healthy premature infants of matched gestational age and weight (LaFranchi, 1999). TSH values are low in these infants. Treatment is not warranted (Osborn, 2001; Valerio et al, 2004).

IODINE DEFICIENCY

Severe iodine deficiency is associated with cretinism. Iodine deficiency is a rare cause of transient hypothyroidism in North America but may occur in women who are dieting, and thus not eating bread or using salt. Many countries have initiated salt iodination.

Iodine is a critical component of thyroid hormone synthesis; therefore, even mild to moderate forms of iodine deficiency can result in adverse outcome for the fetus. Although the mother with iodine deficiency may be clinically euthyroid with normal T_3 levels, maternal T_4 is low in iodine deficiency. An increase in type II MDI is detected in the fetus in response to iodine deficiency. Because normal development of the fetal neocortex is dependent on maternal T_4, which is the primary source of cerebral T_3, low levels of maternal T_4 place the infants at risk for neurologic cretinism. The fetus can suffer several neurologic manifestations such as deafness, motor deficits (spasticity, trunk rigidity, flexion dystonia, and muscle wasting), and mental retardation. Therefore, it is imperative for the pregnant mother to receive an adequate supply of iodine early in pregnancy to avoid brain damage in the fetus (Abalovich et al, 2007; Bernal, 1999). Prenatal vitamins should be used that contain at least 250 μg iodine daily (Abalovich et al, 2007).

Preterm infants are at increased risk of iodine deficiency. The premature separation from maternal supply of iodine and thyroid hormone prevents the preterm infant from accumulating adequate amounts of intrathyroidal hormone. Therefore, the infant is unable to keep up with postnatal thyroid hormone demands. The biochemical profile of iodine deficiency in the newborn comprises low T_4 and elevated TSH. Iodine deficiency is more common in preterm infants and can lead to a transient state of thyroid dysfunction.

DISORDERS OF THYROID HORMONE CARRIER PROTEINS

Thyroid hormones are linked to carrier proteins (TBG, transthyretin and TBPA) in serum as previously discussed. TBG, the main thyroid hormone transport protein, is a glycoprotein synthesized by the liver. Its gene is located on the Xq21-22 chromosomal region, and thus inherited defects in TBG are X-linked (Trent et al, 1987). TBG abnormalities manifest fully in homozygous males and partially in heterozygous females. Because 75% of T_4 and T_3 are bound to TBG, abnormalities in the affinity or capacity of TBG can alter the total thyroid hormone concentration. Because the bound form is in equilibrium with the free hormone, these patients are euthyroid and do not need treatment. The advent of newborn screening has allowed for earlier identification of abnormal thyroxine levels. The newborn screen can be misleading. TBG defects may be inappropriately diagnosed as hypo- or hyperthyroidism, and infants are unnecessarily started on treatment.

THYROXINE-BINDING GLOBULIN DEFICIENCY

The prevalence of TBG deficiency varies from 1 in 2500 to 1 in 5000 newborns (Bhatkar et al, 2004; Mandel et al, 1993). The frequency in males is much higher, 1 in 2400 to 1 in 2800 males, because it is transmitted as an X-linked trait (Mandel et al, 1993). TBG deficiency has no clinical importance but leads to abnormal laboratory tests. Serum TBG levels are very low in affected males and are approximately half of normal in carrier females. In about half of the families with this trait, the TBG level shown by radioimmunoassay (RIA) is very low. In the other half, the defect is partial; serum T_4 levels vary similarly. Affected persons are euthyroid, with normal serum TSH responses to exogenous TRH. Treatment is not indicated (Bhatkar et al, 2004).

As many as 26 different mutations have been reported in the *TBG* gene. Two novel mutations in the *TBG* gene identified most recently include a T insertion at the beginning of intron 1 between nucleotide 2 and 3, and a T deletion in exon 1 leading to a truncated protein. Both mutations fail to produce a functional TBG molecule (Mannavola et al, 2006).

The biochemical profile of TBG deficiency can vary between females, who tend to have partial TBG deficiency, compared to males, who generally have complete TBG deficiency. A partial deficiency comprises reduced TBG levels and normal TSH and FT_4, with T_4 values at the lower limit of normal. A complete deficiency comprises undetectable TBG levels with normal TSH, normal FT_4, and low levels of T_4. Another useful laboratory tool is T_3RU, which is elevated with TBG deficiency (Noguchi et al, 1993). However, this is an indirect measure of TBG levels.

THYROXINE-BINDING GLOBULIN EXCESS

The prevalence of TBG excess is estimated to be 1 in 15,000 to 1 in 25,000 individuals; TBG excess is also transmitted as an X-linked trait (Bhatkar et al, 2004). Persons with increased levels of TBG have increased total serum T_4 concentrations with normal TSH and FT_4 levels. Serum T_3 concentrations are modestly increased. In these persons, as in those with low TBG, TBG production rates and serum levels are correlated, suggesting that the mechanism for high TBG is increased production, presumably by the liver. TBG levels are increased four- to fivefold in affected persons. Studies are compatible with an X-linked mode of inheritance (Bhatkar et al, 2004).

FAMILIAL DYSALBUMINEMIC HYPERTHYROXINEMIA

Familial dysalbuminemic hyperthyroxinemia is characterized by almost a 60-fold increase in the affinity of albumin for T_4, but not for T_3. Mutations in the *ALB* (albumin) gene are transmitted as an X-linked trait (Cartwright et al, 2009). The biochemical profile comprises increased serum T_4 concentrations, but normal FT_4, total serum T_3, and TSH levels. Although binding of T_4 to albumin is increased, T_3 is less avidly bound, accounting for the preferential increase in serum T_4 concentration. Patients with the disorder are euthyroid, with normal thyroid hormone production rates (Cartwright et al, 2009).

Diagnosis is confirmed by protein electrophoresis of serum containing labeled T_4. The fraction of T_4 label associated with TBG, TBPA, or albumin is measured, and the albumin-bound T_4 can be calculated and related to normal values. Measurements of TBG and TBPA concentrations are also useful. Antithyroid therapy is not necessary in these patients, but it is important to make the diagnosis to avoid a misdiagnosis of hyperthyroidism (Stockigt et al, 1986).

THERAPY OF HYPOTHYROIDISM

Treatment of hypothyroidism relies on replacement with exogenous thyroid hormone. Levothyroxine (T_4) is the drug of choice because of its uniform potency and reliable absorption (Rose et al, 2006). Appropriate doses of synthetic T_4 produce normal serum levels of T_3 via peripheral conversion. The best guide to adequacy of therapy is periodic measurement of circulating levels of T_4, FT_4, and TSH. History and physical examination are important in the follow-up evaluation, but mild hypothyroidism or hyperthyroidism cannot always be excluded on clinical grounds. The usual starting dose of thyroid hormone for hypothyroid infants is 10 to 15 μg/kg/day, which approximates 100 μg/m² per day. Recent studies have reported neurodevelopmental benefits of quick normalization of T_4 and FT_4 levels within 3 days of initiation of thyroid hormone with high-dose treatment. Thyroid hormone requirements, however, quickly drop after 2 weeks, and therefore close monitoring of growth and development along with thyroid function tests is necessary (Salerno et al, 2002; Selva et al, 2002). The treatment of each patient must be individualized. Adequate dosage of thyroid hormone in the 1st year usually ranges between 25 and 50 μg thyroid hormone daily. The tablet is crushed and given orally in a small amount of liquid. Using thyroid hormone for treatment, the goal of therapy is to maintain serum T_4 or FT_4 in the upper part of the normal range, which should result in a TSH of 0.5 to 4 mU/L (Baloch et al, 2003). The thyroid hormone-pituitary feedback set point is altered in rare infants with congenital hypothyroidism, and in such infants serum TSH concentration remains elevated in the face of a normal or even elevated serum T_4 level (Fisher et al, 2000).

Infants with presumably transient hypothyroidism resulting from maternal goitrogenic drugs need not be treated unless the low serum T_4 and elevated TSH levels persist beyond 2 weeks of age. Infants with TRBAb-induced hypothyroidism may require treatment for as long as 6 months.

In treatment of infants with severe myxedema associated with fluid retention, possible complications should be kept in mind. Cardiac insufficiency caused by overtaxing the myxedematous heart, through too rapid a mobilization of the myxedema fluid into the circulation, is well known in the adult. This complication in older children and adults is prevented by administering a small dose of thyroid hormone at first and gradually increasing the dosage. However, infants generally tolerate a rapid restoration to the euthyroid state better than adults, and a prompt restoration of T_4 to a normal value is important for the recovery of brain development and maturation. Nevertheless, excessive thyroid hormone therapy must be avoided, and the dose must be adjusted judiciously if there is evidence of severe myxedema, particularly of the heart.

After initiation of therapy with levothyroxine, growth rate should accelerate. Any growth deficit is commonly restored within a few months. Bone age is a sensitive index of thyroid deficiency; however, radiographs are not routinely obtained in the newborn period. Overtreatment can induce tachycardia, excessive nervousness, disturbed sleep patterns, and other problems suggesting thyrotoxicosis. Excessive thyroid hormone administered over a long period can produce premature synostosis of cranial sutures and undue advancement of bone age.

During the first years of life, patients should be monitored frequently: at least every 2 months during the first 6 months of life, every 3 months during the next 2 years, and then twice a year, to assess clinical progress, T_4, FT_4, and TSH (Box 93-1) (Rose et al, 2006). Because poor compliance and noncompliance have major sequelae, the initial and ongoing counseling of parents is of great importance.

Clinical observation should be supplemented with monitoring of the growth curve, T_4, FT_4, and TSH. Patients

---

BOX 93-1 Management of CH

Initial work-up
  Detailed history and physical examination
  Referral to pediatric endocrinologist
  Recheck serum TSH and FT_4
  Thyroid ultrasonography and/or thyroid scan (see text for recommendations)
Medications
  L-T_4: 10–15 μg/kg by mouth once daily
Monitoring
  Recheck T_4, TSH
  2–4 wk after initial treatment is begun
  Every 1–2 mo in the first 6 mo
  Every 3–4 mo between 6 mo and 3 y of age
  Every 6–12 mo from 3 y of age to end of growth
Goal of therapy
  Normalize TSH and maintain T_4 and FT_4 in upper half of reference range
Assess permanence of CH
  If initial thyroid scan shows ectopic/absent gland, CH is permanent
  If initial TSH is <50 mU/L and there is no increase in TSH after newborn period, then trial off therapy at 3 y of age
  If TSH increases off therapy, consider permanent CH

From Rose SR, Brown RS, Foley T, et al: Update of newborn screening and therapy for congenital hypothyroidism, *Pediatrics* 117:2290-2303, 2006. Reproduced with permission from *Pediatrics*, Vol. 117, p. 2297, Copyright 2006 by the American Academy of Pediatrics.

---

with permanent CH (e.g., dysgenesis, dyshormonogenesis) require lifetime substitution therapy. After age 3 years, if there is uncertainty about whether the disease is permanent or transient or if the dose of T_4 has not required an increase (TSH has remained in the target range of 0.5 to 4.0 mU/L), discontinuation of T_4 therapy for 4 to 6 weeks, with close monitoring of the TSH, should distinguish transient from permanent CH. Recent reports indicate that treatment for CH is discontinued within 3 years in more than one third of children being treated for CH. This is inconsistent with current guidelines; however, it remains unknown how many of the children who discontinued treatment prematurely experience adverse effects or require continued treatment.

HYPERTHYROIDISM

The overall incidence of neonatal hyperthyroidism is low. It occurs more commonly in pregnancies complicated by Graves' disease. Of the offspring born to women with Graves' disease, 1% are affected with hyperthyroidism (Polak, 1998). The thyroid dysfunction in the fetus and newborn is associated with transplacental passage of TSH receptor-stimulating antibodies/thyroid-stimulating immunuglobulins (TSA/TSI), not transfer of maternal thyroid hormone. The antibodies stimulate the fetal and neonatal thyroid gland to produce a state of thyroid hormone. It is generally a transient state that clinically resolves by 4 months of age with the clearance of maternal antibodies from the infant's circulation (Polak, 1998). The underlying etiologies are more commonly maternal autoimmune thyroid dysfunction associated with active or inactive Graves' disease or, less commonly, Hashimoto thyroiditis. Other rare nonautoimmune causes of neonatal hyperthyroidism include activating mutations of the stimulatory G protein, as in McCune-Albright syndrome, or an activating mutation of the TSH receptor (Chester et al, 2008; Guerin et al, 2004). A subset of patients can have persistent hyperthyroidism; however, these patients tend to either have a strong family history of Graves' disease or have activating mutations of the TSH receptor (Chester et al, 2008; Zimmerman, 1999).

In pregnancies complicated by maternal Graves' disease, the fetal levels of TSA approximate those of the mother at 30 weeks' gestation. Therefore, fetal thyrotoxicosis generally manifests in the third trimester with fetal tachycardia, fetal goiter, and intrauterine growth retardation. Fetuses of mothers with TSA levels greater than 250% of the upper limit are at increased risk for thyrotoxicosis. Therefore, these fetuses need to be monitored more closely (Zimmerman, 1999).

Graves' disease in the newborn is manifested by irritability, flushing, diarrhea, vomiting, tachycardia, hypertension, poor weight gain, thyroid enlargement, and exophthalmos. Thrombocytopenia, hepatosplenomegaly, jaundice, and hyperviscosity syndrome also have been observed. Arrhythmias, congestive heart failure, and death may occur if thyrotoxicity is severe and the treatment is inadequate. In some infants, the onset of symptoms and signs may be delayed as long as 8 to 14 days. Late onset of neonatal disease can occur for at least two reasons: (1) postnatal depletion of transplacentally acquired blocking doses of maternal antithyroid drugs and the abrupt increase in conversion of T_4 to active T_3 shortly after birth in the newborn, and (2) presence of maternal TRBAb, which can block the effect of TSA for several weeks (Zimmerman, 1999).

The diagnosis is confirmed by measuring high levels of T_4, free T_4, and T_3 in postnatal blood. Cord blood values may be normal or near normal, whereas levels at 2 to 5 days may be markedly increased; the serum TSH is suppressed below normal levels. Neonatal Graves' disease resolves spontaneously as maternal TSA in the newborn are degraded. The usual clinical course of neonatal Graves' disease is 3 to 12 weeks.

Fetal thyrotoxicosis is treated by administering antithyroid agents to the mother. PTU is recommended during pregnancy, because it is associated with a lower rate of fetal malformations than that with methimazole. PTU crosses the placenta to inhibit the fetal production of excess thyroid hormone (Aslam and Inayat, 2008). Hyperthyroid mothers on antithyroid drugs may breastfeed their infants, because the concentration of drug in breast milk is very low. Treatment of hyperthyroidism in the newborn period includes multiple medications depending on the severity of illness. Iodide or antithyroid agents are administered to decrease thyroid hormone secretion. These drugs have additive effects with regard to inhibition of hormone synthesis. In addition, iodide rapidly inhibits hormone release.

Lugol's solution (5% iodine and 10% potassium iodide, containing 126 mg/mL of iodine) is given in a dose of 1 drop (8 mg of iodine) three times daily. Antithyroid agents such as methimazole or carbimazole are administered in doses of 0.5 to 1 mg/kg/day, divided, at 8-hour intervals. PTU is no longer recommended for use in children because of increasing rates of PTU-induced liver failure (Rivkees and Mattison, 2009). Propranolol can be given in a dose of 2 mg/kg/day to decrease β-adrenergic symptoms and inhibit deiodination of T_4 to T_3. A therapeutic response should be observed within 24 to 36 hours. If a satisfactory response is not observed, the dose of antithyroid drug and iodide can be increased by 50%.

More severe cases may require corticosteroids in antiinflammatory doses (1 to 2 mg/kg/day). Steroids suppress deiodination of T_4 to T_3. Digoxin treatment is useful if cardiac failure is present. If hyperthyroidism persists (as in cases with a strong family history of Graves' disease, an activating mutation of the stimulatory G protein, or an activating mutation of the TSH receptor), ablative therapy such as thyroidectomy must be performed (Chester et al, 2008).

Care must be taken to maintain euthyroidism (to avoid inducing hypothyroidism) in the infant. Frequent monitoring to adjust methimazole doses is indicated. Consideration can be given to suppressing thyroid production and adding back levothyroxine to achieve T_4 or FT_4 just above the mean to ensure euthyroidism.

SUGGESTED READINGS

Abalovich M, Amino N, Barbour LA, et al: Management of thyroid dysfunction during pregnancy and postpartum: an Endocrine Society Clinical Practice Guideline, *J Clin Endocrinol Metab* 92:S1-S4, 2007.

Corbetta C, Weber G, Cortinovis F, et al: A 7-year experience with low blood TSH cutoff levels for neonatal screening reveals an unsuspected frequency of congenital hypothyroidism, *Clin Endocrinol (Oxf)* 71:739-745, 2009.

Gruters A, Krude H: Update on the management of congenital hypothyroidism, *Horm Res* 68:107-111, 2007.

Kester MH, Martinez de Mena R, Obregon MJ, et al: Iodothyronine levels in the human developing brain: major regulatory roles of iodothyronine deiodinases in different areas, *J Clin Endocrinol Metab* 89:3117-3128, 2004.

Kooistra L, Crawford S, van Baar AL, et al: Neonatal effects of maternal hypothyroxinemia during early pregnancy, *Pediatrics* 117:161-167, 2006.

Osborn DA: Thyroid hormones for preventing neurodevelopmental impairment in preterm infants, *Cochrane Database Syst Rev* 4:CD001070, 2001.

Polak M: Hyperthyroidism in early infancy: pathogenesis, clinical features and diagnosis with a focus on neonatal hyperthyroidism, *Thyroid* 8:1171-1177, 1998.

Rose SR, Brown RS, Foley T, et al: Update of newborn screening and therapy for congenital hypothyroidism, *Pediatrics* 117:2290-2303, 2006.

Salerno M, Militerni R, Bravaccio C, et al: Effect of different starting doses of levothyroxine on growth and intellectual outcome at four years of age in congenital hypothyroidism, *Thyroid* 12:45-52, 2002.

Selva KA, Mandel SH, Rien L, et al: Initial treatment dose of L-thyroxine in congenital hypothyroidism, *J Pediatr* 141:786-792, 2002.

van Tijn DA, de Vijlder JJ, Vulsma T: Role of the thyrotropin-releasing hormone stimulation test in diagnosis of congenital central hypothyroidism in infants, *J Clin Endocrinol Metab* 93:410-419, 2008.

Van Vliet G, Larroque B, Bubuteishvili L, et al: Sex-specific impact of congenital hypothyroidism due to thyroid dysgenesis on skeletal maturation in term newborns, *J Clin Endocrinol Metab* 88:2009-2013, 2003.

Zimmerman D: Fetal and neonatal hyperthyroidism, *Thyroid* 9:727-733, 1999.

Complete references and supplemental color images used in this text can be found online at www.expertconsult.com

DISORDERS OF CARBOHYDRATE METABOLISM

Vandana Jain, Ming Chen, and Ram K. Menon

One of the most difficult and complex challenges faced by the newborn at birth is the almost instantaneous transition from total dependence on maternal glucose supply via the umbilical artery to complete independence for glucose homeostasis after the severing of the umbilical cord. Thus the newborn is faced with a metabolic milieu characterized by intermittent supply of exogenous glucose with variable periods of fasting during which the newborn is dependent on endogenous glucose production for maintenance of glucose homeostasis. This challenge is compounded by the fact that, on a per body weight basis, the glucose needs of the newborn are three to four times higher than those of the adult. The increased glucose utilization rate in the newborn is primarily due to higher rates of cerebral glucose utilization as a result of the increased proportion of brain size compared with body weight in the newborn (Menon and Sperling, 1988). Glucose homeostasis in neonates is maintained by a complex balance between glucose utilization and production controlled by coordinated changes in the concentrations of insulin and the counterregulatory hormones, principally growth hormone, cortisol, glucagon, and catecholamines. After birth, there is an abrupt fall with subsequent rise in blood glucose concentrations within 1 to 2 hours as the pathways of glycogenolysis and gluconeogenesis are activated in response to increased circulating levels of cortisol, glucagon, and catecholamines. Over the first few days of life, with establishment of regular enteral feeding and continued maturation of hepatic gluconeogenesis, blood glucose levels further stabilize.

Transient disturbances in glucose homeostasis, especially hypoglycemia, are frequently observed in the neonate because of developmental immaturity of the glucose homeostatic pathways. Neonatal hypoglycemia is a more frequent occurrence when glycogen reserves are low, as in preterm babies and neonates with intrauterine growth restriction, or when energy demands are increased, as in sepsis, hypothermia, and birth asphyxia. Persistent hypoglycemia in the neonatal period is relatively less common and either is caused by congenital endocrine disorders, such as congenital hyperinsulinemia or hypopituitarism, or is secondary to inborn errors in the enzymatic pathways of glycogenolysis, gluconeogenesis, or ketogenesis. Hypoglycemia in neonates can manifest with seizures in the short term and can lead to significant neuromorbidity in the long term. Hence, hypoglycemia constitutes a neonatal emergency requiring urgent diagnostic evaluation and appropriate therapeutic intervention.

This chapter reviews the definition, pathophysiology, diagnostic work-up, and treatment of neonatal hypoglycemia. Also discussed are the less commonly seen conditions of transient and permanent neonatal diabetes.

DEFINITION OF HYPOGLYCEMIA

A consensus among experts regarding the precise definition of hypoglycemia remains elusive. Attempts have been made to identify a reliable evidence-based operational threshold at which intervention should be considered for neonatal hypoglycemia to prevent neurologic sequelae. In a population-based metaanalysis of plasma glucose levels among healthy full-term newborns, Alkalay et al (2006) estimated the lower threshold (<5th percentile) at 1 to 2, 3 to 23, 24 to 47, and 48 to 72 hours after birth to be 28, 40, 41, and 48 mg/dL, respectively. It should be noted that plasma glucose values are higher than those in whole blood by approximately 13.5% and should be factored in when comparing whole blood and plasma glucose thresholds.

The risk of hypoglycemic injury to the brain is modified by factors including the availability of alternative fuels such as ketones and lactate and the presence of comorbidities such as hypoxia and sepsis. Operational blood glucose concentration thresholds for therapeutic intervention that factor these variables into consideration have also been proposed: for example, <45 mg/dL for newborns with abnormal clinical signs and symptoms, <63 mg/dL for newborns with hyperinsulinemia (taking into account the low levels of alternative fuels in this cohort), and <36 mg/dL for at-risk neonates assessed as being healthy with absence of clinical signs and symptoms of hypoglycemia (Hussain, 2005). However, some experts contend that the sensitivity to hypoglycemia of a neonate's brain may not be less than that of older children, and therefore the threshold for hypoglycemia in the neonate should be 60 mg/dL (Stanley at al, 1999). In our opinion, in general a plasma glucose level of <50 mg/dL is a practical, reasonable, and safe threshold for assessing a newborn for hypoglycemia (Sperling and Menon, 2004).

SIGNS AND SYMPTOMS

Signs and symptoms of hypoglycemia in neonates are nonspecific and include jitteriness, lethargy, poor feeding, apnea, cyanotic spells, respiratory distress, myoclonic or multifocal clonic seizures, and, rarely, coma. Many neonates are asymptomatic or display minimal signs and symptoms, and therefore the detection of hypoglycemia requires a high index of suspicion, especially in at-risk neonates.

MEASUREMENT OF BLOOD GLUCOSE

The ideal method of blood glucose estimation should be accurate, rapid, and inexpensive; require small sample volume; and be available as a point-of-care test. However, none of the available methods fulfill all of these criteria.

Laboratory techniques based on the hexokinase method for estimation of glucose in serum or plasma are usually accepted as the reference method. Reagent strips and glucose reflectance meters are commonly used in newborn units but lack necessary reproducibility and accuracy. The use of skin-cleansing agents, variations in hematocrit, and operator technique (placing too little or too much blood on the strip) are common sources of error (Ho et al, 2004; Reynolds et al, 1993). Glucose biosensors that measure the molality of glucose in the water phase of blood or plasma are present in most blood glucose and electrolyte analyzer machines. Whereas the glucose biosensor method has not been extensively evaluated, a recent study reported good agreement between a potentiometric glucose oxidase sensor incorporated in a multianalyte analyzer and a laboratory-based reference method (Newman et al, 2002).

Another newer methodology of special relevance to preterm babies who require intensive glucose monitoring for prolonged periods is the continuous glucose monitor using a subcutaneously implanted catheter that continuously measures the concentration of small molecules (including glucose) in the interstitial fluid by microdialysis (Baumeister et al, 2001). Use of this method also reduces the discomfort and blood loss associated with the conventional methods; however, the accuracy of this method at low levels of blood glucose remains to be established.

NEWBORNS REQUIRING GLUCOSE MONITORING

It is essential that glucose monitoring at appropriate intervals be instituted in newborns at increased risk of hypoglycemia. Box 94-1 (modified from Deshpande and Ward Platt, 2005) summarizes the maternal and neonatal conditions that place the newborn at risk of hypoglycemia.

BOX 94-1   Maternal and Neonatal Conditions That Increase the Risk of Neonatal Hypoglycemia

MATERNAL CONDITIONS
Diabetes (gestational or pre-gestational)
Administration of drugs (β sympathomimetics, e.g., terbutaline, oral hypoglycemic agents)
Intrapartum dextrose infusion
Hypertension/ pre-eclampsia

NEONATAL CONDITIONS
Prematurity
Intrauterine growth restriction
Hypoxia-ischemia
Large/small for gestational age
Sepsis
Hypothermia
Polycythemia
Presence of syndromic features (microphallus, midline defects, Beckwith-Wiedemann syndrome)

Modified from Deshpande S, Ward Platt M: The investigation and management of neonatal hypoglycaemia, *Semin Fetal Neonatal Med* 10:351-361, 2005.

CLASSIFICATION OF NEONATAL HYPOGLYCEMIA

Neonatal hypoglycemia is classified (Box 94-2) as transient when it lasts days to weeks after birth and persistent when hypoglycemia continues in infancy.

TRANSIENT HYPOGLYCEMIA

The fetus receives a constant transplacental supply of maternal glucose via insulin-independent GLUT-1 and GLUT-3 glucose transporter mediated diffusion (Bier et al, 1977). This glucose is utilized for meeting the energy demands of the fetus and for assimilation of glycogen and fat stores. The doubling of fetal weight from an average of 1700 grams at 32 weeks to 3400 grams at term is chiefly contributed by the accrual of hepatic glycogen and adipose tissue fat depots.

Transient hypoglycemia is common in neonates if feeding is delayed because of the physiologic immaturity of pathways of glucose homeostasis. In healthy term, appropriate-for-gestational-age newborns, when feeding is delayed to 6 to 8 hours after birth, plasma glucose falls below 50 mg/dL in 30% and below 30 mg/dL in 10% (Lubchenco and Bard, 1971). This propensity for decrease in blood sugar concentrations is believed to be primarily due to developmental immaturity in the pathways of

---

BOX 94-2   Classification of Neonatal Hypoglycemia

TRANSIENT (DAYS)
Developmental immaturity in adaptation to fasting: prematurity, small for gestational age (SGA)
Stress in peripartum/postnatal period: trauma, asphyxia, hypothermia
Transient hyperinsulinemia: infants of diabetic mothers, intrapartum dextrose infusion to mother
Increased metabolic expenditure: sepsis, erythroblastosis fetalis, polycythemia
Other maternal conditions: toxemia, administration of tocolytics (β sympathomimetics)

TRANSIENT (WEEKS TO MONTHS)
Hyperinsulinism in SGA infants and infants with birth asphyxia

PERSISTENT
Hyperinsulinemic
  K_{ATP} channel defects
  Glutamate dehydrogenase (GLUD1)-activating mutation
  Glucokinase-activating mutation
  Short-chain 3-hydroxyacyl coA dehydrogenase (SCHAD) mutation
  Beckwith-Wiedemann syndrome (BWS)
  Hyperinsulinism in congenital disorders of glycosylation
  β-cell adenoma—MEN1
  Undefined
3. Normoinsulinemic
  Counterregulatory hormone deficiency
  Inborn errors of metabolism
  Glycogen storage disease (I, III, VI)
  Disorders of gluconeogenesis
  Defects in fatty acid catabolism and ketogenesis
  Organic acidurias
  Galactosemia
  Hereditary fructose intolerance

gluconeogenesis and ketogenesis wherein some of the key enzymes are not expressed at birth. The expression of these enzymes and the subsequent maturation of these pathways for adaptation to fasting occur rapidly in the postnatal period, usually within the first 24 hours of life.

Major causes of transient hypoglycemia in neonates are listed in Box 94-2, and some of the important causes are discussed in the following sections.

Hypoglycemia in Premature and Small for Gestational Age Infants

Preterm and small for gestational age infants are at increased risk of hypoglycemia because the developmental immaturity in fasting adaptation is coupled with inadequate reserves of glycogen and fat that serve as substrates for gluconeogenesis and ketogenesis. Management of hypoglycemia in these newborns consists of frequent blood glucose monitoring, frequent oral or nasogastric feeding, and intravenous dextrose infusion if enteral feeds are not tolerated. Glucose homeostasis is achieved usually within the first few days of life after establishment of regular feeding and activation of the relevant enzymatic pathways.

Hypoglycemia in Infants of Diabetic Mothers

These infants are characteristically macrosomic and have excess glycogen and fat reserves due to hyperglycemia in the fetal period. However, an elevated circulating level of insulin prevents these infants from appropriately mobilizing these reserves during the early postnatal period. This state of hyperinsulinism generally resolves within the 1st week of life with reestablishment of glucose homeostasis. Maintenance of maternal euglycemia, especially in the third trimester and the intrapartum period, decreases the incidence of hypoglycemia in the newborn (Andersen et al, 1985; Taylor et al, 2002). Management of the hypoglycemia consists of frequent feeding and supplementation with intravenous dextrose if required. The rate of dextrose infusion is titrated to maintain euglycemia. Decrements in dextrose infusion should be instituted in a stepwise manner to prevent rebound hypoglycemia precipitated by sustained insulin secretion after abrupt discontinuation of high rates of glucose infusion.

Transient Hyperinsulinism in Asphyxiated or Small for Gestational Age Infants

Hypoglycemia lasting from several days to a few weeks or months is occasionally observed in infants with birth asphyxia or intrauterine growth retardation. Hyperinsulinism, and possibly an associated deficiency of glucagon, is implicated in the pathogenesis of hypoglycemia. In these infants, exogenous dextrose requirement may exceed 20 mg/kg/minute, and the hypoglycemia is unresponsive to glucocorticoid administration. Most infants show good response to drugs useful in hyperinsulinism, such as diazoxide, octreotide, and glucagon (Bhowmick and Levandowski, 1989; Clark and O'Donovan, 2001). Oral diazoxide is the usual regimen of choice and is administered until resolution of the hyperinsulinism.

PERSISTENT HYPOGLYCEMIA

Hyperinsulinemic Hypoglycemia

Hyperinsulinism characterized by inappropriate insulin secretion in the presence of low plasma glucose is the most common cause of persistent hypoglycemia in the neonate. This entity was first described in 1954 by McQuarrie as "idiopathic hypoglycemia of infancy" and subsequently referred to by various names such as nesidioblastosis, islet dysregulation syndrome, and persistent hyperinsulinemic hypoglycemia of infancy. Currently the preferred term is congenital hyperinsulinism of infancy (CHI). Worldwide the incidence of CHI is 1 in 30,000 to 1 in 50,000 live births. A particularly high incidence of 1 in 2500 has been reported from the Arabian Peninsula and is attributed to high rates of consanguinity (al-Rabeeah et al, 1995; Bin-Abbas et al, 2003).

The commonest and the most severe genetic defects responsible for CHI are mutations in genes coding the two subunits of the ATP-sensitive potassium (K_{ATP}) channel, the SUR1 and Kir6.2 proteins (Doyle et al, 1998; Thomas et al, 1995, 1996). Mutations in other genes that can also manifest as CHI are those coding for glucokinase, glutamate dehydrogenase (GDH), and the mitochondrial enzyme L-3-hydroxyacyl CoA dehydrogenase (HADH) proteins. A brief overview of these conditions is presented in Table 94-1. Hyperinsulinism is also observed in less common disorders such as Beckwith-Wiedemann syndrome (BWS) and congenital disorders of glycosylation. The salient causes of persistent hyperinsulinism in the newborn are discussed in greater detail in the following sections.

K_{ATP} Channel Defects

The commonest mechanism underlying CHI is dysfunction of the ATP-sensitive potassium channel located on the β-cell membrane. This channel has two subunits, the potassium inward rectifying (Kir6.2) pore and the sulfonylurea receptor regulatory subunit (SUR1). The Kir6.2 is encoded by the *KCNJ11* gene and the SUR1 subunit by the *ABCC8* gene, both located in the 11p15.1 region. In the unstimulated (resting) state, the ATP/ADP ratio is low and the channel remains open. This allows the β cell to maintain a polarized state with a resting membrane potential of approximately −65mV. When there is uptake and metabolism of glucose in the β cell, the concentration of ATP increases and that of ADP decreases. This causes the K_{ATP} channels to close, leading to depolarization of the cell membrane. Depolarization leads to opening of the voltage-gated Ca^{2+} channels with resultant influx of calcium and exocytosis of insulin (Figure 94-1) (Sperling and Menon, 2004). Inactivating (loss of function) mutations in the *KCNJ11/ABCC8* gene result in persistent closure of the channel, leading to depolarization of cell membrane, influx of calcium, and inappropriate release of insulin. More than 100 distinct mutations have been described in the SUR1 encoding *ABCC8* gene and are responsible for 50% to 60% of all cases of CHI. Mutations in the Kir6.2 encoding *KCNJ11* gene are responsible for 10% to 15% of all cases of CHI (Dunne et al, 2004).

TABLE 94-1 An Overview of the Genetic Causes of CHI

Inheritance	Molecular Defect	Chromosome	Histology	Clinical Features	Treatment	Outcome
Sporadic	Paternally inherited ABCC8/KCNJ11 mutation with loss of heterozygosity	11p15	Focal	Macrosomia, moderate to severe hypoglycemia in first few days to weeks of life	Poor response to diazoxide, local resection for focal and near-total pancreatectomy for diffuse form	Good in focal and guarded in diffuse
	De novo mutation in ABCC8/KCNJ11		Diffuse			
AR	ABCC8/KCNJ11 (inactivating)	11p15	Diffuse	Macrosomia, onset in first few days to weeks of life, family history or consanguinity may be present	Near-total pancreatectomy	Guarded
AD	ABCC8/KCNJ11 (inactivating)	11p15	Diffuse	Milder symptoms, may manifest in late infancy	Usually responsive to diazoxide	Good
AD	GLUD1 (activating)	10q	Diffuse	Modest hyperinsulinemia and hyperammonemia, onset usually >6 months	Diazoxide, restriction of leucine in diet	Good
AD	GCK (activating)	7p	Diffuse	Modest hyperinsulinemia, onset usually >6 months	Diazoxide	Good
AR	HADH	4q	Diffuse	Variable clinical presentation, abnormal acylcarnitine profile	Diazoxide	Fair

Modified from Sperling MA, Menon RK: Differential diagnosis and management of neonatal hypoglycemia, *Pediatr Clin North Am* 51:703-723, 2004.
ABCC8, ATP-binding cassette subfamily C, member 8; *AD*, autosomal dominant; *AR*, autosomal recessive; ; *GCK*, glucokinase; *GLUD1*, glutamate dehydrogenase 1; *HADH*, L-3-hydroxyacyl coenzyme A dehydrogenase hyperinsulinism; *KCNJ11*, potassium inward rectifying channel subfamily J, member 11.

Pancreatic β cell

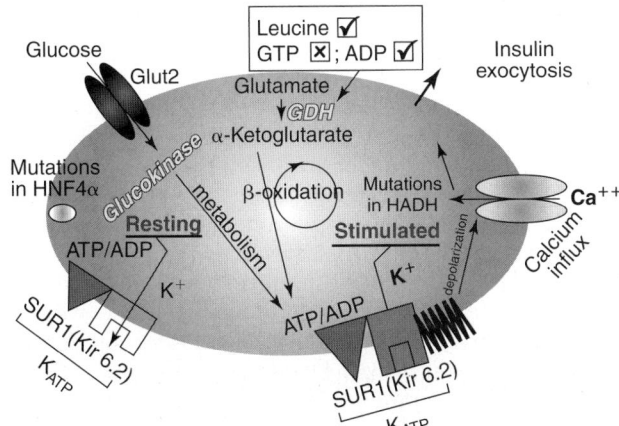

FIGURE 94-1 **Mechanisms of insulin secretion by the β cell of pancreas.** Glucose transported into the β cell by the insulin-dependent glucose transporter, GLUT 2, undergoes phosphorylation by glucokinase and subsequent metabolism, resulting in an increase in the intracellular ATP:ADP ratio. The increase in the ATP:ADP ratio closes the K_{ATP} channel and initiates the cascade of events characterized by increase in intracellular K concentration, membrane depolarization, calcium influx, and release of insulin from storage granules. Leucine stimulates insulin secretion by allosterically activating glutamate dehydrogenase (GDH) and by increasing the oxidation of glutamate, thereby increasing the ATP:ADP ratio and closure of the KATP channel. Mutations in the HADH gene, which codes for the mitochondrial enzyme L-3-hydroxyacyl-coenzyme A dehydrogenase that catalyzes the penultimate step in the fatty acid β-oxidation pathway, is also associated with CHI. Mutations in HNF4α cause multiple defects in glucose stimulated insulin secretion. x, inhibition; √, stimulation. (*Modified from Sperling MA, Menon RK: Differential diagnosis and management of neonatal hypoglycemia, Pediatr Clin North Am 51:703-723, 2004.*)

Histologically, CHI can be classified as either diffuse involvement of the pancreas or focal adenomatous hyperplasia (Kloppel et al, 1999). An estimated 40% to 65% of CHI is characterized as focal and the remainder as the diffuse form. In the diffuse form, the β cells have abundant cytoplasm and large nuclei throughout the pancreas, whereas in the focal form, the lesion is less than 10 mm in size with confluent proliferation of β cells that are normal in size and shape with intermingling of exocrine acinar cells (Figure 94-2, *A* and *B*). Both the forms manifest with similar clinical features, with no correlation between the severity of hypoglycemia and histologic classification. The molecular defect underlying the focal form is most commonly a paternally inherited mutation in SUR1 or Kir6.2 with loss of the 11p15 maternal allele in the pancreatic β cells (loss of heterozygosity). Since the loss of heterozygosity is a somatic defect, focal CHI always manifests as a sporadic event. The underlying defect in cases of diffuse CHI are more varied and include *de novo*, autosomal recessively or dominantly inherited mutations in *KCNJ11* or *ABCC8* genes and less commonly mutations involving β-cell enzymes as discussed later (De Lonlay et al, 2007).

Activating Mutation of the Glutamate Dehydrogenase (GLUD1) Gene

Glutamate dehydrogenase (*GLUD1*) activating mutation, also referred to as hyperinsulinemia hyperammonemia (HIHA) syndrome, is the second commonest cause of CHI. Glutamate dehydrogenase (GDH) is a mitochondrial enzyme that is normally activated by leucine and ADP and inhibited by GTP and ATP. GDH increases the oxidative deamination of glutamate to α-ketoglutarate

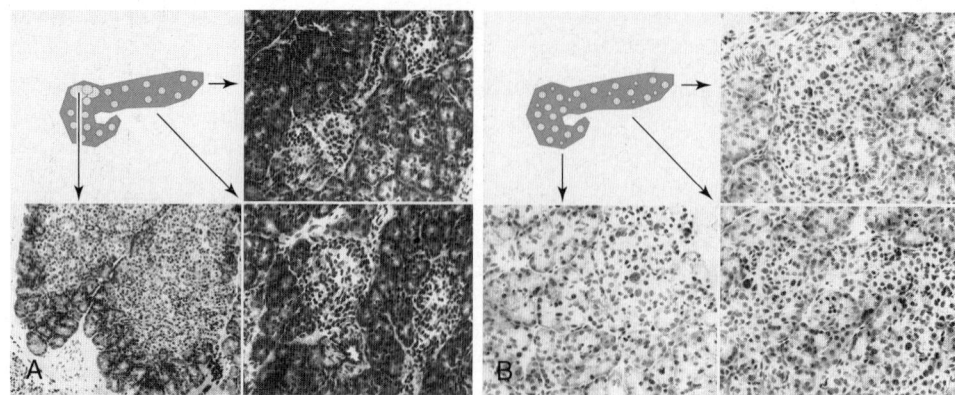

FIGURE 94-2 *(Supplemental color version of this figure is available online at www.expertconsult.com.)* **A,** Representation of frozen sections obtained from three pancreatic sites during surgery for a focal form of hyperinsulinism in the head. Specimens taken from tail and body show islets of Langerhans at rest with little cytoplasm, leading to crowded nuclei, whereas the focal form aspect from the head is that of multilobular involvement with local signs of β-cell hyperactivity: abundant cytoplasm and large, abnormal nuclei (toluidine blue stain; original magnifications ×200 and ×100). **B,** Representation of frozen sections obtained from three pancreatic sites during surgery for diffuse form of hyperinsulinism. On each biopsy, there is one islet showing hyperfunctional signs with abundant cytoplasm and irregular nuclei more than 4 times the size of the acinar nuclei nearby taken as internal control. The disease involves the whole pancreas and, in consequence, can be called diffuse, which does not mean that all islets are involved in the same manner (toluidine blue stain; original magnification ×200). *(Reproduced from Delonlay P, Simon A, Galmiche-Rolland L, et al: Neonatal hyperinsulinism: clinicopathologic correlation,* Hum Pathol 38:387-399, 2007.)

and ammonia, thereby raising the ATP/ADP ratio, which results in closure of the K_{ATP} channel and release of insulin. This form of CHI usually presents beyond 6 months of age with recurrent hypoglycemia and persistent mild hyperammonemia (serum ammonia levels 2–5 times normal). The hypoglycemia is usually less severe than that in the K_{ATP} channel defects and is usually controllable by diazoxide therapy (Stanley et al, 1998).

Activating Mutation of the Glucokinase Gene

This rare form of CHI is caused by an activating mutation in the *GCK* gene resulting in increased affinity of glucokinase for glucose with resultant inappropriate insulin secretion (Glaser et al, 1998).

HADH (L-3-Hydroxyacyl-Coenzyme A Dehydrogenase) Gene Mutation

Mutations in the *HADH* gene, which codes for the mitochondrial enzyme L-3-hydroxyacyl-coenzyme A dehydrogenase (previously referred to as short-chain 3-hydroxyacyl dehydrogenase, SCHAD) that catalyzes the penultimate step in the fatty acid β-oxidation pathway, are also associated with CHI. The exact mechanism of increased insulin secretion in patients with this mutation is not clear. The clinical presentation can vary from severe neonatal-onset to mild late-onset hypoglycemia, but all forms show good response to treatment with diazoxide (Clayton et al, 2001; Eaton et al, 2003).

Beckwith-Wiedemann Syndrome

BWS is characterized by somatic overgrowth, macroglossia, visceromegaly, hemihypertrophy, transverse ear lobe creases, renal tract abnormalities, and predisposition to development of tumors. This condition is sporadic in approximately 85% of cases and inherited in an autosomal dominant manner in the remaining 15%. Several genetic and epigenetic alterations in the 11p15 region such as paternal isodisomy, methylation of H19/ IGF2, and mutations in *CDKN1C* gene have been described (Li et al,

1998). Hypoglycemia of varying severity is seen in 50% of infants and is transient in the vast majority of patients. In persistent cases, the response to treatment is variable. Good control of hypoglycemia with diazoxide is achieved in some patients, with other patients requiring partial pancreatectomy for control of hypoglycemia. The molecular mechanism(s) for hyperinsulinism in BWS has not been clearly defined (DeBaun et al, 2000).

Hyperinsulinism in Congenital Disorders of Glycosylation

Congenital disorders of glycosylation (CDG) are a family of disorders characterized by defects in glycosylation of various glycoproteins, with symptoms affecting multiple systems including brain, liver, gastrointestinal system, and skeleton. Hyperinsulinemic hypoglycemia has been described in CDG-Ia (phosphomannose mutase deficiency) in conjunction with neurologic symptoms (Bohles et al, 2001); CDG-Ib (phosphomannose isomerase deficiency) in association with protein-losing enteropathy and liver disease (Babovic-Vuksanovic et al, 1999); and rarely in CDG-Id (Sun et al, 2005). The pathophysiology of hyperinsulinism in these rare syndromes is not well understood. Hypoglycosylation of SUR1 or other proteins involved in insulin secretion has been postulated to be the responsible mechanism.

Dominant Heterozygous Mutations in the HNF4 α gene

Hepatocyte nuclear factor 4α (HNF4α) is a transcription factor belonging to the nuclear hormone receptor superfamily. This gene is expressed in liver, gut, kidney, and pancreatic islets. In the β cell, HNF4α regulates several key genes involved in glucose-stimulated insulin secretion. Heterozygote mutations in the human *HNF4A* gene generally present as maturity onset diabetes of the young subtype 1 (MODY1). However, recent reports have implicated mutations in the HNF4α gene as causing both transient and persistent CHI (Kapoor et al, 2008).

Diagnosis of Hyperinsulinism

The diagnosis of hyperinsulinism is based on clues from history, physical examination, and laboratory tests performed on a critical blood sample and complemented by molecular diagnosis by genetic testing when available. Infants with hyperinsulinism generally present with severe and persistent hypoglycemia within 4 to 5 hours of fasting, with seizures, lethargy, and apnea, and have high glucose requirements (usually greater than 10 mg/kg/minute). Macrosomia may be a feature in some newborns. Diagnosis is based on evidence of inadequate suppression of insulin secretion on a critical blood sample drawn during an episode of hypoglycemia. Presence of low levels of plasma free fatty acids and ketones (insulin suppresses lipolysis and ketogenesis) and a glycemic response (within 30 minutes of administration of glucagon at the time of the hypoglycemic event) of greater than 30 mg/dL indicating the presence of adequate hepatic glycogen stores are strong evidence of hyperinsulinism (Stanley and Baker, 1976). The diagnostic criteria for hyperinsulinism based on laboratory analysis of a critical blood sample are presented in Box 94-3. Other tests such as serum ammonia for HIHA caused by activating mutation of GDH and plasma acylcarnitine profile and urinary organic acids (increased plasma 3-hydroxybutyrylcarnitine and urine 3-hydroxyglutarate) for CHI caused by mutation in SCHAD enzyme may also be indicated in individual cases. Genetic testing for molecular diagnosis of several forms of CHI is also commercially available.

Differentiation between Focal Adenomatous and Diffuse Pancreatic Hyperplasia

Differentiation between infants with focal and diffuse forms of CHI preoperatively is very helpful in formulating the management strategy and prognosticating the outcome.

BOX 94-3   Diagnostic Criteria for Hyperinsulinism Based on Critical Sample at Time of Hypoglycemia

- Plasma insulin >2μU/ml
- Plasma free fatty acids <1.5 mmol/L
- Plasma β-hydroxybutyrate <2.0 μmol/L
- Glycemic response to 0.1 mg/kg intravenous glucagon >30 mg/dL

The focal form is curable with partial pancreatectomy and has an excellent prognosis, whereas diffuse disease requires near-total (95% to 98%) pancreatectomy with subsequent development of diabetes mellitus in approximately half and persistence of hypoglycemia in a third of the affected infants. Until recently, this differentiation was based on technically difficult and invasive methods with low reliability, such as intrahepatic portal venous sampling and selective pancreatic intraarterial calcium stimulation with venous sampling. Recently positron emission tomography (PET) scans with fluorine-18–L-3,4-dihydroxyphenylalanine (^{18}F-fluoro-L-DOPA) have been successfully used to accurately discriminate focal from diffuse CHI (Otonkoski et al, 2006). This test is based on the fact that β cells take up L-DOPA and convert it to dopamine via DOPA decarboxylase present in islet cells. In cases of focal CHI, there is localized accumulation of ^{18}F-fluoro-L-DOPA, and co-registration of PET and magnetic resonance (MR) images allows anatomic localization of the lesion (Mohnike et al, 2006).

Management

Table 94-2 provides a summary of drugs used in the management of hyperinsulinism. As described earlier, the syndromic, metabolic, and milder form of K_{ATP} channel defects (autosomal dominant with late onset) are usually responsive to diazoxide, which is the first line of treatment. The response should be evaluated after at least 5 days of therapy (based on diazoxide's half-life of 9.5 to 24 hours) and defined as maintenance of plasma glucose >70 mg/dL after 3 to 4 hours of fasting (deLeon and Stanley, 2007). In those infants who fail to respond, octreotide is tried as the second-line drug. Octreotide is a long-acting somatostatin analogue that inhibits insulin secretion. Most infants show an initial response to octreotide but develop tachyphylaxis after a few days. Thus, octreotide's major clinical role is in short-term management of infants awaiting surgery (deLeon and Stanley, 2007). Nifedipine, a calcium channel antagonist, has been reported to be effective in a limited number of cases (Muller et al, 2004), but long-term experience is lacking. Further, this drug can cause life-threatening hypotension in the newborn period and therefore avoided. Glucagon is useful in short-term management of infants awaiting surgery (Hussain et al, 2004).

TABLE 94-2   Drugs Used in the Management of Neonatal Hyperinsulinism

Drug	Dose/Route	Mechanism of Action	Adverse Effects
Diazoxide	5–20 mg/kg/d in three divided doses orally	Binds to SUR1 subunit, opens K_{ATP} channel	Fluid retention, hypertrichosis, rarely eosinophilia, leukopenia, hypotension
Chlorthiazide (in conjunction with diazoxide to decrease fluid retention)	7–10 mg/kg/d in two divided doses orally	Synergistic response to diazoxide	Hyponatremia, hypokalemia
Octreotide	5–25 μg/kg/d 6–8 hourly SC injection or IV infusion	Inhibits insulin secretion by binding to somatostatin receptors and inducing hyperpolarization of β-cells, direct inhibition of voltage-dependent calcium channels	Anorexia, nausea, abdominal pain, diarrhea, tachyphylaxis
Glucagon	1–20 μg/kg/h, SC or IV infusion	Increases glycogenolysis and gluconeogenesis	Nausea, vomiting, paradoxical insulin secretion at high dose
Nifedipine	0.25–2.5 mg/kg/d in three divided doses orally	Calcium channel blocker	Hypotension

IV, Intravenous; *SC,* subcutaneous.

Surgical therapy is required in those infants who fail to respond to medical management. In focal CHI, resection of the lesion will "cure" the infant. Infants with diffuse disease require a near-total (95% to 98%) pancreatectomy and may also require additional therapy with diazoxide, octreotide, and frequent feeding to maintain euglycemia.

Normoinsulinemic Hypoglycemia
Counterregulatory Hormone Deficiency

This is the second most frequent cause of persistent hypoglycemia presenting in the neonatal period. Hypopituitarism causing varying degrees of adrenocorticotrophic hormone (and hence cortisol) and growth hormone (GH) deficiencies may present with hypoglycemia in the neonatal period due to unopposed effects of insulin. Clues to hypopituitarism in the affected neonate are midline facial defects, cholestasis, nystagmus due to optic nerve hypoplasia, and microphallus in the male neonate (reflecting the role of pituitary gonadotropin action in the development of the external male genitalia). In the neonatal period, ketones are absent or low in affected babies, whereas in later infancy ketone levels are usually elevated. Diagnosis is established by demonstrating GH levels to be less than 10 ng/mL during an episode of hypoglycemia (Sperling and Menon, 2004). Provocative testing is not required because the average plasma concentration of GH in normal newborns ranges from 16 to 76 ng/mL in the first few weeks of life (Cornblath et al, 1965).

Primary adrenal insufficiency as in enzymatic deficiency of steroid biosynthesis (congenital adrenal hyperplasia), congenital X-linked adrenal hypoplasia, and adrenal hemorrhage can also present with hypoglycemia in the neonatal period. Presence of dyselectrolytemia (hyponatremia, hyperkalemia) or ambiguous genitalia (in congenital adrenal hyperplasia) may provide a clue to the diagnosis of adrenal insufficiency in the newborn. Familial glucocorticoid deficiency caused by adrenocorticotrophic hormone receptor defects manifests with hypoglycemia and hyperpigmentation without electrolyte disturbance because aldosterone secretion is unaffected. Diagnosis of adrenal insufficiency is established by demonstration of low serum cortisol concentration (<5μg/dL) during hypoglycemia.

Inborn Errors of Metabolism

Inborn errors in the enzymatic pathways of glycogen synthesis or breakdown, gluconeogenesis, and fatty acid oxidation can occur with hypoglycemia. However, these disorders rarely manifest in the neonatal period because several hours of fasting is needed for hypoglycemia to manifest, an unlikely situation in newborns, unless breastfed infants encounter latching-on difficulties. These disorders usually present in later infancy when feeding interval has increased and the infant has started sleeping through the night or during intercurrent illness with reduced oral intake. Some of the major inborn errors of metabolism presenting with hypoglycemia are discussed briefly in the following sections. The key metabolic pathways of intermediary metabolism are presented in Figure 94-3.

Glycogen Storage Diseases

Hypoglycemia is seen with several of the glycogen storage diseases (GSDs), most notably GSD1 caused by glucose-6-phosphatase deficiency. This is a key enzyme in the pathways of glycogenolysis as well as gluconeogenesis. Affected infants have hypertriglyceridemia, hyperuricemia, hypophosphatemia, and elevated levels of ketones and lactate with metabolic acidosis. Frequent feeding and high levels of alternate fuels for cerebral metabolism usually preclude the development of symptomatic hypoglycemia in the neonatal period. GSD3 is caused by the deficiency of amylo-1,6-glucosidase (debrancher enzyme) and has a phenotype similar to that of GSD1. Other forms of GSD such as liver phosphorylase and phosphorylase kinase deficiency (GSD types 6 and 9) and glycogen synthase deficiency (GSD type 0) are rare causes of hypoglycemia in infancy (Wolfsdorf et al, 1999; Wolfsdorf and Weinstein, 2003).

Disorders of Gluconeogenesis

Fructose 1,6-diphosphatase deficiency results in blockage of gluconeogenesis from all possible precursors below the level of fructose 1,6-diphosphate (see Figure 94-3). However, disorders of gluconeogenesis are likely to manifest with hypoglycemia only after prolonged caloric deprivation and are therefore unlikely to manifest in the neonatal period (Stanley et al, 2002).

Disorders of Fatty Acid Catabolism and Ketogenesis

Disorders of fatty acid oxidation represent errors in the uptake, activation, and mitochondrial oxidation of fatty acids. These disorders usually appear after prolonged caloric deprivation (6 to 8 hours in infants <1 year and 10 to 12 hours in older infants), as may occur during intercurrent illness. The phenotype may range from a severe Reye-like syndrome with coma and death to milder forms with varying degrees of involvement of liver, skeletal, and cardiac muscle. The clinical findings may include hepatomegaly, vomiting, hypotonia, muscle weakness, and cardiomyopathy. This group of disorders is characterized by low or absent plasma and urine ketones. The primary diagnostic tool in the evaluation of these disorders is determination of plasma acylcarnitine profile by tandem mass spectrometry. Specific abnormalities of the plasma acylcarnitines are seen in different disorders of fatty acid oxidation (Stanley, 1998).

Galactosemia

Galactosemia is caused by deficiency of the enzyme galactose-1-phosphate uridyl transferase. Deficiency of UDP-galactose-4-epimerase also has a similar clinical presentation. Affected infants present with vomiting, diarrhea, jaundice, and hepatomegaly in addition to hypoglycemia. Escherichia coli sepsis commonly occurs in affected infants. Cataracts, liver dysfunction, renal tubular defects, intellectual impairment, and ovarian failure are other clinical manifestations. Diagnosis is suspected in infants with non-glucose reducing substance in urine and confirmed by assay for galactose-1-phosphate uridyl transferase and epimerase enzymes. Management consists of dietary galactose restriction (Stanley et al, 2002).

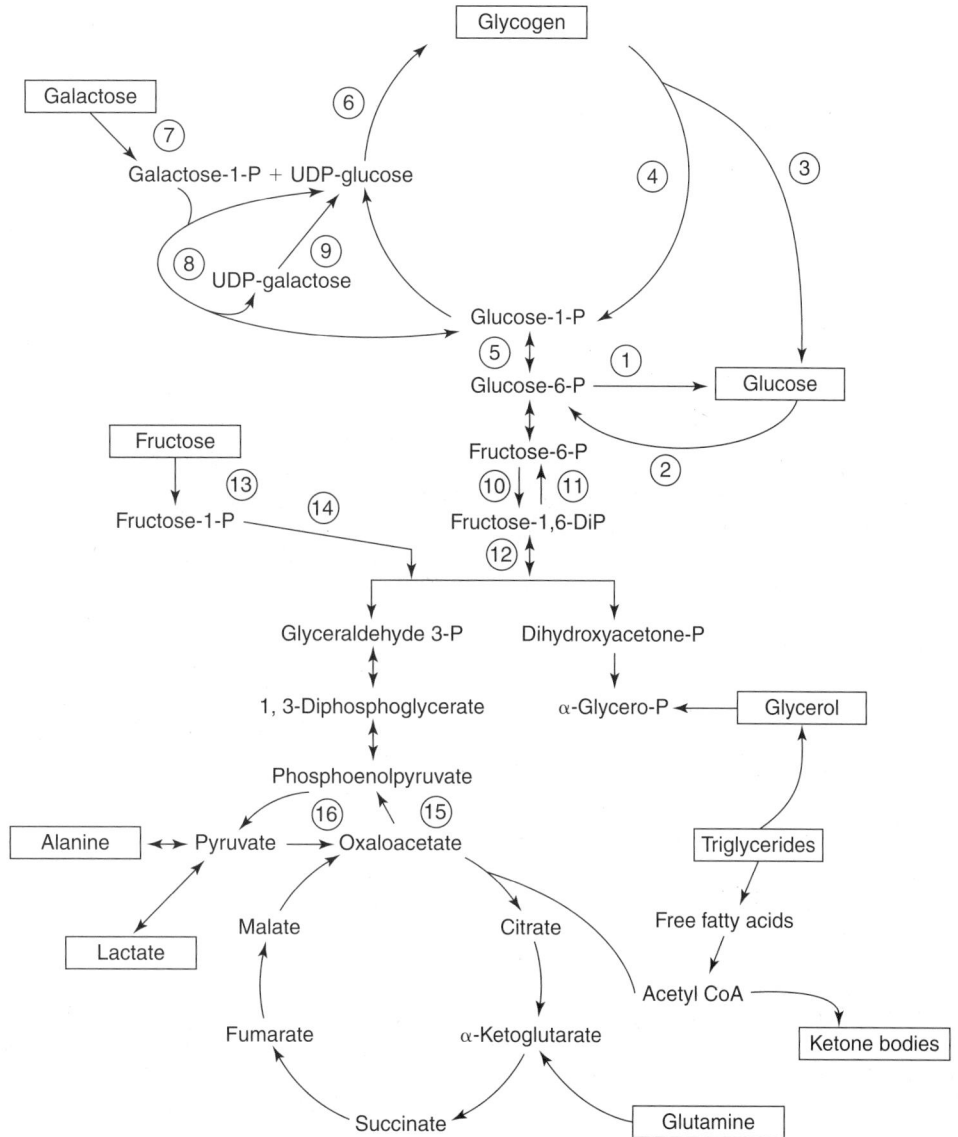

FIGURE 94-3 Key metabolic pathways of intermediary metabolism. *1,* Glucose 6-phosphatase; *2,* glucokinase; *3,* amylo-1,6-glucosidase; *4,* phosphorylase; *5,* phosphoglucomutase; *6,* glycogen synthetase; *7,* galactokinase; *8,* galactose-1-phosphate uridyl transferase; *9,* uridine diphospho-galactose-4-epimerase; *10,* phosphofructokinase; *11,* fructose-1,6-diphosphatase; *12,* fructose-1,6-diphosphate aldolase; *13,* fructokinase; *14,* fructose-1-phosphate aldolase; *15,* phosphoenolpyruvate carboxykinase; *16,* pyruvate carboxylase; *UDP,* uridine diphosphate. *(Modified from Sperling MA, Menon RK: Differential diagnosis and management of neonatal hypoglycemia,* Pediatr Clin North Am *51:703-723, 2004.)*

Hereditary Fructose Intolerance

Hereditary fructose intolerance is caused by deficiency of the enzyme fructose-1-phosphate aldolase and manifests only after inclusion of fructose in the diet. In infants fed with fructose- or sucrose-containing formulas, there is acute postprandial hypoglycemia along with vomiting and abdominal distention. The hypoglycemia is caused by an acute inhibition of glycogenolysis and gluconeogenesis by the accumulation of fructose-1-phosphate (Stanley et al, 2002).

HYPERGLYCEMIA IN THE NEONATE

DEFINITION

Whereas the upper limit of blood sugar levels in healthy newborns has not been clearly defined, it is customary to consider the threshold for diagnosing hyperglycemia in the neonate to be similar (126 mg/dL) to that for children and adults. Blood sugar concentration >180 mg/dL or presence of glycosuria with osmotic diuresis is generally considered an indication for intervention.

ETIOLOGY

Transient hyperglycemia is generally an incidental finding during routine blood sugar monitoring in sick/preterm or SGA neonates. A common cause for this abnormality in glucose homeostasis is iatrogenic glucose overload. Other mechanisms for transient hyperglycemia in the newborn include impaired insulin secretion, insulin resistance, and immaturity of the hepatic enzymes involved in glucose homeostasis. Rarely the hyperglycemia may be due to neonatal diabetes (incidence 1 in 400,000) (Shield, 2007), which is discussed in the subsequent section.

The differential diagnoses of neonatal hyperglycemia are presented in Box 94-4.

Neonatal Diabetes

Onset of diabetes before the age of 6 months is usually referred to as neonatal diabetes. In contrast to classic type 1 diabetes in children and adolescents, neonatal diabetes is not an autoimmune disease, and specific gene defects are the most common cause of neonatal diabetes. Neonatal diabetes is further classified as transient or permanent (Polak, 2007).

Transient Neonatal Diabetes Mellitus

In a recent report by Flanagan et al (2007), among a cohort of 97 patients with transient neonatal diabetes mellitus (TNDM), anomalies in the 6q24 chromosomal region were seen in 69, KCNJ11 mutations in 12, and ABCC8 mutations in 13 patients; only 3 patients had none of these genetic defects. A brief outline of the common causes of TNDM is presented next.

Chromosome 6q24 Anomalies

A majority of cases of TNDM result from anomalies in the imprinted region of 6q24 containing the *ZAC* (*z*inc, *a*poptosis and *c*ycle) and *HYMAI* (for *h*ydatidiform *m*ole *a*ssociated and *i*mprinted) genes. In general, expression of a gene is similar whether the gene is inherited from the female parent (the maternal allele) or the male parent (the paternal allele). However, for a small subset of genes, differences in expression levels are observed when the maternal and paternal alleles are measured separately. This biased expression of one parental allele over the other is termed *genomic imprinting*. Paternal uniparental isodisomy of chromosome 6, unbalanced duplication of paternal 6q24, and loss of imprinting of maternal 6q24 are the three genetic defects that have been associated with TNDM and are believed to result in overexpression of *ZAC* and *HYMAI* genes and consequent inhibition of β-cell proliferation and impairment of glucose-stimulated insulin secretion (Cave et al, 2000).

Diabetes due to 6q24 anomalies usually manifests within the 1st week of life with severe hyperglycemia and dehydration with mild or no ketosis. The majority of affected infants have significant intrauterine growth retardation

reflecting insulinopenia during the intrauterine period as well. The associated diabetes generally resolves within the first 3 months of life but reappears in more than half of patients at puberty or during the stress of intercurrent illness (Temple et al, 2000).

K_{ATP} Channel Defects

Recent reports have identified patients with TNDM bearing activating mutations in *KCNJ11* or *ABCC8* genes that code for the K_{ATP} channel subunits Kir6.2 and SUR1, respectively (Babenko et al, 2006; Gloyn et al, 2005). These activating mutations keep the K_{ATP} channel open even in the presence of increased ATP/ADP ratio, resulting in hyperpolarization of the cell membrane, reduced calcium influx, and reduced exocytosis of insulin vesicles. It is noteworthy that activating K_{ATP} channel mutations are more commonly associated with the permanent form of neonatal diabetes. It is speculated that the less severe mutations may manifest as TNDM where β-cell dysfunction is compensated over time by increase in islet mass. In most patients, however, the clinical course is biphasic, with recurrence of diabetes in adolescence or adulthood.

Infants with TNDM due to K_{ATP} channel defects usually have a less severe impairment of fetal growth as compared to those with 6q24 anomalies, present at a later age (at 4 weeks vs. 1st week), and achieve remission at a later age (35 weeks vs. 13 weeks) (Flanagan et al, 2007). However, the spectrum of presentation in both these etiologies significantly overlaps, and a distinction between these two entities cannot be made solely on the basis of clinical features.

Permanent Neonatal Diabetes Mellitus

In a recent report of 279 patients with permanent neonatal diabetes mellitus (PNDM), genetic mutations could be detected in 53% of patients, with *KCNJ11*, *ABCC8*, and *INS* gene mutations accounting for 31%, 10%, and 12%, respectively (Edghill et al, 2008). A synopsis of the common causes of PNDM is presented next.

K_{ATP} Channel Defects

Heterozygous activating mutations in *KCNJ11* gene, which encodes the Kir6.2 subunit of the K_{ATP} channel, are the commonest cause of PNDM. Because of the mutation, the K_{ATP} channel becomes insensitive to the inhibitory effect of increased ATP:ADP ratio and remains persistently open with ensuing efflux of potassium. Thus, the β-cell membrane remains hyperpolarized, the voltage gated-calcium channels remain closed, and insulin secretion is reduced (Hattersley et al, 2005).

The median age at presentation of patients with this genetic defect is 3 to 4 weeks and their mean birthweight is between the 10th and 25th percentiles. Ketoacidosis is present in approximately 30% of infants at presentation. About 20% of the affected infants have associated neurologic disease in the form of developmental delay with or without epilepsy or muscle weakness, reflecting the importance of the K_{ATP} channel in neuronal physiology. The severest form of neurologic involvement due to a K_{ATP} channel defect is seen in the DEND (developmental delay, epilepsy, and neonatal diabetes) syndrome (Proks et al, 2005). Sulfonylureas close the K_{ATP} channel by binding to the SUR1 subunit, and a majority of patients with PNDM due to *KCNJ11* mutations respond to therapy with this group of drugs (Koster et al, 2005).

Heterozygous activating and compound homozygous activating/inactivating mutations in the *ABCC8* gene that encodes the SUR1 subunit of the K_{ATP} channel also cause PNDM. Similar to PNDM patients with *KCNJ11* mutations, the vast majority of patients with PNDM due to ABCC8 mutations can also be successfully transitioned to sulfonylurea therapy.

INS Gene Mutations

Heterozygous mutations in the insulin (*INS*) gene are the second commonest cause of PNDM. The identified mutations affect the region of preproinsulin critical for normal protein folding. The abnormally folded proinsulin molecule undergoes degeneration in the endoplasmic reticulum (ER), leading to ER stress and increased β-cell death, leading to progressive reduction in islet mass and diabetes (Stoy et al, 2007).

Other Rare Genetic/Syndromic Causes of PNDM

Homozygous IPF-1 Gene Mutation

Insulin promoter factor-1 (IPF-1) plays an important role in the development of pancreas as well as regulation of expression of insulin and somatostatin genes. Homozygous single nucleotide deletion within IPF-1 gene has been reported to present with pancreatic agenesis with neonatal diabetes and severe exocrine pancreatic insufficiency (Stoffers et al, 1997; Thomas et al, 2009). Heterozygous mutations result in MODY 4.

Homozygous Mutations in Glucokinase Gene

PNDM resulting from homozygous mutations in the glucokinase (*GCK*) gene with complete failure of glycolysis in the β cell is a rare entity (Njolstad et al, 2001). The more commonly occurring heterozygous mutations result in impaired fasting glucose (MODY 2).

IPEX Syndrome

IPEX or immune dysregulation, polyendocrinopathy, enteropathy, X-linked is a rare syndrome caused by mutation in the *FOXP3* gene, which plays a role in the normal regulation of T-cell production. The clinical features of this syndrome are failure to thrive, chronic diarrhea, neonatal diabetes, eczema, thyroiditis, hemolytic anemia, and thrombocytopenia (Wildin et al, 2002).

Wolcott-Rallison Syndrome

This is an autosomal recessive syndrome characterized by onset of diabetes in infancy and spondyloepiphyseal dysplasia. This syndrome is caused by a mutation in the *EIF2AK3* gene, which regulates protein synthesis in the endoplasmic reticulum. Mutations in this gene lead to unregulated protein synthesis with accumulation of malfolded proteins in the ER and increase in β-cell apoptosis (Senee et al, 2004).

TREATMENT

Transient Neonatal Hyperglycemia

Transient neonatal hyperglycemia usually resolves in a few days, and hence the treatment strategy should be conservative.
- Treat underlying cause such as sepsis.
- Minimize exogenous glucose infusion rate to 3–5 mg/kg/minute.
- In the presence of blood sugar >180 mg/dL or if osmotic diuresis manifests, treatment with insulin infusion (starting with 0.03 to 0.05 unit/kg/hour) with frequent blood sugar monitoring should be instituted as a last resort.

Neonatal Diabetes

Control of blood sugar is initially achieved by intravenous insulin infusion, starting at a rate of 0.03 to 0.05 unit/kg/hour and titrated according to blood sugar monitoring. Subsequently, these neonates should ideally be managed by pediatric diabetologists. The treatment options are either continuous subcutaneous insulin infusion (CSII) using an insulin pump or one to two subcutaneous injections per day of an intermediate-acting insulin such as NPH or an ultralong-acting insulin analogue such as glargine or determir.

Early genetic testing should be done in all neonates with diabetes. In those patients determined to harbor mutations in the *KCNJ11* or *ABCC8* genes, an attempt should be made to transition from insulin to oral sulfonylurea regimens.

SUGGESTED READINGS

De Leon DD, Stanley CA: Mechanisms of disease: advances in diagnosis and treatment of hyperinsulinism in neonates, *Nat Clin Pract Endocrinol Metab* 3:57-68, 2007.

Doyle DA, Morais Cabral J, Pfuetzner RA, et al: The structure of the potassium channel: molecular basis of K+ conduction and selectivity, *Science* 280:69-77, 1998.

Flanagan SE, Patch AM, Mackay DJ, et al: Mutations in ATP-sensitive K+ channel genes cause transient neonatal diabetes and permanent diabetes in childhood or adulthood, *Diabetes* 56:1930-1937, 2007.

Hattersley AT, Ashcroft FM: Activating mutations in Kir6.2 and neonatal diabetes: new clinical syndromes, new scientific insights, and new therapy, *Diabetes* 54:2503-2513, 2005.

Hussain K, Aynsley-Green A, Stanley CA: Medications used in the treatment of hypoglycemia due to congenital hyperinsulinism of infancy (HI), *Pediatr Endocrinol Rev* 2:163-167, 2004.

Menon RK, Sperling MA: Carbohydrate metabolism, *Semin Perinatol* 12:157-162, 1988.

Mohnike K, Blankenstein O, Christesen HT, et al: Proposal for a standardized protocol for 18F-DOPA-PET (PET/CT) in congenital hyperinsulinism, *Horm Res* 66:40-42, 2006.

Polak M, Cave H: Neonatal diabetes mellitus: a disease linked to multiple mechanisms, *Orphanet J Rare Dis* 2:12, 2007.

Sperling MA, Menon RK: Hyperinsulinemic hypoglycemia of infancy. Recent insights into ATP-sensitive potassium channels, sulfonylurea receptors, molecular mechanisms, and treatment, *Endocrinol Metab Clin North Am* 28:695-708, 1999.

Sperling MA, Menon RK: Differential diagnosis and management of neonatal hypoglycemia, *Pediatr Clin North Am* 51:703-723, 2004.

Stanley CA, Thornton PS, Finegold DN, Sperling MA: Hypoglycemia in neonates and infants, In Sperling MA, editor: *Pediatric endocrinology*, ed 2, Philadelphia, 2002, Saunders, pp 135-159.

Complete references and supplemental color images used in this text can be found online at www.expertconsult.com

CHAPTER

95

CRANIOFACIAL MALFORMATIONS

Kelly Evans, Anne V. Hing, and Michael Cunningham

The neonatologist is often the first point of contact for a child born with a craniofacial malformation. Abnormalities of the face and head can be very distressing to a new parent, who is immediately wondering, "Is my child going to look, feel, and develop normally?" Having a basic understanding of the relationship between craniofacial abnormalities and feeding, hearing, vision, speech and overall development will help the neonatologist begin to counsel a family. Airway compromise is well described in multiple craniofacial syndromes, and early identification can be lifesaving. Prompt recognition of a constellation of anomalies pointing toward a syndrome or diagnosis will result in better targeted evaluations and therapies for that patient. (See Tables 95-1 and 95-2 for a concise presentation of potential ICU issues that may be encountered with certain craniofacial malformations and syndromes.) This chapter highlights the most relevant craniofacial malformations that a neonatologist will encounter. We describe here the epidemiology, genetics, diagnosis, phenotype and potential ICU issues as well as basic management recommendations to help guide the neonatologist in caring for an infant with craniofacial malformations.

MICROGNATHIA/ROBIN SEQUENCE

EPIDEMIOLOGY

The triad of micrognathia, glossoptosis and airway obstruction, originally described in 1923 by Pierre Robin, is known as Robin Sequence (or Pierre Robin Sequence [PRS]), Online Mendelian Inheritance in Man (OMIM) database classification number 261800. Whether cleft palate is an obligatory feature of PRS is debatable. Approximately one quarter of infants with cleft palate (CP) were found to have Robin sequence in a multi-site, population-based, case-control study (Genisca et al, 2009). The tremendous heterogeneity and lack of uniformly accepted diagnostic criteria for, or definitions of, PRS make it challenging to know the true prevalence. However, estimates of birth prevalence range from 1:8500 to 1:20,000 births (Breugem and Mink van der Molen, 2009).

PHENOTYPE

Robin sequence is an etiologically and phenotypically heterogeneous disorder. Over half of children with PRS have an associated syndrome with Stickler syndrome being the

most common. While there is great variation in severity, PRS is characterized by the following phenotypic features: micrognathia (small and symmetrically receded mandible), glossoptosis (tongue of variable size falls backwards into the postpharyngeal space), and cleft palate (U-shaped more common than V-shaped) (Figure 95-1, *A* and *B*). Caouette-Laberge et al (1994) described cleft palate (U or V-shaped) in 90% of 125 individuals with PRS. Infants with PRS often have airway obstruction, feeding difficulties, and challenges gaining weight, and they may have associated anomalies, including hypotonia and limb reduction defects. Congenital heart defects are present in up to 25% of babies with PRS who die in early infancy (Gorlin et al, 2001b). Patent ductus arteriosus is the most common, followed by atrial septal defects, ventricular septal defects, and coarctation of the aorta. It has been reported that more than 20% of individuals will have developmental delay or cognitive impairment, and overall morbidity and mortality are higher in syndromic PRS or PRS with associated anomalies compared with isolated PRS (Caouette-Laberge et al, 1994).

ICU CONCERNS

In infants with PRS, the tongue is displaced toward the posterior pharyngeal wall, resulting in obstruction at the level of the epiglottis. The tongue can act as a ball valve, leading to inspiratory obstruction. In addition to micrognathia, other mechanisms may contribute to airway obstruction in individuals with PRS, such as pharyngeal hypotonia and airway inflammation from associated gastroesophageal reflux. The principal physiologic sequela of PRS is the inability to effectively feed and/or breathe due to airway obstruction. Patients with PRS may present in the immediate neonatal period with increased inspiratory work of breathing, cyanosis, and apnea. Obstruction is more common in the supine position and can be exacerbated during feeding and in sleep, or any state where there is loss of pharyngeal tone. Chronic obstruction can lead to failure to thrive, carbon dioxide retention, pulmonary hypertension, and eventually right-sided heart failure (cor pulmonale).

Airway obstruction is the main cause of feeding and growth issues in infants with PRS. Feeding problems can also be related to inadequate tongue control or pharyngeal hypotonia and complicated by presence of a cleft palate. Increased energy expenditures due to increased work of breathing may lead to failure to thrive if the infant is not

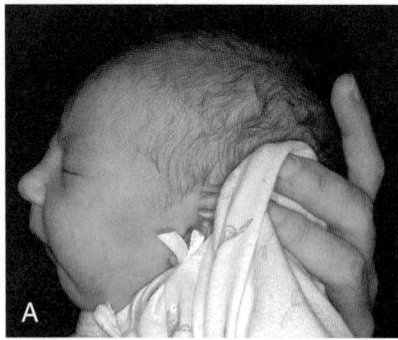 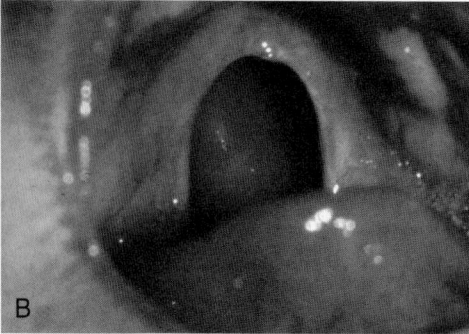 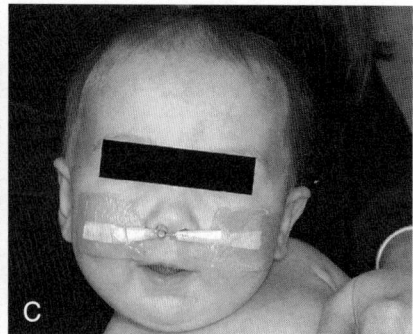

FIGURE 95-1 *(See also Color Plate 38.)* **A,** Infant with Pierre Robin syndrome (PRS) and significant micrognathia. **B,** U-shaped cleft palate. **C,** Infant with PRS and a nasopharyngeal tube in place.

receiving adequate caloric intake. Gastroesophageal reflux is common in PRS, as it is with other infants who have increased work of breathing.

MANAGEMENT

First and foremost, the airway must be addressed. Placement of a nasal trumpet or endotracheal tube may be required in an emergency, and it is important to realize that severe, life-threatening airway obstruction can present in the delivery room. Though uncommon, a prenatal diagnosis of micrognathia allows for involvement of neonatologists and otolaryngologists in the delivery room.

A number of therapeutic maneuvers can be used to stabilize the upper airway in PRS, ranging from positioning to surgery. Placing the baby in the prone or lateral decubitus position will often open up the airway and decrease the degree of obstruction. This may improve airway patency and air exchange, which decreases the work of breathing and may also improve tolerance of oral feeding. When prone positioning fails to provide adequate airway patency, alternative approaches include the use of a nasopharyngeal airway, treatment with tongue-lip adhesion (TLA), and mandibular distraction. Tracheostomy may be necessary to provide a safe and secure airway in some infants. Treatment protocols vary across institutions; however, most providers agree that the majority of neonates with PRS can be managed non-surgically (Schaefer et al, 2004).

A nasopharyngeal (NP) airway provides a temporary way to bypass the infant's airway obstruction (see Figure 95-1, *C*). An endotracheal tube can be modified so that it can be passed through the nares into the hypopharynx above the epiglottis, allowing oxygenation/ventilation by bypassing the obstruction at the base of the tongue (Parhizkan et al, 2010). The NP airway may prevent the need for more invasive procedures and allows the team to address oral skills and feeding (Wagener et al, 2003). In some institutions, the infant is discharged home with an NP airway in place. Children are monitored with oximetry and parents are taught NP airway maintenance (suctioning) and replacement. The NP tube is typically in place for 4 to 6 months or less if symptoms improve or other interventions become necessary.

When airway obstruction is localized to the tongue base and positioning has not improved breathing and feeding, a TLA (attachment of the anterior tongue to the lower lip) may be a temporizing measure to minimize obstruction while allowing for mandibular growth (Schaefer and Gosain, 2003). In some institutions, TLA has been shown to have a high initial success rate for correction of airway obstruction in a neonate. However, long-term follow-up indicates that many infants require secondary interventions to manage their feeding and airway and eventually their orthognathic issues (Denny et al, 2004).

The infant's clinical status, perceived need for long-term respiratory support, and failure of less invasive interventions will determine whether more invasive surgery is indicated (Evans et al, 2011). For some neonates, mandibular distraction osteogenesis may be an alternative to tracheostomy. Endoscopy may help delineate the level of obstruction, and computed tomographic (CT) imaging of the mandibular structures can assist in assessment of jaw anatomy before distraction. Recognition of other airway anomalies or issues, such as laryngotracheomalacia or subglottic stenosis, will also affect decision making regarding airway management. Children with PRS associated with syndromes, skeletal dysplasia, or neurologic conditions may have more than one factor contributing to their airway obstruction such that a tracheostomy may be indicated. Thus, infants with PRS who have airway obstruction unresponsive to positional techniques (side or prone) for whom surgical options are being considered (mandibular distraction versus tracheostomy) should have a comprehensive evaluation of their airway as well as an evaluation for diagnosis of an underlying syndrome and/or associated malformations that might impact respiratory status.

Nutrition can be maintained with a hypercaloric formula and/or fortified breast milk given by side-lying feeding using a cleft feeder, via nasogastric feeding tube, or via gastrostomy tube. Oral feeding can and should be introduced when the airway is stable. Oral stimulation is important to prevent oral aversion. As tone improves, the child gains better control of the tongue, and growth ensues, feeding will become less of a problem. Close observation for any symptoms of gastroesophageal reflux with proactive pharmacologic treatment can minimize airway inflammation.

Given the association with cognitive and motor delay, close monitoring of development and referral to early intervention services, such as a Birth to Three program, are recommended.

STICKLER SYNDROME

More than 50% of infants born with PRS will have an associated syndrome diagnosis, chromosomal abnormality, additional anomalies, or other medical concerns.

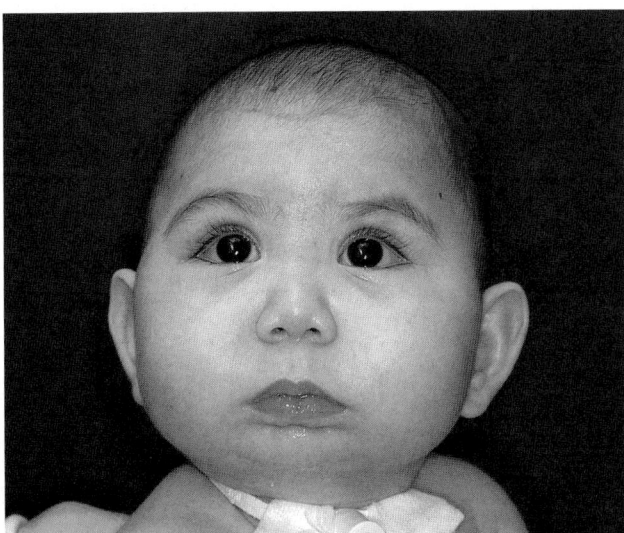

FIGURE 95-2 Infant with Stickler syndrome, showing a flat face, depressed nasal bridge, and epicanthal folds. This infant also has PRS and required tracheostomy.

Therefore, all infants with PRS should be evaluated for associated malformations, chromosomal abnormalities, and syndromic diagnoses and should be considered for genetic testing (Gorlin et al, 2001b). The most common associated syndromes are Stickler syndrome and 22q11.2 deletion syndrome. Thirty percent of individuals with PRS will have Stickler syndrome (Shprintzen, 1988). Stickler syndrome is an autosomal dominant (with variable expressivity) connective tissue disorder with predominantly ophthalmic, orofacial, auditory, and articular manifestations and has been divided into three types (type 1 and 2 have ocular findings, type 3 is nonocular). Type 1 Stickler (OMIM 108300) represents 75% of this syndrome.

Stickler syndrome is characterized by cleft palate, hearing loss, arthropathy, joint hypermobility, reduced height and eye abnormalities including myopia, cataracts, glaucoma and retinal detachment. The myopia of Stickler syndrome is usually congenital, nonprogressive, and of high degree. Facial features include flat midface with depressed nasal bridge, short nose, anteverted nares, and micrognathia, telecanthus, and epicanthal folds (profile appears scooped out; Figure 95-2). Sensorineural hearing loss is more common in type 2 Stickler syndrome.

The diagnosis of Stickler syndrome should be considered in any neonate with PRS or a U-shaped cleft, especially when associated with myopia or hearing loss. Spondyloepiphyseal dysplasia is not usually apparent in the newborn period. Mutations affecting one of four genes (COL2A1, COL9A1, COL11A1, and COL11A2) have been associated with Stickler syndrome, and clinical molecular testing by sequence analysis is available for all three types. The mutation detection rate for type 1 and 2 (COL2A1 and COL11A1 respectively) is approximately 90% (Robin et al, 2009). The diagnosis should also be considered in any newborn with a family history of PRS or Stickler syndrome.

In addition to appropriate management of feeding, breathing and growth (as described earlier in PRS), management of Stickler syndrome includes active detection of myopia because of the risk of retinal detachment and

blindness, which are preventable. An initial ophthalmology evaluation is recommended for all children with PRS between 6 and 12 months of age or at the time of a definitive molecular diagnosis of Stickler syndrome, and then routine surveillance thereafter.

OROFACIAL CLEFTING

EPIDEMIOLOGY

Orofacial clefts of the primary and secondary palate are among the most common congenital anomalies. Classified as either cleft lip with or without cleft palate (CL±P) or cleft palate only (CPO), these two phenotypes are thought to be distinct in etiology. One case of orofacial cleft occurs in approximately every 500 to 550 births, and on an average day in the United States, 20 infants are born with an orofacial cleft (Tolarova and Cervenka, 1998). Cleft lip and palate (CLP) is the most common type of orofacial clefting, followed by cleft lip (CL), then CPO, and less prevalent are atypical clefts (macrostomia or lateral cleft, oblique and midline clefts). Unilateral CL±P is more common than bilateral involvement (Genisca et al, 2009). Clefting of the uvula can be a normal variant, found in 1 of 80 white births and, but can also be a sign of an associated submucous cleft palate, which can have the same functional impact as an overt CP (Gorlin et al, 2001b).

The causes of most orofacial clefts are unknown and are nonsyndromic (isolated) in 75% of infants with CL±P and approximately 50% of those with CPO (Tolarova and Cervenka, 1998). Neonates with orofacial clefting who are born prematurely or have low birthweight may have a higher incidence of associated congenital malformations (Milerad et al, 1997). Racial and ethnic variation in the prevalence of clefts has been described, with the highest prevalence of CL±P found in Native Americans, followed by whites and Hispanics, and the lowest overall prevalence of CL±P demonstrated in African Americans (Croen et al, 1998). The etiology of nonsyndromic clefts is complex and multifactorial, likely resulting from interaction between environmental and genetic factors. Recognition of contributing genetic factors such as the Van der Woude gene (IRF6) is increasing, and the impact of folate supplementation as an environmental modulator is under investigation. Although many candidate genes have been described, there is no routinely recommended genetic testing for a child with isolated CL±P in the absence of a family history. Recurrence risk information for the parents of a child with CL±P or for the affected individual is dependent either on the specific syndrome/genetic diagnosis or on empiric risks for those with nonsyndromic clefting. For a family with just one child affected with CL±P, the recurrence risk is 2% to 5% for a subsequent child, and increasing to 10% to 15% if there are other family members with clefts. The recurrence risk is slightly less if the child has CPO (Harper, 2004).

ANATOMY

The embryologic development of the primary palate begins very early in gestation, and the upper lip and primary palate have usually fused by the 7th week of gestation. A failure of fusion of the medial and lateral nasal processes with

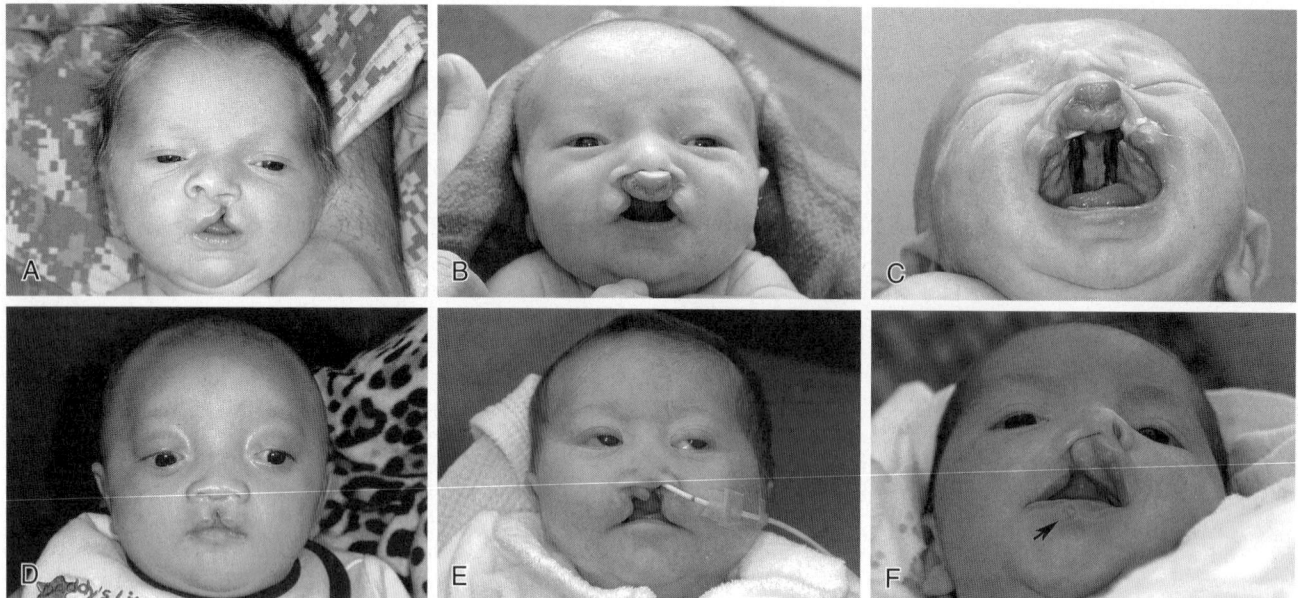

FIGURE 95-3 **A,** Infant with a unilateral incomplete cleft lip. **B** and **C,** Infant with bilateral complete cleft lip and palate. **D,** Infant with midline cleft and hypertelorism. He also has a frontonasal encephalocele. **E,** Infant with premaxillary agenesis and holoprosencephaly. **F,** Infant with Van der Woude syndrome with unilateral complete cleft lip and a lip pit (*arrow*).

maxillary process produces cleft lip with or without cleft palate. Clefts can affect the primary palate (lip, alveolus, or anterior portion of the hard palate that extends to the incisive foramen) and secondary palate (posterior hard palate and soft palate). Clefts of the primary and secondary palate can be unilateral or bilateral and complete or incomplete. A complete cleft of the primary palate leaves no residual tissue between the alar base and the lip, whereas an incomplete cleft does not extend through the floor of the nose (Figure 95-3, *A* to *C*, *F*).

PHENOTYPE

The cleft of the primary and secondary palate will affect facial growth, causing reduced facial height, flat facial profile, midfacial retrusion, increased nasopharyngeal width, and shorter mandible (see Figure 95-3, *A–C*). Children with cleft palate are at increased risk for eustachian tube dysfunction, recurrent otitis media, and acquired hearing loss, as well as speech issues later in childhood. Associated dental findings include hypodontia and, less commonly, natal teeth. Feeding difficulties, nasal regurgitation of feeds, and difficulty gaining weight may occur in infants with a cleft palate (submucous and overt clefts of the palate).

Lateral facial clefting or macrostomia is associated with syndromes, including craniofacial microsomia and Treacher Collins syndrome. Amniotic rupture sequence can be associated with oblique facial clefts and may be associated with underlying central nervous system (CNS) malformations and transverse limb anomalies.

A true median cleft of the upper lip is the rarest type of facial clefting (see Figure 95-3, *D*). Midline clefting can be associated with other congenital defects as can be seen in orofaciodigital syndrome and frontonasal dysplasia. Some midline clefts are not true clefts, but actually represent hypoplasia or agenesis of the primary palate or premaxillary agenesis, which can be associated with holoprosencephaly

(HPE) sequence (see Figure 95-3, *E*). Infants with a median cleft and HPE often have a depressed nasal tip and a short columella and appear hypoteloric (compared to frontonasal dysplasia or frontonasal encephalocele, where midline clefting may be present, but the infant has a broad nasal tip and/or columella and hypertelorism).

Orofacial clefting is rarely associated with clefting of the airway structures, such as cleft larynx or extension of clefting into the trachea. X-linked Opitz G/BBB syndrome (OMIM 145410) is a multiple congenital anomaly syndrome characterized by facial anomalies (100% will be hyperteloric and 50% will have CL±P), genitourinary abnormalities (90% will have hypospadias) and laryngotracheoesophageal (LTE) defects (present in 70%) (Meroni, 2007). Pallister-Hall syndrome (PHS; OMIM 146510) is characterized by a constellation of findings that include hypothalamic hamartoma (resulting in seizures and pituitary dysfunction), polydactyly, airway clefting, and other anomalies (genitourinary, renal, pulmonary, and imperforate anus). Bifid epiglottis is the most common airway manifestation in PHS, although LTE clefts have been reported. LTE defects may vary from LTE dysmotility in mild forms to laryngeal or tracheoesophageal clefts in more severe forms. Clefting of the larynx may result in stridor, a hoarse cry, respiratory distress, swallowing dysfunction, feeding difficulties, regurgitation, and aspiration.

ICU CONCERNS

The majority of infants with CL±P do not require ICU care. Thus, an infant with an apparently isolated cleft who develops significant respiratory or electrolyte abnormalities requiring ICU care should be considered syndromic until proven otherwise. In these infants, a genetics consultation should be considered.

The newborn with a midline cleft or premaxillary agenesis is at risk of serious underlying CNS anomalies, including HPE. In the presence of HPE, detection of associated medical issues is important. Endocrine abnormalities can arise because the midline malformation affects the development of the hypothalamus and the pituitary gland. Clinical manifestations can include growth hormone deficiency, adrenal hypoplasia, hypogonadism, diabetes insipidus, and thyroid deficiency. Neurologic manifestations that warrant close attention include seizures, hypotonia, spasticity, autonomic dysfunction and developmental delays.

With an LTE cleft, there is longitudinal communication between the airway and the esophagus, allowing for tracheal aspiration of oral contents, including saliva and feeds. LTE defects may result in choking or coughing with feeds, aspiration, hypoxia, recurrent pneumonias, and eventually severe respiratory compromise if unrecognized. An infant boy with hypertelorism, hypospadias, orofacial clefting, and symptoms of airway obstruction or aspiration should be evaluated for Opitz syndrome. Infants with PHS may also have respiratory distress due to airway clefting, as well as other potentially life-threatening clinical manifestations such as seizures and severe panhypopituitarism. Genetic evaluation and consideration of molecular testing for Opitz syndrome and PHS can be coordinated through a geneticist.

MANAGEMENT

The specifics of management of orofacial clefting are center specific. Because of the potential impact of the orofacial cleft on breathing, eating, hearing, speech, facial growth, and dental health, it is recommended that infants and children with clefts be referred to a multidisciplinary care team for long-term management. In remote areas, the nearest cleft team may be found through the Cleft Palate Foundation website. Box 95-1 outlines one example of the multidisciplinary team of providers that might contribute to the care of a child born with a craniofacial malformation. Overview of recommended team care for cleft patients can be found at the American Cleft Palate-Craniofacial Association website (2009; Team CLPC, 2006).

On the initial assessment, the provider should assess the cleft and examine the infant for dysmorphic features and other anomalies. Hearing should be evaluated by evoked otoacoustic emissions, or by brainstem auditory evoked response if the newborn does not pass the initial hearing screen. A neonate with a complete cleft lip should be evaluated by a craniofacial or cleft team in the first 2 weeks of life, and some centers offer taping or presurgical molding (nasoalveolar molding) that can be initiated in this time period.

Many mothers will be able to breastfeed an infant born with an isolated cleft lip. Breastfeeding a baby with cleft palate (with or without cleft lip) will prove extremely challenging because the open palate will not generate the negative pressure needed for sucking. Thus, infants with cleft palate ± cleft lip should be offered expressed breast milk or infant formula using a specialized cleft feeder. There are a variety of cleft nipples/bottles that have been devised to allow for oral feeding including the cleft palate nurser (squeeze bottle), Haberman feeder, and Pigeon bottle (www.cleftline.org/parents/feeding_your_baby). Infants with cleft palate tend to swallow a lot of air during feedings. Make sure the child is feeding in an upright position, as gravity will help prevent nasal regurgitation. If the child is still having difficulty feeding, consult a feeding specialist. Adequate weight gain is important, because these children will undergo multiple surgeries in the 1st year of life. Newborns with clefts are considered nutritionally high risk, and a dietitian should be consulted to help determine caloric needs and to closely monitor growth.

In general, surgical closure of the lip and nasal deformity is done within the first 3 to 6 months of life. Palatoplasty typically occurs between 9 and 12 months of age to optimize speech and language development.

If there are concerns about airway clefting or anomalies of the larynx or trachea, a chest x-ray should be obtained and the airway evaluated, in addition to appropriate evaluation of associated anomalies. Microlaryngoscopy under general anesthesia remains the gold standard in the diagnosis of a laryngeal cleft (Rahbar et al, 2006). Given the risk for gastrointestinal manifestations such as gastroesophageal reflux, dysmotility, and risk for aspiration, antireflux precautions should be initiated in infants with suspected or confirmed LTE defects. Early diagnosis and proper repair of the laryngeal cleft are essential to prevent injury to the lungs. Significant LTE defects will need to be managed surgically, and tracheostomy may be necessary initially to ensure an adequate airway.

In the presence of a midline cleft, it is important to evaluate for underlying CNS malformations such as HPE. In any child with a midline cleft or facial features consistent with premaxillary agenesis/hypoplasia, CNS imaging with a CT scan is recommended. Consultation with a geneticist or genetic counselor may provide insight into the genetics, molecular testing options, and recurrence risk of HPE. Treatment of HPE is supportive and based on symptoms. The outcome depends on the severity of HPE and the associated medical and neurologic manifestations.

SYNDROMES ASSOCIATED WITH CLEFT LIP AND/OR PALATE

It is estimated that there are more than 400 syndromes associated with orofacial clefts (Gorlin et al, 2001b). The frequency with which associated malformations are encountered with CL±P is approximately 25% (Genisca et al, 2009). In approaching diagnosis of a syndrome, it is important to categorize the type of cleft (lip with or without palate, U-shaped or V-shaped cleft palate, or more atypical orofacial cleft) and to look for any other malformations. Table 95-1 describes the syndromes most commonly associated with clefting and the key features,

TABLE 95-1   Craniofacial Syndromes Commonly Associated With Cleft Lip or Palate

Syndrome	Phenotype	ICU issues	OMIM#
Robin sequence*	Micrognathia, glossoptosis, cleft palate, airway obstruction	Airway obstruction, feeding difficulties	261800
Stickler syndrome*	Cleft palate, micrognathia, glossoptosis, severe myopia, risk of retinal detachment and blindness, midfacial hypoplasia, hearing impairment, arthropathy, pectus, short fourth and fifth metacarpals	Airway obstruction, feeding difficulties	180300; 604841; 184840; 609508
Chromosome 22q11.2 deletion syndrome (velocardiofacial syndrome, VCFS, DiGeorge syndrome) *	Robin sequence, cleft palate, small mouth, myopathic facies, retrognathia, prominent nose with squared-off nasal tip, hypoplastic nasal alae, short stature, slender tapering digits	Cardiac anomalies, airway obstruction	192430
Opitz oculogenitallaryngeal syndrome (Opitz BBB/G syndrome) *	Hypertelorism, telecanthus, cleft lip and/or palate, dysphagia, esophageal dysmotility, laryngotracheoesophageal cleft (aspiration), hypospadias, bifid scrotum, cryptorchidism, agenesis of the corpus callosum, congenital heart disease, mental retardation	Laryngotracheoesophageal clefting (stridor, feeding difficulties, choking, aspiration)	145410
Pallister-Hall syndrome*	Cleft palate, flat nasal bridge, short nose, multiple buccal frenula, microglossia, micrognathia, malformed ears, hypothalamic hamartoblastoma, hypopituitarism, postaxial polydactyly with short arms, imperforate anus, GU anomalies, IUGR	Laryngotracheoesophageal clefting (stridor, feeding difficulties, choking, aspiration), panhypopituitarism	146510
IRF6-related disorders (including Van der Woude and Popliteal pterygium syndrome)	CL±P, CPO, lower lip pits or cysts, ankyloglossia; PPS will also have popliteal pterygia, bifid scrotum, cryptorchidism, finger and/or toe syndactyly, abnormalities of the skin around the nails, syngnathia and ankyloblepharon	Not anticipated	119300; 119500; 607199
CHARGE syndrome*	*C*oloboma of the eye, *H*eart malformations, choanal *A*tresia, growth *R*etardation, *G*enital anomalies, *E*ar abnormalities and/or deafness, facial palsy, cleft palate, dysphagia	Airway obstruction in bilateral choanal atresia, cardiac anomalies, feeding difficulties, aspiration	214800
Smith-Lemli-Opitz syndrome*	Cleft palate, micrognathia, short nose, ptosis, high square forehead, microcephaly, hypospadias, cryptorchidism, VSD, TOF, hypotonia, mental retardation, postaxial polydactyly, 2- to 3-toe syndactyly, defect in cholesterol biosynthesis	Cardiac anomalies, airway hypotonia/obstruction	270400
Ectrodactyly ectodermal dysplasia and clefting syndrome (EEC1, EEC2)	Cleft lip and/or palate, split-hand/split-foot, ectodermal dysplasia (sparse hair, dysplastic nails, hypohydrosis, hypodontia), genitourinary anomalies	Not anticipated	129900; 602077; 603273
Ankyloblepharon ectodermal dysplasia and clefting syndrome (AEC)	CL±P, CPO, intraoral alveolar bands, maxillary hypoplasia, ankyloblepharon (eyelid fusion), ectodermal dysplasia (sparse hair, dysplastic nails, hypohydrosis, anodontia)	Not anticipated	106260
Orofacialdigital syndrome	Median cleft of upper lip, cleft palate, accessory oral frenula, lobulated tongue with hamartomas, broad nasal root, small nostrils, syndactyly, brachydactyly, postaxial polydactyly, polycystic renal disease, agenesis of the corpus callosum	Not anticipated	311200
Kabuki syndrome*	Cleft palate, arched eyebrow, long palpebral fissures, eversion of lateral third of lower eyelid, brachydactyly, short fifth metacarpal, cardiac anomalies, postnatal growth deficiency/dwarfism, mental retardation	Cardiac anomalies	147920
Fryns syndrome*	Cleft lip ± palate, micrognathia, coarse facies, diaphragmatic hernia, distal limb hypoplasia, malformations of the cardiovascular, gastrointestinal, genitourinary and central nervous systems	Congenital diaphragmatic hernia, pulmonary hypoplasia; cardiac anomalies	229850
Miller syndrome*	Cleft palate (more than cleft lip), malar and mandibular hypoplasia, downslanting palpebral fissures, lower eyelid coloboma, microtia/atresia, conductive hearing loss, postaxial limb deficiency, absent fifth digit	Airway obstruction	263750

TABLE 95-1 Craniofacial Syndromes Commonly Associated With Cleft Lip and/or Palate—cont'd

Syndrome	Phenotype	ICU issues	OMIM#
Treacher Collins syndrome (mandibulofacial dysostosis)*	Cleft palate, malar and mandibular hypoplasia, downslanting palpebral fissures, lower eyelid coloboma (missing medial lower lid lashes), microtia/atresia, conductive hearing loss	Airway obstruction	154500
Aarskog syndrome (faciodig-italgenital syndrome)	Hypertelorism, widow's peak, ptosis, down slant-ing palpebral fissures, strabismus, maxillary hypoplasia, broad nasal bridge with anteverted nostrils, occasional cleft lip and/or palate, floppy ears, brachydactyly, clinodactyly, joint laxity, shawl scrotum	Not anticipated	100050
Wolf-Hirschhorn syndrome (4p deletion syndrome)*	Cleft lip and palate, coloboma, hypertelorism, growth deficiency, microcephaly, mental retar-dation, cardiac septal defects	Congenital diaphragmatic hernia, cardiac anomalies, seizures, airway hypotonia/obstruction	194190
Amnion rupture sequence*	Cleft lip and palate, oblique facial clefts, focal areas of scalp aplasia, constriction bands with terminal limb amputations and syndactylies, occasional anencephaly, encephalocele, and ectopia cordis	Encephalocele, oropharyngeal/airway deformation	217100

*Potential ICU issues.

potential ICU issues, and OMIM database classification. The Online Mendelian Inheritance in Man (OMIM) database at the National Library of Medicine is a com-prehensive collection of more than 12,000 human genes and genetic phenotypes. A referral to a clinical geneticist is recommended when an underlying diagnosis is suspected but not established.

Chromosome 22q11.2 Deletion Syndrome
Epidemiology and Genetics

22q11.2 deletion syndrome (22q11.2DS) is a genetic con-dition with an estimated prevalence of one in 4,000 births in which affected individuals are missing a region (typically 3 megabases) on one copy of chromosome 22 (Devriendt et al, 1998). Before the availability of genetic testing for this condition, individuals with clinical features of 22q11.2DS were classified under a range of other clini-cal syndromes, such as DiGeorge syndrome, velocardiofa-cial syndrome (VCFS), and Shprintzen syndrome, among others (McDonald-McGinn et al, 2005). Subsequently, a subset of children with overlapping features in these con-ditions (such as congenital heart disease and cleft palate) was also noted to share a deletion on chromosome 22q. Investigators later discovered that the majority of children clinically diagnosed with either DiGeorge or VCFS share the deletion on one copy of chromosome 22 (Carlson et al, 1997; Kerstjens-Frederikse et al, 1999; Shaikh et al, 2000; Robin and Shprintzen, 2005). It has been estimated that more than 90% of individuals with "classic" features of the 22q11.2DS have a detectable 22q deletion (McDonald-McGinn et al, 2005). Clinical testing can be performed via fluorescent in situ hybridization using DNA probes. In addition, many of the clinical comparative genome hybridization platforms are designed to detect deletions in this region. 22q11.2 deletion syndrome is associated with more than 180 clinical features, and phenotypic variation is a hallmark of this genetic condition (Robin and Shprint-zen, 2005).

Phenotype

Neonates with 22q11.2DS present in various ways. Some infants with this condition are diagnosed prenatally. Testing may occur as part of the evaluation for fetuses with congen-ital heart disease, or due to parental history of 22q11.2DS. The clinical indications for genetic testing for this condi-tion in neonates frequently include congenital heart mal-formations (particularly conotruncal anomalies), seizures secondary to hypocalcemia, dysphagia, cleft palate, and/or respiratory distress secondary to upper airway obstruction. In this section, we focus on the evaluation of infants with craniofacial characteristics suggestive of 22q11.2DS.

More than 25 craniofacial features have been observed in individuals with 22q11.2DS (Robin and Shprintzen, 2005); however, many of these are subtle and may not be apparent in the newborn period. Common features iden-tified on the newborn physical exam include cleft palate, small, overfolded helices, and tapered fingers. Other clues to the diagnosis include dysphagia and/or nasal regurgita-tion (even in the absence of an overt cleft palate), congeni-tal heart disease (most commonly conotruncal anomalies), and hypocalcemia (with or without seizures).

An estimated 8% of infants with cleft palate have 22q11.2DS (Gorlin et al, 2001c). For this reason, recom-mendations vary regarding routine testing of infants with isolated cleft palate. Most agree, however, that molecu-lar testing is indicated for children with a cleft palate in combination with any of the other features that can be observed in 22q11.2DS. As high as 13% of children with PRS have been reported to have 22q11.2DS (Shprint-zen, 1988). Thus, testing for 22q11.2 deletion should be considered for infants with PRS and other features of 22q11.2DS.

Evaluation and Management

Infants for whom there is a high clinical suspicion and those testing positive for this deletion should receive genetic counseling in addition to studies to identify associated health concerns. These screening evaluations

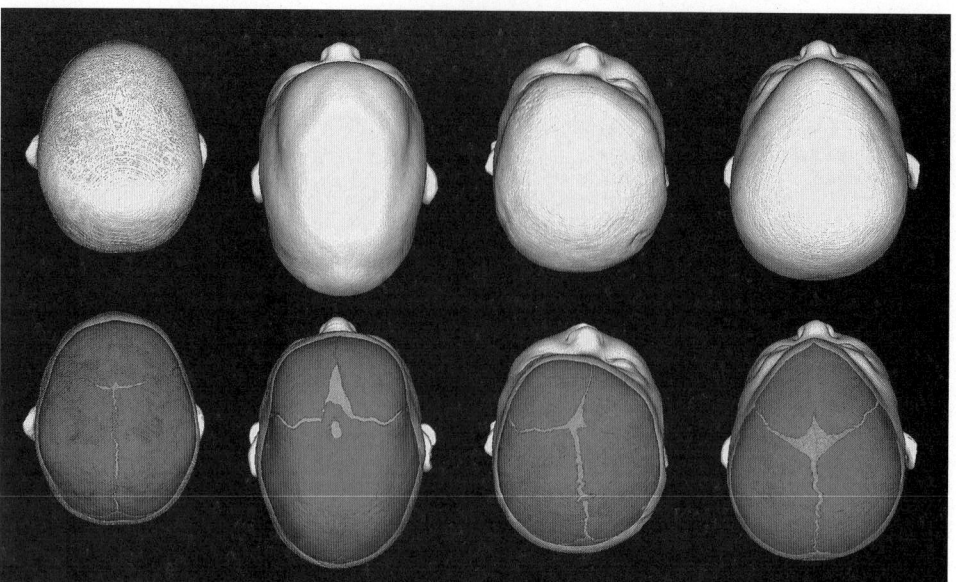

FIGURE 95-4 Representation of head shapes in single suture synostosis. *Left to right:* normal head shape, sagittal synostosis, coronal synostosis, and metopic synostosis.

include a total lymphocyte count, hematocrit, and platelet count and total and ionized calcium levels to screen for hypocalcemia. Additional studies include echocardiogram to evaluate for congenital heart malformations and renal ultrasound. Newborns should have a palatal exam to evaluate for overt or submucous clefting, as well as a diagnostic audiogram. Infants with evidence of dysphagia (even in the absence of a palatal cleft) would likely benefit from an evaluation by a feeding specialist to determine if a cleft bottle would be helpful. Additional recommendations for screening evaluations and management can be found at the GeneTests website (McDonald-McGinn et al, 2005).

CRANIOSYNOSTOSIS

DEFINITIONS/EPIDEMIOLOGY

Craniosynostosis refers to the premature fusion of one or more cranial sutures (metopic, sagittal, right or left coronal, or right or left lambdoid) that normally separate the bony plates of the cranium. Birth prevalence of all craniosynostoses is estimated to be 300 to 400 of every 1 million live births (Cohen, 2000a). In normal infants, open sutures allow the cranium to expand as the brain grows, producing the normal head shape. If one or more sutures fuse prematurely, there is restricted growth perpendicular to the fused sutures and compensatory growth in the patent sutures, producing abnormal head shape. Craniosynostosis is a heterogeneous disorder with significant health consequences that range from an abnormal head shape to secondary visual and intellectual impairments. Known causes of primary craniosynostosis include monogenic and chromosomal abnormalities as well as environmental factors. Nonsyndromic single suture craniosynostosis accounts for 85% of patients. Syndromic craniosynostosis may involve single or multiple fused sutures and additional anomalies (such as limb, cardiac, CNS, and tracheal malformations) or developmental delay. Multiple suture involvement is

usually considered syndromic even when it does not fit a classic pattern of anomalies. Advances in molecular genetics are permitting the identification of defective genes and their pathways in describing these congenital anomalies. The genetic etiology of syndromic craniosynostosis in humans is only partially understood. However, for a subset, identification of the primary genetic cause and contributing factors is possible using clinically available molecular tests (targeted sequencing of FGFR1, FGFR2, FGFR3, TWIST1, MSX2, and EFNB1 genes noted later).

SINGLE SUTURE SYNOSTOSIS

Sagittal synostosis is the most common single suture synostosis (50% to 60%) with a prevalence of 1 in 4200 births (Cohen, 2000a). Known risk factors include male gender, intrauterine head constraint, twin gestation, and maternal smoking. Although uncommon, the most frequently encountered associated anomalies include congenital heart defects and genitourinary tract malformations. Syndromes with synostosis involving only the sagittal suture are rare. Premature union of the sagittal sutures hinders normal calvarial expansion, leading to scaphocephaly, an elongated, narrow calvaria, decreased bitemporal diameter, and frontal and occipital bossing (Figure 95-4). Premature fusion of the suture before birth leads to abnormal head shape in the newborn period. A breech-positioned neonate can have scaphocephaly or dolichocephaly that may be concerning for sagittal synostosis. However, in sagittal synostosis, frontal bossing progresses, whereas the head shape in a breech infant will normalize over time. There is a concern that children with isolated sagittal synostosis are at risk for elevations in intracranial pressure (ICP), local brain injury, and later developmental delays, although this is not completely understood (Kapp-Simon et al, 2007).

Coronal synostosis is the second most common single suture synostosis (20% to 30%) with a prevalence of one in 10,000 births (Cohen, 2000a). The skull is notable for a flat supraorbital rim and orbit that appears lower on the

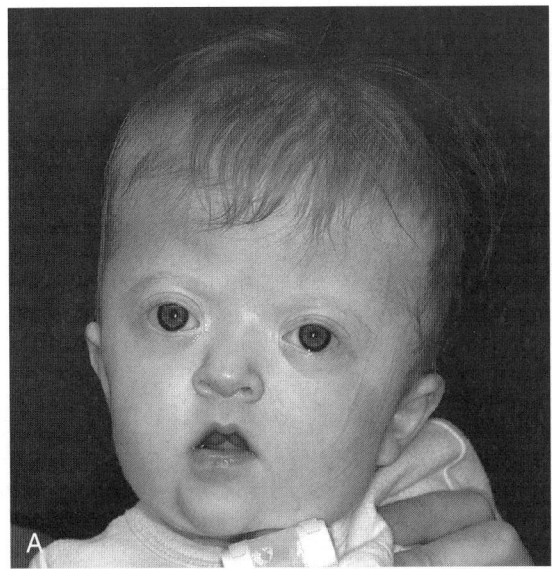
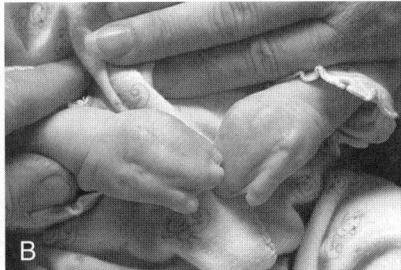
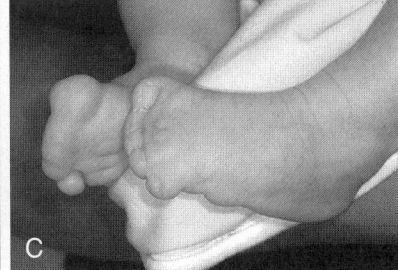

FIGURE 95-5 A, Infant with Apert syndrome, a high and full forehead, proptosis and exotropia, midface hypoplasia, and a trapezoid-shaped mouth. **B** and **C,** Hands and feet in Apert syndrome. Note the syndactyly symmetrically affecting hands and feet. All five digits may be webbed, or a single toe, finger, or thumb may be free.

affected side with a frontal bulge on the contralateral side (see Figure 95-4). The face appears to twist away from the coronal fusion. Genetic syndromes are more frequently seen in individuals with coronal synostosis, including Saethre-Chotzen syndrome, Muenke syndrome, and craniofrontonasal dysplasia. All children with coronal synostosis should be offered genetic consultation and/or genetic testing to include FGFR2, FGFR3, TWIST, and EFNB1 based on clinical examination.

Metopic synostosis (15% to 20% of single suture craniosynostosis) has a prevalence of 1 in 15,000 births (Cohen, 2000a), although recent reports suggest that metopic synostosis may be as common as coronal synostosis (van der Meulen et al, 2009). Risk factors include male gender, twin gestation, and in utero exposure to valproate. Syndromes, associated anomalies, and chromosomal abnormalities occur in approximately one fourth of individuals with metopic synostosis (Azimi et al, 2003; Lajeunie et al, 1998). Premature fusion of the metopic suture results in a triangular head shape, or trigonocephaly, which features a midline forehead ridge, frontotemporal narrowing, hypotelorism, and an increased biparietal diameter (see Figure 95-4). Isolated metopic ridging is common in infancy and is not necessarily associated with metopic synostosis.

Lambdoid synostosis (3% of single suture craniosynostosis) is the least common. It is characterized by flattening of the ipsilateral occiput, posterior-inferior displacement of the ear, and bulge of the mastoid process on the fused side and an asymmetric and tilted skull base.

MULTIPLE SUTURE SYNOSTOSIS

Multiple suture (or multisuture) synostosis describes patients who have two or more fused sutures. Although children with multisuture synostosis are more likely to have a known syndromic form of craniosynostosis such as Apert's or Crouzon's syndrome, some have chromosome aberrations or patterns of craniosynostosis with birth defects and/or developmental delay not previously described. Here we briefly discuss select major syndromes with craniosynostosis that may have medical issues in the newborn period. Please refer to Table 95-2 for description of key phenotypic features and potential airway compromise.

Apert syndrome (OMIM 101200) was initially described as acrocephaly with four-limb syndactyly. It accounts for 4.5% of all craniosynostosis (Gorlin et al, 2001d) (Figure 95-5, *A* to *C*). Apert syndrome is an autosomal dominant condition associated with advanced paternal age. Neurocognitive outcomes vary, but a moderate to severe degree of cognitive impairment is most common. Four mutations in fibroblast growth factor receptor 2 (FGFR2) causing Apert syndrome have been identified.

Crouzon syndrome (OMIM 123500) is an autosomal dominant condition that demonstrates wide phenotypic variability. Shallow orbits (or proptosis) are an important diagnostic feature, although this feature may be more subtle in the newborn (Figure 95-6, *A* and *B*). Significant abnormalities involving the CNS include presence of a Chiari 1 malformation, progressive hydrocephalus, chronic cerebellar herniation, and intracranial hypertension. Compared with Apert syndrome, Crouzon syndrome is associated with more extensive suture involvement, smaller cranial volume, and more severe intracranial constraint. Like Apert's syndrome, Crouzon is caused by mutations in FGFR2. A less common form of Crouzon with acanthosis nigricans skin findings developing in the first 2 years of life is caused by a transmembrane mutation in FGFR3 (OMIM 612247).

Pfeiffer syndrome (OMIM 101600) is a hereditary craniosynostosis that shares significant overlap, both phenotypically and genetically, with Crouzon syndrome. Pfeiffer syndrome is an autosomal dominant inherited disorder that associates craniosynostosis, proptosis, broad and deviated thumbs and big toes, and partial syndactyly of the hands and feet (Figure 95-7, *A* to *C*). Mutations in FGFR1 and FGFR2 cause Pfeiffer syndrome. Type 1 (i.e., classic) Pfeiffer syndrome involves mild manifestations including brachycephaly, midface hypoplasia, and digital malformations. Type

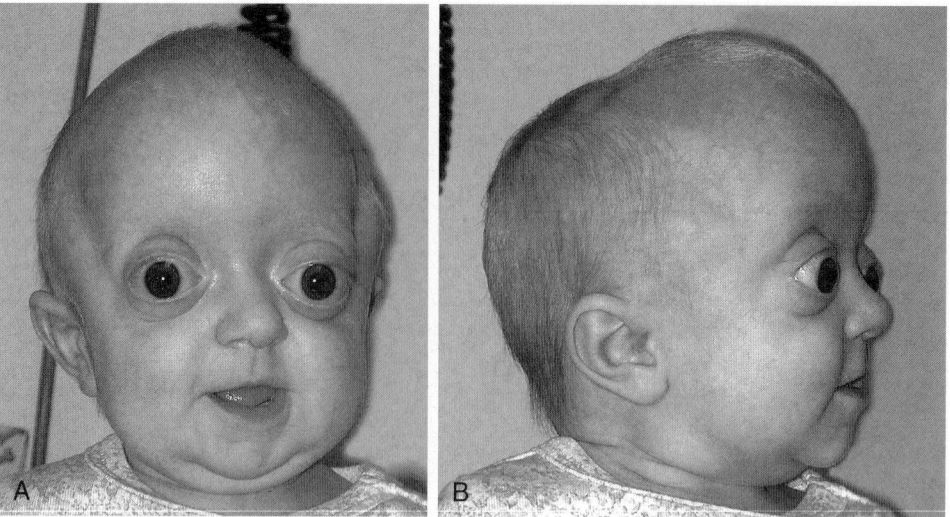

FIGURE 95-6 A, Infant with Crouzon syndrome with brachycephaly. **B,** Proptosis is seen in the lateral view.

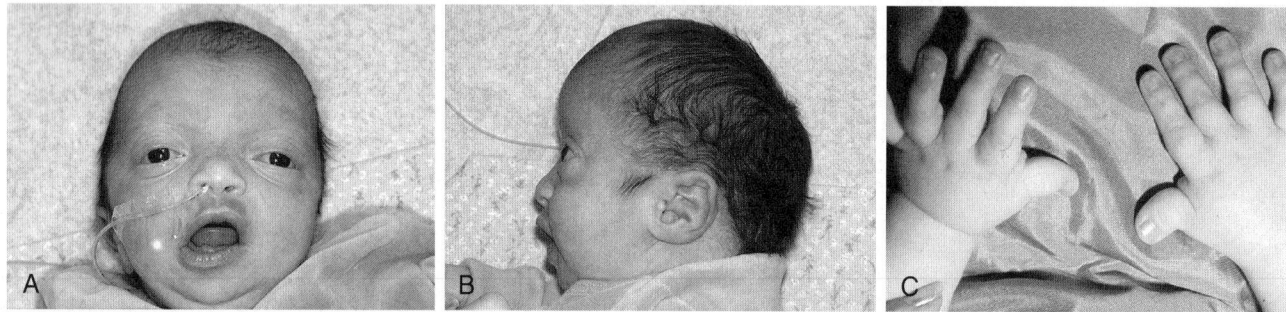

FIGURE 95-7 A and **B,** Infant with Pfeiffer syndrome, brachycephaly, a high forehead, midface hypoplasia, proptosis and ocular hypertelorism. **C,** An older child with Pfeiffer syndrome and the typical broad thumbs with radial deviation.

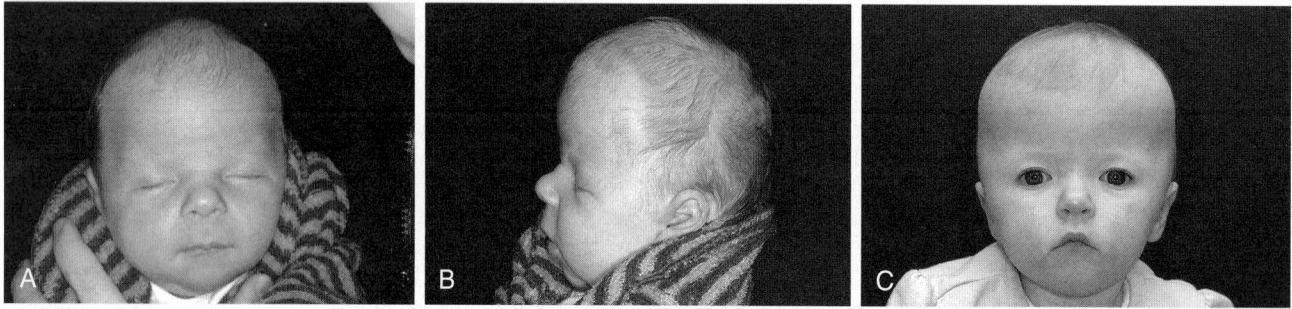

FIGURE 95-8 A and **B,** Infant with Muenke syndrome, acrobrachycephaly due to bicoronal synostosis, absence of proptosis. **C,** Sibling of this infant also affected by Muenke syndrome; note the downslanting palpebral fissures.

2 consists of cloverleaf skull, extreme proptosis, digital malformations, elbow ankylosis, developmental delay, and neurological complications. Type 3 is similar to type 2 but without a cloverleaf skull. There is some debate regarding our classification of syndromes by phenotype when molecular pathogenesis is understood (Cunningham et al, 2007).

Muenke syndrome (OMIM 602849) is a relatively recently described autosomal dominant syndrome caused by a single P250R mutation in the FGFR3 gene. Like Apert syndrome, Muenke syndrome is associated with advanced paternal age. Individuals with Muenke syndrome have coronal (unilateral or bilateral) craniosynostosis or macrocephaly and variable degrees of proptosis, without significant midface hypoplasia (Figure 95-8, *A* to *C*).

Saethre-Chotzen syndrome (SCS, OMIM 101400) is caused by a mutation in the TWIST gene on chromosome 7. The inheritance is autosomal dominant, and many children diagnosed with SCS will have an affected parent. In addition to craniosynostosis, affected individuals commonly have a low frontal hairline, ptosis, 2,3 syndactyly of the fingers, and duplicated halluces. Although learning difficulties may be noted, mental retardation is not typical of SCS. Children with deletions rather than point mutations often demonstrate cognitive impairment.

TABLE 95-2 Craniosynostosis Syndromes and Potential Airway Compromise

Syndrome	Key Features	Tracheal Abnormalities	Midface Hypoplasia	OMIM#
Apert syndrome*	Craniosynostosis (coronal > lambdoid > sagittal), acrobrachycephaly (steep, wide forehead and flat occiput), proptosis, hypertelorism, exotropia, trapezoid-shaped mouth, prognathism, invariable symmetric syndactyly of hands and feet, radiohumeral fusion, cognitive impairment, narrow palate with lateral palatal swellings, widely patent sagittal suture connecting anterior and posterior fontanels	Tracheoesophageal fistula, tracheal cartilaginous sleeve less common	Significant maxillary hypoplasia, obstructive sleep apnea syndrome	101200
Crouzon syndrome*	Craniosynostosis (coronal > lambdoid > sagittal), brachycephaly, prognathism, exophthalmos, papilledema, hypermetropia, divergent strabismus, atresia of auditory canals, Chiari 1 malformation and hydrocephalus	Solid cartilaginous trachea or tracheal cartilaginous sleeve	Significant maxillary hypoplasia, obstructive sleep apnea syndrome	123500
Pfeiffer syndrome types I, II, III*	Craniosynostosis (coronal>sagittal>lambdoid), brachycephaly, hypertelorism, proptosis, broad 1st digits with radial deviation, variable syndactyly, cloverleaf skull	Solid cartilaginous trachea or tracheal cartilaginous sleeve	Significant maxillary hypoplasia, obstructive sleep apnea syndrome	101600
Muenke syndrome	Unilateral or bilateral coronal craniosynostosis, brachydactyly, downslanting palpebral fissures, thimble-like middle phalanges, coned epiphysis, carpal and tarsal fusions, sensorineural hearing loss, Klippel-Feil anomaly		Mild maxillary hypoplasia, no airway compromise anticipated	602849
Saethre-Chotzen syndrome*	Unilateral or bilateral coronal craniosynostosis, acrocephaly, brachycephaly, low frontal hairline, hypertelorism, facial asymmetry, ptosis, characteristic ear (small pinna with a prominent crus), 5th finger clinodactyly, partial 2-3 syndactyly of the fingers, duplicated halluces		Maxillary hypoplasia	101400
Carpenter syndrome	Craniosynostosis (coronal > lambdoid > sagittal), hypertelorism, proptosis, brachycephaly, brachydactyly, preaxial polysyndactyly, mental retardation		Maxillary hypoplasia	201000
Jackson-Weiss syndrome	Craniosynostosis (coronal), acrocephaly, hypertelorism, proptosis, midface hypoplasia, radiographic abnormalities of the foot including fusion of the tarsal and metatarsal bones, 2-3 syndactyly, broad short first metatarsals and broad proximal phalanges		Maxillary hypoplasia	123150

*Significant risk of airway morbidity.

Cloverleaf skull can result from multisuture craniosynostosis. The skull forms a trilobular appearance, as the cerebrum bulges through the sagittal and squamosal sutures, due to craniosynostosis affecting the coronal, metopic and lambdoid sutures. Cloverleaf skull can be isolated or more commonly associated with a syndrome, and it is estimated that up to 20% represent Pfeiffer syndrome.

ICU CONCERNS

The most significant concerns for the newborn with craniosynostosis are airway compromise (specifically, upper airway obstruction) and intracranial hypertension.

Midface hypoplasia and tracheal anomalies which may be present in syndromic craniosynostosis can lead to significant airway compromise (Table 95-2). With midface hypoplasia, there is decreased nasopharyngeal/oropharyngeal space due to posterior displacement of soft tissues and hypoplasia of maxilla, hypopharyngeal obstruction (at level of posterior choanae), leading to breathing problems, obstructive sleep apnea, asphyxia and even death if untreated (Figure 95-9). Obstructive sleep apnea is common in Apert, Pfeiffer, and Crouzon syndromes.

Cartilaginous tracheal abnormalities can be present in multisuture craniosynostosis syndromes. Vertically fused tracheal cartilage (also referred to as tracheal cartilaginous sleeve, solid cartilaginous trachea, and stovepipe trachea)

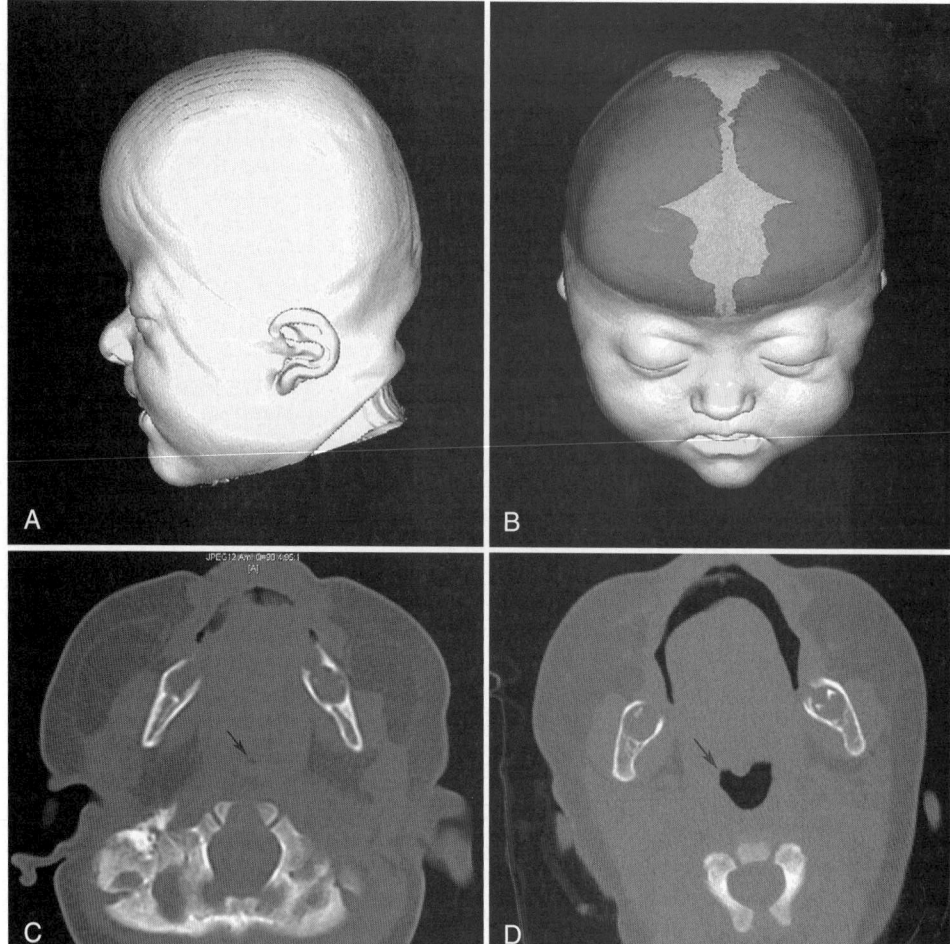

FIGURE 95-9 A and **B,** Three-dimensional reconstruction of a child with Apert syndrome with significant midface hypoplasia, leading to upper airway obstruction. Also notable is acrobrachycephaly due to bicoronal synostosis and the typical pattern of sagittal suture patency. **C,** CT scan axial slice at the level of the skull base in a newborn with Apert syndrome. *Arrow* pointing to airway illustrates significant airway obstruction. **D,** CT scan of a newborn illustrating a normal airway.

in Crouzon and Pfeiffer syndromes may produce a rigid trachea resulting in upper airway stenosis, inability to clear secretions, and increased risk of injury due to decreased distensibility. Characteristic tracheal cartilaginous rings are fused to form a continuous sleeve of cartilage, which may extend from below the subglottis to the carina or bronchus; rarely, the cartilaginous sleeve can begin more proximally, at the level of the cricoid cartilage. Infants with congenital tracheal anomalies may present with fixed stridor, apnea, cyanosis, or increased work of breathing due to the narrowing of the airway.

Neurologic abnormalities such as hydrocephalus and increased ICP may arise, especially in multisuture craniosynostosis. Increased ICP due to constraint of the growing brain within a restricted calvarium is usually low-grade and chronic, causing symptomatic intracranial hypertension when brain growth is accelerated in the first 2 years of life. ICP issues in the neonate are not usually life threatening, given the open fontanel and compensatory splaying of normal sutures or erosion of the calvarium, but brain injury and cognitive impairment may result if a cranioplasty is not performed.

Hydrocephalus, which is more common in Crouzon and Pfeiffer syndromes compared to other multisuture synostosis syndromes, can occur as a result of obstruction of cerebrospinal fluid at the basal cistern, aqueductal stenosis, impeded venous flow, or when there is an associated Chiari malformation. Hydrocephalus is extremely common in cloverleaf skull. Individuals with multisuture craniosynostosis (particularly Apert syndrome) more commonly have nonprogressive distortion ventriculomegaly or compensated hydrocephalus, which does not require shunting (Collmann et al, 2005). Abnormalities of the corpus callosum and septum pellucidum have been described in Apert syndrome, with no true relationship to neurocognitive outcomes (Reiner et al, 1996; Yacubian-Fernandes et al, 2005). Seizures presenting in multisuture craniosynostosis syndromes are usually due to encephalopathy, rather than increased ICP. Epilepsy is more common with increasing number of sutures involved, and seizures are found in approximately 10% of individuals with Crouzon syndrome (Cohen, 2000c).

Conductive and mixed hearing loss, most commonly due to middle ear disease, ossicular abnormalities, and abnormalities in the external auditory canal, can be present in syndromic craniosynostosis. Profound sensorineural hearing loss has been described in Seathre-Chotzen syndrome (Lee et al, 2002).

EVALUATION

The evaluation of the patient with craniosynostosis includes identification of the type of suture fusion, clinical syndrome diagnosis, evaluation for associated anomalies, and preparedness for surgical repair. A craniofacial team made up of the appropriate specialties allows for proper planning and cooperation so that the patient may receive the best possible care.

A careful family history, prenatal history, possible teratogen exposure, maternal hyperthyroidism, and any possible constraint factors (oligohydramnios, twins, fetal movement) and birth history should be ascertained specifically looking for risk factors.

A detailed physical exam should be performed as part of the initial evaluation, looking for any other anomalies with specific attention to cleft palate, limb defects, heart defects, and ear anomalies. The assessment of cranial and face shape, mobility of the calvaria, presence of sutural ridging, skull base, and ear position are important. Facial appearance with particular attention to degree of maxillary hypoplasia is important in determining the risk for airway compromise due to midface hypoplasia. If concerning sleep symptoms are present, such as snoring or apnea, consultation with a sleep specialist and polysomnography may help to quantify the presence and severity of obstructive sleep apnea. Close monitoring for any symptoms of airway obstruction, specifically tracheal malformations, such as vertically fused tracheal cartilage, is crucial in some craniosynostosis syndromes. With the increased awareness of this condition, the diagnosis of these tracheal malformations is increasingly made on direct laryngoscopy/bronchoscopy or with magnetic resonance imaging (MRI).

Neurologic assessment includes ascertaining a history, brain imaging, an audiologic evaluation (early screening for hearing loss in conjunction with frequent otologic examinations), ophthalmologic evaluation, and ongoing developmental assessments. In multisuture craniosynostosis, it is important to monitor for any signs or symptoms of increased ICP. Evaluation for hydrocephalus should be a part of the initial assessment of all children with multisuture craniosynostosis. A CT with three-dimensional reconstruction will ultimately help confirm the diagnosis and delineate the degree of suture involvement in preoperative planning. An MRI may be helpful in defining any associated CNS anomalies. Ophthalmology consultation is valuable in management of proptosis, strabismus, or nystagmus and in determining risk for optic atrophy.

In addition to the foregoing general recommendations, syndrome-specific recommendations are outlined as follows. In Apert syndrome, a cardiac and genitourinary evaluation is recommended. If proptosis is present, as can occur in Apert, Crouzon, and Pfeiffer syndromes, ocular lubricants may be helpful in prevention of exposure keratopathy. In Apert and Saethre-Chotzen syndromes, associated vertebral anomalies, particularly fusions, may be present and can be detected on spine radiographs (Cohen, 2000b). If any limb abnormalities are seen, as in Apert, Jackson-Weiss, Pfeiffer, and Saethre-Chotzen syndromes, radiographs with orthopedic consultation should be obtained.

All individuals with single suture synostosis and developmental delay or associated birth defects should be evaluated by a geneticist to determine association with a clinical syndrome and role for genetic testing. Children with multisuture synostosis due to known classic craniosynostosis syndrome should be offered appropriate genetic testing and genetic counseling. The remaining children with multisuture synostosis in the absence of a known syndromic form should be offered genetic consultation and comparative genomic hybridization (CGH) array testing.

MANAGEMENT

As with all children with functional craniofacial malformations, management with an established craniofacial team is recommended (see Box 95-1). Although specific timing of surgical craniotomy may vary between teams, it is generally accepted that individuals with synostosis should undergo cranioplasty in the 1st year of life. Cranioplasty involves release of fused sutures and repositioning and reconstruction of the calvaria, in order to prevent increased ICP and progressive abnormal craniofacial development.

Early recognition of tracheal malformations can be life saving. Awareness of potential airway compromise and proactive airway management are crucial in many craniofacial syndromes. Temporizing measures to bypass airway obstruction include placement of nasal stents, endotracheal intubation, and ultimately tracheostomy. Specific airway management in syndromic craniosynostosis will depend on the level of obstruction. Serious caution must be extended in the placement and care of tracheostomies in patients with tracheal cartilaginous sleeve malformation because of abnormal tissue healing and granulation tissue formation. Surgical cartilaginous sleeve reduction has been proposed as a cure for some forms of the tracheal anomaly (Noorily et al, 1999).

Midfacial surgery may be necessary in some children who have problems with swallowing, feeding, and dental malocclusion. This is usually performed later in childhood.

For individuals with craniosynostosis, we recommend involvement of a craniofacial team, including pediatrics, neurosurgery, ophthalmology, oral surgery, orthodontics, otolaryngology, nursing, nutrition, plastic surgery, and social work.

DISORDERS OF FIRST AND SECOND BRANCHIAL ARCHES
CRANIOFACIAL MICROSOMIA

Epidemiology and Genetics

Craniofacial microsomia (CFM, OMIM 164210), a congenital malformation in which there is asymmetric deficiency in skeletal and soft tissue on one or both sides of the face, is the most frequently encountered form of facial asymmetry. CFM affects approximately 1 in 5600 births (Grabb, 1965). Individuals with features of CFM have been classified under a variety of different diagnoses (hemifacial microsomia, oculo-aural-vertebral spectrum, facioauricular-vertebral syndrome, first and second branchial arch syndrome, otomandibular dysostosis, Goldenhar

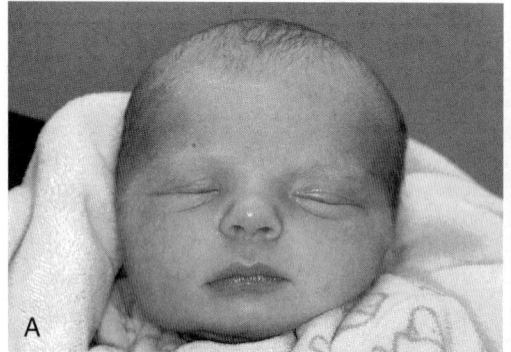
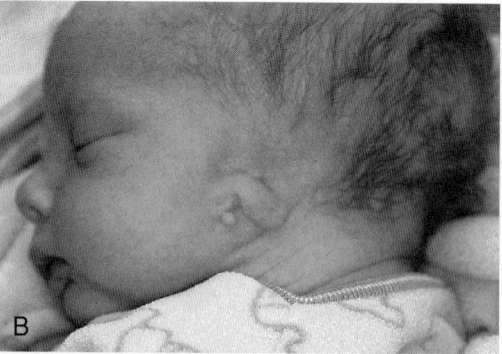
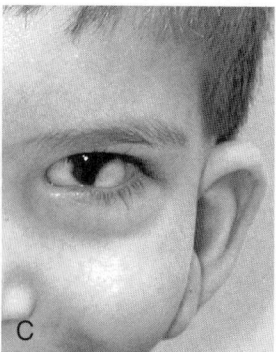

FIGURE 95-10 **A** and **B,** Infant with craniofacial microsomia, mandibular asymmetry, and left-sided microtia. **C,** *(See also Color Plate 39.)* Child with an epibulbar lipodermoid and craniofacial microsomia.

syndrome, lateral facial dysplasia) attesting to the phenotypic variability of disorders associated with mandibular hypoplasia. Most often CFM is a sporadic condition with recurrence risk of approximately 2% for future pregnancies, unless there is a known family history of microtia or CFM (Heike and Hing, 2009). Various causes, both environmental and heritable, have been studied, and for most, the etiology is thought to be multifactorial.

Phenotype

CFM is primarily is a syndrome of the first or second branchial arches, resulting in underdevelopment of the ear, temporomandibular joint, mandibular ramus, mandibular body, and mastication muscles. The affected ear may have an external soft-tissue malformation with or without preauricular tags and may be lower in position compared to the contralateral side. Hearing loss may result from maldevelopment of the ossicular chain and a stenotic or atretic external auditory canal. Second branchial arch defects can involve the facial nerve and muscles of facial expression, which can exacerbate the appearance of facial asymmetry. Even with bilateral facial involvement, there is usually asymmetry (Figure 95-10, *A*). The presence of microtia can be associated with significant risk for hearing loss on the affected side and increased risk of hearing loss in the opposite ear (Figure 95-10, *B*). Infants with CFM are often born small for gestational age, and the perinatal history may include polyhydramnios due to fetal swallowing dysfunction.

A common classification system for CFM is the OMENS Plus system, which characterizes the degree of involvement of facial structures: *O*rbital distortion, *M*andibular hypoplasia, *E*ar anomaly, *N*erve involvement, *S*oft tissue deficiency (Gougoutas et al, 2007). Extracraniofacial anomalies associated with CFM, including renal, cardiac, and vertebral anomalies, are common and will affect recommendations for screening and surveillance.

There can be extreme variability of phenotypic expression ranging from isolated microtia to significant mandibular hypoplasia, bilateral microtia, clefting and extracranial involvement. Isolated microtia may represent a forme fruste of CFM. Other craniofacial features include unilateral macrostomia (the most common form of orofacial clefting in CFM), cleft lip and/or palate, temporomandibular joint (TMJ) ankylosis, ankyloglossia, facial pits (most

common in the distribution of the facial nerve), midface hypoplasia and malocclusion, epibulbar lipodermoids (Figure 95-10, *C*), microphthalmia, eyelid coloboma, facial palsy, and seventh nerve paresis. Goldenhar syndrome appears to be a subgroup variant of CFM characterized by vertebral anomalies and epibibular dermoids in addition to the ear and jaw findings. In CFM, deficient growth of the hypoplastic mandible and the compensatory growth of the contralateral maxilla and zygoma contributes to significant facial asymmetry that progresses with growth (Kearns et al, 2000).

OTHER BRANCHIAL ARCH MALFORMATIONS

Moebius Syndrome

Moebius syndrome (OMIM 157900) is a rare congenital condition affecting approximately 2000 people worldwide (Broussard and Borazjani, 2008). The sixth and seventh cranial nerves are universally affected. Sixth nerve palsy leads to inability to abduct eyes beyond midline. This is usually bilateral but may be unilateral or asymmetric. Paralysis of facial muscles results from the seventh nerve palsy. Newborns may have a masklike facies but can go unrecognized in the newborn period. Feeding difficulties may result from swallowing and sucking problems, aspiration, and palatal weakness presumed to be related to more widespread cranial nerve involvement. There have been associations with chest wall abnormalities including absence of the pectoralis muscle, suggesting a pathogenic relationship to the Poland anomaly (OMIM 173800). Exposure conjunctivitis and keratopathy can occur in facial paralysis and should be treated with appropriate ocular lubricants. Limb defects occur in half of children with Moebius syndrome, most commonly talipes deformity; however, transverse limb anomalies are also seen. Individuals with hypoglossia-hypodactylia or Hanhart's syndrome can have severe limb deformities, ankyloglossia, and TMJ ankylosis, in addition to Moebius-like features and micrognathia, and are at risk for significant swallowing dysfunction and airway compromise (Yasuda et al, 2003).

Treacher Collins Syndrome

Treacher Collins syndrome (TCS, OMIM 154500) is an autosomal dominant disorder of craniofacial development that affects approximately 1 in 50,000 live births (Rovin

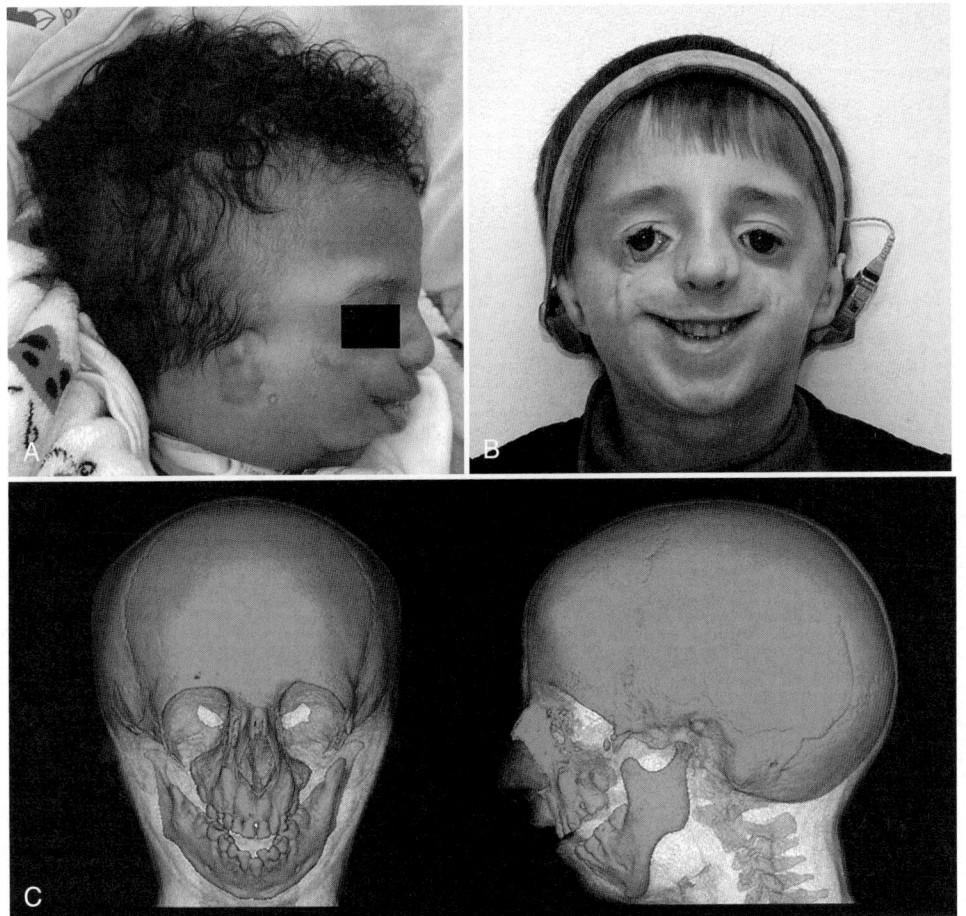

FIGURE 95-11 A, Infant with Treacher Collins syndrome, microtia, severe mandibular and zygomatic hypoplasia, and airway obstruction requiring tracheostomy. **B,** An older child with TCS, downslanting palpebral fissures, eyelid colobomas, and bilateral microtia, wearing a hearing augmentation device. **C,** Three-dimensional reconstruction of TCS. Note the severe mandibular and zygomatic hypoplasia, which may lead to significant airway compromise. Also notable are the orbital defects seen in TCS.

et al, 1964). Like CFM, the tissues affected in TCS arise from the first and second branchial arches. The major clinical features of TCS include hypoplasia of facial bones (particularly the mandible and zygoma), external ear anomalies or microtia, external auditory canal atresia, bilateral conductive hearing loss, lateral downward sloping palpebral fissures, and lower eyelid colobomas (Figure 95-11 *A, B*). Hearing loss is present in up to 50% of individuals with TCS (Dixon et al, 2007). In severe cases, the zygomatic arch may be absent and cleft palate may occur. Extracraniofacial features are rare in TCS. TCOF1 gene mutations, the majority of which occur de novo, have high penetrance with marked phenotypic variability. Diagnosis of TCS is usually made clinically and can be confirmed with genetic testing for the TCOF1 gene (loss of function mutation).

In newborns with TCS, airway management may be required to address narrowing of the airway or extreme shortening of the mandible (Figure 95-11, *C*). When compared to CFM, the mandibular hypoplasia in TCS is usually bilateral and symmetric, leading to increased risk of upper airway obstruction, increased need for tracheostomy, and risk of death in the neonatal period. Choanal atresia and stenosis or severe micrognathia with glossoptosis can lead to airway obstruction in the infant with TCS (Katsanis et al, 2006).

ICU CONCERNS

Mandibular hypoplasia can lead to upper airway obstruction that may be obvious on physical exam, presenting with stridor or stertor concerning for and increased work of breathing, or may be more subtle, as with snoring obstructive sleep apnea. Airway compromise is a particular risk with bilateral severe mandibular and malar involvement as in Treacher Collins syndrome.

Infants with CFM may have feeding difficulties that may be related to palate dysfunction, or more commonly swallow coordination issues and dysphagia related to hypoglossal dysfunction and muscular and bony underdevelopment. Infants with Moebius syndrome may have cranial nerve palsies that affect swallow and oral coordination. These infants are at higher risk for aspiration and should be monitored clinically, especially if they are failing to thrive or developing any concerns for aspiration or lower respiratory disease.

MANAGEMENT

In newborns with suspected CFM, an evaluation should be undertaken for any associated anomalies. All children with external ear anomalies or any evidence of first or second branchial arch abnormalities should undergo a diagnostic audiologic evaluation in the newborn period with follow-up audiometry in the 1st year of life. If there is any hearing loss, ongoing monitoring of hearing is routine. It is also important to monitor ear health and eustachian tube function in the patent/hearing ear. CT imaging to assess middle and inner ear anatomy is not recommended in the neonatal period. Consultation for ear reconstruction and atresia repair should occur by 4 years of age, although aural augmentation and habilitation in conductive hearing loss can be initiated earlier.

Renal ultrasound and cardiac examination (echocardiogram) should be undertaken in infancy to identify any serious structural malformations. Ophthalmology consultation should be sought for appropriate management of epibulbar lipodermoids (if present) and risk for exposure keratopathy. Malocclusion and dental issues will need to be addressed as the child gets older. Children should undergo cervical spine screening radiographs to identify vertebral defects in segmentation. If the newborn has no symptoms of C-spine abnormality, screening four-view cervical spine films can be deferred until the child is 2 to 3 years old, when cervical vertebrae are more easily imaged.

Mild airway obstruction in CFM may be improved or minimized with prone positioning. However, infants with severe mandibular hypoplasia may have significant airway compromise and require tracheostomy placement or early mandibular distraction/advancement. In cases with significant airway compromise, referral to a craniofacial center to evaluate for distraction should be considered.

Oral feeding should be introduced when the airway is stable. Oral stimulation is important to prevent oral aversion. Given the risk of feeding difficulty and aspiration in infants with malformations of the first and second branchial arches, early consultation with both a dietitian and a feeding therapist is recommended.

Mandibular distraction to reconstruct the hypoplastic mandible has been well described (McCarthy et al, 1998). The surgery consists of surgical osteotomy and placement of distraction device that slowly increases mandibular length and ramus height. The timing of surgery is dependent on the degree of mandibular hypoplasia, mandibular growth, and airway involvement. Infants with severe mandibular hypoplasia leading to airway compromise may be candidates for distraction during infancy; however, in those with severe hypoplasia of the mandible, bone grafting may be necessary for reconstruction before distraction.

CHARGE SYNDROME

EPIDEMIOLOGY AND GENETICS

The acronym CHARGE association (*C*oloboma, *H*eart defect, *A*tresia choanae, *R*etarded growth and development, *G*enital hypoplasia, *E*ar anomalies/deafness) was first coined by Pagon, given the observation that the associated malformations occurred more frequently together than one would expect on the basis of chance (Pagon et al, 1981). Over time, the facial features and associated malformations were better characterized as a syndrome, with mutations in at least one major gene described (OMIM 214800).

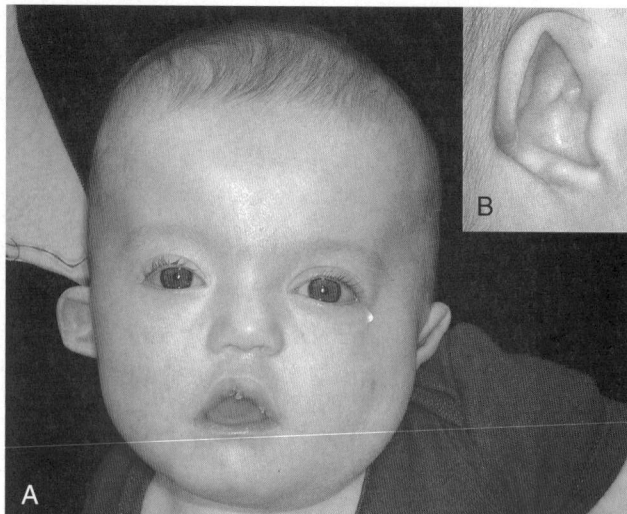

FIGURE 95-12 A and **B,** Child with CHARGE syndrome, with classic ear malformation—hypoplastic lobes, cupped and low-set.

This multiple malformation condition has a prevalence of approximately 1 in 10,000 births (Blake and Prasad, 2006). Although multiple chromosomal aberrations have been reported in children with the phenotype of CHARGE syndrome, mutations in the CHD7 gene account for 60% to 65% of cases. When the diagnosis of CHARGE syndrome is suspected, molecular testing for mutations in the CHD7 gene can be sent to confirm the diagnosis and provide more information to assist in counseling for the parents and the patient. For children in whom CHD7 gene testing is normal, evaluation for chromosomal abnormalities is possible using CGH array technology (Lalani et al, 2007).

PHENOTYPE

The diagnosis of CHARGE syndrome is based on a combination of major and minor clinical criteria, but the diagnosis should be suspected in any neonate with any of the major characteristics: ocular coloboma (80% to 90%), choanal atresia or stenosis (50% to 60%), cranial nerve dysfunction or facial palsy (40% to 90%, depending on which cranial nerve is involved), or classic CHARGE ears (90–100%) (Lalani et al, 2007). Polyhydramnios is commonly present prenatally when bilateral choanal atresia is present.

Distinctive ear anomalies (hypoplastic lobes, cupped or lop, position is often low-set and posteriorly rotated) or deafness occur in most individuals with CHARGE (Figure 95-12, *A, B*). Hearing loss can be a combination of conductive and sensorineural. Other craniofacial features include square face with malar flattening, broad forehead, facial asymmetry, pinched nostrils, full nasal tip, long philtrum, and cleft palate (40%). Ocular colobomas can range from a coloboma of the iris to anophthalmia. Cardiac defects can be a major source of morbidity in infants with CHARGE and are found approximately 80% of the time. Conotruncal and aortic arch anomalies are the most common congenital heart defects, but atrioseptal defects, ventriculoseptal defects, patent ductus arteriosus, hypoplastic left heart, and vascular rings have also been described (Lalani et al, 2007).

ICU CONCERNS

The most important postnatal emergency in CHARGE is bilateral posterior choanal atresia (Blake et al, 2009). Neonates with bilateral choanal atresia will have breathing difficulty and cyanosis within the 1st hour of life. As with all forms of nasal obstruction, crying relieves the cyanosis because it allows the obligate nose breather to take in air through the mouth; feeding exacerbates respiratory distress. Left untreated, the newborn with bilateral choanal atresia can asphyxiate and die. Symptoms of bilateral choanal stenosis or unilateral atresia may not present until after the newborn period with chronic rhinorrhea or breathing problems associated with respiratory infections. Respiratory distress in a newborn with CHARGE syndrome is usually due to choanal atresia, but other features, such as reflux and swallowing dysfunction, can contribute to aspiration and lower respiratory disease. These infants may also have micrognathia and glossoptosis, putting them at risk for airway obstruction at the level of the pharynx/hypopharynx. Infants with CHARGE may require multiple surgeries and procedures over the 1st year of life and are at increased risk for postoperative airway events (Blake et al, 2009).

Cyanotic heart disease may present in the immediate newborn period because of tetralogy of Fallot, outflow tract anomalies, and interrupted aortic arch. Awareness and recognition of the association of CHARGE and congenital heart defects is crucial.

A significant cause of morbidity is feeding difficulty. Feeding and secondary growth problems are common in early infancy and may be attributed to swallowing dysfunction, pharyngeal incoordination, gastroesophageal reflux, and aspiration. Cranial nerve palsies (specifically cranial nerves V, IX, and X) may contribute to swallowing dysfunction, and tracheoesophageal fistula (TEF) contributes to aspiration risk. Although it is well described that infants with CHARGE who survive the newborn period are more likely to survive childhood, the risk of death in infancy remains significant. Male gender, bilateral choanal atresia, TEF, cyanotic heart disease, atrioventricular septal defects, CNS malformations, and ventriculomegaly have all been associated with reduced life expectancy in infants with CHARGE syndrome (Blake et al, 2009; Issekutz et al, 2005; Tellier et al, 1998). A study of 77 individuals with CHARGE found mortality to be 13% (Issekutz et al, 2005).

MANAGEMENT

Children with CHARGE syndrome may require intensive medical management as well as surgical interventions. The primary management targets should be airway stabilization and circulatory support. With this in mind, neonates with CHARGE require immediate evaluation of their airway and cardiac structure and function. An oral airway should be placed if bilateral choanal atresia is suspected. This will allow stabilization of the airway by bypassing the choanal obstruction so that a confirmatory CT scan of the nasal passages can be obtained. A CT of the temporal bones can be included in conjunction with the facial CT and may reveal the characteristic inner ear findings

(Mondini malformation of the cochlea and/or absent or hypoplastic semicircular canals) of CHARGE syndrome. If the oral airway does not allow for adequate air entry, endotracheal intubation may be required. In consultation with a pediatric otolaryngologist, transnasal stents may be placed to keep nasal passages patent in choanal stenosis (and postoperatively after choanal atresia repair). Given the significant risk for cyanotic heart defects, an echocardiogram and cardiology consultation should be obtained to assist in management (Blake and Prasad, 2006).

Infants with CHARGE should also have early audiologic and ophthalmologic evaluations in the neonatal period and should eventually be referred to Birth to Three/early intervention services.

Consultations with both a feeding specialist and dietitian are recommended in the newborn period. If an oral feeding evaluation or videofluoroscopic swallow study are concerning for swallowing dysfunction or aspiration, nasogastric feeding should be initiated. With prolonged feeding issues, gastrostomy tube feeding is often necessary. Infants with severe gastroesophageal reflux may be candidates for Nissen fundoplication at the time of gastrostomy tube placement.

MACROGLOSSIA/ BECKWITH-WIEDEMANN SYNDROME

EPIDEMIOLOGY AND GENETICS

The true prevalence is unknown, but it has been estimated that Beckwith-Wiedemann syndrome (BWS) (OMIM 130650) affects 1 in 13,700 births (Thorburn et al, 1970). This is probably an underestimate, given that there are mild cases of BWS that go undetected. The genetics of BWS is complex and variable. Most cases are sporadic and may result from chromosomal rearrangement, mutations, or epigenetic effects (DNA methylation changes) affecting imprinted genes on chromosome 11p15.5. Although there are no consensus criteria for diagnosis of BWS, the presence of macroglossia, overgrowth, and abdominal wall defects suggests the diagnosis of BWS. Data has suggested a possible link between imprinting disorders and assisted reproduction, and thus infants conceived by in vitro fertilization may be at higher risk for BWS (Maher et al, 2003). If there are features of BWS present or there is a family history of BWS, geneticists may suggest obtaining methylation or chromosome studies to detect abnormalities localized to 11p15. Although this may provide confirmation of diagnosis, sensitivity is not 100%, and thus management is based on the clinical diagnosis.

PHENOTYPE

BWS is a disorder of overgrowth with multiple features, including macrosomia, macroglossia, visceromegaly (involving the kidneys, pancreas, liver, spleen, or adrenal glands), abdominal wall defects (including rectus diastasis, umbilical hernia, and omphalocele), hemihyperplasia (asymmetric overgrowth of one or more regions of the body), renal anomalies (structural anomalies and nephrocalcinosis), and adrenocortical cytomegaly (Figure 95-13). Macroglossia is the most frequent and most

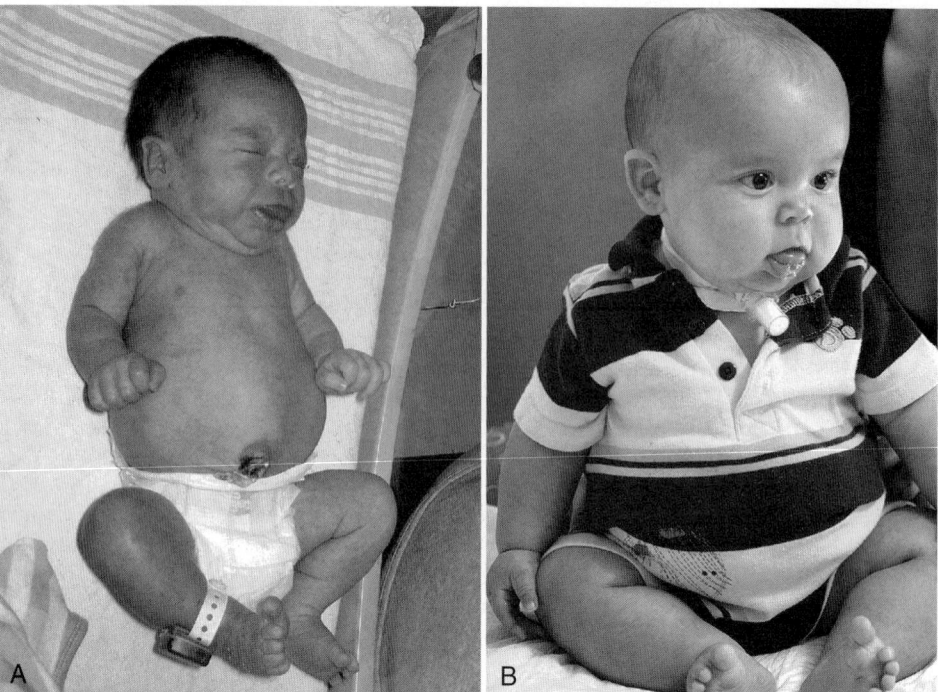

FIGURE 95-13 *(See also Color Plate 40.)* **A,** Premature newborn with Beckwith-Wiedemann syndrome, macroglossia, and rectus diastasis. **B,** Same child at 6 months of age. Macroglossia has increased and he now has a tracheostomy.

obvious manifestation of BWS (present more than 95% of the time) (Elliott et al, 1994). Other craniofacial features include capillary nevus flammeus, metopic ridge, large fontanel, mandibular prognathism, prominent eyes, anterior earlobe linear creases, and posterior helical pits. Less common findings in BWS include cleft palate, cryptorchidism, and cardiac defects (isolated cardiomegaly is more common than cardiomyopathy). Risk of embryonal tumors (Wilms' tumor, hepatoblastoma, neuroblastoma, or rhabdomyosarcoma) in childhood is estimated to be 7.5%, of which 95% present in the first 8 years of life, leading to recommendations for tumor surveillance (Firth and Hurst, 2005).

Some features suggestive of BWS may be present antenatally, including polyhydramnios (due to swallowing dysfunction), preeclampsia, fetal macrosomia, and a large placenta. Prematurity has been reported in 50% of births (Elliott et al, 1994), and in addition to complications of prematurity, the neonate with BWS may develop hypoglycemia and polycythemia.

ICU CONCERNS

Hypoglycemia due to hyperinsulinemia and islet cell hyperplasia occurs in up to 50% of neonates with BWS and usually develops in the first few days of life (Munns and Batch, 2001). It is critical to detect and treat hypoglycemia in any neonate with features of BWS in order to prevent seizures and CNS sequelae. Polycythemia can occur and may need to be treated in the early neonatal period.

Clinical symptoms related to macroglossia may present in the newborn period if macroglossia is severe. However, airway obstruction more commonly presents later in infancy, outside the newborn period. The enlarged tongue can occlude the airway at the level of the hypopharynx,

leading to respiratory distress, apnea, and hypoxia. This may be averted by placing the baby on the side or prone. If the infant requires endotracheal intubation, it is important to exercise caution, because macroglossia can affect visibility of airway structures. A large tongue can also contribute to feeding issues, dysphagia and aspiration.

Infant mortality among infants with BWS has been reported as high as 21% and is related to complications of prematurity and macroglossia (Shurman et al, 2005).

MANAGEMENT

Hypoglycemia in newborns should be managed according to standard protocols for treating neonatal hypoglycemia. If hypoglycemia persists or is refractory to therapy, consider consultation with an endocrinologist. Neonates with an omphalocele may require surgery in the first few days of life.

There is no definitive approach to the management of macroglossia. If macroglossia results in significant airway obstruction or prolonged intubation, tracheostomy may be needed as a temporizing measure to bypass the obstruction. Tongue growth will slow over time, and as jaw growth accelerates, airway compromise should decrease. Some children may benefit from surgical reduction of the tongue, which is usually performed between 2 and 4 years of age, but may be offered as early as 3 to 6 months at some centers.

Referrals to an infant feeding specialist and dietitian are recommended in the infant with severe macroglossia or if the infant is not gaining weight. Although some infants are able to orally feed, others will benefit form nasogastric tube feeds and may go on to need gastrostomy tube feeds.

Although cardiac defects are rare, it is important to do a thorough cardiac evaluation, including electrocardiogram and echocardiogram if any cardiac abnormalities are suspected.

Surveillance for tumors begins in the first months of life. An abdominal ultrasound to assess for organomegaly and a baseline CT or MRI of the abdomen should be performed. Abdominal ultrasounds every 3 months are recommended through 8 years of age. In conjunction, staggered serial serum alpha-fetoprotein measurements (every 6 to 12 weeks) are recommended through 4 years of age to assist in identifying hepatoblastomas before detection by screening ultrasound.

Referral to a craniofacial team may be helpful in the management of the airway obstruction in BWS, including evaluation for tongue reduction and facial hemihypertrophy. A geneticist and genetic counselor may recommend genetic testing for confirmation of diagnosis and/or recurrence risk counseling.

FRONTONASAL DYSPLASIA, HYPERTELORISM, ENCEPHALOCELE

EMBRYOLOGY

Frontonasal dysplasia (FND; also known as frontonasal malformation, median cleft face syndrome, and frontal nasal syndrome) is a malformation resulting from abnormal morphogenesis of the frontonasal process. The development of the facial midline is abnormal, leading to ocular hypertelorism and associated craniofacial features. Most cases of FND are sporadic (OMIM 136760).

PHENOTYPE

FND has been defined phenotypically as containing two or more of the following craniofacial features: ocular hypertelorism; broadening of the nasal root; midline facial cleft affecting the nose, lip, or palate; unilateral or bilateral clefting of the alae nasi; hypoplastic nasal tip; anterior cranium bifidum; and a V-shaped frontal hairline (Wu et al, 2007). Grading of hypertelorism is best achieved by measuring the interpupillary distance. In a term newborn, interpupillary distance greater than 4.5 cm is considered hyperteloric (Jones, 2006).

In addition to hypertelorism, eye anomalies, including epibulbar dermoids, colobomas, ptosis, nystagmus, or cataracts, may be present in FND and are associated with a more severe phenotype and an increased incidence of CNS abnormalities (Wu et al, 2007). Associated CNS manifestations include encephalocele, agenesis of the corpus callosum, and abnormal neuronal migration. Developmental delay is a significant risk, especially when there are CNS malformations. When FND is associated with extracephalic anomalies or when ocular hypertelorism is more severe, there is an increased association with cognitive impairment (Gorlin et al, 2001d). Encephaloceles may occur in isolation or may be associated with a syndrome. Frontonasal encephaloceles (and meningoceles) are the most common encephaloceles in FND (Gorlin et al, 2001a) (Figure 95-14).

A subpopulation of patients with frontonasal malformation also have coronal craniosynostosis and variable skeletal and ectodermal defects and have an X-linked condition

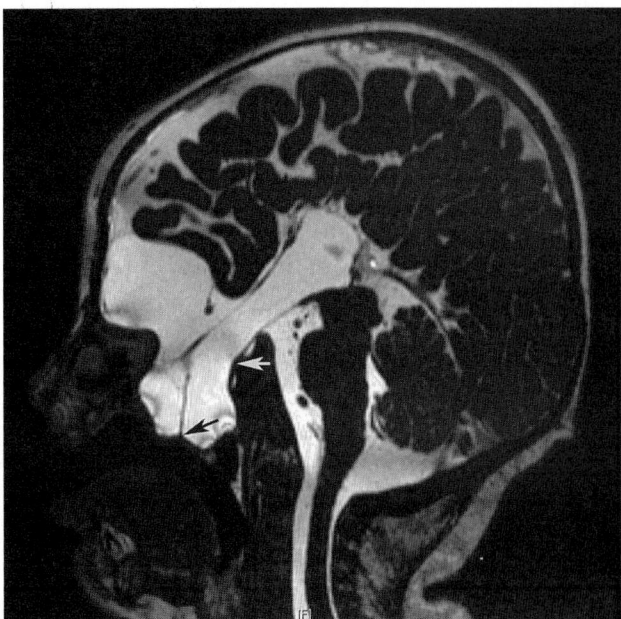

FIGURE 95-14 **MRI of an infant with frontonasal dysplasia and a midline cleft lip.** The scan reveals a moderate-sized meningocele extending into the posterior nasopharynx. *White arrow* points to midbrain meningocele coming through the cribriform plate; *black arrow* points to the intraoral meningocele.

termed craniofrontonasal syndrome (CFNS, OMIM 304110). Similar to FND, facial features include hypertelorism, frontal bossing, broad nasal bridge, and a bifid nasal tip. Children with CFNS often have significant facial asymmetry due to unicoronal synostosis. In this X-linked condition, females are affected more severely than males (and typically have hypertelorism and grooved nails), and mutations are detected in the EFNB1 gene. Affected individuals usually have normal intelligence.

ICU CONCERNS

Intracranial abnormalities associated with FND may put the infant at risk for CNS manifestations such as hydrocephalus or seizures. If the pituitary gland is involved or deficient, as can be seen with HPE sequence, there can be serious endocrine abnormalities (as discussed in the section on orofacial clefting). Also, frontonasal encephalocele may contribute to upper airway compromise.

MANAGEMENT

In any infant with hypertelorism or features that raise suspicion for FND, awareness of potential underlying malformations is critical, and cranial imaging by CT scan or MRI should be considered. Placement of a nasogastric tube or suction catheter should be avoided or used with caution until the CNS anatomy has been delineated. Because infants with FND have a high incidence of frontonasal encephalocele or meningocele, routine placement of these catheters could lead to brain injury. If an infant with FND needs urgent or emergent endotracheal intubation, intraoral structures should be examined carefully to prevent injury to herniating CNS structures if present. Management of seizures or any electrolyte derangements should be managed as per the NICU standard protocol. Consultation with a craniofacial team, including ophthalmology, can be helpful in understanding the work-up and management (including potential surgical interventions) for individuals with FND.

PRENATAL SCREENING FOR FETAL FACE ANOMALIES

The exact role of fetal face examination with ultrasound in a low-risk pregnancy is under evaluation. Routine obstetric surveillance includes a midtrimester anatomic ultrasound (US) at 18–22 weeks' gestation. Most studies looking at the recognition rate and incidence of ultrasonographic diagnosis of orofacial clefting focus on this anatomic examination. Adequate evaluation of the facial structures with ultrasonography can be achieved by 16 to 17 weeks' gestation. The following facial features can be visualized with two-dimensional (2D) routine US at 18 weeks' gestation with standard facial views (which include coronal images of the nose, lips' and orbits and sagittal profile views): orbital size and position, eye size including microphthalmia and anophthalmia, shape of nose, nasal hypoplasia, length of the philtrum, clefts of the upper lip, frontal bossing, retrognathia, micrognathia, macroglossia, and soft tissue abnormalities. Cleft lip with or without cleft palate can be detected by antenatal ultrasound, whereas isolated cleft palate, which is not typically associated with a cleft of the alveolus, may be obscured by the tongue, which has the same echogenicity as the secondary palate, thus making prenatal diagnosis of CPO more difficult. A retrospective study in a low-risk population demonstrated that routine prenatal ultrasound with standard facial views performed at 18 weeks estimated gestational age detected 93% of cases of CL+P, 67% of cases of isolated CL, and 22% of cases of CPO (Cash et al, 2001).

Although the diagnosis is not definitive, prenatal diagnosis is particularly valuable in allowing for appropriate prenatal counseling. Families who have the opportunity to meet with members from a craniofacial team before delivery often appreciate having some understanding of what to expect in the newborn period.

SUGGESTED READINGS

American Cleft Palate and Craniofacial Association ACPA core curriculum. This core curriculum was created by the Education Committee of ACPA to be used as a guide for educators in the various disciplines, when planning the essential parts of their curriculum related to cleft and craniofacial anomalies. http://www.acpa-cpf.org/educmeetings/education.htm. Accessed August 31, 2009.

Blake KD, Prasad C: CHARGE syndrome, *Orphanet J Rare Dis* 1:34, 2006.

Cohen MM: Apert syndrome. In Cohen MM, Maclean RE, editors: *Craniosynostosis: diagnosis, evaluation, and management*, ed 2, New York, 2000, Oxford University Press, pp 877-911.

Elliott M, Bayly R, Cole T, et al: Clinical features and natural history of Beckwith-Wiedemann syndrome: presentation of 74 new cases, *Clin Genet* 46:168-174, 1994.

Evans KN, Sie KC, Hopper RA, et al: Robin sequence: from diagnosis to development of an effective management plan, *Pediatrics* 127:936-948, 2011.

Gorlin RJ, Cohen MM, Hennekam RCM: Orofacial clefting syndromes: common syndromes. In *Syndromes of the head and neck*, ed 4, New York, 2001, Oxford University Press, pp 877-911.

Heike CL, Hing AV: *Medical Genetics Information Resource (online database)*. http://www.genetests.org. 1997-2009Accessed August 21, 2009.

Jones KL: *Smith's recognizable patterns of human malformations*, ed 6, Philadelphia, 2006, Elsevier Saunders.

Katsanis SH, Cutting GR: Treacher Collins syndrome. *GeneReviews at GeneTests: Medical Genetics Information Resource (online database)*, Seattle, October 27, 2006, University of Washington, pp 1997-2009 http://www.genetests.org. Accessed September 15, 2009.

Rahbar R, Rouillon I, Roger G, et al: The presentation and management of laryngeal cleft: a 10-year experience, *Arch Otolaryngol Head Neck Surg* 132:1335-1341, 2006.

Robin NH, Moran RT, Warman M, Ala-Kokko L: Stickler syndrome. *GeneReviews at GeneTests: Medical Genetics Information Resource (online database)*, Seattle, August 20, 2009, University of Washington, pp 1997-2009. http://www.genetests.org. Accessed August 25, 2009.

Robin NH, Shprintzen RJ: Defining the clinical spectrum of deletion 22q11.2, *J Pediatr* 147:90-96, 2005.

Complete references and supplemental color images used in this text can be found online at www.expertconsult.com

COMMON NEONATAL ORTHOPEDIC AILMENTS

Klane K. White and Michael J. Goldberg

Although orthopedic afflictions of the newborn generally are not life threatening, they do have the potential to significantly impair functional performance, even when diagnosed and treated early. This chapter discusses the most commonly encountered of these orthopedic problems.

DEVELOPMENTAL DYSPLASIA OF THE HIP

The term *developmental dysplasia of the hip* (DDH) encompasses a spectrum of pathology from acetabular dysplasia, to "located" hips that are unstable (femoral head can be moved in and out of the confines of the acetabulum), to frankly dislocated hips in which there is a complete loss of contact between the femoral head and acetabulum. DDH occurs in 11.5 of 1000 infants, with frank dislocations occurring in 1 to 2 per 1000 (American Academy of Pediatrics, 2000; Guille et al, 2000). Risk factors for a positive newborn screening examination include female gender (19 per 1000 risk), positive family history (boys, 9.4 per 1000; girls, 44 per 1000), and breech presentation (boys, 26 per 1000; girls, 120 per 1000) (American Academy of Pediatrics, 2009). The left hip alone is affected in 60%, the right hip in 20%, and both hips in 20% of infants (Guille et al, 2000).

Dislocations can be divided into two groups: syndromic and typical. *Syndromic* dislocations are most frequently associated with neuromuscular conditions such as myelodysplasia and arthrogryposis or with dysmorphic syndromes such as Larsen's syndrome. These abnormalities probably occur in either week 12 or 18 of gestation (American Academy of Pediatrics, 2000). *Typical* dislocations occur in otherwise healthy infants in the prenatal or postnatal period.

Congruent reduction and stability of the femoral head are necessary for normal growth and development of the hip joint. The natural history of untreated DDH is controversial, because newborn instability may resolve or progress to subluxation or dislocation. In cases that progress, infants have significantly increased risk of developing precocious arthritis with moderate to severe hip pain as young adults (Cooperman et al, 1983; Wedge and Wasylenko, 1979). This pain can be debilitating. Early detection and treatment of DDH are therefore important in avoiding the devastating sequelae of a late diagnosis.

There are no pathognomonic signs of a dislocated hip. The physical examination requires patience on the part of the examiner and may be facilitated by having the baby feed from a bottle. Evaluation for asymmetry is perhaps the most important key to the evaluation for DDH, although asymmetry may not be evident in bilateral dislocations. Presence of asymmetric abduction is suggestive of a dislocation, as is a Galeazzi sign. The presence of asymmetric thigh folds may be indicative of DDH but is often present in unaffected infants. The Galeazzi sign is

elicited with the baby placed supine on an examining table so that the pelvis is level, with the hips and knees flexed to 90 degrees. With the baby's hips in neutral abduction, the examiner determines if the knees are at the same height. If one femur appears shorter, the hip may be dislocated posteriorly (Figure 96-1). Limitations in hip abduction in babies older than 12 weeks is the most reliable examination finding suggestive of DDH. Adduction of 30 degrees and abduction of 75 degrees should be possible in most newborns. Side-to-side variations should be noted. Each of these signs, individually or in combination, may serve to increase the index of suspicion of the examiner and lower the threshold for further diagnostic studies or referral to a pediatric orthopedist.

There are two common ways of assessing hip stability in the newborn. The Ortolani test is performed on one leg at a time, with the calm newborn supine on the examining table. The index and middle fingers of the examiner are placed along the greater trochanter, while the thumb is placed on the medial aspect of the thigh. The pelvis is stabilized by placing the thumb and ring or long finger of the opposite hand on top of both anterior iliac crests simultaneously. Alternatively, the opposite thigh may be held in the same manner as the examined side while the hip is held in abduction. The hip is flexed to 90 degrees and gently abducted while the leg is lifted with the hip in neutral external/internal rotation. A palpable clunk is felt as the dislocated femoral head reduces into the acetabulum. This finding is reported as the Ortolani sign (positive result on the Ortolani test). The Barlow test is an attempt to dislocate or subluxate a located but unstable hip. The thigh is held and the pelvis stabilized in the same manner as for the Ortolani test. With the hip in neutral external/internal rotation and at 90 degrees of flexion, the leg is then gently adducted with a mild posteriorly directed pressure applied to the knee. A palpable clunk or sensation of posterior movement constitutes a positive result (i.e., the Barlow sign). Each hip should be examined separately. High-pitched clicks are frequently elicited with hip range of motion. These sounds are most frequently attributed to snapping of the iliotibial band over the greater trochanter and are not associated with dysplasia (Bond et al, 1997). With progressive soft tissue contractures, both the Ortolani and Barlow tests become unreliable after 3 months of age.

Imaging of the immature hip can be a valuable adjunct to the physical examination. An anteroposterior (AP) radiograph of the pelvis is difficult to interpret before age 4 to 5 months. The femoral head is composed entirely of cartilage until the secondary center of ossification appears. Before the appearance of the secondary center, ultrasound examination is the method of choice for visualizing the cartilaginous femoral head and acetabulum. Static ultrasound images allow visualization of acetabular and femoral head anatomy, while the complementary dynamic

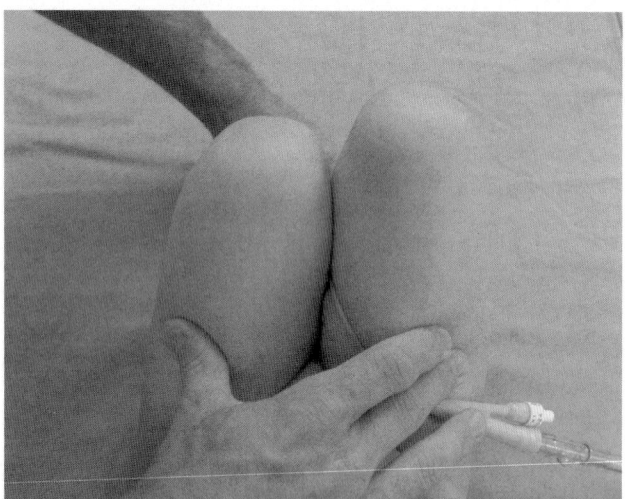

FIGURE 96-1 Presence of Galeazzi sign.

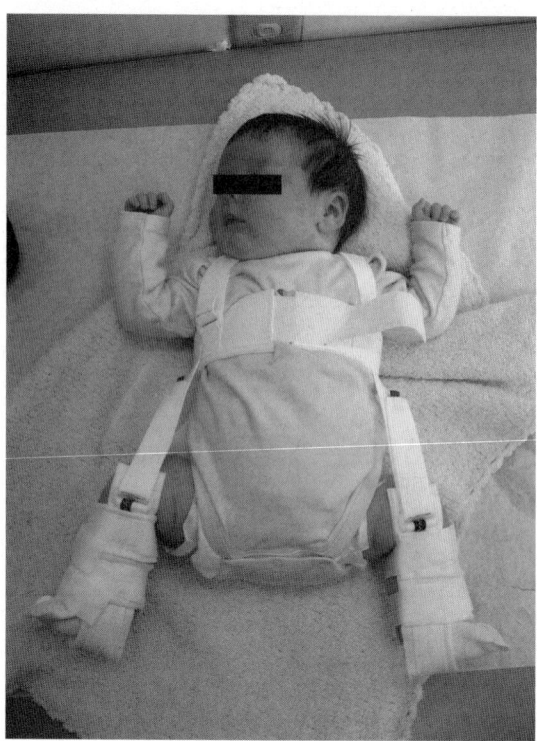

FIGURE 96-2 The Pavlik harness.

images give information on the stability of the hip joint (Clarke et al, 1985; Graf, 1984). The primary limitation of hip ultrasonography is that results are dependent on the experience and skill of the operator, especially when performed within the first 3 weeks of life (Marks et al, 1994). For these reasons ultrasonography is recommended as an adjunct to clinical evaluation rather than as a screening tool (American Academy of Pediatrics, 2000). Studies conducted before 4 weeks of life maybe useful for confirming equivocal physical exam findings and for monitoring treatment of hips with known dislocations. Clinicians must be aware, however, that ultrasound images in this age group often reveal minor degrees of dysplasia that usually resolve spontaneously and may lead to overtreatment of physiological hip variations. Ultrasonography is the technique of choice for assessing infants at high risk for DDH after 4 to 6 weeks of age and, again, is useful in following the results of intervention. After 4 months of age, the gold standard remains the AP pelvic radiograph.

The American Academy of Pediatrics has published a revised clinical practice guideline to aid in the early diagnosis and initiation of appropriate intervention of DDH (American Academy of Pediatrics, 2009). All newborns should be screened for DDH by a properly trained health care provider by physical examination. Risk factors for DDH should be determined by the treating physician. These include the presence of a positive Ortolani or Barlow exam, breech presentation, and positive family history. If there are no risk factors, then serial examinations are recommended according to a standard periodicity schedule until the child is an established walker. If during these periodic visits physical findings raise suspicion of DDH, or if a parental concern suggests hip disease, confirmation is required by an expert physical examination, by referral to a pediatric orthopedist (or other practitioner with expertise in medical and surgical management of newborn hip disease), or by age-appropriate imaging. When a positive Ortolani or Barlow test is present at birth and persists beyond the usual age of spontaneous resolution (4 weeks), the infant should be referred to an orthopedist for management. However, if the positive Ortolani or Barlow test disappears by 4 weeks, then age-appropriate

imaging (ultrasonography at 6 weeks or radiograph at 4 months) is warranted. If the baby has positive risk factors, such as female breech or positive family history, but a stable hip exam, then age appropriate imaging is recommended (ultrasonography at 6 weeks or radiograph at 4 months).

As previously recommended, triple diapering is not an accepted form of treatment in DDH, and communication between providers is encouraged if the practitioner examining the newborn in the hospital is different from the 2-week follow-up examiner. Despite newborn screening programs, 1 in 5000 will have a dislocated hip detected at 18 months of age or older (Dezateux and Godward, 1995). It is important to appreciate that not all dislocated hips are present at birth, and not all hips dislocated at birth are detectable in the newborn period.

Treatment of DDH is dependent on the age at presentation. For children 0 to 6 months of age, a reducible hip is treated in a Pavlik harness. The Pavlik is a dynamic splint that allows the infant to actively move the hips through a sphere of motion that encourages deepening and stabilization of the acetabulum (Figure 96-2). The harness is applied as soon as possible after the diagnosis of DDH is made. The length of treatment is dependent on age at presentation. Progress is judged by serial physical examinations and static and dynamic ultrasonography. In the case of a frankly dislocated hip, treatment is abandoned if no improvement is noted within 4 weeks of splint application. Closed reduction under general anesthesia, usually with arthrographic evaluation and subsequent spica casting, is then attempted at 4 to 5 months of age. For a persistently irreducible dislocation, which is unusual in the 0- to 6-month age group, open operative reduction of the hip with subsequent spica casting is undertaken. The success of Pavlik harness treatment is variable and correlates with the severity of the hip dysplasia. Treatment is successful in nearly 100% of stable hips, greater than 90% in dislocatable (Barlow positive) hips, 61% to 93% in dislocated but reducible (Ortolani positive) hips, and as low as 40% in irreducible dislocations (Hangen et al, 1995; Lerman et al, 2001; Sucato et al, 1999; Swaroop and Mubarak, 2009; Viere et al, 1990).

TORTICOLLIS

Congenital muscular torticollis (CMT) manifests at birth or soon thereafter and is the most frequent cause of wryneck. However, other conditions, some more serious, may cause torticollis. These include congenital anomalies of the vertebra and skull (e.g., Klippel-Feil syndrome, hemivertebrae, basilar invagination, craniosynostosis) (Dubousset, 1986; Hensinger et al, 1974; Raco et al, 1999); abnormalities of the central nervous system (CNS; e.g., syringomyelia, tumors) (Kiwak et al, 1983); Chiari malformations (Dure et al, 1989); ocular abnormalities (Bixenman, 1981); pharyngeal abscess; and gastroesophageal reflux (e.g., Sandifer's syndrome) (Ramenofsky et al, 1978). Patients with CMT can be divided into those who demonstrate a sternocleidomastoid muscle (SCM) "pseudotumor," those with tightness or fibrosis of the SCM without pseudotumor (termed *muscular torticollis*), and those with all of the characteristic features of congenital torticollis without evidence of contracture or fibrosis of muscle (termed *postural torticollis*) (Cheng et al, 2001). CMT has been estimated to occur in 0.3% to 2.0% of live births (Cheng et al, 2001). It is usually discovered between 6 and 8 weeks of life. The infant presents with a cock robin appearance, with the head tilted toward and chin rotated away from the affected SCM. Twenty percent to 30% of patients will have a palpable pseudotumor present in the middle to inferior aspect of the affected SCM, which spontaneously regresses with time, leaving a fibrous band (Herring, 2002). More than half will have facial asymmetry. The left and right SCMs are affected in equal proportions. CMT probably results from ischemia within the SCM, leading to fibrosis (Davids et al, 1993). The cause of the ischemia is unknown, but intrauterine crowding may play a role, inasmuch as some authors have reported an association of torticollis with other deformations such as DDH and metatarsus adductus (Morrison and MacEwen, 1982; Tien et al, 2001).

Excellent results with a manual stretching program can be attained in children first seen before 1 year of age (Morrison and MacEwen, 1982). Initially, the parents are instructed in the technique of stretching the contracted SCM by rotating the infant's chin toward the affected SCM while simultaneously tilting the head away from it. This is completed 10 times each session and held for a count of 10 at least 10 times per day. Unfortunately, compliance may be an issue. If the child fails to improve substantially within 3 to 4 weeks, a physical therapist is enlisted to see the child two or three times weekly to supervise the program and reinforce the home therapy. Additionally, the parents are instructed to configure the infant's crib and toys in such a manner as to encourage active rotation toward the involved side. There is no justification to undertake surgery in any child less than 1 year of age or in any child who has not completed a minimum of 6 months of therapy

(Cheng et al, 2001; Morrison and MacEwen, 1982). In a prospective study of 821 children with muscular torticollis, only 8% of patients with the history of a pseudotumor, and 3% of those without, required surgical intervention following a well-structured stretching program (Cheng et al, 2001). Because of the difficulty of monitoring exercise programs, because parental compliance is always in question, and because surgical intervention is infrequent, it is possible that many patients resolve spontaneously. No patients with postural torticollis require surgery. Risk factors for surgery include late initial presentation, presence of a pseudotumor, and rotation deficit of greater than 15 degrees.

The timing of surgical intervention remains controversial. In patients with significant plagiocephaly and facial asymmetry, surgery should be considered just before 2 years of age in order to maximize the chance for complete remodeling. For those with either no or mild facial asymmetry, good to excellent results can be expected with surgery up to 6 years of age (Ling, 1976). Acceptable results are reported as late as 12 years of age, but the ability to remodel facial asymmetry appears diminished (Lee et al, 1986). Surgery entails either release or lengthening of the SCM through cosmetically pleasing incisions (Ferkel et al, 1983). The use of a molded helmet to promote facial and skull remodeling is common in some centers. Prospective studies that establish the effectiveness of helmets are lacking.

A less frequent cause of congenital torticollis is osseous fusion between bones in the cervical spine. These fusions may be between the skull and C1 and/or C2 or in the lower cervical spine. They result from failure of the bones to properly segment during embryogenesis. These abnormalities, in combination with a low posterior hairline and a short webbed neck with limited range of motion and head tilt, constitute the triad referred to as *Klippel-Feil syndrome* (Copley and Dormans, 1998). These congenital bone fusions can range from involvement of two segments to involvement of the entire cervical spine. Colloquially, Klippel-Feil syndrome has come to refer to any congenital malformation in the cervical spine with or without other elements of the triad. In infants and young children, the neck may remain quite flexible despite the bone abnormalities. In a newborn with torticollis who does not improve with passive stretching exercises, radiologic evaluation is mandatory. Cervical spine films are not recommended in all patients initially presenting with neonatal torticollis, as these films are quite difficult to interpret in this age group because of the predominance of cartilage in the bones of the neck. Furthermore, many neonates would be subjected to unnecessary ionizing radiation.

The natural history of Klippel-Feil in most cases is quite favorable, requiring nothing more than periodic observation. In patients with severe involvement, however, the consequences of this disorder can include early spondylosis with the development of pain or stenosis, the development of progressive torticollis and scoliosis, and the occurrence of neurologic compromise and sudden death secondary to even minimal trauma (Herring, 2002). Despite these potentially devastating sequelae, the greatest advantage to early detection of Klippel-Feil syndrome is in being alerted to commonly associated disorders including congenital heart disease (14% to 29%), renal anomalies (25% to 35%), scoliosis (60%), audiologic anomalies (80%), deafness (15% to 35%), synkinesis (15% to 20%), and, less commonly, posterior fossa desmoid tumors (Herring, 2002; Muzumdar and Goel, 2001). The recognition of a Klippel-Feil anomaly should prompt a thorough evaluation for these associations. Treatment for Klippel-Feil most often involves periodic observation with activity modification. In the face of progression of deformity or severe deformity, spinal fusion may be warranted.

Sandifer's syndrome (gastroesophageal reflux) also can cause a torticollis. With this syndrome, the torticollis is intermittent and may alternate directions, and there is no tightness of the SCM, with normal findings on radiographs (Ramenofsky et al, 1978).

Hemiatlas, or the failure of formation of a portion of the first cervical vertebra, is also a rare cause of torticollis (Dubousset, 1986). In the infant, the neck may be quite flexible and the torticollis passively correctable. An open-mouth (odontoid view) cervical spine radiograph reveals this deformity. If the torticollis is progressive or severe, gradual correction of the deformity with a halo vest followed by posterior occiput-to-cervical spine fusion is necessary. Other potential causes of torticollis in the neonate include CNS tumors and syringomyelia. If radiographs appear normal, a thorough neurologic examination and referral to a neurologist are recommended.

FOOT DEFORMITIES

Congenital deformities of the foot are relatively common but often overlooked in newborns. Consequently, the true incidence of the milder, self-limited deformities is unknown. For identification purposes, congenital foot abnormalities can be divided into those that result in the toes pointing upward (calcaneovalgus) and those that result in the toes pointing inward (metatarsus adductus, clubfoot).

Calcaneovalgus is thought to be a postural deformity secondary to intrauterine positioning in which the dorsum of the foot is, or can be, directly apposed to the anterior aspect of the leg. In the calcaneovalgus foot, the hindfoot is in the dorsiflexed position (calcaneus position) so that the plantar aspect of the forefoot is collinear with it. Plantar flexion of the foot is often limited from contracture of the anterior ankle soft tissues. The estimated incidence of calcaneovalgus is 0.4 per 1000 to 1 per 1000 live births (Nunes and Dutra, 1986; Wynne-Davies, 1964). It appears to be more common in girls and after breech deliveries (Nunes and Dutra, 1986). There may be an increased association with hip dysplasia, so a thorough hip examination is warranted, as outlined in the previous section on DDH. The prognosis for complete resolution with gentle stretching exercises conducted by the parents with each diaper change is excellent in the vast majority of cases. Complete resolution generally occurs by 3 to 6 months of age. Calcaneovalgus may be seen in conjunction with external rotation of the tibia, so that the toes appear to be rotated upward and outward. Additionally, a common association occurs with posteromedial bowing of the tibia, a unilateral deformity. Posterior medial bowing is likely to resolve slowly but may eventually lead to a leg length inequality necessitating

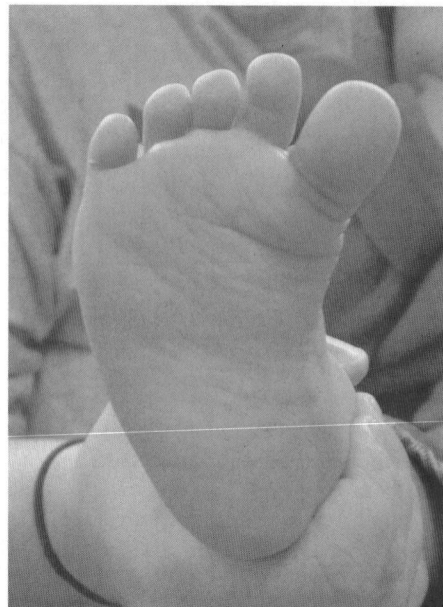

FIGURE 96-3 The appearance of the foot with metatarsus adductus.

limb equalization surgery. Occasionally, in the most severe cases of calcaneovalgus, the foot requires serial casting to facilitate correction. A deformity failing to resolve mandates referral to a pediatric orthopedist.

Calcaneovalgus needs to be differentiated from congenital vertical talus, a rarer condition that frequently is associated with neuromuscular conditions and syndromes. Congenital vertical talus can be differentiated from calcaneovalgus by viewing the hindfoot. If the hindfoot is fixed in equinus (plantar flexion), the foot will demonstrate a "rocker bottom" appearance characteristic of congenital vertical talus, due to dorsal dislocation of the midfoot at Chopart's joint (talonavicular and calcaneocuboid joints). In instances where the midfoot can be reduced (as demonstrated radiographically), the condition is referred to as an *oblique talus.* Treatment during infancy consists of serial casting to stretch dorsal soft tissues and potentially reduce the midfoot. After reduction, through either casting or surgical release, the Achilles tendon is lengthened to treat the hindfoot equinus (Dobbs et al, 2006).

The two common neonatal foot deformities resulting in medial deviation of the toes are metatarsus adductus and talipes equinovarus (clubfoot). *Metatarsus adductus* is present at birth but frequently diagnosed later during the 1st year of life. It has been estimated to occur in 1 in 100 births (Widhe et al, 1988). The pathogenesis is unproved, but the condition is thought to result from intrauterine crowding. Characteristic features include a concave medial border of the foot with a curved lateral border, a "bean-shaped" sole of the foot, a higher-than-normal-appearing arch, fixed adductus of the forefoot when the hindfoot is held in neutral position, separation of the first and second toes, and spontaneous medial deviation of the foot with active movement by the infant (Figure 96-3) (Kite, 1967). Metatarsus adductus can be classified into cases that passively correct and those that do not. Feet in which passive correction is possible are best left alone and will improve spontaneously. Feet in which passive correction cannot be obtained

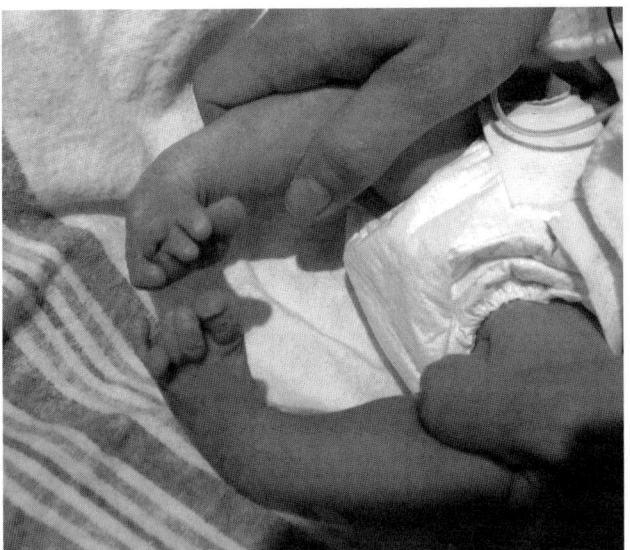

FIGURE 96-4 The appearance of an untreated newborn clubfoot.

should be treated with manipulation and serial casting. The corrections can then be maintained with straight-last shoes if necessary or with nighttime bivalved casts. Operative treatment should be considered only in children older than 3 years of age who have a rigid deformity and have failed to respond to a manipulation and serial casting program (Weinstein, 2000). Farsetti et al (1994) reported on 45 feet demonstrating metatarsus adductus, with an average follow-up period of 33 years. The 16 feet in which the deformities were passively correctible, and in which no intervention was undertaken, were all rated as good, demonstrating spontaneous resolution of the metatarsus adductus. The 29 feet with deformities initially deemed partially correctible or rigid were treated with manipulation and casting. At follow-up examination, 26 feet (90%) were reported as good. None required surgery. The difficulty in treating metatarsus adductus is in convincing the parents and grandparents of the affected infant that the condition will resolve without intervention. Frequently, reverse-last and straight-last shoes are prescribed for benefit of the parent rather than the child.

The term *clubfoot* describes a foot demonstrating hindfoot equinus (plantar flexion) with adduction and supination of the forefoot (Figure 96-4). Clubfoot represents a spectrum of congenital deformity that ranges from the mild "postural" clubfoot to the severe arthrogrypotic clubfoot. It occurs in 1 in 1000 to 2 in 1000 live births (Herring, 2002). Three prominent theories for the etiology of clubfoot have emerged. An arrest in embryonic development in the 6- to 8-week fetus (Bohm, 1929) secondary to connective tissue abnormalities, a primary germ plasm defect (Brockman, 1930), and a neuromuscular defect (Handelsman and Badalamente, 1982) have been proposed. A recently documented risk factor for clubfoot is early amniocentesis (11 to 13 weeks' gestation), which is hypothesized to cause decreased fetal movement during a critical phase of foot development (Tredwell et al, 2001). Although the etiology of clubfoot remains unproved, there appears to be dysplasia of all osseous, muscular, tendinous, cartilaginous, skin, and neurovascular tissues

distal to the knee in the affected limb. On the mild end of the spectrum, postural clubfoot appears to represent a packaging problem due to intrauterine positioning. Postural clubfoot is passively correctible, lacks deep medial creasing, demonstrates minimal or no calf atrophy, and responds quickly to a stretching and casting regimen. At the opposite end of the spectrum is the arthrogrypotic or neuromuscular clubfoot that demonstrates severe rigidity; absence of skin creases, suggesting early in utero affliction; and failure to respond to nonoperative therapies. Between these two extremes lies the classic clubfoot deformity. The anatomic deformities in clubfoot are numerous, complex, and somewhat controversial. Although the specific anatomic abnormalities are well beyond the scope of this chapter, the most notable abnormalities include a small, contracted heel cord complex; medial subluxation of the navicular bone on the talar head so that it abuts or nearly abuts the medial malleolus; and parallelism between the calcaneus and talus bones when these are viewed radiographically from the lateral aspect and from an anterior-to-posterior perspective. Clinically, the foot demonstrates a medial crease, with the toes pointed toward the midline, the sole of the foot angulated medially, the hindfoot plantar flexed with a deep, single, posterior crease, and a smaller foot and calf than on the contralateral side (see Figure 96-4).

All clubfoot deformities should be referred to a pediatric orthopedist for treatment. Initial treatment for all cases of congenital clubfoot is nonoperative. Untreated clubfoot has a poor natural history, with development of early degenerative changes in the foot joints. Historically, good, early results were achieved with operative methods in 85% of cases (Weinstein, 2000). Early surgical correction, however, has yielded poor long-term results and a high recurrence rate. Despite adept surgical correction, approximately 15% of cases of clubfoot have demonstrated recurrence necessitating further surgical intervention. Consequently, this approach has been abandoned.

Some surgeons have advocated a completely nonoperative approach to clubfoot correction (Kite, 1964; Ponseti, 1996; Seringe and Atia, 1990) based on observations that in operated cases of clubfoot, the feet are often stiff and gradually develop scarring, which diminishes the result. These programs vary in the specifics of treatment but share a labor-intensive approach. Although many forms of nonoperative clubfoot treatment exist, the Ponseti method of cast correction has achieved preeminence in this regard (Ponseti, 1992). The Ponseti method uses a specific set of manipulations and serial corrective long-leg casts, followed by a prolonged period of bracing. The "French Functional Method" has also been successfully duplicated at at least one U.S. hospital with good results (Faulks and Richards, 2009; Herring, 2002). This method necessitates daily manipulations by a trained physical therapist for 8 weeks, with the addition of continuous passive motion during the first 4 weeks. This is followed by strapping and continued bracing. Both the Ponseti and the French "nonoperative" methods frequently employ Achilles tenotomy and, at times, tendon transfers to attain the ultimate desired result. Recurrences of deformity are common (16% to 37%), requiring further casting. A smaller percentage of patients (8% to 16%) require surgical release

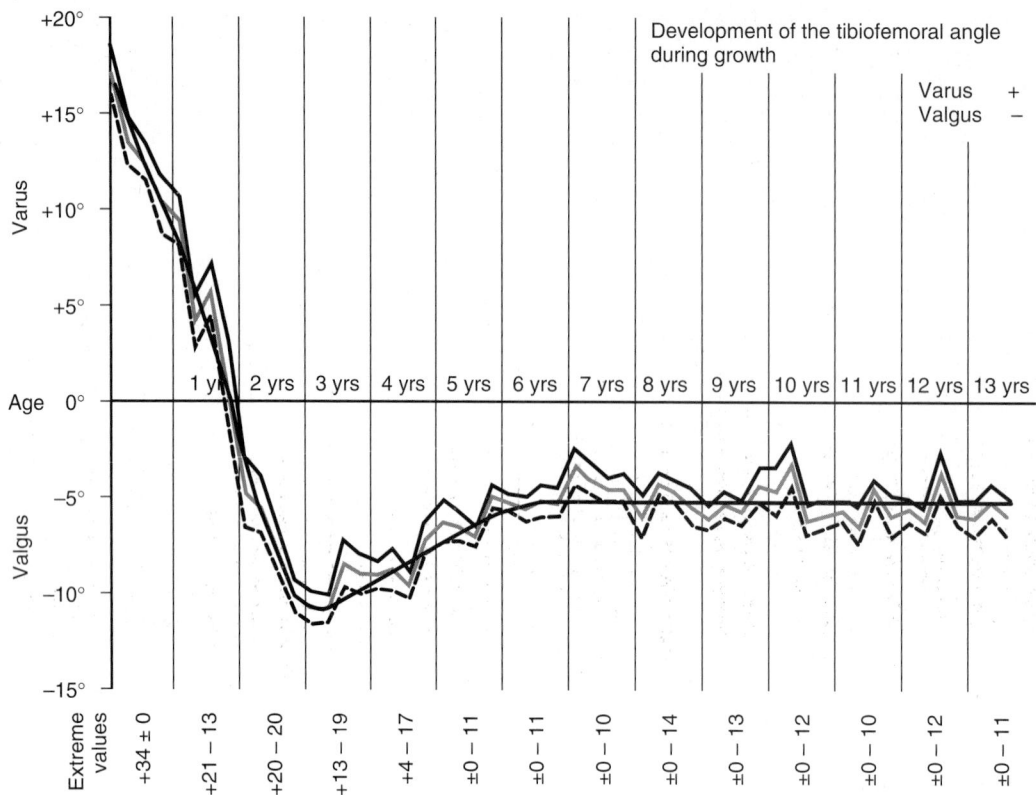

FIGURE 96-5 Development of the tibiofemoral angle during growth. *(Data from Salenius P, Vankka GK: The development of the tibiofemoral angle in children,* J Bone Joint Surg Am *57:259-261, 1975.)*

of the hindfoot to varying degrees (Faulks and Richards, 2009; Janicki et al, 2009).

With the Ponseti method, treatment is ideally commenced within the first few weeks of life, but successful treatment is commonly achieved when treatment is initiated up to 1 year of age (Dobbs, 2004). We prefer to initiate treatment after discharge from the hospital in most cases, allowing parental adjustment to the new child in their lives. Initial treatment usually consists of a manipulation and serial casting or taping program (Faulks and Richards, 2009; Janicki et al, 2009). In the Ponseti method, manipulation of the foot is carried out, and the correction is maintained with a long-leg cast. The casts are changed at 5- to 7-day intervals, with repeated manipulation and casting over 1 to 3 months, averaging four casts in the idiopathic clubfoot (Dobbs et al, 2006). This is followed by Achilles tenotomy in the majority of patients and 3 further weeks of casting. Children are then placed into a foot abduction orthosis full-time for a period of 3 months, and then part time, while sleeping, until approximately age 4 years.

ANGULAR DEFORMITIES OF THE LOWER EXTREMITIES

Torsional and angular deformities of the legs constitute the most frequent nontraumatic reason for referral to a children's orthopedist. Torsional deformities of the lower extremities rarely come to the attention of the physician before the child reaches walking age. Occasionally a neonate demonstrates bowing of the legs, or *genu varum*, of a

sufficient degree to concern parents or grandparents. The true incidence of genu varum is unknown, but based on our experience, it is extremely common. The overwhelming majority of cases of genu varum resolve spontaneously, with a small minority of affected children manifesting a pathologic condition.

The legs of most neonates are bowed. This results from a combination of an external rotation contracture of the hips and internal tibial torsion. The apex anterior bowing of the femora in conjunction with the external rotation contractures of both hips allow the femoral bowing to be seen tangentially when the baby is viewed from the front. These contractures may not resolve until after walking age. Internal tibial torsion is nearly universal in neonates and spontaneously resolves between 2 and 3 years of age. Internal tibial torsion imparts an appearance of bowing to the tibia. When tibial bowing is viewed in combination with the apparent femoral bowing, a striking amount of leg bowing may be present. This is often concerning to both parent and physician.

Genu varum is physiologic up to the age of 2 years. Salenius and Vankka (1975) documented the tibiofemoral angles both clinically and roentgenographically in 979 children on the basis of 1408 examinations between birth and 16 years of age. They noted that newborns demonstrate a mean varus alignment of 15 degrees, which increases and becomes maximal at 6 months of age and then decreases to neutral at approximately 18 months. The maximum valgus of 12 degrees is then achieved by 3 to 4 years. By age 7, normal adult valgus alignment is achieved (Figure 96-5). Natural history studies have demonstrated that physiologic genu varum is a self-limited process. Genu varum with angulation greater than 30 degrees has been shown to correct spontaneously with growth (Heath and Staheli, 1993).

Physical examination should include evaluation of the torsional profile (Staheli, 1977), which includes measurements of internal and external rotation of the hips and the thigh-foot angle. Measurement of the thigh-foot angle is performed with the child in the prone position and is an indicator of tibial torsion. The examiner should look for evidence of rhizomelic shortening, and genu varum, which may herald a diagnosis of achondroplasia or other skeletal dysplasia. Finally, note is made of whether onset of the varus of the lower extremities is gradual or abrupt. If it was abrupt, can the deformity be localized to the distal femur, the proximal tibia, or the midportion of the tibia? Considerations in the differential diagnosis of genu varum include focal fibrocartilage dysplasia, skeletal dysplasias such as achondroplasia, osteogenesis imperfecta, and metabolic bone disease such as vitamin D–resistant rickets, renal osteodystrophy, and tibia vara (infantile Blount disease). Blount disease does not occur before walking age, and most clinicians agree that this diagnosis cannot be made before 2 years of age.

Radiographs are indicated only with asymmetric deformities, with short stature, or in infants with progressive deformities. Photographs are the preferred method of follow-up evaluation for progression. Management of physiologic genu varum and tibial torsion consists of serial observation, reassurance, and parental education. Treatment with orthotics such as the Denis Browne splint is not indicated and in fact may be harmful to the ligaments of the knee.

Focal fibrocartilaginous dysplasia (FFD) involving the medial aspect of the proximal tibial metaphysis is a relatively rare cause of tibia vara in the newborn and infant. It was first reported in 1985 by Bell et al and continues to be recognized in scattered case reports. The pathophysiologic basis for the disease may be abnormal development of fibrocartilage at the insertion of the pes anserinus (sartorius, gracilis, and semitendinosus tendons). Children with FFD present before 1 year of age with unilateral bowing of the tibia that has prompted radiologic evaluation. The radiographs demonstrate a lytic defect in the proximal medial metaphysis of the tibia with surrounding sclerosis. The natural history of the deformity is that of progression until 2 years of age, with subsequent resolution by 4 years of age. During the progression, the deformity can become quite pronounced and unsettling. Up to 1 cm of tibial length discrepancy is likely. Use of orthotics is not indicated. Surgery is indicated only in patients older than 4 years without evidence of spontaneous resolution (Zayer, 1980).

Tibial bowing can be the cause of angular deformities in the shaft of the tibia. Two major types of bowing can be identified according to the direction of the apex of the bow. Posteromedial bowing has been previously described in conjunction with calcaneovalgus foot position in the neonate. Its etiology is unknown, but numerous hypotheses have been proffered, including intrauterine fracture with malunion and in utero malpositioning with subsequent growth retardation and soft tissue contractures (Thompson, 2001). The deformity is unilateral and evident at birth. There is an associated calcaneovalgus foot deformity. Other features include shortening of the tibia and a smaller calf circumference and smaller foot relative to the contralateral side. Frequently there is a dimple at the apex of the deformity. Radiographic examination of the entire extremity from hip to ankle should be performed. Radiographs demonstrate the degree of bowing well. Other radiographic findings include a normal proximal tibia with thickening and sclerosis of the diaphyseal cortices on the compression side of the deformity with obliteration of the intramedullary canal. There is no increased fracture risk associated with the deformity. Posteromedial bowing tends to resolve with growth, so that much of the deformity resolves by 2 years of age, with continued gradual correction beyond that. The shortening of the tibia and fibula persists, however, and progressively worsens during growth. Leg length inequality at skeletal maturity averages 4.1 cm (Hofmann and Wenger, 1981). Early referral to and serial follow-up assessments by a pediatric orthopedist are necessary to appropriately time epiphysiodesis surgery of the normal longer leg to allow for equal leg lengths at skeletal maturity. The foot deformity generally resolves by 9 to 12 months with stretching.

The second and most serious type of tibial bowing is anterolateral. It is usually identified at the newborn examination. It most frequently is associated with congenital pseudoarthrosis of the tibia but also can be associated with congenital longitudinal deficiency of the tibia or the fibula. Although its etiology is unknown, congenital pseudoarthrosis of the tibia is associated with neurofibromatosis (NF1) in 40% to 80% of cases (Masserman et al, 1974; Paterson, 1989; Thompson, 2001). It is arguably the most challenging congenital malformation to treat in orthopedics. It is estimated to occur in 1 in 140,000 live births (Crawford and Schorry, 1999). "Congenital pseudoarthrosis" implies that there is a nonunited fracture, which usually is not the case, so the term *congenital tibial dysplasia* (CTD) has been suggested (Crawford and Schorry, 1999). The newborn examination is notable for anterolateral bowing, which is unilateral. Other, cutaneous signs of NF1 may be evident. If they are not, NF1 should remain a consideration, because café au lait spots and other cutaneous manifestations may not be present in the newborn, and the child should be followed expectantly. If fracture has occurred, motion at the pseudoarthrosis site will be apparent. The foot may be normal or slightly small. The ankle may be in slight valgus to compensate for the bowing.

The natural history of congenital pseudoarthrosis of the tibia is that of fracture with nonunion and repeated surgical attempts at obtaining union. Most of these attempts fail; if one such procedure succeeds, however, repeat fracture is likely, and the cycle begins again. Frequently, amputation is the end result. Because of this possibility, efforts are best directed at prevention of initial fracture. Orthopedic consultation is imperative. In the preambulatory child, a total-contact (clamshell) ankle-foot orthosis should be fabricated and worn at all times except for bathing, to diminish the chance of fracture. When the child begins to walk, the orthosis may be extended above the knee with a drop-lock hinge to allow sitting. Bracing is continued until skeletal maturity is attained. Although definite proof that long-term bracing affects the natural history of this condition is lacking, most orthopedists consider that bracing is warranted. Under no circumstances should an osteotomy to correct the bowing of an unfractured tibia be undertaken because development of a pseudoarthrosis is likely to result.

Many treatment options exist once a documented pseudoarthrosis occurs. Long-term immobilization, external fixation, internal fixation, bone transport, bone grafting, microvascular bone transfer, and electrical stimulation have been attempted, all with a high incidence of failure (Crawford and Schorry, 1999). When union is achieved, there is concern over its quality and longevity. Amputation has been advocated as a salvage procedure after failed attempts at union and as primary treatment for the initial pseudoarthrosis (Jacobsen et al, 1983). Herring et al (1986) reported that children who underwent Symes amputation (none of whom had CTD as the surgical indication, however) had better psychological and orthopedic functioning than that described in children who underwent numerous corrective surgical procedures. Similar results were reported by other authors (Davidson and Bohne, 1975).

CONGENITAL VERTEBRAL MALFORMATIONS

Congenital vertebral malformations occur in 0.5 to 1 in 1000 live births. Although a minority of cases may be due to genetic inheritance, there are no established gene defects that solely account for these disorders. Syndromes associated with them include Klippel-Feil, Goldenhar's, and VATER (VACTERL) sequence. Likewise, many congenital vertebral malformations occur in isolation and may be due to intrauterine exposures such as hyperglycemia, carbon monoxide, or antiepileptic drugs. The ultimate concern with congenital vertebral anomalies is their potential to result in significant spinal deformity, namely scoliosis, kyphosis, or a combination of the two. Many, however, remain asymptomatic throughout life.

Defects can be attributed to a failure of formation, a failure of segmentation, or both. Failures of formation result from asymmetric vertebral body formation and ensuing development of a hemivertebra. Hemivertebrae can be incomplete, with partial retention of the affected side, or complete. When partial retention of the pedicle occurs, a wedge vertebra develops. Complete hemivertebra can be further categorized. Radiographically, the presence of open disk spaces signifies the presence of growth plates and therefore growth potential. Unsegmented hemivertebrae, in which the segment is fused to one or both adjacent vertebrae, have less growth potential and therefore less deformity potential. Fully segmented hemivertebrae retain full growth potential from both the cranial and caudal ends and consequently much greater propensity to result in significant deformity. Failures of segmentation are characterized by bony fusions (bars) between adjacent vertebrae. Bilateral bars result in "block vertebrae" that, because of their symmetry, have minimal potential for deformity.

The propensity to result in a clinically significant deformity depends on the location of the defect, the type of defect, and the age of the patient (Hedequist and Emans, 2007). Curves at the lumbrosacral and cervicothoracic junctions may result in more clinically apparent

deformities. Prediction of progression is largely driven by the presence of unbalanced defects. In order of severity, the risk of progression in congenital spinal deformities is associated with the following defects: unilateral bar with contralateral hemivertebra, unilateral bar, hemivertebra, wedge vertebra, and block vertebra. Additionally, the presence of multiple anomalies at multiple levels (e.g., multiple hemivertebra) can result in additional risk for progression when on the ipsilateral side or, conversely, may result in balanced growth when on contralateral sides of the spine.

All patients with known congenital spinal deformities should be evaluated for associated cardiac and renal anomalies. Cardiac anomalies are found in approximately 15% of these children and are usually clinically evident. Routine screening with an echocardiogram is not recommended unless clinical findings are suggestive (Prybis et al, 2007). Renal anomalies, on the other hand, are often clinically silent and have been reported in up to 37% of children with known congenital spinal anomalies (Riccio et al, 2007). Thus, routine sonography of the urinary tract system is recommended for all children with congenital spinal malformations.

Occult intraspinal anomalies are found in up to 30% of children with congenital spinal malformations. These include Chiari malformations, syringomyelia, tethered cord, reduced spinal cord diameter, or diastematomyelia. Associated physical examination findings are those consistent with occult dysraphism, such as dimpling of the skin, pigmentation changes, or the presence of hairy patches or skin tags in the lower back or intergluteal cleft. Changes to the lower extremities such as atrophy, foot deformities, and asymmetric or pathologic reflexes are also suggestive of intraspinal defects.

Infants with congenital spine anomalies should initially be evaluated with dedicated plain radiographs of the whole spine. Coned-down views of affected parts of the spine may offer additional information about the anatomy of interest. Rib anomalies should be noted, because they are commonly associated with thoracic spine malformations and may have significant long-term implications with regard to restrictive lung disease (Campbell and Hell-Vocke, 2003). The position of the scapula should also be evaluated, because Sprengel's deformity is found in up to 50% of children with congenital cervical spine anomalies (Hensinger et al, 1974). The use of magnetic resonance imaging is reserved for those children preparing to undergo surgical intervention or those with clinical evidence of neurologic abnormality (Hedequist and Emans, 2007). Cutaneous anomalies of the lumbar spine in the newborn may be evaluated by ultrasonography. This is a particularly effective method for determining the level of the conus medullaris and thus the presence of tethered cord. Computed tomography is typically not indicated in the newborn owing to concerns of unneeded radiation exposure, but if done for other reasons, it can give additional detail on spinal anatomy.

OBSTETRICAL TRAUMA

Birth trauma can be divided into two categories: fractures and neurologic injuries. *Birth fractures* most commonly involve the clavicle, with clavicular fractures occurring in 2 per 1000 to 35 per 1000 vaginal births (Cohen and Otto, 1980; Farkas and Levine, 1950; Kaplan et al, 1998; Sanford, 1931). Birth fractures also occur in the proximal humerus (Broker and Burbach, 1990; Fisher et al, 1995), the femur (0.13 per 1000 births) (Morris et al, 2002), and even the thoracic spine. It is important to note that clavicular fracture can be seen in combination with a proximal humeral physeal separation or in combination with a brachial plexus injury. Reported risk factors for upper extremity birth fractures include large size of the baby, limited experience of the obstetrician, and a midforceps delivery (Cohen and Otto, 1980); risk factors for femoral fracture include twin gestation, breech presentation, prematurity, and osteoporosis (Morris et al, 2002). Nadas et al (1993) have reported an association of long-bone fractures with cesarean section, breech delivery with assistance, and low birthweight. The natural history of isolated birth fractures to the extremities is that of uneventful rapid healing without untoward sequelae. Clavicle fractures may be difficult to diagnose, because the neonate may be asymptomatic. In a study of 300 newborns, radiographs revealed 5 unsuspected clavicle fractures (Farkas and Levine, 1950). Newborns with either a clavicle fracture or a proximal humeral physeal separation often present with pseudoparalysis of the upper extremity. Considerations in the differential diagnosis include an obstetric brachial plexus palsy and hematogenous metaphyseal osteomyelitis of the humerus with septic glenohumeral arthritis. Pain with direct palpation of the clavicle may be present with obvious deformity. Pain with motion of the shoulder joint and with palpation of the proximal humerus may be caused by either fracture or infection. Eliciting neonatal reflexes such as the Moro reflex and asymmetric tonic neck reflex (ATNR) may be helpful in evaluating active upper extremity muscle function (Sanford, 1931). Radiographs should be obtained. Ultrasound evaluation of the proximal humerus may be helpful because the proximal humeral epiphysis is entirely cartilaginous at birth and therefore radiolucent. Ultrasound examination can detect proximal physeal separation, metaphyseal osteomyelitis, and septic shoulder arthritis (Broker and Burbach, 1990; Fisher et al, 1995).

Asymptomatic birth fractures of the clavicle and humerus in neonates can be observed. The fracture will unite in short order, with remodeling of bone with growth. Symptomatic fractures in which the child exhibits pseudoparalysis of the upper extremity should be treated with 7 to 10 days of immobilization in a soft dressing or until symptoms subside. Femoral birth fractures can be treated with a Pavlik harness with good results (Morris et al, 2002). This device provides a simple means of immobilization that is accepted well by new parents. Excellent outcomes with no residual deformities or limb length inequalities can be expected.

The presence of multiple long-bone and rib fractures at birth may herald the presence of osteogenesis imperfecta (OI). Prenatal diagnosis is commonly made at ultrasonographic screening, as early as 13 to 14 weeks' gestation on the basis of deformity (Cheung and Glorieux, 2008). OI is typically classified by the Sillence classification, with OI type II and type III being the most common types identified in the perinatal period (Sillence et al, 1979). Type II OI is lethal in the neonatal period, whereas most

children with type III survive into adulthood with considerable short stature and fracture-related morbidity. Thus, prompt genetic consultation is critical to establish a diagnosis and prognosis for an affected child. Infants with type III OI often require substantial respiratory support and pain management because of rib fractures, with respiratory failure being identified as the most common cause of death in the neonatal period. Treatment of long fractures is primarily to support pain management and can be achieved by custom splints or merely soft supports, such as pillows or blankets. Patients with multiple fractures at birth who are expected to survive the neonatal period should be considered for bisphosphonate treatment (Shapiro and Sponsellor, 2009).

Brachial plexus injuries represent the second category of birth trauma afflicting newborns. The brachial plexus receives contributions from the anterior spinal nerve roots of C5 through T1. The various nerve roots combine to form trunks, which combine in turn to form divisions, which combine to form cords, which combine and divide to form the peripheral nerves that supply the motor innervation to the upper extremity. The mechanism of injury is a separation of the head from the shoulder by lateral bending of the neck with simultaneous shoulder depression during vaginal delivery resulting in a stretching of the brachial plexus. These injuries occur in 1 per 1000 to 4 per 1000 live births (Greenwald et al, 1984; Hardy, 1981). Obstetric brachial plexus palsies are most common in vertex deliveries with shoulder dystocia, in large-birthweight babies (in whom the increased size usually is secondary to maternal diabetes), and in multiparous pregnancies (Waters, 1997). It is rarely seen in cesarean section deliveries. Not all cases can be reliably predicted prepartum or prevented. Three major injuries are encountered. The most frequent injury is to the upper trunk that involves the C5 and C6 nerve roots primarily and results in an *Erb's palsy*. Affected infants lack external rotation and abduction of the shoulder. Hand function is preserved. The next most frequently occurring injury is a *global plexus palsy* involving the C5 through T1 nerve roots. This results in flaccid paralysis of the involved upper extremity, including the hand. An isolated lower plexus injury involving the C8 and T1 nerve roots, termed *Klumpke's palsy*, is the least common and may be a manifestation of a recovered global plexus injury (Waters, 1997).

The physical examination has proved to be the most reliable method of assessing the level and severity of the neural injury and thereby predicting the potential for spontaneous recovery (Noetzel et al, 2001; Waters, 1997). Myelography, computed tomographic myelography, magnetic resonance imaging, and electrodiagnostic studies have not proved useful in predicting recovery (Waters, 1997). Active shoulder, elbow, wrist, and finger motion need to be assessed. Frequently, such assessment can be facilitated by eliciting some primitive reflexes that are transiently present in normal newborns. The *hand grasp reflex* is normal in all newborns and disappears between 2 and 4 months. The examiner's little finger is placed on the ulnar aspect of the infant's palm, and the infant's fingers reflexively flex and grasp the examiner's finger. The *Moro reflex* begins to fade at 3 months of age. It is elicited by holding the newborn's hands while raising the baby off the table and then suddenly releasing them. In response, the newborn extends the spine, abducts and extends all four limbs and digits, and then subsequently adducts and flexes the limbs and digits. Last, the ATNR, or *fencing reflex*, can be elicited in a normal newborn until the age of 4 months. With the infant lying supine on an examining table, the head is rotated to one side by the examiner. The infant should respond by extending the elbow on the side toward which the face is looking and by flexing the opposite elbow. In newborns with a brachial plexus injury, some of these reflexes will be abnormal because of lack of motor control. For instance, the newborn with an Erb's palsy will, most notably, not be able to actively flex at the elbow during the ATNR or the Moro. The presence or absence of Horner's syndrome also must be noted. The infant needs repeat serial examinations until 6 months of age.

Return of biceps function by 3 months is the most important indicator of brachial plexus recovery (Michelow et al, 1994). When biceps recovery is combined with the return of shoulder abduction, wrist extension, and finger extension, there is a 95% chance of normal function (Michelow et al, 1994). When biceps function recovers later than 3 months, it is rare for the child to have complete recovery of normal function (Waters, 1999). A total plexus palsy or the presence of Horner's syndrome also heralds a poor prognosis (Michelow et al, 1994; Waters, 1997). In one study of 142 patients with obstetric brachial plexus palsies, 50% demonstrated biceps recovery by 6 weeks, with the remainder demonstrating recovery at varying intervals beyond 6 weeks. At final follow-up evaluation, 67% had excellent shoulder function, 12% good, 5% fair, and 10% poor (Benson et al, 1996). In a similar prospective study, Waters (1999) found that 22 patients of 66 studied had return of biceps function by 3 months. Each of these went on to have normal function. Infants in whom recovery was delayed until the 4th to 6th month had significantly worse function.

The initial treatment for obstetric brachial plexus injury is aimed at avoiding contractures of the shoulder, elbow, forearm, and hand during the observation-for-recovery phase. Secondary treatment involves nerve repair and grafts to restore neurologic function that will not recover spontaneously. Finally, augmenting weak muscles, improving functional ranges of motion, and improving the appearance of residual deformities should be undertaken in children without full neurologic recovery.

Each neonate with an obstetric brachial plexus birth palsy must be referred to a pediatric orthopedist or upper extremity surgeon for early evaluation. Referral to a qualified therapist for passive range of motion exercises also is suggested. Monthly examinations by the orthopedist are undertaken. Brachial plexus exploration with subsequent reconstruction is indicated for infants with total plexus involvement, Horner syndrome, and no return of biceps function at 3 months, and for infants with a C5 to C6 (Erb's) plexopathy and no return of biceps function at 3 to 6 months (Waters, 1997). Surgery is undertaken between 3 and 6 months of age. Using this algorithm prospectively, Waters (1999) operated on 6 infants at 6 months and found that their results were better than those for the 15 patients with biceps recovery at 5 months but worse than those for the 11 patients with biceps recovery at 4 months. Despite treatment as outlined, some children

will have residual deficits. Secondary reconstruction, for chronic brachial plexopathy resulting in a dysfunctional shoulder, can be achieved with a tendon transfer of the latissimus dorsi and teres major to the rotator cuff, or by derotational osteotomy of the humerus. These procedures and others designed to correct limitations in hand and forearm function are undertaken after the true scope of the disability has been assessed.

NEONATAL OSTEOMYELITIS AND SEPTIC ARTHRITIS

Osteomyelitis refers to a bacterial infection of bone, and *septic arthritis* is a pyogenic infection of a diarthrodial joint. Incidence rates of 0.12 per 1000 live births and 0.67 per 1000 neonatal intensive care unit (NICU) admissions (Ho et al, 1989) have been reported for septic arthritis. The mortality rate is reported to be 7.3% (Caksen et al, 2000). The hip, knee, and shoulder joints are involved most frequently. Neonates are particularly susceptible to osteomyelitis and septic arthritis, because of an immature immune response resulting in vulnerability to organisms that are not ordinarily virulent in infants and children, and a delay in expressing the classic physical findings associated with these conditions (Morrissy, 2001). Two subgroups of neonates are affected: premature neonates requiring prolonged hospitalization and otherwise healthy newborns who present within 2 to 4 weeks of discharge (Morrissy, 2001).

Most cases of neonatal osteomyelitis and septic arthritis result from hematogenous spread, but some occur from direct inoculation during percutaneous arterial blood sampling (especially from the femoral artery). Acute hematogenous osteomyelitis (AHO) and septic arthritis in hospitalized neonates usually occur in premature infants undergoing frequent blood drawing, invasive monitoring, intravenous feedings, and intravenous drug administration, especially in those with indwelling umbilical vessel catheters (Lim et al, 1977). These infections are frequently caused by *Staphylococcus aureus* or gram-negative organisms (10% to 15%). Up to 40% of these patients may demonstrate multiple areas of involvement characterized by swelling and tenderness and are systemically ill (Bergdahl et al, 1985; Fox and Sprunt, 1978). This contrasts with the typical out-of-hospital newborn with AHO and septic arthritis, who presents in weeks 2 to 4 of life with swelling, pseudoparalysis, and tenderness of the extremity and who feeds well and is not systemically ill (Morrissy, 2001). *S. aureus* and group B streptococci are the most common organisms encountered in this latter population.

Because of the immature immune response, neonates with AHO and septic arthritis frequently do not demonstrate fever, leukocytosis, or elevation in their erythrocyte sedimentation rates (Scott et al, 1990). However, C-reactive protein appears to be a reasonable indicator of AHO and septic arthritis (Pulliam et al, 2001; Unkila-Kallio et al, 1994). Blood cultures are positive in only 50% of patients; cultures of synovial aspirates identify an organism in only 30% (Lyon and Evanich, 1999). Plain radiographs demonstrate soft tissue swelling by 3 days, but bone changes are not present for a week after the onset of symptoms (Dormans and Drummond, 1994; Jackson and

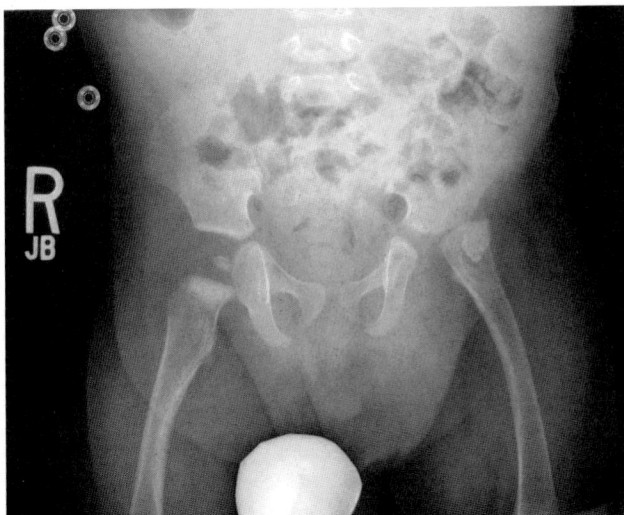

FIGURE 96-6 Unrecognized neonatal hip sepsis can result in complete dissolution of the femoral head as demonstrated in this child's left hip radiograph. This is a devastating complication, in which reconstructive options are limited.

common sites of neonatal septic arthritis, have intraarticular metaphyses, allowing for a subperiosteal route of decompression for pus into the joint. Because of this unique ability to spread from the metaphysis through the growth plate into the joint, early detection and treatment are necessary to avoid permanent damage to each of these structures. The proteolytic enzymes released by the host response to infection can result in destruction of the growth cartilage and articular cartilage in short order, resulting in growth disturbances and precocious arthritis. When an area of involvement is suspected, aspiration should be undertaken (Morrissy, 2001). This may confirm the diagnosis and provide fluid for Gram stain and culture in order to better direct treatment. If pus is discovered in the neonate, surgical debridement in the operating room is required (Figure 96-6).

Nelson, 1982). Bone scan is positive in only 32% of foci of osteomyelitis in neonates due to the usual location of infection near the growth plate (Ash and Gilday, 1980). Ultrasound examination has been advocated as a useful method for the diagnosis and assessment of osteomyelitis (Mah et al, 1994) and is our preferred radiologic method for evaluating the neonate with suspected AHO and/or septic arthritis.

AHO and septic arthritis coexist in up to 76% of neonates as a result of the unique blood supply of the chondroepiphysis (Bergdahl et al, 1985; Fox and Sprunt, 1978), which changes with growth. Infection begins in the metaphyseal veins. Vascular canals traverse the growth plate in the neonate, allowing for rapid spreading of the infection to the cartilaginous chondroepiphysis with subsequent abscess formation. These abscesses frequently rupture into the joint (Ogden, 1979). The growth plate becomes a barrier to the spread of infection in the older child. Additionally, the hip and shoulder, two of the more

SUGGESTED READINGS

American Academy of Pediatrics Subcommittee on Developmental Dysplasia of the Hip: Committee on Quality Improvement: Clinical practice guideline: early detection of developmental dysplasia of the hip, *Pediatrics* 105:896-905, 2000.

Cheng JC, Wong MW, Tang SP, et al: Clinical determinants in the outcome of manual stretching in the treatment of congenital muscular torticollis in infants: a prospective study of 821 cases, *J Bone Joint Surg Am* 83:679-687, 2001.

Cheung MS, Glorieux FH: Osteogenesis imperfecta: update on presentation and management, *Rev Endocr Metab Disord* 9:153-160, 2008.

Davids JR, Wenger DR, Mubarak SJ: Congenital muscular torticollis: sequela of intrauterine or perinatal compartment syndrome, *J Pediatr Orthop* 13:141-147, 1993.

Dobbs MB, Purcell DB, Nunley R, Morcuende JA: Early results of a new method of treatment for idiopathic congenital vertical talus, *J Bone Joint Surg Am* 88:1192-1200, 2006.

Farsetti P, Weinstein SL, Ponseti IV: The long-term functional and radiographic outcomes of untreated and non-operatively treated metatarsus adductus, *J Bone Joint Surg Am* 76:257-265, 1994.

Faulks S, Richards BS: Clubfoot treatment: Ponseti and French functional methods are equally effective, *Clin Orthop Relat Res* 467:1278-1282, 2009.

Hedequist D, Emans J: Congenital scoliosis: a review and update, *J Pediatr Orthop* 27:106-116, 2007.

Salenius P, Vankka GK: The development of the tibio-femoral angle in children, *J Bone Joint Surg Am* 57:259-261, 1975.

Staheli LT: Torsional deformity, *Pediatr Clin North Am* 24:799-811, 1977.

Viere RG, Birch JG, Herring JA, et al: Use of the Pavlik harness in congenital dislocation of the hip. An analysis of failures of treatment, *J Bone Joint Surg Am* 72:238-244, 1990.

Waters PM: Comparison of the natural history, the outcome of microsurgical repair, and the outcome of operative reconstruction in brachial plexus birth palsy, *J Bone Joint Surg Am* 81:649-659, 1999.

Complete references used in this text can be found online at www.expertconsult.com

PART XX

DERMATOLOGIC CONDITIONS

CHAPTER 97

NEWBORN SKIN: DEVELOPMENT AND BASIC CONCEPTS

Bernard A. Cohen and Katherine B. Püttgen

SKIN DEVELOPMENT

Skin is the interface between an organism and its environment. It plays an important role in fluid balance and temperature regulation and provides a barrier against invading microbes and systemic absorption of topically applied agents. This chapter provides an overview of skin development. Emphasis is placed on factors that influence the clinical management of premature infants and the prenatal diagnosis of heritable skin diseases.

The study of skin ontogenesis has been organized primarily on the basis of the development of individual components: epidermis, basement membrane zone, dermis, immigrant cells, and appendageal structures. However, the initiation, differentiation, and growth of all of its components are intimately related. Prenatal skin biopsy for early diagnosis of severe genodermatoses is a useful procedure that depends on precise knowledge of the details of skin development. Disorders of keratinization, basement membrane integrity, melanocytes, and epidermal appendages have been detected as early as 16 weeks' gestation using this technique. In turn, fetal skin biopsy has helped to further clarify the details of epidermal development (Holbrook, 1991; Holbrook et al, 1993). Recent discoveries of genetic markers for many genodermatoses have also allowed for rapid and precise prenatal and neonatal diagnoses, and they have added to the understanding of molecular mechanisms of disease.

EPIDERMIS

The epidermis consists of ectodermally derived, stratified squamous cells with localized proliferations that form the appendages: hair follicles, sebaceous glands, eccrine sweat glands, apocrine glands, and the nail matrix. Melanocytes migrate into the epidermis from the neural crest, and Langerhans cells migrate from mesoderm. The epidermis forms initially as a single layer of indifferent ectoderm and then differentiates into two layers of epidermal cells by 6 weeks' gestation. The outermost layer, called *periderm*, covers the basal layer stem cells. During the next 2 weeks, the basal cells give rise to an intermediate layer beneath the periderm. By 8 weeks' gestation, epithelial cells are capable of expressing keratins, the major cytoskeletal proteins of the epidermis. K5 and K14 are the high-molecular-weight keratins expressed primarily by basal-layer cells, whereas intermediate-layer cells express K1 and K10 (Smack et al,

1994). Genetic abnormalities of these cytoskeletal components give rise to a spectrum of inherited scaling skin diseases that can be diagnosed by detection of specific genetic mutations and characteristic features on histologic examination and electron microscopy of skin specimens obtained by fetal skin biopsy, amniocentesis, and chorionic villus biopsy.

The 3rd month of gestation is an important period in skin development. Differentiation of the epidermis begins as two or three more layers of intermediate cells are added between the basal cells and periderm, while coordinated maturation progresses within other strata of the skin. By 22 to 24 weeks' gestation, granular cells have formed beneath the periderm. Granular cells are named for their prominent organelles, the keratohyalin granules. These granules contain a high-molecular-weight protein called *profilaggrin*, which has a crucial role in terminal differentiation of keratinocytes in the stratum corneum. Cornified cells first appear within the pilosebaceous follicle as early as 15 weeks' gestation. Interfollicular keratinization follows at 24 to 26 weeks' gestation. At 28 weeks' gestation the stratum corneum consists of two or three cell layers. By 32 weeks' gestation there are more than 15 layers of corneocytes, equivalent to that of adult skin (Holbrook, 1991).

BASEMENT MEMBRANE ZONE

Components of the basement membrane zone appear with the first epidermal cells at 35 days' gestation. Important components of the dermoepidermal junction, such as hemidesmosomes, anchoring filaments, and anchoring fibrils, are completely formed by 8 to 10 weeks' gestation. The epidermis and basement membrane generally are flat during fetal development. The undulating rete ridges that expand the surface area of the dermoepidermal junction do not appear until the third trimester and are not fully developed until 6 months after birth, which coincides with the accumulation of dermal matrix (Holbrook, 1991).

DERMIS

A network of stellate mesodermal cells is present beneath the epidermis of a 1- to 2-month embryo. The primary matrix secreted by these cells is composed of glycosaminoglycans. Hyaluronic acid is the predominant glycosaminoglycan during the first trimester. Matrix proteins also are synthesized in the first trimester, including immature fibers resembling elastin and collagen types I, III, V, and VI. Type III and type V collagens are increased in quantity compared with adult dermis. In the 3rd month, the dermis is transformed from a cellular to a fibrous tissue, which coincides with epidermal differentiation. During months 3 to 5, the size and quantity of the matrix proteins increase, and the composition of the glycosaminoglycans changes. Immigrant cells, including Schwann cells, Merkel cells, melanoblasts, pericytes, and mast cells, are found in the dermis by the 5th month. The dermis continues to mature for approximately 6 months postnatally (Holbrook, 1991).

IMMIGRANT CELLS

Melanocytes from the neural crest and mesenchymally derived Langerhans cells migrate to the epidermis by week 8, but do not develop their characteristic organelles until after 65 days' gestation. Melanin production and transfer to adjacent keratinocytes occurs during the fourth to the fifth months, but melanin production is relatively low, even at birth. The antigen-presenting function of Langerhans cells has not been documented in utero (Holbrook, 1991).

EPIDERMAL APPENDAGES

Primordia of hair follicles, apocrine glands, eccrine sweat glands, and nails first appear at 10 to 12 weeks' gestation. The pilosebaceous unit is formed, hair is keratinized, and sebum is synthesized as early as 16 to 18 weeks' gestation. Sebum production and secretion are greatly increased in the third trimester under the influence of fetal and maternal androgens. The number of lipid-filled sebocytes in amniotic fluid has been used to assess fetal maturity. Sebaceous lipids, squalane, and wax esters constitute most of the vernix caseosa, especially in male infants. The vernix of female infants has a slightly higher proportion of cholesterol and cholesterol esters, which are lipids derived from keratinocytes (Holbrook, 1991; Nazzaro-Porro et al, 1979). Apocrine gland formation follows that of the sebaceous glands by 8 weeks' gestation. Apocrine secretion has been detected during the third trimester but not in the neonatal period. The palmoplantar eccrine sweat ducts are the first portion of the apparatus to develop. By 22 weeks' gestation, they open to the skin surface and join the differentiated secretory cells of the eccrine sweat gland. Maturation of the eccrine apparatus elsewhere on the body follows at 24 to 26 weeks' gestation. Neither the morphology of the glandular coil cells nor eccrine gland function is fully developed in the premature infant, but the full complement of the sweat glands and hair follicles is completely formed in utero, making them more densely distributed in infant than in adult skin. However, even in the full-term infant, thermal stress–induced sweating requires a greater stimulus than is needed to induce sweating in older children and adults. This functional response to heat improves with postnatal age (Green and Behrendt, 1973; Harpin and Rutter, 1982). Nail primordia begin to form at 8 to 10 weeks' gestation. Nail plate formation is

initiated at 17 weeks' gestation and is complete by the 5th month (Holbrook, 1991).

FETAL SKIN: WOUND HEALING

Human fetal skin wounds reportedly heal without scarring. This clinical observation, first made by surgeons who were pioneering antenatal diagnosis and treatment, has been followed by an explosion of experimental data elucidating the unique aspects of fetal wound healing (Buchanan et al, 2009; Coolen et al, 2010; Dostal and Gamelli, 1993; Longaker and Adzick, 1991; Mast et al, 1992). Wound healing in the fetus differs from that in the adult in several ways, including nature of tissue environment, inflammatory response, and components of the dermal extracellular matrix (Table 97-1). Wounds can cause scars in some human infants (Cartlidge et al, 1990; Den Ouden et al, 1986), but prospective examination of sternotomy scars (Lista and Thomson, 1988) and bacille Calmette-Guérin vaccination sites (Sivarajah et al, 1990) in children found a direct correlation between increasing age and more prominent scarring.

NEWBORN SKIN

The most clinically significant difference between the skin of premature and term infants is in the structure of the stratum corneum. Infants born before 32 weeks' gestation have a thin stratum corneum, which gives rise to a variety of problems (Rutter, 1988). The primary functions of the stratum corneum are conservation of body water and barrier protection. In premature infants the stratum corneum does not effectively prevent transepidermal water loss, percutaneous absorption of exogenously applied compounds, or invasion of microbes. In the dry postnatal environment, the premature infant experiences excessive losses of body fluid and heat (Baumgart, 1982; Rutter and Hull, 1979; Shwayder and Akland, 2005). A variety of seemingly benign clinical interventions can dramatically increase these losses. Desiccated skin is even more easily injured, providing a portal of entry for invading microbes and increasing the risk of disseminated infection (Baumgart, 1982; Gunnar et al, 1985; Harper and Rutter, 1983; Rosen et al, 1995; Rutter, 1988). A premature infant's increased ratio of body surface area to body weight, diminished metabolic capacity, and decreased immune responses compound these problems.

TABLE 97-1   Comparison of Fetal and Adult Wound Repair

Feature	Fetus (<24 wk old)	Adult
Tissue environment	Amniotic fluid rich in growth factors and hyaluronic acid, relative hypoxemia, sterile	Air
Inflammatory infiltrate	Limited neutrophils and lymphocytes predominate	Macrophages predominate
Extracellular matrix	Nonexcessive deposition of types III and V collagen organized into a reticular pattern; increased amount of hyaluronic acid	Abundant type I collagen deposited into disorganized bundles

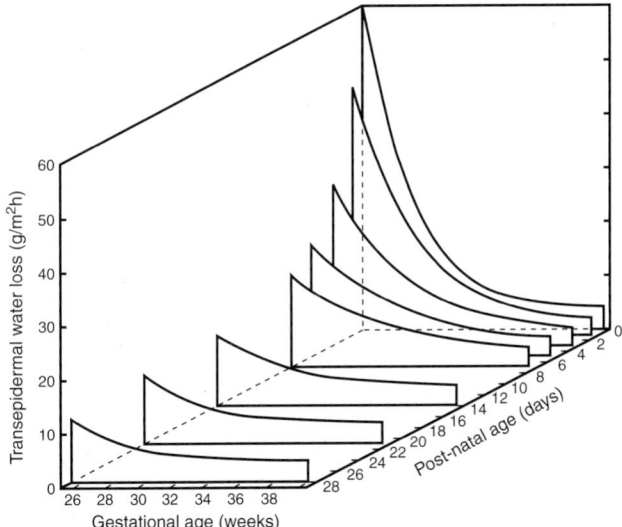

FIGURE 97-1 Transepidermal water loss in relation to gestational age at different postnatal ages in appropriate-for-gestational-age infants. *(From Hammarlund K, Sedin G, Stromberg B: Transepidermal water loss in newborn infants: VIII. Relation to gestational age and postnatal age in appropriate and small for gestational age infants,* Acta Paediatr Scand 72:721, *1983.)*

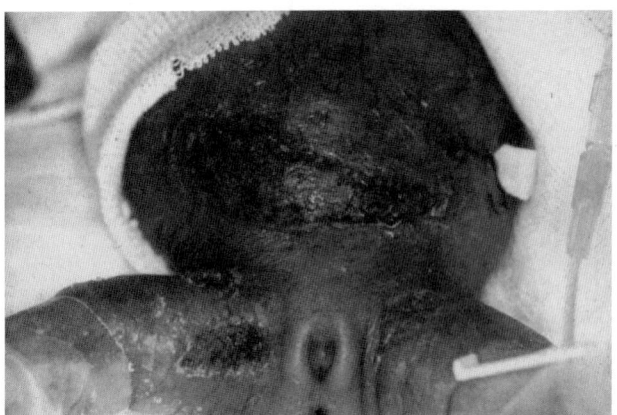

FIGURE 97-2 The cause of this full-thickness skin injury in a 26-week-old infant was innocuous enough to elude identification.

Rates of transepidermal water loss (TEWL) are objective measures of stratum corneum integrity. TEWL has been well studied in premature infants, using the evaporimeter, which provides direct measurements (Gunnar et al, 1985; Nonato and Lund, 2001). During the first 4 weeks after birth, there is an exponential relationship between TEWL and gestational age in appropriate-for-gestational-age (AGA) infants. TEWL is up to 15-fold higher in 1-day-old infants born at 25 weeks' gestation than in term neonates. In very low-birthweight infants, this TEWL can translate into a fluid loss of up to 30% of total body weight in 24 hours. As the stratum corneum develops, TEWL gradually decreases, but at 4 weeks after gestation, TEWL from an infant born at 26 weeks' gestation is still twice that of a term infant (Figure 97-1).

Loss of body water is accompanied by evaporative heat loss at a rate of 2.4×10^3 J/g (or 576 calories of body heat for every milliliter of water) (Hammarlund and Sedin, 1982; Smack et al, 1994). Evaporative losses are greatest in younger, more premature infants. Routine clinical interventions can exacerbate TEWL. Maintaining normal body temperature on an open radiant warmer bed in a nursery with low ambient humidity results in high evaporative loss of body water and heat (LeBlanc, 1991). Higher ambient temperatures are required to maintain normal body temperature under these conditions (Hammarlund and Sedin, 1982; Shwayder and Akland, 2005).

Traditional efforts to minimize these losses have centered on intravascular fluid replacement and modification of the infant's hospital bed. These approaches have inherent problems. Evaporative losses originate as free water from the extracellular compartment. Replacement has been conventionally determined by calculation based on standardized maintenance fluid requirements and measured changes of body weight and extracellular electrolytes, which have a typical lag time of several hours. Replacement fluids given in the form of isotonic

intravenous solutions can result in sodium and glucose overload. Enclosed incubators with high ambient humidity carry a risk of colonization with pathogenic bacteria, although an increased incidence of infection has not been documented (LeBlanc, 1991). Shielding devices used on open radiant warmer beds limit access to infants. Furthermore, some materials used for shielding (e.g., glass, Plexiglas, Lucite, Perspex) absorb infrared energy and block overhead transmission of heat to the infant (Baumgart, 1990; LeBlanc, 1991) (see Chapter 30). Pure polyethylene plastic wraps (e.g., GLAD Wrap) are transparent to infrared heat, but plastic wrap made of more complex polymers can retain heat and have the potential to burn contacted skin (LeBlanc, 1991). More recent data have focused on limiting skin injury and developing methods to improve the cutaneous barrier.

Clinically occult skin injury accompanies routine care. Skin stripping by removal of adhesive-backed products causes acute injury as well as the potential for secondary infection and significant scarring (Baharestani, 2007; Cartlidge et al, 1990). Removal of a piece of tape or an adhesive-backed electrode will markedly compromise the stratum corneum (Cartlidge and Rutter, 1987; Harper and Rutter, 1983), an observation that has been used in a positive way to facilitate transcutaneous monitoring of serum glucose in newborns (De Boer et al, 1994). There have been several cases of full-thickness skin injuries from presumed innocuous local application of pressure or thermal heat (Figure 97-2). The precise causes of this type of wound are often difficult to identify and remain unreported. Ultraviolet light burns have occurred in association with white-light phototherapy for jaundice, from relatively limited inadvertent exposure to near-ultraviolet A (UVA) light, which is 1000 times less erythemogenic than ultraviolet B light (Siegfried et al, 1992). A Plexiglas safety shield, placed in front of daylight fluorescent bulbs, will filter out the ultraviolet A light. However, white-light phototherapy also is a source of infrared heat, and heat stress will exacerbate TEWL. In contrast, phototherapy delivered with blue light alone does not increase TEWL (see Chapter 79) (Kjartansson et al, 1992).

Increased percutaneous absorption of topically applied compounds through an immature stratum corneum has been both advantageous and hazardous to neonates, although there has been little research on this topic in the past decade (Spray and Siegfried, 2001). A finding described in 1971 as "raccoon facies" is a visible periorbital ring of pallor from cutaneous vasoconstriction after the application of phenylephrine eye drops (Rutter, 1987). This effect can be quantified and is directly proportional to measurements of TEWL. Both methods have been established as useful markers of stratum corneum integrity in infants (Plantin et al, 1992; Rutter, 1987). Transdermal delivery may be the optimal route of administration for theophylline (Cartwright et al, 1990; Rutter, 1987) and diamorphine (Barrett et al, 1993) in premature infants. Lidocaine applied topically to premature skin probably is much more effective than after application to mature skin (Barrett and Rutter, 1994). Supplemental oxygen has been administered percutaneously to very small preterm infants with poor pulmonary function (Cartlidge and Rutter, 1988a, 1988b).

In contradistinction, numerous reports have described percutaneous toxicity in infants caused by absorption of topically applied agents (Lane, 1987; Rutter, 1987). Published accounts serve to document the most severe cases of toxicity, often manifested as nursery epidemics of obvious clinical signs or deaths (Table 97-2). The potential for subclinical toxicity must be considered by everyone caring for small newborns (Table 97-3). When several topical therapeutic options are available, the one with the least potential for toxicity should be used. *Poisindex* is an extensive, frequently updated, computer-based reference source for the identification of potentially toxic compounds (Micromedex, 2002). The information from this database and current published literature indicates a lower risk of

percutaneous or systemic toxicity from chlorhexidine skin antisepsis than from povidone-iodine.

The important role of nutrition in skin maturation and wound healing can be overlooked in small, sick infants who receive maintenance nutrition with varying amounts of complex parenteral fluids. Acquired deficiencies and those resulting from inborn errors of metabolism (Table 97-4) are associated with classic cutaneous findings. Deficiencies of protein, essential fatty acids, zinc, biotin, vitamins A and C, and several B vitamins are possible. Daily requirements for most of these nutrients are higher in premature than in term infants (Table 97-5).

Attention to skin integrity will help to control translocation of water through the skin of premature neonates. Appropriate hydration of keratinocytes is essential for normal skin maturation (Rawlings et al, 1994), an optimized barrier against exogenous assault, and maintenance of thermal, fluid, and electrolyte balance. A successful basic skin care regimen should also allow easy access to and handling of infants. Therapeutic goals include minimizing postnatal trauma and providing an artificial barrier until the stratum corneum matures. Currently there is no uniformly defined or accepted standard of care for the skin of premature infants. Formal clinical investigation has been limited. A few studies have verified the safety and efficacy of semiocclusive, adhesive-backed polyurethane membrane barriers in preventing fluid losses (Barak et al, 1989; Knauth et al, 1989; Mancini et al, 1994; Vernon et al, 1990). However, these dressings are not widely used because they are difficult to apply and are thought to limit available area for surface monitors. Neonatal intensive care unit staff members often provide

TABLE 97-2 Reported Hazards of Percutaneous Absorption in the Newborn

Compound	Reference	Product	Toxicity
Aniline	Rutter, 1987	Dye used as a laundry marker	Methemoglobinemia,* death
Mercury	Dinehart et al, 1988	Diaper rinses, teething powders	Rash, hypotonia
Phenolic Compounds			
Pentachlorophenol	West et al, 1981	Laundry disinfectant	Tachycardia, sweating, hepatomegaly, metabolic acidosis, death
Hexachlorophene	—	Topical antiseptic (pHisoHex)	Vacuolar encephalopathy, death
Resorcinol	West et al, 1981	Topical antiseptic	Methemoglobinemia*
Boric acid	Goldbloom and Goldbloom, 1953	Baby powder	Vomiting, diarrhea, erythroderma, seizures, death
Lindane	Rutter, 1987; West et al, 1981	Scabicide	Neurotoxicity
Salicylic acid	Abidel-Magid and El Awad Ahmed, 1994; West et al, 1981	Keratolytic emollient	Metabolic acidosis, salicylism
Isopropyl alcohol (underocclusion)	Rutter, 1987	Topical antiseptic	Cutaneous hemorrhagic necrosis
Silver sulfadiazine	Payne et al, 1992	Topical antibiotic (Silvadene)	Kernicterus (sulfa component), argyria (silver component)
Povidine-iodine	Rutter, 1987; West et al, 1981	Topical antiseptic (Betadine)	Hypothyroidism, goiter
Neomycin	Rutter, 1987	Topical antibiotic	Neural deafness
Corticosteroids	Rutter, 1987; West et al, 1981	Topical antiinflammatory (Lotrisone)	Skin atrophy, adrenal suppression
Benzocaine	Gelman et al, 1996	Mucosal anesthetic (teething products)	Methemoglobinemia*
Prilocaine	Frayling et al, 1990; Reynolds, 1996	Epidermal anesthetic (EMLA)	Methemoglobinemia*

*Heritable glucose-6-phosphate deficiencies are associated with an increased susceptibility to methemoglobinemia, as is coadministration of several drugs such as sulfonamides, acetaminophen, nitroprusside, phenobarbital, and phenytoin.

topical emollient therapy to infants in a random way. The risks and benefits of the use of commercially available topical emollients have not been well defined. Concerns include the risk of systemic absorption and resulting toxicity, overgrowth of microbes, and secondary heat accumulation that could increase surface and core temperature.

There have been many studies of the mechanism of action and benefits of emollients on injured and diseased skin in adults. Petroleum wax–based ointment emollients (e.g., Vaseline petroleum jelly) act primarily by decreasing TEWL and accelerating barrier recovery (Ghadially and Elias, 1992). Some oils, such as safflower oil, contain essential fatty acids, which greatly influence cutaneous structure and function (Schurer et al, 1991; Ziboh and Chapkin, 1987). However, topical application of safflower oil does not prevent essential fatty acid deficiencies in preterm infants (Lee et al, 1993). Oils, oil- and water-based creams, and lotion emollients have greater tactile acceptance than has been identified for greasy ointments. However, these preparations provide a less effective moisture barrier than is conferred by ointment emollients (Lane and Drost, 1993). In addition, formulation of a cream or lotion emulsion requires the addition of several potentially irritating or toxic ingredients. Eucerin Creme is an emollient that has been studied for use in the nursery (Lane and Drost, 1993). It contains water, petrolatum, mineral oil, ceresin, lanolin alcohol, and methylchloroisothiazolinone/methylisothiazolinone (CMI/MI). Although susceptibility of premature infants to allergic contact sensitization is unknown, CMI/MI has been associated with allergic contact sensitization in up to 10% of exposed adults (Frosch et al, 1994). Aquaphor ointment contains essentially two ingredients: petrolatum in ointment—liquid (mineral oil) and solid (mineral wax) phases—and wool wax alcohol. One study documented that application of Aquaphor every 12 hours reduced TEWL, improved skin integrity, did not alter skin flora, and was associated with a significant reduction of the incidence of sepsis. No adverse effects were reported (Nopper et al, 1994). Skin surface temperature was stable, and there was no evidence of hyperthermia or burns after

application of the petroleum-based emollient used under infrared warmers, even in infants receiving concomitant white-light phototherapy, confirming the results of a previous pilot study (Shwayder and Hetzel, 1989). These findings were also corroborated by Pabst et al (1999) in their study of 19 infants between 26 and 30 weeks' gestational age. Recent studies have confirmed the effectiveness and safety of topical emollients in the management of skin integrity of premature infants (Brandon et al, 2010). This study also showed that a novel noncytotoxic liquid film was as effective as the emollients, but with less manipulation of infant skin. Ahmed et al (2007) showed that inexpensive oils used on neonatal skin in the developing world may be as safe and useful as proprietary products marketed in North America and Europe. Increased understanding of the mechanisms contributing to skin development may one day provide therapy to accelerate barrier maturation in very premature infants. Until that time, therapy should be directed toward providing a safe, temporary barrier and minimizing additional skin injury. Proposed recommendations for newborn skin care are outlined in Box 97-1. A summary of dressing materials is outlined in Table 97-6.

DIFFERENTIAL DIAGNOSIS BY CUTANEOUS MORPHOLOGY

Diagnosis of skin disease is based on recognition of definitive morphology of the cutaneous examination. Dermatologists are trained to interpret the important features, including color, shape, texture, and distribution, while ignoring unimportant or misleading features. Skin disease is often categorized into morphologic groups based on the most prominent primary lesion. Use of this classification scheme helps in formulating a differential diagnosis and in directing further investigation. Important morphologic groups in neonatal dermatology are vesicles and pustules, erythroderma, collodion baby, nonblanching violaceous papules and plaques, vascular defects, pigmented lesions, and midline anomalies. Subsequent chapters in this section present more detailed information on specific disorders.

TABLE 97-3 Topically Applied Products That Should Be Used With Caution in the Newborn

Compound	Product	Concern
Triclosan	Lever 2000, liquid deodorant soaps	Risk of toxicities seen with other phenolic compounds
Propylene glycol	Emollients, cleansing agents (Cetaphil lotion)	Excessive enteral and parenteral administration has caused hyperosmolality and seizures in infants
Benzethonium chloride	Skin cleansers	Poisoning by ingestion, carcinogenesis
Glycerin	Emollients, cleansing agents (Aquanil lotion)	Hyperosmolality, seizures
Ammonium lactate	Keratolytic emollient (Lac-Hydrin)	Possible lactic acidosis
Coal tar	Shampoos, topical anti-inflammatory ointments	Excessive use of polycyclic aromatic hydrocarbons is associated with an increased risk of cancer

TABLE 97-4 Metabolic and Nutritional Disorders Manifesting With Dermatitis

Disorder	Reference
Acrodermatitis enteropathica	Goskowics and Eichenfield, 1993
Biotin-dependent multiple carboxylase deficiency	Wolf and Heard, 1991
Prolidase deficiency	Bissonnette et al, 1993
Methylmalonic acidemia	Bodemer et al, 1994; De Raeve et al, 1994
Maple syrup urine disease	Giacoia and Berry, 1993
Propionic acidemia	Bodemer et al, 1994; De Raeve et al, 1994
Citrullinemia	Goldblum et al, 1986
Cystic fibrosis	Darmstadt et al, 1992
Gaucher's disease	Sherer et al, 1993; Sidransky et al, 1992
Kwashiorkor	Goskowics and Eichenfield, 1993

TABLE 97-5 Nutritional Requirements and Cutaneous Signs of Deficiency in Infants

Nutrient	Infant's Daily Requirement		Cutaneous Signs
	Premature	Term	
Protein (g/kg/day)	2.7-3.0	2.5-2.7	"Flaky paint" scaling, hypopigmentation, peripheral edema
Linoleic acid (g/kg/day)	1.2	0.3-0.8	Alopecia, erythema with coarse scaling, erosive intertriginous dermatitis, poor wound healing
Zinc (g/kg/day)	400	100	Alopecia, acral and periorificial erosive, pustular dermatitis, poor wound healing
Biotin (g/kg/day)	6.0	5.0 (not >20)	Alopecia, intertriginous and periorificial dermatitis, generalized scaling
Vitamin C (mg/kg/day)	25	20 (not >80)	Perifollicular hemorrhages, poor wound healing, friable gums
Vitamin A (g/kg/day)	500	175 (not >700)	Generalized scaling
Riboflavin (mg/kg/day)	0.15	0.35* (not >1.4)	Intertriginous and periorificial dermatitis, mucositis
Pyridoxine (mg/kg/day)	0.18	0.25* (not >1.0)	Intertriginous and periorificial dermatitis, mucositis
Niacin (mg/kg/day)	6.8	4.25* (not >17)	Mucositis, symmetrical hyperpigmented plaques at sun-exposed sites

Adapted from Greene HL, Hambridge KM, Schanler R, Tsang RC: Guidelines for the use of vitamins, trace elements, calcium, magnesium, and phosphorus in infants and children receiving total parenteral nutrition: Report of the Subcommittee on Pediatric Parenteral Nutrient Requirements from the Committee on Clinical Practice Issues of the American Society for Clinical Nutrition 1-3, *Am J Clin Nutr* 48:1324, 1988; and Miler SJ: Nutritional deficiency and the skin, *J Am Acad Dermatol* 21:1, 1989. Used with permission.

*For full-term infants, the recommended doses of some water-soluble vitamins are probably high because toxicity has not been reported.

BOX 97-1 Proposed Guidelines for Basic Skin Care in the Newborn

Use adhesives sparingly.
- Place protective dressing (e.g., DuoDerm or Tegaderm) at sites of frequent taping (endotracheal tube and nasogastric tube placement).
- Use nonadhesive electrodes and change them only when they become nonfunctional (Cartlidge and Rutter, 1987).

Limit bathing
- Defer initial cleansing until body temperature has stabilized.
- Avoid cleansing agents for the first 2 weeks.
- Use warm water and moistened cotton pledgets in a humid environment.
- Surface cleansing is required no more than twice per week.
- If antimicrobial skin preparation is required, use short-contact chlorhexidine (except on the face).

Be aware of the composition and quantity of all topically applied agents.
- These agents include antimicrobial cleansers, diaper wipes, adhesive removers, and perineal products.
- Dispense from single-use containers, if possible.

Ensure adequate intake of protein, essential fatty acids, zinc, biotin, and vitamins A, D, and B.
- Erosive periorificial dermatitis is a sign of nutritional deficiency.

Apply a simple cream or ointment emollient every 8 hours (Nopper et al, 1994).

Guard against excessive thermal and ultraviolet exposure.
- Use thermally controlled water for bathing.
- Avoid surface monitors with metal contacts.
- Use Plexiglas shielding over daylight fluorescent phototherapy.

Protect sites of cutaneous injury with the appropriate occlusive dressing.
- Use a film dressing on nonexudative sites (Barak et al, 1989; Knauth et al, 1989; Vernon et al, 1990).
- Use a hydrogel dressing on exudative wounds.
- Maintain appropriate hydration at the skin-dressing interface.
- Remove necrotic debris with each dressing change.

TABLE 97-6 Occlusive Dressing Materials

Class	Examples	Indications
Films		
Polyurethane with out without adhesive backing	Tegaderm, Op-Site, Bioclusive, Omniderm	Superficial, non-exudative wounds, sites of friction
Microporous Teflon or silicone	Silon	
Hydrocolloids		
Hydrophilic colloidal particles in polyurethane foam	DuoDerm, Cutinova hydro, Restore	Exudative wounds, sites of friction
Hydrogels		
Cross-linked polyvinyl or other polymer; 80%-99% water	Vigilon, Cutinova gel, Biofilm	Exudative wounds, fragile skin, sites of friction

Reprinted from Kannon GA, Garrett AB: Moist wound healing with occlusive dressings, *Dermatol Surg* 21:583, 1995. Copyright 1995, with permission from Elsevier Science.

are filled with purulent fluid. Diseases in this category range from totally innocuous and self-limited to severe and life-threatening.

A directed history, including family history of blistering diseases, and physical examination, including examination of the placenta, can focus the differential diagnosis. Small lesions in an otherwise healthy infant usually suggest a purely cutaneous process. Bullae and widespread involvement should prompt a more aggressive workup.

The initial diagnostic workup should include the following:

- Fluid aspirate taken from an intact vesicle, pustule, or scraping of the base of a ruptured vesicle or pustule for Gram stain, Wright stain, and fungal, viral, and bacterial cultures as well as for double fluorescent antibody or polymerase chain reaction when available

VESICLES AND PUSTULES

Many conditions cause blisters and pustules in the newborn. Vesicles are small intraepidermal or subepidermal pockets of clear fluid. If the lesions are large (greater than 1 cm in diameter), they are referred to as *bullae*. Pustules

- Potassium hydroxide (KOH) preparation (or calcofluor white immunofluorescence) of the blister roof
- Scraping from the base of the blister for herpes viral culture or Tzanck smear
- Scraping from a carefully selected intact lesion, mounted in mineral oil, for scabies preparation
- Skin biopsy as indicated, depending on the morphology and extent of the lesions, and results of other evaluations

Differential Diagnosis

Infections Localized to Skin

- Candidiasis: KOH (or calcofluor white) preparation of the blister roof reveals pseudohyphae.
- Bullous impetigo: Wright stain reveals polymorphonuclear neutrophil leukocytes (PMNs); Gram stain shows gram-positive cocci.
- Gram-positive folliculitis: Wright stain reveals PMNs; Gram stain shows gram-positive cocci.
- Pityrosporum folliculitis: KOH preparation reveals short hyphae and spores.
- Neonatal herpes: Tzanck smear reveals viral cytopathic changes; polymerase chain reaction and immunohistochemical marker assays are highly sensitive studies and can be performed using a smear on glass slides submitted to the laboratory. Viral cultures are still the gold standard with high sensitivity and specificity. Only a small amount of blister fluid on a swab inoculated into transport media is necessary, and results may be available within 12 hours.
- Scabies: Mineral oil preparation reveals mites, ova, and feces.

Transient Noninfectious Causes

- Erythema toxicum neonatorum: Wright stain shows eosinophils.
- Neonatal pustular melanosis: Wright stain shows keratinous debris with PMNs; results of a Gram stain are negative.
- Neonatal acne: Close inspection reveals comedones.
- Milia: Wright stain shows keratinocytes only.
- Miliaria crystallina: These tiny, superficial noninflammatory vesicles represent obstruction of the sweat duct.
- Infantile acropustulosis: This pruritic condition mimics infantile scabies, but the vesicles are usually rounded, rather than elongated like burrows.
- Eosinophilic pustular folliculitis: Wright stain shows eosinophils.

Bullae and Extensive Blistering

- The bullous diseases may be life-threatening and may be impossible to distinguish from one another without skin biopsy. Appropriate therapy depends on correct diagnosis.
- Staphylococcal scalded skin syndrome: Skin biopsy reveals a split in the superficial epidermis. Culture of blister contents is negative; the locus of infection is nasopharyngeal, perianal, focus of impetigo, or abscess; mucous membranes may be red but not blistered or eroded, because the target of the staphylococcal exfoliative toxin is not present in mucous membranes.

- Congenital herpes simplex virus infection: Skin, eye, or mouth lesions are presenting signs in one third of infants. In newborns, the presenting part at delivery is most commonly affected.
- Toxic epidermal necrolysis: Skin biopsy reveals a split at the dermoepidermal junction; mucous membranes are diffusely eroded, unlike staphylococcal scalded skin syndrome.
- Bullous mastocytosis: Stroking will produce a wheal and flare (Darier's sign), and a Tzanck smear may show mast cells.
- Genetic disorders: These disorders vary in severity and probability of long-term sequelae. Early diagnosis and genetic counseling are important aspects of management.
- Epidermolysis bullosa: Blisters are most prominent at sites of friction. Familial forms are classified as epidermolytic or simplex, junctional, and dermolytic or dystrophic, based on the skin cleavage plane. Electron microscopic analysis or immunofluorescence mapping or both are required for precise diagnosis. Recently, genetic markers are being used to make a specific diagnosis in selected patients.
- Epidermolytic hyperkeratosis: Widespread erythema and blistering may be present at birth, causing confusion with epidermolysis bullosa and other blistering dermatoses. Thick, greasy, foul-smelling scales accentuated in skin creases may not become apparent until later in the 1st year of life.
- Incontinentia pigmenti: Vesicular skin lesions have a characteristic distribution along the lines of Blaschko. This striking pattern is seen with a variety of cutaneous abnormalities as a result of genetic mosaicism. Tzanck smear may show eosinophils but no multinucleate giant cells, and results of Gram staining are negative for organisms.

ERYTHRODERMA

Generalized redness and scaling in infancy have an alarming appearance and are often clinically and histologically nonspecific. An infant's general state of well-being is an important clue to the extent of the disease. Definitive diagnosis may be possible only after a period of observation. The newborn with erythroderma will have increased insensible heat and water loss requiring careful monitoring of weight, fluid and electrolytes, and body temperature. A neutrothermal and humidified environment may be necessary for the first few days of life. Topical emollients may help to control transepidermal water loss and lower the risk of infection.

Careful history, family history, physical examination, and directed laboratory evaluation may help to clarify the cause. The spectrum of disease includes common conditions limited to skin, infections, nutritional deficiencies, and immunologic disorders.

Infectious causes of erythroderma should always be considered first. The infant's skin should be carefully examined for more specific primary skin lesions. Laboratory evaluation should include complete blood cell count, KOH preparation (or calcofluor white immunofluorescence technique), Tzanck smear, and surveillance cultures of the nasopharynx, rectum, umbilicus, conjunctivae, urine, and blood. Syphilis serologic studies and human immunodeficiency virus (HIV) assay should be considered in epidemiologically relevant locales, with initiation of empiric therapy as needed.

The diagnostic evaluation should be more aggressive in any infant who is not thriving, to search for metabolic or immunologic abnormalities. Components of the investigation should include dietary history, electrolytes, protein, albumin, alkaline phosphatase, microscopic examination of hair, and a sweat test. The results of these screening tests can suggest the need for further laboratory evaluation.

More directed laboratory evaluation includes blood smear to look for leukocyte vacuoles, HIV screening, plasma zinc determination, measurement of serum linoleic and arachidonic acids, amino acid profile, specific assays for biotinidase activity, antinuclear antibody (SS-A and SS-B) titers, quantitative immunoglobulins, tests of cell-mediated immunity, skeletal survey, hair examination, and skin biopsy.

Differential Diagnosis

Systemic infections associated with erythroderma are:

- Candidiasis
- Staphylococcal scalded skin syndrome
- Syphilis
- Acquired immunodeficiency syndrome (AIDS)

Primary Cutaneous Conditions

- Atopic dermatitis: Pruritus and involvement of the face and extensor extremities with marked sparing of the diaper area are helpful diagnostic clues.
- Seborrheic dermatitis: The diaper area and skinfolds are often prominently involved, and the eruption is asymptomatic or minimally pruritic.
- Psoriasis: Skin lesions are often sharply circumscribed, but scale may not be prominent. Psoriasis may clinically overlap seborrheic dermatitis.

Genodermatoses

Skin biopsy helps to distinguish among the ichthyosis-associated abnormalities disorders: lamellar ichthyosis, congenital nonbullous ichthyosiform erythroderma, epidermolytic hyperkeratosis, X-linked ichthyosis, multiple sulfatase deficiency, neutral lipid storage disease, Sjögren-Larsson syndrome, trichothiodystrophy, Netherton syndrome, and X-linked dominant chondrodysplasia punctata. The Foundation for Ichthyosis and Related Skin Types (www.scalyskin.org) is a useful source of information and will assist in the genetic evaluation of patients. Genetic markers for many of these disorders have been identified and may be useful for definitive diagnosis.

Ectodermal Dysplasias

Ectodermal dysplasias are a group of disorders involving abnormalities of the skin and its appendages. Excessive desquamation resembling that seen with postmaturity is a characteristic finding. The most well-recognized form is X-linked recessive hypohidrotic ectodermal dysplasia. Infants with this disorder have a decreased ability to sweat and a tendency toward hyperthermia. Clues include nail and hair anomalies as well as dysmorphic facies.

Immunologic Disorders Associated With Erythroderma

A clinical syndrome of erythroderma, diarrhea, and failure to thrive in infancy was first described in 1908 by Leiner, in association with nonsupplemented breast-feeding. Subsequently, similar signs have been reported in infants with increased susceptibility to infection. A defect in yeast opsonization was found in two infants with Leiner disease in 1972; however, this defect, present in 5% of the general population, does not define the disease. Other patients experienced dramatic clinical improvement after infusion of fresh plasma or a purified preparation containing the fifth component of complement, C5. Consequently, Leiner disease has been associated with C5 dysfunction. More recently, a variety of immunologic abnormalities with varied underlying defects have been reported in infants with similar clinical presentation; this condition has been called *syndrome of erythroderma, failure to thrive*, and *diarrhea in infancy* to avoid confusion (Glover et al, 1988). Other defined disorders in this category include the following:

- Primary immunodeficiencies (e.g., severe combined immunodeficiency [SCID], Wiskott-Aldrich syndrome, hyper-immunoglobulin E syndrome, Omenn syndrome)
- Secondary immunodeficiencies (AIDS, graft-versus-host disease)
- Langerhans cell histiocytosis
- Neonatal lupus
- Diffuse cutaneous mastocytosis

Metabolic and Nutritional Disorders Associated With Erythroderma

Patients with metabolic and nutritional disorders associated with erythroderma often exhibit erosive, periorificial dermatitis (see Table 97-5).

COLLODION BABY

Collodion baby represents a distinct subset of neonatal erythroderma that can be a clinical marker of a variety of underlying abnormalities. The phenotype includes parchmentlike hyperkeratosis, pseudocontractures, ectropion, eclabium, absence of eyebrows, and sparse hair. These infants have defective cutaneous barrier function, with resultant losses of free water and thermal energy. They are extremely susceptible to hypothermia, hypernatremic dehydration, and percutaneous infection. Although the collodion membrane desquamates in 15% of affected infants, leaving normal skin, the majority develop one of the ichthyosis variants (Oji and Traupe, 2009).

NONBLANCHING VIOLACEOUS PAPULES AND PLAQUES

Nonblanching violaceous papules and plaques may be localized or disseminated. Infants with widespread lesions have been described as *blueberry muffin babies*. The diseases in this category represent a variety of processes; most require aggressive evaluation and treatment.

Initial evaluation of a blueberry muffin infant should include complete blood cell count with white blood cell differential; platelet count; reticulocyte count; liver function tests; maternal and neonatal TORCH (toxoplasmosis, other infections, rubella, cytomegalovirus infection, and herpes simplex) infectious agent titers; rapid plasma reagin (RPR) or similar syphilis assay; blood cultures for bacteria; urine, nasopharyngeal swab, and rectal swab samples for viral cultures; and ophthalmologic examination.

A skin biopsy specimen is necessary to distinguish simple hemorrhage into the dermis (purpura) from other infiltrative conditions (e.g., dermal hematopoiesis, tumor) manifesting in the neonatal period.

Differential Diagnosis

Purpura

Ecchymoses: These lesions constitute traumatic purpura, usually secondary to labor and delivery.

Bland thrombosis: Conditions in this category that can occur in the neonatal period include the following:

- Embolization of foreign material: this has been noted in infants receiving extracorporeal membrane oxygenation (ECMO).
- Purpura fulminans: neonatal purpura fulminans is most often associated with homozygous protein C or protein S deficiency (Knoebl, 2008; Marlar et al, 1989)
- Cryoglobulinemia: rarely occurs as a result of transplacental transfer of a monoclonal immunoglobulin G cryoglobulin (Laugel et al, 2004)

Infectious vasculitis: Purpuric lesions represent infectious, inflammatory microemboli, most commonly associated with the following:

- Gram-negative bacterial sepsis, including that due to *Escherichia coli* or meningococci, and ecthyma gangrenosum (*Pseudomonas* spp.)
- Listeriosis
- Aspergillosis

Thrombocytopenia, usually manifested by widely scattered petechiae

Isoimmune thrombocytopenic purpura

Maternal isoimmune thrombocytopenic purpura

Disseminated intravascular coagulopathy

Dermal Hematopoiesis

Dermal hematopoiesis is the histologic basis for the blueberry muffin skin lesions. Before 34 weeks' gestation, the skin serves as a hematopoietic center. It has yet to be shown whether blueberry muffin lesions are due to persistence or recurrence of this fetal potential.

- Rubella
- Cytomegalovirus infection
- Syphilis
- Other viral infections (e.g., coxsackievirus B2 infection)
- Twin-to-twin transfusion syndrome
- Rh hemolytic disease of the newborn

Malignancy

- Congenital leukemia
- Langerhans cell histiocytosis
- Neuroblastoma

VASCULAR DEFECTS

Although it can be difficult to distinguish among the various cutaneous vascular lesions in the neonatal period, attention to morphologic findings, location, distribution, patterns, and clinical course usually allows for a specific diagnosis. Lesions that lack distinctive findings can be diagnosed by gathering additional data from ultrasound imaging, magnetic resonance imaging, and skin biopsy.

Differential Diagnosis

Hemangioma

Hemangioma is the most common tumor of infancy. It usually becomes apparent during the first 2 to 4 weeks after birth and exhibits a characteristic rapid growth phase, peaking at 3 to 6 months in most infants followed by slow involution over the next 5 to 10 years. Although these lesions usually are not associated with extracutaneous findings, hemangiomas in special locations require further evaluation (Guggisberg et al, 2004):

- Lumbosacral and anogenital examination to exclude lumbosacral spine anomalies
- Large facial, scalp, neck, thoracic (PHACES syndrome) examination to exclude cardiac and posterior fossa anomalies
- Beard distribution to monitor and evaluate the airway
- Large segmental examination to evaluate for vascular and soft tissue anomalies of the involved area.

Vascular Malformations

Vascular malformations are a group of lesions, usually apparent at birth, that do not generally grow or involute. Salmon patches occur in 80% of infants in characteristic locations and usually fade or become camouflaged by normal pigment or hair. Port wine birthmarks, present in 0.3% of newborns, are capillary malformations that persist in childhood and become more prominent in later adolescence and adult life. Venous malformations are also present at birth and have a baglike or wormlike texture because of the larger vessels involved and their typical location in the deeper dermis and/or subcutaneous fat. Arteriovenous and lymphatic malformations are much less common and may pose difficult management problems.

Some vascular malformations are associated with characteristic extracutaneous abnormalities:

- Nevus flammeus (port wine stain)
- Klippel-Trénaunay syndrome
- Cobb syndrome
- Arterial, lymph, venous, or mixed malformations
- Cutis marmorata telangiectatica congenita

Lesions That Mimic Vascular Birthmarks

- Pilomatrixoma
- Giant juvenile xanthogranuloma
- Langerhans cell histiocytosis
- Congenital myofibromatosis

PIGMENTED LESIONS

Although a skin biopsy specimen may be necessary to distinguish these lesions, morphologic clues often aid in clinical diagnosis. Most of these lesions are benign, but some require careful monitoring. In general, skin biopsy of a congenital pigmented lesion can be postponed until after the neonatal period. The one exception is a nodular lesion suggestive of melanoma (see Chapter 101).

Differential Diagnosis

- Congenital nevocellular nevus: tend to have fuzzy borders, variable pigmentation and texture, and may have areas with coarse dark hair
- Café au lait macule: sharp edges, uniform pigmentation, no texture
- Nevus spilus (speckled lentiginous nevus): café au lait background component with variably pigmented and textured darker papules scattered throughout
- Mongolian spot: fuzzy borders, flat patches, blue-green-gray color
- Smooth muscle hamartoma: café au lait pigmentation with increased hair
- Plexiform neurofibroma: large soft compressible spongy mass often overlying large café au lait macule
- Nevus of Ota: Mongolian spot on the face particularly around the eye; unlike mongolian spots, these lesions often do not fade
- Epidermal nevus: warty linear plaques that follow the lines of Blaschko

- Urticaria pigmentosa, solitary mastocytoma: golden brown papules with fuzzy borders, leathery texture that urticate with rubbing (Darier's sign)
- Lentigines: large dark freckles that do not fade in the winter

MIDLINE FACIAL LESIONS

See Chapter 101 for a more detailed discussion of midline facial lesions. The main types are as follows:
- Dermoid: firm rubbery nodules typically in a baseball cap distribution on the forehead or scalp
- Nasal glioma: spongy mass arising from the base of the nose; mimics a hemangioma and communicates with the central nervous system
- Encephalocele: direct communication with the central nervous system; may be anywhere along the midline scalp or neck

SUGGESTED READINGS

Cohen BA: *Pediatric dermatology*, Philadelphia, 2005, Elsevier.
Eichenfield LF, Frieden IJ, Esterly NB: *Textbook of neonatal dermatology*, Philadelphia, 2008, WB Saunders.
Harper JH, Orange A, Prose NS: *Textbook of pediatric dermatology*, Mass, 2006, Blackwell.
Schachner LA, Hansen KC: *Pediatric dermatology: expert consult*, St. Louis, 2011, Elsevier.

Complete references and supplemental color images used in this text can be found online at www.expertconsult.com

CONGENITAL AND HEREDITARY DISORDERS OF THE SKIN*

Mark M. Tran and Bernard A. Cohen

The heritable disorders of skin—the genodermatoses—feature diverse aberrations of color, texture, and structural integrity of the epidermis, epidermal appendages, and connective tissue. Some of these diseases are cutaneous only; others are associated with anomalies of multiple organ systems. Many genodermatoses can be diagnosed prenatally by skin biopsy (Holbrook et al, 1993) (Box 98-1). This technique is being replaced, however, by molecular diagnostic methods as the genetic nature of most of these disorders is identified. Enormous progress has been made in the last few years in elucidating the molecular genetics responsible for many of the dermatoses in this chapter. The National Institutes of Health manages databases of genetic diseases through the National Center for Biotechnology Information that can be accessed online, including the Online Mendelian Inheritance in Man (www.ncbi.nlm.nih.gov/omim) and Entrez Gene (www.ncbi.nlm.nih.gov/gene). GeneDx is a private company that specializes in genetic testing for rare hereditary disorders (www.genedx.com). With these exciting new discoveries comes the hope for novel and more efficacious therapies.

GENODERMATOSES AND MOSAICISM

A genetic mosaic is an organism composed of two or more genetically different populations of cells that originate from one zygote. When the skin is involved, unique patterning is seen, reflecting the cellular heterogeneity. Variations of this striking pattern were clinically described and mapped in 1901 by Alfred Blaschko. The distribution is known as *Blaschko's lines*. Blaschko's lines are distinct from dermatomes, skin tension lines, and lines of lymphatic drainage. The pattern is linear and whorled and may be bilaterally symmetric, with a midline demarcation (Figure 98-1). An anatomic equivalent has been described in the eyes and teeth (Bolognia, 1994).

Several diseases are expressed in this fashion. The first to be recognized were X-linked disorders. Affected females are obligate heterozygotes because of the Lyon effect of X-inactivation. Examples include female carriers of the X-linked recessive disorder hypohidrotic ectodermal dysplasia and females with the X-linked dominant disorders, incontinentia pigmenti, chondrodysplasia punctata, CHILD syndrome (see later), and focal dermal hypoplasia. These conditions are seen almost exclusively in females, presumably because they are lethal in males. Autosomal mosaicism is not heritable unless the germ cells are affected (Happle, 1993).

SPECIFIC GENODERMATOSES

ICHTHYOSES

The *ichthyoses* are a diverse group of heritable and acquired skin disorders that share the primary problem of widespread scaly, dry skin. Several distinct types of ichthyosis have been described on the basis of their clinical and histologic features and by their patterns of genetic transmission (Krug, 2009; Williams, 1983, 1986); however, nosology is constantly evolving. Several types of ichthyoses are primary disorders of cornification, with manifestations confined to the skin. Ichthyosiform syndromes have characteristic extracutaneous manifestations. More precise diagnostic criteria and better treatments are being recognized through collaborative research efforts, including genetic analysis. The National Registry for Ichthyosis and Related Disorders was created in 1995 to aid in this effort and can be contacted by telephone at (800) 595-1265. The Foundation for Ichthyosis and Related Skin Types is a privately funded national organization providing information and support for families with these disorders (for contact information, see Box 98-2).

Ichthyoses That Manifest in the Neonatal Period

Three ichthyosiform conditions have alarming presentations at birth. Two of these, the collodion baby and harlequin ichthyosis, have been historically described as distinct entities based on the associated striking and unique clinical appearance. Long-term survival of affected infants and more refined diagnostic studies have permitted identification of these conditions as phenotypically distinct but genotypically heterogeneous. A third condition, epidermolytic hyperkeratosis (autosomal dominant bullous congenital ichthyosiform erythroderma), has an equally striking neonatal appearance. Another severe category of infantile ichthyosis, congenital nonbullous ichthyosiform erythroderma–lamellar ichthyosis, presents a difficult diagnostic and management problem. Recognition of these conditions and appropriate management are vital to the survival of these infants.

Collodion Baby

Neonates affected with the uncommon condition termed *collodion baby* have a pathognomonic appearance. With time, they usually manifest more specific features of one of the ichthyoses.

Clinical Findings

Collodion babies are often premature and small for gestational age. Their skin is parchmentlike, shiny, and thickened at birth, distorting their facial features with ectropion and

---

*This chapter includes material from a chapter in the previous edition, to which Elaine C. Siegfried and Nancy B. Esterly contributed.

eclabium, flattening the ears, and resulting in pseudocontractures of the digits (Figure 98-2). Histologic examination of the skin at this stage has been nonspecific, revealing a markedly thickened, compact stratum corneum. Nonetheless, these infants have an ineffective barrier against transepidermal water loss and invasion of pathogenic microbes, with accompanying temperature instability.

Causes

Several genetically distinct outcomes have been reported for the collodion baby phenotype (Table 98-1). Two thirds of these infants have nonbullous ichthyosiform erythroderma. Fifty-five percent of patients have mutations in the transglutaminase-1 gene (Farasat et al, 2009). Fifty percent of affected infants have no family history suggestive of ichthyosis (Pongprasit, 1993).

Diagnosis

Skin biopsy can be helpful, but is not likely to be specific until after the collodion appearance has resolved. Diagnostic studies should be carefully selected, based on the evolution of the cutaneous findings, associated abnormalities, and family history (see Table 98-1). Several outcomes have been reported,

---

BOX 98-1   Genodermatoses Diagnosed Prenatally Using Fetal Skin Samples

- Epidermolysis bullosa
  - Junctional
  - Recessive dystrophic
  - Dominant dystrophic
  - Epidermolysis bullosa simplex (general)
  - Epidermolysis bullosa simplex—Dowling-Meara
  - Unidentified forms
- Keratinization disorders
  - Bullous congenital ichthyosiform erythroderma
  - Nonbullous congenital ichthyosiform erythroderma/lamellar ichthyosis
  - Harlequin ichthyosis
  - Sjögren-Larsson syndrome
- Pigment disorders
  - Tyrosinase-negative oculocutaneous albinism
  - Congenital nevus
  - Incontinentia pigmenti
- Disorders of epidermal appendages
  - X-linked hypohidrotic ectodermal dysplasia
  - Autosomal-recessive anhidrotic ectodermal dysplasia
- Other disorders
  - Tay syndrome
  - Chédiak-Higashi syndrome
  - Griscelli syndrome
  - Restrictive dermopathy

Adapted from Holbrook KA, Smith LT, Elias S: Prenatal diagnosis of genetic skin disease using fetal skin biopsy samples, *Arch Dermatol* 129:1437-1454, 1993.

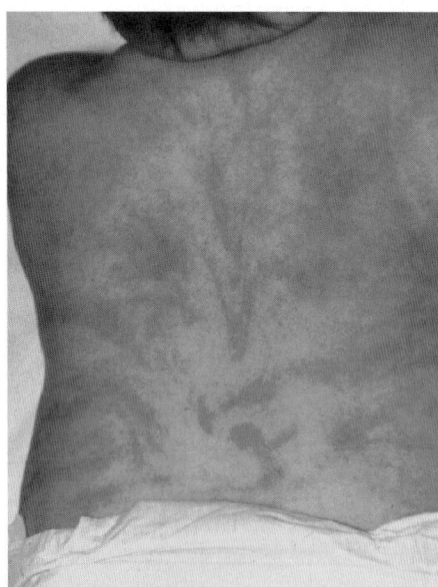

FIGURE 98-1 Lines of Blaschko are a distinct linear and whorled pattern, to be distinguished from dermatomes or skin tension lines, characterized by midline demarcation with a central V. This pattern is the cutaneous clinical manifestation of a variety of mosaic genetic conditions.

BOX 98-2   Resources for Families With Genodermatoses

ICHTHYOSIS

Foundation for Ichthyosis and Related Skin Types
  www.firstskinfoundation.org

OCULOCUTANEOUS ALBINISM

National Organization for Albinism and Hypopigmentation: www.albinism.org

INCONTINENTIA PIGMENTI

Incontinentia Pigmenti International Foundation
  www.ipif.org
Incontinentia Pigmenti Support Network
  Telephone: (313) 729-7912

GENETIC TESTING

Medical Genetics Laboratory, Baylor College of Medicine, Houston, Texas
  www.bcm.edu/geneticlabs

EHLERS-DANLOS SYNDROME

Ehlers-Danlos National Foundation
  www.ednf.org

EPIDERMOLYSIS BULLOSA

National Epidermolysis Bullosa Registry
  c/o Jo-David Fine, MD, Principal Investigator or c/o Lorraine B. Johnson, ScD, Coordinator
  Department of Dermatology, University of North Carolina at Chapel Hill, Chapel Hill, North Carolina
  Telephone: (919) 966-6383
West Coast Registry
  Lexie Nall, MD
  Stanford University Medical Center
  Telephone: (415) 725-8839
Dystrophic Epidermolysis Bullosa Research Association of America
  www.debra.org

NEONATAL LUPUS ERYTHEMATOSUS

North American Collaborative Study of NLE
  c/o Earl Silverman, MD
  The Hospital for Sick Children, Toronto, Ontario, Canada
  Telephone: (416) 813-6249

ECTODERMAL DYSPLASIA

National Foundation for Ectodermal Dysplasias
  www.nfed.org

including complete healing without sequelae (Frenk and de Techtermann, 1992; Shwayder and Ott, 1991). A prolonged period of observation may be required to determine the precise diagnosis and prognosis. Genetic counseling should be provided as soon as a definite diagnosis has been made.

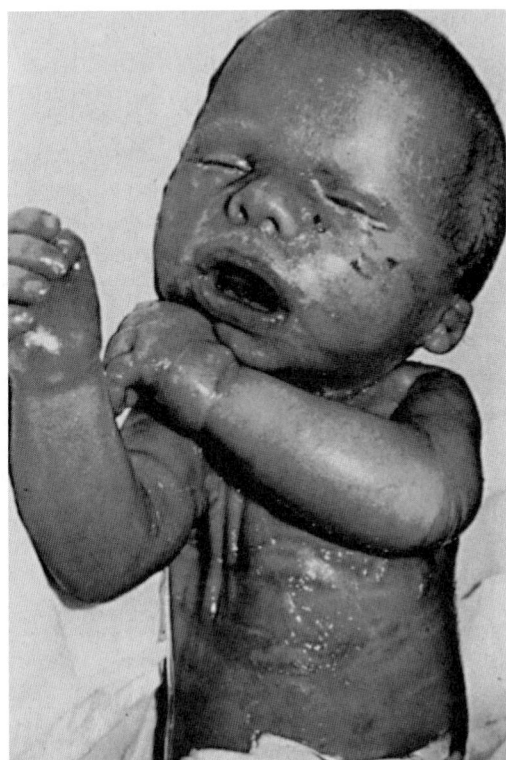

FIGURE 98-2 Collodion baby. Note the ectropion, eclabium, and areas of rupture in the membrane over the anterior thorax.

Treatment

Complications include marked temperature instability, defective barrier function, increased insensible water loss predisposing to hypernatremic dehydration (Buyse et al, 1993), pneumonia secondary to aspiration of squamous material in the amniotic fluid, and cutaneous infections from gram-positive organisms and *Candida albicans*.

Treatment consists of aggressive supportive care. Infants must be placed in a highly humidified incubator. Fluid and electrolyte balance must be monitored closely. A high index of suspicion must be maintained for signs of cutaneous or systemic infection; however, overzealous administration of antibiotics can lead to gram-negative infections and subsequent septicemia. Topical skin care should include application of a bland, occlusive ointment emollient every 6 to 8 hours until the hyperkeratosis has resolved. Potentially toxic topical agents should be avoided because of the increased risk of percutaneous absorption. Manual debridement is not indicated. The eyes should be protected with a bland lubricating ointment; aggressive surgical management of ectropion is almost never necessary. Systemic retinoids have not been useful (Waisman et al, 1989). With optimal supportive care, the thickened stratum corneum usually resolves in 2 to 4 weeks but can persist, especially in infants with lamellar ichthyosis.

Harlequin Ichthyosis

Harlequin ichthyosis is a rare congenital abnormality with more striking appearance and a graver prognosis than for collodion baby. Most infants are stillborn or die in infancy. Survival beyond infancy has been possible only recently. The harlequin phenotype is inherited as

TABLE 98-1   Collodion Baby: Differential Diagnosis and Laboratory Evaluation

Diagnosis	Inheritance	Associated Abnormalities	Diagnostic Tests*
Nonbullous ichthyosiform erythroderma (>60%)	AD, AR	—	Histologic findings are nonspecific; fetal skin biopsy is unreliable; the gene defect has not been identified
Lamellar ichthyosis	AD, AR	Persistent ectropion	Histologic findings are nonspecific; fetal skin biopsy is unreliable; the gene defect has been identified
X-linked ichthyosis	X-linked recessive	Maternal failure to initiate labor; hypogonadism, undescended testes; corneal opacities (carrier females and affected males)	Histologic findings are nonspecific; decreased serum cholesterol sulfate and steroid sulfatase activity; the gene defect has been mapped to Xp22.3
Netherton syndrome	Sporadic	Ichthyosis linearis circumflexa, atopic diathesis, impaired cellular immunity	Histologic findings are nonspecific; microscopic examination of hair shaft reveals pathognomonic trichorrhexis invagina
Gaucher disease	AR	Hepatosplenomegaly, thrombocytopenia, neurologic abnormalities	Liver biopsy; β-glucocerebroside activity; the gene defect has been mapped to 1q21 and sequenced
Trichothiodystrophy (Tay syndrome)	AR	Progeric facies, neurologic abnormalities, hypogonadism, cataracts, dental problems	Hair analyses: polarizing light microscopic examination reveals characteristic banding; there is decreased content of sulfur-rich matrix proteins
Sjögren-Larsson syndrome	AR	Spasticity, retardation, seizures	Pathognomonic retinal changes; fibroblast culture for fatty alcohol oxidoreductase activity
No detectable abnormality (lamellar exfoliation of the newborn)	AR, sporadic	—	Watchful waiting

Data on diagnostic tests from Paller AS: Laboratory tests for ichthyosis, *Derm Clinics* 12:99-107, 1994.
AD, Autosomal dominant; *AR*, autosomal recessive.
*In the immediate neonatal period, skin biopsy findings may be nonspecific. Histologic evaluation can be postponed until after age 3 to 6 months.

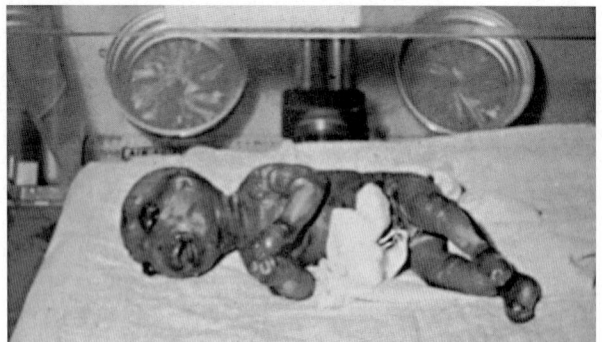

FIGURE 98-3 Harlequin fetus. (*Courtesy Marvin Cornblath.*)

an autosomal recessive trait; several biochemical defects probably underlie the clinical condition. *ABCA12* mutations have been identified in patients in recent investigations (Thomas et al, 2006).

Clinical Findings

The cutaneous scale is firm and platelike, distorting and flattening the nose and ears. Skin rigidity also causes deep fissures, marked ectropion, eclabium, and pseudocontractures of all joints. Chemosis of the conjunctivae obscures the globes. The nails and hair are hypoplastic or absent (Figure 98-3). Primary extracutaneous abnormalities are not prominent.

Diagnosis

The diagnosis is made by the pathognomonic appearance. The light microscopic examination always demonstrates compact hyperkeratosis. Additional light and electron microscopic abnormalities of the stratum corneum have not been identified consistently, supporting the theory that harlequin ichthyosis represents a common phenotype for several different genetic errors of cornification (Hashimoto et al, 1993).

Causes

The cause of harlequin ichthyosis is unknown. Although abnormalities of keratinization and epidermal lipid metabolism have been reported, few affected infants have been studied (Dale and Kam, 1993) with one recent report of a de novo deletion of 18q21 (Smith et al, 2001).

Prognosis and Treatment

Treatment consists of supportive care in a humid, temperature-controlled environment and frequent application of topical emollients to the skin and mucosal surfaces, as for collodion baby (Prasad et al, 1994). Nevertheless, infants given these therapies almost invariably succumb to their disease from sepsis, inability to feed, and inadequate ventilation. Survival beyond 6 weeks was extremely unusual before the use of oral retinoids. Recent reports have documented successful therapy of several affected infants using oral retinoids, with improved quality of life and survival well into childhood. Etretinate has been used most often in the past, at doses of 1 mg/kg/day. Although approval of this drug has been withdrawn by the U.S. Food and Drug Administration, isotretinoin has been used at a dose of

0.5 mg/kg. Infants receiving retinoids must be monitored for toxic effects (Harvey et al, 2010). All survivors have had severe ichthyosis as an outcome; some have intellectual impairment. Genetic counseling for the families of these infants is mandatory. Prenatal diagnosis may be made with a fetal skin biopsy specimen (Holbrook et al, 1993).

Epidermolytic Hyperkeratosis (Congenital Bullous Ichthyosiform Erythroderma)

Epidermolytic hyperkeratosis (EHK) is rare, with an estimated incidence of 1 in 250,000 births. Neonates with EHK are born with generalized erythroderma and blistering. The clinical appearance shares cutaneous features of other infantile bullous disorders, especially epidermolysis bullosa (EB). Molecular defects responsible for EHK have recently been identified with mutations found to be associated with the keratin *K1* and *K10* genes (Covaciu et al, 2010; Morais et al, 2009).

Clinical Findings

Infants may be born with generalized erythroderma and blistering. Hyperkeratosis may not be readily apparent. The neonatal course is complicated by temperature instability, susceptibility to hypernatremia, and sepsis, as in the other severe neonatal ichthyoses. With time, the skin changes evolve to include characteristic ridged scales, accentuated in the flexural areas. Palms and soles usually are involved. Excessive bacterial colonization often causes a distressingly foul odor. There are no extracutaneous manifestations.

Diagnosis

There is significant clinical similarity to other bullous disorders of infancy, including EB, toxic epidermal necrosis, and staphylococcal scalded skin syndrome (Cheng et al, 2009). Precise diagnosis can be lifesaving. Skin biopsy should be performed emergently, with examination of frozen sections. The histologic features of EHK are distinctive, showing intercellular edema and coarse, clumped material in the upper granular layers of the epidermis. Prenatal diagnosis is possible with a fetal skin biopsy specimen (Holbrook et al, 1993).

Causes

EHK is transmitted in an autosomal dominant fashion, with a high rate of spontaneous mutation. Ultrastructural analysis of skin from affected patients suggests an abnormality of keratin filaments in the suprabasal cells. Molecular analysis of affected families has identified genetic mutations in the genes encoding the synthesis of the keratin filaments that are preferentially expressed in the superficial epidermis, *K1* (located within the type I keratin gene cluster at chromosome 17q) and *K10* (located within the type II keratin gene cluster at chromosome 12q) (Francis, 1994; Nirunsuksiri et al, 1995; Smack et al, 1994; Steijlen et al, 1994a). A recent study has shown that these genetic mutations were due to a splice site and deletion mutations of the types I and 10 of keratin (Virtanen et al, 2003). The disorder also can be expressed in mosaic fashion as an epidermal nevus oriented along the lines of Blaschko (Paller, 1994). Prenatal studies for EHK may

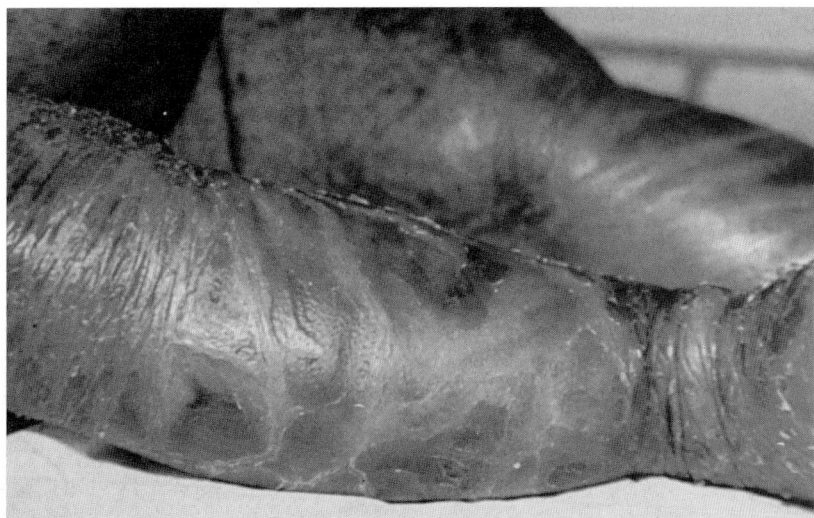

FIGURE 98-4 Large dark scales characteristic of lamellar ichthyosis on the leg of an affected infant.

be indicated for the offspring of parents with extensive epidermal nevi.

Prognosis and Treatment

Infants with widespread blistering should be managed according to the same principles and techniques used for collodion babies. Attention to gentle handling will minimize further trauma. Application of a nonadhesive biooc-clusive dressing (e.g., hydrogel, foam) will promote healing of denuded areas. Infants should be monitored closely for the development of secondary infection.

Nonbullous Congenital Ichthyosiform Erythroderma (Lamellar Ichthyosis)

The nonbullous form of infantile ichthyosiform skin disease, as distinct from the bullous variety (i.e., EHK), initially was characterized by its severity and autosomal recessive inheritance pattern. The term *nonbullous congenital ichthyosiform erythroderma* (NCIE) generally refers to a milder clinical variant. Recent studies suggest the mutation in NCIE lies in the *ALOX12B* gene encoding lipoxygenase (Akiyama et al, 2010). Ultrastructural differences have been described in skin biopsy specimens. The phenotypically more severe lamellar ichthyosis has proved to be genetically distinct, characterized by a defect in the transglutaminase-1 gene (Russell et al, 1995).

Clinical Findings

These conditions are characterized by congenital erythroderma and a varying degree of generalized scaling. The face, flexural sites, palms, and soles are also involved. A majority of collodion babies have these types of ichthyosis. In lamellar ichthyosis, the scales evolve to be thick, dark, and plate-like (Figure 98-4). Facial involvement causes chronic ectropion. Hair growth may be sparse, and nails may be dystrophic. Children with NCIE have generalized erythema with finer, white scales. There is no associated ectropion. Secondary cutaneous infections with bacteria, yeasts, and dermatophytes are common complications.

Diagnosis

Before genetic advances, the diagnosis of these forms of ichthyosis had been based on clinical features alone. Findings from a skin biopsy specimen are nonspecific; a normal granular layer is present. The differential diagnosis includes other causes of erythroderma and collodion baby (see Chapter 97). Prenatal diagnosis is possible for affected families (Holbrook et al, 1993). For patients without a previously defined family history, the appropriate laboratory assessment can be arranged through the National Registry for Ichthyosis and Related Disorders.

Causes

A majority of cases are inherited in an autosomal recessive fashion, but an autosomal dominant form of lamellar ichthyosis also has been described. Russell et al (1995) identified a common locus of genetic mutations identified in several families with recessive lamellar ichthyosis. The linked defects, located on chromosome 14, result in production of abnormal transglutaminase-1. This enzyme normally promotes cross-linking of intracellular proteins in the stratum corneum during terminal differentiation (Huber et al, 1995). New research has revealed genetic heterogeneity with two other loci on chromosomes 2 and 19. In addition, a locus on chromosome 3 was identified that was clinically consistent with NCIE (Fischer et al, 2000).

Prognosis and Treatment

The same management principles recommended for neonates presenting with the collodion baby phenotype can be applied to infants with erythroderma, although their neonatal course is marked by fewer complications. The mainstay of therapy for children with lamellar ichthyosis is the use of topical emollients and keratolytic agents. Successful treatment with topical calcipotriol has been described previously (Delfino et al, 1994; Russell and Young, 1994). Any topically applied agent will be transcutaneously absorbed to a much higher degree than through normal skin; dosing must be monitored carefully (Abdel-Magid and el-Awad, 1994; Lucker, 1994). Treatment with systemic retinoids has had variable success (Steijlen et al, 1994b; Waisman et al, 1989).

Ichthyosiform Syndromes

Several syndromes manifesting in the neonatal period have ichthyosis as a major feature.

Recessive X-linked Ichthyosis

Recessive X-linked ichthyosis (RXLI) is an uncommon condition, affecting 1 in 6000 males. Signs of the disorder are present at birth in one fifth of affected infants; 85% develop skin changes by 3 months of age. The characteristic cutaneous finding is coarse, brownish scaling, most prominent on the neck and extensor extremities. The palms and soles are spared. Extracutaneous manifestations include hypogonadism and cryptorchidism, present in up to 25% of affected males. Severely affected males may have short stature and mental retardation, a variant that has been referred to as *Rud syndrome*. Characteristic corneal opacities are seen in affected males and heterozygote females, but usually not until late childhood or adolescence. Carrier females experience failure to initiate labor or prolonged labor. Light microscopic and ultrastructural findings in skin biopsy specimens are unremarkable. The pathogenesis of recessive X-linked ichthyosis is aberrant production of the enzyme steroid sulfatase (a form of arylsulfatase C), with accumulation of cholesterol sulfate (Cañueto et al, 2010; Williams, 1986). The genetic abnormality has been localized to the distal short arm of the X chromosome (Xp22.3), and prenatal diagnosis can be made with fluorescence in situ hybridization analysis (Watanabe et al, 2003).

Netherton Syndrome/Ichthyosis Linearis Circumflexa

Netherton syndrome is a rare, autosomal recessive condition. It often manifests at birth as ichthyosiform erythroderma with flexural accentuation. The characteristic migratory, polycyclic lesions with a peripheral double-edged scale, referred to as *ichthyosis linearis circumflexa*, do not appear until after 2 years of age. The syndrome is characterized by congenital ichthyosis, hair shaft defects (principally trichorrhexis invaginata), and atopic features (pruritus, hay fever, facial angioedema, and elevated immunoglobulin E), but until the advent of genetic testing, diagnosis in affected children often was not possible for the first several years of life (Judge et al, 1994b). Generalized aminoaciduria and impaired cellular immunity also have been reported. This distinctive pattern of ichthyosis linearis circumflexa can also manifest as an isolated cutaneous condition. Recently, pathogenic mutations in Netherton syndrome were localized to the *SPINK5* gene at chromosomal locus 5q32, which encodes the serine protease inhibitor LEKTI (Chavanas et al, 2000; Hewett et al, 2005). Subsequently, prenatal testing for the disorder was successfully attempted (Müller et al, 2002; Sprecher et al, 2001).

Sjögren-Larsson Syndrome

Sjögren-Larsson syndrome, inherited as an autosomal recessive disorder, usually manifests at birth with ichthyosiform erythroderma. The syndrome includes features that become evident only after the neonatal period: spastic diplegia, characteristic retinal lesions ("glistening dots"), and mental retardation. The diagnosis is supported by finding reduced or absent enzymatic activity of fatty aldehyde dehydrogenase from cultured skin fibroblasts, amniocytes, or chorionic cells (van den Brink, 2004). The genetic disorder that causes Sjögren-Larsson syndrome has been mapped to a locus on chromosome 17p11.2 that codes for a fatty aldehyde dehydrogenase (De Laurenzi, 1996).

Chondrodysplasia Punctata Syndromes (Conradi and Conradi-Hünermann Syndromes)

The chondroplasia punctata syndromes are a loosely defined group of syndromes sharing distinctive skin and bone abnormalities that are present at birth but may disappear with time. The skin lesions consist of patterned hyperkeratosis along the lines of Blaschko. Orthopedic abnormalities (including asymmetrical shortening of the long bones) prompt radiologic evaluation that reveals chondrodysplasia punctata, characterized by punctate calcifications of the epiphyses and cartilage. Abnormal facies and cataracts are associated features. Autosomal dominant, autosomal recessive, and X-linked dominant forms have been reported, and variable expressivity may reflect different patterns of X-inactivation (Ausavarat et al, 2008). The genetic abnormality associated with X-linked dominant Conradi syndrome has now been mapped to the *EBP* gene locus at Xp11.22-p11.23, which codes for a sterol isomerase (Braverman et al, 1999; Derry et al, 1999). Plasma sterol analysis has been found to be a highly specific and sensitive indicator of the presence of an EBP mutation in females with possible chondroplasia punctata syndrome (Herman et al, 2002).

CHILD Syndrome

CHILD syndrome is characterized by a striking phenotype consisting of *c*ongenital *h*emidysplasia, unilateral *i*chthyosiform erythroderma, and *l*imb *d*efects and also is known as *unilateral congenital ichthyosiform erythroderma*. CHILD syndrome is an X-linked disorder that shares some features with the X-linked dominant Conradi syndrome, with CHILD syndrome classically showing extreme lateralization and asymmetric skin lesions compared to the Conradi syndromes (Konig et al, 2002). Most cases of CHILD syndrome are caused by a mutation of the NADPH steroid dehydrogenase–like (NSDHL) protein gene, which has been mapped to Xq28 (Grange et al, 2000; Konig et al, 2000). This steroid dehydrogenase functions upstream of the sterol isomerase, which is defective in X-linked dominant Conradi syndrome in the cholesterol biosynthesis pathway. There have also been cases of mutations in the same *EBP* gene of X-linked Conradi syndrome that also included CHILD syndrome (Traupe and Has, 2000).

Keratitis-Ichthyosis-Deafness Syndrome

Keratitis-ichthyosis-deafness syndrome is a rare disorder of autosomal dominant inheritance (Wilson et al, 1991) that consists of congenital ichthyosiform erythroderma with characteristic pebbly palmoplantar thickening; abnormalities of the nails, hair, and teeth; vascularizing keratitis; and sensorineural deafness (Messmer et al, 2005). A few affected patients have died in infancy from overwhelming sepsis (Caceres-Rios et al, 1996) or in adulthood from malignant proliferating pilar tumors (Nyquist et al, 2007). Recent evidence points to a mutation in connexin 26, encoded by the *GJB2* gene, as the pathogenesis of this disorder (Titeux et al, 2009; van Steensel et al, 2002).

Neutral Lipid Storage Disease

Neutral lipid storage disease, or Chanarin-Dorfman syndrome (CDS), consists of nonbullous congenital ichthyosiform erythroderma, myopathy, neurosensory deafness, and cataracts. Inheritance is autosomal recessive. Vacuolated leukocytes from lipid droplets, seen on peripheral smear, help to establish the diagnosis (Judge et al, 1994a). This disease is characterized by an intracellular accumulation of triacylglycerol droplets. Mutations in a newly discovered protein of the esterase-lipase-thioesterase subfamily, CGI-58, encoded by the *CDS* locus at 3p21, appear to be the cause of this disease (Lefèvre et al, 2001).

Trichothiodystrophy

Trichothiodystrophy (TTD) is a disorder of autosomal recessive inheritance that includes a spectrum of ectodermal abnormalities: congenital ichthyosis (sometimes manifesting initially as collodion baby), brittle hair, and short stature (Kousseff, 1991). More severely affected patients have a constellation of features that has been referred to as *Tay syndrome*. These features include abnormal dentition, cataracts, nail dystrophy, progeric facies, and photosensitivity, with an increased incidence of skin cancers and a wide variety of central nervous system (CNS) abnormalities (Faghri et al, 2008). Diagnosis is supported by detection of characteristic alternating light and dark bands within the hair shaft on examination under polarizing microscopy. Further analyses of hair and nails reveal a decrease in the sulfur-rich proteins (Itin and Pittelkow, 1990).

The genetic mutations that cause TTD are the subject of active research. Two genes implicated in TTD, *XPB* and *XPD*, have been found to encode DNA helicase subunits. Other mutations in these two genes can result in xeroderma pigmentosum, or Cockayne's syndrome. *XPB* has been localized to 2q21, and *XPD* has been localized to 19q13.2-q13.3. There is also evidence that a mutation in an unlocalized third gene, *TTDA*, also may cause TTD (van Brabant et al, 2000).

Primary Cutaneous Ichthyoses

Primary cutaneous ichthyoses are a group of familial disorders that have no prominent extracutaneous manifestations. Lamellar ichthyosis, congenital nonbullous ichthyosiform erythroderma, and EHK are also primary cutaneous ichthyoses.

Ichthyosis Vulgaris

Ichthyosis vulgaris is the most common form of ichthyosis, with an estimated incidence of 1 in 250 births. It is inherited as an autosomal dominant trait. Onset is usually after the first 3 months of life. Scaling is most prominent on the extensor surfaces of the limbs. The palms and soles also are affected. Affected persons often have coexisting keratosis pilaris and atopic dermatitis (Rabinowitz and Esterly, 1994). Skin biopsy distinguishes ichthyosis vulgaris from the other forms of ichthyosis by revealing small or absent

keratohyalin granules. A major component of these granules, profilaggrin, is reduced or undetectable in the skin of affected persons (Nirunsuksiri et al, 1995). Recent molecular genetic investigations of the filaggrin gene have revealed the *R501X* mutation in European patients (Smith et al, 2006) versus the *S2554X* and *3321delA* mutations in Japanese patients (Nomura et al, 2007).

Erythrokeratodermia Variabilis

Erythrokeratodermia variabilis also is a rare type of ichthyosis that can manifest in infancy. It usually is inherited in an autosomal dominant fashion, although a probable case of autosomal recessive inheritance has been reported (Armstrong et al, 1997). Affected persons have transient migratory areas of discrete macular erythema and fixed hyperkeratotic plaques. A mutation in the connexin 31 gene, which codes for the gap junction protein β3, was reported as the cause of erythrokeratodermia variabilis, but a subsequent case did not have a mutated connexin 31 gene (Wilgoss et al, 1999). Studies have confirmed genetic heterogeneity in erythrokeratodermia variabilis affected by the intercellular communication mediated by both connexin 31 and connexin 30.3 genes in epidermal differentiation (Richard et al, 2003).

Prognosis and Treatment for the Ichthyoses

It is important to distinguish among the various forms of ichthyosis so that the physician can offer a prognosis and appropriate genetic counseling to the family. The prognosis is related to the severity of the condition and the type of ichthyosis. The clinical signs and pedigree data sometimes provide sufficient information to make a diagnosis. Skin biopsy for light microscopy is diagnostic only for EHK and ichthyosis vulgaris. Other general screening laboratory tests are equally nonspecific. Unfortunately, a period of observation beyond the first 4 weeks of life is frequently needed, and laboratory confirmation of the correct diagnosis requires specialized studies (Holbrook et al, 1993).

Standard therapy begins with topical care designed to hydrate the stratum corneum. Frequent, brief baths in tepid water should be followed immediately by liberal application of a bland ointment or cream emollient, such as petrolatum, Aquaphor, or Eucerin. Emollients containing keratolytics such as urea (10% to 25%), salicylic acid, propylene glycol, and α-hydroxy acids also are effective but are recommended only after infancy because of the risk of toxicity associated with increased percutaneous absorption. Irritating soaps and detergents should be avoided. Topical calcipotriol has been safe and effective as an agent for short-term therapy in adults with a variety of ichthyoses (Kragballe, 1995).

OCULOCUTANEOUS ALBINISM

The term *oculocutaneous albinism* (OCA) refers to a group of congenital disorders that are clinically manifested by an absence of pigment of the skin, hair, and eyes, with associated photophobia and nystagmus. All races are affected; estimates of gene frequency vary depending on the population under consideration. As with many genetic disorders, the incidence of affected persons is increased in certain racial isolates in which there is a high percentage of consanguineous marriages (Witkop et al, 1989).

Causes

All forms of OCA but one are inherited in an autosomal recessive fashion. The characteristic pigmentary changes are due to a spectrum of biochemical defects that interfere with melanin synthesis or transport. Three types of oculocutaneous albinism have been mapped to specific chromosomal regions that code for regulatory proteins in the transport and synthesis of tyrosine, a precursor in the melanin synthesis pathway (Oetting and King, 1994). OCA type 1 results from mutations in the gene that codes for tyrosinase (locus 11q14-q21). Tyrosinase is a copper-containing enzyme that catalyzes the two rate-limiting steps in the melanin biosynthetic pathway, and patients with homozygous mutations have a lifelong inability to produce melanin in the eyes, hair, and skin. More than 90 different mutations have been identified (Nakamura, 2002). OCA type 2, the most common form of OCA, results from mutations in the *P* gene. Recent findings suggest that the P protein has a major role in modulating the intracellular transport of tyrosinase (Toyofuku et al, 2002). OCA type 3 is caused by mutations in the tyrosinase-related protein 1 gene (*Tyrp1*). The encoded protein functions to maintain stability of tyrosinase (Sarangarajan and Boissy, 2001). Recent research suggests that other genetic mutations cause a fourth form of OCA (Newton et al, 2001).

Diagnosis

OCA type 1 can be distinguished from OCA types 2 and 3 on the basis of subtle clinical differences and the presence or absence of tyrosinase activity. OCA type 1 is the tyrosinase-negative variant and can be diagnosed prenatally with a fetal skin biopsy specimen (Holbrook et al, 1993). It results from any of several defects in the tyrosinase gene (Tomita, 1994). In type 2 and type 3 OCA, tyrosinase activity is positive. Genetic testing of tyrosinase and *P* genes may be necessary to distinguish OCA type 2 from type 3 (King et al, 2003). Oculocutaneous albinism should be distinguished from simple ocular albinism, which has sex-linked, autosomal dominant, and autosomal recessive forms.

Clinical Findings

Affected infants, regardless of their familial skin type, have a decrease in skin pigment. Hair and iris pigmentation can vary, depending on the genotype. Photophobia and nystagmus of varying degrees are also type-specific. Visual acuity is almost always impaired. Patients with tyrosine-negative OCA have the most severe form of visual impairment. Associated abnormalities may include hemorrhagic diathesis (Hermansky-Pudlak syndrome), small stature, and defective mentation. Deafness can occur in association with oculocutaneous albinism and with a number of other pigmentary disorders (Konigsmark, 1972).

Prognosis and Treatment

The most significant associated problems are visual impairment and the increased risk of sun-induced carcinogenesis. Treatment is supportive. Religious use of broad-spectrum sunblock with the highest available sun protection factor (SPF) is mandatory to protect against excessive exposure to sunlight. The safest approach for infants is zinc oxide ointment, sun-protective clothing, and sun avoidance. Persons with tyrosinase-positive albinism accumulate pigment with increasing age, decreasing the risk of sun-induced complications. The National Organization for Albinism and Hypopigmentation can provide additional information and support for affected families (see Box 98-2).

PIEBALDISM

Piebaldism is an autosomal dominant congenital leukoderma, characterized by a white forelock. Histologic studies show an absence of melanocytes in the depigmented areas of skin and normal melanocytes in the uninvolved skin (Jimbow et al, 1975). The molecular basis of the disease has been identified as a defect of the C-kit protooncogene. This gene encodes the cell surface receptor transmembrane tyrosine kinase for an embryonic growth factor. When c-*kit* function is reduced, the migration of melanocytes is curtailed during embryogenesis (Tomita, 1994). c-*kit* in a minority of affected patients is unaffected, but instead has mutations in the *SNAI2* gene (Sanchez-Martin et al, 2003).

Clinical Findings

A white forelock is present in 90% of cases. Other areas of the ventral skin may also be devoid of pigment, including the central forehead, chin, and trunk, with relative sparing of the dorsal surface. Eyebrows and midarm and midleg skin may also be depigmented. Within these areas, smaller, normally pigmented or hyperpigmented patches may be evident (Figure 98-5).

Diagnosis

Piebaldism is readily differentiated from albinism, in which the absence of pigment is uniform. Vitiligo may have a similar appearance, but it is not congenital and usually does not remain fixed. Occasional families may have associated defects such as sensorineural deafness and mental retardation (Telfer et al, 1971). Piebaldism is unrelated to Waardenburg's syndrome, an autosomal dominant condition that features a white forelock, widened nasal bridge, and cochlear deafness.

Prognosis and Treatment

The leukoderma and white forelock remain constant throughout life. Cosmetic camouflage is a treatment option suitable for infants and children. Surgical options are evolving.

APLASIA CUTIS CONGENITA

The congenital absence of skin is a cutaneous anomaly most often affecting the scalp, but occasionally involving the trunk and extremities.

Causes

Several distinct subtypes of aplasia cutis have been described based on the distribution, mode of inheritance, and associated abnormalities (Frieden, 1986). Most cases

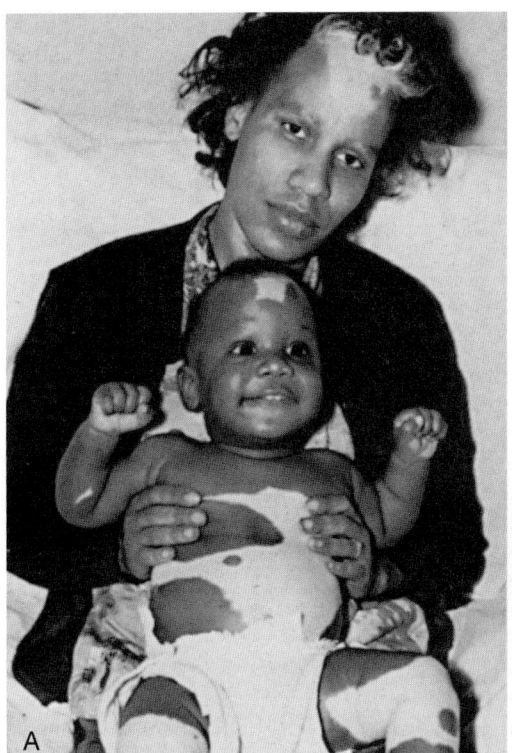
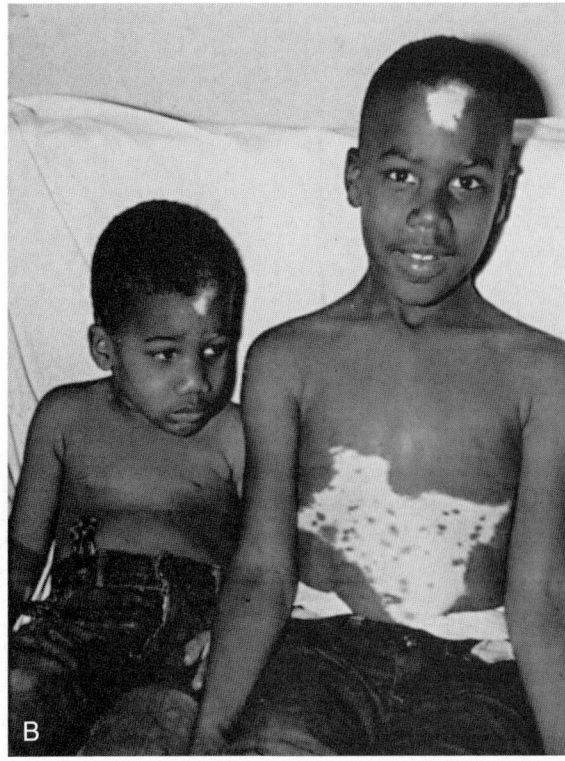

FIGURE 98-5 **A,** Mother and child with piebaldism. Both have patches on the forehead, although of different sizes and shapes. The areas of non-pigmentation on the infant's trunk and extremities are unusually extensive. **B,** Siblings with different degrees of piebaldism. *(From Jahn HM, McIntire MS: Piebaldness, of familial white skin spotting; partial albinism, Am J Dis Child 88:471-480, 1954. Copyright the American Medical Association.)*

of aplasia cutis congenita occur sporadically; autosomal dominant and autosomal recessive modes of transmission also have been well documented (Sybert, 1985). Associated abnormalities include cleft lip and palate, limb anomalies, cutaneous organoid nevi, and EB. Aplasia cutis may overlie embryologic malformations such as meningomyelocele and spinal dysraphia, omphalocele, and gastroschisis (Frieden, 1986; Sybert, 1985). In addition, scalp defects are associated with specific teratogens (methimazole, intrauterine varicella, herpes simplex) and malformation syndromes (trisomy 13, Johanson-Blizzard syndrome, amniotic band disruption complex, and the ectodermal dysplasias). Extensive aplasia cutis has been associated with elevated α-fetoprotein in maternal serum and amniotic fluid (Gerber et al, 1993).

The cause of aplasia cutis congenita is unknown. Basically, it is a phenotypic physical finding signifying disruption of the skin in utero and is attributable to any of a number of causes. Findings of a twin fetus papyraceus or a placental infarct have suggested vascular thrombosis as a cause in infants with lesions on the trunk and limbs (Levin et al, 1980).

Clinical Findings

The defect is usually along the midline of the scalp in the parietal or occipital area. Lesions are sharply marginated and may manifest as ulcers, bullae, or scars. Lesions may be solitary or multiple, measuring up to several centimeters in diameter (Figure 98-6). Up to 30% of affected

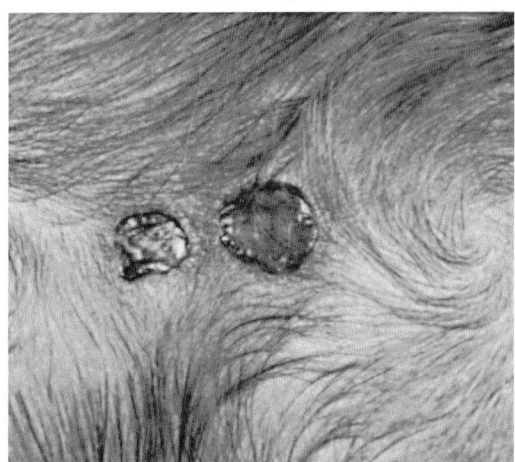

FIGURE 98-6 Skin is absent in two sharply marginated areas on the scalp of a normal newborn male infant whose mother's labor and delivery were normal. The defects extended to the subcutaneous tissue and healed in 3 weeks with the formation of thin, white atrophic scars.

infants have underlying defects of the calvaria. Multiple defects, particularly those on the trunk and extremities, may be strikingly symmetric in distribution (Levin et al, 1980). Larger defects are often deeper and can extend to the dura or meninges. These defects can be complicated by meningitis, hemorrhage (which can be fatal), or venous thrombosis.

Histologic examination of tissue from the defect demonstrates an absence of epidermis and a diminished number of appendageal structures and dermal elastic fibers or, in deeper lesions, the absence of all layers of the integument. There is no evidence of inflammation or pathogenic organisms.

Prognosis and Treatment

Cutaneous and bony lesions can heal spontaneously over a period of weeks to months. A hypertrophic or atrophic patch of alopecia remains. Patients with larger and deeper lesions must be observed for the possibility of a complicating meningitis. Prophylactic excision with repair should be considered in these cases. Lesions that fail to heal or produce cosmetically unacceptable scars can be excised with primary closure (Kosnik and Sayers, 1975).

INCONTINENTIA PIGMENTI

Incontinentia pigmenti (IP), also known as the Bloch-Sulzberger syndrome, is a disorder of the developing neuroectoderm, characterized by three distinctive, transient stages of cutaneous lesions and variable persistent abnormalities of the CNS, eyes, teeth, hair, and nails.

Causes

IP is inherited in an X-linked dominant fashion. Surviving females are mosaics, whereas most hemizygous males do not survive embryogenesis. Molecular research indicates mutations at one genetic locus at Xq28 as the cause of all true cases of IP. Eighty percent of IP cases were found to result from a single mutation (Berlin et al, 2002). The mutation has been associated with the nuclear factor kB essential modulator gene (*NEMO*), which encodes for a transcription factor (Gautheron et al, 2010).

Clinical Findings

The diagnosis of IP is made by cutaneous examination. Most patients exhibit three stages of skin lesions that persist for varying periods (O'Brien and Feingold, 1985). The vesiculobullous phase manifests at birth and generally lasts for several months. It is characterized by widespread inflammatory vesicular lesions on the scalp, trunk, and extremities in a whorled and linear distribution along the lines of Blaschko (Figure 98-7, *A*). The infant is otherwise well, although markedly elevated leukocyte counts and peripheral eosinophilia with as much as 79% eosinophils may be associated (Berlin et al, 2002). Several pediatric cases of late recurrences of the first-stage of IP have been reported, often precipitated by infections, and have been presumed to be due to the persistence of mutant *NEMO* keratinocytes in the sites of previous lesions (Bodak et al, 2003). The vesicular phase evolves into a *verrucous* phase, in which warty lesions appear in roughly the same distribution as the blisters, but are most pronounced on the hands and feet. The third stage is characterized by macular gray or brown pigmentation distributed along the lines of Blaschko, independent of the sites of previous lesions (see Figure 98-7, *B*). The pigmentary lesions usually fade in later years and may disappear by adulthood. Rarely the stage-three pigmentary changes are present at birth,

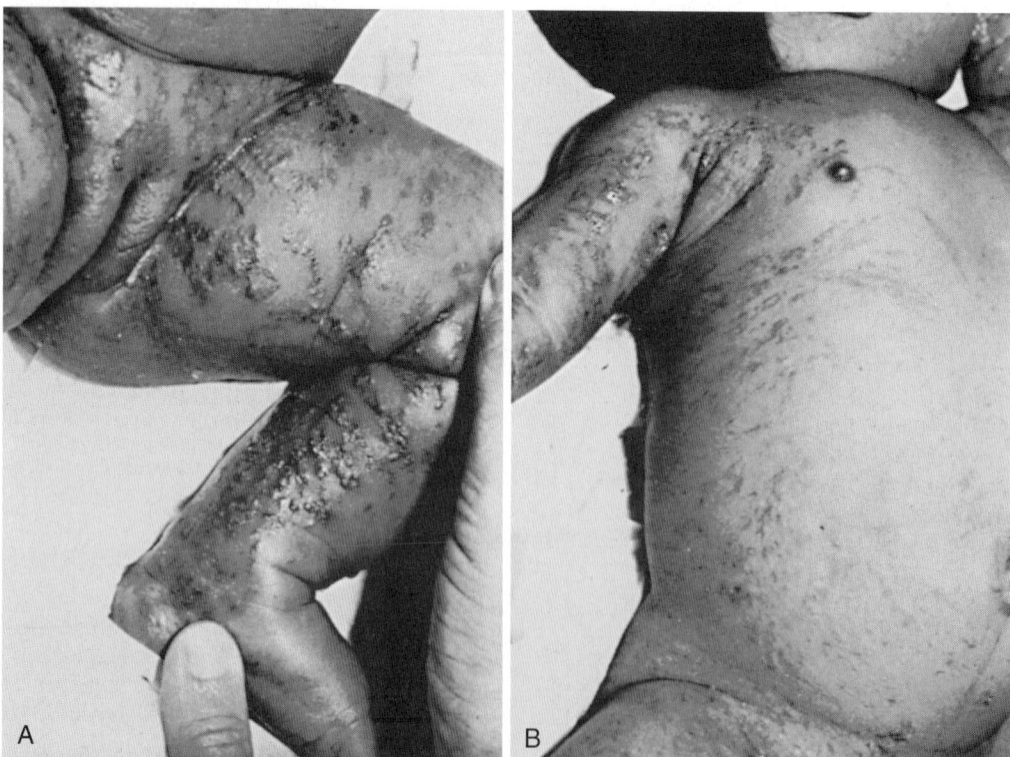

FIGURE 98-7 Incontinentia pigmenti. A, Inflammatory vesicular and crusted lesions on the legs. **B,** Whorled pigmentation developing on the trunk of a 1-month-old infant who still has inflammatory lesions on the limbs.

and the first two stages are never evident (Lerer, 1973). Fourth-stage lesions, seen in some affected women, consist of hypopigmented, atrophic, anhidrotic streaks, usually localized to the legs (Moss and Ince, 1987).

Eighty percent of affected persons have extracutaneous involvement, including CNS aberrations (seizures, microcephaly, retardation, and spastic paralysis), patchy alopecia, defective dentition, ocular abnormalities, and less commonly, bone defects (Carney, 1976).

Diagnosis

Infants with IP usually have blisters. The linear distribution of blisters is often so characteristic that it permits instant recognition of the disorder, but other causes of blisters must be considered in the differential diagnosis (see Chapter 99). Skin biopsy during the bullous phase will show intraepidermal vesicles filled with eosinophils. These features are not pathognomonic but help to exclude more ominous causes of neonatal blistering. Clinicians should refer patients for genetic testing to the DNA Diagnostic Laboratory at Baylor College of Medicine (see Incontinentia Pigmenti in Box 98-2).

Prognosis and Treatment

Treatment of the skin lesions is not necessary. Occasionally vesicular lesions become extremely inflamed or secondarily infected. Patients should be monitored for the development of other anomalies, especially of the eyes, teeth, and CNS. Genetic counseling is indicated. Two IP support groups for patients and their families are the Incontinentia Pigmenti International Foundation and the Incontinentia Pigmenti Support Network (see Box 98-2).

CUTIS LAXA

Cutis laxa is a rare, heterogeneous group of genetic abnormalities of connective tissue with striking cutaneous features. Autosomal dominant, autosomal recessive, and X-linked forms have been described (Beighton, 1972; Byers et al, 1980). Cutis laxa–like skin changes can also be found in other disorders (e.g., combined immunodeficiency disease, the Prader-Willi and Langer-Giedion syndromes).

Clinical Features

Cutis laxa–like skin hangs in pendulous folds, producing a facies with a hooked nose, everted nostrils, a long upper lip, sagging cheeks, and a prematurely aged appearance (Figure 98-8). The infant may have a hoarse cry because of redundant laryngeal tissue. Persons with the autosomal dominant form of cutis laxa suffer few ill effects, apart from their altered appearance, and enjoy good health and a normal life span. Pulmonary and cardiovascular manifestations are absent or minimal. In contrast, patients with the recessive form of the disorder are often seriously compromised and may die in childhood of pulmonary or cardiovascular complications. Systemic manifestations include diverticula of the gastrointestinal and urogenital tracts, rectal prolapse, multiple hernias, pulmonary emphysema,

and cardiac disease (Mehregan et al, 1978). A few infants have been reported who manifested additional defects, such as skeletal anomalies, dislocation of the hips, and intrauterine growth restriction (Sakati et al, 1983).

Diagnosis

The clinical manifestations of cutis laxa can be attributed to abnormalities of elastin, associated with a combined defect in N- and O-glycosylation because of the *ATP6V0A2* gene (Kornak et al, 2008). Elastic fibers are diminished in the papillary and upper dermis, whereas those in the lower dermis undergo fragmentation and granular degeneration (Mehregan et al, 1978). Similar changes occur in the elastic tissue of affected viscera. Autosomal recessive cutis laxa has been associated with a deficiency of lysyl oxidase, a copper-dependent enzyme mapped to chromosome 5 (Debret et al, 2010; Khakoo et al, 1997). The X-linked form has been associated with abnormal intracellular copper metabolism, with a decrease in the activity of lysyl oxidase. This form of cutis laxa, once classified as type IX Ehlers-Danlos syndrome, was redefined as occipital horn syndrome, an X-linked recessive condition allelic to Menkes syndrome (Beighton et al, 1988; Byers, 1994; Goldsmith, 1990) (see Figure 98-8).

Treatment

Plastic surgery can improve the physical appearance of patients with cutis laxa (Thomas et al, 1993). The internal manifestations are not amenable to therapy.

EHLERS-DANLOS SYNDROME

Ehlers-Danlos syndrome (EDS) is another heterogeneous group of inherited connective tissue disorders that share the common features of skin hyperextensibility, articular hypermobility, and tissue fragility (Beighton, 1993). In contrast to patients with cutis laxa, those with EDS have skin that is hyperextensible rather than loose; when stretched, the skin readily snaps back into place (Farmer et al, 2010). Skin fragility is another feature, leading to easy bruising and bleeding, gaping wounds, and numerous

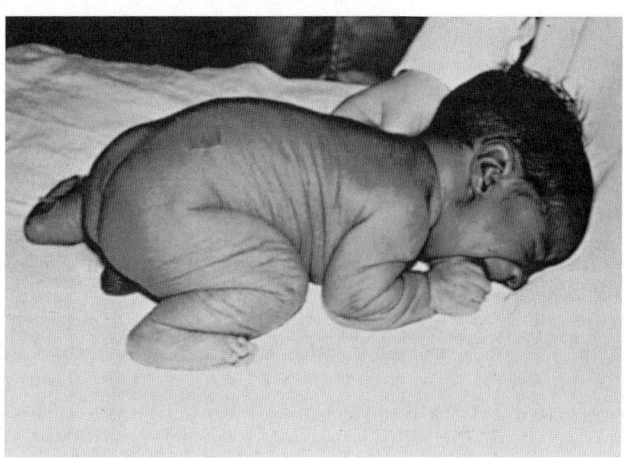

FIGURE 98-8 Newborn infant with clinical features of Menkes syndrome and cutis laxa.

cigarette paper–like scars. Joint hypermobility is another major manifestation. The classification of EDS is evolving, and the latest classification scheme identifies six major types: classic, hypermobility, vascular, kyphoscoliosis, arthrochalasia, and dermatosparaxis. The kyphoscoliosis and dermatosparaxis types are inherited in an autosomal recessive fashion, whereas inheritance for the other four types is autosomal dominant. In addition, there are other known cases of EDS that do not fit into one of these types and await further characterization (Beighton et al, 1998). Persons with the vascular type of EDS (type IV by previous classification) can be easily distinguished from those with the other forms by their thin, translucent skin, marked bruising, and normal range of motion. It is especially important to identify this group because of its life-threatening complications (Byers, 1994).

Causes

All forms of EDS are believed to be due to defects in the biogenesis of collagen. The vascular type is characterized by a variety of defects in the synthesis of type III collagen, the kyphoscoliosis type by lysyl hydroxylase deficiency, the arthrochalasia type by defective processing of type I collagen, and the dermatosparaxis type by procollagen N-proteinase deficiency. These specific defects can be identified by culture of dermal fibroblasts from a skin biopsy.

Treatment

Recognition of the correct subtype is important for prognosis. The vascular type of EDS is particularly important to identify because of the life-threatening association with arterial, bowel, and uterine ruptures. There is no effective treatment for the various forms of EDS. Affected patients tolerate surgical procedures poorly because of difficulty in healing and frequent dehiscence of surgical wounds. Repair of cutaneous wounds may require the services of a plastic surgeon, and progressive joint disease will require ongoing orthopedic care. The Ehlers-Danlos National Foundation can provide additional information and support for affected families (see Box 98-2).

EPIDERMOLYSIS BULLOSA

EB is a diverse group of diseases that is characterized by skin blistering (Sawamura et al, 2010). Classification is based on clinical characteristics, inheritance pattern, and the level of cleavage within the skin, as determined by skin biopsy. This prominent histologic feature defines three main groups: simplex (cleavage within the basal cells of the epidermis), junctional (within the lamina lucida of the basement membrane zone), and dystrophic (beneath the lamina densa of the basement membrane). At each level, there are several protein components that contribute to skin integrity. These molecules all are expressed in utero during the first trimester, allowing prenatal diagnosis by skin biopsy (Holbrook et al, 1993). Further progress in the field has led to a simplified classification system that recognizes 10 major subtypes; three major EB types: epidermolysis bullosa simplex (EBS), junctional epidermolysis bullosa (JEB), and dystrophic epidermolysis bullosa; and

11 minor subtypes (Fine et al, 2000). Research efforts have been greatly enhanced by the Dystrophic Epidermolysis Bullosa Research Association of America (DEBRA) and the National Epidermolysis Bullosa Registry (see Box 98-2) (Fine, 1994). Identification of the molecular basis of a number of EB genotypes has facilitated prenatal and postnatal diagnoses and has also provided insight into the pathogenesis of blistering diseases, as well as the basic mechanisms of epithelial and basement membrane integrity (Uitto et al, 2010).

Epidermolysis Bullosa Simplex

EB simplex features blisters that arise within the basal layer of the epidermis. For this reason, the lesions of EB simplex do not scar. Four major subtypes and several minor subtypes have been recognized (Fine et al, 2000). The molecular defects of EB simplex have been localized to the genes encoding specific keratins, *K14* (located on chromosome 17) and *K5* (located on chromosome 12), except for EB with muscular dystrophy, which is due to a defect in plectin. Keratins K5 and K14 are expressed predominantly in the basal cells of the epidermis, and these disorders are closely related to epidermolytic hyperkeratosis (Francis, 1994) (see discussion under Ichthyoses That Manifest in the Neonatal Period). The four major subtypes are described next.

Epidermolysis Bullosa Simplex, Koebner Subtype

ES simplex, Koebner subtype, inherited as an autosomal dominant trait and is present at birth or early in infancy. Bullae arise most frequently over pressure points, such as the elbows and knees, as well as on the legs, feet, and hands. Mucous membrane involvement occurs primarily during infancy. The extensive erosions that sometimes result from the trauma of birth can be mistaken for aplasia cutis. Nails may be lost but almost always regrow. The prognosis is relatively good, and the propensity to blister may decrease with age.

Epidermolysis Bullosa Simplex, Dowling-Meara Subtype

EB simplex, Dowling-Meara subtype (EBS-DM), is inherited as an autosomal dominant trait and causes generalized, often extensive blistering in the neonatal period and early years of life. Herpetiform grouping of the blisters is characteristic. Additional findings include nail dystrophy, palmoplantar keratoderma as a late feature, and improvement with age. Molecular genetics studies reveal KRT5 and KRT14 mutations underlying patients with EBS-DM (Petek et al, 2010; Pfendner et al, 2005).

Epidermolysis Bullosa Simplex, Weber-Cockayne Subtype

EB simplex, Weber-Cockayne subtype, is inherited in autosomal dominant fashion and usually does not manifest during the neonatal period. The blisters in this disease usually are limited to the hands and feet, although they occasionally occur elsewhere on the body. The gene defects are associated with keratin 5 and keratin 10 (Müller et al, 1998).

Epidermolysis Bullosa Simplex With Muscular Dystrophy

EB simplex with muscular dystrophy (EBS-MD) is a rare variant that is inherited in an autosomal recessive fashion. Affected persons usually demonstrate blisters on the skin and mucous membranes at birth or shortly thereafter. EBS-MD is associated with tooth enamel hypoplasia and nail dystrophy. Progressive muscular dystrophy usually occurs later in life (Shimizu et al, 1999). Recent molecular studies identified plectin as the gene defect (Chiavérini, 2010).

Junctional Epidermolysis Bullosa

JEB is characterized by cleavage within the lamina lucida of the basement membrane zone. Three major subtypes are now recognized: JEB, Herlitz subtype; JEB, non-Herlitz subtype; and JEB with pyloric atresia. Molecular defects have been recognized within several proteins found in the basement membrane zone, including laminin-5, type XVII collagen, and the α_6,β_4-integrin complex. Several subtypes of JEB are relatively localized and benign (Fine et al, 2000). The major subtypes are described next.

Junctional Epidermolysis Bullosa, Herlitz Subtype

JEB, Herlitz subtype (JEB-H), was formerly known as *EB gravis* or *letalis* because many affected patients die in infancy. Generalized blistering is noted at birth. Persons with this form of JEB can, however, exhibit a spectrum of severity. Bullae and moist erosions occur on the scalp, in the perioral area, and over pressure points elsewhere on the body (Figure 98-9, *A*). Some of these erosions become the sites of vegetating granulomas, a pathognomonic finding. The hands and feet are relatively spared, and digital fusion, inevitable in the recessive dystrophic type of EB, does not occur. Nails are affected and may be lost permanently. Defective dentition is the rule, but mucous membrane erosions are inconspicuous and rarely cause

problems. Laryngeal involvement can occur in childhood, manifested as hoarseness or stridor. These patients grow poorly, appear malnourished, and have chronic recalcitrant anemia. Mutations of any of the three α, β, and γ subunits of the *laminin 332* gene can produce the JEB Herlitz phenotype (Varki et al, 2006).

Junctional Epidermolysis Bullosa, Non-Herlitz Subtype

JEB, non-Herlitz subtype, is a disorder of autosomal recessive inheritance that carries the best prognosis of the major subtypes, with affected persons often surviving into adulthood. Onset is usually at birth, with generalized blistering; dystrophic nails or absence of nails is common (Fine et al, 2000).

Junctional Epidermolysis Bullosa with Pyloric Atresia

JEB with pyloric atresia is a rare, autosomal recessively inherited disease characterized by mucocutaneous fragility. JEB with pyloric atresia is usually fatal in the first few weeks of life, although mild cases have been reported. Polyhydramnios seen at ultrasound examination may be the first clue to gastric outlet obstruction. Generalized blistering and ulcerations of skin and mucous membranes usually are evident at birth. The urinary tract frequently is involved, stenosis being a common complication for survivors (Mellerio et al, 1998).

Dystrophic Epidermolysis Bullosa

Dystrophic EB is characterized by subepidermal blistering, below the level of the lamina densa of the basement membrane. The anchoring fibrils that link the lower part of the basement membrane to the papillary dermis are composed of type VII collagen. Mutations of the gene that codes for type VII collagen have been identified in most forms of dystrophic EB. This group of diseases is characterized clinically by milia and scarring at the sites of healed

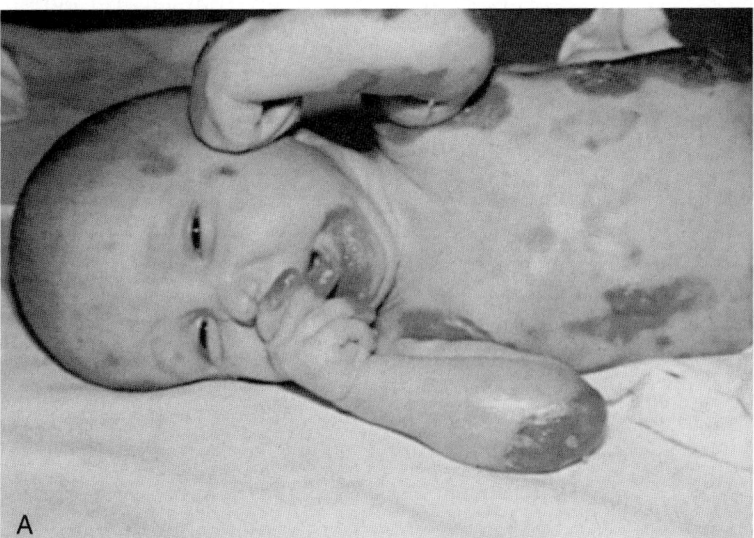
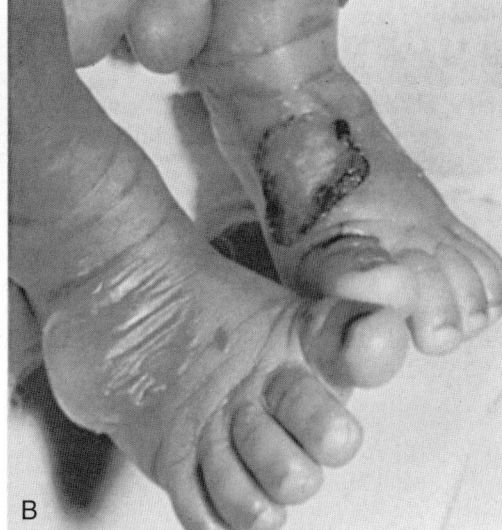

FIGURE 98-9 A, Multiple moist erosions characteristic of junctional epidermolysis bullosa. Note the involvement of fingers and perioral skin. **B,** Large bullae on the feet of an infant with a scarring form of epidermolysis bullosa.

blisters. There are three major subtypes and several minor subtypes. All are present at birth (Fine et al, 1991). Prenatal diagnosis as early as 8 to 10 weeks' gestation is possible by molecular techniques for some families. The three major subtypes are described next, as well as one of the more distinctive minor subtypes.

Dominant Dystrophic Epidermolysis Bullosa

Dominant dystrophic EB is a relatively mild form, inherited as an autosomal dominant trait. Generalized blistering usually is noted at birth. In some cases, blistering may appear only on the hands, feet, elbows, or knees; this pattern usually is due to mechanical trauma. Rarely does scarring cause immobility and deformity of the hands and feet. Small cysts or milia are seen at sites of scarring. There may be mild involvement of the mucous membranes; nails may be thick, dystrophic, or destroyed. Some persons affected by this form of EB may note the presence of small, firm, flesh-colored, or white skin elevations that appear spontaneously on the trunk and extremities, called *albopapuloid lesions*. Genetics studies of affected patients have indicated the collagen type VII alterations due to the *COL7A1* gene (Varki et al, 2007).

The Cockayne-Touraine and Pasini types of EB formerly were considered to represent two generalized forms of dominant dystrophic EB, but they are now included within dominant dystrophic EB in the new classification system. The bullae are subepidermal and heal with scarring, but the process may be relatively limited, involving mainly the hands, feet (see Figure 98-9, *B*), and skin over bony protuberances, or it may be generalized, particularly in the Pasini variant. Nails may be lost. Milia are common and may appear in profusion in the soft, wrinkled scars; pigmentary changes also are common. Mucous membrane lesions, if present, are mild and general health may be unimpaired. The appearance of albopapuloid lesions on the trunk during adolescence is a unique feature of the Pasini variant.

Transient Bullous Dermolysis of the Newborn

The rare variant transient bullous dermolysis of the newborn was first reported in 1985 (Hashimoto et al, 1985). Autosomal dominant and recessive forms have been described. The dominant form is now thought to be a form of dominant dystrophic EB. Affected neonates exhibit alarming acral or generalized blistering that heals with scars. Histologic analyses have localized the abnormality to the precursors of the anchoring fibrils, and genetic studies have shown mutations in a gene that codes for type VII collagen in some cases (Hammami-Hauasli et al, 1998). This condition is unique among the subsets of EB, because it spontaneously resolves within the first years of life.

Recessive Dystrophic Epidermolysis Bullosa, Hallopeau-Siemens Subtype

Recessive dystrophic EB, Hallopeau-Siemens subtype, is the more severe form of recessive dystrophic EB. Infants with Hallopeau-Siemens EB often have extensive denuded lesions at birth and during the neonatal period. Bullae may be hemorrhagic and occur on all surfaces, including the hands and feet; loss of the nails is common. Over subsequent years the mobility of the fingers and toes becomes severely impaired as fusion of digits, bone resorption, and the inevitable mitten-like deformity of the hands and feet ensue. Mucous membrane involvement can be severe, resulting in esophageal strictures and serious impairment of nutrition because of the restriction of oral intake. These bullae are subepidermal and always eventuate in scarring. Affected persons have a markedly increased risk of skin cancer, with a 39.6% cumulative risk of developing squamous cell carcinoma and a 2.5% cumulative risk of developing malignant melanoma by age 30 (Fine et al, 2000). Electron microscopy reveals diminished or absent anchoring fibrils associated with marked degeneration of type VII collagen in the papillary portion of the dermis. Also evident is excess abnormal collagenase in fibroblast cultures.

Recessive Dystrophic Epidermolysis Bullosa, Non–Hallopeau-Siemens Subtype

Recessive dystrophic EB, non–Hallopeau-Siemens subtype, is the less severe form of recessive dystrophic EB. It is characterized by onset at birth, generalized blisters that include the mucosal surfaces, atrophic scarring over bony prominences, and either nail loss or nail dystrophy. Milia, mild finger flexion contractures, albopapuloid lesions, dental disease, and external ear involvement also are often seen. According to one report, affected patients also have an increased risk of squamous cell carcinoma of approximately 14% by age 30 (Fine et al, 2000).

Diagnosis and Treatment of Epidermolysis Bullosa

Diagnosis

Arriving at the correct diagnosis can be difficult, especially in the neonatal period. The differential diagnosis includes the spectrum of blisters and bullae outlined in Chapter 97. The distribution of blisters can be a clue. In EB, the earliest lesions occur on points of friction, such as the heels, wrists, knees, and sacrum. The fluid within the bullae is likely to be clear or hemorrhagic, rather than purulent. A careful family history for blistering diseases should be obtained. The most precise diagnostic tool is a carefully performed skin biopsy to obtain specimens for immunofluorescence mapping and ultrastructural study. The sample for immunofluorescence should be obtained from normal or perilesional skin, excluding the palms or soles, and placed in Zeus or Michel transport medium. The ideal specimen for electron microscopy is a new spontaneous or induced blister preserved in glutaraldehyde (Fine et al, 1994). After the diagnosis of simplex, junctional, or dystrophic EB is made, further subclassification can be difficult during infancy for subsets without a defined genotype. In these patients without a relevant family history, distinguishing clinical features may take months or years to develop.

Treatment

To date, the mainstay of therapy for this group of disorders is supportive. The infant should be protected from frictional trauma; direct pressure is tolerated. Latex gloves can stick to the skin and should be lubricated with petrolatum. Bedding should be of a soft material. Dressing changes should be performed daily. Adequate premedication for pain control should be given. Bathing may have to be restricted to avoid excessive handling. Compresses with normal saline or Burow's solution for eroded areas may be helpful in some instances. Tepid compresses should be used, because warm temperatures increase the tendency to blister. Intact blisters should be lanced with an adequate incision to drain the fluid, while the roof is maintained as a "biologic dressing." Wounds should be covered with petrolatum-impregnated gauze. Topical antibiotics may promote healing, but content and quantity should be carefully monitored in young infants. Topical mupirocin is the antibiotic of choice at several EB centers; bacterial resistance has been reported in chronic users with EB. Commercially available nonadhesive dressings are simpler to use and more effective than plain gauze wraps. Exudry pads, secured with SurgiNet or conforming gauze, are recommended for draining wounds on the body. Omiderm (Doak Pharmaceuticals) is a nonadhesive polyurethane dressing that provides an excellent barrier for moist wounds on the face and hands. Adhesive tape should never be applied, because large areas of epidermis may be torn off with its removal. Dressing should be applied to blistered areas only to maximize the infant's tactile stimulation. For the newborn, environmental temperature must be carefully monitored; overheating can result in extensive blistering. For patients with mucous membrane involvement, soft nipples, bulb syringes, and devices used for feeding infants with cleft palates should be used. Chronic serosanguineous drainage and gastrointestinal involvement often result in poor nutritional status. Iron deficiency anemia is another common complication in infants with severe disease. Routine use of aggressive nutritional supplementation is recommended. After discharge, cribs, high chairs, and infant seats should be well padded, and only soft toys should be offered for play (Gibbons, 1990).

Caregivers should be given anticipatory guidance about protective measures, wound care, and nutrition. The practitioner should encourage contact with DEBRA, a privately funded organization that is an excellent resource for affected families. DEBRA can provide practical information for day-to-day care and direct families to the appropriate regional center for specialized care (see Box 98-2). To register newly diagnosed patients, clinicians should contact the National Epidermolysis Bullosa Registry (see Box 98-2).

NEONATAL LUPUS ERYTHEMATOSUS

Neonatal lupus erythematosus (NLE) is an uncommon immune-mediated disease that results from transplacental transfer of maternal immunoglobulin G antinuclear antibodies. It manifests within the first 2 months of life. Infants exhibit a spectrum of signs, including transient cutaneous lesions, thrombocytopenia, hepatitis, and congenital heart blocks (Kim et al, 2009). All affected infants have serologic evidence of lupus erythematosus during the first few months of life (Lee, 1993; Lee and Weston, 1984; Provost et al, 1987).

Causes

NLE is always marked by the presence of anti-Ro (SS-A), anti-La (SS-B), or anti-U_1RNP autoantibodies in the mother and infant. With the exception of congenital heart block, most of the manifestations of neonatal lupus resolve with the disappearance of maternal antibodies, suggesting an important role for these antibodies in pathogenesis. An association with HLA-DR3 in the mother but not the infant also has been documented (Lee and Weston, 1984). Ro-positive HLA-DR2 mothers, in contrast, produce unaffected infants (Provost, 1987).

Clinical Findings

Half of the affected infants have skin lesions. These may be present with or without evidence of systemic disease (Hardy, 1979). Skin lesions are typically annular erythematous scaling plaques (Figure 98-10), with a predilection for sun-exposed areas. These lesions begin to resolve at approximately 6 months of age, concurrent with the disappearance of maternal antibodies. Persistent telangiectatic matting in a characteristic distribution, involving the scalp, lips, and vulva, also has been described (Figure 98-11) (Thornton et al, 1995).

Diagnosis

The skin lesions of NLE can be mistaken for several cutaneous disorders including syphilis, seborrheic dermatitis, dermatophytosis, atopic dermatitis, and psoriasis. A skin biopsy specimen may demonstrate the histopathologic features of lupus. More reliable, however, is the detection of Ro (SS-A) or La (SS-B) antibody, or both, in serum from the infant and the mother.

The North American Collaborative Study of NLE is an ongoing prospective study of all aspects of the disease. To arrange for enrollment and serologic testing of patients, clinicians should contact study investigators (see under Neonatal Lupus Erythematosus in Box 98-2).

Prognosis and Treatment

Affected infants should be protected from sources of ultraviolet light (e.g., sunlight, daylight fluorescent bulbs) by application of a broad-spectrum sunscreen such as titanium

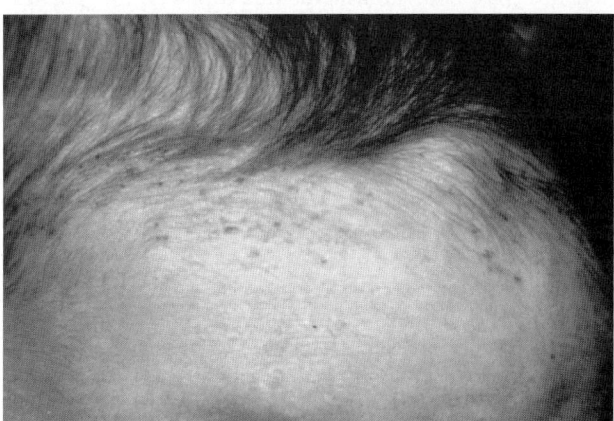

FIGURE 98-10 Newborn with cutaneous lesions of neonatal lupus erythematosus.

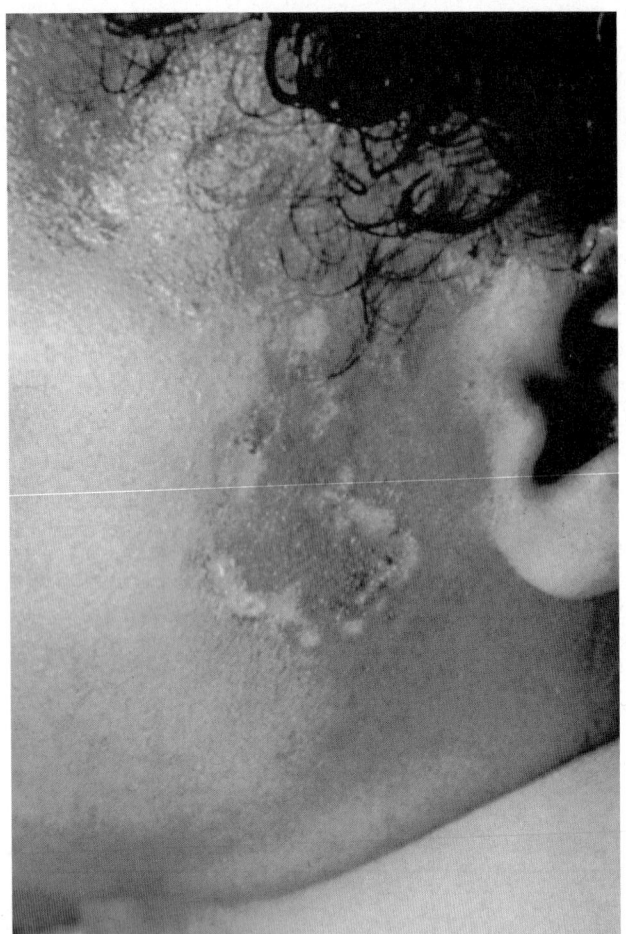

FIGURE 98-11 Telangiectatic matting of the scalp, lips, and groin is a recently recognized cutaneous marker of neonatal lupus.

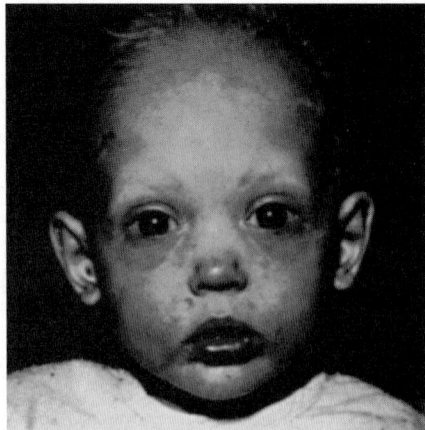

FIGURE 98-12 Girl with fully expressed anhidrotic ectodermal dysplasia. Note the sparse wispy hair, hyperpigmentation around the eyes, depressed nasal bridge, and protruding lips and ears.

dioxide, zinc oxide, and sun-protective clothing. Active skin lesions can be treated with a topical corticosteroid.

The prognosis is excellent, except in affected infants who develop congenital heart block. Most infants with congenital heart block will require a pacemaker, and death will occur in approximately 20% of patients (Tseng and Buyon, 1997).

It is important to recognize that asymptomatic mothers are at risk for development of disorders associated with their serologic abnormalities (e.g., Sjögren syndrome, subacute cutaneous lupus, systemic lupus erythematosus). There is a 25% risk of involvement for each subsequent pregnancy (Gawkrodger and Beveridge, 1984; McCune, 1987).

ECTODERMAL DYSPLASIAS

The ectodermal dysplasias (EDs) are a heterogeneous group of inherited disorders characterized by defects in the development of two or more structures of ectodermal origin. The major structures involved are hair follicles, nails, teeth, and sweat glands; sebaceous glands, conjunctivae, and the lens also may be affected. A formal classification system has been created for the EDs, based on the specific structures affected (Pinheiro and Freire-Maia, 1994). One hundred fifty-four syndromes have been included in this grouping. Several of these, such as incontinentia

pigmenti and syndromes associated with ichthyosis, have not been traditionally regarded as ED. Many others have been reported rarely. The National Foundation for Ectodermal Dysplasias (NFED) is a privately funded organization committed to locating affected families and providing them with information and support (see Box 98-2). The NFED also coordinates and funds research efforts. Three of the more well-characterized types of ED are described next.

Hypohidrotic Ectodermal Dysplasia

Hypohidrotic ED, inherited as an X-linked recessive disorder, was the first type of ED described as Christ-Siemens-Touraine syndrome. It was previously referred to as being *anhidrotic*, but affected persons may have a limited capacity to sweat, and the preferred descriptor is *hypohidrotic*. This type of ED occurs in 1 in 100,000 male births and manifests during the 1st year of life. The most serious problem is diminution of the sweating response because of rudimentary or absent eccrine sweat glands, which results in marked heat intolerance and episodes of hyperpyrexia, frequently misinterpreted as fever of unknown origin (Richards and Kaplan, 1969). If ED is not considered in the differential diagnosis, these infants may be subjected to numerous unnecessary hospitalizations and tests. Recent studies demonstrate genetic mutations in the EDA gene (Lexner et al, 2008).

Clinical Features

Patients with hypohidrotic ED have several characteristic features that may be subtle in the newborn. One common neonatal sign is severe peeling or scaling skin. This skin change, which can be misconstrued as an indication of postmaturity, may provide a valuable clue to the diagnosis (Executive and Scientific Advisory Boards of the National Foundation for Ectodermal Dysplasia, 1989). Thereafter the skin may appear relatively pale and dry, with a prominent venous pattern over most of the body, but hyperpigmented and wrinkled in the periorbital area (Figure 98-12).

The craniofacial characteristics of frontal bossing, depression of the midface, flattened nasal bridge, thick protruding lips, and prominent chin may not be readily apparent in the newborn. The sparse, unruly, light-colored hair and scanty brows and lashes also are difficult to appreciate in the first few months. The changes in dentition cannot, of course, be detected until late infancy. Hypodontia with conical, poorly formed teeth is the rule; these changes can be identified on dental panoramic radiographs before eruption of the teeth. Atrophic rhinitis, diminished lacrimation, hoarseness, and hypoplasia or absence of mucous glands in nasotracheobronchial passages are also frequent findings in these patients (Reed et al, 1970). If the diagnosis is in doubt, palmar skin biopsy may demonstrate absent or hypoplastic eccrine sweat glands. Techniques used to elicit sweating, such as pilocarpine iontophoresis or examination of the sweat pores on the palm with *O*-phthalaldehyde, also can be used to demonstrate the defect (Esterly et al, 1973). Atopic dermatitis occurs frequently in these children (Reed et al, 1970), as well as a decrease in T cell function (Davis and Solomon, 1976).

Hypohidrotic ED is transmitted as an X-linked recessive trait. The gene has been localized to Xq11.21.1. First-trimester prenatal diagnosis is possible (Zonana et al, 1990). All affected males fully express the disease, whereas carrier females have variable expression of the clinical signs. This expression can be explained by the inactivation of a random percentage of abnormal X chromosomes. In these females, hypohidrosis can be demonstrated in areas of skin marking the lines of Blaschko (see the section on mosaicism) (Bolognia et al, 1994; Crump and Danks, 1971; Esterly et al, 1973; Gorlin et al, 1970).

Once the diagnosis is made, it is important to educate parents so that these children are protected from overheating. Defective lacrimation can be palliated by the use of artificial tears. The nasal mucosa should be treated with saline drops or irrigation followed by application of petrolatum. Regular dental evaluations should be started early in life, and dentures should be fitted to promote good nutrition, articulation, and normal appearance before the child starts school. Some of these children also choose a wig and reconstructive procedures later in life to improve facial configuration.

Hidrotic Ectodermal Dysplasia

Hidrotic ED, also known as *Clouston's syndrome*, is an autosomal dominant condition. Affected individuals have characteristic abnormalities of skin, hair, and nails, whereas eccrine and sebaceous functions and dentition are normal. The phenotype is easily recognizable in early childhood, with features including thickened, conical nails and widening of the distal periungual area with cerebriform furrowing. The skin over the joints often is hyperpigmented. The degree of alopecia is variable. The genetic abnormality in hidrotic ED has been mapped to the *GJB6* gene at 13q11-q12.1 encoding connexin 30 (Lamartine et al, 2000).

Ectodermal Dysplasia–Ectrodactyly–Cleft Lip/Palate Syndrome

The ectodermal dysplasia–ectrodactyly–cleft lip/palate (EEC) syndrome is an autosomal dominant condition featuring ectodermal dysplasia (including dental, ocular, nail, and hair defects), ectrodactyly (lobster-claw deformity of the hand), and cleft lip with or without cleft palate. The cutaneous and appendageal anomalies include diffuse hypopigmentation affecting both skin and hair, scanty scalp hair and eyebrows, dystrophic nails, and small teeth with enamel hypoplasia. Sweating appears to be intact, and sweat glands are present in a skin biopsy specimen. The clefting of the lip is usually complete and bilateral, and the palate has a median cleft. Dry granulomatous lesions in the corners of the mouth often are secondarily infected with *Candida albicans*. Other findings include lacrimal duct scarring, blepharitis and conjunctivitis, xerostomia, conductive hearing loss, and mental retardation. EEC syndrome is caused by a mutation in the *p63* gene located at 3q27 (Chiu et al, 2009). The *p63* gene, a homologue of the tumor suppressor *TP53* gene, is highly expressed in the basal layer of many epithelial tissues (Celli et al, 1999).

SUGGESTED READINGS

Armstrong DK, Hutchinson TH, Walsh MY, et al: Autosomal recessive inheritance of erythrokeratoderma variabilis, *Pediatr Dermatol* 14:355-358, 1997.

Beighton P: The Ehlers-Danlos syndromes. In Beighton P, editor: *McKusick's heritable disorders of connective tissue*, ed 5, St Louis, 1993, Mosby, pp 189-251.

Buyse L, Marks R, Wijeyesekera K, et al: Collodion baby dehydration: the danger of high transepidermal water loss, *Br J Dermatol* 129:86-88, 1993.

Carney RG Jr: Incontinentia pigmenti: a world statistical analysis, *Arch Dermatol* 112:535-542, 1976.

Esterly NB, Pashayan HM, West CE: Concurrent hypohidrotic ectodermal dysplasia and X-linked ichthyosis, *Am J Dis Child* 126:539-543, 1973.

Executive and Scientific Advisory Boards of the National Foundation for Ectodermal Dysplasia: Scaling skin in the newborn: a clue to the early diagnosis of X-linked hypohidrotic ectodermal dysplasia (Christ-Siemens-Touraine syndrome), *J Pediatr* 114:600-602, 1989.

Faghri S, Tamura D, Kraemer KH, DiGiovanna JJ: Trichothiodystrophy: a systematic review of 112 published cases characterises a wide spectrum of clinical manifestations, *J Med Genet* 45:609-621, 2008.

Fine JD, Eady RA, Bauer EA, et al: Revised classification system for inherited epidermolysis bullosa: report of the Second International Consensus Meeting on Diagnosis and Classification of Epidermolysis Bullosa, *J Am Acad Dermatol* 42:1051-1066, 2000.

Fine JD, Johnson LB, Wright JT: Inherited blistering diseases of the skin, *Pediatrician* 18:175-187, 1991.

Happle R: Mosaicism in human skin, *Arch Dermatol* 129:1460-1470, 1993.

Pinheiro M, Freire-Maia N: Ectodermal dysplasia: a clinical classification and a casual review, *Am J Med Genet* 53:153-162, 1994.

Sawamura D, Nakano H, Matsuzaki Y: Overview of epidermolysis bullosa, *J Dermatol* 37:214-219, 2010.

Complete references used in this text can be found online at www.expertconsult.com

INFECTIONS OF THE SKIN

Dakara Rucker Wright and Bernard A. Cohen

CHAPTER 99

As a group of potentially life-threatening and often easily treatable diseases, infections are often suspected first in a neonate with skin lesions. Recognition of characteristic morphologic features, aided by a few easily performed tests, will greatly enhance correct diagnosis and early initiation of appropriate therapy of the most common cutaneous infections. In this chapter, the focus is on disease caused by the most common pathogens responsible for neonatal infections that manifest with skin lesions: *Staphylococcus aureus*, *Streptococcus* spp. *Candida albicans*, and herpes simplex virus (HSV).

STAPHYLOCOCCUS AUREUS INFECTIONS

S. aureus is a ubiquitous organism, harbored as a commensal organism by greater than 30% of the general population (Ladhani, 2000). Colonization of the anterior nares and perineum is common, with frequent hand carriage (Dancer and Noble, 1991). This bacterial species is responsible for a variety of skin lesions. Infants become colonized with *S. aureus* during the first few weeks of life, following inoculation at the perineum or from handling. Cutaneous signs of *S. aureus* infection are mediated by local or circulating bacterial toxins that act directly on components of the epidermal keratinocytes, or as "superantigens" to stimulate exuberant immunologic responses (Tokura et al, 1994).

BULLOUS IMPETIGO

Impetigo is a group of superficial skin infections caused by group A streptococci or *S. aureus*, or both. However, neonatal bullous impetigo is primarily caused by coagulase-positive *S. aureus*. This form of impetigo can occur in nursery-based, epidemic patterns, often attributed to nasal carriage of *S. aureus*.

Clinical Findings

Impetigo is one of the most common neonatal skin infections. It occurs during the latter part of the first week or as late as the second week of life, manifested as vesicles or pustules on an erythematous base, most often seen in the periumbilical area, diaper area, or skin folds. Because the blisters are superficial, intact lesions are usually less than 1 cm in diameter. Larger lesions are flaccid and rupture so easily that they are usually seen as erosions, with a red moist base that develops a thin, varnish-like crust (Figure 99-1). These lesions heal rapidly without scarring. Lesions

are usually not closely grouped, differentiating them from the vesicles of herpes simplex infection.

Etiology

S. aureus is the primary cause of both bullous and nonbullous impetigo. Group A streptococci usually are associated with the nonbullous form, especially affecting patients with atopic dermatitis. Bullous impetigo is caused by toxigenic strains of coagulase-positive hemolytic *S. aureus*. Most often, the organism can be classified as one of the group II phage types (71 and 55). The incubation period is 1 to 10 days. Skin lesions are the result of local production of an epidermolytic exotoxin that cleaves a desmosomal protein connecting cells in the granular layer of the epidermis, producing superficial blisters. This is the same toxin produced in staphylococcal scalded skin syndrome (Amagi et al, 2000; Yamaguchi et al, 2002).

Epidemiology

Persons with skin lesions are highly contagious, but the disease also can be transmitted by asymptomatic carriers. The anterior nares of 30% of the general population are colonized with *S. aureus*, providing a reservoir for hand carriage and nosocomial spread (Doebbeling, 1994; Kragballe et al, 1995). Colonization of health care workers by strains of methicillin-resistant *Staphylococcus aureus* (MRSA) poses a potentially serious problem, and outbreaks of MRSA have occurred in neonatal intensive care units (NICUs) caused by an MRSA strain previously found in the community (Regev-Yochay, 2005; Yamaguchi et al, 2002).

Sporadic cases of impetigo are common, but many nursery epidemics have been reported and should be treated aggressively (Dave et al, 1994). Infected infants may not develop skin lesions until after discharge, so infection control surveillance should include all exposed patients. Overcrowding, insufficient nursery personnel, and inadequate hand washing contribute to nosocomial spread. Treatment of the umbilical cord with an antimicrobial agent has been shown to control epidemic *S. aureus* infections in the NICU (Haley et al, 1995). In the setting of an outbreak, nursery personnel should be surveyed for colonization of the hands and nares. Application of mupirocin ointment to the anterior nares twice daily for 5 days will eliminate nasal carriage for up to 1 year (Doebbeling et al, 1994). Effective hand washing can prevent nosocomial spread; chlorhexidine is among the safest and most effective antimicrobial cleansers for hospital use (Doebbeling et al, 1992). The use of antiseptic hand rub has also been shown to be as or more effective than washing with soap. A study by Girou et al in 2002 showed that during routine patient care, hand rubbing with an alcohol-based solution was significantly more efficient in reducing bacterial counts than hand washing with antiseptic soap.

This chapter includes material from the previous editions, to which Nancy B. Esterly, Elisabeth G. Richard, and Elaine C. Siegfried, contributed.

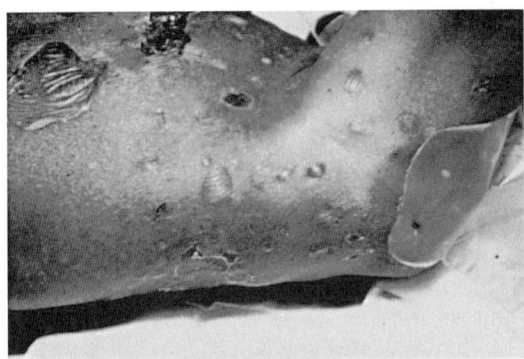

FIGURE 99-1 Bullous impetigo. Multiple intact and ruptured bullae on the abdomen, hip, and thigh of a newborn infant. No underlying erythema is present.

Diagnosis

The diagnosis is supported by the presence of gram-positive cocci in clusters on Gram stain of the fluid from a pustule or vesicle or under crusted plaque of impetigo. Confirmation is made by bacterial culture taken from blood, skin, and soft tissues, especially in the case of suspected MRSA.

Treatment

Bullous impetigo is benign if treated early, but local proliferation with exotoxin production or dissemination can be life-threatening. Treatment should be instituted promptly and isolation maintained until the lesions have resolved. Infants should be closely monitored and a high index of suspicion maintained for evidence of systemic disease. Infants with periumbilical lesions are at risk for bacterial omphalitis. Extremely limited infections may be treated with topical mupirocin, but this form of therapy should be used with caution in neonates. More extensive lesions require a systemically (most recommend parenterally) administered penicillinase-resistant antibiotic for 7 to 10 days. Sensitivities of the organism cultured should ultimately determine the choice of antibiotics, especially with the rising incidence of MRSA. In this case vancomycin or linezolid would be considered.

STAPHYLOCOCCAL SCALDED SKIN SYNDROME

Staphylococcal scalded skin syndrome (SSSS) occurs as a generalized manifestation of a circulating toxin produced by *S. aureus* that specifically cleaves cell-to-cell adhesion proteins in the epidermis. Affected infants are erythrodermic, a striking cutaneous finding that suggests a long list of differential diagnostic possibilities. Early diagnosis and treatment of SSSS can be lifesaving.

Clinical Findings

Affected infants demonstrate abrupt onset of temperature instability and irritability with generalized skin tenderness and erythema that most often starts on the face and spreads rapidly. Erythema often is accentuated in skin folds. Facial edema, conjunctivitis, and crusting around the eyes, nose,

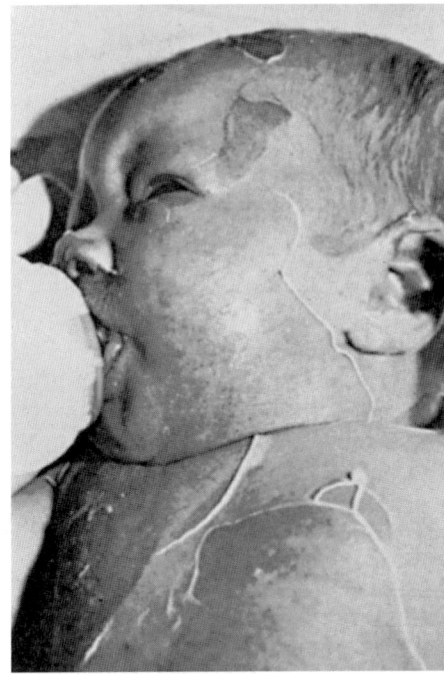

FIGURE 99-2 Staphylococcal scalded skin syndrome (Ritter's disease). Intense erythema and peeling of large areas of epidermis are seen.

and mouth give the infant a characteristic "sad mask" appearance. Flaccid bullae may develop, followed by widespread exfoliation (Figure 99-2) involving the entire skin surface within hours to days. Hypopigmentation may follow exfoliation in darker races that will repigment in time. Blistering is easily elicited by light stroking of intact skin, a diagnostic feature referred to as a Nikolsky sign. When blisters rupture, the skin peels off in sheets, leaving a painful moist, red base. Widespread skin involvement can exacerbate fluid and electrolyte problems (Frieden, 1989). Whereas in bullous impetigo *S. aureus* is identifiable in the blisters, in SSSS *S. aureus* is present at a primary distant site such as the nose, mouth, or conjunctiva.

SSSS must be distinguished from toxic epidermal necrolysis (TEN), a life-threatening condition involving full-thickness epidermal necrosis, most commonly due to a drug reaction. In SSSS, mucosal erythema may be seen but there are no intraoral blisters, whereas in TEN, mucosal blistering is present.

Etiology

The signs and symptoms of SSSS are the result of circulating epidermolytic toxin, produced from an often subclinical focus of *S. aureus* infection. Fresh skin lesions do not contain bacteria, and the blisters are culture-negative. Two distinct epidermolytic toxins have been identified in SSSS, produced by toxigenic strains of *S. aureus*, phage group I, II, or III. Approximately 5% of *S. aureus* isolates produce the toxins (Farrell, 1999). The exotoxin cleaves desmosomal proteins within the epidermal granular layer, resulting in blisters (Amagi et al, 2002; Resnick, 1992). Superantigenic stimulation of cytokine production also has been demonstrated (Dave et al, 1994).

Diagnosis

If the diagnosis is in doubt, skin biopsy prepared for frozen section can be examined emergently. The presence of an intraepidermal rather than full-thickness blister will distinguish SSSS from TEN, allowing rapid initiation of appropriate therapy. Other conditions can be ruled out by examination of formalin-fixed sections. If the clinical impression is strong, surveillance samples will define the primary focus of infection. Gram staining may be performed emergently; cultures will confirm the diagnosis. Common sites of primary infection are the nasopharynx, umbilicus, and ocular conjunctivae; the urine also may demonstrate organisms. Bullous lesions do not contain organisms. Blood culture specimens should be obtained because sepsis, although uncommon, may occur. Phage typing may be of interest in epidemics.

Treatment

Systemic administration of a penicillinase-resistant penicillin is the therapy of choice. Fluid and electrolyte replacement and measures for maintenance of normal body temperature may be required. Approximately 2 to 3 days after initiation of therapy, the denuded areas become dry, and a flaky desquamation ensues. Crusted and denuded areas may be treated with compresses of Burow or normal saline solution. Application of a bland ointment emollient may accelerate the return of the skin to normal during the flaky desquamative phase. Resolution occurs in another 3 to 5 days. Because the intraepidermal cleavage plane is at the level of the granular layer, scarring occurs only in instances of secondary complications (Frieden, 1989).

STREPTOCOCCUS SPP INFECTIONS

Cutaneous streptococcal infections occur in the newborn but are less common than staphylococcal infections. Group A streptococci have been reported to cause disease of epidemic proportions (Dillon, 1966; Peter and Hazard, 1975) following the introduction of the organism into the nursery by maternal carriers or nursery personnel. The umbilicus (omphalitis) is a frequent site of infection. Conjunctivitis, paronychia, vaginitis, and an erysipelas-like eruption also have been described (Dillon, 1966; Geil et al, 1970; Isenberg et al, 1984). Because sepsis and meningitis may result, infected infants should be treated promptly, and strict isolation should be instituted. As with staphylococcal infection, serious efforts should be made to identify the source of the organism. Several nursery outbreaks have been difficult to terminate because colonized infants may show little evidence of disease (Lehtonen et al, 1984). Isolation and treatment of infected infants, disinfection of the umbilical stump as the most likely reservoir of the organism, and penicillin prophylaxis for carriers and exposed infants have been the most effective measures. The infections respond readily to penicillin, which should be administered over a 10-day course.

Group B streptococci are now one of the most frequently encountered pathogens in the newborn nursery. Early-onset disease (during the 1st week of life), probably acquired in utero or during delivery, most commonly becomes manifest as septicemia with respiratory distress and shock. Late-onset disease (7 days to 3 months) is acquired postpartum and more often takes on the form of meningitis. Patients with early-onset disease may harbor the organism on the skin; however, the presence of this agent on the skin is short-lived compared with other sites (Baker, 1977).

Skin infections caused by group B streptococci are uncommon but have been documented (Belgaumkar, 1975; Hebert and Esterly, 1986; Howard and McCrackin, 1974). The most common skin manifestation of GBS is cellulitis, usually of the face (Shet and Ferrieri, 2004). Vesiculopustular lesions and small abscesses and necrotizing fasciitis all have been noted. A 10-day course of procaine penicillin or clindamycin is considered the treatment of choice.

OMPHALITIS

CLINICAL FINDINGS

Omphalitis is infection of the umbilical stump that presents around day 3 of life. Clinically there is erythema, edema, and tenderness around the umbilicus with or without discharge. Infection can extend into the subcutis or along the abdominal wall causing necrotizing fasciitis.

ETIOLOGY

S. aureus, *Escherichia coli*, *Klebsiella* spp., and *S. pyogenes* are common organisms that cause omphalitis. Preterm infants, low-birthweight infants, and infants from home births and complicated deliveries are at increased risk (Sawardekar, 2004).

DIAGNOSIS

Gram stain and bacterial culture from moist umbilical stump fluid can be obtained, but because this area can be contaminated easily, clinical correlation is needed. True infection must be differentiated from embryonic duct remnants or umbilical papilloma.

TREATMENT

Ampicillin and gentamicin can be used initially until culture and sensitivities are obtained. Intravenous antibiotics can be switched to enteral once the skin improves clinically. In a Cochrane review, no difference was demonstrated in cord and other skin infections within 6 weeks of observation between cords treated with antiseptics as compared with dry cord care or placebo. However, there was a trend toward reduced colonization with antibiotics compared to antiseptics and no treatment (Zupan et al, 2004).

CANDIDA ALBICANS INFECTIONS

C. albicans is a frequent pathogen of the female genital tract, especially during pregnancy. Infantile infection may be acquired in utero, during delivery, or postnatally.

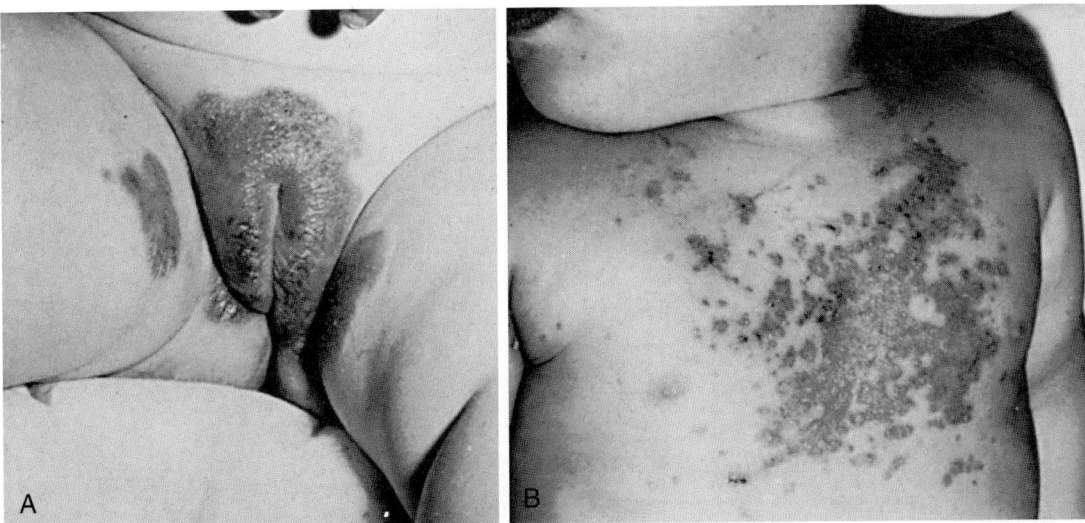

FIGURE 99-3 **A,** Sharply demarcated erythematous, scaly candidal rash in the groin. **B,** Candidal eruption on the central chest of an infant.

LOCALIZED *CANDIDA* INFECTION (PRIMARY CUTANEOUS)

Oral Candidiasis (Thrush)

C. albicans colonizes the oral cavity and gastrointestinal tract of most neonates, with peak incidence of thrush occurring at 4 weeks of age (Russell and Lay, 1973). The lesions are readily recognized as asymptomatic to moderately painful plaques of white, friable material on an erythematous base over the tongue, palate, buccal mucosa, and gingivae.

Diaper Dermatitis

Localized cutaneous candidal infections are common in infants, with peak incidence at 3 to 4 months of age. Characteristic primary lesions are tiny vesicopustules that erode and merge, forming bright, erythematous plaques often with a scalloped edge in the moist intertriginous areas of the perineum and perianal and inguinal creases (Figure 99-3). White scale and "satellite" pustules may be seen along the periphery. Thrush may also be present in conjunction with *Candida* diaper dermatitis. Other intertriginous areas such as the neck folds and axillae can also be infected with *Candida*, as well as the nails.

Diagnosis of Localized Cutaneous *Candida*

Presumptive diagnosis often is made by physical examination and history, but microscopic examination of scrapings suspended in 10% potassium hydroxide for yeast and pseudohyphal forms is useful. The diagnosis may be confirmed by identification of the organism on culture.

Treatment

Nystatin is an antibiotic derived from *Streptomyces noursei* with activity against *Candida* but not dermatophytes. Oral lesions usually respond promptly to a course of nystatin suspension, 100,000 to 200,000 units, administered by mouth four times daily for 14 to 21 days. In refractory cases, an increased dosage of nystatin or systemic therapy may have to be instituted (Hebert and Esterly, 1986). Localized cutaneous candidiasis in an otherwise healthy infant is most easily treated with a topical candidicidal agent, such as nystatin, one of the imidazoles (e.g., miconazole, clotrimazole, ketoconazole), or ciclopirox olamine (Gibney and Siegfried, 1996). Nystatin in an ointment vehicle may be the least irritating. If the breastfeeding mother is affected, treatment of the mother with nystatin cream or oral fluconazole may be indicated. Gentian (crystal) violet is a triphenylmethane antiseptic dye effective against *Candida* species. In a 0.5% or 1% aqueous solution it has been a time-honored, safe, and effective treatment for thrush. Gentian violet is infamous for deep purple staining of the skin, which is transient. Prolonged use of gentian violet has been associated with nausea, vomiting, diarrhea, and mucosal ulceration. Carcinogenicity in mice has been reported (Rosenkranz and Carr, 1971).

CONGENITAL (INTRAUTERINE) CANDIDIASIS

Congenital candidiasis is *Candida* infection acquired in utero from an ascending infection, crossing the fetal membrane and infecting surfaces that come in contact with amniotic fluid and manifests with symptoms in the first days of life. Even though the rate of vaginal colonization is 33%, congenital candidiasis is uncommon. Risk factors include the presence of a foreign body in the maternal uterus or cervix. Systemic dissemination of yeast is rare in the majority of term infants.

Clinical Findings

Lesions of congenital candidiasis can be seen on the placenta and fetal membranes, including characteristic granulomas of the umbilical cord (Hebert and Esterly, 1986; Schirar et al, 1974). The cord lesions are multiple yellow-white papules, usually measuring 1 to 3 mm in diameter. The cutaneous eruption of congenital cutaneous candidiasis may be sparse or widespread and consists of papules and

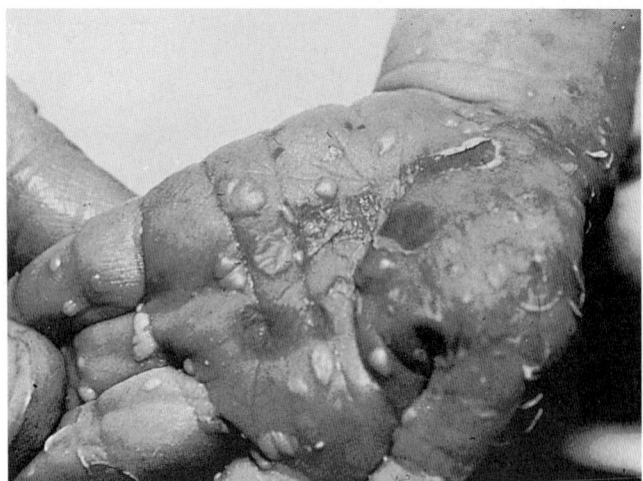

FIGURE 99-4 Congenital cutaneous candidiasis, pustular stage, in a 6-day-old infant. A maculopapular rash was present at birth. *(Courtesy P. J. Kozinn, N. Rudolf, A. A. Tariq, M. R. Reale, and P. K. Goldberg.)*

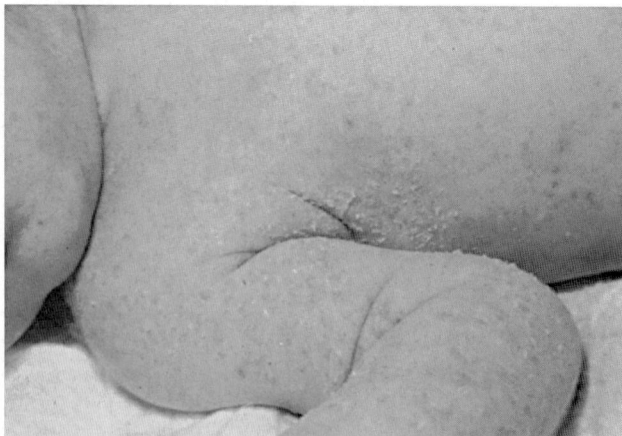

FIGURE 99-5 An 8-day-old infant with a generalized erythematous, scaly eruption sparing only the face and scalp. Oral mucosa was not involved. Hyphae and budding yeasts were seen on potassium hydroxide preparation, and *Candida albicans* was cultured from the lesions. The infant's mother had candidal vaginitis during the pregnancy.

vesicopustules on an intensely erythematous base. The face is relatively spared, as are the oral mucous membranes, and there is no predilection for the diaper area. Palmar and plantar pustules, paronychia, and nail dystrophy help distinguish this condition from more common, benign neonatal dermatoses (Figure 99-4). Bullae and desquamation usually are late features (Figure 99-5). Skin lesions usually resolve with desquamation within 1 to 2 weeks (Darmstadt et al, 2000). The prognosis is good in full-term infants. Topical treatment may be used.

Very low-birthweight infants may present with a less specific, scalded skin–like or erosive dermatitis owing to the organism's penetration of the immature, compromised epidermal barrier, leading to invasive disease. Generalized scaling is the dominant feature, but a careful search may reveal primary vesicopustules and periungual or nail involvement as helpful diagnostic clues (Gibney and Siegfried, 1996).

Diagnosis

The differential diagnosis includes conditions that cause blisters and pustules. Napkin psoriasis is also on differential. A potassium hydroxide preparation that reveals budding yeasts and pseudohyphal forms is the easiest and most cost-effective initial step in establishing the diagnosis. Calcofluor white stain and immunofluorescence microscopy is a more sensitive rapid technique. Positive results on cultures from an intact pustule, skin scrapings, or skin biopsy tissue also support the diagnosis. Cultures of blood, urine, and cerebrospinal fluid are usually negative; however, they are indicated when systemic disease is suspected and in all preterm infants.

SYSTEMIC/DISSEMINATED CANDIDIASIS

Systemic candidiasis infection (*Candida* infection in an otherwise sterile body fluid such as blood, urine, or cerebrospinal fluid) affects very low-birthweight infants more commonly than full-term infants. Most neonatal fungal infections are caused by *C. albicans* and *Candida parapsilosis.*

Systemic or disseminated candidiasis can be due to congenital candidiasis (acquired in utero) in very low-birthweight infants, untreated localized *Candida* infection in preterm infants, or nosocomial spread. Risk factors for congenital systemic infection include birthweight of less than 1500 g, indwelling catheters, broad-spectrum antibiotic therapy, steroid administration, and hyperalimentation. Approximately 10% of NICU infants become colonized in the 1st week of life. *Candida* septicemia represents 10% to 16% of all cases of sepsis in the NICU, and early recognition and appropriate therapy are lifesaving (Gibney and Siegfried, 1996; Leibovitz, 2002). The estimated crude mortality rate for candidemia is 38% to 75% (Lupetti et al, 2002).

Clinical

Skin manifestations may occur in 60% of infants, which include burnlike dermatitis followed by desquamation, progressive diaper dermatitis with papules and pustules, and abscess. Systemic involvement occurs via hematogenous or lymphatic spread, most frequently involving the kidney, central nervous system (CNS), and skeletal system. Pneumonia may result from aspiration of infected amniotic fluid and manifests with respiratory distress. Other systemic signs include apnea, bradycardia, temperature instability, hypotension, guaiac-positive stools, and abdominal distention. Laboratory features include an elevated white blood cell count with a left shift reaching the level of a leukemoid reaction (e.g., 120,000/mm^3). In addition, persistent hyperglycemia and glycosuria may be present (Darmstadt et al, 2000).

Diagnosis

The differential diagnosis includes several other neonatal vesiculopustular eruptions that range from benign, self-limited cutaneous processes to rapidly progressive, life-threatening disease. Early and correct diagnosis is essential. Organisms from skin usually are demonstrable on potassium hydroxide or calcofluor white preparations and cultures of scrapings from involved skin. Disseminated disease can be difficult to diagnose. Respiratory distress and infiltrates on chest radiograph will obscure evidence of *Candida* pneumonia because hyaline membrane disease often occurs in the same patient population. Ophthalmologic examination, chest radiograph, and blood, urine, and cerebrospinal fluid cultures may be helpful, but negative findings are not uncommon in disseminated candidiasis (Johnson et al, 1984). Histologic examination of specimens from the placenta and umbilical cord prepared with the appropriate stains may demonstrate fungal elements. Urinalysis positive for budding yeast or urine culture positive for *C. albicans* may be quickly dismissed as being due to contaminants, but such findings are strongly associated with systemic disease in infants at risk. The diagnosis of disseminated candidiasis can be expedited by a positive touch preparation of a punch biopsy specimen. Using this technique, the practitioner firmly imprints the dermal side of the specimen on a microscope slide and then looks for yeast after potassium hydroxide preparation or Gram staining (Held et al, 1988).

Prognosis and Treatment

Systemic infection with *C. albicans* in premature infants is a serious infection with high morbidity and mortality rates (Johnson et al, 1984). Congenital or acquired candidiasis warrants parenteral antifungal therapy (e.g., with amphotericin B) for infants with any of the following risk factors for disseminated disease: (1) evidence of respiratory distress or sepsis in the immediate neonatal period; (2) birthweight less than 1500 g; (3) treatment with broad-spectrum antibiotics or corticosteroids; (4) extensive instrumentation during delivery or invasive procedures in the neonatal period; (5) positive systemic cultures; (6) evidence of altered immune response; and (7) birth at less than 27 weeks of gestational age. A critical factor for survival in systemic candidiasis is not limited extent of infection but the early initiation of antifungal therapy (Botas et al, 1995; Johnson et al, 1984). A few single-center studies have demonstrated the efficacy of fluconazole in the prevention of both colonization and infection by *Candida* spp. (Kaufman et al, 2001; Manzoni et al, 2006), and a multicenter, prospective, randomized clinical trial has shown the safety and efficacy of fluconazole in preterm and very low-birthweight infants (Kicklighter et al, 2001).

HERPES SIMPLEX VIRUS INFECTION

Early recognition and prompt initiation of therapy for neonatal herpes are critical. The consequences of delaying antiviral therapy can be devastating.

CLINICAL FINDINGS

Onset of symptoms usually occurs at 1 to 2 weeks for most neonates, but congenital lesions have been reported (Salvador et al, 1994). Infection is categorized by extent of disease, as follows: skin-eye-mucosae (SEM) disease, CNS disease, and disseminated disease. Neonatal HSV infection often presents with a sepsis-like syndrome or with a new onset of seizures. Skin or mucosal lesions may appear only late in the disease course, or not at all. Only one

third of infants present with cutaneous involvement (Frieden, 1989), although more than 80% develop typical skin lesions during the course of their disease (Overall, 1994).

Characteristic skin lesions begin as isolated or grouped, tense vesicles on an erythematous base and evolve into pustules, crusts, or small erosions over several days. Forty percent of infected infants have SEM disease. With early treatment, these infants have an excellent prognosis; if the infection is left untreated, it will progress in 75% of cases (Arvin and Prober, 1992). Thirty-five percent of infected infants have CNS disease, with a high incidence of developmental abnormalities. One fourth of the infants present with evidence of disseminated disease (e.g., sepsis, liver dysfunction, coagulopathy, respiratory distress). For this group, the prognosis is poor, with a 60% mortality rate and a 40% risk of long-term neurologic impairment in survivors (Arvin and Prober, 1992; Whitley, 1994).

Infants infected in utero have a distinctive clinical presentation. Skin lesions are almost always present at birth and include widespread erosions and bullae, scars, and scalp lesions that resemble those of aplasia cutis. Other frequent findings include chorioretinitis, microcephaly, hydranencephaly, and microphthalmia (Arvin and Prober, 1992).

ETIOLOGY

A majority of cases of neonatal herpes simplex are the result of vertical transmission. Two thirds of cases are caused by HSV-2 and one third by HSV-1. The usual route of infection is via intrapartum contact with genital mucosa, but ascending infection accounts for 5% of cases of neonatal herpes. Infants who become infected in utero are more often premature or small for gestational age, with more widespread and severe disease (Arvin and Prober, 1992).

EPIDEMIOLOGY

Prospective, single-center studies in the United States have shown rates of neonatal HSV infection as high as 31.2 cases per 100,000 (1 in 3200) live births (Corey and Wald, 2009). Most cases of maternal-fetal transmission involve women with undiagnosed genital herpes, many of whom have acquired primary HSV-1 or HSV-2 near delivery. One half of infected infants are born to mothers with primary infections. These women, who are usually without active lesions, have a 25% to 50% risk of transmitting disease to their newborns (Corey and Wald, 2009). One half of infants with neonatal herpes are born to mothers with recurrent genital herpes, generally from HSV-2. Most of these women also are asymptomatic at the time of delivery and may have no known history of genital herpes. In this group, the risk of transmitting infection is around 2.5%.

DIAGNOSIS

A high index of suspicion is required. The differential diagnosis includes the causes of vesicles and pustules in the newborn outlined in Chapter 97. Tzanck smears, viral cultures, and direct fluorescent antibody detection are the most widely used tests to detect herpes infection. The diagnostic yield for each is variable, largely influenced by the age, quality, and handling of the specimen. Optimally, skin scrapings should be obtained from the base of a fresh vesicle. Other sites should be sampled as well, especially in infants suspected of having CNS or disseminated disease. Tzanck smear analysis is rapid and readily available but will reveal characteristic multinucleated giant cells in only 50% of HSV infections (Nahass et al, 1995). Immunofluorescence is 90% to 95% sensitive and specific but requires a specialized laboratory. IgM assays are not reliable. Viral culture is the diagnostic gold standard and yields positive results for 80% of specimens by 24 hours and for 90% by 48 hours, under optimal conditions of handling and transport. Molecular diagnosis by polymerase chain reaction assay can detect HSV from specimens that would be suboptimal for the other methods (e.g., Tzanck smears, crusts, paraffin-fixed biopsy specimens). Diagnostic polymerase chain reaction assay may be the easiest means of diagnosing HSV infection in the future; however, limitations include the lack of standardization of methodologies, adversely affecting the clinician's ability to interpret results (Kimberlin, 2001; Nahass et al, 1992, 1995).

TREATMENT

Early treatment with antiviral agents is critical to decrease the risk of serious complications and death. All cases of presumptive neonatal HSV infection should be treated with intravenous acyclovir. The standard dose of acyclovir has been 30 mg/kg/day divided every 8 hours. However, the higher dose of 60 mg/kg/day divided every 8 hours could significantly improve the outcome of infants with HSV CNS or disseminated disease (Corey and Wald, 2009; Kimberlin et al, 2001). In the Kimberlin et al study, 79 neonates with HSV disease were studied and treated with either 45 mg/kg/day or 60 mg/kg/day and compared with infants treated with 30 mg/kg/day for 10 days in the original National Institute of Allergy and Infectious Diseases (NIAID) Collaborative Antiviral Study Group trial. Those with disseminated disease who received the higher dose were three times as likely to survive and more than 6 times as likely to be developmentally normal. The only noted side effect was transient neutropenia, which occurred in 21% of those treated with the higher dose (Kimberlin et al, 2001). Vidarabine also is effective in preventing severe disease in infants with SEM disease but not for treatment of infants with more widespread herpes infection (Arvin and Prober, 1992). Morbidity in CNS disease and disseminated disease remains high, with corresponding mortality rates of 15% and 57%, respectively (Jacobs, 1998). Antiviral therapy with intravenous acyclovir reduces mortality from 85% to 31% among infants with disseminated disease and from 50% to 6% among infants with CNS disease (Corey and Wald, 2009). Concomitant administration of immunoglobulin products may improve disease outcome for these infants (Whitley, 1994).

Strategies to decrease risk of vertical transmission include cesarean delivery, serologic screening of pregnant women, prophylactic antiviral therapy, and maternal vaccination development. Delivery via cesarean section for women with active lesions or prodromal symptoms and prophylactic antiviral treatment for women with gestational HSV are some accepted approaches (Enright and Prober, 2002). Suppressive acyclovir reduces the frequency of genital lesions near term and the frequency of cesarean delivery, but there are no data to suggest that it reduces the risk of neonatal herpes. Because a direct correlation exists between the development of neurologic deficits and the frequency of recurrent cutaneous HSV, the use of suppressive oral acyclovir therapy after acute neonatal SEM disease may limit long-term morbidity (Kimberlin et al, 1996).

SUGGESTED READINGS

AAP Committee on the Fetus and Newborn: Guidelines for perinatal care. In ACOG Committee on Obstetrics: *Maternal and fetal medicine*, ed 2, Elk Grove Village, Ill, 1988, American Academy of Pediatrics.

Adachi J, Endo K, Fukuzumi T, et al: Increasing incidence of streptococcal impetigo in atopic dermatitis, *J Dermatol Sci* 17:45-53, 1998.

Albert S, Baldwin R, Czekajewski S, et al: Bullous impetigo due to group II, *Staphylococcus aureus, Am J Dis Child* 120:10-13, 1970.

Anthony BF, Giuliano DM, Oh W: Nursery outbreak of staphylococcal scalded skin syndrome, *Am J Dis Child* 124:41-44, 1972.

Curran JP, Al-Salihi FL: Neonatal staphylococcal scalded skin syndrome: massive outbreak due to an unusual phage type, *Pediatrics* 66:285-290, 1980.

Elias PM, Fritsch P, Epstein EH Jr: Staphylococcal scalded skin syndrome: clinical features, pathogenesis, and recent microbiological and biochemical developments, *Arch Dermatol* 113:207-219, 1977.

Elias PM, Mittermayer H, Tappeiner G, et al: Staphylococcal toxic epidermal necrolysis (TEN): the expanded mouse model, *J Invest Dermatol* 63:467-475, 1974.

Gehlbach SH, Gutman LT, Wilfert CM, et al: Recurrence of skin disease in a nursery: ineffectuality of hexachlorophene bathing, *Pediatrics* 55:422-424, 1975.

Johnson DE, Thompson TR, Ferrieri P: Congenital candidiasis, *Am J Dis Child* 135:273-275, 1981.

Kam LA, Giacoia GP: Congenital cutaneous candidiasis, *Am J Dis Child* 129:1215-1218, 1975.

Melish ME, Glasgow LA: Staphylococcal scalded skin syndrome: the expanded clinical syndrome, *J Pediatr* 78:958-967, 1971.

Melish ME, Glasgow LA: Staphylococcal scalded skin syndrome—development of an experimental model, *N Engl J Med* 282:1114-1119, 1970.

Overturf BD, Balfour G: Osteomyelitis and sepsis: severe complications of fetal monitoring, *Pediatrics* 55:244-247, 1975.

Rubenstein AD, Mesher DM: Epidemic boric acid poisoning simulating staphylococcal toxic epidermal necrolysis of the newborn infant: Ritter's disease, *J Pediatr* 77:884-887, 1970.

Rudolph N, Tariq AA, Reale MR, et al: Congenital cutaneous candidiasis, *Arch Dermatol* 113:1101-1103, 1977.

Rudolph RI, Schwartz W, Leyden JJ: Treatment of staphylococcal toxic epidermal necrolysis, *Arch Dermatol* 110:559-562, 1974.

Sheagren JN: *Staphylococcus aureus*: the persistent pathogen (Parts I and II), *N Engl J Med* 310:1368-1373, 1437-1442, 1984.

Stulberg DL: Common bacterial skin infections, *Am Fam Physician* 66:119-124, 2002.

Wagner MM, Rycheck RR, Yee RB, et al: Septic dermatitis of the neonatal scalp and maternal endomyometritis with intrapartum internal fetal monitoring, *Pediatrics* 74:81-85, 1984.

Complete references used in this text can be found online at www.expertconsult.com

CHAPTER

100

COMMON NEWBORN DERMATOSES*

Dakara Rucker Wright and Bernard A. Cohen

This chapter describes a group of cutaneous disorders that are unique to neonates. All of these disorders have well-recognized clinical and histologic features. Most are asymptomatic and self-limited, and rigorous searches have not been made for precise pathogenetic mechanisms or definitive therapies. It is important to recognize these common neonatal dermatoses so that they are not mistaken for more serious diseases, thus obviating the initiation of aggressive workup and treatment. However, distinguishing these common neonatal dermatoses from more serious neonatal dermatoses can be lifesaving. Important considerations in the differential diagnosis based on clinical morphology are outlined in Chapter 97.

ERYTHEMA TOXICUM NEONATORUM

CLINICAL FINDINGS

Erythema toxicum is an inflammatory cutaneous disease of unknown origin that affects approximately half of all full-term newborns (Berg and Solomon, 1987). It occurs less frequently among preterm infants (Carr et al, 1966; Taylor and Bondurant, 1957). In a majority of infants, the lesions develop between 1 and 3 days of age, but they may appear as late as 3 weeks. No predilection of the disorder for race, gender, season, or geographic location has been reported.

Affected infants appear healthy. The basic skin lesions are small (1 to 3 mm in diameter) erythematous macules that evolve into tiny white pustules, with a prominent halo of erythema, and can look similar to a flea bite. Individual lesions may persist for only a few hours, but the eruption lasts for several days or, rarely, for several weeks. The number of lesions present can vary from a few to dozens. The trunk is the most frequent site of predilection, but the face and extremities also may be involved. Palms and soles are almost always spared. Several lesions may coalesce into plaques measuring several centimeters in diameter (Figure 100-1).

DIAGNOSIS

A Wright-stained smear of pustule contents reveals large numbers of eosinophils, which supports the diagnosis. Skin biopsy may be necessary in clinically atypical cases. Histologic features consist of eosinophil-filled intraepidermal vesicles and a mixed intradermal inflammatory infiltrate that tends to localize around the superficial portion of the pilosebaceous follicle.

Considerations in the differential diagnosis include other benign, self-limited disorders such as transient neonatal pustular melanosis, miliaria, infantile acropustulosis, and eosinophilic pustular folliculitis. Acropustulosis of

infancy is a pruritic eruption and is characterized by recurrent, itchy vesiculopustular lesions primarily on the palms, soles, and a few lesions on the dorsal distal extremities. Rarely lesions may be on the face and scalp. The etiology is unclear, but in some cases there may be an association with a preceding scabies infestation. Eosinophilic pustular folliculitis in infants typically occurs on the scalp and extremities, recurring in crops similar to acropustulosis of infancy. Infants may also have peripheral eosinophilia. The infantile type is, however, distinct from human immunodeficiency virus (HIV)-related eosinophilic pustular folliculitis (Adam, 2008; Humphrey et al, 2006).

Infections such as bacterial folliculitis, bullous impetigo, candidiasis, herpes, and scabies are also included in the differential and need to be ruled out. The early stage of incontinentia pigmenti can also be mistaken for erythema toxicum. The diagnostic workup outlined in Chapter 97 can differentiate among these conditions.

ETIOLOGY

The etiology of erythema toxicum is unknown. The eosinophilic infiltrate suggests that erythema toxicum is a hypersensitivity response, but studies attempting to incriminate chemical or microbiologic substances, acquired either transplacentally or vaginally from the mother (e.g., drugs, topical irritants, sebum, milk), have failed to provide support for this hypothesis (Bassukas, 1992). At a molecular level, there appears to be an accumulation and activation of immune cells in these lesions as seen by immunohistochemical staining of punch biopsy specimens from cutaneous lesions. Monoclonal antibodies placed in skin with lesions detected E-selectin in the vessel wall as well as dendritic cells, eosinophils, macrophages,

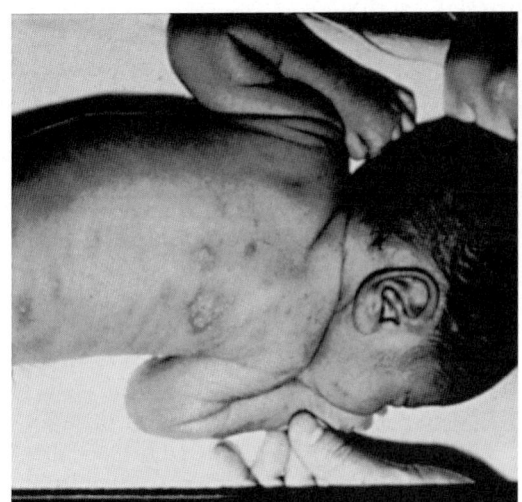

FIGURE 100-1 Florid lesions of erythema toxicum on the back of a newborn infant. The pustules are large and surrounded by an erythematous halo. Smears of the pustular contents showed only eosinophils.

---

*This chapter includes material from the previous edition, to which Nancy B. Esterly, Elaine C. Siegfried, and Rebecca A. Kazin contributed.

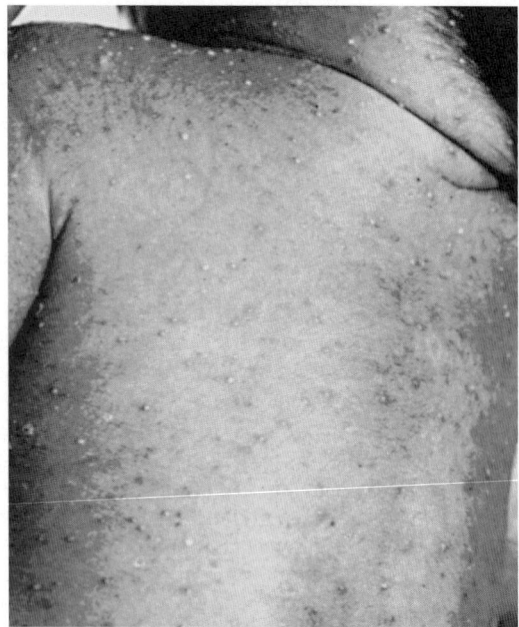

FIGURE 100-2 Numerous superficial pustules on the neck and back of a 1-day-old infant. A few pustules have ruptured, leaving a collarette of scales.

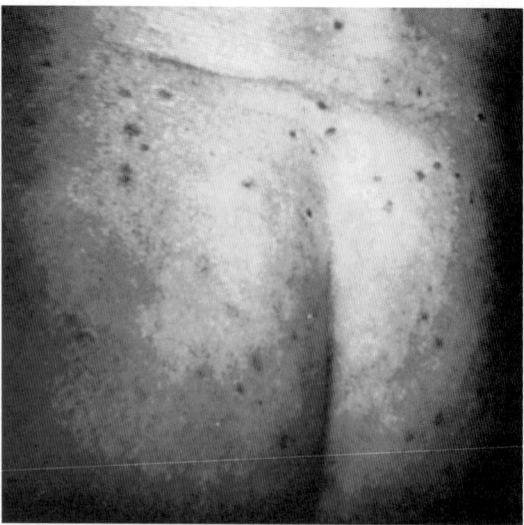

FIGURE 100-3 Transient neonatal pustular melanosis. Hyperpigmented macules on the lower back and buttocks, some of which are encircled by scales. *(From Ramamurthy RS, Reveri M, Esterly NB, et al: Transient neonatal pustular melanosis,* J Pediatr *88:831, 1976.)*

and E-selectin–expressing cells in these affected areas, whereas uninvolved skin demonstrated reduced or absent immunologic activity (Marchini et al, 2001).

TREATMENT AND PROGNOSIS

Erythema toxicum is asymptomatic, resolves spontaneously, and requires no treatment. A prolonged course and recurrence are rare. Once the diagnosis is confirmed, anticipatory guidance and reassurance should be provided to parents.

TRANSIENT NEONATAL PUSTULAR MELANOSIS

CLINICAL FINDINGS

This benign disorder was present at birth in 5% of African American and in 1% of white infants in one older study (Ramamurthy et al, 1976). Characteristic lesions are small, superficial pustules that rupture easily, leaving a collarette of fine scale and hyperpigmented macules that fade over several weeks to months (Figure 100-2). The lesions may be profuse or sparse and can involve all body surfaces, including the palms, soles, and scalp (Figure 100-3). The pustules last approximately 48 hours, but the macules can persist for several months.

DIAGNOSIS

Affected infants are otherwise healthy. A Wright-stained smear of pustule contents revealing keratinous debris and variable numbers of polymorphonuclear neutrophils with few or no eosinophils supports the diagnosis. Gram staining and bacterial cultures obtained from intact pustules uniformly fail to disclose the presence of organisms. The

differential diagnosis includes the conditions listed for erythema toxicum.

ETIOLOGY

The cause of transient neonatal pustular melanosis is unknown. A prospective study reported that 17 infants with typical congenital lesions subsequently developed lesions of erythema toxicum, linking the two conditions (Ferrandiz et al, 1992).

TREATMENT

The disorder is asymptomatic and self-limited. Once the diagnosis is confirmed, further therapy is not required.

MILIA, EPSTEIN PEARLS, AND SEBACEOUS HYPERPLASIA

CLINICAL FINDINGS

Milia (a single lesion is a milium) are found in 40% of full-term infants (Gordon, 1949). They are single or sparsely scattered pearly (1 to 2 mm) lesions that occur on the face. The sites of predilection are the cheeks, forehead, and chin (Figure 100-4). Large milia (greater than 2 mm in diameter) are found in infants with type I oral-facial-digital syndrome (Solomon et al, 1970). Rarely, milia can occur in unusual sites, such as on the arms, legs, or foreskin.

Epstein pearls are milia that occur on the midline of the hard palate, and Bohn's nodules are on the gum margins. These tiny cystic lesions occur in approximately 85% of newborn infants. They usually are grouped, firm, and movable and appear opaque and white.

ETIOLOGY

Milia are due to retention of keratin within the dermis.

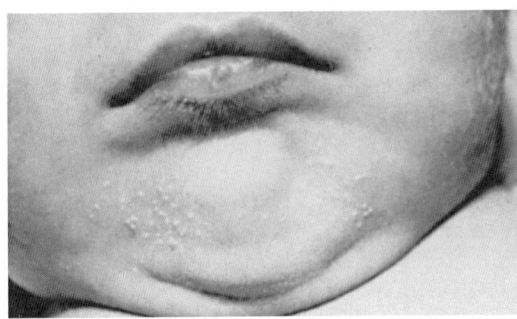

FIGURE 100-4 Numerous grouped milia on the chin of a newborn infant.

DIAGNOSIS

Histologically, a milium is an invagination of epidermal tissue, arising from the pilosebaceous apparatus of vellus hair, which forms a cyst filled with several layers of keratin-producing cells. The expressed contents of milial cysts resembles tiny white pearls and consists mostly of keratinocyte debris, a useful diagnostic feature.

Milia can be mistaken for sebaceous gland hyperplasia, which occurs in the same distribution. The papules of sebaceous gland hyperplasia are smaller (pinpoint) and more yellow and contain sebaceous lipids.

TREATMENT

Treatment is unnecessary because milia usually exfoliate spontaneously within 1 month. Epstein pearls are self-limited, but can take several months to resolve. Sebaceous hyperplasia also resolves spontaneously within the first few weeks of life.

MILIARIA

CLINICAL FINDINGS

Miliaria neonatorum is a vesicular or pustular dermatitis arising from the eccrine duct. Four clinical variants have been described, and their appearances are influenced by the site of obstruction within the duct. Miliaria crystallina (sudamina) consists of superficial, clear, thin-walled, noninflammatory vesicles that rupture easily. The vesicle is localized within the stratum corneum. Miliaria rubra (prickly heat) consists of small, erythematous, grouped papules often localized to skin folds and areas covered by clothing. These lesions arise within the deeper levels of the epidermis and are accompanied by inflammation. The papules can become pustular if there is a prominent inflammatory component or secondary bacterial infection, a condition sometimes referred to as *miliaria pustulosa*. Miliaria profunda is a mildly inflammatory papular eruption that arises within the deeper, dermal portion of the eccrine duct.

ETIOLOGY

Miliaria is believed to be caused by sweat accumulation within obstructed eccrine ducts. Obstruction of the eccrine duct in adults has been reported to result from a variety of triggers such as cutaneous injury, excessive hydration of the stratum corneum, or overgrowth of microbes (Fitzpatrick, 1990). Premature and even full-term neonates have a full complement of immature eccrine glands that are incompletely canalized which may predispose the newborn to miliaria (Straka et al, 1991). Overheating from excessive bundling and from phototherapy probably contributes to its pathogenesis. The widespread availability of environmental temperature control probably has decreased the incidence of this condition.

Recurrent episodes of pustular miliaria rubra could signal the rare condition type I pseudohypoaldosteronism. This potentially fatal condition, of autosomal recessive inheritance, is a disorder of mineralocorticoid resistance that leads to salt-wasting crises through the eccrine ducts. If this condition is suspected, an appropriate serologic workup should be initiated (Urbatsch and Paller, 2002).

DIAGNOSIS

The differential diagnosis for miliaria includes the conditions listed previously for erythema toxicum. Wright staining of vesicle contents from miliaria crystallina will show few cells; that of miliaria rubra will usually reveal a majority of lymphocytes. If screening studies are nondiagnostic, a skin biopsy analysis will be confirmatory (Fitzpatrick, 1990).

TREATMENT

Lesions rapidly resolve after the infant's environmental temperature is reduced. Application of occlusive emollients can exacerbate the eruption.

ACNE

CLINICAL FINDINGS

The appearance of acne in infancy is similar to that of typical acne vulgaris of adolescence. The spectrum of lesions includes comedones, inflammatory papules, pustules, and rarely cysts, generally limited to the face (Figure 100-5). Comedones are an easily recognized, pathognomonic feature of acne.

The condition occurs in up to 20% of infants and is more common in boys. Acne occurs in a bimodal distribution during infancy. Early-onset neonatal acne appears after 1 to 2 weeks of age and usually resolves spontaneously by 3 months. Infantile acne appears after 3 to 6 months and can persist for years.

ETIOLOGY

The pathophysiologic features of acne are similar at all ages. Important components are the increased size and activity of sebaceous glands, which are influenced by circulating levels of adrenal and gonadal androgens, of both endogenous and maternal origins. The role of *Propionibacterium acnes* in the pathogenesis of infantile acne has not been studied. This lipophilic, anaerobic, gram-positive rod has an important role in the pathogenesis of inflammatory lesions in adolescent acne. A family history of acne is

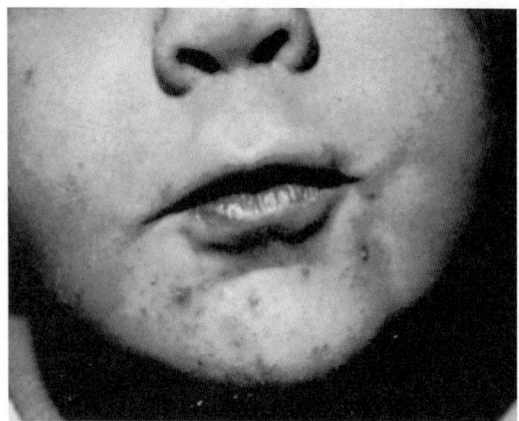

FIGURE 100-5 Papules, pustules, and comedones (diagnostic of acne) on the chin and cheeks of a male infant.

common, and affected infants have a higher risk of developing severe acne later in life (Hellier, 1954), suggesting a genetic predisposition (Forest et al, 1973).

In the past few years a potential etiologic factor of noncomedonal neonatal acne, or cephalic pustulosis, has been identified. *Malassezia* spp. is a lipophilic yeast that is part of the normal flora of adult skin. A variety of factors, including sebaceous gland activity, humidity, heredity, and corticosteroid treatment, may be influential in allowing it to become an opportunistic pathogen. Recently, several investigators have examined the connection between *Malassezia* spp. and neonatal acne. Findings include the rapid progressive skin colonization of neonates by *Malassezia* spp. as seen on smear and culture examination, specifically *Malassezia sympodialis* and *Malassezia globosa*; higher rates of skin colonization by *Malassezia* spp. in more severe cases of cephalic pustulosis; and isolation of *M. sympodialis* in the neonatal pustules (Bernier et al, 2002; Niamba et al, 1998). In a study conducted to explore this association, 8 of 13 patients (61%) with pustules testing positive for *Malassezia* spp. showed a favorable response to treatment with 2% ketoconazole (Rapelanoro et al, 1996.)

However, contrary evidence exists, including the lack of a complete correlation between *Malassezia* spp. and neonatal acne. Other studies have identified patients with neonatal acne in whom *Malassezia* spp. infection was not found, as well as patients without acne whose pustule cultures were positive for *Malassezia* spp. (Katsambas et al, 1999). As a result, further investigation is needed to clarify cephalic pustulosis and neonatal acne and to specifically address the possibility that these inconsistencies could be explained by methodologic or pathologic variation, or that *Malassezia* spp. may be one part of a multifactorial process, or that some cases of neonatal acne are not cephalic pustulosis but true comedonal disease (Bergman and Eichenfield, 2002.)

DIAGNOSIS

Considerations in the differential diagnosis include the papular and pustular disorders listed previously, but the diagnosis of acne can almost always be made by clinical inspection. No other disorder features comedones. Infants with severe or persistent acne should be evaluated for androgenic endocrinopathy.

TREATMENT

Aggressive treatment of neonatal acne is rarely required. For initial therapy, topical 2% erythromycin or 2.5% or 5% benzoyl peroxide can be applied daily. Tretinoin and more potent formulations of benzoyl peroxide may be too irritating. In more severe cases, a course of systemic erythromycin can be added, in divided doses of 30 to 50 mg/kg/day. Creams, ointments, and topical steroids may exacerbate the condition. If *Malassezia* spp. is isolated or suspected, an antifungal agent may be effective (Rapelanoro et al, 1996.)

ECZEMA

The term *eczema* is derived from a Greek term meaning "to boil over." It refers to a clinical and histologic cutaneous phenotype characterized by erythema, edema, and scaling, often accompanied by crusting and, in severe cases, blistering. The histologic hallmark of acute eczema is epidermal intercellular edema (i.e., spongiosis). Epidermal thickening is present in chronic eczema. A mixed perivascular inflammatory infiltrate usually is seen within the papillary dermis.

Different types of eczema can be defined by a spectrum of unifying clinical features. When an infant exhibits widespread eczema, a precise diagnosis sometimes requires a period of observation. Two eczematous conditions that manifest in otherwise healthy infants are seborrheic dermatitis and atopic dermatitis. These diseases differ in pathogenesis, distribution of skin involvement, prognosis, and therapeutic options. Infants with widespread eczema who are not otherwise healthy and those with prominent, erosive periorificial and diaper involvement should be evaluated for associated nutritional, metabolic, or immunologic abnormalities. A more extensive differential diagnosis is detailed under Erythroderma in Chapter 97.

SEBORRHEIC DERMATITIS

CLINICAL FINDINGS

Infantile seborrheic dermatitis is characterized by greasy yellow scales on an erythematous base and minimal pruritus. Onset usually is within the first 2 months of life. The most common sites of involvement are the face, scalp, and diaper area. The condition may be localized or disseminated. Flexural areas such as the posterior auricular sulcus, neck, axillae, and inguinal folds also can be affected. Hypopigmentation is often striking in dark-skinned infants (Figure 100-6). In severe cases, fissures may develop and become secondarily infected.

ETIOLOGY

Pityrosporum ovale is a lipophilic yeast that is commonly present on normal skin, increasing in density during and after puberty. The mycelial form has been identified as a causative agent in tinea versicolor. For a century, the yeast form has been linked to adult seborrheic dermatitis. Therapeutic trials with yeast-inhibiting agents have supported a causal role (Straka et al, 1991). There is a higher incidence of seborrheic

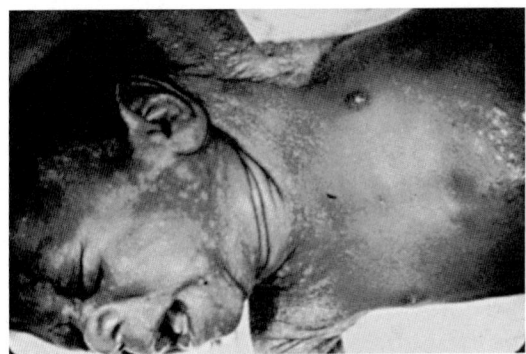

FIGURE 100-6 Infant with seborrheic eczema on the face and neck and in the axillae. Note the scaling and hypopigmentation. Temporary hypopigmentation is common in African American infants with this disorder.

dermatitis in immunocompromised patients, especially those with AIDS (Prose, 1991). The association between *P. ovale* and infantile seborrheic dermatitis also has been confirmed (Broberg and Faergemann, 1989; Ruiz-Maldonado et al, 1989). The pathogenesis of the disorder, and the reasons that carriers remain asymptomatic and immunocompromised persons can be more severely affected, remain unclear.

DIAGNOSIS

The diagnosis is usually made clinically, although skin biopsy can be obtained to differentiate between psoriasis and Langerhans cell histiocytosis, which is a more severe condition. Because seborrhea typically occurs in skin folds, *Candida* spp. infection should be ruled out with a fungal culture. Atopic dermatitis can sometimes overlap with seborrhea dermatitis, but atopic dermatitis causes much more itching.

TREATMENT

Infantile seborrheic dermatitis spontaneously resolves by the end of the 1st year of life. For infants with disfiguring or symptomatic disease, there are several therapeutic alternatives. Topical agents effective against *P. ovale* include topical ketoconazole in a cream or shampoo base (Cutsem et al, 1990), shampoos containing 1% zinc pyrithione or 1% to 2.5% selenium sulfide, and propylene glycol (Faergemann, 1988). Propylene glycol is a hygroscopic preservative, with antimycotic activity against *P. ovale*, that has been widely used for more than a century in foods and cosmetics, but can also rarely cause a contact dermatitis. The safety and efficacy of these products have not been established in infants. Nevertheless, widespread availability and popular use have not produced reports of toxicity. Brief application with daily bathing usually is effective and limits excessive percutaneous absorption. Daily application of 0.5% to 1% hydrocortisone cream is another short-term alternative.

ATOPIC DERMATITIS

CLINICAL FINDINGS

Atopic dermatitis (AD) is a chronic, relapsing, severely pruritic disorder defined by a spectrum of defined cutaneous and extracutaneous manifestations (Hanifin, 1991;

Paller, 1991) that affects 15% to 20% of the population, particularly in industrialized areas. In 60% of cases, onset of signs and symptoms is in infancy; up to 10% of 1-year-old children are affected (Kay et al, 1994). The most easily recognized of the diagnostic criteria for AD may not be present until early childhood. These criteria include onset of rash before the age 2 years, flexural skin lesions, asthma or hay fever, and generalized dry skin (Williams et al, 1994). AD and seborrheic dermatitis share clinical features, often making correct diagnosis difficult during the neonatal period. A common feature that may distinguish one from the other form is involvement of the diaper area. This area is often dramatically spared in infants with AD and is primarily involved in infants with seborrheic dermatitis.

ETIOLOGY

Atopic disease has been clinically recognized since 1916; however, the pathogenesis remains elusive. Previous investigations of the mechanisms and treatment of AD have focused on immune alterations. There is an imbalance of T cell subsets, with inhibition of the cells that produce interferon-γ (T_H1 helper T cells) and a relative activation of the cells that produce IL-4 (T_H2 helper T cells). This can potentiate a vicious cycle of enhanced production of IgE, eosinophilia, mast cell proliferation, release of histamine by basophils and mast cells, and further expansion of T_H2 cells (Hanifin, 1991; Hanifin et al, 1993). Chronic AD shifts toward T_H1 inflammatory responses. Other in vitro immune abnormalities have been described, including alterations in monocyte cyclic AMP production, increased histamine release by basophils and mast cells, abnormal differentiation of antigen-presenting cells, increased serum levels of eosinophil cationic protein and interleukin-4 (IL-4), and diminished production of interferon-γ by circulating lymphocytes (Hanifin, 1991; Hanifin et al, 1993). Recently, filaggrin loss-of-function mutations have been linked to families with AD, particularly early-onset and persistent atopic dermatitis (Brown and Irvine, 2008; Palmer et al, 2006). Filaggrin is a protein in the top layers of the skin which play a role in epidermal differentiation and skin barrier maintenance. It is also present in the oral, esophageal, and nasal vestibulum but not in the bronchial mucosa (Brown and Irvine, 2008; Weidinger et al, 2008; Ying et al, 2006). This discovery helps to classify atopic dermatitis as a skin barrier abnormality for which the skin's function as an immunologic organ is compromised.

Staphylococcus aureus has an important role in the exacerbation of AD. Seventy-six percent to almost 100% of patients with AD carry this microbe on their skin. Staphylococcal exotoxins act as superantigens capable of stimulating a wide variety of T cell responses (Leung et al, 1995). The inflammatory cytokines suppress endogenous antimicrobial peptides, which are already decreased in AD (Huang et al, 2009).

Food and environmental allergens have a role in a minority of patients (Hanifin, 1991). Some authors report that prolonged breastfeeding and delayed exposure to diverse solid foods may protect against AD, especially in infants with a strong family history of atopic disease (Zeiger, 1994).

TREATMENT

The goal of treatment is to control signs and symptoms. A definitive cure is not yet available, but spontaneous improvement occurs before puberty in 40% of patients (Hanifin, 1991). Maintenance therapy aims to hydrate and moisturize the skin, reduce inflammation, control pruritus, and eliminate inciting factors. Bathing daily with a mild cleanser followed by liberal application of a bland ointment emollient is part of skin care. Topical corticosteroids are to be used for flares, but long-term continuous use or inappropriate use can lead to skin atrophy, striae, folliculitis, systemic absorption, hypertrichosis, telangiectasias, bruising, and hypopigmentation.

Both tacrolimus 0.03% ointment and pimecrolimus 1% cream, nonsteroidal selective inhibitors of inflammatory cytokines, have been approved for the treatment of atopic dermatitis in children older than 24 months. However, although studies support the safe use of both agents in infants as young as 3 months, there is a black box warning label about the theoretical risk of lymphoma and skin malignancies. These agents are best used for maintenance. They are also useful for the face and skin folds, because they do not have the same local side effects that corticosteroids have.

Systemic antistaphylococcal antibiotics or topical mupirocin, or both, are sometimes necessary for superinfections or flares. Dilute sodium hypochlorite (bleach) baths have also been shown to decrease infection rates with *S. aureus* as well as disease severity (Huang et al, 2009).

Infants with AD have a relative cutaneous anergy and are at increased risk for the development of cutaneous bacterial, yeast, fungal, and viral infections. A high index of suspicion for secondary infection must be maintained.

DIAPER DERMATITIS

CLINICAL FINDINGS

This disorder is the most common neonatal skin condition, developing in approximately 25% of infants. Most affected infants are healthy, but occasionally diaper dermatitis may provide clues to underlying systemic disorders. Involvement of other skin sites may be helpful in establishing a specific diagnosis. The skin in the area most in contact with the diaper becomes inflamed by the presence of irritants exacerbated by friction and microorganisms. These irritants include moisture from urine and feces, fecal enzymes, and cleansing materials, as well as irritants within the diapers. The usual presentation is thus one of an irritant contact dermatitis with erythema and mild scaling of the gluteal crease, buttocks, convex surfaces of the pubic area (mons pubis, labia majora, scrotum), and perianal rim (Figure 100-7). Shiny plaques or erosions may also be present, particularly in more severe cases. The lower abdomen and upper thighs may also be involved; conversely, there may be relative sparing of the skin folds in the diaper region. The condition is self-limiting and episodic with a typical rash lasting 3 to 5 days (Nield and Kamat, 2007; Scheinfeld, 2005; Shin, 2005).

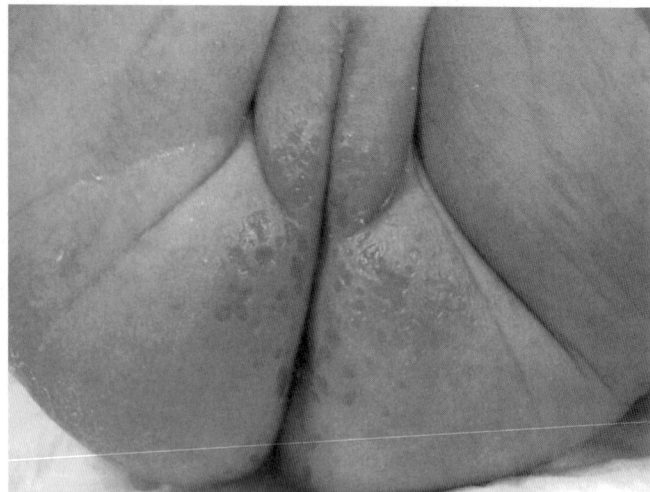

FIGURE 100-7 Erosive diaper dermatitis occurred in this four-month-old following a course of oral antibiotics. *(From www.dermatlas.org. Reproduced with permission.)*

ETIOLOGY

Although diaper dermatitis, described over a century ago, has been widely studied, the cause, true prevalence, and optimal treatment are still issues of debate. Most infants have episodes of diaper dermatitis, usually between 6 and 12 months of age (Jordan and Blaney, 1982). For decades, the condition was believed to be due primarily to the effects of ammonia. However, objective studies did not support this theory (Leyden et al, 1977). Many factors contribute to the pathogenesis of diaper dermatitis, but the nidus of the problem begins with occlusion, excessive hydration, friction, and maceration. Once skin barrier function has been compromised, irritants (urine, fecal lipases, proteases, bile salts) and microorganisms (urease-splitting bacteria, *S. aureus*, beta-hemolytic streptococci, *Pseudomonas* spp., *Candida albicans*) exacerbate the problem. Exogenous irritants, such as soaps, commercial diaper wipes, and a myriad of over-the-counter topical products, can perpetuate the process in susceptible infants.

DIAGNOSIS

Diaper dermatitis is a clinical diagnosis. There is limited histopathology of the condition and thus, no specific diagnostic test (Montes, 1978). Other skin eruptions in the diaper area which should be considered and excluded include both non-infectious and infectious skin conditions. Non-infectious causes of skin eruptions in the diaper area are infantile seborrheic dermatitis, allergic contact dermatitis, Langerhans cell histiocytosis, epidermolysis bullosa, acrodermatitis enteropathica (zinc deficiency), and certain metabolic disorders such as maple syrup urine disease or cystic fibrosis (Nield and Kamat, 2007; Scheinfeld, 2005; Shin, 2005). A distinguishing feature of these conditions is that there are often similar skin lesions in non-diapered areas. Infectious causes of skin eruptions in the diaper area are *Candida* or other fungal infections, *Staphylococcal* scalded skin syndrome, congenital syphilis, herpes simplex, and HIV infection (Scheinfeld, 2005). Similar to the non-infectious causes, skin lesions associated with these infectious are typically also found elsewhere in non-diapered areas. The rash of *Candida* diaper dermatitis is clinically distinct from that of primary irritant diaper dermatitis. The rash associated with Candida is intensely erythematous and is often accompanied by satellite lesions (papules and pustules) which are typically seen in the groin region and perianal rim. Diaper rashes associated with *Staphylococcus aureus* and Group A *Streptococcus* infections are also clinically distinct, with the former typically presenting as bullous impetigo with scattered vesicles and bullae, and the latter as an erythematous perianal patch (Nield and Kamat, 2007). Once any of these infectious or non-infectious causes of diaper dermatitis are suspected, specific diagnostic tests can be done to rule them in or out. Because there is no specific diagnostic test for primary contact or irritant diaper dermatitis, the diagnosis is thus one of exclusion.

TREATMENT

Clearly the most important steps in preventing diaper dermatitis are maintaining skin barrier function and hygiene and preventing irritation. Traditionally, an effective but labor-intensive approach has been frequent diaper changes with gentle cleansing, thorough drying, and limited use of occlusive plastic or rubber diaper covers. This practice has been greatly simplified by the introduction of disposable diapers.

The first disposable diapers were marketed in 1963. Initially, the absorbent core was composed primarily of cellulose fluff. Subsequently, several conflicting studies were done to evaluate the incidence of diaper dermatitis in infants wearing cloth versus disposable diapers (Jordan and Blaney, 1982). In the mid 1980s, a superabsorbent core material was developed, containing a cross-linked sodium polyacrylate. Upon contact with fluid, this material undergoes a transformation to allow it to hold fluid within a gel and has the capacity to absorb many times its own weight. Several studies have concluded that superabsorbent diapers are superior to cloth diapers in preventing diaper dermatitis (Lane et al, 1990). In addition, superabsorbent diapers can prevent occult fecal contamination of clothing and fomites in daycare settings (Rory et al, 1991).

Routine use of topical preparations to prevent diaper dermatitis is not necessary in infants with healthy skin. For some of these products, additional risks have been recognized. Additives have the potential to cause contact sensitization or irritation. Powders applied vigorously enough to raise a cloud pose an aspiration hazard. This is especially true for talc, which can cause irritant pneumonitis. Talc (mainly hydrous magnesium silicate) also may cause granulomatous reactions when applied to wounds.

Appropriate treatment of diaper dermatitis begins with correct diagnosis of the underlying cause. Most infants develop acute diaper dermatitis as a result of the factors described previously. However, other primary pathologic processes must be considered for any infant with chronic, severe, or recurrent diaper rash. Primary cutaneous diseases that can manifest with diaper rash include allergic contact dermatitis, seborrheic dermatitis, psoriasis,

and candidiasis. Uncommon causes of diaper dermatitis such as histiocytosis, congenital syphilis, cystic fibrosis, acrodermatitis enteropathica, bullous pemphigoid, and staphylococcal scalded skin syndrome have serious clinical implications (Kazaks and Lane, 2000).

Mild to moderate, common diaper dermatitis should be treated initially with traditional frequent diaper changes, leaving the area exposed, or both. All potential irritants or sensitizers should be discontinued. Commercial diaper wipes are an often overlooked and common source of these substances. Washcloths, dampened paper towels, and mineral oil–soaked cotton balls are safe alternatives. Zinc oxide ointment and zinc paste are inexpensive, bland, protective agents with antiseptic and astringent properties. Zinc also can have a role in wound healing (Maitra and Dorani, 1992; Okada et al, 1990; Rackett et al, 1993). Some caregivers may object to the difficulty in removing zinc oxide preparations. They should be reassured that it is not necessary to remove the salve. If a parent or clinician needs to remove zinc oxide to assess the skin, this can be easily accomplished with the help of mineral oil.

If there is no objective evidence of candidiasis, such as erythematous papules in skin folds, a short course of a topical low-potency corticosteroid may be beneficial. A topical anticandidal agent should be used when potassium hydroxide preparation or culture suggests yeast infection. Combination products containing potent topical corticosteroids and antifungal agents are less effective than an antifungal used alone (Reynolds et al, 1991). Widespread use of one such product combining a potent, fluorinated topical corticosteroid, 0.05% betamethasone dipropionate, with 1% clotrimazole (Lotrisone), applied under the occlusion of a diaper, has resulted in reports of skin atrophy, striae, and adrenal suppression (Barkley, 1987). Clotrimazole and a similar product combining 0.1% triamcinolone acetonide and nystatin (Mycolog II) are contraindicated for the treatment of diaper dermatitis.

HARLEQUIN COLOR CHANGE

Harlequin color change should not be confused with an entirely different disorder called *harlequin fetus*. Harlequin color change, first described in 1952, usually occurs during the first 4 days of life (Mortensen and Stougard-Andresen, 1959). It is characterized by reddening of one half of the body and simultaneous blanching of the other half. A sharp, midline demarcation runs from the center of the forehead down the face and trunk. Occasionally, the line of demarcation may be incomplete, sparing the face and genitalia. Turning the body from one side to the other accentuates blanching of the upper half and reddening of the lower half. There is no accompanying change in respiratory rate, pupillary reflexes, muscle tone, or response to external stimuli. The total duration of these episodes may range from a few minutes to several hours. Harlequin color change occurs most frequently in low-birthweight infants, but may be seen in up to 10% of term infants. The physiologic basis of the phenomenon has not been defined. It has no pathologic significance, requires no treatment, and can be expected to disappear no later than the 3rd week of life.

SUBCUTANEOUS FAT NECROSIS

CLINICAL FINDINGS

Subcutaneous fat necrosis affects full-term infants who have experienced perinatal distress. Lesions usually appear within the first 2 weeks of life; they may be single or multiple, are poorly circumscribed, and often are tender nodules or plaques that are initially firm with a dusky reddish-purple hue. The lesions are located most often in areas in which a fat pad is present: buttocks, back, arms, and thighs (Figure 100-8). With time, subcutaneous calcification may develop, with subsequent drainage and resultant scarring. The most serious association is hypercalcemia. Infants with hypercalcemia may be asymptomatic, so the incidence and time course have not been well documented (Cook and Stone, 1992). Clinical manifestations include irritability, vomiting, poor feeding, and failure to thrive.

ETIOLOGY

The development of subcutaneous fat necrosis has been related to ischemic injury from perinatal trauma, intrauterine asphyxia (Chen et al, 1981), and hypothermia.

DIAGNOSIS

The differential diagnosis includes sclerema neonatorum (see the following section). A skin biopsy from a well-developed lesion of subcutaneous fat necrosis of the newborn will reveal a subcutaneous granulomatous infiltrate with multinucleated giant cells. Damaged lipocytes contain characteristic needle-shaped clefts. Soft tissue necrosis and inflammation may stimulate local production of 1,25-dihydroxyvitamin D_3, resulting in hypercalcemia (Cook and Stone, 1992).

TREATMENT

In most infants, the process is self-limited; resolution occurs over a period of weeks to months. Infants should be followed closely for the development of hypercalcemia for several months. Hypercalcemic infants should be managed initially with hydration and furosemide-induced diuresis. Low calcium intake, vitamin D restriction, and sometimes systemic corticosteroids may be necessary (Cook and Stone, 1992; Norwood-Galloway et al, 1987). However, this approach may be only partially successful, and persistent hypercalcemia with its associated morbidity may ensue. Bisphosphonate agents, specifically etidronate, have recently been discussed for use as possible agents of last resort to control the persistent hypercalcemia that can be secondary to subcutaneous fat necrosis. In one case report, a newborn with subcutaneous fat necrosis refractory to conservative management had etidronate added to his regimen. After initiation of the drug, the patient's urinary calcium levels soon normalized. It was postulated that the mechanism of lowering the serum and urinary calcium by etidronate was primarily a decrease in bone resorption (Rice and Rivkees, 1999).

Other investigators have commented on the limited use of bisphosphonates in children and question whether

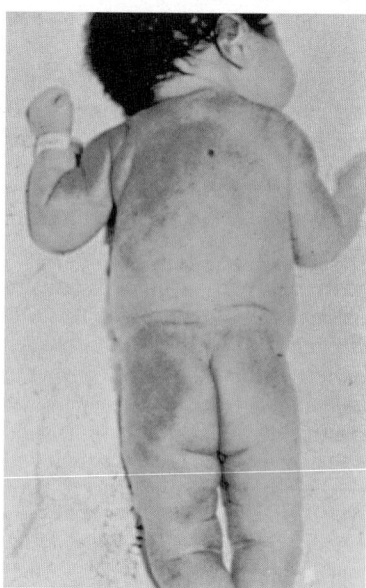

FIGURE 100-8 Rear view of a newborn showing several large discolored areas of subcutaneous fat necrosis. They were irregular in size and shape, felt firm to palpation, and were not hot or tender.

the hypercalcemia of subcutaneous fat necrosis is secondary to enhanced bone resorption or intestinal absorption. Controlled trials have been recommended before the use of these agents for this indication can be recommended (Bachrach and Lum, 1999). In the one case study, etidronate had to be stopped because of a rash severe enough to be of clinical concern. Physicians must be aware of possible bisphosphonate-induced hypersensitivity reactions and stop the agent if suspected (Rice and Rivkees, 1999).

SCLEREMA NEONATORUM

CLINICAL FINDINGS

Sclerema neonatorum is a rare disorder that typically affects severely ill, preterm neonates in the first week of life. It is now classified under the Panniculitides which are inflammatory diseases involving subcutaneous adipose tissue (Zeb and Darmstadt, 2008). It manifests with widespread, stone-hard, non-pitting cutaneous induration, typically beginning in the buttocks, thighs, or trunk but spreading to involve any part of the body except the palms, soles, and genitalia. The skin appears pale and waxy, shaping the face into a masklike expression (Figure 100-9). The involved area may be discolored with a reddened or violaceous hue and the joints are stiff. The hardening hinders movement, feeding, and respiration. Associated metabolic acidosis, hypoglycemia, hyperkalemia, hyponatremia, and azotemia can occur. Sclerema neonatorum is a diffuse, systemic process with a grave prognosis (Fretzin and Arias, 1987; Zeb and Darmstadt, 2008).

ETIOLOGY

The mechanism responsible for sclerema neonatorum is unknown. In a recent review article on the disorder, Zeb and Darmstadt summarized the various theories on its pathogenesis into the following four categories: 1) unique

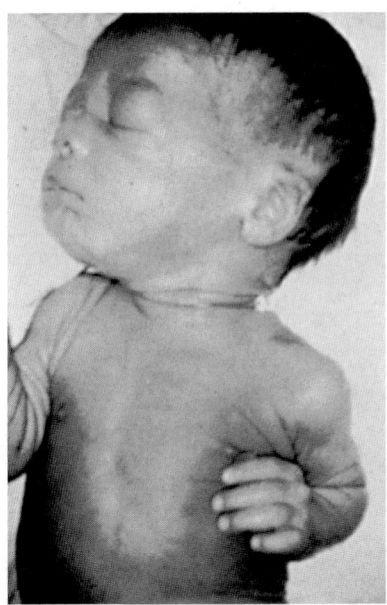

FIGURE 100-9 Sclerema neonatorum. Note the masklike facial expression, pseudotrismus of the partially immobilized mouth, and thickening of the skin over the face, arms, and hands. *(From the Collection of the American Academy of Pediatrics. Reproduced with permission of the officers of the Academy.)*

composition of neonatal fat; 2) defects in neonatal fat metabolism; 3) sign of severe toxicity of grave underlying disorder; 4) special form of edema affecting connective tissue septa (Zeb and Darmstadt, 2008). The disorder has been associated with prematurity, low birthweight, perinatal asphyxia, hypothermia, and sepsis (Ji et al, 1993; Zeb and Darmstadt, 2008).

DIAGNOSIS

The differential diagnosis of sclerema neonatorum includes subcutaneous fat necrosis (described earlier in this chapter), which occurs in healthy term or post-term infants, and scleredema, which occurs in preterm infants and usually involves pitting edema of the lower extremities. Zeb and Darmstadt (2008) summarized the history of the nomenclature of sclerema neonatorum as well as the clinical features, histopathology, and treatment of these three conditions, highlighting the diagnostic confusion

which has existed over the years. The histologic changes of sclerema are not specific. Fat necrosis with crystallization may be seen, but thinning of the epidermis, dermal and subcutaneous fibrosis with edema, and thickening of the interlobular septa or trabeculae which support the subcutaneous adipose tissue are more conspicuous features (Dasgupta et al, 1993). There is usually sparse inflammatory infiltration of lymphocytes, histiocytes, and multinucleated giant cells and less inflammation surrounding the fat lobules than in subcutaneous fat necrosis.

TREATMENT

The treatment of sclerema neonatorum is primarily supportive care and treatment of any underlying disease, such as sepsis. Local therapy or warming the body have not proved to be beneficial. Steroid use has not improved survival but may limit the spread of lesions. The use of exchange transfusion for septic neonates with sclerema neonatorum has also been studied over the past several decades and results have been promising, particularly when done repeatedly and early in the course of the disease (Zeb and Darmstadt, 2008).

SUGGESTED READINGS

Bergman J, Eichenfield L: Neonatal acne and cephalic pustulosis: Is Malassezia the whole story? [editorial], *Arch Dermatol* 138:255-257, 2002.

Hurwitz S: A visual guide to neonatal skin eruptions, *Contemp Pediatr* 82-92, 1985 September.

Kazaks EL, Lane AT: Diaper dermatitis, *Pediatr Clin North Am* 47:909-919, 2000.

Marchini G, Ulfgren AK, Loré K, et al: Erythema toxicum neonatorum: an immunohistochemical analysis, *Pediatr Dermatol* 18:177-187, 2001.

Neligan GW, Strang LB: A "harlequin" colour change in the newborn, *Lancet* 2:1005, 1952.

Norwood-Galloway A, Lebwohl M, Phelps RG, et al: Subcutaneous fat necrosis of the newborn and hypercalcemia, *J Am Acad Dermatol* 16:435-439, 1987.

Ramamurthy RS, Reveri M, Esterly NB, et al: Transient neonatal pustular melanosis, *J Pediatr* 88:831-835, 1976.

Scheinfeld N: Diaper dermatitis: a review and brief survey of eruptions of the diaper area, *Am J Clin Dermatol* 6:273-281, 2005.

Solomon LM, Esterly NB: *Eczema in neonatal dermatology*, Philadelphia, 1973, WB Saunders, p 125.

Straka BF, Cooper PH, Greer K: Congenital miliaria crystallina, *Cutis* 47:103-106, 1991.

Zeb A, Darmstadt GL: Sclerema neonatorum: a review of nomenclature, clinical presentation, histological features, differential diagnoses and management, *J Perinatol* 28:453-460, 2008.

Zeiger RS: Dietary manipulations in infants and their mothers and the natural course of atopic disease, *Pediatr Allergy Immunol* 5:26-28, 1994.

Complete references used in this text can be found online at www.expertconsult.com

CUTANEOUS CONGENITAL DEFECTS*

Katherine B. Püttgen and Bernard A. Cohen

The spectrum of congenital cutaneous defects can be organized by tissue of origin or location within the skin. This spectrum is summarized in Box 101-1. However, in many cases the clinical appearance is not diagnostic for the specific condition or even the tissue type. An overview of differential diagnosis by clinical appearance is included in Chapter 97.

This chapter presents information on the most common and clinically significant congenital cutaneous defects.

VASCULAR ANOMALIES

Precise diagnosis and appropriate management of cutaneous vascular anomalies have been confounded by tremendous confusion in nomenclature and poor understanding of the pathogenesis of the different conditions within this group. For example, the term *hemangioma* has been used indiscriminately to refer to lesions that differ considerably in morphology, behavior, and prognosis. A classification system originally proposed by Mulliken and Glowacki in 1982 and updated in 1996 by the International Society for the Study of Vascular Anomalies (ISSVA) to include infantile hemangioma (IH) variants, other benign vascular tumors, and combined lesions is accepted as the official classification scheme by the ISSVA (Enjolras and Mulliken, 1997; Hand and Frieden, 2002). This scheme separates vascular lesions of infants and children into two major categories: vascular tumors, the most common of which is IHs and vascular malformations. An *infantile hemangioma*, by definition, is a benign tumor of vascular endothelium, characterized by a proliferative phase and an involutional phase (Figure 101-1, *A*). In contrast, a *vascular malformation* is a developmental anomaly generated from a single vascular component or from a combination of vascular components: capillary, venous, arterial, or lymphatic. These two groups can be further differentiated according to clinical, cellular, hematologic, radiologic, and skeletal characteristics (Table 101-1).

INFANTILE HEMANGIOMAS

IHs are the most common tumors of infancy; mature lesions have been noted in 10% to 12% of 1-year-old infants, with more than double this incidence in preterm infants weighing less than 1000 g (Amir et al, 1986). They occur sporadically, most often as single lesions. Low birthweight is the single most important predictor of IH; the risk of IH increases by 40% for every 500-g decrease in birthweight (Drolet et al, 2008). Additional risk factors include prematurity, female sex, white ethnicity, multiple-gestation pregnancy, advanced maternal age, and placental abnormalities including placenta previa (Haggstrom et al, 2007). The male-to-female ratio in term infants is 1:3 (Esterly, 1995).

CLINICAL FINDINGS

Typically, hemangiomas are not clinically apparent at birth but manifest within the first 6 weeks of life as a faint blush or area of pallor, a change known as a *precursor lesion*. They follow a triphasic pattern of growth, marked by proliferation, plateau, and a long, slow period of involution. In the first 2 months of life, nearly all IHs double in size, and most IHs reach 80% of their maximum size between 3 and 5 months of age (Chang et al, 2008). The growth phase usually slows after 5 months and ends by 12 months of age, if not before. The end of involution does not necessarily indicate resolution, and up to 40% of lesions have residual textural changes and scarring characterized by fibrofatty residuum. The clinical appearance is dictated by the depth of the tumor. Superficial lesions are cherry red and sharply circumscribed. Though such terminology should be avoided because it is imprecise, these superficial IHs are often referred to as "strawberry" or "capillary" hemangiomas. Lesions that are confined to the deep dermis and subcutis appear bluish and dome-shaped. Most lesions are mixed and have both superficial and deep components. The head and neck regions are involved most commonly (60% of cases), followed by the trunk (25%), and extremities (15%) (Finn et al, 1983). Lesions can be designated as focal and seem to grow from a single point. Segmental hemangiomas comprise an apparent developmental unit and are thought to arise from embryonic developmental units or placodes, but their exact origin is not fully understood. Indeterminate lesions likely occupy part of a segment. Segmental and deep IHs are known to have a longer proliferative phase. Flattening occurs by age 5 in half of cases and by age 9 in an additional 40% (Esterly, 1995). Parents are frequently concerned about the risk of hemorrhage and should be reassured that significant bleeding rarely occurs. Several other complications are possible, however, and the more serious sequelae are described next.

Obstruction

A hemangioma that obstructs just one eye can pose a significant threat to visual development by limiting the visual field or compressing the globe. Permanent damage to vision can occur in a relatively short period of time. Obstruction of bilateral—but generally not unilateral—external ear canals will impair development of hearing. A lesion encompassing the chin, lower cheeks, and jaw, now referred to as segment 3 or the "beard" area, may indicate upper airway involvement, which can be life-threatening.

---

*This chapter includes material from previous editions, to which Nancy B. Esterly, MD, Elaine C. Siegfried, MD, and Allison Z. Young, MD, contributed.

BOX 101-1   Spectrum of Congenital Cutaneous Defects

VASCULAR DEFECTS

Hemangiomas
Malformations: lymphatic, venous, arterial, capillary, mixed

HYPOPIGMENTED LESIONS

Ash-leaf macules, confetti-like macules
Linear and whorled hypomelanosis
Nevus depigmentosis
Nevus anemicus
Hemangioma precursor

MELANIN-CONTAINING LESIONS

Nevocellular nevi
Melanoma
Lentigines
Café-au-lait macules
Nevus spilus
Mongolian spots
Nevus of Ota and nevus of Ito

TUMORS OF EPITHELIAL ORIGIN

Epidermal (keratinocytic) nevi/sebaceous nevi—nevus unius lateris, nevus verrucosis, ichthyosis hystrix
Nevus comedonicus
Pilomatrixoma
Porokeratosis of Mibelli

DERMAL TUMORS

Connective tissue nevi: collagen, elastic tissue
Digital fibroma

TUMORS OF EXTRACUTANEOUS ORIGIN

Cutaneous mastocytosis: urticaria pigmentosa, solitary mastocytoma, diffuse cutaneous mastocytosis
Juvenile xanthogranuloma
Lipoma
Osteoma cutis
Nasal glioma
Dermoid cyst
Meningioma

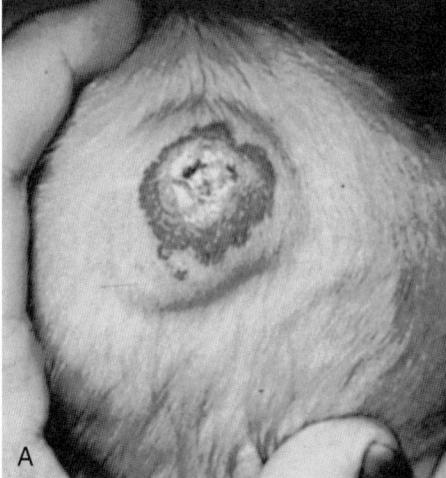

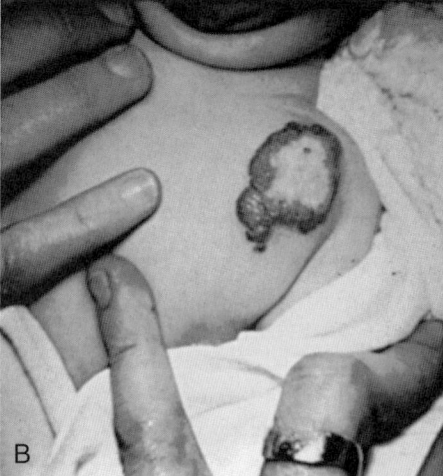

FIGURE 101-1 A, Hemangioma with small central ulceration on the scalp of an infant. **B,** Involuting hemangioma with central gray fibrotic area.

Ulceration

Ulceration occurs in up to 10% of hemangiomas and is more commonly seen in large lesions, those with segmental morphology, and with both superficial and deep components (Chamlin et al, 2007; Morelli et al, 1991, 1994; Mulliken et al, 1995). Areas of friction and chronic exposure to moisture such as the lip, neck, and diaper area are most likely to ulcerate. Ulcerated hemangiomas are painful and at risk for secondary infection. Those at highest risk for ulcer formation are large, of mixed clinical type, segmental in morphology type, and located on the lower lip, neck, or anogenital region. Ulceration most often occurs during the proliferative phase, in younger infants.

Disfigurement

During the 1st year of life, the presence of a prominent hemangioma can elicit a disturbing amount of unwanted attention. Many parents require emotional support through this time. In addition to the transient disfigurement, lesions of the central face and those with a significant superficial component predispose the affected child

to permanent scarring. Disfigurement alone, regardless of threat to function, may be a reasonable indication for medical therapy in certain cases, if surgical reconstruction is likely to be problematic.

Kasabach-Merritt Syndrome

Though originally thought to be associated with IH, Kasabach-Merritt syndrome is now known to be associated with either kaposiform hemangioendothelioma or tufted angiomas, much rarer vascular tumors (Cooper et al, 2002). It is not seen in conjunction with IHs. The lesion consists of a rapidly expanding vascular tumor with compression and invasion of surrounding structures as well as primary platelet trapping and resultant consumptive coagulopathy. The mortality rate is 30% to 40%.

Central Nervous System Anomalies

Large facial hemangiomas may be associated with anomalies of the central nervous system (CNS) (Frieden et al, 1996). PHACE syndrome is a combination of *p*osterior fossa malformations, *h*emangiomas, *a*rterial anomalies, *c*oarctation of the aorta, and *e*ye abnormalities. Sternal cleft and supraumbilical raphe can also be seen, and the disorder is therefore sometimes referred to as PHACES. The

TABLE 101-1   Characteristics of Hemangiomas Versus Vascular Malformations

Hemangioma	Vascular Malformation
Clinical	
Usually nothing seen at birth, 30% manifest as red macule	All present at birth; may not be evident
Rapid postnatal proliferation and slow involution	Commensurate growth; may expand as a result of trauma, sepsis, hormonal modulation
Female to male 3:1	Female:male 1:1
Cellular	
Plump endothelium, increased turnover	Flat endothelium, slow turnover
Increased mast cells	Normal mast cell count
Multilaminated basement membrane	Normal thin basement membrane
Capillary tubule formation in vitro	Poor endothelial growth in vitro
Hematologic	
No specific abnormality	Primary stasis (venous); localized intravascular coagulation (LIC)
Radiologic	
High flow	Angiographic findings: diffuse, no parenchyma
Ultrasound: variable echogenicity, high vessel density, high flow, low resistance, little/no AV shunting	Low-flow (e.g., venous malformation): phleboliths, ectatic channels; MRI: T2 hyperintense, patchy/avid enhancement
MRI: T1 isointense, T2 hyperintense, homogeneously enhancing soft tissue mass. Flow voids in and around lesion	High-flow (e.g., arteriovenous malformation): enlarged, tortuous arteries with arteriovenous shunting; MRI: multiple enlarged flow voids, no soft tissue mass
Skeletal	
Infrequent "mass effect" on adjacent bone; hypertrophy rare	Low-flow: distortion, hypertrophy, or hypoplasia
	High-flow: destruction, distortion, or hypertrophy

Adapted from Mulliken JB, Young AE: *Vascular birthmarks, hemangiomas and malformations*, Philadelphia, 1988, WB Saunders, p 35.

diagnostic criteria for PHACE were recently formalized by a concensus panel, and clinical features grouped into major criteria. Definitive diagnosis of PHACE requires a facial segmental IH or an IH larger than 5 centimeters on face or scalp in addition to one major or two minor criteria. (Metry et al, 2009). For unknown reasons, the female to male ratio for PHACE is a striking 9:1. Because of associated anomalies, patients suspected of having PHACE syndrome are most likely to require imaging. Children with frontotemporal and frontonasal IH (known as segments 1 and 4) have a higher correlation with structural cerebral and cerebrovascular anomalies, whereas those with mandibular (segment 3) or "beard" distribution lesions are at higher risk for cardiac abnormalities and IH in the airway (Waner et al, 2003). The maxillary face (segment 2) appears to be a lower-risk segment for IH involvement. The most common and potentially devastating sequelae of PHACE syndrome are neurologic; these can be structural brain anomalies and abnormalities of cerebral vasculature. Progressive stenoses and occlusions of cerebral arteries can also be seen. Both moya-moya–like vasculopathy and arterial ischemic strokes have been reported (Drolet et al, 2006; Heyer et al, 2006).

Spinal Dysraphism and Genitourinary Abnormalities

Sacral and lumbar hemangiomas may reveal spinal dysraphism, including tethered spinal cord, lipomyelomeningocele, imperforate anus, renal anomalies, or abnormal external genitalia. (Albright et al, 1989; Goldberg et al, 1986; Laurent et al, 1998; Tavafoghi et al, 1978). Perineal

lesions should also be imaged to rule out underlying abnormalities, especially those that are segmental in nature. In recent years, both SACRAL (*s*pinal dysraphism, *a*nogenital, *c*utaneous, *r*enal and urologic anomalies, associated with an *a*ngioma of *l*umbosacral localization) syndrome and PELVIS (*p*erineal hemangioma, *e*xternal genitalia malformations, *l*ipomyelomeningocele, *v*esicorenal abnormalities, *i*mperforate anus, and *s*kin tag) syndrome have been described to emphasize the potential for underlying spinal and genitourinary abnormalities in association with lumbosacral and perineal hemangiomas (Girard et al, 2006; Stockman et al, 2007).

Visceral Involvement

Diffuse neonatal hemangiomatosis manifests as widely scattered, small superficial hemangiomas. Infants with this pattern of cutaneous involvement may have lesions limited to the skin, known as benign neonatal hemangiomatosis. However, associated hemangiomatosis of the liver, gastrointestinal tract, lungs, and/or CNS can be complicated by visceral hemorrhage, hepatomegaly, high-output cardiac failure, or unexplained anemia or thrombocytopenia, with a significant mortality rate (Byard et al, 1991). Congestive heart failure can also occur with a large, isolated cutaneous hemangioma (Mulliken et al, 1995).

DIAGNOSIS

In most cases, a hemangioma can be diagnosed by its clinical appearance and pattern of evolution. A vascular lesion that is not obvious at birth, begins as a precursor noted during the 1st month of life, and exhibits rapid growth is undoubtedly a hemangioma. A lesion that deviates from this typical picture presents a diagnostic dilemma. Considerations in the differential diagnosis include IH, vascular malformation, and a nonvascular mimic. Doppler ultrasound examination is an easily performed test that may help to distinguish between a hemangioma and a low-flow malformation. Other imaging modalities—magnetic resonance imaging (MRI) or angiography—may be indicated for large or obstructive lesions (e.g., ocular, upper airway) to help define the extent of involvement or associated abnormalities (Baker et al, 1993; Esterly, 1995). Skin biopsy is diagnostic for nonvascular tumors, which can mimic vascular birthmarks (e.g., pilomatricoma, juvenile xanthogranuloma, Langerhans cell histiocytosis, infantile myofibromatosis). Differentiating among various vascular tumors and malformations can be quite challenging even to experienced pathologists. GLUT1 is an immunohistochemical marker, highly selective and specific for IH, that is also expressed at the blood-brain barrier and in placental tissue. Its discovery has helped to make correct diagnosis of these challenging lesions more feasible, especially in cases with atypical presentations (North et al, 2000).

PATHOGENESIS

Hemangiomas in the proliferative phase are composed of syncytial aggregates of endothelial cells. These cells, like mature endothelial cells, express alkaline phosphatase, factor VIII antigen, and CD31 PECAM (platelet endothelial cell adhesion molecule), as well as Weibel-Palade bodies on electron microscopy, but ^{3}H labeling demonstrates active proliferation. Other histologic features that distinguish proliferating hemangiomas from malformations are the presence of multilaminate basement membranes bordering the endothelial syncytia, large numbers of mast cells (Esterly, 1995), and increased expression of other immunohistochemical markers, including proliferating cell nuclear antigen, vascular endothelial cell growth factor, type IV collagenase, urokinase, and basic fibroblast growth factor (bFGF) (Takahashi et al, 1994). Elevated bFGF can be detected in urine from infants with hemangiomas (Mulliken et al, 1995). Angiogenesis is a process that allows new blood vessel formation. It plays an important role in the growth of all vascular tumors, including hemangiomas. Identification of the basic processes that contribute to angiogenesis and effective angiogenesis inhibitors will provide insight into the pathogenesis and a more ideal therapy for hemangiomas (Morelli, 1993; Mulliken, 1991; O'Reilly et al, 1995).

It appears that hemangiomas constitute clonal expansions of endothelial cells, suggesting that these tumors are caused by somatic mutations in one or more genes regulating endothelial cell proliferation (Boye et al, 2001). It has been shown that Tie2 and its ligands angiopoietin-1 and angiopoietin-2 may be involved in the pathogenesis of hemangiomas (Yu et al, 2001).

TREATMENT

Eighty percent of hemangiomas are ultimately uncomplicated, and it is difficult to predict which ones will develop problems (Mulliken et al, 1995). For a majority of lesions, the initial treatment of choice is "active nonintervention." During the phase of rapid proliferation, patients with uncomplicated hemangiomas should be examined at 2- to 4-week intervals to evaluate degree of growth and development of problems. During this phase, parents often are anxious and require ongoing, directed anticipatory guidance. A common concern is the risk of significant hemorrhage. This is rare. Minor episodes of bleeding can result from trauma and respond to short-term compression, like any superficial wound. Demonstration of before-and-after photographs of growing and involuted lesions in other children helps diminish concern.

Decades of aggressive therapy followed by suboptimal outcome from the 1940s through the 1960s were followed by a passive approach to the treatment of minimally complicated hemangiomas. The dogma has been to avoid treatment because children whose hemangiomas were allowed to involute spontaneously had less severe scarring than those subjected to excision or ionizing radiation. However, up to 40% of hemangiomas leave permanent skin changes that can be disfiguring (Enjolras and Mulliken, 1993). Psychological and social problems may result from facial or other visible deformities. Early intervention should be considered for lesions with a higher potential for complications. Such lesions include hemangiomas of the periorbital area, central face, skin folds, and hands and those with a pattern suggestive of visceral involvement. Newer therapeutic approaches are aimed at minimizing growth or speeding resolution without the risk of additional scarring. At present, the benefits of newer approaches to therapy outweigh the risks in many cases. Early initiation of therapy, aimed at preventing growth, is more effective than therapy that is delayed until maximal growth has been reached. Treatment options include oral or intralesional corticosteroids and pulsed dye laser; most recently, use of the nonselective beta-blocker propranolol has been suggested as an addition to the therapeutic armamentarium. Because of the up to 20% risk of often irreversible spastic diplegia in infants treated with α-interferon, this therapy has fallen out of favor (Barlow et al, 1998; Deb et al, 1999; Wörle et al, 1999). Vincristine has been used in life-threatening IH but has multiple limitations, including placement of an indwelling catheter, slow time to response, and immune suppression.

Pulsed dye laser was postulated in the late 1980s and 1990s in a number of small case series and case reports to have the potential to halt the growth of superficial IHs and cause dramatic improvement in the appearance of these lesions at a young age (Ashinoff and Geronemus, 1991, 1993; Barlow et al, 1996; Garden et al, 1992; Glassberg et al, 1989; Haywood et al, 2000; Poetke et al, 2000; Scheepers and Quaba, 1995; Sherwood and Tan, 1990; Waner et al, 1994; Wheeland, 1995). However, a randomized prospective controlled trial of 121 infants found that pulsed-dye laser treatment in uncomplicated hemangiomas is no better than watchful waiting and that the primary difference noted after 1 year of treatment was that infants treated with laser were more likely to exhibit skin atrophy and hypopigmentation when compared to untreated infants (Batta et al, 2002). Pulsed-dye laser cannot prevent the preprogrammed growth pattern of hemangiomas and has a limited role during the proliferative phase. In contrast, it is quite useful during involution, if there is residual redness or telangiectasias but relatively little fibrofatty residuum.

Corticosteroids may be administered by topical application, intralesional injection, or enteral/parenteral dosing. Each route utilizes corticosteroid preparations of different potency and duration of action. True comparative efficacy studies would be impossible. Experience is greatest with systemic administration, considered to be the optimal regimen by some experts; the recommended regimen is oral prednisone or prednisolone, 2 to 3 mg/kg/day as a single morning dose or in divided doses (Esterly, 1995; Mulliken et al, 1995). Within 1 to 2 weeks, 30% of hemangiomas will show dramatic response; 40% will respond equivocally. In patients with slower-responding lesions, slowly tapering therapy is required through the proliferative phase. If no response is detected, the medication should be rapidly tapered after 2 weeks.

Intralesional injections may be preferred for well-localized hemangiomas, including those involving the eyelid. Colloidal suspensions of triamcinolone and dexamethasone or betamethasone in 1:1 mixtures are used. Large doses are administered, in the range of 40 mg triamcinolone plus 6 mg of betamethasone in 2 mL of suspension (Kushner, 1979). Administration of this dose to a 5-kg infant is equivalent to 20 mg/kg of prednisone given as a single dose, which may ultimately allow for a lower total systemic dose. Complications include cutaneous atrophy, skin necrosis, ophthalmic artery occlusion, and blindness. Thus, periocular intralesional steroid injection should be performed only by experienced pediatric ophthalmologists. Simultaneous indirect ophthalmoscopy should be considered during the time of the injection to aid in prevention of complications (Egbert et al, 1996).

The paucity of information on the treatment of hemangiomas with topical steroids suggests that this route of administration is minimally effective in comparison with other treatment modalities and likely useful in only very superficial lesions (Ranchod et al, 2005). One retrospective study of ultrapotent topical corticosteroid use in proliferating hemangiomas found that 35% showed good response and 38% showed partial response, and growth ceased before the anticipated end of the proliferative phase based on the patients' age. Thin superficial lesions responded most markedly, with thicker lesions showing minimal improvement (Garzon et al, 2005).

Several small case series and case reports have been published suggesting the improved relative safety and efficacy of the nonselective beta-blocker propranolol as compared with other medical therapies, but at this time there are no data from randomized, controlled clinical trials to fully justify this therapy as the standard of care. Currently, clinical practice varies widely in the use of propranolol versus corticosteroids. Early results appear to be encouraging but more data is needed. The drug is administered as an oral suspension in divided doses every 8 hours; total daily dosing between 2 and 3 mg/kg/day is generally used. Monitoring for potential side effects of hypotension, bradycardia, hypoglycemia, and bronchospasm is necessary (Leaute-Labreze and Taieb, 2008; Leaute-Labreze et al, 2008; Sans et al, 2009).

Ulceration is a therapeutic challenge that may be treated initially with the appropriate occlusive dressing. The choice of dressing and frequency of changes are dictated by the amount of exudate produced. Coban dressing is ideally suited for secure dressings over hemangiomas on the extremities (Kaplan and Paller, 1995). For sites that are difficult to dress, frequent, liberal application of zinc oxide paste or petrolatum jelly is effective. To inspect the skin, zinc oxide is easily removed with mineral oil. There are few prospective trials examining treatment of ulcerated hemangiomas. Various dressing materials including petrolatum impregnated gauze and seaweed-derived alginate dressings are often recommended. Off label use of becaplermin gel, a recombinant human platelet-derived growth factor, has been reported to show dramatic healing in small case series. The product now carries a boxed warning from the FDA, which must now be taken into consideration before its use (Metz et al, 2004; Yan, 2008). Agents for pain control should be prescribed. Alternating doses of acetaminophen and ibuprofen usually are sufficient, but overuse of the latter may increase the risk of bleeding and cause pain from gastrointestinal upset that can be difficult to distinguish from the pain associated with ulceration. A high index of suspicion should be maintained for secondary infection, with a low threshold for use of either topical or systemic antibiotic therapy. If conservative therapy is unsuccessful, yellow-light laser may relieve pain and speed reepithelialization (Achauer and Vander Kam, 1991; Morelli et al, 1991, 1994). The ulcers will heal but will inevitably leave scars.

A hemangioma that interferes with the visual axis should be treated aggressively. Evaluation by an experienced pediatric ophthalmologist is recommended. A hemangioma that limits the visual field but does not distort the globe may be treated by patching the contralateral eye. More complicated lesions may be treated initially with propranolol or corticosteroids: topical, enterally administered, or intralesional. The intralesional route of administration carries the risk of embolic occlusion of the retinal arteries. This tragic adverse effect can occur ipsilaterally, contralaterally, or bilaterally (Brown et al, 1972; Fost and Esterly, 1968; Zuniga et al, 1987) (Figure 101-2). Surgical excision should be considered for vision-threatening hemangiomas that fail to respond to medical management (Mulliken et al, 1995; Walker et al, 1994).

There is no uniformly successful therapy for seriously complicated or life-threatening hemangiomas. Reported treatment options include high-dose corticosteroids, propranolol, aspirin, dipyridamole, interferon-α, cold steel excision, sclerotherapy, arterial embolization, cyclophosphamide, bleomycin, and vincristine (Enjolras et al, 1990; Esterly, 1995; Leaute-Labreze et al, 2008; Mulliken et al, 1995; Payarols et al, 1995; Sarihan et al, 1997;). All carry significant risks.

VASCULAR MALFORMATIONS

Vascular malformations may be indistinguishable from hemangiomas by clinical and light microscopic examination; however, they are biologically distinct lesions.

CLINICAL FINDINGS

Malformations are true structural anomalies, composed of one or more types of vessels—capillaries, veins, arteries, and/or lymphatics. Unlike hemangiomas, they are always present at birth, although in certain cases they may not be noted until later in life. They affect males and females equally. Growth is commensurate with the child's growth, although the lesion may expand as a result of local thrombosis or inflammation. Primary platelet trapping with consumptive coagulopathy (e.g., Kasabach-Merritt syndrome) does not occur, but recurrent episodes of localized intravascular coagulopathy are a potential serious long-term problem (Dompmartin et al, 2008; Mazoyer et al, 2008).

Local skeletal or soft tissue destruction or hypertrophy is common. Spontaneous resolution is not expected except in one specific malformation, the salmon patch. Vascular malformations occur either as isolated cutaneous defects or in association with a variety of well-defined syndromes. The more common variations are described next.

Salmon Patch

The glabellar salmon patch (nevus simplex or nevus flammeus), also known in the vernacular as an "angel's kiss," is a bilaterally symmetric superficial capillary defect. It is

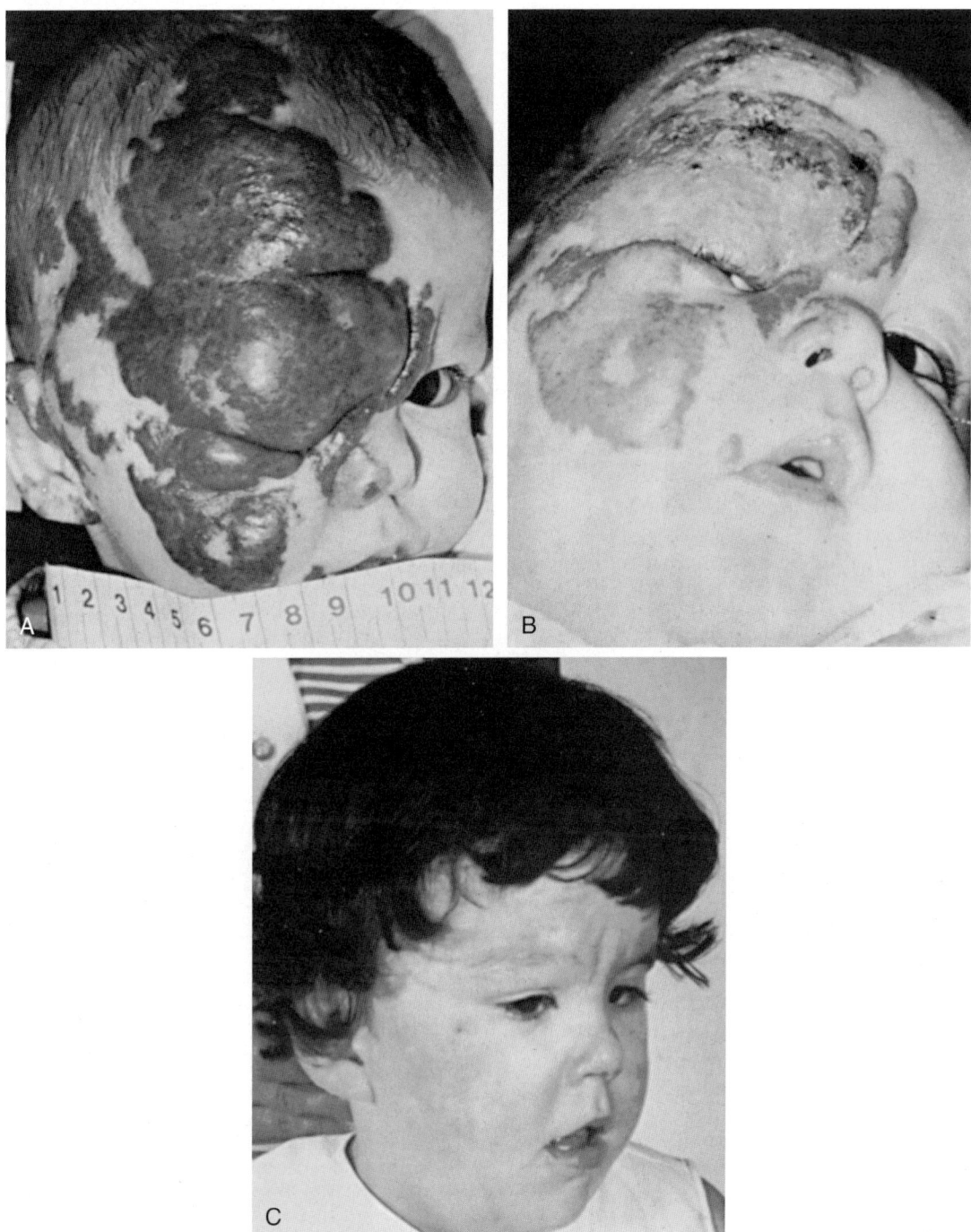

FIGURE 101-2 A, A flat hemangioma was noted at birth; by 3 weeks of age, the lesion had expanded, as shown. **B,** After 11 weeks of prednisone (20 mg/day), the lesion had regressed. **C,** Nearly complete regression is evident by age 4 years. The patient was a normally intelligent child whose only residual problem was strabismus.

the most common vascular malformation and the only one that almost always fades spontaneously. A similar lesion in the nuchal area, colloquially known as the "stork bite," usually is persistent. Large lesions may also involve the eyelids and alae nasi. Prominent glabellar salmon patches are associated with dysmorphic syndromes including Beckwith-Wiedemann syndrome and fetal alcohol syndrome (Burns et al, 1991).

Capillary Malformation (Port-Wine Stain)

Port-wine stain is an asymmetrical postcapillary venule malformation that occurs in 0.3% of neonates. A majority are isolated cutaneous lesions. At birth they are pink, macular, and blanchable. With time, most lesions darken; papulonodular surface change and ipsilateral soft tissue or even bone hypertrophy may occur in adulthood. Facial capillary malformation is a distribution that includes the forehead or upper eyelid and may be associated with buphthalmos or glaucoma. Complete ophthalmologic examination is indicated for affected infants.

Sturge-Weber syndrome (SWS) is a triad of facial capillary malformation, leptomeningeal vascular malformation, and glaucoma that occurs sporadically. The classic finding of double-contoured (tramline) calcifications on a skull film is not seen during infancy; this sign develops during childhood. CNS lesions are most reliably detected by MRI after 6 months of age. SWS occurs in less than 30% of infants with facial port-wine stains; the risk is increased in infants with more extensive lesions (Tallman et al, 1991). The degree of CNS involvement is variable in SWS, ranging from subclinical lesions to intractable seizures and intellectual impairment.

Two national organizations have been established to serve the needs of patients and their families:

The Vascular Birthmarks Foundation, PO Box 106, Latham, NY 12110; telephone 877-VBF-4646; *www.birthmark.org*

The Sturge-Weber Foundation, P.O. Box 418, Mt. Freedom, NJ 07970; telephone 973-895-4445 or 800-627-5482; *www.sturge-weber.org*

Arterial/Lymphatic/Venous Malformation

The arterial/lymphatic/venous malformation category includes a spectrum of isolated cutaneous vascular anomalies that have been given a variety of clinically descriptive names. Rather than relying extensively on eponymous names for a majority of malformations, it is recommended that each malformation be described by the vessel types that exist within it, as seen on radiologic imaging (Enjolras and Mulliken, 1997; Mulliken and Young, 1988).

These lesions do not resolve spontaneously. Corticosteroid therapy is not beneficial. Complications are related to the flow rate and extent of the lesion. Localized thrombosis and phlebitis occur in low-flow lesions; high-flow lesions can cause significant bleeding, destructive interosseous changes, and high-output cardiac failure. Many centers now have collaborative multidisciplinary groups to help manage the most complicated vascular malformations and vascular tumors, which typically require treatment by physicians in many specialties.

Cutis Marmorata Telangiectatica Congenita

Cutis marmorata telangiectatica congenita (CMTC) is a distinct, reticulated capillary-venous malformation that primarily affects the lower extremities (Figure 101-3). CMTC can occur as a single isolated patch or involve an extensive area. With time, associated atrophy and ulceration may occur. Larger lesions may be associated with ipsilateral hypertrophy or hypotrophy of the affected limb.

Klippel-Trénaunay and Parkes Weber Syndromes

Klippel-Trénaunay and Parkes Weber syndromes are clinically defined, sporadic conditions consisting of extensive capillary malformation, most often occurring unilaterally on the lower extremity, associated with underlying venous and lymphatic malformations, and marked by progressive ipsilateral limb hypertrophy. Parkes Weber syndrome is defined by an overlying capillary malformation and underlying arteriovenous malformation or fistula and its associated constellation of complications.

Cobb Syndrome

Cobb syndrome is a sporadic condition consisting of a posterior truncal nevus flammeus overlying a vascular abnormality that involves the spinal cord.

Bonnet-Dechaume-Blanc Syndrome

Bonnet-Dechaume-Blanc syndrome (also known as *Wyburn-Mason syndrome*) consists of a facial port-wine stain overlying a retinal and intracranial arteriovenous malformation. The retinal lesion appears as dilated, tortuous retinal vessels on routine ophthalmoscopy. Cranial bruit, mild proptosis, and conjunctival hyperemia may be present.

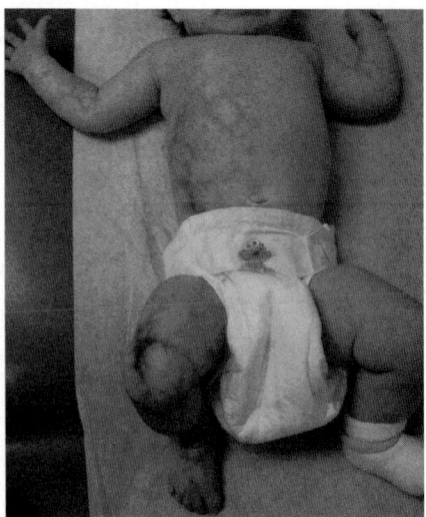

FIGURE 101-3 Cutis marmorata telangiectatica congenita. Note the striking network of dilated vessels, most distinct over the extremities. *(From Humphries JM: J Pediatr 40:486, 1952.)*

Blue Rubber Bleb Nevus Syndrome [OMIM 112200]

Blue rubber bleb nevus syndrome condition, inherited as an autosomal dominant trait, is characterized by venous malformations of the skin and gastrointestinal tract associated with bleeding and iron deficiency anemia. Numerous lesions may be present at birth. They are blue macules or nodules that range in size from 1 mm to several centimeters, resembling the "blueberry muffin" lesions of congenital TORCH (*t*oxoplasmosis, *o*ther infections, *r*ubella, *c*ytomegalovirus, *h*erpes simplex) infection, but are easily compressible. They may be tender to palpation or surmounted by droplets of sweat. An underlying large venous malformation of the lower extremities or pelvis is often present, and patients should undergo magnetic resonance imaging.

Maffucci's Syndrome

Maffucci's syndrome is a sporadic condition that consists of mixed vascular malformations and characteristic enchondromas. Chrondosarcomas are the most common malignancy seen in this syndrome. In 25% of cases, manifestations are present at birth or in early infancy.

PTEN Hamartoma Tumor Syndrome

The hamartomatous tumor group comprises two clinically distinct genetic syndromes caused by mutations in the PTEN (phosphate and tensin homologue deleted on chromosome 10) tumor suppressor gene-Cowden and Bannayan-Riley-Ruvalcaba. There are reports of a Proteus-like syndrome with PTEN mutation (Smith et al, 2002; Thiffault, 2004; Zhou et al, 2000, 2001). Proteus syndrome is now thought to not be related to PTEN mutations. To date, only Cowden syndrome is associated with increased risk of malignancy, but all patients are recommended to undergo periodic cancer screening (Hobert and Eng, 2009).

Cowden syndrome [OMIM 15835], inherited in an autosomal dominant fashion, is characterized by trichilemmomas, papillomatous papules, and acral and plantar keratoses. These benign growths are rarely seen before adulthood. Lhermitte-Duclos disease, macrocephaly, megencephaly and dolichocephaly manifest in childhood. Patients are at increased risk for breast, thyroid, and endometrial cancers.

Bannayan-Riley-Ruvalcaba syndrome [OMIM 15348] manifests with macrocephaly, lipomatosis, hemangiomas, intestinal polyps, penile lentigines, macrosomia, myopathy of proximal muscles, and bony abnormalities. Developmental delay and intellectual impairment is seen in half of patients.

Proteus-like syndrome is characterized by the extensive malformations and hamartomas with striking overgrowth, connective tissue and epidermal nevi, and hyperostosis.

Lymphedema

Lymphedema is a term used to describe diffuse soft tissue swelling characterized by firm, pitting edema. Lymphedema can occur in the setting of anomalous lymphatic drainage. Congenital variants have been reported. Females are affected more frequently than males. The lower limbs are the most commonly affected sites, but other sites also may be involved, and rarely, chylothorax or ascites may be present. *Milroy's disease* is an autosomal dominant condition that manifests with progressive lymphedema of the lower extremities. Lymphedema of the extremities occurs in *Turner (XO) syndrome*.

TREATMENT

Treatment for an uncomplicated capillary malformation is aimed at minimizing disfigurement. With time, these lesions thicken and develop irregular surface changes, often with friable nodules. In 1986, the yellow-light pulsed-dye laser was approved by the U.S. Food and Drug Administration (FDA) for the treatment of capillary malformations, as early as the neonatal period. The copper vapor laser and the argon-pumped tunable dye laser also are yellow-light lasers, but because of increased risk of scarring in comparison with pulsed-dye laser, these lasers are rarely used today. Most of the published data on laser treatment of port-wine stains in children is from studies utilizing the pulsed-dye laser. Children require an average of 5 to 10 pulsed-dye laser treatments for maximal lightening. The best results have been seen in children younger than 4 years of age. In this age group, 20% can expect 95% clearing (Goldman et al, 1993). Pulsed-dye laser therapy is less effective for facial port-wine stains that are close to midline or those on the extremities (Garden and Bakus, 1993; Renfro and Geronemus, 1993). A recent study comparing the effects of the pulsed-dye laser with those of the argon pumped-dye laser for the treatment of port-wine stains has shown that the pulsed-dye laser is clinically superior to the argon pumped-dye laser (Edstrom et al, 2002). Laser therapy can yield remarkable improvement for many port-wine stains, minimizing the emotional pain that accompanies facial disfigurement. Unfortunately, none of the currently available lasers is capable of permanently erasing port-wine stains in a majority of patients. There are also reports of redarkening of port-wine stains many years after effective lightening (Huikeshoven et al, 2007). Attempts to optimize laser treatment efficacy include using the pulsed-dye laser at higher fluences in conjunction with cryogen spray cooling (Kelly et al, 2002). A laser is also available that combines the 595-nanometer pulsed-dye laser with a 1064-nanometer neodymium-doped-yttrium aluminum-garnet (YAG) laser based on the theory that the longer wavelength of the second laser may be able to better target deeper vessels. The range of skin conditions that may benefit from yellow-light laser therapy is expanding rapidly to include a variety of skin lesions with vascular components.

HYPOPIGMENTED LESIONS

Localized areas of hypopigmentation on the skin of the newborn infant may be isolated phenomena, or they may be markers of extracutaneous abnormalities. The degree of hypopigmentation and the distribution of the defect help distinguish among the different conditions.

DEFINITION

A distinction must first be made between complete *depigmentation* and *hypopigmentation*. A depigmenting condition produces pure white lesions that are devoid of normal melanocytes. Even in fair-skinned infants, the lesions can often be easily seen in ordinary daylight. This group of disorders includes tyrosinase-negative albinism and piebaldism, as well as vitiligo, which is rarely seen in infancy. A hypopigmented lesion often is subtly lighter in color than the surrounding skin. Histologic examination reveals a normal number of melanocytes. In fair-skinned children, these lesions may require Wood's lamp illumination to become obvious. This group includes anomalies with a deficient amount of either of the skin's pigments: melanin or hemoglobin. The ash-leaf macules and "confetti-like" lesions of tuberous sclerosis (Figure 101-4), the linear and whorled patterning associated with hypomelanosis of Ito (Figure 101-5, *A*), and simple nevus depigmentosus are hypomelanotic lesions (see Figure 101-5, *B*). Nevus anemicus and hemangioma precursors are areas of pallor that result from diminished superficial blood flow.

ASH-LEAF MACULES

Ash-leaf macules are small oval areas of hypopigmentation, named for their similarity in size and shape to a leaflet from a European mountain ash tree. They are one

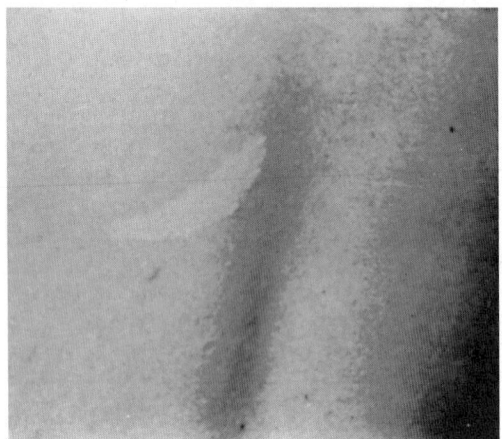

FIGURE 101-4 White ash-leaf macule on the back of a patient with tuberous sclerosis.

of the few congenital markers for infants with tuberous sclerosis. Tuberous sclerosis complex (TSC) is a disorder of autosomal dominant inheritance with variable clinical manifestations characterized by the development of benign and malignant tumors in a variety of tissues: skin, CNS, and kidney. Serious complications of tuberous sclerosis include hamartomas of the lung and kidney and congenital rhabdomyomas of the heart. The diagnosis is currently made by meeting a set of diagnostic criteria, but a majority of manifestations are not present in infancy (Gomez, 1991; Janniger and Schwartz, 1993; Schwartz et al, 2007; Zvulunov and Esterly, 1995). Abnormalities at two different genetic loci have been identified in kindreds with TSC (Wienecke et al, 1995). The two genetic loci are *TSC1* on 9q and *TSC2* on 16p, and the gene products are hamartin and tuberin, respectively. Both hamartin and tuberin are expressed in neurons and astrocytes, where they physically interact (Gutmann et al, 2000).

HYPOMELANOSIS OF ITO

The term *hypomelanosis of Ito* has been used as a diagnosis for a genetic disorder marked by a striking linear and whorled pattern of cutaneous pigment change oriented along the lines of Blaschko. Affected persons may have areas that are hyperpigmented or hypopigmented, or both. The pattern may be congenital or become apparent after birth.

This condition is a form of genetic mosaicism. In a subset of affected persons, karyotype abnormalities are demonstrable in tissue from affected sites. In a majority of reported cases, the patients have extracutaneous abnormalities (CNS, ocular, cardiac, and skeletal) (Alvarez et al, 1993; Dereser-Dennl et al, 2000; Devriendt et al, 1998; Tunca et al, 2000). Patterned pigment change confined to skin probably is a more common occurrence. For persons so affected, the term *linear and whorled nevoid melanosis* may be more appropriate. Chromosomal analysis from

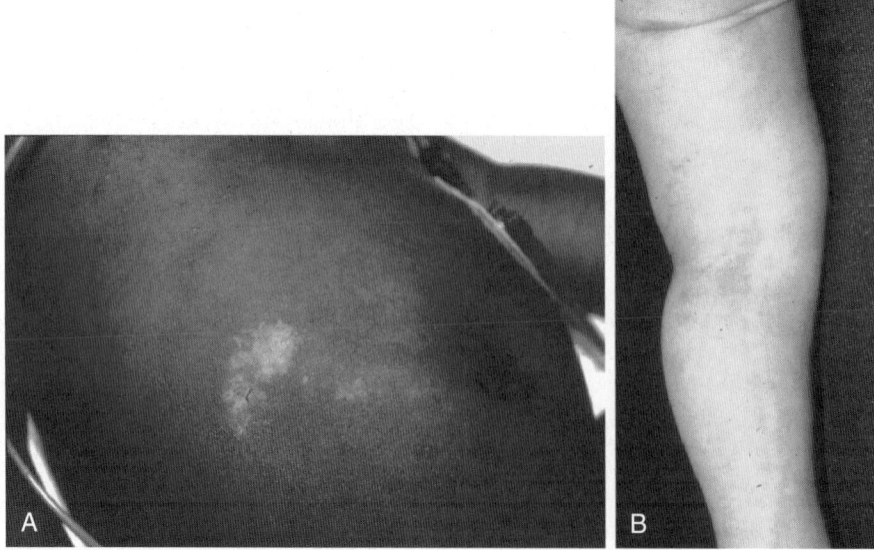

FIGURE 101-5 Nevus depigmentosus is an isolated congenital skin lesion that manifests as a hypomelanotic polygonal macule **(A)** or in a linear Blaschko distribution **(B)**.

separate tissues (e.g., blood, skin) is indicated for children with extensive skin lesions or evidence of extracutaneous involvement (Sybert, 1994).

MELANIN-CONTAINING LESIONS

Brown lesions usually reflect an increased number of melanocytic cells or an excess of melanin. Brown coloration also can be associated with a thickened epidermis. It may be difficult to distinguish among the lesions in this category without histopathologic examination. A majority of congenital brown lesions are isolated and benign, but it is important to recognize those that are syndrome-associated or potentially life-threatening (see Chapter 97 for a differential diagnosis).

In general, skin biopsy of a congenital pigmented lesion can be postponed until after the neonatal period. The one exception is a nodular lesion suggestive of melanoma.

NEVOCELLULAR NEVI

The category of nevocellular nevi includes congenital or acquired nevomelanocytic neoplasms. Nevomelanocytes are dendritic cells of neural crest origin. Nevocellular nevi traditionally have been categorized by the histologic position of the tumor nests within the skin. *Junctional nevi* are the most superficial, located at the junction between the epidermis and dermis. These lesions appear clinically as macules. *Intradermal nevi* are located deep to the dermoepidermal junction and are usually papular. *"Blue" nevi* are a variant located in the deep dermis, made up of cells that have elongated, neural features. *Compound nevi* have both junctional and dermal nests of nevomelanocytes.

Melanocytic nevi can be further divided into categories based on the size they are expected to attain by adulthood: small (less than 1.5 cm in greatest diameter), medium (1.5 to 19.9 cm), large (greater than 20 cm), and giant (greater than 50 cm); and time of onset: congenital, early-onset (before the age of 2 years), and acquired (Kovalyshyn et al, 2009). Diagnostic histologic features have been described for congenital and acquired lesions, but these features may be found in both types.

Large, multiple, or congenital melanocytic nevi have been reported in association with several syndromes (Marghoob et al, 1993) (Table 101-2).

CONGENITAL NEVOCELLULAR NEVI

Congenital nevocytic nevi are common and generally of little or no consequence. However, the infrequent but devastating association with malignant melanoma has made management a controversial issue.

Because size delineations are based on adult data, conversion factors have been developed to help predict ultimate size; for congenital melanocytic nevi (CMN) on the head, multiply size by factor of 1.7, lower extremities by 3.3, and trunk, upper extremities, and feet by 2.8 (Marghoob et al, 1996). Truly congenital lesions are present in 1% of white infants and in 2% to 3% of African American infants surveyed in the nursery (Osburn et al, 1987). Medium CMNs are seen in 1 in 1000 infants, large in 1 in 20,000, and giant

in 1 in 500,000 (Castilla et al, 1981). There is a risk of malignancy associated with small nevi, but it may never be well defined. A distinct subset of melanocytic nevi in children, "early-onset nevi," has recently been recognized. These lesions are not necessarily congenital, appearing during the first 2 years of life. Early-onset nevi have been observed in 25% of children specifically examined for them. Twenty percent to 50% of melanomas arising in children and young adults may be associated with this type of nevus (Williams, 1993; Williams and Pennella, 1994). The frequency of CMN is paradoxically increased in African Americans, who have a much lower risk of melanoma (Shpall et al, 1994). The risk of melanoma associated with these very common pigmented skin lesions must be well below that in children with giant congenital nevi and

TABLE 101-2 Syndromes Associated With Melanocytic Nevi

Associated With:	Other Key Features
Congenital Nevi	
Carney syndrome (including LAMB and NAME syndromes)	Cardiac and cutaneous myxomas, endocrine abnormalities
Epidermal (linear sebaceous) nevus syndrome	Linear epidermal/sebaceous nevi, central nervous system and musculoskeletal defects
Neurocutaneous melanosis	Leptomeningeal melanocytosis and obstructive hydrocephalus
Neurofibromatosis type I	Cutaneous and plexiform neurofibromas, café-au-lait spots, Lisch nodules
Premature aging syndrome	Premature aging, short stature, birdlike facies, deafness
Occult spinal dysraphism/tethered cord	Spinal cord abnormalities, lipomas, vascular malformations
Malformations associated with congenital melanocytic nevi	
Acquired Nevi	
Dysplastic nevus (atypical mole) syndrome	Increased incidence of cutaneous melanoma
Langer-Giedion syndrome	Distinctive facies, cone-shaped epiphyses, multiple exostoses
Congenital and/or Acquired Nevi	
EEC syndrome	Ectrodactyly, ectodermal dysplasia, cleft lip/palate, ocular abnormalities
Goeminne syndrome	Muscular torticollis, spontaneous keloids, genitourinary abnormalities
Kuskokwim syndrome	Skeletal abnormalities, joint contractures, muscle atrophy/hypertrophy
Noonan syndrome	Webbed neck, heart defects, multiple other anomalies
Turner syndrome	Webbed neck, heart defects, multiple other anomalies, X-chromosome defect
Tricho-odonto-onychial dysplasia	Hypotrichosis, enamel defects, nail dystrophy

From Marghoob AA, Orlo SJ, Kopf AW: Syndromes associated with melanocytic nevi, *J Am Acad Dermatol* 29:373-388, 1993.

possibly no higher than the 1% lifetime risk of malignant melanoma in the general white population. Decisions about surgical removal of these lesions must be made on a case-by-case basis (Figure 101-6).

Large, giant (i.e., bathing trunk or garment) congenital nevi are rare and have a much greater potential for malignant degeneration (Figure 101-7). The cumulative risk of malignancy is estimated to be 2% to 15% over a lifetime, with 70% of melanomas diagnosed before the age of 10 years. Based on newer data, lifetime risk is probably closer to 6% (Kuflik and Janniger, 1994; Marghoob et al, 1996; Tannous et al, 2005; Williams and Pennella, 1994).

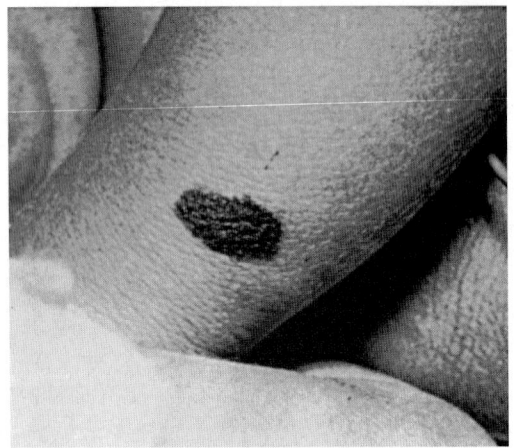

FIGURE 101-6 Dark brown irregular congenital nevus on the limb of an infant.

Conservative management of large congenital nevi by surveillance alone is complicated by the presence of features that strongly suggest melanoma. Most of these nevi have an irregular surface appearance from birth and are variably thickened, hairy, verrucous, or nodular. Smaller, widely scattered "satellite lesions" are almost always present. Extracutaneous lesions also have been detected in several sites, including the meninges, lymph nodes, and placental villi. Often, these nevi have atypical histologic features as well. For children who develop malignant melanoma within a giant nevus, the prognosis is very poor. However, many of the lesions with an alarming appearance from birth do not exhibit malignant behavior or produce widespread metastases, or cause death. In fact, congenital melanoma is very rare and is associated with congenital nevi in less than 50% of reported cases (Williams and Pennella, 1994).

The management of CMN remains controversial, with advocates for and against prophylactic excision. Newly published data question the rationale for routine excision. Nevertheless, case reports of melanoma arising in smaller CMNs, as early as 6 months of age, continue to dramatize the issue (Ceballos et al, 1995; De Raeve et al, 1993; Ozturkcan et al, 1994). To date, the incidence of melanoma arising in small CMNs remains unclear. A 3- to 21-fold increased relative risk for malignant transformation in both small and medium-sized lesions later in life has been reported, depending on the method of study (Richardson et al, 2002).

The least controversial recommendation has been for surgical excision of large or multiple CMNs during infancy (Casson and Colen, 1993). However, surgical removal

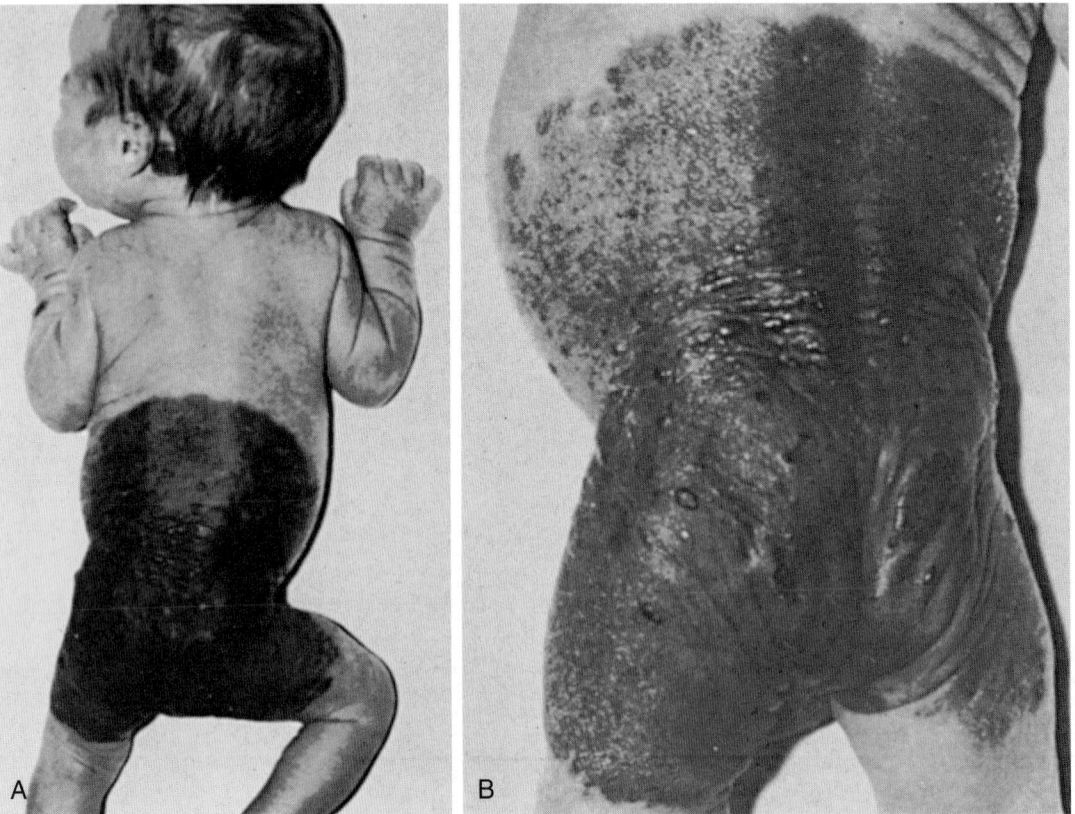

FIGURE 101-7 A, Newborn infant with large black nevus covering the "bathing trunk area." **B,** The closer view permits visualization of the nodular surface typical of giant nevi.

is never an easy option. Multiple procedures usually are required, with the attendant high risks of significant morbidity, sometimes yielding results that are more disfiguring than the birthmark. Newer techniques performed in early childhood, such as tissue expansion (Vergnes et al, 1993) and partial-thickness resection (Sandsmark et al, 1993), may improve the aesthetic outcome. The efficacy of such approaches in the prevention of malignancy has never been documented.

A Congenital Nevocytic Nevus Registry was established at the New York University Medical Center in 1978 to prospectively study the natural history of giant CMN (Gari et al, 1988; Kopf et al, 1979). To participate by mail, clinicians should contact the Skin and Cancer Unit, Department of Dermatology, New York University Medical Center, 550 First Ave., New York, NY 10016; telephone: (212) 340-5260.

Families with an affected child may benefit from information provided by the Nevus Network, a national support group founded by Dr. Bari Joan Bett, a physician with a giant congenital nevus. To receive information, contact The Nevus Network, The Congenital Nevus Support Group, PO Box 305 West Salem, OH 44287; telephone (419) 853-4525 (405) 377-3403. The website is *www.nevusnetwork.org*.

Neurocutaneous melanosis (NCM) is a congenital syndrome characterized by pigment cell tumors of the leptomeninges in patients with large or multiple (at least three) CMNs of the head, neck, or posterior midline (Kadonaga and Frieden, 1991). Symptomatic NCM manifests with signs or symptoms of increased intracranial pressure and carries a poor prognosis (Frieden et al, 1994; Sandsmark et al, 1994). MRI can aid in the diagnosis of NCM (Barkovich et al, 1994). Although initial reports emphasized thickening of the leptomeninges, the most common MRI sign of NCM is actually spin-lattice (T1) nuclear magnetic relaxation time in the parenchyma of the cerebellum or anterior temporal lobes (sometimes accompanied by spin-spin [T2] relaxation time). Radiologic identification of malignant degeneration is difficult. Roughly half of asymptomatic infants and children with giant CMN have evidence of NCM on MRI (Frieden et al, 1994), a finding suggesting that numerous and extensive operations to remove the cutaneous lesion may not be justified in these patients.

Other issues have been raised that challenge the interpretation of signs that have been accepted as ominous. The risk of melanoma in early infancy may have been overestimated by misinterpretation of the histologic findings and extent of the lesions. Neither cellular atypia nor widespread involvement, including lymph nodes and placenta, proves malignancy (Carroll et al, 1994; Hara, 1993). Attempts to further define the risk of malignant degeneration in these lesions have not been insightful (Barnhill et al, 1994; Heimann et al, 1993).

LENTIGINES

Lentigines are small tan-to-dark brown macules that most commonly appear sporadically in adulthood. They are distinguished from other pigmented lesions by histologic examination that reveals elongated rete ridges, an increased number of singly dispersed melanocytes along

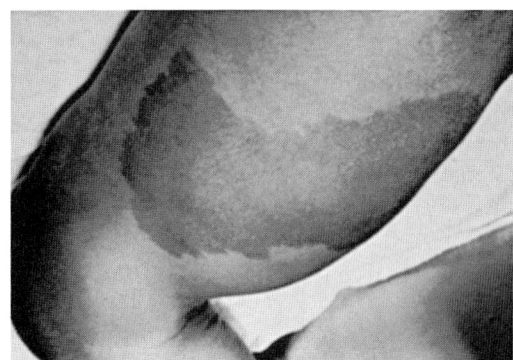

FIGURE 101-8 Large café-au-lait spot on the trunk of a newborn infant.

the basal layer, and increased melanization of the basal keratinocytes. Multiple or congenital lentigines are features of several syndromes.

Carney Complex, Type 1 (Including NAME and LAMB) [OMIM 160980]

Carney complex is an autosomal dominant multiple neoplasia syndrome due to a mutation in the protein kinase A regulatory subunit-1-alpha gene (PRKAR1A) on 17q. Cardiac, endocrine, cutaneous, and myxomatous neural tumors occur. The related phenotypes designated NAME and LAMB share the features of *a*trial *myxoma* and pigmented skin lesions. NAME includes *n*evi and *e*phelides, whereas LAMB includes *l*entigines and *b*lue nevi. Pigmented lesions are present at birth.

LEOPARD Syndrome [OMIM 151100]

Leopard syndrome is an autosomal dominant disorder due to mutations in the PTPN11 gene that includes multiple *l*entigines, *e*lectrocardiographic defects, *o*cular hypertelorism, *p*ulmonic stenosis, *a*bnormal genitalia, growth *r*etardation/restriction, and sensorineural *d*eafness. Skin lesions do not appear until after the 1st year of life.

Peutz-Jeghers Syndrome [OMIM 175200]

Peutz-Jeghers syndrome, a disorder of autosomal dominant inheritance, is due to mutations in the serine/threonine kinase STK11 gene and includes mucocutaneous pigmented macules and intestinal polyposis. The pigmented lesions may be congenital and usually appear on the lips, buccal and gingival mucosae, and dorsa of the fingers and toes.

CAFÉ-AU-LAIT MACULES

Café-au-lait macules (CALMs) are light brown macules that vary in size, ranging from several millimeters to several centimeters in diameter (Figure 101-8). They cannot always be distinguished from nevocellular nevi on clinical grounds, but histologic examination is diagnostic, showing increased melanin within the basal keratinocytes, without melanocyte proliferation. CALMs are present in 2% of white infants and in up to 12% of African-American infants. Large or multiple CALMs in the neonatal period may be an isolated finding but should alert the physician to the possibility of an associated syndrome (Box 101-2).

NEUROFIBROMATOSIS

Neurofibromatosis (NF) consists of a group of variable multisystem disorders that includes cutaneous neurofibromas and multiple CALMs. Several subtypes exist, and NF1 and NF2 (discussed here) are the most well defined. Segmental NF1, familial CALMs, and schwannomatosis are considered within the rubric of neurofibromatosis. A cutaneous disorder of multiple CALMs and axillary freckling, due to mutations in the *SPRED1* gene, was described in 2007 (Brems et al, 2007).

The great majority of patients with NF have subtype 1 (NF-1) [OMIM 162200], or von Recklinghausen's disease. NF-1 is a relatively common autosomal dominant disorder, due to mutations in the *NF1* gene, which is a large gene with a high rate of new mutation. It occurs in 1 in 3500 people. Mutational analysis is available and can be used both for prenatal diagnosis and for individuals who do not meet complete diagnostic criteria. The diagnosis has traditionally been made by fulfilling a set of diagnostic criteria; the presence of six or more CALMs is the most common manifestation, occurring before age 6 years in 99% of affected persons (Boyd et al, 2009; Zvulunov and Esterly, 1995). CALMs may be present at birth but often arise and grow during childhood. Other diagnostic cutaneous findings are axillary or inguinal freckling (Crowe sign) and cutaneous neurofibromas, which may be present at birth. Bony dysplasias (sphenoid wing dysplasia, pretibial pseudarthrosis) also can be detected at birth in a minority of patients. Symptomatic CNS involvement (developmental delay, learning disabilities, seizures) occurs in about one third of patients with NF-1. The most ominous complication of NF-1 is the development of malignant tumors (neurosarcoma, pheochromocytoma, and juvenile chronic myelogenous leukemia) (Zvulunov and Esterly, 1995). A rare triple association of leukemia, NF-1, and cutaneous juvenile xanthogranuloma has been reported (see later discussion).

The genetic defects for NF-1 have been localized to chromosomal region 17q11;2. Most mutations occur on the paternally derived chromosome. "Sporadic" cases may be the result of paternal transmission from a mosaic mutation of a fraction of spermatozoa from a clinically normal father (Lazaro et al, 1994). A portion of the *NF1* gene has homology with mammalian genes that code for guanosine triphosphate–activating proteins. These proteins function to regulate cell proliferation. Therefore, a functional mutation of the *NF1* gene would result in unsuppressed cellular proliferation (i.e., tumorigenesis).

Type 2 neurofibromatosis (NF-2) [OMIM 101000] is an autosomal dominant disorder caused by mutations in the *NF2* gene which encodes neurofibromin-2, also called merlin. It has an incidence of about 1 in 25,000. It is characterized by bilateral acoustic neuromas, meningiomas, and schwannomas of the dorsal roots of the spinal cord. CALMs are not as prominent or numerous as in NF-1, occurring in less than 40% of affected persons (Zvulunov and Esterly, 1995).

McCUNE-ALBRIGHT SYNDROME [OMIM 174800]

McCune-Albright syndrome is a sporadic disease characterized by polyostotic fibrous dysplasia, sexual precocity and other hyperfunctional endocrinopathies, and large café-au-lait spots (Schwindinger et al, 1992; Shenker et al, 1993). It is due to early postzygotic somatic activating mutations in the *GNAS1* gene, which encodes the stimulatory G subunit of adenylate cyclase. In contrast with the CALMs seen in NF-1, those in this syndrome may be unilateral with irregular borders, in a distribution that suggests the lines of Blashchko and genetic mosaicism (Rieger et al, 1994).

NEVUS SPILUS

Nevus spilus (speckled lentiginous nevus) is a hyperpigmented lesion that consists of focal proliferation of melanocytes along the basal layer of the epidermis (the dark spots) within a café-au-lait spot. It may be disfiguring but has no other associated abnormalities.

BLUE-GRAY MACULE OF INFANCY

More than 90% of African American infants, 81% of Asians, and 10% of whites (Pratt, 1953) are born with blue-gray macule of infancy, formerly called *mongolian spot*. These are brown, gray, or blue macules, most commonly located on the lumbosacral area, but they can occur anywhere. The macules may be single or multiple and range in size from a few millimeters to several centimeters in diameter. They often fade within the first few years of life. Extensive lesions have been mistakenly attributed to abuse. Histologically, blue-gray macule of infancy is a collection of spindle-shaped melanocytes located deep in the dermis. Malignant change has never been reported.

NEVUS OF OTA/ITO

Nevus of Ota is a unilateral blue or gray discoloration involving the orbital and zygomatic areas, including the sclera and fundus. It is a sporadic condition, but it occurs with the highest frequency in Asians, affecting up to 1% of persons in Japan (Kopf and Weidman, 1962). The discoloration is detected at birth in 60% of cases. Glaucoma is a frequent complication. A similar lesion, located in the deltotrapezius area, is called *nevus of Ito*. Histologically, these lesions cannot be distinguished from blue-gray macule of infancy. However, spontaneous resolution is not common, and rare association with malignant melanoma has been reported. Successful treatment has been achieved with Q-switched ruby and Q-switched YAG laser surgery.

TUMORS OF EPITHELIAL ORIGIN

EPIDERMAL NEVUS/NEVUS SEBACEUS

Epidermal nevus may manifest in the newborn period as a smooth hyperpigmented patch or rough, skin-colored plaque, most often on the trunk or extremities, frequently oriented along the lines of Blaschko. With time, epidermal nevi may enlarge; most become verrucous. Nevus sebaceus has a yellow hue, occurs most often on the head, and may be nodular at birth and again after puberty, flattening during childhood. A variety of neoplasms, both benign and malignant, including basal cell carcinoma, develop in up to 15% of patients with sebaceous nevi. Development of neoplasms rarely occurs before puberty.

Like other mosaic disorders, epidermal and sebaceous nevi are believed to be localized manifestations of somatic genetic mutations that would be lethal if fully expressed. A subset of patients with epidermal nevi are genetic mosaics for an autosomal dominant form of ichthyosis called *epidermolytic hyperkeratosis* (or bullous ichthyosiform erythroderma) (Paller et al, 1994). These persons may be at risk for having offspring with total body involvement. The striking appearance of epidermal nevi has inspired descriptive nomenclature. *Nevus verrucosus* is a solitary plaque. *Nevus unius lateris* (Figure 101-9) is an extensive linear lesion that is unilateral, following the lines of Blaschko. Both keratinocytic and sebaceous components may occur in the same patient, the former more commonly involving the trunk and extremities and the latter more often involving the head and neck.

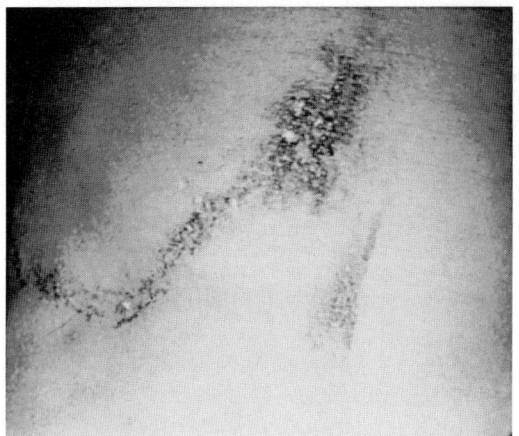

FIGURE 101-9 Linear hyperkeratotic epidermal nevus (*nevus unius lateris*) on the back and lateral aspect of the thorax.

The term *ichthyosis hystrix* refers to extensive, bilateral involvement with epidermal nevus.

Skin biopsy will rule out other conditions, distinguish between epidermal nevus and nevus sebaceus, and detect the diagnostic histologic features of epidermolytic hyperkeratosis. Small epidermal nevi do not require treatment. Nevus sebaceus carries a small risk of malignant degeneration. It may be excised in infancy, childhood, or adolescence, depending on the size of the lesion and the preference of the patient and family. Recent studies suggest that the risk of basal cell carcinoma, the most common malignancy to arise in nevus sebaceus, is closer to 1%, much lower than was reported in the past (Cribier et al, 2000).

There is no optimal therapy for larger lesions or those that are disfiguring. Full-thickness excision, including the subcutaneous tissue, is recommended to decrease the risk of recurrence. Laser therapy holds promise for the future. Topically applied keratolytic agents may be palliative. Genetic counseling about the risk for offspring of fully expressed disease should be considered for persons with epidermal nevi that reveal the histologic features of epidermolytic hyperkeratosis.

EPIDERMAL (LINEAR SEBACEOUS) NEVUS SYNDROME

In less than 10% of affected people, epidermal nevi and sebaceous nevi (especially those involving the head) are associated with a variety of extracutaneous abnormalities, mainly ocular (in 33% of cases), neurologic (in 50%), and skeletal (in 70%), a condition referred to as *epidermal nevus syndrome*. Bone abnormalities include vertebral anomalies, kyphoscoliosis, limb shortening, and hemihypertrophy. CNS disorders include seizures, mental retardation, and hemiparesis; ocular abnormalities include eyelid/conjunctival nevus, coloboma, corneal opacity, and nystagmus. Malignancies also occur in this syndrome with a greater-than-expected frequency, including Wilms' tumor, nephroblastoma, gastrointestinal carcinomas, and rhabdomyosarcoma (Marghoob et al, 1993).

DERMAL TUMORS

JUVENILE XANTHOGRANULOMA

Juvenile xanthogranuloma (JXG) is a benign, self-healing, non-Langerhans cell histiocytic tumor of infancy. JXG may be congenital; a majority of tumors manifest by 6 months of age (Nomland, 1959). Cutaneous lesions vary in color from red-brown to yellow. They occur most often on the upper half of the body (Figure 101-10), may be solitary or multiple, and range from several millimeters to several centimeters in diameter (see Figure 101-5). JXG also may be localized to the eye or mucous membranes (De Raeve et al, 1994).

Skin biopsy usually is diagnostic, revealing characteristic foamy histiocytes and Touton giant cells within the dermis.

The vast majority of infants with JXG are otherwise healthy. Giant JXG can have an alarming appearance and may be confused with other types of histiocytic tumors (Magana et al, 1994). JXG have two clinically significant associations; the first is with ocular JXG and its associated complications. Fewer than 0.5% of children with skin lesions have ocular involvement, but one half of children with ocular JXG have cutaneous lesions (Chang et al, 1996). Ocular tumors may manifest as unilateral glaucoma, uveitis, heterochromia iridis, or proptosis; ocular JXG is the most common cause of hyphema in infancy (Gaynes and Cohen, 1967; Zimmerman, 1965). The iris is the most frequently affected ocular tissue (Hamdani et al, 2000). There are also reports of a rare triad of JXG, juvenile myelomonocytic leukemia (JMML), and NF-1. The appearance of JXG usually preceded the diagnosis of leukemia; the NF, marked by multiple CALMs, was often missed (Sherer et al, 1993). Routine screening for JMML is not recommended in NF-1 patients with or without JXG, but evidence of hepatosplenomegaly, lymphadenopathy, or pallor should prompt appropriate work-up (Burgdorf and Zelger, 2004). Fewer than 20 patients with

intracranial JXG without cutaneous manifestations have been described (Bostrom et al, 2000; Schultz et al, 1997).

A majority of cases of JXG are asymptomatic and self-limited. Giant lesions have a similar prognosis (Magana et al, 1994). Ophthalmologic evaluation is indicated for children who present in the first 2 years of life with multiple lesions. Parents should be provided with anticipatory guidance about the ocular complications (Chang et al, 1996). JXG typically involutes within 3 to 6 years (Hansen, 1992). Recurrence has been documented after surgical excision; this form of therapy is indicated only for lesions that are frequently traumatized or are more disfiguring than the resultant scar would be.

MASTOCYTOSIS

Mastocytosis comprises a group of disorders characterized by increased numbers of tissue mast cells. The skin is the most common site of involvement, but the lymphoreticular system, gastrointestinal tract, and bone marrow also may be affected. Symptoms result from the local or generalized effects after the release of histamine and other mast cell mediators. Pruritus, edema, blistering, and flushing are common. Abdominal pain, diarrhea, and vomiting are unusual. Hypotension is rare (Kettelhut and Metcalfe, 1991). If rubbed or traumatized, skin affected by mastocytosis will develop a diagnostic wheal (Darier sign). The site may blister or become hemorrhagic in a neonate.

Urticaria pigmentosa is the name given to the most common form of mastocytosis in infants, featuring multiple, small (1 to 3 cm in diameter) papules usually located on the trunk (Figure 101-11). The disease may be congenital but usually manifests within the first 6 months of life (Kettelhut and Metcalfe, 1991). A single, localized lesion is known as a solitary mastocytoma. These tumors can vary in size from approximately 2 to 6 centimeters. Diffuse cutaneous mastocytosis is an unusual condition that may manifest at birth with widespread blistering or diffuse thickening of the skin

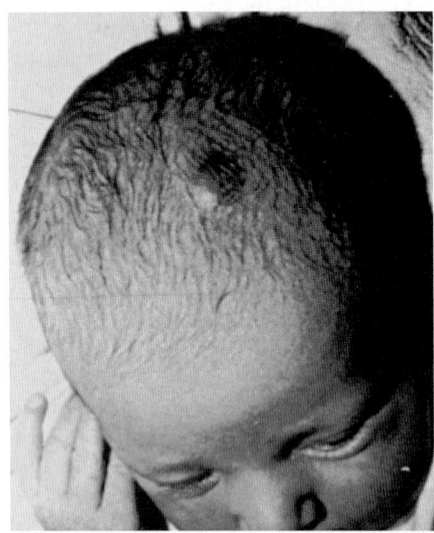

FIGURE 101-10 Solitary juvenile xanthogranuloma on the scalp, a typical site for these lesions.

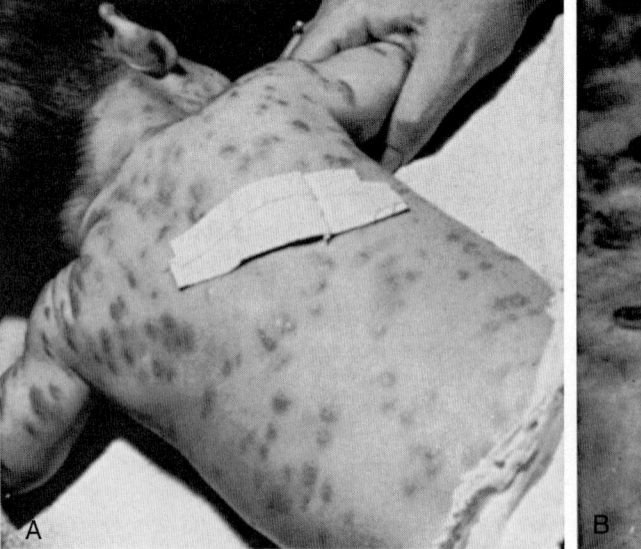 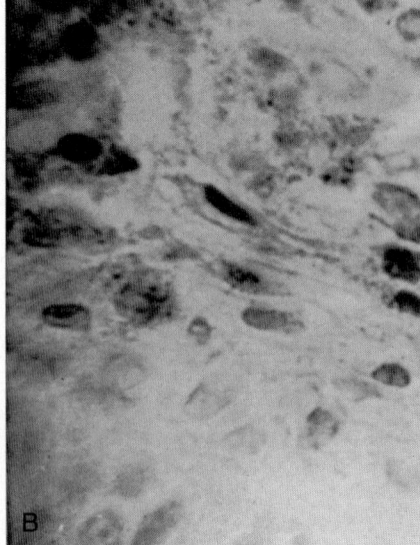

FIGURE 101-11 **A,** Deeply pigmented nodules and macules on the back of an infant with urticaria pigmentosa. A group of vesicles is visible just below the bandage that covers the biopsy site. **B,** Microscopic section from the biopsy specimen, stained with Giemsa stain. The mast cells can be identified as spindle-shaped cells containing granules that are located in the upper dermis.

(Sagher and Evan-Paz, 1967; Solomon and Esterly, 1973). Systemic mastocytosis is more commonly seen in adults and is defined by multifocal lesions in the bone marrow or other extracutaneous organs, together with signs of systemic disease. It is further divided into indolent systemic mastocytosis, systemic mastocytosis with an associated clonal hematologic non–mast cell lineage disease, aggressive systemic mastocytosis, and mast cell leukemia (Valent et al, 2001).

The diagnosis may be confirmed by a skin biopsy, which reveals mast cell hyperplasia within the dermis. Aminocaproate esterase is the most specific enzyme marker for identification of mast cells. Immunohistochemical stains for tryptase and *KIT* also are sensitive and specific markers for mast cells (Li, 2001). Mutations in c-*kit*, the gene encoding the receptor for stem cell factor, may play a significant role in the biology of mast cell malignancies (Gupta et al, 2002). Plasma histamine levels are elevated in a majority of children with mastocytosis, sometimes to remarkably high levels. Further work-up for evidence of systemic involvement should be limited to pediatric patients with extracutaneous signs and symptoms or those who require general anesthesia (Kettelhut and Metcalfe, 1991).

Caregivers should be educated to avoid exposing infants to factors that trigger mast cell degranulation, such as friction, pressure, temperature extremes, and substances that promote mast cell degranulation (aspirin, alcohol, narcotics, amphotericin B, or iodine-containing contrast media). If general anesthesia is required, perioperative administration of histamine receptor blockers is recommended (Lerno et al, 1990).

For patients with limited skin involvement, application of potent topical corticosteroids may hasten involution of lesions. Symptomatic patients may benefit from a classic histamine H_1 receptor blocker such as hydroxyzine or cyproheptadine. An H_2 blocker, such as ranitidine, or oral disodium cromoglycate may be added in the presence of gastrointestinal symptoms. Hypotension requires corticosteroids in addition to H_1 and H_2 antihistamines and intensive supportive care. Solitary mastocytomas usually involute by school age. Lesions of urticaria pigmentosa typically resolve by puberty.

MIDLINE ANOMALIES

Congenital midline defects are a distinct group of diagnostically and therapeutically challenging conditions. These anomalies are located deep to the dermis, occurring at the cranial or caudal midline. Some of these lesions mark an underlying CNS problem or an intracranial connection. Considerations in the differential diagnosis include lesions that occasionally occur in the midline by serendipity; hemangiomas are the most common. Vascular malformations, hair tufts, dimples, and lipomas also may occur at the cranial or caudal midline and can mark a CNS or spinal malformation (Hayashi et al, 1984; Martinez-Lage et al, 1992). A midline mass in the nasal area may represent a dermoid cyst, encephalocele, or glioma (Paller et al, 1991). Occipital lesions include aplasia cutis congenita, encephalocele, and heterotopic brain tissue. The "hair collar sign" may mark ectopic neural tissue and underlying CNS malformations (Commens et al, 1989; Drolet et al, 1995). Biopsy of a midline mass should not be performed unless an imaging study has been obtained to help clarify the nature of the lesion. If the possibility of an intracranial connection exists, referral to a neurosurgeon is indicated (Martinez-Lage et al, 1992).

SUGGESTED READINGS

Boyd KP, Korf BR, Theos A: Neurofibromatosis type 1, *J Am Acad Dermatol* 61:1-14, 2009.
Chang MW, Frieden IJ, Good W: The risk intraocular juvenile xanthogranuloma: survey of current practices and assessment of risk, *J Am Acad Dermatol* 34:445-449, 1996.
Chang LC, Haggstrom AN, Drolet BA, et al: Growth characteristics of infantile hemangiomas: implications for management, *Pediatrics* 122:360-367, 2008.
Drolet BA, Swanson EA, Frieden IJ: Hemangioma Investigator Group: Infantile hemangiomas: an emerging health issue linked to an increased rate of low birth weight infants, *J Pediatr* 153:712-715, 2008.
Drolet BA, Clowry L, McTigue K, et al: The hair collar sign: marker for cranial dysraphism, *Pediatrics* 96:309-313, 1995.
Enjolras O, Mulliken JB: Vascular tumors and vascular malformations (new issues), *Adv Dermatol* 13:375-423, 1997.
Haggstrom AN, Drolet BA, Baselga E, et al: Prospective study of infantile hemangiomas: demographic, prenatal, and perinatal characteristics, *J Pediatr* 150:291-294, 2007.
Kettelhut BV, Metcalfe DD: Pediatric mastocytosis, *J Invest Dermatol* 96:15-18S, 1991.
Metry D, Heyer G, Hess C, et al: Consensus statement on diagnostic criteria for PHACE syndrome, *Pediatrics* 124:1447-1456, 2009.
Paller AS, Syder AJ, Chan YM, et al: Genetic and clinical mosaicism in a type of epidermal nevus, *N Engl J Med* 331:1408-1415, 1994.
Schwartz RA, Fernandez G, Kotulska K, et al: Tuberous sclerosis complex: advances in diagnosis, genetics, and management, *J Am Acad Dermatol* 57:189-202, 2007.

Complete references used in this text can be found online at www.expertconsult.com

CHAPTER
102

DISORDERS OF THE EYE

Alejandra G. de Alba Campomanes, Gil Binenbaum, and Graham E. Quinn

The fast pace of development of the visual system in the neonatal period makes the recognition of ocular abnormalities extremely important. As early as 4 to 6 months after birth, some visual functions are permanently set and if impaired cannot be fully restored to normalcy. For example, a visually significant congenital cataract must be surgically addressed before the 3rd month of life to avoid potentially irreversible vision loss. This urgency makes the neonatal physician an invaluable player in the recognition and management of neonatal eye disease. Screening eye examinations are important in all infants, regardless of gestational age and whether in the neonatal intensive care unit (NICU), the nursery, or the office. Health care professionals taking care of newborns need to be familiar with indications for referral to a pediatric ophthalmologist, and in premature infants, the added risk of retinopathy of prematurity (ROP) mandates that neonatologists ensure timely diagnostic examinations by an ophthalmologist.

GENERAL EXAMINATION TECHNIQUES

THE NEWBORN EYE EXAMINATION: APPROACH AND EQUIPMENT

Effective physical examination of the newborn eye begins with familiarity with eye anatomy. Armed with a baseline understanding of "normal," the pediatrician can identify abnormalities or asymmetries in structure or function of the eyes by following a simple exam framework: I-ARM (Inspection, Acuity, Red Reflex, and Motility) (Simon and Calhoun, 1998). Detailed information on each of these components follows a discussion of general considerations when examining the eyes of a young infant.

A thorough eye examination, although necessary, can be stressful for a newborn or young infant. Swaddling, nesting, nonnutritive sucking, and oral sucrose before, during, and after an examination can be very helpful in this regard, particularly for premature babies undergoing an ROP exam for which an eyelid speculum is being used (Boyle et al, 2006; Grabskaet al, 2005; Marsh et al, 2005; Stevin et al, 1997). Gal et al (2005) undertook a randomized, double-blinded, placebo-controlled, cross-over study using the Premature Infant Pain Profile (PIPP), a previously validated scale, and found 2 mL of 24% oral sucrose to be more effective than placebo in reducing the immediate pain response during ROP exam using a lid speculum and topical anesthetic. Boyle et al investigated both nonnutrient

sucking and 1 mL of 33% sucrose versus placebo in a two-by-two factorial design; they found use of a pacifier to be effective but there was no synergistic effect with sucrose (Boyle et al, 2006). The most distressing aspects of the eye examination are generally the bright light of the ophthalmoscope and the use of a speculum, the pain of which appears to result primarily from stretching of the eyelids. The use of a topical anesthetic, such as proparacaine HCl 0.5%, reduces the discomfort of the speculum but is not always sufficient and should be supplemented with other measures, such as sucrose, pacifiers, and nesting (Marsh et al, 2005). In addition, NICU and office staff should be aware that the chronic use of topical anesthetics can result in corneal ulceration and melting, so bottles should be properly disposed of and not confused with other medications, such as topical lubricants or antibiotics. Use of an indirect ophthalmoscope without a speculum produces significantly less pain response than that noted with examination with a speculum or with a contact fundus camera, such as the RetCam (Clarity Medical Systems, Pleasanton, Calif.) (Mehta et al, 2005). Nevertheless, a speculum is often necessary to adequately visualize ocular structures and should always be used if adequate visualization of the fundus is otherwise not possible. In the experience of the authors, it is extremely rare for a properly supported infant to be unable to tolerate a quick fundus examination, the discomfort of any observers notwithstanding. Finally, particular note should be made of the oculocardiac reflex, a dysrhythmia, typically bradycardia, resulting from direct manipulation of the eye; monitoring by an assistant during the examination is therefore important.

The infant is often best examined lying supine. If he or she is in an incubator, the top must be raised to allow the examiner to examine the eyes closely and from different directions. A parent or a nurse may cradle the baby for examination as well. In slightly older infants, visual tracking and motility are best assessed in an upright position. It usually takes more than one set of hands to examine an infant's eyes. As discussed earlier, assistance with comforting the baby and monitoring vital signs is important. In addition, the head and body of the infant may need to be securely held to allow both a detailed and safe anatomic examination. Such restraint should be applied carefully but firmly and is best left to the end of the examination, because once the child is upset, it will become difficult to assess certain parts of the ophthalmologic examination such as visual function, motility, or intraocular pressure. Under some circumstances, it may become necessary for an ophthalmologist to perform an examination under sedation or general anesthesia.

Newborn eyelid skin is thin and delicate and must be handled gently. Proper technique can ensure that the eyelid fissures are open wide enough to adequately visualize the eyes, while minimizing eyelid trauma. Ideally, tips of the fingers are placed on the eyelid margins and gentle pressure is placed in upward and downward directions to separate the eyelids by their ends. Care must be taken not to abrade the surface of the eye, and the examiner's fingernails should be groomed short. Pulling the lids apart by pulling on the skin of the eyelids does not open the lids as well and may be more uncomfortable for the baby; however, this method is simpler and requires less skill than using the eyelid margins method. If the eyelids are slippery, placing gauze on the skin helps improve traction. Finally, use of an eyelid speculum is sometimes the quickest, most efficient, and even safest method of opening the lids for the skilled examiner. Care must be taken to ensure that the baby cannot grab the speculum while it is in place.

Examination of the eye requires adequate light and magnification. Even a simple flashlight or penlight and a magnifying glass are helpful and worth using if specialized instrumentation is not available. The ideal light source provides a variable, very bright and focused beam. The portable slit lamp microscope combines such a light source in combination with excellent binocular magnification. The light beam width is controllable, allowing three-dimensional cross sections of the anterior segment structures of the eye, including the conjunctiva, cornea, anterior chamber, iris, and lens. Although the slit lamp is an extremely useful instrument, it is expensive, and some degree of practice is needed to develop facility. Again, any simple magnifier and bright light source will prove invaluable for an eye examination in the NICU, emergency room, or pediatrician's office. The direct ophthalmoscope, typically available in all three settings, can serve this purpose and is discussed in the next paragraph. An additional method to identify pathology of the ocular surface is application of fluorescein ophthalmic solution, which will stain areas of denuded corneal and conjunctival epithelium. Once the solution is applied, a blue light source must be shone on the eye, and the examiner can identify corneal abrasions, which appear as patches of staining; corneal dryness, which appears as punctate staining; and multiple other conditions, such as dendritic herpetic lesions, more typical in older children. Most direct ophthalmoscopes have a blue light source, which may be used in conjunction with a magnifier. Alternatively, a Woods lamp may be used.

The direct ophthalmoscope is an important instrument for examining a newborn's or infant's eyes. It provides a light source to evaluate light perception and pupillary reactivity and to use together with a magnifier for examining the anterior structures of the eye. Red reflex testing with a direct ophthalmoscope (described in detail later) is a mandatory element of all newborn and well-baby physical examinations. Numerous vision-threatening and even life-threatening ocular diseases are primarily identified by a pediatrician checking red reflexes, and this technique is the pediatrician's principal method of detecting pathology in the posterior segment of the eye. The direct ophthalmoscope may of course be used to directly visualize the optic nerve head

and retina, but particular considerations and limitations must be kept in mind. Pupil size must be maximal; typically this means pharmacologic dilatation (discussed later). If mydriatics are not used, dimming ambient light and, in older children, having the child fixate in the distance will maximize pupil dilation. The examiner must be very close to the infant (a few centimeters at most). Approaching from a slightly lateral angle and following the "arrows" of branching vessels back to the nerve head will help to identify the optic disk. Most important, the field of view or "spot size" of the direct ophthalmoscope is approximately the size of the optic nerve head, which represents but a tiny fraction of the ocular fundus. Therefore, it is not possible to adequately evaluate the retina for ROP or other pathology with a direct ophthalmoscope. The indirect ophthalmoscope requires both greater skill and a handheld lens to use but provides binocular viewing with depth perception and a much wider field of view, perhaps four disk diameters in size. Pharmacologically dilated funduscopic examination with an indirect ophthalmoscope is required for ROP and other retinal diagnostic examinations, such as for retinoblastoma or retinal hemorrhage in suspected abusive head trauma.

Pharmacologic dilatation with mydriatic eye drops is commonly performed by consulting ophthalmologists, typically on all new patient evaluations and at all ROP examinations. Occasionally, a pediatrician may find it helpful to dilate the pupils to better visualize the red reflex or optic nerve head. Drops are better deferred if an ophthalmology consultation will be requested, because dilating the pupils may make it difficult or impossible to accurately assess the pupils, ocular alignment, intraocular pressure, or iris. Dilating eye drops include sympathomimetics (e.g., phenylephrine) and anticholinergic drugs (e.g., tropicamide, cyclopentolate, atropine). Potential side effects of these drugs include elevated blood pressure, increased heart rate, cardiac arrhythmias, feeding intolerance, slowed gastric emptying, urticaria, contact dermatitis, and seizures (Bonthala et al, 2000; Chew et al, 2005; De mayo and Reidenberg, 2004; Fitzgerald et al, 1990; Isenberg et al, 1985; Wright, 1992). These authors typically use tropicamide 1% and phenylephrine 2.5% and avoid the use of cyclopentolate in children less than 6 months of age. Adverse effects are potentially of greater concern in preterm infants, who are of lower weight and typically require multiple doses to achieve adequate dilatation, as do many children with dark irides. Therefore, it may be prudent to use reduced concentrations of mydriatics in premature infants, particularly cyclopentolate. In a randomized masked trial, Chew et al concluded that cyclopentolate 0.2% + phenylephrine 2.5% is the mydriatic of choice in preterm infants with dark irides, because higher concentrations of cyclopentolate (0.5%, 1.0%) were more likely to result in increased mean blood pressure or feeding intolerance.[9] In all children, systemic absorption of eye drops can be minimized by compressing the lacrimal sac for a few minutes after instillation.

INSPECTION (THE I IN "I-ARM")

Inspection of anatomy is a key method of detecting eye disease. The eyes should be closely examined with proper lighting and magnification (as described earlier), and the periocular and ocular structures approached in a systematic manner. One option is to begin with the external structures and work inward and posteriorly, looking at each eye carefully and comparing the two eyes with each other. As a guideline, any abnormality or asymmetry noted on examination should be referred to a pediatric ophthalmologist for further management. The urgency with which to seek consultation depends on the specific finding, and guidelines appear throughout this chapter. However, one should err on the side of urgency, because the neonatal period represents a critical period in visual development. To adequately inspect the eyes, familiarity with normal anatomy is required. A general overview of these structures follows (Figure 102-1).

The eyelids protect the eyes. The eyelids contain numerous glands, which continually produce tears to keep the ocular surface well lubricated, and blinking actively pumps the tears into the lacrimal drainage system. An inability to adequately close the eyes presents a major problem and can result in surface drying, corneal epithelial breakdown, and vision- or eye-threatening complications, such as ulceration, infection, or scarring. The lacrimal glands actually produce reflex tears. The nasolacrimal duct provides a means of egress for tears, which pass through the puncta, canalicula, and lacrimal sac to the duct. The duct can be blocked at birth in 5% to 10% of newborns, resulting in epiphora and discharge in an otherwise white and quiet eye; 90% of such blockages clear by 1 year of age, after which surgical probing is undertaken. Of note, congenital glaucoma can manifest with epiphora as well (see later discussion of corneal clouding).

The conjunctiva is a translucent membrane that overlies the surface of the eye and the inside of the eyelids. The sclera is the white fibrous wall of the eye. It is relatively flexible at birth and gradually toughens over the first few years of life. The cornea is continuous with the sclera, which it meets at the limbus, and is a clear dome-shaped structure in the center of the globe (eye). It is commonly overlooked by the casual observer, because it is normally transparent. The cornea provides two-thirds of the refractive power of the eye, is richly supplied with sensory nerves, and must be kept well lubricated to prevent surface breakdown. The cornea is a multilayered structure approximately 0.5 mm

thick. It is kept clear by active pumping out of fluid by its endothelium. Any process that affects the clarity or integrity of the cornea can result in loss of vision.

The iris is a donut-shaped structure posterior to the cornea. The anterior chamber of the eye lies between the cornea and iris and is best visualized with slit lamp examination (see earlier discussion). The anterior chamber angle lies at the juncture of the cornea and iris peripherally and contains the aqueous fluid drainage structures of the eye; if these structures are occluded, a rapid rise in intraocular pressure and sight-threatening glaucoma can ensue. The iris contains muscle structures to constrict and dilate the pupil, which is a central aperture that is under nonvoluntary control and changes size with variations in incident light, focusing effort (accommodation), emotions, and medications. The iris is an immature structure at birth. The color tends to be gray or blue and may become darker as the pigmented layer of the iris stroma becomes more fully developed, which typically occurs by about 6 months of age. Heterochromia refers to differences in the color of the iris between or within eyes and can be seen in congenital Horner's syndrome (with mild ptosis and a poorly dilating miotic pupil), as well as syndromic conditions such as Waardenburg's syndrome or Hirschsprung's disease.

Behind the iris lies the crystalline lens, which provides one third of the eye's refractive power. The lens width and therefore refractive power can be varied by contraction of the ciliary muscle of the eye to provide accommodation or "focusing in" ability. An opacity in the lens is referred to as a cataract (see later section on leukocoria). The uvea is composed of the iris, the ciliary body, and the choroid. Inflammation of the uvea, uveitis, is diagnosable with slit-lamp and dilated-fundus examination by directly visualizing white blood cells and proteinaceous flare in the anterior chamber, as well as multiple other signs in the anterior and posterior segments of the eye. The ciliary body produces aqueous humor, which maintains eye pressure and nourishes the anterior segment structures. The choroid is a vascular structure that lies between the sclera and the retina; it supplies the retina and is in fact the most densely packed blood supply in the body.

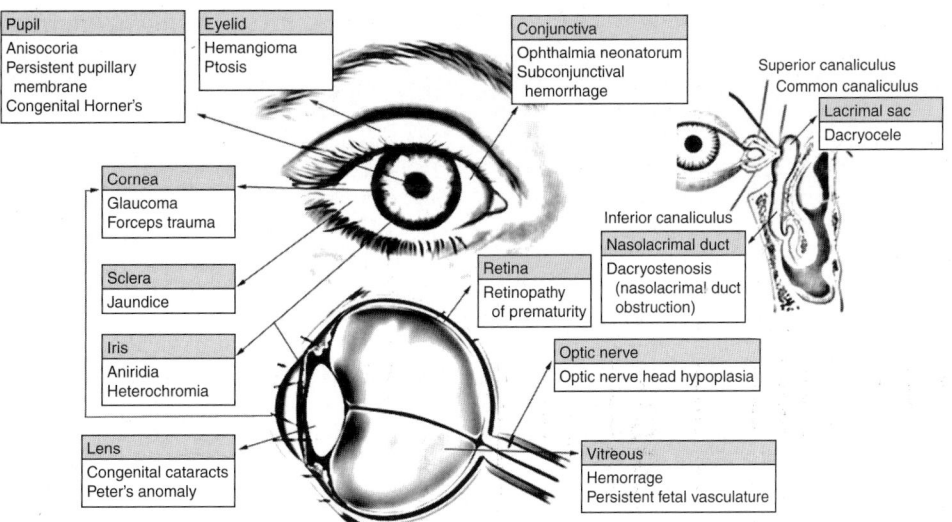

FIGURE 102-1 Anatomic structures and common neonatal pathology.

The retina is a multilayered, complex, highly metabolically active structure that lines the inside surface of the globe and contains photoreceptors that receive light and generate neuronal signals that are ultimately perceived as visual images. The macula is the central, posterior retina, between the superior and inferior temporal retinal vascular arcades, and the fovea is the very central retina containing the highest concentration of photoreceptors and producing central, high-resolution vision. Visual signals are transmitted through the optic nerve, whose cell bodies lie in the most anterior retina and which is actually composed of approximately 1 million individual nerve fibers. The proximal end of the optic nerve is visible as a normally golden disk approximately 15 degrees nasal and just superior to the fovea. The optic nerves lead to the optic chiasm and continuing visual and pupillary pathways in the brain. The anterior portion of the eye contains aqueous humor and the posterior segment contains vitreous humor, which is well formed at birth, but which undergoes gradual liquefaction (synersis) with age. The vitreous is composed primarily of water, collagen, and hyaluronic acid. It is attached to the retina throughout the fundus (posterior inner surface of the eye), all the way to the retina's anterior extent or ora serrata, where the retina meets the ciliary body; however, it has particularly strong attachments at the ora serrata (vitreous base), optic nerve head, and along the retinal vessels in the most superficial layers of the retina.

ACUITY AND VISUAL DEVELOPMENT (THE A IN "I-ARM")

The visual system is very immature at birth. The fovea is not completely differentiated until 15 to 45 months (Hendrickson and Yuodelis, 1984), and myelination of the optic nerve is not completed until about 1 year of age (Magoon and Robb, 1981). The eye continues to develop synapses in the visual cortex during the first 10 years after birth, and although visual acuity reaches normal adult ranges by 2 years of age, this period continues to be important because any abnormality can lead to amblyopia (Isenberg, 1989).

Because of the immaturity of the system at birth, qualitatively estimating the vision of a newborn is seldom attempted. However, clinical and laboratory techniques can be used to grossly estimate vision in special situations. These include eliciting a nystagmus response with optokinetic targets (stripped patterns), preferential forced looking, visual evoked potentials, and electroretinograms. It is estimated that the visual acuity of a full-term infant is approximately 20/400. Other clues to the status of visual function are more commonly used. For example, visual fixation should be present at birth, although it is not well developed until after the 2nd month. A blink response to light is present at 26 weeks' postmenstrual age (Robinson and Fielder, 1990) and a blink in response to an approaching object (visual threat response) develops at approximately 16 weeks' postnatal age. Visually directed reaching should be seen around 8 weeks' postnatal age, and a failure to smile by 6 weeks' postnatal age may signify a serious visual defect (Levene and Chervenak, 2009). The absence of visual responsiveness by the age of 2 months should be taken seriously and prompt an ophthalmologic evaluation.

The knowledge of normal eye structures and certain growth parameters in the newborn is important because a deviation from these averages can be associated with significant pathology. For example, in congenital glaucoma, the corneal diameter is increased, and the axial length (sagittal length) of the eye is a parameter that is carefully followed to determine if the intraocular pressure is adequately controlled. At birth, the eyeball is 70% of the adult size (average axial length 17 mm) and reaches 95% of the adult size by age 3 years. The corneal horizontal diameter is usually 9.5 mm at birth, which is 80% of the adult diameter. These parameters can be assessed by simple bedside examination and with the aid of ultrasonography.

Poor vision or blindness should be suspected in any newborn with absent or poor pupillary responses, paradoxic pupillary response (the pupil dilates instead of constricting in response to a bright light), and nystagmus or searching eye movements, although these are not usually present until 2 to 3 months of age. Constant poking or rubbing the eyes can also be a sign of poor vision.

Causes of congenital blindness or poor vision include Leber's congenital amaurosis, other retinal dystrophies, congenital cataracts, glaucoma, optic nerve abnormalities, uveal colobomas, high refractive errors, and congenital infections. In most babies, the cause of poor vision is obvious after clinical examination. Occasionally, further investigation is necessary; this may include consultation with a pediatric neurologist, electrophysiologic testing, and neuroimaging. Babies affected with cerebral visual impairment (CVI), also known as cortical visual impairment, have a normal eye exam, including normal pupillary responses and no nystagmus. This term is used to describe children with visual impairment due to neurologic disease, which may be congenital or acquired. Perinatal causes include intrauterine infections, cerebral dysgenesis, asphyxia, hypoglycemia, intracranial hemorrhages, periventricular leukomalacia, hydrocephalus, trauma, meningitis, and encephalitis. In developed countries, CVI is the single greatest cause of visual impairment in children, and most of these children have an associated neurologic deficit (usually epilepsy or cerebral palsy), which places a major burden on children's special services in these countries (Taylor and Hoyt, 2005).

Amblyopia is defined as a reduction in vision that cannot be attributed directly to any structural abnormality of the eye or visual pathway. It is caused by abnormal visual experience early in life, and accordingly it is divided in three etiologic categories. Deprivational amblyopia results from obstruction at any point in the visual axis that causes the retina to perceive poor-quality, distorted, or no images. Causes of deprivational amblyopia include congenital or acquired cataracts, corneal opacities, ptosis, and vitreous hemorrhages. Strabismic amblyopia results from a child's preferring one eye over the other when the visual axes are misaligned. Refractive amblyopia is a consequence of a significant inequality of the refractive error in each eye. Any of these forms of amblyopia can be encountered in the first few months of postnatal life. Because amblyopia is responsible for more cases of unilaterally reduced vision in childhood than all other causes combined, and because it is preventable with early detection and treatment, all newborns and infants suspected to have any of these conditions should be referred promptly to an ophthalmologist.

PUPILLARY RESPONSE AND THE RED REFLEX (THE R IN "I-ARM")

The onset of the pupillary light reflex (constriction in response to light) occurs around 30 to 34 weeks' gestation (Robinson and Fielder, 1990) and is not fully developed until the 1st month after birth. The pupils should be examined for size, shape, symmetry, reactivity to light, and afferent defects.

As the light passes through the pupils and is reflected through the normal clear media of the anterior and posterior segments of the eye, a characteristic red reflex is produced. The red reflex test is vital for early detection of vision and potentially life-threatening abnormalities such as cataracts, glaucoma, retinoblastoma, retinal abnormalities, systemic diseases with ocular manifestations, and high refractive errors. Red reflex assessment is an essential component of the neonatal and infant physical examination. The American Academy of Pediatrics currently recommends that all neonates have an examination of the red reflex before discharge from the neonatal nursery. In addition, the test should be performed during all subsequent routine health supervision visits (American Academy of Pediatrics 2008).

The red reflex test should be performed in a darkened room, projecting the bright light of a direct ophthalmoscope onto both eyes of the child simultaneously, from approximately 18 inches away. It is not necessary to pharmacologically dilate the pupils. The symmetry of the color, clarity, and intensity of the red reflex between eyes is usually more useful than the qualitative assessment of each red reflex independently, as there may be significant variation in normalcy. A markedly diminished reflex, the presence of a white reflex (leukocoria) or dark spots, or an asymmetric reflex are all indications of immediate referral to an ophthalmologist who is experienced in the examination of children (American Academy of Pediatrics 2008). The exception to this rule is a transient opacity from mucus or a foreign body in the tear film that is mobile and completely disappears with blinking or manually opening and closing the eyelids. Unequal or high-refractive errors (need for glasses) and strabismus may also produce abnormal or asymmetric red reflexes. An expanded observation is the position of the light reflex on the corneal surface. Asymmetric positioning of this reflex can indicate misalignment of the eyes (strabismus).

In addition, the shape and regularity of each pupillary aperture should be assessed to look for colobomas and other congenital abnormalities (see Common Diagnostic Problems, later). Asymmetry of pupil size (anisocoria) can be a sign of Horner's syndrome, trauma, or a congenital 3rd nerve palsy. The tunica vasculosa lentis is a plexus of vessels that crosses the pupil, visible in preterm babies up to 34 weeks postmenstrual age. A failure of these vessels to regress can occasionally be seen as a persisting pupillary membrane.

MOTILITY AND ALIGNMENT (THE M IN "I-ARM")

Although the extraocular muscles are fully formed by 12 weeks' gestation and fetal eye movements can be detected as early as 16 weeks' gestation, the supranuclear eye movement system is not fully developed until after birth in full-term neonates.

The eyes of a healthy full-term neonate commonly appear misaligned. It is not unusual to see the eyes shift from orthotropia to esotropia to exotropia. Transient deviations (neonatal ocular misalignments) occur very commonly in the 1st month of life in visually normal infants. At this age, it is not possible to distinguish those infants who will progress to develop pathologic strabismus from those who will subsequently develop normal binocular vision (Horwood, 2003a). Exotropia is commonly observed in newborn nurseries and has been reported to occur in up to 33% of infants (Nixon et al, 1985); however, most exodeviations will usually resolve with development of the fixation reflex and are rarely observed beyond 6 months of age (Sondhi et al, 1988). In contrast, transient esodeviations in patients who do not go on to develop infantile esotropia do not usually persist beyond 10 weeks of age (Horwood, 2003b; Sondhi et al, 1988). Most full-term infants establish normal ocular alignment within the first 8 weeks of life. In some babies, the epicanthal folds of the upper eyelids hide the medial aspect of the sclera, creating the appearance of strabismus; however, in these cases the visual axes are not misaligned. This common condition is referred to as pseudostrabismus and can be confirmed by directing a bright light to both eyes simultaneously and observing that the reflection of the light on the corneas appears in the center of each pupil. When in doubt, any apparent misalignment after 2 to 3 months of age should be considered pathologic and referred (see later discussion).

It is recommended that all newborns have an ocular motility assessment (American Academy of Pediatrics, 2003). This is also important because vision assessment in young nonverbal children is accomplished by evaluating the child's ability to fix on and follow objects. This assessment should be performed binocularly and then monocularly in an awake and alert child. If poor fixation and following are noted after 3 months of age, a significant eye or brain abnormality is suspected, and referral is advisable (American Academy of Pediatrics, 2003).

COMMON DIAGNOSTIC PROBLEMS

LEUKOCORIA

The term *leukocoria* means "white pupil." It is often used more broadly to encompass a spectrum of opacities and abnormalities. On inspection, the pediatrician may grossly visualize a white lesion in the pupillary space or identify an abnormal red reflex. The differential diagnosis for leukocoria includes vision- and life-threatening conditions, and leukocoria in an infant or older child requires urgent ophthalmologic evaluation. These conditions include cataract, retinoblastoma, chorioretinal or optic nerve head coloboma, retinal detachment, retinopathy of prematurity, persistent fetal vasculature, Coats' disease, familial exudative vitreoretinopathy, toxocariasis, and uveitis. The distribution varies widely with the population studied. In one series, 60% of 71 children less than age 10 who presented to a tertiary referral center with leukocoria had cataracts and 28% had retinoblastoma (Haider et al, 2008).

CATARACT

A cataract is any opacification of the normally clear crystalline lens of the eye (Figure 102-2). Although some congenital cataracts are small and nonprogressive, dense

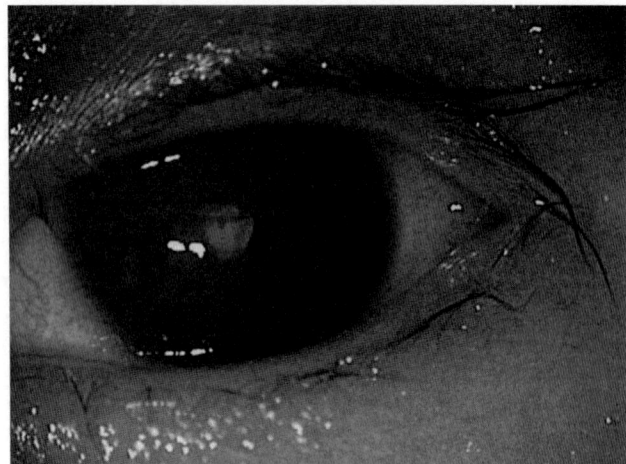

FIGURE 102-2 Congenital cataract. Note central dense opacity surrounded by clearer lens and poor pupillary dilation.

central opacities greater than 3 mm typically are visually significant. In contrast with adult-onset cataracts, which in most cases are removed at the preference of the patient, visually significant congenital cataracts must be surgically removed before 6 to 8 weeks of age to prevent irreversible vision loss from dense amblyopia (see the earlier discussion of visual development) (Birch et al, 2009; Lundvall and Kugelberg, 2002). Therefore, it is essential that all newborns and young infants have screening eye examinations by a pediatrician, because visual prognosis is directly tied to timely ophthalmologic referral. Cataracts can develop or progress with time, so examination for an abnormal red reflex should be repeated at each well-child visit even if prior exam findings appeared normal. Nystagmus may develop when there is a delay in presentation. Nystagmus is an ominous sign of poor visual prognosis and adds even greater urgency for surgical intervention.

Treatment does not end with surgery, because these infants are left aphakic (without a lens) and must receive optical correction with special contact lenses. Glasses, including bifocals, may be required in addition to aphakic contacts but may produce excessive optical aberrations when used as the sole means of refractive correction. Compliance with contacts, glasses, and, in the case of monocular cataracts, aggressive amblyopia treatment is essential for a successful visual outcome. Such children are also at risk for developing aphakic glaucoma, which may present after years, can be very difficult to treat, and is sight-threatening. There is evidence that very early cataract surgery increases the risk of glaucoma, and the optimal timing may lie between 3 and 6 weeks of age (Chak and Rahi, 2008; Khan and A1-Dahmesh, 2009; Michaelides et al, 2007; Swamy et al, 2007).

The etiologic distribution of congenital cataracts is approximately one third inherited; one third associated with systemic genetic, metabolic, or maternal infectious disorders; and one third idiopathic. Genetic inheritance is most commonly autosomal dominant and rarely autosomal or X-linked recessive (Francis et al, 2000; Hejtmancik and Smaoui, 2003). Multiple genes are involved in lens development, and numerous genetic loci have been identified (Hejtmancik and Smaoui, 2003). Marked variability can be present even within the same pedigree, and children with

a family history should be examined early by a pediatric ophthalmologist. The same is true of children diagnosed with one of the numerous systemic conditions associated with cataracts. Examples include intrauterine infections (rubella, varicella); metabolic and endocrine disorders (galactosemia, neonatal hypoglycemia, diabetes mellitus, and hypoparathyroidism); fetal alcohol syndrome; chromosomal disorders (trisomy 21, Turner's syndrome, trisomies 13 and 15); craniofacial syndromes; dermatologic diseases (congenital ichthyosis, ectodermal dysplasia); skeletal and connective tissue disorders (Smith-Lemli-Opitz, Marfan, Conradi's, and Weill-Marchesani syndromes); renal disorders (Lowe, Alport's, and Hallermann-Streiff-Francois syndromes); neurofibromatosis; and myotonic dystrophy. A selective work-up may be pursued in infants diagnosed with cataract, particularly bilateral cataracts, and may include TORCH titers (including syphilis); urine tests for reducing substance (galactosemia), protein, amino acids, and pH (Lowe syndrome); blood glucose, calcium, and phosphate; quantitative amino acids and red blood cell enzyme levels (galactokinase, gal-1-uridyltransferase); genetic consultation; chromosome analysis; and ocular examination of parents and siblings.

RETINOBLASTOMA

Retinoblastoma is the most common ocular malignancy of childhood and accounts for 3% of all childhood cancers. The incidence is between 1 in 15,000 and 1 in 20,000 live births, with approximately 350 newly diagnosed cases in the United States per year (Moll et al, 1997; Seregard et al, 2004). Untreated retinoblastoma is almost uniformly fatal, and long-term survival for disease diagnosed after it has spread outside the eye is under 50% (Chantada et al, 1999; Leander et al, 2007). In contrast, 5-year survival rates are greater than 90% when timely recognition and referral to centers specializing in retinoblastoma treatment occur (Abramson, 1982; Abramson et al, 2003; MacCarthy et al, 2006; Moll et al, 1997; Sanders et al, 1988; Seregard et al, 2004). Abramson et al (2003) reviewed 1831 consecutive cases of retinoblastoma. The most common presenting sign was leukocoria (54%), followed by strabismus (19%), poor vision (4%), family history with request for early exam (5%), and red eye (5%). The mean age at diagnosis was 19.7 months overall, but 7.7 months among those with a known family history receiving screening examinations by an ocular oncologist. In most reports, a majority of cases are diagnosed between 1 and 2 years of age, but the earliest reported date has been in utero, and in a series of 400 cases reported by Shield et al, 8.7% of the patients were older than age 5 years (Maat-Kievit et al, 1993; Shields and Shields, 2004; Shields et al, 1991). In the series reported by Abramson et al (2003), the disease presenting sign was identified first by a family member or friend in 80% of cases, a pediatrician in 8%, and an ophthalmologist in 10%. Among patients presenting with leukocoria, the sign was first identified by the family in 90% of cases. These findings stress the importance of routine red reflex testing for all children seen by pediatricians, beginning with newborns. Any child found to have leukocoria should be referred to an ophthalmologist for urgent evaluation.

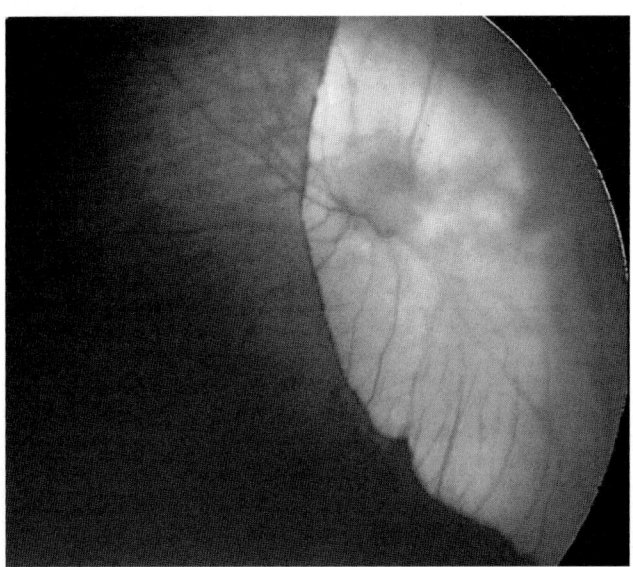

FIGURE 102-3 Chorioretinal and optic nerve head coloboma.

Once referral occurs, diagnosis of retinoblastoma can often be made by visualization using indirect ophthalmoscopy with scleral depression, frequently during examination under anesthesia. Imaging studies may provide useful information, including ocular ultrasonography to identify mass lesions and calcifications; magnetic resonance imagine (MRI) to image the globes and identify orbital and central nervous system (CNS) involvement; and computed tomography (CT) scans to identify calcification, although MRI is now favored over CT for its ability to image soft tissues and avoid ionizing radiation (Balmer et al, 2006; Maat-Kievit et al, 1993). Treatment modalities include enucleation, chemotherapy, focal destructive therapies such as retinal laser photocoagulation or cryotherapy, and radiation, including brachytherapy, stereotactic conformal radiotherapy, and accelerated proton beam irradiation (Balmer et al, 2006). External beam radiotherapy is now much less commonly used.

The retinoblastoma gene, *RB1*, located on chromosomal region 13q14, was the first tumor suppressor gene to be described. Forty percent of patients have an inherited, disease-causing germline mutation, which acts in an autosomal dominant fashion with 90% penetrance (Balmer et al, 2006). Such children, as well as those with spontaneous germline mutations, are also at increased risk of developing nonocular tumors at a rate of 1% per year, or 50% by 50 years of age (Abramson, 1999). A discussion of the risk of retinoblastoma in relatives of affected parents or children is beyond the scope of this chapter. However, children with a positive family history may require serial examinations under anesthesia by an ophthalmologist and referral for genetic counseling.

COLOBOMA

An ocular coloboma is a congenital anatomic defect or cleft that results from failure of part of the optic vesicle fissure to close during embryogenesis (Figure 102-3) (Gregory-Evans et al, 2004). The result is essentially an area of missing tissue in the eye, most commonly in the inferonasal quadrant. Involved structures can include the cornea, iris, ciliary body, lens, retina, choroid, and optic nerve (Gregory-Evans et al, 2004). An iris coloboma appears as an irregular "keyhole," or "cat's-eye" pupil. A chorioretinal or optic nerve head coloboma, depending on the size, will appear as an abnormal red reflex or leukocoria. The affected eye(s) may be microphthalmic. The visual prognosis depends on whether the central macula is involved, and children may have good central vision despite upper visual field defects if the macula is spared. Long term, there is a variable risk of complicating retinal detachment or choroidal neovascularization associated with retinal and optic nerve colobomas (Daufenbach et al, 1998; Gregory-Evans et al, 2004; Guirgis and Lueder, 2003). There are numerous genetic loci, chromosomal aberrations, ocular abnormalities, and systemic findings associated with coloboma. Examples are CHARGE association; 22q11 deletion; Treacher Collins, Walker-Wardburg, and Aicardi's syndromes; and many others. OMIM at www.ncbi.nlm.nih.gov/omim is a good first resource for more detailed information.

PERSISTENT HYPERPLASTIC PRIMARY VITREOUS

During embryogenesis and fetal development, the "primary vitreous" contains the hyaloid vasculature system, which fills the posterior segment of the eye and comes forward to surround the lens. This system normally disappears, and a spectrum of abnormalities can be seen when these structures fail to regress, ranging from persistent pupillary strands to a vascular stalk remnant to a retrolenticular membrane and retinal disorganization or detachment (Dass and Trese, 1999). Involved eyes are typically microphthalmic, and an abnormal red reflex or leukocoria may be identifiable. Depending on extent, surgical intervention may help to avoid recurrent hemorrhage, glaucoma, and phthisis bulbi (atrophy and degeneration of a blind eye, which can become painful), and in some cases useful vision can be achieved (Alexandrakis et al, 2000; Dass and Trese, 1999). In 500 consecutive patients examined by Shields et al at an ocular oncology practice, 288 had retinoblastoma and 212 had lesions that simulate retinoblastoma, the most frequent of which was persistent hyperplastic primary vitreous (PHPV) (38% of 212) (Shields et al, 1991). The next most common retinoblastoma-simulating lesions were Coats' disease (16%) and presumed ocular toxocariasis (16%), with cataract and ROP being less common.

CORNEAL CLOUDING

Opacification of the cornea in a newborn may be the result of congenital glaucoma; corneal dystrophies; developmental abnormalities of the cornea and or other anterior segment structures; infection; iatrogenic trauma; or metabolic disorders (Nischal, 2007). Close inspection with magnification will identify opacification in a focal, regional, or diffuse pattern, depending on the etiology. The cornea is normally clear all the way to its border with the sclera (the limbus), with iris details easily visible. An abnormality centrally may also result in an abnormal red reflex. When identified, congenital corneal opacification requires urgent ophthalmologic evaluation to rule out congenital glaucoma, an infection that could worsen to become eye- or life-threatening, or an opacification that is amenable to surgical correction during the early critical period in visual development.

Glaucoma is an optic neuropathy usually associated with raised intraocular pressure. In contrast with adult- or juvenile-onset glaucoma, which may be successfully managed medically, congenital glaucoma is a surgical disease that requires prompt intervention, frequently in the neonatal period. Vision loss from glaucoma is typically irreversible. Key signs to identify include corneal clouding; corneal and eye enlargement (buphthalmos), even with a clear cornea; tearing; blepharospasm (blinking); Haab's striae (tears in Descemet's membrane, seen as linearities in the red reflex); and photophobia. It is worth highlighting that tearing is a sign of glaucoma, not just of a blocked tear duct, and that "large, beautiful eyes" require an evaluation to rule out glaucoma. Finally, congenital glaucoma has multiple systemic associations, such as Sturge-Weber, neurofibromatosis, Lowe syndrome, congenital rubella, and Rubenstein-Taybi disease.

Sclerocornea is characterized by cornea that is opacified and white like the sclera, with which it is developmentally continuous. Typically, these opaque areas are located at an indistinct corneoscleral limbus (border), can extend centrally, and contain superficial vascularization. Nischal differentiates between isolated sclerocornea and complex sclerocornea, which is associated with cataract, microphthalmos, and/or infantile glaucoma (Nischal, 2007). In contrast with sclerocornea, *Peters' anomaly* classically has a central corneal opacity with clear cornea peripherally, absence of posterior corneal stroma, and variable attachments between the posterior corneal surface and the iris and or lens (Yang et al, 2009). Glaucoma is a potential complication, and the long-term visual outcomes of surgical management with corneal transplantation are highly variable (Rao et al, 2008; Yang et al, 2009; Zaidman et al, 2007). Nischal recently claimed that the diagnosis of Peters' anomaly is imprecise and has proposed a more complex classification for congenital corneal opacities that requires anterior segment imaging with ocular coherence tomography or high-frequency ultrasound (Nischal, 2007). This classification is more specific with regard to pathogenesis, enables more accurate surgical prognostication, and explains the variability in surgical outcomes. Therefore, Peters' anomaly may soon no longer be considered a distinct clinical entity.

Infectious keratitis can be herpetic, resulting in a keratoconjunctivitis, characteristic epithelial dendritic keratitis, and stromal keratitis, all requiring topical and systemic antiviral medications in the newborn period. Of note, infection can occur despite cesarean delivery and intact membranes (Gallardo et al, 2005). *Bacterial keratitis* is less common in countries that practice routine administration of conjunctivitis prophylaxis at birth. However, a bacterial corneal ulcer can begin as a corneal abrasion (see later discussion) and then quickly enlarge, resulting in corneal thinning or perforation, endophthalmitis, and even bacterial sepsis. In the authors' experience, this chain of events can also occur in reverse, with bacteremia seeding the eyes and ultimately manifesting as a keratitis. Findings include a white corneal stromal infiltrate with an overlying corneal epithelial defect that stains with fluorescein. Aggressive topical

and sometimes systemic antibiotics are required, and any infant with a red eye and suspicious corneal signs should be referred for immediate ophthalmologic evaluation.

Iatrogenic trauma may result in corneal injury and be the result of amniocentesis or forceps delivery. Injuries from the latter are characterized by linear breaks in Descemet's membrane, which are more likely vertical or diagonal than to be the horizontal breaks seen with glaucoma, and may be accompanied by other signs of trauma. Corneal dystrophies, such as congenital hereditary endothelial dystrophy and posterior polymorphous dystrophy, may also result in cloudy corneas. The former always manifests at birth, whereas the latter may or may not be present at birth (Nischal, 2007). Metabolic disorders, such as some mucopolysaccharidoses, may cause progressive clouding but often only later in life and rarely during the neonatal period.

RED EYE/EYE DISCHARGE

The most common and important causes of a red eye in neonates include infectious conjunctivitis, subconjunctival hemorrhages, foreign bodies, and vascular malformations.

The incidence of neonatal conjunctivitis (ophthalmia neonatorum) has decreased dramatically since the issuance of prophylaxis in 1881. Despite this, ophthalmia neonatorum still blinds approximately 10,000 babies annually worldwide (Isenberg et al, 1996). The etiologic cause of conjunctivitis in the newborn can be chemical, bacterial, or viral (Table 102-1). Although infections are usually transmitted to the infant by direct contact during passage through the birth canal, organisms can ascend to the uterus so that even infants delivered via cesarean section can be infected, particularly in the setting of prolonged rupture of membranes. Prophylactic agents include 1% silver nitrate, 0.5% erythromycin, 1% tetracycline ointment, and 2.5% povidone-iodine (Isenberg et al, 1995, 1996). No prophylactic agent completely eliminates the risk of developing an infection, and a high index of suspicion should be maintained, in particular in those patients with risk factors (maternal infection, lack of prenatal care, or premature rupture of membranes).

Despite common teaching, the onset of conjunctivitis is not a reliable diagnostic sign, because significant overlap exists among the different etiologic agents. For this reason, conjunctival cultures (in Thayer-Martin, blood agar, and chocolate agar media) and conjunctival scraping for Gram and Giemsa staining are mandatory and should be performed without delay. It is not necessary to wait for an ophthalmologic consultation to initiate laboratory investigation and treatment, because delays in treatment of gonococcal conjunctivitis can have devastating consequences. *Neisseria gonorrhoeae* can penetrate an intact corneal epithelium, rapidly leading to perforation of the globe within hours if treatment is not initiated; therefore, all forms of conjunctivitis must be considered bacterial until proven otherwise. Appropriate treatment should be instituted once the results of cultures are known but should never be delayed (Figure 102-4).

The infant with mucopurulent discharge must be distinguished from the infant who exhibits only excessive tearing and a relatively white eye. The latter is most likely to have nasolacrimal duct obstruction (NLDO), although the

TABLE 102-1   Diagnostic Features and Management of Neonatal Conjunctivitis

Etiologic Agent	Onset	Clinical Characteristics	Diagnosis	Treatment
Chemical	24 hours	Noninfectious Lid edema, watery discharge	History of exposure, self-limited in <48 hours	None
Gonococcal (see Figure 102-4)	3–4 days	Bilateral, hyperacute purulent conjunctivitis, marked lid edema, copious discharge Can perforate cornea	Cell culture and Gram stain Gram-negative intracellular diplococci	Ceftriaxone 25–50 mg/kg/day IV Topical irrigation Topical antibiotics only useful if corneal ulcer present
Chlamydia trachomatis (most common)	5–7 days	Mild mucopurulent nonfollicular conjunctivitis, lid edema, pseudo-membrane formation Pneumonitis after 3–12 weeks	Cell culture, Giemsa stain, direct immunofluorescent assay, enzyme-linked immunoassay, PCR Basophilic intracytoplasmic inclusions in epithelial cells	Oral erythromycin 12.5 mg/kg every 6 hours for 2 weeks or Azithromycin suspension 20 mg/kg PO daily for 3 days
Staphylococcus, *Streptococcus*, and other bacteria	5–14 days	Nosocomial, mucoid discharge, conjunctival hyperemia and chemosis	Cell cultures, Gram stain	Broad-spectrum topical antibiotic (e.g., polymyxin B–trimethoprim 1 drop every 4 hours for 7 days)
Herpes simplex virus	6–14 days	Unilateral or bilateral conjunctivitis (nonfollicular), serous discharge, associated lid vesicles and occasionally, corneal epithelial dendritic defects that stain with fluorescein ± systemic involvement	Cell cultures, direct fluorescent antibody staining, enzyme immunoassay detection, PCR Multinucleated giant cells with intracytoplasmic inclusions	Acyclovir 60 mg/kg per day in 3 divided doses × 2 weeks (3 weeks if CNS or disseminated disease) + topical drops (1% trifluridine, 0.1% iododeoxyuridine, or 3% vidarabine)

CNS, Central nervous system; *IV*, intravenous; *PCR*, polymerase chain reaction; *PO*, by mouth.

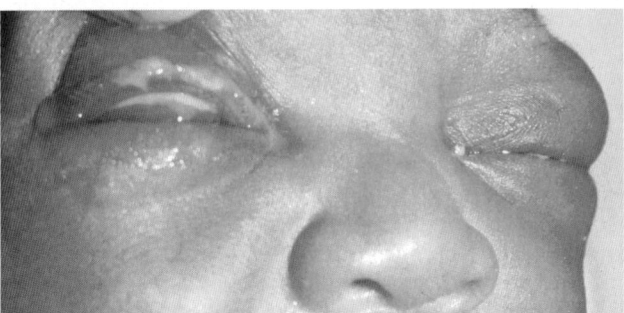

FIGURE 102-4 A 6-day-old newborn with gonococcal conjunctivitis. Note the marked lid edema and copious purulent eye discharge.

possibility of congenital glaucoma must always be ruled out. Congenital obstruction of the nasolacrimal duct is present in 5% to 6% of infants (Paul and Shepherd, 1994) but usually resolves spontaneously by 12 months of age. Usually a thin mucosal membrane at the distal end of the nasolacrimal duct is the cause. Symptoms usually become manifest by 1 month of age in 80% of cases, with tearing or sticky mucoid discharge. As a consequence of chronic obstruction, secondary infection in the lacrimal sac may occur, a condition known as dacryocystitis. This manifests as a tender, erythematous swelling of the skin overlying the lacrimal sac and periocular skin. Pressure on the lacrimal sac causes a reflux of mucopurulent material from the punctum (see Figure 102-1). Acute and chronic conjunctivitis may also develop. NLDO usually resolved spontaneously within the 1st year of life; conservative management is indicated in uncomplicated cases and consists of digital massage downward from the lacrimal sac over the nasolacrimal duct on the side of the nose. The massage empties the sac, reducing the opportunity for bacterial growth, and at the same time it applies hydrostatic pressure to the obstruction, which occasionally opens the obstruction. Topical broad-spectrum antibiotic drops can be used if there is

conjunctival injection and discharge. Referral to an ophthalmologist should be considered if the condition has not resolved toward the end of the 1st year, because probing and/or intubation of the lacrimal sac is sometimes necessary to relieve the obstruction (Katowitz and Welsh, 1987).

Orbital and preseptal cellulitis can also manifest with conjunctival injection, chemosis, and discharge. In addition, orbital cellulitis has altered ocular motility and pupillary reflexes and proptosis. Both are almost always unilateral and can rarely occur in the 1st month of life, sometimes secondary to acute dacryocystitis.

A subconjunctival hemorrhage is seen as a bright red discoloration under the conjunctiva obscuring the white scleral background and is common in the perinatal period. In a majority of cases it is caused by elevated venous pressure in the head and neck produced by compression during uterine contractions. Later in life, subconjunctival hemorrhages may be a feature of child abuse, although they can also occur spontaneously. Subconjunctival hemorrhages in isolation are completely innocuous and usually resolve in 10 to 14 days.

MOTILITY ABNORMALITIES AND NYSTAGMUS

Various eye motility and alignment abnormalities can be present in the 1st month of life. It is sometimes useful to determine whether it is a paralytic or restrictive problem, where the eye movements are evidently limited in one or several directions of gaze (incomitant strabismus) versus a comitant problem where the deviation is the same in every direction of gaze and there is no obvious restriction or motility deficit.

The most common form of strabismus in early infancy is infantile or essential esotropia. This form of convergent comitant strabismus is rarely congenital, so this term has been abandoned. It is usually present by age 3 to 4 months and is characterized by a large angle deviation. These children tend to cross-fixate (use the left eye to view the right visual field and vice versa), simulating an abduction deficit, because it is hard to get the child to follow an object to the ipsilateral field. This can easily be mistaken for bilateral 6th nerve palsy. However, 6th nerve palsies in the neonatal period are extremely rare, and an abduction movement can sometimes be elicited by patching one of the child's eyes to force the other eye to abduct in search of an object or by using the doll's-eye (the eyes lag behind the turning of the head from side to side) or optokinetic nystagmus (OKN) maneuvers. Infantile esotropia is a condition that is not likely to spontaneously resolve without surgical correction. Because of a high associated risk of amblyopia, prompt referral of these patients to a pediatric ophthalmologist within the first few months of life is appropriate. Even if the child's age or systemic condition is not appropriate for surgical correction, patching and other treatments should be initiated as early as possible.

Congenital nystagmus (infantile nystagmus syndrome) is an involuntary, bilateral, conjugate oscillation of the eyes that develops within the first 6 months of life. Despite the name, the eye movement abnormalities are rarely noticed at birth. Disorders of the visual pathways resulting in blindness or severe visual deprivation before the age of 2 to 3 months can also result in nystagmus (sensory nystagmus) which can be manifest as large-amplitude "wandering" eye movements or with a smaller-amplitude, faster movement that resemble the congenital motor form. Any form of bilateral (and sometimes unilateral) visual deprivation, including cataracts, corneal abnormalities, glaucoma, optic nerve problems, and chorioretinal colobomas, can manifest with nystagmus, and a prompt ophthalmic evaluation is needed to rule out these conditions, which are treatable in some cases. Other conditions such as albinism, achromatopsia (congenital absence of the retinal cones), and aniridia can also result in nystagmus, but the ocular findings in these conditions are more subtle and easily missed. In these cases additional testing, including electroretinography, may be recommended.

Because of this overlap, motor nystagmus should always be considered a diagnosis of exclusion, as other ocular and neurologic disorders can manifest with the same clinical characteristics. Certain specific forms of nystagmus are commonly associated with neurologic dysfunction; these include upbeat nystagmus, see-saw nystagmus, and even monocular nystagmus. However, these forms have all been associated with sensory loss, and an ophthalmologic exam is necessary even when neuroimaging studies rule out intracranial pathology.

Other transient disorders of the ocular motor system include opsoclonus, or flutter-like, high-frequency, small-amplitude movements that in newborns may be self-limiting and resolve spontaneously within the first few weeks of life. Some infants can also present with transient downward deviation of the eyes. This disorder can be distinguished from the more serious sun-setting sign, associated with hydrocephalus, by demonstrating intact upgaze using vestibular-ocular responses. Neuroimaging fails to demonstrate any underlying neurologic disorder, and the deviation tends to improve gradually over the following months.

PTOSIS AND OTHER EYELID AND LACRIMAL ABNORMALITIES

External inspection of the eyes and eyelids should be performed in every newborn. The eyelids are fused usually until 25 weeks' gestation, but they may rarely remain fused until 30 weeks. Eyelid colobomas are rare congenital full-thickness defects, usually involving the upper eyelid border. Eyelid colobomas are commonly associated with Goldenhar's syndrome.

Most cases of congenital ptosis are cause by an isolated developmental anomaly of the levator palpebrae muscle. Other causes include congenital 3rd nerve palsy, Horner's syndrome, blepharophimosis syndrome, and Marcus-Gunn jaw-winking ptosis, which is a synkinesis between the levator palpebrae and the mastication muscles. This type of ptosis is characterized by elevation of the lid associated with sucking or chewing.

Because form deprivation amblyopia can occur as a result of complete obstruction of the visual axis, this condition must be managed aggressively by an ophthalmologist familiar with the treatment of lid disorders and amblyopia. Even though this type of amblyopia is the most severe and concerning to the neonatologist, it is important to remember that even without complete obstruction of the pupil, amblyopia can occur secondary to the blur induced by astigmatism produced by the ptotic eyelid on the cornea. If vision is not threatened, surgery may be deferred until 4 to 5 years of age, although some surgeons have argued the benefits of earlier surgery (Katowitz, 2002).

A number of eyelid tumors can be present at birth or shortly thereafter. Capillary hemangiomas can manifest as a localized area of dimpled, red skin that resembles a strawberry or as a deep diffuse purplish mass a few weeks after birth. Typically they progress over the first 5 to 8 months of life and then stabilize, regress, and involute over several years. They are amblyogenic because they can cause mechanical ptosis, obstruct the visual axis, or cause significant astigmatism. A variety of treatment options exist, including topical, intralesional, or systemic steroids; interferon-α; vincristine; and surgical resection. Favorable results have been reported recently with systemic nonselective beta-blockers (e.g., propranolol) (Leaute-Labreze et al, 2008).

Capillary hemangiomas should be distinguished from other capillary vascular malformations (such as port-wine stains) that are present at birth and do not exhibit regression. These are sharply circumscribed lesions that are usually unilateral. In these patients, Sturge-Weber syndrome should be suspected. When the skin lesion involves the eyelid, an ophthalmologic consultation should be requested to rule out glaucoma (occurring in about 50% of patients) and vascular abnormalities of the choroid.

A dacryocystocele is formed when a proximal and a distal obstruction coexist in the lacrimal sac and the lacrimal sac becomes distended. Clinically it is manifested as a bluish, nontender mass just inferior and nasal to the medial canthus (see Figure 102-1). The bulging of the mucosa at the lower end of the nasolacrimal duct into the nasal cavity can significantly compromise the airway and should be ruled out by inspection of the nasal passage (Paysse et al, 2000). A secondary infection of the distended sac is not uncommon and can have potentially serious consequences in a neonate, including meningitis and septicemia. Intravenous antibiotics should be administered followed by decompression of the sac after 24 to 48 hours if the dacryocystitis shows no improvement. A dacryocystocele should be distinguished from a frontal encephalocele and can occasionally be confused with a hemangioma or a dermoid cyst.

OCULAR TRAUMA IN THE NEONATAL PERIOD

Newborns may suffer injuries to the eye as a result of birth, more commonly difficult births, such as those involving prolonged delivery, cephalopelvic disproportion, or forceps use. Intrauterine injuries may result from amniocentesis with discovery at birth. Some common injuries will heal without long-term visual or ocular sequelae (Holden et al, 1992). However, identification of birth-related eye trauma necessitates an ophthalmologic consultation to perform a complete dilated examination, identify all injuries, and assess the need for treatment.

Subconjunctival hemorrhage results from rupture of blood vessels on the surface of the eye. It is distinguished from conjunctival injection from an inflammatory or infectious cause by characteristically well-demarcated borders between spots of blood underneath the conjunctiva and completely white sclera directly adjacent to the blood. Subconjunctival hemorrhage will resolve spontaneously with time and does not require treatment. However, such hemorrhage can often be a sign of more significant trauma underneath the hemorrhage or within the eye, and a complete eye examination, including dilated funduscopic examination, is required. Recurrent subconjunctival hemorrhage could be a sign of a coagulopathy or platelet abnormality, and an appropriate work-up should be pursued in such cases.

Hyphema is the presence of red blood cells in the anterior chamber of the eye (the space between the cornea and the iris), most commonly the result of trauma, including birth trauma. It is often associated with ocular injuries. Clot or hemorrhage of varying magnitude may be seen on close inspection, ranging from a subtle crescent of blood at the corneoscleral limbus to an eye completely filled with blood, obscuring any view of the structures underneath. The red reflex is commonly abnormal. Hyphema is a potentially vision-threatening condition and requires close management by an ophthalmologist. The immediate concern is obstruction of the aqueous fluid drainage angle structures, resulting in an acute rise in intraocular pressure (IOP) or acute glaucoma. High IOP is painful enough to cause vomiting in children and adults and may manifest as crying, irritability, grimacing, poor feeding, or emesis in an infant. If the IOP is high enough for any prolonged period of time, irreversible optic nerve damage can ensue, with permanent vision loss. Corneal blood staining may also result and can take a year or more to clear, resulting in amblyopia. Often, IOP spikes occur with rebleeds, for which the greatest risk is during the first 5 days after an injury. Therefore, management includes full eye examination, daily monitoring, eye shield, avoidance of antiplatelet agents, bed rest in older children, sickle cell testing (portends higher risk of glaucoma), topical and systemic glaucoma medications, and possible surgical intervention to wash out the anterior chamber.

Traumatic hyphema is associated with delayed glaucoma, which may only manifest years after the acute incident, so these children require long-term ophthalmic follow-up.

An open globe injury refers to a full-thickness break in the eyewall (e.g., sclera, cornea). These injuries can occur as a laceration or as a rupture, in which pressure is applied to the front of the eye and the eye wall breaks open at its weakest points, such as the corneoscleral limbus or extraocular muscle insertion sites. Key signs include an obvious break with the protrusion of intraocular contents (e.g., the iris), extensive subconjunctival hemorrhage, a flat anterior chamber (the iris and cornea have come together), hyphema, vitreous hemorrhage (seen as a poor red reflex), and abnormal eye contour or intraocular foreign body on orbital imaging. An open globe represents a surgical eye emergency. Management consists of shielding the eye, aborting any further examination, NPO status, intravenous antibiotics, antiemetics or sedation to minimize Valsalva straining, and exploration and repair in the operating room.

A corneal abrasion is an epithelial defect on the corneal surface. Staining with fluorescein will identify areas of missing epithelium, which appear green under a blue light source and magnification. Treatment includes an urgent, complete ophthalmologic examination to rule out other ocular injuries, topical antibiotics, and close follow-up to ensure complete healing and monitor for the development of bacterial keratitis (see the earlier discussion of corneal clouding). In a neonate, a corneal abrasion must be taken very seriously, because complications have included the sequential development of keratitis, endophthalmitis, septicemia, and meningitis (O'Keefe et al, 2005). Therefore, corneal abrasions should be managed by an ophthalmologist.

Other injuries include retinal hemorrhages (RH; see later discussion); corneal trauma from forceps, resulting in tears of the Descemet's membrane, visible as vertical or circumferential lines on red reflex examination, corneal thickening and opacification from edema, and corneal scarring; eyelid or adnexal injuries requiring surgical repair; choroidal rupture, which requires dilated fundus examination for diagnosis; and even traumatic optic neuropathy (Estafanous et al, 2000; Khalil et al, 2003; Lauer and Rimmer, 1998; Yang et al, 2005).

RETINAL HEMORRHAGES AND ABUSIVE HEAD INJURY

Retinal hemorrhage from birth is very common. The incidence is estimated to be between 10% and 40% of all newborns, depending on the examiner, time from birth, and specific population studied (Anteby et al, 2001; Critchley, 1968; Egge et al, 1980; Emerson et al, 2001; Hughes et al, 2006). The rate in children born through vacuum-assisted delivery is even higher, at 75% to 78% (Emerson et al, 2001; Hughes et al, 2006). The association between vacuum delivery and RH supports a role for mechanical trauma to the retinal vessels, for example from direct compression of the globe; however, there are likely additional factors involved, because head circumference and duration of labor are not significant factors, and RH occurs with cesarean section, albeit at decreased frequency (7%) (Emerson et al, 2001). Adequate description of retinal findings requires dilated funduscopic examination with an indirect ophthalmoscope. However, some RH may be identified with a direct ophthalmoscope, and an abnormal red reflex may be noted in some cases.

Birth-related RH rarely has a long-term visual consequence. However, it is important to understand the characteristics that distinguish birth-related RH from those associated with abusive head trauma, as there may be considerable overlap. The great majority of birth-related RH is intraretinal; subretinal and preretinal hemorrhages are less frequent. Such hemorrhages include superficial flame and deeper blot hemorrhages, and larger hemorrhages may frequently contain white centers (Egge et al, 1980; Emerson et al, 2001; Hughes et al, 2006). Although commonly located in the posterior pole of the eye, they may also extend to the mid- and far- retinal peripheries and range in number from a few to too numerous to count (Emerson et al, 2001; Hughes et al, 2006). They may be bilateral, unilateral, or asymmetric.

The preceding characteristics are similar to the RH seen in abusive head trauma (see later discussion), although severity ranges higher in abuse. A key characteristic, therefore, is the time to resolution of birth-related RH. A majority of intraretinal hemorrhages clear within the first 2 or 3 weeks of life, some within the first few days (Anteby et al, 2001; Emerson et al, 2001; Hughes et al, 2006; Kaur and Taylor, 1992). In most series, all intraretinal hemorrhages have cleared by age 4 weeks, whereas preretinal or subretinal hemorrhages may take up to 6 weeks to clear (Emerson et al, 2001). Of note, Hughes et al (2006) reported two children who had isolated discrete, dense foveal and or peripheral RH that took up to 7 weeks to resolve and which they described as intraretinal. However, in their series, which included 18 infants with birth-related RH, all multiple, confluent intraretinal hemorrhages had cleared by 17 days; the persistent RH showed signs of resolving on photographs taken at 30 days, so that such RH has a different appearance from acute hemorrhage; and again, the persistent hemorrhages were single and isolated (Hughes et al, 2006). Therefore, multiple intraretinal hemorrhages present past 1 month of age should be considered not related to birth. Isolated, resolving intraretinal hemorrhage or persistent pre- or subretinal hemorrhage past 1 month of age may rarely be related to birth, but such RH would not at any age by itself be considered specific for any cause, including abuse.

Pediatric abusive head trauma (AHT) is a leading cause of death in infancy (Billmire and Myers, 1985; Brenner et al 1999; Centers for Disease Control, 1990; Duhaime et al, 1992; Overpeck et al, 1998). Previous names have included the shaken baby syndrome (SBS), inflicted or nonaccidental head trauma, and inflicted childhood neurotrauma (Duhaime et al, 1998; Forbes et al, 2004; Reece, 2003). AHT is characterized by intracranial hemorrhage with or without retinal hemorrhages and or additional injuries, including bony fractures (Duhaime et al, 1998). Affected children are under 3 years of age, with the great majority under a year (Binenbaum et al, 2009; Duhaime et al 1992, 1998). The mechanism of trauma is believed to be repetitive acceleration-deceleration of an infant with or without blunt impact. Based on numerous perpetrator confessions and a frequent lack of scalp and soft tissue injuries, a majority of child abuse experts believe that it is

possible to produce this constellation of findings with shaking alone; however, most fatal and severe injuries include evidence of impact. Biomechanical models of infant head trauma are still in development and have known limitations (Duhaime et al, 1987, 1998; Gill et al, 2009; Prange et al, 2003; Raghupathi and Margulies, 2002; Raghupathi et al, 2004; Starling et al, 2004). Therefore, the term *abusive head trauma* has been adopted by the American Academy of Pediatrics as a term more inclusive of all mechanisms of injury and is preferable to "shaken baby syndrome" (Christian and Block, 2009).

RHs are present in 50% to 100% of victims of abusive head trauma (Altman et al, 1998; Binenbaum et al, 2009; Duhaime et al, 1992, 1998; Green et al, 1996; Kivlin, 2001; Morad et al, 2002).

Of note, however, this designation has been used indiscriminately by clinicians and investigators to describe a spectrum of findings. The presence of any RH in an infant is highly associated with abuse, and increasing RH severity correlates with increasing likelihood of abuse (Binenbaum et al, 2009; Bechtel et al, 2004; Christian et al, 1999; Forbes et al, 2004; Maguire et al, 2009; Morad et al, 2002). In AHT, RH may range from none to a few intraretinal hemorrhages confined to the posterior pole to bilateral, too numerous to count, intra-, sub-, and preretinal hemorrhages, extending to the far periphery or ora serrata (termination of the retina). The hemorrhages may be unilateral or markedly asymmetric. Macular retinal folds and hemorrhagic macular retinoschisis (splitting of the retinal layers) may be seen at the severe end of the spectrum. In comparison, RH associated with accidental head trauma typically are few in number, intraretinal, and limited to the posterior pole (Bechtel et al, 2004; Binenbaum, 2009; Buys et al, 1992; Christian et al, 1999; Duhaime et al, 1992; Forbes et al, 2004). However, more severe RH and even retinal folds may be seen with severe accidental trauma, such as fatal motor vehicle crashes (Kivlin et al, 2008). To date, hemorrhagic macular retinoschisis specifically has been reported only in abusive injury.

In addition to accidental head trauma, the differential diagnosis of RH in infancy includes birth-related RH (see earlier discussion), coagulopathy, septicemia, leukemia, anemia, and glutaric aciduria. These conditions are diagnosable through various diagnostic tests. Terson's syndrome refers simply to RH associated with subarachnoid hemorrhage; its etiology is not established, and it may in fact be a feature of AHT in some cases. Studies have demonstrated that prolonged chest compression with cardiopulmonary resuscitation very rarely results in RH, and when present, these RH are a few isolated posterior pole intraretinal hemorrhages (Odom et al, 1997). RH from convulsions are even rarer, and severe coughing has been reported not to result in RH (Goldman et al, 2006; Mei-Zahav et al, 2002; Sandramouli et al, 1997; Tyagi et al, 1998). RH associated with papilledema (swollen optic nerve head secondary to raised intracranial pressure) is limited to small splinter hemorrhages on the disk with moderate disk swelling or flame-shaped hemorrhages directly around the disk when papilledema is severe.

Children with AHT may present with a history of minor blunt head trauma, such as a short fall, or no trauma history at all and exhibit lethargy, seizures, increased or decreased tone, vomiting, poor feeding, breathing difficulties, or apnea (Duhaime et al, 1998). Head CT identifies subdural or subarachnoid hemorrhage, sometimes with a combination of chronic and acute features, but very rarely may initially be normal; brain MRI provides a better look at the soft tissue and brain parenchyma to identify features such as hypoxic ischemic injury; plain film radiographs may reveal a skull fracture; and a skeletal survey is a critical modality for identifying other bony injuries (Duhaime et al, 1998; Ichord et al, 2007; Morad et al, 2004; Parizel et al, 2003). Because the provided history is often vague or unreliable, a high index of suspicion and low threshold for obtaining diagnostic tests and specialist consultation must be maintained.

Ophthalmologic examination should occur within 48 hours, preferably within 24 hours, because RH can begin to resolve within days. A dilated fundus examination with an indirect ophthalmoscope and, when indicated, scleral depression are required to adequately visualize the retina. Ophthalmologic consultation should not be delayed because of an inability to pharmacologically dilate the pupils due to neurologic pupil exam checks; the ophthalmologist can still attempt to view a portion of the retina and return for a dilated examination later. It is very important to document the type(s), number, location(s), and laterality of all RHs, both using explicit descriptive terms and through diagrams. Fundus photographs, for example with a RetCam camera, should be obtained when possible (Nakagawa and Skrinska, 2001; Saleh et al, 2009). Such photographs are important documentation and are often easily obtained at the time of sedation administered for MRI or other tests. However, the authors stress that the presence of RH is not descriptive enough, and the extent and detailed characteristics of the hemorrhages are vitally important. Such cameras may identify and characterize some posterior pole RH, but they do not consistently provide adequate visualization of the retinal periphery and are not a substitute for an indirect exam. RH have been reported as a result of RetCam use in a premature infant undergoing ROP screening (Adams et al, 2004). Notably, this 25-week-gestational-age infant was less than 34 weeks postmenstrual age at the time of exam and had immature retinal vasculature, without smooth muscle, elastin, or collagen layers and poor autoregulation, unlike the mature vasculature of a few-months-old infant evaluated for AHT (Adams et al, 2004). Further, other investigators have failed to identify any RH with the routine use of the RetCam for ROP screening (Azad et al, 2005). Nevertheless, whenever possible an indirect ophthalmoscopic exam should be completed and documented before using a contact fundus camera.

Visual impairment in children with AHT is most often related to cortical damage. However, persistent macular or vitreous hemorrhage, retinoschisis, and other scarring conditions may result in significant deprivation amblyopia, induced myopia and anisometropic amblyopia, or photoreceptor damage limiting visual function. The overall mortality rate in AHT has been reported to be between 13% and 36% (Barlow et al, 2005; Duhaime et al, 1987). Approximately two-thirds of the survivors have long-term neurologic deficits. In a prospective study of 25 children with a mean 5 years follow-up, Barlow et al found that 68% had neurologic and cognitive impairment, and one-half of

these had severe disabilities and were totally dependent (Barlow et al, 2005).

RETINOPATHY OF PREMATURITY

Retinopathy of prematurity, a disease of the developing retinal vasculature, first became a significant cause of blindness in children in the 1940s and 1950s with increased survival of premature infants due to improved neonatal care, in particular the use of supplemental oxygen in industrialized countries (Patz, 1952, 1954, 1969, 1975). This episode has been termed the "first epidemic," and hyperoxia was determined to be the dominant risk factor (Campbell, 1951), a finding that was substantiated by both basic science and clinical trials (Flynn et al, 1992; Lanman and Guy, 1954). With restriction of oxygen in the mid-1950s, there was a reduction in the blindness from ROP, but this was associated with increased rates of mortality and cerebral palsy in premature babies (Cross, 1973). During the late 1960s, NICUs were introduced with use of oxygen with increasingly accurate methods of monitoring supplementation and improved management of neonatal and perinatal complications. However, because smaller and less mature babies were surviving, blindness from ROP began to reemerge (the "second epidemic) (Flynn et al, 1992). Surgical treatment of established disease (Cryotherapy for Retinopathy of Prematurity Cooperative Group 1988, 1990a; Tasman, 1985;) and improved neonatal care are probably the major factors responsible for reduction of blinding ROP observed during the 1980s and 1990s (Gibson et al, 1989).

Classification of Retinopathy of Prematurity

The International Classification of Retinopathy of Prematurity (ICROP) was published in 1984 (ICROP, 1984) and revised in 1987 (ICROP, 1987), providing a standard nomenclature for clinical findings in acute-phase ROP. As shown in Table 102-2, this classification takes into account four components of the ocular findings: anterior-posterior location of the retinopathy (zone), severity (stage), extent of the disease at the circumference of the vascularized retina (in clock hours), and the presence or absence of so-called plus disease. *Plus disease* is defined as engorged and tortuous vessels of the posterior pole and indicates a more serious form of ROP. The ROP status of an eye is determined by the highest stage and the lowest zone observed, along with noting the presence or absence of plus disease.

In ICROP, the retinal surface is divided into three concentric "zones" centered on the optic nerve (Figure 102-5). Most severe retinopathy occurs in zone I or posterior zone II, most retinopathy occurs in zone II, and ROP that occurs in zone III tends to be mild. The zone in which ROP occurs has important prognostic significance (Good et al, 2005; Palmer et al, 1991). Severity of retinopathy is designated on a scale of 1 to 3 by "staging" the retinopathy at the junction between vascular and avascular retina (Figure 102-6). The first two stages indicate mild disease; the extension of vessels into the vitreous indicates stage 3 ROP, a more serious disease. Stages 4 and 5 indicate the

TABLE 102-2 International Classification of Retinopathy of Prematurity—Revisited (2005)

Anterior-posterior location		Zone I: retinal area within a circle centered on the disk and with a radius of twice the estimated disk-foveal distance Zone II: retinal area extending from the edge of zone I to a circle with a radius from the disk to the nasal ora serrata Zone III: a crescent-shaped retinal area extending beyond zone II to the ora serrata
Severity	Stage of ROP	Stage 1: a thin, sharp line of demarcation between vascularized central retina and more peripheral avascular retina Stage 2: an intraretinal elevation (ridge) at the junction between vascularized and avascular retina Stage 3: a ridge with fibrovascular extension into the vitreous Stage 4: partial retinal detachment; 4A, does not involve the fovea; 4B: involves the fovea Stage 5: total retinal detachment
	AP-ROP	Aggressive posterior ROP recognized by: 1. marked dilation and tortuosity of posterior pole vessels 2. difficulty in documenting the stage of ROP at junction between vascularized and avascular retina 3. occurs in zone I or zone II
Extent		Number of clock hours of ROP along the circumference of the vascularized retina
Posterior pole vascular abnormalities	Plus disease	Presence of dilated and tortuous vessels of the posterior pole present in two or more quadrants
	Preplus disease	Abnormal vascular dilation and tortuosity that is insufficient for diagnosis of plus disease present in two or more quadrants

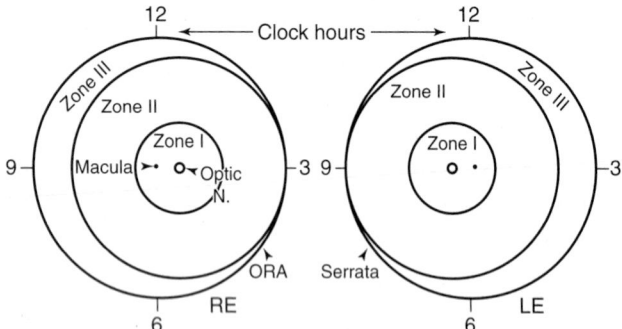

FIGURE 102-5 Scheme of retina of right eye *(RE)* and left eye *(LE)* showing zone borders and clock hours used to describe location and extent of retinopathy of prematurity. *(Reproduced from* Archives of Ophthalmology, *with permission.)*

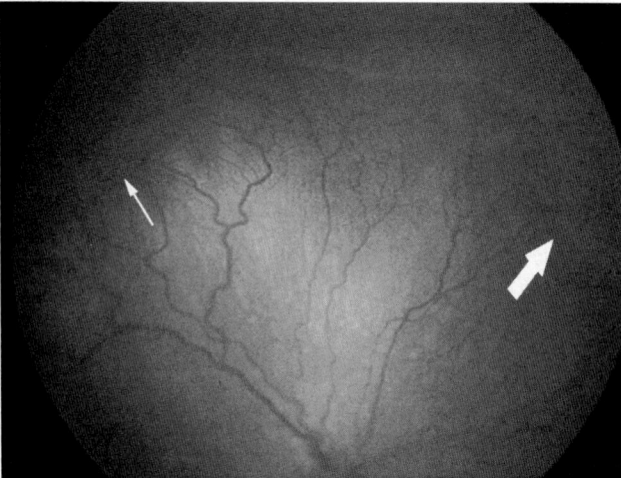

FIGURE 102-6 Fundus photograph showing the ridge between vascularized and avascular retina characteristic of stage 2 retinopathy of prematurity *(large arrow)*. Stage 3 retinopathy of prematurity is present in the left-hand portion of the photograph *(small arrow)*.

presence of retinal detachment. The term plus disease, a clinical diagnosis made by comparing to reference photographs used in clinical treatment trials in the United States (Cryotherapy for Retinopathy of Prematurity Cooperative Group, 1988; Good et al, 2005) indicates marked tortuosity and/or dilation of the peripapillary arterioles and venules in at least two quadrants. Preplus disease designates the presence of vessels that are not normal appearing but are not sufficiently abnormal to be designated as plus disease. Other signs that frequently accompany serious ROP include vitreous haze, iris vascular engorgement, and pupillary rigidity, but these signs are not required to make the diagnosis of plus disease.

In 2005 aggressive posterior ROP (AP-ROP) was added to ICROP, defining the observation of a particularly aggressive form of ROP observed with increasing frequency in the smallest premature babies and that may be more difficult to recognize, because the peripheral retinopathy is not as remarkable even though the posterior pole vascular abnormalities of dilation and tortuosity are quite marked (International Committee for the Classification of ROP, 2005).

Prevalence and Incidence of Retinopathy of Prematurity

Large natural history studies have shown that, in most cases, ROP begins at 31 to 32 weeks postmenstrual age (Fielder et al, 1992; Good et al, 2005; Palmer et al, 1991; Reynolds et al, 2002) with progression over the next 2 to 5 weeks. Spontaneous regression commonly occurs in eyes with stages 1 and 2 and early stage 3 (Palmer et al, 1991; Repka et al, 2000). Blindness or severe visual impairment commonly results from progression of the retinopathy to retinal detachment or severe distortion of the posterior retina (Dobson et al, 1995; Gilbert et al, 1992a, 1992b, 1996; Reynolds et al, 1993).

ROP occurs in a majority of babies with birthweights of less than 1500 g (very low-birthweight [VLBW]) with an even greater proportion of babies developing ROP in the less than 1000 g birthweight category (extremely low-birthweight, ELBW) and in the less than 750 g birthweight infants (Cryotherapy for Retinopathy of Prematurity Cooperative Group, 1991; Darlow et al, 1992, 2005; Fielder et al, 1992; Good et al, 2005). ROP is also more likely to occur in males than females (Darlow et al, 2005) As neonatal services continue to improve, a greater proportion of VLBW and ELBW babies survive, with a resultant increase in the population of babies at risk (Gilbert et al, 2005).

Many case control studies have been undertaken to elucidate risk factors for ROP, and all identify preterm birth and low birthweight as the major risk factors. Other factors associated with the development of ROP (but not necessarily causally associated) include hyperoxia, hypoxia, acidosis, intraventricular hemorrhage, exposure to light, vitamin E deficiency, and septicemia. Progression to advanced, blinding disease seems to be determined by immaturity of the retina and the degree of early insult.

Prevention of Retinopathy of Prematurity

Medical treatment to prevent ROP holds the promise to markedly decrease development of serious ROP. Interventions such as systemic steroids given immediately before preterm birth and surfactant administered shortly after birth decrease the incidence of respiratory distress syndrome, which would be expected to decrease the incidence of serious ROP. However, these medical advances also increase the survival rate of low-birthweight babies (Soll, 2000). Several randomized clinical trials were undertaken in the 1970s and 1980s to determine whether supplementation with the antioxidant vitamin E might prevent development of ROP. Individually, these studies do not demonstrate a significant positive benefit, but a detailed metaanalysis of randomized trials suggested that more investigation is warranted (Raju et al, 1997).

In 2001, Hellstrom and co-investigators showed in a cohort of babies in Sweden that insulin-like growth factor-1 (IGF-1) was deficient in premature infants almost immediately after birth, and they observed that children who were slow to recover to normal serum levels of IGF-1 were more likely to develop ROP (Hellstrom et al, 2001). In several careful follow-up studies, these investigators demonstrated that determining the rate of weight gain, essentially a noninvasive surrogate for growth hormone level, was effective in stratifying the risk of developing serious ROP even before the retinopathy is manifest (Hellstrom et al, 2003; Lofqvist et al, 2006, 2009). Using a risk model (WINROP) (Lofqvist et al, 2009), individual infants could be targeted for more intensive examinations, and infants at little risk would require fewer diagnostic examinations. These approaches, supplemented by extensive work in murine models of oxygen-induced retinopathy by Smith et al (2003, 2008), open the way for potential medical therapies that can be offered to high-risk babies that may prevent ROP or at least modulate its severity (Chen and Smith, 2007; Heidary et al, 2009; Lofqvist et al, 2009; Mantagos et al, 2009).

Detection of Serious Disease

Because the benefit of treatment of serious ROP (as variously defined in clinical trials) has been shown in randomized clinical trials (Cryotherapy for Retinopathy of Prematurity Cooperative Group, 1988; Early Treatment for Retinopathy of Prematurity Cooperative, 2003), it is essential to identify the at-risk baby so that timely examinations can be performed to prevent blindness, or at least decrease its likelihood. In the United States, the recommended guidelines for detection of serious ROP indicate that diagnostic examinations should be performed on infants with birthweights <1500 g or 30 weeks' gestation, along with those high-risk babies in the 1501 to 2000 g birthweight group (American Academy of Pediatrics, 2006). In Latin American countries and in urban centers of newly industrializing countries in Asia and Eastern Europe, the same screening criteria likely do not apply, because evidence suggests that larger, older babies are also at risk in these settings, and national or regional guidelines need to be developed (Azad and Chandra, 2003; Fortes Filho et al, 2007; Trinavarat et al, 2004; Varughese et al, 2008; Vedantham, 2007).

The first examination should generally occur between 31 and 33 weeks postmenstrual age, but not before age 4 weeks (American Academy of Pediatrics, 2006; Reynolds et al, 2002). Examinations usually continue on an every-other-week basis unless ROP develops, at which time examination frequency may be increased. The indications for discontinuing surveillance are not clear at this point, but, in general, examinations continue until ROP is observed to regress, ROP progresses to treatment severity, or vessels are observed on at least two occasions to have progressed into zone III in the absence of ROP. Coordination of this schedule among neonatology, ophthalmology, and nursing is essential. If outpatient appointments are not kept or proper information is not conveyed when the baby is transferred to another facility, potentially treatable disease may be missed, with disastrous consequences (Mills, 2009).

Treatment of Established Retinopathy of Prematurity

Peripheral retinal ablation for eyes with serious ROP can prevent progression to blinding disease. The multicenter Cryotherapy for ROP (CRYO-ROP) study, which enrolled babies in 1986 and 1987, randomly assigned babies with bilateral "threshold" disease (i.e., 5 or more contiguous clock hours of stage 3 "plus" disease, or 8 or more clock hours of noncontiguous disease) to receive cryotherapy in one eye, and the fellow eye served as a control. For those babies with threshold ROP in one eye as the worst ROP, that eye was randomly assigned to undergo cryotherapy or not. During the study, approximately 15% of all babies born in the United States with birthweights of less than 1251 g were enrolled. Results documented a beneficial effect on both visual function and structure in eyes assigned to receive cryotherapy (Cryotherapy for Retinopathy of Prematurity Cooperative Group, 1988a, 1988b), a benefit that persisted through the last study examination at age 15 years (Cryotherapy for Retinopathy of Prematurity Cooperative Group, 1990b, 1990c, 1993, 1996, 2001; Palmer et al, 2005).

Still, almost half of eyes treated with cryotherapy had a visual acuity of worse than 20/200 at age 15 years (Palmer et al, 2005), and earlier intervention was considered in the multicenter Early Treatment for ROP trial (ETROP)

(Early Treatment for Retinopathy of Prematurity Cooperative, 2003). A risk model was based on the results of the CRYO-ROP study to determine which eyes were "high risk" for developing a poor outcome (Hardy et al, 2003). The model included not only the ROP status of the eye but also demographic characteristics and pace of ROP development. The ETROP was a randomized, controlled clinical trial with eyes that were determined to be at high risk for poor outcome assigned either to receive retinal ablative therapy at the diagnosis of high-risk retinopathy or to be followed and treated if the eye developed classic "threshold" ROP. A beneficial effect in both visual acuity and retinal structure was documented in high-risk eyes that underwent peripheral retinal ablation at the diagnosis of high risk compared to the cohort of eyes that were treated at "threshold" ROP if it developed (Early Treatment for Retinopathy of Prematurity Cooperative, 2003).

In the ETROP study, laser photocoagulation was more likely to be used than cryotherapy because of the advantages of using laser, including less discomfort intraoperatively and postoperatively, less pigmentation resulting from the therapy, and direct visualization of the area during treatment (Foroozan et al, 2001; McNamara, 1993; Tasman, 1995).

Follow-up studies of vitreoretinal surgical treatment for advanced disease (i.e., stages 4 and 5) have shown mixed results that very likely depend on whether the detachment is total and/or long-standing (Andrews et al, 1999; Hirose et al, 1993; Jabbour et al, 1987; Trese, 1994;). For eyes with total detachment, it appears that although surgery may give good anatomic results, good functional outcome is not likely to be achieved (Hirose et al, 1993; Quinn et al, 1991, 1996).

There has been a recent and serious interest in the use of anti–vascular endothelial growth factor (VEGF) drugs, with good results reported in babies with ROP (Mintz-Hittner and Best, 2009; Mintz-Hittner and Kuffel, 2008; Quiroz-Mercado et al, 2008). However, clinical trials must be undertaken before this modality is used in babies in whom vasculogenesis is incomplete not only in the eye but in other organs. Long-term systemic effects must be monitored in these children (Darlow et al, 2009).

COMMON OPHTHALMIC MANIFESTATIONS OF SYSTEMIC DISEASES

See Tables 102-3 through 102-5.

Role of the Neonatologist and Pediatrician

Neonatal health care providers clearly play a central role in the ophthalmologic care of the newborn and young infant. The first few weeks of life constitute a critical period of visual development in the brain, and the opportunity and responsibility to screen for ocular disease rests in the hands of the neonatologist and primary medical provider, whether pediatrician, family physician, or nurse practitioner. Using the I-ARM (Inspection, Acuity, Red Reflex, Motility) framework described previously as a guide, referral to a pediatric ophthalmologist should be made for any abnormality or asymmetry in an atomic structure or visual function. Some conditions require particularly urgent

referral, such as an abnormal red reflex, cloudy cornea, and ocular infection or trauma. Identification of a sight-threatening cataract or life-threatening retinoblastoma is most commonly made by an astute pediatric clinician in the NICU, nursery, or primary care office who carefully evaluates the red reflex in both eyes. In the case of neonatal conjunctivitis, diagnostic cultures and treatment should be undertaken without delay, but ophthalmology consultation is still necessary to rule out intraocular involvement. Premature infants at risk for ROP represent a particularly vulnerable population. It is the neonatologist's clinical and medicolegal responsibility to arrange timely diagnostic ROP examinations in the NICU and to communicate to parents the absolute necessity of keeping ophthalmologist outpatient appointments after the infant is discharged from the hospital. Such appointments should be scheduled before discharge. A delay in care by even a week could result in a visually disastrous outcome. ROP examinations should be performed by an ophthalmologist with experience in ROP.

The neonatal health and primary care pediatric health teams should provide ongoing eye-related education and support. Reducing the risk of pediatric abusive head trauma is one important topic to be discussed with all parents and caregivers. Viewing of educational videos on shaken baby syndrome is mandatory in an increasing number of municipalities, and reductions in AHT incidence have been demonstrated. Pediatricians should discuss crying and parental stress at office visits during the first few months of life; the Period of PURPLE Crying educational materials (see Additional Resources, later) are very useful in this regard. Pediatricians can also provide support for the families of children with visual impairment, ensuring early, anticipatory referral to state commissions for the blind and early intervention services, and ongoing encouragement for parents to maximally utilize such resources when available.

Rapid visual development occurs in the months following the neonatal period. Primary care eye examinations and vision assessments continue to be vital for the detection of conditions that may result in visual impairment or blindness, lead to problems with school or social performance, signal the presence of a serious systemic disease, or threaten the child's life (American Academy of Pediatrics, 2003). Children should have an eye examination at each well-child visit. Children at high risk for eye disease should be referred for examination by a pediatric ophthalmologist, including children with a history of prematurity or metabolic or genetic diseases; significant developmental delay or neurologic problems; systemic diseases associated with eye abnormalities; a family history positive for retinoblastoma, childhood cataracts or glaucoma, inherited retinal disorders, or blindness in childhood; and those whose parents needed glasses at a very young age.

Additional Resources

In addition to texts, clinical guidebooks, and online medical literature search engines (such as www.pubmed.org), the following Web-based resources can provide useful information related to newborn eye disease.

Website of the American Academy of Pediatrics, for policy statements on eye-related topics and other

TABLE 102-3 Ophthalmic Manifestations of Systemic Diseases With Neonatal Findings

Etiologic Disorder	Inheritance	Ophthalmic Manifestations
Aicardi's syndrome	X-linked dominant disorder characterized by triad of callosal agenesis, infantile spasms, and chorioretinal lacunae OMIM #304050	Bilateral or unilateral, multiple, chorioretinal lacunae (most constant feature), optic disk/retinal/iris colobomas, optic nerve head hypoplasia, microphthalmos, retinal detachment (Aicardi, 2005)
Alagille syndrome (ALGS 1 and 2)	Autosomal dominant disorders characterized by neonatal jaundice secondary to hepatic cholestasis OMIM #118450 and OMIM #610205	Posterior embryotoxon, optic disk drusen, and retinal pigmentary changes sometimes in associations with rod-cone dystrophy
Albinism	Heterogenous disorder of melanin metabolism associated with abnormal development of the retina and visual pathways Ocular forms: OA1 (X-linked) Oculocutaneous forms: OCA1-4, ADOC, Hermansky-Pudlak and Chediak-Higashi syndromes (autosomal recessive, autosomal dominant) More than 13 genes involved	Reduced vision, delayed visual maturation, nystagmus, strabismus, iris transillumination, fundus hypopigmentation, foveal hypoplasia, misrouting of optic nerve fibers, anomalous optic chiasm
CHARGE syndrome (*c*oloboma, *h*eart defect, *a*tresia choane, *r*etarded growth, *g*enital hypoplasia, and *e*ar anomalies)	Nonrandom cluster of congenital abnormalities Mutation of CHD7 on 8q12.1 (Vissers et al, 2004; Jongmans et al, 2006) OMIM #214800	Unilateral or bilateral uveal colobomas (retinal more frequent than iris), microphthalmos, Bell's palsy
Chromosome 22q11.2 deletion syndrome	Contiguous gene deletion syndrome (encompasses DiGeorge syndrome, velocardiofacial syndrome, conotruncal-anomaly-face syndromes) Autosomal dominant	Posterior embryotoxon, tortuous retinal vessels, eyelid hooding, strabismus, ptosis, sclerocornea (Binenbaum et al, 2008; Forbes et al, 2007)
Down syndrome	Trisomy 21 OMIM #19605	NLDO, refractive errors, nystagmus, strabismus, retinal abnormalities, keratoconus, cataracts (Creavin and Brown, 2009)
de Morsier's syndrome (septo-optic dysplasia)	Heterogeneous disorder defined by the combination of optic nerve hypoplasia, pituitary dysfunction, and midline abnormalities of the brain (absence of the corpus callosum and septum pellucidum) OMIM #182230	Optic nerve hypoplasia (unilateral or bilateral), strabismus, nystagmus, optic chiasm hypoplasia. Severe cases may have microphthalmos or anophthalmos
Galactosemia (classic)	Metabolic disorder due to mutation in the galactose-1-phosphate uridyltransferase gene OMIM#230400	Congenital cataracts ("oil-droplet cataracts")
Goldenhar's syndrome (oculo-auriculovertebral dysplasia, hemifacial microsomia)	Craniofacial birth defect involving first and second branchial arch derivatives OMIM #164210	Epibulbar dermoid (unilateral or bilateral), coloboma of the upper lid, ptosis, strabismus, microphthalmos, nasolacrimal duct obstructions
Homocystinuria	Autosomal recessive metabolic disorder due to cystathionine beta-synthetase deficiency OMIM #236200	Progressive ectopia lentis (lens subluxation), pupil block glaucoma, progressive myopia, optic atrophy, retinal detachment (Harrison et al, 1998)
Kabuki syndrome	Congenital mental retardation syndrome OMIM #147920	Long palpebral fissures with eversion of the lateral third of the lower eyelids, ptosis, strabismus
Möbius sequence	Sporadic disorder characterized by congenital facial weakness and abduction deficits OMIM #157900	Abnormal tearing, esotropia with limited abduction (unilateral or bilateral), horizontal gaze palsy, other CN palsies (III, IV,V), ptosis
Myasthenic syndromes (congenital and neonatal myasthenia gravis)	Neuromuscular disorders. The congenital form is a nonautoimmune autosomal dominant disorder. The neonatal form is secondary to maternal antibodies.	Bilateral ptosis, strabismus, limited ocular motility
Incontinentia pigmenti (Bloch-Sulzberger syndrome)	X-linked dominant disorder with characteristic skin lesions OMIM #308300	Strabismus, nystagmus, cataracts, optic atrophy, corneal abnormalities, retinovascular abnormalities (may resemble ROP), retinal detachment
PHACES syndrome (*p*osterior fossa brain malformations, *h*emangiomas of the face, *a*rterial cerebrovascular anomalies, *c*ardiovascular anomalies, *e*ye anomalies, *s*ternal defects)	Heterogeneous associations that occur in patients with large segmental cervicofacial hemangiomas OMIM #606519	Microphthalmos, Horner's syndrome, retinal vascular abnormalities, optic nerve atrophy, iris hypoplasia, cataracts, sclerocornea, lens coloboma, strabismus, choroidal hemangiomas, congenital 3rd nerve palsy, morning glory deformity, and glaucoma (Coats et al, 1999; Hartemink et al, 2009)
Stickler's syndrome (hereditary arthro-ophthalmopathy) (STL1 and 2)	Autosomal dominant disorder of collagen synthesis OMIM #108300 and #604841	Congenital myopia, vitreous abnormalities, cataracts, retinal detachment
Trisomy 13 (Patau's syndrome)	Chromosomal abnormality most consistently associated with severe ocular defects	Anophthalmos, cyclopia, microphthalmos, uveal colobomas, cataracts, corneal opacities, retinal dysplasia, intraocular cartilage

Continued

TABLE 102-3 Ophthalmic Manifestations of Systemic Diseases With Neonatal Findings—cont'd

Etiologic Disorder	Inheritance	Ophthalmic Manifestations
Trisomy 18	Chromosomal abnormality with frequent ocular defects	Microphthalmos, short palpebral fissures, ptosis, hypertelorism, iris coloboma, corneal opacities, cataracts
Tuberous sclerosis	Autosomal dominant multisystem disease characterized by hamartomatous growths in multiple organs OMIM #191100, #605284	Retinal hamartomas, vitreous hemorrhage, chorioretinal punched-out lesions, papilledema, optic nerve atrophy, strabismus (Rowley et al, 2001)

TABLE 102-4 Eye Manifestations of Intrauterine and Perinatal Infections

Infection	Ophthalmic Findings		Diagnosis
Toxoplasmosis (*Toxoplasma gondii*)	Retinitis, vitritis, choroiditis and anterior uveitis; flat atrophic retinal scars	Present in 75% of newborns with toxoplasmosis, 10% have only ocular findings	Clinical ELISA Positive IgM assay (maternal IgM does not cross the placenta)
Syphilis (*Treponema pallidum*)	Chorioretinitis (salt-and-pepper appearance or pseudoretinitis pigmentosa), anterior uveitis, glaucoma, interstitial keratitis	Bilateral interstitial keratitis is the classic ophthalmic finding, it occurs in 10% of patients but manifests later in childhood or adulthood.	Positive VDRL, FTA-ABS tests
Rubella virus	Nuclear cataracts, glaucoma, uveitis, microphthalmos, retinopathy with "salt-and-pepper" appearance, pseudoretinitis pigmentosa	50% of children with rubella have ocular findings, bilateral 70% Severe postoperative inflammation after cataract surgery	
Cytomegalovirus	Retinochoroiditis, optic nerve atrophy, microphthalmos, cataracts, uveitis, strabismus (Coats et al, 2000)	Most common intrauterine viral infection in the United States Only 10% of infants show clinical features of CMV infection with ophthalmologic abnormalities in lessthan 30% of these	CMV IgM, urine culture, PCR detection of CMV DNA in blood
Herpesvirus (HSV 1 and 2, EBV)	Vesicular skin lesions, keratoconjunctivitis, retinochoroiditis, cataracts		Cultures from conjunctival or corneal swabs

CMV, cytomegalovirus; *EBV*, Epstein-Barr virus; *ELISA*, enzyme-linked immunosorbent assay; *FTA-ABS*, fluorescent treponemal antibody absorption; *HSV*, herpes simplex virus; *PCR*, polymerase chain reaction; *VDRL*, Venereal Disease Research Laboratory.

TABLE 102-5 Eye Findings after in Utero Exposure to Teratogens

Teratogen	Ophthalmic Manifestations
Alcohol (fetal alcohol syndrome)	Short palpebral fissures, microphthalmos, epicanthal folds, optic nerve head hypoplasia, tortuosity of retinal vasculature, strabismus, cataracts (Stromland and Hellstrom, 1996)
Cocaine	Optic nerve abnormalities, delayed visual maturation, ROP-like fundus abnormalities (Teske and Trese, 1987), prolonged eyelid edema (Good et al, 1992)
Anticonvulsants (fetal hydantoin syndrome)	Ptosis, trichomegaly, hypertelorism, strabismus, retinal coloboma, microphthalmos, optic nerve head hypoplasia
Warfarin	Optic atrophy, cataracts, microphthalmos
Thalidomide	Strabismus, Duane's syndrome, ptosis, paradoxic gustolacrimal tearing, Möbius sequence (Miller et al, 2009)
Misoprostol	Möbius sequence (Miller et al, 2009)

resources: www.aap.org. The following policy statements are available at this website:

Red Reflex Examination in Neonates, Infants, and Children. Policy Statement. American Academy of Pediatrics, *Pediatrics* 122:1401-1404, 2008.

Eye Examination in Infants, Children, and Young Adults by Pediatricians. Policy Statement. American Academy of Pediatrics, *Pediatrics* 111:902-907, 2003.

Website of the American Association of Pediatric Ophthalmology and Strabismus (AAPOS), for information on numerous topics and locating a pediatric ophthalmologist: www.aapos.org

Information on the Period of PURPLE Crying and prevention of abusive head trauma: www.dontshake.org

Online Mendelian Inheritance in Man (OMIM), for information on genetic eye disease: www.ncbi.nlm.nih.gov/omim/

NCBI's Gene Tests website, for expert-authored peer-reviewed disease descriptions, international directories of genetic testing laboratories and genetics and prenatal diagnosis clinics, and educational materials, including illustrated glossary, information on genetic services, PowerPoint presentations, and annotated Internet resources: www.ncbi.nlm.nih.gov/sites/GeneTests/

Numerous free online eye atlases are available to provide images of normal and abnormal ocular anatomy and ophthalmologic diseases, by searching "Eye Atlas" on the Internet.

Complete references and supplemental color images used in this text can be found online at www.expertconsult.com

INDEX

A

Aarskog syndrome, cleft lip and/or palate with, 1336t–1337t

ABCA3 gene, in neonatal lung disease, 735

Abdomen
assessment of, 294–295, 294f
examination of, for dysmorphology, 189–190

Abdominal mass, postnatal evaluation of, 1178

Abdominal wall defects, 1007–1012. *See also specific defect.*
transport of neonate with, 355

Abnormal ductus venosus blood flow, prenatal screening for, 182–183

ABO blood group incompatibility, 311, 1126
hemolytic anemia due to, 1091, 1091t
hemolytic disease related to, 1131–1132

Abrasion, corneal, 1431

Abruptio placentae, 1086–1087

Abscess, *Citrobacter*, neonatal neuroimaging of, 838, 840f

Absent nasal bone, 182

Absorption of drugs, 417–418

Abuse, substance. *See* Substance abuse; *specific substance.*

Abusive head trauma (AHT), 1431–1433
visual impairment in, 1433

Acetaminophen
for circumcision, 437
for pain and stress, 438

Achondrogenesis
type IB, 270, 271f
features of, 259t–261t
type II–hypochondrogenesis, 268–269, 269f
features of, 259t–261t

Achondroplasia
differential diagnosis of, 266
etiology of, 266
features of, 259t–261t
inheritance of, 266
management of, 266
presentation of, 264, 265f
radiologic features of, 264–265, 265f

Acid-base balance, 383–389
disturbances of, 384–389. *See also* Metabolic acidosis; Metabolic alkalosis; Respiratory acidosis; Respiratory alkalosis.

Acid-base balance *(Continued)*
general principles in, 384–385, 385f, 385t
simple, 384
transitional, after birth, 385
regulation of, 383–384, 1172

Acidemia
glutaric, type2, 230–231
isovaleric, 228–229
methylmalonic, 226–228
propionic, 228

Acidosis
lactic
early lethal, 238
primary, 234–238
metabolic. *See* Metabolic acidosis
renal tubular. *See* Renal tubular acidosis

Aciduria, glutaric, type II, 1190

Acne, 1399–1400, 1400f
neonatal, 285, 285f

Acquired immunodeficiency syndrome (AIDS). *See* HIV/AIDS.

Acuity, 1424

Acute kidney injury (AKI), 1205–1215
AKIN classification of, 1205
causes of, 1208b
chronic kidney disease due to, 1215
definition of, 1205–1206, 1206f, 1206t
epidemiology of, 1206–1208
evaluation of, 1210–1211, 1210t
in neonatal population, 1207
intrinsic, 1208
vs. prerenal azotemia, 1210t
ischemic, 1208–1209, 1209f
management of, 1211–1214, 1213t
dialysis in, 1213–1214
hemodialysis in, 1214
peritoneal dialysis in, 1214
nephrotoxic, 1209–1210
obstructive, 1210
pathophysiology of, 1208–1210, 1208b, 1209f
RIFLE classification of, 1205

Acute Kidney Injury Network (AKIN) classification, of acute kidney injury, 1205

Acute phase reactants, in bacterial sepsis, 544–546

Acyclovir
for conjunctivitis, 1429t
for HSV infection, 473, 474t, 1396
for VZV infection, 474t, 477
nephrotoxic effects of, 1210

Acylcarnitine translocase deficiency, 233

Acyl-CoA dehydrogenase deficiency(ies), multiple, 1190

Adaptive immunity, 454–461
B cells in, 457
immunoglobulins in, 458–461, 458t, 459f, 460t. *See also* Immunoglobin *entries.*
T cells in
adaptive, 454–456, 454f–455f
regulatory, 456–457

Adefovir, for hepatitis B, 474t

Adenosine, for supraventricular tachycardia, 794, 795f

Adenovirus infection, 503, 503f

Adhesives, application and removal of, in extremely-low-birth-weight infants, 395, 396t

Administration, of neonatal transport program, 345

Admission criteria, for late preterm infants, 414, 415b

Adolescence, function in, neurodevelopmental outcome and, 928

Adrenal crisis, management of, 1284–1285
initial, 1284
maintenance therapy in, 1284
stress replacement therapy in, 1284–1285

Adrenal enzyme deficiency, steroidogenic defects caused by, 1277–1282

Adrenal gland(s), 1274–1277
development of, 1250, 1250f
abnormalities of, 1282–1284
molecular basis for, 1276
disorders of. *See also specific disorder.*
primary, 1277–1285
secondary and tertiary, 1283–1284
embryology of, 1274
function of
assessment of, in neonate, 1276–1277
fetal and adult, 1274–1276, 1275f
glucocorticoid production and, control of, 1276
mineralocorticoid production and, control of, 1276
morphology of, 1274

Page numbers followed by *b*, indicate box; *f*, figure; *t*, table.

1441

H

HADH gene mutation, in congenital hyperinsulinism of infancy, activation of, 1324

Half-life, of drugs, 421, 421f

Halogenated agents, inhaled, for obstetric anesthesia, 170

Halothane, for obstetric anesthesia, 170

Hamartoma(s), renal, 1189–1190

Hamartoma tumor syndrome, 1412

Hand(s), examination of, for dysmorphology, 190, 190f, 192f

Hand grasp reflex, 1359–1360

Hand hygiene, 559–562
    clinical indications for, 560, 560b
    compliance with, 561–562, 562b
    guidelines for, in neonatal intensive care unit, 560–561
    historical perspectives of, 559–560
    preparations for, 561, 561t

HapMap project, 176

Harlequin color change, 1403

Harlequin ichthyosis, 1375–1376, 1376f

Hashimoto's thyroiditis, 90

Head
    assessment of, 282, 288–290, 289f
    circumference of
        at birth, 804
        vs. standard growth data, 281, 299f
    examination of, for dysmorphology, 188–189, 188f, 190f
    molding of, 883

Head box, oxygen delivery via, 614

Head trauma, abusive, 1431–1433
    visual impairment in, 1433

Health, neurodevelopmental outcome and, 931–932

Health and disease hypothesis, developmental origins of, 1253

Health care–acquired infections, in nursery, 551. *See also* Nosocomial infections.

Health informatics, 10–11

Health Insurance Portability and Accountability Act (HIPPA), 13

Health policy, regarding maternal substance abuse, 113

Health record, electronic, 13–15. *See also* Electronic health record.

Hearing assessment, 290, 296

Hearing loss
    CMV-induced, 480–481
    in craniosynostosis syndromes, 1342

Hearing screening, of neonates, 302

Heart. *See also* Cardiac; Cardio- *entries; specific part.*
    anatomy of, segmental approach to, 762–764
    anomalies of, neonatal, 312
    auscultation of, 293

Heart *(Continued)*
    cell types within, 701–702, 701f
    development of, 699, 700f. *See also* Cardiovascular system, development of.

Heart disease
    acquired, 719
    congenital. *See* Congenital heart disease (CHD).
    nonimmune hydrops associated with, 68t, 69
    structural, congenital AV block associated with, 793–794

Heart failure, congestive, signs of, 764

Heart murmurs
    assessment of, 294
    congenital cardiac lesions causing, 766–772
    pathologic, 294

Heart rate
    circulatory compromise and, 721–724
    monitoring of, 612
    neonatal, 293

Heart sounds, assessment of, 293

Heart surgery, effect of, on brain, 804–805, 805b

Heart transplantation, 788, 788t

Heart tube
    embryonic, formation of, 702, 702f
    laterality of, 702–703, 703f

Heart valves, formation of, 707–708, 707f

Heart-lung interactions, 605–611
    effects on lung in, 607–609
        congenital pulmonary lymphangiectasis and, 609
        decreased lymphatic drainage and, 609
        increased driving pressure and, 607–608, 608f, 608b
        increased permeability and, 608–609
        pulmonary edema and, 607, 608f
            symptoms of, 609–610, 610f
            treatment of, 610
        pulmonary hemorrhage and, 610–611
    lung effects on heart in, 605
        inflation on pulmonary vascular resistance and, 607, 607f
        intrathoracic pressure changes and, 605–607
            negative pressure, 605–606, 606f
            positive pressure, 606–607, 606f

Heat loss
    partitioning of heat losses and heat gains and, 359–360, 360f
    physical routes of, 357, 358f

Heat rash, 284–285

Heel sticks, pain management strategies for, 436–437

HELLP syndrome, in pregnancy, 64, 109–110

Hemangioendothelioma, hepatic, 1044, 1161

Hemangioma, 287–288, 1371
    capillary, 1430
    hepatic, 1044
    infantile, 1405, 1406f
        clinical findings in, 1405–1407
        CNS anomalies associated with, 1406–1407
        definition of, 1405
        diagnosis of, 1407–1408
        disfigurement in, 1406
        genitourinary anomalies associated with, 1407
        Kasabach-Merritt syndrome associated with, 1406
        obstruction in, 1405
        pathogenesis of, 1408
        spinal dysraphism associated with, 1407
        ulceration in, 1406
        visceral involvement in, 1407
    salivary gland, 979
    subglottic, congenital, 674–675

Hematocrit
    during cardiopulmonary bypass, 805
    in anemia, 1083, 1083t

Hematologic system
    bilirubin metabolism and, 1053
    cytokines and, 1055
    developmental biology of, 1047
    embryonic hematopoiesis and, 1047, 1048f
    erythropoiesis and, developmental aspects of, 1048–1052, 1049f
    granulocytopoiesis and, developmental aspects of, 1054–1055
    megakaryocytopoiesis and, developmental aspects of, 1053–1054
    platelet transfusion and, 1054
    red blood cell transfusion and, 1052–1053
    stem cell biology and, 1047–1048

Hematopoiesis, 1108–1111
    dermal, 1371
    embryonic, 1047, 1048f
    extramedullary, 1050
    fetal, 1108
    growth factors and, 1108, 1109f
    negative regulators of, 1117–1121
    neonatal, 1108

Hematuria, postnatal, 1180

Hemiatlas, torticollis due to, 1354

Hemimegalencephaly, 861–862, 862f

Hemochorial placentation, 37. *See also* Placenta.

Hemochromatosis, neonatal, 1043

Hemodialysis. *See also* Dialysis; Peritoneal dialysis
    for acute kidney injury, 1214
    for chronic kidney disease, 1219–1220